ONCOLOGY OF INFANCY AND CHILDHOOD

ONCOLOGY OF INFANCY AND CHILDHOOD

Stuart H. Orkin, MD
David G. Nathan Professor of Pediatrics
Harvard Medical School
Chief, Department of Pediatric Oncology
Dana-Farber Cancer Institute
Investigator, Howard Hughes Medical Institute
Boston, Massachusetts

David E. Fisher, MD, PhD
Professor of Pediatrics
Edward Wigglesworth Professor of Dermatology
Harvard Medical School
Chief, Department of Dermatology
Massachusetts General Hospital
Boston, Massachusetts

A. Thomas Look, MD
Professor of Pediatrics
Harvard Medical School
Vice Chair for Research
Department of Pediatric Oncology
Dana-Farber Cancer Institute
Boston, Massachusetts

Samuel E. Lux IV, MD
Robert A. Stranahan Professor of Pediatrics
Harvard Medical School
Vice Chair for Research
Chief Emeritus, Division of Hematology/
    Oncology
Children's Hospital Boston
Boston, Massachusetts

David Ginsburg, MD
James V. Neel Distinguished University Professor
Departments of Internal Medicine, Pediatrics and
    Communicable Diseases, and Human Genetics
Investigator, Howard Hughes Medical Institute
University of Michigan Medical School
Ann Arbor, Michigan

David G. Nathan, MD
Robert A. Stranahan Distinguished Professor of
    Pediatrics
Harvard Medical School
Physician-in-Chief Emeritus
Children's Hospital Boston
President Emeritus, Dana-Farber Cancer Institute
Boston, Massachusetts

Managing Editor: *Cathryn J. Lantigua*

SAUNDERS

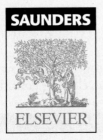

ELSEVIER

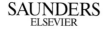

SAUNDERS
ELSEVIER

1600 John F. Kennedy Blvd.
Suite 1800
Philadelphia, PA 19103-2899

Notice

Knowledge and best practice in this field are constantly changing. As new research and experience broaden our knowledge, changes in practice, treatment and drug therapy may become necessary or appropriate. Readers are advised to check the most current information provided (i) on procedures featured or (ii) by the manufacturer of each product to be administered, to verify the recommended dose or formula, the method and duration of administration, and contraindications. It is the responsibility of the practitioner, relying on their own experience and knowledge of the patient, to make diagnoses, to determine dosages and the best treatment for each individual patient, and to take all appropriate safety precautions. To the fullest extent of the law, neither the Publisher nor the Editors assumes any liability for any injury and/or damage to persons or property arising out of or related to any use of the material contained in this book.

The Publisher

Library of Congress Cataloging-in-Publication Data

Oncology of infancy and childhood / Stuart H. Orkin ... [et al.]. – 1st ed.
   p. ; cm.
  Includes bibliographical references.
  ISBN 978-1-4160-3431-5
  1. Cancer in children.   I. Orkin, Stuart H.
[DNLM: 1. Neoplasms. 2. Child. 3. Infant. QZ 275 O58 2009]
RC281.C4O533 2009
618.92'994–dc22   2009001550

Acquisitions Editor: Dolores Meloni
Developmental Editor: Ann Anderson
Publishing Services Manager: Frank Polizzano
Senior Project Manager: Robin E. Hayward
Design Direction: Karen O'Keefe-Owens

Printed in China

Last digit is the print number: 9 8 7 6 5 4 3 2 1

Contributors

Karen Albritton, MD
Instructor, Harvard Medical School; Director, Adolescent and Young Adult Oncology Program, Dana-Farber Cancer Institute, Boston, Massachusetts
Rare Tumors of Childhood

James F. Amatruda, MD, PhD
Assistant Professor of Pediatrics, Molecular Biology and Internal Medicine, University of Texas Southwestern Medical Center; Attending Physician, Children's Medical Center, Dallas, Texas
Pediatric Germ Cell Tumors

Megan E. Anderson, MD
Instructor in Orthopedics, Harvard Medical School; Orthopedic Surgeon, Children's Hospital Boston, Beth Israel Deaconess Medical Center, Boston, Massachusetts
Pediatric Surgical Oncology

Pedram Argani, MD
Professor of Pathology and Oncology, Johns Hopkins University School of Medicine; Staff Pathologist, Johns Hopkins Hospital, Baltimore, Maryland
Pediatric Renal Tumors

Scott A. Armstrong, MD, PhD
Assistant Professor of Pediatrics, Harvard Medical School; Associate Physician in Medicine, Children's Hospital Boston, Boston, Massachusetts
Infant Leukemias

Sharyn D. Baker, PharmD, PhD
Associate Professor of Clinical Pharmacy and Pharmaceutical Sciences, College of Pharmacy, University of Tennessee, Memphis; Associate Member, St. Jude's Children's Research Hospital, Memphis, Tennessee
Chemotherapy in the Pediatric Patient

Raymond C. Barfield, MD, PhD
Associate Professor of Pediatrics and Christian Philosophy, Duke University School of Medicine, Durham, North Carolina
Ethical Considerations in Pediatric Oncology Clinical Trials

Frederic G. Barr, MD, PhD
Associate Professor of Pathology and Laboratory Medicine, University of Pennsylvania School of Medicine; Attending Pathologist, Hospital of the University of Pennsylvania, Philadelphia, Pennsylvania
Rhabdomyosarcoma

Charles B. Berde, MD, PhD
Professor of Anesthesia (Pediatrics), Harvard Medical School; Sara Paige Mayo Chair in Pediatric Pain Medicine, Chief, Division of Pain Medicine, Department of Anesthesiology, Perioperative and Pain Medicine, Children's Hospital Boston, Boston, Massachusetts
Symptom Management in Children with Cancer

Jason N. Berman, MD
Assistant Professor of Pediatric Hematology/Oncology, Departments of Pediatrics and Microbiology/Immunology, Dalhousie University; MSC Clinician Scientist in Pediatric Oncology, IWK Health Centre, Halifax, Nova Scotia, Canada
Myeloid Leukemia, Myelodysplasia, and Myeloproliferative Disease in Children

Mark L. Bernstein, MD
Professor of Pediatrics, Dalhousie University; Head, Division of Pediatric Hematology/Oncology, IWK Health Centre, Halifax, Nova Scotia, Canada
Osteosarcoma

Smita Bhatia, MD, MPH
Chair and Professor of Population Sciences, Staff Physician, Department of Pediatrics, City of Hope, Duarte, California
Epidemiology of Leukemia in Childhood

Amy Louise Billett, MD

Assistant Professor of Pediatrics, Harvard Medical School; Dana-Farber Cancer Institute, Children's Hospital Boston, Boston, Massachusetts

Symptom Management in Children with Cancer

Samuel Blackman, MD, PhD

Associate Director, Experimental Medicine, Merck & Co., Inc., North Wales, Pennsylvania

Tumors of the Brain and Spinal Cord

Patricia A. Branowicki, RN, NEA-BC

Director, Nursing/Patient Care Services, Pediatric Oncology, Dana-Farber Cancer Institute; Vice President, Medical Patient Services, Children's Hospital Boston, Boston, Massachusetts

Nursing Care of Patients with Childhood Cancer

Robert L. Casey, PhD

Instructor in Psychology, Harvard Medical School; Clinical Psychologist, Dana-Farber Cancer Institute, Boston, Massachusetts

Psychosocial Care of Children and Families

Susan N. Chi, MD

Pediatrics, Harvard Medical School; Pediatric Oncology, Dana-Farber Cancer Institute, Children's Hospital Boston, Boston, Massachusetts

Tumors of the Brain and Spinal Cord

Jennifer J. Clark, MD

Pediatric Hematologist/Oncologist, Rocky Mountain Pediatric Hematology/Oncology, Denver, Colorado

Myeloid Leukemia, Myelodysplasia, and Myeloproliferative Disease in Children

Susanne B. Conley, RN, MSN, CPON, NEA-BC

Clinical Instructor, University of Massachusetts; Clinical Nurse Specialist, Dana-Farber Cancer Institute, Boston, Massachusetts

Nursing Care of Patients with Childhood Cancer

Ian J. Davis, MD, PhD

Denman Hammond Assistant Professor of Pediatric Oncology, Departments of Pediatrics and Genetics, University of North Carolina School of Medicine; Lineberger Comprehensive Cancer Center, North Carolina Children's Hospital, Chapel Hill, North Carolina

Nonrhabdomyosarcomas and Other Soft Tissue Tumors

Barbara A. Degar, MD

Instructor, Harvard Medical School; Attending Physician, Dana-Farber Cancer Institute, Children's Hospital Boston, Boston, Massachusetts

Histocytoses

Kenneth B. DeSantes, MD

Associate Professor of Pediatrics, University of Wisconsin School of Medicine and Public Health; Clinical Director, Division of Pediatric Hematology/Oncology, American Family Children's Hospital, Madison, Wisconsin

Immunotherapy of Cancer

Lisa Diller, MD

Associate Professor of Pediatrics, Harvard Medical School; Clinical Director, Pediatric Oncology, Dana-Farber Cancer Institute, Children's Hospital Boston, Boston, Massachusetts

Childhood Cancer Survivorship

Jeffrey S. Dome, MD

Associate Professor of Pediatrics, George Washington University School of Medicine and Health Sciences; Chief, Division of Oncology, Center for Cancer and Blood Disorders, Children's National Medical Center, Washington, DC

Pediatric Renal Tumors

Steven G. DuBois, MD

Assistant Professor of Pediatrics, University of California, San Francisco, School of Medicine; UCSF Children's Hospital, San Francisco, California

Ewing's Sarcoma

Janet Duncan, MSN, CPNP, CPON

Nursing Director, Pediatric Advanced Care Team, Children's Hospital Boston, Boston, Massachusetts

Palliative Care in Pediatric Oncology

Ian F. Dunn, MD

Clinical Fellow in Surgery, Harvard Medical School; Postdoctoral Fellow and Resident in Neurosurgery, Dana-Farber Cancer Institute, Brigham and Women's Hospital, Boston, Massachusetts

Molecular Basis of Human Malignancy

Elana E. Evan, PhD

Assistant Research Professor, Department of Pediatrics, David Geffen School of Medicine at UCLA; Director, UCLA Children's Comfort Care Program, Mattel Children's Hospital at UCLA, Los Angeles, California

Palliative Care in Pediatric Oncology

William E. Evans, PharmD

Professor of Clinical Pharmacy and Pharmaceutical
Sciences, College of Pharmacy, University of
Tennessee, Memphis; Director and CEO, St. Jude's
Children's Research Hospital, Memphis, Tennessee

Chemotherapy in the Pediatric Patient

Carolyn A. Felix, MD

Professor of Pediatrics, University of Pennsylvania
School of Medicine; Division of Oncology, Children's
Hospital of Philadelphia, Philadelphia, Pennsylvania

Cytogenetic and Molecular Pathology of Pediatric Cancer

Adolfo A. Ferrando, MD, PhD

Assistant Professor of Pathology and Pediatrics,
Institute for Cancer Genetics, Columbia University
Medical Center, New York, New York

Malignant Lymphomas and Lymphadenopathies

David E. Fisher, MD, PhD

Professor of Pediatrics, Edward Wigglesworth Professor
of Dermatology, Harvard Medical School; Chief,
Department of Dermatology, Massachusetts General
Hospital, Boston, Massachusetts

Nonrhabdomyosarcomas and Other Soft Tissue Tumors

Mark D. Fleming, MD, DPhil

Associate Professor of Pathology, Harvard Medical
School; Interim Pathologist-in-Chief, Children's
Hospital Boston, Boston, Massachusetts

Histocytoses

Jonathan A. Fletcher, MD

Associate Professor of Pathology and Pediatrics,
Harvard Medical School; Director, Tumor
Cytogenetics, Brigham and Women's Hospital, Boston,
Massachusetts

Cytogenetic and Molecular Pathology of Pediatric Cancer

Judah Folkman, MD*

Professor of Cell Biology and Andrus Professor of
Pediatric Surgery, Harvard Medical School; Surgeon-
in-Chief, Emeritus and Director, Vascular Biology
Program, Children's Hospital Boston, Boston,
Massachusetts

Angiogenesis

A. Lindsay Frazier, MD

Associate Professor of Pediatrics, Harvard Medical
School; Attending Physician, Dana-Farber Cancer
Institute, Boston, Massachusetts

Pediatric Germ Cell Tumors

Mark C. Gebhardt, MD

Frederick W. and Jane M. Ilfeld Professor of
Orthopedics, Harvard Medical School; Children's
Hospital Boston; Chief, Department of Orthopedics,
Beth Israel Deaconess Medical Center, Boston,
Massachusetts

Pediatric Surgical Oncology

Rani E. George, MD, PhD

Assistant Professor of Pediatrics, Harvard Medical
School; Attending Physician, Pediatric Hematology/
Oncology, Dana-Farber Cancer Institute, Children's
Hospital Boston, Boston, Massachusetts

Neuroblastoma

John M. Goldberg, MD

Assistant Professor of Clinical Pediatrics, University of
Miami Miller School of Medicine; Director, Pediatric
Oncology Early Phase Clinical Trials Program,
Sylvester Comprehensive Cancer Center, Miami,
Florida

Rare Tumors of Childhood

Richard Gorlick, MD

Associate Professor of Molecular Pharmacology and
Pediatrics, Albert Einstein College of Medicine of
Yeshiva University; Vice-Chair, Department of
Pediatrics, and Chief, Division of Pediatric
Hematology-Oncology, The Children's Hospital at
Montefiore, Bronx, New York

Osteosarcoma

Eric F. Grabowski, MD, ScD

Associate Professor of Pediatrics, Harvard Medical
School; Pediatrician, Massachusetts General Hospital,
Boston, Massachusetts

Retinoblastoma

Holcombe E. Grier, MD

Associate Professor of Pediatrics, Harvard Medical
School; Dana-Farber Cancer Institute, Children's
Hospital Boston, Boston, Massachusetts

Ewing's Sarcoma

Daphne Haas-Kogan, MD

Professor and Vice Chair of Radiation Oncology and
Professor of Neurological Surgery, University of
California, San Francisco, School of Medicine, San
Francisco, California

Pediatric Radiation Oncology

---

*Deceased

William C. Hahn, MD, PhD

Associate Professor of Medicine, Harvard Medical School; Dana-Farber Cancer Institute, Boston, Massachusetts

Molecular Basis of Human Malignancy

Betsy Herrington, MD

Instructor, Pediatric Oncology, Dana-Farber Cancer Institute, Boston, Massachusetts

Tumors of the Brain and Spinal Cord

Kathleen E. Houlahan, RN

Nurse Manager, Pediatric Oncology, Dana-Farber Cancer Institute; Director, Nursing/Patient Care Services, Pediatric Hematology, Oncology, and Stem Cell Transplantation, Children's Hospital Boston, Boston, Massachusetts

Nursing Care of Patients with Childhood Cancer

Joseph E. Italiano, Jr., PhD

Assistant Professor of Medicine, Harvard Medical School; Department of Medicine, Brigham and Women's Hospital; Department of Surgery, Children's Hospital Boston, Boston, Massachusetts

Angiogenesis

Katherine A. Janeway, MD

Instructor in Pediatrics, Harvard Medical School; Attending Physician, Pediatric Hematology/Oncology, Dana-Farber Cancer Institute, Children's Hospital Boston, Boston, Massachusetts

Osteosarcoma

Lisa B. Kenney, MD, MPH

Instructor in Pediatrics, Harvard Medical School; Pediatric Oncologist, Dana-Farber Cancer Institute, Children's Hospital Boston, Boston, Massachusetts

Childhood Cancer Survivorship

Mark W. Kieran, MD, PhD

Associate Professor of Pediatrics, Harvard Medical School; Director, Pediatric Neuro-Oncology, Dana-Farber Cancer Institute, Children's Hospital Boston, Boston, Massachusetts

Tumors of the Brain and Spinal Cord

Heung Bae Kim, MD

Assistant Professor of Surgery, Harvard Medical School; Director, Pediatric Transplant Center, Children's Hospital Boston, Boston, Massachusetts

Hepatoblastomas and Other Liver Tumors

Szilárd Kiss, MD

Clinical Fellow in Ophthalmology, Harvard Medical School; Massachusetts Eye and Ear Infirmary, Boston, Massachusetts

Retinoblastoma

Eric Kodish, MD

F. J. O'Neill Professor and Chair, Department of Bioethics, Cleveland Clinic; Professor of Pediatrics, Cleveland Clinic Lerner College of Medicine, Case Western Reserve University, Cleveland, Ohio

Ethical Considerations in Pediatric Oncology Clinical Trials

Andrew Y. Koh, MD

Instructor in Pediatrics, Harvard Medical School; Assistant in Medicine, Division of Hematology/ Oncology and Infectious Diseases, Dana-Farber Cancer Institute, Children's Hospital Boston, Boston, Massachusetts

Infectious Diseases in Pediatric Cancer

Mirna Lechpammer, MD, PhD

Clinical Fellow in Neuropathology, Harvard Medical School; Brigham and Women's Hospital; Children's Hospital Boston, Boston, Massachusetts

Tumors of the Brain and Spinal Cord

Yannek I. Leiderman, MD, PhD

Resident in Ophthalmology, Harvard Medical School; Massachusetts Eye and Ear Infirmary, Boston, Massachusetts

Retinoblastoma

Stephen L. Lessnick, MD, PhD

Assistant Professor of Pediatrics, University of Utah School of Medicine; Investigator, Huntsman Cancer Institute, Salt Lake City, Utah

Ewing's Sarcoma

A. Thomas Look, MD

Professor of Pediatrics, Harvard Medical School; Vice Chair for Research, Department of Pediatric Oncology, Dana-Farber Cancer Institute, Boston, Massachusetts

Myeloid Leukemia, Myelodysplasia, and Myeloproliferative Disease in Children

Jennifer W. Mack, MD, MPH

Assistant Professor, Harvard Medical School; Attending Physician, Dana-Farber Cancer Institute, Children's Hospital Boston, Boston, Massachusetts

Palliative Care in Pediatric Oncology

Karen J. Marcus, MD
Associate Professor of Radiation Oncology, Harvard
Medical School; Division Chief, Radiation Oncology,
Children's Hospital Boston, Boston, Massachusetts
*Pediatric Radiation Oncology; Tumors of the Brain
and Spinal Cord*

Shizuo Mukai, MD
Assistant Professor in Ophthalmology, Harvard
Medical School; Surgeon, Massachusetts Eye and Ear
Infirmary, Boston, Massachusetts
Retinoblastoma

Elizabeth Mullen, MD
Instructor, Harvard Medical School; Attending
Physician, Dana-Farber Cancer Institute, Children's
Hospital Boston, Boston, Massachusetts
Oncologic Emergencies

Maureen J. O'Sullivan, MBBC, MD
Senior Lecturer, Trinity College School of Medicine;
Consultant Pediatric Pathologist, Our Lady's
Children's Hospital, Dublin, Ireland
Cytogenetic and Molecular Pathology of Pediatric Cancer

Alberto Pappo, MD
Professor of Pediatrics, Baylor College of Medicine;
Head, Solid Tumor Section, Texas Children's Cancer
Center and Hematology Service, Houston, Texas
Rare Tumors of Childhood

Antonio R. Perez-Atayde, MD, PhD
Associate Professor of Pathology, Harvard Medical
School; Staff Pathologist, Children's Hospital Boston,
Boston, Massachusetts
Nonrhabdomyosarcomas and Other Soft Tissue Tumors

Philip A. Pizzo, MD
Carl and Elizabeth Naumann Dean, Professor of
Pediatrics and Microbiology and Immunology,
Stanford University School of Medicine; Medical Staff,
Department of Pediatrics–Hematology/Oncology,
Stanford Hospital and Clinics, Stanford, California
Infectious Diseases in Pediatric Cancer

Sanjay P. Prabhu, MBBS
Clinical Fellow, Pediatric Radiology, Harvard
School; Pediatric Neuroradiology, Children's Hospital
Boston, Boston, Massachusetts
Tumors of the Brain and Spinal Cord

Christopher J. Recklitis, PhD, MPH
Assistant Professor of Pediatrics, Harvard Medical
School; Director, Research and Support Services,
Perini Family Survivors' Center, Dana-Farber Cancer
Institute, Boston, Massachusetts
Psychosocial Care of Children and Families

Alfred Reiter, MD, PhD
Head, Pediatric Hematology and Oncology, Justus-
Liebig-University; Children's University Hospital,
Geissen, Germany
Malignant Lymphomas and Lymphadenopathies

Charles W. M. Roberts, MD, PhD
Assistant Professor, Harvard Medical School; Dana-
Farber Cancer Institute, Boston, Massachusetts
Pediatric Renal Tumors

Leslie L. Robison, PhD
Chair, Department of Epidemiology and Cancer
Control, St. Jude Children's Research Hospital,
Memphis, Tennessee
Epidemiology of Leukemia in Childhood

Barrett J. Rollins, MD, PhD
Professor of Medicine, Harvard Medical School; Chief
Scientific Officer, Dana-Farber Cancer Institute,
Brigham and Women's Hospital, Boston,
Massachusetts
Histocytoses

David Samuel, MB, ChB
Clinical Fellow, Department of Pediatric Neuro-
Oncology, Harvard Medical School; Dana-Farber
Cancer Institute, Boston, Massachusetts
Tumors of the Brain and Spinal Cord

Krysta D. Schlis, MD
Instructor in Pediatrics, Harvard Medical School;
Assistant in Medicine, Division of Hematology/
Oncology, Children's Hospital Boston, Boston,
Massachusetts
Infant Leukemias

Rosalind A. Segal, MD, PhD
Neurobiology, Harvard Medical School; Pediatric
Oncology, Dana-Farber Cancer Institute, Boston,
Massachusetts
Tumors of the Brain and Spinal Cord

William R. Sellers, MD

Vice President, Global Head Oncology Research, The Novartis Institutes for Biomedical Research, Cambridge, Massachusetts

Targeted Approaches to Drug Development

Robert C. Shamberger, MD

Robert E. Gross Professor of Surgery, Harvard Medical School; Chief, Department of Surgery, Children's Hospital Boston, Boston, Massachusetts

Pediatric Surgical Oncology

Suzanne Shusterman, MD

Assistant Professor of Pediatrics, Harvard Medical School; Attending Physician, Dana-Farber Cancer Institute, Children's Hospital Boston, Boston, Massachusetts

Neuroblastoma

Lewis B. Silverman, MD

Assistant Professor of Pediatrics, Harvard Medical School; Director, Pediatric Hematologic Malignancy Service and Pediatric Oncology Clinic, Dana-Farber Cancer Institute, Children's Hospital Boston, Boston, Massachusetts

Acute Lymphoblastic Leukemia

Paul M. Sondel, MD, PhD

Walker Professor of Pediatrics and Human Oncology, University of Wisconsin School of Medicine and Public Health; Head, Division of Pediatric Hematology/ Oncology, Vice Chair (Research), Department of Pediatrics, Associate Director (Translational Research), UW Paul P. Carbone Comprehensive Cancer Center, American Family Children's Hospital, Madison, Wisconsin

Immunotherapy of Cancer

Alex Sparreboom, PhD

Associate Professor of Clinical Pharmacy and Pharmaceutical Sciences, College of Pharmacy, University of Tennessee, Memphis; Associate Member, St. Jude's Children's Research Hospital, Memphis, Tennessee

Chemotherapy in the Pediatric Patient

Kimberly Stegmaier, MD

Assistant Professor of Pediatrics, Harvard Medical School; Assistant in Medicine, Dana-Farber Cancer Institute, Children's Hospital Boston, Boston, Massachusetts

Targeted Approaches to Drug Development

Gail E. Tomlinson, MD, PhD

Professor of Pediatrics, Greehey Distinguished Chair in Genetics and Cancer, University of Texas Health Science Center at San Antonio; Director, Pediatric Hematology-Oncology, CHRISTUS Santa Rosa Children's Hospital, San Antonio, Texas

Hepatoblastomas and Other Liver Tumors

Christopher Turner, MD

Instructor in Pediatrics, Harvard Medical School; Attending Physician, Neuro-Oncology, Dana-Farber Cancer Institute, Children's Hospital Boston, Boston, Massachusetts

Tumors of the Brain and Spinal Cord

Christina K. Ullrich, MD, MPH

Instructor in Pediatrics, Harvard Medical School; Attending Physician, Pediatric Oncology and Pediatric Palliative Care, Dana-Farber Cancer Institute, Children's Hospital Boston, Boston, Massachusetts

Symptom Management in Children with Cancer

Stephan D. Voss, MD, PhD

Assistant Professor of Radiology, Harvard Medical School; Staff Radiologist, Children's Hospital Boston, Boston, Massachusetts

Diagnostic Imaging in the Evaluation of Childhood Cancer

Lynda M. Vrooman, MD

Instructor in Pediatrics, Harvard Medical School; Staff Physician, Dana-Farber Cancer Institute, Children's Hospital Boston, Boston, Massachusetts

Oncologic Emergencies

Christopher B. Weldon, MD, PhD

Instructor in Surgery, Harvard Medical School; Assistant in Surgery, Children's Hospital Boston, Boston, Massachusetts

Pediatric Surgical Oncology

Jennifer Whangbo, MD, PhD

Instructor in Pediatrics, Harvard Medical School; Staff Physician, Dana-Farber Cancer Institute, Children's Hospital Boston, Boston, Massachusetts

Oncologic Emergencies

Joanne Wolfe, MD, MPH

Assistant Professor, Harvard Medical School; Director, Pediatric Palliative Care, Dana-Farber Cancer Institute, Children's Hospital Boston, Boston, Massachusetts

Palliative Care in Pediatric Oncology

Richard B. Womer, MD
Professor of Pediatrics, University of Pennsylvania
School of Medicine; Senior Oncologist, Children's
Hospital of Philadelphia, Philadelphia, Pennsylvania
Rhabdomyosarcoma

Lonnie Zeltzer, MD
Professor of Pediatrics, Anesthesiology, Psychiatry, and
Behavioral Sciences, David Geffen School of Medicine
at UCLA; Director, Pediatric Pain Program, Mattel
Children's Hospital at UCLA, Los Angeles, California
Psychosocial Care of Children and Families

Preface

The decision to create a separate oncology volume for the seventh edition of *Nathan and Oski's Hematology of Infancy and Childhood* was not difficult. Many readers of the sixth edition view pediatric hematology and oncology as one discipline, but nevertheless had to look elsewhere for comprehensive information on the nonhematologic cancers of childhood. Previous efforts to bridge this gap with a single, lengthy chapter on solid tumors fell woefully short, because of the exponentially expanding base of knowledge, which simply could not be captured in the pages we had formerly allotted. Thus, David Fisher and Thomas Look were charged by our coeditors, Stuart Orkin, David Nathan, David Ginsburg, and Sam Lux, and by our publishers and editors at Elsevier, especially Dolores Meloni and Ann Ruzycka Anderson, to expand the existing chapters on hematologic malignancies in *Hematology of Infancy and Childhood* and complement them with new chapters on malignant solid tumors and the supportive care of childhood cancer patients.

We believe the final product, *Oncology of Infancy and Childhood*, justifies our decision to launch a new textbook of this scope. The reworked format, although retaining updated and indispensable chapters from the sixth edition, is structured to accommodate emerging research developments in cancer biology and therapeutics, both globally and in specific pediatric tumors. To preserve the marriage of clinical practice to basic pathophysiology so central to the success of earlier editions of the Nathan and Oski textbook, we recruited a mix of clinical investigators as authors who we felt would maintain a consistent balance between fundamental disease processes and the principles of effective management of cancer patients. The inclusion of in-depth molecular pathophysiology provides more than an academic curiosity. As with pediatric hematology, many of the molecular-genetic lesions first discovered in childhood cancers gave birth to deep scientific insights of very broad importance in modern biology. And these lesions also are guiding the gradual transformation of oncology therapeutics toward a discipline guided by focused, molecularly-targeted therapies. At all times during the creation of this book, we remained keenly aware that the effects of cancer and its treatment are not restricted by time but extend from the earliest symptoms to the rehabilitation period and well beyond, leaving their imprint on both the patient and his or her family. To provide readers with an in-depth understanding of the issues raised by acute and chronic cancer sequelae in children, we have added a supportive care section written by authors who represent critical subdisciplines involved in this important branch of pediatric oncology.

This volume was organized and written to meet the needs of a diverse readership: clinical specialists and researchers who must stay abreast of a rapidly expanding information base; students, trainees, and junior faculty who are just learning about or entering the field of pediatric oncology; and practitioners in other disciplines who increasingly are called upon to recognize and deal with the delayed effects of treatment. It is our sincere hope that *Oncology of Infancy and Childhood* will earn a reputation as more than an educational tool. If we have performed our task well, this volume should also stimulate the next generation of physicians and biologists to tackle the many outstanding challenges presented by childhood cancer. Our greatest hope is that this volume will require frequent and major revisions, as new and improved therapies continue to reach our patients.

Tragically, one of the world's most brilliant biomedical researchers, and a contributor to this book, died early in 2008. The ideas of M. Judah Folkman founded and energized the entire field of tumor angiogenesis and have led directly to the development of cancer drugs that may act by directly blocking the formation of new blood vessels in tumors. In the words of his good friend David Nathan, "[Judah] was indefatigable and unquenchable. There was no such thing in his lexicon as a defeat—only a learning point." We will deeply miss him and the enthusiasm he brought to bear on contemporary cancer research.

We could not have completed this task without the help of Dolores Meloni, Ann Ruzycka Anderson, and Robin Hayward of Elsevier and our managing editor, Cathy Lantigua. We thank all our authors, old and new, for meeting their responsibilities in a timely fashion and for producing manuscripts that required only a modicum of editing. Our apologies to readers for any redundancies that have occurred due to the need for completeness within individual chapters and for any inconsistencies in nomenclature that developed from the efforts of different groups to generate logical systems of terminology in the face of an exploding database.

We dedicate this book to our parents, spouses, children and mentors, and to childhood cancer patients worldwide, whose courage in the face of devastating illness has inspired remarkable discoveries in the biology and therapy of childhood leukemias and solid tumors.

A. Thomas Look, MD
David E. Fisher, MD, PhD

Contents

I Biology of Cancer

1 Epidemiology of Leukemia in Childhood

Smita Bhatia and Leslie L. Robison

Leukemias of childhood are a highly heterogeneous group of diseases. In reviewing the descriptive and analytic epidemiology of these malignancies, we have, when possible, emphasized specific subgroups, as defined by morphologic, cytogenetic, or molecular features. In selected cases, there is evidence that specific subgroups of leukemia may have distinct causes and that molecular abnormalities associated with particular subgroups may be linked with specific causal mechanisms. In assessing risk factors, studies of the childhood leukemias present several methodologic advantages over those addressing adult leukemias. The interval between exposure to putative risk factors and the onset of leukemia is shorter; therefore, recall of exposures is likely to be more accurate, and intervening factors are less likely to be of importance than those associated with adult leukemias. These characteristics of childhood leukemia lend themselves better to an approach that includes population studies and molecular epidemiologic techniques, permitting the design of studies to assess gene-environment interactions. However, in striking contrast to the impressive advances in the treatment and biology of childhood leukemia, remarkably little has been achieved regarding our understanding of the cause of this most common form of childhood malignancy.

DESCRIPTIVE EPIDEMIOLOGY

Leukemias are the most common cancers affecting children, accounting for 32% of all occurrences of cancer in children younger than 15 years and 27% of occurrences of cancer in children younger than 20 years.[1] In the United States, leukemia is diagnosed in approximately 3540 children younger than 20 years annually. Of these, acute lymphoblastic leukemia (ALL) accounts for 73%, acute myeloid leukemia (AML) accounts for approximately 18%, and chronic myeloid leukemia (CML) is rarely seen, accounting for less than 4%.

International Patterns

There is a wide variation in the incidence of childhood leukemia by geographic location. The highest annual incidence rates are reported in Costa Rica, Ecuador, Hong Kong, Denmark, and Singapore (57.9 to 51.0/million population), whereas some of the lowest rates are found in Zimbabwe, India, Israel, and Algeria (23.1 to 26.0/million).[1] The annual incidence of childhood leukemia for many regions, including North America, Australia, Northern and Western Europe, China, Japan, the Philippines and Singapore, ranges between 35 and 50/million (Table 1-1). When evaluating geographic variation in disease incidence, there are always concerns regarding quality and completeness of reporting. Ecologic studies of childhood leukemia incidence according to annual per capita gross national income have demonstrated substantial variation in low-income countries and a much narrower range in middle- and high-income countries.[2] In addition, there exists a significant correlation between the incidence of childhood leukemia and population mortality rates in those younger than 5 years in low- and middle-income countries. Some of the lowest reported childhood leukemia rates are in countries with high mortality rates for children younger than 5 years, suggesting that children in some low-income countries with undiagnosed leukemia may die with anemia or fever attributed to infectious disease.

Age-Specific Incidence and Male-to-Female Ratio

The incidence rate for all leukemias is highest in children younger than 5 years of age and decreases with age.[3] The age-

TABLE 1-1	Incidence of All Childhood Leukemias, ALL, and AML in Selected International Sites*		
	ANNUAL INCIDENCE RATE (PER MILLION POPULATION)		
Country	**Leukemia**	**ALL**	**AML**
Costa Rica	57.9	46.3	8.9
Ecuador	56.3	39.6	9.1
Hong Kong	53.9	40.6	3.9
Denmark	53.0	42.8	8.4
Singapore	51.0	39.5	6.9
Canada	50.8	41.0	6.3
Finland	49.9	41.9	5.4
Australia	49.9	39.9	8.0
Italy	49.1	37.9	7.9
Sweden	48.7	40.1	6.7
Norway	48.6	38.3	8.0
Philippines	48.1	25.2	8.6
United States (white)	46.9	38.0	6.0
Germany	46.6	39.0	6.7
Uruguay	44.0	29.3	7.4
Colombia	42.8	31.5	6.4
United Kingdom	40.8	32.8	6.3
France	40.5	31.7	6.1
China	40.3	17.4	6.7
Netherlands	40.1	30.9	5.8
Japan	38.5	22.6	7.2
Korea	38.1	20.2	8.7
Cuba	37.7	25.4	5.7
Czech Republic	37.1	28.4	5.1
India (Delhi)	36.0	23.1	6.1
Peru	35.9	25.4	6.9
Brazil	33.7	21.9	5.3
Thailand	29.8	19.8	5.8
United States (black)	29.4	20.8	6.2
Algeria	26.0	14.3	5.7
Israel	25.7	18.6	5.3
India (Bombay)	25.4	16.0	4.8
Zimbabwe	23.1	11.6	11.0

*Children 0-14 years of age.
ALL, acute lymphocytic leukemia; AML, acute myeloid leukemia.
Data from Parkin DM, Kramarova PE, Draper GJ, et al (eds). International Incidence of Childhood Cancer, vol II (Publication No. 144). Lyon, France, International Agency for Research on Cancer, 1998.

adjusted incidence for boys exceeds that for girls, with a male-to-female ratio typically between 1.1:1 and 1.4:1.[1]

Acute Lymphoblastic Leukemia

In developed countries, the age-incidence curve for ALL is characterized by a peak between the ages of 1 and 4 years (Fig. 1-1).[4] Thus, a sharp peak in ALL incidence is seen in 2- to 3-year-olds (more than 100/million), which decreases to a rate of 20/million for 8- to 10-year-olds. The incidence of ALL in 2- to 3-year-olds is approximately fourfold greater than that for infants and is nearly tenfold greater than that for 19-year-olds. Although this age distribution is well recognized and attributable to common ALL (cALL),[5] it has not always been present. It was first observed in England and Wales in the 1920s,[6] American whites in the 1940s,[6] African Americans[7] and in Japan in the 1960s,[8,9] and Jews and non-Jews in Israel in the 1970s.[10] In Kuwait, where the incidence was low during the 1970s, the age peak has recently been observed, whereas in

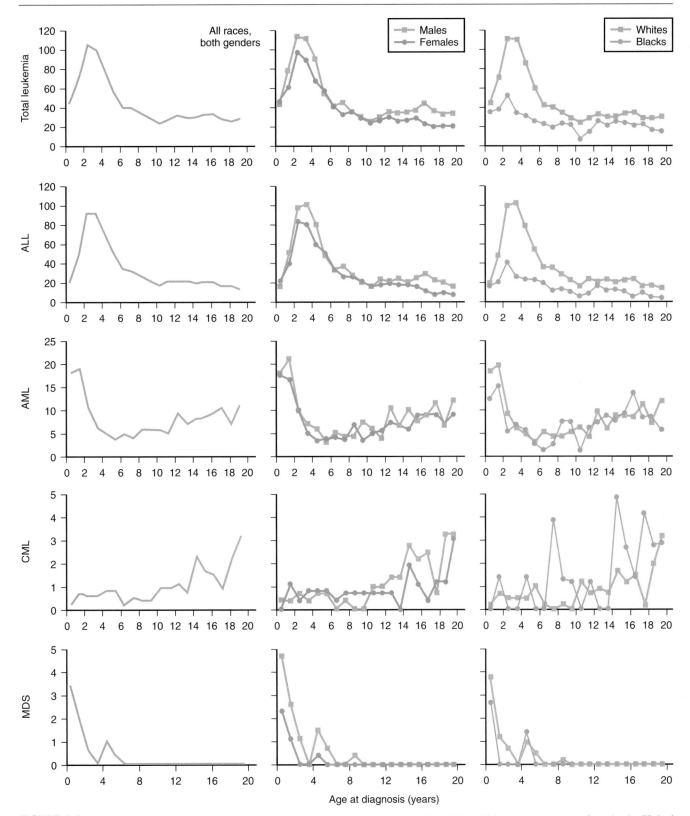

FIGURE 1-1. Age-, gender-, and race-specific annual incidence rates (per million population) for children 0 to 19 years of age in the United States, 2000-2004. ALL, acute lymphocytic leukemia; AML, acute myeloid leukemia; CML, chronic myeloid leukemia; MDS, myelodysplastic syndrome and other myeloproliferative diseases. *(From National Cancer Institute. SEER: Surveillance, Epidemiology, and End Results, 2008. Available at http://www.seer.cancer.gov/seerstat.)*

the African series, in which the incidence is also low, the peak has not been reported yet.[11]

An exaggerated peak incidence in 2- to 3-year-olds, with a very low incidence of ALL in older children, was observed in certain areas of England and Wales and in the rural north of Scotland, and coincided with a high socioeconomic status. These observations have led to a hypothesis that an elevated risk of ALL is influenced by community characteristics such as isolation, high socioeconomic status, and population mixing,[12] which in turn are related to immunologic isolation in infancy; this influences patterns of exposure to common infectious agents in the early years of life, before the appearance of leukemia.[13] These hypotheses are discussed in detail later. The ratio of incidence rates of ALL for boys and girls ranges between 1.1:1 and 1.3:1.[11]

Acute Myeloid Leukemia

In children, the incidence rates for AML are highest in infancy and are fairly uniform in older children (see Fig. 1-1).[4] In the United States, from 1986 to 1995, the incidence in the 0- to 4-year-old age group was 10.3/million, and in the 5- to 9-year-old and 10- to 14-year-old age groups were 5.0 and 6.2/million, respectively. Comparable rates have been reported elsewhere in Europe and in England. The male-to-female ratio is close to 1 for AML.[14]

Chronic Myeloid Leukemia

The incidence rates for CML in one of the largest series originating from the United Kingdom were 1.2/million for infants and 1.6, 0.5, and 0.7 for children aged 1 to 4, 5 to 9, and 10 to 14 years, respectively,[14] comparable to rates observed in the United States for these age ranges.[4] The rate for CML increases during the 15 to 19 year age interval. The male-to-female ratio is 1.6:1.[1]

Myelodysplastic Syndrome and Other Myeloproliferative Diseases

The International Classification of Childhood Cancer[15] includes a classification for MDS (myelodysplastic syndrome and other myeloproliferative diseases). In the 0- to 19-year age group, rates for MDS are similar to those for CML; however, in contrast, the incidence of MDS is highest in infants and drops essentially to 0 by age 8 years.[4] The incidence is almost twice as high in males.

Ethnic Origin

In the United States, there is substantial variation in the incidence rates of ALL by ethnicity. The highest rates have been reported in Hispanics, Filipinos, and Chinese and the lowest rates in African Americans.[4] The incidence rates in whites are moderate to high by international standards, whereas those for Native Americans are somewhat lower.

Conversely, two studies have investigated the incidence of childhood cancer by ethnicity in England, but results were negative. The lack of variation in the incidence of ALL in ethnic groups in England, in conjunction with the markedly lower incidence of ALL in the Indian subcontinent and Africa than in England, suggests that the incidence of ALL depends to some extent on environmental factors in association with geographic location. The contrast between the ethnic variations in incidence could be a reflection of the socioeconomic differences by ethnicity (or the lack thereof) in the two countries.[14] A recent report from the Malaysia-Singapore Leukemia Study Group

has described differences in prognostically important chromosomal abnormalities in an unselected multiethnic Asian population.[16] Ethnic groups differed significantly with regard to the proportion of ALL patients with T-cell ALL (T-ALL) (higher in Chinese and Indians), *TEL-AML1* (lower in Chinese), and *BRC-ABL* (lower in Indian patients). Beyond ethnic differences in the occurrence of childhood ALL, race and ethnicity have been well documented to be associated with prognosis.[17] The black-to-white ratio of the incidence of AML in the United States is 0.85. The rates are highest in Hispanics.[1,18] This higher rate of AML is contributed to by the higher incidence of acute promyelocytic leukemia seen in Hispanics than in non-Hispanics, thus raising the question of genetic predisposition to acute promyelocytic leukemia or exposure to distinct environmental factors.[19] As with ALL, race and ethnicity also have prognostic importance.[20]

Socioeconomic Status

Socioeconomic factors have been proposed as an explanation for the age peak in childhood leukemia.[21] Thus, it has been hypothesized that with economic development, poorer communities move from a situation in which leukemia is rare (T-ALL is the predominant type of ALL), through an intermediate stage in which cALL begins to appear, to a state of high socioeconomic status associated with a high incidence of ALL and cALL. There are a number of descriptive studies that have investigated the relationship between leukemia and socioeconomic status.[22-28] In the vast majority of these, the area of residence of the patients (or those who died) was used as a measure of socioeconomic status. Other measures used included household income and years of schooling. In most of these studies, a weak positive association between leukemia and high socioeconomic status was observed, with a few exceptions.[24,27,29-31] In contrast, several investigators have examined the relationship between AML and socioeconomic status and have failed to show an association.[23]

Time Trends

Several investigators have examined temporal trends for leukemia, but the findings are difficult to interpret.[32-36] This is primarily because of the varying time periods covered and different methods of analysis used. Some investigators analyzed the 0- to 14-year-old age group as a whole, whereas others examined trends in specific age groups. Some have reported trends for each gender, whereas others combined both genders in their analyses. In some analyses, all leukemias were grouped together, whereas others conducted their studies by leukemia subtype. In addition, diagnostic improvements have led to more accurate and precise classification of leukemias over time, which could contribute to the observed temporal trends in incidence.

In the studies reporting an increase in the incidence of ALL, the increase is fairly modest and confined to the 0- to 4-year-old age group. Moreover, in some reports, the increase in incidence of ALL appeared to be accompanied by a decrease in the incidence of AML or other leukemias, which could reflect diagnostic shifts and more accurate and precise classification.[37-40] A temporal increase in the incidence of childhood ALL has been reported in England[41] and attributed to an increase in the precursor B-cell subtype.[42] Between 1974 and 2000, the average annual increase in childhood ALL was 0.7% overall, but 1.4% for cALL. Similarly, analyses of childhood ALL time trends in Italy have demonstrated increases, some related to maternal time variables, including maternal age and maternal birth cohort, which were considered to be consistent with an infectious cause.[43,44] On the other hand, in another study, Linet and associates[45] have reported no substantial change in the incidence of childhood leukemia diagnosed in the United States between 1975 and 1995. The Czech national registries have reported a 1.5-fold increase in childhood ALL incidence between the ages of 1 and 4 years, during the period of substantial socioeconomic transition in European postcommunist countries.[46]

Clustering of Leukemia in Space and Time

Spatial clustering of childhood leukemia has been observed to varying degrees in England,[47,48] France,[49] and Greece,[50] but not in the United States.[51-55] Where spacial clustering was identified, it was strongest for leukemias diagnosed in younger children. Although spatial clustering was confirmed to sparsely populated areas in England, such clustering was found only in urban areas in Greece. Birch and colleagues[56] have addressed the issue of space-time clustering by using the Manchester Children's Tumor Registry. All methods showed highly significant evidence of space-time clustering on the basis of place of birth and time of diagnosis of childhood leukemia. The authors concluded that the results are consistent with an infection hypothesis (see later). Furthermore, the investigators found an excess of cases in males versus females in space-time pairs, thus suggesting gender-specific susceptibility to infections. More recently, they have reported statistically significant cross-clustering in childhood leukemia and CNS tumors and between ALL and astrocytoma, suggesting possible common causes, possibly of an infectious nature.[57] The correlation between childhood leukemias and CNS tumors is of interest, given the recently reported correlation in international rates for these two pediatric cancers.[58]

Historically, clusters of childhood leukemia have been observed where the number of cases observed exceed those expected within a given time and geographic location. Investigation of these clusters has typically not identified any causal agent. A rather recent leukemia cluster in the United States has gained substantial public and scientific attention because of the marked excess observed in a small population.[59] Comprehensive investigation, including biologic samples from individuals in the population analyzed for chemicals, viral markers, and genetic polymorphisms, in conjunction with air, water, soil, and dust sampling, failed to identify any leukemia risk factors.[60]

GENETIC FACTORS AND FAMILIAL AGGREGATION

Certain genetic syndromes are associated with an increased susceptibility to leukemia.[61] These include Down syndrome,[62] neurofibromatosis type 1,[63] and chromosome breakage syndromes, such as ataxia telangiectasia,[64] Bloom syndrome,[65] Shwachman's syndrome,[66,67] Fanconi's anemia, and Langerhans cell histiocytosis.[68] Shaw and associates[69] have reported an association between Klinefelter syndrome and childhood leukemia on the basis of an observation of two children with ALL with a 47,XXY karyotype. However, Hasle and colleagues[70] subsequently have reported no increase in the incidence of childhood leukemia in a cohort of 696 men with Klinefelter syndrome. A recent study of malformation syndromes in children with cancer has reported an association between Bardet-Biedl syndrome and ALL.[71]

Although specific associations have been described mainly as case reports, data on the proportion of instances of leukemia known to have a genetic cause or associated with specific genetic syndromes are limited. In a study from England, 2.6%

of children with leukemia were reported to have a recognized genetic condition, and this was almost entirely accounted for by Down syndrome (2.3% of all leukemias).[72] This proportion is similar to that found in studies from the United States and Scandinavian countries.[73-75]

Population-based studies using record-linkage approaches have documented that approximately 97% of cancers occurring in children with Down syndrome are leukemia.[76] Individuals with Down syndrome have an estimated 56-fold increase in leukemia between the ages of 0 and 4 years, which declines to 10-fold for leukemia risk in those between 5 and 29 years. More recently, there has been increasing interest in identification of environmental factors that may contribute to the development of leukemia in patients with Down syndrome.[77] Case-control investigations comparing Down syndrome patients with leukemia to Down syndrome patients without leukemia have identified a reduced risk of leukemia to be associated with maternal vitamin supplementation in the periconceptional period and have reported a history of infection in the first 2 years of life.[78,79]

Concordance of Childhood Leukemia in Twins

Assessment of concordance for childhood leukemia in twins may provide clues about cause. If childhood leukemia were to have a predominantly genetic cause, monozygotic twins would be expected to be concordant for leukemia more often than dizygotic twins because of their genetic similarity. If childhood leukemia were caused by an abnormal intrauterine environment, it would be expected that if one member of a dizygotic twin pair were affected, the other would be affected more often than a nontwin sibling, because of the shared environment. In a study of leukemia in a pooled series from the United States, Canada, and England, only three concordant pairs (1.5%) were found in 197 pairs in which one or both twins had leukemia, with the concordance rate for monozygotic twins reported to be 3.9% (95% confidence interval [CI] = 0.8 to 11.1).[80] Although the concordance rate in twins of like gender (probably monozygotic twins) is higher than the zero concordance rate reported for twins of unlike gender (dizygotic twins), the concordance rate in twins of like gender is variable.[80,81] This suggests that inherited genetic factors most likely play a relatively small part in the cause of childhood leukemia.

The occurrence of concordant leukemic pairs has been hypothesized to be caused by parallel expansions of clones descended from a single, ancestral cell transformed in utero, with a malignant clone arising in one monozygotic twin and entering the circulation of the co-twin through anatomizing placental vessels. This would account for the early and similar age of onset of leukemia and the similar cytogenetic findings.[82,83] Support for this hypothesis is provided by the observation of shared clonal but nonconstitutional mixed-lineage leukemia gene (*MLL*) rearrangements in the leukemic cells of three pairs of monozygotic twins concordant for infant acute leukemia.[84] The rearrangements were not observed in nonleukemic cells of the twins and were not present in the maternal or paternal blood of two of the three twins.

Leukemia and Cancer in the Families of Children with Leukemia

In studies of leukemias of all types combined, no excess of cancer was observed in siblings, parents, or offspring.[85-91] In studies focusing on acute leukemia, an excess of acute leukemia was observed in siblings, in whom the expected rates were extremely low.[92-94] Limitations of these studies include the inclusion of distant relatives, in whom verification of cancer becomes problematic, incomplete follow-up, and, finally, the inclusion of families with a history of consanguinity.

Cancer in Offspring of Patients Treated for Childhood Leukemia

There have been few studies reporting the rate of occurrence of cancer in the offspring of patients treated for childhood leukemia. Only recently have enough patients survived so that the number of their offspring permitted estimates of their risk of development of malignant neoplasms. On review of the literature, Hawkins and associates[89] have estimated that the proportion of heritable cases in survivors is unlikely to exceed 5%, assuming that the age of onset of all heritable cases is 15 years or younger and that the diseases have a penetrance of 70% or more. Chromosomal instability was examined in 20 apparently healthy children of survivors of childhood malignancy. Compared with control subjects, no increases in spontaneous or bleomycin-induced aberrations were found in these index children. The results suggest that the offspring of subjects who previously received chemotherapy, radiotherapy, or both for childhood malignancy probably have no increased risk of latent chromosomal instability.[95]

Other Conditions in Relatives of Patients with Leukemia

Savitz and Ananth[96] have reported an excess of major birth defects in the siblings of patients with ALL (relative risk [RR] of 3.2, 95% CI 1.3 to 7.7, adjusted for age at diagnosis, gender, and year of diagnosis). Mann and colleagues[97] have reported an excess of congenital defects in parents, uncles, aunts, and other distant relatives of patients with ALL compared with community control subjects. Buckley and associates[98] have reported an excess of a number of conditions in siblings, parents, and grandparents of index patients with various types of ALL. These conditions included musculoskeletal disorders in relatives of patients with the common cell type, gastrointestinal, hematologic, and musculoskeletal disorders and allergies for those with the pre–B-cell type, an excess of gastrointestinal disorders for those with the T-cell type, and an excess of congenital heart and lung disease for those with the null cell type. The offspring of adult survivors of childhood ALL were not found to have an increased risk of occurrence of congenital anomalies compared with the offspring of sibling control subjects.[98] Similarly, Kenney and colleagues[99] have reported no excess of congenital anomalies in the offspring of adult survivors of childhood cancer compared with the offspring of sibling control subjects.

Susceptibility to Childhood Acute Lymphoblastic Leukemia

Association with Human Leukocyte Antigen–DR

Both genetic and environmental factors could possibly play an interactive role in the development of childhood ALL. Because of the demonstration of the influence of major histocompatibility complex (MHC) on mouse leukemia, a human leukocyte antigen (HLA) association has been considered as a possible genetic risk factor. Dorak and associates[100] have demonstrated a moderate association with the most common allele in the HLA-DR53 group, HLA-DRB1*04, which was stronger in males. In addition, homozygosity for HLA-DRB4*01, encoding the HLA-DR53 specificity, was increased in patients. Confounding these associations was a male-specific increase in homozygosity for HLADRB4*01. The cross-reactivity among HLA-DR53 and H-2Ek, extensive mimicry of the immunodominant epitope of HLA-DR53 by several carcinogenic viruses, and the extra amount of DNA in the vicinity of the HLA-DRB4 gene argue for the case that HLA-DRB4*01 may be one of the genetic risk factors for childhood ALL. Comparison of *DQAl* and *DQBl* alleles in 60 children with ALL and 78 newborn infants (control subjects) has revealed that male but not female patients have a higher rate of occurrence of DQA1*0101/*0104 and DQB1*0501 than appropriate control subjects.[101] The authors concluded that this represents a male-associated susceptibility haplotype in ALL, supporting an infectious cause. Additional British investigations have suggested that cALL in children may be associated with HLA-DPB1 through a mechanism that involves the presentation of specific antigenic peptides, possibly derived from infectious agents, which leads to the activation of helper T cells mediating proliferative stress on preleukemic cells.[102]

Genetic Polymorphisms

In the search for gene-environment interactions in the cause of childhood leukemia, investigations have focused on the genetic variability in xenobiotic metabolism, DNA repair pathways, and cell-cycle checkpoint functions that might interact with environmental factors to influence leukemia risk. Although much of the research in this area has been limited by small sample size, there are data that suggest a potential role for polymorphisms in genes encoding cytochrome P450, glutathione S-transferase, reduced nicotinamide adenine dinucleotide (NADPH), quinone oxidoreductase (NQ01), methylenetetrahydrofolate reductase (MTHFR), cycle-cycle inhibitors, and DNA repair polymorphisms.[103-111]

In general, there have been few reports addressing the potential role of these polymorphic genes in childhood leukemia and often they have indicated contradictory findings. This is particularly true with regard to studies of GSTM1 and GSTT1 and CYP-P450 enzymes.[112,113] Low folate intake or alterations in folate metabolism as a result of polymorphisms in the enzyme MTHFR have been associated with neural tube defects and some cancers.[114] Polymorphic variants of MTHFR lead to enhanced thymidine pools and better quality DNA synthesis, which might afford some protection from the development of leukemias, particularly those with translocations. Wiemels and coworkers[103] and Smith and colleagues[111] have reported an association of MTHFR polymorphisms in infant leukemias with *MLL* gene rearrangements and childhood leukemia with either *TEL-AMLl* fusions or hyperdiploid karyotypes. These studies have provided evidence that molecularly defined subgroups of childhood leukemias may have different causes and also suggest a role for folate in the development of childhood leukemia. In a case-control study, MTHFR genotypes TT677/AA1298 and CC677/CCC1298 were associated with a reduced risk of childhood ALL.[112] Moreover, their findings suggested a gene-environment interaction based on the timing of implementation of folic acid supplementation in a Canadian population. To date, no direct gene-environment associations have been established convincingly. When considering the potential significance of the prenatal origin of childhood leukemia, it becomes important to consider the genotypic profile of the mother with respect to metabolizing enzymes. Investigation of maternally mediated genetic effects through NQO1 did not show any effect on risk for childhood ALL.[115]

PRENATAL ORIGIN OF CHILDHOOD ACUTE LYMPHOBLASTIC LEUKEMIA

As noted, molecular studies on several pairs of identical twins, aged between 2 months and 14 years at diagnosis, first provided strong evidence that concordant ALL arises in monozygotic twins after mutation and clonal expansion of one cell in one fetus in utero.[84,116-119] Because the disease in the twins is not clinically or biologically different from that in singletons, Greaves and associates[119] have hypothesized that some of the singletons are likely to have a prenatal initiation of their leukemia. They further hypothesized that an additional event or exposure postnatally results in clinically overt leukemia at a variable time after birth. To test these hypotheses, they used the neonatal blood spots or Guthrie cards[119] to identify the presence of clonotypic or patient-specific leukemia fusion-gene sequences (*TEL-AML1*).[120] The association between the t(12;21) and deletion of the nontranslocated allele of *TEL* is among the most frequent abnormalities observed in B-lineage ALLs.[121] Neonatal blood samples are routinely used to screen for inherited metabolic disorders. By reverse transcriptase polymerase chain reaction (PCR) screening of blood or bone marrow, they identified *TEL-AML1* fusion in 12 children and a pair of identical twins, aged 2 to 5 years, with newly diagnosed ALL. They identified *TEL-AML1* fusion sequences in blood spots from the identical twins and in 6 of 9 studied *TEL-AML1*–positive patients. Greaves concluded that childhood ALL is often initiated by a chromosome translocation event in utero.

This important observation has been more extensively investigated and characterized.[122,123] Screening of neonatal cord blood samples has revealed a putative leukemia clone with the *TEL-AML1* fusion gene in 1% of newborn infants.[124] This represents a frequency 100 times greater than the prevalence of ALL defined by this fusion gene later in childhood. In chil-

dren with cALL who have a *TEL-AML1* fusion gene, deletion of the unrearranged or normal *TEL* allele is a common secondary occurrence. The causal events that lead to the initial *TEL-AML1* fusion in utero and any postnatal secondary mutations are unknown.[125] Some epidemiologic data have provided support for the idea that an abnormal immunologic response under particular social conditions could account for certain critical postnatal events.[13,126] Further epidemiologic studies need to focus on in utero exposures that could result in the initial *TEL-AML1* fusion, and postnatal exposures or events that could explain the secondary mutations.

INFECTION

Considerable interest and research has focused on the potential role of infection in the cause of childhood ALL through a mechanism of stimulation of an inappropriate immune response or via a direct transformation.[127] This avenue of research, proposed and spearheaded by British researchers, reflects two different but conceptually-related, hypothesized mechanisms (Fig. 1-2).

Residence in Areas with High Population Mixing

In 1988, Kinlen[128] hypothesized that the excess of leukemia in children in the vicinity of the Sellafield and Dounreay nuclear reprocessing plants in England could be caused by a rare response to some unidentified mild and subclinical infection, the transmission of which is facilitated by contacts between large numbers of people. An influx of people of diverse origin into a previously isolated area would particularly facilitate transmission. Thus, an excess of leukemia in childhood would be expected in isolated areas into which there had been a significant influx of people. The hypothesis was first tested in an area in Scotland. Glenrothes New Town was identified a priori as an area where, after relative isolation, there was a sudden burst of in-migration in 1964 because of the opening of the

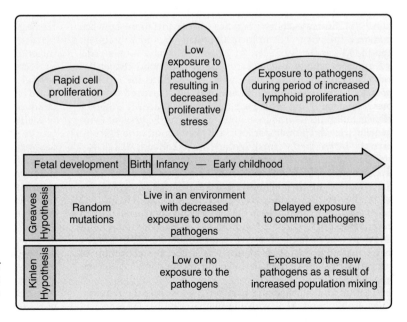

FIGURE 1-2. Proposed models for the potential role of infection associated with the development of childhood acute lymphocytic leukemia through a mechanism of stimulation of an inappropriate immune response.

Forth Road bridge.[128] A significant excess of individuals younger than 25 years who died of leukemia was identified during the period from 1951 to 1967. There was no excess in the period from 1968 to 1985, when the community became much less isolated. The hypothesis has been tested in a number of other situations in England, France, and other parts of Europe and Hong Kong.[6,12,25,49,129-140] A 3.6-fold increase in childhood leukemia was observed in the wartime cohort compared with national Scottish rates in Orkney and Shetland (England's northernmost islands) during World War II, when the local residents were outnumbered by servicemen stationed there. The rates normalized to the national rates in the postwar period.[141] An analysis of the U.S. Surveillance Epidemiology and End Results (SEER) data has also provided confirmatory evidence for the population-mixing hypothesis, findings that changes in rural county population sizes from 1980 to 1989 are associated with incidence rates for childhood ALL.[142]

Critical Event During Index Pregnancy

Infections

An alternative model for the cause of childhood ALL places the critical infectious event during pregnancy rather than early childhood. In this model, the causative agent of the primary infection in the mother is transmitted to the fetus and, as a consequence of this in utero infection, the child is at an increased risk of developing ALL before the age of 5 years. The characteristics that the causative infectious agent should possess include the following: (1) the ability to induce genomic instability; (2) specific effects on B lymphocytes and not on T lymphocytes; (3) higher rates of infection in regions with lower socioeconomic status; (4) limited general oncogenic potential; (5) minimal symptoms associated with the primary infection; and (6) ability to cross the placenta and infect the fetus but not result in severe fetal abnormalities. A virus that meets several of these criteria is the JC virus, a member of the polyomavirus family.[143]

The possibility that maternal infection during pregnancy could potentially be leukemogenic is supported by the observation that leukemia in cats is caused by a feline virus transmitted from the mother to the fetus.[144] Three cohort studies of maternal infection during pregnancy and subsequent childhood cancer have revealed an excess of cancer in these children compared with the age- and gender-matched general population.[145-147] In case-control studies, no association between maternal infection with influenza or varicella and subsequent childhood cancer was seen.[98,148-153] With regard to maternal infection in general, a twofold excess of childhood cancer has been reported. However, the studies are small or the reported prevalence of exposure is low, and may be attributed to recall bias. Neonatal blood spots have been used to identify evidence of selected in utero viral infections.[154,155] Investigations of cytomegalovirus and human parvovirus B19 infection have failed to identify DNA in the small groups of childhood ALL cases compared with healthy controls. First-trimester serum samples from mothers of childhood ALL cases derived from large maternal cohorts in Finland and Iceland have been tested for antibodies to *Chlamydia*, *Helicobacter pylori*, and *Mycoplasma pneumoniae*.[156] Comparison of ALL cases to controls identified an increased risk associated with *M. pneumoniae* immunoglobulin M and, in Iceland, *H. pylori* immunoglobulin G. Within the same maternal cohort, evidence was found for activation of maternal Epstein-Barr virus infection in childhood ALL and non-AML cases.[157]

Smith and colleagues[158] have sought to assess the relationship of childhood ALL with hygiene conditions, an aspect of socioeconomic development affecting rates of exposure to infectious agents. The data suggested that improved public hygiene conditions measured by decreased prevalence of hepatitis A virus infection (an agent with a fecal-oral route of transmission) were associated with high childhood ALL incidence rates. The model presented in this study supports the plausibility of the hypothesis that decreased childhood exposure to a leukemia-inducing agent associated with hygiene conditions leads to higher rates of ALL in children. This occurs by an increase in the incidence of in utero transmission caused by primary infection during pregnancy, or by increasing the number of those infected in early infancy because of lack of protective antibodies.

Antibiotic Use and Immunizations

No association between antibiotic use during pregnancy and leukemia has been identified.[148,150,152,159-161] No consistent association has been reported between vaccination during pregnancy and leukemia. Salonen and Saxen[162] have found a positive association between leukemia and maternal polio vaccination during pregnancy. Similarly, Gilman and colleagues[160] have reported a positive association between total childhood deaths and vaccination during pregnancy, largely accounted for by neoplasms of the reticuloendothelial system. However, in a population-based study in the Netherlands, there was no association between vaccination during pregnancy and ALL.[150]

Factors Related to the Immune System

It has been proposed that some cases of pediatric ALL arise as a rare response to a common childhood infection and that the leukemia-inducing potential of the agent is related to the timing of infection, with a greater leukemogenic effect for later infections compared with those occurring during infancy.[163] In this context, factors related to the child's immune system are of special interest. Several investigators have sought to identify factors such as birth order and breast-feeding that might be used as markers of infections or confer protection against infection before diagnosis of leukemia.[164]

Breast-Feeding

Breast-feeding is well known to have a protective effect against infection in infants.[165] Data on the association between breast-feeding and subsequent childhood leukemia are important because of the proposed hypothesis about the causative role of infections, taking into consideration the fact that breast-feeding protects against infections. This association was examined in several studies, with mixed results. Whereas some researchers failed to show any association between breast-feeding and childhood leukemia,[152,166-172] others have shown that a protective effect is offered by breast-feeding.[174] A report of a large North American case-control study has revealed that breast-feeding is associated with a reduced risk of childhood acute leukemia.[173] The inverse association was stronger with a longer duration of breast-feeding for patients with ALL and AML. A recent meta-analysis has suggested that breast-feeding of any duration is associated with a 9% lower risk of ALL, but there was little evidence of an association for risk of childhood AML.[174]

Immunizations

Previous studies have suggested that vaccinations during infancy may reduce the risk of subsequent childhood leukemia. No consistent association between leukemia and immunization has been identified, although two studies have suggested that early immunization against *Haemophilus influenzae* type b may reduce the incidence of childhood leukemia.[175,176] Groves and associates[176] have compared the vaccination histories of 439 children in whom ALL was diagnosed and 439 community control subjects matched to patients by age, race, and telephone exchange. No association was demonstrated between most infant vaccinations, such as oral poliovirus, diphtheria-pertussis-tetanus, and measles-mumps-rubella. However, infants receiving the conjugate *H. influenzae* type b vaccine had a reduced risk for subsequent childhood ALL. Confirmatory studies are needed.

Sibship Size

Sibship size might be an indirect indicator of exposure to common childhood infections. However, although there is no consistent association between ALL and sibship size,[177] a study from Canada has reported that when all variables defining family structure are included in a model, having older siblings at the time of diagnosis is a risk factor in children in whom ALL was diagnosed before 4 years of age, whereas having older siblings in the first year of life is a protective factor in children in whom ALL was diagnosed at 4 years of age or later.[171] More recently, analysis of the Swedish Family-Cancer Database has demonstrated that having three or more older siblings is associated with a significantly reduced risk of childhood AML and ALL.[178]

Early Child Care and Preschool Experiences

Day care of the index child and siblings has been used as a proxy measure of exposure to infections. The findings of case-control studies have been inconsistent regarding association between attendance at day care centers and risk of leukemia.[177,179-185] The recent study, conducted by the UKCCS investigators, was specifically designed to test the early infection hypothesis, including the role of day care. They found that increasing levels of social activity are associated with reductions in risk of ALL in a dose-response manner.[185]

Related Exposures During Index Child's Lifetime

Studies of an association between childhood cancer and postnatal infection of the index child are problematic because of the difficulty in assessing whether the episodes of infectious disease were a possible cause of the childhood cancer or represented a prediagnostic sign of the disease. Some investigators have attempted to overcome this concern by restricting attention to infection during the first year or first 6 months of life, or by considering infections reported only during a specified period before diagnosis in patients and during a reference time in control subjects. Specifically, investigators have explored the role of parvovirus B19, with its hematotropic effects and the potential to precipitate varying forms of cytopenia, in patients before or after the diagnosis of ALL,[186] but failed to find an association between parvovirus B19 and childhood ALL. Other epidemiologic studies have provided inconsistent findings for an association between leukemia and recorded or reported infections in early life.[98,149,153,167,186-191] The UKCCS investigation, which used general practitioner records for visits during the first year of life, found that children with ALL diagnosed between the ages of 2 and 5 years had significantly more clinically diagnosed infectious episodes in infancy.[191] Another case-control study from the UKCCS explored the relationship between childhood leukemia, infant infection, and three markers of infection exposure—birth order, infant day care attendance, and area-based deprivation. The study findings have indicated that immune dysregulation in children who develop ALL is detectable from an early age.[192] Moreover, epidemiologic data have indicated that the risk of cALL is increased by higher socioeconomic status, isolation, and other community characteristics suggestive of abnormal patterns of infection during infancy,[13] and population-based incidence patterns have identified small peaks in the incidence of childhood ALL that coincide with years immediately following influenza epidemics.[42]

Chloramphenicol

Chloramphenicol can cause bone marrow suppression and could potentially play an causative role in childhood leukemia. Shu and coworkers[193] have reported a positive association with the use of chloramphenicol from a study conducted in Shanghai. The risk of leukemia associated with chloramphenicol use increased with increasing total number of reported days of use. The association was stronger for AML than for ALL. A major limitation of the study was the long interval between diagnosis (1974 to 1986) and interview (1985 to 1986) for the patients, whereas the control subjects were recruited in the 2-year period from 1985 to 1986.

Contact with Animals

Although there has been considerable interest in a possible role of feline leukemia virus because of similarities between human and feline ALL in clinical findings, laboratory data, and response to treatment,[194] evidence is lacking for a biologic association.[195]

Bovine leukemia virus has also been studied for a possible causative role in human leukemia. A case-control study of 131 children with leukemia and 136 regional population control subjects was conducted to investigate this association. However, none of the DNA samples from patients or control subjects hybridized with a bovine leukemia virus DNA probe, providing strong evidence that genomic integration of bovine leukemia virus is not a factor in childhood ALL.[196]

Buckley and colleagues[98] have reported a positive association with mother's, father's, and index child's exposure to farm animals, compared with control subjects with other types of cancer or with community control subjects. However, no overall association with cat ownership was identified. A large case-control study has failed to show any association between pet ownership and childhood acute leukemia.[197]

Leukemia and Bacillus Calmette-Guérin Vaccination

Laboratory evidence that tubercle bacilli of the Calmette-Guérin strain (BCG) can prevent or suppress challenge from leukemia or tumor grafts in laboratory animals[198] has led investigators to explore whether BCG vaccination might reduce the incidence of cancer in humans and of leukemia in particular. However, no consistent association between BCG vaccination and the subsequent risk of leukemia was found.[198-201]

Seasonal Variations in Childhood Leukemia Onset

Seasonal variations in onset of disease could provide supportive evidence of an infectious cause. Westerbeek and associates[202] have demonstrated significant seasonal variation in the date of the first symptom of childhood ALL, with peaks occurring in November. However, a larger study of 15,835 patients with childhood leukemia has failed to reveal any evidence of seasonality in either month of birth or month of diagnosis overall or in any subgroups by age, gender, histologic analysis, or immunophenotype.[203] The study did, however, find a statistically significant February peak in month of birth for patients born before 1960 and an August peak in month of diagnosis for patients in whom leukemia was diagnosed before 1962. Although these findings may be caused by chance, they are also consistent with changes over time in the seasonality of exposure or immunologic response to a relevant infection. Changes in the seasonal variation in the fatality rate of a preleukemic illness, such as pneumonia, could be another explanation. Ross and coworkers[204] have examined the data from the Children's Cancer Group and the Pediatric Oncology Group for seasonal variation patterns. There was a statistically significant seasonal variation for ALL (peak in the summer). Biologic mechanisms underlying these seasonal patterns are probably multifactorial and need to be investigated.

ENVIRONMENTAL EXPOSURES

Although there is a large body of literature describing the associations between various environmental exposures and childhood leukemia, there is insufficient evidence for a causal relationship in most exposure studies, with the exception of those for ionizing radiation. The retrospective studies are limited because of the reliance placed on parental self-report of the exposure in the context of a case-control study design, which can be hampered by recall bias. In addition, the nonspecific nature of the exposure being assessed makes it hard to explore causal mechanisms involved with the associations. Moreover, most of the exposure assessment has focused on paternal exposures, with little emphasis placed on maternal exposures. To evaluate the importance of these exposures more clearly in future investigations, improvement is needed in the following areas: (1) importance given to maternal exposures; (2) sophisticated exposure techniques used; (3) attention paid to the mechanism, timing, and route of exposure; and (4) evidence provided that the exposure is actually transferred to the child's environment.

Radiation Exposure

In utero exposure to radiation has been reported to be associated with a small yet statistically significantly increased risk of development of childhood leukemia in numerous case-control studies.[166,205-213] Reported estimated risks generally ranged from 1.1 to 2.0, with most of the risk ratios being equal to or lower than 1.6. It is reasonable to expect that in utero levels of exposure to radiation would have declined substantially over time, given the knowledge of health-related risks associated with radiation exposure and the reduced level of radiation required for diagnostic procedures. Studies from Sweden, England, and the United States have demonstrated higher risk estimates in children born in earlier eras (e.g., 1930s to 1950s) compared with more recent time periods.[213-216] Nonetheless, the potential role of in utero exposure to radiation in childhood leukemia has remained controversial. Much of the debate has focused on the lack of an observed association in offspring of mothers who were exposed while pregnant at the time of the Hiroshima and Nagasaki atomic bombs,[217,218] coupled with concerns regarding the lack of good exposure assessment and the potential for

recall bias in case-control studies of the topic. Results from a large case-control study in North America did not identify an overall increased risk associated with in utero pelvimetric diagnostic x-rays, nor associations within subgroups defined by immunophenotype.[219] It is likely that the reduced rate and dose of exposure in North America has resulted in an inability to detect the small risk that may exist.

In contrast to the in utero data, postnatal exposure to radiation has not been consistently associated with an increased risk of childhood leukemia.[166,207,212] Regardless, even if leukemia risk is increased, the potential number of instances of leukemia that currently might be attributed to in utero or postnatal exposure to radiation would probably be very small when one considers the modest magnitude of risk and limited level of exposure. Results of a case-control study of 302 cases of infant leukemia have suggested that paternal low-level radiation exposure before conception is associated with an increased risk of infant leukemia, although the nature of this association needs to be evaluated further.[220]

A number of investigations of environmental exposures of children to sources of radiation from nuclear detonations and power plants have been conducted to determine the potential impact on leukemia risk. In studies of children who survived the atomic bombs of Hiroshima and Nagasaki, an increased occurrence of leukemia 5 to 15 years later was seen.[221] Leukemia risk was positively correlated with the dose of radiation in the atomic bomb survivors. Reports relating to follow-up of nuclear accidents at Three Mile Island and early reports from Chernobyl did not provide strong evidence of an increased risk of childhood leukemia. Analyses that included residents in the area surrounding the Three Mile Island facility did not reveal an increase in the ratio of observed to expected incidence of leukemia.[222] Similarly, investigation of specific regions of the former Soviet Union did not reveal increased rates of childhood leukemia within the first 5 years after the Chernobyl accident.[223] Because of the widespread fallout from Chernobyl, a series of investigations were undertaken in affected countries, including Sweden,[224] Finland,[225] England,[226] Scotland,[227] Germany,[228] and Greece.[229] With the exception of higher rates in Scotland and an observed excess of infant leukemia (i.e., younger than 1 year) in Greece,[230] results were generally negative for an observed increase after the accident. The most recent investigation of the acute and long-term risks for childhood leukemia resulting from radiation exposure (median estimated dose less than 10 mGy) following the Chernobyl power station accident has identified a significant increase in leukemia risk with increasing radiation dose to the bone marrow.[231] However, the potential overestimate of childhood leukemia risk in one region has raised serious concerns regarding conclusions that could be drawn about the level of risk resulting from the Chernobyl accident.

During the 1950s, testing of nuclear weapons took place in Nevada, with nuclear fallout affecting regions of Nevada and Utah. Studies were carried out in Utah to determine the potential impact on childhood leukemia, using geographic region–specific radiation dose estimates to the bone marrow. No significant trend between estimated dose and risk of leukemia mortality was found.[232] However, the risk of death from leukemia was found to be higher in those exposed at the highest dose level (6 to 30 mGy) compared with those in the lowest dose group (0 to 2.9 mGy).

During the past several decades, there has been considerable interest in the potential impact of nuclear facilities—nuclear energy plants or nuclear reprocessing plants—on cancer risk in surrounding residents. Studies addressing childhood leukemia have been conducted in England,[233,234] France,[235,236] United States,[237,238] Germany,[239] and Canada.[240] In aggregate, these investigations have not provided strong evidence of an increased occurrence of childhood leukemia, although several have reported increases in incidence and mortality.

Although the biologic plausibility of indoor radon exposure and the cause of childhood leukemia are speculative[241] and debatable,[242] studies have been conducted to address the topic. Ecologic investigations have provided some evidence for a correlation,[241-243] but case-control studies incorporating measurement of indoor radon levels have not found higher levels in homes of children with ALL[244] and AML.[244,245]

Parental Occupational Exposures

Occupational exposure of parents and its association with childhood leukemia have been the subject of several investigations.[246-249] Occupations and exposures of fathers were investigated more often than those of the mother. Detailed assessment, using a job exposure matrix to classify occupational exposures, identified increased risk for childhood AML to be associated with maternal exposure to 1,1,1-tricholorethane, toluene, mineral spirits, alkanes, and mononuclear aromatic hydrocarbons, although dose-response associations were not present.[249] Exposure in the home was not associated with increased risk. Investigation by the U.K. Childhood Cancer Study has identified small but statistically significant increased risks in childhood ALL patients whose fathers were exposed to exhaust fumes, driving, and/or inhaled particulate hydrocarbons.[248] The studies have several limitations related to the quality of exposure assessment, small numbers of exposed children, multiple comparisons, and possible bias toward the reporting of positive results. Although there is some evidence for an association between childhood leukemia and paternal exposure to solvents, paint, and employment in motor vehicle–related occupations, clearly established associations between parental occupation and childhood leukemia are lacking.

Exposure to Chemicals and Dust

Pesticides

There is considerable interest in the association among pesticides, including insecticides, fungicides and herbicides, and childhood leukemia, primarily because of the observed higher incidence of leukemia in rural areas and because of the biologic activity of these chemicals. Leiss and Savitz[250] have reported a positive association between the use of pest strips and childhood leukemia. The insecticide used in pest strips was dichlorvos, an organophosphate that has been associated with adult-onset leukemia in men.[251] Another study has reported an association between the use of pesticides in gardens and farms and childhood leukemia.[252] There was no association of leukemia with reported home pest extermination in this study. A positive association between maternal exposure during pregnancy and lactation and paternal exposure while the mother was pregnant to household pesticides and garden pesticides or herbicides was reported by Lowengart and colleagues.[253] One report has provided further evidence for an association between an increased risk of leukemia and rural residence and use of household pesticides.[254] Several other studies have reported an association between pesticide exposure and childhood leukemia.[255,256]

In a multicenter study of 404 patients with ALL and individually matched community control subjects, Buckley and associates[98] have reported a positive association between ALL and both paternal exposure (RR = 2.8, $P < .001$) and exposure of the index child (RR = 5.0, $P < .001$) to insecticides. The strongest associations for both paternal exposure and exposure of the index child were apparent for T-cell and common cell ALL.

In another case-control study consisting of 204 patients with AML and matched community control subjects, Buckley and coworkers[257] reported a positive association with maternal occupational exposure to pesticides before, during, and after pregnancy and paternal occupational exposure during the same time period. In addition, there was an independent association of maternal exposure to household fly sprays, pesticides, and garden and agricultural sprays and treatment of the house by insect exterminators in the month before the last menstrual cycle and during the index pregnancy, and direct exposure of the index child to household and garden insecticides. These associations were independent of parental occupational exposure.

Thus, although there is a large body of literature on the association between pesticide exposure and childhood leukemia,[255,256] these studies are limited by the nonspecific nature of the exposure, their reliance on parental self-report, and the lack of sufficient evidence for a causal relationship. Moreover, use of pesticides may be an indicator of rural isolation; thus, there is a possible confounding effect because of the patterns of exposure to infection that may be associated with population mixing.

Agent Orange

Wen and colleagues[258] have reported a small increase in the risk of AML being diagnosed before age 2 in offspring of veterans who had served in Cambodia or Vietnam. The causative importance of these observations remains to be determined. Exposure to Agent Orange was evaluated in this study, but no association was identified. Other studies have also concluded that exposure to the herbicides in Agent Orange is not associated with an increased risk of childhood leukemia in the children born to veterans reporting the exposure.[259]

Hydrocarbons and Solvents

Parental exposure to hydrocarbons at work has been investigated as a potential risk factor for childhood leukemia, with no consistent association between paternal or maternal occupational exposure to hydrocarbons and leukemia (all types, specifically ALL).[260-264] Similarly, no association between paternal exposure to benzene and leukemia has been found.[253,257,262-265] Maternal occupational exposure has been less well studied but, in two of the three studies, a positive association, with maternal occupational exposure to hydrocarbons was found that is compatible with the observation that exposure to benzene is associated with AML in adults.[162,193,257] Two studies have indicated that maternal exposures to hydrocarbons during the preconception period, pregnancy, and the postnatal period are related to an increased risk of ALL.[266] A positive association between ALL and paternal exposure to hydrocarbons during the preconception period was also found.

No clear association with residential proximity to industrial sources of hydrocarbons has been observed,[267,268] although one study has reported an increased risk of childhood leukemia, and AML in particular, associated with living near gas stations and/or repair garages.[264] An increased risk of childhood leukemia associated with paternal occupational exposure to chlorinated solvents has been reported by several investigators.[253,257,263] The risk has been assessed for exposure during the periods of 1 year before pregnancy, during pregnancy, and after delivery.[257] Several investigators have reported a positive association with postnatal exposure of the index child to solvents.[98,153] No consistent association with maternal exposure to solvents was apparent.[269] One report has revealed a significant association between substantial participation by household members in some common household activities involving organic solvents and childhood leukemia,[270] but these findings need further substantiation.

Metal Dusts and Fumes

A positive association between total reported duration of paternal occupational exposure to lead and AML has been reported by Buckley and associates.[257] In the same study, they reported an association between maternal occupational exposure to "metal dusts and fumes." Similar findings were reported by Shu and coworkers.[193] In their study in Shanghai, maternal occupational exposure to lead was associated with an increased risk of acute leukemia. A positive association between maternal exposure to molten metal and ALL (null cell and T cell) and a positive association between paternal exposure to metals and T-cell ALL have been reported.[98] However, ecologic studies have failed to show an association between leukemia and proximity to industrial facilities with an increased exposure to metal or metal fumes.[271,272]

Wood Dust

An association between maternal occupational exposure to wood dust before conception of the index child and childhood leukemia and non-Hodgkin lymphoma has been reported. A few women were exposed during or after pregnancy.[263] Significantly elevated relative risks have been reported for paternal occupational exposure to wood dust before conception, during the periconceptional and gestational periods, and postnatally.[246] The association of exposure to wood dust and leukemia was studied by Buckley and coworkers.[98,257] They found that the risk is elevated compared with that for other cancers and for community control subjects.

Traffic

Occupational exposure to elevated concentrations of benzene is a known cause of leukemia in adults. Concentrations of benzene from motor vehicle exhaust fumes could be elevated along highly trafficked streets. The hypothesis that exposure to traffic-related air pollution increases the risk of development of childhood cancer has been examined by several investigators.[273-275] Results indicate that there might be an association between residence on a busy street and childhood leukemia. However, these results need to be viewed with caution, because most of the results are based on ecologic studies, with an imperfect assessment of individual exposure.

Electromagnetic and Radiofrequency Field Exposure

An initial report in 1979 suggested an association between childhood leukemia and residential proximity to sources of electric and magnetic fields, as assessed by wiring configurations.[276] Subsequently, a large number of investigations have been conducted to evaluate the hypothesis further that exposure to extremely low-level electric and magnetic fields may influence the risk of childhood leukemia and other pediatric malignancies.[228,277-289] These studies, although they provide some consistent findings, are difficult to interpret, given the inconsistencies observed in associations between inferred exposure (i.e., wire configuration) compared with measured fields.

Moreover, many of these studies are limited by small sample size and the inability to consider potential confounding factors in the analysis adequately. The more recently reported investigations from the United States,[287] Canada,[288] England,[289,290] and Japan[291] have provided rather convincing evidence that electric and magnetic field exposure is not associated with a significantly increased risk of childhood ALL. Nonetheless, results of meta-analyses[292,293] have been interpreted to suggest that risk may be increased at the highest exposure levels (i.e., more than $0.4\ \mu T$). However, it is important to note that even if there is an increased risk at this highest exposure level, the proportion of the population exposed is extremely small and thus the attributable risk would be negligible. Beyond investigation of risk for leukemia, there are reports of possible associations between electric and magnetic field exposure and prognosis.[294,295]

Although not as extensively studied as electric and magnetic fields, radiofrequency exposure has been suggested as a possible cancer-related risk factor.[296] A recent report investigating radiofrequency exposure in 1928 childhood leukemia patients has observed a twofold increased risk associated with living within 2 km of an AM radio transmitter, which was statistically significant in a dose-dependent fashion for childhood ALL.[297]

LIFESTYLE

A number of associations have been made between lifestyle risk factors and the development of cancer.

Diet and Vitamin Supplements

Maternal Diet and Vitamin Supplement Use During Pregnancy

Diet and use of vitamin supplements have been shown to be associated with the risk of several cancers in adults. In pediatric malignancies, research has focused primarily on use of vitamin supplements during pregnancy, with little attention given to diet.[159,298] Investigation of maternal diet during pregnancy of children with ALL between the ages of 1 and 5 years has found that ALL risk is statistically significantly lower with increased consumption of fruits, vegetables, and fish (seafood), and a significantly higher risk is related to increased maternal intake of sugar and syrups and meat products, but these findings will require confirmation in other populations.[299]

In the available studies of childhood leukemia and maternal consumption of vitamin supplements during pregnancy, no association was found,[159,162,298] with the exception of one study reporting a decrease in risk of ALL in mothers taking iron supplements during the index pregnancy.[300]

Almost 80% of infants with leukemia have a specific genetic abnormality in their leukemic blast cells involving the *MLL* gene on chromosome band 11q23.[301] Abnormalities involving 11q23 have also been reported in secondary AML after exposure to topoisomerase inhibitors. Therefore, Ross and colleagues[301] have hypothesized that infant leukemias involving 11q23 may result from exposure to naturally occurring topoisomerase inhibitors. These agents include caffeine and various fruits and vegetables. A subset of mothers of infants with leukemia diagnosed at 1 year of age or younger and control children selected by random digit dialing included in three multicenter case-control studies of childhood leukemia in the United States[257,298] was revisited to obtain additional information on maternal diet during the index pregnancy.[302] On the basis of data from a food frequency questionnaire assessing consumption of 26 food items during the index pregnancy, there was no association between total estimated dietary intake of topoisomerase II inhibitors and leukemia of all types combined or ALL. However, there was a statistically significant positive association for AML with increasing consumption of dietary topoisomerase II inhibitors. One study has identified bioflavonoids, natural substances in food and in dietary supplements, that cause site-specific DNA cleavage in the *MLL* breakpoint cluster region in vivo.[303] These results suggest that maternal ingestion of bioflavonoids may induce *MLL* breaks and potentially induce translocations in utero, leading to infant leukemia. In utero exposures and their association with infant acute leukemia have been assessed by Alexander and associates.[304] Use of cigarettes and alcohol, the ingestion of certain herbal medicines, and drugs classified as "DNA damaging" and exposure to pesticides were associated with an increased risk of leukemias associated with alterations in *MLL*.

Postnatal Diet of Index Child and Use of Vitamin Supplements

The role of diet of the index child in the development of childhood leukemia has not been the subject of intensive investigation. Results of investigations exploring the association between the intake of certain food items thought to be precursors or inhibitors of *N*-nitroso compounds have been controversial. Some investigators have reported a positive association with hot dogs,[253] whereas others have failed to show any association with consumption of hot dogs or other cured meats.[298] No associations have been reported with postnatal use of vitamins by the index child,[98] consumption of fish, dried milk, fruit juice, or canned foods.[208]

Tobacco Smoking by Parents

Parental smoking and its association with childhood leukemia have been the focus of several investigations. However, issues such as publication bias (greater likelihood of positive associations being published) limit the quality of the data. In summary, the literature has shown no consistent association between childhood leukemia and parental exposure to tobacco.

Furthermore, no consistent association between maternal smoking during pregnancy and leukemia has been found.[305-308] No consistent association between paternal smoking and all types of leukemia combined or AML has been found. In most studies, the period of exposure considered has been up to the birth of the index child. Although a positive association between paternal smoking and ALL has been reported by several investigators,[309-312] others have failed to show any association.[305-308,313,314] The largest investigation of maternal smoking and risk of childhood leukemia, conducted in Sweden, included over 1.4 million children born between 1983 and 1997.[315] This study found that maternal smoking is associated with a lower risk of ALL but a higher risk of AML, particularly in heavy smokers. Sandler and coworkers[316] have evaluated the cancer risk from cumulative household exposure to cigarette smoke in a case-control study. Cancer risk was greater for those exposed during childhood and adulthood than for those exposed during only one period. There is some evidence that the effect of parental smoking could be modified to some extent by variant alleles of the *CYP1A1* gene.[306]

An earlier study has reported an association between AML (M4 or M5) and reported use of mind-altering drugs (primarily marijuana) by the mother in the year before or during the index pregnancy.[159] However, a subsequent study by the same investigators, designed to test the hypothesis of maternal marijuana exposure, failed to reproduce the association.[317] Thus, overall, maternal smoking during pregnancy or exposure of infants to cigarette smoke shortly after birth is unlikely to contribute substantially to the risk of childhood leukemia. Moreover, it seems unlikely that passive smoke inhalation during childhood strongly affects the risk of development of childhood leukemia. However, the demonstration of genotoxic effects on the fetus of exposure to metabolites of tobacco smoke should lead to strong recommendations aimed at fully protecting fetuses, newborns, and infants from tobacco smoke.

Alcohol

Most studies relate solely to alcohol consumption by the mother and only to consumption during the pregnancy leading to the birth of the index child. No consistent associations have been found between maternal alcohol consumption before or during the index pregnancy and leukemia of all types combined or ALL.[149,161,193,310] A recent report has indicated that maternal alcohol consumption before (OR = 1.37; 95% CI, 0.99 to 1.9) or during pregnancy (OR = 1.39; 95% CI, 1.01 to 1.93) may contribute to an increased risk of childhood leukemia.[318] There is, however, some evidence from a number of studies of an association between maternal alcohol consumption and AML, primarily in those in whom leukemia was diagnosed early in life. Severson and colleagues[305] have reported an increased risk of AML in children in whom leukemia was diagnosed at or before 2 years of age and whose mothers reported consuming alcohol during their pregnancies. The association was particularly pronounced in patients with monocytic and myelomonocytic leukemia. However, the authors advised cautious interpretation of the data because of the small number of subjects included in the subgroup analysis. A positive association between alcohol consumption and AML has also been reported by others.[161,310] The risk appears to be increased for alcohol consumption during each of the three trimesters of pregnancy and for each type of beverage. There is also a suggestion of a dose-response relationship.[305,310] No association between paternal alcohol consumption and childhood leukemia has been found.[193,305,310]

MATERNAL REPRODUCTIVE HISTORY

Maternal Age and Birth Order

Accumulation of chromosomal aberrations and mutations during the maturation of germ cells are mechanisms hypothesized for the association between increasing maternal age and cancer in offspring. Most studies have failed to show an association between leukemia and maternal age.[193,319-322] However, a report using the Swedish Family-Cancer Database has revealed a maternal age effect for childhood leukemia (about 50% greater in those older than 35 years).[323]

Most studies based on index cases do not show a positive association with first birth. However, one of the largest of these studies has revealed a decreasing trend with increasing birth order for children in whom ALL was diagnosed between the ages of 0 and 4 years.[322] This study also has shown a positive association between AML and birth order, adjusted for age, gender, calendar period, and maternal age at birth of child. This association was also reported from a combined analysis of data for children with AML that was diagnosed before 1 year of age in the United States.[319]

Prior Fetal Loss

The association between childhood leukemia and prior fetal loss has been examined by many investigators, with the reported relative risks ranging from 0.3 to 1.8.[153,319,320] Data from a Children's Cancer Group case-control study were analyzed to test the hypothesis that this association depends on the number of previous fetal losses and age at leukemia diagnosis. Overall, a modestly increased risk of leukemia was found to be associated with a history of fetal loss. Stratification by age at diagnosis of leukemia has shown that this association is significant only for patients in whom ALL and AML was diagnosed before 4 years of age and most significant in patients in whom leukemia was diagnosed before 2 years of age.[324] Ross and associates[319] also have reported a positive association between infantile AML and prior fetal loss. These reports suggested that childhood acute leukemia occurring at younger ages may be associated with an underlying genetic abnormality or chronic environmental exposure, which can be lethal to the developing fetus or mutagenic, resulting in the development of acute leukemia.

Oral Contraceptives

McKinney and coworkers[152] have reported no association between leukemia and an interval of less than 3 months between when a woman stops taking oral contraceptives and conception. Van Steensel-Moll and colleagues[150] have reported no association between childhood leukemia and any use of oral contraceptives.

Maternal Illness and Use of Medications During Index Pregnancy

Ever since diethylstilbestrol treatment of the mother during pregnancy was causally linked with clear cell adenocarcinoma of the vagina and cervix, several investigators have explored a possible association between use of medications during pregnancy and childhood cancer.

Van Steensel-Moll and colleagues[150] have reported a significant positive association with "threatened miscarriage" and "drugs to maintain pregnancy." Another study has reported a positive association with hormonal treatment for infertility in the preconception period and reported infertility investigations.[148] However, Kobayashi and associates[325] from Japan have shown that no case of maternal ovulation induction was recorded for the mothers of 2301 children with leukemia. The Northern California Childhood Leukemia Study has observed a significantly increased risk of ALL in mothers reporting influenza or pneumonia during the index pregnancy.[300] Lastly, the Children's Oncology Group study of 1840 childhood ALL cases has reported significant associations with parental use of amphetamines or diet pills and mind-altering drugs before and during the index pregnancy.[326]

Other Studies

Ultrasound Examinations

No association has been found between routine ultrasound exposure in pregnancy and childhood leukemia.[219,327-329]

Anesthesia During Labor

No consistent association has been found between childhood leukemia and cesarean section, which is an indication for anesthesia during labor.[148,190,321] McKinney and associates[152] have found a positive association between leukemia and the use of narcotic and opioid analgesics, mainly dextropropoxyphene hydrochloride, and between leukemia and the use of barbiturates in labor, whereas other investigators have failed to show any association.[148]

MEDICAL HISTORY OF THE INDEX CHILD

Wen and coworkers[330] have investigated the association between childhood ALL and allergic disorders (e.g., asthma, hay fever, food or drug allergies, eczema, hives) using a case-control study design. The results of this study agreed with those of most previous studies of adult cancer, suggesting that allergic disorders may be associated with a reduced risk of childhood ALL.

Congenital Anomalies

The presence of cancer and congenital anomalies in the same child may sometimes be explained by an underlying genetic abnormality. An investigation of these associations might provide clues to the identification of genes important to a study of the causes of childhood leukemia. The excess risk of leukemia associated with congenital anomalies appears to be accounted for largely by those with Down syndrome.[331] Children with Down syndrome have a 30-fold increased risk of developing childhood leukemia, with the proportion of leukemia attributable to Down syndrome by age 14 estimated to be 2.7%.[332] To evaluate the risk of leukemia associated with congenital anomalies, a series of matched case-control studies was carried out by the Children's Cancer Group.[333] A total of 2117 children in whom ALL was diagnosed and 605 children in whom AML was diagnosed were compared with matched regional population control subjects. Data on congenital anomalies in the index child were collected by telephone interview with the biologic mother. More congenital anomalies were reported in index case patients with ALL than in control subjects and included statistically significant increases in multiple birthmarks, Down syndrome, congenital heart defects, and gastrointestinal anomalies. Similarly, birth defects were reported more often in index case patients with AML than in control subjects and included a significant increase in multiple birthmarks, Down syndrome, mental retardation, and congenital heart defects. Exclusion of patients with Down syndrome from the analysis did not change the statistically significant excess of gastrointestinal anomalies in patients with ALL or the excess of birthmarks in patients with AML. However, most of the observed associations with congenital anomalies occurred in children with Down syndrome.

In a study of 20,029 children with cancer in England between 1971 and 1986, the occurrence of congenital anomalies was significantly lower in children with leukemia or lymphoma (2.6%) than in those with solid cancers (4.4%).[334] This finding is compatible with the hypothesis that mutations leading to the development of leukemias and lymphomas occur at a much later stage in development in the cells committed to hematopoiesis.

Birth Weight and Length at Birth

Birth weight might serve as an indirect indicator of intrauterine stresses to the fetus, and therefore has been studied by numerous investigators for its association with leukemia.[98,319,322,324,335-339] The accumulating literature on high birth weight and risk of childhood ALL, particularly at younger ages, is becoming increasingly convincing, as demonstrated in a meta-analysis.[340] High levels of insulin-like growth factor-1, which might produce a larger baby and contribute to leukemogenesis, has been postulated as an explanation for this association.[341] No consistent association has been reported between length of child at birth and leukemia.[152,321]

Vitamin K

Several studies have explored the association between vitamin K administered in the neonatal period and leukemia, with inconsistent results.[148,342-347] The initial studies by Golding and associates[342,343] from England have shown an association between intramuscularly but not orally administered vitamin K and childhood leukemia. The biologic basis for the association between vitamin K and childhood leukemia was the observation that concentrations of vitamin K in the infants 12 to 24 hours after injection have been shown to increase sister chromatid exchanges in human placental lymphocytes in vitro and sheep fetal lymphocytes in vitro.[348] However, in vivo studies in human neonates did not substantiate this observation.[349] Moreover, the positive association between leukemia of all types and vitamin K reported by Golding and coworkers has not been confirmed by analytical studies in England,[346] Germany,[345] Denmark,[350] Sweden[344] and the United States.[351] Parker and colleagues[352] have reported a positive association between parenterally administered vitamin K and childhood ALL diagnosed between the ages of 1 and 6 years, although no association was seen in a cohort-based study. The authors stated that a definitive conclusion regarding the relationship between vitamin K and childhood leukemia has not yet been reached. Thus, the relationship between vitamin K and childhood leukemia is tenuous at best, and the attributable risk is extremely small, with some as yet unidentifiable biologic predisposition placing patients at increased risk of developing childhood leukemia.[353]

FUTURE DIRECTIONS

The occurrence of cancer during childhood remains one of the leading causes of childhood mortality, even with the marked improvements in the treatment and cure of pediatric malignancies over the past 3 to 4 decades. Although the volume of epidemiologic research addressing the cause of childhood cancer is considerable, relatively little has been achieved regarding our understanding of the causes of childhood leukemia, which would have a direct impact on potential future prevention strategies. The absence of progress is not the result of a lack of research in global populations directed toward investigation of environmental and genetic factors. This body of research involves large case-control epidemiologic studies including thousands of pediatric leukemia cases, with many incorporating state-of-the-art clinical and biologic characterization, along with environmental sampling designed to enhance exposure assessment. Future research in this, the most common malignancy of childhood, will probably need to focus on patients with a common primary genetic lesion, such as those with *BRC-ABL*, *MML-AF4*, or *TEL-AML1* fusion, or hyperdiploidy. By investigating those in such well-defined groups, the potential exists to identify common environmental and genetic factors that result in the specific genetic lesion.

REFERENCES

1. Parkin DM, Kramarova PE, Draper GJ, et al (eds). International Incidence of Childhood Cancer, vol II (Publication No. 144). Lyon, France, International Agency for Research on Cancer, 1998.
2. Howard SC, Metzger ML, Wilimas JA, et al. Childhood cancer epidemiology in low-income countries. Cancer. 2008;112:461-472.
3. Linet MS, Devesa SS. Descriptive epidemiology of childhood leukaemia. Br J Cancer. 1991;63:424-429.
4. National Cancer Institute. SEER: Surveillance, Epidemiology, and End Results, 2008. Available at http://www.seer.cancer.gov/seerstat.
5. Greaves MF, Colman SM, Beard ME, et al. Geographic distribution of acute lymphoblastic leukaemia subtypes: second report of the collaborative group study. Leukemia. 1993;7:27-34.
6. Alexander FE, Chan LC, Lam TH, et al. Clustering of childhood leukaemia in Hong Kong: association with the childhood peak and common acute lymphoblastic leukaemia and with population mixing. Br J Cancer. 1997;75:457-463.
7. Ross JA, Davies SM, Potter JD, Robison LL. Epidemiology of childhood leukemia, with a focus on infants. Epidemiol Rev. 1994;16:243-272.
8. Court Brown WM, Doll R. Leukaemia in childhood and young adult life. Trends in mortality in relation to aetiology. BMJ. 1961;1:981-988.
9. Ajiki W, Hanai A, Tsukuma H, et al. Incidence of childhood cancer in Osaka, Japan, 1971-1988: reclassification of registered cases by Birch's scheme using information on clinical diagnosis, histology and primary site. Jpn J Cancer Res. 1994;85:139-146.
10. Katz L, Steinitz R. Israel Cancer Registry, 1970-1979. Lyon, France, International Agency for Research on Cancer, 1988.
11. Parkin DM, Stiller CA, Draper GJ, Bieber CA. The international incidence of childhood cancer. Int J Cancer. 1988;42:511-520.
12. Kinlen LJ, Petridou E. Childhood leukemia and rural population movements: Greece, Italy, and other countries. Cancer Causes Control. 1995;6:445-450.
13. Greaves MF, Alexander FE. An infectious etiology for common acute lymphoblastic leukemia in childhood? Leukemia. 1993;7:349-360.
14. Stiller CA, McKinney PA, Bunch KJ, et al. Childhood cancer and ethnic group in Britain: a United Kingdom children's Cancer Study Group (UKCCSG) study. Br J Cancer. 1991;64:543-548.
15. Steliarova-Foucher E, Stiller C, Lacour B, Kaatsch P. International Classification of Childhood Cancer, 3rd ed. Cancer. 2005;103:1457-1467.
16. Ariffin H, Chen SP, Kwok CS, et al. Ethnic differences in the frequency of subtypes of childhood acute lymphoblastic leukemia: results of the Malaysia-Singapore Leukemia Study Group. J Pediatr Hematol Oncol. 2007;29:27-31.
17. Bhatia S, Sather HN, Heerema NA, et al. Racial and ethnic differences in survival of children with acute lymphoblastic leukemia. Blood. 2002;100:1957-1964.
18. Glazer ER, Perkins CI, Young JL Jr, et al. Cancer in Hispanic children in California, 1988-1994: comparison with non-Hispanic white children. Cancer. 1999;86:1070-1079.
19. Douer D, Preston-Martin S, Chang E, et al. High frequency of acute promyelocytic leukemia in Latinos with acute myeloid leukemia. Blood. 1996;87:308-313.

20. Aplenc R, Alonzo TA, Gerbing RB, et al. Ethnicity and survival in childhood acute myeloid leukemia: a report from the Children's Oncology Group. Blood. 2006;108:74-80.

21. Ramot B, Magrath I. Hypothesis: the environment is a major determinant of the immunological sub-type of lymphoma and acute lymphoblastic leukaemia in children. Br J Haematol. 1982;50:183-189.

22. Alexander FE, Ricketts TJ, McKinney PA, Cartwright RA. Community lifestyle characteristics and risk of acute lymphoblastic leukaemia in children. Lancet. 1990;336:1461-1465.

23. Draper GJ, Vincent TJ, O'Connor CM, et al. Socio-economic factors and variations in incidence rates between county districts. In Draper GJ (ed). The Geographic Epidemiology of Childhood Leukemia and Non-Hodgkin's Lymphomas in Great Britain, 1966-83, Studies on Medical and Population Subjects. London, Her Majesty's Stationery Office, 1991, pp 37-45.

24. Muirhead CR. Childhood leukemia in metropolitan regions in the United States: a possible relation to population density? Cancer Causes Control. 1995;6:383-388.

25. Stiller CA, Boyle PJ. Effect of population mixing and socioeconomic status in England and Wales, 1979-85, on lymphoblastic leukaemia in children. BMJ. 1996;313:1297-1300.

26. Rodrigues L, Hills M, McGale P, et al. Socio-economic factors in relation to childhood leukaemia and non-Hodgkin lymphomas: an analysis based on small area statistics for census tracts. In Draper GJ (ed). The Geographic Epidemiology of Childhood Leukaemia and Non-Hodgkin's Lymphomas in Great Britain, 1966-83, Studies on Medical and Population Subjects, vol 53. London, Her Majesty's Stationery Office, 1991, pp 47-56.

27. Swensen AR, Ross JA, Severson RK, et al. The age peak in childhood acute lymphoblastic leukemia: exploring the potential relationship with socioeconomic status. Cancer. 1997;79:2045-2051.

28. McWhirter WR. The relationship of incidence of childhood lymphoblastic leukaemia to social class. Br J Cancer. 1982;46:640-645.

29. Knox G. Epidemiology of childhood leukaemia in Northumberland and Durham. Br J Prev Soc Med. 1964;18:17-24.

30. Borugian MJ, Spinelli JJ, Mezei G, et al. Childhood leukemia and socioeconomic status in Canada. Epidemiology. 2005;16:526-531.

31. Birch JM, Swindell R, Marsden HB, et al. Childhood leukaemia in North West England 1954-1977: epidemiology, incidence and survival. Br J Cancer. 1981;43:324-329.

32. Gurney JG, Davis S, Severson RK, et al. Trends in cancer incidence in children in the U.S. Cancer. 1996;78:532-541.

33. McCredie M, Hoyer A, Coates M, et al. Trends in cancer incidence and mortality in New South Wales 1972-1989. New South Wales Central Cancer Registry. Sydney, Australia, 1992, pp 98-101.

34. Giles G, Waters K, Thursfield V, Farrugia H. Childhood cancer in Victoria, Australia, 1970-1989. Int J Cancer. 1995;63:794-797.

35. Dockerty JD, Cox B, Cockburn MG. Childhood leukaemias in New Zealand: time trends and ethnic differences. Br J Cancer. 1996;73:1141-1147.

36. Parkin DM, Clayton D, Black RJ, et al. Childhood leukaemia in Europe after Chernobyl: 5 year follow-up. Br J Cancer. 1996;73:1006-1012.

37. Gordis L, Szklo M, Thompson B, et al. An apparent increase in the incidence of acute nonlymphocytic leukemia in black children. Cancer. 1981;47:2763-2768.

38. McNally RJ, Cairns DP, Eden OB, et al. Examination of temporal trends in the incidence of childhood leukaemias and lymphomas provides aetiological clues. Leukemia. 2001;15:1612-1618.

39. Bunin GR, Feuer EJ, Witman PA, Meadows AT. Increasing incidence of childhood cancer: report of 20 years experience from the greater Delaware Valley Pediatric Tumor Registry. Paediatr Perinat Epidemiol. 1996;10:319-338.

40. McWhirter WR, Dobson C, Ring I. Childhood cancer incidence in Australia, 1982-1991. Int J Cancer. 1996;65:34-38.

41. McNally RJ, Birch JM, Taylor GM, Eden OB. Incidence of childhood precursor B-cell acute lymphoblastic leukaemia in northwest England. Lancet. 2000;356:485-486.

42. Kroll ME, Draper GJ, Stiller CA, Murphy MF. Childhood leukemia incidence in Britain, 1974-2000: time trends and possible relation to influenza epidemics. J Natl Cancer Inst. 2006;98:417-420.

43. Maule MM, Zuccolo L, Magnani C, et al. Bayesian methods for early detection of changes in childhood cancer incidence: trends for acute lymphoblastic leukaemia are consistent with an infectious aetiology. Eur J Cancer. 2006;42:78-83.

44. Maule MM, Merletti F, Pastore G, et al. Effects of maternal age and cohort of birth on incidence time trends of childhood acute lymphoblastic leukemia. Cancer Epidemiol Biomarkers Prev. 2007;16:347-351.

45. Linet MS, Ries LA, Smith MA, et al. Cancer surveillance series: recent trends in childhood cancer incidence and mortality in the United States. J Natl Cancer Inst. 1999;91:1051-1058.

46. Hrusak O, Trka J, Zuna J, et al. Acute lymphoblastic leukemia incidence during socioeconomic transition: selective increase in children from 1 to 4 years. Leukemia. 2002;16:720-725.

47. Mainwaring D. Epidemiology of acute leukaemia of childhood in the Liverpool area. Br J Prev Soc Med. 1966;20:189-194.

48. Gilman EA, Knox EG. Temporal-spatial distribution of childhood leukaemias and non-Hodgkin's lymphomas in Great Britain. In Draper GJ (ed). The Geographic Epidemiology of Childhood Leukaemia and Non-Hodgkin's Lymphomas in Great Britain, 1966-83, Studies on Medical and Population Subjects, vol 53. London, Her Majesty's Stationery Office, 1991, pp 77-99.

49. Bellec S, Hemon D, Rudant J, et al. Spatial and space-time clustering of childhood acute leukaemia in France from 1990 to 2000: a nationwide study. Br J Cancer. 2006;94:763-770.

50. Petridou E, Revinthi K, Alexander FE, et al. Space-time clustering of childhood leukaemia in Greece: evidence supporting a viral acause. Br J Cancer. 1996;73:1278-1283.

51. Fraumeni JF Jr, Ederer F, Handy VH. Temporal-spatial distribution of childhood leukemia in New York State. Special reference to case clustering by year of birth. Cancer. 1966;19:996-1000.

52. Morris V. Space-time interactions in childhood cancers. J Epidemiol Community Health. 1990;44:55-58.

53. Stark CR, Mantel N. Temporal-spatial distribution of birth dates for Michigan children with leukemia. Cancer Res. 1967;27:1749-1755.

54. Evatt BL, Chase GA, Heath CW Jr. Time-space clustering in cases of acute leukemia in two Georgia counties. Blood. 1973;41:265-272.

55. Larsen RJ, Holmes CL, Heath CW Jr. A statistical test for measuring unimodal clustering: a description of the test and of its application to cases of acute leukemia in metropolitan Atlanta, Georgia. Biometrics. 1973;29:301-309.

56. Birch JM, Alexander FE, Blair V, et al. Space-time clustering patterns in childhood leukaemia support a role for infection. Br J Cancer. 2000;82:1571-1576.

57. McNally RJ, Eden TO, Alexander FE, et al. Is there a common aetiology for certain childhood malignancies? Results of cross-space-time clustering analyses. Eur J Cancer. 2005;41:2911-2916.

58. Hepworth SJ, Feltbower RG, McKinney PA. Childhood leukaemias and CNS tumours: correlation of international incidence rates. Eur J Cancer. 2006;42:509-513.

59. Steinmaus C, Lu M, Todd RL, Smith AH. Probability estimates for the unique childhood leukemia cluster in Fallon, Nevada, and risks near other U.S. military aviation facilities. Environ Health Perspect. 2004;112:766-771.

60. Rubin CS, Holmes AK, Belson MG, et al. Investigating childhood leukemia in Churchill County, Nevada. Environ Health Perspect. 2007;115:151-157.
61. Shannon K. Genetic predispositions and childhood cancer. Environ Health Perspect. 1998;106(Suppl 3):801-806.
62. Zipursky A, Poon A, Doyle J. Leukemia in Down syndrome: a review. Pediatr Hematol Oncol. 1992;9:139-149.
63. Stiller CA, Chessells JM, Fitchett M. Neurofibromatosis and childhood leukaemia/lymphoma: a population-based UKCCSG study. Br J Cancer. 1994;70:969-972.
64. Hecht F, Hecht BK. Cancer in ataxia-telangiectasia patients. Cancer Genet Cytogenet. 1990;46:9-19.
65. German J, Bloom D, Passarge E. Bloom's syndrome. V. Surveillance for cancer in affected families. Clin Genet. 1977;12:162-168.
66. Harnden DG. Inherited factors in leukaemia and lymphoma. Leuk Res. 1985;9:705-707.
67. Pendergrass TW. Epidemiology of acute lymphoblastic leukemia. Semin Oncol. 1985;12:80-91.
68. Egeler RM, Neglia JP, Arico M, et al. Acute leukemia in association with Langerhans cell histiocytosis. Med Pediatr Oncol. 1994;23:81-85.
69. Shaw MP, Eden OB, Grace E, Ellis PM. Acute lymphoblastic leukemia and Klinefelter's syndrome. Pediatr Hematol Oncol. 1992;9:81-85.
70. Hasle H, Mellemgaard A, Nielsen J, Hansen J. Cancer incidence in men with Klinefelter syndrome. Br J Cancer. 1995;71:416-420.
71. Merks JH, Caron HN, Hennekam RC. High incidence of malformation syndromes in a series of 1,073 children with cancer. Am J Med Genet. 2005;134A:132-143.
72. Narod SA, Stiller C, Lenoir GM. An estimate of the heritable fraction of childhood cancer. Br J Cancer. 1991;63:993-999.
73. Robison LL, Nesbit ME Jr, Sather HN, et al. Down syndrome and acute leukemia in children: a 10-year retrospective survey from Childrens Cancer Study Group. J Pediatr. 1984;105:235-242.
74. Watson MS, Carroll AJ, Shuster JJ, et al. Trisomy 21 in childhood acute lymphoblastic leukemia: a Pediatric Oncology Group study (8602). Blood. 1993;82:3098-3102.
75. Zeller B, Gustafsson G, Forestier E, et al. Acute leukaemia in children with Down syndrome: a population-based Nordic study. Br J Haematol. 2005;128:797-804.
76. Hasle H, Clemmensen IH, Mikkelsen M. Risks of leukaemia and solid tumours in individuals with Down's syndrome. Lancet. 2000;355:165-169.
77. Mejia-Arangure JM, Fajardo-Gutierrez A, Flores-Aguilar H, et al. Environmental factors contributing to the development of childhood leukemia in children with Down's syndrome. Leukemia. 2003;17:1905-1907.
78. Canfield KN, Spector LG, Robison LL, et al. Childhood and maternal infections and risk of acute leukaemia in children with Down syndrome: a report from the Children's Oncology Group. Br J Cancer. 2004;91:1866-1872.
79. Ross JA, Blair CK, Olshan AF, et al. Periconceptional vitamin use and leukemia risk in children with Down syndrome: a Children's Oncology Group study. Cancer. 2005;104:405-410.
80. Buckley JD, Buckley CM, Breslow NE, et al. Concordance for childhood cancer in twins. Med Pediatr Oncol. 1996;26:223-229.
81. Inskip PD, Harvey EB, Boice JD Jr, et al. Incidence of childhood cancer in twins. Cancer Causes Control. 1991;2:315-324.
82. Chaganti RS, Miller DR, Meyers PA, German J. Cytogenetic evidence of the intrauterine origin of acute leukemia in monozygotic twins. N Engl J Med. 1979;300:1032-1034.
83. Hartley SE, Sainsbury C. Acute leukaemia and the same chromosome abnormality in monozygotic twins. Hum Genet. 1981;58:408-410.
84. Ford AM, Ridge SA, Cabrera ME, et al. In utero rearrangements in the trithorax-related oncogene in infant leukaemias. Nature. 1993;363:358-360.
85. Miller RW. Deaths from childhood leukemia and solid tumors in twins and other sibs in the United States, 1960-67. J Natl Cancer Inst. 1971;46:203-209.
86. Draper GJ, Heaf MM, Kinnier Wilson LM. Occurrence of childhood cancers in sibs and estimation of familial risks. J Med Genet. 1977;14:81-90.
87. Thompson EN, Dallimore NS, Brook DL. Parental cancer in an unselected cohort of children with cancer referred to a single centre. Br J Cancer. 1988;57:127-129.
88. Olsen JH, Boice JD Jr, Seersholm N, et al. Cancer in the parents of children with cancer. N Engl J Med. 1995;333:1594-1599.
89. Hawkins MM, Draper GJ, Winter DL. Cancer in the offspring of survivors of childhood leukaemia and non-Hodgkin lymphomas. Br J Cancer. 1995;71:1335-1339.
90. Winther JF, Sankila R, Boice JD, et al. Cancer in siblings of children with cancer in the Nordic countries: a population-based cohort study. Lancet. 2001;358:711-717.
91. Rudant J, Menegaux F, Leverger G, et al. Family history of cancer in children with acute leukemia, Hodgkin's lymphoma or non-Hodgkin's lymphoma: the ESCALE study (SFCE). Int J Cancer. 2007;121:119-126.
92. Steinberg AG. The genetics of acute leukemia in children. Cancer. 1960;13:985-999.
93. Hafez M, El-Tahan H, El-Morsi A, et al. Genetic-environmental interaction in acute lymphatic leukemia. In Muller H, Weber W (eds). Familial Cancer, First International Research Conference. Basel, Switzerland, Karger, 1985, pp 161-166.
94. Perkkio M, Lie SO, Ekelund H, et al. Four pairs of siblings with acute leukemia during 1966-1985 in the Nordic countries: indication of an elevated familial risk? Pediatr Hematol Oncol. 1990;7:159-163.
95. Bajnoczky K, Khezri S, Kajtar P, et al. No chromosomal instability in offspring of survivors of childhood malignancy. Cancer Genet Cytogenet. 1999;109:79-80.
96. Savitz DA, Ananth CV. Birth characteristics of childhood cancer cases, controls, and their siblings. Pediatr Hematol Oncol. 1994;11:587-599.
97. Mann JR, Dodd HE, Draper GJ, et al. Congenital abnormalities in children with cancer and their relatives: results from a case-control study (IRESCC). Br J Cancer. 1993;68:357-363.
98. Buckley JD, Buckley CM, Ruccione K, et al. Epidemiological characteristics of childhood acute lymphocytic leukemia. Analysis by immunophenotype. The Childrens Cancer Group. Leukemia. 1994;8:856-864.
99. Kenney LB, Nicholson HS, Brasseux C, et al. Birth defects in offspring of adult survivors of childhood acute lymphoblastic leukemia. A Childrens Cancer Group/National Institutes of Health Report. Cancer. 1996;78:169-176.
100. Dorak MT, Lawson T, Machulla HK, et al. Unravelling an HLA-DR association in childhood acute lymphoblastic leukemia. Blood. 1999;94:694-700.
101. Taylor GM, Robinson MD, Binchy A, et al. Preliminary evidence of an association between HLA-DPB1*0201 and childhood common acute lymphoblastic leukaemia supports an infectious aetiology. Leukemia. 1995;9:440-443.
102. Taylor GM, Dearden S, Ravetto P, et al. Genetic susceptibility to childhood common acute lymphoblastic leukaemia is associated with polymorphic peptide-binding pocket profiles in HLA-DPB1*0201. Hum Mol Genet. 2002;11:1585-1597.
103. Wiemels JL, Smith RN, Taylor GM, et al. Methylenetetrahydrofolate reductase (MTHFR) polymorphisms and risk of molecularly defined subtypes of childhood acute leukemia. Proc Natl Acad Sci U S A. 2001;98:4004-4009.
104. Krajinovic M, Labuda D, Richer C, et al. Susceptibility to childhood acute lymphoblastic leukemia: influence of CYP1A1,

CYP2D6, GSTM1, and GSTT1 genetic polymorphisms. Blood. 1999;93:1496-1501.

105. Davies SM, Robison LL, Buckley JD, et al. Glutathione S-transferase polymorphisms in children with myeloid leukemia: a Children's Cancer Group study. Cancer Epidemiol Biomarkers Prev. 2000;9:563-566.

106. Lanciotti M, Dufour C, Corral L, et al. Genetic polymorphism of NAD(P)H:quinone oxidoreductase is associated with an increased risk of infant acute lymphoblastic leukemia without MLL gene rearrangements. Leukemia. 2005;19:214-216.

107. Krajinovic M, Labuda D, Sinnett D. Glutathione S-transferase P1 genetic polymorphisms and susceptibility to childhood acute lymphoblastic leukaemia. Pharmacogenetics. 2002;12:655-658.

108. Skibola CF, Smith MT, Kane E, et al. Polymorphisms in the methylenetetrahydrofolate reductase gene are associated with susceptibility to acute leukemia in adults. Proc Natl Acad Sci U S A. 1999;96:12810-12815.

109. Healy J, Belanger H, Beaulieu P, et al. Promoter SNPs in G1/S checkpoint regulators and their impact on the susceptibility to childhood leukemia. Blood. 2007;109:683-692.

110. Gast A, Bermejo JL, Flohr T, et al. Folate metabolic gene polymorphisms and childhood acute lymphoblastic leukemia: a case-control study. Leukemia. 2007;21:320-325.

111. Smith MT, Wang Y, Skibola CF, et al. Low NAD(P)H:quinone oxidoreductase activity is associated with increased risk of leukemia with MLL translocations in infants and children. Blood. 2002;100:4590-4593.

112. Alves S, Amorim A, Ferreira F, et al. The GSTM1 and GSTT1 genetic polymorphisms and susceptibility to acute lymphoblastic leukemia in children from north Portugal. Leukemia. 2002;16:1565-1567.

113. Aplenc R. Genetic polymorphisms of CYP1A1, CYP2D6, GSTM1, and GSTT1 and susceptibility to acute lymphoblastic leukemia in Indian children. Pediatr Blood Cancer. 2004;43:539-541.

114. Krajinovic M, Lamothe S, Labuda D, et al. Role of MTHFR genetic polymorphisms in the susceptibility to childhood acute lymphoblastic leukemia. Blood. 2004;103:252-257.

115. Infante-Rivard C, Vermunt JK, Weinberg CR. Excess transmission of the NAD(P)H:quinone oxidoreductase 1 (NQO1) C609T polymorphism in families of children with acute lymphoblastic leukemia. Am J Epidemiol. 2007;165:1248-1254.

116. Ford AM, Pombo-de-Oliveira MS, McCarthy KP, et al. Monoclonal origin of concordant T-cell malignancy in identical twins. Blood. 1997;89:281-285.

117. Ford AM, Bennett CA, Price CM, et al. Fetal origins of the TEL-AML1 fusion gene in identical twins with leukemia. Proc Natl Acad Sci U S A. 1998;95:4584-4588.

118. Wiemels JL, Ford AM, Van Wering ER, et al. Protracted and variable latency of acute lymphoblastic leukemia after TEL-AML1 gene fusion in utero. Blood. 1999;94:1057-1062.

119. Gale KB, Ford AM, Repp R, et al. Backtracking leukemia to birth: identification of clonotypic gene fusion sequences in neonatal blood spots. Proc Natl Acad Sci U S A. 1997;94:13950-13954.

120. Maia AT, van der Velden VH, Harrison CJ, et al. Prenatal origin of hyperdiploid acute lymphoblastic leukemia in identical twins. Leukemia. 2003;17:2202-2206.

121. Raynaud S, Cave H, Baens M, et al. The 12;21 translocation involving TEL and deletion of the other TEL allele: two frequently associated alterations found in childhood acute lymphoblastic leukemia. Blood. 1996;87:2891-2899.

122. Hong D, Gupta R, Ancliff P, et al. Initiating and cancer-propagating cells in TEL-AML1-associated childhood leukemia. Science. 2008;319:336-339.

123. McHale CM, Wiemels JL, Zhang L, et al. Prenatal origin of TEL-AML1-positive acute lymphoblastic leukemia in children born in California. Genes Chromosomes Cancer. 2003;37:36-43.

124. Mori H, Colman SM, Xiao Z, et al. Chromosome translocations and covert leukemic clones are generated during normal fetal development. Proc Natl Acad Sci U S A. 2002;99:8242-8247.

125. Greaves MF, Wiemels J. Origins of chromosome translocations in childhood leukaemia. Nat Rev Cancer. 2003;3:639-649.

126. Kinlen LJ. Epidemiological evidence for an infective basis in childhood leukaemia. Br J Cancer. 1995;71:1-5.

127. McNally RJ, Eden TO. An infectious aetiology for childhood acute leukaemia: a review of the evidence. Br J Haematol. 2004;127:243-263.

128. Kinlen L. Evidence for an infective cause of childhood leukaemia: comparison of a Scottish new town with nuclear reprocessing sites in Britain. Lancet. 1988;2:1323-1327.

129. Kinlen LJ, Clarke K, Hudson C. Evidence from population mixing in British New Towns 1946-85 of an infective basis for childhood leukaemia. Lancet. 1990;336:577-582.

130. Langford I, Bentham G. Infectious aetiology of childhood leukaemia. Lancet. 1990;336:944-945.

131. Langford I. Childhood leukaemia mortality and population change in England and Wales 1969-73. Soc Sci Med. 1991;33:435-440.

132. Laplanche A, de Vathaire F. Leukaemia mortality in French communes (administrative units) with a large and rapid population increase. Br J Cancer. 1994;69:110-113.

133. Kinlen LJ, Hudson C. Childhood leukaemia and poliomyelitis in relation to military encampments in England and Wales in the period of national military service, 1950-63. BMJ. 1991;303:1357-1362.

134. Petridou E, Hsieh CC, Kotsifakis G, et al. Absence of leukaemia clustering on Greek islands. Lancet. 1991;338:1204-1205.

135. Kinlen LJ, O'Brien F, Clarke K, et al. Rural population mixing and childhood leukaemia: effects of the North Sea oil industry in Scotland, including the area near Dounreay nuclear site. BMJ. 1993;306:743-748.

136. Kinlen LJ, John SM. Wartime evacuation and mortality from childhood leukaemia in England and Wales in 1945-9. BMJ. 1994;309:1197-1202.

137. Rudant J, Baccaini B, Ripert M, et al. Population-mixing at the place of residence at the time of birth and incidence of childhood leukaemia in France. Eur J Cancer. 2006;42:927-933.

138. Clark BR, Ferketich AK, Fisher JL, et al. Evidence of population mixing based on the geographic distribution of childhood leukemia in Ohio. Pediatr Blood Cancer. 2007;49:797-802.

139. Nyari TA, Kajtar P, Bartyik K, et al. Childhood acute lymphoblastic leukaemia in relation to population mixing around the time of birth in South Hungary. Pediatr Blood Cancer. 2006;47:944-948.

140. Stiller CA, Kroll ME, Boyle PJ, Feng Z. Population mixing, socioeconomic status and incidence of childhood acute lymphoblastic leukaemia in England and Wales: analysis by census ward. Br J Cancer. 2008;98:1006-1011.

141. Kinlen LJ, Balkwill A. Infective cause of childhood leukaemia and wartime population mixing in Orkney and Shetland, UK. Lancet. 2001;357:858.

142. Wartenberg D, Schneider D, Brown S. Childhood leukaemia incidence and the population mixing hypothesis in U.S. SEER data. Br J Cancer. 2004;90:1771-1776.

143. Smith M. Considerations on a possible viral etiology for B-precursor acute lymphoblastic leukemia of childhood. J Immunother. 1997;20:89-100.

144. Knox EG, Stewart A, Kneale G. Childhood leukaemia and mother-foetus infection. Br J Cancer. 1980;42:158-161.

145. Fine PE, Adelstein AM, Snowman J, et al. Long-term effects of exposure to viral infections in utero. Br Med J (Clin Res Ed). 1985;290:509-511.

146. Fedrick J, Alberman ED. have reported influenza in pregnancy and subsequent cancer in the child. BMJ. 1972;2:485-488.

147. Vianna NJ, Polan AK. Childhood lymphatic leukemia: prenatal seasonality and possible association with congenital varicella. Am J Epidemiol. 1976;103:321-332.

148. Roman E, Ansell P, Bull D. Leukaemia and non-Hodgkin's lymphoma in children and young adults: are prenatal and neonatal factors important determinants of disease? Br J Cancer. 1997;76:406-415.

149. Nishi M, Miyake H. A case-control study of non-T cell acute lymphoblastic leukaemia of children in Hokkaido, Japan. J Epidemiol Community Health. 1989;43:352-355.

150. van Steensel-Moll HA, Valkenburg HA, Vandenbroucke JP, van Zanen GE. Are maternal fertility problems related to childhood leukaemia? Int J Epidemiol. 1985;14:555-559.

151. Till M, Rapson N, Smith PG. Family studies in acute leukaemia in childhood: a possible association with autoimmune disease. Br J Cancer. 1979;40:62-71.

152. McKinney PA, Cartwright RA, Saiu JM, et al. The inter-regional epidemiological study of childhood cancer (IRESCC): a case control study of aetiological factors in leukaemia and lymphoma. Arch Dis Child. 1987;62:279-287.

153. Fajardo-Gutierrez A, Garduno-Espinosa J, Yamamoto-Kimura L, et al. [Risk factors associated with the development of leukemia in children.] Bol Med Hosp Infant Mex. 1993;50:248-257.

154. Gustafsson B, Jernberg AG, Priftakis P, Bogdanovic G. No CMV DNA in Guthrie cards from children who later developed ALL. Pediatr Hematol Oncol. 2006;23:199-205.

155. Isa A, Priftakis P, Broliden K, Gustafsson B. Human parvovirus B19 DNA is not detected in Guthrie cards from children who have developed acute lymphoblastic leukemia. Pediatr Blood Cancer. 2004;42:357-360.

156. Lehtinen M, Ogmundsdottir HM, Bloigu A, et al. Associations between three types of maternal bacterial infection and risk of leukemia in the offspring. Am J Epidemiol. 2005;162:662-667.

157. Tedeschi R, Bloigu A, Ogmundsdottir HM, et al. Activation of maternal Epstein-Barr virus infection and risk of acute leukemia in the offspring. Am J Epidemiol. 2007;165:134-137.

158. Smith MA, Simon R, Strickler HD, et al. Evidence that childhood acute lymphoblastic leukemia is associated with an infectious agent linked to hygiene conditions. Cancer Causes Control. 1998;9:285-298.

159. Robison LL, Buckley JD, Daigle AE, et al. Maternal drug use and risk of childhood nonlymphoblastic leukemia in offspring. An epidemiologic investigation implicating marijuana (a report from the Children's Cancer Study Group). Cancer. 1989; 63:1904-1911.

160. Gilman EA, Wilson LM, Kneale GW, Waterhouse JA. Childhood cancers and their association with pregnancy drugs and illnesses. Paediatr Perinat Epidemiol. 1989;3:66-94.

161. van Duijn CM, van Steensel-Moll HA, Coebergh JW, van Zanen GE. Risk factors for childhood acute non-lymphocytic leukemia: an association with maternal alcohol consumption during pregnancy? Cancer Epidemiol Biomarkers Prev. 1994;3:457-460.

162. Salonen T, Saxen L. Risk indicators in childhood malignancies. Int J Cancer. 1975;15:941-946.

163. Greaves MF. Aetiology of acute leukaemia. Lancet. 1997;349: 344-349.

164. Schuz J, Kaletsch U, Meinert R, et al. Association of childhood leukaemia with factors related to the immune system. Br J Cancer. 1999;80:585-590.

165. Davis MK, Savitz DA, Graubard BI. Infant feeding and childhood cancer. Lancet. 1988;2:365-368.

166. Kwan M, Buffer P. Breast-feeding and risk of childhood acute lymphoblastic leukemia: Results and commentary from a case-control study (abstract). Ann Epidemiol. 2002;12:495.

167. van Steensel-Moll HA, Valkenburg HA, van Zanen GE. Childhood leukaemia and infectious diseases in the first year of life: a register-based case-control study. Am J Epidemiol. 1986;124: 590-594.

168. Shu XO, Clemens J, Zheng W, et al. Infant breastfeeding and the risk of childhood lymphoma and leukaemia. Int J Epidemiol. 1995;24:27-32.

169. Hartley AL, Birch JM, McKinney PA, et al. The Inter-Regional Epidemiological Study of Childhood Cancer (IRESCC): past medical history in children with cancer. J Epidemiol Community Health. 1988;42:235-242.

170. Mathur GP, Gupta N, Mathur S, et al. Breastfeeding and childhood cancer. Indian Pediatr. 1993;30:651-657.

171. Infante-Rivard C, Fortier I, Olson E. Markers of infection, breastfeeding and childhood acute lymphoblastic leukaemia. Br J Cancer. 2000;83:1559-1564.

172. Kwan ML, Buffler PA, Wiemels JL, et al. Breastfeeding patterns and risk of childhood acute lymphoblastic leukaemia. Br J Cancer. 2005;93:379-384.

173. Shu XO, Linet MS, Steinbuch M, et al. Breast-feeding and risk of childhood acute leukemia. J Natl Cancer Inst. 1999;91: 1765-1772.

174. Martin RM, Gunnell D, Owen CG, Smith GD. Breast-feeding and childhood cancer: a systematic review with metaanalysis. Int J Cancer. 2005;117:1020-1031.

175. Groves FD, Gridley G, Wacholder S, et al. Infant vaccinations and risk of childhood acute lymphoblastic leukaemia in the USA. Br J Cancer. 1999;81:175-178.

176. Auvinen A, Hakulinen T, Groves F. Haemophilus influenzae type B vaccination and risk of childhood leukaemia in a vaccine trial in Finland. Br J Cancer. 2000;83:956-958.

177. Neglia JP, Linet MS, Shu XO, et al. Patterns of infection and day care utilization and risk of childhood acute lymphoblastic leukaemia. Br J Cancer. 2000;82:234-240.

178. Altieri A, Castro F, Bermejo JL, Hemminki K. Number of siblings and the risk of lymphoma, leukemia, and myeloma by histopathology. Cancer Epidemiol Biomarkers Prev. 2006;15: 1281-1286.

179. Perrillat F, Clavel J, Auclerc MF, et al. Day-care, early common infections and childhood acute leukaemia: a multicentre French case-control study. Br J Cancer. 2002;86:1064-1069.

180. Petridou E, Kassimos D, Kalmanti M, et al. Age of exposure to infections and risk of childhood leukaemia. BMJ. 1993;307:774.

181. Roman E, Watson A, Bull D, Baker K. Leukaemia risk and social contact in children aged 0-4 years in southern England. J Epidemiol Community Health. 1994;48:601-602.

182. Rosenbaum PF, Buck GM, Brecher ML. Early child-care and preschool experiences and the risk of childhood acute lymphoblastic leukemia. Am J Epidemiol. 2000;152:1136-1144.

183. Ma X, Buffler PA, Wiemels JL, et al. Ethnic difference in daycare attendance, early infections, and risk of childhood acute lymphoblastic leukemia. Cancer Epidemiol Biomarkers Prev. 2005;14: 1928-1934.

184. Jourdan-Da Silva N, Perel Y, Mechinaud F, et al. Infectious diseases in the first year of life, perinatal characteristics and childhood acute leukaemia. Br J Cancer. 2004;90:139-145.

185. Gilham C, Peto J, Simpson J, et al. Day care in infancy and risk of childhood acute lymphoblastic leukaemia: findings from UK case-control study. BMJ. 2005;330:1294.

186. Heegaard ED, Jensen L, Hornsleth A, Schmiegelow K. The role of parvovirus B19 infection in childhood acute lymphoblastic leukemia. Pediatr Hematol Oncol. 1999;16:329-334.

187. McKinney PA, Juszczak E, Findlay E, et al. Pre- and perinatal risk factors for childhood leukaemia and other malignancies: a Scottish case control study. Br J Cancer. 1999;80:1844-1851.

188. Dockerty JD, Skegg DC, Elwood JM, et al. Infections, vaccinations, and the risk of childhood leukaemia. Br J Cancer. 1999;80:1483-1489.

189. Memon A, Doll R. A search for unknown blood-borne oncogenic viruses. Int J Cancer. 1994;58:366-368.

190. Cnattingius S, Zack MM, Ekbom A, et al. Prenatal and neonatal risk factors for childhood lymphatic leukemia. J Natl Cancer Inst. 1995;87:908-914.

191. Roman E, Simpson J, Ansell P, et al. Childhood acute lympho-blastic leukemia and infections in the first year of life: a report from the United Kingdom Childhood Cancer Study. Am J Epidemiol. 2007;165:496-504.

192. Simpson J, Smith A, Ansell P, Roman E. Childhood leukaemia and infectious exposure: a report from the United Kingdom Childhood Cancer Study (UKCCS). Eur J Cancer. 2007;43: 2396-2403.

193. Shu XO, Gao YT, Brinton LA, et al. A population-based case-control study of childhood leukemia in Shanghai. Cancer. 1988;62:635-644.

194. Malone GE, Roseman J, Crist WM, et al. A review of evidence that the feline leukemia virus (FeLV) might be causative in child-hood acute lymphocytic leukemia (ALL). In Humphrey GB, Grindey GB, Dehner LP (eds). Adrenal and Endocrine Tumors in Children. Boston, Martinus Nijhoff, 1983, pp 45-65.

195. Donaldson LJ, Rankin J, Proctor S. Is it possible to catch leukae-mia from a cat? Lancet. 1994;344:971-972.

196. Bender AP, Robison LL, Kashmiri SV, et al. No involvement of bovine leukemia virus in childhood acute lymphoblastic leukemia and non-Hodgkin's lymphoma. Cancer Res. 1988;48: 2919-2922.

197. Swensen AR, Ross JA, Shu XO, et al. Pet ownership and child-hood acute leukemia (USA and Canada). Cancer Causes Control. 2001;12:301-303.

198. Hoover RN. Bacillus Calmette-Guerin vaccination and cancer prevention: a critical review of the human experience. Cancer Res. 1976;36:652-654.

199. Comstock GW. Leukaemia and B.C.G. A controlled trial. Lancet. 1971;2:1062-1063.

200. Snider DE, Comstock GW, Martinez I, Caras GJ. Efficacy of BCG vaccination in prevention of cancer: an update. J Natl Cancer Inst. 1978;60:785-788.

201. Ambrosch F, Wiederman G, Krepler P. Studies on the influence of BCG vaccination on infantile leukaemia. International Sympo-sium of BCG Vaccines and Tuberculins, Budapest, Hungary, 1983. Dev Biol Stand. 1986;58:419-424.

202. Westerbeek RM, Blair V, Eden OB, et al. Seasonal variations in the onset of childhood leukaemia and lymphoma. Br J Cancer. 1998;78:119-124.

203. Higgins CD, dos Santos-Silva I, Stiller CA, Swerdlow AJ. Season of birth and diagnosis of children with leukaemia: an analysis of over 15 000 UK cases occurring from 1953-95. Br J Cancer. 2001;84:406-412.

204. Ross JA, Severson RK, Swensen AR, et al. Seasonal variations in the diagnosis of childhood cancer in the United States. Br J Cancer. 1999;81:549-553.

205. Macmahon B. Prenatal x-ray exposure and childhood cancer. J Natl Cancer Inst. 1962;28:1173-1191.

206. Graham S, Levin ML, Lilienfeld AM, et al. Preconception, intra-uterine, and postnatal irradiation as related to leukemia. Natl Cancer Inst Monogr. 1966;19:347-371.

207. Stewart A, Webb J, Hewitt D. A survey of childhood malignan-cies. Br Med J. 1958;1:1495-1508.

208. Bithell JF, Stewart AM. Pre-natal irradiation and childhood malignancy: a review of British data from the Oxford Survey. Br J Cancer. 1975;31:271-287.

209. Murray R, Heckel P, Hempelmann LH. Leukemia in children exposed to ionizing radiation. N Engl J Med. 1959;261: 585-589.

210. Ager EA, Schuman LM, Wallace HM, et al. An epidemiological study of childhood leukemia. J Chronic Dis. 1965;18:113-132.

211. Hopton PA, McKinney PA, Cartwright RA, et al. X-rays in pregnancy and the risk of childhood cancer. Lancet. 1985;2:773.

212. Shu XO, Jin F, Linet MS, et al. Diagnostic X-ray and ultrasound exposure and risk of childhood cancer. Br J Cancer. 1994;70:531-536.

213. Harvey EB, Boice JD Jr, Honeyman M, Flannery JT. Prenatal x-ray exposure and childhood cancer in twins. N Engl J Med. 1985;312:541-545.

214. Rodvall Y, Pershagen G, Hrubec Z, et al. Prenatal X-ray exposure and childhood cancer in Swedish twins. Int J Cancer. 1990;46:362-365.

215. Mole RH. Radon and leukaemia. Lancet. 1990;335:1336-1340.

216. Monson RR, MacMahon B. Pre-natal x-ray exposure and cancer in children. In Boice JD, Fraumeni JF Jr (eds). Radiation Carci-nogenesis: Epidemiology and Biological Significance. New York, Raven Press, 1984, pp 97-105.

217. Yoshimoto Y, Kato H, Schull WJ. Risk of cancer in children exposed in utero to A-bomb radiations, 1950-84. Lancet. 1988;2:665-669.

218. Boice JD Jr. Studies of atomic bomb survivors. Understanding radiation effects. JAMA. 1990;264:622-623.

219. Shu XO, Potter JD, Linet MS, et al. Diagnostic X-rays and ultrasound exposure and risk of childhood acute lymphoblastic leukemia by immunophenotype. Cancer Epidemiol Biomarkers Prev. 2002;11:177-185.

220. Shu XO, Reaman GH, Lampkin B, et al. Association of paternal diagnostic X-ray exposure with risk of infant leukemia. Investiga-tors of the Children's Cancer Group. Cancer Epidemiol Biomark-ers Prev. 1994;3:645-653.

221. Jablon S, Tachikawa K, Belsky JL, Steer A. Cancer in Japanese exposed as children to atomic bombs. Lancet. 1971;1:927-932.

222. Hatch M, Susser M. Background gamma radiation and childhood cancers within ten miles of a US nuclear plant. Int J Epidemiol. 1990;19:546-552.

223. Ivanov EP, Tolochko G, Lazarev VS, Shuvaeva L. Child leukae-mia after Chernobyl. Nature. 1993;365:702.

224. Hjalmars U, Kulldorff M, Gustafsson G. Risk of acute childhood leukaemia in Sweden after the Chernobyl reactor accident. Swedish Child Leukaemia Group. BMJ. 1994;309:154-157.

225. Auvinen A, Hakama M, Arvela H, et al. Fallout from Chernobyl and incidence of childhood leukaemia in Finland, 1976-92. BMJ. 1994;309:151-154.

226. Cartwright RA, McKinney PA, Alexander FE, Ricketts J. Leuke-mia in young children. Lancet. 1988;2:960.

227. Gibson BE, Eden OB, Barrett A, et al. Leukaemia in young chil-dren in Scotland. Lancet. 1988;2:630.

228. Michaelis J, Schuz J, Meinert R, et al. Childhood leukemia and electromagnetic fields: results of a population-based case-control study in Germany. Cancer Causes Control. 1997;8:167-174.

229. Petridou E, Proukakis C, Tong D, et al. Trends and geographic distribution of childhood leukemia in Greece in relation to the Chernobyl accident. Scand J Soc Med. 1994;22:127-131.

230. Petridou E, Trichopoulos D, Dessypris N, et al. Infant leukaemia after in utero exposure to radiation from Chernobyl. Nature. 1996;382:352-353.

231. Davis S, Day RW, Kopecky KJ, et al. Childhood leukaemia in Belarus, Russia, and Ukraine following the Chernobyl power station accident: results from an international collaborative population-based case-control study. Int J Epidemiol. 2006;35: 386-396.

232. Stevens W, Thomas DC, Lyon JL, et al. Leukemia in Utah and radioactive fallout from the Nevada test site. A case-control study. JAMA. 1990;264:585-591.

233. Cook-Mozaffari PJ, Darby SC, Doll R, et al. Geographic variation in mortality from leukaemia and other cancers in England and Wales in relation to proximity to nuclear installations, 1969-78. Br J Cancer. 1989;59:476-485.

234. Bithell JF, Dutton SJ, Draper GJ, Neary NM. Distribution of childhood leukaemias and non-Hodgkin's lymphomas near

nuclear installations in England and Wales. BMJ. 1994;309: 501-505.

235. Hill C, Laplanche A. Overall mortality and cancer mortality around French nuclear sites. Nature. 1990;347:755-757.

236. Evrard AS, Hemon D, Morin A, et al. Childhood leukaemia incidence around French nuclear installations using geographic zoning based on gaseous discharge dose estimates. Br J Cancer. 2006;94:1342-1347.

237. Jablon S, Hrubec Z, Boice JD Jr, et al. Cancer in Populations Living Near Nuclear Facilities (NIB Publication No. 90-874). Bethesda, Md, U.S. Public Health Service, Department of Health and Human Services, 1990.

238. Jablon S, Hrubec Z, Boice JD Jr. Cancer in populations living near nuclear facilities. A survey of mortality nationwide and incidence in two states. JAMA. 1991;265:1403-1408.

239. Michaelis J, Keller B, Haaf G, Kaatsch P. Incidence of childhood malignancies in the vicinity of West German nuclear power plants. Cancer Causes Control. 1992;3:255-263.

240. Clarke EA, McLaughlin J, Andersen TW. Childhood Leukaemia Around Canadian Nuclear Facilities—Phase II. Final Report. Ottawa, Canada, Atomic Energy Control Board, 1991.

241. Henshaw DL, Eatough JP, Richardson RB. Radon as a causative factor in induction of myeloid leukaemia and other cancers. Lancet. 1990;335:1008-1012.

242. Radon and leukaemia. Lancet. 1990;335:1336-1340.

243. Evrard AS, Hemon D, Billon S, et al. Childhood leukemia incidence and exposure to indoor radon, terrestrial and cosmic gamma radiation. Health Phys. 2006;90:569-579.

244. Lubin JH, Linet MS, Boice JD Jr, et al. Case-control study of childhood acute lymphoblastic leukemia and residential radon exposure. J Natl Cancer Inst. 1998;90:294-300.

245. Steinbuch M, Weinberg CR, Buckley JD, et al. Indoor residential radon exposure and risk of childhood acute myeloid leukemia. Br J Cancer. 1999;81:900-906.

246. Feychting M, Plato N, Nise G, et al. Parental occupation and childhood cancer, a cohort study. Epidemiology. 1999;10:1210.

247. Feychting M, Plato N, Nise G, Ahlbom A. Paternal occupational exposures and childhood cancer. Environ Health Perspect. 2001;109:193-196.

248. McKinney PA, Fear NT, Stockton D. Parental occupation at periconception: findings from the United Kingdom Childhood Cancer Study. Occup Environ Med. 2003;60:901-909.

249. Infante-Rivard C, Siemiatycki J, Lakhani R, Nadon L. Maternal exposure to occupational solvents and childhood leukemia. Environ Health Perspect. 2005;113:787-792.

250. Leiss JK, Savitz DA. Home pesticide use and childhood cancer: a case-control study. Am J Public Health. 1995;85:249-252.

251. Brown LM, Blair A, Gibson R, et al. Pesticide exposures and other agricultural risk factors for leukemia in men in Iowa and Minnesota. Cancer Res. 1990;50:6585-6591.

252. Meinert R, Kaatsch P, Kaletsch U, et al. Childhood leukaemia and exposure to pesticides: results of a case-control study in northern Germany. Eur J Cancer. 1996;32A:1943-1948.

253. Lowengart RA, Peters JM, Cicioni C, et al. Childhood leukemia and parents' occupational and home exposures. J Natl Cancer Inst. 1987;79:39-46.

254. Meinert R, Schuz J, Kaletsch U, et al. Leukemia and non-Hodgkin's lymphoma in childhood and exposure to pesticides: results of a register-based case-control study in Germany. Am J Epidemiol. 2000;151:639-646.

255. Zahm SH. Childhood leukemia and pesticides. Epidemiology. 1999;10:473-475.

256. Daniels JL, Olshan AF, Savitz DA. Pesticides and childhood cancers. Environ Health Perspect. 1997;105:1068-1077.

257. Buckley JD, Robison LL, Swotinsky R, et al. Occupational exposures of parents of children with acute nonlymphocytic leukemia: a report from the Children's Cancer Study Group. Cancer Res. 1989;49:4030-4037.

258. Wen WQ, Shu XO, Steinbuch M, et al. Paternal military service and risk for childhood leukemia in offspring. Am J Epidemiol. 2000;151:231-240.

259. Health status of Vietnam veterans. III. Reproductive outcomes and child health. The Centers for Disease Control Vietnam Experience Study. JAMA. 1988;259:2715-2719.

260. Sanders BM, White GC, Draper GJ. Occupations of fathers of children dying from neoplasms. J Epidemiol Community Health. 1981;35:245-250.

261. Gold EB, Diener MD, Szklo M. Parental occupations and cancer in children—a case-control study and review of the methodologic issues. J Occup Med. 1982;24:578-584.

262. Shaw G, Lavey R, Jackson R, Austin D. Association of childhood leukemia with maternal age, birth order, and paternal occupation. A case-control study. Am J Epidemiol. 1984;119:788-795.

263. McKinney PA, Alexander FE, Cartwright RA, Parker L. Parental occupations of children with leukaemia in west Cumbria, north Humberside, and Gateshead. BMJ. 1991;302:681-687.

264. Steffen C, Auclerc MF, Auvrignon A, et al. Acute childhood leukaemia and environmental exposure to potential sources of benzene and other hydrocarbons; a case-control study. Occup Environ Med. 2004;61:773-778.

265. Feingold L, Savitz DA, John EM. Use of a job-exposure matrix to evaluate parental occupation and childhood cancer. Cancer Causes Control. 1992;3:161-169.

266. Schuz J, Kaletsch U, Meinert R, et al. Risk of childhood leukemia and parental self-reported occupational exposure to chemicals, dusts, and fumes: results from pooled analyses of German population-based case-control studies. Cancer Epidemiol Biomarkers Prev. 2000;9:835-838.

267. Lyons RA, Monaghan SP, Heaven M, et al. Incidence of leukaemia and lymphoma in young people in the vicinity of the petrochemical plant at Baglan Bay, South Wales, 1974 to 1991. Occup Environ Med. 1995;52:225-228.

268. Knox EG. Leukaemia clusters in childhood: geographic analysis in Britain. J Epidemiol Community Health. 1994;48:369-376.

269. Infante-Rivard C, Mur P, Armstrong B, et al. Acute lymphoblastic leukaemia in Spanish children and mothers' occupation: a case-control study. J Epidemiol Community Health. 1991;45:11-15.

270. Freedman DM, Stewart P, Kleinerman RA, et al. Household solvent exposures and childhood acute lymphoblastic leukemia. Am J Public Health. 2001;91:564-567.

271. Alexander F, Cartwright R, McKinney PA, Ricketts TJ. Investigation of spacial clustering of rare diseases: childhood malignancies in North Humberside. J Epidemiol Community Health. 1990;44:39-46.

272. Wulff M, Hogberg U, Sandstrom A. Cancer incidence for children born in a smelting community. Acta Oncol. 1996;35:179-183.

273. Raaschou-Nielsen O, Olsen JH, Hertel O, et al. Exposure of Danish children to traffic exhaust fumes. Sci Total Environ. 1996;189-190:51-55.

274. Pearson RL, Wachtel H, Ebi KL. Distance-weighted traffic density in proximity to a home is a risk factor for leukemia and other childhood cancers. J Air Waste Manag Assoc. 2000;50:175-180.

275. Savitz DA, Feingold L. Association of childhood cancer with residential traffic density. Scand J Work Environ Health. 1989;15:360-363.

276. Wertheimer N, Leeper E. Electrical wiring configurations and childhood cancer. Am J Epidemiol. 1979;109:273-284.

277. Fulton JP, Cobb S, Preble L, et al. Electrical wiring configurations and childhood leukemia in Rhode Island. Am J Epidemiol. 1980;111:292-296.

278. Tomenius L. 50-Hz electromagnetic environment and the incidence of childhood tumors in Stockholm County. Bioelectromagnetics. 1986;7:191-207.

279. Savitz DA, Wachtel H, Barnes FA, et al. Case-control study of childhood cancer and exposure to 60-Hz magnetic fields. Am J Epidemiol. 1988;128:21-38.

280. Coleman MP, Bell CM, Taylor HL, Primic-Zakelj M. Leukaemia and residence near electricity transmission equipment: a case-control study. Br J Cancer. 1989;60:793-798.

281. Myers A, Clayden AD, Cartwright RA, Cartwright SC. Childhood cancer and overhead powerlines: a case-control study. Br J Cancer. 1990;62:1008-1014.

282. London SJ, Thomas DC, Bowman JD, et al. Exposure to residential electric and magnetic fields and risk of childhood leukemia. Am J Epidemiol. 1991;134:923-937.

283. Feychting M, Ahlborn A. Magnetic Fields and Cancer in People Residing Near Swedish High Voltage Power Lines. Stockholm, Karolinska Institute, 1992.

284. Olsen JH, Nielsen A, Schulgen G. Residence near high-voltage facilities and risk of cancer in children. BMJ. 1993;307:891-895.

285. Verkasalo PK, Pukkala E, Hongisto MY, et al. Risk of cancer in Finnish children living close to power lines. BMJ. 1993;307:895-899.

286. Tynes T, Haldorsen T. Electromagnetic fields and cancer in children residing near Norwegian high-voltage power lines. Am J Epidemiol. 1997;145:219-226.

287. Linet MS, Hatch EE, Kleinerman RA, et al. Residential exposure to magnetic fields and acute lymphoblastic leukemia in children. N Engl J Med. 1997;337:1-7.

288. McBride ML, Gallagher RP, Theriault G, et al. Power-frequency electric and magnetic fields and risk of childhood leukemia in Canada. Am J Epidemiol. 1999;149:831-842.

289. Cheng KK, Day N, Cartwright R, et al. Exposure to power-frequency magnetic fields and the risk of childhood cancer. UK Childhood Cancer Study Investigators. Lancet. 1999;354:1925-1931.

290. Skinner J, Mee TJ, Blackwell RP, et al. Exposure to power frequency electric fields and the risk of childhood cancer in the UK. Br J Cancer. 2002;87:1257-1266.

291. Kabuto M, Nitta H, Yamamoto S, et al. Childhood leukemia and magnetic fields in Japan: a case-control study of childhood leukemia and residential power-frequency magnetic fields in Japan. Int J Cancer. 2006;119:643-650.

292. Ahlbom A, Day N, Feychting M, et al. A pooled analysis of magnetic fields and childhood leukaemia. Br J Cancer. 2000;83:692-698.

293. Greenland S, Sheppard AR, Kaune WT, et al. A pooled analysis of magnetic fields, wire codes, and childhood leukemia. Childhood Leukemia-EMF Study Group. Epidemiology. 2000;11:624-634.

294. Foliart DE, Pollock BH, Mezei G, et al. Magnetic field exposure and long-term survival in children with leukaemia. Br J Cancer. 2006;94:161-164.

295. Svendsen AL, Weihkopf T, Kaatsch P, Schuz J. Exposure to magnetic fields and survival after diagnosis of childhood leukemia: a German cohort study. Cancer Epidemiol Biomarkers Prev. 2007;16:1167-1171.

296. Ahlbom A, Green A, Kheifets L, et al. Epidemiology of health effects of radiofrequency exposure. Environ Health Perspect. 2004;112:1741-1754.

297. Ha M, Im H, Lee M, et al. Radio-frequency radiation exposure from AM radio transmitters and childhood leukemia and brain cancer. Am J Epidemiol. 2007;166:270-279.

298. Sarasua S, Savitz DA. Cured and broiled meat consumption in relation to childhood cancer: Denver, Colorado (United States). Cancer Causes Control. 1994;5:141-148.

299. Petridou E, Ntouvelis E, Dessypris N, et al. Maternal diet and acute lymphoblastic leukemia in young children. Cancer Epidemiol Biomarkers Prev. 2005;14:1935-1939.

300. Kwan ML, Metayer C, Crouse V, Buffler PA. Maternal illness and drug/medication use during the period surrounding pregnancy and risk of childhood leukemia in offspring. Am J Epidemiol. 2007;165:27-35.

301. Ross JA, Potter JD, Robison LL. Infant leukemia, topoisomerase II inhibitors, and the MLL gene. J Natl Cancer Inst. 1994;86:1678-1680.

302. Ross JA, Potter JD, Reaman GH, et al. Maternal exposure to potential inhibitors of DNA topoisomerase II and infant leukemia (United States): a report from the Children's Cancer Group. Cancer Causes Control. 1996;7:581-590.

303. Strick R, Strissel PL, Borgers S, et al. Dietary bioflavonoids induce cleavage in the MLL gene and may contribute to infant leukemia. Proc Natl Acad Sci U S A. 2000;97:4790-4795.

304. Alexander FE, Patheal SL, Biondi A, et al. Transplacental chemical exposure and risk of infant leukemia with MLL gene fusion. Cancer Res. 2001;61:2542-2546.

305. Severson RK, Buckley JD, Woods WG, et al. Cigarette smoking and alcohol consumption by parents of children with acute myeloid leukemia: an analysis within morphological subgroups—a report from the Children's Cancer Group. Cancer Epidemiol Biomarkers Prev. 1993;2:433-439.

306. Infante-Rivard C, Krajinovic M, Labuda D, Sinnett D. Parental smoking, CYP1A1 genetic polymorphisms and childhood leukemia (Quebec, Canada). Cancer Causes Control. 2000;11:547-553.

307. Boffetta P, Tredaniel J, Greco A. Risk of childhood cancer and adult lung cancer after childhood exposure to passive smoke: A meta-analysis. Environ Health Perspect. 2000;108:73-82.

308. Brondum J, Shu XO, Steinbuch M, et al. Parental cigarette smoking and the risk of acute leukemia in children. Cancer. 1999;85:1380-1388.

309. Sorahan T, Lancashire R, Prior P, et al. Childhood cancer and parental use of alcohol and tobacco. Ann Epidemiol. 1995;5:354-359.

310. Shu XO, Ross JA, Pendergrass TW, et al. Parental alcohol consumption, cigarette smoking, and risk of infant leukemia: a Children's Cancer Group study. J Natl Cancer Inst. 1996;88:24-31.

311. Ji BT, Shu XO, Linet MS, et al. Paternal cigarette smoking and the risk of childhood cancer in offspring of nonsmoking mothers. J Natl Cancer Inst. 1997;89:238-244.

312. Sasco AJ, Vainio H. From in utero and childhood exposure to parental smoking to childhood cancer: a possible link and the need for action. Hum Exp Toxicol. 1999;18:192-201.

313. John EM, Savitz DA, Sandler DP. Prenatal exposure to parents' smoking and childhood cancer. Am J Epidemiol. 1991;133:123-132.

314. Chang JS, Selvin S, Metayer C, et al. Parental smoking and the risk of childhood leukemia. Am J Epidemiol. 2006;163:1091-1100.

315. Mucci LA, Granath F, Cnattingius S. Maternal smoking and childhood leukemia and lymphoma risk in 1,440,542 Swedish children. Cancer Epidemiol Biomarkers Prev. 2004;13:1528-1533.

316. Sandler DP, Wilcox AJ, Everson RB. Cumulative effects of lifetime passive smoking on cancer risk. Lancet. 1985;1:312-315.

317. Trivers KF, Mertens AC, Ross JA, et al. Parental marijuana use and risk of childhood acute myeloid leukaemia: a report from the Children's Cancer Group (United States and Canada). Paediatr Perinat Epidemiol. 2006;20:110-118.

318. MacArthur AC, McBride ML, Spinelli JJ, et al. Risk of childhood leukemia associated with parental smoking and alcohol consumption prior to conception and during pregnancy: the cross-Canada childhood leukemia study. Cancer Causes Control. 2008;19:283-295.

319. Ross JA, Potter JD, Shu XO, et al. Evaluating the relationships in maternal reproductive history, birth characteristics, and infant leukemia: a report from the Children's Cancer Group. Ann Epidemiol. 1997;7:172-179.

320. Kaye SA, Robison LL, Smithson WA, et al. Maternal reproductive history and birth characteristics in childhood acute lymphoblastic leukemia. Cancer. 1991;68:1351-1355.

321. Zack M, Adami HO, Ericson A. Maternal and perinatal risk factors for childhood leukemia. Cancer Res. 1991;51:3696-3701.

322. Westergaard T, Andersen PK, Pedersen JB, et al. Birth characteristics, sibling patterns, and acute leukemia risk in childhood: a population-based cohort study. J Natl Cancer Inst. 1997;89:939-947.

323. Hemminki K, Kyyronen P, Vaittinen P. Parental age as a risk factor of childhood leukemia and brain cancer in offspring. Epidemiology. 1999;10:271-275.

324. Yeazel MW, Ross JA, Buckley JD, et al. High birth weight and risk of specific childhood cancers: a report from the Children's Cancer Group. J Pediatr. 1997;131:671-677.

325. Kobayashi N, Matsui I, Tanimura M, et al. Childhood neuroectodermal tumours and malignant lymphoma after maternal ovulation induction. Lancet. 1991;338:955.

326. Wen W, Shu XO, Potter JD, et al. Parental medication use and risk of childhood acute lymphoblastic leukemia. Cancer. 2002;95:1786-1794.

327. Cartwright RA, McKinney PA, Hopton PA, et al. Ultrasound examinations in pregnancy and childhood cancer. Lancet. 1984;2:999-1000.

328. Kinnier Wilson LM, Waterhouse JA. Obstetric ultrasound and childhood malignancies. Lancet. 1984;2:997-999.

329. Sorahan T, Lancashire R, Stewart A, Peck I. Pregnancy ultrasound and childhood cancer: a second report from the Oxford Survey of Childhood Cancers. Br J Obstet Gynaecol. 1995;102:831-832.

330. Wen W, Shu XO, Linet MS, et al. Allergic disorders and the risk of childhood acute lymphoblastic leukemia (United States). Cancer Causes Control. 2000;11:303-307.

331. Nishi M, Miyake H, Takeda T, Hatae Y. Congenital malformations and childhood cancer. Med Pediatr Oncol. 2000;34:250-254.

332. Windham GC, Bjerkedal T, Langmark F. A population-based study of cancer incidence in twins and in children with congenital malformations or low birth weight, Norway, 1967-1980. Am J Epidemiol. 1985;121:49-56.

333. Mertens AC, Wen W, Davies SM, et al. Congenital abnormalities in children with acute leukemia: a report from the Children's Cancer Group. J Pediatr. 1998;133:617-623.

334. Narod SA, Hawkins MM, Robertson CM, Stiller CA. Congenital anomalies and childhood cancer in Great Britain. Am J Hum Genet. 1997;60:474-485.

335. Hjalgrim LL, Rostgaard K, Hjalgrim H, et al. Birth weight and risk for childhood leukemia in Denmark, Sweden, Norway, and Iceland. J Natl Cancer Inst. 2004;96:1549-1556.

336. McLaughlin CC, Baptiste MS, Schymura MJ, et al. Birth weight, maternal weight and childhood leukaemia. Br J Cancer. 2006;94:1738-1744.

337. Hirayama T. Descriptive and analytical epidemiology of childhood malignancy in Japan. In Kobayashi N: Recent Advances in Managements of Children with Cancer. Tokyo, The Children's Cancer Association of Japan, 1979, pp 27-43.

338. Daling JR, Starzyk P, Olshan AF, Weiss NS. Birth weight and the incidence of childhood cancer. J Natl Cancer Inst. 1984;72:1039-1041.

339. Robison LL, Codd M, Gunderson P, et al. Birth weight as a risk factor for childhood acute lymphoblastic leukemia. Pediatr Hematol Oncol. 1987;4:63-72.

340. Hjalgrim LL, Westergaard T, Rostgaard K, et al. Birth weight as a risk factor for childhood leukemia: a meta-analysis of 18 epidemiologic studies. Am J Epidemiol. 2003;158:724-735.

341. Ross JA, Perentesis JP, Robison LL, Davies SM. Big babies and infant leukemia: a role for insulin-like growth factor-1? Cancer Causes Control. 1996;7:553-559.

342. Golding J, Paterson M, Kinlen LJ. Factors associated with childhood cancer in a national cohort study. Br J Cancer. 1990;62:304-308.

343. Golding J, Greenwood R, Birmingham K, Mott M. Childhood cancer, intramuscular vitamin K, and pethidine given during labour. BMJ. 1992;305:341-346.

344. Ekelund H, Finnstrom O, Gunnarskog J, et al. Administration of vitamin K to newborn infants and childhood cancer. BMJ. 1993;307:89-91.

345. von Kries R, Gobel U, Hachmeister A, et al. Vitamin K and childhood cancer: a population based case-control study in Lower Saxony, Germany. BMJ. 1996;313:199-203.

346. Ansell P, Bull D, Roman E. Childhood leukaemia and intramuscular vitamin K: findings from a case-control study. BMJ. 1996;313:204-205.

347. Miller RW. Childhood leukemia and neonatal exposure to lighting in nurseries. Cancer Causes Control. 1992;3:581-582.

348. Israels LG, Friesen E, Jansen AH, Israels ED. Vitamin K$_1$ increases sister chromatid exchange in vitro in human leukocytes and in vivo in fetal sheep cells: a possible role for "vitamin K deficiency" in the fetus. Pediatr Res. 1987;22:405-408.

349. Cornelissen M, Smeets D, Merkx G, et al. Analysis of chromosome aberrations and sister chromatid exchanges in peripheral blood lymphocytes of newborns after vitamin K prophylaxis at birth. Pediatr Res. 1991;30:550-553.

350. Olsen JH, Hertz H, Blinkenberg K, Verder H. Vitamin K regimens and incidence of childhood cancer in Denmark. BMJ. 1994;308:895-896.

351. Klebanoff MA, Read JS, Mills JL, Shiono PH. The risk of childhood cancer after neonatal exposure to vitamin K. N Engl J Med. 1993;329:905-908.

352. Parker L, Cole M, Craft AW, Hey EN. Neonatal vitamin K administration and childhood cancer in the north of England: retrospective case-control study. BMJ. 1998;316:189-193.

353. Ross JA, Davies SM. Vitamin K prophylaxis and childhood cancer. Med Pediatr Oncol. 2000;34:434-437.

2 Angiogenesis

Judah Folkman and Joseph E. Italiano, Jr.

Blood vessels and their development have excited the imagination of scientists since the beginning of medical history. The vasculature plays a major role in distributing blood cells, nutrients, gases, metabolites, and various chemical mediators. The interior of the blood vessel wall is lined with endothelium, comprised of more than 10^{12} endothelial cells and covering a surface area of about 500 mm^2. Normally quiescent, with cell turnover measured on the order of years, endothelial cells have a remarkable capacity to proliferate and vascularize tissues in physiologic and pathologic situations. Angiogenesis is the physiologic process involving the growth of new blood vessels from preexisting ones.

This chapter is divided into three major sections. In the first section, the basic concepts and molecular players involved in angiogenesis are summarized. Although angiogenesis is a normal process in development and growth, it is also a fundamental step in the transition of tumors from a dormant to a malignant state. Because it is now generally accepted that for a tumor to grow beyond 1 mm it must recruit new blood vessels, we begin this section by reviewing the original concepts of tumor angiogenesis. The molecular basis of angiogenesis, which has unfolded dramatically over the past several years, is reviewed. Several proangiogenic and antiangiogenic proteins that regulate new vessel development have been identified, and their stimulatory and inhibitory activities are discussed. Finally, the prevailing evidence is presented, which suggests that the relative balance of stimulators and inhibitors of angiogenesis can activate an angiogenic switch.

In the second section, the role of angiogenesis in hematologic malignancy is evaluated. Although the early work on angiogenesis was based on solid tumors, evidence indicates that angiogenesis also plays a significant role in hematologic malignancies. After a discussion on the role of angiogenesis in these specific hematologic malignancies, we discuss the antiangiogenic therapy of cancer. Multiple strategies for inhibiting angiogenesis are outlined and their effectiveness for treating specific cancers is considered.

The third section of this chapter discusses how angiogenesis is modulated by proteins and cells from the hemostatic system. It is becoming increasingly clear that hemostasis and angiogenesis are interrelated. Because it is now apparent that platelets can contribute to tumor growth, we review the angiogenic properties of these cells. Finally, we demonstrate that the capacity of platelets to store and selectively release angiogenesis regulatory proteins provides a new conceptual framework for understanding how angiogenesis is linked to hemostasis in physiologic and pathophysiologic settings.

PRINCIPLES OF ANGIOGENESIS

Angiogenesis is the process of new blood vessel growth. The term is generally applied to the growth of microvessels that are the size of capillary blood vessels. Physiologic angiogenesis is a fundamental biologic mechanism that occurs in embryonic development, because the formation of a vascular system is one of the initial events in organogenesis. Nevertheless, it also occurs in adults during wound healing, in the placenta during pregnancy, in the cycling ovary, and during restoration of blood flow to damaged tissues. Angiogenesis is regulated by a very sensitive interplay of growth factors and inhibitors, and their imbalance can lead to disease. In cancer, diabetic eye disease, age-related macular degeneration, cutaneous and gastric ulcers, and rheumatoid arthritis, aberrant angiogenesis feeds diseased tissue and damages normal tissue. On the other hand, insufficient angiogenesis underlies conditions such as coronary heart disease, stroke, and delayed wound healing, in which limited

vessel growth leads to poor circulation. It is currently estimated that 500 million people worldwide would benefit from either pro- or antiangiogenic therapies.[1]

Cancer and Angiogenesis

The most well-known and best-studied example of pathologic angiogenesis is that of tumor progression. Over a century ago, scientists had observed that the growth of human tumors often coincides with an increase in vasculature.[2] This observation led to the concept that a key aspect of cancer is a disease of the blood vessels. The existence of factors that may be secreted from the tumor and would promote new vessel growth was proposed in 1939. Several years later it was proposed that tumor development is critically dependent on new blood vessel formation.[3,4] In 1971 it was hypothesized that blocking new vessel development (anti-angiogenesis) would be an effective approach to treat cancer, launching an active search for stimulators and inhibitors of angiogenesis.[5] It is now widely accepted that the biogenesis of a tumor represents an interaction between the tumor and its microenvironment (Fig. 2-1). Like all solid tissues, tumor cells require a blood vessel system to provide nutrients, oxygen, and a means of waste disposal.

Molecular Players That Regulate Angiogenesis

Numerous angiogenesis regulatory factors have been reported to regulate new blood vessel development in positive and negative manners. The existence and potency of angiogenic factors were first revealed by implanting small pieces of tumors on the cornea or ears of laboratory animals.[6] Within several days, dense networks of capillaries were observed to converge on the tumors.[7,8] Over the past 25 years, more than 20 angiogenic growth factors have been identified and characterized (Box 2-1).

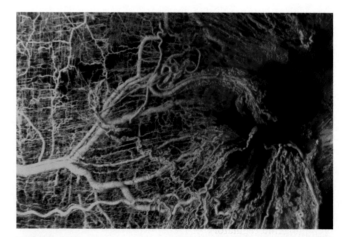

FIGURE 2-1. Organization of tumor-associated vasculature. This image, generated by injecting a resin into blood vessels before fixation of the tissue, demonstrates that the blood vessels feeding a tumor mass (dark area in the upper right corner) are tortuous and highly disorganized, in contrast to the well-organized vessels (top left). *(Courtesy of L. Heiser and R. Ackland, University of Louisville, Louisville, Ky.)*

Box 2-1	Stimulators and Inhibitors of Angiogenesis

Angiogenic factors
  Vascular endothelial growth factor (VEGF)
  Acidic and basic fibroblast growth factors (FGFs)
  Placenta growth factor (PLGF)
  Platelet-derived growth factor (PDGF)
  Transforming growth factor (TGF)
  Epidermal growth factor (EGF)
  Hepatocyte growth factor (HGF)
  Platelet-activating factor
  Tumor necrosis factor
  Insulin-like growth factor
  Angiogenin
  Angiopoietin-1
  Granulocyte-macrophage colony-stimulating factor (GM-CSF)
  Granulocyte colony-stimulating factor (G-CSF)
  Interleukin-2
  Interleukin-6
  Interleukin-8
  Prostaglandins E1, E2
  Vascular integrin (Vitaxin)
  Matrix metalloproteinases
Antiangiogenic factors
  Arresten
Thrombospondin
  Fibronectin
  Angiostatin
  Endostatin
  Interferon
  Interleukin-1
  Interleukin-12
Angiopoietin-2
Tissue inhibitors of metalloproteinases (TIMPs)—platelet factor 4
Retinoic acid

Stimulators of Angiogenesis

Once researchers established that tumor cells could secrete molecules that stimulate the process of angiogenesis, the challenge became to find and study these angiogenesis-stimulating molecules. It first became possible to isolate angiogenic factors when a chick chorioallantoic membrane was used, together with bioassays based on endothelial cell migration and proliferation in vitro and with corneal neovascularization in vivo.[9-17] The first proangiogenic regulatory factor was purified from a tumor in 1984 using heparin affinity chromatography, called basic fibroblast growth factor (bFGF).[18] bFGF is one of the most potent stimulators of angiogenesis and promotes endothelial cell proliferation and the organization of endothelial cells into tube-like structures. Vascular endothelial growth factor (VEGF), which is undoubtedly one of the most important proangiogenic regulatory proteins, was discovered in 1989 by Napoleone Ferrara of Genentech.[19]

VEGF is the most significant promotor of angiogenesis in physiologic and pathologic conditions, increasing the number of capillaries in a given network. It is thought to play an essential role in driving tumor angiogenesis. Overexpression of VEGF is a hallmark feature in most malignant diseases and is typically an indicator of poor prognosis. There is increasing evidence that upregulation of proangiogenic factors is a key process in hematologic malignancies, and VEGF appears to be one of the major regulators. Six different members of the VEGF family have been identified—VEGF-A (also known as vascular permeability factor), VEGF-B, VEGF-C, VEGF-D, VEGF-E, and placental growth factor (PLGF).[20-26] Three members of the receptor tyrosine kinase family, VEGF-R1, VEGF-R2, and VEGF-R3, bind to VEGF isoforms. Neuropilin-1 and neuropilin-2 function as coreceptors for VEGF. VEGF functions by promoting the survival of endothelial cells, proliferation, cell migration, and increased vascular permeability. VEGF also mobilizes progenitor cells from the marrow to the areas of new vessel growth.[27] Although VEGF is upregulated by a variety of growth factors, the most important factor is hypoxia.[28] Hypoxia-inducible factor (HIF), a transcription factor that works in concert with the product of the von Hippel-Lindau (VHL) tumor suppressor gene, plays a crucial role in this process.

How do proangiogenic regulatory proteins stimulate angiogenesis? Angiogenic regulatory proteins, such as VEGF and bFGF, may first be synthesized by the tumor cell and released into the surrounding tissue. Inflammatory cells, stromal cells, and endothelial cells may also release angiogenic regulatory proteins. These angiogenesis-stimulating proteins then bind to specific receptors on the surface of endothelial cells. The binding of bFGF or VEGF to its specific receptor activates a signaling cascade that relays a signal into the nucleus of the endothelial cell, ultimately leading to the synthesis of new molecules essential for the growth of endothelial cells.

Whereas VEGF and FGF are major regulators of angiogenesis, they are only two of a large cohort of natural stimulators of angiogenesis. The angiopoietins Ang1 and Ang2 promote endothelial cell survival and are essential for the formation of mature blood vessels.[29-31] Matrix metalloproteinases (MMPs) play an important role in degrading proteins that keep the vessel walls solid. This proteolytic event allows endothelial cells to escape into the matrix.

Inhibitors of Angiogenesis

In most adult physiologic settings, proangiogenic regulatory proteins are balanced by antiangiogenic regulatory proteins (see Box 2-1). The existence of endogenous antiangiogenesis factors has long been suspected by surgeons who noticed that after large primary tumors were removed, a substantial amount of metastases would suddenly grow at a rapid rate. These observations suggested that the primary tumor was secreting an inhibitory factor that blocked angiogenesis in the secondary tumors.

The isolation of these factors has been under active investigation for over 33 years. The first angiogenesis inhibitor was discovered in cartilage in 1975.[32] One of the most well-characterized inhibitors of angiogenesis is endostatin, which is a naturally occurring 20-kD fragment that arises from the cleavage product of the C-terminal of collagen XVIII, a component of the extracellular matrix.[33,34] Endostatin is a broad-spectrum angiogenesis inhibitor that inhibits the growth of 65 different tumor types and modifies 12% of the human genome to downregulate pathologic angiogenesis.[35] Endostatin was originally found in conditioned media from a murine endothelial tumor cell line, hemangioendothelioma.[36,37] It functions to inhibit endothelial cell migration in vitro and induces endothelial cell apoptosis.

Thrombospondin-1 (TSP-1) is another major regulator of new vessel development, with potent antiangiogenic effects. TSP-1 was first isolated from platelets that were activated with thrombin and was thus given the name thrombin-sensitive protein. TSP-1 forms homodimers and binds to the receptor

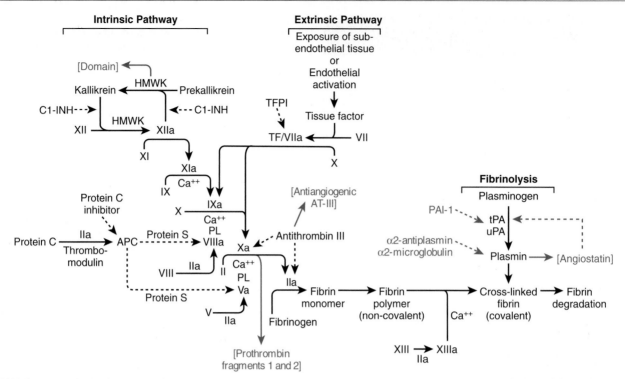

FIGURE 2-2. Cryptic antiangiogenic fragments derived from the hemostatic system. Cryptic fragments generated from coagulation and fibrinolytic proteins which suppress angiogenesis are indicated in red. Coagulation factors are depicted by Roman numerals. The coagulation cascade and fibrinolytic pathway inhibitors are indicated by a dashed arrow. a = activation; AT = antithrombin; C1-INH = complement factor-1 esterase inhibitor; HMWK = high-molecular-weight kininogen; PAI-1 = plasminogen activator inhibitor 1; PL = anionic phospholipids; TF = tissue factor; TFPI = tissue factor pathway inhibitor; tPA = tissue-type plasminogen activator; uPA = urinary plasminogen activator. *(Adapted from Browder T, Folkman J, Pirie-Shepherd S. The hemostatic system as a regulator of angiogenesis. J Biol Chem. 2000;275:1521-1524.)*

CD36, which is located on the plasma membrane of endothelial cells. TSP-1 is a large multifunctional glycoprotein that is secreted by most endothelial cells in the extracellular matrix. TSP-1 inhibits the proliferation and migration of endothelial cells by interacting with CD36. The role of TSP-1 in tumor progression has been studied in great detail. Loss of p53, which is observed in almost all tumors, leads to a significant decrease in TSP-1 and results in an increase in angiogenesis. Because tumors overexpressing TSP-1 typically exhibit less angiogenesis, have fewer metastases, and generally grow slower, TSP-1 is an attractive biologic mediator for cancer therapy.

One important theme that extends throughout this chapter is that angiogenesis and hemostasis share several characteristics. In particular, both processes share certain proteins. Among the approximately 40 proteins that regulate the hemostatic system, there are at least six proteins that contain cryptic angiogenic regulators (Fig. 2-2). The antiangiogenic factor called tumstatin is a product of the cleavage of collagen IV. Cleavage of the amino terminus of plasminogen yields the angiogenesis inhibitor angiostatin.[38] Tissue inhibitors of metalloproteinases (TIMPs) counterbalance the proangiogenic effects of MMPs and prevent elongating capillaries from invading through the extracellular matrix.

Tipping the Balance: The Angiogenic Switch

The capacity to induce new blood vessel growth is a characteristic that many cells within tumors initially lack and must acquire as the tumor progresses. When tumors develop the capacity to stimulate blood vessel growth, these small tumor cells are said to undergo an angiogenic switch, allowing them to multiply rapidly. This angiogenic switch is a necessary phe-

notype of a successful tumor. In this sense, by constraining angiogenesis, the normal microenvironment can be considered to function as a tumor suppressor. Under these normal conditions, there is a balance between endogenous angiogenesis inducers and inhibitors that keep the angiogenic process in check and prevent inappropriate tissue vascularization (Fig. 2-3). It is thought that the phenotypic switch to angiogenesis is usually accomplished by a subset of tumor cells that induce new capillaries, which then converge toward the tumor. The switch is thought to be the result of the synthesis or release of angiogenic factors. Specifically, the balance is altered by increasing the gene expression of stimulators, altering the activity of stimulators, or decreasing the concentrations of endogenous angiogenesis regulatory proteins via gene expression or processing.[39,40] Different types of tumor cells appear to use distinct strategies to flip the angiogenic switch.[41] Identification of the mechanisms that trip the angiogenic switch should yield strategies to treat cancer.

ROLE OF ANGIOGENESIS IN HEMATOLOGIC MALIGNANCY

Hematologic Malignancies Are Angiogenic

It was long thought that leukemia and other hematologic malignancies vary from solid tumors by neither stimulating nor requiring new vessel development. However, this view has completely changed over the past decade.[42] Because the proangiogenic regulatory protein bFGF was abnormally elevated in the urine of patients with leukemia, it was initially postulated that

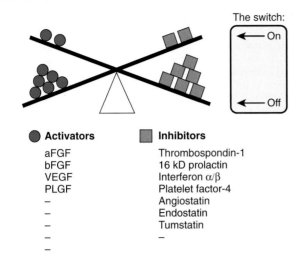

The switch:

On

Off

● **Activators**   ■ **Inhibitors**

aFGF	Thrombospondin-1
bFGF	16 kD prolactin
VEGF	Interferon α/β
PLGF	Platelet factor-4
–	Angiostatin
–	Endostatin
–	Tumstatin
–	–
–	

FIGURE 2-3. The balancing act of angiogenesis. The normally quiescent vasculature can be stimulated to sprout new capillaries (angiogenesis), a process controlled by an angiogenic switch mechanism. This diagram presents the major regulators that function to stimulate or inhibit angiogenesis. It is the balance between two groups of regulators that determine whether and when angiogenesis is turned on. In some tissues, the absence of angiogenesis inducers may keep the switch off, whereas in others the angiogenesis inducers are present but held in check by higher levels of angiogenesis inhibitors. aFGF = acidic fibroblast growth factor. *(Adapted from Hanahan D, Folkman J. Patterns and emerging mechanisms of the angiogenic switch during tumorigenesis. Cell. 1996;86:353-364.)*

leukemias may stimulate angiogenesis.[43,44] These findings were soon followed by a study that demonstrated that the bone marrow is angiogenic in multiple myeloma patients. In fact, this quantitative study showed that microvessel density was five times higher than normal levels.[45] By 1995, it was reported that angiogenesis was increased in B-cell leukemia and soon thereafter it was revealed that children with acute lymphoblastic leukemia have a six- to sevenfold increase in microvessel density.[46,47] bFGF levels in the urine were sevenfold higher than controls, providing further evidence that this disease is associated with angiogenesis. It is now clear that malignant cells in these diseases may recruit new vessels by similar molecular pathways as cells in solid tumors.

Leukemia

Acute myeloid leukemia (AML) is a cancer of the blood or bone marrow characterized by the abnormal proliferation of blood cells. Leukemias originate from hematopoietic stem cells that are blocked in development at different stages of maturation and differentiation. Acute leukemia is characterized by the rapid proliferation of immature hematopoietic stem cells. This crowding inhibits the bone marrow from generating healthy blood cells. A large amount of clinical data has indicated that angiogenesis plays a critical role in the development of AML. Dilly and Jagger first postulated a role for angiogenesis in liquid tumors by demonstrating that there is an abrupt increase in the number of endothelial cells found in the bone marrow of leukemia patients.[48] Microvessel density (MVD) measurements of bone marrow from AML patients are significantly higher than controls, and MVD levels decrease significantly in patients who respond after chemotherapy.[49] Others have used MVD as a means of establishing prognosis, whereby more microvessel

density within the bone marrow signals increased bone marrow myeloblasts.[47] Proangiogenic VEGF and bFGF levels in blood are increased in patients with AML.[50] Furthermore, VEGF levels appear to function as a prognostic indicator in patients with AML.[51] Recently, the VEGF gene and its polymorphisms were found to be helpful in predicting the prognosis of acute leukemias.[52]

In addition to functioning as a prognostic factor in AML, VEGF may also have an essential role in propagating the disease. In addition to synthesizing VEGF, AML cells also display VEGF receptors, forming an autocrine loop that promotes tumor growth and survival.[53] Angiopoietin-1 and its antagonist angiopoietin-2 also appear to play a role in the pathophysiology of AML. Levels of angiopoietin-2 are significantly elevated in AML patients. Angiopoietin-2 also functions as a prognostic indicator for overall survival.[54,55] Although we do not fully understand the mechanism, elevation of angiopoietin-2 in patients treated with polychemotherapy indicates a more positive prognosis. Acute lymphocytic leukemia is the most common type of leukemia in young children. The 5-year survival rate is 85% in children and 50% in adults. Angiogenic regulatory proteins also appear to play a role in acute lymphoblastic leukemia (ALL), because patients with a poor response to chemotherapy had higher VEGF levels than responders.[56]

Chronic leukemia is distinguished by the excessive buildup of mature hematopoietic stem cells. Typically taking months to years to progress, the cells are produced at an elevated rate compared with normal cells. Chronic lymphocytic leukemia (CLL) usually occurs in older individuals and the 5-year survival rate is 75%. Elevated levels of new blood vessel development in bone marrow and lymph nodes have been observed in CLL. In particular, biologic markers of angiogenesis have been shown to be of prognostic relevance in CLL.[57] Molica and colleagues[58] have demonstrated that CLL patients who presented with early stage disease but showed elevated levels of VEGF were more likely to have a poorer prognosis. CLL cells contain receptors for VEGF and secrete VEGF, suggesting an autocrine loop may propagate the survival of cells.[59]

Enhancement of angiogenesis is also one of the hallmarks of chronic myeloid leukemia (CML). This disease occurs mainly in adults and the 5-year survival rate is 90%. VEGF appears to function as a key regulator of disease, as increased levels of VEGF indicate a poor prognosis. In particular, higher VEGF and VEGF receptor levels correlate with shorter survival of patients in chronic CML.[60]

Lymphoma

Lymphoma is a cancer derived from lymphocytes that accounts for approximately 5% of all cases of cancer in the United States. Enhanced angiogenesis is a characteristic of lymphoma and an increased vascular density is highly associated with higher grade malignant variants of the disease.[61] Expression of both VEGF-D and its receptor, VEGFR-3, have been found to be present on B cells and in the capillaries of the bone marrow in a variety of lymphomas as well as leukemias.[62] Plasma levels of bFGF and VEGF are increased in non-Hodgkin's lymphoma (NHL) patients when they are untreated. Patients with the shortest overall survival exhibit concurrent increases of bFGF and VEGF.[63,64]

Myelodysplastic Syndrome

Myelodysplastic syndrome (MDS) is a group of hematologic disorders characterized by ineffective production of blood cells. In MDS, stem cells do not mature into healthy platelets, red cells, and white blood cells. Instead the immature blood cells, called blasts, die in the marrow or soon after they enter circulation. Although the specific pathogenesis of MDS is not fully understood, it may involve elevated levels of cytokines that promote immune-mediated suppression of hematopoiesis, apoptosis of intramedullary hematopoietic cells, or increased angiogenesis in the bone marrow. Several studies have suggested that angiogenic factors may have a direct effect on marrow vascularity in myelodysplastic syndromes.[65] A significant increase in the number of blood vessels is observed in MDS patients, as well as increases in angiogenic factors, including bFGF, VEGF, TNF-α, and HGF. Progressive increases in microvessel density are observed according to the stages of MDS, with highest microvessel densities observed in secondary AML and CML and lowest in refractory anemia. Dynamic magnetic resonance imaging (DMRI) of bone marrow has also demonstrated increased vascularity in patients with MDS.[66] Also, Bellamy and colleagues[67] have shown that the blasts of patients with MDS exhibit overexpression of the VEGF receptor, further supporting the role of angiogenesis in MDS.

Multiple Myeloma

Multiple myeloma (MM) is a type of cancer of the plasma cells, which are immune cells that produce antibodies. A growing body of evidence supports new vessel growth as having an important role in the pathophysiology of multiple myeloma. Increased microvessel density in the bone marrow has been detected with patients with MM, which appears to function as an indicator of poor prognosis.[45,68-70] As observed in solid tumors, the angiogenic switch also appears to play a key role in multiple myeloma.[71] Whereas VEGF is also frequently overexpressed in advanced stage MM, it does not appear to function as a prognostic indicator. Bone marrow endothelial cells from patients with MM do contain elevated VEGF receptor-2 and VEGF, suggesting that an autocrine loop could be a major mechanism in the disease.[72]

Antiangiogenic Therapy of Cancer

Although many angiogenesis inhibitors were discovered in the 1980s, it was not until the mid-1990s that new drugs with antiangiogenic activity entered clinical trials. These drugs began to receive U.S. Food and Drug Administration (FDA) approval in the United States by 2003. Bevacizumab (Avastin), which received FDA approval for the treatment of colorectal cancer in 2004, was the first drug developed exclusively as an angiogenesis inhibitor. Since then, several new drugs with antiangiogenic activity have been approved by the FDA and by equivalent approval agencies in 30 other countries for the treatment of cancer and age-related macular degeneration (Table 2-1).[73] The majority of these drugs target VEGF or one of its receptors. Most of the FDA-approved drugs, as well as those in phase III clinical trials, target one proangiogenic protein. There are approximately 30 drugs with antiangiogenic properties that are in phase III clinical trials for the treatment of cancer, and many of these target more than a single proangiogenic protein (Table 2-2). The reported increased vascularity in pediatric ALL, AML, and MDS, along with the increased presence of proangiogenic factors, suggest that angiogenesis may have a role in the pathophysiology of hematologic malignancies and that antiangiogenesis therapy could have an anticancer effect.[74]

Targeting the Vascular Endothelial Growth Factor Pathway

Inhibitors of the VEGF pathway are the most clinically advanced. The inhibitors currently being tested include a variety of agents with diverse mechanisms of action. Strategies to inhibit VEGF pathways include monoclonal antibodies that bind to VEGF-A or VEGF receptors, soluble receptors such as VEGF trap that sequester the growth factor, and aptamers that bind the heparin-binding domain VEGF165.[75] This class of inhibitors arrests endothelial cell proliferation and prevents

TABLE 2-1	Angiogenesis Inhibitors for Treatment of Cancer and Macular Degeneration*		
Date Approved	**Drug (Generic Name)**	**Where Approved**	**Disease**
May 2003	Bortezomib (Velcade)	United States (FDA)	Multiple myeloma
December 2003	Thalidomide	Australia	Multiple myeloma
February 2004	Bevacizumab (Avastin)	United States (FDA)	Colorectal cancer
February 2004	Cetuximab (Erbitux)	United States (FDA)	Colorectal cancer
November 2004	Erlotinib (Tarceva)	United States (FDA)	Lung cancer
December 2004	Bevacizumab (Avastin)	Switzerland	Colorectal cancer
December 2004	Pegaptanib (Macugen)	United States (FDA)	Macular degeneration
January 2005	Bevacizumab (Avastin)	European Union (27 countries)	Colorectal cancer
September 2005	Endostatin (Endostar)	China (SFDA)	Lung cancer
December 2005	Sorafenib (Nexavar)	United States (FDA)	Kidney cancer
December 2005	Lenalidomide (Revlimid)	United States (FDA)	Myelodysplastic syndrome
January 2006	Sunitinib (Sutent)	United States (FDA)	Gastrointestinal stromal tumor
June 2006	Ranibizumab (Lucentis)	United States (FDA)	Macular degeneration
June 2006	Lenalidomide (Revlimid)	United States (FDA)	Multiple myeloma
August 2006	Ranibizumab (Lucentis)	Switzerland	Macular degeneration
September 2006	Ranibizumab (Lucentis)	India	Macular degeneration
October 2006	Bevacizumab (Avastin)	United States (FDA)	Lung cancer
January 2007	Ranibizumab (Lucentis)	European Union (27 countries)	Macular degeneration
March 2007	Bevacizumab (Avastin)	European Union, Iceland, Norway	Metastatic breast cancer
April 2007	Bevacizumab (Avastin)	Japan	Colorectal cancer
May 2007	Temsirolimus (Torisel, CCI-779)	United States (FDA)	Kidney cancer

*Approved by the U.S. Food and Drug Administration (FDA) and by equivalent agencies in 30 other countries. SFDA = State Food and Drug Administration.

From Folkman J. Angiogenesis: an organizing principle for drug discovery? Nat Rev Drug Discov. 2007;6:273-286.

TABLE 2-2   **Drugs with Antiangiogenic Activity and Varying Degrees of Other Activities***

Agent	Target
AG3340 (Agouron Pharmaceuticals)	MMP inhibitor
Avastin (Genentech)	VEGF
AZD2171 (AstraZeneca)	VEGFR-1, -2, -3, PDGFR
BMS-275291 (Bristol Myers Squibb)	MMP inhibitor
CCI-779 (Wyeth)	VEGFR, mTOR inhibitor
Ceflatonin (homoharringtonine) (ChemGenex)	VEGFR-2/KDR
Celecoxib (Celebrex) (Pfizer)	Increases endostatin
GW786034 (GlaxoSmithKline)	VEGFR
LY317615 (Eli Lilly)	VEGF
Neovastat (Benefin, AE941) (Aeterna Zentaris)	MMP inhibitor
Sorafenib (Nexavar, BAY439006) (Bayer/Onyx)	VEGFR-2 and PDGFR-beta
Vatalanib (PTK787) (Novartis)	VEGFR-1, 2, PDGFR
Everolimus (RAD001) (Novartis)	VEGFR/mTOR
Lenalidomide (Revlimid, CC5013) (Celgene)	VEGF, precursor endothelial cells
Suramin (NCI)	IGF-1, EGFR, PDGFR, TGF-β; inhibits VEGF and bFGF
Sutent (SU11248) (Pfizer)	VEGFR-1, 2, 3, PDGFR
Erlotinib (Tarceva), OSI774) (Genentech, OSI)	HER1, EGFR
Tetrathiomolybdate (TM) (University of Michigan)	VEGF, copper chelator
Thalidomide (Celgene)	VEGF, precursor endothelial cells
VEGF Trap (Regeneron Pharmaceuticals)	VEGF
Bortezomib (Velcade, PS341) (Millennium Pharmaceuticals)	VEGF
Vandetnibib (Zactima, ZD6474) (AstraZeneca)	VEGFR-2, EGFR

*In phase III trial for cancer treatment—February 2007, not yet FDA approved.

bFGF = basic fibroblast growth factor; EGFR = epidermal growth factor receptor (HER1); IGF-1 = insulin-like growth factor 1; KDR = kinase insert domain receptor; MMP = matrix metalloproteinase; mTOR = mammalian target of rapamycin (sirolimus); PDGFR = platelet-derived growth factor receptor; TGF-β = transforming growth factor β; VEGF = vascular endothelial growth factor; VEGFR = VEGF receptor.

From Folkman J. Angiogenesis: an organizing principle for drug discovery? Nat Rev Drug Discov. 2007;6:273-286.

vessel growth, as well as stimulating regression of existing blood vessels by increasing endothelial cell death. Bevacizumab is a recombinant humanized monoclonal antibody to VEGF. The FDA approved bevacizumab after a large, randomized, double-blind, phase III study in which the drug was administered in combination with a bolus IFL (*i*rinotecan, 5-*f*luorouracil [5-FU], and *l*eucovorin) chemotherapy for metastatic colorectal cancer.[76] Median survival increased from 15.6 months in the bolus IFL plus placebo arm of the trial to 20.3 months in the bolus IFL plus bevacizumab arm.

Clinical studies using inhibitors of the VEGF pathway appear to be promising treatments for malignancies with VEGF receptor expression on tumor cells, such as MM and AML. A significant clinical response was observed in an AML patient on VEGF–tyrosine kinase inhibitor SU5416.[77] A phase II clinical trial of bevacizumab administered following chemotherapy to adults with refractory or relapsed AML has been described.[77a] Cytotoxic chemotherapy followed by bevacizumab resulted in a favorable complete remission rate and duration in patients with AML resistant to traditional treatments.

Despite the promising results of targeting the VEGF pathway, anti–VEGF antibody only provides an overall survival benefit in breast, colorectal, and lung cancer patients when combined with conventional chemotherapy. One limitation of this treatment is that tumors may become refractory to antiangiogenic therapy, especially if it targets only a single angiogenic regulatory protein (i.e., VEGF)—in other words, a monoantiangiogenic therapy.[35] Although VEGF is expressed by up to 60% of human tumors, most tumors also express five to eight other angiogenic regulatory proteins. For example, human breast cancers can express up to six angiogenic proteins. When one angiogenic protein is suppressed for an extended period, others may emerge. The mechanism of this compensatory response is unclear. Some angiogenesis inhibitors target up to three angiogenic proteins, and others target an even broader spectrum of angiogenic proteins. These are less likely to promote the development of resistance.

Antiangiogenic Chemotherapy

The concept that chemotherapeutics can cause endothelial damage has been known for some time.[78-80] Browder and colleagues[81] first reported that when murine tumors are made drug-resistant to cyclophosphamide, and cyclophosphamide is administered on a conventional chemotherapy maximum tolerated dose schedule, all mice died of larger tumors. However, if cyclophosphamide was given more frequently at a lower dose, the tumors were potently inhibited because of programmed cell death of endothelial cells. If an angiogenesis inhibitor was added that by itself could only inhibit the tumors by 50%, the drug-resistant tumors were eliminated. This experiment demonstrated a new principle—a cytotoxic chemotherapeutic agent could be redirected to an endothelial target by altering its dose and frequency of administration. This approach was confirmed using a second chemotherapeutic agent.[82] It was further demonstrated that levels of an inhibitor of angiogenesis, TSP-1, increase during antiangiogenic therapy, and that deletion of TSP-1 gene in mice completely nullified the antitumor effect of this antiangiogenic therapy.[83] This optimization of chemotherapy to treat vascular endothelium in the tumor bed has been termed *metronomic therapy*.[84] Metronomic chemotherapy has entered clinical trial. Kieran and associates[85] reported a recent study of children with different types of brain tumors refractory to surgery, radiotherapy, and chemotherapy who were treated for 6 months with daily oral thalidomide and celecoxib, plus daily low-dose oral cyclophosphamide alternated every 3 weeks with daily low-dose oral etoposide. Of all patients, 25% were progression free for more than 2.5 years from starting therapy; 40% of patients completed the 6 months of therapy, which resulted in prolonged or constant disease-free status. Only elevated TSP-1 levels in the blood correlated with prolonged response, which is consistent with the elevated circulating TSP-1 levels observed in tumor-bearing mice treated with antiangiogenic metronomic cyclophosphamide.[82]

Thalidomide

Thalidomide has both in vitro and in vivo antiangiogenic properties.[86-90] Corneal neovascularization in rabbits induced by bFGF or VEGF was blocked by orally administered thalidomide. Thalidomide is a very weak inhibitor of TNF-α, but experimental evidence suggests that the antiangiogenic activity is not related to TNF-α inhibition. In addition to the antiangiogenic activity, thalidomide has a direct effect on myeloma cells and the immune system. Therefore, the exact mechanism whereby thalidomide functions is not fully understood. The first report of thalidomide therapy for multiple myeloma was in 1999.[89] A 32% response was observed in patients with disease refractory to all other therapy. Response was monitored by the reduction of myeloma protein in serum or Bence Jones protein in urine that lasted for at least 6 weeks.[91-94] Thalidomide is considered one of the most active drugs in relapsed myeloma. Clinical studies using thalidomide to treat multiple myeloma have resulted in a 37% remission in poor-risk patients.[86] Thalidomide can be used for frontline therapy and maintenance therapy.[95-96] In addition to being tested for almost all types of multiple myeloma, thalidomide has also been found to be effective in myeloproliferative disorders and leukemia.[97,98]

HEMOSTATIC SYSTEM AS A REGULATOR OF ANGIOGENESIS

Blood Platelets and Cancer

The hemostatic system as a whole, and platelets in particular, have a close association with the development of cancer.[99] A survey of the literature reveals the reciprocal nature of the tumor-platelet relationship—whereas numerous platelet abnormalities have been identified in cancer patients, platelet activity, in turn, appears to influence the development of cancer. Over 140 years ago, Trousseau described a close association between cancer and hemostasis.[100] Gasic and coworkers[101,102] later established that thrombocytopenia induced by injecting neuraminidase into mice causes a marked reduction in metastasis formation when ascites tumor cells are injected.[103] A significant number of cancer patients have very high platelet counts, which is associated with a poor prognosis.[104,105] In addition, these patients are at risk of venous thromboembolism and have raised levels of von Willebrand factor and fibrin degradation products.[106] Increased numbers of activated platelets and increased expression of platelet adhesion receptors are common findings in cancer patients.[107] The correlation between platelet numbers and tumor development has recently been demonstrated in a mouse model. Camerer and colleagues[108] have shown that when melanoma cells are intravenously injected into nuclear factor (erythroid-derived 2) (NF-E2)–deficient mice that contain almost no circulating platelets, an almost complete absence of surface tumors in lungs and marked protection against hematogenous metastasis is observed. In 1998, Pinedo and associates[109] have proposed that platelets play a crucial role in tumor angiogenesis by releasing angiogenic regulatory proteins during platelet activation. Some tumor cells can activate platelets and increase aggregation, which stimulates the release of angiogenic factors, thereby directly affecting the tumor endo-

thelium.[110-112] Interestingly, inhibition of the fibrinogen receptor, GPIIb/IIIa, has also been shown to decrease metastasis formation.[110,113] The strongest molecular conclusion from this body of data is that platelets have the capacity to contribute to tumor development.

Platelets and Angiogenesis

Most experimental and clinical data suggest that platelets contribute to tumor development by functioning as a transport and delivery system of angiogenic regulatory proteins.[109,114,115] Almost 1 trillion platelets circulate in an adult human. Because of their small size and the rheology of flowing blood, platelets are thrust against the endothelium by larger blood cells. The proximity and ability to interact with the endothelium are key factors that allow platelets to modulate angiogenesis. Some of the first evidence suggesting that platelets influence new blood vessel development was reported by Gimbrone and coworkers,[116] who showed that the perfusion of plasma depleted of platelets resulted in instability of the endothelial layer and hemorrhages. By adding back platelets, they demonstrated that they could rescue this injurious effect. Additional studies in animals went on to show that absence of platelets (thrombocytopenia) leads to elevated vascular permeability, the likely result of large spaces between endothelial cells.[117,118] Pipili-Synetos and colleagues[119] definitively have shown that platelets influence angiogenesis by demonstrating that platelets stimulate the formation of tubes and capillary-like structures when added to human umbilical vein endothelial cells in vitro. They further noted that the soluble platelet factors by themselves do not promote capillary formation. This demonstrates that the interaction between the platelet and endothelial surface is essential for the stimulation of capillary-like structures. These results dovetail with the recent finding that the adhesion function of platelets, as mediated by the GPIb α-glycoprotein receptor, significantly contributes to the angiogenic properties of platelets.[120]

Although platelets have been presumed to contribute to tumor development by providing numerous pro- and antiangiogenic regulatory proteins, the regulatory role of platelets in this process is still poorly understood.[115] Platelets contain numerous regulators of angiogenesis, which can be delivered to the endothelium during platelet activation (Table 2-3). The proangiogenic regulatory proteins VEGF, bFGF, epidermal growth factor (EGF), platelet-derived growth factor (PDGF), sphingosine 1-phosphate, and metalloproteinases have all been identified in platelets.[44,121-134] The stimulators in platelets are counterbalanced by the platelet angiogenesis inhibitors, including endostatin, TSP-1, platelet factor 4, angiostatin, and TIMPs.[135-142]

Most angiogenic regulatory proteins identified in platelets have been localized to alpha granules, the major storage granule of platelets. Each human platelet contains 40 to 80 alpha granules, which are from 200 to 500 nm in diameter (Fig. 2-4). In essence, alpha granules function like small sepharose beads, concentrating the angiogenic regulatory proteins into a small compartment. By adhering to the endothelium of injured organs and tissues and then secreting their contents, platelets deposit high concentrations of angiogenic regulatory proteins in a localized manner. Many proteins localized to alpha granules have been shown to be synthesized solely by megakaryocytes. However, other proteins, such as fibrinogen, are synthesized by other cells and must be taken up via endocytosis by megakaryocytes and platelets. It has been assumed by the hematology community that alpha granules are composed of a homogeneous population with respect to their contents.

The levels of these angiogenic regulatory proteins in platelets appear to play a role in tumor angiogenesis. Klement and colleagues[82] have reported that when a microscopic-sized human tumor is present in a mouse, circulating platelets take up and sequester specific angiogenesis regulatory proteins, such as platelet factor 4, VEGF, connective tissue–activating peptide (CTAP), and basic fibroblast growth factor (FGF). The angiogenic regulatory proteins are sequestered in the platelets at a significantly higher concentration than observed in the plasma. In fact, when radiolabeled VEGF is implanted subcutaneously in a Matrigel pellet in mice, platelet lysates contain almost all the VEGF. This new platelet property, quantifiable by mass spectrometry of platelet lysates, may lead to the development of a biomarker for very early detection of tumor recurrence.[143]

Capacity of Platelets to Regulate Angiogenesis

This ability evolves from the structure of platelets. An association between angiogenesis and platelets has long been recognized, but the cause-and-effect relationship linking the two has been unclear. A new structural property of platelets now provides a mechanistic explanation as to how platelets can selectively promote or inhibit angiogenesis. Given that platelets contain both stimulators and inhibitors of angiogenesis packaged into a homogeneous population of alpha granules, the question becomes, how can you attain a proangiogenic or antiangiogenic effect? The release of a mixture of both pro- and antiangiogenic regulatory proteins from platelets should cancel the effects of each other. We have recently discovered that angiogenesis regulatory proteins are in fact segregated among distinct sets of alpha granules in platelets—the major proangiogenic regulatory protein VEGF is housed in one set of alpha granules, and the major antiangiogenic regulatory protein endostatin is packaged into another set of alpha granules (Fig. 2-5).[144] Double immunofluorescence labeling of VEGF (an angiogenesis stimulator) and endostatin (an angiogenesis inhibitor), or of TSP-1 and basic FGF, confirms the segregation of stimulators and inhibitors into separate and distinct alpha granules. These observations have led to the hypothesis that distinct populations of alpha granules could undergo selective release. The treatment of human platelets with the selective protease-activated receptor 4 (PAR-4) agonist results in the release of endostatin-containing but not VEGF-containing granules, whereas the selective PAR-1 agonist liberates VEGF-containing but not endostatin-containing granules. These observations have demonstrated that separate packaging of angiogenesis regulators into pharmacologically and morphologically distinct populations of alpha granules in megakaryocytes and platelets provides a mechanism whereby platelets can locally stimulate

TABLE 2-3	Positive and Negative Regulators of Angiogenesis Reported in Platelets
Positive	**Negative**
VEGF-A	PF4
VEGF-C	Thrombospondin
bFGF	NK1, NK2, NK3 fragments of HGF
HGF	TGF-β1
Angiopoietin-1	Plasminogen (angiostatin)
PDGF	High-molecular-weight kininogen (domain 5)
EGF	Fibronectin (45-kD fragment)
IGF-1	EGF (fragment)
IGF BP-3	Alpha-2 antiplasmin (fragment)
Vitronectin	Beta-thromboglobulin
Fibronectin	Endostatin
Fibrinogen	
Heparinase	

bFGF = basic fibroblast growth factor; BP-3 = murine BP-3 antigen; EGF = epidermal growth factor; HGF = hematopoietic growth factor; IGF-1 = insulin-like growth factor 1; NK = natural killer (cell); PDGF = platelet-derived growth factor; PF4 = platelet factor 4; TGF-β1 = transforming growth factor β1; VEGF = vascular endothelial growth factor; VEGF-A = vascular endothelial growth factor A.

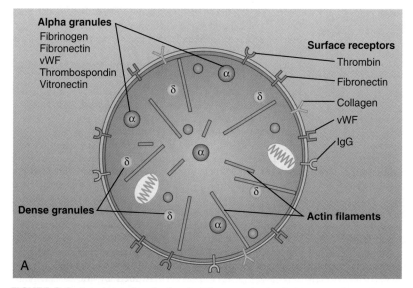
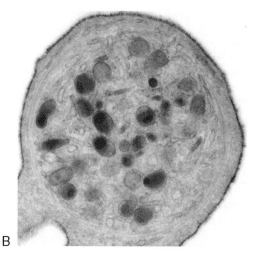

FIGURE 2-4. Structure of a platelet. A, Diagram of subcellular organelles and secretory granules of platelets. This schematic rendering of the subcellular organization of the resting platelet is based on electron microscopy (B). The marginal microtubule band encircles the cytoplasm of the platelet. The alpha granules constitute the majority of storage granules, interspersed with dense granules, peroxisomes, and lysosomes. IgG = immunoglobulin G; vWF = von Willebrand factor.

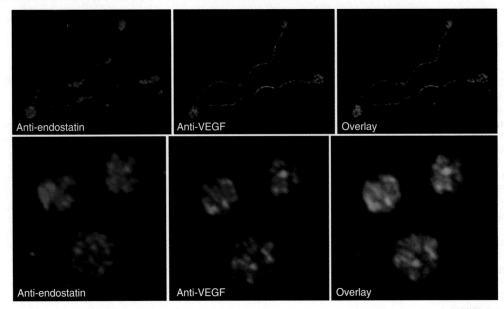

FIGURE 2-5. Vascular endothelial growth factor (VEGF; green) and endostatin (red) present in megakaryocytes and resting platelets are observed in separate and distinct alpha granules.

or inhibit angiogenesis. This heretofore unknown function of platelets provides a mechanistic link to the process of angiogenesis.

A new opportunity lies ahead to determine how platelets release proangiogenic proteins at a wound site and then later release antiangiogenic proteins. Furthermore, the putative role of platelet secretion of angiogenesis regulatory proteins in tumors now remains to be elucidated. It is well established that certain tumors trap platelets and put them in a position to deliver angiogenic regulatory proteins to the growing mass. Recently, it was reported that in cancer patients receiving bevacizumab (Avastin), the anti–VEGF antibody was taken up by platelets where it was bound to VEGF in the alpha granules.[145] These findings raise the possibility that bevacizumab could be functioning in part through platelets. The capacity of certain tumors to trap platelets may lead to the delivery of bevacizumab to the tumor.

CONCLUSION

Three concepts have emerged in the field of angiogenesis research:

1. Angiogenesis is regulated by a sensitive interplay of growth factors and inhibitors, and their imbalance can contribute to diseases such as cancer. A major goal should be continued research into characterizing the signal transduction pathways and molecules that influence new blood vessel growth.
2. Hematologic malignancies are angiogenesis-dependent. Continued efforts to find a role for specific angiogenic factors in these liquid tumor systems should lead to advances in antiangiogenic treatment.
3. The capacity of the hemostatic system to store and deliver proteins that regulate angiogenesis provides a new conceptual framework to understand how angiogenesis is regulated.

A better understanding of the mechanisms by which platelets release angiogenic regulatory proteins should yield new therapeutic strategies.

REFERENCES

1. Carmeliet P. Angiogenesis in life, disease and medicine. Nature. 2005;438:932-936.
2. Ferrara N. VEGF and the quest for tumour angiogenesis factors. Nat Rev Cancer. 2002;2:795-803.
3. Ide AG, Baker NH, Warren SL. Vascularization of the Brown-Pearce rabbit epithelioma transplant as seen in the transparent ear chamber. Am J Roentgenol. 1939;42:891-899.
4. Algire GH, Chalkely HW, Legallais FY, Park H. Vascular reactions of normal and malignant tumors in vivo. I. Vascular reactions of mice to wounds and to normal and neoplastic transplants. J Natl Cancer Inst. 1945;6:73-85.
5. Folkman J. Tumor angiogenesis: therapeutic implications. N Engl J Med. 1971;285:1182-1186.
6. Peterson GL. Review of the Folin phenol protein quantitation method of Lowry, Rosebrough, Farr and Randall. Anal Biochem. 1979;100:201-220.
7. Leunig M, Yuan F, Menger MD, et al. Angiogenesis, microvascular architecture, microhemodynamics, and interstitial fluid pressure during early growth of human adenocarcinoma LS174T in SCID mice. Cancer Research. 1992;52:6553-6560.
8. Wedge SR, Ogilvie DJ, Dukes M, et al. ZD6474 inhibits vascular endothelial growth factor signaling, angiogenesis, and tumor growth following oral administration. Cancer Res. 2002;62:4645-4655.
9. Folkman J, Long DM. The use of silicone rubber as a carrier for prolonged drug therapy. J Surg Res. 1964;4:139-142.
10. Muthukkaruppan V, Auerbach R. Angiogenesis in the mouse cornea. Science. 1979;205:1416-1418.
11. Gimbrone MA Jr, Cotran RS, Folkman J. Endothelial regeneration: studies with human endothelial cells in culture. Ser Haematol. 1973;6:453-455.

12. Gimbrone MA Jr, Cotran RS, Leapman SB, Folkman J. Tumor growth and neovascularization: an experimental model using the rabbit cornea. J Natl Cancer Inst. 1974;52:413-427.

13. Gimbrone MA Jr, Cotran RS, Folkman J. Human vascular endothelial cells in culture. Growth and DNA synthesis. J Cell Biol. 1974;60:673-684.

14. Jaffe EA, Nachman RL, Becker CG, Minick CR. Culture of human endothelial cells derived from umbilical veins. Identification by morphologic and immunologic criteria. J Clin Invest. 1973;52:2745-2756.

15. Auerbach R, Kubai L, Knighton D, Folkman J. A simple procedure for the long-term cultivation of chicken embryos. Dev Biol. 1974;41:391-394.

16. Ausprunk DH, Knighton DR, Folkman J. Differentiation of vascular endothelium in the chick chorioallantois: a structural and autoradiographic study. Dev Biol. 1974;38:237-248.

17. Folkman J, Haudenschild C. Angiogenesis in vitro. Nature. 1980;288:551-556.

18. Shing Y, Folkman J, Sullivan R, et al. Heparin affinity: purification of a tumor-derived capillary endothelial cell growth factor. Science. 1984;223:1296-1299.

19. Ferrara N, Henzel WJ. Pituitary follicular cells secrete a novel heparin-binding growth factor specific for vascular endothelial cells. Biochem Biophys Res Commun. 1989;161:851-858.

20. Beck L, D'Amore PA. Vascular development: cellular and molecular regulation. FASEB J. 1997;11:365-373.

21. Bussolino F, Albini A, Camussi G, et al. Role of soluble mediators in angiogenesis. Eur J Cancer. 1996;32A:2401-2412.

22. Olofsson B, Pajusola K, Kaipainen A, et al. Vascular endothelial growth factor B, a novel growth factor for endothelial cells. Proc Natl Acad Sci U S A. 1996;93:2576-2581.

23. Jeltsch M, Kaipainen A, Joukov V, et al. Hyperplasia of lymphatic vessels in VEGF-C transgenic mice. Science. 1997;276:1423-1425.

24. Yamada Y, Nezu J, Shimane M, Hirata Y. Molecular cloning of a novel vascular endothelial growth factor, VEGF-D. Genomics. 1997;42:483-488.

25. Klagsbrun M, Takashima S, Mamluk R. The role of neuropilin in vascular and tumor biology. Adv Exp Med Biol. 2002;515:33-48.

26. Larrivee B, Karsan A. Signaling pathways induced by vascular endothelial growth factor (review). Int J Mol Med. 2000;5:447-456.

27. Hicklin DJ, Ellis LM. Role of the vascular endothelial growth factor pathway in tumor growth and angiogenesis. J Clin Oncol. 2005;23:1011-1027.

28. Safran M, Kaelin WG Jr. HIF hydroxylation and the mammalian oxygen-sensing pathway. J Clin Invest. 2003;111:779-783.

29. Davis S, Aldrich TH, Jones PF, et al. Isolation of angiopoietin-1, a ligand for the TIE2 receptor, by secretion-trap expression cloning. Cell. 1996;87:1161-1169.

30. Suri C, Jones PF, Patan S, et al. Requisite role of angiopoietin-1, a ligand for the TIE2 receptor, during embryonic angiogenesis. Cell. 1996;87:1171-1180.

31. Maisonpierre PC, Suri C, Jones PF, et al. Angiopoietin-2, a natural antagonist for Tie2 that disrupts in vivo angiogenesis. Science. 1997;277:55-60.

32. Brem H, Folkman J. Inhibition of tumor angiogenesis mediated by cartilage. J Exp Med. 1975;141:427-439.

33. Bloch W, Huggel K, Sasaki T, et al. The angiogenesis inhibitor endostatin impairs blood vessel maturation during wound healing. FASEB J. 2000;14:2373-2376.

34. Sasaki T, Larsson H, Tisi D, et al. Endostatins derived from collagens XV and XVIII differ in structural and binding properties, tissue distribution and antiangiogenic activity. J Mol Biol. 2000;301:1179-1190.

35. Folkman J. Antiangiogenesis in cancer therapy—endostatin and its mechanisms of action. Exp Cell Res. 2006;312:594-607.

36. Zatterstrom UK, Felbor U, Fukai N, Olsen BR. Collagen XVIII/endostatin structure and functional role in angiogenesis. Cell Struct Funct. 2000;25:97-101.

37. O'Reilly MS, Boehm T, Shing Y, et al. Endostatin: an endogenous inhibitor of angiogenesis and tumor growth. Cell. 1997;88:277-285.

38. Cao Y, Ji RW, Davidson D, et al. Kringle domains of human angiostatin. Characterization of the anti-proliferative activity on endothelial cells. J Biol Chem. 1996;271:29461-29467.

39. Hanahan D, Folkman J. Patterns and emerging mechanisms of the angiogenic switch during tumorigenesis. Cell. 1996;86:353-364.

40. Bouck N, Stellmach V, Hsu SC. How tumors become angiogenic. Adv Cancer Res. 1996;69:135-174.

41. Ribatti D, Nico B, Crivellato E, et al. The history of the angiogenic switch concept. Leukemia. 2007;21:44-52.

42. Moehler TM, Ho AD, Goldschmidt H, Barlogie B. Angiogenesis in hematologic malignancies. Crit Rev Oncol Hematol. 2003;45:227-244.

43. Nguyen M, Watanabe H, Budson AE, et al. Elevated levels of an angiogenic peptide, basic fibroblast growth factor, in the urine of patients with a wide spectrum of cancers. J Natl Cancer Inst. 1994;86:356-361.

44. Brunner G, Nguyen H, Gabrilove J, et al. Basic fibroblast growth factor expression in human bone marrow and peripheral blood cells. Blood. 1993;81:631-638.

45. Vacca A, Ribatti D, Roncali L, et al. Bone marrow angiogenesis and progression in multiple myeloma. Br J Haematol. 1994;87:503-508.

46. Vacca A, Ribatti D, Roncali L, Dammacco F. Angiogenesis in B cell lymphoproliferative diseases. Biologic and clinical studies. Leuk Lymphoma. 1995;20:27-38.

47. Perez-Atayde AR, Sallan SE, Tedrow U, et al. Spectrum of tumor angiogenesis in the bone marrow of children with acute lymphoblastic leukemia. Am J Pathol. 1997;150:815-821.

48. Dickson DJ, Shami PJ. Angiogenesis in acute and chronic leukemias. Leuk Lymphoma. 2001;42:847-853.

49. Kuzu I, Beksac M, Arat M, et al. Bone marrow microvessel density (MVD) in adult acute myeloid leukemia (AML): therapy induced changes and effects on survival. Leuk Lymphoma. 2004;45:1185-1190.

50. Aguayo A, Kantarjian HM, Estey EH, et al. Plasma vascular endothelial growth factor levels have prognostic significance in patients with acute myeloid leukemia but not in patients with myelodysplastic syndromes. Cancer. 2002;95:1923-1930.

51. Bieker R, Padro T, Kramer J, et al. Overexpression of basic fibroblast growth factor and autocrine stimulation in acute myeloid leukemia. Cancer Res. 2003;63:7241-7246.

52. Kim DH, Lee NY, Lee MH, et al. Vascular endothelial growth factor (VEGF) gene (VEGFA) polymorphism can predict the prognosis in acute myeloid leukaemia patients. Br J Haematol. 2008;140:71-79.

53. Zhang H, Li Y, Li H, et al. Inhibition of both the autocrine and the paracrine growth of human leukemia with a fully human antibody directed against vascular endothelial growth factor receptor 2. Leuk Lymphoma. 2004;45:1887-1897.

54. Schliemann C, Bieker R, Padro T, et al. Expression of angiopoietins and their receptor Tie2 in the bone marrow of patients with acute myeloid leukemia. Haematologica. 2006;91:1203-1211.

55. Loges S, Heil G, Bruweleit M, et al. Analysis of concerted expression of angiogenic growth factors in acute myeloid leukemia: expression of angiopoietin-2 represents an independent prognostic factor for overall survival. J Clin Oncol. 2005;23:1109-1117.

56. Faderl S, Do KA, Johnson MM, et al. Angiogenic factors may have a different prognostic role in adult acute lymphoblastic leukemia. Blood. 2005;106:4303-4307.

57. Letilovic T, Vrhovac R, Verstovsek S, et al. Role of angiogenesis in chronic lymphocytic leukemia. Cancer. 2006;107:925-934.

58. Molica S, Vitelli G, Levato D, et al. Increased serum levels of vascular endothelial growth factor predict risk of progression in early B-cell chronic lymphocytic leukaemia. Br J Haematol. 1999;107:605-610.

59. Bairey O, Boycov O, Kaganovsky E, et al. All three receptors for vascular endothelial growth factor (VEGF) are expressed on B-chronic lymphocytic leukemia (CLL) cells. Leuk Res. 2004;28:243-248.

60. Verstovsek S, Kantarjian H, Manshouri T, et al. Prognostic significance of cellular vascular endothelial growth factor expression in chronic phase chronic myeloid leukemia. Blood. 2002;99: 2265-2267.

61. Vacca A, Ribatti D, Ruco L, et al. Angiogenesis extent and macrophage density increase simultaneously with pathologic progression in B-cell non-Hodgkin's lymphomas. Br J Cancer. 1999;79:965-970.

62. Bardelli M, Leucci E, Schurfeld K, et al. VEGF-D is expressed in activated lymphoid cells and in tumors of hematopoietic and lymphoid tissues. Leuk Lymphoma. 2007;48:2014-2021.

63. Salven P, Orpana A, Teerenhovi L, Joensuu H. Simultaneous elevation in the serum concentrations of the angiogenic growth factors VEGF and bFGF is an independent predictor of poor prognosis in non-Hodgkin lymphoma: a single-institution study of 200 patients. Blood. 2000;96:3712-3718.

64. Salven P, Teerenhovi L, Joensuu H. A high pretreatment serum vascular endothelial growth factor concentration is associated with poor outcome in non-Hodgkin's lymphoma. Blood. 1997;90:3167-3172.

65. Aguayo A, Kantarjian H, Manshouri T, et al. Angiogenesis in acute and chronic leukemias and myelodysplastic syndromes. Blood. 2000;96:2240-2245.

66. Scherer A. Dynamic magnetic resonance imaging of the lumbar spine for the evaluation of microcirculation during antiangiogenic therapy in patients with myelodysplastic syndrome. Fortschr Roentgenstr. 2002;174:164-169.

67. Bellamy WT, Richter L, Sirjani D, et al. Vascular endothelial cell growth factor (VEGF) is an autocrine promoter of abnormal localized immature myeloid precursors (ALIP) and leukemia progenitor formation in myelodysplastic syndromes. Blood. 2001;98:1272-1273.

68. Rajkumar SV, Leong T, Roche PC, et al. Prognostic value of bone marrow angiogenesis in multiple myeloma. Clin Cancer Res. 2000;6:3111-3116.

69. Munshi NC, Wilson C. Increased bone marrow microvessel density in newly diagnosed multiple myeloma carries a poor prognosis. Semin Oncol. 2001;28:565-569.

70. Vacca A, Ribatti D, Presta M, et al. Bone marrow neovascularization, plasma cell angiogenic potential, and matrix metalloproteinase-2 secretion parallel progression of human multiple myeloma. Blood. 1999;93:3064-3073.

71. Asosingh K, De Raeve H, Menu E, et al. Angiogenic switch during 5T2MM murine myeloma tumorigenesis: role of CD45 heterogeneity. Blood. 2004;103:3131-3137.

72. Ria R, Vacca A, Russo F, et al. A VEGF-dependent autocrine loop mediates proliferation and capillarogenesis in bone marrow endothelial cells of patients with multiple myeloma. Thromb Haemost. 2004;92:1438-1445.

73. Folkman J. Angiogenesis: an organizing principle for drug discovery? Nat Rev Drug Discov. 2007;6:273-286.

74. Yee KWL, Giles FJ. Antiangiogenic therapy for hematologic malignancies. In Davis DW, Herbst RS, Abbruzzese JL (eds). Antiangiogenic Cancer Therapy. Boca Raton, Fla, CRC Press, 2008, pp 655-732.

75. Ferrara N, Kerbel RS. Angiogenesis as a therapeutic target. Nature. 2005;438:967-974.

76. Hurwitz H, Fehrenbacher L, Novotny W, et al. Bevacizumab plus irinotecan, fluorouracil, and leucovorin for metastatic colorectal cancer. N Engl J Med. 2004;350:2335.

77. Mesters RM, Padro T, Bieker R, et al. Stable remission after administration of the receptor tyrosine kinase inhibitor SU5416 in a patient with refractory acute myeloid leukemia. Blood. 2001;98:241-243.

77a. Karp JE, Gojo I, Pili R, et al. Targeting vascular endothelial growth factor for relapsed and refractory adult acute myelogenous leukemias: Therapy with sequential 1-beta-D-arabinofuranosyl-cytosine, mitoxantrone, and bevacizumab. Clin Cancer Res. 2004;10:3577-3585

78. Dias S, Hattori K, Zhu Z, et al. Autocrine stimulation of VEGFR-2 activates human leukemic cell growth and migration. J Clin Invest. 2000;106:511-521.

79. Levine MN, Gent M, Hirsh J, et al. The thrombogenic effect of anticancer drug therapy in women with stage II breast cancer. N Engl J Med. 1988;318:404-407.

80. Lorenzo E, Ruiz-Ruiz C, Quesada AJ, et al. Doxorubicin induces apoptosis and CD95 gene expression in human primary endothelial cells through a p53-dependent mechanism. J Biol Chem. 2002;277:10883-10892.

81. Browder T, Butterfield CE, Kraling BM, et al. Antiangiogenic scheduling of chemotherapy improves efficacy against experimental drug-resistant cancer. Cancer Res. 2000;60:1878-1886.

82. Klement G, Kikuchi L, Kieran M, et al. Early tumor detection using platelet uptake of angiogenesis regulators. Blood (ASH Annual Meeting Abstracts). 2004;104:839a.

83. Bocci G, Francia G, Man S, et al. Thrombospondin 1, a mediator of the antiangiogenic effects of low-dose metronomic chemotherapy. Proc Natl Acad Sci U S A. 2003;100:12917-12922.

84. Hanahan D, Bergers G, Bergsland E. Less is more, regularly: metronomic dosing of cytotoxic drugs can target tumor angiogenesis in mice. J Clin Invest. 2000;105:1045-1047.

85. Kieran MW, Turner CD, Rubin JB, et al. A feasibility trial of antiangiogenic (metronomic) chemotherapy in pediatric patients with recurrent or progressive cancer. J Pediatr Hematol Oncol. 2005; 27:573-581.

86. Barlogie B, Desikan R, Eddlemon P, et al. Extended survival in advanced and refractory multiple myeloma after single-agent thalidomide: identification of prognostic factors in a phase 2 study of 169 patients. Blood. 2001;98:492-494.

87. D'Amato RJ, Loughnan MS, Flynn E, Folkman J. Thalidomide is an inhibitor of angiogenesis. Proc Natl Acad Sci U S A. 1994;91:4082-4085.

88. Neben K, Moehler T, Kraemer A, et al. Response to thalidomide in progressive multiple myeloma is not mediated by inhibition of angiogenic cytokine secretion. Br J Haematol. 2001;115:605-608.

89. Singhal S, Mehta J, Desikan R, et al. Antitumor activity of thalidomide in refractory multiple myeloma. N Engl J Med. 1999;341:1565-1571.

90. Juliusson G, Celsing F, Turesson I, et al. Frequent good partial remissions from thalidomide including best response ever in patients with advanced refractory and relapsed myeloma. Br J Haematol. 2000;109:89-96.

91. Rajkumar SV, Witzig TE. A review of angiogenesis and antiangiogenic therapy with thalidomide in multiple myeloma. Cancer Treat Rev. 2000;26:351-362.

92. Hideshima T, Chauhan D, Shima Y, et al. Thalidomide and its analogs overcome drug resistance of human multiple myeloma cells to conventional therapy. Blood. 2000;96:2943-2950.

93. Rajkumar SV, Fonseca R, Dispenzieri A, et al. Thalidomide in the treatment of relapsed multiple myeloma. Mayo Clin Proc. 2000;75:897-901.

94. Zomas A, Anagnostopoulos N, Dimopoulos MA. Successful treatment of multiple myeloma relapsing after high-dose therapy

and autologous transplantation with thalidomide as a single agent. Bone Marrow Transplant. 2000;25:1319-1320.

95. Harousseau JL. Thalidomide in multiple myeloma: past, present and future. Future Oncol. 2006;2:577-589.

96. Cibeira MT, Rosinol L, Ramiro L, et al. Long-term results of thalidomide in refractory and relapsed multiple myeloma with emphasis on response duration. Eur J Haematol. 2006;77:486-492.

97. Maier SK, Hammond JM. Role of lenalidomide in the treatment of multiple myeloma and myelodysplastic syndrome. Ann Pharmacother. 2006;40:286-289.

98. Chanan-Khan A, Miller KC, Takeshita K, et al. Results of a phase 1 clinical trial of thalidomide in combination with fludarabine as initial therapy for patients with treatment-requiring chronic lymphocytic leukemia (CLL). Blood. 2005;106:3348-3352.

99. Nierodzik ML, Karpatkin S. Tumor growth and metastasis. In Michelson AD (ed). Platelets. Oxford, England, Elsevier, 2007, pp 769-778.

100. Trousseau A. Phlegmasia alba dolens. Clinique medicale de l'Hotel-Dieu Paris. Paris, Baillière, 1865, pp 94-96.

101. Gasic GJ, Gasic TB, Stewart CC. Antimetastatic effects associated with platelet reduction. Proc Natl Acad Sci U S A. 1968;61:46-52.

102. Gasic GJ. Role of plasma, platelets, and endothelial cells in tumor metastasis. Cancer Metastasis Rev. 1984;3:99-114.

103. Greenberg J, Packham MA, Cazenave JP, et al. Effects on platelet function of removal of platelet sialic acid by neuraminidase. Lab Invest. 1975;32:476-484.

104. Pederson LM, Milman N. Prognostic significance of thrombocytosis in patients with primary lung cancer. Eur Respir J. 1996;9:1826-1830.

105. Ikeda M, Furukawa H, Imamura H, et al. Poor prognosis associated with thrombocytosis in patients with gastric cancer. Ann Surg Oncol. 2002;9:287-291.

106. Lip GY, Chin BS, Blann AD. Cancer and the prothrombotic state. Lancet Oncol. 2002;3:27-34.

107. Sierko E, Wojtukiewicz MZ. Platelets and angiogenesis in malignancy. Semin Thromb Hemost. 2004;30:95-108.

108. Camerer E, Qazi AA, Duong DN, et al. Platelets, protease-activated receptors, and fibrinogen in hematogenous metastasis. Blood. 2004;104:397-401.

109. Pinedo HM, Verheul HM, D'Amato RJ, Folkman J. Involvement of platelets in tumour angiogenesis? Lancet. 1998; 352:1775-1777.

110. Nierodzik ML, Klepfish A, Karpatkin S. Role of platelets, thrombin, integrin IIb-IIIa, fibronectin and von Willebrand factor on tumor adhesion in vitro and metastasis in vivo. Thromb Haemost. 1995;74:282-290.

111. Zacharski LR, Rickles FR, Henderson WG, et al. Platelets and malignancy. Rationale and experimental design for the VA Cooperative Study of RA-233 in the treatment of cancer. Am J Clin Oncol. 1982;5:593-609.

112. Mehta P. Potential role of platelets in the pathogenesis of tumor metastasis. Blood. 1984;63:55-63.

113. Karpatkin S, Pearlstein E, Ambrogio C, Coller BS. Role of adhesive proteins in platelet tumor interaction in vitro and metastasis formation in vivo. J Clin Invest. 1988;81:1012-1019.

114. Verheul HM, Hoekman K, Luykx-de Bakker S, et al. Platelet: transporter of vascular endothelial growth factor. Clin Cancer Res. 1997;3:2187-2190.

115. Brill A, Varon D. Angiogenesis. In Michelson AD (ed). Platelets. Oxford, England, Elsevier; 2007, pp 757-768.

116. Gimbrone MA Jr, Aster RH, Cotran RS, et al. Preservation of vascular integrity in organs perfused in vitro with a platelet-rich medium. Nature. 1969;221:33-36.

117. Gore I, Takada M, Austin J. Ultrastructural basis of experimental thrombocytopenic purpura. Arch Pathol. 1970;90:197-205.

118. Kitchens CS, Weiss L. Ultrastructural changes of endothelium associated with thrombocytopenia. Blood. 1975;46:567-578.

119. Pipili-Synetos E, Papadimitriou E, Maragoudakis ME. Evidence that platelets promote tube formation by endothelial cells on matrigel. Br J Pharmacol. 1998;125:1252-1257.

120. Kisucka J, Butterfield CE, Duda DG, et al. Platelets and platelet adhesion support angiogenesis while preventing excessive hemorrhage. Proc Natl Acad Sci U S A. 2006;103:855-860.

121. Browder T, Folkman J, Pirie-Shepherd S. The hemostatic system as a regulator of angiogenesis. J Biol Chem. 2000; 275:1521-1524.

122. Mohle R, Green D, Moore MA, et al. Constitutive production and thrombin-induced release of vascular endothelial growth factor by human megakaryocytes and platelets. Proc Natl Acad Sci U S A. 1997;94:663-668.

123. Wartiovaara U, Salven P, Mikkola H, et al. Peripheral blood platelets express VEGF-C and VEGF which are released during platelet activation. Thromb Haemost. 1998;80:171-175.

124. Heldin CH, Westermark B, Wasteson A. Platelet-derived growth factor. Isolation by a large-scale procedure and analysis of subunit composition. Biochem J. 1981;193:907-913.

125. Bar RS, Boes M, Booth BA, et al. The effects of platelet-derived growth factor in cultured microvessel endothelial cells. Endocrinology. 1989;124:1841-1848.

126. Kaplan DR, Chao FC, Stiles CD, et al. Platelet alpha granules contain a growth factor for fibroblasts. Blood. 1979;53:1043-1052.

127. Nakamura T, Tomita Y, Hirai R, et al. Inhibitory effect of transforming growth factor-beta on DNA synthesis of adult rat hepatocytes in primary culture. Biochem Biophys Res Commun. 1985;133:1042-1050.

128. Karey KP, Sirbasku DA. Human platelet-derived mitogens. II. Subcellular localization of insulinlike growth factor I to the alpha-granule and release in response to thrombin. Blood. 1989;74:1093-1100.

129. White RR, Shan S, Rusconi CP, et al. Inhibition of rat corneal angiogenesis by a nuclease-resistant RNA aptamer specific for angiopoietin-2. Proc Natl Acad Sci U S A. 2003;100:5028-5033.

130. English D, Welch Z, Kovala AT, et al. Sphingosine 1-phosphate released from platelets during clotting accounts for the potent endothelial cell chemotactic activity of blood serum and provides a novel link between hemostasis and angiogenesis. FASEB J. 2000;14:2255-2265.

131. Hla T. Physiologic and pathologic actions of sphingosine 1-phosphate. Semin Cell Dev Biol. 2004;15:513-520.

132. Galt SW, Lindemann S, Allen L, et al. Outside-in signals delivered by matrix metalloproteinase-1 regulate platelet function. Circ Res. 2002;90:1093-1099.

133. Fernandez-Patron C, Martinez-Cuesta MA, Salas E, et al. Differential regulation of platelet aggregation by matrix metalloproteinases-9 and -2. Thromb Haemost. 1999;82:1730-1735.

134. Jurasz P, Chung AW, Radomski A, Radomski MW. Nonremodeling properties of matrix metalloproteinases: the platelet connection. Circ Res. 2002;90:1041-1043.

135. Iruela-Arispe ML, Bornstein P, Sage H. Thrombospondin exerts an antiangiogenic effect on cord formation by endothelial cells in vitro. Proc Natl Acad Sci U S A. 1991;88:5026-5030.

136. Streit M, Velasco P, Riccardi L, et al. Thrombospondin-1 suppresses wound healing and granulation tissue formation in the skin of transgenic mice. EMBO J. 2000;19:3272-3282.

137. Maione TE, Gray GS, Petro J, et al. Inhibition of angiogenesis by recombinant human platelet factor-4 and related peptides. Science. 1990;247:77-79.

138. Sharpe RJ, Byers HR, Scott CF, et al. Growth inhibition of murine melanoma and human colon carcinoma by recombinant human platelet factor 4. J Natl Cancer Inst. 1990;82:848-853.

139. Kolber DL, Knisely TL, Maione TE. Inhibition of development of murine melanoma lung metastases by systemic administration of recombinant platelet factor 4. J Natl Cancer Inst. 1995; 87:304-309.

140. Tanaka T, Manome Y, Wen P, et al. Viral vector-mediated transduction of a modified platelet factor 4 cDNA inhibits angiogenesis and tumor growth. Nat Med. 1997;3:437-442.

141. Jurasz P, Santos-Martinez MJ, Radomska A, Radomski MW. Generation of platelet angiostatin mediated by urokinase plasminogen activator: effects on angiogenesis. J Thromb Haemost. 2006;4:1095-1106.

142. Radomski A, Jurasz P, Sanders EJ, et al. Identification, regulation and role of tissue inhibitor of metalloproteinases-4 (TIMP-4) in human platelets. Br J Pharmacol. 2002;137:1330-1338.

143. Cervi D, Yip TT, Bhattacharya N, et al. Platelet-associated PF-4 as a biomarker of early tumor growth. Blood. 2008;111:1201-1207.

144. Italiano JE Jr, Richardson JL, Patel-Hett S, et al. Angiogenesis is regulated by a novel mechanism: pro- and antiangiogenic proteins are organized into separate platelet alpha granules and differentially released. Blood. 2008;111:1227-1233.

145. Verheul HM, Lolkema MP, Qian DZ, et al. Platelets take up the monoclonal antibody bevacizumab. Clin Cancer Res. 2007;13:5341-5347.

3 Molecular Basis of Human Malignancy

Ian F. Dunn and William C. Hahn

Cancer arises from the accumulation of mutations in genes that program the malignant phenotype. Work from many laboratories has now defined the key classes of genes that normally regulate physiologic processes but when mutated or dysregulated contribute to the development of cancer. Indeed, almost all cancers show evidence of activation of mutant versions of proto-oncogenes and the inactivation of tumor suppressor genes. With the advent of technologies that now enable whole-genome interrogation of genes altered in cancer, enumeration of all the mutations in specific tumors may soon be possible.

At the same time, it is apparent that most, if not all, human cancers share core biologic phenotypes.[1-3] Some of these characteristics occur primarily within the developing tumor cell and can thus be considered as cell-intrinsic. These traits include infinite proliferative capacity, autonomous proliferative potential, insensitivity to antigrowth and apoptotic signals, and inherent genetic instability. Beyond these cell intrinsic properties, other hallmarks of the malignant state involve interactions with the tumor cell microenvironment. These cell-extrinsic properties include angiogenic potential, the capacity to invade surrounding tissue and metastasize,[3] and the ability to evade the immune system. In this chapter, we will review our current understanding of the molecular basis of cancer, with an emphasis on the salient cell-intrinsic principles that govern the development of human cancers.

CELL OF ORIGIN

Although an increasing number of the mutated genes that are being identified initiate tumor formation and drive cancer progression, the identity of the cell population(s) susceptible to such transforming events remains undefined for most human cancers. Recent work has indicated that a small population of cells endowed with unique self-renewal properties and tumorigenic potential is present in some and perhaps all tumors.[4] These self-renewing cell populations, called tumor-initiating cells or cancer stem cells, have been described in acute myelogenous leukemia (AML),[5] glioblastoma,[6] and breast and colon cancers.[7-9] Tumor-initiating cells exhibit several defining characteristics, including the capacity for self-renewal, the ability to differentiate, easily detectable telomerase activity, activation of antiapoptotic pathways and, in some cases, the ability to migrate and metastasize.[10-12]

Although our understanding of the biology of these putative cancer stem cells remains rudimentary, the existence of such cells has implications for current conceptualizations of malignant transformation and therapeutic approaches to cancer. Indeed, the notion that a small population of cancer-initiating cells is responsible for both cancer initiation and progression challenges prior models, which suggested that cancers are derived from the accumulation of mutations in fully differentiated cells. The idea that cancers are formed from a stem cell population would explain some observations in human cancer specimens and cell lines that are difficult to reconcile with a model in which mutations occur only in differentiated cells. For example, the terminally differentiated cells rarely proliferate, making it unlikely that any single mature cell could accumulate the necessary set of mutations for tumor initiation. In addition, most human tumors exhibit considerable cellular heterogeneity and are composed of cells at various stages of differentiation and transformation. Although cancer-associated mutations may induce an epithelial to mesenchymal transition (EMT) in more differentiated cells, work in hematopoietic cancers has indicated that an undifferentiated stem cell population can give rise to tumor cell types in varying stages of maturity.[4] In addition, recent work has indicated that many signaling pathways thought to be involved in the maintenance of normal stem cells are found to be mutated in human cancers,[4] including those regulated by Wnt, β-catenin, phosphatase and tensin homologue (PTEN), transforming growth factor β (TGF-β), Hedgehog, Notch, and Bmi-1.[13-19]

Furthermore, cancer stem cells exhibit a more tumorigenic phenotype in experimental models of tumor formation than established cancer cell lines. Although the injection of a few hundred cancer stem cells suffices to induce tumors in animal models,[7] a substantially greater number of cells from established cell lines are needed to form tumors in similar experiments.[20,21] Moreover, the tumors in these models derived from transplanted stem cells appear to replicate the heterogeneity observed in human cancer specimens with greater fidelity than those formed by tumor-derived cell lines.

These experimental approaches implicate cancer stem cells in tumor initiation, but putative tumor-initiating cells comprise only a small fraction of human tumors. Further isolation and molecular characterization of cancer stem cells should clarify their roles in tumor initiation, maintenance, and progression. The refinement of the stem cell hypothesis will likely complement rather than replace existing hypotheses that cancer originates from more differentiated cells, because it remains likely that aberrant genetic events in stem cells or differentiated cells may also initiate or contribute to tumor progression. Particular types of cancers may arise from tumor-initiating cells, whereas others may begin in more differentiated cells. Importantly, the molecular events that initiate and drive cancer progression will likely be relevant in either model.

Cell-Intrinsic Events

Two complementary experimental approaches have provided insights into the molecular basis of cancer—the detailed study of tumors derived from patients and the manipulation of experimental models of cancer. These approaches have established the genetic nature of cancer, identified some mutations present in cancer genomes and, in a few cases, led to a molecular understanding of how specific mutations initiate cancer development. In particular, the investigation of specific mutations in manipulated cells and animal models now provides an outline of the complex process whereby a normal cell is converted into a cancer cell.

Clinically, with a few notable exceptions, pediatric and adult malignancies exhibit clear differences, including clinical presentation, prevalence and types of common cancers, and overall efficacy of treatment regimens. These disparities in clinical parameters are likely the consequence of fundamental differences in the molecular events that drive pediatric and adult cancers. Most childhood solid and hematologic cancers are characterized by signature karyotypic abnormalities, such as balanced translocations, as compared with the karyotypic chaos observed in most adult epithelial cancers. This dichotomy in chromosomal alterations implies that a smaller number of mutations may be required to drive most pediatric malignancies. Although the reasons behind this difference remain unclear, it is possible that pediatric cancers are more closely linked to the dysregulation of developmental pathways in susceptible tissues. Despite these apparent differences in childhood and adult cancers, the core principles of tumorigenesis and many of the genetic participants are shared. In this section, we will review the cell-intrinsic processes that drive uncontrolled cell proliferation and tumor growth.

Immortalization

Early evidence that transformation is driven by a defined number of altered genes came from the discovery that avian and murine retroviruses contain proto-oncogenes related to normal cellular genes.[22,23] Following this finding, many oncogenes were discovered within the genomes of transforming viruses. These sequences were derived from sequences found in host cells, including a wide range of genes whose protein products are involved in proliferation and differentiation.[23] Similarly, transfection of genomic DNA derived from human tumors[24] or from chemically transformed rodent cells[25] led to the identification of single oncogenes that were able to transform National Institutes of Health (NIH) 3T3 cells, an immortal established murine fibroblast line. Subsequent studies have identified many classes of oncogenes, including growth factors, growth factor receptors, components of signal transduction pathways, and transcription factors. Subsequently, alterations in these genes were detected in spontaneously arising tumors where they are activated by mechanisms such as promoter hypomethylation, mutation, gene amplification, and chromosomal translocation.

Although these oncogenes were identified by their ability to transform immortal rodent cells, further studies have shown that the introduction of single oncogenes alone rarely induced the transformed phenotype in primary cells. Instead, a combination of two oncogenes, such as *myc* and H-*ras* or E1A and H-*ras*, led to morphologic and functional transformation.[26,27] Eventually, several combinations of cooperating oncogenes were found that led to rodent cell transformation.[28] However, unlike rodent cells, the introduction of these same combinations of oncogenes into human cells led to cells with a limited cell life span that were not tumorigenic, suggesting that additional steps beyond those required to transform rodent cells are necessary to convert human cells to tumorigenesis.[29] These studies have suggested that immortalization is an essential aspect of cell transformation.

Limitless Replicative Potential: Telomerase, p53, and Rb

More than 40 years ago, Hayflick and Moorhead determined that normal human cells have a limited proliferative capacity in culture in comparison with cancer cell lines, which generally exhibited an immortal phenotype.[30] This seminal observation suggested that alterations in the mechanisms that regulate cell life span are altered in human cancer cells. Following a defined number of population doublings, normal cells undergo a process known as senescence.[31] Senescence is an irreversible state of cell cycle arrest accompanied by overt changes in cell morphology and metabolism. More recently, senescence has been attributed to cell physiologic insults, such as oxidative stress and DNA damage, which may be induced by oncogenes or chemical or physical agents,[32-34] suggesting that senescence serves as a general mechanism to suppress malignant transformation. If cells sustain mutations that permit them to bypass senescence, they hit a second regulatory barrier termed *crisis*, which results in widespread cell death of most of the culture (Fig. 3-1). Although rodent cells readily bypass both of these barriers to become immortalized, human cells rarely undergo spontaneous immortalization. One report has defined the molecular events that allow human cells to bypass senescence and crisis to become immortalized.[35] In particular, these studies highlight the importance of telomere maintenance and the p53 and retinoblastoma (Rb) tumor suppressor pathways in regulating cell life span.

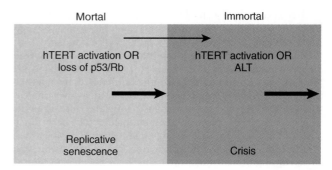

FIGURE 3-1. Barriers to immortalization. Human cells must overcome both replicative senescence and crisis to become immortal. Replicative senescence may be overcome by the inactivation of Rb and p53 pathways or by telomerase activation in some cell types. Telomere maintenance—by telomerase or alternative lengthening of telomeres—allows cells to avoid crisis.

Telomeres and Telomerase in Human Cancer

Telomeres are composed of repeated DNA elements and DNA-binding proteins at the ends of eukaryotic chromosomes. In mammals, the telomeric complex consists of 4 to 10 kb of TTAGGG repeats bound to a number of telomere-binding proteins, including telomeric repeat binding factor 1 (TRF1), TRF2, and protection of telomeres 1 (POT1).[36-38] Additional proteins bind these telomere-binding proteins to form a complex termed *shelterin*.[39] Disruption of the telomeric complex leading to an inability to maintain telomere structure leads to the formation of end-to-end chromosomal fusions.[40-43] These illegitimate chromosomal arrangements activate a DNA damage response that leads to cell cycle arrest or apoptosis.[44-47] Proteins known to participate in the cell's response to DNA damage, including the Mre11 and Ku complex, also congregate at the telomere, particularly under conditions during which telomere maintenance is compromised.[48-50]

In almost all human cancer cells, the maintenance of telomeres is accomplished by the reverse transcriptase telomerase or by an alternative mechanism, termed alternative *lengthening of telomeres* (ALT). Telomerase is a specialized RNA-dependent DNA polymerase composed of two essential subunits, a telomerase RNA component (hTERC) and telomerase catalytic component (hTERT).[51,52] In human cells, hTERC is expressed ubiquitously, whereas hTERT is only expressed in cells that exhibit telomerase activity, suggesting that hTERT is the rate-limiting component of telomerase.[53-55] A significant minority of cancers maintain telomeres through a second pathway that operates independently of telomerase, ALT.[56] ALT appears to be more commonly activated in subsets of neuroepithelial or mesenchymal tumors, including astrocytomas, soft tissue sarcomas, and osteosarcomas.[56,57] Several lines of evidence have indicated that telomere maintenance by ALT likely involves recombination between telomeres. In *Saccharomyces cerevisiae*, the ALT phenotype is dependent on Rad52, which participates in DNA recombination,[58] and in an immortalized human fibroblast line that lacks telomerase, marker DNA sequences were shown to be copied from telomere to telomere.[59] These observations have implicated telomere maintenance as an important mechanism to regulate genomic stability. Supporting this view, cells at crisis harbor extremely short telomeres and evidence of increased genomic instability.[60] The loss of telomere end protection is likely to play an important role in destabilizing cancer genomes, thus promoting the acquisition of mutations that drive cancer progression.

However, studies have indicated that telomere maintenance plays an equally important role in human cancer by regulating replicative life span. Although most human cancer cells exhibit stable telomere lengths with passage in culture, telomeres in normal human cells shorten with accumulated cell division.[61] Corresponding with this difference in telomere length maintenance, telomerase is expressed at low or undetectable levels in normal cells, whereas telomerase activity or the ALT phenotype is found in most human cancer cells. These observations suggest that the telomere attrition observed in normal human cells is a molecular clock that limits the life span of primary somatic human cells to 50 to 80 cell divisions.[62] Indeed, overexpression of hTERT in some normal human cells such as fibroblasts, endothelial cells, and mesothelial cells[63-66] not only induces high constitutive levels of telomerase activity, which stabilizes telomere lengths, but also suffices to immortalize these cells. Together, these observations suggest that the stable telomere lengths observed in most cancer cell lines contribute directly to their immortal phenotype in culture. Consistent with this view, inhibition of telomerase activity in telomerase-expressing cancer cell lines leads to telomere shortening and cell death,[41,67] whereas constitutive expression of telomerase, together with oncogenes, induces cell transformation and tumorigenicity.[68]

Roles of p53 and Rb Tumor Suppressor Pathways in Senescence and Immortalization

Although telomere maintenance plays a central role in regulating cell life span and replicative senescence, the p53 and Rb tumor suppressor pathways are also critical regulators of these processes. Thus, these three molecular pathways work in concert to regulate entry into senescence. The functions of p53 and Rb may be perturbed at several points (see later); two ways to inactivate both pathways experimentally are through the expression of the simian virus 40 (SV40) large T antigen (LT) or human papillomavirus E6 and E7 oncoproteins.[69,70] These viral oncoproteins bind to and inactivate the p53 and Rb tumor suppressor proteins, albeit by different mechanisms.

As noted, constitutive expression of telomerase leading to telomere maintenance suffices to confer unlimited replicative potential in some cell types, allowing such telomerase-expressing cells to bypass replicative senescence. However, in many types of epithelial cells, expression of telomerase alone fails to induce immortalization, but instead facilitates immortalization if the Rb and p53 tumor suppressor pathways are also inactivated.[64,71] In addition, even in the absence of constitutive telomerase expression, inactivation of the p53 and Rb tumor suppressor pathways also permits cells to bypass replicative senescence.[64,71-73] However, these postsenescent cells experience progressive telomere shortening with continued cell division and, in contrast to cells that exhibit stable telomere lengths, reach a second barrier to continued cell proliferation termed *M2* or *crisis*, a period of widespread chromosomal instability and cell death (see Fig. 3-1). The genetic catastrophe associated with crisis triggers apoptosis in most cells; the rare cells that survive exhibit aneuploidy and nonreciprocal translocations,[74] supporting the concept that telomeres play an essential role in protecting chromosomes from degradation and recombination.

Thus, the p53, Rb, and telomere maintenance pathways are pivotal players in regulating entry into replicative senescence. Because the Rb, p53, and telomere maintenance pathways are disrupted in most cancers, these findings suggest that immortalization contributes directly to the transformed state. Consistent with this view, the experimental transformation of a wide range of human cells requires disruption of each of these pathways.[75,76]

Roles of p53 and Rb in Tumor Suppression. Although it is clear that Rb and p53 play an essential role in regulating cell life span, these two tumor suppressor genes control several key homeostatic mechanisms that regulate cell proliferation and survival. These two genes were among the first tumor suppressor genes identified, based in part on the finding that kindreds that harbor a single mutated allele exhibit highly penetrant, increased susceptibility to early cancer development. Because cancers derived from such patients show inactivation of the remaining wild-type allele, the concept that emerged from the study of these two genes is that biallelic inactivation is necessary to bypass the homeostatic function of tumor suppressor genes. Although discovered in rare cancer–susceptible populations, biallelic mutations or loss of heterozygosity of these two genes or genes in the pathways that they control have been found in most, if not all, human cancers.[77-79] Based on a large body of work, it is now clear that the pathways regulated by Rb and p53 play critical roles in suppressing cancer development by integrating the signals from intrinsic and extrinsic sources and regulating key steps in cell proliferation and survival. Here we review the current understanding of these pathways (Fig. 3-2).

p53. The p53 protein was first discovered in complexes with the SV40 large T antigen.[80,81] *TP53* mutations were first reported in osteogenic sarcomas,[82] and over 15,000 mutant *TP53* alleles have now been identified.[83] A significant percentage of families that show a syndrome of early-onset cancers, the Li-Fraumeni familial cancer syndrome,[84] harbor inactivating mutations of *TP53*, and tumors from such patients show loss of the remaining allele. Consistent with these findings in cancer-susceptible populations, p53 was subsequently shown to be lost in many human colorectal carcinomas.[85]

p53 is a transcription factor and functions in a protective role, inducing a G_1 cell cycle arrest and/or apoptosis in response to cellular insults such as telomere shortening, nutrient deprivation, hypoxia, oncogene activation, and DNA damage.[86-88] In response, p53 may activate a spectrum of downstream pathways to trigger apoptosis cell cycle arrest, survival, DNA repair, genomic stability, and senescence.[89] One of the best studied targets of p53 is p21[CIP1], an inhibitor of the cyclin-dependent kinases necessary for progression through the cell cycle. Increased expression of p21[CIP1] induces cell cycle arrest.

p53 levels are regulated in part by MDM2 and the tumor suppressor p14[ARF]. MDM2 is a ubiquitin ligase that binds p53 and marks it for degradation through ubiquitination.[90] In turn, p14[ARF] binds and inactivates MDM2.[91] Because MDM2 is amplified in up to 7% of human cancers in the absence of p53 mutation, and deletions or mutations of *ARF* also occur in a mutually exclusive manner with p53 mutation, most, if not all, human cancers likely harbor mutations in the p53 pathway.

Although loss of p53 confers an increased susceptibility to tumor formation, recent studies have suggested that restoration of wild-type p53 function reverses this phenotype. Reactivation of wild-type p53 function in conditional murine models of p53 loss with hepatocellular cancer, as well as sarcomas and lymphomas, leads to striking degrees of tumor regression.[78,79,92] Interestingly, restoring p53 function has lineage-specific effects—p53 induces apoptosis in lymphoma, whereas reactivating p53 expression in sarcoma and hepatocellular carcinoma cells induces cellular senescence. Tumors in which p53 function is restored demonstrate increased rates of p53 mutation as well as inactivation of modulators of p53 function, such as p19[ARF].[92]

Mutations in *TP53* account for approximately 50% of cases of p53 dysfunction. Interestingly, mutations in p53 appear to behave differently than inactivating mutations in some other tumor suppressor genes. Conventionally, cancer cells select

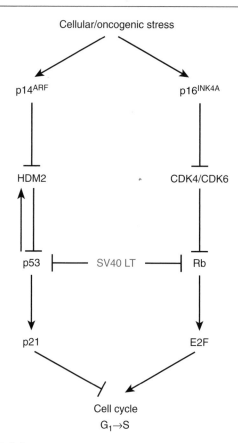

FIGURE 3-2. Rb and p53 tumor suppressor pathways. Mutations affecting the function of these pathways are found in most human cancers and affect the G₁ to S cell cycle transition. The viral oncoprotein SV40 large T antigen (LT) inactivates both the Rb and p53 pathways. The human *INK4A* and *ARF* genes encoding the tumor suppressor proteins p16 and p14, respectively, are encoded in alternative reading frames by the same locus, *CDKN2A*, and target different tumor suppressor pathways.

tumor suppressor mutations that result in a loss of the wild-type protein expression or function. However, mutant p53 protein is often retained, and cancer cells with mutant p53 accumulate high levels of the mutant protein[93]; mutant p53 may acquire novel biologic activities that may impair the function of closely related proteins p63 and p73. Such interactions may enhance malignant and metastatic tumor potential.[94-96]

Rb. Like p53, the Rb pathway plays a critical role in determining the response to oncogenic stress, and Rb loss is a frequent event in human cancers. First described based on epidemiologic studies of retinoblastoma and Wilms' tumor, the observation that sequential inactivation of one copy of the *Rb* gene in the germline and of the remaining copy in somatic tumor tissue provided the molecular basis for Knudson's two-hit hypothesis.[97] Although loss of function *Rb* mutations is the primary molecular alteration in pediatric retinoblastoma, *Rb* is also subject to somatic inactivation in several other human cancers, including a large fraction of osteosarcomas, soft tissue sarcomas, and small cell lung carcinomas.[98] When phosphorylated, several viral oncoproteins bind and inactivate Rb, including SV40 LT, adenovirus E1A, and human papillomavirus (HPV) E7.[99-101] The binding of these viral oncoproteins to Rb is essential for the transforming activity of these viruses, and

mechanistic studies have led to key insights into the function and regulation of the Rb pathway.

Rb regulates the G₁-S cell cycle transition, a critical restriction point that governs the initiation of cell proliferation.[102] Rb controls S-phase entry by altering the function of the E2F transcription factors. Moreover, dephosphorylated Rb recruits histone deacetylases (HDACs) and other chromatin remodeling factors to repress the expression of genes required for cell cycle progression.[103,104] In response to appropriate mitogenic stimulation, Rb is phosphorylated by the G₁ cyclin-dependent kinases complexes CDK4/CDK6-cyclin D1 and CDK2-cyclin E, rendering Rb unable to bind E2F transcription factors.[105] Thus, the phosphorylation status of Rb plays an essential role in regulating cell cycle progression.

Similar to what has been observed for p53, some cancers show evidence of Rb inactivation but a larger set of cancers exhibit mutations that affect proteins that regulate Rb. In retinoblastomas, osteosarcomas, and small cell lung carcinomas, biallelic *Rb* mutations result in loss of functional Rb.[106] In many cervical carcinomas, the Rb protein is sequestered and marked for degradation by the HPV E7 oncoprotein.[107] In breast cancer, cyclin D1 or cyclin E overexpression disrupts the regulation of phosphorylation and causes functional inactivation of Rb.[108,109] In mantle cell lymphoma, the t(11:14) translocation places the immunoglobulin heavy-chain promoter upstream of cyclin D1, leading to constitutive activation of cyclin D transcription.[110] Alternatively, genetic or epigenetic inactivation of the cyclin-dependent inhibitor p16^INK4a, described later, may indirectly lead to Rb inactivation through effects on the CDK4-cyclin D1 and CDK2-cyclin E kinases. These alterations, all of which converge on the loss of growth suppression by Rb, are therefore present in a diverse array of human cancers.[106]

INK4a/ARF. The *INK4a-ARF* locus, *CDKN2A* in humans, harbors two tumor suppressor genes that regulate Rb and p53 function. This single locus encodes two alternative transcripts initiated at different promoters and spliced to shared downstream exon sequences that are translated in alternative reading frames.[91] The protein products of these transcripts, p16^INK4A and p14^ARF in humans, are structurally unrelated and regulate the Rb and p53 pathways, respectively. p16^INK4A accumulates as cells are passaged in culture and induces a G₁ cell cycle arrest, culminating in senescence by associating with CDK4 and CDK6, thereby blocking the phosphorylation and inactivation of the Rb protein. p14^ARF is also a potent tumor suppressor that activates p53 by binding directly to and inactivating MDM2 (HDM2 in humans).[111] The relationship between p53, Rb, p14^ARF, and p16^INK4A is shown in Figure 3-2.

Most commonly, *INK4a* is inactivated by gene deletion, point mutation, or transcriptional silencing by epigenetic methylation of promoter sequences.[112] Loss of p16^INK4A through point mutation or deletion of *INK4a* is a common event in human cancer.[113,114] In children, mutations or deletions of this locus have been described in a wide spectrum of cancers, including acute lymphoblastic leukemia (ALL),[115] rhabdomyosarcoma,[116] and osteosarcoma.[117] Alternatively, amplification of *CDK4* or mutation of *CDK4* so that it can no longer be regulated by p16[118] also occurs; Rb is hyperphosphorylated in each of these contexts. Loss of Rb, inactivation of *INK4a*, and amplification or mutation of *CDK4* are usually mutually exclusive events,[119] suggesting that dysregulation of the Rb pathway is the common functional consequence of all these mutations.

Transformation

Although alterations in the p53 and Rb pathways and telomere maintenance pathways facilitate cell immortalization,

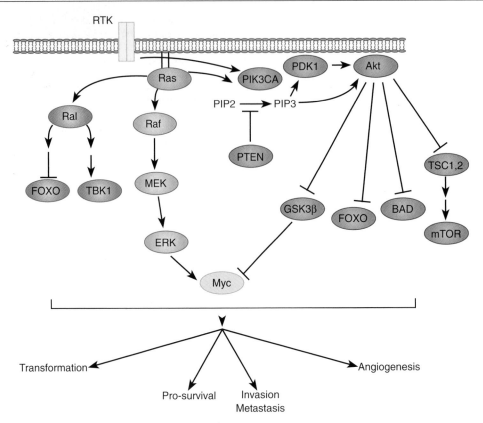

FIGURE 3-3. Ras signaling. Once activated by a receptor tyrosine kinase (RTK) mutation or otherwise, Ras signals through such downstream effectors as Ral, Raf, and phosphatidylinositol 3′-kinase (PI3K). The Raf and PI3K pathways are more clearly defined. Raf signaling is mediated by MEK, ERK, and Myc. PI3K, antagonized by PTEN, activates Akt to initiate multiple downstream signaling pathways engaging mTOR, BAD, FOXO transcription factors, and GSK3β, among others. GSK3β = glycogen synthase kinase 3β; TSC1,2 = tuberous sclerosis 1, 2.

perturbing these pathways alone fails to render cells tumorigenic. For example, immortal cells that have bypassed replicative senescence and crisis do not form tumors in animal hosts.[68] These observations suggest that additional genetic modifications are required to confer the tumorigenic phenotype. Recent work has begun to define the additional cooperating events required for a fully malignant phenotype. In human cells immortalized by the expression of telomerase, together with ablation of the p53 and Rb pathways, the additional expression of oncogenic forms of *RAS* and the SV40 small t antigen (SV40 ST) are required to convert immortalized cells to tumorigenicity.[1,2,68,75] This combination of genetic elements can convert a wide range of different types of normal human cells into cells capable of tumorigenic growth in immunodeficient hosts[120-125] without aneuploidy,[126] providing an experimental platform in which to identify the minimal requirements for cell transformation.

Although these experimental models do not fully recapitulate the process whereby spontaneous cancers occur, the genetic alterations that suffice to drive malignant transformation in such models are the same as those found in many human cancers. Thus, understanding the pathways perturbed in the process of in vitro transformation provides insight into the pathways involved in true human cancers. Here we review specific oncogene and tumor suppressor pathways involved in cell transformation in vitro and in vivo (Fig. 3-3).

Ras

The Ras proteins—N-Ras, H-Ras, and K-Ras—are small guanosine triphosphate (GTP)–binding proteins that integrate a diverse set of mitogenic stimuli.[127] In response to physiologic or aberrant upstream signaling (e.g., from receptor tyrosine kinases such as the epidermal growth factor receptor, EGFR), Ras guanine nucleotide exchange factors (GEFs) are activated and catalyze the exchange of GTP for guanosine diphosphate (GDP), thereby activating Ras. A separate class of proteins, the Ras-GTPase–activating proteins (GAPs), act in opposition to regulate Ras activity; neurofibromin 1 (NF1) is a member of this family of proteins and its loss in patients harboring biallelic mutations of *NF1* also activates the Ras signaling pathway.

Ras was one of the first oncogenes identified. The Harvey (H-*ras*) and Kirsten (K-*ras*) rat sarcoma retroviruses were shown to harbor mutant, activated versions of *Ras*, and the canvassing of human tumor genomes in search of oncogenic elements from human bladder carcinomas has identified a mutant allele of H-*Ras*.[128,129] The most common *Ras* mutation produces a glycine to valine substitution at codon 12 (*Ras^V12*),[128] but mutations in codons 13, 59, and 61 are also found in human tumors.[130] Extensive experimentation has indicated that over 25% of human cancers contain a mutant form of *Ras* itself, and a significantly greater percentage of human tumors rely on aberrant signaling driven through the Ras pathway via alterations in upstream or downstream pathway members.

Aberrant Ras activation in cancer may be derived from mutations of upstream regulatory molecules or downstream Ras effectors; common upstream proteins that signal through Ras and other downstream cascades include the receptor tyrosine kinases (RTKs). Aberrant activation of RTKs occurs in many cancers. In malignant cells, RTK signaling may be deregulated by aberrant autocrine or paracrine pathways or through genetic alteration, leading to enhanced signaling through downstream mediators and contributing to malignant transformation. Mutations and/or amplifications in RTKs, such as *HER2* in breast cancer[131] and *EGFR* in glioma[132] and non–small cell lung carcinoma,[133] lead to constitutive signaling through Ras. Targeting these RTKs by antibodies or small-molecule kinase inhibitors induces clinical responses in tumors that harbor RTK mutations, demonstrating the importance of these signaling pathways for tumor maintenance.[134]

Ras regulates several downstream effector pathways, including the Raf, RalGEF, and phosphatidylinositol 3′-kinase (PI3K) pathways. The Raf family of serine-threonine kinases consists of three members, c-RAF, BRAF, and ARAF. These kinases trigger a cascade of signaling events involving the mitogen-activated protein kinase–extracellular signal-regulated kinase (MAPK/ERK) family. Consequences of activating this signaling pathway are cell cycle progression and activation of cell-extrinsic processes, including angiogenesis and invasion. Somatic mutations of *BRAF* occur in approximately 7% of human cancers, whereas *CRAF* and *ARAF* mutations are rare.[135-137] A study has indicated that *BRAF* mutations are found in up to 70% of melanomas and 12% of colon cancers.[138] In particular, substitution of glutamic acid for valine at position 600 (V600E) accounts for over 90% of *BRAF* mutations and results in constitutive activation of the RAF-MEK-ERK pathway.

Other Ras effectors are RalGEFs, which regulate a family of GTPases, the Ras-like GTPases A and B (RalA, RalB). Although much less is known about this pathway, recent work has suggested that RalA and RalB play important roles in malignant transformation, particularly in human cells.[139] Specifically, Ral GTPase activity is essential for Ras-mediated cell transformation in a broad variety of human epithelial cells, driving tumorigenesis in concert with the SV40 small T antigen in an immortalized background.[140] RalA and RalB regulate a wide range of cell processes and signaling pathways[141] and it is not yet clear which of these pathways is important for cell transformation. Studies have indicated that RalB may activate the tank-binding kinase 1 (TBK1),[139] and Ral family members have been shown to inhibit the FOXO family of Forkhead transcription factors.[142] FOXO transcription factors themselves regulate a wide range of cell functions, including cell cycle progression through the induction of p27[KIP1] and apoptosis through the regulation of the BH3-only protein Bim.[143]

PIK3CA, a class Ia PI3K, was first discovered through its association with viral oncoproteins,[144] and the catalytic subunit p110α was later identified as an avian retrovirus–encoded oncogene capable of transforming chick embryo fibroblasts.[145] Class I PI3Ks are heterodimers composed of a p85 regulatory subunit and a p110α catalytic subunit; they are activated by Ras or by recruitment to the cell surface by activated growth factor receptors, including the platelet-derived growth factor (PDGF), Met proto-oncogene (Met), and EGFR. Once active, PI3K converts phosphatidylinositol 4,5-bisphosphate (PIP2) to phosphatidylinositol 3,4,5-triphosphate (PIP3), which leads to the recruitment of pleckstrin homology (PH)–containing proteins. Two of the best characterized pleckstrin homology proteins are Akt and phosphatidylinositol-dependent kinase 1 (PDK1).[146] Akt is activated by PDK1 at the membrane and phosphorylates and inactivates such targets as tuberin to activate the mammalian target of rapamycin (mTOR) pathway, GSK3β, p27[KIP1], and FOXO proteins to drive cell cycle progression, and BAD to resist apoptosis (see Fig. 3-3).[147,148]

The tumor suppressor phosphatase with tensin homology (*PTEN*) is deleted or mutated biallelically in a wide range of human cancers and antagonizes signaling driven by *PIK3CA* activation.[149-151] Thus, *PTEN* acts as a tumor suppressor that inhibits PI3K signaling.

Accumulating evidence has shown that mutations of *PIK3CA* occur in over 25% of colorectal, gastric, and breast cancers and glioblastomas.[152] Infrequent mutations are found in neuroblastoma,[153] medulloblastoma,[154] and certain hematopoietic cancers.[155] Interestingly, more than 80% of *PIK3CA* mutations cluster in two small conserved regions within the helical and kinase domains. These hot-spot mutations result in enzymatic gain of function[156,157] reminiscent of activating mutations described in *RAS* and *BRAF*.

Host Cell Pathways Perturbed by SV40 Small t Antigen

In experimental systems, introduction of the SV40 small t (ST) antigen or manipulation of its downstream signaling pathways is essential for transformation of human cells by oncogenic alleles of *Ras* in the context of LT and hTERT expression.[125,158,159] The primary binding partner of ST is the protein phosphatase 2A (PP2A) family of serine-threonine phosphatases.[160] Because PP2A is the most abundant serine-threonine phosphatase in human cells, perturbation of PP2A activity may affect the phosphorylation status of a broad range of signaling molecules (reviewed by Arroyo and Hahn[161]). Long-term treatment of mice with the selective PP2A inhibitor okadaic acid (OA) leads to cancer development, suggesting that PP2A inhibition contributes to malignant transformation.[162,163] Studies have indicated that expression of ST or mutations in the PP2A Aα subunit found in colon, breast, and lung cancers selectively deplete PP2A complexes containing the PP2A B56γ subunit, indicating that PP2A complexes that contain this subunit mediate cell transformation.[164-166]

PP2A regulates the activity of many signaling pathways (reviewed by Arroyo and Hahn[161] and Millward and colleagues[167]), and we lack a complete understanding of which of these pathways is involved in malignant transformation. Recent work suggests that loss of function of PP2A contributes to cell transformation by activating the PI3K pathway. Activated alleles of *PIK3CA* or a combination of the PI3K substrates Akt and Rac1 substitute for ST in human cell transformation,[168] and inhibiting PP2A phosphatase activity[169] or expression of ST induces Akt activation.[168,170] In addition, inhibition of PP2A by expression of ST leads to stabilization of the *c-Myc* oncogene.[171]

Myc

The *Myc* family—*c-Myc, N-Myc, L-Myc, S-myc*, and *B-myc*—are also well-characterized oncogenes.[172] Myc proteins are transcription factors that exist in a variety of heterodimeric complexes that regulate the expression of a large number of genes. For example, complexes of Myc and Max promotes cell survival and proliferation[172-174] by regulating a diverse array of genes, including *CCND1, CCND2, CDK4*, and *E2F2*.[175-178] Alternatively, when complexed with other binding proteins such as Mad1, Mad2, or Mnt, Myc promotes cell death.

Abundant data in human tumors confirm that Myc plays a central role in many cancer types. For example, *c-Myc* is translocated and overexpressed in almost 100% of cases of Burkitt's lymphoma.[179] The signature chromosomal translocation in Burkitt's lymphoma results brings *c-Myc* under the control of an immunoglobulin (Ig) enhancer and leads to constitutive expression of high levels of *c-Myc*.[180] Chromosomal rearrangements involving *Myc* are also found in diffuse large cell lymphoma (DLCL), ALL, multiple myeloma (MM), and primary plasma cell leukemia (PCL).[181-183] In solid tumors, aberrant *Myc* expression occurs more commonly from gene amplification or overexpression. Of retinoblastomas, 10% to 20% harbor *N-myc* amplification,[184] whereas 10% to 30% of neuroblastomas and rhabdomyosarcomas show evidence of N-*myc* amplification.[185,186]

Cell Lineage and Transforming Gene Combinations

Studies from a number of laboratories have now shown that the introduction of genes that disrupt the pathways described lead to the transformation of a wide range of cell types.[120-125] These studies suggest that a finite set of pathways suffices to mediate malignant transformation. However, more recent work indicates that specific types of cancers may exhibit different requirements for cell transformation.

For example, although inactivation of Rb and p53, together with expression of hTERT, ST, and H-Ras, lead to the transformation of fibroblasts, embryonic kidney (HEK) cells, and mammary epithelial cells (HMEC), each of these cell types exhibits differences in their dependence on specific Ras effector pathways necessary to achieve cell transformation. In human fibroblasts, activation of the Raf and Ral-GEF pathways suffice to achieve cell transformation, whereas tumorigenic growth of HEK cells depends on the activation of the PI3K and Ral-GEF pathways. Moreover, transformation of HMEC requires the coordinate activation of Raf, PI3K, and Ral-GEFs.[159] These observations indicate that although perturbation of a defined set of pathways can drive transformation, the specific pathways activated in particular types of cancer may depend on cell lineage.

Consistent with this view, although human melanocytes can be rendered transformed by the introduction of the same set of genes that transforms fibroblasts or HMEC, expression of a constitutively active Met replaced Ras to drive the formation of melanomas,[187] suggesting that Met may play an important role in the genesis of malignant melanoma. Moreover, recent work in melanocytes has indicated that cell lineage and local environment both play important roles in malignant transformation. Using an orthotopic approach, genetic alterations associated with human melanoma were introduced into human melanocytes.[188] Of the different gene combinations tested, the coexpression of activated *Ras* and *hTERT* with the disruption of the Rb and p53 pathways produced tumors that shared many of the clinical and histologic features of melanoma. Coexpression of either CDK4 to disable the Rb pathway or inactivation of the p53 pathway with oncogenic *Ras* and *hTERT* induced invasive melanocytic lesions, indicating that transformation of melanocytes may not require the coordinate inactivation of the Rb and p53 pathway. Moreover, activation of the PI3K pathway but not expression of the B-Raf[V599E] mutant substituted for Ras in this model.[188] Together, these observations indicate that different types of cells require the perturbation of specific pathways to induce malignant transformation, perhaps in part explaining the association of specific mutations with particular types of cancers.

Although further work is required to define the specific combinations of genetic alterations critical for specific cancer subtypes, work from many laboratories has supported the notion that despite the requirement for multiple genetic events to program the fully malignant phenotype, cancer cells exhibit a striking dependence on particular mutations. One hypothesis to explain this observation is that once oncogenic signaling is engaged, tumor cells become excessively dependent on these activated signaling pathways, a state referred to as oncogene addiction.[189] Alternatively, persistent deregulation of prosurvival mechanisms that operate during the development of specific cellular lineages may render cancers dependent on lineage-specific pathways. For example, the microphthalmia-associated transcription factor (MITF) in melanocytes, FMS-related tyrosine kinase 3 (FLT3) in the myeloid lineage, and the androgen receptor in the prostate[190] represent lineage-specific genes that

participate directly in cancer development. Improved understanding of essential pathways for specific oncogenes and cell lineages will facilitate the development of rational approaches to target these pathways therapeutically.

Epigenetics and Genomic Instability

Epigenetics

Although genetic alterations such as mutation, amplification, and deletion play a direct role in malignant transformation, changes in gene expression mediated by events that do not affect the primary DNA sequence, or epigenetic changes, also contribute to cancer initiation, maintenance, and progression.[191] Epigenetic regulation of gene expression can involve each component of the DNA packaging and chromatin remodeling machinery. The three primary epigenetic mechanisms include DNA methylation by DNA methyltransferases (DNMTs), nucleosome remodeling by complex nucleosomal remodeling factors (NURFs), and histone modifications by histone deacetylases (HDACs) and histone methyltransferases (HMTs).[192]

The best understood epigenetic modification is the aberrant methylation of CpG islands in the promoters of tumor suppressors. CpG islands are regions of at least 200 bases with a (G + C) content of at least 50% and a ratio of observed to expected CpG frequency of at least 0.6.[193] Methylation in these promoter regions effectively silences associated genes and serves as an alternative mechanism to mutation or deletion events in the repression of aberrant growth control pathways.

It has long been recognized that cancer genomes exhibit both aberrant *hyper*methylation and *hypo*methylation.[111,192,194,195] For example, aberrant DNA methylation of CpG islands has been widely observed in human colorectal tumors and is associated with gene silencing. A subset of colorectal tumors has an exceptionally high frequency of methylation of some CpG islands, leading to the suggestion of a distinct trait referred to as CpG island methylator phenotype, or CIMP.[196] This phenotype has also been observed in several other cancer types, including AML.[197-199] Epigenetic allelic inactivation of a tumor suppressor gene by hypermethylation may have the same phenotypic effect as deletion or inactivating mutation; *INK4a* hypermethylation occurs in preinvasive lesions of the breast, colon, and other cancers.[200-202]

Although it is clear that further work is necessary to understand the full role of epigenetic changes in cancer development and progression, recent work suggests that such events are potentially reversible and as such offer opportunities for therapeutic intervention. For example, DNMT inhibitors such as 5-azacytidine (Vidaza, Pharmion, Boulder, Colo) and HDAC inhibitors[203] such as vorinostat, have shown particular promise in early trials for specific types of cancers such as cutaneous T-cell lymphoma.

Genetic Instability

Most epithelial cancers show widespread karyotypic chaos, suggesting that such tumors have experienced a period of genetic instability. Aneuploidy has long been recognized in human cancers[203-205] and often serves as a prognostic indicator. For example, hyperdiploidy of 51 to 60 chromosomes is present in the leukemic blasts of 25% of early B lineage ALL patients and is usually characterized by nonrandom gains of chromosomes 4, 6, 10, 14, 17, 18, 21, and X.[206,207] In childhood early B lineage ALL, the presence of aneuploid blasts is associated with a better prognosis, with some studies suggesting that aneuploid blasts are more susceptible to spontaneous and chemotherapy-induced apoptosis than their diploid counterparts.[208,209] Aneuploidy is uncommon in ALL derived from the T-cell lineage and, when present, does not appear to affect survival.[210]

Furthermore, mutations in genes involved in the regulation of genome integrity are implicated in cancer susceptibility syndromes. Examples of familial cancer syndromes and their associated genetic mutations include Li-Fraumeni syndrome (*TP53*), Fanconi's anemia (*FANCI/FANCD2*),[211] hereditary nonpolyposis coli conferring increased risk of colorectal carcinoma (*MSH/MLH*), and hereditary breast and ovarian cancer syndromes (*BRCA1, BRCA2*). Mosaic variegated aneuploidy (MVA), associated with germline mutations in *BUB1B*,[212] is characterized by mosaic aneuploidy and by increased risk of rhabdomyosarcoma, Wilms' tumor, and ALL.[213] Collectively, these syndromes involving germline mutations in genes governing chromosomal stability support a causal link between aneuploidy and cancer development.

At least two distinct classes of genetic instability are found in human malignancies: microsatellite instability (MIN) or chromosomal instability (CIN). Microsatellite instability involves the inactivation of DNA mismatch repair (MMR) genes such as *MSH2 or MLH*,[214] which compromises the mechanisms that repair naturally occurring replication errors. The consequence of MIN is the accumulation of single nucleotide mutations throughout the genome, without gross alterations in chromosome number or configuration.[215,216] The presence of MIN can be detected by analyzing the number and variation of short sequences of DNA repeats scattered throughout the genome, called microsatellites.[217,218]

In contrast to MIN, many cancers exhibit widespread karyotypic alterations. Although the causes of CIN are incompletely understood, in some cases CIN has been shown to be the consequence of aberrant mitotic checkpoint control or DNA damage repair (DDR) mechanisms. The mitotic checkpoint prevents chromosome mis-segregation and aneuploidy by inhibiting the irreversible transition to anaphase until all the replicated chromosomes have made productive attachments to spindle microtubules. Vogelstein and colleagues have reported mutations in two mitotic checkpoint genes in a small subset of colorectal cancer cell lines[219]; since then, mutations in a large number of genes whose protein products participate in mitotic checkpoint control have been identified (reviewed by Weaver and associates[205]).

Although genome-wide instability may contribute to tumorigenesis in a wide spectrum of cancers, pediatric malignancies often exhibit the presence of balanced translocations in which portions of two nonhomologous chromosomes are exchanged. Balanced translocations may result in the placement of a particular gene under the control of a nonphysiologic promoter, such as the t(8;14) translocation in Burkitt's lymphoma, in which *Myc* is juxtaposed with the immunoglobulin heavy chain (*IgH*) promoter or may yield novel oncogenic fusion proteins, such as the BCR-ABL fusion protein formed from the t(9;22) translocation in chronic myelogenous leukemia (CML). Translocations are best characterized in hematologic malignancies; 267 balanced translocations have been described in AML to date.[220] Rarely, specific translocations occur in almost every tumor of a particular histopathologic subtype. Examples include *BCR-ABL1* in CML, *IGH-CCND1* in mantle cell lymphoma, *IGH-MYC* in Burkitt's lymphoma, and the *PML-RARA* in acute promyelocytic leukemia (APML).[220] Whereas hematologic malignancies contain the overwhelming majority of translocation events, over 70 unique translocations have been described in solid tumors, in particular childhood sarcomas. For example, Ewing's sarcomas harbor high rates of rearrangements involving the *EWSR1* gene.[220-222] Alveolar rhabdomyosarcomas are characterized by the *PAX3-FKHR* translocation, and almost all synovial sarcomas feature a t(X;18) translocation, producing *SYT* fusions with *SSX1, SSX2,* or *SSX4*.[220]

Cell-Extrinsic Events in Tumor Growth: Cancer and Its Microenvironment

In addition to the cell-intrinsic alterations that occur within the nascent cancer cell, accumulating evidence suggests that interactions between cancer cells and the tumor microenvironment also play an important role in some cancers. Such cell-extrinsic characteristics include angiogenic capacity, metastasis, and immune evasion and are defined by unique interactions between cells of the tumor and cells of distinct host compartments. In this section, we review some of these cell-cell interactions important for cancer development and/or progression.

Angiogenic Potential

As tumors increase in size, they must create new blood vessels or co-opt existing vessels to permit sustained tumor growth beyond 1 to 2 mm^3.[223] The acquisition of proangiogenic properties has been termed the *angiogenic switch*,[224] and likely represents a state in which proangiogenic factors overwhelm endogenous inhibitors and permit the development of new tumor vasculature. The acquisition of a blood supply to growing tumors not only provides a system for nutrient delivery, but may also facilitate the migration of tumor cells into the host circulation.[225]

A complex interplay between proangiogenic factors and angiogenic inhibitors appears to govern angiogenesis in cancer. One major proangiogenic factor is the vascular endothelial growth factor (VEGF). The VEGF family of proteins were originally identified as inducers of proliferation and migration of endothelial cells in vitro, and blood vessel permeabilization and angiogenesis in vivo.[226] VEGF elaborated by tumor cells binds primarily to two receptor tyrosine kinases, VEGF receptor-1 (VEGFR1/Flt1) and VEGFR2/KDR/Flk1, to stimulate endothelial cell proliferation. VEGFR-2 plays a critical role in blood vessel formation, whereas VEGFR-1 appears to play a more important role in the proper organization of newly formed vasculature.[227,228] Studies with monoclonal antibodies and small molecules targeting VEGF and its receptors underscore the importance of these pathways in cancer development.

Cancer Cell Invasion and Metastasis

Although we now understand many of the pathways involved in tumor initiation and maintenance, most cancer patients die from complications of metastatic disease.[229] Metastasis is a complex biologic process, likely composed of several discrete steps, including loss of local cellular adhesion, increased motility and invasiveness, entry and survival of tumor cells in the host circulation, exit from the bloodstream, and colonization of a new distant tissue site.[230,231] The prevailing view is that tumor cells acquire an invasive phenotype, in part through the expression of a mesenchymal program that operates during embryogenesis. For epithelial cancers, this process has been termed *epithelial-mesenchymal transition* (EMT), characterized initially by diminished intercellular adhesiveness of tumor cells to each other and increased motility on activation of specific transcription factors such as snail, twist, and slug, which are active in embryogenesis.[232]

A complex interplay between cancer cell and extracellular matrix (ECM) is mediated by GTPases Rho, cdc42, and Rac, integrins and focal adhesion complexes, and proteases. The interaction of cancer cells with these various components may serve as barriers to the spread of cancer cells. For example, recent observations have indicated that pediatric neuroblastoma cells, which exhibit deficient caspase 8 activity, are markedly more invasive and metastatic,[233] suggesting that defects in apoptosis may facilitate metastatic potential.[234]

In addition, the stroma surrounding tumors may enhance or suppress the advancement of a tumor's invasive front. Studies have suggested that fibroblasts surrounding primary breast cancers secrete the chemokine CXCL12, which enhances tumor migration and angiogenesis.[235,236] In addition, other studies have suggested that hematopoietic precursor cells expressing VEGFR1 may exit the bone marrow and colonize potential metastatic foci prior to the arrival of metastasizing tumor cells, forming a premetastatic niche.[237,238] Consistent with this view, in animal models, VEGFR1 inhibition or depletion of VEGR1+ cells from the bone marrow eliminates the metastatic potential of primary tumor cells. Taken together, these and other observations suggest that studies of the interactions between cancer cells and their microenvironment will provide insights into the initiation, maintenance, and progression of cancer.

CONCLUSION

Cancer is clearly a genetic disease, driven by alterations in multiple genes that cooperate to drive the malignant state. Although many of the best characterized genetic alterations change cell-intrinsic tumor cell physiology, accumulating evidence indicates that some of these alterations alter cell-cell interactions and that cell-extrinsic mechanisms also play important, although incompletely understood, roles in tumor progression.

Although we still lack a comprehensive knowledge of all the changes that cooperate to program the malignant state of any particular cancer, current technologies promise to make it possible to enumerate such changes for many cancers. By gaining a deeper understanding of the molecular changes that drive malignant transformation, the rational design of therapies will eventually be possible, and treatment will be dictated by specific molecular characteristics.

REFERENCES

1. Hahn WC, Weinberg RA. Modelling the molecular circuitry of cancer. Nat Rev Cancer. 2002;2:331-341.
2. Hahn WC, Weinberg RA. Rules for making human tumor cells. N Engl J Med. 2002;347:1593-1603.
3. Hanahan D, Weinberg RA. The hallmarks of cancer. Cell. 2000;100:57-70.
4. Polyak K, Hahn WC. Roots and stems: stem cells in cancer. Nat Med. 2006;12:296-300.
5. Bonnet D, Dick JE. Human acute myeloid leukemia is organized as a hierarchy that originates from a primitive hematopoietic cell. Nat Med. 1997;3:730-737.
6. Singh SK, Hawkins C, Clarke ID, et al. Identification of human brain tumour initiating cells. Nature. 2004;432:396-401.
7. Al-Hajj M, Wicha MS, Benito-Hernandez A, et al. Prospective identification of tumorigenic breast cancer cells. Proc Natl Acad Sci U S A. 2003;100:3983-3988.
8. O'Brien CA, Pollett A, Gallinger S, Dick JE. A human colon cancer cell capable of initiating tumour growth in immunodeficient mice. Nature. 2007;445:106-110.
9. Ricci-Vitiani L, Lombardi DG, Pilozzi E, et al. Identification and expansion of human colon cancer-initiating cells. Nature. 2007;445:111-115.
10. Dontu G, Abdallah WM, Foley JM, et al. In vitro propagation and transcriptional profiling of human mammary stem/progenitor cells. Genes Dev. 2003;17:1253-1270.
11. Reynolds BA, Weiss S. Clonal and population analyses demonstrate that an EGF-responsive mammalian embryonic CNS precursor is a stem cell. Dev Biol. 1996;175:1-13.
12. Weiss S, Reynolds BA, Vescovi AL, et al. Is there a neural stem cell in the mammalian forebrain? Trends Neurosci. 1996;19:387-393.
13. Beachy PA, Karhadkar SS, Berman DM. Tissue repair and stem cell renewal in carcinogenesis. Nature. 2004;432:324-331.
14. Crowe DL, Parsa B, Sinha UK. Relationships between stem cells and cancer stem cells. Histol Histopathol. 2004;19:505-509.
15. Miller SJ, Lavker RM, Sun TT. Interpreting epithelial cancer biology in the context of stem cells: tumor properties and therapeutic implications. Biochim Biophys Acta. 2005;1756:25-52.
16. Tsai RY. A molecular view of stem cell and cancer cell self-renewal. Int J Biochem Cell Biol. 2004;36:684-694.
17. Valk-Lingbeek ME, Bruggeman SW, van Lohuizen M. Stem cells and cancer; the polycomb connection. Cell. 2004;118:409-418.
18. Woodward WA, Chen MS, Behbod F, Rosen JM. On mammary stem cells. J Cell Sci. 2005;118(Pt 16):3585-3594.
19. Young HE, Duplaa C, Romero-Ramos M, et al. Adult reserve stem cells and their potential for tissue engineering. Cell Biochem Biophys. 2004;40:1-80.
20. Al-Hajj M, Clarke MF. Self-renewal and solid tumor stem cells. Oncogene. 2004;23:7274-7282.
21. Masters JR. Human cancer cell lines: fact and fantasy. Nat Rev Mol Cell Biol. 2000;1:233-236.
22. Stehelin D, Varmus HE, Bishop JM, Vogt PK. DNA related to the transforming gene(s) of avian sarcoma viruses is present in normal avian DNA. Nature. 1976;260:170-173.
23. Bishop JM. Viral oncogenes. Cell. 1985;42:23-38.
24. Shih C, Weinberg RA. Isolation of a transforming sequence from a human bladder carcinoma cell line. Cell. 1982;29:161-169.
25. Shih C, Shilo BZ, Goldfarb MP, et al. Passage of phenotypes of chemically transformed cells via transfection of DNA and chromatin. Proc Natl Acad Sci U S A. 1979;76:5714-5718.
26. Land H, Parada LF, Weinberg RA. Tumorigenic conversion of primary embryo fibroblasts requires at least two cooperating oncogenes. Nature. 1983;304:596-602.
27. Ruley HE. Adenovirus early region 1A enables viral and cellular transforming genes to transform primary cells in culture. Nature. 1983;304:602-606.
28. Hunter T. Cooperation between oncogenes. Cell. 1991;64:249-270.
29. Stevenson M, Volsky DJ. Activated v-myc and v-ras oncogenes do not transform normal human lymphocytes. Mol Cell Biol. 1986;6:3410-3417.
30. Hayflick L, Moorhead PS. The serial cultivation of human diploid cell strains. Exp Cell Res. 1961;25:585-621.
31. Sager R. Senescence as a mode of tumor suppression. Environ Health Perspect. 1991;93:59-62.
32. Bartkova J, Rezaei N, Liontos M, et al. Oncogene-induced senescence is part of the tumorigenesis barrier imposed by DNA damage checkpoints. Nature. 2006;444:633-637.
33. Chua KF, Mostoslavsky R, Lombard DB, et al. Mammalian SIRT1 limits replicative life span in response to chronic genotoxic stress. Cell Metab. 2005;2:67-76.
34. Lombard DB, Chua KF, Mostoslavsky R, et al. DNA repair, genome stability, and aging. Cell. 2005;120:497-512.
35. Blackburn EH. Telomeres and telomerase. Keio J Med. 2000;49:59-65.
36. Bilaud T, Brun C, Ancelin K, et al. Telomeric localization of TRF2, a novel human telobox protein. Nat Genet. 1997;17:236-239.

37. Broccoli D, Smogorzewska A, Chong L, de Lange T. Human telomeres contain two distinct Myb-related proteins, TRF1 and TRF2. Nat Genet. 1997;17:231-235.

38. Chong L, van Steensel B, Broccoli D, et al. A human telomeric protein. Science. 1995;270:1663-1667.

39. de Lange T. Shelterin: the protein complex that shapes and safeguards human telomeres. Genes Dev. 2005;19:2100-2110.

40. Blasco MA, Lee HW, Hande MP, et al. Telomere shortening and tumor formation by mouse cells lacking telomerase RNA. Cell. 1997;91:25-34.

41. Hahn WC, Stewart SA, Brooks MW, et al. Inhibition of telomerase limits the growth of human cancer cells. Nat Med. 1999;5:1164-1170.

42. Karlseder J, Broccoli D, Dai Y, et al. p53- and ATM-dependent apoptosis induced by telomeres lacking TRF2. Science. 1999;283:1321-1325.

43. Yu GL, Bradley JD, Attardi LD, Blackburn EH. In vivo alteration of telomere sequences and senescence caused by mutated Tetrahymena telomerase RNAs. Nature. 1990;344:126-132.

44. d'Adda di Fagagna F, Reaper PM, Clay-Farrace L, et al. A DNA damage checkpoint response in telomere-initiated senescence. Nature. 2003;426:194-198.

45. Hao LY, Strong MA, Greider CW. Phosphorylation of H2AX at short telomeres in T cells and fibroblasts. J Biol Chem. 2004;279:45148-45154.

46. Hemann MT, Rudolph KL, Strong MA, et al. Telomere dysfunction triggers developmentally regulated germ cell apoptosis. Mol Biol Cell. 2001;12:2023-2030.

47. Lee HW, Blasco MA, Gottlieb GJ, et al. Essential role of mouse telomerase in highly proliferative organs. Nature. 1998;392:569-574.

48. Hsu HL, Gilley D, Blackburn EH, Chen DJ. Ku is associated with the telomere in mammals. Proc Natl Acad Sci U S A. 1999;96:12454-12458.

49. Hsu HL, Gilley D, Galande SA, et al. Ku acts in a unique way at the mammalian telomere to prevent end joining. Genes Dev. 2000;14:2807-2812.

50. Zhu XD, Kuster B, Mann M, et al. Cell-cycle-regulated association of RAD50/MRE11/NBS1 with TRF2 and human telomeres. Nat Genet. 2000;25:347-352.

51. Meyerson M. Role of telomerase in normal and cancer cells. J Clin Oncol. 2000;18:2626-2634.

52. Nakamura TM, Cech TR. Reversing time: origin of telomerase. Cell. 1998;92:587-590.

53. Harrington L, Zhou W, McPhail T, et al. Human telomerase contains evolutionarily conserved catalytic and structural subunits. Genes Dev. 1997;11:3109-3115.

54. Meyerson M, Counter CM, Eaton EN, et al. hEST2, the putative human telomerase catalytic subunit gene, is up-regulated in tumor cells and during immortalization. Cell. 1997;90:785-795.

55. Nakamura TM, Morin GB, Chapman KB, et al. Telomerase catalytic subunit homologs from fission yeast and human. Science. 1997;277:955-959.

56. Bryan TM, Englezou A, Dalla-Pozza L, et al. Evidence for an alternative mechanism for maintaining telomere length in human tumors and tumor-derived cell lines. Nat Med. 1997;3:1271-1274.

57. Muntoni A, Reddel RR. The first molecular details of ALT in human tumor cells. Hum Mol Genet. 2005;14 Spec No. 2:R191-196.

58. Lundblad V, Blackburn EH. An alternative pathway for yeast telomere maintenance rescues est1-senescence. Cell. 1993;73:347-360.

59. Dunham MA, Neumann AA, Fasching CL, Reddel RR. Telomere maintenance by recombination in human cells. Nat Genet. 2000;26:447-450.

60. Counter CM. The roles of telomeres and telomerase in cell life span. Mutat Res. 1996;366:45-63.

61. Harley CB, Futcher AB, Greider CW. Telomeres shorten during ageing of human fibroblasts. Nature. 1990;345:458-460.

62. Harley CB, Kim NW, Prowse KR, et al. Telomerase, cell immortality, and cancer. Cold Spring Harb Symp Quant Biol. 1994;59:307-315.

63. Bodnar AG, Ouellette M, Frolkis M, et al. Extension of life-span by introduction of telomerase into normal human cells. Science. 1998;279:349-352.

64. Dickson MA, Hahn WC, Ino Y, et al. Human keratinocytes that express hTERT and also bypass a p16(INK4a)-enforced mechanism that limits life span become immortal yet retain normal growth and differentiation characteristics. Mol Cell Biol. 2000;20:1436-1447.

65. Vaziri H, Benchimol S. Reconstitution of telomerase activity in normal human cells leads to elongation of telomeres and extended replicative life span. Curr Biol. 1998;8:279-282.

66. Yang J, Chang E, Cherry AM, et al. Human endothelial cell life extension by telomerase expression. J Biol Chem. 1999;274:26141-26148.

67. Zhang X, Mar V, Zhou W, et al. Telomere shortening and apoptosis in telomerase-inhibited human tumor cells. Genes Dev. 1999;13:2388-2399.

68. Hahn WC, Counter CM, Lundberg AS, et al. Creation of human tumour cells with defined genetic elements. Nature. 1999;400:464-468.

69. Ali SH, DeCaprio JA. Cellular transformation by SV40 large T antigen: interaction with host proteins. Semin Cancer Biol. 2001;11:15-23.

70. Shay JW, Wright WE, Werbin H. Defining the molecular mechanisms of human cell immortalization. Biochim Biophys Acta. 1991;1072:1-7.

71. Kiyono T, Foster SA, Koop JI, et al. Both Rb/p16INK4a inactivation and telomerase activity are required to immortalize human epithelial cells. Nature. 1998;396:84-88.

72. DiRenzo J, Signoretti S, Nakamura N, et al. Growth factor requirements and basal phenotype of an immortalized mammary epithelial cell line. Cancer Res. 2002;62:89-98.

73. Shay JW, Wright WE. Quantitation of the frequency of immortalization of normal human diploid fibroblasts by SV40 large T-antigen. Exp Cell Res. 1989;184:109-118.

74. Hahn WC. Immortalization and transformation of human cells. Mol Cells. 2002;13:351-361.

75. Boehm JS, Hession MT, Bulmer SE, Hahn WC. Transformation of human and murine fibroblasts without viral oncoproteins. Mol Cell Biol. 2005;25:6464-6474.

76. Zhao JJ, Roberts TM, Hahn WC. Functional genetics and experimental models of human cancer. Trends Mol Med. 2004;10:344-350.

77. Sherr CJ. Principles of tumor suppression. Cell. 2004;116:235-246.

78. Ventura A, Kirsch DG, McLaughlin ME, et al. Restoration of p53 function leads to tumour regression in vivo. Nature. 2007;445:661-665.

79. Xue W, Zender L, Miething C, et al. Senescence and tumour clearance is triggered by p53 restoration in murine liver carcinomas. Nature. 2007;445:656-660.

80. Lane DP, Crawford LV. T antigen is bound to a host protein in SV40-transformed cells. Nature. 1979;278:261-263.

81. Linzer DI, Levine AJ. Characterization of a 54K dalton cellular SV40 tumor antigen present in SV40-transformed cells and uninfected embryonal carcinoma cells. Cell. 1979;17:43-52.

82. Masuda H, Miller C, Koeffler HP, et al. Rearrangement of the p53 gene in human osteogenic sarcomas. Proc Natl Acad Sci U S A. 1987;84:7716-7719.

83. Olivier M, Eeles R, Hollstein M, et al. The IARC TP53 database: new online mutation analysis and recommendations to users. Hum Mutat. 2002;19:607-614.

84. Malkin D, Li FP, Strong LC, et al. Germ line p53 mutations in a familial syndrome of breast cancer, sarcomas, and other neoplasms. Science. 1990;250:1233-1238.

85. Nigro JM, Baker SJ, Preisinger AC, et al. Mutations in the p53 gene occur in diverse human tumour types. Nature. 1989;342:705-708.

86. Jacks T, Weinberg RA. Cell-cycle control and its watchman. Nature. 1996;381:643-644.

87. Kastan MB, Onyekwere O, Sidransky D, et al. Participation of p53 protein in the cellular response to DNA damage. Cancer Res. 1991;51(Pt 1):6304-6311.

88. Lowe SW. Activation of p53 by oncogenes. Endocr Relat Cancer. 1999;6:45-48.

89. Vousden KH, Lane DP. p53 in health and disease. Nat Rev Mol Cell Biol. 2007;8:275-283.

90. Momand J, Jung D, Wilczynski S, Niland J. The MDM2 gene amplification database. Nucleic Acids Res. 1998;26:3453-3459.

91. Sherr CJ. The INK4a/ARF network in tumour suppression. Nat Rev Mol Cell Biol. 2001;2:731-737.

92. Martins CP, Brown-Swigart L, Evan GI. Modeling the therapeutic efficacy of p53 restoration in tumors. Cell. 2006;127:1323-1334.

93. Soussi T, Lozano G. p53 mutation heterogeneity in cancer. Biochem Biophys Res Commun. 2005;331:834-842.

94. Lang GA, Iwakuma T, Suh YA, et al. Gain of function of a p53 hot spot mutation in a mouse model of Li-Fraumeni syndrome. Cell. 2004;119:861-872.

95. Olive KP, Tuveson DA, Ruhe ZC, et al. Mutant p53 gain of function in two mouse models of Li-Fraumeni syndrome. Cell. 2004;119:847-860.

96. Sigal A, Rotter V. Oncogenic mutations of the p53 tumor suppressor: the demons of the guardian of the genome. Cancer Res. 2000;60:6788-6793.

97. Knudson AG Jr. Mutation and cancer: statistical study of retinoblastoma. Proc Natl Acad Sci U S A. 1971;68:820-823.

98. Bookstein R, Lee WH. Molecular genetics of the retinoblastoma suppressor gene. Crit Rev Oncog. 1991;2:211-227.

99. Foster SA, Galloway DA. Human papillomavirus type 16 E7 alleviates a proliferation block in early passage human mammary epithelial cells. Oncogene. 1996;12:1773-1779.

100. Ludlow JW, Shon J, Pipas JM, et al. The retinoblastoma susceptibility gene product undergoes cell cycle-dependent dephosphorylation and binding to and release from SV40 large T. Cell. 1990;60:387-396.

101. Moran E, Mathews MB. Multiple functional domains in the adenovirus E1A gene. Cell. 1987;48:177-178.

102. Weinberg RA. The retinoblastoma protein and cell cycle control. Cell. 1995;81:323-330.

103. Ogawa H, Ishiguro K, Gaubatz S, et al. A complex with chromatin modifiers that occupies E2F- and Myc-responsive genes in G0 cells. Science. 2002;296:1132-1136.

104. Rayman JB, Takahashi Y, Indjeian VB, et al. E2F mediates cell cycle-dependent transcriptional repression in vivo by recruitment of an HDAC1/mSin3B corepressor complex. Genes Dev. 2002;16:933-947.

105. Trimarchi JM, Lees JA. Sibling rivalry in the E2F family. Nat Rev Mol Cell Biol. 2002;3:11-20.

106. Sellers WR, Kaelin WG Jr. Role of the retinoblastoma protein in the pathogenesis of human cancer. J Clin Oncol. 1997;15:3301-3312.

107. zur Hausen H. Papillomaviruses and cancer: from basic studies to clinical application. Nat Rev Cancer. 2002;2:342-350.

108. Jacks T, Weinberg RA. The expanding role of cell cycle regulators. Science. 1998;280:1035-1036.

109. Sicinski P, Weinberg RA. A specific role for cyclin D1 in mammary gland development. J Mammary Gland Biol Neoplasia. 1997;2:335-342.

110. Rimokh R, Berger F, Bastard C, et al. Rearrangement of CCND1 (BCL1/PRAD1) 3′ untranslated region in mantle-cell lymphomas and t(11q13)-associated leukemias. Blood. 1994;83:3689-3696.

111. Kamijo T, Zindy F, Roussel MF, et al. Tumor suppression at the mouse INK4a locus mediated by the alternative reading frame product p19ARF. Cell. 1997;91:649-659.

112. Shapiro GI, Park JE, Edwards CD, et al. Multiple mechanisms of p16INK4A inactivation in non-small cell lung cancer cell lines. Cancer Res. 1995;55:6200-6209.

113. Ruas M, Peters G. The p16INK4a/CDKN2A tumor suppressor and its relatives. Biochim Biophys Acta. 1998;1378:F115-177.

114. Forbes S, Clements J, Dawson E, et al. Cosmic 2005. Br J Cancer. 2006;94:318-322.

115. Carter TL, Watt PM, Kumar R, et al. Hemizygous p16(INK4A) deletion in pediatric acute lymphoblastic leukemia predicts independent risk of relapse. Blood. 2001;97:572-574.

116. Iolascon A, Faienza MF, Coppola B, et al. Homozygous deletions of cyclin-dependent kinase inhibitor genes, p16(INK4A) and p18, in childhood T cell lineage acute lymphoblastic leukemias. Leukemia. 1996;10:255-260.

117. Benassi MS, Molendini L, Gamberi G, et al. Alteration of pRb/p16/cdk4 regulation in human osteosarcoma. Int J Cancer. 1999;84:489-493.

118. Wolfel T, Hauer M, Schneider J, et al. A p16INK4a-insensitive CDK4 mutant targeted by cytolytic T lymphocytes in a human melanoma. Science. 1995;269:1281-1284.

119. He J, Allen JR, Collins VP, et al. CDK4 amplification is an alternative mechanism to p16 gene homozygous deletion in glioma cell lines. Cancer Res. 1994;54:5804-5807.

120. Berger R, Febbo PG, Majumder PK, et al. Androgen-induced differentiation and tumorigenicity of human prostate epithelial cells. Cancer Res. 2004;64:8867-8875.

121. Elenbaas B, Spirio L, Koerner F, et al. Human breast cancer cells generated by oncogenic transformation of primary mammary epithelial cells. Genes Dev. 2001;15:50-65.

122. Lundberg AS, Randell SH, Stewart SA, et al. Immortalization and transformation of primary human airway epithelial cells by gene transfer. Oncogene. 2002;21:4577-4586.

123. MacKenzie KL, Franco S, Naiyer AJ, et al. Multiple stages of malignant transformation of human endothelial cells modelled by co-expression of telomerase reverse transcriptase, SV40 T antigen and oncogenic N-ras. Oncogene. 2002;21:4200-4211.

124. Rich JN, Guo C, McLendon RE, et al. A genetically tractable model of human glioma formation. Cancer Res. 2001;61:3556-3560.

125. Yu J, Boyapati A, Rundell K. Critical role for SV40 small-t antigen in human cell transformation. Virology. 2001;290:192-198.

126. Zimonjic D, Brooks MW, Popescu N, et al. Derivation of human tumor cells in vitro without widespread genomic instability. Cancer Res. 2001;61:8838-8844.

127. Downward J. Targeting RAS signalling pathways in cancer therapy. Nat Rev Cancer. 2003;3:11-22.

128. Barbacid M. ras genes. Annu Rev Biochem. 1987;56:779-827.

129. Parada LF, Tabin CJ, Shih C, Weinberg RA. Human EJ bladder carcinoma oncogene is homologue of Harvey sarcoma virus ras gene. Nature. 1982;297:474-478.

130. Bos JL. ras oncogenes in human cancer: a review. Cancer Res. 1989;49:4682-4689.

131. Slamon DJ, Clark GM, Wong SG, et al. Human breast cancer: correlation of relapse and survival with amplification of the HER-2/neu oncogene. Science. 1987;235:177-182.

132. Libermann TA, Nusbaum HR, Razon N, et al. Amplification, enhanced expression and possible rearrangement of EGF receptor gene in primary human brain tumours of glial origin. Nature. 1985;313:144-147.

133. Paez JG, Janne PA, Lee JC, et al. EGFR mutations in lung cancer: correlation with clinical response to gefitinib therapy. Science. 2004;304:1497-1500.

134. Zwick E, Bange J, Ullrich A. Receptor tyrosine kinases as targets for anticancer drugs. Trends Mol Med. 2002;8:17-23.

135. Emuss V, Garnett M, Mason C, Marais R. Mutations of C-RAF are rare in human cancer because C-RAF has a low basal kinase activity compared with B-RAF. Cancer Res. 2005;65:9719-9726.

136. Garnett MJ, Marais R. Guilty as charged: B-RAF is a human oncogene. Cancer Cell. 2004;6:313-319.

137. Zebisch A, Staber PB, Delavar A, et al. Two transforming C-RAF germ-line mutations identified in patients with therapy-related acute myeloid leukemia. Cancer Res. 2006;66:3401-3408.

138. Davies H, Bignell GR, Cox C, et al. Mutations of the BRAF gene in human cancer. Nature. 2002;417:949-954.

139. Chien Y, Kim S, Bumeister R, et al. RalB GTPase-mediated activation of the IkappaB family kinase TBK1 couples innate immune signaling to tumor cell survival. Cell. 2006;127:157-170.

140. Lim KH, Baines AT, Fiordalisi JJ, et al. Activation of RalA is critical for Ras-induced tumorigenesis of human cells. Cancer Cell. 2005;7:533-545.

141. Feig LA. Ral-GTPases: approaching their 15 minutes of fame. Trends Cell Biol. 2003;13:419-425.

142. Essers MA, Weijzen S, de Vries-Smits AM, et al. FOXO transcription factor activation by oxidative stress mediated by the small GTPase Ral and JNK. EMBO J. 2004;23:4802-4812.

143. De Ruiter ND, Burgering BM, Bos JL. Regulation of the Forkhead transcription factor AFX by Ral-dependent phosphorylation of threonines 447 and 451. Mol Cell Biol. 2001;21:8225-8235.

144. Sugimoto Y, Whitman M, Cantley LC, Erikson RL. Evidence that the Rous sarcoma virus transforming gene product phosphorylates phosphatidylinositol and diacylglycerol. Proc Natl Acad Sci U S A. 1984;81:2117-2121.

145. Chang HW, Aoki M, Fruman D, et al. Transformation of chicken cells by the gene encoding the catalytic subunit of PI 3-kinase. Science. 1997;276:1848-1850.

146. Vanhaesebroeck B, Alessi DR. The PI3K-PDK1 connection: more than just a road to PKB. Biochem J. 2000;346(Pt 3):561-576.

147. Engelman JA, Luo J, Cantley LC. The evolution of phosphatidylinositol 3-kinases as regulators of growth and metabolism. Nat Rev Genet. 2006;7:606-619.

148. Sansal I, Sellers WR. The biology and clinical relevance of the PTEN tumor suppressor pathway. J Clin Oncol. 2004;22:2954-2963.

149. Li J, Yen C, Liaw D, et al. PTEN, a putative protein tyrosine phosphatase gene mutated in human brain, breast, and prostate cancer. Science. 1997;275:1943-1947.

150. Liaw D, Marsh DJ, Li J, et al. Germline mutations of the PTEN gene in Cowden disease, an inherited breast and thyroid cancer syndrome. Nat Genet. 1997;16:64-67.

151. Steck PA, Pershouse MA, Jasser SA, et al. Identification of a candidate tumour suppressor gene, MMAC1, at chromosome 10q23.3 that is mutated in multiple advanced cancers. Nat Genet. 1997;15:356-362.

152. Samuels Y, Wang Z, Bardelli A, et al. High frequency of mutations of the PIK3CA gene in human cancers. Science. 2004;304:554.

153. Dam V, Morgan BT, Mazanek P, Hogarty MD. Mutations in PIK3CA are infrequent in neuroblastoma. BMC Cancer. 2006;6:177.

154. Broderick DK, Di C, Parrett TJ, et al. Mutations of PIK3CA in anaplastic oligodendrogliomas, high-grade astrocytomas, and medulloblastomas. Cancer Res. 2004;64:5048-5050.

155. Muller CI, Miller CW, Hofmann WK, et al. Rare mutations of the PIK3CA gene in malignancies of the hematopoietic system as well as endometrium, ovary, prostate and osteosarcomas, and discovery of a PIK3CA pseudogene. Leuk Res. 2007;31:27-32.

156. Bader AG, Kang S, Vogt PK. Cancer-specific mutations in PIK3CA are oncogenic in vivo. Proc Natl Acad Sci U S A. 2006;103:1475-1479.

157. Samuels Y, Diaz LA Jr, Schmidt-Kittler O, et al. Mutant PIK3CA promotes cell growth and invasion of human cancer cells. Cancer Cell. 2005;7:561-573.

158. Hahn WC, Dessain SK, Brooks MW, et al. Enumeration of the simian virus 40 early region elements necessary for human cell transformation. Mol Cell Biol. 2002;22:2111-2123.

159. Rangarajan A, Hong SJ, Gifford A, Weinberg RA. Species- and cell type-specific requirements for cellular transformation. Cancer Cell. 2004;6:171-183.

160. Pallas DC, Shahrik LK, Martin BL, et al. Polyoma small and middle T antigens and SV40 small t antigen form stable complexes with protein phosphatase 2A. Cell. 1990;60:167-176.

161. Arroyo JD, Hahn WC. Involvement of PP2A in viral and cellular transformation. Oncogene. 2005;24:7746-7755.

162. Bialojan C, Takai A. Inhibitory effect of a marine-sponge toxin, okadaic acid, on protein phosphatases. Specificity and kinetics. Biochem J. 1988;256:283-290.

163. Suganuma M, Fujiki H, Suguri H, et al. Okadaic acid: an additional non-phorbol-12-tetradecanoate-13-acetate-type tumor promoter. Proc Natl Acad Sci U S A. 1988;85:1768-1771.

164. Chen W, Arroyo JD, Timmons JC, et al. Cancer-associated PP2A Aalpha subunits induce functional haploinsufficiency and tumorigenicity. Cancer Res. 2005;65:8183-8192.

165. Chen W, Possemato R, Campbell KT, et al. Identification of specific PP2A complexes involved in human cell transformation. Cancer Cell. 2004;5:127-136.

166. Ruediger R, Pham HT, Walter G. Disruption of protein phosphatase 2A subunit interaction in human cancers with mutations in the A alpha subunit gene. Oncogene. 2001;20:10-15.

167. Millward TA, Zolnierowicz S, Hemmings BA. Regulation of protein kinase cascades by protein phosphatase 2A. Trends Biochem Sci. 1999;24:186-191.

168. Zhao JJ, Gjoerup OV, Subramanian RR, et al. Human mammary epithelial cell transformation through the activation of phosphatidylinositol 3-kinase. Cancer Cell. 2003;3:483-495.

169. Andjelkovic M, Jakubowicz T, Cron P, et al. Activation and phosphorylation of a pleckstrin homology domain containing protein kinase (RAC-PK/PKB) promoted by serum and protein phosphatase inhibitors. Proc Natl Acad Sci U S A. 1996;93:5699-5704.

170. Yuan H, Veldman T, Rundell K, Schlegel R. Simian virus 40 small tumor antigen activates AKT and telomerase and induces anchorage-independent growth of human epithelial cells. J Virol. 2002;76:10685-10691.

171. Yeh E, Cunningham M, Arnold H, et al. A signalling pathway controlling c-Myc degradation that impacts oncogenic transformation of human cells. Nat Cell Biol. 2004;6:308-318.

172. Adhikary S, Eilers M. Transcriptional regulation and transformation by Myc proteins. Nat Rev Mol Cell Biol. 2005;6:635-645.

173. Blackwood EM, Eisenman RN. Max: a helix-loop-helix zipper protein that forms a sequence-specific DNA-binding complex with Myc. Science. 1991;251:1211-1217.

174. Blackwood EM, Luscher B, Kretzner L, Eisenman RN. The Myc:Max protein complex and cell growth regulation. Cold Spring Harb Symp Quant Biol. 1991;56:109-117.

175. Hermeking H, Rago C, Schuhmacher M, et al. Identification of CDK4 as a target of c-MYC. Proc Natl Acad Sci U S A. 2000;97:2229-2234.

176. Seoane J, Pouponnot C, Staller P, et al. TGFbeta influences Myc, Miz-1 and Smad to control the CDK inhibitor p15INK4b. Nat Cell Biol. 2001;3:400-408.

177. Staller P, Peukert K, Kiermaier A, et al. Repression of p15INK4b expression by Myc through association with Miz-1. Nat Cell Biol. 2001;3:392-399.

178. Wilson A, Murphy MJ, Oskarsson T, et al. c-Myc controls the balance between hematopoietic stem cell self-renewal and differentiation. Genes Dev. 2004;18:2747-2763.

179. Boxer LM, Dang CV. Translocations involving c-myc and c-myc function. Oncogene. 2001;20:5595-5610.

180. Nesbit CE, Tersak JM, Prochownik EV. MYC oncogenes and human neoplastic disease. Oncogene. 1999;18:3004-3016.

181. Avet-Loiseau H, Gerson F, Magrangeas F, et al. Rearrangements of the c-myc oncogene are present in 15% of primary human multiple myeloma tumors. Blood. 2001;98:3082-3086.

182. Burmeister T, Schwartz S, Horst HA, et al. Molecular heterogeneity of sporadic adult Burkitt-type leukemia/lymphoma as revealed by PCR and cytogenetics: correlation with morphology, immunology and clinical features. Leukemia. 2005;19:1391-1398.

183. Frost M, Newell J, Lones MA, et al. Comparative immunohistochemical analysis of pediatric Burkitt lymphoma and diffuse large B-cell lymphoma. Am J Clin Pathol. 2004;121:384-392.

184. Lee WH, Murphree AL, Benedict WF. Expression and amplification of the N-myc gene in primary retinoblastoma. Nature. 1984;309:458-460.

185. Brodeur GM, Seeger RC, Schwab M, et al. Amplification of N-myc in untreated human neuroblastomas correlates with advanced disease stage. Science. 1984;224:1121-1124.

186. Schwab M. MYCN in neuronal tumours. Cancer Lett. 2004;204:179-187.

187. Gupta PB, Kuperwasser C, Brunet JP, et al. The melanocyte differentiation program predisposes to metastasis after neoplastic transformation. Nat Genet. 2005;37:1047-1054.

188. Chudnovsky Y, Adams AE, Robbins PB, et al. Use of human tissue to assess the oncogenic activity of melanoma-associated mutations. Nat Genet. 2005;37:745-749.

189. Weinstein IB. Cancer. Addiction to oncogenes—the Achilles heel of cancer. Science. 2002;297:63-64.

190. Garraway LA, Sellers WR. Lineage dependency and lineage-survival oncogenes in human cancer. Nat Rev Cancer. 2006;6:593-602.

191. Baylin SB, Ohm JE. Epigenetic gene silencing in cancer—a mechanism for early oncogenic pathway addiction? Nat Rev Cancer. 2006;6:107-116.

192. Jones PA, Baylin SB. The epigenomics of cancer. Cell. 2007;128:683-692.

193. Gardiner-Garden M, Frommer M. CpG islands in vertebrate genomes. J Mol Biol. 1987;196:261-282.

194. Feinberg AP, Tycko B. The history of cancer epigenetics. Nat Rev Cancer. 2004;4:143-153.

195. Herman JG, Baylin SB. Promoter-region hypermethylation and gene silencing in human cancer. Curr Top Microbiol Immunol. 2000;249:35-54.

196. Weisenberger DJ, Siegmund KD, Campan M, et al. CpG island methylator phenotype underlies sporadic microsatellite instability and is tightly associated with BRAF mutation in colorectal cancer. Nat Genet. 2006;38:787-793.

197. Garcia-Manero G, Daniel J, Smith TL, et al. DNA methylation of multiple promoter-associated CpG islands in adult acute lymphocytic leukemia. Clin Cancer Res. 2002;8:2217-2224.

198. Issa JP. CpG island methylator phenotype in cancer. Nat Rev Cancer. 2004;4:988-993.

199. Toyota M, Kopecky KJ, Toyota MO, et al. Methylation profiling in acute myeloid leukemia. Blood. 2001;97:2823-2829.

200. Belinsky SA, Nikula KJ, Palmisano WA, et al. Aberrant methylation of p16(INK4a) is an early event in lung cancer and a potential biomarker for early diagnosis. Proc Natl Acad Sci U S A. 1998;95:11891-11896.

201. McDermott KM, Zhang J, Holst CR, et al. p16(INK4a) prevents centrosome dysfunction and genomic instability in primary cells. PLoS Biol. 2006;4:e51.

202. Reynolds PA, Sigaroudinia M, Zardo G, et al. Tumor suppressor p16INK4A regulates polycomb-mediated DNA hypermethylation in human mammary epithelial cells. J Biol Chem. 2006;281:24790-24802.

203. Marks PA, Breslow R. Dimethyl sulfoxide to vorinostat: development of this histone deacetylase inhibitor as an anticancer drug. Nat Biotechnol. 2007;25:84-90.

204. Weaver BA, Cleveland DW. Does aneuploidy cause cancer? Curr Opin Cell Biol. 2006;18:658-667.

205. Weaver BA, Silk AD, Cleveland DW. Cell biology: nondisjunction, aneuploidy and tetraploidy. Nature. 2006;442:E9-E10.

206. Mertens F, Johansson B, Mitelman F. Dichotomy of hyperdiploid acute lymphoblastic leukemia on the basis of the distribution of gained chromosomes. Cancer Genet Cytogenet. 1996;92:8-10.

207. Raimondi SC, Pui CH, Hancock ML, et al. Heterogeneity of hyperdiploid (51-67) childhood acute lymphoblastic leukemia. Leukemia. 1996;10:213-224.

208. Ito C, Kumagai M, Manabe A, et al. Hyperdiploid acute lymphoblastic leukemia with 51 to 65 chromosomes: a distinct biological entity with a marked propensity to undergo apoptosis. Blood. 1999;93:315-320.

209. Zhang Y, Lu J, van den Berghe J, Lee SH. Increased incidence of spontaneous apoptosis in the bone marrow of hyperdiploid childhood acute lymphoblastic leukemia. Exp Hematol. 2002;30:333-339.

210. Schneider NR, Carroll AJ, Shuster JJ, et al. New recurring cytogenetic abnormalities and association of blast cell karyotypes with prognosis in childhood T-cell acute lymphoblastic leukemia: a pediatric oncology group report of 343 cases. Blood. 2000;96:2543-2549.

211. Smogorzewska A, Matsuoka S, Vinciguerra P, et al. Identification of the FANCI protein, a monoubiquitinated FANCD2 paralog required for DNA repair. Cell. 2007;129:289-301.

212. Hanks S, Coleman K, Reid S, et al. Constitutional aneuploidy and cancer predisposition caused by biallelic mutations in BUB1B. Nat Genet. 2004;36:1159-1161.

213. Jacquemont S, Boceno M, Rival JM, et al. High risk of malignancy in mosaic variegated aneuploidy syndrome. Am J Med Genet. 2002;109:17-21.

214. Peltomaki P, de la Chapelle A. Mutations predisposing to hereditary nonpolyposis colorectal cancer. Adv Cancer Res. 1997;71:93-119.

215. Eshleman JR, Lang EZ, Bowerfind GK, et al. Increased mutation rate at the hprt locus accompanies microsatellite instability in colon cancer. Oncogene. 1995;10(1):33-37.

216. Parsons R, Li GM, Longley MJ, et al. Hypermutability and mismatch repair deficiency in RER+ tumor cells. Cell. 1993;75:1227-1236.

217. Cahill DP, Kinzler KW, Vogelstein B, Lengauer C. Genetic instability and darwinian selection in tumours. Trends Cell Biol. 1999;9:M57-60.

218. Ionov Y, Peinado MA, Malkhosyan S, et al. Ubiquitous somatic mutations in simple repeated sequences reveal a new mechanism for colonic carcinogenesis. Nature. 1993;363:558-561.

219. Cahill DP, Lengauer C, Yu J, et al. Mutations of mitotic checkpoint genes in human cancers. Nature. 1998;392:300-303.

220. Mitelman F, Johansson B, Mertens F. The impact of translocations and gene fusions on cancer causation. Nat Rev Cancer. 2007;7:233-245.

221. Rabbitts TH. Chromosomal translocations in human cancer. Nature. 1994;372:143-149.

222. Rowley JD. Chromosome translocations: dangerous liaisons revisited. Nat Rev Cancer. 2001;1:245-250.

223. Folkman J. What is the evidence that tumors are angiogenesis dependent? J Natl Cancer Inst. 1990;82:4-6.

224. Folkman J, Watson K, Ingber D, Hanahan D. Induction of angiogenesis during the transition from hyperplasia to neoplasia. Nature. 1989;339:58-61.

225. Folkman J. Angiogenesis. Annu Rev Med. 2006;57:1-18.

226. Neufeld G, Cohen T, Gengrinovitch S, Poltorak Z. Vascular endothelial growth factor (VEGF) and its receptors. FASEB J. 1999;13:9-22.

227. Fong GH, Klingensmith J, Wood CR, et al. Regulation of flt-1 expression during mouse embryogenesis suggests a role in the establishment of vascular endothelium. Dev Dyn. 1996;207: 1-10.

228. Shalaby F, Rossant J, Yamaguchi TP, et al. Failure of blood-island formation and vasculogenesis in Flk-1-deficient mice. Nature. 1995;376:62-66.

229. Gupta GP, Massague J. Cancer metastasis: building a framework. Cell. 2006;127:679-695.

230. Chambers AF, Groom AC, MacDonald IC. Dissemination and growth of cancer cells in metastatic sites. Nat Rev Cancer. 2002;2:563-572.

231. Fidler IJ. The pathogenesis of cancer metastasis: the "seed and soil" hypothesis revisited. Nat Rev Cancer. 2003;3:453-458.

232. Cavallaro U, Christofori G. Cell adhesion and signalling by cadherins and Ig-CAMs in cancer. Nat Rev Cancer. 2004; 4:118-132.

233. Stupack DG, Teitz T, Potter MD, et al. Potentiation of neuroblastoma metastasis by loss of caspase-8. Nature. 2006;439: 95-99.

234. Mehlen P, Puisieux A. Metastasis: a question of life or death. Nat Rev Cancer. 2006;6:449-458.

235. Allinen M, Beroukhim R, Cai L, et al. Molecular characterization of the tumor microenvironment in breast cancer. Cancer Cell. 2004;6:17-32.

236. Orimo A, Gupta PB, Sgroi DC, et al. Stromal fibroblasts present in invasive human breast carcinomas promote tumor growth and angiogenesis through elevated SDF-1/CXCL12 secretion. Cell. 2005;121:335-348.

237. Kaplan RN, Psaila B, Lyden D. Bone marrow cells in the "premetastatic niche": within bone and beyond. Cancer Metastasis Rev. 2006;25:521-529.

238. Kaplan RN, Riba RD, Zacharoulis S, et al. VEGFR1-positive haematopoietic bone marrow progenitors initiate the pre-metastatic niche. Nature. 2005;438:820-827.

4 Targeted Approaches to Drug Development

Kimberly Stegmaier and William R. Sellers

With the discovery of nitrogen mustard as an anticancer agent in the 1940s, medicinal and hence systemic cancer therapy became a reality. The identification and application of cytotoxic agents dominated the next 60 years of cancer treatment. Today, we are embarking on a new era of targeted therapy, heralded by the success of imatinib for BCR-ABL rearranged chronic myelogenous leukemia (CML). There is much to learn from the 60-year experience in empirically based therapy that should be directly applicable in the development of molecularly targeted therapy. Cytotoxic chemotherapy, although often regarded as largely unsuccessful, has led to substantial cure rates for a number of well-defined malignancies. In this chapter, we will discuss the fundamental concepts, advantages, and disadvantages of cytotoxic cancer therapy and their relevance to targeted drug therapy for malignancy. We will define targeted therapy, including its advantages and disadvantages, discuss the credentialing of targets, and provide a system for categorizing classes of targets and classes of therapies. We will then focus on particular lessons learned in the early development and testing of new targeted therapies for adult malignancies, with examples from each of the target classes. Our intent is to highlight illustrative examples rather than provide an exhaustive list of all targeted therapies in development. We will conclude with a discussion of the challenges regarding the development of targeted therapies for children and highlight emerging pediatric cancer-based targets.

TRADITIONAL CHEMOTHERAPY

Conventional Chemotherapeutic Approaches

Although we tend to view conventional chemotherapy agents as nonspecific cytotoxics, over the years we have gained insight about the mechanism of action in killing tumor cells. In general, these agents were designed to interfere with molecular pathways required for nucleotide synthesis, DNA replication, and the mechanics of cell division. Thus, these agents have significant, but often predictable, or at least stereotypical, morbidity related to the suppression of hematopoiesis or of the cell division process required for the homeostasis of other organ systems. Following is a brief description of common classes of cytotoxic chemotherapeutic agents widely used in pediatric oncology.

Alkylating Agents

The alkylating agents are chemically reactive compounds that bind covalently to alkyl groups, particularly those on DNA, forming DNA-DNA and DNA-protein cross-links. These compounds can be monofunctional or bifunctional alkylators, which elicit a DNA damage response resulting in apoptosis. Commonly used alkylating agents in pediatric oncology include the nitrogen mustard analogues (cyclophosphamide, ifosfamide, and melphalan), the nitrosoureas (carmustine and lomustine), and busulfan. Other known conventional chemotherapy agents with a similar mechanism of action are the platinum compounds, including the commonly used agents cisplatin and carboplatin. These drugs are heavy metal coordination complexes that form reactive aquated intermediates in solution that then bind to DNA and initiate intra- and interstrand cross-links.

Antimetabolites

The antimetabolites are agents that inhibit the synthesis of RNA or DNA or are incorporated into DNA and RNA, creating defective products. Commonly used antimetabolites for pediatric cancer fall into two main categories:

1. Structural analogues of intermediates in the biosynthesis of nucleotides, such as purine analogues (mercaptopurine and thioguanine) and pyrimidine analogues (cytarabine, gemcitabine, and fluorouracil).
2. Structural analogues of vital cofactors in the synthesis of nucleotides, such as the folic acid analogue methotrexate. Methotrexate inhibits dihydrofolate reductase, the enzyme that converts folate to the active tetrahydrofolate form.

Topoisomerase Inhibitors

Most of the topoisomerase inhibitors now clinically available were not identified by rational approaches designed to target this enzyme class. Rather, they were identified as cytotoxic agents with anticancer activity and then later characterized to have this mechanism of action. One example is camptothecin. The anticancer activity of camptothecin was discovered in 1966, but its activity as a topoisomerase I inhibitor was not discovered until 1980.[1]

Topoisomerases are nuclear enzymes that alter the supercoiling of DNA. Their activities are essential to the replication, repair, and transcription of DNA. Topoisomerase I changes the degree of supercoiling by cleaving one strand and religating, whereas topoisomerase II cleaves both strands of DNA. Normally, topoisomerase strand breaks are present at a low steady-state level in the cell. Conditions that increase the level of these topoisomerase–DNA cleavage complexes are injurious to the cell.[2] Camptothecin binds to topoisomerase I, stabilizes the topoisomerase I–DNA cleavage complex that forms during replication, and prevents religation. The collision of the replication fork with the cleaved strand of DNA causes an irreversible double-strand break, an event that can trigger cell death.[3] Irinotecan and topotecan, two commonly used topoisomerase I inhibitors, were identified as analogues of camptothecin in a search to identify compounds with better aqueous solubility and reduced toxicity.

The topoisomerase II inhibitors increase the steady state of the topoisomerase II–DNA cleavage complexes and thus poison the cell by excess complex formation, leading to apoptosis. The topoisomerase II inhibitors are thought to work either by enhancing the forward rate of DNA cleavage complex formation or by inhibiting the ability of the enzyme to religate DNA.[4] One example is the anthracycline class (doxorubicin and daunorubicin), which represents some of the earlier drugs used to treat malignancy. The anthracyclines are cytotoxic antibiotics produced by the microorganism *Streptomyces*. Their cytotoxic effects are likely multifactorial. In part, these compounds may exert their damaging effects on cells by mediating free radical formation, with subsequent damage to cell membranes and DNA. More recently, however, their inhibition of topoisomerase activity has been characterized.[5] The anthracyclines intercalate into DNA and subsequently interfere with the activity of topoisomerase II, producing DNA strand breaks. Mitoxantrone and dactinomycin are two other antibiotic cytotoxics that bind to DNA and have topoisomerase-mediated DNA breaks as their mechanism of action. Epidophyllotoxins (etoposide and teniposide) are another class of agents that inhibit topoisomerase II. These are semisynthetic analogues of the natural product, podophyllotoxin. They stabilize the covalent bond between DNA and topoisomerase II and impair the ability of the enzyme to religate DNA.

Inhibitors of Microtubule Formation

Disruption of microtubule formation interferes with several cellular processes, including mitotic spindle formation, leading to metaphase arrest during mitosis, as well as cell migration and axonal transport. The *Vinca* alkaloids, derived from leaf extracts of the periwinkle plant, including vincristine and vinblastine, are mitotic inhibitors that bind to tubulin, disrupting its polymerization and the formation of microtubules. In contrast, paclitaxel, a diterpene derivative isolated from the bark of the Western Yew, *Taxus brevifolia*, binds to and stabilizes the microtubule, hence preventing depolymerization.[6]

Lessons Learned from Cytotoxic Chemotherapy

Although the use of cytotoxic chemotherapeutic agents is an imperfect science, we have learned many lessons over the years about the medicinal treatment of cancer that should be strongly considered in the development of targeted therapy (Box 4-1).

Combination Therapy: Required for Cure

There are several goals of combination therapy. First, because it is difficult to predict which single agent will be most effective against an individual patient's tumor, the use of multiple drugs increases the potential for an initial complete response. Second, combination therapy can prevent the development of tumor resistance. Third, drug combinations may have additive or synergistic interactions, increasing the total activity of the drugs and potentially enabling lower dosing and less toxicity. One example is the successful dose reduction of cytotoxic chemotherapy with the addition of all-*trans* retinoic acid (ATRA) for the treatment of patients with acute promyelocytic leukemia (APL).[7,8] With few exceptions, curative systemic therapy has required the combination of highly active agents rather than combinations of active and inactive agents.

The need for multiagent therapy was first appreciated in the treatment of acute lymphoblastic leukemia (ALL). Estimates are that at best, 60% of patients will achieve complete remission with single-agent chemotherapy. Despite continued use, almost all patients will relapse within 6 to 9 months with single-agent therapy. However, complete remission rates exceed 95% in patients treated with combination chemotherapy, and cure rates today for children with ALL exceed 80% with multiagent treatment regimens.[9,10] Similarly, patients with acute promyelocytic leukemia (APL) had very poor remission and cure rates until the discovery of ATRA differentiation therapy for this disease. ATRA achieved a high complete remission rate in use as a single agent, but almost all patients ultimately relapsed.[11,12] It was not until the combination of cytotoxic chemotherapy with ATRA that these patients achieved the best long-term survival rates of any acute myeloblastic leukemia (AML) subtype.[7] Furthermore, even with already existing three-drug regimens, the addition of new agents can enhance long-term survival. This is well illustrated with the improvement of relapse-free survival for patients with Ewing's sarcoma

through the addition of etoposide and ifosfamide to the backbone of cyclophosphamide, doxorubicin (Adriamycin), and vincristine treatment regimens. In this case, the 5-year event-free survival increased from 54% to 69%.[13]

Appropriate Dose for Improved Outcome

A guiding principle in the delivery of cytotoxic chemotherapeutic agents is the concept of the maximum tolerated dose (MTD), the simple idea that more is better. Drugs are delivered at the maximum dose possible, a dose above which unacceptable toxicity is encountered. Here, without a clear cellular biomarker of cytotoxic activity, it is not possible to relate the maximum molecular effect to maximum achievable efficacy. Thus, cytotoxic drugs are first evaluated in phase I studies with the primary study goal of establishing the maximum tolerated dose. Subsequent phase II and III trials are then based on this dosing schedule. MTD assumes that some toxicity is acceptable and, in fact, expected in the pursuit of cure. The most extreme example of this concept has been the use of autologous stem cell transplantation to deliver what otherwise would be lethal doses of chemotherapy. In this case, the MTD is surpassed by replacing the dose-limiting factor, the hematopoietic system, with stem cells harvested from the patient prior to delivery of the conditioning chemotherapy. Although a brute force approach in its nature, the MTD paradigm also established an important corollary—significant side effects can be tolerated when therapy is administered with curative intent (see later).

Many retrospective studies of chemotherapy dose intensity and outcome have supported this premise, particularly in the pediatric setting. In high-stage neuroblastoma, the addition of dose intensification with stem cell transplantation has improved the outcome for patients with metastatic disease.[14-17] In pediatric ALL, several studies have suggested that dose intensification is important for long-term outcome, including one randomized study comparing standard versus dose-reduced methotrexate and mercaptopurine.[18-21] In contrast to the results of retrospective studies, fewer prospective studies have been performed to address the issue of dose intensity and outcome for pediatric tumors. Importantly, as these studies begin to emerge, some of our prior concepts about MTD have come into question. For example, retrospective studies have supported the notion that doxorubicin and/or methotrexate dose intensity is important for outcome in patients with localized high-grade osteosarcoma.[22,23] However, recent prospective studies involving large patient numbers have called into question the role of further dose intensification for this disease.[24,25] Furthermore, randomized trials for malignancies such as breast cancer have demonstrated that massively increasing dose with stem cell transplantation does not always improve long-term survival.[26,27] Conducting well-controlled prospective trials is critical to address the issue of dose intensification, even for cytotoxic agents.

Toxicity Acceptable with Curative Therapy

The oncology community has accepted toxicity as inherent in the mission of cure. With the implementation of dose-intensive regimens, however, comes additional toxicity. Because of the relatively nonspecific nature of traditional chemotherapy, morbidity from these treatment regimens is significant. Acute toxicity takes the form of infection, transfusion dependence, renal injury, and hepatic injury. There are also the potential long-term consequences such as cardiac injury, infertility, chronic renal insufficiency, hearing loss, skeletal injury, and secondary malignancies.[28] Ongoing efforts are focused on decreasing these short- and long-term side effects. For example, to minimize acute toxicity, chemotherapy dosing is usually individualized based on body surface area (mg/m^2). For some cytotoxic agents such as methotrexate and busulfan, drug levels can be monitored to minimize toxicity. In the case of busulfan, adjustments can be made to subsequent dosing. For methotrexate, hydration can be increased to facilitate drug clearance, and leucovorin (folinic acid) can be adjusted to rescue normal cells from toxicity. Dose intensity can also be achieved with regional tumor delivery, growth factor support, or rescue with stem cells. Furthermore, better supportive care, such as infection prophylaxis, has enabled tolerance of prolonged immunosuppression. To decrease long-term morbidity, safe maximum cumulative doses are being established, such as maximum cumulative doxorubicin to minimize late cardiac effects. Furthermore, new supportive agents are in development and have been incorporated into clinical practice, such as dexrazoxane used with anthracyclines to prevent long-term cardiac toxicity.[29,30] Although toxicity can be tolerated, it is essential that the level of toxicity be commensurate with the level of benefit. Marginally effective therapeutic regimens that result in substantial toxicity should not become accepted standards.

Establishment of Curative Regimens with Attempts to Reduce Toxicity.

Most of the pediatric malignancies, including ALL and the solid tumors, have used disease stratification to decrease dose in treatment regimens. A dose-intensive regimen is initially used to establish efficacy. Then, good-prognosis patients are treated with less intensive regimens with the goal of comparable disease-free outcomes but decreased treatment-related morbidity. This is particularly important for pediatric disease, in which the long-term toxicity of treatment is experienced over a lifetime. Historically, these stratifications were based on features such as age, stage, and histology, but now include molecular genetic markers, such as N-myc amplification in neuroblastoma, and mixed-lineage leukemia (MLL) rearrangement in pediatric ALL. For example, the National Wilms' Tumor Study (NWTS3) evaluated a half-dose chemotherapy regimen for infants with low-risk disease in an attempt to decrease the incidence of toxic deaths without compromising long-term survival. The infants had acceptable toxicity, with no toxic deaths, and long-term survival was not compromised.[31] A similar approach has been taken with infants and young children with low-stage neuroblastoma.[32,33]

As our understanding of the molecular basis of malignancy improves, so will our ability to develop fine-grained prognostic categories and patient-tailored treatment regimens, perhaps even for traditional chemotherapy agents. As we implement targeted therapy, it is expected that disease stratification and patient selection will be based on molecular genetic findings related to the credentialed target. In the clinical development of targeted therapies, we must continue to consider these key concepts—combination therapy, appropriate dose intensification, tolerance of toxicity for substantial efficacy and cure, and treatment adjustment in established favorable prognostic groups.

Inadequacies of Cytotoxic Chemotherapy

Although we have made great strides with the current cytotoxic armamentarium, further strides in the treatment of cancer are limited with this approach alone. Several shortcomings of this approach are intimately related to the lack of specific target knowledge (Box 4-2):

1. Toxicity is significant.
2. Optimization of anticancer effect versus side effects is difficult.

Box 4-2	**Shortcomings of Cytotoxic Chemotherapy**

Toxicity is significant.
Optimization of anticancer effect versus side effects is difficult.
Mechanistic understanding of nonresponding and resistant disease is lacking.
Predictors of patient response to a specific drug are poor.
Cytotoxics have explored a narrow range of cellular and molecular mechanisms.

---

3. Mechanistic understanding of nonresponding and resistant disease is lacking.
4. Predictors of patient response to a specific drug are poor.
5. To date, cytotoxics have explored a narrow range of cellular and molecular mechanisms.

One major shortcoming of cytotoxic therapy is morbidity. Because these agents are relatively nonspecific, there is significant toxicity to normal host cells. Patients can expect to experience short- and long-term morbidity from these drugs and even incur the risk of therapy-related fatality. Furthermore, because the most relevant targets of these drugs are poorly understood, it is difficult to optimize the anticancer effect versus the toxicity, and it is difficult to separate on-target from off-target toxicities. Often, there is no relationship between the administered dose (pharmacokinetics) or the maximum tolerated dose and inhibition of the putative target (pharmacodynamics). Developing a strong correlation between the pharmacokinetics of a drug and its pharmacodynamic effect is obviously impossible when the target of a drug is frankly unknown. Similarly, in the absence of target knowledge, our understanding of resistant or refractory disease is poor at best, and it is very difficult to predict a priori who will respond to a given treatment. This has necessitated long clinical development programs with large trials to identify responsive subpopulations of patients and then follow-up trials to investigate responses in this patient subset more thoroughly. Targeted therapy has the potential to address these shortcomings, enable more rational tumor specific therapy with less morbidity, and explore previously unexploited cancer-related molecular mechanisms. With the sequencing of the human genome, the development of high-throughput genomic technologies, and an ever-increasing understanding of the molecular pathogenesis of cancer, this promise is likely to be realized.

INTRODUCTION TO TARGETED THERAPY

What is Targeted Therapy?

Targeted therapy can be defined as a therapeutic modality whose preclinical development focused on the modulation of a single molecular target, typically inhibition but occasionally activation of the molecular entity. Targeted therapy relies on the concept of cancer cell dependence—that is, the malignant cell or tumor as a whole is dependent for its survival or proliferation on the particular gene product or pathway. The discovery of targeted therapy differs significantly from that of cytotoxic therapy. Historically, cytotoxic therapy discovery relied on simple, phenotypic cell death assays, in which small molecule libraries were screened in vitro against a panel of cancer cell lines. Because cytotoxic compounds are believed to cause

Box 4-3	Advantages of Targeted Therapy

Improved patient selection is enabled.

Drug efficacy and target inhibition are linked, enabling rational dosing.

Side effects are more predictable.

Understanding of target and pathway increases options for the subsequent development of therapeutics with improved efficacy.

The mechanisms of resistance may, in some cases, be more readily discovered and interdicted with second-generation therapeutics.

Rational pathway-based combination regimens can be tested.

nonspecific cell death, effective compounds should theoretically have activity in all cancer types. In practice, however, this has not proven to be the case. Thus, although phenotypic screens may be of significant value in identifying molecules with complex mechanisms of action, the direct prediction of clinical efficacy from limited in vitro testing remains problematic. This is in sharp contrast to the concept of targeted therapy.

There are three critical elements to the implementation of targeted therapy. First, based on available data, a hypothesis is generated suggesting a causal or pathogenic link between a specific protein or gene (the potential drug target) and cancer. Then, experiments are performed and data generated to test the validity of this hypothesis. Is this candidate target relevant to oncogenesis or the maintenance of the malignant phenotype? Second, there must be a valid therapeutic approach to interfering with the target activity through small molecules, antibodies, or protein-based biologicals. Third, one must estimate the likely impact of target manipulation on a relevant clinical application. For example, a targeted therapeutic may have limited clinical application if the disease state is already readily cured. The process of evaluating potential targets that emerge is target validation.

Advantages of Targeted Therapy

Targeted therapy offers several potential advantages over nonspecific cytotoxic treatments (Box 4-3):

1. Improved patient selection is enabled.
2. Drug efficacy and target inhibition are linked, enabling rational dosing.
3. Side effects are more predictable.
4. Understanding of target and pathway increases options for the subsequent development of therapeutics with improved efficacy.
5. The mechanisms of resistance may, in some cases, be more readily discovered and interdicted with second generation therapeutics.
6. Rational pathway-based combination regimens can be tested.

For example, hormone therapy has become the standard of care for patients with estrogen receptor–positive breast cancer. In this case, there is a lineage-dependent target in the malignant cell, the estrogen receptor (ER), and antiestrogen agents, such as tamoxifen, have been developed to inhibit competitive binding of estrogen to the estrogen receptor. Numerous studies exploring estrogen antagonist therapy with tamoxifen for patients with ER-positive versus ER-negative disease have

demonstrated benefit only in the ER-positive patients.[34-37] In conjunction with diagnostic tools to identify hormone receptor status, patients are now rationally chosen for therapy, thus eliminating exposure to drug toxicity for patients not likely to respond and enhancing the apparent efficacy.

A second advantage of targeted therapy is the strong link between the target inhibition and efficacy. The dosing goal is achievement of complete target inhibition, not a maximum tolerated dose. Thus, there is no need to suffer undue toxicity in the achievement of an MTD. Studies have shown that tamoxifen treatment responses do not correlate with serum levels and that higher doses do not necessarily increase efficacy.[38,38a]

A related third advantage of targeted therapy is that the side effects can generally be anticipated and serve as a marker for on-target inhibition. For example, the side effects of tamoxifen are predominantly related to the antiestrogen effects of this drug—vaginal dryness, hot flashes, and irregular menses. Because this drug also has proestrogen effects, thromboses and endometrial cancer can be seen.

A fourth advantage of targeted therapy is that understanding of the target and pathway increases the possibilities for therapy design. In the case of modifying estrogen receptor signaling, there are several methods to accomplish this other than direct ER antagonism. One method is to decrease ovarian production of estrogen with luteinizing hormone–releasing factor (LHRF) agonists, which induces a medical ovarian ablation. A second method of interfering with estrogen receptor signaling is to decrease estrogen production via inhibition of aromatase activity. Aromatase belongs to the group of cytochrome P-450 enzymes involved in steroid biosynthesis in muscle, fat, liver, and breast tumor cells and is the final enzyme in estrogen synthesis, converting the androgens androstenedione and testosterone to the estrogens estrone and estradiol. Aromatase inhibitors work by decreasing this conversion, thus decreasing circulating estrogens, and have been shown to have efficacy in breast cancer. Aromatase inhibitors have improved efficacy over tamoxifen and have the advantage of fewer side effects in terms of hot flashes, endometrial disease, and ischemic cerebrovascular effects.[39,40] However, they do have the on-target side effects of bone fractures and musculoskeletal disorders.[41,42] Because of the clear dependence of some breast cancers on estrogen receptors, and detailed knowledge regarding estrogen biosynthesis and signaling, multiple agents could be developed to inhibit this pathway.

The fifth advantage of targeted therapeutics is the ability to understand the molecular mechanisms associated with resistance more readily. Although this has not been the case in understanding the resistance to hormone therapy in breast cancer, the success of targeted inhibition of BCR-ABL in CML and of epidermal growth factor receptor (EGFR) in lung cancer was rapidly followed by the specific elucidation of direct resistance mutations in the target, leading to decreased activity of the relevant small-molecule inhibitors imatinib, erlotinib, or gefitinib, respectively.[43,44] In the case of CML, new agents were soon developed to treat resistant patients by specifically interfering with the mutant BCR-ABL proteins.[45]

The final advantage of targeted therapies may be their ability to generate rational and novel combination regimens. Currently, the vast majority of combination strategies are based on combining a novel agent with components of existing standards of care, without regard to mechanism. This strategy is largely based on clinical expedience, existing clinical efficacy (for the standard of care), and tolerability. The difficulty of empirically discovering new synergistic combinations stems from the large number of permutations required to test all possible combinations against multiple in vitro and in vivo models, or multiple cancer types. Targeted therapeutics are often related to one another in the context of a pathway. This allows specific pathway-related hypotheses to be tested. For example, combinations might target upstream and downstream components of the same pathway to defeat feedback mechanisms, target components of parallel pathways to defeat pathway redundancy, or target distinct antiproliferative and prosurvival pathways. The ongoing clinical development of combinations of inhibitors of mTOR with anti–vascular endothelial growth factor receptor (VEGF) or anti-KDR therapeutics is an example of a rational combination attacking upstream and downstream components of the hypoxia-signaling cascades.

Classes of Targets

Much current cancer therapy development focuses on specific changes that alter the malignant cell, setting it apart from its normal counterpart and creating distinct molecular or pathway dependence for cell survival and replication. These may be genetic mutations, gene rearrangements, epigenetic modifications such as altered patterns of methylation or acetylation, lineage legacies, or other metabolic liabilities. Genes whose expression and activation have been increased, resulting in a cancer-dependent state, are prime targets for therapy development. On the basis of cancer dependencies, cancer targets can be categorized into four classes: genetic, lineage, host, and synthetic lethal or empirical (Box 4-4).[46] Some targets may cross over from one class to another, but this classification may be useful for the design of clinical trials and elucidation of the parallel biomarker strategy.

Genetics Track

The genetics track relies on the idea that a cancer develops from a finite number of genetic alterations, these alterations give the malignant cell a selective advantage, and these genetic changes are passed on during malignant cell replication. Furthermore, the malignant cell becomes dependent on a set of these changes for continued survival, a process sometimes termed *oncogene addiction*.[47,48] This cancer cell dependence or addiction should provide a window for drug specificity for the malignant cell compared with normal cells. Targeted therapeutics that take advantage of genetic abnormalities should, in theory, be more injurious to the malignant cell than to the normal cellular counterpart. Advances in cytogenetic studies, high-throughput gene sequencing, detection of copy number alteration, whole genome expression profiling, and proteomic approaches have revolutionized candidate genetic target discovery. Now, tens of thousands of genes in hundreds of tumor samples can be analyzed simultaneously. These candidate targets must then be carefully credentialed for their suitability as a drug target. Is there cancer cell dependence on the genetic abnormality, and can the target be pharmacologically manipulated? Imatinib is one of a number of examples of clinically validated targeted therapeutics that exploit a genetic dependence, in this case the dependence of CML on the activity of the Abelson kinase (ABL). The very existence of the cancer dependent state is dramatically illus-

trated by the emergence of resistance mechanisms that largely appear to restore Abelson activity (see later).

Lineage Track

Cancer cells often maintain developmental features of the lineage from which they were derived. This is well supported with gene expression studies that have reported tumor cells more closely resembling the normal lineage counterpart than tumors of a different cell type. The notion that lineage or legacy features of a tumor cell may be exploited with targeted therapy is known as lineage addiction.[49] One of the earliest examples of the success of this approach has been the antagonism of estrogen receptor and its signaling pathway in patients with ER-positive breast cancer. Similarly, the vast majority of patients with prostate cancer derive significant benefit from antagonism of the androgen receptor (AR). In both ER-positive breast cancer and in prostate cancer, almost all of which express AR, the emergence of hormone-refractory disease largely appears to rely on mechanisms that restore steroid receptor signaling.[50] Thus, as in the case of imatinib resistance, the dependent state is illustrated by these resistance mechanisms.

Host Track

The importance of tumor cell environment to the development and maintenance of the malignant state has become increasingly recognized and represents another potential inroad to targeted therapy. It is possible that tumors, by evolving in a particular environmental context, may become dependent on certain growth factors or neighboring cells for survival in that niche. Two tumor-environment interactions have been exploited clinically to date. Preclinical evidence has suggested that many tumors require new blood vessel development for their growth and maintenance. The identification of these angiogenetic factors has enabled the development of modifiers of the angiogenetic process, leading to the successful clinical application of bevacizumab, an anti-VEGF antibody, for patients with colorectal cancer and the approval of KDR inhibitors (sunitinib and sorafenib) in renal cell carcinoma (see later). The interaction of tumors with the bone microenvironment has been targeted using inhibitors of osteoclastogenesis. Here, multiple bisphosphonate agents have been approved for the prevention of cancer-related fractures.[51]

Synthetic Lethal or Empirical Track

A number of highly efficacious anticancer agents do not conveniently map to the first three categories. The understanding of their mechanisms of efficacy remains opaque. Nonetheless, it is likely that these agents, including many of the cytotoxic agents described, take advantage of aspects of cancer cell biology that remain unknown, but may be broadly categorized as synthetic lethal interactions. Synthetic lethal genetic interactions are defined as mutations that are lethal in combination but that do not produce a lethal phenotype as a single event. Similarly, gain-of-fitness alterations in a malignant cell that give the cell a survival advantage may sensitize the cell to other stresses that have no consequence in a normal state but may be lethal with the malignancy-promoting alteration. Thus, cancer-promoting mutations give the malignant cell a survival advantage but may also incur a distinct liability that can be exploited therapeutically. Rather than two synthetic lethal genetic events, one can also apply synthetic lethal concepts to a preceding cancer-related molecular alteration followed by the application of a therapeutic modality. For example, many cancer cells have lost protective apoptotic signals in the process of becoming tumorigenic, such as with the overexpression of the antiapoptotic protein B-cell leukemia–lymphoma 2 (BCL2) family members. In this case, in which the cells are exquisitely sensitive to the antiapoptotic signal, restoration of the normal apoptotic pathway may result in selective death of these tumor cells.[52]

More recently, a striking synthetic lethal relationship was discovered between the loss of BRCA1 or BRCA2 function and inhibition of the poly(ADP-ribose) polymerase (PARP) I enzyme. Here, the loss of PARP1 was found to induce double-strand DNA breaks that required the recruitment of the RAD51 homologous recombination repair complex to the site of these breaks for effective repair. Because it was known that BRCA1 and 2 were required for RAD51 recruitment to such complexes, it was hypothesized that the loss of BRCA1 or BRCA2 would create sensitivity to PARP inhibition. This was demonstrated both with small interfering RNA (siRNA) and small-molecule inhibitors of PARP.[53] Moreover, clinical activity of PARP inhibitors has now been seen in BRCA1 and BRCA2 patients with ovarian or breast cancer in early clinical trials.[54]

Additional emerging examples of synergy in cancer therapy relates to novel agents that have specific cellular targets present in both cancer and in normal cells, but selectively induce cell death in cancer cells by unknown mechanisms. Examples of these include agents that modify epigenetic phenomena, such as histone deacetylase (HDAC) inhibitors and hypomethylating agents, proteosome inhibitors, and heat shock protein 90 (HSP90) inhibitors. In the case of the proteosome inhibitor bortezomib for multiple myeloma, it has been hypothesized that these malignant cells are highly dependent on the activity of nuclear factor-κB (NF-κB) and that inhibition of NF-κB with bortezomib inhibits cell growth and promotes death.[55] An alternative synthetic lethal hypothesis attempts to explain bortezomib activity as taking advantage of the high rates of protein production, and hence high dependence on folding and degradation pathways in myeloma cells.[56]

Credentialing Targets

By the strictest of measures, a drug target is not validated until a selective inhibitor of the target of interest has proven clinical activity and when resistance emerges through specific alterations in the direct target. Although few cancer targets have achieved this degree of validation, we can envision preclinical experimental methods that will allow one to credential a target for further drug discovery efforts. Toward this end, the goals are to build data sets proving or disproving certain target-based hypotheses and to use them to prioritize target selection for future drug discovery efforts. Three key questions regarding the relevance of any given target to anticancer therapy may be considered:

1. Is the activity of the target required for the development and maintenance of the cancer-dependent state?
2. Can a strategy be identified for developing a therapeutic agent for the target of interest?
3. Is there a clinical application for the eventual therapeutic agent?

We will focus on the approaches relevant to addressing the role of a given target in cancer dependence. There are two general sources of information: the study of a target in human cancers (target epidemiology) and the functional study of a target in model systems of tumor biology (functional validation; Box 4-5).

Target Epidemiology

Preclinical models of cancer are limited in number and in their qualitative relationship to human cancers. Comprehensive col-

---

Box 4-5	Credentialing Targets

TARGET EPIDEMIOLOGY: STUDY OF A TARGET IN HUMAN CANCERS

Target Expression
Genetic Alteration

Gain of function
  Translocation
  Activating point mutations
  Copy number gain
Loss of function
  Translocation
  Inactivating point mutations
  Deletion: Homozygous, heterozygous, loss of heterozygosity

Protein Epidemiology

FUNCTIONAL VALIDATION: STUDY OF A TARGET IN A MODEL SYSTEM OF TUMOR BIOLOGY

Gain of function: Address sufficiency of target
Loss of function: Address necessity of target

---

lections of human tumor specimens could, in theory, be used to study a given target in a large array of samples, broadly covering tissue distribution and stage distribution (primary versus metastatic sites). In practice, however, there are limited sets of comprehensive tumor collections and generally the largest tumor-type specific collections are limited to fixed, paraffin-embedded specimens. The availability of tissue samples paired with robust clinical data remains limited. Furthermore, the vast majority of human cancer collections come from surgical resection samples, which do not necessarily reflect the disease state in which a therapeutic agent will be initially tested. Despite these limitations, molecular epidemiology studies in tissue samples, enabled by emerging technologies, including tissue microarrays, single nucleotide polymorphism (SNP) arrays, expression microarrays, and reverse protein arrays, remain critical to establishing the cancer relevance of a given target.

Target Expression

The desire to discover genes selectively expressed in cancer led first to the development of differential expression methods, including the subtractive hybridization cDNA libraries, differential display, and serial analysis of gene expression (SAGE).[57,58] Following the elucidation of the human genome sequence and the development of DNA-based microarrays, comparative expression profiling largely replaced difference methods. In all cases, the basic premise has been to identify genes overexpressed in cancer based on the concept that overexpression will equate with increased sensitivity to target inhibition and hence serve to improve the therapeutic index. This idea, however, must be challenged and carefully considered for each target, because resistance to therapeutic agents can similarly be engendered through overexpression. Based on standard biochemical principles, increased target expression should shift inhibitory drug concentrations in the adverse direction. This is clearly the case in the amplification of dihydrofolate reductase (DHFR) in generating resistance to methotrexate.[59] Similarly, studies have suggested that increased expression of AR can lead to resistance to AR blockade.[50] Thus, caution is required before proceeding with target selection based solely on expression data in the absence of a demonstrated causal or functional link to the maintenance of a cancer state.

When overexpression is determined, there can be technical problems in the array-based approaches. Mean differences in the expression levels or values of genes determined when comparing tumor tissue with normal tissue is confounded by gene expression differences that arise from changes in the state of differentiation, changes in the extent of epithelial cells versus stromal cells in cancer samples,[60] and lack of an appropriate normal sample for comparison. This latter confounder is exemplified in ovarian cancer in which the normal cellular counterpart is a mesothelial cell rather than a germ cell taken from the bulk of the normal ovary. An advance in the use of gene expression profiles is the use of gene sets rather than single genes to interrogate array-based data.[61] Gene set enrichment analysis, for example, has been used to discover pathway activities upregulated in cancer when single-gene analysis did not provide the necessary biologic insight.[62] Another approach, known as outlier analysis, has been applied to the analysis of existing data sets searching for extreme expression differences in cancer subsets (i.e., a within-cancer comparison rather than normal cancer comparisons). In one remarkable example, cancer outlier profile analysis (COPA) allowed for the identification of novel translocations and oncogenes in prostate cancer, suggesting that such methods may be particularly useful for finding functionally relevant genes.[63]

Genetic Alterations

As illustrated by the success of all-*trans* retinoic acid (ATRA), trastuzumab, and imatinib, direct genetic alteration leading to gene activation of a given drug target remains perhaps the best evidence for the causal role of a given gene in carcinogenesis. Genetic alterations that occur frequently in a given tumor type and are present in most cells are a strong indicator of causality. In the era of large-scale resequencing projects, it is critical that one distinguishes driver mutations (causal mutations) from so-called passenger mutations.[64] In addition, driver mutations that arise late in the course of disease that are present in a minor fraction of the tumors, or that are present in only a fraction of tumor cells in a given single tumor, must be given less weight. These findings would suggest a reduced likelihood of this lesion possessing a strong causal link to the initiation of the disease state. The types of genetic alterations (e.g., point mutations, focal amplifications, broad amplifications, and translocations) are also distinguished with respect to the extent to which they can be used to establish causality or to infer dependence.

Gain-of-Function Genetic Alterations

Gain-of-function genetic alterations include translocations, activating point mutations, and increases in gene copy number. Translocations were among the earliest discovered genetic alterations initially described using chromosome spreads. This technique has enabled the discovery in hematologic malignancies, but discovery has been slower in solid tumors. New approaches to the discovery of chromosomal rearrangements include exon microarrays, which can potentially detect imbalanced or amplified translocations, COPA (see earlier), paired-end resequencing of BAC clones from a genomic library (giving a structural map of a cancer genome),[65] and new methods of single-molecule sequencing (see later). Translocations are highly informative with respect to causality because they typically alter only two genes and because background or random translocation events are rare.

Amplifications are now routinely detected by the methods of DNA copy number analyses—array comparative genomic hybridization (CGH) and high-density single nucleotide poly-

morphism (SNP) arrays. There are two general types of increases in gene copy, focal amplifications and broad copy number increases covering an entire chromosome or chromosome arm. With sufficient sample numbers, one can often discern one to several genes contained in a focal amplicon. Typically, the minimal region of amplification is a guide. However, newer methods for copy number alterations (i.e., genomic identification of significant targets in cancer [GISTIC]) also use the amplitude of amplification as an important parameter.[66] Although not definitive proof, amplification lends evidence to a causal relationship between a given gene within an amplicon and a cancer state. In some amplicons, multiple genes remain strong candidates for oncogenes targeted by the amplification. One notable example is the 11q13 amplification with genes, including *Cyclin D1*, *FGF3*, and *FGF4*.[67] In this case and other cases certain amplifications may require the upregulation of more than one gene. Noteworthy in this regard is the finding in mice that knockin of an activated Her2 allele results in breast cancers associated with amplification of the knocked-in allele and the coamplification of a number of genes, including *ERBB2* (*Her2*) itself, *GRB7* and *CAB1*, all of which are syntenic and amplified in Her2-positive breast cancer.[68]

Larger scale chromosomal alterations leading to trisomy or gain of an entire chromosome arm are frequent but more difficult to study. As such, identifying single genes (or drug targets) within such broad regions remains a challenge. In this case, the number of genes implicated in such large-scale alterations is so large that almost no importance can be ascribed to the cancer relevance of a gene contained in such broad chromosomal level alterations. Outlier analysis may begin to allow the elucidation of multigene targeting by such broad regions, and is illustrated by the analysis of trisomy 7 in glioma revealing a dependence on cMET and its ligand hepatocyte growth factor (HGF), both located on chromosome 7 (Fig. 4-1).[69]

Subtle nucleic acid level alterations, including point mutations and small insertions and deletions, are an important mechanism for the activation of oncogenes. Point mutations leading to the constitutive guanosine triphosphate (GTP)-bound and hence activated form of N-Ras and K-Ras,[70] as well as point mutations leading to activation of the BRAF kinase in melanoma, thyroid cancer, and colorectal cancer,[71] are examples of this mechanism. The initiation of large-scale sequencing projects has unveiled new mutations, activating oncogenes such as *EGFR*[44] and phosphatidylinositol 3-kinase catalytic subunit alpha (*PIK3CA*).[72] However, it has become apparent that the detection of so-called passenger mutations, constituting the background rate of mutation, can be a significant challenge. These passenger mutations must be separated from the more prevalent and recurrent driver mutations.[64] Such passenger mutations may be exceedingly high in certain types of tumors, particularly those bearing mutations in mismatch repair genes. In one case, inactivating mutations in the mismatch repair gene *MSH6* were discovered in glioma tumors recurring after treatment with temozolomide. Here, the sequencing of *MSH6* was triggered by the very high rate of observed passenger mutations in treated versus untreated tumors.[73,74] These data suggest that cautious interpretation of low-frequency events is warranted when considering mutation analysis from larger scale modalities. Sequencing technology itself is also advancing rapidly. Newer single-molecule sequencing platforms are now being developed by 454 Biotechnology[75] and Illumina/Solexa.[76] These methods provide extraordinary throughput and promise to allow the much deeper analysis of larger tumor and gene sets.

Loss-of-Function Genetic Alterations

Loss-of-function alterations usually do not directly indicate or point to a specific gene as a candidate drug target. However,

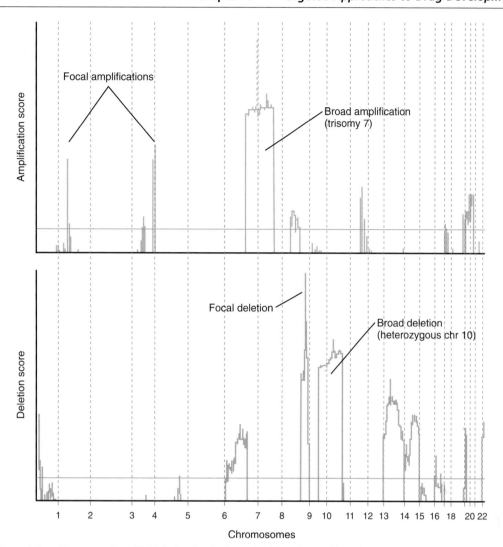

FIGURE 4-1. Determining glioma genetics with high-density single nucleotide polymorphism (SNP) analysis. High-density SNP arrays (Affymetrix) were used to derive DNA copy number information from a set of ~100 malignant glioma tumors. The panels show the amplification and deletion scores derived across the entire data set using a method known as GISTIC (genomic identification of significant targets in cancer). The y axis indicates the amplification or deletion score (roughly the frequency of each event multiplied by the amplitude) for each genome marker (or each SNP) and the x axis is a nonproportional ordering of the genome markers across the genome. The centromeres are represented by the dashed vertical lines. Examples of broad or focal amplifications and deletions are indicated in the figure. (Data from Beroukhim R, Getz G, Nghiemphu L, *et al.* Assessing the significance of chromosomal aberrations in cancer: methodology and application to glioma. Proc Natl Acad Sci U S A 2007;104:20007-20012.)

such alterations may predict sensitivity to agents acting against protein targets contained within downstream or parallel pathways. For example, clinical trials are underway testing inhibitors of mTOR function against sporadic tumors or hereditable cancer predisposition syndromes resulting from loss of the tumor suppressors phosphatase and tensin homologue (*PTEN*) and tuberous sclerosis 1 (*TSC1*) or *TSC2*. In both cases, loss-of-function mutations in these tumor suppressor genes are thought to lead to constitutive activation and hence constitutive dependence on mTOR (see later for the rationale).

Similarly, in the hedgehog pathway, a key development pathway regulating cell patterning, deletions, or mutations in the gene encoding the Patched receptor (PTCH) are associated with hereditary and sporadic basal cell carcinomas and sporadic medulloblastoma.[77-79] Loss of PTCH, a receptor for the ligands in the hedgehog family, leads to constitutive activation of the atypical G-protein–coupled receptor (GPCR)-like protein Smoothened (Smo).[80] Cyclopamine, a naturally derived inhibi-

tor of Smo, has significant activity in preclinical models lacking *PTCH* gene function.[81] These examples illustrate that identification of loss-of-function mutations can reveal downstream target molecules in critical cancer pathways.

Translocations are typically thought of as gain-of-function genetic events in that they act dominantly. However, they can functionally inactivate endogenous genes through the creation of dominant-negative protein fusions. For example, the PML-RARα fusion protein is believed to act, at least in part, as a dominant-negative inhibitor of endogenous RARα function.[82] This type of molecular action can be difficult to elucidate in functional experiments. Nonetheless, it is worth remembering this possibility when evaluating proteins or genes as drug targets when they are involved in new or existing translocations.

Chromosomal level alterations leading to loss-of-function events include homozygous deletions, heterozygous deletions, and loss of heterozygosity. Homozygous deletions are generally highly focal in their nature. When the boundaries are defined with large sample sets, often only a few genes are found in the overlapping region. For example, in the case of focal deletions on 9p, the typical minimal deleted regions in tumors such as melanoma contain only *INK4a* and *INK4b*.[83] Heterozygous deletions are typically larger and usually involve entire chromosomes or chromosome arms. As is the case with amplifications, such large-scale broad genetic alterations make it difficult to ascertain the cancer relevance of any single gene contained within a larger region. Loss of heterozygosity (LOH) can occur as an event associated with heterozygous deletion, leaving only one parental chromosome behind, which is thus homozygous. LOH can also occur in the setting of duplication of the remaining parental chromosome, creating a situation known as uniparental disomy. This may indicate preservation of a mutated allele, leading to two mutant alleles of a given gene. In the case of the tumor suppressor gene p53, copy-neutral LOH is common.

Inactivating point mutations are a common means for gene inactivation. In this case, stop codons are the most efficient mechanism for disrupting gene function. As a result, tumor suppressor gene mutations often are enriched for stop or truncating mutations. This creates certain technical and cost difficulties in sequencing genes for inactivating mutations because one needs to sequence all coding exons, consider sequencing of the regulatory elements governing splicing, and consider the detection of promoter mutations. As a result of these difficulties, there is an inherent underreporting bias for mutations in tumor suppressor genes.

Protein Molecular Epidemiology by Immunohistochemistry

It is important to understand the relationship between the expression or activity of a gene product and patient outcome or other clinicopathologic data. Whereas establishing a relationship between protein expression and clinical data (i.e., survival) does not provide a causal link to cancer, such linkage to patient outcome likely indicates a nonrandom association with cancer behavior. Here one should be careful to consider the relationship between protein expression and the state of differentiation of the cancer. Because the degree of cancer differentiation state, frequently referred to as grade, is usually already linked to patient prognosis, candidate drug targets whose protein levels vary with differentiation state may be secondarily linked to patient outcome. Thus, an independent association between a protein's expression and patient outcome should be sought in multivariate analysis. In the case of the targeted disruption of HER2 in patients with breast cancer, the association of *HER2* amplification with poor outcome has provided a significant motivation for the development of trastuzumab, an anti-HER2 monoclonal antibody.[84]

The ability to perform larger scale epidemiology analyses typically relies on archived tissue for which longer term clinical follow-up is available. This largely dictates that target epidemiology be carried out in paraffin-embedded fixed tissue. Here, RNA and DNA can be examined by in situ hybridization (ISH) or fluorescence in situ hybridization (FISH). However, the most common method for interrogating human tissue samples is protein-based immunohistochemistry (IHC). These studies have recently been expedited by the advent of tissue microarrays. These arrays align hundreds of tumor samples on a single slide, facilitating the experimental procedures. IHC is primarily limited by the quality of the antibody reagents used and the care with which such reagents are subject to rigorous validation. Too often, poorly described or unvalidated antibodies are used in IHC studies after a quality assessment based solely on the observed staining pattern in tissue sections. Whenever IHC is used, the controls should include experimental, fixed cell blocks derived from negative control cells or tissues known to lack the antigen of interest or from positive control cells or tissue known to harbor the antigen of interest. These controls can generally be obtained from blocks created from cell lines in which the negative controls can be generated using short hairpin RNAs (shRNAs). A common misconception is that preabsorption with immune peptide provides an appropriate negative control. Unfortunately, peptide blocking will block specific and nonspecific binding of the primary antibody and only controls for background staining of the secondary antibody.

Functional Studies to Address Cancer Dependence

Ideally, the functional relevance of a putative cancer target should be elucidated prior to embarking on the lengthy process of drug discovery. Here, the simple concept is that one would rather fail or invalidate a putative target in preclinical studies than fail later in clinical trials. Although there are a number of reasons for the failure of a given therapeutic agent in clinical development, presumably one should avoid failure because the drug is made against an irrelevant target. Hence, one should develop a robust understanding of the science surrounding a given drug target and relate this to cancer-relevant processes. It is useful to consider two questions in the context of designing experiments for functional validation. First, is the putative cancer target necessary for the maintenance of a cancer-related phenotype? Second, is the putative cancer target sufficient for inducing a cancer or transformation-related phenotype? These questions are generally addressed by experiments directed at inducing loss of function of the target (addressing necessity) or at inducing gain of function (addressing sufficiency).

Gain-of-Function Experiments

Gain of function of a given protein typically involves overexpression of the cDNA or of an activated allele generated by mutation. The functional consequences of gene activation are assayed first in in vitro growth assays, transformation assays, and cotransformation experiments. Typically, gain of function in transformation assays would be assessed in murine embryonic fibroblasts, immortalized NIH3T3 cells, or Rat1a fibroblasts. More recently, the ability to transform human primary epithelial cells has been made possible through the use of telomerase and has provided a set of new assays that can be used to measure the ability of a given gene to induce transformation in human cells.[85]

Short-term validation experiments using in vivo systems have become more attractive with the advent of tissue reconstitution murine models, enabling rapid genetic manipulation. Examples of this approach include the use of murine hematopoietic cells or murine fetal hepatoblast cells. In each case, retroviruses directing the expression of the relevant candidate oncogene can be introduced into the respective primary cells, which are then reintroduced into host animals. In the case of the hematopoietic reconstitution, host irradiation is required prior to reimplantation. For example, mutations in JAK2 discovered in myeloproliferative syndromes recapitulate the disease entity when reintroduced in retroviral vectors into the hematopoietic reconstitution system.[86-88] Similarly, the use of hepatoblasts has been useful in demonstrating that certain gene activation events can induce hepatocellular carcinoma.[89,90] These systems provide some of the speed and flexibility of in vitro systems but maintain the more authentic relationship between stroma and the generated tumor cells.

Fully genetically engineered models, including transgenic mice, can be useful in studying gene activation in the specific tissue of origin, depending on the extent to which promoter regulation can be used to direct gene expression to the indicated cell. More recently, knock-in animals have been generated in which mutant Ras alleles are reintroduced into the endogenous murine Ras gene locus.[91] These animals, generated through homologous recombination, can then be crossed with transgenic mice expressing Cre recombinase (Cre) in a tissue-specific manner or by exposure to Cre activity through the introduction of adenoviruses directing the expression of Cre in infected tissues. Cre-mediated activation of mutant Ras in knock-in mice bearing K-Ras mutations has been used to demonstrate sufficiency of K-Ras for the induction of lung adenocarcinomas,[91] carcinomas of the pancreas,[92] and myeloproliferative disease.[93] These engineered models also provide a stable resource for testing candidate drug compounds in highly defined mechanistically driven models.

Loss-of-Function Experiments

For many years, there were no feasible methods for readily inducing loss-of-function alterations in mammalian systems. Consequently, the elaboration of a cell-penetrating small molecule inhibitor or tool compound was one of the only ways to achieve the desired inhibitory effect. The development of robust siRNA methods, taking advantage of the endogenous siRNA processing systems, now allows for transient, stable, or regulated knockdown of almost any mammalian gene product.[94,95] This powerful tool is complemented by existing methods for loss of function, including the use of inhibitory antibodies for extracellular targets, soluble protein traps for extracellular ligands and receptors, dominant-negative proteins expressed from cDNAs, murine germline knockouts, and inducible knockouts. Generally, loss-of-function experiments would be attempted first in human cancer cell line models. Increasingly, cell line models are being characterized in greater genetic detail, enabling more rational selection of models for functional inactivation experiments. More recently, shRNAs have been merged with the bone marrow transplantation and the hepatoblast tissue reconstruction models described earlier (Fig. 4-2).[96] Finally, regulated germline shRNAs can now be engineered in the mouse as a rapid method for generating tissue-specific and temporally regulated gene knockdowns.[97]

Genetic Studies in Lower Organisms

The topic of genetic studies in lower organisms is too broad for a complete discussion in this chapter. However, it is worth noting the emerging usefulness of defining genetic dependence in the context of highly conserved pathways that are shared between mammals, flies (*Drosophila melanogaster*) and worms (*Caenorhabditis elegans*). In some cases, lower organisms have a reduced set of homologues for any given pathway member, and thus the necessity of a single gene can be tested directly. Although the relationship between a gene and cancer phenotype in these organisms cannot usually be established, the genetic dependence or epistatic relationships elucidated in such model systems have proven highly informative for human studies. A notable example is the discovery of the relationship between loss-of-function mutations in the TSC genes and activation of the mTOR and S6K (ribosomal S6 kinase) pathways. Specifically, loss-of-function studies have revealed that alterations in the function of the *TSC1* and *TSC2* genes, which give rise to the proteins hamartin and tuberin, are associated with the induction of a large-cell phenotype reminiscent of cell growth control problems elicited by the activation of S6K.[98-100] Moreover, additional studies have shown that loss-of-function mutations in S6K could complement and reverse the phenotype induced by the loss of *TSC2*.[98] These studies gave rise to the concept that mTOR inhibitors, which were known to block

S6K activity, might be capable of altering the tuberous sclerosis phenotype in humans. Clinical trials testing available mTOR inhibitors, including rapamycin, are underway and are beginning to show promise. Although many mammalian cell-based experiments helped solidify these results, the first and most important observation came from the genetic experiments carried out in *Drosophila*.

Target Credentialing Summary

The credentialing of drug targets ultimately must be thought of as a set of hypotheses to be tested experimentally. In each case, these hypotheses must be built around the relevant biology. Importantly, one must distinguish targets with cell autonomous effects versus those in which the interaction between cancer cell and host factors is critical. In the case of drug targets encoded by human oncogenes with definitive genetic alterations, one can have a high degree of confidence in the likely therapeutic effect of inhibitory molecules. Unfortunately, this group is the minority of drug targets for consideration. The intent of credentialing is therefore to enable a rational stratification of potential drug targets and a rational application of resources to specific drug discovery efforts.

Classes of Targeted Therapies

Targeted therapies can be divided into two main classes—drugs (small molecules, natural products, antisense, and siRNA) and biologicals (antibodies and proteins or peptides) (Box 4-6). Biologicals, as defined by the U.S. Food and Drug Administration (FDA), include a wide range of products, such as vaccines, blood and blood components, somatic cells, gene therapy, tissues, and recombinant therapeutic proteins. They can be composed of sugars, proteins, or nucleic acids or complex combinations of these substances, or may be living entities, such as cells and tissues. Biologicals are isolated from a variety of natural sources—human, animal, or microorganism—and may be produced by biotechnology methods. From a practical point of view, drugs entering the market require the filing of a new drug application (NDA) whereas biologicals require the filing of a biologic license application (BLA).

Drugs

Small molecules are defined as carbon-containing compounds that usually have a molecular weight less than 2000 g/mol. These small organic compounds have the advantage of purity, high permeability into target cells, ease of manufacturing, and

Box 4-6	**Classes of Therapies**
DRUGS	
Small molecules	
Natural products	
Antisense oligonucleotides	
RNA interference	
BIOLOGICALS	
Antibody	
Protein	
Whole protein	
Peptides	
Soluble receptors	

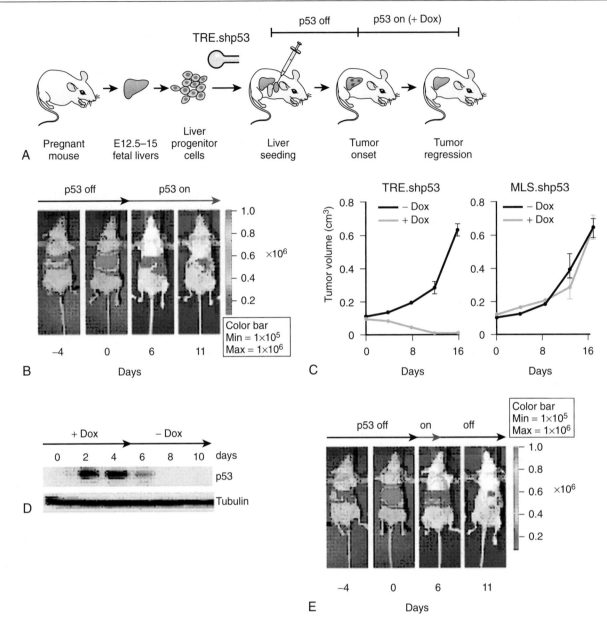

FIGURE 4-2. Reactivation of p53 results in liver tumor regression. **A,** Embryonic liver progenitor cells were transduced with a tetracycline-regulatable p53 shRNA (TRE.shp53), tTA, and H-rasV12. After onset of liver tumors, p53 expression could be restored by doxycycline (Dox) treatment. **B,** Reactivation of p53 leads to rapid tumor regression. Tumor-bearing mice were treated with Dox starting at day 0 and imaged at the indicated time points ($N = 9$). **C,** Subcutaneous tumors derived from ras-transformed liver progenitor cells with tet-off shRNA (TRE.shp53) or a nonregulatable shRNA (MLS.shp53) were grown in nude mice. Values represent mean SD ($N = 4$). **D,** p53 reactivation is reversed by Dox withdrawal. Protein lysates from liver progenitor cells pulse-treated with Dox for 4 days were immunoblotted for p53. **E,** Representative mice ($N = 6$) as in **B** were pulse-treated with Dox for 4 days and imaged at the indicated time. *(Adapted from Xue W, Zender L, Miething C, et al. Senescence and tumour clearance is triggered by p53 restoration in murine liver carcinomas. Nature. 2007;445:656-660.)*

stability, and remain the primary class amenable to oral delivery. However, there can be the disadvantages of insufficient selectivity, resulting in off-target toxicity, including cardiotoxicity, challenges with poor bioavailability, and challenges with metabolism of the molecule. Over the last decade, synthetic methods have been developed for producing a diversity of chemical structures using directed medicinal chemistry approaches or combinatorial chemistry, the synthesis of numerous organic compounds by combining variations of each of the building blocks that comprise the compounds.[101] More recently, the synthesis of small-molecule libraries exploring chemical

space more broadly has been undertaken through diversity-oriented synthesis (DOS). With DOS, chemists design branched reactions that provide diversity in the skeleton and stereochemical complexity of the small molecule in only three to four transformations.[102,103] In parallel, there has been the elaboration of a diverse set of methods for identifying the initial small-molecule hits against a desired target. High-throughput screening involves the in vitro assay of target activity against chemical libraries ranging in size from 1 to 4 million. In silico screening can be used to dock millions of compounds into known or modeled three-dimensional structures of a given target. Fragment-based screening uses x-ray or nuclear magnetic resonance (NMR)–based structural approaches to identify very-low-molecular-weight fragments that can interrogate the binding surface of a new target.[104] Finally, target-specific cell-based screening can be used to identify cell-penetrating small molecules perturbing a target-specific reporter or phenotype.

Natural products have been important in the development of drugs and have played a dominant role in cancer therapy.[105] Approximately 75% of the current anticancer drugs are natural products or natural product–derived.[106] The chemical diversity of natural products complements that of synthetic libraries. As a result of a long evolutionary process, natural products tend to be sterically complex, with greater diversity of ring systems compared with synthetic and combinatorial libraries. They also contain more carbon, hydrogen, and oxygen, and less nitrogen and other elements than synthetic library compounds, and have higher molecular masses.

Natural products are classified according to shared scaffolding elements and can be divided into several structural classes, such as terpenes, alkaloids, polyketides, and nonribosomal peptides. The building blocks for the natural products are usually monomeric components of primary metabolic pathways that are then shunted into secondary metabolic pathways. Plants and soil microbes are traditional sources of natural products, with new sources, such as fungi and marine life forms (i.e., sponges and algae), under active exploration.[107]

Drug development with natural products may have specific advantages over that of synthetic molecules. The complexity of natural products may lead to greater specificity. In addition, unanticipated mechanisms of action may be discovered that would be difficult to engineer into a small molecule. For example, rapamycin, derived from a soil fungus from Easter Island (Rapa Nui), creates a novel protein-drug-protein interaction between the protein FKBP12, rapamycin, and the mTOR kinase, resulting in an exquisitely selective inhibition of mTOR.[108,109] However, although the natural products have been developed into successful drugs, there are several disadvantages to these libraries. First, natural product extracts are generally impure, and hence identifying the active compound can be difficult. Second, the synthesis of these compounds in production-level quantities for medicinal purposes can be challenging. Third, subsequent optimization of the lead natural product can be difficult in the absence of a complete in vitro synthesis of the relevant natural product. New high-throughput strategies are under development to tackle roadblocks to the use of natural products for medicinal purposes.

Antisense oligonucleotides are single strands of short deoxynucleotide sequences (18 to 21 oligomers) that bind to a target mRNA sequence by Watson-Crick hybridization and induce transcript destruction. They interact with the target transcript with sequence specificity and inhibit production of the target protein by several potential mechanisms. First, they activate endogenous nucleases, such as RNAse H, which then cleave the RNA strand of an RNA-DNA heteroduplex. A second potential mechanism of antisense activity is a noncatalytic effect with steric inhibition of the translational machinery, with induction of translational arrest and inhibition of protein synthesis. A third mechanism is interference with normal RNA splicing, resulting in the inhibition of specific splice variants. Antisense therapeutics held the promise of pharmacologically inhibiting targets that had been intractable with small-molecule approaches. In theory, almost any gene can be targeted with antisense approaches with an expectation of high target selectivity. However, the development of antisense therapy has faced many challenges, and this approach has not yet realized significant clinical benefit. Early antisense therapy faced the problems of poor solubility, limited intracellular uptake, and rapid degradation. To overcome these issues, subsequent antisense therapy focused on modification of the backbone to which the nucleoside bases are attached. Such modifications include substitutions of the nonbridging oxygen atoms in the phosphodiester bond with a sulfur atom (phosphorothioates), modification of the sugar moiety to increase nuclease resistance and target RNA affinity, replacement of the deoxyribose phosphate backbone with a peptide-based backbone creating peptic nucleic acid (PNA) oligonucleotides, and replacement of the deoxyribose with a six-membered morpholino ring, together with the replacement of the charged phosphodiester linkages with a nonionic phosphorodiamidate backbone, creating so-called morpholino oligonucleotides.[110-112]

Despite these efforts, the use of antisense therapy for cancer has been disappointing. However, there have been some responses seen in clinical trials. Oblimersen (Genasense), a phosphorothioate antisense therapy targeting Bcl-2, has shown some activity in patients with heavily pretreated chronic lymphocytic leukemia (CLL).[113] Furthermore, recent studies from a randomized phase III trial for patients with relapsed or refractory CLL comparing fludarabine plus cyclophosphamide with or without oblimersen have demonstrated an increase in complete response and nodular partial response in patients in the oblimersen arm, particularly for those patients with fludarabine-sensitive disease.[114]

RNA interference (RNAi) is a more recent approach to nucleic acid-based therapy. Similar to antisense therapy, RNAi may have therapeutic application, particularly for targets that have been considered intractable by traditional drug discovery approaches. RNAi is a double-stranded RNA (dsRNA)–induced mechanism of gene silencing naturally occurring in plants and animals. Over the last few years, it has become possible to target almost any gene in the genome for knockdown with small dsRNA gene silencing using siRNAs or expressed shRNAs. The RNAi pathway is hypothesized to have evolved early in eukaryotes as a protection against viral and genetic pathogens. Double-stranded RNA viruses and genetic elements are subject to RNAi-dependent gene silencing as a means of cell-based immunity. Furthermore, endogenously expressed shRNAs may regulate gene expression during development through the RNAi pathway.[94,95]

RNAi begins with the conversion of dsRNA and shRNA into siRNAs by Dicer, an RNase III family nuclease, and then incorporation into a multiprotein-RNA complex called RISC (RNA-induced silencing complex).[115] This RNA-RISC complex then locates an mRNA sequence within the cytoplasm with homologous nucleotide sequence and induces cleavage of the mRNA. If exploited as a potential cancer therapy, RNAi has the following potential advantages: (1) relative specificity for a particular gene target; (2) efficiency with the potential to achieve over 90% knockdown; and (3) widespread applicability with the potential of targeting any gene in the human genome. Unlike antisense oligonucleotides, RNAi takes advantage of a naturally occurring cellular mechanism for gene silencing.

As is the case with oligonucleotides, there are obstacles to the development of RNAi-based therapies, including the difficulty of delivering large nucleic acid molecules to intracellular targets in humans. Unmodified siRNAs have a short half-life in human plasma and are rapidly excreted by the kidneys. Furthermore, to have activity, the siRNA or shRNA must reach the cytoplasm of the targeted cell, and naked siRNAs are not efficiently taken up by mammalian cells unaided. One method of delivering shRNA that is commonly used in the laboratory to develop stable knockdown is the use of viral vectors. However, with viral vector delivery, there remains significant concern regarding insertional mutagenesis, carcinogenesis, direct cellular toxicity, and short-lived on-target effects.[116-119] Other nonviral methods of delivery are actively under exploration. One possibility is to modify the siRNA chemically to increase its stability with modifications such as locked nucleic acid (LNA) residues[120,121] or phosphorothioates.[122] A second approach to increase the stability of the siRNA is to package it in liposomes[123] or other nanoparticles such as the cationic polymer polyethylenimine,[124] or to use cholesterol modifications.[125] These packaging systems can also be modified to contain tissue-specific homing signals, such as the attachment of specific antibodies. Despite the problems with delivery and stability of RNAi, novel therapeutics using RNAi have entered clinical trials. RNAi-based phase I trials have been initiated for respiratory syncytial virus (RSV) by Alnylam Pharmaceuticals and for age-related macular degeneration by Sirna Therapeutics and Acuity Pharmaceuticals.

Biologicals

Antibody therapy with monoclonal antibodies (MAbs) is an increasingly important mode of targeted therapy for cancer. Early attempts at antibody-based therapy with murine MAbs were limited by immunogenicity, short half-life in humans, and poor ability to activate human immune effector mechanisms. With the evolution of recombinant DNA technology, it now has become possible to create chimeric and humanized MAbs. This technology combines antibody-variable domains (murine, humanized, or human) involved in antigen recognition to human antibody-constant regions. Recombinant antibodies with human crystallizable fragment (Fc) regions are much less immunogenic in humans than murine MAbs and can facilitate the activation of immune effector mechanisms. Thus, recombinant MAbs may have the dual mechanism of anticancer activity secondary to the specificity of epitope targeting with the antigen-binding fragment (Fab) and the recruitment of immune effectors with the Fc region. As a direct effect of the MAb variable domain binding to the target, they can have antagonist effects on receptor-ligand interactions and receptor-receptor interactions or agonistic effects on the target's biologic activity. Second, if engineered to be of the immunoglobulin G1 (IgG1) subclass and contain an Fc region, they induce immune effector function against the target cell following their interactions with complement or with receptors for the Fc region, such as FcγR, a class of surface glycoproteins expressed predominantly on white blood cells. The Fc region interactions with FcγR can induce antibody-dependent cell cytotoxicity (ADCC), phagocytosis, endocytosis of immune complexes followed by antigen presentation, and release of inflammatory mediators.[126] Finally, antibodies can be linked to chemical moieties with additional antitumor activity, such as in gemtuzumab ozogamicin, in which an antibody to CD33 is conjugated to the antitumor antibiotic calicheamicin (see later).

Antibody-based therapy has several advantages when compared with small molecule–based treatment (Box 4-7). First, there is a high degree of specificity for the target of interest, resulting in reduced off-target effects. Second, from a development and production perspective, the bulk of the molecule is the same from one antibody-based product to another, with differences predominantly in the target-specific Fab region. This feature facilitates more rapid development of any new therapeutic MAb because most of the molecule has previously been optimized. Third, pharmacokinetic properties are similar from one antibody product to another, with the half-life of an infused antibody generally lasting 2 weeks. Unlike the case of small molecules, there is little antibody metabolism, thus eliminating a highly variable aspect of low-molecular-weight (LMW) drug development. Fourth, the spectrum of targets amenable to antibody-based therapeutics is largely distinct from small molecules and includes large extracellular domains and secreted ligands, which otherwise are undruggable.

On the other hand, there are several disadvantages of antibody-based therapy compared with small-molecule therapy. In its current conception, antibody-based therapies are generally delivered via an intravenous (IV) route of administration. Patients require IV access, with its inherent risks, and often require hospitalization or a clinic visit for treatment. However, with an increasing acceptance of home IV infusion therapy, this may become less of a disadvantage. A second disadvantage is that preclinical in vivo studies can be difficult to conduct.[127] One must address whether the antibody in development will recognize the appropriate antigen in the animal model being tested. In some cases, only primates conserve the relevant human epitope, limiting the selection of species available for toxicology studies. Efficacy studies, in particular against stromal or host factors, may require generation of a murine-equivalent antibody, although equivalence is difficult to quantitate. The robust evaluation of host effector function elicited by an antibody and the role of this function in antitumor activity is also difficult to assess in a typical human tumor xenotransplant study in rodents. A third challenge with antibody-based therapy is that the patient can develop neutralizing antibodies to the therapy. This has been particularly problematic with murine-based antibody therapy. Fourth, antibodies cannot access intracellular antigens. Fifth, the volume of distribution of antibodies is limited by the large molecular weight, and there is thus a theoretical concern regarding tumor penetration. Finally, there is generally a higher cost of production associated with antibody-based treatment compared with small-molecule therapy.

Targeted Therapy: Lessons Learned from Adult Oncology

With rare exceptions, most drugs are first tested in adults before evaluation in children. This has been true for targeted agents as well. In the following section, we discuss several examples of successful targeted therapies for the treatment of adult patients with cancer. We will focus our attention on particular lessons learned in the development and testing of these early agents. They will be categorized based on the previously discussed structures of four target classes—genetics, lineage, host, and synthetic lethal-empirical.

Genetic Examples of Targeted Therapy

Treatment of Acute Promyelocytic Leukemia with ATRA

The successful treatment of patients with M3-AML (APL) with ATRA is one of the earliest examples of targeted therapy in the genetic class. This therapeutic discovery was serendipitous. The observation that myeloid blasts differentiate in response to retinoic acid derivatives preceded the discovery of the retinoic acid receptor's involvement in the pathogenesis of APL.[128,129] ATRA treatment is one example of how the discovery of a compound inducing a phenotypic alteration can lead to greater understanding of the mechanisms underlying the change in state. By morphologic examination, APL is characterized by a predominance of malignant hypergranular cells blocked at the promyelocyte stage of differentiation. At the molecular level, a reciprocal translocation involving the retinoic acid receptor α gene (RARα) on chromosome 17q21 is invariably present. This translocation most commonly fuses RARα to the PML gene on chromosome 15q22. RARα is a hormone-dependent, DNA-binding nuclear receptor transcription factor that can act as a transcriptional activator or inhibitor.[82,130,131] In the presence of physiologic amounts of retinoic acid, it normally functions as a transcriptional activator. Abnormal RARα fusion proteins function as transcriptional repressors, enhancing interactions with the corepressor complex.[132,133] Pharmacologic doses of ATRA appear to overcome the PML-RARα–induced transcriptional repression by dissociating the corepressors from PML-RARα and restoring normal ATRA-mediated myeloid differentiation.[134] Furthermore, the PML-RARα protein undergoes proteolytic cleavage in APL cells after ATRA treatment.[135] ATRA treatment increases the fraction of differentiated cells with functional characteristics of neutrophils, induces a mature membrane phenotype, inhibits leukemia cell proliferation, and ultimately induces apoptosis. Historically, APL was among the most fatal subtypes of AML. However, with the addition of ATRA to APL chemotherapy regimens, the overall 2-year survival is more than 75%. APL now has the highest cure rate of the AML subtypes.[7,11,136]

The success of ATRA in the treatment of PML-RARα–rearranged AML illustrates several important issues regarding targeted therapy. First, specific somatic rearrangements, such as PML-RARα, can be exploited with targeted therapy, and the specific underlying genetic event predicts response, not the phenotype. For example, other RARα rearrangements, such as promyelocytic leukemia zinc finger (PLZF) protein–RARα, are associated with an APL phenotype. However, the PLZF-RARα fusion protein is associated with nuclear corepressor interactions resistant to ATRA therapy. Patients with the PLZF-RARα rearrangement are resistant to ATRA therapy.[137] A second important concept that emerges from the success of ATRA is that differentiation therapy is feasible for some malignancies. In general, terminally differentiated cells lose the capacity to divide and ultimately undergo apoptosis. This is the case for APL cells treated with ATRA, raising the possibility that such approaches may be more broadly applicable. A third important lesson from this example is that modulation of transcription factors is therapeutically feasible. Rearrangements involving transcription factors are a common event in the acute leukemias and pediatric solid tumors. Although well-characterized contributors to the malignant state, these transcription factor abnormalities have been considered undruggable or pharmacologically intractable because there is no obvious

approach to inhibiting their function. However, ATRA therapy for the genetic lesion PML-RARα lends credence to the hypothesis that these lesions can be targeted and that their modulation can have therapeutic efficacy. Finally, this example reinforces the importance of combination therapy, not only for cytotoxic agents but also for targeted therapy. Although most patients with APL in early trials achieved complete remission with ATRA as a single agent, it was only in combination with conventional chemotherapy that the long-term cure rates experienced today have been achieved.[12,136,138]

Imatinib in Chronic Myelogenous Leukemia

The development of imatinib for the treatment of CML stands out as the first example of a designed small-molecule inhibitor developed for the purpose of targeting an activated oncogene. Moreover, its dramatic single-agent activity in its initial phase I and II trials, along with the rapid path to registration, has provided the impetus for attempting to identify highly responsive patient populations during preclinical and early clinical development. In 1960, Nowell and Hungerford[139] first detected the presence of the then-named Philadelphia chromosome (Ph) in almost all patients with CML.[139] This aberrant chromosome, resulting from the fusion of chromosomes 9 and 22, was subsequently shown to encode a fusion protein linking a gene of unknown function (BCR or breakpoint cluster region) to the product of the Abelson gene—the cellular homologue of an oncoprotein activated by the Abelson leukemia virus. The discovery that the Abelson gene product (ABL) could function as a protein tyrosine kinase and that the normal autoregulatory domain of ABL was replaced with coding sequences from BCR led to the idea that constitutive activation of ABL kinase activity was likely a causal genetic event in chronic myelogenous leukemia.[140-142] In animal models, production of BCR-ABL was sufficient to induce acute and chronic leukemia.[143] These data, along with the presence of a catalytic domain, made BCR-ABL kinase an attractive drug target. Based on these elements, a drug discovery program was launched culminating in the discovery and clinical testing of imatinib (Gleevec), a small-molecule inhibitor of BCR-ABL, with preclinical activity against models of BCR-ABL–driven CML.[144-147]

In the initial phase I trial by Druker and colleagues,[148] 83 patients with interferon-refractory CML were enrolled and treated with doses of imatinib ranging from 25 to 1000 mg/day. No MTD was reached, and nausea, myalgias, edema, and diarrhea were the most frequent side effects. Remarkably, at a dose of 140 mg or more, all patients had a hematologic response. At doses of 300 mg/day or greater, 53 of 54 patients had complete hematologic responses, 17 had major cytogenetic responses, and 7 had complete cytogenetic remissions (Fig. 4-3).[148] In a separate dose escalation study, imatinib was tested in patients with CML in lymphoid or myeloid blast crisis or with Ph-positive ALL in doses ranging from 300 to 1000 mg.[148a] The overall response rate was 55%, including 70% in ALL or lymphoid blast crisis, although responses were shorter in duration. Responses occurred in 21 of 38 patients (55%) with a myeloid–blast crisis phenotype; 4 of these 21 patients had a complete hematologic response. Of 20 patients with lymphoid blast crisis or ALL, 14 (70%) had a response, including 4 who had complete responses.[148a] Subsequently, 532 patients with interferon-α (IFN-α)–refractory CML were treated with imatinib, 400 mg PO daily, in a phase II trial. Of the initial population, the diagnosis of chronic stage CML was confirmed by central review in 454 patients. In this group, complete cytogenetic response was observed in 41%, major cytogenetic responses in 60% and a complete hematologic response in 95% of patients.[149]

In a phase II trial of 235 CML patients, of whom 181 had a confirmed diagnosis of accelerated phase, patients were

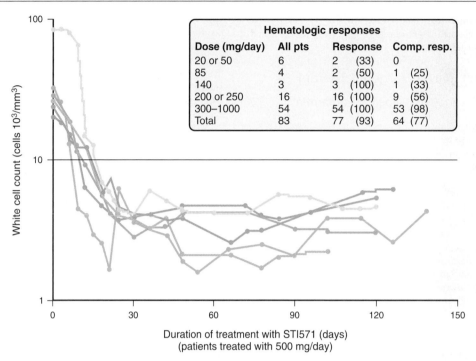

The inset table reads:

Hematologic responses			
Dose (mg/day)	All pts	Response	Comp. resp.
20 or 50	6	2 (33)	0
85	4	2 (50)	1 (25)
140	3	3 (100)	1 (33)
200 or 250	16	16 (100)	9 (56)
300–1000	54	54 (100)	53 (98)
Total	83	77 (93)	64 (77)

FIGURE 4-3. Phase I study of imatinib for chronic myelogenous leukemia. Representative results from the phase I trial of imatinib are shown in two forms. **Inset** (box), response and complete responses for all patients treated with imatinib by dose level. The percentage response rates are shown in parentheses. The response of individual patients treated with 500 mg of imatinib (STI571) is shown: the y axis represents the white blood cell count (log scale) and the x axis shows days on treatment. Each colored line represents an individual patient. *(Adapted from Druker BJ, Talpaz M, Resta DJ, et al. Efficacy and safety of a specific inhibitor of the BCR-ABL tyrosine kinase in chronic myeloid leukemia. N Engl J Med. 2001;344:1031-1037.)*

treated with 400 or 600 mg/day of imatinib. Here, hematologic responses were seen in 82%, complete hematologic responses in 34%, major cytogenetic responses in 24%, and complete cytogenetic responses in 17% of patients. Data from this trial also suggested that a daily dose of 600 mg was more effective than 400 mg.[150] In phase II testing in blast crisis, patients treated with 400 or 600 mg of imatinib/day demonstrated a hematologic response in 52%, a complete hematologic response in 8%, and major cytogenetic responses in 16% of patients.[151]

Most recently, the 5-year results of the randomized crossover IRIS (International Randomized Study of Interferon and STI571) trial of imatinib versus IFN-α plus cytarabine were reported. Here, 1106 patients were randomized to imatinib (553 patients) or to IFN-α (553 patients) along with low-dose cytarabine. Crossover to the alternative treatment was allowed with specified criteria. In the imatinib arm, 69% remained on treatment compared with 3% in the interferon arm. At 5 years of follow-up for those patients who started on imatinib, the complete cytogenetic response was 87% and overall survival at 5 years was 89%. Too few patients were left on the interferon arm for 5-year data from this portion of the trial.[152,153] To estimate the magnitude of the benefit, the results from this randomized prospective trial were compared with the long-term outcome of a randomized trial conducted prior to the introduction of imatinib—the CML91, in which patients were treated with interferon and cytosine arabinoside (Ara-C), but in which crossover to imatinib was not possible. Comparing these trials at 3 years, the complete cytogenetic response rate with imatinib was 87% versus 43% for IFN-α–Ara-C, and transformation-free survival and overall survival favored imatinib.[154]

Based on these data, imatinib is now the gold standard for first-line therapy of CML. Of significant interest is that the annual rate of relapse drops to less than 1%/year for patients who have been on continuous therapy for 5 years, strongly suggesting sustained benefit. Nonetheless, resistance to imatinib does occur. In vitro experiments conducted using randomly mutagenized *ABL* cDNA libraries inserted into sensitive CML cells have revealed that a defined spectrum of mutations in the *ABL* gene itself could preserve kinase activity but could disrupt binding to imatinib.[155] More importantly, sequencing of the *ABL* kinase domain in patients relapsing on imatinib revealed a similar spectrum of mutations in patient samples.[156,157] When these mutations were isolated and placed into ABL kinase constructs and reinserted into sensitive CML cells in vitro, these mutant ABL constructs also rescued lethality induced by imatinib inhibition. These data, although initially of concern regarding the potential for long-term control of the CML disease state, definitively demonstrated in humans the absolute requirement for ABL kinase activity in CML and closed the loop on the concept of a fully validated drug target. Moreover, the identification of such mutants provided the impetus for testing second-generation inhibitors that might overcome these resistance alleles. Here, two separate approaches were considered. First, although imatinib is a fairly selective inhibitor, it is not a particularly potent inhibitor. Because many mutations shifted the IC_{50} of the kinase activity, it remained possible that a more potent inhibitor might be able to overcome or prevent the emergence of these resistance alleles. Nilotinib is a second-generation inhibitor designed to target BCR-ABL and preserve the interaction with the inhibited form of the ABL kinase, the type II binding mode.[158] Nilotinib is more potent in biochemical and cellular assays of ABL activity, and in phase I and phase II trials has significant activity in imatinib-resistant CML.[159] Dasatinib, initially developed as an Src kinase inhibitor, binds to the active form of its kinase targets. Src kinases are highly

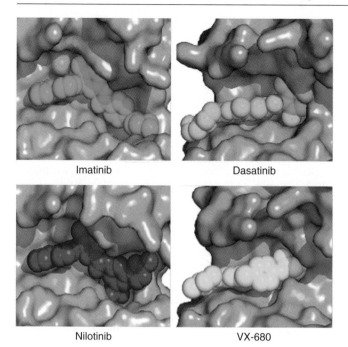

FIGURE 4-4. Abl inhibitors. Shown are representative structural images of the indicated small molecule inhibitors (colored) bound to the ABL kinase domain (gray). Imatinib and nilotinib are type II inhibitors and contain molecular components that occupy the hydrophobic pocket, which is exposed when the kinase is in an inactive conformation. Dasatinib and VX-680 are type I inhibitors and do not have extended interactions with the hydrophobic pocket; instead, they bind to the active conformation of the kinase. *(Courtesy of Sandra Jacobson, Novartis Institutes for BioMedical Research, Cambridge, Mass.)*

related to ABL kinase activity, and in vitro testing has shown that dasatinib has activity against imatinib-resistant alleles.[160] In phase I and II trials, dasatinib has shown significant activity in imatinib-resistant patients[161] and has gained FDA approval in imatinib-resistant patients in CML and CML accelerated phase and blast crisis.

Unfortunately, both nilotinib and dasatinib lack activity against a common, yet difficult to target, *ABL* mutation, the T315I or gatekeeper mutation. This mutation creates a steric problem in the ATP binding domain. This particular kinase domain conformation creates challenges in the drug design process. Notably, it has been difficult to make potent and selective inhibitors of this conformation inhibition. Recently, the inhibitor VX-680, initially developed as an IV-administered Aurora kinase inhibitor, was demonstrated to have activity against ABL and was cocrystallized with the ABL kinase domain containing the gatekeeper mutation (Fig. 4-4).[162] This molecule is now in clinical development. In a phase I trial, three T315I-bearing CML patients were treated. In this phase I trial, doses of VX-680 were administered by continuous IV infusion over 5 days every 2 to 3 weeks, from 8 to 32 mg/m²/hr dose. The three patients with T315I-mutated CML or Ph-positive ALL had clinical responses to VX-680 and were continuing on therapy at the time of the report. Cytogenetic responses were not reported.[163]

Imatinib and Gastrointestinal Stromal Tumors

In addition to rearrangements in gene sequence leading to aberrant protein expression, direct point mutations, gene insertions, and gene deletions can lead to abnormal protein products. For example, activating mutations of the proto-oncogene c-KIT receptor tyrosine kinase (CD117) in patients with gastrointestinal stromal tumors (GISTs) are found in up to 92% of patients with GIST.[164,165] Those lacking c-KIT mutations harbor activation mutations in platelet-derived growth factor receptor α (PDGFRα).[166] Moreover, germline mutations in c-KIT have been described and are associated with a hereditable form of gastrointestinal stromal tumor.[167] These latter data suggest that c-KIT mutation is likely an initiating event in this disease. Of perhaps greater interest is the change in the rate of diagnosis of GIST once a molecular hallmark had been discovered. The incidence of GIST has increased over time, likely as a result of the reclassification (or resolution) of relatively heterogeneous sarcomas, such as smooth muscle tumors, into a more precise molecularly defined cancer (c-KIT mutant GIST). For example, in a retrospective study conducted in Sweden of tumors that might be candidates for GIST, 650 patients' tumors were identified for immunohistochemical staining, primarily looking at anti-CD117 (c-KIT) staining.[168] Primary GISTs were identified in 288 patients, of which the original primary diagnosis of GIST was made in only 28% of patients. Common misdiagnoses included leiomyoma (34%), leiomyoblastoma, (13%), leiomyosarcoma (18%), and others (7%). These data are in keeping with results from the SEER registry in the United States, in which a 25-fold age-adjusted increase in the incidence of GIST was found from 1992 to 2002, from 0.028 to 0.688/100,000.[169] Thus, the ability to understand the molecular underpinnings of this tumor has led to a new molecular definition of this tumor subtype.

Imatinib, in addition to inhibiting ABL kinase activity, also has activity against activated c-KIT and PDGFR. In preclinical cell line models, it showed significant efficacy in vitro and in murine xenograft models.[170] Based on these early preclinical findings, a patient with inoperable recurrent and treatment refractory GIST was treated with imatinib, 400 mg/day. After 4 weeks of therapy, the fluorodeoxyglucose–positron emission tomography (FDG-PET) scan showed a complete resolution of tracer uptake compared with the pretreatment scan and, over the ensuing 8 months, the patient had a progressive diminution in tumor volume.[171] In a phase I study of imatinib, 40 patients, of whom 36 had GISTs, were treated with imatinib at doses of 400 mg/day, or 300, 400, or 500 mg twice daily. Dose-limiting toxicities were observed at 500 mg twice daily. In patients with GIST, 32 patients had tumor responses, with 19 partial responses; 29 patients were still on treatment after 9 months.[172] In a randomized phase II trial, 147 patients with inoperable GIST were randomized to 400 or 600 mg of imatinib/day. With a median follow-up of 288 days, 120 patients remained in the study and partial responses were achieved in 54% of patients. An additional 28% of patients had stable disease and 14% of patients had early resistance to imatinib.[173]

With greater clinical experience with imatinib treatment in GIST, the longer term data have indicated that patients achieve a greater response over time and that there is an increase in the percentage of patients achieving a durable response (reviewed by Siddiqui and associates[174]). Moreover, recent studies have compared the use of imatinib in the postsurgical adjuvant setting and showed a relapse-free survival at 1 year of 96% compared with 33% for the control arm.[175]

Beyond Chronic Myelogenous Leukemia and Gastrointestinal Stromal Tumors

The activity of imatinib against PDGFR or KIT has enabled clinical development in diseases recently characterized as harboring specific genetic alterations activating these receptors. In the case of dermatofibrosarcoma, the majority of patient lesions harbor translocations between chromosomes 17 and 22, fusing the *PDGFB* ligand gene downstream of the Col1a promoter.[176] This translocation leads to constitutive ligand production and constitutive receptor activation and to sensitivity to imatinib in in vitro models and in transplantable primary tumors from patients.[177,178] The first patient with this disease treated with imatinib had a metastatic unresectable dermatofibrosarcoma. With 400 mg PO of imatinib twice daily, this patient had a complete response, with no viable remaining tumor in the residual mass at surgical resection.[179] In a larger series, of eight patients with locally advanced disease, all harboring the t(17;22) translocation, four had complete responses. In the two patients with metastatic disease, one patient was t(17;22) positive and had a partial response and one patient was t(17;22) negative and did not respond.[180] A number of additional complete responses of significant duration have been reported in this disease, including those in patients with metastatic disease.[181]

In hypereosinophilic syndrome (HES), Schaller and Burkland[182] have reported that empirical imatinib treatment of a patient with HES induces a complete and rapid remission of the disease. Similarly, Gleich and coworkers[183] have reported the empirical treatment of five HES patients, four of whom had a prompt and sustained response to imatinib, with a resolution of the eosinophilia. In a slightly larger study, nine patients with HES were treated initially with 100 mg imatinib PO daily. Doses for patients with no hematological response after 4 weeks were increased to 400 mg PO daily. Five patients responded, four with a complete response.[184] The basis for these dramatic observations was uncovered in 2003, when Cools and colleagues[185] reported the discovery of an intrachromosomal deletion that placed the PDGFRα downstream of the promoter of the *FIP1L1* gene, resulting in constitutive upregulation of the receptor.

The remarkable finding in the examples of CML, GIST, dermatofibrosarcoma (DFS), and HES is that in each case, a specific genetic event leads to constitutive activation of a molecular target of imatinib and, in each case, a high degree of efficacy is achieved. Moreover, we have learned that efficacy is identified rapidly in selected patient populations with dramatic responses, even in phase I. MTD does not necessarily set the appropriate effective dose and MTD end points were not reached in a number of the early phase I trials.

Epithelial Growth Factor Receptor Inhibition for Non–Small Cell Lung Cancer

With the success of imatinib for the treatment of patients with CML, a high bar was set for subsequent small-molecule kinase inhibitors. Much excitement was generated about the possibilities of using this targeted approach for the poorly treated adult epithelial malignancies. The EGFR pathway is thought to be important in the development, maintenance, and proliferation of many malignancies, and EGFR is frequently overexpressed in epithelial solid tumors. For these reasons, EGFR was an attractive target for small-molecule inhibition. Gefitinib (Iressa) and erlotinib (Tarceva), both orally administered tyrosine kinase inhibitors, were developed to bind competitively at the adenosine triphosphate pocket of EGFR, inhibiting autophosphorylation and suppressing downstream EGFR signaling. Surprisingly, these EGFR inhibitors have been ineffective in the treatment of solid tumors, with one exception—the treatment of a subset of patients with non–small cell lung cancer (NSCLC).[186] In two large phase II trials (IDEAL trials), patients with refractory NSCLC were randomized to 250 versus 500 mg of gefitinib daily.[187,188] The objective response rate and 1-year overall survival were 18% and 27%, respectively, in IDEAL-1 and 10% and 35%, respectively, in IDEAL-2, results similar to that seen with cytotoxic chemotherapy. In these studies, no difference was seen in efficacy with the chosen doses, but increased toxicity was encountered at 500 mg. Importantly, although in a minority of patients, a subset of patients did have dramatic and durable response. These IDEAL trials led to FDA-accelerated approval of gefitinib as third-line therapy for NSCLC in May 2003.

Subsequent randomized trials comparing gefitinib, 250 mg, to placebo (ISEL study) did not show a survival difference, and the FDA subsequently restricted the use of gefitinib to patients on clinical trials or to patients who had already demonstrated response to the drug.[189] In contrast, erlotinib in a randomized, placebo-controlled trial (BR.21) demonstrated a survival advantage with a median survival of 6.7 months for erlotinib and 4.7 months for placebo.[190] On the basis of the BR.21 study, erlotinib was approved by the FDA in November 2004 for second- and third-line treatment of NSCLC. Interestingly, this trial used erlotinib at the maximum tolerated dose, a possible explanation for the outcome difference seen in these trials using two very similar drugs. It has been hypothesized that the higher dose of erlotinib enabled the inhibition of wild-type EGFR in addition to mutant EGFR (see later). These results require further consideration. Ideally, one would seek to achieve optimal target inhibition (i.e., mutant EGFR). However, in the absence of reliable measures of target inhibition and limited ability to relate quantitative and temporal patterns of target inhibition with drug efficacy, the MTD may still be a prudent initial testing dose.

Following these initial clinical studies, numerous reports have characterized the clinical predictors of tumor response, as opposed to survival. It was soon apparent that these patients frequently shared similar demographic features—a nonsmoking history, a well-differentiated adenocarcinoma histology, female gender, and Asian origin, although the underlying genetic reason for these response differences was not known.[189-191] One hypothesis was that expression levels of EGFR correlated with these clinical characteristics and hence with the response. However, these initial clinical trials failed to identify a correlation between receptor expression and clinical outcome.

Later, in 2004, two research groups independently identified a correlation between mutations in the tyrosine kinase domain of the EGFR and patient responders.[44,192] These EGFR mutations enhance ligand-dependent EGFR activation and sensitivity to gefitinib-erlotinib and are more common in nonsmokers, women, Asians, and patients with adenocarcinoma. Approximately 90% of these mutations occur in a few amino acids. Of the mutations, 45% to 50% are in-frame deletions of exon 19 (codons 746 to 750), and 35% to 45% of mutations are missense mutation leucine to arginine at codon 858 (L858R) in exon 21.[193-196] Several studies have also reported that patients with EGFR mutant tumors have a longer survival when treated with EGFR small-molecule inhibitors compared with patients with wild-type EGFR tumors.[195,197-199]

The question of whether EGFR copy number determined by FISH or EGFR protein overexpression measured by IHC predicts clinical outcome remains controversial. Many challenges have made this question difficult to address. First, there are technical difficulties in performing assays to determine overexpression. Furthermore, there have been inconsistencies in the assays used by different investigators, making direct comparisons difficult. Second, there is the problem of poor sample quality and few numbers of biologic samples to enable statistical significance. Third, there is the observation that a single EGFR allele can undergo mutation and amplification, requiring the simultaneous study of expression level and mutational status.[44,196] Although not yet conclusive, recent reports have suggested an improved response and survival with gefitinib treatment for patients with overexpression.[198,200,201]

Another lesson learned from the experience with small-molecule EGFR inhibitors is the continued importance of combination therapy. Although a subset of patients has a dramatic response to these tyrosine kinase inhibitors (TKIs), even these patients almost always relapse, often with a second somatic mutation in EGFR (T790M).[202-204] It is not yet clear that dramatic response to a single-agent EGFR inhibitor is associated with improved overall survival. Newer EGFR inhibitors, with irreversible binding to the EGFR, may have efficacy for these patients with the T790M who comprise approximately 50% of those with an initial response to TKIs but ultimately develop resistance. However, it is unlikely that all patients with progressive disease will respond to these new inhibitors. A recent study has demonstrated that in a subset of tumors initially responsive to EGFR TKIs, *MET* oncogene amplification accounts for resistance. These tumors maintain activation of ERBB3-PI3K-Akt signaling in the presence of gefitinib. *MET* amplification was detected in approximately 20% of lung cancer specimens that had become resistant to gefitinib or erlotinib.[205] This work suggests that more potent inhibitors of EGFR alone will not have efficacy for this subset of patients. In this case, a combination of an EGFR inhibitor with an MET inhibitor should be considered. The initial EGFR mutations, subsequent EGFR resistance mutations, and MET amplifications all appear to induce phosphorylation of ERBB3, recruiting and activating the lipid kinase phosphoinositide 3'-kinase (PI3K). Inhibitors of MET kinase are just entering clinical trials and could be used in combination with EGFR inhibitors. Another combination that has been considered is that of TKIs with conventional chemotherapy. Unfortunately, these studies have yielded disappointing results. Trials testing gefitinib or erlotinib and cytotoxic chemotherapy have failed to show a survival benefit with the addition of the targeted therapy.[206-209]

This work underscores the importance of developing a molecular understanding of disease and response. The molecular characterization of EGFR abnormalities in NSCLC and their relationship to response to TKIs have been illuminating for the clinical application of targeted therapy. This work underscores the potential of genotype-targeted molecular therapy, as well as the challenges. In the future, improved biologic sample collection, optimized mutational and expression analyses, and adequately powered prospective clinical trials incorporating these elements will be necessary to realize the power of genotype-directed targeted therapy fully.

Lineage Dependence Examples of Targeted Therapy

Several successful targeted cancer therapies capitalize on the lineage dependency of the tumor. Two successful modalities are antibody-based therapy directed against cancers with hematologic lineage markers, rituximab (Rituxan) and gemtuzumab ozogamicin (Mylotarg). These therapies have the advantage of target specificity, with predictability of side effects based on the expression pattern of the lineage marker.

Rituximab Therapy for Non-Hodgkin's Lymphoma

In 1997, rituximab became the first monoclonal antibody approved by the FDA for the treatment of malignancy (non-Hodgkin's lymphoma [NHL]). It is a chimeric, anti-CD20 monoclonal antibody composed of murine variable regions fused with human IgG1 heavy and kappa light chains. CD20 is a 35-kD transmembrane protein expressed on normal and malignant mature B lymphocytes.[210] Its normal physiologic role is poorly understood, but it is hypothesized to be important in calcium transportation and to be involved in B-cell activation, differentiation, and growth regulation.[211] CD20 was an appealing target for therapy development because it is not shed and is not modulated or internalized with antibody binding.[212,213] Rituximab binds to CD20 and induces a depletion of CD20-positive B cells in the circulation and in lymph nodes. Its activity is postulated to occur from multiple mechanisms—antibody-dependent cellular cytotoxicity (ADCC), complement-dependent cytotoxicity (CDC), and inhibition of cell growth.[214,215]

Previously, the gold standard for treating patients with aggressive NHL was CHOP (cyclophosphamide, doxorubicin, vincristine [Oncovin], and prednisone), with a cure rate of approximately 50%.[216,217] Because CHOP alone is curative for patients with aggressive NHL, the first trials evaluating rituximab were in patients with indolent lymphoma for whom no curative therapy exists. The pivotal multicenter trial evaluated four doses of rituximab for patients with relapsed low-grade or follicular lymphoma and demonstrated an overall response rate of 50% and a complete remission rate of 6%. These results were comparable with the best single-agent cytotoxic therapy for relapsed follicular lymphoma.[218]

Subsequent trials have evaluated retreatment or maintenance therapy with rituximab in patients with low-grade or follicular NHL. One study evaluating rituximab retreatment of patients with multiply relapsed low-grade or follicular NHL has shown an overall response rate of 40% and complete response rate of 11%.[219] Trials evaluating extended rituximab treatment demonstrated prolonged event-free survival with maintenance rituximab compared with the historical control of standard 4-week therapy.[220] Another randomized trial compared extended rituximab treatment to the standard 4-week schedule (rituximab, 375 mg/m²/week × 4) in 202 patients with newly diagnosed or refractory or relapsed follicular lymphoma. In 185 evaluable patients, the overall response rate was 67% in newly diagnosed patients and 46% in pretreated patients. At 12 weeks, patients responding or with stable disease were randomized to no further treatment or to extended rituximab therapy (375 mg/m² every 2 months for four doses). The median event-free survival in the no further treatment group was 12 months, and 23 months in the prolonged treatment group.[221] Another group compared maintenance therapy with rituximab versus retreatment at progression in a phase II trial for patients with indolent NHL. In this trial, overall and complete response rates were improved with maintenance therapy, and there was a significant difference in progression-free survival with maintenance therapy versus retreatment (31.3 vs. 7.4 months, $P = 0.007$). However, the median duration of rituximab benefit was similar for these two groups at the time of publication (31.3 vs. 27.4 months).[222]

Rituximab has also been evaluated in combination with cytotoxic chemotherapy. One of the earliest studies, published in 1999, evaluated 40 patients with low-grade or follicular lymphoma treated with six cycles of CHOP and rituximab (R-CHOP). The initial report suggested an additive benefit of rituximab with no additional toxicity when these two therapies are used in combination.[223] The overall response rate was 95% and the complete response rate was 55% in the intent to treat group. The 9-year follow-up study of these patients showed that 16 patients were still in remission 6 to 9 years after treatment and 3 of these 16 had received prior therapy.[224] Another study evaluated CHOP and rituximab for aggressive NHL. In this study, the overall response rate was 94% and the complete response rate was 61%, at least comparable with CHOP alone and with no significant added toxicity.[225] In a randomized phase III study comparing CHOP to R-CHOP in older patients with diffuse large B-cell lymphoma the rate of complete response was higher in the group receiving R-CHOP (76% vs. 63%; $P = 0.005$). Furthermore, at 2 years, event-free and overall survival were higher in the R-CHOP arm, with no significant additional toxicity.[226]

Toxicity from rituximab with short-term use is primarily infusion-related—chills, fever, hypotension, dyspnea, hypoxia, and arrhythmias. These symptoms occur twice as often during the first infusion compared with subsequent infusions, occur more frequently in older patients, and can often be attenuated with premedication, such as acetaminophen and diphenhydramine. These symptoms are mediated by the release of inflammatory cytokines, such as tumor necrosis factor-alpha (TNF-α), interleukin-8, and interferon-γ, both secondary to B-cell destruction and macrophage activation.[227] Studies in patients receiving chronic rituximab therapy for autoimmune disorders have raised the potential for infectious complications, such as reactivation of hepatitis and the development of progressive multifocal leukoencephalopathy from John Cunningham (JC) virus reactivation.[228-230]

It is clear from the experience with rituximab that the reduced toxicities associated with highly specific, and in this case unconjugated, antibodies can allow for direct addition to already complex chemotherapeutic regimens. In this case, the combination improved efficacy without changing overall toxicity. Thus, R-CHOP is now considered to be the standard of care for the first-line treatment of CD20-positive diffuse large B-cell lymphoma and for CD20-positive follicular B-cell NHL in combination with CVP (*c*yclophosphamide, *v*incristine, and *p*rednisolone) chemotherapy. Rituximab is also indicated for the treatment of patients with relapsed or refractory CD20-positive low-grade or follicular NHL.

Gemtuzumab Ozogamicin for Acute Myelogenous Leukemia

Gemtuzumab ozogamicin (GO) is another example of a successful monoclonal antibody–targeted cancer therapy. In contrast to rituximab, GO is a recombinant, humanized anti-CD33 antibody linked to calicheamicin, a potent antitumor antibiotic. Approximately 90% of patients with AML express CD33 antigen on their leukemic blasts. CD33 is a 67-kD transmembrane sialoglycoprotein involved in cell-cell interactions and signaling in the hematopoietic and immune systems. It is a member of an immunoglobulin superfamily subset of sialic acid–binding immunoglobulin-related lectins.[231] CD33 is expressed on normal, early-multilineage hematopoietic progenitors, myelomonocytic precursors, and more mature myeloid cells, such as monocytes, macrophages, and dendritic cells.[232-234] It is also expressed on hepatocytes.[235] However, it is absent from normal pluripotent hematopoietic stem cells.[236] On binding of GO to CD33, under the control of the CD33 cytoplasmic immunoreceptor tyrosine-based inhibitory motifs, the antibody is internalized and calicheamicin is released inside the acidic environment of the lysosome.[237] Once released, calicheamicin binds to DNA, causes double-strand breaks, and induces apoptosis.[238,239]

GO therapy is approved in the United States for the treatment of older adults with relapsed AML who are not considered as candidates for further cytotoxic chemotherapy.[240] One landmark multicenter trial evaluated GO monotherapy at a dose of 9 mg/m^2 on days 1 and 15 for patients with a median age of 61 years.[241,242] The final report from this trial included 277 patients.[243] In patients older than 60 years, the complete response (CR) rate was 12%. An additional 12% of patients sustained a complete response without full platelet recovery (CRp). In patients younger than 60, the CR was 13% and the CRp was 14%. For those patients who received at least two doses of GO, the median overall survival was 12.2 months for patients who achieved CR and 12.9 months for patients with CRp. Additional phase II trials testing GO for patients with refractory or relapsed disease have demonstrated similar results.[244] Treatment of APL with GO has become of particular

interest because APL cells express high levels of CD33.[245,246] For these patients, GO has shown significant single-agent and combination activity with other chemotherapeutic agents, including ATRA. It has had activity in the relapsed setting as well as in de novo APL treatment.[247-251]

Several small studies have tested GO as monotherapy in previously untreated patients with poor-risk AML. One study has reported the use of a standard dose of GO for induction, followed by GO, 6 mg/m^2, given 45 to 60 days after induction, and then 3 mg/m^2 every 4 weeks for maintenance therapy for 4 times. Twelve patients 65 years or older were evaluated. The response rate was 27% and the median response duration was 7.6 months, with cardiotoxicity in some patients.[252] Another study by GIMEMA-EORTC evaluated GO as a monotherapy in 40 patients older than 60 years who were ineligible for cytotoxic chemotherapy, using two doses of GO, 9 mg/m^2, separated by 2 weeks. The response rate was 33% in patients 60 to 75 years but only 5% in patients older than 75 years, and toxicity was deemed unacceptable at this dosing.[253] More recently, a study has reported using GO, 6 and 9 mg/m^2, in 38 patients with AML, including new diagnoses and relapse. In this study, the best results were observed in newly diagnosed patients, with a 47% overall response versus 22% in the relapsed group.[254]

Notable toxicity with GO monotherapy includes infusion-related fever, chills, or hypotension, myelosuppression, infection, hepatic enzyme or bilirubin elevation, and veno-occlusive disease (VOD). VOD was a problem, particularly for patients who went on to transplantation within 3 months of GO therapy.[255] These toxicities have made it more difficult to combine GO with standard cytotoxic chemotherapy. GO therapy has been tested in combination with other chemotherapy in an attempt to achieve a higher CR and relapse-free survival (RFS) in patients with newly diagnosed and relapsed disease. Some of these studies, such as one that tested GO with fludarabine, cytarabine, and cyclosporine for patients with relapsed disease, had a higher CR rate than other previously reported salvage regimens (30% vs. 17% to 20%).[256] However, many GO combination trials were associated with unacceptable toxicity, including fatal infections and hepatic VOD.[257-259] Further investigation is needed to determine the most effective and least toxic regimens incorporating GO therapy. Several cooperative group phase III studies combining GO with standard chemotherapy are ongoing.

Host Track

Bevacizumab and Colorectal Cancer

Angiogenesis plays an important role in tumor formation. Continued tumor growth is dependent on new blood vessels for the supply of oxygen and critical nutrients. Moreover, certain somatic and germline alterations, including those disrupting the function of the von Hippel-Lindau (VHL) tumor suppressor gene, appear to act largely by triggering dysregulated hypoxic and angiogenic responses.[260-263] Over the last several years, numerous angiogenic growth factors have been characterized, including vascular endothelial growth factor (VEGF). VEGF is a member of a large family of dimeric glycoproteins acting as growth factors. It is essential for the normal development of blood vessels and is a growth factor for vascular endothelium.[264,265] VEGF binds to the transmembrane tyrosine kinase receptors VEGFR1, VEGFR2, and VEGFR3. In the malignant state, VEGF secreted by the tumor or surrounding stroma leads to endothelial cell proliferation and migration. Because VEGF and its receptors play a critical role in tumor formation, progression, and maintenance, VEGF or VEGFR inhibition has become a focus of targeted antiangiogenesis therapy.[266] Several approaches are ongoing, but the two with the most success to date are the following: (1) neutralizing antibodies that inhibit the binding of VEGF to its receptors; and (2) small-molecule tyrosine kinase inhibitors that block downstream signaling from the VEGFR.

Bevacizumab (Avastin) is a recombinant, humanized monoclonal antibody that binds to VEGF-A, preventing its interaction with the VEGF receptors. It is believed that bevacizumab affects tumor vasculature by several mechanisms: (1) induces regression of tumor vasculature; (2) normalizes the tumor vasculature; (3) inhibits new blood vessel formation; and (4) prevents recruitment of progenitor cells from the marrow. It may also improve chemotherapy delivery by its alteration of tumor vasculature and by decreasing interstitial pressure.[267] Bevacizumab was approved by the FDA for first-line (2004) and second-line (2006) treatment of patients with metastatic colorectal cancer and nonsquamous metastatic lung cancer.

Prior to the development of targeted therapies, metastatic colorectal cancer was treated with a combination of 5-fluorouracil (5-FU) modulated by leucovorin, combined with irinotecan or oxaliplatin. Overall survival was reported as approximately 18 to 21 months with these regimens. A landmark phase III bevacizumab trial randomized 813 patients with newly diagnosed metastatic colorectal cancer to receive irinotecan, bolus 5-FU, and leucovorin, and either placebo or bevacizumab.[268] The median duration to progression was 10.6 months in the bevacizumab group versus 6.2 months in the placebo group, and the median duration of survival was 20.3 months in the bevacizumab group versus 15.6 months in the placebo group. Several other trials have demonstrated similar results for patients receiving up-front therapy.[269-271] Bevacizumab was also tested in patients with previously treated colorectal cancer. In the phase III trial reported in 2007, 829 patients with previously treated metastatic colon cancer (fluoropyrimidine and irinotecan) were randomly assigned to one of three treatment groups: oxaliplatin, fluorouracil, and leucovorin (FOLFOX4) with or without bevacizumab, or bevacizumab alone.[272] The primary end point was overall survival. The median duration of survival was 12.9 months for FOLFOX4 with bevacizumab, 10.8 months for FOLFOX4 alone, and 10.2 months for bevacizumab alone. The median progression-free survival was 7.3 months for FOLFOX4 with bevacizumab, 4.7 months for FOLFOX4, and 2.7 months for bevacizumab alone. Numerous other studies are ongoing to establish the optimal combination of chemotherapy and bevacizumab.

As with most of the targeted therapies, many of the side effects of bevacizumab are predictable. Some reported side effects include hypertension, proteinuria, arterial thromboembolic events, bleeding, poor wound healing, gastrointestinal perforation, and reversible posterior leukoencephalopathy syndrome (RPLS). Most of these side effects are predictable from the known activity of VEGF. For example, VEGF is a homeostatic factor for regulating blood pressure. Blocking of VEGF or VEGFR leads to increased vascular tension and thus problems with hypertension and RPLS. It is interesting to note that the side effects of VEGF inhibition are similar to the signs of preeclampsia or eclampsia (hypertension, proteinuria, and mental status changes), a disease in which soluble VEGFR 1 (sVEGFR-1), which antagonizes VEGF functions, has been implicated.[273,274] Other toxicities have been more puzzling. For example, the mechanism of gastrointestinal perforation remains unclear. It has been hypothesized that bevacizumab leads to impaired platelet function, with subsequent impairment of wound healing and bleeding.[275]

Other VEGFR pathway inhibitor development has focused on the inhibition of the kinase activity of the VEGF receptor. In December 2005, the FDA approved the drug sorafenib (Nexavar), a small-molecule VEGFR inhibitor, for the treatment of patients with advanced renal cell carcinoma and, in January 2006, the FDA approved the multitargeted inhibitor (including VEGFR and KIT) sunitinib (Sutent) for the treatment of patients with advanced renal cell carcinoma or GIST who are intolerant of or who have had disease progression with imatinib treatment.

The success of bevacizumab for colorectal cancer is a humbling one for drug development. In reality, there is still much room for improvement when the successful drug extends overall survival by less than 6 months. In pediatric cancer care, this would hardly be deemed a victory. However, much has been learned from this experience. One is that antiangiogenesis-directed therapy can play a role in some disease treatments. A second is the continued importance of combination therapy, even for targeted therapy. Bevacizumab alone has very little activity. It was in combination with standard cytotoxic agents that a clinical benefit was demonstrated. Third, careful evaluation of targeted therapy benefits and toxicities may provide new insight into human disease.

Empirical or Synthetic Lethal

As noted, classic chemotherapy is likely to exploit cancer-dependent states that are not fully understood. For example, microtubule inhibitors such as the taxanes specifically interact with protein components of microtubules and are efficacious in a number of cancers, although there is no current scientific rationale for understanding their selective efficacy. A number of emerging therapeutics target highly selective protein targets involved in diverse basic cellular processes and have been elaborated based on specific synthetic lethal hypotheses.

Heat Shock Protein 90 Inhibitors

Heat shock protein 90 (Hsp90) is a ubiquitous and highly abundant chaperone protein required for the proper folding of a large number of cellular proteins. In studies in yeast, Hsp90 appears to play a capacitor role in allowing for the tolerance of coding mutations and thus can play a role in facilitating the emergence of fungal resistance to antifungal therapeutics. Hsp90 has also been argued to play a role in allowing for mutation-based evolution.

In some cancers, Hsp90 was found to be overexpressed[276] and in complex with v-Src and Raf oncoproteins.[277,278] It now appears that a number of oncoproteins activated by mutation directly in the oncogene or by the loss of function of a tumor suppressor are dependent to a greater extent than other cellular proteins on Hsp90 activity.[279] Inhibition of Hsp90 leads to a loss of folding activity and rapid proteasome-mediated degradation of these client proteins. The understanding of the role for Hsp90 in cancer has emerged, at least in part, through efforts to characterize the anticancer properties of geldanamycin, a naturally derived ansamycin antibiotic. Although first thought to act as a kinase inhibitor with activity against malignant cells, Whitesell and associates[280] have demonstrated that geldanamycin can bind to and disrupt the Hsp90 chaperone complex and dissociate the complex from Src. This mechanism was confirmed by the elucidation of the structure of the Hsp90 chaperone bound to geldanamycin.[281] Derivatization of geldanamycin led to the elaboration of 17-AAG (17-allylamino-17-demethoxygeldanamycin), which has reduced hepatotoxicity compared with geldanamycin.[282] The results of five phase I studies have been reported testing IV infusion given on days 1, 8, and 15 in a 28-day cycle, given on days 1, 4, 8, and 11 of a 21-day cycle, or given on days 1, 4, 8, 11, 15, and 18 of a 28-day cycle.[283-287] Most of these trials reported dose-limiting toxicity involving liver transaminase and occasional bilirubin elevation. In the phase I trials, one patient with hepatoblastoma had a reduction in α-fetoprotein and stable disease over three cycles. No partial or complete responses were otherwise noted. A single phase II study in renal cell carcinoma was reported, in which 12 patients with clear cell carcinoma and 8 patients with papillary renal cell carcinoma were treated with 17-AAG, 220 mg/m² IV twice weekly for 2 weeks followed by 1 week off. No responses were seen.[288] 17-AAG has poor aqueous solubility and thus is difficult to formulate for IV delivery. 17-DMAG (dimethylaminoethylamino-17-demethoxygeldanamycin) has improved aqueous solubility and improved oral availability.[289] Phase I trials for this derivative are currently underway.

More recently, a derivative of 17-AAG (IPI-504), which allows for improved formulation, has entered phase I clinical trials. In this case, a selected phase I trial in GIST patients was conducted using PET response as an ancillary biomarker. IPI-504 was administered to 21 patients with progressive GIST on days 1, 4, 8, and 11 of a 21-day cycle, at 5 dose levels ranging from 90 to 400 mg/m². Although the MTD was not reached, PET responses were seen that demonstrated decreases in tumor FDG avidity in 8 of the 18 evaluable patients, suggesting clinical activity in this disease.[290]

Histone Deacetylase Inhibitors

Histone deacetylase inhibitors are a second example of emerging empirically acting targeted agents. In the 1990s, the emerging genetic understanding of AML indicated two classes of cooperating oncogenic events. The first class consisted of activated kinases typified by BCR-ABL or TEL-PDGFR, in which constitutive kinase activity was enacted through protein fusions. The second class consisted of inhibitory transcription factor translocations that appeared to act, at least in part, through transcriptional repression.[291] Both the PML-RARα and AML-ETO translocations appear to function through this molecular mechanism.[132,133,137,292] In animal models, activating kinase lesions induced a proliferative disorder, but when introduced with a mutation from the second class, a full-blown acute leukemia would result.[293,294] These data also appeared to recapitulate the genetics required for the transforming activity of the avian erythroblastosis virus, in which the oncogene *ErbB* constitutes an activated kinase (EGFR) whereas *ErbA* is a constitutive repressor derived from the thyroid receptor.[295,296] The elucidation of the repression function of *ErbA* has perhaps provided the first direct evidence that transcriptional repression is an important mechanism underlying certain modes of cellular transformation.

Transcriptional repression and transcriptional activation partly reflect the balance of histone modification of chromatin structures surrounding gene regulatory regions. Histone acetylation is of particular importance. In many cases, transcriptional activators recruit histone acetylase activity to gene regulatory regions, whereas transcriptional repression complexes typically recruit histone deacetylase to the same regions. In keeping with the notion that repression might underlie the function of oncogenic transcription factor translocations, histone deacetylase enzymes are recruited to the critical promoters by *ErbA* and by various translocation partners, including RARα and ETO. These data provide a compelling rationale for the development and testing of HDAC inhibitors. In keeping with the underlying concept of synthetic lethality, one can hypothesize an enhanced dependence on, or constitutive requirement for, histone deacetylase enzymes by the aforementioned repressive oncogenes. Although the original therapeutic concept evolved from a link between leukemogenesis and transcriptional repression, a large array of proteins are now known to be modulated through acetylation by 11 related

HDACs.[297] This will invariably create difficulty in elucidating the underlying therapeutic mechanisms linked to the anticancer activity now being observed in the clinic with relatively broadly acting HDAC inhibitors.

An array of HDAC inhibitors targeting the major classes of HDAC enzymes are now in clinical trials. Most of these inhibitors have a core hydroxamate structure that sits deep in the enzymatic pocket, making contacts with a key coordinated zinc atom in the enzyme. The most advanced of these compounds, vorinostat (suberoylanilide hydroxamic acid, SAHA), has been approved for the treatment of cutaneous T-cell leukemia (CTLC).[298] Vorinostat emerged from an attempt to understand the prodifferentiation effects of dimethylsulfoxide (DMSO), which in turn led to the generation of hexamethylene bisacetamide (HMBA) and eventually to vorinostat. Only the structural similarity between vorinostat and trichostatin A, a then recently discovered histone deacetylase inhibitor,[299] allowed for the identification of HDACs as targets for vorinostat. HMBA does not inhibit HDACs.[300] In initial phase I studies, vorinostat was dose-escalated when administered IV for 3 consecutive days on a 21-day cycle or when administered for 5 consecutive days given for 3 weeks (here, escalation from 1 to 2 to 3 weeks was carried out first). In this latter part of the trial, an MTD of 300 mg/m²/day × 5 days for 3 weeks was reached for patients with hematological malignancies.[301] Subsequently, oral administration of vorinostat, in which an MTD of 400 mg daily or 200 mg PO twice daily was reached in a phase I study, indicated that diarrhea, anorexia, dehydration, and fatigue were the limiting side effects. Thrombocytopenia was also frequent, with grade 3 or 4 events occurring in 21% of patients treated daily and 36% of patients treated twice daily. Complete and partial responses were seen in patients with diffuse large-cell lymphoma and partial responses (two) were seen in laryngeal and thyroid cancers.[302] Similar toxicities were seen in an additional oral and IV phase I study that focused on hematopoietic malignancies. Here, one complete response was seen in a patient with diffuse large-cell lymphoma and several partial responses were seen in patients with Hodgkin's disease (one), diffuse large-cell lymphoma (two), and CTCL (one).[303] Based on early evidence of efficacy in CTCL patients, a phase II trial of vorinostat was conducted that explored three dose levels: 400 mg daily, 300 mg twice daily 3 consecutive days/week, and 300 mg twice daily for 14 days with 7 days rest followed by 200 mg twice daily.[304] Eight of 33 patients achieved a partial response. The most common side effects were fatigue, diarrhea, nausea, and thrombocytopenia, with thrombocytopenia and dehydration as the most common grade 3 or 4 drug-related events. A phase IIB multicenter trial was conducted testing 400 mg PO daily and allowing for dose reductions to 300 mg PO daily for 7 days or 300 mg PO daily for 5 days. In this trial of 74 patients, who had all progressed or relapsed on at least two prior treatment regimens, 30% achieved an objective response and 77% of patients had some measure of disease improvement. One patient achieved a complete response.[305] These data provided the basis for the FDA approval of vorinostat for CTCL in 2006.

Depsipeptide (FR901228, FK228; romidepsin) is a natural product, bicyclic depsipeptide, originally isolated from a broth culture of *Chromobacterium violaceum* and shown to have antitumor activity against Ras-transformed cells and to inhibit the growth of xenograft tumors grown in nude mice.[306,307] In a screen for activators of SV40 transcription, FR901228 was discovered to have potent transcriptional activation properties and was a potent inhibitor of HDAC enzymatic activity.[308] In the first reported clinical experience, patients were treated with increasing doses of depsipeptide administered by IV infusion on days 1 and 5 of a 21-day cycle. An MTD of 17.8 mg/m² was identified, with dose-limiting toxicities that included fatigue, nausea, vomiting, and thrombocytopenia. In addition, electrocardiographic abnormalities were observed.[309] In the same trial, three patients with cutaneous T-cell lymphoma sustained partial responses, and one patient with a peripheral T-cell lymphoma had a complete response.[310] These trials provided the motivation for testing additional HDAC inhibitors, including vorinostat, in this disease. Another phase I study has addressed concerns over cardiac safety and treated patients with IV infusions weekly for 3 weeks with 1 week rest, reaching an MTD of 13.3 mg/m^2, and finding minimal electrocardiographic changes and DLTs of thrombocytopenia and fatigue.[311] On this schedule, 10 patients with CLL and 10 patients with AML were treated, resulting in similar side effects of fatigue and nausea but no partial or complete responses.[312] A phase I trial conducted in pediatric patients tested depsipeptide administered as a 4-hour IV infusion at doses ranging from 10 to 22 mg/m^2 given for 3 weeks, with 1 week off. Here, the MTD was 17 mg/m^2 and dose-limiting toxicities were T-wave inversions and transient sick sinus syndrome, which were asymptomatic.[313]

In phase II trials, depsipeptide was tested in 15 patients with neuroendocrine tumors, 14 mg/m^2, and in metastatic renal cell carcinoma, 13 mg/m^2, on days 1, 8, and 15 of a 28-day cycle. The neuroendocrine study was terminated because of serious cardiac adverse events, including ventricular arrhythmias and prolonged QTc interval.[314] In the renal cancer trial, a prolonged QTc interval (two patients), grade 3 atrial fibrillation and tachycardia (one patient), and sudden death (one patient) were observed.[315] There was insufficient antitumor activity to warrant further study for these indications. Phase II registration trials of depsipeptide in patients with CTCL are ongoing and have reported an overall response rate of 32% (12 of 38), including 8% complete responses in the interim data from one trial and a 26% overall response rate (18 of 70), with a 7% complete response rate in the interim data from the second trial.[316]

LBH589 is a synthetic hydroxamic acid–based small-molecule inhibitor that was specifically designed as part of a drug discovery effort directed at producing a pan-HDAC inhibitor. LBH589, as with other HDAC inhibitors, has preclinical antitumor activity. It has been tested in phase I trials in solid tumors and non-Hodgkin's lymphoma. In a phase I trial for the IV formulation, 15 patients were treated with LBH589, 4.8 to 14 mg/m^2, on days 1 and 7 of a 21-day cycle. Four dose-limiting toxicities were observed, consisting of QTc prolongation. Other treatment-related toxicities included nausea, diarrhea, vomiting, hypokalemia, and thrombocytopenia (13%). In 8 of 11 patients with leukemia with peripheral blasts, transient reductions occurred with a rebound following the 7-day treatment period.[317] Sharma and colleagues[318] have tested LBH580 in advanced solid tumors and lymphoma, administered IV once weekly for 3 of 4 weeks. One DLT of thrombocytopenia was found at 20 mg/m^2. Two patients had QT prolongation at 20 mg/m^2. Finally, in their open-label phase I trial of oral LBH589, Prince and associates[319] have found an MTD of 20 mg, given PO three times/week. Of the 10 CTCL patients treated, 2 patients achieved complete responses, 4 achieved a partial response, and 2 were found to have stable disease.

It is clear from the summation of these current studies that HDAC inhibition results in significant activity in CTCL, although the mechanisms of action for this empirical observation remain obscure. HDAC inhibitors are now being tested more widely in other solid tumor and hematologic malignancies. The key to these studies will be the elucidation of effective but well-tolerated dosing regimens.

Box 4-8	**Special Considerations in Pediatric Targeted Therapy Development**

Majority of children with cancer are cured
Pediatric cancer is rare
Reduced market incentive
Clinical trial design and accrual difficult
Limited number of agents can be reasonably tested
Toxicity may be specific to developmental stage
Ethical considerations are more difficult
Informed consent for experimental therapy
Informed consent for participation in biologic studies

NEW AND EMERGING OPPORTUNITIES IN PEDIATRIC CANCER

Targeted therapies have been introduced into the pediatric cancer therapeutic arsenal. Almost all these agents have already been tested in adult patients. Several have had success in the pediatric setting, in which the potential target is shared by the phenotypically identical adult and pediatric tumors—for example, ATRA for children with APL,[320,321] imatinib for BCR-ABL–rearranged CML,[322] GO for AML,[323,324] and rituximab for lymphoma.[325,326] There are many targets shared by adult and pediatric malignancies and targets specific to pediatric cancers that have not yet been thoroughly explored with targeted approaches. In the following sections, we will discuss these new and emerging targets, as well as the special considerations in bringing targeted therapy to the pediatric setting (Box 4-8).

Special Considerations in Targeted Therapy Development for Children

Cure Achieved in Most Children with Cancer

There are numerous special considerations in the development of targeted therapy for pediatric cancer. In contrast to cancer in the adult, most children with cancer will be cured of the malignancy, making the selection of pediatric patients for testing of new targeted therapies more challenging and raising the required level of activity necessary for success. For example, in de novo pediatric pre–B-cell ALL, with cure rates over 80%, it is difficult to introduce a new targeted agent for fear of detracting from an already excellent cure rate by diluting curative agents. Thus, although there are many new interesting targets emerging, such as PAX5 and other genes important in B-cell developmental pathways,[327] it would be difficult to justify the inclusion of up-front novel targeted therapy in patients with this excellent outcome. Hence, it is likely in the relapsed setting, or in de novo disease with poor outcome, that novel targeted therapies will undergo initial testing. If efficacy and safety are demonstrated, incorporation into up-front clinical trials may then be considered.

Rarity of Pediatric Cancer

It was estimated that in 1998, 12,400 children in the United States younger than 20 years were diagnosed with cancer and 2500 died of cancer, ranking cancer as the fourth leading cause of death in this age group.[328] In contrast, it was estimated that 1,444,920 adult men and women (766,860 men and 678,060 women) in the United States would be diagnosed with cancer and 559,650 men and women would die of all types of cancer in 2007.[329] Thus, the pediatric cancers are rare in comparison with adult malignancies, and there is a reduced market incentive for pediatric-specific targeted drug development by the pharmaceutical industry. Furthermore, there has been hesitancy to test new drugs in children. Therefore, there are almost no drugs that have been developed specifically for pediatric malignancies. Even when a common target has been identified in adult and pediatric cancers, it may be years before a drug reaches a pediatric trial. For example, mutations in FLT3 in MLL-rearranged infant ALL were reported in 2003, and several FLT3 inhibitors have been tested in adults with AML.[330,331] However, there have been no reported trials testing an FLT3 inhibitor for infants with MLL-rearranged ALL. Because the pediatric cancers are rare, even with drugs available for testing, clinical trials are difficult. A rare disease incidence means a slow accrual of patients and necessitates large cooperative groups to power the trial with appropriate patient numbers. Limited numbers of patients also precludes testing of all possible new agents. New methods are needed to choose novel targeted agents for testing in children more rationally.

One attempt to prioritize the selection of new agents for testing in children with cancer was the development of the Pediatric Preclinical Testing Program (PPTP) by the National Cancer Institute. This group prospectively tested new agents against a panel of xenografts and genetic models of pediatric cancer, such as neuroblastoma, rhabdomyosarcoma, osteosarcoma, and ALL. The PPTP built on prior work that demonstrated the ability of preclinical testing of new agents in rhabdomyosarcoma and neuroblastoma xenografts to predict in vivo activity in children with these malignancies.[332,333] The development of new genetically engineered models of pediatric cancer should also facilitate preclinical evaluation of targeted therapies and better prioritization of new agents for clinical trials, particularly for diseases such as Ewing's sarcoma, for which limited such models exist.[333a]

Developmental and Ethical Considerations in Targeted Therapy for Children

Developmental Considerations

Children may tolerate targeted therapies differently from adults secondary to age-specific differences in physiology that result in altered pharmacokinetics or to drug interference with critical developmental pathways. For example, concern has been raised about the potential adverse effects of antiangiogenic agents on longitudinal bone growth in the developing child, particularly in light of the effects of the antiangiogenic agent, thalidomide, on limb development during embryogenesis.[334] In normal development, vascularization of cartilage is prominent during embryogenesis and during periods of growth when neoangiogenesis occurs at growth plates.[335,336] Inhibition of VEGF signaling has been reported in animal models to result in thickening of the epiphyseal growth plates secondary to an expansion of the hypertrophic chondrocyte zone.[337,338] These findings have been attributed to a delayed vascular invasion of the epiphyseal growth plate, with a subsequent reduced rate of chondrocyte apoptosis. Inhibition of VEGF signaling has also been reported to impair trabecular bone formation, induce dental dysplasia, and ovarian atrophy.[339] Although the animal study results are of concern, the actual long-term effects of this class of drug on children is unknown.

Ethical Considerations

The testing of drugs in children raises issues universal to cytotoxic and targeted therapies, as well as challenges more specific to targeted treatments. Adults can make informed decisions about the risk and potential benefits of experimental therapies and biologic studies, and can actively participate in treatment decisions. Particularly for young children, however, true informed consent from patients for experimental therapies cannot be obtained; it is the parent or legal guardian who makes decisions about participation in a trial. Considering this potential conflict of interest, special regulations have been instituted to afford additional protection to children. These include the Code of Federal Regulations, Part 46, Protection of Human Subjects, Subpart D, and the related FDA regulation, Part 50, Protection of Human Subjects, Subpart D. These regulations outline allowable research in children based on the risk to the child, potential benefit to the child or other children, and alternative therapies. In the testing of targeted therapies, pharmacodynamic studies with sampling of tumor tissue prior to and following therapy initiation become more critical. For obvious reasons, these studies can be difficult, if not impossible, to perform with the current regulations, particularly for solid tumors or brain tumors. In general, tissue collection in children for the purpose of biologic studies must be considered to be no greater than a minor increase in minimal risk. Innovative methods are needed to evaluate pharmacodynamic response, such as new imaging technologies, and better techniques are needed to assess surrogate tissues.

Emerging Genetic Targets in Pediatric Cancer

Significant progress has been made in our understanding of the pediatric leukemias and solid tumors. Numerous potential genetic targets have emerged over the past 10 years. With the excellent cure rates for some pediatric malignancies, it might be difficult to incorporate target-directed therapies associated with good-outcome genetic lesions, such as TEL-AML1 in pediatric ALL. In these early stages of targeted therapy for pediatric malignancies, the focus will likely be on lesions associated with poor outcome. Here we discuss some of these genetic lesions with the potential for therapeutic targeting.

Fms-Like Tyrosine Kinase 3 and Acute Leukemias

Although much progress has been made in the treatment of childhood ALL, one subgroup of patients who continue to have a poor prognosis are children with mixed-lineage leukemia (MLL) rearrangements involving chromosome 11q23. MLL rearrangements are identified in 80% of infants with ALL and in 5% of childhood ALLs. Prognosis for these children is poor, particularly for infants, for whom overall survival is reported as 20% to 35%, despite intensive chemotherapy.[340-345] Alternative noncytotoxic treatment approaches are needed for this disease subset. One possible target for these patients is the MLL fusion itself. However, MLL is a transcription factor, and DNA binding proteins have been difficult to inhibit with small molecules. A second therapeutic approach has emerged from the identification of a role for menin in MLL-dependent oncogenesis. Studies have suggested that disruption of the MLL-menin protein-protein interaction might reverse the oncogenic function of MLL fusions.[346] A third recently revealed target is the Fms-like tyrosine kinase 3, FLT-3. Gene expression profiling studies comparing MLL-rearranged ALL to all other ALL and AML have demonstrated a unique expression profile for MLL-rearranged leukemia. FLT-3 is the gene most frequently overexpressed in MLL as compared with the other acute leukemias.[347,348]

FLT-3 is a class III receptor tyrosine kinase with structural homology to PDGFR, C-Kit, and C-Fms. On binding the FLT-3 ligand, wild-type receptors dimerize and become activated by phosphorylation, leading to activation of downstream signal transduction pathways. Mutations in FLT-3 can be identified in blasts from 30% of patients with AML with constitutive activation of the kinase resulting from internal tandem duplications (ITDs) in the juxtamembrane domain or point mutations in the activation loop.[349] An initial study has reported mutations in FLT-3 in approximately 15% of samples of MLL-rearranged ALL. All these were point mutations in the activation loop, including mutations not previously reported in patients with AML (deletion of isoleucine 836). These mutations lead to constitutive activation of the kinase and increased sensitivity to small-molecule inhibitors of FLT-3 in vitro, in cell lines and primary patient samples, and in a xenograft model of MLL. Furthermore, MLL-rearranged lymphoblasts with high levels of wild-type FLT-3 were sensitive to the FLT-3 inhibitor PKC412.[330] Subsequent studies have reported an incidence of FLT-3 mutations in infant MLL samples ranging from 3% to 18%. These studies also confirmed increased expression of FLT-3 in MLL-rearranged infant ALL compared with infant and noninfant patients with germline MLL. Even in the absence of documented mutation, high levels of FLT-3 expression were associated with FLT-3 ligand independence and with increased sensitivity to the FLT-3 inhibitor PKC412.[350,351] In addition to MLL-rearranged ALL, FLT-3 is a potential target in children with T-cell ALL, and up to 25% of children with hyperdiploid ALL have been reported to have FLT-3 mutations.[351,352] Furthermore, FLT-3 ITDs are present in 15% of pediatric AML patients and FLT-3 point mutations in 7%. Children with FLT-3 ITDs have a particularly poor prognosis.[353]

Several FLT-3 inhibitors have been tested in clinical trials for adults with AML—CEP-701, MLN-518, PKC412, SU5416, and SU11248.[354-359] Most of the trials testing these compounds have had some transient responders, with decreased peripheral blood or marrow blasts, and the compounds have generally been well tolerated. However, few patients enter complete remission and most patients do not respond. Moreover, it is not yet clear whether demonstrated responses are actually a result of FLT-3 inhibition. None of these inhibitors is specific for FLT-3; each has other receptor tyrosine kinase targets, confounding the interpretation of clinical responses. In addition, responses have been reported for patients with wild-type FLT-3 and those with mutant FLT-3. The most convincing evidence that FLT-3 is the actual in vivo target of these inhibitors would be the identification of a FLT-3 inhibitor–resistant FLT-3 mutant, analogous to BCR-ABL or c-KIT mutants that confer imatinib resistance. No trials testing FLT-3 inhibitors in children with leukemia have been reported. However, there is an ongoing Children's Oncology Group trial to test the efficacy of a FLT-3 inhibitor (lestaurtinib [CEP-701]) in pediatric AML.

Notch1 in T-Cell Acute Lymphoblastic Leukemia

With intensive chemotherapy, most children with T-cell acute lymphoblastic leukemia (T-ALL) will be cured. However, ALL is still the leading cause of death from cancer in children, and intensive chemotherapy is not without toxicity. An emerging target for T-ALL is Notch1. Notch1 was initially discovered through the analysis of a rare (7;9) translocation in T-ALL.[360] Enforced Notch signaling induces T-ALL in mice.[361] Notch1 encodes a transmembrane receptor required for T-cell differentiation and for the assembly of pre–T-cell receptor complexes in immature thymocytes (Fig. 4-5). Notch is activated by the binding of ligands of the delta-serrate-lag2 (DSL) family, which

triggers a series of proteolytic cleavages. ADAM metalloprotease cleavage, at a site just external to the transmembrane domain of Notch, produces a short-lived Notch intermediate, NTM. The second cleavage, catalyzed by the gamma-secretase complex, releases the intracellular domain of Notch (ICN) into the cytoplasm, for subsequent translocation to the nucleus. Once in the nucleus, Notch acts as a transcriptional activator complexed with the DNA-binding protein CSL (CBF1, suppressor of hairless, lag-1) and the transcriptional coactivators of the Mastermind-like gene family (MAM1).[362,363] Only a limited number of targets of Notch have been identified, such as the hairy enhancer of split (Hes) and c-Myc.[364-366]

Mutations in Notch have been discovered in 50% to 60% of T-ALL samples.[367,368] Mutations of Notch have also been reported in numerous murine models of T-ALL.[369-371] In humans, these mutations are activating mutations that involve the heterodimerization domain and/or the PEST domain of Notch. Inhibition of gamma-secretase is one possible approach to inhibiting Notch signaling. Gamma-secretase inhibitors (GSIs) were initially developed because of their potential therapeutic role in Alzheimer's disease in cleaving amyloid precursor protein.[372] However, they were tested in Notch-dependent cancers in an attempt to block the production of the processed nuclear form of Notch.[373] Many human T-ALL cell lines with Notch mutation have shown a G_0-G_1 cell cycle arrest in response to a GSI.[367] A Notch pathway inhibitor clinical trial with MK-0752 was initiated in 2005 for patients with refractory T-ALL.[374] The drug was tolerated in a limited number of patients at doses below 300 mg/m^2 once daily. However, further dose escalation by continuous infusion was discontinued secondary to diarrhea. This toxicity is likely to be secondary to the effects of GSI on all four Notch receptors, not only to the effects on Notch1. Furthermore, there has been concern about the lack of T-ALL cell death, even in vitro, with GSI. Rather, cell cycle arrest has been reported. Thus, more basic and preclinical work is needed if the potential of Notch pathway inhibition for T-ALL is to be realized. It is likely that clinical efficacy will be obtained only if multiple agents are used in combination. A recent study has suggested that Notch signals positively regulate mTOR pathway activity in T-ALL and that GSIs and rapamycin, an mTOR inhibitor, have highly synergistic effects on GSI-sensitive T-ALL growth in vitro. In addition, GSIs have augmented the suppressive effects of rapamycin on GSI-resistant cell lines.[375]

Sonic Hedgehog Signaling and Medulloblastoma

Medulloblastoma is the most common malignant pediatric brain tumor. The Sonic hedgehog signaling pathway, implicated in the pathogenesis of this disease, is a potential pathway for targeted therapy. Aberrant Sonic hedgehog signaling was first implicated in the pathogenesis of medulloblastoma with the discovery of germline mutations in the Sonic hedgehog (Shh) receptor Patched-1 (PTCH1) in patients with Gorlin's syndrome (basal cell nevus syndrome) who have an underlying predisposition to develop medulloblastoma.[77,78] Heterozygous loss of PTCH1 occurs in approximately 10% of sporadic medulloblastomas. Mutations in the downstream members of the Hedgehog pathway, Smoothened (Smo) and Suppressor of fused (Sufu), have also been reported.[376-381] Furthermore, the Hedgehog pathway is activated in approximately 30% of human medulloblastomas based on gene expression studies.[382]

PTCH1 is a transmembrane receptor for the ligand Shh (Fig. 4-6). In the absence of Shh, PTCH1 inhibits Smo, a transmembrane protein with homology to G protein-coupled receptors. On Shh (ligand) binding to PTCH1, the repression is relieved and signal is transduced through Smo to the nucleus.

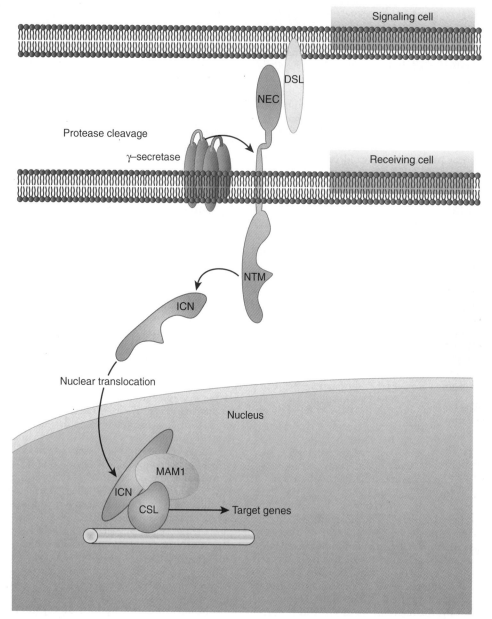

FIGURE 4-5. Notch1 signaling. Notch is activated by binding of the ligands of the DSL family, which triggers a series of proteolytic cleavages. Notch receptors are cleaved by ADAM metalloproteases, producing two noncovalently associated subunits, NEC and NTM. Next, cleavage by gamma-secretase releases the intracellular domain of Notch (ICN), which translocates to the nucleus and forms a transcriptional activation complex with CSL and Mastermind-like (MAM1) cofactors. CSL = CBF1, suppressor of hairless, lag-1.

This activity upregulates the Gli transcription factors, which in turn induces a set of transcriptional targets, including cyclin D1, PTCH1, and Gli1 themselves. Sufu appears to have a role in the repression of Hedgehog signaling by interacting with Gli proteins in the cytoplasm and nucleus.[383-385] The Hedgehog pathway is critical for the development of the cerebellum and regulates the proliferation of granule neuron precursor cells in the cerebellum. Medulloblastomas are thought to originate from these immature granule cells.[379]

Inhibitors of the Hedgehog pathway have already been identified. Cyclopamine is a plant-derived alkaloid from *Veratrum calcificornicum* initially described because of its causal role in the development of holoprosencephaly in livestock ingesting the plant.[386,387] Cyclopamine inhibits Hedgehog signaling by binding to Smo and influencing the balance of active and inac-

tive Smo. It has been demonstrated to inhibit the growth of medulloblastoma in vitro and in xenograft models of medulloblastoma.[81,388,389] Genetically engineered mouse models of medulloblastoma have been created with mice heterozygous for the *PCTH1* gene and null for *p53*. These animals develop medulloblastoma as early as week 2 and die from the disease by week 16.[390] In this animal model of medulloblastoma, a benzimidazole derivative, Hh-Antag691, with Hedgehog inhibitory activity via binding to Smo, led to a dose-dependent downregulation of Hedgehog pathway members, decreased tumor burden, and increased disease-free survival in treated mice.[391] Preclinical evidence has suggested that inhibiting the Hedgehog pathway should have therapeutic efficacy for children with medulloblastoma. Cyclopamine-derivatives and other Smo-directed compounds are now entering phase I testing.

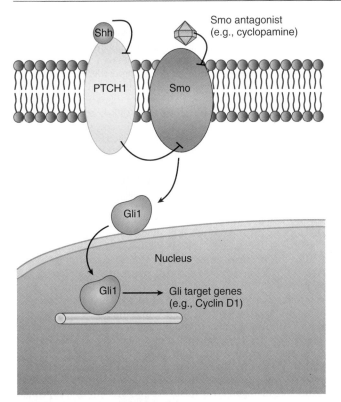

FIGURE 4-6. Hedgehog signaling. Patched (PTCH1) is a transmembrane receptor for the ligand Sonic hedgehog (Shh). In the absence of Shh, PTCH1 inhibits Smoothened (Smo), a transmembrane protein with homology to G protein–coupled receptors. On Shh binding to Smo, this repression is relieved and signal is transduced through Smo to the nucleus, upregulating Gli transcription factors, which turn on a host of other transcriptional targets, including cyclin D1. *(Courtesy of Curtis Glavin and William Sellers.)*

Hopefully, in the next few years, we will address whether these preclinical findings translate to clinical efficacy in children with medulloblastoma.

Transcription Factors and Pediatric Cancer

Abnormalities of transcription factors are a common genetic theme in the development of pediatric solid tumors as well as leukemia. Often, the transcription factor is involved in a translocation, rendering a new protein with aberrant transcriptional activity. Some examples of common transcription factor rearrangements include Ewing's sarcoma (EWS-FLI, EWS-ERG), alveolar rhabdomyosarcoma (PAX3-FKHR, PAX7-FKHR), infantile fibrosarcoma (TEL-NTRK3), ALL (TEL-AML1, MLL rearrangements, E2A-PBX), AML (PML-RARα, AML1-ETO, CBFβ-MYH11, MLL rearrangements). Although initially not thought to play a role in the development of adult carcinomas, emerging evidence has suggested that cryptic rearrangements of transcription factors in adult solid tumors may be common. Recent studies have identified ETS rearrangements in most adult prostate tumors.[63,392,393] The high frequency of these abnormalities and the tumor cell specificity make these genetic lesions attractive targets. However, transcription factors have been considered undruggable. Unlike enzymatic targets, such as kinases, transcription factors are not easily amenable to high-throughput screening assays. With the exception of the treatment of PML-RARα–rearranged APL, no current therapy directly targets these transcription factor abnor-

malities. Alternative approaches to small-molecule discoveries are needed. New technologies, such as RNAi, may facilitate therapeutic targeting of oncogenic transcription factors as better delivery methods are developed. Furthermore, these evolving technologies have enabled the development of new methods for small-molecule library screening.

One approach to address the challenges to transcription factor targeting exploits gene expression signatures (Fig. 4-7). With this method, gene expression signatures, defined using genome-wide expression profiling, are used to define different biologic states. Then, a small-molecule library is screened with a low-cost, higher throughput assay to identify compounds that induce the change in gene expression signature from state A to state B. The gene expression signature definition, amplification, and detection are generic. Furthermore, a priori knowledge of a target is not needed. The gene expression signature serves as a surrogate for the biologic state in question. The method is thus well suited for discovery of modulators of oncogenic transcription factors in which the mutant transcription factor's transforming mechanism is unknown.

One recently developed method, gene expression–based high-throughput screening (GE-HTS), uses Affymetrix microarrays to define expression signatures of the two biologic states of interest. From these high-complexity arrays, up to 100 genes are selected as marker genes for each state. These signature genes are then amplified and detected with a high-throughput assay.[394,395] This approach was successfully used in a proof of concept experiment to identify inducers of AML differentiation. It was then extended to the modulation of transcription factors in an effort to identify small-molecule modulators of EWS-FLI in Ewing's sarcoma.[396] First, the transcriptional profile of A673 Ewing's sarcoma cells in the presence or absence of a shRNA directed against the endogenous EWS-FLI transcript was established. Then, an EWS-FLI rescue system, in which loss of oncogenic transformation with shRNA directed against the 3'-untranslated region (3'-UTR) could be rescued by ectopic expression of an EWS-FLI cDNA lacking the 3'-UTR, was profiled. From these two data sets, a signature for EWS-FLI–on versus EWS-FLI–off was developed. Next, a small-molecule library was screened for compounds that induce the EWS-FLI–off signature in A673 cells. The top hit from this screen, Ara-C, decreased EWS-FLI protein levels, inhibited cell growth, induced apoptosis, and attenuated transformation in multiple Ewing's sarcoma cell lines positive for EWS-FLI. Based on this work, Ara-C was tested in a phase II Children's Oncology Group trial for pediatric patients with relapsed or refractory Ewing's sarcoma. Unfortunately, Ara-C at the dose and schedule utilized in the trial resulted in hematological toxicity that limited delivery, and the regimen had minimal activity in this group of patients.[396a] In principle, however, this approach can be used to identify modulators of any oncoprotein simply by defining a signature of the oncoprotein's activity. With an ever-expanding list of undruggable oncoproteins critical in the development of cancer, such as the discovery of ETS transcription factor rearrangements in most patients with prostate cancer, it will be increasingly important to explore alternative small-molecule discovery platforms. GE-HTS provides an avenue for identifying tool compounds for the study of these genetic lesions and for identifying therapeutic leads. Avalon Pharmaceuticals is leading an industry-based effort to use gene expression fingerprints for drug discovery.

A second signature-based approach to address this problem uses a reference collection of gene expression profiles from cells treated with bioactive small molecules. This approach was initially demonstrated as being feasible in yeast by a pivotal study that confirmed that gene expression data could be used to annotate small molecules and genes functionally.[397] More recently, a pilot study has demonstrated the feasibility of this

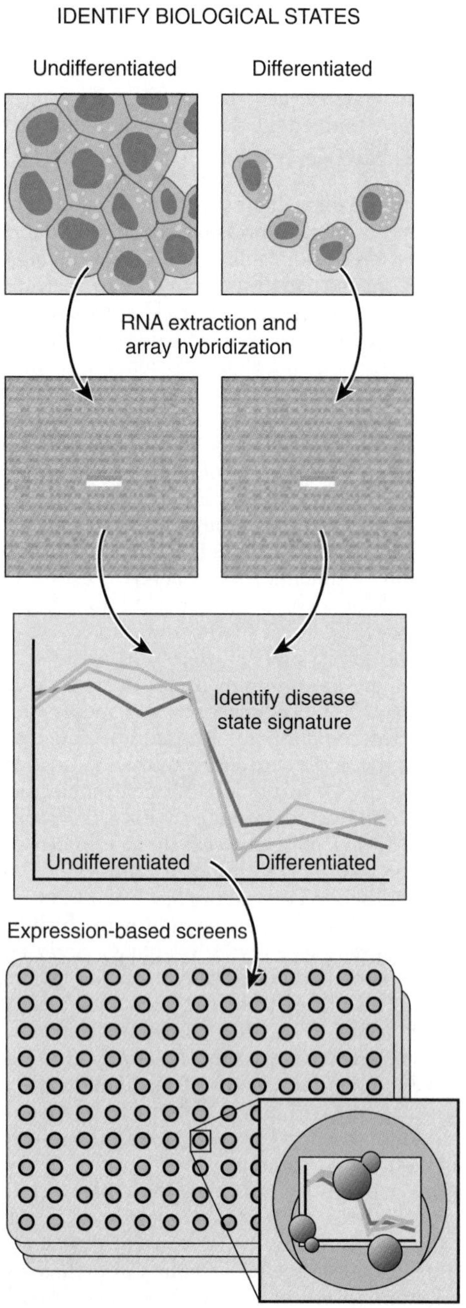

IDENTIFY BIOLOGICAL STATES

FIGURE 4-7. Gene expression-based high-throughput screening (GE-HTS). With this approach, any cellular state of interest can be defined by a gene expression signature and small molecules screened for the ability to modulate this signature. The first step in this signature-based approach to compound discovery is the genome-wide profiling of two biologic states with microarrays. Using these complex data, marker genes distinguishing the two states of interest are identified. Then, small-molecule libraries are screened with a high-throughput assay for compounds inducing the desired gene expression signature.

approach in human cell lines with the expression profiling of 164 distinct small-molecule perturbagens, including many FDA-approved drugs and known bioactive compounds. Here, the goal was to create an in silico tool (the connectivity map, or C-Map) for discovering the relationships among diseases, physiologic processes, and small-molecule interventions (Fig.

4-8).[398,399] One pertinent study of pediatric leukemia has identified rapamycin as a small-molecule candidate to reverse dexamethasone resistance in ALL.[400] In this example, the C-Map was screened for molecules whose profile overlapped with a gene expression signature of glucocorticoid (GC) sensitivity or resistance in ALL cells. The screen indicated that the mTOR inhibitor rapamycin profile matched the signature of GC sensitivity. Rapamycin sensitized ALL to GC-induced apoptosis via modulation of antiapoptotic MCL1. The study indicated that MCL1 is an important regulator of GC-induced apoptosis and that the combination of rapamycin and glucocorticoids has potential usefulness for lymphoid malignancies. A clinical trial testing this hypothesis for patients with relapsed ALL has been initiated.

These two signature-based approaches (GE-HTS and C-Map) can also complement each other. One study has used GE-HTS to discover small molecules that induce a signature of androgen receptor activation inhibition and the C-Map to identify the mechanism of action of these compounds in this activity.[399] Gedunin and celastrol, structurally similar natural products with a history of anticancer and medicinal use, have been identified as top hits from the GE-HTS screen. To investigate the target activity of these compounds, the C-Map was used to connect the activities of celastrol and gedunin to drugs with known biologic activity at the gene expression level. A genome-wide expression signature was characterized for these compounds using Affymetrix microarrays. This gene expression signature was subsequently used as a C-Map query. Both compounds invoke gene expression signatures that recapitulate gene expression signatures of known Hsp90 inhibitors. This prediction has been validated by work demonstrating that celastrol and gedunin inhibit Hsp90 activity and Hsp90 clients, including the androgen receptor.

There still remains the desire to inhibit the activity of a given transcription factor directly. One potential approach to achieving this goal might use stapled protein technology applied to the activation of apoptosis using a hydrocarbon-stapled BH3 peptide.[401,402] BCL-2 is the founding member of a family of proteins with proapoptotic (BAX, BAK, BID, BAD) and anti-apoptotic function (BCL-2, BCL-XL). The interaction between BCL-2 family members is mediated through the amphipathic, alpha-helical BH3 segment, an essential death domain.[403] In theory, helical peptides might be used to interfere with protein-protein interactions. However, the efficacy of helical motifs has been limited because of the loss of secondary structure in solution, susceptibility to degradation, and poor penetration of intact cells. In this new approach, hydrocarbon stapling was used to generate peptides designed to mimic the BH3 domain of BID, with favorable pharmacologic properties. The stapled peptides proved to be helical, protease-resistant, cell-permeable molecules that bound with increased affinity to multidomain BCL-2 member pockets. A stapled peptide of the BH3 domain from the BID protein specifically activated the apoptotic pathway to kill leukemia and effectively inhibited human leukemia xenografts. Hydrocarbon stapling of native peptides may provide a useful strategy for experimental and therapeutic modulation of protein-protein interactions, especially in disrupting transcription factor homodimers and heterodimers requiring extended helical interaction surfaces, as is the case for the myc family.

A second peptide-based approach might interfere with the interface between proteins involved in transcriptional regulation. One example is the use of specific peptide interference with BCL6 (B-cell lymphoma 6) transcriptional mechanisms in B-cell lymphoma.[404] Regulatory elements of the *BCL6* gene are frequently mutated in human diffuse large B-cell lymphoma, leading to sustained expression of BCL6.[405,406] This is thought to enhance B-cell survival, proliferation, and block

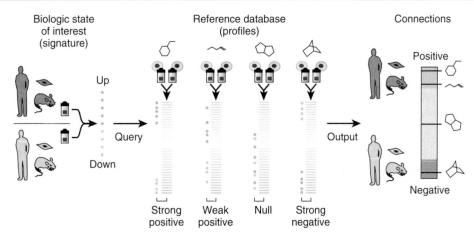

FIGURE 4-8. The connectivity map. Gene expression profiles derived from the treatment of cultured human cells with a large number of perturbagens populate a reference database. Gene expression signatures represent any induced or organic cell state of interest (*left*). Pattern matching algorithms score each reference profile for the direction and strength of enrichment with the query signature (*center*). Perturbagens are ranked by this connectivity score. Those at the top (positive) and bottom (negative) are functionally connected with the query state (*right*) through the transitory feature of common gene expression changes. (*Adapted from Lamb J, Crawford ED, Peck D, et al. The Connectivity Map: using gene-expression signatures to connect small molecules, genes, and disease. Science. 2006;313:1929-1935.*)

differentiation. BCL6 possesses an N-terminal BTB-POZ (Bric-a-brac, Tramtrack, broad complex–poxvirus zinc finger) domain, and the BTB domain recruits the corepressors SMRT (silencing mediator of retinoid and thyroid receptors), NCoR (nuclear receptor corepressor), and BCoR (BCL6 corepressor).[407] The interface through which BCL6 recruits corepressor proteins has been characterized with x-ray crystallography and, based on this structure, a peptide inhibitor blocking the interaction of these proteins has been designed.[408] This peptide disrupted BCL6-mediated repression and reactivated the expression of BCL6 target genes. Furthermore, in B-cell lymphoma cells positive for BCL6, the peptide caused apoptosis and cell cycle arrest. With improved methods of delivering peptides to cells, peptide therapy has become more feasible. One method fuses the peptide with protein transduction domains (PTDs). PTDs mediate receptor-independent cell penetration by binding the peptide to lipid rafts and triggering macropynocytosis.[409]

Emerging Lineage-Dependent Targets in Pediatric Cancer

Antidisialoganglioside and Neuroblastoma

Cure rates for children with high-stage neuroblastoma have improved with the dose intensity of chemotherapy. However, even with double autologous stem cell transplantation, most children with stage 4 disease will relapse. For long-term survivors, therapy-related morbidity is high. Alternative approaches to cytotoxic therapy are clearly needed. One approach to targeted therapy for this disease has exploited the high-density expression of the neuronal lineage marker disialoganglioside (GD2) on neuroblastoma cells.[410] Several anti-GD2 monoclonal antibodies have been developed and tested in clinical trials. One of the first was a murine immunoglobulin G3 (IgG3) monoclonal antibody, 3F8, directed at GD2. 3F8 is reported to mediate neuroblastoma cell death by human complement activation and by activation of lymphocytes, monocytes, and neutrophils.[411-413] In one review of the use of 3F8, 34 children were treated with 3F8 after receiving chemotherapy and radiation for stage 4 neuroblastoma.[414] All 34 patients had stable or minimal disease at the time of initiation of 3F8 treatment, and 25 had evidence of minimal residual disease by at least one measurement. There was evidence of response by bone marrow PCR studies (7 of 12) and marrow immunocytology (6 of 9). At the time of study follow-up, 14 patients were alive and 13 were without disease progression 40 to 130 months after the initiation of treatment with 3F8. Side effects included those common to antibody therapy, such as allergic reactions with anaphylaxis, as well as those specific to GD2 lineage, such as severe pain.

Subsequent studies have evaluated whether the addition of granulocyte macrophage–colony-stimulating factor (GM-CSF) to 3F8 would increase response by increasing the number of granulocytes and by priming effector cells for greater cytotoxicity. Forty-five patients with high-stage disease not in remission were enrolled.[415] In this study, 80% of 15 patients with refractory bone marrow disease had a CR in bone marrow; 11 patients were treated for recurrent neuroblastoma that was refractory to salvage therapy; 5 of 10 with marrow disease had CR in the marrow, but the only patient with soft tissue disease progressed. Additionally, the 15 patients treated for progressive disease did poorly, with all continuing to progress. The combination of GM-CSF and 3F8 was well tolerated; the principal side effects were pain and rash. It was concluded that 3F8 and GM-CSF is well tolerated and shows promise for the treatment of minimal residual neuroblastoma in the bone marrow. Subsequent studies have evaluated potential predictors of clinical outcome and markers for monitoring minimal residual disease. One study has identified GD2 synthase mRNA as a sensitive marker for minimal residual disease, with potential use as an early predictor of disease progression with 3F8–GM-CSF immunotherapy.[416] A second study has identified the *FCGR2A* polymorphism as correlated with clinical outcome after this immunotherapy regimen.[417] GM-CSF enhances phagocyte-mediated ADCC, and ADCC is mediated by Fcγ receptors. Thus, it is not surprising that different Fcγ receptors' alleles might correlate with different responses to antibody-based therapy.

Another anti-GD2 antibody is 14.G2a, a murine monoclonal IgG2a antibody, that has been tested in clinical trials.[418,419] In an attempt to improve this antibody, a chimeric human–murine anti-GD2 monoclonal antibody (ch14.18) was developed and tested in phase I clinical trials, with some encouraging results.[420,421] This construct uses the 14.G2a variable region's heavy and light chains and human constant region genes for IgG1 heavy chains and kappa light chains. However, a large retrospective study that included 334 assessable children older than 1 year (166 received ch14.18 consolidation treatment, 99 received 12-month low-dose maintenance chemotherapy, and 69 had no additional treatment) failed to demonstrate an advantage to ch14.18 in event-free survival (EFS) or overall survival (OS) with multivariate analysis.[422] Similarly, an analysis of infants younger than 1 year failed to show a difference in outcome with ch14.18 consolidation therapy.[423]

Ch14.18 was also tested in combination with GM-CSF in a phase I study with manageable toxicities, including pain, urticaria, and emesis.[424] Testing was performed with humanized ch14.18 linked to interleukin-2 (IL-2) with the hypothesis that IL-2 would augment activation of preexisting antigen-specific T cells, enhancing destruction of tumor cells and activation of natural killer cells. A phase I trial demonstrated manageable side effects—hypotension, allergic reaction, fever, pain, marrow suppression, and blurred vision. Out of 27 patients, 3 experienced some antitumor activity, with decreased tumor burden in the bone marrow.[425]

Although treatment with anti-GD2-based immunotherapy is not curative for patients with neuroblastoma, there may be a role for its use in bone marrow and minimal residual disease. Although the overall evidence remains unclear, many of the clinical trials have demonstrated some evidence of marrow response in patients with minimal tumor burden. A phase III trial evaluating ch14.18–IL2 with GM-CSF and 13-*cis*-retinoic acid versus retinoic acid alone for patients post–stem cell transplantation is ongoing.

Stromal Dependence

Vascular Endothelial Growth Factor Receptor and Ewing's Sarcoma

As with adult epithelial tumors, angiogenic factors are likely important in the growth and progression of pediatric tumors. In particular, there is specific interest in antiangiogenesis agents for Ewing's sarcoma. Ewing's sarcoma cell lines have been reported to express high levels of VEGF compared with normal osteoblasts.[426] This cell line–based evidence is supported by human in vivo studies, in which serum VEGF levels were elevated in children with Ewing's sarcoma, lymphoma, medulloblastoma, and Langerhans cell histiocytosis. These levels declined with treatment of the tumor with chemotherapy.[427] Another study has confirmed that serum levels of VEGF are higher in patients with Ewing's sarcoma, but not in patients with osteosarcoma or chondrosarcoma.[428] High levels of VEGF in Ewing's sarcoma have been associated with poor outcome, and data suggest that EWS-FLI may activate the expression of VEGF.[429] Furthermore, increased expression of VEGF has been reported in human fibroblasts engineered to express the EWS-FLI fusion.[430]

Chemical, antibody, and genetic manipulation of VEGF or VEGFR in Ewing's tumors have been demonstrated to induce antitumor activity. One group of investigators found downregulated VEGF expression following transfection with the adenovirus type 5 early region 1A (E1A). Specifically, in mice bearing a Ewing's xenograft, intratumoral injection of this adenoviral vector containing E1A decreased expression of VEGF, decreased tumor growth, decreased blood vessel density, and increased the survival rates of the mice.[426] Furthermore, direct inhibition of VEGF with siRNA inhibited Ewing's sarcoma tumor growth in a xenograft model.[431] Initial preclinical testing of the VEGF inhibitor, AZD2171, indicated broad inhibitory activity in multiple xenograft solid tumors, including Ewing's sarcoma, but only rare tumor regression, suggesting an antiangiogenic effect.[432] A new Children's Oncology Group trial, testing cytoxan and topotecan with or without bevacizumab, is ongoing.

Synthetic Lethal or Empirical Track

Insulin-like Growth Factor Receptor Signaling and Pediatric Solid Tumors

Over 10 years ago, the insulin-like growth factor-1 receptor (IGF-1R) signaling pathway was implicated in Ewing's sarcoma. It has also been implicated in other pediatric and adult tumors.[433] With the evolution of small-molecule inhibitors of receptor tyrosine kinases and the development of antibody-based therapy, therapeutic inhibition of this pathway has become a reality. The IGF-1R is a heterodimeric receptor with an alpha subunit containing the extracellular ligand binding domain and the beta subunit containing the transmembrane and intracellular tyrosine kinase domains. IGF-I and IGF-II and, to a lesser extent, insulin, bind to IGF-1R, leading to receptor activation, autophosphorylation, and phosphorylation of downstream targets. The receptor is important for development, cell growth, transformation, and prevention of apoptosis.

One early study has demonstrated that IGF-1 mRNA is expressed in 90% of Ewing's tumor samples positive for the EWS-FLI translocation. Furthermore, it demonstrated that blockade of the IGF-1R with a monoclonal antibody inhibits serum-free growth in a Ewing's cell line.[434] Next, it was demonstrated that IGF-1R is essential for EWS-FLI transformation of fibroblasts and that expression of the EWS-FLI fusion may alter the IGF-1R signaling pathway.[435] In addition, the expression of insulin-like growth factor binding protein (IGFBP-3) is strongly induced with siRNA against EWS-FLI, and EWS-FLI can bind the IGFBP-3 promoter and repress its activity, suggesting that dysregulation of IGFBP-3 contributes to the development of Ewing's sarcoma.[436,437] More recent work has demonstrated that a small-molecule inhibitor of IGF-1R, NVP-AEW541, a pyrrolopyrimidine derivative with selectivity for IGF-1R versus insulin receptor, has activity in in vitro and in vivo models of Ewing's sarcoma.[438,439] Furthermore, a dominant negative mutant IGF-1R inhibits tumorigenesis and induces apoptosis in Ewing's sarcoma cells.[440]

In addition to Ewing's sarcoma, IGF-1R has been implicated in a number of other pediatric solid tumors. One study has reported inhibition of proliferation in several pediatric cancer–related cell lines (neuroblastoma, rhabdomyosarcoma, and osteosarcoma) with an antagonistic, monoclonal antibody (EM164) directed against IGF-1R.[441] Other evidence implicating IGF-related signaling in rhabdomyosarcoma, particularly for alveolar, includes upregulation of IGF-II in cell lines, cooperation of IGFII and PAX3-FKHR, and inhibition of rhabdomyosarcoma growth with overexpression of IGFBP6, an inhibitor of IGF-II.[442-444] In osteosarcoma, expression of IGF-1R has been reported in canine and human cells.[445] In neuroblastoma, the small-molecule inhibitor NVP-AEW541 has in vitro and in vivo activity,[446] and evidence suggests that IGF-1R expression may regulate metastases to bone.[447]

An ongoing phase I trial in adults is testing AMG479, a fully human monoclonal antibody against IGF-1R, in patients with advanced cancer. Activity has been reported in an initial abstract presentation at the American Society of Clinical Oncology meeting in 2007.[448] Trials are now ongoing testing monoclonal antibodies against IGF-1R in pediatric patients.

CONCLUSION

Tremendous progress has been made in the treatment of pediatric cancer over the last century. The empirical combination of cytotoxic agents has proven curative for many patients, but at the expense of toxicity. Over the last decade, heralded by the success of targeting BCR-ABL in CML, we have entered a new era of drug discovery, with an emphasis on target-based treatment that holds promise for improved cure rates and decreased toxicity. New and developing high-throughput genomic and proteomic technologies are dramatically altering the landscape of research, enabling the identification and credentialing of new targets with a speed previously unfathomable. In this chapter, we have provided a framework for classifying and credentialing new targets. We have highlighted examples of successful targeted approaches for the treatment of adults with cancer and have discussed emerging targets for pediatric cancer. Although it is an exciting time in cancer therapy, there are many sobering challenges that lie ahead in the development of targeted therapy, particularly for pediatric cancer. Continued advancement will require innovative approaches to intractable targets (e.g., transcription factors), rational approaches to combination therapy, and collaborative efforts between industry and academic centers to identify new pediatric targets, along with target-specific drugs. For maximal progress in the treatment of children with cancer, we will need to address the issues that confront the clinical development of novel therapeutics collectively. Trials that allow for biopsies, genetic profiling of tumors, and "window treatment" periods may be necessary to bring targeted therapies into the pediatric realm.

REFERENCES

1. Eng WK, Faucette L, Johnson RK, Sternglanz R. Evidence that DNA topoisomerase I is necessary for the cytotoxic effects of camptothecin. Mol Pharmacol. 1988;34:755-760.
2. Rothenberg ML. Topoisomerase I inhibitors: review and update. Ann Oncol. 1997;8:837-855.
3. Avemann K, Knippers R, Koller T, Sogo JM. Camptothecin, a specific inhibitor of type I DNA topoisomerase, induces DNA breakage at replication forks. Mol Cell Biol. 1988;8:3026-3034.
4. Burden DA, Osheroff N. Mechanism of action of eukaryotic topoisomerase II and drugs targeted to the enzyme. Biochim Biophys Acta. 1998;1400:139-154.
5. Zunino F, Capranico G. DNA topoisomerase II as the primary target of anti-tumor anthracyclines. Anticancer Drug Des. 1990;5:307-317.
6. Kumar N. Taxol-induced polymerization of purified tubulin. Mechanism of action. J Biol Chem. 1981;256:10435-10441.
7. Fenaux P, Chastang C, Chevret S, et al. A randomized comparison of all-transretinoic acid (ATRA) followed by chemotherapy and ATRA plus chemotherapy and the role of maintenance therapy in newly diagnosed acute promyelocytic leukemia. The European APL Group. Blood. 1999;94:1192-1200.
8. Sanz MA, Martin G, Lo Coco F. Choice of chemotherapy in induction, consolidation and maintenance in acute promyelocytic leukaemia. Best Pract Res Clin Haematol. 2003;16:433-451.
9. Moghrabi A, Levy DE, Asselin B, et al. Results of the Dana-Farber Cancer Institute ALL Consortium Protocol 95-01 for children with acute lymphoblastic leukemia. Blood. 2007;109:896-904.
10. Chauvenet AR, Martin PL, Devidas M, et al. Anti-metabolite therapy for lesser risk B-lineage acute lymphoblastic leukemia of childhood: a report from Children's Oncology Group Study P9201. Blood. 2007;110:1105-1111.
11. Chen ZX, Xue YQ, Zhang R, et al. A clinical and experimental study on all-trans retinoic acid-treated acute promyelocytic leukemia patients. Blood. 1991;78:1413-1419.
12. Huang ME, Ye YC, Chen SR, et al. Use of all-trans retinoic acid in the treatment of acute promyelocytic leukemia. Blood. 1988;72:567-572.
13. Grier HE, Krailo MD, Tarbell NJ, et al. Addition of ifosfamide and etoposide to standard chemotherapy for Ewing's sarcoma and primitive neuroectodermal tumor of bone. N Engl J Med. 2003;348:694-701.
14. Cheung NV, Heller G. Chemotherapy dose intensity correlates strongly with response: median survival, and median progression-free survival in metastatic neuroblastoma. J Clin Oncol. 1991;9:1050-1058.
15. Matthay KK, Villablanca JG, Seeger RC, et al. Treatment of high-risk neuroblastoma with intensive chemotherapy, radiotherapy, autologous bone marrow transplantation, and 13-cis-retinoic acid. Children's Cancer Group. N Engl J Med. 1999;341:1165-1173.
16. Grupp SA, Stern JW, Bunin N, et al. Tandem high-dose therapy in rapid sequence for children with high-risk neuroblastoma. J Clin Oncol. 2000;18:2567-2575.
17. George RE, Li S, Medeiros-Nancarrow C, et al. High-risk neuroblastoma treated with tandem autologous peripheral-blood stem cell-supported transplantation: long-term survival update. J Clin Oncol. 2006;24:2891-2896.
18. Pinkel D, Hernandez K, Borella L, et al. Drug dosage and remission duration in childhood lymphocytic leukemia. Cancer. 1971;27:247-256.
19. Silverman LB, Gelber RD, Dalton VK, et al. Improved outcome for children with acute lymphoblastic leukemia: results of Dana-Farber Consortium Protocol 91-01. Blood. 2001;97:1211-1218.
20. Gaynon PS, Steinherz PG, Bleyer WA, et al. Association of delivered drug dose and outcome for children with acute lymphoblastic leukemia and unfavorable presenting features. Med Pediatr Oncol. 1991;19:221-227.
21. Childhood ALL Collaborative Group. Duration and intensity of maintenance chemotherapy in acute lymphoblastic leukaemia: overview of 42 trials involving 12 000 randomised children. Lancet. 1996;347:1783-1788.
22. Delepine N, Delepine G, Bacci G, et al. Influence of methotrexate dose intensity on outcome of patients with high grade osteogenic osteosarcoma. Analysis of the literature. Cancer. 1996;78:2127-2135.
23. Bacci G, Ferrari S, Longhi A, et al. Relationship between dose-intensity of treatment and outcome for patients with osteosarcoma of the extremity treated with neoadjuvant chemotherapy. Oncol Rep. 2001;8:883-888.
24. Lewis IJ, Nooij MA, Whelan J, et al. Improvement in histologic response but not survival in osteosarcoma patients treated with intensified chemotherapy: a randomized phase III trial of the European Osteosarcoma Intergroup. J Natl Cancer Inst. 2007;99:112-128.
25. Eselgrim M, Grunert H, Kuhne T, et al. Dose intensity of chemotherapy for osteosarcoma and outcome in the Cooperative Osteosarcoma Study Group (COSS) trials. Pediatr Blood Cancer. 2006;47:42-50.
26. Moore HC, Green SJ, Gralow JR, et al. Intensive dose-dense compared with high-dose adjuvant chemotherapy for high-risk operable breast cancer: Southwest Oncology Group/Intergroup study 9623. J Clin Oncol. 2007;25:1677-1682.
27. Kroger N, Frick M, Gluz O, et al. Randomized trial of single compared with tandem high-dose chemotherapy followed by autologous stem-cell transplantation in patients with chemotherapy-sensitive metastatic breast cancer. J Clin Oncol. 2006;24:3919-3926.
28. Meadows AT. Pediatric cancer survivorship: research and clinical care. J Clin Oncol. 2006;24:5160-5165.

29. Swain SM. Adult multicenter trials using dexrazoxane to protect against cardiac toxicity. Semin Oncol. 1998;25:43-47.

30. Lipshultz SE, Rifai N, Dalton VM, et al. The effect of dexrazoxane on myocardial injury in doxorubicin-treated children with acute lymphoblastic leukemia. N Engl J Med. 2004;351:145-153.

31. Corn BW, Goldwein JW, Evans I, D'Angio GJ. Outcomes in low-risk babies treated with half-dose chemotherapy according to the Third National Wilms' Tumor Study. J Clin Oncol. 1992;10:1305-1309.

32. Rubie H, Coze C, Plantaz D, et al. Localised and unresectable neuroblastoma in infants: excellent outcome with low-dose primary chemotherapy. Br J Cancer. 2003;89:1605-1609.

33. Evans AE, Silber JH, Shpilsky A, D'Angio GJ. Successful management of low-stage neuroblastoma without adjuvant therapies: a comparison of two decades, 1972 through 1981 and 1982 through 1992, in a single institution. J Clin Oncol. 1996;14:2504-2510.

34. Rutqvist LE, Cedermark B, Glas U, et al. Randomized trial of adjuvant tamoxifen in node negative postmenopausal breast cancer. Stockholm Breast Cancer Study Group. Acta Oncol. 1992;31:265-270.

35. Early Breast Cancer Trialists' Collaborative Group (EBCTCG). Effects of chemotherapy and hormonal therapy for early breast cancer on recurrence and 15-year survival: an overview of the randomised trials. Lancet. 2005;365:1687-1717.

36. Jones KL, Buzdar AU. A review of adjuvant hormonal therapy in breast cancer. Endocr Relat Cancer. 2004;11:391-406.

37. Osborne CK. Tamoxifen in the treatment of breast cancer. N Engl J Med. 1998;339:1609-1618.

38. Tormey DC, Simon RM, Lippman ME, et al. Evaluation of tamoxifen dose in advanced breast cancer: a progress report. Cancer Treat Rep. 1976;60:1451-1459.

38a. Bratherton DG, Brown CH, Buchanan R, et al. A comparison of two doses of tamoxifen (Nolvadex) in postmenopausal women with advanced breast cancer: 10 mg bd versus 20 mg bd. Br J Cancer. 1984;50:199-205.

39. Coombes RC, Hall E, Gibson LJ, et al. A randomized trial of exemestane after two to three years of tamoxifen therapy in postmenopausal women with primary breast cancer. N Engl J Med. 2004;350:1081-1092.

40. Coombes RC, Kilburn LS, Snowdon CF, et al. Survival and safety of exemestane versus tamoxifen after 2-3 years' tamoxifen treatment (Intergroup Exemestane Study): a randomised controlled trial. Lancet. 2007;369:559-570.

41. Baum M, Buzdar A, Cuzick J, et al. Anastrozole alone or in combination with tamoxifen versus tamoxifen alone for adjuvant treatment of postmenopausal women with early-stage breast cancer: results of the ATAC (Arimidex, Tamoxifen Alone or in Combination) trial efficacy and safety update analyses. Cancer. 2003;98:1802-1810.

42. Coleman RE, Banks LM, Girgis SI, et al. Skeletal effects of exemestane on bone-mineral density, bone biomarkers, and fracture incidence in postmenopausal women with early breast cancer participating in the Intergroup Exemestane Study (IES): a randomised controlled study. Lancet Oncol. 2007;8:119-127.

43. Gorre ME, Mohammed M, Ellwood K, et al. Clinical resistance to STI-571 cancer therapy caused by BCR-ABL gene mutation or amplification. Science. 2001;293:876-880.

44. Paez JG, Janne PA, Lee JC, et al. EGFR mutations in lung cancer: correlation with clinical response to gefitinib therapy. Science. 2004;304:1497-1500.

45. Weisberg E, Manley PW, Cowan-Jacob SW, et al. Second generation inhibitors of BCR-ABL for the treatment of imatinib-resistant chronic myeloid leukaemia. Nat Rev Cancer. 2007;7:345-356.

46. Benson JD, Chen YN, Cornell-Kennon SA, et al. Validating cancer drug targets. Nature. 2006;441:451-456.

47. Weinstein IB. Cancer. Addiction to oncogenes—the Achilles heal of cancer. Science. 2002;297:63-64.

48. Sawyers CL. Opportunities and challenges in the development of kinase inhibitor therapy for cancer. Genes Dev. 2003;17:2998-3010.

49. Garraway LA, Sellers WR. Lineage dependency and lineage-survival oncogenes in human cancer. Nat Rev Cancer. 2006;6:593-602.

50. Chen CD, Welsbie DS, Tran C, et al. Molecular determinants of resistance to antiandrogen therapy. Nat Med. 2004;10:33-39.

51. Michaelson MD, Smith MR. Bisphosphonates for treatment and prevention of bone metastases. J Clin Oncol. 2005;23:8219-8224.

52. O'Neill J, Manion M, Schwartz P, Hockenbery DM. Promises and challenges of targeting Bcl-2 anti-apoptotic proteins for cancer therapy. Biochim Biophys Acta. 2004;1705:43-51.

53. Farmer H, McCabe N, Lord CJ, et al. Targeting the DNA repair defect in BRCA mutant cells as a therapeutic strategy. Nature. 2005;434:917-921.

54. Yap TA, Boss DS, Fong PC, et al. First in human phase I pharmacokinetic (PK) and pharmacodynamic (PD) study of KU-0059436 (Ku), a small molecule inhibitor of poly ADP-ribose polymerase (PARP) in cancer patients (p), including BRCA1/2 mutation carriers. Abstract 3529. American Society of Clinical Oncology Meeting Proceedings, Part I. J Clin Oncol. 2007;25:145s.

55. Rajkumar SV, Richardson PG, Hideshima T, Anderson KC. Proteasome inhibition as a novel therapeutic target in human cancer. J Clin Oncol. 2005;23:630-639.

56. Obeng EA, Carlson LM, Gutman DM, et al. Proteasome inhibitors induce a terminal unfolded protein response in multiple myeloma cells. Blood. 2006;107:4907-4916.

57. Liang P, Pardee AB. Differential display of eukaryotic messenger RNA by means of the polymerase chain reaction. Science. 1992;257:967-971.

58. Velculescu VE, Zhang L, Vogelstein B, Kinzler KW. Serial analysis of gene expression. Science. 1995;270:484-487.

59. Schimke RT, Kaufman RJ, Alt FW, Kellems RF. Gene amplification and drug resistance in cultured murine cells. Science. 1978;202:1051-1055.

60. Febbo PG, Sellers WR. Use of expression analysis to predict outcome after radical prostatectomy. J Urol. 2003;170:S11-S19.

61. Mootha VK, Lindgren CM, Eriksson KF, et al. PGC-1alpha-responsive genes involved in oxidative phosphorylation are coordinately downregulated in human diabetes. Nat Genet. 2003;34:267-273.

62. Subramanian A, Tamayo P, Mootha VK, et al. Gene set enrichment analysis: a knowledge-based approach for interpreting genome-wide expression profiles. Proc Natl Acad Sci U S A. 2005;102:15545-15550.

63. Tomlins SA, Rhodes DR, Perner S, et al. Recurrent fusion of TMPRSS2 and ETS transcription factor genes in prostate cancer. Science. 2005;310:644-648.

64. Greenman C, Stephens P, Smith R, et al. Patterns of somatic mutation in human cancer genomes. Nature. 2007;446:153-158.

65. Volik S, Zhao S, Chin K, et al. End-sequence profiling: sequence-based analysis of aberrant genomes. Proc Natl Acad Sci U S A. 2003;100:7696-7701.

66. Takeyama K, Monti S, Manis JP, et al. Integrative analysis reveals 53BP1 copy loss and decreased expression in a subset of human diffuse large B-cell lymphomas. Oncogene. 2007;27:318-22.

67. Zaharieva BM, Simon R, Diener PA, et al. High-throughput tissue microarray analysis of 11q13 gene amplification (CCND1, FGF3, FGF4, EMS1) in urinary bladder cancer. J Pathol. 2003;201:603-608.

68. Ursini-Siegel J, Schade B, Cardiff RD, Muller WJ. Insights from transgenic mouse models of ERBB2-induced breast cancer. Nat Rev Cancer. 2007;7:389-397.

69. Beroukhim R, Getz G, Nghiemphu L, et al. Assessing the significance of chromosomal aberrations in cancer: methodology and application to glioma. Proc Natl Acad Sci U S A. 2007;104(50):20007-20012.

70. Bos JL. ras oncogenes in human cancer: a review. Cancer Res. 1989;49:4682-4689.

71. Davies H, Bignell GR, Cox C, et al. Mutations of the BRAF gene in human cancer. Nature. 2002;417:949-954.

72. Samuels Y, Wang Z, Bardelli A, et al. High frequency of mutations of the PIK3CA gene in human cancers. Science. 2004;304:554.

73. Cahill DP, Levine KK, Betensky RA, et al. Loss of the mismatch repair protein MSH6 in human glioblastomas is associated with tumor progression during temozolomide treatment. Clin Cancer Res. 2007;13:2038-2045.

74. Hunter C, Smith R, Cahill DP, et al. A hypermutation phenotype and somatic MSH6 mutations in recurrent human malignant gliomas after alkylator chemotherapy. Cancer Res. 2006;66:3987-3991.

75. Margulies M, Egholm M, Altman WE, et al. Genome sequencing in microfabricated high-density picolitre reactors. Nature. 2005;437:376-380.

76. Bentley DR. Whole-genome re-sequencing. Curr Opin Genet Dev. 2006;16:545-552.

77. Johnson RL, Rothman AL, Xie J, et al. Human homolog of patched, a candidate gene for the basal cell nevus syndrome. Science. 1996;272:1668-1671.

78. Hahn H, Wicking C, Zaphiropoulous PG, et al. Mutations of the human homolog of Drosophila patched in the nevoid basal cell carcinoma syndrome. Cell. 1996;85:841-851.

79. Gailani MR, Stahle-Backdahl M, Leffell DJ, et al. The role of the human homologue of Drosophila patched in sporadic basal cell carcinomas. Nat Genet. 1996;14:78-81.

80. Stone DM, Hynes M, Armanini M, et al. The tumour-suppressor gene patched encodes a candidate receptor for Sonic hedgehog. Nature. 1996;384:129-134.

81. Taipale J, Chen JK, Cooper MK, et al. Effects of oncogenic mutations in Smoothened and Patched can be reversed by cyclopamine. Nature. 2000;406:1005-1009.

82. Kakizuka A, Miller WH Jr, Umesono K, et al. Chromosomal translocation t(15;17) in human acute promyelocytic leukemia fuses RAR alpha with a novel putative transcription factor, PML. Cell. 1991;66:663-674.

83. Walker GJ, Flores JF, Glendening JM, et al. Almost 100% of melanoma cell lines harbor alterations at the DNA level within CDKN2A, CDKN2B, or one of their downstream targets. Genes Chromosomes Cancer. 1998;22:157-163.

84. Slamon DJ, Godolphin W, Jones LA, et al. Studies of the HER-2/neu proto-oncogene in human breast and ovarian cancer. Science. 1989;244:707-712.

85. Hahn WC, Counter CM, Lundberg AS, et al. Creation of human tumour cells with defined genetic elements. Nature. 1999;400:464-468.

86. James C, Ugo V, Le Couedic JP, et al. A unique clonal JAK2 mutation leading to constitutive signalling causes polycythaemia vera. Nature. 2005;434:1144-1148.

87. Kralovics R, Passamonti F, Buser AS, et al. A gain-of-function mutation of JAK2 in myeloproliferative disorders. N Engl J Med. 2005;352:1779-1790.

88. Levine RL, Wadleigh M, Cools J, et al. Activating mutation in the tyrosine kinase JAK2 in polycythemia vera, essential thrombocythemia, and myeloid metaplasia with myelofibrosis. Cancer Cell. 2005;7:387-397.

89. Zender L, Spector MS, Xue W, et al. Identification and validation of oncogenes in liver cancer using an integrative oncogenomic approach. Cell. 2006;125:1253-1267.

90. Zender L, Xue W, Cordon-Cardo C, et al. Generation and analysis of genetically defined liver carcinomas derived from bipotential liver progenitors. Cold Spring Harb Symp Quant Biol. 2005;70:251-261.

91. Johnson L, Mercer K, Greenbaum D, et al. Somatic activation of the K-ras oncogene causes early onset lung cancer in mice. Nature. 2001;410:1111-1116.

92. Hingorani SR, Petricoin EF, Maitra A, et al. Preinvasive and invasive ductal pancreatic cancer and its early detection in the mouse. Cancer Cell. 2003;4:437-450.

93. Chan IT, Kutok JL, Williams IR, et al. Conditional expression of oncogenic K-ras from its endogenous promoter induces a myeloproliferative disease. J Clin Invest. 2004;113:528-538.

94. Hannon GJ. RNA interference. Nature. 2002;418:244-251.

95. Paddison PJ, Hannon GJ. RNA interference: the new somatic cell genetics? Cancer Cell. 2002;2:17-23.

96. Xue W, Zender L, Miething C, et al. Senescence and tumour clearance is triggered by p53 restoration in murine liver carcinomas. Nature. 2007;445:656-660.

97. Dickins RA, McJunkin K, Hernando E, et al. Tissue-specific and reversible RNA interference in transgenic mice. Nat Genet. 2007;39:914-921.

98. Potter CJ, Huang H, Xu T. Drosophila Tsc1 functions with Tsc2 to antagonize insulin signaling in regulating cell growth, cell proliferation, and organ size. Cell. 2001;105:357-368.

99. Tapon N, Ito N, Dickson BJ, et al. The Drosophila tuberous sclerosis complex gene homologs restrict cell growth and cell proliferation. Cell. 2001;105:345-355.

100. Ito N, Rubin GM. gigas, a Drosophila homolog of tuberous sclerosis gene product-2, regulates the cell cycle. Cell. 1999;96:529-539.

101. Stockwell BR. Chemical genetics: ligand-based discovery of gene function. Nat Rev Genet. 2000;1:116-125.

102. Burke MD, Berger EM, Schreiber SL. Generating diverse skeletons of small molecules combinatorially. Science. 2003;302:613-618.

103. Burke MD, Schreiber SL. A planning strategy for diversity-oriented synthesis. Angew Chem Int Ed Engl. 2004;43:46-58.

104. Shuker SB, Hajduk PJ, Meadows RP, Fesik SW. Discovering high-affinity ligands for proteins: SAR by NMR. Science. 1996;274:1531-1534.

105. Newman DJ, Cragg GM, Snader KM. Natural products as sources of new drugs over the period 1981-2002. J Nat Prod. 2003;66:1022-1037.

106. Tan G, Gyllenhaal C, Soejarto DD. Biodiversity as a source of anticancer drugs. Curr Drug Targets. 2006;7:265-277.

107. Clardy J, Walsh C. Lessons from natural molecules. Nature. 2004;432:829-837.

108. Bierer BE, Somers PK, Wandless TJ, et al. Probing immunosuppressant action with a nonnatural immunophilin ligand. Science. 1990;250:556-559.

109. Zheng XF, Florentino D, Chen J, et al. TOR kinase domains are required for two distinct functions, only one of which is inhibited by rapamycin. Cell. 1995;82:121-130.

110. Vidal L, Blagden S, Attard G, de Bono J. Making sense of antisense. Eur J Cancer. 2005;41:2812-2818.

111. Stein CA, Benimetskaya L, Mani S. Antisense strategies for oncogene inactivation. Semin Oncol. 2005;32:563-572.

112. Kurreck J. Antisense technologies. Improvement through novel chemical modifications. Eur J Biochem. 2003;270:1628-1644.

113. O'Brien SM, Cunningham CC, Golenkov AK, et al. Phase I to II multicenter study of oblimersen sodium, a Bcl-2 antisense oligonucleotide, in patients with advanced chronic lymphocytic leukemia. J Clin Oncol. 2005;23:7697-7702.

114. O'Brien S, Moore JO, Boyd TE, et al. Randomized phase III trial of fludarabine plus cyclophosphamide with or without oblimersen sodium (Bcl-2 antisense) in patients with relapsed or refractory chronic lymphocytic leukemia. J Clin Oncol. 2007;25:1114-1120.

115. Bernstein E, Caudy AA, Hammond SM, Hannon GJ. Role for a bidentate ribonuclease in the initiation step of RNA interference. Nature. 2001;409:363-366.

116. Li CX, Parker A, Menocal E, et al. Delivery of RNA interference. Cell Cycle. 2006;5:2103-2109.

117. Hacein-Bey-Abina S, von Kalle C, Schmidt M, et al. A serious adverse event after successful gene therapy for X-linked severe combined immunodeficiency. N Engl J Med. 2003;348:255-256.

118. Hacein-Bey-Abina S, Von Kalle C, Schmidt M, et al. LMO2-associated clonal T cell proliferation in two patients after gene therapy for SCID-X1. Science. 2003;302:415-419.

119. Noureddini SC, Curiel DT. Genetic targeting strategies for adenovirus. Mol Pharm. 2005;2:341-347.

120. Braasch DA, Jensen S, Liu Y, et al. RNA interference in mammalian cells by chemically-modified RNA. Biochemistry. 2003;42:7967-7975.

121. Elmen J, Thonberg H, Ljungberg K, et al. Locked nucleic acid (LNA) mediated improvements in siRNA stability and functionality. Nucleic Acids Res. 2005;33:439-447.

122. Nawrot B, Sipa K. Chemical and structural diversity of siRNA molecules. Curr Top Med Chem. 2006;6:913-925.

123. Landen CN Jr, Chavez-Reyes A, Bucana C, et al. Therapeutic EphA2 gene targeting in vivo using neutral liposomal small interfering RNA delivery. Cancer Res. 2005;65:6910-6918.

124. Urban-Klein B, Werth S, Abuharbeid S, et al. RNAi-mediated gene-targeting through systemic application of polyethylenimine (PEI)-complexed siRNA in vivo. Gene Ther. 2005;12:461-466.

125. Spagnou S, Miller AD, Keller M. Lipidic carriers of siRNA: differences in the formulation, cellular uptake, and delivery with plasmid DNA. Biochemistry. 2004;43:13348-13356.

126. Siberil S, Dutertre CA, Fridman WH, Teillaud JL. FcgammaR: The key to optimize therapeutic antibodies? Crit Rev Oncol Hematol. 2007;62:26-33.

127. Loisel S, Ohresser M, Pallardy M, et al. Relevance, advantages and limitations of animal models used in the development of monoclonal antibodies for cancer treatment. Crit Rev Oncol Hematol. 2007;62:34-42.

128. Breitman TR, Selonick SE, Collins SJ. Induction of differentiation of the human promyelocytic leukemia cell line (HL-60) by retinoic acid. Proc Natl Acad Sci U S A. 1980;77:2936-2940.

129. Kogan SC, Bishop JM. Acute promyelocytic leukemia: from treatment to genetics and back. Oncogene. 1999;18:5261-5267.

130. Grignani F, Ferrucci PF, Testa U, et al. The acute promyelocytic leukemia-specific PML-RAR alpha fusion protein inhibits differentiation and promotes survival of myeloid precursor cells. Cell. 1993;74:423-431.

131. Melnick A, Licht JD. Deconstructing a disease: RARalpha, its fusion partners, and their roles in the pathogenesis of acute promyelocytic leukemia. Blood. 1999;93:3167-3215.

132. Grignani F, De Matteis S, Nervi C, et al. Fusion proteins of the retinoic acid receptor-alpha recruit histone deacetylase in promyelocytic leukaemia. Nature. 1998;391:815-818.

133. Lin RJ, Nagy L, Inoue S, et al. Role of the histone deacetylase complex in acute promyelocytic leukaemia. Nature. 1998;391:811-814.

134. Lo Coco F, Avvisati G, Diverio D, et al. Molecular evaluation of response to all-trans-retinoic acid therapy in patients with acute promyelocytic leukemia. Blood. 1991;77:1657-1659.

135. Yoshida H, Kitamura K, Tanaka K, et al. Accelerated degradation of PML-retinoic acid receptor alpha (PML-RARA) oncoprotein by all-trans-retinoic acid in acute promyelocytic leukemia: possible role of the proteasome pathway. Cancer Res. 1996;56:2945-2948.

136. Warrell RP Jr, Frankel SR, Miller WH Jr, et al. Differentiation therapy of acute promyelocytic leukemia with tretinoin (all-trans-retinoic acid). N Engl J Med. 1991;324:1385-1393.

137. He LZ, Guidez F, Triboli C, et al. Distinct interactions of PML-RARalpha and PLZF-RARalpha with co-repressors determine differential responses to RA in APL. Nat Genet. 1998;18:126-135.

138. Sanz MA. Recent advances in the treatment of APL. Clin Adv Hematol Oncol. 2006;4:727-729.

139. Nowell PC, Hungerford DA. Chromosome studies on normal and leukemic human leukocytes. J Natl Cancer Inst. 1960;25:85-109.

140. Shtivelman E, Lifshitz B, Gale RP, Canaani E. Fused transcript of abl and bcr genes in chronic myelogenous leukaemia. Nature. 1985;315:550-554.

141. Ben-Neriah Y, Daley GQ, Mes-Masson AM, et al. The chronic myelogenous leukemia-specific P210 protein is the product of the bcr/abl hybrid gene. Science. 1986;233:212-214.

142. Davis RL, Konopka JB, Witte ON. Activation of the c-abl oncogene by viral transduction or chromosomal translocation generates altered c-abl proteins with similar in vitro kinase properties. Mol Cell Biol. 1985;5:204-213.

143. Daley GQ, Van Etten RA, Baltimore D. Induction of chronic myelogenous leukemia in mice by the P210bcr/abl gene of the Philadelphia chromosome. Science. 1990;247:824-830.

144. Buchdunger E, Zimmermann J, Mett H, et al. Inhibition of the Abl protein-tyrosine kinase in vitro and in vivo by a 2-phenylaminopyrimidine derivative. Cancer Res. 1996;56:100-104.

145. Druker BJ, Tamura S, Buchdunger E, et al. Effects of a selective inhibitor of the Abl tyrosine kinase on the growth of Bcr-Abl positive cells. Nat Med. 1996;2:561-566.

146. Deininger MW, Goldman JM, Lydon N, Melo JV. The tyrosine kinase inhibitor CGP57148B selectively inhibits the growth of BCR-ABL-positive cells. Blood. 1997;90:3691-3698.

147. Gambacorti-Passerini C, le Coutre P, Mologni L, et al. Inhibition of the ABL kinase activity blocks the proliferation of BCR/ABL+ leukemic cells and induces apoptosis. Blood Cells Mol Dis. 1997;23:380-394.

148. Druker BJ, Talpaz M, Resta DJ, et al. Efficacy and safety of a specific inhibitor of the BCR-ABL tyrosine kinase in chronic myeloid leukemia. N Engl J Med. 2001;344:1031-1037.

148a. Druker BJ, Sawyers CL, Kantarjian H, et al. Activity of a specific inhibitor of the BCR-ABL tyrosine kinase in the blast crisis of chronic myeloid leukemia and acute lymphoblastic leukemia with the Philadelphia chromosome. N Engl J Med 2001;344:1038-1042.

149. Kantarjian H, Sawyers C, Hochhaus A, et al. Hematologic and cytogenetic responses to imatinib mesylate in chronic myelogenous leukemia. N Engl J Med. 2002;346:645-652.

150. Talpaz M, Silver RT, Druker BJ, et al. Imatinib induces durable hematologic and cytogenetic responses in patients with accelerated phase chronic myeloid leukemia: results of a phase 2 study. Blood. 2002;99:1928-1937.

151. Sawyers CL, Hochhaus A, Feldman E, et al. Imatinib induces hematologic and cytogenetic responses in patients with chronic myelogenous leukemia in myeloid blast crisis: results of a phase II study. Blood. 2002;99:3530-3539.

152. Druker BJ, Guilhot F, O'Brien SG, et al. Five-year follow-up of patients receiving imatinib for chronic myeloid leukemia. N Engl J Med. 2006;355:2408-2417.

153. O'Brien SG, Guilhot F, Larson RA, et al. Imatinib compared with interferon and low-dose cytarabine for newly diagnosed chronic-phase chronic myeloid leukemia. N Engl J Med. 2003;348:994-1004.

154. Roy L, Guilhot J, Krahnke T, et al. Survival advantage from imatinib compared with the combination interferon-alpha plus cytarabine in chronic-phase chronic myelogenous leukemia: historical comparison between two phase 3 trials. Blood. 2006;108:1478-1484.

155. Azam M, Latek RR, Daley GQ. Mechanisms of autoinhibition and STI-571/imatinib resistance revealed by mutagenesis of BCR-ABL. Cell. 2003;112:831-843.

156. Shah NP, Nicoll JM, Nagar B, et al. Multiple BCR-ABL kinase domain mutations confer polyclonal resistance to the tyrosine kinase inhibitor imatinib (STI571) in chronic phase and blast crisis chronic myeloid leukemia. Cancer Cell. 2002;2:117-125.

157. Roumiantsev S, Shah NP, Gorre ME, et al. Clinical resistance to the kinase inhibitor STI-571 in chronic myeloid leukemia by mutation of Tyr-253 in the Abl kinase domain P-loop. Proc Natl Acad Sci U S A. 2002;99:10700-10705.

158. Weisberg E, Manley PW, Breitenstein W, et al. Characterization of AMN107, a selective inhibitor of native and mutant Bcr-Abl. Cancer Cell. 2005;7:129-141.

159. Kantarjian H, Giles F, Wunderle L, et al. Nilotinib in imatinib-resistant CML and Philadelphia chromosome-positive ALL. N Engl J Med. 2006;354:2542-2551.

160. Shah NP, Tran C, Lee FY, et al. Overriding imatinib resistance with a novel ABL kinase inhibitor. Science. 2004;305:399-401.

161. Talpaz M, Shah NP, Kantarjian H, et al. Dasatinib in imatinib-resistant Philadelphia chromosome-positive leukemias. N Engl J Med. 2006;354:2531-2541.

162. Young MA, Shah NP, Chao LH, et al. Structure of the kinase domain of an imatinib-resistant Abl mutant in complex with the Aurora kinase inhibitor VX-680. Cancer Res. 2006;66:1007-1014.

163. Giles FJ, Cortes J, Jones D, et al. MK-0457, a novel kinase inhibitor, is active in patients with chronic myeloid leukemia or acute lymphocytic leukemia with the T315I BCR-ABL mutation. Blood. 2007;109:500-502.

164. Nakahara M, Isozaki K, Hirota S, et al. A novel gain-of-function mutation of c-kit gene in gastrointestinal stromal tumors. Gastroenterology. 1998;115:1090-1095.

165. Rubin BP, Singer S, Tsao C, et al. KIT activation is a ubiquitous feature of gastrointestinal stromal tumors. Cancer Res. 2001;61:8118-8121.

166. Heinrich MC, Corless CL, Demetri GD, et al. Kinase mutations and imatinib response in patients with metastatic gastrointestinal stromal tumor. J Clin Oncol. 2003;21:4342-4349.

167. Li FP, Fletcher JA, Heinrich MC, et al. Familial gastrointestinal stromal tumor syndrome: phenotypic and molecular features in a kindred. J Clin Oncol. 2005;23:2735-2743.

168. Nilsson B, Bumming P, Meis-Kindblom JM, et al. Gastrointestinal stromal tumors: the incidence, prevalence, clinical course, and prognostication in the preimatinib mesylate era—a population-based study in western Sweden. Cancer. 2005;103:821-829.

169. Perez EA, Livingstone AS, Franceschi D, et al. Current incidence and outcomes of gastrointestinal mesenchymal tumors including gastrointestinal stromal tumors. J Am Coll Surg. 2006;202:623-629.

170. Tuveson DA, Willis NA, Jacks T, et al. STI571 inactivation of the gastrointestinal stromal tumor c-KIT oncoprotein: biological and clinical implications. Oncogene. 2001;20:5054-5058.

171. Joensuu H, Roberts PJ, Sarlomo-Rikala M, et al. Effect of the tyrosine kinase inhibitor STI571 in a patient with a metastatic gastrointestinal stromal tumor. N Engl J Med. 2001;344:1052-1056.

172. van Oosterom AT, Judson I, Verweij J, et al. Safety and efficacy of imatinib (STI571) in metastatic gastrointestinal stromal tumours: a phase I study. Lancet. 2001;358:1421-1423.

173. Demetri GD, von Mehren M, Blanke CD, et al. Efficacy and safety of imatinib mesylate in advanced gastrointestinal stromal tumors. N Engl J Med. 2002;347:472-480.

174. Siddiqui M, Asif A, Scott LJ. Imatinib: A review of its use in the management of gastrointestinal stromal tumours. Drugs. 2007;67:805-820.

175. Nilsson B, Sjolund K, Kindblom LG, et al. Adjuvant imatinib treatment improves recurrence-free survival in patients with high-risk gastrointestinal stromal tumours (GIST). Br J Cancer. 2007;96:1656-1658.

176. Shimizu A, O'Brien KP, Sjoblom T, et al. The dermatofibrosarcoma protuberans-associated collagen type I alpha1/platelet-derived growth factor (PDGF) B-chain fusion gene generates a transforming protein that is processed to functional PDGF-BB. Cancer Res. 1999;59:3719-3723.

177. Sjoblom T, Shimizu A, O'Brien KP, et al. Growth inhibition of dermatofibrosarcoma protuberans tumors by the platelet-derived growth factor receptor antagonist STI571 through induction of apoptosis. Cancer Res. 2001;61:5778-5783.

178. Greco A, Roccato E, Miranda C, et al. Growth-inhibitory effect of STI571 on cells transformed by the COL1A1/PDGFB rearrangement. Int J Cancer. 2001;92:354-360.

179. Rubin BP, Schuetze SM, Eary JF, et al. Molecular targeting of platelet-derived growth factor B by imatinib mesylate in a patient with metastatic dermatofibrosarcoma protuberans. J Clin Oncol. 2002;20:3586-3591.

180. McArthur GA, Demetri GD, van Oosterom A, et al. Molecular and clinical analysis of locally advanced dermatofibrosarcoma protuberans treated with imatinib: Imatinib Target Exploration Consortium Study B2225. J Clin Oncol. 2005;23:866-873.

181. Kasper B, Lossignol D, Gil T, et al. Imatinib mesylate in a patient with metastatic disease originating from a dermatofibrosarcoma protuberans of the scalp. Anticancer Drugs. 2006;17:1223-1225.

182. Schaller JL, Burkland GA. Case report: rapid and complete control of idiopathic hypereosinophilia with imatinib mesylate. Med Gen Med. 2001;3:9.

183. Gleich GJ, Leiferman KM, Pardanani A, et al. Treatment of hypereosinophilic syndrome with imatinib mesilate. Lancet. 2002;359:1577-1578.

184. Cortes J, Ault P, Koller C, et al. Efficacy of imatinib mesylate in the treatment of idiopathic hypereosinophilic syndrome. Blood. 2003;101:4714-4716.

185. Cools J, DeAngelo DJ, Gotlib J, et al. A tyrosine kinase created by fusion of the PDGFRA and FIP1L1 genes as a therapeutic target of imatinib in idiopathic hypereosinophilic syndrome. N Engl J Med. 2003;348:1201-1214.

186. Sequist LV, Bell DW, Lynch TJ, Haber DA. Molecular predictors of response to epidermal growth factor receptor antagonists in non-small-cell lung cancer. J Clin Oncol. 2007;25:587-595.

187. Fukuoka M, Yano S, Giaccone G, et al. Multi-institutional randomized phase II trial of gefitinib for previously treated patients with advanced non-small-cell lung cancer (The IDEAL 1 Trial) [corrected]. J Clin Oncol. 2003;21:2237-2246.

188. Kris MG, Natale RB, Herbst RS, et al. Efficacy of gefitinib, an inhibitor of the epidermal growth factor receptor tyrosine kinase, in symptomatic patients with non-small cell lung cancer: a randomized trial. JAMA. 2003;290:2149-2158.

189. Thatcher N, Chang A, Parikh P, et al. Gefitinib plus best supportive care in previously treated patients with refractory advanced non-small-cell lung cancer: results from a randomised, placebo-controlled, multicentre study (Iressa Survival Evaluation in Lung Cancer). Lancet. 2005;366:1527-1537.

190. Shepherd FA, Rodrigues Pereira J, Ciuleanu T, et al. Erlotinib in previously treated non-small-cell lung cancer. N Engl J Med. 2005;353:123-132.

191. West HL, Franklin WA, McCoy J, et al. Gefitinib therapy in advanced bronchioloalveolar carcinoma: Southwest Oncology Group Study S0126. J Clin Oncol. 2006;24:1807-1813.

192. Lynch TJ, Bell DW, Sordella R, et al. Activating mutations in the epidermal growth factor receptor underlying responsiveness of non-small-cell lung cancer to gefitinib. N Engl J Med. 2004;350:2129-2139.

193. Shigematsu H, Lin L, Takahashi T, et al. Clinical and biological features associated with epidermal growth factor receptor gene mutations in lung cancers. J Natl Cancer Inst. 2005;97:339-346.

194. Marchetti A, Martella C, Felicioni L, et al. EGFR mutations in non-small-cell lung cancer: analysis of a large series of cases and development of a rapid and sensitive method for diagnostic screening with potential implications on pharmacologic treatment. J Clin Oncol. 2005;23:857-865.

195. Mitsudomi T, Kosaka T, Endoh H, et al. Mutations of the epidermal growth factor receptor gene predict prolonged survival after gefitinib treatment in patients with non-small-cell lung cancer with postoperative recurrence. J Clin Oncol. 2005;23:2513-2520.

196. Kosaka T, Yatabe Y, Endoh H, et al. Mutations of the epidermal growth factor receptor gene in lung cancer: biological and clinical implications. Cancer Res. 2004;64:8919-8923.

197. Han SW, Kim TY, Hwang PG, et al. Predictive and prognostic impact of epidermal growth factor receptor mutation in non-small-cell lung cancer patients treated with gefitinib. J Clin Oncol. 2005;23:2493-2501.

198. Cappuzzo F, Hirsch FR, Rossi E, et al. Epidermal growth factor receptor gene and protein and gefitinib sensitivity in non-small-cell lung cancer. J Natl Cancer Inst. 2005;97:643-655.

199. Takano T, Ohe Y, Sakamoto H, et al. Epidermal growth factor receptor gene mutations and increased copy numbers predict gefitinib sensitivity in patients with recurrent non-small-cell lung cancer. J Clin Oncol. 2005;23:6829-6837.

200. Hirsch FR, Varella-Garcia M, McCoy J, et al. Increased epidermal growth factor receptor gene copy number detected by fluorescence in situ hybridization associates with increased sensitivity to gefitinib in patients with bronchioloalveolar carcinoma subtypes: a Southwest Oncology Group Study. J Clin Oncol. 2005;23:6838-6845.

201. Hirsch FR, Varella-Garcia M, Cappuzzo F, et al. Combination of EGFR gene copy number and protein expression predicts outcome for advanced non-small-cell lung cancer patients treated with gefitinib. Ann Oncol. 2007;18:752-760.

202. Kobayashi S, Boggon TJ, Dayaram T, et al. EGFR mutation and resistance of non-small-cell lung cancer to gefitinib. N Engl J Med. 2005;352:786-792.

203. Pao W, Miller VA, Politi KA, et al. Acquired resistance of lung adenocarcinomas to gefitinib or erlotinib is associated with a second mutation in the EGFR kinase domain. PLoS Med. 2005;2:e73.

204. Balak MN, Gong Y, Riely GJ, et al. Novel D761Y and common secondary T790M mutations in epidermal growth factor receptor-mutant lung adenocarcinomas with acquired resistance to kinase inhibitors. Clin Cancer Res. 2006;12:6494-6501.

205. Engelman JA, Zejnullahu K, Mitsudomi T, et al. MET amplification leads to gefitinib resistance in lung cancer by activating ERBB3 signaling. Science. 2007;316:1039-1043.

206. Giaccone G, Herbst RS, Manegold C, et al. Gefitinib in combination with gemcitabine and cisplatin in advanced non-small-cell lung cancer: a phase III trial—INTACT 1. J Clin Oncol. 2004;22:777-784.

207. Herbst RS, Giaccone G, Schiller JH, et al. Gefitinib in combination with paclitaxel and carboplatin in advanced non-small-cell lung cancer: a phase III trial—INTACT 2. J Clin Oncol. 2004;22:785-794.

208. Herbst RS, Prager D, Hermann R, et al. TRIBUTE: a phase III trial of erlotinib hydrochloride (OSI-774) combined with carboplatin and paclitaxel chemotherapy in advanced non-small-cell lung cancer. J Clin Oncol. 2005;23:5892-5899.

209. Gatzemeier U, Pluzanska A, Szczesna A, et al. Phase III study of erlotinib in combination with cisplatin and gemcitabine in advanced non-small-cell lung cancer: the Tarceva Lung Cancer Investigation Trial. J Clin Oncol. 2007;25:1545-1552.

210. Einfeld DA, Brown JP, Valentine MA, et al. Molecular cloning of the human B cell CD20 receptor predicts a hydrophobic protein with multiple transmembrane domains. EMBO J. 1988;7:711-717.

211. Bubien JK, Zhou LJ, Bell PD, et al. Transfection of the CD20 cell surface molecule into ectopic cell types generates a Ca2+ conductance found constitutively in B lymphocytes. J Cell Biol. 1993;121:1121-1132.

212. Press OW, Appelbaum F, Ledbetter JA, et al. Monoclonal antibody 1F5 (anti-CD20) serotherapy of human B cell lymphomas. Blood. 1987;69:584-591.

213. Liu AY, Robinson RR, Murray ED Jr, et al. Production of a mouse-human chimeric monoclonal antibody to CD20 with potent Fc-dependent biologic activity. J Immunol. 1987;139:3521-3526.

214. van Meerten T, van Rijn RS, Hol S, et al. Complement-induced cell death by rituximab depends on CD20 expression level and acts complementary to antibody-dependent cellular cytotoxicity. Clin Cancer Res. 2006;12:4027-4035.

215. Bonavida B. Rituximab-induced inhibition of antiapoptotic cell survival pathways: implications in chemo/immunoresistance, rituximab unresponsiveness, prognostic and novel therapeutic interventions. Oncogene. 2007;26:3629-3636.

216. Fisher RI, Gaynor ER, Dahlberg S, et al. Comparison of a standard regimen (CHOP) with three intensive chemotherapy regimens for advanced non-Hodgkin's lymphoma. N Engl J Med. 1993;328:1002-1006.

217. Fisher RI, Gaynor ER, Dahlberg S, et al. A phase III comparison of CHOP vs. m-BACOD vs. ProMACE-CytaBOM vs. MACOP-B in patients with intermediate- or high-grade non-Hodgkin's lymphoma: results of SWOG-8516 (Intergroup 0067), the National High-Priority Lymphoma Study. Ann Oncol. 1994;5(suppl 2):91-95.

218. McLaughlin P, Grillo-Lopez AJ, Link BK, et al. Rituximab chimeric anti-CD20 monoclonal antibody therapy for relapsed indolent lymphoma: half of patients respond to a four-dose treatment program. J Clin Oncol. 1998;16:2825-2833.

219. Davis TA, Grillo-Lopez AJ, White CA, et al. Rituximab anti-CD20 monoclonal antibody therapy in non-Hodgkin's lymphoma: safety and efficacy of re-treatment. J Clin Oncol. 2000;18:3135-3143.

220. Hainsworth JD, Litchy S, Burris HA 3rd, et al. Rituximab as first-line and maintenance therapy for patients with indolent non-Hodgkin's lymphoma. J Clin Oncol. 2002;20:4261-4267.

221. Ghielmini M, Schmitz SF, Cogliatti SB, et al. Prolonged treatment with rituximab in patients with follicular lymphoma significantly increases event-free survival and response duration compared with the standard weekly ×4 schedule. Blood. 2004;103:4416-4423.

222. Hainsworth JD, Litchy S, Shaffer DW, et al. Maximizing therapeutic benefit of rituximab: maintenance therapy versus re-treatment at progression in patients with indolent non-Hodgkin's lymphoma—a randomized phase II trial of the Minnie Pearl Cancer Research Network. J Clin Oncol. 2005;23:1088-1095.

223. Czuczman MS, Grillo-Lopez AJ, White CA, et al. Treatment of patients with low-grade B-cell lymphoma with the combination of chimeric anti-CD20 monoclonal antibody and CHOP chemotherapy. J Clin Oncol. 1999;17:268-276.

224. Czuczman MS, Weaver R, Alkuzweny B, et al. Prolonged clinical and molecular remission in patients with low-grade or follicular non-Hodgkin's lymphoma treated with rituximab plus CHOP chemotherapy: 9-year follow-up. J Clin Oncol. 2004;22:4711-4716.

225. Vose JM, Link BK, Grossbard ML, et al. Phase II study of rituximab in combination with chop chemotherapy in patients with previously untreated, aggressive non-Hodgkin's lymphoma. J Clin Oncol. 2001;19:389-397.

226. Coiffier B, Lepage E, Briere J, et al. CHOP chemotherapy plus rituximab compared with CHOP alone in elderly patients with diffuse large-B-cell lymphoma. N Engl J Med. 2002;346:235-242.

227. Byrd JC, Murphy T, Howard RS, et al. Rituximab using a thrice weekly dosing schedule in B-cell chronic lymphocytic leukemia and small lymphocytic lymphoma demonstrates clinical activity and acceptable toxicity. J Clin Oncol. 2001;19:2153-2164.

228. Freim Wahl SG, Folvik MR, Torp SH. Progressive multifocal leukoencephalopathy in a lymphoma patient with complete remission after treatment with cytostatics and rituximab: case report and review of the literature. Clin Neuropathol. 2007;26:68-73.

229. Matteucci P, Magni M, Di Nicola M, et al. Leukoencephalopathy and papovavirus infection after treatment with chemotherapy and anti-CD20 monoclonal antibody. Blood. 2002;100:1104-1105.

230. Dervite I, Hober D, Morel P. Acute hepatitis B in a patient with antibodies to hepatitis B surface antigen who was receiving rituximab. N Engl J Med. 2001;344:68-69.

231. Crocker PR. Siglecs: sialic-acid-binding immunoglobulin-like lectins in cell-cell interactions and signalling. Curr Opin Struct Biol. 2002;12:609-615.

232. Andrews RG, Takahashi M, Segal GM, et al. The L4F3 antigen is expressed by unipotent and multipotent colony-forming cells but not by their precursors. Blood. 1986;68:1030-1035.

233. Andrews RG, Torok-Storb B, Bernstein ID. Myeloid-associated differentiation antigens on stem cells and their progeny identified by monoclonal antibodies. Blood. 1983;62:124-132.

234. Griffin JD, Linch D, Sabbath K, et al. A monoclonal antibody reactive with normal and leukemic human myeloid progenitor cells. Leuk Res. 1984;8:521-534.

235. Tchilian EZ, Beverley PC, Young BD, Watt SM. Molecular cloning of two isoforms of the murine homolog of the myeloid CD33 antigen. Blood. 1994;83:3188-3198.

236. Robertson MJ, Soiffer RJ, Freedman AS, et al. Human bone marrow depleted of CD33-positive cells mediates delayed but durable reconstitution of hematopoiesis: clinical trial of MY9 monoclonal antibody-purged autografts for the treatment of acute myeloid leukemia. Blood. 1992;79:2229-2236.

237. Walter RB, Raden BW, Kamikura DM, et al. Influence of CD33 expression levels and ITIM-dependent internalization on gemtuzumab ozogamicin-induced cytotoxicity. Blood. 2005;105:1295-1302.

238. Zein N, Poncin M, Nilakantan R, Ellestad GA. Calicheamicin gamma 1I and DNA: molecular recognition process responsible for site-specificity. Science. 1989;244:697-699.

239. Hinman LM, Hamann PR, Wallace R, et al. Preparation and characterization of monoclonal antibody conjugates of the calicheamicins: a novel and potent family of antitumor antibiotics. Cancer Res. 1993;53:3336-3342.

240. Bross PF, Beitz J, Chen G, et al. Approval summary: gemtuzumab ozogamicin in relapsed acute myeloid leukemia. Clin Cancer Res. 2001;7:1490-1496.

241. Sievers EL, Larson RA, Stadtmauer EA, et al. Efficacy and safety of gemtuzumab ozogamicin in patients with CD33-positive acute myeloid leukemia in first relapse. J Clin Oncol. 2001;19:3244-3254.

242. Larson RA, Boogaerts M, Estey E, et al. Antibody-targeted chemotherapy of older patients with acute myeloid leukemia in first relapse using Mylotarg (gemtuzumab ozogamicin). Leukemia. 2002;16:1627-1636.

243. Larson RA, Sievers EL, Stadtmauer EA, et al. Final report of the efficacy and safety of gemtuzumab ozogamicin (Mylotarg) in patients with CD33-positive acute myeloid leukemia in first recurrence. Cancer. 2005;104:1442-1452.

244. Piccaluga PP, Martinelli G, Rondoni M, et al. Gemtuzumab ozogamicin for relapsed and refractory acute myeloid leukemia and myeloid sarcomas. Leuk Lymphoma. 2004;45:1791-1795.

245. Guglielmi C, Martelli MP, Diverio D, et al. Immunophenotype of adult and childhood acute promyelocytic leukaemia: correlation with morphology, type of PML gene breakpoint and clinical outcome. A cooperative Italian study on 196 cases. Br J Haematol. 1998;102:1035-1041.

246. Paietta E. Expression of cell-surface antigens in acute promyelocytic leukaemia. Best Pract Res Clin Haematol. 2003;16:369-385.

247. Aribi A, Kantarjian HM, Estey EH, et al. Combination therapy with arsenic trioxide, all-trans retinoic acid, and gemtuzumab ozogamicin in recurrent acute promyelocytic leukemia. Cancer. 2007;109:1355-1359.

248. Petti MC, Pinazzi MB, Diverio D, et al. Prolonged molecular remission in advanced acute promyelocytic leukaemia after treatment with gemtuzumab ozogamicin (Mylotarg CMA-676). Br J Haematol. 2001;115:63-65.

249. Lo-Coco F, Cimino G, Breccia M, et al. Gemtuzumab ozogamicin (Mylotarg) as a single agent for molecularly relapsed acute promyelocytic leukemia. Blood. 2004;104:1995-1999.

250. Estey E, Garcia-Manero G, Ferrajoli A, et al. Use of all-trans retinoic acid plus arsenic trioxide as an alternative to chemotherapy in untreated acute promyelocytic leukemia. Blood. 2006;107:3469-3473.

251. Takeshita A, Shinjo K, Naito K, et al. Two patients with all-trans retinoic acid-resistant acute promyelocytic leukemia treated successfully with gemtuzumab ozogamicin as a single agent. Int J Hematol. 2005;82:445-448.

252. Nabhan C, Rundhaugen LM, Riley MB, et al. Phase II pilot trial of gemtuzumab ozogamicin (GO) as first line therapy in acute myeloid leukemia patients age 65 or older. Leuk Res. 2005;29:53-57.

253. Amadori S, Suciu S, Stasi R, et al. Gemtuzumab ozogamicin (Mylotarg) as single-agent treatment for frail patients 61 years of age and older with acute myeloid leukemia: final results of AML-15B, a phase 2 study of the European Organisation for Research and Treatment of Cancer and Gruppo Italiano Malattie Ematologiche dell'Adulto Leukemia Groups. Leukemia. 2005;19:1768-1773.

254. van der Heiden PL, Jedema I, Willemze R, Barge RM. Efficacy and toxicity of gemtuzumab ozogamicin in patients with acute myeloid leukemia. Eur J Haematol. 2006;76:409-413.

255. Wadleigh M, Richardson PG, Zahrieh D, et al. Prior gemtuzumab ozogamicin exposure significantly increases the risk of veno-occlusive disease in patients who undergo myeloablative allogeneic stem cell transplantation. Blood. 2003;102:1578-1582.

256. Tsimberidou A, Cortes J, Thomas D, et al. Gemtuzumab ozogamicin, fludarabine, cytarabine and cyclosporine combination regimen in patients with CD33+ primary resistant or relapsed acute myeloid leukemia. Leuk Res. 2003;27:893-897.

257. Cortes J, Tsimberidou AM, Alvarez R, et al. Mylotarg combined with topotecan and cytarabine in patients with refractory acute myelogenous leukemia. Cancer Chemother Pharmacol. 2002;50:497-500.

258. Alvarado Y, Tsimberidou A, Kantarjian H, et al. Pilot study of Mylotarg, idarubicin and cytarabine combination regimen in patients with primary resistant or relapsed acute myeloid leukemia. Cancer Chemother Pharmacol. 2003;51:87-90.

259. Chevallier P, Roland V, Mahe B, et al. Administration of mylotarg 4 days after beginning of a chemotherapy including intermediate-dose aracytin and mitoxantrone (MIDAM regimen) produces a high rate of complete hematologic remission in patients with CD33+ primary resistant or relapsed acute myeloid leukemia. Leuk Res. 2005;29:1003-1007.

260. Kaelin WG, Jr. Molecular basis of the VHL hereditary cancer syndrome. Nat Rev Cancer. 2002;2:673-682.

261. George DJ, Kaelin WG Jr. The von Hippel-Lindau protein, vascular endothelial growth factor, and kidney cancer. N Engl J Med. 2003;349:419-421.

262. Kim WY, Kaelin WG. Role of VHL gene mutation in human cancer. J Clin Oncol. 2004;22:4991-5004.

263. Li L, Zhang L, Zhang X, et al. Hypoxia-inducible factor linked to differential kidney cancer risk seen with type 2A and type 2B VHL mutations. Mol Cell Biol. 2007;27:5381-5392.

264. Carmeliet P, Ferreira V, Breier G, et al. Abnormal blood vessel development and lethality in embryos lacking a single VEGF allele. Nature. 1996;380:435-439.

265. Ferrara N, Carver-Moore K, Chen H, et al. Heterozygous embryonic lethality induced by targeted inactivation of the VEGF gene. Nature. 1996;380:439-442.

266. Ferrara N, Gerber HP, LeCouter J. The biology of VEGF and its receptors. Nat Med. 2003;9:669-676.

267. Willett CG, Boucher Y, di Tomaso E, et al. Direct evidence that the VEGF-specific antibody bevacizumab has antivascular effects in human rectal cancer. Nat Med. 2004;10:145-147.

268. Hurwitz H, Fehrenbacher L, Novotny W, et al. Bevacizumab plus irinotecan, fluorouracil, and leucovorin for metastatic colorectal cancer. N Engl J Med. 2004;350:2335-2342.

269. Kabbinavar F, Hurwitz HI, Fehrenbacher L, et al. Phase II, randomized trial comparing bevacizumab plus fluorouracil (FU)/leucovorin (LV) with FU/LV alone in patients with metastatic colorectal cancer. J Clin Oncol. 2003;21:60-65.

270. Kabbinavar FF, Schulz J, McCleod M, et al. Addition of bevacizumab to bolus fluorouracil and leucovorin in first-line metastatic colorectal cancer: results of a randomized phase II trial. J Clin Oncol. 2005;23:3697-3705.

271. Giantonio BJ, Levy DE, O'Dwyer PJ, et al. A phase II study of high-dose bevacizumab in combination with irinotecan, 5-fluorouracil, leucovorin, as initial therapy for advanced colorectal cancer: results from the Eastern Cooperative Oncology Group study E2200. Ann Oncol. 2006;17:1399-1403.

272. Giantonio BJ, Catalano PJ, Meropol NJ, et al. Bevacizumab in combination with oxaliplatin, fluorouracil, and leucovorin (FOLFOX4) for previously treated metastatic colorectal cancer: results from the Eastern Cooperative Oncology Group Study E3200. J Clin Oncol. 2007;25:1539-1544.

273. Chaiworapongsa T, Romero R, Espinoza J, et al. Evidence supporting a role for blockade of the vascular endothelial growth factor system in the pathophysiology of preeclampsia. Young Investigator Award. Am J Obstet Gynecol. 2004;190:1541-1547; discussion 1547-1550.

274. Venkatesha S, Toporsian M, Lam C, et al. Soluble endoglin contributes to the pathogenesis of preeclampsia. Nat Med. 2006;12:642-649.

275. Verheul HM, Hoekman K, Luykx-de Bakker S, et al. Platelet: transporter of vascular endothelial growth factor. Clin Cancer Res. 1997;3:2187-2190.

276. Yufu Y, Nishimura J, Nawata H. High constitutive expression of heat shock protein 90 alpha in human acute leukemia cells. Leuk Res. 1992;16:597-605.

277. Xu Y, Lindquist S. Heat-shock protein hsp90 governs the activity of pp60v-src kinase. Proc Natl Acad Sci U S A. 1993;90:7074-7078.

278. Stancato LF, Silverstein AM, Owens-Grillo JK, et al. The hsp90-binding antibiotic geldanamycin decreases Raf levels and epidermal growth factor signaling without disrupting formation of signaling complexes or reducing the specific enzymatic activity of Raf kinase. J Biol Chem. 1997;272:4013-4020.

279. Whitesell L, Lindquist SL. Hsp90 and the chaperoning of cancer. Nat Rev Cancer. 2005;5:761-772.

280. Whitesell L, Mimnaugh EG, De Costa B, et al. Inhibition of heat shock protein Hsp90-pp60v-src heteroprotein complex formation by benzoquinone ansamycins: essential role for stress proteins in oncogenic transformation. Proc Natl Acad Sci U S A. 1994;91:8324-8328.

281. Stebbins CE, Russo AA, Schneider C, et al. Crystal structure of an Hsp90-geldanamycin complex: targeting of a protein chaperone by an antitumor agent. Cell. 1997;89:239-250.

282. Schulte TW, Neckers LM. The benzoquinone ansamycin 17-allylamino-17-demethoxygeldanamycin binds to Hsp90 and shares important biologic activities with geldanamycin. Cancer Chemother Pharmacol. 1998;42:273-279.

283. Goetz MP, Toft D, Reid J, et al. Phase I trial of 17-allylamino-17-demethoxygeldanamycin in patients with advanced cancer. J Clin Oncol. 2005;23:1078-1087.

284. Nowakowski GS, McCollum AK, Ames MM, et al. A phase I trial of twice-weekly 17-allylamino-demethoxy-geldanamycin in patients with advanced cancer. Clin Cancer Res. 2006; 12:6087-6093.

285. Bagatell R, Gore L, Egorin MJ, et al. Phase I pharmacokinetic and pharmacodynamic study of 17-N-allylamino-17-demethoxygeldanamycin in pediatric patients with recurrent or refractory solid tumors: a pediatric oncology experimental therapeutics investigators consortium study. Clin Cancer Res. 2007;13:1783-1788.

286. Weigel BJ, Blaney SM, Reid JM, et al. A phase I study of 17-allylaminogeldanamycin in relapsed/refractory pediatric patients with solid tumors: a Children's Oncology Group study. Clin Cancer Res. 2007;13:1789-1793.

287. Ramanathan RK, Egorin MJ, Eiseman JL, et al. Phase I and pharmacodynamic study of 17-(allylamino)-17-demethoxygeldanamycin in adult patients with refractory advanced cancers. Clin Cancer Res. 2007;13:1769-1774.

288. Ronnen EA, Kondagunta GV, Ishill N, et al. A phase II trial of 17-(allylamino)-17-demethoxygeldanamycin in patients with papillary and clear cell renal cell carcinoma. Invest New Drugs. 2006;24:543-546.

289. Egorin MJ, Lagattuta TF, Hamburger DR, et al. Pharmacokinetics, tissue distribution, and metabolism of 17-(dimethylaminoethylamino)-17-demethoxygeldanamycin (NSC 707545) in CD2F1 mice and Fischer 344 rats. Cancer Chemother Pharmacol. 2002;49:7-19.

290. Demetri GD, George S, Morgan JA, et al. Inhibition of the heat shock protein 90 (Hsp90) chaperone with the novel agent IPI-504 to overcome resistance to tyrosine kinase inhibitors (TKIs) in metastatic GIST: updated results of phase I trial. Abstract 10024. American Society of Clinical Oncology Meeting Proceedings, Part 1. J Clin Oncol. 2007;25:551s.

291. Deguchi K, Gilliland DG. Cooperativity between mutations in tyrosine kinases and in hematopoietic transcription factors in AML. Leukemia. 2002;16:740-744.

292. Wang J, Hoshino T, Redner RL, et al. ETO, fusion partner in t(8;21) acute myeloid leukemia, represses transcription by interaction with the human N-CoR/mSin3/HDAC1 complex. Proc Natl Acad Sci U S A. 1998;95:10860-10865.

293. Cuenco GM, Nucifora G, Ren R. Human AML1/MDS1/EVI1 fusion protein induces an acute myelogenous leukemia (AML) in mice: a model for human AML. Proc Natl Acad Sci U S A. 2000;97:1760-1765.

294. Dash AB, Williams IR, Kutok JL, et al. A murine model of CML blast crisis induced by cooperation between BCR/ABL and NUP98/HOXA9. Proc Natl Acad Sci U S A. 2002;99: 7622-7627.

295. Damm K, Thompson CC, Evans RM. Protein encoded by v-erbA functions as a thyroid-hormone receptor antagonist. Nature. 1989;339:593-597.

296. Zenke M, Munoz A, Sap J, et al. v-erbA oncogene activation entails the loss of hormone-dependent regulator activity of c-erbA. Cell. 1990;61:1035-1049.

297. Bolden JE, Peart MJ, Johnstone RW. Anticancer activities of histone deacetylase inhibitors. Nat Rev Drug Discov. 2006;5: 769-784.

298. Duvic M, Vu J. Vorinostat: a new oral histone deacetylase inhibitor approved for cutaneous T-cell lymphoma. Expert Opin Investig Drugs. 2007;16:1111-1120.

299. Yoshida M, Kijima M, Akita M, Beppu T. Potent and specific inhibition of mammalian histone deacetylase both in vivo and in vitro by trichostatin A. J Biol Chem. 1990;265:17174-17179.

300. Marks PA, Breslow R. Dimethyl sulfoxide to vorinostat: development of this histone deacetylase inhibitor as an anticancer drug. Nat Biotechnol. 2007;25:84-90.

301. Kelly WK, Richon VM, O'Connor O, et al. Phase I clinical trial of histone deacetylase inhibitor: suberoylanilide hydroxamic acid administered intravenously. Clin Cancer Res. 2003;9: 3578-3588.

302. Kelly WK, O'Connor OA, Krug LM, et al. Phase I study of an oral histone deacetylase inhibitor, suberoylanilide hydroxamic acid, in patients with advanced cancer. J Clin Oncol. 2005; 23:3923-3931.

303. O'Connor OA, Heaney ML, Schwartz L, et al. Clinical experience with intravenous and oral formulations of the novel histone deacetylase inhibitor suberoylanilide hydroxamic acid in patients with advanced hematologic malignancies. J Clin Oncol. 2006; 24:166-173.

304. Duvic M, Talpur R, Ni X, et al. Phase 2 trial of oral vorinostat (suberoylanilide hydroxamic acid, SAHA) for refractory cutaneous T-cell lymphoma (CTCL). Blood. 2007;109:31-39.

305. Olsen EA, Kim YH, Kuzel TM, et al. Phase IIb multicenter trial of vorinostat in patients with persistent, progressive, or treatment refractory cutaneous T-cell lymphoma. J Clin Oncol. 2007;25: 3109-3115.

306. Ueda H, Nakajima H, Hori Y, et al. FR901228, a novel antitumor bicyclic depsipeptide produced by Chromobacterium violaceum No. 968. I. Taxonomy, fermentation, isolation, physico-chemical and biological properties, and antitumor activity. J Antibiot (Tokyo). 1994;47:301-310.

307. Ueda H, Manda T, Matsumoto S, et al. FR901228, a novel antitumor bicyclic depsipeptide produced by Chromobacterium violaceum No. 968. III. Antitumor activities on experimental tumors in mice. J Antibiot (Tokyo). 1994;47:315-323.

308. Nakajima H, Kim YB, Terano H, et al. FR901228, a potent antitumor antibiotic, is a novel histone deacetylase inhibitor. Exp Cell Res. 1998;241:126-133.

309. Sandor V, Bakke S, Robey RW, et al. Phase I trial of the histone deacetylase inhibitor, depsipeptide (FR901228, NSC 630176), in patients with refractory neoplasms. Clin Cancer Res. 2002; 8:718-728.

310. Piekarz RL, Robey R, Sandor V, et al. Inhibitor of histone deacetylation, depsipeptide (FR901228), in the treatment of peripheral and cutaneous T-cell lymphoma: a case report. Blood. 2001;98:2865-2868.

311. Marshall JL, Rizvi N, Kauh J, et al. A phase I trial of depsipeptide (FR901228) in patients with advanced cancer. J Exp Ther Oncol. 2002;2:325-332.

312. Byrd JC, Marcucci G, Parthun MR, et al. A phase 1 and pharmacodynamic study of depsipeptide (FK228) in chronic lymphocytic leukemia and acute myeloid leukemia. Blood. 2005; 105:959-967.

313. Fouladi M, Furman WL, Chin T, et al. Phase I study of depsipeptide in pediatric patients with refractory solid tumors: a Children's Oncology Group report. J Clin Oncol. 2006;24:3678-3685.

314. Shah MH, Binkley P, Chan K, et al. Cardiotoxicity of histone deacetylase inhibitor depsipeptide in patients with metastatic neuroendocrine tumors. Clin Cancer Res. 2006;12:3997-4003.

315. Stadler WM, Margolin K, Ferber S, et al. A phase II study of depsipeptide in refractory metastatic renal cell cancer. Clin Genitourin Cancer. 2006;5:57-60.

316. Piekarz R, Frye R, Wright J, et al. Update of the NCI multiinstitutional phase II trial of romidepsin, FK228, for patients with cutaneous or peripheral T-cell lymphoma. Abstract 8027. American Society of Clinical Oncology Meeting Proceedings, Part 1. J Clin Oncol. 2007;25:447s.

317. Giles F, Fischer T, Cortes J, et al. A phase I study of intravenous LBH589, a novel cinnamic hydroxamic acid analogue histone deacetylase inhibitor, in patients with refractory hematologic malignancies. Clin Cancer Res. 2006;12:4628-4635.

318. Sharma S, Vogelzang NJ, Beck J, et al. Phase I pharmacokinetic (PK) and pharmacodynamic (PD) study of LBH589, a novel deacetylase (DAC) inhibitor given intravenously on a new once-weekly schedule. Abstract 14019. American Society of Clinical Oncology Meeting Proceedings, Part 1. J Clin Oncol. 2007;25: 613s.

319. Prince HM, George D, Patnaik A, et al. Phase I study of oral LBH589, a novel deacetylase (DAC) inhibitor in advanced solid tumors and non-Hodgkin's lymphoma. Abstract 3500. American Society of Clinical Oncology Meeting Proceedings, Part 1. J Clin Oncol. 2007;25:138s.

320. Testi AM, Biondi A, Lo Coco F, et al. GIMEMA-AIEOPAIDA protocol for the treatment of newly diagnosed acute promyelocytic leukemia (APL) in children. Blood. 2005;106:447-453.

321. Ortega JJ, Madero L, Martin G, et al. Treatment with all-trans retinoic acid and anthracycline monochemotherapy for children with acute promyelocytic leukemia: a multicenter study by the PETHEMA Group. J Clin Oncol. 2005;23:7632-7640.

322. Kolb EA, Pan Q, Ladanyi M, Steinherz PG. Imatinib mesylate in Philadelphia chromosome-positive leukemia of childhood. Cancer. 2003;98:2643-2650.

323. Zwaan CM, Reinhardt D, Corbacioglu S, et al. Gemtuzumab ozogamicin: first clinical experiences in children with relapsed/refractory acute myeloid leukemia treated on compassionate-use basis. Blood. 2003;101:3868-3871.

324. Arceci RJ, Sande J, Lange B, et al. Safety and efficacy of gemtuzumab ozogamicin in pediatric patients with advanced CD33+ acute myeloid leukemia. Blood. 2005;106:1183-1188.

325. Jetsrisuparb A, Wiangnon S, Komvilaisak P, et al. Rituximab combined with CHOP for successful treatment of aggressive recurrent, pediatric B-cell large cell non-Hodgkin's lymphoma. J Pediatr Hematol Oncol. 2005;27:223-226.

326. Giulino LB, Bussel JB, Neufeld EJ. Treatment with rituximab in benign and malignant hematologic disorders in children. J Pediatr. 2007;150:338-344.

327. Mullighan CG, Goorha S, Radtke I, et al. Genome-wide analysis of genetic alterations in acute lymphoblastic leukaemia. Nature. 2007;446:758-764.

328. Ries LAG, Percy CL, Bunin GR. Introduction. In Gloeckler Ries LA, Smith MA, Gurney JG, et al (eds). Cancer Incidence and Survival Among Children and Adolescents:United States SEER Program 1975-1995. Bethesda, Md, National Cancer Institute, Cancer Statistics Branch, 1999, pp 1-16.

329. Gloeckler Ries LA, Melbert D, Krapcho M, et al. Cancer Stat Fact Sheets. SEER Cancer Statistics Review, 1975-2004. Bethesda, Md, National Cancer Institute, 1999.

330. Armstrong SA, Kung AL, Mabon ME, et al. Inhibition of FLT3 in MLL. Validation of a therapeutic target identified by gene expression based classification. Cancer Cell. 2003;3: 173-183.

331. Sawyers CL. Finding the next Gleevec: FLT3 targeted kinase inhibitor therapy for acute myeloid leukemia. Cancer Cell. 2002;1:413-415.

332. Furman WL, Stewart CF, Poquette CA, et al. Direct translation of a protracted irinotecan schedule from a xenograft model to a phase I trial in children. J Clin Oncol. 1999;17:1815-1824.

333. Zamboni WC, Stewart CF, Thompson J, et al. Relationship between topotecan systemic exposure and tumor response in human neuroblastoma xenografts. J Natl Cancer Inst. 1998; 90:505-511.

333a. Lin PP, Pandey MK, Jin F, et al. EWS-FLI1 induces developmental abnormalities and accelerates sarcoma formation in a transgenic mouse model. Cancer Res 2008;68:8968-8975.

334. D'Amato RJ, Loughnan MS, Flynn E, Folkman J. Thalidomide is an inhibitor of angiogenesis. Proc Natl Acad Sci U S A. 1994;91:4082-4085.

335. Gerber HP, Vu TH, Ryan AM, et al. VEGF couples hypertrophic cartilage remodeling, ossification and angiogenesis during endochondral bone formation. Nat Med. 1999;5:623-628.

336. Gerber HP, Ferrara N. Angiogenesis and bone growth. Trends Cardiovasc Med. 2000;10:223-228.

337. Gerber HP, Hillan KJ, Ryan AM, et al. VEGF is required for growth and survival in neonatal mice. Development. 1999; 126:1149-1159.

338. Wedge SR, Ogilvie DJ, Dukes M, et al. ZD4190: an orally active inhibitor of vascular endothelial growth factor signaling with broad-spectrum antitumor efficacy. Cancer Res. 2000;60: 970-975.

339. Hall AP, Westwood FR, Wadsworth PF. Review of the effects of anti-angiogenic compounds on the epiphyseal growth plate. Toxicol Pathol. 2006;34:131-147.

340. Chen CS, Sorensen PH, Domer PH, et al. Molecular rearrangements on chromosome 11q23 predominate in infant acute lymphoblastic leukemia and are associated with specific biologic variables and poor outcome. Blood. 1993;81:2386-2393.

341. Pui CH, Behm FG, Downing JR, et al. 11q23/MLL rearrangement confers a poor prognosis in infants with acute lymphoblastic leukemia. J Clin Oncol. 1994;12:909-915.

342. Heerema NA, Sather HN, Ge J, et al. Cytogenetic studies of infant acute lymphoblastic leukemia: poor prognosis of infants with t(4;11)—a report of the Children's Cancer Group. Leukemia. 1999;13:679-686.

343. Reaman GH, Sposto R, Sensel MG, et al. Treatment outcome and prognostic factors for infants with acute lymphoblastic leukemia treated on two consecutive trials of the Children's Cancer Group. J Clin Oncol. 1999;17:445-455.

344. Pui CH, Chessells JM, Camitta B, et al. Clinical heterogeneity in childhood acute lymphoblastic leukemia with 11q23 rearrangements. Leukemia. 2003;17:700-706.

345. Pui CH, Gaynon PS, Boyett JM, et al. Outcome of treatment in childhood acute lymphoblastic leukaemia with rearrangements of the 11q23 chromosomal region. Lancet. 2002;359:1909-1915.

346. Yokoyama A, Somerville TC, Smith KS, et al. The menin tumor suppressor protein is an essential oncogenic cofactor for MLL-associated leukemogenesis. Cell. 2005;123:207-218.

347. Armstrong SA, Staunton JE, Silverman LB, et al. MLL translocations specify a distinct gene expression profile that distinguishes a unique leukemia. Nat Genet. 2002;30:41-47.

348. Armstrong SA, Golub TR, Korsmeyer SJ. MLL-rearranged leukemias: insights from gene expression profiling. Semin Hematol. 2003;40:268-273.

349. Gilliland DG, Griffin JD. The roles of FLT3 in hematopoiesis and leukemia. Blood. 2002;100:1532-1542.

350. Stam RW, den Boer ML, Schneider P, et al. Targeting FLT3 in primary MLL-gene-rearranged infant acute lymphoblastic leukemia. Blood. 2005;106:2484-2490.

351. Armstrong SA, Mabon ME, Silverman LB, et al. FLT3 mutations in childhood acute lymphoblastic leukemia. Blood. 2004; 103:3544-3546.

352. Van Vlierberghe P, Meijerink JP, Stam RW, et al. Activating FLT3 mutations in CD4+/CD8- pediatric T-cell acute lymphoblastic leukemias. Blood. 2005;106:4414-4415.

353. Meshinchi S, Alonzo TA, Stirewalt DL, et al. Clinical implications of FLT3 mutations in pediatric AML. Blood. 2006; 108:3654-3661.

354. Smith BD, Levis M, Beran M, et al. Single-agent CEP-701, a novel FLT3 inhibitor, shows biologic and clinical activity in patients with relapsed or refractory acute myeloid leukemia. Blood. 2004;103:3669-3676.

355. DeAngelo DJ, Stone RM, Heaney ML, et al. Phase 1 clinical results with tandutinib (MLN518), a novel FLT3 antagonist, in patients with acute myelogenous leukemia or high-risk myelodysplastic syndrome: safety, pharmacokinetics, and pharmacodynamics. Blood. 2006;108:3674-3681.

356. Stone RM, DeAngelo DJ, Klimek V, et al. Patients with acute myeloid leukemia and an activating mutation in FLT3 respond to a small-molecule FLT3 tyrosine kinase inhibitor, PKC412. Blood. 2005;105:54-60.

357. Fiedler W, Mesters R, Tinnefeld H, et al. A phase 2 clinical study of SU5416 in patients with refractory acute myeloid leukemia. Blood. 2003;102:2763-2767.

358. O'Farrell AM, Foran JM, Fiedler W, et al. An innovative phase I clinical study demonstrates inhibition of FLT3 phosphorylation by SU11248 in acute myeloid leukemia patients. Clin Cancer Res. 2003;9:5465-5476.

359. Fiedler W, Serve H, Dohner H, et al. A phase 1 study of SU11248 in the treatment of patients with refractory or resistant acute myeloid leukemia (AML) or not amenable to conventional therapy for the disease. Blood. 2005;105:986-993.

360. Ellisen LW, Bird J, West DC, et al. TAN-1, the human homolog of the Drosophila notch gene, is broken by chromosomal translocations in T lymphoblastic neoplasms. Cell. 1991;66:649-661.

361. Pear WS, Aster JC, Scott ML, et al. Exclusive development of T cell neoplasms in mice transplanted with bone marrow expressing activated Notch alleles. J Exp Med. 1996;183:2283-2291.

362. Artavanis-Tsakonas S, Rand MD, Lake RJ. Notch signaling: cell fate control and signal integration in development. Science. 1999;284:770-776.

363. Hansson EM, Lendahl U, Chapman G. Notch signaling in development and disease. Semin Cancer Biol. 2004;14:320-328.

364. Jarriault S, Brou C, Logeat F, et al. Signalling downstream of activated mammalian Notch. Nature. 1995;377:355-358.

365. Palomero T, Lim WK, Odom DT, et al. NOTCH1 directly regulates c-MYC and activates a feed-forward-loop transcriptional network promoting leukemic cell growth. Proc Natl Acad Sci U S A. 2006;103:18261-18266.

366. Weng AP, Millholland JM, Yashiro-Ohtani Y, et al. c-Myc is an important direct target of Notch1 in T-cell acute lymphoblastic leukemia/lymphoma. Genes Dev. 2006;20:2096-2109.

367. Weng AP, Ferrando AA, Lee W, et al. Activating mutations of NOTCH1 in human T cell acute lymphoblastic leukemia. Science. 2004;306:269-271.

368. Breit S, Stanulla M, Flohr T, et al. Activating NOTCH1 mutations predict favorable early treatment response and long-term outcome in childhood precursor T-cell lymphoblastic leukemia. Blood. 2006;108:1151-1157.

369. Dumortier A, Jeannet R, Kirstetter P, et al. Notch activation is an early and critical event during T-Cell leukemogenesis in Ikaros-deficient mice. Mol Cell Biol. 2006;26:209-220.

370. Lin YW, Nichols RA, Letterio JJ, Aplan PD. Notch1 mutations are important for leukemic transformation in murine models of precursor-T leukemia/lymphoma. Blood. 2006;107:2540-2543.

371. O'Neil J, Calvo J, McKenna K, et al. Activating Notch1 mutations in mouse models of T-ALL. Blood. 2006;107:781-785.

372. Wolfe MS. Therapeutic strategies for Alzheimer's disease. Nat Rev Drug Discov. 2002;1:859-866.

373. Shih Ie M, Wang TL. Notch signaling, gamma-secretase inhibitors, and cancer therapy. Cancer Res. 2007;67:1879-1882.

374. De Angelo DJ, Stone RM, Silverman LB, et al. a phase I clinical trial of the notch inhibitor MK-0752 in patients with T-Cell acute lymphoblastic leukemia/lymphoma (T-ALL) and other leukemias. American Society of Clinical Oncology Meeting Proceedings, Part I. J Clin Oncol. 2006;24:3575.

375. Chan SM, Weng AP, Tibshirani R, et al. Notch signals positively regulate activity of the mTOR pathway in T-cell acute lymphoblastic leukemia. Blood. 2007;110:278-286.

376. Raffel C, Jenkins RB, Frederick L, et al. Sporadic medulloblastomas contain PTCH mutations. Cancer Res. 1997;57:842-845.

377. Louis DN, Pomeroy SL, Cairncross JG. Focus on central nervous system neoplasia. Cancer Cell. 2002;1:125-128.

378. Lee Y, Miller HL, Jensen P, et al. A molecular fingerprint for medulloblastoma. Cancer Res. 2003;63:5428-5437.

379. Wechsler-Reya R, Scott MP. The developmental biology of brain tumors. Annu Rev Neurosci. 2001;24:385-428.

380. Reifenberger J, Wolter M, Weber RG, et al. Missense mutations in SMOH in sporadic basal cell carcinomas of the skin and primitive neuroectodermal tumors of the central nervous system. Cancer Res. 1998;58:1798-1803.

381. Taylor MD, Liu L, Raffel C, et al. Mutations in SUFU predispose to medulloblastoma. Nat Genet. 2002;31:306-310.

382. Thompson MC, Fuller C, Hogg TL, et al. Genomics identifies medulloblastoma subgroups that are enriched for specific genetic alterations. J Clin Oncol. 2006;24:1924-1931.

383. Ingham PW, McMahon AP. Hedgehog signaling in animal development: paradigms and principles. Genes Dev. 2001;15:3059-3087.

384. Dunaeva M, Michelson P, Kogerman P, Toftgard R. Characterization of the physical interaction of Gli proteins with SUFU proteins. J Biol Chem. 2003;278:5116-5122.

385. Merchant M, Vajdos FF, Ultsch M, et al. Suppressor of fused regulates Gli activity through a dual binding mechanism. Mol Cell Biol. 2004;24:8627-8641.

386. Binns W, James LF, Shupe JL, Thacker EJ. Cyclopian-type malformation in lambs. Arch Environ Health. 1962;5:106-108.

387. Keeler RF, Binns W. Teratogenic compounds of Veratrum californicum (Durand). V. Comparison of cyclopian effects of steroidal alkaloids from the plant and structurally related compounds from other sources. Teratology. 1968;1:5-10.

388. Berman DM, Karhadkar SS, Hallahan AR, et al. Medulloblastoma growth inhibition by hedgehog pathway blockade. Science. 2002;297:1559-1561.

389. Chen JK, Taipale J, Cooper MK, Beachy PA. Inhibition of Hedgehog signaling by direct binding of cyclopamine to Smoothened. Genes Dev. 2002;16:2743-2748.

390. Wetmore C, Eberhart DE, Curran T. Loss of p53 but not ARF accelerates medulloblastoma in mice heterozygous for patched. Cancer Res. 2001;61:513-516.

391. Romer JT, Kimura H, Magdaleno S, et al. Suppression of the Shh pathway using a small molecule inhibitor eliminates medulloblastoma in Ptc1(+/-)p53(-/-) mice. Cancer Cell. 2004;6:229-240.

392. Tomlins SA, Mehra R, Rhodes DR, et al. TMPRSS2:ETV4 gene fusions define a third molecular subtype of prostate cancer. Cancer Res. 2006;66:3396-3400.

393. Tomlins SA, Mehra R, Rhodes DR, et al. Integrative molecular concept modeling of prostate cancer progression. Nat Genet. 2007;39:41-51.

394. Stegmaier K, Ross KN, Colavito SA, et al. Gene expression-based high-throughput screening(GE-HTS) and application to leukemia differentiation. Nat Genet. 2004;36:257-263.

395. Peck D, Crawford ED, Ross KN, et al. A method for high-throughput gene expression signature analysis. Genome Biol. 2006;7:R61.

396. Stegmaier K, Wong JS, Ross KN, et al. Signature-based small molecule screening identifies cytosine arabinoside as an EWS/FLI modulator in Ewing sarcoma. PLoS Med. 2007;4:e122.

396a. Dubois SG, Krailo MD, Lessnick SL, et al. Phase II study of intermediate-dose cytarabine in patients with relapsed or refractory Ewing sarcoma: A report from the Children's Oncology Group. Pediatr Blood Cancer. 2008. Epub ahead of print.

397. Hughes TR, Marton MJ, Jones AR, et al. Functional discovery via a compendium of expression profiles. Cell. 2000;102:109-126.

398. Lamb J, Crawford ED, Peck D, et al. The connectivity map: using gene-expression signatures to connect small molecules, genes, and disease. Science. 2006;313:1929-1935.

399. Hieronymus H, Lamb J, Ross KN, et al. Gene expression signature-based chemical genomic prediction identifies a novel class of Hsp90 pathway modulators. Cancer Cell. 2006;10:321-330.

400. Wei G, Twomey D, Lamb J, et al. Gene expression-based chemical genomics identifies rapamycin as a modulator of MCL1 and glucocorticoid resistance. Cancer Cell. 2006;10:331-342.

401. Walensky LD, Kung AL, Escher I, et al. Activation of apoptosis in vivo by a hydrocarbon-stapled BH3 helix. Science. 2004;305:1466-1470.

402. Walensky LD, Pitter K, Morash J, et al. A stapled BID BH3 helix directly binds and activates BAX. Mol Cell. 2006;24:199-210.

403. Danial NN, Korsmeyer SJ. Cell death: critical control points. Cell. 2004;116:205-219.

404. Polo JM, Dell'Oso T, Ranuncolo SM, et al. Specific peptide interference reveals BCL6 transcriptional and oncogenic mechanisms in B-cell lymphoma cells. Nat Med. 2004;10:1329-1335.

405. Niu H. The proto-oncogene BCL-6 in normal and malignant B cell development. Hematol Oncol. 2002;20:155-166.

406. Dalla-Favera R, Migliazza A, Chang CC, et al. Molecular pathogenesis of B cell malignancy: the role of BCL-6. Curr Top Microbiol Immunol. 1999;246:257-263.

407. Melnick A, Carlile G, Ahmad KF, et al. Critical residues within the BTB domain of PLZF and Bcl-6 modulate interaction with corepressors. Mol Cell Biol. 2002;22:1804-1818.

408. Ahmad KF, Melnick A, Lax S, et al. Mechanism of SMRT corepressor recruitment by the BCL6 BTB domain. Mol Cell. 2003;12:1551-1564.

409. Wadia JS, Stan RV, Dowdy SF. Transducible TAT-HA fusogenic peptide enhances escape of TAT-fusion proteins after lipid raft macropinocytosis. Nat Med. 2004;10:310-315.

410. Wu ZL, Schwartz E, Seeger R, Ladisch S. Expression of GD2 ganglioside by untreated primary human neuroblastomas. Cancer Res. 1986;46:440-443.

411. Munn DH, Cheung NK. Interleukin-2 enhancement of monoclonal antibody-mediated cellular cytotoxicity against human melanoma. Cancer Res. 1987;47:6600-6605.

412. Kushner BH, Cheung NK. GM-CSF enhances 3F8 monoclonal antibody-dependent cellular cytotoxicity against human melanoma and neuroblastoma. Blood. 1989;73:1936-1941.

413. Kushner BH, Cheung NK. Clinically effective monoclonal antibody 3F8 mediates nonoxidative lysis of human neuroectodermal tumor cells by polymorphonuclear leukocytes. Cancer Res. 1991;51:4865-4870.

414. Cheung NK, Kushner BH, Cheung IY, et al. Anti-G(D2) antibody treatment of minimal residual stage 4 neuroblastoma diagnosed at more than 1 year of age. J Clin Oncol. 1998;16:3053-3060.

415. Kushner BH, Kramer K, Cheung NK. Phase II trial of the anti-G(D2) monoclonal antibody 3F8 and granulocyte-macrophage colony-stimulating factor for neuroblastoma. J Clin Oncol. 2001;19:4189-4194.

416. Cheung IY, Lo Piccolo MS, Kushner BH, Cheung NK. Early molecular response of marrow disease to biologic therapy is highly prognostic in neuroblastoma. J Clin Oncol. 2003;21:3853-3858.

417. Cheung NK, Sowers R, Vickers AJ, et al. FCGR2A polymorphism is correlated with clinical outcome after immunotherapy of neuroblastoma with anti-GD2 antibody and granulocyte macrophage colony-stimulating factor. J Clin Oncol. 2006;24:2885-2890.

418. Murray JL, Cunningham JE, Brewer H, et al. Phase I trial of murine monoclonal antibody 14G2a administered by prolonged intravenous infusion in patients with neuroectodermal tumors. J Clin Oncol. 1994;12:184-193.

419. Frost JD, Hank JA, Reaman GH, et al. A phase I/IB trial of murine monoclonal anti-GD2 antibody 14.G2a plus interleukin-

2 in children with refractory neuroblastoma: a report of the Children's Cancer Group. Cancer. 1997;80:317-333.

420. Yu AL, Uttenreuther-Fischer MM, Huang CS, et al. Phase I trial of a human-mouse chimeric anti-disialoganglioside monoclonal antibody ch14.18 in patients with refractory neuroblastoma and osteosarcoma. J Clin Oncol. 1998;16:2169-2180.

421. Handgretinger R, Anderson K, Lang P, et al. A phase I study of human/mouse chimeric antiganglioside GD2 antibody ch14.18 in patients with neuroblastoma. Eur J Cancer. 1995;31A:261-267.

422. Simon T, Hero B, Faldum A, et al. Consolidation treatment with chimeric anti-GD2-antibody ch14.18 in children older than 1 year with metastatic neuroblastoma. J Clin Oncol. 2004;22:3549-3557.

423. Simon T, Hero B, Faldum A, et al. Infants with stage 4 neuroblastoma: the impact of the chimeric anti-GD2-antibody ch14.18 consolidation therapy. Klin Padiatr. 2005;217:147-152.

424. Ozkaynak MF, Sondel PM, Krailo MD, et al. Phase I study of chimeric human/murine anti-ganglioside G(D2) monoclonal antibody (ch14.18) with granulocyte-macrophage colony-stimulating factor in children with neuroblastoma immediately after hematopoietic stem-cell transplantation: a Children's Cancer Group Study. J Clin Oncol. 2000;18:4077-4085.

425. Osenga KL, Hank JA, Albertini MR, et al. A phase I clinical trial of the hu14.18-IL2 (EMD 273063) as a treatment for children with refractory or recurrent neuroblastoma and melanoma: a study of the Children's Oncology Group. Clin Cancer Res. 2006;12:1750-1759.

426. Zhou Z, Zhou RR, Guan H, et al. E1A gene therapy inhibits angiogenesis in a Ewing's sarcoma animal model. Mol Cancer Ther. 2003;2:1313-1319.

427. Pavlakovic H, Von Schutz V, Rossler J, et al. Quantification of angiogenesis stimulators in children with solid malignancies. Int J Cancer. 2001;92:756-760.

428. Holzer G, Obermair A, Koschat M, et al. Concentration of vascular endothelial growth factor (VEGF) in the serum of patients with malignant bone tumors. Med Pediatr Oncol. 2001;36:601-604.

429. Fuchs B, Inwards CY, Janknecht R. Vascular endothelial growth factor expression is up-regulated by EWS-ETS oncoproteins and Sp1 and may represent an independent predictor of survival in Ewing's sarcoma. Clin Cancer Res. 2004;10:1344-1353.

430. Lessnick SL, Dacwag CS, Golub TR. The Ewing's sarcoma oncoprotein EWS/FLI induces a p53-dependent growth arrest in primary human fibroblasts. Cancer Cell. 2002;1:393-401.

431. Guan H, Zhou Z, Wang H, et al. A small interfering RNA targeting vascular endothelial growth factor inhibits Ewing's sarcoma growth in a xenograft mouse model. Clin Cancer Res. 2005;11:2662-2669.

432. Maris JM, Courtright J, Houghton PJ, et al. Initial testing of the VEGFR inhibitor AZD2171 by the pediatric preclinical testing program. Pediatr Blood Cancer. 2008;50:581-587.

433. LeRoith D, Roberts CT Jr. The insulin-like growth factor system and cancer. Cancer Lett. 2003;195:127-137.

434. Yee D, Favoni RE, Lebovic GS, et al. Insulin-like growth factor I expression by tumors of neuroectodermal origin with the t(11;22) chromosomal translocation. A potential autocrine growth factor. J Clin Invest. 1990;86:1806-1814.

435. Toretsky JA, Kalebic T, Blakesley V, et al. The insulin-like growth factor-I receptor is required for EWS/FLI-1 transformation of fibroblasts. J Biol Chem. 1997;272:30822-30827.

436. Prieur A, Tirode F, Cohen P, Delattre O. EWS/FLI-1 silencing and gene profiling of Ewing cells reveal downstream oncogenic pathways and a crucial role for repression of insulin-like growth factor binding protein 3. Mol Cell Biol. 2004;24: 7275-7283.

437. Benini S, Zuntini M, Manara MC, et al. Insulin-like growth factor binding protein 3 as an anticancer molecule in Ewing's sarcoma. Int J Cancer. 2006;119:1039-1046.

438. Scotlandi K, Manara MC, Nicoletti G, et al. Antitumor activity of the insulin-like growth factor-I receptor kinase inhibitor NVP-AEW541 in musculoskeletal tumors. Cancer Res. 2005; 65:3868-3876.

439. Manara MC, Landuzzi L, Nanni P, et al. Preclinical in vivo study of new insulin-like growth factor-I receptor—specific inhibitor in Ewing's sarcoma. Clin Cancer Res. 2007;13:1322-1330.

440. Scotlandi K, Avnet S, Benini S, et al. Expression of an IGF-I receptor dominant negative mutant induces apoptosis, inhibits tumorigenesis and enhances chemosensitivity in Ewing's sarcoma cells. Int J Cancer. 2002;101:11-16.

441. Maloney EK, McLaughlin JL, Dagdigian NE, et al. An anti-insulin-like growth factor I receptor antibody that is a potent inhibitor of cancer cell proliferation. Cancer Res. 2003;63: 5073-5083.

442. Wang W, Kumar P, Wang W, et al. Insulin-like growth factor II and PAX3-FKHR cooperate in the oncogenesis of rhabdomyosarcoma. Cancer Res. 1998;58:4426-4433.

443. Wang W, Slevin M, Kumar S, Kumar P. The cooperative transforming effects of PAX3-FKHR and IGF-II on mouse myoblasts. Int J Oncol. 2005;27:1087-1096.

444. Gallicchio MA, Kneen M, Hall C, et al. Overexpression of insulin-like growth factor binding protein-6 inhibits rhabdomyosarcoma growth in vivo. Int J Cancer. 2001;94:645-651.

445. MacEwen EG, Pastor J, Kutzke J, et al. IGF-1 receptor contributes to the malignant phenotype in human and canine osteosarcoma. J Cell Biochem. 2004;92:77-91.

446. Tanno B, Mancini C, Vitali R, et al. Down-regulation of insulin-like growth factor I receptor activity by NVP-AEW541 has an antitumor effect on neuroblastoma cells in vitro and in vivo. Clin Cancer Res. 2006;12:6772-6780.

447. van Golen CM, Schwab TS, Kim B, et al. Insulin-like growth factor-I receptor expression regulates neuroblastoma metastasis to bone. Cancer Res. 2006;66:6570-6578.

448. Tolcher AW, Rothenberg ML, Rodon J, et al. A phase I pharmacokinetic and pharmacodynamic study of AMG 479, a fully human monoclonal antibody against insulin-like growth factor type 1 receptor (IGF-1R), in advanced solid tumors. Abstract 3002. American Society of Clinical Oncology Meeting Proceedings, Part I. J Clin Oncol. 2007;25:118s.

5

Cytogenetic and Molecular Pathology of Pediatric Cancer

Maureen J. O'Sullivan, Jonathan A. Fletcher, and Carolyn A. Felix

Cytogenetic and molecular analyses have provided pivotal biologic and clinical insights into pediatric neoplasia. It is increasingly evident that genetic assays of various types can provide essential diagnostic or prognostic information about pediatric solid tumors (Tables 5-1 and 5-2) and hematologic malignancies (Tables 5-3 through 5-5). This chapter offers an overview of the methods in use for the analysis of cytogenetic and molecular aberrations (Table 5-6) in pediatric cancers together with their relative attributes, discusses the causes of these genetic aberrations, and summarizes their diagnostic and predictive relevance in clinical practice.

CYTOGENETIC AND MOLECULAR METHODOLOGIES

The pathognomonic genetic aberrations in pediatric cancer can be evaluated by various methods. Because each of these methods has a different profile of substrate requirements, sensitivity, and specificity (see Table 5-6), the optimal approach must be tailored individually in regard to both the nature and quantity of material available and to the precise information being sought.

Karyotyping

The traditional karyotype provides a low-resolution snapshot of the entire genome. Cells are cultured, arrested in metaphase, and then subjected to staining of the chromosomes to produce characteristic banding patterns,[1-4] which are described using standardized nomenclature (Box 5-1). Probably the major advantage of karyotypic analysis is the provision of a global overview of the chromosomal composition of a cultured cellular population without any requirement for preknowledge, especially enabling the identification of completely novel aberrations (Fig. 5-1). However, karyotyping has distinct limitations, including the requirement for fresh material in sufficient amounts and slow turnaround because of time required for tumor cell growth.

Need for Sufficient Viable Tumor

Solid tumors may comprise substantial nonviable or hypocellular regions containing few neoplastic cells. Such regions may be extensively necrotic because the tumor cells have died, having outstripped their blood supply. Other regions of a tumor mass may be composed largely of blood (hemorrhage) or scar tissue (fibrosis). Therefore, in the case of solid tumor

Text continues on p. 105

TABLE 5-1   Typical Genetic Aberrations in Soft Tissue and Bone Tumors

Histologic Findings		Cytogenetic Events	Molecular Events	Frequency (%)
Alveolar soft part sarcoma		t(X;17)(p11;q25)	*ASPL-TFE3* fusion	>90
Aneurysmal bone cyst (extraosseous)		16q22 and 17p13 rearrangements	*USP6* fusion genes	>50
Angiomatoid fibrous histiocytoma		t(12;16)(q13;p11)	*FUS-ATF1* fusion	10
			EWS-GREB1 fusion	80
Chondromyxoid fibroma		Deletion of 6q		>75
Chondrosarcoma				
	Skeletal	Complex*		>75
	Extraskeletal myxoid	t(9;22)(q22;q12)	*EWS-NR4A3* fusion	>75
		t(9;17)(q22;q11)	*TAF2N-NR4A3* fusion	<10
		t(9;15)(q22;q21)	*TCF12-NR4A3* fusion	<10
Clear cell sarcoma–melanoma of soft parts		t(12;22)(q13;q12)	*EWS-ATF1* fusion	>75
Dermatofibrosarcoma protuberans		Ring form of chromosomes 17 and 22	*COL1A1-PDGFB* fusion	>75
		t(17;22)(q21;q13)	*COL1A1-PDGFB* fusion	10
Desmoplastic small round cell tumor		t(11;22)(p13;q12)	*EWS-WT1* fusion	>75
Endometrial stromal tumor		t(7;17)(p15;q21)	*JAZF1-JJAZ1*	30
Ewing's sarcoma		t(11;22)(q24;q12)	*EWS-FLI1* fusion	>80
		t(21;22)(q12;q12)	*EWS-ERG* fusion	5-10
		t(2;22)(q33;q12)	*EWS-FEV* fusion	<5
		t(7;22)(p22;q12)	*EWS-ETV1* fusion	<5
		t(17;22)(q12;q12)	*EWS-E1AF* fusion	<5
		t(16;21)(p11;q12)	*FUS-ERG* fusion	<5
		t(2;16)(q33;p11)	*FUS-FEV* fusion	<5
		inv(22)(q12q12)	*EWS-ZSG* fusion	<5
Fibromatosis (desmoid)		Trisomies 8 and 20		30
		Deletion of 5q	*APC* inactivation	10
			Beta-catenin mutation	70
Fibromyxoid sarcoma, low-grade		t(7;16)(q33;p11)	*FUS-BBF2H7* fusion	50
Fibrosarcoma, infantile		t(12;15)(p13;q26)	*TEL-NTRK3* fusion	>75
		Trisomies 8, 11, 17, and 20		>75
Gastrointestinal stromal tumor		Monosomies 14 and 22		>75
		Deletion of 1p		>25
			KIT or *PDGFRA* mutation	>90
Giant cell tumor				
	Bone	Telomeric associations		>50
	Tenosynovial	Trisomies 5 and 7		>25
		t(1;2)(p13;q35)	*CSF1-COL6A3* fusion	25

TABLE 5-1	Typical Genetic Aberrations in Soft Tissue and Bone Tumors—cont'd		
Histologic Findings		**Cytogenetic Events**	**Molecular Events**	**Frequency (%)**
Hibernoma		11q13 rearrangement		>50
Inflammatory myofibroblastic tumor		2p23 rearrangement	*ALK* fusion genes	50
Leiomyoma				
	Uterine	t(12;14)(q15;q24) or deletion of 7q	*HMGIC* rearrangement	40
	Extrauterine	Deletion of 1p		?
Leiomyosarcoma		Deletion of 1p		>50
Lipoblastoma		8q12 rearrangement or polysomy 8	*PLAG1* oncogenes	>80
Lipoma				
	Typical	12q15 rearrangement	*HMGIC* rearrangement	60
	Spindle cell or pleomorphic	Deletion of 13q or 16q		>75
	Chondroid	t(11;16)(q13;p12-13)		?
Liposarcoma				
	Well-differentiated	Ring form of chromosome 12		>75
	Myxoid, round cell	t(12;16)(q13;p11)	*FUS-CHOP* fusion	>75
		t(12;22)(q13;q12)	*EWS-CHOP* fusion	<5
	Pleomorphic	Complex★		90
Malignant fibrous histiocytoma				
	Myxoid	Ring form of chromosome 12		?
	High-grade	Complex★		>90
Myxofibrosarcoma		(see "Malignant fibrous histiocytoma")		
Malignant peripheral nerve sheath tumor		(see "Schwannoma")		
Mesothelioma		Deletion of 1p	?*BCL10* inactivation	>50
		Deletion of 9p	*p15*, *p16*, and *p19* inactivation	>75
		Deletion of 22q	*NF2* inactivation	>50
		Deletions of 3p and 6q		>50
Neuroblastoma				
	Good prognosis	Hyperdiploid, no 1p deletion		40
	Poor prognosis	1p deletion		40
		Double-minute chromosomes	N-*myc* amplification	>25
Osteochondroma		Deletion of 8q	*EXT1* inactivation	>25
Osteosarcoma				
	Low-grade	Ring chromosomes		>50
	High-grade	Complex★	Rb and p53 inactivation	>80
Pericytoma		t(7;12)(p22;q13-15)	*GLI-ACTB* fusion	?
		(see "Giant cell tumor: Tenosynovial")		
Pigmented villonodular synovitis				
Primitive neuroectodermal tumor		(see "Ewing's sarcoma")		
Rhabdoid tumor		Deletion of 22q	*INI1* inactivation	>90
Rhabdomyosarcoma				
	Alveolar	t(2;13)(q35;q14)	*PAX3-FKHR* fusion	60
		t(1;13)(p36;q14), double minutes	*PAX7-FKHR* fusion	10-20
	Embryonal	Trisomies 2q, 8 and 20		>75
			Loss of heterozygosity at 11p15	>75
Schwannoma	Benign	Deletion of 22q	*NF2* inactivation	>80
	Malignant, low-grade	None		
	Malignant, high-grade	Complex★		>90
Synovial sarcoma				
	Monophasic	t(X;18)(p11;q11)	*SYT-SSX1* or *SYT-SSX2* fusion	>90
	Biphasic	t(X;18)(p11;q11)	*SYT-SSX1* fusion	>90

★Indicates presence of complicated numeric and structural chromosomal aberrations.

TABLE 5-2   Genetic Aberrations of Ancillary Predictive or Therapeutic Relevance in Pediatric Solid Tumors

Histologic Findings	Cytogenetic Aberration	Molecular Events	Other Possible Clinical Relevance
Dermatofibrosarcoma protuberans	Ring form of chromosomes 17 and 22	*COL1A1-PDGFB* fusion	PDGFRB therapeutic inhibition
	t(17;22)(q21;q13)	*COL1A1-PDGFB* fusion	PDGFRB therapeutic inhibition
Fibromatosis (desmoid)	Deletion of 5q	*APC* inactivation	Association with germline *APC* mutation and familial adenomatous polyposis
Fibrosarcoma, infantile	t(12;15)(p13;q26)	*TEL-NTRK3* fusion	NTRK3 therapeutic inhibition
Gastrointestinal stromal tumor		*KIT* or *PDGFRA* mutation	KIT-PDGFRA therapeutic inhibition
Giant cell tumor, tenosynovial	t(1;2)(p13;q35)	*CSF1-COL6A3* fusion	CSF1R therapeutic inhibition
Inflammatory myofibroblastic tumor	2p23 rearrangement	*ALK* fusion genes	ALK therapeutic inhibition
Liposarcoma—myxoid, round cell	t(12;16)(q13;p11)	*FUS-CHOP* fusion	Trabectedin therapeutic response
Neuroblastoma	Hyperdiploid, no 1p deletion		Favorable prognosis
	1p deletion		Unfavorable prognosis
	Double-minute chromosomes	N-*myc* amplification	Unfavorable prognosis
Rhabdomyosarcoma, alveolar	t(2;13)(q35;q14)	*PAX3-FKHR* fusion	Prognosis
	t(1;13)(p36;q14), double minutes	*PAX7-FKHR* fusion	Prognosis
Synovial sarcoma			
Monophasic	t(X;18)(p11;q11)	*SYT-SSX1* or *SYT-SSX2* fusion	Prognosis
Biphasic	t(X;18)(p11;q11)	*SYT-SSX1* fusion	
Oligodendroglioma	Deletion of 1p and 19q		Therapeutic response to CDDP
Wilms' tumor	Deletion 11p13	*WT1* inactivation	Association with syndromic Wilms' tumor
	1p deletion		Adverse prognosis in low-stage FH
	16q deletion		Adverse prognosis in low-stage FH
	1q gain		Increased relapse risk

CDDP, *cis*-diaminedichloroplatinum; FH, favorable histology; PDGFRA, platelet-derived growth factor receptor alpha; PDGFRB, platelet-derived growth factor receptor beta.

TABLE 5-3   Typical Genetic Aberrations in Pediatric Lymphomas

Histologic Findings	Cytogenetic Events	Molecular Events	Frequency (%)
Hodgkin's, classic	Complex*	Clonal Ig rearrangements	95
		Clonal *IGH* translocations	17
		Clonal *IGK* translocations	1
		Clonal *IGL* translocations	3
		Clonal *TCR* rearrangements	1-2
Hodgkin's, nodular lymphocyte–predominance	t(3;14)(q27;q32)	*BCL6* rearrangement	50
Burkitt's	t(8;14)(q24;q32)	*IGH-MYC* rearrangement	80
	t(2;8)(p11;q24)	*IGK-MYC* rearrangement	5
	t(8;22)(q24;q11)	*IGL-MYC* rearrangement	15
Lymphoblastic (see Table 5-4) ALL			
Anaplastic large cell	t(2;5)(p23;q35)	*NPM-ALK* fusion	80
	Various inversions and translocations	*ALK* fusions with *TPM3, ATIC, CLTC* and others	10-20
Diffuse large B-cell	Complex*		
Subcutaneous panniculitic T-cell		Clonal T-cell receptor rearrangements	
Hepatosplenic T-cell	Isochromosome 7q; trisomy 8	Clonal T-cell receptor rearrangements	>75

*Indicates presence of complicated numeric and structural chromosomal aberrations.

TABLE 5-4   Typical Genetic Aberrations in Pediatric Leukemias and Myeloproliferative Disorders

Histologic Findings	Cytogenetic Events	Molecular Events	Frequency
T-cell ALL	t(1;14)(p34;q11)	SCL(TAL1)-TCR alpha-delta locus fusions or SIL-SCL rearrangements	30% T-cell ALL
	t(1;3)(p34;p21)	SCL-TCTA fusion	Rare
	Chromosome band 11p13 translocations	LMO2-TCR loci fusions	10%-20% T-cell ALL
	Chromosome band 11p15, 19p13.2, or 10q24 translocations	LMO1, LYL1. HOX11(TLX1)-TCR loci fusions	?
	t(7;9)(q34;q34)	TCRB-NOTCH1 fusion	<1% T-cell ALL
	t(6;7)(q23;q34)	TCRB-MYB fusion	
		Activating NOTCH1 mutations	50% T-cell ALL
		PTEN gene mutation	8% T-cell ALL
T-cell ALL, precursor B-cell ALL	Translocations, inversions involving chromosome bands 14q32, 14q11, 7q34, 7p14	Hybrid antigen receptor gene rearrangements	?
	Chromosome band 9p21 deletion	CDKN2A [p16 (INK4A)/p14 (ARF)] deletion/variable CDKN2B [p15 (INK4B)] deletion	60% T-cell ALL, 20% childhood precursor B-cell ALL
Precursor B-cell ALL	Chomosome band 11q23 translocations	MLL gene rearrangements	80% of infant ALL
	Hyperdiploidy		30% precursor B-cell ALL
	Hypodiploidy		6%-8% precursor B-cell ALL
	t(12;21)(p13;q21) (cryptic; detectable by FISH only)	TEL-AML1 fusion	25% of "common" ALL
	t(9;22)(q34;q11)	BCR-ABL1 fusion	5% precursor B-cell ALL
	t(1;19)(q23;p13.3)	E2A-PBX1 fusion	~4% Precursor B-cell ALL; 25% cIg+ cases; <1% cIg- cases
	t(17;19)(q22;p13.3)	E2A-HLF fusion	1% precursor B-cell ALL
	t(5;14)(q31;q32)	IGH-IL3 fusion	<1% precursor B-cell ALL
	t(6;14)(p22.3;q32)	IGH-ID4 fusion	?
	t(1;19)(q23;p13.3)	MEF2D-DAZAP1 fusion	?
		FLT3 point mutation	5% childhood precursor B-cell ALL, 16% infant ALL, ~21%-28% high hyperdiploid ALL, 18% MLL-rearranged ALL
		FLT3/ITD	2% precursor B-cell ALL
B-cell ALL	t(8;14)(q24;q32)	IGH-MYC fusion	Rare
	t(2;8)(p12;q24)	IGK-MYC fusion	Rare
	t(8;22)(q24;q11)	IGL-MYC fusion	Rare
AML	t(8;21)(q22;q22)	AML1-ETO fusion	~12% pediatric AML
	Chromosome band 11q23 translocations	MLL gene rearrangements	80% myelomonocytic-monoblastic AML in infants and young children; ~7%-18% pediatric AML
	inv(16)(p13q22) or t(16;16)(p13;q22)	CBF-MYH11 fusion	~7% pediatric AML
	t(8;16)(p11;p13)	MOZ-CBP fusion	Rare
	t(6;9)(p23;q34)	DEK-CAN fusion	Rare
	May be associated with t(8;21) or inv(16)	KIT mutation	37% CBF AML
		NPM mutation	~7%-8% pediatric AML
		FLT3 point mutation	7%-9% pediatric AML
		FLT3/ITD	~12%-15% pediatric AML
APL	t(15;17)(q22;q21)	PML-RARA fusion	~12% pediatric AML
	t(11;17)(q23;q21)	PLZF-RARA fusion	Rare
		FLT3/ITD	~30% pediatric APL
Therapy-related MDS/AML, de novo MDS/AML	Monosomy 7/del(7q)		~40% pediatric MDS, 49% RC, 4%-5% pediatric AML
De novo or therapy-related AML, ALL, MDS	Chromosome band 11p15 translocations	NUP98 gene rearrangements	?
Therapy-related MDS/AML	Monosomy 5, del(5q)		
	May be associated with segmental jumping translocations	TP53 mutation	? (more common in therapy-related than de novo MDS, AML)

Continues

TABLE 5-4 Typical Genetic Aberrations in Pediatric Leukemias and Myeloproliferative Disorders—cont'd

Histologic Findings	Cytogenetic Events	Molecular Events	Frequency
Therapy related ALL and AML after exposure to topoisomerase II poisons	Chomosome band 11q23 translocations	*MLL* gene rearrangements	
5q– syndrome, refractory anemia	del(5q)	*RPS14* deletion	?—not described in children
JMML, AML, MDS, precursor B-cell ALL		*PTPN11* mutation	30%-35% of JMML, 4% of AML, 18% of FAB M5 AML
JMML	May be associated with monosomy 7	*NF1* mutation	~30% of JMML, ~50% of JMML in constitutional NF1 syndrome
JMML, AML, MDS	May be associated with monosomy 7 in JMML/MDS or with t(8;21) or inv(16) in AML	*KRAS* or *NRAS* mutation	20%-30% JMML, ~20%-30% pediatric AML, 30% monosomy 7 MDS
CMML	t(5;12)(q33;p13)	*TEL-PDGFRB* fusion	Rare
TAM, AMKL	May be associated with +8 if progression to AMKL	*GATA-1* mutations	
Non–Down syndrome AMKL	t(1;22)(p13;q13)	*OTT-MAL* fusion	Rare
Refractory cytopenia (RC)	Trisomy 8		9% of RC

ALL, acute lymphocytic leukemia; AMKL, acute megakaryoblastic leukemia; AML, acute myeloid leukemia; APL, acute promyelocytic leukemia; CBF, core-binding factor; CMML, chronic myelomonocytic leukemia; ITD, internal tandem duplication; JMML, juvenile myelomonocytic leukemia; MDS, myelodysplastic syndrome; TAM, transient abnormal myelopoiesis.

TABLE 5-5 Genetic Aberrations of Ancillary Predictive or Therapeutic Relevance in Pediatric Leukemias and Myeloproliferative Disorders

Histologic Findings	Cytogenetic Aberration	Molecular Events	Other Possible Clinical Relevance
T-cell ALL	t(10;14)(q24;q11)	*HOX11(TLX1)* overexpression, *HOX11(TLX1)-TCRD* fusion	Favorable prognosis
	t(6;7)(q23;q34)	*TCRB-cMYB* fusion	Associated with young age
	t(7;9)(q34;q34)	*TCRB-NOTCH1* fusion, activating *NOTCH1* mutations	Gamma secretase inhibitor sensitivity
T-cell ALL	None	*PTEN* mutation	Associated with disease progression
Precursor B-cell ALL	t(5;14)(q31;q32)	*IGH-IL3* fusion	Peripheral eosinophilia
Precursor B-cell ALL	t(6;14)(p22.3;q32.22)	*IGH-ID4* fusion	Favorable prognosis
Precursor B-cell ALL	t(12;21)(p13;q21) (cryptic; detectable by FISH only)	*TEL-AML1* fusion	Favorable prognosis
Precursor B-cell ALL	t(1;19)(q23;p13.3)	*E2A-PBX1* fusion	Poor prognosis in cIg+ cases
Precursor B-cell ALL	t(17;19)(q22;p13.3)	*E2A-HLF* fusion	Coagulopathy, poor prognosis
Precursor B-cell ALL	t(9;22)(q34;q11)	*BCR-ABL1* fusion	Poor prognosis, associated with older age, imatinib mesylate sensitivity
Precursor B-cell ALL, AML, therapy-related AML and ALL	Chromosome band 11q23 translocations	*MLL* gene rearrangements	Poor prognosis especially in ALL and therapy-related cases, associated with FAB M4, FAB M5, other AML morphologies, leukemia cutis, extramedullary involvement, topoisomerase II poison exposure
Precursor B-cell ALL	Hyperdiploidy		Favorable prognosis if >50 chromosomes and specific trisomies
Precursor B-cell ALL	Hypodiploidy		Unfavorable prognosis if <44 chromosomes, –7, dicentric chromosome
Precursor B-cell ALL, AML		*FLT3*-ITD, *FLT3* point mutation	Poor prognosis, increased FLT3-ITD allelic ratio associated with AML relapse, sensitivity to FLT3 tyrosine kinase inhibition
Precursor B-cell ALL, T-cell ALL	Chromosome band 9p21 deletion	*CDKN2A [p16 (INK4A-p14 (ARF)]* deletion; variable *CDKN2B [p15 (INK4B)]* deletion	Associated with relapse, poor prognosis
AML, therapy-related AML	t(8;21)(q22;q22)	*AML1-ETO* fusion	Associated with FAB M2 morphology, granulocytic sarcoma presentation, favorable prognosis

TABLE 5-5   Genetic Aberrations of Ancillary Predictive or Therapeutic Relevance in Pediatric Leukemias and Myeloproliferative Disorders—cont'd

Histologic Findings	Cytogenetic Aberration	Molecular Events	Other Possible Clinical Relevance
AML, therapy-related AML	inv(16)(p13;q22) or t(16;16)(p13;q22)	*CBFB-MYH11* fusion	Associated with abnormal eosinophils (adults), FAB M2 or M4 AML without eosinophilia (pediatrics), favorable prognosis
APL, therapy-related APL	t(15;17)(q22;q21)	*PML-RARA* fusion	Favorable prognosis, ATRA sensitivity, arsenic trioxide sensitivity
APL	t(11;17)(q23;q21)	*PLZF-RARA* fusion	Insensitive to ATRA
AML	t(8;16)(p11;p13)	*MOZ-CBP* fusion	Unfavorable prognosis, erythrophagocytosis, coagulopathy, associated with leukemia cutis and spontaneous remission in neonates
AML	t(6;9)(p23;q34)	*DEK-CAN* fusion	Unfavorable prognosis
Therapy-related MDS, AML	Monosomy 7, del(7q)		Alkylating agent exposure, associated with disease progression, poor prognosis, can be familial
Therapy-related MDS, AML	Monosomy 5, del(5q)		Alkylating agent exposure
5q– syndrome, refractory anemia	del(5q)	*RPS14* deletion	Lenalidomide sensitivity
JMML	None (may be associated with monosomy 7)	*NF1* mutation	Associated with constitutional NF1 syndrome
JMML	None	*PTPN11* mutation	Associated with Noonan syndrome
CMML	t(5;12)(q33;p13)	*TEL-PDGFRB* fusion	Associated with eosinophilia, progression to AML
TAM, AMKL	None	*GATA-1* mutations	Associated with Down syndrome
Non–Down syndrome AMKL	t(1;22)(p13;q13)	*OTT-MAL* fusion	Found in neonates
AML	None; may be associated with t(8;21) or inv(16)	*KIT* mutation	Sensitivity to imatinib, sensitivity to FLT3 tyrosine kinase inhibition
Therapy-related MDS or AML	None (may be associated with segmental jumping translocations)	*TP53* mutation	Alkylating agent exposure, associated with AML in Li-Fraumeni syndrome
AML	None	*NPM* mutation	Favorable prognosis in absence of *FLT3* ITD

ALL, acute lymphocytic leukemia; AMKL, acute megakaryoblastic leukemia; AML, acute myeloid leukemia; APL, acute promyelocytic leukemia; ATRA, all-trans-retinoic acid; CMML, chronic myelomonocytic leukemia; FAB, French-American-British; FISH, fluorescence in situ hybridization; ITD, internal tandem duplication; JMML, juvenile myelomonocytic leukemia; MDS, myelodysplastic syndrome; TAM, transient abnormal myelopoiesis.

TABLE 5-6   Complementary Nature of Cytogenetic and Molecular Assays

Assay Consideration	METHOD				
	Karyotyping	FISH	CGH	SNP	PCR Sequencing
Cost of assay	High	Low	High	High	Low
What types of tumor material can be used?	Fresh	Any	Fresh, frozen*	Fresh, frozen*	Any
Does assay detect translocations?	Yes	Yes	No	No	Yes
Does assay detect point mutations?	No	No	No	No	Yes
Does assay detect deletions?	Yes	Yes	Yes	Yes	Yes, if qPCR
Does assay detect amplifications?	Yes	Yes	Yes	Yes	Yes, if qPCR
Does assay detect low-frequency mutations?	No	Yes; 1 in 100	No	No	Yes; 1 in 10,000
Does assay permit genome-wide evaluation?	Yes	No	Yes	Yes	No

*Can be performed using DNA extracted from paraffin materials, but with some loss of resolution.

CGH, comparative genomic hybridization; FISH, fluorescence in situ hybridization; PCR, polymerase chain reacion; qPCR, quantitative PCR; SNP, single-nucleotide polymorphism analysis.

karyotyping, it is crucial that the pathologist select a maximally viable region for analysis.

Unpredictable Tumor Cell Growth in Culture

Even when tumor tissue has been selected from an optimal region, the unpredictable growth of neoplastic cells in culture remains a major consideration. Benign tumors often contain only few mitotic cells and so one generally has to wait several days before such specimens proliferate actively in culture. In the meantime, the culture may become overgrown by non-neoplastic cells, such as fibroblasts. Perhaps surprisingly, even highly malignant solid tumors may grow poorly in tissue culture, despite the fact that they grew well in the patient. Such tumor cultures may occasionally be stimulated by the use of specialized culture media or growth factors,[5] but it is impractical in most clinical cytogenetic laboratories to trouble-shoot tissue cultures to optimize the growth of each tumor type. Therefore, in practice, it may be challenging to culture and karyotype certain types of pediatric tumors in the clinical laboratory. In the case of bone marrow cytogenetics, it is well known that post-therapy specimens can be difficult to analyze, being hypo-

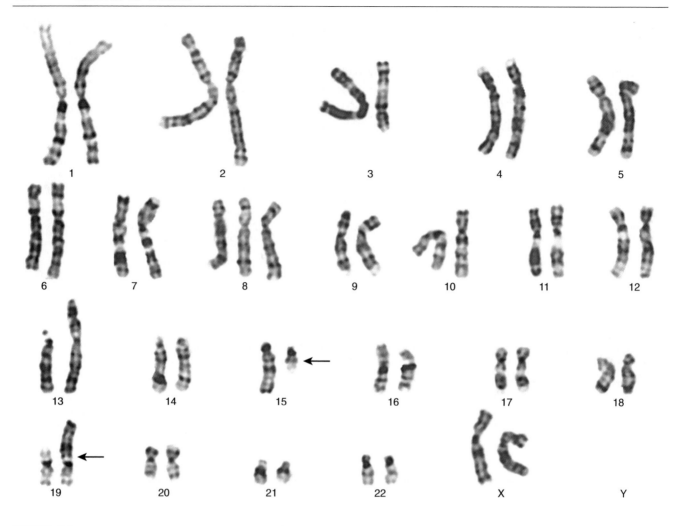

FIGURE 5-1. Giemsa-banded karyotype of highly lethal NUT midline carcinoma, demonstrating balanced t(15;19) with arrows indicating the translocation breakpoints. Other cytogenetic findings, including chromosome 3 and 13 rearrangements and trisomy 8, are secondary aberrations.

cellular and containing cells—reactive and/or neoplastic—that have been temporarily growth-arrested by therapy and therefore fail to give rise to metaphases in culture.

Nonrepresentative Cell Culture

It is also important to recognize that only a subpopulation of cells within a given sample might be capable of growing under a particular set of culture conditions. Therefore, one cannot necessarily assume that a clonally abnormal karyotype is representative of the overall neoplastic process. For example, in a given tumor, the final karyotype might be representative of the components of the tumor that were more or less clinically aggressive, depending on which component was best suited for growth under the particular culture conditions used at that time.

Culture Overgrowth by Non-neoplastic Cells

All tumor samples contain mixtures of neoplastic and non-neoplastic cells. The non-neoplastic elements may include hematopoietic cells, fibroblasts, normal epithelial cells, endothelial cells, or glial cells, depending on the type and location of the tumor. Any of these reactive or support cell types might proliferate more successfully than the neoplastic cells in culture. Invariably, when a pediatric cancer submitted for cytogenetic

analysis is reported to have a normal karyotype, the normal karyotype is a false-negative result, only signifying that the culture was overgrown by normal cells. Therefore, the cytogenetic analysis must always be timed carefully, so that metaphases are analyzed at a point at which the neoplastic population is actively dividing. This technical challenge can, in the case of solid tumors, be met if the cytogeneticist develops familiarity with the distinctive morphologies of the various neoplastic and reactive cell types, and then inspects the tissue cultures daily to determine when the neoplastic cells have the proliferative advantage.[5]

Complex Karyotype

Beyond the initial challenges incurred at the culture stage, various additional considerations influence the success of cytogenetic evaluation in different types of pediatric cancer. For example, conventional karyotyping can be challenging in many high-grade solid tumors, in which the karyotypes are often complex compared with those seen in leukemias and lymphomas. A single metaphase cell from such cancers can contain dozens of clonal and nonclonal chromosomal aberrations, making it impractical to characterize the exact mechanisms of rearrangement responsible for each chromosomal aberration or to estimate the relative significance of any of these abnormalities.

Technical Limitations in Detecting Aberrations

There are certain aberrations that cannot be detected by karyotyping, because the resolution is too low. These include smaller deletions or amplifications and point mutations, but also cryptic or masked aberrations, which include, for example, the chromosomal translocation t(12;15) characteristic of congenital

Box 5-1	**Cytogenetic Abbreviations and Definitions**

cDNA: complementary DNA

cen: centromere

CGH: comparative genomic hybridization

CISH: chromogenic in situ hybridization

del: deletion

dmin; double minute chromosome (extrachromosomal amplicon)

FISH: fluorescence in situ hybridization

hsr: homogeneously staining region (intrachromosomal amplicon)

ins: insertion within chromosome

inv: inversion of chromosome segment

ISH: in situ hybridization

mar: marker chromosome (aberrant chromosome whose origin cannot be ascertained)

p: chromosome short arm

q: chromosome long arm

r: ring chromosome

SKY: spectral karyotyping

t: translocation

tel: telomere

or infantile fibrosarcoma, congenital cellular mesoblastic nephroma, secretory breast carcinomas, and a subset of acute myelogenous leukemias (Fig. 5-2).[6,7] Another translocation that cannot be resolved by conventional karyotype analysis is the t(12;21), which is the most common translocation in pediatric leukemia. It is found in a large fraction of common acute lymphoblastic leukemia (ALL) in children and fuses the *TEL* (*ETV6*) and *AML1* (*RUNX1*) genes.

In essence, then, the major advantage of karyotypic evaluation of solid tumors is the breadth of the data provided. Notable challenges include the successful culture of representative tumor cells, particularly because this is essentially a one-shot approach, with no opportunity to return to the specimen, because the window of opportunity for culture is confined to the short period of viability of fresh cells following biopsy. Even when culture is successful, meaningful interpretation of the findings on karyotype may represent a further challenge, depending on the number and nature of the aberrations.

Although solid tumors are less readily accessible for biopsy compared with hematologic neoplasms, minimally invasive sampling by a percutaneous approach is becoming more common. Needle biopsy is often performed under ultrasound or computer tomography (CT) guidance, and can involve fine-needle aspiration or needle core biopsy of the tumor. Solid tumor samples obtained by these methods can be karyotyped successfully,[8-11] but the small amount of starting material is a constraint in that fewer cultures can be established. Because the successful cytogenetic evaluation of tumors in standard practice is limited by these factors, alternative, more robust methods are needed for the successful routine demonstration of genetic aberrations. Traditionally, these have included FISH (fluorescence in situ hybridization) and PCR (polymerase chain reaction) techniques, which have the distinct advantage of applicability to fixed material and therefore to large cohorts of archival cases also. Both FISH and molecular analyses can be straightforward also in fine-needle specimens.[12,13]

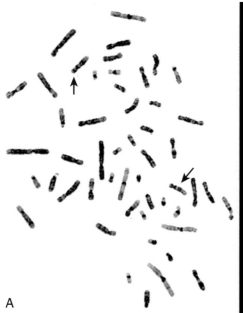 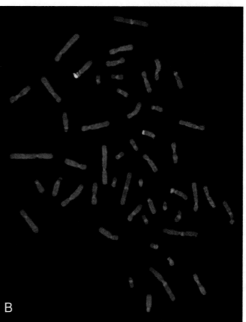

FIGURE 5-2. **A,** Giemsa banding studies in infantile fibrosarcoma do not reveal the characteristic, but cytogenetically cryptic t(12;15), associated with *TEL-NTRK3* oncogenic fusion. Black arrows indicate the normal (*top*) and rearranged (*middle*) copies of chromosome 12, as demonstrated by *TEL* break-apart fluorescence in situ hybridization (FISH). **B,** The FISH studies reveal yellow probe fusion signal on the normal chromosome 12, whereas the t(12;15) results in split red and green FISH signals on rearranged chromosomes 12 and 15, respectively.

Molecular Cytogenetics

Recombinant DNA technologies

Southern Blot Analysis

In pediatric solid tumors, leukemias, and lymphomas, recombinant DNA technologies, including Southern blot analyses of candidate genes relevant to particular disease states, can overcome limitations of conventional karyotype analysis for the detection of chromosomal aberrations (Fig. 5-3). Although no longer used extensively in most clinical diagnostic laboratories, Southern blotting has served an important role in gene discovery. That is, genomic Southern blot analyses, coupled with PCR-based molecular cloning and gene sequencing strategies, have identified unknown partner genes fused to various known genes in chromosomal translocations. For example, the demonstration of IG and TCR loci rearrangements in leukemias and lymphomas, as evidenced by altered size of restriction enzyme fragments on genomic Southern blot analyses, has been essential in highlighting crucial regions that could be studied by molecular cloning strategies, and that characterize the genomic translocation breakpoint junction sequences that define these tumors. The molecular principles that provide the basis for current clinical molecular cytogenetic diagnostic strategies (e.g., FISH) in pediatric leukemias and solid tumors are not substantially different from the recombinant DNA concepts used in Southern blotting. Some seminal examples of gene rearrangements characterized originally by Southern blotting and now detected routinely by FISH include *MYC* gene rearrangements, involving the IGH or IGL chain loci in Burkitt's lymphoma,[14] and *MLL* rearrangements, of which the first characterized type was associated with t(4;11), resulting in *MLL-AF4* fusion.[15]

Another application of Southern blot analysis has been in discerning gene copy number variation. One example is *MLL* gene amplification (Fig. 5-4), involving an interlocus DNA rearrangement known as segmental jumping translocation in which the unrearranged *MLL* DNA segment is amplified and translocated to various regions of the genome.[16]

Molecular Cloning

Whereas conventional cytogenetic analyses are performed using staining techniques that highlight chromosomal banding patterns (1;2), the various molecular cytogenetic methods interrogate chromosomal regions of interest by using nucleic acid probes.[17,18] Most molecular cytogenetic methods use some variant of ISH (in situ hybridization), in which DNA probes are hybridized and evaluated in the cellular context. These probes are usually cosmids, containing an approximately 40-kb sequence of interest or bacterial artificial chromosomes (BACs), containing hundreds to a few thousand kilobases of sequence. ISH assays can be performed with fluorescence or enzymatic detection, referred to as FISH and CISH (chromogenic in situ hybridization), respectively (Figs. 5-5 and 5-6).[18]

Flexibility of in Situ Hybridization: Substrate Options. FISH and CISH analyses are performed routinely in cytogenetic preparations (metaphase spreads) and in paraffin sections and other archival pathology preparations. Substantial advantages of using paraffin sections include the following: (1) the abundance of source material for each case permits retrospective and repeat analyses; and (2) the well-preserved cell morphology can guide evaluation of the chromosomal events in the relevant cell populations. However, a drawback in the use of paraffin sections is that the nuclei are generally incomplete, having been sliced through during preparation of the sections by microtomy.[19] This limitation can be addressed by performing the ISH assays with nuclei disaggregated from thick (50- to 60-μ) paraffin sections[20] or from thin cores of the paraffin block.[21]

Resolution. Most ISH studies have a resolution of one to several megabases on metaphase spreads. Notwithstanding the aforementioned problems of interphase FISH on fixed material, the technique offers the advantage of higher resolution, given the less compact arrangement of DNA in interphase nuclei. Higher resolution FISH techniques have been developed in which the DNA is essentially stretched out over a slide, as in DIRVISH (**dir**ect **vis**ual **h**ybridization), resulting in a resolution of between 700 and 5 kb,[22] or fiber FISH, in which the resolution is between 500 kb and just a few kilobases.[23]

Highly Combinatorial Modifications of Fluorescence in Situ Hybridization. Various newer molecular cytogenetic methods have expanded the capabilities of FISH, enabling evaluation of the entire genome or karyotype. Examples include comparative genomic hybridization (CGH)[24,25] and spectral karyotyping (SKY).[26] Comparative genomic hybridization is performed by extracting total genomic DNA from a tumor of interest and from a non-neoplastic control cell population. These DNAs are differentially labeled (e.g., tumor DNA with fluorescein and control DNA with rhodamine), and then cohybridized against normal metaphase cells (metaphase CGH) or against arrays of genomic or complementary DNA (cDNA) clones (array CGH).

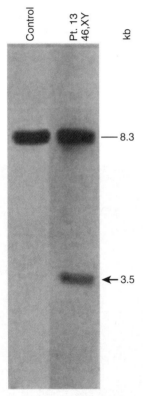

FIGURE 5-3. Detection of cryptic *MLL* bcr rearrangement by Southern blot analysis in treatment-associated acute myelogenous leukemia (AML). The karyotype was normal but the French-American-British (FAB) M4 morphology and clinical history of dactinomycin exposure informed further analysis of *MLL*. The dash indicates the germline pattern and the arrow shows a rearrangement, which panhandle polymerase chain reaction molecular cloning revealed to be an *MLL* internal tandem duplication. (Adapted from Megonigal MD, Rappaport EF, Jones DH, et al. Panhandle PCR strategy to amplify MLL genomic breakpoints in treatment-related leukemias. Proc Natl Acad Sci U S A. 1997;94:11583-11588.)

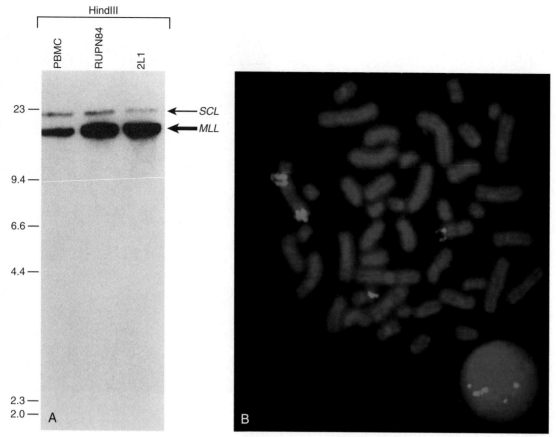

FIGURE 5-4. A, Southern blot analysis indicating *MLL* gene amplification in treatment-related acute myelogenous leukemia (AML). Southern blot analysis of *HindIII*-digested genomic DNA from French-American-British (FAB) M4 AML cells (RUPN84) of a patient whose AML karyotype showed no evidence of chromosome band 11q23 rearrangement that would suggest *MLL* gene rearrangement and a cell line established from the same AML (2L1). Cohybridization with a *MLL* bcr-region probe and a loading control *SCL* probe demonstrates unrearranged but amplified *MLL* with signal intensity of 4.3:1 in the AML compared with normal peripheral blood mononuclear cell (PBMC) control DNA. **B,** Fluorescence in situ hybridization (FISH) confirms *MLL* genomic amplification in RUPN84. (Adapted from Felix CA, Megonigal MD, Chervinsky DS, et al. Association of germline p53 mutation with MLL segmental jumping translocation in treatment-related leukemia. Blood. 1998;91:4451-4456.).

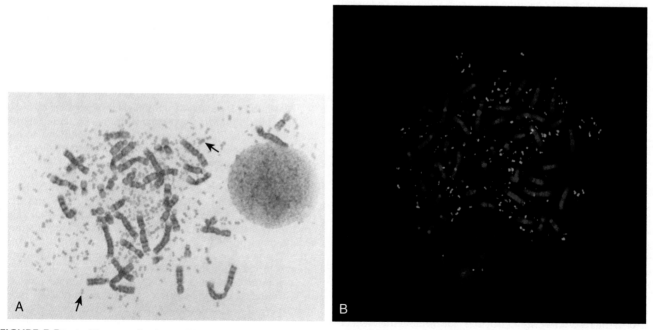

FIGURE 5-5. A, Giemsa-stained neuroblastoma metaphase cell (and with nucleus from a different cell on right) showing hundreds of variably sized double-minute chromosomes (dmin), as indicated by arrows. **B,** *MYCN* (*N-myc*) fluorescence in situ hybridization (FISH) evaluation of neuroblastoma metaphase cell, showing numerous extrachromosomal double minutes containing *MYNC* (*green*) whereas the reference chromosome 2 pericentromeric FISH probe (*red*) shows two copies.

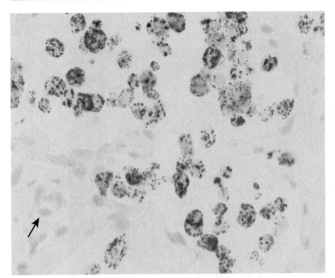

FIGURE 5-6. MYCN (N-myc) chromogenic in situ hybridization (CISH) in a neuroblastoma paraffin section. Peroxidase-DAB detection (*brown*) of MYCN fluorescence in situ hybridization (FISH) probe demonstrates high-level MYCN amplification in neuroblastoma cells, but not in fibrovascular non-neoplastic cells (*arrow*).

Chromosomal regions overrepresented (amplified) or under-represented (deleted) in the tumor DNA relative to normal DNA are manifested as color shifts when the metaphase cells, or arrays, are visualized under fluorescence.

An advantage of comparative genomic hybridization, compared with conventional karyotyping, is that the tumor DNA can be isolated from frozen or even paraffin specimens, without any need for cell culture, thereby avoiding the selection pressures imposed by culture, and instead capturing an overview of the in vivo situation, although diluted by the admixture of support stromal DNA. In addition, the array CGH methods can detect very small deletions, which would be overlooked by traditional cytogenetic banding assays and might even be missed by FISH. However, comparative genomic hybridization does not detect the balanced chromosomal rearrangements, particularly the translocations that are the genetic hallmarks of many pediatric cancers. Furthermore, while detecting chromosomal amplifications and deletions reliably, the technique does not provide a functional assay in terms of expression level changes.

Genome-wide molecular cytogenetics can be performed using spectral karyotyping or M-FISH, in which entire panels of DNA probes are simultaneously hybridized against tumor metaphase cells.[26] Whereas conventional FISH techniques involve hybridization of one or two fluorescence-tagged probes, the spectral karyotyping and M-FISH methods use probes for each chromosome or chromosome arm (24 or more probes). Each probe is then detected combinatorially, using different ratios of fluorescence markers, such as fluorescein and rhodamine. By varying the ratio of fluorescence tags, each chromosome can be visualized with a unique color (Fig. 5-7). Thus, spectral karyotyping enables a comprehensive ISH screen of the entire tumor cell karyotype. Spectral karyotyping and M-FISH are powerful research tools in tumor cytogenetics, and have been useful in identifying rearrangements that are cryptic by conventional cytogenetic banding methods, or highly complex.[27,28] However, these techniques are as yet largely confined to the research realm rather than constituting the basis of standard clinical tumor genetic assays.

Routine Applications of Fluorescence in Situ Hybridization.
Most ISH studies performed in clinical laboratories are focused

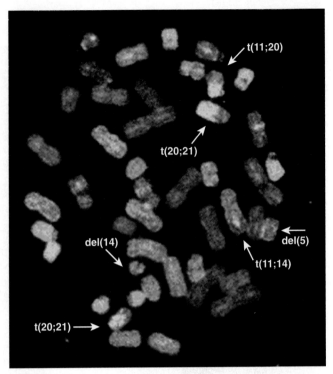

FIGURE 5-7. Metaphase spectral karyotype in treatment-associated acute myelogenous leukemia, showing typical 5q deletion, among other clonal aberrations. (Courtesy of Hesed, National Institutes of Health, Bethesda, Md.)

on investigating deletions, rearrangements, or amplifications of particular gene loci, or chromosomes. The probes used for FISH analysis of chromosomal translocations (and other balanced cytogenetic rearrangements) generally fall into two categories. First, there are those that hybridize to a region spanning a breakpoint on one involved chromosome, producing a split signal in the presence of chromosomal rearrangement (see Fig. 5-2), Second, there are probes designed to come together in the presence of a fusion, in which a probe labeled with one fluorochrome hybridizes to one partner gene and the other, differentially labeled, to its fusion partner, with these producing a fused fluorescent signal only in the presence of a gene rearrangement.

Maximizing Data Yield from Individual Fluorescence in Situ Hybridization Probes for Rearrangements. Judicious selection of break-apart FISH probes can allow applicability to a wide variety of tumors, in which the probe interrogates a frequently rearranged gene such as *EWS* in various solid tumors or *MLL* in leukemias. The *EWS* gene undergoes rearrangement with various *ETS* family genes in Ewing's sarcoma and *EWS* is rearranged in pediatric desmoplastic round cell tumors and clear cell sarcomas of soft parts, among others. Each of these diagnostically useful *EWS* rearrangements can be demonstrated using a single *EWS* break-apart FISH probe (Fig. 5-8), with ultimate diagnosis requiring interpretation of the molecular findings in the context of the histology.

Additional gross genetic aberrations routinely accompanying chromosomal translocation may be exploited to refine interpretation of FISH-based analysis in certain contexts. For example, *FKHR* (*FOXO1*) gene FISH can distinguish the *PAX7-FKHR* and *PAX3-FKHR* oncogenic fusions in alveolar rhabdomyosarcoma, given that the *PAX7-FKHR* (but not the *PAX3-FKHR*) is invariably highly amplified in these tumors. This distinction is warranted because of its prognostic significance. In the typical scenario, in which routine pathologic evaluation by light microscopy of H&E (hematoxylin and eosin)–stained sections with accompanying immunohistochemistry has generated a reasonably narrow differential diagnosis, genetic testing by this type of assay is highly informative and increasingly being used. Generally, this somewhat looser FISH-based assay may be regarded as having optimal attributes, providing perhaps greater sensitivity than karyotypic analysis and being capable of detecting cryptic or masked translocations,[29] while not being burdened by the restrictive specificity of PCR-based assays (see later).

Fluorescence in Situ Hybridization in the Analysis of Gains and Losses. Although quantitative assessment of gene amplifications and deletions can be obtained by quantitative PCR (qPCR) or FISH, in practice such assays are more often conducted in clinical laboratories by FISH-based methods. In the

example of *MYCN* (aka *N-myc*) amplification in neuroblastoma, FISH detection is performed routinely (see Figs. 5-5 and 5-6). Assessment of *MYCN* amplification may alternatively be done by semiquantitative PCR, using a standard PCR assay with normal (unamplified) and known amplified controls and multiplexing the reaction to include a housekeeping gene along with the gene of interest. However, such assessments can be confounded by intratumoral heterogeneity. In neuroblastoma, this heterogeneity may encompass substantial variations in cellular composition and maturation and thus careful selection of tumor tissue for analysis is essential. The analysis of poorly selected tissue for *MYCN* evaluation—for example, submission of schwannian stroma—will otherwise yield a false-negative result.[30] Moreover, contributions of different components of the neuroblastic tumor in the final DNA isolate can dilute out regional (neuroblast-specific) *MYCN* amplification, again yielding false-negative results. In this context, there is a distinct advantage to the FISH assays for *MYCN* amplification, because such methods permit correlation with cytology or morphology for the detection of regional heterogeneity of *MYCN* amplification, particularly when performed in tissue sections or multifocal touch imprints.

Detection of deletions by FISH is a more complex matter and particularly challenging when using the ready resource of fixed tissue, in which the assay is for an absence of signal and one is dealing with interphase nuclei, by definition incomplete (sliced through by microtomy), with an admixture of normal stromal cells further confounding the picture. Where cytogenetically abnormal metaphase spreads are available, these problems are largely circumvented, but there are other potentially more suitable technical strategies that might be used, including PCR-based assays—again with the caveat of normal cell admixture—to establish loss of heterozygosity (LOH). The immunohistochemical stain may provide a ready assay for such detection, as in the case of the *INI1-SNF5* gene on chromosome 22q, commonly deleted in malignant rhabdoid tumors (Fig. 5-9), and atypical teratoid rhabdoid tumors.[31]

Polymerase Chain Reaction–Based Molecular Assays

General Applications of Polymerase Chain Reaction–Based Methods

Since the initial description of the basic PCR assay,[32] critical modifications of the technique have led to massive expansion of the applicability of this technology. The initial methodology

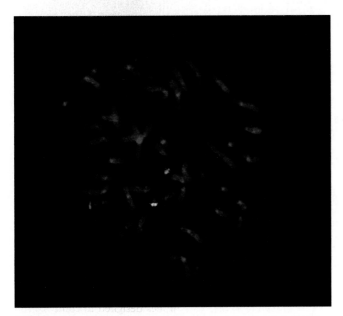

FIGURE 5-8. *EWS* break-apart fluorescence in situ hybridization (FISH) probe, hybridized to Ewing's sarcoma metaphase cell, in which probe components centromeric and telomeric to *EWS* are detected with fluorescein isothiocyanate (FITC) (*green*) and rhodamine (*red*), respectively. *EWS* rearrangement is indicated by the breaking apart of the normal yellow (*green-red fusion*) signal into the red and green components, which localize to different chromosomes as a result of translocation.

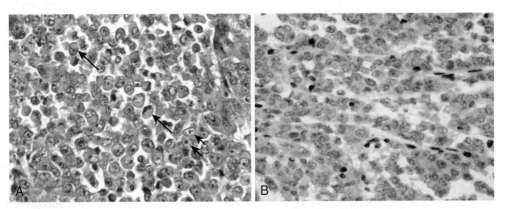

FIGURE 5-9. A, Rhabdoid tumor showing loosely cohesive cells, many containing intracytoplasmic inclusions (*arrows*). Nuclei are vesicular and contain prominent nucleoli (*short arrows*) (H&E stain). **B,** INI1 immunohistochemistry, showing entirely negative reaction in the neoplastic cells, reflecting loss of 22q, and with only the endothelial and occasional admixed inflammatory cells staining positively.

involved the use of a DNA template from which a sequence of interest could selectively be amplified. This methodology provides the basis for testing for LOH, which relies on the natural allelic heterogeneity of repeat sequences in the vicinity of a gene of interest.[33] Where a genomic region is deleted, the concomitant loss of an adjacent allelic repeat sequence results in PCR amplification of only one version of the repeat sequence, thus producing hemizygosity (seeming homozygosity) at that locus.

Reverse Transcriptase Polymerase Chain Reaction

Where a particular question revolves around the presence of a specific transcript, the starting material is RNA, which is subjected to reverse transcriptase PCR (RT-PCR), a highly sensitive technique.[34] The principle is that total RNA extracted from fresh, flash-frozen, or fixed material is reverse-transcribed into first-strand cDNA. This provides the template[34,35] for testing for the presence of fusion oncogene transcripts using primers complementary to the involved partner genes flanking the fusion point in the chimeric transcript, and which cannot therefore generate a product from unrearranged normal tran-

script. The technique is extraordinarily sensitive, able to detect as few as 1 in 10,000 cells bearing a fusion transcript.[36] The presence of just a small neoplastic component within a tissue sample for genetic testing is therefore sufficient for detection. Thus, this PCR-based technology is useful for the detection of minimal residual disease[35] and well suited for the surveillance of hematologic malignancy, in which serial peripheral blood or bone marrow specimens are obtained for routine follow-up of patients. However, this same sensitivity of PCR-based methods carries with it the risk of false-positive results, from cross-contamination of minute amounts of fusion gene templates within assays, or detection of very-low-level biologically insignificant fusion transcripts within specimens. Although moot in the context of demonstrating uniquely tumor-associated aberrations (e.g., fusion products), ideally DNAse I treatment of the RNA substrate should be performed to eliminate the possibility of inadvertent genomic amplification during RT-PCR.

Specificity of Reverse Transcriptase Polymerase Chain Reaction. Breakpoint variability within the genes involved in translocation-generated fusion oncogenes has prognostic impli-

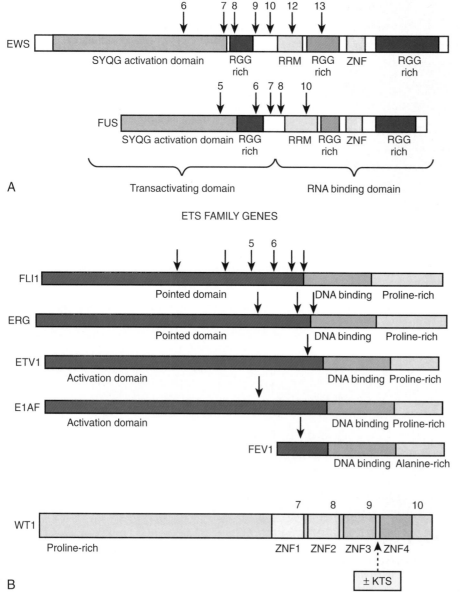

FIGURE 5-10. A, *EWS* and *FUS* genes encode an N-terminal transcriptional activation domain, RGG-rich regions, RNA recognition motif, and a zinc finger. Arrows indicate various breakpoints reported in *EWS* or *FUS* oncogenes. **B, upper panel,** Domains encoded by the various ETS-family genes fused with *EWS* or *FUS* in Ewing's sarcoma. Arrows indicate various breakpoints that have been reported in fusion rearrangements. The most common oncogenic rearrangements in Ewing's sarcoma involve the fusion of the *EWS* exon 7 to *FLI1* exon 6 (type 1 transcript) or exon 5 (type 2 transcript). **Bottom panel,** Domains encoded by the *WT1* gene, which is fused with *EWS* in desmoplastic small round cell tumor. Two WT1 isoforms are produced by an alternative spicing event (±KTS) between zinc fingers 3 and 4.

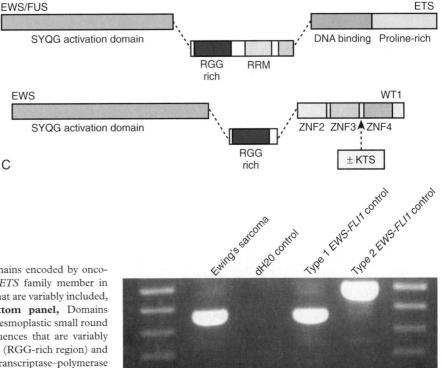

FIGURE 5-10, cont'd. C, upper panel, Domains encoded by oncogenic fusions between *EWS* or *FUS* with an *ETS* family member in Ewing's sarcoma. Dotted lines indicate regions that are variably included, depending on the breakpoint locations. **Bottom panel,** Domains encoded by the *EWS-WT1* fusion oncogene in desmoplastic small round cell tumor. Dotted lines indicate encoded sequences that are variably included, depending on the breakpoint locations (RGG-rich region) and alternative splicing events (KTS). **D,** Reverse transcriptase–polymerase chain reaction (RT-PCR) demonstration of type 1 *EWS-FLI1* transcript in Ewing's sarcoma (lane 1). Positive controls for types 1 and 2 transcripts are in lanes 3 and 4, respectively.

cations in some cases. This is reported for Ewing's sarcoma and synovial sarcoma, in which a favorable prognosis is associated with a type I fusion of *EWS* exon 7 to *FLI1* exon 6 compared with all other combinatorial variations in Ewing's sarcoma (Fig. 5-10).[37-39] *SYT-SSX2* fusion in synovial sarcoma is similarly reportedly associated with better patient outcome.[40,41] Assays may be designed to address breakpoint variability through choice of primers, selectively amplifying only one variant product, or by choosing consensus primers that will amplify several transcripts[42,43] and then sequencing the product to establish the precise nature of the transcript. An indication of transcript type might already have been obtained from gel electrophoresis demonstrating the product size (Fig. 5-11; see Fig. 5-10). PCR-based assays are best suited to the detection of such fine genetic detail, which cannot be detected by karyotypic analysis and only by specifically designed FISH assays. Currently, distinction among variant transcripts generally remains of academic interest because it provides no basis for therapeutic stratification.

In the case of *MLL* translocations, not only can one of more than 50 different partner genes be fused to *MLL*, but it has also been suggested that the various partner genes of *MLL* affect the prognosis.[44] In this case, PCR with gene-specific primers has been one approach to identify fusion transcripts involving some of the more common partner genes of *MLL*, and primer combinations for different *MLL* transcripts can be combined in a multiplex PCR reaction. This is most feasible in acute lymphoblastic leukemia (ALL), where the *MLL* partner genes are less heterogeneous than in acute myeloid leukemia (AML). Alternatively, approaches such as cDNA panhandle PCR can detect the fusion transcript produced by the 5'-*ML* partner gene 3' rearrangement using primer sequences derived from MLL. This is accomplished by the generation of a stem loop template in which a known *MLL* sequence has been attached to the unknown partner sequence by reverse transcribing the first-strand cDNA from total RNA using a 5'-*MLL*-random hexamer adapter-3' primer for the primer extension.[45] cDNA panhandle PCR was also used to characterize fusion transcripts involving new partner genes of the NUP98 gene at chromosome band 11p15 that result from recurring translocations in AML and ALL.[46]

Additionally, genomic panhandle PCR approaches[47-49] and long distance inverse PCR approaches[50,51] are alternatives for characterizing translocations in which the sequence of only one of the involved genes is known. The specificity of conventional PCR-based analysis of tumors in the effort to demonstrate fusion transcripts becomes a drawback when complex or new fusion variants involving different fusion partners or new breakpoints are encountered, because highly specific assays may fail to detect these, generating false-negative results.

One clinical scenario that requires the ability to detect a broad range of chromosomal translocations, including unknown or rare fusion variants, is in surveillance screening for evidence of a preleukemic state in chemotherapy-exposed patients, before these patients manifest frank secondary leukemia.[52] Advances in sensitive molecular PCR-based screening methods and molecular cytogenetic screening methods such as FISH will better enable the prospective detection of chromosomal translocations, which is crucial in such applications. If the abundance of a known transcript is of interest, quantitation of the assay can provide the answer (see below).

Quantitative Polymerase Chain Reaction

Simultaneous PCR of a constitutively expressed housekeeping gene provides an internal control. A standard positive control may be used as a comparator across a series of cases to rank these in a semiquantitative approach.[53] Use of quantitative PCR methods can provide precise information about the actual copy number of oncogene transcripts (gene expression level) by qRT-PCR or gene copy number when genomic DNA is used as template material. Quantitative PCR has advantages of

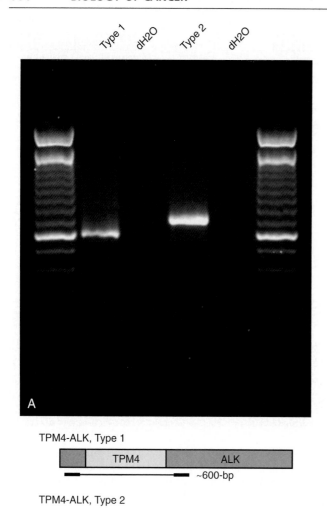

TPM4-ALK, Type 1

TPM4	ALK

~600-bp

TPM4-ALK, Type 2

TPM4	ALK

~715-bp

B

FIGURE 5-11. Reverse transcriptase–polymerase chain reaction (RT-PCR) demonstration of various *TPM4-ALK* fusion oncogene transcripts in inflammatory myofibroblastic tumors, as distinguished by gel electrophoresis of PCR products generated with the same primers **(A)**, with primer hybridization sites as indicated **(B)**.

subject to false positivity because of contamination or detection of primer-dimer; and (2) TaqMan methodology, based on highly specific primer-probe combinations. In TaqMan qPCR, a probe labeled with a fluorescent dye at one end (5′) and a quencher at the other (3′) is designed to bind within the sequence amplified by qPCR. In the unbound state, the proximity of quencher to the fluorescent dye inhibits detection of the fluorescence through Foerster resonance energy transfer (FRET). Once the probe has bound within the amplified sequence, 5′ exonuclease activity of the polymerase enzyme leads to probe cleavage and dissociation of fluorescent dye and quencher, with ensuing accumulation of fluorescence proportional to product amplification (strictly probe cleavage). Multiplexing of reactions is possible with TaqMan but not SYBR green technology.

Other Techniques

In addition to the above-mentioned techniques, high-throughput assays, including cDNA and oligonucleotide arrays, BAC CGH arrays, single-nucleotide polymorphism (SNP) analysis (Fig. 5-12), and highly parallel sequencing have been developed. These techniques are in use primarily in research, however, and still have a limited current role in clinical pediatric cancer genetic work, so they will not be discussed further here.

It might be surmised that the optimal setup of a tumor genetics laboratory in the pediatric context would strive to culture cells from all newly diagnosed tumors. It would largely rely on FISH-based assays to screen for rearrangements or amplifications of commonly involved genes such as *EWS*, *FKHR*, *N-Myc*, *MLL*, and *ALK* but retain expertise in PCR for LOH studies, detection of minimal residual disease, and in recombinant DNA technologies such as genomic Southern blot analysis and PCR-based cloning to identify novel variant rearrangements. Also, it is fully expected that array-based platforms enabling gene expression profiling and the detection of copy number variation will soon be added to the repertoire of routine screening tests, as is already being planned and implemented in some institutions.

GENOMIC MECHANISMS IN PEDIATRIC TUMORS

The cytogenetic aberrations in pediatric tumors can be extremely simple, involving loss or rearrangement of only a single chromosome, or can be highly complex, as manifested by a karyotype showing dozens of abnormal chromosomes. Complexly abnormal pediatric cancer karyotypes, containing 10 or more clonal rearrangements, are most often found in highly malignant solid tumors, such as osteosarcoma. On the other hand, a subset of highly malignant solid tumors, such as Ewing's sarcoma and synovial sarcoma, has noncomplex karyotypes. Therefore, the absence of cytogenetic complexity is not, in itself, a reassuring finding.

Clinically relevant chromosomal aberrations in pediatric tumors result in amplification, translocation, or deletion of various target genes. Amplifications, manifest as intrachromosomal homogeneously staining regions or extrachromosomal double minutes (see Figs. 5-5 and 5-6), are of greatest clinical relevance in neuroblastoma. They are also seen frequently in subsets of rhabdomyosarcoma, osteosarcoma, and central nervous system (CNS) tumors[54,55] and in leukemia, in which DNA segments encompassing various amplified oncogenes can be translocated to different regions of the genome. This

increased reliability and reproducibility over conventional PCR. Because it provides data accrued during the entire cycle, rather than just end point analysis, as in standard PCR, it will discriminate between different assays quantitatively rather than based on product size differences. Additionally, the graphic readout of accumulating fluorescence generated within each tube or well during the reaction is instantaneous (real time) and therefore no delaying additional step for product analysis is required. In conventional PCR, the amplification products must typically be evaluated by gel electrophoresis. Therefore, the assay turnaround time is minimized in qPCR, so that a complete analysis can be performed in only a few hours. qPCR is more sensitive, with an ability to detect twofold changes in expression level as opposed to a 10-fold cutoff for standard PCR assays. If desired, the products can still be subjected to gel electrophoresis—for example, to evaluate product size. Various forms of qPCR are available, including: (1) an SYBR green-based method, detecting double-stranded DNA product accumulation by binding to the minor groove of double-stranded DNA nonspecifically and thus being more readily

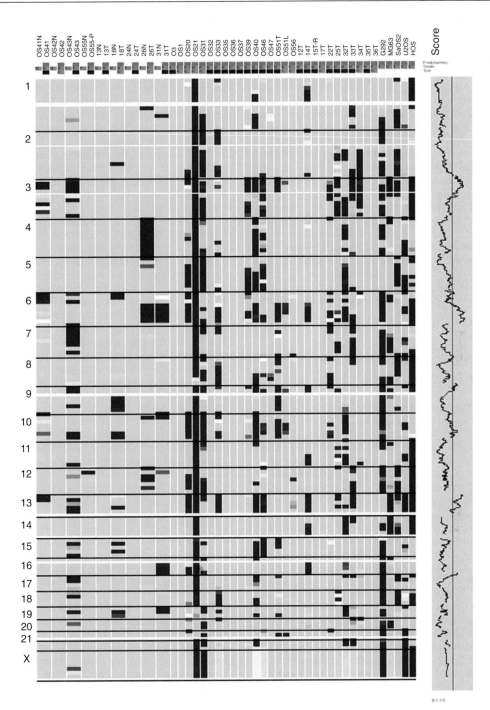

FIGURE 5-12. Genome-wide single-nucleotide polymorphism (SNP) analysis of osteosarcomas, with each column showing data from an individual case and the rows showing SNP data for each chromosome. Most osteosarcomas have numerous regions of SNP loss of heterozygosity, which are indicated in blue, whereas admixed regions of retained heterozygosity are in yellow.

phenomenon is termed *segmental jumping translocation.*[16,56] Deletions are generally thought to target tumor suppressor gene loci. Although of limited ancillary diagnostic value, detection of deletions may have prognostic implications (see Tables 5-2 and 5-5). Chromosomal translocations are particularly frequent in leukemias, lymphomas, and sarcomas, where they typically create fusions of regulatory or coding sequences in genes located at the breakpoints of the participant chromosomes.[57,58] Translocations result from double-strand DNA breaks, which are believed to occur more frequently in cancer cells than in normal cells, presumably as a manifestation of the genetic instability that is characteristic of many cancers. Most random translocations arising in cancer cells do not create functionally significant oncogenes and are therefore not selected for and retained by most of the cells in that cancer. The cytogenetic evidence suggests that at most a limited variety of translocations serve an oncogenic role in any given type of pediatric cancer. Many such recurring translocations have clinical use as diagnostic biomarkers (see Tables 5-1, 5-3, and 5-4) or for identifying tumor-specific therapeutic targets (see Tables 5-2 and 5-5).

Some translocation breakpoints directly interrupt the coding sequences of the target genes, leading to the creation of a fusion oncogene. Other breakpoints are outside of the gene coding sequences, but nonetheless alter transcriptional regulation of the target gene. In the case of coding sequence fusions, important functional domains from the two component genes are generally brought together by the chromosomal rearrangement. For example, fusion kinase oncogenes often result from apposition of the kinase gene catalytic domain with a translocation partner's protein-protein association domain (oligomerization domain). Such fusions lead to constitutive activation of the kinase. In other translocations, the intact coding sequence of a particular gene, usually one expressed at weak to undetectable levels in the non-neoplastic progenitor cell, is overexpressed by translocational juxtaposition to highly active promoter and enhancer sequences. One well-known example occurs in Burkitt's lymphomas, in which *MYC* oncogene expression is increased by translocation into various transcriptionally active immunoglobulin gene regions. The following sections review considerations of causative factors for translocation-associated oncogenes and provide key examples of their structural and functional roles in pediatric cancers.

Causes and Predisposing Factors for Chromosomal Translocations

The underlying mechanisms responsible for the genesis of chromosomal translocations are still poorly understood, but DNA double-strand breakage is a key step in this process. This may be induced by intracellular (endogenous) or extracellular (exogenous) agents. Some endogenous processes associated with double-strand breakage include V(D)J recombinase-mediated intrachromosomal rearrangements at immunoglobulin or T-cell receptor (TCR) loci, meiotic recombination between homologous chromatids, topoisomerase II–mediated changes in DNA topology that are required for DNA strand passage during mitosis and for the relaxation of supercoiled DNA for RNA transcription, and production of DNA-damaging agents (e.g., oxygen free radicals) from spontaneous hydrolysis, which themselves can alter DNA topology. Among the many exogenous insults causing double-stranded DNA breakage, ionizing radiation is the most extensively studied, and has been shown to disrupt hydrogen bonds and sugar-phosphate backbones, damage purine and pyrimidine bases, and induce cross-links between DNA strands. Such damage can lead to single- or double-strand DNA breakage. Notably, the locations of chromosomal breakage induced by ionizing radiation are not entirely random. Rather, smaller chromosomes appear to be disproportionately affected, as are regions rich in GC repeats. Other inducers of chromosomal breakage include ultraviolet A (UVA)–activated psoralens, chemotherapeutic agents, and DNA endonucleases.

One class of chemotherapeutic agents that can induce chromosomal breakage is the alkylating agents, such as nitrogen mustards, mitomycin C, nitrosureas, and platinum compounds, which form DNA adducts and cause intrastrand and interstrand DNA cross-linkage. DNA damage caused by treatment with these agents is associated with secondary myelodysplastic syndrome (MDS) and secondary leukemias, whose salient molecular cytogenetic features include complex numerical and structural abnormalities that often involve loss of chromosome 5, 5q, 7, or 7q. Noteworthy also is that germline and somatic mutations in the TP53 tumor suppressor protein, which is critical for DNA damage recognition, are frequent in secondary leukemias with chromosome 5q abnormalities and a complex karyotype, suggesting that genomic instability caused by loss of TP53 predisposes to this treatment complication.[16,59] The second class of chemotherapeutic agents that can induce chromosomal breakage are the topoisomerase II poisons, which target the nuclear enzyme topoisomerase II (e.g., the epipodophyllotoxins etoposide and teniposide; the anthracyclines doxorubicin, daunorubicin, and idarubicin; the anthracenedione mitoxantrone; and the combined topoisomerase I–topoisomerase II poison dactinomycin).[60]

Studies on genomic instability mechanisms in the yeast *Saccharomyces cerevisiae* have implicated defects in double-strand DNA breakage repair as causative factors in chromosomal translocations.[61] These repair defects can involve homologous recombination repair or nonhomologous end joining. Homologous recombination repair necessitates guidance of the DNA repair mechanism by two homologous sister chromatids, and is therefore more active in the G2 and S phases of the cell cycle. Nonhomologous end joining is intrinsically mutagenic and does not require extensive homology (usually less than 10 base pairs [bp]) between the two sequences that are joined. Nonhomologous end joining does not require the presence of guiding sister chromatids and is therefore most active during the G1 phase of the cell cycle. Malfunction of these DNA repair systems is responsible for the chromosomal instability in some cancer and premature aging syndromes such as Bloom's syndrome, an autosomal recessive disorder caused by inactivating mutations of the *BLM* gene. *BLM* encodes a nuclear protein related to the RecQ family of helicases, DNA-unwinding proteins involved in homologous recombination. Bloom's syndrome patients show increased rates of chromosomal breakage and exhibit sister chromatid exchanges in the form of quadriradials, four-armed structures composed of two chromosomes intersecting at regions of chromatin homology. Bloom's syndrome patients develop various benign and malignant tumors, generally occurring at an earlier age than in the normal population.

Other chromosomal instability syndromes result from defects in RecQ helicase proteins. For example, Werner's and Rothmund-Thompson syndromes are autosomal recessive disorders with germline mutations of *RECQL2* and *RECQL4*, respectively. Affected individuals develop various tumors, with osteosarcomas being particularly characteristic of patients with the Rothmund-Thompson syndrome. Ataxia-telangiectasia is an autosomal recessive disorder conferring exquisite sensitivity to ionizing radiation.[62] Ataxia-telangiectasia generally results from mutations in the *ATM* gene, which encodes a protein kinase that participates in surveillance for double-strand DNA breakage. Lymphocytes from ataxia-telangiectasia patients show increased levels of chromosomal rearrangement.

Nijmegen breakage syndrome shares several features with ataxia-telangiectasia, but is caused by mutations of the *NBS1* gene. The NBS1 protein participates in a complex with apparent roles in homologous recombination repair and nonhomologous end joining. Patients with ataxia-telangiectasia and Nijmegen breakage syndromes are particularly susceptible to the development of leukemias and lymphomas.

Fanconi's anemia is a heterogeneous group of autosomal recessive disorders with predisposition to cancer, particularly leukemias and squamous cell carcinomas. At least eight distinct genes involved in DNA double-strand breakage repair have been implicated in the genesis of Fanconi's anemia.[63] The chromosomes of Fanconi's anemia patients exhibit increased sensitivity to DNA cross-linking agents, such as diepoxybutane, and this feature can be useful in diagnosis of the disease. Fanconi's anemia DNA repair defects can also result from germline mutations of the *BRCA2* gene.

The Li-Fraumeni syndrome is a familial cancer predisposition syndrome that manifests as early onset of a constellation of tumors (rhabdomyosarcoma, breast carcinoma, osteogenic sarcoma, astrocytic brain tumors, adrenal cortical carcinoma, acute myelogenous leukemia) caused by germline mutation in the TP53 tumor suppressor protein.[64]

Certain DNA sequences may be targeted for chromosomal rearrangements. For example, certain sequences within the *MLL* transcription factor gene might comprise topoisomerase II DNA-binding sites that promote leukemia-associated rearrangements, and this has been studied in detail.[65] Notably, *MLL* is typically rearranged in secondary leukemias following exposure to topoisomerase II poisons, including epipodophyllotoxins, and in leukemia in infants in whom maternal-fetal exposures to dietary or environmental topoisomerase II poisons have been implicated.[60] Even though there is not a clear consensus topoisomerase II DNA-binding sequence in *MLL* and the preferred sites of enzyme recognition are modified by specific chemotherapeutic agents, it has been shown that *MLL* translocation breakpoints occur near functional sites of chemotherapy-enhanced topoisomerase II cleavage in in vitro assays.[60] Topoisomerase II is an essential cellular enzyme that relaxes supercoiled DNA by transiently cleaving and religating both strands of the double helix. Topoisomerase II catalyzes the sequential reactions of double-strand DNA cleavage, DNA strand passage, and DNA strand rejoining (religation). The DNA cleavage reaction occurs when each subunit of the topoisomerase II enzyme homodimer covalently attaches to and introduces staggered nicks in the DNA, with the nicked DNA remaining tethered to the enzyme subunits, forming a fleeting topoisomerase II–DNA intermediate called the cleavage complex. Particular anticancer drugs such as etoposide alter the cleavage-religation equilibrium by decreasing the rate of religation, which damages the DNA by increasing cleavage complexes. Chemotherapeutic agents that interact with topoisomerase II in this manner are termed *topoisomerase II poisons* because the enzyme is converted to a cellular toxin that promotes strand breakage. Although sometimes called topoisomerase II inhibitors when used clinically, these agents are distinct in their activity from catalytic inhibitors of this enzyme. The association of various chemotherapeutic topoisomerase II poisons used for anticancer treatment with secondary leukemias characterized by balanced chromosomal translocations has suggested that topoisomerase II has a role in other balanced translocations, such as the t(8;21), t(15;17), and inv(16) in addition to those involving *MLL*.

Other examples of recombination-promoting sequences are the heptamer-nonamer sequences adjacent to translocation breakpoints in many B-cell lymphomas. These sequences serve as sites of V(D)J recombination and are, therefore, recombination signals in the B-cell context. Similarly, the sites of V(D)J recombination also promote translocations of TCR genes with heterologous gene loci in T-cell ALL and T-cell lymphomas.

Physical proximity of genes in interphase nuclei has also been implicated in their incorporation into fusion genes. For example, radiation-induced thyroid carcinomas frequently exhibit rearrangements of the protein tyrosine kinase gene *RET* on chromosome 10q11, which is most often fused with the *H4* locus, telomeric (band 10q21) to *RET* on the same chromosome arm.[66,67] *RET* and *H4* are physically juxtaposed in 35% of normal human thyroid cells, providing a hypothesis as to why these two particular genes are disproportionately likely to be fused after radiation-induced double-strand DNA breakage.[68]

One intriguing aspect of cancer chromosomal translocations is that they are sometimes amplified, providing additional

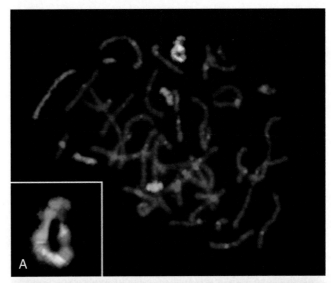

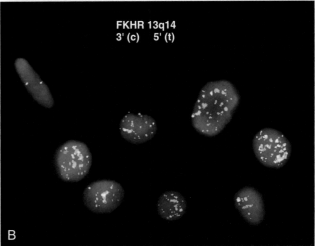

FIGURE 5-13. A, Fluorescence in situ hybridization (FISH), with whole chromosome "painting" probes to chromosomes 17 (*pink*) and 22 (*green*), demonstrates alternating segments of chromosomes 17 and 22 in a dermatofibrosarcoma protuberans ring chromosome (magnified in inset), resulting in threefold amplification of the characteristic *COL1A1-PDGFB* fusion oncogene. **B,** FISH demonstration of highly amplified and rearranged *FKHR* gene (*green*) in an alveolar rhabdomyosarcoma with *PAX7-FKHR* oncogenic fusion. Break-apart probe components 5′ and 3′ to the *FKHR* gene are red and green, respectively. Normal fibroblast nucleus at upper left contains two normal fusion probe signals.

copies of the associated fusion oncogenes. After their formation, the translocation breakpoint regions can be amplified as tandem repeats within the original chromosome, or can be amplified as extrachromosomal structures, such as double-minute chromosomes. One example of intrachromosomal amplification occurs with the typically low-level amplification of *PDGFB* fusion genes in the spindle cell sarcoma dermatofibrosarcoma protuberans (Fig. 5-13A).[69,70] An example of extrachromosomal amplification is found in a subset of alveolar rhabdomyosarcomas, in which double-minute chromosomes contain numerous copies of the *PAX7-FKHR* fusion oncogene (see Fig. 5-13B).[71] In either of these situations, the amplification event suggests that multiple copies of the fusion oncogenes are required to accomplish cellular transformation.

BIOLOGIC CONSEQUENCES OF CHROMOSOMAL TRANSLOCATION

Chromosomal Rearrangements Involving Transcription Factor Genes

Transcription factors are a heterogeneous group of DNA-binding proteins, most of which have domains involved in DNA binding, protein dimerization (for interaction with homologous proteins), and gene transactivation (for activation of gene transcription) or transcriptional repression. There are several classes of transcription factors, primarily relating to the structure of their DNA-binding domains. Some of the major categories include homeodomain proteins, zinc finger proteins, leucine zipper proteins, forkhead proteins, and helix-loop-helix proteins. Transcription factor genes are disrupted by many chromosomal translocations, resulting in their aberrant expression and function. Often, these transcription factor genes control lineage-specific developmental pathways and their abnormal activation can induce ectopic or asynchronous expression of corresponding lineage-specific antigenic markers, which then become a defining aspect of the transformed phenotype.

Many chromosomal translocations involving transcription factors have been described in leukemias and lymphomas. Chromosomal translocations in leukemias often interfere with the normal differentiation program of myeloid and lymphoid lineages,[72] although the presence of a chromosomal translocation per se does not prevent subclone evolution via further lineage-associated differentiation (e.g., progression from IGH gene rearrangement only to IGH plus IGL-chain rearrangement in precursor B-cell ALL). In acute leukemias, the targets for various chromosomal translocations are genes encoding hematopoiesis-related transcription factors, including AML1 (also known as RUNX1) and CBFB (see Fig. 5-12). AML1 is a DNA-binding protein with significant homology to the *Drosophila melanogaster* developmental protein Runt. AML1 binds to the DNA enhancer sequence TGTGGT; the DNA-binding capabilities of AML1 are enhanced through interactions with the non–DNA-binding protein subunit of CBF (core-binding factor) called CBFB, thereby regulating expression of several genes involved in hematopoiesis. One of the most common chromosomal translocations observed in acute myeloid leukemias (approximately 12% of cases) is the t(8;21)(q22;q22), which fuses *AML1* on chromosome 21q to *ETO* on chromosome 8.[73] *ETO* encodes a nuclear phosphoprotein expressed in the nervous system and in CD34+ hematopoietic progenitor cells. ETO is a transforming protein that normally participates in a multiprotein complex involved in chromatin remodeling and transcriptional repression. The fusion protein AML1-ETO retains the Runt domain of AML1 and almost the entire sequence of ETO.[74] It appears that the ETO domains incorporated into the fusion oncoprotein can dominantly repress transcription of certain genes, the expression of which is normally activated by AML1. As an example, the tumor supressor protein p14^{ARF} normally is transcriptionally activated by AML1, but p14^{ARF} is transcriptionally repressed by AML1-ETO.[75,76] AML1 is also involved in several other chromosomal translocations in leukemias and myeloproliferative disorders, including *AML1-MDS1* in myelodysplastic (preleukemic) syndromes, *AML1-EVI1* in chronic myelogenous leukemia in blast crisis, and *TEL(ETV6)-AML1* in pre-B acute lymphoblastic leukemia. All these fusion genes retain the AML1 Runt domain.[77]

Another example of a fusion gene affecting the normal function of the AML1-CBFB DNA-binding transcription factor protein complex is *CBFB-SMMHC*, which results from rearrangement of chromosome 16 in the French-American-British (FAB) M4Eo subtype of acute myelogenous leukemia.[78] *CBFB-SMMHC* can result from translocation or pericentric inversion of chromosome 16, thereby fusing sequences from the 5′ end of *CBFB* to the 3′ end of *SMMHC*. The resultant fusion oncoprotein contains the AML1-binding heterodimerization domain of CBFB juxtaposed to the coiled-coil domains of the SMMHC protein. The fusion protein CBFB-SMMHC binds to the AML1 Runt domain more effectively than the normal CBFB and has a dominant negative effect on the AML1-CBFB complex.[79]

MLL is a transcription factor protein in which the amino and carboxyl aspects contribute transcriptional repression and activation activities, respectively. MLL undergoes post-translational processing so that the transcriptional repression and activation regions are separated by cleavage, but they then reassociate with one another in a large multiprotein chromatin remodeling complex. MLL maintains but does not initiate expression of its target genes via histone methyltransferase activity, which is provided by a SET domain within the MLL carboxyl terminus.[80] A wide range of MLL fusion oncoproteins resulting from translocations of the *MLL* gene at chromosome band 11q23 contain the amino terminus of the MLL transcription factor and the carboxyl terminus of partner proteins that are themselves involved in transcriptional regulation. However, there is substantial diversity in MLL partner protein function, and not all MLL partner proteins are transcription factors.[80]

Chimeric (fusion) transcription factor oncogenes are also featured in many soft tissue tumors. A much-studied example is the *EWS-FLI1* fusion oncogene resulting from the t(11;22)(q24;q12) translocation[81] in Ewing's sarcoma. This translocation fuses *EWS* 5′ sequences to *FLI1* 3′ sequences. *EWS* encodes a ubiquitously expressed protein involved in DNA transcription, and *FLI1* is a member of a large family of DNA transcription factors that contain the highly conserved ETS domain. The *EWS-FLI1* fusion oncogene structure varies, depending on which *EWS* and *FLI1* exons are retained in the chimeric gene (see Fig. 5-10), but the *EWS-FLI1* oncogene resulting from fusion of *EWS* exon 7 to *FLI1* exon 6 is the most common form, referred to as type 1. Type 1 fusions have been associated with improved survival when compared with the other *EWS-FLI1* fusion types.[37-39] *EWS* can be fused with other ETS family members to provide the oncogenic impulse in Ewing's sarcoma, and *FUS* (an EWS family member) can also be fused with ETS family members in Ewing's sarcomas. Similarly, EWS or FUS are fused with other transcriptional regulator genes (not belonging to the ETS family) in various non-Ewing's mesenchymal neoplasms, always resulting in fusion oncoproteins with EWS or FUS at the amino terminal end of the fusion protein. One example is desmoplastic small round cell tumor (DSRCT), which is an exceptionally malignant cancer composed of nests of small round tumor cells sharply delineated by a reactive fibroblastic proliferation. DSRCT is cytogenetically characterized by the translocation t(11;22)(p13;q12), which fuses *EWS* to the *WT1* gene.[82] The EWS-WT1 fusion oncoprotein retains the EWS transactivation domain and the WT1 DNA-binding domain. *WT1* is a tumor suppressor gene located on chromosome 11p13 that encodes a zinc finger transcription factor with crucial roles in genitourinary tract development. Germline *WT1* mutations cause Wilms' tumor syndromes, including Denys-Drash and WAGR (**W**ilms'-**a**niridia-**g**enitourinary abnormalities and mental **r**etardation) syndromes.

Tumors of epithelial differentiation (carcinomas) often have complex karyotypes, which can obfuscate recurrent translocations. However, translocations involving transcriptional regulatory genes have been identified in several pediatric carcinomas, including follicular thyroid carcinomas, renal cell carcinomas, and NUT midline carcinoma.[83,84] Follicular thyroid carcinomas can feature *PAX8-PPARγ* fusion transcription

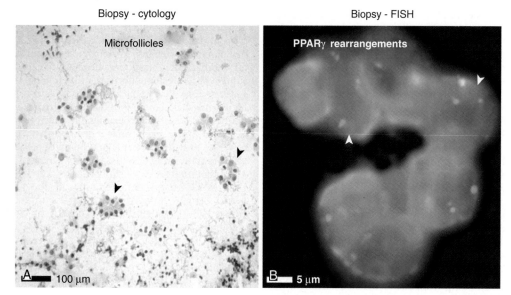

FIGURE 5-14. A, Cytology and fluorescence in situ hybridization (FISH; **B**) of follicular thyroid carcinoma, demonstrating rearrangement of the *PPARγ* gene, using break-apart probe, in microfollicle cells. (Courtesy of Dr. Todd Kroll.)

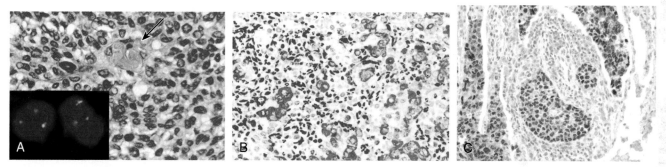

FIGURE 5-15. A, NUT midline carcinoma (sinonasal primary) composed of undifferentiated rounded cells with focal keratinization (*arrow*). Inset, *BRD4* break-apart fluorescence in situ hybridization (FISH) reveals rearrangement. Immunohistochemical study demonstrates reactivity for pan-keratin **(B),** indicating epithelial differentiation (alkaline phosphatase red). The NUT protein **(C)** (peroxidase DAB) is expressed in tumor cells but not in admixed histiocytes and lymphocytes.

factor genes resulting from translocation t(2;3)(q13;p15) (85) (Fig. 5-14), whereas in the highly lethal NUT midline carcinomas, a translocation t(15;19)(q13;p13) (Fig. 5-15) results in oncogenic fusion of the bromodomain transcriptional regulator *BRD4* with a novel testis-restricted gene, *NUT*.[86] Although exhibiting epithelial immunophenotypic features, NUT midline carcinomas typically have a primitive round cell morphology (see Fig. 5-15).

Chromosomal Rearrangements Involving Protein Tyrosine Kinase Genes

Chromosomal translocations in various neoplasms produce protein tyrosine kinase fusion genes, and such oncogenes are of considerable clinical importance. Protein tyrosine kinases comprise a large family of proteins, which are primarily involved in signal transduction. All tyrosine kinase proteins contain a highly conserved kinase (catalytic) domain, which mediates the phosphorylation of tyrosine residues in protein substrates. Phosphorylated tyrosines serve to stabilize various protein-

protein interactions and to enhance kinase activity in those substrates with intrinsic kinase function. Tyrosine kinase fusion oncoproteins resulting from chromosomal translocations in cancer have a consistent structure. The carboxyl-terminal end of these fusion oncoproteins typically contains the entire kinase domain from the tyrosine kinase protein, whereas the amino-terminal end contains an oligomerization domain from the other fusion partner. The oligomerization domain facilitates spontaneous interactions between kinase fusion oncoproteins, and the complexed oncoproteins can then phosphorylate each other, resulting in further upregulation of kinase activity.

The Philadelphia (Ph) chromosome is the cytogenetic hallmark of chronic myelogenous leukemia (CML), and was the first diagnostic translocation identified in a human cancer, also providing the best known example of a fusion tyrosine kinase oncogene.[87] The Ph chromosome results from chromosomal translocation between chromosomes 9 and 22, in which the *BCR* gene on chromosome 22 is fused with the *ABL* kinase gene on chromosome 9. This translocation is found in most CMLs, 25% of acute lymphoblastic leukemia in adults, 5% of acute lymphoblastic leukemias in children and, less often, in AML. *ABL* encodes a 145-kD nonreceptor protein tyrosine kinase that shuttles between the nucleus and cytoplasm and is involved in various cellular processes, such as cell cycle regulation and apoptosis. *BCR* encodes a 160-kD protein with dimerization, serine-threonine kinase, Rho-GEF (guanine nucleotide exchange factor), and Rac–guanosine triphosphatase (GTPase) domains. The BCR-ABL fusion oncoprotein is expressed as three structural variants, depending on the location of the breakpoint in the *BCR* gene. The BCR-ABL fusion transcript types segregate with specific neoplasms so that the 190-, 210-, and 230-kD BCR-ABL proteins are typically expressed in ALL, CML, and chronic neutrophilic leukemia, respectively. In AML, BCR-ABL fusion oncoproteins can be the P210 or P190 form.[88] The BCR-ABL fusion oncoproteins feature constitutive activation of the ABL kinase domain, resulting in autophosphorylation and tyrosine phosphorylation of various substrates. The phosphotyrosine residues serve as binding sites for various signaling proteins, resulting in activation of signaling pathways, such as Ras-MAPK (implicated in cell proliferation) and PI3K-AKT (implicated in cell survival).

Translocation-associated fusion kinase oncogenes are also found in various soft tissue tumors, including congenital fibrosarcoma, a pediatric spindle cell neoplasm with an excellent prognosis. Cytogenetically, congenital fibrosarcoma is characterized by the balanced translocation t(12;15)(p13;q25), which fuses the 5′ end of the transcription factor gene *TEL* to the 3′ end of the *NTRK3* protein tyrosine kinase gene (see Fig. 5-2).[89] The TEL-NTRK3 fusion oncoprotein retains the TEL helix-loop-helix dimerization domain and the NTRK3 kinase domain. *TEL* is also rearranged with other genes, including protein tyrosine kinase genes in various leukemias. The *TEL-NTRK3* fusion gene is seen in pediatric renal tumors known as congenital cellular mesoblastic nephromas, which are histologically similar to congenital fibrosarcoma (Fig. 5-16).[6] This finding suggests that congenital fibrosarcoma and cellular mesoblastic nephroma belong to the same spectrum of tumors. TEL-NTRK3 is also found occasionally in myeloid leukemia,[7] and is one of a few fusion oncogenes known to play transforming roles not only in soft tissue and hematopoietic neoplasms[90] but also in epithelial neoplasia (secretory breast carcinoma).

Inflammatory myofibroblastic tumor (IMT) is an unusual entity that arises predominantly in the abdominal cavity/peritoneum of young patients. Similar to congenital fibrosarcoma, IMT is usually associated with an excellent prognosis and metastases are rare. However, a subset of patients with IMT do develop disseminated disease and it is notable that many IMTs have chromosomal translocations that create activated fusion forms of the *ALK* receptor tyrosine kinase gene detectable by immunohistochemical means (Fig. 5-17).[90] *ALK* oncogenic fusion genes were initially described as a consequence of the chromosomal translocation t(2;5)(p23;q35), which occurs in a subset of anaplastic large cell lymphomas (ALCLs).[91] At least nine *ALK* fusion genes have now been described in IMT and ALCL; in all of them, the resultant fusion oncoproteins contain the ALK kinase domain fused to

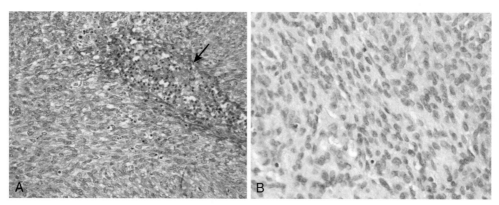

FIGURE 5-16. A, Congenital mesoblastic nephroma and infantile fibrosarcoma **(B)** are histologically indistinguishable tumors composed of mitotically active plump spindle cells, with varying extent of fascicular arrangement and showing islands of spontaneous necrosis as a characteristic feature (*arrow*).

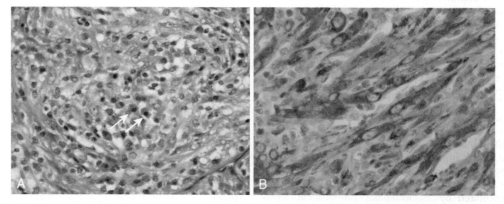

FIGURE 5-17. A, Inflammatory myofibroblastic tumor composed of plump neoplastic spindle cells with a reactive infiltrate featuring abundant plasma cells (*arrows*). **B,** Immunohistochemistry in a case with *TPM4-ALK* fusion, showing diffuse cytoplasmic staining with nuclear sparing in spindle cell (myofibroblastic) component, and absence of immunoreactivity in the inflammatory cell infiltrate.

an oligomerization domain of another protein. Two of the *ALK* fusion genes, *TPM3-ALK* and *CLTC-ALK* , have been found in IMT and ALCL, indicating that an identical oncogenic mechanism can contribute to these different tumors.[90,92] Most recently, *ALK* kinase domain mutations and gene amplification have been demonstrated in hereditary and sporadic neuroblastoma.[92a-c] Other receptor tyrosine kinase translocations in pediatric cancer include those in papillary thyroid cancers, which can target the *RET* or *NTRK1* genes.[93,94] In these fusion oncoproteins, the RET or NTRK1 kinase domains are activated by fusion with various oligomerization-inducing domains.

A further mechanism of protein tyrosine kinase activation by chromosomal translocation is seen in dermatofibrosarcoma protuberans (DFSP).[95] DFSP is a subcutaneous plump spindle cell sarcoma that exhibits high local recurrence rates but rarely metastasizes. Cytogenetically, this tumor is characterized by the chromosomal translocation t(17;22)(q21;q13), often amplified within a circular or ring chromosome (see Fig. 5-13A). The t(17;22) creates a *COL1A1-PDGFB* fusion gene, in which the entire *PDGFB* coding sequence is placed under the transcriptional control of the highly active *COL1A1* promoter in an event referred to as promoter swapping. This mechanism results in *PDGFB* overexpression, with resultant autocrine activation of the *PDGFB* receptor.[95] The same genetic event underlies the development of giant cell fibroblastoma, which is a pediatric tumor thought to be closely related to DFSP.[69,96]

Chromosomal Rearrangements Associated with Transcriptional Upregulation of Nonfusion Oncogenes

Many pediatric lymphomas feature juxtaposition of intact proto-oncogenes to transcriptionally active loci (e.g., the immunoglobulin locus in B-cell lymphomas or the TCR locus in T-cell lymphomas). V(D)J recombination and class switch recombination, which normally occur within the immunoglobulin or TCR loci in lymphocytes, have been implicated in the genesis of these nonfusion genes.[97] V(D)J recombination and class switch recombination mechanisms are exemplified by the nonfusion genes targeting *MYC*, a regulator of cell growth and survival, in many Burkitt's lymphomas. V(D)J recombination facilitates the chromosomal translocation t(8;14)(q24;q32) in endemic Burkitt's lymphomas found in patients from equatorial Africa. This translocation juxtaposes *MYC* to the intronic immunoglobulin heavy chain gene enhancer, leading to MYC overexpression. In contrast, most nonendemic Burkitt's lymphomas have translocation breakpoints downstream elsewhere in the immunoglobulin heavy chain gene locus, juxtaposing *MYC* to other enhancers. Alternatively, *MYC* overexpression can result from juxtaposition to the immunoglobulin kappa or lambda light chain genes resulting from t(2;8) or t(8;22).

Like Burkitt's lymphomas, follicular cell lymphomas of B-cell origin also feature rearrangements of immunoglobulin loci, but with *BCL2* or *BCL6*, rather than *MYC*, typically overexpressed by translocation into the region of an immunoglobulin gene promoter. *BCL2* alterations, conferring well-described antiapoptotic effects, often result from immunoglobulin heavy chain V(D)J recombination, with a breakpoint in exon 3 of *BCL2* becoming fused to the 5′ end of J_H or D-J_H heavy chain segments. These mechanisms result in *BCL2* transcriptional upregulation, mediated by the immunoglobulin heavy chain gene enhancer. Although deregulated BCL2 expression provides a survival advantage in such lymphomas, additional gene mutations are needed for full neoplastic transformation.[98]

However, in the pediatric population, follicular lymphomas are uncommon and the vast majority of cases feature elevated BCL6 expression. Cases with the t(14;18) translocation fusing the IGH chain locus with the BCL2 gene comprise only a small subset of the cases, which is in contrast to adults, but increased BCL2 expression is associated with advanced disease and a poor prognosis in pediatric lymphoma.[99]

TCR locus rearrangements are demonstrable in many T-cell leukemias and lymphomas, resulting in transcriptional upregulation of various translocated genes, similar to the mechanisms involving IG regions in various B-cell malignancies. The T-cell leukemia and lymphoma cytogenetic rearrangements dysregulate expression of transcription factor genes, such as *MYC, HOX11, HOX11L2, TAL-SCL, LYL1, LMO1,* and *LMO2*, by placing these genes under the control of highly active *cis*-acting transcriptional regulatory TCR elements, although dysregulation of these T-cell oncogenes can also occur in the absence of cytogenetic TCR rearrangements.[100,101]

Translocations resulting in nonfusion oncogenes can be seen in pediatric solid tumors; one example is the *PDGFB* fusion gene in DFSP (see earlier). Other examples include translocations of chromosome 8, targeting the *PLAG1* gene, a zinc finger transcription factor, in salivary gland pleomorphic adenoma and the primitive adipose tumor lipoblastoma. In both tumor types, the chromosomal breakpoints occur in the 5′ noncoding regions of the involved genes, resulting in promoter swapping, in which the transcriptionally inactive *PLAG1* promoter is replaced by the highly active promoter of the translocation partner gene, leading to *PLAG1* overexpression.[102-104]

BIOLOGIC BASIS FOR SPECIFICITY OF BALANCED CHROMOSOMAL REARRANGEMENTS: DIAGNOSTIC RELEVANCE

Recurrent chromosomal rearrangements involving specific breakpoint regions are increasingly being used as diagnostic markers in various pediatric cancers. Translocations are the most extensively studied of these rearrangements, but other mechanisms include chromosomal insertions, inversions, and interstitial deletions. Although diagnostic rearrangements, such as those involving chromosome 22 in Ewing's sarcoma, have become useful biomarkers, it is unclear whether most such characteristic rearrangements are initiating tumorigenic events or later events responsible for tumor progression. However, their oncogenic nature is generally convincing in that they can transform cells, as can be demonstrated by expressing the oncogenes in non-neoplastic cells in vitro or in mice. Although *EWS* and its family member *TLS-FUS* are frequently rearranged in chromosomal translocation in sarcomas, the partner gene varies and appears occasionally to dictate the tumor phenotype (see Table 5-1). For example *EWS-WT1* transcripts are found in DSRCT but not Ewing's sarcoma, whereas *EWS-ATF1* fusion occurs in soft tissue clear cell sarcoma but not other sarcomas. It has not yet been clearly established whether it is the partner gene that determines lineage in these tumors, or whether only certain cells, already lineage-committed, might tolerate the presence of these oncogenic transcripts.

Translocations of the *MLL* gene at chromosome band 11q23 are examples of leukemia chromosomal translocations that create potent fusion oncoproteins. *MLL* translocations are believed to be the events that initiate these leukemias.[105] Analogous to *EWS* variant rearrangements in pediatric solid tumors, particular *MLL* partner genes are more likely to occur in ALL than in AML, even though there is some overlap, and leukemias with *MLL* translocations can also exhibit dual lineage or actually switch lineage.[106]

There is substantial evidence that single genetic aberrations are insufficient to produce cancer. Rather, tumor development requires many gene mutations, perturbing different aspects of the cell biology (including apoptosis, proliferation, differentiation, and adhesion), which collectively results in the neoplastic phenotype. Even with *MLL* translocations in which there is a short latency from the in utero occurrence of the translocation to manifestation of disease, which is often in the newborn (younger than 3 months old) or even in the neonate or the fetus,[107] there are characteristic secondary alterations in addition to the translocations.[108]

Some of the same characteristic genetic alterations, including chromosomal translocations, observed in human cancers have been detected at very low levels (e.g., 1 in 10,000 cells) in non-neoplastic cell populations.[109,110] The rare cells containing these alterations are individually at low risk for progression to malignancy, presumably because it is unlikely that they will acquire the other mutations required to result in clinically evident cancer. However, this likely is more pertinent to solid tumors, in which a greater number of events generally is believed to be required for full oncogenesis than in leukemias. Similarly, it is likely that various diagnostic genetic alterations can be detected at very low levels in cancer types in which they are not characteristically encountered, and where they likely are not serving an important transforming role for the vast majority of cells in that cancer. Therefore, when using genetic alterations as diagnostic markers, it is important to have some sense that the alteration is found in most cells in the cancer, rather than being a rare and perhaps trivial event. It is similarly crucial to correlate the genetic findings with the histology, thereby confirming that the molecular diagnosis is credible.

The recurring and relatively specific association of chromosomal translocations with one or a few types of cancer has enabled the development of assays in which the translocations serve as ancillary diagnostic markers. There is a biologic basis to such tumor specificity because the neoplastic phenotype is essentially a symbiotic interaction between cell environment and translocation product, and certain genetic alterations, particularly those resulting from translocations, appear oncogenic in only a limited number of cancer cell environments.[111] Support for this concept is provided by B-cell lymphomas, in which diagnostic translocations often juxtapose oncogenes to the immunoglobulin loci. The immunoglobulin gene promoters are extremely active in the B-cell context, and ectopic placement of oncogenes near these promoters results in striking overexpression of the oncogenes, provided that the chromosomal rearrangement occurs in the B-cell context. By contrast, this same chromosomal rearrangement would presumably be irrelevant in other cell types, in which the immunoglobulin genes are transcriptionally silent. Translocations that occur in B-cell lymphoma have not been found in other varieties of human cancer. Another factor accounting for tumor specificity is the restriction of transforming properties of translocation-associated oncoproteins to certain cell lineages. Fusion oncoproteins always require interactions with other cellular proteins that facilitate and support the effect of that oncoprotein. Therefore, cell lineages lacking the relevant interacting proteins will not be transformed by a given fusion oncoprotein. These concepts are underscored by the observation that the BCR-ABL fusion oncoprotein, which is highly transforming in hematopoietic progenitor cells, fails to transform fibroblast cell lines.[112]

In pediatric tumors, genetic aberrations useful for testing as ancillary diagnostic findings are especially frequent in sarcomas, leukemias, and lymphomas. Interestingly, in contrast to adult tumors, diagnostic alterations are also found in many pediatric carcinomas, including papillary and follicular thyroid carcinomas, renal cell carcinomas, and lethal midline carcinoma. Although cytogenetic and molecular profiles are diagnostic in some pediatric cancers, there are many others that lack specific genetic or cytogenetic aberrations, or have extremely complex karyotypes in which the specific aberrations, if present at all, are difficult to identify.

CYTOGENETIC AND MOLECULAR PATHOLOGY: MAJOR TUMOR TYPES

Cytogenetic and molecular analyses have provided extraordinary insights into the biology and pathogenesis of pediatric cancer and, in some cases, these insights have then formed the basis for more accurate assessment of diagnosis and prognosis. However, neither cytogenetic nor molecular methods are required routinely in the clinical setting. In some pediatric solid tumors, there is not yet a basis for genetic testing because recurrent genetic aberrations are unknown. In others, particularly those that are benign clinically, the histopathology diagnosis and prognosis are generally straightforward and genetic adjuncts are therefore irrelevant. Some pediatric solid tumors, such as high-grade osteosarcoma, have extremely complex karyotypes, so that to date, there is little clinical advantage in genetic analysis, given the formidable task of describing the many genetic aberrations in a given tumor and the questionable prognostic relevance of the individual genetic perturbations. Widespread application of genetic assays in such tumors awaits the identification of key genetic predictors, which might then be determined in tumor interphase cells by molecular cytogenetic assays.

The following sections will highlight applications of cytogenetic and molecular assays in subsets of pediatric tumors, in which the technical challenges of genetic assays are manageable, and in which genetic findings are acknowledged to provide important diagnostic or prognostic information.

Mesenchymal Neoplasms: Soft Tissue and Bone Tumors

Ewing's Sarcoma

Ewing's sarcomas are highly aggressive tumors, characteristically occurring in bone and soft tissue, but also, less commonly, in viscera, in which the neoplastic cells are generally of the small, round, blue cell type. Ewing's sarcoma and peripheral primitive neuroectodermal tumor (pPNET), although historically considered distinct entities, share molecular and morphological features, and are now regarded as essentially the same entity. Ewing's sarcomas typically contain chromosomal translocations involving the Ewing's sarcoma gene (*EWS* or *EWSR1*), which is located on the long arm of chromosome 22. These translocations involve a number of partner genes (see Table 5-1), with the most common translocation being the t(11;22)(q24;q12), resulting in oncogenic fusion of 3′ sequences of the *FLI1* gene on chromosome 11 with 5′ sequences of *EWS*.[113-117] *FLI1* encodes a transcription factor belonging to the *ETS* family of transcription factors, and the oncogenic *EWS-FLI1* fusion gene encodes an activated version of this transcription factor. In variant translocations, *EWS* is fused with alternative *ETS* transcription factor family members (see Fig. 5-10 and Table 5-1)[118-122] and, rarely, the *EWS*-family gene, *FUS*, can also be fused with an *ETS* family gene in Ewing's sarcomas (Fig. 5-18).[123] The *EWS* family and *ETS* family gene translocations are apparently essential for oncogenesis, being found in almost all Ewing's sarcomas. These translocations are

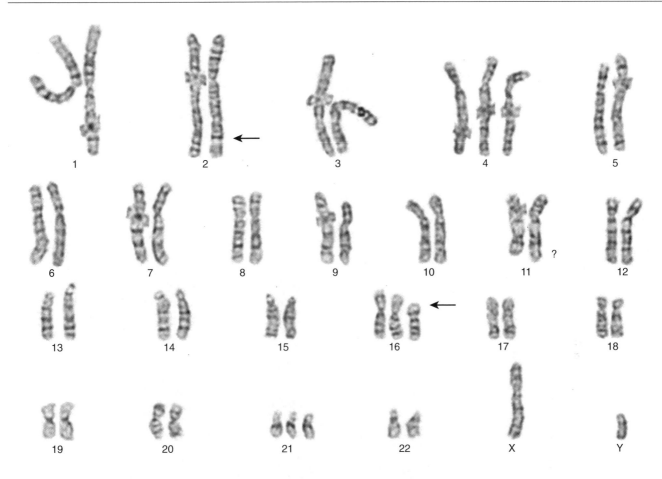

FIGURE 5-18. Ewing's sarcoma with t(2;16)(q35;p11), resulting in oncogenic fusion of the *FEV1* and *FUS* genes (*arrows* indicate translocation breakpoints).

readily detected by conventional cytogenetic methods, even using needle biopsy material, because Ewing's sarcoma cells grow well in tissue culture.[9] The translocations can also be detected by FISH, typically using dual-color probes flanking the *EWS* locus (see Fig. 5-8).[124] Although this does not identify the partner gene fused to *EWS*, that information is generally unnecessary for diagnostic purposes. Another method for detecting these translocations is by RT-PCR.[125] Advantages of PCR include superior sensitivity, identification of the *EWS* fusion partner gene, and identification of the breakpoint locations within the genes. The most common fusion is between *EWS* exon 7 and *FLI1* exon 6, known as type I fusion, whereas type II fusion involves fusion of *EWS* exon 7 with *FLI1* exon 5, and many further variants have been described (see Fig. 5-10). Although several studies have indicated that *EWS-FLI1* breakpoint locations might be prognostic in Ewing's sarcoma,[37,39,126] with tumors bearing the type I transcript doing better than all others, this information is not used routinely to guide therapeutic decisions.

Although histomorphologic and immunohistochemical features are often sufficient to establish the diagnosis of Ewing's sarcoma, genetic corroboration of the diagnosis is highly reassuring in distinguishing Ewing's sarcoma from other small round blue cell tumors, particularly in smaller biopsies, or if tumor cell preservation is compromised and/or immunohistochemistry is suboptimal. Although the cells are essentially undifferentiated, and superficially similar or identical to those in many other small round cell tumors, there are nonetheless

characteristic findings, such as subtle cytologic features and crisp cytoplasmic membrane–associated expression of the CD99 (O13-HBA71, pseudoautosomal gene-encoded membrane glycoprotein) (Fig. 5-19) that aid the diagnosis. Thus, the combined traditional histologic evaluation of H&E stained sections, together with immunohistochemical profiling, enables distinction of Ewing's sarcoma from, for example, a reasonable mimic in alveolar rhabdomyosarcoma by the demonstration of CD99 expression in Ewing's sarcoma versus expression of myogenic markers such as myogenin, MyoD1, and desmin in rhabdomyosarcoma (Fig. 5-20). The characteristic oncogene fusions in Ewing's sarcoma (*EWS-FLI1*) and alveolar rhabdomyosarcoma (*PAX-FKHR*) might contribute to the distinct cell differentiation profiles that separate these two round cell tumors immunophenotypically and morphologically. Evidence to this effect has been obtained from in vitro studies in which *EWS-ETS* oncogenes can induce neuroectodermal differentiation,[127] whereas *PAX-FKHR* induces a myogenic program.[128] Secondary genetic aberrations in Ewing's sarcoma can include *p53* mutation and *CDKN2A* deletion, which are each found in approximately 25% of cases, and are more frequent in cases that are clinically aggressive and poorly chemoresponsive.[129]

Rhabdomyosarcoma

Rhabdomyosarcomas are malignant tumors featuring skeletal muscle differentiation, with several histologic subtypes (see Fig. 5-20). The common varieties are the embryonal and

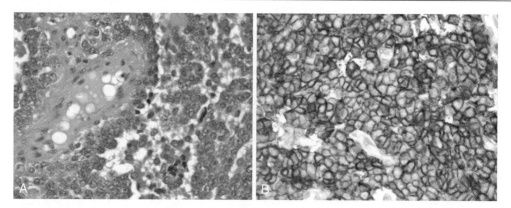

FIGURE 5-19. Ewing's sarcoma composed of undifferentiated round cells **(A)** arranged around thick fibrovascular cores and demonstrating strong and crisp CD99 expression confined to the cell surface **(B)**, producing a mosaic-like effect.

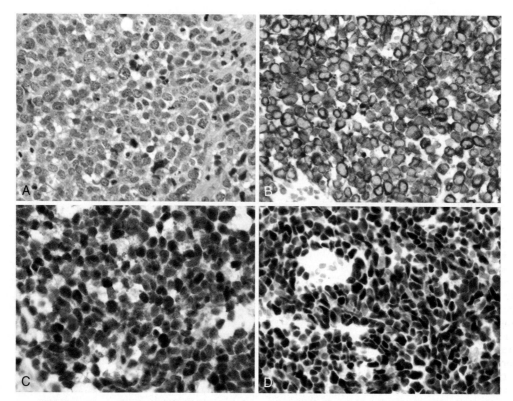

FIGURE 5-20. Solid variant of alveolar rhabdomyosarcoma composed of undifferentiated, moderately pleomorphic round cells histologically **(A)**, but with convincing evidence of myogenic differentiation, as demonstrated by strong and diffuse cytoplasmic expression of desmin **(B)**, and nuclear reactivity for MyoD1 **(C)**, and myogenin **(D)**. Of note, the percentage of nuclei reacting for both myogenin and MyoD1 is very high, as is typical of the alveolar variant of rhabdomyosarcoma.

alveolar subtypes and, although there are classic morphologies of alveolar and embryonal rhabdomyosarcoma, the distinction is not always clear-cut and composite cases occur. Therefore, especially with decreasing biopsy size, traditional morphologic distinction between embryonal and alveolar subtypes of rhabdomyosarcoma is not always a reliable means of subclassifying the tumors, but is essential for appropriate therapeutic stratification of patients with these two biologically different tumors. Alveolar rhabdomyosarcoma exhibits a higher proportional nuclear reactivity for both myogenin and MyoD1 than embryonal rhabdomyosarcoma,[130] but even this feature may be unconvincing in small biopsies and thus be of little value in establishing the diagnosis. The biologically distinct nature of embryonal and

alveolar subtypes is confirmed by genetic studies, which show translocations targeting the chromosome 13 *FKHR-FOXO1A* (forkhead transcription factor) gene in most alveolar rhabdomyosarcomas, and nontranslocation cytogenetic alterations, including 11p deletion, trisomy 8, and trisomy 20, in embryonal rhabdomyosarcomas. About 70% to 80% of alveolar rhabdomyosarcomas show fusion of the *FKHR* gene with the *PAX3* gene on chromosome 2,[131-133] and approximately 10% have fusions of *FKHR* with the *PAX7* gene on chromosome 1.[134] The *PAX7-FKHR* fusion is often highly amplified in the form of double-minute chromosomes (see Fig. 5-13B), whereas the *PAX3-FKHR* fusions are not usually amplified. This difference appears to reflect the lower intrinsic expression of *PAX7-*

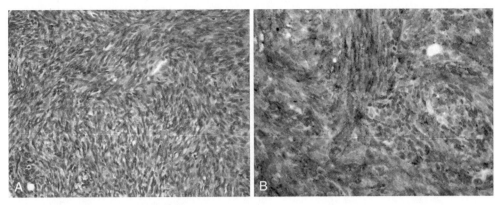

FIGURE 5-21. A, Monophasic synovial sarcoma, with interdigitating fascicular arrangement of fusiform spindle cells. **B,** Weak, patchy immunohistochemical staining for epithelial membrane antigen (EMA) in the spindle cells.

FKHR, relative to that of *PAX3-FKHR,* with genomic amplification therefore required to provide a comparable and sufficient level of oncogenic transcript.[135] The *FKHR, PAX3,* and *PAX7* genes encode transcription factors, and the *PAX3-FKHR* and *PAX7-FKHR* fusion oncogenes encode activated forms of those transcription factors[136,137] which function to induce myogenic differentiation programs.[128] Notably, alveolar rhabdomyosarcomas with *PAX7-FKHR* rearrangements appear to have better prognoses than those with *PAX3-FKHR* when comparing patients presenting with metastatic disease.[138]

Synovial Sarcoma

Synovial sarcomas are monophasic (Fig. 5-21), in which the tumor is predominantly composed of spindle cells, biphasic, in which the tumor contains both spindle cell and epithelioid elements, with the latter exhibiting more convincing epithelial immunophenotypic characteristics or, uncommonly, poorly differentiated, with a primitive round cell morphology reminiscent of Ewing's sarcoma. Synovial sarcomas feature translocation of chromosomes X and 18, t(X;18)(p11;q11).[139,140] t(X;18) is found in more than 90% of synovial sarcomas but not generally in histologic mimics such as hemangiopericytoma, mesothelioma, leiomyosarcoma, or malignant peripheral nerve sheath tumor. The molecular underpinnings of the t(X;18) translocation are complex in that the oncogene on chromosome 18 (*SYT* or *SS18*) can be fused with one of several almost identical genes (generally *SSX1* or *SSX2* and, rarely, *SSX4*) on chromosome X.[141,142] *SSX1* and *SSX2* are adjacent genes and, given their close proximity, it is impossible to distinguish *SYT-SSX1* and *SYT-SSX2* translocations using conventional chromosomal banding methods. However, the alternative *SSX* fusions can be demonstrated by FISH or RT-PCR using specific primers.[143,144] One study has suggested that synovial sarcomas with the *SYT-SSX1* fusion are typically biphasic, whereas those with *SYT-SSX2* can be biphasic or monophasic and have better metastasis-free survival compared with those bearing *SYT-SSX1* fusions.[145] This morphologic-genotypic correlate is substantiated by studies of SYT-SSX1 and SYT-SSX2 interactions with SNAIL and SLUG, both transcriptional repressors of E-cadherin, which mediates mesenchymal to epithelial transition.[146]

Although intriguing aspects of SYT and SYT-SSX function have been elucidated, these insights have not yet provided a more general understanding of the key biologic roles for SYT-SSX in synovial sarcoma. SYT and SSX contribute transcriptional activator and repressor domains to the SYT-SSX fusion proteins and SYT complexes with p300, thereby promoting cell adhesion[147] and perhaps influencing chromatin remodeling

activities.[148] Also, SYT-SSX recruits beta-catenin to the cell nucleus, and interacts with beta-catenin as a transcriptionally active complex.[149] Therefore, SYT-SSX oncoproteins likely regulate gene transcription, although the crucial downstream gene targets in synovial sarcoma have not been identified.

Adipose Tumors

Most subtypes of adipose tumors, whether benign or malignant, contain distinctive genetic aberrations (see Table 5-1). Useful diagnostic markers include 8q rearrangement in lipoblastoma, 12q rearrangement in lipoma, ring chromosomes in well-differentiated and dedifferentiated liposarcoma, and t(12;16) translocations in mxyoid or round cell liposarcoma.

Lipoblastomas are pediatric adipose tumors containing variable numbers of primitive cells (lipoblasts), and generally bearing translocations of the chromosome 8 long arm at bands 8q11-12, resulting in rearrangement of the *PLAG1* zinc finger oncogene.[103] Hibernomas, which contain adipose cells with a brown fat phenotype, generally have rearrangements of the chromosome 11 long arm,[150] although the gene target of that translocation has not been identified.

Another diagnostically useful aberration is the translocation of chromosomes 12 and 16 found in myxoid liposarcomas.[151-153] This translocation is also found in round cell liposarcomas and is retained in myxoid liposarcomas that acquire round cell features and thereby undergo transition to higher histologic grade.[154,155] The t(12;16) translocation results in fusion of the *CHOP* transcription factor gene on chromosome 12 to the *TLS* gene on chromosome 16,[156,157] and the resultant fusion oncoprotein is an activated transcription factor. The t(12;16) translocation has not been found in other subtypes of liposarcoma or in other types of myxoid soft tissue tumors.[158,159] It appears to be relevant therapeutically, in that patients with myxoid or round cell liposarcoma show impressive responses to trabectedin chemotherapy.[160]

Clear Cell Sarcoma: Malignant Melanoma of Soft Parts

Clear cell sarcomas of the soft tissues resemble cutaneous melanomas morphologically, and therefore have been referred to as melanoma of soft parts. Despite their histologic overlaps, clear cell sarcoma and true melanoma are different clinically. Whereas most melanomas are of cutaneous origin, clear cell sarcomas generally present as isolated masses in deep soft tissues, without apparent origin from, or involvement of, skin. More than 75% of clear cell sarcomas contain a chromosomal translocation, t(12;22)(q13;q12), that has never been reported in cutaneous

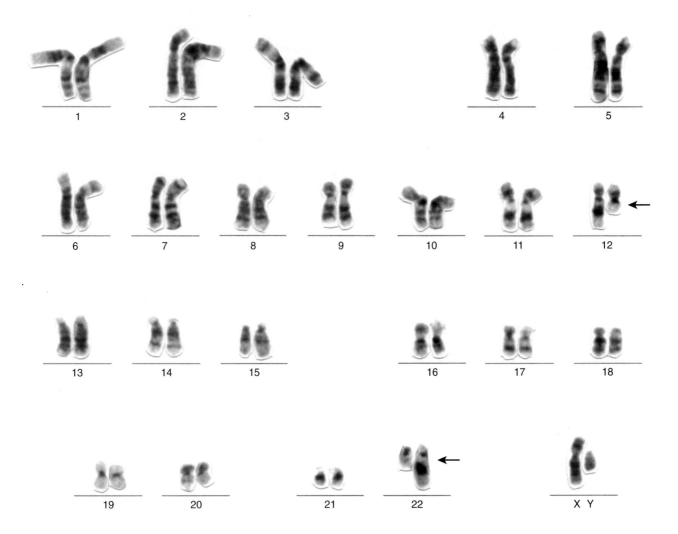

FIGURE 5-22. Clear cell sarcoma karyotype showing balanced translocation, t(12;22), as the only cytogenetic aberration. Arrows indicate translocation breakpoints.

melanoma, and which therefore serves as a reliable marker in distinguishing these two tumor types (Fig. 5-22). The t(12;22) translocation fuses the *ATF1* gene on chromosome 12 with the *EWS* gene on chromosome 22.[161,162] *ATF1* encodes a transcription factor, and the biologic implications of the translocation are probably similar to those in Ewing's sarcoma translocations (see earlier).

Desmoplastic Small Round Cell Tumor

Desmoplastic small round cell tumors are aggressive and chemotherapy-resistant neoplasms that arise most commonly from the peritoneum or intra-abdominal soft tissues, particularly in adolescent males.[163] They are composed of undifferentiated malignant small round cells in a striking desmoplastic reaction, ensnaring sharply demarcated islands of tumor cells (Fig. 5-23).[163] Almost all cases express an *EWS-WT1* fusion oncogene[164,165] resulting from translocation between the chromosome 11 short arm and chromosome 22 long arm.[166,167] The EWS-WT1 oncoproteins are expressed as several isoforms (see Fig. 5-10), each of which is composed of the EWS amino-terminal transactivation region fused to the last three

of four zinc fingers at the WT1 carboxyl-terminal end.[168,169] These oncoproteins result from fusion of *EWS* exon 7, 8, or 9 to *WT1* exon 8. Quantitatively minor secondary transcripts lacking exon 6 of *EWS* and/or exon 9 of *WT1* are also expressed, although the functional relevance of these transcripts is unknown.[168] The *EWS-WT1* fusion results in expression of the C-terminal but not N-terminal aspect of WT1 in DSRCT, which may be detected by immunohistochemistry using appropriate antibodies (see Fig. 5-23). The EWS-WT1 oncoprotein retains an alternative splicing site (±KTS) between the third and fourth WT1 zinc fingers (see Fig. 5-10). The KTS− isoform regulates genes that are thought to have important biologic roles in DSRCTs, including platelet-derived growth factor alpha (PDGFA) and insulin-like growth factor receptor I (IGFR-I), whereas the KTS+ isoform regulates a different set of genes.[170] Notably, only the KTS− isoform has shown transforming activity when evaluated in vitro.[171] PDGFA is known to activate potent receptor (platelet-derived growth factor receptor [PDGFR])–mediated mitogenic signaling pathways in fibroblasts,[172] and EWS-WT1 might therefore induce desmoplastic proliferation via PDGFA transcriptional upregulation.[169]

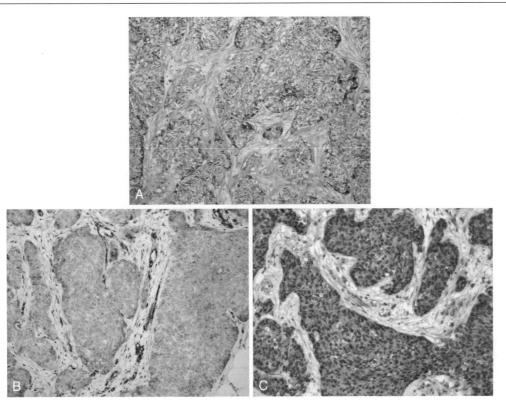

FIGURE 5-23. A, Desmoplastic small round cell tumor with sharply demarcated islands of blue tumor cells separated by pink densely fibrotic "desmoplastic" stroma. Immunoreactivities with antibodies to N-terminal **(B)** and C-terminal **(C)** regions of WT1 are negative and strongly positive, respectively, in the tumor cells, in keeping with EWS-WT1 fusion oncoprotein expression.

Dermatofibrosarcoma Protuberans

DFSP is a low-grade spindle cell tumor, which can occasionally progress to a more aggressive fibrosarcomatous phase. Most DFSPs contain ring chromosomes composed of sequences from chromosomes 17 and 22 (see Fig. 5-13A).[173,174] The ring chromosomes contain multiple copies of a fusion gene, *COL1A1-PDGFB*, in which *COL1A1* (a collagen gene) is contributed from chromosome 17 and *PDGFB* (platelet-derived growth factor beta gene) from chromosome 22.[70,95] Alternatively, DFSP, particularly in pediatric patients, occasionally has t(17;22) translocations, resulting in a single copy of the *COL1A1-PDGFB* fusion gene.[175] The *COL1A1-PDGFB* oncogene results in overexpression of PDGFB, which is a growth factor that activates platelet-derived growth factor receptor beta (PDGFRB) and PDGFRA. This cytogenetic observation has suggested that patients with inoperable DFSP might benefit from treatment with PDGFR inhibitors such as imatinib, and this hypothesis has been confirmed by impressive clinical responses to PDGFRB therapeutic inhibition with imatinib.[176-179] *COL1A1-PDGFB* oncogenic fusion is also seen in giant cell fibroblastoma (GCF), a pediatric neoplasm closely related to DFSP.[96,180] Studies of GCF and composite GCF-DFSP cases have shown the presence of a single translocation t(17;22), and the resultant *COL1A1-PDGFB* fusion, in the GCF component, with acquisition of additional copies of the oncogene being associated with progression to DFSP.[69]

Desmoid Tumors

Desmoid tumors, also known as deep fibromatoses, contain various genetic aberrations, including the *APC* (adenomatous polyposis coli) gene or beta-catenin mutations,[181,182] and triso-mies for chromosomes 8 or 20.[183] Cytogenetic deletions of the chromosome 5 long arm are seen in occasional desmoids, resulting in loss of the *APC* tumor suppressor gene.[184,185] However, the most common mutations, particularly in nonfamilial desmoid tumors, are activating beta-catenin mutations, which are found in at least 50% of cases.[181,182] Both *APC* inactivating and beta-catenin activating mutations result in stabilization and resultant overexpression, of the beta-catenin protein. The cytogenetic aberrations in most desmoid tumors, particularly the trisomies 8 and 20, are mechanisms of progression, and are acquired subsequent to the *APC* or beta-catenin mutations.

Infantile Fibrosarcoma

Infantile fibrosarcomas characteristically present within the first year of life. These are tumors composed of plump fibroblast-like cells (see Fig. 5-16), which often show high mitotic activity, and featuring trisomies of chromosomes 8, 11, 17, and 20.[186] This same group of trisomies occur in the histologically identical pediatric renal tumor, congenital cellular mesoblastic nephroma (see Fig. 5-18).[187] Most infantile fibrosarcomas and congenital cellular mesoblastic nephromas also contain a diagnostic chromosomal translocation, t(12;15)(p13;q26), which is cryptic when studied by traditional cytogenetic banding methods (see Fig. 5-2).[6,89,188] t(12;15)(p13;q26) results in fusion of the *TEL* gene on chromosome 12 to the *NTRK3* receptor tyrosine kinase gene on chromosome 15, producing constitutive tyrosine kinase activation. Although challenging to detect by banding methods, the t(12;15) translocation is demonstrated readily by FISH with a dual-color break-apart TEL probe (see Fig. 5-2) or RT-PCR.[6,89,188]

Inflammatory Myofibroblastic Tumor

Inflammatory myofibroblastic tumors, belonging to the group of inflammatory pseudotumors, are relatively rare tumors occurring primarily in children and young adults. They are composed of myofibroblastic cells admixed with an infiltrate of lymphocytes and plasma cells (see Fig. 5-17). The inflammatory component of these tumors is non-neoplastic, and therefore lacks cytogenetic aberrations, whereas the myofibroblastic cells often contain clonal chromosomal aberrations[189-191] involving rearrangement and oncogenic activation of the *ALK* receptor tyrosine kinase gene at chromosome band 2p23.[90] The *ALK* oncogenes cause constitutive activation of the ALK kinase by enhanced oligomerization resulting from fusion of the ALK kinase domain to the oligomerization domain of the partner gene.[90] *ALK* oncogenic activation is associated with strong, immunohistochemically detectable ALK expression in the IMT spindle cells (see Fig. 5-17).[90] The ALK immunohistochemical staining pattern reflects the fusion type, insofar as fusion of ALK with most of the various partners (TPM3, TPM4, CARS, CLTC, ALO17) produces cytoplasmic staining, whereas ALK-RANBP2 fusion produces nuclear membrane–associated reactivity.[192,193] These immunohistochemical findings can distinguish IMT from its histologic mimics, and demonstration of *ALK* rearrangement can further confirm the diagnosis.

Gastrointestinal Stromal Tumors

Most adult gastrointestinal stromal tumors (GISTs) contain activating mutations of the *KIT* or *PDGFRA* oncogenes.[194-196] These mutations have been targeted with spectacular success using the KIT and PDGFRA inhibitor imatinib (Gleevec).[197,198] In addition, germline (inherited) KIT mutations are responsible for rare syndromes of familial, multifocal, gastrointestinal stromal tumors.[199] However, most pediatric GISTs do not contain *KIT* or *PDGFRA* mutations,[200-202] and pediatric GISTs lack the typical sequential cytogenetic deletions that seem to drive genetic and clinical progression in adult GISTs.[203] Given these biologic differences, it is unclear at this time whether children with metastatic GISTs will benefit from the KIT-PDGFRA kinase inhibitor therapies that have been so successful in adults.

Malignant Peripheral Nerve Sheath Tumors

Benign and malignant peripheral nerve sheath tumors are frequent complications in patients with hereditary neurofibromatosis (NF) syndromes. The NF syndromes are the most common tumor predisposition syndromes, affecting 1 in 3500 individuals worldwide. Neurofibromas and malignant peripheral nerve sheath tumors are common in those with neurofibromatosis type 1, whereas benign schwannomas are common in neurofibromatosis type 2 (central neurofibromatosis). Characterization of the neurofibromatosis syndrome genes has shed substantial light on the pathogenesis of peripheral nerve sheath tumors. The neurofibromatosis type 1 (*NF1*) and type 2 (*NF2*) genes are located on chromosomes 17 and 22, respectively, and both these genes encode tumor suppressor proteins that normally constrain cellular proliferation.[204-209] NF1 protein tumor suppressor mechanisms involve regulation of RAS GTPase activity,[205,206] with *NF1* gene deletion therefore resulting in constitutive RAS activation, suggesting that therapeutics targeting RAS (or downstream signaling intermediates such as RAF and MEK-MAPK) might be useful for clinical management of malignant peripheral nerve sheath tumors (MPNST) and other NF1-associated cancers.[210] MPNST often have *NF1* gene deletions, which can be demonstrated by FISH assay. The *NF1*

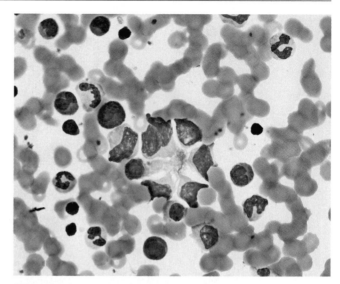

FIGURE 5-24. Bone marrow involvement by disseminated neuroblastoma, showing a classic rosette of tumor cells, with bluish cytoplasm and neuropil. (Courtesy of Marybeth Helfrich, Children's Hospital of Philadelphia.)

gene aberrations are accompanied by a generally complex karyotype, suggesting that genetic instability plays a prominent role in the development of MPNST. Notably, *NF1* gene deletions can also be shown in only the Schwann cell component of neurofibromas.[211] This observation supports the view that neurofibromas are clonal Schwann cell neoplasms, whereas the other admixed cell lineages—including fibroblasts, mast cells, and perineural cells—are reactive.

Neuroblastoma

Most neuroblastomas have distinctive cytogenetic features that correlate with their clinical behavior. Favorable prognosis neuroblastomas, which respond well to chemotherapy and can even undergo spontaneous regression, generally feature near-triploid karyotypes without 1p deletion or *MYCN* (*N-myc*) amplification.[212] Unfavorable prognosis neuroblastomas (Fig. 5-24), by contrast, feature near-diploid or near-tetraploid karyotypes, often accompanied by 1p deletion, 17q amplification, and/or *MYCN* amplification,[213] whereas deletions of 3p and 11q are reportedly predictive of metastasis.[214] *MYCN* amplification, typically manifested as double-minute chromosomes (see Figs. 5-5 and 5-6), is arguably the most ominous of the adverse genetic markers. Children with *MYCN*-amplified neuroblastomas are rarely curable, although complete remission can be achieved through intensive myeloablative chemotherapy. Therefore, genetic parameters can be useful adjuncts for determining appropriate intensity of therapy, particularly for those children whose prognoses are not clear based on clinical parameters alone.[213] Cytogenetic analysis of neuroblastoma has been difficult, however, because the tumor cells from most favorable prognosis neuroblastomas fail to divide in culture.[213] *MYCN* amplification and chromosome 1p deletion can be demonstrated in interphase cells by FISH or CISH (see Fig. 5-6), obviating the need for tumor cell culture.[215,216] It remains unclear whether one or more conventional tumor suppressor genes are targeted by the 1p deletions found in most poor-prognosis neuroblastomas. However, several microRNAs in the critical 1p deletion region function to maintain neuroblastoma survival and activate *MYCN* transcription.[217,218] Recently, *ALK* kinase domain mutations and

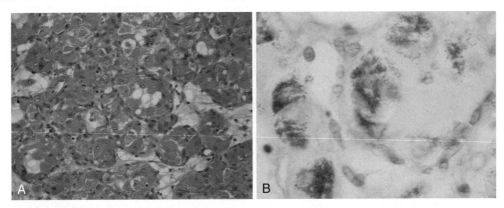

FIGURE 5-25. Characteristic histologic features of alveolar soft part sarcoma include an alveolar-like arrangement of cells with abundant deeply eosinophilic cytoplasm **(A)** and diastase-resistant, periodic acid–Schiff–positive intracytoplasmic crystals **(B)**.

gene amplifications have been demonstrated in hereditary and sporadic neuroblastoma,[92a-c] suggesting that ALK inhibitors might be useful therapeutically in neuroblastoma.

Rhabdoid Tumor

Malignant rhabdoid tumors generally are remarkably aggressive neoplasms clinically and most cases, whether arising in soft tissues, kidney, or CNS, have deletions of the chromosome 22 long arm, targeting the *INI1* tumor suppressor gene. *INI1* (also known as *SNF5*, or *SMARCB1*) encodes a member of the SWI-SNF protein complex involved in chromatin remodeling.[219,220] Chromosome 22 deletion is often the only detectable cytogenetic aberration in rhabdoid tumors, suggesting that *INI1* inactivation is an early event in rhabdoid tumorigenesis.[221,222] Additional evidence of an essential tumorigenic role includes the finding of germline *INI1* mutations in some individuals with rhabdoid tumors[220,223,224] and the development of rhabdoid tumor models in mice with inactivating INI1 mutations.[225] Notably, germline *INI1* mutations are not restricted to rhabdoid tumors, but have been implicated also in familial schwannomatosis[226] and in various nonrhabdoid CNS tumors, including choroid plexus carcinoma and medulloblastoma.[223] INI1 loss of function has been reported to predispose to chromatin instability and leads to polyploidization in malignant rhabdoid tumor cells,[227] but it is unclear if such perturbations are highly relevant in rhabdoid tumors, which generally lack polyploidization.[221] INI1 inhibits cyclin D1 expression by recruiting a histone deacetylase 1 complex to the *CCND1* (cyclin D1) promoter, resulting in G1 cell cycle arrest.[228] The relevance of cyclin D1 in *INI1*-mediated tumorigenesis is underscored by the observation that rhabdoid tumors develop in INI1 +/− mice expressing cyclin D1, whereas INI1 +/− mice with cyclin D1 deficiency (cyclin D1−/−) do not develop rhabdoid tumors.[229] These observations suggest that drugs targeting cyclin D1 might be relevant for rhabdoid tumors.[230]

Rhabdoid tumors are characteristically composed of cells with vesicular nuclei and prominent nucleoli, with the nuclei often being pushed to an eccentric location within the cell by dense intracytoplasmic condensation inclusion (see Fig. 5-9), which, as seen by electron microscopy, consists of a tightly arranged whorl of intermediate filaments. These filaments stain nonspecifically for various markers, giving the tumor a polyphenotypic appearance. Absence of INI1 expression in the tumor cells but not the normal stromal support nuclei, as is readily demonstrable by immunohistochemistry, is useful for diagnosing rhabdoid tumor (see Fig. 5-9).[31,231]

Alveolar Soft Part Sarcoma

Alveolar soft part sarcoma is a rare tumor, occurring mostly in the young, with a predilection for involvement of soft tissues in the head and neck region. However, other soft tissue and even hollow viscera may be involved. Characterized by a distinctive morphology, with nested or alveolar-like growth, the tumor cells are epithelioid, with abundant clear to eosinophilic cytoplasm, sharply defined cellular borders, and diastase-resistant, periodic acid–Schiff (PAS)–positive intracytoplasmic crystals (Fig. 5-25), which on electron microscopic examination are rhomboidal. Alveolar soft part sarcomas generally exhibit indolent behavior, but nonetheless have a high risk for late metastases and no histologic features to predict clinical behavior. The classic cytogenetic feature of ASPS is translocation t(X;17)(p11;q25), producing fusion of the *ASPL* and *TFE3* genes.[232] This same translocation is seen in a subset of pediatric renal cell carcinomas. Antibody raised to the C-terminus of TFE3 produces strong nuclear reactivity in *ASPL-TFE3* fusion-positive tumors.[233]

Epithelial Neoplasms

Renal Tumors

Most pediatric renal tumors contain characteristic cytogenetic aberrations. Deletion of 11p is a well-known aberration in Wilms' tumor, but several other aberrations, including extra copies of chromosome 12, are more frequent and have apparent prognostic relevance, as does LOH of 1p and 16q.[234,235] Another pediatric renal tumor with consistent cytogenetic aberrations is congenital cellular mesoblastic nephroma, in which various chromosomal trisomies and oncogenic fusion of the TEL and NTRK3 proteins are observed reliably.[6,188]

Pediatric Renal Cell Carcinomas with Xp11 or 6p21 Translocations

Pediatric renal cell carcinomas are uncommon and they generally have a papillary morphology, accompanied by translocations involving chromosomes X or 6.[236] By comparison, adult papillary renal cancers typically have a distinctive profile of chromosomal trisomies, although a rare few contain the same translocations seen in pediatric renal cancers. The unifying theme for the pediatric carcinoma translocations is that they target various members of the MiT family of transcription factors. The most frequent translocation is

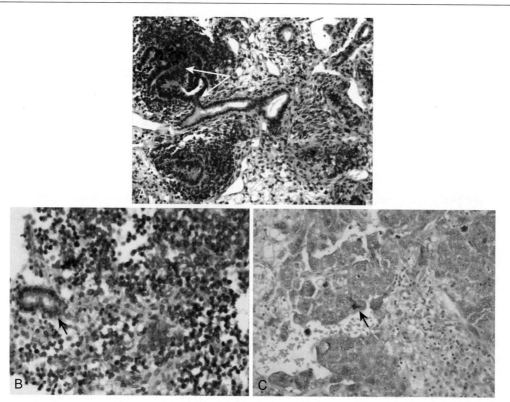

FIGURE 5-26. A, Wilms' tumor with triphasic histology. The tumor recapitulates nephrogenesis with condensation of mesenchyme at tips of tubular branch-points. Here, the blastema is condensed around a focus of tubular differentiation (*arrows*). **B,** High-power image showing undifferentiated blastema, which in the absence of obvious tubular differentiation (*arrow*) might be difficult to distinguish from other undifferentiated small round cell tumors. **C,** Anaplastic Wilms' tumor with bizarre mitoses and massively enlarged hyperchromatic nuclei (*arrow*).

t(X;1)(p11;q21), resulting in fusion of *PRCC* (at chromosome band 1q21) and the MiT family member *TFE3* (at chromosome band Xp11). There are variants of this translocation, including t(X;17)(p11;q25), in which *TFE3* is fused with the *ASPL* gene at chromosome band 17q25.[237] An apparently childhood-restricted translocation, t(6;11)(p21;q13), fuses the MiT family member *TFEB* (at chromosome band 6p21) with the Alpha gene (at chromosome band 11q13).[238]

Wilms' Tumor

Wilms' tumors are the most common type of renal cancer in children. They typically contain primitive blastemal cells that differentiate into tubular epithelial, glomerular and/or mesenchymal populations. The classic triphasic Wilms' tumor contains an admixture of blastemal, epithelial, and mesenchymal components (Fig. 5-26), and all three cell types may contain the same clonal chromosomal aberrations.[239] Various genetic alterations are found in subsets of Wilms' tumors, including trisomies 6, 8, 12, and 18, and deletions of 11p13 (see later). Deletions of 11p15, 1p, and 16q bode ill in patients with low-stage favorable histology tumors and 1q gains are associated with relapse (see Table 5-2).[235,240-242]

Deletion 11p13 is the most extensively characterized cytogenetic aberration in Wilms' tumors. This aberration became the focus of many studies after reports that individuals with the WAGR syndrome often had constitutional deletions at chromosome band 11p13. The Wilms' tumor suppressor gene (*WT1*) is deleted in WAGR syndrome, and this has been cloned and characterized.[243] It appears to play a critical role in urogenital development.[243,244] However, the WAGR phenotype results from deletions of several genes, with the *WT1* gene deletion responsible for predisposition to Wilms' tumors, and deletion

of a neighboring gene, *PAX6*, responsible for aniridia.[245] Although most or all WAGR-associated Wilms' tumors have complete inactivation of *WT1*, such inactivation is found in fewer than 20% of sporadic Wilms' tumors. Approximately 7% to 30% of Wilms' tumors have deletion of the *WTX* gene, which notably is the first putative tumor suppressor gene identified on chromosome X.[246-248] *WTX* deletions result from deletion of the corresponding region on the single copy of chromosome X in males, although there is controversy as to whether the deletion in females invariably involves the active copy of chromosome X.[249,250] There is also controversy as to whether *WT1* and *WTX* mutations are mutually exclusive in Wilms' tumors.[251,252] The WTX protein promotes beta-catenin ubiquitination and degradation,[253] and it is therefore expected that *WTX* gene deletions in Wilms' tumors would hyperactivate WNT–beta-catenin signaling pathways. This concept is in keeping with the finding of beta-catenin activating oncogenic mutations in a subset of Wilms' tumors that lack *WTX* mutations.[254-257]

Various cytogenetic findings are associated with anaplastic histology in Wilms' tumor. Complex karyotypes with chromosome counts in the triploid to tetraploid range are generally found in tumors with diffuse or focal anaplasia.[258] Similarly, Wilms' tumors with p53 tumor suppressor gene mutations generally show anaplasia (see Fig. 5-26),[259] a finding linked more with therapy resistance than to a more biologically aggressive phenotype per se.

Mesoblastic Nephroma

Mesoblastic nephromas are the most common renal tumors diagnosed in infancy, but may rarely also be encountered in older children. Histologically, mesoblastic nephroma falls into

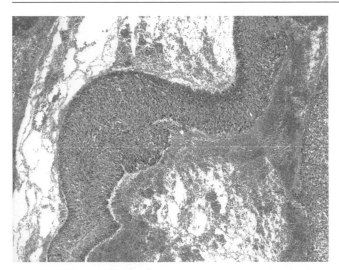

FIGURE 5-27. Cellular congenital mesoblastic nephroma with prominent blood lakes.

two categories; those tumors composed of bland, benign-appearing spindle cells, essentially recapitulating the morphology of fibromatosis, are known as classic mesoblastic nephroma,[260] whereas those with greater cellularity, sometimes in a fascicular arrangement with plump nuclei and with less cytoplasm, more mitoses, blood lakes, and often zonal necrosis, are known as cellular mesoblastic nephroma (Fig. 5-27; see Fig. 5-16).[261] Trisomy 11 is a consistent cytogenetic aberration in mesoblastic nephromas, but is found only in the cellular group.[187,262] Approximately 70% of cellular mesoblastic nephromas contain trisomy 11, often accompanied by trisomies for chromosomes 8 and 17.[187] By contrast, clonal chromosomal aberrations have not been identified in classic mesoblastic nephroma. These findings suggest that trisomy 11, with or without other clonal chromosomal aberrations, is associated with progression from classic to cellular histology in mesoblastic nephroma.[187] Mesoblastic nephromas with trisomy 11 generally also contain a balanced translocation t(12;15)(p13;q26), resulting in oncogenic fusion of the *TEL* and *NTRK3* genes. The t(12;15)(p13;q26) is cryptic by cytogenetic evaluation using chromosomal banding, but is readily demonstrable by FISH or RT-PCR (see Fig. 5-2). These cytogenetic associations have been useful diagnostically, because Wilms' tumors (the entity most likely confused with mesoblastic nephroma on small biopsy when blastema only has been sampled) rarely have trisomy 11, and have not been found to bear t(12;15).[240,241]

NUT Midline Carcinomas

Based on initial case reports, NUT midline carcinoma was considered a malignancy of children and adolescents arising in midline structures, especially upper aerodigestive tract and thymus.[86,263,264] Midline origin below the diaphragm is now well recognized, and the entity may also present in adulthood.[265,266] With the exception of an isolated atypical case,[267] all reported patients have died of disease or treatment complications within months of diagnosis. The histologic appearance is variable, typically including undifferentiated cells but often accompanied by immunohistochemical evidence of epithelial differentiation and, in some cases, with histologically convincing squamous differentiation (see Fig. 5-15). This entity was initially defined by the midline location, undifferentiated carcinoma-like histology, highly lethal course, and characteristic cytogenetic feature of translocation t(15;19) (see Fig. 5-1). The t(15;19) results in oncogenic fusion of the *BRD4* (bromodomain-containing) and

NUT genes on chromosomes 19 and 15, respectively, encoding a BRD4-NUT fusion oncoprotein. A subset of NUT midline carcinomas features similar oncogenic mechanisms in which NUT is fused with BRD3, or with yet unidentified translocation partners.[265] Diagnosis can be confirmed by karyotypic demonstration of the translocation t(15;19), molecular cytogenetic demonstration of *NUT* gene rearrangement, or RT-PCR demonstration of *BRD4-NUT* or *BRD3-NUT* fusion oncogenes.[265,266,268] The oncogenic function of BRD3-4–NUT oncoproteins is not yet well understood and the normal function of NUT is unknown. Interestingly, however, the NUT fusion oncoproteins do appear to block squamous differentiation in epithelial cell precursors.[268]

Thyroid Carcinomas

Thyroid malignancies include medullary carcinoma, which may be sporadic, or familial in the setting of multiple endocrine neoplasia type IIA (MEN-IIA) and MEN-IIB with germline *RET* tyrosine kinase gene mutations. Papillary thyroid carcinomas may also be sporadic, but are encountered with greatly increased frequency in individuals exposed to radiation, including adults post–external beam irradiation, and children exposed to radioactive fallout, as in the Chernobyl disaster. Regardless of the patient's age or exposure to radiation, papillary carcinomas can feature chromosomal rearrangements resulting in oncogenic *RET* fusions.[67,269] *BRAF* mutations, on the other hand, although found in many adult papillary thyroid carcinomas, are uncommon in childhood thyroid carcinomas.[270,271] Follicular thyroid carcinomas are uncommon, but are associated with a diagnostic translocation t(2;3), resulting in oncogenic fusion of the *PAX8* and *PPARγ* genes (see Fig. 5-14).[85]

Blastomas

The central tumorigenic role of RB1 inactivation in retinoblastoma has served as a paradigm for tumor suppressor genes in oncology, but little is known of the other genetic mechanisms responsible for tumor progression in this disease. Similarly, the molecular underpinnings of hepatoblastoma, pancreatoblastoma, and pleuropulmonary blastoma are only poorly understood. Trisomies of chromosomes 2 and 8 are found in many hepatoblastomas and pleuropulmonary blastomas,[272-274] but the genes targeted by these trisomies have not been identified.

CNS Tumors

Distinctive cytogenetic aberrations are found in many of the major subtypes of brain tumors, but karyotyping of brain tumors is not performed routinely in most cytogenetic laboratories. This is partly because many brain tumors do not grow well in tissue culture, particularly when the biopsy material is limited in size or viability. In addition, some of the clinically relevant cytogenetic aberrations are amenable to evaluation by FISH, which can be performed in frozen or paraffin-embedded material once the histologic diagnosis has been established. Examples include the 1p and 19q deletions in oligodendroglioma, the presence of which portends a favorable response to multiagent chemotherapy regimens, at least in adult patients, although the evidence is less than convincing in the pediatric population.[275,276] Other response predictors have been identified in oligodendroglioma. These include amplification of *EGFR* (epidermal growth factor receptor) at 7p12 and homozygous deletion of *CDKN2A* at 9p21, which correlate with poor response to chemotherapy and reduced survival.[275] ErbB2 and

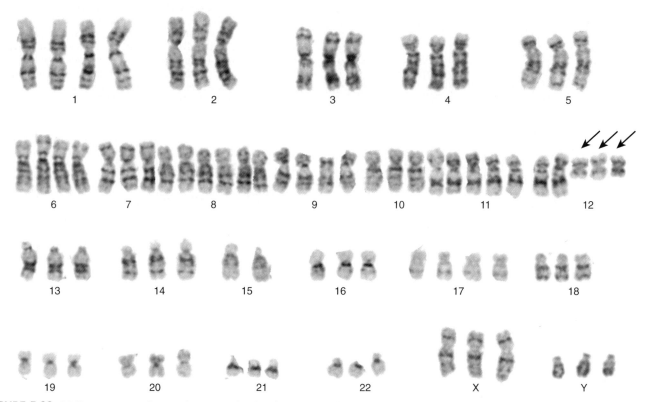

FIGURE 5-28. Malignant germ cell tumor karyotype showing three copies of the pathognomonic isochromosome 12p (*arrows*).

4 amplification observed in ependymomas promises potential therapeutic targetability,[277] and *EGFR* amplification in high-grade gliomas similarly calls for investigation of its role as a molecular therapeutic target in that tumor.[278]

Germ Cell Tumors

Many germ cell tumors contain a diagnostic cytogenetic marker, isochromosome 12p, often found in the context of a moderately complex karyotype, among other clonal chromosomal aberrations (Fig. 5-28).[279] Isochromosome 12p results from duplication of the chromosome 12 short arm on either side of the centromere, and is uncommon in carcinomas and sarcomas.[280] Therefore, demonstration of isochromosome 12p, particularly in any poorly differentiated cancer, should provoke strong suspicion of a germ cell origin.

Hematologic Neoplasms

Hodgkin's Lymphoma

Hodgkin's disease (HD), first described by Thomas Hodgkin in 1832, remained a poorly understood disease for over a century and a half, largely because of the sparse nature of neoplastic cells (typically less than 1%) within the tumor mass, even raising occasional doubt as to the neoplastic nature of the entity. This sparseness of malignant cells, combined with their poor proliferative index, confounded attempts to investigate the molecular basis of HD. Karyotypic evaluations have been challenging, but nonetheless yielded early insights into the nature of HD. The capacity to grow Hodgkin's cells continuously in vitro and the fact that injection of these cells into athymic nude

mice produced tumors supported a neoplastic nature,[281] as did the aneuploid karyotypes demonstrated in Hodgkin's lymphoma (HL) cell cultures.[282]

Light microscopic examination has permitted morphologic assignment of HL into classic and nodular lymphocyte–predominance subtypes,[283-285] a categorization recognized by the World Health Organization (WHO); this provided an attempt at cell of origin classification. The nodular lymphocyte-predominant subtype features a lymphocyte and histiocyte (L&H) neoplastic cell population, also known as popcorn cells (Fig. 5-29), with B-cell immunophenotype—expressing CD45, CD20, and Bcl-6 but lacking CD15 and CD30—whereas classic Hodgkin's–Reed-Sternberg (H-RS) cells show only equivocal expression of the pan B-cell marker CD20 and lack CD45 reactivity but express CD15 and CD30 in a membrane and Golgi staining pattern (Fig. 5-30).[286,287] Classic HL is subclassified into nodular sclerosis, mixed cellularity, lymphocyte-depleted, and lymphocyte-rich variants, depending on the composition of the background non-neoplastic elements in the tumor. The lack of any obvious physiologic counterpart, together with its otherwise noncommittal immunophenotype, initiated a search to reveal the true nature of the H-RS cell, and molecular studies have assisted substantially in these efforts (see later).

Substantial insights into HL pathogenesis have come from single-cell studies showing that L&H and the vast majority of H-RS cells are B cells and clonal in nature.[288] These neoplastic H-RS cells seem to be of germinal center B-cell derivation,[289] with 96% featuring clonal immunoglobulin (Ig) rearrangements but lacking Ig gene transcripts because of defects in Ig gene regulatory elements. These findings apply in both Epstein-Barr virus (EBV)–associated and EBV-unassociated HL.[290] L&H cells express BCL6, in keeping with a germinal center differentiation stage, whereas H-RS cells express CD138 (syndecan),

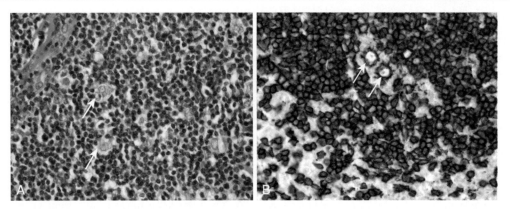

FIGURE 5-29. Nodular lymphocyte–predominance Hodgkin's lymphoma featuring lymphocyte and histiocyte popcorn neoplastic cells (**A,** *arrows*) among small reactive lymphocytic infiltrate, and with immunohistochemical reactivity for the CD20 pan-B marker in both reactive and neoplastic cells (*arrows*) (**B**).

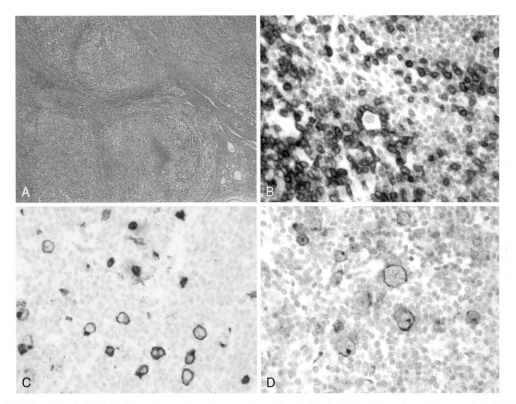

FIGURE 5-30. Nodular sclerosis Hodgkin's lymphoma showing prominent fibrotic bands (**A**) and rimming of characteristic Reed-Sternberg cells by CD57-positive lymphocytes (**B**). The Reed-Sternberg elements show cell membrane and Golgi expression of CD15 (**C**) and CD30 (**D**).

more in keeping with a post–germinal center differentiation stage.[291] Single-cell studies of H-RS cells have shown clonal Ig gene rearrangements supporting a B-cell phenotype in 95% of cases. Even the 15% of HL with H-RS cells expressing T-cell markers generally contain clonal Ig gene rearrangements and, overall, only 1% to 2% of cHL cases have clonal T-cell receptor gene rearrangements.[292-295] Thus, T-cell marker expression is generally considered aberrant in H-RS cells.

Both classic and nodular lymphocyte-predominance HL (NLPHL) are characterized by chromosomal instability, which is manifest by extremely complex cytogenetic aberrations in the neoplastic cells.[296] Molecular cytogenetic studies typically demonstrate chromosomal aberrations in the hyperdiploid range.[297]

Nodular Lymphocyte-Predominance Hodgkin's Lymphoma

The observation that NLPHL corresponds to germinal center stage B-cell differentiation is in keeping with the finding of recurrent IGH-BCL6 fusions, resulting from translocation t(3;14)(q27;q32).[298] HL karyotyping evaluations have not revealed IGH region 14q32 rearrangements in NLPHL; these aberrations are undoubtedly being masked by the overall complexity of the HL karyotypes, with the recurring t(3;14) being cytogenetically cryptic.[299] However, molecular cytogenetic studies have demonstrated BCL6 rearrangements in almost 50% of NLPHL.[298,300-302] Comparative genomic hybridization (CGH) analyses in NLPHL have underscored the genomic complexity of these tumors, with frequent copy number gains involving chromosomes 1, 2q, 3, 4q, 5q, 6, 8q, 11q, 12q, and X and copy number losses for chromosome 17.[303] The copy number gains involving 2q, 4q, 5q, 6, and 11q are otherwise uncommon in hematologic neoplasia, and therefore might signify genomic aberrations of unique importance in the pathogenesis of NLPHL.

Classic Hodgkin's Lymphoma

In classic HL, gains of 2p and 9p are identified in 30% to 50% of cases and 12q aberrations are also noted.[304] FISH studies have confirmed that the aberrations involve the locus of the JAK2 gene at 9p23-24[305] and MDM2 at 12q14-15.[306,307] The 2p copy number gains, which involve the REL gene (encoding one of the five subunits of nuclear factor κB [NF-κB]), might contribute to constitutive NF-κB activation, which is a hallmark of HL.[308]

Evaluations of Ig gene aberrations in classic HL have demonstrated IgH, IgL, and IgK rearrangements in 17%, 3%, and 1% of cases, respectively.[309] These rearrangements juxtaposed the Ig loci with genes at 2p16 (REL), 3q27 (BCL6), 8q24 (MYC), 14q24, 16p13.1, 17q12, and 19q13.2 (BCL3-RELB). IGH-BCL6 fusions were found in 4 of 70 cases, although a previous study had not shown such events in 40 cases of nodular sclerosis and mixed cellularity classic HL.[302] Translocation t(14;18), resulting in the typical IGH-BCL2 fusion, has been reported in one case of follicular lymphoma evolving into Hodgkin's lymphoma.[310]

Non-Hodgkin's Lymphoma

Non-Hodgkin's lymphomas (NHL) account for 7% to 10% of all pediatric malignancies. Cytogenetic and molecular genetic aberrations have been studied extensively in adult NHL, but there have been few comparable studies in pediatric NHL, with the exception of well-characterized MYC gene rearrangements in Burkitt's lymphomas. Most pediatric NHLs belong to one of four overall categories: Burkitt's (40%); lymphoblastic (30%); large B-cell (20%); and anaplastic large cell (10%). Cytogenetic hallmarks include MYC rearrangements in Burkitt's lymphomas, 14q11 rearrangements in T-cell lymphoblastic leukemia and lymphomas, and ALK rearrangements in anaplastic large cell lymphomas.[311] The proposed WHO classification of lymphoid neoplasms incorporates the REAL classification, which takes into account morphologic, immunophenotype, genetic, and clinical features. Notably, there can be marked differences in molecular mechanisms and clinical response when comparing pediatric with adult forms of the same NHL subtype. For example, adult large B-cell lymphomas are heterogeneous entities, many of which have a phenotype suggesting follicular center cell origin and containing IGH region translocations that upregulate the BCL2 or BCL6 genes. Pediatric large B-cell lymphomas, by contrast, generally have gene expression and immunophenotypic features of germinal center cell origin and lack IGH-BCL2 rearrangements, but have a better prognosis than adult cases.[312] Lymphoblastic lymphomas are on a biologic continuum with ALL, and the biology of this subtype is discussed in the Acute Lymphoblastic Leukemia section (see later).

Burkitt's Lymphoma

The cytogenetic underpinnings of Burkitt's lymphoma were first reported in 1972, when Manolov and Manolova described aberrations of the chromosome 14 long arm[313]; these were later shown to represent t(8;14)(q24;q32) translocation, resulting in rearrangement of the IGH gene with the chromosome 8q MYC oncogene region.[14,314] IGH-MYC rearrangements are found in approximately 80% of Burkitt's lymphomas, irrespective of whether the tumors are EBV-positive or EBV-negative, and whether they are sporadic or arise in an endemic region.[315] However, IGH-MYC rearrangement can be found rarely in diffuse large cell lymphomas, so this cytogenetic aberration is not diagnostic of Burkitt's lymphoma. Alternative cytogenetic mechanisms dysregulate MYC transcription by juxtaposing MYC with the kappa or lambda immunoglobulin gene loci.[316] The kappa and lambda Ig rearrangements result from t(2;8) and t(8;22) translocations, which are found in 5% and 15% of Burkitt's lymphomas, respectively.

Burkitt's lymphoma has a characteristic cytomorphologic appearance in which the cells are squared off from each other. A starry sky appearance results from engulfment of cellular apoptotic debris by interspersed macrophages, whereas the actual neoplastic cells have relatively uniform intermediate-sized nuclei and exhibit at least a 99% proliferative index, as demonstrated by immunostaining for Ki-67 (Fig. 5-31). MYC region genomic breakpoints vary between the endemic and sporadic types of Burkitt's lymphoma. The breakpoints in endemic Burkitt's lymphomas can be as much as 300 kb upstream or downstream of the MYC coding sequences, whereas those in sporadic Burkitt's lymphomas typically involve the first exon or first intron of MYC.[316] Despite this considerable variability in genomic breakpoint location, all the rearrangements serve the purpose of dysregulating MYC expression and can be detected by a simple dual-color MYC break-apart FISH assay, in which the probe components are more than 300 kb upstream and downstream of MYC, thereby flanking most MYC region translocation breakpoints (Fig. 5-32). Secondary cytogenetic aberrations occur in conjunction with MYC translocations in some Burkitt's lymphomas. Several of these, particularly 1q duplication and 13q deletion, may be associated with worse prognosis, although the numbers of patients studied have been few.[317]

Follicular Lymphoma

Follicular lymphoma is uncommon in childhood. When diagnosed, it more commonly affects boys and presents with localized disease in lymph nodes or tonsils. Such cases generally lack BCL2 rearrangement and BCL2 expression.[318]

Diffuse Large B-Cell Lymphoma

Diffuse large B-cell lymphomas may be categorized into germinal center, activated B-cell–like, or primary mediastinal types. In children, diffuse large B-cell lymphomas are frequently of the germinal center type, and associated with an overal better prognosis than for adults. Despite the germinal center phenotype, however, diffuse large B-cell lymphomas in children generally lack the t(14;18) seen in a proportion of adult cases of this subtype.[312]

Anaplastic Large Cell Lymphoma

ALCLs are predominantly mature T-cell disorders with excellent prognosis in the pediatric population.[319] ALCL is a diagnostic pitfall for the pathologist, although the morphology is uniquely different from all other hematopoietic malignancies. The cells often appear relatively cohesive and have abundant cytoplasm, so they may mimic an epithelial neoplasm more so than suggesting a lymphoid one; ALCLs, furthermore, classically express epithelial membrane antigen (Fig. 5-33). The cells typically react for CD30 and often also express the anaplastic lymphoma kinase (ALK) receptor tyrosine kinase protein (see Fig. 5-33), which is constitutively activated by oncogenic

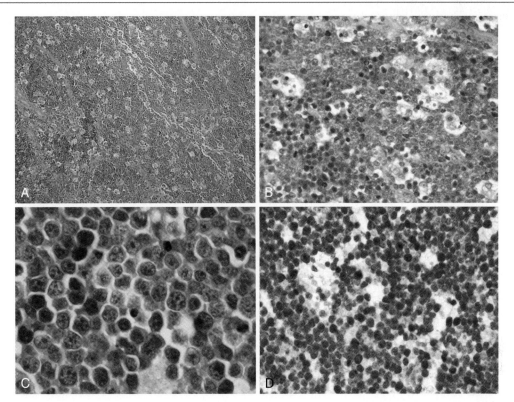

FIGURE 5-31. Burkitt's lymphoma low-power **(A)** and intermediate-power **(B)** views show starry sky appearance resulting from engulfment of cellular apoptotic debris by interspersed macrophages; higher power view shows typical squaring off of cells from one another **(C)**. The Ki-67 proliferation marker is expressed strongly by almost 100% of the lymphoma cells **(D)**.

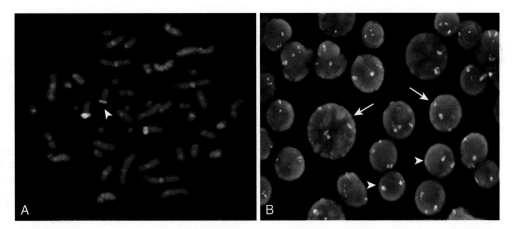

FIGURE 5-32. Burkitt's lymphoma fluorescence in situ hybridization (FISH) using *MYC* break-apart probe in metaphase cell **(A)** and interphase cells **(B)** from malignant pleural effusion in a 5-year-old child. The metaphase cell shows a t(8;14), indicative of *IGH-MYC* fusion, in which the centromeric (*red*) and telomeric (*green*) FISH probe components localize to chromosomes 8 (*arrowhead*) and 14, respectively. The interphase cells include *MYC*-rearranged Burkitt's lymphoma (*arrows*) and reactive non-neoplastic lymphocytes (*arrowheads*).

fusions to various partners containing dimerization domains. The most common of these fusions, found in 80% of ALCLs, results from a translocation t(2;5) fusing the 3′ end of the *ALK* gene to the 5′ end of *NPM*,[320] and serving as a useful diagnostic marker of ALCL. Less common *ALK* fusions involve ATIC, TFG, CTLC, TPM3, TPM4, and MSN.[92,321-323] ALCL occurs in a cutaneous form, which is usually ALK-negative, whereas nodal and extranodal systemic forms express ALK in about 95% of pediatric cases. ALK encodes a receptor tyrosine kinase

that is normally expressed in neural cells of the intestine, testis, and brain but not in non-neoplastic lymphoid cells. A smaller number of pediatric ALCLs are B-cell disorders, and these cases often feature oncogenic fusions of the *ALK* and clathrin genes.[319] The pattern of ALK immunostaining in association with ALK-NPM fusion resulting from t(2;5) is one of nuclear and cytoplasmic staining, with distinctive nucleolar accentuation (see Fig. 5-33). Similarly, other ALK oncoproteins are associated with distinctive immunostaining patterns, including

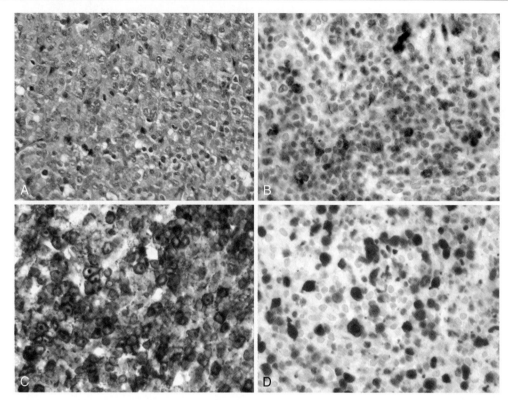

FIGURE 5-33. In anaplastic large cell lymphoma, histologic features include cohesive cells with abundant cytoplasm, imparting an epithelioid appearance **(A)**. Immunohistochemical features include patchy expression of epithelial membrane antigen **(B)**, strong membrane and Golgi reactivity for CD30 **(C)**, and anaplastic lymphoma kinase (ALK) immunostain **(D)**, which in this t(2;5)-positive case shows reactivity in both nuclear and cytoplasmic compartments.

the granular cytoplasmic staining with clathrin-ALK rearrangement, diffuse cytoplasmic staining in the case of TFG-ALK and ATIC-ALK rearrangements, diffuse membranous and cytoplasmic staining with TPM3-ALK, and nuclear membrane staining with RANBP2-ALK rearrangement. However, ALK staining is not specific for ALCL. As noted earlier (see "Mesenchymal Neoplasms: Soft Tissue and Bone Tumors"), ALK oncoprotein expression is characteristic of inflammatory myofibroblastic tumors also. In the hematopoietic group of neoplasms, ALK reactivity as an indicator of clathrin-ALK fusion oncoproteins has been described for large B-cell neoplasms also.[324]

Subcutaneous Panniculitic T-Cell Lymphoma

This lymphoma subtype produces firm nodular infiltrates of skin, which occasionally progress to ulceration. These infiltrates are generally confined to subcutaneous fat, with sparing of the overlying dermis and epidermis. Other helpful histologic features include evidence of cellular atypia and characteristic rimming of adipocytes by the neoplastic cells. In the presence of such histologic features, demonstration of T-cell receptor gene rearrangement confirms the diagnosis.

Hepatosplenic T-Cell Lymphoma

This is an extranodal lymphoma of γ-δ T-cells. Clinical presentation is generally that of hepatosplenomegaly without accompanying lymphadenopathy, although other anatomic locations, typically also extranodal, may be involved. The histologic findings on a diagnostic liver biopsy may mimic those of hepatitis. The neoplastic infiltrate is sinusoidal in distribution, sparing

the portal tracts. Expansion of the sinusoids by a monotonous lymphoid population should prompt consideration of this diagnosis. Demonstration of T-cell γ receptor gene rearrangement is confirmatory, and another helpful genetic feature, seen in many cases, is the cytogenetic finding of isochromosome 7q,[325,326] often accompanied by trisomy 8.[327] Development of hemophagocytic syndrome may ensue and heralds poor outcome.

Acute Lymphoblastic Leukemia

ALL, the most common childhood cancer, comprises a heterogeneous spectrum of diseases characterized by clonal proliferations of lymphoid precursor cells at varying stages of development, but traditionally assigned to one of three FAB subtypes (Fig. 5-34). Classic teaching has been that the ALL cell of origin is a committed lymphoid progenitor, with the particular stage of lymphoid differentiation during which the transforming event occurs being highly variable. However, although controversial, studies have suggested that leukemic transformation in ALL may occur in a more primitive stem cell.[328] Irrespective of whether the non-neoplastic cell that is targeted for transformation is a committed lymphoid cell, the major demonstrable immunophenotypic ALL subsets are B- or, less often, T-cell precursors. About 85% of cases are B-cell precursor ALL, whereas 10% to 15% are T-cell precursors. Expression of the CD10 B-cell differentiation antigen characterizes common ALL, which is the most frequent form of childhood ALL (Fig. 5-35). By contrast, the vast majority of cases of ALL in infants (defined as younger than 1 year old) are negative for CD10 cell surface antigen expression. Burkitt's leukemias, with their characteristic phenotype of mature B-cell

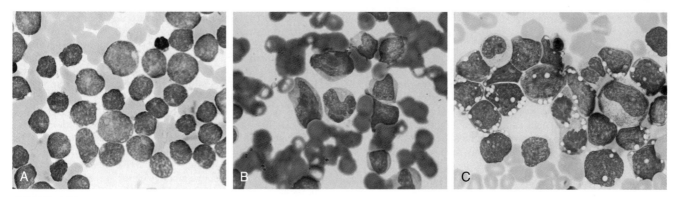

FIGURE 5-34. Acute lymphoblastic leukemia historical French-American-British (FAB) subtypes. **A,** L1, with smaller, more uniform cells, and a high nuclear-to-cytoplasmic ratio. **B,** L2, with somewhat larger cells, and a more varied nuclear-to-cytoplasmic ratio. **C,** L3 (Burkitt's), with larger cells and numerous vacuoles. (Courtesy of Marybeth Helfrich, Children's Hospital of Philadelphia.)

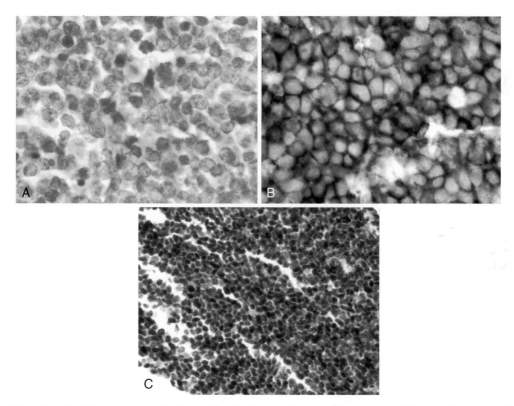

FIGURE 5-35. A, Lymph node infiltration by pre-B-cell acute lymphoblastic leukemia lacking any appreciable cytoplasm and with slightly irregular nuclear contours. The nuclear chromatin is finely dispersed. This case shows typical strong immunohistochemical staining for CD10 (common ALL antigen) **(B)** and nuclear TdT expression **(C)**.

surface Ig expression, account for only approximately 0.5% of cases of childhood ALL.[2] Heterogeneous primary molecular genetic aberrations cause leukemic transformation and are associated with distinctive biologic properties and clinical features in the different major subtypes of childhood ALL.

Intralocus IG and TCR Gene Rearrangements

Historically, the patterns of *IG* and *TCR* gene rearrangements in pediatric ALL have provided insights into the ordered hierarchy of rearrangements of *IG* and *TCR* genes in lymphoid maturation.[329,330] The diversity of rearrangements of variable (V), diversity (D) and joining (J) segments generated within these loci in the human immune response affords a signature of unique markers of lineage, clonality, and maturation stage in each ALL. This is particularly true because *TCR* gene rearrangements can be identified even in precursor B-cell ALL and, conversely, *IG* gene rearrangements can occur in T-cell ALL. Furthermore, *IG* and *TCR* gene rearrangements are not static but can evolve after leukemic transformation via subclone progression (e.g., from D-J to complete V-D-J assembly or from *IGH* to *IGK* light chain gene rearrangement).[331] However, because of the related nature of the ALL subclones in any given patient, *IG* and *TCR* gene rearrangements can serve as sensitive markers for detecting minimal residual disease (MRD) and predicting relapse.[332,333] Comparable sensitivity in detecting minimal residual disease can also be achieved by multiparameter flow cytometric analysis of various antigens, expression of which is restricted to leukemic cells.[334]

One study has suggested that about 25% of cases of B-cell precursor ALL undergo transformation at the pro-B– to pre-B–cell stage, characterized by cytoplasmic mu expression and assembly of the pre-B–cell receptor complex. The pre-B–cell differentiation stage is a critical cell survival checkpoint because most normal B cells cannot form intact immunoglobulin and instead undergo apoptosis.[335] The subset of ALL transitioning from pro-B to pre-B cells exhibits steroid sensitivity.[335]

Interlocus IG and TCR Gene Rearrangements and Translocations

Not only do *IG* and *TCR* genes undergo intralocus rearrangements, but their aberrant recombination also causes interlocus chromosomal translocations and inversions. These chromosomal rearrangements can create hybrid antigen receptor genes when two different antigen receptor loci recombine with each other. A small fraction of pediatric ALLs of B- or T-cell lineage harbor these hybrid antigen receptor gene rearrangements.[336] Alternatively, chromosomal rearrangements can juxtapose transformation-inducing non–*IG*/non–*TCR* genes with the regulatory enhancer and promoter elements of *IG* or *TCR* genes as a second type of interlocus rearrangement. V(D)J recombination errors of this type,[337] causing transcriptional upregulation of the juxtaposed non–*IG*/non–*TCR* genes, occur in subsets of pediatric ALL, especially in T-cell ALL.

SIL-SCL rearrangements and *SCL* translocations disrupting *TCR* genes are present in approximately 30% of cases of T-cell ALL overall. The *SCL(TAL1)* gene at chromosome band 1p34, which encodes a basic helix-loop-helix (bHLH) transcription factor, was first discovered at the t(1;14)(p34;q11) translocation breakpoint junction involving the TCR alpha-delta locus in a stem cell leukemia.[338] Other T-cell ALL cases harbor a different type of *SCL* rearrangement, in which illegitimate V(D)J recombinase activity at recombinase-like signal sequences in *SCL* and *SIL* (SCL-interrupting locus) creates an interstitial deletion on chromosome 1p. The *SIL-SCL* rearrangement causes aberrant regulation of *SCL* expression by the *SIL* promoter.[339,340] The t(1;3)(p34;p21) translocation, fusing *SCL* and the non–antigen receptor gene *TCTA*, is mediated by a similar mechanism of illegitimate V(D)J recombinase activity.[341]

In other recurrent translocations in T-cell ALL, various oncogenic transcription factor genes such as *LMO1, LMO2, LYL1,* and *HOX11(TLX1)* are fused to different *TCR* loci, leading to unscheduled expression of the relevant transcription factor protein.[72] *LMO2* translocations occur in 10% to 20% of T-cell ALLs. Microarray experiments have shown that oncogenic transcription factor genes can be overexpressed in T-cell ALL subsets at distinct maturation stages and are prognostic markers, even when conventional karyotyping studies do not reveal such translocations.[342] For example, dual-color FISH analysis and a ligation-mediated PCR assay have revealed cryptic translocations of the *HOX11(TLX1)* gene with the *TCRD* locus in most T-cell ALLs in which there was high *HOX11* expression.[343] This finding is particularly intriguing because high-level *HOX11* expression in T-cell ALL correlates with a favorable prognosis.[343] In addition, the CD34−, CD1a+, CD4 8 double-positive cortical immunophenotype has suggested that the immature β pre-αβ stage of maturation arrest is associated with high *HOX11* expression.[343] These results have demonstrated that molecular cytogenetics can provide more sensitive and consistent evaluations of ALL oncogenic mechanisms compared with conventional karyotyping.

The most recently identified example of a recurrent *TCR* gene translocation in T-cell ALL is the t(6;7)(q23;q34) translocation, which juxtaposes the *C-MYB* gene at chromosome band 6q23 with the *TCRB* locus.[344] Although the subtelomeric locations of *TCRB* and *C-MYB* precluded recognition of this rearrangement by conventional karyotyping, the rearrangement is readily detectable with methods such as FISH, Southern blotting, or PCR assay.[344] Molecular cloning has revealed a hepatamer-like sequence adjacent to the translocation breakpoint in the *C-MYB* gene, consistent with illegitimate V(D)J recombinase activity as the mechanism of this translocation. In this translocation, placement of *C-MYB* in close proximity with the *TCRB* enhancer regulatory element results in aberrant expression of the translocated *C-MYB* allele and a gene expression signature consistent with upregulation of various proliferation and mitosis genes.[344] The t(6;7) translocation is of clinical interest because the median age of the patients is only 2.2 years old,[344] which is unusual because T-cell ALL is otherwise infrequent in young children. This translocation exemplifies the importance of cooperating mutations in pediatric ALL pathogenesis, because many cases of T-cell ALL with t(6;7) translocation also contain *NOTCH1* mutations and *CDNK2A p16 ARF* deletions.[344] Dysregulated *C-MYB* expression in T-cell ALL of the very young can also result from gene duplications, as demonstrated by molecular and fiber FISH analyses of *C-MYB* gene copy number.[344] *C-MYB* is expressed at high levels in the thymus, and it has been suggested that *C-MYB* deregulation results from sustained rather than ectopic expression[344]; in that sense, it differs from several other transcription factor oncogenes disrupted in T-cell ALL.

Another T-cell ALL translocation, t(7;9)(q34;q34.3), fuses *TCRB* to the gene encoding the NOTCH1 transmembrane receptor protein, which regulates T-cell maturation.[345] This is an extremely uncommon translocation, occurring in less than 1% of cases of T-cell ALL; however, it was more recently shown that at least 50% of T-cell ALL cases have activating intragenic *NOTCH1* mutations, including cases with other major translocations.[346] Activating *NOTCH1* mutations affecting the extracellular heterodimerization (HD) domain result in ligand-independent activation, whereas those affecting the intracellular PEST domain cause increased stability of the protein. The mutant NOTCH1 protein is a potential therapeutic target of gamma secretase inhibitors, which can block NOTCH1-mediated signaling in T-cell ALL.[346] Inhibition of NOTCH1 signaling by gamma secretase inhibitors is associated with upregulation of the phosphatase and tensin homologue (PTEN) tumor suppressor protein.[347] Although a phase 1-2 clinical trial of gamma secretase inhibition did not show efficacy in T-cell ALL, the observed drug resistance could be attributed in part to *PTEN* gene deletion. PTEN inhibits the PI3K-AKT pathway and loss of PTEN function is associated with AKT activation and a switch in oncogene addiction from the NOTCH1 to the AKT signaling pathway. *PTEN* mutational analyses have indicated that a subset of T-cell ALL (8%) harbors mutations of this gene at diagnosis, independently or together with *NOTCH1* mutations or, alternatively, the *PTEN* mutations can be secondary alterations associated with disease progression.

Analogous to the interlocus *TCR* gene rearrangements in T-cell ALL, molecular approaches have also been revealing in precursor B-cell ALL, and recurrent novel translocations that juxtapose *IG* genes with oncogenic transcription factor genes have been identified and characterized. One recent example is the t(6;14)(p22.3;q32.22) that fuses the joining region of the *IGH* gene with the gene encoding ID4.[348] The translocation causes overexpression of the ID4 bHLH transcription factor and is associated with a CD19+, CD10+, HLADR+, TdT+ common precursor B-cell immunophenotype, low-risk clinical features, and favorable prognosis.[348] This translocation is often accompanied by deletion of the chromosome 9p genes, *CDKNA* and *PAX5*, suggesting cooperativity of these alterations in the pathogenesis of this disease.[348] Another example of *IGH* gene rearrangement is seen with the t(5;14), which occurs in less than 1% of cases of precursor B-cell ALL. The t(5;14) places the *IL3* gene under transcriptional regulatory control of the *IGH* locus, resulting in the hallmark clinical feature of peripheral eosinophilia associated with this translocation.[72]

In the rare entity of Burkitt's leukemia, expression of the *MYC* oncogene is altered by translocation into the *IGH* or, less often, the *IGK* or *IGL* light chain locus, but oncogenic transformation at a more mature B-cell developmental stage is reflected by IgM expression on the leukemia cell surface.

Another area of interest has been in the application of molecular approaches to determine the temporal origins of ALL-specific *IG*, *TCR*, or transcription factor gene rearrangements. Studies of ALL in monozygous twins and studies of ALL molecular cytogenetic aberrations in neonatal Guthrie blood spots have been useful in indicating whether various ALL subtypes arise before or after birth. In the case of T-cell ALL, there is recent evidence that the disease is not initiated in utero or that the clonal aberration in most cases is present below the detection sensitivity of PCR at the time of birth.[349] However, these findings are in contrast to PCR-based findings on *TCR* gene rearrangements in two other studies, which were consistent with a prenatal origin of T-cell ALL.[350,351] In one of three cases of T-cell ALL with *NOTCH1* mutation, the *NOTCH1* mutation was detectable in neonatal Guthrie blood spot DNA, whereas the *SIL-SCL* rearrangement in the same case occurred later as a postnatal event.[352] Thus, ALL-specific *IG* and *TCR* gene rearrangements and/or leukemia-associated transcription factor alterations in at least some T-cell ALLs are in utero events, even though the latency to clinically evident disease can be protracted. Most subtypes of precursor B-cell ALL also initiate in utero (see later).

Chromosomal Translocations Not Involving IG or TCR Genes

TEL-AML1 Translocations. Several of the major recurrent chromosomal translocations in pediatric ALL do not involve *IG*, *TCR*, or other genes with obvious V(D)J recombination signal sequences. The most frequent chromosomal translocation in all pediatric cancers[353] is the t(12;21) translocation present in 25% of cases of CD10$^+$ B-lineage common ALL. This translocation is cryptic by conventional Giemsa-banded karyotyping and must be detected by FISH or molecular analyses. The leukemogenic fusion of the *TEL(ETV6)* gene from chromosome band 12p13 to the *CBFA2 (AML1)* gene from chromosome band 21q21 is associated with recruitment of complexes containing histone deacetylases to AML1 target genes, causing aberrant transcriptional repression.[353] There is evidence that the t(12;21) translocation occurs as an in utero event[354,355] in cells that are at a stem or B-cell progenitor developmental stage, before *IG* and *TCR* gene rearrangement. Rearrangement of the immune receptor loci occurs after the initiating *TEL-AML1* translocation.[356] *TEL-AML1* translocations occur in cord blood specimens of healthy newborns at 100 times the incidence of *TEL-AML1* translocations in leukemia, indicating that progression to overt ALL is rare in *TEL-AML1*-positive cells. Similarly, the low concordance (approximately 5% to 10%) of *TEL-AML1* leukemia in monozygous twins has suggested that postnatal mutations are required for transformation of *TEL-AML1*-positive progenitor cells into frank ALL.[357] These additional mutations often include loss of the normal *TEL* allele.[353] The *TEL-AML1* translocation is associated with a favorable outcome.[353]

E2A Gene Translocations. The t(1;19) translocation occurs in approximately 5% of cases of pediatric ALL, fusing the *E2A* gene on chromosome band 19p13.3 to the *PBX1* gene on chromosome band 1q23. This translocation is most often found in cIg+ (pre-B) rather than cIg– B-cell precursor ALL (25% vs. less than 1% of cases).[358] The t(1;19)(q23;p13.3) translocation is associated with a poor prognosis in the cIg+ (pre-B) cases. *E2A* is a critical B-cell developmental gene that encodes an IG enhancer binding protein. The *E2A* gene encodes three different bHLH transcription factors via alternative splicing of the *E2A* transcript. The *PBX1* gene product is a homeobox transcription factor and the t(1;19) translocation results in the production of a fusion oncoprotein from the der(19) chromosome, in which the DNA-binding domain of PBX1 replaces the carboxyl DNA-binding bHLH domain of E2A. The t(1;19)(q23;p13.3) translocation is detectable in neonatal Guthrie cards in only about 10% of cases, suggesting a postnatal origin, and is different in that sense from the other major subtypes of pediatric ALL.[357,359] Split-signal FISH using different color probes for the *E2A* and *PBX1* genes is a useful tool for the definitive identification of this translocation,[360] which is otherwise indistinguishable karyotypically from a different translocation sharing breakpoints in the same chromosome bands. The alternate form of t(1;19)(q23;p13.3) translocation in ALL does not disrupt the *E2A* and *PBX1* genes, but rather fuses the *DAZAP1* RNA-binding protein gene on chromosome band 19p13.3 to the *MEF2D* DNA-binding protein gene on chromosome band 1q23.[361]

A rare t(17;19) *E2A* variant translocation occurs in 1% of cases of childhood B-cell precursor ALL, which creates a *E2A-HLF* (hepatic leukemia factor) fusion gene. The t(17;19) translocation is associated with coagulation abnormalities and has a poor prognosis.[358]

BCR-ABL1 Translocations. About 5% of cases of B-cell precursor ALL harbor the t(9;22)(q34;q11) translocation fusing *BCR* with the *ABL1* tyrosine kinase gene. This translocation is associated with the clinically high-risk features of older age and high white blood cell (WBC) count, and an especially grim prognosis.[72] However, emerging data have indicated that the molecularly targeted ABL kinase inhibitor, imatinib mesylate, has clinical activity against BCR-ABL$^+$ ALL in the pediatric population as well as in adults.[362]

MLL Translocations. Leukemia is the second most common malignancy during infancy. The infant cases comprise 2.5% to 5% of ALLs and 6% to 14% of AMLs in the pediatric population overall. The annual incidence of infant ALL and AML is 19 and 10/million, respectively.[106,363] Infant leukemia is a special subtype of pediatric leukemia characterized by chromosomal translocations that generate fusion oncoproteins, and approximately 80% of cases of infant ALL and myelomonocytic-monoblastic AMLs feature balanced chromosomal translocations of the *MLL* (mixed-lineage leukemia; myeloid lymphoid leukemia) gene at chromosome band 11q23.[364] Cases of ALL with *MLL* translocations often coexpress myeloid-associated surface antigens, especially CD15. Additionally, *MLL* translocations can be associated with true bilineal acute leukemias, in which there are separate lymphoid and myeloid cell populations (Fig. 5-36), and acute leukemias with *MLL* translocations can undergo lineage switch. *MLL* translocations are also found in secondary leukemias in patients treated with chemotherapeutic topoisomerase II poisons.[60] The *MLL* gene encodes a large complex oncoprotein that regulates transcription[15,365-368] and has regional amino acid similarity to that of *Drosophila* trithorax (trx).[105,366,367] Whereas trx is involved in the maintenance of expression of homeotic gene complexes during embryonic development,[369] of relevance to leukemia, MLL maintains

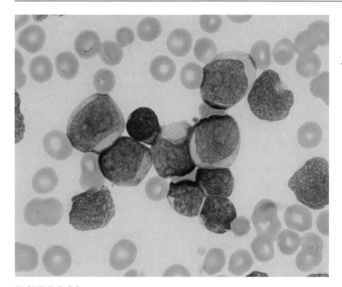

FIGURE 5-36. Infant bilineal acute leukemia with *MLL* translocation showing lymphoid and myeloid blast cell populations. (Courtesy of Marybeth Helfrich, Children's Hospital of Philadelphia.)

HOX gene expression during hematopoiesis.[370] *MLL* translocations in various types of pediatric leukemia disrupt an 8.3-kb breakpoint cluster region and fuse the 5′ portion of *MLL* with one of more than 50 different partner genes, generating diverse leukemogenic fusion oncoproteins containing the amino-terminus of MLL and the carboxyl-terminus of the partner protein.[50,65,80,371]

The native MLL protein has complex transcriptional regulatory functions. MLL undergoes proteolytic cleavage into amino- and carboxyl-segments that reassociate with one another in a mutiprotein complex,[372-374] regulating *HOX* gene expression and epigenetic modifications of nucleosomes and histones.[375] The MLL chimeric oncoproteins resulting from the various *MLL* partner gene rearrangements lack the MLL proteolytic cleavage site and affect leukemogenic transformation through transcriptional dysregulation of MLL target genes.[376] Although many *MLL* partner genes themselves encode important proteins in transcriptional regulation or cell signaling pathways,[105,376] it is unclear how the partner gene disruption contributes to leukemogenesis mediated by *MLL* translocations.

Of the approximately 80% of infant ALL cases with *MLL* translocations, 70% and 13% of cases, respectively, involve the *AF4* (chromosome band 4q21) or *ENL* (chromosome band 19p13) transcription factor partner genes.[377] In AML, the partner genes of *MLL* are much more heterogeneous, including not only genes that encode nuclear transcription factors and transcriptional regulatory proteins but also cytoplasmic proteins and proteins in various cellular organelles.[50]

MLL translocations in infant leukemias exemplify another principle in the molecular cytogenetics of pediatric leukemias—namely, the association of host risk factors and gene-environment interactions with specific aberrations. The *MLL* translocation in infant leukemia is an in utero event, the origin of which has been established by the detection of identical nonconstitutional *MLL* rearrangements in leukemias of monozygous twins,[378,379] as well as the detection of *MLL* translocations in neonatal Guthrie blood spot DNA in nontwin cases.[380] Maternal-fetal exposure from consumption of food containing topoisomerase II interacting substances during pregnancy has been implicated as a risk factor in *MLL*-rearranged infant AML.[381] Moreover, an inactivating polymorphism in the gene encoding reduced nicotinamide adenine dinucleotide phosphate (NADPH) quinone oxidoreductase 1 (NQO1), increases the risk of all *MLL*-rearranged infant acute leukemias, especially cases with t(4;11) fusing *MLL* to *AF4*, which are primarily ALL.[382,383] The inactivating NQO1 polymorphism is a plausible host predisposition factor because the *p*-benzoquinone detoxified by NQO1 is a topoisomerase II poison[384] and four-base 5′ overhangs from topoisomerase II cleavage lend readily to DNA damage resolution by nonhomologous end joining (NHEJ) repair, features of which usually are evident at *MLL* translocation breakpoint junctions.[48,385] Infant leukemia risk is also modulated by a genetic polymorphism in the methylene tetrahydrofolate reductase (MTHFR) gene; it has been suggested that the resultant increased thymidine synthesis, which enhances DNA repair, protects against *MLL* translocations.[386]

Infant ALLs with *MLL* translocations are CD10⁻ early B progenitor cells, but they may have monocytic features and express the myeloid-associated CD15 cell surface antigen.[106] Clinically, *MLL* translocations are important because of their unfavorable prognosis.[377] The *MLL* translocation in infant ALL is associated with a high leukemia burden manifest as marked hyperleukocytosis, massive hepatosplenomegaly, and meningeal involvement.[106] Neonatal leukemia (leukemia in the first month of life) has an annual incidence of 4.7/million live births[387] and comprises an important fraction of leukemia in infants. The clinical manifestations of neonatal leukemia include stillbirth, signs of leukemia at birth, or hematologic abnormalities preceding the leukemia diagnosis within a few weeks.[107] Clinical hallmarks include hepatosplenomegaly, hydrops, and polyhydramnios detected antenatally, and the archetypal marked hyperleukocytosis, hepatosplenomegaly, leukemia cutis and CNS involvement detected after birth.[107] *MLL* translocations in infant and neonatal leukemia have significant adverse effects on response to treatment, especially in cases of early B-lineage ALL.[44,107,377,388] The substantial adverse impact of *MLL* translocations on prognosis places infant ALL at the extreme of pediatric ALL in which outcome is the poorest.[44,107,377,388] However, in AML, in which outcome is less favorable overall than in ALL, *MLL* translocations are not independent prognostic factors. Overexpression of *FLT3* mRNA is a common secondary alteration in infant ALL with *MLL* translocations.[389] In these cases, the *FLT3* gene is often mutated and the FLT3 protein is highly expressed.[108,390,391]

Other Clinically Important Genomic Aberrations in Acute Lymphoblastic Leukemia

***FLT3* Mutations.** Aberrations of the FMS-like tyrosine kinase 3 (FLT3) receptor tyrosine kinase protein are crucial oncogenic events that contribute to cellular proliferation and survival and arrested differentiation in a subset of ALL.[392,393] *FLT3* mutations have been proposed to function as secondary oncogenic events in ALL where there is already a proliferation-inducing primary oncogenic mutation involving another gene.[394] *FLT3* molecular aberration types include in-frame deletions and internal tandem duplications (ITDs) in the juxtamembrane region and point mutations in the activation loop of the kinase domain.[390,394,395] All of these are associated with FLT3 protein overexpression and constitutive activation of FLT3 signaling pathways through STAT5, MAP kinase, and AKT.[394,396] FLT3-ITD mutations are found in approximately 2% of childhood ALL,[397] and FLT3 point mutations are found in approximately 5% and 16% of childhood B-lineage ALL and infant ALL, respectively.[394,397] FLT3 mutations have a predilection for particular molecular/cytogenetic ALL subtypes, being found in approximately 21% to 28% of cases of high hyperdiploid ALL[108,391,394] and in 18% of ALL with *MLL* gene translocations, which consequently also express high levels of constitutively active FLT3 protein.[390,391] Overexpression of the wild-type FLT3 protein is another mechanism of FLT3 activation in leukemias with *MLL* translocations,[108] and microarray analyses have demonstrated increased *FLT3* mRNA expression as a distinguishing feature of ALL cases with *MLL* translocations.[389,398] Alternatively, the expression of FLT3 ligand (FL) by leukemia cells can cause autocrine activation of FLT3 signaling by increasing constitutive FLT3 phosphorylation.[108,391,399] *FLT3* mutations are clinically important in infant ALL because they are associated with a poor prognosis.[394]

Alterations in *BCL2* Expression. In addition to classic oncogenes and tumor suppressor genes, genes that control cell death and survival decisions are clinically important, not only in pediatric ALL but all types of pediatric cancer because they have an impact on chemosensitivity and resistance. The intrinsic (mitochondrial) cell death pathway is regulated by the formation of homo- and heterotypic dimers involving BCL2 and many other BCL2 family protein members with opposing pro- or antiapoptotic actions that collectively determine the apoptosis threshold.[400-404] Almost all cases of pediatric ALL express detectable BCL2 protein.[405] BCL2 mRNA and protein are particularly abundant in infant and pediatric leukemias with t(4;11) or other *MLL* translocations compared with ALL and AML cases without *MLL* translocations,[406] but *BCL2* expression is not exclusively a feature of *MLL* disease.[405,407,408]

***CDKN2* Tumor Suppressor Gene Deletions.** Chromosome band 9p21 is a site of recurring deletions in pediatric ALL. The critical deleted region at chromosome band 9p21 contains the *CDKN2A* gene, which encodes two different tumor suppressor proteins p16 (INK4A) and p14 (ARF). The adjacent gene *CDKN2B* encodes p15 (INK4b) and is often co-deleted with the *CDKN2A* gene.[409] p16 (INK4A) and p15 (INK4b) inhibit the cyclin D–dependent kinases CDK4 and CDK6.[410] Deletions of the p15 and p16 tumor suppressor genes at the *CDKN2* loci are present in 60% and 20% of cases, respectively, of T-cell and B-cell precursor ALL, and the p15 promoter is inactivated by hypermethylation in additional cases. *CDKN2* alterations have been implicated in relapse and poor response to treatment,[409-414] and homozygous loss of p16 (INK4A) is more frequent in pediatric ALL at relapse than at diagnosis, indicating that this aberration portends disease progression.[415] Notably, hemizygous p16 deletion may be constitutional and confer susceptibility to leukemia and other forms of cancer.[416]

***SMAD3* Alterations.** Loss of *SMAD3* expression is important in the pathogenesis of pediatric T-cell ALL.[417] Transforming growth factor β (TGF-β) is a cytokine family composed of three isoforms that have a role in tumor suppression. The *SMAD3* component protein in the TGFβ signaling pathway was discovered to be absent or barely detectable in each of 10 cases of T-cell ALL, but sequencing of the corresponding *MADH3* gene from the leukemia cells of affected patients did not reveal mutations, and the mechanism of loss of *SMAD3* expression is unknown. Nonetheless, the loss of *SMAD3* impairs the growth-suppressive effects of TGF-β on T cells. *SMAD3* loss is apparently restricted to T-cell ALL and is not observed in precursor B-cell ALL or AML.[417] Deletions resulting in haploinsufficiency of the cyclin-dependent kinase inhibitor p27[Kip1] (*CDKN1B*) at chromosome band 12p12 are also recurring abnormalities in T-cell ALL,[418] and *SMAD3* loss has been demonstrated to cooperate with p27[Kip1] (*CDKN1B*) loss in a murine leukemogenesis model.[417]

Numerical Chromosomal Abnormalities. The largest cytogenetic subset of childhood precursor B cell ALL (approximately 30%) is characterized by a hyperdiploid karyotype, which results when nondisjunction of chromosomes causes chromosomal gains. Hyperdiploidy can be of prenatal origin, as evidenced by its presence in cord blood and neonatal Guthrie blood spots, suggesting that hyperdiploidy itself may be the initiating event in this form of ALL.[419,420] High hyperdiploid ALL (more than 50 chromosomes) has a favorable prognosis, especially when there are specific chromosomal trisomies, such as +4, +10, +18[421] or +10, and +17.[72,422] About 25% of cases of high hyperdiploid ALL have *FLT3* mutations, whereas other cases exhibit overexpression of the FLT3 protein through autocrine activation.[108,391]

In contrast, hypodiploidy occurs in only about 6% to 8% of childhood ALL, is frequently associated with chromosomal translocations, and is a poor prognostic factor.[423,424] In one study, the adverse prognosis was especially pronounced in cases with near-haploid karyotypes containing 24 to 28 chromosomes.[424] In a more recent study, there was no difference in outcome when 24 to 29, 33 to 39, or 40 to 43 chromosomes were present.[425] Nonetheless, hypodiploidy with less than 44 chromosomes is generally regarded as a marker of poor prognosis. Patients with ALL containing 44 or 45 chromosomes have a better outcome unless there is monosomy 7 or a dicentric chromosome.[425]

Importantly, the major pediatric ALL leukemia subtypes recognizable at the cytogenetic and molecular levels can now be distinguished based on their unique gene expression profiles. These broad gene expression profile differences provide new insights into ALL biology and predictive markers, and might be useful in identifying novel, molecularly targeted treatments.[426]

MicroRNA Aberrations. A burgeoning class of abnormalities in cancer cells involves changes in gene expression mediated by the aberrant activity of microRNAs, which affect the translation of coding mRNAs into their respective proteins.[427,428] MicroRNAs, which are short noncoding RNAs, originate via the excision of approximately 19 to 25 nucleotide (nt) segments after formation of a hairpin pre-microRNA loop from a larger primary pri-microRNA transcript. The base pairing interactions of microRNAs with protein coding mRNAs[428] result in microRNA-mediated translational repression. Using microRNA profiling arrays, it recently has been possible to discern unique microRNA signatures and microRNA mutations in particular leukemia subtypes.[429] For example, ALL and AML can be distinguished by differential expression of miRNAs. The microRNAs miR-128a and miR-128b are overexpressed and the microRNAs let-7b and miR-223 are underexpressed in ALL compared with AML.[430] miRNAs can regulate oncoprotein expression, as shown by mir-203 regulation of BCR-ABL, as relevant in CML and BCR-ABL⁺ ALL.[431] It has also been suggested that microRNA signatures have prognostic relevance in leukemias in adults.[432,433] Therefore, the further characterization of microRNA mechanisms has important implications for the development of new antileukemia targeted therapeutics.

Acute Myeloid Leukemia

Pediatric AMLs exhibit heterogeneous but characteristic clinical and biologic features, which reflect underlying molecular and cytogenetic abnormalities. Many of the characteristic AML cytogenetic aberrations are similar to those in adult AML, although the relative frequencies of the aberrations differ between pediatric and adult AML. The major FAB morphologic subtypes of AML (Fig. 5-37) are, in general, associated with typical balanced chromosomal translocations.[434] WHO has reclassified AML based on molecular and cytogenetic aberrations, which underlie unique biologic subgroups, have clinical

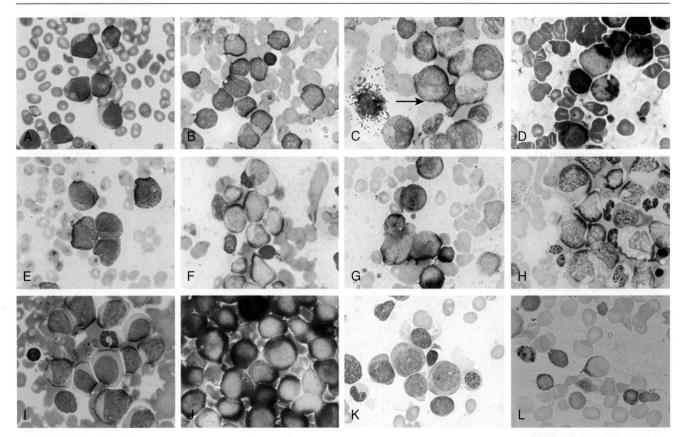

FIGURE 5-37. Major acute myeloid leukemia subtypes. M0 **(A)** and M1 **(B)** have minimal differentiation. **C,** M2 shows greater myeloid differentiation and may feature Auer rods (*arrow*) along with strong myeloperoxidase staining **(D)**. **E,** M3 promyelocytic leukemia with typical coarse cytoplasmic granules. **F,** M4 myelomonocytic leukemia with staining for chloroacetate esterase (*blue*) in the myeloblasts, and nonspecific esterase (*brownish red*) in the monoblasts **(G)**. **H,** M4eo with pronounced eosinophilic features. **I,** M5 monoblastic leukemia with staining for nonspecific esterase **(J)**. **K,** M6 erythroleukemia with staining for periodic acid–Schiff **(L)**. (Courtesy of Marybeth Helfrich, Children's Hospital of Philadelphia.)

importance and form the basis for assignment to appropriate treatment regimens.[435] The current WHO classification system incorporates genetic, immunophenotypic, clinical, and biologic features for diagnosis of the myeloid neoplasms.[435]

Major molecular cytogenetic aberrations in AML recognized in the WHO classification system are the following: AML with t(8;21)(q22;q22), (*AML1-ETO*); AML with abnormal bone marrow eosinophils and inv(16)(p13q22) or t(16;16)(p13;q22), (*CBFB-MYH11*); acute promyelocytic leukemia (APL) with t(15;17)(q22;q21), (*PML-RARA*), and variants; and AML with 11q23 (*MLL*) abnormalities. It has been estimated that the t(8;21), t(15;17), inv(16), and *MLL* translocations are present in 12%, 7%, 12%, and 7% of cases of pediatric AML, respectively.[434,436] However, these frequencies are inexact, with another study using standard cytogenetic analyses finding *MLL* translocations in approximately 18% of cases.[437] Furthermore, other characteristic recurrent molecular cytogenetic aberrations are observed.

Although morphology no longer serves as the diagnostic gold standard for AML, the observation of a dyshesive, monotonous, immature cell population should trigger and guide further investigations by histochemical, immunophenotypic (including flow cytometric) and molecular cytogenetic methods. AML may exhibit morphologic features of any of the various hematopoietic progenitors, or even of several simultaneously. The cytologic features, cytochemical staining pattern, and immunotype all assist in the subclassification of AML morphol-

ogy by the FAB system, which recognizes the eight different subcategories (see Fig. 5-37) described here.

In FAB M0 AML, there are more than 30% blasts with no or minimal features of myeloid differentiation. FAB M0 AML nuclei are generally large, with remarkably fine nuclear chromatin, prominent nucleoli, and high nuclear-to-cytoplasmic ratio.[438] The cytoplasm may exhibit focal granularity, and Sudan black reactivity is typical. Myeloperoxidase (MPO) expression is inapparent by light microscopy, but can be demonstrated by electron microscopy.

In FAB M1 AML, like in FAB M0, there are more than 30% blasts with minimal differentiation but, unlike in FAB M0, MPO expression is readily demonstrable and accompanies Sudan black and chloracetate esterase (CEA) positivity.

The diagnosis of FAB M2 AML is based on the observation of myeloblasts with some maturation, generally requiring more than 30% total blasts, with more than 10% of the blasts showing granulocytic differentiation. FAB M2 AML blasts also exhibit MPO and CEA staining. FAB M2 morphology is typical in AML with t(8;21).[439] Although the typical morphology of AML with inv(16)(p13;q22) is FAB M4eo, in one series, a substantial fraction of pediatric AML with inv(16)(p13;q22) showed FAB M2 morphology.[440]

The classic FAB M3 APL has coarse cytoplasmic granules, the nuclear chromatin is less fine than in myeloblasts, and the nucleus often is eccentric. FAB M3v is an APL microgranular variant in which the cytoplasmic granules are finer than in classic FAB M3 APL, and the nuclei may have irregular contours, appearing reniform or folded. The genetic underpinnings, typically associated with t(15;17), are similar to FAB M3, but FAB M3v APL does not carry the risk of massive hemorrhage during chemotherapy induction that is associated with classic FAB M3 APL.

FAB M4 AML is acute myelomonocytic leukemia, which is composed of myeloblasts, monoblasts, and promonocytes. The monoblast has a substantially lower nuclear-to-cytoplasmic ratio than the myeloblast or promyelocyte; its nucleoli are more prominent and its cytoplasm is more abundant, with fine granularity and occasional vacuolation. Although the promonocyte has similar features, it shows a different cytoplasmic hue. Both monoblasts and promonocytes, whether in FAB M4 or FAB M5 AML, are nonspecific esterase (NSE)–positive. FAB M4 and FAB M5 AMLs also express CAE, MPO, and alpha-naphthol acetate, and some stain with PAS. FAB M4 and FAB M5 AMLs are typically, although not exclusively, associated with *MLL* gene translocations. FAB M4 AML with abnormal bone marrow eosinophils (FAB M4eo) is associated with inv(16)(p13;q22).

FAB M5 acute monocytic leukemias encompass two subcategories; one subcategory with no differentiation is FAB M5a (monoblastic leukemia), whereas the other with differentiation is FAB M5b. Monoblasts predominate in FAB M5a AML, but promonocytes predominate in the FAB M5b morphologic subtype.

FAB M6 AML is acute erythroid leukemia, which generally exhibits a predominance of erythroblasts, but often a substantial myeloblast component also. The erythroblast shows a high nuclear-to-cytoplasmic ratio and a condensed rounded nucleus. The cytoplasm is deeply basophilic and may contain vacuoles. FAB M6 cases express glycophorin and stain for PAS, but not other cytochemical markers.

The FAB M7 category is acute megakaryoblastic leukemia (AMKL). FAB M7 AML may be associated with prominent marrow fibrosis, making aspiration difficult. The cells are pleomorphic (see Fig. 5-39) and the megakaryocytic nature may not be obvious by morphology alone. FAB M7 AMKL cells may express alpha-naphthol acetate. Expression of glycoprotein Ia, IIb, or IIIa or factor VIII can aid in the diagnosis of FAB M7 AMKL. As described in more detail later, AML in Down syndrome is AMKL; however, the t(1;22) is found in some non–Down syndrome cases.[441]

Major Chromosomal Translocations

t(8;21). The archetypal chromosomal translocation in FAB M2 AML is the t(8;21), which fuses the 5′ terminus of the *AML1 (RUNX1, CBFA2)* gene at chromosome band 21q22, with almost the entire *ETO* gene from chromosome band 8q22.[73] In one series, 82% of pediatric AML with this translocation had FAB M2 morphology.[439] These morphologic-cytogenetic correlates, although compelling, are imperfect. Therefore, some classifications have taken account of cytogenetic abnormalities, thereby highlighting crucial biologic pathways and, in some cases, therapeutic targets.[435] The t(8;21) also is strongly associated with extramedullary granulocytic sarcoma presentations.[439,442] Leukemias with this translocation, which disrupt the *AML1* gene encoding the DNA-binding subunit of core binding factor, comprise one of the two subtypes of core binding factor leukemias. The AML1 fusion oncoprotein binds the non–DNA-binding subunit of core binding factor, CBFB, as does native AML1, but the fusion oncoprotein interacts with nuclear corepressors that inhibit AML1-mediated transcriptional activation through the deregulation of histone deacetylation.[73] The t(8;21) has been associated with a favorable

prognosis in studies conducted by the Pediatric Oncology Group[443] and the Children's Cancer Group.[444] The t(8;21) has been associated with a mixed outcome in the experience of St. Jude Children's Research Hospital, but the treatment regimens did not specify repetitive high-dose cytosine arabinoside as did other regimens in which the t(8;21) was associated with a favorable prognosis.[439,444,445] Variant *AML1 (CBFA2)* translocations involving other partner genes have heterogeneous morphologic MDS and AML presentations, but these translocations occur primarily in adult leukemias and tend to be treatment-related rather than to occur de novo.[446]

inv(16) and t(16;16). The second subtype of core binding factor AML has inversions or, less often, translocations fusing the *CBFB* gene encoding the non–DNA-binding subunit of CBF at chromosome band 16p13 to the *MYH11* gene at chromosome band 16q22.[447] The classic morphologic presentation of AMLs with inv(16) and t(16;16) in adults is myelomonocytic leukemia with eosinophilia (FAB M4eo)[448] but many pediatric cases present as FAB M2 or M4 AML, without eosinophilia.[440,449] RT-PCR and FISH are particularly useful and important for the detection of this rearrangement.[450-453] Additionally, the leukemic blast cells may co-express the CD2 T-cell surface antigen.[454] The inv(16) is leukemogenic via a mechanism of dominant transcriptional repression of AML1-regulated genes, so that the pathways involved and the biologic consequences are similar to those resulting from the t(8;21).[73] The outcome associated with this aberration is also favorable in several pediatric series, similar to the t(8;21).[455] In one large study of adults and children, the outcomes were comparable in patients undergoing allotransplantation and receiving high-dose or low-dose cytosine arabinoside, and the outcome was better in the younger patients.[456] Pediatric studies have found that current regimens incorporating intensive high-dose cytosine arabinoside into post-remission treatment are associated with event-free survival rates of approximately 70% or higher.[437,444]

t(15;17). The t(15;17) fusing the *PML* and *RARA* genes at chromosome bands 15q22 and 17q21, respectively, is associated with FAB M3 APL.[457,458] The t(15;17) and variant translocations associated with APL disrupt the function of the retinoic acid receptor α (RARα), also called the RARA protein, which is a ligand-dependent transcription factor important in myeloid differentiation. The RARα protein forms a heterodimer with another ligand-dependent protein, retinoic X receptor protein (RXR). The natural ligand of RARα is all-trans-retinoic acid (ATRA), whereas RXR is responsive to ATRA or 9-*cis*-retinoic acid.[457] In the presence of ligand, the heterodimeric complex interacts with transcriptional co-activators to induce myeloid differentiation. In contrast, the molecular pathogenesis of APL involves the aberrant recruitment of transcriptional co-repressors and the histone deacetylase complex to RARα target genes. Notably, the first molecularly targeted agent ever to be implemented for anti-leukemia treatment was ATRA. Variant translocations fuse *RARA* with partner genes other than *PML*, including *NPM*, *NuMA*, *STAT5b*, *PRKAR1A*, and *PLZF*.[457,459-462] The *PRKAR1A-RARA* fusion was first identified by *RARA* FISH analysis in an ATRA-sensitive adult APL that had normal cytogenetics by conventional karyotype analysis.[462] *PRKAR1A* encodes the regulatory subunit type 1-α of cyclic adenosine monophosphate (cAMP)–dependent protein kinase,[462] and the karyotypically cryptic nature of the translocation highlights the importance of molecular cytogenetic testing. APLs with *PLZF-RARA* translocation are insensitive to ATRA, whereas those with the other *RARA* fusion types are ATRA-responsive.[457]

Mixed-Lineage Leukemia (*MLL*) Gene Translocations. In contrast to ALL, in which *MLL* partner genes are limited and *AF4* is the most common, the partner genes are much more diverse in AML.[463] Nonetheless, *MLL* partner genes in ALL and AML, and in de novo and treatment-related leukemias are at least partially overlapping. Many MLL partner proteins have structural motifs of nuclear transcription factors,[15,105,367] transcriptional regulatory proteins,[464] or other nuclear proteins.[465-467] Others are cytoplasmic proteins or cell membrane proteins.[105,379,468-474] *MLL* also undergoes self-fusion in a type of rearrangement termed *partial tandem duplication*; therefore, in AML, MLL itself is an MLL partner protein.[47,475,476] As in ALL, cDNA panhandle PCR has been applied to detect novel and rare partner genes of *MLL* and covert *MLL* rearrangements in AML.[477-479] There is no obvious functional relationship between the many partner genes of *MLL* but some are members of the same gene families.[379,470-472,480,481] It has been suggested that the nuclear partner proteins mediate transcriptional activation[105,481,482] and that cytoplasmic partner proteins cause forced MLL dimerization or oligomerization.[483] Several MLL partner proteins also interact with one another.[484] Fusion proteins from the der(11) chromosome, which retain the AT hook, SNL, and MT domains of MLL but replace the MLL PHD, transactivation, and SET domains with the carboxyl partner protein, transform hematopoietic progenitors and cause leukemia in mice.[485,486] In murine models, MLL fusion proteins constitutively activate *Hoxa9*, and *Hoxa9* activation is essential for leukemogenesis with some MLL fusion proteins (e.g., MLL-ENL).[376] However, altered *Hox* expression is not essential for leukemogenesis with other MLL fusion proteins, including MLL-AF9 and MLL-GAS7.[487]

As described earlier, balanced *MLL* gene translocations are the primary molecular aberrations underlying most cases of acute leukemia in infants.[364] AML is more common than ALL in neonates, unlike during the rest of infancy and childhood.[107,488] It has been estimated that *MLL* translocations are present in half of all ALLs and AMLs diagnosed during the neonatal period (the first month of infancy).[107] *MLL* translocations also comprise 5% to 10% of acquired chromosomal rearrangements in childhood AML.[489] The particular partner gene fused to *MLL* affects cell lineage and differentiation features, which are reflected in the immunophenotype. *MLL* translocations in AML are often associated with myelomonocytic and monoblastic features.[106] Leukemias with *MLL* translocations can also present as treatment-associated myelodysplastic syndrome or AML[490,491]; this is particularly characteristic of cases with t(11;16) fusing *MLL* with *CBP* (CREB binding protein).[464,492-494] Unlike in ALL, the presence of an *MLL* translocation is not an independent prognostic factor in pediatric AML with current treatment. However, in some series, the *MLL-AF9* fusion resulting from t(9;11) has been associated with a more favorable outcome than other *MLL* translocations[449] (e.g., *MLL-AF10*).[495]

Certain clinical and laboratory features are associated with the archetypal neonatal FAB M4 and FAB M5 leukemias with *MLL* translocations. These features include cutaneous nodules (leukemia cutis), petechiae and ecchymoses, in addition to the hematologic abnormalities (hyperleukocytosis, anemia, thrombocytopenia) and CNS involvement.[107,488,496] Curiously, congenital *MLL*-rearranged AML may be present predominantly in the skin and not in the marrow (aleukemic leukemia cutis) and, on occasion, can undergo spontaneous remission.[496,497] In these situations, molecular analysis of bone marrow and skin biopsy material is warranted because of the propensity for progressive disease when a clonal *MLL* rearrangement is identified.[496,497]

As discussed earlier for infant ALL, the *MLL* translocations in many infant AMLs are in utero events.[379] In some cases,

however, an in utero origin cannot be demonstrated, possibly because the clonotypic sequences of the translocations are present below the detection limit of the PCR assay.[498] The occasional stillbirth presentations[107] and the presentation of monoblastic AML with an *MLL-ELL* rearrangement as a granulocytic sarcoma diagnosed by prenatal ultrasound[499] further substantiate that *MLL* translocations arise in utero in infant AML. However, latency to leukemia underscores that additional secondary alterations are important, and perhaps required, for the development of leukemia with an *MLL* translocation.[105]

t(8;16). The chromosome 16 rearrangement in the t(8;16)(p11;p13) translocation is in the same band (16p13) disrupted by inversions and translocations of the *MYH11* gene in M4Eo AML.[447,500,501] However, the 16p13.3 breakpoints in t(8;16) target a different gene, encoding the transcriptional coactivator CREB binding protein (CBP; CREBBP) at chromosome band 16p13.3, which is fused with the *MOZ (MYST3)* gene on chromosome 8.[502] The CBP protein contains RARA and CREB binding domains, a bromodomain, and E1A and transcription factor IIB (TFIIB) binding regions, whereas MOZ contains zinc finger motifs and a MYST acetyltransferase domain.[502-506] The *CBP-MOZ* fusion transcript encoded by the der(16) chromosome is not in-frame, whereas the *MOZ-CBP* transcript is believed to have transforming properties and clinical relevance.[502,507,508] MOZ-CBP tumorigenic mechanisms have been proposed to involve inhibition of AML1-mediated transcriptional activation.[509] The *MOZ-CBP* rearrangement is associated with a gene expression signature that includes *HOXA9*, *MEIS1*, and *FLT3* overexpression, similar to the gene expression profiles in AML with *MLL* translocations.[510] Notably, *CBP* is also an occasional fusion partner of *MLL* in MDS.[464,492-494] *CBP* oncogenic aberrations can be constitutional, as evidenced by the germline *CBP* point mutations, microdeletions, and translocations that underlie the Rubinstein-Taybi syndrome.[511-513]

The t(8;16) is associated with a prognostically unfavorable subset of FAB M4 and FAB M5 AMLs, other features of which include erythrophagocytosis and coagulopathy.[514,515] Therefore, recognition of this AML subset is clinically important and can be accomplished by molecular cytogenetic detection of the rearrangement. Although a rare translocation, accounting for only approximately 2% of pediatric AML,[516] most AMLs with this translocation have occurred in infants and children.[502,515] The t(8;16) in neonatal AML, like translocations in several other AML subtypes, can be associated with leukemia cutis and spontaneous remission.[517,518]

A variant t(10;16) translocation fuses the *MORF* gene at chromosome band 10q22 to *CBP*, and was discovered in a case of childhood FAB M5a AML.[519] The MORF protein contains zinc fingers, nuclear localization signals, and a histone acetyltransferase domain[519] and, similar to MOZ, contributes to chromatin remodeling.[506] Additional variant translocations result in fusion of *MOZ* with the *TIF2 (NCOA2)* or *p300 (EP300)* genes[520-522]; p300 is related structurally to CBP, and the MOZ-TIF2 oncoprotein recruits CBP. Therefore, CBP-mediated oncogenic transcriptional regulatory functions appear crucial in the several translocation variants that compose this AML molecular cytogenetic subset.

t(6;9). The t(6;9) (p23;q34) translocation is a rare recurrent translocation in AML, primarily seen in adults, the clinical and molecular features of which include myelodysplasia, basophilia, a CD34⁻ immunophenotype and *FLT3* mutations.[523-525] AML with t(6;9) in children and adolescents has had a poor prognosis.[516,526-528] The translocation occurs in various morphologic AML subtypes, including FAB M1, M2, and M4, and fuses the 5′ end of the *DEK* gene (chromosome 6) to the 3′ end of the *CAN* gene (chromosome 9), creating a *DEK-CAN* oncogene.[529-531] The *DEK* gene product is a multimeric chromatin protein, regulated by CK2 kinase, which modifies DNA topology by the introduction of supercoils into closed circular DNA.[532,533] The *CAN* gene at chromosome band 9q34 (also called *CAIN*, because of its chromosomal proximity to *ABL*), encodes the nucleoporin protein NUP214 of the nuclear pore complex. DEK-CAN oncogenic roles in leukemogenesis involve a myeloid lineage–specific increase in protein translation, which occurs in conjunction with increased eIF-4E translation initiation factor phosphorylation.[534] Leukemias with the *DEK-CAN* fusion may have oncogenic mechanisms in common with other AML subtypes, as is suggested by the observation that nucleoporin-specific FG repeats in the fusion oncoprotein can induce transcriptional activation by recruitment of the transcriptional coactivators CBP and p300. Reverse transcriptase and real-time PCR methods have been helpful for AML monitoring in patients with this rearrangement, because the persistence of the fusion transcript identifies patients at risk of relapse.[535-537] A translocation variant resulting in the *SET-CAN* oncogenic fusion gene has been observed in AML of the FAB M0 subtype.[529]

***NUP98* Translocations.** The *NUP98* gene at chromosome band 11p15 encodes a nucleoporin protein that serves as a structural component of nuclear pore complex. The NUP98 protein is located on the nucleoplasmic side of the nuclear pore and provides a docking site for the export of mRNA between the nucleus and cytoplasm.[538,539] Various chromosomal translocations produce *NUP98* oncogenic fusions and, depending on exactly which partner gene is fused with *NUP98*, these translocations can be associated with de novo or treatment-related AML, ALL, or MDS.[540-558] Many of the *NUP98* partner genes encode homeobox transcription factors, but some of the partner genes, including *TOP1* and *TOP2B*, have more diverse functions.[540,549,555] Several *NUP98* fusions, such as those involving *NSD1*, *HOXD13*, and *LEDGF*, are found in infant and pediatric de novo AML.[550,556,557] The t(7;11)(p15;p15), which fuses *NUP98* with *HOXA9*, and the t(10;11)(q23;p15), which fuses *NUP98* with *HHEX*, have been shown to shift the cellular distribution of NUP98 away from the nuclear pore complex and into intranuclear aggregation bodies.[543,551] Because of the substantial variety of *NUP98* partner genes, it is most feasible to detect these rearrangements using a general *NUP98* breakapart FISH strategy.[555,559] cDNA panhandle PCR has also been applied as a gene discovery tool to identify new partner genes in leukemias with *NUP98* translocations.[46]

Therapy-Related Acute Myeloid Leukemias and Myelodysplastic Syndromes

Therapy-related AMLs and MDSs comprise a separate WHO AML subgroup[435] relevant to pediatrics; two major categories have been recognized. Therapy-related leukemias are of increasing concern in children, in whom survivorship—as a percentage of patients diagnosed with cancer—is greater than in the adult cancer population.[560] Therapy-related leukemia or MDS is also well-recognized as a long-term complication after autologous hematopoietic stem cell transplantation.[561-563] The two major categories of chemotherapies associated with leukemia and MDS are alkylating agents and topoisomerase II poisons. The forms of leukemia associated with these agents have distinctive molecular cytogenetic features, which can also be found in subsets of leukemia arising de novo.

All alkylating agents engender some risk of leukemia as a treatment complication, but the risk is variable, depending on the particular agent(s), cumulative dose, patient age, and superimposed effects of radiotherapy.[564-567] The latency period is variable, ranging from 2 to 12 years after exposure, but the peak incidence occurs at approximately 6 years.[568] The archetypal cytogenetic features in alkylating agent–related leukemias are complete or partial deletions of chromosomes 5 and 7 and complex, unbalanced, numeric and structural cytogenetic abnormalities.[569] The chromosome 7 aberrations are the most common cytogenetic events in leukemias after alkylating agent treatment.[570,571] Most cases with chromosome 7q deletions exhibit allelic loss of the chromosomal segment between bands 7q22 and 7q31 but, despite identification of various candidate genes in this genomic region, the exact tumor suppressor gene(s) have not been convincingly identified.[572-576] In treatment-associated MDS and AML lacking chromosome 5 aberrations, the monosomy 7 or del(7q) may be acquired by subclone evolution and accompanied by other key mutational aberrations, including t(3;21), *RAS* mutation, and p15 promoter hypermethylation.[571]

Monosomy 5 and del(5q) are the next most common aberrations in alkylating agent–related MDS and AML. FISH analyses have revealed that the chromosome 5q abnormalities frequently are covert unbalanced translocations.[571] The chromosome 5q abnormalities arise as primary aberrations and not by subclone evolution, and additional aberrations in therapy-related MDS and AML with monosomy 5 or del(5q) can include monosomy 7 or del(7q), *TP53* mutations, and gene duplications, such as *MLL* segmental jumping translocations.[16,571,577] The critical genes targeted by 5q deletion have been difficult to pinpoint because of variable involvement of a large genomic region that encompasses chromosome bands 5q13 to 5q33.[570,578-584] Two recently implicated chromosome 5q31 candidate genes are *CTNNA1* encoding the alpha-catenin protein[585] and the *EGR1* gene,[586] although there have been several others.[570,578-584] Epigenetic dysregulation may also contribute to the pathogenesis, with transcriptional silencing in the retained non-deleted *CTNAA1* allele resulting from promoter methylation and histone deacetylation.[585]

A tumor suppressor gene, *RPS14*, has been identified as the target of 5q– in the syndrome of refractory anemia, in which there is preservation of megakaryopoiesis and myelopoiesis,[587] but the role of *RPS14* in therapy-related MDS and AML remains to be determined. This gene encodes a ribosomal protein required for processing of 18S pre-rRNA.[587] The strategy of screening normal human CD34+ cells with short hairpin RNAs (shRNAs) against various genes in the minimal 5q–deletion region has revealed that *RPS14* silencing causes erythroid maturation block and increased apoptosis in differentiating erythroid cells, similar to the increased apoptosis observed in MDS.[587] Furthermore, lentiviral RPS14 expression restored erythroid differentiation in bone marrow cells from patients with 5q– refractory anemia syndrome.[587] These insights underscore the role of ribosomal genes in anemia, given that other ribosomal genes, *RPS19* and *RPS24*, contribute to Diamond-Blackfan anemia.

Most AMLs developing after autologous hematopoietic stem cell transplantation have complex numeric and structural karyotypic aberrations, including losses of chromosomes 5 and 7; these are also features of AML arising after exposure to alkylating agents.[563,588-590] The secondary AMLs can occur early after transplantation, and the cytogenetic aberrations in these treatment-associated leukemias are often demonstrable in pre-transplantation specimens, suggesting that the genotoxic damage results from the prior therapy.[588,591] On the other hand, such cytogenetic aberrations are not demonstrable in peripheral blood stem cell autografts.[592]

Therapy-related leukemias can be caused by exposure to various chemotherapeutic topoisomerase II poisons, including epipodophyllotoxins and anthracyclines, the anthracenedione mitoxantrone, and the topoisomerase I/II interacting agent dactinomycin.[60] Balanced translocations, often involving the *MLL* gene,[593] are the most typical molecular alterations in leukemias related to topoisomerase II poisons. The typical latency is about 2 to 2½ years after chemotherapy exposure,[490,594] although more protracted latencies of up to 10 years have been described.[477,595] A particularly high risk has been reported in association with high cumulative doses of etoposide and anthracyclines,[596] but other studies have not found a correlation between etoposide cumulative dose and secondary leukemia risk.[597] Intermittent weekly or twice-weekly etoposide dose schedules, and semicontinuous schedules, have also been associated with increased risk of secondary AML.[596,597] The *MLL* translocations in therapy-related AML (as is the case in de novo AML) are often associated with myelomonocytic and monoblastic morphology.[598,599] Other translocations in therapy-related MDS and AML include t(8;21) and its variants,[446,600-609] t(15;17),[593] inv(16) and t(16;16),[594,610-613] t(8;16),[614,615] t(9;22),[615] and various translocations involving the *NUP98* gene at chromosome band 11p15.[540,541,543,554,616-619]

Treatment-related MDS/AML can present with bizarre and highly abnormal morphology in some cases (Fig. 5-38) but, in others, can be insidious and challenging to diagnose, particularly in patients actively receiving treatment, in whom the hematologic features of cytopenia and monocytosis can be indistinguishable from ordinary side effects of chemotherapy and recovery of the marrow. Additionally, some patients with treatment-related MDS and AML, particularly in the early stages, have no obvious peripheral blood cell abnormalities at all.[52,469] Therefore, one front-line pediatric neuroblastoma treatment protocol has specified routine bone marrow surveillance every 3 to 6 months, not only for neuroblastoma relapse, but also for leukemia-associated aberrations.[52] In addition to the insidious nature of the clinical presentations, the spectrum of known molecular cytogenetic abnormalities associated with therapy-related MDS and AML is constantly increasing and is already very large, creating the yet-unmet need for broad molecular cytogenetic screening methods with which to monitor high-risk patients. For example, even though there are few data on patients followed in this manner, it seems that most of the protean *MLL* translocations emerging during treatment, which involve many different partner genes, are harbingers of MDS

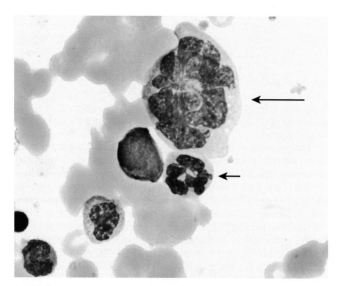

FIGURE 5-38. Therapy-related MDS showing hypersegmented granulocyte (*short arrow*) below an extremely dysplastic hypersegmented neutrophil (*arrow*). (Courtesy of Marybeth Helfrich, Children's Hospital of Philadelphia.)

or AML.[52,469,620] An *MLL-FRYL* translocation that was traced prospectively by molecular cytogenetic testing (FISH, panhandle PCR) caused clonal replacement of the bone marrow without affecting differentiation, only after a long latency culminated in clear-cut therapy-related MDS.[52] However, clinical progression is apparently not inevitable because, in one patient, the morphologically normal clone harboring a *MLL-ARHGEF17* translocation gradually regressed and neither leukemia nor MDS ensued.[621]

Additional challenges for molecular characterization result from the variable locations of *MLL* translocation breakpoints, which can be within or outside a breakpoint hot spot region.* Secondary myeloid disorders are particularly challenging to diagnose in patients previously diagnosed with AML—for example, the *MOZ* oncogenic rearrangement resulting from a novel t(2;8)(p23;p11.2) translocation in treatment-related MDS after AML in a pediatric patient.[624]

Clinically, the molecular cytogenetic features of the therapy-related leukemias are important prognostic factors. Most cases, except those with favorable translocations—t(8;21), inv(16), t(15;17)—are resistant to current treatment strategies, but intensive regimens, including hematopoietic stem cell transplantation, have been more successful. Prognosis is affected further by the reduced tolerance to additional intensive antileukemia therapy after primary cancer treatment.[625] Nonetheless, just as in the de novo leukemias, additional targeted therapy options are emerging from an understanding of the molecular cytogenetic aberrations in these challenging disorders.

Myelodysplasia and Myeloproliferative Diseases

MDS and myeloproliferative diseases comprise a very small fraction (less than 10%) of all hematologic malignancies in children. Incomplete coverage of various unique features of pediatric MDS and myeloproliferative diseases in the current WHO classification system have led to the development of diagnostic guidelines for MDS and myeloproliferative categories applicable specifically to children.[626] To fulfill minimal diagnostic criteria for MDS, at least two of the following four features are required: (1) sustained unexplained cytopenia; (2) bilineage morphologic myelodysplasia; (3) acquired clonal hematopoietic cell cytogenetic abnormality; and (4) 5% or more blasts in the marrow.[626] In contrast to AML, which is defined by a bone marrow blast threshold of 20% and aberrant differentiation, and to MDS, myeloproliferative disorders are characterized by expansion of one or more hematopoietic lineages but retained differentiation.[626,627] Three major categories of MDS and myeloproliferative diseases are applicable to children: (1) a group of myelodysplastic-myeloproliferative disorders comprised primarily of juvenile myelomonocytic leukemia (JMML); (2) myeloid leukemia of Down syndrome; and (3) MDS.[626]

Juvenile Myelomonocytic Leukemia

The constellation of hepatosplenomegaly, lymphadenopathy, pallor, and rash, especially in children younger than 3 years old, are clinical features of JMML, the diagnostic criteria for which include peripheral monocytosis, absence of the *BCR-ABL* rearrangement, less than 20% blasts in the bone marrow, and at least two of the following: increased fetal hemoglobin (HbF), circulating myeloid precursors (Fig. 5-39), WBC more than 10

---

*References 45, 48, 52, 60, 94, 107, 112, 127, 324, 327-331, 464, 469, 622, and 623.

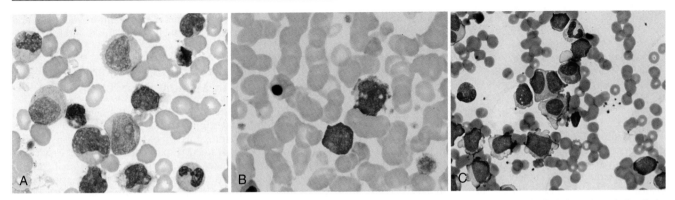

FIGURE 5-39. A, Juvenile myelomonocytic leukemia peripheral blood showing leukocytosis, monocytosis, myeloid left shift, and myelodysplasia. **B,** Down syndrome transient abnormal myelopoiesis (TAM). This peripheral blood specimen shows a megakaryoblast, nucleated red blood cell, and giant platelet. **C,** Acute megakaryoblastic leukemia (FAB M7) featuring pleomorphic blasts and cytoplasmic blebbing. (Courtesy of Marybeth Helfrich, Children's Hospital of Philadelphia.)

$\times 10^9$/L, presence of a clonal cytogenetic abnormality, and in vitro hypersensitivity of myeloid precursors to granulocyte-macrophage colony-stimulating factor (GM-CSF).[627] Children with neurofibromatosis type 1 (NF1) or Noonan syndrome are predisposed to JMML. Notably, several of the key molecular abnormalities contributing to JMML pathogenesis result in RAS signaling pathway hyperactivation.

Many hematopoietic growth factors transduce signals from the cell surface to the nucleus through RAS family proteins, which regulate cellular proliferation and differentiation by cycling between active guanosine triphosphate (GTP)–bound and inactive guanosine diphosphate (GDP)–bound states.[628,629] Somatic mutations in *RAS* oncogenes are one mechanism of RAS pathway activation and are found in 20% to 30% of JMMLs,[629,630] often involving *KRAS* or *NRAS* at codons 12, 13, or 61. Some cases of *RAS*-mutant JMML undergo spontaneous regression,[631] whereas *NRAS*-mutant JMML can progress with loss of the remaining normal *NRAS* allele.[632] Monosomy 7 is also found in some cases of JMML with *RAS* oncogene mutations.[633]

The *NF1* tumor suppressor gene product, neurofibromin, is a GTPase activating protein that accelerates GTP hydrolysis on RAS proteins.[634] Germline mutations in the *NF1* gene, often with accompanying loss of the normal *NF1* allele, result in elevated levels of GTP-bound RAS. Thus, germline *NF1* mutations comprise an alternative mechanism for hyperactivating the RAS signaling pathway, predisposing to JMML.[634,635] Loss of heterozygosity at the *NF1* locus is observed in approximately 50% of JMML arising in patients with NF1.[634] In NF1 kindreds, JMML is seen particularly in boys with maternal transmission of the mutant *NF1* allele.[636] Additional mutations in the *NF1* gene, with or without LOH, occur in sporadic JMML that is not associated with the NF1 syndrome.[637] In some of these cases, the *NF1* mutations are germline, with JMML being the presenting feature of the NF1 syndrome. Overall, it is estimated that *NF1* mutations are present in approximately 30% of all JMMLs.[637] Monosomy 7 occurs in addition to *NF1* mutation in some JMMLs.[634] However, *NF1* and *RAS* mutations in JMMLs are mutually exclusive.[637]

Noonan syndrome is an autosomal dominant disorder associated with germline mutations in the *PTPN11 (SHP2)* gene in approximately 50% of cases and is characterized by JMML, facial dysmorphology, short stature, and cardiac defects.[638] The *PTPN11* gene product, SHP2 phosphatase, regulates RAS-MAPK pathway signaling, but is inactive in its baseline state.[639,640] *PTPN11* mutations in Noonan syndrome result in SHP2 activation and, consequently, hyperactivation of RAS-MAPK signaling.[639] In pediatric patients without Noonan syndrome, *PTPN11* somatic mutations can be found in sporadic cases of JMML, MDS, AML (particularly the FAB M5 subtype), and B-lineage ALL.[641-645] Somatically acquired *PTPN11* mutations are present in 30% to 35% of de novo JMML.[643,645] Generally, the types of *PTPN11* mutations occurring as somatic events in nonsyndromic cases are more strongly activating than the germline *PTPN11* mutations in patients with Noonan syndrome.[627,646] The fact that *PTPN11* mutations are less strongly activating in patients with Noonan syndrome might explain why syndromic JMML is associated with less severe hematologic abnormalities and can resolve spontaneously.[627,645] Thus, dysregulation of the RAS signaling pathway by *RAS, NF1,* or *PTPN11* mutations is instrumental to the aberrant cell growth and differentiation in JMML, and these three mechanisms of RAS dysregulation are usually mutually exclusive.[643]

The myeloproliferative disorder known as monosomy 7 syndrome has clinical overlap with JMML and is characterized by myelodysplasia, thrombocytopenia, anemia, and hepatosplenomegaly.[647] However, this disorder is not included in the more recent classification system for pediatric MPD/MDS.[626]

Chronic Myelomonocytic Leukemia

Chronic myelomonocytic leukemia (CMML) is a clonal bone marrow stem cell disorder characterized by monocytosis, myelodysplasia, and absence of *BCR-ABL* fusion.[41,435] The t(5;12)(q33;p13) translocation, which generates the *TEL-PDGFRB* fusion product, is a recurring but rare rearrangement in CMML.[435] The case in which the fusion transcript was first described occurred in an adolescent patient.[648] The t(5;12) is associated with eosinophilia and progression to AML on acquisition of additional cytogenetic changes.[648] However, only secondary and not de novo CMML is included as a diagnostic category in the pediatric adaptation of the WHO classification of myelodysplastic and myeloproliferative diseases.[626]

Transient Abnormal Myelopoiesis and Acute Megakaryoblastic Leukemia of Down Syndrome

Ten percent to 20% of neonates with Down syndrome are affected with transient abnormal myelopoiesis (TAM), and approximately 20% to 30% of TAM will progress to AMKL by 4 years of age (see Fig. 5-39).[649-651] Several laboratories have identified truncating *GATA-1* point mutations as in utero mutational oncogenic events that initiate both TAM and AMKL.[649,652] GATA-1 is a hematopoietic transcription factor that, via interactions with the FOG-1 cofactor and GATA-2, regulates erythroid and megakaryocyte maturation.[649] However, whereas the *GATA-1* mutation is sufficient for TAM, postnatal secondary changes such as *TP53* mutation and/or trisomy 8 are required for subsequent clonal expansion, a prerequisite for disease progression to AMKL.[653] In many cases of TAM, however, there is no disease progression because the clone with *GATA-1* mutation is ultimately extinguished in the absence of requisite secondary alterations.[649] The TAM and AMKL in Down syndrome have distinct gene expression profiles.[650]

Several chromosome 21 genes, including *CBS* (cystathionine beta-synthase), at band 21q22 may contribute to the unique forms of leukemogenesis in Down syndrome.[654] The *CBS* gene is overexpressed, above and beyond the levels predicted based on the trisomy 21 increased gene dosage. This up-regulation seems to result from mechanisms involving transcriptional up-regulation through the *CBS* promoter.[654] Consequences of *CBS* over-expression include reduced levels of plasma homocysteine, methionine, *S*-adenosylmethionine and *S*-adenosylhomocysteine, resulting in altered CpG methylation and consequent dysregulation of gene expression. Other effects include perturbed folate metabolism and genetic instability (increased DNA mutations), which may predispose to accumulation of the secondary genetic mutations in AMKL.[654] Another consequence of *CBS* overexpression is increased cytosine arabinoside sensitivity,[654] which contributes to increased treatment-related toxicities and to the more favorable outcome associated with myeloid leukemia of Down syndrome.[655]

The t(1;22)(p13;q13) translocation fusing *OTT* and *MAL* is associated with non–Down syndrome AMKL, another distinct form of AMKL peculiar to neonates.[107,364,656]

Myelodysplastic Syndrome

The three MDS morphologic subtypes of greatest relevance in pediatrics are refractory cytopenia, refractory anemia with excess blasts (RAEB), and RAEB in transformation (RAEB-T).[626] Monosomy 7 or del(7q) occurs in approximately 40% of cases and is the most commonly acquired cytogenetic aberration in pediatric MDS.[657] In cases of refractory cytopenia, monosomy 7 is associated with disease progression and poor outcome.[626,658] Similarly, monosomy 7, with or without other cytogenetic abnormalities, is a frequent finding in RAEB-T.[657] Despite the generally poor prognosis of –7/del(7q) in MDS, spontaneous and durable hematologic remissions have been described in some children diagnosed with MDS characterized by this cytogenetic feature.[659] Rarely, MDS with monosomy 7 is familial and observed in siblings.[636,660] In one study of refractory anemia of childhood, which is a form of refractory cytopenia, cytogenetic analyses have demonstrated monosomy 7 in 49% of cases, whereas trisomy 8 was the next most common abnormality, found in 9% of cases.[658] The 5q– syndrome associated with an indolent refractory anemia but with preservation of megakaryopoiesis and myelopoiesis[587] has not been described in children.[626] FISH analysis with chromosome specific probes in combination with immunophenotyping has enabled characterization of the cell lineages affected by the clonal aberrations in MDS[661] as well as evaluation of the lineages affected by MDS clonal expansion.[662] MDS secondary to prior therapy has been discussed earlier. As is true for adults,[569] pediatric patients with MDS secondary to cytotoxic therapies (see earlier) often have chromosome 5 and 7 abnormalities.[663] Constitutional disorders

associated with congenital bone marrow failure syndromes and acquired aplastic anemia are included in the differential diagnosis of MDS in children.[626]

Other Clinically Important Genomic Aberrations in Myeloid Disorders

It has been proposed that in addition to the major chromosomal aberrations that underlie the various AML morphologic subtypes, cooperating mutations affecting proliferation and differentiation are essential in AML pathogenesis,[364] and may affect prognosis and treatment. The balanced chromosomal translocations that disrupt major hematopoietic transcription factor genes are generally regarded as the primary molecular alterations in the associated AML morphologic subsets. Translocations that disrupt major hematopoietic transcription factor genes generally alter differentiation,[364] whereas additional aberrations, including kinase or RAS-RAF pathway gene mutations, often contribute to hyperproliferative behavior.

FLT3 *Alterations*

Although less common than in adult AML, *FLT3* mutations are nonetheless found in a considerable minority of pediatric AML cases, with juxtamembrane region ITD and activation loop point mutations identified in approximately 12% to 15% and 7% to 9% of pediatric cases, respectively.[397,664,665] Indeed, *FLT3* mutations might represent the most frequently occurring molecular abnormalities in AML. *FLT3* mutations are common in pediatric AML with *MLL* translocations; 23% of *MLL*-rearranged AML in one large series harbored either *FLT3* ITD or kinase domain mutations.[397] Also, *FLT3* mutations are particularly common in AMLs with normal karyotypes, in which they are demonstrable in up to 60% of cases.[397] Another subset of AML features autocrine FLT3 activation caused by the expression of FLT3 ligand, resulting in constitutive FLT3 phosphorylation and signaling.[665] *FLT3* ITD mutations in pediatric AML are associated with poor outcomes, similar to those in adult cases.[665-667] An increased *FLT3* ITD allelic ratio is associated with relapse, and molecular diagnostic tests have been developed to detect *FLT3* mutations and quantify *FLT3* ITD allelic ratio.[668,669] *FLT3* ITD mutations occur in approximately 30% of childhood APL.[669a] *FLT3* ITD mutations, although common in de novo AML, are infrequent in treatment-related cases, as reported in an adult series.[670]

KIT *Mutations*

Mutations in the *KIT* receptor tyrosine kinase gene are also common in pediatric AML and occur most often in cases with t(8;21) or inv(16), which disrupt DNA or non–DNA-binding subunits of CBF.[671] The *KIT* mutations are associated with constitutive, ligand-independent activation of the KIT protein. One recent study has estimated that 37% of all AML in children with either t(8;21) or inv(16) harbor *KIT* mutations. *KIT* mutations do not affect prognosis but are nonetheless significant because preclinical studies have indicated that AML with *KIT* mutations are sensitive to imatinib mesylate and FLT3 inhibition.[671]

RAS *Mutations*

It has long been recognized that the RAS oncogene family members can be activated by mutations in myeloid neoplasms,[672] although these mutations do not usually have prognostic relevance.[671] Mutations of *NRAS* or *KRAS* codons 12, 13, or 16 have been described in approximately 20% of pediatric AMLs with *MLL* translocation,[673] and in approximately 30% of pediatric AMLs with t(8;21) or inv(16).[671] *RAS* mutations are also found in about one third of MDS with monosomy 7.[674] In secondary AML, *RAS* mutations are less common than in de novo disease,[675,676] but are seen more often in alkylating agent–related cases, especially cases with monosomy 7, than in AML arising after exposure to topoisomerase II poisons. Additional evidence of RAS pathway oncogenic roles is seen in the germline *C-RAF* mutations in adult therapy-related AML.[677] C-RAF is activated by RAS binding and participates in RAS signaling.

PTPN11 *Mutations*

The RAS-RAF-MEK-ERK signaling pathway can also be activated by mutations in the SHP2 phosphatase gene, *PTPN11*. Although somatic *PTPN11* mutations are uncommon, and occur in only approximately 4% of childhood AMLs overall, *PTPN11* mutations have a predilection for the FAB M5 morphologic subtype, in which they are found in approximately 18% of cases.[644]

PI3K-AKT-mTOR *Pathway Aberrations*

The PI3K-AKT-mammalian target of rapamycin (mTOR) pathway is a signaling pathway that promotes cell proliferation and survival in leukemia. In adults, constitutive AKT activation, leading to downstream mTOR activation, contributes to the progression of MDS to AML.[678,679]

PTEN is a tumor suppressor protein that inhibits the PI3K-AKT-mTOR signaling pathway. Although *PTEN* gene mutations and loss of heterozygosity are uncommon in AML, aberrant *PTEN* mRNA splicing has been demonstrated, primarily in adult AML.[680] Constitutive PTEN phosphorylation, which results in PTEN inactivation, may contribute to AML,[681,682] whereas reduced PTEN expression may be important in MDS progression.[678] These oncogenic mechanisms may impede normal PTEN functions, which include not only attenuation of PI3-K survival signaling but also promotion of hematopoietic stem cell quiescence and preservation of the self-renewal capacity of the hematopoietic stem cell compartment.[683]

TP53 *Mutations*

TP53 is a crucial cell cycle regulatory tumor suppressor protein that senses and responds to DNA damage by regulation of the G1-S cell cycle checkpoint. *TP53* mutations are features of alkylating agent–related leukemias in adults and children.[16,59,676,684] In contrast to *RAS* mutations, *TP53* mutations are more common in therapy-related than de novo cases.[676] Segmental jumping translocations are chromosomal abnormalities in which multiple copies of various oncogenes are dispersed extrachromosomally and throughout the genome.[16] Gene amplification accompanies loss of wild-type TP53 after exposure to genotoxic agents, and *TP53* mutations and *MLL* segmental jumping translocations are strongly associated, with both occurring after alkylating agent treatment.[577] The *TP53* mutations may be of germline origin.[16,685] Similarly, *TP53* gene mutations are associated with *AML1* gene amplification or duplication in MDS and AML after alkylating agent treatment.[686] *TP53* mutations occur in de novo AML in patients affected with the Li-Fraumeni syndrome.[64,687]

NPM1 *(Nucleophosmin) Mutations*

The *NPM1* gene encodes a nucleolar shuttle protein with multiple functions in protein trafficking, preribosomal assembly, and ARF-TP53 pathway regulation.[688,689] The t(5;17) variant translocation in APL involves fusion of the *NPM1* gene to *RARA*,[460] and *NPM1* is fused to *ALK* in a subset of anaplastic large cell lymphomas.[320] Identification of *NPM1* point mutations in adult AML without karyotypic abnormalities has led to the recent analysis and discovery of *NPM1* mutations in childhood AML. The mutations cause loss of nucleolar localization with accumulation of nucleophosmin in the cytoplasm. Leukemic cells with *NPM1* mutations have a particular gene expression signature of *HOXB2*, *HOXB3*, *HOXB6*, and *HOXD4* upregulation.[690] In contrast to adult AML, in which *NPM1* mutations are present in approximately 25% to 35% of cases, and even in up to 60% of cases with a normal karyotype, the frequency of *NPM1* mutations in pediatric AML is only approximately 7% to 8%. Similar to adult AML, however, *NPM1* mutations are concentrated in patients with normal cytogenetics and, in the absence of *FLT3* ITD mutations, *NPM1* mutations are associated with an especially good prognosis.[688,689] *NPM1* mutations in AML are more common in older than younger children and in girls than boys.[689] In addition, *NPM1* mutations are significant because they may facilitate risk stratification and allow for MRD detection in cases in which no other molecular cytogenetic markers are available.[688]

Monosomy 7 and del(7q)

Monosomy 7 or del(7q) occurs with or without other cytogenetic aberrations in only approximately 4% to 5% of pediatric AMLs, but in 40% of pediatric MDSs.[657] Because of the infrequency of these aberrations, an international retrospective study was conducted to characterize –7 and del(7q) in pediatric AML and MDS. del(7q) is more common than –7 in AML cases with favorable cytogenetic features, such as t(8;21), inv(16), t(15;17), or t(9;11), whereas –7 is more common in cases with inv(3), t(9;22), i(17q), or +21. Further subgroup analysis, which was enabled by the size of the study, has demonstrated that –7 is associated with inferior survival compared with del(7q), and that survival is worse in the del(7q) subgroup without other favorable cytogenetic features compared with the del(7q) group having other favorable cytogenetic features.[657]

MicroRNA Abnormalities

Levels of a particular microRNA (miRNA), miR-223, are low in AML with the t(8;21) translocation.[430] The underlying mechanism was shown to involve epigenetic transcriptional silencing of miR-223 by the AML1-ETO fusion oncoprotein through the recruitment of several chromatin-remodeling enzymes, including DNA methyltransferases and HDAC1 to the pre–miR-223 gene.[691] The age of the patients studied was not specified (they were presumably adults), but t(8;21) is a feature of AML in adult and pediatric patients.

RELEVANCE OF GENETIC ABERRATIONS FOR TARGETED THERAPIES

The role of cancer gene alterations as therapeutic targets has been shown for various leukemias, most notably in the *BCR-ABL* oncogenic fusion in chronic myelogenous leukemia and the *PML-RARA* fusion in APL. The molecular and cytogenetic subclassification of leukemias, which also underlies their distinct biologic behaviors, forms the basis for assigning patients to appropriate treatment regimens. Examples of how molecular and cytogenetic testing have an impact on diagnosis and therapeutic decision making in pediatric ALL are highlighted in Figure 5-40. Aberrations in the leukemic blast cells influencing risk-adapted treatment encompass not only structural but also numeric karyotypic abnormalities, so much so that children with hypodiploid ALL are stratified to receive ultrahigh-risk post-induction treatment.[425] Studies of modal chromosome number by several pediatric cooperative groups have revealed an inferior outcome in hypodiploid ALL with less than 44 chromosomes, comprising the majority of hypodiploid cases, compared with hypodiploid ALL with 44 chromosomes without monosomy 7 or a dicentric chromosome.[425,692]

Analyses of MRD by quantitative real-time PCR and flow cytometry performed at the end of induction therapy are highly predictive of the risk of relapse. Therefore, MRD is used as an indication for the intensification of post-induction treatment.[693] Gene expression profiling of childhood ALL leukemic blast cells at the time of diagnosis has identified genes involved in mitotic spindle assembly, cell cycle progression, and apoptosis regulation, decreased expression of which is predictive of MRD during and following induction. It has been proposed that assays for the expression level of these genes should be incorporated into pediatric ALL risk stratification in the near future.[694,695] Similarly, AML risk stratification for treatment purposes and disease monitoring is dependent on molecular and cytogenetic testing. For example, cases of APL with t(15;17) and variants warrant special therapy, whereas inv(16) or t(16;16), and t(8;21) define a low-risk category, and the presence of monosomy 7 is considered high risk.

Advances in unraveling the cytogenetic and molecular pathology of pediatric cancer have also led to the development of several efficacious, molecularly targeted agents with a low toxicity profile. These hold promise to improve outcomes for subsets of pediatric cancers that have to date been refractory to more conventional treatments. Many new molecularly targeted agents have been developed for anti-cancer treatments over the last 10 to 15 years; their mechanisms of action targeting specific signaling cascades differ from more general mechanisms of action of conventional chemotherapy. Appropriate clinical choices are increasingly reliant on molecular cytogenetic testing for the relevant target aberrations. In addition, molecular characterization has become important for elucidating mechanisms of resistance to certain targeted treatments, which may result from reactivating mutations within a specific target (e.g., BCL-ABL),[696-698] activation of a parallel signaling pathway (e.g., as

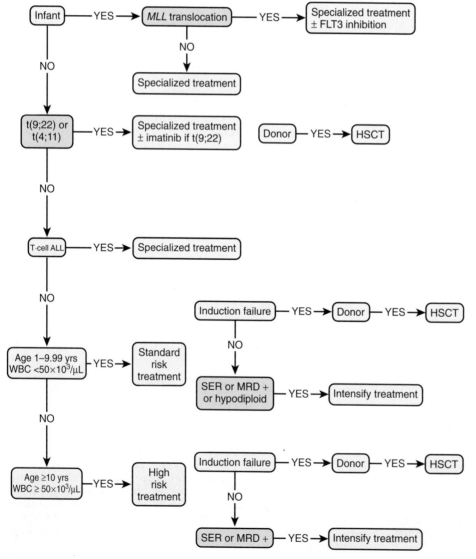

FIGURE 5-40. Molecular and cytogenetic determinants for therapeutic decisions in pediatric acute myeloid leukemia. ALL, acute lymphoblastic leukemia; HSCT, hematopoietic stem cell transplantation; WBC, white blood cell count; MRD, minimal residual disease; SER, slow early response.

is seen with FLT3 tyrosine kinase inhibition),[396] or acquisition of a tumor suppressor gene mutation[347,699] or a mutation affecting downstream signaling. Future challenges and opportunities for the field of targeted therapeutics will be in the identification not only of primary oncogenic mutations but also co-existing and acquired resistance mechanisms. Identification of the latter might then be exploited for the development of new agents. The use of automated platforms for the detection of biomarkers of responsiveness to specific targeted agents[700] is expected to become routine oncology practice soon. Although not exhaustive in scope, a discussion of molecularly targeted agents at varying stages of development follows.

All-*Trans*-Retinoic Acid

ATRA is the ligand of the RARA receptor. In the late 1980s, even before the *PML-RARA* fusion gene was characterized, it was shown in clinical trials that ATRA in pharmacologic doses comprised a highly efficacious therapy for induction of differentiation in APL, and that APL was uniquely sensitive to the therapeutic benefit of this agent.[701] The molecular basis for this responsiveness to ATRA became apparent when the *RARA* gene at chromosome band 17q21 was shown to be disrupted by the t(15;17) translocations occurring in APL.[702-704] RARA is a member of the steroid–thyroid receptor superfamily of nuclear hormone receptors that heterodimerize with retinoic X receptors (RXRs). In the presence of physiologic concentrations of retinoic acid, the RARA-RXR complex recruits co-activator proteins with histone acetyltransferase activity and functions as a transcriptional activator. In contrast, PML-RARA seems to function as a transcriptional repressor through recruitment of co-repressors with histone deacetylase activity. ATRA displaces co-repressors from the complex and recruits co-activators, restoring the granulocytic differentiation program.[705] Thus, ATRA was not only among the first molecularly targeted anticancer agents, but also the first anti-cancer agent to restore differentiation.[703,705] Furthermore, the usefulness of molecular evaluation of patient responsiveness to ATRA became apparent early.[706] More recently, it has been suggested that ATRA treatment upregulates the expression of the miRNAs miR-107 and miR-223, which are important for granulocytic differentiation, and also that ATRA treatment results in increased expression of let-7a and miR-15a–miR-16-1, which are involved in the regulation of *RAS* and *BCL-2* expression.[707] Widespread successful use of ATRA in clinical trials has led to the consideration that t(15;17) is a favorable translocation, and underscores the necessity for molecular cytogenetics in leukemia diagnosis and treatment decisions.[458] ATRA combined with anthracyclines is highly efficacious front-line treatment and has improved survival rates for children with APL.[708-710] APL is a clonal proliferative disorder of myeloid cells arrested at the promyelocytic stage of differentiation, and is highly responsive to ATRA-induced differentiation. At least five variant chromosomal translocations involving the retinoic acid receptor (*RARA*) gene have been found in APL in addition to the classic t(15;17).[457,459-462,705] The molecular cytogenetic distinction of which *RARA* fusion is involved is critical when considering ATRA treatment because APL with the t(11;17) variant translocation fusing the *PLZF* gene to *RARA* is insensitive to ATRA treatment.[457]

Arsenic Trioxide

Arsenic trioxide also exhibits therapeutic efficacy in APL. It has long been known from preclinical experiments on APL that arsenic trioxide stimulates apoptosis at high concentrations,

but promotes differentiation at lower concentrations, and similar effects have been observed in patients.[711,712] Durable remissions have even been achieved with minimal toxicities using single-agent arsenic trioxide in adult and pediatric APL, both at relapse and as front-line therapy.[713,714] ATRA primarily has been combined with chemotherapy for treating APL. The combination of ATRA and arsenic trioxide, with reliance on molecular monitoring by RT-PCR, has been incorporated into front-line APL treatment as an alternative to ATRA-chemotherapy combinations in adult APL.[715] Recently, it was discovered that the effects of arsenic trioxide on apoptosis are negatively regulated by the AKT-mTOR signaling pathway, suggesting that the anti-leukemic effects of arsenic trioxide might be enhanced even further by combining arsenic trioxide with mTOR inhibitors.[716]

Rapamycin

The mTOR protein is a pivotal signaling protein that is downstream of AKT in the PI3K-AKT-mTOR signal transduction pathway. AKT activates mTOR via the release of mTOR from repression by the tumor suppressor tuberous sclerosis proteins (TSC1 and TSC2).[717] mTOR activation, in turn, leads to phosphorylation of downstream signaling molecules, which leads to activation of the translation initiation factor eIF-4E[717] and thus to mRNA translation. Therapeutic inhibition of mTOR by rapamycin and related compounds appears to be relevant in both ALL and myeloid neoplasia.[717] In precursor B-cell ALL, rapamycin inhibits interleukin-7 (IL-7)–mediated growth signaling, which occurs through the p70 S6 kinase, a downstream target of mTOR phosphorylation.[718] Consistent with this observation, testing by the Pediatric Preclinical Testing Program (PPTP) has found high activity of single-agent rapamycin against ALL xenografts.[719] Clinical trials evaluating rapamycin and related compounds are ongoing in adult AML and other hematopoietic cancers.[717,720]

Imatinib Mesylate

Imatinib mesylate (Gleevec) is the prototype of the ever-expanding group of small-molecule drugs designed to inhibit tyrosine kinase function, finding its initial application in adults with Ph+ CML.[721] Imatinib inhibits ABL and several PDGFR-family tyrosine kinase proteins by occupying the ATP-binding pocket of the kinase domain, thereby preventing substrate phosphorylation. Imatinib is highly efficacious in CML, with complete cytogenetic responses in more than 80% of patients and improved survival.[721] Major molecular responses, defined as 1000-fold reduction in *BCR-ABL1* transcript copy number, or complete molecular responses defined as reduction of *BCR-ABL1* transcript copy number to below reverse transcriptase PCR detection, occur in more than 50% of patients with a complete response at the cytogenetic level[722,723] and are associated with a less than 1% per year risk of disease progression.[722]

Even though Ph+ leukemia is uncommon in children, the pediatric clinical experience also indicates that Ph+ leukemia, including chronic phase, advanced phase, and refractory CML, ALL, and therapy-related CML, are responsive to imatinib.[362,724-726] Therefore, the U.S. Food and Drug Administration (FDA) has approved the use of imatinib for CML in children.[727] CMML with t(5;12)(q33;p13) translocation, which generates a *TEL-PDGFRB* kinase oncogene, has also been successfully treated with imatinib.[728] The TEL-PDGFRB kinase oncoprotein is exquisitely sensitive to imatinib inhibition.[729,730]

The knowledge that secondary *BCR-ABL* kinase domain mutations underlie treatment failures associated with imatinib resistance has led to the development of the dual SRC and ABL tyrosine kinase inhibitor dasatinib.[696-698] This second-generation tyrosine kinase inhibitor is active against many imatinib-resistant BCR-ABL oncoproteins, except for cases with particular *BCR-ABL* kinase domain mutations. The use of dasatinib has been approved for adult imatinib-resistant CML[697] and this agent has the added advantage of superior CNS penetration.[731] The specific mechanisms of resistance to imatinib and dasatinib have implications for the integration of detailed molecular cytogenetic testing into clinical practice.[697,698] Importantly, the adult experience has suggested that dasatinib can also induce cytogenetic responses in Ph+ ALL.[732] When the PPTP evaluated the potential usefulness of dasatinib by screening in xenograft tumor models, the most significant activity was in Ph+ ALL.[733]

FLT3 Inhibitors

Aberrant FLT3 signaling in various forms of leukemia has prompted the development of agents to silence this protein. There has been substantial progress in testing FLT3 inhibitors in vitro and in murine models.[108,398,665,666,734,735] The demonstration that FLT3 inhibition selectively kills childhood ALL cells with high levels of FLT3 expression and exhibits synergy with anti-leukemia cytotoxic drugs[391,736] has formed the basis for a Children's Oncology Group clinical trial incorporating FLT3 inhibition into combination chemotherapy for the front-line treatment of infant ALL. The molecular characterization of specific FLT3 alterations is important because leukemias with different types of FLT3 alterations exhibit different sensitivities to the various small-molecule inhibitors targeting this protein.[395] Another approach to silencing FLT3 signaling currently in development involves the use of anti-FLT3 monoclonal antibodies, offering the added benefit of NK cell–mediated antibody-dependent cytotoxicity in leukemias with increased FLT3 expression.[737]

SHP2 Inhibitors

Drug screening performed via computer simulation has recently identified a small-molecule inhibitor that binds to the catalytic site of the SHP2 protein tyrosine phosphatase and blocks SHP2-dependent phosphorylation of the Erk1/2 MAP kinases. This agent is expected to be developed for the treatment of myeloid diseases with *PTPN11 (SHP2)* mutations.[738]

Pro-apoptotic Agents

Alterations in the intrinsic (mitochondrial) cell death pathway are relevant because various molecularly targeted strategies directed at this pathway are already in clinical development in adults and are now in preclinical development for pediatric cancer.[406,739,740] The interaction of a multi-domain anti-apoptotic BCL-2 family protein with conserved BH3 sequence motifs of a pro-apoptotic BH3-only BCL-2 family protein inhibits the biologic activity of both binding partners.[741-745] Ongoing efforts of the PPTP have suggested that potent cytotoxicity can be achieved in pediatric ALL using a BH3 mimetic (ABT 263) as a single agent in vitro and in pediatric ALL xenograft murine models.[739] Of particular interest, when the in vitro activity of the related compound ABT 737 was evaluated in T-cell ALL and pre-B ALL cell lines, including one cell line with t(4;11), synergistic cytotoxicity was observed with antileukemic chemotherapy combinations, and chemosensitization could sometimes be achieved where there was resistance to the chemotherapy alone.[740]

Gemtuzumab Ozogamicin

Gemtuzumab ozogamicin consists of a humanized anti-CD33 antibody linked to the antitumor antibiotic calicheamicin. CD33 positivity is observed in most subtypes of pediatric AML. The results of clinical testing of gemtuzumab ozogamicin for the induction of remission and in conjunction with intensive post-induction therapy for relapsed or refractory CD33+ AML in children are encouraging.[746,747] This agent will be tested further during standard induction therapy for pediatric AML.[747] CD33 might also serve as a therapeutic target in certain subtypes of refractory CD33+ pediatric ALL, including those with *MLL* gene rearrangements, which express myeloid surface markers.[746]

Lenalidomide

Although more relevant to adults than children, the thalidomide analogue lenalidomide was recently shown to induce a gene expression signature similar to *RPS14* knockdown, and lenalidomide is now specifically indicated for MDS characterized by the 5q– syndrome.[748] Importantly, the characteristic refractory anemia of patients likely to benefit from this agent can be identified by a particular gene expression profile.[748]

REFERENCES

1. Seabright M. A rapid banding technique for human chromosomes. Lancet. 1971;2:971-972.
2. Sperling K, Wiesner R. A rapid banding technique for routine use in human and comparative cytogenetics. Humangenetik. 1972;15:349-353.
3. Yunis JJ, Sanchez O. G-banding and chromosome structure. Chromosoma. 1973;44:15-23.
4. Reeves BR. Cytogenetics of malignant lymphomas. Studies utilising a Giemsa-banding technique. Humangenetik. 1973;20:231-250.
5. Fletcher JA, Kozakewich HP, Hoffer FA, et al. Diagnostic relevance of clonal cytogenetic aberrations in malignant soft-tissue tumors. N Engl J Med. 1991;324:436-442.
6. Rubin BP, Chen CJ, Morgan TW, et al. Congenital mesoblastic nephroma t(12;15) is associated with ETV6- NTRK3 gene fusion: cytogenetic and molecular relationship to congenital (infantile) fibrosarcoma. Am J Pathol. 1998;153:1451-1458.
7. Eguchi M, Eguchi-Ishimae M, Tojo A, et al. Fusion of ETV6 to neurotrophin-3 receptor TRKC in acute myeloid leukemia with t(12;15)(p13;q25). Blood. 1999;93:1355-1363.
8. Sreekantaiah C, Appaji L, Hazarika D. Cytogenetic characterisation of small round cell tumours using fine needle aspiration. J Clin Pathol. 1992;45:728-730.
9. Akerman M, Dreinhofer K, Rydholm A, et al. Cytogenetic studies on fine-needle aspiration samples from osteosarcoma and Ewing's sarcoma. Diagn Cytopathol. 1996;15:17-22.
10. Hoffer FA, Gianturco LE, Fletcher JA, Grier HE. Percutaneous biopsy of peripheral primitive neuroectodermal tumors and Ewing's sarcomas for cytogenetic analysis. Am J Roentgenol. 1994;162:1141-1142.

11. Saboorian MH, Ashfaq R, Vandersteenhoven JJ, Schneider NR. Cytogenetics as an adjunct in establishing a definitive diagnosis of synovial sarcoma by fine-needle aspiration. Cancer. 1997;81: 187-192.

12. Cajulis RS, Frias-Hidvegi D. Detection of numerical chromosomal abnormalities in malignant cells in fine needle aspirates by fluorescence in situ hybridization of interphase cell nuclei with chromosome-specific probes. Acta Cytol. 1993;37:391-396.

13. Cajulis RS, Kotliar S, Haines GK, et al. Comparative study of interphase cytogenetics, flow cytometric analysis, and nuclear grade of fine-needle aspirates of breast carcinoma. Diagn Cytopathol. 1994;11:151-158.

14. Taub R, Kirsch I, Morton C, et al. Translocation of the c-myc gene into the immunoglobulin heavy chain locus in human Burkitt lymphoma and murine plasmacytoma cells. Proc Natl Acad Sci U S A. 1982;79:7837-7841.

15. Gu Y, Cimino G, Alder H, et al. The (4;11)(q21;q23) chromosome translocations in acute leukemias involve the VDJ recombinase. Proc Natl Acad Sci U S A. 1992;89:10464-10468.

16. Felix CA, Megonigal MD, Chervinsky DS, et al. Association of germline p53 mutation with *MLL* segmental jumping translocation in treatment-related leukemia. Blood. 1998;91:4451-4456.

17. Ried T. Interphase cytogenetics and its role in molecular diagnostics of solid tumors. Am J Pathol. 1998;152:325-327.

18. Hsi BL, Xiao S, Fletcher JA. Chromogenic in situ hybridization and FISH in pathology. Methods Mol Biol. 2002;204:343-351.

19. Kim SY, Lee JS, Ro JY, et al. Interphase cytogenetics in paraffin sections of lung tumors by non- isotopic in situ hybridization. Mapping genotype/phenotype heterogeneity. Am J Pathol. 1993;142:307-317.

20. Schofield DE, Fletcher JA. Trisomy 12 in pediatric granulosa-stromal cell tumors. Demonstration by a modified method of fluorescence in situ hybridization on paraffin-embedded material. Am J Pathol. 1992;141:1265-1269.

21. Paternoster SF, Brockman SR, McClure RF, et al. A new method to extract nuclei from paraffin-embedded tissue to study lymphomas using interphase fluorescence in situ hybridization. Am J Pathol. 2002;160:1967-1972.

22. Maarek O, Thomas G, Aurias A. Importance of the DIRVISH technique for detecting microdeletions. Ann Genet. 1996;39: 173-175.

23. Heng HH, Tsui LC. High resolution free chromatin/DNA fiber fluorescent in situ hybridization. J Chromatogr A. 1998;806: 219-229.

24. Kallioniemi A, Kallioniemi OP, Sudar D, et al. Comparative genomic hybridization for molecular cytogenetic analysis of solid tumors. Science. 1992;258:818-821.

25. Albertson DG, Ylstra B, Segraves R, et al. Quantitative mapping of amplicon structure by array CGH identifies CYP24 as a candidate oncogene. Nat Genet. 2000;25:144-146.

26. Schrock E, du Manoir S, Veldman T, et al. Multicolor spectral karyotyping of human chromosomes. Science. 1996;273:494-497.

27. Veldman T, Vignon C, Schrock E, et al. Hidden chromosome abnormalities in haematological malignancies detected by multicolour spectral karyotyping. Nat Genet. 1997;15:406-410.

28. Macville M, Schrock E, Padilla-Nash H, et al. Comprehensive and definitive molecular cytogenetic characterization of HeLa cells by spectral karyotyping. Cancer Res. 1999;59:141-150.

29. Geurts van Kessel A, de Bruijn D, Hermsen L, et al. Masked t(X;18)(p11;q11) in a biphasic synovial sarcoma revealed by FISH and RT-PCR. Genes Chromosomes Cancer. 1998;23: 198-201.

30. Ambros IM, Benard J, Boavida M, et al. Quality assessment of genetic markers used for therapy stratification. J Clin Oncol. 2003;21:2077-2084.

31. Bourdeaut F, Freneaux P, Thuille B, et al. hSNF5/INI1-deficient tumours and rhabdoid tumours are convergent but not fully overlapping entities. J Pathol. 2007;211:323-330.

32. Mullis K, Faloona F, Scharf S, et al. Specific enzymatic amplification of DNA in vitro: the polymerase chain reaction. Cold Spring Harb Symp Quant Biol. 1986;51(Pt 1):263-273.

33. Gruis NA, Abeln EC, Bardoel AF, et al. PCR-based microsatellite polymorphisms in the detection of loss of heterozygosity in fresh and archival tumour tissue. Br J Cancer. 1993;68:308-313.

34. Simpson D, Crosby RM, Skopek TR. A method for specific cloning and sequencing of human hprt cDNA for mutation analysis. Biochem Biophys Res Commun. 1988;151:487-492.

35. Miller WH Jr, Kakizuka A, Frankel SR, et al. Reverse transcription polymerase chain reaction for the rearranged retinoic acid receptor alpha clarifies diagnosis and detects minimal residual disease in acute promyelocytic leukemia. Proc Natl Acad Sci U S A. 1992;89:2694-2698.

36. Downing JR, Head DR, Curcio-Brint AM, et al. An AML1/ETO fusion transcript is consistently detected by RNA- based polymerase chain reaction in acute myelogenous leukemia containing the (8;21)(q22;q22) translocation. Blood. 1993;81:2860-2865.

37. de Alava E, Kawai A, Healey JH, et al. EWS-FLI1 fusion transcript structure is an independent determinant of prognosis in Ewing's sarcoma. J Clin Oncol. 1998;16:1248-1255.

38. Lin PP, Brody RI, Hamelin AC, et al. Differential transactivation by alternative EWS-FLI1 fusion proteins correlates with clinical heterogeneity in Ewing's sarcoma. Cancer Res. 1999;59:1428-1432.

39. Zoubek A, Dockhorn-Dworniczak B, Delattre O, et al. Does expression of different EWS chimeric transcripts define clinically distinct risk groups of Ewing's tumor patients? J Clin Oncol. 1996;14:1245-1251.

40. Mezzelani A, Mariani L, Tamborini E, et al. SYT-SSX fusion genes and prognosis in synovial sarcoma. Br J Cancer. 2001;85:1535-1539.

41. Ladanyi M, Antonescu CR, Leung DH, et al. Impact of SYT-SSX fusion type on the clinical behavior of synovial sarcoma: a multi-institutional retrospective study of 243 patients. Cancer Res. 2002;62:135-140.

42. Morishita T, Bolander ME, Zhang K, et al. A method for accurate detection of translocation junctions in Ewing's family of tumors. Mol Biotechnol. 2001;18:97-104.

43. Strehl S, Konig M, Meyer C, et al. Molecular dissection of t(11;17) in acute myeloid leukemia reveals a variety of gene fusions with heterogeneous fusion transcripts and multiple splice variants. Genes Chromosomes Cancer. 2006;45:1041-1049.

44. Hilden JM, Dinndorf PA, Meerbaum SO, et al. Analysis of prognostic factors of acute lymphoblastic leukemia in infants: report on CCG 1953 from the Children's Oncology Group. Blood. 2006;108:441-451.

45. Megonigal MD, Rappaport EF, Wilson RB, et al. Panhandle PCR for cDNA: a rapid method for isolation of *MLL* fusion transcripts involving unknown partner genes. Proc Natl Acad Sci U S A. 2000;97:9597-9602.

46. Taketani T, Taki T, Shibuya N, et al. The *HOXD11* gene is fused to the *NUP98* gene in acute myeloid leukemia with t(2;11)(q31;p15). Cancer Res. 2002;62:33-37.

47. Megonigal MD, Rappaport EF, Jones DH, et al. Panhandle PCR strategy to amplify *MLL* genomic breakpoints in treatment-related leukemias. Proc Natl Acad Sci U S A. 1997;94:11583-11588.

48. Raffini LJ, Slater DJ, Rappaport EF, et al. Panhandle and reverse-panhandle PCR enable cloning of der(11) and der(other) genomic breakpoint junctions of *MLL* translocations and identify complex translocation of *MLL, AF-4,* and *CDK6.* Proc Natl Acad Sci U S A. 2002;99:4568-4573.

49. Robinson BW, Slater DJ, Felix CA. BglII-based panhandle and reverse panhandle PCR approaches increase capability for cloning der(II) and der(other) genomic breakpoint junctions of MLL translocations. Genes Chromosomes Cancer. 2006;45:740-753.

50. Meyer C, Schneider B, Jakob S, et al. The MLL recombinome of acute leukemias. Leukemia. 2006;20:777-784.

51. Meyer C, Schneider B, Reichel M, et al. Diagnostic tool for the identification of MLL rearrangements including unknown partner genes. Proc Natl Acad Sci U S A. 2005;102:449-454.

52. Robinson BW, Cheung NK, Kolaris CP, et al. Prospective tracing of MLL-FRYL clone with low MEIS1 expression from emergence during neuroblastoma treatment to diagnosis of myelodysplastic syndrome. Blood. 2008;111:3802-3812.

53. Pernas-Alonso R, Morelli F, di Porzio U, Perrone-Capano C. Multiplex semi-quantitative reverse transcriptase-polymerase chain reaction of low abundance neuronal mRNAs. Brain Res Brain Res Protoc. 1999;4:395-406.

54. Look AT, Hayes FA, Shuster JJ, et al. Clinical relevance of tumor cell ploidy and N-myc gene amplification in childhood neuroblastoma: a Pediatric Oncology Group study. J Clin Oncol. 1991;9:581-591.

55. Ross JS, Fletcher JA, Linette GP, et al. The Her-2/neu gene and protein in breast cancer 2003: biomarker and target of therapy. Oncologist. 2003;8:307-325.

56. Tanaka K, Arif M, Eguchi M, Kyo T, et al. Frequent jumping translocations of chromosomal segments involving the ABL oncogene alone or in combination with CD3-MLL genes in secondary leukemias. Blood. 1997;89:596-600.

57. Mackall CL, Meltzer PS, Helman LJ. Focus on sarcomas. Cancer Cell. 2002;2:175-178.

58. Oliveira AM, Fletcher JA. Translocation Breakpoints in Cancer. Encyclopedia of the Human Genome. London, Nature Publishing, 2002,

59. Christiansen DH, Andersen MK, Pedersen-Bjergaard J. Mutations with loss of heterozygosity of p53 are common in therapy-related myelodysplasia and acute myeloid leukemia after exposure to alkylating agents and significantly associated with deletion or loss of 5q, a complex karyotype, and a poor prognosis. J Clin Oncol. 2001;19:1405-1413.

60. Felix CA, Kolaris CP, Osheroff N. Topoisomerase II and the etiology of chromosomal translocations. DNA Repair (Amst). 2006;5:1093-1108.

61. van G, Hoeijmakers JH, Kanaar R. Chromosomal stability and the DNA double-stranded break connection. Nat Rev Genet. 2001;2:196-206.

62. Rotman G, Shiloh Y. ATM: from gene to function. Hum Mol Genet. 1998;7:1555-1563.

63. Ahmad SI, Hanaoka F, Kirk SH. Molecular biology of Fanconi anaemia—an old problem, a new insight. Bioessays. 2002;24:439-448.

64. Malkin D, Li FP, Strong LC, et al. Germ line p53 mutations in a familial syndrome of breast cancer, sarcomas, and other neoplasms. Science. 1990;250:1233-1238.

65. Rowley JD. The critical role of chromosome translocations in human leukemias. Annu Rev Genet. 1998;32:495-519.

66. Fugazzola L, Pilotti S, Pinchera A, et al. Oncogenic rearrangements of the RET proto-oncogene in papillary thyroid carcinomas from children exposed to the Chernobyl nuclear accident. Cancer Res. 1995;55:5617-5620.

67. Sadetzki S, Calderon-Margalit R, Modan B, et al. Ret/PTC activation in benign and malignant thyroid tumors arising in a population exposed to low-dose external-beam irradiation in childhood. J Clin Endocrinol Metab. 2004;89:2281-2289.

68. Nikiforova MN, Stringer JR, Blough R, et al. Proximity of chromosomal loci that participate in radiation-induced rearrangements in human cells. Science. 2000;290:138-141.

69. Macarenco RS, Zamolyi R, Franco MF, et al. Genomic gains of COL1A1-PDFGB occur in the histologic evolution of giant cell fibroblastoma into dermatofibrosarcoma protuberans. Genes Chromosomes Cancer. 2008;47:260-265.

70. O'Brien KP, Seroussi E, Dal Cin P, et al. Various regions within the alpha-helical domain of the COL1A1 gene are fused to the second exon of the PDGFB gene in dermatofibrosarcomas and giant-cell fibroblastomas. Genes Chromosomes Cancer. 1998;23:187-193.

71. Barr FG. Gene fusions involving PAX and FOX family members in alveolar rhabdomyosarcoma. Oncogene. 2001;20:5736-5746.

72. Look AT. Oncogenic transcription factors in the human acute leukemias. Science. 1997;278:1059-1064.

73. Linggi BE, Brandt SJ, Sun ZW, Hiebert SW. Translating the histone code into leukemia. J Cell Biochem. 2005;96:938-950.

74. Meyers S, Downing JR, Hiebert SW. Identification of AML-1 and the (8;21) translocation protein (AML- 1/ETO) as sequence-specific DNA-binding proteins: the runt homology domain is required for DNA binding and protein-protein interactions. Mol Cell Biol. 1993;13:6336-6345.

75. Hiebert SW, Reed-Inderbitzin EF, Amann J, et al. The t(8;21) fusion protein contacts co-repressors and histone deacetylases to repress the transcription of the p14ARF tumor suppressor. Blood Cells Mol Dis. 2003;30:177-183.

76. Linggi B, Muller-Tidow C, van de LL, et al. The t(8;21) fusion protein, AML1 ETO, specifically represses the transcription of the p14(ARF) tumor suppressor in acute myeloid leukemia. Nat Med. 2002;8:743-750.

77. Ito Y. RUNX genes in development and cancer: regulation of viral gene expression and the discovery of RUNX family genes. Adv Cancer Res. 2008;99:33-76.

78. Alcalay M, Orleth A, Sebastiani C, et al. Common themes in the pathogenesis of acute myeloid leukemia. Oncogene. 2001;20:5680-5694.

79. Huang G, Shigesada K, Wee HJ, et al. Molecular basis for a dominant inactivation of RUNX1/AML1 by the leukemogenic inversion 16 chimera. Blood. 2004;103:3200-3207.

80. Hess JL. MLL: a histone methyltransferase disrupted in leukemia. Trends Mol Med. 2004;10:500-507.

81. Arvand A, Denny CT. Biology of EWS/ETS fusions in Ewing's family tumors. Oncogene. 2001;20:5747-5754.

82. Gerald WL, Rosai J, Ladanyi M. Characterization of the genomic breakpoint and chimeric transcripts in the EWS-WT1 gene fusion of desmoplastic small round cell tumor. Proc Natl Acad Sci U S A. 1995;92:1028-1032.

83. Sozzi G, Bongarzone I, Miozzo M, et al. A t(10;17) translocation creates the RET/PTC2 chimeric transforming sequence in papillary thyroid carcinoma. Genes Chromosomes Cancer. 1994;9:244-250.

84. Argani P, Ladanyi M. Translocation carcinomas of the kidney. Clin Lab Med. 2005;25:363-378.

85. Kroll TG, Sarraf P, Pecciarini L, et al. PAX8-PPARgamma1 fusion oncogene in human thyroid carcinoma. Science. 2000;289:1357-1360.

86. French CA, Kutok JL, Faquin WC, et al. Midline carcinoma of children and young adults with NUT rearrangement. J Clin Oncol. 2004;22:4135-4139.

87. Deininger MW, Goldman JM, Melo JV. The molecular biology of chronic myeloid leukemia. Blood. 2000;96:3343-3356.

88. Yoshida A, Kishi S, Kita K, et al. Molecular analysis of a case of Philadelphia chromosome-positive acute myeloid leukemia. Anticancer Res. 1997;17:625-628.

89. Knezevich SR, McFadden DE, Tao W, et al. A novel ETV6-NTRK3 gene fusion in congenital fibrosarcoma. Nat Genet. 1998;18:184-187.

90. Lawrence B, Perez-Atayde A, Hibbard MK, et al. TPM3-ALK and TPM4-ALK oncogenes in inflammatory myofibroblastic tumors. Am J Pathol. 2000;157:377-384.

91. Falini B. Anaplastic large cell lymphoma: pathological, molecular and clinical features. Br J Haematol. 2001;114:741-760.

92. Bridge JA, Kanamori M, Ma Z, et al. Fusion of the ALK gene to the clathrin heavy chain gene, CLTC, in inflammatory myofibroblastic tumor. Am J Pathol. 2001;159:411-415.

92a. George RE, Sanda T, Hanna M, et al. Activating mutations in ALK provide a therapeutic target in neuroblastoma. Nature. 2008;455:975-978.

92b. Janoueix-Lerosey I, Lequin D, Brugières L, et al. Somatic and germline activating mutations of the ALK kinase receptor in neuroblastoma. Nature. 2008;455:967-970.

92c. Mossé YP, Laudenslager M, Longo L, et al. Identification of ALK as a major familial neuroblastoma predisposition gene. Nature. 2008;455:930-935.

93. Pierotti MA, Vigneri P, Bongarzone I. Rearrangements of RET and NTRK1 tyrosine kinase receptors in papillary thyroid carcinomas. Recent Results Cancer Res. 1998;154:237-247.

94. Greco A, Roccato E, Pierotti MA. TRK oncogenes in papillary thyroid carcinoma. Cancer Treat Res. 2004;122:207-219.

95. Simon MP, Pedeutour F, Sirvent N, et al. Deregulation of the platelet-derived growth factor B-chain gene via fusion with collagen gene COL1A1 in dermatofibrosarcoma protuberans and giant-cell fibroblastoma. Nat Genet. 1997;15:95-98.

96. Shmookler BM, Enzinger FM, Weiss SW. Giant cell fibroblastoma. A juvenile form of dermatofibrosarcoma protuberans. Cancer. 1989;64:2154-2161.

97. Kuppers R, la-Favera R. Mechanisms of chromosomal translocations in B cell lymphomas. Oncogene. 2001;20:5580-5594.

98. Stamatopoulos K, Kosmas C, Belessi C, et al. Molecular insights into the immunopathogenesis of follicular lymphoma. Immunol Today. 2000;21:298-305.

99. Lorsbach RB, Shay-Seymore D, Moore J, et al. Clinicopathologic analysis of follicular lymphoma occurring in children. Blood. 2002;99:1959-1964.

100. Pui CH, Robison LL, Look AT. Acute lymphoblastic leukaemia. Lancet. 2008;371:1030-1043.

101. Ferrando AA, Herblot S, Palomero T, et al. Biallelic transcriptional activation of oncogenic transcription factors in T-cell acute lymphoblastic leukemia. Blood. 2004;103:1909-1911.

102. Voz ML, Agten NS, Van de Ven WJ, Kas K. PLAG1, the main translocation target in pleomorphic adenoma of the salivary glands, is a positive regulator of IGF-II. Cancer Res. 2000;60:106-113.

103. Hibbard MK, Kozakewich HP, Dal Cin P, et al. PLAG1 fusion oncogenes in lipoblastoma. Cancer Res. 2000;60:4869-4872.

104. Gisselsson D, Hibbard MK, Dal CP, et al. PLAG1 alterations in lipoblastoma: involvement in varied mesenchymal cell types and evidence for alternative oncogenic mechanisms. Am J Pathol. 2001;159:955-962.

105. Ayton PM, Cleary ML. Molecular mechanisms of leukemogenesis mediated by MLL fusion proteins. Oncogene. 2001;20:5695-5707.

106. Pui CH, Kane JR, Crist WM. Biology and treatment of infant leukemias. Leukemia. 1995;9:762-769.

107. Isaacs H Jr. Fetal and neonatal leukemia. J Pediatr Hematol Oncol. 2003;25:348-361.

108. Armstrong SA, Kung AL, Mabon ME, et al. Inhibition of FLT3 in MLL. Validation of a therapeutic target identified by gene expression based classification. Cancer Cell. 2003;3:173-183.

109. Limpens J, Stad R, Vos C, et al. Lymphoma-associated translocation t(14;18) in blood B cells of normal individuals. Blood. 1995;85:2528-2536.

110. Limpens J, de Jong D, van Krieken JH, et al. Bcl-2/JH rearrangements in benign lymphoid tissues with follicular hyperplasia. Oncogene. 1991;6:2271-2276.

111. Barr FG. Translocations, cancer and the puzzle of specificity. Nat Genet. 1998;19:121-124.

112. Daley GQ, McLaughlin J, Witte ON, Baltimore D. The CML-specific P210 bcr/abl protein, unlike v-abl, does not transform NIH/3T3 cells. Science. 1987;237:532-535.

113. Delattre O, Zucman J, Plougastel B, et al. Gene fusion with an ETS DNA-binding domain caused by chromosome translocation in human tumours. Nature. 1992;359:162-165.

114. Turc-Carel C, Philip I, Berger MP, et al. Chromosome study of Ewing's sarcoma (ES) cell lines. Consistency of a reciprocal translocation t(11;22)(q24;q12). Cancer Genet Cytogenet. 1984;12:1-19.

115. Turc-Carel C, Aurias A, Mugneret F, et al. Chromosomes in Ewing's sarcoma. I. An evaluation of 85 cases of remarkable consistency of t(11;22)(q24;q12). Cancer Genet Cytogenet. 1988;32:229-238.

116. Ewen ME, Ludlow JW, Marsilio E, et al. An N-terminal transformation-governing sequence of SV40 large T antigen contributes to the binding of both p110Rb and a second cellular protein, p120. Cell. 1989;58:257-267.

117. Janknecht R: EWS-ETS oncoproteins: the linchpins of Ewing tumors. Gene. 2005;363:1-14.

118. Buckler AJ, Chang DD, Graw SL, et al. Exon amplification: a strategy to isolate mammalian genes based on RNA splicing. Proc Natl Acad Sci U S A. 1991;88:4005-4009.

119. Jeon IS, Davis JN, Braun BS, et al. A variant Ewing's sarcoma translocation (7;22) fuses the EWS gene to the ETS gene ETV1. Oncogene. 1995;10:1229-1234.

120. Peter M, Couturier J, Pacquement H, et al. A new member of the ETS family fused to EWS in Ewing tumors. Oncogene. 1997;14:1159-1164.

121. Kaneko Y, Yoshida K, Handa M, et al. Fusion of an ETS-family gene, EIAF, to EWS by t(17;22)(q12;q12) chromosome translocation in an undifferentiated sarcoma of infancy. Genes Chromosomes Cancer. 1996;15:115-121.

122. Ishida S, Yoshida K, Kaneko Y, et al. The genomic breakpoint and chimeric transcripts in the EWSR1- ETV4/E1AF gene fusion in Ewing sarcoma. Cytogenet Cell Genet. 1998;82:278-283.

123. Ng TL, O'Sullivan MJ, Pallen CJ, et al. Ewing sarcoma with novel translocation t(2;16) producing an in-frame fusion of FUS and FEV. J Mol Diagn. 2007;9:459-463.

124. Davison JM, Morgan TW, Hsi BL, et al. Subtracted, unique-sequence, in situ hybridization: experimental and diagnostic applications. Am J Pathol. 1998;153:1401-1409.

125. Barr FG, Chatten J, D'Cruz CM, et al. Molecular assays for chromosomal translocations in the diagnosis of pediatric soft tissue sarcomas. JAMA. 1995;273:553-557.

126. Fletcher JA. Ewing's sarcoma oncogene structure: a novel prognostic marker? J Clin Oncol. 1998;16:1241-1243.

127. Teitell MA, Thompson AD, Sorensen PH, et al. EWS/ETS fusion genes induce epithelial and neuroectodermal differentiation in NIH 3T3 fibroblasts. Lab Invest. 1999;79:1535-1543.

128. Khan J, Bittner ML, Saal LH, et al. cDNA microarrays detect activation of a myogenic transcription program by the PAX3-FKHR fusion oncogene. Proc Natl Acad Sci U S A. 1999;96:13264-13269.

129. Huang HY, Illei PB, Zhao Z, et al. Ewing sarcomas with p53 mutation or p16/p14ARF homozygous deletion: a highly lethal subset associated with poor chemoresponse. J Clin Oncol. 2005;23:548-558.

130. Sebire NJ, Malone M. Myogenin and MyoD1 expression in paediatric rhabdomyosarcomas. J Clin Pathol. 2003;56:412-416.

131. Galili N, Davis RJ, Fredericks WJ, et al. Fusion of a fork head domain gene to PAX3 in the solid tumour alveolar rhabdomyosarcoma. Nat Genet. 1993;5:230-235.

132. Barr FG, Galili N, Holick J, et al. Rearrangement of the PAX3 paired box gene in the paediatric solid tumour alveolar rhabdomyosarcoma. Nat Genet. 1993;3:113-117.

133. Shapiro DN, Sublett JE, Li B, et al. Fusion of PAX3 to a member of the forkhead family of transcription factors in human alveolar rhabdomyosarcoma. Cancer Res. 1993;53:5108-5112.

134. Davis RJ, D'Cruz CM, Lovell MA, et al. Fusion of PAX7 to FKHR by the variant t(1;13)(p36;q14) translocation in alveolar rhabdomyosarcoma. Cancer Res. 1994;54:2869-2872.

135. Davis RJ, Barr FG. Fusion genes resulting from alternative chromosomal translocations are overexpressed by gene-specific mechanisms in alveolar rhabdomyosarcoma. Proc Natl Acad Sci U S A. 1997;94:8047-8051.

136. Fredericks WJ, Galili N, Mukhopadhyay S, et al. The PAX3-FKHR fusion protein created by the t(2;13) translocation in alveolar rhabdomyosarcomas is a more potent transcriptional activator than PAX3. Mol Cell Biol. 1995;15:1522-1535.

137. Bennicelli JL, Fredericks WJ, Wilson RB, et al. Wild type PAX3 protein and the PAX3-FKHR fusion protein of alveolar rhabdomyosarcoma contain potent, structurally distinct transcriptional activation domains. Oncogene. 1995;11:119-130.

138. Sorensen PH, Lynch JC, Qualman SJ, et al. PAX3-FKHR and PAX7-FKHR gene fusions are prognostic indicators in alveolar rhabdomyosarcoma: a report from the children's oncology group. J Clin Oncol. 2002;20:2672-2679.

139. Turc-Carel C, Dal Cin P, Limon J, et al. Involvement of chromosome X in primary cytogenetic change in human neoplasia: nonrandom translocation in synovial sarcoma. Proc Natl Acad Sci U S A. 1987;84:1981-1985.

140. Limon J, Mrozek K, Mandahl N, et al: Cytogenetics of synovial sarcoma: presentation of ten new cases and review of the literature. Genes Chromosom Cancer. 1991;3:338-345.

141. Clark J, Rocques PJ, Crew AJ, et al. Identification of novel genes, SYT and SSX, involved in the t(X;18)(p11.2;q11.2) translocation found in human synovial sarcoma. Nat Genet. 1994;7:502-508.

142. Tornkvist M, Brodin B, Bartolazzi A, Larsson O. A novel type of SYT/SSX fusion: methodological and biological implications. Mod Pathol. 2002;15:679-685.

143. Janz M, de Leeuw B, Weghuis DO, et al. Interphase cytogenetic analysis of distinct X-chromosomal translocation breakpoints in synovial sarcoma. J Pathol. 1995;175:391-396.

144. Shipley JM, Clark J, Crew AJ, et al: The t(X;18)(p11.2;q11.2) translocation found in human synovial sarcomas involves two distinct loci on the X chromosome. Oncogene. 1994;9:1447-1453.

145. Kawai A, Woodruff J, Healey JH, et al. SYT-SSX gene fusion as a determinant of morphology and prognosis in synovial sarcoma. N Engl J Med. 1998;338:153-160.

146. Saito T, Nagai M, Ladanyi M. SYT-SSX1 and SYT-SSX2 interfere with repression of E-cadherin by snail and slug: a potential mechanism for aberrant mesenchymal to epithelial transition in human synovial sarcoma. Cancer Res. 2006;66:6919-6927.

147. Eid JE, Kung AL, Scully R, Livingston DM. p300 interacts with the nuclear proto-oncoprotein SYT as part of the active control of cell adhesion. Cell. 2000;102:839-848.

148. Kato H, Tjernberg A, Zhang W, et al. SYT associates with human SNF/SWI complexes and the C-terminal region of its fusion partner SSX1 targets histones. J Biol Chem. 2002;277:5498-5505.

149. Pretto D, Barco R, Rivera J, et al. The synovial sarcoma translocation protein SYT-SSX2 recruits beta-catenin to the nucleus and associates with it in an active complex. Oncogene. 2006;25:3661-3669.

150. Mrozek K, Karakousis CP, Bloomfield CD. Band 11q13 is nonrandomly rearranged in hibernomas. Genes Chromosom Cancer. 1994;9:145-147.

151. Turc-Carel C, Limon J, Dal Cin P, et al. Cytogenetic studies of adipose tissue tumors. II. Recurrent reciprocal translocation t(12;16)(q13;p11) in myxoid liposarcomas. Cancer Genet Cytogenet. 1986;23:291-299.

152. Sreekantaiah C, Karakousis CP, Leong SP, Sandberg AA. Cytogenetic findings in liposarcoma correlate with histopathologic subtypes. Cancer. 1992;69:2484-2495.

153. Fletcher CD, Akerman M, Dal Cin P, et al. Correlation between clinicopathological features and karyotype in lipomatous tumors. A report of 178 cases from the Chromosomes and Morphology (CHAMP) Collaborative Study Group. Am J Pathol. 1996;148:623-630.

154. Hisaoka M, Tsuji S, Morimitsu Y, et al. Detection of TLS/FUS-CHOP fusion transcripts in myxoid and round cell liposarcomas by nested reverse transcription-polymerase chain reaction using archival paraffin-embedded tissues. Diagn Mol Pathol. 1998;7:96-101.

155. Kuroda M, Ishida T, Horiuchi H, et al. Chimeric TLS/FUS-CHOP gene expression and the heterogeneity of its junction in human myxoid and round cell liposarcoma. Am J Pathol. 1995;147:1221-1227.

156. Aman P, Ron D, Mandahl N, et al. Rearrangement of the transcription factor gene CHOP in myxoid liposarcomas with t(12;16)(q13;p11). Genes Chromosom Cancer. 1992;5:278-285.

157. Crozat A, Aman P, Mandahl N, Ron D. Fusion of CHOP to a novel RNA-binding protein in human myxoid liposarcoma. Nature. 1993;363:640-644.

158. Mandahl N, Heim S, Arheden K, et al. Rings, dicentrics, and telomeric association in histiocytomas. Cancer Genet Cytogenet. 1988;30:23-33.

159. Turc-Carel C, Dal Cin P, Rao U, et al. Recurrent breakpoints at 9q31 and 22q12.2 in extraskeletal myxoid chondrosarcoma. Cancer Genet Cytogenet. 1988;30:145-150.

160. Grosso F, Jones RL, Demetri GD, et al. Efficacy of trabectedin (ecteinascidin-743) in advanced pretreated myxoid liposarcomas: a retrospective study. Lancet Oncol. 2007;8:595-602.

161. Zucman J, Delattre O, Desmaze C, et al. EWS and ATF-1 gene fusion induced by t(12;22) translocation in malignant melanoma of soft parts. Nat Genet. 1993;4:341-345.

162. Brown AD, Lopez-Terrada D, Denny C, Lee KA. Promoters containing ATF-binding sites are de-regulated in cells that express the EWS/ATF1 oncogene. Oncogene. 1995;10:1749-1756.

163. Gerald WL, Miller HK, Battifora H, et al. Intra-abdominal desmoplastic small round-cell tumor. Report of 19 cases of a distinctive type of high-grade polyphenotypic malignancy affecting young individuals. Am J Surg Pathol. 1991;15:499-513.

164. Ladanyi M, Gerald W. Fusion of the EWS and WT1 genes in the desmoplastic small round cell tumor. Cancer Res. 1994;54:2837-2840.

165. Gerald WL, Ladanyi M, de Alava E, et al. Clinical, pathologic, and molecular spectrum of tumors associated with t(11;22)(p13;q12): desmoplastic small round-cell tumor and its variants. J Clin Oncol. 1998;16:3028-3036.

166. Rodriguez E, Sreekantaiah C, Gerald W, et al. A recurring translocation, t(11;22)(p13;q11.2), characterizes intra-abdominal desmoplastic small round-cell tumors. Cancer Genet Cytogenet. 1993;69:17-21.

167. Biegel JA, Conard K, Brooks JJ. Translocation (11;22)(p13;q12): primary change in intra-abdominal desmoplastic small round cell tumor. Genes Chromosom Cancer. 1993;7:119-121.

168. Liu J, Nau MM, Yeh JC, et al. Molecular heterogeneity and function of EWS-WT1 fusion transcripts in desmoplastic small round cell tumors. Clin Cancer Res. 2000;6:3522-3529.

169. Lee SB, Kolquist KA, Nichols K, et al. The EWS-WT1 translocation product induces PDGFA in desmoplastic small round-cell tumour. Nat Genet. 1997;17:309-313.

170. Li H, Smolen GA, Beers LF, et al. Adenosine transporter ENT4 is a direct target of EWS/WT1 translocation product and is highly expressed in desmoplastic small round cell tumor. PLoS ONE. 2008;3:e2353.

171. Kim J, Lee K, Pelletier J. The desmoplastic small round cell tumor t(11;22) translocation produces EWS/WT1 isoforms with differing oncogenic properties. Oncogene. 1998;16:1973-1979.

172. Kelly JD, Haldeman BA, Grant FJ, et al. Platelet-derived growth factor (PDGF) stimulates PDGF receptor subunit dimerization and intersubunit trans-phosphorylation. J Biol Chem. 1991;266: 8987-8992.

173. Pedeutour F, Simon MP, Minoletti F, et al. Ring 22 chromosomes in dermatofibrosarcoma protuberans are low- level amplifiers of chromosome 17 and 22 sequences. Cancer Res. 1995;55: 2400-2403.

174. Naeem R, Lux ML, Huang SF, et al. Ring chromosomes in dermatofibrosarcoma protuberans are composed of interspersed sequences from chromosomes 17 and 22. Am J Pathol. 1995;147: 1553-1558.

175. Pedeutour F, Simon MP, Minoletti F, et al. Translocation, t(17;22)(q22;q13), in dermatofibrosarcoma protuberans: a new tumor-associated chromosome rearrangement. Cytogenet Cell Genet. 1996;72:171-174.

176. Maki RG, Awan RA, Dixon RH, et al. Differential sensitivity to imatinib of 2 patients with metastatic sarcoma arising from dermatofibrosarcoma protuberans. Int J Cancer. 2002;100:623-626.

177. Rubin BP, Schuetze SM, Eary JF, et al. Molecular targeting of platelet-derived growth factor B by imatinib mesylate in a patient with metastatic dermatofibrosarcoma protuberans. J Clin Oncol. 2002;20:3586-3591.

178. McArthur GA, Demetri GD, van Oosterom A, et al. Molecular and clinical analysis of locally advanced dermatofibrosarcoma protuberans treated with imatinib: Imatinib Target Exploration Consortium Study B2225. J Clin Oncol. 2005;23:866-873.

179. Labropoulos SV, Fletcher JA, Oliveira AM, et al. Sustained complete remission of metastatic dermatofibrosarcoma protuberans with imatinib mesylate. Anticancer Drugs. 2005;16: 461-466.

180. Cin PD, Sciot R, de Wever I, et al. Cytogenetic and immunohistochemical evidence that giant cell fibroblastoma is related to dermatofibrosarcoma protuberans. Genes Chromosomes Cancer. 1996;15:73-75.

181. Alman BA, Li C, Pajerski ME, et al. Increased beta-catenin protein and somatic APC mutations in sporadic aggressive fibromatoses (desmoid tumors). Am J Pathol. 1997;151:329-334.

182. Tejpar S, Nollet F, Li C, et al. Predominance of beta-catenin mutations and beta-catenin dysregulation in sporadic aggressive fibromatosis (desmoid tumor). Oncogene. 1999;18:6615-6620.

183. Fletcher JA, Naeem R, Xiao S, Corson JM. Chromosome aberrations in desmoid tumors. Trisomy 8 may be a predictor of recurrence. Cancer Genet Cytogenet. 1995;79:139-143.

184. Miyaki M, Konishi M, Kikuchi-Yanoshita R, et al. Coexistence of somatic and germ-line mutations of APC gene in desmoid tumors from patients with familial adenomatous polyposis. Cancer Res. 1993;53:5079-5082.

185. Sen-Gupta S, Van der Luijt RB, Bowles LV, et al. Somatic mutation of APC gene in desmoid tumour in familial adenomatous polyposis. Lancet. 1993;342:552-553.

186. Schofield DE, Fletcher JA, Grier HE, Yunis EJ. Fibrosarcoma in infants and children. Application of new techniques. Am J Surg Pathol. 1994;18:14-24.

187. Schofield DE, Yunis EJ, Fletcher JA. Chromosome aberrations in mesoblastic nephroma. Am J Pathol. 1993;143:714-724.

188. Knezevich SR, Garnett MJ, Pysher TJ, et al. ETV6-NTRK3 gene fusions and trisomy 11 establish a histogenetic link between mesoblastic nephroma and congenital fibrosarcoma. Cancer Res. 1998;58:5046-5048.

189. Treissman SP, Gillis DA, Lee CL, et al. Omental-mesenteric inflammatory pseudotumor. Cytogenetic demonstration of genetic changes and monoclonality in one tumor. Cancer. 1994;73: 1433-1437.

190. Snyder CS, Dell'Aquila M, Haghighi P, et al. Clonal changes in inflammatory pseudotumor of the lung: a case report. Cancer. 1995;76:1545-1549.

191. Su LD, Atayde-Perez A, Sheldon S, et al. Inflammatory myofibroblastic tumor: cytogenetic evidence supporting clonal origin. Mod Pathol. 1998;11:364-368.

192. Cools J, Wlodarska I, Somers R, et al. Identification of novel fusion partners of ALK, the anaplastic lymphoma kinase, in anaplastic large-cell lymphoma and inflammatory myofibroblastic tumor. Genes Chromosomes Cancer. 2002;34:354-362.

193. Ma Z, Hill DA, Collins MH, et al. Fusion of ALK to the Ran-binding protein 2 (RANBP2) gene in inflammatory myofibroblastic tumor. Genes Chromosomes Cancer. 2003;37:98-105.

194. Hirota S, Isozaki K, Moriyama Y, et al. Gain-of-function mutations of c-kit in human gastrointestinal stromal tumors. Science. 1998;279:577-580.

195. Rubin BP, Singer S, Tsao C, et al. KIT Activation Is a Ubiquitous Feature of Gastrointestinal Stromal Tumors. Cancer Res. 2001;61:8118-8121.

196. Heinrich MC, Corless CL, Duensing A, et al. PDGFRA activating mutations in gastrointestinal stromal tumors. Science. 2003;299:708-710.

197. Demetri GD, von Mehren M, Blanke CD, et al. Efficacy and safety of imatinib mesylate in advanced gastrointestinal stromal tumors. N Engl J Med. 2002;347:472-480.

198. van Oosterom AT, Judson I, Verweij J, et al. Safety and efficacy of imatinib (STI571) in metastatic gastrointestinal stromal tumours: a phase I study. Lancet. 2001;358:1421-1423.

199. Nishida T, Hirota S, Taniguchi M, et al. Familial gastrointestinal stromal tumours with germline mutation of the KIT gene. Nat Genet. 1998;19:323-324.

200. O'Sullivan MJ, McCabe A, Gillett P, et al. Multiple gastric stromal tumors in a child without syndromic association lacks common KIT or PDGFRalpha mutations. Pediatr Dev Pathol. 2005;8:685-689.

201. Price VE, Zielenska M, Chilton-MacNeill S, et al. Clinical and molecular characteristics of pediatric gastrointestinal stromal tumors (GISTs). Pediatr Blood Cancer. 2005;45:20-24.

202. Prakash S, Sarran L, Socci N, et al. Gastrointestinal stromal tumors in children and young adults: a clinicopathologic, molecular, and genomic study of 15 cases and review of the literature. J Pediatr Hematol Oncol. 2005;27:179-187.

203. Janeway KA, Liegl B, Harlow A, et al. Pediatric KIT wild-type and platelet-derived growth factor receptor alpha-wild-type gastrointestinal stromal tumors share KIT activation but not mechanisms of genetic progression with adult gastrointestinal stromal tumors. Cancer Res. 2007;67:9084-9088.

204. Legius E, Marchuk DA, Collins FS, Glover TW. Somatic deletion of the neurofibromatosis type 1 gene in a neurofibrosarcoma supports a tumour suppressor gene hypothesis. Nat Genet. 1993;3:122-126.

205. Basu TN, Gutmann DH, Fletcher JA, et al. Aberrant regulation of ras proteins in malignant tumour cells from type 1 neurofibromatosis patients. Nature. 1992;356:713-715.

206. DeClue JE, Papageorge AG, Fletcher JA, et al. Abnormal regulation of mammalian p21ras contributes to malignant tumor growth in von Recklinghausen (type 1) neurofibromatosis. Cell. 1992;69: 265-273.

207. Rouleau GA, Merel P, Lutchman M, et al. Alteration in a new gene encoding a putative membrane-organizing protein causes neuro-fibromatosis type 2. Nature. 1993;363:515-521.

208. Twist EC, Ruttledge MH, Rousseau M, et al. The neurofibromatosis type 2 gene is inactivated in schwannomas. Hum Mol Genet. 1994;3:147-151.

209. Lutchman M, Rouleau GA. The neurofibromatosis type 2 gene product, schwannomin, suppresses growth of NIH 3T3 cells. Cancer Res. 1995;55:2270-2274.

210. Yan N, Ricca C, Fletcher J, Glover T, et al. Farnesyltransferase inhibitors block the neurofibromatosis type I (NF1) malignant phenotype. Cancer Res. 1995;55:3569-3575.

211. Kluwe L, Friedrich R, Mautner V-F. Loss of *NF1* allele in Schwann cells but not in fibroblasts dervied from an NF1-associated neurofibroma. Genes Chromosomes Cancer. 1999; 24:283-285.

212. Hayashi Y, Inaba T, Hanada R, Yamamoto K. Chromosome findings and prognosis in 15 patients with neuroblastoma found by VMA mass screening. J Pediatr. 1988;112:567-571.

213. Brodeur GM, Azar C, Brother M, et al: Neuroblastoma. Effect of genetic factors on prognosis and treatment. Cancer. 1992; 70:1685-1694.

214. Maris JM. The biologic basis for neuroblastoma heterogeneity and risk stratification. Curr Opin Pediatr. 2005;17:7-13.

215. Shapiro DN, Valentine MB, Rowe ST, et al. Detection of N-myc gene amplification by fluorescence in situ hybridization. Diagnostic utility for neuroblastoma. Am J Pathol. 1993;142:1339-1346.

216. Komuro H, Valentine MB, Rowe ST, et al. Fluorescence in situ hybridization analysis of chromosome 1p36 deletions in human MYCN amplified neuroblastoma. J Pediatr Surg. 1998;33: 1695-1698.

217. Cole KA, Attiyeh EF, Mosse YP, et al. A Functional Screen Identifies miR-34a as a Candidate Neuroblastoma Tumor Suppressor Gene. Mol Cancer Res. 2008;6:735-742.

218. Wei JS, Song YK, Durinck S, et al. The MYCN oncogene is a direct target of miR-34a. Oncogene. 2008;27:5204-5213.

219. Versteege I, Sevenet N, Lange J, et al. Truncating mutations of hSNF5/INI1 in aggressive paediatric cancer. Nature. 1998;394: 203-206.

220. Biegel JA, Zhou JY, Rorke LB, et al. Germ-line and acquired mutations of INI1 in atypical teratoid and rhabdoid tumors. Cancer Res. 1999;59:74-79.

221. Biegel JA, Rorke LB, Packer RJ, Emanuel BS. Monosomy 22 in rhabdoid or atypical tumors of the brain. J Neurosurg. 1990; 73:710-714.

222. Schofield DE, Beckwith JB, Sklar J. Loss of heterozygosity at chromosome regions 22q11-12 and 11p15.5 in renal rhabdoid tumors. Genes Chromosomes Cancer. 1996;15:10-17.

223. Sevenet N, Sheridan E, Amram D, et al. Constitutional mutations of the hSNF5/INI1 gene predispose to a variety of cancers. Am J Hum Genet. 1999;65:1342-1348.

224. Janson K, Nedzi LA, David O, et al. Predisposition to atypical teratoid/rhabdoid tumor due to an inherited INI1 mutation. Pediatr Blood Cancer. 2006;47:279-284.

225. Roberts CW, Galusha SA, McMenamin ME, et al. Haploinsufficiency of Snf5 (integrase interactor 1) predisposes to malignant rhabdoid tumors in mice. Proc Natl Acad Sci U S A. 2000;97: 13796-13800.

226. Hulsebos TJ, Plomp AS, Wolterman RA, et al. Germline mutation of INI1/SMARCB1 in familial schwannomatosis. Am J Hum Genet. 2007;80:805-810.

227. Vries RG, Bezrookove V, Zuijderduijn LM, et al. Cancer-associated mutations in chromatin remodeler hSNF5 promote chromosomal instability by compromising the mitotic checkpoint. Genes Dev. 2005;19:665-670.

228. Zhang ZK, Davies KP, Allen J, et al. Cell cycle arrest and repression of cyclin D1 transcription by INI1/hSNF5. Mol Cell Biol. 2002;22:5975-5988.

229. Tsikitis M, Zhang Z, Edelman W, et al. Genetic ablation of Cyclin D1 abrogates genesis of rhabdoid tumors resulting from Ini1 loss. Proc Natl Acad Sci U S A. 2005;102:12129-12134.

230. Alarcon-Vargas D, Zhang Z, Agarwal B, et al. Targeting cyclin D1, a downstream effector of INI1/hSNF5, in rhabdoid tumors. Oncogene. 2006;25:722-734.

231. Sigauke E, Rakheja D, Maddox DL, et al. Absence of expression of SMARCB1/INI1 in malignant rhabdoid tumors of the central nervous system, kidneys and soft tissue: an immunohistochemical study with implications for diagnosis. Mod Pathol. 2006 19:717-725.

232. Ladanyi M, Lui MY, Antonescu CR, et al. The der(17)t(X;17)(p11;q25) of human alveolar soft part sarcoma fuses the TFE3 transcription factor gene to ASPL, a novel gene at 17q25. Oncogene. 2001;20:48-57.

233. Vistica DT, Krosky PM, Kenney S, et al. Immunohistochemical discrimination between the ASPL-TFE3 fusion proteins of alveolar soft part sarcoma. J Pediatr Hematol Oncol. 2008;30: 46-52.

234. Kaneko Y, Homma C, Maseki N, et al. Correlation of chromosome abnormalities with histological and clinical features in Wilms' and other childhood renal tumors. Cancer Res. 1991; 51:5937-5942.

235. Grundy PE, Telzerow PE, Breslow N, et al. Loss of heterozygosity for chromosomes 16q and 1p in Wilms' tumors predicts an adverse outcome. Cancer Res. 1994;54:2331-2333.

236. Meloni AM, Dobbs RM, Pontes JE, Sandberg AA. Translocation (X;1) in papillary renal cell carcinoma. A new cytogenetic subtype. Cancer Genet Cytogenet. 1993;65:1-6.

237. Argani P, Antonescu CR, Illei PB, et al. Primary renal neoplasms with the ASPL-TFE3 gene fusion of alveolar soft part sarcoma: a distinctive tumor entity previously included among renal cell carcinomas of children and adolescents. Am J Pathol. 2001; 159:179-192.

238. Davis IJ, Hsi BL, Arroyo JD, et al. Cloning of an alpha-TFEB fusion in renal tumors harboring the t(6;11)(p21;q13) chromosome translocation. Proc Natl Acad Sci U S A. 2003;100:6051-6056.

239. Weremowicz S, Kozakewich HP, Haber D, et al. Identification of genetically aberrant cell lineages in Wilms' tumors. Genes Chromosomes Cancer. 1994;10:40-48.

240. Solis V, Pritchard J, Cowell JK. Cytogenetic changes in Wilms' tumors. Cancer Genet Cytogenet. 1988;34:223-234.

241. Slater RM, Mannens MM. Cytogenetics and molecular genetics of Wilms' tumor of childhood. Cancer Genet Cytogenet. 1992; 61:111-121.

242. Lu YJ, Hing S, Williams R, et al. Chromosome 1q expression profiling and relapse in Wilms' tumour. Lancet. 2002;360: 385-386.

243. Haber DA, Buckler AJ, Glaser T, et al. An internal deletion within an 11p13 zinc finger gene contributes to the development of Wilms' tumor. Cell. 1990;61:1257-1269.

244. Bruening W, Bardeesy N, Silverman BL, et al. Germline intronic and exonic mutations in the Wilms' tumour gene (WT1) affecting urogenital development. Nature Genetics. 1992;1:144-148.

245. Ton CC, Hirvonen H, Miwa H, et al. Positional cloning and characterization of a paired box- and homeobox-containing gene from the aniridia region. Cell. 1991;67:1059-1074.

246. Rivera MN, Kim WJ, Wells J, et al. An X chromosome gene, WTX, is commonly inactivated in Wilms tumor. Science. 2007;315:642-645.

247. Perotti D, Gamba B, Sardella M, et al. Functional inactivation of the WTX gene is not a frequent event in Wilms' tumors. Oncogene. 2008;27:4625-4632.

248. Ruteshouser EC, Robinson SM, Huff V. Wilms tumor genetics: mutations in WT1, WTX, and CTNNB1 account for only about one-third of tumors. Genes Chromosomes Cancer. 2008;47:461-470.

249. Rivera MN, Kim WJ, Wells J, et al. An X chromosome gene, WTX, is commonly inactivated in Wilms tumor. Science. 2007;315:642-645.

250. Perotti D, Gamba B, Sardella M, et al. Functional inactivation of the WTX gene is not a frequent event in Wilms' tumors. Oncogene. 2008;27:4625-4632.

251. Rivera MN, Kim WJ, Wells J, et al. An X chromosome gene, WTX, is commonly inactivated in Wilms tumor. Science. 2007;315:642-645.

252. Ruteshouser EC, Robinson SM, Huff V. Wilms tumor genetics: mutations in WT1, WTX, and CTNNB1 account for only about

one-third of tumors. Genes Chromosomes Cancer. 2008;47:461-470.

253. Major MB, Camp ND, Berndt JD, et al. Wilms tumor suppressor WTX negatively regulates WNT/beta-catenin signaling. Science. 2007;316:1043-1046.

254. Koesters R, Ridder R, Kopp-Schneider A, et al. Mutational activation of the beta-catenin proto-oncogene is a common event in the development of Wilms' tumors. Cancer Res. 1999;59:3880-3882.

255. Maiti S, Alam R, Amos CI, Huff V. Frequent association of beta-catenin and WT1 mutations in Wilms tumors. Cancer Res. 2000;60:6288-6292.

256. Tycko B, Li CM, Buttyan R. The Wnt/beta-catenin pathway in Wilms tumors and prostate cancers. Curr Mol Med. 2007;7:479-489.

257. Ruteshouser EC, Robinson SM, Huff V. Wilms tumor genetics: mutations in WT1, WTX, and CTNNB1 account for only about one-third of tumors. Genes Chromosomes Cancer. 2008;47:461-470.

258. Douglass EC, Look AT, Webber B, et al. Hyperdiploidy and chromosomal rearrangements define the anaplastic variant of Wilms' tumor. J Clin Oncol. 1986;4:975-981.

259. Bardeesy N, Falkoff D, Petruzzi MJ, et al. Anaplastic Wilms' tumour, a subtype displaying poor prognosis, harbours p53 gene mutations. Nat Genet. 1994;7:91-97.

260. Bolande RP, Brough AJ, Izant RJ Jr. Congenital mesoblastic nephroma of infancy. A report of eight cases and the relationship to Wilms' tumor. Pediatrics. 1967;40:272-278.

261. Pettinato G, Manivel JC, Wick MR, Dehner LP. Classical and cellular (atypical) congenital mesoblastic nephroma: a clinicopathologic, ultrastructural, immunohistochemical, and flow cytometric study. Hum Pathol. 1989;20:682-690.

262. Mascarello JT, Cajulis TR, Krous HF, Carpenter PM. Presence or absence of trisomy 11 is correlated with histologic subtype in congenital mesoblastic nephroma. Cancer Genet Cytogenet. 1994;77:50-54.

263. French CA, Miyoshi I, Aster JC, et al. BRD4 bromodomain gene rearrangement in aggressive carcinoma with translocation t(15;19). Am J Pathol. 2001;159:1987-1992.

264. Vargas SO, French CA, Faul PN, et al. Upper respiratory tract carcinoma with chromosomal translocation 15;19: evidence for a distinct disease entity of young patients with a rapidly fatal course. Cancer. 2001;92:1195-1203.

265. French CA. Molecular pathology of NUT midline carcinomas. J Clin Pathol. 2008;Jun 13. [Epub ahead of print].

266. Stelow EB, Bellizzi AM, Taneja K, et al. NUT rearrangement in undifferentiated carcinomas of the upper aerodigestive tract. Am J Surg Pathol. 2008;32:828-834.

267. Mertens F, Wiebe T, Adlercreutz C, et al. Successful treatment of a child with t(15;19)-positive tumor. Pediatr Blood Cancer. 2006;46:476-481.

268. French CA, Ramirez CL, Kolmakova J, et al. BRD-NUT oncoproteins: a family of closely related nuclear proteins that block epithelial differentiation and maintain the growth of carcinoma cells. Oncogene. 2008;27:2237-2242.

269. Fenton CL, Lukes Y, Nicholson D, et al. The ret/PTC mutations are common in sporadic papillary thyroid carcinoma of children and young adults. J Clin Endocrinol Metab. 2000;85:1170-1175.

270. Kumagai A, Namba H, Saenko VA, et al. Low frequency of BRAFT1796A mutations in childhood thyroid carcinomas. J Clin Endocrinol Metab. 2004;89:4280-4284.

271. Rosenbaum E, Hosler G, Zahurak M, et al. Mutational activation of BRAF is not a major event in sporadic childhood papillary thyroid carcinoma. Mod Pathol. 2005;18:898-902.

272. Sciot R, Dal Cin P, Brock P, et al. Pleuropulmonary blastoma (pulmonary blastoma of childhood): genetic link with other embryonal malignancies? Histopathology. 1994;24:559-563.

273. Fletcher JA, Kozakewich HP, Pavelka K, et al. Consistent cytogenetic aberrations in hepatoblastoma: a common pathway of genetic alterations in embryonal liver and skeletal muscle malignancies? Genes Chromosomes Cancer. 1991;3:37-43.

274. Vargas SO, Nose V, Fletcher JA, Perez-Atayde AR. Gains of chromosome 8 are confined to mesenchymal components in pleuropulmonary blastoma. Pediatr Dev Pathol. 2001;4:434-445.

275. Reifenberger G, Louis DN. Oligodendroglioma: toward molecular definitions in diagnostic neuro-oncology. J Neuropathol Exp Neurol. 2003;62:111-126.

276. Ino Y, Betensky RA, Zlatescu MC, et al. Molecular subtypes of anaplastic oligodendroglioma: implications for patient management at diagnosis. Clin Cancer Res. 2001;7:839-845.

277. Gilbertson RJ, Bentley L, Hernan R, et al. ERBB receptor signaling promotes ependymoma cell proliferation and represents a potential novel therapeutic target for this disease. Clin Cancer Res. 2002;8:3054-3064.

278. Bredel M, Pollack IF, Hamilton RL, James CD. Epidermal growth factor receptor expression and gene amplification in high-grade non-brainstem gliomas of childhood. Clin Cancer Res. 1999;5:1786-1792.

279. Bosl GJ, Ilson DH, Rodriguez E, et al. Clinical relevance of the i(12p) marker chromosome in germ cell tumors. J Natl Cancer Inst. 1994;86:349-355.

280. Mertens F, Johansson B, Mitelman F. Isochromosomes in neoplasia. Genes Chromosom Cancer. 1994;10:221-230.

281. Zamecnik PC, Long JC. Growth of cultured cells from patients with Hodgkin's disease and transplantation into nude mice. Proc Natl Acad Sci U S A. 1977;74:754-758.

282. Long JC, Zamecnik PC, Aisenberg AC, Atkins L. Tissue culture studies in Hodgkin's disease: Morphologic, cytogenetic, cell surface, and enzymatic properties of cultures derived from splenic tumors. J Exp Med. 1977;145:1484-1500.

283. Harris NL, Jaffe ES, Stein H, et al. A revised European-American classification of lymphoid neoplasms: a proposal from the International Lymphoma Study Group. Blood. 1994;84:1361-1392.

284. Jaffe ES, Harris NL, Diebold J, Muller-Hermelink HK. World Health Organization classification of lymphomas: a work in progress. Ann Oncol. 1998;9(Suppl 5):S25-S30.

285. Harris NL. Hodgkin's disease: classification and differential diagnosis. Mod Pathol. 1999;12:159-175.

286. Kuppers R, Klein U, Schwering I, et al. Identification of Hodgkin and Reed-Sternberg cell-specific genes by gene expression profiling. J Clin Invest. 2003;111:529-537.

287. Schwering I, Brauninger A, Klein U, et al. Loss of the B-lineage-specific gene expression program in Hodgkin and Reed-Sternberg cells of Hodgkin lymphoma. Blood. 2003;101:1505-1512.

288. Kuppers R, Rajewsky K, Zhao M, et al. Hodgkin disease: Hodgkin and Reed-Sternberg cells picked from histological sections show clonal immunoglobulin gene rearrangements and appear to be derived from B cells at various stages of development. Proc Natl Acad Sci U S A. 1994;91:10962-10966.

289. Cossman J, Annunziata CM, Barash S, et al. Reed-Sternberg cell genome expression supports a B-cell lineage. Blood. 1999;94:411-416.

290. Marafioti T, Hummel M, Foss HD, et al. Hodgkin and Reed-Sternberg cells represent an expansion of a single clone originating from a germinal center B-cell with functional immunoglobulin gene rearrangements but defective immunoglobulin transcription. Blood. 2000;95:1443-1450.

291. Carbone A, Gloghini A, Gaidano G, et al. Expression status of BCL-6 and syndecan-1 identifies distinct histogenetic subtypes of Hodgkin's disease. Blood. 1998;92:2220-2228.

292. Seitz V, Hummel M, Marafioti T, et al. Detection of clonal T-cell receptor gamma-chain gene rearrangements in Reed-Sternberg cells of classic Hodgkin disease. Blood. 2000;95:3020-3024.

293. Aguilera NS, Chen J, Bijwaard KE, et al. Gene rearrangement and comparative genomic hybridization studies of classic Hodgkin

lymphoma expressing T-cell antigens. Arch Pathol Lab Med. 2006;130:1772-1779.

294. Tzankov A, Bourgau C, Kaiser A, et al. Rare expression of T-cell markers in classical Hodgkin's lymphoma. Mod Pathol. 2005;18:1542-1549.

295. Daus H, Trumper L, Roth J, et al. Hodgkin and Reed-Sternberg cells do not carry T-cell receptor gamma gene rearrangements: evidence from single-cell polymerase chain reaction examination. Blood. 1995;85:1590-1595.

296. Re D, Zander T, Diehl V, Wolf J. Genetic instability in Hodgkin's lymphoma. Ann Oncol. 2002;13(Suppl 1):19-22.

297. Weber-Matthiesen K, Deerberg J, Poetsch M, et al. Numerical chromosome aberrations are present within the CD30+ Hodgkin and Reed-Sternberg cells in 100% of analyzed cases of Hodgkin's disease. Blood. 1995;86:1464-1468.

298. Renne C, Martin-Subero JI, Hansmann ML, Siebert R. Molecular cytogenetic analyses of immunoglobulin loci in nodular lymphocyte predominant Hodgkin's lymphoma reveal a recurrent IGH-BCL6 juxtaposition. J Mol Diagn. 2005;7:352-356.

299. vet-Loiseau H, Brigaudeau C, Morineau N, et al. High incidence of cryptic translocations involving the Ig heavy chain gene in multiple myeloma, as shown by fluorescence in situ hybridization. Genes Chromosomes Cancer. 1999;24:9-15.

300. Falzetti D, Crescenzi B, Matteuci C, et al. Genomic instability and recurrent breakpoints are main cytogenetic findings in Hodgkin's disease. Haematologica. 1999;84:298-305.

301. Liang R, Chan WP, Chan AC, Ho FC. Rearrangement of the bcl-6 gene in Hodgkin's disease, lymphocyte predominant type. Am J Hematol. 1996;52:63-64.

302. Wlodarska I, Nooyen P, Maes B, et al. Frequent occurrence of BCL6 rearrangements in nodular lymphocyte predominance Hodgkin lymphoma but not in classical Hodgkin lymphoma. Blood. 2003;101:706-710.

303. Franke S, Wlodarska I, Maes B, et al. Lymphocyte predominance Hodgkin disease is characterized by recurrent genomic imbalances. Blood. 2001;97:1845-1853.

304. Joos S, Menz CK, Wrobel G, et al. Classical Hodgkin lymphoma is characterized by recurrent copy number gains of the short arm of chromosome 2. Blood. 2002;99:1381-1387.

305. Joos S, Kupper M, Ohl S, et al. Genomic imbalances including amplification of the tyrosine kinase gene JAK2 in CD30+ Hodgkin cells. Cancer Res. 2000;60:549-552.

306. Küpper M, Joos S, von Bonin F, et al. MDM2 gene amplification and lack of p53 point mutations in Hodgkin and Reed-Sternberg cells: results from single-cell polymerase chain reaction and molecular cytogenetic studies. Br J Haematol. 2001;112:768-775.

307. Vassilev LT, Vu BT, Graves B, et al. In vivo activation of the p53 pathway by small-molecule antagonists of MDM2. Science. 2004;303:844-848.

308. Martin-Subero JI, Gesk S, Harder L, et al. Recurrent involvement of the REL and BCL11A loci in classical Hodgkin lymphoma. Blood. 2002;99:1474-1477.

309. Martin-Subero JI, Klapper W, Sotnikova A, et al. Chromosomal breakpoints affecting immunoglobulin loci are recurrent in Hodgkin and Reed-Sternberg cells of classical Hodgkin lymphoma. Cancer Res. 2006;66:10332-10338.

310. Nakamura N, Ohshima K, Abe M, Osamura Y. Demonstration of chimeric DNA of bcl-2 and immunoglobulin heavy chain in follicular lymphoma and subsequent Hodgkin lymphoma from the same patient. J Clin Exp Hematop. 2007;47:9-13.

311. Heerema NA, Bernheim A, Lim MS, et al. State of the Art and Future Needs in Cytogenetic/Molecular Genetics/Arrays in childhood lymphoma: summary report of workshop at the First International Symposium on childhood and adolescent non-Hodgkin lymphoma, April 9, 2003, New York. Pediatr Blood Cancer. 2005;45:616-622.

312. Oschlies I, Klapper W, Zimmermann M, et al. Diffuse large B-cell lymphoma in pediatric patients belongs predominantly to the germinal-center type B-cell lymphomas: a clinicopathologic analysis of cases included in the German BFM (Berlin-Frankfurt-Munster) Multicenter Trial. Blood. 2006;107:4047-4052.

313. Manolov G, Manolova Y. Marker band in one chromosome 14 from Burkitt lymphomas. Nature. 1972;237:33-34.

314. Dalla-Favera R, Bregni M, Erikson J, et al. Human c-myc onc gene is located on the region of chromosome 8 that is translocated in Burkitt lymphoma cells. Proc Natl Acad Sci U S A. 1982;79: 7824-7827.

315. Kaiser-McCaw B, Epstein AL, Kaplan HS, Hecht F. Chromosome 14 translocation in African and North American Burkitt's lymphoma. Int J Cancer. 1977;19:482-486.

316. Haluska FG, Tsujimoto Y, Croce CM. Oncogene activation by chromosome translocation in human malignancy. Annu Rev Genet. 1987;21:321-345.

317. Lones MA, Sanger WG, Le Beau MM, et al. Chromosome abnormalities may correlate with prognosis in Burkitt/Burkitt-like lymphomas of children and adolescents: a report from Children's Cancer Group Study CCG-E08. J Pediatr Hematol Oncol. 2004;26:169-178.

318. Swerdlow SH. Pediatric follicular lymphomas, marginal zone lymphomas, and marginal zone hyperplasia. Am J Clin Pathol. 2004;122(Suppl):S98-109.

319. Jaffe ES. Mature T-cell and NK-cell lymphomas in the pediatric age group. Am J Clin Pathol. 2004;122(Suppl):S110-S121.

320. Morris SW, Kirstein MN, Valentine MB, et al. Fusion of a kinase gene, ALK, to a nucleolar protein gene, NPM, in non-Hodgkin's lymphoma. Science. 1994;263:1281-1284.

321. Colleoni GW, Bridge JA, Garicochea B, et al. ATIC-ALK: A novel variant ALK gene fusion in anaplastic large cell lymphoma resulting from the recurrent cryptic chromosomal inversion, inv(2)(p23q35). Am J Pathol. 2000;156:781-789.

322. Tort F, Pinyol M, Pulford K, et al. Molecular characterization of a new ALK translocation involving moesin (MSN-ALK) in anaplastic large cell lymphoma. Lab Invest. 2001;81:419-426.

323. Hernandez L, Pinyol M, Hernandez S, et al. TRK-fused gene (TFG) is a new partner of ALK in anaplastic large cell lymphoma producing two structurally different TFG-ALK translocations. Blood. 1999;94:3265-3268.

324. Gascoyne RD, Lamant L, Martin-Subero JI, et al. ALK-positive diffuse large B-cell lymphoma is associated with Clathrin-ALK rearrangements: report of 6 cases. Blood. 2003;102:2568-2573.

325. Alonsozana EL, Stamberg J, Kumar D, et al. Isochromosome 7q: the primary cytogenetic abnormality in hepatosplenic gammadelta T cell lymphoma. Leukemia. 1997;11:1367-1372.

326. Wlodarska I, Martin-Garcia N, Achten R, et al. Fluorescence in situ hybridization study of chromosome 7 aberrations in hepatosplenic T-cell lymphoma: isochromosome 7q as a common abnormality accumulating in forms with features of cytologic progression. Genes Chromosomes Cancer. 2002;33:243-251.

327. Chin M, Mugishima H, Takamura M, et al. Hemophagocytic syndrome and hepatosplenic gammadelta T-cell lymphoma with isochromosome 7q and 8 trisomy. J Pediatr Hematol Oncol. 2004;26:375-378.

328. Cox CV, Evely RS, Oakhill A, et al. Characterization of acute lymphoblastic leukemia progenitor cells. Blood. 2004;104: 2919-2925.

329. Korsmeyer SJ, Arnold A, Bakhshi A, et al. Immunoglobulin gene rearrangement and cell surface antigen expression in acute lymphocytic leukemias of T cell and B cell precursor origins. J Clin Invest. 1983;71:301-313.

330. Felix CA, Wright JJ, Poplack DG, et al. T cell receptor alpha-, beta-, and gamma-genes in T cell and pre-B cell acute lymphoblastic leukemia. J Clin Invest. 1987;80:545-556.

331. Wright JJ, Poplack DG, Bakhshi A, et al. Gene rearrangements as markers of clonal variation and minimal residual disease in acute lymphoblastic leukemia. J Clin Oncol. 1987;5:735-741.

332. Yamada M, Wasserman R, Lange B, et al. Minimal residual disease in childhood B-lineage lymphoblastic leukemia. Persistence of leukemic cells during the first 18 months of treatment. N Engl J Med. 1990;323:448-455.

333. Wasserman R, Galili N, Ito Y, et al. Residual disease at the end of induction therapy as a predictor of relapse during therapy in childhood B-lineage acute lymphoblastic leukemia. J Clin Oncol. 1992;10:1879-1888.

334. Coustan-Smith E, Sancho J, Behm FG, et al. Prognostic importance of measuring early clearance of leukemic cells by flow cytometry in childhood acute lymphoblastic leukemia. Blood. 2002;100:52-58.

335. Kim JM, Fang J, Rheingold S, et al. Cytoplasmic μ heavy chain confers sensitivity to dexamethasone-induced apoptosis in early B-lineage acute lymphoblastic leukemia. Cancer Res. 2002;62:4212-4216.

336. Denny CT, Hollis GF, Hecht F, et al. Common mechanism of chromosome inversion in B- and T-cell tumors: relevance to lymphoid development. Science. 1986;234:197-200.

337. Raghavan SC, Kirsch IR, Lieber MR. Analysis of the V(D)J recombination efficiency at lymphoid chromosomal translocation breakpoints. J Biol Chem. 2001;276:29126-29133.

338. Begley CG, Aplan PD, Denning SM, et al. The gene *SCL* is expressed during early hematopoiesis and encodes a differentiation-related DNA-binding motif. Proc Natl Acad Sci U S A. 1989;86:10128-10132.

339. Aplan PD, Lombardi DP, Ginsberg AM, et al. Disruption of the human *SCL* locus by "illegitimate" V-(D)-J recombinase activity. Science. 1990;250:1426-1429.

340. Aplan PD, Lombardi DP, Reaman GH, et al. Involvement of the putative hematopoietic transcription factor SCL in T-cell acute lymphoblastic leukemia. Blood. 1992;79:1327-1333.

341. Aplan PD, Johnson BE, Russell E, et al. Cloning and characterization of *TCTA*, a gene located at the site of a t(1;3) translocation. Cancer Res. 1995;55:1917-1921.

342. Ferrando AA, Neuberg DS, Staunton J, et al. Gene expression signatures define novel oncogenic pathways in T cell acute lymphoblastic leukemia. Cancer Cell. 2002;1:75-87.

343. Bergeron J, Clappier E, Radford I, et al. Prognostic and oncogenic relevance of *TLX1/HOX11* expression level in T-ALLs. Blood. 2007;110:2324-2330.

344. Clappier E, Cuccuini W, Kalota A, et al. The *C-MYB* locus is involved in chromosomal translocation and genomic duplications in human T-cell acute leukemia (T-ALL), the translocation defining a new T-ALL subtype in very young children. Blood. 2007;110:1251-1261.

345. Ellisen LW, Bird J, West DC, et al. *TAN-1*, the human homolog of the Drosophila notch gene, is broken by chromosomal translocations in T lymphoblastic neoplasms. Cell. 1991;66:649-661.

346. Weng AP, Ferrando AA, Lee W, et al. Activating mutations of NOTCH1 in human T cell acute lymphoblastic leukemia. Science. 2004;306:269-271.

347. Palomero T, Sulis ML, Cortina M, et al. Mutational loss of PTEN induces resistance to NOTCH1 inhibition in T-cell leukemia. Nat Med. 2007;13:1203-1210.

348. Russell LJ, Akasaka T, Majid A, et al. t(6;14)(p22;q32): a new recurrent *IGH@* translocation involving *ID4* in B-cell precursor acute lymphoblastic leukemia (BCP-ALL). Blood. 2008;111:387-391.

349. Fischer S, Mann G, Konrad M, et al. Screening for leukemia- and clone-specific markers at birth in children with T-cell precursor ALL suggests a predominantly postnatal origin. Blood. 2007;110:3036-3038.

350. Ford AM, Pombo-de-Oliveira MS, McCarthy KP, et al. Monoclonal origin of concordant T-cell malignancy in identical twins. Blood. 1997;89:281-285.

351. Fasching K, Panzer S, Haas OA, et al. Presence of clone-specific antigen receptor gene rearrangements at birth indicates an in utero origin of diverse types of early childhood acute lymphoblastic leukemia. Blood. 2000;95:2722-2724.

352. Eguchi-Ishimae M, Eguchi M, Kempski H, Greaves M. NOTCH1 mutation can be an early, prenatal genetic event in T-ALL. Blood. 2008;111:376-378.

353. Zelent A, Greaves M, Enver T. Role of the *TEL-AML1* fusion gene in the molecular pathogenesis of childhood acute lymphoblastic leukaemia. Oncogene. 2004;23:4275-4283.

354. Wiemels JL, Cazzaniga G, Daniotti M, et al. Prenatal origin of acute lymphoblastic leukaemia in children. Lancet. 1999;354:1499-1503.

355. Ford AM, Bennett CA, Price CM, et al. Fetal origins of the *TEL-AML1* fusion gene in identical twins with leukemia. Proc Natl Acad Sci U S A. 1998;95:4584-4588.

356. Pine SR, Wiemels JL, Jayabose S, Sandoval C. *TEL-AML1* fusion precedes differentiation to pre-B cells in childhood acute lymphoblastic leukemia. Leuk Res. 2003;27:155-164.

357. Greaves MF, Wiemels J. Origins of chromosome translocations in childhood leukaemia. Nat Rev Cancer. 2003;3:639-649.

358. Hunger SP. Chromosomal translocations involving the *E2A* gene in acute lymphoblastic leukemia: clinical features and molecular pathogenesis. Blood. 1996;87:1211-1224.

359. Wiemels JL, Leonard BC, Wang Y, et al. Site-specific translocation and evidence of postnatal origin of the t(1;19) *E2A-PBX1* fusion in childhood acute lymphoblastic leukemia. Proc Natl Acad Sci U S A. 2002;99:15101-15106.

360. van der BM, Poulsen TS, Hunger SP, et al. Split-signal FISH for detection of chromosome aberrations in acute lymphoblastic leukemia. Leukemia. 2004;18:895-908.

361. Prima V, Gore L, Caires A, et al. Cloning and functional characterization of MEF2D/DAZAP1 and DAZAP1/MEF2D fusion proteins created by a variant t(1;19)(q23;p13.3) in acute lymphoblastic leukemia. Leukemia. 2005;19:806-813.

362. Kolb EA, Pan Q, Ladanyi M, Steinherz PG. Imatinib mesylate in Philadelphia chromosome-positive leukemia of childhood. Cancer. 2003;98:2643-2650.

363. Gurney JG, Ross JA, Wall DA, et al. Infant cancer in the U.S.: histology-specific incidence and trends, 1973 to 1992. J Pediatr Hematol Oncol. 1997;19:428-432.

364. Gilliland DG, Jordan CT, Felix CA. The molecular basis of leukemia. Hematology (Am Soc Hematol Educ Program). 2004;80-97.

365. Rasio D, Schichman SA, Negrini M, et al. Complete exon structure of the ALL1 gene. Cancer Res. 1996;56:1766-1769.

366. Djabali M, Selleri L, Parry P, et al. A trithorax-like gene is interrupted by chromosome 11q23 translocations in acute leukaemias. Nat Genet. 1992; 2:113-118.

367. Tkachuk DC, Kohler S, Cleary ML. Involvement of a homolog of Drosophila trithorax by 11q23 chromosomal translocations in acute leukemias. Cell. 1992;71:691-700.

368. Ma Q, Alder H, Nelson KK, et al. Analysis of the murine *All-1* gene reveals conserved domains with human *ALL-1* and identifies a motif shared with DNA methyltransferases. Proc Natl Acad Sci U S A. 1993;90:6350-6354.

369. Hanson RD, Hess JL, Yu BD, et al. Mammalian trithorax and polycomb-group homologues are antagonistic regulators of homeotic development. Proc Natl Acad Sci U S A. 1999;96:14372-14377.

370. Yu BD, Hess JL, Horning SE, et al. Altered Hox expression and segmental identity in Mll-mutant mice. Nature. 1995;378:505-508.

371. Harrison CJ, Cuneo A, Clark R, et al. Ten novel 11q23 chromosomal partner sites. European 11q23 Workshop participants. Leukemia. 1998;12:811-822.

372. Yokoyama A, Kitabayashi I, Ayton PM, et al. Leukemia protooncoprotein MLL is proteolytically processed into 2 fragments with opposite transcriptional properties. Blood. 2002;100:3710-3718.

373. Hsieh JJ, Cheng EH, Korsmeyer SJ. Taspase1: a threonine aspartase required for cleavage of MLL and proper *HOX* gene expression. Cell. 2003;115:293-303.

374. Hsieh JJ, Ernst P, Erdjument-Bromage H, et al. Proteolytic cleavage of MLL generates a complex of N- and C-terminal fragments that confers protein stability and subnuclear localization. Mol Cell Biol. 2003;23:186-194.

375. Milne TA, Briggs SD, Brock HW, et al. MLL targets SET domain methyltransferase activity to Hox gene promoters. Mol Cell. 2002;10:1107-1117.

376. Ayton PM, Cleary ML. Transformation of myeloid progenitors by MLL oncoproteins is dependent on Hoxa7 and Hoxa9. Genes Dev. 2003;17:2298-2307.

377. Pui CH, Gaynon PS, Boyett JM, et al. Outcome of treatment in childhood acute lymphoblastic leukaemia with rearrangements of the 11q23 chromosomal region. Lancet. 2002;359:1909-1915.

378. Ford AM, Ridge SA, Cabrera ME, et al. In utero rearrangements in the trithorax-related oncogene in infant leukaemias. Nature. 1993;363:358-360.

379. Megonigal MD, Rappaport EF, Jones DH, et al. t(11;22)(q23;q11.2) In acute myeloid leukemia of infant twins fuses *MLL* with *hCDCrel*, a cell division cycle gene in the genomic region of deletion in DiGeorge and velocardiofacial syndromes. Proc Natl Acad Sci U S A. 1998;95:6413-6418.

380. Gale KB, Ford AM, Repp R, et al. Backtracking leukemia to birth: identification of clonotypic gene fusion sequences in neonatal blood spots. Proc Natl Acad Sci U S A. 1997;94:13950-13954.

381. Spector LG, Xie Y, Robison LL, et al. Maternal diet and infant leukemia: the DNA topoisomerase II inhibitor hypothesis: a report from the children's oncology group. Cancer Epidemiol Biomarkers Prev. 2005;14:651-655.

382. Wiemels JL, Pagnamenta A, Taylor GM, et al. A lack of a functional NAD(P)H:quinone oxidoreductase allele is selectively associated with pediatric leukemias that have *MLL* fusions. United Kingdom Childhood Cancer Study Investigators. Cancer Res. 1999;59:4095-4099.

383. Smith MT, Wang Y, Skibola CF, et al. Low NAD(P)H:quinone oxidoreductase activity is associated with increased risk of leukemia with *MLL* translocations in infants and children. Blood. 2002;100:4590-4593.

384. Lindsey RH Jr, Bromberg KD, Felix CA, Osheroff N. 1,4-Benzoquinone is a topoisomerase II poison. Biochemistry. 2004; 43:7563-7574.

385. Reichel M, Gillert E, Breitenlohner I, et al. Rapid isolation of chromosomal breakpoints from patients with t(4;11) acute lymphoblastic leukemia: implications for basic and clinical research. Cancer Res. 1999;59:3357-3362.

386. Wiemels JL, Smith RN, Taylor GM, et al. Methylenetetrahydrofolate reductase (MTHFR) polymorphisms and risk of molecularly defined subtypes of childhood acute leukemia. Proc Natl Acad Sci U S A. 2001;98:4004-4009.

387. Sande JE, Arceci RJ, Lampkin BC. Congenital and neonatal leukemia. Semin Perinatol. 1999;23:274-285.

388. Pieters R, Schrappe M, De LP, et al. A treatment protocol for infants younger than 1 year with acute lymphoblastic leukaemia (Interfant-99): an observational study and a multicentre randomised trial. Lancet. 2007;370:240-250.

389. Armstrong SA, Staunton JE, Silverman LB, et al. MLL translocations specify a distinct gene expression profile that distinguishes a unique leukemia. Nat Genet. 2002;30:41-47.

390. Armstrong SA, Mabon ME, Silverman LB, et al. *FLT3* mutations in childhood acute lymphoblastic leukemia. Blood. 2004;103:3544-3546.

391. Brown P, Levis M, Shurtleff S, et al. FLT3 inhibition selectively kills childhood acute lymphoblastic leukemia cells with high levels of FLT3 expression. Blood. 2005;105:812-820.

392. Zheng R, Friedman AD, Levis M, et al. Internal tandem duplication mutation of *FLT3* blocks myeloid differentiation through suppression of C/EBPalpha expression. Blood. 2004;103:1883-1890.

393. Drexler HG, Quentmeier H. FLT3: receptor and ligand. Growth Factors. 2004;22:71-73.

394. Taketani T, Taki T, Sugita K, et al. *FLT3* mutations in the activation loop of tyrosine kinase domain are frequently found in infant ALL with *MLL* rearrangements and pediatric ALL with hyperdiploidy. Blood. 2004;103:1085-1088.

395. Grundler R, Thiede C, Miething C, et al. Sensitivity toward tyrosine kinase inhibitors varies between different activating mutations of the FLT3 receptor. Blood. 2003;102:646-651.

396. Piloto O, Wright M, Brown P, et al. Prolonged exposure to FLT3 inhibitors leads to resistance via activation of parallel signaling pathways. Blood. 2007;109:1643-1652.

397. Andersson A, Paulsson K, Lilljebjorn H, et al. *FLT3* mutations in a 10 year consecutive series of 177 childhood acute leukemias and their impact on global gene expression patterns. Genes Chromosomes Cancer. 2008;47:64-70.

398. Stam RW, Den Boer ML, Schneider P, et al. Targeting FLT3 in primary MLL-gene-rearranged infant acute lymphoblastic leukemia. Blood. 2005;106:2484-2490.

399. Zheng R, Levis M, Piloto O, et al. FLT3 ligand causes autocrine signaling in acute myeloid leukemia cells. Blood. 2004;103:267-274.

400. Reed JC, Miyashita T, Takayama S, et al. BCL-2 family proteins: regulators of cell death involved in the pathogenesis of cancer and resistance to therapy. J Cell Biochem. 1996;60:23-32.

401. Nicholson DW. From bench to clinic with apoptosis-based therapeutic agents. Nature. 2000;407:810-816.

402. Danial NN, Korsmeyer SJ. Cell death: critical control points. Cell. 2004;116:205-219.

403. Certo M, Del Gaizo Moore V, Nishino M, et al. Mitochondria primed by death signals determine cellular addiction to antiapoptotic BCL-2 family members. Cancer Cell. 2006;9:351-365.

404. Letai A, Scorrano L. Laying the foundations of programmed cell death. Cell Death Differ. 2006;13:1245-1247.

405. Coustan-Smith E, Kitanaka A, Pui CH, et al. Clinical relevance of BCL-2 overexpression in childhood acute lymphoblastic leukemia. Blood. 1996;87:1140-1146.

406. Robinson BW, Behling KC, Gupta M, et al. Abundant anti-apoptotic BCL-2 is a molecular target in leukaemias with t(4;11) translocation. Br J Haematol. 2008;141:827-839.

407. Uckun FM, Yang Z, Sather H, et al. Cellular expression of anti-apoptotic BCL-2 oncoprotein in newly diagnosed childhood acute lymphoblastic leukemia: a Children's Cancer Group Study. Blood. 1997;89:3769-3777.

408. Maung ZT, MacLean FR, Reid MM, et al. The relationship between bcl-2 expression and response to chemotherapy in acute leukaemia. Br J Haematol. 1994;88:105-109.

409. Bertin R, Acquaviva C, Mirebeau D, et al. *CDKN2A, CDKN2B,* and *MTAP* gene dosage permits precise characterization of mono- and bi-allelic 9p21 deletions in childhood acute lymphoblastic leukemia. Genes Chromosomes Cancer. 2003;37:44-57.

410. Okuda T, Shurtleff SA, Valentine MB, et al. Frequent deletion of *p16INK4a/MTS1* and *p15INK4b/MTS2* in pediatric acute lymphoblastic leukemia. Blood. 1995;85:2321-2330.

411. van Zutven LJ, van DE, de Bont JM, et al. *CDKN2* deletions have no prognostic value in childhood precursor-B acute lymphoblastic leukaemia. Leukemia. 2005;19:1281-1284.

412. Kees UR, Burton PR, Lu C, Baker DL. Homozygous deletion of the *p16/MTS1* gene in pediatric acute lymphoblastic leukemia is associated with unfavorable clinical outcome. Blood. 1997;89:4161-4166.

413. Calero Moreno TM, Gustafsson G, Garwicz S, et al. Deletion of the Ink4-locus (the *p16ink4a, p14ARF* and *p15ink4b* genes) pre-

dicts relapse in children with ALL treated according to the Nordic protocols NOPHO-86 and NOPHO-92. Leukemia. 2002;16: 2037-2045.

414. Carter TL, Watt PM, Kumar R, et al. Hemizygous *p16(INK4A)* deletion in pediatric acute lymphoblastic leukemia predicts independent risk of relapse. Blood. 2001;97:572-574.

415. Carter TL, Reaman GH, Kees UR. INK4A/ARF deletions are acquired at relapse in childhood acute lymphoblastic leukaemia: a paired study on 25 patients using real-time polymerase chain reaction. Br J Haematol. 2001;113:323-328.

416. Carter TL, Terry P, Gottardo N, et al. Deletion of one copy of the p16INK4A tumor suppressor gene is implicated as a predisposing factor in pediatric leukemia. Biochem Biophys Res Commun. 2004;318:852-855.

417. Wolfraim LA, Fernandez TM, Mamura M, et al. Loss of Smad3 in acute T-cell lymphoblastic leukemia. N Engl J Med. 2004;351:552-559.

418. Komuro H, Valentine MB, Rubnitz JE, et al. p27KIP1 deletions in childhood acute lymphoblastic leukemia. Neoplasia. 1999;1: 253-261.

419. Maia AT, van der Velden VH, Harrison CJ, et al. Prenatal origin of hyperdiploid acute lymphoblastic leukemia in identical twins. Leukemia. 2003;17:2202-2206.

420. Maia AT, Tussiwand R, Cazzaniga G, et al. Identification of pre-leukemic precursors of hyperdiploid acute lymphoblastic leukemia in cord blood. Genes Chromosomes Cancer. 2004;40:38-43.

421. Moorman AV, Richards SM, Martineau M, et al. Outcome heterogeneity in childhood high-hyperdiploid acute lymphoblastic leukemia. Blood. 2003;102:2756-2762.

422. Heerema NA, Sather HN, Sensel MG, et al. Prognostic impact of trisomies of chromosomes 10, 17, and 5 among children with acute lymphoblastic leukemia and high hyperdiploidy (> 50 chromosomes). J Clin Oncol. 2000;18:1876-1887.

423. Pui CH, Williams DL, Raimondi SC, et al. Hypodiploidy is associated with a poor prognosis in childhood acute lymphoblastic leukemia. Blood. 1987;70:247-253.

424. Heerema NA, Nachman JB, Sather HN, et al. Hypodiploidy with less than 45 chromosomes confers adverse risk in childhood acute lymphoblastic leukemia: a report from the children's cancer group. Blood. 1999;94:4036-4045.

425. Nachman JB, Heerema NA, Sather H, et al. Outcome of treatment in children with hypodiploid acute lymphoblastic leukemia. Blood. 2007;110:1112-1115.

426. Yeoh EJ, Ross ME, Shurtleff SA, et al. Classification, subtype discovery, and prediction of outcome in pediatric acute lymphoblastic leukemia by gene expression profiling. Cancer Cell. 2002;1:133-143.

427. Bartel DP. MicroRNAs: genomics, biogenesis, mechanism, and function. Cell. 2004;116:281-297.

428. Kertesz M, Iovino N, Unnerstall U, et al. The role of site accessibility in microRNA target recognition. Nat Genet. 2007;39: 1278-1284.

429. Calin GA, Ferracin M, Cimmino A, et al. A MicroRNA signature associated with prognosis and progression in chronic lymphocytic leukemia. N Engl J Med. 2005;353:1793-1801.

430. Mi S, Lu J, Sun M, et al. MicroRNA expression signatures accurately discriminate acute lymphoblastic leukemia from acute myeloid leukemia. Proc Natl Acad Sci U S A. 2007;104:19971-19976.

431. Bueno MJ, Pérez de Castro I, Gómez de Cedrón M, et al. Genetic and epigenetic silencing of microRNA-203 enhances ABL1 and BCR-ABL1 oncogene expression. Cancer Cell. 2008;13:496-506.

432. Lowenberg B. Diagnosis and prognosis in acute myeloid leukemia—the art of distinction. N Engl J Med. 2008;358:1960-1962.

433. Marcucci G, Radmacher MD, Maharry K, et al. MicroRNA expression in cytogenetically normal acute myeloid leukemia. N Engl J Med. 2008;358:1919-1928.

434. Martinez-Climent JA. Molecular cytogenetics of childhood hematologic malignancies. Leukemia. 1997;11:1999-2021.

435. Vardiman JW, Harris NL, Brunning RD. The World Health Organization (WHO) classification of the myeloid neoplasms. Blood. 2002;100:2292-2302.

436. Grimwade D, Walker H, Oliver F, et al. The importance of diagnostic cytogenetics on outcome in AML: analysis of 1,612 patients entered into the MRC AML 10 trial. The Medical Research Council Adult and Children's Leukaemia Working Parties. Blood. 1998;92:2322-2333.

437. Raimondi SC, Chang MN, Ravindranath Y, et al. Chromosomal abnormalities in 478 children with acute myeloid leukemia: clinical characteristics and treatment outcome in a cooperative Pediatric Oncology Group study-POG 8821. Blood. 1999;94: 3707-3716.

438. Kaleem Z, White G. Diagnostic criteria for minimally differentiated acute myeloid leukemia (AML-M0). Evaluation and a proposal. Am J Clin Pathol. 2001;115:876-884.

439. Rubnitz JE, Raimondi SC, Halbert AR, et al. Characteristics and outcome of t(8;21)-positive childhood acute myeloid leukemia: a single institution's experience. Leukemia. 2002;16:2072-2077.

440. Chan NP, Wong WS, Ng MH, et al. Childhood acute myeloid leukemia with CBFbeta-MYH11 rearrangement: study of incidence, morphology, cytogenetics, and clinical outcomes of Chinese in Hong Kong. Am J Hematol. 2004;76:300-303.

441. Duchayne E, Fenneteau O, Pages MP, et al. Acute megakaryoblastic leukaemia: a national clinical and biological study of 53 adult and childhood cases by the Groupe Francais d'Hematologie Cellulaire (GFHC). Leuk Lymphoma. 2003;44:49-58.

442. Schwyzer R, Sherman GG, Cohn RJ, et al. Granulocytic sarcoma in children with acute myeloblastic leukemia and t(8;21). Med Pediatr Oncol. 1998;31:144-149.

443. Chang M, Raimondi SC, Ravindranath Y, et al. Prognostic factors in children and adolescents with acute myeloid leukemia (excluding children with Down syndrome and acute promyelocytic leukemia): univariate and recursive partitioning analysis of patients treated on Pediatric Oncology Group (POG) Study 8821. Leukemia. 2000;14:1201-1207.

444. Woods WG, Neudorf S, Gold S, et al. A comparison of allogeneic bone marrow transplantation, autologous bone marrow transplantation, and aggressive chemotherapy in children with acute myeloid leukemia in remission. Blood. 2001;97:56-62.

445. Byrd JC, Ruppert AS, Mrozek K, et al. Repetitive cycles of high-dose cytarabine benefit patients with acute myeloid leukemia and inv(16);(p13q22) or t(16;16)(p13;q22): results from CALGB 8461. J Clin Oncol. 2004;22:1087-1094.

446. Roulston D, Espinosa R III, Nucifora G, et al. *CBFA2(AML1)* translocations with novel partner chromosomes in myeloid leukemias: association with prior therapy. Blood. 1998;92:2879-2885.

447. Kundu M, Chen A, Anderson S, et al. Role of Cbfb in hematopoiesis and perturbations resulting from expression of the leukemogenic fusion gene *Cbfb-MYH11*. Blood. 2002;100:2449-2456.

448. Larson RA, Williams SF, Le Beau MM, et al. Acute myelomonocytic leukemia with abnormal eosinophils and inv(16) or t(16;16) has a favorable prognosis. Blood. 1986;68:1242-1249.

449. Kalwinsky DK, Raimondi SC, Schell MJ, et al. Prognostic importance of cytogenetic subgroups in de novo pediatric acute non-lymphocytic leukemia. J Clin Oncol. 1990;8:75-83.

450. van der Reijden BA, Lombardo M, Dauwerse HG, et al. RT-PCR diagnosis of patients with acute nonlymphocytic leukemia and inv(16)(p13;q22) and identification of new alternative splicing in *CBFB-MYH11* transcripts. Blood. 1995;86:277-282.

451. Vance GH, Kim H, Hicks GA, et al. Utility of interphase FISH to stratify patients into cytogenetic risk categories at diagnosis of AML in an Eastern Cooperative Oncology Group (ECOG) clinical trial (E1900). Leuk Res. 2007;31:605-609.

452. Cox MC, Panetta P, Venditti A, et al. Comparison between conventional banding analysis and FISH screening with an AML-specific set of probes in 260 patients. Hematol J. 2003;4:263-270.

453. Merchant SH, Haines S, Hall B, et al. Fluorescence in situ hybridization identifies cryptic t(16;16)(p13;q22) masked by del(16)(q22) in a case of AML-M4 Eo. J Mol Diagn. 2004;6:271-274.

454. Zhou HF, Li JY, Wu YJ, et al. Immunophenotypic and cytogenetic features of acute myelomonocytic leukemia. Ai Zheng. 2006;25:1252-1255.

455. Martinez-Climent JA, Lane NJ, Rubin CM, et al. Clinical and prognostic significance of chromosomal abnormalities in childhood acute myeloid leukemia de novo. Leukemia. 1995;9:95-101.

456. Delaunay J, Vey N, Leblanc T, et al. Prognosis of inv(16)/t(16;16) acute myeloid leukemia (AML): a survey of 110 cases from the French AML Intergroup. Blood. 2003;102:462-469.

457. Melnick A, Licht JD. Deconstructing a disease: RARalpha, its fusion partners, and their roles in the pathogenesis of acute promyelocytic leukemia. Blood. 1999;93:3167-3215.

458. Mistry AR, Pedersen EW, Solomon E, Grimwade D. The molecular pathogenesis of acute promyelocytic leukaemia: implications for the clinical management of the disease. Blood Rev. 2003;17:71-97.

459. Arnould C, Philippe C, Bourdon V, et al. The signal transducer and activator of transcription *STAT5b* gene is a new partner of retinoic acid receptor alpha in acute promyelocytic-like leukaemia. Hum Mol Genet. 1999;8:1741-1749.

460. Redner RL, Rush EA, Faas S, et al. The t(5;17) variant of acute promyelocytic leukemia expresses a nucleophosmin-retinoic acid receptor fusion. Blood. 1996;87:882-886.

461. Chen Z, Brand NJ, Chen A, et al. Fusion between a novel Kruppel-like zinc finger gene and the retinoic acid receptor-alpha locus due to a variant t(11;17) translocation associated with acute promyelocytic leukaemia. EMBO J. 1993;12:1161-1167.

462. Catalano A, Dawson MA, Somana K, et al. The *PRKAR1A* gene is fused to *RARA* in a new variant acute promyelocytic leukemia. Blood. 2007;110:4073-4076.

463. Secker-Walker LM. General report on the European Union Concerted Action Workshop on 11q23, London, UK, May 1997. Leukemia. 1998;12:776-778.

464. Sobulo OM, Borrow J, Tomek R, et al. *MLL* is fused to *CBP*, a histone acetyltransferase, in therapy-related acute myeloid leukemia with a t(11;16)(q23;p13.3). Proc Natl Acad Sci U S A. 1997;94:8732-8737.

465. Ono R, Taki T, Taketani T, et al. *LCX*, leukemia-associated protein with a CXXC domain, is fused to *MLL* in acute myeloid leukemia with trilineage dysplasia having t(10;11)(q22;q23). Cancer Res. 2002;62:4075-4080.

466. Lorsbach RB, Moore J, Mathew S, et al. *TET1*, a member of a novel protein family, is fused to *MLL* in acute myeloid leukemia containing the t(10;11)(q22;q23). Leukemia. 2003;17:637-641.

467. Hayette S, Tigaud I, Vanier A, et al. *AF15q14*, a novel partner gene fused to the MLL gene in an acute myeloid leukaemia with a t(11;15)(q23;q14). Oncogene. 2000;19:4446-4450.

468. Bernard OA, Mauchauffe M, Mecucci C, et al. A novel gene, *AF-1p*, fused to HRX in t(1;11)(p32;q23), is not related to *AF-4*, *AF-9* nor *ENL*. Oncogene. 1994;9:1039-1045.

469. Megonigal MD, Cheung NK, Rappaport EF, et al. Detection of leukemia-associated *MLL-GAS7* translocation early during chemotherapy with DNA topoisomerase II inhibitors. Proc Natl Acad Sci U S A. 2000;97:2814-2819.

470. Osaka M, Rowley JD, Zeleznik-Le NJ. *MSF* (MLL septin-like fusion), a fusion partner gene of *MLL*, in a therapy-related acute myeloid leukemia with a t(11;17)(q23;q25). Proc Natl Acad Sci U S A. 1999;96:6428-6433.

471. Taki T, Ohnishi H, Shinohara K, et al. *AF17q25*, a putative septin family gene, fuses the *MLL* gene in acute myeloid leukemia with t(11;17)(q23;q25). Cancer Res. 1999;59:4261-4265.

472. Borkhardt A, Teigler-Schlegel A, Fuchs U, et al. An ins(X;11)(q24;q23) fuses the MLL and the *Septin6/KIAA0128* gene in an infant with AML-M2. Genes Chromosomes Cancer. 2001;32:82-88.

473. Wechsler DS, Engstrom LD, Alexander BM, et al. A novel chromosomal inversion at 11q23 in infant acute myeloid leukemia fuses *MLL* to *CALM*, a gene that encodes a clathrin assembly protein. Genes Chromosomes Cancer. 2003;36:26-36.

474. Kourlas PJ, Strout MP, Becknell B, et al. Identification of a gene at 11q23 encoding a guanine nucleotide exchange factor: evidence for its fusion with MLL in acute myeloid leukemia. Proc Natl Acad Sci U S A. 2000;97:2145-2150.

475. Schichman SA, Caligiuri MA, Gu Y, et al. *ALL-1* partial duplication in acute leukemia. Proc Natl Acad Sci U S A. 1994;91:6236-6239.

476. Caligiuri MA, Strout MP, Schichman SA, et al. Partial tandem duplication of *ALL-1* as a recurrent molecular defect in acute myeloid leukemia with trisomy 11. Cancer Res. 1996;56:1418-1425.

477. Pegram LD, Megonigal MD, Lange BJ, et al. t(3;11) translocation in treatment-related acute myeloid leukemia fuses *MLL* with the *GMPS* (*GUANOSINE 5' MONOPHOSPHATE SYNTHETASE*) gene. Blood. 2000;96:4360-4362.

478. Shih LY, Liang DC, Fu JF, et al. Characterization of fusion partner genes in 114 patients with de novo acute myeloid leukemia and MLL rearrangement. Leukemia. 2006;20:218-223.

479. Fu JF, Hsu HC, Shih LY. *MLL* is fused to *EB1* (*MAPRE1*), which encodes a microtubule-associated protein, in a patient with acute lymphoblastic leukemia. Genes Chromosomes Cancer. 2005;43:206-210.

480. Taki T, Kano H, Taniwaki M, et al. AF5q31, a newly identified *AF4*-related gene, is fused to *MLL* in infant acute lymphoblastic leukemia with ins(5;11)(q31;q13q23). Proc Natl Acad Sci U S A. 1999;96:14535-14540.

481. So CW, Cleary ML. Common mechanism for oncogenic activation of MLL by forkhead family proteins. Blood. 2003;101:633-639.

482. Zeisig BB, Schreiner S, Garcia-Cuellar MP, Slany RK. Transcriptional activation is a key function encoded by MLL fusion partners. Leukemia. 2003;17:359-365.

483. So CW, Lin M, Ayton PM, et al. Dimerization contributes to oncogenic activation of MLL chimeras in acute leukemias. Cancer Cell. 2003;4:99-110.

484. Erfurth F, Hemenway CS, de Erkenez AC, Domer PH. MLL fusion partners AF4 and AF9 interact at subnuclear foci. Leukemia. 2004;18:92-102.

485. Corral J, Lavenir I, Impey H, et al. An *Mll-AF9* fusion gene made by homologous recombination causes acute leukemia in chimeric mice: a method to create fusion oncogenes. Cell. 1996;85:853-861.

486. So CW, Karsunky H, Passegue E, et al. MLL-GAS7 transforms multipotent hematopoietic progenitors and induces mixed lineage leukemias in mice. Cancer Cell. 2003;3:161-171.

487. So CW, Karsunky H, Wong P, et al. Leukemic transformation of hematopoietic progenitors by MLL-GAS7 in the absence of Hoxa7 or Hoxa9. Blood. 2004;103:3192-3199.

488. Bresters D, Reus AC, Veerman AJ, et al. Congenital leukaemia: the Dutch experience and review of the literature. Br J Haematol. 2002;117:513-524.

489. Bacher U, Kern W, Schnittger S, et al. Population-based age-specific incidences of cytogenetic subgroups of acute myeloid leukemia. Haematologica. 2005;90:1502-1510.

490. Smith MA, Rubinstein L, Ungerleider RS. Therapy-related acute myeloid leukemia following treatment with epipodophyllotoxins: estimating the risks. Med Pediatr Oncol. 1994;23:86-98.

491. Winick N, Buchanan GR, Kamen BA. Secondary acute myeloid leukemia in Hispanic children. J Clin Oncol. 1993;11:1433.

492. Rowley JD, Reshmi S, Sobulo O, et al. All patients with the T(11;16)(q23;p13.3) that involves *MLL* and *CBP* have treatment-related hematologic disorders. Blood. 1997;90:535-541.

493. Satake N, Ishida Y, Otoh Y, et al. Novel *MLL-CBP* fusion transcript in therapy-related chronic myelomonocytic leukemia with a t(11;16)(q23;p13) chromosome translocation. Genes Chromosomes Cancer. 1997;20:60-63.

494. Taki T, Sako M, Tsuchida M, Hayashi Y. The t(11;16)(q23;p13) translocation in myelodysplastic syndrome fuses the *MLL* gene to the *CBP* gene. Blood. 1997;89:3945-3950.

495. Dreyling MH, Schrader K, Fonatsch C, et al. *MLL* and *CALM* are fused to *AF10* in morphologically distinct subsets of acute leukemia with translocation t(10;11): both rearrangements are associated with a poor prognosis. Blood. 1998;91:4662-4667.

496. Burnett MM, Huang MS, Seliem RM. Case records of the Massachusetts General Hospital. Case 29-2007. Case 39-2007. A 5-month-old girl with skin lesions. N Engl J Med. 2007;357: 2616-2623.

497. Grundy RG, Martinez A, Kempski H, et al. Spontaneous remission of congenital leukemia: a case for conservative treatment. J Pediatr Hematol Oncol. 2000;22:252-255.

498. Burjanivova T, Madzo J, Muzikova K, et al. Prenatal origin of childhood AML occurs less frequently than in childhood ALL. BMC Cancer. 2006;6:100.

499. Bayoumy M, Wynn T, Jamil A, et al. Prenatal presentation supports the in utero development of congenital leukemia: a case report. J Pediatr Hematol Oncol. 2003;25:148-152.

500. Giles RH, Dauwerse JG, Higgins C, et al. Detection of *CBP* rearrangements in acute myelogenous leukemia with t(8;16). Leukemia. 1997;11:2087-2096.

501. Wessels JW, Mollevanger P, Dauwerse JG, et al. Two distinct loci on the short arm of chromosome 16 are involved in myeloid leukemia. Blood. 1991;77:1555-1559.

502. Borrow J, Stanton VP, Andresen M, et al. The translocation t(8;16)(p11;p13) of acute myeloid leukaemia fuses a putative acetyltransferase to the CREB-binding protein. Nat Genet. 1996;14:33-41.

503. Pelletier N, Champagne N, Lim H, Yang XJ. Expression, purification, and analysis of MOZ and MORF histone acetyltransferases. Methods. 2003;31:24-32.

504. Pelletier N, Champagne N, Stifani S, Yang XJ. MOZ and MORF histone acetyltransferases interact with the Runt-domain transcription factor Runx2. Oncogene. 2002;21:2729-2740.

505. Champagne N, Bertos NR, Pelletier N, et al. Identification of a human histone acetyltransferase related to monocytic leukemia zinc finger protein. J Biol Chem. 1999;274:28528-28536.

506. Champagne N, Pelletier N, Yang XJ. The monocytic leukemia zinc finger protein MOZ is a histone acetyltransferase. Oncogene. 2001;20:404-409.

507. Panagopoulos I, Isaksson M, Lindvall C, et al. RT-PCR analysis of the *MOZ-CBP* and *CBP-MOZ* chimeric transcripts in acute myeloid leukemias with t(8;16)(p11;p13). Genes Chromosomes Cancer. 2000;28:415-424.

508. Panagopoulos I, Fioretos T, Isaksson M, et al. RT-PCR analysis of acute myeloid leukemia with t(8;16)(p11;p13): identification of a novel *MOZ/CBP* transcript and absence of *CBP/MOZ* expression. Genes Chromosomes Cancer. 2002;35:372-374.

509. Kitabayashi I, Aikawa Y, Nguyen LA, et al. Activation of AML1-mediated transcription by MOZ and inhibition by the MOZ-CBP fusion protein. EMBO J. 2001;20:7184-7196.

510. Camos M, Esteve J, Jares P, et al. Gene expression profiling of acute myeloid leukemia with translocation t(8;16)(p11;p13) and *MYST3-CREBBP* rearrangement reveals a distinctive signature with a specific pattern of *HOX* gene expression. Cancer Res. 2006;66:6947-6954.

511. Petrij F, Giles RH, Dauwerse HG, et al. Rubinstein-Taybi syndrome caused by mutations in the transcriptional co-activator CBP. Nature. 1995;376:348-351.

512. Taine L, Goizet C, Wen ZQ, et al. Submicroscopic deletion of chromosome 16p13.3 in patients with Rubinstein-Taybi syndrome. Am J Med Genet. 1998;78:267-270.

513. Petrij F, Dorsman JC, Dauwerse HG, et al. Rubinstein-Taybi syndrome caused by a de novo reciprocal translocation t(2;16)(q36.3;p13.3). Am J Med Genet. 2000;92:47-52.

514. Schmidt HH, Strehl S, Thaler D, et al. RT-PCR and FISH analysis of acute myeloid leukemia with t(8;16)(p11;p13) and chimeric *MOZ* and *CBP* transcripts: breakpoint cluster region and clinical implications. Leukemia. 2004;18:1115-1121.

515. Stark B, Resnitzky P, Jeison M, et al. A distinct subtype of M4/M5 acute myeloblastic leukemia (AML) associated with t(8;16)(p11;p13), in a patient with the variant t(8;19)(p11: q13)—case report and review of the literature. Leuk Res. 1995;19:367-379.

516. Stark B, Jeison M, Gabay LG, et al. Classical and molecular cytogenetic abnormalities and outcome of childhood acute myeloid leukaemia: report from a referral centre in Israel. Br J Haematol. 2004;126:320-337.

517. Sainati L, Bolcato S, Cocito MG, et al. Transient acute monoblastic leukemia with reciprocal (8;16)(p11;p13) translocation. Pediatr Hematol Oncol. 1996;13:151-157.

518. Weintraub M, Kaplinsky C, Amariglio N, et al. Spontaneous regression of congenital leukaemia with an 8;16 translocation. Br J Haematol. 2000;111:641-643.

519. Panagopoulos I, Fioretos T, Isaksson M, et al. Fusion of the *MORF* and *CBP* genes in acute myeloid leukemia with the t(10;16)(q22;p13). Hum Mol Genet. 2001;10:395-404.

520. Carapeti M, Aguiar RC, Goldman JM, Cross NC. A novel fusion between MOZ and the nuclear receptor coactivator TIF2 in acute myeloid leukemia. Blood. 1998;91:3127-3133.

521. Deguchi K, Ayton PM, Carapeti M, et al. *MOZ-TIF2*-induced acute myeloid leukemia requires the MOZ nucleosome binding motif and TIF2-mediated recruitment of CBP. Cancer Cell. 2003;3:259-271.

522. Kitabayashi I, Aikawa Y, Yokoyama A, et al. Fusion of *MOZ* and *p300* histone acetyltransferases in acute monocytic leukemia with a t(8;22)(p11;q13) chromosome translocation. Leukemia. 2001;15:89-94.

523. Lillington DM, MacCallum PK, Lister TA, Gibbons B. Translocation t(6;9)(p23;q34) in acute myeloid leukemia without myelodysplasia or basophilia: two cases and a review of the literature. Leukemia. 1993;7:527-531.

524. Alsabeh R, Brynes RK, Slovak ML, Arber DA. Acute myeloid leukemia with t(6;9) (p23;q34): association with myelodysplasia, basophilia, and initial CD34 negative immunophenotype. Am J Clin Pathol. 1997;107:430-437.

525. Oyarzo MP, Lin P, Glassman A, et al. Acute myeloid leukemia with t(6;9)(p23;q34) is associated with dysplasia and a high frequency of flt3 gene mutations. Am J Clin Pathol. 2004; 122:348-358.

526. Nakano H, Shimamoto Y, Suga K, Kobayashi M. Detection of minimal residual disease in a patient with acute myeloid leukemia and t(6;9) at the time of peripheral blood stem cell transplantation. Acta Haematol. 1995;94:139-141.

527. Barnard DR, Kalousek DK, Wiersma SR, et al. Morphologic, immunologic, and cytogenetic classification of acute myeloid leukemia and myelodysplastic syndrome in childhood: a report from the Childrens Cancer Group. Leukemia. 1996;10:5-12.

528. Boer J, Mahmoud H, Raimondi S, et al. Loss of the *DEK-CAN* fusion transcript in a child with t(6;9) acute myeloid leukemia following chemotherapy and allogeneic bone marrow transplantation. Leukemia. 1997;11:299-300.

529. von Lindern M, Breems D, van Baal S, et al. Characterization of the translocation breakpoint sequences of two *DEK-CAN* fusion

genes present in t(6;9) acute myeloid leukemia and a *SET-CAN* fusion gene found in a case of acute undifferentiated leukemia. Genes Chromosomes Cancer. 1992;5:227-234.

530. von Lindern M, Fornerod M, van Baal S, et al. The translocation (6;9), associated with a specific subtype of acute myeloid leukemia, results in the fusion of two genes, dek and can, and the expression of a chimeric, leukemia-specific dek-can mRNA. Mol Cell Biol. 1992;12:1687-1697.

531. von Lindern M, Poustka A, Lerach H, Grosveld G. The (6;9) chromosome translocation, associated with a specific subtype of acute nonlymphocytic leukemia, leads to aberrant transcription of a target gene on 9q34. Mol Cell Biol. 1990;10:4016-4026.

532. Kappes F, Scholten I, Richter N, et al. Functional domains of the ubiquitous chromatin protein DEK. Mol Cell Biol. 2004;24:6000-6010.

533. Waldmann T, Scholten I, Kappes F, et al. The DEK protein—an abundant and ubiquitous constituent of mammalian chromatin. Gene. 2004;343:1-9.

534. Ageberg M, Drott K, Olofsson T, et al. Identification of a novel and myeloid specific role of the leukemia-associated fusion protein DEK-NUP214 leading to increased protein synthesis. Genes Chromosomes Cancer. 2008;47:276-287.

535. Garcon L, Libura M, Delabesse E, et al. *DEK-CAN* molecular monitoring of myeloid malignancies could aid therapeutic stratification. Leukemia. 2005;19:1338-1344.

536. Ostergaard M, Stentoft J, Hokland P. A real-time quantitative RT-PCR assay for monitoring *DEK-CAN* fusion transcripts arising from translocation t(6;9) in acute myeloid leukemia. Leuk Res. 2004;28:1213-1215.

537. Tobal K, Frost L, Liu Yin JA. Quantification of *DEK-CAN* fusion transcript by real-time reverse transcription polymerase reaction in patients with t(6;9) acute myeloid leukemia. Haematologica. 2004;89:1267-1269.

538. Radu A, Moore MS, Blobel G. The peptide repeat domain of nucleoporin Nup98 functions as a docking site in transport across the nuclear pore complex. Cell. 1995;81:215-222.

539. Moore MA, Chung KY, Plasilova M, et al. NUP98 dysregulation in myeloid leukemogenesis. Ann N Y Acad Sci. 2007;1106:114-142.

540. Ahuja HG, Felix CA, Aplan PD. The t(11;20)(p15;q11) chromosomal translocation associated with therapy-related myelodysplastic syndrome results in an *NUP98-TOP1* fusion. Blood. 1999;94:3258-3261.

541. Arai Y, Hosoda F, Kobayashi H, et al. The inv(11)(p15q22) chromosome translocation of de novo and therapy-related myeloid malignancies results in fusion of the nucleoporin gene, *NUP98*, with the putative RNA helicase gene, *DDX10*. Blood. 1997;89:3936-3944.

542. Arai Y, Kyo T, Miwa H, et al. Heterogeneous fusion transcripts involving the NUP98 gene and *HOXD13* gene activation in a case of acute myeloid leukemia with the t(2;11)(q31;p15) translocation. Leukemia. 2000;14:1621-1629.

543. Borrow J, Shearman AM, Stanton VP Jr, et al. The t(7;11)(p15;p15) translocation in acute myeloid leukaemia fuses the genes for nucleoporin NUP98 and class I homeoprotein HOXA9. Nat Genet. 1996;12:159-167.

544. Cerveira N, Correia C, Doria S, et al. Frequency of *NUP98-NSD1* fusion transcript in childhood acute myeloid leukaemia. Leukemia. 2003;17:2244-2247.

545. Cimino G, Sprovieri T, Rapanotti MC, et al. Molecular evaluation of the *NUP98/RAP1GDS1* gene frequency in adults with T-acute lymphoblastic leukemia. Haematologica. 2001;86:436-439.

546. Hussey DJ, Moore S, Nicola M, Dobrovic A. Fusion of the *NUP98* gene with the *LEDGF*/p52 gene defines a recurrent acute myeloid leukemia translocation. BMC Genet. 2001;2:20.

547. Hussey DJ, Nicola M, Moore S, et al. The (4;11)(q21;p15) translocation fuses the *NUP98* and *RAP1GDS1* genes and is recurrent in T-cell acute lymphocytic leukemia. Blood. 1999;94:2072-2079.

548. Ikeda T, Ikeda K, Sasaki K, et al. The inv(11)(p15;q22) chromosome translocation of therapy-related myelodysplasia with *NUP98-DDX10* and *DDX10-NUP98* fusion transcripts. Int J Hematol. 1999;69:160-164.

549. Iwase S, Akiyama N, Sekikawa T, et al. Both *NUP98/TOP1* and *TOP1/NUP98* transcripts are detected in a de novo AML with t(11;20)(p15;q11). Genes Chromosomes Cancer. 2003;38:102-105.

550. Jaju RJ, Fidler C, Haas OA, et al. A novel gene, *NSD1*, is fused to *NUP98* in the t(5;11)(q35;p15.5) in de novo childhood acute myeloid leukemia. Blood. 2001;98:1264-1267.

551. Jankovic D, Gorello P, Liu T, et al. Leukemogenic mechanisms and targets of a *NUP98/HHEX* fusion in acute myeloid leukemia. Blood. 2008;111:5672-5682.

552. Kobzev YN, Martinez-Climent J, Lee S, et al. Analysis of translocations that involve the *NUP98* gene in patients with 11p15 chromosomal rearrangements. Genes Chromosomes Cancer. 2004;41:339-352.

553. Mecucci C, La Starza R, Negrini M, et al. t(4;11)(q21;p15) translocation involving *NUP98* and *RAP1GDS1* genes: characterization of a new subset of T acute lymphoblastic leukaemia. Br J Haematol. 2000;109:788-793.

554. Nishiyama M, Arai Y, Tsunematsu Y, et al. 11p15 translocations involving the NUP98 gene in childhood therapy-related acute myeloid leukemia/myelodysplastic syndrome. Genes Chromosomes Cancer. 1999;26:215-220.

555. Nebral K, Schmidt HH, Haas OA, Strehl S. *NUP98* is fused to topoisomerase (DNA) IIbeta 180 kDa (*TOP2B*) in a patient with acute myeloid leukemia with a new t(3;11)(p24;p15). Clin Cancer Res. 2005;11:6489-6494.

556. Shimada H, Arai Y, Sekiguchi S, et al. Generation of the *NUP98-HOXD13* fusion transcript by a rare translocation, t(2;11)(q31;p15), in a case of infant leukaemia. Br J Haematol. 2000;110:210-213.

557. Morerio C, Acquila M, Rosanda C, et al. t(9;11)(p22;p15) with *NUP98-LEDGF* fusion gene in pediatric acute myeloid leukemia. Leuk Res. 2005;29:467-470.

558. Pan Q, Zhu YJ, Gu BW, et al. A new fusion gene *NUP98-IQCG* identified in an acute T-lymphoid/myeloid leukemia with a t(3;11)(q29q13;p15)del(3)(q29) translocation. Oncogene. 2008;27:3414-3423.

559. Romana SP, Radford-Weiss I, Ben AR, et al. *NUP98* rearrangements in hematopoietic malignancies: a study of the Groupe Francophone de Cytogenetique Hematologique. Leukemia. 2006;20:696-706.

560. Smith MA, McCaffrey RP, Karp JE. The secondary leukemias: challenges and research directions. JNCI. 1996;88:407-418.

561. Miller JS, Arthur DC, Litz CE, et al. Myelodysplastic syndrome after autologous bone marrow transplantation: an additional late complication of curative cancer therapy. Blood. 1994;83:3780-3786.

562. Stone RM, Neuberg D, Soiffer R, et al. Myelodysplastic syndrome as a late complication following autologous bone marrow transplantation for non-Hodgkin's lymphoma. J Clin Oncol. 1994;12:2535-2542.

563. Rege KP, Janes SL, Saso R, et al. Secondary leukaemia characterised by monosomy 7 occurring post-autologous stem cell transplantation for AML. Bone Marrow Transplant. 1998;21:853-855.

564. Smith SM, Le Beau MM, Huo D, et al. Clinical-cytogenetic associations in 306 patients with therapy-related myelodysplasia and myeloid leukemia: the University of Chicago series. Blood. 2003;102:43-52.

565. Davies SM. Therapy-related leukemia associated with alkylating agents. Med Pediatr Oncol. 2001;36:536-540.

566. Meadows AT, Obringer AC, Marrero O, et al. Second malignant neoplasms following childhood Hodgkin's disease: treatment and splenectomy as risk factors. Med Pediatr Oncol. 1989;17: 477-484.

567. Greene MH, Harris EL, Gershenson DM, et al. Melphalan may be a more potent leukemogen than cyclophosphamide. Ann Intern Med. 1986;105:360-367.

568. Blayney DW, Longo DL, Young RC, et al. Decreasing risk of leukemia with prolonged follow-up after chemotherapy and radiotherapy for Hodgkin's disease. N Engl J Med. 1987;316: 710-714.

569. Pedersen-Bjergaard J, Pedersen M, Roulston D, Philip P. Different genetic pathways in leukemogenesis for patients presenting with therapy-related myelodysplasia and therapy-related acute myeloid leukemia. Blood. 1995;86:3542-3552.

570. Willman CL. Molecular genetic features of myelodysplastic syndromes (MDS). Leukemia. 1998;12(Suppl 1): S2-S6.

571. Pedersen-Bjergaard J, Andersen MK, Christiansen DH, Nerlov C. Genetic pathways in therapy-related myelodysplasia and acute myeloid leukemia. Blood. 2002;99:1909-1912.

572. Liang H, Fairman J, Claxton DF, et al. Molecular anatomy of chromosome 7q deletions in myeloid neoplasms: evidence for multiple critical loci. Proc Natl Acad Sci U S A. 1998;95:3781-3785.

573. Bodner SM, Naeve CW, Rakestraw KM, et al. Cloning and chromosomal localization of the gene encoding human cyclin D-binding Myb-like protein (hDMP1). Gene. 1999;229:223-228.

574. Emerling BM, Bonifas J, Kratz CP, et al. *MLL5*, a homolog of Drosophila trithorax located within a segment of chromosome band 7q22 implicated in myeloid leukemia. Oncogene. 2002;21: 4849-4854.

575. Kratz CP, Emerling BM, Bonifas J, et al. Genomic structure of the *PIK3CG* gene on chromosome band 7q22 and evaluation as a candidate myeloid tumor suppressor. Blood. 2002;99:372-374.

576. Kratz CP, Emerling BM, Donovan S, et al. Candidate gene isolation and comparative analysis of a commonly deleted segment of 7q22 implicated in myeloid malignancies. Genomics. 2001;77: 171-180.

577. Andersen MK, Christiansen DH, Kirchhoff M, Pedersen-Bjergaard J. Duplication or amplification of chromosome band 11q23, including the unrearranged *MLL* gene, is a recurrent abnormality in therapy-related MDS and AML, and is closely related to mutation of the *TP53* gene and to previous therapy with alkylating agents. Genes Chromosomes Cancer. 2001;31: 33-41.

578. Willman CL, Sever CE, Pallavicini MG, et al. Deletion of *IRF-1*, mapping to chromosome 5q31.1, in human leukemia and preleukemic myelodysplasia. Science. 1993;259:968-971.

579. Boultwood J, Lewis S, Wainscoat JS. The 5q-syndrome. Blood. 1994;84:3253-3260.

580. Zhao N, Stoffel A, Wang PW, et al. Molecular delineation of the smallest commonly deleted region of chromosome 5 in malignant myeloid diseases to 1-1.5 Mb and preparation of a PAC-based physical map. Proc Natl Acad Sci U S A. 1997;94: 6948-6953.

581. Lezon-Geyda K, Najfeld V, Johnson EM. Deletions of *PURA*, at 5q31, and *PURB*, at 7p13, in myelodysplastic syndrome and progression to acute myelogenous leukemia. Leukemia. 2001;15:954-962.

582. Fairman J, Wang RY, Liang H, et al. Translocations and deletions of 5q13.1 in myelodysplasia and acute myelogenous leukemia: evidence for a novel critical locus. Blood. 1996;88: 2259-2266.

583. Castro P, Liang H, Liang JC, Nagarajan L. A novel, evolutionarily conserved gene family with putative sequence-specific single-stranded DNA-binding activity. Genomics. 2002;80:78-85.

584. Castro PD, Liang JC, Nagarajan L. Deletions of chromosome 5q13.3 and 17p loci cooperate in myeloid neoplasms. Blood. 2000;95:2138-2143.

585. Liu TX, Becker MW, Jelinek J, et al. Chromosome 5q deletion and epigenetic suppression of the gene encoding alpha-catenin (CTNNA1) in myeloid cell transformation. Nat Med. 2007; 13:78-83.

586. Joslin JM, Fernald AA, Tennant TR, et al. Haploinsufficiency of *EGR1*, a candidate gene in the del(5q), leads to the development of myeloid disorders. Blood. 2007;110:719-726.

587. Ebert BL, Pretz J, Bosco J, et al. Identification of *RPS14* as a 5q- syndrome gene by RNA interference screen. Nature. 2008;451:335-339.

588. Deeg HJ, Socie G. Malignancies after hematopoietic stem cell transplantation: many questions, some answers. Blood. 1998;91: 1833-1844.

589. Pedersen-Bjergaard J, Andersen MK, Christiansen DH. Therapy-related acute myeloid leukemia and myelodysplasia after high-dose chemotherapy and autologous stem cell transplantation. Blood. 2000;95:3273-3279.

590. Micallef IN, Lillington DM, Apostolidis J, et al. Therapy-related myelodysplasia and secondary acute myelogenous leukemia after high-dose therapy with autologous hematopoietic progenitor-cell support for lymphoid malignancies. J Clin Oncol. 2000;18: 947-955.

591. Abruzzese E, Radford JE, Miller JS, et al. Detection of abnormal pretransplant clones in progenitor cells of patients who developed myelodysplasia after autologous transplantation. Blood. 1999;94: 1814-1819.

592. Weber MH, Wenzel U, Thiel E, Knauf WU. Chromosomal aberrations characteristic for sAML/sMDS are not detectable by random screening using FISH in peripheral blood-derived grafts used for autologous transplantation. J Hematother Stem Cell Res. 2000;9:861-865.

593. Rowley JD, Olney HJ. International workshop on the relationship of prior therapy to balanced chromosome aberrations in therapy-related myelodysplastic syndromes and acute leukemia: overview report. Genes Chromosomes Cancer. 2002;33:331-345.

594. Pedersen-Bjergaard J, Rowley JD. The balanced and the unbalanced chromosome aberrations of acute myeloid leukemia may develop in different ways and may contribute differently to malignant transformation. Blood. 1994;83:2780-2786.

595. Sano K, Hayakawa A, Piao JH, et al. Novel SH3 protein encoded by the AF3p21 gene is fused to the mixed lineage leukemia protein in a therapy-related leukemia with t(3;11)(p21;q23). Blood. 2000;95:1066-1068.

596. Le Deley MC, Leblanc T, Shamsaldin A, et al. Risk of secondary leukemia after a solid tumor in childhood according to the dose of epipodophyllotoxins and anthracyclines: a case-control study by the Societe Francaise d'Oncologie Pediatrique. J Clin Oncol. 2003;21:1074-1081.

597. Smith MA, Rubinstein L, Anderson JR, et al. Secondary leukemia or myelodysplastic syndrome after treatment with epipodophyllotoxins. J Clin Oncol. 1999;17:569-577.

598. Ratain MJ, Kaminer LS, Bitran JD, et al. Acute nonlymphocytic leukemia following etoposide and cisplatin combination chemotherapy for advanced non-small-cell carcinoma of the lung. Blood. 1987;70:1412-1417.

599. Pui CH, Kalwinsky DK, Schell MJ, et al. Acute nonlymphoblastic leukemia in infants: clinical presentation and outcome. J Clin Oncol. 1988;6:1008-1013.

600. Pedersen-Bjergaard J, Daugaard G, Hansen SW, et al. Increased risk of myelodysplasia and leukaemia after etoposide, cisplatin, and bleomycin for germ-cell tumours. Lancet. 1991;338: 359-363.

601. Pedersen-Bjergaard J, Philip P. Balanced translocations involving chromosome bands 11q23 and 21q22 are highly characteristic of myelodysplasia and leukemia following therapy with cytostatic

agents targeting at DNA-topoisomerase II. Blood. 1991;78: 1147-1148.

602. Pui CH, Hancock ML, Raimondi SC, et al. Myeloid neoplasia in children treated for solid tumours. Lancet. 1990;336: 417-421.

603. Sandoval C, Pui CH, Bowman LC, et al. Secondary acute myeloid leukemia in children previously treated with alkylating agents, intercalating topoisomerase II inhibitors, and irradiation. J Clin Oncol. 1993;11:1039-1045.

604. Kantarjian HM, Keating MJ, Walters RS, et al. The association of specific "favorable" cytogenetic abnormalities with secondary leukemia. Cancer. 1986;58:924-927.

605. Pedersen-Bjergaard J, Andersen MK, Andersen MT, Christiansen DH. Genetics of therapy-related myelodysplasia and acute myeloid leukemia. Leukemia. 2008;22:240-248.

606. Nucifora G, Birn DJ, Espinosa R III, et al. Involvement of the AML1 gene in the t(3;21) in therapy-related leukemia and in chronic myeloid leukemia in blast crisis. Blood. 1993;81: 2728-2734.

607. Larson RA, Le Beau M, Ratain MJ, Rowley JD. Balanced translocations involving chromosome bands 11q23 and 21q22 in therapy-related leukemia. Blood. 1992;79:1892-1893.

608. Rubin CM, Larson RA, Anastasi J, et al. t(3;21)(q26;q22): a recurring chromosomal abnormality in therapy-related myelodysplastic syndrome and acute myeloid leukemia. Blood. 1990;76: 2594-2598.

609. Slovak ML, Bedell V, Popplewell L, et al. 21q22 balanced chromosome aberrations in therapy-related hematopoietic disorders: report from an international workshop. Genes Chromosomes Cancer. 2002;33:379-394.

610. Pedersen-Bjergaard J, Andersen MK, Johansson B. Balanced chromosome aberrations in leukemias following chemotherapy with DNA-topoisomerase II inhibitors. J Clin Oncol. 1998;16: 1897-1898.

611. Andersen MK, Larson RA, Mauritzson N, et al. Balanced chromosome abnormalities inv(16) and t(15;17) in therapy-related myelodysplastic syndromes and acute leukemia: report from an international workshop. Genes Chromosomes Cancer. 2002;33: 395-400.

612. Fenaux P, Lucidarme D, Lai JL, Bauters F. Favorable cytogenetic abnormalities in secondary leukemia. Cancer. 1989;63:2505-2508.

613. Dissing M, Le Beau MM, Pedersen-Bjergaard J. Inversion of chromosome 16 and uncommon rearrangements of the CBFB and MYH11 genes in therapy-related acute myeloid leukemia: rare events related to DNA-topoisomerase II inhibitors? J Clin Oncol. 1998;16:1890-1896.

614. Quesnel B, Kantarjian H, Bjergaard JP, et al. Therapy-related acute myeloid leukemia with t(8;21), inv(16), and t(8;16): a report on 25 cases and review of the literature. J Clin Oncol. 1993;11:2370-2379.

615. Block AW, Carroll AJ, Hagemeijer A, et al. Rare recurring balanced chromosome abnormalities in therapy-related myelodysplastic syndromes and acute leukemia: report from an international workshop. Genes Chromosomes Cancer. 2002;33:401-412.

616. Nakamura T, Largaespada DA, Lee MP, et al. Fusion of the nucleoporin gene NUP98 to HOXA9 by the chromosome translocation t(7;11)(p15;p15) in human myeloid leukaemia. Nat Genet. 1996;12:154-158.

617. Stark B, Jeison M, Shohat M, et al. Involvement of 11p15 and 3q21q26 in therapy-related myeloid leukemia (t-ML) in children. Case reports and review of the literature. Cancer Genet Cytogenet. 1994;75:11-22.

618. Kobayashi H, Arai Y, Hosoda F, et al. Inversion of chromosome 11 inv(11)(p15q22), as a recurring chromosomal aberration associated with de novo and secondary myeloid malignancies: identification of a P1 clone spanning the 11q22 breakpoint. Genes Chromosomes Cancer. 1997;19:150-155.

619. Nakamura T, Yamazaki Y, Hatano Y, Miura I. NUP98 is fused to PMX1 homeobox gene in human acute myelogenous leukemia with chromosome translocation t(1;11)(q23;p15). Blood. 1999; 94:741-747.

620. Blanco JG, Dervieux T, Edick MJ, et al. Molecular emergence of acute myeloid leukemia during treatment for acute lymphoblastic leukemia. Proc Natl Acad Sci U S A. 2001;98:10338-10343.

621. Teuffel O, Betts DR, Thali M, et al. Clonal expansion of a new MLL rearrangement in the absence of leukemia. Blood. 2005;105:4151-4152.

622. Domer PH, Head DR, Renganathan N, et al. Molecular analysis of 13 cases of MLL/11q23 secondary acute leukemia and identification of topoisomerase II consensus-binding sequences near the chromosomal breakpoint of a secondary leukemia with the t(4;11). Leukemia. 1995;9:1305-1312.

623. Atlas M, Head D, Behm F, et al. Cloning and sequence analysis of four t(9;11) therapy-related leukemia breakpoints. Leukemia. 1998;12:1895-1902.

624. Imamura T, Kakazu N, Hibi S, et al. Rearrangement of the MOZ gene in pediatric therapy-related myelodysplastic syndrome with a novel chromosomal translocation t(2;8)(p23;p11). Genes Chromosomes Cancer. 2003;36:413-419.

625. Barnard DR, Lange B, Alonzo TA, et al. Acute myeloid leukemia and myelodysplastic syndrome in children treated for cancer: comparison with primary presentation. Blood. 2002;100: 427-434.

626. Hasle H, Niemeyer CM, Chessells JM, et al. A pediatric approach to the WHO classification of myelodysplastic and myeloproliferative diseases. Leukemia. 2003;17:277-282.

627. Lauchle JO, Braun BS, Loh ML, Shannon K. Inherited predispositions and hyperactive Ras in myeloid leukemogenesis. Pediatr Blood Cancer. 2006;46:579-585.

628. Bourne HR, Sanders DA, McCormick F. The GTPase superfamily: a conserved switch for diverse cell functions. Nature. 1990;348:125-132.

629. Kalra R, Paderanga DC, Olson K, Shannon KM. Genetic analysis is consistent with the hypothesis that NF1 limits myeloid cell growth through p21ras. Blood. 1994;84:3435-3439.

630. Miyauchi J, Asada M, Sasaki M, et al. Mutations of the N-ras gene in juvenile chronic myelogenous leukemia. Blood. 1994;83:2248-2254.

631. Matsuda K, Shimada A, Yoshida N, et al. Spontaneous improvement of hematologic abnormalities in patients having juvenile myelomonocytic leukemia with specific RAS mutations. Blood. 2007;109:5477-5480.

632. Matsuda K, Nakazawa Y, Sakashita K, et al. Acquisition of loss of the wild-type NRAS locus with aggressive disease progression in a patient with juvenile myelomonocytic leukemia and a heterozygous NRAS mutation. Haematologica. 2007;92:1576-1578.

633. Neubauer A, Shannon K, Liu E. Mutations of the ras protooncogenes in childhood monosomy 7. Blood. 1991;77:594-598.

634. Shannon KM, O'Connell P, Martin GA, et al. Loss of the normal NF1 allele from the bone marrow of children with type 1 neurofibromatosis and malignant myeloid disorders. N Engl J Med. 1994;330:597-601.

635. Bollag G, Clapp DW, Shih S, et al. Loss of NF1 results in activation of the Ras signaling pathway and leads to aberrant growth in haematopoietic cells. Nat Genet. 1996;12:144-148.

636. Shannon KM, Watterson J, Johnson P, et al. Monosomy 7 myeloproliferative disease in children with neurofibromatosis, type 1: epidemiology and molecular analysis. Blood. 1992;79:1311-1318.

637. Side LE, Emanuel PD, Taylor B, et al. Mutations of the NF1 gene in children with juvenile myelomonocytic leukemia without clinical evidence of neurofibromatosis, type 1. Blood. 1998;92: 267-272.

638. Tartaglia M, Mehler EL, Goldberg R, et al. Mutations in PTPN11, encoding the protein tyrosine phosphatase SHP-2, cause Noonan syndrome. Nat Genet. 2001;29:465-468.

639. Fragale A, Tartaglia M, Wu J, Gelb BD. Noonan syndrome-associated *SHP2/PTPN11* mutants cause EGF-dependent prolonged GAB1 binding and sustained ERK2/MAPK1 activation. Hum Mutat. 2004;23:267-277.

640. Gelb BD, Tartaglia M. Noonan syndrome and related disorders: dysregulated RAS-mitogen activated protein kinase signal transduction. Hum Mol Genet. 2006;15(Spec No 2):R220-R226.

641. Tartaglia M, Niemeyer CM, Fragale A, et al. Somatic mutations in *PTPN11* in juvenile myelomonocytic leukemia, myelodysplastic syndromes and acute myeloid leukemia. Nat Genet. 2003;34:148-150.

642. Tartaglia M, Martinelli S, Cazzaniga G, et al. Genetic evidence for lineage-related and differentiation stage-related contribution of somatic *PTPN11* mutations to leukemogenesis in childhood acute leukemia. Blood. 2004;104:307-313.

643. Loh ML, Vattikuti S, Schubbert S, et al. Mutations in *PTPN11* implicate the SHP-2 phosphatase in leukemogenesis. Blood. 2004;103:2325-2331.

644. Tartaglia M, Martinelli S, Iavarone I, et al. Somatic *PTPN11* mutations in childhood acute myeloid leukaemia. Br J Haematol. 2005;129:333-339.

645. Kratz CP, Niemeyer CM, Castleberry RP, et al. The mutational spectrum of *PTPN11* in juvenile myelomonocytic leukemia and Noonan syndrome/myeloproliferative disease. Blood. 2005;106:2183-2185.

646. Tartaglia M, Martinelli S, Stella L, et al. Diversity and functional consequences of germline and somatic *PTPN11* mutations in human disease. Am J Hum Genet. 2006;78:279-290.

647. Luna-Fineman S, Shannon KM, Lange BJ. Childhood monosomy 7: epidemiology, biology, and mechanistic implications. Blood. 1995;85:1985-1999.

648. Golub TR, Barker GF, Lovett M, Gilliland DG. Fusion of PDGF receptor beta to a novel ets-like gene, tel, in chronic myelomonocytic leukemia with t(5;12) chromosomal translocation. Cell. 1994;77:307-316.

649. Gurbuxani S, Vyas P, Crispino JD. Recent insights into the mechanisms of myeloid leukemogenesis in Down syndrome. Blood. 2004;103:399-406.

650. Lightfoot J, Hitzler JK, Zipursky A, et al. Distinct gene signatures of transient and acute megakaryoblastic leukemia in Down syndrome. Leukemia. 2004;18:1617-1623.

651. Hitzler JK. Acute megakaryoblastic leukemia in Down syndrome. Pediatr Blood Cancer. 2007;49:1066-1069.

652. Hitzler JK, Cheung J, Li Y, et al. *GATA1* mutations in transient leukemia and acute megakaryoblastic leukemia of Down syndrome. Blood. 2003;101:4301-4304.

653. Malkin D, Brown EJ, Zipursky A. The role of p53 in megakaryocyte differentiation and the megakaryocytic leukemias of Down syndrome. Cancer Genet Cytogenet. 2000;116:1-5.

654. Ge Y, Jensen TL, Matherly LH, Taub JW. Transcriptional regulation of the cystathionine-beta -synthase gene in Down syndrome and non-Down syndrome megakaryocytic leukemia cell lines. Blood. 2003;101:1551-1557.

655. Gamis AS. Acute myeloid leukemia and Down syndrome evolution of modern therapy—state of the art review. Pediatr Blood Cancer. 2005;44:13-20.

656. Mercher T, Busson-Le Coniat M, Khac FN, et al. Recurrence of OTT-MAL fusion in t(1;22) of infant AML-M7. Genes Chromosomes Cancer. 2002;33:22-28.

657. Hasle H, Alonzo TA, Auvrignon A, et al. Monosomy 7 and deletion 7q in children and adolescents with acute myeloid leukemia: an international retrospective study. Blood. 2007;109:4641-4647.

658. Kardos G, Baumann I, Passmore SJ, et al. Refractory anemia in childhood: a retrospective analysis of 67 patients with particular reference to monosomy 7. Blood. 2003;102:1997-2003.

659. Mantadakis E, Shannon KM, Singer DA, et al. Transient monosomy 7: a case series in children and review of the literature. Cancer. 1999;85:2655-2661.

660. Shannon KM, Turhan AG, Chang SS, et al. Familial bone marrow monosomy 7. Evidence that the predisposing locus is not on the long arm of chromosome 7. J Clin Invest. 1989;84:984-989.

661. Van Lom K, Hagemeijer A, Smit E, , et al. Cytogenetic clonality analysis in myelodysplastic syndrome: monosomy 7 can be demonstrated in the myeloid and in the lymphoid lineage. Leukemia. 1995;9:1818-1821.

662. Anastasi J, Feng J, Le Beau MM, et al. Cytogenetic clonality in myelodysplastic syndromes studied with fluorescence in situ hybridization: lineage, response to growth factor therapy, and clone expansion. Blood. 1993;81:1580-1585.

663. Rubin CM, Arthur DC, Woods WG, et al. Therapy-related myelodysplastic syndrome and acute myeloid leukemia in children: correlation between chromosomal abnormalities and prior therapy. Blood. 1991;78:2982-2988.

664. Zwaan CM, Meshinchi S, Radich JP, et al. *FLT3* internal tandem duplication in 234 children with acute myeloid leukemia: prognostic significance and relation to cellular drug resistance. Blood. 2003;102:2387-2394.

665. Brown P, Meshinchi S, Levis M, et al. Pediatric AML primary samples with *FLT3/ITD* mutations are preferentially killed by FLT3 inhibition. Blood. 2004;104:1841-1849.

666. Brown P, Small D. FLT3 inhibitors: a paradigm for the development of targeted therapeutics for paediatric cancer. Eur J Cancer. 2004;40:707-721.

667. Levis M, Small D. FLT3: ITDoes matter in leukemia. Leukemia. 2003;17:1738-1752.

668. Meshinchi S, Alonzo TA, Stirewalt DL, et al. Clinical implications of *FLT3* mutations in pediatric AML. Blood. 2006;108:3654-3661.

669. Murphy KM, Levis M, Hafez MJ, et al. Detection of *FLT3* internal tandem duplication and D835 mutations by a multiplex polymerase chain reaction and capillary electrophoresis assay. J Mol Diagn. 2003;5:96-102.

669a. Stubbs MC, Armstrong SA. FLT3 as a therapeutic target in childhood leukemia. Curr Drug Targets. 2007;8:703-714.

670. Christiansen DH, Pedersen-Bjergaard J. Internal tandem duplications of the *FLT3* and *MLL* genes are mainly observed in atypical cases of therapy-related acute myeloid leukemia with a normal karyotype and are unrelated to type of previous therapy. Leukemia. 2001;15:1848-1851.

671. Goemans BF, Zwaan CM, Miller M, et al. Mutations in *KIT* and *RAS* are frequent events in pediatric core-binding factor acute myeloid leukemia. Leukemia. 2005;19:1536-1542.

672. Vogelstein B, Civin CI, Preisinger AC, et al. *RAS* gene mutations in childhood acute myeloid leukemia: a Pediatric Oncology Group study. Genes Chromosomes Cancer. 1990;2:159-162.

673. Mahgoub N, Parker RI, Hosler MR, et al. *RAS* mutations in pediatric leukemias with *MLL* gene rearrangements. Genes Chromosomes Cancer. 1998;21:270-275.

674. Lubbert M, Mirro J Jr, Kitchingman G, et al. Prevalence of *N-ras* mutations in children with myelodysplastic syndromes and acute myeloid leukemia. Oncogene. 1992;7:263-268.

675. Misawa S, Horiike S, Kaneko H, et al. Significance of chromosomal alterations and mutations of the *N-RAS* and *TP53* genes in relation to leukemogenesis of acute myeloid leukemia. Leuk Res. 1998;22:631-637.

676. Side LE, Curtiss NP, Teel K, et al. *RAS, FLT3,* and *TP53* mutations in therapy-related myeloid malignancies with abnormalities of chromosomes 5 and 7. Genes Chromosomes Cancer. 2004;39:217-223.

677. Zebisch A, Staber PB, Delavar A, et al. Two transforming *C-RAF* germ-line mutations identified in patients with therapy-related acute myeloid leukemia. Cancer Res. 2006;66:3401-3408.

678. Nyakern M, Tazzari PL, Finelli C, et al. Frequent elevation of Akt kinase phosphorylation in blood marrow and peripheral blood

mononuclear cells from high-risk myelodysplastic syndrome patients. Leukemia. 2006;20:230-238.

679. Follo MY, Mongiorgi S, Bosi C, et al. The Akt/mammalian target of rapamycin signal transduction pathway is activated in high-risk myelodysplastic syndromes and influences cell survival and proliferation. Cancer Res. 2007;67:4287-4294.

680. Liu TC, Lin PM, Chang JG, et al. Mutation analysis of *PTEN/MMAC1* in acute myeloid leukemia. Am J Hematol. 2000;63:170-175.

681. Cheong JW, Eom JI, Maeng HY, et al. Phosphatase and tensin homologue phosphorylation in the C-terminal regulatory domain is frequently observed in acute myeloid leukaemia and associated with poor clinical outcome. Br J Haematol. 2003;122:454-456.

682. Min YH, Cheong JW, Lee MH, et al. Elevated S-phase kinase-associated protein 2 protein expression in acute myelogenous leukemia: its association with constitutive phosphorylation of phosphatase and tensin homologue protein and poor prognosis. Clin Cancer Res. 2004;10:5123-5130.

683. Rossi DJ, Weissman IL. Pten, tumorigenesis, and stem cell self-renewal. Cell. 2006;125:229-231.

684. Felix CA, Hosler MR, Provisor D, et al. The p53 gene in pediatric therapy-related leukemia and myelodysplasia. Blood. 1996;87:4376-4381.

685. Dockhorn-Dworniczak B, Wolff J, Poremba C, et al. A new germline *TP53* gene mutation in a family with Li-Fraumeni syndrome. Eur J Cancer. 1996;32A:1359-1365.

686. Andersen MK, Christiansen DH, Pedersen-Bjergaard J. Amplification or duplication of chromosome band 21q22 with multiple copies of the *AML1* gene and mutation of the *TP53* gene in therapy-related MDS and AML. Leukemia. 2005;19:197-200.

687. Nichols KE, Malkin D, Garber JE, et al. Germ-line p53 mutations predispose to a wide spectrum of early-onset cancers. Cancer Epidemiol Biomarkers Prev. 2001;10:83-87.

688. Cazzaniga G, Dell'oro MG, Mecucci C, et al. Nucleophosmin mutations in childhood acute myelogenous leukemia with normal karyotype. Blood. 2005;106:1419-1422.

689. Brown P, McIntyre E, Rau R, et al. The incidence and clinical significance of nucleophosmin mutations in childhood AML. Blood. 2007;110:979-985.

690. Mullighan CG, Kennedy A, Zhou X, et al. Pediatric acute myeloid leukemia with *NPM1* mutations is characterized by a gene expression profile with dysregulated *HOX* gene expression distinct from *MLL*-rearranged leukemias. Leukemia. 2007;21:2000-2009.

691. Fazi F, Racanicchi S, Zardo G, et al. Epigenetic silencing of the myelopoiesis regulator microRNA-223 by the AML1/ETO oncoprotein. Cancer Cell. 2007;12:457-466.

692. Heerema NA, Nachman JB, Sather HN, et al. Deletion of 7p or monosomy 7 in pediatric acute lymphoblastic leukemia is an adverse prognostic factor: a report from the Children's Cancer Group. Leukemia. 2004;18:939-947.

693. Zhou J, Goldwasser MA, Li A, et al. Quantitative analysis of minimal residual disease predicts relapse in children with B-lineage acute lymphoblastic leukemia in DFCI ALL Consortium Protocol 95-01. Blood. 2007;110:1607-1611.

694. Flotho C, Coustan-Smith E, Pei D, et al. A set of genes that regulate cell proliferation predicts treatment outcome in childhood acute lymphoblastic leukemia. Blood. 2007;110:1271-1277.

695. Flotho C, Coustan-Smith E, Pei D, et al. Genes contributing to minimal residual disease in childhood acute lymphoblastic leukemia: prognostic significance of CASP8AP2. Blood. 2006;108:1050-1057.

696. Cortes J, Jabbour E, Kantarjian H, et al. Dynamics of *BCR-ABL* kinase domain mutations in chronic myeloid leukemia after sequential treatment with multiple tyrosine kinase inhibitors. Blood. 2007;110:4005-4011.

697. O'Hare T, Eide CA, Deininger MW. Bcr-Abl kinase domain mutations, drug resistance, and the road to a cure for chronic myeloid leukemia. Blood. 2007;110:2242-2249.

698. Goldman JM. How I treat chronic myeloid leukemia in the imatinib era. Blood. 2007;110:2828-2837.

699. Palomero T, Dominguez M, Ferrando AA. The role of the PTEN/AKT pathway in NOTCH1-induced leukemia. Cell Cycle. 2008;7:965-970.

700. McDermott U, Iafrate AJ, Gray NS, et al. Genomic alterations of anaplastic lymphoma kinase may sensitize tumors to anaplastic lymphoma kinase inhibitors. Cancer Res. 2008;68:3389-3395.

701. Huang ME, Ye YC, Chen SR, et al. Use of all-trans retinoic acid in the treatment of acute promyelocytic leukemia. Blood. 1988;72:567-572.

702. Alcalay M, Zangrilli D, Pandolfi PP, et al. Translocation breakpoint of acute promyelocytic leukemia lies within the retinoic acid receptor alpha locus. Proc Natl Acad Sci U S A. 1991;88:1977-1981.

703. Grignani F, Fagioli M, Alcalay M, et al. Acute promyelocytic leukemia: from genetics to treatment. Blood. 1994;83:10-25.

704. Warrell RP Jr, de Thé H, Wang ZY, Degos L. Acute promyelocytic leukemia. N Engl J Med. 1993;329:177-189.

705. Zelent A, Guidez F, Melnick A, et al. Translocations of the *RARalpha* gene in acute promyelocytic leukemia. Oncogene. 2001;20:7186-7203.

706. Lo Coco F, Avvisati G, Diverio D, et al. Molecular evaluation of response to all-trans-retinoic acid therapy in patients with acute promyelocytic leukemia. Blood. 1991;77:1657-1659.

707. Garzon R, Pichiorri F, Palumbo T, et al. MicroRNA gene expression during retinoic acid-induced differentiation of human acute promyelocytic leukemia. Oncogene. 2007;26:4148-4157.

708. de Botton S, Coiteux V, Chevret S, et al. Outcome of childhood acute promyelocytic leukemia with all-trans-retinoic acid and chemotherapy. J Clin Oncol. 2004;22:1404-1412.

709. Testi AM, Biondi A, Lo Coco F, et al. GIMEMA-AIEOPAIDA protocol for the treatment of newly diagnosed acute promyelocytic leukemia (APL) in children. Blood. 2005;106:447-453.

710. da Costa Moraes CA, Trompieri NM, Cavalcante Felix FH. Pediatric acute promyelocytic leukemia: all-transretinoic acid therapy in a Brazilian pediatric hospital. J Pediatr Hematol Oncol. 2008;30:387-390.

711. Chen GQ, Shi XG, Tang W, et al. Use of arsenic trioxide (As$_2$O$_3$) in the treatment of acute promyelocytic leukemia (APL): I. As$_2$O$_3$ exerts dose-dependent dual effects on APL cells. Blood. 1997;89:3345-3353.

712. Rojewski MT, Baldus C, Knauf W, et al. Dual effects of arsenic trioxide (As$_2$O$_3$) on non-acute promyelocytic leukaemia myeloid cell lines: induction of apoptosis and inhibition of proliferation. Br J Haematol. 2002;116:555-563.

713. Mathews V, George B, Lakshmi KM, et al. Single-agent arsenic trioxide in the treatment of newly diagnosed acute promyelocytic leukemia: durable remissions with minimal toxicity. Blood. 2006;107:2627-2632.

714. Fox E, Razzouk BI, Widemann BC, et al. Phase 1 trial and pharmacokinetic study of arsenic trioxide in children and adolescents with refractory or relapsed acute leukemia, including acute promyelocytic leukemia or lymphoma. Blood. 2008;111:566-573.

715. Estey E, Garcia-Manero G, Ferrajoli A, et al. Use of all-trans retinoic acid plus arsenic trioxide as an alternative to chemotherapy in untreated acute promyelocytic leukemia. Blood. 2006;107:3469-3473.

716. Altman JK, Yoon P, Katsoulidis E, et al. Regulatory effects of mammalian target of rapamycin-mediated signals in the generation of arsenic trioxide responses. J Biol Chem. 2008;283:1992-2001.

717. Altman JK, Platanias LC. Exploiting the mammalian target of rapamycin pathway in hematologic malignancies. Curr Opin Hematol. 2008;15:88-94.

718. Brown VI, Fang J, Alcorn K, et al. Rapamycin is active against B-precursor leukemia in vitro and in vivo, an effect that is modulated by IL-7-mediated signaling. Proc Natl Acad Sci U S A. 2003;100:15113-15118.

719. Houghton PJ, Morton CL, Kolb EA, et al. Initial testing (stage 1) of the mTOR inhibitor rapamycin by the Pediatric Preclinical Testing Program. Pediatr Blood Cancer. 2008;50:799-805.

720. Rizzieri DA, Feldman E, Dipersio JF, et al. A phase 2 clinical trial of deforolimus (AP23573, MK-8669), a novel mammalian target of rapamycin inhibitor, in patients with relapsed or refractory hematologic malignancies. Clin Cancer Res. 2008;14:2756-2762.

721. O'Brien SG, Guilhot F, Larson RA, et al. Imatinib compared with interferon and low-dose cytarabine for newly diagnosed chronic-phase chronic myeloid leukemia. N Engl J Med. 2003;348:994-1004.

722. Hughes TP, Kaeda J, Branford S, et al. Frequency of major molecular responses to imatinib or interferon alfa plus cytarabine in newly diagnosed chronic myeloid leukemia. N Engl J Med. 2003;349:1423-1432.

723. Cortes J, Talpaz M, O'Brien S, et al. Molecular responses in patients with chronic myelogenous leukemia in chronic phase treated with imatinib mesylate. Clin Cancer Res. 2005;11:3425-3432.

724. Waldman D, Weintraub M, Freeman A, et al. Favorable early response of secondary chronic myeloid leukemia to imatinib. Am J Hematol. 2004;75:217-219.

725. Champagne MA, Capdeville R, Krailo M, et al. Imatinib mesylate (STI571) for treatment of children with Philadelphia chromosome-positive leukemia: results from a Children's Oncology Group phase 1 study. Blood. 2004;104:2655-2660.

726. Millot F, Guilhot J, Nelken B, et al. Imatinib mesylate is effective in children with chronic myelogenous leukemia in late chronic and advanced phase and in relapse after stem cell transplantation. Leukemia. 2006;20:187-192.

727. FDA approves Gleevec for pediatric leukemia. FDA Consum. 2003;37:6.

728. Wittman B, Horan J, Baxter J, et al. A 2-year-old with atypical CML with a t(5;12)(q33;p13) treated successfully with imatinib mesylate. Leuk Res. 2004;28(Suppl 1):S65-S69.

729. David M, Cross NC, Burgstaller S, et al. Durable responses to imatinib in patients with *PDGFRB* fusion gene-positive and *BCR-ABL*-negative chronic myeloproliferative disorders. Blood. 2007;109:61-64.

730. Apperley JF, Gardembas M, Melo JV, et al. Response to imatinib mesylate in patients with chronic myeloproliferative diseases with rearrangements of the platelet-derived growth factor receptor beta. N Engl J Med. 2002;347:481-487.

731. Porkka K, Koskenvesa P, Lundan T, et al. Dasatinib crosses the blood-brain barrier and is an efficient therapy for central nervous system Philadelphia chromosome-positive leukemia. Blood. 2008;112:1005-1012.

732. Ottmann O, Dombret H, Martinelli G, et al. Dasatinib induces rapid hematologic and cytogenetic responses in adult patients with Philadelphia chromosome positive acute lymphoblastic leukemia with resistance or intolerance to imatinib: interim results of a phase 2 study. Blood. 2007;110:2309-2315.

733. Kolb EA, Gorlick R, Houghton PJ, et al. Initial testing of dasatinib by the Pediatric Preclinical Testing Program. Pediatr Blood Cancer. 2008;50:1198-1206.

734. Albert DH, Tapang P, Magoc TJ, et al. Preclinical activity of ABT-869, a multitargeted receptor tyrosine kinase inhibitor. Mol Cancer Ther. 2006;5:995-1006.

735. Yee KW, O'Farrell AM, Smolich BD, et al. SU5416 and SU5614 inhibit kinase activity of wild-type and mutant FLT3 receptor tyrosine kinase. Blood. 2002;100:2941-2949.

736. Brown P, Levis M, McIntyre E, et al. Combinations of the FLT3 inhibitor CEP-701 and chemotherapy synergistically kill infant and childhood MLL-rearranged ALL cells in a sequence-dependent manner. Leukemia. 2006;20:1368-1376.

737. Piloto O, Nguyen B, Huso D, et al. IMC-EB10, an anti-FLT3 monoclonal antibody, prolongs survival and reduces nonobese diabetic/severe combined immunodeficient engraftment of some acute lymphoblastic leukemia cell lines and primary leukemic samples. Cancer Res. 2006;66:4843-4851.

738. Hellmuth K, Grosskopf S, Lum CT, et al. Specific inhibitors of the protein tyrosine phosphatase Shp2 identified by high-throughput docking. Proc Natl Acad Sci U S A. 2008;105:7275-7280.

739. Lock R, Carol H, Houghton PJ, et al. Initial testing (stage 1) of the BH3 mimetic ABT-263 by the Pediatric Preclinical Testing Program. Pediatr Blood Cancer. 2008;50:1181-1189.

740. Kang MH, Kang YH, Szymanska B, et al. Activity of vincristine, L-ASP, and dexamethasone against acute lymphoblastic leukemia is enhanced by the BH3-mimetic ABT-737 in vitro and in vivo. Blood. 2007;110:2057-2066.

741. Muchmore SW, Sattler M, Liang H, et al. X-ray and NMR structure of human Bcl-xL, an inhibitor of programmed cell death. Nature. 1996;381:335-341.

742. Sattler M, Liang H, Nettesheim D, et al. Structure of Bcl-xL-Bak peptide complex: recognition between regulators of apoptosis. Science. 1997;275:983-986.

743. Zha J, Harada H, Osipov K, et al. BH3 domain of BAD is required for heterodimerization with BCL-XL and pro-apoptotic activity. J Biol Chem. 1997;272:24101-24104.

744. Zha H, Aimé-Sempé C, Sato T, Reed JC. Proapoptotic protein Bax heterodimerizes with Bcl-2 and homodimerizes with Bax via a novel domain (BH3) distinct from BH1 and BH2. J Biol Chem. 1996;271:7440-7444.

745. Reed JC, Zha H, Aimé-Sempé C, et al. Structure-function analysis of Bcl-2 family proteins. Regulators of programmed cell death. Adv Exp Med Biol. 1996;406:99-112.

746. Zwaan CM, Reinhardt D, Corbacioglu S, et al. Gemtuzumab ozogamicin: first clinical experiences in children with relapsed/refractory acute myeloid leukemia treated on compassionate-use basis. Blood. 2003;101:3868-3871.

747. Arceci RJ, Sande J, Lange B, et al. Safety and efficacy of gemtuzumab ozogamicin in pediatric patients with advanced CD33+ acute myeloid leukemia. Blood. 2005;106:1183-1188.

748. Ebert BL, Galili N, Tamayo P, et al. An erythroid differentiation signature predicts response to lenalidomide in myelodysplastic syndrome. PLoS Med. 2008;5:e35.

II Pediatric Cancer Therapeutics

6

Chemotherapy in the Pediatric Patient

Alex Sparreboom, William E. Evans, and Sharyn D. Baker

For most primary tumors the treatment of choice is surgery and/or radiotherapy. These measures can be effective for controlling localized tumors. However, at the time of diagnosis, most cancers have already microscopically metastasized throughout the body, leading to recurrent disease in 60% to 70% of cancer patients. Thus, systemic chemotherapy with anticancer drugs is required to control the outgrowth of metastases. Although chemotherapy might be administered up front to allow better surgery for some locally invasive tumors at advanced disease stages, cancer chemotherapy is primarily the treatment of metastases, or other widespread disease, such as in hematologic malignancies.

During the last 2 decades, a significant number of drugs has become available to treat a wide variety of neoplastic diseases, and the whole field of anticancer drug discovery and development has changed substantially. Not only are we now dealing with highly innovative and distinct classes of molecules in terms of mechanism of action and chemical structure, but also an impressive array of new techniques and ideas is being deployed. Moreover, our emerging understanding of the relationships between pharmacokinetics—the quantitative study of the concentration-time profile of the drug in the body, incorporating absorption, distribution, metabolism, and excretion—and pharmacodynamics—the quantitative study of the effects on the body, including efficacy and toxicity—is encouraging a more systematic and rigorous analysis of the potential role of pharmacology in the daily management of cancer patients.[1,2] It has become widely appreciated at the same time that the narrow therapeutic index (i.e., the ratio of the theoretical minimum effective dose to the maximum tolerated dose) of most anticancer drugs demands that a rigorous effort be made to optimize their regimens (Fig. 6-1). Effective systemic treatment for cancer requires the use of cytotoxic drugs with modest differences in their toxic effects on normal cells and their therapeutic, lethal effects on malignant cells. Exploiting this narrow thera-

peutic margin of anticancer agents has been a major challenge for pediatric oncologists and pharmacologists who have attacked the problem on multiple fronts, including the use of drug combinations with different dose-limiting toxicities, the rescue or reconstitution of normal tissues (e.g., administration of reduced folates following methotrexate, the use of growth factors or bone marrow transplantation after high-dose chemotherapy), and the use of biologic modifiers to overcome specific mechanisms of cancer cell resistance. In this chapter, we will review the principles of chemotherapy in children, highlight causes of variability in their response to chemotherapeutic treatment, and discuss the implementation of pharmacokinetic, pharmacodynamic, and/or pharmacogenetic principles in the design of clinical trials that allow tailor-made therapy for individual patients.

CHEMOTHERAPEUTIC DRUGS

The roles of chemotherapy in the management of cancer include induction chemotherapy, which denotes its use as primary therapy when there is no alternative treatment available or subsequently, even after tumor response, such as for hematologic malignancies in which the disease is systemic. After induction therapy, for some cancers such as leukemia, chemotherapy may be administered subsequently over a prolonged period as continuation therapy. Chemotherapy is an adjuvant in combined modality therapy, when systemic treatment is applied after the tumor has been controlled by an alternative modality, such as surgery or radiotherapy, or neoadjuvant (primary) when localized cancer will otherwise not be optimally managed if systemic chemotherapy is not used before definitive local therapy.

The arsenal of anticancer drugs used in pediatric malignancies is generally similar to that available for the treatment of adult diseases; they can be classified into conventional cytotoxic agents and molecularly targeted agents. The former class can be further subdivided into two large groups based on the dependence of their mechanism of action on the cell cycle. Cell cycle–nonspecific agents, which include alkylating agents, platinum agents, and most antitumor antibiotics, kill both resting and cycling tumor cells. Examples of cell cycle–specific agents include antimetabolites and tubulin and topoisomerase interactive agents. Table 6-1 provides an overview of drugs used in the treatment of childhood cancers, along with their key pharmacologic features.

RATIONALE FOR CHEMOTHERAPY OPTIMIZATION

The current concept that chemotherapeutic agents should be administered at a maximum dose that the patient can tolerate before the onset of unacceptable toxicity is still in wide clinical use. This approach is based on a series of retrospective analyses, which have indicated that the higher the dose intensity (i.e., the dose delivered over a standard interval of time) of an anticancer drug, the better the outcome.[3-5] However, the therapeutic range for most anticancer agents is extremely narrow and, in most cases, no information is available on the intrinsic sensitivity of a patient's tumor to a particular agent and the patient's tolerability of a given dose prior to therapy. Hence, the dosage of chemotherapeutic agents remains largely empirical, and is basically derived from the type of information shown in Figure 6-2. Because the effect of a therapeutic agent in the body is generally

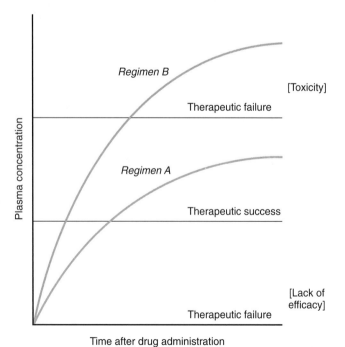

FIGURE 6-1. When a drug is given at a fixed dose and at fixed time intervals, it accumulates within the body until a plateau is reached. With regimen A, therapeutic success is achieved, although not initially. With regimen B, the therapeutic objective is achieved more quickly, but the plasma concentration is ultimately too high.

Text continues on page 182.

TABLE 6-1 Key Features of Drugs Used in Pediatric Oncology

Drug (Trade Name; Chemical Class)	Mechanism of Action	Antitumor Activity	Route of Administration	Primary Pathway of Elimination	Enzymes and Transporters	Principal Side Effects
ALKYLATING AGENTS						
Mechlorethamine (Mustargen; nitrogen mustard, mustine, HN2)	Alkylation; DNA cross-linking	Hodgkin's disease (MOPP)	IV injection	Hydrolysis; liver	N-demethylation (CYP)	A, M, N&V, Mu, HU, Derm, V, Phleb, G, SM
Melphalan (Alkeran; mechlorethamine analogue)	Alkylation; DNA cross-linking	HDCT	IV injection or infusion; oral	Hydrolysis; renal	NA	A, M, N&V, D, Mu, Derm, Vas, Phleb, SIADH, G, SM
Chlorambucil (Leukeran; mechlorethamine analogue)	Alkylation; DNA cross-linking	Hodgkin's disease (ChlVPP)	Oral	Hydrolysis	ABCC2	A, M, N&V, HU, P, S, G, SM
Cyclophosphamide (Cytoxan; mechlorethamine analogue)	Alkylation (prodrug); DNA cross-linking	Leukemias, lymphomas, neuroblastoma, sarcoma	IV infusion; oral	Hydrolysis; liver	CYP2B6, CYP2C9, CYP3A4	A, M, N&V, Cy, SIADH, C, P, G, SM
Ifosfamide (Ifex; mechlorethamine analogue)	Alkylation (prodrug); DNA cross-linking	Sarcomas, germ cell	IV infusion	Hydrolysis; liver	CYP2B6, CYP3A4	A, M, N&V, Met, Cy, SIADH, NT, C, P, R, G, SM
Thiotepa (Thioplex; aziridine)	Alkylation; DNA cross-linking	HDCT	IV injection or infusion; intrathecal, intravesical	Liver	NA	A, M, N&V, HU, Derm, Cy, G, SM
Busulfan (Myleran; alkyl alkane sulfonate)	Alkylation; DNA cross-linking	HDCT	IV infusion; oral	Conjugation with glutathione; liver	CYP3A4	A, M, N&V, Mu, Derm, HU, AI, NT, VOD, P, S, G, SM
Carmustine (BiCNU; BCNU, nitrosourea)	Alkylation; DNA cross-linking; carbamoylation	Brain tumors, Hodgkin's disease, lymphoma	IV infusion; wafer implant (glioblastoma)	Chemical hydrolysis; liver	CYP	M, N&V, Phleb, S (wafer), C, H, P, R, G, SM
Lomustine (CeeNU; CCNU, nitrosourea)	Alkylation; DNA cross-linking; carbamoylation	Brain tumors, Hodgkin's disease, lymphoma	Oral	Chemical hydrolysis; liver	NA	M, N&V, NT, C, H, P, R, G, SM
Dacarbazine (DTIC, DTIC-Dome; imidazole-carboxamide)	Methylation inhibition (prodrug)	Hodgkin's disease, neuroblastoma, sarcomas	IV infusion	Chemical hydrolysis; liver, renal	N-demethylation (CYP); CYP2E1	M, N&V, Flu, H
Procarbazine (Mutulane; imidazole-carboxamide)	Methylation inhibition (prodrug)	Brain tumors; Hodgkin's disease (ChlVPP)	Oral	Chemical hydrolysis; liver, renal	CYP, MAO	M, N&V, Mu, Flu, NT, Derm, G, SM
Temozolomide (Temodar; imidazole-carboxamide)	Methylation inhibition (prodrug)	Brain tumors	Oral	Chemical hydrolysis	CYP (minor)	M, N&V, NT, PE, H
ANTIMETABOLITES						
Cytarabine (Cytosar; Ara-C, cytosine arabinoside; cytidine analogue)	Incorporated into DNA; inhibits DNA polymerase; terminates DNA chain elongation	Leukemias	IV injection or infusion; intrathecal; SC	Activated to triphosphate; deamination	Cytidine deaminase	M, N&V, Mu, GI, HU, Derm, HFS, PE, Conj, NT, H, PE

Continues

TABLE 6-1   Key Features of Drugs Used in Pediatric Oncology—cont'd

Drug (Trade Name; Chemical Class)	Mechanism of Action	Antitumor Activity	Route of Administration	Primary Pathway of Elimination	Enzymes and Transporters	Principal Side Effects
Azacytidine (Vidaza; cytidine analogue)	Hypomethylation of DNA (low dose)	MDS, in development	SC	Activated to triphosphate; chemical degradation; deamination	Cytidine deaminase	M, N&V, F, Mu, D, Inj, Derm
Decitabine (Dacogen; cytidine analogue)	Hypomethylation of DNA (low dose)	MDS, in development	IV infusion	Activated to triphosphate; chemical degradation; deamination	Cytidine deaminase	M, N&V, F, Mu, D, Derm
Gemcitabine (Gemzar; cytidine analogue)	Incorporated into DNA; inhibits DNA polymerase; terminates DNA chain elongation; inhibits ribonucleotide reductase (prodrug)	Solid tumors, lymphoma (in development)	IV infusion	Activated to triphosphate; deamination	Cytidine deaminase	M, N&V, Mu, D, F, Flu, Derm, NT, PE, H, R
Cladribine (Leustatin; adenosine analogue)	Incorporated into DNA; inhibits DNA polymerase; terminates DNA chain elongation; inhibits ribonucleotide reductase (prodrug)	Leukemias	IV infusion	Activated to triphosphate; renal; liver	Oxidative cleavage, oxidation, conjugation	M, N&V, D, Derm, NT
Clofarabine (Clolar; adenosine analogue)	Incorporated into DNA; inhibits DNA polymerase; terminates DNA chain elongation; inhibits ribonucleotide reductase (prodrug)	Leukemias	IV infusion	Activated to triphosphate; extrahepatic	NA	M, N&V, D, C, H, R
Fludarabine (Fludara; adenosine analogue)	Incorporated into DNA; inhibits DNA polymerase; terminates DNA chain elongation; inhibits ribonucleotide reductase (prodrug)	AML, CML, indolent lymphomas	IV infusion	Activated to triphosphate; renal	NA	M, HA, Derm, fever, L, NT, TLS
6-Mercaptopurine (Purinethol; hypoxanthine analogue)	Incorporated into DNA, RNA; blocks purine synthesis (prodrug)	ALL, AML	Oral	Liver, renal (high dose)	TPMT, HGPRT	M, L, Mu, N&V, HU, crystalluria, GI
6-Thioguanine (guanine analogue)	Incorporated into DNA, RNA; blocks purine synthesis (prodrug)	ALL, AML	Oral	Liver	TPMT, HGPRT	M, L, Mu, N&V, HU, crystalluria
5-Fluorouracil (fluoropyrimidine)	Incorporated into RNA, DNA; inhibits thymidine synthase (prodrug of 5'-DFUR)	Carcinomas, hepatic tumors	IV injection or infusion	Liver	DPD	M, Mu, N&V, HFS, D, Derm, NT, C

Drug	Mechanism	Indication	Route	Elimination	Genes	Toxicities
Capecitabine (Xeloda; fluoropyrimidine)	Incorporated into RNA, DNA; inhibits thymidine synthase (prodrug of 5'-DFUR)	Colorectal cancer (in development)	Oral	Urine	CES2, CES1A1, cytidine deaminase, thymidine phosphorylase, DPD	M, Mu, N&V, HFS, D, Derm, NT, C
Methotrexate (Trexall; antifolate)	Interferes with folate metabolism	Leukemias, lymphomas, osteosarcoma	Oral; IM; SC; IV injection; intrathecal	Renal	OATP1A2, OAT1/3, ABCC1, ABCC2, ABCG2	M, Mu, Derm, L, R, NT
Pemetrexed (Alimta; antifolate)	Interferes with folate metabolism	Various (in development)	IV infusion	Renal	NA	M, fatigue, Mu, HFS, Derm
ANTITUMOR ANTIBIOTICS						
Bleomycin (Blenoxane)	Free radical-mediated DNA strand breaks	Lymphomas, testicular cancer	IV injection; IM, SC	Renal	NA	P, Derm, fever, Mu, A, HSR, N&V
Mitomycin C (Neulasta)	DNA cross-linking	Various (in development)	IV injection or infusion; intravesical	Liver	NA	M, N&V, Mu, HU, anemia, VOD
Daunorubicin (Daunomycin; anthracycline)	DNA strand breaks (topo II)	ALL, ANLL, lymphomas	IV injection or infusion	Renal, liver	ABCB1, aldoketoreductase	M, Mu, N&V, D, A, C, V
Doxorubicin (Adriamycin; anthracycline)	DNA strand breaks (topo II)	ALL, ANLL, lymphomas, solid tumors	IV infusion	Liver	ABCB1, aldoketoreductase	M, Mu, N&V, A, D, C, V
Epirubicin (Ellence; anthracycline)	DNA strand breaks (topo II)	Various (in development)	IV infusion	Renal, liver	ABCB1, aldoketoreductase	M, Mu, N&V, A, C, V
Idarubicin (Idamycin; anthracycline)	DNA strand breaks (topo II)	ALL, ANLL, lymphomas	IV injection or infusion; oral	Renal, liver	ABCB1, aldoketoreductase	M, Mu, N&V, D, A, C, V
Mitoxantrone (Novantrone; anthracenedione)	DNA strand breaks (topo II)	ALL, ANLL, lymphomas	IV infusion; IP	Renal, liver	ABCB1, ABCG2	M, Mu, N&V, A, urine, veins and nail discoloration
ASPARAGINASES						
L-Asparaginase (Elspar, Kidrolase; native asparaginase from *Escherichia coli*)	Depletion of plasma asparagine	ALL	IV infusion (>30 min)	Nonrenal	NA	HSR, thrombosis, GI, glucose intolerance, coagulopathy, hyperglycemia, L
Crisantaspase (Erwinase; Erwinia L-asparaginase, native asparaginase from *Erwinia chrysanthemi*)	Depletion of plasma asparagine	ALL (in development)	IV infusion (>30 min)	Nonrenal	NA	HSR, thrombosis, GI, glucose intolerance, coagulopathy, hyperglycemia, L
Pegasparaginase (Oncospar; PEG-asparaginase, from *Escherichia coli*)	Depletion of plasma asparagine	ALL	IV infusion (1-2 hours)	Nonrenal	NA	HSR, thrombosis, GI, glucose intolerance, coagulopathy, hyperglycemia, L
CORTICOSTEROIDS						
Dexamethasone (Decadron)	Receptor-mediated lympholysis	Leukemias, lymphomas	Oral, IV injection; IM	Liver	CYP3A4, CYP17	Muscle weakness, osteoporosis, Derm, hypertension, N&V, headache

Continues

TABLE 6-1   Key Features of Drugs Used in Pediatric Oncology—cont'd

Drug (Trade Name; Chemical Class)	Mechanism of Action	Antitumor Activity	Route of Administration	Primary Pathway of Elimination	Enzymes and Transporters	Principal Side Effects
Prednisolone (Orapred OTD, Pediapred)	Receptor-mediated lympholysis	Leukemias, lymphomas	Oral; IV injection	Renal, liver	CYP3A4, sulfation, glucuronidation	Muscle weakness, osteoporosis, Derm, hypertension, N&V, headache
Prednisone (Deltasone)	Receptor-mediated lympholysis (prodrug)	Leukemias, lymphomas	Oral	Renal, liver	CYP3A4, sulfation, glucuronidation	Muscle weakness, osteoporosis, Derm, hypertension, N&V, headache
PLATINUM COMPOUNDS						
Carboplatin (Paraplatin)	Platination; DNA cross-linking	Brain tumors, neuroblastoma, sarcomas	IV infusion	Renal	NA; glomerular filtration	M, N&V, NT, EA, HSR
Cisplatin (Platinol)	Platination; DNA cross-linking	Testicular, brain tumors, osteosarcoma, neuroblastoma	IV infusion	Renal	OCT2	N&V, R, NT, M, EA, O, HSR
Oxaliplatin (Eloxatin)	Platination; DNA cross-linking	Colorectal cancer (in development)	IV infusion	Renal	OCT2	NT, N&V, D, M, R, HSR
RETINOIDS						
All-*trans*-retinoic acid (ATRA; Vesanoid; retinoin; retinol derivative)	Differentiation agent	Acute promyelocytic leukemia	Oral	Liver	CYP3A7, CYP1A1, CYP2C8	Retinoic acid syndrome, pseudotumor cerebri, cheilitis
13-*cis*-retinoic acid (Accutane; retinol derivative)	Differentiation agent	Neuroblastoma	Oral	Liver	CYP2B6, CYP2C8, CYP3A4/5, CYP2A6	Cheilitis, conjunctivitis, dry mouth, xerosis, pruritus, headache
TOPOISOMERASE-INTERACTIVE AGENTS						
Etoposide (VePesid; VP-16)	DNA strand breaks (topo II)	ALL, ANLL, lymphomas, neuroblastoma, sarcomas, brain tumors	IV infusion	Renal, liver	CYP3A4, CYP1A2, CYP2E1, UGT1A1, ABCB1, ABCC1, ABCC2	M, N&V, hypotension, HSR, SM
Teniposide (Vumon; VM-26)	DNA strand breaks (topo II)	ALL	IV infusion; oral	Liver	CYP3A4, ABCB1	M, N&V, HSR, hypotension, SM
Irinotecan (Camptosar; CPT-11; camptothecin analogue)	DNA strand breaks (topo I; prodrug of SN-38)	Rhabdomyosarcoma, solid tumors	IV infusion	Renal, liver	OATP1B1, CYP3A4, CYP3A5, CES2, UGT1A, ABCB1, ABCC2, ABCG2	M, D, N&V, A, L
Topotecan (Hycamptin; camptothecin analogue)	DNA strand breaks (topo I)	Neuroblastoma; rhabdomyosarcoma	IV infusion	Renal	ABCB1, ABCG2	M, Mu, D, N&V, A, Derm, L

TUBULIN-INTERACTIVE AGENTS

Docetaxel (Taxotere; taxanes)	Microtubule depolarization inhibitor	Ewing's sarcoma (in development)	IV infusion	Liver	OATP1B3, CYP3A4/5, CYP2C8, ABCB1, ABCC2	M, HSR, A, NT, Derm, Mu
Paclitaxel (Taxol; Abraxane; taxane)	Microtubule depolarization inhibitor	Solid tumors (in development)	IV infusion	Liver	CYP2C8, CYP3A4/5, ABCB1, ABCC2	M, HSR, A, NT, M, C
Vinblastine (Velban; *Vinca* alkaloid)	Microtubule polarization inhibitor	Histiocytosis, Hodgkin's disease, testicular cancer	IV push or infusion	Liver	CYP3A4, CYP2D6, ABCB1	M, A, Mu, NT, V
Vincristine (Oncovin; *Vinca* alkaloid)	Microtubule polarization inhibitor	ALL, lymphomas, solid tumors	IV injection	Liver	CYP3A5, CYP3A4, ABCB1	NT, A, SIADH hypotension, V
Vinorelbine (Navelbine; *Vinca* alkaloid)	Microtubule polarization inhibitor	In development	IV injection of infusion	Liver	CYP3A4	M, NT, A, V

TYROSINE KINASE INHIBITORS

Imatinib (Gleevec; STI-571, benzamide analogue)	Bcr-Abl inhibitor	Ph+ CML	Oral	Liver	CYP3A4/5, CYP2D6, CYP2C9, CYP2C19, ABCB1, ABCG2	N&V, F, D, H, M
Dasatinib (Sprycel; carboxamide analogue)	Scr-Abl inhibitor	In development	Oral	Liver	CYP3A4, FMO3	M, D, N&V, Derm, fatigue, headache
Sunitinib (Sutent; carboxamide analogue)	VEGFR, PDGFR inhibitor	In development	Oral	Liver	CYP3A4, CYP1A2, ABCB1	M, D, Derm, anorexia, hypertension, fatigue, headache
Sorafenib (Nexavar; carboxamide analogue)	C-Raf inhibitor	In development	Oral	Liver	CYP3A4, UGT1A9	M, D, Derm, anorexia, hypertension, fatigue, headache
Erlotinib (Tarceva; OSI-774, quinazolinamine analogue)	EGFR inhibitor	In development	Oral	Liver	CYP3A4/5, CYP1A2, ABCG2	Derm, D, anorexia, fatigue, N&V, dyspnea, fatigue
Gefitinib (Iressa; ZD1839, anilinoquinazoline analogue)	EGFR inhibitor	In development	Oral	Liver	CYP3A4/5, CYP2D6, ABCB1, ABCG2	D, Derm, N&V

A, alopecia; ABC, ATP-binding cassette transporter; AI, adrenal insufficiency; ANC, absolute neutrophil count; AS, addisonian syndrome; C, cardiac toxicity; ChIVPP, chemotherapy regimen consisting of chlorambucil, vinblastine, procarbazine, and prednisolone; CML, chronic myelogenous leukemia; MDS, myelodysplastic syndrome; Conj, conjunctivitis; Cy, cystitis; CYP, cytochrome P-450 enzyme; D, diarrhea; Derm, dermatologic toxicity (skin rash and/or nail changes); EA, electrolyte abnormalities; F, fever; Flu, flu-like syndrome; FMO3, flavin-containing monooxygenase 3; G, gonadal toxicity; GI, gastrointestinal (ulcers, pancreatitis); H, hepatic; HA, hemolytic syndrome; HDCT, high-dose chemotherapy; HFS, hand-foot syndrome; HU, hyperuricemia; IM, intramuscular injection; Inj, injection site reaction or irritation; IP, intraperitoneal injection; IV, intravenous; M, myelosuppression; Met, metabolic acidosis; MOA, monoamine oxidase; MOPP, chemotherapy regimen consisting of mechlorethamine, vincristine, prednisone, and procarbazine; Mu, mucositis; NA, information not available; N&V, nausea and vomiting; NT, neurotoxicity; O, ototoxicity; OAT, organic anion transporter; OATP, organic anion–transporting polypeptide; P, pulmonary toxicity; PE, peripheral edema; Ph+, Philadelphia chromosome–positive; Phleb, phlebitis; Plt, platelets; R, renal toxicity; S, seizures; SC, subcutaneous injection; SIADH, syndrome of inappropriate antidiuretic hormone; SM, secondary malignancy; TLS, tumor lysis syndrome; UGT, uridine diphosphate glucuronosyltransferase; V, vesicant; Vas, vasculitis; VOD, veno-occlusive disease.

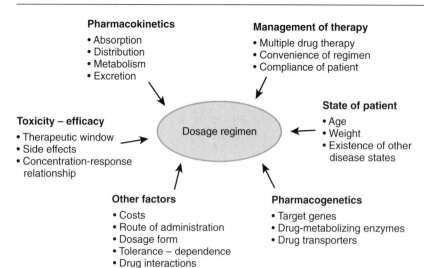

FIGURE 6-2. Determinants of a dosage regimen for an anticancer drug.

TABLE 6-2   **Factors Contributing to Variability in Drug Response**

Parameter	Source of Variability
Dose selection	Physician's preference; patient's condition (performance status)
Dose administration	Noncompliance; medication error; pharmaceutical formulation
Systemic exposure	Age; concomitant drugs; food effects; gender; route of administration; altered organ function; enzyme polymorphisms (pharmacogenetics)
Active site drug levels	Cellular uptake; intracellular activation; tumor sensitivity
Pharmacologic effect	Host sensitivity (e.g., previous treatments)

a function of its concentration at the (molecular) site of action, a description of the spatial-temporal behavior of the drug in the body is helpful, if not essential, for understanding and predicting normal tissue toxicity and optimizing tumor response. Considering the multiple factors that can cause drug concentrations to vary after administration of a fixed dose (Table 6-2), it is clearly more meaningful to have knowledge of drug exposure measures, usually expressed as the area under the concentration-time curve (AUC), rather than of just the absolute dose. Ideally, this would be at the molecular locus of action or at least at the tissue or tumor level but, with the exception of leukemias, drug concentrations are usually only measured in plasma, which is the only readily accessible surrogate.

There is often a marked variation in drug handling among individual patients, resulting in variability in AUC and clearance. Figure 6-3 illustrates interindividual variability in drug clearance, expressed as the coefficient of variation, for selected anticancer agents. Variation in drug clearance often leads to variability in the pharmacodynamic effects of a given dose of a drug. That is, an identical dose of drug may result in acceptable toxicity in one patient, but an unacceptable and possibly life-threatening toxicity in another. A combination of physiologic variables, genetic characteristics, and environmental factors is known to alter the relationship between the absolute dose and the concentration-time profile in plasma. The correlation between, for example, the AUC of a drug in plasma and the

intensity of pharmacodynamic effects is commonly better than that between absolute dose and such effects.[2] The definition of the relationships between the pharmacokinetic variables of a drug and the drug's pharmacodynamic end points may allow the administration of the optimum dosage of that drug in any given patient. The optimum dosage is the dose that maximizes the likelihood of response and simultaneously minimizes the likelihood of toxicity in a particular patient. In incidental cases, it is possible to define the optimum dosage to achieve a required drug exposure measure a priori for an individual patient from measurable physiologic variables, such as renal or hepatic function. In most cases, however, dose adjustments will be required in the light of pharmacokinetic or pharmacodynamic data obtained after administration of an initial dose and possibly subsequent doses of the drug in the individual patient.

PHARMACOKINETIC CHANGES IN CHILDREN

Changes in body composition and organ function at the extremes of age can affect drug disposition and drug effect.[6,7] Maturational processes in infancy may alter absorption and distribution of drugs, as well as change the capacity for drug metabolism and excretion. The importance of understanding the influence of age on the pharmacokinetics and pharmacodynamics of individual anticancer agents has increased steadily as treatment for the malignancies of infants has advanced. Although the influence of age has been evaluated formally for a limited number of cytotoxic drugs, reevaluating our current understanding of how maturation from birth to young adulthood and subsequent senescence influences the approaches for individualizing drug treatment to enhance the chance of therapeutic success. Although pediatric cancer remains a rare disease compared with cancer in adults, optimizing treatment in a patient group with a high cure rate and a long expected survival becomes critical to minimize the incidence of preventable late complications while maintaining efficacy.

Absorption Changes

Gastric emptying time varies with gestational age and may be prolonged in premature infants and neonates compared with older children.[8] Gastric pH is neutral in the first few weeks after

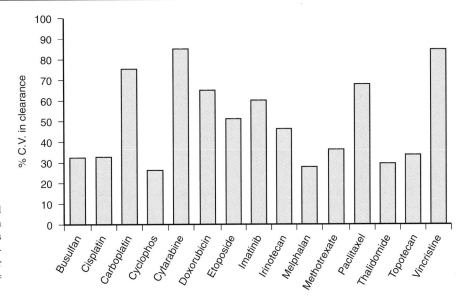

FIGURE 6-3. Examples of interindividual pharmacokinetic variability of drugs in pediatric oncology. Data are expressed as the coefficient of variation (% C.V.) for systemic clearance (or apparent clearance for orally administered drugs). cyclophos = cyclophosphamide.

birth, and gradually declines to adult values by the age of 2, which may affect the bioavailability of compounds.[9,10] Methotrexate absorption, for example, is significantly reduced by coadministration with milk.[11] The implication of higher pH is a delay in the absorption of weak acids and an increased absorption of weak bases. In addition, drugs may be administered in altered forms to small children. For example, crushed tablets in food or slurries administered by nasogastric tube may alter their rate and extent of absorption.

Volume of Distribution Changes

Changes in body composition between birth and adolescence may alter pharmacokinetic parameters. Skeletal muscle mass and subcutaneous fat are reduced in the newborn compared with the older infant. Changes in the proportion of body water compartments, particularly extracellular fluid volume, are dramatic between birth and adulthood; extracellular fluid volume represents 50% of body weight for premature infants, 35% for infants 4 to 6 months old, and 20% of adolescent and adult volume.[12-14] Polar drugs, which distribute primarily in body water, will therefore have a larger volume of distribution in infants compared with older children and adults. The net result of an isolated increase in volume of distribution is a lower peak concentration and prolonged terminal half-life, which occurs if the drug clearance remains unchanged.

Drug distribution may also be affected by alterations in plasma proteins. Protein binding may be reduced because of persistence of fetal albumin and reduced plasma protein content, particularly low levels of gamma globulin. Although adult values of protein for binding of acidic drugs may be achieved between 1 and 2 years of age, adult values for gamma globulin are not reached until age 7 to 12 years.[15]

Additional changes in body composition, particularly changes that differ in boys and girls, occur with the onset of puberty. In adolescence, boys actually lose body fat (to a mean of 12% of body weight), whereas girls increase the proportion of body weight caused by fat, up to 25%. These changes suggest that during adolescence, gender-related differences in volume of distribution and clearance could be more prominent than in children or older adults.

One unique aspect of the immature infant is the gradual maturation of specific organs. For example, the myelin content of the brain is lower in newborns. Because of incomplete maturation of the blood-brain barrier, membrane permeability is greater in the infant, and the brain-to-plasma ratio of some drugs has been shown to vary with age.[16,17] Similarly, renal tubular function develops later than glomerular filtration, so that drugs that undergo substantial tubular resorption in older children and adults may have a larger clearance than expected in the infant.

Renal Changes

The immature kidney has a diminished glomerular filtration rate (GFR). For full-term infants, the GFR is 40 mL/min/1.73 m^2, with substantial interindividual variability.[18] The GFR decreases to maximal values between the age of 6 and 12 months. Tubular function and passive resorption may also be significantly lower in the neonate. Because tubular resorption matures at a slower rate than glomerular filtration, toddlers may have remarkably high clearance rates for compounds that undergo tubular resorption in older children.

The glomerular filtration rate assessed by ^{99m}Tc-diethylenetriaminepentaacetic acid (DTPA) in children between 2 months and 17 years was correlated with body surface area (BSA), but when GFR was normalized to BSA, there was no correlation between GFR and age.[19] Premature and term infants require dose adjustments based on measurements or estimation of GFR for drugs eliminated primarily by glomerular filtration, such as carboplatin. Formulas are available for the estimation of creatinine clearance for infants and older children based on creatinine and height,[20,21] or by using some other endogenous surrogate marker of GFR, such as cystatin C,[22] but height can be difficult to measure accurately in infants.

Hepatic Metabolism

Immature organ systems in preterm and term infants and young children can cause altered disposition for many classes of drugs, including antibiotics, anticonvulsants, and antineoplastic agents.[6,13,23,24] Although the activity of cytochrome P-450 (CYP) microsomal enzymes responsible for the oxidation may be low in neonates, a dramatic increase in the metabolic capacity occurs between 8 weeks and 3 years, with rates increasing from 20% of adult clearance to two- to sixfold higher rates than adults. Values then decline gradually to reach adult clearance rates in puberty.[25] Glucuronidation enzymes increase from birth to 30% of adult activity by the age of 3 months.[26] Esterase activity, metabolically important for agents such as irinotecan and capecitabine, gradually increases during the first year of life; reduced hydrolysis rates have been reported for drugs such as procaine in premature infants and neonates, with normal activity measurable by 12 months.[27] Studies of hepatic metabolism and elimination in adolescents are limited. In general, however, adolescents have clearances that are intermediate between the high clearance rates observed in toddlers and the lower clearance rates measured in adults.[28]

Influence of Underlying Disease on Metabolism

Pathophysiologic changes associated with particular malignancies in children may also cause alterations in drug disposition. For example, increases in the clearance of antipyrine and lorazepam were noted after remission induction compared with time of diagnosis in children with acute lymphoblastic leukemia (ALL).[29] The clearance of unbound teniposide is lower in children with ALL in relapse than during first remission.[30] Because leukemic infiltration of the liver at the time of diagnosis is common, drugs metabolized by the liver may have a reduced clearance, as has been documented in preclinical models.[31]

Like adults, children who have undergone extensive prior therapy for malignancy may have cumulative organ toxicity that may alter drug clearance. Studies of high doses of etoposide and carboplatin in children as part of the preparative regimen for bone marrow transplantation (BMT) have reported 50% to 80% lower clearances than adults.[32,33] In mouse models, certain tumors elicited an acute phase response that coincided with downregulation of human CYP3A4 in the liver, as well as the mouse orthologue Cyp3a11.[34] The reduction of murine hepatic Cyp3a gene expression in tumor-bearing mice has resulted in decreased Cyp3a protein expression and consequently a significant reduction in Cyp3a-mediated metabolism of midazolam. These findings support the possibility that tumor-derived inflammation may alter the pharmacokinetic and pharmacodynamic properties of CYP3A4 substrates, leading to reduced metabolism of drugs in humans.[34]

Influence of Age on Drug Effects

Pediatric experience dictates that children tolerate the conventional toxicities of chemotherapy better than adults, and that children experience a very low regimen-related mortality, except for neonates. This may be partly explained by undocumented, relatively low drug exposure, because of higher drug clearance, rather than altered pharmacodynamics. Lower exposures can explain shorter periods of neutropenia, the rarity of hepatic veno-occlusive disease, diminished mucositis, and treatment failures, such as failure to engraft. However, the immature organ systems of the very young may be more susceptible to certain aspects of toxicity, including late development of cardiomyopathy, increased risk of neuron developmental disorders, delayed puberty, growth plate arrest, and infertility.

For example, children seem more sensitive to the cardiotoxic effects of doxorubicin.[35] Follow-up studies have shown that months or years after completion of treatment for central nervous system (CNS) leukemia with intrathecal methotrexate, cranial irradiation, and systemic chemotherapy, a chronic demyelinating encephalopathy may develop.[36] Furthermore, the latent effects of chemotherapy on fertility appear to vary with age of the patient at treatment. Treatment of leukemia and lymphoma in prepubertal boys, for example, does not appear to produce sustained damage to the testis unless large cumulative doses of alkylating agents are used.[36-41] Treatment during puberty is more likely to result in permanent damage to the germinal epithelium, although sexual maturation proceeds within a normal time frame.[42] In prepubertal girls treated with antimetabolites for leukemia, most achieve menarche and progress through puberty.[43,44] Even the alkylating agents used for Hodgkin's lymphoma are unlikely to damage ovarian function. However, almost 70% of girls with brain tumors treated with procarbazine and/or nitrosoureas had evidence of ovarian hormonal failure.[45]

PHARMACOKINETIC-PHARMACODYNAMIC RELATIONSHIPS

Preclinical Development

In general, the preclinical data available before a candidate anticancer drug is entered into clinical trials include the in vitro cytotoxic activity in various animal and human tumor cell lines, and the in vivo antitumor activity in mouse tumor models or in human tumors xenografted in nude mice. In addition to these antitumor evaluations, toxicologic studies are conducted in various species to determine toxicity, such as the lethal dose for 10% of the animals (LD_{10}). These in vitro evaluations clearly have value in defining target plasma drug concentrations, although direct extrapolation is often difficult because of oversimplification of these models, because usually no correction is applied for the lack of metabolic transformation (or any other form of drug elimination) and/or the presence of physiologic barriers. Nonetheless, these studies may guide the choice of administration schedules and starting dosage in phase I clinical trials. For example, if drug cytotoxic activity is S-phase specific, prolonged exposure may be required that would be better achieved using a prolonged IV infusion if that agent has a relatively short terminal half-life. Preclinical data have also shown to be valuable in defining a therapeutic window to be reached in patients. Theoretically, it is possible to define two-dimensional plasma concentration time windows, the lower limit (or threshold concentration) of which is associated with antitumor activity, and the upper (or toxic concentration) with an unacceptable degree of toxic side effects.[46] This approach is the basis of therapeutic drug monitoring, which is also widely used and accepted for numerous noncancer drugs, including calcineurin inhibitors and antiretroviral agents.[47]

Clinical Development

Choice of Starting Dose

Historically, the empirical starting dose for anticancer agents is based on toxicologic studies in rodents (mice and rats) and dogs, and 10% of the murine LD_{10} is often chosen for the first dose level to be used in patients because at this dose, intolerable toxicity is rarely encountered.[48] Based on theoretical considerations in addition to an extensive review of preclinical toxicologic studies from literature data, it has been proposed that limited toxicologic models using mouse and rat data only can appropriately and safely be used for anticancer drug development.[49,50] It is important to realize, however, that compared with patients, much higher plasma concentrations of (experimental) anticancer agents can generally be achieved in animals, which cannot always be explained by a proportionally higher drug clearance. When trying to extrapolate results from efficacy studies performed in tumor-bearing animals to the clinical situation, it should thus be taken into consideration that tumors are exposed to drug levels that can, in most cases, never be achieved in patients. Clearly, this is particularly relevant when the relationships between plasma levels and antitumor effects are poorly understood.

Dose Escalation Schemes

If the starting dose is not severely toxic in patients, further dose escalation is usually based on the modified Fibonacci sequence, in which escalating steps have decreasing relative increments (e.g., 100%, 67%, 50%). Each succeeding step is typically continued in cohorts of three patients until dose-limiting toxicity is reached. The major limitations of this standard design related to ethical considerations and efficiency have been reviewed,[49] and numerous alternative methodologies have been proposed. One of these approaches was designed to accelerate dose escalation rationally by using preclinical pharmacologic data. This process of pharmacokinetically guided dose escalation assumes that for agents showing no major differences in target cell sensitivity, schedule dependence, or toxicity between animals and patients, the AUC at the murine LD_{10} and the AUC at the human maximum tolerated dose should be similar. This approach has proven useful in saving dose levels to be studied in trials of several agents over the past decade, including flavone acetic acid, hexamethylene bisacetamide, piroxantrone, and iododeoxydoxorubicin,[49] thereby reducing the number of patients exposed to theoretically subtherapeutic dosages of the drug involved.

Other groups have advocated similar approaches to escalate systemic exposure measures rather than dose to determine the maximum tolerated systemic exposure, and have used it in trials with various agents, including topotecan, teniposide, carboplatin, and paclitaxel.[51,52] Both concepts have value in reducing the number of patients required for the trials, but have proven difficult to adopt in the clinical setting because of a number of pitfalls, including the assumption of linear pharmacokinetics between species, the substantial interpatient variability in results, and logistic issues in obtaining real-time data that enable subsequent escalation steps. Currently, there is clearly a need for more in vitro and in vivo preclinical pharmacologic studies in an effort to rationalize the transition between animals and patients, which still remains a difficult and hazardous task and a rather empirical exercise. Because of this, even the most recently proposed dose escalation methods are still largely based on empirical experience.[53]

Parameter Estimates

Pharmacokinetic studies performed during early clinical development should be applied to define pharmacokinetic parameters at different dose levels, including peak concentration, drug clearance, half-lives, volume of distribution, and metabolic profiles. This information can be used subsequently to design more rational schedules of administration and define the therapeutic window of the agent, and may provide clues about potentially cumulative toxicity or specific toxicity associated with organ dysfunction. The detection of metabolites and the description of their pharmacokinetic behavior are also extremely important, particularly for agents that require metabolic activation, such as irinotecan and cyclophosphamide. The generated parameters are tentatively correlated with the observed clinical outcome, particularly in terms of toxicity, in an effort to define pharmacokinetic-pharmacodynamic relationships that may be of use in further clinical testing of the agent involved. In addition, dose-effect relationships, at least in terms of toxicity, can best be assessed at this early step in clinical development, in which a wide range of doses is being administered to patients, rather than during the other clinical phases of drug development.

Once a dose is selected, the same dose is usually maintained throughout treatment unless serious toxicity occurs, in which case the dose is empirically decreased for subsequent treatment courses. In contrast, the dose of chemotherapy is rarely increased in the absence of toxicity, even though this might be a reason for treatment failure. Although wide interpatient variability has been demonstrated in all aspects of anticancer drug pharmacokinetics, several studies have demonstrated reasonably predictive relationships between some measure of drug exposure and toxicity or antitumor efficacy in pediatric patients (Table 6-3), which would add to the argument to increase the dose in case of limited toxicity. To analyze the relationship between drug concentration and pharmacologic effects of anticancer agents, various mathematical models have been used, such as the modified Hill equation or the E_{max} model—the maximum effect a drug produces. The Hill equation reflects a sigmoidal relationship between AUC, steady state or threshold concentrations, and pharmacologic response, usually hematologic toxicity, transformed in percentage. This type of relationship has been demonstrated for a number of commonly used anticancer drugs, including carboplatin, doxorubicin, etoposide, 5-fluorouracil, paclitaxel, and vinblastine.[54] When nonhematologic toxicities are dose-limiting, they become more difficult to model because of the subjective nature of grading these types of toxicity in contrast to hematologic toxicity, which is a more quantitative and continuous variable. However, efforts to model these side effects have yielded useful correlations between nephrotoxicity and cisplatin AUC, for example, and gastrointestinal toxicity and glucuronidation rates of the irinotecan metabolite, SN-38.[55]

DRUG INTERACTIONS

Coadministration of Other Chemotherapeutic Drugs

The vast majority of pharmacologic studies of anticancer agents have modeled the effects of a single drug. However, as a consequence of somatic mutations, tumor cell kill tends to decrease with subsequent courses of treatment, and because genetically-resistant cell types are selected out, single-agent treatment is rarely curative. Therefore, and for other reasons (see later), cancer chemotherapy is most frequently given as a combination of different drugs. Favorable and unfavorable interactions between drugs must be considered in developing such combination regimens. These interactions may influence the effectiveness of each of the components of the combination. To take optimal advantage of combination chemotherapy theoretically, it has been proposed that several prerequisites must be met:

- Drugs with at least activity as a single agent should be selected. Because of primary resistance, which is frequent for any single agent, even in the most responsive tumors, single-agent complete response rates rarely exceed 20%.
- Drugs with different mechanisms of action should be combined. The various anticancer agent classes have different

TABLE 6-3   Some Pharmacokinetic-Pharmacodynamic Relationships for Anticancer Drugs

Drug	Toxicity/efficacy (disease)	Pharmacokinetic parameter
Busulfan	Hepatotoxicity	AUC
Carboplatin	Thrombocytopenia	AUC
Cisplatin	Nephrotoxicity	C_{max} (unbound drug)
	Neurotoxicity	C_{max} (unbound drug)
Cyclophosphamide	Cardiotoxicity	AUC
Docetaxel	Neutropenia	AUC
Doxorubicin	ANLL	C_{3-hr}
	Leukocytopenia	AUC
	Thrombocytopenia	doxorubicinol AUC
5-Fluorouracil	Mucositis	AUC > 30 µg.h/ml
	Leukocytopenia	AUC and C_{ss}
Irinotecan	Neutropenia	AUC
	Diarrhea	Biliary index
6-Mercaptopurine	ALL	AUC; RBC 6-TGN levels
Methotrexate	Mucositis, myelosuppression	$C_{48\ hr}$ > 0.9 µM
Paclitaxel	Neutropenia	Time above 0.05 µM
Teniposide	Lymphoma, leukemia	C_{ss} and CL
Topotecan	Myelosuppression	Lactone AUC
Vinblastine	Neutropenia	C_{ss}
Vincristine	Neurotoxicity	AUC

AUC, area under the plasma concentration-time curve; ANLL, acute nonlymphocytic leukemia; C_{3-hr}, plasma concentration at 3 hours after IV bolus administration; $C_{48\ hrs}$ plasma concentration at 48 hours; C_{max}, peak plasma concentration; C_{ss}, plasma concentration at steady-state; CL, total plasma clearance; ALL, acute lymphocytic leukemia; RBC, red blood cell; 6-TGN, 6-thioguanine nucleotide (intracellular active metabolites of 6-mercaptopurine).

targets in the cell. The use of multiple agents with different mechanisms of action enables independent cell killing by each agent. Cells resistant to one agent might still be sensitive to the other drug(s) in the regimen, and might thus still be killed. Known patterns of cross resistance must be taken into consideration in the design of drug combinations.

- Drugs with different mechanisms of resistance should be combined. Resistance to many agents may be the result of mutational changes unique to those agents. However, in other circumstances, a single mutational change may lead to resistance to various different drugs. The number of potential mechanisms of resistance is continuously increasing and partly drug-dependent. Because of the presence of drug-resistant mutants at the time of clinical diagnosis, the earliest possible use of non–cross-resistant drugs is recommended to avoid the selection of double mutants by sequential chemotherapy. Adequate cytotoxic doses of drugs have to be administered as frequently as possible to achieve maximal kill of sensitive and moderately resistant cells.
- If possible, drugs with different dose-limiting toxicities should be combined. For drugs with nonoverlapping toxicity, it is more likely that each drug can be used at full dose and thus the effectiveness of each agent will be maintained in the combination.

As noted, multiple-drug therapy can give rise to clinically important drug-drug interactions, which typically occur when the pharmacokinetic behavior of one drug is altered by the other. These interactions are important in the design of drug combinations because, occasionally, the outcome of concurrent drug administration is diminished therapeutic efficacy or increased toxicity of one or more of the administered drugs. Pharmacokinetic interactions between chemotherapeutic agents are usually evaluated and identified in phase I and II trials.

In addition to pharmacokinetic interactions, combinations of drugs might also show pharmacodynamic interactions that cannot be explained by altered pharmacokinetic profiles. Some of these interactions are at the cellular level or are cell cycle–related and can be classified as synergistic, additive, or antagonistic. Provided that the drugs used are active in a particular disease, knowledge of cellular kinetics can be used to consider therapy initiation with non–cell cycle phase-specific agents (e.g., alkylating agents), first to reduce tumor bulk and second to recruit slowly dividing cells into active DNA synthesis. Once the latter is achieved, treatment can be continued within the same cycle of treatment by cell cycle phase-specific agents (e.g., methotrexate or fluoropyrimidines), which mainly affect cells during DNA synthesis. Further, repeated courses with S-phase specific drugs, such as cytarabine and methotrexate, that block cells during the period of DNA synthesis, are most effective if they are administered during the rebound rapid recovery of DNA synthesis that follows the period of suppression of DNA synthesis.[56] If pharmacokinetic and pharmacodynamic interactions exist, the drug doses and sequence of administration that allows safe administration of combination chemotherapy are typically defined during early clinical evaluation.

Coadministration of Nonchemotherapeutic Drugs

Many prescription and over-the-counter medications have the potential to interact pharmacokinetically with anticancer agents, altering their pharmacokinetic characteristics and leading to clinically significant interactions. Over 100,000 deaths/year in the United States alone can be attributed to such drug-drug interactions, placing these interactions between the fourth and sixth leading causes of death.[57] It is obvious that all aspects of pharmacokinetics might be affected when a drug is given in combination with another drug, including absorption (resulting in altered absorption rate or oral bioavailability), distribution (mostly caused by protein-binding displacement), metabolism, and excretion. However, most known drug-drug interactions are caused by changes in metabolic routes related to altered

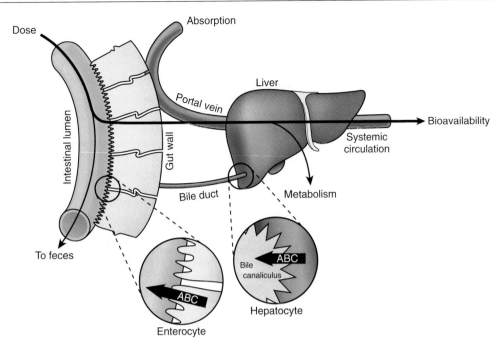

FIGURE 6-4. Role of active transport directed toward the gut lumen and bile by ATP binding-cassette transporters expressed in the intestinal epithelium and liver, respectively, in drug absorption and elimination. ABC = ATP-binding cassette transporters.

expression or functionality of CYP isozymes. This class of enzymes, particularly the CYP3A4 isoform, is responsible for the oxidation of most currently prescribed anticancer drugs, resulting in more polar and usually inactive metabolites. Elevated CYP activity (induction), translated into a more rapid metabolic rate, may result in a decrease in plasma concentrations and thus a loss of therapeutic effect. For example, anticonvulsant drugs (e.g., phenytoin, phenobarbital, carbamazepine) induce drug-metabolizing enzymes and thereby increase the clearance in children of various anticancer agents, including teniposide[58] and irinotecan.[59] Moreover, anticonvulsant therapy has been related to worse event-free survival, hematologic relapse, and CNS relapse in patients with acute lymphoblastic leukemia.[60] Conversely, suppression (inhibition) of CYP activity may trigger a rise in plasma concentrations and lead to exaggerated toxicity commensurate with overdose (http://www.druginteractions.com).

It should be noted that several pharmacokinetic parameters could be altered simultaneously. Oral bioavailability plays a crucial role, especially in the development of anticancer agents given by the oral route.[61] This parameter is contingent on adequate intestinal absorption and the circumvention of intestinal and, subsequently, hepatic metabolism of the drug. A principal mechanism that can explain interactions with anticancer agents given orally is the affinity for adenosine triphosphate (ATP)–binding cassette transporters expressed in the intestinal epithelium and directed toward the gut lumen (Fig. 6-4). The three major classes of drug transporters, referred to as P-glycoprotein (ABCB1), multidrug resistance–associated protein-1 (MRP1, ABCC1) and its homologue MRP2 (cMOAT, ABCC2), and breast cancer resistance protein (BCRP, ABCG2), may play a significant role in mediating transmembrane transport of anticancer drugs.[62] Extraction of anticancer drugs by extensive metabolism in the gut wall and/or the liver during first pass (i.e., prior to reaching the systemic circulation) is another potential mechanism involved in suspected interactions among various agents. An ideal chemotherapeutic drug would have an adequate absolute bioavailability

and little interpatient and intrapatient variability in absorption. For the most commonly used oral agents, such as etoposide, cyclophosphamide, and methotrexate, however, these criteria are not met. The generally narrow therapeutic index of these agents means that significant inter- and intrapatient variability would predispose some individuals to excessive toxicity or, conversely, inadequate efficacy.

Coadministration of Complementary and Alternative Medicine

In recent years, interest in complementary and alternative medicine (CAM) has grown rapidly in the industrialized world. Some reasons for this increase relate to dissatisfaction with conventional allopathic therapies, a desire of parents (and patients) to be involved more actively in their children's health care, and because parents and patients find these alternatives to be more congruent with their own lifestyle.[63] Surveys within the past decade have estimated the prevalence of CAM use in pediatric oncology to be between 31% and 87% and, in many cases, the treating physician is unaware of the patient's CAM use. With a larger number of children using herbal treatments,[64] such as garlic supplementation and echinacea,[65] combined with allopathic therapies, the risk for herb-drug interactions is a growing concern, and there is an increasing need to understand possible adverse drug-drug interactions in oncology. This is of particular relevance to pediatric cancer patients because CAM use is more common in this group than in the general population.[64]

During the last decade, a wealth of evidence has been generated from in vitro and in vivo studies showing that many herbal preparations interact extensively with drug-metabolizing enzymes and drug transporters. A number of clinically important pharmacokinetic interactions have now been recognized, although causal relationships have not always been established and confirmatory studies in children are currently lacking. Most

TABLE 6-4   **Predicted Effects of Commonly Used Herbs on Activity of Enzymes and Transporters in Humans**

Herb	Effect
Asian ginseng (*Panax ginseng*)	Weak inhibition of CYP2D6, CYP3A4; no influence on CYP1A2, CYP2E1
Balloon vine (*Cardiospermum halicacabum*)	Potential inhibition of CYP1A2
Bitter orange (*Citrus aurantium*)	No influence on CYP1A2, CYP2D6, CYP2E1, or CYP3A4
Black cohosh (*Actaea racemosa*)	Weak inhibition of CYP2D6; no influence on CYP1A2, CYP2E1, CYP3A4, ABCB1
Black pepper (*Piper nigrum*)	Potential inhibition of CYP3A4, ABCB1
Bloodwort (*Sanguisorba officinalis*)	Potential induction of CYP1A2
Boldo (*Peumus boldus*)	Potential inhibition of CYP2C9
Chinese skullcap (*Scutellaria baicalensis*)	Potential inhibition of CYP3A4, ABCB1
Cranberry (*Vaccinium macrocarpon*)	No influence on CYP2C9, CYP3A4, ABCB1
Dandelion (*Taraxacum mongolicum*)	Potential induction of CYP1A2
Danshen (*Salvia miltiorrhiza*)	Potential inhibition of CYP2C9; potential induction of CYP3A4
Devil's claw (*Harpagophytum procumbens*)	No conclusive data available
Dogbane (*Apocynum venetum*)	No influence on CYP3A4, ABCB1
Dong quai (*Angelica sinensis*)	Potential inhibition of CYP2C9
Echinacea (*Echinacea* spp.)	Potential induction of CYP3A4; no influence on CYP1A2, CYP2D6, CYP2E1
Fennel (*Foeniculum vulgare*)	Potential induction of CYP1A2
Feverfew (*Tanacetum parthenium*)	No conclusive data available
Fo-ti (*Polygonum multiflorum*)	No conclusive data available
Garlic (*Allium sativum*)	Weak inhibition of CYP3A4, CYP2E1, ABCB1; weak induction of *N*-acetyltransferase
Ginger (*Zingiber officinalis*)	No influence on CYP2C9
Ginkgo (*Ginkgo biloba*)	Strong induction of CYP2C19; weak inhibition of CYP3A4; no influence on CYP2C9
Goldenseal (*Hydrastis canadensis*)	Strong inhibition of CYP2D6 and CYP3A4
Grapefruit juice (*Citrus paradise*)	Strong inhibition of (intestinal) CYP3A4
Grape seed (*Vitis vinifera*)	Potential induction of (hepatic) CYP3A4
Green tea (*Camellia sinensis*)	No influence on CYP2D6, CYP3A4; potential induction of CYP1A2
Guar gum (*Cyamopsis tetragonoloba*)	No influence on ABCB1
Guggul tree (*Commiphora mukul*)	Potential induction of CYP3A4
Horny goat weed (*Epimedium* spp.)	No conclusive data available
Japanese arrowroot (*Pueraria lobata*)	Potential inhibition of ABCC and OAT transporters
Kangen-Karyu	Potential inhibition of CYP2C9
Kava kava (*Piper methysticum*)	Strong inhibition of CYP2E1; strong induction of CYP3A4
Licorice (*Glycyrrhiza uralensis*)	Potential inhibition of CYP3A4; potential induction of CYP2C9, CYP3A4
Milk thistle (*Silybum marianum*)	No influence on CYP1A2, CYP2D6, CYP2E1, CYP3A4, ABCB1
Peppermint oil (*Mentha piperita*)	Weak inhibition of CYP3A4
Pomelo juice (*Citrus grandis*)	Weak inhibition of CYP3A4 or ABCB1 (or both)
Red clover (*Trifolium pratense*)	No conclusive data available
Saw palmetto (*Serenoa repens*)	No influence on CYP1A2, CYP2D6, CYP2E1, CYP3A4
Shoseiryuto (includes *Ephedra sinica, Schisandra,* cinnamon)	No influence on CYP3A4
Siberian ginseng (*Panax quinquefolius*)	No influence on CYP2D6, CYP3A4
Soy (*Glycine max*)	No influence on CYP3A4
St. John's wort (*Hypericum perforatum*)	Strong induction of CYP1A2, CYP2C8, CYP2C9, CYP2C19, CYP2E1, CYP3A4, ABCB1
Tanner's Cassia (*Cassia auriculata*)	Potential inhibition of CYP1A2
Tortoise shell (quilinggao)	Potential induction of CYP2C9
Turmeric (*Curcuma longa*)	No influence on CYP3A4, ABCB1
Valerian (*Valeriana officinalis*)	No influence on CYP1A2, CYP2D6, CYP2E1, CYP3A4
Wheat bran (*Triticum aestivum*)	No influence on ABCB1; potential inhibition of CYP3A4
White peony (*Radix paeoniae alba*)	No influence on CYP3A4
Wolfberry (*Lycium barbarum*)	Potential inhibition of CYP2C9
Wu wei zi (*Schisandra chinensis*)	Potential induction of CYP2C9, CYP3A4
Wu chu yu (*Evodia rutaecarpa*)	Potential induction of CYP1A2

of the observed interactions point to the herbs affecting several isoforms of the CYP family, through inhibition or induction. These enzymes have a crucial role in the elimination of various anticancer drugs, and concurrent use of some herbs with chemotherapy is destined to have serious clinical and toxicologic implications. Therefore, rigorous testing for possible pharmacokinetic interactions of anticancer drugs with widely used herbs is urgently required.

In the context of chemotherapeutic drugs, only St. John's wort (*Hypericum perforatum*),[66] garlic (*Allium sativum*),[67] and milk thistle (*Silybum marianum*)[68] have been formally evaluated for their drug-drug interaction potential in vivo. However, various other herbs have the potential to significantly modulate the expression and/or activity of drug-metabolizing enzymes and drug transporters, including ginkgo (*Ginkgo biloba*), echinacea (*Echinacea purpurea*), ginseng (*Panax ginseng*), and kava (*Piper methysticum*) (Table 6-4). An additional consideration for cancer chemotherapy is that herb-mediated induction of various enzymes and transporters may also take place in tumor cells, and subsequently result in resistance to anthracyclines, epi-

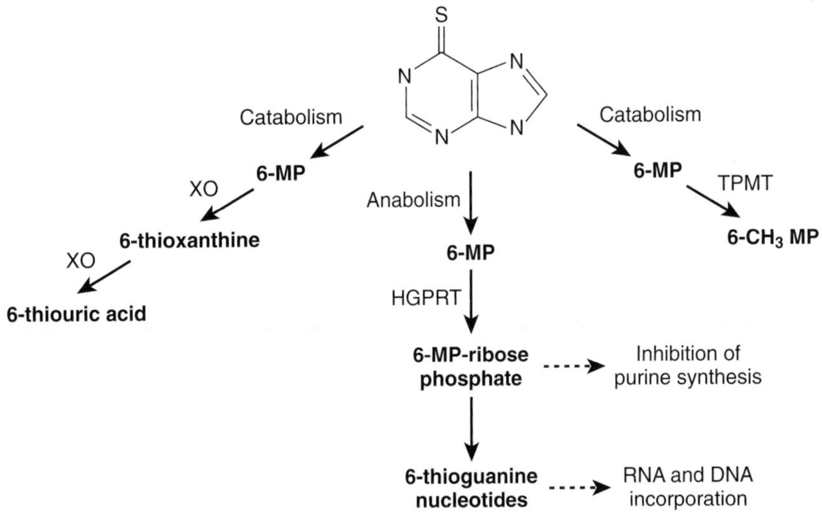

FIGURE 6-5. Simplified schematic of metabolic pathways of 6-mercaptopurine (6-MP). HGPRT = hypoxanthine-guanine phosphoribosyltransferase; TPMT = thiopurine *S*-methyltransferase; XO = xanthine oxidase.

podophyllotoxins, taxanes and *Vinca* alkaloids. Similarly, catalytic inhibition of topoisomerase II-alpha in tumor cells by some herbs[69] might diminish therapeutic responses to anthracyclines, dactinomycin, and etoposide.[70] Because of the high prevalence of herbal medicine use in the United States, physicians should include herb usage in their routine drug histories so they can review which potential hazards should be taken into consideration with individual patients.

PHARMACOGENETICS

The discipline of pharmacogenetics describes differences in the pharmacokinetics and pharmacodynamics of drugs as a result of inherited variation in drug-metabolizing enzymes, drug transporters, and drug targets among patients.[71,72] These inherited differences in enzymes and receptors are one of the major factors responsible for interpatient variability in drug disposition (systemic exposure) and effects (normal tissue and tumor exposure). Severe toxicity might occur in the absence of typical metabolism of active compounds, whereas the therapeutic effect of a drug could be diminished in the case of absence of activation of a prodrug. The importance and detectability of polymorphisms for a given enzyme depend on the contribution of the variant gene product to pharmacologic response, the availability of alternative pathways of metabolism, and the frequency of occurrence of the least common variant allele. Although many substrates have been identified for the known polymorphic drug-metabolizing enzymes and transporters, the contribution of a genetically determined source of variability has been established for only a few cancer chemotherapeutic agents. Some of these proteins are known to be involved in anticancer agent metabolism and excretion (see Table 6-1), and are responsible for extensive interindividual variability in anticancer drug pharmacokinetics.

Drug-Metabolizing Enzymes

Thiopurine *S*-Methyltransferase

The *TPMT* genetic polymorphism probably best illustrates the huge potential impact of pharmacogenetics on pediatric oncology.[73] Thiopurine *S*-methyltransferase (TPMT) plays an important role in the metabolism of the thiopurine drugs 6-mercaptopurine (6-MP), 6-thioguanine, and azathioprine. These prodrugs require metabolic activation by hypoxanthine phosphoribosyltransferase to form thiopurine nucleotides, which undergo incorporation into DNA and/or inhibit de novo purine synthesis. TPMT catalyzes the transfer of the methyl group from *S*-adenosyl methionine (SAM) to the sulfur atoms of thiopurines, which is the predominant inactivation pathway of these agents in hematopoietic tissue. A simplified schematic of the various metabolic pathways of 6-MP is shown in Figure 6-5.

Polymorphic TPMT activity in erythrocytes, which correlates well with that in other tissues, was first described in 1980[74] and its genetic basis is now well understood. TPMT activity displays a trimodal distribution, with approximately 90% of individuals having high enzyme activity, 10% having intermediate activity because of heterozygosity, and 0.3% having low or no detectable enzyme activity because they inherit two nonfunctional *TPMT* alleles. *TPMT*3C, TPMT*3A*, and *TPMT*2* are the predominant variant alleles accounting for over 95% of inherited TPMT deficiency.[75] Considerable differences in the types and frequencies of TPMT alleles have been observed among different ethnic groups, with *TPMT*3A* being the most common in white populations, whereas *TPMT*3C* is the most prevalent among Asian, African, and African American populations.

TPMT-deficient patients accumulate excessive concentrations of thioguanine nucleotides following conventional dosing of thiopurines, leading to severe and potentially fatal hematologic toxicity.[76-78] Heterozygous patients have an intermediate risk of toxicity and typically require only a modest dose reduction (up to 50%),[79,80] whereas patients inheriting two nonfunctional alleles require a 90% to 95% dose reduction to as little as 5% to 10% of the standard dose. Pretreatment knowledge of a patient's TPMT status is now being used for dose optimization to reduce the likelihood of toxicity. A radiochemical of high-performance liquid chromatographic assay can be used to measure TPMT activity in erythrocytes, and rapid *TPMT* genotyping methods—for example, those based on DNA microchips[81]—are now available to make the diagnosis based on genotype. When thiopurines are administered according to genotype, comparable cellular thioguanine nucleotide concentrations are achieved; therefore, all patients, regardless of *TPMT*

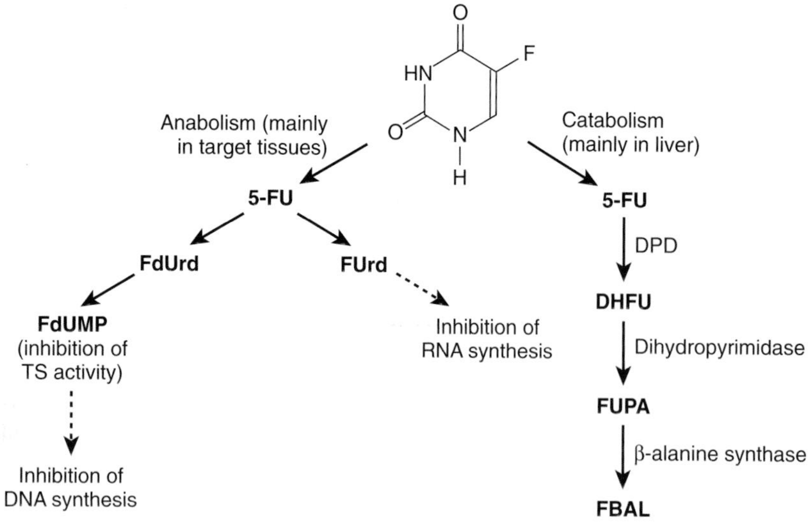

FIGURE 6-6. Simplified schematic of metabolic pathways of 5-fluorouracil (5-FU). DHFU = 5′,6′-dihydroxyfluorouracil; DPD = dihydropyrimidine dehydrogenase; FBAL = 5-fluoro-β-alanine; FdUMP = fluorodeoxyuridine monophosphate; FdUrd = fluorodeoxyuridine; FUPA = α-fluoro-β-ureidopropionic acid; FUrd = fluorouridine; TS = thymidylate synthase.

phenotypes, can be treated without adverse effects and without compromising efficacy.[82]

Dihydropyrimidine Dehydrogenase

Dihydropyrimidine dehydrogenase (DPD) is the initial and rate-limiting enzyme in the catabolic pathway of the naturally occurring pyrimidines uracil and thymine, and is also responsible for the degradation of the anticancer agent 5-fluorouracil (5-FU; Fig. 6-6). The relationship between DPD and the efficacy and toxicity of 5-FU has been reviewed.[83] 5-FU is widely used as a single agent and in combination therapies for the treatment of various pediatric malignancies. The antitumor activity and cytotoxicity of 5-FU depend on its anabolism to cytotoxic nucleotides, which incorporate into RNA and/or DNA and inhibit thymidylate synthase. DPD essentially regulates the availability of 5-FU for anabolism. More than 80% of an administered dose of 5-FU is inactivated by DPD.[84] Furthermore, studies have shown an inverse correlation between the circadian rhythm of DPD activity and plasma levels of 5-FU in patients receiving a continuous infusion.[85]

Deficiency of DPD is an autosomal recessive disorder, with a variable phenotype that ranges from partial to complete loss of enzyme activity. Patients with DPD deficiency have a reduced capacity to degrade 5-FU, so are at risk of developing severe to life-threatening toxicity following 5-FU administration.[86-90] To date, 39 different mutations and polymorphisms have been identified in the human DPD gene (*DYPD*).[83] Of these, 14 have been identified in patients experiencing excessive 5-FU–associated toxicity, the most common one being a G to A point mutation in the invariant splice donor site (*IVS14 + 1G > A* mutation). This mutation is present in Dutch, German, Finnish, Turkish, and Taiwanese populations but has not been detected in Japanese or African-American populations. One study has detected the IVS14 + 1G > A mutation in 24% to 28% of patients suffering from severe 5-FU toxicity,[88] but further studies have suggested that 5-FU toxicity resulting from reduced DPD activity cannot be entirely explained by this or other known polymorphisms.[91]

The identification of patients with an increased risk of developing severe toxicity following 5-FU administration would allow dose reduction or the selection of alternative anticancer therapies. Several methods have been developed to screen for *DYPD* mutations or assess DPD activity prior to therapy.[92-95] However, genotyping tests for *DYPD* mutations have low sensitivity in identifying high-risk patients, and current methods for assessing DPD activity are laborious and not convenient for routinely screening cancer patients who are going to receive 5-FU–based therapy. The most recently published method to identify DPD-deficient cancer patients makes use of a simple, rapid, and noninvasive 2-^{13}C-uracil breath test.[96] The clinical usefulness of this procedure as an a priori approach to administer 5-FU–based treatment modalities in patients with cancer remains to be established.

Cytochrome P-450 Isozymes

The CYP superfamily consists of over 60 enzymes that have been grouped into several families and subfamilies. These enzymes are responsible for the oxidative metabolism of over 90% of drugs in clinical use, including several anticancer agents. Obviously, for pharmacogenetic screening to be effective, it is important that the CYP enzyme contributes significantly to the metabolism of the specific drug, that there is a genetic polymorphism known that affects the metabolic activity of the enzyme to a major extent, and that such a polymorphism occurs frequently enough to warrant screening. Given current knowledge, clinically relevant associations between CYP polymorphisms and anticancer therapy are most likely to be discovered for *CYP2B6*, *CYP2C8*, and *CYP3A5*, the latter of which is also relevant to many, but not all, the drugs that are metabolized by CYP3A4.

CYP2B6

CYP2B6 is expressed in the liver and extrahepatic tissues. Activity of this isozyme varies considerably among individuals and has recently been demonstrated to be 1.7-fold higher in females compared to males.[97] Based on *S*-mephenytoin *N*-demethylation, 7% of females and 20% of males have proved to be CYP2B6 poor metabolizers (PMs).[97] For the *CYP2B6* gene, located on chromosome 19q13.2, nine SNPs composing variant alleles *1 through *7 have been described.[98] The *1459C > T* genetic polymorphism (Arg487Cys), present in *5 and *7 alleles, corresponds to lower CYP2B6 protein levels in heterozygous and homozygous variant individuals when compared with *CYP2B6*1* wild types.[98] According to Hiratsuka and colleagues,[99] the allele frequencies in whites are 11% and 3% for *CYP2B6*5* (Arg487Cys) and *7 alleles (Gln172His, Lys262Arg, Arg487Cys), respectively, whereas in the Japanese they are 1%

and 0%. Other groups have reported allele frequencies of 14%[98] and 13%[97] for the *1459C > T* polymorphism in whites. Interestingly, a correlation has been demonstrated between the *1459C > T* single nucleotide polymorphism (SNP) (*5 and *7 alleles) and CYP2B6 activity in white females but not in males.[97] Other groups have shown that *CYP2B6*6/*6* homozygous individuals (Gln172His, Lys262Arg) have low CYP2B6 protein levels.[100] An allelic frequency of 26% (whites) and 16% (Japanese) was found for the *CYP2B6*6* allele.[99] However, it is unclear whether the overall effect of the *CYP2B6*6* genotype will be reduced activity caused by decreased protein expression or higher activity caused by increased catalytic potential.[101] Interestingly, the *CYP2B6*4* variant allele (*785A > G*, Lys262Arg) has been associated with an increase in enzymatic activity, as measured by bupropion hydroxylation.[102] Population kinetic analysis in that study showed that the CYP2B6-dependent hydroxylation does not differ among the *CYP2B6*1*, *2, *5, and *6 alleles, but that clearance by *CYP2B6*4* allele carriers (CYP2B6*1/*4 heterozygotes) was 1.6-fold higher compared with wild-type *CYP2B6*1/*1* individuals. Both the *4 and *6 variant allele carry the *785A > G* mutation (encoding Lys268Arg), which may be responsible for the increase in enzymatic activity. The additional Gln172His mutation in the *CYP2B6*6* allele decreases protein expression whereby the net effect on CYP2B6 activity is compensated in this allele. The allelic frequency reported for white males was 5.0% for *CYP2B6*4*, 9.5% for *CYP2B6*5*, 25% for *CYP2B6*6*, and 0% for *CYP2B6*7*.[102] A *CYP2B6*4* allele frequency of 5% was also reported by Lamba and associates,[97] although others have reported an allelic frequency in whites of 32.6%.[98] However, the clinical impact of this genetic polymorphism remains to be determined.

CYP2B6 is involved in the metabolism of various anticancer agents, including cyclophosphamide and ifosfamide.[100] The aforementioned difference in CYP2B6 activity between males and females was reflected by a twofold higher *N*-dechloroethylation of ifosfamide in microsomes obtained from females compared with males.[103] Regarding the conversion of cyclophosphamide to 4-hydroxycyclophosphamide as a function of total CYP-450 protein, however, no difference was observed between *CYP2B6*1/*1* individuals compared with *CYP2B6*6/*6* individuals,[100] thus arguing against *CYP2B6*6* screening prior to cyclophosphamide treatment. For the *1459C > T* SNP, present in the *CYP2B6*5* and *7 alleles, correlation with low activity in vivo requires further study, as does the increased activity of the *CYP2B6*4* allele. Reported allele frequencies differ significantly among studies, but are high enough to warrant further investigation.

CYP2C8, CYP2C9, and CYP2C19

The CYP2C subfamily is responsible for the metabolism of approximately 20% of clinically used drugs. It consists of four members—CYP2C8, CYP2C9, CYP2C18 and CYP2C19—and the corresponding genes are clustered on chromosome 10q24. Polymorphisms in the *CYP2C8, 2C9,* and *2C19* genes have been shown to result in toxicity of certain anticancer drugs in affected individuals.[104]

For CYP2C8, the decreased activity allele *CYP2C8*2* (*805A > T*; Ile269Phe) was found predominantly in African Americans (allele frequency 18%) but not in whites (0%). In contrast, the variant *CYP2C8*3* allele (*416G > A* and *1196A > G*; Arg139Lys and Lys399Arg) had allele frequencies of 13% in whites and 2% in African Americans. Decreased activity of recombinant CYP2C8.2 and CYP2C8.3 enzymes was demonstrated in metabolism studies of the anticancer drug paclitaxel, which undergoes CYP2C8-mediated hydroxylation.[105] Preliminary investigations have suggested that the *CYP2C8*3* variant is associated with reduced plasma concentrations of the

CYP2C8 substrate drug repaglinide,[106] but not paclitaxel.[107] A *CYP2C8*4* (*792C > G*; Ile264Met) allele with decreased activity has been reported.[108] Furthermore, a potentially inactive *CYP2C8*5* allele (*475delA*; frameshift) was found in one Japanese individual. The clinical consequences of these variant alleles, particularly in relation to the clinical pharmacology of paclitaxel, are yet to be determined.

For CYP2C9, which is the principal CYP2C in human liver,[109] 11 variant alleles (*2 through *12) have been described. *CYP2C9*2* (*430C > T;* Arg144Cys) and *CYP2C9*3* (*1075A > C;* Ile359Leu) have been shown to affect CYP2C9 metabolism in vivo and occur in 11% and 3% to 16% of whites, respectively, and in 3% and 1.3% of African Americans, respectively.[110] The *CYP2C9*3* genotype seems to be associated with the largest change in catalytic activity; *CYP2C9*3/*3* polymorphisms among whites occur at a frequency of approximately 0.3%.[111] The *CYP2C9*4* allele (*1076T > C;* Ile359Thr) and *CYP2C9*5* (Asp360Glu) allele displays altered metabolism of diclofenac in vitro.[112,113] The *CYP2C9*4* allele is a rare allele that has been identified in one Japanese subject[114] but has not been found in whites, African Americans, or Chinese. The *5 allele was found with a frequency of 1.7% in African Americans and is absent or extremely rare in whites.[112] Interestingly, the nucleotide changes in the *CYP2C9*3, *4,* and *5 alleles affect two amino acids close together, 359 and 360. The *CYP2C9*6* allele (*818delA*) encodes a frameshift and is therefore a true CYP2C9 null allele. This allele, identified in an African American exhibiting severe drug toxicity on normal phenytoin dosages, was found in 0.6% of African Americans but not in whites.[115] With respect to anticancer therapy, a threefold lower intrinsic clearance of cyclophosphamide in a yeast expression system was observed with recombinant CYP2C9.2 and CYP2C9.3 protein when compared with CYP2C9.1 reference protein.[110] However, no significant differences in cyclophosphamide metabolism by human microsomes obtained from *CYP2C9*2* or *3 individuals compared with those from *CYP2C9*1* homozygotes was demonstrated.[110]

The first genetic polymorphism in *CYP2C19* was discovered because of abnormal metabolism of the anticonvulsant drug mephenytoin, for which 3% to 5% of whites and 12% to 23% of Asians appear to be PMs. A splice site mutation in exon 5 (*CYP2C19*2*) and a premature stop codon in exon 4 (*CYP2C19*3*) represent the two most predominant null alleles.[116] To date, 15 variant alleles have been described (http://www.imm.ki.se/CYPalleles/), of which 7 (*CYP2C19*2* through *8) encode no enzyme activity. With respect to anticancer therapy, CYP2C19 plays a role in the metabolism of cyclophosphamide, ifosfamide, teniposide, and thalidomide.[117-119]

CYP2D6

The observation of considerable interindividual variation in the metabolism of the antihypertensive drug debrisoquine[120] has led to the identification of a genetic variant allele for CYP2D6, the *CYP2D6*4* allele.[121,122] Currently, the *CYP2D6* gene (located on chromosome 22q13.1) is one of the most extensively studied members of the CYP450 superfamily, with over 40 variant alleles (*1 through *43) identified, which includes 26 null alleles (encoding nonfunctional CYP2D6) and 6 alleles encoding enzymes with decreased activity (http://www.imm.ki.se/CYPalleles). In addition, *CYP2D6* gene duplication has been described and correlated with ultrarapid metabolism.[123] This duplication is present in 1% to 2% of the Swedish white population,[124] and increases to 3.6% in Germany,[125] 7% to 10% in Spain,[126] and 10% in the south of Italy.[127] The incidence of gene duplication is even higher in Saudi Arabians and black Ethiopians, 20% and 29%, respectively.[128,129] Interestingly, the ultrarapid phenotype in Ethiopians with the *CYP2D6* duplication (metabolic ratio for debrisoquine of 0.1 to 1) is not as extreme as in whites (metabolic ratio of 0.01 to 0.02).[130] In general, 71% of CYP2D6 alleles in whites are functional alleles, whereas 26% are non-functional. In contrast, only around 50% of the CYP2D6 alleles are functional in Asians.

The reduced function allele CYP2D6*10 has an allelic frequency of approximately 40% in Asians, causing a population shift toward lower mean CYP2D6 activity. For African Americans and Africans, reduced function alleles represent 35% of CYP2D6 genes, with CYP2D6*17 being the main contributor.[130]

Because alleles encoding nonfunctional or decreased function enzymes affect CYP2D6 metabolic potential, knowledge of CYP2D6 genetic makeup may help in optimizing therapy. The genetic variant that needs to be taken into consideration is an important question and the described interethnic differences in variant alleles complicate the answer. For whites, the nonfunctional CYP2D6*4 (allele frequency, 20%) is carried by 75% of CYP2D6 PMs. Screening whites for the presence of the nonfunctional alleles *3 (allele frequency 1% to 2%), *4 (20%), *5 (3.8%), and *6 (1%) will identify more than 98% of CYP2D6 PMs. For Asians and African Americans, the reduced function alleles CYP2D6*10 and *17 should also be evaluated. Homozygosity for nonfunctional CYP2D6 alleles will predict PMs but, given that many CYP2D6 variant alleles exist, it may become evident that the absence of nonfunctional alleles only decreases the chance of being a PM without excluding it completely. A new approach for screening whites has been described in which the (−1584)C > G polymorphism in the 5′-untranslated region seemed to predict non-PMs, with a positive predictive value of 1.0. When heterozygous (−1584)CG or homozygous (−1584)GG, there was a 12% chance of being a poor metabolizer.[131]

With respect to cancer chemotherapy, CYP2D6 does not seem to play a major role in anticancer drug metabolism. For tamoxifen treatment, however, CYP2D6 activity might be of importance. Tamoxifen can either be converted to the inactive N-desmethyl tamoxifen by CYP3A4 (approximately 90% of metabolism) or be activated by CYP2D6 to 4-hydroxytamoxifen (approximately 10% of metabolism), which has 50- to 100-fold higher activity than the parent compound.[132] It appears that CYP2D6 poor metabolizers perform less well on tamoxifen therapy.[133-135] In the context of pediatric oncology, CYP2D6 genotyping might have relevance in relation to the use of serotonin 5-hydroxytryptamine type 3 receptor antagonists like tropisetron or ondansetron, which are used to ameliorate nausea and vomiting in cancer chemotherapy.[136]

CYP3A4 and CYP3A5

The CYP3A subfamily, which represents most CYP protein in the human liver, is responsible for the metabolism of many endogenous compounds and over 30% of all currently used oncology drugs.[137] Four human CYP3A genes have been identified (CYP3A4, CYP3A5, CYP3A7 and CYP3A43), which cluster on chromosome 7.[138] Based on the amount of protein and catalytic potential, CYP3A4 is the most important member of the CYP3A subfamily. CYP3A4 activity in vivo shows extensive interindividual variation, up to 14–fold, which may be caused by health status or environmental, hormonal, or genetic factors.[139] It is thought that genetic differences may explain up to 90% of the observed variation in drug-metabolizing capacity of patients,[140] although only a single very rare "null" allele for CYP3A4 has been described to date.[141] Over 30 SNPs for CYP3A4 have been reported, representing alleles *1 through *20, most of which occur with allele frequencies lower than 5%. The first genetic CYP3A4 polymorphism to be described was the promoter variant allele CYP3A4*1B (−392A > G, originally

referred to as −290A > G), identified by linkage to a worse presentation of prostate cancer.[142] The allele frequency showed a large interethnic variation—2% to 9% in whites, 35% to 67% in African Americans, 0% in Taiwanese, and 0% in Chinese.[143] Although the CYP3A4*1B allele was initially shown to have a 1.5-fold increase in transcription in vitro,[144] it is now generally considered to be not associated with functional changes. Currently, 20 alleles encoding amino acid changes are known (http://www.imm.ki.se/CYPalleles). Decreased CYP3A4 activity has been demonstrated for the CYP3A4*17 allele (566T > C; Phe189Ser) in vitro.[145] There are also indications that the CYP3A4*4 (352A > G; Ile118Val), *5 (653 C > G; Pro218Arg), and *6 (831insA; frameshift) alleles encode proteins with decreased catalytic activity.[145] The impact of these alleles on in vivo CYP3A4 activity, however, remains unclear.[145,146]

The next important member of the CYP3A subfamily is CYP3A5,[145,147] which is expressed in only 10% to 40% of whites. A genetic polymorphism in intron 3 of the CYP3A5 gene (6986A > G, which was named the CYP3A5*3 allele) was found to be responsible for this lack of expression.[148] It was demonstrated that 80% of whites and 30% of African Americans are homozygous for this inactive CYP3A5 allele, and thus are deficient in CYP3A5 activity.[148] In addition, the CYP3A5*5 (12952T > C) and *6 (14690C > A) alleles both encode frameshifts and therefore may also represent null alleles, although with much lower allelic frequency (0.0% and 0.1%, respectively).[148,149] In some individuals, CYP3A5 protein expression may contribute to more than 50% of total CYP3A protein in the liver.[148,150] Consequently, some believe that the CYP3A5 genetic polymorphism will have an important contribution toward predicting liver CYP3A activity, whereas others debate this finding.[151,152] Because there is a large overlap in substrate specificity between CYP3A4 and CYP3A5, the contribution of each isozyme to total CYP3A activity will depend on the drug under investigation and a patient's genotype. In addition, CYP3A5 is expressed extrahepatically in the prostate, kidney, and adrenal and pituitary glands,[153] whereas CYP3A4 activity is more restricted to the liver and intestine.[154] Consequently, depending on the site of action of a drug, the role of CYP3A5 may be larger than anticipated. The identification of anticancer drugs that may benefit from CYP3A5 genetic screening was indicated with the discovery of an allele (CYP3A5*3) that encodes the absence of a protein and occurs with a high frequency in an enzyme family known to be involved in the metabolism of many drugs. One of the first examples indicating this was the metabolism of agents that have higher intrinsic clearance for CYP3A5 compared with CYP3A4, such as the immunosuppressive drug tacrolimus and the Vinca alkaloid vincristine.[155,156] For most drugs, however, including prototypical phenotyping probe drugs such as midazolam and erythromycin, the common polymorphisms in CYP3A4 and CYP3A5 do not appear to have important functional significance.[137,139,157]

As noted, the CYP3A family is involved in the metabolism of many anticancer drugs. For example, both CYP3A4 and CYP3A5 are involved in the biotransformation of docetaxel, with an estimated contribution of 64% to 93% to total metabolism. CYP3A4 and CYP3A5 have shown comparable V_{max} values (1.17 and 1.36 m^{-1}, respectively) but differed by a factor of 10 in K_m value (0.91 μM vs. 9.28 μM, respectively).[158] Furthermore, the clearance of docetaxel is potentially correlated with CYP3A activity, as measured by the CYP3A-specific drug midazolam,[159] the erythromycin breath test,[160] urinary excretion of cortisol,[161] or dexamethasone pharmacokinetic parameters.[162] Similar association analyses have been described for irinotecan,[163] gefitinib,[164] and vinorelbine.[165]

Even though CYP3A4 and CYP3A5 variants may not (completely) explain variation in CYP3A activity and altered pharmacokinetics of anticancer drug substrates, such as etoposide,[166] paclitaxel,[107] imatinib,[167] and irinotecan,[168] a consensus is building that human variation in CYP3A activity might also be caused by polymorphisms in transcription factors that regulate enzyme expression, such as the pregnane X receptor (PXR) and the constitutive androstane receptor (CAR).[169] Several variants in the human PXR gene, *NR1I2*, have been identified, with altered transactivation activity.[170,171] However, these variants are extremely rare in African-American and white populations (allelic frequency, 0% to 1.6%), and it is therefore unlikely that they account for a substantial degree of variation in CYP3A4 and CYP3A5 expression.

Uridine Diphosphate Glucuronosyltransferases

Uridine diphosphate glucuronosyltransferases (UGTs) represent one of the major classes of enzymes involved in phase II conjugative metabolism. These enzymes catalyze the transfer of a glucuronic acid moiety from uridine diphosphoglucuronic acid to various endogenous and xenobiotic substrates of diverse chemical structure. This results in the formation of glucuronide conjugates, which are more polar than the parent compounds, thus facilitating their excretion in the bile or urine. Knowledge of UGTs, including their molecular genetics, substrate specificity, and tissue distribution, has increased considerably in recent years.[172] The liver represents one of the major sites of glucuronidation; however, UGTs are also expressed in extrahepatic tissues, including those of the gastrointestinal tract, kidney, and brain. More than 16 UGTs have been characterized to date, classified into two families, UGT1 and UGT2, which are further divided based on sequence similarities into the subfamilies UGT1A, UGT2A, and UGT2B.

A number of polymorphisms have been described for *UGT1* and *UGT2B* gene families. However, only a few of potential clinical relevance have been described to date.[173] Most efforts have focused on genetic alterations of the *UGT1A1* gene; over 60 have been reported so far and many of these influence its expression and functional properties. UGT1A1 is the major isoform responsible for the glucuronidation of bilirubin in humans, and its genetic variation has been extensively investigated in relation to hyperbilirubinemic syndromes. These disorders, which include Crigler-Najjar syndrome types 1 and 2 and Gilbert's syndrome, are characterized by decreased or absent UGT1A1 activity as a result of *UGT1A1* promoter or coding region polymorphisms.[174-177] Of the known genetic variants, *UGT1A1*28*, which results from a dinucleotide (TA) insertion in the $(TA)_6TAA$ element of the *UGT1A1* promoter region, is the most common. This variant allele, with seven TA repeats, is associated with reduced gene expression and a decrease in function.[178,179] The frequency of these polymorphic alleles varies considerably in different ethnic groups, with the promoter variant being most prevalent among whites and African Americans, whereas missense mutations in the *UGT1A1* coding region are more common in Asians.[180]

With respect to anticancer therapy, the *UGT1A1* polymorphism is of greatest importance in the metabolism of irinotecan.[181] Irinotecan can also be converted by human carboxylesterase 2 (hCE2) to its active metabolite 7-ethyl-10-hydroxy-camptothecin (SN-38), which shows considerably greater (1000-fold) potency than the parent compound (Fig. 6-7).[182] SN-38 subsequently undergoes glucuronide conjugation by the polymorphic UGT1A1 and UGT1A9 isoforms to form the inactive metabolite SN-38 glucuronide (SN-38G),[183] which is eliminated mainly in the bile by the transporter protein ABCG2 (MRP2).[184,185] Although irinotecan has shown antitumor activity in various pediatric malignancies, it can cause also severe toxicities, including diarrhea and neutropenia, which are typically observed in 20% to 35% of those treated.

Several studies have confirmed the relationship between *UGT1A1*28* genotype and irinotecan pharmacokinetics and toxicity. These investigations have found that grade 4 neutropenia is more common in homozygous (50%) than heterozygous patients (12.5%) and that none of the patients with the reference alleles experienced toxicity. Furthermore, those patients with the 7/7 genotype had a higher risk of developing severe neutropenia[186] or diarrhea,[187] although the possibility of a dose reduction for irinotecan in patients with a *UGT1A1*28* polymorphism is not supported by the result of larger studies performed in white[188] or Asian populations.[189] The clinical implications of genetic variability in the *UGT1A1* gene for treatment with irinotecan in children are currently under investigation.

Drug Transporters

In addition to drug metabolism, pharmacokinetic processes are highly dependent on the interplay with drug transport in organs such as the intestine, kidney, and liver. Genetically determined variation in drug transporter function or expression is now increasingly recognized to have a significant role as a determinant of intersubject variability in response to commonly prescribed drugs.[190] The most extensively studied class of drug transporters are those encoded by the family of ATP-binding cassette (ABC) genes, which also play a role in the resistance of malignant cells to anticancer agents. Among the 48 known ABC gene products, ABCB1 (P-glycoprotein), ABCC1 (multidrug resistance–associated protein-1 [MRP1]) and its homologue ABCC2 (MRP2, cMOAT), and ABCG2 (breast cancer resistance protein [BCRP]) are known to influence the oral absorption and disposition of a wide variety of drugs.[191] As a result, the expression levels of these proteins in humans have important consequences for an individual's susceptibility to certain anticancer drug-induced side effects, interactions, and treatment efficacy. In recent years, various naturally occurring variants in these ABC transporter genes have been identified that might affect the function and/or expression of the corresponding proteins.[191-193]

Similar to the discoveries of functional genetic variations in drug efflux transporters of the ABC family, there have been considerable advances in the identification of SNPs in transporters that facilitate cellular drug uptake in tissues that play an important role in drug elimination, such as the liver and kidney (Fig. 6-8). Among these, members of the organic anion-transporting polypeptides (OATPs), organic anion transporters (OATs), and organic cation transporters (OCTs) can mediate the cellular uptake of a large number of structurally divergent compounds.[194,195] Accordingly, functionally relevant polymorphisms in these influx transporters may contribute to interindividual and interethnic variability in drug disposition and response.[196] In the context of cancer chemotherapy, however, clinically relevant associations between transporter polymorphisms and anticancer drugs have only been critically evaluated for *ABCB1* and *ABCG2*, which are involved in the absorption and elimination of numerous investigational and approved agents.

ABCB1

Formerly known as *MDR1* or *PGY1*, *ABCB1* was the first human ABC transporter gene cloned and characterized through its ability to confer a multidrug resistance phenotype to cancer cells that had developed resistance to certain chemotherapy drugs. The gene product ABCB1 (P-glycoprotein) has been shown to be a promiscuous transporter of a large number of hydrophobic substrates from diverse therapeutic classes, includ-

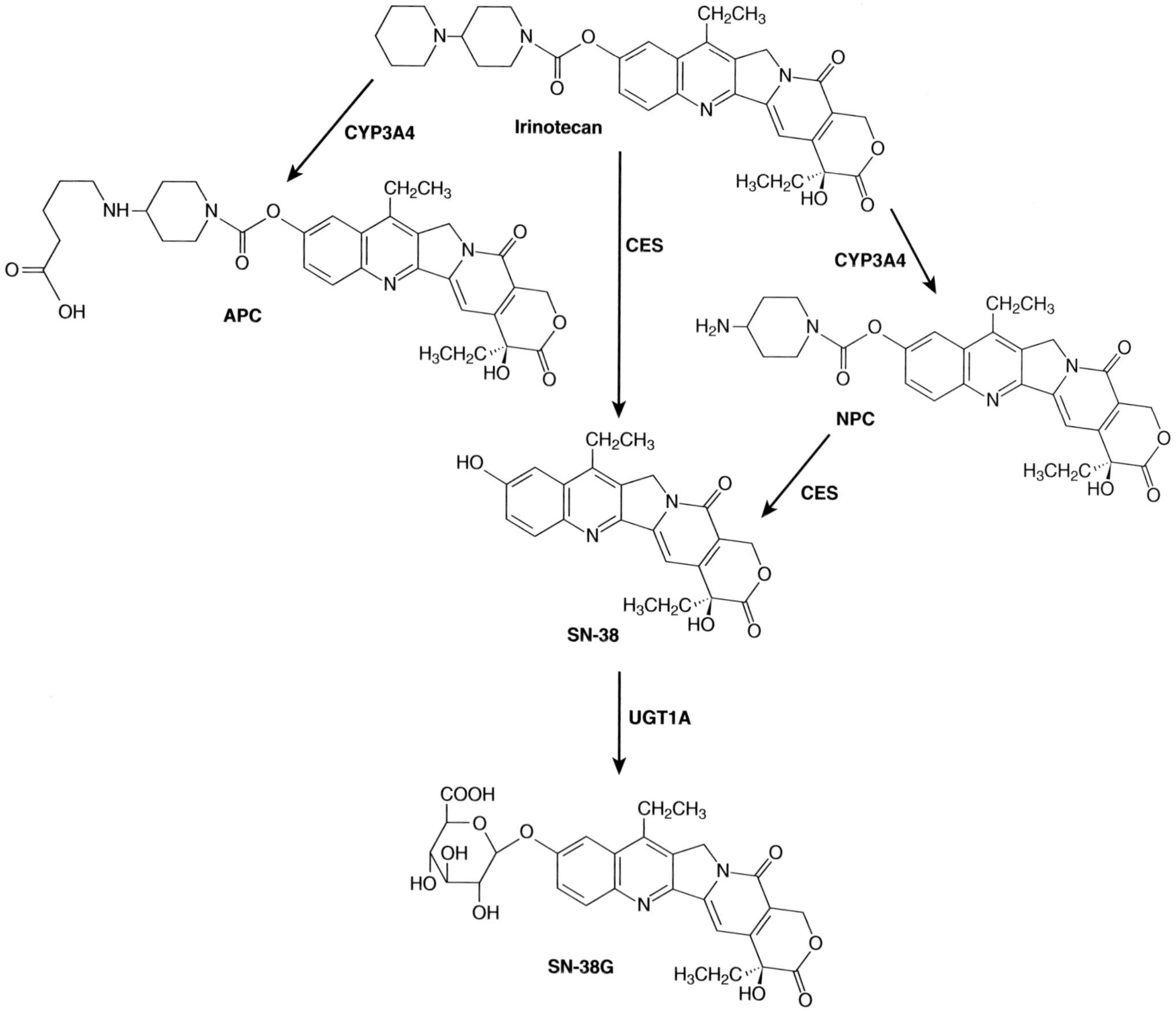

FIGURE 6-7. Simplified schematic of metabolic pathways of irinotecan. APC/NPC = oxidative metabolites; CES = carboxylesterase; CYP3A4 = cytochrome P-450 3A4; SN-38G = β-glucuronide metabolite of SN-38; UGT1A = UDP glucuronosyltransferase 1A isoform.

ing a multitude of anticancer drugs that include anthracyclines, taxanes, and *Vinca* alkaloids.[191]

A systematic screen of the *ABCB1* gene for the presence of SNPs was first performed by Hoffmeyer and colleagues.[197] In this study, sequencing the *ABCB1* genes from 188 white volunteers revealed 15 polymorphisms (in 8 exons and 7 introns). A detailed analysis of the potential functional consequences of different *ABCB1* variants has not yet been evaluated, except for some of the most common synonymous and nonsynonymous coding SNPs (e.g., Asn21Asp, Phe103Leu, Ser400Asn, Ala893Ser/Thr, and Ala998Thr).[198,199] Transport studies of several tested substrates have indicated that the substrate specificity of the protein is not substantially affected by any of these SNPs, whereas cell surface expression and function of even double mutants show no difference from the wild-type protein. This suggests that these SNPs result in mutant proteins, with a distribution and function similar to those of the wild-type protein.

The most extensively studied *ABCB1* variant to date is a common synonymous mutation at the transition C to T at

position 3435 (*3435C > T*) at a wobble position in exon 26. Although this transition does not change its encoded Ile amino acid (i.e., a silent mutation), it has been associated with altered protein expression in duodenum biopsies, as well as with altered oral absorption of certain ABCB1 substrate drugs given orally, such as digoxin.[62] Nonetheless, the association of the *3435C > T* polymorphism with ABCB1 protein expression and function remains controversial in vivo, even though it has associated with mRNA stability[200] and altered substrate specificity in vitro.[201]

As far as anticancer drugs are concerned, studies investigating the clinical consequences of the *ABCB1* polymorphisms in terms of their ability to modulate the pharmacokinetic profile of substrates in adults are still scarce, and have been essentially negative.[62] Interestingly, a weak but statistically significant association between irinotecan pharmacokinetics and the *ABCB1* *1236C > T* polymorphism has been described,[168] which was later independently confirmed.[163,202] Similarly, the *ABCB1* *1236C > T* genotype was associated with the systemic exposure to the farnesyltransferase inhibitor tipifarnib (R115777,

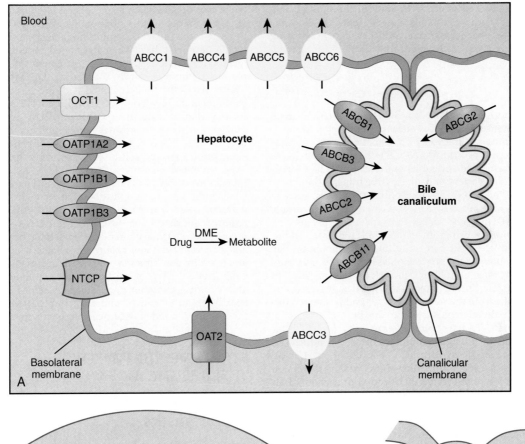

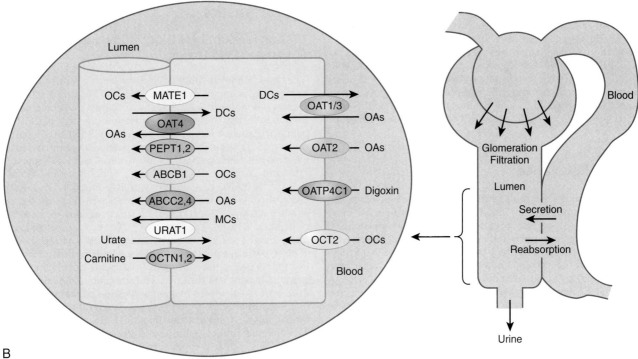

FIGURE 6-8. Common mechanisms involved in anticancer drug elimination through the liver (A) and kidney (B). ABC = ATP-binding cassette transporter; DCs = dicarboxylates; DME = drug-metabolizing enzyme(s); MATE = mutidrug and toxic extrusion transporter; MCs = monocarboxylates; NTCP = (Na⁺)-taurocholate cotransporting polypeptide; OAs = organic anions; OAT = organic anion transporter; OATP = organic anion-transporting polypeptide; OCs = organic cations; OCT = organic cation transporter; OCTN = novel organic cation transporter; PEPT = peptide transporter; URAT = urate transporter.

Zarnestra) administered orally.[203] In spite of the limited data currently available, these findings suggest that ABCB1 may play a role in the pharmacokinetic profile of anticancer drug substrates that are given orally and/or undergo substantial renal excretion.

ABCG2

The *ABCG2* (formerly known as *BCRP/MXR/ABCP*) gene encodes a half-transporter with a nucleotide-binding fold transmembrane orientation. Analyses of cell lines resistant to mitoxantrone that do not overexpress ABCB1 or related proteins of the ABCC subfamily led several laboratories in the late 1990s to identify *ABCG2* as a gene encoding a drug transporter almost simultaneously.[204] ABCG2 can transport several dyes, such as rhodamine 123 and Hoechst 33462, as well as a structurally diverse group of anticancer drugs that include mitoxantrone, methotrexate, 9-aminocamptothecin, SN-38, topotecan, diflomotecan (BN80915), gefitinib, erlotinib, and imatinib. The gene is highly expressed in the trophoblast cells of the placenta and, in the intestine and liver,[205] restricts the exposure to ingested carcinogens and potentially toxic anticancer drugs by decreasing uptake from the gut lumen,[206,207] and is able to concentrate drugs and carcinogenic xenotoxins into milk.[208]

To date, *ABCG2* has been systematically screened for genetic variations in different ethnic groups,[209-211] and several genetic variants have been identified. The common *ABCG2 421C > A* allele in exon 5, in which the C to A transversion results in an amino acid change of Lys to Glu at codon 141, has been associated with low ABCG2 expression levels[212,213] as well as altered sensitivity to and transport of several anticancer drugs in vitro as compared with the wild-type protein.[214,215] This allele is carried by 46% of normal Japanese,[212] by 10% to 12% in European whites, but at only very low frequencies or not at all in African Americans and Africans.[209,211]

The *ABCG2 421C > A* polymorphism has also been linked recently with altered exposure or toxicity in vivo to various anticancer drugs, including the campothecin analogues diflomotecan,[216] topotecan,[213] and irinotecan,[217] as well as the epithelial growth factor receptor (EGFR) tyrosine kinase inhibitor gefitinib.[218]

Clinical Relevance

The TPMT and DPD polymorphisms perhaps best illustrate the issues involved in how this information can be used in a clinical setting—for example, in defining the relative advantages and disadvantages of phenotyping and genotyping. At present, a clinically convenient method of phenotyping for the TPMT polymorphism is available and, although the DNA sequences of several variant alleles are known, many are yet to be discovered. Hence, many patients will be misdiagnosed with molecular techniques that focus only on known DNA sequence variants. The metabolism, dose requirements, and tolerance of 6-mercaptopurine among 180 pediatric patients with different TPMT phenotypes have been studied.[80] It was shown that erythrocyte concentrations of thioguanine nucleotides were inversely related to TPMT enzyme activity in TPMT homozygous wild-type, heterozygous, and homozygous-deficient patients. Thus, lowering doses of 6-mercaptopurine in TPMT heterozygotes and in deficient patients allows the administration of full protocol doses of other chemotherapeutic agents while maintaining high thioguanine nucleotide concentrations.

Once it became clear that a genetically mediated deficiency of DPD was responsible for some cases of 5-FU toxicity, attempts were made to confirm the diagnosis on easily accessible tissues or cells, such as peripheral blood mononuclear cells. However, frequency distribution histograms of DPD activity in these cells did not show a multimodal distribution. Thus, genotyping strategies have been developed based on DNA-based techniques combined with measurement of urinary and/or plasma pyrimidine levels to identify DPD heterozygotes.[219] These diagnostic tools, coupled with increased understanding of the genetic regulation of TPMT and DPD, will enable us to individualize anticancer treatment. It is expected that, for example, in case of irinotecan chemotherapeutic treatment, dose adjustments based on genotyping for genes involved in its elimination pathway will be possible in the near future. Similarly, as noted, various techniques have been developed as specific measures of CYP3A4 activity.[220] These techniques are most commonly based on probes that recognize that each metabolic pathway can vary independently. Further studies are required to determine whether these tests can adequately predict the pharmacokinetics of substrate drugs in question, and also whether these probes have value when the substrates are used in combination chemotherapy regimens. Presently, many studies are ongoing to evaluate the interindividual variability in drug-metabolizing enzyme systems in relation to toxicity[221,222] and efficacy[223] and their implications for improving the therapeutic index of anticancer agents in children.

STRATEGIES TO IMPROVE THERAPEUTIC INDEX

Dose Adjustment Based on Patient Characteristics

Conventional Method: Body Surface Area–Based Dosing

The traditional method of individualizing anticancer drug dosage is by using body surface area.[224] There are a number of considerations as to why BSA has become the single variable for determining the dose of anticancer agents, especially in pediatric patients. First, it has been established that a correlation exists between BSA and some particular characteristics of each patient, such as GFR, blood volume, and basal metabolic rate, and certainly this provides a condition to individualize doses.[225] A similar relationship with liver function has not been established, which is particularly noteworthy, because the metabolic pathways of most drugs are strictly related to the activity of hepatic enzymes (see Table 6-1). However, these basic principles have been somewhat questioned by a study in which a poor correlation between BSA and GFR was reported.[226] Second, as noted, the starting dose of agents calculated in phase I studies is based on data derived from animal models in which drug dose is calculated relative to weight (mg/kg) or BSA (mg/m^2). In animals, doses are usually tested until the LD$_{10}$, and in human phase I studies the first dose used is 10% of LD$_{10}$. Third, some studies published in the 1950s have suggested a role of BSA in drug dose calculation, when attempts were made to define a more accurate method for the administration of cytotoxic drugs to children. In 1958, Pinkel[227] reported the results of a retrospective analysis applying a BSA-based formula for adults and children and Meeh's formula for animals to determine the conventional pediatric and adult doses of five cytotoxic drugs (mercaptopurine, methotrexate, mechlorethamine, triethylene thiophosphoramide, and actinomycin). The doses per unit surface area were calculated and similar values were found for all agents tested in children and adults, except for mercaptopurine, and normalizing the doses of cytotoxic agents using BSA was recommended.

TABLE 6-5	Patient Characteristics Affecting Anticancer Drug Pharmacokinetics In Children
Parameter	**Anticancer Drug**
Renal function	Bleomycin, carboplatin, cisplatin, cyclophosphamide, etoposide, methotrexate, topotecan
Hepatic function	Doxorubicin, epirubicin, vinblastine, vincristine
Serum albumin	Etoposide
Third spaces	Methotrexate
Obesity	Cyclophosphamide, doxorubicin, 6-mercaptopurine, methotrexate
Cancer cachexia	5-Fluorouracil, methotrexate

BSA is commonly estimated using a formula that was derived primarily for its use of basal metabolism determination by the use of weight and height alone, and more recently, it has been confirmed that the original formula was surprisingly accurate considering the small sample size used in its derivation.[224] The usefulness of normalizing anticancer drug dose to BSA in adults has been questioned recently, since it clearly has been shown that for most drugs, there is no relationship between BSA and anticancer drug clearance in adults.[228] It should be pointed out that BSA is probably a much more important consideration in drug dose calculation for pediatric patients as compared to adults, because of the larger size range in the former population.[229]

Pathophysiologic Status

As discussed, most pharmacologic studies of anticancer agents have shown important interindividual as well as intraindividual variability in pharmacokinetic behavior. In some cases, this is due to changing pathophysiologic status of cancer patients due to the disease itself or to dysfunction of specific organs involved in drug elimination (Table 6-5). For example, if urinary excretion is an important elimination route for a given drug, any decrement in renal function could lead to decreased drug clearance and may result in drug accumulation and toxicity. It would therefore be logical to decrease the drug dose relative to the degree of impaired renal function, to maintain plasma concentrations within a target therapeutic window, which is well documented for bleomycin, cisplatin, cyclophosphamide, etoposide, methotrexate and topotecan.[230] Still the best known example of this a priori dose adjustment of an anticancer agent is carboplatin, which is excreted renally almost entirely by glomerular filtration. Various strategies have been developed to estimate carboplatin doses based on renal function among patients, either using creatinine clearance[231] or glomerular filtration rates as measured by a radioisotope method.[232] Application of these procedures has led to a substantial reduction in pharmacokinetic variability, such that carboplatin is currently one of the few drugs routinely administered to achieve a target exposure rather than on a mg/m² or mg/kg basis.

In contrast to the predictable decline in renal clearance of drugs when glomerular filtration is impaired, it is not as easy to make a general prediction on the effect of impaired liver function on drug clearance. The major problem is that hepatic enzymes are typically not good indicators of metabolizing activity and alternative hepatic function tests, such as indocyanine green and antipyrine, have limited value in predicting anticancer drug pharmacokinetics (and metabolism). An alternative

dynamic measure of liver function has been proposed which is based on totaled values (scored to the WHO grading system) of serum bilirubin, alkaline phosphatase, and either alanine aminotransferase or aspartate aminotransferase to give a hepatic dysfunction score.[233] Based on carefully conducted pharmacokinetic studies in patients with normal and impaired hepatic function, guidelines have been proposed for dose adjustments of several agents when administered to patients with liver dysfunction, including anthracyclines (doxorubicin and epirubicin), etoposide, docetaxel, and some *Vinca* alkaloids (vinblastine and vincristine).[1]

The binding of drugs to plasma proteins, particularly those that are highly bound, may also have significant clinical implications for therapeutic outcome.[234] Although protein binding is a major determinant of drug action, it is clearly only one of a myriad of factors that influence drug disposition. The extent of protein binding is a function of drug and protein concentrations, the affinity constants for the drug-protein interaction and the number of protein-binding sites per class of binding site. Because only the unbound (or free) drug in plasma water is available for diffusion from the vascular compartment to the tumor interstitium, the therapeutic response will correlate with free drug concentration rather than total drug concentration. Several clinical situations, including liver and renal disease, can significantly decrease the extent of plasma binding and may lead to higher free drug concentrations and possible risk of unexpected toxicity, although the total (free plus bound forms) plasma drug concentrations are unaltered.[235] It is important to realize, however, that after therapeutic doses of most anticancer drugs, plasma binding is drug concentration-independent, suggesting that the total plasma concentration is reflective of the unbound concentration. Thus, other physiologic changes, for instance decreased renal and hepatic function, generally produce more clinically significant alterations in drug disposition than that seen with alterations in plasma protein binding. For some anticancer agents, including etoposide[236,237] and paclitaxel,[238] it has been shown that protein binding is highly dependent on dose- and schedule-varying plasma concentrations. Indeed, by taking into consideration protein binding of etoposide it has been reported that prospective pharmacokinetic monitoring allows an increase in dose intensity without a parallel increase in toxicity.[239] It should also be pointed out that very few studies have been performed to evaluate the pharmacokinetics of anticancer drugs in neonates. In most cases, aging could not be considered as an independent feature of drug disposition, since it is characterized by a conjunction of physiologic alterations that may occur simultaneously. It appears, therefore, that dose adaptation as a function of individual physiology is better than adaptation as a function of age.

Adjusting the dosage a posteriori based on a patient's tolerance is also a widely used approach, even though it might result in dose reductions, which can compromise dose intensity and lead to treatment failure. Clearly, the seriousness of the first side effect is the major determinant of whether it can or cannot be used as an end point. Examples of this type of dose adjustments are the platelet nadir-directed dosage approach to individualizing carboplatin dosage,[240] or leukopenia-targeted dosing of methotrexate and mercaptopurine in patients with childhood ALL.[241]

Dose Adaptation Using Pharmacokinetic-Pharmacodynamic Principles

Therapeutic Drug Monitoring

Prolonged infusion schedules of anticancer drugs offer a very convenient setting for dose adaptation in individual patients.

At the time required to achieve steady-state concentration, it is then possible to modify the infusion rate for the remainder of the treatment course if a relationship is known between this steady-state concentration and a desired pharmacodynamic end point. This method has been successfully used to adapt the dose during continuous infusions of 5-FU and etoposide, and for repeated oral administration of etoposide or repeated IV administration of cisplatin.[1] Methotrexate plasma concentrations are monitored routinely to identify patients at high risk of toxicity and to adjust leucovorin rescue in patients with delayed drug excretion. This monitoring has significantly reduced the incidence of serious toxicity (including toxic death) and in fact, improved outcome by eliminating unacceptably low systemic exposure levels.[242] Therapeutic drug monitoring has also been applied to or is currently under investigation for 5-FU, etoposide, melphalan, busulfan, cisplatin, and topotecan.[243,244]

Feedback Controlled-Dosing

It remains to be seen how information on variability can be used eventually to devise an optimal dosage regimen of a drug for the treatment of a given disease in an individual patient. Obviously, the desired objective would be most efficiently achieved if the individual's dosage requirements could be calculated prior to administering the drug. While this ideal can not be met completely in clinical practice, with the notable exception of carboplatin, as described above, some success may be achieved by adopting feedback-controlled dosing. In the adaptive dosage with feedback control, population-based predictive models are used initially, but allow the possibility of dosage alteration based on feedback revision. In this approach, patients are first treated with standard dose and then during treatment pharmacokinetic information is estimated by a limited-sampling strategy and compared with that predicted from the population model with which dosage was initiated. On the basis of the comparison, more patient-specific pharmacokinetic parameters are calculated, and dosage is adjusted accordingly to maintain the target exposure measure producing the desired pharmacodynamic effect. It has been proposed that, despite its mathematical complexity, this approach may be the only way to deliver the desired precise exposure of an anticancer agent. However, the use of population pharmacokinetic models is increasingly studied, in an attempt to accommodate as much of the pharmacokinetic variability as possible in terms of measurable characteristics. This type of analysis has been conducted for a number of clinically important anticancer drugs, including carboplatin,[245] docetaxel,[246] and topotecan,[247] and provided mathematical equations based on BSA, gender, and protein levels, for example, to predict drug clearance with an acceptable degree of precision.

Circadian Rhythm-Based Dosing

It has been suggested that administration at certain times of the day can improve the therapeutic index of several anticancer drugs.[248,249] For example, a significant improvement in survival has been demonstrated for children with leukemia who received 6-mercaptopurine in the evening compared with those who received the drug in the morning.[250] Such findings led to the assumption of a coupling between tolerability rhythms and the rest-activity cycle in cancer patients. Indeed, an improved tolerability of chronotherapy schedules based upon this concept was shown in several clinical trials for other anticancer drugs including busulfan, carboplatin, docetaxel, 5-FU, and oxaliplatin.[251-253] Furthermore, the chronotherapy principle was validated in 2 randomized multicenter phase III trials involving a total of 278 patients receiving a 5-FU containing regimen. A 5-fold reduction in the incidence of severe mucositis, a 2-fold decrease in peripheral neuropathy, and a near doubling of objective response rate resulted from delivering 5-FU and oxaliplatin at experimentally determined circadian times, i.e., at 4:00 AM and at 4:00 PM, respectively, compared with constant rate infusion.[254,255] The precise mechanisms by which these agents are more effective at certain times of the day is still unknown, but pharmacokinetic as well as pharmacodynamic explanations have been proposed (including a circadian-dependency of hematopoiesis). Whether the potential benefits will justify the major inconvenience related to drug administration in the middle of the night is yet unclear.

Intentional Biomodulation

Pharmacodynamic Alterations

The use of specific agents co-administered with anticancer drugs to increase the therapeutic index of chemotherapeutic treatment has made a substantial impact on certain diseases. One of the most widely used biomodulating agents is leucovorin, a reduced folate that is used in combination with both methotrexate and 5-FU. This agent has been shown to decrease methotrexate-induced toxicity to various normal tissues and enhance 5-FU-mediated cytotoxicity to tumor cells by inhibition of thymidylate synthase, thereby allowing escalation of the anticancer drug dose without affecting its disposition profile.[256] Other examples of agents interfering with anticancer drug pharmacodynamics include: (1) the use of amifostine to reduce cisplatin-associated myelosuppression, nephrotoxicity, and neurotoxicity[257]; (2) dexrazoxane to decrease anthracycline-induced cardiotoxicity[258,259]; and (3) coadministration of cefixime to ameliorate irinotecan-induced diarrhea.[260]

The concept of pharmacodynamic biomodulation has also been extensively studied with ABCB1-blocking agents, in an attempt to improve the therapeutic index of anticancer agents.[261] As mentioned previously, this multidrug-resistant protein is a drug-efflux transporter encoded by the *ABCB1* gene, and is abundantly present in various types of human cancer. Studies performed over the last several years have shown that intrinsic and acquired expression of ABCB1 might play a role in clinical drug resistance in specific hematologic malignancies. Consequently, clinical trials have been performed worldwide, in which ABCB1 blockers such as verapamil and cyclosporin A have been given to patients along with anticancer drugs, with the intent of attenuating carrier-mediated tumor cell drug resistance in patients. Unfortunately, in these trials decreased systemic clearance of the anticancer drugs became a serious problem and necessitated substantial dose reductions, thereby losing all the potential benefits in terms of antitumor activity as compared to normal dosages given without the addition of these blockers.[261] In most cases, the pharmacokinetic interference appears to be the result of competition for enzymes (mainly CYP3A4) involved in drug metabolism.[262] A new generation of P-glycoprotein blockers is now available for efficacy testing in clinical trials for reversal of multidrug resistance, and these modulators have been demonstrated not to interfere with anticancer drug pharmacokinetics. Theoretically, the use of these agents will allow assessment of the contribution of ABCB1 to the toxicity and antitumor activity of chemotherapeutic regimens for multidrug resistance reversal, although improved therapeutic specificity and efficacy have yet to be demonstrated in any disease.[263]

Pharmacokinetic Alterations

One of the best-studied examples of pharmacokinetic biomodulation is the co-administration of eniluracil, an inactivator of

DPD, with 5-FU.[264] As indicated, DPD is the initial rate-limiting enzyme in the catabolism of 5-FU. The high variation in the population in DPD activity accounts for much of the variability observed with the therapeutic use of 5-FU, including variable drug levels, variable bioavailability, and inconsistent toxicity and activity profiles. Eniluracil has been shown to improve the efficacy of 5-FU in preclinical models through the selective, irreversible inhibition of DPD-mediated metabolism.[265] In a subsequent clinical study, eniluracil prolonged the half-life of intravenously administered 5-FU and reduced its clearance.[266] Eniluracil also enabled the oral administration of 5-FU by inhibiting the intestinal DPD activity,[267] thereby increasing the oral availability and diminishing the variability in absorption.[268,269]

Intestinal metabolic systems and drug efflux pumps located in the intestinal mucosa represent another limitation in the bioavailability of oral drugs.[270] Several enzymes located in the enterocyte, such as CYP3A4, are involved in the presystemic metabolism of many cytotoxic agents, including cyclophosphamide, etoposide, paclitaxel, irinotecan, and vinorelbine, thereby limiting the oral absorption of these drugs.[271] The bioavailability of these drugs might be substantially enhanced by pharmacologic modulation of enteric CYP3A4 activity. Several investigators confirmed recently, that by co-administration of specific inhibitors such as erythromycin, quinidine, ketoconazole, and cyclosporin A to inhibit CYP3A4 activity, the oral bioavailability of various anticancer agents such as etoposide could be improved, while also diminishing the variability in absorption.[272] Similarly, ABCB1, which is also abundantly present in the gastrointestinal tract, has been shown to limit the intestinal absorption of numerous (anticancer) agents, including paclitaxel, etoposide, and vinblastine.[273] Combined inhibition of intestinal ABCB1 and CYP3A4 by cyclosporin A was shown to substantially increase the systemic exposure to oral paclitaxel in cancer patients,[274] suggesting that modulation of these transports simultaneously could be considered for anticancer agents given by the oral route that have poor bioavailability.

Even though intentional biomodulation can be beneficial in pediatric cancer patients, prospective pharmacokinetic and pharmacodynamic studies will need to be conducted to determine at which level (i.e., kinetics or dynamics) the interaction takes place and whether biomodulation ultimately improves the therapeutic index of anticancer agents.

Drug Scheduling and Administration Sequencing

The antitumor activity of certain chemotherapeutic agents is highly schedule-dependent. For these drugs, the dose fractionated over several days can produce a different antitumor response or toxicity profile compared with the same dose given over a shorter period. In the first definitive demonstration of etoposide schedule-dependency in oncology, investigators documented markedly increased efficacy in patients with small-cell lung cancer when an identical total dose of etoposide was administered by a 5-day divided-dose schedule rather than a 24-hour infusion.[275] Pharmacokinetic analysis in that study showed that both schedules produced very similar overall drug exposure (as measured by AUC), but that the divided-dose schedule produced twice the duration of exposure to an etoposide plasma concentration of >1 µg/ml. This observation was consistent with preclinical data, and the authors speculated that exposure to this threshold concentration was important in achieving clinical efficacy, while exposure to higher plasma concentrations augmented drug-induced toxicity. Subsequently, this finding has led to the use of prolonged oral administration of etoposide to treat patients with cancer.[276] Similar

schedule-dependency has also been demonstrated for a number of other anticancer agents, notably paclitaxel[277] and topotecan.[278] For both these agents, the variability in clinically tested treatment schedules is enormous, ranging from short IV infusions of less than 30 min to 21-day or even 7-week continuous infusion administrations, with large differences in toxicity profiles. In most cases, the mechanisms underlying the schedule dependencies are not completely understood, and further investigation will be essential to define the underlying basis as well as the optimal durations of drug administration. An opposite effect has been observed with the administration of purine and pyrimidine analogues, where toxicity is accentuated by prolonged infusions as compared to shorter infusions.

The combination of anticancer drugs can also exhibit schedule-dependent toxicity or antitumor activity either through pharmacokinetic or pharmacodynamic modulation. An example of a metabolic interaction is shown by the experimental demonstration that the sequence of 5-FU and methotrexate seems crucial to the cytotoxicity of this combination. In vitro, if methotrexate precedes 5-FU by at least one hour, synergistic results are obtained.[279] This may be due to an increased activation of 5-FU to its nucleotide form. The opposite sequence of drug administration leads to antagonism due to block of the thymidylate synthase pathway induced by 5-FU. Through this block the intracellular folates are preserved in their active tetrahydrofolate form which diminishes the effect of the methotrexate block of dihydrofolate reductase.

Interactions have also been described for other classes of drugs that cannot be explained by alterations in pharmacokinetics (Table 6-6). An example of this is the combination of cisplatin and topoisomerase I inhibitors. DNA topoisomerase I is a nuclear enzyme involved in cellular replication and transcription. By forming a covalent adduct between topoisomerase I and DNA, called the cleavable complex, topoisomerase I inhibitors interfere with the process of DNA breakage and resealing during DNA synthesis. The stabilized cleavable complex blocks the progress of the replication fork, resulting in

TABLE 6-6	Sequence-Dependent Drug-Drug Interactions between Anticancer Agents
Drugs	**Effect(s)**
Docetaxel-ifosfamide	CL_I increased in D → I sequence
Docetaxel-methotrexate	M → D sequence more myelotoxic; PK unchanged
Gemcitabine-pemetrexed	P → G sequence more myelotoxic; PK unchanged
Irinotecan-cisplatin	C → I sequence more myelotoxic; PK unchanged
Paclitaxel-cisplatin	C → P sequence more myelotoxic; CL_P reduced
Paclitaxel-cyclophosphamide	P → C sequence more myelotoxic; PK unchanged
Paclitaxel-anthracyclines	P → A sequence more myelotoxic; CL_A reduced
Paclitaxel-etoposide	CL_E reduced in P → E sequence
Topotecan (IV)-cisplatin	C → T sequence more myelotoxic; CL_T reduced
Topotecan (PO)-cisplatin	C → T sequence more myelotoxic; PK unchanged

CL, total plasma clearance; PK, pharmacokinetics.

TABLE 6-7	Strategies to Improve Therapeutic Index of Anticancer Drugs in Children
Dose Adjustment Type	**Example**
BASED ON PATIENT CHARACTERISTICS	
Body surface area	All drugs
Pathophysiologic status (renal function)	Carboplatin
BASED ON PHARMACOKINETIC-DYNAMIC PRINCIPLES	
Therapeutic drug monitoring	Methotrexate
Feedback-controlled dosing	Carboplatin
Circadian rhythm–based dosing	6-Mercaptopurine
Biomodulation	
Pharmacokinetic modulation	5-Fluorouracil–leucovorin
Pharmacodynamic modulation	Docetaxel-R101933
Drug scheduling	Etoposide
Drug administration sequence	Methotrexate–5-fluorouracil 5-Fluorouracil–DPD
BASED ON PHARMACOGENETIC PRINCIPLES	

DPD, dihydropyridine dehydrogenase.

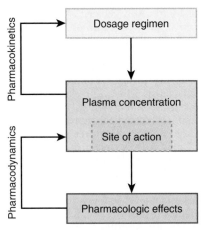

FIGURE 6-9. Schematic representation of an alternative approach to the design of a dosage regimen. The pharmacokinetics and pharmacodynamics of the drug are determined first. Then, either the plasma drug concentration-time data or the effects produced, via pharmacokinetics, are used as feedback (solid lines) to modify the dosage regimen to achieve optimal therapy.

irreversible DNA double-strand breaks leading to cell death.[280] Based on their mechanism of action, synergy was suspected for the combination of topoisomerase I inhibitors and DNA damaging agents such as cisplatin. Preclinical studies confirmed this hypothesis. However, the observed interaction seemed to depend on the cell line studied and the individual schedule of administration of camptothecin-type topoisomerase I inhibitors combined with cisplatin.[281] As mentioned previously, phase I and II dose-escalation trials evaluating combination chemotherapy typically uncover relevant pharmacokinetic and pharmacodynamic interactions and define drug doses and sequence of administrations that can be safely administered.

CONCLUSION AND PERSPECTIVES

Substantial progress in the optimization of cancer chemotherapy has been made in recent years with the use of pharmacokinetics, pharmacodynamics, and pharmacogenetics, although some aspects of anticancer drug pharmacology will require more work before they become more useful clinically. The incorporation of pharmacologic principles in drug development and clinical trials is essential to maximize the clinical potential of new anticancer agents. For example, improvements in outcome have been observed using these principles to individualize anticancer drug administration for methotrexate and carboplatin (Table 6-7). Careful attention to pharmacokinetics and pharmacodynamics will also be essential for the rational development of new agents designed to specifically target the products of oncogenes, tumor suppressor genes and related signal transduction pathways, including apoptosis, as well as for the optimal use of agents designed for chemoprevention or to inhibit invasion, angiogenesis and metastasis (Fig. 6-9).[282,283] Specifically targeted agents may require an especially careful and imaginative choice of dosage regimens to maintain active but nontoxic dose (and concentration) levels. Pharmacogenomic studies now include the application of gene expression microarrays as prognostic tests,[284,285] and the inherited nature of differences in drug disposition and pharmacodynamic effects

is now being elucidated, which will provide a stronger scientific basis for optimizing drug therapy on the basis of each patient's genetic constitution.[30,286] Furthermore, the development of various technologies like genomics, high-throughput screening, and combinatorial chemistry is likely to result in an exponential increase in the number of targets and candidate compounds to explore, and it is expected that a deeper understanding of each compound's pharmacologic properties in the exploratory stage of drug development will be mandatory.[287] In addition, the use of computer simulation to guide clinical trials has evolved over the past two decades to yield pharmacologically sound, realistic outcomes, which will definitively impact on pharmacologically guided trial design in the future.[288,289] Over the next several years, anticancer chemotherapy should become much more targeted to exploit the genetic abnormalities found in individual tumors, while toxicity is reduced through judicious analysis of constitutional features that control the metabolism and excretion of these new drugs.

REFERENCES

1. Canal P, Chatelut E, Guichard S. Practical treatment guide for dose individualisation in cancer chemotherapy. Drugs. 1998;56: 1019-1038.
2. Masson E, Zamboni WC. Pharmacokinetic optimisation of cancer chemotherapy. Effect on outcomes. Clin Pharmacokinet. 1997;32: 324-343.
3. Hryniuk WM, Figueredo A, Goodyear M. Applications of dose intensity to problems in chemotherapy of breast and colorectal cancer. Semin Oncol. 1987;14:3-11.
4. Hryniuk WM. More is better. J Clin Oncol. 1988;6:1365-1367.
5. Tannock IF, Boyd NF, DeBoer G, et al. A randomized trial of two dose levels of cyclophosphamide, methotrexate, and fluorouracil chemotherapy for patients with metastatic breast cancer. J Clin Oncol. 1988;6:1377-1387.
6. McLeod HL, Relling MV, Crom WR, et al. Disposition of antineoplastic agents in the very young child. Br J Cancer Suppl. 1992;18:S23-S29.
7. Rodman JH, Relling MV, Stewart CF, et al. Clinical pharmacokinetics and pharmacodynamics of anticancer drugs in children. Semin Oncol. 1993;20:18-29.

8. Strolin BM, Whomsley R, Baltes EL. Differences in absorption, distribution, metabolism and excretion of xenobiotics between the paediatric and adult populations. Expert Opin Drug Metab Toxicol. 2005;1:447-471.

9. Strolin BM, Baltes EL. Drug metabolism and disposition in children. Fundam Clin Pharmacol. 2003;17:281-299.

10. Tetelbaum M, Finkelstein Y, Nava-Ocampo AA, Koren G. Back to basics: understanding drugs in children: pharmacokinetic maturation. Pediatr Rev. 2005;26:321-328.

11. Pinkerton CR, Welshman SG, Glasgow JF, Bridges JM. Can food influence the absorption of methotrexate in children with acute lymphoblastic leukaemia? Lancet. 1980;2:944-946.

12. Friis-Hansen B. Body composition during growth. In vivo measurements and biochemical data correlated to differential anatomical growth. Pediatrics. 1971;47(1Suppl 2):264.

13. Morselli PL, Franco-Morselli R, Bossi L. Clinical pharmacokinetics in newborns and infants. Age-related differences and therapeutic implications. Clin Pharmacokinet. 1980;5:485-527.

14. Widdowson EM. Changes in the composition of the body at birth and their bearing on function and food requirements. Maandschr Kindergeneeskd. 1964;32:211-223.

15. Ehrnebo M, Agurell S, Jalling B, Boreus LO. Age differences in drug binding by plasma proteins: studies on human foetuses, neonates and adults. Eur J Clin Pharmacol. 1971;3:189-193.

16. Assael BM. Pharmacokinetics and drug distribution during postnatal development. Pharmacol Ther. 1982;18:159-197.

17. Cornford EM, Pardridge WM, Braun LD, Oldendorf WH. Increased blood-brain barrier transport of protein-bound anticonvulsant drugs in the newborn. J Cereb Blood Flow Metab. 1983;3:280-286.

18. Milsap RL, Jusko WJ. Pharmacokinetics in the infant. Environ Health Perspect. 1994;102(Suppl 11):107-110.

19. Rodman JH, Maneval DC, Magill HL, Sunderland M. Measurement of Tc-99m DTPA serum clearance for estimating glomerular filtration rate in children with cancer. Pharmacotherapy. 1993;13:10-16.

20. Schwartz GJ, Haycock GB, Edelmann CM Jr, Spitzer A. A simple estimate of glomerular filtration rate in children derived from body length and plasma creatinine. Pediatrics. 1976;58:259-263.

21. Schwartz GJ, Feld LG, Langford DJ. A simple estimate of glomerular filtration rate in full-term infants during the first year of life. J Pediatr. 1984;104:849-854.

22. Gretz N, Schock D, Sadick M, Pill J. Bias and precision of estimated glomerular filtration rate in children. Pediatr Nephrol. 2007;22:167-169.

23. Besunder JB, Reed MD, Blumer JL. Principles of drug biodisposition in the neonate. A critical evaluation of the pharmacokinetic-pharmacodynamic interface (Part II). Clin Pharmacokinet. 1988;14:261-286.

24. Besunder JB, Reed MD, Blumer JL. Principles of drug biodisposition in the neonate. A critical evaluation of the pharmacokinetic-pharmacodynamic interface (Part I). Clin Pharmacokinet. 1988;14:189-216.

25. Boreus LO. The role of therapeutic drug monitoring in children. Clin Pharmacokinet. 1989;17(Suppl 1):4-12.

26. Coughtrie MW, Burchell B, Leakey JE, Hume R. The inadequacy of perinatal glucuronidation: immunoblot analysis of the developmental expression of individual UDP-glucuronosyltransferase isoenzymes in rat and human liver microsomes. Mol Pharmacol. 1988;34:729-735.

27. Ecobichon DJ, Stephens DS. Perinatal development of human blood esterases. Clin Pharmacol Ther. 1973;14:41-47.

28. Crom WR, Relling MV, Christensen ML, et al. Age-related differences in hepatic drug clearance in children: studies with lorazepam and antipyrine. Clin Pharmacol Ther. 1991;50:132-140.

29. Relling MV, Crom WR, Pieper JA, et al. Hepatic drug clearance in children with leukemia: changes in clearance of model substrates during remission-induction therapy. Clin Pharmacol Ther. 1987;41:651-660.

30. Evans WE, Rodman JH, Relling MV, et al. Differences in teniposide disposition and pharmacodynamics in patients with newly diagnosed and relapsed acute lymphocytic leukemia. J Pharmacol Exp Ther. 1992;260:71-77.

31. Powis G, Harris RN, Basseches PJ, Santone KS. Effects of advanced leukemia on hepatic drug-metabolizing activity in the mouse. Cancer Chemother Pharmacol. 1986;16:43-49.

32. Marsoni S, Ungerleider RS, Hurson SB, et al. Tolerance to antineoplastic agents in children and adults. Cancer Treat Rep. 1985;69:1263-1269.

33. Rodman JH, Murry DJ, Madden T, Santana VM. Altered etoposide pharmacokinetics and time to engraftment in pediatric patients undergoing autologous bone marrow transplantation. J Clin Oncol. 1994;12:2390-2397.

34. Charles KA, Rivory LP, Brown SL, et al. Transcriptional repression of hepatic cytochrome P450 3A4 gene in the presence of cancer. Clin Cancer Res. 2006;12:7492-7497.

35. Lipshultz SE, Colan SD, Gelber RD, et al. Late cardiac effects of doxorubicin therapy for acute lymphoblastic leukemia in childhood. N Engl J Med. 1991;324:808-815.

36. Paakko E, Vainionpaa L, Lanning M, et al. White matter changes in children treated for acute lymphoblastic leukemia. Cancer. 1992;70:2728-2733.

37. Aubier F, Flamant F, Brauner R, et al. Male gonadal function after chemotherapy for solid tumors in childhood. J Clin Oncol. 1989;7:304-309.

38. Matus-Ridley M, Nicosia SV, Meadows AT. Gonadal effects of cancer therapy in boys. Cancer. 1985;55:2353-2363.

39. Nicosia SV, Matus-Ridley M, Meadows AT. Gonadal effects of cancer therapy in girls. Cancer. 1985;55:2364-2372.

40. Ortin TT, Shostak CA, Donaldson SS. Gonadal status and reproductive function following treatment for Hodgkin's disease in childhood: the Stanford experience. Int J Radiat Oncol Biol Phys. 1990;19:873-880.

41. Wallace WH, Shalet SM, Lendon M, Morris-Jones PH. Male fertility in long-term survivors of childhood acute lymphoblastic leukaemia. Int J Androl. 1991;14:312-319.

42. Whitehead E, Shalet SM, Jones PH, et al. Gonadal function after combination chemotherapy for Hodgkin's disease in childhood. Arch Dis Child. 1982;57:287-291.

43. Damewood MD, Grochow LB. Prospects for fertility after chemotherapy or radiation for neoplastic disease. Fertil Steril. 1986;45:443-459.

44. Siris ES, Leventhal BG, Vaitukaitis JL. Effects of childhood leukemia and chemotherapy on puberty and reproductive function in girls. N Engl J Med. 1976;294:1143-1146.

45. Clayton PE, Shalet SM, Price DA, Jones PH. Ovarian function following chemotherapy for childhood brain tumours. Med Pediatr Oncol. 1989;17:92-96.

46. Collins JM, Zaharko DS, Dedrick RL, Chabner BA. Potential roles for preclinical pharmacology in phase I clinical trials. Cancer Treat Rep. 1986;70:73-80.

47. Jaquenoud SE, van der Velden JW, Rentsch K, et al. Therapeutic drug monitoring and pharmacogenetic tests as tools in pharmacovigilance. Drug Saf. 2006;29:735-768.

48. Mahmood I, Balian JD. The pharmacokinetic principles behind scaling from preclinical results to phase I protocols. Clin Pharmacokinet. 1999;36:1-11.

49. Eisenhauer EA, O'Dwyer PJ, Christian M, Humphrey JS. Phase I clinical trial design in cancer drug development. J Clin Oncol. 2000;18:684-692.

50. Newell DR, Burtles SS, Fox BW, et al. Evaluation of rodent-only toxicology for early clinical trials with novel cancer therapeutics. Br J Cancer. 1999;81:760-768.

51. Evans WE, Rodman JH, Relling MV, et al. Concept of maximum tolerated systemic exposure and its application to phase I-II

studies of anticancer drugs. Med Pediatr Oncol. 1991;19:153-159.

52. Woo MH, Relling MV, Sonnichsen DS, et al. Phase I targeted systemic exposure study of paclitaxel in children with refractory acute leukemias. Clin Cancer Res. 1999;5:543-549.

53. Simon R, Freidlin B, Rubinstein L, et al. Accelerated titration designs for phase I clinical trials in oncology. J Natl Cancer Inst. 1997;89:1138-1147.

54. Kobayashi K, Jodrell DI, Ratain MJ. Pharmacodynamic-pharmacokinetic relationships and therapeutic drug monitoring. Cancer Surv. 1993;17:51-78.

55. Gupta E, Lestingi TM, Mick R, et al. Metabolic fate of irinotecan in humans: correlation of glucuronidation with diarrhea. Cancer Res. 1994;54:3723-3725.

56. Vaughan WP, Karp JE, Burke PJ. Two-cycle timed-sequential chemotherapy for adult acute nonlymphocytic leukemia. Blood. 1984;64:975-980.

57. Lazarou J, Pomeranz B, Corey P. Incidence of adverse drug reactions in hospitalized patients: a meta-analysis of prospective studies. JAMA. 1998;279:1200-1205.

58. Baker DK, Relling MV, Pui CH, et al. Increased teniposide clearance with concomitant anticonvulsant therapy. J Clin Oncol. 1992;10:311-315.

59. Crews KR, Stewart CF, Jones-Wallace D, et al. Altered irinotecan pharmacokinetics in pediatric high-grade glioma patients receiving enzyme-inducing anticonvulsant therapy. Clin Cancer Res. 2002;8:2202-2209.

60. Relling MV, Pui CH, Sandlund JT, et al. Adverse effect of anticonvulsants on efficacy of chemotherapy for acute lymphoblastic leukaemia. Lancet. 2000;356:285-290.

61. DeMario MD, Ratain MJ. Oral chemotherapy: rationale and future directions. J Clin Oncol. 1998;16:2557-2567.

62. Lepper ER, Nooter K, Verweij J, et al. Mechanisms of resistance to anticancer drugs: the role of the polymorphic ABC transporters ABCB1 and ABCG2. Pharmacogenomics. 2005;6:115-138.

63. Sparreboom A, Cox MC, Acharya MR, Figg WD. Herbal remedies in the United States: potential adverse interactions with anticancer agents. J Clin Oncol. 2004;22:2489-2503.

64. McLean TW, Kemper KJ. Complementary and alternative medicine therapies in pediatric oncology patients. J Soc Integr Oncol. 2006;4:40-45.

65. Kelly KM. Complementary and alternative medical therapies for children with cancer. Eur J Cancer. 2004;40:2041-2046.

66. Mathijssen RH, Verweij J, De Bruijn P, et al. Effects of St. John's wort on irinotecan metabolism. J Natl Cancer Inst. 2002;94:1247-1249.

67. Cox MC, Low J, Lee J, et al. Influence of garlic (Allium sativum) on the pharmacokinetics of docetaxel. Clin Cancer Res. 2006;12:4636-4640.

68. van Erp NP, Baker SD, Zhao M, et al. Effect of milk thistle (Silybum marianum) on the pharmacokinetics of irinotecan. Clin Cancer Res. 2005;11:7800-7806.

69. Peebles KA, Baker RK, Kurz EU, et al. Catalytic inhibition of human DNA topoisomerase II alpha by hypericin, a naphthodianthrone from St. John's wort (Hypericum perforatum). Biochem Pharmacol. 2001;62:1059-1070.

70. Mansky PJ, Straus SE. St. John's Wort: more implications for cancer patients. J Natl Cancer Inst. 2002;94:1187-1188.

71. Boddy AV, Ratain MJ. Pharmacogenetics in cancer etiology and chemotherapy. Clin Cancer Res. 1997;3:1025-1030.

72. Marsh S, McLeod HL. Cancer pharmacogenetics. Br J Cancer. 2004;90:8-11.

73. Krynetski E, Evans WE. Drug methylation in cancer therapy: lessons from the TPMT polymorphism. Oncogene. 2003;22:7403-7413.

74. Weinshilboum RM, Sladek SL. Mercaptopurine pharmacogenetics: monogenic inheritance of erythrocyte thiopurine methyltransferase activity. Am J Hum Genet. 1980;32:651-662.

75. McLeod HL, Siva C. The thiopurine S-methyltransferase gene locus—implications for clinical pharmacogenomics. Pharmacogenomics. 2002;3:89-98.

76. Evans WE, Horner M, Chu YQ, et al. Altered mercaptopurine metabolism, toxic effects, and dosage requirement in a thiopurine methyltransferase-deficient child with acute lymphocytic leukemia. J Pediatr. 1991;119:985-989.

77. McLeod HL, Miller DR, Evans WE. Azathioprine-induced myelosuppression in thiopurine methyltransferase deficient heart transplant recipient. Lancet. 1993;341:1151.

78. Schutz E, Gummert J, Mohr F, Oellerich M. Azathioprine-induced myelosuppression in thiopurine methyltransferase deficient heart transplant recipient. Lancet. 1993;341:436.

79. Black AJ, McLeod HL, Capell HA, et al. Thiopurine methyltransferase genotype predicts therapy-limiting severe toxicity from azathioprine. Ann Intern Med. 1998;129:716-718.

80. Relling MV, Hancock ML, Rivera GK, et al. Mercaptopurine therapy intolerance and heterozygosity at the thiopurine S-methyltransferase gene locus. J Natl Cancer Inst. 1999;91:2001-2008.

81. Nasedkina TV, Fedorova OE, Glotov AS, et al. Rapid genotyping of common deficient thiopurine S-methyltransferase alleles using the DNA-microchip technique. Eur J Hum Genet. 2006;14:991-998.

82. Relling MV, Pui CH, Cheng C, Evans WE. Thiopurine methyltransferase in acute lymphoblastic leukemia. Blood. 2006;107:843-844.

83. van Kuilenburg AB. Dihydropyrimidine dehydrogenase and the efficacy and toxicity of 5-fluorouracil. Eur J Cancer. 2004;40:939-950.

84. Heggie GD, Sommadossi JP, Cross DS, et al. Clinical pharmacokinetics of 5-fluorouracil and its metabolites in plasma, urine, and bile. Cancer Res. 1987;47:2203-2206.

85. Harris BE, Song R, Soong SJ, Diasio RB. Relationship between dihydropyrimidine dehydrogenase activity and plasma 5-fluorouracil levels with evidence for circadian variation of enzyme activity and plasma drug levels in cancer patients receiving 5-fluorouracil by protracted continuous infusion. Cancer Res. 1990;50:197-201.

86. Maring JG, van Kuilenburg AB, Haasjes J, et al. Reduced 5-FU clearance in a patient with low DPD activity due to heterozygosity for a mutant allele of the DPYD gene. Br J Cancer. 2002;86:1028-1033.

87. van Kuilenburg AB, Muller EW, Haasjes J, et al. Lethal outcome of a patient with a complete dihydropyrimidine dehydrogenase (DPD) deficiency after administration of 5-fluorouracil: frequency of the common IVS14+1G>A mutation causing DPD deficiency. Clin Cancer Res. 2001;7:1149-1153.

88. van Kuilenburg AB, Meinsma R, Zoetekouw L, Van Gennip AH. High prevalence of the IVS14 + 1G>A mutation in the dihydropyrimidine dehydrogenase gene of patients with severe 5-fluorouracil-associated toxicity. Pharmacogenetics. 2002;12:555-558.

89. van Kuilenburg AB, Meinsma R, Zoetekouw L, Van Gennip AH. Increased risk of grade IV neutropenia after administration of 5-fluorouracil due to a dihydropyrimidine dehydrogenase deficiency: high prevalence of the IVS14+1g>a mutation. Int J Cancer. 2002;101:253-258.

90. van Kuilenburg AB, Baars JW, Meinsma R, Van Gennip AH. Lethal 5-fluorouracil toxicity associated with a novel mutation in the dihydropyrimidine dehydrogenase gene. Ann Oncol. 2003;14:341-342.

91. Collie-Duguid ES, Etienne MC, Milano G, McLeod HL. Known variant DPYD alleles do not explain DPD deficiency in cancer patients. Pharmacogenetics. 2000;10:217-223.

92. Ezzeldin H, Okamoto Y, Johnson MR, Diasio RB. A high-throughput denaturing high-performance liquid chromatography method for the identification of variant alleles associated with

dihydropyrimidine dehydrogenase deficiency. Anal Biochem. 2002;306:63-73.

93. Fernandez-Salguero P, Gonzalez FJ, Etienne MC, et al. Correlation between catalytic activity and protein content for the polymorphically expressed dihydropyrimidine dehydrogenase in human lymphocytes. Biochem Pharmacol. 1995;50:1015-1020.

94. Johnson MR, Yan J, Shao L, et al. Semi-automated radioassay for determination of dihydropyrimidine dehydrogenase (DPD) activity. Screening cancer patients for DPD deficiency, a condition associated with 5-fluorouracil toxicity. J Chromatogr B Biomed Sci Appl. 1997;696:183-191.

95. Kuhara T, Ohdoi C, Ohse M, et al. Rapid gas chromatographic-mass spectrometric diagnosis of dihydropyrimidine dehydrogenase deficiency and dihydropyrimidinase deficiency. J Chromatogr B Analyt Technol Biomed Life Sci. 2003;792:107-115.

96. Mattison LK, Ezzeldin H, Carpenter M, et al. Rapid identification of dihydropyrimidine dehydrogenase deficiency by using a novel 2-13C-uracil breath test. Clin Cancer Res. 2004;10:2652-2658.

97. Lamba V, Lamba J, Yasuda K, et al. Hepatic CYP2B6 expression: gender and ethnic differences and relationship to CYP2B6 genotype and CAR (constitutive androstane receptor) expression. J Pharmacol Exp Ther. 2003;307:906-922.

98. Lang T, Klein K, Fischer J, et al. Extensive genetic polymorphism in the human CYP2B6 gene with impact on expression and function in human liver. Pharmacogenetics. 2001;11:399-415.

99. Hiratsuka M, Takekuma Y, Endo N, et al. Allele and genotype frequencies of CYP2B6 and CYP3A5 in the Japanese population. Eur J Clin Pharmacol. 2002;58:417-421.

100. Xie HJ, Yasar U, Lundgren S, et al. Role of polymorphic human CYP2B6 in cyclophosphamide bioactivation. Pharmacogenomics J. 2003;3:53-61.

101. Ariyoshi N, Miyazaki M, Toide K, et al. A single nucleotide polymorphism of CYP2b6 found in Japanese enhances catalytic activity by autoactivation. Biochem Biophys Res Commun. 2001;281:1256-1260.

102. Kirchheiner J, Klein C, Meineke I, et al. Bupropion and 4-OH-bupropion pharmacokinetics in relation to genetic polymorphisms in CYP2B6. Pharmacogenetics. 2003;13:619-626.

103. Schmidt R, Baumann F, Hanschmann H, et al. Gender difference in ifosfamide metabolism by human liver microsomes. Eur J Drug Metab Pharmacokinet. 2001;26:193-200.

104. Goldstein JA. Clinical relevance of genetic polymorphisms in the human CYP2C subfamily. Br J Clin Pharmacol. 2001;52:349-355.

105. Dai D, Zeldin DC, Blaisdell JA, et al. Polymorphisms in human CYP2C8 decrease metabolism of the anticancer drug paclitaxel and arachidonic acid. Pharmacogenetics. 2001;11:597-607.

106. Niemi M, Leathart JB, Neuvonen M, et al. Polymorphism in CYP2C8 is associated with reduced plasma concentrations of repaglinide. Clin Pharmacol Ther. 2003;74:380-387.

107. Henningsson A, Marsh S, Loos WJ, et al. Association of CYP2C8, CYP3A4, CYP3A5, and ABCB1 polymorphisms with the pharmacokinetics of paclitaxel. Clin Cancer Res. 2005;11:8097-8104.

108. Bahadur N, Leathart JB, Mutch E, et al. CYP2C8 polymorphisms in whites and their relationship with paclitaxel 6alpha-hydroxylase activity in human liver microsomes. Biochem Pharmacol. 2002;64:1579-1589.

109. Goldstein JA, de Morais SM. Biochemistry and molecular biology of the human CYP2C subfamily. Pharmacogenetics. 1994;4:285-299.

110. Xie HG, Prasad HC, Kim RB, Stein CM. CYP2C9 allelic variants: ethnic distribution and functional significance. Adv Drug Deliv Rev. 2002;54:1257-1270.

111. Sullivan-Klose TH, Ghanayem BI, Bell DA, et al. The role of the CYP2C9-Leu359 allelic variant in the tolbutamide polymorphism. Pharmacogenetics. 1996;6:341-349.

112. Dickmann LJ, Rettie AE, Kneller MB, et al. Identification and functional characterization of a new CYP2C9 variant (CYP2C9*5) expressed among African Americans. Mol Pharmacol. 2001; 60:382-387.

113. Ieiri I, Tainaka H, Morita T, et al. Catalytic activity of three variants (Ile, Leu, and Thr) at amino acid residue 359 in human CYP2C9 gene and simultaneous detection using single-strand conformation polymorphism analysis. Ther Drug Monit. 2000;22:237-244.

114. Imai J, Ieiri I, Mamiya K, et al. Polymorphism of the cytochrome P450 (CYP) 2C9 gene in Japanese epileptic patients: genetic analysis of the CYP2C9 locus. Pharmacogenetics. 2000;10: 85-89.

115. Kidd RS, Curry TB, Gallagher S, et al. Identification of a null allele of CYP2C9 in an African-American exhibiting toxicity to phenytoin. Pharmacogenetics. 2001;11:803-808.

116. de Morais SM, Wilkinson GR, Blaisdell J, et al. Identification of a new genetic defect responsible for the polymorphism of (S)-mephenytoin metabolism in Japanese. Mol Pharmacol. 1994;46:594-598.

117. Ando Y, Fuse E, Figg WD. Thalidomide metabolism by the CYP2C subfamily. Clin Cancer Res. 2002;8:1964-1973.

118. Ando Y, Price DK, Dahut WL, et al. Pharmacogenetic associations of CYP2C19 genotype with in vivo metabolisms and pharmacologic effects of thalidomide. Cancer Biol Ther. 2002;1: 669-673.

119. Relling MV, Evans WE, Fonne-Pfister R, Meyer UA. Anticancer drugs as inhibitors of two polymorphic cytochrome P450 enzymes, debrisoquin and mephenytoin hydroxylase, in human liver microsomes. Cancer Res. 1989;49:68-71.

120. Mahgoub A, Idle JR, Dring LG, et al. Polymorphic hydroxylation of Debrisoquine in man. Lancet. 1977;2:584-586.

121. Gonzalez FJ, Skoda RC, Kimura S, et al. Characterization of the common genetic defect in humans deficient in debrisoquine metabolism. Nature. 1988;331:442-446.

122. Skoda RC, Gonzalez FJ, Demierre A, Meyer UA. Two mutant alleles of the human cytochrome P-450db1 gene (P450C2D1) associated with genetically deficient metabolism of debrisoquine and other drugs. Proc Natl Acad Sci U S A. 1988;85:5240-5243.

123. Johansson I, Lundqvist E, Bertilsson L, et al. Inherited amplification of an active gene in the cytochrome P450 CYP2D locus as a cause of ultrarapid metabolism of debrisoquine. Proc Natl Acad Sci U S A. 1993;90:11825-11829.

124. Dahl ML, Johansson I, Bertilsson L, et al. Ultrarapid hydroxylation of debrisoquine in a Swedish population. Analysis of the molecular genetic basis. J Pharmacol Exp Ther. 1995;274:516-520.

125. Sachse C, Brockmoller J, Bauer S, Roots I. Cytochrome P450 2D6 variants in a white population: allele frequencies and phenotypic consequences. Am J Hum Genet. 1997;60:284-295.

126. Agundez JA, Ledesma MC, Ladero JM, Benitez J. Prevalence of CYP2D6 gene duplication and its repercussion on the oxidative phenotype in a white population. Clin Pharmacol Ther. 1995; 57:265-269.

127. Scordo MG, Spina E, Facciola G, et al. Cytochrome P450 2D6 genotype and steady state plasma levels of risperidone and 9-hydroxyrisperidone. Psychopharmacology (Berl). 1999;147:300-305.

128. Aklillu E, Persson I, Bertilsson L, et al. Frequent distribution of ultrarapid metabolizers of debrisoquine in an Ethiopian population carrying duplicated and multiduplicated functional CYP2D6 alleles. J Pharmacol Exp Ther. 1996;278:441-446.

129. McLellan RA, Oscarson M, Seidegard J, et al. Frequent occurrence of CYP2D6 gene duplication in Saudi Arabians. Pharmacogenetics. 1997;7:187-191.

130. Bradford LD. CYP2D6 allele frequency in European whites, Asians, Africans and their descendants. Pharmacogenomics. 2002;3:229-243.

131. Gaedigk A, Ryder DL, Bradford LD, Leeder JS. CYP2D6 poor metabolizer status can be ruled out by a single genotyping assay for the -1584G promoter polymorphism. Clin Chem. 2003;49:1008-1011.

132. Dehal SS, Kupfer D. CYP2D6 catalyzes tamoxifen 4-hydroxylation in human liver. Cancer Res. 1997;57:3402-3406.

133. Bonanni B, Macis D, Maisonneuve P, et al. Polymorphism in the CYP2D6 tamoxifen-metabolizing gene influences clinical effect but not hot flashes: data from the Italian Tamoxifen Trial. J Clin Oncol. 2006;24:3708-3709.

134. Goetz MP, Rae JM, Suman VJ, et al. Pharmacogenetics of tamoxifen biotransformation is associated with clinical outcomes of efficacy and hot flashes. J Clin Oncol. 2005;23:9312-9318.

135. Jin Y, Desta Z, Stearns V, et al. CYP2D6 genotype, antidepressant use, and tamoxifen metabolism during adjuvant breast cancer treatment. J Natl Cancer Inst. 2005;97:30-39.

136. Kaiser R, Sezer O, Papies A, et al. Patient-tailored antiemetic treatment with 5-hydroxytryptamine type 3 receptor antagonists according to cytochrome P-450 2D6 genotypes. J Clin Oncol. 2002;20:2805-2811.

137. Lepper ER, Baker SD, Permenter M, et al. Effect of common CYP3A4 and CYP3A5 variants on the pharmacokinetics of the cytochrome P450 3A phenotyping probe midazolam in cancer patients. Clin Cancer Res. 2005;11:7398-7404.

138. Gellner K, Eiselt R, Hustert E, et al. Genomic organization of the human CYP3A locus: identification of a new, inducible CYP3A gene. Pharmacogenetics. 2001;11:111-121.

139. Baker SD, van Schaik RH, Rivory LP, et al. Factors affecting cytochrome P-450 3A activity in cancer patients. Clin Cancer Res. 2004;10:8341-8350.

140. Ozdemir V, Kalowa W, Tang BK, et al. Evaluation of the genetic component of variability in CYP3A4 activity: a repeated drug administration method. Pharmacogenetics. 2000;10:373-388.

141. Westlind-Johnsson A, Hermann R, Huennemeyer A, et al. Identification and characterization of CYP3A4*20, a novel rare CYP3A4 allele without functional activity. Clin Pharmacol Ther. 2006;79:339-349.

142. Rebbeck TR, Jaffe JM, Walker AH, et al. Modification of clinical presentation of prostate tumors by a novel genetic variant in CYP3A4. J Natl Cancer Inst. 1998;90:1225-1229.

143. Lamba JK, Lin YS, Thummel K, et al. Common allelic variants of cytochrome P4503A4 and their prevalence in different populations. Pharmacogenetics. 2002;12:121-132.

144. Amirimani B, Walker AH, Weber BL, Rebbeck TR. Response: re: modification of clinical presentation of prostate tumors by a novel genetic variant in CYP3A4. J Natl Cancer Inst. 1999;91:1588-1590.

145. Hsieh KP, Lin YY, Cheng CL, et al. Novel mutations of CYP3A4 in Chinese. Drug Metab Dispos. 2001;29:268-273.

146. He P, Court MH, Greenblatt DJ, Von Moltke LL. Genotype-phenotype associations of cytochrome P450 3A4 and 3A5 polymorphism with midazolam clearance in vivo. Clin Pharmacol Ther. 2005;77:373-387.

147. Schuetz EG, Relling MV, Kishi S, et al. PharmGKB Update: II. CYP3A5, cytochrome P450, family 3, subfamily A, polypeptide 5. Pharmacol Rev. 2004;56:159.

148. Kuehl P, Zhang J, Lin Y, et al. Sequence diversity in CYP3A promoters and characterization of the genetic basis of polymorphic CYP3A5 expression. Nat Genet. 2001;27:383-391.

149. Hustert E, Haberl M, Burk O, et al. The genetic determinants of the CYP3A5 polymorphism. Pharmacogenetics. 2001;11:773-779.

150. Tateishi T, Watanabe M, Moriya H, et al. No ethnic difference between white and Japanese hepatic samples in the expression frequency of CYP3A5 and CYP3A7 proteins. Biochem Pharmacol. 1999;57:935-939.

151. Thummel KE. Does the CYP3A5*3 polymorphism affect in vivo drug elimination? Pharmacogenetics. 2003;13:585-587.

152. Westlind-Johnsson A, Malmebo S, Johansson A, et al. Comparative analysis of CYP3A expression in human liver suggests only a minor role for CYP3A5 in drug metabolism. Drug Metab Dispos. 2003;31:755-761.

153. Koch I, Weil R, Wolbold R, et al. Interindividual variability and tissue-specificity in the expression of cytochrome P450 3A mRNA. Drug Metab Dispos. 2002;30:1108-1114.

154. de Wildt SN, Kearns GL, Leeder JS, van den Anker JN. Cytochrome P450 3A: ontogeny and drug disposition. Clin Pharmacokinet. 1999;37:485-505.

155. Dennison JB, Kulanthaivel P, Barbuch RJ, et al. Selective metabolism of vincristine in vitro by CYP3A5. Drug Metab Dispos. 2006;34:1317-1327.

156. Hesselink DA, van Schaik RH, van der Heiden IP, et al. Genetic polymorphisms of the CYP3A4, CYP3A5, and MDR-1 genes and pharmacokinetics of the calcineurin inhibitors cyclosporine and tacrolimus. Clin Pharmacol Ther. 2003;74:245-254.

157. Floyd MD, Gervasini G, Masica AL, et al. Genotype-phenotype associations for common CYP3A4 and CYP3A5 variants in the basal and induced metabolism of midazolam in European- and African-American men and women. Pharmacogenetics. 2003;13:595-606.

158. Shou M, Martinet M, Korzekwa KR, et al. Role of human cytochrome P450 3A4 and 3A5 in the metabolism of taxotere and its derivatives: enzyme specificity, interindividual distribution and metabolic contribution in human liver. Pharmacogenetics. 1998;8:391-401.

159. Goh BC, Lee SC, Wang LZ, et al. Explaining interindividual variability of docetaxel pharmacokinetics and pharmacodynamics in Asians through phenotyping and genotyping strategies. J Clin Oncol. 2002;20:3683-3690.

160. Hirth J, Watkins PB, Strawderman M, et al. The effect of an individual's cytochrome CYP3A4 activity on docetaxel clearance. Clin Cancer Res. 2000;6:1255-1258.

161. Yamamoto N, Tamura T, Kamiya Y, et al. Correlation between docetaxel clearance and estimated cytochrome P450 activity by urinary metabolite of exogenous cortisol. J Clin Oncol. 2000;18:2301-2308.

162. Puisset F, Chatelut E, Dalenc F, et al. Dexamethasone as a probe for docetaxel clearance. Cancer Chemother Pharmacol. 2004;54(3):265-272.

163. Mathijssen RH, De Jong FA, van Schaik RH, et al. Prediction of irinotecan pharmacokinetics using cytochrome P450 3A4 phenotyping probes. J Natl Cancer Inst. 2004;96(21):1585-1592.

164. Li J, Karlsson MO, Brahmer J, et al. CYP3A phenotyping approach to predict systemic exposure to EGFR tyrosine kinase inhibitors. J Natl Cancer Inst. 2006;98:1714-1723.

165. Wong M, Balleine RL, Blair EY, et al. Predictors of vinorelbine pharmacokinetics and pharmacodynamics in patients with cancer. J Clin Oncol. 2006;24:2448-2455.

166. Kishi S, Yang W, Boureau B, et al. Effects of prednisone and genetic polymorphisms on etoposide disposition in children with acute lymphoblastic leukemia. Blood. 2004;103:67-72.

167. Gardner ER, Burger H, van Schaik RH, et al. Association of enzyme and transporter genotypes with the pharmacokinetics of imatinib. Clin Pharmacol Ther. 2006;80:192-201.

168. Mathijssen RH, Marsh S, Karlsson MO, et al. Irinotecan pathway genotype analysis to predict pharmacokinetics. Clin Cancer Res. 2003;9:3246-3253.

169. Schuetz EG. Lessons from the CYP3A4 promoter. Mol Pharmacol. 2004;65:279-281.

170. Hustert E, Zibat A, Presecan-Siedel E, et al. Natural protein variants of pregnane X receptor with altered transactivation

activity toward CYP3A4. Drug Metab Dispos. 2001;29:1454-1459.

171. Zhang J, Kuehl P, Green ED, et al. The human pregnane X receptor: genomic structure and identification and functional characterization of natural allelic variants. Pharmacogenetics. 2001;11:555-572.

172. Tukey RH, Strassburg CP. Human UDP-glucuronosyltransferases: metabolism, expression, and disease. Annu Rev Pharmacol Toxicol. 2000;40:581-616.

173. Guillemette C. Pharmacogenomics of human UDP-glucuronosyltransferase enzymes. Pharmacogenomics J. 2003;3:136-158.

174. Aono S, Yamada Y, Keino H, et al. Identification of defect in the genes for bilirubin UDP-glucuronosyl-transferase in a patient with Crigler-Najjar syndrome type II. Biochem Biophys Res Commun. 1993;197:1239-1244.

175. Aono S, Yamada Y, Keino H, et al. A new type of defect in the gene for bilirubin uridine 5′-diphosphate-glucuronosyltransferase in a patient with Crigler-Najjar syndrome type I. Pediatr Res. 1994;35:629-632.

176. Aono S, Adachi Y, Uyama E, et al. Analysis of genes for bilirubin UDP-glucuronosyltransferase in Gilbert's syndrome. Lancet. 1995;345:958-959.

177. Bosma PJ, Chowdhury JR, Bakker C, et al. The genetic basis of the reduced expression of bilirubin UDP-glucuronosyltransferase 1 in Gilbert's syndrome. N Engl J Med. 1995;333:1171-1175.

178. Iyer L, King CD, Whitington PF, et al. Genetic predisposition to the metabolism of irinotecan (CPT-11). Role of uridine diphosphate glucuronosyltransferase isoform 1A1 in the glucuronidation of its active metabolite (SN-38) in human liver microsomes. J Clin Invest. 1998;101:847-854.

179. Iyer L, Hall D, Das S, et al. Phenotype-genotype correlation of in vitro SN-38 (active metabolite of irinotecan) and bilirubin glucuronidation in human liver tissue with UGT1A1 promoter polymorphism. Clin Pharmacol Ther. 1999;65:576-582.

180. Desai AA, Innocenti F, Ratain MJ. UGT pharmacogenomics: implications for cancer risk and cancer therapeutics. Pharmacogenetics. 2003;13:517-523.

181. Smith NF, Figg WD, Sparreboom A. Pharmacogenetics of irinotecan metabolism and transport: an update. Toxicol In Vitro. 2006;20:163-175.

182. Mathijssen RH, van Alphen RJ, Verweij J, et al. Clinical pharmacokinetics and metabolism of irinotecan (CPT-11). Clin Cancer Res. 2001;7:2182-2194.

183. Paoluzzi L, Singh A, Price DK, et al. Influence of genetic variants in UGT1A1 and UGT1A9 on the in vivo glucuronidation of SN-38. J Clin Pharmacol 2004;44(8):854-860.

184. De Jong FA, Kitzen JJ, de Bruin P, et al. Hepatic transport, metabolism and biliary excretion of irinotecan in a cancer patient with an external bile drain. Cancer Biol Ther. 2006;5:1105-1110.

185. De Jong FA, Scott-Horton TJ, Kroetz DL, et al. Irinotecan-induced diarrhea: functional significance of the polymorphic ABCC2 transporter protein. Clin Pharmacol Ther. 2007;81:42-49.

186. Innocenti F, Undevia SD, Iyer L, et al. Genetic variants in the UDP-glucuronosyltransferase 1A1 gene predict the risk of severe neutropenia of irinotecan. J Clin Oncol. 2004;22:1382-1388.

187. De Jong FA, Kehrer DF, Mathijssen RH, et al. Prophylaxis of irinotecan-induced diarrhea with neomycin and potential role for UGT1A1*28 genotype screening: a double-blind, randomized, placebo-controlled study. Oncologist. 2006;11:944-954.

188. Toffoli G, Cecchin E, Corona G, et al. The role of UGT1A1*28 polymorphism in the pharmacodynamics and pharmacokinetics of irinotecan in patients with metastatic colorectal cancer. J Clin Oncol. 2006;24:3061-3068.

189. Han JY, Lim HS, Shin ES, et al. Comprehensive analysis of UGT1A polymorphisms predictive for pharmacokinetics and treatment outcome in patients with non–small-cell lung cancer treated with irinotecan and cisplatin. J Clin Oncol. 2006;24:2237-2244.

190. Evans WE, McLeod HL. Pharmacogenomics—drug disposition, drug targets, and side effects. N Engl J Med. 2003;348:538-549.

191. Sparreboom A, Danesi R, Ando Y, et al. Pharmacogenomics of ABC transporters and its role in cancer chemotherapy. Drug Resist Updat. 2003;6:71-84.

192. Lockhart AC, Tirona RG, Kim RB. Pharmacogenetics of ATP-binding cassette transporters in cancer and chemotherapy. Mol Cancer Ther. 2003;2:685-698.

193. Marzolini C, Paus E, Buclin T, Kim RB. Polymorphisms in human MDR1 (P-glycoprotein): recent advances and clinical relevance. Clin Pharmacol Ther. 2004;75:13-33.

194. Kim RB. Organic anion-transporting polypeptide (OATP) transporter family and drug disposition. Eur J Clin Invest. 2003;33 (Suppl 2):1-5.

195. Smith NF, Figg WD, Sparreboom A. Role of the liver-specific transporters OATP1B1 and OATP1B3 in governing drug elimination. Expert Opin Drug Metab Toxicol. 2005;1:429-445.

196. Marzolini C, Tirona RG, Kim RB. Pharmacogenomics of the OATP and OAT families. Pharmacogenomics. 2004;5:273-282.

197. Hoffmeyer S, Burk O, von Richter O, et al. Functional polymorphisms of the human multidrug-resistance gene: multiple sequence variations and correlation of one allele with P-glycoprotein expression and activity in vivo. Proc Natl Acad Sci U S A. 2000;97:3473-3478.

198. Kimchi-Sarfaty C, Gribar JJ, Gottesman MM. Functional characterization of coding polymorphisms in the human MDR1 gene using a vaccinia virus expression system. Mol Pharmacol. 2002;62:1-6.

199. Kroetz DL, Pauli-Magnus C, Hodges LM, et al. Sequence diversity and haplotype structure in the human ABCB1 (MDR1, multidrug resistance transporter) gene. Pharmacogenetics. 2003;13:481-494.

200. Wang D, Johnson AD, Papp AC, et al. Multidrug resistance polypeptide 1 (MDR1, ABCB1) variant 3435C>T affects mRNA stability. Pharmacogenet Genomics. 2005;15:693-704.

201. Kimchi-Sarfaty C, Oh JM, Kim IW, et al. A "silent" polymorphism in the MDR1 gene changes substrate specificity. Science. 2007;315:525-528.

202. Sai K, Kaniwa N, Itoda M, et al. Haplotype analysis of ABCB1/MDR1 blocks in a Japanese population reveals genotype-dependent renal clearance of irinotecan. Pharmacogenetics. 2003;13:741-757.

203. Sparreboom A, Marsh S, Mathijssen RH, et al. Pharmacogenetics of tipifarnib (R115777) transport and metabolism in cancer patients. Invest New Drugs. 2004;22:285-289.

204. Gardner ER, Figg WD, Sparreboom A. Pharmacogenomics of the human ATP-binding cassette transporter ABCG2. Current Pharmacogenomics. 2004;4:331-344.

205. Maliepaard M, Scheffer GL, Faneyte IF, et al. Subcellular localization and distribution of the breast cancer resistance protein transporter in normal human tissues. Cancer Res. 2001;61:3458-3464.

206. Jonker JW, Buitelaar M, Wagenaar E, et al. The breast cancer resistance protein protects against a major chlorophyll-derived dietary phototoxin and protoporphyria. Proc Natl Acad Sci U S A. 2002;99:15649-15654.

207. van Herwaarden AE, Jonker JW, Wagenaar E, et al. The breast cancer resistance protein (Bcrp1/Abcg2) restricts exposure to the dietary carcinogen 2-amino-1-methyl-6-phenylimidazo[4,5-b]pyridine. Cancer Res. 2003;63:6447-6452.

208. Jonker JW, Merino G, Musters S, et al. The breast cancer resistance protein BCRP (ABCG2) concentrates drugs and carcinogenic xenotoxins into milk. Nat Med. 2005;11:127-129.

209. De Jong FA, Marsh S, Mathijssen RH, et al. ABCG2 pharmacogenetics: ethnic differences in allele frequency, and assessment of influence on irinotecan disposition. Clin Cancer Res. 2004; 10(17):5889-5894.

210. Iida A, Saito S, Sekine A, et al. Catalog of 605 single-nucleotide polymorphisms (SNPs) among 13 genes encoding human ATP-binding cassette transporters: ABCA4, ABCA7, ABCA8, ABCD1, ABCD3, ABCD4, ABCE1, ABCF1, ABCG1, ABCG2, ABCG4, ABCG5, and ABCG8. J Hum Genet. 2002;47:285-310.

211. Zamber CP, Lamba JK, Yasuda K, et al. Natural allelic variants of breast cancer resistance protein (BCRP) and their relationship to BCRP expression in human intestine. Pharmacogenetics. 2003;13:19-28.

212. Imai Y, Nakane M, Kage K, et al. C421A polymorphism in the human breast cancer resistance protein gene is associated with low expression of Q141K protein and low-level drug resistance. Mol Cancer Ther. 2002;1:611-616.

213. Sparreboom A, Loos WJ, Burger H, et al. Effect of ABCG2 genotype on the oral bioavailability of topotecan. Cancer Biol Ther. 2005;4:650-658.

214. Mizuarai S, Aozasa N, Kotani H. Single nucleotide polymorphisms result in impaired membrane localization and reduced atpase activity in multidrug transporter ABCG2. Int J Cancer. 2004;109:238-246.

215. Morisaki K, Robey RW, Ozvegy-Laczka C, et al. Single nucleotide polymorphisms modify the transporter activity of ABCG2. Cancer Chemother Pharmacol. 2005;56:161-172.

216. Sparreboom A, Gelderblom H, Marsh S, et al. Diflomotecan pharmacokinetics in relation to ABCG2 421C>A genotype. Clin Pharmacol Ther. 2004;76:38-44.

217. Zhou Q, Sparreboom A, Tan EH, et al. Pharmacogenetic profiling across the irinotecan pathway in Asian patients with cancer. Br J Clin Pharmacol. 2005;59:415-424.

218. Cusatis G, Gregorc V, Li J, et al. Pharmacogenetics of ABCG2 and adverse reactions to gefitinib. J Natl Cancer Inst. 2006;98: 1739-1742.

219. Milano G, McLeod HL. Can dihydropyrimidine dehydrogenase impact 5-fluorouracil-based treatment? Eur J Cancer. 2000;36: 37-42.

220. Watkins PB. Noninvasive tests of CYP3A enzymes. Pharmacogenetics. 1994;4:171-184.

221. Kishi S, Cheng C, French D, et al. Ancestry and pharmacogenetics of antileukemic drug toxicity. Blood. 2007;109:4151-4157.

222. Relling MV, Yang W, Das S, et al. Pharmacogenetic risk factors for osteonecrosis of the hip among children with leukemia. J Clin Oncol. 2004;22:3930-3936.

223. Rocha JC, Cheng C, Liu W, et al. Pharmacogenetics of outcome in children with acute lymphoblastic leukemia. Blood. 2005;105:4752-4758.

224. Gurney H. Dose calculation of anticancer drugs: a review of the current practice and introduction of an alternative. J Clin Oncol. 1996;14:2590-2611.

225. Felici A, Verweij J, Sparreboom A. Dosing strategies for anticancer drugs: the good, the bad and body-surface area. Eur J Cancer. 2002;38:1677-1684.

226. Dooley MJ, Poole SG. Poor correlation between body surface area and glomerular filtration rate. Cancer Chemother Pharmacol. 2000;46:523-526.

227. Pinkel D. The use of body surface area as a criterion of drug dosage in cancer chemotherapy. Cancer Res. 1958;18:853-856.

228. Baker SD, Verweij J, Rowinsky EK, et al. Role of body surface area in dosing of investigational anticancer agents in adults, 1991-2001. J Natl Cancer Inst. 2002;94:1883-1888.

229. Bartelink IH, Rademaker CM, Schobben AF, van den Anker JN. Guidelines on paediatric dosing on the basis of developmental physiology and pharmacokinetic considerations. Clin Pharmacokinet. 2006;45:1077-1097.

230. Kintzel PE, Dorr RT. Anticancer drug renal toxicity and elimination: dosing guidelines for altered renal function. Cancer Treat Rev. 1995;21:33-64.

231. Egorin MJ, Van Echo DA, Olman EA, et al. Prospective validation of a pharmacologically based dosing scheme for the cis-diamminedichloroplatinum(II) analogue diamminecyclobutanedicarboxylatoplatinum. Cancer Res. 1985;45:6502-6506.

232. Calvert AH, Newell DR, Gumbrell LA, et al. Carboplatin dosage: prospective evaluation of a simple formula based on renal function. J Clin Oncol. 1989;7:1748-1756.

233. Twelves C, Glynne-Jones R, Cassidy J, et al. Effect of hepatic dysfunction due to liver metastases on the pharmacokinetics of capecitabine and its metabolites. Clin Cancer Res. 1999;5: 1696-1702.

234. Grandison MK, Boudinot FD. Age-related changes in protein binding of drugs: implications for therapy. Clin Pharmacokinet. 2000;38:271-290.

235. Sparreboom A, Nooter K, Loos WJ, Verweij J. The (ir)relevance of plasma protein binding of anticancer drugs. Neth J Med. 2001;59:196-207.

236. Perdaems N, Bachaud JM, Rouzaud P, et al. Relation between unbound plasma concentrations and toxicity in a prolonged oral etoposide schedule. Eur J Clin Pharmacol. 1998;54:677-683.

237. Stewart CF, Arbuck SG, Fleming RA, Evans WE. Relation of systemic exposure to unbound etoposide and hematologic toxicity. Clin Pharmacol Ther. 1991;50:385-393.

238. Sparreboom A, van Zuylen L, Brouwer E, et al. Cremophor EL-mediated alteration of paclitaxel distribution in human blood: clinical pharmacokinetic implications. Cancer Res. 1999;59:1454-1457.

239. Ratain MJ, Mick R, Schilsky RL, et al. Pharmacologically based dosing of etoposide: a means of safely increasing dose intensity. J Clin Oncol. 1991;9:1480-1486.

240. Egorin MJ. Overview of recent topics in clinical pharmacology of anticancer agents. Cancer Chemother Pharmacol. 1998;42 (Suppl):S22-S30.

241. Schmiegelow K, Schroder H, Gustafsson G, et al. Risk of relapse in childhood acute lymphoblastic leukemia is related to RBC methotrexate and mercaptopurine metabolites during maintenance chemotherapy. Nordic Society for Pediatric Hematology and Oncology. J Clin Oncol. 1995;13:345-351.

242. Evans WE, Relling MV, Rodman JH, et al. Conventional compared with individualized chemotherapy for childhood acute lymphoblastic leukemia. N Engl J Med. 1998;338:499-505.

243. Santana VM, Furman WL, Billups CA, et al. Improved response in high-risk neuroblastoma with protracted topotecan administration using a pharmacokinetically guided dosing approach. J Clin Oncol. 2005;23:4039-4047.

244. Stewart CF, Iacono LC, Chintagumpala M, et al. Results of a phase II upfront window of pharmacokinetically guided topotecan in high-risk medulloblastoma and supratentorial primitive neuroectodermal tumor. J Clin Oncol. 2004;22:3357-3365.

245. Chatelut E, Canal P, Brunner V, et al. Prediction of carboplatin clearance from standard morphologic and biologic patient characteristics. J Natl Cancer Inst. 1995;87:573-580.

246. Bruno R, Hille D, Riva A, et al. Population pharmacokinetics/pharmacodynamics of docetaxel in phase II studies in patients with cancer. J Clin Oncol. 1998;16:187-196.

247. Gallo JM, Laub PB, Rowinsky EK, et al. Population pharmacokinetic model for topotecan derived from phase I clinical trials. J Clin Oncol. 2000;18:2459-2467.

248. Hrushesky WJ. Circadian timing of cancer chemotherapy. Science. 1985;228:73-75.

249. Hrushesky WJ, Bjarnason GA. Circadian cancer therapy. J Clin Oncol. 1993;11:1403-1417.

250. Rivard GE, Infante-Rivard C, Hoyoux C, Champagne J. Maintenance chemotherapy for childhood acute lymphoblastic leukaemia: better in the evening. Lancet. 1985;2:1264-1266.

251. Giacchetti S, Perpoint B, Zidani R, et al. Phase III multicenter randomized trial of oxaliplatin added to chronomodulated fluorouracil-leucovorin as first-line treatment of metastatic colorectal cancer. J Clin Oncol. 2000;18:136-147.

252. Levi F, Metzger G, Massari C, Milano G. Oxaliplatin: pharmacokinetics and chronopharmacologic aspects. Clin Pharmacokinet. 2000;38:1-21.

253. Tampellini M, Filipski E, Liu XH, et al. Docetaxel chronopharmacology in mice. Cancer Res. 1998;58:3896-3904.

254. Levi F. Chronotherapeutics: the relevance of timing in cancer therapy. Cancer Causes Control. 2006;17:611-621.

255. Levi FA, Zidani R, Vannetzel JM, et al. Chronomodulated versus fixed-infusion-rate delivery of ambulatory chemotherapy with oxaliplatin, fluorouracil, and folinic acid (leucovorin) in patients with colorectal cancer metastases: a randomized multiinstitutional trial. J Natl Cancer Inst. 1994;86:1608-1617.

256. Papamichael D. The use of thymidylate synthase inhibitors in the treatment of advanced colorectal cancer: current status. Oncologist. 1999;4:478-487.

257. O'Dwyer PJ, Stevenson JP, Johnson SW. Clinical pharmacokinetics and administration of established platinum drugs. Drugs. 2000;59(Suppl 4):19-27.

258. Hensley ML, Schuchter LM, Lindley C, et al. American Society of Clinical Oncology clinical practice guidelines for the use of chemotherapy and radiotherapy protectants. J Clin Oncol. 1999;17:3333-3355.

259. Pai VB, Nahata MC. Cardiotoxicity of chemotherapeutic agents: incidence, treatment and prevention. Drug Saf. 2000;22:263-302.

260. Furman WL, Crews KR, Billups C, et al. Cefixime allows greater dose escalation of oral irinotecan: a phase I study in pediatric patients with refractory solid tumors. J Clin Oncol. 2006;24: 563-570.

261. van Zuylen L, Nooter K, Sparreboom A, Verweij J. Development of multidrug-resistance convertors: sense or nonsense? Invest New Drugs. 2000;18:205-220.

262. Sparreboom A, Nooter K. Does P-glycoprotein play a role in anticancer drug pharmacokinetics? Drug Resist Updat. 2000;3:357-363.

263. Teodori E, Dei S, Martelli C, et al. The functions and structure of ABC transporters: implications for the design of new inhibitors of Pgp and MRP1 to control multidrug resistance (MDR). Curr Drug Targets. 2006;7:893-909.

264. Baccanari DP, Davis ST, Knick VC, Spector T. 5-Ethynyluracil (776C85): a potent modulator of the pharmacokinetics and antitumor efficacy of 5-fluorouracil. Proc Natl Acad Sci U S A. 1993;90:11064-11068.

265. Cao S, Rustum YM, Spector T. 5-Ethynyluracil (776C85): modulation of 5-fluorouracil efficacy and therapeutic index in rats bearing advanced colorectal carcinoma. Cancer Res. 1994;54: 1507-1510.

266. Schilsky RL, Hohneker J, Ratain MJ, et al. Phase I clinical and pharmacologic study of eniluracil plus fluorouracil in patients with advanced cancer. J Clin Oncol. 1998;16:1450-1457.

267. Ahmed FY, Johnston SJ, Cassidy J, et al. Eniluracil treatment completely inactivates dihydropyrimidine dehydrogenase in colorectal tumors. J Clin Oncol. 1999;17:2439-2445.

268. Baker SD, Khor SP, Adjei AA, et al. Pharmacokinetic, oral bioavailability, and safety study of fluorouracil in patients treated with 776C85, an inactivator of dihydropyrimidine dehydrogenase. J Clin Oncol. 1996;14:3085-3096.

269. Baker SD, Diasio RB, O'Reilly S, et al. Phase I and pharmacologic study of oral fluorouracil on a chronic daily schedule in combination with the dihydropyrimidine dehydrogenase inactivator eniluracil. J Clin Oncol. 2000;18:915-926.

270. Benet LZ, Izumi T, Zhang Y, et al. Intestinal MDR transport proteins and P-450 enzymes as barriers to oral drug delivery. J Control Release. 1999;62:25-31.

271. de Jonge ME, Huitema AD, Schellens JH, et al. Individualised cancer chemotherapy: strategies and performance of prospective studies on therapeutic drug monitoring with dose adaptation: a review. Clin Pharmacokinet. 2005;44:147-173.

272. Yong WP, Desai AA, Innocenti F, et al. Pharmacokinetic modulation of oral etoposide by ketoconazole in patients with advanced cancer. Cancer Chemother Pharmacol. 2007;60(6):811-819.

273. Sparreboom A, van Asperen J, Mayer U, et al. Limited oral bioavailability and active epithelial excretion of paclitaxel (Taxol) caused by P-glycoprotein in the intestine. Proc Natl Acad Sci U S A. 1997;94:2031-2035.

274. Meerum Terwogt JM, Malingre MM, Beijnen JH, et al. Coadministration of oral cyclosporin A enables oral therapy with paclitaxel. Clin Cancer Res. 1999;5:3379-3384.

275. Slevin ML, Clark PI, Joel SP, et al. A randomized trial to evaluate the effect of schedule on the activity of etoposide in small-cell lung cancer. J Clin Oncol. 1989;7:1333-1340.

276. Hainsworth JD. Extended-schedule oral etoposide in selected neoplasms and overview of administration and scheduling issues. Drugs. 1999;58(Suppl 3):51-56.

277. Verweij J, Clavel M, Chevalier B. Paclitaxel (Taxol) and docetaxel (Taxotere): not simply two of a kind. Ann Oncol. 1994;5:495-505.

278. Gerrits CJ, de Jonge MJ, Schellens JH, et al. Topoisomerase I inhibitors: the relevance of prolonged exposure for present clinical development. Br J Cancer. 1997;76:952-962.

279. Cadman E, Heimer R, Davis L. Enhanced 5-fluorouracil nucleotide formation after methotrexate administration: explanation for drug synergism. Science. 1979;205:1135-1137.

280. Hsiang YH, Lihou MG, Liu LF. Arrest of replication forks by drug-stabilized topoisomerase I-DNA cleavable complexes as a mechanism of cell killing by camptothecin. Cancer Res. 1989;49: 5077-5082.

281. de Jonge MJ, Loos WJ, Gelderblom H, et al. Phase I pharmacologic study of oral topotecan and intravenous cisplatin: sequence-dependent hematologic side effects. J Clin Oncol. 2000;18: 2104-2115.

282. Boral AL, Dessain S, Chabner BA. Clinical evaluation of biologically targeted drugs: obstacles and opportunities. Cancer Chemother Pharmacol. 1998;42(Suppl):S3-S21.

283. Gelmon KA, Eisenhauer EA, Harris AL, et al. Anticancer agents targeting signaling molecules and cancer cell environment: challenges for drug development? J Natl Cancer Inst. 1999;91: 1281-1287.

284. Evans WE. Gene expression microarrays as a prognostic test. Clin Adv Hematol Oncol. 2005;3:902-904.

285. Holleman A, Cheok MH, den Boer ML, et al. Geneexpression patterns in drug-resistant acute lymphoblastic leukemia cells and response to treatment. N Engl J Med. 2004;351: 533-542.

286. Evans WE, Relling MV. Moving towards individualized medicine with pharmacogenomics. Nature. 2004;429:464-468.

287. Kummar S, Kinders R, Rubinstein L, et al. Compressing drug development timelines in oncology using phase '0' trials. Nat Rev Cancer. 2007;7:131-139.

288. Holford NH, Kimko HC, Monteleone JP, Peck CC. Simulation of clinical trials. Annu Rev Pharmacol Toxicol. 2000;40: 209-234.

289. Sheiner LB, Steimer JL. Pharmacokinetic/pharmacodynamic modeling in drug development. Annu Rev Pharmacol Toxicol. 2000;40:67-95.

7

Immunotherapy of Cancer

Kenneth B. DeSantes and Paul M. Sondel

INTRODUCTION

Chemotherapy and radiation have proven to be highly effective weapons in the war against pediatric cancer. However, the use of these modalities is currently limited by acute toxicities, concerns regarding late sequelae, and the ability of tumors to acquire a drug-resistant phenotype or to become insensitive to radiation-induced DNA damage. Clearly, new strategies are required to improve cure rates and reduce the morbidity of current therapies. The creation of small molecular inhibitors of oncogenesis such as imatinib mesylate represents a major breakthrough in the treatment of certain cancers. Indeed, imatinib mesylate has proven to be a highly effective and well-tolerated therapy for chronic myeloid leukemia. Unfortunately, further development of these reagents for pediatric oncology is hindered by an incomplete understanding of the pathogenesis of most childhood malignancies. Another approach is to use immunologic mechanisms to eradicate tumor. The inherent specificity of the immune system and the potential to mediate tumor cytotoxicity utilizing pathways that are non–cross-resistant with chemotherapy and radiation provide compelling rationales to explore this potentially powerful anticancer modality. The immune system consists of humoral and cellular components that function in an integrative manner to protect the host against infection and possibly against neoplasia.

Immunotherapeutic strategies that rely primarily on humoral reagents may act by targeting a specific tumor antigen or pathway (e.g., monoclonal antibodies; MoAbs) or may nonspecifically enhance immune effector cell function (e.g., cytokines). Similarly, cellular immunotherapeutic strategies may be directed against specific tumor targets (e.g., adoptive transfer of T cells, cancer vaccines) or may employ effector cells lacking antigen recognition capabilities (e.g., adoptive transfer of natural killer [NK] cells). This chapter reviews the progress that has been made in the field of cancer immunotherapy, outlines obstacles that must be overcome to improve efficacy, and discusses future directions of research. The next two sections present an overview of the cellular and humoral components of an immune response, with emphasis on their potential roles in cancer immunotherapy and on the molecules that immune responses may recognize on tumor cells. The subsequent sections focus on how various components of the immune system are being used in the setting of clinical cancer immunotherapy, with an emphasis on applications to childhood malignancies.

COMPONENTS OF THE IMMUNE SYSTEM IMPORTANT IN TUMOR IMMUNOLOGY

The Humoral Arm of the Immune System

Monoclonal Antibodies

The humoral arm of the immune system consists of soluble reagents, including antibodies and a wide array of cytokines. Antibody molecules are composed of two heavy chains: γ, δ, α, μ, or ε, depending on the antibody subclass; and two light chains: λ or κ (Fig. 7-1). The Fab portion of an antibody contains the antigen recognition site, which is composed of one constant and one variable domain from each of the heavy and light chains. The Fc portion of the molecule is composed of

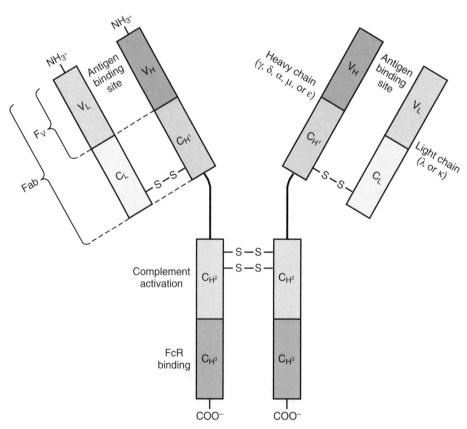

FIGURE 7-1. Schematic representation of an antibody molecule. C_H, constant heavy chain; C_L, constant light chain; V_H, variable heavy chain; V_L, variable light chain.

two heavy chains and mediates complement fixation or binds to Fc receptors (FcRs) present on effector cells, resulting in activation or inhibition of effector cell function. Monoclonal antibodies (MoAbs) recognize a single antigenic determinant, whereas polyclonal antibodies demonstrate multiple specificities. Unconjugated, or naked, MoAbs may kill tumor cells by a variety of mechanisms, including complement fixation, blockade of growth factor receptors, induction of apoptosis, or by antibody-dependent cell-mediated cytotoxicity (ADCC; Fig. 7-2). The last phenomenon involves the binding of the MoAb Fc component to FcRs present on dendritic cells, neutrophils, macrophages, and NK cells, resulting in opsonization or cytolysis of the antigenic target. FcRs are members of the immunoglobin superfamily and may be activating or inhibitory (Fig. 7-3).[1] Activating FcRs contain a cytoplasmic immunoreceptor tyrosine activation motif (ITAM), whereas inhibitory receptors contain a cytoplasmic immunoreceptor tyrosine inhibitor motif (ITIM). Human activating FcRs include FcγRI (macrophages, neutrophils, and dendritic cells); FcγRII-A (macrophages, neutrophils); and FcγRIII-A (macrophages, neutrophils, and NK cells). Human inhibitory FcRs include FcγRII-B1 (B cells) and FcγRII-B2 (macrophages, neutrophils). It is likely that coengagement of activating and inhibitory FcRs by antibody serves to modulate the immune response and provides an important checkpoint for immune activation.[2]

The antitumor efficacy of naked MoAbs is often dependent on activation of host immune effector mechanisms. However, MoAbs may also be conjugated to highly lethal molecules, such as radionuclides and plant or bacterial toxins, thereby serving as guided missiles that transport their cytotoxic moiety directly to the tumor bed or to metastatic sites. Radionuclides that have been conjugated to MoAbs for the treatment of human cancer include ^{131}I, ^{125}I, ^{90}Y, ^{186}Re, ^{111}In, and ^{177}Lu.[3] Radioimmunoconjugates are attractive immunotherapeutic agents because they do not require cellular internalization to mediate cytotoxicity. Furthermore, radioimmunoconjugates may establish a lattice of energy within the tumor bed, resulting in the destruction of cancer cells not directly bound to antibody (the innocent bystander effect; Fig. 7-4). A disadvantage of utilizing radioimmunoconjugates relates to the difficulty of handling radioactive materials and waste, as well as radiation safety concerns to family members and hospital personnel.

Immunotoxins are tumor-reactive MoAbs bound to potent cellular poisons. A small number of these molecules are generally sufficient to kill a malignant cell. However, these compounds require internalization in order to damage the intracellular processes that ultimately result in cell death (Fig. 7-5). Consequently, they must be linked to MoAbs that induce internalization when bound to antigen on tumor. In addition, because immunotoxins are large molecules, they generally do not penetrate well into solid tumors and may be better suited for the treatment of leukemias. Examples of plant and bacterial toxins that have been conjugated to MoAbs for clinical trials include ricin A chain, diphtheria toxin, and *Pseudomonas* exotoxin.[4]

MoAbs may also be conjugated to immunomodulating agents such as interleukin-2 (IL-2), which augment effector cell function, leading to enhanced tumor killing by ADCC. These MoAb-cytokine conjugates have been designated immunocytokines. Utilizing immunocytokines for cancer therapy is potentially more effective than administering the MoAb and cytokine separately because the conjugate allows for higher concentrations of cytokine to accumulate within the tumor microenvironment, thus favoring the activation of an immune response. As with naked MoAbs, immunocytokines rely on host effector mechanisms to eradicate tumor.

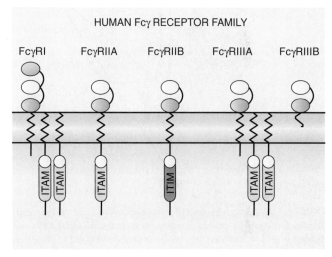

FIGURE 7-3. The family of FcRs includes several activating receptors (that bear ITAM motifs) and inhibitory receptors that bear ITIM motifs or function as "decoys." *(Courtesy of Dr. R. Clynes, Columbia University, New York.)*

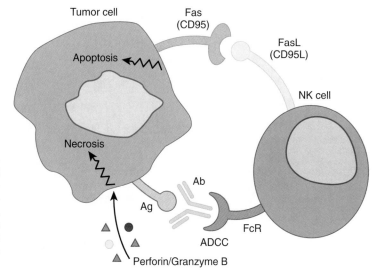

FIGURE 7-2. Antibody-dependent cell-mediated cytotoxicity. ADCC involves cells of the innate immune system bearing activating FcRs to interact with the Fc end of immunoglobulins binding to a target cell. If sufficient activation of the FcRs occurs, the effector cells are triggered to mediate target cell destruction, using membrane-bound and -released molecules that induce target cell apoptosis and necrosis. *(Redrawn from Mitra R, Singh S, Khar A. Antitumour immune responses. Exp Rev Mo Med. 2003;5. © 2003, Cambridge University Press.)*

Cytokines

Cytokines are soluble intercellular signaling proteins that are generally produced by leukocytes and mediate a wide variety of cellular functions relating to immunity, inflammation, and hematopoiesis. Cytokines have been grouped into various classes, including interleukins, interferons, chemokines, and hematopoietic growth factors, on the basis of their presumed functions. A number of cytokines have been used as cancer therapeutic agents, though clinical responses have generally been modest. However, cytokines will likely play an important adjuvant role when combined with other immunotherapeutics, such as vaccines or MoAbs.

The Cellular Arm of the Immune System

T Cells

T cells are part of the adaptive immune system, and they recognize specific tumor antigenic peptides in association with class I or class II major histocompatibility complex (MHC) molecules via the heterodimeric T-cell receptor (TCR), which consists of an α and a β chain, each of which has gone through somatic genetic recombination and editing. This editing occurs in the thymus, resulting in a complete T-cell repertoire. Cytotoxic T cells (CTLs), generally bearing the CD8 surface molecule, recognize tumor antigen associated with class I MHC molecules expressed on all nucleated cells. CTLs are capable of mediating tumor cell lysis by releasing perforin/granzyme B or by inducing apoptosis through Fas/Fas ligand (FasL) interactions (Fig. 7-6). In addition to engagement of the TCR, T cells must receive costimulatory signals from antigen-processing cells (APCs), which typically are mediated by interactions between CD28 on the T cell and B7 family proteins (CD80 or CD86) on the APC. Other costimulatory molecules on the APC may be required for T-cell activation, including CD40 and the cellular adhesion proteins ICAM-1 (CD54) and LFA-3 (CD58). Absence of costimulation may result in an anergic response upon further ligation of the TCR with its cognate antigen. The molecular interface between T cells and APCs has been referred to as the immune synapse (Fig. 7-7).

Helper T cells (T_Hs), which generally bear the CD4 surface molecule, recognize tumor antigen associated with class II MHC molecules expressed on B cells, macrophages, and other antigen-presenting cells. T_H lymphocytes do not directly mediate lysis of tumor cells, but they do produce cytokines that significantly influence immune function. T_Hs may be divided into two subtypes, T_H1 and T_H2, based on their cytokine-

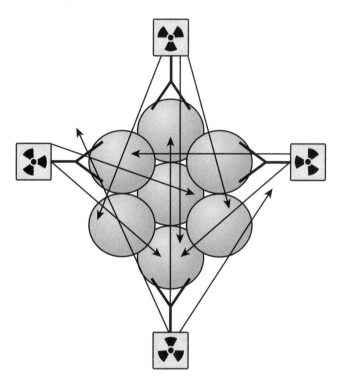

FIGURE 7-4. Radioimmunoconjugates recognize tumor surface antigens and establish a lattice of energy that can kill cancer cells not directly bound to antibody (the innocent-bystander effect).

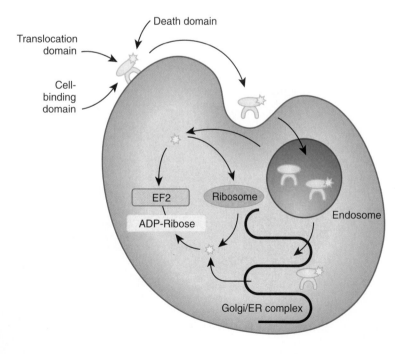

FIGURE 7-5. Immunotoxins consist of a cell-binding domain that recognizes a tumor surface antigen; a translocation domain that facilitates transport of the compound through the cell membrane by endocytosis; and a death domain that poisons intracellular processes, resulting in apoptosis. Upon entering the cytosol, the immunotoxin is sequestered within an endosome where the acidic environment may promote translocation of the toxin moiety across the endocytic membrane. Some toxins (e.g., diphtheria toxin) may then mediate adenosine diphosphate (ADP) ribosylation of elongation factor 2 (EF2), thereby arresting protein synthesis. Other toxins (e.g., ricin A chain) disrupt protein synthesis by cleaving ribosomal RNA. Certain immunotoxins (e.g., ricin A chain, *Pseudomonas* exotoxin) are processed through the Golgi complex and endoplasmic reticulum (ER), where translocation into the cytosol occurs, allowing for disruption of protein synthesis.

secretion profiles. CD4$^+$ T cells mediating a T$_H$1 response (also designated a type 1 response) produce proinflammatory cytokines such as interferon-gamma (IFN-γ) and tumor necrosis factor (TNF), which enhance the function of macrophages and CTLs and promote the secretion of other immunostimulatory cytokines, such as IL-12. Helper T cells mediating a T$_H$2 response (also designated a type 2 response), induce antibody

production by B cells and promote antibody class switching, but they also produce inhibitory cytokines such as IL-4, IL-10, and IL-13, thereby downregulating the cellular immune response. Regulatory T cells (T$_{regs}$) represent another subclass of CD4$^+$ T cells that serve to inhibit immune activation and induce self-tolerance. These lymphocytes are identified by their surface expression of CD25 (the IL-2 receptor α chain) and the FOXP3 transcription factor. The elimination of T$_{regs}$ may be an important step in facilitating a cellular immune response against tumor.

T-cell adoptive immunotherapy is most commonly performed in the context of hematopoietic stem cell transplantation (HSCT) because mature T lymphocytes are transferred from the donor to the patient at the time of transplantation. In addition, T cells may be infused post-transplant (donor lymphocyte infusion; DLI) for the prevention or treatment of leukemic relapse. This strategy is especially effective in the setting of minimal residual disease, such as a patient with chronic myelogenous leukemia (CML) in molecular relapse. Advances in cell biology have also allowed for the ex vivo isolation, activation, and expansion of autologous T-cell clones with specificities against tumor epitopes. T cells may be derived from the peripheral blood by leukopheresis or directly from the tumor bed (tumor infiltrating lymphocytes, TIL). However, because most tumors are weakly immunogenic, the efficacy of this approach has often been enhanced by using T cells genetically engineered to improve their antigen recognition capabilities, facilitate trafficking to tumor, increase survival, or potentiate cellular mechanisms of cytotoxicity.

$\gamma\delta$ T Cells

$\gamma\delta$ T cells are a unique subclass of T lymphocytes that reflect a minority of circulating T cells (<5%). They use a heterodimeric TCR consisting of a γ and a δ chain, each of which has gone through somatic genetic recombination and editing. $\gamma\delta$ T cells recognize nonpeptide antigens in an MHC-independent fashion and are thought to play an important role in protecting against certain microbial pathogens, such as *Mycobacterium tuberculosis* and malarial parasites, but may also be involved with tumor immunosurveillance. $\gamma\delta$ T cells may kill tumor either by recognition of specific antigenic determinants

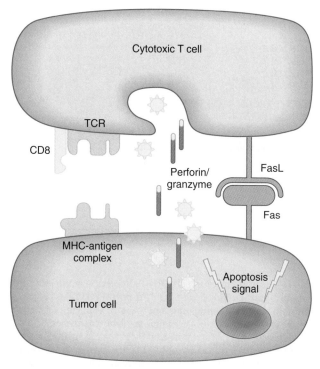

FIGURE 7-6. Cytotoxic T cells generally express surface CD8 and recognize tumor antigenic peptides in association with class I MHC molecules. Following engagement of the TCRs, CTLs can kill tumor targets by releasing perforin/granzyme B or can facilitate apoptosis through Fas/FasL interactions.

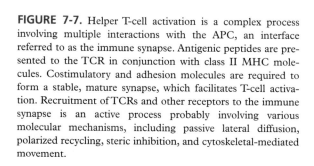

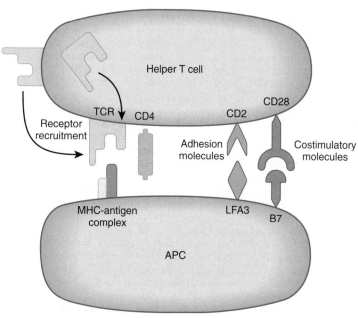

FIGURE 7-7. Helper T-cell activation is a complex process involving multiple interactions with the APC, an interface referred to as the immune synapse. Antigenic peptides are presented to the TCR in conjunction with class II MHC molecules. Costimulatory and adhesion molecules are required to form a stable, mature synapse, which facilitates T-cell activation. Recruitment of TCRs and other receptors to the immune synapse is an active process probably involving various molecular mechanisms, including passive lateral diffusion, polarized recycling, steric inhibition, and cytoskeletal-mediated movement.

through the TCR or by a TCR-independent pathway similar to that of NK cells. As such, γδ T cells serve as a bridge between the innate and adaptive immune system.

Natural Killer T Cells

Natural killer T (NKT) cells represent a small subset of T lymphocytes that demonstrate a highly restricted TCR repertoire and recognize certain glycolipid antigens such as α-galactosylceramide in conjunction with CD1d, a nonclassical MHC class I antigen presenting molecule. Several lines of evidence suggest an important role for NKT cells in promoting an immunologic response against tumor. Preclinical murine models utilizing adoptively transferred NKT cells have shown activity against sarcomas and melanoma.[5] In humans, both quantitative and qualitative defects in the NKT pool have been described in patients with melanoma, squamous cell carcinoma, prostate, colon, lung, and breast cancer.[6] In addition, low numbers of tumor-infiltrating NKT cells have been associated with a poor prognosis in children with neuroblastoma.[7] The antitumor activity of NKT cells may be due primarily to their capacity to rapidly produce large amounts of T_H1 type cytokines, especially IFN-γ. Secretion of IFN-γ results in effector cell activation and promotes dendritic cell maturation and the production of IL-12. It is interesting to note that NKT cells also produce T_H2 type cytokines and thereby may serve as important regulators of immune activation.

Natural Killer Cells

NK cells are a component of the innate immune system and do not require recognition of cognate antigen to mediate cytotoxicity, nor are they capable of developing immunologic memory. These sentinel cells are capable of rapid killing and represent an early line of defense against infection or neoplastic transformation. Our knowledge regarding NK cell biology has improved greatly in recent years. The function of NK cells is tightly regulated by complex interactions between inhibitory and activating receptors, which generally recognize MHC class I molecules as well as separate class-I-like molecules. Perhaps the best characterized are the killer Ig-like receptors (KIRs), which are transmembrane proteins structurally composed of two or three extracellular Ig-like domains and a cytoplasmic tail containing an ITIM or ITAM, depending on whether the receptor is inhibitory or activating, respectively. Examples of inhibitory NK cell receptors and their ligand specificities are presented in Table 7-1. When an inhibitory NK cell receptor binds to its corresponding ligand, it generates a signal; that signal impedes cytolytic activity. If, however, the inhibitory ligand is absent, a situation that is referred to as KIR-KIR ligand incompatibility, the NK cell may mediate destruction of the target cell, provided that appropriate activating signals are also present (Fig. 7-8). Examples of activating KIRs include KIR2DS1, KIR2DS2, and KIR2DS3, which all recognize human leukocyte antigen (HLA)-C alleles. Another class of activating receptors is the natural cytotoxicity receptors (NCRs), including NKp30, NKp46, and NKp44. The NCRs are expressed early in NK cell development and mediate cytotoxicity against MHC class I deficient cells. NKp30 and NKp46 are constitutively expressed on all circulating NK cells, whereas NKp44 is expressed on IL-2 activated NK cells. Target ligands for the NCRs include viral hemagglutinins and possibly heat shock protein 72 (HSP72). NKG2D is another activation receptor expressed on most NK cells, and also mediates cytotoxicity against MHC class I deficient targets. The activating ligands on human cells for NKG2D include MHC-class-I-polypeptide-related sequence A (MICA), MHC-class-I-polypeptide-related sequence B (MICB), and cytomegalovirus (CMV)

TABLE 7-1	Human Inhibitory Natural Killer Cell Receptors
Receptor	**Ligand Specificity**
KILLER CELL IMMUNOGLOBULIN-LIKE RECEPTORS	
KIR2DL1 (CD158a)	Group 2 HLA-C Asn77Lys80 (w2, w4, w5, w6, and related alleles)
KIR2DL2 (CD158b)	Group 1 HLA-C Ser77Asn80 (w1, w3, w7, w8, and related alleles)
KIR2DL3 (CD158b)	Group 1 HLA-C Ser77Asn80 (w1, w3, w7, w8, and related alleles)
KIR2DL5	Unknown
KIR3DL1	HLA-Bw4
KIR3DL2	HLA-A3, -A11
KIR3DL7	Unknown
C-TYPE LECTIN RECEPTORS	
CD94/NKG2A/B	HLA-E (loaded with HLA-A, -B, -C, -G leader peptides)
IMMUNOGLOBULIN-LIKE TRANSCRIPTS	
ILT-2 (LIR-1)	Unknown
OTHERS	
P75/AIRM	Unknown (sialic acid dependent)
IRp60	Unknown
LAIR-1	Ep-CAM

UL-16 binding protein (ULBP). These activating receptors probably play an important role in empowering NK cells to eliminate targets manifesting aberrant MHC expression secondary to viral infection or malignant transformation.

NK cells may destroy tumor by a variety of mechanisms. Rapid induction of cytotoxicity occurs primarily through a perforin/granzyme B-dependent pathway. However, NK cells may also mediate apoptosis utilizing FasL or a separate tumor necrosis factor–related apoptosis–inducing ligand (designated TRAIL). In addition, activated NK cells may secrete a wide array of cytokines, including granulocyte-macrophage colony-stimulating factor (GM-CSF), IFN-γ, and TNF-α, that modulate the immune response. Finally, most NK cells express FcRIII (CD16) and can therefore participate in ADCC.

NK cells may be activated in vivo by the systemic administration of cytokines such as IL-2 or may be activated ex vivo and then used for autologous infusions. However, given the inhibitory signals transmitted by autologous cells, immunotherapy employing allogeneic NK cells may potentially be associated with a greater anti-tumor effect. Indeed, NK cells have been shown to mediate a potent graft versus leukemia (GVL) effect in allogeneic HSCT recipients. Adoptive immunotherapy using allogeneic NK cells in non-HSCT patients has also been explored, although survival of the infused NK cells in this setting is limited.

Dendritic Cells

Dendritic cells (DCs) are professional APCs that process and present antigeneic peptides to naïve T cells in association with class I or II MHC molecules and can migrate from sites of antigen to the paracortex and medullary regions of lymph nodes. Two broad types of DCs have been described on the basis of their presumed lineage: lymphoid (also known as plasmacytoid) DCs and myeloid DCs. Lymphoid DCs are thought to be derived from the thymus and to promote negative selection of autoreactive T cell clones, possibly through Fas-

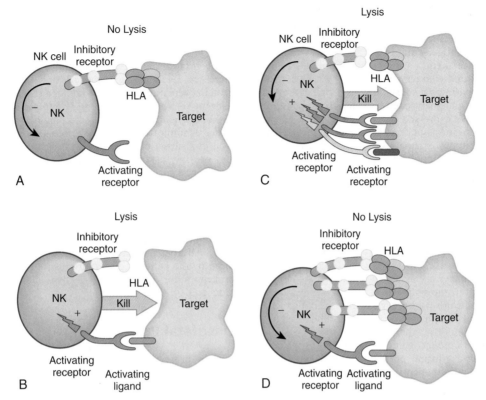

FIGURE 7-8. NK cell activity is regulated by a combination of inhibitory and activating signals. NK cells may kill tumor targets after engagement of activating ligands, provided inhibitory signals are absent or minimized. *(Redrawn from Farag SS, Fehniger TA, Ruggeri L, et al. Natural killer cell receptors: new biology and insights into the graft-versus-leukemia effect. Blood. 2002;100:1935-1947.)*

mediated apoptosis. Lymphoid DCs may also preferentially activate a T_H2 type response, thereby serving as important regulators of immune activation. Myeloid DCs initially exist in a resting or immature state and are unable to stimulate T-cell responses. Upon activation by inflammatory cytokines or microbial products, myeloid DCs upregulate the expression of MHC and costimulatory molecules, such as CD40, CD54, CD58, CD80, and CD86, and produce abundant amounts of IL-12 and various chemokines. These mature DCs can then present antigen to T cells and provide the costimulatory signals required for T-cell activation.

The function of DCs may be augmented in vivo by the administration of cytokines such as GM-CSF. However, the primary use of DCs for cancer immunotherapy has been their incorporation into cancer vaccines. DCs may be isolated from the peripheral blood, expanded ex vivo, and then loaded or pulsed with specific tumor antigens or tumor cell lysates. DCs used for cancer vaccines may also be genetically modified to augment their antigen presentation or costimulatory functions.

Neutrophils

Neutrophils are noted for their ability to mediate rapid destruction of pathogens, particularly bacterial, fungal, and certain parasitic organisms, but these cells may also be involved in antitumor activities of the immune system.[8] Neutrophils bear FcRs and thus can be involved in antibody dependent tumor cell cytotoxicity through ADCC. In addition, activation of neutrophils at sites of tumor or tumor antigen by local administration of soluble activators (such as GM-CSF) may play a role in causing degradation of the tumor cells and subsequent

enhancement of antigen presentation by macrophages and DCs.[9]

Macrophages-Monocytes

Although DCs are currently considered "professional" antigen-presenting cells, monocytes and their derivatives are able to ingest apoptotic cells, digest them, and present their peptidic components in an immunogenic way as well. Furthermore, activated macrophages prominently secrete cytokines such as IL-12, which may be critical in activating local immune responses by NK cells and T cells. Macrophages are found as a common component of the "non-neoplastic" cells in the stroma of many solid tumors; in certain diseases, the degree of infiltration of macrophages into the tumor correlates inversely with prognosis.[10] This may be because macrophages may be induced to have either M1 or M2 phenotypes and activity, corresponding roughly to the T_H1 and T_H2 phenotypes of T_H cells. M1 macrophages induce cytolytic and inflammatory responses, whereas M2 macrophages induce angiogenesis, wound healing, and fibroblastic growth. Thus, it appears that most macrophages found in growing tumors have the M2 phenotype. Of interest is the ability of activated M1 macrophages to have potent direct antitumor effects in vitro and in tumor-bearing mice.[11]

TUMOR TARGET ANTIGENS

Tumor target antigens are molecules that enable selective tumor recognition by components of the immune system.

In the 1980s it was observed that tumor-infiltrating lymphocytes obtained from melanoma patients were capable of lysing HLA-matched melanoma cell lines, suggesting the presence of shared tumor antigens that could be used as targets for immunotherapy. Since then, a wide array of tumor antigens have been identified and characterized, and they may be classified into various subgroups according to their origins. Proteins found exclusively on malignant cells are referred to as tumor-specific antigens; those expressed on both tumor and normal tissues are termed tumor-associated antigens. Tumor-specific antigens include epitopes arising from mutated oncogenes, clonally rearranged immunoglobulin genes, and oncoviral processes. Tumor-associated antigens arise from overexpressed normal proteins, oncofetal proteins, lineage-restricted proteins, histocompatibility molecules, and proteins normally expressed in immune-privileged sites.

Antigens Arising from Mutated Proteins

A number of malignancies are associated with specific genetic alterations that result in the synthesis of novel proteins. These novel mutated proteins are commonly involved in inducing or maintaining the neoplastic phenotype and should be foreign to the host's immune response, thereby representing potential target antigens for immune recognition. Examples of such antigens include the bcr/abl fusion protein created by a t(9:22) translocation, as seen in patients with CML and in some patients with acute lymphoblastic leukemia (ALL); the EWS-FLI fusion protein resulting from a t(11:22) translocation characteristic of Ewing's sarcoma; and mutated ras or p53 gene products seen in a variety of tumors.

Clonally Rearranged Immunoglobulin Genes

Patients with B-cell malignancies, such as B-cell non-Hodgkin lymphomas and multiple myeloma, harbor tumor clones that manifest unique idiotypic immunoglobulin gene rearrangements. These idiotypes may serve as targets for immunotherapy that uses anti-idiotypic MoAbs or T cells that recognize the idiotypic determinant.

Oncoviral Proteins

Viral infections are thought to play a causal role in the development of several types of cancer that result in the cell surface expression of immunogenic viral proteins. These antigens may serve as targets for adoptive immunotherapy using T cells with TCRs specific for virus-derived epitopes; they may also be the focus of vaccine-based strategies. Examples are the Epstein-Barr virus (EBV) antigens EBNA-1, EBNA-3, LMP-1, and LMP-2, expressed in post-transplant lymphoproliferative disorder (PTLD) and in some Hodgkin's lymphomas, as well as the human papillomavirus antigens E6 and E7, found in some cases of cervical cancer. Other viruses implicated in causing human cancers include the human T-cell leukemia viruses (HTLVs), associated with a form of adult T-cell leukemia seen particularly in Asia; the human herpes virus-6 family, associated with Kaposi's sarcoma in immunodeficient individuals; and the hepatitis B virus (HBV), associated with hepatocellular carcinoma. Vaccination against oncogenic viruses, such as the human papillomavirus and the HBV, has been implemented as a strategy to protect against cervical cancer and hepatocellular carcinoma, respectively.

Normal Proteins Overexpressed in Tumor Tissue

Some tumors demonstrate amplification of normal genes or increased levels of gene transcription that result in aberrant protein overexpression by the malignant cells. The best example relevant to pediatric oncology is genetic amplification of the N-MYC oncogene seen in some patients with neuroblastoma. Other examples include overexpression of Her2/neu, which is seen in a subset of patients with breast cancer, ovarian cancer, and possibly osteogenic sarcoma, and overexpression of telomerase and survivin, both of which are seen in several pediatric tumors.[12-14] Because these molecules are expressed on certain normal tissues, the patient's immune system should be tolerant of them and choose to ignore them. However, these molecules might be targets for recognition by passively administered immunotherapy (i.e., MoAbs or adoptively transferred immune cells). Alternatively, these antigens potentially might be recognized by the patient's own immune system; if tolerance can be broken, a form of tumor-selective autoimmunity could be induced.

Oncofetal Proteins

Certain proteins that are normally expressed at high levels during ontogeny may be aberrantly expressed by tumors. Examples include the carcinoembryonic antigen (CEA) seen in colorectal cancer and the α-fetoprotein seen in patients with hepatoblastoma and germ cell tumors.

Lineage-Specific Tumor Antigens

Tumors often express differentiation antigens related to their tissue of origin. These antigens are lineage restricted, although not tumor specific. Examples include hematopoietic differentiation antigens such as the CD19 and CD22 in pre-B cell ALL; the MART-1, gp100, and tyrosinase seen in melanoma; and the prostate-specific antigen seen in prostate cancer. These molecules may or may not be overexpressed on tumor cells compared to their expression on the normal tissue of origin. The decision to induce an immune response against them for therapeutic purposes would be made on the basis of the level of expression on the tumor and the importance of the normal tissue that also expresses them. For example, inducing potent immunity against a prostate-associated antigen might be seen as an effective treatment for prostate cancer, even if it is associated with immune destruction of all normal prostate cells. In contrast, inducing potent immunity against a lung-specific antigen might effectively destroy lung cancer but at the expense of fatal autoimmunity to pulmonary tissue.

Normal Proteins Expressed in Immune-Privileged Sites

Tumors may synthesize nonmutated proteins that arise from germ line–associated genes normally expressed in immune-privileged sites such as the testes. These antigens are promising immunotherapeutic targets because their tissue distribution is highly restricted and they may elicit a potent immune response. Examples include MAGE, BAGE, RAGE, and NY-ESO, which are expressed on a wide variety of human cancers. Although tolerance might have to be broken to induce immunity against these antigens, the resulting immune response would be relatively tumor specific.

Histocompatibility Antigens

Histocompatibility antigens expressed widely on normal tissues may serve as immunologic targets for T cells in the context of allogeneic HSCT. In cases of HLA-matched sibling transplantation, minor histocompatibility antigens (mHAs) may generate a graft-versus-leukemia (GVL) response. HA-1 and HA-2 represent mHA expressed only on hematopoietic cells and are appealing targets for adoptive immunotherapy because donor CTLs directed against these antigens will not damage nonhematopoietic host tissue and cause graft-versus-host disease (GVHD). Other mHAs, such as HA-3 and H-Y, have been identified in humans and may also be expressed on tumors, thereby serving as targets for donor T cells after allogeneic transplantation.

Molecules That Activate Recognition of the Innate Immune System

Certain cell membrane molecules demonstrate cell damage, or stress, and activate recognition by cells of the innate immune system. When normal tissues are infected by virus or stressed to near apoptotic conditions by physical or chemical damage, their membranes are modified in ways that can induce recognition by cells of the innate immune system (γδT cells, NKT cells, NK cells, neutrophils, and monocytes-macrophages). These changes in membrane conformation might not be recognized by endogenous T or B cells, and thus might not be considered antigenic, but they can still induce potent recognition and destruction by cells of the innate immune system.[15] The molecules expressed by these infected or stressed cells, which are only recently being evaluated and characterized, are often expressed at low levels on normal cells. As such, the structure of the molecules expressed, and the cell membrane pattern of their expression, may play roles in signaling activation of the innate immune system. The initiation of tumor cell destruction by cells of the innate immune system suggests that under certain conditions, the process of oncogenesis might induce expression of membrane structures or patterns that can trigger an immune response. This is a relatively new and developing field.

The remaining sections of this chapter present the clinical applications of all these principles as they are currently being applied to pediatric cancer immunotherapy. A key question guiding this research is how might immunotherapy, using components of the adaptive and innate immune system, best target structures recognizable on pediatric cancers to induce clinically meaningful immune-mediated antitumor effects?

TUMOR VACCINES

Rationale and Physiology

The clinical application of prophylactic immunization has had far-reaching, worldwide effects on the prevention of smallpox, polio, measles, and other important communicable diseases. This successful use of immunization was a strong stimulus for attempts to use similar vaccine strategies in the treatment of malignancy. Since the widespread application of the polio vaccine in 1955, basic immunology research has provided important detailed characterizations of the cells and molecules participating in effective protective responses induced by prophylactic vaccination.[16] These responses include the roles of T cells and their subsets, B cells, antigen-presenting DCs, inflammatory cells (neutrophils and macrophages), and NK cells. When an immunocompetent individual is exposed to a vaccine consisting of the specific molecule to be recognized (the

antigen) and the appropriate molecular signals able to incite a danger signal (often referred to as adjuvants), the cells of the immune system become involved in a well-orchestrated and comprehensive response that releases molecular signals: cytokines, lymphokines, and mediators of inflammation.[17-22] These complex interactions produce the following ultimate results: (1) activation of macrophages and NK cells that can mediate destruction of cells that appear stressed; (2) activation of memory T cells that are able to recognize peptides from the specific antigen, as presented by class I and class II MHC molecules, including CTL, and are able to destroy cells expressing that antigen presented by surface MHC molecules; and (3) activation of B cells that will continue to secrete protective immunoglobulin (Ig) able to recognize the immunizing antigen and thereby opsonize pathogens that express the antigen on their surface, leading to their rapid destruction on future clinical exposures.[23] In vivo testing of this immunization approach as a form of cancer prevention or treatment during the first half of the past century included a variety of novel strategies.[24-32] For the most part, they were ineffective in patients and in animal models largely because of major conceptual holes in the understanding of the cellular and molecular components of an effective immune response. In particular, these early efforts were undertaken without an appreciation of the importance of histocompatibility molecules in regulating responses to allogeneic tissues and in regulating responses to altered autologous tissues.[31]

Eventually, immunization of mice with irradiated or inactivated syngeneic neoplastic tissue was shown to induce immune responses that appeared to be directed against antigens expressed primarily on the tumor cells. The reactions included immune responses to sarcomas, breast cancers, and leukemias that were experimentally induced in mice.[33-35] In some studies, healthy tumor-free mice could be immunized against particular tumor antigens and could be shown to undergo a potent T-cell response to the relevant antigen. These immunized mice would reject a subsequent challenge of tumor cells (bearing the relevant antigen) that would have grown in naïve, nonimmunized mice. Although such a strategy may be relevant to potential cancer prevention (as for human papillomavirus and hepatitis B virus, described earlier), this strategy does not appear to be useful for therapy in patients already diagnosed with cancer. Separate studies generated tumor-reactive T cells, either by in vivo or in vitro immunization and expansion techniques, and infused them into animals bearing small amounts of established tumors; some degree of antitumor activity was noted. This is designated adoptive immunotherapy and is described later in this chapter in the discussion of autologous and allogeneic infusions of immune cells. Finally, under certain experimental conditions, mice bearing established (usually very small) tumors could be treated with tumor vaccines (using a variety of vaccination strategies) and generate effective antitumor immune responses that slowed or eradicated the existing tumor cells. The potential benefits of such vaccine strategies have generated much enthusiasm, and many clinical trials have attempted to translate the antitumor effects obtained in certain animal models[36] into clinical antitumor efficacy. However, to date, the benefits of these vaccine strategies have been relatively modest in patients with established cancers. Analyses of preclinical studies led to the following generalized conclusions regarding the requirements for antitumor efficacy:

1. Immunization is most effective if the tumor antigen to be recognized is foreign to the host's immune system. If it is not (i.e., if the tumor antigen is a self antigen), potent vaccine strategies are needed to break tolerance.
2. Immunization is best done when the animal has an intact immune system that is not suppressed owing to administra-

tion of immunosuppressive drugs or the immunosuppressive effects of the cancer itself.

3. Complete tumor eradication is best achieved when an antitumor immune response is activated (or autologous/syngeneic antitumor immune cells are adoptively transferred) at a time when the host has a relatively small burden of tumor cells.

These principles have had an important influence on the translation of findings from experimental models to clinical testing in cancer patients.

Translating Data from Animal Models to Clinical Testing

The ideal cancer vaccine for use in the clinical setting should be able to simulate the molecular, cellular, and clinical conditions required for antitumor efficacy identified in experimental animal models. However, many clear discrepancies between the best-studied animal models and the typical clinical setting prevent easy extrapolation. First, the majority of human malignancies are not caused by foreign viruses whose proteins are expressed as foreign target antigens in the neoplastic cells. Second, there are many mechanisms whereby progressive, newly diagnosed malignancies can cause profound immune suppression, making any vaccine less effective in activating the desired host-immune response.[37] Third, to lower the tumor burden to levels potentially controllable by immune responses, more conventional antitumor treatments (i.e., chemotherapy, radiation therapy, surgery) are needed; they are usually quite immunosuppressive.[38,39] Thus, despite much research, there are still relatively few examples of effective vaccine regimens designed to immunize a tumor-bearing patient that have had a positive impact on human malignancies. The following material provides examples of two broad types of human cancer vaccine strategies: immunization against tumor antigens and immunization against tumor cells.

Immunization to Tumor Antigens

Many human cancers have been studied and found to express molecules that are unique to the cancer, are overexpressed by the cancer, or are selectively expressed on the cancer (with minimal expression on normal tissues). Once such putative tumor antigens have been identified, a variety of strategies can be used in efforts to vaccinate the patient against the antigen of interest. The goal is to induce a strong response by the adaptive immune system, resulting in potent antitumor T- and B-cell responses. The hope is that these primed immune effectors will eradicate any remaining cancer cells in vivo.[40] Clinical trials of these concepts have used a great variety of vaccine strategies to induce potent immunity to the tumor antigen of interest. In general, these strategies have attempted to present the tumor antigen in an immunogenic way, often by means of repeated booster immunizations, and to use coadministration of APC activators (termed immune adjuvants) to help induce potent immunity. For any known putative tumor antigen, the delivery of the antigen itself usually involves injection (most often intradermally or subcutaneously) of a molecule that represents the antigen of interest. Clinical trials have used purified antigenic proteins, purified peptides representing the most immunogenic epitopes of the protein, DNA vectors that encode for the entire antigenic protein, as well as DNA vectors that contain a "mini gene" that encodes the immunogenic peptide from the protein. These tumor immunizations are usually coadministered with adjuvants, such as crude or partially purified preparations of immunostimulatory material from microbes

(i.e., incomplete Freund's adjuvant or lipopolysaccharide derivatives); immunostimulatory viruses (vaccinia or fowlpox); cytokines that activate antigen presentation (i.e., GM-CSF); or ex vivo cultured and activated antigen-presenting cells. In general, detailed immunologic monitoring of patients treated with these tumor antigen vaccines has been able to demonstrate that at least some treated patients develop a population of T cells or B cells with the specific ability to recognize the immunizing tumor antigen. However, even in the face of a tumor-specific T- or B-cell immune response, the vast majority of treated patients are not demonstrating clinically meaningful antitumor effects. This may be because the treated patients have too large a tumor burden for the immune response to overcome; because the tumor may have lost the functional ability to express the tumor antigen; or because of a variety of local or systemic immunosuppressive mechanisms that may interfere with mounting a clinically meaningful antitumor response.

One example of tumor-specific antigenic vaccination has appeared to induce some degree of clinical activity in adult patients and might in the future apply to pediatric patients. The unique Ig gene rearrangement pattern within each clone of mature B cells allows each clone of B cells to express a clonally unique Ig variable region (the Fab component) on its set of secreted Igs and on its Igs that are displayed as receptors on the cell surface. This unique sequence is termed the immunoglobulin idiotype.[41] Thus, it is possible to raise anti-idiotypic antibodies against the idiotype on a MoAb (Fig. 7-9). Because all monoclonal B-cell malignancies are derived from an initial clone, every malignant cell in that clone will express the identical Ig gene rearrangement and hence the same monoclonal idiotype. Thus, one can generate anti-idiotypic antibodies against the idiotype on a patient's B-cell tumor. Efforts have included the immunization of mice to create such anti-idiotypic antibodies (see later section on MoAbs). More recently, T cells from patients with B-cell lymphoma have been activated to recognize peptides from idiotypic Ig of the malignant clone, as presented by HLA class I molecules.

This concept has been extensively developed by Ron Levy and his colleagues from Stanford, and by his former fellow, Lawrence Kwak, while at the National Cancer Institute and, more recently, at MD Anderson in Houston.[40-44] First, in vitro studies were performed to show that T cells occasionally could recognize the unique peptide sequence of the malignant idiotype, as presented by class I HLA molecules. This group then demonstrated in a clinical trial that some patients could be immunized by their own purified idiotypic peptide, which was obtained by cloning the genes responsible for the malignant idiotype from their autologous lymphoma. When this autologous idiotypic protein was used as a vaccine, some patients developed anti-idiotypic antibodies, and some developed T cells able to recognize their lymphoma cells in vitro. Nevertheless, most immunized patients in the initial phase I study had bulky progressive lymphoma and few developed tumor-specific cytotoxic T cells after vaccination. Several changes were then made to improve the immunologic efficacy of this approach. First, the idiotypic protein was fused to a carrier protein (KLH) to enhance in vivo T-cell interactions. Second, it was injected along with GM-CSF to further activate endogenous APCs at the site of the vaccine. Third, and probably most important, the vaccine was given to patients with low-grade follicular lymphoma who had a very high risk for developing progressive, refractory lymphoma but in whom clinical remission had been achieved through chemotherapy. These patients were given 6 months of rest after their chemotherapy before the vaccine regimen was initiated. These 6 months were provided to allow recovery of immune vigor and repertoire after the immunosuppressive chemotherapy used to induce clinical remission. Because these patients had a low-grade lymphoma

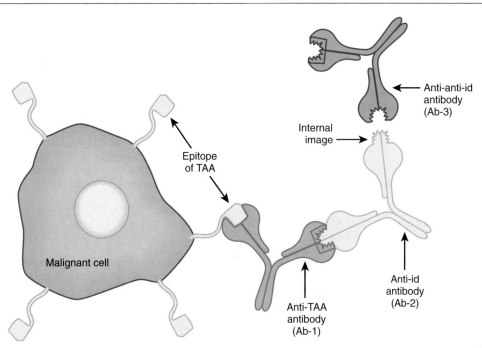

FIGURE 7-9. Mimicry of tumor-associated antigens (TAA) by anti-idiotypic (anti-id) antibodies. An epitope of a TAA is shown schematically by the box attached to a glycoprotein on the membrane of the tumor cell. A monoclonal antibody was made in mice against this TAA. This anti-TAA antibody (Ab-1) has antigen-binding ends (Fab) that allow tight binding of the TAA epitope. When Ab-1 is used as an immunogen, it can induce an antibody directed against it. This anti-idiotypic antibody (Ab-2) has antigen-binding sites that can bind to the antigen binding sites of Ab-1. Thus, the antigen-binding sites of Ab-2 may interact with the antigen-binding sites of Ab-1 in the same way that the antigen-binding sites of Ab-1 interact with the TAA itself. Thus, the antigen-binding sites of Ab-2 and the TAA are both recognized by Ab-1, and the antigen binding sites of Ab-2 may be immunologically similar in structure to the TAA of the malignant cell. This similarity in structure is referred to as internal image. If the Ab-2 molecule is recognized as an antigen, the antibody directed against it is an anti-anti-id antibody (Ab-3). As the Ab-3 recognizes the internal image of the TAA found on Ab-2, the Ab-3 antibody may directly recognize the TAA itself. This is the rationale behind. using an anti-id (Ab-2) to induce an immune response (Ab-3) able to recognize a TAA. *(Redrawn from Sondel PM, Rakhmilevich AL, deJong J, et al. Cellular immunity and cytokines. In Mendelsohn J, Howley PM, Israel MA, et al (eds). The Molecular Basis of Cancer. Philadelphia, WB Saunders, 2001, p 561.)*

that commonly recurs but grows slowly, it was possible for them to complete the initial scheduled chemotherapy with the anticipation that remission would last for the 6 months required for immune recovery. Clearly, this waiting period of 6 months would not be possible for many patients with high-grade lymphomas or for most children with hematologic malignancies. All patients treated with this anti-idiotypic vaccine regimen developed anti-idiotypic antibodies, and 17 of 20 patients developed idiotype-specific cytotoxic T cells. Furthermore, 11 of these 20 patients had a molecular marker from the t(14:18) translocation associated with this malignancy that was detectable by polymerase chain reaction (PCR). Blood samples obtained at diagnosis and after completion of chemotherapy from all 11 of these patients showed tumor cells that were detectable by PCR despite the patients' having achieved a clinically complete response status. Of these 11 patients, 8 had negative PCR results after vaccination, and in all of the 8, PCR results remained negative for more than 18 months of follow-up. Results in the 3 patients who continued to have positive PCR results after vaccination, including at least 1 patient who did not develop a CD8 T-cell response, remained positive, and at least one has relapsed. This study suggests that the patients' own idiotypic vaccine induced an effective T-cell response in most patients and that this T-cell response was responsible for inducing the molecular remissions detected by PCR. Additional follow-up of these patients is needed to determine whether these molecular remissions correspond to long-term lymphoma-free survival. In addition, randomized trials of this approach are underway to further test these exciting results.[41]

This clinical model replicates conditions in which tumor vaccinations have been most effective in animal models and provides important leads for vaccine studies of other human malignancies for which tumor-specific antigens have been identified. The results also strongly imply that vaccine efficacy will be optimal if it is tested in the setting of minimal residual disease, at a time when the patient's immune system is not suppressed by bulky malignancy or by cytotoxic treatment. Furthermore, in small nonrandomized studies, the use of molecular markers (detected by PCR) as surrogate measurements of disease status provides an important parameter for evaluating antineoplastic effects.

Certain pediatric cancers have been found to express tumor-specific or tumor-associated antigens, but relatively few clinical trials have used these antigens in attempting to induce beneficial antitumor effects via tumor-antigen vaccines. One recent important study has been published by the pediatric oncology team at the National Cancer Institute, led by Crystal Mackall. Patients with Ewing's sarcoma bear a common translocation that represents a putative cancer-specific antigen. The team immunized patients to the immunodominant peptide in this tumor-specific fusion protein and also administered influenza vaccines.[45] In an effort to maximize T-cell reactivity, patients received an immunosuppressive dose of cyclophosphamide (to induce in vivo lymphopoiesis) and also received infusions of autologous banked T cells obtained earlier, with or without IL-2. Most patients did show induction of immune responses to influenza, but the immune reactivity induced against the immunodominant tumor peptide was weak or limited in most vaccinated patients. Furthermore, the most striking finding was the induction of a large cohort of suppressive T-regulatory cells (T_{regs}) following the vaccination. Somewhat surprisingly, these T_{regs} were further expanded by the IL-2 infusions, resulting in greater immune suppression, rather than the anticipated augmentation of antitumor immunity. These important studies have led to the design of a successor study by the same team, using a modified, more immunogenic form of the vaccine as well as in vivo treatment designed to prevent the outgrowth of T_{regs}.

Immunization to Tumor Cells

Immunization strategies using specific tumor antigens are based on the concept that certain well-defined molecules shared by cancers in distinct patients might be good targets for immune attack. An alternative approach is that tumor cells might express a variety of potential antigenic determinants that are not well defined or well characterized. The only way to use these uncharacterized antigens for induction of antitumor immunity involves vaccination with the tumor itself, rather than with highly purified individual antigens from the tumor. Preclinical data have suggested that tumors of similar histology may share antigens that can be recognized by MHC-restricted T cells. This type of research has enabled the characterization of some of these antigens on human tumors. The concept of the sharing of uncharacterized antigens has led to the use of allogeneic tumor cells or tumor cell lines as sources of vaccines. This has been most widely tested in the setting of melanoma vaccination. A mixture of allogeneic melanoma cells is pooled, and a crude extract is obtained from them and used as a vaccine in combination with adjuvant. Various trials of this concept have suggested some potential benefit, particularly in small subsets of analyzed patients.[46,47] However, the overall results in large phase III trials of patients in remission have not confirmed benefit.

An alternative concept is that the most immunodominant of tumor antigens are likely to be private antigens, unique to each patient's tumor and not shared with other patients' tumors. This hypothesis is well supported by analyses of spontaneous and chemical carcinogen–induced tumors in mice. In syngeneic mice, tumors that result from the same chemical carcinogen may show virtually identical histology yet show distinct tumor antigens. Immunizing to one tumor generates a protective immune response only to that one tumor, not to a syngeneic tumor arising independently, even of identical histology. This concept, developed initially by Prehn, is that each independent tumor has its own unique tumor-specific antigens.[48] The clinical extrapolation of this concept would require that any vaccination strategy mandate immunization by antigens obtained from a patient's own cancer in an individualized vaccine preparation. Clinical trials in adults have used crude extracts obtained from autologous tumors as vaccines. These have been mixed with adjuvants or used to pulse autologous (or allogeneic HLA-matched) DCs prior to vaccination. An alternative approach involves growing autologous tumor cells in vitro and transfecting them with immunostimulatory cytokine genes (such as GM-CSF or IL-12). These cytokine-gene–modified autologous tumor cells are then irradiated (to prevent their in vivo growth) and injected as an antitumor vaccine. Preclinical data show compelling evidence that these approaches can be effective in eradicating minimal residual disease.[49] However, most clinical trials of this concept have tested the strategy in the setting of detectable tumor, and measurable antitumor effects have been modest.[50] Because the nature of the immunodominant antigens in these autologous vaccines is not known, the only way to monitor the patients for induction of tumor-specific immunity involves testing them for immune reactions (in vitro or in vivo)

to the autologous tumor preparation itself, a somewhat complex laboratory challenge. In the setting of measurable disease, some patients treated with these autologous vaccines have shown clinical signs of antitumor response, but they are anecdotal and often involve histologic evidence of inflammatory cell infiltrates into the tumor after the vaccines rather than clinical disappearance of measurable lesions. In the setting of minimal residual disease, two separate trials, one with renal cell cancer, and one with prostate cancer, have shown some evidence of clinical benefit.[51,52] Because of the difficulty in obtaining sufficient autologous tumor tissue at the appropriate time for creation of these autologous vaccines, this concept has had relatively little testing in the pediatric setting.[53]

CYTOKINES

The cellular components of the immune system interact via cellular contact and by communication through the exchange of soluble signals that are recognized by specific receptors. The soluble signals include an array of proteins that can act to stimulate diverse cells that may be near or far from the cell releasing the signaling molecule (paracrine stimulation) or can act directly on the secreting cell by stimulating the receptors it expresses that are able to recognize the stimulatory molecule (autocrine stimulation). The interaction of the stimulatory molecule and its specific receptor (usually at the cell membrane) results in the activation of signaling molecules in the cytoplasm. These immune-stimulating molecules are produced in cells and thus are termed cytokines. Many of them are made by leukocytes and function selectively to stimulate leukocytes, so are designated interleukins. More than 30 human interleukins have been identified and cloned so far,[54] and many other cytokines have been identified. Many of them are being used in clinical trials. Figure 7-10 shows how some cells of the immune system interact via cytokines.[55,56] These cytokines play an essential role in the maintenance of immune function and in the orchestration of the immune response. In particular, the use of hematopoietic cytokines has become part of the standard treatment for a variety of dysfunctional states of bone marrow, including the stimulation of hematopoietic recovery after myelosuppressive chemotherapy. Ongoing investigations of clinical cytokine therapy are also focused on the antitumor effects that can be mediated directly by these cytokines or by the immunologic reactions that these cytokines can activate. In this section the use and testing of selected cytokines to generate antitumor effects in children with cancer are summarized.

The Interferons

Interferons (IFNs) are a class of molecules that were investigated initially for their ability to interfere with viral infections. They are released by cells of the immune system and other cells upon viral infection. IFN-γ is an essential cytokine involved in the activation of immune effectors in all T_H1-type immune responses. Interferons can also mediate a direct antiproliferative effect on cells with appropriate interferon receptors, including many types of neoplastic cells. Thus, IFNs have been tested as a clinical treatment for cancers on the basis of their immunologic, antiangiogenic, and antiproliferative properties.[57-59] Clinically meaningful activity of IFNs was shown against CML in vitro and in vivo. Thus, IFN has been used as a standard therapy for many patients with this disorder. Daily injection (subcutaneous. or intramuscular) of 2.5 to 5.0 mIU/m²/day of recombinant IFN-α has been used effectively for children with adult-type Ph⁺ CML.[60] Fever, chills, and other flu-like side

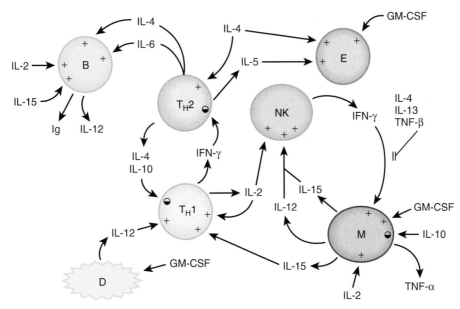

FIGURE 7-10. Interactions between cytokines and cells of the immune system. B, B cell; D, dendritic cell; E, eosinophil; Ig, immunoglobulin; M, monocyte/macrophage; NK, natural killer cell; T$_H$1, type 1 helper T cell; T$_H$2, type 2 helper T cell; TNF, tumor necrosis factor. (*Redrawn from Sondel PM, Rakhmilevich AL, deJong J, et al. Cellular immunity and cytokines. In Mendelsohn J, Howley PM, Israel MA, et al (eds). The Molecular Basis of Cancer. Philadelphia, WB Saunders, 2001, p 550.*)

effects are common, and doses are modified on the basis of patient tolerance and response. As specific kinase inhibitors have shown greater efficacy for Ph⁺ CML, the role of IFN has been curtailed, but its potential in multimodality regimens for treating this neoplastic disease of myeloid stem cells remains for further study.

Interleukin-2

IL-2 is one of the most well-studied cytokines. It is a 15-kD protein released by T$_H$1 cells early in an immune response, and it acts on a variety of cells in the immune system, particularly T cells, macrophages, and B cells.[61] These cells respond to IL-2 by means of a cell surface receptor consisting of a 75-kD β chain, a 64-kD γ chain, and a 55-kD α chain. The bimolecular βγ complex is considered an intermediate affinity receptor and requires substantial concentrations of IL-2 to induce a cellular response through this signal. The trimolecular αβγ-receptor complex is a high-affinity receptor and can trigger cells when exposed to relatively low concentrations of IL-2. Only these two bimolecular or trimolecular complexes on the cell surface are able to mediate functionally meaningful IL-2 binding in vivo or cell signaling in response to IL-2. Cells of the immune system can regulate their responsiveness to IL-2 by modulating their surface expression of α-, β-, or γ-receptor molecules. Resting T cells express functional levels of βγ receptors but are induced to produce α chains when they are activated. This allows them to respond to small concentrations of IL-2 via the high-affinity αβγ receptors they produce.[62] Thus, the use of a MoAbs that recognizes the IL-2 receptor (IL-2R) α chain has been effective in preventing activated T cells from responding to IL-2 and has been clinically useful in preventing organ allograft rejection and in treating severe GVHD.[63] Some malignant T cells express high levels of IL-2R αβγ high-affinity receptors and can preferentially bind IL-2 at very low concentrations. Thus IL-2 directly conjugated with diphtheria toxin is being used to treat patients with T-cell lymphoma.[64]

The most widely used clinical application of IL-2 has been to activate IL-2–responsive immune cells (primarily NK cells

and T cells) in vivo. The activated NK and T cells, in certain clinical situations, have been able to mediate direct destruction of neoplastic cells in vivo. In animal models, IL-2 treatment is able to induce antitumor effects against a variety of neoplasms, including lymphoid and myeloid malignancies. When human peripheral blood lymphocytes are stimulated by IL-2 in vitro, the resulting activated cells can mediate destruction of several leukemic cell lines and some level of destruction of freshly obtained leukemia and lymphoma cells as well as a variety of solid tumors. Thus, human recombinant IL-2 has been tested for its ability to turn on antitumor effector mechanisms in patients with a variety of malignancies. Provided that patients did not have a primary immunodeficiency or ongoing treatment by immunosuppressive drugs, virtually all patients who received immunostimulatory doses of IL-2 for a long enough time (i.e., 4.5×10^6 IU/m²/day for 4 days) demonstrated some degree of immune activation. This included lymphocytosis, increased numbers and function of circulating NK cells, increased numbers of circulating T cells bearing IL-2R α receptors, and increased serum levels of soluble IL-2R α chains. In retrospect, it appears that some of the T cells that are being activated are likely to be T$_{regs}$ and may be inducing immune suppression. The immune activation associated with IL-2 treatment also caused dose-dependent physiologic changes, including fever, rash, and capillary leakage. In addition, for some patients with measurable tumors, this IL-2 treatment resulted in measurable responses. Most striking were the complete and partial responses noted in approximately 10% to 15% of adults with melanoma and renal cell cancer treated with IL-2.[61] Some patients with lymphoma or acute myeloid leukemia (AML) also showed evidence of antitumor response.[65] These measurable responses were the first examples of antitumor effects in patients induced by drugs that have no known direct action against the tumor cells themselves but rather act indirectly, activating the patients' own immune cells to mediate attacks against the patients' tumors. This proof that the patients' own immune systems could be activated to make clinically meaningful responses to the patients' own tumors led to the approval of IL-2 for standard clinical use and to expanded testing of this agent.[66]

In murine models, the immune activation induced by IL-2 often provides the best effects in survival of tumor-bearing mice if the IL-2 treatment is given at a time of relatively minimal tumor burden. Several nonrandomized pilot studies have suggested a benefit of this approach in patients with AML after autologous marrow transplant, but these studies involved comparisons to historical control subjects.[67-69] A randomized comparison did not demonstrate any advantage for a patient receiving IL-2 postengraftment after an autologous stem cell transplant when the acute leukemia was in remission.[70]

A similar approach has recently been tested by the Children's Oncology Group (COG) in patients with AML. After all scheduled chemotherapy was completed for patients who had not received an allogeneic transplant, those still in remission were randomly assigned to receive a brief treatment regimen of IL-2,[71,72] similar to that developed by Fefer and associates,[67] or to be observed only. Data for this study are still in analysis, but the initial early review did not demonstrate any disease-free survival advantage for the cohort randomized to receive IL-2.

Because IL-2 is a potent immunostimulatory factor, it has also been used in combination with cellular immunotherapy approaches. A variety of experimental strategies have been effective in murine models and are being tested clinically. IL-2 has been used to treat peripheral blood lymphocytes as well as bone marrow cells in vitro before in vivo infusion[73] to augment cellular immune reactivity to the neoplastic cells. Relatively few data support the clinical efficacy of this approach. In part, this may reflect the fact that treatment with IL-2 alone activates NK cells and T cells but does not preferentially expand or activate cells able to selectively recognize tumor cells. Thus, IL-2 has been combined with approaches that may be able to better direct the cells responsive to IL-2 toward tumor-selective recognition and destruction.

IL-2 has been used in combination with allogeneic DLIs. Because the allogeneic T cells are responsive to IL-2, this approach might be expected to cause more instances of graft-versus-host disease (GVHD) and also to produce more GVL effects.[74] Anecdotal reports have identified patients with leukemia in whom an initial DLI did not produce remission but in whom remission was achieved when another DLI was given in combination with in vivo IL-2 treatments. Finally, autologous T-cell lines and clones, activated by IL-2 and propagated in vitro, that are able to mediate antigen-specific T-cell reactivity have been identified. This reactivity has included T cells reactive with CMV antigens, T cells reactive with EBV-associated antigens expressed in EBV PTLDs, and other clinically relevant antigens.[75] These in vitro propagated T cells often appear to become dependent on IL-2. Thus, in regimens in which in vitro propagated T cells are being administered, IL-2 infusions are commonly provided to maintain the in vivo function of the infused T cells.

Because IL-2-activated NK cells and macrophages have Fc receptors and can mediate ADCC, IL-2 infusions have been combined with tumor-reactive MoAbs to facilitate in vivo ADCC. This combined MoAb plus IL-2 approach has a greater antitumor effect in murine models than does treatment with IL-2 or a MoAb alone.[76-78] In clinical studies, IL-2 infusions are being combined with antibodies selectively able to recognize a variety of tumor types. In the pediatric setting, these studies have focused largely on the use of IL-2 in combination with anti-GD2 MoAbs reactive with neuroblastoma. Separate studies are under way to evaluate the use of IL-2 with MoAbs that recognize hematopoietic malignancies to facilitate ADCC against the tumor cells.[79] The antitumor MoAb that is combined with IL-2 must be reactive to the malignant cells but not able to recognize an antigen that is expressed by the effector cells. For example, some lymphoid malignancies express surface molecules that are also expressed by normal NK cells. If such an NK cell–reactive MoAb were to be given along with a therapeutic IL-2 infusion, this anti-NK cell MoAb would result in NK cells mediating ADCC against one another, thereby diminishing their ability to mediate ADCC against the malignant cells.

Many other cytokines are known to act on cells of the immune system and induce activity that can result in antitumor effects in animal models. IL-12, IL-15, and IL-18 are all excellent candidates for induction of antitumor effector cells in clinical testing based on studies in murine models, as are synthetic oligonucleotides that stimulate the release of these cytokines.[80-84] IL-7 is a recently tested cytokine that can induce the expansion and activation of T cells. It is being tested in the pediatric setting as a means of augmenting overall T-cell function, with the hope of inducing tumor-reactive T cells. Clinical studies of these cytokines, particularly in the treatment of pediatric malignancies, will require substantial time and development before it is clear whether these or others will become parts of standard treatment regimens.

MONOCLONAL ANTIBODIES

At the turn of the 20th century Paul Ehrlich described antibodies and introduced the concept of a "magic bullet" to cure infectious diseases. He reasoned that it should be possible to develop molecules that have specific affinities with pathogenic organisms, and these agents could be used to mediate cytotoxicity against the recognized target. It was not until 1975, when George Kohler and Cesar Milstein developed the methodology to generate hybridomas and create monoclonal antibodies, that this principle could be applied to the field of cancer immunotherapy.[85] The first clinical trial that used monoclonal antibodies to treat malignancy was reported in 1981 by Ritz and colleagues, who administered J-5, a murine anti-CD10 MoAb, to a small cohort of children and young adults with ALL.[86] Although rapid clearance of circulating blasts was achieved after treatment with J-5, no clinical benefit was documented, at least partly because of antigenic modulation induced by the antibody therapy. The following year, however, Levy and colleagues reported obtaining significant clinical responses in patients with B-cell lymphoma who were treated with tumor-specific murine anti-idiotypic antibodies.[87] However, production of these MoAbs proved cumbersome because a unique reagent had to be created for each patient. Furthermore, it has become evident that murine MoAbs are not ideally suited for human immunotherapy. Murine MoAbs are foreign proteins and consequently can generate neutralizing human antimouse antibodies following administration to patients. In addition, the mouse Fc antibody component does not interact optimally with human Fc receptors, preventing efficient activation of human immune effector mechanisms required to eliminate tumor targets. A major breakthrough in MoAb therapy has resulted from advances in genetic engineering, which have allowed for the synthesis of chimeric or humanized antibodies.[88] Chimeric MoAbs contain mouse variable sequences, but the constant regions consist primarily of human protein. Humanized MoAbs are composed entirely of human protein, except for the complementarity-determining regions, which are responsible for epitope recognition. Compared to murine MoAbs, chimeric or humanized antibodies are less immunogenic, are more effective in mediating ADCC and complement fixation, and are generally less toxic because they induce fewer allergic reactions. However, there are other obstacles associated with the use of MoAbs for cancer immunotherapy, and they must be taken into consideration. They include the inability of antibodies to penetrate bulky tumors, the antigenic modulation or shedding by malignant cells, the development of antigen-negative tumor variants, the inadequacy of host effector mechanisms, and the acquisition of resistance to those effector pathways. Despite these concerns, MoAbs have proven to be valuable antineoplastic agents for leukemia, lymphoma, and some solid tumors.[89] As with other immunotherapeutic strategies, the use of MoAbs will probably prove most beneficial in the setting of MRD.

Naked Monoclonal Antibodies

The first MoAb to be approved by the Federal Drug Administration for the treatment of malignancy was the chimeric anti-CD20 antibody, rituximab. CD20 is a transmembrane protein expressed in the vast majority of B-cell lymphomas. When used as a single agent, rituximab may kill $CD20^+$ targets by the induction of ADCC or by complement fixation.[90] Analyses of FcR polymorphisms have shown a greater likelihood for antitumor benefit when rituximab is used in patients with FcRs that have high affinity for the antibody's Fc component. They include analyses of polymorphisms for $Fc\gamma II$ (largely on polymorphonuclear cells [PMNs] and macrophages) and $Fc\gamma III$ (largely on NK cells), suggesting that PMNs, macrophages, and NK cells may all be involved in mediating the in vivo antitumor effects of rituximab.[91] In addition, ligation of CD20 by rituximab results in the aggregation of this protein into specialized plasma membrane microdomains, referred to as rafts, which is thought to induce apoptosis.[90] Rituximab may also synergize with chemotherapy by inhibiting the activity of P-glycoprotein, thereby reducing the efflux of certain chemotherapeutic agents from cancer cells, or through downregulation of IL-10, which leads to decreased production of the antiapoptosis protein bcl-2.[92]

Rituximab has been administered as a single agent to adult lymphoma patients as front-line therapy or at relapse. McLaughlin and colleagues reported a response rate of 48% in 166 patients with recurrent indolent lymphomas.[93] When used as front-line therapy, a response rate of 73%, including a 26% complete recovery (CR), was demonstrated in 50 patients with follicular lymphoma.[94] Multiple randomized studies have documented that combining rituximab with chemotherapy has improved CR rates and event-free survival rates in adult patients with follicular or diffuse large B-cell lymphomas.[95-99] There are considerably fewer data addressing the use of rituximab to treat pediatric malignancies. A phase-two study using rituximab in combination with ifosfamide, carboplatin, and etoposide for patients with recurrent $CD20^+$ non-Hodgkin's lymphoma (NHL) and ALL was conducted through the COG. Of 20 evaluable patients, there were 7 with complete response and 5 with partial response. Administration of rituximab was associated with manageable infusion-related toxicities and did not appear to increase infection risk. Rituximab has also been incorporated into a COG chemotherapy trial in children with newly diagnosed $CD20^+$ leukemias and lymphomas, but results of this study are not yet available. Rituximab has proven to be a valuable agent in the treatment of PTLD, which is seen in HSCT and solid organ transplant recipients. PTLD results from an uncontrolled proliferation of B cells caused by EBV infection in an immunocompromised host. Giulino and colleagues reviewed the results in 71 children with PTLD who were treated with weekly doses of rituximab for 1 to 9 weeks, and they noted a 70% CR rate.[100] A phase-two COG study combining rituximab with cyclophosphamide and prednisone for the treatment of PTLD is currently under way.

Neuroblastoma cells constitutively express a surface ganglioside, GD2, which has been the target of several MoAb-based immunotherapy trials. Kushner and colleagues used 3F8, an anti-GD2 IgG_3 murine MoAb, in combination with GM-CSF, to treat 19 neuroblastoma patients who had failed to achieve CR with induction chemotherapy.[101] Following the 3F8 + GM-CSF treatment, neuroblastoma cells were eradicated from the bone marrow in 80% of patients with marrow involvement. Of the 19 patients, 11 developed progressive disease, and 8 remained progression-free in a median follow-up of 15 months. Cheung and colleagues reported treating 136 neuroblastoma patients with multiagent chemotherapy followed by immunotherapy with 3F8 and GM-CSF.[102] Allelic polymorphisms for $Fc\gamma RII$-A were also characterized on the basis of which amino acid was present at position 131. Using an enzyme-linked immunosorbent assay, 3F8 demonstrated preferential binding to the $Fc\gamma RII$-A-R131 (R, arginine) allotype, compared with the $Fc\gamma RII$-A-H131 (H, histidine) allotype. Patients could be classified into three different genotypes (H/H, H/R, or R/R) depending on their inherited $Fc\gamma RII$-A alleles. It is interesting that the 5-year progression-free survival rate was 52% for patients with the R/R genotype compared to 29% for patients bearing the H/H or H/R genotype. When the analysis was restricted to a subgroup of patients who had not relapsed prior to study entry, the progression-free survival rate was 65% for R/R patients compared to 36% for H/H or H/R patients. These data suggest that treatment with 3F8 and GM-CSF was associated with an antitumor effect, possibly mediated by the induction of ADCC by GM-CSF–stimulated PMNs and macrophages.

A phase 2 study using the chimeric anti-GD2 MoAb, ch14.18, in combination with GM-CSF, was conducted through the Pediatric Oncology Group. Thirty patients with neuroblastoma were enrolled in the study; all of them had been heavily pretreated. The 1-year event-free survival and overall survival rates were 17% and 33%, respectively. One child achieved CR, three achieved partial responses, and two had mixed responses. Toxicities were manageable and included neuropathic pain, fever, rash, and transient thrombocytopenia. Collectively, data concerning 3F8 and ch14.18 support the use of anti-GD2 MoAb therapy in children with neuroblastoma but also suggest that this treatment is most effective if administered prior to disease progression, ideally in the setting of MRD. This approach was piloted by the COG in the setting of autologous stem cell transplant using ch14.18 together with GM-CSF and IL-2.[103,104] Currently, patients with high-risk neuroblastoma who have undergone intensive cytoreduction by chemotherapy, surgery, radiation therapy, and autologous HSCT are eligible to participate in a phase 3 COG trial of ch14.18 given in alternating cycles with GM-CSF or IL-2. This study should help to determine the clinical value of incorporating anti-GD2 immunotherapy into the initial treatment regimen for children with high-risk neuroblastoma.

Epratuzumab is an IgG_1 humanized anti-CD22 MoAb that is being evaluated in children and adults for the treatment of B cell malignancies. CD22 is a transmembrane sialoglycoprotein that is expressed on B-lineage lymphocytes. It appears to be involved with CD19 and B-cell antigen receptor (BCR) signal transduction and cell death induced by B-cell antigen receptors, and it serves as an intercellular adhesion molecule.[105] Consequently, CD22 helps regulate B-cell function, proliferation, and survival and is an appealing target for antibody-based immunotherapy. Preclinical studies have shown that epratuzumab is able to induce phosphorylation of CD22, modulate the BCR, and facilitate moderate ADCC. In addition, modulation of CD22 upon binding to anti-CD22 MoAbs may induce apoptosis.[106,107] Hence, the therapeutic efficacy of epratuzumab may be related to alteration of B-cell function or direct elimination of B cells by induction of apoptosis. Epratuzumab has been tested as a single agent and in combination with chemotherapy in adult patients with recurrent aggressive and indolent B-cell NHL and in newly diagnosed patients with diffuse large B-cell lymphoma.[105] Epratuzumab has also been used with rituximab to treat B-cell malignancies. Micallef and colleagues reported administering epratuzumab and rituximab in combination with CHOP (cyclophosphamide, doxorubicin, vincristine, and prednisone) chemotherapy to 15 patients with diffuse large B-cell lymphoma.[108] The 2-year disease-free survival (DFS) was 86% in this small patient cohort. Because CD22 is widely expressed on B-cell precursor ALL, epratuzumab is currently undergoing phase 2 testing in a COG trial for relapsed childhood CD22+ ALL. The MoAb is being administered as a single agent every 4 days for four doses during a reduction phase, followed by four additional doses in combination with induction chemotherapy. Preliminary data demonstrate that epratuzumab is well tolerated when administered alone and in combination with chemotherapy. Of 12 patients completing the reduction phase of therapy, 8 had stable disease, 2 had minimal responses, and 2 progressed. Flow cytometry performed within 24 hours of drug administration revealed absence of CD22+ leukemic blasts in the peripheral blood, demonstrating effective targeting of CD22 by epratuzumab.

Human epidermal growth factor receptor 2 (HER2) is a proto-oncogene that encodes a transmembrane tyrosine kinase, which is overexpressed in a number of adult malignancies, including breast and ovarian carcinoma. Amplification of HER2/*neu* has been associated with an aggressive tumor phenotype and poor overall survival rates. Signal transduction by HER2 is thought primarily to involve the phosphatidylinositol 3-kinase (PI3K) and mitogen-activated protein kinase (MAPK) cascades.[109,110] Signaling through HER2 also appears to reduce expression of cyclin D and c-myc, resulting in decreased levels of the cyclin-dependent kinase inhibitor p27kip1 and increased cellular proliferation.[111,112] Trastuzumab is a recombinant humanized MoAb that recognizes an extracellular epitope on the HER2 protein. Binding of trastuzumab to HER2 + tumor cells causes internalization of the HER2 receptor, with consequent inhibition of downstream signaling through the PI3K and MAPK cascades. Trastuzumab may also eliminate tumor targets by facilitating ADCC. Several clinical trials for patients with metastatic breast cancer have documented responses to trastuzumab when used as a single agent, although the MoAb appears to be more effective when combined with chemotherapy. Furthermore, incorporation of trastuzumab into the treatment regimen of early-stage breast cancer has led to improved rates of freedom from disease and improved overall survival rates.[113] The relevance to pediatric oncology stems from the observation that some patients with osteosarcoma appear to overexpress HER2. The clinical significance of HER2 amplification in osteosarcoma remains controversial; some, but not all, analyses demonstrate that HER2 expression is inversely associated with response to chemotherapy and survival.[114,115] A phase 2 trial using trastuzumab in combination with cisplatin, doxorubicin, methotrexate, ifosfamide, and etoposide in patients with metastatic HER2-amplified osteosarcoma was recently conducted through the COG. After a loading dose of 4 mg/kg, trastuzumab was administered weekly at a dose of 2 mg/kg for up to 34 weeks. Efficacy data from this study are not yet available, but the trastuzumab was well tolerated, with only 1 of 41 patients developing a transient, asymptomatic decrease in cardiac function. Further prospective studies will be required to elucidate the role of trastuzumab in the treatment of HER2-amplified osteosarcoma.

Immunotoxins

Immunotoxins (see Fig. 7-5) combine the specificity of MoAbs with powerful cellular poisons that usually are derived from plants or microorganisms. They consist of a cellular recognition domain (the antibody moiety); a translocation domain that facilitates migration through the cell membrane into the cytosol; and a death domain that arrests protein synthesis, typically by damaging ribosomes or inactivating elongation factor 2. Initially, immunotoxins were produced by chemically conjugating native toxins to MoAbs.[116] The resulting molecules were heterogeneous and relatively unstable, and they demonstrated undesirable binding to normal tissue. Second-generation immunotoxins were also created by chemical conjugation, but removal of the toxins' native cell recognition domain resulted in reduced nonspecific binding and improved tolerability. Third-generation immunotoxins use recombinant DNA technology to replace the toxins' cell-binding domain with the MoAb antigen-recognition moiety, resulting in highly homogeneous reagents. Immunotoxins are large molecules that diffuse poorly into solid tumors, so their main utility may lie in the treatment of leukemias and lymphomas. Immunotoxins have been developed to target a variety of hematopoietic tissue antigens, including the IL-2 and GM-CSF receptors, CD19, CD22, CD30, and CD33. Two immunotoxins relevant to pediatric oncology are Combotox and gemtuzumab ozogamicin.

Combotox is a 1:1 mixture of 2 immunotoxins prepared from deglycosylated ricin A chain (dgA) conjugated to monoclonal antibodies directed against CD22 (RFB4-dgA) and CD19 (HD37-dgA). Combining the two immunotoxins was more effective than either agent administered separately in a severe combined immunodeficiency (SCID) mouse model for disseminated B-cell lymphoma,[117] possibly by preventing the emergence of antigen-negative clones. A phase 1 trial of Combotox was conducted in 22 adult patients with refractory B-cell lymphoma.[118] The drug was administered as a continuous infusion over 8 days at a dose of 10, 20, or 30 mg/m^2. Patients who had circulating lymphoma cells (>50/mm^3) tolerated the highest dose level, whereas a safe dose level could not be established in patients not harboring circulating tumor. The main toxicities reported were vascular leak syndrome and hemolytic uremic syndrome, which accounted for two deaths. A strong association was observed between risk for mortality and prior stem cell transplantation or exposure to radiotherapy. Conceivably, prior treatment with high-dose chemotherapy or radiation caused endothelial injury that increased the risk for vascular leak syndrome and hemolytic uremic syndrome following immunotoxin therapy. Two patients achieved partial responses and five had minor responses to the Combotox regimen. A clinical trial incorporating Combotox into the treatment schema for recurrent pediatric ALL is currently being planned by the COG.

Gemtuzumab ozogamicin (GO; Mylotarg) is a recombinant humanized IgG4 murine anti-CD33 MoAb (hP67.6) that has been chemically linked to calicheamicin, a highly cytotoxic antibiotic. Upon binding to CD33+ cells, GO is rapidly internalized, the calicheamicin is released and mediates sequence-specific DNA double-stranded breaks, resulting in cell death. CD33 is expressed on approximately 90% of AML blasts but not on resting hematopoietic stem cells or other nonhematopoietic tissues.[119] Sievers and colleagues conducted a phase I trial in 40 patients with relapsed or refractory AML and determined the maximum tolerated dose to be 9 mg/m^2.[120] Toxicities included myelosuppression and infusion-related fever and chills. Phase 2 studies were conducted in 142 patients with AML in first relapse, and the overall response rate was 30%.[121] Myelosuppression was commonly observed, and 30% of patients developed infectious complications. Hepatic toxicity also occurred; veno-occlusive disease occurred in 3% of patients (and was fatal in two cases). GO is currently approved by the Food and Drug Administration as monotherapy for elderly patients with relapsed AML. In pediatric oncology, investigations have focused on combining GO with chemotherapy for children with recurrent and newly diagnosed CD33+ AML. A phase 1 study was conducted through the COG for children with recurrent or refractory AML.[122] A single dose of GO was given together with high doses of cytarabine (ARA-C, 12 gm/m^2) and L-asparaginase (6000 IU/m^2) or ARA-C (8 gm/m^2) and mitoxantrone (48 mg/m^2). The maximum tolerated dose of GO was 2 mg/m^2 when combined with high-dose ARA-C/L-asparaginase, and it was 3 mg/m^2 when combined with mitoxantrone/ARA-C. CR plus complete response with partial recovery of platelet count rates of 52% and 40% ware observed in the mitoxantrone/ARA-C and high-dose ARA-C/L-asparaginase arms, respectively. The COG also completed a pilot trial in which patients newly diagnosed with AML were treated with GO in combination with Medical Research Council-based chemotherapy. GO (3 mg/m^2) was administered during the induction and consolidation phases of chemotherapy (two doses total). A CR rate of 84% was documented at the end of induction, and appeared superior to that achieved in the prior AML trial (COG 2961), although a longer follow-up period is required before any definitive conclusions can be drawn. The treatment-related mortality rate was lower than expected, and the incidence of veno-occlusive disease was 3%. A phase 3 trial examining the use of GO in patients newly diagnosed with AML is currently being conducted by the COG, and it should help to elucidate the role of this immunotoxin for the treatment of de novo AML.

Denileukin diftitox (Ontak) is classified as an immunotoxin, even though it is created by replacing the cell-binding domain of diphtheria toxin with IL-2, and therefore targets cells expressing high levels of the IL-2 receptor. It has been used mainly to treat adults with hematologic malignancies, including cutaneous T-cell lymphoma, chronic lymphocytic leukemia, B- and T-cell NHL, and mycosis fungoides.[123-127] Denileukin diftitox has also been used to bolster the immune response to cancer vaccines through the elimination of T_{regs}. Another use of denileukin diftitox has been in the treatment of steroid-refractory acute GVHD; complete response rates of 50% to 59% were reported.[128,129]

Radioimmunoconjugates

Clinical experience with radioimmunoconjugates in pediatric oncology is quite limited, although they have many attractive attributes as anticancer reagents. The antibody directs radioactivity to the tumor bed and to metastatic sites, and there is relative sparing of normal tissues. In addition, radioimmunoconjugates do not rely upon host effector mechanisms or require cellular internalization to mediate cytotoxicity. Furthermore, antigen-negative cancer cells can be eliminated through an innocent-bystander effect caused by radiation crossfiring (see Fig. 7-4). Beta emitters, such as iodine-131 (^{131}I) and yttrium-90 (^{90}Y), have often been used for radioimmunotherapy because they produce particle emissions ranging from approximately 1 to 5 mm, which is suitable for the treatment of macroscopic disease. ^{131}I was one of the first radionuclides used for radioimmunotherapy because it is readily available, and techniques for iodinating antibodies have been well established. An advantage of ^{131}I antibody conjugates is that they emit both γ and β particles and can therefore be used for tumor detection and dosimetry in addition to radioimmunotherapy. A disadvantage of using ^{131}I radioimmunoconjugates to treat cancer is that they undergo enzymatic dehalogenation after patient infusion, resulting in free ^{131}I that can accumulate in normal tissues, such as thyroid, stomach, and salivary glands. In addition, if the radioimmunoconjugate induces antigenic modulation, further dehalogenation and exocytosis will occur, thereby reducing the radiation dose delivered to tumor. ^{90}Y radioimmunoconjugates are more stable and have a longer path length (5 mm vs. 1 mm)

and a higher energy (2.3 MeV vs. 0.6 MeV) than iodinated conjugates, theoretically making them better suited to treat larger tumor volumes. However, the longer particle length of ^{90}Y may increase radiation exposure of normal tissues, especially when targeting microscopic disease, and accumulation in cortical bone and liver has resulted in dose-limiting toxicities. Furthermore, ^{90}Y emits only β particles and is therefore not suitable for tumor imaging or dosimetry. Consequently, a surrogate isotope such as indium-111 must be used for these purposes. More recently, ^{64}Cu, a positron emission tomography contrast isotope, has been conjugated with a novel chelator to tumor reactive MoAbs and used preclinically for very precise immunolocalization and diagnostic studies.[130]

Some pediatric experience using radioimmunoconjugates has been in the treatment of neuroblastoma. A phase 1 trial of ^{131}I-3F8 was conducted at Memorial Sloan-Kettering Cancer Center.[131] The main toxicity encountered was myelosuppression; 22 of 23 patients required autologous stem cell support. Other side effects included infusion-related pain, fever, and diarrhea. The average radiation dose to tumor was calculated to be 150 rad/mCi/kg, and the total body radiation dose was estimated to be 500 to 700 cGy. Of 10 patients evaluable for response, 2 achieved CR from bone marrow disease and 2 achieved partial responses of soft tissue disease. This radioimmunoconjugate was subsequently incorporated into the initial treatment regimen for children with newly diagnosed high-risk neuroblastoma.[131] Patients received intensive multiagent chemotherapy, surgery, hyperfractionated external beam radiotherapy, radioimmunology using ^{131}I-3F8 at a dose of 20 mCi/kg followed by autologous stem cell rescue, and subsequent treatment with unlabeled 3F8. Of 42 patients enrolled, 35 completed radioimmunology. The main toxicities associated with ^{131}I-3F8 included myelosuppression, fever, and hypothyroidism. The overall survival rate was 40% in this very high-risk patient population.

Radionuclides have also been conjugated to anti-CD20 MoAbs for the treatment of B-cell lymphomas. ^{90}Y ibritumomab (^{90}Y Zevalin) was approved by the Food and Drug Administration in 2002 for the treatment of relapsed or refractory B-cell non-Hodgkin's lymphoma. In a phase 1/2 trial, Witzig and colleagues determined the maximum tolerated dose of ^{90}Y ibritumomab to be 0.4 mCi/kg (0.3 mCi/kg for patients with mild thrombocytopenia).[132] The overall response rate for patients with low-grade NHL was 82%; the rate of complete cure was 26%. A phase 3 trial was conducted comparing ^{90}Y ibritumomab to rituximab in 143 patients with relapsed or refractory follicular lymphoma, low-grade nonfollicular lymphoma, or transformed lymphoma.[133] The overall response rate was superior in the ^{90}Y ibritumomab arm (80% vs. 56%, $P = 0.002$), although the median time to progression and response duration were similar for both treatment groups. A phase 1 trial for pediatric patients with relapsed or refractory CD20$^+$ lymphomas was conducted through the COG. Patients were pretreated with rituximab 250 mg/m^2 (to eliminate normal CD20$^+$ cells); that was followed by infusion of ^{111}In ibritumomab for dosimetry. Patients who achieved a radiation dose of less than 2000 cGy to normal organs and less than 300 cGy to bone marrow, based on dosimetry calculations, were given a second dose of rituximab followed by ^{90}Y ibritumomab 1 day later. Children estimated to have good marrow reserves (and normal platelet counts) received a dose of 0.4 mCi/kg, whereas children who previously had undergone a stem cell transplant received a dose of 0.1 mCi/kg. All five patients enrolled in the study were able to receive their planned therapeutic doses of ^{90}Y ibritumomab, and dose-limiting toxicities were not observed. Unfortunately, the study was closed prematurely because of slow accrual.

^{131}I tositumomab (Bexxar) has also been used to treat patients with relapsed or refractory NHL. Vose and colleagues reported a phase 2 multicenter study in which ^{131}I tositumomab was administered to 57 heavily pretreated patients with indolent or transformed NHL.[134] An overall response rate of 57% was observed; with a CR rate of 32%. Of the patients achieving CR, the median response duration was 19.9 months. When administered to less heavily pretreated patients with indolent or transformed NHL in first or second relapse, ^{131}I tositumomab produced overall and complete response rates of 76% and 49%, respectively. Of patients achieving CR, the median remission duration exceeded 3.1 years. Notably, these responses were achieved following a treatment regimen completed in little more than 1 week. A phase 3 study conducted in 78 relapsed NHL patients compared ^{131}I tositumomab to unlabeled tositumomab.[135] As might be expected, patients treated with ^{131}I tositumomab had overall and complete response rates (55% and 33%) that were superior to those of patients treated with the naked antibody (33% and 8%). The use of ^{131}I tositumomab has thus far not been reported in pediatric patients.

Other radioimmunoconjugates that could potentially be used to treat pediatric hematologic malignancies include ^{131}I HD37 (anti-CD19, ALL); ^{131}I or ^{90}Y epratuzumab (anti-CD22, ALL); ^{131}I BC8 (anti-CD45, AML, and ALL); ^{131}I or [90]Y HuM195 (anti-CD33, AML); and ^{131}I or [90]Y Lym-1 (anti-HLA-DR, NHL). Radioimmunoconjugates that could be used to treat pediatric solid tumors include ^{131}I IMMU-30 (anti-α fetoprotein, hepatoblastoma, and germ cell tumors); ^{131}I UJ181 (anti-L1, primitive neuroectodermal tumors); and [131]I 81C6 (antitenascin, high-grade gliomas).

Immunocytokines

Tumor-reactive MoAbs have also been linked to cytokines, such as IL-2, GM-CSF, and IL-12, to activate effector cells at the microenvironment of tumors in vivo because the cytokines are delivered by the antibody.[136-138] In preclinical studies these reagents mediate far greater antitumor effects than equimolar amounts of the MoAb and the cytokine infused simultaneously but not conjugated. These preclinical data indicate that the MoAb-cytokine fusion protein brings the cytokine to the tumor microenvironment, where it can act locally and further activate antitumor effector cells. Preclinical and clinical testing has proceeded with an immunocytokine that has linked IL-2 to a MoAb that recognizes the epithelial cell adhesion molecule expressed on adult epithelial cancers (KS-IL2),[139] and a separate immunocytokine that has linked IL-2 to a humanized anti-GD2 MoAb (hu14.18-IL2).[140] The latter has been used in phase 1 trials in melanoma and neuroblastoma[141,142] and is currently being evaluated by the COG in an ongoing phase 2 trial.[143]

Bifunctional and Trifunctional Monoclonal Antibodies

A separate strategy has created antibody conjugates that link two separate MoAbs together. One MoAb recognizes the tumor-associated antigen on the tumor cell. The other MoAb recognizes an activating determinant on effector cells, such as CD3 on T cells or CD-16 on NK cells.[144,145] When these antibody conjugates bind simultaneously to tumor and effector cells, they induce membrane contact between the two cells and effector activation of lytic pathways that cause destruction of the tumor cell. These bifunctional reagents can be made by conjugating the two separate MoAbs together. Alternatively, some bifunctional antibodies are made by fusing two separate hybridomas to create a "quadroma." These quadromas produce each individual MoAb as well as the bifunctional heteroantibody, consisting of an immunoglobulin that has one heavy chain from one hybridoma and a second heavy chain from the other. When these bifunctional antibodies are purified, they have a functional Fc component, and thus have been designated trifunctional reagents.[146] Clinical trials have used these bifunctional reagents as drugs that can be infused. Alternatively, they have been used to arm effector cells (T cells or NK cells) ex vivo, prior to their infusion.

Nonmonoclonal Antibody Immunoconjugates

Several fusion proteins that are being entered into clinical tests involve toxins selectively carried to tumor cells by recognition molecules other than MoAbs. These include hormones and growth factors that are specifically recognized by receptors on tumor cells. For example, a truncated diphtheria toxin can be linked to human granulocyte-macrophage colony–stimulating factor (GM-CSF), maintaining the binding specificity of the GM-CSF to its receptor and the toxic activity of the diphtheria toxin for cells that internalize it.[147] These molecules are able to mediate selective destruction in vitro and in vivo of cells with GM-CSF receptors, including AML cells. Clinical testing of these molecules and those like them (e.g., IL-2 linked to diphtheria toxin for IL-2 receptor-bearing T-cell malignancies) are under way.[148]

Use of Monoclonal Antibodies to Redirect Effector Cells

The goal of the bifunctional and trifunctional MoAbs just described is to redirect T cells and NK cells to mediate destruction of tumors recognized by the antibody. This same goal can be achieved through the genetic engineering of endogenous T or NK cells. Originally proposed by Eshhar and colleagues as T-cell bodies,[149] several teams have transfected T cells or NK cells with plasmids that have linked the Fab component of a tumor reactive MoAb to the transmembrane and cytoplasmic domain of the CD3 or CD16 triggering receptor. The resultant T cells or NK cells can use these newly acquired artificial receptors to recognize the tumor antigen seen by the MoAb and then trigger the antitumor effector mechanisms of the T cell or NK cell. Clinical approaches to this concept are being tested, particularly in the setting of neuroblastoma.[150-155] These trials require ex vivo transfection of the endogenous T or NK cells, followed by ex vivo propagation and activation prior to their in vivo use. The infusion of this large population of autologous effector cells into cancer patients can be considered a form of adoptive immunotherapy, a treatment modality that is receiving increasing attention in both the autologous and allogeneic settings.

ADOPTIVE CELLULAR IMMUNOTHERAPY: AUTOLOGOUS

Adoptive T-Cell Therapy

The generation of cytotoxic lymphocytes (CTLs) against autologous tumor antigens has proven to be a complex and difficult task. Most tumors are weakly immunogenic, exist in a microenvironment that may impede immune function, and can develop multiple pathways of resistance to immune-mediated cytolysis. Using CTLs for cancer immunotherapy requires the isolation, activation (to break self-tolerance), and expansion of immune effector cells, while preserving their specificity and function. This approach has greatly benefited from the genetic modification of T cells to enhance antigen recognition, costimulation, trafficking to tumor, and survival.

Autologous lymphocytes may be obtained directly from the tumor, from the peripheral blood by leukopheresis, or from draining lymph nodes. Selection of T-cell clones demonstrating antitumor reactivity may be achieved by flow cytometry or by magnetic cell sorting using bispecific antibodies and peptide-MHC tetramers.[156] Alternatively, generation of T cells for adoptive immunotherapy may be accomplished by repetitive stimulation of peripheral blood mononuclear cells by APCs that have been pulsed with antigenic peptides, recombinant proteins, or tumor lysates or transfected by genes encoding tumor antigens. T cells may also be genetically modified to alter their antigen specificity by introducing genes encoding the α and β chains of the TCR. A limitation of this approach is that tumor recognition is still mediated by the MHC-restricted TCR, and neoplasms can thereby evade immune destruction through downregulation of class I and II HLA molecules. Furthermore, the TCR recognizes only protein antigens, whereas tumors may display important glycolipid or carbohydrate moieties that could be used as targets for immunotherapy. To overcome these obstacles, T cells have been transfected with genes encoding chimeric antigen receptors, which consist of a tumor antigen-recognition domain and an intracellular signaling domain capable of inducing T-cell activation. Chimeric antigen receptors have been developed to target a wide variety of cancers, including B-cell malignancies and neuroblastoma.[157]

T cells may be modified in other ways to augment their cytolytic function, proliferation, and survival. T-cell function can be enhanced by increasing expression of co-stimulatory molecules, such as CD28 and OX40, or by down-regulating inhibitory receptors, such as the transforming growth factor-β (TGF-β) receptor.[158-162] TGF-β mediates T-cell growth arrest, inhibits effector cell function, and promotes the development of T_{regs}, which collectively dampen the immune response.[163] T cells can be modified to express dominant-negative TGF-β receptors, rendering them less susceptible to inhibition by TGF-β–mediated pathways. The adoptive transfer of murine T cells, transduced with dominant-negative TGF-β receptors into TGF-β–expressing tumor-bearing mice, resulted in preferential tumor infiltration and persistence of the modified clones.[164]

T-cell proliferative capacity may be improved by transducing T cells with genes encoding stimulatory cytokines, such as IL-2.[165] In fact, the use of IL-2 transduced tumor infiltrating lymphocytes by Rosenberg and colleagues was perhaps the first clinical application of genetically modified T cells to treat patients who have cancer.[166] T-cell survival has been enhanced by inhibition of Fas expression through genetic transfer of small interfering RNA, which can render T cells resistant to apoptosis by tumors expressing Fas ligand.[167] Other manipulations that may enhance T-cell survival include transduction with anti-apoptotic genes, such as Bcl-2 and Bcl-$_{XL}$ or with genes encoding cytokines that promote survival (e.g., IL-7, IL-15, IL-21).[168-170] Hsu demonstrated that T cells engineered with a codon-optimized IL-15 gene maintained expression of Bcl-2 and Bcl-$_{XL}$ and were resistant to apoptosis after withdrawal of IL-2.[171]

Once CTLs have been isolated, they must be expanded ex vivo in order to obtain sufficient cells for clinical use. This has traditionally been accomplished by incubation with cytokines (e.g., IL-2) and stimulatory molecules such as CD3 and CD28. It is important that the expansion process not significantly impair T-cell specificity, function, survival, or trafficking to tumor. Once infused, it may be possible to augment the antitumor activity of adoptively transferred cells by modifying the hosts' immunologic milieu. One strategy being explored involves

the elimination of T_{regs} utilizing MoAbs that target T_{reg}-associated molecules, including the glucocorticoid-induced TNF receptor family molecule (GITR) and CD25.[163] Another approach under investigation exploits endogenous host mechanisms to maintain lymphocyte homeostasis. Lymphodepletion of the patient prior to adoptive immunotherapy creates an environment favoring proliferation of the infused cells, possibly through increased availability of homeostatic cytokines, such as IL-7 and IL-15, by reducing the number of host cells consuming these molecules (cytokine sinks). Lymphodepletion may be accomplished by the administration of immunosuppressive chemotherapeutic agents such as cyclophosphamide and fludarabine, radiation, or by the use of MoAbs targeting antigens ubiquitously expressed on leukocytes (i.e., CD45). It is interesting to note that Wrzesinski and colleagues recently described a murine model in which the administration of hematopoietic stem cells to lymphodepleted hosts promoted the function and expansion of infused CTLs with antitumor specificity.[172] The authors postulated that increased production of cytokines by the stem cells promoted expansion of CTLs, but it is possible that other mechanisms such as the generation of APCs derived from hematopoietic stem cells were involved.[173]

Adoptive T-Cell Therapy to Treat Pediatric Malignancies

There have been very few clinical trials using autologous T cells to treat pediatric cancer. One disorder affecting children that is associated with a strong antigenic target is PTLD, which is caused by EBV reactivation in profoundly immunodeficient patients, including immunosuppressed recipients of allogeneic organ transplants (i.e., bone marrow, kidney, liver, heart, and lung). The B-cell lymphoid proliferations in this disorder appear to be morphologically malignant and often start as oligoclonal expansions of transformed B cells. If an effective T-cell immune system were present, EBV-reactive T cells would readily recognize the numerous strong peptide antigens encoded by the EBV genome and expressed in these transformed B cells, thereby destroying them. Thus, for patients receiving immunosuppressive drugs who develop an EBV-induced PTLD, the first step toward controlling the neoplasia is tapering the immunosuppressive therapy. For some, this has allowed reactivation of T cells able to recognize and destroy the transformed B-cell clones. If the patient's immunosuppressive therapy cannot be adequately decreased, efforts to expand the number of EBV-reactive T cells in vitro, followed by their clinical infusion, has provided antitumor reactivity and clinical protection in some trials. Savoldo and colleagues generated CTLs against the EBV from the PBMC of 35 solid-organ transplant recipients, the majority of whom were children, for the prophylaxis or treatment of PTLD.[174] None of the 10 patients who received prophylactic EBV-CTL developed PTLD, despite being classified as being at high risk for this complication, and 2 patients treated for PTLD showed evidence of clinical response. The use of cytotoxic MoAbs directed against B-cell antigens, such as CD20, has also helped to eradicate EBV-transformed B cells in patients with PTLD (see the earlier material concerning Naked MoAbs).

An EBV-targeted strategy has also been used for patients with EBV-associated Hodgkin's disease. Bollard and colleagues reported infusing autologous EBV-CTL into 14 mainly adult patients with relapsed EBV-positive Hodgkin's disease.[175] Gene-marking studies demonstrated that the infused CTLs expanded several logs in vivo, trafficked to tumor, and persisted for up to 1 year. Of the 14 patients, 5 remain in CR, with a median follow-up of 27 months, and 2 of them had measurable lymphoma at the time CTLs were infused. One additional patient achieved a partial response, and 5 experienced disease stabilization for varying amounts of time.

Adoptive Therapy Using Natural Killer Cells

In the 1980s and 1990s investigators explored the use of lymphokine-activated killer (LAK) cells to treat a variety of malignancies. LAK cells, which consist mainly of CD56+ NK cells, were activated in vitro with IL-2, infused into patients, and then maintained in an activated state by in vivo administration of IL-2. Some patients with metastatic melanoma or renal cell carcinoma responded quite well to this type of adoptive immunotherapy, although the approach was not very effective against most other cancers, and significant toxicities were encountered. The lack of clinical efficacy possibly was related to inhibition of NK-cell function mediated by KIR-KIR (killer cell immunoglobulin-like receptor) ligand interactions, lack of stimulatory signals, and the ability of tumors to develop resistance to perforin/granzyme and other cytotoxic pathways used by NK cells. Interest in autologous LAK-cell therapy has waned, but this approach may still prove useful for cancer treatment when combined with other immunotherapeutic strategies. For example, Berdeja and colleagues administered LAK cells, IL-2, and rituximab to patients with CD20+ lymphomas who were known to be resistant to rituximab therapy.[176] LAK-cell infusions augmented ADCC and prevented the decline in ADCC seen after rituximab treatment when the MoAb was used alone.

It is possible that autologous NK cell therapy may prove most beneficial for patients bearing specific immunogenetic phenotypes. The genes encoding KIRs and their corresponding HLA class I ligands segregate independently, so some patients may express a KIR gene but not its cognate ligand. The NK cells of such individuals would potentially be more autoreactive and perhaps better equipped to eradicate tumor. Leung and colleagues evaluated KIR and HLA class I typing in 16 children with lymphoma or solid tumor undergoing autologous HSCT.[177] The probability of post-transplant disease recurrence was 83% for patients exhibiting no KIR-KIR ligand mismatching, compared to 50% and 0% for patients lacking one or two of the corresponding KIR ligands, respectively. These data suggest that NK cells facilitate elimination of minimal residual disease in autologous transplant recipients, but the ability to mediate tumor eradication is largely dependent on the patient's KIR-KIR ligand phenotype.

Adoptive Therapy Using Cytokine-Induced Killer Cells

Cytokine-induced killer (CIK) cells are CD3+ CD56+ cells generated from bone marrow or PBMC by culturing lymphocytes with IFN-γ, OKT-3 (anti-CD3), and IL-2. They are derived from T lymphocytes, rather than from de novo NKT cells, and can mediate non-MHC restricted killing of leukemia, lymphoma, and some solid tumor cell lines.[178] CIK cells generated from patients with AML and CML show cytolytic activity against autologous blasts.[179,180] In a SCID mouse model for CML, animals infused with CIK cells demonstrated a markedly improved clearance of bcr-abl+ tumor compared to control animals not receiving immunotherapy. Unfortunately, ALL cells appeared to be relatively resistant to CIK-mediated killing. However, Marin and colleagues generated CIK cells from the bone marrow of children with B-lineage ALL and then transfected the cells with anti-CD19 chimeric receptor retroviral vectors.[181] CIK cells transfected with anti-CD19 and costimulatory molecules such as CD28 or 4-1BB demonstrated potent cytotoxic activity against ALL cell lines.

Clinical experience in using CIK cells for cancer therapy is currently limited. Leemhuis and colleagues conducted a phase 1 study using CIK cells in nine patients with Hodgkin's disease or NHL who failed autologous HSCT.[182] Four patients achieved partial responses or stabilization of disease, and toxicity was minimal. A trial using IL-2–transfected CIK cells in patients with metastatic colon cancer, renal cell carcinoma, or lymphoma was reported; one patient achieved CR.[183] CIK cells have also been administered to patients with gastric cancer and hepatocellular carcinoma.[184,185]

ALLOGENEIC

The Graft Versus Leukemia Reaction

Bone marrow transplantation has frequently been used to treat patients with very high-risk or relapsed hematologic malignancies. Initially, it was believed the transplanted cells served only to reconstitute hematopoiesis after patients were treated with ablative chemoradiotherapy. However, as early as 1956, Barnes and colleagues noted that allogeneic recognition of leukemia cells might be required to cure animals in a murine transplant model.[186] In 1979, Weiden and colleagues observed that patients who had undergone bone marrow transplantation and developed GVHD had a significantly lower risk for leukemic relapse than did patients who did not develop this complication, suggesting that immunologic mechanisms mediated by donor-derived effector cells could facilitate the eradication of tumor.[187] The existence of a GVL effect in humans was confirmed by retrospectively analyzing data from the International Bone Marrow Transplant Registry. Horowitz and co-workers reported a higher risk for leukemic relapse in recipients of identical twin (syngeneic) grafts than in patients receiving HLA-matched allogeneic grafts (Fig. 7-11).[188] An increased probability of leukemic relapse was also noted in patients who did not develop clinically significant GVHD and in recipients of T-cell–depleted grafts. Collectively, these data indicated that T lymphocytes contained within the stem cell graft were capable of recognizing alloantigen presented by leukemia cells and of mounting a potent cytotoxic response that reduced the incidence of leukemic relapse. It is interesting to note that although the probability of relapse inversely correlated with the extent of GVHD, overall survival was lower among patients with severe (grades III or IV) GVHD because of increased transplant-related mortality rates. However, the development of mild GVHD was associated with superior survival, underscoring the delicate balance between immune-mediated tumor destruction by donor cells and the morbidity and mortality resulting from recognition of alloantigen on normal tissues. Separation of GVL from GVHD has been the focus of much scientific investigation, yet it remains an elusive goal.

Although many different lymphocyte populations are likely to be involved in the GVL response, several lines of evidence suggest that helper T cells play a pivotal role. CD4 cells isolated from patients or donors after allogeneic bone marrow transplantation are capable of lysing cryopreserved allogeneic leukemia cells.[189,190] In addition, transplants utilizing CD8-depleted marrow grafts have been associated with a lower risk for GVHD without a concomitant increase in leukemic relapse.[191] Moreover, patients with CML relapsing after allogeneic transplantation commonly achieved a second CR following treatment by CD8-depleted donor lymphocyte infusions or by escalating doses of donor CD4 cells.[192,193] However, several murine transplant models also support a role for CD8 cells in promoting

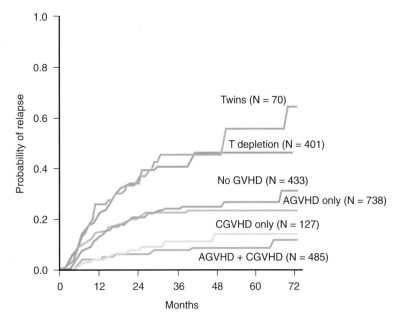

FIGURE 7-11. Actuarial probability of relapse after bone marrow transplantation for leukemia based on the type of graft and development of acute graft-versus-host disease (AGVHD) or chronic graft-versus-host disease (CGVHD). Patients who received syngeneic (identical twin) or T-cell-depleted grafts and those who did not develop GVHD had a significantly increased risk for post-transplant recurrence of their leukemias. Patients who developed both AGVHD and CGVHD had the lowest probability of relapse. Collectively, these data strongly support the existence of a graft-versus-leukemia effect and suggest that donor-derived T lymphocytes are important mediators of this phenomenon. *(Redrawn from Horowitz MM, Gale RP, Sondel PM, et al. Graft versus leukemia reactions after bone marrow transplantation. Blood.1990;75:555-562.)*

GVL activity. Animals receiving CD8-depleted grafts had a higher risk for post-transplant leukemic relapse, whereas the addition of highly purified CD8 cells augmented the GVL effect.[194-196] Furthermore, alloreactive CD8 lymphocytes have been generated in humans, and they demonstrate significant antileukemic activity.[197] γδ T lymphocytes are also capable of destroying leukemia cells and may participate in the GVL phenomenon. Clones of γδ T cells that have been isolated from patients with ALL exhibit potent cytotoxicity against autologous tumor cells.[198] In addition, Malkovska and colleagues reported that infusions of human γδ T cells into SCID mice previously injected with lethal doses of Daudi lymphoma cells significantly prolonged the survival of the animals.[199]

The close association between GVL and GVHD suggests that mHAs play an important role in the immune recognition of leukemic cells following HLA-matched allogeneic transplantation. The mHAs HA-3 and H-Y are expressed on skin-derived fibroblasts, keratinocytes, and hematopoietic tissue and could therefore be responsible for both GVHD and GVL reactions. Other mHAs, such as HA-1 and HA-2, show lineage-restricted expression on hematopoietic tissue and could serve as targets for GVL but would not be expected to trigger GVHD.[200] CTLs generated against such antigens would be attractive reagents for adoptive immunotherapy. Mutis and colleagues were able to create CTLs against HA-1 and HA-2 from healthy donors by using DCs pulsed with synthetic peptides.[201] These clones could be expanded ex vivo and were capable of lysing allogeneic AML and ALL targets. Hematopoietic differentiation antigens, such as CD5, CD19, and CD22, could also potentially initiate a GVL response if aberrantly expressed on leukemia cells. Furthermore, it is conceivable that allelic variations of these antigens could stimulate alloreactivity of donor T cells with consequent immune activation. Leukemia cells may also express neoantigens resulting from chromosomal translocations or point mutations directly involved in leukemogenesis. Examples of such antigens include the PML/RARA and bcr-abl fusion proteins seen in acute promyelocytic leukemia and CML, respectively. Although it is tempting to speculate that such tumor-specific molecules may initiate a GVL reaction, it remains uncertain to what extent these antigens are capable of inducing a clinically meaningful immune response.

Once antigenic determinants on a leukemic clone are recognized by the donor's immune system, tumor-cell eradication can occur through a variety of mechanisms. Both CD4 and CD8 lymphocytes are capable of directly mediating cytotoxicity utilizing perforin/granzyme-B or fas/fas-ligand pathways. CML cells have a greater density of fas molecules on their surface than do normal hematopoietic stem cells, and for this reason they might be especially vulnerable to T-cell–mediated killing.[202,203] CD4 cells can also indirectly facilitate tumor cytotoxicity by secreting cytokines that recruit and activate other immune effectors capable of inducing leukemic cell death. T_H1 cells produce cytokines such as IFN-γ and TNF-α that can directly impede tumor cell growth, but they also secrete IL-2 and IL-12, which activate NK cells and augment their cytolytic function. IL-2 also stimulates T cells in an autocrine loop, which promotes expansion of the alloreactive clones. T_H2 cells function in a helper-regulatory capacity and secrete cytokines such as IL-3, IL-4, and GM-CSF. GM-CSF activates macrophages and monocytes, thereby facilitating antigen presentation and enhancing ADCC.

It is clear that T lymphocytes are important mediators of the GVL phenomenon, but other immune effectors may help to eliminate leukemia cells after allogeneic HSCT, especially when T cells have been depleted from the graft. In a seminal paper, Ruggeri and colleagues reported that patients with AML who received T-cell depleted haploidentical grafts had a markedly improved survival rate if donor NK cells could recognize and attack recipient tissue, a situation referred to as KIR ligand incompatibility.[204] Patients with AML who were KIR ligand mismatched with their donors had a lower probability of leukemic relapse (0% vs. 75%), a lower rate of clinically significant GVHD (0% vs. 14%) and a lower risk for graft rejection (0% vs. 15%). Presumably, donor-derived NK cells not encountering inhibitory KIR ligands were capable of targeting residual leukemia cells, and eradicated recipient APC and lymphocytes resulting in lower rates of GVHD and graft rejection. In this trial, the survival benefit associated with KIR ligand mismatching was restricted to patients afflicted with myeloid malignancies. Leung and colleagues evaluated donor KIR repertoire and host KIR ligand expression in 36 pediatric patients undergoing haploidentical HSCT for hematologic malignancies.[205] Patients whose HLA class I expression would be expected to inhibit donor NK cell activity were classified as being at high risk, whereas patients lacking inhibitory KIR ligands were classified as being at low risk. High-risk patients had a significantly greater probability of leukemic relapse than did low-risk patients (54% vs. 13%). Remarkably, this difference was even more striking when the analysis was limited to patients with ALL (75% vs. 15%; Fig. 7-12), which provides evidence for a potent antileukemic effect mediated by NK cells against both myeloid and lymphoid malignancies.

Although the benefits associated with NK cell alloreactivity appear more pronounced for patients receiving extensively T-cell–depleted haploidentical grafts, NK cells may also influence the outcome of HLA-matched sibling and unrelated donor transplants. Higher numbers of NK cells in the graft have been associated with decreased infection risk, faster immune reconstitution, and improved survival rates for recipients of HLA-matched sibling transplants.[206] The influence of KIR-KIR ligand matching was examined in 178 patients receiving HLA-matched sibling transplants for hematologic malignancies.[207] KIR-KIR ligand compatibility did not appear to affect outcome for patients with ALL or CML; however, a significant effect was seen in patients with AML and myelodysplastic syndrome. The probability of DFS in this cohort directly correlated with the extent of KIR-KIR ligand mismatching. The impact of NK-cell alloreactivity has also been evaluated in 130 patients receiving unrelated donor transplants for hematologic malignancies.[208] The probabilities of overall survival and DFS were 87% and 87% for KIR-ligand–incompatible donor-recipient pairs, compared to 48% and 39% for patients transplanted with KIR-ligand–compatible donors. Furthermore, patients receiving KIR-ligand–incompatible grafts demonstrated a significant reduction in transplant-related mortality rates (6% vs. 40%), at least partly explained by a lower risk for severe GVHD.

It should be noted that not all studies have demonstrated a favorable effect of KIR-ligand mismatching for allogeneic transplant recipients.[209] Variability in study outcomes is probably explained by differences in the modeling systems used to identify NK-cell alloreactivity (e.g., ligand-ligand vs. receptor-ligand) as well as by the methodologies employed to identify KIR expression. For example, the St. Jude team identified a discrepancy between KIR genotyping and phenotyping in 25% of patients tested.[210] Another important factor that appears to modulate the influence of NK-cell alloreactivity is the number of T cells present in the graft. The beneficial effect of activating donor NK cells may be overridden by the deleterious consequences of GVHD resulting from priming donor T cells against class I HLA antigens (Fig. 7-13).

The realization that donor immune effector mechanisms significantly contribute to disease eradication in patients undergoing transplantation for leukemia and lymphoma has led to the use of reduced-intensity conditioning regimens and the infusion of donor lymphocytes post-transplant to prevent relapse or to treat disease recurrence.

Nonmyeloablative Transplants for Leukemia and Lymphoma

Goals of the pretransplant conditioning regimen have traditionally included elimination of malignancy, immunosuppression (to prevent graft rejection), and creation of space within the host's marrow microenvironment to allow for donor stem cell expansion. Unfortunately, the conditioning regimen also causes substantial nonhematopoietic toxicity, which increases transplant-related morbidity and mortality rates. Furthermore, the toxicity of the conditioning regimen limits the ability to offer allogeneic transplantation to elderly patients and those with significant comorbidities. Consequently, many centers have explored the use of reduced-intensity conditioning (RIC) regimens, which are usually nonmyeloablative and cause significantly less damage to normal tissues, resulting in decreased transplant-related morbidity and fewer fatalities.[211,212] The agents utilized in RIC regimens typically have antineoplastic effects, but the main objective is to induce a state of profound immune suppression to facilitate engraftment. Reliance on the GVL effect to control disease requires expansion of antineoplastic alloreactive clones and maturation of the donor's immune system within the transplanted host. The latter process occurs gradually, so the use of nonmyeloablative transplants is generally limited to patients with slowly progressing malignancies or those who have undergone transplantation in a state of minimal residual disease. Most RIC regimens have used low-dose total-body irradiation or reduced doses of alkylating agents in combination with potent immunosuppressive drugs such as fludarabine, with or without anti–T-cell antibodies. Mobilized peripheral blood stem cells are typically used for the transplant in order to maximize the stem cell dose and facilitate engraftment. Donor lymphocyte infusions may be required post-

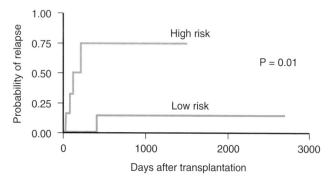

FIGURE 7-12. The actuarial probability of relapse in children with lymphoid malignancies treated by haploidentical stem cell transplantation is markedly diminished if patients lack inhibitory KIR ligands. These data provide compelling evidence for a GVL effect against lymphoblasts mediated by donor NK cells. (*Redrawn from Leung W, Iyengar R, Turner V, et al. Determinants of antileukemia effects of allogeneic NK cells. J Immunol. 2004;172:644-650.*)

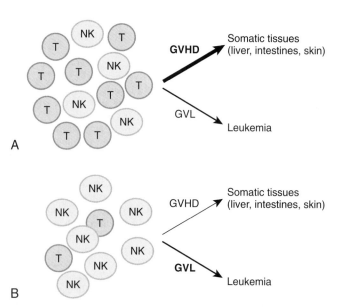

FIGURE 7-13. A, In T-cell–replete transplants, the risk for GVHD may outweigh the benefits derived from a GVL effect, especially if donor and recipient are HLA disparate. B, In T-cell–depleted transplants, the risk of GVHD is significantly reduced, but alloreactive NK cells may still mediate potent GVL activity.

transplant to promote full donor chimerism, which has been associated with a reduced risk for relapse.[213] Immunosuppressive medications, such as cyclosporine and mycophenolate mofetil, are administered for GVHD prophylaxis, but these drugs are tapered rapidly to enhance the GVL effect. RIC transplants may cause less acute GVHD than conventional HSCT transplantation, although the incidence of chronic GVHD appears to be similar.[214] The development of chronic GVHD has been associated with a decreased relapse risk and improved disease-free survival.[213]

Several pediatric malignancies have been treated with RIC regimens. Hegenbart and colleagues reported treating 122 patients who had AML with related (*n* = 58) or unrelated (*n* = 64) donor HSCT using an RIC regimen consisting of fludarabine and 2 Gy total-body irradiation.[215] Overall and progression-free survival at 2 years was 48% and 44%, respectively. Patients in first CR who received transplants from unrelated donors had a significantly lower risk for relapse and improved survival rates than recipients of related-donor grafts, suggesting the greater HLA disparity associated with unrelated-donor transplantation resulted in a stronger antitumor effect. Peggs and colleagues reported treating 49 patients who had Hodgkin's disease using alemtuzumab (Campath 1H), fludarabine, and melphalan.[216] The median number of prior treatment regimens was five, and 44 patients had failed a prior autologous transplant. Beginning 3 months post-transplant, DLI was administered to patients with persistent or progressive disease. Of 16 patients so treated, there were 7 complete and 2 partial responses, providing strong evidence of a therapeutic effect mediated by the donors' immune systems. Overall and DFS probabilities at 4 years were 59% and 39%. The ability to promote engraftment using RIC regimens, which reduce morbidity and transplant-related mortality rates, has led to a renewed interest in exploring the efficacy of allogeneic HSCT to treat patients with solid tumors.

Nonmyeloablative Transplants for Solid Tumors

Most investigations using allogeneic HSCT to treat solid tumors have focused on adult patients with renal cell carcinoma, melanoma or breast cancer. Childs and colleagues treated 19 patients who had refractory metastatic renal cell carcinoma with an RIC regimen consisting of cyclophosphamide and fludarabine, followed by mobilized peripheral blood stem cells from a related donor.[217] Tumor regression was documented in 10 patients, included 3 who had CR. The development of acute GVHD was strongly associated with antitumor responses, providing proof of the principle that allogeneic HSCT can promote regression of solid tumors. Multiple studies have now been conducted using nonmyeloablative HSCT to treat patients with metastatic renal cell carcinoma; response rates range from 0% to 57%.[218] Nonmyeloablative HSCT has also been used to treat patients with metastatic melanoma, but minimal benefit has been documented.[219] Response rates for women with metastatic breast cancer have ranged from 17% to 37%, although relatively few patients achieved durable CR.[220,221] Improving the efficacy of nonmyeloablative HSCT to treat solid tumors is likely to depend on enhancing the graft-versus-tumor response by using post-transplant vaccination strategies or ex vivo expansion and infusion of donor-derived T-cell clones with antitumor specificities (or alloreactive NK cells). In addition, treating patients at the early stages of disease will probably improve outcomes.

Relatively little data exist regarding the use of allogeneic HSCT for the treatment of pediatric solid tumors. Matthay and colleagues treated patients who had high-risk neuroblastomas with myeloablative chemoradiotherapy followed by autologous or allogeneic (for patients with HLA-matched siblings) HSCT.[222] It is surprising to note that allograft recipients did not demonstrate a decreased risk for post-transplant relapse, though no attempt was made to augment a graft-versus-tumor effect by rapid tapering of immunosuppressive therapy or infusion of donor lymphocytes. Case reports successfully using allogeneic HSCT to treat pediatric solid tumors have been published for Ewing's sarcoma and osteogenic sarcoma.[223,224] Lang and colleagues reported the results of a pilot study employing an RIC regimen and haploidentical HSCT to treat six children with metastatic neuroblastoma (*n* = 4), Ewing's sarcoma (*n* = 1), or rhabdomyosarcoma (*n* = 1) who relapsed after autologous transplantation.[225] All patients harbored significant tumor burdens at the time of allogeneic transplant. Four patients died of disease progression and two were surviving at a median follow-up of 6 months. Given the extremely poor prognosis associated with certain metastatic and recurrent pediatric tumors, this novel approach deserves further investigation.

Donor Lymphocyte Infusions

The infusion of "buffy coats" from the donor into allogeneic transplant recipients was first described by the Seattle team as a means to reduce the risk for graft rejection in patients who had aplastic anemia.[226] Donor lymphocytes can target host immune effector cells and impede their ability to reject the allograft. This approach is commonly employed following nonmyeloablative HSCT in order to achieve full donor chimerism, as discussed earlier. However, DLI is also an effective therapeutic intervention for treating selected patients with hematologic malignancies who have relapsed after allogeneic HSCT. Previously, the only potentially curative option for such individuals was to undergo a second myeloablative transplant. Unfortunately, this resulted in a high risk for early transplant-related mortality and often failed to eradicate the underlying malignancy.[227] In 1990, Kolb and colleagues reported that three patients with CML who relapsed following allogeneic transplants achieved second remissions after receiving leukocyte transfusions from their donors.[228] Early studies conducted by Slavin and others demonstrated that a variety of hematologic malignancies were responsive to DLI, and durable remissions could be obtained in some cases.[229,230] Patients with CML are most likely to benefit from this approach, although efficacy is inversely related to tumor burden at the time of relapse. For example, the remission induction rate for patients with CML who were treated in cytogenetic or early hematologic relapse is approximately 80%, compared to only 12% for patients receiving DLI in the accelerated phase or blast crisis.[230] Responses achieved in patients with CML tend to be durable, and the combined use of DLI and imatinib mesylate may act synergistically to further improve survival rates.[231-234]

The use of DLI for patients with acute leukemia who relapse after HSCT has not been as effective, with early trials demonstrating CR rates of 17% and 25% for ALL and AML patients, respectively.[231,232,235] These less favorable results may be caused partially by high tumor burdens at the time of relapse and the increased proliferative capacity of acute leukemias. The rate of disease progression could overwhelm the ability of donor immune mechanisms to eradicate leukemic clones. Consequently, cytoreductive chemotherapy has sometimes been administered prior to DLI to reduce the leukemic burden and provide critical time for the activation and expansion of alloreactive donor cells. Choi and colleagues treated 10 patients with ALL who had relapsed after HSCT with cytarabine, idarubicin, and etoposide, followed by granulocyte colony-stimulating factor (G-CSF)– mobilized DLI.[236] Mobilized DLIs containing hematopoietic stem cells were used to reduce the risk for marrow aplasia following chemotherapy. Of the 10 patients, 7 achieved CR, but in only two cases were the responses durable. Two responding patients died during CR as the result of complications of GVHD. Collins and colleagues reviewed the clinical course of 44 relapsed patients with ALL who were treated with DLI, of whom 28 had received prior chemotherapy. The overall survival rate at 3 years was 13%, and the use of cytoreductive chemotherapy did not significantly improve outcome.[237] It seems likely that ALL is inherently less susceptible to T-cell–mediated cytotoxicity, possibly because of decreased surface expression of HLA class I and II antigens or inadequate presentation of costimulatory or adhesion molecules.[237] Nonetheless, some ALL patients respond to this therapy, and improved efficacy might be achieved by administering DLI prior to overt hematologic relapse or by modulating immune activation to augment the GVL effect. Sanchez and colleagues used multiparameter flow cytometry to monitor minimal residual disease in 40 patients with ALL who underwent allogeneic HSCT.[238] Six of these patients received DLI, but a sustained remission was achieved only when donor cells were infused prior to overt relapse. Porter and colleagues conducted a novel clinical trial utilizing ex vivo–activated DLI to treat 18 patients relapsing after HSCT. Donor lymphocytes were activated by beads coated with anti-CD3 and anti-CD28. Eight patients achieved CR, including four of the seven patients with ALL, although most of these responses were not durable. IL-2 has also been used in combination with allogeneic DLI to activate immune effectors and augment the GVL effect.[239]

Patients with AML may be somewhat more amenable to treatment with DLI. Choi reported that 10 of 16 AML patients with AML who relapsed after an allogeneic transplant achieved CR following administration of chemotherapy and G-CSF– mobilized DLI.[240] The 2-year overall survival rate was 31%, and 4 patients attained durable remissions.

Although DLI has proven efficacious in some patients, toxicities associated with this procedure have not been trivial and include GVHD and marrow aplasia. The treatment-related mortality rate is estimated to be 12% to 22%.[230,241,242] The incidence and severity of GVHD correlate with the T-cell dose administered as well as with the degree of HLA disparity between donor and host. For recipients of unrelated-donor grafts, infusing a given T-cell dose results in more extensive GVHD than occurs in patients receiving DLI from an HLA-matched sibling.[241] Consequently, different lymphocyte dosing regimens have sometimes been used for related- and unrelated-donor transplants.[243] Because the optimal dose of T cells for DLI may also vary among patients, using intrapatient dose escalation might minimize the risk of severe GVHD while retaining the desired antileukemic effect. Implementation of this strategy is supported by the preclinical observation that sequential infusions of progressively increasing numbers of allogeneic T cells may not cause GVHD, whereas a single infusion of a moderate dose of T cells can induce severe GVHD. Bacigalupo and colleagues reported that patients with relapsed CML who received a single DLI containing $>1 \times 10^8$ cells/kg had a significantly higher risk for developing GVHD and had lower survival probability than did patients receiving multiple infusions containing fewer cells and given in an escalated fashion.[242] A similar observation was made by Dazzi et al., who compared patients receiving a single DLI, to those treated with escalated doses of donor lymphocytes administered 12 to 33 weeks apart. The latter group experienced lower incidences of GVHD and higher cytogenetic remission rates, despite receiving the same total doses of lymphocytes.[243]

An alternative approach to reducing the risk for GVHD associated with DLI, while retaining a GVL effect, is the infusion of CD8-depleted cell products, as discussed earlier. Other potential strategies include the use of immunomodulatory cytokines such as IL-12, which may inhibit GVHD without dampening GVL activity, as well as the ex vivo generation of tumor-specific CTLs or CTLs directed against hematopoietic lineage-restricted mHA (e.g., HA-1 and HA-2).[244-246]

Another complication associated with DLI is marrow aplasia, which has been reported in 5% to 50% of patients.[229] Myelosuppression may be a direct consequence of donor T cells targeting donor-derived hematopoietic tissue presenting passively acquired host antigens, or myelosuppression may be secondary to inhibitory growth factors released after the initiation of GVHD. The risk for aplasia is inversely related to the degree of donor chimerism at the time DLI is instituted. Hence, the patients at greatest risk for developing pancytopenia following DLI are those exhibiting predominantly host hematopoiesis, such as patients with CML in hematologic relapse.[232] Conversely, early implementation of DLI, prior to loss of donor engraftment or hematopoietic overgrowth by host-derived malignant cells, minimizes the risk for aplasia. The use of mobilized DLI, as discussed earlier, provides additional donor stem cells that promote hematopoiesis and reduce the risk for marrow dysfunction.

Adoptive T-Cell Therapy for Virus-Related Diseases

The use of donor-derived virus-specific CTLs has been highly effective as a means of preventing or controlling viruses and virus-associated diseases in HSCT recipients. The main viruses that have been targeted are the CMV and the EBV. Riddell and colleagues generated and infused donor-derived CTLs directed against CMV proteins into 14 HSCT patients for prophylaxis of CMV. Restoration of cellular immunity against CMV was achieved in all patients, and there were no cases of CMV viremia or disease. Persistence of CMV-specific CTLs was dependent on recovery of endogenous CD4 cells.[247]

A similar approach has been employed for the prophylaxis or treatment of PTLD in HSCT recipients. Rooney and colleagues administered donor-derived EBV-specific CTLs into 60 HSCT patients as prophylaxis for PTLD.[248] None of these patients developed PTLD, whereas there was a 12% incidence in a historical control group. Moreover, 5 of 6 patients with established PTLD who were treated with EBV-specific CTL clones achieved CR.

One drawback to using donor-derived CTLs for HSCT patients is the need to establish individual CTL clones for each donor-recipient pair. However, Haque and colleagues recently reported the results of a multicenter trial using off-the-shelf CTLs generated from EBV seropositive blood donors to treat PTLD in 33 allogeneic HSCT recipients.[249] CTL clones were chosen for each patient based on the best available HLA match and in vitro cytotoxicity testing. Of the patients, 14 achieved CR, 3 showed partial responses, 16 had no responses, and 5 died before completing treatment. Factors having a favorable impact on response included closer HLA matching between the CTL donor and the recipient and a higher CD4 content in the infused cell product. No adverse effects of the CTL infusions were documented.

Allogeneic Natural Killer-Cell Infusions

Most investigators have focused on the use of T lymphocytes for adoptive immunotherapy, but increased recognition that allogeneic NK cells are capable of mediating potent antileukemic effects has led to renewed interest in using these effectors to treat cancer. Miller and colleagues infused NK cells isolated from the peripheral blood mononuclear cells of haploidentical donors into 43 patients suffering from a variety of malignancies.[250] Patients were treated with immunosuppressive therapy prior to the NK-cell infusions to facilitate engraftment of donor cells. Two different regimens were tested: (1) low-dose cyclophosphamide and methylprednisolone; and (2) high-dose cyclophosphamide and fludarabine. All patients received subcutaneous IL-2 after the NK-cell infusions to augment NK-cell activity. Transient persistence of donor cells was documented in patients pretreated with low-dose immunosuppressive therapy. However, patients receiving the more intensive immunosuppressive regimen demonstrated in vivo expansion of allogeneic NK cells, and 5 of 19 patients with AML achieved CR. It is likely that NK cell–mediated cytotoxicity contributed to the anti-leukemic effect in this trial since 75% of AML patients demonstrating KIR ligand mismatching with the donor achieved CR, compared to only 13% of patients lacking NK cell–alloreactivity. The use of NK cell–selected DLI following haploidentical HSCT for pediatric patients with recurrent leukemia or solid tumors is currently being explored at the University of Wisconsin's American Family Children's Hospital.

Allogeneic Cytokine-Induced Killer Cells

CIK cells may be attractive candidates for allogeneic cell therapy because they have a reduced capacity to induce GVHD and readily migrate into leukemia-infiltrated tissue One potentially novel application of CIK cells would be their use in DLI following umbilical cord blood (UCB) transplantation. CIK cells have been generated from UCB and expanded in vitro with IL-2. These cells were cytotoxic against B and T cell lymphoma and myeloid leukemia cell lines, as well as fresh leukemic blasts.[251] The production of CIK cells from umbilical cord blood would allow for prophylactic or therapeutic administration of DLI to recipients of umbilical cord blood grafts, an option currently unavailable to these patients.

MECHANISMS OF TUMOR EVASION AND ESCAPE FROM IMMUNOTHERAPY

As neoplastic cells demonstrate genetic and gene expression instability, individual neoplastic cells and their clonal progeny can often demonstrate phenotypic changes. This is particularly evident when any selective pressure is applied. As such, a variety of molecular mechanisms have been described to account for the outgrowth of variant subclones of cancer that acquire resistance to chemotherapeutic agents that were effective against the parent neoplastic clone.[252] Similar mechanisms have also been found for cancer variants that become resistant to immunotherapy; numerous preclinical examples have been well characterized, and several clinical examples have now been described.[253,254] First, tumors may lose expression of the antigens that a form of immunotherapy uses to distinguish them as tumor cells. For example, a tumor recognized by a monoclonal antibody (e.g., an anti-idiotypic antibody) might lose expression of that idiotypic antigen. Second, when antigen recognition by T cells requires presentation by MHC class I or class II molecules, the tumor might downregulate, or mutate to lose MHC expression. This may actually occur during the process of oncogenesis. A number of tumors at the time of diagnosis are missing HLA class I molecules entirely or are missing a specific allele.[254] This suggests that an antitumor immune response may have been acting on the incipient neoplastic cells during oncogenesis; the result is a new tumor that has already been selected for poor recognition by T cells. Third, and in contrast to T-cell recognition, for immunotherapy that is mediated by NK cells, the presence of MHC class I molecules can turn off the NK cells through their inhibitory-KIR receptors.[255] This may explain why some tumors that have recurred following NK-mediated immunotherapy appear to express a dramatic upregulation of their MHC class I molecules. Finally, immune-mediated destruction involves certain effector pathways important to the immune system; such as complement, Fas-ligand, granzymes, perforin, or TNF. Some tumors appear to escape from immunotherapy by modifying their phenotypes in ways that block or circumvent these immune-destroying pathways.

In the setting of effective cancer chemotherapy, using multiple agents that act through separate pathways is a strategy that has been effective in preventing outgrowth of resistant cancer variants. Although tumors may modify their phenotypes to escape effectively from one type of treatment, it is difficult simultaneously to modify phenotype to avoid three or four separate destructive pathways in combination. For these reasons, more recent approaches for developing immunotherapy have been using combination treatments. They include combining immunotherapy with more conventional treatments or combining two or more distinct forms of immunotherapy with each other.

CHALLENGES AND FUTURE DIRECTIONS

In this chapter current clinical uses of immunotherapies and trials under way in the setting of childhood cancer are summarized. Preclinical data in murine models have shown that strategies using allogeneic T-cell therapy, adoptive autologous immunotherapy, MoAbs, vaccines, cytokines, gene therapies, or genetically engineered variations of these approaches may be effective. For the most part, to emphasize the technical and conceptual differences among these strategies, we have presented each strategy as a distinct clinical approach and have emphasized regimens that have been shown to have clinical efficacy or are being tested for efficacy in clinical trials. In fact, the goals of all these strategies are similar—to enable components of the immune system selectively to recognize and destroy clinical malignancies in patients so as to prolong survival and reduce the risk for disease recurrence. In many of these clinical treatments a combined immunotherapeutic approach is used. In vitro–propagated clones of tumor-reactive T cells may require coadministration of IL-2 to maintain their viability and functionality in vivo. GVL induced by donor lymphocyte infusions may be best maintained, in the absence of GVHD, by also providing IL-2 infusions. Preclinical data suggest that further combinations will be even more effective. The combination of cytokines, such as IL-2 and GM-CSF, that activate cells able to mediate ADCC (such as NK cells and neutrophils) with tumor-reactive MoAbs may allow better in vivo tumor ADCC and is being tested in a phase 3 clinical trial for patients with neuroblastoma. Linking cytokine administration to antitumor MoAb in the form of immunocytokines is itself a form of combined immunotherapy. Preclinical data from the lab of Laurence Cooper suggest that the use of an immunocytokine can dramatically enhance the survival and antitumor efficacy of genetically engineered tumor reactive T cells.[256] Preclinical data suggested that combining vaccine approaches that activate T-cell responses with MoAb approaches that use NK cells to mediate ADCC may be a strategy for preventing the escape of tumor variants after T-cell– or NK-cell–based immunotherapy.[257] Combining genetic vaccination approaches with cytokine infusions or adoptive immunotherapy may help these methods to be more effective in patients with cancer. Finally, a novel approach taken by Jensen and colleagues has combined the T-cell-body approach of transfecting T cells (for autologous adoptive therapy) with an artificial receptor, based on the concept of cytokine-targeted delivery. Because certain CNS tumors overexpress the IL-13α2 receptor, Jensen has created a construct that links IL-13 to the extracellular domain of a chimeric T-cell receptor gene (designated IL-13-zetakine).[258] This construct thus binds to the tumor, triggers the T cell, and then induces tumor apoptosis. Constructs confer steroid resistance on these transfected T cells, making them potentially useful even in patients requiring ongoing steroid treatment. His very recent data document that the first two glioma patients receiving intracranial infusions of these genetically modified autologous T cells have shown induction of CRs.[259]

In summary, several forms of immunotherapy are clinically effective and are becoming part of standard pediatric oncology care. They include the use of rituximab for PTLD, the use of allogeneic T-cell infusions after hematopoietic stem cell transplant, and the use of viral vaccines as cancer preventives. Several other approaches that have shown encouraging results when used as single-agent therapies are now being integrated into standard cancer care. Furthermore, there are numerous ways in which the forms of clinical immunotherapy that are effective in animal models might be combined to test for additive or synergistic antitumor effects. It is imperative that these clinical trials test the immunotherapeutic strategies in clinical conditions that attempt to simulate the conditions that have demonstrated efficacy in the preclinical models. From this perspective, it is equally important that investigations of experimental immunotherapy in animal models attempt to test clinical strategies under conditions that best simulate, within experimental limitations, conditions that may be occurring in the setting of clinical cancer. After these combined approaches have been proved to be effective in laboratory testing, the most promising will continue to be moved into the clinical testing arena.

REFERENCES

1. Clynes R. Antitumor antibodies in the treatment of cancer: Fc receptors link opsonic antibody with cellular immunity. Hematol Oncol Clin North Am. 2006;20:585-612.
2. Boruchov A, Heller G, Veri M, et al. Activating and inhibitory IgG Fc receptors on human DCs mediate opposing functions. J Clin Invest. 2005;115:2914-2923.
3. Wong J. Systemic targeted radionuclide therapy: potential new areas. Int J Radiat Oncol Biol Phys. 2006;66:S74-S82.
4. Pastan I, Hassan R, FitzGerald D, et al. Immunotoxin therapy of cancer. Annu Rev Med. 2007;58:1-37.
5. Crowe N, Coquet J, Berzins S, et al. Differential antitumor immunity mediated by NKT cell subsets in vivo. J Ex Med. 2005;202:1279-1288.
6. van derVliet H, Molling J, Blomberg B, et al. The immunoregulatory role of CD1d-restricted natural killer T cells in disease. Clin Immunol. 2004;112:8-23.
7. Metelitsa L, Wu H, Wang H, et al. Natural killer T cells infiltrate neuroblastomas expressing the chemokine CCL2. J Exp Med. 2004;199:1213-1221.
8. Koga Y, Matsuzaki A, Suminoe A, et al. Neutrophil-derived TNF-related apoptosis-inducing ligand (TRAIL): a novel mechanism of antitumor effect by neutrophils. Cancer Res. 2004;64:1037-1043.
9. Di Carlo E, Forni G, Musiani P. Neutrophils in the antitumoral immune response. Chem Immunol Allergy. 2003;83:182-203.
10. Leek RD, Harris AL. Tumor-associated macrophages in breast cancer. J Mammary Gland Biol Neoplasia. 2002;7:177-189
11. Buhtoiarov IN, Lum H, Berke G, et al. CD40 ligation activates murine macrophages via an IFN-gamma-dependent mechanism resulting in tumor cell destruction in vitro. J Immunol. 2005;174:6013-6022.
12. Scotlandi K, Manara MC, Hattinger CM, et al. Prognostic and therapeutic relevance of HER2 expression in osteosarcoma and Ewing's sarcoma. Eur J Cancer. 2005;41:1349-1361.
13. Coughlin CM, Fleming MD, Carroll RG, et al. Immunosurveillance and surviving-specific T-cell immunity in children with high-risk neuroblastoma. J Clin Oncol. 2006;24:5725-5734.
14. Polychronopoulou S, Koutroumba P. Telomere length and telomerase activity: variations with advancing age and potential role in childhood malignancies. J Pediatr Hematol Oncol. 2004;26:342-350.
15. Beppu M, Hayashi T, Hasegawa T, et al. Recognition of sialo-saccharide chains of glycophorin on damaged erythrocytes by macrophage scavenger receptors. Biochim Biophys Acta. 1995;1268:9-19.
16. Kufe DW. Smallpox, polio and now a cancer vaccine? Nat Med. 2000;6:252-253.
17. Matzinger P. Tolerance, danger, and the extended family. Annu Rev Immunol. 1994;12:991-1045.
18. Moretta L, Biassoni R, Bottino C. Human NK-cell receptors. Immunol Today. 2000;21:420-422.
19. Wu J, Song Y, Bakker ABH. An activating immunoreceptor complex formed by NKG2D and DAP10. Science. 1999;285:730-732.
20. Fisch P, Moris A, Rammensee HG. Inhibitory MHC class 1 receptors on γδ T cells in tumour immunity and autoimmunity. Immunol Today. 2000;21:187-191.
21. Koh CY, Blazar BR, George T. Augmentation of antitumor effects by NK cell inhibitory receptor blockade in vitro and in vivo. Blood. 2001;97:3132-3137.
22. Gupta RK, Silber GR. Adjuvants for human vaccines: current status, problems and future prospects. Vaccine. 1995;13:1263-1276.
23. Halloran ME, Anderson RM, Azevedo-Neto RS, et al. Population biology, evolution and immunology of vaccination and vaccination programs. Am J Med Sci. 1998;315:76-86.
24. Coley WB. Late results of the treatment of inoperable sarcoma by the mixed toxins of erysipelas and *Bacillus prodigiosus*. Am J Med Sci. 1906;131:373.
25. Everson TC, Cole WH. Spontaneous regression of cancer: preliminary report. Ann Surg. 1956;144:366.
26. Woodruff MFA. Immunological aspects of cancer. Lancet. 1964;2:265.
27. Burnet FM. Immunologic surveillance in neoplasia. Transplant Rev. 1971;7:3-25.
28. Evans AE, Gerson J, Schnaufer L. Spontaneous regression of neuroblastoma. J Natl Cancer Inst Monogr. 1976;44:4.
29. Old LJ. Tumor immunology: the first century. Curr Opin Immunol. 1992;4:603-607.
30. Bach FJ, Bach ML, Sondel PM. Differential function of major histocompatibility complex antigens in T lymphocyte activation. Nature. 1976;259:273.
31. Zinkernagel RM, Doherty PC. MHC-restricted cytotoxic T cells: studies on the biological role of polymorphic major transplantation antigens determining T cell restriction-specificity, function and responsiveness. Adv Immunol. 1979;27:51.
32. Davis MM, Bjorkman PJ. T-cell antigen receptor genes and T-cell recognition. Nature. 1988;334:395-402.
33. Klein G, Klein E. Genetic studies of the relationship of tumor-host cells. Nature. 1956;178:1389.
34. Prehn RT, Main J. Immunity of methylcholanthrene-induced sarcomas. J Natl Cancer Inst. 1957;18:769.

35. Gross L. Intradermal immunization of C3H mice against a sarcoma that originated in an animal of the same line. Cancer Res. 1943;3:326.

36. Schreiber H, Ward PL, Rowley DA, et al. Unique tumor-specific antigens. Annu Rev Immunol. 1988;6:465-483.

37. Wojtowicz-Praga S. Reversal of tumor induced immunosuppression: a new approach to cancer therapy. J Immunother. 1997;20:165-177.

38. Finke J, Ferrone S, Frey A, et al. Where have all the T cells gone? Mechanisms of immune evasion by tumors. Immunol Today. 1999;20:158-160.

39. Mackall CL, Fleisher TA, Brown MR, et al. Lymphocyte depletion during treatment with intensive chemotherapy for cancer. Blood. 1994;84:2221-2228.

40. Kessler JH, Melief CJ. Identification of T-cell epitopes for cancer immunotherapy. Leukemia. 2007;21:1859-1874.

41. Kim SB, Kwak LW. The use of idiotype as a target for clinical immunotherapy of B cell malignancies. In Giaccone G, Schilsky R, Sondel P (eds). Cancer Chemotherapy and Biological Response Modifiers. Amsterdam, Elsevier, 2001, pp 289-296.

42. Kwak LW, Taub DD, Duffey PL, et al. Transfer of myeloma idiotype-specific immunity from an actively immunised marrow donor. Lancet. 1995;345:1016-1020.

43. Bendandi M, Gocke CD, Kobrin CB, et al. Complete molecular remissions induced by patient-specific vaccination plus granulocyte-monocyte colony-stimulating factor against lymphoma. Nat Med. 1999;5:1171-1177.

44. De Gruijl TD, Curiel DT. Cancer vaccine strategies get bigger and better. Nat Med. 1999;5:1124-1125.

45. Zhang H, Chua KS, Guimond M, et al. Lymphopenia and interleukin-2 therapy alter homeostasis of CD4+CD25+ regulatory T cells. Nat Med. 2005;11:1238-1243.

46. Sondak VK, Sosman JA. Results of clinical trials with an allogenic melanoma tumor cell lysate vaccine: melacine. Semin Cancer Biol. 2003;13:409-415.

47. Terando AM, Faries MB, Morton DL. Vaccine therapy for melanoma: current status and future directions. Vaccine. 2007;25(suppl 2):B4-B16.

48. Yu P, Lee Y, Wang Y, et al. Targeting the primary tumor to generate CTL for the effective eradication of spontaneous metastases. J Immunol. 2007;179:1960-1968.

49. Hege KM, Jooss K, Pardoll D. GM-CSF gene-modifed cancer cell immunotherapies: of mice and men. Int Rev Immunol. 2006;25:321-352.

50. Soiffer R, Hodi FS, Haluska F, et al. Vaccination with irradiated, autologous melanoma cells engineered to secrete granulocyte-macrophage colony-stimulating factor by adenoviral-mediated gene transfer augments antitumor immunity in patients with metastatic melanoma. J Clin Oncol. 2003;21:3343-3350.

51. Harzstark AL, Small EJ. Immunotherapy for prostate cancer using antigen-loaded antigen-presenting cells: APC8015 (Provenge). Expert Opin Biol Ther. 2007;7:1275-1280.

52. Wierecky J, Müller MR, Wirths S, et al. Immunologic and clinical responses after vaccinations with peptide-pulsed dendritic cells in metastatic renal cancer patients. Cancer Res. 2006;6:5910-5918.

53. Geiger JD, Hutchinson RJ, Hohenkirk LF, et al. Vaccination of pediatric solid tumor patients with tumor lysate-pulsed dendritic cells can expand specific T cells and mediate tumor regression. Cancer Res. 2001;61:8513-8519.

54. Huising MO, Kruiswijk CP, Flik G. Phylogeny and evolution of class-I helical cytokines. J Endocrinol. 2006;189:1-25.

55. Sondel PM, Mackall CL. Tumor immunology and pediatric cancer. In Pizzo PA, Poplack DG (eds). Principles and Practice of Pediatric Oncology, ed 4. Philadelphia, Lippincott Raven, 2002, pp 21-148.

56. Sondel PM, Rakhmilevich AL, deJong J, et al. Cellular immunity and cytokines. In Mendelsohn J, Howley PM, Israel MA, et al

(eds). The Molecular Basis of Cancer. Philadelphia, WB Saunders, 2001, pp 535-572.

57. Kaplan DH, Shankaran V, Dighe AS, et al. Demonstration of an interferon gamma-dependent tumor surveillance system in immunocompetent mice. Proc Natl Acad Sci U S A. 1998;95:7556-7561.

58. Boehm U, Klamp T, Groot M, et al. Cellular responses to interferon-gamma. Annu Rev Immunol. 1997;15:749-795.

59. Kurzrock R, Gutterman JU, Kantarjian H, et al. Therapy of chronic myelogenous leukemia with interferon. Cancer Invest. 1989;7:83-91.

60. Dow LW, Raimondi SC, Culbert SJ, et al. Response to alpha-interferon in children with Philadelphia chromosome-positive chronic myelocytic leukemia. Cancer. 1991;68:1678-1684.

61. Farner NL, Hank JA, Sondel PM. Molecular and clinical aspects of interleukin 2. In Cytokines in Health and Disease, ed 2. New York, Marcel Dekker, 1997, pp 29-40.

62. Voss SD, Hong R, Sondel PM. Severe combined immunodeficiency, interleukin-2 (IL-2), and the IL-2 receptor: experiments of nature continue to point the way. Blood. 1994;83:626-635.

63. Willenbacher W, Basara N, Blau IW. Treatment of steroid refractory acute and chronic graft-versus-host disease with daclizumab. Br J Haematol. 2001;112:820-823.

64. Waldmann TA. IL-2R and IL-15R: targets for immunotherapy of leukemia/lymphoma and autoimmune disease and for the prevention of organ allograft rejection. Hematology, Am Soc Hematol Educ Program Book. 2000;395-397.

65. Malkovska V, Sondel PM. Prospects for Interleukin-2 therapy in hematologic malignant neoplasms. J Natl Cancer Inst Monogr. 1990;10:69-72.

66. Rosenberg SA. Interleukin-2 and the development of immunotherapy for the treatment of patients with cancer. Cancer J. 2000;6(suppl 1):S200-S207.

67. Benyunes MC, Massumoto C, York A, et al. IL2 with or without LAK cells as consolidative immunotherapy after autologous BMT for AML. Bone Marrow Transplant. 1993;12:159-163.

68. Goldberg SL, Pecora AL, Rosenbluth RJ, et al. Treatment of leukemic relapse following unrelated umbilical cord blood transplantation with interleukin-2: potential for augmenting graft-versus-leukemia and graft-versus-host effects with cytokines. Bone Marrow Transplant. 2000;26:353-355.

69. Margolin KA, Van Besien K, Wright C, et al. Interleukin-2 activated autologous bone marrow and peripheral blood stem cells in the treatment of acute leukemia and lymphoma. Biol Blood Marrow Transplant. 1999;5:36-45.

70. Blaise D, Attal M, Reiffers J, et al. Randomized study of recombinant interleukin-2 after autologous bone marrow transplantation for acute leukemia in first complete remission. Eur Cytokine Netw. 2001;11:91-98.

71. Sievers EL, Lange BJ, Sondel PM, et al. Feasibility, toxicity and biologic response of interleukin-2 after consolidation chemotherapy for acute myelogenous leukemia: a report from the Children's Cancer Group. J Clin Oncol. 1998;16:914-919.

72. Cortes JE, Kantarjian HM, O'Brien S, et al. A pilot study of interleukin-2 for adult patients with acute myelogenous leukemia in first complete remission. Cancer. 1999;85:1506-1513.

73. Areman EM, Rhodes PL, Mazumder A, et al. Differential effects of IL-2 incubation on hematopoietic potential of autologous bone marrow and mobilized PBSC from patients with hematologic malignancies. J Hematother. 1999;8:39-44.

74. Slavin S. Donor lymphocyte infusions for hematopoietic malignancy. In Giaccone G, Schilsky R, Sondel P (eds). Cancer Chemotherapy and Biological Response Modifiers. Amsterdam, Elsevier; 2002, pp 291-300.

75. Riddell SR, Warren EH, Gavin MA, et al. Immunotherapy of human viral and malignant diseases with genetically modified T-cell clones. Cancer J. 2000;6(suppl 3):S250-S258.

76. Bernstein N, Starnes C, Levy R. Specific enhancement of the therapeutic effect of anti-idiotype antibodies on a murine B cell lymphoma by IL2. J Immunol. 1988;140:2839-2845.

77. Shiloni E, Eisenthal A, Sachs D, et al. Antibody-dependent cellular cytotoxicity mediated by murine lymphocytes activated in recombinant interleukin-2. J Immunol. 1987;138:1992-1998.

78. Sondel PM, Hank JH. Combination of interleukin-2 with anti-tumor monoclonal antibodies. Cancer J. 1997;3:5121-5127.

79. Kossman SE, Scheinberg DA, Jurcic JG, et al. A phase I trial of humanized monoclonal antibody HuM195 (anti-CD33) with low-dose interleukin 2 in acute myelogenous leukemia. Clin Cancer Res. 1999;5:2748-2755.

80. Gollob JA, Meir JW, Atkins MB. Clinical use of systemic IL-12 therapy. In Giaccone G, Schilsky R, Sondel P (eds). Cancer Chemotherapy and Biological Response Modifiers. Amsterdam, Elsevier, 2001, pp 353-370.

81. Trinchieri G. Interleukin-12: a cytokine at the interface of inflammation and immunity. Adv Immunol. 1998;70:183-243.

82. Caux C, Dezutter-Dambuyant C, Schmitt D, et al. GM-CSF and TNF-α cooperate in the generation of dendritic Langerhans cells. Nature. 1992;360:258.

83. Houtenbos I, Bracho F, Davenport V, et al. Autologous bone marrow transplantation for childhood acute lymphoblastic leukemia: a novel combined approach consisting of ex vivo marrow purging, modulation of multi-drug resistance, induction of autograft vs leukemia effect, and post-transplant immuno- and chemotherapy (PTIC). Bone Marrow Transplant. 2001;27:145-153.

84. Blazar BR, Krieg AM, Taylor PA. Synthetic unmethylated cytosine-phosphate-guanosine oligodeoxynucleotides are potent stimulators of antileukemia responses in naive and bone marrow transplant recipients. Blood. 2001;98:1217-1225.

85. Kohler G, Milstein C. Continuous culture of fused cells secreting antibody of predefined specificity. Nature. 1975;256:495-497.

86. Ritz J, Pasando J, Sallan S, et al. Serotherapy of acute lymphoblastic leukemia with monoclonal antibody. Blood. 1981;58:141-152.

87. Miller R, Maloney D, Warnke R, et al. Treatment of B-cell lymphoma with monoclonal antiidiotype antibody. N Engl J Med. 1982;4:517-522.

88. Jain M, Kamal N, Batra SK. Engineering antibodies for clinical applications. Trends Biotechnol. 2007;25:307-316.

89. López-Guillermo A, Mercadal S. The clinical use of antibodies in haematological malignances. Ann Oncol. 2007;18(suppl 9):ix 51-57.

90. Coiffier B. Rituximab therapy in malignant lymphoma. Oncogene. 2007;26:3603-3613.

91. Weng W, Levy R. Two immunoglobulin G fragment C receptor polymorphisms independently predict response to rituximab in patients with follicular lymphoma. J Clin Oncol. 2003;21:3940-3947.

92. Bonavida B. Rituximab-induced inhibition of antiapoptotic cell survival pathways: implications in chemo/immunoresistance, rituximab unresponsiveness, prognostic and novel therapeutic interventions. Oncogene. 2007;26:3629-3636.

93. McLaughlin P, Grillolopez A, Link B, et al. Rituximab chimeric anti-Cd20 monoclonal antibody therapy for relapsed indolent lymphoma: half of patients respond to a four-dose treatment program. J Clin Oncol. 1998;16:2825-2833.

94. Colombat P, Salles G, Brousse N, et al. Rituximab (anti-CD20 monoclonal antibody) as single first-line therapy for patients with follicular lymphoma with a low tumor burden: clinical and molecular evaluation. Blood. 2001;97:101-106.

95. Hiddemann W, Kneba M, Dreyling M, et al. Frontline therapy with rituximab added to the combination of cyclophosphamide, doxorubicin, vincristine, and prednisone (CHOP) significantly improves the outcome for patients with advanced-stage follicular lymphoma compared with therapy with CHOP alone: results of a prospective randomized study of the German Low-Grade Lymphoma Study Group. Blood. 2005;106:3725-3732.

96. Marcus R, Imrie K, Belch A, et al. CVP chemotherapy plus rituximab compared with CVP as first-line treatment for advanced follicular lymphoma. Blood. 2005;105:1417-1423.

97. Coiffier B, Lepage E, Briere J, et al. CHOP chemotherapy plus rituximab compared with CHOP alone in elderly patients with diffuse large-B-cell lymphoma. N Engl J Med. 2002;346:235-242.

98. Feugier P, Van Hoof A, Sebban C, et al. Long-term results of the R-CHOP study in the treatment of elderly patients with diffuse large B-cell lymphoma: a study by the Groupe d'Etude des Lymphomes de l'Adulte. J Clin Oncol. 2005;23:4117-4126.

99. Pfreundschuh M, Trumper L, Osterborg A, et al. CHOP-like chemotherapy plus rituximab versus CHOP-like chemotherapy alone in young patients with good-prognosis diffuse-large-B-cell lymphoma: a randomised controlled trial by the Mab Thera International Trial (MInT) Group. Lancet Oncol. 2006;7:379-391.

100. Giulino L, Bussel J, Neufeld E, et al. Treatment with rituximab in benign and malignant hematologic disorders in children. J Pediatr. 2007;150:338-344.

101. Kushner B, Kramer K, Cheung N-K. Phase II trial of the anti-GD2 monoclonal antibody 3F8 and granulocyte-macrophage colony-stimulating factor for neuroblastoma. J Clin Oncol. 2001;219:4189-4194.

102. Cheung N-K, Sowers R, Vickers AJ, et al. FCGR2A polymorphism is correlated with clinical outcome after immunotherapy of neuroblastoma with anti-GD2 antibody and granulocyte macrophage colony-stimulating factor. J Clin Oncol. 2006;24:2885-2890.

103. Ozkaynak M, Sondel P, Krailo M, et al. Phase I study of chimeric human/murine anti-ganglioside G(D2) monoclonal antibody (ch14.18) with granulocyte-macrophage colony-stimulating factor in children with neuroblastoma immediately after hematopoietic stem-cell transplantation: a Children's Cancer Group Study. J Clin Oncol. 2000;18:4077-4085.

104. Gilman AL, Ozkaynak F, Matthay K, et al. Phase I study of ch14.18 with GM-CSF and IL-2 in children with neuroblastoma following autologous bone marrow transplant or stem cell rescue: a report from the Children's Oncology Group. J Clin Oncol. 2008 (in press).

105. Leonard J, Goldenberg D. Preclinical and clinical evaluation of epratuzumab (anti-CD22 IgG) in B-cell malignancies Oncogene. 2007;26:3704-3713.

106. Tuscano J, Riva A, Toscano S, et al. CD22 cross-linking generates B-cell antigen receptor-dependent signals that activate the JNK/SAPK signaling cascade. Blood. 1999;94:1382-1392.

107. Tuscano J, O'Donnell R, Miers L, et al. Anti-CD22 ligand-blocking antibody HB22.7 has independent lymphomacidal properties and augments the efficacy of 90Y-DOTA-pedtide-Lym-1 in lymphoma xenografts. Blood. 2003;101:3641-3647.

108. Micallef I, Kahl B, Maurer M, et al. A pilot study of epratuzumab and rituximab in combination withcyclophosphamide, doxorubicin, vincristine, and prednisone chemotherapy in patients with previously untreated, diffuse large B-cell lymphoma. Cancer. 2006;107:2826-2832.

109. Sliwkowski M, Lofgren J, Lewis G, et al. Nonclinical studies addressing the mechanism of action of trastuzumab (Herceptin). Semin Oncol. 1999;26(suppl 12):60-70.

110. Baselga J, Albanell J, Molina MA, et al. Mechanism of action of trastuzumab and scientific update. Semin Oncol. 2001;28(suppl 16):4-11.

111. Lane H, Beuvink I, Motoyama A, et al. ErbB2 potentiates breast tumor proliferation through modulation of p27(Kip1)-Cdk2 complex formation: receptor overexpression does not determine growth dependency. Mol Cell Biol. 2000;20:3210-3223.

112. Neve R, Sutterluty H, Pullen N, et al. Effects of oncogenic ErbB2 on G1 cell cycle regulators in breast tumour cells. Oncogene. 2000;19:1647-1656.

113. Nahta R, Esteva F. Trastuzumab: triumphs and tribulations. Oncogene. 2007;26:3637-3643.

114. Scotlandi K, Manara M, Hattinger C, et al. Prognostic and therapeutic relevance of HER2 expression in osteosarcoma and Ewing's sarcoma. Eur J Cancer. 2005;41:1349-1361.

115. Fellenberg J, Krauthoff A, Pollandt K, et al. Evaluation of the predictive value of Her-2/neu gene expression on osteosarcoma therapy in laser-microdissected paraffin-embedded tissue. Lab Invest. 2004;84:4-5.

116. Pastan I, Hassan R, FitzGerald D, Kreitman RJ, et al. Immunotoxin treatment of cancer. Annu Rev Med. 2007;58:221-237.

117. Ghetie M, Tucker K, Richardson J, et al. The antitumor activity of an anti-CD22 immunotoxin in SCID mice with disseminated Daudi lymphoma is enhanced by either an anti-CD19 antibody or an anti-CD19 immunotoxin. Blood. 1992;80:2315-2320.

118. Messmann R, Vitetta E, Headlee D, et al. A phase I study of combination therapy with immunotoxins IgGHD37-deglycosylated ricin A chain (dgA) and IgG-RFB4-dgA (Combotox) in patients with refractory CD19+,CD22+ B cell lymphoma. Clin Cancer Res. 2000;6:1302-1313.

119. Pagano L, Fianchi L, Caira M, et al. The role of gemtuzumab ozogamicin in the leukemia patients. Oncogene. 2007;26:3679-3690.

120. Sievers E, Appelbaum F, Spielberger R, et al. Selective ablation of acute myeloid leukemia using antibody-targeted chemotherapy: a phase I study of an anti-CD33 calicheamicin immunoconjugate. Blood. 1999;93:3678-3684.

121. Sievers E, Larson R, Stadtmauer E, et al. Efficacy and safety of gemtuzumab ozogamicin in patients with CD33-positive acute myeloid leukemia in first relapse. J Clin Oncol. 2001;19:3244-3254.

122. Aplenc R, Alonzo T, Gerbing R, et al. Treatment of children with relapsed acute myeloid leukemia with gemtuzumab in combination with mitoxantrone and cytarabine. Blood. 2005;106:239b (abstract).

123. Carretero-Margolis C, Fivenson, D. A complete and durable response to denileukin diftitox in a patient with mycosis fungoides. J Am Acad Derm. 2003;48:275-276.

124. Olsen E, Duvic M, Frankel A, et al. Pivotal phase III trial of two dose levels of denileukin diftitox for the treatment of cutaneous T-cell lymphoma. J Clin Oncol. 2001;19:376-388.

125. Dang H, Hagemeister F, Pro B, et al. Phase II study of denileukin diftitox for relapsed/refractory B-cell non-Hodgkin's lymphoma. J Clin Oncol. 2004;22:4095-4102.

126. Frankel E, Fleming D, Hall P, et al. A phase II study of DT fusion protein denileukin diftitox in patients with fludarabine-refractory chronic lymphocytic leukemia. Clin Can Res. 2003;9:3555-3561.

127. Dang N, Pro B, Hagemeister F, et al. Phase II trial of denileukin diftitox for relapsed/refractory T-cell non-Hodgkin lymphoma. Br J Haematol. 2006;136:439-447.

128. Ho V, Zahrieh D, Hochberg E, et al. Safety and efficacy of denileukin diftitox in patients with steroid-refractory acute graft-versus-host disease after allogeneic hematopoietic stem cell transplantation. Blood. 2004;104:1224-1226.

129. Shaughnessy P, Bachier C, Grimley M, et al. Denileukin diftitox for the treatment of steroid-resistant acute graft-versus-host disease. Biol Blood Marrow Transplant. 2005;11:188-193.

130. Voss S, Smith S, Dibartolo N, et al. Positron emission tomography (PET) imaging of neuroblastoma and melanoma with 64Cu-SarAr immuno-conjugates. Proc Natl Acad Sci U S A. 2007;104:17489-17493.

131. Modak S, Cheung N-K. Antibody-based targeted radiation to pediatric tumors. J Nucl Med. 2005;46:157S-163S.

132. Witzig T, White C, Gordon L, et al. Safety of yttrium-90 ibritumomab tiuxetan radioimmunotherapy for relapsed low-grade, follicular, or transformed non-Hodgkin's lymphoma. J Clin Oncol. 2003;21:1263-1270.

133. Witzig T, Gordon L, Cabanillas F, et al. Randomized controlled trial of yttrium-90-labeled ibritumomab tiuxetan radioimmunotherapy versus rituximab immunotherapy for patients with relapsed or refractory low-grade, follicular, or transformed B-cell non-Hodgkin's lymphoma. J Clin Oncol. 2002;20:2453-2463.

134. Vose J, Wahl R, Saleh M, et al. Multicenter phase II study of iodine-131 tositumomab for chemotherapy-relapsed/refractory low-grade and transformed low-grade B-cell non-Hodgkin's lymphomas. J Clin Oncol. 2000;18:1316-1323.

135. Davies A, Rohatiner A, Howell S, et al. Tositumomab and iodine I 131 tositumomab for recurrent indolent and transformed B-cell non-Hodgkin's lymphoma. J Clin Oncol. 2004;22:1469-1479.

136. Hank JA, Surfus JE, Gan J, et al. Activation of human effector cells by a tumor reactive recombinant anti-ganglioside GD2 interleukin-2 fusion protein (ch14.18-IL2). Clin Cancer Res. 1996;2:1951-1959.

137. Lode HN, Xiang R, Varki NM, et al. Targeted interleukin-2 therapy of spontaneous neuroblastoma to bone marrow. J Natl Cancer Inst. 1997;89:1586.

138. Batova A, Kamps A, Gillies SD, et al. The Ch14.18-GM-CSF fusion protein is effective at mediating antibody-dependent cellular cytotoxicity and complement-dependent cytotoxicity in vitro. Clin Cancer Res. 1999;5:4259-4263.

139. Connor J, Felder M, Hank JA, et al. Ex-vivo evaluation of anti-EpCAM immunocytokine KS-IL2 in ovarian cancer. J Immunother. 2004;27:211-219.

140. Neal ZC, Yang JC, Rakhmilevich AL, et al. Enhanced activity of hu14.18-IL2 immunocytokine against the murine NXS2 neuroblastoma when combined with IL2 therapy. Clin Cancer Res. 2004;10:4839-4847.

141. King DM, Albertini MR, Schalch H, et al. A phase I clinical trial of the immunocytokine EMD 273063 (hu14.18-IL2) in patients with melanoma. J Clin Oncol. 2004;22:4463-4473.

142. Osenga KL, Hank JA, Albertini MR, et al. A phase I clinical trial of Hu14.18-IL2 (EMD 273063) as a treatment for children with refractory or recurrent neuroblastoma and melanoma: a study of the Children's Oncology Group. Clin Cancer Res. 2006;12:1750-1759.

143. Shusterman S, London WB, Gilles S, et al. Anti-neuroblastoma activity of hu14.18-IL2 against minimal residual disease in a Children's Oncology Group (COG) phase II study. J Clin Oncol. 2008;26(15s) (abstract 3002):132S.

144. DeGast GC, vandeWindel JG, Bast BE. Clinical perspectives of bispecific antibodies in cancer. Cancer Immunol Immunother. 1997;45:171-173.

145. Weiner LM, Alpaugh RK, vonMehren M. Redirected cellular cytotoxicity employing bispecific antibodies and other multifunctional bending proteins. Cancer Immunol Immunother. 1997;45:190-192.

146. Morecki S, Lindhofer H, Yacovlev E, et al. Use of trifunctional bispecific antibodies to prevent graft-versus-host disease induced by allogeneic lymphocytes. Blood. 2006;107:1564-1569.

147. Frankel AE, Powell BL, Lilly MB. Diphtheria toxin conjugate therapy of cancer. In Giaccone G, Schilsky R, Sondel P (eds). Cancer Chemotherapy and Biological Response Modifiers. Amsterdam, Elsevier, 2002, pp 301-315.

148. Dang NH, Pro B, Hagemeister FB, et al. Phase II trial of denileukin diftitox for relapsed/refractory T-cell non-Hodgkin lymphoma. Br J Haematol. 2007;136:439-447.

149. Eshhar Z. The T-body approach: redirecting T cells with antibody specificity. Handb Exp Pharmacol. 2008;181:329-342.

150. Rossig C, Brenner MK. Genetic modification of T lymphocytes for adoptive immunotherapy. Mol Ther. 2004;10:5-18.

151. Rossig C, Bollard CM, Nuchtern JG, et al. Targeting of GD2-positive tumor cells by human T lymphoctyes engineered to express chimeric T-cell receptor genes. Int J Cancer. 2001;94:228-236.

152. Gonzalez S, Naranjo A, Serrano LM, et al. Genetic engineering of cytotoxic T lymphocytes for adoptive T-cell therapy of neuroblastoma. J Gene Med. 2004;6:704-711.

153. Park JR, Digiusto DL, Slovak M, et al. Adoptive transfer of chimeric antigen receptor redirected cytotoxic T lymphocyte clones in patients with neuroblastoma. Mol Ther. 2007;15:825-833.

154. Jensen MC, Clarke P, Tan G, et al. Human T lymphocyte genetic modification with naked DNA. Mol Ther. 2000;1:49-55.

155. Serrano LM, Pfeiffer T, Olivares S, et al. Differentiation of naïve cord-blood T cells into CD19-specific cytolytic effectors for post-transplantation adoptive immunotherapy. Blood. 2006;107:2643-2652.

156. Riddell S. Finding a place for tumor-specific T Cells in targeted cancer therapy. J Exp Med. 2004;200:1533-1537.

157. Sadelain M, Rivière I, Brentjens R. Targeting tumors with genetically enhanced T lymphocytes. Nat Rev Cancer. 2003;3:35-45.

158. Maher J, Brentjens R, Gunset G, et al. Human T-lymphocyte cytotoxicity and proliferation directed by a single chimeric TCRζ/CD28 receptor. Nat Biotechnol. 2002;20:70-75.

159. Haynes N, Trapani J, Teng M, et al. Rejection of syngeneic colon carcinoma by CTLs expressing single-chain antibody receptors codelivering CD28 costimulation. J Immunol. 2002;169:5780-5786.

160. Pule M, Straathof K, Dotti G, et al. A chimeric T cell antigen receptor that augments cytokine release and supports clonal expansion of primary human T cells. Mol Ther. 2005;12:933-941.

161. Finney H, Akbar A, Lawson A. Activation of resting human primary T cells with chimeric receptors: costimulation from CD28, inducible costimulator, CD134, and CD137 in series with signals from the TCRζ chain. J Immunol. 2004;172:104-113.

162. Imai C, Mihara K, Andreansky M, et al. Chimeric receptors with 4-1BB signaling capacity provoke potent cytotoxicity against acute lymphoblastic leukemia. Leukemia. 2004;18:676-684.

163. Leen A, Ronney C, Foster A. Improving T cell therapy for cancer. Annu Rev Immunol. 2007;25:243-265.

164. Zhang Q, Yang X, Pins M, et al. Adoptive transfer of tumor-reactive transforming growth factor-ß-insensitive CD8+ T cells: eradication of autologous mouse prostate cancer. Cancer Res. 2005;65:1761-1769.

165. Liu K, Rosenberg S. Transduction of an IL-2 gene into human melanoma- reactivelymphocytes results in their continued growth in the absence of exogenous IL-2 and maintenance of specific antitumor activity. J Immunol. 2001;167:6356-6365.

166. Hwu P, Rosenberg SA. The use of gene-modified tumor-infiltrating lymphocytes for cancer therapy. Ann N Y Acad Sci. 1994;716:188-197.

167. Dotti G, Savoldo B, Pule M, et al. Human cytotoxic T lymphocytes with reduced sensitivity to Fas-induced apoptosis. Blood. 2005;105:4677-4684.

168. Charo J, Finkelstein S, Grewal N, et al. Bcl-2 overexpression enhances tumor-specific T-cell survival. Cancer Res. 2005;65:2001-2008.

169. Eaton D, Gilham D, O'Neill A, et al. Retroviral transduction of human peripheral blood lymphocytes with bcl-XL promotes in vitro lymphocyte survival in proapoptotic conditions. Gene Ther. 2002;9:527-535.

170. Gattinoni L, Powell D, Rosenberg S, et al. Adoptive immunotherapy for cancer: building on success. Nat Rev Immunol. 2006;6:383-393.

171. Hsu C, Hughes M, Zheng Z, et al. Primary human T lymphocytes engineered with a codon-optimized IL-15 gene resist cytokine withdrawal-induced apoptosis and persist long-term in the absence of exogenous cytokine. J Immunol. 2005;175:7226-7234.

172. Wrzesinski C, Paulos C, Gattinoni L, et al. Hematopoietic stem cells promote the expansion and function of adoptively transferred antitumor CD8+ T cells. J Clin Invest. 2007;117:492-501.

173. Anasetti C, Mulé J. To ablate or not to ablate? HSCs in the T cell driver's seat. J Clin Invest. 2007;117:306-310.

174. Savoldo B, Goss J, Hammer M, et al. Treatment of solid organ transplant recipients with autologous Epstein-Barr virus-specific cytotoxic T lymphocytes (CTLs). Blood. 2006;108:2942-2949.

175. Bollard C, Aguilar L, Straathof K, et al. Cytotoxic T lymphocyte therapy for Epstein-Barr virus + Hodgkin's disease. J Ex Med. 2004;200:1623-1633.

176. Berdeja G, Hess A, Lucas D, et al. Systemic interleukin-2 and adoptive transfer of lymphokine-activated killer cells improves antibody-dependent cellular cytotoxicity in patients with relapsed B-cell lymphoma treated with rituximab. Clin Cancer Res. 2007;13:2392-2399.

177. Leung W, Handgretinger R, Iyengar R, et al. Inhibitory KIR-HLA receptor-ligand mismatch in autologous haematopoietic stem cell transplantation for solid tumour and lymphoma. Br J Cancer. 2007;97:539-542.

178. Linn Y, Hui K. Cytokine-induced killer cells: NK-like T cells with cytolytic specificity against leukemia. Leuk Lymphoma. 2003;44:1457-1462.

179. Hoyle C, Bangs C, Chang P, et al. Expansion of Philadelphia chromosome-negative CD3+CD56+ cytotoxic cells from chronic myeloid leukemia patients: in vitro and in vivo efficacy in severe combined immunodeficiency disease mice. Blood. 1998;92:3318-3327.

180. Linn YC, Lau LC, Hui KM. Generation of cytokine-induced killer cells from leukaemic samples with in vitro cytotoxicity against autologous and allogeneic leukaemic blasts. Br J Haematol. 2002;116:78-86.

181. Marina V, Kakudab H, Dandera E, et al. Enhancement of the anti-leukemic activity of cytokine induced killer cells with an anti-CD19 chimeric receptor delivering a 4-1BB-z activating signal. Exp Hematol. 2007;35:1388-1397.

182. Leemhuis T, Wells S, Horn P, et al. Autologous cytokine-induced killer cells for the treatment of relapsed Hodgkin's disease and non-Hodgkin's lymphoma. Blood. 2000;abstract #3624.

183. Schmidt-Wolf I, Finke S, Trojaneck B, et al. Phase I clinical study applying autologous immunological effector cells transfected with the interleukin-2 gene in patients with metastatic renal cancer, colorectal cancer and lymphoma. Br J Cancer. 1999;81:1009-1016.

184. Jiang J, Xu N, Wu C, et al. Treatment of advanced gastric cancer by chemotherapy combined with autologous cytokine-induced killer cells. Anticancer Res. 2006;26:2237-2242.

185. Shi M, Zhang B, Tang Z, et al. Autologous cytokine-induced killer cell therapy in clinical trial phase I is safe in patients with primary hepatocellular carcinoma. World J Gastroenterol. 2004;10:1146-1151.

186. Barnes D, Loutit J, Neal F. Treatment of murine leukemia with x-rays and homologous bone marrow. BMJ. 1956;2:626-627.

187. Weiden P, Fluornoy N, Thomas E, et al. Anti-leukemic effects of graft versus host disease in human recipients of allogeneic marrow grafts. N Engl J Med. 1979;300:1068-1073.

188. Horowitz M, Gale R, Sondel P, et al. Graft versus leukemia reactions after bone marrow transplantation. Blood. 1990;75:555-562.

189. Sosman J, Oettel K, Smith S, et al. Specific recognition of human leukemic cells by allogeneic T cells. II. Evidence of HLA-D restricted determinants on leukemic cells that are crossreactive with determinants present on unrelated nonleukemic cells. Blood. 1990;75:2005-2016.

190. Faber L, van Luxemburg-Heijs S, Veenhof W, et al. Generation of cd4+ cytotoxic lymphocyte clones from a patient with severe graft-versus-host disease after allogeneic bone marrow trans-

plantation: implications for graft-versus-leukemia activity. Blood. 1995;86:2821-2828.

191. Nimer S, Giorgi J, Gajewski J, et al. Selective depletion of CD8+ cells for preventkion of graft-versus-host disease after bone marrow transplantation. A randomized controlled trial. Transplantation. 1994;57:82-87.

192. Giralt S, Hester J, Huh Y, et al. CD8-depleted donor lymphocyte infusions as treatment for relapsed chronic myelogenous leukemia after allogeneic bone marrow transplantation. Blood. 1995;86: 4337-4343.

193. Alyea E, Soiffer R, Canning C, et al. Toxicity and efficacy of defined doses of CD4+ donor lymphocytes for treatment of relapse after allogeneic bone marrow transplantation. Blood. 1998;91:3671-3680.

194. O'Kunewick J, Kociban D, Machen L, et al. Effect of selective donor T cell depletion on the graft-versus-leukemia reaction in allogeneic marrow transplantation. Transplant Proc. 1992;24: 2998-2999.

195. Truitt R, Atasoylu A. Contribution of CD4+ and CD8+ T cells to graft-versus-host disease and graft-versus-leukemia reactivity after transplantation of MHC-compatible bone marrow. Bone Marrow Transplant. 1991;8:51-58.

196. Palathumpat V, Dejbakhsh-Jones S, Strober S. The role of purified CD8+ T cells in graft-versus-leukemia activity and engraftment after allogeneic bone marrow transplantation. Transplantation. 1995;60:355-361.

197. Faber L, van der Hoeven J, Goulmy E, et al. Recognition of clonogenic leukemia cells, remission bone marrow and HLA-identical donor bone marrow by CD8+ or CD4+ minor histocompatibility antigen-specific cytotoxic T lymphocytes. J Clin Invest. 1995;96:877-883.

198. Bensussan A, Lagabrielle J, Degos L. TCR gamma delta bearing lymphocyte clones with lymphokine-activated killer activity against autologous leukemia cells. Blood. 1989;73:2077-2080.

199. Malkovska V, Cigel F, Armstrong N, et al. Antilymphoma activity of human gamma delta T cells in mice with severe combined immune deficiency. Cancer Res. 1992;52:5610-5616.

200. de Bueger M, Bakker A, Van Rood J, et al. Tissue distribution of minor histocompatibility antigens. Ubiquitous versus restricted tissue distribution indicates heterogeneity among human cytotoxic T lymphocyte-defined non-MHC antigens. J Immunol. 1992;149:1788-1794.

201. Mutis T, Verdijk R, Schrama E, et al. Feasibility of immunotherapy of relapsed leukemia wiyh ex vivo-generated cytotoxic T lymphocytes specific for hematopoietic system-restricted minor histocompatibility antigens. Blood. 1999;93:2336-2341.

202. Jiang Y, Mavroudis D, Dermime S, et al. Alloreactive CD4+ T lymphocytes can exert cytotoxicity to chronic myeloid leukemia cells processing and presenting exogenous antigen. Br J Haematol. 1996;93:606-612.

203. Munker R, Lubbert M, Yonehara S, et al. Expression of Fas antigen on primary human leukemia cells. Ann Hematol. 1995;70:15-17.

204. Ruggeri L, Capanni M, Urbani E, et al. Effectiveness of donor natural killer cell alloreactivity in mismatched hematopoietic transplants. Science. 2002; 295:2097-2100.

205. Leung W, Iyengar R, Turner V, et al. Determinants of antileukemic effects of allogeneic NK cells. J Immunol. 2004;172:644-650.

206. Kim D, Sohn S, Lee N, et al. Transplantation with higher dose of natural killer cells associated with better outcomes in terms of non-relapse mortality and infectious events after allogeneic peripheral blood stem cell transplantation from HLA-matched sibling donors. Eur J Haematol. 2005;75:299-308.

207. Hsu K, Keever-Taylor C, Wilton A, et al. Improved outcome in HLA-identical sibling hematopoietic stem-cell transplantation for acute myelogenous leukemia predicted by KIR and HLA genotypes. Blood. 2005;105:4878-4884.

208. Giebel S, Locatelli F, Lamparelli T, et al. Survival advantage with KIR ligand incompatibility in hematopoietic stem cell transplantation from unrelated donors. Blood. 2003;102:814-819.

209. Davies S, Ruggeri L, DeFor T, et al. An evaluation of KIR ligand incompatibility in mismatched unrelated donor hematopoietic transplants. Blood. 2002;100:3825-3827.

210. Leung W, Iyengar R, Triplett B, et al. Comparison of killer Ig-like receptor genotyping and phenotyping for selection of allogeneic blood stem cell donors. J Immunol. 2005;174:6540-6545.

211. Fukuda T, Hackman R, Guthrie K, et al. Risks and outcome of idiopathic pneumonia syndrome after nonmyeloablative and conventional conditioning regimens for allogeneic hematopoietic stem cell transplantation. Blood. 2003;102:2777-2785.

212. Hogan W, Maris M, Storer B, et al. Hepatic injury after nonmyeloablative conditioning followed by hematopoietic stem cell transplantation: a study of 193 patients. Blood. 2004;103:73-84.

213. Baron F, Maris M, Sandmaier B, et al. Graft-versus-tumor effects after allogeneic hematopoietic cell transplantation with nonmyeloablative conditioning. J Clin Oncol. 2005;23:1993-2003.

214. Mielcarek M, Martin P, Leisenring W, et al. Graft-versus-host disease after nonmyeloablative versus conventional hematopoietic stem cell transplantation. Blood. 2003;102:756-762.

215. Hegenbart U, Niederwieser D, Sandmaier B, et al. Treatment of acute myelogenous leukemia by low-dose total-body irradiation-based conditioning and hematopoietic stem cell transplantation from related and unrelated donors. J Clin Oncol. 2006;24: 444-453.

216. Peggs K, Sureda A, Qian W, et al. Reduced-intensity conditioning for allogeneic haematopoietic stem cell transplantation in relapsed and refractory Hodgkin lymphoma: impact of alemtuzumab and donor lymphocyte infusions on long-term outcomes. Br J Haematol. 2007;139:70-80.

217. Childs R, Chernoff A, Contentin N, et al. Regression of metastatic renal-cell carcinoma after nonmyeloablative allogeneic peripheral-blood stem-cell transplantation. N Engl J Med. 2000;343:750-758.

218. Sandmaier B, Mackinnon S, Childs R. Reduced intensity conditioning for allogeneic hematopoietic cell transplantation: current perspectives. Biol Blood Marrow Transplant. 2007;13:87-97.

219. Lundqvist A, Childs R. Allogeneic hematopoietic cell transplantation as immunotherapy for solid tumors: current status and future directions. J Immunother. 2005;28:281-288.

220. Blaise D, Bay J, Faucher C, et al. Reduced-intensity preparative regimen and allogeneic stem cell transplantation for advanced solid tumors. Blood. 2004;103:435-441.

221. Bishop M, Fowler D, Marchigiani D, et al. Allogeneic lymphocytes induce tumor regression of advanced metastatic breast cancer. J Clin Oncol. 2004;22:3886-3892.

222. Matthay K, Seeger R, Reynolds C, et al. Allogeneic versus autologous purged bone marrow transplantation for neuroblastoma: a report from the Children's Cancer Group. J Clin Oncol. 1994;12:2382-2389.

223. Koscielniak E, Gross-Wieltsch U, Treuner J, et al. Graft-versus-Ewing sarcoma effect and long-term remission induced by haploidentical stem-cell transplantation in a patient with relapse of metastatic disease. J Clin Oncol. 2005;23:242-244.

224. Goi K, Sugita K, Tezuka T, et al. A successful case of allogeneic bone marrow transplantation for osteosarcoma with multiple metastases of lung and bone. Bone Marrow Transplant. 2006;37:115-116.

225. Lang P, Pfeiffer M, Müller I, et al. Haploidentical stem cell transplantation in patients with pediatric solid tumors: preliminary results of a pilot study and analysis of graft versus tumor effects. Klin Padiatr. 2006;218:321-326.

226. Storb R, Doney K, Thomas E, et al. Marrow transplantation with or without donor buffy-coat cells for 65 transfused aplastic anemia patients. Blood. 1982;59:236-246.

227. Radich J, Sanders J, Buckner C, et al. Second allogeneic marrow transplantation for patients with recurrent leukemia after initial transplant with total-body irradiation-containing regimens. J Clin Oncol. 1993;11:304-313.

228. Kolb H, Mittermuller J, Clemm C, et al. Donor leukocyte transfusions for treatment of recurrent chronic myelogenous leukemia in marrow transplant patients. Blood. 1990;76:2462-2465.

229. Slavin S, Naparstek E, Nagler A, et al. Allogeneic cell therapy for relapsed leukemia after bone marrow transplantation with donor peripheral blood lymphocytes. Exp Hematol. 1995;23:1553-1562.

230. Kolb H, Schattebberg A, Goldman J, et al. Graft-versus-leukemia effect of donor lymphocyte transfusions in marrow grafted patients. European Group for Blood and Marrow Transplantation Working Party Chronic Leukemia. Blood. 1995;86:2041-2050.

231. Porter D, Antin JH. The graft-versus-leukemia effects of allogeneic cell therapy. Annu Rev Med. 1999;50:369-386.

232. Kolb H. Donor leukocyte transfusions for treatment of leukemic relapse after bone marrow transplantation. EBMT Immunology and Chronic Leukemia Working Parties. Vox Sang. 1998;74(suppl 2):321-329.

233. Porter D, Collins R, Shpilberg O, et al. Long-term follow-up of patients who achieved complete remission after donor leukocyte infusions. Biol Blood Marrow Transplant. 1999;5:253-261.

234. Savani1 B, Montero1 A, Kurlander R, et al. Imatinib synergizes with donor lymphocyte infusions to achieve rapid molecular remission of CML relapsing after allogeneic stem cell transplantation. Bone Marrow Transplant. 2005;36:1009-1015.

235. Shiobara1 S, Nakao S, Ueda M, et al. Donor leukocyte infusion for Japanese patients with relapsed leukemia after allogeneic bone marrow transplantation: lower incidence of acute graft-versus-host disease and improved outcome. Bone Marrow Transplant. 2000;26:769-774.

236. Choi S, Lee J, Lee J, et al. Treatment of relapsed acute lymphoblastic leukemia after allogeneic bone marrow transplantation with chemotherapy followed by G-CSF-primed donor leukocyte infusion: a prospective study. Bone Marrow Transplant. 2005;36:163-169.

237. Collins R, Goldstein S, Giralt S, et al. Donor leukocyte infusions in acute lymphocytic leukemia. Bone Marrow Transplant. 2000;26:511-516.

238. Sánchez J, Serrano J, Gómez P, et al. Clinical value of immunological monitoring of minimal residual disease in acute lymphoblastic leukaemia after allogeneic transplantation. Br J Haematol. 2002;116:686-694.

239. Slavin S. Donor lymphocyte infusions for hematopoietic malignancy. In Giaccone G, Schilsky R, Sondel P (eds). Cancer Chemotherapy and Biologic Response Modifiers. Amsterdam, Elsevier, 2002, pp 291-300.

240. Choi S, Lee J, Lee J, et al. Treatment of relapsed acute myeloid leukemia after allogeneic bone marrow transplantation with chemotherapy followed by G-CSF-primed donor leukocyte infusion: a high incidence of isolated extramedullary relapse. Leukemia. 2004;18:1789-1797.

241. van Rhee F, Savage D, Blackwell J, et al. Adoptive immunotherapy for relapse of chronic myeloid leukemia after allogeneic bone marrow transplant: equal efficacy of lymphocytes from sibling and matched unrelated donors. Bone Marrow Transplant. 1998;21:1055-1061.

242. Bacigalupo A, Soracco M, Vassallo F, et al. Donor lymphocyte infusions (DLI) in patients with chronic myeloid leukemia following allogeneic bone marrow transplantation. Bone Marrow Transplant. 1997;19:927-932.

243. Dazzi F, Szydlo R, Craddock C, et al. Comparison of single-dose and escalating-dose regimens of donor lymphocyte infusion for relapse after allografting for chronic myeloid leukemia. Blood. 2000;95:67-71.

244. Sykes M, Harty M, Szot G, et al. Interleukin-2 inhibits graft-versus-host disease-promoting activity of CD4+ cells while preserving CD4- and CD8-mediated graft-versus-leukemia effects. Blood. 1994;83:2560-2569.

245. Mutis T, Verdijk R, Schrama E, et al. Feasibility of immunotherapy of relapsed leukemia with ex vivo-generated cytotoxic T lymphocytes specific for hematopoietic system-restricted minor histocompatibility antigens. Blood. 1999;93:2336-2341.

246. Yang Y, Sykes M. The role of interleukin-12 in preserving the graft-versus-leukemia effect of allogeneic CD8 T cells independently of GVHD. Leuk Lymphoma. 1999;33:409-420.

247. Walter E, Greenberg P, Gilbert M, et al. Reconstitution of cellular immunity against cytomegalovirus in recipients of allogeneic bone marrow by transfer of T-Cell clones from the donor. N Engl J Med. 1995;333:1038-1044.

248. Rooney C, Smith C, Ng C, et al. Use of gene-modified virus-specific T lymphocytes to control Epstein-Barr virus-related lymphoproliferation. Lancet. 1995;345:9-13.

249. Haque T, Wilkie G, Jones M, et al. Allogeneic cytotoxic T-cell therapy for EBV-positive posttransplantation lymphoproliferative disease: results of a phase 2 multicenter clinical trial. Blood. 2007;110:1123-1131.

250. Miller J, Soignier Y, Panoskaltsis-Mortari A, et al. Haploidentical NK cells in patients with cancer. Blood. 2005;105:3051-3057.

251. Introna M, Franceschetti M, Ciocca A, et al. Rapid and massive expansion of cord blood-derived cytokine-induced killer cells: an innovative proposal for the treatment of leukemia relapse after cord blood transplantation. Bone Marrow Transplant. 2006;38:621-627.

252. Choi S, Henderson MJ, Kwan E, et al. Relapse in children with acute lymphoblastic leukemia involving selection of a preexisting drug-resistant subclone. Blood. 2007;110:632-639.

253. Bui JD, Schreiber RD. Cancer immunosurveillance, immunoediting and inflammation: independent or interdependent processes? Curr Opin Immunol. 2007;19:203-208.

254. Demanet C, Mulder A, Deneys V, et al. Down-regulation of HLA-A and HLA-Bw6, but not HLA-Bw4, allospecificities in leukemic cells: an escape mechanism from CTL and NK attack? Blood. 2004;103:3122-3130.

255. Neal ZC, Imboden M, Rakhmilevich AL, et al. NXS2 murine neuroblastomas express increased levels of MHC class I antigens upon recurrence following NK-dependent immunotherapy. Cancer Immunol Immunother. 2004;53:41-52.

256. Singh H, Serrano LM, Pfeiffer T, et al. Combining adoptive cellular and immunocytokine therapies to improve treatment of B-lineage malignancy. Cancer Res. 2007;67:2872-2880.

257. Neal ZC, Sondel PM, Bates MK, et al. Flt3-L gene therapy enhances immunocytokine-mediated antitumor effects and induces long-term memory. Cancer Immunol Immunother. 2007;56:1765-1774.

258. Kahlon KS, Brown C, Cooper LJ, et al. Specific recognition and killing of glioblastoma multiforme by interleukin 13-zetakine redirected cytolytic T cells. Cancer Res. 2004;64:9160-9166.

259. Aranceli N, Wagner JR, Bautista CD, et al. Engineering cytolytic effector cells for glioma immunotherapy using gene insertion and zinc finger nuclease genomic editing. J Immunother. 2007;30:857-858.

8 Pediatric Radiation Oncology

Karen J. Marcus and Daphne Haas-Kogan

PRINCIPLES OF RADIATION ONCOLOGY

A significant proportion of children with cancer receive radiation therapy at some point during the clinical course. As advances in surgery, chemotherapy, and radiotherapy enter clinical practice, multimodality therapy has become the norm. For any given tumor, the incorporation of radiation therapy into such multimodality treatment must consider the timing of radiation, the most appropriate radiation modality, the short- and long-term toxicities both for radiation alone and in conjunction with chemotherapy and, finally, the integration of novel antineoplastic agents with radiation.

THE PHYSICAL BASIS OF RADIATION THERAPY

Radiation has been present throughout the evolution of life on Earth; it is not a new technologic advance. However, with the discovery of x-rays in 1895 by the German physicist Wilhelm Konrad Röntgen and of radioactivity in 1898 by Henri Becquerel, the biologic effects of radiation were soon recognized.[1] By the early part of the 20th century, ionizing radiation had rapidly come into use to treat malignant and benign conditions. At the 1922 International Congress of Oncology in Paris, Coutard presented the first evidence of the use of fractionated radiotherapy to cure advanced laryngeal cancer without disastrous sequelae.[2]

This event marked the beginning of the field of radiation oncology. Ionizing radiation produces ionizations and excitations during the absorption of energy in exposed tissue. Ionizing radiation includes both particulate radiation and electromagnetic waves. Electromagnetic waves are part of a broad spectrum that includes radio waves, microwaves, visible light, x-rays, and gamma rays. In therapeutic radiation oncology, x-rays, gamma rays, and particulate radiation are used. Gamma rays and x-rays share similar general properties, differing in their source and their energies. X-rays are produced when charged particles, generally electrons, are accelerated and bombard a high-density target. The target, most commonly tungsten, emits photons of varying energies up to the peak energy of the accelerated electrons. The energy of the photons is determined using the relationship $E = h\nu$, where h is the constant of proportionality known as Planck's constant, and ν is the frequency of the wave. Substituting for the frequency, the equation becomes $E = hc/\lambda$, where c is the speed of light and λ is the wavelength.

Radiation may be directly ionizing or indirectly ionizing. Direct ionization results in a direct disruption of the atomic or molecular structure of tissue through which the beam of radiation passes. This disruption causes biochemical and molecular damage. Particle beams are directly ionizing. Electromagnetic waves and neutrons are indirectly ionizing so that when they are absorbed in tissue they give up their energy by producing fast-moving charged particles. These charged particles directly damage tissue. In tissue, photons interact in several different ways, including the Compton effect, the photoelectric effect, coherent scattering, pair production, and photodisintegration. The dominant reaction is governed by the energy of the photons. The predominant reaction in radiation therapy is the Compton effect. This process, shown in Figure 8-1, involves the interaction of the photon with a loosely bound orbital electron. Part of the energy of the incident photon is transferred to the electron as kinetic energy. This Compton electron may then interact with electrons in the surrounding tissue. The remaining energy is carried away by another photon that is less energetic than the original photon. The probability of Compton interac-

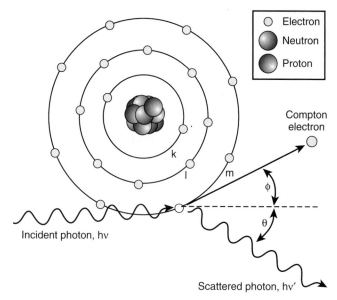

FIGURE 8-1. The Compton effect.

tions is independent of the atomic number of the target tissue.

Protons, neutrons, and other heavy particles interact with the nuclei of atoms rather than with orbital electrons, as do photons. Heavy particles also cause showers of lower energy densely ionizing protons, neutrons, and other particles, depositing large amounts of energy over a very short distance. This is referred to as linear energy transfer (LET) and depends on the type of radiation used. Photons and electrons have a low rate of energy transfer. Heavy particles tend to deposit their energy in a track over a relatively short distance; this process is considered high-LET radiation.

External beam radiation treatment machines produce ionizing radiation by radioactive decay of a nuclide, most commonly Cobalt-60, or electronically through the acceleration of electrons or other charged particles such as protons. In a linear accelerator, electrons are accelerated down a waveguide by the use of alternating microwave fields. In a Cobalt-60 unit, the source is always on in that radioactive decay occurs continuously. The source is moved to an unshielded position to initiate a treatment. In a linear accelerator, no source is present until the unit is energized and there is an *on* switch and an *off* switch. The energy spectra are different for the two types of treatment units. Cobalt-60 units emit two monoenergetic gamma rays with each decay, producing a discrete spectrum with peaks at 1.17 and 1.33 MeV. A linear accelerator produces a continuous x-ray spectrum with a maximum energy of E_{max} (the accelerating potential) and all other photon energies down to zero. An average x-ray produces the energy of approximately one-third E_{max}. A linear accelerator can produce a treatment beam of electrons as well as photons. The accelerated electron beam exits the treatment unit under controlled conditions of scatter.

The basic components of the treatment machine include a radiation source, a collimating system to form and direct the beam, inherent shielding for protection, a light field to delineate visibly the area being treated, a control system to turn the beam on and off, a system to rotate the beam, and a support apparatus for the patient. Modern treatment machines are assembled with isocentric geometry. The isocenter is a point in space at which all of the treatment machine's rotational axes intersect.

Any mechanical rotation occurs around an axis that passes through the isocenter.

The amount of energy deposited per unit mass represents the absorbed dose of radiation. The official unit of dose is the gray, in honor of L. H. Gray, the noted British radiobiologist who discovered the oxygen effect; it replaces the older unit, rad. One joule per kilogram is called a gray (Gy) and 1 gray equals 100 cGy. Clinical radiation therapy uses external radiation beam delivery, most often x-rays (photons) or electrons. Linear accelerators accelerate electrons to the desired energy, generally 4 to 25 MeV; the electrons bombard a target, usually tungsten, resulting in the formation of an x-ray beam. The x-ray beams contain photons of varying energies up to the peak of the accelerated electrons.

The linear accelerator has many degrees of geometric movement and can produce a treatment field in almost any orientation relative to the patient. The beam source is also mounted on a gantry that rotates fully about the patient. The patient is on a treatment couch that can pivot with respect to the plane of gantry rotation. This degree of movement allows multiple fields to approach the target volume. In addition, the collimation assembly mounted on the gantry allows the radiation treatment field to be geometrically conformed to the target volume intersection. Further field shaping is provided by apertures that block the radiation from specific areas. Multileaf collimators are used for intensity-modulated radiation therapy (IMRT), an important technology that is explained later. The multileaf collimator is a device that has a number of opposing leaves that span the field and can be individually adjusted to provide unique blocking patterns. Radiotherapy treatment generally involves multiple nonoverlapping conformal treatment fields. This approach reduces the dose delivered to uninvolved tissue. Further discussion of new technologies may be found in the section of this chapter designated Technologic Advances in Radiation Oncology.

In addition to external-beam radiation therapy, other radiation therapy delivery modalities are used in specific circumstances. Implanting radioactive sources directly into a tumor is known as brachytherapy, from the Greek *brachys*, meaning short. Brachytherapy can involve the placement of encapsulated sources into a body cavity (intracavitary), or directly into the tumor or adjacent tissue (interstitial implants), or on the surface adjacent to the tumor (plaque therapy). Permanent implants in the form of radioactive seeds are placed under the guidance of ultrasound, computed tomography, or magnetic resonance imaging. Temporary implants are performed using hollow catheters or loading devices inserted at the time of surgery and then subsequently loaded with radioactive sources. The chief advantage of this technique is to deliver a high dose to the target tissue while sparing the nearby normal tissue. Iridium-192 and Iodine-125 are the most commonly used radionuclides. Radionuclides are embedded in seeds and sealed in thin plastic strands that can be inserted into after-loading catheters. Iodine-125, with a relatively short half-life of 57 days, is often used in permanent implants. The other feature of Iodine-125, which makes it appealing for use in pediatrics, is the lower energy photons emitted, making the radiation safety concerns far simpler than those involved with Iridium-192. There are radiobiologic differences between brachytherapy and external-beam radiation therapy. Implants deliver continuous doses of 30 to 100 cGy per hour to the target tissue over the duration of the implant. This is in contrast to external-beam treatment in which the target tissue receives a short pulse of approximately 200 cGy daily, at a dose rate of 100 cGy per minute, over many weeks. Decreasing the dose rate may reduce the cell kill rate of a given dose because repair of sublethal damage continues throughout the protracted exposure. High-dose-rate brachytherapy techniques are becoming more widely used, although late complications increase with higher dose rates.[3] For dose rates exceeding 1 Gy per hour, a reduction in the total dose is considered. In addition, fractionation of high-dose rates can help to diminish the late complications of high-dose-rate delivery.

RADIOBIOLOGY

Mechanisms of Radiation Damage

The biologic effects of ionizing radiation result primarily from the formation of double-strand breaks in cellular DNA. Although most single-strand breaks in DNA caused by radiation are repaired, double-strand breaks can result in irreparable damage that leads to mitotic cell death. Photon radiation (x-rays or gamma rays) can cause damage via direct interaction with the DNA molecule or via the formation of free radicals that subsequently damage the DNA (indirect damage). Charged particles, such as helium, carbon, and neon, cause damage predominantly through direct interactions. High-energy neutrons interact with the nucleus of an atom, resulting in the creation of densely ionizing recoil protons, alpha particles, and nuclear fragments.[4] LET measures the average energy deposited in tissue per unit distance traveled by a particle or photon. Conventional radiation is sparsely ionizing (low LET), whereas fast neutrons and heavy particles are more densely ionizing (high LET).[4]

Radiation causes complex cascades of molecular events that affect cell cycle checkpoints, apoptosis, DNA damage response, and DNA repair. These effects offer many potential approaches to enhancing radiation damage of tumor cells and to protecting normal tissues. These techniques are discussed in this chapter.

Clonogenic Survival Curves

A typical clonogenic survival curve is shown in Figure 8-2. The surviving fraction is plotted on a logarithmic scale and the dose of radiation on a linear scale. The resulting cell survival curve has two distinct regions. In the initial "shoulder" portion of the curve, the fraction of cells killed increases slightly with increasing radiation doses. Killing then becomes exponential, which means that a given dose increment kills a constant fraction of cells. The slope of the exponential portion of the survival curve is called the D_0. This term is related to the inherent radiosensitivity of the cell. The smaller the D_0, the more sensitive the cells are to radiation. This is in contrast to radioresponsiveness, which refers only to the rate of disappearance of a tumor after irradiation and has no correlation with the innate sensitivity of the cells. The D_0 for mammalian cells in vitro generally falls between 1 and 2 Gy. The relatively narrow range of values for widely varying types of cells is striking. The initial nonexponential portion of the curve is believed to result from the capacity of most mammalian cells to repair nonlethal radiation injury. Saturation of the repair capability is thought to occur at the point where killing becomes exponential.[4]

Additional mathematical models have been used to characterize the cellular response to ionizing radiation. One of the most commonly used models, the linear-quadratic survival model, is routinely used to investigate how different tumor repopulation kinetics between radiation treatments influence the scheduling of radiation treatment. As various fractionation schemes have been examined clinically, including hyperfractionation, accelerated fractionation, and combined modality therapy (chemoradiation), the linear-quadratic model has been

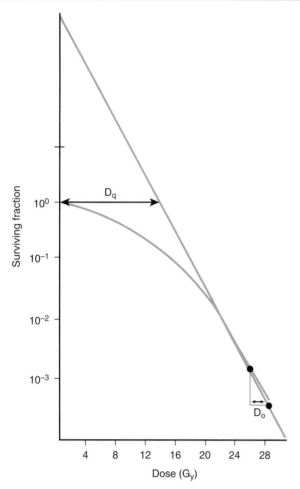

FIGURE 8-2. Idealized radiation cell survival curve. The fraction of surviving cells is plotted on a logarithmic scale against dose on a linear scale. The D_0 is the dose necessary to reduce the surviving fraction to 0.38 of e^{-1}. The smaller the D_0, the more sensitive the cells are to radiation. The D_q is the quasithreshold dose and is a quantitative measure of the sublethal repair capability. *(Modified from Hall EJ. Radiobiology for the Radiologist, 2nd ed. Hagerstown, Md, Harper Row, 1978.)*

used to calculate the tolerability of specific tissues to various radiation schedules.[5] The concept of the biologically effective dose, a tool offered by the linear-quadratic model, allows quantification of the effects of radiation schedules on tumors and on normal structures.[6] Although this model has been helpful when applying alternative fractionation schemes to patient treatment, caution must be exercised in its application because features such as faster tumor growth rate and higher repair capacity result in greater variations in the outcome of the survival fraction. Gaps in treatment, planned or unplanned, also accentuate the differences in the survival fraction under varying growth dynamics.[7] These limitations notwithstanding, mathematical modeling of the cellular response to radiation has contributed greatly to the clinical application of radiation to combating malignancies.

The Oxygen Effect

Tissue oxygenation influences the response of tumors and normal tissues to ionizing radiation. Poorly oxygenated tissues

are two to three times more resistant to radiation than are normally oxygenated tissues. Oxygen is thought to mediate indirect damage, combining with free radicals to make DNA damage irreversible. The effect of oxygenation is measured by the oxygen enhancement ratio. This is the ratio of doses under hypoxic versus aerated conditions required to produce a given level of cell kill. As LET increases, the effect of oxygen enhancement decreases.[4]

Stabilization of the hypoxia-inducible factor-1 plays a key role in the cellular response to hypoxic stress and the resultant resistance to radiation.[8] Subtleties in the effects of hypoxia on radiation resistance have emerged. Martinive and colleagues demonstrated that intermittent hypoxia stabilizes the hypoxia-inducible factor-1 more effectively than does chronic hypoxia.[9] Furthermore, this research suggests that intermittent hypoxia mediates radiation resistance by enhancing the growth and survival of vascular endothelial cells. Such cutting-edge investigations have propelled enthusiasm for agents that sensitize cells to radiation by targeting the hypoxia-inducible factor-1 in general and specifically by inhibiting hypoxia-inducible factor-1's promoter activity.[10]

Radiation Interactions with Chemotherapeutic Agents

A number of chemical substances may alter the radiation response of a cell.[11] The effects may be additive, such as those of most alkylating agents and antimetabolites, or they may be synergistic, such as those of the antibiotic dactinomycin.[12] Doxorubicin and dactinomycin markedly reduce the shoulder region of the radiation cell survival curve.[12] Dactinomycin also steepens the slope of the exponential portion of the cell survival curve and potentiates the radiation effect; thus it is thought to be a true radiation sensitizer.

Combining radiation and chemotherapy can achieve better clinical outcomes than either modality alone, but can also potentiate toxicities to normal tissues. Hepatic veno-occlusive disease (VOD) is a case in point. VOD of the liver is a nonthrombotic obliteration of the lumina of small intrahepatic veins that results in occlusion of hepatic venous outflow and postsinusoidal intrahepatic hypertension. Clinically, hepatic VOD is manifested by jaundice, weight gain, ascites, and painful hepatomegaly, and historically, VOD has occurred in 20% to 50% of patients receiving combined therapy.[13] Cooperative group studies of patients with Wilms' tumors have highlighted the interaction between radiation and dactinomycin in increasing the risk for VOD. The National Wilms' Tumor Study-4 randomized children into groups; in one, the children received single-dose dactinomycin; in another, the children received divided-dose dactinomycin. Severe hepatic toxicity occurred in 14.3% of children on the single-dose schedule of dactinomycin administration. However, even in the two remaining groups receiving lower doses of dactinomycin, the frequency of severe hepatic toxicity was tenfold higher than the 0.4% observed in similar nonirradiated patients in the National Wilms' Tumor Study-3.[14]

Interactions between chemotherapy and radiation can increase the risk for toxicity in normal tissues, even when the two modalities are temporally spaced. An interesting yet enigmatic phenomenon termed radiation recall was first described in 1959 by Dr. G. J. D'Angio. It is important that all those treating children with cancer be aware of this phenomenon because it influences many aspects of multimodality therapy. Radiation recall describes the remembering, or reemergence, of an inflammatory reaction that occurs within the radiation field and is prompted by the administration of particular agents days to years after initial radiation exposure. In the original case described by D'Angio, dermatitis emerged within the radiation field after application to the skin of actinomycin D.[12] Although radiation recall is most commonly documented as skin reactions, other tissues and organs are also susceptible to this phenomenon, including oral and intestinal mucosa, larynx, lungs, muscles, and the central nervous system.[15]

The cause of radiation recall remains poorly understood. Although timing and dosing factors clearly impact the risk and severity of the recall reaction, there is no clear radiation dose threshold. In addition, oral drugs generally have a longer latency of recall reaction than intravenous agents, reflecting differences in their systemic uptake and bioavailability. Recall reactions generally appear after first exposure to a recall-eliciting drug, and repeat exposure causes yet another recall reaction only occasionally.

Typically, radiation recall occurs after treatment with megavoltage radiotherapy, and it occurs 3 days to 2 months after administration of the triggering agent. However, recall reactions have been described over a range of minutes to years after radiation therapy.

MOLECULAR TARGETS FOR RADIOSENSITIZATION

Receptor Tyrosine Kinases

Receptor tyrosine kinases (RTKs) play pleiotropic roles in maintaining the homeostasis of individual cells as well as that of entire organisms. They regulate cellular proliferation, survival, adhesion, and differentiation, and their function is therefore tightly regulated. A family of RTKs includes molecules with a ligand-binding extracellular portion, a transmembrane section, and an intracellular portion that contains the tyrosine kinase catalytic domain.[16-18] This family includes the epidermal growth factor receptor (EGFR), platelet-derived growth factor receptor (PDGFR), vascular endothelial growth factor receptor, fibroblast growth factor receptor, stem-cell factor receptor, and nerve growth factor receptor. Inactivating mutations that confer ligand-independent phosphorylation and activation of the kinases occur in various domains of the protein, including the cytoplasmic juxtamembrane, extracellular, and kinase domains.[19] Several human malignancies develop as direct consequences of tyrosine kinase activation, and such aberrations can influence prognosis.[20,21]

Distinct domains of RTKs are targets not only of activating mutations but also of pharmacologic inhibitors directed at either the extracellular or the intracellular domain. Agents that inhibit protein tyrosine kinases fall into two main categories: monoclonal antibodies and small-molecule inhibitors.

Monoclonal antibodies can block signaling through growth factor receptors by preventing the binding of ligands and impeding the ensuing phosphorylation loop.[22,23] Advances in antibody construction have helped to alleviate problems such as the detrimental antibodies that patients develop against rodent antibodies.[24] Small-molecule inhibitors generally block signaling through RTKs by competing with adenosine triphosphate for its binding site on the receptor.[17] Both strategies of RTK inhibition—monoclonal antibodies and small pharmacologic agents—significantly impact the antineoplastic effects of ionizing radiation. Inhibitors of several RTKs cause radiosensitization of cancer cells, and their incorporation into radiation regimens is imminent.

Epidermal Growth Factor Receptor Family Inhibitors

The EGFR family consists of four different receptors: ErbB-1 (also known as EGFR); ErbB-2 (also known as HER2/*neu*); ErbB-3 (also known as HER3); and ErbB-4 (also known as HER4).[25-27] EGFR, located on chromosome 7p12, plays a key role in the oncogenesis of glioblastoma multiformes. Mechanisms of EGFR activation include amplification, overexpression, and expression of a truncated constitutively active form. It is the most commonly amplified oncogene in glioblastoma multiformes, with amplification seen in 40% of tumors.[28-30] One third of glioblastoma multiformes in which EGFR is amplified contain a mutant form, most commonly the EGFRvIII mutant, in which deletion in the extracellular domain results in constitutive tyrosine kinase activity.[31,32]

Small-molecule inhibitors of EGFRs have entered clinical trials for gliomas. Two such inhibitors are ZD1839 and CP-358,774, which inhibit EGFR signaling by targeting the adenosine triphosphate binding site of the receptor.[33-35] Both are oral drugs that exhibit great specificity and promise in ongoing clinical trials.

Inhibition of EGFR signaling has been accomplished not only by pharmacologic agents but also by monoclonal antibodies raised against the extracellular domain of EGFR. Human/murine chimeric antibodies offer the advantage of reduced immunogenicity while preserving potency. MAb-C225 is such an antibody whose administration in animal models delays growth of xenograft tumors resulting from overexpression of ErbB-1.[36]

Platelet-Derived Growth Factor Receptor Inhibitors

STI571 is a small-molecule drug that rather specifically inhibits the tyrosine kinases Abl, PDGFRs, and Kit.[37] Clinical trials have documented the efficacy of STI571 in the treatment of chronic myeloid leukemia, a malignancy driven by constitutive activation of Abl resulting from a chromosomal translocation called Bcr-Abl. The relevance of STI571 for glioma therapy rests in molecular aberrations involving PDGF (platelet-derived growth factor) and PDGFRs. PDGFR-α and PDGFR-β are two distinct receptors that bind the PDGF ligand which, in turn, consists of various dimers of PDGF-α and PDGF-β chains. Overexpression of the PDGF ligand and receptor are seen in all grades of gliomas, suggesting activation of an autocrine loop that drives glioma proliferation.[38,39] The mechanism of such overexpression is unknown, although in the minority of cases amplification of the PDGF-α gene underlies overexpression.

Aberrant PDGFR signaling in low-grade as well as high-grade gliomas suggests a role for this signaling cascade in the initiation and progression of gliomas. These molecular aberrations establish the rationale for treating gliomas of all grades with PDGF inhibitors. STI571 has already entered clinical protocols for the treatment of gliomas.

Vascular Endothelial Growth Factor Receptor Inhibitors

Uncontrolled tumor growth relies not only on uncontrolled cell proliferation and survival but also on the concomitant development of blood vessels to support the enlarging mass. Molecules that block or promote angiogenesis have been isolated. The best-described proangiogenic factors are vascular endothelial growth factors (VEGFs), which transmit their signals through Flt-1 (also known as VEGF-R1) and Flk-1/KDR (also known as VEGF-R2) receptors.[40] Whereas VEGF ligands are secreted by tumor and stromal cells, VEGF receptors are expressed mostly by endothelial cells.

As with other RTKs, strategies to block signaling through VEGF receptors consist of small-molecule inhibitors and antibodies directed against receptors or ligands. SU5416 selectively inhibits Flk-1/KDR and Flt-1.[41] A second pharmacologic molecule, SU6668, exhibits wider specificity toward potentially proangiogenic RTKs, including Flk-1/KDR, PDGF, and fibroblast growth factor receptors.[42] Antibodies directed against VEGF or its receptor have entered clinical trials as well. Studies of anti-VEGF agents have focused on human solid tumors because solid malignancies rely on robust blood supplies. Gliomas exemplify such tumors; vascularity increases with glioma grade, and endothelial proliferation helps to define the highest grade of glioma. Phase 1 clinical trials employing VEGF inhibitors as single agents report disease stabilization but not objective tumor responses.

Farnesyltransferase Inhibitors

Signaling cascades emanating from engagement of growth factor receptors use intermediate molecules to propagate their signals to downstream pathways. The Ras proteins are such intermediaries. Ras is a GTPase that cycles between its active guanosine 5′-triphosphate–bound state and its inactive guanosine 5′-biphosphate–bound state. Ras mediates many functions, including proliferation, survival, cytoskeletal organization, differentiation, and membrane trafficking. Ras activities depend on its association with the inner surface of the plasma membrane.[43-45] Ras proteins are synthesized as cytosolic precursors and are converted to membrane-bound forms through posttranslational modifications. Such post-translational modifications begin with the addition of a 15-carbon farnesyl moiety (an isoprene lipid) to a specific motif at the carboxyl terminus of Ras proteins. Farnesyltransferase catalyzes the transfer of a farnesyl group from farnesyl diphosphate to a cysteine residue within the CAAX box (A is an aliphatic amino acid and X is methionine or serine) of Ras.[46]

Farnesyltransferase inhibitors (FTIs) can directly block the function of Ras but may also interrupt the effects of RTKs that signal through Ras. Thus, although gliomas rarely contain mutated, oncogenic forms of Ras, common genetic aberrations such as EGFR overexpression may be susceptible to therapeutic targeting by FTIs. However, the precise mode of FTI action remains unclear because the mutational status of Ras does not consistently correlate with the response of cells to FTI treatment. Furthermore, an enlarging body of evidence suggests that FTI activity is mediated in part through inhibition of farnesylation of other Ras family members such as RhoB.[47-49] With such unresolved uncertainties, it remains difficult to delineate precisely which tumors represent the most promising cohort for FTI treatment. These ambiguities notwithstanding, treatment of gliomas in vitro with FTI results in decreased proliferation and induction of apoptosis. Glioma cells overexpressing EGFR may exhibit enhanced sensitivity to such FTI treatment.

Histone Deacetylase Inhibitors

Histone modification has emerged as a central regulator of gene expression in a variety of cancers. A dynamic equilibrium between histone acetyltransferase and histone deacetylase controls levels of acetylated histones in nuclear chromatin.[50] By inducing acetylation of the nuclear histones H3 and H4, histone deacetylase inhibitors (HDACIs) cause relaxation of the chromatin structure, allowing access of transcription factors and thus modulating the expression of several genes. HDACIs play a major role in regulating gene expression, growth arrest, and the differentiation and apoptosis of tumor cells.[51-53] A number of HDACIs are in preclinical and clinical development, including short or aromatic fatty acids and their derivatives (Pivanex, also known as AN-9,[54]); hydroxamic acids (SAHA, TSA[55,56]); and phenylbutyrate.[57,58]

Preclinical and clinical studies are evaluating several HDACIs, including a prodrug of butyric acid (BA), pivaloylomethyl butyrate (AN-9), hydroxamic acids suberoylanilide hydroxamic acid [SAHA] and trichostatin A [TSA], benzamide derivatives (MS-275 and CI-994), cyclic peptides (trapoxin, apicidin, and depsipeptide), and valproic acid.[59,60] Studies have revealed the radiosensitizing abilities of various HDACIs, including MS-275,[61] SAHA,[62] valproic acid,[63] TSA,[64] and BA.[65]

Although HDACIs result in cell differentiation, apoptosis, or growth arrest, depending on the cell system, these agents are cytostatic in most solid tumors. Thus HDACIs are most likely to improve patient survival rates in combination with other agents. Indeed, several laboratories have documented that HDACIs sensitize various cancers to radiation, in vitro and in vivo. Studies examining mechanisms of HDACI-radiation interactions suggest that enhanced induction of DNA damage underlies the documented radiosensitization.[61,63,66] These studies highlight the potential for incorporating HDACIs into multimodality treatment of cancer, and such studies are sure to be tested by cooperative groups.

Combining Molecularly Targeted Therapies with Conventional Antineoplastic Treatments

Inhibitors of cell signaling, whether antibodies or small-molecule drugs, are most likely to impact the treatment of human cancers when combined with standard forms of antineoplastic therapy, such as chemotherapy and radiation. Such clinical impact is maximized if novel inhibitors sensitize human malignancies to standard cytotoxic agents. Many studies, most commonly of cell lines in vitro or xenograft tumor models in rodents, indicate that treatment with signaling inhibitors augments tumor responses to radiation and chemotherapy.[67] Molecular mechanisms implicated in radiosensitization associated with signaling inhibitors include effects on cell proliferation, survival, migration, invasion, angiogenesis, and DNA repair. The precise molecular mechanisms, however, remain elusive.

The strongest data for radiosensitization exist for agents that block EGFR signaling. EGFR overexpression correlates with resistance to radiation in vitro and in vivo.[68-71] EGFR overexpression also correlates with the radiographically measured radiation responses of the human glomerular basement membrane in vivo.[72] In a model of human squamous cell carcinoma cells grown in mice, administration of MAb-C225 together with radiation resulted in complete regression of established xenograft tumors.[73,74] Such impressive efficacy of concurrent MAb-C225 and radiation has also been documented in intracranial tumors of human glioma cells grown as xenografts in athymic mice. Small-molecule inhibitors of EGFR similarly sensitize human malignancies to radiation in cell lines in vitro and in animal models of human malignancies in vivo. ZD1839 sensitizes several human cell lines to radiation, as does an additional pharmacologic tyrosine kinase inhibitor, CI-1033, which blocks activities of all four types of ErbB receptors.[26] These studies establish the rationale for current clinical trials that are examining concurrent administration of ZD183 and radiation in the treatment of adult and pediatric gliomas.

There is great appeal to the use of double-edged swords such as EGFR inhibitors that may block tumor growth and sensitize resistant tumors to radiation. Similarly, promising results indicate that treatment with FTIs sensitizes human cancer cell lines to irradiation. FTIs reversed the radiation resistance of cell lines containing mutant Ras without affecting the radiosensitivity of cells expressing wild-type Ras.[75] A critical unanswered question is whether FTIs will also preferentially radiosensitize cells with aberrant signaling cascades that rely on Ras as an intermediary.

Direct evidence is lacking for radiosensitization by signaling inhibitors that target other RTKs, such as PDGF and VEGF receptors. However, laboratory investigations offer encouraging evidence that additional signaling inhibitors will augment the radiation response. For example, studies in which VEGF mediates resistance to radiation predict that blocking VEGF signaling will augment the cytotoxic effects of radiation. Furthermore, antiangiogenic drugs synergize with radiation to block tumor growth in vivo.[76] Such promising preliminary studies provide the impetus for designing innovative studies in which molecularly targeted agents are administered together with radiation or chemotherapy.

Targeting Tumor-Host Components

Studies to date have focused on the cancer cell itself and agents that act as radiosensitizers. A new approach has now come into focus—that of targeting host components such as the tumor microvasculature.[77] Indeed, the antineoplastic effects of radiation are enhanced when it is combined with protein tyrosine kinase inhibitors (TKIs), partially because of increased damage to tumor vasculature.[78] TKIs with such antiangiogenic effects include inhibitors of VEGF, PDGF, and fibroblast growth factors. These TKIs destroy tumor vasculature and enhance the effects of radiation by inhibiting phosphoinositide 3-kinase (PI3-kinase), a key mediator of growth-factor signaling.[78]

It is therefore not surprising that preclinical studies have suggested clinical benefit of combining radiation with antiangiogenic agents, a benefit that is probably mediated through enhanced destruction of tumor vasculature.[79,80] Future designs of clinical trials combining radiation and antiangiogenic agents will benefit from elucidation of several issues, including biologically effective doses, appropriate sequencing, and validated surrogate markers of biologic responses and clinical efficacy. Given the data that indicate that PI3-kinase mediates the antiangiogenic effects of TKIs and their radiosensitizing functions, perhaps the most promising target for therapeutic inhibition is PI3-kinase itself.[77]

p53 Tumor-Suppressor Protein

p53 stands at the crossroads of cell death, growth, and differentiation and therefore sustains the homeostasis of individual cells, specific tissues, and entire organisms. p53 regulates apoptosis, proliferation, differentiation, angiogenesis, and cell-matrix interactions.[81,82] Each individual tissue and cell lineage incorporates a distinct balance among the various biologic processes mediated by p53.[83] For example, p53-dependent apoptosis dominates the behavior of hematologic cells, so irradiation of hematologic malignancies, such as leukemia and lymphoma, produces rapid apoptosis. A clinical corollary of this laboratory

observation is that radiation of hematologic malignancies produces rapid and durable responses when treated by radiation therapy. Similarly, in many pediatric tissues, apoptosis plays a key role during organogenesis, and pediatric solid tumors, such as Wilms' tumor and neuroblastoma, exhibit significant apoptosis and excellent cure rates when treated by radiation. In contradistinction, in many adult solid tumors apoptosis plays a minor role, and the balance of p53-mediated functions tilts toward proliferation and differentiation. Thus, documentation of p53-mediated apoptosis in vivo following irradiation of adult solid tumors such as glioblastoma multiforme and sarcomas has remained elusive.

Despite these complex considerations, the presence of p53 mutations in more than half of human cancers has provided enthusiasm for harnessing p53 to overcome tumor resistance to conventional therapies such as radiation.[84] The expression of p53 in cells lacking wild-type p53 enhances cellular sensitivity to ionizing radiation.

In the quest to restore wild-type p53 function and overcome resistance to radiation, two main approaches have been used: gene therapy and pharmacologic molecules that confer wild-type p53 function on mutant forms of p53.[85] Genetic introduction of wild-type p53 with viral or nonviral vectors may restore physiologic roles of p53 and such functions, particularly p53-mediated apoptosis, may radiosensitize human tumors to radiation. However, many impediments to gene therapy have arisen, including inefficient delivery and detrimental immune responses.

Pharmacologic agents that impinge on p53 functions hold great promise for translational clinical practice. Some mutated forms of p53 are amenable to treatment with either synthetic peptides or monoclonal antibodies that can restore wild-type p53 function. Furthermore, large libraries of pharmacologic compounds can be rapidly screened for their ability to reinstate transcriptional transactivating abilities of mutant p53. As such novel agents enter clinical trials, the prospect of overcoming the radiation resistance of gliomas appears to be within reach.

TECHNOLOGIC ADVANCES IN RADIATION ONCOLOGY

Modern Treatment Approaches

Conformal radiotherapy describes treatment that delivers a high-dose volume that is shaped to conform to the target volume while minimizing the dose to critical normal tissues in the adjacent area. Because conformal radiotherapy attempts to conform the dose to the target, careful and accurate delineation of the target is critical. Patient immobilization for setup accuracy and to limit patient motion is critical to minimize the dose to normal tissue but not miss the target. The International Commission on Radiological Units and Measurements-50 defined target volumes that are currently used in treatment planning.[86] The gross tumor volume is the volume of macroscopic tumor that is visualized on imaging studies. The clinical target volume is the volume that should be treated to high dose, typically incorporating both the gross tumor volume and the surrounding tissues assumed to be at risk because of microscopic spread of the disease. The planning target volume is the volume that should be treated in order to ensure that the clinical target volume is appropriately covered; this takes into account systematic and random setup errors between treatments and during treatment (Fig. 8-3A and B). The treated volume is the volume of tissue enclosed by a specific isodose line. The treated volume is greater than the planning target volume.

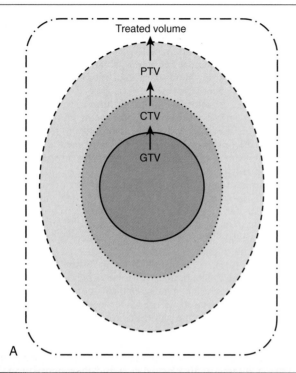

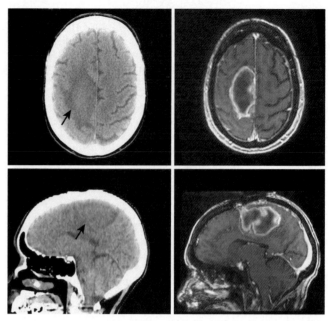

FIGURE 8-4. Magnetic resonance image fusion with planning computed tomography, demonstrating improved tumor delineation by magnetic resonance imaging.

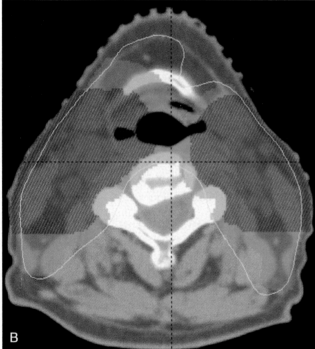

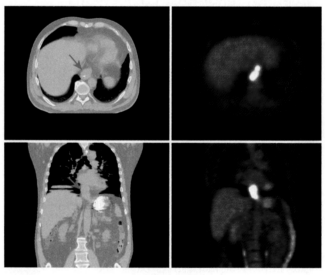

FIGURE 8-5. Computed tomography and positron emission tomography fusion to delineate active tumor.

FIGURE 8-3. A, Target volumes for treatment planning. CVT, clinical target volume; GTV, gross tumor volume; PVT, planning target volume. **B,** Gross tumor volume shown in pink; expanded clinical target volume is hatched; the planning target volume is green. The yellow line delineates the treated volume.

Conformal radiotherapy requires imaging that allows careful delineation of the tumor as well as of critical structures. Computed tomography, magnetic resonance imaging, and functional nuclear imaging all are useful in defining these volumes (Fig. 8-4). The conformal treatment plan can be used only when such target delineation is available and patient immobilization can be ensured. Dataset registration and fusion of multiple imaging modalities, including magnetic resonance imaging and positron emission tomography, and computed tomography, are extremely useful in defining tumor and normal tissue (Fig. 8-5).

Intensity-Modulated Radiation Therapy

Sophisticated planning techniques have significantly improved the ability to tailor the radiation field to the desired treatment region. IMRT is one such novel technique that allows the radiation oncologist optimally to manipulate the intensities of individual rays within each beam. IMRT requires highly specialized technology and software that are not available at every radiation oncology center.

IMRT offers a new approach to delivering high doses to the tumor while sparing normal tissues in the body. The precise position of the tumor may change, both during a given treatment session and between days of treatment. Such movement may result from shifting internal organs such as during breathing or digestion and may result from small alterations in the exact position of the patient on the treatment table. Tumor movement may cause portions of the tumor to receive less radiation than prescribed or may cause normal structures to receive more radiation than intended.

Therefore, key to effective use of IMRT is accurate demarcation of the tumor and normal structures and immobilization of the patient. To address patient immobilization and daily positioning, some centers are using image-guided techniques. These new approaches allow the radiation oncologist to confirm the tumor's location every day. One of the most exciting techniques for minimizing tumor and patient movement is the use of a computed tomography image of the patient using the cone beam technique, which allows the generation of an image of the tumor and all surrounding normal structures using the same linear accelerator with which the patient is being treated. Appropriate adjustments can then be made daily to ensure that the tumor is receiving the appropriate dose of radiation and normal tissues are receiving doses within their tolerance ranges.

The emerging concept of image-guided motion management is taking hold within the radiation oncology community, and many centers are learning not only to optimize patient immobilization techniques but also to use novel technology to ensure ever-increasing accuracy in radiation delivery.

PARTICLE BEAM THERAPY

Proton Beam Radiation Therapy

Charged particles deposit energy in tissue through multiple interactions with electrons in the atoms of cells; a small amount of energy is also transferred to tissue through collisions with the nuclei of atoms. The particle range is determined by the energy of the incoming particles. Particle beams, such as proton beams and heavier ion beams, show an increase in energy deposition with penetration depth that rises to a sharp maximum at the ends of their ranges. The energy loss per unit path length is constant and relatively small until near the end of the range of the particle, where the residual energy is lost over a short distance. This results in a steep rise in the absorbed dose. This portion of the particle track, where the particle loses energy rapidly over a very short distance, is known as the Bragg peak. There is an initial low-dose region prior to the Bragg peak referred to as the plateau of the dose distribution curve; the plateau is about 30% of the maximum during the Bragg peak. The Bragg peak is narrow and to be clinically useful must be modulated to deliver a uniform dose over a larger distance. The extended dose region is called the spread-out Bragg peak and does increase the entrance dose somewhat. The proton dose distribution is characterized by a lower dose region in normal tissue proximal to the tumor. Favorable dose distributions with the steep dose falloff at the field borders allow for more precise dose localization when using particle beams than when using photon beams.

The LET is the rate of energy loss by the particle in the tissue. Charged particles are characterized as having either high or low LET. Photons (gamma and x-rays), protons, and helium ions are considered low-LET radiation. Heavier charged particles, such as neon and carbon, are considered high-LET radiation. The LET influences the biologic impact.[87] High-LET radiation is less influenced by tissue oxygenation and less sensitive to variations in the cell cycle. However, despite the higher LET of protons compared to photons, their radiobiologic properties do not differ substantially. For clinical applications, the absorbed dose is multiplied by a factor of 1.1 to express the biologic effective dose in cobalt gray equivalents. Heavier particle beams such as carbon ions share the physical properties of protons but have a biologic advantage in that their biologic efficiency increases at the end of the beam's range, whereas it is low along the entrance path. When tumors are surrounded by radiosensitive normal tissue, the relative biologic effectiveness (RBE) of these heavy particle beams can be as high as 4.[88]

Protons are now among the most widely used of the charged particles in radiotherapy. Based on the favorable beam profile of the absence of exit dose and the reduction in the integral dose to normal tissue achieved by using protons, more proton facilities are under development. A variety of tumors have been successfully treated by proton beam radiotherapy, including uveal melanoma, sarcomas of the skull base and spine, prostate carcinoma, acoustic neuromas, optic gliomas, and other astrocytomas and medulloblastomas.[89-92,93-95] Outcomes following proton radiotherapy compare favorably with the results of precision photon therapy.[96-98] In the treatment of pediatric patients, protons can have a particular advantage over photons by sparing the dose to normal structures, as in the treatment of orbital rhabdomyosarcoma and retroperitoneal tumors. A number of ongoing trials of proton beam radiation therapy are in progress worldwide. Comparisons of standard conformal photon treatment plans, intensity-modulated radiation therapy, photon plans, and proton plans for a variety of tumor locations demonstrate the substantial sparing of normal tissue that can be achieved by using protons (Figs. 8-6 and 8-7).[93]

Carbon Ions

Carbon ion radiotherapy provides a particle-therapy modality that combines the physical advantages of proton beams with favorable biologic properties. Compared with photons, heavy charged particles have a favorable physical beam profile in which the dose increases with depth, and then the energy is lost at a specified depth. Carbon ions provide higher RBE within the Bragg peak compared to the entrance dose. This increased RBE within the Bragg peak is advantageous for treating slow-growing tumors. Such tumors are often less sensitive to conventional radiotherapy. Carbon ions, like protons, provide higher physical selectivity because of their finite range in tissue. Carbon ions have the advantage over protons and photons of RBE within the Bragg, as shown in Figure 8-8.[99] These advantages of greater RBE and better dose distributions permit dose escalation within the target and optimal sparing of nearby normal tissue. The biologic advantages of carbon ions over protons are expected to be most significant for tumors that are not particularly radiosensitive and in particular when such tumors are surrounded by radiosensitive normal tissue.[99] Although the therapeutic use of carbon ions is relatively recent and relatively limited, more than 2100 patients have been treated at more than 25 centers in China, Germany, and Japan. The Gesellschaft fur Schwerionenforschung in Germany has reported that patients treated with carbon ions for skull-based chordomas, low-grade chondrosarcomas, and adenoid cystic carcinomas demonstrated excellent local control and low toxicity.[100-102]

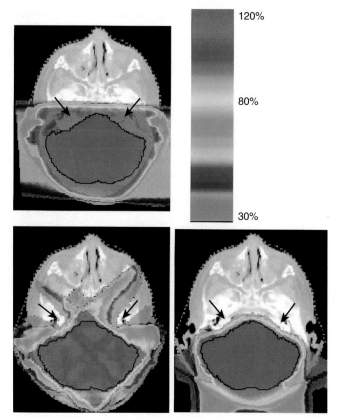

FIGURE 8-6. Isodose distributions comparing opposed lateral photons, IMRT, and proton dose distributions. *(From St. Clair WH, Adams JA, Bus M, et al. Advantages of protons compared to conventional x-rays or IMRT in the treatment of a pediatric patient with medulloblastoma. Int J Radiat Oncol Biol Physiol. 2004;58:727-734.)*

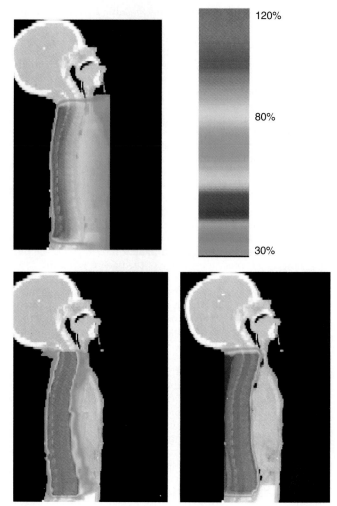

FIGURE 8-7. Isodose distributions comparing single-field photons, IMRT, and protons. *(From St. Clair WH, Adams JA, Bus M, et al. Advantages of protons compared to conventional x-rays or IMRT in the treatment of a pediatric patient with medulloblastoma. Int J Radiat Oncol Biol Physiol. 2004;58:727-734.)*

Clinical Applications

Along with chemotherapy and surgery, therapeutic radiation remains one of the primary modalities for treating cancer, including those that occur in children. Malignant cells differ little from normal cells in their responses to ionizing radiation. Most cells have the capacity to undergo repair of sublethal damage. Malignant tumors do differ in radiosensitivity, although cell survival curves suggest that various cell types have some inherent differences in radiosensitivity. The differences in sensitivity among tumors are the result of many factors, including the inherent sensitivity, the hypoxic fraction, the vascularity, and the surrounding normal tissue. Although the term *radiosensitivity* has been used to describe how rapidly a tumor shrinks following irradiation, the more appropriate term would be *radioresponsiveness*. Shrinkage of tumor is more a factor of cell removal or cell loss and is not related to radiosensitivity at the cellular level.

Both normal and malignant tumors have sigmoid dose-response curves such that a certain dose must be reached before a response is seen; after that, the rate of response increases rapidly and is followed by a diminished rate of response. The probability of complications increases with increased doses as is shown in Figure 8-6. The probability of tumor control and the probability of normal tissue complications are both a sigmoid function of dose; if the two curves are well separated, it is possible to achieve a high rate of tumor control with a small rate of complications. Fractionated radiotherapy generally shifts the curve of normal tissue complications to the right of the

curve of tumor control. When the curves are closer together, the favorable condition of good control with minimal complications does not apply. The balance between tumor control and normal tissue complications is referred to as the therapeutic ratio. In general, at doses that result in no normal tissue complications, the cure rates are low, whereas at doses that result in very high tumor control rates, unacceptable morbidity may also result. Therefore, in clinical practice, intermediate doses are used; they represent a balance between toxicity and benefit. When the potential complications are likely to result in severe morbidity, such as radiation myelitis or pneumonitis, the dose or field of radiation is limited to avoid these toxicities, even at the cost of decreased likelihood of tumor control. In cases in which the role of radiotherapy is short-term palliation of symptoms with no expectation of cure, doses that cause limited morbidity are used.

A number of treatment parameters can be varied, including the volume irradiated, the total dose, the fraction size, and the dose rate. All of these parameters influence tumor control as well as normal tissue complications. In general, the doses of radiotherapy are not based on the age of the patient but on the tumor type. However, the decision to use radiotherapy in a child is influenced by the age of the child, the tumor, and the

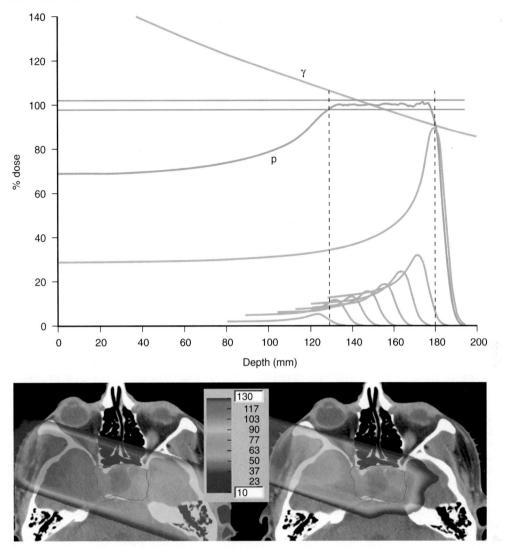

FIGURE 8-8. Depth dose curves (top) for a single spread-out Bragg peak (SOBP) field of protons (p) and a single photon field (γ). The single-field SOBP curve shows a constant plateau of dose (the green lines indicate +/− 2% of dose) whose length can be selected by the user to achieve coverage in depth of the target. The SOBP shows the proton characteristic distal fall-off. The single photon field cannot achieve uniform target volume coverage and if normalized to the target volume center would, of course, deliver unacceptable dose to the proximal tissues. This effect is also illustrated in the bottom panels for a single photon field (left) and single proton field (right). Only an ensemble of photon fields can achieve an acceptable homogeneity of dose across a target volume. The blue curves in the top panel are the individual proton pristine Bragg peaks that are delivered to achieve the homogeneous plateau in the SOBP.

site of disease. The normal tissue tolerances that are used for children are similar to those established for adults (Table 8-1). However, whether these critical organs in young children are more or less vulnerable to the effects of irradiation is not well established. The dose that can be delivered to a particular tumor may be limited by several factors: the anatomic location of the tumor, the size of the radiotherapy field, and the age of the patient. The long-term toxicities in children are different from those in adults, leading to adjustments in doses even at the cost of decreased chance of tumor control. The late effects of radiotherapy are discussed subsequently.

The indications for radiotherapy vary greatly in pediatric cancers. Radiotherapy, like surgery, is considered a local treatment rather than a systemic treatment. Solid tumors generally require some form of local treatment; radiotherapy may be indicated when surgical resection is not possible or has been

TABLE 8-1	Normal Tissue Tolerance Doses
Organ	**Dose Limit (Gy)**
Optic nerve and chiasm	46.8
Lacrimal gland	41.4
Small bowel	45.0
Spinal cord	45.0
Lung (when > ⅓ but < ½ of total lung volume is in the PTV)	18.0
Lung (when > ½ of total lung volume is in the PTV)	15.0
Whole kidney	19.8
Whole liver	23.4

PTV, planning target volume

incomplete. Soft tissue and bone sarcomas, including Ewing's, rhabdomyosarcoma, and other soft tissue sarcomas, require radiation therapy as part of local tumor control if there is microscopic or gross residual disease following surgery. Rhabdomyosarcomas and Ewing's sarcomas require systemic chemotherapy, but local control can be accomplished successfully with radiotherapy and no surgery. Wilms' tumor, advanced neuroblastoma, Hodgkin's disease, and nasopharyngeal carcinoma also require systemic chemotherapy, but radiotherapy is often needed for local control.

Acute leukemia in children is the most common childhood malignancy. Radiotherapy is indicated as part of central nervous system prophylaxis in children with high-risk features, such as T-cell phenotype or very high counts of white blood cells. Total body irradiation is used in stem cell transplantation in children with relapsed leukemia. Brain tumors are the most common solid tumor in children. Radiotherapy is used in the management of many of these tumors. The volume of treatment as well as the dose vary according to the histology of the tumor and clinical factors such as age of the patient and the extent of the disease.

The treatment of childhood tumors is best determined by large clinical trials that are designed to improve the outcome and minimize the toxicities. When radiotherapy is part of the treatment of a tumor, these trials may seek to arrive at the appropriate indications and doses or to eliminate radiotherapy. Detailed discussions of the indications and doses of radiation therapy by tumor type are included in the respective chapters discussing each tumor.

As a result of the recognized toxicities associated with radiation therapy, current trials strive to limit the dose or eliminate radiotherapy whenever possible. The role of radiotherapy has been diminishing for some pediatric tumors as we gain both greater understanding of tumor biology and which tumors can be successfully treated using less aggressive treatment. This is the case with the treatment of lymphoblastic leukemia, in which more intensive chemotherapy has been able to replace radiotherapy in central nervous system prophylaxis in children with standard-risk leukemia, but radiotherapy continues to be used for patients with some high-risk features.

Oncologic emergencies are potentially life-threatening situations in which a tumor could be encroaching on the airway or the spinal cord or causing uncontrolled bleeding. A mediastinal mass from lymphoblastic lymphoma can cause respiratory distress as well as compression of the superior vena cava. Radiotherapy is a modality often considered for urgent life-threatening symptoms of malignancy. Spinal cord compression resulting from a growing paraspinal or intraspinal tumor results in permanent paraplegia unless the spinal cord can be decompressed rapidly. The neurosurgeon and the radiation oncologist are consulted to act urgently, according to the clinical situation. Airway compromise caused by a mass in the mediastinum can rapidly lead to cardiorespiratory arrest, and the radiation oncologist must be available immediately. If a diagnosis can be made, chemotherapy can be administered and radiotherapy withheld. Even if a pathologic diagnosis has not been made, in the majority of cases, clinical impressions are sufficient to initiate chemotherapy.[103]

In addition to its role in oncologic emergencies, radiotherapy is an important modality for palliation of symptoms in children for whom there may be no expectation of cure. Painful bony metastases and other painful metastases are well treated by a course of radiotherapy. Metastatic lesions that cause spinal cord compression or airway obstruction are also situations in which a short course of radiotherapy can improve the quality of life, even if there is no expectation of long-term survival. Palliative treatment will not necessarily extend the life of a child but may well make his remaining time more tolerable.

Sequelae of Treatment

Although the goal of therapeutic radiation is to eradicate tumors, tumors are not isolated in petri dishes but occur in the human body, in the midst of normal tissues that are susceptible to damage by irradiation. This normal tissue damage occurs during the course of treatment or long after the treatment has been given. The term *acute effects* refers to reactions during or very soon after treatment; reactions occurring more than 3 months after treatment are termed *late effects*. Normal tissue tolerance to fractionated treatment is a function of the volume of the organ or tissue, the total dose, and the time course over which treatment is given. When chemotherapy is given concurrently with radiotherapy, some acute and late toxicities may be enhanced. Acute and late effects are generally restricted to tissues within the radiation field or at least to tissues having received some dose of radiation therapy. The one exception to this is the systemic toxicity of fatigue, which is experienced by some patients undergoing treatment.

The most typical acute effects are those on skin, on the mucosa of the aerodigestive tract, and on bone marrow. Most acute effects require supportive care, such as topical creams for skin reactions; ongoing hydration; topical anesthetics; and narcotics for severe mucositis. Abdominal irradiation can cause nausea, vomiting, and diarrhea. These toxicities are managed with antiemetics, hydration, and antidiarrheal agents if symptoms are severe. Acute toxicities can be severe and occasionally require treatment breaks. However, prolonged breaks are undesirable because the overall treatment time is an important factor in tumor control.

The mechanisms of late complications resulting from radiotherapy, though not precisely known, are speculated to be caused by vascular endothelial damage or by damage to parenchymal stem cells or to DNA. The normal tissue tolerance doses for the various bodily organs have been well studied.[104] The tolerance doses for adult normal tissue are applied in children with some exceptions, as discussed later. Late effects are dependent on the total dose and fraction size.[105] The potential for late toxicity is one of the most important factors in the decisions regarding dose and volume, and it is a major concern in the treatment of children with cancer. In children, treatment before full development has been reached can cause abnormal or arrested development. The severity of the effect on musculoskeletal development depends upon the dose of irradiation, the area treated, and the age of the patient. Doses of irradiation to the growth plate that are above 20 Gy are likely to have significant effects.[106,107] The age of the patient influences the severity of the damage. Younger children with greater growth potential are more profoundly affected. Irradiation of the pituitary gland and hypothalamus can lead to short stature by decreasing the production of growth hormone.[108] Spinal irradiation in the treatment of medulloblastoma in prepubertal children causes a shortened spine.[109]

The neurocognitive sequelae of brain irradiation are among the most serious late effects when radiation therapy is used in children.[110,111] The age of the patient, the dose, and the volume of brain treated influence the severity of these toxicities.[110,112,113]

One of the most devastating late toxicities of radiation therapy is the development of a second cancer associated with the prior treatment.[114,115] Radiation-associated second tumors occur within the prior radiotherapy field, are of a different histology from the primary tumor, and appear after a latency period, generally, of at least several years. A number of factors are involved in the development of second tumors, including the patient's underlying genetic predisposition, the dose of radiation, the age and sex of the patient, and the specific tissue irradiated. For example, following radiotherapy to the chest for Hodgkin's disease, teenage girls have a markedly increased risk for developing breast cancer.[116,117] Further discussion of the late effects of treatment appears in Chapter 32.

REFERENCES

1. Röntgen WC. On a new kind of rays. Science. 1896;3:227-231.
2. Coutard H. Roentgen therapy of epitheliomas of the tonsillar regional hypopharynx and larynx from 1920 to 1926. Am J Roentgenol Radium Ther Nucl Med. 1932;28:313-331.
3. Mazeron JJ, Simon JM, Crook J, et al. Influence of dose rate on local control of breast carcinoma treated by external beam irradiation plus iridium 192 implant. Int J Radiat Oncol Biol Phys. 1991;21:1173-1177.
4. Hall EJ. Radiobiology for the Radiologist, 5th ed. Philadelphia, Lippincott Williams & Wilkins, 2000.
5. Fowler JF, Harari PM, Leborgne F, Leborgne JH. Acute radiation reactions in oral and pharyngeal mucosa: tolerable levels in altered fractionation schedules. Radiother Oncol. 2003;69: 161-168.
6. Plataniotis GA, Dale RG. Radiobiologic modeling of cytoprotection effects in radiotherapy. Int J Radiat Oncol Biol Phys. 2007;68:236-242.
7. McAneney H, O'Rourke SF. Investigation of various growth mechanisms of solid tumour growth within the linear-quadratic model for radiotherapy. Phys Med Biol. 2007;52:1039-1054.
8. Dewhirst MW. Intermittent hypoxia furthers the rationale for hypoxia-inducible factor-1 targeting. Cancer Res. 2007;67:854-855.
9. Martinive P, Defresne F, Bouzin C, et al. Preconditioning of the tumor vasculature and tumor cells by intermittent hypoxia: implications for anticancer therapies. Cancer Res. 2006;66:11736-11744.
10. Giaccia A, Siim BG, Johnson RS. HIF-1 as a target for drug development. Nat Rev Drug Discov. 2003;2:803-811.
11. Bentzen SM, Harari PM, Bernier J. Exploitable mechanisms for combining drugs with radiation: concepts, achievements and future directions. Nat Clin Pract Oncol. 2007;4:172-180.
12. D'Angio GJ. Clinical and biologic studies of actinomycin D and roentgen irradiation. Am J Roentgenol Radium Ther Nucl Med. 1962;87:106-109.
13. Carreras E, Granena A, Rozman C. Hepatic veno-occlusive disease after bone marrow transplant. Blood Rev. 1993;7:43-51.
14. Green DM, Norkool P, Breslow NE, et al. Severe hepatic toxicity after treatment with vincristine and dactinomycin using single-dose or divided-dose schedules: a report from the National Wilms' Tumor Study. J Clin Oncol. 1990;8:1525-1530.
15. Caloglu M, Yurut-Caloglu V, Cosar-Alas R, et al. An ambiguous phenomenon of radiation and drugs: recall reactions. Onkologie. 2007;30:209-214.
16. Porter AC, Vaillancourt RR. Tyrosine kinase receptor-activated signal transduction pathways which lead to oncogenesis. Oncogene. 1998;17:1343-1352.
17. Levitzki A, Gazit A. Tyrosine kinase inhibition: an approach to drug development. Science. 1995;267:1782-1788.
18. Hunter T. Signaling—2000 and beyond. Cell. 2000;100:113-127.
19. Demetri GD. Targeting c-kit mutations in solid tumors: scientific rationale and novel therapeutic options. Semin Oncol. 2001;28: 19-26.
20. Taniguchi M, Nishida T, Hirota S, et al. Effect of c-kit mutation on prognosis of gastrointestinal stromal tumors. Cancer Res. 1999;59:4297-4300.
21. Lasota J, Jasinski M, Sarlomo-Rikala M, Miettinen M. Mutations in exon 11 of c-Kit occur preferentially in malignant versus benign gastrointestinal stromal tumors and do not occur in leiomyomas or leiomyosarcomas. Am J Pathol. 1999;154:53-60.
22. Drebin JA, Link VC, Stern DF, et al. Down-modulation of an oncogene protein product and reversion of the transformed phenotype by monoclonal antibodies. Cell. 1985;41:697-706.
23. Drebin JA, Link VC, Weinberg RA, Greene MI. Inhibition of tumor growth by a monoclonal antibody reactive with an oncogene-encoded tumor antigen. Proc Natl Acad Sci U S A. 1986;83: 9129-9133.
24. Fan Z, Mendelsohn J. Therapeutic application of anti-growth factor receptor antibodies. Curr Opin Oncol. 1998;10:67-73.
25. Klapper LN, Kirschbaum MH, Sela M, Yarden Y. Biochemical and clinical implications of the ErbB/HER signaling network of growth factor receptors. Adv Cancer Res. 2000;77:25-79.
26. Mendelsohn J, Baselga J. The EGF receptor family as targets for cancer therapy. Oncogene. 2000;19:6550-6565.
27. Olayioye MA, Neve RM, Lane HA, Hynes NE. The ErbB signaling network: receptor heterodimerization in development and cancer. EMBO J. 2000;19:3159-3167.
28. Wong AJ, Bigner SH, Bigner DD, et al. Increased expression of the epidermal growth factor receptor gene in malignant gliomas is invariably associated with gene amplification. Proc Natl Acad Sci U S A. 1987;84:6899-6903.
29. Ekstrand AJ, James CD, Cavenee WK, et al. Genes for epidermal growth factor receptor, transforming growth factor alpha, and epidermal growth factor and their expression in human gliomas in vivo. Cancer Res. 1991;51:2164-2172.
30. von Deimling A, Louis DN, von Ammon K, et al. Association of epidermal growth factor receptor gene amplification with loss of chromosome 10 in human glioblastoma multiforme. J Neurosurg. 1992;77:295-301.
31. Ekstrand AJ, Sugawa N, James CD, Collins VP. Amplified and rearranged epidermal growth factor receptor genes in human glioblastomas reveal deletions of sequences encoding portions of the N- and/or C-terminal tails. Proc Natl Acad Sci U S A. 1992;89:4309-4313.
32. Wikstrand CJ, McLendon RE, Friedman AH, Bigner DD. Cell surface localization and density of the tumor-associated variant of the epidermal growth factor receptor, EGFRvIII. Cancer Res. 1997;57:4130-4140.
33. Fan S, Smith ML, Rivet DJ 2nd, et al. Disruption of p53 function sensitizes breast cancer MCF-7 cells to cisplatin and pentoxifylline. Cancer Res. 1995;55:1649-1654.
34. Fry DW, Kraker AJ, McMichael A, et al. A specific inhibitor of the epidermal growth factor receptor tyrosine kinase. Science. 1994;265:1093-1095.
35. Klohs WD, Fry DW, Kraker AJ. Inhibitors of tyrosine kinase. Curr Opin Oncol. 1997;9:562-568.
36. Goldstein NI, Prewett M, Zuklys K, et al. Biological efficacy of a chimeric antibody to the epidermal growth factor receptor in a human tumor xenograft model. Clin Cancer Res. 1995;1:1311-1318.
37. Sawyers CL. Rational therapeutic intervention in cancer: kinases as drug targets. Curr Opin Genet Dev. 2002;12:111-115.
38. Hermanson M, Funa K, Koopmann J, et al. Association of loss of heterozygosity on chromosome 17p with high platelet-derived growth factor alpha receptor expression in human malignant gliomas. Cancer Res. 1996;56:164-171.
39. Westermark B, Heldin CH, Nistér M. Platelet-derived growth factor in human glioma. Glia. 1995;15:257-263.
40. Carmeliet P, Jain RK. Angiogenesis in cancer and other diseases. Nature. 2000;407:249-257.
41. Fong TA, Shawver LK, Sun L, et al. SU5416 is a potent and selective inhibitor of the vascular endothelial growth factor receptor (Flk-1/KDR) that inhibits tyrosine kinase catalysis, tumor vascularization, and growth of multiple tumor types. Cancer Res. 1999;59:99-106.
42. Laird AD, Vajkoczy P, Shawver LK, et al. SU6668 is a potent antiangiogenic and antitumor agent that induces regression of established tumors. Cancer Res. 2000;60:4152-4160.

43. Bourne HR, Sanders DA, McCormick F. The GTPase super-family: a conserved switch for diverse cell functions. Nature. 1990;348:125-132.

44. Downward J. Control of ras activation. Cancer Surv. 1996; 27:87-100.

45. Lowy DR, Willumsen BM. Function and regulation of ras. Annu Rev Biochem. 1993;62:851-891.

46. Rowinsky EK, Windle JJ, Von Hoff DD. Ras protein farnesyl-transferase: a strategic target for anticancer therapeutic development. J Clin Oncol. 1999;17:3631-3652.

47. Du W, Lebowitz PF, Prendergast GC. Cell growth inhibition by farnesyltransferase inhibitors is mediated by gain of geranylgera-nylated RhoB. Mol Cell Biol. 1999;19:1831-1840.

48. Reuter CW, Morgan MA, Bergmann L. Targeting the Ras signaling pathway: a rational, mechanism-based treatment for hematologic malignancies? Blood. 2000;96:1655-1669.

49. Lebowitz PF, Prendergast GC. Non-Ras targets of farnesyl-transferase inhibitors: focus on Rho. Oncogene. 1998;17:1439-1445.

50. Kuo MH, Allis CD. Roles of histone acetyltransferases and deacetylases in gene regulation. Bioessays. 1998;20:615-626.

51. Marks PA, Richon VM, Breslow R, Rifkind RA. Histone deacety-lase inhibitors as new cancer drugs. Curr Opin Oncol. 2001;13:477-483.

52. Vigushin DM, Coombes RC. Histone deacetylase inhibitors in cancer treatment. Anticancer Drugs. 2002;13:1-13.

53. Jung M. Inhibitors of histone deacetylase as new anticancer agents. Curr Med Chem. 2001;8:1505-1511.

54. Reid T, Valone F, Lipera W, et al. Phase II trial of the histone deacetylase inhibitor pivaloyloxymethyl butyrate (Pivanex, AN-9) in advanced non-small cell lung cancer. Lung Cancer. 2004;45:381-386.

55. Butler LM, Agus DB, Scher HI, et al. Suberoylanilide hydroxamic acid, an inhibitor of histone deacetylase, suppresses the growth of prostate cancer cells in vitro and in vivo. Cancer Res. 2000;60:5165-5170.

56. Desai D, Das A, Cohen L, et al. Chemopreventive efficacy of suberoylanilide hydroxamic acid (SAHA) against 4-(methylnitrosamino)-1-(3-pyridyl)-1-butanone (NNK)-induced lung tumorigenesis in female A/J mice. Anticancer Res. 2003;23:499-503.

57. Gilbert J, Baker SD, Bowling MK, et al. A phase I dose escalation and bioavailability study of oral sodium phenylbutyrate in patients with refractory solid tumor malignancies. Clin Cancer Res. 2001;7:2292-2300.

58. Pelidis MA, Carducci MA, Simons JW. Cytotoxic effects of sodium phenylbutyrate on human neuroblastoma cell lines. Int J Oncol. 1998;12:889-893.

59. Liu T, Kuljaca S, Tee A, Marshall GM. Histone deacetylase inhibitors: multifunctional anticancer agents. Cancer Treat Rev. 2006;32:157-165.

60. Garcia-Manero G, Issa JP. Histone deacetylase inhibitors: a review of their clinical status as antineoplastic agents. Cancer Invest. 2005;23:635-642.

61. Camphausen K, Scott T, Sproull M, Tofilon PJ. Enhancement of xenograft tumor radiosensitivity by the histone deacetylase inhibitor MS-275 and correlation with histone hyperacetylation. Clin Cancer Res. 2004;10:6066-6071.

62. Zhang X, Wei L, Yang Y, Yu Q. Sodium 4-phenylbutyrate induces apoptosis of human lung carcinoma cells through activating JNK pathway. J Cell Biochem. 2004;93:819-829.

63. Camphausen K, Cerna D, Scott T, et al. Enhancement of in vitro and in vivo tumor cell radiosensitivity by valproic acid. Int J Cancer. 2005;114:380-386.

64. Tang XX, Robinson ME, Riceberg JS, et al. Favorable neuro-blastoma genes and molecular therapeutics of neuroblastoma. Clin Cancer Res. 2004;10:5837-5844.

65. Munshi A, Kurland JF, Nishikawa T, et al. Histone deacetylase inhibitors radiosensitize human melanoma cells by suppressing DNA repair activity. Clin Cancer Res. 2005;11:4912-4922.

66. Entin-Meer M, Rephaeli A, Yang X, et al. Butyric acid prodrugs are histone deacetylase inhibitors that show antineoplastic activity and radiosensitizing capacity in the treatment of malignant gliomas. Mol Cancer Ther. 2005;4:1952-1961.

67. Jones PF, Jakubowicz T, Pitossi FJ, et al. Molecular cloning and identification of a serine/threonine protein kinase of the second-messenger subfamily. Proc Natl Acad Sci U S A. 1991;88:4171-4175.

68. Pillai MR, Jayaprakash PG, Nair MK. Tumour-proliferative fraction and growth factor expression as markers of tumour response to radiotherapy in cancer of the uterine cervix. J Cancer Res Clin Oncol. 1998;124:456-461.

69. Miyaguchi M, Takeuchi T, Morimoto K, Kubo T. Correlation of epidermal growth factor receptor and radiosensitivity in human maxillary carcinoma cell lines. Acta Otolaryngol. 1998;118:428-431.

70. Sheridan MT, O'Dwyer T, Seymour CB, Mothersill CE. Potential indicators of radiosensitivity in squamous cell carcinoma of the head and neck. Radiat Oncol Investig. 1997;5:180-186.

71. Wollman R, Yahalom J, Maxy R, et al. Effect of epidermal growth factor on the growth and radiation sensitivity of human breast cancer cells in vitro. Int J Radiat Oncol Biol Phys. 1994;30:91-98.

72. Barker FG 2nd, Simmons ML, Chang SM, et al. EGFR overex-pression and radiation response in glioblastoma multiforme. Int J Radiat Oncol Biol Phys. 2001;51:410-418.

73. Huang SM, Bock JM, Harari PM. Epidermal growth factor receptor blockade with C225 modulates proliferation, apoptosis, and radiosensitivity in squamous cell carcinomas of the head and neck. Cancer Res. 1999;59:1935-1940.

74. Milas L, Mason K, Hunter N, et al. In vivo enhancement of tumor radioresponse by C225 antiepidermal growth factor receptor antibody. Clin Cancer Res. 2000;6:701-708.

75. Jones HA, Hahn SM, Bernhard E, McKenna WG. Ras inhibitors and radiation therapy. Semin Radiat Oncol. 2001;11:328-337.

76. Gorski DH, Beckett MA, Jaskowiak NT, et al. Blockage of the vascular endothelial growth factor stress response increases the antitumor effects of ionizing radiation. Cancer Res. 1999;59:3374-3378.

77. Kim DW, Huamani J, Fu A, Hallahan DE. Molecular strategies targeting the host component of cancer to enhance tumor response to radiation therapy. Int J Radiat Oncol Biol Phys. 2006;64:38-46.

78. Lu B, Shinohara ET, Edwards E, et al. The use of tyrosine kinase inhibitors in modifying the response of tumor microvascu-lature to radiotherapy. Technol Cancer Res Treat. 2005;4:691-698.

79. Wachsberger P, Burd R, Dicker AP. Improving tumor response to radiotherapy by targeting angiogenesis signaling pathways. Hematol Oncol Clin North Am. 2004;18:1039-1057, viii.

80. Wachsberger P, Burd R, Dicker AP. Tumor response to ionizing radiation combined with antiangiogenesis or vascular targeting agents: exploring mechanisms of interaction. Clin Cancer Res. 2003;9:1957-1971.

81. Lane DP. Cancer. p53, guardian of the genome. Nature. 1992;358:15-16.

82. Kastan MB, Zhan Q, el-Deiry WS, et al. A mammalian cell cycle checkpoint pathway utilizing p53 and GADD45 is defective in ataxia-telangiectasia. Cell. 1992;71:587-597.

83. Schmitt CA, Fridman JS, Yang M, et al. Dissecting p53 tumor suppressor functions in vivo. Cancer Cell. 2002;1:289-298.

84. Brown JM, Wouters BG. Apoptosis, p53, and tumor cell sensitivity to anticancer agents. Cancer Res. 1999;59:1391-1399.

85. Pruschy M, Rocha S, Zaugg K, et al. Key targets for the execution of radiation-induced tumor cell apoptosis: the role of p53 and caspases. Int J Radiat Oncol Biol Phys. 2001;49:561-567.

86. ICRU Report 50: Prescribing, Recording and Reporting Photon Beam Therapy. Bethesda, Md: International Commission on Radiation Units and Measurements; 1993.

87. Demizu Y, Kagawa K, Ejima Y, et al. Cell biological basis for combination radiotherapy using heavy-ion beams and high-energy X-rays. Radiother Oncol. 2004;71:207-211.

88. Ando K, Koike S, Uzawa A, et al. Biological gain of carbon-ion radiotherapy for the early response of tumor growth delay and against early response of skin reaction in mice. J Radiat Res (Tokyo). 2005;46:51-57.

89. Munzenrider JE, Liebsch NJ. Proton therapy for tumors of the skull base. Strahlenther Onkol. 1999;175(suppl 2):57-63.

90. Munzenrider JE. Proton therapy for uveal melanomas and other eye lesions. Strahlenther Onkol. 1999;175(suppl 2):68-73.

91. Terahara A, Niemierko A, Goitein M, et al. Analysis of the relationship between tumor dose inhomogeneity and local control in patients with skull base chordoma. Int J Radiat Oncol Biol Phys. 1999;45:351-358.

92. Bush DA, McAllister CJ, Loredo LN, et al. Fractionated proton beam radiotherapy for acoustic neuroma. Neurosurgery. 2002; 50:270-273; discussion 273-275.

93. St Clair WH, Adams JA, Bues M, et al. Advantage of protons compared to conventional X-ray or IMRT in the treatment of a pediatric patient with medulloblastoma. Int J Radiat Oncol Biol Phys. 2004;58:727-734.

94. Shipley WU, Verhey LJ, Munzenrider JE, et al. Advanced prostate cancer: the results of a randomized comparative trial of high dose irradiation boosting with conformal protons compared with conventional dose irradiation using photons alone. Int J Radiat Oncol Biol Phys. 1995;32:3-12.

95. Egger E, Zografos L, Schalenbourg A, et al. Eye retention after proton beam radiotherapy for uveal melanoma. Int J Radiat Oncol Biol Phys. 2003;55:867-880.

96. Yuh GE, Loredo LN, Yonemoto LT, et al. Reducing toxicity from craniospinal irradiation: using proton beams to treat medulloblastoma in young children. Cancer J. 2004;10:386-390.

97. Hug EB, Sweeney RA, Nurre PM, et al. Proton radiotherapy in management of pediatric base of skull tumors. Int J Radiat Oncol Biol Phys. 2002;52:1017-1024.

98. Hug EB, Muenter MW, Archambeau JO, et al. Conformal proton radiation therapy for pediatric low-grade astrocytomas. Strahlenther Onkol. 2002;178:10-17.

99. Schulz-Ertner D, Tsujii H. Particle radiation therapy using proton and heavier ion beams. J Clin Oncol. 2007;25:953-964.

100. Schulz-Ertner D, Nikoghosyan A, Thilmann C, et al. Results of carbon ion radiotherapy in 152 patients. Int J Radiat Oncol Biol Phys. 2004;58:631-640.

101. Schulz-Ertner D, Nikoghosyan A, Hof H, et al. Carbon ion radiotherapy of skull base chondrosarcomas. Int J Radiat Oncol Biol Phys. 2007;67:171-177.

102. Schulz-Ertner D, Karger CP, Feuerhake A, et al. Effectiveness of carbon ion radiotherapy in the treatment of skull-base chordomas. Int J Radiat Oncol Biol Phys. 2007;68:449-457.

103. Loeffler JS, Leopold KA, Recht A, et al. Emergency prebiopsy radiation for mediastinal masses: impact on subsequent pathologic diagnosis and outcome. J Clin Oncol. 1986;4:716-721.

104. Hall EJ. Radiobiology for the Radiologist. 4th ed. Philadelphia: JB Lippincott; 1994.

105. Withers H, Peters L. The pathobiology of late effects of radiation. In: Meyn R, Wither H, eds. Radiation Biology in Cancer Research. New York: Raven Press; 1980:439-448.

106. Probert JC, Parker BR, Kaplan HS. Growth retardation in children after megavoltage irradiation of the spine. Cancer. 1973; 32:634-639.

107. Probert JC, Parker BR. The effects of radiation therapy on bone growth. Radiology. 1975;114:155-162.

108. Merchant TE, Goloubeva O, Pritchard DL, et al. Radiation dose-volume effects on growth hormone secretion. Int J Radiat Oncol Biol Phys. 2002;52:1264-1270.

109. Silber JH, Littman PS, Meadows AT. Stature loss following skeletal irradiation for childhood cancer. J Clin Oncol. 1990;8: 304-312.

110. Merchant TE, Kiehna EN, Li C, et al. Radiation dosimetry predicts IQ after conformal radiation therapy in pediatric patients with localized ependymoma. Int J Radiat Oncol Biol Phys. 2005; 63:1546-1554.

111. Merchant TE, Kiehna EN, Li C, et al. Modeling radiation dosimetry to predict cognitive outcomes in pediatric patients with CNS embryonal tumors including medulloblastoma. Int J Radiat Oncol Biol Phys. 2006;65:210-221.

112. Mulhern RK, Palmer SL, Merchant TE, et al. Neurocognitive consequences of risk-adapted therapy for childhood medulloblastoma. J Clin Oncol. 2005;23:5511-5519.

113. Mulhern RK, Merchant TE, Gajjar A, et al. Late neurocognitive sequelae in survivors of brain tumours in childhood. Lancet Oncol. 2004;5:399-408.

114. Tucker MA, D'Angio GJ, Boice JD Jr, et al. Bone sarcomas linked to radiotherapy and chemotherapy in children. N Engl J Med. 1987;317:588-593.

115. Eng C, Li FP, Abramson DH, et al. Mortality from second tumors among long-term survivors of retinoblastoma. J Natl Cancer Inst. 1993;85:1121-1128.

116. Tarbell NJ, Gelber RD, Weinstein HJ, Mauch P. Sex differences in risk of second malignant tumours after Hodgkin's disease in childhood. Lancet. 1993;341:1428-1432.

117. Ng AK, Bernardo MV, Weller E, et al. Second malignancy after Hodgkin disease treated with radiation therapy with or without chemotherapy: long-term risks and risk factors. Blood. 2002;100: 1989-1996.

9 Pediatric Surgical Oncology

Christopher B. Weldon, Megan E. Anderson, Mark C. Gebhardt, and Robert C. Shamberger

INTRODUCTION

Successful treatment of pediatric solid tumors requires collaborative management by the disciplines of surgery, oncology, and radiotherapy. Multimodal therapy achieves the highest rate of cure in many solid tumors and often minimizes the long-term morbidity. Smooth collaboration provides optimal care. The role of the surgeon varies greatly, depending on the primary tumor, its site, and the presence or absence of metastatic disease. Surgeons should be involved in decisions regarding primary resection versus biopsy with neoadjuvant chemotherapy and delayed resection. The surgeon's knowledge of the risks involved in primary resection is critical. The method of biopsy is also very important. Inappropriate initial excisional biopsies with positive pathologic margins will require more extensive subsequent resection than if an initial incisional biopsy had been performed. Similarly, inappropriate biopsies, such as a thoracoscopic biopsy of chest wall Ewing's sarcoma or a percutaneous or open biopsy of Wilms' tumor, needlessly contaminate the thoracic and abdominal cavities, respectively, and require more intensive therapies, particularly the use of radiation therapy. A growing emphasis on minimizing the morbidity of therapy is required because the survival rate of infants and children with solid tumors is quite high. We must, therefore, avoid any diagnostic or therapeutic missteps that require more intensive therapy.

Surgery is critical in the staging of pediatric solid tumors. This is well established in cases of Wilms' tumor. In a classic study by Beimann Othersen and the National Wilms' Tumor Study Group (NWTSG), surgeons had a 31.3% false-negative rate in their clinical assessment of lymph node involvement with tumor by gross inspection and a false-positive rate of 18.1%.[1] It should be stressed that in cases of Wilms' tumors, the protocols of the NWTSG and the Children's Oncology Group determine the intensity of chemotherapy and whether abdominal radiotherapy is used based on local stage. Patients with pulmonary metastases (stage IV) with local stage I or stage II tumors receive intensified chemotherapy and pulmonary radiation but no abdominal radiation.

The vital importance of adequate lymph node biopsy has been demonstrated in several studies. An increased incidence of local relapse occurred in children enrolled in the NWTSG-4 if no biopsy was performed of the abdominal lymph nodes, particularly in stage I cases.[2] This finding suggested that undertreatment of local disease in children without lymph node biopsy resulted in an increased frequency of local relapse. Although lymph node biopsy is essential in children with Wilms' tumors, an extensive retroperitoneal lymph node resection has not been demonstrated to improve local control.[3]

Lymph node biopsy in patients with rhabdomyosarcoma is critical as well. The occurrence of lymph node involvement in rhabdomyosarcoma is determined by the primary site. Children presenting without evidence of distant metastases have an overall 10% incidence of lymph node involvement. It is most common in tumors arising in the prostate (41%), the paratesticular (26%), and the genitourinary sites (24%).[4] Lesions in the extremities have an intermediate frequency of 12%, whereas the orbit (0%), the truncal sites (3%), and the nonorbital head and neck sites (7%) are the least common sites of lymphatic dissemination. In the extremity and genitourinary sites, assessment of lymph node involvement is essential to ensure that radiation fields are appropriately designed and sufficiently inclusive. Whether the sentinel lymph node biopsy technique will optimize the identification of nodal spread in rhabdomyosarcoma has not been established. Although lymph node biopsy is critical to identifying the extent of spread, a lymph node dissection should generally not be performed because it may produce lymphedema, which will complicate radiotherapy and subsequent surgical resection of the primary tumor.

Radiographic assessment is inadequate for staging rhabdomyosarcoma as it is in cases of Wilms' tumor. In Intergroup Rhabdomyosarcoma III, 121 boys with paratesticular rhabdomyosarcoma underwent retroperitoneal lymph node dissection to evaluate nodal status.[5] The lymph nodes were assessed to be clinically negative based on computed tomography (CT) scans in 18% of the boys, 14% of whom had positive nodes when biopsy or retroperitoneal lymph node dissection was performed. In the boys with clinically positive lymph nodes based on the CT scans, 94% were confirmed to be positive pathologically. Retroperitoneal relapse occurred in only 2 of the 121 boys, one of whom had pathologically negative lymph nodes and did not receive radiotherapy. Thus, CT was very accurate if lymph node abnormalities were identified, but it was not extremely sensitive in identifying nodal involvement. In a subsequent study, Weiner and colleagues reported an increased incidence of retroperitoneal relapse in children treated during Intergroup Rhabdomyosarcoma-IV. The use of abdominal radiation in this study was based on thin-cut CT scans in 98% of cases as compared with children treated during the preceding Intergroup Rhabdomyosarcoma-III, in which 94% had retroperitoneal biopsy or lymph node dissection. In the subsequent study, Intergroup Rhabdomyosarcoma-IV, a decrease in stage-II disease (positive lymph nodes) from 35% to 17% occurred when the staging was based on radiographic findings. This resulted in a decrease in the use of abdominal radiation in this cohort. The result was a fourfold increase in retroperitoneal lymph node relapse. This is another example of how critical adequate staging is to avoid local failure.[6]

In this chapter we present some of the critical surgical issues in the treatment of infants, children, and adolescents who have solid tumors. We discuss the use of anesthesia in a patient who has an anterior mediastinal mass, appropriate methods of biopsy, the role of neoadjuvant chemotherapy, and the management of pulmonary metastases.

ANESTHESIA IN A PATIENT WITH AN ANTERIOR MEDIASTINAL MASS

A patient presenting with an anterior mediastinal mass poses a therapeutic challenge to the anesthesiologist and the surgeon. Correct diagnosis of the tumor will provide the greatest chance for cure. There are, however, a plethora of reports in the anesthesia and surgical literature of patients with anterior mediastinal masses suffering respiratory collapse upon the induction of general anesthesia. This occurrence has led to an understandable reluctance among anesthesiologists to use general anesthesia in this setting. Respiratory symptoms are a poor index of the risk for respiratory collapse, with the clear exception of orthopnea, which suggests a high risk that respiratory collapse will occur. An initial attempt to establish the radiographic parameters that would correlate with respiratory collapse upon induction of general anesthesia involved a retrospective evaluation of 74 adults with Hodgkin's disease.[7] In this study the authors used the ratio of the transverse diameter of the mediastinal mass to the transverse diameter of the chest as the critical parameter. They found the incidence of respiratory collapse was 2.1% with a mediastinal mass less than 31% of the transverse diameter compared with 10.5% for a mass with a ratio of 32% to 44% and 33.3% for a mass with a ratio greater than 45%. Similar results were reported by Turoff and associates.[8]

Thorne Griscom and colleagues demonstrated that CT scans can accurately determine the tracheal dimensions in chil-

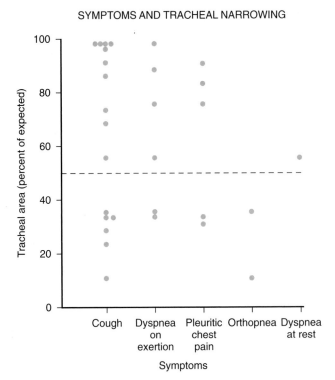

SYMPTOMS AND TRACHEAL NARROWING

FIGURE 9-1. Correlation of symptoms with tracheal areas in a cohort of 42 children and adolescents with anterior mediastinal masses. *(Redrawn from Shamberger RC, Holtzman RS, Griscom NT, et al. CT quantitation of tracheal cross-sectional areas as a guide to the surgical anesthetic management of children with anterior mediastinal masses. J Pediatr Surg. 1991;26:138-142. By permission of WB Saunders.)*

dren and adolescents, and he established the normative values in children.[9,10] Azizkhan first used this methodology in reviewing 50 children with anterior mediastinal masses.[11] He found that 15 patients in his cohort had "marked" tracheal compression that was defined as a tracheal cross-sectional area of less than 66% of predicted mass. When general anesthesia was induced in 8 of these 13 patients, total airway obstruction occurred in 5, all of whom had 50% or less of the predicted tracheal area. It was suggested, based on these findings, that general anesthesia should be avoided in children with less than 66% of the predicted tracheal area.

In a retrospective study at Children's Hospital Boston, 42 patients were identified who had anterior mediastinal masses and who had CT scans and underwent surgical procedures. These patients were divided into those whose masses were more than 75% of the expected area (19 cases); those whose masses were 50% to 75% of the predicted area (16 cases); those whose masses were 25% to 50% of the predicted area (5 cases); and those whose masses were less than 25% of the predicted area (2 cases).[12] One clear finding of that study was that the presence or absence of respiratory symptoms did not correlate well with the degree of tracheal narrowing shown by CT scan, except in cases of orthopnea (Fig. 9-1). General anesthesia with spontaneous ventilation was performed in 4 patients (who had tracheal areas 33%, 73%, 76%, and 98% of the predicted percentage). General endotracheal anesthesia with paralysis was used in the remaining 32 patients, only 3 of whom had tracheal areas less than 50% of the predicted areas (30%, 26%, and 24%). One patient received preoperative radiation therapy (26%). None of these 32 patients had symptoms of orthopnea or dyspnea at rest and only 1 had dyspnea on exertion. All tol-

erated anesthesia without difficulty, and no patients suffered respiratory or cardiovascular collapse. Adequate material for pathologic diagnosis was obtained in all cases. It was concluded in this study that general anesthesia was safe in patients with tracheal areas greater than or equal to 50% of the predicted areas.

In a subsequent prospective study, 31 children with mediastinal masses were evaluated by both CT scan and pulmonary function tests.[13] Although the use of pulmonary function tests had been proposed by many investigators as a method for assessing the risks involved in anesthesia, few evaluations of this modality had been performed. Miller and Hyatt evaluated the flow-volume loop curves in a series of patients with intrathoracic and extrathoracic obstructions resulting from strictures of the trachea, malignant tumors, or bilateral vocal cord paralysis.[14] The predominant distortion of the flow loops in intrathoracic obstruction was a marked reduction in the maximum expiratory flow rate. Hence, in this prospective study, the peak expiratory flow rate was used as a critical factor. Patients with either a peak expiratory flow rate of less than 50% of predicted or a tracheal area of less than 50% of predicted were given local anesthesia for their procedures. General endotracheal anesthesia was used only in patients with greater than 50% of predicted for both parameters. All patients in this study did well when general anesthesia was applied (Fig. 9-2). Further analysis of this cohort revealed that patients with tracheal areas greater than 50% but peak expiratory flow rates less than 50% had one of two problems: either a very low total lung capacity (38% and 55% of predicted) resulting from the massive size of the tumor or moderate to severe bronchial narrowing based on qualitative estimation (four of these five patients; Fig. 9-3A, B).

In a subsequent study by King and coauthors, 51 children with Hodgkin's and non-Hodgkin's lymphoma were evaluated. Respiratory symptoms were present in 49% of the children in this series and are more common in children with non-Hodgkin's lymphoma (76%) than in those with Hodgkin's disease (30%). The extent of aberration in the pulmonary function test was also worse in those with non-Hodgkin's lymphoma. The forced expiratory volume (FEV_1) was more strongly affected in the group with non-Hodgkin's lymphoma (mean value of 63% ± 27% of predicted) than in the group with Hodgkin's disease (mean value of 87% ± 16% of predicted).

Patients with severe obstruction have one of three therapeutic options. Patients can be treated in a preliminary fashion with either radiation therapy or steroids and chemotherapy for the most likely diagnosis based on the clinical findings (Fig. 9-4A, B). In a series of young adults who underwent postradiation biopsy of an anterior mediastinal mass, a histologic diagnosis could not be obtained in 8 of 10 patients because of extensive necrosis.[15] In some cases, one area of tumor can be shielded for subsequent biopsy while the bulk of the tumor receives radiation. Non-Hodgkin's lymphoma is also extremely responsive to steroid therapy. Pretreatment with steroids often obscures the histologic diagnosis.[16,17]

The second option is aspiration of a pleural effusion if it is present. Patients with lymphoblastic lymphoma have higher incidences of associated pleural effusions (71%) than do children with Hodgkin's disease (11.4%).[18] Aspiration of the effusion in patients with lymphoblastic lymphoma is often diagnostic. Cells in the effusion can be assayed by immunocytochemical studies as well as by cytogenetic evaluation, immunophenotyping, and cytology.

The third option, in children with significant respiratory compromise and no pleural effusion and no lymph nodes palpable outside the chest, is either a percutaneous needle biopsy under radiographic guidance or an open anterior thoracotomy (Chamberlain procedure). Both can be performed successfully under local anesthesia. Children should be seated

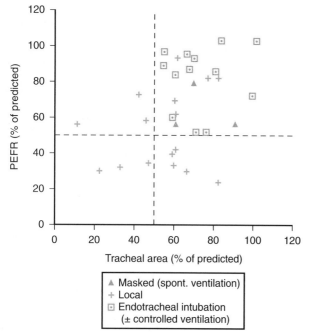

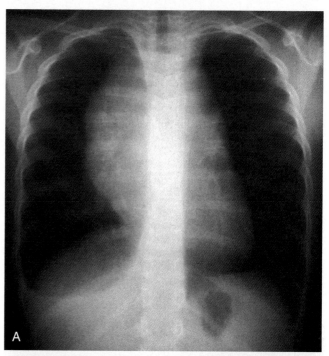

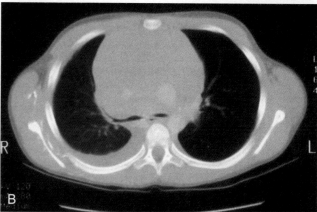

FIGURE 9-2. The relationship between peak expiratory flow rate (PEFR) and tracheal area in a cohort of 31 children prospectively evaluated with anterior mediastinal masses. Children with PEFRs or tracheal areas less than 50% of predicted (below or to the left of the dotted lines) received local anesthesia and did well. Children with PEFRs and tracheal areas greater than 50% of predicted received predominantly general anesthesia and did well (right upper quadrant). The five children with tracheal areas greater than 50% of predicted but with peak PEFR less than 50% of predicted (in lower right box) might have been considered for general anesthesia if the tracheal area had been the only parameter considered in assessing risk. Although the study could not demonstrate that these children would have had problems with anesthesia, it did confirm that the parameters of greater than 50% PEFR and tracheal areas greater than 50% of predicted were safe for the administration of general anesthesia. *(Redrawn from Shamberger RC, Holzman RS, Griscom NT, et al. Prospective evaluation of computed tomography and pulmonary function tests of children with mediastinal masses. Surgery. 1995;118:468-471. By permission of Mosby-Year Book.)*

FIGURE 9-3. A, Chest radiograph of an 11-year-old female who presented with a several-week history of a cough and dyspnea on exertion as well as puffy eyes and orthopnea. Radiography revealed an anterior mediastinal mass. **B,** A CT scan showed a tracheal area that was 82% of predicted but revealed marked narrowing of the bronchi. The peak expiratory flow rate was only 42% of predicted while sitting and 24% of predicted while supine. Aspiration of her pleural effusion confirmed the diagnosis of lymphoblastic lymphoma. *(From Shamberger RC. Preanesthetic evaluation of children with anterior mediastinal masses. Semin Pediatr Surg. 1999;8;61-68.).*

in a semi-upright position and should be ventilating spontaneously to maximize their pulmonary function (Fig. 9-5). This position also decreases venous congestion if it is present. Spontaneous ventilation minimizes collapse of the trachea because of the negative pressure exerted by the chest wall. Following these guidelines for the use of general and local anesthesia and the biopsy techniques discussed, a biopsy can be obtained safely in essentially all children and adolescents with anterior mediastinal masses.

METHODS OF BIOPSY

A biopsy serves as the basis of diagnosis and treatment of a tumor. It establishes the prognosis and defines the multimodality therapy required for cure. Beyond establishing the diagnosis, a biopsy may be required for several other important purposes in the delivery of modern oncologic care: to confirm the presence of metastatic disease, to determine the response to treatment, and to document the presence of complications resulting from treatment, especially suspicious lesions that may be infec-

tious in nature and that pose significant risks for an immunosuppressed patient.

The Five Principles

Five principles must be followed when considering a biopsy.

First, to minimize the psychological and physical stress for the patient and family, the need for a biopsy, how it will be performed, and the possible complications must be discussed with the patient and the family.

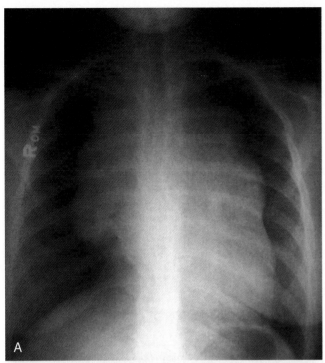

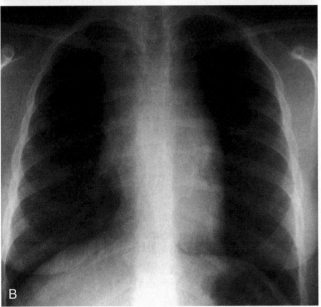

FIGURE 9-4. A 14-year-old girl presented with a nonproductive cough, retrosternal pain, a 19-pound weight loss, and orthopnea. **A,** Chest radiograph showed a large anterior mediastinal mass. A biopsy was obtained in the suprasternal notch, revealing lymphoblastic lymphoma. She received two courses of radiotherapy (250 cGy/per dose) over 2 days. **B,** The chest radiograph obtained 7 days later showed a remarkable response by the tumor to the radiation. *(From Shamberger RC. Preanesthetic evaluation of children with anterior mediastinal masses. Semin Pediatr Surg. 1999;8;61-68.)*

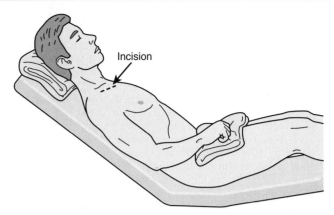

FIGURE 9-5. The proper position for a patient with airway compromise for obtaining a biopsy of an anterior mediastinal mass. The semiupright position optimizes pulmonary function and facilitates ventilation as well as venous drainage from potentially engorged vessels. *(Redrawn from Shamberger RC. Preanesthetic evaluation of children with anterior mediastinal masses. Semin Pediatr Surg. 1999;8;61-68.)*

chemical analysis) to provide the maximum amount of information.

Third, the precise biopsy route and site must be selected to facilitate future therapy. The wrong incision or biopsy site can greatly complicate the subsequent local therapy, whether it be resection or radiotherapy. Factors that must be considered are local tissue trauma, risk for tumor spillage or hemorrhage, and minimal violation of anatomic planes.

Fourth, the patient's general state of health and medical history and immune status must also be considered to fully assess the physiologic impact of anesthesia and biopsy, including risk for hemorrhagic and respiratory collapse.

Last, the possibility of combining several invasive procedures into one administration of anesthesia should be considered. For example, a patient who requires biopsy of a lesion may also need central venous access or a bone marrow biopsy and aspiration, and these procedures could be combined. Although the grouping of procedures is not always possible, it is an option the oncologic team should discuss in advance so as to present a uniform plan to the patient and parents.

Method of Biopsy Overview

The type of biopsy a patient requires varies greatly and is dependent on the site of the mass, the characteristics of the lesion itself (cystic or solid), the condition of the patient, and the diagnostic possibilities. Once the decision has been made to proceed with a biopsy, the first technical question that must be answered is the amount of tissue required and which biopsy technique will avoid increasing the stage of the patient or complicate future therapy. The fundamental techniques may be divided into biopsies that remove small or large specimens.

Small Specimen Biopsies

Small specimen biopsies are those that are acquired by the use of hollow needles that sample an aspirate (fine needle aspiration; FNA) or the core (core needle biopsy; CNB) of the tissue. They are often obtained using imaging assistance (ultrasound, fluoroscopy, or CT). The advantages of small specimen biopsies are that they can commonly be performed with minimal or

Second, a preprocedure conference among the oncologist, pathologist, radiologist, and surgeon must take place to determine the best biopsy technique for obtaining the required amount of tissue and to ensure that the tissue is processed appropriately (light microscopy, electron microscopy, cytogenetic and other biogenic marker evaluation, or immunohisto-

no anesthesia and are less invasive than open procedures. Cost is also generally less for this approach, and recovery time for the patient is quicker. The disadvantages to this approach, however, are that the amount of tissue returned is quite small, and this may create challenges in establishing a diagnosis or by providing an inadequate amount of tissue to complete the necessary secondary tests required to define the lesion adequately. Furthermore, if imaging modalities are used to assist in this form of biopsy, radiation exposure occurs if CT or fluoroscopy is used, rather than magnetic resonance imaging (MRI) or ultrasound. This issue of radiation exposure is of extreme importance in the pediatric population because there is an increased risk for developing a malignancy as the result of radiation exposure.[19,20] In addition, there is the possibility of tumor spread in needle tracks or hemorrhage.[21-23] The risk that there might be sampling error in which the specimen harvested may not adequately represent the entirety of the mass is always a concern with biopsies, and the smaller the sample, the larger the concern. Despite these limitations, small specimen biopsies are an accepted standard of practice in pediatric oncology, and their use is described in detail.

Fine Needle Aspiration and Core Needle Biopsy

FNA specimens are acquired using a 20- to 25-gauge needle connected to a standard syringe with the plunger partially withdrawn (Fig. 9-6). The needle is inserted directly into the lesion, guided by palpation or by image guidance (Fig. 9-7A-F). Multiple passes are made into the lesion as suction is applied to the syringe. Upon removing the needle, the contents of the syringe and needle are placed directly onto slides for cytologic analysis.

Multiple biopsies (three, on average) can be taken from the same lesion at the same time using this approach, and the cytologic results are available for almost immediate review. However, no histologic assessment is possible using this technique, thus causing difficulty in diagnosing certain tumors whose cytologic appearances are similar, such as the small, round, blue cell tumors.

Histopathologic analysis is possible when taking a CNB. Specimens taken by CNB are retrieved by using larger, hollow-bore needles (13- to 20-gauge) attached to spring-loaded devices that allow for one-step tissue harvest and extraction (Fig. 9-8). Image guidance is commonly employed during this procedure, as it is for the acquisition of FNA samples. The CNB device is commonly inserted through a coaxial sheath or cylinder that allows the operator to instill a coagulant into the tissue defects made by the CNB device so as to reduce the incidence of hemorrhage and tumor spillage (Fig. 9-9). Generally, multiple specimens (10 or more) are gathered from various areas of the lesion to minimize sampling error and to provide more tissue for complete pathologic analysis.[24-26] Representa-

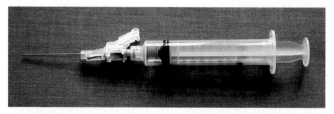

FIGURE 9-6. A standard FNA device with a 22-gauge needle attached to a 10-mL syringe that has the plunger partially withdrawn to facilitate the removal of the aspirate.

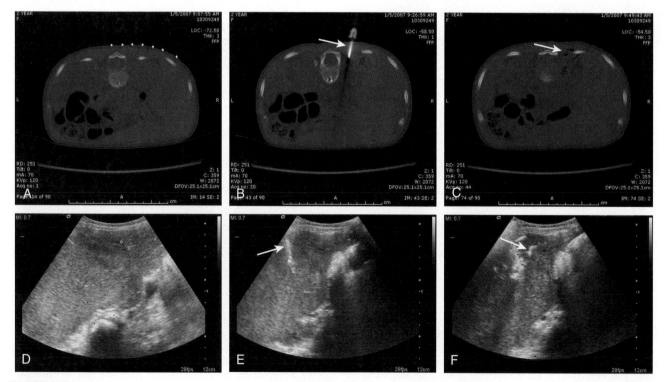

FIGURE 9-7. A, The prebiopsy CT of a retroperitoneal mass with external grid for biopsy marking. **B,** The same patient with the needle in the retroperitoneal mass *(arrow)*. **C,** Postbiopsy CT with air in the mass and soft tissues *(arrow)* from the biopsy procedure. **D,** Prebiopsy ultrasound of a liver mass. **E,** The ultrasound-guided biopsy of a liver mass *(arrow)*. **F,** Postbiopsy hemorrhage in the mass *(arrow)*.

tive examples of the microscopic appearances of biopsy specimens taken by FNA and CNB are shown in Figure 9-10A-D. Imaging techniques can often distinguish areas that have viable versus necrotic tissue to help identify the areas best to biopsy.

The results and outcomes of small specimen biopsies taken from almost any organ in the body have been reported extensively in adult patients, and they show excellent diagnostic accuracy and minimal procedural morbidity. However, small specimen biopsy techniques and the comparison of these techniques in pediatric oncology patients, especially in cases of

abdominal lesions, have only recently gained widespread acceptance and usage.[26-32]

Hugosson and colleagues in 1999 reviewed their series of image-guided percutaneous small specimen biopsies in children between 1992 and 1996.[28] A total of 90 biopsies (53 FNA, 37 CNB) were taken in 75 patients (mean age, 6.9 years). The authors compared the use of FNA to CNB (1.2 mm core

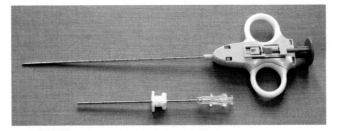

FIGURE 9-9. An automated 16-gauge CNB device with a 15-gauge coaxial sheath (Coaxial Temno Evolution, Allegiance Healthcare, McGraw Park, IL).

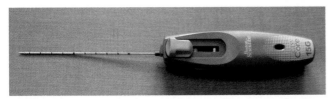

FIGURE 9-8. An automated 15-gauge CNB device (Easy Core Biopsy System, Boston Scientific, Natick, MA).

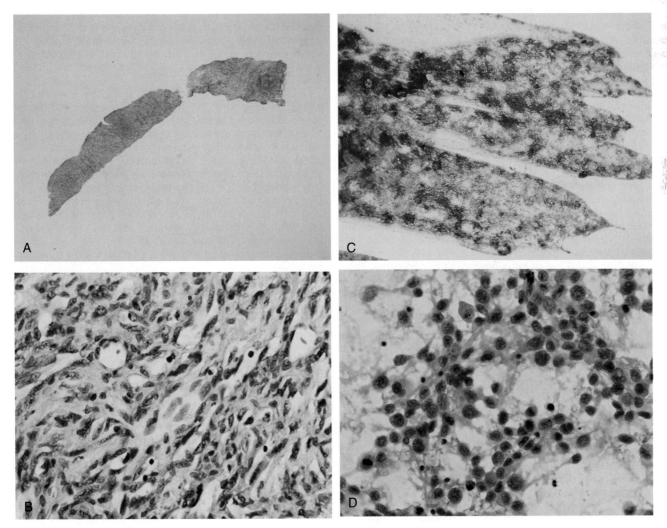

FIGURE 9-10. A, The CNB specimen of a liver mass at 2× (angiosarcoma). **B,** 600× (CNB) with sheets of moderately pleomorphic spindled cells and lumina formation. **C,** FNA specimen from a submandibular lymph node at 2× (nasopharyngeal alveolar rhabdomyosarcoma). **D,** Specimen at 600×, revealing round and elongated pleomorphic tumor cells with marked apoptosis.

specimens) under ultrasound guidance. Their cohort had many different malignant processes, and they obtained biopsies from liver, kidney, adrenal gland, spleen, pelvic masses, and enlarged abdominal lymph nodes. The diagnostic accuracy rate of FNA was 77% (73% for malignant lesions and 83% for benign lesions) and was 95% for CNB (93% malignant lesions and 100% for benign lesions). The complication rate was 8%. They concluded that CNB is a more accurate technique and that it has a complication rate similar to that of FNA. These results were echoed by Hussain and colleagues, who examined their institutional experience with image-guided percutaneous biopsies (CNBs) in children (mean age, 4 years).[29] Of their cohort, 94% had abdominal or pelvic masses. Their reported diagnostic accuracy rate was 88%, and the initial diagnosis was subsequently confirmed by whole-specimen pathologic analysis. Their complication rate was approximately 8%, and they too concluded that CNB was generally successful in diagnosing tumors in children.

Sklair-Levy and colleagues published their institution's 10-year experience in small specimen biopsies in pediatric patients.[30] They performed 69 biopsies (62 CNBs) in 57 patients, using image guidance. Their diagnostic accuracy rate was 88.7% (55/62 patients). For malignant lesions, CNB had an accuracy rate of 98% as an isolated diagnostic technique in solid malignant tumors, although seven CNBs had to be repeated because the initial results were nondiagnostic. All seven repeat CNBs were correct on subsequent evaluation. They performed seven FNAs that showed a diagnostic accuracy rate of only 28%, and these patients then underwent surgical excision of the lesion in question. Though this accuracy rate is far lower than previously reported,[28] none of the lesions in question were abdominal or pelvic masses, and the majority of the lesions were enlarged lymph nodes. Therefore, direct comparison of the utility and diagnostic accuracy of FNA in this situation is not possible. The accuracy of FNAs in diagnosing primary, metastatic, and recurrent lesions was in excess of 94% for all tumor types save lymphomas, in which they were correct only 60% of the time. It is interesting that there was not a single complication.

A more comprehensive study was published by Skoldenberg and colleagues. They examined their institution's results in 147 CNBs in 110 children (mean age, 4 years) and in all anatomic sites (there were 61 abdominal and pelvic lesions in the 110 children).[31] An overall accuracy rate of 89% was achieved for the CNBs performed. Of the 110, 24 children required 37 additional biopsies because of nondiagnostic first specimens (12), a question of recurrence (22), or an insufficient quantity of tissue for all the diagnostic studies needed (3). This study reported a sensitivity rate of 82% and a positive predictive value rate of 98.8%. A complication rate of 7% (10/141 cases) was seen; half were hemorrhagic in nature. Of the patients, 14 required narcotics for pain management postprocedure. A statistically significant difference in the occurrence of postprocedure pain was noted in older children. The authors strongly encourage the use of CNB in the diagnosis of pediatric malignancy, and they tout its superiority to FNA.

Finally, researchers at St. Jude's Children's Research Hospital published their experience with CNB in pediatric solid tumors over a 5-year period.[27] Under image guidance and anesthesia, 202 CNBs were performed. Ultrasound was the predominant mode of imaging assistance (124/202), and the biopsies were performed to evaluate both primary and metastatic sites of disease. Of the 202, 103 primary CNBs were performed with a 96.9% rate of sensitivity, 100% specificity, and an accuracy rate of 98%. For metastatic or recurrent lesions, they measured a sensitivity rate of 83.1%, a specificity of 100%, and an accuracy rate of 87.9%. There were no false-positive results. In the cohort of patients with abdominal and pelvic tumors, the sensitivity and accuracy of CNB was 100%. They had a complication rate of 13.4%, with hemorrhage being the most common. Their results and experience across all anatomic regions and pathologic lesions demonstrate that small specimen biopsies should be considered as the initial diagnostic procedure of choice. Therefore, solid masses in the pediatric population should be approached where indicated with image-guided small specimen biopsies, especially using the CNB technique.

Large Specimen Biopsies

Large specimen tissue biopsies involve the removal of all (excisional biopsy) or part (incisional biopsy) of a lesion, using an open or minimally invasive surgical technique. This method of biopsy should not be confused with a formal extirpative procedure because the surgeon does not remove either part of the mass or the entire mass with concerns about adequate margins of resection. The goal of these procedures is to remove a piece or all of the mass in question to provide tissue for diagnosis, not for local control of the primary site. Large specimen biopsies are also performed in anatomic areas and on lesions in which image-guided small specimen biopsies are difficult because of proximity to major vessels or nerves, the lesions are very vascular, or the lesions cannot be reached without damaging overlying organs and structures (for example, retroperitoneal lymph nodes). A large specimen biopsy may be performed sequentially with a small specimen biopsy while the patient is under the same anesthetic if there is any doubt regarding the adequacy for a histopathologic diagnosis of the FNA or CNB.

The disadvantages of large specimen biopsies are that they require a longer procedural time, anesthetic time, and recovery time and require hospitalization. They can delay the initiation of adjuvant therapies and are more costly. Assuming there are no complications, the vast majority of pediatric patients in whom a small specimen biopsy has been performed on a solid abdominal mass do not remain hospitalized for more than 8 hours postprocedure, as shown by recent large studies.[27,29-33] The same cannot be said for large specimen biopsies. Finally, operative exploration for large specimen sampling can complicate definitive local control therapies, especially from an operative standpoint. Violating the thoracic or peritoneal cavities induces adhesion formation that can complicate the subsequent resection.

Although significant disadvantages of large specimen biopsies exist, there are marked advantages. First, large biopsy samples are obtained and multiple areas are sampled within the lesion, decreasing the likelihood of sampling error. Second, a detailed macroscopic evaluation of the lesion in question and all surrounding structures can be performed to search for extension of or metastasis by the tumor. Third, radiation exposure of the patient and the health care team is avoided. Finally, hemostasis and tumor sampling are controlled and confirmed directly, before closing the incision, so as to minimize the complications of tumor spillage and hemorrhage.

In the past decade, several groups have reported success in using a minimally invasive surgical (MIS) approach for either incisional or excisional large specimen biopsies. The MIS approach relies on the same basic tenets of surgical discipline as does an open procedure, but it uses smaller incisions and advanced technology to achieve these goals. An operating telescope capable of excellent image resolution and magnification is used to display a picture on closed-circuit monitors. Dissection and biopsy are performed using long, fine instruments that are introduced through percutaneously placed 2- to 12-mm cannulas. When operating in the peritoneal cavity, carbon dioxide gas (CO_2) is introduced through an insufflation apparatus that distends the abdominal wall to provide adequate space for assessment of the abdominal structures. The pressure is kept as low as possible consistent with adequate exposure. An important point that must be discussed with the anesthesiologist is the degree of respiratory impairment that CO_2 insufflation may induce, especially in pediatric patients with extremely compliant diaphragms. If at any point the child becomes physiologically unstable, the CO_2 gas is released and the procedure terminated. Advantages of the MIS approach are decreased postoperative pain because of the small incisions, a shorter postoperative stay, improved cosmetic results, and an earlier return of bowel function.[32,34] Complication rates in the pediatric population of 4% or less have been reported in a recent large series, but this rate is clearly related to the experience of the surgeon.[34]

Some 34 years ago, Gans and Berci described their successful experiences with MIS in pediatric patients, but their procedures were not related to tumors.[35] In fact, it was not until Holcomb and colleagues' report from the Surgical Discipline Committee of the Children's Cancer Group in 1995 that the MIS approach was formally reviewed for its efficacy in oncology.[36] In this study involving 15 participating centers, 25 abdominal and 63 thoracic explorations were undertaken for the purposes of diagnosis (primary, relapsed, and metastatic lesions), staging, assessment of resectability, and evaluation of treatment complications. All abdominal lesions (16), and 50 of 51 thoracic lesions that required biopsy were successfully diagnosed. There were no perioperative mortalities, and only 7 complications—all in the thoracic cohort.

A prospective trial sponsored by the National Institutes of Health concerning the use of MIS in pediatric oncology patients was begun by the combined Surgical Discipline Committees of the Children's Cancer Group (CCG) and the Pediatric Oncology Group (POG) in 1996.[36] The study failed for lack of accrual, and it was closed after 2 years. A questionnaire soliciting reasons for the failure of this study documented that lack of familiarity with the MIS technique by both the surgeons and the institutions, surgeon and pediatric oncologist bias against the MIS technique, and the failure to submit the necessary paperwork to local institutional review boards for study approval were statistically significant factors in the study's failure. Despite these results, MIS is gaining acceptance in pediatric oncology, especially for the diagnosis of lesions.

Spurbeck and colleagues at the St. Jude's Children's Research Hospital published their experience with MIS in pediatric oncology patients from 1995 to 2000.[37] In the study, 101 patients underwent 113 operations (64 abdominal and 49 thoracic procedures). Abdominal biopsies were attempted in 25 patients and were successful in 23 (92%). Evaluation of resectability was determined successfully in two other cases, and seven extirpative procedures were performed. There were three complications in the abdominal group, and four MIS procedures were converted to open procedures. Three complications were reported in the abdominal cohort. The thoracoscopic procedures had similar rates of success, conversion, and complications. They reported no port-site recurrences or metastases in their study, in either the abdominal or the thoracic cohorts, although a feared complication, the incidence of port site recurrence, is rare in thoracic cases (there is a single report by Sartorelli and colleagues).[38] Abdominal port site recurrence rates are higher, but they are determined by the tumor involved.[39-42] Needless to say, these are retrospective data spanning many institutions, surgeons, tumors, and techniques. The conclusions reached by Spurbeck and colleagues attest to the safety and efficacy of MIS techniques in the successful diagnosis of pediatric tumors, but their use in the formal extirpation of tumors remains to be established.

Extremity Tumors

Biopsy of a soft tissue or bone tumor in an extremity should be considered the first interventional procedure in limb salvage. Although the technical aspects are quite simple, the decision-making process is not. At risk are not only the patient's limb but also overall disease control and outcome.

Biopsy is truly a multidisciplinary process involving medical oncologists, surgeons, radiologists, pathologists, and radiation oncologists. The accuracy and outcome of biopsy procedures are improved when each of these specialists has a knowledge of musculoskeletal tumors and limb salvage principles. This is commonly best accomplished at tertiary centers with experience in the management of sarcomas.[43,44]

The first step in planning a biopsy is performing a complete workup. Based on history and physical exam findings, suspicion is raised about a tumor. Plain radiographs are often diagnostic of a bone malignancy and are crucial. MRI is also essential for both bone and soft tissue tumors to define the extent of the tumor itself and the involvement of neighboring compartments and neurovascular structures. It should be performed prior to biopsy to avoid artifact signal. Ultrasound is helpful to determine whether a soft tissue mass is cystic or solid, but MRI is the gold standard for the evaluation of a suspicious mass.

Based on the findings of the workup, a differential diagnosis can be established through collaboration at a multidisciplinary conference. All the specialists involved should be aware of the potential of a malignancy so that proper techniques are used for the procedure itself and for the handling of the tissue. The biopsy approach is selected by the surgeon on the basis of knowledge of limb salvage surgery. The biopsy track should be along the planned incision for limb salvage so that the entire track can be excised later with the resection of the tumor. This is critical because errors in placement of the biopsy incision can contaminate neurovascular and other important structures, making limb salvage impossible or necessitating large soft tissue flaps for coverage.[43,44] The tumor should be attained by the most direct approach and through a muscle, not in between muscles, to decrease contamination of normal tissue.

Biopsy of an extremity tumor can be performed by an open or a closed (CNB) technique (Table 9-1). Open biopsy offers the advantage of a larger tissue sample so that adequate pathologic evaluation can be performed. However, the major disadvantages are higher risks for contamination of critical structures and complications, such as bleeding, infection, and pathologic fracture. It is also more expensive and requires more time. Incisional biopsy is performed by entering into the tumor itself and removing a small section of it. The pseudocapsule is repaired and careful hemostasis is obtained in an effort to decrease tumor cell spillage or the creation of a hematoma. Excisional biopsy involves removing the whole tumor in one piece. This is rarely indicated for extremity tumors because resection surgery for malignant tumors is so vastly different

TABLE 9-1	**Comparison of Open and Needle Biopsy**	
	Open	**Needle**
Sample size	Larger	Smaller
Accuracy	Higher	Lower
Morbidity	Higher	Lower
Risk for contamination	Higher	Lower
Complications	Higher	Lower

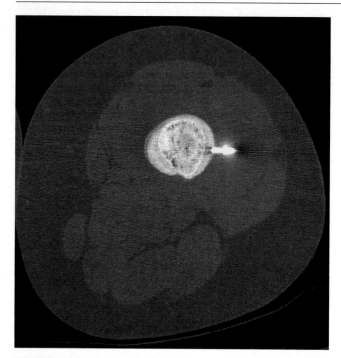

FIGURE 9-11. Core needle biopsy of an osteosarcoma of the femur under guidance by CT.

from that for benign tumors. Also, most musculoskeletal tumors are treated with neoadjuvant therapy prior to excision. This approach is used for two reasons. First, it increases the ability to perform limb salvage surgery. Second, it provides an in vivo assay of response to standard chemotherapy (please see the section concerning adjuvant therapy).

Needle biopsy, on the other hand, is associated with less morbidity for the patient. It carries a lower risk for complications and contamination and is often simpler to perform. However, the smaller tissue sample size is a disadvantage and decreases the accuracy rate of the diagnosis. Using a large-bore needle to remove a core of the tumor is thus usually more advantageous than using a fine needle for aspiration, as previously discussed. Sampling error is another disadvantage of CNB. Image guidance using CT (Fig. 9-11) or ultrasound improves accuracy and decreases sampling error, but it is imperative that the surgeon discuss the approach with the radiologist performing the procedure. There is a risk for local recurrence if the needle biopsy track is not excised with the tumor, but the risk is probably less than exists with open biopsy.

Pathologic analysis also requires specific knowledge of musculoskeletal tumors, especially with smaller sample sizes. The specialist obtaining the biopsy should discuss the case with the pathologist. A frozen section at the time of biopsy is essential, not for definitive diagnosis but to ensure that sufficient neoplastic tissue is available to the pathologist to make a diagnosis. Proper tissue handling is also crucial so the pathologist can arrive at the correct diagnosis. Hematoxylin and eosin staining as well as most immunohistochemistry can be performed on tissue placed in standard formaldehyde. However, electron microscopy, cytogenetic investigation, tissue culture, flow cytometry, and immunofluorescence require special handling and often require fresh tissue. The discovery of specific cytogenetic abnormalities in certain tumors—for example, t(11;22) in Ewing's sarcoma and t(2;13) in alveolar rhabdomyosarcoma—has increased the ability of pathologists to make

the diagnosis with small tissue samples, but they must be processed in the correct manner.

Combined discussion of the pathology completes the biopsy process. The multidisciplinary team caring for the patient can then review all of the staging studies with the known diagnosis in mind and arrive at a recommendation for treatment.

NEOADJUVANT THERAPY FOR SOLID TUMORS

Wilms' Tumor

Cooperative group trials by the NWTSG in North America, the Société Internationale d'Oncologie Pédiatrique (SIOP) in Europe, and the United Kingdom Children's Cancer Group have provided a great wealth of information regarding the optimal management of Wilms' tumors. A major difference in approach exists between SIOP and the NWTSG. In North America, primary resection followed by chemotherapy and radiotherapy is generally used. In the SIOP studies, children generally first receive either chemotherapy or radiotherapy, followed by resection. This approach has been driven by a high incidence of operative tumor rupture in their early series. In SIOP 1, the use of preoperative radiation therapy (20 Gy) was randomized versus primary resection. The rate of intraoperative rupture decreased from 33% to 4% with the use of radiation.[45] Survival was not affected and the incidence of local recurrence was not reported. The frequency of operative rupture that occurred in the NWTSG 1 and 2 were 22% and 12%, respectively.[46,47] In a subsequent SIOP study, preoperative therapy was randomized between abdominal radiation (20 Gy) and actinomycin-D compared with those receiving vincristine and actinomycin-D. The frequency of rupture was 9% and 6%, respectively.[48]

In SIOP-6, which started in 1980, all patients received initial preoperative chemotherapy (vincristine and actinomycin-D). Radiotherapy was given after resection to children with stage-II NI and stage III disease. Children with stage-II N0 (lymph node negative) were randomized to receive either 20 Gy abdominal radiotherapy or no radiation. All children received vincristine and actinomycin-D for 38 weeks. The radiotherapy randomization was halted after 123 children were randomized, 64 to radiotherapy and 59 to chemotherapy alone. Of the recurrences in the 59 children who did not receive radiotherapy, 6 children had local recurrences, whereas no recurrences occurred in the group who did receive radiotherapy. These findings suggested that prenephrectomy treatment altered the pathologic findings that would have led to a diagnosis of stage II NI or stage III disease (i.e., lymph node involvement or capsular penetration) and resulted in the standard administration of local radiation. No statistical difference in survival rates has been seen in these children on extended follow-up because those who relapsed had treatment alternatives.[49,50]

In SIOP-9, which began in 1987, preoperative therapy was randomized between 4 and 8 weeks' duration. The goal was to produce a larger proportion of stage-I tumors.[51] In this study, postoperative radiotherapy for stage II node-negative children was replaced by an anthracycline (epirubicin or doxorubicin). Preoperative treatment for patients without distant metastases consisted of four weekly courses of vincristine and three 2-day courses of actinomycin-D every 2 weeks versus 8 weeks of the identical therapy. No advantage was seen in the extended therapy in terms of staging at resection (stage I, 64%, versus 62%) or in intraoperative tumor rupture (1% versus 3%). Therapy after resection was based on the pathologic findings.

In SIOP-9, the surgery-related complications were reported to be 8%.[52]

In the NWTSG protocols and now in those of the Children's Oncology Group, primary surgical resection is generally recommended. There are certain generally accepted situations in which preoperative therapy is appropriate. These include the occurrence of Wilms' tumor in a solitary kidney, bilateral renal tumors, tumor in a horseshoe kidney, and respiratory distress resulting from extensive metastatic disease in the lungs. In these cases, pretreatment biopsy should be obtained and percutaneous biopsies are often used. Although needle track seeding has been reported, this is quite rare. The aim of neoadjuvant treatment in bilateral tumors, the solitary kidney, and the horseshoe kidney is to preserve the maximum amount of renal parenchyma and function.

The efficacy of preoperative treatment in achieving partial nephrectomy in patients with unilateral Wilms' tumors has been evaluated by several centers. McLorie and associates in Toronto obtained percutaneous biopsy in 31 children with Wilms' tumors. Multiagent chemotherapy was then administered for 4 to 6 weeks. Partial nephrectomy was performed in 9 children (4 with unilateral tumors and 5 with bilateral tumors).[53] Two of these children suffered intra-abdominal relapse and only 4 of the 30 unilateral tumors (13.3%) were amenable to partial nephrectomy. Hence, in unilateral cases not identified by prospective radiographic imaging in patients with syndromes, partial nephrectomy is rarely possible, even with preoperative therapy. Another assessment of the feasibility of partial nephrectomies was performed at St. Jude Children's Research Hospital.[54] The preoperative CT scans of 43 children with nonmetastatic unilateral Wilms' tumors were reviewed. The criteria used to define those tumors suitable for partial nephrectomy were involvement by the tumor of one pole and less than one third of the kidney, a functioning kidney, no involvement of the collecting system or renal vein, and clear margins between the tumor and surrounding structures. Only 2 of 43 scans (4.7%) met these criteria, suggesting that partial nephrectomy was feasible. The primary concerns regarding the administration of preoperative chemotherapy, as in the studies of Kozzi and associates and Moorman-Voestermans and coworkers, are to create "resectable" small tumors and that these children may be curable by surgical resection alone without subjecting them to the toxicity of additional treatments.[55,56]

The surgical resectability of Wilms' tumors has been poorly correlated with radiographic studies. In fact, extremely large tumors can be stage II lesions and can be fairly safely resected (Fig. 9-12). The surgical recommendations in the NWTSG studies have been that if resection of the tumor would involve resection of adjacent organs (i.e., liver, pancreas, or spleen because of adherence), biopsies should be obtained and subsequent chemotherapy applied prior to resection because such resections are associated with increased likelihood of complication (Fig. 9-13A, B). Complications in the most recently reported NWTSG-4 study have been assessed.[57] Complications occurred in 12.7% of a random sample of 534 of the 3335 patients enrolled in the study. Intestinal obstruction was the most common complication (5.1%), followed by extensive hemorrhage (1.9%), wound infection (1.9%), and vascular injury (1.5%). Factors associated with increased incidence of complication included intravascular extension into the inferior vena cava or atrium and nephrectomy performed through a flank or paramedian incision. Tumor diameter greater than or equal to 10 cm was also associated with increased complications. In SIOP-9, complications occurred in 8% of 598 patients. These patients were pretreated with vincristine, actinomycin-D, and epirubicin or doxorubicin before nephrectomy.[52] Their complications included small bowel obstruction in 3.7% and

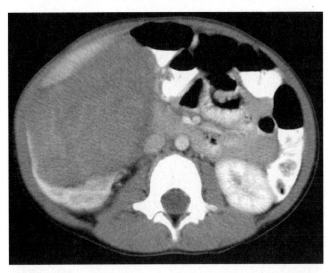

FIGURE 9-12. CT scan in a girl 4 years, 10 months old, who presented with a palpable abdominal mass. The study revealed a large tumor and a very thin renal capsule. A primary resection was performed, and the tumor was stage II with favorable histology. She went on to receive double-agent therapy with vincristine and actinomycin-D.

tumor rupture in 2.8%. The latter is not reported as a complication in the NWTSG reviews.

Neuroblastoma

Surgery plays a primary role in the treatment of low-stage neuroblastoma. Tumors the surgeon deems readily resectable should generally have primary resection for staging and to establish the diagnosis and the biologic risk factors of the tumor. In many children with small tumors and favorable biologic factors, surgery is the only therapy required. Resection is generally accepted prior to administration of chemotherapy for most thoracic, pelvic, and cervical primaries and limited abdominal lesions that do not extend across the midline. This approach is used to avoid the toxicity of chemotherapy, and in many patients with low-stage favorable biology tumors, resection alone is curative. In situations in which resection would entail removal of vital organs, or there is extensive lymph node extension, preliminary treatment by adjuvant chemotherapy, particularly in the biologically adverse tumors, would be most appropriate. In patients with favorable biologic features, even subtotal resection may be the only therapy required.[58]

It is regrettable that the majority of infants and children present with metastatic disease at diagnosis. In these cases, the diagnosis and biologic features must be established. Tissue may be obtained by laparotomy or thoracotomy as well as by laparoscopy and thoracoscopy. In older patients with metastatic disease, when Shimada staging is not required to determine the patient's treatment, needle biopsy from bone marrow or the primary metastatic tumor provides adequate material for both pathology and biologic grading. For patients in whom the Shimada criteria are critical for determining therapeutic treatment, open or minimal-access surgery is required to obtain adequate tissue.

In patients with extensive abdominal primaries, adjuvant therapy has been useful. It is well recognized by surgeons that preoperative chemotherapy decreases the vascularity and friability of the tumor and facilitates resection, particularly in

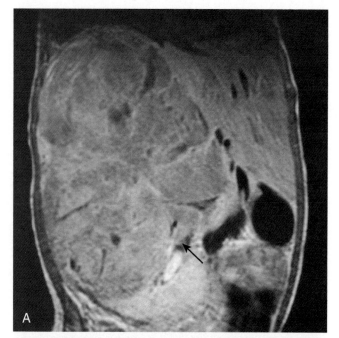

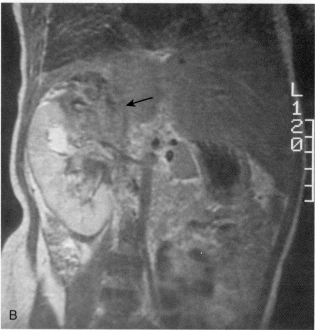

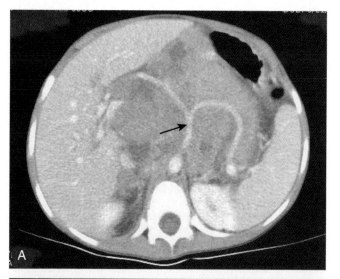

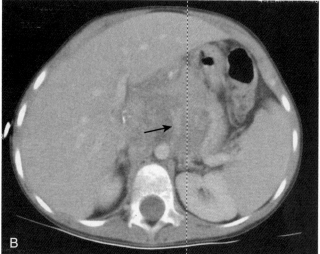

FIGURE 9-14. A 4-year-old presented with bone pain and a palpable abdominal mass. **A,** A CT scan showed an extensive mass arising from the adrenal gland. This scan shows extensive involvement of the lymph nodes around the aorta, with the celiac axis *(arrow)* projecting anteriorly and surrounded by tumor. In this section, the splenic artery as well as the hepatic artery are shown surrounded by tumor. **B,** Subsequent CT scan after four courses of multiagent chemotherapy revealed marked resolution in the size of the mass, although it was still surrounding the superior mesenteric artery *(arrow)*.

FIGURE 9-13. A, An MRI scan of a 2½-year-old girl first seen with a massive right-sided abdominal mass *(arrow)* that appeared to arise from the kidney. A chest radiograph revealed pulmonary nodules as well, making her stage IV. Because of the size of the primary tumor and the presence of metastatic disease, she received neoadjuvant chemotherapy after needle biopsy demonstrated a standard-risk tumor (diffuse blastemal subtype). She first received three courses of actinomycin-D, vincristine, and Cytoxan, which achieved some shrinkage of the tumor. At attempted resection, the extensive tumor was densely adherent to the posterior aspect of the liver and the vena cava. The attempted resection was halted at that time because it was clear that a portion of the liver would have to be resected with the nephrectomy. Repeat biopsies again demonstrated a standard-histology Wilms' tumor with tumor invasion into the liver. She then received more intensive therapy involving cisplatin and VP-16, as well as abdominal and thoracic radiation. **B,** MRI after additional therapy showed remarkable shrinkage of the tumor, allowing a less extensive and safer resection. A plane could be developed between the liver and kidney at this point and hepatectomy was not required.

developing the dissection plane between the tumor and the great vessels.[59] Lymph node involvement surrounding the aorta, vena cava, or renal vessels is commonly seen in children with advanced-stage abdominal, adrenal, or paravertebral primaries (Fig. 9-14A, B).

Although two studies have shown no differences in the surgical complication rates between initial and postinduction resection, other studies have demonstrated higher incidences of complications, including nephrectomy in the group undergoing primary resection.[60-65]

In patients with high-risk tumors, who commonly require autologous bone marrow transplants, preservation of the ipsilateral kidney during the resection is critical.[66] The neoadjuvant approach has contributed to decreased operative complications requiring nephrectomy.[67]

A multi-institutional review of children treated over an 11-year interval demonstrated a 14.9% incidence of nephrectomy or renal infarction as a result of surgery for local control (52 of 349 children). There was a 25% incidence among those with initial resection (29 children) and a 9.9% incidence in postchemotherapy resection (23 children). Children with initial resection had more than a twofold increase in their risk for nephrectomy. Hence, the approach to neuroblastomas regarding primary lesions is quite different from the approach to Wilms' tumors. The other determining factor is that the pathologic staging information is not as critical to determining local control in neuroblastomas as it is in Wilms' tumors, and essentially all of the children with large primary lesions require adjuvant chemotherapy and radiation. Hence, administration preoperatively in no way increases the likelihood that chemotherapy will be required and is generally recommended in most current protocols.

Hepatoblastoma

Surgery is the cornerstone in the treatment of hepatoblastoma, and children are rarely cured without resection. Neoadjuvant and adjuvant chemotherapy facilitates its feasibility and success rate. Historically, resection with complete removal of all radiographically identifiable disease cured only 25% of children; 50% of children who presented with hepatoblastoma had resectable lesions and of those, only 50% survived.[68,69] Failure was attributed to occult metastatic disease not identified radiographically,[70] and Weinblatt and colleagues[71] reported the early success of neoadjuvant chemotherapy to convert unresectable liver tumors into resectable lesions; more than 75% of the lesions became resectable in both series (Fig. 9-15A, B). Subsequent reports document the utility of various chemotherapeutic regimens in hepatoblastoma to treat unresectable lesions or residual disease.[72-78] These reports establish the efficacy of doxorubicin, cisplatin, vincristine, and 5-fluorouracil alone or in various combinations. Furthermore, both adjuvant and neoadjuvant regimens in combination with surgery achieved survival rates of greater than 65%, and tumor response rates of greater than 90%. Although the regimens varied, most patients received at least two cycles before definitive surgery. The critical need for resection of the primary tumor prior to the development of chemoresistance was demonstrated by von Schweinitz and colleagues.[76] They documented tumor regrowth as early as after the fourth course of therapy in 6 of 11 patients. The 5-year survival rates for all patients with hepatoblastoma had increased in just 2 decades to more than 85% with the use of neoadjuvant and adjuvant chemotherapy.

In the past decade, a defined treatment protocol consisting of neoadjuvant chemotherapy and surgical resection or early orthotopic transplant evaluation for patients with tumors that are too extensive to resect has been developed and reported by the International Society of Pediatric Oncology Liver Tumor Group (SIOPEL).[79,80] This regimen was termed PLADO, and it consisted of pretreatment; an imaging-defined staging protocol (pretreatment extent of disease; PRETEXT); pretreatment diagnostic biopsy (core needle or incisional biopsy); neoadjuvant chemotherapy of continuous infusion cisplatin (day 1) followed by continuous infusion of doxorubicin (days 2 and 3); surgical resection after 4 to 6 cycles 12 to 20 weeks from diagnosis; and orthotopic liver transplant evaluation and referral for tumors confined to the liver that remained unresectable despite chemotherapy. The only tumors resected primarily were those deemed to be confined to a single section (i.e., right anterior, right posterior, left medial, left lateral) of the liver (PRETEXT I). The overall 5-year survival rate was 75% for the entire cohort, and 85% for those following the

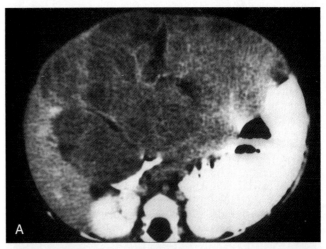

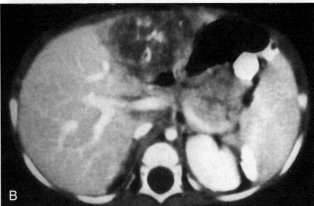

FIGURE 9-15. A 9-month-old female presented with a palpable abdominal mass extending to below her umbilicus. **A,** A CT scan revealed an extensive mass in her liver. **B,** A CT scan after four courses of chemotherapy showed remarkable resolution of the mass, which was subsequently resected by a left trisegmentectomy.

complete protocol, including neoadjuvant chemotherapy regardless of PRETEXT stage. PRETEXT stages I through IV had overall survival rates of 100%, 91%, 58%, and 57%, respectively, which compare favorably to survival rates achieved by Ortega and colleagues[81] through a CCG/POG cooperative trial comparing multimodality treatment protocols using various chemotherapeutic regimens. The surgical mortality rate was 6%, and the overall mortality rate was 24%. Of the patients, 20% presented with pulmonary metastases; 92% of the patients had complete resection under this protocol, and there were 10 patients who relapsed—5 with local recurrences and 5 with pulmonary metastases. SIOPEL's use of orthotopic liver transplant (OLTX) as the primary treatment for local control was recently published by Otte and colleagues.[82] Patients whose tumors involved all sectors of the liver or were intimately involved with either the hepatic or portal veins but showed no evidence of metastatic disease and demonstrated some response to neoadjuvant chemotherapy were considered for a primary OLTX. Another cohort of patients who had intrahepatic recurrences of disease after resection or incomplete resection was eligible for rescue OLTX. The 10-year survival rates of the primary and rescue OLTX groups were 85% and 40%, respectively. The authors advocated, based on their results, the following: (1) total resection of all gross disease, including the retrohepatic vena cavae, if necessary; (2)

the use of preoperative chemotherapy to control extrahepatic micrometastases and promote primary tumor regression; (3) transplantation in patients with synchronous pulmonary metastases if they had responded to neoadjuvant therapy; (4) no transplantation in patients with evidence of metastatic disease present at surgery; (5) limiting the interval between diagnosis and OLTX to account for the rise of chemoresistance and the availability of donors (cadaveric or living); and (5) questioning the need for post-OLTX chemotherapy in an immunosuppressed patient. Although their cohort was small (12), they reviewed the world's experience with OLTX for hepatoblastoma in the same report, and the results were similar. As a corollary to this report, Austin and colleagues[83] reported on the experience of the United Network of Organ Sharing for 152 orthotopic liver transplants performed in 135 patients in the setting of hepatoblastoma. Their actuarial 1-, 5-, and 10-year survival rates were 79%, 69%, and 66%, respectively. More than 54% of patients died of recurrent disease, and the only statistically significant predictors of favorable outcome were the preoperative conditions of the patients (hospitalization in the intensive care unit, hospitalization outside of the intensive care unit, or no hospitalization), and the era when the patient received the transplant (before or after December 31, 1994). These reports document not only the feasibility but also the success of orthotopic liver transplant as a component in the multimodality treatment of hepatoblastoma.

Rhabdomyosarcoma

Except for Wilms' tumor, no other pediatric solid tumor has benefited so greatly from the combined efforts of oncologists of all disciplines in forming multimodality protocols designed to diagnose, stage, treat, and surveil a lesion adequately as has rhabdomyosarcoma. The 5-year survival of children with this disease was less than 25% prior to 1972, when the Intergroup Rhabdomyosarcoma Study Group was formed.[83,84] Over the next 3 decades, this figure has increased almost threefold to 70%.[85-87] Because rhabdomyosarcoma is a tumor of mesenchymal origin, it may appear almost anywhere in the body and be situated in almost any organ. Treatment protocols and outcomes vary greatly depending on the site and stage of the tumor. Initial pretreatment evaluations document the characteristics of the primary lesions and the regional lymph node basins. If an extremity lesion is excised with positive margins and proves to be a rhabdomyosarcoma, it has been shown that pretreatment reexcision with generous margins (0.5 cm or greater) of uninvolved tissues and local lymph node sampling results in improved survival rates.[88] Debilitating resections producing loss of function are not currently warranted, except in cases with residual disease after adjuvant radiotherapy and chemotherapy. Regional and distant lymphadenopathy diagnosed clinically or radiographically must be biopsied to establish the presence or absence of tumor, which will impact treatment strategies and prognosis.[89] Aggressive lymphadenectomies are not warranted, but a stepwise progression of draining lymph node basins should be sampled to determine the lymph node status of these contiguous basins and, hence, the extent of regional radiotherapy. Finally, so-called second-look operations performed on the primary site in the Intergroup Rhabdomyosarcoma Study Group III proved useful in the excision of residual tumor, the confirmation of the effectiveness of adjuvant therapies, and the improved prognosis of all tumors save pelvic sites, which had pathologically confirmed complete responses to therapy.[90] These principles of complete resection of the primary tumor and lymph node biopsy determine postoperative clinical groupings that determine adjuvant treatment therapies and prognosis.

Radiotherapy is a core modality of treatment for local control, and its field is based on the size of the mass before resection. Patients receive a radiation field with at least a 2 cm margin around the primary mass. It is generally begun 8 to 12 weeks after the initiation of chemotherapy and continues for 5 to 6 weeks. All histopathologic subtypes receive radiation therapy, except for group I embryonal disease.[87] All other groups and rhabdomyosarcoma variants receive at least 4000 rads for microscopic residual disease and up to 5000 rads for macroscopic residual disease,[87,91,92] providing a strong basis for primary resection if safely feasible.

Adjuvant chemotherapy is critical, and its use is based on a risk stratification schema that incorporates site of tumor origin, tumor histopathology, TNM staging, and the postoperative clinical grouping. Patients are stratified into low-risk, intermediate-risk, or high-risk categories. Low-risk patients typically receive a three-drug regimen of vincristine, dactinomycin, and cyclophosphamide. Intermediate-risk patients generally receive the same three-drug regimen, but those with tumors in favorable sites and those with completely resected tumors in unfavorable sites receive dose-intensified cyclophosphamide.[92] High-risk patients, however, should receive a two-drug regimen of ifosfamide with etoposide or doxorubicin.[93,94] Metastatic disease or alveolar subtypes should also receive topotecan or irinotecan in addition to standard therapy.[95,96] Ideally, neoadjuvant chemotherapy can reduce tumor burden and convert unresectable lesions to resectable ones that allow for decreased morbidity in patients (Fig. 9-16A, B).

Osteosarcoma, Ewing's Sarcoma

The single most important factor in improved survival rates for patients with osteosarcoma or Ewing's sarcoma has been the development of effective chemotherapy. Prior to 1970, patients with osteosarcoma had an overall survival rate of about 10%. Prior to the 1960s, survival rates were even lower than 10% for patients with Ewing's sarcoma. Ablative surgery and radiation were the only modalities available at that time. Local control, however, was not the issue. Patients succumbed primarily to metastatic disease, believed to be present at diagnosis, although it could not be demonstrated radiographically. Systemic treatment was necessary to achieve improved survival rates and cure. Medications were identified and successfully applied in cooperative multi-institutional trials. With modern chemotherapy protocols, the overall survival rate for patients with osteosarcoma is now 60% or better, and it approaches 60% for Ewing's sarcoma. Please see the individual chapters concerning each of these topics for more detail.

Current protocols for osteosarcoma involve neoadjuvant chemotherapy, surgery, then further adjuvant chemotherapy. Protocols are similar for Ewing's sarcoma, except that radiation can be used in combination with surgery or alone as local treatment. The advantages of this approach are that tumor cells in the primary tumor and in micrometastatic form are treated immediately and that histologic response to the chemotherapy can be assessed. The potential advantage of making limb-salvage surgery safer is debatable but, certainly, any reduction in size of the primary tumor improves the feasibility of surgical resection (Fig. 9-17A, B). The disadvantages are that in patients who do not respond to the usual drugs, the disease may progress, and drug resistance may develop. Response to chemotherapy has been identified as one of the more important prognostic factors, with potential implications for changes in therapy, so this overall approach is used in the majority of trials. The reality, though, is that no new drugs or changes in therapy have been shown to improve survival rates to any great extent in poor responders. Efforts to improve survival rates for poor

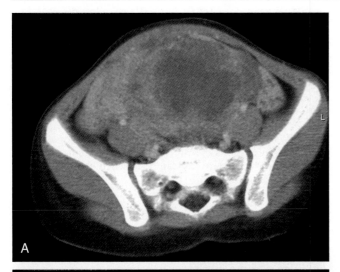

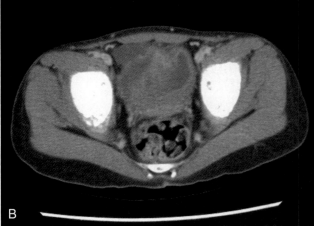

FIGURE 9-16. A, A 7-year-old patient with a large bladder rhabdomyosarcoma prechemotherapy. **B,** A significant decrease in the size of the tumor is seen.

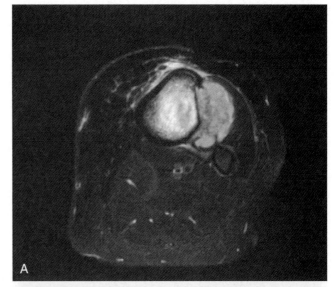

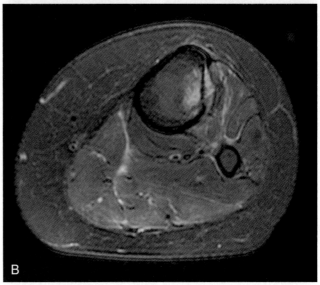

FIGURE 9-17. Ewing's sarcoma of the proximal tibia: T2-weighted sequence with fat saturation, axial MRI. **A,** At initial diagnosis, there was a large anterolateral soft tissue extension outside of the bone. **B,** After neoadjuvant chemotherapy, the soft tissue mass had noticeably decreased in size, making surgery, especially dissection around the atrial trifurcation, less difficult.

responders and for patients who relapse are the focus of current protocols and research.

LIMB SALVAGE PROCEDURES

Surgical Principles

The surgical treatment of bone sarcomas has evolved since the prechemotherapy era when all patients underwent amputations, radiation therapy, or both, to the current practice, in which 80% or more of patients receive limb salvage resection.[97] The resection can be thought of in two phases: wide resection of the tumor and involved bone and reconstruction, for which there are multiple alternatives. A "safe" resection requires complete excision of the involved bone and soft tissues, leaving a cuff of normal tissue surrounding the entire specimen, a so-called wide margin. The necessary thickness of this cuff of tissue and the length of normal marrow away from the tumor is not precisely known,[98-102] but at a minimum, there should not be "ink on tumor." As experience with these operations grows, most surgeons now accept soft tissue margins of 2 to 5 mm of normal soft tissue and 1 to 2 cm of marrow margin, but there is no evidence-based minimum margin that has been docu-

mented to be safe with respect to local recurrence. Neoadjuvant chemotherapy probably lessens the likelihood of local recurrence.[103-106] Recent data suggest that a wide margin in a patient with a good response to chemotherapy has a low likelihood of local recurrence.[107-109] Resections with narrower margins (marginal or intralesional) and those with poor responses to chemotherapy have higher risk for local recurrence. It is clear that local recurrence is associated with poor prognosis for survival.[110-113]

The decision to perform a resection rather than an amputation and the type of reconstruction to be made require careful evaluation of the imaging studies by a multidisciplinary team that includes an experienced musculoskeletal radiologist and involves a detailed discussion with the patient and family regarding the alternatives. Although most patients would prefer to save the limb if it is possible to do so, it should be understood that current reconstruction options cannot create a normal limb, and most are not meant to return the patient to athletic activities. Patients with lower extremity primaries who want to continue contact and running sports are better served by amputation or rotationplasty.

The resection requires careful analysis of the radiograph and MRI. The entire bone should be imaged to exclude the possibility of skip metastases. MRI is the best study for assessing the extent of the tumor within the bone and soft tissue (Fig. 9-18A-D).[114-118] Osteosarcomas may cross growth plates to involve the epiphysis of the bone, but they rarely cross the articular cartilage unless there has been a fracture.[114,116] Adjacent joint involvement is rare, but if present requires an extra-articular resection. Tumors may enter the joint by extending along the joint capsule (e.g., in the proximal humerus, the metaphysis is partially intra-articular) or cruciate ligaments (knee), or ligamentum teres (hip). The major nerves and vessels must be uninvolved or resectable to achieve the required margin. Finally, there must be sufficient muscle remaining after the resection to allow soft tissue coverage of the reconstruction and to power the limb. At times rotational flaps or free tissue transfers may be indicated to obtain soft tissue coverage and lessen the likelihood of wound complication.[119,120] For all resection types, infection is the worst immediate complication, and the chances of its occurrence can be lessened by adequate soft tissue closure.

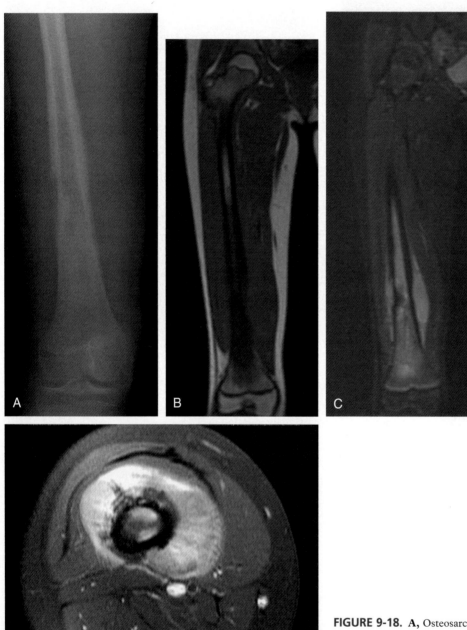

FIGURE 9-18. A, Osteosarcoma of the femur showing ill-defined bone destruction in the metaphysis and soft tissue mass. **B,** Coronal T1-weighted image shows the extent of the tumor in the medullary canal. **C** and **D,** Coronal and axial images show the extent of the soft tissue mass and the relationship to the femoral artery and vein.

Once the resection has been completed, the pathologist should examine the specimen grossly to ensure complete resection. The use of frozen section analysis of the marrow margins is a routine and accepted practice but is of uncertain value.[121] Bisecting the specimen using a band saw and visualizing it will reassure the surgeon that an adequate resection has been accomplished.

Types of Reconstruction in Children

Reconstruction options include the use of metallic endoprostheses, bone allografts, and rotationplasty. Some sites require no bony reconstruction. These "expendable" bones include the fibula, clavicle, rib, and iliac wing (if the acetabulum can be preserved). Most osteosarcomas are located around the knee, hip, or shoulder and involve resection of the distal femoral, proximal tibial, proximal femoral, or proximal humeral metaphysis and epiphysis. In addition to the bony defect, a major growth center is included; in the lower extremity this adds complexity to the reconstruction that is not encountered in adults. For patients close to skeletal maturity (10 to 12 years of age in girls and 14 to 16 years of age in boys) this is seldom a major issue and can be addressed by reconstruction that uses a slightly longer implant than the length resected. Limb length discrepancies of 2 cm or less are seldom a clinical problem and can be treated with a simple shoe lift. For tumors in the vicinity of the knee in younger patients, limb length must be addressed by the reconstruction chosen. The alternatives include the use of expandable prostheses, bone allografts, and rotationplasty. Each has advantages and disadvantages. An expandable prosthesis, in theory, allows "growth" of the prosthesis over time but will have to be revised to an adult prosthesis at skeletal maturity.[122-126] Some of these prostheses require frequent operations to achieve lengthening,[126] whereas others have nonoperative mechanisms of expansion.[122] They are expensive, complex prostheses that involve many potential complications. Children younger than 8 years of age have difficulty cooperating with physical therapy, so joint contractures are a problem. In addition, mechanical failure of the prosthesis, metal debris, loosening, and infection can be significant problems.[127] Bone allografts have the advantage of preserving the adjacent bone and its growth plate (i.e., the proximal tibia can be preserved following distal femoral resection), but obviously have no capacity to grow. There are also issues concerning finding an allograft of appropriate size and shape, but if a suitable bone is available, length equalization can be addressed by inserting a graft 1 to 2 cm longer than the length resected and addressing limb length subsequently by means of standard pediatric orthopedic techniques of contralateral epiphyseodesis. At skeletal maturity, closed femoral shortening and limb lengthening techniques are also available. Rotationplasty addresses this issue because the prosthesis can be adjusted to the desired length as the child grows.

Bone Allografts

Bone allografts are employed to reconstruct defects primarily at the distal femur, proximal tibia, proximal femur, and proximal humerus.[128-132] The obvious concern is transmission of bacterial and viral disease, but bone banks are now accredited by the American Association of Tissue Banks, and the safety record of these grafts has been quite good since better testing for HIV and hepatitis has become available.[133-135] The advantages for young patients are that they restore bone stock and joint structures (articular cartilage, ligaments, and joint capsules) and delay the need for metallic prostheses. In theory,

they restore bone stock, but experience has shown that the grafts are only partially replaced by host bone, and it is likely that most osteoarticular grafts will require joint arthroplasty at some time (5 to 20 years after the index procedure). Delaying the placement of artificial joints until adulthood is probably advantageous for long-term salvage of the limb. In a young child, a major advantage of an osteoarticular allograft is the avoidance of resection or placing an implant across the adjacent growth plate. These are complex operations, and they require the availability of a tissue bank and surgical expertise in the use of allografts; and the procedure is associated with a significant complication rate. Infection, reported in the range of 0 to 20%,[128-132] is the worst complication and usually requires removal of the graft. Nonunion of the allograft-host junction (reported to occur overall in 17% of cases) is higher (27%) in patients receiving chemotherapy[136] but can usually be addressed by revision of the fixation and bone grafting of the osteosynthesis site. Fracture is a later complication and occurs in about 15% of patients.[128,130-132,136-138] Occasionally the fracture will heal with conservative means but more commonly, revision to another allograft, augmentation with a vascularized fibular graft,[139] or conversion to an endoprosthesis is required.[140] Postoperative management includes closed suction drains for 24 to 48 hours; pre- and postoperative antibiotic coverage (there are no data regarding the necessary length of antibiotic coverage); venous thrombosis prophylaxis; and initial immobilization. Physical therapy to start joint motion is begun at 6 weeks, and the limbs are protected by the use of crutches and bracing until the osteosynthesis site heals (approximately 6 to 9 months in patients receiving chemotherapy).

Endoprostheses

Metallic prostheses were initially custom-made to fit the expected bone resection defect. Currently, there are a number of available modular systems that allow the surgeon to reconstruct the defect on the operating table.[141-148] In older children who are close to skeletal maturity, adult prostheses can be used. Most reconstructions of the knee employ a rotating hinge construct that reduces the forces that are transmitted to the host-prosthesis interface, and this design is believed to increase the longevity of the implants because of delayed loosening of the stems. Modern stem designs include the option of cemented or uncemented stems, and in the femur there are curved and straight stem designs. In theory, uncemented stems offer the advantage of avoiding osteolysis and loosening, but whether bony ingrowth is reduced in patients receiving adjuvant therapies is uncertain at this time.[143,144,149,150] The main advantage of endoprostheses is that they are as stable and functional as they will ever be as soon as the wound heals, so return to function is more rapid than it is with allografts. Patients do not need to wait for an osteosynthesis to heal, and early weight bearing and range of motion is permitted. The disadvantages include infection (although the reported rates are lower than those reported with allografts); loosening or mechanical failure of the implants; the presence of metal debris; and decreased longevity.[148,149,151-153] Because 70% to 80% of children who have bone sarcomas now survive, it is unlikely that these implants will last the lifetime of the patient. Revision is possible, but multiple revisions over time may limit the options and lead to amputation. The longevity (not function) of the implants is about 60% to 80% at 5 years and 50% to 80% at 10 years for lower extremity implants, depending on the specific series.[126,144,146-152,154-157] The expandable endoprostheses are more complex and are likely to have higher complication rates.[122-127,158-160]

Examples by Anatomic Site

Distal Femur and Proximal Tibia

Tumors in the vicinity of the knee can be reconstructed by any of the methods discussed. A few examples are provided. Figure 9-19 shows an example of the use of an endoprosthesis in the distal femur. The implant is a modular prosthesis that is cemented into the remaining femur and proximal tibia following an intra-articular resection. The initial function of these constructs is quite good, but it is expected that loosening will occur sometime in the future. It is known from adult arthroplasty and early experience using custom and modular prostheses that the interface between the cement and the bone will fail over time, in part because of particulate debris and the biologic response to it. Design improvements such as ingrowth surfaces near the stem-implant junction that allow bony or soft tissue ingrowth may delay or prevent loosening.[154] Uncemented stems may also offer longevity advantages. A further concern is stress shielding. The stem takes the mechanical load from the adjacent bone and the host responds by resorbing the corti-

cal bone over time. The concern is that in future revisions, insufficient bone stock will remain. There are newer stem devices that load the bone to avoid stress shielding and offer the hope of greater longevity. The early data concerning these stems are encouraging. Unfortunately, there are no direct comparisons between osteoarticular allografts (Fig. 9-20) and endoprostheses at this site, but the current literature suggests that for the distal femur, an endoprosthesis is superior.[157] Some surgeons believe that in the skeletally immature, it is still advantageous to use allografts at this site for the reasons stated earlier.

In the proximal tibia, an osteoarticular allograft offers the advantage of providing a site for attachment of the patellar tendon. This is much more difficult to achieve in an endoprosthesis. As shown in Figure 9-21A-F, an intra-articular proximal tibial resection is achieved, including the host menisci (although they can be preserved, depending on the extent of the tumor). The reconstruction allows repair of the cruciate ligaments, joint capsule, and patellar tendon. A gastrocnemius flap is sometimes required for soft tissue coverage and is always required to augment soft tissue attachment of the patellar tendon if an

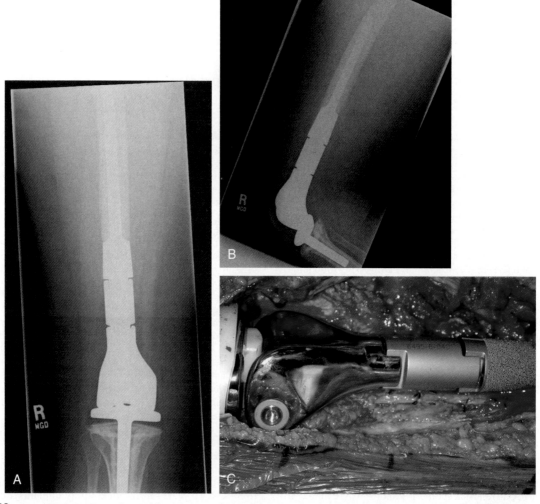

FIGURE 9-19. A and **B,** Anteroposterior and lateral views of a modular tumor prosthesis used for reconstruction following a resection for distal femoral osteosarcoma. A rotating hinge design is used, and the modular nature of the prosthesis can be appreciated. **C,** The prosthesis after insertion at operation.

endoprosthesis is used. Fixation is achieved by using the standard plates and screws used to treat fractures. Plates that span the entire length of the allograft or intramedullary fixation are desirable to lessen the likelihood of fracture. Intramedullary rods require supplemental plate fixation to control rotation at the osteosynthesis site. Newer locking plate designs may lessen the incidence of nonunion and fracture.[161] A variation of this construct is to combine an allograft and standard total knee prosthesis, usually a rotating hinge design for stability (Fig. 9-22). This allows a stable knee construct initially and a site

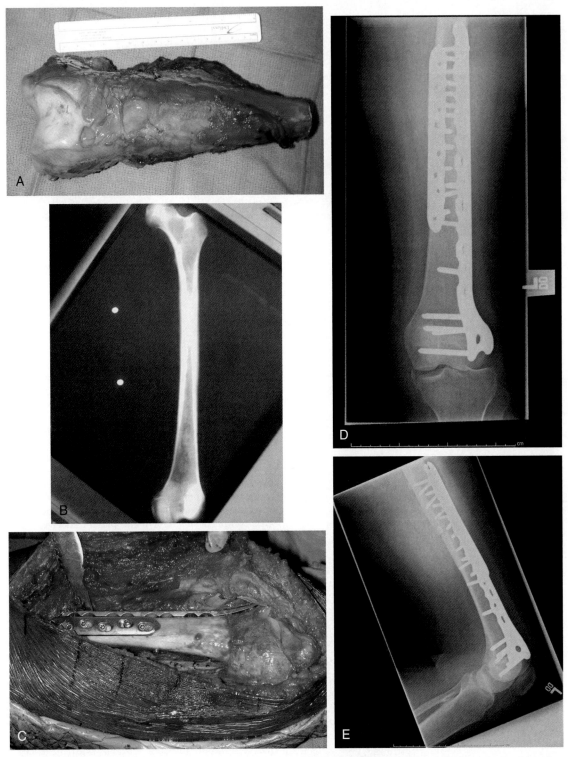

FIGURE 9-20. A, A resection specimen following intra-articular resection of the distal femur for osteosarcoma; a margin of muscle surrounding the tumor is shown. **B,** An osteoarticular allograft from a bone bank is thawed and then cut to fit the defect created. **C,** An intraoperative photograph shows the graft being held in place by dynamic compression plates following ligament reconstruction. **D** and **E,** The postoperative appearance on radiographs.

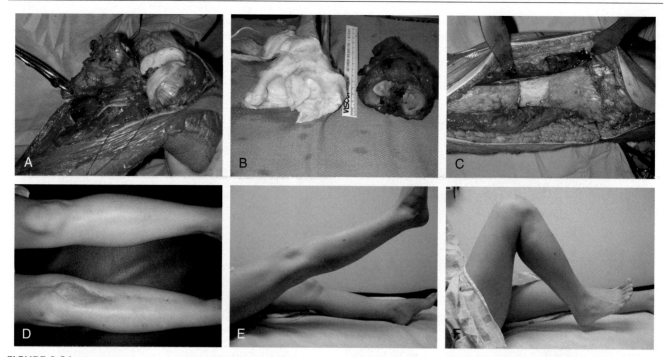

FIGURE 9-21. A, Resection of a proximal tibial osteosarcoma with preservation of the tibial vessels and sacrifice of the menisci. **B,** Comparison of the resected specimen with menisci (right) and the allograft (left). **C,** The allograft is in place after plate fixation and ligament reconstruction. The sutures in the patellar tendon are evident. **D,** Postoperative photograph showing a rotational gastrocnemius flap and skin graft. **E and F,** The function of a patient is demonstrated by full extension and straight-leg raising **(E)** and the flexion arc **(F).**

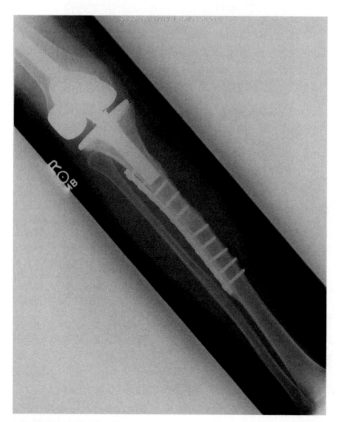

FIGURE 9-22. The radiographic appearance of an allograft prosthetic composite of the proximal tibia.

for reattachment of the patellar tendon. It has the disadvantage in a skeletally immature patient of placing an implant across the adjacent (distal femoral) growth plate, creating a greater potential for limb length discrepancy.

A further option at the knee is an expandable prosthesis (Figs. 9-23A-D and 9-24A-C). These can be used for the distal femur and proximal tibia; an example of each is shown. Many parents are now aware of these devices and are requesting them, but their long-term outcomes are still uncertain. One could argue that an attempt at this procedure is reasonable if the alternative is amputation or rotationplasty. One can plan to deal with complications later if the patient survives. The downside is that it restricts young children from normal activities, including sports; if they pursue sports, the likelihood of failure of the prosthesis is higher.

Rotationplasty

For large tumors of the distal femur and in very young patients with distal femoral sarcomas, rotationplasty is an excellent alternative to amputation.[162-164] A rotationplasty preserves the distal leg, foot, and ankle and places it at the level of the contralateral knee (Fig. 9-25A-F). The tibia replaces the femoral shaft, and by rotating the limb 180 degrees, the ankle and foot act like a knee, making the construct function like a below-knee amputation rather than a high-thigh amputation. A modification of this procedure can be performed for proximal tibial and proximal femoral sarcomas.[165-167] The margin achieved is wider than a standard resection because with the exception of the sciatic nerve, no other structures have to be saved. The vessels can be dissected and coiled like the nerve at closure, or they can be resected and anastomosed after the osteosynthesis has been achieved. This procedure may be more suitable for a

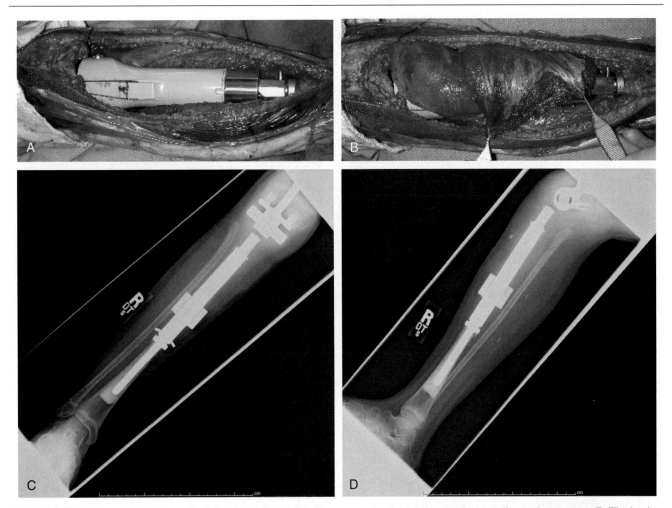

FIGURE 9-23. A, An expandable prosthesis for the proximal tibia. The sutures for the attachment of the patellar tendon are seen. **B,** The implant has been covered by a gastrocnemius and soleus flap that aid in anchoring the patellar tendon and in wound healing. This particular prosthesis allows for lengthening without an operation. **C** and **D,** Anteroposterior and lateral views show the radiographic appearance of the prosthesis in place. The spring mechanism allows for the expansion after an electromagnetic field transiently melts a restraint to expansion.

patient with a pathologic fracture because of the wider margin it achieves, but if the patient has a widely displaced fracture and a large sarcoma at diagnosis and requires spica immobilization during preoperative chemotherapy, there is a higher risk that the anastomosis will fail because of venous congestion in the leg (personal observation). Rotationplasty has the advantage of avoiding phantom pain because the sciatic nerve and its branches are preserved, and growth is not an issue because the prosthesis can be adjusted as the patient grows. It usually requires a single operation, has a low complication rate, and allows the child to participate fully in activities. The functional results are rewarding. The main drawback is the cosmetic appearance. Patients must be carefully selected, and it is essential that the child and the parents meet a patient that has had a rotationplasty and work with an experienced therapist preoperatively so that they fully understand the operation. Many patients, parents, and surgeons refuse this option because it is distasteful, but those that accept it do extremely well functionally and emotionally. This success has been documented in long-term studies.[162,168-174]

Proximal Femur

Resection of the proximal femur requires careful assessment of the hip joint (Fig. 9-26A-G, Fig. 9-27). If an intra-articular

reconstruction can be achieved, the reconstruction options include either a metallic prosthesis or an allograft.[143,147,175,176] The likelihood that an allograft will fit perfectly into the acetabulum is low, so most allografts at this site are allograft-prosthetic composites. If the acetabulum requires resection, the reconstruction is much more complex. An allograft offers the theoretical advantage of a site for reattachment of the abductor muscles hence lessening the abductor lurch during gait, but attaching the abductors to a metallic prosthesis or to the iliotibial band has been shown to be quite successful and is probably equivalent. The decision about whether to do a total hip prosthesis or a hemiarthroplasty is more difficult. Although the hemiarthroplasty is easier and more stable than a total hip arthroplasty, recent data in children suggest that they may subluxate as the child grows and the acetabulum develops, necessitating revision to a total joint arthroplasty.[177]

Pelvis

In general, patients with sarcomas in the pelvis have worse prognoses than patients who have sarcomas in the extremities.[178-183] Assessment of response to chemotherapy is critical. For Ewing's sarcoma, the alternative of irradiation for local control is available, but for osteosarcoma, surgical resection is required, even if it means hemipelvectomy, if the goal is cure.

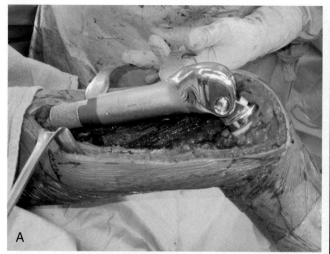

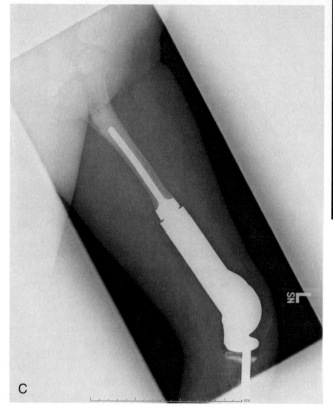

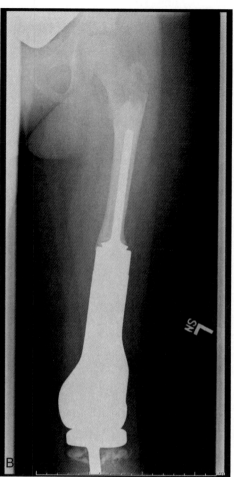

FIGURE 9-24. A, The intraoperative appearance of another expandable prosthesis of the distal femur. This prosthesis requires an open procedure to lengthen it. **B** and **C,** The radiographic appearance of the prosthesis cemented in place. An uncemented, smooth stem placed across the tibial physis allows that physis to grow.

Resections are difficult and commonly require the expertise of an orthopedic oncologist, a surgical oncologist and, at times, a vascular surgeon or urologist. The site of the tumor is critical. Tumors of the iliac wing can be resected without much functional loss if the acetabulum can be preserved (Fig. 9-28A-C). Bone grafts are sometimes used to restore the pelvic ring. Likewise, tumors involving the pubic rami can be resected and require little reconstruction other than synthetic mesh to prevent herniation of the abdominal contents (Fig. 9-29A,B). The difficult area is the acetabulum. Resection of the acetabulum or other areas of the pelvis that include the acetabulum result in complex reconstruction challenges. Frequently, the best alternative is to leave the hip flail (Fig. 9-30A,B). Significant shortening will occur, but function is better than an ampu-

tation, even if a major nerve is sacrificed. Attempts at arthrodesis of the proximal femur to the remaining pelvis can be considered, but arthrodesis is difficult to achieve. Allografts have been employed, but are reported to cause significant morbidity, including a high infection rate and long-term mechanical problems, including fracture.[184-187] Custom metallic replacements have also been used,[188] but they require careful planning and have a high failure rate. All of these considerations are amplified if the adjacent sacrum requires resection as well. The multidisciplinary team and the family must have a careful discussion of the goals, resection options, reconstruction alternatives, and other treatment strategies before the pelvic resection is undertaken. Surgical expertise in the intraoperative and postoperative management of these patients is essential for success.

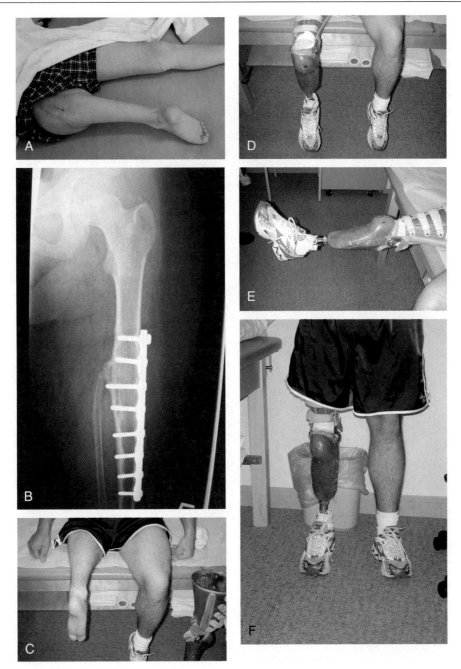

FIGURE 9-25. A, The appearance of a patient with a rotationplasty for a distal femoral osteosarcoma. **B,** The radiographic image reveals the osteosynthesis of the tibia to the femur. **C,** The appearance of the patient with the prosthesis off. **D,** The patient with the prosthesis on. **E,** Demonstration of the ability of the patient to extend the knee actively against gravity. **F,** The patient's appearance in stance.

Proximal Humerus

All attempts should be made to avoid amputation in patients with upper extremity tumors. Unlike the lower extremity, there are no prostheses that replicate the function of the hand. Limb length in the upper extremity is usually not a major concern. A resection of the proximal humerus and scapula en bloc (a Tikhoff-Lindberg resection) is preferable to a forequarter amputation and is usually possible.[189-194]

In patients with proximal humeral sarcomas that are amenable to intra-articular resections, reconstruction can be accomplished by using metallic prostheses (Fig. 9-31A, B),[147,152,195-198]

osteoarticular allografts (Fig. 9-32), or allograft-prosthesis composites.[128,199-201] Function is a result primarily of whether the deltoid muscle, axillary nerve, and rotator cuff can be preserved. A flail shoulder is superior to an amputation if all these muscles must be resected. In cases of high-grade sarcomas, the deltoid is commonly resected, but some active motion can be preserved if all or part of the rotator cuff can be preserved. Allografts provide sites for attachment of these motors, but metallic prostheses combined with synthetic materials surrounding the prostheses and synthetic suture materials can result in active motion as well. Even tumors that require resection of the radial nerve can be reconstructed, and the resultant

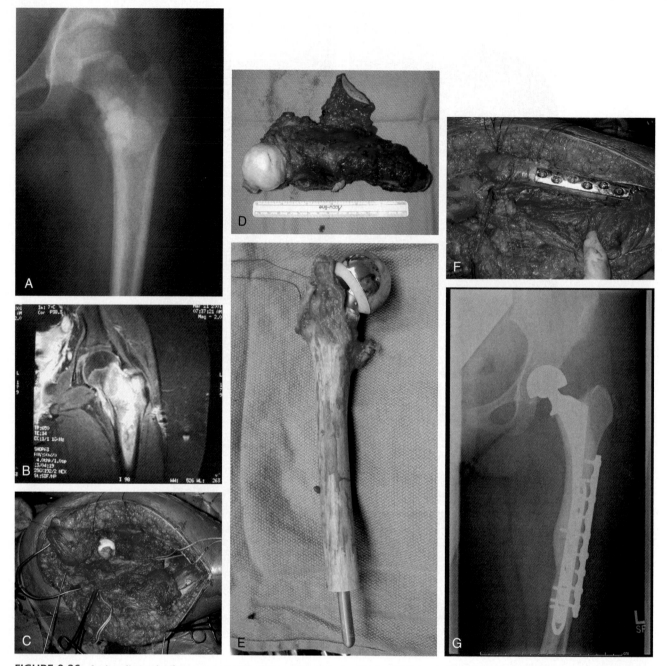

FIGURE 9-26. **A,** A radiograph of an osteosarcoma of the proximal femur. **B,** An MRI shows that the hip joint is not involved. **C,** The intraoperative findings following resection. The acetabulum can be seen, and sutures are retracting the gluteus medius and minimus. **D,** The resected specimen with the biopsy track included. **E,** The allograft after a bipolar, long-stem prosthesis has been cemented into it. **F,** Intraoperative photograph after the allograft has been fixed to the host bone. A unicortical plate is used for rotational control. The hip abductors have been sutured to the corresponding sites on the allograft. **G,** The postoperative appearance.

nerve deficit can be treated by nerve graft or by tendon transfers to restore radial nerve function in the hand. If the joint is involved, an extra-articular resection that includes the glenoid can be performed. The choice is between the constructs mentioned and an arthrodesis using allografts, with or without vascularized fibular grafts.[132,199,200,202] The latter allows for a stable shoulder, which is useful in a laborer but is difficult to achieve.

Outcomes

Although the goal of preserving a limb is laudable, and with experience the success rate of restoring functional limbs is improving, limb-sparing procedures are complex operations and the short- and long-term complications are not trivial. It should also be remembered that young patients with amputations of a lower extremity do quite well with modern prostheses.

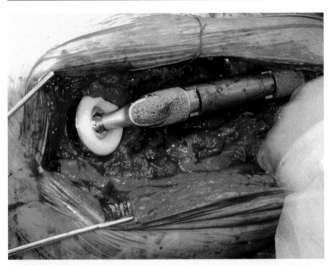

FIGURE 9-27. The intraoperative appearance of a modular metallic, bipolar prosthesis with sites for sutures to secure the abductors. The rough surface is designed to allow tissue ingrowth with time. Distally, a similar surface allows placement of bone graft to seal the bone-cement interface and retard loosening.

We are only beginning to assess the quality of life and functional outcomes following these reconstructions, and the tools we have to assess the parameters are limited. The data that exist suggest that the energy cost of walking is lower in the presence of a metallic prosthesis than in an above-knee amputation.[203] A rotationplasty is similar to a below-knee amputation in that regard.[204] Most of the outcome studies report function using the Musculoskeletal Tumor Society rating system that has not been validated and is based on a surgeon's assessment. Other outcome tools like the Short Form–36 (SF-36) or the Toronto Extremity Salvage Score (TESS) are patient driven and are not specific to sarcomas or a rare measure of disability.[205] The data we have suggest that there is little difference in outcome and quality of life for amputees and limb salvage patients, and there is even less difference among those who have undergone various types of reconstruction; however, the data are meager, and no controlled studies have been performed. This is an area that requires further study and development as the reconstruction options and prostheses continue to evolve. Much progress has been made in the ability to treat pediatric bone sarcomas and to preserve limbs, but better reconstruction options are still needed, including further development of tissue engineering.

MANAGEMENT OF PULMONARY METASTASIS IN PEDIATRIC SOLID TUMORS

The value of the pediatric surgical oncologist in the locoregional control of malignant lesions in children was established well before the advent of chemotherapy or radiotherapy. However, the same cannot be said of the treatment of tumor metastases, especially in the lung. An excellent review of the evolution and disease-specific implementation of pediatric pulmonary metastasectomy has been published.[206] The past five decades have seen rapid expansion of the use of pulmonary metastasectomy in pediatric cancers, but evidence-based proof of its efficacy is limited. This is the result of a general lack of tumor-specific, prospective, randomized clinical trials critically evaluating this therapeutic intervention. Reported studies come primarily from a single institution, are retrospective in nature,

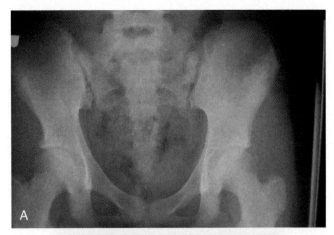

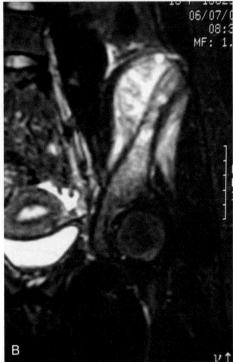

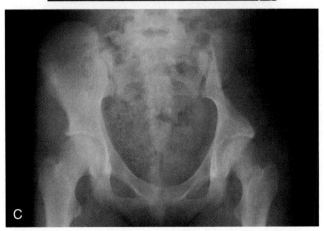

FIGURE 9-28. A, A radiograph of Ewing's sarcoma of the iliac wing. **B,** MRI reveals the extent of the soft tissue mass. **C,** Following chemotherapy, the soft tissue mass was smaller, and resection was possible. The acetabulum was preserved, allowing reasonable function with a mild abductor lurch.

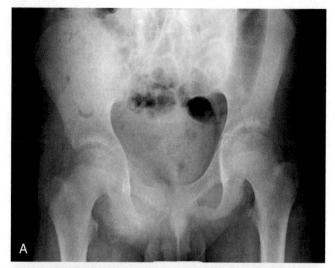

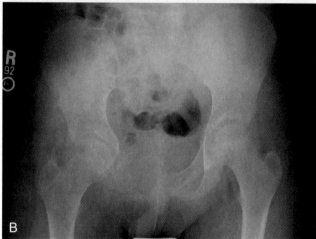

FIGURE 9-29. **A,** Preoperative radiograph of an osteosarcoma of the pubic rami. **B,** The appearance following resection, showing preservation of the acetabulum. Function in these situations is nearly normal, although hernia formation may be a problem.

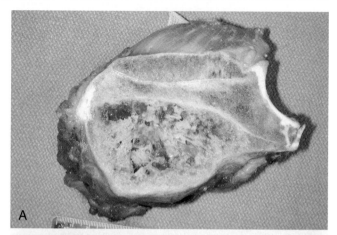

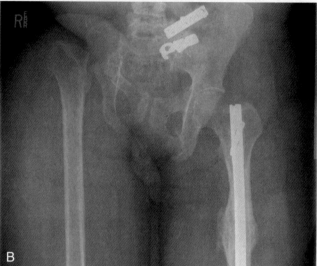

FIGURE 9-30. **A,** A specimen following resection of the iliac crest, including the acetabulum, because of osteosarcoma. Function after these procedures is poor but better than it is after an external hemipelvectomy. **B,** Radiograph of another patient more than 20 years after resection of her right ilium and acetabulum for osteosarcoma. She has had a closed femoral shortening on the left side to partially balance limb lengths. Despite her disabilities, she works full time and has a family.

and span years to decades and multiple treatment protocols. The studies also generally clump multiple tumors, weakening the strength of any recommendations. Despite these limitations, some general principles and lesion-specific recommendations can be made.

The Four Principles

When considering the management of a suspected metastatic pulmonary lesion, four principles must be addressed in each patient. First, the primary tumor diagnosis must be established. The response of pulmonary lesions to chemotherapy and radiotherapy is linked not only to the primary diagnosis but also to the biologic subtype involved (i.e., favorable versus anaplastic Wilms' tumor).

Second, the primary tumor must be controlled. A surgeon should not consider pulmonary metastasectomy prior to achieving local control of the primary lesion. However, biopsy to establish the presence of metastasis is required in some settings because it will determine the intensity of therapy.

Third, the therapeutic benefit of surgical resection must be assessed, and this is clearly dependent on the specific tumor. Ideally, the cancer should be chemoresponsive so as to control residual micrometastases. The lack of effective adjuvant therapy may temper the enthusiasm for pulmonary metastasectomy.

Finally, the extent of the pulmonary resection required to remove all metastatic disease should be assessed. The extent of the resection must be balanced with the therapeutic benefit achieved. An aggressive resection creating pulmonary impairment is difficult to support in the presence of chemotherapy-resistant disease, particularly in the presence of multiple lesions. Some cancers (osteosarcoma, adrenocorticocarcinoma) require aggressive operative approaches to remove all gross evidence of disease resulting from limited response to chemotherapy in an attempt to provide an improved overall and disease-free survival.

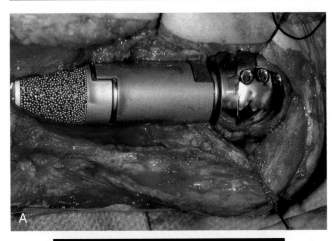

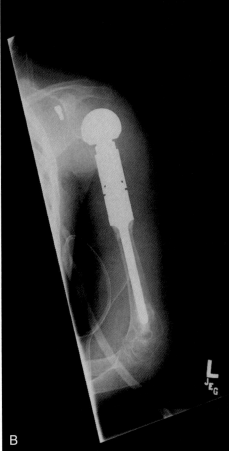

FIGURE 9-31. A, The intraoperative photograph of a metallic prosthesis used to reconstruct a patient with Ewing's sarcoma who had a local recurrence following intercalary resection and allograft reconstruction. **B,** A postoperative radiograph of the prosthesis. Active abduction is limited, but she has normal hand and elbow function.

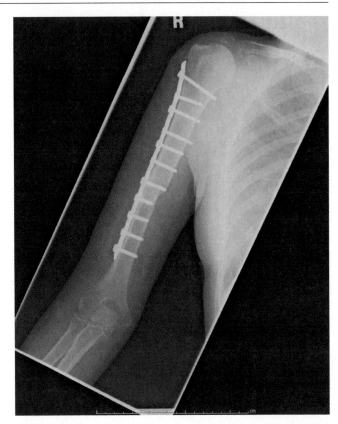

FIGURE 9-32. A proximal humeral osteoarticular allograft was used to reconstruct an intra-articular resection of the proximal humerus.

Metastasis Localization

Depending on the cancer involved, a combination of radiographic studies and nuclear imaging modalities are used to identify metastases, especially in the lungs. Multidetector computed tomography (MDCT) is the mainstay for identifying pulmonary lesions today, and nuclear imaging is used for osseous lesions. More than 80% of lesions 3 mm or larger can be readily identified by this imaging modality,[207,208] but increasing sensitivity comes with decreasing specificity. Many lesions identified on MDCT may not be malignant. It is useful to understand the appearance and location of the lesions, but peripheral lesions that are smooth and well circumscribed are more likely to be malignant, so biopsy is required for small lesions. Also, multiple lesions are more likely to be malignant than isolated lesions.[209] Beyond this modality, nuclear medicine studies have been used for specific tumors with some success. Nuclear medicine studies exploit the biologic pathways of substrate molecules unique to specific tumors to identify these lesions as hot spots on subsequent whole-body scanning. These studies seldom stand alone as the only means of identifying metastases, and they routinely act as corollary or confirmatory tests for lesions identified by MDCT. For example, bone scintigraphy has been used to identify lesions in osteosarcoma,[206] but it is taken up only by large and biologically active lesions. Iodine-131 total body scans are routinely used in the evaluation and identification of pulmonary or osseous metastases in differentiated thyroid cancer, and it appears to be very sensitive and specific.[210-217] Finally, whole-body positron emission scanning using fluorodeoxyglucose has been reported to have a sensitivity of 87% to 89% and a specificity of 100% in sarcomatous[218,219] and carcinomatous[219] pulmonary metastases, but this technique has limited assessment value in pediatric primary malignancies, let alone metastases.

Biomarkers may be confirmatory tests for suspicious lesions found by MDCT or nuclear scintigraphy. Examples of tumor types with such markers that are routinely followed are adrenocorticol carcinoma, differentiated thyroid carcinoma, germ cell carcinoma, and hepatoblastoma.

Technical Considerations

Pulmonary metastasectomy can be performed safely and with minimal morbidity. A mortality rate of less than 1% is documented in the International Registry of Lung Metastases.[219] The type of pulmonary resection can be either anatomic or nonanatomic (wedge) despite early reports to the contrary,[220] but the vast majority of pulmonary metastasectomies performed are wedge resections, in which the lesion is removed with a small rim of normal lung parenchyma (5 to 10 mm). Collective studies document the success of this procedure; it eliminates the need for a formal lung resection along anatomic boundaries.[209,219,221,222-224]

The use of MIS approaches for the resection of pulmonary lesions has been described in several studies.[225-230] It has become an established technique, except in cases of osteosarcoma, in which MDCT scanning has been shown to underestimate the number of lesions, and formal thoracotomy has been recommended.[231] A cohort of patients with osteosarcoma and unilateral, metachronous pulmonary metastases confirmed by MDCT within 2 years of the primary lesion were found to have occult metastases on the contralateral side in 78% of cases.[232] Therefore, staged or sequential bilateral thoracotomies are recommended by some authors for patients with osteosarcoma, although in a prospective study, this approach has not been shown to prolong either event-free survival or overall survival.

Selected Pediatric Malignancies

Adrenocortical Carcinomas

Pulmonary metastases of adrenocortical carcinoma should be considered for complete surgical removal because effective chemotherapy is not available. A recent review of the International Pediatric Adrenocortical Tumor Registry revealed that the mean age at presentation was 3.2 years, with more than 90% of the lesions being functional tumors (84% virilizing).[233] The rate of 5-year event-free survival was 54%, and the incidence of pulmonary metastases was 7% at presentation. Prognosis was better for younger patients with completely resected, small (<200 g), early-stage tumors with virilizing symptoms. Separate analysis of the patients with lung metastases could not be performed because of the small number of patients. Isolated case reports in the literature document long-term survival in patients after pulmonary metastasectomy for adrenocortical carcinoma.[234,235] If one examines the adult studies addressing this question, the role of complete tumor excision becomes readily apparent. Kwauk and colleagues examined their series of 24 primarily adult patients with adrenocorticol carcinoma and pulmonary metastases.[236] They noted that complete surgical excision of all metastatic disease achieved a 5-year survival rate of 71%, as opposed to 0 for those with unresected disease. Although the patient cohort was small and not randomized, they concluded that in the light of ineffective chemotherapy, complete pulmonary metastasectomy was not only indicated but mandatory to achieve long-term survival.

Schulick and colleagues echoed these results and sentiments when analyzing their institution's results with metastatic adrenocortical carcinoma in predominantly adult patients.[237] In fact, they advocate not only for an initial pulmonary metastasectomy, but for repeated resections as well. Some patients in their series had as many as seven resections for recurrent disease. This may seem overly aggressive, but they note that for every reoperation, the median survival time was longer for groups that underwent complete rather than incomplete resec-

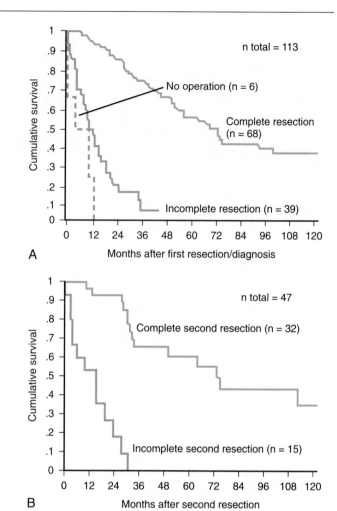

FIGURE 9-33. A and **B,** Disease-specific survival rates for patients undergoing complete versus incomplete primary resections for adrenocortical carcinoma. *(Redrawn from Schulick RD, Brennan MF. Long-term survival after complete resection and repeat resection in patients with adrenocortical carcinoma. Ann Surg Oncol. 1999;6:719-726. By permission of Lippincott Williams and Wilkins.)*

tions, which is probably a function of the biology of the tumor involved and the anatomic limits of resection as opposed to the operation performed (Fig 9-33A, B). Furthermore, the majority of metastatic resections performed were for pulmonary disease. Thus, the data confirm the important role of surgery in the treatment of adrenocortical carcinoma metastatic to the lungs and in resectable disease when increased rates of survival and cure can be achieved.

Differentiated Thyroid Cancers

Pulmonary metastases from differentiated thyroid cancer should not be treated by surgical excision except in cases in which there is indecision about the nature of the diagnosis, especially after treatment. Despite the presence of disseminated disease to the lungs, prognosis is still quite good. Unlike skeletal and pleural involvement, patients with pulmonary metastases have mortality rates ranging from 0 to 6%.[212,213,215-217,237] Studies have reported the incidence of pulmonary metastases to be 6% to 25%.[213-217] It is interesting that these studies have also documented that the pulmonary metastases are very responsive to radioactive iodine treatment. They are seen more commonly in younger patients and can first appear more than 10 years after the initial diagnosis.

A recent comprehensive review of the treatment of thyroid cancers in children exposed to radiation by the collapse of the Chernobyl nuclear power station is the largest series focused on pediatric thyroid carcinoma.[217] There were 740 cases of thyroid cancer in 681 children who had had direct exposure to the accident. There were 131 cases (17.7%) of pulmonary disease that were diagnosed by radionuclide scan, with a mean presentation time of 19 months after the primary diagnosis. Only 2.3% of the cases of pulmonary metastases were found on chest radiograph; hence, they recommend the use of radioactive iodine scanning as the procedure of choice because of its increased sensitivity and specificity. The risk factors for metastatic disease were female gender, younger age at diagnosis, and the presence of clinical symptoms. The children were treated with radioactive iodine for the initial pulmonary metastasis. With the administration of therapeutic radioactive iodine for pulmonary metastases, 28.9% showed a complete response (negative nuclear imaging and thyroglobulin <1 ng/L); 47.7% showed a partial but stable response (negative nuclear imaging and thyroglobulin 1 to 10 ng/L); and 23.4% showed a partial response. The 5- and 10-year survival rates were 99.5% and 98.8%, respectively, and only five children died of distant metastases (three medullary, one follicular, and one papillary); there was a mean follow-up of 115 months. This study and others document the success of medical therapy. Surgery is required only for diagnosis if the lesions fail to take up iodine.

Germ Cell Tumors (Gonadal)

Pulmonary metastases from gonadal germ cell tumors should be biopsied only if their origin is in question. This tumor is very responsive to chemotherapy, so resection is performed only after treatment if radiographic abnormalities persist. Germ cell tumors comprise a broad range of tumors of which 20% are malignant.[238] The malignant lesions are chemosensitive and with the advent of cisplatin-based regimens, long-term survival rates have increased to 90%.[239] However, residual disease after adjuvant therapies may harbor viable tumor,[239-243] with the lung being the most common site of distant metastasis.[240] Synchronous pulmonary metastases are found in 50% of patients with retroperitoneal lymphadenopathy and in 10% of patients without adenopathy.[239] Therefore, the role of pulmonary metastasectomy is primarily to define the presence of viable tumor in residual lesions after chemotherapy. This would establish a basis for further therapy.

Several groups have examined their data concerning the role and utility of pulmonary metastasectomy. Cagini and colleagues examined their cohort of 141 patients who had both pulmonary and mediastinal involvement over a 17-year period; 51% of patients had isolated pulmonary disease, 24% had pulmonary and mediastinal disease, and 24% had mediastinal disease alone.[239] Roughly one third of patients had a single lesion, one third had two to three lesions, and one third had more than three lesions. Of these patients, 87% underwent complete resection, and histologic analysis revealed that 23% of the lesions had only necrosis or fibrosis, 45% had mature teratoma, and 32% were malignant. Biomarker analysis in these patients was not helpful because 23% of patients with malignant disease had negative biomarkers. A second recurrence occurred in 47% of patients. The overall mortality rate was 19% for the entire group. Actuarial survival after pulmonary

metastasectomy was 78% at 5 years, 76% at 10 years, and 66% at 15 years post treatment. Statistically significant prognostic factors were the pathology of the specimen (complete necrosis or fibrosis of the specimen as opposed to the presence of viable tumor); presence of residual disease (mediastinal disease alone showed better outcomes than pulmonary disease with or without mediastinal disease); and the number of resected lesions.

These results were echoed by Liu and colleagues, who examined their cohort of 157 patients with isolated pulmonary metastases after chemotherapy over a 28-year period.[239] The majority of patients had multiple lesions (72%), and 89% of patients underwent nonanatomic resections. The mortality rate was 0.6%, and the morbidity rate was 6%. Pathologic analysis revealed viable tumor in 44% of the cohort, and 37% of the cohort had subsequent recurrence of disease in the chest; 56% of these died. The overall mortality rate was 32%. Statistically significant negative prognostic factors were age greater than 25, no cisplatin-based chemotherapy, the presence of viable tumor when the lesions were resected post therapy, and the existence of metastatic disease outside of the thorax or retroperitoneum. The authors concluded that surgery plays a critical role in determining the patients who would benefit from further therapy. These results are also confirmed by other groups,[241-243] but patient selection is an important criterion. Ultimately, surgical salvage using pulmonary metastasectomy is a viable alternative for patients with residual, radiographically identifiable lesions to determine the chemoresponsiveness of these tumors and to provide for increased long-term survival with complete surgical resection.

Hepatoblastomas

Pulmonary metastases from hepatoblastomas should be treated first with adjuvant chemotherapy, and only then should any residual lesions be resected. Data to support this concept have appeared over the past several decades; the initial report was written by Black and colleagues.[244] They reported four patients who were long-term survivors, and they stressed the need for complete local control and adjuvant chemotherapy. Furthermore, they correlated the need to perform the pulmonary metastasectomy with the patient's α-fetoprotein levels, advocating early surgery especially for patients with rising titers during appropriate therapy.

Feusner and colleagues,[245] representing the Children's Cancer Group, published their results, and they confirmed the premises outlined by Black and colleagues. Of their cohort of six patients with pulmonary recurrence, four had complete remission and three survived for more than 5 years. Their approach was to combine adjuvant chemotherapy with aggressive pulmonary resections. Some caution is appropriate, however, when it is recognized that the overall survival rates and event-free survival rates of patients presenting with stage IV disease in hepatoblastoma is 16%, and patients with relapse generally do worse if they have already received the primary therapies. Beyond these North American results, two reports from the International Society of Pediatric Oncology on Childhood Liver Tumors have documented their results in hepatoblastoma and pulmonary metastases. The first, a report by Perilongo and colleagues[246] in 2000, documented the results of SIOPEL-1: 20% of patients with hepatoblastoma presented with pulmonary metastases, and they achieved a 5-year event-free survival rate of only 28%. A sustained remission of 26% of the cohort with metastatic pulmonary lesions was achieved by using chemotherapy alone. Schnater and colleagues[80] analyzed the surgical approach in SIOPEL-1 and documented that

41% of patients who presented with pulmonary metastases were long-term survivors, but only four patients who underwent surgery and chemotherapy to treat their pulmonary metastases were alive at data analysis (a minimum of 2.5 years post-treatment). In a nonrandomized study, the apparent difference in outcome may result from selection factors. Their data also suggest that recurrent pulmonary disease could be cured by surgery and chemotherapy as long as there is local control of the tumor. Thus, these studies cumulatively support a possible role for pulmonary metastasectomy for hepatoblastoma in selected residual lesions.

Neuroblastomas

Pulmonary metastases from neuroblastomas are rare, and they should not be treated by surgical excision except in cases in which there is indecision about the nature of the lesion, especially after or during treatment. The incidence of pulmonary metastases from neuroblastomas has been reported to occur in 1% to 23% of cases,[247-251] but most large studies report rates of 5% or less.[249-251] They can be synchronous or metachronous, and they are usually multiple, bilateral, subcentimeter, and peripheral. Patients with pulmonary metastases from neuroblastomas have poor prognoses, a high association with unfavorable Shimada histology, MYCN amplification, and a lower event-free survival rate.[250,251] Hence, the utility of performing resections except to confirm the diagnosis has not been established.

Wilms' Tumors

Pulmonary metastases from nephroblastomas should generally not be resected, and suspected lesions should only be biopsied. Some authors[222,252] have advocated for primary pulmonary metastasectomy to spare the effects of radiotherapy on patients,[253] but North American centers, under the protocols established by the NWTSG, have demonstrated the efficacy of chemotherapy and radiotherapy in the treatment of pulmonary metastases over chemotherapy and surgical excision, regardless of pathologic subtype.[254-256] Specifically, Green and colleagues, in 1991, examined patients enrolled in NWTSG's studies 1 through 3 who had pulmonary recurrences. Of the patients meeting the study's criteria, the resection of pulmonary metastases within 30 days of diagnosis did not affect 4-year survival outcomes in favorable or unfavorable histopathologic cohorts. Furthermore, Green and colleagues[256] reported results from NWTS-4, in which pulmonary metastasectomy had almost no role in the treatment of patients with stage IV disease. It was performed to deal with residual lesions after chemotherapy and radiotherapy, but it did not affect the overall survival rates, which were 75% to 90%. The importance of biopsy for suspicious lesions, especially small lesions (<1 cm) found only on CT, was confirmed by Ehrlich and colleagues,[257] who reviewed children enrolled in NWTS-5. Of those who received radiotherapy, 33% had had a prior biopsy that was negative for tumor, so they were overtreated. These results were for patients with both isolated and multiple lesions. These studies collectively confirm the general success of combined chemotherapy and radiotherapy in the treatment of pulmonary metastases of nephroblastomas. Whether, in fact, the children with metastatic disease that is seen only on MDCT and that resolve with chemotherapy need pulmonary radiotherapy remains an unanswered question. Finally, surgical intervention for pulmonary lesions in nephroblastomas should be used only to confirm the existence of malignancy in MDCT-defined masses prior to administering therapy.

Sarcomas

Pulmonary metastases from sarcomatous pediatric tumors should be biopsied at least, and complete resections should be performed on the basis of the precise histologic subtype. The most comprehensive reports concerning this topic are by Temeck and colleagues from the National Cancer Institute. They published two reports in the 1990s that documented the results of initial[258] and recurrent[259] pulmonary metastasectomies. Their initial report examined 152 patients who underwent 258 thoracotomies over 18 years. The lesions included osteosarcoma (50%); nonrhabdomyosarcoma soft tissue sarcomas (27%); Ewing's sarcoma (18%); and rhabdomyosarcoma (3%). Of the patients, 80% underwent complete resection, and the cohort had morbidity and mortality rates of approximately 6% and 1.3%, respectively. The highest median survival rate occurred in the osteosarcoma group (3.1 years), and the lowest occurred in patients with rhabdomyosarcomas (0.4 year). Statistically significant poor-prognosis factors included the presence of three or more metastases, a diagnosis other than osteosarcoma, and an incomplete resection. The follow-up study of recurrent lesions further documented the importance of histologic subtypes; no patients with rhabdomyosarcoma were eligible for evaluation. The authors also documented that CT missed 39% of lesions, of which 24% were found to be malignant, supporting the need for thorough evaluation of the thorax by means of an open approach. Furthermore, they documented a complete resection rate of 77%, with a 5.6% morbidity rate and a 1% mortality rate. Finally, they documented a statistically significant improved survival rate in patients who underwent complete resections, regardless of the number of recurrences. In fact, this survival advantage was 8 to 20 times greater, depending on the number of recurrences. These data, although encouraging for sarcomas in general, must be considered in the light of individual histologic variants. The one sarcomatous variant that may benefit from pulmonary metastasectomy is osteosarcoma.

The usefulness of complete, recurrent pulmonary metastasectomy in cases of osteosarcoma was ushered in by the report by Martini and colleagues describing their experience in 1971.[260] They reported a 45% survival rate in patients who had had complete pulmonary metastasectomies; this rate is four times greater than that achieved by chemotherapy alone. Reports from the past decade[206,225,232,261-276] have not only confirmed these results but have also clarified the therapeutic approach to pulmonary metastases in osteosarcoma. First, osteosarcoma should be treated by a multiagent regimen that addresses synchronous pulmonary lesions at the time of local control. Second, pulmonary lesions should undergo repeated complete resections because this provides the best chance for long-term disease-free and overall survival. Third, extirpation of extrapulmonary metastases does not confer the same survival benefits as does pulmonary metastasectomy, and they are commonly less feasible because many of these lesions are osseous. Fourth, CT imaging does not identify all pulmonary lesions, and most lesions are not calcified. Therefore, staged bilateral thoracotomies are suggested by some for complete evaluation and resection of all pulmonary disease. Fifth, once metachronous lesions have been identified and treated surgically, most patients will have at least one pulmonary recurrence, and most of them occur within 12 months of the first resection. Therefore, continued surveillance and frequent, repeat imaging is essential. Finally, although tumor burden was and still is an important prognostic factor in the determination of outcome, several biologic features—disease-free intervals and percentage of tumor necrosis on histopathologic evaluation—have become even more significant, according to reviews. Hence, aggressive, repeated, and complete resection of pulmonary metastases is critical to the successful treatment of patients with osteosarcomas.

REFERENCES

1. Othersen B, Delorimer A, Harbrovsky E. Surgical evaluation of lymph node metastases in Wilms' tumor. J Pediatr Surg. 1990;25:330-331.
2. Shamberger RC, Guthrie KA, Ritchey ML, et al. Surgery-related factors and local recurrence of Wilms' tumor in National Wilms' Tumor Study 4. Ann Surg. 1999;229:292-297.
3. Jeb B, Tournade M, Lemerle J. Lymph node invasion and prognosis in nephroblastoma. Cancer. 1980;45:1632-1636.
4. Lawrence W Jr, Hayes DM, Moon TE. Lymphatic metastases with childhood rhabmyosarcoma. Cancer. 1977;39:556-559.
5. Weiner E, Lawrence W, Hays D, et al. Retroperitoneal lymph node biopsy in paratesticular rhabdomyosarcoma. J Pediatr Surg. 1994;29:171-177 (discussion 178).
6. Weiner E, Anderson J, Ojimba J, et al. Controversies in the management of peri-testicular rhabdomyosarcoma: is staging retroperitoneal lymph node dissection necessary for adolescents with resected peri-testicular rhabdomyosarcoma? Semin Pediatr Surg. 2001;10:146-152.
7. Piro A, Weiss D, Hellman S. Mediastinal Hodgkin's disease: a possible danger for intubation anesthesia. Int J Radit Oncol Biol Physiol. 1976;1:415-419.
8. Turoff R, Gomes G, Berjian R, et al. Postoperative respiratory complications in patients with Hodgkin's disease: relationship to the size of the mediastinal tumor. Eur J Cancer Clin Oncol. 1985;21:1043-1046.
9. Griscom NT. Computed tomographic determination of tracheal dimensions in children and adolescents. Radiology. 1982;145:361-364.
10. Griscom NT. CT measurement of the tracheal lumen in children and adolescents. AJR Am J Roentgenol. 1991;156:371-372.
11. Aziz Khan RG, Dudgeon DL, Buck JP, et al. Life-threatening airway obstruction as a complication to the management of mediastinal masses in children. J Pediatr Surg. 1985;20:816-822.
12. Shamberger RC, Holzman RS, Griscom NT, et al. CT quantitation of tracheal cross-sectional area as a guide to the surgical and anesthetic management of children with anterior mediastinal masses. J Pediatr Surg. 1991;26:138-142.
13. Shamberger RC, Holzman RS, Griscom NT, et al. Prospective evaluation by computed tomography and pulmonary function tests of children with mediastinal masses. Surgery. 1995;118:468-471.
14. Miller RD, Hyatt RE. Evaluation of obstructing lesions of the trachea and larynx by flow-volume loops. Am Rev Respir Dis. 1973;108:475-481.
15. Loeffler JS, Leopold KA, Recht A, et al. Emergency prebiopsy radiation for mediastinal masses: impact on subsequent pathologic diagnosis and outcome. J Clin Oncol. 1986;4:716-721.
16. Halpern S, Chatten J, Meadows AT, et al. Anterior mediastinal masses: anesthesia hazards and other problems. J Pediatr. 1983;102:407-410.
17. Borenstein SH, Gerstle T, Malkin D, et al. The effects of prebiopsy corticosteroid treatment on the diagnosis of mediastinal lymphoma. J Pediatr Surg. 2000;35:973-976.
18. Chaignaud BE, Bonsack TA, Kozakewich HP, Shamberger RC. Pleural effusions in lymphoblastic lymphoma: a diagnostic alternative. J Pediatr Surg. 1998;33:1355-1357.
19. Frush D, Donnelly L, Rosen N. Computed tomography and radiation risks: what pediatric health care providers should know. Pediatrics. 2003;112:971-972.
20. Brenner J, Elliston C, Hall E, Berdon W. Estimated risks of radiation-induced fatal cancer from pediatric CT. AJR Am J Roentgenol. 2001;176:289-296.
21. Smith E. Complications of percutaneous abdominal fine-needle biopsy. Radiology. 1991;178:253-258 (review).
22. Lundstedt C, Strideck H, Anderson R, et al. Tumor seeding occurring after fine-needle biopsy of abdominal malignancies. Acta Radiol. 1991;32:518-520.
23. Ayar D, Golla B, Lee J, Nath H. Needle-track metastasis after transthoracic needle biopsy. J Thorac Imaging. 1998;13:2-6.
24. Hoffer F, Gianturco L, Fletcher J, Grier H. Percutaneous biopsy of peripheral primitiveneuroectodermal tumors and Ewing's sarcoma for cytogenetic analysis. AJR Am J Roentgenol. 1994;162:1141-1142.
25. Fletcher J, Kozakewich H, Hoffer F, et al. Diagnostic relevance of clonal cytogenetic aberrations in malignant soft-tissue tumors. N Engl J Med. 1991;324:436-442.
26. Hoffer F, Chung T, Diller L, et al. Percutaneous biopsy for prognostic testing of neuroblastoma. Radiology. 1996;200:213-216.
27. Garrett K, Fuller C, Santana V, et al. Percutaneous biopsy of pediatric solid tumor. Cancer. 2005;104:644-652.
28. Hugosson C, Nyman R, Cappelton-Smith J, et al. Ultrasound-guided biopsy of abdominal and pelvic lesions in children. A comparison between fine-needle aspiration and 1.2 mm-needle core biopsy. Pediatr Radiol. 1999;29:31-36.
29. Hussain H, Kingston J, Domizio P, et al. Imaging-guided core biopsy for the diagnosis of malignant tumors in pediatic patients. Am J Roentgenol. 2001;176:43-47.
30. Sklair-Levy M, Lebensart PD, Applbaum Y, et al. Percutaneous image-guided needle biopsy in children: summary of our experience with 57children. Pediatr Radiol. 2001;31:732-736.
31. Skoldenberg E, Jakobson A, Elvin A, et al. Diagnosing childhood tumors: a review of 147 cutting needle biopsies in children. J Pediatr Surg. 2002;37:50-56.
32. Amaral J, Schwartz J, Chait P, et al. Sonographically guided percutaneous liver biopsy in infants: a retrospective review. Am J Roentgenol. 2006;187:W644-W649.
33. Stewart C, Coldewey J, Stewart I. Comparison of fine needle aspiration cytology and needle core biopsy in the diagnosis of radiographically detected abdominal lesions. J Clin Pathol. 2002;55:93-97.
34. Chen M, Schropp K, Lobe T. Complication of minimal-access surgery in children. J Pediatr Surg. 1996;31:1161-1165.
35. Gans S, Berci G. Peritoneoscopy in infants and children. J Pediatr Surg. 1973;8:399-405.
36. Holcomb G, Tomita S, Haase G, et al. Minimally invasive surgery in children with cancer. Cancer. 1995;76:121-128.
37. Spurbeck WW, Davidoff AM, Lobe TE, et al. Minimally invasive surgery in pediatric cancer patients. Ann Surg Oncol. 2004;11:340-343.
38. Sartorelli K, Patrick D, Meagher DJ. Port-site recurrence after thoracoscopic resection of pulmonary metastasis owing to osteogenic sarcoma. J Pediatr Surg. 1996;31:1443-1444.
39. Iwanaka T, Arai M, Yamamoto H, et al. No incidence of port-site recurrence after endosurgical procedure for pediatric malignancies. Pediatr Surg Int. 2003;19:200-203.
40. Paolucci V, Schaeff B, Schneider M, Gutt C. Tumor seeding following laparoscopy: international survey. World J Surg. 1999;23:989-995.
41. Fleshman J, Nelson H, Peters W, et al. Early results of laparoscopic surgery for colorectal cancer: retrospective analysis of 372 patients treated by Clinical Outcomes of Surgical Therapy (COST) Study Group. Dis Colon Rectum. 1996;39(suppl):S53-S58.
42. Pearlstone D, Mansfield P, Curley S, et al. Laparoscopy in 533 patients with abdominal malignancy. Surgery. 1999;125:67-72.
43. Mankin H, Lange T, Spanier S. The hazards of biopsy in patients with malignant primary bone and soft-tissue tumors. J Bone Joint Surg Am. 1982;64:1121-1127.

44. Mankin H, Mankin C, Simon M. The hazards of biopsy, revisited. J Bone Joint Surg Am. 1996;78:639-643.

45. Lemerle J, Voute P, Tourade M, et al. Preoperative versus postoperative radiotherapy, single versus multiple courses of actinomycin D in the treatment of Wilms' tumor. Preliminary results of a controlled clinical trial conducted by the International Society of Pediatric Oncology (SIOP). Cancer. 1976;38:647-654.

46. D'Angio GJ, Evans AE, Breslow N, et al. The treatment of Wilms' tumor: results of the national Wilms' tumor study. Cancer. 1976;38:633-646.

47. D'Angio GJ, Evans AE, Breslow N, et al. The treatment of Wilms' tumor: results of the second national Wilms' tumor study. Cancer. 1981;47:2302-2311.

48. Lemerle J, Voute PA, Tournade MF, et al. Effectiveness of preoperative chemotherapy in Wilms' tumor: results of an International Society of Paediatric Oncology (SIOP) clinical trial. J Clin Oncol. 1983;1:604-609.

49. Tournade MF, Com-Nougue C, Voute PA, et al. Results of the Sixth International Society of Pediatric Oncology Wilms' Tumor Trial and Study: a risk-adapted therapeutic approach in Wilms' tumor. J Clin Oncol. 1993;11:1014-1023.

50. Jereb B, Burgers JM, Tournade MF, et al. Radiotherapy in the SIOP (International Society of Pediatric Oncology) nephroblastoma studies: a review. Med Pediatr Oncol. 1994;22:221-227.

51. Tournade MF, Com-Nougue C, de Kraker J, et al. Optimal duration of preoperative therapy in unilateral and nonmetastatic Wilms' tumor in children older than 6 months: results of the Ninth International Society of Pediatric Oncology Wilms' Tumor Trial and Study. J Clin Oncol. 2001;19:488-500.

52. Godzinski J, Tournade MF, deKraker J, et al. Rarity of surgical complications after postchemotherapy nephrectomy for nephroblastoma. Experience of the International Society of Paediatric Oncology-Trial and Study SIOP-9. International Society of Paediatric Oncology Nephroblastoma Trial and Study Committee. Eur J Pediatr Surg. 1998;8:83-86.

53. McLorie GA, McKenna PH, Greenberg M, et al. Reduction in tumor burden allowing partial nephrectomy following preoperative chemotherapy in biopsy proved Wilms' tumor. J Urol. 1991;146:509-513.

54. Wilimas JA, Magill L, Parham DM, et al. Is renal salvage feasible in unilateral Wilms' tumor? Proposed computed tomographic criteria and their relation to surgical pathologic findings. J Pediatr Hematol Oncol. 1990;12:164-167.

55. Kozzi F, Schiavetti A, Bonanini M, et al. Enucleative surgery for stage 1 nephroblastoma with a normal contralateral kidney. J Urol. 1996;156:1788-1791.

56. Moorman-Voestermans CG, Aronson DC, Staalman CR, et al. Is partial nephrectomy appropriate treatment for unilateral Wilms' tumor? J Pediatr Surg. 1998;33:165-170.

57. Ritchey ML, Shamberger RC, Haase G, et al. Surgical complications after primary nephrectomy for Wilms' tumor: report from the National Wilms' Tumor Study Group. J Am Coll Surg. 2001;192:63-68; quiz 146.

58. Kushner BH, Cheung NK, LaQuaglia MP, et al. Survival from locally invasive or widespread neuroblastoma without cytotoxic therapy. J Clin Oncol. 1996;14:373-381.

59. Smith E, Krous H, Tunell W, et al. The impact of chemotherapy and radiology therapy on secondary operations for neuroblastoma. Ann Surg. 1979;191:561-569.

60. Haase GM, O'Leary MC, Ramsay NK, et al. Aggressive surgery combined with intensive chemotherapy improves survival in poor-risk neuroblastoma. J Pediatr Surg. 1991;26:1119-1123; discussion 1123-1124.

61. Berthold F, Utsch S, Holschneider AM. The aim of preoperative chemotherapy on resectibility of primary tumour and complication rate of metastatic neuroblastoma. Z Kinderchir. 1989;41:21-24.

62. Smith E, Shockett S, Hayes F, et al. Results and lessons for the future from the Pediatric Oncology Group Studies (8104-844 from the surgical viewpoint. Pediatr Oncol (Japan). 1988;25:71-80.

63. Shamberger RC, Allarde-Segundo A, Kozakewich HP, Grier HE. Surgical management of stage III and IV neuroblastoma: resection before or after chemotherapy? J Pediatr Surg. 1991;26:1113-1117; discussion 1117-1118.

64. DeCou JM, Bowman LC, Rao BN, et al. Infants with metastatic neuroblastoma have improved survival with resection of the primary tumor. J Pediatr Surg. 1995;30:937-940; discussion 940-941.

65. Siddiqui AM, Shamberger RC, Filler RM, et al. Enteric duplications of the pancreatic head: definitive management by local resection. J Pediatr Surg. 1998;33:1117-1120; discussion 1120-1121.

66. Hota Y, Uchino J, Sasaki F, et al. Kidney-preserving radical tumor resection in advanced neuroblastoma. J Pediatr Surg. 1989;24:382.

67. Shamberger RC, Smith EI, Joshi VV, et al. The risk of nephrectomy during local control in abdominal neuroblastoma. J Pediatr Surg. 1998;33:161-164.

68. Exelby P, Filler R, Grosfeld J. Liver tumors in children in the particular reference to hepatoblastoma and hepatocellular carcinoma: American Academy of Pediatrics Surgical Section Survey, 1974. J Pediatr Surg. 1975;10:329-337.

69. Giacomantonio M, Ein S, Mancer K, Stephens C. Thirty years of experience with pediatric primary malignant liver tumors. J Pediatr Surg. 1984;19:523-526.

70. Andrassy R, Brennan L, Siegel M, Weitzman J. Preoperative chemotherapy for hepatoblastoma in children: report of six cases. J Pediatr Surg. 1980;15:517-522.

71. Weinblatt M, Siegel S, Siegel M, et al. Preoperative chemotherapy for unresectable primary hepatic malignancies in children. Cancer. 1982;50:1061-1064.

72. Ortega J, Krailo M, Haas J, et al. Effective treatment of unresectable or metastatic hepatoblastoma with cisplatin and continuous-infusion doxorubicin chemotherapy: a report from the Childrens Cancer Study Group. J Clin Oncol. 1991;9:2167-2176.

73. King D, Ortega J, Campbell J, et al. The surgical management of children with incompletely resected hepatic cancer is facilitated by intensive chemotherapy. J Pediatr Surg. 1991;26:1074-1080.

74. Filler R, Ehrlich P, Greenberg M, Babyn P. Preoperative chemotherapy in hepatoblastoma. Surgery. 1991;110:591-597.

75. Reynolds M, Douglass E, Finegold M, et al. Chemotherapy can convert unresectable hepatoblastoma. J Pediatr Surg. 1992;27:1080-1084.

76. von Schweinitz D, Hecker H, Harms D, et al. Complete resection before development of drug resistance is essential for survival from advanced hepatoblastoma: a report from the German Cooperative Pediatric Liver Tumor Study HB-89. J Pediatr Surg. 1995;30:845-852.

77. Seo T, Ando H, Watanabe Y, et al. Treatment of hepatoblastoma: less extensive hepatectomy after effective preoperative chemotherapy with cisplatin and adriamycin. Surgery. 1998;123:407-414.

78. Ehrlich P, Greenberg M, Filler R. Improved long-term survival with preoperative chemotherapy for hepatoblastoma. J Pediatr Surg. 1997;32:999-1003.

79. Pritchard J, Brown J, Shafford E, et al. Cisplatin, doxorubicin, and delayed surgery for childhood hepatoblastoma: a successful approach—results of the first prospective study of the International Society of Pediatric Oncology. J Clin Oncol. 2000;18:3819-3828.

80. Schnater J, Aronson D, Plaschkes J, et al. Surgical view of the treatment of patients with hepatoblastoma: results from the first prospective trial of the International Society of Pediatric Oncology Liver Tumor Study Group. Cancer. 2002;94:1111-1120.

81. Ortega J, Douglass E, Feusner J, et al. Randomized comparison of cisplatin/viscristine/fluouracil and cisplatin/continuous infusion doxorubicin for treatment of pediatric hepatoblastoma: a report from the Children's Cancer Group. J Clin Oncol. 2000;18:2665-2675.

82. Otte JB, Pritchard J, Aronson DC, et al. Liver transplantation for hepatoblastoma: results from the International Society of Pediatric Oncology (SIOP) study SIOPEL-1 and review of the world experience. Pediatr Blood Cancer. 2004;42:74-83.

83. Austin M, Leys C, Feurer Iea. Liver transplantation for childhood hepatic malignancy: a review of the United Network for Organ Sharing (UNOS) database. J Pediatr Surg. 2006;41:182-186.

84. Sutow W, Sullivan M, Ried H, et al. Prognosis in childhood rhabdomyosarcoma. Cancer. 1970;25:1384-1390.

85. Crist W, Anderson J, Meza J, et al. Intergroup rhabdomyosarcoma study-IV: results for patients with nonmetastatic disease. J Clin Oncol. 2001;19:3091-3102.

86. Maurer H, Veltangady M, Gehan E, et al. The Intergroup Rhabdomyosarcoma Study-I: a final report. Cancer. 1988;61:209-220.

87. Maurer H, Gehan E, Beltangady M, et al. The Intergroup Rhabdomyosarcoma Study-II. Cancer. 1993;71:1904-1922.

88. Crist W, Gehan E, Ragab A, et al. The Third Intergroup Rhabdomyosarcoma Study. J Clin Oncol. 1995;13:610-630.

89. Crist W, Garnsey L, Beltangady M, et al. Prognosis in children with rhabdomyosarcoma: a report of the intergroup rhabdomyosarcoma studies I and II. Intergroup Rhabdomyosarcoma Committee. J Clin Oncol. 1990;8(3):443-452.

90. Weiner E, Lawrence W, Hays D, et al. Complete response or not complete response? Second-look operations are the answer in children with rhabdomyosarcoma. Proc Am Soc Clin Oncol. 1991;10:316.

91. Wolden S, Anderson J, Crist W, et al. Indications for radiotherapy and chemotherapy after complete resection in rhabdomyosarcoma: a report from the Intergroup Rhabdomyosarcoma Studies I to III. J Clin Oncol. 1999;17:3468-3475.

92. Donaldson S, Meza J, Breneman J, et al. Results from the IRS-IV randomized trial of hyperfractionated radiotherapy in children with rhabdomyosarcoma: a report from the IRSG. Int J Radiat Oncol. 2001;51:718-728.

93. Breitfeld P, Lyden E, Raney R, et al. Ifosfamide and etoposide are superior to vincristine and melphalan for pediatric metastatic rhabdomyosarcoma when administered with irradiation and combination chemotheraopy: a report from the Intergroup Rhabdomyosarcoma Study Group. J Pedatr Hematol Oncol. 2001;23:225-233.

94. Sandler E, Lyden E, Ruymann F, et al. Efficacy of ifosfamide and doxorubicin given as a phase II window in children with newly diagnosed metastatic rhabdomyosarcoma: a report from the Intergroup Rhabdomyosarcoma Study Group. Med Pediatr Oncol. 2001;37:442-448.

95. Pappo A, Lyden E, Breneman J, et al. Up-front window trial of topotecan in previously untreated children and adolescents with metastatic rhabdomyosarcoma: an intergroup rhabdomyosarcoma study. J Clin Oncol 2001;19:213-219.

96. Cosetti M, Wexler L, Calleja E, et al. Irinotecan for pediatric solid tumors: the Memorial Sloan-Kettering experience. J Pedatr Hematol Oncol. 2002;24:101-105.

97. Grimer R. Surgical options for children with osteosarcoma. Lancet Oncol. 2005;6:85-92.

98. Kotz R, Dominkus M, Zettl T, et al. Advances in bone tumour treatment in 30 years with respect to survival and limb salvage. Int Orthop. 2002;26:197-202.

99. Grimer R, Taminiau A, Cannon S. Surgical outcomes in osteosarcoma. J Bone Joint Surg Br. 2002;84:395-400.

100. Kumta S, Cheng J, Li C, et al. Scope and limitations of limb-sparing surgery in childhood sarcomas. J Pediatr Orthop. 2002; 22:244-248.

101. Sluga M, Windhager R, Lang S, et al. The role of surgery and resection margins in the treatment of Ewing's sarcoma. Clin Orthop Relat Res. 2001;392:394-399.

102. Bacci G, Longhi A, Briccoli A, et al. The role of surgical margins in treatment of Ewing's sarcoma family tumors: experience of a single institution with 512 patients treated with adjuvant and neoadjuvant chemotherapy. Int Radiat Oncol Biol Phys. 2006;65:766-772.

103. Ferrari S, Smeland S, Mercuri M, et al. Neoadjuvant chemotherapy with high-dose ifosfamide, high-dose methotrexate, cisplatin, and doxorubicin for patients with localized osteosarcoma of the extremity: a joint study by the Italian and Scandinavian sarcoma groups. J Clin Oncol. 2005;23:8845-8852.

104. Bacci G, Briccoli A, Ferrari S, et al. Neoadjuvant chemotherapy for osteosarcoma of the extremity: long-term results of the Rizzoli 4th protocol. Eur J Cancer. 2001;37:2030-2039.

105. Ferguson W, Goorin A. Current treatment of osteosarcoma. Cancer Invest. 2001;19:292-315.

106. Bacci G, Ferrari S, Longhi A, et al. Neoadjuvant chemotherapy for high-grade osteosarcoma of the extremities: long-term results for patients treated according to the Rizzoli ior/os-3b protocol. J Chemother. 2001;13:93-99.

107. Gherlinzoni F, Picci P, Bacci G, Campanacci D. Limb sparing versus amputation in osteosarcoma: correlation between local control, surgical margins and tumor necrosis: Instituto Rizzoli experience. Ann Oncol. 1992;3(suppl 2):S23-S27.

108. Picci P, Sangiorgi L, Rougraff B, et al. Relationship of chemotherapy-induced necrosis and surgical margins to local recurrence in osteosarcoma. J Clin Oncol. 1994;12:2699-2705.

109. Picci P, Sangiorgi L, Bahamonde Lea. Risk factors for local recurrences after limb-salvage surgery for high-grade osteosarcoma of the extremities. Ann Oncol. 1997;8:899-903.

110. Rodrigues-Galindo C, Shah N, McCarville M, et al. Outcome after local recurrences of osteosarcoma: The St. Jude Children's Research Hospital experience. Cancer. 2004;100:1928-1935.

111. Bacci G, Longhi A, Cesari M, Bertoni F. Influence of local recurrence on survival in patients with extremity osteosarcoma treated with neoadjuvant chemotherapy: the experience of a single institution with 44 patients. Cancer. 2006;106:2701-2706.

112. Bacci G, Longhi A, Versari M, et al. Prognostic factors for osteosarcoma of the extremity treated with neoadjuvant chemotherapy: 15-year experience in 789 patients treated at a single instituion. Cancer. 2006;106:1154-1161.

113. Kempf-Bielack B, Bielack S, Jurgens H, et al. Osteosarcoma relapse after combined modality therapy: an anlysis of unselected patients in the cooperative osteosarcoma study group (COSS). J Clin Oncol. 2005;23:559-568.

114. Hoffer F, Nikanorov A, Reddick W, et al. Accuracy of MR imaging for detecting epiphyseal extension of osteosarcoma. Pediatr Radiol. 2000;30:289-298.

115. Kager L, Zoubeck A, Kastner U, et al. Skip metastases in osteosarcoma: experience of the cooperative osteosarcoma study group. J Clin Oncol. 2006;24:1535-1541.

116. Quan G, Slavin J, Schlicht S, et al. Osteosarcoma near joints: assessment and implications. J Surg Oncol. 2005; 91:159-166.

117. Yamaguchi H, Minami A, Kaneda K, et al. Comparison of magnetic resonance imaging and computed tomography in the local assessment of osteosarcoma. Int Orthop. 1992;16:285-290.

118. Sundaram M, McGuire M, Herbold D. Magnetic resonance imaging of osteosarcoma. Skeletal Radiol. 1987;16:23-29.

119. Wallace R, Davoudi M, Neel M, Lachica R. The role of the pediatric plastic surgeon in limb salvage surgery for osteosarcoma of the lower extremity. J Craniofac Surg. 2003;14:680-686.

120. Mastorakos D, Disa J, Athanasian E, et al. Soft-tissue flap coverage maximizes limb salvage after allograft bone extremity reconstruction. Plast Reconstr Surg. 2002;109:1567-1573.

121. Meyer M, Spanier S, Moser M, Scarborough M. Evaluating marrow margins for resection of osteosarcoma: a modern approach. Clin Orthop Relat Res. 1999;363:170-175.

122. Gupta A, Meswania J, Pollock R, et al. Non-invasive distal femoral expandable endoprosthesis for limb-salvage surgery in paediatric tumours. J Bone Joint Surg Br. 2006;88:649-654.

123. Gitelis S, Neel M, Wilkins R, et al. The use of a closed expandable prosthesis for pediatric sarcomas. Chir Organi Mov. 2003; 88:327-333.

124. Neel M, Wilkins R, Rao BN, Kelly C. Early multicenter experience with a noninvasive expandable prosthesis. Clin Orthop Relat Res. 2003;415:72-81.

125. Wilkins R, Soubieran A. The Phenix expandable prosthesis: early American experience. Clin Orthop Relat Res. 2001;382:51-58.

126. Eckardt J, Kabo J, Kelley C, et al. Expandable endoprosthesis recostruction in skeletally immature patients with tumors. Clin Orthop Relat Res. 2000;373:51-61.

127. Jeys L, Grimer R, Carter S, Tillman R. Periprosthetic infection in patients treated for an orthopaedic oncological condition. J Bone Joint Surg Am. 2005;87:842-849.

128. Rodl R, Ozaki T, Hoffmann C, et al. Osteoarticular allograft in surgery for high-grade malignant tumours of bone. J Bone Joint Surg Br. 2000;82:1006-1010.

129. Donati D, Di Liddo M, Zavatta M, et al. Massive bone allograft reconstruction in high-grade osteosarcoma. Clin Orthop Relat Res. 2000;377:186-194.

130. Muscolo D, Ayerza M, Apongte-Tinao L, Ranalletta M. Use of distal femoral osteoarticular allografts in limb salvage surgery.: surgical technique. Bone Joint Surg Am. 2006;88(suppl 1):305-321.

131. Brigman BE, Hornicek FJ, Gebhardt MC, Mankin HJ. Allografts about the knee in young patients with high-grade sarcoma. Clin Orthop Relat Res. 2004;421:232-239.

132. Donati D, Giacomini S, Gozzi E, et al. Allograft arthrodesis treatment of bone tumors: a two-center study. Clin Orthop Relat Res. 2002;400:217-224.

133. Boyce T, Edwards J, Scarborough N. Allograft bone. The influence of processing on safety and performance. Orthop Clin North Am. 1999;30:571-581.

134. Joyce M. Safety and FDA regulations for musculoskeletal allografts: perspective of an orthopaedic surgeon. Clin Orthop Relat Res. 2005;435:22-30.

135. Kainer M, Linden J, Whaley D, et al. Clostridium infections associated with musculoskeletal-tissue allografts. N Engl J Med. 2004;350:2564-2571.

136. Hornicek F, Gebhardt M, Wea T, et al. Factors affecting nonunion of the allograft-host junction. Clin Orthop Relat Res. 2001;382:87-98.

137. Lietman SA, Tomford WW, Gebhardt MC, et al. Complications of irradiated allografts in orthopaedic tumor surgery. Clin Orthop Relat Res. 2000;375:214-217.

138. Muscolo D, Ayerza M, Aponte-Tinao L. Survivorship and radiographic analysis of knee osteoarticular allografts. Clin Orthop Relat Res. 2000;373:73-79.

139. Bae D, Waters P, Gebhardt M. Results of free vascularized fibula grafting for allograft nonunion after limb salvage surgery for malignant bone tumors. J Pediatr Orthop. 2006;26:809-814.

140. Wang J, Temple H, Pitcher J, et al. Salvage of failed massive allograft reconstruction with endoprosthesis. Clin Orthop Relat Res. 2006;443:296-301.

141. Ilyas I, Pant R, Kurar A, et al. Modular megaprosthesis for proximal femoral tumors. Int Orthop. 2002;26:170-173.

142. Ilyas I, Kurar A, Moreau P, Younge D. Modular megaprosthesis for distal femoral tumors. Int Orthop. 2001;25:375-377.

143. Donati D, Zavatta M, Gozzi E, et al. Modular prosthetic replacement of the proximal femur after resection of a bone tumour: a long-term follow-up. J Bone Joint Surg Br. 2001;83:1156-1160.

144. Mittermayer F, Krepler P, Dominkus M, et al. Long-term follow-up of uncemented tumor endoprosthesis for the lower extremity. Clin Orthop Relat Res. 2001;388:167-177.

145. Malo M, Davis A, Wunder J, et al. Functional evaluation in distal femoral endoprosthetic replacement for bone sarcoma. Clin Orthop Relat Res. 2001;389:173-180.

146. Zeegen EN, Aponte-Tinao LA, Hornicek FJ, et al. Survivorship analysis of 141 modular metallic endoprostheses at early follow-up. Clin Orthop Relat Res. 2004;420:239-250.

147. Menendez L, Ahlmann E, Kerani C, Gotha H. Endoprosthetic reconstruction for neoplasms of the proximal femur. Clin Orthop Relat Res. 2006;450:39-45.

148. Morgan H, Cizik A, Leopold S, et al. Survival of tumor megaprostheses replacements about the knee. Clin Orthop Relat Res. 2006;450:39-45.

149. Griffin A, Parsons J, Davis A, et al. Uncemented tumor endoprostheses at the knee: root causes of failure. Clin Orthop Relat Res. 2005;438:71-79.

150. Flint M, Griffin A, Bell R, et al. Aseptic loosening is uncommon with uncemented proximal tibia tumor prostheses. Clin Orthop Relat Res. 2006;450:164-171.

151. Gosheger G, Gebert C, Ahrens H, et al. Endoprosthetic reconstruction in 250 patients with sarcoma. Clin Orthop Relat Res. 2006;450:164-171.

152. Torbert J, Fox E, Hosalkar H, et al. Endoprosthetic reconstructions: results of long-term follow-up of 139 patients. Clin Orthop Relat Res. 2005;438:51-59.

153. Wilkins R, Miller C. Reoperation after limb preservation surgery for sarcomas of the knee in children. Clin Orthop Relat Res. 2003;412:153-161.

154. Chao E, Fuchs B, Rowland C, et al. Long-term results of segmental prosthesis fixation by extracortical bone-bridging and ingrowth. J Bone Joint Surg Am. 2004;86A:948-955.

155. Sharma S, Turcotte R, Isler M, Wong C. Cemented rotating hinge endoprosthesis for limb salvage of distal femur tumors. Clin Orthop Relat Res. 2006;450:28-32.

156. San-Julian M, Dolz R, Garcia-Barrecheguren E, et al. Limb salvage in bone sarcomas in patients younger than age 10: a 20-year experience. J Pediatr Orthop. 2003;23:753-762.

157. Wunder J, Leitch KG, Davis A, Bell R. Comparison of two methods of reconstruction for primary malignant tumors at the knee: a sequential cohort study. J Surg Oncol. 2001;77:89-99.

158. Grimer R, Belthur M, Carter S, et al. Extendible replacements of the proximal tibia for bone tumours. J Bone Joint Surg Br. 2000;82:255-260.

159. Bickels J, Wittig J, Kollender Y, et al. Distal femur resection with endoprosthetic reconstruction: a long-term follow-up study. Clin Orthop Relat Res. 2002;400:225-235.

160. Neel M, Heck R, Britton L, et al. Use of a smooth press-fit stem preserves physeal growth after tumor resection. Clin Orthop Relat Res. 2004;426:125-128.

161. Buecker PJ, Berenstein M, Gebhardt MC, et al. Locking versus standard plates for allograft fixation after tumor resection in children and adolescents. J Pediatr Orthop. 2006;26:680-685.

162. Fuchs B, Kotajarvi BR, Kaufman KR, Sim FH. Functional outcome of patients with rotationplasty about the knee. Clin Orthop Relat Res. 2003;4:52-58.

163. Merkel KD, Gebhardt M, Springfield DS. Rotationplasty as a reconstructive operation after tumor resection. Clin Orthop Relat Res. 1991;270:231-236.

164. Kotz R, Salzer M. Rotation-plasty for childhood osteosarcoma of the distal part of the femur. J Bone Joint Surg Am. 1982;64: 959-969.

165. Winkelmann WW. Type-B-IIIa hip rotationplasty: an alternative operation for the treatment of malignant tumors of the femur in early childhood. J Bone Joint Surg Am. 2000;82:814-828.

166. Hillmann A, Rosenbaum D, Gosheger G, et al. Rotationplasty type B IIIa according to Winkelmann: electromyography and gait analysis. Clin Orthop Relat Res. 2001;384:224-231.

167. Krajbich JI. Modified Van Ness rotationplasty in the treatment of malignant neoplasms in the lower extremities of children. Clin Orthop Relat Res. 1991;262:74-77.

168. Hopyan S, Tan JW, Graham HK, Torode IP. Function and upright time following limb salvage, amputation, and rotationplasty for pediatric sarcoma of bone. J Pediatr Orthop. 2006;26:405-408.

169. Veenstra KM, Sprangers MA, van der Eyken JW, Taminiau AH. Quality of life in survivors with a van Ness-Borggreve rotationplasty after bone tumour resection. J Surg Oncol. 2000;73:192-197.

170. Rodl RW, Pohlmann U, Gosheger G, et al. Rotationplasty: quality of life after 10 years in 22 patients. Acta Orthop Scand. 2002;73:85-88.

171. Hanlon M, Krajbich JI. Rotationplasty in skeletally immature patients. Long-term follow-up results. Clin Orthop Relat Res. 1999;358:75-82.

172. Catani F, Capanna R, Benedetti MG, et al. Gait analysis in patients after van Ness rotationplasty. Clin Orthop Relat Res. 1993; 296:270-277.

173. Miller G, Krystolovich P, MacMillan K. Rehabilitation following a van Ness rotation arthroplasty. Can Nurse. 1987;83:24-25.

174. Murray MP, Jacobs PA, Gore DR, et al. Functional performance after tibial rotationplasty. J Bone Joint Surg Am. 1985;67:392-399.

175. Donati D, Albisinni U, Zavatta M, et al. Long-term roentgenographic evaluation of proximal femur prosthesis after tumor resection. Chir Organi Mov. 2004;89:191-203.

176. Donati D, Giacomini S, Gozzi E, Mercuri M. Proximal femur reconstruction by an allograft prosthesis composite. Clin Orthop Relat Res. 2002;394:192-200.

177. Manoso MW, Boland PJ, Healey JH, et al. Acetabular development after bipolar hemiarthroplasty for osteosarcoma in children. J Bone Joint Surg Br. 2005;87:1658-1662.

178. Rodl RW, Hoffmann C, Gosheger G, et al. Ewing's sarcoma of the pelvis: combined surgery and radiotherapy treatment. J Surg Oncol. 2003;83:154-160.

179. Ham SJ, Kroon HM, Koops HS, Hoekstra HJ. Osteosarcoma of the pelvis: oncological results of 40 patients registered by The Netherlands Committee on Bone Tumours. Eur J Surg Oncol. 2000;26:53-60.

180. Sucato DJ, Rougraff B, McGrath BE, et al. Ewing's sarcoma of the pelvis: long-term survival and functional outcome. Clin Orthop Relat Res. 2000;373:193-201.

181. Saab R, Rao BN, Rodriguez-Galindo C, et al. Osteosarcoma of the pelvis in children and young adults: the St. Jude Children's Research Hospital experience. Cancer. 2005;103:1468-1474.

182. Yock TI, Krailo M, Fryer CJ, et al. Local control in pelvic Ewing sarcoma: analysis from INT-0091: a report from the Children's Oncology Group. J Clin Oncol. 2006;24:3838-3843.

183. Grier HE, Krailo MD, Tarbell NJ, et al. Addition of ifosfamide and etoposide to standard chemotherapy for Ewing's sarcoma and primitive neuroectodermal tumor of bone. N Engl J Med. 2003;348:694-701.

184. Schwameis E, Dominkus M, Krepler P, et al. Reconstruction of the pelvis after tumor resection in children and adolescents. Clin Orthop Relat Res. 2002;402:220-35.

185. Langlais F, Lambotte JC, Thomazeau H. Long-term results of hemipelvis reconstruction with allografts. Clin Orthop Relat Res. 2001;388:178-186.

186. Hillmann A, Hoffmann C, Gosheger G, et al. Tumors of the pelvis: complications after reconstruction. Arch Orthop Trauma Surg. 2003;123:340-344.

187. Verma NN, Kuo KN, Gitelis S. Acetabular osteoarticular allograft after Ewing's sarcoma resection. Clin Orthop Relat Res. 2004; 419:149-154.

188. Krettek C, Geerling J, Bastian L, et al. Computer-aided tumor resection in the pelvis. Injury. 2004;35(suppl 1):S-A79-A83.

189. Sandy G, Shores J, Reeves M. Tikhoff-Linberg procedure and chest wall resection for recurrent sarcoma of the shoulder girdle involving the chest wall. J Surg Oncol. 2005;89:91-94.

190. Voggenreiter G, Assenmacher S, Schmit-Neuerburg KP. Tikhoff-Linberg procedure for bone and soft tissue tumors of the shoulder girdle. Arch Surg. 1999;134:252-257.

191. Volpe CM, Pell M, Doerr RJ, Karakousis CP. Radical scapulectomy with limb salvage for shoulder girdle soft tissue sarcoma. Surg Oncol. 1996;5:43-48.

192. Hahn SB, Kim NH, Choi NH. Treatment of bone tumors around the shoulder joint by the Tikhoff-Linberg procedure. Yonsei Med J. 1990;31:110-122.

193. Capanna R, van Horn JR, Biagini R, et al. The Tikhoff-Linberg procedure for bone tumors of the proximal humerus: the classical "extensive" technique versus a modified "transglenoid" resection. Arch Orthop Trauma Surg. 1990;109:63-67.

194. Malawer MM, Sugarbaker PH, Lampert M, et al. The Tikhoff-Linberg procedure: report of ten patients and presentation of a modified technique for tumors of the proximal humerus. Surgery. 1985;97:518-528.

195. Capanna R, Van Horn JR, Biagini R, et al. A humeral modular prostheses for bone tumour surgery: a study of 56 cases. Int Orthop. 1986;10:231-238.

196. Gosheger G, Hardes J, Ahrens H, et al. Endoprosthetic replacement of the humerus combined with trapezius and latissimus dorsi transfer: a report of three patients. Arch Orthop Trauma Surg. 2005;125:62-65.

197. Manili M, Fredella N, Santori FS. Shoulder prosthesis in reconstruction of the scapulohumeral girdle after wide resection to treat malignant neoformation of the proximal humerus. Chir Organi Mov. 2002;87:25-33.

198. Ayoub KS, Fiorenza F, Grimer RJ, et al. Extensible endoprostheses of the humerus after resection of bone tumours. J Bone Joint Surg Br. 1999;81:495-500.

199. O'Connor MI, Sim FH, Chao EY. Limb salvage for neoplasms of the shoulder girdle. Intermediate reconstructive and functional results. J Bone Joint Surg Am. 1996;78:1872-1888.

200. Cheng EY, Gebhardt MC. Allograft reconstructions of the shoulder after bone tumor resections. Orthop Clin North Am. 1991;22:37-48.

201. Gebhardt MC, Roth YF, Mankin HJ. Osteoarticular allografts for reconstruction in the proximal part of the humerus after excision of a musculoskeletal tumor. J Bone Joint Surg Am. 1990;72:334-345.

202. Fuchs B, O'Connor MI, Padgett DJ, et al. Arthrodesis of the shoulder after tumor resection. Clin Orthop Relat Res. 2005; 436:202-207.

203. Otis JC, Lane JM, Kroll MA. Energy cost during gait in osteosarcoma patients after resection and knee replacement and after above-the-knee amputation. J Bone Joint Surg Am. 1985;67:606-611.

204. van der Windt DA, Pieterson I, van der Eijken JW, et al. Energy expenditure during walking in subjects with tibial rotationplasty, above-knee amputation, or hip disarticulation. Arch Phys Med Rehabil. 1992;73:1174-1180.

205. Gebhardt MC. What's new in musculoskeletal oncology. J Bone Joint Surg Am. 2002;84A:694-701.

206. Kayton ML. Pulmonary metastasectomy in pediatric patients. Thorac Surg Clin. 2006;16:167-183, vi.

207. Chang AE, Schaner EG, Conkle DM, et al. Evaluation of computed tomography in the detection of pulmonary metastases: a prospective study. Cancer. 1979;43:913-916.

208. Mintzer RA, Malave SR, Neiman HL, et al. Computed vs. conventional tomography in evaluation of primary and secondary pulmonary neoplasms. Radiology. 1979;132:653-659.

209. Rusch VW. Pulmonary metastasectomy. Current indications. Chest. 1995;107 9(suppl):322S-331S.

210. Yeh SD, La Quaglia MP. [131]I therapy for pediatric thyroid cancer. Semin Pediatr Surg. 1997;6:128-133.

211. Vassilopoulou-Sellin R, Klein M, Smith T, et al. Pulmonary metastases in children and young adults with differentiated thyroid cancer. Cancer. 1993;71:1348-1352.

212. Newman KD, Black T, Heller G, et al. Differentiated thyroid cancer: determinants of disease progression in patients <21 years of age at diagnosis: a report from the Surgical Discipline Committee of the Children's Cancer Group. Ann Surg. 1998;227:533-541.

213. Vassilopoulou-Sellin R, Goepfert H, Raney B, Schultz PN. Differentiated thyroid cancer in children and adolescents: clinical outcome and mortality after long-term follow-up. Head Neck. 1998;20:549-555.

214. Okada T, Sasaki F, Takahashi H, et al. Management of childhood and adolescent thyroid carcinoma: long-term follow-up and clinical characteristics. Eur J Pediatr Surg. 2006;16:8-13.

215. Spinelli C, Bertocchini A, Antonelli A, Miccoli P. Surgical therapy of the thyroid papillary carcinoma in children: experience with 56 patients < or = 16 years old. J Pediatr Surg. 2004;39:1500-1505.

216. Chaukar DA, Rangarajan V, Nair N, et al. Pediatric thyroid cancer. J Surg Oncol. 2005;92:130-133.

217. Demidchik YE, Demidchik EP, Reiners C, et al. Comprehensive clinical assessment of 740 cases of surgically treated thyroid cancer in children of Belarus. Ann Surg. 2006;243:525-532.

218. Lucas JD, O'Doherty MJ, Wong JC, et al. Evaluation of fluorodeoxyglucose positron emission tomography in the management of soft-tissue sarcomas. J Bone Joint Surg Br. 1998;80:441-447.

219. Pastorino U. History of the surgical management of pulmonary metastases and development of the International Registry. Semin Thorac Cardiovasc Surg. 2002;14:18-28.

220. Ballantine TV, Wiseman NE, Filler RM. Assessment of pulmonary wedge resection for the treatment of lung metastases. J Pediatr Surg. 1975;10:671-676.

221. Kilman JW, Kronenberg MW, O'Neill JA Jr, Klassen KP. Surgical resection for pulmonary metastases in children. Arch Surg. 1969;99:158-165.

222. Baldeyrou P, Lemoine G, Zucker JM, Schweisguth O. Pulmonary metastases in children: the place of surgery: a study of 134 patients. J Pediatr Surg. 1984;19:121-125.

223. Karnak I, Emin Senocak M, Kutluk T, et al. Pulmonary metastases in children: an analysis of surgical spectrum. Eur J Pediatr Surg. 2002;12:151-158.

224. Abel RM, Brown J, Moreland B, Parikh D. Pulmonary metastasectomy for pediatric solid tumors. Pediatr Surg Int. 2004;20:630-632.

225. Gilbert JC, Powell DM, Hartman GE, et al. Video-assisted thoracic surgery (VATS) for children with pulmonary metastases from osteosarcoma. Ann Surg Oncol. 1996;3:539-542.

226. Hardaway BW, Hoffer FA, Rao BN. Needle localization of small pediatric tumors for surgical biopsy. Pediatr Radiol. 2000;30:318-322.

227. Waldhausen JH, Shaw DW, Hall DG, Sawin RS. Needle localization for thoracoscopic resection of small pulmonary nodules in children. J Pediatr Surg. 1997;32:1624-1625.

228. Partrick DA, Bensard DD, Teitelbaum DH, et al. Successful thoracoscopic lung biopsy in children utilizing preoperative CT-guided localization. J Pediatr Surg. 2002;37:970-973; discussion 970-973.

229. Scorpio RJ, Stokes K, Grattan-Smith D, Tiedemann K. Percutaneous localization of small pulmonary metastases, enabling limited resection. J Pediatr Surg. 1994;29:685-687.

230. McConnell PI, Feola GP, Meyers RL. Methylene blue-stained autologous blood for needle localization and thoracoscopic resection of deep pulmonary nodules. J Pediatr Surg. 2002;37:1729-1731.

231. Kayton ML, Huvos AG, Casher J, et al. Computed tomographic scan of the chest underestimates the number of metastatic lesions in osteosarcoma. J Pediatr Surg. 2006;41:200-206; discussion 200-206.

232. Su WT, Chewning J, Abramson S, et al. Surgical management and outcome of osteosarcoma patients with unilateral pulmonary metastases. J Pediatr Surg. 2004;39:418-423; discussion 418-423.

233. Michalkiewicz E, Sandrini R, Figueiredo B, et al. Clinical and outcome characteristics of children with adrenocortical tumors: a report from the International Pediatric Adrenocortical Tumor Registry. J Clin Oncol. 2004;22:838-845.

234. Appelqvist P, Kostianinen S. Multiple thoracotomy combined with chemotherapy in metastatic adrenal cortical carcinoma: a case report and review of the literature. J Surg Oncol. 1983;24:1-4.

235. De Leon DD, Lange BJ, Walterhouse D, Moshang T. Long-term (15 years) outcome in an infant with metastatic adrenocortical carcinoma. J Clin Endocrinol Metab. 2002;87:4452-4456.

236. Kwauk S, Burt M. Pulmonary metastases from adrenal cortical carcinoma: results of resection. J Surg Oncol. 1993;53:243-246.

237. Schulick RD, Brennan MF. Long-term survival after complete resection and repeat resection in patients with adrenocortical carcinoma. Ann Surg Oncol. 1999;6:719-726.

238. Lo Curto M, Lumia F, Alaggio R, et al. Malignant germ cell tumors in childhood: results of the first Italian cooperative study TCG 91. Med Pediatr Oncol. 2003;41:417-425.

239. Cagini L, Nicholson AG, Horwich A, et al. Thoracic metastasectomy for germ cell tumours: long-term survival and prognostic factors. Ann Oncol. 1998;9:1185-1191.

240. Liu D, Abolhoda A, Burt ME, et al. Pulmonary metastasectomy for testicular germ cell tumors: a 28-year experience. Ann Thorac Surg. 1998;66:1709-1714.

241. Horvath LG, McCaughan BC, Stockle M, Boyer MJ. Resection of residual pulmonary masses after chemotherapy in patients with metastatic non-seminomatous germ cell tumours. Intern Med J. 2002;32:79-83.

242. Kesler KA, Wilson JL, Cosgrove JA, et al. Surgical salvage therapy for malignant intrathoracic metastases from nonseminomatous germ cell cancer of testicular origin: analysis of a single-institution experience. J Thorac Cardiovasc Surg. 2005;130:408-415.

243. Pfannschmidt J, Zabeck H, Muley T, et al. Pulmonary metastasectomy following chemotherapy in patients with testicular tumors: experience in 52 patients. Thorac Cardiovasc Surg. 2006;54:484-488.

244. Black CT, Luck SR, Musemeche CA, Andrassy RJ. Aggressive excision of pulmonary metastases is warranted in the management of childhood hepatic tumors. J Pediatr Surg. 1991;26:1082-1085; discussion 1085-1086.

245. Feusner JH, Krailo MD, Haas JE, et al. Treatment of pulmonary metastases of initial stage I hepatoblastoma in childhood. Report from the Children's Cancer Group. Cancer. 1993;71:859-864.

246. Perilongo G, Brown J, Shafford E, et al. Hepatoblastoma presenting with lung metastases: treatment results of the first cooperative, prospective study of the International Society of Paediatric Oncology on childhood liver tumors. Cancer. 2000;89:1845-1853.

247. Towbin R, Gruppo RA. Pulmonary metastases in neuroblastoma. AJR Am J Roentgenol. 1982;138:75-78.

248. Furuya K, Okamura J, Koga M, et al. Unusual pulmonary metastasis of neuroblastoma: a case report. Radiat Med. 1996;14:283-285.

249. Cowie F, Corbett R, Pinkerton CR. Lung involvement in neuroblastoma: incidence and characteristics. Med Pediatr Oncol. 1997;28:429-432.

250. DuBois SG, Kalika Y, Lukens JN, et al. Metastatic sites in stage IV and IVS neuroblastoma correlate with age, tumor biology, and survival. J Pediatr Hematol Oncol. 1999;21:181-189.

251. Kammen BF, Matthay KK, Pacharn P, et al. Pulmonary metastases at diagnosis of neuroblastoma in pediatric patients: CT findings and prognosis. AJR Am J Roentgenol. 2001;176:755-759.

252. de Kraker J, Lemerle J, Voute PA, et al. Wilm's tumor with pulmonary metastases at diagnosis: the significance of primary chemotherapy. International Society of Pediatric Oncology Nephroblastoma Trial and Study Committee. J Clin Oncol. 1990;8:1187-1190.

253. Green DM, Finklestein JZ, Tefft ME, Norkool P. Diffuse interstitial pneumonitis after pulmonary irradiation for metastatic Wilms' tumor: a report from the National Wilms' Tumor Study. Cancer. 1989;63:450-453.

254. Green DM, Breslow NE, Ii Y, et al. The role of surgical excision in the management of relapsed Wilms' tumor patients with pulmonary metastases: a report from the National Wilms' Tumor Study. J Pediatr Surg. 1991;26:728-733.

255. Green DM, Beckwith JB, Breslow NE, et al. Treatment of children with stages II to IV anaplastic Wilms' tumor: a report from the National Wilms' Tumor Study Group. J Clin Oncol. 1994;12:2126-2131.

256. Green DM, Breslow NE, Beckwith JB, et al. Comparison between single-dose and divided-dose administration of dactinomycin and doxorubicin for patients with Wilms' tumor: a report from the National Wilms' Tumor Study Group. J Clin Oncol. 1998;16:237-245.

257. Ehrlich PF, Hamilton TE, Grundy P, et al. The value of surgery in directing therapy for patients with Wilms' tumor with pulmonary disease: a report from the National Wilms' Tumor Study Group (National Wilms' Tumor Study 5). J Pediatr Surg. 2006;41:162-167; discussion 162-167.

258. Temeck BK, Wexler LH, Steinberg SM, et al. Reoperative pulmonary metastasectomy for sarcomatous pediatric histologies. Ann Thorac Surg. 1998;66:908-912; discussion 913.

259. Temeck BK, Wexler LH, Steinberg SM, et al. Metastasectomy for sarcomatous pediatric histologies: results and prognostic factors. Ann Thorac Surg. 1995;59:1385-1389; discussion 1390.

260. Martini N, Huvos AG, Mike V, et al. Multiple pulmonary resections in the treatment of osteogenic sarcoma. Ann Thorac Surg. 1971;12:271-280.

261. Meyers PA, Heller G, Healey JH, et al. Osteogenic sarcoma with clinically detectable metastasis at initial presentation. J Clin Oncol. 1993;11:449-453.

262. Bacci G, Mercuri M, Briccoli A, et al. Osteogenic sarcoma of the extremity with detectable lung metastases at presentation: results

of treatment of 23 patients with chemotherapy followed by simultaneous resection of primary and metastatic lesions. Cancer. 1997;79:245-254.

263. La Quaglia MP. Osteosarcoma. Specific tumor management and results. Chest Surg Clin North Am. 1998;8:77-95.

264. Antunes M, Bernardo J, Salete M, et al. Excision of pulmonary metastases of osteogenic sarcoma of the limbs. Eur J Cardiothorac Surg. 1999;15:592-596.

265. Kaste SC, Pratt CB, Cain AM, et al. Metastases detected at the time of diagnosis of primary pediatric extremity osteosarcoma at diagnosis: imaging features. Cancer. 1999;86:1602-1608.

266. Horan TA, Santiago FF, Araujo LM. The benefit of pulmonary metastectomy for bone and soft tissue sarcomas. Int Surg. 2000;85:185-189.

267. McCarville MB, Kaste SC, Cain AM, et al. Prognostic factors and imaging patterns of recurrent pulmonary nodules after thoracotomy in children with osteosarcoma. Cancer. 2001;91:1170-1176.

268. Tsuchiya H, Kanazawa Y, Abdel-Wanis ME, et al. Effect of timing of pulmonary metastases identification on prognosis of patients with osteosarcoma: the Japanese Musculoskeletal Oncology Group study. J Clin Oncol. 2002;20:3470-3477.

269. Hawkins DS, Arndt CA. Pattern of disease recurrence and prognostic factors in patients with osteosarcoma treated with contemporary chemotherapy. Cancer. 2003;98:2447-2456.

270. Kager L, Zoubek A, Potschger U, et al. Primary metastatic osteosarcoma: presentation and outcome of patients treated on neoadjuvant Cooperative Osteosarcoma Study Group protocols. J Clin Oncol. 2003;21:2011-2018.

271. Briccoli A, Rocca M, Salone M, et al. Resection of recurrent pulmonary metastases in patients with osteosarcoma. Cancer. 2005;104:1721-1725.

272. Mialou V, Philip T, Kalifa C, et al. Metastatic osteosarcoma at diagnosis: prognostic factors and long-term outcome: the French pediatric experience. Cancer. 2005;104:1100-1109.

273. Harting MT, Blakely ML. Management of osteosarcoma pulmonary metastases. Semin Pediatr Surg. 2006;15:25-29.

274. Pfannschmidt J, Klode J, Muley T, et al. Pulmonary resection for metastatic osteosarcomas: a retrospective analysis of 21 patients. Thorac Cardiovasc Surg. 2006;54:120-123.

275. Suzuki M, Iwata T, Ando S, et al. Predictors of long-term survival with pulmonary metastasectomy for osteosarcomas and soft tissue sarcomas. J Cardiovasc Surg (Torino). 2006;47:603-608.

276. Harting MT, Blakely ML, Jaffe N, et al. Long-term survival after aggressive resection of pulmonary metastases among children and adolescents with osteosarcoma. J Pediatr Surg. 2006;41:194-199.

III Hematologic Malignancy

10 Acute Lymphoblastic Leukemia

Lewis B. Silverman

The acute leukemias of childhood are rare diseases that collectively represent about 30% of malignancies in children younger than 15 years.[1] Approximately 3000 new cases of childhood leukemia occur annually in the United States, 80% of which are acute lymphoblastic leukemia (ALL). Between the 1960s and 1990s, the prognosis for children with ALL improved dramatically. With current multiagent chemotherapy regimens, approximately 80% of children with ALL are long-term relapse-free survivors.[2-4] In this chapter, childhood ALL is reviewed with respect to classification, pathophysiology, clinical presentation, laboratory findings, differential diagnosis, treatment strategies, prognosis, and late effects of therapy. Causative and epidemiologic considerations, including the incidence, prevalence, and life span of afflicted individuals, are discussed in Chapter 1. Discussion of the cytogenetic aspects of the leukemias appears in Chapter 5, and molecular genetics and oncogenes are considered in Chapter 3. Details concerning the various chemotherapeutic agents are provided in Chapter 6, and myelogenous leukemias and myeloproliferative disorders are discussed in Chapter 11.

CLASSIFICATION

The childhood leukemias can be classified as acute or chronic. Acute leukemia is characterized by clonal expansion of immature hematopoietic or lymphoid precursors, whereas chronic leukemia refers to conditions characterized by the expansion of mature marrow elements. Congenital leukemia refers to leukemias diagnosed within the first 4 weeks of life.

Acute leukemia is characterized by replacement of normal marrow elements with malignant blast cells, relatively undifferentiated cells with diffusely distributed nuclear chromatin, one or more nucleoli, and basophilic cytoplasm. A number of methods exist for characterizing malignant blast cells, including morphology, cytochemistry, and immunophenotype, as well as chromosomal and molecular genetic aberrations. Approximately 80% of cases of childhood acute leukemia are lymphoblastic (ALL).

Morphologic and Cytochemical Classification

The production of blast forms is part of the normal maturational sequence of hematopoietic and lymphoid elements. Blast cells are primitive precursors, lacking many of the features of differentiation. Under normal conditions, blast forms constitute fewer than 5% of the nucleated cells of the bone marrow. Blast cells are usually not observed in the peripheral blood, except during periods of profound overproduction of blood cells in response to infection or bleeding, or bone marrow invasion by granulomas, fibrosis, or tumor cells (leukoerythroblastosis). Leukemic blast cells can be difficult to distinguish morphologically from normal, nonmalignant blasts, although the finding of more than 5% blast forms in the marrow, or the presence of blast cells in the peripheral blood, should raise the suspicion of leukemia. In acute leukemia, patients often present with a marrow that is almost fully replaced by blast forms.

Once the diagnosis of leukemia is made, it is sometimes difficult to differentiate a lymphoid from a myeloid blast. Figure 10-1 displays the morphologic characteristics of lymphoblasts. Wright-Giemsa–stained lymphoblasts have smooth, homogeneous nuclear material with indistinct nucleoli and only a small rim of light blue–staining cytoplasm, generally without

granules. Granular ALL has been described as a rare variant in only 3% to 4.5% of cases.[5] In contrast, myeloblasts differ from lymphoblasts in that the former have a lower nuclear-to-cytoplasmic ratio, more finely developed nuclear chromatin, and more distinct punched-out nucleoli. Cytoplasmic granules are often present in myeloblasts, and the detection of eosinophilic Auer rods is pathognomonic. However, small myeloblasts may be confused with lymphoblasts morphologically, although they can usually be distinguished by cytochemical and/or flow cytometric studies.

A standardized morphologic classification system devised by the French-American-British (FAB) Cooperative Working Group is generally used to categorize the appearance of leukemic blasts.[6] Using this system, ALL can be subdivided into three morphologic categories, L1, L2, and L3 (see Fig. 10-1). L1 is the most common subtype, observed in about 90% of cases of childhood ALL. L1 lymphoblasts are small cells characterized by a high nuclear-to-cytoplasmic ratio. The pale blue cytoplasm is scanty and limited to a small portion of the perimeter of the cell. The cells have indistinct nucleoli and nuclear membranes that vary from round to clefted. Cells in the L2 category, found in 5% to 15% of pediatric cases, are larger than those classified as L1, show marked variability in size, and have prominent nucleoli and more abundant cytoplasm. They may be indistinguishable from the M1 variant of myeloid leukemia; the differentiation must be made by cytochemical staining and cell surface markers. Only 1% to 2% of ALL pediatric patients have L3 lymphoblasts, which appear identical to Burkitt's lymphoma cells, with deeply basophilic cytoplasm and prominent cytoplasmic vacuolization. Although L3 ALL is almost always associated with mature B-cell immunophenotype, L1 and L2 lymphoblasts do not differ significantly in terms of cell surface markers or genetic abnormalities.[7] Historically, results from some clinical trials have suggested that L2 morphology conveyed a worse prognosis than L1 morphology,[8] although when patients are treated with more intensive regimens, FAB classification no longer appears to be an independent prognostic variable.[9,10] Most investigators no longer consider the distinction between the L1 and L2 subtypes when risk-stratifying patients. However, patients with L3 morphology and mature B-cell phenotype should be treated with regimens for advanced-stage Burkitt's lymphoma rather than ALL.[11,12] Other morphologic variants of ALL, including ALL with hand mirror cells or granules, have been described but do not appear to have prognostic significance.[10]

Various cytochemical stains can distinguish ALL from AML. In approximately 80% of cases of ALL, lymphoblasts react positively with periodic acid–Schiff (PAS), which stains cytoplasmic glycogen.[13] Myeloid-specific stains, such as myeloperoxidase, specific and nonspecific esterase, and Sudan black (a cytoplasmic lipid stain) are usually negative in ALL. In contrast, myeloblasts are myeloperoxidase-positive in 75% of patients. Terminal deoxynucleotidyl transferase (TdT), an enzyme that catalyzes the polymerization of deoxynucleoside monophosphates into a single-strand DNA primer, can be demonstrated in the nuclei of both T- and B-cell lymphoblasts, but is rarely present in cases of myeloid leukemia.[14,15]

Immunophenotype

Identification of immunophenotypic subtypes of ALL in the 1970s allowed a classification that was more precise and biologically oriented than the morphologic approach.[16,17] ALL has been subcategorized based on the expression of lineage- and maturation-specific antigens present on the cell surface and in the cytoplasm of lymphoblasts. In addition, immunophenotypic studies of lymphoblasts have provided important insights into

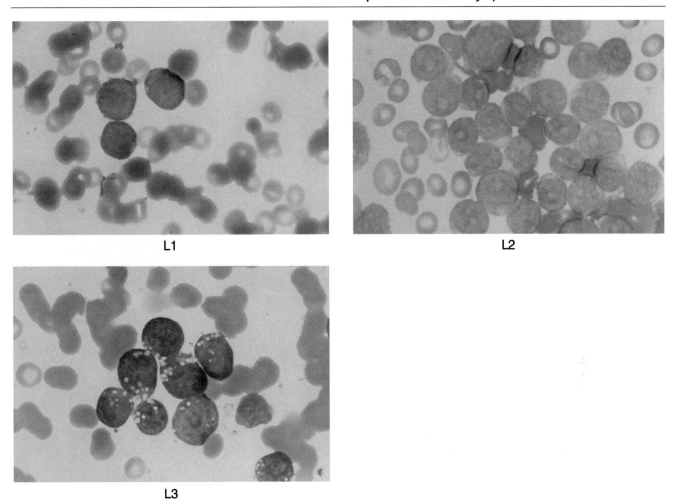

FIGURE 10-1. The French-American-British (FAB) classification system of acute leukemia. **L1,** Acute lymphoblastic leukemia. Note the high nuclear-to-cytoplasmic ratio and lack of distinct nucleoli. **L2,** Acute lymphoblastic leukemia. Note the large nucleoli and increased amount of cytoplasm. **L3,** Acute lymphoblastic leukemia. This subtype is associated with surface immunoglobulin. Note the dark blue cytoplasm and vacuoles. *(Courtesy of Pearl Leavitt.)*

the differentiation and maturation of normal B and T lymphocytes. Because the leukemic blast represents the neoplastic expansion of a lymphoid progenitor cell, many phenotypic and genotypic features of the lymphoblast mimic those of the normal lymphoid cell counterpart of specific lineage and maturational stage.[18,19] Figure 10-2 depicts a simplified schematic overview of lymphoid cell differentiation.[20]

Based on reactivity with a panel of lineage-associated antibodies, ALL has been subclassified into three broad categories—B-precursor, mature B-cell, and T-cell. The immunophenotypic subsets are associated with distinctive clinical features (Table 10-1).[21,22]

B-Precursor Cell Acute Lymphoblastic Leukemia

Approximately 80% to 85% of children with ALL present with B-precursor phenotype. These leukemia cells are characterized by reactivity with monoclonal antibodies specific for B-cell–associated antigens (e.g., CD9, CD19, and CD20) and are distinguished from mature B-cell ALL by the absence of surface immunoglobulin. The vast majority (80% to 90%) of B-precursor ALL cells express CD10, also known as the common ALL antigen (CALLA).[17]

Over 90% of cases of B-precursor ALL have evidence of immunoglobulin gene rearrangements, predominantly involving the immunoglobulin heavy chain (IgH).[23] The pattern of immunoglobulin gene rearrangements in ALL cells may indicate the degree of differentiation of the B-precursor cell from which it derives, because normal B-cell maturation is characterized by sequential rearrangements of the IgH, kappa, and then lambda light chain rearrangements.[24] However, many B-precursor ALL cells display an immunoglobulin gene rearrangement profile that is not consistent with any known stage of normal B-cell development, reflecting the disordered nature of the leukemic cell genome.[25] Moreover, T-cell receptor gene

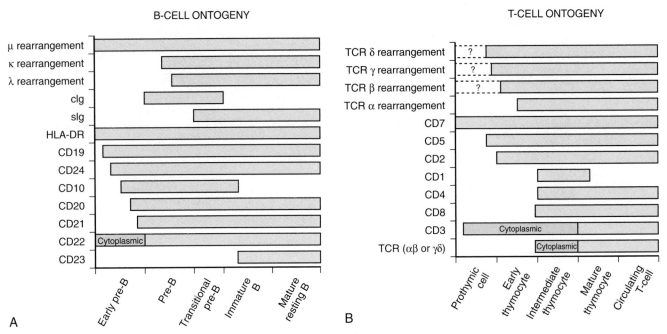

FIGURE 10-2. Schematic representation of human lymphoid differentiation. **A,** Hypothetical schema of marker expression and gene rearrangement during normal B-cell ontogeny. **B,** Hypothetical schema of marker expression and gene rearrangement during normal T-cell ontogeny. *(Adapted from Pui CH, Behm FG, Crist WM: Clinical and biologic relevance of immunologic marker studies in childhood acute lymphoblastic leukemia. Blood 1993;82:343-362.)*

TABLE 10-1   Correlation of Immunophenotype with Clinical Characteristics

Parameter	Early Pro-B, CD10⁻	Early Pro-B, CD10⁺	Pro-B (cIgM+)	T-cell
No. of patients	52	635	156	124
Gender (% male)	39%	53%	50%	75%
Age (yr)				
<1 (%)	33%	1%	6%	1%
1 to <10 (%)	50%	82%	80%	62%
≥10 (%)	17%	17%	14%	37%
Leukocyte count (× 10⁹/L)				
≤20 (%)	38%	75%	53%	23%
>50 (%)	44%	11%	21%	57%
Platelet count ≤ 100 × 10⁹/L (%)	77%	75%	81%	56%
Hemoglobin ≤ 8 g/dL (%)	58%	40%	60%	15%
Splenomegaly (%)★	50%	34%	46%	57%
Hepatomegaly (%)★	56%	46%	48%	61%
Mediastinal mass (%)	0%	0%	1%	72%
Lymphadenopathy	35%	36%	41%	78%
CNS-positive (CNS-3)†	10%	1%	1%	11%

★>4 cm below the costal margin; †CNS-3, diagnostic cerebrospinal fluid specimen with 5 or more white blood cells/high-power field and lymphoblasts seen on cytospin preparation.

cIgM+, intracytoplasmic immunoglobulin M–positive; CNS, central nervous system.

From Reiter A, Schrappe M, Ludwig WD, et al. Chemotherapy in 998 unselected childhood acute lymphoblastic leukemia patients. Results and conclusions of the multicenter trial ALL-BFM 86. Blood. 1994;84:3122-3133; and H. Riehm, personal communication, 1996.

rearrangements occur frequently in B-precursor ALL, and IgH gene rearrangements have been observed in T-cell ALL.[23] Thus, the pattern of immunoglobulin and T-cell receptor gene rearrangements is insufficient to categorize the lineage and/or degree of differentiation of an individual patient's lymphoblasts.

The presence of intracytoplasmic immunoglobulin (cIg) and various cell surface markers has been used to distinguish different subsets of B-precursor cell ALL based on their level of differentiation. These subsets include pro-B ALL (3% to 4% of pediatric patients), early pre-B ALL (60% to 70% of pediatric patients) and pre-B ALL (20% to 30% of pediatric patients):[26]

- Pro-B ALL, thought to be derived from a very immature B-cell precursor, is characterized by CD10-negative immunophenotype and the absence of cIg. It is most frequently observed in infants with ALL, especially those with abnormalities involving chromosome 11q23 (*MLL* gene locus).[27-29]
- Early pre-B ALL is the most common subtype of B-precursor ALL in children. It is thought to be derived from a more mature B-cell precursor than pro-B ALL. Early pre-B cells frequently express CD10, but still lack cIg. CD10 (CALLA)-positive leukemias without cytoplasmic immunoglobulin are also referred to as common ALL (c-ALL).[30]
- Pre-B cell ALL is characterized by the presence of cIg.[31] It is thought to derive from an intermediate B-precursor cell, more mature than those lacking cIg (early pre-B cells) but not as mature as those with surface immunoglobulin (mature B cells). Like early pre-B cells, pre-B lymphoblasts typically express CD10 and human leukocyte antigen (HLA)–DR. Approximately 25% of cases of pre-B (cIg+) ALL have the chromosomal translocation t(1;19)(q23;p13), which fuses the *E2A* gene on chromosome 19 with the *PBX1* gene on chromosome 1.[31] This translocation is observed in only 1% of cases of early pre-B (or common) ALL. Whereas initial studies have suggested that patients with pre-B ALL (cIg+) had a worse outcome than those with early pre-B ALL (cIg–),[32] subsequent reports have indicated that the adverse outcome of pre-B ALL is a result of the subset with the t(1;19) translocation.[33] With more intensive regimens, even pre-B cases with this translocation do not appear to have an inferior outcome.[34,35]

Mature B-Cell Acute Lymphoblastic Leukemia

Mature B-cell ALL accounts for 1% to 2% of childhood ALL cases.[21] It is characterized by the presence of surface immunoglobulin, most often IgM, which is monoclonal for kappa or lambda light chains. The cells generally express other B-cell antigens, including CD19, CD20, and HLA-DR. Morphologically, the blasts tend to have FAB L3 features, with intensely staining cytoplasmic basophilia similar to that of erythroblasts. Cases of mature B-cell ALL without L3 morphologic features have been reported, but are rare.[36] Almost all cases of B-cell ALL are associated with one of three nonrandom chromosomal translocations—t(8;14)(q24;q32) or less commonly, t(2;8)(p12;q24) or t(8;22)(q24;q11).[37,38] The chromosomal breakpoints involve the *MYC* oncogene on chromosome 8 and the genes for the immunoglobulin heavy chain (chromosome 14), kappa light chain (chromosome 2), or lambda light chain (chromosome 22). Mature B-cell ALL is clinically indistinguishable from disseminated Burkitt's lymphoma, and is much more successfully treated with regimens used for that disease than when treated with conventional childhood ALL therapy.[11,12]

T-Cell Acute Lymphoblastic Leukemia

Approximately 10% to 15% of children with ALL present with the T-cell immunophenotype.[3,39] Compared with B-precursor ALL, T-cell ALL is more frequently associated with older age at diagnosis, higher presenting leukocyte counts, and bulky extramedullary disease (including lymphadenopathy, hepatosplenomegaly, overt CNS leukemia, and an anterior mediastinal thymic mass).[26] Historically, patients with T-cell ALL had an inferior outcome compared with those with B-precursor ALL,[40] although this prognostic difference is not observed when more intensive regimens are used.[39,41] However, the time period in which relapses occur differs between the two immunophenotypic subtypes, with earlier relapses observed more frequently in T-cell ALL.[39]

T-cell ALL can be subclassified by using monoclonal antibodies that recognize surface antigens expressed during discrete stages of normal T-cell development.[42] The clinical relevance, if any, of subclassifying T-cell ALL in this way remains controversial.[43-45]

Mixed-Lineage Expression

In some instances, individual leukemic cells simultaneously express lymphoid and myeloid surface antigens. These leukemias have been referred to as mixed-lineage or biphenotypic leukemia. Mixed-lineage leukemia may arise from a transformed pluripotent stem cell capable of differentiation in the lymphoid or myeloid pathway, or from aberrant gene regulation in a precursor cell not representative of normal hematopoiesis (lineage infidelity).[46,47] Myeloid antigen coexpression has been reported in up to 20% of cases of ALL.[48,49] Biphenotypic ALL is associated with young age at diagnosis (younger than 12 months), pro-B (CD10-negative) immunophenotype, and certain chromosomal abnormalities, such as rearrangements of chromosome 11q23 (frequently observed in infants with ALL), the Philadelphia chromosome [t(9;22)], and the *TEL/AML1* [t(12;21)] fusion.[50-53] Older studies suggested that patients with biphenotypic ALL had a worse prognosis,[54] but more recent reports have indicated that myeloid antigen coexpression lacks independent prognostic significance.[48,49,53]

Cytogenetics and Molecular Genetics

Childhood ALL can also be subclassified in terms of the genetic abnormalities observed in lymphoblasts at the time of diagnosis. Abnormalities exist in chromosome number (ploidy) and structure (translocations). Increasingly, these recurrent, nonrandom chromosomal abnormalities have been shown to have prognostic significance (see later). This topic is discussed in detail in Chapter 5.

CLINICAL MANIFESTATIONS

ALL may present insidiously or acutely, as an incidental finding on a routine blood cell count of an asymptomatic child or as a life-threatening hemorrhage, infection, or episode of respiratory distress. Common presenting symptoms include fever, pallor, bruising, petechiae, bone pain (presumably secondary to stretching of the periosteum or joint capsule by leukemic infiltration), and limp.

Although ALL is primarily a disease of the bone marrow and peripheral blood, any organ or tissue may be infiltrated by the abnormal cells. Such infiltration may be clinically apparent

TABLE 10-2   Presenting Features by Age in 5181 Children and Adolescents with Acute Lymphoblastic Leukemia (ALL) treated on ALL-BFM Trials (1986-1999)

Presenting Feature	AGE (yr)		
	<1 (2.5% of Patients)	1 to <10 (79% of Patients)	10-18 (18.5% of Patients)
Gender			
Male	52%	56%	61%
Female	48%	44%	39%
WBC ≥ 100 × 10⁹/L	59%	10%	15%
Phenotype			
B-precursor	96%	90%	73%
T-ALL	4%	10%	27%
CNS-positive*	21%	2.3%	3.9%
High hyperdiploidy†	1.5%	27%	15%
TEL/AML1 fusion†	4.5%	27%	11%
t(9;22) BCR-ABL†	0%	2.2%	5.1%

*CNS-3, diagnostic cerebrospinal fluid specimen with 5 or more white blood cells (WBCs)/high-power field and lymphoblasts seen on cytopsin preparation.
†Results for B-precursor cases only.
CNS, central nervous system; WBC, white blood cell count.
Adapted from Moricke A, Zimmermann M, Reiter A, et al. Prognostic impact of age in children and adolescents with acute lymphoblastic leukemia: data from the trials ALL-BFM 86, 90, and 95. Klin Pediatr. 2005;217:310-320.

by physical examination. At initial diagnosis, 30% to 50% of children have enlargement of the liver or spleen, with organs palpable more than 4 cm below the costal margins (see Table 10-1). Lymphadenopathy caused by leukemic infiltration is an equally frequent presenting sign. Generally, the degree of organ infiltration correlates with peripheral blood blast count, thus reflecting the total leukemic mass. Leukemic invasion of tissues may, however, be occult and detectable only by histologic sampling.

Peripheral Blood

Clinical laboratory data often provide a broad spectrum of abnormal findings at the time of diagnosis of leukemia. Anemia, abnormal leukocyte counts and differential, and thrombocytopenia are common (see Table 10-1). However, some children with ALL may have normal peripheral blood cell counts at the time of diagnosis, even when the bone marrow is replaced by leukemic cells.

The red blood cells are usually normochromic and normocytic. Failure of erythroid production is manifested by a low reticulocyte count. Peripheral blood smear may reveal teardrop forms and nucleated red cells, consistent with marrow invasion.

Platelet counts may vary from normal to extremely low. Most children have fewer than 100,000 cells/mm³ at presentation, and the platelets are usually of normal size. In contrast to idiopathic thrombocytopenic purpura (ITP), thrombocytopenia at the time of ALL diagnosis is usually accompanied by other hematologic or physical manifestations of leukemia.[55]

There is a wide range of leukocyte counts observed at the time of diagnosis, from extremely low to more than 1 million cells/mm³. Approximately 20% of children with ALL present with leukocyte counts of more than 50,000 cells/mm³.[56] Even with high presenting leukocyte counts, absolute granulocytopenia is common. Blast forms may not be present on routine smears of peripheral blood, especially in leukopenic patients. Even when present, peripheral blast cells may be misleading, and the definitive diagnosis of leukemia cannot be made from the peripheral blood. For example, myeloblasts may be detected

in the peripheral blood when the marrow has been infiltrated by various disorders, including osteopetrosis, myelofibrosis, granulomatous infections, sarcoidosis, metastatic tumor, and even ALL. Additionally, in patients with leukemia, the morphologic appearance of leukemic blast cells in the peripheral blood may differ from that of the marrow.

Hypereosinophilia has been described in association with ALL.[57] The eosinophilia may precede the diagnosis of ALL, appear at presentation, and then disappear with successful remission induction.[57,58] Eosinophilia in B-precursor ALL has been associated with the t(5;14)(q31;q32) translocation, involving the IL-3 gene on chromosome 5 and the immunoglobulin heavy chain gene on chromosome 14.[59,60]

In regard to hyperleukocytosis, approximately 10% of children with ALL present with extremely high leukocyte counts (more than 100,000 cells/mm³) (Table 10-2).[2,3] In patients with markedly elevated leukocyte counts, blood flow in the microcirculation can be impeded by intravascular clumping of the poorly deformable blasts.[61] This may result in local hypoxemia, endothelial damage, hemorrhage, and infarction, especially in the central nervous system (CNS) and lung. Clinically significant leukostasis, resulting in intracerebral hemorrhage or respiratory failure, is more common with hyperleukocytosis in acute myelogenous leukemia (AML) than in ALL.[62] In one series, neurologic and/or pulmonary symptoms were observed in 5% to 10% of children with ALL and a presenting leukocyte count higher than 200,000 cells/mm³, and CNS hemorrhage was diagnosed in 2% of those patients (all of whom had leukocyte counts higher than 400 × 10⁹/L).[63] Treatment of hyperleukocytosis consists of vigorous intravenous hydration. Red blood cell transfusions should be administered cautiously to avoid increasing whole blood viscosity and worsening symptoms. For patients with very high presenting leukocyte counts and symptomatic leukostasis, leukapheresis or exchange transfusion may prevent hyperviscosity and lysis-related problems.[62,63]

Bone Marrow

Evaluation of the bone marrow by aspiration and biopsy is essential for making the diagnosis of leukemia. The marrow specimen is usually hypercellular and characterized by a homogeneous population of cells. Leukemia should be suspected in patients whose marrows contain more than 5% blasts, but the diagnosis should not be made on the basis of a single marrow smear with fewer than 25% blasts. In most cases of ALL, the marrow generally has more than 50% blasts.

A bone marrow aspirate may be difficult to obtain at the time of diagnosis. This is usually caused by the density of blast forms in the marrow, but it may be caused by marrow fibrosis or necrosis.[64,65] In such cases, a diagnosis can be made by bone marrow biopsy. "Touch preps" of the biopsy specimen can be helpful in elucidating morphology when aspiration is not successful.

Differences may occur in leukemic involvement found in marrow aspirates derived from widely separated sites. Patchy marrow involvement of leukemic infiltration has been reported at diagnosis and relapse.[66,67] If clinical findings suggest leukemia, but a single-site bone marrow specimen is normal, the marrow should be sampled at additional sites.

The distinction between ALL with lymph node involvement and non-Hodgkin's lymphoblastic lymphoma with bone marrow invasion (stage IV) is arbitrary. Commonly, the disease is classified as ALL when there are more than 25% lymphoblasts in the marrow and as stage IV non-Hodgkin's lymphoblastic lymphoma when there are fewer than 25% lymphoblasts in the marrow. Although the lymphoblasts of ALL and lymphoblastic lymphoma appear morphologically and immunophenotypically indistinguishable, gene expression profiling studies have suggested that there may be differences in underlying biology between these two diagnoses.[68] However, the distinction may not be clinically important because advanced-stage lymphoblastic lymphoma and ALL respond similarly to intensive ALL-type therapy.[39,69,70]

Extramedullary Leukemia

Although marrow replacement is the major cause of symptoms of leukemia, many important syndromes result from extramedullary invasion. These are discussed in this section.

Central Nervous System Manifestations

Up to 20% of children will have blast cells visible on a cytocentrifuged cerebrospinal fluid (CSF) specimen at diagnosis.[71,72] These cells can usually be identified by the use of cytocentrifugation and Wright-Giemsa staining. Such morphologic evaluation is necessary to distinguish the pleocytosis of leukemic meningitis from that induced as a result of intrathecal chemotherapeutic agents (arachnoiditis) or from CNS infections.[73] Contamination of the CSF with peripheral blood, as indicated by the presence of erythrocytes, can make interpretation of the results difficult, and may adversely affect prognosis.[72,74]

Clinical symptoms related to CNS involvement at the time of diagnosis are uncommon, even in children with detectable CSF lymphoblasts. Symptomatic patients may present with diffuse or focal neurologic signs and symptoms, including manifestations of increased intracranial pressure (vomiting, headache, papilledema, and lethargy), seizures, and nuchal rigidity. Cranial nerve palsies are rare, with the facial nerve being the most frequently involved.[75,76] When it is affected, unilateral facial nerve paralysis may precede the symptoms and signs of increased intracranial pressure. CNS leukemia rarely presents as hypothalamic involvement, resulting in excessive weight gain, behavior disturbances, and hirsutism.[77] Other rare manifestations of CNS leukemia include central

pontine myelinosis,[78] cerebellar involvement, multifocal leukoencephalopathy,[79] and diabetes insipidus.[80] Clinically significant spinal cord involvement has been reported in ALL, manifesting as a localized epidural leukemic infiltrate compressing the cord.[81]

Anterior Mediastinal Mass

Leukemic infiltration of the thymus appears as an anterior mediastinal mass on a chest radiograph. It is observed in about 10% of newly diagnosed patients and is almost always associated with T-cell immunophenotype (see Table 10-1). Leukemic infiltration of the mediastinal structures may cause life-threatening tracheobronchial or cardiovascular compression. Pleural effusion may also be associated with thymic enlargement, which can exacerbate respiratory distress. Prompt initiation of systemic chemotherapy (e.g., corticosteroids) is necessary to handle such emergencies and, rarely, emergent radiation may be indicated.

Genitourinary Tract Manifestations

Testicular Enlargement. The clinical presentation of testicular ALL is a painless enlargement of one or both testes. Clinically detectable testicular leukemia is uncommon at diagnosis, occurring in 1% to 2% of boys, and does not appear to have prognostic significance.[82,83] Occult testicular involvement at diagnosis is more common, especially in the presence of a high tumor burden. In a study in which testicular biopsies were performed in boys with newly diagnosed ALL, approximately 20% had microscopic leukemic involvement.[84] However, this finding does not appear to have any prognostic significance, and routine testicular biopsies at the time of diagnosis to document occult disease are not recommended.

Other Genitourinary Tract Sites of Involvement. Ultrasonographically enlarged kidneys have been observed in children with ALL at the time of diagnosis and are thought to be primarily caused by leukemic infiltration.[85] Renal enlargement in acute leukemia may also be related to hyperuricemia, hemorrhage, and pyelonephritis. Hypertension is more commonly associated with the treatment of leukemia, especially with the prolonged use of corticosteroids, than with renal involvement. Occasionally, urolithiasis is observed at presentation or during therapy for ALL. Most renal stones in ALL patients are calcium-based in composition, and occur most frequently during phases of therapy that include corticosteroids.[86] Although leukemic bladder infiltration may rarely result in hematuria,[87] the latter is most often associated with thrombocytopenia or hemorrhagic cystitis induced by cyclophosphamide.

Priapism is rare and usually associated with an elevated white blood cell count.[88] The pathogenesis may be caused by involvement of sacral nerve roots or it may be related to mechanical obstruction of the corpora cavernosa and dorsal veins by leukemic infiltration or leukostasis.

Ovarian involvement has been found at the time of autopsy in 30% of girls with leukemia.[89] Reports of isolated ovarian involvement are rare and most of the girls had other extramedullary sites involved as well.[90,91] Leukemic involvement of the fallopian tubes, uterus, broad ligaments, and pelvic lymph nodes has been described.[90]

Bone and Joint Manifestations

As many as 40% of patients with childhood leukemia initially present with a limp or painful bones or joints.[92-94] Bone pain may be the result of direct leukemic infiltration of the periosteum, periosteal elevation of underlying cortical disease, bone infarction, and/or expansion of the marrow cavity by the leukemic cells. Pain and swelling of the joint are less frequent but may be presenting manifestations of disease and can initially cause confusion in the diagnosis.[95,96] Migratory joint pain accompanied by swelling and tenderness can be misdiagnosed as juvenile rheumatoid arthritis or rheumatic fever.[93,96]

Up to 25% of children with ALL have characteristic radiographic changes such as osteopenia and fracture at diagnosis, including vertebral compression fractures.[93,94,97] Some patients have radiographic changes in the absence of bone pain, whereas others have bone pain unaccompanied by radiographic changes. Radiographic changes are most often seen in the long bones, especially around the areas of rapid growth (e.g., the knees, wrists, and ankles), and include subperiosteal new bone formation, transverse metaphyseal radiolucent bands, osteolytic lesions involving the medullary cavity and cortex, diffuse demineralization, and transverse metaphyseal lines of increased density (growth arrest lines).[98,99] The latter probably represent regions of growth arrest during active phases of the disease rather than direct infiltration by leukemic cells.

Gastrointestinal Manifestations

The most common gastrointestinal manifestation of leukemia is bleeding, as reflected by gross or occult blood in the stool. This is usually secondary to thrombocytopenia, disseminated intravascular coagulopathy, or the toxic effects of chemotherapy on the gastrointestinal mucosa. Leukemic infiltrates in the lower gastrointestinal tract are commonly observed at autopsy but rarely cause clinical problems, except in the terminally ill relapsed patient. Such individuals may develop symptoms of an acute abdomen secondary to perforation, infarction, or infection of the infiltrated bowel wall. Severe hepatic dysfunction, presumably from leukemic infiltration, has been observed at diagnosis in some children with ALL and can complicate initial therapy, because many induction agents are hepatically metabolized and/or hepatotoxic.[100,101]

Ocular Manifestations

Ophthalmic manifestations of leukemia can be observed in more than a third of all newly diagnosed patients.[102] Leukemia can involve almost all ocular structures. Retinal hemorrhages, the most frequent ocular abnormality, are presumably caused by thrombocytopenia or anemia.[103] However, local infiltration of the capillary vessel walls with subsequent rupture and hemorrhage also may occur, especially in patients with very high leukocyte counts. Ocular motor palsies and papilledema are indicative of meningeal leukemia. Occasionally, the optic nerve may be directly involved by leukemic infiltration.[104] In such situations, visual acuity may be markedly affected, and patients may present with monocular blindness. Prompt radiation therapy may be necessary to salvage useful vision. Leukemic infiltration of the anterior chamber with hypopyon and iritis has also been reported, and can be the first manifestation of relapse.[105] Symptoms include conjunctival injection, photophobia, pain, blurring, and decreased vision.

Pulmonary Manifestations

Pulmonary complications in leukemia are most often of infectious origin, but pulmonary leukemic infiltration may occur with high presenting leukocyte counts. Pulmonary leukostasis, which can lead to respiratory failure, is much more common in AML than in ALL.[62,63] Radiographic distinction among infection, leukemic infiltration, and hemorrhage may be difficult.

Dermatologic Manifestations

Skin infiltration is uncommon in childhood leukemia, with the exception of congenital leukemia (both AML and ALL).[106] Leukemia cutis typically manifests as red or violaceous papules, nodules, or plaques.

DIFFERENTIAL DIAGNOSIS AND PROGNOSIS

A careful history and physical examination, together with an examination of the peripheral blood and bone marrow, result in a straightforward diagnosis of leukemia in the vast majority of cases. However, at times, ALL may present with the signs and symptoms of other conditions. These include ITP, aplastic anemia, juvenile rheumatoid arthritis, infectious mononucleosis and other infections, and metastatic solid tumors.

Differential Diagnosis

Idiopathic Thrombocytopenic Purpura

ITP is the most common cause of the acute onset of petechiae and purpura in children. Patients with ITP usually present with isolated thrombocytopenia, often with large platelets seen on a blood smear, contrasting sharply with the more generalized blood cell abnormalities and small platelets typically observed in patients with ALL.[55] Physical findings in ITP are usually limited to bruising or bleeding associated with thrombocytopenia. An occasional patient develops modest splenomegaly, probably caused by a recent viral infection. In most cases, the leukocyte level and differential count are unremarkable, and there is no anemia unless bleeding has been substantial or an unrelated anemia is present. Bone marrow examination is rarely necessary in uncomplicated cases of pediatric ITP (i.e., children with otherwise normal blood counts, consistent peripheral blood smear, and absence of adenopathy, hepatosplenomegaly, or other concerning findings on physical examination). However, if the diagnosis of ITP is in question or any of these concerning findings are present, clinicians should consider marrow evaluation to rule out leukemia before starting corticosteroids to avoid partially treating occult ALL.[107] The bone marrow aspirate is usually diagnostic because the marrow elements in ITP appear normal or show increased megakaryocytes.

Aplastic Anemia, Myelodysplasia, and Myeloproliferative Disorders

Like patients with leukemia, those with aplastic anemia, myelodysplasia, and myeloproliferative disease may present with pancytopenia and have fevers or infections associated with granulocytopenia. Lymphadenopathy and hepatosplenomegaly are unusual in those with aplastic anemia. The radiographic skeletal changes sometimes seen in leukemia do not occur in aplastic anemia.[108] To differentiate acute leukemia from these other disorders, biopsy of the marrow is mandatory and usually revealing. Rarely, patients with ALL present with pancytopenia and have areas of bone marrow that are fibrotic and empty, impeding diagnosis. Repeated bone marrow aspirates or biopsies establish the correct diagnosis by demonstrating areas of marrow that are infiltrated with lymphoblasts.

Rarely, patients with ALL present with a transient pancytopenia preceding the leukemic phase.[109] The pancytopenic period may persist for a few days or weeks and be accompanied by high fevers. Spontaneous recovery with a period of normal blood counts often occurs prior to the onset of ALL.[109] In those cases, ALL typically occurs within 6 months of the aplasia. However, ALL may also develop after a period of aplasia, without any recovery of blood counts.[110] Distinguishing pre-ALL pancytopenia from aplastic anemia may be difficult. The pathogenesis of the preleukemic pancytopenia prodrome is unclear. The pancytopenic presentation of ALL is more often seen in girls and does not appear to be prognostically significant.[109,110]

Juvenile Rheumatoid Arthritis and Connective Tissue Disease

Because ALL often presents primarily with joint or extremity complaints (especially limp, arthritis, or arthralgia), it may be confused with juvenile rheumatoid arthritis (JRA) or other autoimmune disorders.[93,96] Children with JRA can manifest fever, pallor, splenomegaly, and anemia, and patients with ALL can present with a positive test for antinuclear antibody (ANA), highlighting how difficult it may be to distinguish these conditions from each other.[96] Because of this difficulty, bone marrow aspiration should be considered before initiating corticosteroid therapy in children with presumed JRA.

Infectious Mononucleosis and Other Viral Infections

Childhood infectious mononucleosis and other viral illnesses can masquerade as leukemia. Patients may have generalized lymphadenopathy, splenomegaly, rash, fevers, and peripheral blood lymphocytosis. The atypical lymphocytes observed in infectious mononucleosis and other viral infections can sometimes be confused with peripheral leukemic blasts, because they are larger than normal lymphocytes. Usually, viral infections can be differentiated from leukemia without bone marrow aspiration, but the procedure is sometimes necessary for accurate diagnosis. The detection of Epstein-Barr virus infection by serology or polymerase chain reaction testing may be helpful in establishing the correct diagnosis.

Metastatic Solid Tumors

ALL and neuroblastoma may have similar presenting signs and symptoms, including fever, bone pain, and pancytopenia. Children with neuroblastoma frequently have malignant involvement of liver, lymph nodes, bone, or bone marrow; the marrow involvement may be extensive. Occasionally, neuroblasts are found on a peripheral blood smear, and their appearance may resemble that of lymphoblasts. In the bone marrow, neuroblasts tend to cluster and form pseudorosettes, in contrast to the diffuse involvement generally observed in ALL. The diagnosis of neuroblastoma can be confirmed by measurement of urinary catecholamines and radiographic demonstration of an abdominal nonhepatic mass. Other tumors with extensive marrow involvement, including rhabdomyosarcoma and Ewing's sarcoma, can also rarely be confused with leukemia. If questions remain after the examination of marrow morphology, other studies, such as immunophenotype and cytogenetics, may be helpful in distinguishing leukemia from a metastatic solid tumor.

Prognostic Factors

An array of clinical and biologic features have been identified as prognostically significant in childhood ALL, including age, presenting leukocyte count, immunophenotype, chromosomal abnormalities (ploidy, translocations), the presence of overt

CNS leukemia at diagnosis, and the rapidity with which patients respond to initial induction chemotherapy.[56] Ultimately, the prognostic significance of any factor is treatment-dependent, and the importance of a particular presenting feature in predicting outcome may vary, depending on the therapy delivered to that patient.

Age

The age of patients with ALL significantly correlates with clinical outcome. In childhood ALL, infants and adolescents have a worse prognosis than patients in the intermediate age group (aged 1 to 10 years).[111] ALL in infancy (younger than 1 year at diagnosis) is associated with high presenting leukocyte counts, increased frequency of central nervous system leukemia at presentation, and a high incidence of rearrangements of the *MLL* gene on chromosome 11q23 (see Table 10-2).[28,29,111] Even when treated with intensified regimens, infants with *MLL* gene rearrangements have a dismal prognosis, with long-term event-free survival rates ranging from 10% to 30%.[111-115]

Adolescents (10 to 21 years of age) with ALL also have a less favorable outcome than children aged 1 to 10 years, although not as poor as infants. Adolescents with ALL more frequently present with adverse features at diagnosis, including T-cell immunophenotype, higher presenting leukocyte counts, and a lower incidence of potentially favorable cytogenetic abnormalities, including high hyperdiploidy and the *TEL/AML1* gene fusion (see Table 10-2).[111,116]

Leukocyte Count

The initial peripheral blood leukocyte count is a significant predictor of treatment outcome, with worsening outcomes as the leukocyte count increases.[56] Since 1996, based on the recommendation of the Cancer Therapy Evaluation Program (CTEP) of the National Cancer Institute (NCI), many investigators have considered a leukocyte count of 50,000 cells/mm^3 as the level separating patients with a higher risk of relapse from those with a more favorable prognosis.[56]

Immunophenotype

Historically, immunophenotype was considered an important prognostic factor, with inferior outcomes observed in patients with mature B-cell and T-cell disease. However, if they are treated with more intensive regimens, children with T-cell phenotype fare as well as those with B-precursor disease.[39] As noted earlier, mature B-cell ALL is more effectively treated with the same therapy used for advanced-stage Burkitt's lymphoma.[11,12]

Some investigators have reported prognostic differences within subsets of patients with B-precursor ALL. Initial studies have suggested that patients with pre-B ALL (cIg+) have a worse outcome than those with early pre-B ALL (cIg–).[32] Subsequent reports indicated that the adverse outcome of patients with pre-B ALL was caused by the subset with the t(1;19) translocation.[33] However, with greater treatment intensity, even patients with this cytogenetic abnormality may not have an adverse prognosis.[34,35]

In approximately 15% to 30% of patients with newly diagnosed ALL, flow cytometry reveals coexpression of at least one myeloid antigen on the cell surface of the lymphoblasts.[49,53,54] Myeloid antigen coexpression has been associated with several genetic abnormalities, including the *TEL/AML1* fusion [t(12;21)], *MLL* gene (11q23) rearrangements, and the Philadelphia chromosome (*BCR/ABL* rearrangement), but is almost never observed in high hyperdiploid ALL (51-65 chromosomes).[53,117,118] Preliminary findings suggested that patients with myeloid antigen coexpression fared less well than other patients with ALL[54]; however, more recent reports have indicated that myeloid antigen coexpression is not an independent prognostic factor.[49,53,119]

Chromosomal Abnormalities

Several recurrent chromosomal abnormalities are important prognostic factors in childhood ALL. Two abnormalities, high hyperdiploidy (51 to 65 chromosomes or a DNA index greater than or equal to 1.16) and the cryptic t(12;21) (*TEL/AML1* fusion), have been associated with a favorable prognosis.[120-123] High hyperdiploidy is observed in 25% to 30% of cases of childhood ALL and is more common in younger (non-infant) children with B-precursor phenotype and low leukocyte counts.[124] The most favorable outcomes in high hyperdiploid ALL patients have been associated with the presence of trisomies of chromosomes 4, 10, and 17.[125-127]

The *TEL/AML1* fusion, which is rarely detected by karyotypic analysis, has been identified in approximately 20% of children with ALL using other more sensitive techniques, such as fluorescence in situ hybridization (FISH) and the reverse transcriptase–polymerase chain reaction (RT-PCR) assay.[128,122] Like high hyperdiploidy, the *TEL/AML1* fusion is more common in younger (non-infant) patients with low leukocyte counts and is observed almost exclusively in patients with B-precursor phenotype. Up to 80% of children with B-precursor ALL diagnosed between the ages of 2 and 7 years have high hyperdiploidy or the *TEL/AML1* fusion,[129] although never both; these two chromosomal abnormalities appear to be mutually exclusive.[130,131] Whereas the results of retrospective and prospective studies have confirmed that children with *TEL/AML1*-positive ALL have favorable event-free survival rates, there are conflicting data about whether the presence of this fusion has independent prognostic significance.[122,123,132-136] When relapses are observed in children with *TEL/AML1*-positive ALL, they tend to occur relatively late and may be more responsive to post-relapse salvage therapy.[122,135,137]

Chromosomal abnormalities associated with an adverse prognosis include hypodiploidy (fewer than 44 or 45 chromosomes),[138-140] rearrangements of the *MLL* gene on chromosome 11q23,[112,138,141] and the Philadelphia chromosome [t(9;22)].[138,142-145] *MLL* gene rearrangements are more frequent in infants than in older children with ALL.[141] The incidence of Philadelphia chromosome–positive ALL increases with age at diagnosis, and is more common in adolescents and young adults.[142,144] Intrachromosomal amplification of the *AML1* gene on chromosome 21, detected in 1% to 2% of children with ALL, may also be associated with an inferior outcome.[124] The adverse prognostic significance of the t(1;19) translocation appears to be abrogated with more intensive therapy.[34,35] Chromosomal abnormalities in childhood ALL are reviewed in depth in Chapter 5.

Overt Central Nervous System Disease at Diagnosis

Approximately 15% to 20% of children with ALL present with detectable lymphoblasts in their cerebrospinal fluid.[71,72] Some children, such as those diagnosed within the first 12 months of life and those with T-cell ALL, have a higher incidence of CNS leukemia at diagnosis.[111]

Most investigators consider the presence of overt CNS disease at diagnosis to be an adverse prognostic indicator, and these patients are usually treated with more aggressive therapy. CNS status at presentation is usually classified as CNS-1 (no blast cells), CNS-2 (fewer than five leukocytes per microliter with blast cells), and CNS-3 (more than five leukocytes per microliter with blast cells or cranial nerve palsy).[56] Historically,

CNS leukemia was defined as CNS-3 status (observed in approximately 5% of patients at diagnosis).[71,72] CNS-3 status at diagnosis is associated with a lower probability of event-free survival.[72] Several investigators have reported that patients with CNS-2 status also have a higher risk of relapse, although it does not appear to be as high as in patients with CNS-3 status at diagnosis.[71,72] Intensification of CNS-directed therapy (e.g., increasing the frequency of intrathecal chemotherapeutic treatments) may abrogate the adverse prognostic significance of CNS-2 status.[146] Thus, patients with CNS-2 status at diagnosis usually receive extra doses of intrathecal chemotherapy without other changes in treatment, whereas those with CNS-3 status are typically classified as higher risk and receive more intensive systemic and CNS-directed therapies.

Traumatic lumbar punctures (defined as 10 or more red blood cells per microliter) with lymphoblasts on cytospin have also been associated with an adverse prognosis.[72,74] Like patients with CNS-2 status, those with traumatic lumbar punctures with lymphoblasts at diagnosis may also benefit from additional doses of intrathecal chemotherapy.[72]

Early Response to Induction Chemotherapy

The rapidity with which a patient responds to initial chemotherapy is a significant predictor of long-term outcome.[147] Early response to therapy has been evaluated using morphologic measures (residual microscopic leukemia) and more sensitive techniques, such as PCR and flow cytometry.

Morphologic Response to Therapy. Patients who require two or more cycles of induction chemotherapy to achieve complete remission (CR) have a much worse prognosis than those who achieve CR within 1 month of diagnosis.[148,149] The Berlin-Frankfurt-Munster (BFM) group treats patients with one week of corticosteroid monotherapy (and one dose of intrathecal methotrexate) prior to beginning multiagent induction chemotherapy, and has reported that poor peripheral blood response at the end of that week (defined as an absolute blast count of $1000/mm^3$) is an independent predictor of adverse outcome.[150] Others have reported that the rate of clearance of blasts from the peripheral blood after multiagent chemotherapy is also an independent predictor of relapse.[151-153] Similarly, the persistence of leukemia in bone marrow specimens obtained 7 or 14 days after beginning multiagent chemotherapy strongly correlates with poor outcome,[147] although intensification of therapy can abrogate the adverse prognostic significance of slow early response.[154]

Minimal Residual Disease. Minimal residual disease (MRD) evaluation involves the measurement of very low levels of leukemia using sensitive techniques, such as PCR or specialized multiparameter flow cytometry. Leukemic cells are identified using targets identified at diagnosis, including leukemia-specific immunophenotypes (for flow cytometry–based assays), chromosomal translocations, or lymphoblast-specific immunoglobulin or T-cell antigen receptor gene rearrangements (for PCR-based assays). Using these techniques, leukemia cells have been identified at levels as low as 1 in 1000 to 1 in 100,000 cells.[155-158]

Many studies have demonstrated that MRD levels early in therapy are a significant and independent predictor of long-term outcome.[155,159-163] For patients achieving a morphologic remission at the end of induction therapy, those with higher levels of MRD at that time-point have a higher risk of relapse than those with lower or undetectable MRD.[155,159-161,163,164] The risk of relapse directly correlates with MRD level—that is, those with the highest MRD levels at the end of remission induction have the worst prognosis. High levels of MRD detected soon after commencing with postinduction therapy (weeks 12 to 14 of treatment) have also been associated with an increased risk of relapse,[155,159,160] as have high levels measured as early as day 15 of induction therapy.[162,165]

Other Prognostic Factors

Gender and Race. Some investigators have reported that males fare worse than female patients.[166,167] This observation had been attributed, in part, to the risk of testicular relapse,[166] although higher relapse rates in males have been observed even when testicular relapse rates were low.[167] Race may also influence outcome, with lower event-free survival (EFS) rates reported for African American and Hispanic patients, even after adjustment for differences in prognostically significant presenting features.[168,169] The reasons why patients of different gender or race have varying responses to therapy on certain regimens have not been fully elucidated, but may in part be related to differences in pharmacogenomics.

Pharmacogenomics. Several studies have suggested that outcome may be affected by how rapidly and effectively an individual patient metabolizes certain chemotherapeutic agents. Polymorphisms in genes involved in chemotherapy drug metabolism have been associated with risk of relapse.[170] More favorable long-term outcomes have been reported in patients with mutant thiopurine methyltransferase phenotypes involved in the metabolism of thioguanines, such as 6-mercaptopurine,[171,172] although such patients may also be at higher risk of developing significant treatment-related toxicities, including low blood counts, infection, liver dysfunction, and second malignancies.[173,174] Investigations of other genes, such as the glutathione S-transferase genes (encoding enzymes involved in the intracellular detoxification of various compounds)[175,176] and the folate metabolism genes (e.g., thymidylate synthase, methylenetetrahydrofolate reductase, and methylenetetrahydrofolate dehydrogenase)[177-179] have led to conflicting results, without clear consensus regarding the prognostic significance of various polymorphisms.

THERAPY

Historical Background

Over the last 50 years, there has been a dramatic improvement in the prognosis of children with ALL (Fig. 10-3). Prior to 1947, when the first complete remission in childhood ALL was attained by Farber and colleagues,[180] the median duration of survival from the time of diagnosis was 2 months.[181] During the 1950s, drugs such as 6-mercaptopurine, methotrexate, and corticosteroids were found to be active in leukemia-bearing mice and subsequently in human leukemias.[182,183] The first controlled clinical trials were conducted by Frei and associates,[184] who ushered in the era of single-agent (and soon thereafter combination-agent) antileukemic chemotherapy trials.[184,185] Active drugs introduced in the 1960s and 1970s included the anthracyclines (doxorubicin and daunorubicin), asparaginase, and the epipodophyllotoxins (etoposide and teniposide).[186-188]

With current regimens for the treatment of childhood ALL, more than 95% of patients achieve complete remission and approximately 80% are long-term event-free survivors (Table 10-3 and Fig. 10-4).[2-4] This is true despite the fact that with few exceptions, the drugs used for the treatment of ALL today were all available by the late 1960s. Improvement in outcome over the last 30 to 40 years can be attributed to many factors, including the following: (1) the development of complex

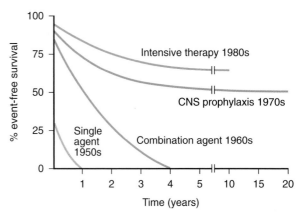

FIGURE 10-3. Historical perspective of the treatment of childhood acute lymphoblastic leukemia. The single-agent era resulted in few complete remissions and no cures. The combination-agent era without adequate central nervous system (CNS) treatment resulted in high complete remission rates but almost uniform mortality. Between the mid-1960s and 1970s, combination chemotherapy and CNS treatment resulted in prolonged, disease-free survival for approximately 50% of children. Intensive therapy in the 1980s and 1990s resulted in an event-free survival of 75% to 80% of children.

chemotherapeutic regimens designed to achieve clonal eradication; (2) improvements in supportive care; (3) recognition of the central nervous system as a sanctuary site; and (4) application of risk-directed therapy.

Risk-Adapted Therapy

After the addition of CNS-directed therapy improved cure rates to approximately 50% in the 1970s, investigators compared presenting features in patients who were cured and those who relapsed to establish clinically relevant prognostic factors. Subsequent clinical trials used these prognostic factors to stratify therapy. More intensive therapy was administered to those patients considered to be at the highest risk of relapse. In contrast, some of the more morbid components of therapy were modified or eliminated for those children considered to have the best prognosis. The goal of risk-adapted therapy is to treat away adverse presenting features, so that high-risk and low-risk patients have similar cure rates. For example, on DFCI ALL Consortium protocols, children with T-cell ALL (historically, a subgroup with an inferior prognosis) are treated as high-risk patients (receiving higher cumulative dosages of anthracycline and corticosteroid than lower risk patients); with that therapy, their outcomes are as favorable as those with B-precursor disease.[39]

For many years, pediatric cooperative groups and institutions applied prognostic factors differently when defining risk categories for clinical trials. A more uniform approach to risk classification was proposed and agreed on at an NCI-sponsored workshop held in 1993.[56] For patients with B-precursor ALL, the standard-risk category was defined as age between 12 months and younger than 10 years and initial leukocyte count lower than 50,000/mm³. The remaining patients were considered to have high-risk ALL. Other characteristics used by the various cooperative groups to classify patients as high risk include T-cell phenotype, certain cytogenetic abnormalities (e.g., Philadelphia chromosome, *MLL* gene rearrangements, and hypodiploidy), CNS-3 status at diagnosis, and slow early response to induction chemotherapy, as measured by morphology and/or MRD.[56,189] These various prognostic factors are

TABLE 10-3   **Outcome by Presenting Features of 491 Children and Adolescents (Ages 0-18 years) Treated on Dana-Farber Cancer Institute ALL Consortium Protocol 95-01 (1996-2000)**

Presenting Feature	No. of Patients	5-year EFS (±SE)
Overall	491	82 ± 2
Age at diagnosis (yr)		
<1	14	42 ± 13
1-9	385	84 ± 2
≥10	92	75 ± 5
WBC (× 10^9/L)		
<20	318	87 ± 2
20-49	76	71 ± 5
50-99	43	79 ± 6
≥100	54	66 ± 7
Immunophenotype		
B precursor	434	81 ± 2
T cell	52	85 ± 5
Central nervous system (CNS) leukemia		
CNS-1	403	83 ± 2
CNS-2	49	72 ± 7
CNS-3	12	75 ± 13
Traumatic	19	68 ± 11
Gender		
Male	274	79 ± 3
Female	217	84 ± 3
B-precursor cell National Cancer Institute Risk Group		
Standard	299	86 ± 2
High	121	70 ± 4

EFS, event-free survival; SE, standard error.

Adapted from Moghrabi A, Levy DE, Asselin B, et al. Results of the Dana-Farber Cancer Institute ALL Consortium Protocol 95-01 for children with acute lymphoblastic leukemia. Blood. 2007;109:896-904.

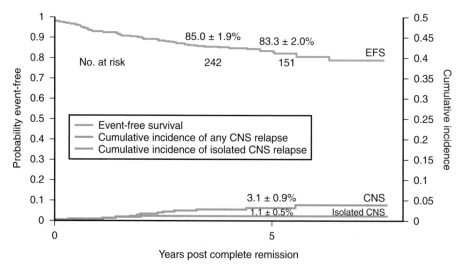

FIGURE 10-4. Event-free survival and cumulative incidence of any CNS relapse and of isolated CNS relapse for 377 patients treated on DFCI ALL Consortium protocol 91-01, conducted from 1991 to 1995. Median follow-up was 5 years.[2,41] *(Adapted from Silverman LB, Declerck L, Gelber RD, et al. Results of Dana-Farber Cancer Institute Consortium protocols for children with newly diagnosed acute lymphoblastic leukemia [1981-1995]. Leukemia. 2000;14:2247-2256.)*

discussed earlier. Ultimately, treatment is the most important prognostic factor, and those factors used to risk-stratify patients on one regimen may be irrelevant for patients treated on a different regimen.

Phases of Therapy

In general, treatment regimens for children with newly diagnosed ALL include four phases: remission induction,

CNS-directed therapy, intensification (or consolidation), and continuation (or maintenance). The remission induction phase of therapy is designed to destroy measurable leukemia cells rapidly and minimize residual leukemia burden (i.e., the total number of leukemic cells in the body). The CNS treatment phase is used to address the issue of pharmacologic sanctuary sites (i.e., areas of the body, such as the brain and spinal cord, that are not well penetrated by conventional doses of most antileukemic drugs). The intensification or consolidation phase is designed to reduce the total body leukemia cell burden further and address issues of antileukemic drug resistance. The continuation or maintenance phase, consisting of low-dose chemotherapy, is designed to eradicate the residual leukemia cell burden.

Remission Induction

After the diagnosis of ALL has been established and any urgent medical issues, such as metabolic imbalances, have been addressed, antileukemic chemotherapy should be initiated without delay.

The initial phase of treatment, remission induction, is designed to reduce the leukemic cell burden to a clinically and hematologically undetectable level. Hematologic remission is defined as attainment of a normocellular bone marrow with 5% or fewer blasts, and peripheral blood without lymphoblasts, with a granulocyte count exceeding 500 to 1000/mm^3 and a platelet count exceeding 100,000/mm^3. Complete remission is defined as achievement of these criteria plus the absence of any signs and symptoms of extramedullary leukemia. A complete remission must be induced before the next component of therapy is begun. The duration of most induction regimens is 4 to 6 weeks.

Clinical trials in the 1960s demonstrated that combinations of two agents were consistently superior to single agents for inducing complete remission in children with ALL. Vincristine and prednisone produced complete remission in approximately 90% of pediatric patients with ALL.[190,191] Addition of a third drug increased both the number of patients who achieved complete remission and the long-term relapse-free survival.[192,193] Current induction regimens, therefore, consist of at least three agents, most often L-asparaginase or an anthracycline, in addition to vincristine and prednisone.

Many groups have further intensified induction regimens to include four or more agents. In theory, these more intensive induction regimens may prevent the emergence of drug-resistant leukemic clones by an initial leukemic cell lysis of greater rapidity and magnitude.[194] The benefit in terms of long-term survival of using four drugs during induction therapy (vincristine, prednisone, asparaginase, and an anthracycline) is widely accepted in higher risk patients[195] but less clear in lower risk patients.[196] Other agents that have been added to induction regimens include epipodophyllotoxins (teniposide, etoposide)[197] and antimetabolites (e.g., methotrexate).[41] Intensive induction regimens may enhance long-term survival, but can result in increased short-term morbidity, especially from infections during periods of granulocytopenia. However, even with intensive induction regimens, few toxic deaths are reported.[2,3,198]

The initiation of CNS treatment is an integral component of induction therapy. After the diagnosis of ALL has been established by bone marrow examination, a lumbar puncture is performed for diagnostic and therapeutic purposes. It is generally recommended that intrathecal chemotherapy be given with the first diagnostic lumbar puncture to reduce the theoretical risk of inadvertently seeding the meninges with peripheral blood lymphoblasts.[74] In addition to the diagnostic lumbar puncture, intrathecal chemotherapy is usually administered at least one more time during the first month of treatment. Patients with lymphoblasts present on their initial CSF specimen (CNS-2 or CNS-3 status, or traumatic lumbar puncture with blasts) typically receive more doses of intrathecal chemotherapy during the induction phase than those without any detectable CSF lymphoblasts (CNS-1 status).[72]

Failure to achieve remission after one month of therapy (induction failure) is uncommon, occurring in fewer than 5% of patients.[148,149] Induction failure is observed more commonly in patients with high presenting leukocyte counts, T-cell phenotype, slow early morphologic response (measured 7 to 14 days after starting treatment), and/or the Philadelphia chromosome.[148,149] Successful treatment of refractory ALL has been reported with the use of drugs such as cytarabine, epipodophyllotoxins (e.g., etoposide, teniposide), and anthracyclines (e.g., idarubicin).[199-201] Nelarabine (ara-G) has been shown to induce remissions in patients with refractory T-cell ALL.[202,203] Ultimately, 80% to 90% of children with initially refractory disease are able to achieve a complete remission.[148,149] Despite this relatively high complete remission rate, overall survival for patients with a history of initial induction failure is poor (20% to 30%).[148,149] Allogeneic stem cell transplantation in first remission may improve the outcome for patients with initial induction failure.[204]

Central Nervous System Treatment

In the 1960s, as systemic chemotherapy became more effective in prolonging the duration of hematologic remission in patients with ALL, the incidence of central nervous system leukemia as an initial site of relapse became progressively more common.[205,206] It was hypothesized that leukemia cells, even if subclinical, were present in the CNS in all patients, and that these cells were protected by the blood-brain barrier from systemically administered chemotherapy. Thus, the concept of the CNS as a "pharmacologic sanctuary" (i.e., an anatomic space that is poorly penetrated by systemically administered chemotherapeutic agents) emerged. The introduction of radiation therapy to treat subclinical CNS leukemia in the 1970s was a pivotal step in boosting long-term disease-free survival rates in childhood ALL to 50%.[207] Although most pediatric patients are now treated without prophylactic cranial radiation, the importance of effectively treating subclinical CNS leukemia is undisputed for childhood ALL.

All successful treatment regimens for ALL include therapy directed at treating central nervous system leukemia. Options for CNS-directed therapies include cranial radiation, intrathecal chemotherapy, and CNS penetrant systemic chemotherapy.

Radiation therapy was the first modality successfully used to prevent CNS relapses. The use of radiation as CNS treatment was based on experiments demonstrating that L1210 murine leukemia could be cured when cranial radiation was added to systemic treatment with cyclophosphamide.[208] In the 1960s and 1970s, studies performed at St. Jude Children's Research Hospital (SJCRH) documented the effectiveness of CNS radiation as preventive therapy in children with ALL.[209] In one study, patients were randomized to receive 2400 cGy craniospinal radiation or no radiation. The difference in CNS relapse rates was striking: only 2 of 45 irradiated patients (4%) had their initial complete remissions ended by meningeal relapse, compared with 33 of 49 nonirradiated patients (67%).[210] Moreover, 31 of the patients who received prophylactic radiation remained alive after 18 to 20 years, compared with only 10 patients in the nonirradiated group. Subsequent studies demonstrated that 2400 cGy cranial radiation with intrathecal methotrexate is as effective in preventing CNS relapse as 2400 cGy craniospinal radiation without intrathecal chemotherapy.[211,212] Because craniospinal radiation was associated with increased toxicity, including excessive myelosuppression and spinal growth retardation, radiation directed only to the cranium administered with intrathecal chemotherapy became the standard form of CNS treatment in the 1970s.

Although 2400 cGy cranial radiation (with intrathecal chemotherapy) effectively prevents CNS relapses in children with ALL, it is also associated with subsequent learning disabilities, growth and neuroendocrinologic abnormalities, and an increased risk of second malignant neoplasms. Thus, many investigators have studied alternative CNS treatments, including lower doses of cranial radiation (1200 to 1800 cGy), high-dose systemic chemotherapy (known to achieve therapeutic levels in cerebrospinal fluid), and/or intrathecal chemotherapy. Current regimens for childhood ALL include some or all of these CNS-directed therapies.

Most pediatric protocols currently restrict the use of cranial radiation to patients with a higher risk of relapse, especially those with T-cell disease, high presenting leukocyte counts, or CNS-3 status at diagnosis.[213] Doses lower than 2400 cGy have been shown to be effective, and therefore are typically used when cranial radiation is administered. For instance, CNS and marrow relapse rates were not significantly different when the dose of cranial radiation was lowered from 2400 to 1800 cGy in consecutive Children's Cancer Study Group trials.[214] The BFM group has successfully used 1200 cGy radiation in the context of an intensive systemic regimen that included high-dose methotrexate (known to penetrate the CNS effectively).[150,215] Irradiated patients also typically receive intermittent intrathecal chemotherapy in addition to cranial radiation as CNS preventive therapy.

Systemic therapy plays an important role in the prevention of central nervous system leukemia. Penetration of the cerebrospinal fluid by drugs has been clearly demonstrated with the use of glucocorticoids[216] and high doses of methotrexate and cytarabine.[217,218] It has also been shown that systemically administered asparaginase, whose efficacy is a function of asparagine depletion, effectively lowers cerebrospinal fluid asparagine levels.[219,220]

Intrathecal chemotherapy, used in conjunction with intensive systemic therapy and/or cranial radiation, is an important component of CNS treatment. Many investigators have attempted to replace cranial radiation with frequent dosing of intrathecal chemotherapy, especially in lower risk patients. The success of these efforts appears to depend on the frequency with which intrathecal chemotherapy is delivered, as well as the intensity and CNS penetration of the systemic chemotherapy administered. Investigators from the Children's Cancer Group (CCG) demonstrated that administering intrathecal methotrexate throughout all phases of therapy was as effective in preventing CNS relapses in lower risk patients as 1800 cGy cranial radiation combined with only 6 months of intrathecal methotrexate, but only in the context of an intensified systemic regimen.[221] When a less intensive systemic regimen was used, more CNS relapses were observed in nonirradiated patients. Similarly, in a Dana-Farber Cancer Institute (DFCI) ALL Consortium study, excessive CNS relapses were observed in standard-risk males when cranial radiation was eliminated without increasing the frequency of intrathecal chemotherapy or the intensity of systemic chemotherapy.[222] However, in a subsequent study conducted by the same group, standard-risk patients who received more frequent doses of intrathecal chemotherapy had as low a CNS relapse rate as irradiated patients.[2] Randomized studies have also demonstrated that the use of dexamethasone instead of prednisone, which is thought to be less CNS penetrant, is associated with a lower rate of isolated CNS relapses in nonirradiated patients.[223,224] Thus, those regimens that have successfully eliminated cranial radiation include extended and/or frequent dosing of intrathecal chemotherapy in conjunction with intensified, more CNS penetrant systemic therapy, including dexamethasone and/or high- or intermediate-dose methotrexate.[2,146,225-228]

The goal of eliminating cranial radiation in pediatric patients is to minimize long-term sequelae (see later). Although several studies have indicated that intrathecal chemotherapy and intensive systemic therapy can be as effective as cranial radiation in preventing CNS relapses, the relative late neurocognitive toxicities of these CNS treatment strategies remains unsettled. Moreover, higher rates of acute neurotoxicity, including seizures, have been observed with regimens that included multiple courses of high-dose methotrexate and frequent doses of intrathecal chemotherapy.[229]

Intensification Therapy

The goals of intensification or consolidation therapy are to reduce the disease burden further and to adjust the intensity of treatment based on the risk of subsequent relapse. As is the case with CNS-directed therapy, most investigators agree that inclusion of an intensification phase is important, but the optimal treatment schedule remains uncertain. A wide variety of agents and schedules have been used during the intensification phase of treatment in pediatric trials. In general, there has been an attempt in lower risk patients to limit exposure to agents associated with significant acute and late toxicities while reserving the use of more intensive therapies for patients at higher risk of relapse. On some protocols, the intensification phase is administered immediately after achieving remission (early intensification), whereas on others it is given after a short period of less intensive therapy (delayed intensification).

Several childhood ALL regimens include a phase of early intensification immediately after remission induction. For example, the DFCI ALL Consortium has demonstrated that early intensification with weekly high-dose asparaginase for 20 to 30 weeks improves event-free survival for all patients.[230] The inclusion of doxorubicin in this early intensification phase has favorably affected the outcome of high-risk patients, including those with T-cell phenotype.[41,230] Several clinical trials have included early intensification with high-dose methotrexate immediately after remission induction for both low- and high-risk patients, often in place of cranial radiation.[150,231-234]

Many pediatric regimens include one or more cycles of delayed intensification, in addition to or instead of an early intensification phase. On protocols that include a delayed intensification phase, patients receive an intensive cycle of chemotherapy administered several weeks after achieving complete remission, often after a period of less intensive chemotherapy (interim maintenance). The BFM and CCG groups have demonstrated that patients with both low- and high-risk ALL benefit from such a strategy. On these protocols, the delayed intensification phase consists of a chemotherapy course almost identical to the initial remission induction phase—including vincristine, corticosteroid, anthracycline, and asparaginase—followed by a consolidation cycle consisting of cyclophosphamide, low-dose cytarabine, and 6-thioguanine or 6-mercaptopurine.[150,195,196,235] Augmentation of this regimen, including the use of two delayed intensification cycles instead of one, has led to improved outcomes for higher risk patients, including those with a slow early morphologic response to initial induction therapy.[154,236-238]

Continuation Therapy

Almost all current treatment regimens for ALL include a phase of continuation or maintenance therapy, in which patients are treated with less intensive chemotherapy to complete at least 2 years of therapy. Most continuation regimens consist of weekly low-dose methotrexate and daily oral 6-mercaptopurine. Some groups have added regular pulses of vincristine and corticosteroid to this regimen, although their benefit remains controversial.[239-241]

Several pharmacologic studies have documented highly variable bioavailability after oral administration of 6-mercaptopurine and methotrexate during the continuation phase.[242-246] This may have important prognostic implications, because lower intracellular levels of thioguanine nucleotides and methotrexate polyglutamates, the major metabolites of 6-mercaptopurine and methotrexate, have been correlated with a higher risk of relapse.[243,246,247] Variable bioavailability may be the result of various factors, including concurrent food, which may interfere with drug absorption.[245] Bioavailability of oral mercaptopurine appears to be improved if it is given in the evening, without food or milk.[245,248,249] Polymorphisms within genes involved in drug metabolism also affect rates of drug activation and clearance.[173] For example, patients with deficiency in the activity of thiopurine methyltransferase (TPMT), an enzyme that inactivates mercaptopurine, have higher rates of toxicity during continuation therapy (but also may have better survival) than patients with normal TPMT activity.[171,173] Most physicians attempt to compensate for the interindividual variations of bioavailability and metabolism by tailoring the dose of both drugs to the leukocyte count. Administration of maximally tolerated doses of methotrexate and 6-mercaptopurine during continuation therapy may improve outcome, as suggested by studies demonstrating that patients with lower leukocyte and/or neutrophil counts during continuation chemotherapy have lower relapse rates.[250,251] Lack of patient compliance with oral medications, as well as physician compliance with protocol dosages, may adversely affect the efficacy of continuation chemotherapy.[252,253]

6-Thioguanine is an alternative thiopurine which, unlike 6-mercaptopurine, does not rely on TPMT for its metabolism, resulting in higher intracellular levels of thioguanine nucleotides.[254] 6-thioguanine also has been shown to be more potent than 6-mercaptopurine in inducing cell death of lymphoblasts in vitro.[255] However, in a randomized clinical trial, there was no difference in event-free or overall survival rates when comparing 6-thioguanine and 6-mercaptopurine.[256] Additionally, the use of 6-thioguanine during the maintenance phase has been associated with significant hepatotoxicity, including veno-occlusive disease and cirrhosis, as well as higher remission death rates, primarily caused by infection.[256,257] Thus, 6-mercaptopurine remains the thiopurine of choice during the continuation phase.

Several investigators have studied the relative efficacy and toxicity of two corticosteroids used during postinduction therapy, prednisone and dexamethasone. Interest in substituting dexamethasone for prednisone stems from studies suggesting that dexamethasone has more potent in vitro antileukemic activity, higher free plasma levels, and enhanced CSF penetration.[216,258-260] In several clinical trials conducted in the 1990s, the nonrandomized substitution of dexamethasone for prednisone appeared to affect outcome favorably.[227,261] This finding was confirmed in a randomized trial conducted by the Children's Cancer Group comparing the two agents in lower risk patients, which indicated that dexamethasone was associated with a superior 5-year EFS.[223] In another randomized trial conducted in the United Kingdom, dexamethasone was associated with a superior EFS and lower incidence of CNS and non-CNS relapses in standard- and high-risk patients.[224] However, dexamethasone may also be associated with increased steroid-related toxicities, including higher rates of bony morbidity and infectious complications, especially in older children and adolescents.[223,224,262,263] Thus, the optimal corticosteroid preparation and dosing have yet to be determined, and may differ based on presenting features (such as age) and risk of relapse.

Attempts to intensify continuation therapy by administering rotating pairs of non–cross-resistant drugs, including many agents not traditionally incorporated during the continuation phase, such as cyclophosphamide, epipodophyllotoxins, and cytarabine, have led to mixed results. In studies conducted by SJCRH, this strategy resulted in improved outcomes for higher risk but not lower risk patients,[264] but also was associated with

high rates of toxicity, including secondary acute myelogenous leukemia.[265] Based on this risk, these agents (especially epipodophyllotoxins) are, in general, no longer administered to most patients during the continuation phase.

Cessation of Treatment

The optimal duration of therapy remains unknown. Most investigators continue to treat patients for 2 to 3 years, based on results of older studies, in which patients received therapy that was less intensive than in current regimens.[266] Randomized studies conducted by CCG have indicated that there was no significant difference in outcome when comparing 5 versus 3 years of therapy.[267,268] In a randomized study of 2 versus 3 years of continuation therapy, the UKALL group observed no significant survival advantage with longer therapy. In that study, patients receiving the shorter duration of therapy had a higher relapse rate, but this was counterbalanced by a higher remission death rate in those receiving 3 years of treatment.[269] Some early studies suggested that the optimal duration of therapy may be different for boys and girls, with boys benefiting from a more prolonged continuation phase,[270] although this finding may be less relevant with current intensive regimens.

Even with intensive regimens, attempts to shorten therapy duration from 2 years have not been successful. The BFM group randomized patients to receive 18 or 24 months of treatment, and observed a higher relapse rate with patients who received the shorter course of treatment.[150] Similarly, high relapse rates were observed in a nonrandomized study conducted by the Tokyo Children's Cancer Study Group, in which patients received intensified therapy for only 12 months, suggesting that truncated therapy, even if intensive, is inadequate for most children with ALL.[271]

Treatment of Special Patient Subsets

Philadelphia Chromosome–Positive Acute Lymphoblastic Leukemia

The Philadelphia chromosome, t(9;22)(q34;q11), which leads to fusion of the *BCR* and *ABL* genes, is detectable in approximately 5% of children and 20% of adults with ALL.[272] When treated on regimens with conventional chemotherapeutic agents, these patients have a dismal prognosis, with long-term EFS rates ranging from 0% to 25%.[142-145] Allogeneic stem cell transplantation in first remission leads to more favorable outcomes and has been considered the treatment of choice for children with Philadelphia chromosome–positive ALL.[273] In one study, which reviewed the outcome of 267 children with Philadelphia chromosome–positive ALL treated by 10 study groups between 1986 and 1996, patients who received a transplant in first remission from an HLA-matched related donor had a disease-free survival (DFS) rate of 65%, significantly better than patients treated with chemotherapy alone (DFS of 25%).[145] Over the last decade, with advances in HLA matching by molecular high-resolution typing, as well as improvements in supportive care, unrelated donor stem cell transplantation in first remission has emerged as a viable therapeutic option for patients with Philadelphia chromosome–positive ALL who lack a matched related donor.[274,275]

Imatinib mesylate is a selective inhibitor of the *BCR-ABL* tyrosine kinase. Phase I and II studies of single-agent imatinib in children and adults with relapsed or refractory Philadelphia chromosome–positive ALL ·have demonstrated relatively high response rates, although these responses tended to be of short duration.[276,277] Results from pilot trials in adults with newly diagnosed Philadelphia chromosome–positive ALL have suggested that the administration of imatinib mesylate in combination with multiagent chemotherapy is feasible and may be associated with higher rates of complete remission.[278,279] Further work is necessary to determine how imatinib should be incorporated into the therapy of pediatric patients.

Infants

Patients diagnosed during the first year of life represent 2% to 4% cases of childhood ALL.[280] The outcome of infants with ALL is significantly worse than that for older children, with reported long-term EFS rates of 20% to 40%.[114,281,282] The major cause of treatment failure is relapse, which tends to occur early, often in the first year after diagnosis.[113,114,283-286] In vitro chemosensitivity assays have indicated that lymphoblasts from infants with ALL are relatively resistant to agents commonly used in childhood ALL regimens, such as corticosteroids and asparaginase.[287] Infants also appear to be more vulnerable to the toxic effects of therapy, especially severe infections.[114,284,288]

The poor outcome of infants appears to be related to the biologic distinctiveness of the disease observed in this age group. Up to 80% of infants with ALL present with molecularly detectable rearrangements of the *MLL* gene on chromosome 11q23.[28,29,114,115] The presence of an *MLL* gene rearrangement is an independent predictor of poor outcome in infant ALL, with the worst outcomes observed in *MLL*-rearranged patients who present at a very young age (younger than 6 months at diagnosis) and with high presenting leukocyte counts.[114,115]

Because of their poor prognosis, infants with ALL are usually treated on separate protocols with intensified therapy. In vitro drug sensitivity testing and small, nonrandomized clinical trials have suggested that high-dose cytarabine, an agent more often used in acute myelogenous leukemia, might benefit infants with ALL.[287,289,288] In the largest clinical trial conducted for infants with ALL, the international Interfant Trials Group tested a cytarabine-intensive regimen, resulting in a 4-year EFS of 47%.[115] Some investigators have treated patients with *MLL*-rearranged infant ALL with allogeneic stem cell transplantation in first remission.[290-292] However, the role of transplantation in first remission for these infants is controversial, without clear-cut evidence that it is associated with a survival benefit.[112,115] Improvement in the outcomes of infants with ALL, especially those with *MLL* gene rearrangements, may depend on the development of novel therapies. Gene expression profiling has led to the identification of several potential therapeutic targets, including FLT3, a tyrosine kinase receptor that is overexpressed and often mutated in *MLL*-rearranged ALL.[293-295] See Chapter 12 for additional information about infant leukemia.

Adolescents

Older children and adolescents (aged 10 to 18 years at diagnosis) have a less favorable outcome than children aged 1 to 10 years at diagnosis, and more aggressive treatments are generally administered to these patients. Adolescents present more frequently with adverse prognostic features, such as a high leukocyte count, T-cell immunophenotype, and the *BCR-ABL* translocation, and a lower frequency of favorable features, such as high hyperdiploidy and the *TEL-AML1* fusion gene.[111,116,296] Adolescents also appear to be at higher risk than younger children for developing treatment-related complications, including osteonecrosis, pancreatitis, and thrombosis.[116,262,297] Several investigators have compared outcomes of older adolescents with ALL (aged 15 to 20 years) treated in pediatric or adult clinical trials, and all have found that these patients fare better with a pediatric regimen.[298-300] The superior outcome of older adolescents treated with pediatric ALL regimens may be related,

in part, to the components and increased intensity of therapy; pediatric regimens tend to include higher cumulative dosages of vincristine, corticosteroid, and asparaginase than treatments designed for adults with ALL.[298]

Down Syndrome

Children with Down syndrome have increased risk for developing both ALL and acute myeloid leukemia (AML). Approximately one half to two thirds of cases of acute leukemia in children with Down syndrome are ALL. Although the vast majority of cases of AML in children with Down syndrome occur before the age of 4 years, ALL in children with Down syndrome has an age distribution similar to that of ALL in non–Down syndrome children.[301,302] Patients with ALL and Down syndrome almost always present with B-precursor phenotype, and have a lower incidence of favorable and unfavorable cytogenetic abnormalities.[303-305] They appear to be at higher risk for developing treatment-related complications, especially those related to methotrexate, such as mucositis and myelosuppression.[306,307] Outcomes for children with Down syndrome and ALL have generally been reported to be less favorable than those of non–Down syndrome patients,[303-305] which may be related to a higher incidence of treatment-related mortality because of infection and a lower frequency of favorable biologic features, such as high hyperdiploidy and the *TEL/AML1* fusion.[302-305]

COMPLICATIONS OF TREATMENT

At Diagnosis and During Treatment

At the time of diagnosis, the major clinical problems are the results of metabolic disturbances secondary to leukemia cell lysis, disrupted hematopoiesis leading to abnormal peripheral blood counts, and leukemic infiltration of nonhematopoietic organs. Initiation of chemotherapy may exacerbate these issues and lead to additional problems, including myelosuppression, increased risk of infections, and mucosal toxicity.

Metabolic Complications

Rapid turnover of leukemia cells prior to and immediately following the initiation of chemotherapy leads to the release of intracellular contents, which can overwhelm the body's normal excretory mechanisms, especially in patients with high presenting leukocyte counts. The resultant metabolic disturbances include hyperkalemia, hyperuricemia, hyperphosphatemia, and hypocalcemia.[308,309] Patients with high levels of uric acid are at risk for the development of acute renal failure secondary to uric acid deposition in the kidney. To ensure that uric acid remains in solution in the renal tubule for optimal excretion, intravenous hydration, usually with bicarbonate-containing intravenous fluid, should be instituted immediately after diagnosis to maintain dilute, alkaline urine. In addition, administration of a xanthine oxidase inhibitor such as allopurinol, which prevents the formation of uric acid during cell lysis, should be started prior to the institution of antileukemic drugs. Recombinant urate oxidase, which catalyzes the breakdown of uric acid to the more soluble allantoin, may be used instead of allopurinol to decrease levels of uric acid rapidly, especially in patients presenting with high uric acid levels, high presenting leukocyte counts, impaired renal function, or in whom aggressive hydration is contraindicated.[310,311]

Hypercalcemia, although uncommon, has been reported in patients with ALL at diagnosis, especially in those with skeletal abnormalities, such as vertebral compression fractures and osteolytic lesions. Hypercalcemia has also been associated with the t(17,19) translocation (*E2A-HLF* fusion), an uncommon chromosomal abnormality that also leads to disseminated intravascular coagulation.[312]

Anemia and Thrombocytopenia

Thrombocytopenia, in association with anemia, is a common presenting feature of ALL[55]; however, active bleeding is a relatively unusual feature at the time of diagnosis. Prophylactic transfusions have frequently been given when platelet counts fall below 15,000 to 20,000/mm³. A study of adults with AML has demonstrated the safety of decreasing the prophylactic platelet transfusion threshold to a platelet count of 10,000/mm³ in clinically stable patients.[313] Any active hemorrhage associated with a platelet count of less than 100,000/mm³ should be treated with platelet transfusions. Similarly, symptomatic anemia should be treated by transfusion of packed red blood cells. Prophylactic transfusions are generally administered for a hematocrit below 20% to 25%. Stabilization of these two hematologic parameters should take no longer than 12 to 24 hours and should therefore not delay the start of antileukemic therapy. Similar transfusion threshold guidelines are used once patients begin therapy and experience chemotherapy-associated myelosuppression.

Coagulation Abnormalities

Disseminated intravascular coagulation (DIC) is infrequently observed in patients with ALL at diagnosis. It is more common in T-cell ALL as a result of thromboplastic substances released from T lymphoblasts.[314] DIC has also been reported in patients with the uncommon t(17;19) translocation, associated with B-precursor immunophenotype.[315] DIC should be treated promptly with infusions of fresh-frozen plasma and cryoprecipitate. L-asparaginase, a major component of therapy for children with ALL, can induce coagulopathy by inhibition of protein synthesis of clot-forming and clot-inhibitory proteins, including antithrombin III, plasminogen, and fibrinogen.[316-320] CNS and peripheral thromboses have been observed in 2% to 4% of patients receiving L-asparaginase for ALL.[2,261,321]

Infection

Life-threatening infection, observed at the time of diagnosis and during therapy, is one of the most frequent complications experienced by patients with ALL. Infections, most often bacterial and often associated with granulocytopenia, are the primary cause of treatment-related mortality in children receiving therapy for ALL.[198] Documented episodes of bacteremia have been reported in 15% to 30% of children receiving chemotherapy for ALL, and deaths caused by serious infection have been reported in up to 3% of patients.[3,198] Any febrile patient receiving therapy for ALL must be considered potentially bacteremic. Cultures should be obtained promptly, and the patient should be begun immediately on broad-spectrum antibiotics with activity against bowel and respiratory organisms while awaiting culture results.[322]

As chemotherapy regimens have become more intensive, fungal disease, including invasive infections of *Candida* and *Aspergillus* species, have also been increasingly observed during the initial treatment of leukemia.[323,324] Viral infections can also cause significant morbidity in children with ALL. Varicella complicated by pneumonitis, hepatitis, or cerebritis can be particularly devastating.[325] Postexposure prophylaxis (within 72 hours) with varicella-zoster immunoglobulin and treatment with acyclovir once symptoms develop have reduced the frequency of severe disease.[326-328] However, even with these interventions, deaths from varicella have been reported in children undergoing therapy for ALL.[329] Rare cases of measles in children with ALL have been accompanied by a high incidence of morbidity and mortality.[330,331]

Pneumocystis carinii can cause a severe, often fatal interstitial pneumonitis in children receiving multiagent chemotherapy. The incidence of *P. carinii* increases with the degree and duration of immunosuppression and thus is usually observed during the later phases of ALL therapy, but it has been observed in the earlier phases as well.[332] Prophylaxis with trimethoprim-sulfamethoxazole markedly reduces the incidence of infection with *P. carinii* and is recommended for all children receiving therapy for ALL.[333]

The use of hematologic growth factors, such as filgrastim (granulocyte colony-stimulating factor [G-CSF]), remains a matter of controversy. In prospective randomized studies, the use of filgrastim in children and adults receiving treatment for ALL was associated with a shorter duration of neutropenia and a tighter adherence to the planned treatment schedule.[334-337] However, although some investigators have reported a significantly decreased incidence in severe infections in patients treated with filgrastim during ALL therapy,[334,337] others have not confirmed this finding.[335,336] Also, filgrastim has not been shown to prolong survival or reduce the cost of supportive care for children with ALL.[335]

Typhlitis

A specific syndrome of right lower quadrant pain with rebound tenderness, abdominal distention, vomiting, and sepsis, referred to as typhlitis or necrotizing enterocolitis, can develop as a consequence of intensive chemotherapy, especially during the remission induction phase.[338,339] Findings on plain abdominal radiographs vary, but frequently show a paucity of air in the right lower quadrant.[338] Ultrasonography or CT may reveal a characteristic thickening of the colonic mucosa.[339-341] The pathogenesis of typhlitis is most likely related to mucosal and bowel wall damage secondary to chemotherapy in the setting of prolonged neutropenia. It has rarely been observed before the institution of chemotherapy.[342,343] Management includes bowel rest, intravenous fluids, and broad-spectrum antibiotics. Surgery is usually not indicated, except in the rare case of perforation or uncontrolled bleeding.[344,345] The differential diagnosis of typhlitis also includes common surgical conditions of childhood, including appendicitis and intussusception, as well as rare problems related to leukemia or antileukemic therapy, such as pancreatitis and acute cholangitis.

Acute Neurologic Toxicity

Intrathecal chemotherapy, high doses of systemic methotrexate, and cranial radiation, either alone or in combination, have been associated with acute neurotoxicity, including seizures.[229,346,347] Some of the highest rates of acute neurotoxicity have been observed in clinical trials that have used frequent dosing of intravenous and intrathecal methotrexate as a substitute for cranial radiation. For example, in a randomized trial conducted by the Pediatric Oncology Group (POG) in children with lower risk B-precursor ALL, the incidence of acute neurotoxicity was approximately 10% in patients receiving repeated courses of intermediate-dose intravenous methotrexate compared with 4% in those receiving low-dose oral methotrexate.[229]

A transient episode of somnolence, anorexia, lethargy, and fever can often be observed 6 to 8 weeks after cranial radiation.[348,349] This "somnolence syndrome" is often accompanied by electroencephalographic changes, cerebrospinal fluid pleocytosis, and fever.[350] Most children recover uneventfully, and it is not clear whether there are any long-term neurologic implications.[350]

Peripheral and autonomic neuropathy secondary to vincristine is frequently seen in children receiving ALL therapy. Signs and symptoms vary in severity, and include constipation, absent deep tendon reflexes, distal muscle weakness, gait abnormalities, parasthesias, and cranial nerve palsie.[351] Rarely, postural hypotension, bladder atony, and the syndrome of inappropriate secretion of antidiuretic hormone can occur.[351,352] Vincristine-associated neurotoxicity is usually reversible after therapy is completed, and long-term sequelae are rare.[351,353]

Other Acute Toxicities

Asparaginase is associated with pancreatitis in 5% to 10% of patients and allergic reaction in up to one third of children.[2,261] Asparaginase has also been associated with transient hyperlipidemia.[354] Complications from corticosteroids include hypertension, hyperglycemia, myopathy, mood and behavioral problems, and an increased incidence of bone fractures.[224,262,355-357]

Late Effects of Treatment

With prolonged survival of children with ALL, late effects related to the disease and its treatment have become increasingly evident. The clinical magnitude of late effects is a function of treatment and host-related factors, such as age at diagnosis. Late effects include neurocognitive deficits, short stature, obesity, bony morbidity, cardiac dysfunction, and second malignant neoplasms.

Central Nervous System Sequelae

There are a number of long-term problems associated with CNS treatment and CNS leukemia. Historically, low and low average intelligence quotients (IQs) were frequent findings in survivors of ALL.[358-360] These learning disabilities were related to a slow speed of processing information, distractibility, and difficulty in dealing with complex or conceptually demanding material.[361,362] With contemporary therapy, the severity of neuropsychological sequelae varies, dependent on treatment and patient characteristics. For example, younger children (younger than 3 to 5 years old at diagnosis) are more vulnerable than older children[358,360,363] and, in some studies, girls are more vulnerable than boys.[361,364-366] Children with meningeal relapse who receive a second course of CNS treatment are at particularly high risk of significant and progressive intellectual loss.[367-369]

Most long-term neuropsychological effects have been attributed to cranial radiation.[358,359,362,366,370] The most severely impaired long-term survivors are those who received cranial radiation doses (24 to 28 Gy), which are higher than doses used in current treatment regimens (12 to 18 Gy).[371,372] Long-term survivors treated with 18 Gy radiation (especially those who were 3 years or older at diagnosis) appear to fare relatively well, with less severe neurocognitive sequelae than children who had received higher doses of radiation. In some studies, this group of survivors does not demonstrate any significant cognitive deficits, although subtle effects are observed with detailed neuropsychological testing.[363,373]

The contribution of systemic and intrathecal chemotherapy to the development of neurocognitive sequelae has not been fully elucidated. There is evidence that cognitive deficits are present in long-term survivors treated without cranial radiation,[373-375] but these deficits do not tend to be severe and overall neurocognitive function is generally within the normal range.[366,376] In most studies of long-term survivors, nonirradiated patients have fewer and less severe impairments than those who received cranial radiation,[360,370] although with current chemotherapy regimens and lower doses of radiation, differences between the two groups may be subtle.[373] Systemic chemotherapy also affects the severity of radiation-associated neuropsychological sequelae. In one study, IQ decline was associated with combined therapy of high-dose systemic methotrexate and 1800 cGy cranial radiation, but not with either therapy alone.[377]

Neuropathologic changes in the CNS have been identified in survivors of childhood ALL. Leukoencephalopathy, a relatively rare phenomenon, is characterized by multifocal demyelination visible on radiographic imaging (CT or magnetic resonance imaging [MRI]).[378] Patients may present with a wide range of neurologic and behavioral problems, including poor school performance, confusion, memory problems, personality changes and, in its most severe form, progressive dementia and coma.[378] Risk factors for the development of leukoencephalopathy include large doses of cranial radiation (2400 cGy or higher) and/or high cumulative doses of systemic and intrathecal methotrexate.[378] In one study, the development of leukoencephalopathy was associated with escalating doses of weekly systemic methotrexate beyond 50 mg/m^2 in previously irradiated children.[379] Microcephaly has also been reported as a late effect of central nervous system treatment and was found to be dependent on the radiation dose.[380] Radiation-induced cavernous hemangiomas and other vasculopathies, sometimes leading to cerebral hemorrhage, have been reported in survivors of childhood ALL.[381,382]

Growth

In several studies, survivors of ALL are shorter than expected for their age.[383-387] Although all survivors of childhood ALL appear to be at increased risk of adult short stature, the greatest impact on final height has been noted in patients treated with 2400 cGy cranial radiation, with less severe growth failure noted in patients whose CNS treatment included 1800 cGy or no cranial radiation.[384,387,388] Young age and female gender are associated with more severe growth impairment.[383,384,386,387] Short stature in survivors of childhood ALL is occasionally associated with growth hormone deficiency,[389-391] suggesting that growth hormone replacement may have a potential therapeutic role in some patients.

Obesity is also prevalent among survivors of childhood ALL and, like short stature, is more frequently observed in girls and in those treated at a young age.[386,392-395] The cause of obesity is not clear; some investigators have reported an increased risk of obesity in survivors who received cranial radiation, especially at higher doses (higher than 20 Gy),[395,396] whereas others have not observed any relationship between body mass index and prior radiation.[386,394,397] Corticosteroids may also play a role in the development of obesity, with increased rates of obesity associated with higher cumulative dosages.[394]

Bony Morbidity

Bony morbidity, including osteopenia, fractures, and osteonecrosis, has been reported to occur in up to 30% of survivors of childhood ALL, and is primarily secondary to corticosteroids.[262] Several investigators have demonstrated that children with ALL have reduced bone mineral density during therapy,[398,399] resulting in an increased risk for fractures during and immediately after treatment.[356,400] However, it appears that bone mineral density improves once therapy is completed, although some degree of residual osteopenia may persist.[401-404] The clinical implications, if any, related to persistent osteopenia in long-term survivors have not yet been fully elucidated.

Osteonecrosis, also known as avascular necrosis, is a disabling bony toxicity, frequently involving multiple joints. Osteonecrosis can lead to significant pain and loss of function, sometimes necessitating total joint replacement.[405-407] Symptomatic osteonecrosis has been observed in 2% to 9% of children treated for ALL, with higher rates associated with higher cumulative dosages of corticosteroids.[262,297,408] Adolescents with ALL are at a much higher risk of developing symptomatic osteonecrosis, with reported cumulative incidence rates of 9% to 14%.[297,408]

Cardiac Sequelae

Echocardiographic abnormalities, particularly increased afterload and decreased contractility, are well-characterized late effects of anthracycline therapy.[409,410] The mechanism of this toxicity is impairment of myocardial growth. The severity of cardiac dysfunction is correlated with higher cumulative doses of anthracycline and higher dose rates.[409-412] Patients treated at a young age, females, and those with Down syndrome appear to be more vulnerable to anthracycline-associated cardiac toxicity.[411,412] Over the last two decades, as patients have received lower cumulative dosages of anthracyclines, symptomatic congestive heart failure has become increasingly uncommon and now only rarely occurs in long-term survivors of childhood ALL.[410,412] In a randomized study of children with high-risk ALL, the cardioprotectant agent dexrazoxane was shown to reduce the incidence of doxorubicin-associated myocardial injury (as measured by cardiac troponin-T) without affecting antileukemic outcomes.[2,413]

Sexual Development and Fertility

Ovarian and testicular function are relatively unaffected by most current childhood ALL regimens,[385,414,415] with the possible exception of programs that use high cumulative dosages of alkylating agents (e.g., cyclophosphamide).[416,417] Prophylactic gonadal radiation can also impair subsequent ovarian or testicular function,[417] but this treatment is no longer included in most regimens. Thus, sexual development is normal and fertility is preserved in the vast majority of survivors of childhood ALL. In a study of 949 female childhood ALL survivors, almost all experienced menarche within the normal range, although prior cranial radiation increased the risk of both early and late menarche.[418] In both genders, normal pubertal growth spurts may be blunted.[385,414] There is currently no evidence that the progeny of survivors of childhood ALL are at increased risk of congenital abnormalities.[419,420]

Cataracts

In one study, small, nonprogressive posterior subcapsular cataracts, which did not impair vision or require surgical treatment, were detected in over 50% of children treated for ALL.[421] Although the cataracts were thought to be related to the administration of high cumulative doses of corticosteroids, these patients had also received cranial radiation, which included treatment of the posterior half of the globes and optic nerves.

Second Malignancies

Long-term survivors of childhood ALL are at increased risk for developing second malignant neoplasms, including AML, brain tumors, non-Hodgkin's lymphomas, and carcinomas of the parotid and thyroid glands.[422-425] The overall cumulative incidence of second malignant neoplasms reported in the literature ranges from 1% to 6%, depending on the treatment regimen and length of follow-up.[422-426] Compared with age-adjusted expected incidence in the general population, survivors of ALL appear to have a 6- to 14-fold increased risk for developing another cancer.[422-426] Risk factors for the development of secondary AML include treatment with epipodophyllotoxins and alkylating agents.[427-429] For example, the cumulative risk of secondary AML was 5% to 6% after treatment with epipodophyllotoxin-containing regimens,[427,428] but less than 1% after therapy lacking both epipodophyllotoxins and alkylators.[426,430] Cranial and craniospinal radiation have been associated with an increased risk for secondary solid tumors, primarily malignant gliomas and meningiomas.[422-425] In several large studies, the long-term cumulative incidence rates of secondary brain tumors in previously irradiated patients ranged from 1.0% to 1.6%.[422,426,431] It is not clear whether radiation dose is correlated with risk of secondary tumor although, in one study, patients who had received 18 Gy cranial radiation appeared to be at lower risk than those who had received 24 Gy radiation.[423] The cumulative incidence of malignant glioma appears to plateau approximately 15 to 20 years after diagnosis although, even with 30 years of follow-up, a plateau in the incidence of meningiomas has not yet been observed.[424]

Other Sequelae

Abnormalities of dental and craniofacial development have been observed after cranial radiation and appear to be related to the age of the patient at the initiation of therapy, with younger patients more severely affected.[432] Elevations of transaminase levels are common while patients are receiving therapy, but are not associated with chronic liver disease once therapy is completed, and late-occurring hepatotoxicity is a rare phenomenon.[433,434] Chronic liver changes, including portal hypertension and cirrhosis, have been reported after the use of 6-thioguanine.[435]

RELAPSED ACUTE LYMPHOBLASTIC LEUKEMIA

Approximately 20% to 25% of children with ALL who achieve remission after initial induction chemotherapy will subsequently relapse. Several factors have been identified that influence the outcome of patients with relapsed ALL, including duration of initial remission, site of relapse, and immunophenotype.

Duration of initial remission is one of the most important prognostic factors, with significantly worse outcomes observed in patients who relapse early—defined as those occurring while on or within 6 months from completion of initial therapy—than in those with longer initial remissions.[436-440] T-lineage immunophenotype and age older than 10 years at initial diagnosis have also been associated with an adverse prognosis after relapse.[437-442] In one study, patients with low presenting leukocyte counts at relapse had a superior prognosis,[443] although others have not confirmed this finding.[436,437] The BFM group has reported that the absence of peripheral blasts at the time of a first late marrow relapse is associated with a more favorable outcome.[444]

Site of relapse also has prognostic importance, with superior outcomes observed for patients experiencing isolated extramedullary relapses compared with marrow relapses.[438,445] Some studies have suggested that patients with combined marrow and extramedullary relapses have a better prognosis than those with isolated marrow relapses,[445,446] although this has not been consistently demonstrated.[438]

By using these prognostic factors, investigators have identified subsets of relapsed patients with a relatively favorable prognosis (e.g., patients experiencing a late extramedullary relapse) who may be able to maintain durable second remissions with conventional-dose chemotherapy. Patients with a less favorable prognosis, such as those experiencing an early marrow relapse, are considered candidates for more intensive therapies, such as allogeneic stem cell transplantation.

Marrow Relapse

Marrow relapse accounts for most recurrences of childhood ALL. Induction of second complete remission can be expected in 70% to 90% of children with relapsed B-precursor ALL, but is lower in children with T-cell immunophenotype and those whose relapses occur early (less than 36 months from initial diagnosis).[439-441,447-449] After a second complete remission has been attained, subsequent treatment may include conventional-dose or high-dose chemotherapy with stem cell transplantation.

Chemotherapy

Most trials of conventional-dose chemotherapy have been unsuccessful at producing long-term survival in the majority of patients who experience a marrow relapse. In large published series, overall survival rates for children treated with chemotherapy alone (without allogeneic transplant) have ranged from 25% to 40%.[439-441]

Duration of initial remission significantly predicts the outcome of children with a marrow relapse who receive chemotherapy alone as salvage therapy. In almost all reported chemotherapy trials, overall survival after an early relapse is less than 20%.[437,440,441,448] The most successful chemotherapy trial results have been achieved with patients whose initial complete remissions exceeded 24 to 36 months. With intensive chemotherapy regimens, the probability of EFS for this subset of patients has ranged from 40% to 60%.[438,440-442] Minimal residual disease (MRD) levels may also help identify patients who might respond favorably to chemotherapy-only regimens after a marrow relapse. Several groups have demonstrated that MRD levels measured at the end of the first month of reinduction therapy predict long-term outcome in patients who have experienced a marrow relapse, with significantly higher survival rates associated with lower levels of MRD.[450,451]

HLA-Matched Sibling Allogeneic Stem Cell Transplantation

HLA-matched sibling allogeneic stem cell transplantation (SCT) is an important treatment option for children with relapsed ALL.[452-456] Transplantation in second remission has generally been more favorable than in a third or subsequent remission.[457] Survival after HLA-matched sibling SCT appears to be better when total body irradiation (TBI) is included in the preparatory regimen.[442,458] In most published reports, the most common cause of failure after allogeneic stem cell transplantation is recurrence of leukemia.[454-456] Therapy-related toxicity, including infections and severe graft-versus-host disease, is also a major cause of death, occurring in 15% to 30% of patients.[452-455,458,459] In recent years, the incidence of treatment-related complications appears to be decreasing with improvements in supportive care.[442]

As has been demonstrated in chemotherapy trials for relapsed ALL, duration of initial remission is an important predictor of outcome after matched sibling SCT, with improved survival observed in patients with longer initial remissions.[442,452] MRD levels, measured at the end of reinduction therapy and just prior to transplantation, also have been shown to predict outcome after matched sibling allogeneic SCT, with poorer survival rates observed for patients with higher levels of pretransplantation MRD.[460-462]

The indications for transplantation in second remission after marrow relapse remain controversial. Several studies have attempted to compare outcomes of patients treated with and without allogeneic SCT; however, there are many potential problems inherent in these analyses, including selection bias in terms of which patients receive a transplant. To address these issues, investigators have used matched pair analyses and other statistical methods to control for time to transplantation and other important prognostic variables when comparing the two treatment modalities. In most of these reports, HLA-matched sibling SCT has been associated with a lower relapse risk and better survival rates compared with chemotherapy-only salvage regimens for patients with early marrow relapse.[442,452,453,456] However, it is less clear that allogeneic SCT is associated with a survival advantage in patients with a late marrow relapse.[442,453]

Unrelated and Autologous Stem Cell Transplantation

Because over 80% of patients do not have histocompatible sibling donors, various methods have been developed to circumvent the lack of a matched related donor. Other potential stem cell sources for transplantation include matched unrelated donors and autologous marrow.

Historically, unrelated donor SCT in children with relapsed ALL was associated with a substantial risk of morbidity, with treatment-related mortality rates as high as 40% to 50% in some reports.[463,464] With improvements in supportive care and more accurate genomic typing of HLA antigens, treatment-related mortality after unrelated donor SCT has decreased significantly, making unrelated donor SCT a more viable treatment option.[465-467] Outcomes after unrelated donor SCT appear to be approaching those observed with HLA-matched sibling SCT. In one nonrandomized study, patients in second remission who received an unrelated SCT had an equivalent EFS to those who received a matched sibling donor SCT.[467] A similar result was reported in a comparison of unrelated cord blood and matched sibling donor SCT in children with relapsed ALL.[468] Despite an increased risk of treatment-related mortality, unrelated donor SCT has been associated with a survival advantage when compared with chemotherapy in children with early marrow relapses.[469]

Autologous transplantation has also been investigated as an option for patients in second or subsequent CR who do not have a matched related donor. Autologous transplantation has been performed in conjunction with ex vivo purging of residual leukemia in harvested marrow via immunologic or pharmacologic techniques.[470-473] For patients with long initial remissions, results achieved after autologous transplantation are comparable to those observed with chemotherapy regimens or after allogeneic SCT, with EFS rates of 40% to 50%.[459,472-474] Patients with short initial remissions fare less well with autologous SCT.[473,474] Relapse is the most common cause of treatment failure after autologous SCT, with a lower incidence of toxicity-related deaths than that observed after allogeneic SCT.[459] It does not appear that autologous SCT offers any advantage over chemotherapy[474] and, in general, it is no longer used in children with marrow relapses.

Isolated Extramedullary Relapses

Isolated extramedullary relapses, occurring either in the CNS or testicle, are less frequent than marrow relapses in ALL. Such relapse may not actually be isolated; using sensitive molecular techniques, submicroscopic marrow disease can be demonstrated in most children at the time of an isolated extramedullary relapse.[475] The level of this submicroscopic marrow disease may predict response to postrelapse therapy.[475]

Isolated CNS relapse occurs in fewer than 10% of patients with ALL (see Fig. 10-4). Although CNS remission can be successfully induced in more than 90% of such patients with CNS-directed therapy, most patients treated without intensive systemic therapy will subsequently develop a bone marrow recurrence.[476,477] Thus, in addition to CNS-directed therapy, usually radiation with intrathecal chemotherapy, patients with isolated CNS relapses are also treated with intensive systemic therapy. Several reports have indicated that intensive chemotherapy regimens in conjunction with cranial or craniospinal radiation may provide adequate postremission therapy for patients with an isolated CNS relapse, with EFS rates as high as 70%.[478-480] From the limited published data, it is not clear that allogeneic SCT is associated with a survival advantage for patients with an isolated CNS relapse. In two published comparisons, outcomes after allogeneic SCT were similar to those achieved with chemotherapy and/or radiation in children with an isolated CNS relapse.[481,482]

As with marrow relapses, patients experiencing late isolated CNS relapses have a better prognosis than those whose relapses occur earlier.[438,439,479,480] On two consecutive clinical trials conducted by the POG, children with B-precursor phenotype and a relatively late isolated CNS relapse (initial remission duration of at least 18 months) had EFS rates of 77% to 83% when treated with intensive chemotherapy and delayed cranial radiation, whereas patients with earlier relapses fared less well with the same regimen.[479,480] Some studies have indicated that patients whose initial CNS prophylaxis included cranial radiation may have a worse prognosis after an isolated CNS relapse than previously unirradiated patients.[478]

Isolated testicular relapses are uncommon, occurring in 0.5% to 1% of boys with ALL.[2,3] For boys with isolated testicular relapses, systemic chemotherapy and testicular radiation have resulted in prolonged second remissions in more than 80% of patients with late-occurring relapses.[483,484] This approach has been less successful in patients whose testicular relapses occurred during or soon after cessation of initial therapy, with long-term EFS ranging from 20% to 43%.[483,485]

Other rare sites of extramedullary relapse include eyes and ovaries. Case reports have indicated successful treatment of these patients with local radiation and intensive systemic therapy.[486,487]

FUTURE DIRECTIONS

Although risk-adapted therapy has resulted in marked improvement in the outcome of children with ALL over the last few decades, survival rates have plateaued over the last decade, suggesting that we may have reached the limits of currently applied clinical risk factors and standard chemotherapeutic agents. Molecular techniques may help identify biologic factors that may supplement or replace the epidemiologic factors currently used to determine risk-based therapy. For example, microarray gene expression studies have identified biologically distinctive and prognostically relevant subtypes of ALL based on distinctive gene expression profiles.[293,488,489] In addition, research focused on pharmacogenomics may identify patient-related factors that affect outcome and help lead to more individualized therapy.[170]

New drug development is essential to improve outcomes. Newer cytotoxic agents, such as clofarabine and nelarabine, may help improve the outcome of some high-risk patients but, like currently available drugs, are associated with significant side effects.[202,490] Imatinib, the selective inhibitor of the BCR-ABL encoded tyrosine kinase, is the prototype of a new type of antileukemic agent that is more specific and less toxic than current chemotherapy.[277] Inhibitors of the FLT3 tyrosine kinase,[295] the antiapoptotic protein BCL-2,[491] and the mammalian target of rapamycin (mTOR) pathway, which has been implicated in glucocorticoid resistance,[492] are examples of targeted therapies under investigation. Monoclonal antibodies directed toward leukemia cell surface antigens are another alternative therapeutic approach under investigation.[493]

As more children with ALL become long-term survivors, there is an increasingly important need to address issues of late sequelae and the physical and emotional costs of cure.[494,495] While awaiting the development of more specific antileukemic therapeutic modalities, the impact of currently available primary and salvage therapies must be better understood so that rational therapeutic decisions can be made, with the ultimate goal of improving survival and minimizing toxicity.

REFERENCES

1. Ries LAG, Smith MA, Gurney JG, et al. Cancer Incidence and Survival Among Children and Adolescents: United States SEER Program 1975-1995. (Publication No. 99-4649). Bethesda, Md, National Cancer Institute, SEER Program, 1999.
2. Moghrabi A, Levy DE, Asselin B, et al. Results of the Dana-Farber Cancer Institute ALL Consortium Protocol 95-01 for children with acute lymphoblastic leukemia. Blood. 2007;109:896-904.
3. Moricke A, Reiter A, Zimmermann M, et al. Risk-adjusted therapy of acute lymphoblastic leukemia can decrease treatment burden and improve survival: treatment results of 2169 unselected pediatric and adolescent patients enrolled in the trial ALL-BFM 95. Blood. 2008;111:4477-4489.
4. Pui CH, Sandlund JT, Pei D, et al. Improved outcome for children with acute lymphoblastic leukemia: results of Total Therapy Study XIIIB at St. Jude Children's Research Hospital. Blood. 2004;104:2690-2696.
5. Invernizzi R, Rosanda C, Basso G, et al. Granular acute lymphoblastic leukemia in children. "Aieop Cooperative Group for Cytology of Acute Leukemias." Haematologica. 1992;77:30-34.
6. Bennett JM, Catovsky D, Daniel MT, et al. Proposals for the classification of the acute leukaemias. French-American-British (FAB) co-operative group. Br J Haematol. 1976;33:451-458.
7. Pui CH. Childhood leukemias. N Engl J Med. 1995;332:1618-1630.
8. Hammond D, Sather H, Nesbit M, et al. Analysis of prognostic factors in acute lymphoblastic leukemia. Med Pediatr Oncol. 1986;14:124-134.
9. van Eys J, Pullen J, Head D, et al. The French-American-British (FAB) classification of leukemia. The Pediatric Oncology Group experience with lymphocytic leukemia. Cancer. 1986;57:1046-1051.
10. Lilleyman JS, Hann IM, Stevens RF, et al. Cytomorphology of childhood lymphoblastic leukaemia: a prospective study of 2000 patients. United Kingdom Medical Research Council's Working Party on Childhood Leukaemia. Br J Haematol. 1992;81:52-57.
11. Patte C, Auperin A, Michon J, et al. The Société Française d'Oncologie Pédiatrique LMB89 protocol: highly effective multiagent chemotherapy tailored to the tumor burden and initial

response in 561 unselected children with B-cell lymphomas and L3 leukemia. Blood. 2001;97:3370-3379.

12. Cairo MS, Gerrard M, Sposto R, et al. Results of a randomized international study of high-risk central nervous system B non-Hodgkin lymphoma and B acute lymphoblastic leukemia in children and adolescents. Blood. 2007;109:2736-2743.

13. Lilleyman JS, Britton JA, Anderson LM, et al. Periodic acid Schiff reaction in childhood lymphoblastic leukaemia. The Medical Research Council Working Party on Childhood Leukaemia. J Clin Pathol. 1994;47:689-692.

14. McCaffrey R, Harrison TA, Parkman R, Baltimore D. Terminal deoxynucleotidyl transferase activity in human leukemic cells and in normal human thymocytes. N Engl J Med. 1975;292:775-780.

15. Hutton JJ, Coleman MS. Terminal deoxynucleotidyl transferase measurements in the differential diagnosis of adult leukaemias. Br J Haematol. 1976;34:447-456.

16. Vogler LB, Crist WM, Bockman DE, et al. Pre-B-cell leukemia. A new phenotype of childhood lymphoblastic leukemia. N Engl J Med. 1978;298:872-878.

17. Nadler LM, Korsmeyer SJ, Anderson KC, et al. B cell origin of non-T cell acute lymphoblastic leukemia. A model for discrete stages of neoplastic and normal pre-B cell differentiation. J Clin Invest. 1984;74:332-340.

18. Greaves MF. Differentiation-linked leukemogenesis in lymphocytes. Science. 1986;234:697-704.

19. Rolink A, Melchers F. Molecular and cellular origins of B lymphocyte diversity. Cell. 1991;66:1081-1094.

20. Pui CH, Behm FG, Crist WM. Clinical and biologic relevance of immunologic marker studies in childhood acute lymphoblastic leukemia. Blood. 1993;82:343-362.

21. Crist WM, Grossi CE, Pullen DJ, et al. Immunologic markers in childhood acute lymphocytic leukemia. Semin Oncol. 1985;12:105-121.

22. Pullen DJ, Boyett JM, Crist WM, et al. Pediatric oncology group utilization of immunologic markers in the designation of acute lymphocytic leukemia subgroups: influence on treatment response. Ann N Y Acad Sci. 1984;428:26-48.

23. Felix CA, Poplack DG, Reaman GH, et al. Characterization of immunoglobulin and T-cell receptor gene patterns in B-cell precursor acute lymphoblastic leukemia of childhood. J Clin Oncol. 1990;8:431-442.

24. Korsmeyer SJ, Hieter PA, Ravetch JV, et al. Developmental hierarchy of immunoglobulin gene rearrangements in human leukemic pre-B-cells. Proc Natl Acad Sci U S A. 1981;78:7096-7100.

25. Hurwitz CA, Loken MR, Graham ML, et al. Asynchronous antigen expression in B lineage acute lymphoblastic leukemia. Blood. 1988;72:299-307.

26. Hann IM, Richards SM, Eden OB, et al. Analysis of the immunophenotype of children treated on the Medical Research Council United Kingdom Acute Lymphoblastic Leukaemia Trial XI (MRC UKALLXI). Medical Research Council Childhood Leukaemia Working Party. Leukemia. 1998;12:1249-1255.

27. Stark B, Vogel R, Cohen IJ, et al. Biologic and cytogenetic characteristics of leukemia in infants. Cancer. 1989;63:117-125.

28. Chen CS, Sorensen PH, Domer PH, et al. Molecular rearrangements on chromosome 11q23 predominate in infant acute lymphoblastic leukemia and are associated with specific biologic variables and poor outcome. Blood. 1993;81:2386-2393.

29. Pui CH, Behm FG, Downing JR, et al. 11q23/MLL rearrangement confers a poor prognosis in infants with acute lymphoblastic leukemia. J Clin Oncol. 1994;12:909-915.

30. Bene MC, Castoldi G, Knapp W, et al. Proposals for the immunological classification of acute leukemias. European Group for the Immunological Characterization of Leukemias (EGIL). Leukemia. 1995;9:1783-1786.

31. Carroll AJ, Crist WM, Parmley RT, et al. Pre-B cell leukemia associated with chromosome translocation 1;19. Blood. 1984;63:721-724.

32. Crist W, Boyett J, Roper M, et al. Pre-B cell leukemia responds poorly to treatment: a pediatric oncology group study. Blood. 1984;63:407-414.

33. Crist WM, Carroll AJ, Shuster JJ, et al. Poor prognosis of children with pre-B acute lymphoblastic leukemia is associated with the t(1;19)(q23;p13): a Pediatric Oncology Group study. Blood. 1990;76:117-122.

34. Raimondi SC, Behm FG, Roberson PK, et al. Cytogenetics of pre-B-cell acute lymphoblastic leukemia with emphasis on prognostic implications of the t(1;19). J Clin Oncol. 1990;8:1380-1388.

35. Uckun FM, Sensel MG, Sather HN, et al. Clinical significance of translocation t(1;19) in childhood acute lymphoblastic leukemia in the context of contemporary therapies: a report from the Children's Cancer Group. J Clin Oncol. 1998;16:527-535.

36. Sullivan MP, Pullen DJ, Crist WM, et al. Clinical and biological heterogeneity of childhood B cell acute lymphocytic leukemia: implications for clinical trials. Leukemia. 1990;4:6-11.

37. Berger R, Bernheim A. Cytogenetic studies on Burkitt's lymphoma-leukemia. Cancer Genet Cytogenet. 1982;7:231-244.

38. Croce CM. Chromosome translocations and human cancer. Cancer Res. 1986;46:6019-6023.

39. Goldberg JM, Silverman LB, Levy DE, et al. Childhood T-cell acute lymphoblastic leukemia: the Dana-Farber Cancer Institute acute lymphoblastic leukemia consortium experience. J Clin Oncol. 2003;21:3616-3622.

40. Sallan SE, Ritz J, Pesando J, et al. Cell surface antigens: prognostic implications in childhood acute lymphoblastic leukemia. Blood. 1980;55:395-402.

41. Silverman LB, Declerck L, Gelber RD, et al. Results of Dana-Farber Cancer Institute Consortium protocols for children with newly diagnosed acute lymphoblastic leukemia (1981-1995). Leukemia. 2000;14:2247-2256.

42. Roper M, Crist WM, Metzgar R, et al. Monoclonal antibody characterization of surface antigens in childhood T-cell lymphoid malignancies. Blood. 1983;61:830-837.

43. Crist WM, Shuster JJ, Falletta J, et al. Clinical features and outcome in childhood T-cell leukemia-lymphoma according to stage of thymocyte differentiation: a Pediatric Oncology Group Study. Blood. 1988;72:1891-1897.

44. Shuster JJ, Falletta JM, Pullen DJ, et al. Prognostic factors in childhood T-cell acute lymphoblastic leukemia: a Pediatric Oncology Group study. Blood. 1990;75:166-173.

45. Uckun FM, Gaynon PS, Sensel MG, et al. Clinical features and treatment outcome of childhood T-lineage acute lymphoblastic leukemia according to the apparent maturational stage of T-lineage leukemic blasts: a Children's Cancer Group study. J Clin Oncol. 1997;15:2214-2221.

46. Smith LJ, Curtis JE, Messner HA, et al. Lineage infidelity in acute leukemia. Blood. 1983;61:1138-1145.

47. Uckun FM, Muraguchi A, Ledbetter JA, et al. Biphenotypic leukemic lymphocyte precursors in CD2+CD19+ acute lymphoblastic leukemia and their putative normal counterparts in human fetal hematopoietic tissues. Blood. 1989;73:1000-1015.

48. Pui CH, Behm FG, Singh B, et al. Myeloid-associated antigen expression lacks prognostic value in childhood acute lymphoblastic leukemia treated with intensive multiagent chemotherapy. Blood. 1990;75:198-202.

49. Uckun FM, Sather HN, Gaynon PS, et al. Clinical features and treatment outcome of children with myeloid antigen positive acute lymphoblastic leukemia: a report from the Children's Cancer Group. Blood. 1997;90:28-35.

50. Ludwig WD, Bartram CR, Harbott J, et al. Phenotypic and genotypic heterogeneity in infant acute leukemia. I. Acute lymphoblastic leukemia. Leukemia. 1989;3:431-439.

51. Hirsch-Ginsberg C, Childs C, Chang KS, et al. Phenotypic and molecular heterogeneity in Philadelphia chromosome-positive acute leukemia. Blood. 1988;71:186-195.

52. Pui CH, Frankel LS, Carroll AJ, et al. Clinical characteristics and treatment outcome of childhood acute lymphoblastic leukemia with the t(4;11)(q21;q23): a collaborative study of 40 cases. Blood. 1991;77:440-447.

53. Pui CH, Rubnitz JE, Hancock ML, et al. Reappraisal of the clinical and biologic significance of myeloid-associated antigen expression in childhood acute lymphoblastic leukemia. J Clin Oncol. 1998;16:3768-3773.

54. Wiersma SR, Ortega J, Sobel E, Weinberg KI. Clinical importance of myeloid-antigen expression in acute lymphoblastic leukemia of childhood. N Engl J Med. 1991;324:800-808.

55. Dubansky AS, Boyett JM, Falletta J, et al. Isolated thrombocytopenia in children with acute lymphoblastic leukemia: a rare event in a Pediatric Oncology Group Study. Pediatrics. 1989;84:1068-1071.

56. Smith M, Arthur D, Camitta B, et al. Uniform approach to risk classification and treatment assignment for children with acute lymphoblastic leukemia. J Clin Oncol. 1996;14:18-24.

57. Nelken RP, Stockman JA 3rd. The hypereosinophilic syndrome in association with acute lymphoblastic leukemia. J Pediatr. 1976;89:771-773.

58. Wimmer RS, Raney RB Jr, Naiman JL. Hypereosinophilia with acute lymphocytic and acute myelocytic leukemia in childhood. J Pediatr. 1978;92:244-246.

59. Grimaldi JC, Meeker TC. The t(5;14) chromosomal translocation in a case of acute lymphocytic leukemia joins the interleukin-3 gene to the immunoglobulin heavy chain gene. Blood. 1989;73:2081-2085.

60. Hogan TF, Koss W, Murgo AJ, et al. Acute lymphoblastic leukemia with chromosomal 5;14 translocation and hypereosinophilia: case report and literature review. J Clin Oncol. 1987;5:382-390.

61. Lichtman MA, Heal J, Rowe JM. Hyperleukocytic leukaemia: rheological and clinical features and management. Baillieres Clin Haematol. 1987;1:725-746.

62. Bunin NJ, Pui CH. Differing complications of hyperleukocytosis in children with acute lymphoblastic or acute nonlymphoblastic leukemia. J Clin Oncol. 1985;3:1590-1595.

63. Lowe EJ, Pui CH, Hancock ML, et al. Early complications in children with acute lymphoblastic leukemia presenting with hyperleukocytosis. Pediatr Blood Cancer. 2005;45:10-15.

64. Hann IM, Evans DI, Marsden HB, et al. Bone marrow fibrosis in acute lymphoblastic leukaemia of childhood. J Clin Pathol. 1978;31:313-315.

65. Eguiguren JM, Pui CH. Bone marrow necrosis and thrombotic complications in childhood acute lymphoblastic leukemia. Med Pediatr Oncol. 1992;20:58-60.

66. Raney RB, McMillan CW. Simultaneous disparity of bone marrow specimens in acute leukemia. Am J Dis Child. 1969;117:548-552.

67. Ragab AH, Crist WM. Morphologic discordance in acute leukemia. N Engl J Med. 1972;287:1134-1135.

68. Raetz EA, Perkins SL, Bhojwani D, et al. Gene expression profiling reveals intrinsic differences between T-cell acute lymphoblastic leukemia and T-cell lymphoblastic lymphoma. Pediatr Blood Cancer. 2006;47:130-140.

69. Reiter A, Schrappe M, Ludwig WD, et al. Intensive ALL-type therapy without local radiotherapy provides a 90% event-free survival for children with T-cell lymphoblastic lymphoma: a BFM group report. Blood. 2000;95:416-421.

70. Neth O, Seidemann K, Jansen P, et al. Precursor B-cell lymphoblastic lymphoma in childhood and adolescence: clinical features, treatment, and results in trials NHL-BFM 86 and 90. Med Pediatr Oncol. 2000;35:20-27.

71. Mahmoud HH, Rivera GK, Hancock ML, et al. Low leukocyte counts with blast cells in cerebrospinal fluid of children with newly diagnosed acute lymphoblastic leukemia. N Engl J Med. 1993;329:314-319.

72. Burger B, Zimmermann M, Mann G, et al. Diagnostic cerebrospinal fluid examination in children with acute lymphoblastic leukemia: significance of low leukocyte counts with blasts or traumatic lumbar puncture. J Clin Oncol. 2003;21:184-188.

73. McIntosh S, Ritchey AK. Diagnostic problems in cerebrospinal fluid of children with lymphoid malignancies. Am J Pediatr Hematol Oncol. 1986;8:28-31.

74. Gajjar A, Harrison PL, Sandlund JT, et al. Traumatic lumbar puncture at diagnosis adversely affects outcome in childhood acute lymphoblastic leukemia. Blood. 2000;96:3381-3384.

75. Ingram LC, Fairclough DL, Furman WL, et al. Cranial nerve palsy in childhood acute lymphoblastic leukemia and non-Hodgkin's lymphoma. Cancer. 1991;67:2262-2268.

76. Krishnamurthy S, Weinstock AL, Smith SH, et al. Facial palsy, an unusual presenting feature of childhood leukemia. Pediatr Neurol. 2002;27:68-70.

77. Greydanus DE, Burgert EO Jr, Gilchrist GS. Hypothalamic syndrome in children with acute lymphocytic leukemia. Mayo Clin Proc. 1978;53:217-220.

78. Rosman NP, Kakulas BA, Richardson EP Jr. Central pontine myelinolysis in a child with leukemia. Arch Neurol. 1966;14:273-280.

79. Kanner SP, Wiernik PH, Serpick AA, et al. CNS leukemia mimicking multifocal leukoencephalopathy. Am J Dis Child. 1970;119:264-266.

80. Miller VI, Campbell WG Jr. Diabetes insipidus as a complication of leukemia. A case report with a literature reviews. Cancer. 1971;28:666-673.

81. Kataoka A, Shimizu K, Matsumoto T, et al. Epidural spinal cord compression as an initial symptom in childhood acute lymphoblastic leukemia: rapid decompression by local irradiation and systemic chemotherapy. Pediatr Hematol Oncol. 1995;12:179-184.

82. Hijiya N, Liu W, Sandlund JT, et al. Overt testicular disease at diagnosis of childhood acute lymphoblastic leukemia: lack of therapeutic role of local irradiation. Leukemia. 2005;19:1399-1403.

83. Sirvent N, Suciu S, Bertrand Y, et al. Overt testicular disease (OTD) at diagnosis is not associated with a poor prognosis in childhood acute lymphoblastic leukemia: results of the EORTC CLG study 58881. Pediatr Blood Cancer. 2007;49:344-348.

84. Kim TH, Hargreaves HK, Chan WC, et al. Sequential testicular biopsies in childhood acute lymphocytic leukemia. Cancer. 1986;57:1038-1041.

85. Goh TS, LeQuesne GW, Wong KY. Severe infiltration of the kidneys with ultrasonic abnormalities in acute lymphoblastic leukemia. Am J Dis Child. 1978;132:1204-1205.

86. Howard SC, Kaplan SD, Razzouk BI, et al. Urolithiasis in pediatric patients with acute lymphoblastic leukemia. Leukemia. 2003;17:541-546.

87. Troup CW, Thatcher G, Hodgson NB. Infiltrative lesion of the bladder presenting as gross hematuria in child with leukemia: case report. J Urol. 1972;107:314-315.

88. Castagnetti M, Sainati L, Giona F, et al. Conservative management of priapism secondary to leukemia. Pediatr Blood Cancer. 2008;51:420-423.

89. Hustu HO, Aur RJ. Extramedullary leukaemia. Clin Haematol. 1978;7:313-337.

90. Cecalupo AJ, Frankel LS, Sullivan MP. Pelvic and ovarian extramedullary leukemic relapse in young girls: a report of four cases and review of the literature. Cancer. 1982;50:587-593.

91. Zarrouk SO, Kim TH, Hargreaves HK, et al. Leukemic involvement of the ovaries in childhood acute lymphocytic leukemia. J Pediatr. 1982;100:422-424.

92. Jonsson OG, Sartain P, Ducore JM, et al. Bone pain as an initial symptom of childhood acute lymphoblastic leukemia: association with almost normal hematologic indexes. J Pediatr. 1990;117: 233-237.

93. Rogalsky RJ, Black GB, Reed MH. Orthopaedic manifestations of leukemia in children. J Bone Joint Surg Am. 1986;68:494-501.

94. Halton JM, Atkinson SA, Fraher L, et al. Mineral homeostasis and bone mass at diagnosis in children with acute lymphoblastic leukemia. J Pediatr. 1995;126:557-564.

95. Saulsbury FT, Sabio H. Acute leukemia presenting as arthritis in children. Clin Pediatr (Phila). 1985;24:625-628.

96. Jones OY, Spencer CH, Bowyer SL, et al. A multicenter case-control study on predictive factors distinguishing childhood leukemia from juvenile rheumatoid arthritis. Pediatrics. 2006; 117:e840-844.

97. Ribeiro RC, Pui CH, Schell MJ. Vertebral compression fracture as a presenting feature of acute lymphoblastic leukemia in children. Cancer. 1988;61:589-592.

98. Kushner DC, Weinstein HJ, Kirkpatrick JA. The radiologic diagnosis of leukemia and lymphoma in children. Semin Roentgenol. 1980;15:316-334.

99. Hughes RG, Kay HE. Major bone lesions in acute lymphoblastic leukaemia. Med Pediatr Oncol. 1982;10:67-70.

100. Belgaumi AF, Hudson MM. Childhood acute lymphoblastic leukemia presenting with severe hepatic dysfunction. Med Pediatr Oncol. 2001;37:142-144.

101. Kelleher JF, Monteleone PM, Steele DA, et al. Hepatic dysfunction as the presenting feature of acute lymphoblastic leukemia. J Pediatr Hematol Oncol. 2001;23:117-121.

102. Schachat AP, Markowitz JA, Guyer DR, et al. Ophthalmic manifestations of leukemia. Arch Ophthalmol. 1989;107:697-700.

103. Guyer DR, Schachat AP, Vitale S, et al. Leukemic retinopathy. Relationship between fundus lesions and hematologic parameters at diagnosis. Ophthalmology. 1989;96:860-864.

104. Schwartz CL, Miller NR, Wharam MD, et al. The optic nerve as the site of initial relapse in childhood acute lymphoblastic leukemia. Cancer. 1989;63:1616-1620.

105. Bunin N, Rivera G, Goode F, et al. Ocular relapse in the anterior chamber in childhood acute lymphoblastic leukemia. J Clin Oncol. 1987;5:299-303.

106. Bresters D, Reus AC, Veerman AJ, et al. Congenital leukaemia: the Dutch experience and review of the literature. Br J Haematol. 2002;117:513-524.

107. Jubelirer SJ, Harpold R. The role of the bone marrow examination in the diagnosis of immune thrombocytopenic purpura: case series and literature review. Clin Appl Thromb Hemost. 2002; 8:73-76.

108. Shackelford GD, Bloomberg G, McAlister WH. The value of roentgenography in differentiating aplastic anemia from leukemia masquerading as aplastic anemia. Am J Roentgenol Radium Ther Nucl Med. 1972;116:651-654.

109. Hasle H, Heim S, Schroeder H, et al. Transient pancytopenia preceding acute lymphoblastic leukemia (pre-ALL). Leukemia. 1995;9:605-608.

110. Matloub YH, Brunning RD, Arthur DC, et al. Severe aplastic anemia preceding acute lymphoblastic leukemia. Cancer. 1993; 71:264-268.

111. Moricke A, Zimmermann M, Reiter A, et al. Prognostic impact of age in children and adolescents with acute lymphoblastic leukemia: data from the trials ALL-BFM 86, 90, and 95. Klin Padiatr. 2005;217:310-320.

112. Pui CH, Gaynon PS, Boyett JM, et al. Outcome of treatment in childhood acute lymphoblastic leukaemia with rearrangements of the 11q23 chromosomal region. Lancet. 2002;359:1909-1915.

113. Chessells JM, Harrison CJ, Watson SL, et al. Treatment of infants with lymphoblastic leukaemia: results of the UK Infant Protocols 1987-1999. Br J Haematol. 2002;117:306-314.

114. Hilden JM, Dinndorf PA, Meerbaum SO, et al. Analysis of prognostic factors of acute lymphoblastic leukemia in infants: report on CCG 1953 from the Children's Oncology Group. Blood. 2006;108:441-451.

115. Pieters R, Schrappe M, De Lorenzo P, et al. A treatment protocol for infants younger than 1 year with acute lymphoblastic leukaemia (Interfant-99): an observational study and a multicentre randomised trial. Lancet. 2007;370:240-250.

116. Barry E, DeAngelo DJ, Neuberg D, et al. Favorable outcome for adolescents with acute lymphoblastic leukemia treated on Dana-Farber Cancer Institute Acute Lymphoblastic Leukemia Consortium Protocols. J Clin Oncol. 2007;25:813-819.

117. Baruchel A, Cayuela JM, Ballerini P, et al. Most myeloid-antigen-positive (My+) childhood B-cell precursor acute lymphoblastic leukaemias express TEL-AML1 fusion transcripts. Br J Haematol. 1997;99:101-106.

118. Carbonell F, Swansbury J, Min T, et al. Cytogenetic findings in acute biphenotypic leukaemia. Leukemia. 1996;10:1283-1287.

119. Putti MC, Rondelli R, Cocito MG, et al. Expression of myeloid markers lacks prognostic impact in children treated for acute lymphoblastic leukemia: Italian experience in AIEOP-ALL 88-91 studies. Blood. 1998;92:795-801.

120. Look AT, Roberson PK, Williams DL, et al. Prognostic importance of blast cell DNA content in childhood acute lymphoblastic leukemia. Blood. 1985;65:1079-1086.

121. Trueworthy R, Shuster J, Look T, et al. Ploidy of lymphoblasts is the strongest predictor of treatment outcome in B-progenitor cell acute lymphoblastic leukemia of childhood: a Pediatric Oncology Group study. J Clin Oncol. 1992;10:606-613.

122. Loh ML, Goldwasser MA, Silverman LB, et al. Prospective analysis of TEL/AML1 positive patients treated on Dana-Farber Cancer Institute Consortium Protocol 95-01. Blood. 2006;107: 4508-4513.

123. Rubnitz JE, Wichlan D, Devidas M, et al. Prospective analysis of TEL gene rearrangements in childhood acute lymphoblastic leukemia: a Children's Oncology Group study. J Clin Oncol. 2008;26:2186-2191.

124. Moorman AV, Richards SM, Robinson HM, et al. Prognosis of children with acute lymphoblastic leukemia (ALL) and intrachromosomal amplification of chromosome 21 (iAMP21). Blood. 2007;109:2327-2330.

125. Harris MB, Shuster JJ, Carroll A, et al. Trisomy of leukemic cell chromosomes 4 and 10 identifies children with B-progenitor cell acute lymphoblastic leukemia with a very low risk of treatment failure: a Pediatric Oncology Group study. Blood. 1992;79: 3316-3324.

126. Heerema NA, Sather HN, Sensel MG, et al. Prognostic impact of trisomies of chromosomes 10, 17, and 5 among children with acute lymphoblastic leukemia and high hyperdiploidy (>50 chromosomes). J Clin Oncol. 2000;18:1876-1887.

127. Sutcliffe MJ, Shuster JJ, Sather HN, et al. High concordance from independent studies by the Children's Cancer Group (CCG) and Pediatric Oncology Group (POG) associating favorable prognosis with combined trisomies 4, 10, and 17 in children with NCI Standard-Risk B-precursor Acute Lymphoblastic Leukemia: a Children's Oncology Group (COG) initiative. Leukemia. 2005; 19:734-740.

128. Harrison CJ, Moorman AV, Barber KE, et al. Interphase molecular cytogenetic screening for chromosomal abnormalities of prognostic significance in childhood acute lymphoblastic leukaemia: a UK Cancer Cytogenetics Group Study. Br J Haematol. 2005;129:520-530.

129. Forestier E, Schmiegelow K. The incidence peaks of the childhood acute leukemias reflect specific cytogenetic aberrations. J Pediatr Hematol Oncol. 2006;28:486-495.

130. Attarbaschi A, Mann G, Konig M, et al. Incidence and relevance of secondary chromosome abnormalities in childhood TEL/

AML1+ acute lymphoblastic leukemia: an interphase FISH analysis. Leukemia. 2004;18:1611-1616.

131. Forestier E, Andersen MK, Autio K, et al. Cytogenetic patterns in ETV6/RUNX1-positive pediatric B-cell precursor acute lymphoblastic leukemia: a Nordic series of 245 cases and review of the literature. Genes Chromosomes Cancer. 2007;46:440-450.

132. McLean TW, Ringold S, Neuberg D, et al. TEL/AML-1 dimerizes and is associated with a favorable outcome in childhood acute lymphoblastic leukemia. Blood. 1996;88:4252-4258.

133. Rubnitz JE, Downing JR, Pui CH, et al. TEL gene rearrangement in acute lymphoblastic leukemia: a new genetic marker with prognostic significance. J Clin Oncol. 1997;15:1150-1157.

134. Harbott J, Viehmann S, Borkhardt A, et al. Incidence of TEL/AML1 fusion gene analyzed consecutively in children with acute lymphoblastic leukemia in relapse. Blood. 1997;90:4933-4937.

135. Seeger K, Adams HP, Buchwald D, et al. TEL-AML1 fusion transcript in relapsed childhood acute lymphoblastic leukemia. The Berlin-Frankfurt-Munster Study Group. Blood. 1998;91:1716-1722.

136. Loh ML, Silverman LB, Young ML, et al. Incidence of TEL/AML1 fusion in children with relapsed acute lymphoblastic leukemia. Blood. 1998;92:4792-4797.

137. Seeger K, von Stackelberg A, Taube T, et al. Relapse of TEL-AML1—positive acute lymphoblastic leukemia in childhood: a matched-pair analysis. J Clin Oncol. 2001;19:3188-3193.

138. Chessels JM, Swansbury GJ, Reeves B, et al. Cytogenetics and prognosis in childhood lymphoblastic leukaemia: results of MRC UKALL X. Medical Research Council Working Party in Childhood Leukaemia. Br J Haematol. 1997;99:93-100.

139. Heerema NA, Nachman JB, Sather HN, et al. Hypodiploidy with less than 45 chromosomes confers adverse risk in childhood acute lymphoblastic leukemia: a report from the children's cancer group. Blood. 1999;94:4036-4045.

140. Nachman JB, Heerema NA, Sather H, et al. Outcome of treatment in children with hypodiploid acute lymphoblastic leukemia. Blood. 2007;110:1112-1115.

141. Behm FG, Raimondi SC, Frestedt JL, et al. Rearrangement of the MLL gene confers a poor prognosis in childhood acute lymphoblastic leukemia, regardless of presenting age. Blood. 1996;87:2870-2877.

142. Crist W, Carroll A, Shuster J, et al. Philadelphia chromosome positive childhood acute lymphoblastic leukemia: clinical and cytogenetic characteristics and treatment outcome. A Pediatric Oncology Group study. Blood. 1990;76:489-494.

143. Fletcher JA, Lynch EA, Kimball VM, Donnelly M, Tantravahi R, Sallan SE. Translocation (9;22) is associated with extremely poor prognosis in intensively treated children with acute lymphoblastic leukemia. Blood. 1991;77:435-439.

144. Uckun FM, Nachman JB, Sather HN, et al. Clinical significance of Philadelphia chromosome positive pediatric acute lymphoblastic leukemia in the context of contemporary intensive therapies: a report from the Children's Cancer Group. Cancer. 1998;83:2030-2039.

145. Arico M, Valsecchi MG, Camitta B, et al. Outcome of treatment in children with Philadelphia chromosome-positive acute lymphoblastic leukemia. N Engl J Med. 2000;342:998-1006.

146. Pui CH, Mahmoud HH, Rivera GK, et al. Early intensification of intrathecal chemotherapy virtually eliminates central nervous system relapse in children with acute lymphoblastic leukemia. Blood. 1998;92:411-415.

147. Gaynon PS, Desai AA, Bostrom BC, et al. Early response to therapy and outcome in childhood acute lymphoblastic leukemia: a review. Cancer. 1997;80:1717-1726.

148. Silverman LB, Gelber RD, Young ML, et al. Induction failure in acute lymphoblastic leukemia of childhood. Cancer. 1999;85:1395-1404.

149. Oudot C, Auclerc MF, Levy V, et al. Prognostic factors for leukemic induction failure in children with acute lymphoblastic leukemia and outcome after salvage therapy: the FRALLE 93 study. J Clin Oncol. 2008;26:1496-1503.

150. Schrappe M, Reiter A, Zimmermann M, et al. Long-term results of four consecutive trials in childhood ALL performed by the ALL-BFM study group from 1981 to 1995. Berlin-Frankfurt-Munster. Leukemia. 2000;14:2205-2222.

151. Rautonen J, Hovi L, Siimes MA. Slow disappearance of peripheral blast cells: an independent risk factor indicating poor prognosis in children with acute lymphoblastic leukemia. Blood. 1988;71:989-991.

152. Gajjar A, Ribeiro R, Hancock ML, et al. Persistence of circulating blasts after 1 week of multiagent chemotherapy confers a poor prognosis in childhood acute lymphoblastic leukemia. Blood. 1995;86:1292-1295.

153. Griffin TC, Shuster JJ, Buchanan GR, et al. Slow disappearance of peripheral blood blasts is an adverse prognostic factor in childhood T cell acute lymphoblastic leukemia: a Pediatric Oncology Group study. Leukemia. 2000;14:792-795.

154. Nachman JB, Sather HN, Sensel MG, et al. Augmented post-induction therapy for children with high-risk acute lymphoblastic leukemia and a slow response to initial therapy. N Engl J Med. 1998;338:1663-1671.

155. van Dongen JJ, Seriu T, Panzer-Grumayer ER, et al. Prognostic value of minimal residual disease in acute lymphoblastic leukaemia in childhood. Lancet. 1998;352:1731-1738.

156. Coustan-Smith E, Behm FG, Sanchez J, et al. Immunological detection of minimal residual disease in children with acute lymphoblastic leukaemia. Lancet. 1998;351:550-554.

157. Weir EG, Cowan K, LeBeau P, et al. A limited antibody panel can distinguish B-precursor acute lymphoblastic leukemia from normal B precursors with four color flow cytometry: implications for residual disease detection. Leukemia. 1999;13:558-567.

158. Li A, Zhou J, Zuckerman D, et al. Sequence analysis of clonal immunoglobulin and T-cell receptor gene rearrangements in children with acute lymphoblastic leukemia at diagnosis and at relapse: implications for pathogenesis and for the clinical utility of PCR-based methods of minimal residual disease detection. Blood. 2003;102:4520-4526.

159. Cave H, van der Werff ten Bosch J, Suciu S, et al. Clinical significance of minimal residual disease in childhood acute lymphoblastic leukemia. European Organization for Research and Treatment of Cancer—Childhood Leukemia Cooperative Group. N Engl J Med. 1998;339:591-598.

160. Coustan-Smith E, Sancho J, Hancock ML, et al. Clinical importance of minimal residual disease in childhood acute lymphoblastic leukemia. Blood. 2000;96:2691-2696.

161. Nyvold C, Madsen HO, Ryder LP, et al. Precise quantification of minimal residual disease at day 29 allows identification of children with acute lymphoblastic leukemia and an excellent outcome. Blood. 2002;99:1253-1258.

162. Panzer-Grümayer ER, Schneider M, et al. Rapid molecular response during early induction chemotherapy predicts a good outcome in childhood acute lymphoblastic leukemia. Blood. 2000;95:790-794.

163. Zhou J, Goldwasser MA, Li A, et al. Quantitative analysis of minimal residual disease predicts relapse in children with B-lineage acute lymphoblastic leukemia in DFCI ALL Consortium Protocol 95-01. Blood. 2007;110:1607-1611.

164. Brisco MJ, Condon J, Hughes E, et al. Outcome prediction in childhood acute lymphoblastic leukaemia by molecular quantification of residual disease at the end of induction. Lancet. 1994;343:196-200.

165. Coustan-Smith E, Sancho J, Behm FG, et al. Prognostic importance of measuring early clearance of leukemic cells by flow cytometry in childhood acute lymphoblastic leukemia. Blood. 2002;100:52-58.

166. Chessells JM, Richards SM, Bailey CC, et al. Gender and treatment outcome in childhood lymphoblastic leukaemia: report

from the MRC UKALL trials. Br J Haematol. 1995;89:364-372.

167. Shuster JJ, Wacker P, Pullen J, et al. Prognostic significance of sex in childhood B-precursor acute lymphoblastic leukemia: a Pediatric Oncology Group Study. J Clin Oncol. 1998;16:2854-2863.

168. Pui CH, Boyett JM, Hancock ML, et al. Outcome of treatment for childhood cancer in black as compared with white children. The St Jude Children's Research Hospital experience, 1962 through 1992. JAMA. 1995;273:633-637.

169. Pollock BH, DeBaun MR, Camitta BM, et al. Racial differences in the survival of childhood B-precursor acute lymphoblastic leukemia: a Pediatric Oncology Group Study. J Clin Oncol. 2000;18:813-823.

170. Kager L, Evans WE. Pharmacogenomics of acute lymphoblastic leukemia. Curr Opin Hematol. 2006;13:260-265.

171. Relling MV, Hancock ML, Boyett JM, et al. Prognostic importance of 6-mercaptopurine dose intensity in acute lymphoblastic leukemia. Blood. 1999;93:2817-2823.

172. Stanulla M, Schaeffeler E, Flohr T, et al. Thiopurine methyltransferase (TPMT) genotype and early treatment response to mercaptopurine in childhood acute lymphoblastic leukemia. JAMA. 2005;293:1485-1489.

173. Relling MV, Hancock ML, Rivera GK, et al. Mercaptopurine therapy intolerance and heterozygosity at the thiopurine S-methyltransferase gene locus. J Natl Cancer Inst. 1999;91:2001-2008.

174. Relling MV, Rubnitz JE, Rivera GK, et al. High incidence of secondary brain tumours after radiotherapy and antimetabolites. Lancet. 1999;354:34-39.

175. Stanulla M, Schrappe M, Brechlin AM, et al. Polymorphisms within glutathione S-transferase genes (GSTM1, GSTT1, GSTP1) and risk of relapse in childhood B-cell precursor acute lymphoblastic leukemia: a case-control study. Blood. 2000;95:1222-1228.

176. Davies SM, Bhatia S, Ross JA, et al. Glutathione S-transferase genotypes, genetic susceptibility, and outcome of therapy in childhood acute lymphoblastic leukemia. Blood. 2002;100:67-71.

177. Krajinovic M, Costea I, Chiasson S. Polymorphism of the thymidylate synthase gene and outcome of acute lymphoblastic leukaemia. Lancet. 2002;359:1033-1034.

178. Krajinovic M, Lemieux-Blanchard E, Chiasson S, et al. Role of polymorphisms in MTHFR and MTHFD1 genes in the outcome of childhood acute lymphoblastic leukemia. Pharmacogenomics J. 2004;4:66-72.

179. Lauten M, Asgedom G, Welte K, et al. Thymidylate synthase gene polymorphism and its association with relapse in childhood B-cell precursor acute lymphoblastic leukemia. Haematologica. 2003;88:353-354.

180. Farber S, Diamond LK, Mercer RD, et al. Temporary remissions in acute leukemia in children produced by folic acid antagonist, 4-aminopteroyl-glutamic acid (aminopterin). N Engl J Med. 1948;238:787-793.

181. Frei E 3rd. Acute leukemia in children. Model for the development of scientific methodology for clinical therapeutic research in cancer. Cancer. 1984;53:2013-2025.

182. Elion GB, Hitchings GH. Metabolic basis for the actions of analogs of purines and pyrimidines. Adv Chemother. 1965;2:91-177.

183. Burchenal JH, Murphy ML, Ellison RR, et al. Clinical evaluation of a new antimetabolite, 6-mercaptopurine, in the treatment of leukemia and allied diseases. Blood. 1953;8:965-999.

184. Frei E 3rd, Holland JF, Schneiderman MA, et al. A comparative study of two regimens of combination chemotherapy in acute leukemia. Blood. 1958;13:1126-1148.

185. Freireich EJ, Frei E 2nd. Recent advances in acute leukemia. Prog Hematol. 1964;4:187-202.

186. Blum RH, Carter SK. Adriamycin. A new anticancer drug with significant clinical activity. Ann Intern Med. 1974;80:249-259.

187. Tallal L, Tan C, Oettgen H, et al. E. coli L-asparaginase in the treatment of leukemia and solid tumors in 131 children. Cancer. 1970;25:306-320.

188. Jaffe N, Traggis D, Das L, et al. Comparison of daily and twice-weekly schedule of L-asparaginase in childhood leukemia. Pediatrics. 1972;49:590-595.

189. Schultz KR, Pullen DJ, Sather HN, et al. Risk- and response-based classification of childhood B-precursor acute lymphoblastic leukemia: a combined analysis of prognostic markers from the Pediatric Oncology Group (POG) and Children's Cancer Group (CCG). Blood. 2007;109:926-935.

190. Holland JF, Glidewell O. Chemotherapy of acute lymphocytic leukemia of childhood. Cancer. 1972;30:1480-1487.

191. Berry DH, Pullen J, George S, et al. Comparison of prednisolone, vincristine, methotrexate, and 6-mercaptopurine vs. vincristine and prednisone induction therapy in childhood acute leukemia. Cancer. 1975;36:98-102.

192. Ortega JA, Nesbit ME Jr, Donaldson MH, et al. L-Asparaginase, vincristine, and prednisone for induction of first remission in acute lymphocytic leukemia. Cancer Res. 1977;37:535-540.

193. Hitchcock-Bryan S, Gelber R, Cassady JR, Sallan SE. The impact of induction anthracycline on long-term failure-free survival in childhood acute lymphoblastic leukemia. Med Pediatr Oncol. 1986;14:211-215.

194. Goldie JH, Coldman AJ, Gudauskas GA. Rationale for the use of alternating non-cross-resistant chemotherapy. Cancer Treat Rep. 1982;66:439-449.

195. Gaynon PS, Steinherz PG, Bleyer WA, et al. Improved therapy for children with acute lymphoblastic leukemia and unfavorable presenting features: a follow-up report of the Children's Cancer Group Study CCG-106. J Clin Oncol. 1993;11:2234-2242.

196. Tubergen DG, Gilchrist GS, O'Brien RT, et al. Improved outcome with delayed intensification for children with acute lymphoblastic leukemia and intermediate presenting features: a Childrens Cancer Group phase III trial. J Clin Oncol. 1993;11:527-537.

197. Pui CH, Boyett JM, Rivera GK, et al. Long-term results of Total Therapy studies 11, 12 and 13A for childhood acute lymphoblastic leukemia at St Jude Children's Research Hospital. Leukemia. 2000;14:2286-2294.

198. Rubnitz JE, Lensing S, Zhou Y, et al. Death during induction therapy and first remission of acute leukemia in childhood: the St. Jude experience. Cancer. 2004;101:1677-1684.

199. Ochs J, Rivera GK, Pollock BH, et al. Teniposide (VM-26) and continuous infusion cytosine arabinoside for initial induction failure in childhood acute lymphoblastic leukemia. A Pediatric Oncology Group pilot study. Cancer. 1990;66:1671-1677.

200. Giona F, Testi AM, Annino L, et al. Treatment of primary refractory and relapsed acute lymphoblastic leukaemia in children and adults: the GIMEMA/AIEOP experience. Gruppo Italiano Malattie Ematologiche Maligne dell'Adulto. Associazione Italiana Ematologia ed Ocologia Pediatrica. Br J Haematol. 1994;86:55-61.

201. Rivera G, Dahl GV, Bowman WP, et al. VM-26 and cytosine arabinoside combination chemotherapy for initial induction failures in childhood lymphocytic leukemia. Cancer. 1980;46:1727-1730.

202. Berg SL, Blaney SM, Devidas M, et al. Phase II study of nelarabine (compound 506U78) in children and young adults with refractory T-cell malignancies: a report from the Children's Oncology Group. J Clin Oncol. 2005;23:3376-3382.

203. DeAngelo DJ, Yu D, Johnson JL, et al. Nelarabine induces complete remissions in adults with relapsed or refractory T-lineage acute lymphoblastic leukemia or lymphoblastic lymphoma: Cancer and Leukemia Group B study 19801. Blood. 2007;109:5136-5142.

204. Balduzzi A, Valsecchi MG, Uderzo C, et al. Chemotherapy versus allogeneic transplantation for very-high-risk childhood acute lymphoblastic leukaemia in first complete remission: comparison by genetic randomisation in an international prospective study. Lancet. 2005;366:635-642.

205. Pinkel D, Hernandez K, Borella L, et al. Drug dosage and remission duration in childhood lymphocytic leukemia. Cancer. 1971; 27:247-256.

206. Evans AE, Gilbert ES, Zandstra R. The increasing incidence of central nervous system leukemia in children. (Children's Cancer Study Group A.) Cancer. 1970;26:404-409.

207. Rivera GK, Pinkel D, Simone JV, et al. Treatment of acute lymphoblastic leukemia. 30 years' experience at St. Jude Children's Research Hospital. N Engl J Med. 1993;329: 1289-1295.

208. Johnson RE. An experimental therapeutic approach to L1210 leukemia in mice: combined chemotherapy and central nervous system irradiation. J Natl Cancer Inst. 1964;32:1333-1341.

209. Hustu HO, Aur RJ, Verzosa MS, et al. Prevention of central nervous system leukemia by irradiation. Cancer. 1973;32: 585-597.

210. Simone J, Aur RJ, Hustu HO, et al. "Total therapy" studies of acute lymphocytic leukemia in children. Current results and prospects for cure. Cancer. 1972;30:1488-1494.

211. Aur RJ, Simone JV, Hustu HO, et al. A comparative study of central nervous system irradiation and intensive chemotherapy early in remission of childhood acute lymphocytic leukemia. Cancer. 1972;29:381-391.

212. Nesbit ME, Sather H, Robison LL, et al. Sanctuary therapy: a randomized trial of 724 children with previously untreated acute lymphoblastic leukemia: a Report from Children's Cancer Study Group. Cancer Res. 1982;42:674-680.

213. Pui CH, Howard SC. Current management and challenges of malignant disease in the CNS in paediatric leukaemia. Lancet Oncol. 2008;9:257-268.

214. Nesbit ME Jr, Sather HN, Robison LL, et al. Presymptomatic central nervous system therapy in previously untreated childhood acute lymphoblastic leukaemia: comparison of 1800 rad and 2400 rad. A report for Children's Cancer Study Group. Lancet. 1981; 1:461-466.

215. Schrappe M, Reiter A, Henze G, et al. Prevention of CNS recurrence in childhood ALL: results with reduced radiotherapy combined with CNS-directed chemotherapy in four consecutive ALL-BFM trials. Klin Padiatr. 1998;210:192-199.

216. Balis FM, Lester CM, Chrousos GP, et al. Differences in cerebrospinal fluid penetration of corticosteroids: possible relationship to the prevention of meningeal leukemia. J Clin Oncol. 1987;5:202-207.

217. Frick J, Ritch PS, Hansen RM, et al. Successful treatment of meningeal leukemia using systemic high-dose cytosine arabinoside. J Clin Oncol. 1984;2:365-368.

218. Wang JJ, Freeman AI, Sinks LF. Treatment of acute lymphocytic leukemia by high-dose intravenous methotrexate. Cancer Res. 1976;36:1441-1444.

219. Dibenedetto SP, Di Cataldo A, Ragusa R, et al. Levels of L-asparagine in CSF after intramuscular administration of asparaginase from Erwinia in children with acute lymphoblastic leukemia. J Clin Oncol. 1995;13:339-344.

220. Woo MH, Hak LJ, Storm MC, et al. Cerebrospinal fluid asparagine concentrations after Escherichia coli asparaginase in children with acute lymphoblastic leukemia. J Clin Oncol. 1999;17:1568-1573.

221. Tubergen DG, Gilchrist GS, O'Brien RT, et al. Prevention of CNS disease in intermediate-risk acute lymphoblastic leukemia: comparison of cranial radiation and intrathecal methotrexate and the importance of systemic therapy: a Childrens Cancer Group report. J Clin Oncol. 1993;11:520-526.

222. LeClerc JM, Billett AL, Gelber RD, et al. Treatment of childhood acute lymphoblastic leukemia: results of Dana-Farber ALL Consortium Protocol 87-01. J Clin Oncol. 2002;20:237-246.

223. Bostrom BC, Sensel MR, Sather HN, et al. Dexamethasone versus prednisone and daily oral versus weekly intravenous mercaptopurine for patients with standard-risk acute lymphoblastic leukemia: a report from the Children's Cancer Group. Blood. 2003;101:3809-3817.

224. Mitchell CD, Richards SM, Kinsey SE, et al.; Council Childhood Leukaemia Working Party. Benefit of dexamethasone compared with prednisolone for childhood acute lymphoblastic leukaemia: results of the UK Medical Research Council ALL97 randomized trial. Br J Haematol. 2005;129:734-745.

225. Pullen J, Boyett J, Shuster J, et al. Extended triple intrathecal chemotherapy trial for prevention of CNS relapse in good-risk and poor-risk patients with B-progenitor acute lymphoblastic leukemia: a Pediatric Oncology Group study. J Clin Oncol. 1993;11:839-849.

226. Conter V, Arico M, Valsecchi MG, et al. Extended intrathecal methotrexate may replace cranial irradiation for prevention of CNS relapse in children with intermediate-risk acute lymphoblastic leukemia treated with Berlin-Frankfurt-Munster-based intensive chemotherapy. The Associazione Italiana di Ematologia ed Oncologia Pediatrica. J Clin Oncol. 1995;13:2497-2502.

227. Veerman AJ, Hahlen K, Kamps WA, et al. High cure rate with a moderately intensive treatment regimen in non-high-risk childhood acute lymphoblastic leukemia. Results of protocol ALL VI from the Dutch Childhood Leukemia Study Group. J Clin Oncol. 1996;14:911-918.

228. Hill FG, Richards S, Gibson B, et al. Successful treatment without cranial radiotherapy of children receiving intensified chemotherapy for acute lymphoblastic leukaemia: results of the risk-stratified randomized central nervous system treatment trial MRC UKALL XI (ISRC TN 16757172). Br J Haematol. 2004;124: 33-46.

229. Mahoney DH Jr, Shuster JJ, Nitschke R, et al. Acute neurotoxicity in children with B-precursor acute lymphoid leukemia: an association with intermediate-dose intravenous methotrexate and intrathecal triple therapy—a Pediatric Oncology Group study. J Clin Oncol. 1998;16:1712-1722.

230. Sallan SE, Hitchcock-Bryan S, Gelber R, et al. Influence of intensive asparaginase in the treatment of childhood non-T-cell acute lymphoblastic leukemia. Cancer Res. 1983;43:5601-5607.

231. Schrappe M, Reiter A, Ludwig WD, et al. Improved outcome in childhood acute lymphoblastic leukemia despite reduced use of anthracyclines and cranial radiotherapy: results of trial ALL-BFM 90. German-Austrian-Swiss ALL-BFM Study Group. Blood. 2000;95:3310-3322.

232. Kamps WA, Veerman AJ, van Wering ER, et al. Long-term follow-up of Dutch Childhood Leukemia Study Group (DCLSG) protocols for children with acute lymphoblastic leukemia, 1984-1991. Leukemia. 2000;14:2240-2246.

233. Gustafsson G, Schmiegelow K, Forestier E, et al. Improving outcome through two decades in childhood ALL in the Nordic countries: the impact of high-dose methotrexate in the reduction of CNS irradiation. Nordic Society of Pediatric Haematology and Oncology (NOPHO). Leukemia. 2000;14:2267-2275.

234. Chauvenet AR, Martin PL, Devidas M, et al. Antimetabolite therapy for lesser-risk B-lineage acute lymphoblastic leukemia of childhood: a report from Children's Oncology Group Study P9201. Blood. 2007;110:1105-1111.

235. Gaynon PS, Trigg ME, Heerema NA, et al. Children's Cancer Group trials in childhood acute lymphoblastic leukemia: 1983-1995. Leukemia. 2000;14:2223-2233.

236. Arico M, Valsecchi MG, Conter V, et al. Improved outcome in high-risk childhood acute lymphoblastic leukemia defined by prednisone-poor response treated with double Berlin-Frankfurt-Muenster protocol II. Blood. 2002;100:420-426.

237. Lange BJ, Bostrom BC, Cherlow JM, et al. Double-delayed intensification improves event-free survival for children with intermediate-risk acute lymphoblastic leukemia: a report from the Children's Cancer Group. Blood. 2002;99:825-833.

238. Seibel NL, Steinherz PG, Sather HN, et al. Early postinduction intensification therapy improves survival for children and adolescents with high-risk acute lymphoblastic leukemia: a report from the Children's Oncology Group. Blood. 2008;111:2548-2555.

239. Bleyer WA, Sather HN, Nickerson HJ, et al. Monthly pulses of vincristine and prednisone prevent bone marrow and testicular relapse in low-risk childhood acute lymphoblastic leukemia: a report of the CCG-161 study by the Childrens Cancer Study Group. J Clin Oncol. 1991;9:1012-1021.

240. Childhood ALL Collaborative Group. Duration and intensity of maintenance chemotherapy in acute lymphoblastic leukaemia: overview of 42 trials involving 12,000 randomised children. Lancet. 1996;347:1783-1788.

241. Conter V, Valsecchi MG, Silvestri D, et al. Pulses of vincristine and dexamethasone in addition to intensive chemotherapy for children with intermediate-risk acute lymphoblastic leukaemia: a multicentre randomised trial. Lancet. 2007;369:123-131.

242. Balis FM, Savitch JL, Bleyer WA. Pharmacokinetics of oral methotrexate in children. Cancer Res 1983;43:2342-2345.

243. Lennard L, Lilleyman JS. Variable mercaptopurine metabolism and treatment outcome in childhood lymphoblastic leukemia. J Clin Oncol. 1989;7:1816-1823.

244. Poplack DG, Balis FM, Zimm S. The pharmacology of orally administered chemotherapy. A reappraisal. Cancer. 1986;58:473-480.

245. Riccardi R, Balis FM, Ferrara P, et al. Influence of food intake on bioavailability of oral 6-mercaptopurine in children with acute lymphoblastic leukemia. Pediatr Hematol Oncol. 1986;3:319-324.

246. Schmiegelow K, Schroder H, Gustafsson G, et al. Risk of relapse in childhood acute lymphoblastic leukemia is related to RBC methotrexate and mercaptopurine metabolites during maintenance chemotherapy. Nordic Society for Pediatric Hematology and Oncology. J Clin Oncol. 1995;13:345-351.

247. Koren G, Ferrazini G, Sulh H, et al. Systemic exposure to mercaptopurine as a prognostic factor in acute lymphocytic leukemia in children. N Engl J Med. 1990;323:17-21.

248. Rivard GE, Infante-Rivard C, Hoyoux C, et al. Maintenance chemotherapy for childhood acute lymphoblastic leukaemia: better in the evening. Lancet. 1985;2:1264-1266.

249. Schmiegelow K, Glomstein A, Kristinsson J, et al. Impact of morning versus evening schedule for oral methotrexate and 6-mercaptopurine on relapse risk for children with acute lymphoblastic leukemia. Nordic Society for Pediatric Hematology and Oncology (NOPHO). J Pediatr Hematol Oncol. 1997;19:102-109.

250. Schmiegelow K, Pulczynska MK. Maintenance chemotherapy for childhood acute lymphoblastic leukemia: should dosage be guided by white blood cell counts? Am J Pediatr Hematol Oncol. 1990;12:462-467.

251. Pearson AD, Amineddine HA, Yule M, et al. The influence of serum methotrexate concentrations and drug dosage on outcome in childhood acute lymphoblastic leukaemia. Br J Cancer. 1991;64:169-173.

252. Lau RC, Matsui D, Greenberg M, Koren G. Electronic measurement of compliance with mercaptopurine in pediatric patients with acute lymphoblastic leukemia. Med Pediatr Oncol. 1998;30:85-90.

253. Peeters M, Koren G, Jakubovicz D, et al. Physician compliance and relapse rates of acute lymphoblastic leukemia in children. Clin Pharmacol Ther. 1988;43:228-232.

254. Erb N, Harms DO, Janka-Schaub G. Pharmacokinetics and metabolism of thiopurines in children with acute lymphoblastic leukemia receiving 6-thioguanine versus 6-mercaptopurine. Cancer Chemother Pharmacol. 1998;42:266-272.

255. Adamson PC, Poplack DG, Balis FM. The cytotoxicity of thioguanine vs mercaptopurine in acute lymphoblastic leukemia. Leuk Res. 1994;18:805-810.

256. Vora A, Mitchell CD, Lennard L, et al. Toxicity and efficacy of 6-thioguanine versus 6-mercaptopurine in childhood lymphoblastic leukaemia: a randomised trial. Lancet. 2006;368:1339-1348.

257. Jacobs SS, Stork LC, Bostrom BC, et al. Substitution of oral and intravenous thioguanine for mercaptopurine in a treatment regimen for children with standard risk acute lymphoblastic leukemia: a collaborative Children's Oncology Group/National Cancer Institute pilot trial (CCG-1942). Pediatr Blood Cancer. 2007;49:250-255.

258. Jones B, Freeman AI, Shuster JJ, et al. Lower incidence of meningeal leukemia when prednisone is replaced by dexamethasone in the treatment of acute lymphocytic leukemia. Med Pediatr Oncol. 1991;19:269-275.

259. Ito C, Evans WE, McNinch L, et al. Comparative cytotoxicity of dexamethasone and prednisolone in childhood acute lymphoblastic leukemia. J Clin Oncol. 1996;14:2370-2376.

260. Kaspers GJ, Veerman AJ, Popp-Snijders C, et al. Comparison of the antileukemic activity in vitro of dexamethasone and prednisolone in childhood acute lymphoblastic leukemia. Med Pediatr Oncol. 1996;27:114-121.

261. Silverman LB, Gelber RD, Dalton VK, et al. Improved outcome for children with acute lymphoblastic leukemia: results of Dana-Farber Consortium Protocol 91-01. Blood. 2001;97:1211-1218.

262. Strauss AJ, Su JT, Dalton VM, et al. Bony morbidity in children treated for acute lymphoblastic leukemia. J Clin Oncol. 2001;19:3066-3072.

263. Hurwitz CA, Silverman LB, Schorin MA, et al. Substituting dexamethasone for prednisone complicates remission induction in children with acute lymphoblastic leukemia. Cancer. 2000;88:1964-1969.

264. Rivera GK, Raimondi SC, Hancock ML, et al. Improved outcome in childhood acute lymphoblastic leukaemia with reinforced early treatment and rotational combination chemotherapy. Lancet. 1991;337:61-66.

265. Pui CH, Ribeiro RC, Hancock ML, et al. Acute myeloid leukemia in children treated with epipodophyllotoxins for acute lymphoblastic leukemia. N Engl J Med. 1991;325:1682-1687.

266. Simone JV, Aur RJ, Hustu HO, et al. Three to ten years after cessation of therapy in children with leukemia. Cancer. 1978;42:839-844.

267. Nesbit ME Jr, Sather HN, Robison LL, et al. Randomized study of 3 years versus 5 years of chemotherapy in childhood acute lymphoblastic leukemia. J Clin Oncol. 1983;1:308-316.

268. Miller DR, Leikin SL, Albo VC, et al. Three versus five years of maintenance therapy are equivalent in childhood acute lymphoblastic leukemia: a report from the Childrens Cancer Study Group. J Clin Oncol. 1989;7:316-325.

269. Eden OB, Lilleyman JS, Richards S, et al. Results of Medical Research Council Childhood Leukaemia Trial UKALL VIII (report to the Medical Research Council on behalf of the Working Party on Leukaemia in Childhood). Br J Haematol. 1991;78:187-196.

270. Ravindranath Y, Soorya DT, Schultz GE, Lusher JM. Long-term survivors of acute lymphoblastic leukemia—risk of relapse after cessation of therapy. Med Pediatr Oncol. 1981;9:209-218.

271. Toyoda Y, Manabe A, Tsuchida M, et al. Six months of maintenance chemotherapy after intensified treatment for acute lymphoblastic leukemia of childhood. J Clin Oncol. 2000;18:1508-1516.

272. Bloomfield CD, Goldman AI, Alimena G, et al. Chromosomal abnormalities identify high-risk and low-risk patients with acute lymphoblastic leukemia. Blood. 1986;67:415-420.

273. Barrett AJ, Horowitz MM, Ash RC, et al. Bone marrow transplantation for Philadelphia chromosome-positive acute lymphoblastic leukemia. Blood. 1992;79:3067-3070.

274. Sierra J, Radich J, Hansen JA, et al. Marrow transplants from unrelated donors for treatment of Philadelphia chromosome-positive acute lymphoblastic leukemia. Blood. 1997;90:1410-1414.

275. Marks DI, Bird JM, Cornish JM, et al. Unrelated donor bone marrow transplantation for children and adolescents with Philadelphia-positive acute lymphoblastic leukemia. J Clin Oncol. 1998;16:931-936.

276. Ottmann OG, Druker BJ, Sawyers CL, et al. A phase 2 study of imatinib in patients with relapsed or refractory Philadelphia chromosome-positive acute lymphoid leukemias. Blood. 2002;100:1965-1971.

277. Champagne MA, Capdeville R, Krailo M, et al. Imatinib mesylate (STI571) for treatment of children with Philadelphia chromosome-positive leukemia: results from a Children's Oncology Group phase 1 study. Blood. 2004;104:2655-2660.

278. Thomas DA, Faderl S, Cortes J, et al. Treatment of Philadelphia chromosome-positive acute lymphocytic leukemia with hyper-CVAD and imatinib mesylate. Blood. 2004;103:4396-4407.

279. de Labarthe A, Rousselot P, Huguet-Rigal F, et al. Imatinib combined with induction or consolidation chemotherapy in patients with de novo Philadelphia chromosome-positive acute lymphoblastic leukemia: results of the GRAAPH-2003 study. Blood. 2007;109:1408-1413.

280. Biondi A, Cimino G, Pieters R, Pui CH. Biological and therapeutic aspects of infant leukemia. Blood. 2000;96:24-33.

281. Chessells JM, Eden OB, Bailey CC, et al. Acute lymphoblastic leukaemia in infancy: experience in MRC UKALL trials. Report from the Medical Research Council Working Party on Childhood Leukaemia. Leukemia. 1994;8:1275-1279.

282. Reaman GH, Sposto R, Sensel MG, et al. Treatment outcome and prognostic factors for infants with acute lymphoblastic leukemia treated on two consecutive trials of the Children's Cancer Group. J Clin Oncol. 1999;17:445-455.

283. Biondi A, Rizzari C, Valsecchi MG, et al. Role of treatment intensification in infants with acute lymphoblastic leukemia: results of two consecutive AIEOP studies. Haematologica. 2006;91:534-537.

284. Frankel LS, Ochs J, Shuster JJ, et al. Therapeutic trial for infant acute lymphoblastic leukemia: the Pediatric Oncology Group experience (POG 8493). J Pediatr Hematol Oncol. 1997;19:35-42.

285. Dordelmann M, Reiter A, Borkhardt A, et al. Prednisone response is the strongest predictor of treatment outcome in infant acute lymphoblastic leukemia. Blood. 1999;94:1209-1217.

286. Isoyama K, Eguchi M, Hibi S, et al. Risk-directed treatment of infant acute lymphoblastic leukaemia based on early assessment of MLL gene status: results of the Japan Infant Leukaemia Study (MLL96). Br J Haematol. 2002;118:999-1010.

287. Pieters R, den Boer ML, Durian M, et al. Relation between age, immunophenotype and in vitro drug resistance in 395 children with acute lymphoblastic leukemia—implications for treatment of infants. Leukemia. 1998;12:1344-1348.

288. Silverman LB, McLean TW, Gelber RD, et al. Intensified therapy for infants with acute lymphoblastic leukemia: results from the Dana-Farber Cancer Institute Consortium. Cancer. 1997;80:2285-2295.

289. Ramakers-van Woerden NL, Beverloo HB, Veerman AJ, et al. In vitro drug-resistance profile in infant acute lymphoblastic leukemia in relation to age, MLL rearrangements and immunophenotype. Leukemia. 2004;18:521-529.

290. Marco F, Bureo E, Ortega JJ, et al. High survival rate in infant acute leukemia treated with early high-dose chemotherapy and stem-cell support. Groupo Espanol de Trasplante de Medula Osea en Ninos. J Clin Oncol. 2000;18:3256-3261.

291. Kosaka Y, Koh K, Kinukawa N, et al. Infant acute lymphoblastic leukemia with MLL gene rearrangements: outcome following intensive chemotherapy and hematopoietic stem cell transplantation. Blood. 2004;104:3527-3534.

292. Sanders JE, Im HJ, Hoffmeister PA, et al. Allogeneic hematopoietic cell transplantation for infants with acute lymphoblastic leukemia. Blood. 2005;105:3749-3756.

293. Armstrong SA, Staunton JE, Silverman LB, et al. MLL translocations specify a distinct gene expression profile that distinguishes a unique leukemia. Nat Genet. 2002;30:41-47.

294. Armstrong SA, Kung AL, Mabon ME, et al. Inhibition of FLT3 in MLL. Validation of a therapeutic target identified by gene expression based classification. Cancer Cell. 2003;3:173-183.

295. Brown P, Levis M, Shurtleff S, et al. FLT3 inhibition selectively kills childhood acute lymphoblastic leukemia cells with high levels of FLT3 expression. Blood. 2005;105:812-820.

296. Santana VM, Dodge RK, Crist WM, et al. Presenting features and treatment outcome of adolescents with acute lymphoblastic leukemia. Leukemia. 1990;4:87-90.

297. Mattano LA Jr, Sather HN, Trigg ME, et al. Osteonecrosis as a complication of treating acute lymphoblastic leukemia in children: a report from the Children's Cancer Group. J Clin Oncol. 2000;18:3262-3272.

298. Boissel N, Auclerc MF, Lheritier V, et al. Should adolescents with acute lymphoblastic leukemia be treated as old children or young adults? Comparison of the French FRALLE-93 and LALA-94 trials. J Clin Oncol. 2003;21:774-780.

299. de Bont JM, Holt B, Dekker AW, et al. Significant difference in outcome for adolescents with acute lymphoblastic leukemia treated on pediatric vs adult protocols in the Netherlands. Leukemia. 2004;18:2032-2035.

300. Hallbook H, Gustafsson G, Smedmyr B, et al. Treatment outcome in young adults and children >10 years of age with acute lymphoblastic leukemia in Sweden: a comparison between a pediatric protocol and an adult protocol. Cancer. 2006;107:1551-1561.

301. Hasle H, Clemmensen IH, Mikkelsen M. Risks of leukaemia and solid tumours in individuals with Down's syndrome. Lancet. 2000;355:165-169.

302. Zeller B, Gustafsson G, Forestier E, et al. Acute leukaemia in children with Down syndrome: a population-based Nordic study. Br J Haematol. 2005;128:797-804.

303. Chessells JM, Harrison G, Richards SM, et al. Down's syndrome and acute lymphoblastic leukaemia: clinical features and response to treatment. Arch Dis Child. 2001;85:321-325.

304. Bassal M, La MK, Whitlock JA, et al. Lymphoblast biology and outcome among children with Down syndrome and ALL treated on CCG-1952. Pediatr Blood Cancer. 2005;44:21-28.

305. Whitlock JA, Sather HN, Gaynon P, et al. Clinical characteristics and outcome of children with Down syndrome and acute lymphoblastic leukemia: a Children's Cancer Group study. Blood. 2005;106:4043-4049.

306. Blatt J, Albo V, Prin W, et al. Excessive chemotherapy-related myelotoxicity in children with Down syndrome and acute lymphoblastic leukaemia. Lancet. 1986;2:914.

307. Peeters MA, Poon A, Zipursky A, et al. Toxicity of leukaemia therapy in children with Down syndrome. Lancet. 1986;2:1279.

308. Davidson MB, Thakkar S, Hix JK, et al. Pathophysiology, clinical consequences, and treatment of tumor lysis syndrome. Am J Med. 2004;116:546-554.

309. Cairo MS, Bishop M. Tumour lysis syndrome: new therapeutic strategies and classification. Br J Haematol. 2004;127:3-11.

310. Pui CH, Mahmoud HH, Wiley JM, et al. Recombinant urate oxidase for the prophylaxis or treatment of hyperuricemia in patients with leukemia or lymphoma. J Clin Oncol. 2001;19:697-704.

311. Goldman SC, Holcenberg JS, Finklestein JZ, et al. A randomized comparison between rasburicase and allopurinol in children with

lymphoma or leukemia at high risk for tumor lysis. Blood. 2001;97:2998-3003.

312. Inukai T, Hirose K, Inaba T, et al. Hypercalcemia in childhood acute lymphoblastic leukemia: frequent implication of parathyroid hormone-related peptide and E2A-HLF from translocation 17;19. Leukemia. 2007;21:288-296.

313. Rebulla P, Finazzi G, Marangoni F, et al. The threshold for prophylactic platelet transfusions in adults with acute myeloid leukemia. Gruppo Italiano Malattie Ematologiche Maligne dell'Adulto. N Engl J Med. 1997;337:1870-1875.

314. Ribeiro RC, Pui CH. The clinical and biological correlates of coagulopathy in children with acute leukemia. J Clin Oncol. 1986;4:1212-1218.

315. Hunger SP. Chromosomal translocations involving the E2A gene in acute lymphoblastic leukemia: clinical features and molecular pathogenesis. Blood. 1996;87:1211-1224.

316. Priest JR, Ramsay NK, Steinherz PG, et al. A syndrome of thrombosis and hemorrhage complicating L-asparaginase therapy for childhood acute lymphoblastic leukemia. J Pediatr. 1982;100:984-989.

317. Kucuk O, Kwaan HC, Gunnar W, et al. Thromboembolic complications associated with L-asparaginase therapy. Etiologic role of low antithrombin III and plasminogen levels and therapeutic correction by fresh frozen plasma. Cancer. 1985;55:702-706.

318. Homans AC, Rybak ME, Baglini RL, et al. Effect of L-asparaginase administration on coagulation and platelet function in children with leukemia. J Clin Oncol. 1987;5:811-817.

319. Shapiro AD, Clarke SL, Christian JM, et al. Thrombosis in children receiving L-asparaginase. Determining patients at risk. Am J Pediatr Hematol Oncol. 1993;15:400-405.

320. Mall V, Thomas KB, Sauter S, et al. Effect of glucocorticoids, E. coli- and Erwinia L-asparaginase on hemostatic proteins in children with acute lymphoblastic leukemia. Klin Padiatr. 1999;211:205-210.

321. Nowak-Gottl U, Ahlke E, Fleischhack G, et al. Thromboembolic events in children with acute lymphoblastic leukemia (BFM protocols): prednisone versus dexamethasone administration. Blood. 2003;101:2529-2533.

322. Pizzo PA. Management of fever in patients with cancer and treatment-induced neutropenia. N Engl J Med. 1993;328:1323-1332.

323. Pizzo PA, Walsh TJ. Fungal infections in the pediatric cancer patient. Semin Oncol. 1990;17:6-9.

324. Chanock SJ, Pizzo PA. Infectious complications of patients undergoing therapy for acute leukemia: current status and future prospects. Semin Oncol. 1997;24:132-140.

325. Feldman S, Hughes WT, Daniel CB. Varicella in children with cancer: Seventy-seven cases. Pediatrics. 1975;56:388-397.

326. Winsnes R. Efficacy of zoster immunoglobulin in prophylaxis of varicella in high-risk patients. Acta Paediatr Scand. 1978;67:77-82.

327. Zaia JA, Levin MJ, Preblud SR, et al. Evaluation of varicella-zoster immune globulin: protection of immunosuppressed children after household exposure to varicella. J Infect Dis. 1983;147:737-743.

328. Balfour HH Jr, Bean B, Laskin OL, et al. Acyclovir halts progression of herpes zoster in immunocompromised patients. N Engl J Med. 1983;308:1448-1453.

329. Hill G, Chauvenet AR, Lovato J, et al. Recent steroid therapy increases severity of varicella infections in children with acute lymphoblastic leukemia. Pediatrics. 2005;116:e525-e529.

330. Gray MM, Hann IM, Glass S, et al. Mortality and morbidity caused by measles in children with malignant disease attending four major treatment centres: a retrospective review. Br Med J (Clin Res Ed). 1987;295:19-22.

331. Hughes I, Jenney ME, Newton RW, et al. Measles encephalitis during immunosuppressive treatment for acute lymphoblastic leukaemia. Arch Dis Child. 1993;68:775-778.

332. Siegel SE, Nesbit ME, Baehner R, et al. Pneumonia during therapy for childhood acute lymphoblastic leukemia. Am J Dis Child. 1980;134:28-34.

333. Hughes WT, Rivera GK, Schell MJ, et al. Successful intermittent chemoprophylaxis for Pneumocystis carinii pneumonitis. N Engl J Med. 1987;316:1627-1632.

334. Welte K, Reiter A, Mempel K, et al. A randomized phase-III study of the efficacy of granulocyte colony- stimulating factor in children with high-risk acute lymphoblastic leukemia. Berlin-Frankfurt-Munster Study Group. Blood. 1996;87:3143-3150.

335. Pui CH, Boyett JM, Hughes WT, et al. Human granulocyte colony-stimulating factor after induction chemotherapy in children with acute lymphoblastic leukemia. N Engl J Med. 1997;336:1781-1787.

336. Ottmann OG, Hoelzer D, Gracien E, et al. Concomitant granulocyte colony-stimulating factor and induction chemoradiotherapy in adult acute lymphoblastic leukemia: a randomized phase III trial. Blood. 1995;86:444-450.

337. Geissler K, Koller E, Hubmann E, et al. Granulocyte colony-stimulating factor as an adjunct to induction chemotherapy for adult acute lymphoblastic leukemia—a randomized phase-III study. Blood. 1997;90:590-596.

338. Katz JA, Wagner ML, Gresik MV, et al. Typhlitis. An 18-year experience and postmortem review. Cancer. 1990;65:1041-1047.

339. McCarville MB, Adelman CS, Li C, et al. Typhlitis in childhood cancer. Cancer. 2005;104:380-387.

340. Ojala AE, Lanning FP, Lanning BM. Abdominal ultrasound findings during and after treatment of childhood acute lymphoblastic leukemia. Med Pediatr Oncol. 1997;29:266-271.

341. Alexander JE, Williamson SL, Seibert JJ, et al. The ultrasonographic diagnosis of typhlitis (neutropenic colitis). Pediatr Radiol. 1988;18:200-204.

342. Quigley MM, Bethel K, Nowacki M, et al. Neutropenic enterocolitis: a rare presenting complication of acute leukemia. Am J Hematol. 2001;66:213-219.

343. Paulino AF, Kenney R, Forman EN, et al. Typhlitis in a patient with acute lymphoblastic leukemia prior to the administration of chemotherapy. Am J Pediatr Hematol Oncol. 1994;16:348-351.

344. Shamberger RC, Weinstein HJ, Delorey MJ, et al. The medical and surgical management of typhlitis in children with acute nonlymphocytic (myelogenous) leukemia. Cancer. 1986;57:603-609.

345. Moir CR, Scudamore CH, Benny WB. Typhlitis: selective surgical management. Am J Surg. 1986;151:563-566.

346. Ochs JJ, Bowman WP, Pui CH, et al. Seizures in childhood lymphoblastic leukaemia patients. Lancet. 1984;2:1422-1424.

347. Winick NJ, Bowman WP, Kamen BA, et al. Unexpected acute neurologic toxicity in the treatment of children with acute lymphoblastic leukemia. J Natl Cancer Inst. 1992;84:252-256.

348. Freeman JE, Johnston PG, Voke JM. Somnolence after prophylactic cranial irradiation in children with acute lymphoblastic leukaemia. BMJ. 1973;4:523-525.

349. Littman P, Rosenstock J, Gale G, et al. The somnolence syndrome in leukemic children following reduced daily dose fractions of cranial radiation. Int J Radiat Oncol Biol Phys. 1984;10:1851-1853.

350. Ch'ien LT, Aur RJ, Stagner S, et al. Long-term neurological implications of somnolence syndrome in children with acute lymphocytic leukemia. Ann Neurol. 1980;8:273-277.

351. Legha SS. Vincristine neurotoxicity. Pathophysiology and management. Med Toxicol. 1986;1:421-427.

352. Stuart MJ, Cuaso C, Miller M, Oski FA. Syndrome of recurrent increased secretion of antidiuretic hormone following multiple doses of vincristine. Blood. 1975;45:315-320.

353. Postma TJ, Benard BA, Huijgens PC, et al. Long-term effects of vincristine on the peripheral nervous system. J Neurooncol. 1993; 15:23-27.

354. Parsons SK, Skapek SX, Neufeld EJ, et al. Asparaginase-associated lipid abnormalities in children with acute lymphoblastic leukemia. Blood. 1997;89:1886-1895.

355. Pui CH, Burghen GA, Bowman WP, et al. Risk factors for hyperglycemia in children with leukemia receiving L-asparaginase and prednisone. J Pediatr. 1981;99:46-50.

356. Hogler W, Wehl G, van Staa T, et al. Incidence of skeletal complications during treatment of childhood acute lymphoblastic leukemia: comparison of fracture risk with the General Practice Research Database. Pediatr Blood Cancer. 2007;48:21-27.

357. Drigan R, Spirito A, Gelber RD. Behavioral effects of corticosteroids in children with acute lymphoblastic leukemia. Med Pediatr Oncol. 1992;20:13-21.

358. Meadows AT, Gordon J, Massari DJ, et al. Declines in IQ scores and cognitive dysfunctions in children with acute lymphocytic leukaemia treated with cranial irradiation. Lancet. 1981;2:1015-1018.

359. Rowland JH, Glidewell OJ, Sibley RF, et al. Effects of different forms of central nervous system prophylaxis on neuropsychologic function in childhood leukemia. J Clin Oncol. 1984;2:1327-1335.

360. Jankovic M, Brouwers P, Valsecchi MG, et al. Association of 1800 cGy cranial irradiation with intellectual function in children with acute lymphoblastic leukaemia. ISPACC. International Study Group on Psychosocial Aspects of Childhood Cancer. Lancet. 1994;344:224-227.

361. Waber DP, Gioia G, Paccia J, et al. Sex differences in cognitive processing in children treated with CNS prophylaxis for acute lymphoblastic leukemia. J Pediatr Psychol. 1990;15:105-122.

362. Butler RW, Hill JM, Steinherz PG, et al. Neuropsychologic effects of cranial irradiation, intrathecal methotrexate, and systemic methotrexate in childhood cancer. J Clin Oncol. 1994; 12:2621-2629.

363. Waber DP, Shapiro BL, Carpentieri SC, et al. Excellent therapeutic efficacy and minimal late neurotoxicity in children treated with 18 grays of cranial radiation therapy for high-risk acute lymphoblastic leukemia: a 7-year follow-up study of the Dana-Farber Cancer Institute Consortium Protocol 87-01. Cancer. 2001;92:15-22.

364. Waber DP, Tarbell NJ, Kahn CM, et al. The relationship of sex and treatment modality to neuropsychologic outcome in childhood acute lymphoblastic leukemia. J Clin Oncol. 1992;10: 810-817.

365. Mulhern RK, Fairclough D, Ochs J. A prospective comparison of neuropsychologic performance of children surviving leukemia who received 18-Gy, 24-Gy, or no cranial irradiation. J Clin Oncol. 1991;9:1348-1356.

366. Harila-Saari AH, Lahteenmaki PM, Pukkala E, et al. Scholastic achievements of childhood leukemia patients: a nationwide, register-based study. J Clin Oncol. 2007;25:3518-3524.

367. Mulhern RK, Ochs J, Fairclough D, et al. Intellectual and academic achievement status after CNS relapse: a retrospective analysis of 40 children treated for acute lymphoblastic leukemia. J Clin Oncol. 1987;5:933-940.

368. Longeway K, Mulhern R, Crisco J, et al. Treatment of meningeal relapse in childhood acute lymphoblastic leukemia: II. A prospective study of intellectual loss specific to CNS relapse and therapy. Am J Pediatr Hematol Oncol. 1990;12:45-50.

369. Kumar P, Mulhern RK, Regine WF, et al. A prospective neurocognitive evaluation of children treated with additional chemotherapy and craniospinal irradiation following isolated central nervous system relapse in acute lymphoblastic leukemia. Int J Radiat Oncol Biol Phys. 1995;31:561-566.

370. Spiegler BJ, Kennedy K, Maze R, et al. Comparison of long-term neurocognitive outcomes in young children with acute lymphoblastic leukemia treated with cranial radiation or high-dose or very high-dose intravenous methotrexate. J Clin Oncol. 2006;24: 3858-3864.

371. Halberg FE, Kramer JH, Moore IM, et al. Prophylactic cranial irradiation dose effects on late cognitive function in children treated for acute lymphoblastic leukemia. Int J Radiat Oncol Biol Phys. 1992;22:13-16.

372. Mulhern RK, Kovnar E, Langston J, et al. Long-term survivors of leukemia treated in infancy: factors associated with neuropsychologic status. J Clin Oncol. 1992;10:1095-1102.

373. Waber DP, Turek J, Catania L, et al. Neuropsychological outcomes from a randomized trial of triple intrathecal chemotherapy compared with 18 Gy cranial radiation as CNS treatment in acute lymphoblastic leukemia: findings from Dana-Farber Cancer Institute ALL Consortium Protocol 95-01. J Clin Oncol. 2007;25:4914-4921.

374. Copeland DR, Moore BD 3rd, Francis DJ, et al. Neuropsychologic effects of chemotherapy on children with cancer: a longitudinal study. J Clin Oncol. 1996;14:2826-2835.

375. Buizer AI, de Sonneville LM, van den Heuvel-Eibrink MM, et al. Behavioral and educational limitations after chemotherapy for childhood acute lymphoblastic leukemia or Wilms tumor. Cancer. 2006;106:2067-2075.

376. Kingma A, van Dommelen RI, Mooyaart EL, et al. Slight cognitive impairment and magnetic resonance imaging abnormalities but normal school levels in children treated for acute lymphoblastic leukemia with chemotherapy only. J Pediatr. 2001;139: 413-420.

377. Waber DP, Tarbell NJ, Fairclough D, et al. Cognitive sequelae of treatment in childhood acute lymphoblastic leukemia: cranial radiation requires an accomplice. J Clin Oncol. 1995;13: 2490-2496.

378. Filley CM, Kleinschmidt-DeMasters BK. Toxic leukoencephalopathy. N Engl J Med. 2001;345:425-432.

379. Aur RJ, Simone JV, Verzosa MS, et al. Childhood acute lymphocytic leukemia: study VIII. Cancer. 1978;42:2123-2134.

380. Waber DP, Urion DK, Tarbell NJ, et al. Late effects of central nervous system treatment of acute lymphoblastic leukemia in childhood are sex-dependent. Dev Med Child Neurol. 1990;32: 238-248.

381. Humpl T, Bruhl K, Bohl J, et al. Cerebral haemorrhage in long-term survivors of childhood acute lymphoblastic leukaemia. Eur J Pediatr. 1997;156:367-370.

382. Heckl S, Aschoff A, Kunze S. Radiation-induced cavernous hemangiomas of the brain: a late effect predominantly in children. Cancer. 2002;94:3285-3291.

383. Schriock EA, Schell MJ, Carter M, et al. Abnormal growth patterns and adult short stature in 115 long-term survivors of childhood leukemia. J Clin Oncol. 1991;9:400-405.

384. Sklar C, Mertens A, Walter A, et al. Final height after treatment for childhood acute lymphoblastic leukemia: comparison of no cranial irradiation with 1800 and 2400 centigrays of cranial irradiation. J Pediatr. 1993;123:59-64.

385. Didcock E, Davies HA, Didi M, et al. Pubertal growth in young adult survivors of childhood leukemia. J Clin Oncol. 1995;13: 2503-2507.

386. Dalton VK, Rue M, Silverman LB, et al. Height and weight in children treated for acute lymphoblastic leukemia: relationship to CNS treatment. J Clin Oncol. 2003;21:2953-2960.

387. Chow EJ, Friedman DL, Yasui Y, et al. Decreased adult height in survivors of childhood acute lymphoblastic leukemia: a report from the Childhood Cancer Survivor Study. J Pediatr. 2007; 150:370-375.

388. Katz JA, Chambers B, Everhart C, et al. Linear growth in children with acute lymphoblastic leukemia treated without cranial irradiation. J Pediatr. 1991;118:575-578.

389. Voorhess ML, Brecher ML, Glicksman AS, et al. Hypothalamic-pituitary function of children with acute lymphocytic leukemia

after three forms of central nervous system prophylaxis. A retrospective study. Cancer. 1986;57:1287-1291.

390. Stubberfield TG, Byrne GC, Jones TW. Growth and growth hormone secretion after treatment for acute lymphoblastic leukemia in childhood. 18-Gy versus 24-Gy cranial irradiation. J Pediatr Hematol Oncol. 1995;17:167-171.

391. Swift PG, Kearney PJ, Dalton RG, et al. Growth and hormonal status of children treated for acute lymphoblastic leukaemia. Arch Dis Child. 1978;53:890-894.

392. Odame I, Reilly JJ, Gibson BE, et al. Patterns of obesity in boys and girls after treatment for acute lymphoblastic leukaemia. Arch Dis Child. 1994;71:147-149.

393. Didi M, Didcock E, Davies HA, et al. High incidence of obesity in young adults after treatment of acute lymphoblastic leukemia in childhood. J Pediatr. 1995;127:63-67.

394. Van Dongen-Melman JE, Hokken-Koelega AC, Hahlen K, et al. Obesity after successful treatment of acute lymphoblastic leukemia in childhood. Pediatr Res. 1995;38:86-90.

395. Oeffinger KC, Mertens AC, Sklar CA, et al. Obesity in adult survivors of childhood acute lymphoblastic leukemia: a report from the Childhood Cancer Survivor Study. J Clin Oncol. 2003;21:1359-1365.

396. Sklar CA, Mertens AC, Walter A, et al. Changes in body mass index and prevalence of overweight in survivors of childhood acute lymphoblastic leukemia: role of cranial irradiation. Med Pediatr Oncol. 2000;35:91-95.

397. Razzouk BI, Rose SR, Hongeng S, et al. Obesity in survivors of childhood acute lymphoblastic leukemia and lymphoma. J Clin Oncol. 2007;25:1183-1189.

398. Halton JM, Atkinson SA, Fraher L, et al. Altered mineral metabolism and bone mass in children during treatment for acute lymphoblastic leukemia. J Bone Miner Res. 1996;11:1774-1783.

399. Arikoski P, Komulainen J, Riikonen P, et al. Reduced bone density at completion of chemotherapy for a malignancy. Arch Dis Child. 1999;80:143-148.

400. van der Sluis IM, van den Heuvel-Eibrink MM, Hahlen K, et al. Altered bone mineral density and body composition, and increased fracture risk in childhood acute lymphoblastic leukemia. J Pediatr. 2002;141:204-210.

401. Arikoski P, Komulainen J, Voutilainen R, et al. Reduced bone mineral density in long-term survivors of childhood acute lymphoblastic leukemia. J Pediatr Hematol Oncol. 1998;20:234-240.

402. Kadan-Lottick N, Marshall JA, Baron AE, et al. Normal bone mineral density after treatment for childhood acute lymphoblastic leukemia diagnosed between 1991 and 1998. J Pediatr. 2001;138:898-904.

403. Mandel K, Atkinson S, Barr RD, et al. Skeletal morbidity in childhood acute lymphoblastic leukemia. J Clin Oncol. 2004;22:1215-1221.

404. Kaste SC, Rai SN, Fleming K, et al. Changes in bone mineral density in survivors of childhood acute lymphoblastic leukemia. Pediatr Blood Cancer. 2006;46:77-87.

405. Hanif I, Mahmoud H, Pui CH. Avascular femoral head necrosis in pediatric cancer patients. Med Pediatr Oncol. 1993;21:655-660.

406. Thornton MJ, O'Sullivan G, Williams MP, et al. Avascular necrosis of bone following an intensified chemotherapy regimen including high dose steroids. Clin Radiol. 1997;52:607-612.

407. Wei SY, Esmail AN, Bunin N, et al. Avascular necrosis in children with acute lymphoblastic leukemia. J Pediatr Orthop. 2000;20:331-335.

408. Burger B, Beier R, Zimmermann M, et al. Osteonecrosis: a treatment related toxicity in childhood acute lymphoblastic leukemia (ALL)—experiences from trial ALL-BFM 95. Pediatr Blood Cancer. 2005;44:220-225.

409. Lipshultz SE, Colan SD, Gelber RD, et al. Late cardiac effects of doxorubicin therapy for acute lymphoblastic leukemia in childhood. N Engl J Med. 1991;324:808-815.

410. Sorensen K, Levitt G, Bull C, et al. Anthracycline dose in childhood acute lymphoblastic leukemia: issues of early survival versus late cardiotoxicity. J Clin Oncol. 1997;15:61-68.

411. Lipshultz SE, Lipsitz SR, Mone SM, et al. Female sex and drug dose as risk factors for late cardiotoxic effects of doxorubicin therapy for childhood cancer. N Engl J Med. 1995;332:1738-1743.

412. Krischer JP, Epstein S, Cuthbertson DD, et al. Clinical cardiotoxicity following anthracycline treatment for childhood cancer: the Pediatric Oncology Group experience. J Clin Oncol. 1997;15:1544-1552.

413. Lipshultz SE, Rifai N, Dalton VM, et al. Dexrazoxane reduces myocardial injury in doxorubicin-treated children with acute lymphoblastic leukemia: results from a randomized trial. N Engl J Med. 2004;351:145-153.

414. Quigley C, Cowell C, Jimenez M, et al. Normal or early development of puberty despite gonadal damage in children treated for acute lymphoblastic leukemia. N Engl J Med. 1989;321:143-151.

415. Blatt J, Poplack DG, Sherins RJ. Testicular function in boys after chemotherapy for acute lymphoblastic leukemia. N Engl J Med. 1981;304:1121-1124.

416. Lendon M, Hann IM, Palmer MK, et al. Testicular histology after combination chemotherapy in childhood for acute lymphoblastic leukaemia. Lancet. 1978;2:439-441.

417. Muller HL, Klinkhammer-Schalke M, Seelbach-Gobel B, et al. Gonadal function of young adults after therapy of malignancies during childhood or adolescence. Eur J Pediatr. 1996;155:763-769.

418. Chow EJ, Friedman DL, Yasui Y, et al. Timing of menarche among survivors of childhood acute lymphoblastic leukemia: a report from the Childhood Cancer Survivor Study. Pediatr Blood Cancer. 2008;50:854-858.

419. Green DM, Hall B, Zevon MA. Pregnancy outcome after treatment for acute lymphoblastic leukemia during childhood or adolescence. Cancer. 1989;64:2335-2339.

420. Kenney LB, Nicholson HS, Brasseux C, et al. Birth defects in offspring of adult survivors of childhood acute lymphoblastic leukemia. A Childrens Cancer Group/National Institutes of Health Report. Cancer. 1996;78:169-176.

421. Hoover DL, Smith LE, Turner SJ, et al. Ophthalmic evaluation of survivors of acute lymphoblastic leukemia. Ophthalmology. 1988;95:151-155.

422. Loning L, Zimmermann M, Reiter A, et al. Secondary neoplasms subsequent to Berlin-Frankfurt-Munster therapy of acute lymphoblastic leukemia in childhood: significantly lower risk without cranial radiotherapy. Blood. 2000;95:2770-2775.

423. Bhatia S, Sather HN, Pabustan OB, et al. Low incidence of second neoplasms among children diagnosed with acute lymphoblastic leukemia after 1983. Blood. 2002;99:4257-4264.

424. Hijiya N, Hudson MM, Lensing S, et al. Cumulative incidence of secondary neoplasms as a first event after childhood acute lymphoblastic leukemia. JAMA. 2007;297:1207-1215.

425. Maule M, Scelo G, Pastore G, et al. Risk of second malignant neoplasms after childhood leukemia and lymphoma: an international study. J Natl Cancer Inst. 2007;99:790-800.

426. Kimball Dalton VM, Gelber RD, Li F, et al. Second malignancies in patients treated for childhood acute lymphoblastic leukemia. J Clin Oncol. 1998;16:2848-2853.

427. Pui CH, Behm FG, Raimondi SC, et al. Secondary acute myeloid leukemia in children treated for acute lymphoid leukemia. N Engl J Med. 1989;321:136-142.

428. Winick NJ, McKenna RW, Shuster JJ, et al. Secondary acute myeloid leukemia in children with acute lymphoblastic leukemia treated with etoposide. J Clin Oncol. 1993;11:209-217.

429. Tucker MA, Meadows AT, Boice JD Jr, et al. Leukemia after therapy with alkylating agents for childhood cancer. J Natl Cancer Inst. 1987;78:459-464.

430. Kreissman SG, Gelber RD, Cohen HJ, et al. Incidence of secondary acute myelogenous leukemia after treatment of childhood acute lymphoblastic leukemia. Cancer. 1992;70:2208-2213.

431. Walter AW, Hancock ML, Pui CH, et al. Secondary brain tumors in children treated for acute lymphoblastic leukemia at St Jude Children's Research Hospital. J Clin Oncol. 1998;16:3761-3767.

432. Sonis AL, Tarbell N, Valachovic RW, et al. Dentofacial development in long-term survivors of acute lymphoblastic leukemia. A comparison of three treatment modalities. Cancer. 1990;66:2645-2652.

433. Nesbit M, Krivit W, Heyn R, et al. Acute and chronic effects of methotrexate on hepatic, pulmonary, and skeletal systems. Cancer. 1976;37:1048-1057.

434. Farrow AC, Buchanan GR, Zwiener RJ, et al. Serum aminotransferase elevation during and following treatment of childhood acute lymphoblastic leukemia. J Clin Oncol. 1997;15:1560-1566.

435. Broxson EH, Dole M, Wong R, et al. Portal hypertension develops in a subset of children with standard risk acute lymphoblastic leukemia treated with oral 6-thioguanine during maintenance therapy. Pediatr Blood Cancer. 2005;44:226-231.

436. Henze G, Fengler R, Hartmann R, et al. Six-year experience with a comprehensive approach to the treatment of recurrent childhood acute lymphoblastic leukemia (ALL-REZ BFM 85). A relapse study of the BFM group. Blood. 1991;78:1166-1172.

437. Wheeler K, Richards S, Bailey C, Chessells J. Comparison of bone marrow transplant and chemotherapy for relapsed childhood acute lymphoblastic leukaemia: the MRC UKALL X experience. Medical Research Council Working Party on Childhood Leukaemia. Br J Haematol. 1998;101:94-103.

438. Gaynon PS, Qu RP, Chappell RJ, et al. Survival after relapse in childhood acute lymphoblastic leukemia: impact of site and time to first relapse—the Children's Cancer Group Experience. Cancer. 1998;82:1387-1395.

439. Roy A, Cargill A, Love S, et al. Outcome after first relapse in childhood acute lymphoblastic leukaemia—lessons from the United Kingdom R2 trial. Br J Haematol. 2005;130:67-75.

440. Einsiedel HG, von Stackelberg A, Hartmann R, et al. Long-term outcome in children with relapsed ALL by risk-stratified salvage therapy: results of trial acute lymphoblastic leukemia-relapse study of the Berlin-Frankfurt-Munster Group 87. J Clin Oncol. 2005;23:7942-7950.

441. Rivera GK, Zhou Y, Hancock ML, et al. Bone marrow recurrence after initial intensive treatment for childhood acute lymphoblastic leukemia. Cancer. 2005;103:368-376.

442. Eapen M, Raetz E, Zhang MJ, et al. Outcomes after HLA-matched sibling transplantation or chemotherapy in children with B-precursor acute lymphoblastic leukemia in a second remission: a collaborative study of the Children's Oncology Group and the Center for International Blood and Marrow Transplant Research. Blood. 2006;107:4961-4967.

443. Giona F, Testi AM, Rondelli R, et al. ALL R-87 protocol in the treatment of children with acute lymphoblastic leukaemia in early bone marrow relapse. Br J Haematol. 1997;99:671-677.

444. Buhrer C, Hartmann R, Fengler R, et al. Peripheral blast counts at diagnosis of late isolated bone marrow relapse of childhood acute lymphoblastic leukemia predict response to salvage chemotherapy and outcome. Berlin-Frankfurt-Munster Relapse Study Group. J Clin Oncol. 1996;14:2812-2817.

445. Buhrer C, Hartmann R, Fengler R, et al. Superior prognosis in combined compared to isolated bone marrow relapses in salvage therapy of childhood acute lymphoblastic leukemia. Med Pediatr Oncol. 1993;21:470-476.

446. Sadowitz PD, Smith SD, Shuster J, et al. Treatment of late bone marrow relapse in children with acute lymphoblastic leukemia: a Pediatric Oncology Group study. Blood. 1993;81:602-609.

447. Abshire TC, Pollock BH, Billett AL, et al. Weekly polyethylene glycol conjugated L-asparaginase compared with biweekly dosing produces superior induction remission rates in childhood relapsed acute lymphoblastic leukemia: a Pediatric Oncology Group Study. Blood. 2000;96:1709-1715.

448. Matsuzaki A, Nagatoshi Y, Inada H, et al. Prognostic factors for relapsed childhood acute lymphoblastic leukemia: impact of allogeneic stem cell transplantation—a report from the Kyushu-Yamaguchi Children's Cancer Study Group. Pediatr Blood Cancer. 2005;45:111-120.

449. Hijiya N, Gajjar A, Zhang Z, et al. Low-dose oral etoposide-based induction regimen for children with acute lymphoblastic leukemia in first bone marrow relapse. Leukemia. 2004;18:1581-1586.

450. Eckert C, Biondi A, Seeger K, et al. Prognostic value of minimal residual disease in relapsed childhood acute lymphoblastic leukaemia. Lancet. 2001;358:1239-1241.

451. Coustan-Smith E, Gajjar A, Hijiya N, et al. Clinical significance of minimal residual disease in childhood acute lymphoblastic leukemia after first relapse. Leukemia. 2004;18:499-504.

452. Barrett AJ, Horowitz MM, Pollock BH, et al. Bone marrow transplants from HLA-identical siblings as compared with chemotherapy for children with acute lymphoblastic leukemia in a second remission. N Engl J Med. 1994;331:1253-1258.

453. Uderzo C, Valsecchi MG, Bacigalupo A, et al. Treatment of childhood acute lymphoblastic leukemia in second remission with allogeneic bone marrow transplantation and chemotherapy: ten-year experience of the Italian Bone Marrow Transplantation Group and the Italian Pediatric Hematology Oncology Association. J Clin Oncol. 1995;13:352-358.

454. Dopfer R, Henze G, Bender-Gotze C, et al. Allogeneic bone marrow transplantation for childhood acute lymphoblastic leukemia in second remission after intensive primary and relapse therapy according to the BFM- and CoALL-protocols: results of the German Cooperative Study. Blood. 1991;78:2780-2784.

455. Weisdorf DJ, Woods WG, Nesbit ME Jr, et al. Allogeneic bone marrow transplantation for acute lymphoblastic leukaemia: risk factors and clinical outcome. Br J Haematol. 1994;86:62-69.

456. Torres A, Alvarez MA, Sanchez J, et al. Allogeneic bone marrow transplantation vs chemotherapy for the treatment of childhood acute lymphoblastic leukaemia in second complete remission (revisited 10 years on). Bone Marrow Transplant. 1999;23:1257-1260.

457. Brochstein JA, Kernan NA, Groshen S, et al. Allogeneic bone marrow transplantation after hyperfractionated total-body irradiation and cyclophosphamide in children with acute leukemia. N Engl J Med. 1987;317:1618-1624.

458. Davies SM, Ramsay NK, Klein JP, et al. Comparison of preparative regimens in transplants for children with acute lymphoblastic leukemia. J Clin Oncol. 2000;18:340-347.

459. Parsons SK, Castellino SM, Lehmann LE, et al. Relapsed acute lymphoblastic leukemia: similar outcomes for autologous and allogeneic marrow transplantation in selected children. Bone Marrow Transplant. 1996;17:763-768.

460. Knechtli CJ, Goulden NJ, Hancock JP, et al. Minimal residual disease status before allogeneic bone marrow transplantation is an important determinant of successful outcome for children and adolescents with acute lymphoblastic leukemia. Blood. 1998;92:4072-4079.

461. Bader P, Hancock J, Kreyenberg H, et al. Minimal residual disease (MRD) status prior to allogeneic stem cell transplantation is a powerful predictor for post-transplant outcome in children with ALL. Leukemia. 2002;16:1668-1672.

462. Sramkova L, Muzikova K, Fronkova E, et al. Detectable minimal residual disease before allogeneic hematopoietic stem cell transplantation predicts extremely poor prognosis in children with

acute lymphoblastic leukemia. Pediatr Blood Cancer. 2007;48: 93-100.

463. Davies SM, Wagner JE, Shu XO, et al. Unrelated donor bone marrow transplantation for children with acute leukemia. J Clin Oncol. 1997;15:557-565.

464. Bunin N, Carston M, Wall D, et al. Unrelated marrow transplantation for children with acute lymphoblastic leukemia in second remission. Blood. 2002;99:3151-3157.

465. Locatelli F, Zecca M, Messina C, et al. Improvement over time in outcome for children with acute lymphoblastic leukemia in second remission given hematopoietic stem cell transplantation from unrelated donors. Leukemia. 2002;16:2228-2237.

466. Woolfrey AE, Anasetti C, Storer B, et al. Factors associated with outcome after unrelated marrow transplantation for treatment of acute lymphoblastic leukemia in children. Blood. 2002;99: 2002-2008.

467. Saarinen-Pihkala UM, Gustafsson G, Ringden O, et al. No disadvantage in outcome of using matched unrelated donors as compared with matched sibling donors for bone marrow transplantation in children with acute lymphoblastic leukemia in second remission. J Clin Oncol. 2001;19:3406-3414.

468. Jacobsohn DA, Hewlett B, Ranalli M, et al. Outcomes of unrelated cord blood transplants and allogeneic-related hematopoietic stem cell transplants in children with high-risk acute lymphocytic leukemia. Bone Marrow Transplant. 2004;34:901-907.

469. Borgmann A, von Stackelberg A, Hartmann R, et al. Unrelated donor stem cell transplantation compared with chemotherapy for children with acute lymphoblastic leukemia in a second remission: a matched-pair analysis. Blood. 2003;101:3835-3839.

470. Busca A, Anasetti C, Anderson G, et al. Unrelated donor or autologous marrow transplantation for treatment of acute leukemia. Blood. 1994;83:3077-3084.

471. Sallan SE, Niemeyer CM, Billett AL, et al. Autologous bone marrow transplantation for acute lymphoblastic leukemia. J Clin Oncol. 1989;7:1594-1601.

472. Billett AL, Kornmehl E, Tarbell NJ, et al. Autologous bone marrow transplantation after a long first remission for children with recurrent acute lymphoblastic leukemia. Blood. 1993;81: 1651-1657.

473. Maldonado MS, Diaz-Heredia C, Badell I, et al. Autologous bone marrow transplantation with monoclonal antibody purged marrow for children with acute lymphoblastic leukemia in second remission. Spanish Working Party for BMT in Children. Bone Marrow Transplant. 1998;22:1043-1047.

474. Borgmann A, Schmid H, Hartmann R, et al. Autologous bone-marrow transplants compared with chemotherapy for children with acute lymphoblastic leukaemia in a second remission: a matched-pair analysis. The Berlin-Frankfurt-Munster Study Group. Lancet. 1995;346:873-876.

475. Hagedorn N, Acquaviva C, Fronkova E, et al. Submicroscopic bone marrow involvement in isolated extramedullary relapses in childhood acute lymphoblastic leukemia: a more precise definition of "isolated" and its possible clinical implications, a collaborative study of the Resistant Disease Committee of the International BFM study group. Blood. 2007;110:4022-4029.

476. George SL, Ochs JJ, Mauer AM, et al. The importance of an isolated central nervous system relapse in children with acute lymphoblastic leukemia. J Clin Oncol. 1985;3:776-781.

477. Behrendt H, van Leeuwen EF, Schuwirth C, et al. The significance of an isolated central nervous system relapse, occurring as first relapse in children with acute lymphoblastic leukemia. Cancer. 1989;63:2066-2072.

478. Ribeiro RC, Rivera GK, Hudson M, et al. An intensive re-treatment protocol for children with an isolated CNS relapse of acute lymphoblastic leukemia. J Clin Oncol. 1995;13:333-338.

479. Ritchey AK, Pollock BH, Lauer SJ, et al. Improved survival of children with isolated CNS relapse of acute lymphoblastic leukemia: a pediatric oncology group study. J Clin Oncol. 1999;17:3745-3752.

480. Barredo JC, Devidas M, Lauer SJ, et al. Isolated CNS relapse of acute lymphoblastic leukemia treated with intensive systemic chemotherapy and delayed CNS radiation: a pediatric oncology group study. J Clin Oncol. 2006;24:3142-3149.

481. Borgmann A, Hartmann R, Schmid H, et al. Isolated extramedullary relapse in children with acute lymphoblastic leukemia: a comparison between treatment results of chemotherapy and bone marrow transplantation. BFM Relapse Study Group. Bone Marrow Transplant. 1995;15:515-521.

482. Eapen M, Zhang MJ, Devidas M, et al. Outcomes after HLA-matched sibling transplantation or chemotherapy in children with acute lymphoblastic leukemia in a second remission after an isolated central nervous system relapse: a collaborative study of the Children's Oncology Group and the Center for International Blood and Marrow Transplant Research. Leukemia. 2008;22: 281-286.

483. Uderzo C, Grazia Zurlo M, Adamoli L, et al. Treatment of isolated testicular relapse in childhood acute lymphoblastic leukemia: an Italian multicenter study. Associazione Italiana Ematologia ed Oncologia Pediatrica. J Clin Oncol. 1990;8:672-677.

484. Wofford MM, Smith SD, Shuster JJ, et al. Treatment of occult or late overt testicular relapse in children with acute lymphoblastic leukemia: a Pediatric Oncology Group study. J Clin Oncol. 1992;10:624-630.

485. Finklestein JZ, Miller DR, Feusner J, et al. Treatment of overt isolated testicular relapse in children on therapy for acute lymphoblastic leukemia. A report from the Childrens Cancer Group. Cancer. 1994;73:219-223.

486. Novakovic P, Kellie SJ, Taylor D. Childhood leukaemia: relapse in the anterior segment of the eye. Br J Ophthalmol. 1989;73: 354-359.

487. Heaton DC, Duff GB. Ovarian relapse in a young woman with acute lymphoblastic leukaemia. Am J Hematol. 1989;30:42-43.

488. Yeoh EJ, Ross ME, Shurtleff SA, et al. Classification, subtype discovery, and prediction of outcome in pediatric acute lymphoblastic leukemia by gene expression profiling. Cancer Cell. 2002;1:133-143.

489. Ferrando AA, Neuberg DS, Staunton J, et al. Gene expression signatures define novel oncogenic pathways in T cell acute lymphoblastic leukemia. Cancer Cell. 2002;1:75-87.

490. Jeha S, Gaynon PS, Razzouk BI, et al. Phase II study of clofarabine in pediatric patients with refractory or relapsed acute lymphoblastic leukemia. J Clin Oncol. 2006;24:1917-1923.

491. Del Gaizo Moore V, Schlis KD, Sallan SE, et al. BCL-2 dependence and ABT-737 sensitivity in acute lymphoblastic leukemia. Blood. 2008;111:2300-2309.

492. Wei G, Twomey D, Lamb J, et al. Gene expression-based chemical genomics identifies rapamycin as a modulator of MCL1 and glucocorticoid resistance. Cancer Cell. 2006;10:331-342.

493. Dijoseph JF, Dougher MM, Armellino DC, et al. Therapeutic potential of CD22-specific antibody-targeted chemotherapy using inotuzumab ozogamicin (CMC-544) for the treatment of acute lymphoblastic leukemia. Leukemia. 2007;21:2240-2245.

494. Pui CH, Cheng C, Leung W, et al. Extended follow-up of long-term survivors of childhood acute lymphoblastic leukemia. N Engl J Med. 2003;349:640-649.

495. Mody R, Li S, Dover DC, et al. Twenty-five-year follow-up among survivors of childhood acute lymphoblastic leukemia: a report from the Childhood Cancer Survivor Study. Blood. 2008;111:5515-5523.

Myeloid Leukemia, Myelodysplasia, and Myeloproliferative Disease in Children

11

Jennifer J. Clark, Jason N. Berman, and A. Thomas Look

ACUTE MYELOGENOUS LEUKEMIA

Acute myelogenous leukemia (AML) comprises a heterogeneous group of disorders characterized by the malignant clonal transformation of a hematopoietic stem or progenitor cell. In recent years, deeper understanding has been gained into the chromosomal changes and specific genetic mutations that precipitate this transformation. AML is a relatively rare disorder in children, with between 500 and 600 newly diagnosed patients in the United States each year. Because of the heterogeneous nature of AML, it has proven difficult to find a treatment strategy that is effective for all patients; thus, overall cure rates for AML have improved only modestly in the past few decades, lagging behind those for acute lymphoblastic leukemia (ALL). Drawing from data from the Medical Research Council (MRC) trials, patients with AML are now risk-stratified. Current ongoing clinical trials are attempting to minimize toxicity for patients with low-risk disease and intensify therapy for patients with high-risk disease. As the molecular genetics behind the biology of AML are better elucidated, there is a pressing need to develop new strategies for targeted therapy to improve outcomes in AML.

Epidemiology and Etiology

According to the National Cancer Institute (NCI) Surveillance Epidemiology and End Results (SEER) data, it was estimated that each year, from 2000 to 2004, approximately 12,000 children younger than 14 years and 5,600 adolescents aged 15 to 20 years were diagnosed with cancer.[1] Leukemias made up 37% of the cancers in children younger than 5 years, but only 14% of cancers in adolescents aged 15 to 20 years.[1,2] The predominant childhood leukemia is ALL. AML comprises only about 16% of childhood leukemias in children younger than 15 years, but 36% of leukemias in adolescents 15 to 20 years, for a total of 500 to 600 new pediatric AML patients annually in the United States. AML has a bimodal distribution, occurring with higher incidence in children younger than 2 years and then again in adolescents 15 to 20 years old.

In ALL, boys are more commonly affected than girls; however, the incidence of AML is similar for all pediatric age groups, regardless of gender.[1,2] Similarly, although the incidence of childhood ALL is higher in white than in black children, the incidence of AML is comparable for both races across all pediatric age groups. With regard to ethnicity, there is a higher incidence of AML in Hispanic versus non-Hispanic children. Of interest, although the incidence of ALL for children younger than 15 years increased from 1977 to 1995, the incidence of AML did not change significantly over this time period.[2]

For a subset of patients with AML, a series of risk factors predisposing to the development of AML has been identified (Box 11-1) These risk factors fall into two general categories, exposures (environmental or toxic) and genetic predisposition. The best understood of the exposures is prior treatment with chemotherapy and radiation. Alkylating agents (e.g., nitrogen mustard, cyclophosphamide, ifosfamide, chlorambucil, and melphalan) are associated with the development of myelodysplastic syndrome (MDS) and secondary AML, with deletions of chromosomes 5 and 7.[3,4] Treatment with topoisomerase II inhibitors such as the epipodophyllotoxins has been linked to a specific type of AML with chromosome band 11q23 translocations, which produce fusion proteins involving the mixed-lineage leukemia (MLL) gene.[5-9] Treatment with anthracyclines in adults with breast cancer, or in children for leukemias and sarcomas such as osteosarcoma, is associated with the development of secondary leukemias, including ALL, AML,

---

Box 11-1 | **Predisposing Factors for the Development of Acute Myelogenous Leukemia or Myelodysplastic Syndromes**

PRENATAL EXPOSURES

Alcohol
Pesticides★
Foods naturally high in topoisomerase II inhibitors★
Viral infections

ENVIRONMENTAL EXPOSURES

Ionizing radiation
Chemotherapeutic agents
Alkylating agents
Epipodophyllotoxins
Anthracyclines
Organic solvents (i.e., benzene)
Radon★
Pesticides★
Viral infections★

HEREDITARY CONDITIONS

Down syndrome
Fanconi's anemia
Bloom's syndrome
Severe congenital neutropenia (i.e., Kostmann's syndrome)
Shwachman-Diamond syndrome
Neurofibromatosis type I
Klinefelter's syndrome (XXY)★

ACQUIRED DISORDERS

Aplastic anemia
Paroxysmal nocturnal hemoglobinuria

★Conflicting or limited data.

---

and chronic myelogenous leukemia (CML).[10,11] Although therapy-related AML generally carries a worse prognosis than de novo AML, there have been reported cases of therapy-related AML harboring the better risk cytogenetic abnormalities: t(8;21), inv(16), t(16;16), and t(15;17), often in conjunction with other cytogenetic abnormalities.[12,13] In the case of therapy-related AML with inv(16) and t(16;16), a rare core-binding factor β (CBFβ)–myosin heavy chain 11 (MYH11) fusion transcript has been reported, with different breakpoints compared with the usual fusion transcript found in better risk de novo AML.[13] Similarly, there is a case report of a patient with therapy-related AML with t(8;21), and the breakpoint at 21q22 was outside the AML1 locus.[14]

Radiation exposure may be acquired from the environment or through medical procedures and is well documented to predispose to leukemia. The increased risk of AML and CML in survivors of nuclear blasts in Japan who were exposed to excessive doses of ionizing radiation has been well documented, and these patients have a higher rate of abnormalities of chromosomes 5 and 7.[15-17] An increased risk of AML and ALL in children exposed to radiation in utero has been described, particularly in the past, when diagnostic x-rays were more common during pregnancy,[18,19] although a retrospective study of children with leukemia in Sweden did not confirm this finding.[20] Nuclear power plant workers have a higher risk of leukemia, although there does not appear to be a higher risk in residents living near such plants.[21-23] Air travel is a source of exposure to cosmic radiation and studies have shown an increase in malignant melanoma and other skin cancers in flight crew members, an increase in breast cancer in female flight crew members, and an increase in AML in male cockpit crew members who logged more than 5000 flight hours annually.[24,25] Studies designed to measure the potential risk of malignancy from residential or occupational exposure to magnetic fields around high-voltage electrical lines have generated conflicting results, and a causal relationship with AML has not been established.[26-33]

There are several other environmental exposures with possible links to AML, some of which have yet to be proven definitively. Benzene exposure, which may occur occupationally or through tobacco smoking, has been shown to increase the risk of AML.[24,25,34,35] Several prenatal exposures have been studied as risk factors for the development of AML, particularly in children younger than 3 years. Maternal alcohol consumption during pregnancy was studied in a Children's Cancer Group (CCG) case-control study and found to have an association with increased rates of childhood AML in a dose-dependent matter, with an odds ratio of 2.64 overall and an odds ratio of 7.62 for M1 (myeloblastic with minimal maturation) and M2 (myeloblastic with maturation) AML; other case-control studies have confirmed this finding.[36,37] Some early studies had suggested an association between maternal tobacco and marijuana use and childhood AML, but more recent analyses have not confirmed this association. A Children's Oncology Group (COG) case-control study looked at maternal consumption of foods such as soy, green and black tea, cocoa, red wine, and certain fruits and vegetables that are naturally high in DNA topoisomerase II inhibitors and found an odds ratio of 1.9 to 3.2 for the development of *MLL*-rearranged AML in the setting of high maternal consumption of these foods.[38] Some studies have suggested an increased risk of childhood AML after high exposure to pesticides, either prenatally or postnatally, up to 3 years of age.[39] There is interest in an association between viral infections and AML, but few data. One case-control study has suggested an increase in childhood AML in offspring of mothers who reactivated Epstein-Barr virus (EBV) during pregnancy.[40] Parvovirus B19 is associated with pure red cell aplasia, and certain human leukocyte antigen (HLA)–DRB1 alleles seem to be associated with symptomatic infection.[41] One study of 16 leukemia patients has suggested an association between parvovirus B19 infection and acute leukemia in 4 of the patients, including 1 patient with AML, all of whom carried these particular HLA-DRB1 alleles, although this association needs further investigation.[42] Several retrospective studies have suggested that breast-feeding may be protective against ALL and AML.[43-45] Risk related to indoor radon exposure is controversial, with one French study showing a higher rate of AML in children with high exposure, but other studies showing no association.[46,47] Rarely used now, chloramphenicol use in children was formerly associated with an increased risk of AML.[48]

An increased incidence of AML has been observed for patients with certain hereditary disorders. Children with congenital disorders of myelopoiesis, such as Kostmann's syndrome, Shwachman-Diamond syndrome, and Diamond-Blackfan anemia, are predisposed to AML.[49-56] Patients with inherited syndromes associated with chromosome fragility and impaired DNA repair mechanisms, such as Fanconi's anemia[57-60] and Bloom's syndrome,[61-63] also have an increased risk for development of AML. Neurofibromatosis type 1, which is caused by mutations in the neurofibromin tumor suppressor gene on chromosome 17, is associated with juvenile myelomonocytic leukemia (JMML).[64-66] Patients with certain constitutional chromosomal abnormalities carry a higher risk for AML.[67,68] Down syndrome is one of the most clinically prominent examples in this category. It is estimated that over 10% of infants with Down syndrome exhibit a transient myeloproliferative disease (TMD) associated with a GATA-1 mutation.[69] Down syndrome patients have a 10 to 20 times higher than average risk of developing acute leukemia. In Down syndrome patients younger than 4 years, AML, usually acute megakaryoblastic (AMKL), is far more common than ALL, with an estimated 1 in 500 Down syndrome patients developing AML.[69,70] In contrast to AMKL in the general pediatric population, which carries an extremely poor prognosis, this disease in Down syndrome patients is extremely chemotherapy-sensitive and will be discussed in detail in a later section of this chapter.[69,70] Although early studies did not suggest a higher risk of AML in patients with Klinefelter's syndrome (XXY), some newer data suggest that these patients may have a higher risk of hematologic malignancy, including AML.[71-73]

Although the predisposing risk factors and genetic conditions described may provide insight into the causative mechanisms that increase the risk of development of AML, most patients with de novo AML have no known predisposing exposures or conditions. Point mutations and chromosomal deletions and translocations occur at a background rate, even in normal healthy individuals, during hematopoietic stem and progenitor cell expansion. The extent to which inherited, expressed, single-nucleotide polymorphisms in the general population alter mutational rates during myelopoiesis and increase the risk of AML and other cancers remains an area of intense investigation.

Biology

Clonal Origin of Myeloid Leukemia Cells

Normal myelopoiesis is a complex differentiation program whereby primitive hematopoietic stem cells develop along a multistep pathway into fully differentiated, functionally active circulating blood cells.[74] This exquisitely controlled process is regulated by the intricate interactions among the expression levels of various transcription factors, growth factors and their receptors, cytokines, enzymes, and still unidentified novel molecules. A series of sequential genetic abnormalities perturbs this normal developmental progression and leads to AML. Although the relationships between specific morphologic subtypes of AML and their specific recurring genetic abnormalities have provided some insight into the mechanisms of leukemogenesis, understanding of the process whereby these fusion gene products interact with normal signal transduction pathways to subvert hematopoietic cell development is incomplete.[75]

Several strong lines of evidence have supported the hypotheses that AML progresses from a single transformed hematopoietic stem or progenitor cell. More than 30 years ago, studies were pioneered by Beutler and colleagues[76] and Fialkow[77] using X inactivation patterns in female patients to establish the clonal origin of human malignancies, including leukemia. By showing the presence of a single glucose-6-hydrogenase (G6PD) isoenzyme in the leukemic myeloblasts of heterozygous females, the clonal origin of myeloid leukemia cells was demonstrated.[78-80] Females who are heterozygous at the G6PD locus express two isoforms of the enzyme. Approximately half of the cells in normal somatic tissue have randomly inactivated one of the X chromosomes, and approximately half of the cells should therefore express each isoform. Unlike normal somatic cells, AML cells of female patients heterozygous for G6PD expressed only one G6PD isoform, indicating cells of clonal origin.[79,80] In the 1980s, Vogelstein and coworkers[81,82] developed a strategy using X chromosome–linked DNA restriction length fragment polymorphisms to determine the clonal origin of human tumors. They established that maturing granulocytic cells arise from the malignant clone in patients with AML.[83] Later, X chromosome inactivation to determine clonality in malignancies was carried out using the polymerase chain reaction (PCR) assay to distinguish X-linked polymorphic genes.[84-86]

Transformation of Stem Cells with Self-Renewal Capacity

These earlier studies, and those performed by Bonnet and Dick and associates in the 1990s,[87,88] led to the insight that leukemia cell populations form a hierarchy in which leukemia stem cells or leukemia-initiating cells (LICs) are responsible for their own self-renewal and for the generation of the more differentiated progeny within the leukemic clone. Whereas AML was the first human cancer in which cancer stem cells were identified, the case has been similarly made more recently in breast cancer,[89] brain tumors,[90-92] and colon cancer.[93] Although the concept that AML stem cells exist is well accepted, the identity of the corresponding normal cell that has been transformed remains controversial. AML is a heterogeneous disease in its clinical manifestations, response to therapy, and molecular genetics; thus, insight into the cell of origin would have important rami-

fications regarding diagnosis and treatment. Dick's group has produced a series of convincing papers[87,88,94] that strongly implicate the primitive, pluripotent hematopoietic stem cell (HSC) as the LIC in most types of AML. Subsequently, the HSC's inherent gene programs ensuring self-renewal, proliferation, and survival become sabotaged through a series of genetic events and ultimately a fully transformed AML LIC is generated, capable of producing a clonal population of leukemia cells. According to this argument, different AML phenotypes often occur as a result of the gene(s) that are altered, leading to differentiation arrest within the progeny of the LIC, but not necessarily reflecting the degree of the commitment of the initially transformed cell (Fig. 11-1).

Support for this hypothesis initially came from several clonality studies in leukemic cells from patients with AML,[95-97] which demonstrated multilineage involvement in a high proportion of cases and implicated a multipotent HSC as the cell of origin.[96] More supportive evidence has come from studies looking at cytogenetic markers and characteristic cell surface antigen expression patterns.[98] Pluripotent hematopoietic stem cells express CD34, but do not express CD38 or HLA-DR, whereas more committed myeloid progenitor cells are CD34+, CD38+, and HLA-DR+.[74,98] Using fluorescence-activated cell sorting (FACS) of leukemic cell populations, the same two subpopulations, CD34+/CD38– and CD34+/CD38+, were isolated from the bone marrow of patients with different AML subtypes. The two subpopulations were then evaluated using fluorescence in situ hybridization (FISH) to determine the presence of cytogenetic abnormalities. The studies detected the same characteristic cytogenetic abnormalities in the CD34+/

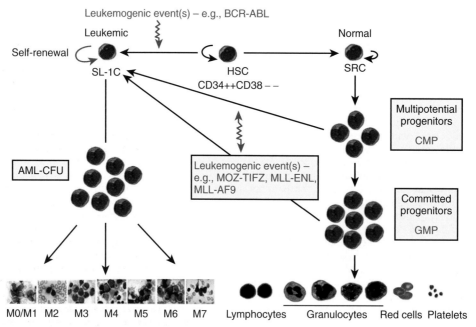

FIGURE 11-1. The hierarchical model of acute myelogenous leukemia (AML) based on the organization of the normal hematopoietic system. A leukemogenic event occurring in a hematopoietic stem cell that inherently has self-renewal capabilities (e.g., BCR-ABL translocation) often results in the disruption of normal lineage development and/or increased proliferation, thus converting that cell into a leukemic stem cell. Additional mutations result in further expansion of the leukemic clone and suppression of normal hematopoiesis. Alternatively, some chimeric transcription factors that confer self-renewal capabilities (e.g., MOZ-TIF2, MLL-ENL, MLL-AF9) can convert a more differentiated cell (e.g., CMP, GMP) into a leukemic stem cell, at least in part by endowing it with the capactiy for self renewal. Again, additional mutations result in further expansion of the leukemic phenotype and suppression of normal hematopoiesis. The nature of the leukemogenic mutations, not the lineage commitment of the leukemia-initiating cell, determines the differentiation program of the leukemic blast. CFU, colony-forming unit; CMP, common myeloid progenitors; GMP, granulocytic-monocytic–restricted progenitor; HSC, hematopoietic stem cell. (Courtesy of Dr. John E. Dick, Princess Margaret Hospital, Toronto; adapted from Zon LI [ed]. Hematopoiesis: A Developmental Approach. New York, Oxford University Press, 2001.)

CD38− stem cell fraction as were present in the original leukemic bone marrow samples, implying origin in a very early HSC compartment.[99,100]

Further evidence supporting the stem cell origin model of AML was derived from transplantation experiments in which purified human AML cells were transplanted into mice with severe combined immunodeficiency (SCID). These experiments defined a SCID mouse leukemia–initiating cell (SL-IC) in the bone marrow of patients with AML and showed that these SL-ICs are CD34+/CD38− and that their engraftment produces large numbers of colony-forming progenitors. The CD34+/CD38+ and CD34− fractions did not engraft.[88] Similar results were obtained through transplantation studies in a modified SCID mouse, the nonobese diabetic mouse with SCID (NOD/SCID), with cells from patients with AML.[87] These studies identified and analyzed AML stem cells from samples of different French-American-British (FAB) subtypes on the basis of their ability to initiate human AML after transplantation in NOD/SCID mice. These SL-ICs were able to proliferate and differentiate after transplantation, producing disease in the mice identical to that in the donor, as well as being able to renew themselves, re-establishing AML in secondary recipients and demonstrating that the SL-ICs are capable of self-renewal. Again, the SL-ICs were found to reside in the CD34+/CD38− fraction and not in the CD34+/CD38+ or CD34− fractions. The SL-IC phenotype was consistent regardless of the FAB subtype (e.g., M1, M2, M4, M5). As few as 2×10^4 CD34+ cells were able to initiate the leukemic clone in recipient mice, whereas 100 times as many CD34− cells failed to engraft. Cells with the CD34 surface antigen were further fractionated on the basis of CD38 expression. Only the CD34+/CD38− fraction contained SL-ICs.[87]

These data strongly support the leukemic stem cell hypothesis for AML, which has gained momentum and acceptance, given the shared functional profile between a normal hematopoietic stem cell and LICs. However, several recent studies have given new credence to an older theory that hypothesized that committed progenitor cells along the pathway of myeloid differentiation are vulnerable to transforming mutations that could alter normal myeloid cell differentiation and confer self-renewal properties to progenitor cells that inherently lack this ability.[101-103] These transformation events would create a LIC capable of generating a population of aberrant cells blocked at the differentiation state at which the initial transforming event occurred.

Several translocations involving the *MLL* gene have been shown to initiate self-renewal in myeloid progenitor cells and to result in an AML phenotype.[102,104] A head-to-head comparison was conducted by retrovirally transducing the human AML-associated *MLL-ENL* fusion gene into murine HSC, common myeloid progenitors (CMPs), and granulocytic-monocytic–restricted progenitors (GMPs) and evaluating the relative transforming ability and resultant phenotype in each cell type. AML developed in mice transplanted with any of the three transduced cell populations and, in each case, displayed an identical myelomonocytic phenotype as assessed by morphology and flow cytometry.[102] Similarly, the *MOZ-TIF2* fusion gene was able to confer self-renewal properties to committed myeloid progenitor cells and result in AML when transplanted into irradiated mice.[103] This AML phenotypically recapitulated human *MOZ-TIF2* AML, including myelomonocytic morphology, diffuse organ infiltration, and the presence of chloromas. Although the fusion genes *MLL-ENL* and *MOZ-TIF2* appear to impart leukemogenic capabilities to committed progenitor cells convincingly, other fusion genes such as *BCR-ABL* can induce leukemic transformation only when expressed in an HSC, but not a more mature myeloid cell (see Fig. 11-1).

These findings point to the differing transforming abilities of different oncogenes that are likely cell-type and cell-context specific.[105] Hence, both cell-of-origin hypotheses may be correct, depending on the specific oncogene or tumor suppressor that provides the initiating genetic lesion. Increased proliferation, survival, and self-renewal are all necessary attributes of a leukemia stem cell. Some genetic abnormalities, such as *MLL-ENL* and *MOZ-TIF2*, may be capable of inducing self-renewal and thus are able to transform a more differentiated myeloid cell into a LIC, whereas other oncogene fusions, such as *BCR-ABL*, may be able to induce proliferation and survival signals. However, these do not possess self-renewal capabilities and thus require a cell that inherently has this characteristic—namely, the HSC. Undoubtedly, further studies will continue to elucidate the transforming ability of other AML-associated oncogenes and tumor suppressors.

Molecular Genetics

Molecular genetics has played a major role in understanding the mechanisms of leukemogenesis and has evolved from scientific discoveries into the field of molecular hematopathology, which is an essential modality for the classification of disease and the determination of prognosis. Recent AML protocols have incorporated current knowledge regarding the significance of specific genetic abnormalities as part of a new risk-based approach to treatment. These clonal, nonrandom, chromosomal abnormalities identifiable on cytogenetic examination of the blast cells are associated with specific subtypes of both adult and pediatric AML (Fig. 11-2).[106,107] Careful analysis of these recurring abnormalities in leukemia patients has had a profound impact on our understanding of the molecular genetic basis of leukemia. Although many chromosomal abnormalities from AML blast cells have been identified and studied extensively, no single mutation has been shown to be sufficient to cause acute leukemia. Gilliland and colleagues[108-111] have proposed a compelling model of the leukemic transformation of AML resulting from distinct but collaborative sequential mutations in parallel molecular pathways that affect cell survival, proliferation, differentiation, and self-renewal. At a minimum, two distinct classes of mutations are required. Class I mutations frequently involve an activated receptor or cytoplasmic=nuclear tyrosine kinase and confer proliferative and/or survival abilities to a specific cell, but do not affect differentiation. By contrast, class II mutations specifically result in differentiation arrest and/or self-renewal and often involve key transcription factor oncogenes, but alone do not confer a proliferative advantage. Although this model attempts to represent what occurs in primary AML, support for these two classes of mutations and their phenotypes is provided by studies of secondary AML following the premalignant MDSs and myeloproliferative diseases (MPDs; see later). MDS is a heterogeneous disease, but subtypes share the features of impaired differentiation and dysplastic-appearing cells and are often associated with chromosomal deletions affecting tumor suppressor genes. MDS frequently progresses to AML following the acquisition of additional genetic abnormalities, presumably those that subsequently induce a proliferation advantage. By contrast, MPD consists of several different entities, including CML, polycythemia vera, essential thrombocythemia and mastocytosis, which have all been found to have activated tyrosine kinases and present as the expansion of a mature differentiated cell type. These diseases may also progress to AML following additional mutations that impair differentiation. Although this two-hit model of AML is attractive, it likely represents an oversimplification and additional mutations that affect self-renewal are required, such as those targeting critical regulatory pathways (e.g., WNT,[112,113]

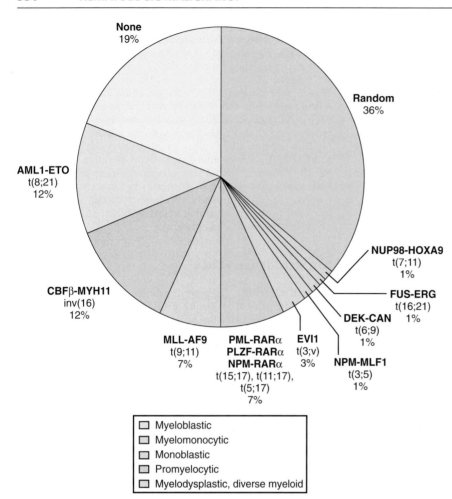

FIGURE 11-2. Distribution of the translocation-generated fusion genes in the various FAB subtypes of pediatric acute myeloid leukemia (AML). (Adapted from Look AT. Oncogenic transcription factors in the human acute leukemias. Science. 1997;278:1059.)

NOTCH,[114-116] and HOX[117-119] pathways). Additionally, key tumor suppressor genes such as p53[120] may play important roles in the progression of AML with complex aberrant karyotypes (Fig. 11-3).

Class I Mutations

Among the earliest examples of class I mutations, *RAS* mutations were described in the early 1980s. There are three functional RAS gene family members, *NRAS*, *KRAS* and *HRAS*, which all act as guanosine nucleotide phosphate (GTP) binding proteins.[110] Mutations of *NRAS* are the most prominent RAS mutations in AML and have been found in up to 30% of adult patients with AML.[121] Mutations, most frequently in codons 12, 13, and 61, result in the retention of the RAS protein in its active GTP-bound state and lead to the constitutive activation of downstream effector proteins, which causes the transcriptional activation of various target genes that direct cellular differentiation, proliferation, and survival (Fig. 11-4).[122] RAS proteins may be alternatively activated by mutations in genes encoding a number of regulatory factors. Activating point mutations in the *SHP-2/PTPN11* phosphatase provide a stimulatory signal through guanine nucleotide exchange factors, such as "Son of Sevenless" (SOS), resulting in downstream RAS pathway signaling, as do inactivating mutations of neurofibromin-1 (*NF-1*), a GTPase-activating protein (GAP).[123,124] NF-1, normally functions, at least in part, by increasing the GTPase activity of RAS, thereby inactivating RAS-GTP by converting it into the inactive RAS-GDP form.[125] These three types of

mutations function independently to activate RAS signaling and lead to disturbances in hematopoietic cell differentiation and proliferation that may ultimately contribute to the development of MDS, MPD, and AML (see Fig. 11-4).[126-128] Mutations in *NF-1* and *PTPN11* have been particularly associated with JMML (see later).[124,129]

There has been significant disagreement regarding the prognostic implications of *RAS* mutations in MDS and AML. Several studies have demonstrated that *RAS* mutations in patients with MDS confer a poor prognosis and increase the risk of progression to acute leukemia.[130-137] Other studies have reported no difference in survival in AML patients who carried *RAS* mutations compared with patients without *RAS* mutations[134]; some have suggested improved survival in patients with AML and *NRAS* mutations.[135] A recent large study of over 2500 patients with AML demonstrated no difference in prognosis in patients with or without *RAS* mutations. This study also demonstrated an association between *RAS* mutations and a leukemia karyotype containing inv(16), a class II mutation resulting in the CBFβ-MYH11 fusion protein and altered function of the CBF transcriptional complex.[138] This association further supports the model of class I and II mutations collaborating in the pathogenesis of AML.

Another group of class I mutations involves constitutive activation of receptor or cytoplasmic-nuclear tyrosine kinases. The BCR-ABL translocation that is the sine qua non of CML is an example of a class I mutation causing the activation of the ABL tyrosine kinase. Similarly, receptor tyrosine kinase mutations activate the human proto-oncogenes *KIT* and *FLT3* in

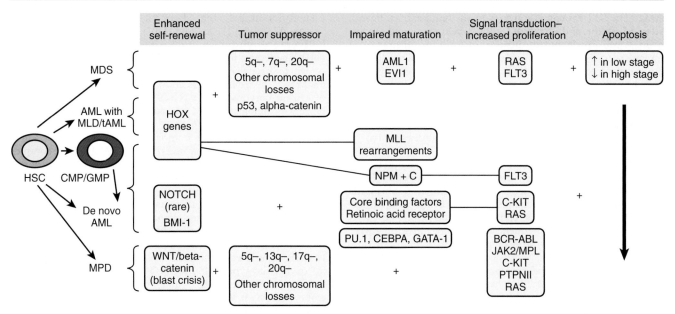

FIGURE 11-3. Mutations that collaborate in the development of acute myeloid leukemia (AML). AML may result de novo or secondarily following prior treatment (tAML) or a premalignant syndrome, myelodysplastic syndrome (MDS) or myeloproliferative disease (MPD). A number of collaborating genetic abnormalities in different pathways are necessary for the development of overt AML. The involved genes or chromosomes have been grouped into five general categories—enhanced self-renewal, tumor suppressor genes, impaired maturation, signal transduction/increased proliferation, and apoptosis. Some of these genetic abnormalities are shared by different subtypes of AML and are indicated by an extended box. The lines signify relationships that have been demonstrated between two genetic abnormalities.

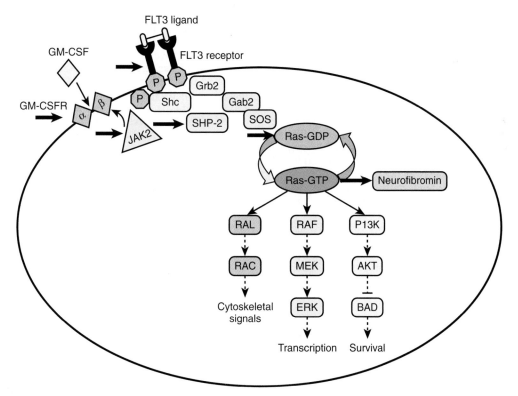

FIGURE 11-4. Constitutive activation of the RAS pathway is central to myeloid leukemogenesis. RAS pathway signaling may be constitutively activated via a number of mutually exclusive mechanisms (indicated by the horizontal black arrows). These include the following: mutations in the GM-CSF or FLT3 surface receptors, resulting in ligand independent activation (found primarily in de novo AML); activating mutations in JAK2 (found in PV, ET, and AMM) or SHP-2 (found in JMML); activating mutations in RAS itself (found in all types of AML); or inactivating mutations in neurofibromin (found in JMML). AMM, agnogenic myelofibrosis with myeloid metaplasia; ET, essential thrombocytosis; FLT3, fms-like tyrosine kinase 3; GM-CSF, granulocyte-macrophage colony-stimulating factor; JAK2, Janus 2 kinase; JMML, juvenile myelomonocytic leukemia; PV, polycythemia vera. (Adapted from Loh ML, Vattikuti S, Schubert S, et al. Mutations in PTPN11 implicate the SHP-2 phosphatase in leukemogenesis. Blood. 2004;103:2325-2331.)

AML. The KIT protein is activated by the binding of its ligand, stem cell factor, and is critical for the development and growth of mast cells, melanocytes, hematopoietic stem cells, and the interstitial cells of Cajal.[139] Mutations in *KIT* allow ligand-independent activation of KIT and confer factor-free growth and tumorigenicity in hematopoietic cell lines.[140,141] Blasts from patients with AML express KIT on their cell surfaces in most cases.[142-144] Deletional and insertional mutations of *KIT* have been identified in the blast cells of patients with AML, often in association with the CBF abnormalities inv(16) or t8;21.[145]

The *FLT3* gene encodes a class III fms-like receptor tyrosine kinase expressed in early hematopoietic progenitors. *FLT3* mutations occur in two varieties, internal tandem duplications (ITDs) in the juxtamembrane region and activation loop mutations (ALMs), primarily at codons 835 and 836. The *FLT3* ITD is one of the most frequent abnormalities in adult AML, documented in 25% to 30% of patients,[146-150] and generally confers a poor prognosis.[151,152] By contrast, ALMs occur in only 10% of adult patients and have not been associated with inferior survival rates. *FLT3* ITDs have been observed in 5% to 16% of pediatric AML cases and ALMs in 2% to 5% of cases. Paralleling the adult studies, *FLT3* ITDs, but not ALMs, were associated with a poor prognosis in children.[153-156] *FLT3* ITDs result in the constitutive activation of FLT3 and cause interleukin-3 (IL-3)–independent growth in Ba/F3 and 32D cells.[146,149,157] This activation, in turn, results in the signaling of multiple downstream pathways, including the aforementioned RAS pathway, and the inhibition of caspase-mediated apoptosis through the stimulation of PI3 kinase and AKT (see Fig. 11-4). However, mice transplanted with FLT3-transformed hematopoietic cells develop a myeloproliferative disorder characterized by splenomegaly and leukocytosis, but they do not develop AML.[158] Additional mutations that impair hematopoietic differentiation are required for the development of acute myeloid leukemia.

Class II Mutations

In class II mutations, the molecular defect appears to be at the level of transcriptional activation, whereby transcriptional repressors cause a dominant negative inhibition of normal hematopoietic cell differentiation. AML can be subtyped based on the type of class II mutations in the blast cells of patients. Type 1 mutations occur in patients with de novo AML. These are typical chromosomal translocations resulting in chimeric oncoproteins that cause the inhibition of differentiation. Type 2 mutations usually are found in patients with AML arising after a prodrome of MDS and manifest more commonly in older adults or in patients who have received previous chemotherapy. Cytogenetic studies of the blast cell populations in these patients have complex karyotypes, lacking translocations but harboring deletions such as 5q–, monosomy 7, and 20q–.

Type 1 Mutations

Translocations Involving Core-Binding Factor Complex. Several of the translocations that have been identified in adult and childhood de novo AML involve the CBF complex. The CBF complex is the most frequent target of chromosomal translocations in the human leukemias. The CBF regulatory complex consists of a DNA-binding subunit, RUNX1 (also called CBFα or AML1) and CBFβ, a subunit that does not bind DNA independently but heterodimerizes with RUNX1 or one of its closely related family members.[159] Chromosomal translocations that modify the CBF complex in AML include the following: t(8;21)(q22;q22), which generates the AML1-ETO fusion protein (Fig. 11-5); t(3;21)(q26;q22), which gives rise to AML1-EVI1; and inv(16)(p11;q22), which fuses the CBFβ to smooth muscle myosin heavy chain (SMMHC). The *AML1* gene was inactivated in the germline of mice and was shown to be essential for definitive hematopoiesis of all cell lineages.[160,161] Homozygous animals die early in embryogenesis of central nervous system (CNS) hemorrhage, but they have normal morphogenesis and yolk sac hematopoiesis lineages.[160,161] Inactivation of the *CBFβ* gene in the mouse has shown a similar phenotype in the homozygous null mice.[159,162] These experiments have demonstrated that the AML1/CBFα complex is essential for normal hematopoiesis and that chromosomal rearrangements involving this complex may interfere with its regulatory function in ways that lead to disruption of cellular differentiation, and eventually malignant transformation.

Evidence primarily from knock-in studies in mice has supported the hypothesis that the AML1-ETO fusion protein functions as a dominant negative inhibitor of wild-type functions.[163-165] In these experiments, the *AML1-ETO* fusion gene is "knocked in" to the wild-type *AML1* locus. The phenotype of these mice is identical to the *AML1* knock-out; the mice die early in embryogenesis from CNS hemorrhage and lack any evidence of definitive hematopoiesis, although the rare cells that survive and express AML1-ETO have an increased capacity for self-renewal.[165] Biochemical experiments have shown that the ETO portion of the AML1-ETO chimeric protein recruits nuclear corepressor complexes to the CBF promoters, resulting in transcriptional inhibition of target genes normally activated by the AML1/CBFβ heterodimeric complex (see Fig. 11-5D).[166,167] Subsequent studies using inducible murine model systems to bypass the embryonic lethality of *AML1-ETO* overexpression have demonstrated that overexpression of this transgene at later developmental time points confers enhanced self-renewal capacity to bone marrow progenitors, as demonstrated by serial culture experiments. Importantly, the mice do not develop AML, but appear to be predisposed to leukemogenesis. Thus, following treatment with *N*-ethyl-*N*- nitrosourea (ENU), the mice developed rapid onset of AML compared with similarly exposed wild-type mice. Moreover, as noted, there is an association in myeloid leukemia of AML1-ETO translocations and mutant tyrosine kinases, such as KIT.[117,168]

Translocations Involving the Retinoic Acid Receptor-α. Reciprocal chromosomal translocations involving the retinoic acid receptor-α (*RARA*) gene locus on chromosome 17 are the defining molecular features of acute promyelocytic leukemia (APL). Before the RARA translocations were described, retinoic acid was known to induce myeloid differentiation in vitro,[169] and therapy with all-trans retinoic acid (ATRA) in patients with APL was shown to induce complete remission.[170] The intense investigation of the *RARA* gene triggered by these observations culminated in identification of the promyelocytic leukemia PML–RARA translocation breakpoint, t(15;17)(q22;q11), reported simultaneously by several groups.[171-176] Although most APL cases have the associated t(15;17), other reciprocal translocations involving the *RARA* gene have been identified in which the gene is fused to other gene partners. The most common of these include the promyelocytic leukemia zinc finger (*PLZF*) gene on chromosome 11 in t(11;17)(p13;q11) and the nucleophosmin gene (*NPM*) on chromosome 5 in t(5;17)(q31;q11).[177,178]

Normally, RARA functions as a ligand-dependent activator of transcription.[179] It forms a heterodimer with the related protein, retinoid X receptor (RXR)[180] and binds through its zinc finger domain to a specific promoter sequence; in the presence of the retinoic acid ligand, the RARA-RXR heterodimer activates transcription of retinoic acid responsive genes.[173] This process is accomplished in concert with a coactivator complex

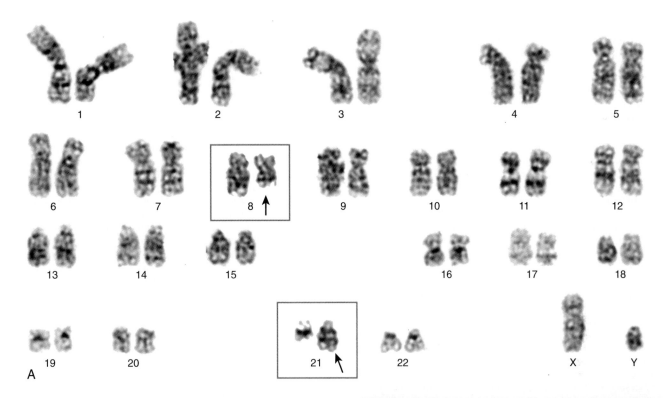

A

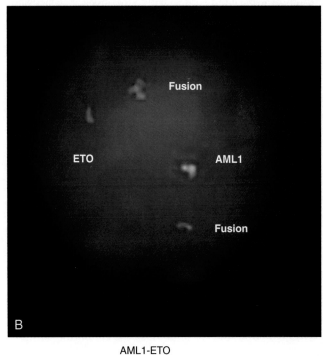

B

FIGURE 11-5. Consequences of the t(8;21) AML1-ETO translocation. **A,** Karyotype demonstrating the reciprocal t(8;21)(q22;q22) translocation in an affected patient. **B,** Interphase fluorescence in situ hybridization (FISH) using the AML1/ETO dual-color, dual–fusion, Vysis probe demonstrates the novel AML1-ETO fusion by the presence of linked green AML1 and red ETO signals. **C,** The normal AML1-CBFβ transcription factor complex. **D,** The molecular consequences of the AML1-ETO fusion—namely, disrupted DNA binding and transcription repression. (A and B courtesy of Dr. Barbara Morash, Cytogenetics, IWK Health Centre, Halifax, Nova Scotia, Canada; D adapted from Downing JR. The core-binding factor leukemias: lessons learned from murine models. Curr Opin Genet Dev. 2003:13;48-54.)

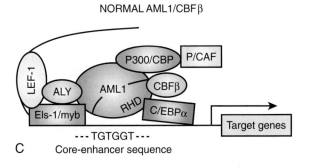

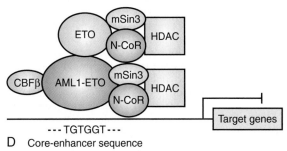

that includes proteins such as p300 and pCAF. In the absence of retinoic acid, a corepressor complex is recruited, comprised of N-CoR (nuclear receptor corepressor) or SMRT (silencing mediator of retinoid and thyroid receptors), which binds to another protein called Sin3 and then to HDAC1.[178,181-183] HDAC1 is a histone deacetylase protein, which epigenetically alters histones to keep DNA in an untranscribable form. The expression of retinoic acid–responsive genes is essential for normal myeloid development.[184]

Much evidence supports the hypothesis that the PML-RARA fusion protein functions as a dominant negative inhibitor of the PML protein and RXR. PML proteins are normally located in macromolecular nuclear organelles, called PML oncogenic domains (PODs).[185] The PML-RARA fusion protein disrupts the PODs, causing normal PML, RXR, and other nuclear proteins to disperse in an abnormal pattern.[186,187] ATRA and arsenic trioxide (As_2O_3)[188] have shown activity in APL blast cells and in patients with APL, and studies of these drugs have afforded important insights into the mechanisms of leukemogenesis in APL.[170,189] ATRA and As_2O_3 appear to act through different biochemical pathways, and promyelocytes resistant to ATRA are often sensitive to treatment with As_2O_3. Both drugs induce degradation of the PML-RARA fusion protein but through different mechanisms. Retinoic acid binding to wild-type retinoic acid receptors (RARs) in the cell nucleus causes degradation of the PML-RARA protein through the ubiquitin-proteosome and caspase systems, thus allowing for the terminal differentiation of leukemic promyelocytes.[190-192] This binding also results in N-CoR being dissociated from the PML-RARA fusion protein and, subsequently, the nuclear coactivator complex is recruited to reverse histone deacetylase-mediated repression. PODs are relocated back to the normal nuclear pattern.[187,193] By contrast, As_2O_3 appears to target the PML portion of the PML-RARA fusion protein preferentially and causes its degradation by inducing apoptosis,[194] potentially through downregulation of the antiapoptotic factor BCL-2.[195,190,195,196] The activity of these agents has led to the inferences that fusion proteins may interfere with normal myeloid cell development in several ways—through inhibitory effects on assembly of the PODs that contain PML or through dominant inhibitory effects on transcriptional targets of dimeric complexes with normal retinoid receptors, leading to arrest of differentiation at the promyelocyte stage.

Studies using transgenic mice have shown that the PML-RARA fusion product is involved in the development of leukemia. Transgenic mice generated with the PML-RARA fusion protein specifically expressed in the myeloid-promyelocytic lineage develop a myelodysplastic-like disorder during the first year of life.[197,198] A subset of these mice then develops a form of acute leukemia that closely mimics human APL and responds to ATRA. Given the relatively long latency period and the development of leukemia in only a fraction of the mice, it is likely that the PML-RARA translocation is insufficient by itself to cause APL, and that second mutations are necessary for leukemic transformation.

Mixed-Lineage Leukemia Gene Translocations. Transcriptional coactivators and corepressors have been implicated in leukemogenesis.[108] An example is the myeloid-lymphoid or MLL protein, a large protein containing transcriptional activation and repression domains, which is thought to act epigenetically to modulate gene expression through its effects on chromatin structure and configuration. Wild-type MLL is required for normal hematopoiesis and hematopoietic stem cell development.[199] Mice deficient in MLL die on embryonic day 10.5 and have numerous skeletal, neural, and hematologic deficits. Heterozygous mice have defects in embryonic segmentation and yolk sac hematopoiesis, and adults demonstrate a

mild anemia and thrombocytopenia.[200,201] Chromosomal translocations of the MLL gene on chromosome segment 11q23 have been identified in human AML and ALL and confer a poor prognosis.[202,203] Many gene partners have been identified that are involved in these translocations, including AF4, AF9, ENL, AF6, ELL, and AF10. In most cases, the fusion proteins incorporate the 5′ end of MLL and the 3′ end of the partner.[204,205] Despite the number of different fusion partners, leukemias with MLL translocations tend to possess a distinct genetic signature compared with AML and ALL samples lacking an MLL translocation. This genetic signature includes the upregulation of a number of specific HOX family genes, including HOXA9, HOXA7, and MEIS1.[202,206-208] Wild-type MLL is known to play a major role in HOX gene transcriptional regulation.[209] In turn, HOX genes play critical roles in embryonic development and normal hematopoiesis. A number of studies have clearly demonstrated that overexpression of specific major HOX genes in mouse models and human bone marrow samples, whether by involvement in reciprocal translocations or by gene upregulation, is linked to the transformation of malignant hematopoietic stem cells in AML.[210-218] The mechanism whereby MLL fusion proteins upregulate HOX gene expression may differ, depending on whether the fusion partner encodes a nuclear partner with direct transcriptional activity or a cytoplasmic protein that results in MLL protein dimerization and subsequent transcriptional activation.[104]

Transcriptional control may be mediated through the modification of histone proteins, which function to maintain chromatin structure. The MLL gene is rearranged in up to 20% of pediatric cases of AML.[219] Translocations of MLL are the single most common genetic alteration in infants with acute leukemia, regardless of phenotype, and account for approximately 70% of all cases of AML and ALL in infants.[220] In pediatric and adult cases of AML, the presence of the 11q23 translocation is generally associated with an unfavorable prognosis.[221]

Although less common than MLL translocations, the MLL gene can possess partial tandem duplications (PTDs) of particular exons. These PTDs occur in adult and pediatric AMLs with a normal karyotype, as well as those with trisomy 11. Like MLL fusions, the MLL PTD tends to be associated with a poor prognosis and often with the presence of a FLT3 mutation. The mechanisms underlying MLL PTD leukemogenesis have not yet been elucidated, but appear to be different than those of MLL fusions.[205,222] Interestingly, MLL PTD appears to repress wild-type MLL expression, which may be an important feature underlying the leukemogenic potential of this abnormality.[222]

Type 2 Mutations

The leukemogenic mutations discussed in the previous sections involve balanced translocations, duplications, or substitutions that appear to disrupt regulatory mechanisms controlling hematopoiesis and result in dysregulated cell differentiation. Another group of mutations involve unbalanced chromosome rearrangements, such as chromosome loss (e.g., monosomy 5, monosomy 7) or large chromosomal deletions (e.g., 5q–, 7q–, 20q–).[223,224] These mutations may lead to leukemic transformation by the loss of a tumor suppressor gene (or genes), which then confers a differentiation block and growth advantage to the mutated cells.[225] Identification of these putative tumor suppressor genes has been problematic because the deleted regions are usually large and include many candidate genes. Moreover, leukemogenesis is triggered by the gene's inactivation rather than by altered structure, making the abnormal gene difficult to identify. However, alpha-catenin has recently been identified by our group as a novel tumor suppressor gene on the proximal region of the long arm of chromosome 5.[226] Non–therapy-related AML with these chromosomal losses or deletions occurs most commonly in older patients and is often associated with the prodrome of MDS. In the pediatric population, this class of cytogenetic abnormality is uncommon and is also frequently preceded by MDS.[227] Monosomy 7 is the most frequent chromosomal abnormality documented in children with MDS and is sometimes the sole detectable cytogenetic abnormality.[228,229] Overall, chromosome loss represents about half of the chromosomal abnormalities identified in MDS.[227]

Therapy-related Acute Myelogenous Leukemia. Chromosomal loss and large chromosomal deletions are common in therapy-related AML in the adult and pediatric populations. Although most cases of MDS and AML arise de novo, without evidence of any leukemogenic exposure, in 10% to 20% of patients, the disease arises after previous exposure, particularly to topoisomerase II inhibitors, alkylating agents, and ionizing radiation.[230] The 11q23 translocation is also a common cytogenetic abnormality in patients who develop AML after therapy with topoisomerase II inhibitors (e.g., epipodophyllotoxins).[5,6,231] AML developing after the use of topoisomerase II inhibitors has a short median latency period of 30 to 34 months, is usually FAB M4 or M5, and lacks the antecedent prodrome of MDS.[232] The blast cells of patients with AML or MDS occurring after exposure to alkylating agents often have large chromosomal losses or deletions and have a poor prognosis.[230,233,234] The most common chromosomal abnormalities in such cases involve chromosome 7 and chromosome 5. In contrast to the therapy-related AML with MLL fusion genes that develops after treatment with topoisomerase II inhibitors, MDS or AML related to therapy with alkylating agents typically develops after a longer median latency period, 3 to 5 years from the alkylator exposure.

Acute Myelogenous Leukemia with a Normal Karyotype. Chromosomal abnormalities have provided some understanding of the mechanisms of malignant transformation in leukemia. However, in many cases of de novo leukemia, no chromosomal abnormality can be detected, and the mechanism behind leukemogenesis in these cases is unknown. Because AML involves a block in myeloid differentiation, evidence for mutations in key transcription factors involved in normal myelopoiesis has been sought. Mutations in the early myeloid transcription factors, PU.1 and CCAAT/enhancer-binding protein α (C/EBPα), have been identified in a number of AML subtypes and are generally not associated with a known chromosomal translocation.[235] More recently, mouse models have demonstrated that the degree of transcription factor knockdown is critical to the particular phenotype. Mice expressing PU.1 at 20% of normal levels develop AML, whereas those with complete knockdown or 50% of normal levels do not.[236] GATA-1, a critical transcription factor for erythrocyte and megakaryocyte development, is mutated in nearly all cases of acute megakaryoblastic leukemia associated with Down syndrome (see later).[237]

Expression profiling using microarrays first used to distinguish prognostic tumor subclasses in breast carcinoma[238-241] and large B-cell lymphoma[242] has also been applied to leukemia.[210] Using this technology, a set of 50 genes was sufficient to discriminate ALL from AML. More recent validation of this technique in AML has demonstrated the correlation between gene expression profiling studies and the prognostic classification of human AML based on cytogenetic abnormalities.[243] Gene expression profiling has provided valuable new insights into the identification of prognostic subclasses in adult[244] and pediatric[245] AML with a normal karyotype. These studies have validated genes previously shown to have prognostic significance

(e.g., *CEBPα*, favorable; *HOX* genes, unfavorable), demonstrated new gene associations suggesting potential interactions and identified novel genes not previously known to be involved in AML pathogenesis. AML with a normal karyotype has remained a heterogeneous group with regard to prognosis. Further efforts are currently underway to establish and refine subsets defined by genetic signatures in normal karyotype AML, which may be informative for the design of specific custom-tailored treatment approaches.

Recently, our understanding of the molecular mechanisms underlying de novo AML with a normal karyotype was advanced by the finding of mutations involving the *NPM* gene in 35% of cases of adult AML and 60% of cases with a normal karyotype.[246] This frequency supersedes the incidence of *FLT3* mutations and has established *NPM* mutations as the most frequent genetic abnormality in adult AML. The frequency of *NPM* mutations is lower in pediatric AML, occurring in only 6% to 8% of all pediatric patients with AML, but also occurs in a higher number of pediatric patients with a normal karyotype (approximately 27%).[247,248] The *NPM* gene on chromosome 5q was previously well known as a partner in a number of oncogenic translocations, including *NPM*–anaplastic lymphoma kinase (*ALK*) in anaplastic large cell lymphoma and *NPM-RARA* in APL. NPM is a molecular chaperone that shuttles between the cytoplasm and nucleus, but is found most prominently in nucleoli. It has been shown to function in the prevention of protein aggregation in the nucleolus and the regulation of preribosomal particles through the nuclear membrane. It has also been shown to play a role in the regulation of the alternate reading frame (ARF)-p53 tumor suppressor pathway. *NPM* mutations are heterogeneous but occur predominantly in exon 12, uniformly affecting the C-terminal of the protein and causing the formation of a neomorphic nuclear export signal in the resulting NPMc protein. This results in a shift of NPM localization, sequestering it exclusively to the cytoplasm. *NPM* mutations occur more frequently in children older than 10 years and, as is the case in adults, tend to be associated with a good prognosis. However, there has been a strong association established between patients with *NPM* mutations and *FLT3* ITDs, which portend a poor prognosis. Patients with both these abnormalities do not fare as well as those with *NPM* mutations alone.

Morphology and Cytochemistry

The initial diagnosis of AML relies on accurate interpretation of the cellular morphology of the bone marrow smears. The diagnosis usually can be made based on the morphologic characteristics of the blasts in a Wright-Giemsa–stained bone marrow smear (Fig. 11-6). In addition to general morphology, the diagnosis can be confirmed in cases exhibiting Auer rods (thin, needle-shaped cytoplasmic deposits that stain pink with Wright-Giemsa and are strongly myeloperoxidase [MPO]-positive). In addition to examination of the morphology of the blasts, the Wright-Giemsa stain is also used to assess for dysplastic features in erythroid, myeloid, and megakaryocytic cell lines.

Additional cytochemical stains are important for the accurate diagnosis of AML. MPO and Sudan black B (SBB) are cytochemical stains for granulocyte, eosinophil, and monocyte lineages. Peroxidase is present in the primary granules of myeloid cells, beginning at the promyelocyte stage and throughout subsequent maturation. Typically, leukemic myeloblasts are also strongly peroxidase-positive. MPO staining of Auer rods is particularly robust in leukemic blasts and can demonstrate Auer rods not recognized using the Wright-Giemsa stain. By contrast, the MPO staining of monoblasts shows a fine

Text continues on p. 346

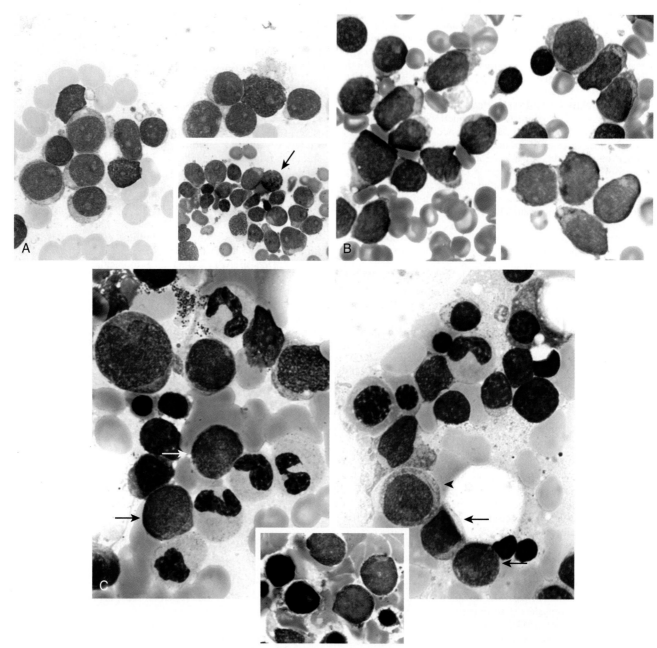

FIGURE 11-6. Subtypes of acute myeloid leukemia. All images are from Wright-Giemsa–stained bone marrow aspirate smears, except where otherwise designated. **A,** Acute myeloblastic leukemia, minimally differentiated. The blasts may vary in size, but have round to oval nuclei, variably prominent single or multiple small nucleoli, and scant cytoplasm that is agranular. **Inset,** The blasts here show no reactivity for myeloperoxidase, although rare reactivity (<3% blasts) may be seen; a neutrophil (*arrow*) serves as a positive internal control. **B,** Acute myeloblastic leukemia, without maturation. Blasts generally predominate within the marrow and comprise 90% or more of nonerythroid cells. The blasts may contain cytoplasmic granules and occasional Auer rods or may resemble lymphoblasts. **Inset,** Myeloperoxidase positivity is present in >3% of blasts, although the reactivity itself is of varied intensity. **C,** Acute myeloblastic leukemia, with maturation. Blasts comprise 20% or more of marrow cellularity (*arrows*), whereas maturing neutrophils (e.g., promyelocytes, myelocytes, metamyelocytes, bands and neutrophils) constitute 10% or more of nucleated elements. Dysmyelopoiesis may be evident. Auer rods are commonly present and may be long and tapered in appearance (*arrowhead*). **Inset,** Myeloperoxidase shows variable reactivity in a subset of the blasts (>3%) and strong reactivity in the maturing neutrophilic forms.

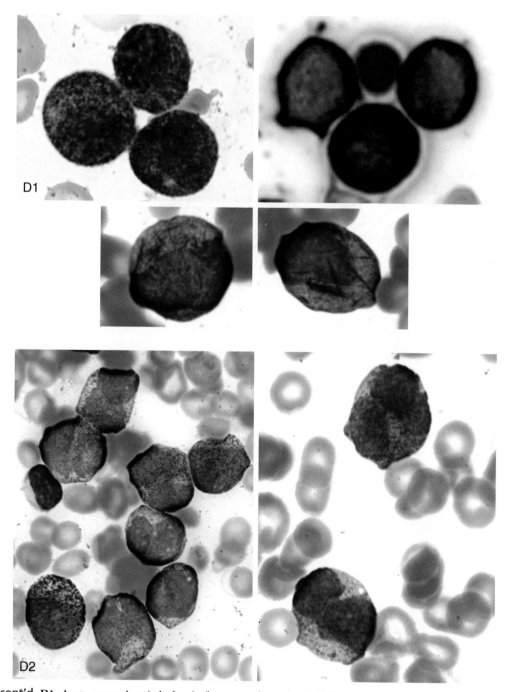

FIGURE 11-6, cont'd. D1, Acute promyelocytic leukemia (hypergranular variant). Malignant promyelocytes have eccentric nuclei, prominent nucleoli, and abundant cytoplasm, with intense azurophilic granules. Varied numbers of promyelocytes may contain multiple Auer rods, a characteristic finding (*lower panels*). Myeloperoxidase shows intense reactivity in the promyelocytes that largely obscures the nucleus (*upper right panel*). **D2,** Acute promyelocytic leukemia (microgranular variant). These malignant promyelocytes have a bilobed or butterfly-shaped nucleus, fine chromatin, variably prominent nucleoli, and abundant cytoplasm, with sparse to numerous azurophilic granules. Myeloperoxidase shows intense reactivity in these variants similar to that seen in the hypergranular forms.

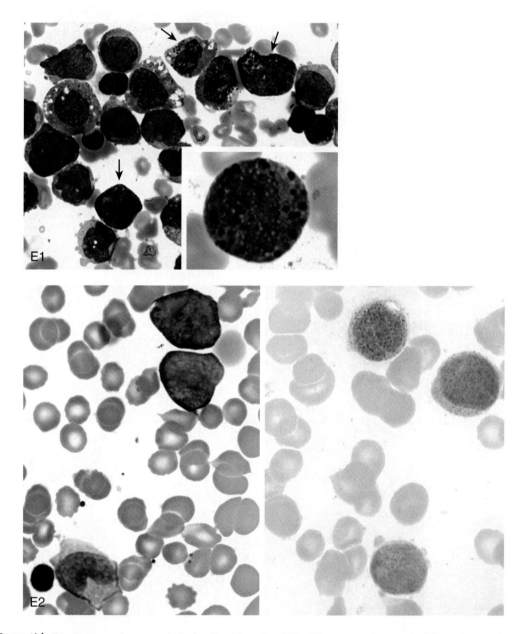

FIGURE 11-6, cont'd. E1, Acute myelomonocytic leukemia with eosinophilia. Blasts, maturing neutrophils, and maturing monocytes each constitute 20% or more of marrow cellularity. Additionally, abnormal eosinophils are present in all stages of maturation and contain enlarged granules that are purple-violet in appearance as opposed to orangeophilic (*arrows; inset*). **E2,** Acute myelomonocytic leukemia with eosinophilia (cytochemistries). At least 3% of blasts show myeloperoxidase reactivity (*left*), whereas monoblasts, promonocytes, and monocytes exhibit nonspecific esterase reactivity that may be weak, as seen in this case (*right*).

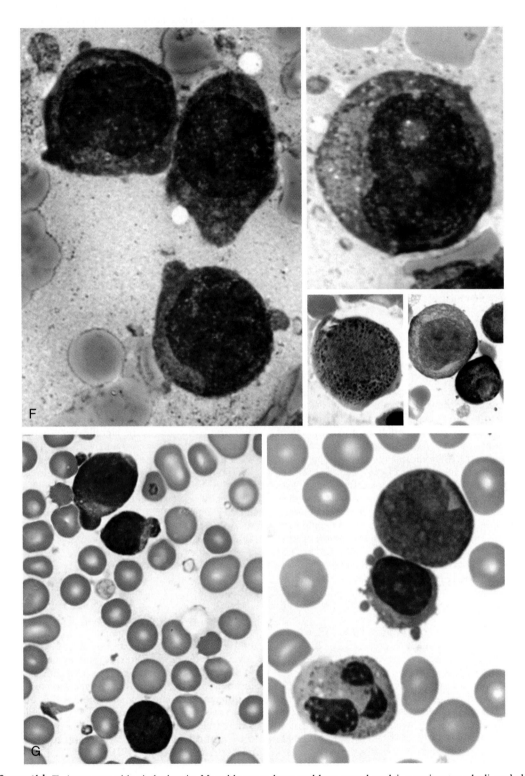

FIGURE 11-6, cont'd. F, Acute monoblastic leukemia. Monoblasts are large and have round nuclei, prominent nucleoli, and abundant deeply basophilic cytoplasm, which may contain fine granules and/or vacuoles. Monoblasts show strong reactivity for nonspecific esterase (*lower right, left inset*) and are typically myeloperoxidase negative (*lower right, right inset*). **G,** Acute megakaryoblastic leukemia. Megakaryoblasts are varied in size and have round, slightly indented or markedly irregular nuclear contours as well as fine chromatin, single to multiple small nucleoli, and scant to moderate basophilic (agranular or granular) cytoplasm, often with cytoplasmic blebs or pseudopod formation. (Courtesy of Dr. Jo-Anne Vergilio, Assistant Professor in Pathology, Harvard Medical School.)

granular pattern in the monoblast cytoplasm. The staining pattern of SBB is similar to that of peroxidase, particularly in myeloblasts and in the detection of Auer rods. Monoblasts either do not stain or show a weakly positive, diffuse pattern with SBB.

The esterase stains are useful for distinguishing granulocytic cells from cells of the monocytic lineage. Chloroacetate esterase is a specific stain for granulocytes and mast cells. Results of staining of early myeloblasts are often negative, but promyelocytes and later granulocytic lineage cells stain strongly, as do Auer rods. Monoblasts do not stain with chloroacetate esterase. In contrast, the nonspecific esterases (NSEs) such as α-naphthyl butyrate esterase and α-naphthyl acetate esterase stain monoblasts and monocytes strongly. Granulocytic and lymphoid cells do not stain with the nonspecific esterases. The blast cells of AML-M4 (i.e., myelomonocytic leukemia) should demonstrate positive chloroacetate esterase activity and α-naphthyl butyrate esterase or α-naphthyl acetate activity; this finding is important for making the diagnosis. The periodic acid–Schiff (PAS) reaction is not as informative as the previously described stains, but it can be useful, particularly in the diagnosis of AML-M6 (i.e., erythroleukemia). Leukemic erythroblasts can stain strongly with PAS, whereas normal erythroid precursors generally demonstrate no PAS activity.

Immunophenotype

Since the 1980s, multiparameter flow cytometric analysis has become an important element in the diagnosis and classification of leukemia. More recently, multiparameter flow cytometry has been used as a tool to detect minimal residual disease in acute myeloid leukemia and is being incorporated into clinical trials to clarify prognostic groups and help make treatment decisions.[249-258] Immunophenotyping using a large panel of monoclonal antibodies to myeloid and lymphoid lineage and progenitor cell–associated antigens has been used to discriminate myeloid or lymphoid differentiation correctly in up to 98% of patients.[259,260] Monoclonal antibodies have been classified based on their reactivity with the lineage or differentiation-associated antigens on the surfaces of normal and malignant cells. Because the monoclonal antibodies are not leukemia cell–specific and most of the hematopoietic antibodies are not strictly lineage-specific, it is necessary to use panels of antibodies on blast cell populations and to incorporate the immunophenotypic information with the clinical findings and other morphologic, cytochemical, and cytogenetic results for accurate leukemia cell classification.

Blasts of myeloid origin generally express HLA-DR, CD33, and CD34. Monocytic cells usually express HLA-DR at all stages of maturation, whereas promyelocytes and more mature cells of the granulocyte lineage do not. CD33 and CD13 are expressed on neutrophil and monocyte precursors, but CD33 is absent on mature neutrophils. CD14 is relatively specific for cells of the monocytic lineage. As myeloid differentiation continues, CD15 expression increases, whereas CD34 expression decreases. Megakaryocytic cells and platelets express CD41, CD42, and CD61.

Immunophenotyping has been particularly valuable for lineage assignment in undifferentiated leukemias (i.e., AML-M0), identification of acute megakaryocytic leukemia, and characterization of the MLLs.[261-266]

Cytogenetics

Cytogenetic analysis is an essential component in the diagnosis and treatment of AML. The chromosomal aberrations detected by cytogenetic testing also have prognostic value and may be used as tumor markers. In the World Health Organization (WHO) classification of hematologic malignancies, specific cytogenetic abnormalities have been included in the diagnostic and prognostic criteria for differentiating subclasses of AML.[267]

Cytogenetic analyses of bone marrow samples have revealed chromosomal abnormalities in most patients with AML.[268-275] In the pediatric population, the incidence of cytogenetic abnormalities is even higher than that in adults.[219,268,276] However, the distribution of the specific cytogenetic abnormalities is different in the various age groups. In infants with AML, the most common chromosomal aberrations are translocations involving the *MLL* gene (band 11q23).[277-279] The incidence of 11q23 translocations is as high as 40% in AML blasts of children younger than 2 years. After age 2, the frequency of 11q23 translocations decreases with age, and the translocation is detectable in AML blasts from less than 10% of older children and adults.[107,219,268,276] One rare chromosomal abnormality, the t(1;22)(p13;q13), is found almost exclusively in non–Down syndrome infants with acute megakaryocytic leukemia. In a published review of 39 patients with this translocation, 95% were younger than 2 years, and it was not identified in adults with AML.[280] This translocation is now known to result in aberrant expression of the *OTT-MAL* fusion gene.[281]

There are two classification systems for AML (see next section). The French-American-British (FAB) classification is based exclusively on morphology. However, there are some morphologic subtypes such as M3 and M4eo that are always associated with particular cytogenetic changes—that is, *RARA* rearrangements for the former and inv(16) or t(16;16) in the latter. In addition, there are certain cytogenetic changes that are often (if not exclusively) associated with a particular subtype and that carry prognostic significance, such as the good prognosis t(8;21) often associated with the M2 subtype or *MLL* rearrangements often associated with the M5 subtype. The WHO classification system takes this into account and has a category of "acute myeloid leukemia with recurrent genetic abnormalities," which includes t(8;21), inv(16) or t(16;16), t(15;17), and 11q23. The fusion proteins thus generated are discussed in more detail earlier (see "Acute Myelogenous Leukemia: Biology"). Some of the more common chromosomal abnormalities and their associated FAB and WHO subtypes are shown in Table 11-1 and Box 11-2. The prognostic significance of certain cytogenetic abnormalities is discussed later (see "Prognosis").

French-American-British Classification

In 1976, the FAB group proposed a system of classification of AML based on morphologic and cytochemical features (see Table 11-1). The system divides AML into seven subtypes, M1 through M7.[263,282,283] An M0 subtype was later added to describe undifferentiated leukemia and, since 1976, immunophenotypic data have also been included.[262,263,284] In general, AML can be differentiated from ALL based on morphologic features and cytochemical stains. Cells of myeloid origin should stain with myeloperoxidase and SBB. Cells of monocytic derivation usually stain with nonspecific esterase. AML blasts usually do not have PAS activity, except for erythroblasts in AML-M6 and eosinophils of the M4Eo subtype.

M0: Acute Myeloblastic Leukemia with Minimal Differentiation

In patients with AML-M0, the bone marrow is usually hypercellular and more than 90% of the cells are blasts. Most blast cells lack cytoplasmic granules, nucleoli, or Auer rods and

TABLE 11-1 FAB Classification of AML with Corresponding Cytogenetic and Immunophenotype Characteristics

FAB Subtype	MPO	SBB	NSE	PAS	MYELOID							ERYTHROID		MEGAKARYOCYTIC			T-CELL LINEAGE				OTHER		Translocations and Rearrangements	Genes Involved
					CD 11b	CD 13	CD 14	CD 15	CD 33	CD 34	CD 65	Glycophorin A	CD 41/61	CD 42	CD 36	CD 2	CD 3	CD 4	CD 7	CD 56	HLA-DR	CD 117		
M0	-	-	-	-	-	++	±	±	++	++	-	±	±	±	-	+	-	+-	+-	±	++	++	11q23	MLL rearrangements
M1	+	+	-	-	-	+	-	+	++	++	-	-	-	±	-	+	-	-	+	±	++	++	trisomy 4, 8,13, -5, -7; t(8;21)(q22;q22); t(9;22)(q34;q11)	AML1-ETO; BCR-ABL
M2	+	+	-	-	±	+	-	+	++	++	-	-	-	±		+	-	+	+	±	++	+	trisomy 8, -5, -7; t(8;21)(q22;q22); t(6;9); inv3(q21;q26), t(3:3) (q21;q26)	AML1-ETO; DEK-CAN; EVI1
M3	+	+	-	-	+	+	-	++	+	++	-	-	-			+	-		+	±	±	+	trisomy 8, -5, -7; t(15;17)(q22;q12); t(11;17)(q23;q12), t(5;17) (q32;q12)	PML-RARA; PLZF-RARA; NPM-RARA
M4	+	+	+	-	++	++	++	+	+	±	-	-	-	++	+	+	-	++	+	+	+++	+	t(6;9); inv3(q21;q26), t(3:3) (q21;q26); t(9;11)(p22;q23); 11q23	DEK-CAN; EVI1; AF9-MLL; MLL rearrangements
(M4eo)	+	+	+	+	++	++	++	+	+	±	-	-	-	++	-	+	-	++	+	+	++	+	inv16(p13;q22), t(16:16)	MYH11-CBFβ
M5	-	-	+	-	++	++	++	++	+	++		-	-	++	-	+	-	++	+	+	+++	±	t(11;17)(q23;q21); 11q23; 11q23,t(9;11)(p22;q23) [M5a]; t(8;16), t(10;11) (p12;q23) [M5b]	MLL-AF17; MLL; MLL, AF9-MLL; MOZ-CBP; AF10-MLL
M6	+	+	-	+	-	+	-	-	+	++	++	-	-	++	-	-	-	-	+	±	-	±	trisomy 8, -5, -7	
M7	-	-	+	+	-	+	-	-	+	+	-	++	++	++	++	-	-	+	+	+	+	+	t(1;22)(p13;q13)	OTT-MAL
M7 (DS)	-	-	+	+	-	+	-	-	+	+	-	++	++	++	++	++	-	+	+	+	+	+	trisomy 21	GATA-1

AML, acute myelogenous leuemia; DS, Down syndrome; FAB, French-American-British; MLL, mixed-lineage leukemia; MPO, myeloperoxidase; NSE, nonspecific esterase; PAS, periodic acid–Schiff; SBB, Sudan black B.

results with MPO and SBB stains are negative.[262] Immunophenotypic analysis shows the presence of myeloid or monocytic cell antigens (i.e., CD13, CD14, CD33, or CD34) that are detectable on the cell surface of most AML-M0 blasts, but some AML-M0 blasts express terminal deoxynucleotidyl transferase, an enzyme usually associated with ALL. AML-M0 is associated with a high incidence of cytogenetic abnormalities, most of which are complex and often involve chromosomes 5 and 7, trisomy 8, or MLL rearrangements.[260,285]

M1: Acute Myeloblastic Leukemia without Maturation

The bone marrow of patients with AML-M1 is hypercellular and filled with myeloblasts (more than 90% blasts). Most blasts stain with MPO and SBB. The blast cells in this subtype display minimal myeloid differentiation. Morphologically, the blast cells may contain scant gray-blue cytoplasm and few or no azurophilic granules or Auer rods. Prominent nucleoli are usually detectable. Flow cytometric analysis usually shows that the blast cells of AML-M1 express HLA-DR, CD13, CD33,

and CD34. Cytogenetic abnormalities for this subclass often include monosomy 5 or 7 or trisomy 8.

M2: Acute Myeloblastic Leukemia with Maturation

The bone marrow of patients with AML-M2 usually shows evidence of some maturation beyond the myeloblast, with evidence of maturation beyond the promyelocyte stage in more than 10% of nonerythroid cells. Myeloblasts must represent more than 30% of the bone marrow cells but less than 90% of nonerythroid cells. The blasts generally have a few clusters of primary granules, and stain with MPO and SBB. Auer rods and prominent nucleoli are common. Immunophenotypic expression of HLA-DR, CD13, CD33, CD11, and CD15 is typical. This subtype may exhibit monosomy 5 or 7, trisomy 8, t(8;21), t(6;9), or abnormalities of chromosome 3.

M3: Acute Promyelocytic Leukemia

There are two types of AML-M3. The more common type is the hypergranular variant, in which more than 30% of the blasts are promyelocytes and myeloblasts. Most promyelocytes have heavy granulation. Auer rods and Auer rod bundles are common. In the rare microgranular variant, the cells exhibit fine cytoplasmic granules, which are not distinguishable by light microscopy and nuclear morphologic irregularities (i.e., microgranular M3 or M3v). The cells of both subtypes stain strongly with MPO and SBB and also with chloroacetate esterase. The promyelocytes usually do not show PAS and NSE activity. The blasts express CD13, CD33, CD11, and CD15, but they are HLA-DR– and CD14–. This subtype exclusively exhibits RARA rearrangements, the vast majority of which are t(15;17) leading to *PML-RARA*.

M4: Acute Myelomonocytic Leukemia

The M4 subtype is defined by the presence of blast cells with both granulocytic and monocytic features. The bone marrow in these patients has more than 30% infiltration by immature myeloid precursors, and there is often extramedullary involvement and a peripheral blood monocytosis. The blasts are usually pleomorphic with regard to size, amount of cytoplasm, granularity, and nuclear morphologic features. Some Auer rods can be seen, and prominent nucleoli are usually present. Staining is variable, with some of the blast cells showing positivity for MPO, SBB, and NSE. M4 AML may be associated with t(6;9), abnormalities of chromosome 3, and *MLL* gene rearrangements, in particular t(9;11). A small proportion of patients with AML-M4 have a moderate eosinophilia in their bone marrow (M4Eo). The eosinophils are notable for the presence of basophilic and eosinophilic granules and stain with chloroacetate esterase and PAS. Cell surface antigen expression includes CD13, CD15, CD33, CD4, CD11c, CD14, CD64, and HLA-DR. M4eo AML exhibits an inv(16) or t(16;16).

M5: Acute Monocytic Leukemia

More that 80% of the nonerythroid bone marrow cells in patients with AML-M5 are monocytic. There are two subtypes, M5a (undifferentiated) and M5b (differentiated). In AML-M5a, more than 80% of the cells are monoblasts. Patients with AML-M5a tend to be younger, have higher presenting white blood cell (WBC) counts, and have a poorer prognosis. In AML-M5b, fewer than 80% of the monocytic cells are monoblasts, and most of the cells are recognizable as monocytes or promonocytes. The peripheral blood in patients with AML-M5b exhibits a profound monocytosis. In both subtypes, the blasts demonstrate strong NSE activity. MPO and SBB staining results are usually negative. Cell surface antigen expression includes CD13, CD15, CD33, CD4, CD11c, CD14, CD64, and HLA-DR. M5 AML often exhibits MLL rearrangement, t(9;11) or t(11;17) in M5a and t(10;11) in M5b.

M6: Acute Erythrocytic Leukemia

AML-M6 is an uncommon form of AML overall and is rare in children. This form of leukemia is defined by a more than 50% erythroblast infiltration of the bone marrow. M6 AML may exhibit monosomy 5 or 7 or trisomy 8.

M7: Acute Megakaryoblastic Leukemia

The bone marrow exhibits an infiltration with pleomorphic megakaryoblasts that often display cytoplasmic budding and may appear in clusters. M7 blasts generally do not stain with MPO and SBB but show activity with PAS. Immunophenotyping is usually required to distinguish AML-M7 from ALL-L2, documenting the presence of the megakaryocytic antigens, glycoprotein Ib, glycoprotein IIb/IIIa, or factor VIII. Non–Down syndrome infants with M7 AML often exhibit a t(1;22). Down syndrome patients have a very high incidence of M7 AML with a particularly good prognosis, which is in contrast to the poor prognosis of M7 AML in non–Down syndrome children and adults.

World Health Organization Classification

The discovery of cytogenetic and molecular genetic abnormalities in malignant disease has had a significant impact on our understanding of malignant transformation. In myeloid malignancies, some genetic abnormalities have prognostic significance, whereas others appear to define specific disease subtypes. The WHO has proposed a classification system for neoplastic diseases of the hematopoietic and lymphoid tissues that includes a classification for AML (see Box 11-2 and Fig. 11-6) This classification uses the traditional FAB type morphologic categories of disease and includes additional entities such as immunophenotype, molecular genetic, and clinical characteristics that make the system more clinically relevant for diagnosis, prognosis, and treatment.[286] The WHO classification system divides myeloid diseases into four major subtypes—myeloproliferative diseases, myelodysplastic-myeloproliferative diseases, MDS, and AML. Within the category of AML, four additional subtypes are defined—AML with recurrent cytogenetic translocations, AML with myelodysplasia-related features, therapy-related AML and MDS, and AML not otherwise specified.

Within the subtype containing recurrent cytogenetic translocations, four additional categories have been described:

1. AML with t(8;21)(q22;q22), *AML1-ETO*
2. APL (AML with t(15;17)(q22;q11-12) and variants *PML-RARA*, *PLZF-RARA*, and *NPM-RARA*
3. AML with abnormal bone marrow eosinophils and inv(16)(p13;q22) or t(16;16(p(13;q22), *CBFB-MYH11*
4. AML with 11q23 (*MLL* gene) abnormalities

The FAB standard used to define AML had been 30% replacement of the bone marrow by the blast cells, but later studies have shown that patients with 20% to 30% blasts (previously classified as refractory anemia with excess blasts in transformation [RAEB-T]) have a prognosis similar

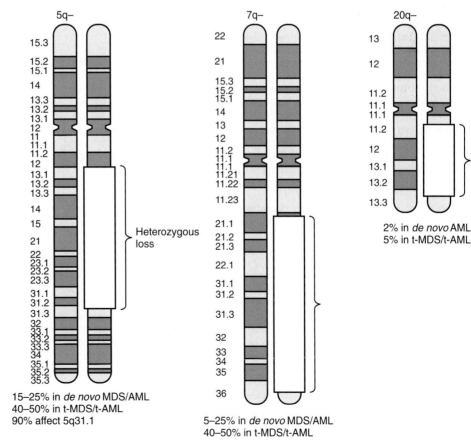

FIGURE 11-7. The hallmark of myelodysplastic syndrome (MDS) is the loss of specific chromosomal regions. Deletions of the long arm of chromosomes 5 and 7 (5q–, 7q–) occur in de novo MDS and acute myelogenous leukemia (AML), but much more frequently in t-MDS and t-AML following treatment with alkylating agents. 20q– abnormalities are less common but also occur in both de novo MDS and AML and following prior chemotherapy. (Data from Heaney ML, Golde DW. Myelodysplasia. N Engl J Med. 1999;340: 1649-1660; Hofmann WK, Lubbert M, Hoelzer D, Phillip Koeffler H. Myelodysplastic syndromes. Hematol J. 2004;5:1-8; Pedersen-Bjergaard J, Andersen MT, Andersen MK. Genetic pathways in the pathogenesis of therapy-related myelodysplasia and acute myeloid leukemia. Hematology Am Soc Hematol Educ Program. 2007; 2007:392-397.)

to that of patients with more than 30% blasts. The blast count for the diagnosis of AML in the WHO classification was therefore changed to 20%, and the category of RAEB-T was eliminated.

Certain specific and recurrent cytogenetic abnormalities are common in MDS, in alkylating agent–related AML, and in de novo AML with a poor prognosis. These abnormalities include 3q–, –5, 5q–, –7, 7q–, +8, +9, 11q–, 12p–, –8, –19, 20q–, +21, t(1;7), t(2;11), and complex karyotypes. In the classification scheme, these cytogenetic abnormalities were considered to indicate a poor prognosis. Prior therapy with topoisomerase II inhibitors (i.e., epipodophyllotoxins and doxorubicin [Adriamycin]) was also associated with a poor prognosis. Typically, patients in whom AML develops after exposure to these agents have translocations involving 11q23 (MLL). The WHO classification includes these patients in the poor-prognosis category but distinguishes them from alkylating agent–related secondary leukemia.

A separate category was defined for MDS with multilineage dysplasia. Evidence has shown that patients with MDS with fewer than 5% blasts, but significant dysplasia involving granulocytic and megakaryocytic lines, have a worse prognosis and are more likely to die of marrow failure or to develop acute leukemia than those lacking these features, and a separate category was recognized.

Clinical Presentation

The presenting signs and symptoms of AML result from leukemic blast cell infiltration of the bone marrow. The leukemia cells overwhelm the processes of normal hematopoiesis, resulting in anemia, thrombocytopenia, and neutropenia. It is rare for AML to be diagnosed incidentally on a routine medical evaluation, but there is considerable variability in the range of presenting signs and symptoms in patients with de novo AML. Usually, patients seek medical attention for fever, fatigue, pallor, skin or mucosal bleeding, bone pain, or infections not responding to appropriate antibiotic therapy.[287] Bone pain is a common symptom, and patients may present with a limp, rib pain, or back pain.[287]

The WBC count of patients with newly diagnosed AML can range from less than 1,000/μL to more than 500,000/μL.[287-289] The leukocyte count is more than 100,000/μL in approximately 25% of pediatric patients with AML, and an elevated count is more common in those with the M4 and M5 subtypes and in those with FLT3-ITD mutations.[155,156,287,290,291] The number of circulating granulocytes is often critically decreased, regardless of the total leukocyte count and, because their function is usually impaired, the risk of overwhelming bacterial infection in patients with newly diagnosed AML is markedly increased. Patients with AML who have a fever require immediate treatment with broad-spectrum antibiotics after appropriate culture samples have been obtained. The hemoglobin level is occasionally normal but is usually less than 9 g/dL, and levels as low as 3 g/dL at diagnosis are not uncommon. About half of children with new-onset AML have platelet counts of 50,000/μL or less, which increases the risk of life-threatening bleeding.[287]

Disseminated intravascular coagulation (DIC) has been observed in patients with all FAB subtypes of AML, but is most common in acute promyelocytic leukemia (APL; see later). APL cells express abnormally high levels of annexin II, which increases the production of plasmin, a fibrinolytic protein, and may lead to DIC in these patients.[292] Before the development of ATRA, treatment with low-dose heparin during induction was initiated for patients with AML-M3 to prevent DIC.[293,294]

The later addition of ATRA to induction therapy rapidly resolved DIC in patients with AML-M3 and markedly reduced early mortality.[170,295-298]

Patients with hyperleukocytosis have an increased risk of mortality from leukostasis, particularly in the brain or lung, and urgent leukapheresis may be necessary.[299,300] Routine pheresis for patients with a WBC count more than 100,000/μL has resulted in lower mortality rates during induction compared with historical controls and, in one study, patients who achieved a more than 30% decrease in total WBCs through pheresis had a higher complete remission rate than those who achieved less than a 30% decrease.[299,301,302] Extramedullary leukemia occurs in approximately 20% to 25% of children with AML and may include chloromas (tumor nodules), skin infiltration, central nervous system disease, gingival infiltration, hepatosplenomegaly, or testicular involvement.[287,303] Chloromas (e.g., myeloblastomas and granulocytic sarcomas), are solid tumors of myeloblasts that may occur in any area of the body, but are most common in the orbit and epidural area.[304] Skin infiltration, leukemia cutis, usually presents as slightly purple lesions (i.e., "blueberry muffin" spots), is more common in infants with monocytic leukemia, and may be the initial sign of disease.[305] CNS involvement at diagnosis is more common in AML than in ALL. Up to 15% of patients with AML have myeloblasts in the cerebrospinal fluid at diagnosis.[306-309] Gingival infiltration may present as hyperplasia, often accompanied by bleeding.[310] Severe extramedullary disease with massive hepatosplenomegaly is also a more common finding in infants.[305] Extramedullary involvement of the testes can also be documented, but is less common than in ALL.[311,312] Extramedullary infiltration, particularly gingival involvement, is more common with the M4 and M5 (acute myelomonocytic and acute monoblastic and monocytic) leukemias.[310,313,314] Chloromas and CNS disease are more common in AMLs with the t(8;21). Extramedullary infiltration in pediatric patients is not clearly associated with worse prognosis unless accompanied by a high presenting WBC count.

Treatment

As is true for any pediatric cancer, the goal of therapy for children with AML is to eradicate the disease while limiting treatment toxicity. In general, therapy for AML includes immediate supportive care measures followed by intensive remission induction and consolidation chemotherapy. At any given time, several large, multicenter phase III clinical trials are ongoing, each aimed to improve overall survival through randomized comparisons of treatment options while minimizing short- and long-term toxicities.

Remission Induction

During the past 40 years, survival rates for patients with AML have risen from less than 10% to more than 50% of patients because of intensification of chemotherapy, use of hematopoietic stem cell transplantation (HSCT), and improved supportive care. The first phase of chemotherapy is termed *induction* and consists of two to four cycles of intensive chemotherapy with the goal of inducing remission. Morphologic remission is defined as the presence of fewer than 5% blasts visible on bone marrow aspirate obtained after recovery of counts. Patients may also achieve cytogenetic and FISH-negative remission, as defined by the absence of a previously detected leukemic clone–associated cytogenetic abnormality in the bone marrow cells. Remission is now often also being defined by the absence of minimal residual disease assessed by multiparameter flow cytometry, designed to detect as few as 0.1% leukemic blasts in the marrow.

Induction chemotherapy should be initiated as soon as the diagnosis of AML is confirmed, preferably by morphologic, immunophenotypic, and cytogenetic studies of the bone marrow. In some cases, particularly in patients presenting with hyperleukocytosis, the patient may be too unstable for bone marrow evaluation, in which case the diagnosis can often be confirmed on studies of the peripheral blood. Induction chemotherapy regimens consist of high-dose myelosuppressive cytotoxic agents that result in prolonged pancytopenia. The period of bone marrow hypoplasia generally lasts from 21 to 30 days from the initiation of therapy, but may last considerably longer. During this period, patients have a high risk for life-threatening infection and bleeding. Aggressive supportive care is necessary (see later).

The basis of modern induction therapy for AML is a combination of cytarabine (cytosine arabinoside) and an anthracycline. The most commonly used combination therapy is the so-called 7 + 3 regimen, which consists of a continuous 7-day intravenous infusion of cytarabine at 100 to 200 mg/m²/day and 3 days of bolus infusions of daunorubicin at 45 to 60 mg/m² daily. Remission is achieved in approximately 60% to 70% of patients with newly diagnosed AML using this regimen.[315-317] In children, several strategies have been used to intensify this regimen to achieve higher rates of complete remission. CCG trial 213 added etoposide, thioguanine, and dexamethasone to the traditional 7 + 3 regimen to create the five-drug Denver regimen. The Denver and 7 + 3 regimens were compared in a randomized fashion and there was no significant difference in complete remission (CR) rate, with 79% of children achieving CR with 7 + 3 and 76% achieving CR with Denver regimen.[318]

In CCG trial 2891, the same drugs were used, but the timing was intensified in an attempt to improve CR. The hypothesis was that leukemia cells may be recruited synchronously into the cell cycle after chemotherapy, and therefore reexposure at an earlier time point may affect cells while more of them are at a sensitive phase in the cell cycle. In the CCG trial 2981, the Denver regimen was modified into the five-drug DCTER regimen, again consisting of *d*examethasone, *c*ytarabine, *t*hioguanine, *e*toposide, and *R*ubidomycin (daunorubicin). Induction consisted of a total of four cycles of chemotherapy and patients were randomized to standard or intensive timing. For standard timing, each cycle of induction began with count recovery from the previous cycle. With intensive timing, cycles 2 and 4 began at day 10 after the start of cycles 1 or 3, respectively, regardless of hematologic status. Not surprisingly, the intensive timing resulted in far greater toxicity, with 11% of patients in this arm dying from toxicity compared with only 4% of patients dying from toxicity in the standard timing arm.[319] Because of this, better supportive care measures were instituted for the intensive timing arm, including more aggressive empirical antibiotic and antifungal coverage and the use of granulocyte colony-stimulating factor (G-CSF). Interestingly, the CR rates were similar for the two arms, 75% for intensive timing and 70% for standard timing, but the reason for failure to achieve remission was different, with 11% toxic death and only 14% resistant disease in the intensive timing arm versus only 4% toxic death but 26% resistant disease in the standard timing arm. The most dramatic results, however, came later, when it was shown for those patients who achieved a CR that there was a 3-year disease-free survival (DFS) of 55% for those who had been treated in the intensive timing arm versus a DFS of only 37% for those who had received standard timing. For this reason, the standard timing arm was closed early and an intensive timing DCTER/DCTER schedule became the new

standard combination therapy for newly diagnosed AML patients.

In the meantime, a comprehensive review of five randomized trials comparing idarubicin to daunorubicin as induction therapy for AML had shown improved remission induction rates and overall survival for patients receiving idarubicin.[320] For this reason, the CCG pilot trial 2941 tried to intensify therapy further by using idarubicin in place of daunorubicin in each cycle of the intensively timed regimen. Because of unacceptably high toxicity, with a toxic death rate of 14%, this was modified to idarubicin only in cycles 1 and 3, and more strict supportive care guidelines were put into place, including mandatory hospitalization during neutropenia, and stricter infection prophylaxis (see later, "Supportive Therapy at Diagnosis and During Therapy").[321] The addition of idarubicin showed no advantage in remission induction or event-free survival, but did show a decrease in marrow blasts at day 14 of induction. CCG trial 2961 continued to use the hybrid idaDCTER/DCTER intensive timing induction regimen and has resulted in induction remission rates of 89%, which were similar to historical controls. Most of the improvement was thought to be related to better supportive care rather than the change in chemotherapy.

Medical Research Council Trials (MRC10 and MRC12)

During this period, data emerged from the British Medical Research Council (MRC) trials that seemed to show better survival and less toxicity. MRC10 induction chemotherapy randomized DAT (daunorubicin, cytarabine, thioguanine) to ADE (cytarabine, daunorubicin, etoposide) in a 10-day cycle of chemotherapy followed by an 8-day cycle of the same drugs on count recovery. The CR rate for children in this study was 93%, with a 4% rate of toxic death and a 3% rate of resistant disease.[322] Early data suggested a benefit for pediatric patients using ADE versus DAT, but the later data have shown no difference in 10-year overall survival (DAT, 57%; ADE, 51%; P = .3), disease-free survival (DAT, 53%; ADE, 48%; P = .3) or event-free survival (DAT, 48%; ADE, 45%; P = .5).[322,323] Because of the early results possibly favoring ADE, MRC12 compared ADE with MAE (mitoxantrone, cytarabine, etoposide) in a 10-day cycle followed by an 8-day cycle on count recovery. The CR rates were similar for the two groups (ADE, 92%; MAE, 90%; P = .3) with a slight increase in toxic deaths for the MAE group (ADE, 3%; MAE, 6%), but a better DFS rate for the MAE group (ADE, 59%; MAE, 68%; P = .04) although the estimated 5-year overall-survival rate is not significantly different (ADE, 64%; MAE, 70%; P = .1).[322]

Current U.S. Trials

The next series of U.S. trials built on the data from MRC10, and currently ongoing is a COG trial and a trial from St. Jude Children's Research Hospital (SJCRH). Two cycles of ADE are used as the backbone of induction chemotherapy in both trials, but each trial has come up with a different strategy for trying to intensify this therapy further. The COG pilot AAML03P1 used a strategy of adding targeted therapy to induction. Gemtuzumab ozogamicin (GMTZ, GO, Mylotarg) is a recombinant humanized anti-CD33 monoclonal agent linked to the tumor antibiotic calicheamicin. Because CD33 is expressed on most AML cells but not on pluripotent hematopoietic stem cells or other tissues, this drug can target leukemia cells more specifically.[324,325] The COG pilot trial AAML03P1 assessed the safety of adding a single dose of GMTZ to the first cycle of ADE chemotherapy. Toxicity in this pilot study appeared acceptable, and now COG trial AAML0531 is open, which is a phase III randomized trial designed to test the safety and efficacy of the addition of GMTZ to induction chemotherapy. The SJCRH trial randomizes patients to standard low- or high-dose cytarabine during the first cycle of induction. High-dose cytarabine has been used successfully in induction regimens in adults and children, although the toxicity appears higher than with regimens using standard-dose cytarabine. A difference in CR rates has not been observed between high- and standard-dose cytarabine groups, but there is a trend toward longer remissions and fewer relapses in those who received high-dose cytarabine during induction.[326,327] The SJCRH trial also uses minimal residual disease (MRD) measurements during induction to guide therapy. Persistent MRD by multidimensional flow cytometry is associated with a higher risk of relapse.[258,328,329] Therefore, in the SJCRH trial, GMTZ is added to induction therapy for those patients who have significant MRD at day 21 after the first induction round.

Postremission Therapy

Several randomized studies have demonstrated that without postremission therapy, almost all patients with newly diagnosed AML suffer a relapse within 2 years.[330-332] The strategies for postremission therapy include autologous HSCT, allogeneic HSCT, or continued courses of chemotherapy. The CCG trials have shown no benefit to autologous HSCT over continued cycles of chemotherapy so, although that strategy continues to be used in some European trials, autologous HSCT is not part of the current U.S. trials.[323,333-339] Most studies have shown a lower relapse rate for AML patients treated with matched related donor HSCT versus chemotherapy, but the overall survival is often no better because of the significant morbidity and mortality of HSCT.[336,338-351] For this reason, until the most recent trials, unrelated donor HSCT was thought to be too morbid for patients in first remission and so trials used a genetic randomization, wherein all patients with a matched related donor proceeded to HSCT and all those without proceeded with further cycles of chemotherapy.[338,340,341]

The most recent British MRC trials, however, have had better results with chemotherapy alone than had been demonstrated in any of the previous U.S. trials.[322,323,341] In addition, the MRC trials were used to establish a risk stratification system for patients with AML using a combination of cytogenetic characteristics and response to therapy.[352] MRC10 has shown that patients in the good-risk group have a 78% survival from CR and a surprisingly high 61% survival from relapse, suggesting that these patients may not require HSCT in first remission.[352] The standard-risk group also had a reasonably high survival of 60% from CR but a much worse survival of only 17% from relapse. Patients in the poor-risk group had a poor survival of only 33% from CR and no patients survived after relapse, suggesting that a more aggressive or more targeted approach is needed in these patients. Once the U.S. trials moved to using the MRC backbone for chemotherapy, these data were used to formulate a more rational approach to recommending HSCT. In both the current COG and SJCRH trials, HSCT, even from a matched related donor, is not recommended for patients with low-risk disease. This is defined by COG as the presence of a t(8;21) or inv(16) in the leukemic clone at diagnosis and defined by SJCRH to include both these groups, plus patients with the t(9;11), because this group has been shown to have better than average survival in previous SJCRH trials.[219,268,269,353-359] For patients in either trial with standard-risk disease, defined as the absence of good- or poor-risk characteristics, HSCT is recommended if the patient has a matched family donor. With recent advances in supportive care and improved therapy to prevent and treat graft-versus-host

disease (GVHD), outcomes have improved for matched related and matched unrelated donor HSCT.[336,345,346,348] Therefore, for patients with high-risk disease, both trials recommend HSCT in first CR using an unrelated donor if no matched family donor is identified. The COG trial has classified high-risk disease as monosomy 7, −5/5q−, or more than 15% blasts in the marrow after one course of induction chemotherapy.[106,229,268,279,323,353,360] The SJCRH trial high-risk criteria includes monosomy 7, t(6;9), FAB M6 or M7, treatment-related AML, AML arising from prior MDS, RAEB-T, or a FLT3-ITD in the leukemic clone, as well as those patients who do not respond to the first cycle of induction.[*] Again based on the MRC data, patients in both these trials with both high- and low-risk features were treated as low risk and did not receive HSCT.[352] The optimal number of cycles of chemotherapy prior to HSCT to balance minimizing toxicity while minimizing MRD is variable, with the MRC10 trial using four cycles, the SJCRH trial two cycles, and the COG trial three cycles prior to HSCT.[322,323]

For patients who do not proceed to HSCT, there is controversy as to how many courses of chemotherapy are needed and what chemotherapy should be included. Several trials have shown that cycles of high-dose cytarabine postremission are associated with improved long-term survival.[269,274,344,349,365-369] MRC12 randomized patients to receive four versus five total cycles of chemotherapy, with early results suggesting that five cycles are superior; thus, that strategy has been used in the current U.S. trials.[352] The current COG trial tries to mimic the MRC trials closely with postinduction cycles of cytarabine and etoposide; cytarabine and mitoxantrone with or without GMTZ (randomization); and cytarabine and asparaginase (Capizzi II).[368-371] The SJCRH trial has tried to make up for the lack of amsacrine by tailoring the first postinduction cycle based on the patient's AML subtype and cytogenetics. Patients with t(9;11) or inv(16) AML receive cytarabine and cladribine; patients with M4/M5 AML receive cytarabine and etoposide; and patients with t(8;21) and all others receive high-dose cytarabine and mitoxantrone.[269,358,372-376] All patients subsequently receive two further courses consisting of cytarabine and asparaginase (Capizzi II) followed by cytarabine and mitoxantrone.[368-371]

CNS leukemia in patients with AML is highly sensitive to chemotherapy, and the addition of cranial irradiation does not decrease CNS relapse compared with treatment with systemic and intrathecal chemotherapy. Therefore, cranial irradiation is no longer part of the therapy for patients with AML.[377] Furthermore, in pediatrics, the addition of prolonged low-intensity maintenance therapy is associated with lower overall survival because of more resistant disease at relapse, so maintenance therapy is not used in the current U.S. trials.[378-380]

Supportive Therapy at Diagnosis and During Therapy

The diagnosis and treatment of childhood AML require a multidisciplinary approach involving pediatric oncologists, hematopathologists, pediatric surgeons, infectious disease specialists, pediatric intensivists, and pediatric nurses. While studies and procedures are initiated to make the diagnosis, special care must be taken to prevent and treat the life-threatening consequences of leukemia and accompanying pancytopenia. The most serious complications of leukemia at diagnosis are infection, bleeding, tumor lysis syndrome, and leukostasis. The most common causes of death once remission is achieved are relapse,

---

*References 151-155, 219, 228, 229, 231, 232, 268, and 361-364.

infection, hemorrhage, and cardiac events.[340,381] The improvement in overall survival of patients with AML over the past several decades is attributable as much to better support care efforts as to more effective treatment regimens.[382]

Infectious Complications

At the time of initial presentation, up to 40% of patients with leukemia exhibit fever, and most of these patients are neutropenic or have impaired neutrophil function.[287] During remission induction and subsequent cycles of chemotherapy, all AML patients experience profound prolonged neutropenia and are at high risk of life-threatening bacterial infections, particularly viridans group streptococcal infections.[381,383-385] Almost all AML patients experience at least one febrile neutropenic episode during therapy, and approximately 40% of these patients will have a documented infection, most commonly bacterial infections, followed by viral infections and then fungal infections. Infections account for nearly two thirds of deaths in remission.[340,381,385] Therefore, supportive care during induction and postremission therapy must pay particular attention to prophylactic, empirical, and treatment coverage for infectious complications. Several strategies are used to prevent infection or decrease mortality from infection. Some centers isolate patients receiving AML therapy in laminar airflow rooms during episodes of neutropenia.[381,386] The supportive care guidelines for the CCG-2961 study included mandatory hospitalization for all patients, whether febrile or not, until the absolute phagocyte count (APC) has risen. This recommendation has been continued in the current COG trial AAML0531. To decrease the rate of bacterial infections, some programs routinely prescribe the use of gut decontamination, mouthwashes, or prophylactic antibiotics.[340,382] This remains an area of controversy because, in some studies, it has been shown to decrease the rate of bacterial infection but may also be associated with an increase in drug-resistant organisms, and further investigation is indicated in a prospective randomized fashion before it is widely adopted.[381,386-393] However, patients who are febrile at initial presentation and patients who experience febrile neutropenia during therapy should be immediately started empirically on broad-spectrum antibiotics, including vancomycin, once cultures have been obtained.[394-396] In many centers, vancomycin is discontinued after 48 to 72 hours if there is no evidence of gram-positive bacteremia.[381] Typhlitis, or generalized bacterial infection of the cecum, is more common in children than in adults and is more common in patients treated with doxorubicin instead of daunorubicin.[397,398] Although this is a potentially life-threatening complication, conservative management with broad-spectrum antibiotics and nothing by mouth is generally preferable to surgical treatment in the setting of profound neutropenia.[399]

AML patients are at high risk for invasive fungal infection, which carries a high risk of mortality. The routine use of fungal prophylaxis is becoming more widely accepted. Some early studies have shown a decrease in some *Candida* species with fluconazole prophylaxis, but an increase in *C. krusei* infections was documented, with no decrease in infection by invasive molds.[400-402] Two meta-analyses have concluded that there is a reduction in morbidity because of invasive fungal infections when prophylaxis is used for those with prolonged neutropenia and post-HSCT patients.[403,404] A randomized controlled trial of posaconazole versus fluconazole or itraconazole as fungal prophylaxis in neutropenic patients with AML or MDS has shown a lower rate of invasive fungal infections and improved overall survival in the posaconazole group.[405] Voriconazole is also being studied as a prophylactic agent that has activity against both yeast and aspergillus.

A test to detect galactomannan-containing *Aspergillus* antigens in the sera of immunocompromised patients has become commercially available. At this point, the galactomannan assay has been used most advantageously to follow the status of invasive aspergillosis and its response to therapy.[406,407] However, some centers do not use fungal prophylaxis during AML therapy, but rather screen twice weekly with the galactomannan assay and use a low threshold for CT scanning to detect early invasive disease.[408,409] Whether or not fungal prophylaxis is used, empirical fungal therapy should be initiated for neutropenic patients who remain febrile for longer than 72 hours. Patients who need empirical fungal therapy should be routinely scanned during neutropenia and after the recovery of circulating neutrophils to screen for evidence of fungal disease, and the diagnosis of fungal infection should be made by biopsy whenever feasible. Amphotericin has long been the antifungal of choice for empirical therapy, and the liposomal forms appear to be equivalent in efficacy and less toxic to renal function.[410,411] One prospective randomized trial has shown that caspofungin as empirical fungal therapy is as effective as liposomal amphotericin B and is generally better tolerated.[412] Voriconazole as empirical fungal therapy was compared with amphotericin in a prospective randomized trial and found to provide comparable coverage with less renal toxicity, but with more visual changes and hallucinations.[413]

All patients undergoing AML therapy should receive prophylaxis against *Pneumocystis carinii* (now called *P. jiroveci*) pneumonia (PCP). The first-line agent in PCP prophylaxis is trimethoprim-sulfamethoxazole, but in some patients this is associated with significant allergic reaction or prolonged bone marrow suppression.[414-416] Dapsone is also effective as PCP prophylaxis in pediatric oncology patients, but is associated with significant hemolysis and methemoglobinemia in some patients.[417] Atovaquone has recently been shown to be highly effective as PCP prophylaxis for pediatric leukemia patients, although it may be associated with gastrointestinal side effects, including pancreatitis.[418] Aerosolized pentamidine has also been shown to be effective as PCP prophylaxis in children with leukemia, although it may be associated with significant bronchospasm.[419]

Viral infections can be a significant cause of morbidity and mortality in AML patients as well. CCG2961 and the current COG AAML0531 advocate intravenous immune serum globulin (IVIG) administration for low IgG levels and some centers also recommend respiratory syncytial virus (RSV) prophylaxis for infants. All blood products transfused should be leukoreduced and cytomegalovirus (CMV)-negative whenever possible. Acyclovir may be required for patients with recurrent zoster or mucocutaneous herpes simplex.[420]

Growth factors, such G-CSF and granulocyte-macrophage stimulating factor, have been used in the past, both as priming agents to synchronize the cell cycle prior to chemotherapy and as supportive care to decrease the duration of neutropenia after chemotherapy. Trials have shown that although G-CSF does shorten the duration of neutropenia, its use does not lead to fewer episodes of febrile neutropenia, fewer microbiologically documented infections, less infection-related mortality, or improved overall survival.[382,421-424] Based on these data, most centers no longer advocate the routine use of growth factors as supportive care during AML therapy.

Bleeding Complications

Severe thrombocytopenia is not unusual in leukemia patients, and hemorrhage is one of the leading causes of early mortality in these patients.[425-427] AML patients who present with bleeding and thrombocytopenia should be treated with platelet transfusions. In patients who are thrombocytopenic but do not have active bleeding, concern still remains about spontaneous bleeding, particularly intracranial, which can be catastrophic and have irreversible sequelae. The level of thrombocytopenia that warrants prophylactic platelet transfusion to prevent bleeding, however, is controversial. Some early observations had suggested that platelet counts less than 20,000/μL predispose to increased bleeding, and that number became a standard threshold for transfusion.[428] However, this was primarily in patients also receiving aspirin therapy, and subsequent studies have shown spontaneous bleeding occurs at a similar rate with platelet counts of less than 10,000 or 20,000/μL and many centers have adopted 10,000/μL as the new threshold for transfusion.[429-435] The threshold for platelet transfusion in patients undergoing procedures such as line placement or lumbar puncture has also not been well studied and the accepted standard threshold of 50,000/μL may be higher than is necessary.[428,436] All blood products should be leukoreduced or CMV-negative to prevent CMV infection and irradiated to prevent transfusion-related GVHD.[437-439] Menstruating women may require hormonal menstrual suppression for the duration of therapy with expected platelet drops to less than 50,000/μL.

Patients with AML, particularly FAB subtype M3 (acute promyelocytic), may also present with DIC and coagulation studies should be a routine part of the initial workup in a patient with AML.[440,441] In acute promyelocytic leukemia, blasts express high levels of annexin II, causing increased production of the fibrinolytic protein plasmin, which may be part of the cause of DIC in these patients.[292] Patients whose leukemic cells are successfully treated will exhibit resolution of DIC with the reduction in blast cells but, as the blast count is decreasing, DIC should be treated with fresh-frozen plasma, cryoprecipitate, or recombinant factor VIIa as needed to prevent bleeding. For patients with acute promyelocytic leukemia, the initiation of ATRA prior to chemotherapy leads to rapid resolution of DIC and has markedly reduced the early mortality previously associated with APL.[296-298,442] Since the development of ATRA, patients with APL are no longer treated with low-dose heparin to prevent DIC.[293,294]

Hyperleukocytosis Complications

Patients with AML, particularly those with high presenting leukocyte counts, have an increased risk for tumor lysis syndrome. In patients with leukemia, the rate of blast cell turnover can exceed the body's ability to metabolize and excrete the contents of dying cells, leading to life-threatening metabolic derangements.[443] Hyperuricemia resulting from the metabolism of excessive amounts of released nucleic acids can cause renal failure. The ensuing hyperkalemia may lead to fatal cardiac arrhythmias, and hyperphosphatemia and hypocalcemia may cause seizures and worsen the renal failure. Elevated blood urea nitrogen levels cause platelet dysfunction, which may exacerbate an existing coagulopathy. Vigorous intravenous hydration and administration of bicarbonate and other agents, such as intravenous allopurinol or recombinant urate oxidase, should be started immediately to decrease formation and increase the solubility and renal excretion of insoluble urate.[444-446] Recombinant urate oxidase can dramatically decrease uric acid levels within a few hours but, in patients with G6PD deficiency, it can cause methemoglobinemia and life-threatening hemolysis.[447,448]

Patients with leukocyte counts higher than 100,000/μL have an increased risk of leukostasis. Leukostasis causes intravascular clumping of blasts, leading to sluggish blood flow and subsequent hypoxia, hemorrhage, and infarction of tissue.[288,289,299,300,449] Leukostasis can be life-threatening when it occurs in the organs at greatest risk, the brain and lungs. Patients with pulmonary leukostasis present with significant hypoxia and tachypnea, which may progress rapidly to respiratory failure. CNS leukostasis may produce symptoms of confusion, headache, and somnolence and can lead to coma, stroke, and death. Hydration and hydroxyurea are therapies that can be initiated immediately to decrease the blast count. Leukapheresis or exchange transfusion can reduce the number of circulating blasts quickly, although this effect is transient, and therapy with cytoreductive drugs should be started as soon as possible.[449] Routine pheresis for patients with a WBC count higher than 100,000/μL has resulted in lower mortality rates during induction compared with historical controls. In one study, patients who achieved a higher than 30% decrease in total WBCs through pheresis had a higher complete remission rate than those who achieved less than a 30% decrease.[299,301,302] Other retrospective reviews have shown a decrease in early mortality after leukapheresis, but not an improvement in overall survival. Cytoreductive chemotherapy should be initiated as rapidly as possible, because other measures to reduce leukemic blast numbers have only temporary effectiveness.[450,451]

Chemotherapy Complications

High-dose cytarabine is associated with chemical conjunctivitis, and dexamethasone or prednisolone eyedrops should be used to prevent this.[452,453] High-dose cytarabine is also associated with neurotoxicity, including seizures and cerebellar dysfunction, which may not be reversible.[454-456] Patients should be monitored with frequent neurologic examinations and high-dose cytarabine should be immediately discontinued if cerebellar signs develop. Cytarabine may also be associated with an impressive febrile response, which is difficult to distinguish from an infection-related febrile response.[457,458] AML chemotherapy is associated with significant nausea and vomiting, and aggressive antiemetic regimens should be instituted. However, because of the high risk of fungal infection in these patients, dexamethasone should not be used as an antiemetic.[459-461] Mucositis is a significant toxicity during AML therapy, and almost all patients require parenteral pain medication and nutrition. Malnutrition at the time of diagnosis appears to carry a worse prognosis in children with leukemia and, even in those who are well-nourished at diagnosis, weight loss during chemotherapy should be monitored closely, followed by the initiation of parenteral or enteral feedings in those who lose more than 10% of their initial body weight.[462]

Renal toxicity during AML therapy is common and may be caused by a combination of chemotherapy, tumor lysis syndrome, sepsis, or treatment with antibacterial, antifungal, and antiviral agents. A creatinine clearance or glomerular filtration rate (GFR) should be checked in patients with abnormal creatinine or prolonged use of medications with renal toxicity. For patients with a creatinine clearance lower than 60 mL/min/1.73 m², high-dose cytarabine, etoposide, and other renally cleared chemotherapy agents are usually given at reduced dosages. Significant liver toxicity can also be observed during therapy for AML, particularly for regimens containing the humanized anti-CD33 monoclonal antibody GMTZ. GMTZ has been associated with sinusoidal obstructive syndrome and veno-occlusive disease, most commonly when used as a component of combination therapy or in patients who are heavily pretreated or who have undergone prior HSCT or undergo subsequent HSCT within 3 months of treatment with GMTZ.[463]

AML regimens rely heavily on anthracyclines and their derivatives. The cumulative anthracycline dose in these regimens is often 300 mg/m² or higher in doxorubicin equivalents, and therefore carries a high risk of cardiac toxicity. Cardiac deaths are one of the top three causes of death in remission for

AML patients.[340,382] All patients should undergo cardiac assessment prior to administration of chemotherapy cycles containing anthracyclines and yearly after chemotherapy is complete, until growth is completed in adulthood. In vitro evidence has suggested that the cardioprotectant dexrazoxane works synergistically, not antagonistically, with anthracyclines against AML blasts, and there is increasing interest in incorporating this medication into AML clinical trials.[464-466]

Extramedullary Disease

Between 20% and 40% of children with AML have evidence of extramedullary disease at the time of diagnosis.[310,313] The most common manifestations of extramedullary disease are skin infiltrates, soft tissue or bone involvement, gingival infiltration, and CNS involvement. Some patients, particularly infants, may have isolated extramedullary leukemia without other evidence of disease, but bone marrow infiltration invariably occurs in these patients without systemic therapy.

Central Nervous System Involvement

CNS involvement is more common in AML patients with high presenting WBC counts, favorable cytogenetic changes—t(9;11), t(8;21), and inv(16)—and children younger than 2 years.[306,377,467] AML patients with CNS disease at diagnosis have a higher risk of CNS relapse, but they often have a better overall prognosis because CNS disease is more common in the favorable-risk cytogenetic groups, which carry a lower risk of systemic relapse.[467,468] Specific CNS-directed therapy in AML may also be less important than in ALL because several AML chemotherapy agents, including high-dose cytarabine and cladribine, have excellent CNS penetrance. Cranial radiation was previously used in AML patients as prophylaxis against CNS relapse, but because of concerns about the myriad side effects of CNS radiation, including secondary malignancy, endocrine and growth impairment, and neurocognitive toxicity, later trials attempted to minimize radiation.[469,470] In the BFM-87 study, all patients received intrathecal cytarabine, but the low-risk patients were randomized to additional therapy with cranial radiation or no further CNS treatment. An interim analysis has shown no increase in CNS relapse in the group that did not receive cranial radiation, so the radiation arm was closed early.[309] Intrathecal chemotherapy with cytarabine alone, methotrexate alone, or triple intrathecal therapy with cytarabine, methotrexate, and hydrocortisone have all been reported to be effective as CNS treatment and prophylaxis.[377,467,471,472] As prophylaxis for CNS negative patients, the current COG study AAML0531 uses intrathecal cytarabine alone at the start of each cycle, except for the Capizzi II cycle, which includes 3 g/m^2 of systemic cytarabine. For patients who have CNS disease at diagnosis, twice-weekly intrathecal therapy with cytarabine alone is used until the CSF is clear, plus an additional two doses, with a minimum of four doses and a maximum of six doses. If more than six doses are required, the patient is taken off study for refractory CNS disease. The SJCRH AML2002 trial uses a prophylaxis regimen of triple intrathecal chemotherapy with cytarabine, methotrexate, and hydrocortisone given at the start of each cycle, but separated by at least 24 hours from systemic cytarabine dosages ≥ 1 g/m^2, to prevent neurotoxicity. Patients with CNS disease at diagnosis receive once-weekly triple intrathecal chemotherapy for four doses. To decrease mucosal toxicity from the methotrexate, all patients receive leucovorin rescue at 24 and 30 hours after the intrathecal administration.

CNS relapse occurs in 2% to 8.8% of patients with AML.[368,377,473] Most AML patients who suffer a CNS relapse will simultaneously or soon thereafter develop a bone marrow relapse. Truly isolated CNS relapse is rare, and is associated with age younger than 2 years, hepatosplenomegaly at diagnosis, elevated presenting WBC count, M5 AML, and chromosome 11 abnormalities.[468] For those with a truly isolated CNS relapse, the optimum treatment plan is unclear. There have been survivors reported after treatment with intrathecal chemotherapy alone, combined intrathecal and systemic chemotherapy, radiation therapy, and HSCT.[306,468]

Chloromas

Extramedullary infiltrations of the soft tissue, also known as chloromas, myelosarcomas, or granulocytic sarcomas, occur in approximately 4% to 5% of children with AML.[304,310,474] They may also be documented in patients with CML, MDS, or rarely in ALL, and may be initially confused with non-Hodgkin's lymphoma.[475] Chloromas most often present simultaneously with AML or shortly before the systemic evidence of disease, but they may be isolated. The prognostic significance of extramedullary disease is not clear. Some groups have reported an unfavorable prognosis associated with chloromas,[337] but others have demonstrated a more favorable outcome.[366,473] Blast cells from patients with chloromas often exhibit the relatively favorable t(8;21).[313,314,476] Most studies from Europe, Saudi Arabia, Japan, and the United States have reported no influence of chloromas on the overall survival of children with AML.[303,310,337,342,368,477] Accordingly, most centers treat patients who have chloromas with standard AML regimens, because there is no consistent evidence supporting more intensive therapy.[310] A beneficial role for radiation therapy in the treatment of chloromas has not been demonstrated.[477] In a CCG trial, patients with chloromas were treated with local irradiation in addition to systemic therapy. There was no difference in event-free survival or in the incidence of local recurrence compared with the chemotherapy-only regimen. However, chloromas arising in the orbit or CNS may cause loss of vision or cord compression, and emergency radiation therapy as well as chemotherapy is indicated in these situations.[477]

Prognosis

There are several major prognostic factors for patients with AML, and new data are constantly emerging. Some information about prognosis can be gleaned simply by the morphologic subtype of AML, although prognosis is most likely actually related to the underlying genetic changes as opposed to the morphology itself. FAB subtype M0, which commonly harbors a complex karyotype, abnormalities of 5 or 7, or trisomy 8, is associated with a poor prognosis.[478] M7 AML, often associated with monosomy 7, carries a poor prognosis.[479-483] M3 AML with the t(15;17) was previously one of the poor-prognosis groups but, with the addition of ATRA to chemotherapy regimens, this has become a favorable subtype.[484-487] M2 AML with t(8;21) and M4eo AML with inv(16) are both favorable subtypes.[488,489]

Demographic Risk Factors

Age younger than 10 years has been reported to carry a favorable prognosis in the more recent trials at SJRCH utilizing more intensive therapy.[490] Race and ethnicity play a role in prognosis as well. Patients on CCG2891 who received chemotherapy alone had an overall survival of 48% for white children versus only 37% for Hispanic children ($P = .016$) and 34% for black children ($P = .007$).[491] AML-97, one of the more recent AML trials at SJCRH, has also shown a trend toward inferior outcomes for black compared with white children (hazard ratio [HR] = 1.61; 95% confidence interval [CI] = 0.76 to 3.42; P = 0.22 with 5-year survival rates of 55.6% vs. 27.3%).[491a] In these trials, there was no difference in other prognostic variables between the groups, and these patients were hospitalized and received intravenous chemotherapy, received the same supportive care, and had the same compliance rates. Therefore, the observed differences may be attributable to pharmacogenomic differences that affect response to and toxicity from chemotherapy.[479,491] Patients who are overweight (body mass index [BMI] ≥ 95th percentile) or underweight (≤10th percentile) also carry a worse prognosis and are less likely to survive and more likely to suffer treatment-related mortality.[492]

Cytogenetic Factors

Probably the single most important prognostic factor is the result of cytogenetic analysis of the AML blasts. Results of several large multicenter trials have confirmed the correlation between certain cytogenetic abnormalities and clinical outcome and have shown that karyotype in AML represents an independent prognostic variable for attainment of complete response and overall survival.[268,270,271,274,493] In children and adults, the highest complete response rates and longest survival times have been linked to the t(8;21) and inv(16) or t(16;16).[488,489] These translocations result in modifications to the core-binding complex, a group of proteins that appear to play a vital role in hematopoiesis. AML cells with inv(16) have increased incorporation of cytarabine into nuclear DNA and are more susceptible to cytarabine chemotherapy in vitro.[494] Patients with APL and the t(15;17) previously represented a poor-risk group but, since the advent of ATRA therapy (see later), now represent a group with a favorable prognosis.[484-487] Other cytogenetic aberrations have been associated with an unfavorable outcome. These include monosomy 5, del(5q), monosomy 7, abnormalities of 3q, aberrations of 12p, and complex cytogenetic abnormalities.[268,273,495] For pediatric patients with monosomy 7, several studies have shown better overall survival when HSCT is used as consolidation therapy as opposed to conventional chemotherapy.[481-483] Patients with normal karyotypes have traditionally been grouped together in an intermediate-prognosis group, but now that mutations in genes such as *FLT3* (poor prognosis) and *NPM* (good prognosis) are being recognized in these patients, they are no longer being considered as a single category.[362] Abnormal karyotypes linked with an intermediate prognosis include del(7q), 11q23 translocations, +21, +8, +22, and del(9q).[268,362] As more studies with large numbers of patients undergoing cytogenetic evaluation are completed, certain groups of karyotype aberrations are showing heterogeneity in their prognostic significance. For example, all 11q23 translocations were previously grouped together in the intermediate- to poor-prognosis category. However, studies have shown that the 11q23 aberration may be subdivided into groups of lesser and greater prognostic risk. Patients with the t(9;11)(p22;q23) have significantly longer event-free and overall survival times than patients with other 11q23 translocations.[221,270,272,273,362,493] In the MRC AML-10 trial, patients with the t(9;11) had a more favorable outcome than those with the t(10;11)(p12;q23).[268] This finding was confirmed in several large clinical trials enrolling children, in which the presence of the t(9;11) predicted a significantly improved prognosis compared with that observed with other 11q23 translocations. These results were also documented in children younger than 2 years.[220,278,496,497] As new therapeutic agents are developed that target the specific molecular aberrations identified by cytogenetic analysis, accurate detection of these abnormalities becomes even more important.[362]

Molecular Genetic Factors

Analysis of molecular genetics is emerging as an invaluable tool in prognostic determination for patients with AML, as well as for providing insight into the pathogenesis of AML and elucidating possibilities for targeted therapy.[110] *Ras* mutations have been identified in pediatric AML patients, with *NRAS* mutations in 14.7% and *KRAS* mutations in 3.3% of patients.[498] As in adults, these mutations are more common in children with the CBF leukemias although, unlike the adult population, the increase is not only for inv(16) (25% of children, 36% of adults), but also t(8;21) (36.4% of children, 8% of adults).[498,499] Thus far, *Ras* mutations have shown no significant impact on prognosis.[135,364,498,500-503] *c-Kit* mutations have been identified in 11.3% of pediatric AML patients, again predominantly in the CBF leukemias, with mutations in 54.5% of patients with inv(16) and 31.3% of pediatric patients with t(8;21).[498] The role of *c-Kit* mutations in prognosis is unclear; in some series, the *c-Kit* mutations do not seem to have prognostic significance, in others, *c-Kit* mutations have been shown to confer worse prognosis in patients with t(8;21) but not in patients with inv(16) and, in still other trials, *c-Kit* mutations confer a worse prognosis in all subsets of CBF leukemias.[498,499,504,505]

As noted, *FLT3* mutations include ITDs in the juxtamembrane domain and point mutations in the activation loop (ALM). *FLT3* ITDs have a worse prognosis, particularly when present in a high allelic ratio,[155,506-509] whereas *FLT3* ALMs seem to have no impact on prognosis.[155,506,509] Partial tandem duplications of the *MLL* gene have also been reported in 13% of pediatric AML patients and are associated with a worse prognosis in adult and pediatric patients.[205,506,510,511] Frame shift mutations in *NPM1* lead to cytoplasmic localization of nucleophosmin and have been identified in 6% to 8% of all children with AML, and 25% to 30% of pediatric AML patients with normal cytogenetics.[247,248] When identified as an isolated mutation in adults and children, it is associated with improved prognosis, but when found in conjunction with a *FLT3* ITD, the poor prognostic impact of the *FLT* ITD prevails.[247,248,512-514] *PTPN11* mutations are only found in 4% of pediatric patients with AML (4%), and 18% to 36% of the *PTPN11* mutations are seen in M5 AML. In pediatrics, this mutation does not appear to have prognostic importance.[124,515] The Wilms' tumor gene (*WT1*) is aberrantly expressed in AML; in adults, high expression levels of WT1 at diagnosis have been associated with a poor prognosis in many studies.[516-521] In pediatric patients, however, the available data are contradictory. One small study of 47 patients has shown that low levels of WT1 at diagnosis are associated with good outcome,[522] whereas another small study of 41 patients has shown that high levels of WT1 are more commonly seen in association with the t(8;21) and inv(16) favorable prognosis cytogenetic findings, and therefore associated with a better prognosis.[523]

Relapsed or Refractory Disease

The prognosis is grave for children with disease refractory to induction chemotherapy or who have a disease relapse. Although 80% to 90% of pediatric patients with AML will achieve remission, 30% to 40% will later recur, and the overall survival remains only 40% to 60%.[322,471,472,479,524-528] The bone marrow is the most common site of relapse in AML and isolated CNS relapse is an uncommon finding.[341,468]

Prognosis in Relapsed or Refractory Disease

A durable remission is less likely to be achieved and maintained in patients with relapsed or refractory AML than in patients with newly diagnosed AML, but the salvage rate in these patients has improved in recent years.[479,528,529] The single most important prognostic indicator after relapse is duration of first remission, with less than 1 year to relapse carrying an overall survival rate of 0% to 21%, and longer than 1 year to relapse carrying an overall survival rate of 33% to 62%.[341,479,528,530-534] Other characteristics that have been associated with better prognosis after relapse are male gender, good-risk cytogenetic features of t(8;21) and inv(16), chemotherapy alone without HSCT as consolidation during first CR, and the use of HSCT as part of relapse therapy. The characteristics associated with worse prognosis after relapse are early recurrence, M5 or M7 morphology, poor-risk cytogenetics, and HSCT during first CR.

Conventional Therapy for Relapsed or Refractory Disease

There is no accepted standard therapy for adult or pediatric patients with relapsed or refractory AML. However, several researchers have demonstrated activity of high-dose cytarabine in patients with relapsed disease, even in those who had been exposed to cytarabine during prior treatment.[535] High-dose cytarabine has been used in combination with other agents, such as mitoxantrone, asparaginase, etoposide, fludarabine, cladribine, and clofarabine.[531,536-541] The combination of cytarabine and mitoxantrone was particularly effective as reinduction with a remission rate of 76%, but now that this regimen has been incorporated into the current standard first-line regimens, its use as a reinduction regimen may provide too much cumulative anthracycline for many patients.[531] Fludarabine, cladribine, and clofarabine are all deoxyadenosine analogues that have been used for the treatment of AML. Trials using high-dose cytarabine in combination with fludarabine and G-CSF (i.e., the FLAG regimen) have demonstrated a 70% remission rate in patients with relapsed AML.[542-544] The addition of idarubicin to the FLAG regimen has resulted in longer lasting remissions in some studies, but it was also associated with more significant toxicity.[545-548] The combination of cytarabine and cladribine has been successful as a relapse regimen in some trials for adult patients and pediatric patients with de novo AML, particularly those with the M5 subtype.[374,549-554] However, this combination seems to be of little benefit in pediatric patients with relapsed or refractory AML.[555] Clofarabine was found to be effective as a single agent in relapsed ALL and AML and was subsequently approved by the U.S. Food and Drug Administration (FDA) for use in relapsed ALL.[539,556] Clofarabine has now been shown to be safe and effective in combination with cytarabine in regimens for adult patients and is currently in clinical trials for pediatric patients with relapsed or refractory AML.[540,541] For patients who cannot tolerate high-dose cytarabine or further anthracyclines, one alternative regimen that has been used at the Memorial Sloan-Kettering Cancer Center is topotecan, vinorelbine, thiotepa, dexamethasone, and gemcitabine (TVTG), with five of nine AML patients responding to this therapy.[557]

Long-term remission for patients with relapsed or refractory disease requires consolidation therapy with allogeneic HSCT.[318,547] Traditionally, this has included matched family members or matched unrelated donors, but the more recent use of alternative hematopoietic stem cell sources, such as banked umbilical cord blood or haploidentical family donors, has increased the number of patients with a potential marrow source. It is possible to cure patients who have persistent, refractory disease at the time of allogeneic HSCT, particularly if they have less than 20% blasts in the marrow and a total body irradiation (TBI)–based regimen is used, although the cure rate in this group is uniformly less than 25%.[558-563] For patients who

have had a long first remission and proceed to HSCT in a second CR, the overall survival rates are much better and may be as high as 40% to 62%.[479,528,563] The graft-versus-leukemia (GVL) effect is an important component in the curative role of allogeneic HSCT for AML. This effect is difficult to measure directly, but has been indirectly inferred from the presence of GVHD. The presence of acute and chronic GVHD has been associated with lower relapse rates in AML.[564-570] Donor lymphocyte infusions (DLIs) have been used successfully to induce GVL effect in patients with CML who relapse after allogeneic HSCT, but this strategy is much less effective in patients with AML who relapse after allogeneic HSCT.[571,572]

There can be GVL effect without GVHD, however, as evidenced by lower relapse rates in patients receiving HSCT from a matched sibling versus an identical twin, even in the absence of GVHD.[573] There is much interest in maximizing the GVL effect and recent studies have concentrated on the role of alloreactive natural killer (NK) cells in this process. Donors who are mismatched at the killer immunoglobulin-like receptor (KIR) ligand produce NK cells that recognize and destroy host AML cells in response to the lack of expression of a self class I ligand on the AML cells.[574-576] Deliberate KIR mismatching through haploidentical HSCT has been shown in small studies to decrease the relapse rate without increasing GVHD, therefore resulting in improved long-term survival. This strategy is being used in clinical trials for patients with high-risk de novo AML or relapsed and refractory disease, and is currently being incorporated into ongoing pediatric trials of the COG and SJCRH.[575]

Novel Agents and Targeted Therapy

Conventional therapy for AML is predominantly a "shotgun" approach in which leukemia cells, as well as normal hematopoietic stem and progenitor cells and many other normal tissues, are injured, with the hope that the normal cells will recover faster and more completely than the leukemia cells. As discussed earlier, this approach has not resulted in superior cure rates in AML and the intensity has been increased to the point that most patients suffer toxicity and treatment-related morbidity; a substantial fraction of patients suffer treatment-related mortality. As the molecular pathogenesis of AML has been elucidated, opportunities have appeared for the development of novel and targeted agents that preferentially destroy leukemia cells, with far less significant effects on normal hematopoietic cells and other normal tissues.[577,578]

Antibody Therapy with Gemtuzumab Ozogamicin

Gemtuzumab ozogamicin (also discussed earlier in the induction chemotherapy section) is a recombinant, humanized anti-CD33 monoclonal antibody linked to the tumor antibiotic calicheamicin. CD33 is expressed on most AML cells but not on pluripotent hematopoietic stem cells or other tissues, thus making it possible to target leukemia cells more specifically.[324,325] GMTZ has been used successfully as a single agent for adults and children in relapse, with infusional side effects of fever and chills, hematologic toxicity resulting from pancytopenia, including some cases of prolonged thrombocytopenia, and hepatic toxicity ranging from transient liver function abnormalities to fatal veno-occlusive disease, particularly when used within 3 months of HSCT.[463,579-586] Gemtuzumab as a single agent is not a particularly strong reinduction regimen, but it has now been used successfully in combination with cytarabine-mitoxantrone and cytarabine-asparaginase as part of a reinduction regimen.[491,578,585,587-591] It was also successfully piloted in a COG trial as part of an induction regimen for de novo AML with acceptable toxicity; it now is included in the induction regimens of the currently open COG and SJCRH AML trials.

Receptor Tyrosine Kinase Inhibitors

FLT3 (discussed in detail earlier) is a receptor tyrosine kinase that is upregulated in the AML cells of most patients. There are also two types of activating mutations in *FLT3* and, in pediatric patients with AML, ITDs are present in 5% to 16% and ALMs are present in 2% to 5% of cases.[153-156] Several small-molecule inhibitors of the FLT3 tyrosine kinase have been developed, some of which are effective against only the ITDs and some of which are effective against both the ITDs and the ALMs.[592,593] These inhibitors are now in various phases of clinical trials. Overall, they appear to be well tolerated and to induce a decrease in blasts, but as single agents they generally do not result in durable remissions.[153-156,594] Clinical trials are currently underway to combine FLT3 inhibitors with chemotherapy, including an open COG pilot study of CEP-701 (lestaurtinib) in combination with high-dose cytarabine for patients with relapsed or refractory *FLT3*-mutant AML.

Farnesyltransferase Inhibitors

Mutations in *RAS* itself, as well as perturbations in the RAS pathway, are associated with AML. The RAS protein requires isoprenylation by farnesyltransferase to bind to the plasma membrane properly and be fully active. Several farnesyltransferase inhibitors have been developed with the goal of inhibiting upregulated or dysregulated RAS activity. Because these drugs do not specifically target a known mutation in *RAS* and have effect on other proteins that also require farnesylation, they can be effective in patients with or without *RAS* mutations. Tipifarnib (R115777, Zarnestra) as an oral agent has shown activity in adult patients with refractory AML and in older adult patients with de novo AML, with a few transient complete responses, even when used as a single agent.[595-598] The drug was generally well tolerated with toxicities of myelosuppression, neurotoxicity, and reversible renal toxicity.[595,597] In pediatrics, a phase I trial of tipifarnib for refractory solid tumors and neurofibromatosis type 1–related plexiform neurofibromas and a phase II trial for brain tumors both have shown that the drug was tolerated well overall, with dose-limiting toxicities of myelosuppression, rash, nausea, and vomiting; one patient also developed a seizure.[599,600] A phase I trial in patients with refractory leukemia was completed by COG in 2005. The drug has also been used safely in combination with capecitabine for children with advanced solid tumors. Currently, there are ongoing trials combining tipifarnib with chemotherapy for adults with AML as well as a COG trial combining tipifarnib with *cis*-retinoic acid, cytarabine, and fludarabine with HSCT for children with JMML.[601] Two other farnesyltransferase inhibitors, lonafarnib (Sarasar, SCH66336) and BMS-214662 have also shown some promise in adults with myeloid disorders, but there are as yet no data for pediatric AML.[602]

Histone Deacetylase Inhibitors

Double-stranded DNA binds to histones to form compact nucleosomes when the DNA is not being actively transcribed. Acetylation of lysine residues by histone acetyltransferases (HATs) allows the release of DNA from histones for transcription. Deacetylation by histone deacetylase (HDAC) reverses the process. Inappropriate recruitment of HDACs leading to gene silencing has been demonstrated in the CBF leukemic cells bearing translocations t(8;21) and inv(16), as well as in APL cells bearing the t(15;17).[603-608] The use of HDAC inhibitors may allow for renewed expression of silenced genes that when activated can induce differentiation or cell death.[609,610] Several HDAC inhibitors have been tested in clinical trials in AML patients, including the antiseizure medication valproic acid. It has been used in clinical trials for adults with MDS or AML as monotherapy and in combination with ATRA, 5-aza-2′-deoxycytidine (DAC), as well as 5-azacytidine and ATRA together.[577,611,612] It was generally well tolerated, with toxicities of myelosuppression, neurotoxicity, and sedation. Some transient responses were seen, even when valproic acid was used as monotherapy, but it was most effective when used in combination with ATRA and 5-azacytidine.[577,611,612] A more potent HDAC, depsipeptide, has been used in clinical trials and has had more toxicity, including fatigue, nausea, and constitutional symptoms. In these trials, it has shown some promise in T-cell lymphoma but thus far only modest antileukemia activity.[613,614]

DNA Methylation Inhibitors

Hypermethylation of DNA also leads to gene inactivation. Several hypermethylated genes have been identified in AML blasts, leading to interest in DNA methyltransferase inhibitors as a therapeutic strategy.[615-620] 5-Azacytidine is a DNA methyltransferase inhibitor that is FDA-approved for the treatment of MDS.[621] Higher doses have been used successfully to induce transient remission in adults with AML who were not candidates for more aggressive chemotherapy.[622] Decitabine is another DNA methyltransferase inhibitor that has been used successfully, with limited nonhematologic toxicity in AML patients, possibly by inducing differentiation of leukemic blasts.[623-625] There has also been interest in HDAC inhibitors and DNA methyltransferase inhibitors as combination therapy. In some trials, this seems to be a safe and effective strategy[626] but, in at least one trial using decitabine and valproic acid, the combination did not show an improved response rate over decitabine alone and proved too toxic because of encephalopathy.[627]

Proteosome Inhibitors

The proteosome is a multiprotein complex that mediates the destruction of most intracellular proteins.[628-630] Through inhibition of the ubiquitin proteosome pathway, proteosome inhibitors inhibit nuclear factor κB (NF-κB) and induce apoptosis in malignant cells.[631] Bortezomib (Velcade, PS-341) is a selective reversible inhibitor of the proteosome complex that is FDA-approved for use in multiple myeloma. In AML cell lines, bortezomib alone induces apoptosis of blasts and the effect is synergistic when used in combination with cytarabine and daunorubicin or with tipifarnib.[632-635] In a phase I study in adults with AML, bortezomib was added to an induction regimen of idarubicin and cytarabine and was found to be safe, with nonhematologic toxicities of hypoxia, hyperbilirubinemia, and elevated transaminase levels.[636] A phase I trial of bortezomib in pediatric patients with refractory leukemias has been completed through COG, but the results are not yet available.

Apoptosis inhibitors

BCL-2 is an inhibitor of apoptosis that is highly expressed in some patients with AML and is associated with a poor prognosis.[637-639] A BCL-2 antisense oligonucleotide has been tested as a single agent and shown to induce transient remission in some AML patients.[640] It has also been shown to be safe and effective in combination with cytarabine and daunorubicin.[641] This agent is now being used in clinical trials of AML through the Cancer and Leukemia Group B (CALGB) as part of combination therapy during induction and consolidation.[578]

ACUTE PROMYELOCYTIC LEUKEMIA

Pathobiology

APL or M3 AML is a subtype of AML defined by a specific morphology, a balanced translocation involving the RARA gene, and a characteristic coagulopathy.[173,283,642,643] Although most patients with APL have the classic t(15;17) resulting in the *PML-RARA* fusion gene, up to 8% do not. Approximately 5% of patients have a *PML-RARA* because of an insertion or other variant, 1% of patients have a t(11;17) resulting in a *PLZF-RARA*, another 1% have a t(5;17) resulting in an *NPM-RARA* or a t(11;17) resulting in a *NuMA-RARA* or a *STAT5b-RARA*, and 1% of patients do not have an identifiable *RARA* rearrangement.[644] APL provides a clear example of the proposed two-hit model for AML (see earlier, "Molecular Genetics"). The fusion protein resulting from the pathognomonic translocation in APL, the PML-*RARA* protein, is an example of a class II mutation, resulting in a block in differentiation. As detailed earlier (see "Biology"), this protein has been shown to interfere with normal myeloid cell development through dominant inhibitory mechanisms that cause differentiation arrest at the promyelocyte stage.[645-647] Mutations in the receptor tyrosine kinase *FLT3* occur in up to 43% of cases of APL, and these mutations are classic examples of class I mutations, conferring a proliferative advantage.[648,649] At diagnosis, APL patients with *FLT3* mutations more often present with hyperleukocytosis, microgranular variant morphology, and the bcr3 PML breakpoint.[146,648-653] Although *FLT3* ITDs clearly confer a worse prognosis in other subtypes of AML, their role in prognosis for APL is less clear. Some groups have reported a worse prognosis for APL patients with a *FLT3* ITD, whereas other groups have found no statistically significant impact on the generally favorable risk outcome of this disease.[648,649,653-655]

Clinical Presentation

APL is more common in girls and obese children. Compared with adults, children with APL have a higher incidence of hyperleukocytosis at presentation, microgranular variant morphology, and PML-RARA isoforms bcr2 and bcr3.[656] A presenting WBC count higher than 10,000/µL has been repeatedly shown to carry a worse prognosis.[484,657-659] Patients with APL often present with a characteristic life-threatening coagulopathy that results from DIC and plasmin-dependent fibrinolysis. Before the 1970s, bleeding complications caused significant mortality for patients with APL. Measures that have been used successfully to manage the coagulopathy include platelet and cryoprecipitate transfusions, use of low-dose heparin, and prompt initiation of anthracycline-based chemotherapy.[293,294,314,643] However, the most dramatic decrease in early and induction-related deaths has been the result of the addition of ATRA to the induction regimen, which rapidly leads to the resolution of DIC, and therefore has markedly reduced early mortality.[170,295-298]

Treatment

All-Trans-Retinoic Acid

With the introduction of ATRA, the treatment and outcome of APL have changed dramatically. ATRA induces differentiation in the APL blasts in vivo and in vitro and, as a single agent, can induce remission in up to 90% of patients with newly diagnosed APL.[170,296,660-662] However, without further chemotherapy, the duration of remission is short. Treatment combin-

ing ATRA with conventional chemotherapy has dramatically improved the prognosis for patients with APL compared with chemotherapy alone.[486,663-667] A long-term analysis has demonstrated significantly higher actuarial event-free survival rates, lower relapse rates, and improved overall survival in the group treated with both ATRA and chemotherapy.[668] The addition of ATRA to the chemotherapy regimen has been particularly effective for pediatric patients. The APL93 trial used ATRA in combination with daunorubicin and cytarabine in induction, and the children in this trial had a CR rate of 97%.[669] The PETHEMA and GIMEMA-AIEOPAIDA groups have completed pediatric trials using ATRA and idarubicin as induction chemotherapy, with reported CR rates of 92% to 96%.[670,671]

One potentially life-threatening complication of ATRA therapy is the retinoic acid syndrome. This syndrome occurs in approximately 25% of patients and is characterized by fever, respiratory distress, pleural or pericardial effusions, edema, hypotension and, in some cases, renal failure.[442,672-674] In most patients, the symptoms are preceded by an increasing WBC count.[661,673] Retinoic acid syndrome can be life-threatening, and the mortality rate ranges from 8% to 15% in different reports.[664,665,673,675] The syndrome is also associated with a higher risk of bone marrow and extramedullary relapse.[672,676] The use of chemotherapy concurrently with ATRA therapy during induction, particularly in patients with high presenting WBC counts, results in a significantly lower incidence of fatal retinoic acid syndrome.[677] The use of high-dose corticosteroids at the first sign of symptoms has also been shown to be effective in preventing ATRA syndrome and reducing its mortality rate. Another serious complication of ATRA therapy is pseudotumor cerebri, presenting as headache and papilledema. True pseudotumor cerebri is observed in up to 16% of children, and an additional 39% of children develop headaches without other signs of increased intracranial pressure.[669,671] Pseudotumor cerebri may require treatment with diuretics such as acetazolamide or serial lumbar punctures to reduce intracranial pressure and, in some cases, discontinuation or dose reduction of ATRA is required.[678] Close follow-up with an ophthalmologist is advised because these patients may suffer visual loss, which in rare cases may be irreversible.[679] Because of the high rate of ATRA-related side effects, the AML-BFM study group studied dose reduction of ATRA during induction from 45 to 25 mg/m^2/day. They found that this dose was still effective, although in pediatric patients, there was still a very high rate of CNS side effects, with 57% of children exhibiting headache, increased intracranial pressure, or frank pseudotumor cerebri.[680,681] The recently closed CALGB trial C9710 included pediatric patients and used the higher dose of ATRA, but consideration is being given to using lower dosages in future pediatric trials through the COG.

Arsenic Trioxide

Arsenic trioxide (As_2O_3, ATO) has been used for decades in China as treatment for leukemia. The precise mechanism of action is actively being studied, but ATO appears to induce both differentiation and apoptosis of APL blasts and to degrade the PML-RARA fusion protein.[190,195,682] ATO appears to induce nonterminal differentiation followed by apoptosis via the caspase pathway.[190,195,682-684] When ATO was used as a single agent in patients with APL, remission rates of 65% to 85% were reported and the 10-year survival was as high as 30%.[442] Later studies done in China and the United States showed favorable results, with moderate toxicity, using ATO in patients with relapsed APL who had previously received ATRA therapy.[189,683,685-687] More recently, several studies have shown promising results using ATO in remission induction and consolidation therapy for patients with newly diagnosed APL.[688-690]

One small series of 11 children with newly diagnosed APL treated with ATO as a single agent showed mild toxicity, including leukocytosis, skin changes, and mild neuropathy.[690] CR was induced in 91% of these patients, with 1 patient dying of cerebral hemorrhage during induction. With a relatively short median follow-up of 30 months, the relapse-free survival was 81% with only 1 relapse; the patient who relapsed achieved a second CR and thus the overall survival rate remains 91%.[690] ATO was used in a randomized fashion during consolidation in the recently closed CALGB trial that included pediatric patients through the COG, but data from this trial are not yet available. ATRA and ATO have been used safely together as induction therapy in children and adults.[190,195,682,691-693] The drugs may have a synergistic effect when used together, with one study showing a shorter median time to CR in the group receiving the combination (40.5 days for ATRA alone, 31 days for ATO alone, 25.5 days for ATRA with ATO).[693] The combination also provided longer duration of remission in this study. With a short median follow-up of 18 months, there were also 0 of 20 relapses in the combination group compared with 7 of 37 relapses in the monotherapy groups.[693] Because of these promising data, several groups are interested in using ATO as part of induction or consolidation therapy for newly diagnosed pediatric APL patients, with the hope of reducing the total cumulative dose of anthracycline exposure.

ATO therapy is generally well tolerated, often with only minimal and reversible toxicity.[690,694,695] However, care must be taken with its use, because it can produce a prolonged QTc interval, which may be asymptomatic but can progress to torsades de pointes and fatal cardiac arrhythmia.[695-698] In one retrospective analysis, the rate of arrhythmia was significantly higher in African American patients (3 of 4) versus non–African-American patients (1 of 73).[699] QTc intervals should be followed closely by electrocardiography, and hypokalemia and hypomagnesemia should be meticulously avoided.[700] Because of the induction of cellular differentiation, ATO commonly results in a condition similar to retinoic acid syndrome, most often characterized by fluid retention and pleural and pericardial effusions.[701] This may be successfully treated in the same way as ATRA-induced retinoic acid syndrome. ATO can also cause a significant polyneuropathy, particularly when given in repeated courses.[702] Less dangerous side effects include skin changes with rash, hyperpigmentation, keratosis, and transient liver function test abnormalities. In a COG phase I study of ATO in children with refractory or relapsed acute leukemia, dose-limiting toxicities included prolonged QTc, pneumonitis, and neuropathic pain, whereas non–dose-limiting toxicities included elevated liver function test results, nausea, vomiting, abdominal pain, constipation, electrolyte changes, hyperglycemia, dermatitis, and headache.[703]

Cytarabine

Although cytarabine is the backbone of induction chemotherapy for other subtypes of AML, its role in APL has been less clear.[298] The PETHEMA group completed a pediatric trial using ATRA and idarubicin as induction chemotherapy without cytarabine and the CR rate was 92%.[670] The GIMEMA-AIEOPAIDA protocol also used ATRA and idarubicin during induction without cytarabine and showed a 96% CR rate in children.[671] However, this question was subsequently studied in a randomized clinical trial in which patients younger than 60 years and with a presenting WBC count less than 10,000/μL were randomly assigned in induction to ATRA and daunorubicin, with or without cytarabine. CR rates were comparably high for the two groups—99% with cytarabine and 94% without—however, in the cytarabine arm, the relapse rate was significantly lower (4.7% vs. 15.9%; $P = .011$), the event-free

survival higher (93.3% vs. 77.2%; $P = .0021$), and the overall survival higher (97.9% vs 89.6%; $P = .0066$). Of note, the current trials all use high cumulative anthracycline doses to achieve excellent overall survival rates, but there is concern about long-term cardiac toxicity, particularly in pediatric patients.[704] Considering the improved results with the addition of cytarabine to the induction and consolidation regimens, several groups are interested in studying the use of more cytarabine with less anthracycline in pediatric patients with APL.

Maintenance Therapy

Another difference between APL and other subtypes of AML is that patients with APL clearly benefit from maintenance therapy. The APL93 trial randomized pediatric patients after consolidation to an arm with no further therapy or to arms with 2 years of intermittent ATRA, continuous chemotherapy with 6-mercaptopurine and methotrexate, or both ATRA and chemotherapy. Although 23% of pediatric patients in this trial relapsed, none of the patients who received both chemotherapy and ATRA during maintenance therapy relapsed.[669] In this trial, all relapsed patients achieved a second CR. The 5-year event-free survival was 71% and overall survival was 90%. The PETHEMA group also used ATRA plus 6-mercaptopurine and methotrexate during 2 years of maintenance therapy for pediatric patients and demonstrated a disease-free survival of 82% and overall survival of 87%.[670] Since these earlier studies, all current and planned trials for APL include a maintenance phase of therapy, although the ideal schedule of drugs and length of treatment during the maintenance phase remains unclear.

Targeted Therapy

With the use of ATRA and ATO, targeted therapy for APL is already a reality. Other targeted agents are also being used successfully in APL. Gemtuzumab ozogamicin (GMTZ; see earlier) is a recombinant, humanized, anti-CD33 monoclonal antibody linked to the tumor antibiotic calicheamicin. APL cells express very high levels of CD33, making them an attractive target for GMTZ.[705] GMTZ has been used successfully as a single agent to induce remission in patients with multiply relapsed APL.[706,707] In a small series of 12 patients, GMTZ was used safely in combination with ATRA with or without idarubicin, depending on the extent of MRD, as induction therapy for patients with de novo APL with a CR rate of 84%.[708] Some groups are now studying the use of GMTZ as induction therapy in larger numbers of patients.

As discussed earlier, mutations in *FLT3* have been identified in up to 43% of patients with APL, making the use of FLT3 inhibitors an attractive option. Most FLT3 inhibitors are oral agents with little toxicity. In one mouse model of APL with the *FLT3* mutation, treatment with doxorubicin alone had no impact on survival, but treatment with the FLT3 inhibitor SU11657, with or without doxorubicin, resulted in prolonged survival.[709] In another mouse model, treatment with ATRA and SU11657 resulted in the rapid regression of APL.[710] There is considerable interest in using FLT3 inhibitors in combination with ATRA and other targeted agents to improve therapy for patients with APL.

Hematopoietic Stem Cell Transplantation

Because the combination of chemotherapy and ATRA results in such high cure rates for APL, HSCT is not recommended for patients in first CR, even with a matched sibling donor. There is evidence for prolonged remission without HSCT, even after relapse for patients treated with agents such as ATRA, ATO, and GMTZ, especially when combined with chemotherapy.[189,683,685-687,706,707,711] Both autologous and allogeneic HSCT have been used successfully in patients with relapsed APL. For autologous HSCT to be successful, peripheral blood stem cells or bone marrow cells must be harvested once the patient has achieved negative MRD by PCR assay.[712,713] The GVL effect appears to play a role in the allogeneic HSCT treatment of APL, as evidenced by the fact that relapse rates are significantly lower after allogeneic HSCT compared with autologous HSCT and that patients who suffer a molecular relapse after allogeneic HSCT may achieve remission after the withdrawal of immunosuppression.[713-715] However, despite the lower relapse rate, because of significantly higher transplantation-related mortality (TRM) after allogeneic HSCT, overall survival in adults is higher after autologous HSCT than after allogeneic HSCT (postallogeneic HSCT: RFS 92.3%; EFS 52.2%; OS 51.8%; TRM 39%; postautologous HSCT with negative preharvest PCR: RFS 87.3%; EFS 76.5%; OS 75.3%; TRM 6%).[713] In pediatric patients, allogeneic HSCT is much better tolerated, and a recent retrospective analysis has shown no difference in overall survival after allogeneic HSCT versus autologous HSCT, although the allogeneic HSCT group had a lower relapse rate and higher TRM (postallogeneic HSCT: RR 10%; EFS 71%; OS 76%; TRM 19%; postautologous HSCT: RR 27%; EFS 73%; OS 82%; TRM 0%).[714] Given these data, in adults, autologous HSCT is usually the preferred choice over allogeneic HSCT for patients in second CR, whereas in children, allogeneic HSCT is often the preferred choice, particularly if a fully matched sibling donor is available.

Central Nervous System Involvement

In patients with APL, CNS disease at the time of diagnosis is rare and, because of coagulopathy, diagnostic lumbar puncture prior to the initiation of therapy is not safe for most patients. In the pre-ATRA era, CNS relapse was rarely observed in APL patients. However, as the survival rate for APL improved dramatically with the introduction of ATRA, an increasing number of CNS relapses were reported. Unlike other subtypes of AML, most APL regimens did not include CNS prophylaxis. CNS relapse is more common in patients with a presenting WBC count higher than 10,000/μL, with microgranular variant morphology, and with bcr3 PML-RARA isoform, all of which are also associated with the presence of a FLT3 ITD and all of which are more common in pediatric patients.[146,648-653,656,669,705,716,717] Although there was initially concern that ATRA itself was contributing to CNS relapses, it now seems that ATRA does not penetrate the CNS well and, with more patients surviving APL therapy, this likely contributes to the higher rate of CNS relapse currently observed.[716-719] Several groups have now initiated a screening lumbar puncture at the time of CR and use prophylactic intrathecal chemotherapy, usually with cytarabine and methotrexate, for patients at high risk for CNS relapse.[717,720] As discussed earlier, more groups are also considering the addition of high-dose cytarabine to APL regimens, and this will also provide better CNS coverage.

Minimal Residual Disease Monitoring

Detection of the *PML-RARA* fusion gene by reverse transcription PCR (RT-PCR) has become a valuable tool for measuring MRD in APL. RT-PCR positivity at the end of induction does not seem to portend a higher risk of relapse, but RT-PCR positivity after consolidation does carry a significantly higher risk for relapse, and RT-PCR positivity during maintenance or after therapy is indicative of impending relapse in almost all patients.[671,721,722] MRD analysis is being used to identify high-risk groups that require more intensive therapy for cure.[671] When detected early by RT-PCR, molecular relapse may also be easier to treat than frank morphologic relapse because of the lower disease burden and the treatment of a healthier asymptomatic patient.[723] In many studies, RT-PCR analysis is carried out on bone marrow cells and evidence regarding analysis of peripheral blood is not as clear.[724] There is also controversy over the threshold for a "positive" result; some groups do not consider a result a true positive unless there are two positive results separated by 2 to 4 weeks.

DOWN SYNDROME WITH TRANSIENT MYELOPROLIFERATIVE DISORDER AND ACUTE MYELOGENOUS LEUKEMIA

Down Syndrome with Transient Myeloproliferative Disorder

Pathobiology

Down syndrome, characterized by trisomy 21, is the most common congenital chromosomal abnormality, occurring in an estimated 1 in 600 to 1000 live births.[725,726] Up to 10% of infants with Down syndrome are born with a TMD. TMD is characterized by the presence of immature megakaryoblasts in the liver, bone marrow, and peripheral blood. The disorder usually spontaneously regresses within 3 months.[69,727-729] By morphology, TMD blasts are identical to AMKL blasts and, even though in most cases they regress, up to 30% of Down syndrome infants with TMD subsequently develop AMKL within 3 years.[730,731] Studies have shown that TMD blasts are clonal and that the same clone subsequently evolves into AMKL in a subset of patients.[732-735]

In 2002, Wechsler and colleagues[237] first reported mutations in exon 2 of *GATA-1* in Down syndrome associated AMKL. Soon thereafter, several groups reported that *GATA-1* mutations were detectable in almost all patients with Down syndrome–associated TMD.[736-741] Interestingly, *GATA-1* mutations have also been detected in approximately 10% of Down syndrome patients who have never been diagnosed with a hematologic abnormality.[742] It is not clear whether these patients have a history of subclinical TMD that regressed without detection or if the mutation simply did not result in the TMD phenotype in these cases. Normal GATA-1 plays a vital role in the maturation of erythroid cells and megakaryocytes.[743] The *GATA-1* mutations in Down syndrome TMD and AMKL result in GATA-1s, a truncated protein lacking the N-terminal activation domain.[739,744,745] GATA-1s appears to be a normal isoform of GATA-1 and has been detected in human hematopoietic cell lines and mouse fetal liver. However, because *GATA-1* is an X-linked gene, only the truncated GATA-1s is expressed in Down syndrome TMD and AMKL blasts. It has been hypothesized that the presence of a trisomy 21 in conjunction with a GATA-1s allows abnormal proliferation of megakaryoblasts, but only in the fetal hematopoietic system (i.e., the fetal liver); thus, TMD resolves with the loss of fetal hematopoiesis.[727,746] Although the combination of trisomy 21 and a *GATA-1* mutation appears sufficient to result in TMD, this is not sufficient to result in frank leukemia, and only if additional mutations are accumulated over time will the disease progress to frank AMKL.

Wilms' tumor gene (*WT1*) levels detected by PCR assay are elevated in patients with TMD. Levels normalized in four of five patients studied who had regression of TMD, with no further sequelae, but did not normalize in the fifth, who went on to develop AMKL at 11 months of age, making this an attractive marker for MRD and prognosis.[747] Both gain- and loss-of-function mutations in Janus kinase 3 (*JAK3*) have been identified in a subset of patients with TMD, although the prognostic relevance of this is not yet known.[748,749]

Clinical Presentation

Because Down syndrome infants with TMD are often asymptomatic, the incidence of 10% may be an underestimate, because many patients may have TMD that spontaneously regresses, without ever being detected.[735,750-753] For this reason, many physicians obtain a routine screening complete blood cell (CBC) count at birth for all infants with known or suspected Down syndrome. However, some infants with Down syndrome have a dramatic presentation of TMD at or shortly after birth, with hydrops fetalis, pleural and pericardial effusions, ascites, and massive hepatosplenomegaly, and these patients may rapidly progress to liver fibrosis or multisystem organ failure, both of which are most often fatal.[729,754-757] In the Pediatric Oncology Group (POG) trial 9481, 48 children with TMD were followed prospectively; 19% developed life-threatening disease with hepatic fibrosis or cardiopulmonary failure, with an overall mortality at 3 months of age of 10.4%.[729] Another recent retrospective analysis from Japan has shown that 22.9% of patients with TMD die before the age of 6 months, and the main causes of death were hepatic or cardiopulmonary failure.[758] In this study, early gestational age, WBC count ≥ 100,000/μL, high percentage of peripheral blasts, elevated aspartate transaminase (AST), elevated direct bilirubin, and low Apgar score were significantly associated with poor survival. They noted that only 7.7% of term Down syndrome infants with WBC less than 100,000/μL died, whereas 54.5% of preterm infants with WBC higher than 100,000/μL died, suggesting that risk stratification may be possible to determine high-risk subgroups of patients who require earlier and more aggressive therapy.

Treatment

Because most patients with TMD will exhibit spontaneous regression, treatment often consists of supportive care only. Many groups, including COG protocol 2971, which closed in 2004, have recommended supportive care only for TMD patients unless they exhibit signs or symptoms of life-threatening disease, including hyperviscosity, with a total blast count higher than 100,000/μL, organomegaly causing respiratory compromise, congestive heart failure not caused by a congenital heart defect, hydrops fetalis, symptomatic hepatic or renal dysfunction, or DIC.[729,759] For patients who require therapy, the choices include leukapheresis, exchange transfusion, or low dose cytarabine.[754] Low-dose cytarabine has been effective when used early in critically ill patients.[760] In patients with hyperleukocytosis or who require therapy with cytarabine, treatment to prevent the consequences of rapid tumor lysis (see earlier) should be promptly initiated.

Down Syndrome with Acute Myelogenous Leukemia

Pathobiology

Children with Down syndrome have a markedly increased risk of leukemia during the first 10 years of life. Acute leukemia is 10 to 20 times more common in children with Down syndrome than in children in the general population, and leukemia in Down syndrome patients younger than 4 years is most commonly AML (specifically AMKL), whereas leukemia in older children with Down syndrome is most commonly ALL.[361,730,761-769] The ratio of ALL to AML is approximately 1:1 in children with Down syndrome but in the first 4 years of life, AML is 100 times more common than ALL.[70] Although AMKL is a rare subtype of AML in the general population, it is the predominant form of AML in children with Down syndrome, making Down syndrome patients 500 times more likely than other children to develop AMKL. Unlike other children with AML, AMKL in children with Down syndrome often manifests after a period of myelodysplasia, usually characterized by months of thrombocytopenia and later by anemia.[70,770,771] Most cases of AMKL in Down syndrome patients are preceded by TMD.[742] Several studies have confirmed that when there is a proven antecedent TMD, it is the same TMD clone that subsequently evolves into AMKL.[736,738,772,773]

Also characteristic of AMKL in Down syndrome are *GATA-1* mutations (see earlier). Because *GATA-1* encodes a transcription factor essential for megakaryocyte development, samples from patients with AMKL were studied for evidence of *GATA-1* mutations.[237] Mutations in exon 2 of GATA-1 were detected in AMKL blasts from Down syndrome patients, but not in other subtypes of AML in Down syndrome patients or in AMKL blasts from non–Down syndrome patients. Several subsequent studies have confirmed *GATA-1* mutations leading to a premature stop codon in almost all cases of Down syndrome–associated AMKL.[736-741] *GATA-1* mutations have been identified in the blood spots of three of four Down syndrome patients with AMKL who had not been previously diagnosed with TMD, suggesting that in most, if not all cases of AMKL, the mutation has been present since birth.[738,742,772,773] Down syndrome patients who develop AML after the age of 4 do not usually have *GATA-1*–mutated AMKL, but have AML more typical of the general pediatric population. This disease is not as sensitive to chemotherapy and does not carry the exceptionally good prognosis carried by Down syndrome AMKL (see later).[774-776]

Additional mutations beyond the *GATA-1* mutation in the presence of trisomy 21 are necessary to produce AMKL. The good-risk translocations common in other forms of pediatric AML, including t(8;21), t(15;17), inv(16), and t(9;11), are almost never seen in Down syndrome AMKL, although they are more commonly reported in Down syndrome patients who develop AML after the age of 4.[764,766,776-778] Other than trisomy 21, trisomy 8 is the most common cytogenetic abnormality in Down syndrome AMKL. Other translocations commonly reported in AMKL in the absence of Down syndrome, including t(1;22) and t(1;3), are only rarely documented in Down syndrome AMKL.[779] Monosomy 7 may be seen but does not seem to carry the same poor prognosis as in non–Down syndrome patients.[780] Approximately 25% of patients have no cytogenetic abnormalities other than the constitutional trisomy 21, although some patients will exhibit tetrasomy 21. As in TMD, overexpression of *WT1* and mutations in *JAK3* have been reported in Down syndrome AMKL.[747-749]

Clinical Presentation

Children with Down syndrome who develop AML present at a younger age than average for childhood AML, with 60% to 70% of patients diagnosed when they are younger than 2 years.[70,764,766,774,777,778] Down syndrome patients generally present with lower total WBC counts (median, 7-10,000/μL) and lower platelet counts (median, 25-30,000/μL) than other children. Hepatosplenomegaly is more common in

Down syndrome patients with AML than in other children, whereas lymphadenopathy and CNS involvement are less common. Down syndrome AMKL is frequently preceded by TMD, which is almost absent in non–Down syndrome patients, or MDS, which is far less common in non–Down syndrome patients. Older Down syndrome patients with AML have presenting signs and symptoms that more closely mirror those of the general population, reflecting the virtual lack of AMKL with *GATA-1* mutations in patients older than 5 years.

Treatment

Many children with Down syndrome have been entered into large clinical trials since 1982, when legislation was passed that prohibits withholding medical intervention from children with disabilities.[70] In the early clinical trials that included patients with Down syndrome and AML, the outcome was poor because of excessive toxicity. The associated congenital abnormalities, increased susceptibility to infection, and altered drug metabolism in patients with Down syndrome made it challenging to find appropriate therapy for this group. However, as general medical care for children with Down syndrome has improved, the outcome for children with AML and Down syndrome has also inproved. Multiple studies from around the world have consistently demonstrated that Down syndrome AML patients have a better overall prognosis than children with AML in the general population.[471,764,766,774,777,778,781] A remarkable feature of AML in children with Down syndrome is its extraordinary responsiveness to AML chemotherapy.[70,765] Down syndrome AMKL blasts are significantly more sensitive to chemotherapy agents than other AML blasts, including cytarabine (12-fold), anthracyclines (2- to 7-fold), mitoxantrone (9-fold), amsacrine (16-fold), etoposide (20-fold), 6-thioguanine (3-fold), busulfan (5-fold), and vincristine (23-fold).[782] The increased sensitivity of Down syndrome AML blasts to cytarabine may partly be the result of overexpression of the chromosome 21 gene encoding cystathionine β-synthase (CBS), resulting in altered metabolism of cytarabine and rendering the cells 10-fold more sensitive to the drug.[783-785] In addition, the cytidine deaminase (CDA) levels in Down syndrome AMKL blasts are low, leading also to increased sensitivity to cytarabine. The CDA promoter contains several binding sites for GATA-1, suggesting that *GATA-1* mutations may contribute to the sensitivity of these blasts.[785]

Multiple studies have illustrated that Down syndrome patients with AML fare better with less intensive therapy than that required for other patients with AML. Down syndrome patients exhibit excessive toxicity, particularly infectious complications, in intense AML protocols and, because their disease is so sensitive to chemotherapy, this level of intensity is not required for disease control. In the German collaborative AML-BFM93 protocol, children with Down syndrome fared worse than other patients because of an increased frequency of infectious complications, but none of the patients relapsed and EFS was approximately 70%.[776,786] Therefore, in the subsequent AML-BFM98 protocol, Down syndrome patients received a reduced intensity regimen and the EFS improved dramatically, to almost 90%. In a Japanese collaborative study, 33 children with Down syndrome and AML or MDS were treated with a reduced intensity regimen consisting of daunorubicin, cytarabine, and etoposide. Complete remission was achieved in all patients, and the estimated 8-year event-free survival rate was 80%.[787] In the Nordic Society for Paediatric Haematology and Oncology-Acute Myeloid Leukaemia (NOPHO-AML) trials, the earlier, more intensive NOPHO-AML88 trial showed a high death rate from infectious complications for Down syndrome patients with AML, with an

EFS of only 47%, compared with much better outcomes in the later, less intensive NOPHO-AML93 trial, with an EFS of 85% (76% for those who received full-dose therapy and 92% for those who received reduced-dose therapy).[788] The MRC trials showed similar results with Down syndrome patients receiving the same standard therapy as other patients, resulting in a higher rate of death from toxicity, but lower relapse rate when compared with other children.[789] Perhaps the most striking example comes from the CCG 2891 study. In this study, all children were randomly assigned to receive induction chemotherapy with intensive timing (i.e., proceeding with the second cycle, regardless of counts) versus standard timing (i.e., awaiting count recovery before initiating the second cycle). The Down syndrome patients in the intensive timing arm suffered a 32% mortality rate compared with an 11% mortality rate for the remainder of the patients, prompting early closure of that arm for Down syndrome patients.[766] Standard timing induction for Down syndrome patients resulted in an impressively high CR rate of 95% (2.4% with toxic death and 2.4% with resistant disease).[766] Postremission consolidation with allogeneic HSCT in this trial also resulted in an unacceptably high treatment-related mortality for Down syndrome patients, with only 33% survival at 4 years.[766] In this study, standard timing induction followed by consolidation with chemotherapy was clearly the superior treatment for Down syndrome patients, with a 4-year DFS of 88% compared with a DFS of only 42% for this regimen in the non–Down syndrome patients.[766]

Given these collective data, COG trial A2971 used a less intensive approach for Down syndrome patients, with four cycles of standard timing low-dose cytarabine, daunorubicin, and thioguanine, followed by a cycle of high-dose cytarabine with asparaginase (Capizzi II) and then intrathecal therapy.[790] This trial closed in 2004 and the results have not been published. Of note, on retrospective analysis of several trials, it has become clear that Down syndrome AML patients older than 4 years do not appear to have the same good prognosis that younger patients have, and their disease appears to behave more like AML in the general pediatric population. In the BFM-93 trial, 3 of 4 patients older than 4 years lacked the typical AMKL of Down syndrome and only 1 of the 3 survived.[776] In a combined analysis of European trials, 17 of 317 Down syndrome patients diagnosed with AML were older than 4 years.[775] DNA was available from blasts of 10 of these patients and, of these, 3 children younger than 7 years had the characteristic AMKL and 1 additional younger child had M0 AML with a *GATA-1* mutation. Of the 6 remaining patients without AMKL or a *GATA-1* mutation, all were 7 years of age or older, and 4 relapsed. In CCG trial 2891, Down syndrome patients with AML older than 2 years had lower CR rates and higher rates of resistant disease than those 2 years of age or younger, and the trend worsened when only those 4 years of age or older were considered.[774] Given these data, the current COG trial AAML0431 with reduced-intensity therapy includes only those Down syndrome patients younger than 4 years. Given the high rate of congenital cardiac anomalies in Down syndrome patients, there is also considerable interest in reducing their anthracycline exposure. In the POG study 9421, 42% of the enrolled Down syndrome patients had congenital heart defects, and 17.5% of Down syndrome patients developed symptomatic cardiomyopathy.[791] Interestingly, only half of patients who developed cardiomyopathy had a previously diagnosed congenital heart defect, making it difficult to predict which patients were more susceptible. Accordingly, COG trial AAML0431 has decreased the cumulative anthracycline for Down syndrome patients (daunorubicin, 240 instead of 375 mg/m^2) in an attempt to minimize cardiac toxicity.

MYELODYSPLASTIC SYNDROMES

The myelodysplastic syndromes are a heterogeneous group of clonal hematologic disorders characterized by ineffective hematopoiesis, progressive cytopenias, dysplastic transformation of hematopoietic cells, and a propensity for transformation into AML.[792] MDS is most common in patients older than 60 years, but at the same time is an unusual but clinically important disease of childhood.

Diagnosis and Classification

Morphology

The morphologic features of MDS include bone marrow dysplastic changes involving all three cell lineages (i.e., trilineage dysplasia). A common theme underlying these features is asynchrony between the usual cytoplasmic and nuclear differentiation programs, so that nuclei appear abnormal and less mature than the features of the surrounding cytoplasm. Typical erythrocytic abnormalities include megaloblastoid changes, perinuclear ringlike deposits of iron (i.e., ringed sideroblasts), multinucleation, nuclear budding and fragmentation, and an increased percentage of immature forms. Dysmegakaryopoiesis is characterized by micromegakaryocytes, abnormal nuclei, and abnormal nuclear lobulation. The dysplastic features of the granulocytic cells comprise immature forms, hypogranulation, and the Pelger-Huet–type abnormality. Monocytic dysplasia includes increased numbers of bone marrow monocytes, abnormal granulation with increased azurophilic granules, hemophagocytosis, abnormal nuclei, and giant forms. Bone marrow cellularity is usually normal or increased, and the reticulin concentration is increased in most cases.

Patients with MDS may present initially with a single peripheral blood cytopenia, which usually progresses to pancytopenia with anemia, leukopenia, and thrombocytopenia. The anemia in MDS is caused by ineffective erythropoiesis with low reticulocyte counts and macrocytosis, teardrop cell formation, and moderate poikilocytosis. In addition, megaloblastoid circulating nucleated red blood cells are frequently detected. Peripheral blood dysgranulopoiesis manifests as circulating myeloblasts, progranulocytes, and Pelger-Huet cells. Thus, early signs may be a falling hematocrit with increasing mean corpuscular volume (MCV) or unexplained thrombocytopenia. The peripheral blood may also exhibit increased numbers of monocytes and monoblasts.

Cytogenetics

Cytogenetic abnormalities are common in children with MDS and were reported in 59% of 227 children tested in one study.[793] Chromosomal deletions are the hallmark of MDS and frequently involve the long arms of chromosomes 5, 7, and 20 (see Fig. 11-7) Other common cytogenetic abnormalities include trisomy 8, del(17p), +21, inv(1), and t(7;16).[227,794,795] These chromosomal abnormalities are accompanied by other complex karyotypic changes in many cases. Other abnormalities that have been reported in pediatric cases of MDS include +6, +9, and +11, whereas deletions of chromosomes 11, 12, and 13 and Y are rare.[796] Common balanced chromosomal translocations found in AML, such as t(8;21), t(15;17), and inv(16), are not usually detected in MDS.[797]

Classification

In 1982, the FAB cooperative group defined five categories for the adult myelodysplastic and myeloproliferative syndromes—refractory anemia (RA), RA with ringed sideroblasts (RARS), RA with excess blasts (RAEB), RA with excess blasts in transformation (RAEB-T), and chronic myelomonocytic leukemia (CMML).[282,283,798,799] Classification of childhood MDS into defined FAB subcategories is not always straightforward. Many children show overlapping features of MPD and MDS, particularly patients with JMML and infant monosomy 7 syndrome.[228] The classification of pediatric MDS is also complicated by the fact that some children develop MDS in the context of inherited predispositions such as neurofibromatosis type 1, severe congenital neutropenia, and Down syndrome.[228] Using the FAB system of classification, the most common subtypes of MDS in children are RAEB and RAEB-T, whereas RA and RARS are uncommon and CMML is rare.

The WHO proposed a revised classification of MDS in 1997. The WHO system includes the following changes to the FAB criteria: elimination of the RAEB-T subtype through a reduction in the marrow blast count to 20% for the diagnosis of AML and the division of the RAEB subtype into RAEB-I, consisting of 5% to 10% marrow blasts, and RAEB-II, comprising 11% to 20% blasts.[267,286,800] Other WHO recommendations include two new categories for patients with refractory cytopenias with multilineage dysplasia and a new category for unclassified MDS. In the new system, CMML is removed completely and reclassified as a myeloproliferative disorder.

A third classification system is used in parallel with the FAB and WHO systems, the IPSS Scoring System.[801] This system assigns a numeric value to each of the number of cytopenias, cytogenetic abnormalities, and percentage of bone marrow blasts, and a higher score is associated with a poor prognosis. The value of the IPSS for pediatric MDS patients remains to be proven.[802]

Pathophysiology

Evidence for clonality in MDS comes primarily from nonrandom X-inactivation studies (see earlier) performed on the bone marrow cells of female patients with MDS. These studies have demonstrated clonal involvement of hematopoietic cells in this disorder.[803-805] The trilineage dysplasia that characterizes MDS strongly suggests that the cell of origin resides within the compartment containing early hematopoietic progenitors or stem cells with multilineage potential.[806] Early mutations in stem cells may cause a failure in myeloid cell maturation, as well as enhanced apoptosis, leading to dysplasia, whereas subsequent defects affecting myeloid cell proliferation and the development of antiapoptotic signals may cause the clonal expansion of aberrant cells and frank leukemia. An increased level of apoptosis has been documented in early MDS, which is followed by decreased blast cell apoptosis in patients whose disease transforms to AML. MDS cells have been found to overexpress certain cell surface death receptors and their ligands, which may be induced as a result of signals from inflammatory cells present in the hematopoietic microenvironment.[797] Patients with more advanced MDS (FAB RAEB) have decreased levels of death receptor expression compared with early-stage MDS and increased expression levels of antiapoptotic factors, such as BCL-2.[807,808]

The most common chromosomal abnormalities in childhood MDS involve large deletions, but little is known about the genes contained in the deleted segment[794,809-811] and whether these large genetic aberrations are inciting events leading to the development of MDS or represent secondary events. Recently, Ebert and colleagues[812] have used an RNA interference screen to identify a putative gene deleted from the distal end of the long arm of chromosome 5 in 5q– syndrome, a subtype of MDS commonly encountered in older women, but uncommon in pediatric patients. They found that haploinsufficiency of *RPS14*, a gene which codes for a component of the 40S ribosomal subunit results in the characteristic phenotype of selectively diminished erythropoiesis, with preservation of megakaryocyte maturation. Moreover, the introduction of a lentiviral vector expressing *RPS14* into CD34+ cells of MDS patients demonstrates restored erythroid differentiation exclusively in those with a 5q– genotype. These elegant studies convincingly identified a specific genetic lesion underlying the 5q– syndrome and also established this ribosomal protein as critical in erythroid development.[812] This finding is in keeping with the elucidated role of other ribosomal proteins in a number of bone marrow failure syndromes, such as Diamond-Blackfan anemia.[813]

5q– syndrome has a reasonably favorable outcome because of its natural history of slower progression to AML and sensitivity to treatment with lenalidomide, an analogue of thalidomide.[814,815] In this select population, lenalidomide (Revlimid) reduces the need for red cell transfusions and induces significant cytogenetic responses, which has resulted in its recent approval by the FDA for the treatment of MDS patients with 5q– syndrome.[816] Although this therapy has demonstrated impressive efficacy in this condition, deletion of this distal region of 5q is relatively rare. Only a minority of MDS patients without this cytogenetic abnormality respond to lenalidomide and responders possess no distinguishing clinical or laboratory characteristics compared with nonresponders.[817] However, other studies[818] have suggested that responders have a unique genetic signature consisting of low expression levels of genes typically involved in terminal erythroid differentiation. These results have implicated that restoration of normal red cell development underlies lenalidomide's mechanism of action, which would account for the successful response in 5q– syndrome. Clinically, this suggests that genetic profiling could be used to select a group of MDS patients without 5q– deletions who would be more likely to respond to this agent.

These large deletions also likely contain certain important tumor suppressor genes, whose elimination contributes to MDS pathogenesis. For example, we have recently completed a detailed analysis of the more proximally deleted region of the long arm of chromosome 5 and identified alpha-catenin as a novel tumor suppressor gene in MDS.[226] In both primary patient samples and AML cell lines with a deletion of 5q-, alpha-catenin expression levels were found to be specifically and substantially decreased through the combination of a deletion on one chromosome and epigenetic silencing by hypermethylation and histone deacetylation of the promoter of the second allele. Another group has identified the WT-1 transcription factor, early growth response 1 (*EGR1*), as a putative candidate gene in this same region and demonstrated that haploinsufficiency of this tumor suppressor gene can result in MDS or MPD following treatment with an alkylating agent.[819]

In addition to gene deletions, a number of other genes have been found to contribute to MDS pathogenesis. Balanced translocations, such as those seen in de novo AML, are uncommon in MDS, but some of the same genes may be involved. Other genetic lesions appear to be specific for MDS. We and others have shown that certain HOX genes, most notably *HOXA9*, are overexpressed in the hematopoietic stem cells of patients with MDS.[820-822] Translocations involving HOX genes and the nucleoporin gene (*NUP98*) on chromosome 11 including *NUP98-HOXA9*[823] and *NUP98-HOXA13*[824] have been found in rare patients with MDS. Certain genetic abnormalities are more characteristic following prior treatment with chemotherapy. Overexpression of the *EVI1* transcription factor on chromosome 3, either through gene rearrangements or rare translocations, has been associated with MDS following

chemotherapy.[825-827] Similarly, nucleophosmin and myeloid leukemia factor 1 (*NPM-MLF1*) fusion gene, formed as a result of a t(3;5) chromosomal translocation, occurs in rare cases of MDS or AML arising from MDS.[828,829] Mutations in *RAS* and *FLT3*, such as those seen in de novo AML, are found in patients with MDS, particularly those with 7q– and often after treatment with alkylating agents.[830] These patients may also have mutations in the *AML1* gene, whereas the *AML1-ETO* translocation is rare in MDS.[831,832] Prior treatment with alkylators can also lead to MDS with 5q– and these patients often have a mutation in *p53*, a gene that is also frequently mutated in AML cases with a complex aberrant karyotype, which include a 5q deletion, but rarely in classic de novo AML.[831-833]

Inherited and Environmental Predisposing Factors

Several environmental exposures and inherited conditions are associated with an increased risk of MDS and AML. As noted, alkylating agents and topoisomerase II inhibitors can predispose to MDS and AML, which can occur as treatment-related second malignancies in patients treated for ALL and many other types of cancer. Secondary disease associated with alkylating agent chemotherapy tends to occur from 3 to 11 years following treatment, after which the incidence appears to plateau.[834-836] The disease often presents as MDS and an underlying predisposition may involve defective DNA repair mechanisms. Commonly, there are deletions of chromosomes 5 or 7.[835] *MLL* gene rearrangements are often found in AML cases that arise following treatment with topoisomerase II inhibitors such as etoposide, but these patients tend to present with frank AML after a short latency of 1 to 3 years from therapy and without an MDS prodrome.[835,837]

A number of genetic conditions are associated with an increased risk of MDS and subsequent AML, particularly the bone marrow failure syndromes and chromosomal breakage disorders. Some disorders, such as Fanconi's anemia, in which patients demonstrate both pancytopenia and increased sensitivity to DNA damage, suggest that impaired DNA repair may be a mechanism for malignant transformation. However, other marrow failure syndromes are not characterized by increased susceptibility to chromosomal breakage and present predominantly with a single cytopenia, such as neutropenia in Shwachman-Diamond syndrome, anemia in Diamond-Blackfan anemia, and low platelets in amegakaryocytic thrombocytopenia. The evolution of MDS in these conditions is variable (30% in Shwachman-Diamond compared with 5% in Diamond-Blackfan anemia) and the mechanism remains elusive, although defective ribosomal processing may be involved, given the identified functions of the target proteins involved in a number of these conditions.[797]

Clinical Presentation

Children with MDS generally present with the signs and symptoms associated with bone marrow failure. Abnormalities in the peripheral blood may also be detected on routine medical examinations in asymptomatic children. Symptomatic children often present with some degree of fatigue, fever, malaise, or infections. Physical examination frequently reveals pallor, easy bruising, and petechiae. Splenomegaly, hepatomegaly, and lymphadenopathy are uncommon findings. The peripheral blood counts usually reveal anemia, neutropenia, and thrombocytopenia.

Differential Diagnosis

With a careful history and physical examination, as well as the evaluation of peripheral blood and a bone marrow aspirate, biopsy, and cytogenetics, a diagnosis of MDS can be made. Severe nutritional deficiencies of vitamin B_{12} and folate should be excluded, because they may impart a megaloblastic appearance to the bone marrow. Other nutritional deficiencies such as thiamine, pyridoxine, iron, and riboflavin can also present with some degree of bone marrow dysplasia and should be considered in the differential diagnosis. Occasionally, severe aplastic anemia can be difficult to distinguish from MDS, although a bone marrow biopsy should resolve this question. Certain viral infections (e.g., human immunodeficiency virus, parvovirus B19, EBV, human herpes virus 6, cytomegalovirus) and exposures (e.g., irradiation, chemotherapy, organic solvents) are associated with bone marrow failure and should be considered before making the diagnosis of MDS. The bone marrow cell karyotype should be determined to identify any clonal abnormalities. In addition, evidence has suggested that whole genome scan by single nucleotide polymorphism (SNP) analysis may detect clonal abnormalities in some patients with a normal bone marrow cell karyotype.[838,839]

Treatment

The rarity and heterogeneity of MDS in children, the lack of consensus on nomenclature, and the need for a risk-based classification system specific for pediatric MDS have hindered the development of appropriate therapy for pediatric MDS. Most clinical trials studying MDS have enrolled adults, in whom the disease may be different, and there have been few meaningful trials enrolling children. Regardless of treatment, the overall clinical outcome of children with MDS is guarded.

The only proven curative treatment for MDS is allogeneic HSCT. Prior to HSCT, or if an appropriate donor was not available, treatment primarily consisted of supportive care with packed red blood cell or platelet transfusions, parenteral antibiotics, and hydration. Other noncytotoxic therapies, including hormone therapy (e.g., androgens, glucocorticoids), recombinant hematopoietic growth factors (e.g., G-CSF, granulocyte-macrophage colony-stimulating factor [GM-CSF], erythropoietin), and differentiating agents (e.g., 13-cis-retinoic acid, ATRA), have been used in adults and have shown minimal benefit.[840-850] Low-dose chemotherapy has been used in an attempt to promote differentiation of the malignant hematopoietic clone. Although studies using low-dose cytarabine have shown improvement in peripheral counts and decreased marrow blast percentages in some patients with MDS, the responses have not been sustained.[851] Other agents, such as melphalan, hydroxyurea, etoposide, topotecan, 6-mercaptopurine, and busulfan, have been used with only partial or temporary responses in small numbers of patients.

More recently, a number of new agents have emerged for the treatment of pediatric MDS following randomized clinical trials in adult patients. These therapies have evolved out of a growing interest in the field of epigenetics and the concept that the repression of key tumor suppressor genes in MDS may occur because of aberrant methylation and histone deacetylation, instead of or in concert with gene deletions and mutations.[226] Studies involving the p15INK4B tumor suppressor have demonstrated evidence of methylated CpG islands in the promoter region, preventing gene transcription and leading to gene repression.[852,853] Since these initial studies, a number of other genes have been found to have reduced expression because of DNA methylation, thus prompting clinical trials of demethylating agents in MDS.[854,855] Based on the impressive

response rates and delayed progression to AML compared with supportive care, two demethylating agents, 5-azacytidine and decitabine, have both been FDA-approved for the treatment of MDS in adults.[856,857] These agents have shown greatest efficacy in low-risk MDS. They are given in a low dosage schedule and patients may need to be treated for several months before a clinical response is achieved. Although these agents have improved the time to progression in adult MDS, they cannot cure the disease. The role of these therapies in pediatric MDS is currently under active investigation. As indicated earlier, lenalidomide is now approved for the treatment of patients with MDS with the 5q– cytogenetic abnormality, and appears to work best in those whose MDS clone lacks any other cytogenetic abnormalites.[814]

For children with MDS, allogeneic HSCT remains the treatment of choice. In the absence of a sibling donor, a matched unrelated donor should be sought. Children with lower risk MDS are frequently treated with allogeneic HSCT without prior chemotherapy, particularly if a matched sibling is available, to avoid the need for large numbers of transfusions. In more advanced MDS (WHO RAEB1 and 2), AML-type chemotherapy is administered to induce a remission or to reduce the disease burden prior to HSCT. At the Fred Hutchinson Cancer Research Center in Seattle, 251 children and adults with MDS received HLA-matched HSCTs between 1981 and 1996.[858,859] The preparative regimens and donor sources varied in this study. Most patients received HLA-matched or partially matched, related donor HSCTs, and a minority had HLA-matched, unrelated donor HSCTs. The preparative ablative regimen varied, with most patients receiving total-body irradiation and chemotherapy and others receiving a busulfan-based regimen. Higher survival rates for patients correlated with decreased marrow blasts, intermediate or favorable cytogenetics, younger age, shorter disease duration, and a matched sibling donor for the HSCT. Patients younger than 20 years had an overall DFS rate of about 60%. A more recent study from the same institution, specifically looking at children with MDS, demonstrated a 3-year survival rate of patients with lower stage MDS of 74% compared with 68% for patients with more advanced disease.[860] The European Working Group on MDS in Children (EWOG-MDS) has reported a 55% 5-year EFS rate for 33 pediatric patients with MDS after HSCT.[861]

MYELOPROLIFERATIVE DISORDERS

Juvenile Myelomonocytic Leukemia

JMML is a rare, clonal, myeloproliferative disorder of the stem cell that usually manifests in the first few years of life. It has also been referred to as juvenile chronic myelomonocytic leukemia (JCML), infantile monosomy 7 syndrome, or juvenile granulocytic leukemia. Although JMML, adult CML, and CMML have some similar features, JMML is a clinically and pathophysiologically distinct disorder of young children. An international consensus panel consisting of the JMML Working Group and the EWOG-MDS has established a set of clinical and laboratory criteria for the diagnosis of JMML (Box 11-3).[862]

Pathobiology

The cause of JMML is unknown. Several recurrent chromosomal abnormalities have been associated with JMML, but their relevance to the pathogenesis of the disease is not well understood. For example, up to 20% of patients meeting the diagnostic criteria for JMML have abnormalities in chromosome 7 (e.g., monosomy 7, 7q–), and the genes involved and their contributions to disease pathogenesis remain an area of intense investigation.[481,862] At the molecular level, one or more defects involving the NF1/RAS signal pathway have been demonstrated in studies of JMML cells, implicating this pathway in the development of the disease. Activating point mutations in *N*- and *K-RAS* genes have been demonstrated in 15% to 30% of patients with JMML.[863,864] Other patients have loss of the neurofibromatosis type 1 gene *(NF1)*, which codes for a RAS GTPase-activating protein involved in the GM-CSF signaling pathway.[66,865] More recently, mutations in *PTPN11* encoding the SHP-2 phosphatase have been found in patients with JMML.[866,867] These mutations are all mutually exclusive. JMML cells grown in culture demonstrate a specific hypersensitivity to the growth factor GM-CSF that is not observed with other growth factors, such as interleukin-3 (IL)3.[868] Knock-out mice lacking expression of *NF1* die at embryonic day 13 or 14, but hematopoietic progenitor cells from these embryos grown in culture also demonstrate a specific hypersensitivity treatment with GM-CSF.[126] Moreover, immunodeficient mice transplanted with these cells develop a myeloproliferative disorder similar to JMML.[128,869]

An increasing body of evidence has suggested that JMML arises from a pluripotent hematopoietic stem cell, but the molecular abnormalities underlying the transformation appear to be distinct from those in the adult-type myeloproliferative disorders.[869] JMML cells maintain their clonality when grown in long-term culture-initiating assays, in contrast to Philadelphia chromosome–positive CML cells, which yield to polyclonal residual normal cells in similar culture assays. Marrow cells from patients with JMML grow in culture and generate granulocyte-macrophage colony-forming units (GM-CFUs) spontaneously, in the absence of added hematopoietic growth factors. In contrast, GM-CFUs from normal individuals and from patients with adult CML only grow when exogenous growth factors are added to the semisolid culture medium.

Clinical Presentation

The presenting signs and symptoms of JMML result from organ infiltration of malignant cells; the most common symptoms are fever, cough, infection, pallor, malaise, hepatosplenomegaly, lymphadenopathy, rash, bleeding, and failure to thrive.[862] Laboratory abnormalities usually include an elevated WBC count with monocytosis, anemia, thrombocytopenia, an elevated fetal hemoglobin level, and hypergammaglobulinemia.[862]

JMML is a progressive and often rapidly fatal disease, particularly in older children. Children younger than 2 years may have a more indolent course, whereas as older patients (older than 2 years) tend to present with lower presenting platelet counts and more complex cytogenetic abnormalities and are predisposed to a rapidly fatal outcome.[870] The accelerated blast phase characteristic of adult CMML is unusual in children with JMML.

Treatment

Several treatment regimens have been used to improve survival, including low-dose chemotherapy, intensive AML-type therapy, and 13-*cis*-retinoic acid.[481,57,871-876] Although durable remissions have been reported in a minority of cases, the response to these agents is usually transient and the long-term survival is poor. The only known curative therapy for JMML is allogeneic HSCT. When an HLA-matched related donor is available, HSCT is the recommended treatment for patients with newly diagnosed disease. Survival rates of 35% to 55% have been reported with HSCT, but treatment-related mortality and relapse rates remain high, particularly for patients who undergo unrelated donor HSCT.[877-880] Several issues remain controversial, including the management of patients without HLA-matched related donors, GVHD prophylaxis, pre-HSCT chemotherapy, and appropriate myeloablative therapy.

Chronic Myelogenous Leukemia Caused by the BCR-ABL Fusion Gene

In 1951, Dameshek first introduced the idea that CML, polycythemia vera (PV), essential thrombocythemia (ET), and agnogenic myeloid metaplasia (AMM) were related myeloproliferative syndromes, even though each has distinct clinical, laboratory, and biologic features.[881,882] A common feature is multilineage clonal proliferation involving the entire spectrum of myeloid cells, suggesting that transformation has occurred in a pluripotent stem cell. More recently, all these conditions, as well as systemic mastocytosis, hypereosinophilic syndrome, chronic eosinophilic leukemia, and chronic myelomonocytic leukemia, have been linked to a specific mutation or translocation resulting in the constitutive activation of a receptor tyrosine kinase. This accounts for the increased hematopoietic stem and progenitor cell proliferation with differentiation that characterizes these disorders. Patients may occasionally present with mixed manifestations rather than a distinct myeloproliferative disorder or, over the course of their illness, develop problems more typical of one of the other disorders.

Chronic myelogenous leukemia was first recognized as early as 1845, with several described cases of splenomegaly, anemia, and massive granulocytosis.[883,884] However, it was not until 1960, with the discovery of the Philadelphia chromosome (Ph), that the disease became better understood.[885] CML constitutes 15% to 20% of all leukemias, but accounts for only 1% to 3% of all childhood leukemias. In children, the disorder may present as one of two distinct clinical syndromes, adult-type

TABLE 11-2 **Clinical Characteristics of Children with Juvenile Myelomonocytic Leukemia (JMML) Versus Adult-type Chronic Myelogenous Leukemia (ACML)**

Characteristics at Diagnosis	JMML	ACML
Age (yr)	Usually <4	Usually >4
Lymphadenopathy	Common	Unusual
Skin lesions	Common	Unusual
Bleeding	Common	Unusual
Bacterial infection	Common	Unusual
White blood cell count >100,000/μL	Unusual	Common
Hemoglobin < 12 g/dL	Common	Variable
Platelets	Usually decreased	Usually increased
Monocytosis	Common	Unusual
Circulating pronormoblasts	Common	Unusual
Increased HgbF	Common	Unusual
Philadelphia chromosome	Absent	>90%
BCR-ABL fusion gene	Absent	Present
Leukocyte alkaline phosphatase decreased	Variable	Common
CLINICAL COURSE		
Median survival (yr)	1-2	4-5
Blast phase	Unusual	Common

CML (ACML), which is the same as the disease in older patients (and herein referred to as CML) and juvenile CML (JCML), now known as JMML, a syndrome described in the previous section that is restricted to children and has distinct clinical, laboratory, and cytogenetic characteristics (Table 11-2). The incidence of CML is less than 1 case/100,000 for patients younger than 20 years and 1 to 2 cases/100,000 for those 20 to 50 years, and it rises slowly thereafter. The median age at diagnosis is 67 years and the male-to-female ratio is 1.8:1. It has been difficult to identify environmental factors associated with the pathogenesis of CML. Ionizing radiation is the only clearly identified risk factor for CML. A sevenfold increase has been documented in the survivors of the nuclear bomb–related exposure to radiation in Japan and, notably, the incidence of CML in this population was highest in young people, especially children younger than 5 years.[886,887]

Pathobiology

The diagnosis of CML is almost always associated with a t(9;22)(q34;q11) chromosomal translocation in bone marrow cells. Currently available tests to diagnose this abnormality include cytogenetic testing, FISH, PCR assay, and Northern or Southern blot analysis of the bone marrow cells. This reciprocal translocation is detected by standard cytogenetic techniques in almost 90% of CML cases.[885,888] However, the presence of Ph in bone marrow cells is not pathognomonic for CML, because Ph is present at diagnosis in 25% to 50% of adult patients, 3% to 5% of children with ALL,[889] and 2% of patients with AML. It is absent in 5% of patients with CML, although these patients' bone marrow cells may harbor a variant of the translocation detectable only by RT-PCR or FISH.[890]

The Philadelphia chromosome of CML involves a reciprocal translocation of the *ABL* gene from its normal position at the end of the q arm of chromosome 9 to a site on the q arm of chromosome 22 within the *bcr* region. The reciprocal t(9;22)

chromosomal translocation creates a fusion *BCR-ABL* gene. The chimeric gene encodes a dysregulated tyrosine kinase that is constitutively active, is expressed in the cytoplasm, and has increased activity compared with the normal ABL protein.[891] In contrast to cytoplasmic BCR-ABL proteins, normal ABL is a nuclear kinase, whose activity is tightly regulated *in vivo*.[892] Although the precise function of normal ABL is not known, available evidence has suggested that it regulates pathways that mediate cell cycle arrest after genotoxic damage.[893-897] The main clinical manifestation of CML is an overabundance of mature myeloid cells from hyperproliferative progenitor cells. Evidence for the role of the *BCR-ABL* translocation in the pathogenesis of CML is confirmed by the observation that BCR-ABL proteins can also induce a CML-like syndrome *in vivo* in mice when they are expressed in hematopoietic progenitors.[898-901] Mechanistic studies of these fusion proteins have shown that RAS signaling is essential for transformation and that multiple accessory molecules, including the adapters GRB2, SHC, and CRKL, are used to couple the activated ABL kinase to RAS, resulting in activation of Jun kinase.[902-904] Oncogenic signaling by BCR-ABL has also been shown to involve the cell cycle–regulated genes *MYC* and cyclin D1.[905,906] Thus, multiple signaling pathways are activated to mediate leukemic transformation by BCR-ABL. Transformation has also been shown to occur in the pluripotent stem cell. Murine experiments in which sorted HSCs were transduced with *BCR-ABL* and transplanted into irradiated recipients developed a CML-like phenotype, whereas the same experiment performed using more differentiated progenitor cells failed to induce a myeloproliferative disease.[103] Moreover, granulocytes, monocytes, erythroid cells, megakaryocytes, and lymphocytes from patients with this disease have been shown to be clonal progeny of a single cell and to harbor the Ph.[907-909] Probably because of some persistent normal hematopoiesis in patients with CML and because of the long life span of some cell types, such as T lymphocytes, all patients do not have demonstrable involvement of all lineages.[908] It is worth emphasizing that the *BCR-ABL* fusion gene is acquired somatically by a hematopoietic stem cell and its expression is restricted to its clonal progeny, so the nonhematopoietic cells of the patient do not contain the translocation.[910,911]

Clinical Presentation

CML can present in one of three phases—chronic phase, accelerated phase, or blast crisis. Most patients present in the chronic phase and may be asymptomatic. When symptoms and signs are present, they are often mild and are caused by the accumulation of mature and immature granulocytic cells. Generalized malaise, weakness, weight loss, fever, pallor, and organomegaly, particularly splenomegaly, are frequent presenting symptoms. Abdominal pain from massive splenomegaly may also bring a patient to medical attention. CNS, retinal, and pulmonary dysfunction can occur, as well as arthritis and priapism. Occasionally, the diagnosis is made from a routine blood cell count.[912] WBC counts usually exceed 100,000/μL, with the appearance of some circulating immature myeloid forms.[913,914] Basophilia and eosinophilia may also occur. In addition, platelet counts above 400,000/μL are frequently observed, although thrombocytopenia may also occur. The WBC and platelet counts in CML patients may fluctuate spontaneously and nonconcordantly, making it difficult to attribute changes to the effects of therapy.[915] The presence of anemia is also variable in CML.[916] Leukostasis, a syndrome caused by hyperleukocytosis and frequently presenting with neurologic symptoms, such as dizziness, confusion, and somnolence, or pulmonary symptoms, including tachypnea, dyspnea and respiratory failure, is observed in AML and ALL secondary to high blast cell counts. However, symptoms of leukostasis are uncommon in adults with CML and are only slightly more common in childhood CML, even in patients with very elevated WBC counts.[917] Skin nodules, representing extramedullary hematopoiesis, may also be present.[918] The bone marrow in CML patients typically demonstrates normal myeloid maturation, with granulocytic hyperplasia and an increased myeloid-to-erythroid ratio. Megakaryocytic hyperplasia may also occur.[912] Dysplastic marrow basophils or eosinophils are common and cells of these lineages may be increased in number. About one in six CML patients has lipid-laden macrophages, sometimes called sea-blue histiocytes, similar to Gaucher's cells.[919] Although an increase in reticulin may occur, myelofibrosis is unusual. By definition, in chronic phase CML, the blast cell percentages in both the peripheral blood and bone marrow are less than 10%, and an increase above these levels may indicate a transition from chronic phase to accelerated phase or blast crisis. Other abnormal laboratory findings in chronic phase CML include low leukocyte alkaline phosphatase (LAP) activity and increased vitamin B_{12} levels. The latter occurs because of the increased white blood cell mass, which produces WBC-derived vitamin B_{12} binding protein. The cause of the low LAP is unclear, but may involve imperfect maturation of CML granulocytes. With therapy, the level of vitamin B_{12} falls to normal, whereas changes in LAP are less predictable.[920]

The accelerated phase is characterized by increased marrow or blood blast cell values of 10% to 19%, peripheral basophilia greater than 20%, persistent thrombocytopenia unrelated to therapy or thrombocytosis unresponsive to therapy, and increasing spleen size or WBC count. If marrow or blood blast cell percentages exceed 19% of total leukocytes, this signifies a transition to blast crisis, which may be myeloid, lymphoid, or mixed. Presentation in blast crisis can mimic an acute leukemia of lymphoid or myeloid lineage, and in this case the cells harbor the Philadelphia chromosome.

Differential Diagnosis

The differential diagnosis of an elevated WBC count (also known as a leukemoid reaction) includes severe infections, congenital heart disease, and metastatic cancer. In disorders other than CML, the peripheral blood rarely contains blasts and promyelocytes, the WBC count is usually somewhat lower, and the LAP scores and cytogenetic studies are normal. In general, patients with CML have a WBC count of more than 100,000/μL, a WBC differential containing promyelocytes and myelocytes (the blood smear often appears similar to a marrow smear), a low LAP, a large spleen, and Ph or molecular detection of the *BCR-ABL* transcript. Because CML patients can present in blast crisis, the patient with Ph-positive ALL presents a problem in differential diagnosis. Determination of the size of the abnormal fusion protein (usually 210 kD in CML and 185 kD in Ph-positive ALL) and the fusion transcript breakpoint by RT-PCR can help, as can the response to therapy. An important distinction is that in ALL, Ph commonly disappears with intensive chemotherapy, whereas in CML presenting in blast crisis, the disease may revert to the chronic phase, with the Philadelphia chromosome persisting in the recovering bone marrow cells.[921]

Clinical Course

Approximately 90% of patients are in the chronic phase at diagnosis. Prior to the advent of imatinib therapy, patients sometimes enjoyed unimpaired lifestyles for periods of many months to years, with minimal therapy during the chronic phase of their disease. However, if untreated, most patients will experience progressive disease from 3 to 8 years after diagnosis.

This is because of the development of the accelerated phase, which progresses to eventual blast crisis, usually within 3 months. Overall, blast crisis will develop in 75% to 85% of all untreated patients with CML. Blast crisis is a clinically high-risk form of CML that is difficult to control with chemotherapy and often leads to death within a short time, usually months.

Although BCR-ABL alone may be able to induce chronic phase CML, evolution to accelerated phase or blast crisis is often accompanied by the acquisition of duplicated Philadelphia chromosome or additional cytogenetic abnormalities in the bone marrow, such as trisomy 8 or abnormalities involving chromosome 7, including the t7;11(p15;p15) that creates the *NUP98-HOXA9* fusion.[922] Transformation to blast crisis appears to follow many of the same multiple mutational steps involved in the molecular pathogenesis of de novo AML or ALL. LAP levels may also rise during the transition to blast crisis. Myeloid blast crisis is somewhat more common and carries a poorer prognosis than lymphoid blast crisis.[921,923-925] About one third of patients have a lymphoblastic crisis, usually B precursor by immunophenotype, although T-lymphoblastic crisis phenotypes can occur.[926,927] Patients with lymphoid blast crisis have a younger median age than patients with myeloid blast crisis.[928] CML blast crisis can also contain subpopulations of blast cells with differing phenotypes (possibly subclones differentiated along both lymphoid and myeloid lineages, biphenotypic leukemias) and blast crisis in which individual cells simultaneously express features of more than one lineage (mixed-lineage leukemias).

Treatment

Historical Chemotherapy

Traditional chemotherapy for CML used busulfan or hydroxyurea.[929] Busulfan is associated with infertility and, rarely, marrow aplasia and interstitial pneumonitis. Hydroxyurea is less toxic, but only induces a decreased granulocyte count. Hydroxyurea does not induce cytogenetic remissions or change the natural history of the disease. Interferon-α (IFN-α) has demonstrated improved rates of hematologic remission over hydroxyurea, with evidence of hematologic control in 70% to 80% of patients and complete cytogenetic responses in 6% to 26% when given as a single agent in different series.[930-932] The normalization of bone marrow cytogenetics was shown to persist for many years in some patients, even after stopping the drug. Interestingly, these patients often remain PCR-positive for the *BCR-ABL* transcript if sensitive techniques are used.[933-935] Despite the efficacy of IFN-α, unwanted side effects are common and include fatigue, myalgias, arthralgias, headaches, weight loss, depression, diarrhea, neurologic symptoms, memory changes, hair thinning, autoimmune diseases, and cardiomyopathy,[936-938] leading 14% to 26% of patients to discontinue therapy.[939-942] Thus, although IFN demonstrated some promise in this disease, the toxicity profile made it intolerable to a large fraction of CML patients.

Tyrosine Kinase Inhibitors

The treatment of chronic phase CML has since been revolutionized with the advent of molecularly targeted therapy that specifically targets the BCR-ABL fusion protein. Imatinib mesylate, also known as STI-571 or Gleevec, is a tyrosine kinase inhibitor that blocks enzymatic activity of several tyrosine kinases, including mainly ABL, PDGFR, and KIT, by binding to the adenosine triphosphate (ATP) binding site. The promising results of phase I and II studies that produced impressive activity in patients who had already failed interferon[943] have led to the International Randomized Study of

Interferon and STI571 (IRIS), which randomized patients to imatinib versus interferon with cytarabine as initial therapy for patients with CML.[944] This study has demonstrated better outcome with longer times to progression and to accelerated phase or blast crisis for patients initially treated with imatinib. Additionally, patients treated with imatinib had higher rates of hematologic and cytogenetic remission and, for the first time, molecular responses were obtained with an undetectable *BCR-ABL* fusion transcript. Treatment with imatinib effectively established new standards for response rates, including complete hematologic response (CHR), implying a normalization of peripheral blood cell counts, major cytogenetic response (MCyR), with the presence of Ph in 1% to 35% bone marrow cells analyzed by metaphase spread, complete cytogenetic response (CCyR), with the absence of Ph, and major molecular response (MMR), demonstrating a 3-log reduction in detection of the *BCR-ABL* transcript in bone marrow cell RNA compared with diagnostic levels. The 5-year outcome of the IRIS study has been published[945] and has convincingly demonstrated the long-term benefit and tolerability of imatinib therapy, with increasing rates of CHR and CCyR over time. Imatinib has excellent oral bioavailability, with minimal systemic effects other than myelosuppression. Other side effects include peripheral and periorbital edema, muscle cramps, gastrointestinal (GI) intolerance, and skin rash. Cardiac complications, including congestive heart failure, are rare, but have been reported.[946] However, imatinib must be continued indefinitely because cessation of the drug is associated with an increase in bone marrow cell *BCR-ABL* transcript levels and eventually hematologic relapse. Thus, imatinib is currently the first-line therapy for adults with chronic phase CML.

Based on the success, promise, and safety profile of imatinib therapy in adults, studies to determine the efficacy of this drug in childhood CML have been undertaken. The Children's Oncology Group has published the results of a phase I trial of imatinib in children with Ph-positive disease who had failed interferon therapy.[947] Imatinib was well tolerated at escalating dose levels up to 570 mg/m^2 and CHR was demonstrated for all 14 chronic phase patients within 1 month of starting therapy. Ten of 12 evaluated patients had achieved a CCyR by a median of 3 months. A Phase 2 European pediatric study[948] has demonstrated equally encouraging results for children with chronic phase CML who failed interferon therapy. These studies and extrapolation from adult data have resulted in imatinib becoming first-line therapy in children with chronic phase CML. Confidence in this approach has been improved by evidence that prior imatinib therapy has no negative impact on the transplantation-related mortality following an allogeneic donor HSCT.[949] Side effects of imatinib in children include GI problems and skin rashes. If signs of leukostasis are present, more urgent therapy must be used. If the WBC count must be lowered quickly, leukapheresis and immediate chemotherapy with high-doses of hydroxyurea may be used. Proper hydration, alkalinization of the urine, and the use of allopurinol are imperative before the rapid lysis of cells is induced with chemotherapy.

Resistance to imatinib mesylate has been demonstrated.[950-954] Mechanisms of resistance include point mutations in *BCR-ABL*, amplification of the *BCR-ABL* gene, overexpression of the BCR-ABL protein, enhanced expression of the multidrug resistance gene, and excessive binding of imatinib by serum proteins. Analysis of a small number of blast crisis patients who relapsed while receiving imatinib has frequently shown either *BCR-ABL* gene amplification or *BCR-ABL* kinase domain mutations.[951] These observations have indicated that resistance to imatinib as a single agent in the treatment of CML involves alterations of the BCR-ABL protein expression level or structure, allowing it to escape

inhibition by the drug, rather than mutations in entirely different genes that might have reduced the malignant cells' dependence on BCR-ABL for transformation. A number of approaches have been suggested as interventions following the identification of imatinib resistance. High-dose imatinib has shown some promise for inducing cytogenetic remissions, despite a lack of efficacy of standard-dose therapy.[955] Additionally, two new tyrosine kinase inhibitors have emerged and are more potent inhibitors of BCR-ABL than imatinib. Nilotinib is a structural derivative of imatinib and effective at lower concentrations,[956] and dasatinib has a completely different structure and binding configuration, making it active against most imatinib-resistant *BCR-ABL* mutations, as well as a host of other tyrosine kinases. Dasatinib is currently FDA-approved for the treatment of imatinib-resistant chronic phase CML.[955]

Hematopoietic Stem Cell Transplantation

Of all malignancies, CML has the most extensive long-term data on the effectiveness of allogeneic HSCT. This approach can provide prolonged DFS in CML and is the only proven curative therapy. The effectiveness of allogeneic HSCT in CML is thought to be caused in part by the effects of the transplanted immune system, rather than solely the result of the high-dose total body irradiation and chemotherapy in the conditioning regimen. The allogeneic graft creates a new immune system that plays an active role in eradicating CML cells. Immune-mediated antileukemic effects are suspected because patients may remain PCR-positive for *BCR-ABL* transcripts for months after HSCT, and yet appear to be cured of their disease and eventually convert to PCR-negativity without further therapy. Furthermore, there is an extremely high relapse rate for autologous, syngeneic, and T-cell–depleted grafts using the same myeloablative conditioning regimens used for standard, non–T-cell–depleted grafts, suggesting that alloreactivity is associated with lower relapse rates.[957-959] Because of the role of immune-mediated cytotoxicity in CML, treatments that combine less than myeloablative chemotherapy with infusions of peripheral blood stem cells in "minitransplants" are currently being tested for efficacy in clinical trials.

The role of allogeneic HSCT in CML provides a moving target in the post-imatinib era. The potential toxicity associated with allogeneic HSCT, especially from a matched unrelated donor, compared with the efficacy and tolerability of imatinib has raised questions regarding the indications and timing for HSCT in CML patients. Although some patients may go on to long-term survival when HSCT is performed in accelerated phase or blast crisis of CML (15% to 30% of cases), results are substantially better when HSCT is performed in the chronic phase.[960] If the procedure is performed while the patient is in chronic phase using a matched sibling donor, 1-year survival rates are 60% to 80%, with a 10-year DFS rate of approximately 50%.[957,961-963] Some studies have demonstrated increased survival outcomes if the HSCT was performed within the first year of diagnosis.[964-966] Prior to imatinib therapy, these data prompted the initiation of allogeneic HSCT early in the course of treatment. However, HSCT has always been limited to patients who can medically tolerate the procedure and have appropriate donors—30% have matched sibling donors, 5% have matches with additional family members, and 50% have matched unrelated donors in donor registries. Imatinib can be safely given pre-HSCT and has no impact on transplantation-related mortality.[949,967] Currently, most adult patients, including even those with sibling donors, are being maintained on imatinib until evidence of resistance develops, which then prompts a change in therapy and consideration of HSCT. In children, the timing of HSCT for CML is even more challenging. Although imatinib has now demonstrated impressive 5-year outcomes, will these be sustained for the many years that a child with CML would be required to take the drug? Allogeneic HSCT still remains the only curative therapy and is generally better tolerated by children, particularly with modern approaches to supportive care.

Between 10% and 15% of recipients of matched sibling HSCT and less than 5% of matched unrelated donor recipients relapse hematologically following allogeneic HSCT. Patients who relapse following HSCT may respond to interferon or withdrawal of immunosuppression.[968-971] Recent evidence has suggested that relapse rates may be reduced with the addition of imatinib therapy post-HSCT, whether or not the patient received imatinib pre-HSCT. However, the recommended duration of imatinib therapy post-HSCT remains uncertain. Patients who relapse post-HSCT may benefit from a second HSCT or from donor-lymphocyte infusions (DLIs). Approximately 60% to 80% of patients who relapse cytogenetically or hematologically and return to chronic phase after HSCT can be salvaged by DLIs, without further cytotoxic chemotherapy.[572,972-974] Unfortunately, acute and chronic GVHD and marrow aplasia remain significant complications after DLI.[975] Approximately 5% to 15% of patients successfully treated with DLI subsequently relapse again, but remissions induced by this modality are durable in the most patients.

Blast Phase Chronic Myelogenous Leukemia

Blast phase CML is generally resistant to chemotherapy.[923] As in acute leukemia, leukostasis is more likely in patients with high blast counts, and rapid institution of therapy to lower the WBC count is indicated after initiating measures to protect the patient from tumor lysis syndrome. The blast cell morphology and surface markers should guide therapy in blast crisis of CML. Lymphoid blast morphology or surface markers predict a good initial response to drugs effective in ALL, such as prednisone and vincristine.[912,928,976] However, patients whose blast cells have a myeloid morphology and immunophenotype respond poorly to most therapies. Median survival is only 2 months after transformation to myeloid blast crisis, compared with 6 months if the blast cells have lymphoblastic characteristics.[977] Allogeneic HSCT in late-stage CML is associated with a poor outcome, primarily because of the high peri-HSCT mortality from regimen-related toxicity and an extremely high relapse rate.

Chronic Myelogenous Leukemia Caused by Other Translocations

Other chromosomal translocations have also been identified in CML. The *TEL* gene belongs to a large family of transcription factors referred to as the *ETS* family. These genes encode related proteins defined by a highly conserved, 90–amino acid, winged helix-turn-helix dimerization motif. This region appears to be an essential requirement for constitutive tyrosine kinase activity and transforming capacity of fusion proteins derived from chromosomal translocations involving *TEL*, generally partnered with a tyrosine kinase gene such as the *PDGF* receptor.[978-980] With the exception of the t(12;21)-associated *TEL-AML1* fusion gene exclusively associated with early B-lineage ALL, *TEL* gene rearrangements are rare in human leukemia. Because of the small numbers of patients with myeloid malignancy who have *TEL* gene fusions, there is insufficient clinical experience to determine their clinical implications. However, there is a trend toward an unfavorable outcome in patients with atypical CML or CMML accompanied by *TEL* gene rearrangements.

Polycythemia Vera

Polycythemia is defined as an increase in numbers of circulating erythrocytes, hemoglobin, and hematocrit. There are three types of polycythemia: (1) polycythemia vera (PV), or primary polycythemia; (2) secondary polycythemia; and (3) relative polycythemia.[981] The first two types are associated with an increase in red blood cell mass, whereas in the third, the red blood cell mass is normal and plasma volume is reduced. Secondary polycythemia can arise from a multitude of causes, including those that result in excessive erythropoietin production caused by decreased tissue oxygenation (physiologically appropriate), inappropriate erythropoietin secretion from a tumor, a mutant hemoglobin with abnormal oxygen affinity, and decreased erythrocyte diphosphoglycerate.

PV is a myeloproliferative disease caused by clonal expansion of an abnormal multipotent stem cell that produces erythroid progenitors that can proliferate in the absence of erythropoietin (EPO).[982,983] In contrast, normal fetal erythroid progenitors and those with mutations in the EPO receptor still require erythropoietin for their function. Growth of erythropoietin-independent erythroid colonies in serum-containing cultures can be a useful diagnostic test.[983] Because this is a hematopoietic stem cell disorder, aberrations in the WBC and platelet counts can accompany the increased red blood cell mass. The diagnosis of PV used to be a diagnosis of exclusion. One had to prove that the elevated red cell mass was not from a secondary cause, such as hypoxia or a high oxygen affinity hemoglobin, and that the *BCR-ABL* transgene was absent. However, in 2005, several groups simultaneously reported the presence of a somatically acquired clonal *V617F* mutation in the Janus 2 kinase (*JAK2*) in more than 90% of cases of sporadic PV in adults.[984-987] This seminal discovery linked PV with the other myeloproliferative disorders, such as CML, by demonstrating a primary mutation in a tyrosine kinase as a causative factor and effectively established *JAK2* mutational analysis as a diagnostic test for PV. Interestingly, this same mutation was found in 50% of cases of essential thrombocythemia (ET; see later) and agnogenic myelofibrosis with myeloid metaplasia (AMM).[984-987] These three different phenotypes caused by the same genotype pose many questions and scientists are currently investigating the role of gene dosage, modifying mutations, or genetic predisposition to account for the difference in disease phenotype. Some studies have suggested that patients with PV have at least a subpopulation of cells that are homozygous for the *JAK2* mutation, whereas patients with ET are heterozygous.[988,989] Moreover, the *JAK2* mutation may be sufficient to induce PV but other mutations are likely required for the development of ET and AMM. Rare cases of familial polycythemia may exhibit autosomal recessive or dominant inheritance, and erythropoietin levels can be low, normal, or elevated.[990] Studies of these families have revealed that the *JAK2* mutation is acquired, suggesting that there is an inherited predisposition allele that has not yet been identified.[991] In some of the families, a mutation in the negative regulatory domain of the erythropoietin receptor gene appears to be involved.[992-994] Most recently, several *JAK2 V617F*-negative patients with PV were found to have a number of different mutations involving exon 12 of *JAK2*.[995]

The WHO previously established strict criteria for the diagnosis of PV, with recent suggestions for revisions to *JAK2* mutational evaluation.[996-998] Evaluation should include a careful history and physical examination, including examination for splenomegaly and measurements of oxygen saturation, a complete blood count, and serum erythropoietin level, *JAK2* mutational analysis, and bone marrow aspirate and biopsy, including cytogenetics to rule out *BCR-ABL* or other translocation-induced fusion genes.

Polycythemia vera is extremely uncommon in children. The median age at presentation is 60 years, and fewer than 1% of PV patients are younger than 25 years.[981,999,1000] Children with PV are also less likely than adults to exhibit the most prevalent *JAK2* mutation. Erythrocytosis can cause cardiac symptoms, such as dyspnea and hypertension, and symptoms of disturbed cerebral circulation, such as dizziness and paresthesias. Abnormal platelet function and thrombocytosis may lead to thrombosis and hemorrhage. Granulocytic proliferation can cause increased histamine turnover, resulting in GI symptoms and pruritus. Hyperuricemia and hypermetabolic symptoms are common, including weakness and weight loss. Most patients have large spleens and may have large livers and increased blood pressure.[981] The marrow shows hypercellularity, an increase in megakaryocyte number, and decreased iron stores. Serum erythropoietin levels are usually normal or decreased.[1001] A total of 10% to 25% of patients have a clonal chromosomal abnormality evident by cytogenetic analysis, most often a 20q– deletion. Box 11-4 lists suggested criteria for the diagnosis of pediatric PV.[1002,1003]

Prolonged survival after the diagnosis of PV is common, but spontaneous remission is rare.[1004] Vascular occlusive episodes related to high hematocrit levels are an important cause of morbidity and mortality.[1005] Other life-threatening complications of polycythemia vera include bleeding, myelofibrosis with pancytopenia, and acute leukemia.[1006] A poorly defined spent phase may occur, characterized by a decrease in hematocrit

---

Box 11-4 **Suggested Criteria for Childhood Polycythemia Vera***

MAJOR CRITERIA

Elevated red cell mass
No cause of secondary erythrocytosis, including:
   a. Absence of familial erythrocytosis (e.g., hereditary mutations of erythropoietin [EPO] receptor)
   b. No elevation of EPO caused by
      i. Hypoxia (arterial PO_2 < 92%)
      ii. High oxygen affinity hemoglobin
      iii. Truncated EPO receptor
      iv. Inappropriate EPO production by tumor

MINOR CRITERIA

Presence of *JAK2 V617F* mutation
Endogenous erythroid colony formation
Hypercellular bone marrow with trilineage proliferation
Low serum EPO levels

---

*Requires the presence of both major and one minor criteria. Adapted from Vardiman JW, Harris NL, Brunning RD. The World Health Organization (WHO) classification of the myeloid neoplasms. Blood. 2002;100:2292-2302; Tefferi A, Thiele J, Orazi A, et al. Proposals and rationale for revision of the World Health Organization diagnostic criteria for polycythemia vera, essential thrombocythemia, and primary myelofibrosis: recommendations from an ad hoc international expert panel. Blood. 2007;110:1092-1097; Teofili L, Giona F, Martini M, et al. Markers of myeloproliferative diseases in childhood polycythemia vera and essential thrombocythemia. J Clin Oncol. 2007;25:1048-1053; and Teofili L, Giona F, Martini M, et al. The revised WHO diagnostic criteria for Ph-negative myeloproliferative diseases are not appropriate for the diagnostic screening of childhood polycythemia vera and essential thrombocythemia. Blood. 2007;110:3384-3386.

(often because of increased plasma volume), variable depression of other blood cell counts, hepatosplenomegaly, and increased bone marrow reticulin and fibrosis.[1007,1008] Patients often benefit from phlebotomy, although isovolumic erythropheresis may be a safer procedure, but this requires specific resources and is not uniformly available.[1009] The highest risk for thrombotic or hemorrhagic complications is observed immediately following phlebotomy. Iron replacement therapy should be given, because iron deficiency can lead to nonhematologic disturbances and an increase in blood viscosity.[1010] Low-dose aspirin is also recommended for adults with PV.[1011] Radioactive phosphorus or chemotherapy can also control the hematocrit in polycythemia vera. However, these treatments have been associated with an increased risk of transformation to AML.[1006] Hydroxyurea, IFN-α, and anagrelide are all agents used in adults to control cell counts and may be useful in pediatric cases.[1012-1014] Hydroxyurea is simpler to administer and has fewer side effects than interferon, and the leukemogenic risk of hydroxyurea appears to be low, as demonstrated by a number of long-term studies in sickle cell anemia patients. However, the risk of transformation to AML is still higher in PV, because patients have a primary clonal stem cell disorder.[1015] The main toxicity from hydroxyurea is neutropenia. Anagrelide is a newer agent that inhibits the action of cyclic AMP phosphodiesterase and primarily targets megakaryocyte differentiation and proliferation. It has resulted in the disappearance of thrombocythemia-related symptoms in 80% of patients with polycythemia vera.[1016] However, it has been found to be inferior to hydroxyurea in ET.[1017] Tarceva (Erlotinib) has been reported to inhibit the mutant JAK2 kinase specifically[1018] and clinical trials of this drug are underway for PV, ET, and AMM.

Essential Thrombocythemia

ET is a myeloproliferative disorder characterized by an increased platelet count not attributable to any other cause; Box 11-5 lists causes of thrombocytosis.[999,1019-1023] Like the other myeloproliferative diseases, ET is a clonal stem cell disorder that also affects other hematopoietic lineages.[1024] The *JAK2 V617F* mutation is found in approximately 50% of cases and other cases may be associated with a mutation affecting the genes encoding thrombopoietin or the thrombopoietin receptor (MPL).[1025-1027] ET may occur in childhood, but rarely,[1000,1025,1028-1030] and it may be familial in some cases.[1031] A number of families have been identified who have ET and/or other myeloproliferative diseases with or without acquisition of the *JAK2 V617F* mutation, demonstrating that other mutations are involved in the pathogenesis of the disease and that there is likely an underlying genetic predisposition that has not yet been elucidated.[991,1032,1033] The requirements for essential thrombocythemia are a platelet count above 600,000/μL (although suggestions have been made to reduce this to 450,000/μL), a hemoglobin concentration not exceeding 13 g/dL (normal red blood cell mass), normal iron stores, a lack of the Philadelphia chromosome by molecular or cytogenetic analysis, the absence of collagen fibrosis of the marrow, and no other identifiable cause of thrombocytosis.[998,1019] Box 11-6 suggests criteria for the diagnosis of pediatric ET.

Essential thrombocythemia may be an incidental finding, or patients may present with venous or arterial thrombosis, bleeding, or symptoms of a hypermetabolic state. The bleeding is generally mild and its cause is unknown, although platelet function is often abnormal.[1034,1035] Splenomegaly is common, as is mild leukocytosis. Bone marrow cytogenetics are usually normal. The clinical course is highly variable and some patients have been followed for 10 years without problems.[1023] In adults, 80% survive more than 100 months, with 5 of 95 patients

Box 11-5	**Causes of Thrombocytosis in Children**

NUTRITIONAL

Iron deficiency
Megaloblastic anemia
Vitamin E deficiency
Metabolic
Hyperadrenalism

INFECTIOUS

Viral factors
Bacterial
Mycobacterial

TRAUMATIC

Surgery
Fracture
Hemorrhage

INFLAMMATORY

Collagen vascular disease
Inflammatory bowel disease
Sarcoidosis
Any inflammatory condition

NEOPLASTIC

Myeloproliferative disease
Hepatoblastoma
Neuroblastoma
Histiocytosis
Lymphoma
Carcinoma

MEDICATION-RELATED

Corticosteroids
Vinca alkaloids
Citrovorum factor

MISCELLANEOUS

Splenectomy, congenital asplenia
Infantile cortical hyperostosis (Caffey's disease)
Cerebrovascular accident
Hemolytic anemia

Data from Addiego JE Jr, Mentzer WC Jr, Dallman PR. Thrombocytosis in infants and children. J Pediatr. 1974;85:805-807; Heath HW, Pearson HA. Thrombocytosis in pediatric outpatients. J Pediatr. 1989;114:805-807; and Chan KW, Kaikov Y, Wadsworth LD. Thrombocytosis in childhood: a survey of 94 patients. Pediatrics. 1989;84: 1064-1067.

Box 11-6	**Suggested Criteria for Childhood Essential Thrombocythemia**

Sustained platelet count > 450,000/μL
Bone marrow biopsy specimen showing proliferation mainly of the megakaryocytic lineage, with increased numbers of enlarged mature megakaryocytes; no significant increase or left shift of neutrophil granulopoiesis or erythropoiesis
Not meeting World Health Organization criteria for polycythemia vera, AMM, chronic myelogenous leukemia, myelodysplastic syndrome, or other myeloid neoplasm (e.g., no Philadelphia chromosome or *BCR-ABL* fusion)
Demonstration of *JAK2 V617F* or of another clonal marker (e.g., MPL mutation), or, in the absence of a clonal marker, no evidence of reactive thrombocytosis

Adapted from Vardiman JW, Harris NL, Brunning RD. The World Health Organization (WHO) classification of the myeloid neoplasms. Blood. 2002;100:2292-2302; Tefferi A, Thiele J, Orazi A, et al. Proposals and rationale for revision of the World Health Organization diagnostic criteria for polycythemia vera, essential thrombocythemia, and primary myelofibrosis: recommendations from an ad hoc international expert panel. Blood. 2007;110:1092-1097; Teofili L, Giona F, Martini M, et al. Markers of myeloproliferative diseases in childhood polycythemia vera and essential thrombocythemia. J Clin Oncol. 2007;25:1048-1053; and Teofili L, Giona F, Martini M, et al. The revised WHO diagnostic criteria for Ph-negative myeloproliferative diseases are not appropriate for the diagnostic screening of childhood polycythemia vera and essential thrombocythemia. Blood. 2007;110:3384-3386.

ultimately experiencing a conversion to AML in one study.[1036] Patients with ET can also develop myelofibrosis. Children appear to have a more benign course than adults.[1000,1025,1037] Asymptomatic children do not need to be treated. Treatment options are similar to those available for PV, including hydroxyurea, anagrelide,[1038-1040] or IFN-α.[1041,1042] Treatment is usually recommended to prevent thrombotic complications in patients with platelet counts higher than 1,000,000/μL or a prior history of thrombohemorrhagic episodes. A randomized clinical trial in adults of hydroxyurea and aspirin or anagrelide and aspirin has demonstrated equal efficacy of these combinations in lowering the platelet count, but a higher incidence of arterial thromboses, significant hemorrhage, and transformation to myelofibrosis in the anagrelide-treated group.[1017] The results have suggested that hydroxyurea and aspirin should remain as frontline therapy for ET and furthermore inferred that a lower platelet count alone is not protective. Anagrelide is fairly platelet-specific, whereas hydroxyurea has more global hematopoietic and vascular effects. which may contribute to the improved outcome.

Agnogenic Myeloid Metaplasia with Myelofibrosis

AMM is a myeloproliferative disease characterized by leukoerythroblastosis, myeloid metaplasia, and varying degrees of myelofibrosis.[1043-1045] The median age at presentation is 60 years, and pediatric cases are rare.[1046] Approximately 22% of patients are younger than 56 years and approximately 11% are younger than 46 years.[1047] Symptoms include malaise, weight loss, night sweats, and discomfort from splenomegaly. Peripheral blood cell counts are varied, and the smears often show Pelger-Huet cells, leukoerythroblastosis, and teardrop formation, along with occasional immature WBC precursors.[1048] Bone marrow cells are difficult to aspirate, and biopsies show fibrosis in most patients.[1048] Cytogenetic abnormalities are common in AMM if enough marrow cells can be obtained for study.[234,1049] AMM is a clonal disease involving all myeloid elements,[1049] and the cause of the associated myelofibrosis is unknown.[1050-1052] However, like PV and ET, the *JAK2 V617F* mutation has been found in approximately 50% of patients. Another 10% of patients have been found to have a *W515L* mutation in the thrombopoietin receptor.[1053] Because this disorder is very rare in children, other causes of myelofibrosis need to be ruled out. These causes include nutritional, inflammatory, infectious, and neoplastic disorders.[1054]

The natural history of AMM can be variable, with patient survival varying from 1.5 to more than 5 years.[1055] Children with AMM may have a more favorable natural history than adults.[1056,1057] Young adults tend to have less severe anemia, higher incidence of splenomegaly, lower frequency of thrombocytosis, and lower frequency of chromosomal abnormalities.[1047] Complications of this disease include bleeding, intercurrent infection, transformation to acute leukemia,[1058] and portal hypertension.[1055] Splenectomy will not cause a further reduction of blood cell counts and therefore should be considered only for mechanical problems, portal hypertension, refractory thrombocytopenia, and hemolytic anemia.[1059] The role of chemotherapy in AMM is ill defined, although hydroxyurea, anagrelide, and IFN-α have been used.[1060]

Mastocytosis

Mastocytosis is a pathologic proliferation and accumulation of mast cells in various tissues in the body.[1061] Mast cells are myeloid cells derived from HSCs but, unlike other lineages, they exit the marrow before they are fully matured and complete their development in the tissues in which they eventually reside.[1062-1064] Given their role in allergic and inflammatory conditions, mast cells are commonly found in vascularized connective tissues such as the skin and the mucosal surfaces of the GI tract and respiratory epithelium.[1065] The cutaneous form of mastocytosis is most common in children and may consist of an isolated mastocytoma or diffuse lesions termed *urticaria pigmentosa*.[1066] This is a generally benign condition, although in rare cases progression to systemic mastocytosis (SM) can occur. SM implies mast cell proliferation in an extracutaneous site, most commonly the bone marrow. SM is a clonal myeloproliferative disease frequently associated with a *D816V* point mutation in the gene encoding the KIT tyrosine kinase and presents with varying degrees of mast cell hyperproliferation and impaired differentiation, depending on the subtype.[1061] SM is further divided into four subtypes—indolent systemic mastocytosis (ISM), systemic mastocytosis with an associated hematopoietic clonal non–mast cell lineage disease (SM-AHNMD), aggressive systemic mastocytosis (ASM), and mast cell leukemia (MCL). Whereas the *KIT* mutations may be sufficient to result in the indolent form of the systemic disease, additional genetic abnormalities appear to be required for progression to the more aggressive forms of the disease.[1061] SM may occur in conjunction with the generally favorable prognostic t(8;21) translocation (*AML1-ETO*) but, in this context, it confers a poor prognosis.[1067,1068] Similarly, mast cell leukemia is associated with a poor outcome.[1069] Treatment strategies include combination therapy with steroids and IFN-α,[1069,1070] cladribine,[1071] and more recently with tyrosine kinase inhibitors.[1072,1073] Imatinib mesylate, which is known to target the KIT tyrosine kinase in addition to BCR-ABL, has been used in patients with SM. Imatinib has shown preferential efficacy for the minority of patients who lack the *D816V* mutation[1074,1075] and has been FDA-approved for this indication. Other tyrosine kinase inhibitors, including dasatinib, have demonstrated some promise with improved responses in imatinib-resistant *D816V*-positive disease.[1076]

CONCLUSIONS

Although considerable progress has been made in improving the remission induction rates in AML, remission is not attained in a significant number of children with newly diagnosed AML. The overall survival of patients with AML is still not optimal, and the toxicity of treatment is often excessive. Myeloid leukemias, myelodysplastic syndromes, and myeloproliferative disorders are heterogeneous in their molecular pathophysiologic course and are often difficult to treat effectively. Significant improvements have been made in the treatment of APL with ATRA and ATO. Similarly, the treatment of CML has been revolutionized with the use of imatinib and other ABL tyrosine kinase inhibitors. As more is understood about the molecular biology of the other types of myeloid malignancies, future studies will emphasize the introduction of new agents that target malignant cells more specifically while sparing normal hematopoietic stem and progenitor cells. This exciting new strategy of targeted therapy will undoubtedly greatly improve the outcome and reduce the toxicity for increasingly large subsets of patients afflicted by myeloid malignancies.

REFERENCES

1. Ries LAG, Melbert D, Krapcho M, et al. SEER Cancer Statistics Review, 1975-2004. Bethesda, Md, National Cancer Institute, 2007. Available at http://seer.cancer.gov/csr/1975_2004.
2. Ries LAG, Smith MA, Gurney JG, et al. Cancer Incidence and Survival in Children and Adolescents: United States SEER Program 1975-1995 (NIH Publication No. 99-4649). Bethesda, Md, National Cancer Institute, 1999.
3. Pedersen-Bjergaard J. Radiotherapy- and chemotherapy-induced myelodysplasia and acute myeloid leukemia. A review. Leuk Res. 1992;16:61-65.
4. Tucker MA, Meadows AT, Boice JD Jr, et al. Leukemia after therapy with alkylating agents for childhood cancer. J Natl Cancer Inst. 1987;78:459-464.
5. Pui CH, Ribeiro RC, Hancock ML, et al. Acute myeloid leukemia in children treated with epipodophyllotoxins for acute lymphoblastic leukemia. N Engl J Med. 1991;325:1682-1687.
6. Pui CH, Behm FG, Raimondi SC, et al. Secondary acute myeloid leukemia in children treated for acute lymphoid leukemia. N Engl J Med. 1989;321:136-142.
7. Andersen MK, Christiansen DH, Jensen BA, et al. Therapy-related acute lymphoblastic leukaemia with MLL rearrangements following DNA topoisomerase II inhibitors, an increasing problem: report on two new cases and review of the literature since 1992. Br J Haematol. 2001;114:539-543.
8. Andersen MK, Christiansen DH, Kirchhoff M, Pedersen-Bjergaard J. Duplication or amplification of chromosome band 11q23, including the unrearranged MLL gene, is a recurrent abnormality in therapy-related MDS and AML, and is closely related to mutation of the TP53 gene and to previous therapy with alkylating agents. Genes Chromosomes Cancer. 2001;31:33-41.
9. Super HJ, McCabe NR, Thirman MJ, et al. Rearrangements of the MLL gene in therapy-related acute myeloid leukemia in patients previously treated with agents targeting DNA-topoisomerase II. Blood. 1993;82:3705-3711.
10. Demuynck H, Verhoef GE, Zachee P, et al. Therapy-related acute myeloid leukemia with t(8;16)(p11;p13) following anthracycline-based therapy for nonmetastatic osteosarcoma. Cancer Genet Cytogenet. 1995;82:103-105.
11. Howard RA, Gilbert ES, Chen BE, et al. Leukemia following breast cancer: an international population-based study of 376,825 women. Breast Cancer Res Treat. 2007;105(3):359-368.

12. Andersen MK, Larson RA, Mauritzson N, et al. Balanced chromosome abnormalities inv(16) and t(15;17) in therapy-related myelodysplastic syndromes and acute leukemia: report from an international workshop. Genes Chromosomes Cancer. 2002;33: 395-400.

13. Schnittger S, Bacher U, Haferlach C, et al. Rare CBFB-MYH11 fusion transcripts in AML with inv(16)/t(16;16) are associated with therapy-related AML M4eo, atypical cytomorphology, atypical immunophenotype, atypical additional chromosomal rearrangements and low white blood cell count: a study on 162 patients. Leukemia. 2007;21:725-731.

14. Kawano S, Miyanishi S, Shimizu K, et al. Genetic analysis of 8;21 chromosomal translocation without AML1 gene involvement in MDS-AML. Br J Haematol. 1997;99:632-640.

15. Kato H, Brown CC, Hoel DG, Schull WJ. Studies of the mortality of A-bomb survivors. Report 7. Mortality, 1950-1978: Part II. Mortality from causes other than cancer and mortality in early entrants. Radiat Res. 1982;91:243-264.

16. Peterson AV Jr, Prentice RL, Ishimaru T, et al. Investigation of circular asymmetry in cancer mortality of Hiroshima and Nagasaki A-bomb survivors. Radiat Res. 1983;93:184-199.

17. Nakanishi M, Tanaka K, Shintani T, et al. Chromosomal instability in acute myelocytic leukemia and myelodysplastic syndrome patients in atomic bomb survivors. J Radiat Res (Tokyo). 1999;40:159-167.

18. Doll R, Wakeford R. Risk of childhood cancer from fetal irradiation. Br J Radiol. 1997;70:130-139.

19. Ross JA, Davies SM, Potter JD, Robison LL. Epidemiology of childhood leukemia, with a focus on infants. Epidemiol Rev. 1994;16:243-272.

20. Naumburg E, Bellocco R, Cnattingius S, et al. Intrauterine exposure to diagnostic X rays and risk of childhood leukemia subtypes. Radiat Res. 2001;156:718-723.

21. von Muhlendahl KE. Chernobyl fallout, nuclear plants and leukaemia: review of recent literature. Eur J Pediatr. 1998;157: 602-604.

22. Estey E, Dohner H. Acute myeloid leukaemia. Lancet. 2006; 368:1894-1907.

23. Cardis E, Gilbert ES, Carpenter L, et al. Effects of low doses and low dose rates of external ionizing radiation: cancer mortality in nuclear industry workers in three countries. Radiat Res. 1995;142:117-132.

24. Aw JJ. Cosmic radiation and commercial air travel. J Travel Med. 2003;10:19-28.

25. Gundestrup M, Storm HH. Radiation-induced acute myeloid leukaemia and other cancers in commercial jet cockpit crew: a population-based cohort study. Lancet. 1999;354:2029-2031.

26. Ahlbom A, Day N, Feychting M, et al. A pooled analysis of magnetic fields and childhood leukaemia. Br J Cancer. 2000;83: 692-698.

27. Ciccone G, Mirabelli D, Levis A, et al. Myeloid leukemias and myelodysplastic syndromes: chemical exposure, histologic subtype and cytogenetics in a case-control study. Cancer Genet Cytogenet. 1993;68:135-139.

28. Kleinerman RA, Linet MS, Hatch EE, et al. Magnetic field exposure assessment in a case-control study of childhood leukemia. Epidemiology. 1997;8:575-583.

29. Linet MS, Hatch EE, Kleinerman RA, et al. Residential exposure to magnetic fields and acute lymphoblastic leukemia in children. N Engl J Med. 1997;337:1-7.

30. Richardson S, Zittoun R, Bastuji-Garin S, et al. Occupational risk factors for acute leukaemia: a case-control study. Int J Epidemiol. 1992;21:1063-1073.

31. Severson RK, Stevens RG, Kaune WT, et al. Acute nonlymphocytic leukemia and residential exposure to power frequency magnetic fields. Am J Epidemiol. 1988;128:10-20.

32. Theriault G, Li CY. Risks of leukaemia in residents close to high voltage transmission electric lines. Occup Environ Med. 1997; 54:625-628.

33. Tynes T, Haldorsen T. Electromagnetic fields and cancer in children residing near Norwegian high-voltage power lines. Am J Epidemiol. 1997;145:219-226.

34. Rinsky RA, Smith AB, Hornung R, et al. Benzene and leukemia. An epidemiologic risk assessment. N Engl J Med. 1987;316: 1044-1050.

35. Zhang L, Rothman N, Wang Y, et al. Increased aneusomy and long arm deletion of chromosomes 5 and 7 in the lymphocytes of Chinese workers exposed to benzene. Carcinogenesis. 1998; 19:1955-1961.

36. Menegaux F, Ripert M, Hemon D, Clavel J. Maternal alcohol and coffee drinking, parental smoking and childhood leukaemia: a French population-based case-control study. Paediatr Perinat Epidemiol. 2007;21:293-299.

37. Shu XO, Ross JA, Pendergrass TW, et al. Parental alcohol consumption, cigarette smoking, and risk of infant leukemia: a Children's Cancer Group study. J Natl Cancer Inst. 1996;88: 24-31.

38. Spector LG, Xie Y, Robison LL, et al. Maternal diet and infant leukemia: the DNA topoisomerase II inhibitor hypothesis: a report from the children's oncology group. Cancer Epidemiol Biomarkers Prev. 2005;14:651-655.

39. Belson M, Kingsley B, Holmes A. Risk factors for acute leukemia in children: a review. Environ Health Perspect. 2007;115: 138-145.

40. Tedeschi R, Bloigu A, Ogmundsdottir HM, et al. Activation of maternal Epstein-Barr virus infection and risk of acute leukemia in the offspring. Am J Epidemiol. 2007;165:134-137.

41. Kerr JR, Mattey DL, Thomson W, et al. Association of symptomatic acute human parvovirus B19 infection with human leukocyte antigen class I and II alleles. J Infect Dis. 2002;186: 447-452.

42. Kerr JR, Barah F, Cunniffe VS, et al. Association of acute parvovirus B19 infection with new onset of acute lymphoblastic and myeloblastic leukemia. J Clin Pathol. 2003;56:873-875.

43. Kwan ML, Buffler PA, Abrams B, Kiley VA. Breastfeeding and the risk of childhood leukemia: a meta-analysis. Public Health Rep. 2004;119:521-535.

44. Altinkaynak S, Selimoglu MA, Turgut A, et al. Breast-feeding duration and childhood acute leukemia and lymphomas in a sample of Turkish children. J Pediatr Gastroenterol Nutr. 2006;42:568-572.

45. Shu XO, Linet MS, Steinbuch M, et al. Breast-feeding and risk of childhood acute leukemia. J Natl Cancer Inst. 1999;91: 1765-1772.

46. Evrard AS, Hemon D, Billon S, et al. Ecological association between indoor radon concentration and childhood leukaemia incidence in France, 1990-1998. Eur J Cancer Prev. 2005;14: 147-157.

47. Steinbuch M, Weinberg CR, Buckley JD, et al. Indoor residential radon exposure and risk of childhood acute myeloid leukaemia. Br J Cancer. 1999;81:900-906.

48. Shu XO, Gao YT, Linet MS, et al. Chloramphenicol use and childhood leukaemia in Shanghai. Lancet. 1987;2:934-937.

49. Woods WG, Roloff JS, Lukens JN, Krivit W. The occurrence of leukemia in patients with the Shwachman syndrome. J Pediatr. 1981;99:425-428.

50. Wasser JS, Yolken R, Miller DR, Diamond L. Congenital hypoplastic anemia (Diamond-Blackfan syndrome) terminating in acute myelogenous leukemia. Blood. 1978;51:991-995.

51. Freedman MH. Diamond-Blackfan anaemia. Baillieres Best Pract Res Clin Haematol. 2000;13:391-406.

52. Freedman MH, Alter BP. Risk of myelodysplastic syndrome and acute myeloid leukemia in congenital neutropenias. Semin Hematol. 2002;39:128-133.

53. Freedman MH, Bonilla MA, Fier C, et al. Myelodysplasia syndrome and acute myeloid leukemia in patients with congenital neutropenia receiving G-CSF therapy. Blood. 2000;96:429-436.

54. Dror Y, Freedman MH. Shwachman-Diamond syndrome: an inherited preleukemic bone marrow failure disorder with aberrant hematopoietic progenitors and faulty marrow microenvironment. Blood. 1999;94:3048-3054.

55. Dong F, Brynes RK, Tidow N, et al. Mutations in the gene for the granulocyte colony-stimulating-factor receptor in patients with acute myeloid leukemia preceded by severe congenital neutropenia. N Engl J Med. 1995;333:487-493.

56. Cipolli M, D'Orazio C, Delmarco A, et al. Shwachman's syndrome: pathomorphosis and long-term outcome. J Pediatr Gastroenterol Nutr. 1999;29:265-272.

57. Faivre L, Guardiola P, Lewis C, et al. Association of complementation group and mutation type with clinical outcome in fanconi anemia. European Fanconi Anemia Research Group. Blood. 2000;96:4064-4070.

58. Cavenagh JD, Richardson DS, Gibson RA, et al. Fanconi's anaemia presenting as acute myeloid leukaemia in adulthood. Br J Haematol. 1996;94:126-128.

59. Lensch MW, Rathbun RK, Olson SB, et al. Selective pressure as an essential force in molecular evolution of myeloid leukemic clones: a view from the window of Fanconi anemia. Leukemia. 1999;13:1784-1789.

60. Auerbach AD, Allen RG. Leukemia and preleukemia in Fanconi anemia patients. A review of the literature and report of the International Fanconi Anemia Registry. Cancer Genet Cytogenet. 1991;51:1-12.

61. Grasemann H, Kremens B, Passarge E. Experience treating a patient with Bloom syndrome and acute myelogenous leukemia. Med Pediatr Oncol. 1998;30:309-310.

62. Poppe B, Van Limbergen H, Van Roy N, et al. Chromosomal aberrations in Bloom syndrome patients with myeloid malignancies. Cancer Genet Cytogenet. 2001;128:39-42.

63. Aktas D, Koc A, Boduroglu K, et al. Myelodysplastic syndrome associated with monosomy 7 in a child with Bloom syndrome. Cancer Genet Cytogenet. 2000;116:44-46.

64. Side L, Taylor B, Cayouette M, et al. Homozygous inactivation of the NF1 gene in bone marrow cells from children with neurofibromatosis type 1 and malignant myeloid disorders. N Engl J Med. 1997;336:1713-1720.

65. Miles DK, Freedman MH, Stephens K, et al. Patterns of hematopoietic lineage involvement in children with neurofibromatosis type 1 and malignant myeloid disorders. Blood. 1996;88:4314-4320.

66. Shannon KM, O'Connell P, Martin GA, et al. Loss of the normal NF1 allele from the bone marrow of children with type 1 neurofibromatosis and malignant myeloid disorders. N Engl J Med. 1994;330:597-601.

67. Hecht F. Risks of hematologic malignancy with constitutional chromosome abnormalities. Cancer Genet Cytogenet. 1987;24:375-377.

68. Welborn J. Constitutional chromosome aberrations as pathogenetic events in hematologic malignancies. Cancer Genet Cytogenet. 2004;149:137-153.

69. Zipursky A. Transient leukaemia—a benign form of leukaemia in newborn infants with trisomy 21. Br J Haematol. 2003;120:930-938.

70. Lange B. The management of neoplastic disorders of haematopoiesis in children with Down's syndrome. Br J Haematol. 2000;110:512-524.

71. Hasle H, Mellemgaard A, Nielsen J, Hansen J. Cancer incidence in men with Klinefelter syndrome. Br J Cancer. 1995;71:416-420.

72. Horsman DE, Pantzar JT, Dill FJ, Kalousek DK. Klinefelter's syndrome and acute leukemia. Cancer Genet Cytogenet. 1987;26:375-376.

73. Price WH, Clayton JF, Wilson J, et al. Causes of death in X chromatin positive males (Klinefelter's syndrome). J Epidemiol Community Health. 1985;39:330-336.

74. Akashi K, Traver D, Miyamoto T, Weissman IL. A clonogenic common myeloid progenitor that gives rise to all myeloid lineages. Nature. 2000;404:193-197.

75. Look AT. Oncogenic transcription factors in the human acute leukemias. Science. 1997;278:1059-1064.

76. Beutler E, Yeh M, Fairbanks VF. The normal human female as a mosaic of X-chromosome activity: studies using the gene for C-6-PD-deficiency as a marker. Proc Natl Acad Sci U S A. 1962;48:9-16.

77. Fialkow PJ. Use of genetic markers to study cellular origin and development of tumors in human females. Adv Cancer Res. 1972;15:191-226.

78. Fialkow PJ, Gartler SM, Yoshida A. Clonal origin of chronic myelocytic leukemia in man. Proc Natl Acad Sci U S A. 1967;58:1468-1471.

79. Fialkow PJ, Singer JW, Adamson JW, et al. Acute nonlymphocytic leukemia: expression in cells restricted to granulocytic and monocytic differentiation. N Engl J Med. 1979;301:1-5.

80. Fialkow PJ, Singer JW, Adamson JW, et al. Acute nonlymphocytic leukemia: heterogeneity of stem cell origin. Blood. 1981;57:1068-1073.

81. Vogelstein B, Fearon ER, Hamilton SR, Feinberg AP. Use of restriction fragment length polymorphisms to determine the clonal origin of human tumors. Science. 1985;227:642-645.

82. Vogelstein B, Fearon ER, Hamilton SR, et al. Clonal analysis using recombinant DNA probes from the X-chromosome. Cancer Res. 1987;47:4806-4813.

83. Fearon ER, Burke PJ, Schiffer CA, et al. Differentiation of leukemia cells to polymorphonuclear leukocytes in patients with acute nonlymphocytic leukemia. N Engl J Med. 1986;315:15-24.

84. Busque L, Gilliland DG, Prchal JT, et al. Clonality in juvenile chronic myelogenous leukemia. Blood. 1995;85:21-30.

85. Gilliland DG, Blanchard KL, Levy J, et al. Clonality in myeloproliferative disorders: analysis by means of the polymerase chain reaction. Proc Natl Acad Sci U S A. 1991;88:6848-6852.

86. Gilliland DG, Blanchard KL, Bunn HF. Clonality in acquired hematologic disorders. Annu Rev Med. 1991;42:491-506.

87. Bonnet D, Dick JE. Human acute myeloid leukemia is organized as a hierarchy that originates from a primitive hematopoietic cell. Nat Med. 1997;3:730-737.

88. Lapidot T, Sirard C, Vormoor J, et al. A cell initiating human acute myeloid leukaemia after transplantation into SCID mice. Nature. 1994;367:645-648.

89. Al-Hajj M, Wicha MS, Benito-Hernandez A, et al. Prospective identification of tumorigenic breast cancer cells. Proc Natl Acad Sci U S A. 2003;100:3983-3988.

90. Singh SK, Clarke ID, Hide T, Dirks PB. Cancer stem cells in nervous system tumors. Oncogene. 2004;23:7267-7273.

91. Singh SK, Clarke ID, Terasaki M, et al. Identification of a cancer stem cell in human brain tumors. Cancer Res. 2003;63:5821-5828.

92. Singh SK, Hawkins C, Clarke ID, et al. Identification of human brain tumour initiating cells. Nature. 2004;432:396-401.

93. O'Brien CA, Pollett A, Gallinger S, Dick JE. A human colon cancer cell capable of initiating tumour growth in immunodeficient mice. Nature. 2007;445:106-110.

94. Hope KJ, Jin L, Dick JE. Human acute myeloid leukemia stem cells. Arch Med Res. 2003;34:507-514.

95. Fialkow PJ, Singer JW, Raskind WH, et al. Clonal development, stem-cell differentiation, and clinical remissions in acute non-lymphocytic leukemia. N Engl J Med. 1987;317:468-473.

96. Keinanen M, Griffin JD, Bloomfield CD, et al. Clonal chromosomal abnormalities showing multiple-cell-lineage involvement in acute myeloid leukemia. N Engl J Med. 1988;318:1153-1158.

97. van Lom K, Hagemeijer A, Vandekerckhove F, et al. Clonality analysis of hematopoietic cell lineages in acute myeloid leukemia and translocation (8;21): only myeloid cells are part of the malignant clone. Leukemia. 1997;11:202-205.

98. Huang S, Terstappen LW. Formation of haematopoietic microenvironment and haematopoietic stem cells from single human bone marrow stem cells. Nature. 1992;360:745-749.

99. Haase D, Feuring-Buske M, Konemann S, et al. Evidence for malignant transformation in acute myeloid leukemia at the level of early hematopoietic stem cells by cytogenetic analysis of CD34+ subpopulations. Blood. 1995;86:2906-2912.

100. Mehrotra B, George TI, Kavanau K, et al. Cytogenetically aberrant cells in the stem cell compartment (CD34+lin-) in acute myeloid leukemia. Blood. 1995;86:1139-1147.

101. So CW, Karsunky H, Passegue E, et al. MLL-GAS7 transforms multipotent hematopoietic progenitors and induces mixed lineage leukemias in mice. Cancer Cell. 2003;3:161-171.

102. Cozzio A, Passegue E, Ayton PM, et al. Similar MLL-associated leukemias arising from self-renewing stem cells and short-lived myeloid progenitors. Genes Dev. 2003;17:3029-3035.

103. Huntly BJ, Shigematsu H, Deguchi K, et al. MOZ-TIF2, but not BCR-ABL, confers properties of leukemic stem cells to committed murine hematopoietic progenitors. Cancer Cell. 2004;6:587-596.

104. So CW, Lin M, Ayton PM, et al. Dimerization contributes to oncogenic activation of MLL chimeras in acute leukemias. Cancer Cell. 2003;4:99-110.

105. Jamieson CH, Weissman IL, Passegue E. Chronic versus acute myelogenous leukemia: a question of self-renewal. Cancer Cell. 2004;6:531-533.

106. Martinez-Climent JA. Molecular cytogenetics of childhood hematological malignancies. Leukemia. 1997;11:1999-2021.

107. Mrozek K, Heinonen K, de la Chapelle A, Bloomfield CD. Clinical significance of cytogenetics in acute myeloid leukemia. Semin Oncol. 1997;24:17-31.

108. Dash A, Gilliland DG. Molecular genetics of acute myeloid leukaemia. Best Pract Res Clin Haematol. 2001;14:49-64.

109. Gilliland DG. Molecular genetics of human leukemias: new insights into therapy. Semin Hematol. 2002;39:6-11.

110. Frohling S, Scholl C, Gilliland DG, Levine RL. Genetics of myeloid malignancies: pathogenetic and clinical implications. J Clin Oncol. 2005;23:6285-6295.

111. Gilliland DG, Jordan CT, Felix CA. The molecular basis of leukemia. Hematology Am Soc Hematol Educ Program. 2004:80-97.

112. Reya T, Duncan AW, Ailles L, et al. A role for Wnt signalling in self-renewal of haematopoietic stem cells. Nature. 2003; 423:409-414.

113. Simon M, Grandage VL, Linch DC, Khwaja A. Constitutive activation of the Wnt/beta-catenin signalling pathway in acute myeloid leukaemia. Oncogene. 2005;24:2410-2420.

114. Palomero T, McKenna K, O-Neil J, et al. Activating mutations in NOTCH1 in acute myeloid leukemia and lineage switch leukemias. Leukemia. 2006;20:1963-1966.

115. Chiaramonte R, Basile A, Tassi E, et al. A wide role for NOTCH1 signaling in acute leukemia. Cancer Lett. 2005;219: 113-120.

116. Tohda S, Nara N. Expression of Notch1 and Jagged1 proteins in acute myeloid leukemia cells. Leuk Lymphoma. 2001;42: 467-472.

117. Moore MA. Converging pathways in leukemogenesis and stem cell self-renewal. Exp Hematol. 2005;33:719-737.

118. Rice KL, Licht JD. HOX deregulation in acute myeloid leukemia. J Clin Invest. 2007;117:865-868.

119. Thorsteinsdottir U, Kroon E, Jerome L, et al. Defining roles for HOX and MEIS1 genes in induction of acute myeloid leukemia. Mol Cell Biol. 2001;21:224-234.

120. Pedersen-Bjergaard J, Christiansen DH, Desta F, Andersen MK. Alternative genetic pathways and cooperating genetic abnormalities in the pathogenesis of therapy-related myelodysplasia and acute myeloid leukemia. Leukemia. 2006;20:1943-1949.

121. Bos JL. ras oncogenes in human cancer: a review. Cancer Res. 1989;49:4682-4689.

122. Byrne JL, Marshall CJ. The molecular pathophysiology of myeloid leukaemias: Ras revisited. Br J Haematol. 1998;100:256-264.

123. Mohi MG, Williams IR, Dearolf CR, et al. Prognostic, therapeutic, and mechanistic implications of a mouse model of leukemia evoked by Shp2 (PTPN11) mutations. Cancer Cell. 2005;7:179-191.

124. Loh ML, Reynolds MG, Vattikuti S, et al. PTPN11 mutations in pediatric patients with acute myeloid leukemia: results from the Children's Cancer Group. Leukemia. 2004;18:1831-1834.

125. Weijzen S, Velders MP, Kast WM. Modulation of the immune response and tumor growth by activated Ras. Leukemia. 1999;13:502-513.

126. Bollag G, Clapp DW, Shih S, et al. Loss of NF1 results in activation of the Ras signaling pathway and leads to aberrant growth in haematopoietic cells. Nat Genet. 1996;12:144-148.

127. Kalra R, Paderanga DC, Olson K, Shannon KM. Genetic analysis is consistent with the hypothesis that NF1 limits myeloid cell growth through p21ras. Blood. 1994;84:3435-3439.

128. Largaespada DA, Brannan CI, Jenkins NA, Copeland NG. Nf1 deficiency causes Ras-mediated granulocyte/macrophage colony stimulating factor hypersensitivity and chronic myeloid leukaemia. Nat Genet. 1996;12:137-143.

129. Tartaglia M, Niemeyer CM, Shannon KM, Loh ML. SHP-2 and myeloid malignancies. Curr Opin Hematol. 2004;11: 44-50.

130. Hirai H, Kobayashi Y, Mano H, et al. A point mutation at codon 13 of the N-ras oncogene in myelodysplastic syndrome. Nature. 1987;327:430-432.

131. Hirai H, Okada M, Mizoguchi H, et al. Relationship between an activated N-ras oncogene and chromosomal abnormality during leukemic progression from myelodysplastic syndrome. Blood. 1988;71:256-258.

132. Lubbert M, Mirro J Jr, Kitchingman G, et al. Prevalence of N-ras mutations in children with myelodysplastic syndromes and acute myeloid leukemia. Oncogene. 1992;7:263-268.

133. Misawa S, Horiike S, Kaneko H, et al. Significance of chromosomal alterations and mutations of the N-RAS and TP53 genes in relation to leukemogenesis of acute myeloid leukemia. Leuk Res. 1998;22:631-637.

134. Nakagawa T, Saitoh S, Imoto S, et al. Multiple point mutation of N-ras and K-ras oncogenes in myelodysplastic syndrome and acute myelogenous leukemia. Oncology. 1992;49:114-122.

135. Neubauer A, Greenberg P, Negrin R, et al. Mutations in the ras proto-oncogenes in patients with myelodysplastic syndromes. Leukemia. 1994;8:638-641.

136. Paquette RL, Landaw EM, Pierre RV, et al. N-ras mutations are associated with poor prognosis and increased risk of leukemia in myelodysplastic syndrome. Blood. 1993;82:590-599.

137. Vogelstein B, Civin CI, Preisinger AC, et al. RAS gene mutations in childhood acute myeloid leukemia: a Pediatric Oncology Group study. Genes Chromosomes Cancer. 1990;2: 159-162.

138. Bacher U, Haferlach T, Schoch C, et al. Implications of NRAS mutations in AML: a study of 2502 patients. Blood. 2006;107: 3847-3853.

139. Longley BJ, Reguera MJ, Ma Y. Classes of c-KIT activating mutations: proposed mechanisms of action and implications for disease classification and therapy. Leuk Res. 2001;25:571-576.

140. Ikeda H, Kanakura Y, Tamaki T, et al. Expression and functional role of the proto-oncogene c-kit in acute myeloblastic leukemia cells. Blood. 1991;78:2962-2968.

141. Kanakura Y, Ikeda H, Kitayama H, et al. Expression, function and activation of the proto-oncogene c-kit product in human leukemia cells. Leuk Lymphoma. 1993;10:35-41.

142. Broudy VC, Smith FO, Lin N, et al. Blasts from patients with acute myelogenous leukemia express functional receptors for stem cell factor. Blood. 1992;80:60-67.

143. Cole SR, Aylett GW, Harvey NL, et al. Increased expression of c-Kit or its ligand Steel Factor is not a common feature of adult acute myeloid leukaemia. Leukemia. 1996;10:288-296.

144. Tajima F, Kawatani T, Ishiga K, et al. Serum soluble c-kit receptor and expression of c-kit protein and mRNA in acute myeloid leukemia. Eur J Haematol. 1998;60:289-296.

145. Beghini A, Peterlongo P, Ripamonti CB, et al. C-kit mutations in core binding factor leukemias. Blood. 2000;95:726-727.

146. Kiyoi H, Naoe T, Yokota S, et al. Internal tandem duplication of FLT3 associated with leukocytosis in acute promyelocytic leukemia. Leukemia Study Group of the Ministry of Health and Welfare (Kohseisho). Leukemia. 1997;11:1447-1452.

147. Nakao M, Yokota S, Iwai T, et al. Internal tandem duplication of the flt3 gene found in acute myeloid leukemia. Leukemia. 1996;10:1911-1918.

148. Small D, Levenstein M, Kim E, et al. STK-1, the human homolog of Flk-2/Flt-3, is selectively expressed in CD34+ human bone marrow cells and is involved in the proliferation of early progenitor/stem cells. Proc Natl Acad Sci U S A. 1994;91: 459-463.

149. Yamamoto Y, Kiyoi H, Nakano Y, et al. Activating mutation of D835 within the activation loop of FLT3 in human hematologic malignancies. Blood. 2001;97:2434-2439.

150. Yokota S, Kiyoi H, Nakao M, et al. Internal tandem duplication of the FLT3 gene is preferentially seen in acute myeloid leukemia and myelodysplastic syndrome in various hematological malignancies. A study on a large series of patients and cell lines. Leukemia. 1997;11:1605-1609.

151. Abu-Duhier FM, Goodeve AC, Wilson GA, et al. FLT3 internal tandem duplication mutations in adult acute myeloid leukaemia define a high-risk group. Br J Haematol. 2000;111:190-195.

152. Kottaridis PD, Gale RE, Frew ME, et al. The presence of a FLT3 internal tandem duplication in patients with acute myeloid leukemia (AML) adds important prognostic information to cytogenetic risk group and response to the first cycle of chemotherapy: analysis of 854 patients from the United Kingdom Medical Research Council AML 10 and 12 trials. Blood. 2001; 98:1752-1759.

153. Iwai T, Yokota S, Nakao M, et al. Internal tandem duplication of the FLT3 gene and clinical evaluation in childhood acute myeloid leukemia. The Children's Cancer and Leukemia Study Group, Japan. Leukemia. 1999;13:38-43.

154. Meshinchi S, Woods WG, Stirewalt DL, et al. Prevalence and prognostic significance of Flt3 internal tandem duplication in pediatric acute myeloid leukemia. Blood. 2001;97:89-94.

155. Meshinchi S, Alonzo TA, Stirewalt DL, et al. Clinical implications of FLT3 mutations in pediatric AML. Blood. 2006;108: 3654-3661.

156. Kang HJ, Hong SH, Kim IH, et al. Prognostic significance of FLT3 mutations in pediatric non-promyelocytic acute myeloid leukemia. Leuk Res. 2005;29:617-623.

157. Mizuki M, Fenski R, Halfter H, et al. Flt3 mutations from patients with acute myeloid leukemia induce transformation of

158. Kelly LM, Liu Q, Kutok JL, et al. FLT3 internal tandem duplication mutations associated with human acute myeloid leukemias induce myeloproliferative disease in a murine bone marrow transplant model. Blood. 2002;99:310-318.

159. Wang Q, Stacy T, Miller JD, et al. The CBFbeta subunit is essential for CBFalpha2 (AML1) function in vivo. Cell. 1996;87:697-708.

160. Okuda T, van Deursen J, Hiebert SW, et al. AML1, the target of multiple chromosomal translocations in human leukemia, is essential for normal fetal liver hematopoiesis. Cell. 1996;84: 321-330.

161. Wang Q, Stacy T, Binder M, et al. Disruption of the Cbfa2 gene causes necrosis and hemorrhaging in the central nervous system and blocks definitive hematopoiesis. Proc Natl Acad Sci U S A. 1996;93:3444-3449.

162. Sasaki K, Yagi H, Bronson RT, et al. Absence of fetal liver hematopoiesis in mice deficient in transcriptional coactivator core binding factor beta. Proc Natl Acad Sci U S A. 1996;93: 12359-12363.

163. Okuda T, Cai Z, Yang S, et al. Expression of a knocked-in AML1-ETO leukemia gene inhibits the establishment of normal definitive hematopoiesis and directly generates dysplastic hematopoietic progenitors. Blood. 1998;91:3134-3143.

164. Rhoades KL, Hetherington CJ, Harakawa N, et al. Analysis of the role of AML1-ETO in leukemogenesis, using an inducible transgenic mouse model. Blood. 2000;96:2108-2115.

165. Yergeau DA, Hetherington CJ, Wang Q, et al. Embryonic lethality and impairment of haematopoiesis in mice heterozygous for an AML1-ETO fusion gene. Nat Genet. 1997;15: 303-306.

166. Gelmetti V, Zhang J, Fanelli M, et al. Aberrant recruitment of the nuclear receptor corepressor-histone deacetylase complex by the acute myeloid leukemia fusion partner ETO. Mol Cell Biol. 1998;18:7185-7191.

167. Westendorf JJ, Yamamoto CM, Lenny N, et al. The t(8;21) fusion product, AML-1-ETO, associates with C/EBP-alpha, inhibits C/EBP-alpha-dependent transcription, and blocks granulocytic differentiation. Mol Cell Biol. 1998;18: 322-333.

168. Schessl C, Rawat VP, Cusan M, et al. The AML1-ETO fusion gene and the FLT3 length mutation collaborate in inducing acute leukemia in mice. J Clin Invest. 2005;115:2159-2168.

169. Elliott S, Taylor K, White S, et al. Proof of differentiative mode of action of all-trans retinoic acid in acute promyelocytic leukemia using X-linked clonal analysis. Blood. 1992;79: 1916-1919.

170. Huang ME, Ye YC, Chen SR, et al. Use of all-trans retinoic acid in the treatment of acute promyelocytic leukemia. Blood. 1988;72:567-572.

171. Chomienne C, Ballerini P, Balitrand N, et al. The retinoic acid receptor alpha gene is rearranged in retinoic acid-sensitive promyelocytic leukemias. Leukemia. 1990;4:802-807.

172. de The H, Chomienne C, Lanotte M, et al. The t(15;17) translocation of acute promyelocytic leukaemia fuses the retinoic acid receptor alpha gene to a novel transcribed locus. Nature. 1990;347:558-561.

173. Kakizuka A, Miller WH Jr, Umesono K, et al. Chromosomal translocation t(15;17) in human acute promyelocytic leukemia fuses RAR alpha with a novel putative transcription factor, PML. Cell. 1991;66:663-674.

174. Lemons RS, Eilender D, Waldmann RA, et al. Cloning and characterization of the t(15;17) translocation breakpoint region in acute promyelocytic leukemia. Genes Chromosomes Cancer. 1990;2:79-87.

175. Longo L, Pandolfi PP, Biondi A, et al. Rearrangements and aberrant expression of the retinoic acid receptor alpha gene in

acute promyelocytic leukemias. J Exp Med. 1990;172:1571-1575.

176. Miller WH Jr, Warrell RP Jr, Frankel SR, et al. Novel retinoic acid receptor-alpha transcripts in acute promyelocytic leukemia responsive to all-trans-retinoic acid. J Natl Cancer Inst. 1990;82:1932-1933.

177. Chen Z, Brand NJ, Chen A, et al. Fusion between a novel Kruppel-like zinc finger gene and the retinoic acid receptor-alpha locus because ofa variant t(11;17) translocation associated with acute promyelocytic leukaemia. EMBO J. 1993;12:1161-1167.

178. Redner RL, Rush EA, Faas S, et al. The t(5;17) variant of acute promyelocytic leukemia expresses a nucleophosmin-retinoic acid receptor fusion. Blood. 1996;87:882-886.

179. Evans RM. The steroid and thyroid hormone receptor superfamily. Science. 1988;240:889-895.

180. Yu VC, Delsert C, Andersen B, et al. RXR beta: a coregulator that enhances binding of retinoic acid, thyroid hormone, and vitamin D receptors to their cognate response elements. Cell. 1991;67:1251-1266.

181. Alland L, Muhle R, Hou H Jr, et al. Role for N-CoR and histone deacetylase in Sin3-mediated transcriptional repression. Nature. 1997;387:49-55.

182. Laherty CD, Yang WM, Sun JM, et al. Histone deacetylases associated with the mSin3 corepressor mediate mad transcriptional repression. Cell. 1997;89:349-356.

183. Heinzel T, Lavinsky RM, Mullen TM, et al. A complex containing N-CoR, mSin3 and histone deacetylase mediates transcriptional repression. Nature. 1997;387:43-48.

184. Tsai S, Collins SJ. A dominant negative retinoic acid receptor blocks neutrophil differentiation at the promyelocyte stage. Proc Natl Acad Sci U S A. 1993;90:7153-7157.

185. Salomoni P, Pandolfi PP. The role of PML in tumor suppression. Cell. 2002;108:165-170.

186. Dyck JA, Maul GG, Miller WH Jr, et al. A novel macromolecular structure is a target of the promyelocyte-retinoic acid receptor oncoprotein. Cell. 1994;76:333-343.

187. Weis K, Rambaud S, Lavau C, et al. Retinoic acid regulates aberrant nuclear localization of PML-RAR alpha in acute promyelocytic leukemia cells. Cell. 1994;76:345-356.

188. Zhang TD, Chen GQ, Wang ZG, et al. Arsenic trioxide, a therapeutic agent for APL. Oncogene. 2001;20:7146-7153.

189. Shen ZX, Chen GQ, Ni JH, et al. Use of arsenic trioxide (As₂O₃) in the treatment of acute promyelocytic leukemia (APL): II. Clinical efficacy and pharmacokinetics in relapsed patients. Blood. 1997;89:3354-3360.

190. Shao W, Fanelli M, Ferrara FF, et al. Arsenic trioxide as an inducer of apoptosis and loss of PML/RAR alpha protein in acute promyelocytic leukemia cells. J Natl Cancer Inst. 1998;90:124-133.

191. Zhu J, Gianni M, Kopf E, et al. Retinoic acid induces proteasome-dependent degradation of retinoic acid receptor alpha (RARalpha) and oncogenic RARalpha fusion proteins. Proc Natl Acad Sci U S A. 1999;96:14807-14812.

192. Liu TX, Zhang JW, Tao J, et al. Gene expression networks underlying retinoic acid-induced differentiation of acute promyelocytic leukemia cells. Blood. 2000;96:1496-1504.

193. Koken MH, Puvion-Dutilleul F, Guillemin MC, et al. The t(15;17) translocation alters a nuclear body in a retinoic acid-reversible fashion. EMBO J. 1994;13:1073-1083.

194. Look AT. Arsenic and apoptosis in the treatment of acute promyelocytic leukemia. J Natl Cancer Inst. 1998;90:86-88.

195. Chen GQ, Zhu J, Shi XG, et al. In vitro studies on cellular and molecular mechanisms of arsenic trioxide (As₂O₃) in the treatment of acute promyelocytic leukemia: As₂O₃ induces NB4 cell apoptosis with downregulation of Bcl-2 expression and modulation of PML-RAR alpha/PML proteins. Blood. 1996;88:1052-1061.

196. Chen GQ, Shi XG, Tang W, et al. Use of arsenic trioxide (As₂O₃) in the treatment of acute promyelocytic leukemia (APL): I. As₂O₃ exerts dose-dependent dual effects on APL cells. Blood. 1997;89:3345-3353.

197. Brown D, Kogan S, Lagasse E, et al. A PMLRARalpha transgene initiates murine acute promyelocytic leukemia. Proc Natl Acad Sci U S A. 1997;94:2551-2556.

198. He LZ, Tribioli C, Rivi R, et al. Acute leukemia with promyelocytic features in PML/RARalpha transgenic mice. Proc Natl Acad Sci U S A. 1997;94:5302-5307.

199. Ernst P, Fisher JK, Avery W, et al. Definitive hematopoiesis requires the mixed-lineage leukemia gene. Dev Cell. 2004;6:437-443.

200. Hess JL, Yu BD, Li B, et al. Defects in yolk sac hematopoiesis in Mll-null embryos. Blood. 1997;90:1799-1806.

201. Yu BD, Hess JL, Horning SE, et al. Altered Hox expression and segmental identity in Mll-mutant mice. Nature. 1995;378:505-508.

202. Armstrong SA, Staunton JE, Silverman LB, et al. MLL translocations specify a distinct gene expression profile that distinguishes a unique leukemia. Nat Genet. 2002;30:41-47.

203. Rowley JD. The role of chromosome translocations in leukemogenesis. Semin Hematol. 1999;36:59-72.

204. Langmuir PB, Aplenc R, Lange BJ. Acute myeloid leukaemia in children. Best Pract Res Clin Haematol. 2001;14:77-93.

205. Basecke J, Whelan JT, Griesinger F, Bertrand FE. The MLL partial tandem duplication in acute myeloid leukaemia. Br J Haematol. 2006;135:438-449.

206. Ferrando AA, Armstrong SA, Neuberg DS, et al. Gene expression signatures in MLL-rearranged T-lineage and B-precursor acute leukemias: dominance of HOX dysregulation. Blood. 2003;102:262-268.

207. Hsu K, Look AT. Turning on a dimer: new insights into MLL chimeras. Cancer Cell. 2003;4:81-83.

208. Ayton PM, Cleary ML. Molecular mechanisms of leukemogenesis mediated by MLL fusion proteins. Oncogene. 2001;20:5695-5707.

209. Milne TA, Briggs SD, Brock HW, et al. MLL targets SET domain methyltransferase activity to Hox gene promoters. Mol Cell. 2002;10:1107-1117.

210. Golub TR, Slonim DK, Tamayo P, et al. Molecular classification of cancer: class discovery and class prediction by gene expression monitoring. Science. 1999;286:531-537.

211. Kroon E, Krosl J, Thorsteinsdottir U, et al. Hoxa9 transforms primary bone marrow cells through specific collaboration with Meis1a but not Pbx1b. Embo J. 1998;17:3714-3725.

212. Kroon E, Thorsteinsdottir U, Mayotte N, et al. NUP98-HOXA9 expression in hemopoietic stem cells induces chronic and acute myeloid leukemias in mice. EMBO J. 2001;20:350-361.

213. Borrow J, Shearman AM, Stanton VP Jr, et al. The t(7;11)(p15;p15) translocation in acute myeloid leukaemia fuses the genes for nucleoporin NUP98 and class I homeoprotein HOXA9. Nat Genet. 1996;12:159-167.

214. Kawagoe H, Humphries RK, Blair A, et al. Expression of HOX genes, HOX cofactors, and MLL in phenotypically and functionally defined subpopulations of leukemic and normal human hematopoietic cells. Leukemia. 1999;13:687-698.

215. Lawrence HJ, Helgason CD, Sauvageau G, et al. Mice bearing a targeted interruption of the homeobox gene HOXA9 have defects in myeloid, erythroid, and lymphoid hematopoiesis. Blood. 1997;89:1922-1930.

216. Soejima K, Ishizaka A, Urano T, et al. Protective effect of B464, a lipid A analog, on endotoxin-induced cellular responses and acute lung injury. Am J Respir Crit Care Med. 1996;154:900-906.

217. Nakamura T, Largaespada DA, Lee MP, et al. Fusion of the nucleoporin gene NUP98 to HOXA9 by the chromosome

translocation t(7;11)(p15;p15) in human myeloid leukaemia. Nat Genet. 1996;12:154-158.

218. Roche J, Zeng C, Baron A, et al. Hox expression in AML identifies a distinct subset of patients with intermediate cytogenetics. Leukemia. 2004;18:1059-1063.

219. Raimondi SC, Chang MN, Ravindranath Y, et al. Chromosomal abnormalities in 478 children with acute myeloid leukemia: clinical characteristics and treatment outcome in a cooperative pediatric oncology group study-POG 8821. Blood. 1999;94: 3707-3716.

220. Martinez-Climent JA, Espinosa R 3rd, Thirman MJ, et al. Abnormalities of chromosome band 11q23 and the MLL gene in pediatric myelomonocytic and monoblastic leukemias. Identification of the t(9;11) as an indicator of long survival. J Pediatr Hematol Oncol. 1995;17:277-283.

221. Cortes J, O'Brien S, Kantarjian H, et al. Abnormalities in the long arm of chromosome 11 (11q) in patients with de novo and secondary acute myelogenous leukemias and myelodysplastic syndromes. Leukemia. 1994;8:2174-2178.

222. Whitman SP, Liu S, Vukosavljevic T, et al. The MLL partial tandem duplication: evidence for recessive gain-of-function in acute myeloid leukemia identifies a novel patient subgroup for molecular-targeted therapy. Blood. 2005;106: 345-352.

223. Roulston D, Espinosa R 3rd, Stoffel M, et al. Molecular genetics of myeloid leukemia: identification of the commonly deleted segment of chromosome 20. Blood. 1993;82:3424-3429.

224. Le Beau MM, Espinosa R 3rd, Neuman WL, et al. Cytogenetic and molecular delineation of the smallest commonly deleted region of chromosome 5 in malignant myeloid diseases. Proc Natl Acad Sci U S A. 1993;90:5484-5488.

225. Johansson B, Mertens F, Mitelman F. Cytogenetic deletion maps of hematologic neoplasms: circumstantial evidence for tumor suppressor loci. Genes Chromosomes Cancer. 1993;8: 205-218.

226. Liu TX, Becker MW, Jelinek J, et al. Chromosome 5q deletion and epigenetic suppression of the gene encoding alpha-catenin (CTNNA1) in myeloid cell transformation. Nat Med. 2007;13: 78-83.

227. Fenaux P, Morel P, Lai JL. Cytogenetics of myelodysplastic syndromes. Semin Hematol. 1996;33:127-138.

228. Luna-Fineman S, Shannon KM, Atwater SK, et al. Myelodysplastic and myeloproliferative disorders of childhood: a study of 167 patients. Blood. 1999;93:459-466.

229. Luna-Fineman S, Shannon KM, Lange BJ. Childhood monosomy 7: epidemiology, biology, and mechanistic implications. Blood. 1995;85:1985-1999.

230. Pedersen-Bjergaard J, Andersen MK, Christiansen DH, Nerlov C. Genetic pathways in therapy-related myelodysplasia and acute myeloid leukemia. Blood. 2002;99:1909-1912.

231. Pui CH, Raimondi SC, Crist WM. Secondary leukaemias after epipodophyllotoxins. Lancet. 1992;340:672-673.

232. Pui CH, Relling MV. Topoisomerase II inhibitor-related acute myeloid leukaemia. Br J Haematol. 2000;109:13-23.

233. Le Beau MM, Albain KS, Larson RA, et al. Clinical and cytogenetic correlations in 63 patients with therapy-related myelodysplastic syndromes and acute nonlymphocytic leukemia: further evidence for characteristic abnormalities of chromosomes no. 5 and 7. J Clin Oncol. 1986;4:325-345.

234. Whang-Peng J, Young RC, Lee EC, et al. Cytogenetic studies in patients with secondary leukemia/dysmyelopoietic syndrome after different treatment modalities. Blood. 1988;71:403-414.

235. Tenen DG. Disruption of differentiation in human cancer: AML shows the way. Nat Rev Cancer. 2003;3:89-101.

236. Rosenbauer F, Wagner K, Kutok JL, et al. Acute myeloid leukemia induced by graded reduction of a lineage-specific transcription factor, PU.1. Nat Genet. 2004;36:624-630.

237. Wechsler J, Greene M, McDevitt MA, et al. Acquired mutations in GATA1 in the megakaryoblastic leukemia of Down syndrome. Nat Genet. 2002;32:148-152.

238. Hedenfalk I, Duggan D, Chen Y, et al. Gene-expression profiles in hereditary breast cancer. N Engl J Med. 2001;344:539-548.

239. Perou CM, Sorlie T, Eisen MB, et al. Molecular portraits of human breast tumours. Nature. 2000;406:747-752.

240. Sorlie T, Perou CM, Tibshirani R, et al. Gene expression patterns of breast carcinomas distinguish tumor subclasses with clinical implications. Proc Natl Acad Sci U S A. 2001;98: 10869-10874.

241. West M, Blanchette C, Dressman H, et al. Predicting the clinical status of human breast cancer by using gene expression profiles. Proc Natl Acad Sci U S A. 2001;98:11462-11467.

242. Alizadeh AA, Eisen MB, Davis RE, et al. Distinct types of diffuse large B-cell lymphoma identified by gene expression profiling. Nature. 2000;403:503-511.

243. Valk PJ, Verhaak RG, Beijen MA, et al. Prognostically useful gene-expression profiles in acute myeloid leukemia. N Engl J Med. 2004;350:1617-1628.

244. Bullinger L, Dohner K, Bair E, et al. Use of gene-expression profiling to identify prognostic subclasses in adult acute myeloid leukemia. N Engl J Med. 2004;350:1605-1616.

245. Yagi T, Morimoto A, Eguchi M, et al. Identification of a gene expression signature associated with pediatric AML prognosis. Blood. 2003;102:1849-1856.

246. Falini B, Mecucci C, Tiacci E, et al. Cytoplasmic nucleophosmin in acute myelogenous leukemia with a normal karyotype. N Engl J Med. 2005;352:254-266.

247. Cazzaniga G, Dell'Oro MG, Mecucci C, et al. Nucleophosmin mutations in childhood acute myelogenous leukemia with normal karyotype. Blood. 2005;106:1419-1422.

248. Brown P, McIntyre E, Rau R, et al. The incidence and clinical significance of nucleophosmin mutations in childhood AML. Blood. 2007;110:979-985.

249. Buccisano F, Maurillo L, Gattei V, et al. The kinetics of reduction of minimal residual disease impacts on duration of response and survival of patients with acute myeloid leukemia. Leukemia. 2006;20:1783-1789.

250. Laane E, Derolf AR, Bjorklund E, et al. The effect of allogeneic stem cell transplantation on outcome in younger acute myeloid leukemia patients with minimal residual disease detected by flow cytometry at the end of post-remission chemotherapy. Haematologica. 2006;91:833-836.

251. Maurillo L, Buccisano F, Spagnoli A, et al. Monitoring of minimal residual disease in adult acute myeloid leukemia using peripheral blood as an alternative source to bone marrow. Haematologica. 2007;92:605-611.

252. Feller N, van der Pol MA, van Stijn A, et al. MRD parameters using immunophenotypic detection methods are highly reliable in predicting survival in acute myeloid leukaemia. Leukemia. 2004;18:1380-1390.

253. Kern W, Voskova D, Schnittger S, et al. Four-fold staining including CD45 gating improves the sensitivity of multiparameter flow cytometric assessment of minimal residual disease in patients with acute myeloid leukemia. Hematol J. 2004;5:410-418.

254. Kern W, Voskova D, Schoch C, et al. Determination of relapse risk based on assessment of minimal residual disease during complete remission by multiparameter flow cytometry in unselected patients with acute myeloid leukemia. Blood. 2004;104:3078-3085.

255. Kern W, Voskova D, Schoch C, et al. Prognostic impact of early response to induction therapy as assessed by multiparameter flow cytometry in acute myeloid leukemia. Haematologica. 2004;89:528-540.

256. Perea G, Lasa A, Aventin A, et al. Prognostic value of minimal residual disease (MRD) in acute myeloid leukemia (AML) with

favorable cytogenetics [t(8;21) and inv(16)]. Leukemia. 2006; 20:87-94.

257. Coustan-Smith E, Ribeiro RC, Rubnitz JE, et al. Clinical significance of residual disease during treatment in childhood acute myeloid leukaemia. Br J Haematol. 2003;123:243-252.

258. Sievers EL, Lange BJ, Alonzo TA, et al. Immunophenotypic evidence of leukemia after induction therapy predicts relapse: results from a prospective Children's Cancer Group study of 252 patients with acute myeloid leukemia. Blood. 2003;101: 3398-3406.

259. Creutzig U, Harbott J, Sperling C, et al. Clinical significance of surface antigen expression in children with acute myeloid leukemia: results of study AML-BFM-87. Blood. 1995;86: 3097-3108.

260. Jennings CD, Foon KA. Recent advances in flow cytometry: application to the diagnosis of hematologic malignancy. Blood. 1997;90:2863-2892.

261. van't Veer MB. The diagnosis of acute leukemia with undifferentiated or minimally differentiated blasts. Ann Hematol. 1992;64:161-165.

262. Bennett JM, Catovsky D, Daniel MT, et al. Proposal for the recognition of minimally differentiated acute myeloid leukaemia (AML-MO). Br J Haematol. 1991;78:325-329.

263. Bennett JM, Catovsky D, Daniel MT, et al. Criteria for the diagnosis of acute leukemia of megakaryocyte lineage (M7). A report of the French-American-British Cooperative Group. Ann Intern Med. 1985;103:460-462.

264. Cuneo A, Ferrant A, Michaux JL, et al. Clinical review on features and cytogenetic patterns in adult acute myeloid leukemia with lymphoid markers. Leuk Lymphoma. 1993;9:285-291.

265. Cuneo A, Michaux JL, Ferrant A, et al. Correlation of cytogenetic patterns and clinicobiological features in adult acute myeloid leukemia expressing lymphoid markers. Blood. 1992;79: 720-727.

266. Paietta E, Van Ness B, Bennett J, et al. Lymphoid lineage-associated features in acute myeloid leukaemia: phenotypic and genotypic correlations. Br J Haematol. 1992;82:324-331.

267. Harris NL, Jaffe ES, Diebold J, et al. The World Health Organization classification of neoplastic diseases of the hematopoietic and lymphoid tissues. Report of the Clinical Advisory Committee meeting, Airlie House, Virginia, November, 1997. Ann Oncol. 1999;10:1419-1432.

268. Grimwade D, Walker H, Oliver F, et al. The importance of diagnostic cytogenetics on outcome in AML: analysis of 1,612 patients entered into the MRC AML 10 trial. The Medical Research Council Adult and Children's Leukaemia Working Parties. Blood. 1998;92:2322-2333.

269. Bloomfield CD, Lawrence D, Byrd JC, et al. Frequency of prolonged remission duration after high-dose cytarabine intensification in acute myeloid leukemia varies by cytogenetic subtype. Cancer Res. 1998;58:4173-4179.

270. Keating MJ, Smith TL, Kantarjian H, et al. Cytogenetic pattern in acute myelogenous leukemia: a major reproducible determinant of outcome. Leukemia. 1988;2:403-412.

271. Fenaux P, Preudhomme C, Lai JL, et al. Cytogenetics and their prognostic value in de novo acute myeloid leukaemia: a report on 283 cases. Br J Haematol. 1989;73:61-67.

272. Marosi C, Koller U, Koller-Weber E, et al. Prognostic impact of karyotype and immunologic phenotype in 125 adult patients with de novo AML. Cancer Genet Cytogenet. 1992;61:14-25.

273. Dastugue N, Payen C, Lafage-Pochitaloff M, et al. Prognostic significance of karyotype in de novo adult acute myeloid leukemia. The BGMT group. Leukemia. 1995;9:1491-1498.

274. Bloomfield CD, Shuma C, Regal L, et al. Long-term survival of patients with acute myeloid leukemia: a third follow-up of the Fourth International Workshop on Chromosomes in Leukemia. Cancer. 1997;80:2191-2198.

275. Mehta J, Powles R, Treleaven J, et al. The impact of karyotype on remission rates in adult patients with de novo acute myeloid leukemia receiving high-dose cytarabine-based induction chemotherapy. Leuk Lymphoma. 1999;34:553-560.

276. Wells RJ, Arthur DC, Srivastava A, et al. Prognostic variables in newly diagnosed children and adolescents with acute myeloid leukemia: Children's Cancer Group Study 213. Leukemia. 2002;16:601-607.

277. Satake N, Maseki N, Nishiyama M, et al. Chromosome abnormalities and MLL rearrangements in acute myeloid leukemia of infants. Leukemia. 1999;13:1013-1017.

278. Pui CH, Raimondi SC, Srivastava DK, et al. Prognostic factors in infants with acute myeloid leukemia. Leukemia. 2000;14: 684-687.

279. Chessells JM, Harrison CJ, Kempski H, et al. Clinical features, cytogenetics and outcome in acute lymphoblastic and myeloid leukaemia of infancy: report from the MRC Childhood Leukaemia working party. Leukemia. 2002;16:776-784.

280. Bernstein ID. Monoclonal antibodies to the myeloid stem cells: therapeutic implications of CMA-676, a humanized anti-CD33 antibody calicheamicin conjugate. Leukemia. 2000;14:474-475.

281. Mercher T, Coniat MB, Monni R, et al. Involvement of a human gene related to the Drosophila spen gene in the recurrent t(1;22) translocation of acute megakaryocytic leukemia. Proc Natl Acad Sci U S A. 2001;98:5776-5779.

282. Bennett JM, Catovsky D, Daniel MT, et al. Proposals for the classification of the acute leukaemias. French-American-British (FAB) co-operative group. Br J Haematol. 1976;33: 451-458.

283. Bennett JM, Catovsky D, Daniel MT, et al. Proposed revised criteria for the classification of acute myeloid leukemia. A report of the French-American-British Cooperative Group. Ann Intern Med. 1985;103:620-625.

284. Drexler HG, Minowada J. The use of monoclonal antibodies for the identification and classification of acute myeloid leukemias. Leuk Res. 1986;10:279-290.

285. Cuneo A, Ferrant A, Michaux JL, et al. Cytogenetic profile of minimally differentiated (FAB M0) acute myeloid leukemia: correlation with clinicobiologic findings. Blood. 1995;85: 3688-3694.

286. Harris NL, Jaffe ES, Diebold J, et al. World Health Organization classification of neoplastic diseases of the hematopoietic and lymphoid tissues: report of the Clinical Advisory Committee meeting-Airlie House, Virginia, November 1997. J Clin Oncol. 1999;17:3835-3849.

287. Choi SI, Simone JV. Acute nonlymphocytic leukemia in 171 children. Med Pediatr Oncol. 1976;2:119-146.

288. Bunin NJ, Kunkel K, Callihan TR. Cytoreductive procedures in the early management in cases of leukemia and hyperleukocytosis in children. Med Pediatr Oncol. 1987;15:232-235.

289. Creutzig U, Ritter J, Budde M, et al. Early deaths because ofhemorrhage and leukostasis in childhood acute myelogenous leukemia. Associations with hyperleukocytosis and acute monocytic leukemia. Cancer. 1987;60:3071-3079.

290. Frohling S, Schlenk RF, Breitruck J, et al. Prognostic significance of activating FLT3 mutations in younger adults (16 to 60 years) with acute myeloid leukemia and normal cytogenetics: a study of the AML Study Group Ulm. Blood. 2002;100: 4372-4380.

291. Gilliland DG, Griffin JD. Role of FLT3 in leukemia. Curr Opin Hematol. 2002;9:274-281.

292. Menell JS, Cesarman GM, Jacovina AT, et al. Annexin II and bleeding in acute promyelocytic leukemia. N Engl J Med. 1999;340:994-1004.

293. Drapkin RL, Gee TS, Dowling MD, et al. Prophylactic heparin therapy in acute promyelocytic leukemia. Cancer. 1978;41: 2484-2490.

294. Gralnick HR, Bagley J, Abrell E. Heparin treatment for the hemorrhagic diathesis of acute promyelocytic leukemia. Am J Med. 1972;52:167-174.

295. Bapna A, Nair R, Tapan KS, et al. All-trans-retinoic acid (ATRA): pediatric acute promyelocytic leukemia. Pediatr Hematol Oncol. 1998;15:243-248.

296. Castaigne S, Chomienne C, Daniel MT, et al. All-trans retinoic acid as a differentiation therapy for acute promyelocytic leukemia. I. Clinical results. Blood. 1990;76:1704-1709.

297. Degos L, Dombret H, Chomienne C, et al. All-trans-retinoic acid as a differentiating agent in the treatment of acute promyelocytic leukemia. Blood. 1995;85:2643-2653.

298. Fenaux P, Chomienne C, Degos L. All-trans retinoic acid and chemotherapy in the treatment of acute promyelocytic leukemia. Semin Hematol. 2001;38:13-25.

299. Cuttner J, Holland JF, Norton L, et al. Therapeutic leukapheresis for hyperleukocytosis in acute myelocytic leukemia. Med Pediatr Oncol. 1983;11:76-78.

300. Ablin AR. Supportive care for children with cancer. Guidelines of the Children's Cancer Study Group. Managing the problem of hyperleukocytosis in acute leukemia. Am J Pediatr Hematol Oncol. 1984;6:287-290.

301. Thiebaut A, Thomas X, Belhabri A, et al. Impact of pre-induction therapy leukapheresis on treatment outcome in adult acute myelogenous leukemia presenting with hyperleukocytosis. Ann Hematol. 2000;79:501-506.

302. Ventura GJ, Hester JP, Smith TL, Keating MJ. Acute myeloblastic leukemia with hyperleukocytosis: risk factors for early mortality in induction. Am J Hematol. 1988;27:34-37.

303. Kobayashi R, Tawa A, Hanada R, et al. Extramedullary infiltration at diagnosis and prognosis in children with acute myelogenous leukemia. Pediatr Blood Cancer. 2007;48:393-398.

304. Brown LM, Daeschner C 3rd, Timms J, Crow W. Granulocytic sarcoma in childhood acute myelogenous leukemia. Pediatr Neurol. 1989;5:173-178.

305. Pui CH, Kalwinsky DK, Schell MJ, et al. Acute nonlymphoblastic leukemia in infants: clinical presentation and outcome. J Clin Oncol. 1988;6:1008-1013.

306. Pui CH, Dahl GV, Kalwinsky DK, et al. Central nervous system leukemia in children with acute nonlymphoblastic leukemia. Blood. 1985;66:1062-1067.

307. Grier HE, Gelber RD, Link MP, et al. Intensive sequential chemotherapy for children with acute myelogenous leukemia: VAPA, 80-035, and HI-C-Daze. Leukemia. 1992;6(Suppl 2): 48-51.

308. Dahl GV, Simone JV, Hustu HO, Mason C. Preventive central nervous system irradiation in children with acute nonlymphocytic leukemia. Cancer. 1978;42:2187-2192.

309. Creutzig U, Ritter J, Zimmermann M, Schellong G. Does cranial irradiation reduce the risk for bone marrow relapse in acute myelogenous leukemia? Unexpected results of the Childhood Acute Myelogenous Leukemia Study BFM-87. J Clin Oncol. 1993;11:279-286.

310. Bisschop MM, Revesz T, Bierings M, et al. Extramedullary infiltrates at diagnosis have no prognostic significance in children with acute myeloid leukaemia. Leukemia. 2001;15:46-49.

311. Economopoulos T, Alexopoulos C, Anagnostou D, et al. Primary granulocytic sarcoma of the testis. Leukemia. 1994;8: 199-200.

312. Giagounidis AA, Hildebrandt B, Braunstein S, et al. Testicular infiltration in acute myeloid leukemia with complex karyotype including t(8;21). Ann Hematol. 2002;81:115-118.

313. Byrd JC, Edenfield WJ, Shields DJ, Dawson NA. Extramedullary myeloid cell tumors in acute nonlymphocytic leukemia: a clinical review. J Clin Oncol. 1995;13:1800-1816.

314. Tallman MS, Hakimian D, Shaw JM, et al. Granulocytic sarcoma is associated with the 8;21 translocation in acute myeloid leukemia. J Clin Oncol. 1993;11:690-697.

315. Rai KR, Holland JF, Glidewell OJ, et al. Treatment of acute myelocytic leukemia: a study by cancer and leukemia group B. Blood. 1981;58:1203-1212.

316. Rowe JM, Tallman MS. Intensifying induction therapy in acute myeloid leukemia: has a new standard of care emerged? Blood. 1997;90:2121-2126.

317. Rowe JM. What is the best induction regimen for acute myelogenous leukemia? Leukemia. 1998;12(Suppl 1):S16-19.

318. Wells RJ, Woods WG, Buckley JD, et al. Treatment of newly diagnosed children and adolescents with acute myeloid leukemia: a Children's Cancer Group study. J Clin Oncol. 1994;12: 2367-2377.

319. Woods WG, Kobrinsky N, Buckley JD, et al. Timed-sequential induction therapy improves postremission outcome in acute myeloid leukemia: a report from the Children's Cancer Group. Blood. 1996;87:4979-4989.

320. AML Collaborative Group. A systematic collaborative overview of randomized trials comparing idarubicin with daunorubicin (or other anthracyclines) as induction therapy for acute myeloid leukaemia. Br J Haematol. 1998;103:100-109.

321. Lange BJ, Dinndorf P, Smith FO, et al. Pilot study of idarubicin-based intensive-timing induction therapy for children with previously untreated acute myeloid leukemia: Children's Cancer Group Study 2941. J Clin Oncol. 2004;22:150-156.

322. Gibson BE, Wheatley K, Hann IM, et al. Treatment strategy and long-term results in paediatric patients treated in consecutive UK AML trials. Leukemia. 2005;19:2130-2138.

323. Stevens RF, Hann IM, Wheatley K, Gray RG. Marked improvements in outcome with chemotherapy alone in paediatric acute myeloid leukemia: results of the United Kingdom Medical Research Council's 10th AML trial. MRC Childhood Leukaemia Working Party. Br J Haematol. 1998;101:130-140.

324. Bernstein ID, Singer JW, Andrews RG, et al. Treatment of acute myeloid leukemia cells in vitro with a monoclonal antibody recognizing a myeloid differentiation antigen allows normal progenitor cells to be expressed. J Clin Invest. 1987;79:1153-1159.

325. Dinndorf PA, Buckley JD, Nesbit ME, et al. Expression of myeloid differentiation antigens in acute nonlymphocytic leukemia: increased concentration of CD33 antigen predicts poor outcome—a report from the Children's Cancer Study Group. Med Pediatr Oncol. 1992;20:192-200.

326. Weick JK, Kopecky KJ, Appelbaum FR, et al. A randomized investigation of high-dose versus standard-dose cytosine arabinoside with daunorubicin in patients with previously untreated acute myeloid leukemia: a Southwest Oncology Group study. Blood. 1996;88:2841-2851.

327. Bishop JF, Matthews JP, Young GA, et al. A randomized study of high-dose cytarabine in induction in acute myeloid leukemia. Blood. 1996;87:1710-1717.

328. San Miguel JF, Vidriales MB, Lopez-Berges C, et al. Early immunophenotypical evaluation of minimal residual disease in acute myeloid leukemia identifies different patient risk groups and may contribute to postinduction treatment stratification. Blood. 2001;98:1746-1751.

329. San Miguel JF, Martinez A, Macedo A, et al. Immunophenotyping investigation of minimal residual disease is a useful approach for predicting relapse in acute myeloid leukemia patients. Blood. 1997;90:2465-2470.

330. Cassileth PA, Andersen JW, Bennett JM, et al. Escalating the intensity of post-remission therapy improves the outcome in acute myeloid leukemia: the ECOG experience. The Eastern Cooperative Oncology Group. Leukemia. 1992;6(Suppl 2): 116-119.

331. Cassileth PA, Begg CB, Silber R, et al. Prolonged unmaintained remission after intensive consolidation therapy in adult acute nonlymphocytic leukemia. Cancer Treat Rep. 1987;71:137-140.

332. Cassileth PA, Lynch E, Hines JD, et al. Varying intensity of postremission therapy in acute myeloid leukemia. Blood. 1992;79:1924-1930.

333. Ball ED, Wilson J, Phelps V, Neudorf S. Autologous bone marrow transplantation for acute myeloid leukemia in remission or first relapse using monoclonal antibody-purged marrow: results of phase II studies with long-term follow-up. Bone Marrow Transplant. 2000;25:823-829.

334. Cassileth PA, Harrington DP, Appelbaum FR, et al. Chemotherapy compared with autologous or allogeneic bone marrow transplantation in the management of acute myeloid leukemia in first remission. N Engl J Med. 1998;339:1649-1656.

335. Ravindranath Y, Yeager AM, Chang MN, et al. Autologous bone marrow transplantation versus intensive consolidation chemotherapy for acute myeloid leukemia in childhood. Pediatric Oncology Group. N Engl J Med. 1996;334:1428-1434.

336. Reiffers J, Stoppa AM, Attal M, et al. Allogeneic vs autologous stem cell transplantation vs chemotherapy in patients with acute myeloid leukemia in first remission: the BGMT 87 study. Leukemia. 1996;10:1874-1882.

337. Woods WG, Kobrinsky N, Buckley J, et al. Intensively timed induction therapy followed by autologous or allogeneic bone marrow transplantation for children with acute myeloid leukemia or myelodysplastic syndrome: a Childrens Cancer Group pilot study. J Clin Oncol. 1993;11:1448-1457.

338. Woods WG, Neudorf S, Gold S, et al. A comparison of allogeneic bone marrow transplantation, autologous bone marrow transplantation, and aggressive chemotherapy in children with acute myeloid leukemia in remission. Blood. 2001;97:56-62.

339. Zittoun RA, Mandelli F, Willemze R, et al. Autologous or allogeneic bone marrow transplantation compared with intensive chemotherapy in acute myelogenous leukemia. European Organization for Research and Treatment of Cancer (EORTC) and the Gruppo Italiano Malattie Ematologiche Maligne dell'Adulto (GIMEMA) Leukemia Cooperative Groups. N Engl J Med. 1995;332:217-223.

340. Riley LC, Hann IM, Wheatley K, Stevens RF. Treatment-related deaths during induction and first remission of acute myeloid leukaemia in children treated on the Tenth Medical Research Council acute myeloid leukaemia trial (MRC AML10). The MCR Childhood Leukaemia Working Party. Br J Haematol. 1999;106:436-444.

341. Webb DK, Wheatley K, Harrison G, et al. Outcome for children with relapsed acute myeloid leukaemia following initial therapy in the Medical Research Council (MRC) AML 10 trial. MRC Childhood Leukaemia Working Party. Leukemia. 1999;13:25-31.

342. Amadori S, Testi AM, Arico M, et al. Prospective comparative study of bone marrow transplantation and postremission chemotherapy for childhood acute myelogenous leukemia. The Associazione Italiana Ematologia ed Oncologia Pediatrica Cooperative Group. J Clin Oncol. 1993;11:1046-1054.

343. Dinndorf P, Bunin N. Bone marrow transplantation for children with acute myelogenous leukemia. J Pediatr Hematol Oncol. 1995;17:211-224.

344. Feig SA, Lampkin B, Nesbit ME, et al. Outcome of BMT during first complete remission of AML: a comparison of two sequential studies by the Children's Cancer Group. Bone Marrow Transplant. 1993;12:65-71.

345. Appelbaum FR. Allogeneic hematopoietic stem cell transplantation for acute leukemia. Semin Oncol. 1997;24:114-123.

346. Blaise D, Maraninchi D, Archimbaud E, et al. Allogeneic bone marrow transplantation for acute myeloid leukemia in first remission: a randomized trial of a busulfan-Cytoxan versus Cytoxan-total body irradiation as preparative regimen: a report from the Group d'Etudes de la Greffe de Moelle Osseuse. Blood. 1992;79:2578-2582.

347. Frassoni F, Labopin M, Gluckman E, et al. Results of allogeneic bone marrow transplantation for acute leukemia have improved in Europe with time—a report of the acute leukemia working party of the European group for blood and marrow transplantation (EBMT). Bone Marrow Transplant. 1996;17:13-18.

348. Jourdan E, Maraninchi D, Reiffers J, et al. Early allogeneic transplantation favorably influences the outcome of adult patients suffering from acute myeloid leukemia. Societe Francaise de Greffe de Moelle (SFGM). Bone Marrow Transplant. 1997;19:875-881.

349. Mayer RJ, Davis RB, Schiffer CA, et al. Intensive postremission chemotherapy in adults with acute myeloid leukemia. Cancer and Leukemia Group B. N Engl J Med. 1994;331:896-903.

350. Appelbaum FR, Fisher LD, Thomas ED. Chemotherapy v marrow transplantation for adults with acute nonlymphocytic leukemia: a five-year follow-up. Blood. 1988;72:179-184.

351. Champlin RE, Ho WG, Gale RP, et al. Treatment of acute myelogenous leukemia. A prospective controlled trial of bone marrow transplantation versus consolidation chemotherapy. Ann Intern Med. 1985;102:285-291.

352. Wheatley K, Burnett AK, Goldstone AH, et al. A simple, robust, validated and highly predictive index for the determination of risk-directed therapy in acute myeloid leukaemia derived from the MRC AML 10 trial. United Kingdom Medical Research Council's Adult and Childhood Leukaemia Working Parties. Br J Haematol. 1999;107:69-79.

353. Byrd JC, Mrozek K, Dodge RK, et al. Pretreatment cytogenetic abnormalities are predictive of induction success, cumulative incidence of relapse, and overall survival in adult patients with de novo acute myeloid leukemia: results from Cancer and Leukemia Group B (CALGB 8461). Blood. 2002;100:4325-4336.

354. Rubnitz JE, Look AT. Molecular genetics of childhood leukemias. J Pediatr Hematol Oncol. 1998;20:1-11.

355. Rubnitz JE, Raimondi SC, Halbert AR, et al. Characteristics and outcome of t(8;21)-positive childhood acute myeloid leukemia: a single institution's experience. Leukemia. 2002;16:2072-2077.

356. Rubnitz JE, Raimondi SC, Tong X, et al. Favorable impact of the t(9;11) in childhood acute myeloid leukemia. J Clin Oncol. 2002;20:2302-2309.

357. Byrd JC, Dodge RK, Carroll A, et al. Patients with t(8;21)(q22;q22) and acute myeloid leukemia have superior failure-free and overall survival when repetitive cycles of high-dose cytarabine are administered. J Clin Oncol. 1999;17:3767-3775.

358. Razzouk BI, Raimondi SC, Srivastava DK, et al. Impact of treatment on the outcome of acute myeloid leukemia with inversion 16: a single institution's experience. Leukemia. 2001;15:1326-1330.

359. Sandoval C, Head DR, Mirro J Jr, et al. Translocation t(9;11)(p21;q23) in pediatric de novo and secondary acute myeloblastic leukemia. Leukemia. 1992;6:513-519.

360. de Nully Brown P, Jurlander J, Pedersen-Bjergaard J, et al. The prognostic significance of chromosomal analysis and immunophenotyping in 117 patients with de novo acute myeloid leukemia. Leuk Res. 1997;21:985-995.

361. Athale UH, Razzouk BI, Raimondi SC, et al. Biology and outcome of childhood acute megakaryoblastic leukemia: a single institution's experience. Blood. 2001;97:3727-3732.

362. Mrozek K, Heinonen K, Bloomfield CD. Clinical importance of cytogenetics in acute myeloid leukaemia. Best Pract Res Clin Haematol. 2001;14:19-47.

363. Whitman SP, Archer KJ, Feng L, et al. Absence of the wild-type allele predicts poor prognosis in adult de novo acute myeloid leukemia with normal cytogenetics and the internal tandem duplication of FLT3: a cancer and leukemia group B study. Cancer Res. 2001;61:7233-7239.

364. Kiyoi H, Naoe T, Nakano Y, et al. Prognostic implication of FLT3 and N-RAS gene mutations in acute myeloid leukemia. Blood. 1999;93:3074-3080.

365. Weinstein HJ, Mayer RJ, Rosenthal DS, et al. Treatment of acute myelogenous leukemia in children and adults. N Engl J Med. 1980;303:473-478.

366. Weinstein HJ, Mayer RJ, Rosenthal DS, et al. Chemotherapy for acute myelogenous leukemia in children and adults: VAPA update. Blood. 1983;62:315-319.

367. Nesbit ME Jr, Buckley JD, Feig SA, et al. Chemotherapy for induction of remission of childhood acute myeloid leukemia followed by marrow transplantation or multiagent chemotherapy: a report from the Childrens Cancer Group. J Clin Oncol. 1994;12:127-135.

368. Ravindranath Y, Steuber CP, Krischer J, et al. High-dose cytarabine for intensification of early therapy of childhood acute myeloid leukemia: a Pediatric Oncology Group study. J Clin Oncol. 1991;9:572-580.

369. Wells RJ, Woods WG, Lampkin BC, et al. Impact of high-dose cytarabine and asparaginase intensification on childhood acute myeloid leukemia: a report from the Childrens Cancer Group. J Clin Oncol. 1993;11:538-545.

370. Buchner T, Hiddemann W, Wormann B, et al. Double induction strategy for acute myeloid leukemia: the effect of high-dose cytarabine with mitoxantrone instead of standard-dose cytarabine with daunorubicin and 6-thioguanine: a randomized trial by the German AML Cooperative Group. Blood. 1999;93:4116-4124.

371. Creutzig U, Ritter J, Zimmermann M, et al. Improved treatment results in high-risk pediatric acute myeloid leukemia patients after intensification with high-dose cytarabine and mitoxantrone: results of Study Acute Myeloid Leukemia-Berlin-Frankfurt-Munster 93. J Clin Oncol. 2001;19:2705-2713.

372. Downing JR. The AML1-ETO chimaeric transcription factor in acute myeloid leukaemia: biology and clinical significance. Br J Haematol. 1999;106:296-308.

373. Lowenberg B, Downing JR, Burnett A. Acute myeloid leukemia. N Engl J Med. 1999;341:1051-1062.

374. Krance RA, Hurwitz CA, Head DR, et al. Experience with 2-chlorodeoxyadenosine in previously untreated children with newly diagnosed acute myeloid leukemia and myelodysplastic diseases. J Clin Oncol. 2001;19:2804-2811.

375. Nishikawa A, Nakamura Y, Nobori U, et al. Acute monocytic leukemia in children. Response to VP-16-213 as a single agent. Cancer. 1987;60:2146-2149.

376. Odom LF, Gordon EM. Acute monoblastic leukemia in infancy and early childhood: successful treatment with an epipodophyllotoxin. Blood. 1984;64:875-882.

377. Abbott BL, Rubnitz JE, Tong X, et al. Clinical significance of central nervous system involvement at diagnosis of pediatric acute myeloid leukemia: a single institution's experience. Leukemia. 2003;17:2090-2096.

378. Perel Y, Auvrignon A, Leblanc T, et al. Maintenance therapy in childhood acute myeloid leukemia. Ann Hematol. 2004;83(Suppl 1):S116-119.

379. Perel Y, Auvrignon A, Leblanc T, et al. Impact of addition of maintenance therapy to intensive induction and consolidation chemotherapy for childhood acute myeloblastic leukemia: results of a prospective randomized trial, LAME 89/91. Leucamie Aique Myeloide Enfant. J Clin Oncol. 2002;20:2774-2782.

380. Miyawaki S, Sakamaki H, Ohtake S, et al. A randomized, post-remission comparison of four courses of standard-dose consolidation therapy without maintenance therapy versus three courses of standard-dose consolidation with maintenance therapy in adults with acute myeloid leukemia: the Japan Adult Leukemia Study Group AML 97 Study. Cancer. 2005;104:2726-2734.

381. Brunet AS, Ploton C, Galambrun C, et al. Low incidence of sepsis because of viridans streptococci in a ten-year retrospective study of pediatric acute myeloid leukemia. Pediatr Blood Cancer. 2006;47:765-772.

382. Creutzig U, Zimmermann M, Reinhardt D, et al. Early deaths and treatment-related mortality in children undergoing therapy for acute myeloid leukemia: analysis of the multicenter clinical trials AML-BFM 93 and AML-BFM 98. J Clin Oncol. 2004;22:4384-4393.

383. Gamis AS, Howells WB, DeSwarte-Wallace J, et al. Alpha hemolytic streptococcal infection during intensive treatment for acute myeloid leukemia: a report from the Children's Cancer Group study CCG-2891. J Clin Oncol. 2000;18:1845-1855.

384. Gassas A, Grant R, Richardson S, et al. Predictors of viridans streptococcal shock syndrome in bacteremic children with cancer and stem-cell transplant recipients. J Clin Oncol. 2004;22:1222-1227.

385. Okamoto Y, Ribeiro RC, Srivastava DK, et al. Viridans streptococcal sepsis: clinical features and complications in childhood acute myeloid leukemia. J Pediatr Hematol Oncol. 2003;25:696-703.

386. Barker GJ, Call SK, Gamis AS. Oral care with vancomycin paste for reduction in incidence of alpha-hemolytic streptococcal sepsis. J Pediatr Hematol Oncol. 1995;17:151-155.

387. Guiot HF, van den Broek PJ, van der Meer JW, van Furth R. Selective antimicrobial modulation of the intestinal flora of patients with acute nonlymphocytic leukemia: a double-blind, placebo-controlled study. J Infect Dis. 1983;147:615-623.

388. Sleijfer DT, Mulder NH, de Vries-Hospers HG, et al. Infection prevention in granulocytopenic patients by selective decontamination of the digestive tract. Eur J Cancer. 1980;16:859-869.

389. Gurwith MJ, Brunton JL, Lank BA, et al. A prospective controlled investigation of prophylactic trimethoprim/sulfamethoxazole in hospitalized granulocytopenic patients. Am J Med. 1979;66:248-256.

390. Weiser B, Lange M, Fialk MA, et al. Prophylactic trimethoprim-sulfamethoxazole during consolidation chemotherapy for acute leukemia: a controlled trial. Ann Intern Med. 1981;95:436-438.

391. Kauffman CA, Liepman MK, Bergman AG, Mioduszewski J. Trimethoprim/sulfamethoxazole prophylaxis in neutropenic patients. Reduction of infections and effect on bacterial and fungal flora. Am J Med. 1983;74:599-607.

392. Wilson JM, Guiney DG. Failure of oral trimethoprim-sulfamethoxazole prophylaxis in acute leukemia: isolation of resistant plasmids from strains of Enterobacteriaceae causing bacteremia. N Engl J Med. 1982;306:16-20.

393. Craig M, Cumpston AD, Hobbs GR, et al. The clinical impact of antibacterial prophylaxis and cycling antibiotics for febrile neutropenia in a hematological malignancy and transplantation unit. Bone Marrow Transplant. 2007;39:477-482.

394. Pizzo PA, Robichaud KJ, Wesley R, Commers JR. Fever in the pediatric and young adult patient with cancer. A prospective study of 1001 episodes. Medicine (Baltimore). 1982;61:153-165.

395. Albano EA, Pizzo PA. Infectious complications in childhood acute leukemias. Pediatr Clin North Am. 1988;35:873-901.

396. Fanci R, Paci C, Martinez RL, et al. Management of fever in neutropenic patients with acute leukemia: current role of ceftazidime plus amikacin as empiric therapy. J Chemother. 2000;12:232-239.

397. Buckley JD, Lampkin BC, Nesbit ME, et al. Remission induction in children with acute non-lymphocytic leukemia using cytosine arabinoside and doxorubicin or daunorubicin: a report from the Children's Cancer Study Group. Med Pediatr Oncol. 1989;17:382-390.

398. Pastore D, Specchia G, Mele G, et al. Typhlitis complicating induction therapy in adult acute myeloid leukemia. Leuk Lymphoma. 2002;43:911-914.

399. Schlatter M, Snyder K, Freyer D. Successful nonoperative management of typhlitis in pediatric oncology patients. J Pediatr Surg. 2002;37:1151-1155.

400. Goodman JL, Winston DJ, Greenfield RA, et al. A controlled trial of fluconazole to prevent fungal infections in patients undergoing bone marrow transplantation. N Engl J Med. 1992;326:845-851.

401. Wingard JR, Merz WG, Rinaldi MG, et al. Increase in Candida krusei infection in patients with bone marrow transplantation and neutropenia treated prophylactically with fluconazole. N Engl J Med. 1991;325:1274-1277.

402. Winston DJ, Chandrasekar PH, Lazarus HM, et al. Fluconazole prophylaxis of fungal infections in patients with acute leukemia. Results of a randomized placebo-controlled, double-blind, multicenter trial. Ann Intern Med. 1993;118:495-503.

403. Bow EJ, Laverdiere M, Lussier N, et al. Antifungal prophylaxis for severely neutropenic chemotherapy recipients: a meta analysis of randomized-controlled clinical trials. Cancer. 2002;94:3230-3246.

404. Kanda Y, Yamamoto R, Chizuka A, et al. Prophylactic action of oral fluconazole against fungal infection in neutropenic patients. A meta-analysis of 16 randomized, controlled trials. Cancer. 2000;89:1611-1625.

405. Cornely OA, Maertens J, Winston DJ, et al. Posaconazole vs. fluconazole or itraconazole prophylaxis in patients with neutropenia. N Engl J Med. 2007;356:348-359.

406. Bretagne S, Marmorat-Khuong A, Kuentz M, et al. Serum Aspergillus galactomannan antigen testing by *sandwich* ELISA: practical use in neutropenic patients. J Infect. 1997;35:7-15.

407. Ulusakarya A, Chachaty E, Vantelon JM, et al. Surveillance of Aspergillus galactomannan antigenemia for in*vasive asper*gillosis by enzyme-linked immunosorbent assay in neutropenic patients treated for hematological malignancies. Hematol J. 2000;1:111-116.

408. De Pauw BE, Donnelly JP. Prophylaxis and aspergillosis—has the principle been proven? N Engl J Med. 2007;356:409-411.

409. Maertens J, Theunissen K, Verhoef G, et al. Galactomannan and computed tomography-based preemptive antifungal therapy in neutropenic patients at high risk for invasive fungal infection: a prospective feasibility study. Clin Infect Dis. 2005;41:1242-1250.

410. Cagnoni PJ. Liposomal amphotericin B versus conventional amphotericin B in the empirical treatment of persistently febrile neutropenic patients. J Antimicrob Chemother. 2002;49(Suppl 1):81-86.

411. Wingard JR, White MH, Anaissie E, et al. A randomized, double-blind comparative trial evaluating the safety of liposomal amphotericin B versus amphotericin B lipid complex in the empirical treatment of febrile neutropenia. L Amph/ABLC Collaborative Study Group. Clin Infect Dis. 2000;31:1155-1163.

412. Walsh TJ, Teppler H, Donowitz GR, et al. Caspofungin versus liposomal amphotericin B for empirical antifungal therapy in patients with persistent fever and neutropenia. N Engl J Med. 2004;351:1391-1402.

413. Walsh TJ, Pappas P, Winston DJ, et al. Voriconazole compared with liposomal amphotericin B for empirical antifungal therapy in patients with neutropenia and persistent fever. N Engl J Med. 2002;346:225-234.

414. Gordin FM, Simon GL, Wofsy CB, Mills J. Adverse reactions to trimethoprim-sulfamethoxazole in patients with the acquired immunodeficiency syndrome. Ann Intern Med. 1984;100:495-499.

415. Hughes WT, Kuhn S, Chaudhary S, et al. Successful chemoprophylaxis for Pneumocystis carinii pneumonitis. N Engl J Med. 1977;297:1419-1426.

416. Hughes WT, Rivera GK, Schell MJ, et al. Successful intermittent chemoprophylaxis for Pneumocystis carinii pneumonitis. N Engl J Med. 1987;316:1627-1632.

417. Williams S, MacDonald P, Hoyer JD, et al. Methemoglobinemia in children with acute lymphoblastic leukemia (ALL) receiving dapsone for pneumocystis carinii pneumonia (PCP) prophylaxis: a correlation with cytochrome b5 reductase (Cb5R) enzyme levels. Pediatr Blood Cancer. 2005;44:55-62.

418. Madden RM, Pui CH, Hughes WT, et al. Prophylaxis of Pneumocystis carinii pneumonia with atovaquone in children with leukemia. Cancer. 2007;109:1654-1658.

419. Weinthal J, Frost JD, Briones G, Cairo MS. Successful Pneumocystis carinii pneumonia prophylaxis using aerosolized pentamidine in children with acute leukemia. J Clin Oncol. 1994;12:136-140.

420. Bergmann OJ, Mogensen SC, Ellermann-Eriksen S, Ellegaard J. Acyclovir prophylaxis and fever during remission-induction therapy of patients with acute myeloid leukemia: a randomized, double-blind, placebo-controlled trial. J Clin Oncol. 1997;15:2269-2274.

421. Alonzo TA, Kobrinsky NL, Aledo A, et al. Impact of granulocyte colony-stimulating factor use during induction for acute myelogenous leukemia in children: a report from the Children's Cancer Group. J Pediatr Hematol Oncol. 2002;24:627-635.

422. Lehrnbecher T, Zimmermann M, Reinhardt D, et al. Prophylactic human granulocyte colony-stimulating factor after induction therapy in pediatric acute myeloid leukemia. Blood. 2007;109:936-943.

423. Creutzig U, Zimmermann M, Lehrnbecher T, et al. Less toxicity by optimizing chemotherapy, but not by addition of granulocyte colony-stimulating factor in children and adolescents with acute myeloid leukemia: results of AML-BFM 98. J Clin Oncol. 2006;24:4499-4506.

424. Lehrnbecher T, Welte K. Haematopoietic growth factors in children with neutropenia. Br J Haematol. 2002;116:28-56.

425. Athale UH, Chan AK. Hemorrhagic complications in pediatric hematologic malignancies. Semin Thromb Hemost. 2007;33:408-415.

426. Green D. Management of bleeding complications of hematologic malignancies. Semin Thromb Hemost. 2007;33:427-434.

427. Heal JM, Blumberg N. Optimizing platelet transfusion therapy. Blood Rev. 2004;18:149-165.

428. Consensus conference. Platelet transfusion therapy. JAMA. 1987;257:1777-1780.

429. Aderka D, Praff G, Santo M, et al. Bleeding because ofthrombocytopenia in acute leukemias and reevaluation of the prophylactic platelet transfusion policy. Am J Med Sci. 1986;291:147-151.

430. Callow CR, Swindell R, Randall W, Chopra R. The frequency of bleeding complications in patients with haematological malignancy following the introduction of a stringent prophylactic platelet transfusion policy. Br J Haematol. 2002;118:677-682.

431. Gmur J, Burger J, Schanz U, et al. Safety of stringent prophylactic platelet transfusion policy for patients with acute leukaemia. Lancet. 1991;338:1223-1226.

432. Lawrence JB, Yomtovian RA, Hammons T, et al. Lowering the prophylactic platelet transfusion threshold: a prospective analysis. Leuk Lymphoma. 2001;41:67-76.

433. Navarro JT, Hernandez JA, Ribera JM, et al. Prophylactic platelet transfusion threshold during therapy for adult acute myeloid leukemia: 10,000/microL versus 20,000/microL. Haematologica. 1998;83:998-1000.

434. Wandt H, Frank M, Ehninger G, et al. Safety and cost effectiveness of a $10 \times 10(9)$/L trigger for prophylactic platelet transfusions compared with the traditional $20 \times 10(9)$/L trigger: a prospective comparative trial in 105 patients with acute myeloid leukemia. Blood. 1998;91:3601-3606.

435. Gil-Fernandez JJ, Alegre A, Fernandez-Villalta MJ, et al. Clinical results of a stringent policy on prophylactic platelet transfusion: non-randomized comparative analysis in 190 bone marrow transplant patients from a single institution. Bone Marrow Transplant. 1996;18:931-935.

436. Friedmann AM, Sengul H, Lehmann H, et al. Do basic laboratory tests or clinical observations predict bleeding in thrombocytopenic oncology patients? A reevaluation of prophylactic platelet transfusions. Transfus Med Rev. 2002;16:34-45.

437. Adler SP. Transfusion-associated cytomegalovirus infections. Rev Infect Dis. 1983;5:977-993.

438. Narvios AB, Przepiorka D, Tarrand J, et al. Transfusion support using filtered unscreened blood products for cytomegalovirus-negative allogeneic marrow transplant recipients. Bone Marrow Transplant. 1998;22:575-577.

439. Orlin JB, Ellis MH. Transfusion-associated graft-versus-host disease. Curr Opin Hematol. 1997;4:442-448.

440. Chojnowski K, Wawrzyniak E, Trelinski J, et al. Assessment of coagulation disorders in patients with acute leukemia before and after cytostatic treatment. Leuk Lymphoma. 1999;36:77-84.

441. Nur S, Anwar M, Saleem M, Ahmad PA. Disseminated intravascular coagulation in acute leukaemias at first diagnosis. Eur J Haematol. 1995;55:78-82.

442. Fenaux P, Chomienne C, Degos L. Treatment of acute promyelocytic leukaemia. Best Pract Res Clin Haematol. 2001;14:153-174.

443. O'Regan S, Carson S, Chesney RW, Drummond KN. Electrolyte and acid-base disturbances in the management of leukemia. Blood. 1977;49:345-353.

444. Jones DP, Stapleton FB, Kalwinsky D, et al. Renal dysfunction and hyperuricemia at presentation and relapse of acute lymphoblastic leukemia. Med Pediatr Oncol. 1990;18:283-286.

445. Pui CH, Relling MV, Lascombes F, et al. Urate oxidase in prevention and treatment of hyperuricemia associated with lymphoid malignancies. Leukemia. 1997;11:1813-1816.

446. Pui CH. Urate oxidase in the prophylaxis or treatment of hyperuricemia: the United States experience. Semin Hematol. 2001;38:13-21.

447. Browning LA, Kruse JA. Hemolysis and methemoglobinemia secondary to rasburicase administration. Ann Pharmacother. 2005;39:1932-1935.

448. Renyi I, Bardi E, Udvardi E, et al. Prevention and treatment of hyperuricemia with rasburicase in children with leukemia and non-Hodgkin's lymphoma. Pathol Oncol Res. 2007;13:57-62.

449. Porcu P, Farag S, Marcucci G, et al. Leukocytoreduction for acute leukemia. Ther Apher. 2002;6:15-23.

450. Giles FJ, Shen Y, Kantarjian HM, et al. Leukapheresis reduces early mortality in patients with acute myeloid leukemia with high white cell counts but does not improve long-term survival. Leuk Lymphoma. 2001;42:67-73.

451. Bug G, Anargyrou K, Tonn T, et al. Impact of leukapheresis on early death rate in adult acute myeloid leukemia presenting with hyperleukocytosis. Transfusion. 2007;47:1843-1850.

452. Matteucci P, Carlo-Stella C, Di Nicola M, et al. Topical prophylaxis of conjunctivitis induced by high-dose cytosine arabinoside. Haematologica. 2006;91:255-257.

453. Higa GM, Gockerman JP, Hunt AL, et al. The use of prophylactic eye drops during high-dose cytosine arabinoside therapy. Cancer. 1991;68:1691-1693.

454. Nand S, Messmore HL Jr, Patel R, et al. Neurotoxicity associated with systemic high-dose cytosine arabinoside. J Clin Oncol. 1986;4:571-575.

455. Grossman L, Baker MA, Sutton DM, Deck JH. Central nervous system toxicity of high-dose cytosine arabinoside. Med Pediatr Oncol. 1983;11:246-250.

456. Dunton SF, Nitschke R, Spruce WE, et al. Progressive ascending paralysis following administration of intrathecal and intrave-nous cytosine arabinoside. A Pediatric Oncology Group study. Cancer. 1986;57:1083-1088.

457. Bensinger TA, Fahey JL, Kellon DB, Beutler E. Febrile response to cytarabine (letter). JAMA. 1974;229:1578.

458. Rose MS, Bateman DN. Pyrexia with cytosine arabinoside. Br Med J. 1972;4:115.

459. Flynn PM, Marina NM, Rivera GK, Hughes WT. Candida tropicalis infections in children with leukemia. Leuk Lymphoma. 1993;10:369-376.

460. Martino P, Girmenia C, Micozzi A, et al. Fungemia in patients with leukemia. Am J Med Sci. 1993;306:225-232.

461. Mantadakis E, Danilatou V, Stiakaki E, Kalmanti M. Infectious toxicity of dexamethasone during all remission-induction chemotherapy: report of two cases and literature review. Pediatr Hematol Oncol. 2004;21:27-35.

462. Sala A, Pencharz P, Barr RD. Children, cancer, and nutrition—A dynamic triangle in review. Cancer. 2004;100:677-687.

463. Wadleigh M, Richardson PG, Zahrieh D, et al. Prior gemtuzumab ozogamicin exposure significantly increases the risk of veno-occlusive disease in patients who undergo myeloablative allogeneic stem cell transplantation. Blood. 2003;102:1578-1582.

464. Budman DR, Calabro A, Kreis W. In vitro effects of dexrazoxane (Zinecard) and classical acute leukemia therapy: time to consider expanded clinical trials? Leukemia. 2001;15:1517-1520.

465. Pearlman M, Jendiroba D, Pagliaro L, et al. Dexrazoxane in combination with anthracyclines lead to a synergistic cytotoxic response in acute myelogenous leukemia cell lines. Leuk Res. 2003;27:617-626.

466. Styczynski J, Wysocki M, Balwierz W, Kowalczyk JR. Dexrazoxane has no impact on sensitivity of childhood leukemic blasts to daunorubicin. Leukemia. 2002;16:820-825.

467. Pui CH, Howard SC. Current management and challenges of malignant disease in the CNS in paediatric leukaemia. Lancet Oncol. 2008;9:257-268.

468. Johnston DL, Alonzo TA, Gerbing RB, et al. Risk factors and therapy for isolated central nervous system relapse of pediatric acute myeloid leukemia. J Clin Oncol. 2005;23:9172-9178.

469. Pui CH, Cheng C, Leung W, et al. Extended follow-up of long-term survivors of childhood acute lymphoblastic leukemia. N Engl J Med. 2003;349:640-649.

470. Hijiya N, Hudson MM, Lensing S, et al. Cumulative incidence of secondary neoplasms as a first event after childhood acute lymphoblastic leukemia. JAMA. 2007;297:1207-1215.

471. Lie SO, Abrahamsson J, Clausen N, et al. Long-term results in children with AML: NOPHO-AML Study Group—report of three consecutive trials. Leukemia. 2005;19:2090-2100.

472. Liang DC, Chan TT, Lin KH, et al. Improved treatment results for childhood acute myeloid leukemia in Taiwan. Leukemia. 2006;20:136-141.

473. Grier HE, Gelber RD, Camitta BM, et al. Prognostic factors in childhood acute myelogenous leukemia. J Clin Oncol. 1987;5:1026-1032.

474. Reinhardt D, Creutzig U. Isolated myelosarcoma in children—update and review. Leuk Lymphoma. 2002;43:565-574.

475. Paydas S, Zorludemir S, Ergin M. Granulocytic sarcoma: 32 cases and review of the literature. Leuk Lymphoma. 2006;47:2527-2541.

476. Schwyzer R, Sherman GG, Cohn RJ, et al. Granulocytic sarcoma in children with acute myeloblastic leukemia and t(8;21). Med Pediatr Oncol. 1998;31:144-149.

477. Jenkin RD, Al-Shabanah M, Al-Nasser A, et al. Extramedullary myeloid tumors in children: the limited value of local treatment. J Pediatr Hematol Oncol. 2000;22:34-40.

478. Barbaric D, Alonzo TA, Gerbing RB, et al. Minimally differentiated acute myeloid leukemia (FAB AML-M0) is associated with

an adverse outcome in children: a report from the Children's Oncology Group, studies CCG-2891 and CCG-2961. Blood. 2007;109:2314-2321.

479. Rubnitz JE, Razzouk BI, Lensing S, et al. Prognostic factors and outcome of recurrence in childhood acute myeloid leukemia. Cancer. 2007;109:157-163.

480. Oki Y, Kantarjian HM, Zhou X, et al. Adult acute megakaryocytic leukemia: an analysis of 37 patients treated at M.D. Anderson Cancer Center. Blood. 2006;107:880-884.

481. Woods WG, Barnard DR, Alonzo TA, et al. Prospective study of 90 children requiring treatment for juvenile myelomonocytic leukemia or myelodysplastic syndrome: a report from the Children's Cancer Group. J Clin Oncol. 2002;20:434-440.

482. Kardos G, Baumann I, Passmore SJ, et al. Refractory anemia in childhood: a retrospective analysis of 67 patients with particular reference to monosomy 7. Blood. 2003;102:1997-2003.

483. Trobaugh-Lotrario AD, Kletzel M, Quinones RR, et al. Monosomy 7 associated with pediatric acute myeloid leukemia (AML) and myelodysplastic syndrome (MDS): successful management by allogeneic hematopoietic stem cell transplant (HSCT). Bone Marrow Transplant. 2005;35:143-149.

484. Burnett AK, Grimwade D, Solomon E, et al. Presenting white blood cell count and kinetics of molecular remission predict prognosis in acute promyelocytic leukemia treated with all-trans retinoic acid: result of the Randomized MRC Trial. Blood. 1999;93:4131-4143.

485. Fenaux P, Chastang C, Degos L. Treatment of newly diagnosed acute promyelocytic leukemia (APL) by a combination of all-trans retinoic acid (ATRA) and chemotherapy. French APL Group. Leukemia. 1994;8(Suppl 2):S42-S47.

486. Tallman MS, Andersen JW, Schiffer CA, et al. All-trans-retinoic acid in acute promyelocytic leukemia. N Engl J Med. 1997; 337:1021-1028.

487. Warrell RP Jr, Maslak P, Eardley A, et al. Treatment of acute promyelocytic leukemia with all-trans retinoic acid: an update of the New York experience. Leukemia. 1994;8: 929-933.

488. Betts DR, Ammann RA, Hirt A, et al. The prognostic significance of cytogenetic aberrations in childhood acute myeloid leukaemia. A study of the Swiss Paediatric Oncology Group (SPOG). Eur J Haematol. 2007;78:468-476.

489. Tomizawa D, Tabuchi K, Kinoshita A, et al. Repetitive cycles of high-dose cytarabine are effective for childhood acute myeloid leukemia: long-term outcome of the children with AML treated on two consecutive trials of Tokyo Children's Cancer Study Group. Pediatr Blood Cancer. 2007;49:127-132.

490. Razzouk BI, Estey E, Pounds S, et al. Impact of age on outcome of pediatric acute myeloid leukemia: a report from 2 institutions. Cancer. 2006;106:2495-2502.

491. Aplenc R, Alonzo TA, Gerbing RB, et al. Ethnicity and survival in childhood acute myeloid leukemia: a report from the Children's Oncology Group. Blood. 2006;108:74-80.

491a. Rubnitz JE, Lensing S, Razzouk BI, et al. Effect of race on outcome of white and black children with acute myeloid leukemia: the St. Jude experience. Pediatr Blood Cancer. 2007;48; 10-15.

492. Lange BJ, Gerbing RB, Feusner J, et al. Mortality in overweight and underweight children with acute myeloid leukemia. JAMA. 2005;293:203-211.

493. Stasi R, Del Poeta G, Masi M, et al. Incidence of chromosome abnormalities and clinical significance of karyotype in de novo acute myeloid leukemia. Cancer Genet Cytogenet. 1993;67: 28-34.

494. Tosi P, Visani G, Ottaviani E, et al. Inv(16) acute myeloid leukemia cells show an increased sensitivity to cytosine arabinoside in vitro. Eur J Haematol. 1998;60:161-165.

495. Visani G, Bernasconi P, Boni M, et al. The prognostic value of cytogenetics is reinforced by the kind of induction/consolidation

therapy in influencing the outcome of acute myeloid leukemia—analysis of 848 patients. Leukemia. 2001;15:903-909.

496. Martinez-Climent JA, Lane NJ, Rubin CM, et al. Clinical and prognostic significance of chromosomal abnormalities in childhood acute myeloid leukemia de novo. Leukemia. 1995;9: 95-101.

497. Kalwinsky DK, Raimondi SC, Schell MJ, et al. Prognostic importance of cytogenetic subgroups in de novo pediatric acute nonlymphocytic leukemia. J Clin Oncol. 1990;8:75-83.

498. Goemans BF, Zwaan CM, Miller M, et al. Mutations in KIT and RAS are frequent events in pediatric core-binding factor acute myeloid leukemia. Leukemia. 2005;19:1536-1542.

499. Boissel N, Leroy H, Brethon B, et al. Incidence and prognostic impact of c-Kit, FLT3, and Ras gene mutations in core binding factor acute myeloid leukemia (CBF-AML). Leukemia. 2006; 20:965-970.

500. Stirewalt DL, Kopecky KJ, Meshinchi S, et al. FLT3, RAS, and TP53 mutations in elderly patients with acute myeloid leukemia. Blood. 2001;97:3589-3595.

501. Coghlan DW, Morley AA, Matthews JP, Bishop JF. The incidence and prognostic significance of mutations in codon 13 of the N-ras gene in acute myeloid leukemia. Leukemia. 1994; 8:1682-1687.

502. Ritter M, Kim TD, Lisske P, et al. Prognostic significance of N-RAS and K-RAS mutations in 232 patients with acute myeloid leukemia. Haematologica. 2004;89:1397-1399.

503. Radich JP, Kopecky KJ, Willman CL, et al. N-ras mutations in adult de novo acute myelogenous leukemia: prevalence and clinical significance. Blood. 1990;76:801-807.

504. Care RS, Valk PJ, Goodeve AC, et al. Incidence and prognosis of c-KIT and FLT3 mutations in core binding factor (CBF) acute myeloid leukaemias. Br J Haematol. 2003;121:775-777.

505. Shimada A, Taki T, Tabuchi K, et al. KIT mutations, and not FLT3 internal tandem duplication, are strongly associated with a poor prognosis in pediatric acute myeloid leukemia with t(8;21): a study of the Japanese Childhood AML Cooperative Study Group. Blood. 2006;107:1806-1809.

506. Shimada A, Taki T, Tabuchi K, et al. Tandem duplications of MLL and FLT3 are correlated with poor prognoses in pediatric acute myeloid leukemia: a study of the Japanese childhood AML Cooperative Study Group. Pediatr Blood Cancer. 2008;50: 264-269.

507. Zwaan CM, Meshinchi S, Radich JP, et al. FLT3 internal tandem duplication in 234 children with acute myeloid leukemia: prognostic significance and relation to cellular drug resistance. Blood. 2003;102:2387-2394.

508. Liang DC, Shih LY, Hung IJ, et al. Clinical relevance of internal tandem duplication of the FLT3 gene in childhood acute myeloid leukemia. Cancer. 2002;94:3292-3298.

509. Liang DC, Shih LY, Hung IJ, et al. FLT3-TKD mutation in childhood acute myeloid leukemia. Leukemia. 2003;17:883-886.

510. Caligiuri MA, Strout MP, Lawrence D, et al. Rearrangement of ALL1 (MLL) in acute myeloid leukemia with normal cytogenetics. Cancer Res. 1998;58:55-59.

511. Dohner K, Tobis K, Ulrich R, et al. Prognostic significance of partial tandem duplications of the MLL gene in adult patients 16 to 60 years old with acute myeloid leukemia and normal cytogenetics: a study of the Acute Myeloid Leukemia Study Group Ulm. J Clin Oncol. 2002;20:3254-3261.

512. Schnittger S, Schoch C, Kern W, et al. Nucleophosmin gene mutations are predictors of favorable prognosis in acute myelogenous leukemia with a normal karyotype. Blood. 2005;106: 3733-3739.

513. Thiede C, Koch S, Creutzig E, et al. Prevalence and prognostic impact of NPM1 mutations in 1485 adult patients with acute myeloid leukemia (AML). Blood. 2006;107:4011-4020.

514. Dohner K, Schlenk RF, Habdank M, et al. Mutant nucleophosmin (NPM1) predicts favorable prognosis in younger adults with acute myeloid leukemia and normal cytogenetics: interaction with other gene mutations. Blood. 2005;106:3740-3746.

515. Tartaglia M, Martinelli S, Iavarone I, et al. Somatic PTPN11 mutations in childhood acute myeloid leukaemia. Br J Haematol. 2005;129:333-339.

516. Menssen HD, Renkl HJ, Rodeck U, et al. Presence of Wilms' tumor gene (wt1) transcripts and the WT1 nuclear protein in the majority of human acute leukemias. Leukemia. 1995;9:1060-1067.

517. Miwa H, Beran M, Saunders GF. Expression of the Wilms' tumor gene (WT1) in human leukemias. Leukemia. 1992;6:405-409.

518. Inoue K, Sugiyama H, Ogawa H, et al. WT1 as a new prognostic factor and a new marker for the detection of minimal residual disease in acute leukemia. Blood. 1994;84:3071-3079.

519. Bergmann L, Miething C, Maurer U, et al. High levels of Wilms' tumor gene (wt1) mRNA in acute myeloid leukemias are associated with a worse long-term outcome. Blood. 1997;90:1217-1225.

520. Garg M, Moore H, Tobal K, Liu Yin JA. Prognostic significance of quantitative analysis of WT1 gene transcripts by competitive reverse transcription polymerase chain reaction in acute leukaemia. Br J Haematol. 2003;123:49-59.

521. Barragan E, Cervera J, Bolufer P, et al. Prognostic implications of Wilms' tumor gene (WT1) expression in patients with de novo acute myeloid leukemia. Haematologica. 2004;89:926-933.

522. Trka J, Kalinova M, Hrusak O, et al. Real-time quantitative PCR detection of WT1 gene expression in children with AML: prognostic significance, correlation with disease status and residual disease detection by flow cytometry. Leukemia. 2002;16:1381-1389.

523. Rodrigues PC, Oliveira SN, Viana MB, et al. Prognostic significance of WT1 gene expression in pediatric acute myeloid leukemia. Pediatr Blood Cancer. 2007;49:133-138.

524. Creutzig U, Zimmermann M, Ritter J, et al. Treatment strategies and long-term results in paediatric patients treated in four consecutive AML-BFM trials. Leukemia. 2005;19:2030-2042.

525. Smith FO, Alonzo TA, Gerbing RB, et al. Long-term results of children with acute myeloid leukemia: a report of three consecutive Phase III trials by the Children's Cancer Group: CCG 251, CCG 213 and CCG 2891. Leukemia. 2005;19:2054-2062.

526. Ravindranath Y, Chang M, Steuber CP, et al. Pediatric Oncology Group (POG) studies of acute myeloid leukemia (AML): a review of four consecutive childhood AML trials conducted between 1981 and 2000. Leukemia. 2005;19:2101-2116.

527. Ribeiro RC, Razzouk BI, Pounds S, et al. Successive clinical trials for childhood acute myeloid leukemia at St. Jude Children's Research Hospital, from 1980 to 2000. Leukemia. 2005;19:2125-2129.

528. Abrahamsson J, Clausen N, Gustafsson G, et al. Improved outcome after relapse in children with acute myeloid leukaemia. Br J Haematol. 2007;136:229-236.

529. Vignetti M, Orsini E, Petti MC, et al. Probability of long-term disease-free survival for acute myeloid leukemia patients after first relapse: A single-centre experience. Ann Oncol. 1996;7:933-938.

530. Aladjidi N, Auvrignon A, Leblanc T, et al. Outcome in children with relapsed acute myeloid leukemia after initial treatment with the French Leucemie Aique Myeloide Enfant (LAME) 89/91 protocol of the French Society of Pediatric Hematology and Immunology. J Clin Oncol. 2003;21:4377-4385.

531. Wells RJ, Adams MT, Alonzo TA, et al. Mitoxantrone and cytarabine induction, high-dose cytarabine, and etoposide intensification for pediatric patients with relapsed or refractory acute myeloid leukemia: Children's Cancer Group Study 2951. J Clin Oncol. 2003;21:2940-2947.

532. Ferrara F, Palmieri S, Mele G. Prognostic factors and therapeutic options for relapsed or refractory acute myeloid leukemia. Haematologica. 2004;89:998-1008.

533. Steuber CP, Krischer J, Holbrook T, et al. Therapy of refractory or recurrent childhood acute myeloid leukemia using amsacrine and etoposide with or without azacitidine: a Pediatric Oncology Group randomized phase II study. J Clin Oncol. 1996;14:1521-1525.

534. Stahnke K, Boos J, Bender-Gotze C, et al. Duration of first remission predicts remission rates and long-term survival in children with relapsed acute myelogenous leukemia. Leukemia. 1998;12:1534-1538.

535. Estey EH. Treatment of relapsed and refractory acute myelogenous leukemia. Leukemia. 2000;14:476-479.

536. Hiddemann W, Kreutzmann H, Straif K, et al. High-dose cytosine arabinoside and mitoxantrone: a highly effective regimen in refractory acute myeloid leukemia. Blood. 1987;69:744-749.

537. Wells RJ, Gold SH, Krill CE, et al. Cytosine arabinoside and mitoxantrone induction chemotherapy followed by bone marrow transplantation or chemotherapy for relapsed or refractory pediatric acute myeloid leukemia. Leukemia. 1994;8:1626-1630.

538. Whitlock JA, Wells RJ, Hord JD, et al. High-dose cytosine arabinoside and etoposide: an effective regimen without anthracyclines for refractory childhood acute non-lymphocytic leukemia. Leukemia. 1997;11:185-189.

539. Jeha S, Gandhi V, Chan KW, et al. Clofarabine, a novel nucleoside analog, is active in pediatric patients with advanced leukemia. Blood. 2004;103:784-789.

540. Faderl S, Gandhi V, O'Brien S, et al. Results of a phase 1-2 study of clofarabine in combination with cytarabine (ara-C) in relapsed and refractory acute leukemias. Blood. 2005;105:940-947.

541. Faderl S, Verstovsek S, Cortes J, et al. Clofarabine and cytarabine combination as induction therapy for acute myeloid leukemia (AML) in patients 50 years or older. Blood. 2006;108:45-51.

542. Visani G, Tosi P, Zinzani PL, et al. FLAG (fludarabine + high-dose cytarabine + G-CSF): an effective and tolerable protocol for the treatment of 'poor risk' acute myeloid leukemias. Leukemia. 1994;8:1842-1846.

543. Montillo M, Mirto S, Petti MC, et al. Fludarabine, cytarabine, and G-CSF (FLAG) for the treatment of poor risk acute myeloid leukemia. Am J Hematol. 1998;58:105-109.

544. Ferrara F, Melillo L, Montillo M, et al. Fludarabine, cytarabine, and G-CSF (FLAG) for the treatment of acute myeloid leukemia relapsing after autologous stem cell transplantation. Ann Hematol. 1999;78:380-384.

545. Leahey A, Kelly K, Rorke LB, Lange B. A phase I/II study of idarubicin (Ida) with continuous infusion fludarabine (F-ara-A) and cytarabine (ara-C) for refractory or recurrent pediatric acute myeloid leukemia (AML). J Pediatr Hematol Oncol. 1997;19:304-308.

546. Parker JE, Pagliuca A, Mijovic A, et al. Fludarabine, cytarabine, G-CSF and idarubicin (FLAG-IDA) for the treatment of poor-risk myelodysplastic syndromes and acute myeloid leukaemia. Br J Haematol. 1997;99:939-944.

547. Fleischhack G, Hasan C, Graf N, et al. IDA-FLAG (idarubicin, fludarabine, cytarabine, G-CSF), an effective remission-induction therapy for poor-prognosis AML of childhood prior to allogeneic or autologous bone marrow transplantation: experiences of a phase II trial. Br J Haematol. 1998;102:647-655.

548. Steinmetz HT, Schulz A, Staib P, et al. Phase-II trial of idarubicin, fludarabine, cytosine arabinoside, and filgrastim (Ida-FLAG) for treatment of refractory, relapsed, and secondary AML. Ann Hematol. 1999;78:418-425.

549. Robak T, Wrzesien-Kus A, Lech-Maranda E, et al. Combination regimen of cladribine (2-chlorodeoxyadenosine), cytarabine

and G-CSF (CLAG) as induction therapy for patients with relapsed or refractory acute myeloid leukemia. Leuk Lymphoma. 2000;39:121-129.

550. Gordon MS, Young ML, Tallman MS, et al. Phase II trial of 2-chlorodeoxyadenosine in patients with relapsed/refractory acute myeloid leukemia: a study of the Eastern Cooperative Oncology Group (ECOG), E5995. Leuk Res. 2000;24:871-875.

551. Wrzesien-Kus A, Robak T, Lech-Maranda E, et al. A multi-center, open, non-comparative, phase II study of the combination of cladribine (2-chlorodeoxyadenosine), cytarabine, and G-CSF as induction therapy in refractory acute myeloid leukemia—a report of the Polish Adult Leukemia Group (PALG). Eur J Haematol. 2003;71:155-162.

552. Santana VM, Mirro J Jr, Harwood FC, et al. A phase I clinical trial of 2-chlorodeoxyadenosine in pediatric patients with acute leukemia. J Clin Oncol. 1991;9:416-422.

553. Santana VM, Mirro J Jr, Kearns C, et al. 2-Chlorodeoxyadenosine produces a high rate of complete hematologic remission in relapsed acute myeloid leukemia. J Clin Oncol. 1992;10:364-370.

554. Santana VM, Hurwitz CA, Blakley RL, et al. Complete hematologic remissions induced by 2-chlorodeoxyadenosine in children with newly diagnosed acute myeloid leukemia. Blood. 1994;84:1237-1242.

555. Rubnitz JE, Razzouk BI, Srivastava DK, et al. Phase II trial of cladribine and cytarabine in relapsed or refractory myeloid malignancies. Leuk Res. 2004;28:349-352.

556. Douer D, Watkins K, Levine AM, et al. Induction of complete remission using single agent clofarabine in a patient with primary refractory acute myeloblaste leukemia. Leuk Lymphoma. 2003;44:2135-2136.

557. Kolb EA, Steinherz PG. A new multidrug reinduction protocol with topotecan, vinorelbine, thiotepa, dexamethasone, and gemcitabine for relapsed or refractory acute leukemia. Leukemia. 2003;17:1967-1972.

558. Zander AR, Dicke KA, Keating M, et al. Allogeneic bone marrow transplantation for acute leukemia refractory to induction chemotherapy. Cancer. 1985;56:1374-1379.

559. Zander AR, Keating M, Dicke K, et al. A comparison of marrow transplantation with chemotherapy for adults with acute leukemia of poor prognosis in first complete remission. J Clin Oncol. 1988;6:1548-1557.

560. Forman SJ, Schmidt GM, Nademanee AP, et al. Allogeneic bone marrow transplantation as therapy for primary induction failure for patients with acute leukemia. J Clin Oncol. 1991;9:1570-1574.

561. Biggs JC, Horowitz MM, Gale RP, et al. Bone marrow transplants may cure patients with acute leukemia never achieving remission with chemotherapy. Blood. 1992;80:1090-1093.

562. Mehta J, Powles R, Horton C, et al. Bone marrow transplantation for primary refractory acute leukaemia. Bone Marrow Transplant. 1994;14:415-418.

563. Nemecek ER, Gooley TA, Woolfrey AE, et al. Outcome of allogeneic bone marrow transplantation for children with advanced acute myeloid leukemia. Bone Marrow Transplant. 2004;34:799-806.

564. Kataoka I, Kami M, Takahashi S, et al. Clinical impact of graft-versus-host disease against leukemias not in remission at the time of allogeneic hematopoietic stem cell transplantation from related donors. The Japan Society for Hematopoietic Cell Transplantation Working Party. Bone Marrow Transplant. 2004;34:711-719.

565. Randolph SS, Gooley TA, Warren EH, et al. Female donors contribute to a selective graft-versus-leukemia effect in male recipients of HLA-matched, related hematopoietic stem cell transplants. Blood. 2004;103:347-352.

566. Valcarcel D, Martino R, Caballero D, et al. Sustained remissions of high-risk acute myeloid leukemia and myelodysplastic syndrome after reduced-intensity conditioning allogeneic hematopoietic transplantation: chronic graft-versus-host disease is the strongest factor improving survival. J Clin Oncol. 2008;26:577-584.

567. Min CK, Eom KS, Lee S, et al. Effect of induced GVHD in leukemia patients relapsing after allogeneic bone marrow transplantation: single-center experience of 33 adult patients. Bone Marrow Transplant. 2001;27:999-1005.

568. Grigg AP, Szer J, Beresford J, et al. Factors affecting the outcome of allogeneic bone marrow transplantation for adult patients with refractory or relapsed acute leukaemia. Br J Haematol. 1999;107:409-418.

569. Elmaagacli AH, Beelen DW, Trenn G, et al. Induction of a graft-versus-leukemia reaction by cyclosporin A withdrawal as immunotherapy for leukemia relapsing after allogeneic bone marrow transplantation. Bone Marrow Transplant. 1999;23:771-777.

570. Singhal S, Powles R, Kulkarni S, et al. Long-term follow-up of relapsed acute leukemia treated with immunotherapy after allogeneic transplantation: the inseparability of graft-versus-host disease and graft-versus-leukemia, and the problem of extramedullary relapse. Leuk Lymphoma. 1999;32:505-512.

571. Shiobara S, Nakao S, Ueda M, et al. Donor leukocyte infusion for Japanese patients with relapsed leukemia after allogeneic bone marrow transplantation: lower incidence of acute graft-versus-host disease and improved outcome. Bone Marrow Transplant. 2000;26:769-774.

572. Porter DL, Collins RH Jr, Hardy C, et al. Treatment of relapsed leukemia after unrelated donor marrow transplantation with unrelated donor leukocyte infusions. Blood. 2000;95:1214-1221.

573. Ringden O, Labopin M, Gorin NC, et al. Is there a graft-versus-leukaemia effect in the absence of graft-versus-host disease in patients undergoing bone marrow transplantation for acute leukaemia? Br J Haematol. 2000;111:1130-1137.

574. Ruggeri L, Mancusi A, Burchielli E, et al. NK cell alloreactivity and allogeneic hematopoietic stem cell transplantation. Blood Cells Mol Dis. 2008;40:84-90.

575. Ruggeri L, Capanni M, Urbani E, et al. Effectiveness of donor natural killer cell alloreactivity in mismatched hematopoietic transplants. Science. 2002;295:2097-2100.

576. Ciccone E, Pende D, Viale O, et al. Evidence of a natural killer (NK) cell repertoire for (allo) antigen recognition: definition of five distinct NK-determined allospecificities in humans. J Exp Med. 1992;175:709-718.

577. Morgan MA, Reuter CW. Molecularly targeted therapies in myelodysplastic syndromes and acute myeloid leukemias. Ann Hematol. 2006;85:139-163.

578. Tallman MS, Gilliland DG, Rowe JM. Drug therapy for acute myeloid leukemia. Blood. 2005;106:1154-1163.

579. Brethon B, Auvrignon A, Galambrun C, et al. Efficacy and tolerability of gemtuzumab ozogamicin (anti-CD33 monoclonal antibody, CMA-676, Mylotarg) in children with relapsed/refractory myeloid leukemia. BMC Cancer. 2006;6:172.

580. Cohen AD, Luger SM, Sickles C, et al. Gemtuzumab ozogamicin (Mylotarg) monotherapy for relapsed AML after hematopoietic stem cell transplant: efficacy and incidence of hepatic venoocclusive disease. Bone Marrow Transplant. 2002;30:23-28.

581. Giles FJ, Kantarjian HM, Kornblau SM, et al. Mylotarg (gemtuzumab ozogamicin) therapy is associated with hepatic venoocclusive disease in patients who have not received stem cell transplantation. Cancer. 2001;92:406-413.

582. Leopold LH, Berger MS, Feingold J. Acute and long-term toxicities associated with gemtuzumab ozogamicin (mylotarg(r)) therapy of acute myeloid leukemia. Clin Lymphoma. 2002;2:S29-34.

583. Sievers EL. Efficacy and safety of gemtuzumab ozogamicin in patients with CD33-positive acute myeloid leukaemia in first relapse. Expert Opin Biol Ther. 2001;1:893-901.

584. Sievers EL. Antibody-targeted chemotherapy of acute myeloid leukemia using gemtuzumab ozogamicin (Mylotarg). Blood Cells Mol Dis. 2003;31:7-10.

585. Sievers EL, Linenberger M. Mylotarg: antibody-targeted chemotherapy comes of age. Curr Opin Oncol. 2001;13:522-527.

586. Zwaan CM, Reinhardt D, Corbacioglu S, et al. Gemtuzumab ozogamicin: first clinical experiences in children with relapsed/refractory acute myeloid leukemia treated on compassionate-use basis. Blood. 2003;101:3868-3871.

587. Specchia G, Pastore D, Carluccio P, et al. Gemtuzumab ozogamicin with cytarabine and mitoxantrone as a third-line treatment in a poor prognosis group of adult acute myeloid leukemia patients: a single-center experience. Ann Hematol. 2007;86:425-428.

588. Brethon B, Auvrignon A, Cayuela JM, et al. Molecular response in two children with relapsed acute myeloid leukemia treated with a combination of gemtuzumab ozogamicin and cytarabine. Haematologica. 2006;91:419-421.

589. Clavio M, Vignolo L, Albarello A, et al. Adding low-dose gemtuzumab ozogamicin to fludarabine, Ara-C and idarubicin (MY-FLAI) may improve disease-free and overall survival in elderly patients with non-M3 acute myeloid leukaemia: results of a prospective, pilot, multi-centre trial and comparison with a historical cohort of patients. Br J Haematol. 2007;138:186-195.

590. Eom KS, Kim HJ, Min WS, et al. Gemtuzumab ozogamicin in combination with attenuated doses of standard induction chemotherapy can successfully induce complete remission without increasing toxicity in patients with acute myeloid leukemia aged 55 or older. Eur J Haematol. 2007;79:398-404.

591. Tsimberidou AM, Giles FJ, Estey E, et al. The role of gemtuzumab ozogamicin in acute leukaemia therapy. Br J Haematol. 2006;132:398-409.

592. Clark JJ, Cools J, Curley DP, et al. Variable sensitivity of FLT3 activation loop mutations to the small molecule tyrosine kinase inhibitor MLN518. Blood. 2004;104:2867-2872.

593. Barry EV, Clark JJ, Cools J, et al. Uniform sensitivity of FLT3 activation loop mutants to the tyrosine kinase inhibitor midostaurin. Blood. 2007;110:4476-4479.

594. Mesters RM, Padro T, Bieker R, et al. Stable remission after administration of the receptor tyrosine kinase inhibitor SU5416 in a patient with refractory acute myeloid leukemia. Blood. 2001;98:241-243.

595. Karp JE. Farnesyl protein transferase inhibitors as targeted therapies for hematologic malignancies. Semin Hematol. 2001;38:16-23.

596. Lancet JE, Gojo I, Gotlib J, et al. A phase 2 study of the farnesyltransferase inhibitor tipifarnib in poor-risk and elderly patients with previously untreated acute myelogenous leukemia. Blood. 2007;109:1387-1394.

597. Harousseau JL, Lancet JE, Reiffers J, et al. A phase 2 study of the oral farnesyltransferase inhibitor tipifarnib in patients with refractory or relapsed acute myeloid leukemia. Blood. 2007;109:5151-5156.

598. Zimmerman TM, Harlin H, Odenike OM, et al. Dose-ranging pharmacodynamic study of tipifarnib (R115777) in patients with relapsed and refractory hematologic malignancies. J Clin Oncol. 2004;22:4816-4822.

599. Widemann BC, Salzer WL, Arceci RJ, et al. Phase I trial and pharmacokinetic study of the farnesyltransferase inhibitor tipifarnib in children with refractory solid tumors or neurofibromatosis type I and plexiform neurofibromas. J Clin Oncol. 2006;24:507-516.

600. Fouladi M, Nicholson HS, Zhou T, et al. A phase II study of the farnesyl transferase inhibitor, tipifarnib, in children with recurrent or progressive high-grade glioma, medulloblastoma/primitive neuroectodermal tumor, or brainstem glioma: a Children's Oncology Group study. Cancer. 2007;110:2535-2541.

601. Gore L, Holden SN, Cohen RB, et al. A phase I safety, pharmacological and biological study of the farnesyl protein transferase inhibitor, tipifarnib and capecitabine in advanced solid tumors. Ann Oncol. 2006;17:1709-1717.

602. Cortes J, Faderl S, Estey E, et al. Phase I study of BMS-214662, a farnesyl transferase inhibitor in patients with acute leukemias and high-risk myelodysplastic syndromes. J Clin Oncol. 2005;23:2805-2812.

603. Peterson LF, Zhang DE. The 8;21 translocation in leukemogenesis. Oncogene. 2004;23:4255-4262.

604. Hart SM, Foroni L. Core binding factor genes and human leukemia. Haematologica. 2002;87:1307-1323.

605. Minucci S, Nervi C, Lo Coco F, Pelicci PG. Histone deacetylases: a common molecular target for differentiation treatment of acute myeloid leukemias? Oncogene. 2001;20:3110-3115.

606. Durst KL, Hiebert SW. Role of RUNX family members in transcriptional repression and gene silencing. Oncogene. 2004;23:4220-4224.

607. Blyth K, Cameron ER, Neil JC. The RUNX genes: gain or loss of function in cancer. Nat Rev Cancer. 2005;5:376-387.

608. Cameron ER, Neil JC. The Runx genes: lineage-specific oncogenes and tumor suppressors. Oncogene. 2004;23:4308-4314.

609. Drummond DC, Noble CO, Kirpotin DB, et al. Clinical development of histone deacetylase inhibitors as anticancer agents. Annu Rev Pharmacol Toxicol. 2005;45:495-528.

610. Marks PA, Richon VM, Breslow R, Rifkind RA. Histone deacetylase inhibitors as new cancer drugs. Curr Opin Oncol. 2001;13:477-483.

611. Soriano AO, Yang H, Faderl S, et al. Safety and clinical activity of the combination of 5-azacytidine, valproic acid, and all-trans retinoic acid in acute myeloid leukemia and myelodysplastic syndrome. Blood. 2007;110:2302-2308.

612. Kuendgen A, Strupp C, Aivado M, et al. Treatment of myelodysplastic syndromes with valproic acid alone or in combination with all-trans retinoic acid. Blood. 2004;104:1266-1269.

613. Piekarz RL, Robey R, Sandor V, et al. Inhibitor of histone deacetylation, depsipeptide (FR901228), in the treatment of peripheral and cutaneous T-cell lymphoma: a case report. Blood. 2001;98:2865-2868.

614. Byrd JC, Marcucci G, Parthun MR, et al. A phase 1 and pharmacodynamic study of depsipeptide (FK228) in chronic lymphocytic leukemia and acute myeloid leukemia. Blood. 2005;105:959-967.

615. Christiansen DH, Andersen MK, Pedersen-Bjergaard J. Methylation of p15INK4B is common, is associated with deletion of genes on chromosome arm 7q and predicts a poor prognosis in therapy-related myelodysplasia and acute myeloid leukemia. Leukemia. 2003;17:1813-1819.

616. Daskalakis M, Nguyen TT, Nguyen C, et al. Demethylation of a hypermethylated P15/INK4B gene in patients with myelodysplastic syndrome by 5-Aza-2'-deoxycytidine (decitabine) treatment. Blood. 2002;100:2957-2964.

617. Hasegawa D, Manabe A, Kubota T, et al. Methylation status of the p15 and p16 genes in paediatric myelodysplastic syndrome and juvenile myelomonocytic leukaemia. Br J Haematol. 2005;128:805-812.

618. Johan MF, Bowen DT, Frew ME, et al. Aberrant methylation of the negative regulators RASSFIA, SHP-1 and SOCS-1 in myelodysplastic syndromes and acute myeloid leukaemia. Br J Haematol. 2005;129:60-65.

619. Leone G, Teofili L, Voso MT, Lubbert M. DNA methylation and demethylating drugs in myelodysplastic syndromes and secondary leukemias. Haematologica. 2002;87:1324-1341.

620. Momparler RL. Cancer epigenetics. Oncogene. 2003;22:6479-6483.

621. Kaminskas E, Farrell A, Abraham S, et al. Approval summary: azacitidine for treatment of myelodysplastic syndrome subtypes. Clin Cancer Res. 2005;11:3604-3608.

622. Sudan N, Rossetti JM, Shadduck RK, et al. Treatment of acute myelogenous leukemia with outpatient azacitidine. Cancer. 2006;107:1839-1843.

623. Issa JP, Garcia-Manero G, Giles FJ, et al. Phase 1 study of low-dose prolonged exposure schedules of the hypomethylating agent 5-aza-2'-deoxycytidine (decitabine) in hematopoietic malignancies. Blood. 2004;103:1635-1640.

624. Petti MC, Mandelli F, Zagonel V, et al. Pilot study of 5-aza-2'-deoxycytidine (Decitabine) in the treatment of poor prognosis acute myelogenous leukemia patients: preliminary results. Leukemia. 1993;7(Suppl 1):36-41.

625. Pinto A, Attadia V, Fusco A, et al. 5-Aza-2'-deoxycytidine induces terminal differentiation of leukemic blasts from patients with acute myeloid leukemias. Blood. 1984;64:922-929.

626. Garcia-Manero G, Kantarjian HM, Sanchez-Gonzalez B, et al. Phase 1/2 study of the combination of 5-aza-2'-deoxycytidine with valproic acid in patients with leukemia. Blood. 2006; 108:3271-3279.

627. Blum W, Klisovic RB, Hackanson B, et al. Phase I study of decitabine alone or in combination with valproic acid in acute myeloid leukemia. J Clin Oncol. 2007;25:3884-3891.

628. Drexler HC. Activation of the cell death program by inhibition of proteasome function. Proc Natl Acad Sci U S A. 1997;94: 855-860.

629. Adams J, Palombella VJ, Sausville EA, et al. Proteasome inhibitors: a novel class of potent and effective antitumor agents. Cancer Res. 1999;59:2615-2622.

630. Kitagawa H, Tani E, Ikemoto H, et al. Proteasome inhibitors induce mitochondria-independent apoptosis in human glioma cells. FEBS Lett. 1999;443:181-186.

631. Hideshima T, Mitsiades C, Akiyama M, et al. Molecular mechanisms mediating antimyeloma activity of proteasome inhibitor PS-341. Blood. 2003;101:1530-1534.

632. Yanamandra N, Colaco NM, Parquet NA, et al. Tipifarnib and bortezomib are synergistic and overcome cell adhesion-mediated drug resistance in multiple myeloma and acute myeloid leukemia. Clin Cancer Res. 2006;12:591-599.

633. Minderman H, Zhou Y, O'Loughlin KL, Baer MR. Bortezomib activity and in vitro interactions with anthracyclines and cytarabine in acute myeloid leukemia cells are independent of multidrug resistance mechanisms and p53 status. Cancer Chemother Pharmacol. 2007;60:245-255.

634. Riccioni R, Senese M, Diverio D, et al. M4 and M5 acute myeloid leukaemias display a high sensitivity to Bortezomib-mediated apoptosis. Br J Haematol. 2007;139:194-205.

635. Colado E, Alvarez-Fernandez S, Maiso P, et al. The effect of the proteasome inhibitor bortezomib on acute myeloid leukemia cells and drug resistance associated with the CD34+ immature phenotype. Haematologica. 2008;93:57-66.

636. Attar EC, De Angelo DJ, Supko JG, et al. Phase I and pharmacokinetic study of bortezomib in combination with idarubicin and cytarabine in patients with acute myelogenous leukemia. Clin Cancer Res. 2008;14:1446-1454.

637. Hess CJ, Berkhof J, Denkers F, et al. Activated intrinsic apoptosis pathway is a key related prognostic parameter in acute myeloid leukemia. J Clin Oncol. 2007;25:1209-1215.

638. Karakas T, Miething CC, Maurer U, et al. The coexpression of the apoptosis-related genes bcl-2 and wt1 in predicting survival in adult acute myeloid leukemia. Leukemia. 2002;16:846-854.

639. Venditti A, Del Poeta G, Maurillo L, et al. Combined analysis of bcl-2 and MDR1 proteins in 256 cases of acute myeloid leukemia. Haematologica. 2004;89:934-939.

640. Marcucci G, Stock W, Dai G, et al. Phase I study of oblimersen sodium, an antisense to Bcl-2, in untreated older patients with acute myeloid leukemia: pharmacokinetics, pharmacodynamics, and clinical activity. J Clin Oncol. 2005;23:3404-3411.

641. Marcucci G, Byrd JC, Dai G, et al. Phase 1 and pharmacodynamic studies of G3139, a Bcl-2 antisense oligonucleotide, in

combination with chemotherapy in refractory or relapsed acute leukemia. Blood. 2003;101:425-432.

642. Tallman MS, Kwaan HC. Reassessing the hemostatic disorder associated with acute promyelocytic leukemia. Blood. 1992;79: 543-553.

643. Dombret H, Scrobohaci ML, Ghorra P, et al. Coagulation disorders associated with acute promyelocytic leukemia: corrective effect of all-trans retinoic acid treatment. Leukemia. 1993;7: 2-9.

644. Grimwade D, Lo Coco F. Acute promyelocytic leukemia: a model for the role of molecular diagnosis and residual disease monitoring in directing treatment approach in acute myeloid leukemia. Leukemia. 2002;16:1959-1973.

645. Pandolfi PP, Alcalay M, Longo L, et al. Molecular genetics of the t(15;17) of acute promyelocytic leukemia (APPL). Leukemia. 1992;6(Suppl 3):120S-122S.

646. Grignani F, Ferrucci PF, Testa U, et al. The acute promyelocytic leukemia-specific PML-RAR alpha fusion protein inhibits differentiation and promotes survival of myeloid precursor cells. Cell. 1993;74:423-431.

647. Grignani F, Valtieri M, Gabbianelli M, et al. PML/RAR alpha fusion protein expression in normal human hematopoietic progenitors dictates myeloid commitment and the promyelocytic phenotype. Blood. 2000;96:1531-1537.

648. Gale RE, Hills R, Pizzey AR, et al. Relationship between FLT3 mutation status, biologic characteristics, and response to targeted therapy in acute promyelocytic leukemia. Blood. 2005; 106:3768-3776.

649. Callens C, Chevret S, Cayuela JM, et al. Prognostic implication of FLT3 and Ras gene mutations in patients with acute promyelocytic leukemia (APL): a retrospective study from the European APL Group. Leukemia. 2005;19:1153-1160.

650. Kainz B, Heintel D, Marculescu R, et al. Variable prognostic value of FLT3 internal tandem duplications in patients with de novo AML and a normal karyotype, t(15;17), t(8;21) or inv(16). Hematol J. 2002;3:283-289.

651. Noguera NI, Breccia M, Divona M, et al. Alterations of the FLT3 gene in acute promyelocytic leukemia: association with diagnostic characteristics and analysis of clinical outcome in patients treated with the Italian AIDA protocol. Leukemia. 2002;16:2185-2189.

652. Shih LY, Kuo MC, Liang DC, et al. Internal tandem duplication and Asp835 mutations of the FMS-like tyrosine kinase 3 (FLT3) gene in acute promyelocytic leukemia. Cancer. 2003;98:1206-1216.

653. Au WY, Fung A, Chim CS, et al. FLT-3 aberrations in acute promyelocytic leukaemia: clinicopathological associations and prognostic impact. Br J Haematol. 2004;125:463-469.

654. Hasan SK, Sazawal S, Dutta P, et al. Impact of FLT3 internal tandem duplications on Indian acute promyelocytic leukemia patients: prognostic implications. Hematology. 2007;12:99-101.

655. Yoo SJ, Park CJ, Jang S, et al. Inferior prognostic outcome in acute promyelocytic leukemia with alterations of FLT3 gene. Leuk Lymphoma. 2006;47:1788-1793.

656. Mantadakis E, Samonis G, Kalmanti M. A comprehensive review of acute promyelocytic leukemia in children. Acta Haematol. 2008;119:73-82.

657. Chou WC, Tang JL, Yao M, et al. Clinical and biological characteristics of acute promyelocytic leukemia in Taiwan: a high relapse rate in patients with high initial and peak white blood cell counts during all-trans retinoic acid treatment. Leukemia. 1997;11:921-928.

658. Asou N, Adachi K, Tamura J, et al. Analysis of prognostic factors in newly diagnosed acute promyelocytic leukemia treated with all-trans retinoic acid and chemotherapy. Japan Adult Leukemia Study Group. J Clin Oncol. 1998;16:78-85.

659. Sanz MA, Lo Coco F, Martin G, et al. Definition of relapse risk and role of nonanthracycline drugs for consolidation in patients with acute promyelocytic leukemia: a joint study of the PETHEMA and GIMEMA cooperative groups. Blood. 2000;96:1247-1253.

660. Chomienne C, Ballerini P, Balitrand N, et al. All-trans retinoic acid in acute promyelocytic leukemias. II. In vitro studies: structure-function relationship. Blood. 1990;76:1710-1717.

661. Warrell RP Jr, Frankel SR, Miller WH Jr, et al. Differentiation therapy of acute promyelocytic leukemia with tretinoin (all-trans-retinoic acid). N Engl J Med. 1991;324:1385-1393.

662. Chen ZX, Xue YQ, Zhang R, et al. A clinical and experimental study on all-trans retinoic acid-treated acute promyelocytic leukemia patients. Blood. 1991;78:1413-1419.

663. Fenaux P, Chastang C, Chevret S, et al. A randomized comparison of all transretinoic acid (ATRA) followed by chemotherapy and ATRA plus chemotherapy and the role of maintenance therapy in newly diagnosed acute promyelocytic leukemia. The European APL Group. Blood. 1999;94: 1192-1200.

664. Fenaux P, Le Deley MC, Castaigne S, et al. Effect of all transretinoic acid in newly diagnosed acute promyelocytic leukemia. Results of a multicenter randomized trial. European APL 91 Group. Blood. 1993;82:3241-3249.

665. Kanamaru A, Takemoto Y, Tanimoto M, et al. All-trans retinoic acid for the treatment of newly diagnosed acute promyelocytic leukemia. Japan Adult Leukemia Study Group. Blood. 1995; 85:1202-1206.

666. Mandelli F, Diverio D, Avvisati G, et al. Molecular remission in PML/RAR alpha-positive acute promyelocytic leukemia by combined all-trans retinoic acid and idarubicin (AIDA) therapy. Gruppo Italiano-Malattie Ematologiche Maligne dell'Adulto and Associazione Italiana di Ematologia ed Oncologia Pediatrica Cooperative Groups. Blood. 1997;90:1014-1021.

667. Sanz MA, Martin G, Rayon C, et al. A modified AIDA protocol with anthracycline-based consolidation results in high antileukemic efficacy and reduced toxicity in newly diagnosed PML/RARalpha-positive acute promyelocytic leukemia. PETHEMA group. Blood. 1999;94:3015-3021.

668. Fenaux P, Chevret S, Guerci A, et al. Long-term follow-up confirms the benefit of all-trans retinoic acid in acute promyelocytic leukemia. European APL group. Leukemia. 2000;14: 1371-1377.

669. de Botton S, Coiteux V, Chevret S, et al. Outcome of childhood acute promyelocytic leukemia with all-trans-retinoic acid and chemotherapy. J Clin Oncol. 2004;22:1404-1412.

670. Ortega JJ, Madero L, Martin G, et al. Treatment with all-trans retinoic acid and anthracycline monochemotherapy for children with acute promyelocytic leukemia: a multicenter study by the PETHEMA Group. J Clin Oncol. 2005;23:7632-7640.

671. Testi AM, Biondi A, Lo Coco F, et al. GIMEMA-AIEOPAIDA protocol for the treatment of newly diagnosed acute promyelocytic leukemia (APL) in children. Blood. 2005;106:447-453.

672. De Botton S, Dombret H, Sanz M, et al. Incidence, clinical features, and outcome of all trans-retinoic acid syndrome in 413 cases of newly diagnosed acute promyelocytic leukemia. The European APL Group. Blood. 1998;92:2712-2718.

673. Frankel SR, Eardley A, Lauwers G, et al. The "retinoic acid syndrome" in acute promyelocytic leukemia. Ann Intern Med. 1992;117:292-296.

674. Tallman MS, Andersen JW, Schiffer CA, et al. Clinical description of 44 patients with acute promyelocytic leukemia who developed the retinoic acid syndrome. Blood. 2000;95:90-95.

675. Vahdat L, Maslak P, Miller WH Jr, et al. Early mortality and the retinoic acid syndrome in acute promyelocytic leukemia: impact of leukocytosis, low-dose chemotherapy, PMN/RAR-alpha isoform, and CD13 expression in patients treated with all-trans retinoic acid. Blood. 1994;84:3843-3849.

676. Ko BS, Tang JL, Chen YC, et al. Extramedullary relapse after all-trans retinoic acid treatment in acute promyelocytic leukemia—the occurrence of retinoic acid syndrome is a risk factor. Leukemia. 1999;13:1406-1408.

677. Fenaux P, Castaigne S, Dombret H, et al. All-transretinoic acid followed by intensive chemotherapy gives a high complete remission rate and may prolong remissions in newly diagnosed acute promyelocytic leukemia: a pilot study on 26 cases. Blood. 1992;80:2176-2181.

678. Wall M. Idiopathic intracranial hypertension (pseudotumor cerebri). Curr Neurol Neurosci Rep. 2008;8:87-93.

679. Agarwal MR, Yoo JH. Optic nerve sheath fenestration for vision preservation in idiopathic intracranial hypertension. Neurosurg Focus. 2007;23:E7.

680. Lanvers C, Reinhardt D, Dubbers A, et al. Pharmacology of all-trans-retinoic acid in children with acute promyelocytic leukemia. Med Pediatr Oncol. 2003;40:293-301.

681. Castaigne S, Lefebvre P, Chomienne C, et al. Effectiveness and pharmacokinetics of low-dose all-trans retinoic acid (25 mg/m2) in acute promyelocytic leukemia. Blood. 1993;82:3560-3563.

682. Zhu J, Koken MH, Quignon F, et al. Arsenic-induced PML targeting onto nuclear bodies: implications for the treatment of acute promyelocytic leukemia. Proc Natl Acad Sci U S A. 1997;94:3978-3983.

683. Soignet SL, Maslak P, Wang ZG, et al. Complete remission after treatment of acute promyelocytic leukemia with arsenic trioxide. N Engl J Med. 1998;339:1341-1348.

684. Konig A, Wrazel L, Warrell RP Jr, et al. Comparative activity of melarsoprol and arsenic trioxide in chronic B-cell leukemia lines. Blood. 1997;90:562-570.

685. Tamm I, Paternostro G, Zapata JM. Treatment of acute promyelocytic leukemia with arsenic trioxide. N Engl J Med. 1999;340:1043; author reply 1044-1045.

686. Niu C, Yan H, Yu T, et al. Studies on treatment of acute promyelocytic leukemia with arsenic trioxide: remission induction, follow-up, and molecular monitoring in 11 newly diagnosed and 47 relapsed acute promyelocytic leukemia patients. Blood. 1999;94:3315-3324.

687. Soignet SL, Frankel SR, Douer D, et al. United States multicenter study of arsenic trioxide in relapsed acute promyelocytic leukemia. J Clin Oncol. 2001;19:3852-3860.

688. Lu DP, Qiu JY, Jiang B, et al. Tetra-arsenic tetra-sulfide for the treatment of acute promyelocytic leukemia: a pilot report. Blood. 2002;99:3136-3143.

689. Zhang P. The use of arsenic trioxide (As_2O_3) in the treatment of acute promyelocytic leukemia. J Biol Regul Homeost Agents. 1999;13:195-200.

690. George B, Mathews V, Poonkuzhali B, et al. Treatment of children with newly diagnosed acute promyelocytic leukemia with arsenic trioxide: a single center experience. Leukemia. 2004;18: 1587-1590.

691. Zhang L, Zhao H, Zhu X, et al. Retrospective analysis of 65 Chinese children with acute promyelocytic leukemia: a single center experience. Pediatr Blood Cancer. 2008;51:210-215.

692. Quezada G, Kopp L, Estey E, Wells RJ. All-trans-retinoic acid and arsenic trioxide as initial therapy for acute promyelocytic leukemia. Pediatr Blood Cancer. 2008;51:133-135.

693. Shen ZX, Shi ZZ, Fang J, et al. All-trans retinoic acid/As_2O_3 combination yields a high quality remission and survival in newly diagnosed acute promyelocytic leukemia. Proc Natl Acad Sci U S A. 2004;101:5328-5335.

694. Mathews V, George B, Lakshmi KM, et al. Single-agent arsenic trioxide in the treatment of newly diagnosed acute promyelocytic leukemia: durable remissions with minimal toxicity. Blood. 2006;107:2627-2632.

695. Ohnishi K, Yoshida H, Shigeno K, et al. Arsenic trioxide therapy for relapsed or refractory Japanese patients with acute promy-

elocytic leukemia: need for careful electrocardiogram monitoring. Leukemia. 2002;16:617-622.

696. Westervelt P, Brown RA, Adkins DR, et al. Sudden death in patients with acute promyelocytic leukemia treated with arsenic trioxide. Blood. 2001;98:266-271.

697. Huang SY, Chang CS, Tang JL, et al. Acute and chronic arsenic poisoning associated with treatment of acute promyelocytic leukaemia. Br J Haematol. 1998;103:1092-1095.

698. Unnikrishnan D, Dutcher JP, Garl S, et al. Cardiac monitoring of patients receiving arsenic trioxide therapy. Br J Haematol. 2004;124:610-617.

699. Patel SP, Garcia-Manero G, Ferrajoli A, et al. Cardiotoxicity in African-American patients treated with arsenic trioxide for acute promyelocytic leukemia. Leuk Res. 2006;30:362-363.

700. Barbey JT, Pezzullo JC, Soignet SL. Effect of arsenic trioxide on QT interval in patients with advanced malignancies. J Clin Oncol. 2003;21:3609-3615.

701. Camacho LH, Soignet SL, Chanel S, et al. Leukocytosis and the retinoic acid syndrome in patients with acute promyelocytic leukemia treated with arsenic trioxide. J Clin Oncol. 2000; 18:2620-2625.

702. Lazo G, Kantarjian H, Estey E, et al. Use of arsenic trioxide (As_2O_3) in the treatment of patients with acute promyelocytic leukemia: the M. D. Anderson experience. Cancer. 2003;97: 2218-2224.

703. Fox E, Razzouk BI, Widemann BC, et al. Phase 1 trial and pharmacokinetic study of arsenic trioxide in children and adolescents with refractory or relapsed acute leukemia, including acute promyelocytic leukemia or lymphoma. Blood. 2008;111: 566-573.

704. Thomas X, Le QH, Fiere D. Anthracycline-related toxicity requiring cardiac transplantation in long-term disease-free survivors with acute promyelocytic leukemia. Ann Hematol. 2002;81:504-507.

705. Guglielmi C, Martelli MP, Diverio D, et al. Immunophenotype of adult and childhood acute promyelocytic leukaemia: correlation with morphology, type of PML gene breakpoint and clinical outcome. A cooperative Italian study on 196 cases. Br J Haematol. 1998;102:1035-1041.

706. Petti MC, Pinazzi MB, Diverio D, et al. Prolonged molecular remission in advanced acute promyelocytic leukaemia after treatment with gemtuzumab ozogamicin (Mylotarg CMA-676). Br J Haematol. 2001;115:63-65.

707. Lo-Coco F, Cimino G, Breccia M, et al. Gemtuzumab ozogamicin (Mylotarg) as a single agent for molecularly relapsed acute promyelocytic leukemia. Blood. 2004;104:1995-1999.

708. Estey EH, Giles FJ, Beran M, et al. Experience with gemtuzumab ozogamycin ("mylotarg") and all-trans retinoic acid in untreated acute promyelocytic leukemia. Blood. 2002;99: 4222-4224.

709. Lee BD, Sevcikova S, Kogan SC. Dual treatment with FLT3 inhibitor SU11657 and doxorubicin increases survival of leukemic mice. Leuk Res. 2007;31:1131-1134.

710. Sohal J, Phan VT, Chan PV, et al. A model of APL with FLT3 mutation is responsive to retinoic acid and a receptor tyrosine kinase inhibitor, SU11657. Blood. 2003;101:3188-3197.

711. Thomas X, Anglaret B, Thiebaut A, et al. Improvement of prognosis in refractory and relapsed acute promyelocytic leukemia over recent years: the role of all-trans retinoic acid therapy. Ann Hematol. 1997;75:195-200.

712. Meloni G, Diverio D, Vignetti M, et al. Autologous bone marrow transplantation for acute promyelocytic leukemia in second remission: prognostic relevance of pretransplant minimal residual disease assessment by reverse-transcription polymerase chain reaction of the PML/RAR alpha fusion gene. Blood. 1997;90:1321-1325.

713. de Botton S, Fawaz A, Chevret S, et al. Autologous and allogeneic stem-cell transplantation as salvage treatment of acute pro-

myelocytic leukemia initially treated with all-trans-retinoic acid: a retrospective analysis of the European acute promyelocytic leukemia group. J Clin Oncol. 2005;23:120-126.

714. Dvorak CC, Agarwal R, Dahl GV, et al. Hematopoietic stem cell transplant for pediatric acute promyelocytic leukemia. Biol Blood Marrow Transplant. 2008;14:824-830.

715. Lo-Coco F, Romano A, Mengarelli A, et al. Allogeneic stem cell transplantation for advanced acute promyelocytic leukemia: results in patients treated in second molecular remission or with molecularly persistent disease. Leukemia. 2003;17:1930-1933.

716. de Botton S, Sanz MA, Chevret S, et al. Extramedullary relapse in acute promyelocytic leukemia treated with all-trans retinoic acid and chemotherapy. Leukemia. 2006;20:35-41.

717. Breccia M, Carmosino I, Diverio D, et al. Early detection of meningeal localization in acute promyelocytic leukaemia patients with high presenting leucocyte count. Br J Haematol. 2003;120: 266-270.

718. Evans GD, Grimwade DJ. Extramedullary disease in acute promyelocytic leukemia. Leuk Lymphoma. 1999;33:219-229.

719. Ravandi F. Prophylactic intrathecal chemotherapy in acute promyelocytic leukemia (APL). Leukemia. 2004;18:879-880.

720. Ohno R, Asou N, Ohnishi K. Treatment of acute promyelocytic leukemia: strategy toward further increase of cure rate. Leukemia. 2003;17:1454-1463.

721. Santamaria C, Chillon MC, Fernandez C, et al. Using quantification of the PML-RARalpha transcript to stratify the risk of relapse in patients with acute promyelocytic leukemia. Haematologica. 2007;92:315-322.

722. Xin L, Wan-jun S, Zeng-jun L, et al. A survival study and prognostic factors analysis on acute promyelocytic leukemia at a single center. Leuk Res. 2007;31:765-771.

723. Reiter A, Lengfelder E, Grimwade D. Pathogenesis, diagnosis and monitoring of residual disease in acute promyelocytic leukaemia. Acta Haematol. 2004;112:55-67.

724. Korninger L, Knobl P, Laczika K, et al. PML-RAR alpha PCR positivity in the bone marrow of patients with APL precedes haematological relapse by 2-3 months. Br J Haematol. 1994;88: 427-431.

725. Weijerman ME, van Furth AM, Vonk Noordegraaf A, et al. Prevalence, neonatal characteristics, and first-year mortality of Down syndrome: a national study. J Pediatr. 2008;152:15-19.

726. Pritchard M, Reeves RH, Dierssen M, et al. Down syndrome and the genes of human chromosome 21: current knowledge and future potentials. Report on the Expert workshop on the biology of chromosome 21 genes: towards gene-phenotype correlations in Down syndrome. Washington DC, September 28-October 1, 2007. Cytogenet Genome Res. 2008;121:67-77.

727. Gamis AS, Hilden JM. Transient myeloproliferative disorder, a disorder with too few data and many unanswered questions: does it contain an important piece of the puzzle to understanding hematopoiesis and acute myelogenous leukemia? J Pediatr Hematol Oncol. 2002;24:2-5.

728. Zipursky A, Rose T, Skidmore M, et al. Hydrops fetalis and neonatal leukemia in Down syndrome. Pediatr Hematol Oncol. 1996;13:81-87.

729. Al-Kasim F, Doyle JJ, Massey GV, et al. Incidence and treatment of potentially lethal diseases in transient leukemia of Down syndrome: Pediatric Oncology Group Study. J Pediatr Hematol Oncol. 2002;24:9-13.

730. Zipursky A, Poon A, Doyle J. Leukemia in Down syndrome: a review. Pediatr Hematol Oncol. 1992;9:139-149.

731. Zipursky A, Brown EJ, Christensen H, Doyle J. Transient myeloproliferative disorder (transient leukemia) and hematologic manifestations of Down syndrome. Clin Lab Med. 1999;19:157-167, vii.

732. Kounami S, Aoyagi N, Tsuno H, et al. Additional chromosome abnormalities in transient abnormal myelopoiesis in Down's syndrome patients. Acta Haematol. 1997;98:109-112.

733. Yamaguchi Y, Fujii H, Kazama H, et al. Acute myeloblastic leukemia associated with trisomy 8 and translocation 8;21 in a child with Down syndrome. Cancer Genet Cytogenet. 1997; 97:32-34.

734. Morgan R, Hecht F, Cleary ML, et al. Leukemia with Down's syndrome: translocation between chromosomes 1 and 19 in acute myelomonocytic leukemia following transient congenital myeloproliferative syndrome. Blood. 1985;66:1466-1468.

735. Wong KY, Jones MM, Srivastava AK, Gruppo RA. Transient myeloproliferative disorder and acute nonlymphoblastic leukemia in Down syndrome. J Pediatr. 1988;112:18-22.

736. Hitzler JK, Cheung J, Li Y, et al. GATA1 mutations in transient leukemia and acute megakaryoblastic leukemia of Down syndrome. Blood. 2003;101:4301-4304.

737. Groet J, McElwaine S, Spinelli M, et al. Acquired mutations in GATA1 in neonates with Down's syndrome with transient myeloid disorder. Lancet. 2003;361:1617-1620.

738. Rainis L, Bercovich D, Strehl S, et al. Mutations in exon 2 of GATA1 are early events in megakaryocytic malignancies associated with trisomy 21. Blood. 2003;102:981-986.

739. Xu G, Nagano M, Kanezaki R, et al. Frequent mutations in the GATA-1 gene in the transient myeloproliferative disorder of Down syndrome. Blood. 2003;102:2960-2968.

740. Mundschau G, Gurbuxani S, Gamis AS, et al. Mutagenesis of GATA1 is an initiating event in Down syndrome leukemogenesis. Blood. 2003;101:4298-4300.

741. Greene ME, Mundschau G, Wechsler J, et al. Mutations in GATA1 in both transient myeloproliferative disorder and acute megakaryoblastic leukemia of Down syndrome. Blood Cells Mol Dis. 2003;31:351-356.

742. Ahmed M, Sternberg A, Hall G, et al. Natural history of GATA1 mutations in Down syndrome. Blood. 2004;103:2480-2489.

743. Cantor AB, Orkin SH. Transcriptional regulation of erythropoiesis: an affair involving multiple partners. Oncogene. 2002; 21:3368-3376.

744. Martin DI, Orkin SH. Transcriptional activation and DNA binding by the erythroid factor GF-1/NF-E1/Eryf 1. Genes Dev. 1990;4:1886-1898.

745. Calligaris R, Bottardi S, Cogoi S, et al. Alternative translation initiation site usage results in two functionally distinct forms of the GATA-1 transcription factor. Proc Natl Acad Sci U S A. 1995;92:11598-11602.

746. Gurbuxani S, Vyas P, Crispino JD. Recent insights into the mechanisms of myeloid leukemogenesis in Down syndrome. Blood. 2004;103:399-406.

747. Hasle H, Lund B, Nyvold CG, et al. WT1 gene expression in children with Down syndrome and transient myeloproliferative disorder. Leuk Res. 2006;30:543-546.

748. De Vita S, Mulligan C, McElwaine S, et al. Loss-of-function JAK3 mutations in TMD and AMKL of Down syndrome. Br J Haematol. 2007;137:337-341.

749. Sato T, Toki T, Kanezaki R, et al. Functional analysis of JAK3 mutations in transient myeloproliferative disorder and acute megakaryoblastic leukaemia accompanying Down syndrome. Br J Haematol. 2008;141:681-688.

750. Massey GV. Transient leukemia in newborns with Down syndrome. Pediatr Blood Cancer. 2005;44:29-32.

751. Schunk GJ, Lehman WL. Mongolism and congenital leukemia. JAMA. 1954;155:250-251.

752. Weinstein HJ. Congenital leukaemia and the neonatal myeloproliferative disorders associated with Down's syndrome. Clin Haematol. 1978;7:147-154.

753. Paolucci G, Rosito P. Neonatal myeloproliferative disorders in Down's syndrome and congenital leukemias. Haematologica. 1987;72:121-125.

754. Nakagawa T, Nishida H, Arai T, et al. Hyperviscosity syndrome with transient abnormal myelopoiesis in Down syndrome. J Pediatr. 1988;112:58-61.

755. Becroft DM, Zwi LJ. Perinatal visceral fibrosis accompanying the megakaryoblastic leukemoid reaction of Down syndrome. Pediatr Pathol. 1990;10:397-406.

756. Ruchelli ED, Uri A, Dimmick JE, et al. Severe perinatal liver disease and Down syndrome: an apparent relationship. Hum Pathol. 1991;22:1274-1280.

757. Miyauchi J, Ito Y, Kawano T, et al. Unusual diffuse liver fibrosis accompanying transient myeloproliferative disorder in Down's syndrome: a report of four autopsy cases and proposal of a hypothesis. Blood. 1992;80:1521-1527.

758. Muramatsu H, Kato K, Watanabe N, et al. Risk factors for early death in neonates with Down syndrome and transient leukaemia. Br J Haematol. 2008 May 28. [Epub ahead of print].

759. Dormann S, Kruger M, Hentschel R, et al. Life-threatening complications of transient abnormal myelopoiesis in neonates with Down syndrome. Eur J Pediatr. 2004;163:374-377.

760. Tchernia G, Lejeune F, Boccara JF, et al. Erythroblastic and/or megakaryoblastic leukemia in Down syndrome: treatment with low-dose arabinosyl cytosine. J Pediatr Hematol Oncol. 1996; 18:59-62.

761. Hitzler JK. Acute megakaryoblastic leukemia in Down syndrome. Pediatr Blood Cancer. 2007;49:1066-1069.

762. Hasle H, Clemmensen IH, Mikkelsen M. Risks of leukaemia and solid tumours in individuals with Down's syndrome. Lancet. 2000;355:165-169.

763. Fong CT, Brodeur GM. Down's syndrome and leukemia: epidemiology, genetics, cytogenetics and mechanisms of leukemogenesis. Cancer Genet Cytogenet. 1987;28:55-76.

764. Creutzig U, Ritter J, Vormoor J, et al. Myelodysplasia and acute myelogenous leukemia in Down's syndrome. A report of 40 children of the AML-BFM Study Group. Leukemia. 1996;10: 1677-1686.

765. Kojima S, Kato K, Matsuyama T, et al. Favorable treatment outcome in children with acute myeloid leukemia and Down syndrome. Blood. 1993;81:3164.

766. Lange BJ, Kobrinsky N, Barnard DR, et al. Distinctive demography, biology, and outcome of acute myeloid leukemia and myelodysplastic syndrome in children with Down syndrome: Children's Cancer Group Studies 2861 and 2891. Blood. 1998;91:608-615.

767. Robison LL, Nesbit ME Jr, Sather HN, et al. Down syndrome and acute leukemia in children: a 10-year retrospective survey from Childrens Cancer Study Group. J Pediatr. 1984;105:235-242.

768. Vormoor J, Ritter J, Creutzig U, et al. Acute myelogenous leukaemia in children under 2 years—experiences of the West German AML studies BFM-78, -83 and -87. AML-BFM Study Group. Br J Cancer Suppl. 1992;18:S63-S67.

769. Zipursky A, Peeters M, Poon A. Megakaryoblastic leukemia and Down's syndrome: a review. Pediatr Hematol Oncol. 1987;4: 211-230.

770. Kojima S, Matsuyama T, Sato T, et al. Down's syndrome and acute leukemia in children: an analysis of phenotype by use of monoclonal antibodies and electron microscopic platelet peroxidase reaction. Blood. 1990;76:2348-2353.

771. Zipursky A, Brown E, Christensen H, et al. Leukemia and/or myeloproliferative syndrome in neonates with Down syndrome. Semin Perinatol. 1997;21:97-101.

772. Duflos-Delaplace D, Lai JL, Nelken B, et al. Transient leukemoid disorder in a newborn with Down syndrome followed 19 months later by an acute myeloid leukemia: demonstration of the same structural change in both instances with clonal evolution. Cancer Genet Cytogenet. 1999;113:166-171.

773. Polski JM, Galambos C, Gale GB, et al. Acute megakaryoblastic leukemia after transient myeloproliferative disorder with clonal karyotype evolution in a phenotypically normal neonate. J Pediatr Hematol Oncol. 2002;24:50-54.

774. Gamis AS, Woods WG, Alonzo TA, et al. Increased age at diagnosis has a significantly negative effect on outcome in children with Down syndrome and acute myeloid leukemia: a report from the Children's Cancer Group Study 2891. J Clin Oncol. 2003;21:3415-3422.

775. Hasle H, Abrahamsson J, Arola M, et al. Myeloid leukemia in children 4 years or older with Down syndrome often lacks GATA1 mutation and cytogenetics and risk of relapse are more akin to sporadic AML. Leukemia. 2008;22:1428-1430.

776. Creutzig U, Reinhardt D, Diekamp S, et al. AML patients with Down syndrome have a high cure rate with AML-BFM therapy with reduced dose intensity. Leukemia. 2005;19:1355-1360.

777. Ravindranath Y, Abella E, Krischer JP, et al. Acute myeloid leukemia (AML) in Down's syndrome is highly responsive to chemotherapy: experience on Pediatric Oncology Group AML Study 8498. Blood. 1992;80:2210-2214.

778. Levitt GA, Stiller CA, Chessells JM. Prognosis of Down's syndrome with acute leukaemia. Arch Dis Child. 1990;65:212-216.

779. Trejo RM, Aguilera RP, Nieto S, Kofman S. A t(1;22)(p13;q13) in four children with acute megakaryoblastic leukemia (M7), two with Down syndrome. Cancer Genet Cytogenet. 2000;120:160-162.

780. Bunin N, Nowell PC, Belasco J, et al. Chromosome 7 abnormalities in children with Down syndrome and preleukemia. Cancer Genet Cytogenet. 1991;54:119-126.

781. Lie SO, Jonmundsson G, Mellander L, et al. A population-based study of 272 children with acute myeloid leukaemia treated on two consecutive protocols with different intensity: best outcome in girls, infants, and children with Down's syndrome. Nordic Society of Paediatric Haematology and Oncology (NOPHO). Br J Haematol. 1996;94:82-88.

782. Zwaan CM, Kaspers GJ, Pieters R, et al. Different drug sensitivity profiles of acute myeloid and lymphoblastic leukemia and normal peripheral blood mononuclear cells in children with and without Down syndrome. Blood. 2002;99:245-251.

783. Taub JW, Huang X, Matherly LH, et al. Expression of chromosome 21-localized genes in acute myeloid leukemia: differences between Down syndrome and non-Down syndrome blast cells and relationship to in vitro sensitivity to cytosine arabinoside and daunorubicin. Blood. 1999;94:1393-1400.

784. Taub JW, Matherly LH, Stout ML, et al. Enhanced metabolism of 1-beta-D-arabinofuranosylcytosine in Down syndrome cells: a contributing factor for the superior event free survival of Down syndrome children with acute myeloid leukemia. Blood. 1996;87:3395-3403.

785. Ge Y, Jensen TL, Stout ML, et al. The role of cytidine deaminase and GATA1 mutations in the increased cytosine arabinoside sensitivity of Down syndrome myeloblasts and leukemia cell lines. Cancer Res. 2004;64:728-735.

786. Zubizarreta P, Felice MS, Alfaro E, et al. Acute myelogenous leukemia in Down's syndrome: report of a single pediatric institution using a BFM treatment strategy. Leuk Res. 1998;22:465-472.

787. Kojima S, Sako M, Kato K, et al. An effective chemotherapeutic regimen for acute myeloid leukemia and myelodysplastic syndrome in children with Down's syndrome. Leukemia. 2000;14:786-791.

788. Abildgaard L, Ellebaek E, Gustafsson G, et al. Optimal treatment intensity in children with Down syndrome and myeloid leukaemia: data from 56 children treated on NOPHO-AML protocols and a review of the literature. Ann Hematol. 2006;85:275-280.

789. Rao A, Hills RK, Stiller C, et al. Treatment for myeloid leukaemia of Down syndrome: population-based experience in the UK and results from the Medical Research Council AML 10 and AML 12 trials. Br J Haematol. 2006;132:576-583.

790. Gamis AS. Acute myeloid leukemia and Down syndrome evolution of modern therapy—state of the art review. Pediatr Blood Cancer. 2005;44:13-20.

791. O'Brien MM, Taub JW, Chang MN, et al. Cardiomyopathy in children with Down syndrome treated for acute myeloid leukemia: a report from the Children's Oncology Group Study POG 9421. J Clin Oncol. 2008;26:414-420.

792. Koeffler HP. Myelodysplastic syndromes. Semin Hematol. 1996;33:87-94.

793. Novitzky N. Myelodysplastic syndromes in children. A critical review of the clinical manifestations and management. Am J Hematol. 2000;63:212-222.

794. Barnard DR, Kalousek DK, Wiersma SR, et al. Morphologic, immunologic, and cytogenetic classification of acute myeloid leukemia and myelodysplastic syndrome in childhood: a report from the Children's Cancer Group. Leukemia. 1996;10:5-12.

795. Heaney ML, Golde DW. Myelodysplasia. N Engl J Med. 1999;340:1649-1660.

796. Look AT. Molecular pathogenesis of MDS. Hematology Am Soc Hematol Educ Program. 2005:156-160.

797. Corey SJ, Minden MD, Barber DL, et al. Myelodysplastic syndromes: the complexity of stem-cell diseases. Nat Rev Cancer. 2007;7:118-129.

798. Bennett JM. Classification of the myelodysplastic syndromes. Clin Haematol. 1986;15:909-923.

799. Bennett JM, Catovsky D, Daniel MT, et al. Proposals for the classification of the myelodysplastic syndromes. Br J Haematol. 1982;51:189-199.

800. Vardiman JW, Harris NL, Brunning RD. The World Health Organization (WHO) classification of the myeloid neoplasms. Blood. 2002;100:2292-2302.

801. Greenberg P, Cox C, LeBeau MM, et al. International scoring system for evaluating prognosis in myelodysplastic syndromes. Blood. 1997;89:2079-2088.

802. Hasle H, Baumann I, Bergstrasser E, et al. The International Prognostic Scoring System (IPSS) for childhood myelodysplastic syndrome (MDS) and juvenile myelomonocytic leukemia (JMML). Leukemia. 2004;18:2008-2014.

803. Abkowitz JL, Fialkow PJ, Niebrugge DJ, et al. Pancytopenia as a clonal disorder of a multipotent hematopoietic stem cell. J Clin Invest. 1984;73:258-261.

804. Raskind WH, Fialkow PJ. The use of cell markers in the study of human hematopoietic neoplasia. Adv Cancer Res. 1987;49:127-167.

805. Raskind WH, Tirumali N, Jacobson R, et al. Evidence for a multistep pathogenesis of a myelodysplastic syndrome. Blood. 1984;63:1318-1323.

806. Nilsson L, Astrand-Grundstrom I, Arvidsson I, et al. Isolation and characterization of hematopoietic progenitor/stem cells in 5q-deleted myelodysplastic syndromes: evidence for involvement at the hematopoietic stem cell level. Blood. 2000;96:2012-2021.

807. Parker JE, Mufti GJ, Rasool F, et al. The role of apoptosis, proliferation, and the Bcl-2-related proteins in the myelodysplastic syndromes and acute myeloid leukemia secondary to MDS. Blood. 2000;96:3932-3938.

808. Boudard D, Sordet O, Vasselon C, et al. Expression and activity of caspases 1 and 3 in myelodysplastic syndromes. Leukemia. 2000;14:2045-2051.

809. Hasle H, Arico M, Basso G, et al. Myelodysplastic syndrome, juvenile myelomonocytic leukemia, and acute myeloid leukemia associated with complete or partial monosomy 7. European Working Group on MDS in Childhood (EWOG-MDS). Leukemia. 1999;13:376-385.

810. Lessard M, Herry A, Berthou C, et al. FISH investigation of 5q and 7q deletions in MDS/AML reveals hidden translocations, insertions and fragmentations of the same chromosomes. Leuk Res. 1998;22:303-312.

811. Martinez-Climent JA, Garcia-Conde J. Chromosomal rearrangements in childhood acute myeloid leukemia and myelodysplastic syndromes. J Pediatr Hematol Oncol. 1999;21:91-102.

812. Ebert BL, Pretz J, Bosco J, et al. Identification of RPS14 as a 5q– syndrome gene by RNA interference screen. Nature. 2008;451:335-339.

813. Gazda HT, Grabowska A, Merida-Long LB, et al. Ribosomal protein S24 gene is mutated in Diamond-Blackfan anemia. Am J Hum Genet. 2006;79:1110-1118.

814. List A, Kurtin S, Roe DJ, et al. Efficacy of lenalidomide in myelodysplastic syndromes. N Engl J Med. 2005;352:549-557.

815. List A, Dewald G, Bennett J, et al. Lenalidomide in the myelodysplastic syndrome with chromosome 5q deletion. N Engl J Med. 2006;355:1456-1465.

816. Giagounidis A, Fenaux P, Mufti GJ, et al. Practical recommendations on the use of lenalidomide in the management of myelodysplastic syndromes. Ann Hematol. 2008;87:345-352.

817. Raza A, Reeves JA, Feldman EJ, et al. Phase 2 study of lenalidomide in transfusion-dependent, low-risk, and intermediate-1 risk myelodysplastic syndromes with karyotypes other than deletion 5q. Blood. 2008;111:86-93.

818. Ebert BL, Galili N, Tamayo P, et al. An erythroid differentiation signature predicts response to lenalidomide in myelodysplastic syndrome. PLoS Med. 2008;5:e35.

819. Joslin JM, Fernald AA, Tennant TR, et al. Haploinsufficiency of EGR1, a candidate gene in the del(5q), leads to the development of myeloid disorders. Blood. 2007;110:719-726.

820. Heinrichs S, Berman JN, Ortiz TM, et al. CD34+ cell selection is required to assess HOXA9 expression levels in patients with myelodysplastic syndrome. Br J Haematol. 2005;130:83-86.

821. Moore MA, Chung KY, Plasilova M, et al. NUP98 dysregulation in myeloid leukemogenesis. Ann N Y Acad Sci. 2007;1106:114-142.

822. Hofmann WK, de Vos S, Komor M, et al. Characterization of gene expression of CD34+ cells from normal and myelodysplastic bone marrow. Blood. 2002;100:3553-3560.

823. Hatano Y, Miura I, Nakamura T, et al. Molecular heterogeneity of the NUP98/HOXA9 fusion transcript in myelodysplastic syndromes associated with t(7;11)(p15;p15). Br J Haematol. 1999;107:600-604.

824. Fujino T, Suzuki A, Ito Y, et al. Single-translocation and double-chimeric transcripts: detection of NUP98-HOXA9 in myeloid leukemias with HOXA11 or HOXA13 breaks of the chromosomal translocation t(7;11)(p15;p15). Blood. 2002;99:1428-1433.

825. Cuenco GM, Nucifora G, Ren R. Human AML1/MDS1/EVI1 fusion protein induces an acute myelogenous leukemia (AML) in mice: a model for human AML. Proc Natl Acad Sci U S A. 2000;97:1760-1765.

826. Nucifora G, Begy CR, Kobayashi H, et al. Consistent intergenic splicing and production of multiple transcripts between AML1 at 21q22 and unrelated genes at 3q26 in (3;21)(q26;q22) translocations. Proc Natl Acad Sci U S A. 1994;91:4004-4008.

827. Nucifora G, Birn DJ, Espinosa R 3rd, et al. Involvement of the AML1 gene in the t(3;21) in therapy-related leukemia and in chronic myeloid leukemia in blast crisis. Blood. 1993;81:2728-2734.

828. Hitzler JK, Witte DP, Jenkins NA, et al. cDNA cloning, expression pattern, and chromosomal localization of Mlf1, murine homologue of a gene involved in myelodysplasia and acute myeloid leukemia. Am J Pathol. 1999;155:53-59.

829. Yoneda-Kato N, Look AT, Kirstein MN, et al. The t(3;5)(q25.1;q34) of myelodysplastic syndrome and acute myeloid leukemia produces a novel fusion gene, NPM-MLF1. Oncogene. 1996;12:265-275.

830. Side LE, Curtiss NP, Teel K, et al. RAS, FLT3, and TP53 mutations in therapy-related myeloid malignancies with abnormalities of chromosomes 5 and 7. Genes Chromosomes Cancer. 2004;39:217-223.

831. Niimi H, Harada H, Harada Y, et al. Hyperactivation of the RAS signaling pathway in myelodysplastic syndrome with AML1/RUNX1 point mutations. Leukemia. 2006;20:635-644.

832. Christiansen DH, Andersen MK, Pedersen-Bjergaard J. Mutations of AML1 are common in therapy-related myelodysplasia following therapy with alkylating agents and are significantly associated with deletion or loss of chromosome arm 7q and with subsequent leukemic transformation. Blood. 2004;104:1474-1481.

833. Horiike S, Misawa S, Kaneko H, et al. Distinct genetic involvement of the TP53 gene in therapy-related leukemia and myelodysplasia with chromosomal losses of Nos 5 and/or 7 and its possible relationship to replication error phenotype. Leukemia. 1999;13:1235-1242.

834. Bhatia S, Robison LL, Oberlin O, et al. Breast cancer and other second neoplasms after childhood Hodgkin's disease. N Engl J Med. 1996;334:745-751.

835. Bhatia S. Cancer survivorship—pediatric issues. Hematology Am Soc Hematol Educ Program. 2005:507-515.

836. Josting A, Wiedenmann S, Franklin J, et al. Secondary myeloid leukemia and myelodysplastic syndromes in patients treated for Hodgkin's disease: a report from the German Hodgkin's Lymphoma Study Group. J Clin Oncol. 2003;21:3440-3446.

837. Smith MA, Rubinstein L, Anderson JR, et al. Secondary leukemia or myelodysplastic syndrome after treatment with epipodophyllotoxins. J Clin Oncol. 1999;17:569-577.

838. Tiu R, Gondek L, O'Keefe C, Maciejewski JP. Clonality of the stem cell compartment during evolution of myelodysplastic syndromes and other bone marrow failure syndromes. Leukemia. 2007;21:1648-1657.

839. Gondek LP, Tiu R, Haddad AS, et al. Single nucleotide polymorphism arrays complement metaphase cytogenetics in detection of new chromosomal lesions in MDS. Leukemia. 2007;21:2058-2061.

840. Bagby GC Jr, Gabourel JD, Linman JW. Glucocorticoid therapy in the preleukemic syndrome (hemopoietic dysplasia): identification of responsive patients using in-vitro techniques. Ann Intern Med. 1980;92:55-58.

841. Negrin RS, Stein R, Doherty K, et al. Maintenance treatment of the anemia of myelodysplastic syndromes with recombinant human granulocyte colony-stimulating factor and erythropoietin: evidence for in vivo synergy. Blood. 1996;87:4076-4081.

842. Negrin RS, Stein R, Vardiman J, et al. Treatment of the anemia of myelodysplastic syndromes using recombinant human granulocyte colony-stimulating factor in combination with erythropoietin. Blood. 1993;82:737-743.

843. Najean Y, Pecking A. Refractory anemia with excess of blast cells: prognostic factors and effect of treatment with androgens or cytosine arabinoside. Results of a prospective trial in 58 patients. Cooperative Group for the Study of Aplastic and Refractory Anemias. Cancer. 1979;44:1976-1982.

844. Letendre L, Levitt R, Pierre RV, et al. Myelodysplastic syndrome treatment with danazol and cis-retinoic acid. Am J Hematol. 1995;48:233-236.

845. Kurzrock R, Estey E, Talpaz M. All-trans retinoic acid: tolerance and biologic effects in myelodysplastic syndrome. J Clin Oncol. 1993;11:1489-1495.

846. Koeffler HP, Heitjan D, Mertelsmann R, et al. Randomized study of 13-cis retinoic acid v placebo in the myelodysplastic disorders. Blood. 1988;71:703-708.

847. Hurtado R, Sosa R, Majluf A, Labardini JR. Refractory anaemia (RA) type I FAB treated with oxymetholone (OXY): long-term results. Br J Haematol. 1993;85:235-236.

848. Hellstrom E, Birgegard G, Lockner D, et al. Treatment of myelodysplastic syndromes with recombinant human erythropoietin. Eur J Haematol. 1991;47:355-360.

849. Clark RE, Ismail SA, Jacobs A, et al. A randomized trial of 13-cis retinoic acid with or without cytosine arabinoside in patients with the myelodysplastic syndrome. Br J Haematol. 1987;66:77-83.

850. Cines DB, Cassileth PA, Kiss JE. Danazol therapy in myelodysplasia. Ann Intern Med. 1985;103:58-60.

851. Cheson BD. Standard and low-dose chemotherapy for the treatment of myelodysplastic syndromes. Leuk Res. 1998;22(Suppl 1):S17-21.

852. Herman JG, Jen J, Merlo A, Baylin SB. Hypermethylation-associated inactivation indicates a tumor suppressor role for p15INK4B. Cancer Res. 1996;56:722-727.

853. Uchida T, Kinoshita T, Nagai H, et al. Hypermethylation of the p15INK4B gene in myelodysplastic syndromes. Blood. 1997;90:1403-1409.

854. Herman JG, Baylin SB. Gene silencing in cancer in association with promoter hypermethylation. N Engl J Med. 2003;349:2042-2054.

855. Issa JP. CpG island methylator phenotype in cancer. Nat Rev Cancer. 2004;4:988-993.

856. Silverman LR, Demakos EP, Peterson BL, et al. Randomized controlled trial of azacitidine in patients with the myelodysplastic syndrome: a study of the cancer and leukemia group B. J Clin Oncol. 2002;20:2429-2440.

857. Kantarjian H, Issa JP, Rosenfeld CS, et al. Decitabine improves patient outcomes in myelodysplastic syndromes: results of a phase III randomized study. Cancer. 2006;106:1794-1803.

858. Anderson JE, Anasetti C, Appelbaum FR, et al. Unrelated donor marrow transplantation for myelodysplasia (MDS) and MDS-related acute myeloid leukaemia. Br J Haematol. 1996;93:59-67.

859. Appelbaum FR, Anderson J. Bone marrow transplantation for myelodysplasia in adults and children: when and who? Leuk Res. 1998;22(Suppl 1):S35-S39.

860. Yusuf U, Frangoul HA, Gooley TA, et al. Allogeneic bone marrow transplantation in children with myelodysplastic syndrome or juvenile myelomonocytic leukemia: the Seattle experience. Bone Marrow Transplant. 2004;33:805-814.

861. Locatelli F, Zecca M, Niemeyer C, et al. Role of allogeneic bone marrow transplantation for the treatment of myelodysplastic syndromes in childhood. The European Working Group on Childhood Myelodysplastic Syndrome (EWOG-MDS) and the Austria-Germany-Italy (AGI) Bone Marrow Transplantation Registry. Bone Marrow Transplant. 1996;18(Suppl 2):63-68.

862. Niemeyer CM, Arico M, Basso G, et al. Chronic myelomonocytic leukemia in childhood: a retrospective analysis of 110 cases. European Working Group on Myelodysplastic Syndromes in Childhood (EWOG-MDS). Blood. 1997;89:3534-3543.

863. Miyauchi J, Asada M, Sasaki M, et al. Mutations of the N-ras gene in juvenile chronic myelogenous leukemia. Blood. 1994;83:2248-2254.

864. Niemeyer CM, Kratz CP. Paediatric myelodysplastic syndromes and juvenile myelomonocytic leukaemia: molecular classification and treatment options. Br J Haematol. 2008;140:610-624.

865. Satoh T, Nakafuku M, Miyajima A, Kaziro Y. Involvement of ras p21 protein in signal-transduction pathways from interleukin 2, interleukin 3, and granulocyte/macrophage colony-stimulating factor, but not from interleukin 4. Proc Natl Acad Sci U S A. 1991;88:3314-3318.

866. Loh ML, Vattikuti S, Schubbert S, et al. Mutations in PTPN11 implicate the SHP-2 phosphatase in leukemogenesis. Blood. 2004;103:2325-2331.

867. Tartaglia M, Niemeyer CM, Fragale A, et al. Somatic mutations in PTPN11 in juvenile myelomonocytic leukemia, myelodysplastic syndromes and acute myeloid leukemia. Nat Genet. 2003;34:148-150.

868. Emanuel PD, Bates LJ, Castleberry RP, et al. Selective hypersensitivity to granulocyte-macrophage colony-stimulating factor by juvenile chronic myeloid leukemia hematopoietic progenitors. Blood. 1991;77:925-929.

869. Emanuel PD. Myelodysplasia and myeloproliferative disorders in childhood: an update. Br J Haematol. 1999;105:852-863.

870. Castro-Malaspina H, Schaison G, Passe S, et al. Subacute and chronic myelomonocytic leukemia in children (juvenile CML). Clinical and hematologic observations, and identification of prognostic factors. Cancer. 1984;54:675-686.

871. Castleberry RP, Emanuel PD, Zuckerman KS, et al. A pilot study of isotretinoin in the treatment of juvenile chronic myelogenous leukemia. N Engl J Med. 1994;331:1680-1684.

872. Chan HS, Estrov Z, Weitzman SS, Freedman MH. The value of intensive combination chemotherapy for juvenile chronic myelogenous leukemia. J Clin Oncol. 1987;5:1960-1967.

873. Diaz de Heredia C, Ortega JJ, Coll MT, et al. Results of intensive chemotherapy in children with juvenile chronic myelomonocytic leukemia: a pilot study. Med Pediatr Oncol. 1998;31:516-520.

874. Festa RS, Shende A, Lanzkowsky P. Juvenile chronic myelocytic leukemia: experience with intensive combination chemotherapy. Med Pediatr Oncol. 1990;18:311-316.

875. Lilleyman JS, Harrison JF, Black JA. Treatment of juvenile chronic myeloid leukemia with sequential subcutaneous cytarabine and oral mercaptopurine. Blood. 1977;49:559-562.

876. Thomas WJ, North RB, Poplack DG, et al. Chronic myelomonocytic leukemia in childhood. Am J Hematol. 1981;10:181-194.

877. Bunin N, Saunders F, Leahey A, et al. Alternative donor bone marrow transplantation for children with juvenile myelomonocytic leukemia. J Pediatr Hematol Oncol. 1999;21:479-485.

878. Bunin NJ, Casper JT, Lawton C, et al. Allogeneic marrow transplantation using T cell depletion for patients with juvenile chronic myelogenous leukemia without HLA-identical siblings. Bone Marrow Transplant. 1992;9:119-122.

879. MacMillan ML, Davies SM, Orchard PJ, et al. Haemopoietic cell transplantation in children with juvenile myelomonocytic leukaemia. Br J Haematol. 1998;103:552-558.

880. Matthes-Martin S, Mann G, Peters C, et al. Allogeneic bone marrow transplantation for juvenile myelomonocytic leukaemia: a single centre experience and review of the literature. Bone Marrow Transplant. 2000;26:377-382.

881. Dameshek W. Some speculations on the myeloproliferative syndromes. Blood. 1951;6:372-375.

882. Adamson JW, Fialkow PJ. The pathogenesis of myeloproliferative syndromes. Br J Haematol. 1978;38:299-303.

883. Craigie D. Case of disease of the spleen, in which death took place in consequence of the purulent matter in the blood. Edinburgh Medical and Surgical Journal. 1845;64:400-413.

884. Bennett J. Case of hypertrophy of the spleen and liver, in which death took place from suppuration of the blood. Edinburgh Medical and Surgical Journal. 1845;64:413-423.

885. Nowell P, Hungerford D. A minute chromosome in human chronic granulocytic leukemia. Science. 1960;132:1497.

886. Bizzozero OJ Jr, Johnson KG, Ciocco A, et al. Radiation-related leukemia in Hiroshima and Nagasaki 1946-1964. II. Ann Intern Med. 1967;66:522-530.

887. Goh KO, Swisher SN, Herman EC Jr. Chronic myelocytic leukemia and identical twins. Additional evidence of the Philadelphia chromosome as postzygotic abnormality. Arch Intern Med. 1967;120:214-219.

888. Rowley JD. A new consistent chromosomal abnormality in chronic myelogenous leukaemia identified by quinacrine fluorescence and Giemsa staining (letter). Nature. 1973;243:290-293.

889. Arico M, Valsecchi MG, Camitta B, et al. Outcome of treatment in children with Philadelphia chromosome-positive acute lymphoblastic leukemia. N Engl J Med. 2000;342:998-1006.

890. Batista DA, Hawkins A, Murphy KM, Griffin CA. BCR/ABL rearrangement in two cases of Philadelphia chromosome negative chronic myeloid leukemia: deletion on the derivative chromosome 9 may or not be present. Cancer Genet Cytogenet. 2005;163:164-167.

891. Konopka JB, Watanabe SM, Witte ON. An alteration of the human c-abl protein in K562 leukemia cells unmasks associated tyrosine kinase activity. Cell. 1984;37:1035-1042.

892. Van Etten RA, Jackson P, Baltimore D. The mouse type IV c-abl gene product is a nuclear protein, and activation of transforming ability is associated with cytoplasmic localization. Cell. 1989;58:669-678.

893. Goga A, Liu X, Hambuch TM, et al. p53 dependent growth suppression by the c-Abl nuclear tyrosine kinase. Oncogene. 1995;11:791-799.

894. Kharbanda S, Ren R, Pandey P, et al. Activation of the c-Abl tyrosine kinase in the stress response to DNA-damaging agents. Nature. 1995;376:785-788.

895. Mattioni T, Jackson PK, Bchini-Hooft van Huijsduijnen O, Picard D. Cell cycle arrest by tyrosine kinase Abl involves altered early mitogenic response. Oncogene. 1995;10:1325-1333.

896. Sawyers CL, McLaughlin J, Goga A, et al. The nuclear tyrosine kinase c-Abl negatively regulates cell growth. Cell. 1994;77: 121-131.

897. Yuan ZM, Huang Y, Whang Y, et al. Role for c-Abl tyrosine kinase in growth arrest response to DNA damage. Nature. 1996;382:272-274.

898. Daley GQ, Baltimore D. Transformation of an interleukin 3-dependent hematopoietic cell line by the chronic myelogenous leukemia-specific P210bcr/abl protein. Proc Natl Acad Sci U S A. 1988;85:9312-9316.

899. Elefanty AG, Hariharan IK, Cory S. bcr-abl, the hallmark of chronic myeloid leukaemia in man, induces multiple haemopoietic neoplasms in mice. EMBO J. 1990;9:1069-1078.

900. Gishizky ML, Johnson-White J, Witte ON. Efficient transplantation of BCR-ABL-induced chronic myelogenous leukemia-like syndrome in mice. Proc Natl Acad Sci U S A. 1993;90:3755-3759.

901. Kelliher M, Knott A, McLaughlin J, et al. Differences in oncogenic potency but not target cell specificity distinguish the two forms of the BCR/ABL oncogene. Mol Cell Biol. 1991;11: 4710-4716.

902. Goga A, McLaughlin J, Afar DE, et al. Alternative signals to RAS for hematopoietic transformation by the BCR-ABL oncogene. Cell. 1995;82:981-988.

903. Raitano AB, Halpern JR, Hambuch TM, Sawyers CL. The Bcr-Abl leukemia oncogene activates Jun kinase and requires Jun for transformation. Proc Natl Acad Sci U S A. 1995;92:11746-11750.

904. Senechal K, Halpern J, Sawyers CL. The CRKL adaptor protein transforms fibroblasts and functions in transformation by the BCR-ABL oncogene. J Biol Chem. 1996;271:23255-23261.

905. Afar DE, Goga A, McLaughlin J, et al. Differential complementation of Bcr-Abl point mutants with c-Myc. Science. 1994;264: 424-426.

906. Afar DE, McLaughlin J, Sherr CJ, et al. Signaling by ABL oncogenes through cyclin D1. Proc Natl Acad Sci U S A. 1995;92:9540-9544.

907. Fauser AA, Kanz L, Bross KJ, Lohr GW. T cells and probably B cells arise from the malignant clone in chronic myelogenous leukemia. J Clin Invest. 1985;75:1080-1082.

908. Fialkow PJ, Denman AM, Jacobson RJ, Lowenthal MN. Chronic myelocytic leukemia. Origin of some lymphocytes from leukemic stem cells. J Clin Invest. 1978;62:815-823.

909. Fialkow PJ, Jacobson RJ, Papayannopoulou T. Chronic myelocytic leukemia: clonal origin in a stem cell common to the granulocyte, erythrocyte, platelet and monocyte/macrophage. Am J Med. 1977;63:125-130.

910. Greenberg BR, Wilson FD, Woo L, Jenks HM. Cytogentics of fibroblastic colonies in Ph1-positive chronic myelogenous leukemia. Blood. 1978;51:1039-1044.

911. Maniatis AK, Amsel S, Mitus WJ, Coleman N. Chromosome pattern of bone marrow fibroblasts in patients with chronic granulocytic leukaemia. Nature. 1969;222:1278-1279.

912. Griffin JD, Todd RF 3rd, Ritz J, et al. Differentiation patterns in the blastic phase of chronic myeloid leukemia. Blood. 1983;61:85-91.

913. Castro-Malaspina H, Schaison G, Briere J, et al. Philadelphia chromosome-positive chronic myelocytic leukemia in children. Survival and prognostic factors. Cancer. 1983;52:721-727.

914. Rowe JM, Lichtman MA. Hyperleukocytosis and leukostasis: common features of childhood chronic myelogenous leukemia. Blood. 1984;63:1230-1234.

915. Vodopick H, Rupp EM, Edwards CL, et al. Spontaneous cyclic leukocytosis and thrombocytosis in chronic granulocytic leukemia. N Engl J Med. 1972;286:284-290.

916. Smith KL, Johnson W. Classification of chronic myelocytic leukemia in children. Cancer. 1974;34:670-679.

917. Suri R, Goldman JM, Catovsky D, et al. Priapism complicating chronic granulocytic leukemia. Am J Hematol. 1980;9: 295-299.

918. Barton JC, Conrad ME, Poon MC. Pseudochloroma: extramedullary hematopoietic nodules in chronic myelogenous leukemia. Ann Intern Med. 1979;91:735-738.

919. Dosik H, Rosner F, Sawitsky A. Acquired lipidosis: Gaucher-like cells and "blue cells" in chronic granulocytic leukemia. Semin Hematol. 1972;9:309-316.

920. Chikkappa G, Corcino J, Greenberg ML, Herbert V. Correlation between various blood white cell pools and the serum B12-binding capaities. Blood. 1971;37:142-151.

921. Goto T, Nishikori M, Arlin Z, et al. Growth characteristics of leukemic and normal hematopoietic cells in Ph' + chronic myelogenous leukemia and effects of intensive treatment. Blood. 1982;59:793-808.

922. Dash AB, Williams IR, Kutok JL, et al. A murine model of CML blast crisis induced by cooperation between BCR/ABL and NUP98/HOXA9. Proc Natl Acad Sci U S A. 2002;99:7622-7627.

923. Kantarjian HM, Smith TL, McCredie KB, et al. Chronic myelogenous leukemia: a multivariate analysis of the associations of patient characteristics and therapy with survival. Blood. 1985;66:1326-1335.

924. Sokal JE, Cox EB, Baccarani M, et al. Prognostic discrimination in "good-risk" chronic granulocytic leukemia. Blood. 1984;63: 789-799.

925. Sokal JE, Gomez GA, Baccarani M, et al. Prognostic significance of additional cytogenetic abnormalities at diagnosis of Philadelphia chromosome-positive chronic granulocytic leukemia. Blood. 1988;72:294-298.

926. Canellos GP. Chronic granulocytic leukemia. Med Clin North Am. 1976;60:1001-1018.

927. Hernandez P, Carnot J, Cruz C. Chronic myeloid leukaemia blast crisis with T-cell features. Br J Haematol. 1982;51:175-177.

928. Janossy G, Woodruff RK, Pippard MJ, et al. Relation of "lymphoid" phenotype and response to chemotherapy incorporating vincristine-prednisolone in the acute phase of Ph1 positive leukemia. Cancer. 1979;43:426-434.

929. Rushing D, Goldman A, Gibbs G, et al. Hydroxyurea versus busulfan in the treatment of chronic myelogenous leukemia. Am J Clin Oncol. 1982;5:307-313.

930. Deaven LL, Van Dilla MA, Bartholdi MF, et al. Construction of human chromosome-specific DNA libraries from flow-sorted chromosomes. Cold Spring Harb Symp Quant Biol. 1986;51 Pt 1:159-167.

931. Niederle N, Kloke O, Osieka R, et al. Interferon alfa-2b in the treatment of chronic myelogenous leukemia. Semin Oncol. 1987;14:29-35.

932. Talpaz M, Kantarjian HM, McCredie K, et al. Hematologic remission and cytogenetic improvement induced by recombinant human interferon alpha A in chronic myelogenous leukemia. N Engl J Med. 1986;314:1065-1069.

933. Chronic granulocytic leukaemia: comparison of radiotherapy and busulphan therapy. Report of the Medical Research Council's working party for therapeutic trials in leukaemia. Br Med J. 1968;1:201-208.

934. Hochhaus A, Lin F, Reiter A, et al. Quantification of residual disease in chronic myelogenous leukemia patients on interferon-alpha therapy by competitive polymerase chain reaction. Blood. 1996;87:1549-1555.

935. Hochhaus A, Lin F, Reiter A, et al. Variable numbers of BCR-ABL transcripts persist in CML patients who achieve complete cytogenetic remission with interferon-alpha. Br J Haematol. 1995;91:126-131.

936. Sacchi S, Kantarjian H, O'Brien S, et al. Immune-mediated and unusual complications during interferon alfa therapy in chronic myelogenous leukemia. J Clin Oncol. 1995;13:2401-2407.

937. Talpaz M, Kantarjian H, Kurzrock R, et al. Interferon-alpha produces sustained cytogenetic responses in chronic myelogenous leukemia. Philadelphia chromosome-positive patients. Ann Intern Med. 1991;114:532-538.

938. Wetzler M, Kantarjian H, Kurzrock R, Talpaz M. Interferon-alpha therapy for chronic myelogenous leukemia. Am J Med. 1995;99:402-411.

939. The Italian Cooperative Study Group on Chronic Myeloid Leukemia. Interferon alfa-2a as compared with conventional chemotherapy for the treatment of chronic myeloid leukemia. N Engl J Med. 1994;330:820-825.

940. Allan NC, Richards SM, Shepherd PC. UK Medical Research Council randomised, multicentre trial of interferon-alpha n1 for chronic myeloid leukaemia: improved survival irrespective of cytogenetic response. The UK Medical Research Council's Working Parties for Therapeutic Trials in Adult Leukaemia. Lancet. 1995;345:1392-1397.

941. Hehlmann R, Heimpel H, Hasford J, et al. Randomized comparison of interferon-alpha with busulfan and hydroxyurea in chronic myelogenous leukemia. The German CML Study Group. Blood. 1994;84:4064-4077.

942. Ohnishi K, Ohno R, Tomonaga M, et al. A randomized trial comparing interferon-alpha with busulfan for newly diagnosed chronic myelogenous leukemia in chronic phase. Blood. 1995; 86:906-916.

943. Druker BJ, Lydon NB. Lessons learned from the development of an abl tyrosine kinase inhibitor for chronic myelogenous leukemia. J Clin Invest. 2000;105:3-7.

944. O'Brien SG, Guilhot F, Larson RA, et al. Imatinib compared with interferon and low-dose cytarabine for newly diagnosed chronic-phase chronic myeloid leukemia. N Engl J Med. 2003;348:994-1004.

945. Druker BJ, Guilhot F, O'Brien SG, et al. Five-year follow-up of patients receiving imatinib for chronic myeloid leukemia. N Engl J Med. 2006;355:2408-2417.

946. Kerkela R, Grazette L, Yacobi R, et al. Cardiotoxicity of the cancer therapeutic agent imatinib mesylate. Nat Med. 2006; 12:908-916.

947. Champagne MA, Capdeville R, Krailo M, et al. Imatinib mesylate (STI571) for treatment of children with Philadelphia chromosome-positive leukemia: results from a Children's Oncology Group phase 1 study. Blood. 2004;104:2655-2660.

948. Millot F, Guilhot J, Nelken B, et al. Imatinib mesylate is effective in children with chronic myelogenous leukemia in late chronic and advanced phase and in relapse after stem cell transplantation. Leukemia. 2006;20:187-192.

949. Deininger M, Schleuning M, Greinix H, et al. The effect of prior exposure to imatinib on transplant-related mortality. Haematologica. 2006;91:452-459.

950. Gambacorti-Passerini C, Barni R, le Coutre P, et al. Role of alpha1 acid glycoprotein in the in vivo resistance of human BCR-ABL(+) leukemic cells to the abl inhibitor STI571. J Natl Cancer Inst. 2000;92:1641-1650.

951. Gorre ME, Mohammed M, Ellwood K, et al. Clinical resistance to STI-571 cancer therapy caused by BCR-ABL gene mutation or amplification. Science. 2001;293:876-880.

952. le Coutre P, Tassi E, Varella-Garcia M, et al. Induction of resistance to the Abelson inhibitor STI571 in human leukemic cells through gene amplification. Blood. 2000;95:1758-1766.

953. Mahon FX, Deininger MW, Schultheis B, et al. Selection and characterization of BCR-ABL positive cell lines with differential sensitivity to the tyrosine kinase inhibitor STI571: diverse mechanisms of resistance. Blood. 2000;96:1070-1079.

954. Weisberg E, Griffin JD. Mechanism of resistance to the ABL tyrosine kinase inhibitor STI571 in BCR/ABL-transformed hematopoietic cell lines. Blood. 2000;95:3498-3505.

955. Kantarjian H, Pasquini R, Hamerschlak N, et al. Dasatinib or high-dose imatinib for chronic-phase chronic myeloid leukemia after failure of first-line imatinib: a randomized phase 2 trial. Blood. 2007;109:5143-5150.

956. Kantarjian H, Giles F, Wunderle L, et al. Nilotinib in imatinib-resistant CML and Philadelphia chromosome-positive ALL. N Engl J Med. 2006;354:2542-2551.

957. van Rhee F, Szydlo RM, Hermans J, et al. Long-term results after allogeneic bone marrow transplantation for chronic myelogenous leukemia in chronic phase: a report from the Chronic Leukemia Working Party of the European Group for Blood and Marrow Transplantation. Bone Marrow Transplant. 1997;20:553-560.

958. Gratwohl A, Hermans J, Apperley J, et al. Acute graft-versus-host disease: grade and outcome in patients with chronic myelogenous leukemia. Working Party Chronic Leukemia of the European Group for Blood and Marrow Transplantation. Blood. 1995;86:813-818.

959. Horowitz MM, Gale RP, Sondel PM, et al. Graft-versus-leukemia reactions after bone marrow transplantation. Blood. 1990;75:555-562.

960. Thomas ED, Clift RA, Fefer A, et al. Marrow transplantation for the treatment of chronic myelogenous leukemia. Ann Intern Med. 1986;104:155-163.

961. Clift RA, Storb R. Marrow transplantation for CML: the Seattle experience. Bone Marrow Transplant. 1996;17(Suppl 3):S1-S3.

962. Gratwohl A, Hermans J. Allogeneic bone marrow transplantation for chronic myeloid leukemia. Working Party Chronic Leukemia of the European Group for Blood and Marrow Transplantation (EBMT). Bone Marrow Transplant. 1996; 17(Suppl 3):S7-S9.

963. Horowitz MM, Rowlings PA, Passweg JR. Allogeneic bone marrow transplantation for CML: a report from the International Bone Marrow Transplant Registry. Bone Marrow Transplant. 1996;17(Suppl 3):S5-S6.

964. Davies SM, DeFor TE, McGlave PB, et al. Equivalent outcomes in patients with chronic myelogenous leukemia after early transplantation of phenotypically matched bone marrow from related or unrelated donors. Am J Med. 2001;110:339-346.

965. Goldman JM, Szydlo R, Horowitz MM, et al. Choice of pretransplant treatment and timing of transplants for chronic myelogenous leukemia in chronic phase. Blood. 1993;82: 2235-2238.

966. Cwynarski K, Roberts IA, Iacobelli S, et al. Stem cell transplantation for chronic myeloid leukemia in children. Blood. 2003;102:1224-1231.

967. Oehler VG, Gooley T, Snyder DS, et al. The effects of imatinib mesylate treatment before allogeneic transplantation for chronic myeloid leukemia. Blood. 2007;109:1782-1789.

968. Arcese W, Goldman JM, D'Arcangelo E, et al. Outcome for patients who relapse after allogeneic bone marrow transplantation for chronic myeloid leukemia. Chronic Leukemia Working Party. European Bone Marrow Transplantation Group. Blood. 1993;82:3211-3219.

969. Higano CS, Chielens D, Raskind W, et al. Use of alpha-2a-interferon to treat cytogenetic relapse of chronic myeloid leukemia after marrow transplantation. Blood. 1997;90:2549-2554.

970. Higano CS, Raskind WH, Singer JW. Use of alpha interferon for the treatment of relapse of chronic myelogenous leukemia in chronic phase after allogeneic bone marrow transplantation. Blood. 1992;80:1437-1442.

971. Steegmann JL, Casado LF, Tomas JF, et al. Interferon alpha for chronic myeloid leukemia relapsing after allogeneic bone marrow transplantation. Bone Marrow Transplant. 1999;23:483-488.

972. Collins RH Jr, Shpilberg O, Drobyski WR, et al. Donor leukocyte infusions in 140 patients with relapsed malignancy after allogeneic bone marrow transplantation. J Clin Oncol. 1997;15:433-444.

973. Kolb HJ, Schattenberg A, Goldman JM, et al. Graft-versus-leukemia effect of donor lymphocyte transfusions in marrow grafted patients. Blood. 1995;86:2041-2050.

974. Porter DL, Roth MS, McGarigle C, et al. Induction of graft-versus-host disease as immunotherapy for relapsed chronic myeloid leukemia. N Engl J Med. 1994;330:100-106.

975. Keil F, Haas OA, Fritsch G, et al. Donor leukocyte infusion for leukemic relapse after allogeneic marrow transplantation: lack of residual donor hematopoiesis predicts aplasia. Blood. 1997;89:3113-3117.

976. Dube ID, Kalousek DK, Coulombel L, et al. Cytogenetic studies of early myeloid progenitor compartments in Ph1-positive chronic myeloid leukemia. II. Long-term culture reveals the persistence of Ph1-negative progenitors in treated as well as newly diagnosed patients. Blood. 1984;63:1172-1177.

977. Rosenthal S, Canellos GP, Whang-Peng J, Gralnick HR. Blast crisis of chronic granulocytic leukemia. Morphologic variants and therapeutic implications. Am J Med. 1977;63:542-547.

978. Golub TR, Barker GF, Stegmaier K, Gilliland DG. The TEL gene contributes to the pathogenesis of myeloid and lymphoid leukemias by diverse molecular genetic mechanisms. Curr Top Microbiol Immunol. 1997;220:67-79.

979. Golub TR, Goga A, Barker GF, et al. Oligomerization of the ABL tyrosine kinase by the Ets protein TEL in human leukemia. Mol Cell Biol. 1996;16:4107-4116.

980. Jousset C, Carron C, Boureux A, et al. A domain of TEL conserved in a subset of ETS proteins defines a specific oligomerization interface essential to the mitogenic properties of the TEL-PDGFR beta oncoprotein. EMBO J. 1997;16:69-82.

981. Berlin NI. Diagnosis and classification of the polycythemias. Semin Hematol. 1975;12:339-351.

982. Fisher MJ, Prchal JF, Prchal JT, D'Andrea AD. Anti-erythropoietin (EPO) receptor monoclonal antibodies distinguish EPO-dependent and EPO-independent erythroid progenitors in polycythemia vera. Blood. 1994;84:1982-1991.

983. Prchal JF, Adamson JW, Murphy S, et al. Polycythemia vera. The in vitro response of normal and abnormal stem cell lines to erythropoietin. J Clin Invest. 1978;61:1044-1047.

984. Kralovics R, Passamonti F, Buser AS, et al. A gain-of-function mutation of JAK2 in myeloproliferative disorders. N Engl J Med. 2005;352:1779-1790.

985. Levine RL, Wadleigh M, Cools J, et al. Activating mutation in the tyrosine kinase JAK2 in polycythemia vera, essential thrombocythemia, and myeloid metaplasia with myelofibrosis. Cancer Cell. 2005;7:387-397.

986. Baxter EJ, Scott LM, Campbell PJ, et al. Acquired mutation of the tyrosine kinase JAK2 in human myeloproliferative disorders. Lancet. 2005;365:1054-1061.

987. James C, Ugo V, Le Couedic JP, et al. A unique clonal JAK2 mutation leading to constitutive signalling causes polycythaemia vera. Nature. 2005;434:1144-1148.

988. Lacout C, Pisani DF, Tulliez M, et al. JAK2V617F expression in murine hematopoietic cells leads to MPD mimicking human PV with secondary myelofibrosis. Blood. 2006;108:1652-1660.

989. Levine RL, Belisle C, Wadleigh M, et al. X-inactivation-based clonality analysis and quantitative JAK2V617F assessment reveal a strong association between clonality and JAK2V617F in PV but not ET/MMM, and identifies a subset of JAK2V617F-negative ET and MMM patients with clonal hematopoiesis. Blood. 2006;107:4139-4141.

990. Prchal JT, Crist WM, Goldwasser E, et al. Autosomal dominant polycythemia. Blood. 1985;66:1208-1214.

991. Bellanne-Chantelot C, Chaumarel I, Labopin M, et al. Genetic and clinical implications of the Val617Phe JAK2 mutation in 72 families with myeloproliferative disorders. Blood. 2006;108:346-352.

992. de la Chapelle A, Sistonen P, Lehvaslaiho H, Ikkala E, Juvonen E. Familial erythrocytosis genetically linked to erythropoietin receptor gene. Lancet. 1993;341:82-84.

993. Sokol L, Luhovy M, Guan Y, et al. Primary familial polycythemia: a frameshift mutation in the erythropoietin receptor gene and increased sensitivity of erythroid progenitors to erythropoietin. Blood. 1995;86:15-22.

994. Sokol L, Prchal JF, D'Andrea, et al. Mutation in the negative regulatory element of the erythropoietin receptor gene in a case of sporadic primary polycythemia. Exp Hematol. 1994;22:447-453.

995. Scott LM, Tong W, Levine RL, et al. JAK2 exon 12 mutations in polycythemia vera and idiopathic erythrocytosis. N Engl J Med. 2007;356:459-468.

996. Thiele J, Kvasnicka HM. A critical reappraisal of the WHO classification of the chronic myeloproliferative disorders. Leuk Lymphoma. 2006;47:381-396.

997. Tefferi A. Classification, diagnosis and management of myeloproliferative disorders in the JAK2V617F era. Hematology Am Soc Hematol Educ Program. 2006:240-245.

998. Tefferi A, Thiele J, Orazi A, et al. Proposals and rationale for revision of the World Health Organization diagnostic criteria for polycythemia vera, essential thrombocythemia, and primary myelofibrosis: recommendations from an ad hoc international expert panel. Blood. 2007;110:1092-1097.

999. Frezzato M, Ruggeri M, Castaman G, Rodeghiero F. Polycythemia vera and essential thrombocythemia in young patients. Haematologica. 1993;78:11-17.

1000. Teofili L, Giona F, Martini M, et al. Markers of myeloproliferative diseases in childhood polycythemia vera and essential thrombocythemia. J Clin Oncol. 2007;25:1048-1053.

1001. de Klerk G, Rosengarten PC, Vet RJ, Goudsmit R. Serum erythropoietin (ESF) titers in polycythemia. Blood. 1981;58:1171-1174.

1002. Berger R, Bernheim A, Le Coniat M, et al. Chromosome studies in polycythemia vera patients. Cancer Genet Cytogenet. 1984;12:217-223.

1003. Testa JR, Kanofsky JR, Rowley JD, et al. Karyotypic patterns and their clinical significance in polycythemia vera. Am J Hematol. 1981;11:29-45.

1004. Cowan DH, Messner HA, Jamal N, et al. Spontaneous remission of polycythemia vera: clinical and cell culture characteristics. Am J Hematol. 1994;46:54-56.

1005. Pearson TC, Wetherley-Mein G. Vascular occlusive episodes and venous haematocrit in primary proliferative polycythaemia. Lancet. 1978;2:1219-1222.

1006. Berk PD, Goldberg JD, Silverstein MN, et al. Increased incidence of acute leukemia in polycythemia vera associated with chlorambucil therapy. N Engl J Med. 1981;304:441-447.

1007. Najean Y, Arrago JP, Rain JD, Dresch C. The 'spent' phase of polycythaemia vera: hypersplenism in the absence of myelofibrosis. Br J Haematol. 1984;56:163-170.

1008. Silverstein MN. The evolution into and the treatment of late stage polycythemia vera. Semin Hematol. 1976;13:79-84.

1009. Rosenthal A, Nathan DG, Marty AT, et al. Acute hemodynamic effects of red cell volume reduction in polycythemia of cyanotic congenital heart disease. Circulation. 1970;42:297-308.

1010. Hutton RD. The effect of iron deficiency on whole blood viscosity in polycythaemic patients. Br J Haematol. 1979;43: 191-199.

1011. Landolfi R, Marchioli R, Kutti J, et al. Efficacy and safety of low-dose aspirin in polycythemia vera. N Engl J Med. 2004; 350:114-124.

1012. Foa P, Massaro P, Ribera S, et al. Role of interferon alpha-2a in the treatment of polycythemia vera. Am J Hematol. 1995; 48:55-57.

1013. Nand S, Stock W, Godwin J, Fisher SG. Leukemogenic risk of hydroxyurea therapy in polycythemia vera, essential thrombocythemia, and myeloid metaplasia with myelofibrosis. Am J Hematol. 1996;52:42-46.

1014. Taylor PC, Dolan G, Ng JP, et al. Efficacy of recombinant interferon-alpha (rIFN-alpha) in polycythaemia vera: a study of 17 patients and an analysis of published data. Br J Haematol. 1996;92:55-59.

1015. McMullin MF, Bareford D, Campbell P, et al. Guidelines for the diagnosis, investigation and management of polycythaemia/ erythrocytosis. Br J Haematol. 2005;130:174-195.

1016. Petrides PE, Beykirch MK, Trapp OM. Anagrelide, a novel platelet lowering option in essential thrombocythaemia: treatment experience in 48 patients in Germany. Eur J Haematol. 1998;61:71-76.

1017. Harrison CN, Campbell PJ, Buck G, et al. Hydroxyurea compared with anagrelide in high-risk essential thrombocythemia. N Engl J Med. 2005;353:33-45.

1018. Li Z, Xu M, Xing S, et al. Erlotinib effectively inhibits JAK2V617F activity and polycythemia vera cell growth. J Biol Chem. 2007;282:3428-3432.

1019. Murphy S, Iland H, Rosenthal D, Laszlo J. Essential thrombocythemia: an interim report from the Polycythemia Vera Study Group. Semin Hematol. 1986;23:177-182.

1020. Silverstein MN. Primary or hemorrhagic thrombocythemia. Arch Intern Med. 1968;122:18-22.

1021. Sutor AH. Thrombocytosis in childhood. Semin Thromb Hemost. 1995;21:330-339.

1022. Tefferi A, Hoagland HC. Issues in the diagnosis and management of essential thrombocythemia. Mayo Clin Proc. 1994;69:651-655.

1023. Tefferi A, Silverstein MN, Hoagland HC. Primary thrombocythemia. Semin Oncol. 1995;22:334-340.

1024. Fialkow PJ, Faguet GB, Jacobson RJ, et al. Evidence that essential thrombocythemia is a clonal disorder with origin in a multipotent stem cell. Blood. 1981;58:916-919.

1025. Hoagland HC, Silverstein MN. Primary thrombocythemia in the young patient. Mayo Clin Proc. 1978;53:578-580.

1026. Pardanani AD, Levine RL, Lasho T, et al. MPL515 mutations in myeloproliferative and other myeloid disorders: a study of 1182 patients. Blood. 2006;108:3472-3476.

1027. Pikman Y, Lee BH, Mercher T, et al. MPLW515L is a novel somatic activating mutation in myelofibrosis with myeloid metaplasia. PLoS Med. 2006;3:e270.

1028. Freedman MH, Olivares RS, McClure PD, Weinstein L. Primary thrombocythemia in a child (letter). J Pediatr. 1973; 83:163-164.

1029. Linch DC, Hutton R, Cowan D, et al. Primary thrombocythaemia in childhood. Scand J Haematol. 1982;28:72-76.

1030. Ozer FL, Traux WE, Miesch DC, Levin WC. Primary hemorrhagic thrombocythemia. Am J Med. 1960;28:807-823.

1031. Kikuchi M, Tayama T, Hayakawa H, et al. Familial thrombocytosis. Br J Haematol. 1995;89:900-902.

1032. Levine RL, Wernig G. Role of JAK-STAT signaling in the pathogenesis of myeloproliferative disorders. Hematology Am Soc Hematol Educ Program. 2006:233-239, 510.

1033. Higgs JR, Sadek I, Neumann PE, et al. Familial essential thrombocythemia with spontaneous megakaryocyte colony formation and acquired JAK2 mutations. Leukemia. 2008;22:1551-1556

1034. Kaywin P, McDonough M, Insel PA, Shattil SJ. Platelet function in essential thrombocythemia. Decreased epinephrine responsiveness associated with a deficiency of platelet alpha-adrenergic receptors. N Engl J Med. 1978;299:505-509.

1035. Weinfeld A, Branehog I, Kutti J. Platelets in the myeloproliferative syndrome. Clin Haematol. 1975;4:373-392.

1036. Bellucci S, Janvier M, Tobelem G, et al. Essential thrombocythemias. Clinical evolutionary and biological data. Cancer. 1986;58:2440-2447.

1037. Addiego JE Jr, Mentzer WC Jr, Dallman PR. Thrombocytosis in infants and children. J Pediatr. 1974;85:805-807.

1038. Anagrelide Study Group. Anagrelide, a therapy for thrombocythemic states: experience in 577 patients. Am J Med. 1992; 92:69-76.

1039. Chintagumpala MM, Kennedy LL, Steuber CP. Treatment of essential thrombocythemia with anagrelide. J Pediatr. 1995; 127:495-498.

1040. Spencer CM, Brogden RN. Anagrelide. A review of its pharmacodynamic and pharmacokinetic properties, and therapeutic potential in the treatment of thrombocythaemia. Drugs. 1994; 47:809-822.

1041. Pogliani EM, Rossini F, Miccolis I, et al. Alpha interferon as initial treatment of essential thrombocythemia. Analysis after two years of follow-up. Tumori. 1995;81:245-248.

1042. Tornebohm-Roche E, Merup M, Lockner D, Paul C. Alpha-2a interferon therapy and antibody formation in patients with essential thrombocythemia and polycythemia vera with thrombocytosis. Am J Hematol. 1995;48:163-167.

1043. Njoku OS, Lewis SM, Catovsky D, Gordon-Smith EC. Anaemia in myelofibrosis: its value in prognosis. Br J Haematol. 1983; 54:79-89.

1044. Tefferi A, Silverstein MN, Noel P. Agnogenic myeloid metaplasia. Semin Oncol. 1995;22:327-333.

1045. Ward HP, Block MH. The natural history of agnogenic myeloid metaplasia (AMM) and a critical evaluation of its relationship with the myeloproliferative syndrome. Medicine (Baltimore). 1971;50:357-420.

1046. Boxer LA, Camitta BM, Berenberg W, Fanning JP. Myelofibrosis-myeloid metaplasia in childhood. Pediatrics. 1975;55:861-865.

1047. Cervantes F, Barosi G, Demory JL, et al. Myelofibrosis with myeloid metaplasia in young individuals: disease characteristics, prognostic factors and identification of risk groups. Br J Haematol. 1998;102:684-690.

1048. Laszlo J. Myeloproliferative disorders (MPD): myelofibrosis, myelosclerosis, extramedullary hematopoiesis, undifferentiated MPD, and hemorrhagic thrombocythemia. Semin Hematol. 1975;12:409-432.

1049. Dewald GW, Wright PI. Chromosome abnormalities in the myeloproliferative disorders. Semin Oncol. 1995;22:341-354.

1050. Castro-Malaspina H, Gay RE, Jhanwar SC, et al. Characteristics of bone marrow fibroblast colony-forming cells (CFU-F) and their progeny in patients with myeloproliferative disorders. Blood. 1982;59:1046-1054.

1051. Golde DW, Hocking WG, Quan SG, et al. Origin of human bone marrow fibroblasts. Br J Haematol. 1980;44:183-187.

1052. Jacobson RJ, Salo A, Fialkow PJ. Agnogenic myeloid metaplasia: a clonal proliferation of hematopoietic stem cells with secondary myelofibrosis. Blood. 1978;51:189-194.

1053. Levine RL, Pardanani A, Tefferi A, Gilliland DG. Role of JAK2 in the pathogenesis and therapy of myeloproliferative disorders. Nat Rev Cancer. 2007;7:673-683.

1054. McCarthy DM. Annotation. Fibrosis of the bone marrow: content and causes. Br J Haematol. 1985;59:1-7.

1055. Varki A, Lottenberg R, Griffith R, Reinhard E. The syndrome of idiopathic myelofibrosis. A clinicopathologic review with emphasis on the prognostic variables predicting survival. Medicine (Baltimore). 1983;62:353-371.

1056. Altura RA, Head DR, Wang WC. Long-term survival of infants with idiopathic myelofibrosis. Br J Haematol. 2000;109:459-462.

1057. Sekhar M, Prentice HG, Popat U, et al. Idiopathic myelofibrosis in children. Br J Haematol. 1996;93:394-397.

1058. Tasaka T, Nagai M, Murao S, et al. CD7, CD34-positive stem cell leukemia arising in agnogenic myeloid metaplasia. Am J Hematol. 1993;44:53-57.

1059. Silverstein MN, Wollaeger EE, Baggenstoss AH. Gastrointestinal and abdominal manifestations of agnogenic myeloid metaplasia. Arch Intern Med. 1973;131:532-537.

1060. Sacchi S. The role of alpha-interferon in essential thrombocythaemia, polycythaemia vera and myelofibrosis with myeloid metaplasia (MMM): a concise update. Leuk Lymphoma. 1995;19:13-20.

1061. Valent P, Akin C, Sperr WR, et al. Mastocytosis: pathology, genetics, and current options for therapy. Leuk Lymphoma. 2005;46:35-48.

1062. Kitamura Y, Shimada M, Hatanaka K, Miyano Y. Development of mast cells from grafted bone marrow cells in irradiated mice. Nature. 1977;268:442-443.

1063. Kirshenbaum AS, Kessler SW, Goff JP, Metcalfe DD. Demonstration of the origin of human mast cells from CD34+ bone marrow progenitor cells. J Immunol. 1991;146:1410-1415.

1064. Okayama Y, Kawakami T. Development, migration, and survival of mast cells. Immunol Res. 2006;34:97-115.

1065. Galli SJ, Nakae S, Tsai M. Mast cells in the development of adaptive immune responses. Nat Immunol. 2005;6:135-142.

1066. Wolff K, Komar M, Petzelbauer P. Clinical and histopathological aspects of cutaneous mastocytosis. Leuk Res. 2001; 25:519-528.

1067. Pullarkat VA, Bueso-Ramos C, Lai R, et al. Systemic mastocytosis with associated clonal hematological non-mast-cell lineage disease: analysis of clinicopathologic features and activating c-kit mutations. Am J Hematol. 2003;73:12-17.

1068. Pullarkat V, Bedell V, Kim Y, et al. Neoplastic mast cells in systemic mastocytosis associated with t(8;21) acute myeloid leukemia are derived from the leukemic clone. Leuk Res. 2007; 31:261-265.

1069. Valent P, Akin C, Sperr WR, et al. Aggressive systemic mastocytosis and related mast cell disorders: current treatment options and proposed response criteria. Leuk Res. 2003;27: 635-641.

1070. Hauswirth AW, Simonitsch-Klupp I, Uffmann M, et al. Response to therapy with interferon alpha-2b and prednisolone in aggressive systemic mastocytosis: report of five cases and review of the literature. Leuk Res. 2004;28:249-257.

1071. Kluin-Nelemans HC, Oldhoff JM, Van Doormaal JJ, et al. Cladribine therapy for systemic mastocytosis. Blood. 2003; 102:4270-4276.

1072. Shah NP, Lee FY, Luo R, et al. Dasatinib (BMS-354825) inhibits KITD816V, an imatinib-resistant activating mutation that triggers neoplastic growth in most patients with systemic mastocytosis. Blood. 2006;108:286-291.

1073. Gotlib J, Berube C, Growney JD, et al. Activity of the tyrosine kinase inhibitor PKC412 in a patient with mast cell leukemia with the D816V KIT mutation. Blood. 2005;106:2865-2870.

1074. Musto P, Falcone A, Sanpaolo G, et al. Inefficacy of imatinib-mesylate in sporadic, aggressive systemic mastocytosis. Leuk Res. 2004;28:421-422.

1075. Droogendijk HJ, Kluin-Nelemans HJ, van Doormaal JJ, et al. Imatinib mesylate in the treatment of systemic mastocytosis: a phase II trial. Cancer. 2006;107:345-351.

1076. Growney JD, Clark JJ, Adelsperger J, et al. Activation mutations of human c-KIT resistant to imatinib mesylate are sensitive to the tyrosine kinase inhibitor PKC412. Blood. 2005;106: 721-724.

12 Infant Leukemias

Krysta D. Schlis and Scott A. Armstrong

The biologic features and clinical characteristics of infant leukemias differ significantly from those of leukemias in older children. Infant leukemias are distinguished not only by the young age of the patients at diagnosis, but by their unique morphologic, immunologic, clinical, and genetic presentation.[1] For example, acute lymphoblastic leukemia (ALL) and acute myeloid leukemia (AML) present in infants with a somewhat unique constellation of clinical features, including hyperleukocytosis, massive organomegaly, and central nervous system (CNS) involvement at diagnosis.[2,3] Biologically, the most notable feature distinguishing infant leukemia from leukemia in older children is the high incidence of rearrangements involving the mixed lineage leukemia gene (*MLL*) located on chromosome band 11q23.[2,4-7] In the case of infant ALL, unique clinical and biologic characteristics are accompanied by an exceptionally poor prognosis, which is in stark contrast to the cure rates achieved for older children with ALL. In this chapter, the epidemiology, biology, clinical features, and treatment of infant ALL and AML will be discussed.

EPIDEMIOLOGY

The annual incidence of leukemia in the first year of life in the United States is approximately 40 cases/million children.[8] Infants account for 2.5% to 5% of ALLs and 6% to 14% of AMLs in childhood.[9] Unlike in older children with leukemia, in whom the percentage of ALL cases is approximately four times that of AML, in infants the ratio of ALL to AML is approximately equal. Furthermore, in contrast to an excess of males among older children with leukemia, there is a slight female predominance in infants with this disease.[8,10,11] Although neuroblastoma represents the most common neoplasm in infants, leukemia is the leading cause of death caused by neoplastic disease in this age group (Table 12-1).[1,8]

PRENATAL ORIGIN OF INFANT LEUKEMIA

The onset of leukemia in infancy strongly suggests a prenatal leukemogenic event, and there is significant molecular and epidemiologic evidence to support this hypothesis. Molecular studies of monozygotic twins with concordant ALL have demonstrated identical clonal, nonconstitutional rearrangements of the *MLL* gene and identical oligoclonal, heavy-chain immunoglobulin gene rearrangements in the peripheral blood of these infants.[12-15] This finding suggests the occurrence of a single in utero leukemogenic event in one twin generating a clone that is passed to the other fetus by intraplacental metastasis. Further evidence of oncogenesis in utero comes from reports of fetal deaths caused by AML with an *MLL* gene rearrangement.[16] Moreover, identical *MLL* fusions have been traced back to neonatal Guthrie genetic screening cards of children who were diagnosed with ALL in their first 2 years of life.[12,17,18] Similarly, leukemia has been diagnosed in fetuses with Down syndrome as early as 33 weeks' gestation, and the characteristic *GATA1* gene mutation associated with megakaryocytic leukemia in young children with Down syndrome has been identified in the neonatal Guthrie genetic screening cards of children who later developed leukemia.[19,20]

RISK FACTORS

As with most cancers, the causes of infant leukemia remain largely unknown. However, several epidemiologic risk factors associated with an increased risk of leukemia in young children have been identified. Given the close temporal relationship between embryogenesis and the clinical diagnosis of cancer, most investigations have focused on maternal characteristics and in utero exposures. Maternal alcohol consumption during pregnancy has been correlated with an increased risk of infant AML.[21] Studies have also shown an increased incidence of infant leukemia, particularly ALL, in infants with birth weights higher than 4000 g.[22-24] It has been speculated that high levels of endogenous insulin-like growth factors associated with high birth weight may contribute to leukemogenesis.[9,22] Other proposed risk factors include maternal pesticide and solvent exposure, in utero radiation exposure, and an adverse maternal reproductive history.[25-29] However, given the rarity of infant leukemia, it has been difficult to connect leukemia development with any of these exposures or clinical features definitively.

Of particular interest is the potential relationship between maternal consumption of naturally occurring DNA topoisomerase II inhibitors and the development of infant leukemia. *MLL* gene rearrangements, similar to those found in many infant leukemias, are common in secondary acute leukemias arising after exposure to DNA topoisomerase II inhibitors, including the epipodophyllotoxins (e.g., etoposide).[30-32] This relationship has led to the hypothesis that transplacental exposure to naturally occurring topoisomerase II inhibitors may be involved in the pathogenesis of infant leukemia.[33] This hypothesis is supported by the finding that both primary infant *MLL*-rearranged leukemias and therapy-related secondary acute leukemias have *MLL* breakpoints that are similarly distributed within the *MLL* breakpoint cluster region.[31] Furthermore, several dietary bioflavonoids, such as quercetin (found in certain fruits and vegetables) and genistein (found in soybeans) are known topoisomerase II inhibitors and have been shown to induce *MLL* cleavage in vitro.[34] A study by the Children's Oncology Group (COG) found that increased maternal consumption of these and other naturally occurring topoisomerase II inhibitors, such as catechins (found in red wine, tea, cocoa), is associated with an increased risk of *MLL*-rearranged infant AML but not infant ALL.[33,35,36] This association, if true, likely only accounts for a small proportion of infant leukemia cases. Furthermore, the fact that many of these foods are commonly consumed and infant leukemia is rare suggests that this association is either weak or requires a combination of factors. Thus, one cannot make recommendations to restrict certain foods to

TABLE 12-1	Incidence of Cancer in Infants*
Histology	**Incidence (per million)**
Neuroblastoma	64.6
Leukemias	40.5
Central nervous system	29.7
Retinoblastoma	26.7
Wilms' tumor	22.5
Germ cell	15.3
Soft tissue	15.2
Hepatic	9.5
Lymphomas	4.4
Epithelial	2.8
Other, unspecified	1.2
Bone	0.5

*SEER, 1976-1984 and 1986-1994.
From Ries LAG, Smith M, Gurney JG, et al (eds). Cancer Incidence and Survival Among Children and Adolescents: United States SEER Program 1975-1995 (NIH Publication No. 99-4649). Bethesda, Md, National Cancer Institute, SEER Program, 1999.

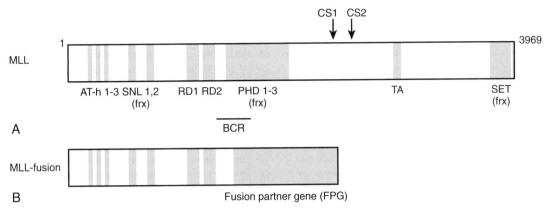

FIGURE 12-1. Schematic representation of the mixed lineage leukemia (MLL) protein and MLL fusions. **A,** The MLL gene is approximately 89 kb long, consists of 37 exons, and encodes a 3969-amino acid nuclear protein with a complex domain structure (unique domains are highlighted). The N terminus contains three short AT hook motifs (AT-h 1-3), which are thought to mediate binding to the minor groove of AT-rich genomic DNA sequences. There are two nuclear localization sites (SNL1 and SNL2) immediately C-terminal to the AT hooks that are followed by a transcriptional repression domain (TRD) consisting of two functional subunits, RD1 and RD2. RD1 contains a DNA methyltransferase (DMT) homology domain. The plant homeodomains (PHD) zinc finger motifs may mediate binding to a number of different proteins or to chromatin. The transcriptional activation domain (TA) recruits the transcriptional coactivator CBP (CREB binding protein) and precedes a C-terminal SET domain that possesses histone H3 lysine 4 (H3K4) methyltransferase activity. The breakpoint cluster region (BCR) spans exons 8 to 13. **B,** Structure of MLL fusion proteins generated by MLL translocations. A typical MLL fusion protein contains the N terminus of MLL encoded by the first 8 to 13 exons and the C terminus of one of over 50 fusion partners.

decrease the likelihood of leukemia development. Moreover, maternal consumption of fruits and vegetables during pregnancy has been associated with a decrease rather than increase in the risk of infant leukemia overall.[36]

Pharmacogenetic differences in the metabolism of topoisomerase II inhibitors have been hypothesized to modulate the relationship between exposure to these chemicals and the occurrence of *MLL* rearrangements. A common structural feature shared by many topoisomerase II inhibitors, including bioflavonoids, is a quinone moiety. Quinone metabolites generated as by-products of these compounds in the fetal liver have been shown to cleave the *MLL* gene.[34] Quinones are normally detoxified by reduced nicotinamide adenine dinucleotide phosphatase (NADPH): quinone oxidoreductase (NQO1). The presence of a low-activity variant of NQO1 has been associated with an increased risk of *MLL*-rearranged infant ALL.[37] However, a similar study has also demonstrated a relationship between this NQO1 polymorphism and infant ALL without *MLL* rearrangements.[38]

BIOLOGY OF MIXED LINEAGE LEUKEMIA TRANSLOCATIONS

The mixed lineage leukemia (*MLL, ALL1, HRX*) gene located on chromosome band 11q23 is commonly altered in infant leukemia in that it is rearranged in 80% of infant ALL and 60% of infant AML cases. These chromosomal abnormalities usually involve reciprocal translocations, which encode chimeric transcripts that give rise to oncogenic fusion proteins with pronounced transforming potential.[39] A number of groups cloned the *MLL-AF4* gene in the early 1990.[40-43] *MLL-AF4* encodes a protein of 2304 amino acids, with the NH$_2$-terminal 1439 amino acids derived from *MLL* on chromosome 11, and COOH-terminal 865 amino acids from the *AF4* gene on chromosome 4. Subsequently, more than 30 different translocations have been identified, all of which appear to produce a fusion

protein possessing the NH$_2$ terminus of MLL fused in-frame to the COOH terminus of the fusion partner (Fig. 12-1).[39]

The *MLL* gene encodes a 3969–amino acid DNA-binding protein that possesses multiple recognizable protein motifs, including an NH$_2$-terminal DNA binding domain, transcriptional activation and repression domains, and a COOH-terminal SET domain that contains histone methyltransferase activity.[44,45] Biochemical studies have identified MLL as a member of a large multiprotein complex that contains members involved in chromatin modification and remodeling. Notably, the complex includes histone deacetylases (HDACs) and members of the Swi/Snf chromatin remodeling complex.[45] Also, MLL is recruited to the promoters of select cell cycle regulatory genes by the protein product of the *MEN1* tumor suppressor gene, suggesting a role for MLL in tumor suppression and cell cycle control.[46,47] These data support the hypothesis that the MLL protein regulates gene expression via chromatin modification.[48]

Analysis of *Mll* knockout mice has suggested that *Mll* plays an important role in development and hematopoiesis through maintenance of appropriate homeotic (*Hox*) gene expression.[49,50] Detailed studies assessing the specific role of Mll in hematopoietic development have shown that Mll is necessary for definitive hematopoiesis and for the expansion of hematopoietic progenitors and stem cells found in the aorta-gonad-mesonephros (AGM) region of the developing embryo.[51,52] The defect in hematopoietic progenitor expansion can be rescued by re-expression of *Hox* genes, confirming the importance of Mll-mediated *Hox* gene expression during hematopoiesis.

Multiple studies have demonstrated the ability of *Hox* genes to induce leukemia in mice,[53] and the t(7;11)(p15;p15) translocation found in some human acute myeloid leukemias results in a fusion of the *HOXA9* gene to the nucleoporin *NUP98.*[54,55] Given the apparent importance of *HOX* genes in leukemogenesis, it seems likely that translocations involving *MLL*, a known regulator of *HOX* genes, alters expression of *HOX* genes that are important for leukemogenesis. Further support for *HOX* genes as central regulators of *MLL*-induced leukemogenesis comes from gene expression studies that have found multiple *HOXA* cluster genes more highly expressed in *MLL*-rearranged myelogenous and lymphoblastic leukemias as compared with *MLL* germline leukemias.[56-59]

The association of *MLL* rearrangements with leukemias of multiple hematopoietic lineages have prompted multiple hypotheses with regard to the cells of origin and mechanisms of oncogenesis of *MLL*-rearranged leukemias.[60,61] These have suggested that *MLL* rearrangements either induce inappropriate expression of lineage-specified genes (i.e., expression of myeloid-associated genes in a lymphoid precursor), or immortalize a hematopoietic progenitor with both myeloid and lymphoid potential. Gene expression studies of human *MLL*-rearranged leukemias combined with studies in mouse models have begun to shed light on this issue.[56,59,62-64]

Gene expression studies of human *MLL*-rearranged B-precursor ALL have demonstrated that hundreds of genes are differentially expressed when compared with other B-precursor ALLs.[56-58,65] Based on the magnitude of the differences in gene expression, it appears that *MLL* translocations specify a unique lymphoblastic leukemia. Other large gene expression studies have also shown that ALLs with distinct chromosomal rearrangements have unique gene expression profiles, providing support for this hypothesis.[58] The genes that are relatively highly expressed in *MLL*-rearranged B-precursor ALL are those associated with hematopoietic progenitors and developing myeloid cells, whereas the genes expressed at lower levels are genes associated with lymphoid identity. Studies have also defined specific gene expression signatures associated with *MLL* translocations in pediatric—and in some cases infant—AML blasts.[59] Of interest, even though there are clear differences in expression of lineage-associated genes between *MLL*-rearranged ALL and *MLL*-rearranged AML, there appears to be a core gene expression profile found in all *MLL*-rearranged human leukemias, independent of the lineage markers.[59] Presumably, MLL fusion proteins directly regulate a subset of these genes. This is further supported by the fact that this *MLL*-associated signature consists of multiple highly expressed *HOX* genes.

The observation that leukemic cells bearing an *MLL* translocation often coexpress both myeloid and lymphoid markers raises the possibility that MLL fusion genes selectively transform hematopoietic stem cells (HSCs). If so, this HSC population would have an inherent self-renewal capacity that could be co-opted for leukemogenesis. Xenograft transplantation studies have demonstrated that a rare subpopulation of CD34$^+$ and CD38$^-$ human myeloid leukemia cells are able to transfer the disease to immunodeficient mice, providing support for HSCs as the normal compartment from which leukemia-initiating cells (leukemia stem cells) might arise.[66] Alternatively, the translocation event between *MLL* and a partner gene may affect a more committed population. In this scenario, the MLL fusion protein might confer a self-renewal and proliferative capacity to these short-lived progenitors and allow them to initiate leukemogenesis. Studies have suggested that Mll fusion proteins and potentially other translocation-associated fusion proteins are capable of inducing leukemia when expressed in fully committed myeloid progenitors, such as granulocyte-macrophage progenitors (GMPs).[62,67] These findings are of particular importance because they suggest that products of chromosomal translocations found in human leukemias are able to induce a program of self-renewal that is not normally present in hematopoietic progenitors.

Mouse models of leukemia predict that multiple genetic events are necessary for the development of acute leukemias. Knock-in models of leukemia have been developed, in which the fusion genes generated by translocations found in human leukemias are under the control of the endogenous promoter. Such models have been generated for a number of Mll fusions. Mice containing an *MLL-AF9* fusion gene under control of the *Mll* promoter spontaneously develop AML, with a latency of 4 months to more than 1 year.[68] This latency is widely interpreted as signifying a requirement for a second genetic event during leukemogenesis. Other models such as an *Mll-Cbp* knock-in or *Aml1-Eto* knock-in model do not spontaneously develop leukemia.[69,70] In these models, either irradiation or chemical mutagenesis is necessary to induce leukemias, thus clearly implicating multiple events for the development of leukemia.

Multiple lines of evidence now point to a multistep pathogenesis of human acute leukemia. Elegant epidemiologic studies have suggested that childhood leukemias require at least two and probably more genetic events to occur for the development of leukemia. In particular, lymphoblastic leukemias with *TEL-AML1* rearrangements appear to develop after a multistep process. *TEL-AML1* rearrangements have been detected in blood taken at birth from a child who then developed ALL 3 to 5 years later. This suggests that *TEL-AML1* rearrangements are the first genetic event, but also that other mutations are required for the development of ALL.[71] Similar studies have been performed on blood spots from children who subsequently developed *MLL*-rearranged ALL, and the *MLL* translocations clearly develop in utero, even though the leukemias become apparent at some point during the first year of life.[12]

Receptor tyrosine kinases are attractive candidates as signaling molecules that may cooperate with translocation-associated fusion proteins during leukemogenesis. Ever-increasing evidence has suggested that activated kinases play a central role in the pathogenesis of leukemias and myeloproliferative syndromes.[72] The most dramatic evidence for such a role is activation of the ABL tyrosine kinase by the BCR-ABL fusion produced by the t(9;22), and its inhibition by imatinib (Gleevec).[73,74] Other mutant kinases frequently identified in AML are the receptor tyrosine kinases FLT3 and c-KIT.[72] Mouse experiments have supported the hypothesis that DNA-binding fusion proteins generated by leukemia-associated translocations perform different functions than activated tyrosine kinases.[67] DNA-binding fusions induce a block in differentiation or activate self-renewal in developing hematopoietic progenitors, whereas activated kinases may provide survival or proliferation signals. This has prompted the hypothesis that at least two different classes of mutations are necessary for leukemogenesis.[75] Further support for this hypothesis has come from studies of *MLL*-rearranged ALL, which have demonstrated high-level expression and frequent mutation of the receptor tyrosine kinase FLT3 in this disease, rendering *MLL*-rearranged ALL cells sensitive to FLT3 inhibitors in vitro and in murine models.[76-79] Studies are underway to assess FLT3 inhibitors in patients with *MLL*-rearranged ALL (see later).

ACUTE LYMPHOBLASTIC LEUKEMIA

Clinical and Biologic Features

ALL in infants is characterized by a high leukocyte count at presentation, marked hepatosplenomegaly, and a relatively high incidence of central nervous system involvement.[2,3,80,81] The immunophenotype of infant ALL is usually that of an immature B-lineage precursor and is characterized by a lack of CD10 expression, as well as by the coexpression of myeloid-associated antigens, such as CD14, CD15, and CDw65. Lack of CD10 expression and coexpression of myeloid markers correlates with the presence of an *MLL* gene rearrangement, which is present in 80% of infants with ALL compared with only 2% to 4% of older children with ALL.[4,6,82-84] *MLL* gene rearrangements are more frequent in younger infants, with approximately 90% of infants younger than 6 months at diagnosis having *MLL* gene rearrangements in their leukemic blasts compared with 30% to 60% of infants aged 6 to 12 months.[4,85,86] The most common *MLL* translocation observed in infant ALL is the t(4;11)(q21;q23), resulting in the MLL-AF4 fusion. This translocation is found in approximately 70% of *MLL*-rearranged infant ALLs. Other common translocations include the t(11;19), resulting in the MLL-ENL fusion, and the t(9;11), resulting in the MLL-AF9 fusion, and occur in 15% and 4% of *MLL*-rearranged infant ALLs, respectively.[6,82-84,87] Infant ALLs without an *MLL* rearrangement generally resemble the more common B-precursor ALL phenotype (CD19+, CD10+) typical of older children with ALL. Chromosomal abnormalities known to be favorable in older children with ALL, such as high hyperdiploidy (51 to 65 chromosomes, or DNA index more than 1.16) and the *TEL-AML1* fusion gene, are notably absent in infants.[81] The distinguishing presenting characteristics of infants with ALL are summarized in Table 12-2.

Prognostic Factors and Outcomes

Despite extraordinary improvements in the cure rates for older children with ALL, the prognosis for infants with this disease remains poor. Historically, infants with ALL treated on standard regimens had less than 20% event-free survival. Over the

last decade, intensified regimens designed especially for infants have resulted in improved rates of event-free survival (EFS), ranging from 28% to 54% (Table 12-3).[81,82,84,86,88-95] This is in contrast to EFS rates of greater than 80% for older children with ALL.[96-99] Although 90% to 95% of infants with ALL achieve remission after initial induction chemotherapy, a favorable outcome is hampered by an exceedingly high relapse rate, typically within the first year after diagnosis.

Several closely related adverse prognostic factors have been identified for infants with ALL, including the presence of an *MLL* gene rearrangement, lack of CD10 expression, coexpression of myeloid markers, age less than 6 months at diagnosis, high white blood cell (WBC) count at presentation, central nervous system involvement, and poor early response to prednisone therapy.[84,92,100,101] In multivariate analyses, the presence of an *MLL* gene rearrangement, age younger than 6 months, and a poor early response to prednisone therapy consistently emerge as the most important adverse prognostic features.[86,93] In many studies, the presence of an *MLL* gene rearrangement is the most important independent predictor of outcome for infants.[85] Long-term event-free survival for infants with *MLL*-rearranged ALL has ranged from 13% to 34% versus 52% to 95% for infants with germline *MLL* (Fig. 12-2).[4,6,84-86,89,92,93,102]

In addition to *MLL* gene status and age, early response to therapy has been shown to be an important predictor of outcome in infants with ALL. The Berlin-Frankfurt-Munster (BFM) group has identified a poor response to prednisone as one of the strongest predictors of outcome for infants with ALL, regardless of *MLL* gene status.[92] Infants with ALL who have a poor response to a 7-day prednisone monotherapy prophase (defined as more than 1000 blasts/μL present in peripheral blood on day 8) had a 6-year EFS of only 15%, compared with 53% for infants with a good response to prednisone. This finding was reproduced in the most recent clinical trial conducted by the Interfant study group (Interfant 99), in which infants with a poor response to steroids had a 30% 4-year EFS, compared with 56% for good responders.[86] Similarly, the Children's Cancer Group (CCG) found a threefold excess risk of treatment failure in infants whose bone marrows contained more than 5% leukemic blast cells after 14 days of multiagent chemotherapy.[93]

It has been suggested that the specific *MLL* fusion partner might also have prognostic significance for infants with ALL.[93,101] However, in a large retrospective study that included data from more than 200 cases of *MLL*-rearranged ALL in infants, there was no significant difference in outcome among cytogenetic subgroups, including the t(4;11), t(9;11), t(11;19), and other 11q23 rearrangements.[87] More recently, the Interfant study group has also failed to find any association between the specific *MLL* translocations and treatment outcome.[86]

TABLE 12-2	Presenting Characteristics of Infants and Older Children with Acute Lymphoblastic Leukemia	
	AGE (yr)	
Characteristic	**0-1 (%)**	**1-18 (%)**
WBC* > 100,000[81]	58	6.3
CNS-positive*[81]	14	1.5
Phenotype		
B lineage	96	86.5
T lineage	4	13.5
CD-10 negative[81]	54.7	3.3
Myeloid antigen coexpression[84a,92]	28	5
DNA index* > 1.16[81]	1.5	24.7
TEL-AML1* rearrangement[81]	4.5	24.1
MLL rearrangement[82-84]	70-80	2-4

*B lineage patients only.
From Silverman LB. Acute lymphoblastic leukemia in infancy. Pediatr Blood Cancer. 2007;49:1070-1073.

TABLE 12-3	Outcomes of Treatment Protocols for Acute Lymphoblastic Leukemia in Infants				
Study	**Publication Date**	**Patients Enrolled**	**CR Rate (%)**	**EFS Time Point (yr)**	**EFS (%)**
DFCI (1985-1995)[87]	1997	23	96	4	54
Interfant-99[94]	2007	482	94	5	45
AIEOP-91, 95[93]	2006	52	96	5	45
BFM 86, 90, 95[81]	1999	129	95	8	43
CCG-1953[84]	2006	115	97	5	42
CCG-1883[91]	1999	135	97	4	39
CCG-107[91]	1999	99	94	4	33
UKALL-92[92]	2002	86	94	5	33
POG 8493[88]	1997	82	93	4	28

CR, complete remission; EFS, event-free survival.

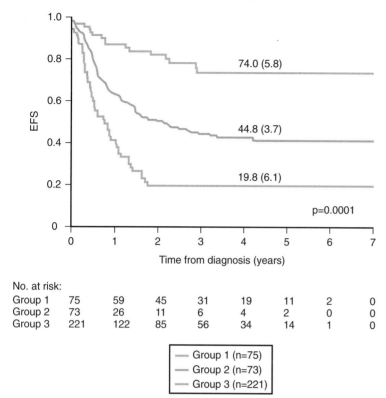

No. at risk:

Group 1	75	59	45	31	19	11	2	0
Group 2	73	26	11	6	4	2	0	0
Group 3	221	122	85	56	34	14	1	0

— Group 1 (n=75)
— Group 2 (n=73)
--- Group 3 (n=221)

FIGURE 12-2. Event-free survival (EFS) for infant ALL patients treated on Interfant-99.[94] Group 1 consisted of patients with germline *MLL* gene. Group 2 consisted of patients with an *MLL* gene rearrangement, age younger than 6 months at diagnosis, and white blood cell count higher than 300×10^9 cells/L at diagnosis. Group 3 consisted of all other patients. *(Adapted from Pieters R, Schrappe M, De Lorenzo P, et al. A treatment protocol for infants younger than 1 year with acute lymphoblastic leukemia (Interfant-99): an observational study and a multicentre randomized trial. Lancet. 2007;370:240-250.)*

Treatment

Attempts to improve clinical outcomes for infants with ALL have generally involved intensifying treatment regimens as well as incorporating chemotherapeutic agents more commonly used in AML therapy. Several preclinical and clinical findings have also informed the development of treatment regimens for infants with ALL, including clinical response to prednisone therapy and in vitro drug sensitivity profiles of infant ALL lymphoblasts.

When compared with cells from older children with ALL, leukemic blasts from infant ALL patients are more often resistant to glucocorticoids (prednisone and dexamethasone) and L-asparaginase in in vitro assays. Importantly, both of these agents are central components of current ALL therapeutic regimens.[92,103-105] Given the prognostic significance of prednisone response in ALL, some infant ALL treatment groups now risk-stratify infants based on prednisone response as well as other common prognostic factors, including *MLL* gene status, age, and diagnostic white blood cell count.[86]

Although infant ALL blasts are relatively resistant to some common ALL therapeutic agents, they are remarkably sensitive to cytosine arabinoside (Ara-C, cytarabine), a drug commonly used in the treatment of AML.[103,104] This increased sensitivity may be related in part to elevated expression of the human equilibrative nucleoside transporter 1 (hENT1), which allows cytarabine to permeate the cell membrane at low to moderate concentrations.[106-109] Clinical data are accumulating to suggest that increased use of cytarabine may benefit infants with ALL.[86,89,93] Investigators from the Dana-Farber Cancer Institute ALL Consortium first reported an improved outcome in a small number of infants treated with intensified therapy that included high-dose cytarabine.[110] Subsequently the cooperative groups, Children's Oncology Group (COG) and Interfant, incorporated high-dose cytarabine into their intensified thera-

peutic regimens, a strategy that is likely to have contributed to the improvements in event-free survival for infants with ALL observed over the past decade.

Hematopoietic Stem Cell Transplantation

The role of hematopoietic stem cell transplantation (HSCT) in first remission for infants with ALL is controversial. Small uncontrolled studies have suggested that HSCT may benefit infants with *MLL* rearrangements.[111-113] Although encouraging, these results must be interpreted with caution, given the small sample sizes and the failure to control for waiting time from diagnosis to transplantation. In contrast, a larger retrospective analysis did not confirm a benefit of HCST for infants with ALL.[87] The most recent Interfant study group trial (Interfant 99) also failed to demonstrate a statistically significant difference in the 4-year EFS between high-risk patients who received stem cell transplants and those who received chemotherapy alone. Similarly, the Children's Oncology group found no benefit of transplantation over intensive chemotherapy alone.[84] Further studies are needed to adequately define the role for stem cell transplantation in infants with ALL.

Toxicity and Central Nervous System–Directed Therapy

A major consideration in the treatment of ALL in infants is the significant potential for short- and long-term toxicity given the intensity of treatment regimens and the lack of pharmacokinetic and pharmacodynamic studies to ensure optimal dosing of chemotherapeutic agents in infants. Of particular concern is the risk of debilitating neuropsychological sequelae, especially in infants receiving cranial radiation. Severe neurologic deficits and learning disabilities have been reported in long-term survivors of infant ALL who received cranial radiation.[3,88,89] In

TABLE 12-4 Outcomes of Treatment Protocols for Acute Myeloid Leukemia in Infants

Study	Study Period	Patients Enrolled	EFS Time Point	EFS (%)
St. Jude (AML80-91)[122]	1980-1987	28	5	32
BFM (AML 93)[131]	1993-1998	112*	5	41
MRC (AML10, 12)[132]	1988-2002	151	5	58
POG (8821)[133]	1988-1993	122*	5	22
Nordic (NOPHO-93)[134]	1993-2001	57*	5	54
CCG 2891[135]	1989-1995	116	8	71
Japan (ANLL91)[136]	1995-1998	35	3	72
French (LAME 89, 91)[137]	1988-1998	42	5	37.3
FHCRC[138]	1995-1998	35*	3	72

*Children 1 to 2 years of age were included.
EFS, event-free survival.

almost all subsequent clinical trials, attempts have been made to reduce neuropsychological complications by minimizing, delaying, or eliminating cranial radiation. Currently, most investigators favor eliminating radiation in infants with ALL, even those with CNS leukemia at diagnosis, relying instead on intensive systemic and intrathecal chemotherapy. Several observations have supported this approach, including outcomes from large cooperative group studies documenting very low CNS relapse rates (3% to 9%) with intensive systemic and intrathecal chemotherapy alone.[86,90,93]

ACUTE MYELOID LEUKEMIA

Clinical and Prognostic Features

Infant AML is characterized by a high incidence of myelomonoblastic (FAB M4) or monoblastic (FAB M5) morphology, frequent CNS involvement, extramedullary disease (including skin involvement) and relatively high leukocyte counts at diagnosis.[2]

MLL gene rearrangements are found in about 60% of infant AML cases, with the most common translocation being the t(9;11), resulting in the MLL-AF9 fusion, followed by the t(11;19), resulting in the MLL-ENL fusion. *MLL* gene rearrangements in infant AML are associated with a FAB M4 or M5 morphology and hyperleukocytosis.[100,114,115] Other cytogenetic abnormalities in infant AML of the FAB M4 or M5 morphologic subtype include inv(16) and monosomy 7. Translocations commonly seen in older children with AML, such as t(8;21) and t(15;17), are rare in infants with AML.[116]

Unlike infant ALL, the prognostic factors that predict outcome for infant AML are not clearly defined. Several studies have identified a variety of potential prognostic factors for infants with AML, including presenting white blood cell count, FAB M4 or M5 morphology, gender, and presence of an *MLL* gene rearrangement, but the findings of these studies have varied widely and are often contradictory.[117-122] The difficulty in clearly identifying consistent prognostic factors in infant AML may point to more biologic heterogeneity in infant AML (as compared with infant ALL), as well as significant variations in the definition of study groups and treatment regimens.

The prognostic significance of *MLL* gene rearrangements in infant AML is unclear. Several studies have found that *MLL* rearrangements lack prognostic significance in childhood AML, whereas at least one study has found a trend toward a worse outcome.[115,117,123-126] Alternatively, several groups have demonstrated that the presence of a specific translocation,

t(9;11)(p22;q22) or MLL-AF9, confers a favorable prognosis.[122,127-130] For example, the investigators at St. Jude found the presence of a t(9;11) to be an important prognostic factor for patients treated in four consecutive pediatric AML trials. The 5-year EFS for infants whose leukemia cells carried the t(9;11) was 70% versus 25% for those with other cytogenetic abnormalities, including other *MLL* rearrangements.[122]

Outcomes and Treatment

Whereas age-associated treatment results are clearly evident in childhood ALL, with infants faring significantly worse, similar age-related differences in outcomes have not been routinely observed in AML. Large clinical trials in children with AML have reported EFS rates for infants of 22% to 73%, which do not differ significantly from outcomes achieved in older children (Table 12-4).[112,122,131-138] Given that treatment outcomes do not differ by age group, there has been no compelling clinical justification for the development of unique treatment strategies for infants with AML. Current therapeutic regimens for infants and older children focus on intensive remission induction and consolidation chemotherapy, with hematopoietic stem cell transplantation reserved for those with matched sibling donors and those with poor prognostic features. Although treatment regimens for infants with AML do not currently differ from those for older children, some potential differences have been proposed. The observation that the t(9;11) may be a favorable prognostic factor in infants with AML has resulted in controversy as to whether bone marrow transplantation in first remission should be considered in this subgroup of patients. Another possible exception includes infants with megakaryoblastic leukemia harboring a t(1;22)(p13;q13), who appear to have a particularly poor prognosis and may be candidates for more aggressive treatment or innovative experimental therapy.[141,142]

Association with Down Syndrome

Several genetic syndromes, including monosomy 7, del (7q) syndromes, Noonan's syndrome, and neurofibromatosis type I, are associated with an increased risk of developing myelodysplasia, myeloproliferative diseases, and myeloid leukemia in infancy. A striking example is the increased incidence of leukemia seen in children with Down syndrome. Individuals with Down syndrome have a 10- to 20-fold increased lifetime risk of developing leukemia, including ALL and AML. The most marked increase is observed in young children with Down syndrome who develop acute megakaryoblastic leukemia (FAB M7, AMKL).[143] The risk of AMKL is estimated to be 500 times higher in children with Down syndrome than in the general population. A transient form of megakaryoblastic leukemia, known as transient leukemia, transient abnormal myelopoiesis, or transient myeloproliferative disorder (TMD), often precedes AMKL in newborn infants with Down syndrome (or trisomy 21 mosaicism). Although the true incidence of TMD is unknown, a small study has found that 10% of neonates with Down syndrome have evidence of TMD on examination of their peripheral blood smears.[144] The true incidence of TMD is likely to be higher, given that fetuses who develop TMD in utero may not be identified and neonates with subtle manifestations of TMD may go unnoticed.[145,146]

Clinically, the presentation of TMD can be variable, from asymptomatic, with an incidental finding of an elevated white blood cell count and circulating blasts in the peripheral blood, to fulminating life-threatening disease, with severe liver dysfunction and liver fibrosis, multiple effusions, and respiratory compromise. TMD has also been associated with intrauterine death and hydrops fetalis.[146,147] Usually, TMD has a relatively benign course, with spontaneous remission within the first 3 months of life. However, 13% to 33% of infants who recover from TMD will go on to develop AMKL by age 3 years.[148-150] Often, the subsequent leukemia is preceded by a myelodysplastic phase, with progressive cytopenias and increasing marrow fibrosis. A prospective study of neonates with TMD conducted by the Children's Oncology Group has found that 64% of infants with TMD experienced a spontaneous and continuous remission, 17% suffered an early death (predominantly because of liver failure), and 19% experienced a spontaneous remission but went on to develop AMKL at a mean age of 20 months.[150]

TMD and AMKL in Down syndrome nicely illustrate the multistep process of leukemic transformation. Biologically, the blasts from TMD and AMKL are morphologically and immunophenotypically similar and consistent with megakaryoblastic progenitors.[151-153] Chromosomal abnormalities are more frequent in AMKL than TMD, with the most common abnormality being trisomy 8.[144,154] The leukemic blasts of TMD and AMKL in patients with Down syndrome have been shown to harbor a unique mutation of the gene encoding the hematopoietic transcription factor GATA1.[155,156] These mutations are found exclusively in Down syndrome–associated TMD and AMKL and have not been found in non-Down syndrome–associated AMKL nor in Down syndrome patients with ALL.[155,157,158] GATA1 has essential functions during normal erythroid and megakaryocytic development.[159,160] Most GATA1 mutations cluster within exon 2 and result in the expression of a truncated mutant protein, GATA1s, which retains its DNA binding zinc fingers but lacks the amino-terminal transcriptional activation domain. Recent studies in model systems have suggested that GATA1 possesses unique activity that leads to expansion of an early megakaryocyte progenitor in the fetal liver, perhaps explaining why GATA1 mutations are only found in infant AMKL from patients with Down syndrome.[161]

Another remarkable characteristic of AMKL in Down syndrome is its extraordinary responsiveness to AML therapy.[119,162-165] In early clinical trials, the outcomes for patients with AML and Down syndrome were not favorable, although poor outcomes were primarily the result of treatment-related toxicity rather than relapsed or refractory disease. Subsequently, patients with Down syndrome and AML treated in a series of large multicenter pediatric trials were found to have a better response to chemotherapy and better survival rates than patients without Down syndrome. EFS rates for children with Down syndrome and AML treated by modern protocols range from 80% to 100%.[119,162,163,165-168] Current treatment protocols for patients with Down syndrome and AML favor less intensive regimens, which aim to maintain high cure rates while minimizing toxicity.

Infant AMKL with t(1;22)

AMKL also occurs in a subset of infants without Down syndrome. AMKL in these infants frequently harbors a t(1;22)(p13;q13).[141,142,169] The t(1;22)(p13;q13) is found almost exclusively in infants and young children with AMKL. This disorder is typically accompanied by significant bone marrow fibrosis and organomegaly and has a poor prognosis, with a median survival of only 8 months. The t(1;22)(p13;q13) characteristic of this malignancy is associated with the fusion of two novel genes, RNA-binding motif protein-15 (*RBMI15*), a RNA recognition motif-encoding gene, and megakaryoblastic leukemia-1 (*MKL1*), a gene encoding an SAP (SAF-A/B, Acinus, and PIAS) DNA binding domain.[170] The mechanism by which this fusion contributes to leukemogenesis is not yet fully understood.

FUTURE DIRECTIONS IN INFANT ACUTE LYMPHOBLASTIC LEUKEMIA TREATMENT

Although morphologic complete remission is achieved in the vast majority of infants with ALL, a favorable outcome is hampered by an exceedingly high relapse rate in the first year following diagnosis. To date, intensification of conventional chemotherapeutic agents has resulted in only incremental improvement in the prognosis of infants with ALL, emphasizing the need for novel, more effective therapies.[171]

Modulators of Glucocorticoid Resistance

Cellular drug resistance may significantly contribute to the poor prognosis of infant ALL.[171] Infants with ALL are more likely to have a poor in vivo response to prednisone than older children with ALL.[92,105] In addition, leukemic blasts from infant ALL patients are highly resistant to glucocorticoids in vitro.[103,104] Both in vivo and in vitro responses to prednisone are highly predictive of clinical outcome in childhood ALL; thus, the mechanisms of glucocorticoid resistance are attractive targets for novel therapeutic agents.[172,173] Gene expression profiling of steroid-resistant and steroid-sensitive lymphoblasts indicates that MCL-1, an antiapoptotic member of the BCL2 family, may be an important modulator of glucocorticoid resistance in ALL.[174,175] Furthermore, a gene expression–based chemical genomics screen has identified the mammalian target of rapamycin (mTOR) inhibitor, sirolimus (more commonly known as rapamycin), as an agent capable of reversing a gene expression signature associated with glucocorticoid resistance. It has also been shown that sirolimus sensitizes lymphoid cells to glucocorticoids via the modulation of MCL-1 levels.[174] Other modulators of MCL-1 have been identified including honokiol, a naturally occurring compound, and synthetic inhibitors, Seliciclib (CYC202, or R-roscovitine) and R-etodolac (SDX-101).[176-179] The potential to overcome glucocorticoid resistance in infant ALL by compounds that modulate MCL-1, or other antiapoptotic molecules such as BCL2, makes agents targeting the apoptotic pathway attractive candidates for further investigation as therapeutic approaches for the treatment of infant ALL.[180]

Nucleoside Analogues

Although infant ALL blasts are relatively resistant to some chemotherapeutic agents, they are more sensitive to the cytidine analogue cytosine arabinoside (Ara-C, cytarabine) when compared with blasts from older children with ALL.[103,104] In addition, infant ALL cells are also highly sensitive to the adenosine analogue 2-CdA (2-chlorodeoxyadenosine, or cladribine).[104] Furthermore, several studies have demonstrated synergistic effects between Ara-C and 2-CdA in vitro, and the addition of 2-CdA to Ara-C–containing regimens has been shown to improve complete remission rates in AML.[181-183] These observations suggest that regimens combining Ara-C and 2-CdA might also provide benefit for infants with ALL. Moreover, given the apparent sensitivity of infant ALL cells to nucleoside analogues, novel nucleoside analogues such as clofarabine, troxacitabine (Troxatyl), and sapacitabine are attractive candidates for further testing in infant ALL.[184-189]

FLT3 Inhibitors

Lymphoblastic leukemias with rearrangements of the *MLL* gene display a unique gene expression profile that distinguishes them from other subgroups of ALL and AML.[56,58,59,65] This distinct gene expression profile has led to the identification of several potential therapeutic targets. One of the most highly expressed genes distinguishing *MLL*-rearranged ALL from other acute leukemias is *FLT3*, the gene encoding Fms-like tyrosine kinase 3.[56,76] *FLT3* mutations resulting in a constitutively active receptor are common in AML. Several small-molecule FLT3 inhibitors have been developed (e.g., CEP-701, PKC412) and clinical trials are underway to evaluate the effectiveness of these compounds in the treatment of AML.[190-192] High levels of *FLT3* expression have also been demonstrated in *MLL*-rearranged ALL. FLT3 inhibitors have been shown to be active against *MLL*-rearranged cell lines overexpressing *FLT3* as well as in primary *MLL*-rearranged lymphoblasts.[76,79,193] Additionally, results from in vitro experiments with *MLL*-rearranged cell lines have suggested that FLT3 inhibitors may work synergistically with several standard chemotherapeutic agents including Ara-C.[78,193] However, the sequence of administration of these agents appears to be important. In vitro studies have found that to achieve maximal synergistic cytotoxicity, the chemotherapeutic agent must be given immediately prior to the FLT3 inhibitor, whereas pretreatment with the FLT3 inhibitor followed by the chemotherapeutic agent results in antagonistic effects.[78,194] The preclinical data demonstrating activity of FLT-3 inhibitors in infant ALL suggest that FLT3 inhibition may represent a novel therapeutic strategy for infant ALL, and clinical testing is underway.

Targeting the MLL Fusion

Finally, given its critical role in leukemogenesis, the ultimate therapeutic target for infant leukemias may be the MLL fusion gene, transcript, or protein. There are preliminary in vitro data to suggest that targeting MLL-AF4 using RNA interference effectively induces apoptosis in treated cells.[195] The same approach may also be effective in targeting other regulators of MLL-induced leukemogenesis, such as *HOX* or other genes controlled by the MLL fusion protein. Small-molecule inhibitors that disrupt critical components of MLL fusion complexes are also promising. Given that wild-type MLL is a histone methyltransferase and at least some MLL fusions recruit other histone methyltransferases,[196] this class of enzymes may also represent interesting targets for future drug development.

The unique clinical and biologic characteristics of the infant leukemias continue to intrigue clinicians and scientists alike. Recent insights into the molecular mechanisms responsible for leukemias in infants provide hope that new, more effective and less toxic therapeutic approaches are on the horizon.

REFERENCES

1. Isaacs H Jr. Fetal and neonatal leukemia. J Pediatr Hematol Oncol. 2003;25:348-361.
2. Pui CH, Kane JR, Crist WM. Biology and treatment of infant leukemias. Leukemia. 1995;9:762-769.
3. Reaman G, Zeltzer P, Bleyer WA, et al. Acute lymphoblastic leukemia in infants less than one year of age: a cumulative experience of the Children's Cancer Study Group. J Clin Oncol. 1985;3:1513-1521.
4. Chen CS, Sorensen PH, Domer PH, et al. Molecular rearrangements on chromosome 11q23 predominate in infant acute lymphoblastic leukemia and are associated with specific biologic variables and poor outcome. Blood. 1993;81:2386-2393.
5. Cimino G, Lo Coco F, Biondi A, et al. ALL-1 gene at chromosome 11q23 is consistently altered in acute leukemia of early infancy. Blood. 1993;82:544-546.
6. Rubnitz JE, Link MP, Shuster JJ, et al. Frequency and prognostic significance of HRX rearrangements in infant acute lymphoblastic leukemia: a Pediatric Oncology Group study. Blood. 1994;84: 570-573.
7. Heerema NA, Arthur DC, Sather H, et al. Cytogenetic features of infants less than 12 months of age at diagnosis of acute lymphoblastic leukemia: impact of the 11q23 breakpoint on outcome: a report of the Childrens Cancer Group. Blood. 1994;83:2274-2284.
8. Ries LAG, Smith M, Gurney JG, et al (eds). Cancer Incidence and Survival Among Children and Adolescents: United States SEER Program 1975-1995 (NIH Publication No. 99-4649). Bethesda, Md, National Cancer Institute, SEER Program, 1999.
9. Biondi A, Cimino G, Pieters R, Pui CH. Biologic and therapeutic aspects of infant leukemia. Blood. 2000;96:24-33.
10. Chessells JM. Leukaemia in the young child. Br J Cancer Suppl. 1992;18:S54-S57.
11. Birch JM, Blair V. The epidemiology of infant cancers. Br J Cancer Suppl. 1992;18:S2-S4.
12. Ford AM, Ridge SA, Cabrera ME, et al. In utero rearrangements in the trithorax-related oncogene in infant leukaemias. Nature. 1993;363:358-360.
13. Bayar E, Kurczynski TW, Robinson MG, et al. Monozygotic twins with congenital acute lymphoblastic leukemia (ALL) and t(4;11)(q21;q23). Cancer Genet Cytogenet. 1996;89:177-180.
14. Greaves MF, Maia AT, Wiemels JL, Ford AM. Leukemia in twins: lessons in natural history. Blood. 2003;102:2321-2333.
15. Mahmoud HH, Ridge SA, Behm FG, et al. Intrauterine monoclonal origin of neonatal concordant acute lymphoblastic leukemia in monozygotic twins. Med Pediatr Oncol. 1995;24: 77-81.
16. Hunger SP, McGavran L, Meltesen L, et al. Oncogenesis in utero: fetal death due to acute myelogenous leukaemia with an MLL translocation. Br J Haematol. 1998;103:539-542.
17. Gale KB, Ford AM, Repp R, et al. Backtracking leukemia to birth: identification of clonotypic gene fusion sequences in neonatal blood spots. Proc Natl Acad Sci U S A. 1997;94:13950-13954.
18. Taub JW, Konrad MA, Ge Y, et al. High frequency of leukemic clones in newborn screening blood samples of children with B-precursor acute lymphoblastic leukemia. Blood. 2002;99:2992-2996.

19. Zerres K, Schwanitz G, Niesen M, et al. Prenatal diagnosis of acute non-lymphoblastic leukaemia in Down syndrome. Lancet. 1990;335:117.

20. Ahmed M, Sternberg A, Hall G, et al. Natural history of GATA1 mutations in Down syndrome. Blood. 2004;103:2480-2489.

21. Shu XO, Ross JA, Pendergrass TW, et al. Parental alcohol consumption, cigarette smoking, and risk of infant leukemia: a Children's Cancer Group study. J Natl Cancer Inst. 1996;88: 24-31.

22. Ross JA, Perentesis JP, Robison LL, Davies SM. Big babies and infant leukemia: a role for insulin-like growth factor-1? Cancer Causes Control. 1996;7:553-559.

23. Hjalgrim LL, Westergaard T, Rostgaard K, et al. Birth weight as a risk factor for childhood leukemia: a meta-analysis of 18 epidemiologic studies. Am J Epidemiol. 2003;158:724-735.

24. Spector LG, Davies SM, Robison LL, et al. Birth characteristics, maternal reproductive history, and the risk of infant leukemia: a report from the Children's Oncology Group. Cancer Epidemiol Biomarkers Prev. 2007;16:128-134.

25. Kaye SA, Robison LL, Smithson WA, et al. Maternal reproductive history and birth characteristics in childhood acute lymphoblastic leukemia. Cancer. 1991;68:1351-1355.

26. Buckley JD. The aetiology of cancer in the very young. Br J Cancer Suppl. 1992;18:S8-S12.

27. Yeazel MW, Buckley JD, Woods WG, et al. History of maternal fetal loss and increased risk of childhood acute leukemia at an early age. A report from the Children's Cancer Group. Cancer. 1995;75:1718-1727.

28. Ross JA, Potter JD, Shu XO, et al. Evaluating the relationships among maternal reproductive history, birth characteristics, and infant leukemia: a report from the Children's Cancer Group. Ann Epidemiol. 1997;7:172-179.

29. Moysich KB, Menezes RJ, Michalek AM. Chernobyl-related ionising radiation exposure and cancer risk: an epidemiologic review. Lancet Oncol. 2002;3:269-279.

30. Felix CA, Hosler MR, Winick NJ, et al. ALL-1 gene rearrangements in DNA topoisomerase II inhibitor-related leukemia in children. Blood. 1995;85:3250-3256.

31. Cimino G, Rapanotti MC, Biondi A, et al. Infant acute leukemias show the same biased distribution of ALL1 gene breaks as topoisomerase II related secondary acute leukemias. Cancer Res. 1997;57:2879-2883.

32. Pui CH, Relling MV, Rivera GK, et al. Epipodophyllotoxin-related acute myeloid leukemia: a study of 35 cases. Leukemia. 1995;9:1990-1996.

33. Ross JA, Potter JD, Robison LL. Infant leukemia, topoisomerase II inhibitors, and the MLL gene. J Natl Cancer Inst. 1994;86: 1678-1680.

34. Strick R, Strissel PL, Borgers S, et al. Dietary bioflavonoids induce cleavage in the MLL gene and may contribute to infant leukemia. Proc Natl Acad Sci U S A. 2000;97:4790-4795.

35. Ross JA, Potter JD, Reaman GH, et al. Maternal exposure to potential inhibitors of DNA topoisomerase II and infant leukemia (United States): a report from the Children's Cancer Group. Cancer Causes Control. 1996;7:581-590.

36. Spector LG, Xie Y, Robison LL, et al. Maternal diet and infant leukemia: the DNA topoisomerase II inhibitor hypothesis: a report from the children's oncology group. Cancer Epidemiol Biomarkers Prev. 2005;14:651-655.

37. Wiemels JL, Pagnamenta A, Taylor GM, et al. A lack of a functional NAD(P)H:quinone oxidoreductase allele is selectively associated with pediatric leukemias that have MLL fusions. United Kingdom Childhood Cancer Study Investigators. Cancer Res. 1999;59:4095-4099.

38. Lanciotti M, Dufour C, Corral L, et al. Genetic polymorphism of NAD(P)H:quinone oxidoreductase is associated with an increased risk of infant acute lymphoblastic leukemia without MLL gene rearrangements. Leukemia. 2005;19:214-216.

39. Ayton PM, Cleary ML. Molecular mechanisms of leukemogenesis mediated by MLL fusion proteins. Oncogene. 2001;20: 5695-5707.

40. Domer PH, Fakharzadeh SS, Chen CS, et al. Acute mixed-lineage leukemia t(4;11)(q21;q23) generates an MLL-AF4 fusion product. Proc Natl Acad Sci U S A. 1993;90:7884-7888.

41. Gu Y, Nakamura T, Alder H, et al. The t(4;11) chromosome translocation of human acute leukemias fuses the ALL-1 gene, related to Drosophila trithorax, to the AF-4 gene. Cell. 1992;71: 701-708.

42. Tkachuk DC, Kohler S, Cleary ML. Involvement of a homolog of Drosophila trithorax by 11q23 chromosomal translocations in acute leukemias. Cell. 1992;71:691-700.

43. Ziemin-van der Poel S, McCabe NR, Gill HJ, et al. Identification of a gene, MLL, that spans the breakpoint in 11q23 translocations associated with human leukemias. Proc Natl Acad Sci U S A. 1991;88:10735-10739.

44. Milne TA, Briggs SD, Brock HW, et al. MLL targets SET domain methyltransferase activity to Hox gene promoters. Mol Cell. 2002;10:1107-1117.

45. Nakamura T, Mori T, Tada S, et al. ALL-1 is a histone methyltransferase that assembles a supercomplex of proteins involved in transcriptional regulation. Mol Cell. 2002;10:1119-1128.

46. Hughes CM, Rozenblatt-Rosen O, Milne TA, et al. Menin associates with a trithorax family histone methyltransferase complex and with the hoxc8 locus. Mol Cell. 2004;13:587-597.

47. Milne TA, Hughes CM, Lloyd R, et al. Menin and MLL cooperatively regulate expression of cyclin-dependent kinase inhibitors. Proc Natl Acad Sci U S A. 2005;102:749-754.

48. Krivtsov AV, Armstrong SA. MLL translocations, histone modifications and leukaemia stem-cell development. Nat Rev Cancer. 2007;7:823-833.

49. Hess JL, Yu BD, Li B, et al. Defects in yolk sac hematopoiesis in Mll-null embryos. Blood. 1997;90:1799-1806.

50. Yu BD, Hess JL, Horning SE, et al. Altered Hox expression and segmental identity in Mll-mutant mice. Nature. 1995;378: 505-508.

51. Ernst P, Fisher JK, Avery W, et al. Definitive hematopoiesis requires the mixed-lineage leukemia gene. Dev Cell. 2004;6: 437-443.

52. Ernst P, Mabon M, Davidson AJ, et al. An Mll-dependent Hox program drives hematopoietic progenitor expansion. Curr Biol. 2004;14:2063-2069.

53. Owens BM, Hawley RG. HOX and non-HOX homeobox genes in leukemic hematopoiesis. Stem Cells. 2002;20:364-379.

54. Borrow J, Shearman AM, Stanton VP Jr, et al. The t(7;11)(p15;p15) translocation in acute myeloid leukaemia fuses the genes for nucleoporin NUP98 and class I homeoprotein HOXA9. Nat Genet. 1996;12:159-167.

55. Nakamura T, Largaespada DA, Lee MP, et al. Fusion of the nucleoporin gene NUP98 to HOXA9 by the chromosome translocation t(7;11)(p15;p15) in human myeloid leukaemia. Nat Genet. 1996;12:154-158.

56. Armstrong SA, Staunton JE, Silverman LB, et al. MLL translocations specify a distinct gene expression profile that distinguishes a unique leukemia. Nat Genet. 2002;30:41-47.

57. Ferrando AA, Armstrong SA, Neuberg DS, et al. Gene expression signatures in MLL-rearranged T-lineage and B-precursor acute leukemias: dominance of HOX dysregulation. Blood. 2003;102:262-268.

58. Yeoh E, Ross M, Shurtleff S, et al. Classification, subtype discovery, and prediction of outcome in pediatric acute lymphoblastic leukemia by gene expression profiling. Cancer Cell. 2002;1:133-143.

59. Ross ME, Mahfouz R, Onciu M, et al. Gene expression profiling of pediatric acute myelogenous leukemia. Blood. 2004;104:3679-3687.

60. McCulloch EA, Smith LJ, Alder S. Cellular lineages in normal and leukemic hemopoiesis. Prog Clin Biol Res. 1983;134:229-244.

61. Greaves MF, Chan LC, Furley AJ, et al. Lineage promiscuity in hemopoietic differentiation and leukemia. Blood. 1986;67:1-11.

62. Cozzio A, Passegue E, Ayton PM, et al. Similar MLL-associated leukemias arising from self-renewing stem cells and short-lived myeloid progenitors. Genes Dev. 2003;17:3029-3035.

63. So CW, Karsunky H, Passegue E, et al. MLL-GAS7 transforms multipotent hematopoietic progenitors and induces mixed lineage leukemias in mice. Cancer Cell. 2003;3:161-171.

64. Cano F, Drynan LF, Pannell R, Rabbitts TH. Leukaemia lineage specification caused by cell-specific Mll-Enl translocations. Oncogene. 2008;27:1945-1950.

65. Ross M, Zhou X, Song G, et al. Classification of pediatric acute lymphoblastic leukemia by gene expression profiling. Blood. 2003;102:2951-2959.

66. Bonnet D, Dick JE. Human acute myeloid leukemia is organized as a hierarchy that originates from a primitive hematopoietic cell. Nat Med. 1997;3:730-737.

67. Huntly BJ, Shigematsu H, Deguchi K, et al. MOZ-TIF2, but not BCR-ABL, confers properties of leukemic stem cells to committed murine hematopoietic progenitors. Cancer Cell. 2004;6:587-596.

68. Corral J, Lavenir I, Impey H, et al. An Mll-AF9 fusion gene made by homologous recombination causes acute leukemia in chimeric mice: a method to create fusion oncogenes. Cell. 1996;85:853-861.

69. Higuchi M, O'Brien D, Kumaravelu P, et al. Expression of a conditional AML1-ETO oncogene bypasses embryonic lethality and establishes a murine model of human t(8;21) acute myeloid leukemia. Cancer Cell. 2002;1:63-74.

70. Wang J, Iwasaki H, Krivtsov A, et al. Conditional MLL-CBP targets GMP and models therapy-related myeloproliferative disease. EMBO J. 2005;24:368-381.

71. Wiemels JL, Cazzaniga G, Daniotti M, et al. Prenatal origin of acute lymphoblastic leukaemia in children. Lancet. 1999;354:1499-1503.

72. Scheijen B, Griffin JD. Tyrosine kinase oncogenes in normal hematopoiesis and hematological disease. Oncogene. 2002;21:3314-3333.

73. Sawyers CL. Rational therapeutic intervention in cancer: kinases as drug targets. Curr Opin Genet Dev. 2002;12:111-115.

74. Druker BJ, Talpaz M, Resta DJ, et al. Efficacy and safety of a specific inhibitor of the BCR-ABL tyrosine kinase in chronic myeloid leukemia. N Engl J Med. 2001;344:1031-1037.

75. Kelly LM, Gilliland DG. Genetics of myeloid leukemias. Annu Rev Genomics Hum Genet. 2002;3:179-198.

76. Armstrong SA, Kung AL, Mabon ME, et al. Inhibition of FLT3 in MLL. Validation of a therapeutic target identified by gene expression based classification. Cancer Cell. 2003;3:173-183.

77. Taketani T, Taki T, Sugita K, et al. FLT3 mutations in the activation loop of tyrosine kinase domain are frequently found in infant ALL with MLL rearrangements and pediatric ALL with hyperdiploidy. Blood. 2004;103:1085-1088.

78. Brown P, Levis M, McIntyre E, et al. Combinations of the FLT3 inhibitor CEP-701 and chemotherapy synergistically kill infant and childhood MLL-rearranged ALL cells in a sequence-dependent manner. Leukemia. 2006;20:1368-1376.

79. Brown P, Levis M, Shurtleff S, et al. FLT3 inhibition selectively kills childhood acute lymphoblastic leukemia cells with high levels of FLT3 expression. Blood. 2005;105:812-820.

80. Chessells JM, Eden OB, Bailey CC, et al. Acute lymphoblastic leukaemia in infancy: experience in MRC UKALL trials. Report from the Medical Research Council Working Party on Childhood Leukaemia. Leukemia. 1994;8:1275-1279.

81. Moricke A, Zimmermann M, Reiter A, et al. Prognostic impact of age in children and adolescents with acute lymphoblastic leukemia: data from the trials ALL-BFM 86, 90, and 95. Klin Padiatr. 2005;217:310-320.

82. Isoyama K, Eguchi M, Hibi S, et al. Risk-directed treatment of infant acute lymphoblastic leukaemia based on early assessment of MLL gene status: results of the Japan Infant Leukaemia Study (MLL96). Br J Haematol. 2002;118:999-1010.

83. Harrison CJ, Moorman AV, Barber KE, et al. Interphase molecular cytogenetic screening for chromosomal abnormalities of prognostic significance in childhood acute lymphoblastic leukaemia: a UK Cancer Cytogenetics Group Study. Br J Haematol. 2005;129:520-530.

84. Hilden JM, Dinndorf PA, Meerbaum SO, et al. Analysis of prognostic factors of acute lymphoblastic leukemia in infants: report on CCG 1953 from the Children's Oncology Group. Blood. 2006;108:441-451.

84a. Reiter A, Schrappe M, Ludwig WD, et al. Chemotherapy in 998 unselected childhood acute lymphoblastic leukemia patients. Results and conclusions of the multicenter trial ALL-BFM 86. Blood. 1994;84:3122-3133.

85. Pui CH, Behm FG, Downing JR, et al. 11q23/MLL rearrangement confers a poor prognosis in infants with acute lymphoblastic leukemia. J Clin Oncol. 1994;12:909-915.

86. Pieters R, Schrappe M, De Lorenzo P, et al. A treatment protocol for infants younger than 1 year with acute lymphoblastic leukaemia (Interfant-99): an observational study and a multicentre randomised trial. Lancet. 2007;370:240-250.

87. Pui CH, Gaynon PS, Boyett JM, et al. Outcome of treatment in childhood acute lymphoblastic leukaemia with rearrangements of the 11q23 chromosomal region. Lancet. 2002;359:1909-1915.

88. Ferster A, Bertrand Y, Benoit Y, et al. Improved survival for acute lymphoblastic leukaemia in infancy: the experience of EORTC-Childhood Leukaemia Cooperative Group. Br J Haematol. 1994;86:284-290.

89. Silverman LB, McLean TW, Gelber RD, et al. Intensified therapy for infants with acute lymphoblastic leukemia: results from the Dana-Farber Cancer Institute Consortium. Cancer. 1997;80:2285-2295.

90. Frankel LS, Ochs J, Shuster JJ, et al. Therapeutic trial for infant acute lymphoblastic leukemia: the Pediatric Oncology Group experience (POG 8493). J Pediatr Hematol Oncol. 1997;19:35-42.

91. Lauer SJ, Camitta BM, Leventhal BG, et al. Intensive alternating drug pairs after remission induction for treatment of infants with acute lymphoblastic leukemia: a Pediatric Oncology Group pilot study. J Pediatr Hematol Oncol. 1998;20:229-233.

92. Dordelmann M, Reiter A, Borkhardt A, et al. Prednisone response is the strongest predictor of treatment outcome in infant acute lymphoblastic leukemia. Blood. 1999;94:1209-1217.

93. Reaman GH, Sposto R, Sensel MG, et al. Treatment outcome and prognostic factors for infants with acute lymphoblastic leukemia treated on two consecutive trials of the Children's Cancer Group. J Clin Oncol. 1999;17:445-455.

94. Chessells JM, Harrison CJ, Watson SL, et al. Treatment of infants with lymphoblastic leukaemia: results of the UK Infant Protocols 1987-1999. Br J Haematol. 2002;117:306-314.

95. Biondi A, Rizzari C, Valsecchi MG, et al. Role of treatment intensification in infants with acute lymphoblastic leukemia: results of two consecutive AIEOP studies. Haematologica. 2006;91:534-537.

96. Moghrabi A, Levy DE, Asselin B, et al. Results of the Dana-Farber Cancer Institute ALL Consortium Protocol 95-01 for children with acute lymphoblastic leukemia. Blood. 2007;109:896-904.

97. Schrappe M, Camitta B, Pui CH, et al. Long-term results of large prospective trials in childhood acute lymphoblastic leukemia. Leukemia. 2000;14:2193-2194.

98. Pui CH, Sandlund JT, Pei D, et al. Improved outcome for children with acute lymphoblastic leukemia: results of Total Therapy

Study XIIIB at St Jude Children's Research Hospital. Blood. 2004;104:2690-2696.

99. Silverman LB, Gelber RD, Dalton VK, et al. Improved outcome for children with acute lymphoblastic leukemia: results of Dana-Farber Consortium Protocol 91-01. Blood. 2001;97:1211-1218.

100. Pui CH, Ribeiro RC, Campana D, et al. Prognostic factors in the acute lymphoid and myeloid leukemias of infants. Leukemia. 1996;10:952-956.

101. Heerema NA, Sather HN, Ge J, et al. Cytogenetic studies of infant acute lymphoblastic leukemia: poor prognosis of infants with t(4;11)—a report of the Children's Cancer Group. Leukemia. 1999;13:679-686.

102. Nagayama J, Tomizawa D, Koh K, et al. Infants with acute lymphoblastic leukemia and a germline MLL gene are highly curable with use of chemotherapy alone: results from the Japan Infant Leukemia Study Group. Blood. 2006;107:4663-4665.

103. Pieters R, den Boer ML, Durian M, et al. Relation between age, immunophenotype and in vitro drug resistance in 395 children with acute lymphoblastic leukemia—implications for treatment of infants. Leukemia. 1998;12:1344-1348.

104. Ramakers-van Woerden NL, Beverloo HB, Veerman AJ, et al. In vitro drug-resistance profile in infant acute lymphoblastic leukemia in relation to age, MLL rearrangements and immunophenotype. Leukemia. 2004;18:521-529.

105. Riehm H, Reiter A, Schrappe M, et al. [Corticosteroid-dependent reduction of leukocyte count in blood as a prognostic factor in acute lymphoblastic leukemia in childhood (therapy study ALL-BFM 83)]. Klin Padiatr. 1987;199:151-160.

106. Stam RW, den Boer ML, Meijerink JP, et al. Differential mRNA expression of Ara-C-metabolizing enzymes explains Ara-C sensitivity in MLL gene-rearranged infant acute lymphoblastic leukemia. Blood. 2003;101:1270-1276.

107. Gati WP, Paterson AR, Larratt LM, et al. Sensitivity of acute leukemia cells to cytarabine is a correlate of cellular es nucleoside transporter site content measured by flow cytometry with SAENTA-fluorescein. Blood. 1997;90:346-353.

108. Wiley JS, Jones SP, Sawyer WH, Paterson AR. Cytosine arabinoside influx and nucleoside transport sites in acute leukemia. J Clin Invest. 1982;69:479-489.

109. White JC, Rathmell JP, Capizzi RL. Membrane transport influences the rate of accumulation of cytosine arabinoside in human leukemia cells. J Clin Invest. 1987;79:380-387.

110. Silverman LB. Acute lymphoblastic leukemia in infancy. Pediatr Blood Cancer. 2007;49:1070-1073.

111. Kosaka Y, Koh K, Kinukawa N, et al. Infant acute lymphoblastic leukemia with MLL gene rearrangements: outcome following intensive chemotherapy and hematopoietic stem cell transplantation. Blood. 2004;104:3527-3534.

112. Marco F, Bureo E, Ortega JJ, et al. High survival rate in infant acute leukemia treated with early high-dose chemotherapy and stem-cell support. Groupo Espanol de Trasplante de Medula Osea en Ninos. J Clin Oncol. 2000;18:3256-3261.

113. Sanders JE, Im HJ, Hoffmeister PA, et al. Allogeneic hematopoietic cell transplantation for infants with acute lymphoblastic leukemia. Blood. 2005;105:3749-3756.

114. Cimino G, Rapanotti MC, Elia L, et al. ALL-1 gene rearrangements in acute myeloid leukemia: association with M4-M5 French-American-British classification subtypes and young age. Cancer Res. 1995;55:1625-1628.

115. Sorensen PH, Chen CS, Smith FO, et al. Molecular rearrangements of the MLL gene are present in most cases of infant acute myeloid leukemia and are strongly correlated with monocytic or myelomonocytic phenotypes. J Clin Invest. 1994;93:429-437.

116. Pui CH, Raimondi SC, Murphy SB, et al. An analysis of leukemic cell chromosomal features in infants. Blood. 1987;69:1289-1293.

117. Grier HE, Gelber RD, Camitta BM, et al. Prognostic factors in childhood acute myelogenous leukemia. J Clin Oncol. 1987;5:1026-1032.

118. Woods WG, Kobrinsky N, Buckley JD, et al. Timed-sequential induction therapy improves postremission outcome in acute myeloid leukemia: a report from the Children's Cancer Group. Blood. 1996;87:4979-4989.

119. Lie SO, Jonmundsson G, Mellander L, et al. A population-based study of 272 children with acute myeloid leukaemia treated on two consecutive protocols with different intensity: best outcome in girls, infants, and children with Down's syndrome. Nordic Society of Paediatric Haematology and Oncology (NOPHO). Br J Haematol. 1996;94:82-88.

120. Stevens RF, Hann IM, Wheatley K, Gray RG. Marked improvements in outcome with chemotherapy alone in paediatric acute myeloid leukaemia: results of the United Kingdom Medical Research Council's 10th AML trial. MRC Childhood Leukaemia Working Party. Br J Haematol. 1998;101:130-140.

121. Creutzig U, Zimmermann M, Ritter J, et al. Definition of a standard-risk group in children with AML. Br J Haematol. 1999;104:630-639.

122. Pui CH, Raimondi SC, Srivastava DK, et al. Prognostic factors in infants with acute myeloid leukemia. Leukemia. 2000;14:684-687.

123. Hilden JM, Smith FO, Frestedt JL, et al. MLL gene rearrangement, cytogenetic 11q23 abnormalities, and expression of the NG2 molecule in infant acute myeloid leukemia. Blood. 1997;89:3801-3805.

124. Satake N, Maseki N, Nishiyama M, et al. Chromosome abnormalities and MLL rearrangements in acute myeloid leukemia of infants. Leukemia. 1999;13:1013-1017.

125. Grimwade D, Walker H, Oliver F, et al. The importance of diagnostic cytogenetics on outcome in AML: analysis of 1,612 patients entered into the MRC AML 10 trial. The Medical Research Council Adult and Children's Leukaemia Working Parties. Blood. 1998;92:2322-2333.

126. Raimondi SC, Chang MN, Ravindranath Y, et al. Chromosomal abnormalities in 478 children with acute myeloid leukemia: clinical characteristics and treatment outcome in a cooperative pediatric oncology group study-POG 8821. Blood. 1999;94:3707-3716.

127. Creutzig U, Ritter J, Schellong G. Identification of two risk groups in childhood acute myelogenous leukemia after therapy intensification in study AML-BFM-83 as compared with study AML-BFM-78. AML-BFM Study Group. Blood. 1990;75:1932-1940.

128. Rubnitz JE, Raimondi SC, Tong X, et al. Favorable impact of the t(9;11) in childhood acute myeloid leukemia. J Clin Oncol. 2002;20:2302-2309.

129. Martinez-Climent JA, Lane NJ, Rubin CM, et al. Clinical and prognostic significance of chromosomal abnormalities in childhood acute myeloid leukemia de novo. Leukemia. 1995;9:95-101.

130. Mrozek K, Heinonen K, Lawrence D, et al. Adult patients with de novo acute myeloid leukemia and t(9; 11)(p22; q23) have a superior outcome to patients with other translocations involving band 11q23: a cancer and leukemia group B study. Blood. 1997;90:4532-4538.

131. Creutzig U, Zimmermann M, Ritter J, et al. Treatment strategies and long-term results in paediatric patients treated in four consecutive AML-BFM trials. Leukemia. 2005;19:2030-2042.

132. Gibson BE, Wheatley K, Hann IM, et al. Treatment strategy and long-term results in paediatric patients treated in consecutive UK AML trials. Leukemia. 2005;19:2130-2138.

133. Ravindranath Y, Chang M, Steuber CP, et al. Pediatric Oncology Group (POG) studies of acute myeloid leukemia (AML): a review of four consecutive childhood AML trials conducted between 1981 and 2000. Leukemia. 2005;19:2101-2116.

134. Lie SO, Abrahamsson J, Clausen N, et al. Long-term results in children with AML: NOPHO-AML Study Group—report of three consecutive trials. Leukemia. 2005;19:2090-2100.

135. Woods WG, Neudorf S, Gold S, et al. A comparison of allogeneic bone marrow transplantation, autologous bone marrow transplantation, and aggressive chemotherapy in children with acute myeloid leukemia in remission. Blood. 2001;97:56-62.

136. Kawasaki H, Isoyama K, Eguchi M, et al. Superior outcome of infant acute myeloid leukemia with intensive chemotherapy: results of the Japan Infant Leukemia Study Group. Blood. 2001;98:3589-3594.

137. Perel Y, Auvrignon A, Leblanc T, et al. Treatment of childhood acute myeloblastic leukemia: dose intensification improves outcome and maintenance therapy is of no benefit—multicenter studies of the French LAME (Leucemie Aigue Myeloblastique Enfant) Cooperative Group. Leukemia. 2005;19:2082-2089.

138. Woolfrey AE, Gooley TA, Sievers EL, et al. Bone marrow transplantation for children less than 2 years of age with acute myelogenous leukemia or myelodysplastic syndrome. Blood. 1998;92:3546-3556.

139. Odom LF, Gordon EM. Acute monoblastic leukemia in infancy and early childhood: successful treatment with an epipodophyllotoxin. Blood. 1984;64:875-882.

140. Wells RJ, Woods WG, Buckley JD, et al. Treatment of newly diagnosed children and adolescents with acute myeloid leukemia: a Children's Cancer Group study. J Clin Oncol. 1994;12:2367-2377.

141. Carroll A, Civin C, Schneider N, et al. The t(1;22) (p13;q13) is nonrandom and restricted to infants with acute megakaryoblastic leukemia: a Pediatric Oncology Group Study. Blood. 1991;78:748-752.

142. Lion T, Haas OA, Harbott J, et al. The translocation t(1;22)(p13;q13) is a nonrandom marker specifically associated with acute megakaryocytic leukemia in young children. Blood. 1992;79:3325-3330.

143. Zipursky A, Peeters M, Poon A. Megakaryoblastic leukemia and Down's syndrome—a review. Prog Clin Biol Res. 1987;246:33-56.

144. Zipursky A, Thorner P, De Harven E, et al. Myelodysplasia and acute megakaryoblastic leukemia in Down's syndrome. Leuk Res. 1994;18:163-171.

145. Smrcek JM, Baschat AA, Germer U, et al. Fetal hydrops and hepatosplenomegaly in the second half of pregnancy: a sign of myeloproliferative disorder in fetuses with trisomy 21. Ultrasound Obstet Gynecol. 2001;17:403-409.

146. Zipursky A, Rose T, Skidmore M, et al. Hydrops fetalis and neonatal leukemia in Down syndrome. Pediatr Hematol Oncol. 1996;13:81-87.

147. Zipursky A. Transient leukaemia—a benign form of leukaemia in newborn infants with trisomy 21. Br J Haematol. 2003;120:930-938.

148. Homans AC, Verissimo AM, Vlacha V. Transient abnormal myelopoiesis of infancy associated with trisomy 21. Am J Pediatr Hematol Oncol. 1993;15:392-399.

149. Al-Kasim F, Doyle JJ, Massey GV, et al. Incidence and treatment of potentially lethal diseases in transient leukemia of Down syndrome: Pediatric Oncology Group Study. J Pediatr Hematol Oncol. 2002;24:9-13.

150. Massey GV, Zipursky A, Chang MN, et al. A prospective study of the natural history of transient leukemia (TL) in neonates with Down syndrome (DS): Children's Oncology Group (COG) study POG-9481. Blood. 2006;107:4606-4613.

151. Zipursky A, Christensen H, De Harven E. Ultrastructural studies of the megakaryoblastic leukemias of Down syndrome. Leuk Lymphoma. 1995;18:341-347.

152. Karandikar NJ, Aquino DB, McKenna RW, Kroft SH. Transient myeloproliferative disorder and acute myeloid leukemia in Down

153. syndrome. An immunophenotypic analysis. Am J Clin Pathol. 2001;116:204-210.

153. Yumura-Yagi K, Hara J, Kurahashi H, et al. Mixed phenotype of blasts in acute megakaryocytic leukaemia and transient abnormal myelopoiesis in Down's syndrome. Br J Haematol. 1992;81:520-525.

154. Athale UH, Razzouk BI, Raimondi SC, et al. Biology and outcome of childhood acute megakaryoblastic leukemia: a single institution's experience. Blood. 2001;97:3727-3732.

155. Wechsler J, Greene M, McDevitt MA, et al. Acquired mutations in GATA1 in the megakaryoblastic leukemia of Down syndrome. Nat Genet. 2002;32:148-152.

156. Xu G, Nagano M, Kanezaki R, et al. Frequent mutations in the GATA-1 gene in the transient myeloproliferative disorder of Down syndrome. Blood. 2003;102:2960-2968.

157. Mundschau G, Gurbuxani S, Gamis AS, et al. Mutagenesis of GATA1 is an initiating event in Down syndrome leukemogenesis. Blood. 2003;101:4298-4300.

158. Hitzler JK, Cheung J, Li Y, et al. GATA1 mutations in transient leukemia and acute megakaryoblastic leukemia of Down syndrome. Blood. 2003;101:4301-4304.

159. Cantor AB, Katz SG, Orkin SH. Distinct domains of the GATA-1 cofactor FOG-1 differentially influence erythroid versus megakaryocytic maturation. Mol Cell Biol. 2002;22:4268-4279.

160. Shivdasani RA. Molecular and transcriptional regulation of megakaryocyte differentiation. Stem Cells. 2001;19:397-407.

161. Li Z, Godinho FJ, Klusmann JH, et al. Developmental stage-selective effect of somatically mutated leukemogenic transcription factor GATA1. Nat Genet. 2005;37:613-619.

162. Kojima S, Kato K, Matsuyama T, et al. Favorable treatment outcome in children with acute myeloid leukemia and Down syndrome. Blood. 1993;81:3164.

163. Lange BJ, Kobrinsky N, Barnard DR, et al. Distinctive demography, biology, and outcome of acute myeloid leukemia and myelodysplastic syndrome in children with Down syndrome: Children's Cancer Group Studies 2861 and 2891. Blood. 1998;91:608-615.

164. Lange B. The management of neoplastic disorders of haematopoiesis in children with Down's syndrome. Br J Haematol. 2000;110:512-524.

165. Ravindranath Y, Abella E, Krischer JP, et al. Acute myeloid leukemia (AML) in Down's syndrome is highly responsive to chemotherapy: experience on Pediatric Oncology Group AML Study 8498. Blood. 1992;80:2210-2214.

166. Ravindranath Y, Yeager AM, Chang MN, et al. Autologous bone marrow transplantation versus intensive consolidation chemotherapy for acute myeloid leukemia in childhood. Pediatric Oncology Group. N Engl J Med. 1996;334:1428-1434.

167. Creutzig U, Reinhardt D, Diekamp S, et al. AML patients with Down syndrome have a high cure rate with AML-BFM therapy with reduced dose intensity. Leukemia. 2005;19:1355-1360.

168. Zeller B, Gustafsson G, Forestier E, et al. Acute leukaemia in children with Down syndrome: a population-based Nordic study. Br J Haematol. 2005;128:797-804.

169. Bernstein J, Dastugue N, Haas OA, et al. Nineteen cases of the t(1;22)(p13;q13) acute megakaryblastic leukaemia of infants/children and a review of 39 cases: report from a t(1;22) study group. Leukemia. 2000;14:216-218.

170. Ma Z, Morris SW, Valentine V, et al. Fusion of two novel genes, RBM15 and MKL1, in the t(1;22)(p13;q13) of acute megakaryoblastic leukemia. Nat Genet. 2001;28:220-221.

171. Stam RW, den Boer ML, Pieters R. Towards targeted therapy for infant acute lymphoblastic leukaemia. Br J Haematol. 2006;132:539-551.

172. Kaspers GJ, Pieters R, Van Zantwijk CH, et al. Prednisolone resistance in childhood acute lymphoblastic leukemia: vitro-vivo

correlations and cross-resistance to other drugs. Blood. 1998;92:259-266.

173. Den Boer ML, Harms DO, Pieters R, et al. Patient stratification based on prednisolone-vincristine-asparaginase resistance profiles in children with acute lymphoblastic leukemia. J Clin Oncol. 2003;21:3262-3268.

174. Wei G, Twomey D, Lamb J, et al. Gene expression-based chemical genomics identifies rapamycin as a modulator of MCL1 and glucocorticoid resistance. Cancer Cell. 2006;10:331-342.

175. Holleman A, Cheok MH, den Boer ML, et al. Gene-expression patterns in drug-resistant acute lymphoblastic leukemia cells and response to treatment. N Engl J Med. 2004;351:533-542.

176. Battle TE, Arbiser J, Frank DA. The natural product honokiol induces caspase-dependent apoptosis in B-cell chronic lymphocytic leukemia (B-CLL) cells. Blood. 2005;106:690-697.

177. Raje N, Kumar S, Hideshima T, et al. Seliciclib (CYC202 or R-roscovitine), a small-molecule cyclin-dependent kinase inhibitor, mediates activity via down-regulation of Mcl-1 in multiple myeloma. Blood. 2005;106:1042-1047.

178. Yasui H, Hideshima T, Hamasaki M, et al. SDX-101, the R-enantiomer of etodolac, induces cytotoxicity, overcomes drug resistance, and enhances the activity of dexamethasone in multiple myeloma. Blood. 2005;106:706-712.

179. Neri P, Yasui H, Hideshima T, et al. In vivo and in vitro cytotoxicity of R-etodolac with dexamethasone in glucocorticoid-resistant multiple myeloma cells. Br J Haematol. 2006;134:37-44.

180. Robinson BW, Behling KC, Gupta M, et al. Abundant anti-apoptotic BCL-2 is a molecular target in leukaemias with t(4;11) translocation. Br J Haematol. 2008;141:827-839.

181. Kristensen J, Nygren P, Liliemark J, et al. Interactions between cladribine (2-chlorodeoxyadenosine) and standard antileukemic drugs in primary cultures of human tumor cells from patients with acute myelocytic leukemia. Leukemia. 1994;8:1712-1717.

182. Chow KU, Boehrer S, Napieralski S, et al. In AML cell lines Ara-C combined with purine analogues is able to exert synergistic as well as antagonistic effects on proliferation, apoptosis and disruption of mitochondrial membrane potential. Leuk Lymphoma. 2003;44:165-173.

183. Holowiecki J, Grosicki S, Robak T, et al. Addition of cladribine to daunorubicin and cytarabine increases complete remission rate after a single course of induction treatment in acute myeloid leukemia. Multicenter, phase III study. Leukemia. 2004;18:989-997.

184. Jeha S, Gandhi V, Chan KW, et al. Clofarabine, a novel nucleoside analog, is active in pediatric patients with advanced leukemia. Blood. 2004;103:784-789.

185. Faderl S, Gandhi V, O'Brien S, et al. Results of a phase 1-2 study of clofarabine in combination with cytarabine (ara-C) in relapsed and refractory acute leukemias. Blood. 2005;105:940-947.

186. Bouffard DY, Jolivet J, Leblond L, et al. Complementary anti-neoplastic activity of the cytosine nucleoside analogues troxacitabine (Troxatyl) and cytarabine in human leukemia cells. Cancer Chemother Pharmacol. 2003;52:497-506.

187. Giles FJ, Garcia-Manero G, Cortes JE, et al. Phase II study of troxacitabine, a novel dioxolane nucleoside analog, in patients with refractory leukemia. J Clin Oncol. 2002;20:656-664.

188. Hanaoka K, Suzuki M, Kobayashi T, et al. Antitumor activity and novel DNA-self-strand-breaking mechanism of CNDAC (1-(2-C-cyano-2-deoxy-beta-D-arabino-pentofuranosyl) cytosine) and its N4-palmitoyl derivative (CS-682). Int J Cancer. 1999;82:226-236.

189. Serova M, Galmarini CM, Ghoul A, et al. Antiproliferative effects of sapacitabine (CYC682), a novel 2'-deoxycytidine-derivative, in human cancer cells. Br J Cancer. 2007;97:628-636.

190. Levis M, Allebach J, Tse KF, et al. A FLT3-targeted tyrosine kinase inhibitor is cytotoxic to leukemia cells in vitro and in vivo. Blood. 2002;99:3885-3891.

191. Weisberg E, Boulton C, Kelly LM, et al. Inhibition of mutant FLT3 receptors in leukemia cells by the small molecule tyrosine kinase inhibitor PKC412. Cancer Cell. 2002;1:433-443.

192. Yee KW, O'Farrell AM, Smolich BD, et al. SU5416 and SU5614 inhibit kinase activity of wild-type and mutant FLT3 receptor tyrosine kinase. Blood. 2002;100:2941-2949.

193. Stam RW, den Boer ML, Schneider P, et al. Targeting FLT3 in primary MLL-gene-rearranged infant acute lymphoblastic leukemia. Blood. 2005;106:2484-2490.

194. Levis M, Pham R, Smith BD, Small D. In vitro studies of a FLT3 inhibitor combined with chemotherapy: sequence of administration is important to achieve synergistic cytotoxic effects. Blood. 2004;104:1145-1150.

195. Thomas M, Gessner A, Vornlocher HP, et al. Targeting MLL-AF4 with short interfering RNAs inhibits clonogenicity and engraftment of t(4;11)-positive human leukemic cells. Blood. 2005;106:3559-3566.

196. Okada Y, Feng Q, Lin Y, et al. hDOT1L links histone methylation to leukemogenesis. Cell. 2005;121:167-178.

13 Malignant Lymphomas and Lymphadenopathies

Alfred Reiter and Adolfo A. Ferrando

The malignant lymphomas (Hodgkin's and non-Hodgkin's lymphoma) constitute the third most commonly diagnosed group of malignancies in children after leukemia and brain tumors. They account for approximately 10% to 12% of all cancers diagnosed in children younger than 15 years and 15% of all malignancies in children and adolescents younger than 20 years.[1] The lymphomas are a diverse collection of malignant diseases affecting the cells and organs of the immune system. Lymphoid cells usually traffic among several major lymphoid organs as well as the lymph nodes, bone marrow, blood, and sites of lymphoid tissue aggregates in the gut, liver, and elsewhere. The constituent cells of the immune system are themselves diverse, deriving from different cell lineages and serving different functions. Understanding the anatomy of the normal immune system and normal lymphocyte maturation is essential for an accurate appreciation of the malignant lymphomas. Conversely, the study of malignant cells has contributed immensely to our understanding of normal lymphocyte differentiation.

The normal lymphoid system is divided among functionally distinct compartments.[2] The marrow stem cells and lymphoid progenitors give rise to precursors for all classes of lymphocytes. The central lymphoid organs are responsible for the development of immature lymphocytes into functional, immunocompetent T or B cells capable of participating in an immune response. Cells committed to lymphoid differentiation arise in the bone marrow from multipotential stem cells. T cells undergo further differentiation in the thymus. The central lymphoid organ associated with B-cell maturation in humans is probably the marrow itself, which in this respect is equivalent to the bursa of Fabricius in birds. The recombination mechanisms used by the immunoglobulin and T-cell receptor genes are the basic biologic processes in precursor B- and T-cell maturation, culminating in the surface expression of immunoglobulin molecules in B cells or receptor molecules in T cells.[3,4] With the expression of surface receptors, the lymphoid cells become competent to respond to antigen. The remaining compartment, the peripheral lymphoid system, contains the lymphocyte populations already programmed by the central lymphoid organs, which are capable of generating an immune response after antigenic challenge and includes the spleen, lymph nodes, and lymphoid tissue of the gut, respiratory tract, and skin. These organs are served by blood and lymphatic circulations facilitating cellular migration and the intermingling of cells involved in the immune response. Malignant transformation can occur in any of the morphologically and functionally distinct subpopulations of lymphoid cells of the immune system and in any of the central or peripheral lymphoid organs, which accounts for the heterogeneity of morphologic, immunologic, and clinical features observed in malignant lymphomas, as well as the diverse findings related to the site and extent of disease. In childhood, about 80% of malignant lymphomas are of B-cell origin and the rest are T-cell malignancies. This appears surprising, given the similar frequency of T and B cells in the human body, but might be understandable considering the specific factors that influence the pathogenesis of B-cell neoplasms.[5]

Our understanding of the biology of the childhood lymphomas has been promoted by enormous advances in the fields of histopathology, immunology, cytogenetics, and molecular biology that have occurred during the past 2 decades. Concurrently, therapy for childhood lymphomas has improved dramatically so that most children with lymphoma can now be cured. The lymphomas of childhood include Hodgkin's lymphoma and the non-Hodgkin's lymphomas (NHLs). The behavior of childhood Hodgkin's lymphoma closely resembles that of its adult counterpart. The evolution of therapy for children with Hodgkin's lymphoma has paralleled advances made in the treatment of adults with this disease, but also reflects the unique features of the growing child as the host. In contrast to Hodgkin's lymphoma, it is now clear that childhood NHL bears little resemblance to adult NHL in terms of clinical behavior and response to therapy. Thus, although the NHLs and Hodgkin's lymphoma are classified together under the rubric of malignant lymphoma, the biology and treatment of childhood Hodgkin's lymphoma and NHL are more different than alike, and these diseases will be considered separately in this chapter.

People with inherited or acquired immunodeficiency are at increased risk of developing lymphoma. Post-transplantation lymphoproliferative disease (PTLD) observed in children with iatrogenic impaired immune function following organ transplantation represents a broad spectrum of disorders; these range from polymorphous and polyclonal early lesions to monoclonal lymphoid neoplasms indistinguishable from lymphomas typically found in those with normal immune systems. The risk of PTLD depends on the degree of immunosuppression, and the course of PTLD can be influenced by the modification of immunosuppressive therapy. Thus, PTLD will be discussed separately. The nonlymphomatous forms of lymphadenopathy will also be discussed separately, because the malignant lymphomas are prominent in the differential diagnosis of lymphadenopathy, and the clinical and histologic features of the malignant lymphomas overlap with those of nonmalignant conditions that cause lymph node enlargement.

HODGKIN'S LYMPHOMA

Definition

Hodgkin's disease was first described in 1832 by Thomas Hodgkin (Fig. 13-1) as a disorder characterized by a peculiar enlargement of the absorbent (lymphatic) glands and spleen, and was so named in 1865 by Sir Samuel Wilks (Box 13-1).[6,7] Sternberg and Reed, in 1898 and 1902, respectively, are credited with the first definitive and thorough description of the binucleate or multinucleated giant cells that, when present, are considered pathognomonic of this disorder (Fig. 13-2).[8,9] The malignant nature of the disease was proven when Seif and Spriggs confirmed the clonal origin of the malignant cell by cytogenetic analysis.[10] Biologic and clinical studies of the last 20 years have increased the understanding of the nature of the disorder. It has been shown that in the vast majority of cases, the malignant cells are B lymphocytes.[11] Thus, in the World Health Organization Classification of Tumors of the Hematopoietic and Lymphoid Tissue (WHO classification), the term *Hodgkin's disease* replaced *Hodgkin's lymphoma*.[12] Moreover, it has been shown that Hodgkin's lymphomas are comprised of two different disease entities, classic Hodgkin's lymphoma (CHL) and nodular lymphocyte-predominant Hodgkin's lymphoma (NLPHL), which differ in their clinical and biologic features.

Histopathology and Classification

The Rye modification of the Lukes-Butler classification of Hodgkin's disease was universally accepted for 25 years for purposes of diagnosis and classification.[13] It divided Hodgkin's disease into four categories: lymphocyte predominance, nodular sclerosis, mixed cellularity, and lymphocyte depletion, which varied by age and demography. More recently, the International Lymphoma Study Group introduced a revised European-American classification of malignant lymphoma, which included some modifications in the classification of Hodgkin's disease.[14] Thereafter, these modifications were incorporated into the WHO classification.[12] This recognizes Hodgkin's disease as a lymphoma and separates NLPHL from CHL in view of its distinct biologic, histologic, and clinical features.

Classic Hodgkin's Lymphoma

CHL is characterized by the presence of mononuclear Hodgkin's and multinucleated Reed-Sternberg cells. Hodgkin's and

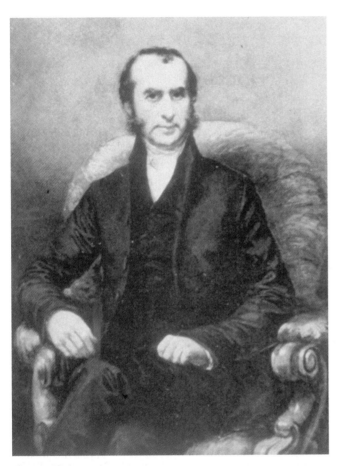

Figure 13-1. Thomas Hodgkin.

Reed-Sternberg cells are usually in the minority, residing in a reactive infiltrate of a variable mixture of non-neoplastic lymphocytes, eosinophils, neutrophils, plasma cells, fibroblasts, and collagen fibers present in response to cytokines produced by the tumor.[12] The Reed-Sternberg cells are large cells, with abundant, slightly basophilic cytoplasm and have at least two nuclear lobes or nuclei containing a prominent inclusion-like eosinophilic nucleolus. Diagnostic Reed-Sternberg cells must have at least two nuclei in two separate lobes (see Fig. 13-2). Mononuclear variants are termed *Hodgkin's cells* and often have a more intense basophilic cytoplasm. Microdissection techniques have enabled the isolation of Reed-Sternberg cells from frozen sections and the investigation of their lineage commitment. In more than 98% of cases, Reed-Sternberg cells are B cells, as defined by monoclonal immunoglobulin gene rearrangements.[11] Only a few cases have shown clonal T-cell receptor (TCR) gene rearrangement in the Reed-Sternberg cells, suggesting T-cell origin.[15] Reed-Sternberg cells of CHL express the B-lineage antigens CD20 and CD79a in variable propor-

Box 13-1	**Milestones in the Description, Classification, and Treatment of Hodgkin's Lymphoma**

- **1832** First description, by Thomas Hodgkin
- **1898** Sternberg and Reed (**1902**) publish descriptions of Reed-Sternberg cells
- **1901** First radiotherapy
- **1946** First chemotherapy with Mustargen (Goodman)
- **1947** First classification, by Jackson and Parker
- **1964/1970** Combination chemotherapy: MOPP (DeVita)
- **1965** Histopathologic classification of Lukes and Butler, Rye
- **1966** Concept of curative radiotherapy (Kaplan)
- **1971** Ann Arbor staging classificatio
- **1974/1980** Combined-modality radio-chemotherapy for children (Donaldson)
- **1982** Risk-adapted chemoradiotherapy (Schellong)
- **1994** HRS cells are clonal B cells (Küppers)
- **2000** WHO classification: Separation of lymphocyte-predominant Hodgkin's lymphoma from classic Hodgkin's lymphoma

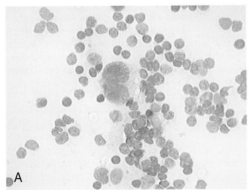
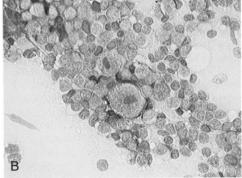

Figure 13-2. A, Reed-Sternberg cell. **B,** Hodgkin's cell. Reed-Sternberg cells are large cells with abundant slightly basophilic cytoplasm and have at least two nuclear lobes or nuclei containing a prominent inclusion-like eosinophilic nucleolus. Mononuclear variants are known as Hodgkin's cells and often have a more intense basophilic cytoplasm.

TABLE 13-1	Immunohistochemical Findings in Tumor Cells of Childhood and Adolescent Hodgkin's Lymphoma and Non-Hodgkin's Lymphoma Subtypes				
Marker	**CHL**	**LRCHL**	**NLPHL**	**TCRLBCL**	**ALCL**
CD30	+	+	−	−	+
CD15	±	±	−	−	Rare
EMA	Rare	Rare	±	±	±
CD45	−	−	+	+	±
CD20	±	±	+	+	−
CD79a	±	±	+	+	−
BSAP	±	±	+	+	−
J chain	−	−	+		
BOB.1	±	±	+	+	−
Oct2	±	±	+	+	−
CD3	−	−	−	−	±
CD2	−	−	−	−	±
Perforin-granzyme B	−	−	−	−	+
Alk	−	−	−	−	>80%
EBV (latency type II)	±	±	−	−	−

ALCL, anaplastic large cell lymphoma; CHL, classic Hodgkin's lymphoma; LRCHL, lymphocyte-rich classic Hodgkin's lymphoma; NLPHL, nodular lymphocyte-predominant Hodgkin's lymphoma; TCRLBCL, T-cell–rich large B-cell lymphoma.

Adapted from Stein H, Delsol G, Peleri S, et al. Nodular lymphocyte predominant Hodgkin lymphoma. In Jaffe ES, Harris NL, Stein H, Vardiman JW (eds). World Health Organization Classification of Tumours. Pathology and Genetics of Tumours of Haematopoetic and Lymphoid Tissues. Lyon, France, IARC Press, 2001, pp 240-243.

tions, whereas the B-cell–specific activator protein (BSAP), a product of the PAX5 gene, is expressed in about 90% of cases (Table 13-1).[16,17] Reed-Sternberg cells are almost invariably positive for the CD30 antigen[18] and usually express the CD15 antigen, whereas the expression of the epithelial membrane antigen (EMA) is rare. In Epstein-Barr virus (EBV)–positive cases of CHL, the Reed-Sternberg cells express the EBV latency type II pattern LMP-1 and EBNA-1, but without EBNA-2.[19] Almost invariably, structural chromosomal aberrations can be identified in Reed-Sternberg cells (see later), but they are not yet diagnostic criteria of the WHO classification of Hodgkin's lymphoma.

Based on the characteristics of the reactive infiltrate and the morphology of the Reed-Sternberg cells, four subtypes of classic Hodgkin's lymphoma are distinguished in the WHO classification[12,16]: lymphocyte-rich Hodgkin's lymphoma (LRHL), lymphocyte-depleted Hodgkin's lymphoma (LDHL), mixed cellularity Hodgkin's lymphoma (MCHL), and nodular sclerosis Hodgkin's lymphoma (NSHL). The immunophenotypic and genetic features of the Reed-Sternberg cells are identical in these histologic subtypes, whereas they differ in clinical features and association with EBV. CHL is associated with overexpression and an abnormal pattern of cytokines and chemokines and their receptors by Reed-Sternberg cells and the cells of the reactive background.[20,21] The abnormal cytokine and chemokine expression most likely accounts for the abundant admixture and pattern of inflammatory cells in CHL lesions as well as for distinct clinical features (see later). For example, overexpression of eotaxin correlates with the extent of eosinophilia within the infiltrate, whereas the expression levels of transforming growth factor β (TGF-β) may account for the extent of fibrosis.[22,23] The NSHL subtype is characterized by a nodal growth pattern, with collagen bands that surround at least one nodule and the formation of clusters of Reed-Sternberg cells and so-called lacunar cells (mononuclear Hodgkin's cells with only moderately prominent nucleoli).[12,16] NSHL can be grade 1 or 2, mainly depending on the number of Reed-Sternberg cells in distinct nodules.[24] The EBV-encoded latent membrane protein 1 (LMP-1) antigen is less frequently expressed than in other subtypes. The MCHL subtype is characterized by scattered classic Reed-Sternberg cells in a diffuse

or vaguely nodular mixed inflammatory background, without sclerosis. The EBV-encoded LMP-1 antigen is more frequently expressed than in NSHL. The LRHL subtype contains scattered Reed-Sternberg cells and a nodular or diffuse background of small lymphocytes, but with an absence of neutrophils and eosinophils. The LDHL subtype is a diffuse form of CHL, rich in Reed-Sternberg cells and/or depleted of non-neoplastic lymphocytes, and often sarcomatoid in appearance.

Nodular Lymphocyte-Predominant Hodgkin's Lymphoma

NLPHL is a monoclonal B-cell neoplasm.[16,25] Although NLPHL appears to have a less aggressive natural course than CHL, it is not a benign disease.[26] The histology is characterized by effacement of the lymph node architecture by a nodular or nodular and diffuse infiltrate of small lymphocytes, with an associated follicular dendritic network and scattered or clustered large cells referred to as lymphocytic and histiocytic (L&H) cells.[12,16] NLPHL corresponds to Hodgkin's paragranuloma of the classification of Jackson and Parker from 1947[27] and to lymphocyte-predominant Hodgkin's disease of the Rye modification of Lukes and Butler.[13] Differentiation of NLPHL from the lymphocyte rich subtype of classic Hodgkin's lymphoma can be difficult in some cases. However, the phenotype of L&H cells (also termed *popcorn cells* because of their often multilobed nuclei) is different than classic Reed-Sternberg cells of the CHL subtypes in that they express CD45 and usually retain most normal markers of B-cell differentiation, such as CD20, CD79a, and the B-cell specific transcription factors BOB.1 and Oct-2, but do not express CD30 and CD15 (see Table 13-1).[12,16] Also, EBV infection is consistently absent from L&H cells of NLPLH.[25] In some patients with NLPHL, progressively transformed germinal centers are observed in association with NPLHL. However, it remains uncertain whether these lesions are truly preneoplastic because most patients with such lesions in reactive lymph node hyperplasia do not develop a lymphoma.

In Western countries, approximately 70% of children and adolescents with Hodgkin's lymphoma show the NSHL subtype, whereas the proportion of patients diagnosed with

TABLE 13-2	Characteristics of Children and Adolescents with Hodgkin's Lymphoma in Different Geographic Regions		
Parameter	**North America[28]**	**India[30]**	**Europe[29,45]**
No. of patients	829	148	1018
Age range, median (yr)	0-21, nd	2.75-14, 8	2-18, nd
Gender ratio (male-to-female)	1.2:1	9.6:1	?
	Rye Classification	**Rye Classification**	**WHO Classification**
HISTOPATHOLOGY			
NSHL	76.8%	7%	68.3%
MCHL	10.2%	86%	21.0%
LDHL	0.3%	2.1%	0.7%
Lymphocyte-predominant	9.4%	2.1%	LRHL, 0.7%; LPHL, 9.3%
Unclassified	3.1%	2.8%	0%
ANN ARBOR STAGE			
I	16%	18.2%	7.4%
II	52%	36.5%	59%
III	15%	39.9%	21.2%
IV	17%	5.4%	12.4%
B symptoms present	26%	54.4%	32%
Mediastinal	65%	45.9%	82%
Spleen	nd	14.9%	23%
Liver	nd	nd	2.2%
Lung involvement	nd	1.4%	16%
Pleura	nd	1.4%	14%
Pericardium	nd	nd	19%
Bone involvement	nd	nd	4.5%
Bone marrow involvement	nd	2.7%	2.3%
CNS involvement	nd	nd	0%
Skin involvement	nd	nd	0.7%
HEMATOLOGIC ABNORMALITIES			
Anemia: Hb < 10.5 g/dL	nd	57.7%	nd
ESR ≥ 40 mm/hr	nd	57.8%	

CNS, central nervous system; ESR, erythrocyte sedimentation rate; Hb, hemoglobin; LDHL, lymphocyte-depleted Hodgkin's lymphoma; LRHL, lymphocyte-rich Hodgkin's lymphoma; LDHL, lymphocyte-depleted Hodgkin's lymphoma; MCHL, mixed cellularity Hodgkin's lymphoma; nd, no data given; NLPHL, nodular lymphocyte-predominant Hodgkin's lymphoma; NSHL, nodular sclerosis Hodgkin's lymphoma.

mixed cellularity varies from 10% to 20%. Both LDHL and LRHL are rare in children and adolescents.[28,29] NLPHL accounts for approximately 10% of cases of Hodgkin's lymphoma and corresponds well to the proportion of lymphocyte-predominant Hodgkin's disease when patients are classified according to the Rye modification of Lukes and Butler (Table 13-2). The distribution of subtypes, however, appears to be significantly different in different geographic regions. Thus, in a well-characterized cohort from India, most pediatric Hodgkin's lymphoma was of the MCHL subtype.[30]

In some patients, distinction between true Hodgkin's lymphoma and certain subtypes of NHL can be difficult. This applies especially to the separation between NLPHL with a diffuse infiltration pattern variant and T-cell–rich, large B-cell lymphoma, even if extended immunohistochemistry markers are examined (see Table 13-1). At present, an overlap between these two entities cannot be completely excluded.[12,16] Other pairs that present diagnostic difficulties are anaplastic large cell lymphoma (ALCL) and LDHL and other classic Hodgkin's lymphoma cases rich in Reed-Sternberg cells. In these cases, investigation of an extended battery of B- and T-lineage specific markers can help disclose the B-cell nature of the true Hodgkin's lymphoma cases and the T-cell origin of the true ALCL cases. Also, ALCL cases are generally negative for EBV antigens.[31] Immunostaining of fixed sections for anaplastic lymphoma kinase (ALK) may be decisive, because more than 80%

of childhood and adolescent cases of ALCL are ALK-positive (see later), whereas Hodgkin's lymphoma is consistently ALK-negative (see Table 13-1). Although recent studies of gene expression profiling have suggested a relationship of NSHL and primary mediastinal (thymic) large B-cell lymphoma with sclerosis,[32,33] the histologic distinction of both entities rarely poses problems.

Epidemiology and Causative Factors

Epidemiologic studies have suggested that Hodgkin's lymphoma is a complex of related conditions that are partly mediated by infectious diseases, immune deficits, and genetic susceptibilities.[34] Different incidence patterns of Hodgkin's lymphoma have been described for different geographic regions and socioeconomic conditions. Data from cancer incidence surveys conducted in five continents have suggested that Hodgkin's lymphoma has a bimodal peak at ages 15 to 34 years and older than 60 years in most European, American, Hispanic, and Australian populations, whereas in Asian populations the incidence is low at a younger age and increases with age, but that the highest rates are only half that of those in Europe.[34,35] In children 0 to 14 years of age, incidence rates were highest in Eastern European countries (1.46 in 100,000/year), 0.5 to 0.6 in Middle or Western European countries, 0.7 as found by the

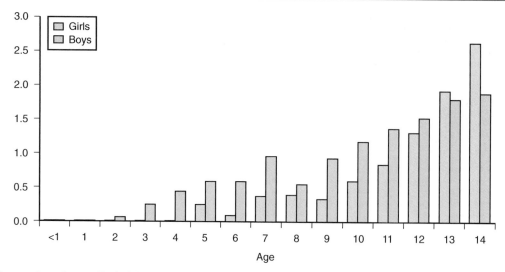

Figure 13-3. Age- and gender-specific incidence rates (per 100,000) of Hodgkin's lymphoma during childhood in Germany, 2000 to 2004. (Adapted from Kaatsch P, Spix C. Annual Report, 2005. German Childhood Cancer Registry. Mainz, Germany, Institut für Medizinische Biometrie, Epidemiologie und Informatik, 2007, p 52.)

U.S. Surveillance, Epidemiology and End Results (SEER) program for whites and 0.62 for blacks, and lowest in Japan. In a more recent analysis confined to Hodgkin's lymphoma in childhood and adolescence, four different patterns of age-related incidence rates were described: (1) low childhood rates and high young adult rates in the United States and Midwestern Europe; (2) a higher rate in childhood in the Eastern European countries than in the United States and Western Europe, and an even higher rate in young adults; (3) a similar rate in Latin America to that in economically developed countries; and (4) uniformly low Hodgkin's lymphoma incidence rates in Asia.[36] In all regions, Hodgkin's lymphoma occurs rarely in children younger than 3 years of age (Fig. 13-3).

Studies on the trend of incidence rates over time in children and adolescents have also exhibited different geographic patterns. In India, Scandinavia, and North America, a significant increase in the incidence of Hodgkin's lymphoma in adolescents was observed, mainly because of an increase in females suffering from NSHL.[37-41] In the United Kingdom, a decrease in the incidence rate was observed in most age groups; in the younger age group, however, it decreased only in females.[42] In the population-based German Childhood Cancer Registry, there was no significant change in the incidence rate for children 0 to 14 years of age between 1983 and 2004.[43] Incidence rates and the male-to-female ratio differ according to the specific childhood age groups (see Fig. 13-3). The incidence rate is generally low during the first 10 years of age and higher in boys compared with girls. Beyond the age of 10 years, the incidence rate increases and the male-to-female ratio becomes more balanced. The differences in the male-to-female ratio according to age most likely reflect differences in the distribution of gender by subtype and the different incidence rates of subtypes according to age. Within the pediatric age group, the mixed cellularity subtype is most commonly diagnosed in children 10 years of age or younger, whereas the nodular sclerosing subtype is the most commonly observed subtype in adolescents and young adults.[44] In NSHL, the male-to-female ratio is almost equal.[45] However, the distribution by gender appears also to vary with the geographic region. Thus, in India, there is a much higher predominance of male Hodgkin's lymphoma patients, although part of the difference may be the result of deficiencies in overall health care for females.[46]

Studies on the space-time clustering of Hodgkin's lymphoma have suggested evidence for an infectious cause, although investigations of possible person-to-person transmission or exposure to a particular environmental factor have not revealed unequivocal conclusions.[34,47-49] A positive association of Hodgkin's lymphoma with higher social class has been reported from studies in children and adolescents.[50,51] An interesting finding in regard to seasonal variation was a significant peak of Hodgkin's lymphoma diagnosis in young men in the United States in February and in the United Kingdom in March.[52,53] In 1966, MacMahon[54] suggested an infectious cause of Hodgkin's lymphoma and, in 1974, Rosdahl and colleagues[55] reported an increased risk of Hodgkin's lymphoma in people with a history of infectious mononucleosis. Since then, numerous studies have substantiated the causative role of EBV in the pathogenesis of Hodgkin's lymphoma. Seroepidemiologic studies have demonstrated an altered pattern of EBV antibodies before the diagnosis of Hodgkin's lymphoma.[56-59] Furthermore, an increased load of EBV viral DNA was observed in the peripheral blood of pediatric patients with Hodgkin's lymphoma.[60] Weiss and associates[61-63] have identified EBV viral genomes in Reed-Sternberg cells of Hodgkin's lymphoma that were monoclonal, implying that the Reed-Sternberg cells were infected before malignant transformation. The proportion of EBV-positive Hodgkin's lymphoma cases seems to vary, however, according to geographic region, age, and histologic subtype but may also vary with the laboratory tests that were used. The proportion of EBV-positive Hodgkin's lymphoma cases is higher in children than adults and generally higher in Africa, Asia, and South America compared with Europe and North America, and patients are more likely to have the mixed cellularity subtype than nodular sclerosis (Table 13-3). A Scandinavian cohort study including more than 38,000 people with a history of infectious mononucleosis (IM) and more than 21,000 controls has supported the assumption of a causal association of IM-related EBV infection and the EBV-positive subgroup of Hodgkin's lymphoma in young adults.[64] Only serologically confirmed EBV IM was associated with increased risk of Hodgkin's lymphoma, whereas there was no increased risk for EBV-negative Hodgkin's lymphoma after IM. The median time from serologically confirmed IM to the diagnosis of EBV-positive HL was 4.1 years. In a recent analysis of more than 800 children

TABLE 13-3   Epstein-Barr Virus (EBV)–Positive Rates in Childhood Hodgkin's Lymphoma*

Region	Country (Study)	EBV Gene Product	All HL (%)	NSHL	MCHL	LDHL	LPHL
Africa	Kenya[657]	LMP	53/53 (100)	25/25 (100)	16/16 (100)	6/6 (100)	1/1 (100)
Asia	China[658]	LMP	67/82 (82)	18/23 (78)	30/33 (91)	—	—
South America	Argentina[659]	EBER	22/41 (54)	0/9 (0)	19/25 (76)	1/1 (100)	2/6 (33)
Europe	United Kingdom[660]	LMP and EBER	37/130 (28)	13/68 (19)	20/42 (48)		—
	Germany[65]	LMP-1	236/840 (31)	122/549 (22)	131/190 (69)	2/6 (33)	LRCHL 3/5 (66); NLPHL 5/90 (5)
North America	United States[661]	EBER	9/25 (36)	2/15 (13)	6/7 (86)	—	0/2
	United States[662]	EBER	15/26 (58)	2/6 (33)	12/17 (71)	1/2 (50)	0/1

*According to geographic region.

EBER, EBV-encoded small RNA; HL, Hodgkin's lymphoma; LDHL, lymphocyte-depleted Hodgkin's lymphoma; LMP-1, latent membrane protein 1; LPHL, lymphocyte-predominant Hodgkin's lymphoma; LRCHL, lymphocyte-rich classic Hodgkin's lymphoma; MCHL, mixed cellularity Hodgkin's lymphoma; NLPHL, nodular lymphocyte-predominant Hodgkin's lymphoma; NSHL, nodular sclerosis Hodgkin's lymphoma.

Adapted from Cartwright RA, Watkins G. Epidemiology of Hodgkin's disease: a review. Hematol Oncol. 2004;22:11-26.

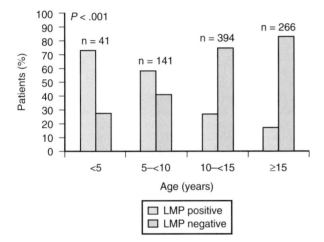

Figure 13-4. Age dependency of latent membrane protein (LMP) status in Hodgkin's lymphoma showing the highest frequency of Epstein-Barr virus (EBV) infection in the age group younger than 5 years. (Adapted from Claviez A, Tiemann M, Luders H, et al. Impact of latent Epstein-Barr virus infection on outcome in children and adolescents with Hodgkin's's lymphoma. J Clin Oncol. 2005;23: 4048-4056.)

and adolescents consecutively enrolled in German-Austrian-Scandinavian multicenter trials of pediatric lymphoma, EBV associated LMP-1 was positive in Reed-Sternberg cells in 31% of cases.[65] EBV infection of Reed-Sternberg cells was correlated with gender (39% male vs. 23% female; $P < .001$), histologic subtype (69% mixed cellularity vs. 22% nodular sclerosis vs. 6% lymphocyte predominance; $P < .001$), and young age (Fig. 13-4). Several studies of the possible involvement of other human herpesviruses (HHVs), including HHV-6, -7, -8, and measles, have not reached conclusive results.[66-68]

Studies of occupational exposures, mainly including adult Hodgkin's lymphoma cases, have revealed little significance for environmental factors involved in the pathogenesis of Hodgkin's lymphoma.[34] A most striking observation, however, was that the regular use of aspirin decreased the risk of Hodgkin's lymphoma significantly in a case-control study.[69] Aspirin inhibits nuclear factor kappa B (NF-κB), which has a vital role in Reed-Sternberg cell survival and resistance to apoptosis.[70]

People with HIV-related immunodeficiency carry a significantly increased risk of developing Hodgkin's lymphoma.[71] In contrast to Kaposi's sarcoma and NHL, the incidence of HL in persons with HIV-AIDS appears to increase after the introduction of highly active antiretroviral therapy (HAART).[72]

Familial aggregation of Hodgkin's lymphoma was first described by Razis and coworkers in 1959[73] and is now well documented.[74-77] The familial risk of Hodgkin's lymphoma ranks among the highest in the population-based Swedish Family-Cancer Database.[78] In an analysis of 28 reports of familial Hodgkin's lymphoma, Ferraris and colleagues[79] found only one major peak between 15 and 34 years of age for familial Hodgkin's lymphoma, instead of the classic bimodal age distribution of sporadic Hodgkin's lymphoma.[79] This corresponds to the findings of two large studies of an increased sevenfold risk in siblings of cases diagnosed at ages younger than 45 and 35 years of age, respectively, but little or no increased risk in siblings of cases diagnosed at older ages.[49,80] The risk for siblings of the same gender was higher than the risk of siblings of different genders, however. Whether familial aggregation of Hodgkin's lymphoma mainly reflects genetic susceptibility or a shared environmental factor, such as shared exposure to infection, remains undetermined. Studies of familial Hodgkin's lymphoma have failed to detect high levels of anti-EBV antibodies in affected relatives and EBER (EBV-encoded small RNA) was infrequently detected in Reed-Sternberg cells of familial Hodgkin's lymphoma.[81,82] From the observation of higher risk of siblings compared to parent-offspring pairs, Altieri and Hemminki[78] have suggested a recessive inheritance component or shared childhood exposures as determinants for familial aggregations of Hodgkin's lymphoma. Strong evidence for a role for genetic susceptibility was provided by the finding that monozygotic twins of Hodgkin's lymphoma patients have a 99-fold increased risk, whereas no increased risk in dizygotic twins was observed.[74] Recent studies have provided evidence that familial aggregation of Hodgkin's lymphoma may reflect inherited abnormalities of the immune response. A familial or personal history of autoimmune conditions and sarcoidosis was found to be strongly associated with an increased risk for Hodgkin's lymphoma,[83,84] and a 51-fold increased risk for Hodgkin's lymphoma was found in kindreds predisposed to the autoimmune lymphoproliferative syndrome, a disorder of lymphocyte homeostasis usually associated with germline *FAS* gene mutations.[85] In patients with ataxia telangiectasia (ATM), the risk of Hodgkin's lymphoma was increased, but its risk was much lower than the risk of NHL.[86] Liberzon and associates[87] have found a low frequency of molecular variants of the ATM gene in Israeli children, suggesting that ATM mutations do not play a major role in pathogenesis.

In 1975, Svejgaard and coworkers first described an association of certain human leukocyte antigen (HLA) loci with an increased risk of Hodgkin's lymphoma, suggesting a disease susceptibility gene within or near the histocompatibility region on chromosome 6.[88,89] Since then, numerous studies have confirmed the association of particular HLA loci in the susceptibility to Hodgkin's lymphoma, including HLA A1, B5, B8, B15, B27, B35, and B37.[90] In a large study on familial Hodgkin's lymphoma, Chakravarti and colleagues[91] have found strong evidence for a recessive mode of inheritance for susceptibility to Hodgkin's lymphoma, and approximately 60% of associations were caused by an HLA-linked susceptibility gene.

Thus, increasing evidence from epidemiologic studies suggests that both genetic susceptibility (HLA-linked and HLA-unlinked) and environmental factors can predispose to the onset of Hodgkin's lymphoma. These associations are highlighted by a recent report of a family in which three of five children developed EBV-positive Hodgkin's lymphoma. All three of these children shared the same maternal and paternal HLA-haplotypes, whereas the two unaffected offspring had different haplotypes.[92]

Molecular and Cellular Biology

The cell of origin of the malignant cells in classic Hodgkin's disease was long a matter of controversy because of the low frequency of Reed-Sternberg cells in the tumors and their unusual immunophenotype in that they lack expression of immunoglobulins and other B-cell markers; rather, they express markers characteristic of dendritic cells, granulocytes, monocytes, and T cells.[93] However, the identification of immunoglobulin gene rearrangement[11,94,95] and somatic hypermutation in microdissected Reed-Sternberg cells in almost all cases of classic Hodgkin's disease has demonstrated that these cells derive from postgerminal B cells. In addition, these studies have demonstrated that about 25% of classic Hodgkin's disease cases carry crippling immunoglobulin rearrangements that destroy the function of the immunoglobulin gene.[11,94] These nonfunctional rearrangements typically induce rapid apoptosis in normal B cells, suggesting that Hodgkin's disease may originate from germinal center B cells that have escaped apoptosis. Analysis of T-cell receptor rearrangements has shown that despite the frequent expression of T-cell markers, CHL originates from T cells in only 1% to 2% of cases.[15]

In NLPHL, the malignant popcorn cells show expression of B-cell markers such as CD20 and CD79a, suggesting a B-cell origin for these tumors as well. As in CHL, the analysis of immunoglobulin genes in microdissected tumors has shown clonal and somatically mutated gene rearrangements.[11,96] In addition, 50% of cases have shown evidence of ongoing somatic hypermutation, which strongly suggests that they derive from germinal center B cells.[11]

Mechanisms of Transformation

Almost 40% of CHL cases show EBV infection of the Reed-Sternberg cell. Importantly, EBV can immortalize human B cells in vitro. Thus, it is likely that EBV contributes to the pathogenesis of CHL. In this regard, *LMP-1*, a virally encoded oncogene expressed in Reed-Sternberg cells, can activate the NF-κB pathway, which is constitutively active in Hodgkin's disease (see later). *LMP-2*, a second viral gene product, mimics B-cell receptor signaling and might play a role in rescuing Reed-Sternberg cells with immunoglobulin crippling mutations from apoptosis.[97]

The most prominent molecular abnormality found in Hodgkin's disease is the constitutive activation of the NF-κB pathway. NF-κB functions as an important survival signaling pathway in B cells in response to the activation of members of the tumor necrosis factor (TNF) receptor family (CD30, CD40). In Hodgkin's disease, somatic mutations in different elements of the NF-κB pathway keep it constitutively activated. Thus, the *REL* gene, which encodes an NF-κB component, is frequently amplified in Reed-Sternberg cells[98] and mutations of the gene encoding NF-κB inhibitors *IKBA* and *IKBE* are found in cases of Hodgkin's disease.[99,100] In addition, activation of TNF signaling by the microenvironment and activation of NF-κB by the *LMP1* EBV oncogene may also contribute to aberrant NF-κB signaling.

Gene amplification of *JAK2* and *MDM2* has been found in Reed-Sternberg cells.[101,102] The JAK2 tyrosine kinase mediates signaling from cytokine receptors through the JAK/STAT pathway and has been shown to be oncogenic in T-cell lymphomas expressing a *TEL-JAK2* fusion oncogene,[103] and in polycythemia vera and essential thrombocytosis caused by the activating mutation *JAK2* V617F.[104] MDM2 regulates the stability of TP53 and plays a central role in the regulation of apoptosis.[105] Overexpression of MDM2 induces active degradation of TP53 in the proteasome and blocks the function of this tumor suppressor.

In contrast to classic Hodgkin's disease, the malignant cells of the lymphocyte-predominant type of Hodgkin's lymphomas are always EBV-negative. The only molecular aberration identified so far in these tumors is the presence of chromosomal translocations involving the *BCL6* oncogene on band 3q27 in 48% of cases.[106] BCL6 is a zinc finger transcription repressor normally expressed only in germinal center B cells. *Bcl6* null mice fail to generate germinal centers in response to immunization, showing that this factor is required for germinal center formation.[107] Dysregulated expression of BCL6 in lymphoma may lead to a developmental block and confer a proliferative advantage. In addition, recent studies have shown that BCL6 may contribute to genomic instability via downregulation of TP53[108] and ATR, a protein kinase involved in sensing DNA damage.[109]

Cellular Microenvironment: Cytokines and Chemokines

The cellular and cytokine microenvironment surrounding the lymphoid cells in Hodgkin's disease plays an essential role in the pathogenesis of this disease. In particular, the expression of soluble factors and their receptors by malignant cells and the reactive microenvironment seems not only to mediate the inflammatory characteristics observed in the histology of Hodgkin's disease, but also to contribute to the proliferation and survival of the malignant clone. Thus, the cellular microenvironment supports and is supported by a network of cytokines secreted in autocrine and paracrine loops, which are essential for the proliferation of Reed-Sternberg cells and the maintenance of a favorable inflammatory environment rich in regulatory T cells and eosinophils.

Both interleukin-13 (IL-13) and the IL-13 receptor IL-13RA1 are expressed in Hodgkin's disease and constitute an important autocrine loop for Reed-Sternberg cells.[110,111] Other cytokines expressed in Hodgkin's disease and thought to influence survival of these cells include IL-4, IL-6, IL-7, IL-9, and IL-15.[20,21]

The vast majority of cells in a tumor biopsy of Hodgkin's disease are not malignant cells, but represent an inflammatory-like cellular infiltrate composed mainly of CD4+ T lymphocytes intermixed with macrophages, eosinophils, plasma cells, and fibroblasts. Most lymphocytes present in this infiltrate are regulatory T cells, which play an important role in protecting the tumor Reed-Sternberg cells from cytotoxic T cells involved in antitumor immune surveillance.[97]

In contrast with the abundance of regulatory T cells, Th1 CD4+ T cells and CD8+ cytotoxic T cells are rare in Hodgkin's disease biopsies and are not detected in the immediate proximity of Reed-Sternberg cells. The recruitment of cells involved in immune tolerance and the exclusion of lymphoid cells responsible for antitumor immune responses are explained by the expression by Reed-Sternberg cells of pro–Th2-associated cytokines, such as IL-4 and IL-13, and anti-Th1 or CD8 cytokines, such as IL-10 and TGF-β.[97] The secretion of these immunosuppressive cytokines creates an immune-privileged microenvironment, allowing the tumor cells to avoid immune surveillance and T-cell–mediated apoptosis.

One of the most prominent features of Reed-Sternberg cells is the expression of CD30. Although coexpression of CD30 and its respective receptor CD153 initially suggested an autocrine mechanism promoting the proliferation of Reed-Sternberg cells via NF-κB, it is now well established that the activation of CD30 is primarily a CD153-independent process.[112] Two additional members of the TNF receptor family, CD40 and RANK, are expressed in Reed-Sternberg cells. Activation of CD40 seems to be mediated by the expression of CD40 ligand (CD40L) on T lymphocytes surrounding the Reed-Sternberg cell.[113,114] Importantly, soluble CD40L induces proliferation and blocks CD95-induced apoptosis in Reed-Sternberg cells.[113-115] Activation of RANK and osteoprotegerin, a member of the TNF receptor superfamily, is triggered by the autocrine expression of RANK ligand (RANKL) in Reed-Sternberg cells. Activation of RANK promotes NF-κB activation and contributes to the maintenance of an inflammatory microenvironment by promoting interferon gamma (IFN-γ) and IL-13 secretion.[97] Overall, the activation of TNF receptors by different mechanisms seems to play an important role in promoting the survival of the Reed-Sternberg cell.

Clinical Characteristics

The most common clinical presentation of Hodgkin's lymphoma in children and adolescents is a persistently enlarged node in the cervical or supraclavicular region. Characteristically, the lymph nodes involved with Hodgkin's lymphoma are not painful or tender but have a "rubbery" firmness on palpation. Enlarged nodes have often been present for weeks or months, increasing and decreasing in size irrespective of whether antibiotic therapy has been given. In approximately 30% of cases, constitutional signs referred to as B symptoms are present, which are defined as the presence of fever (temperature higher than 38° C [100.4° F]) for 3 consecutive days, drenching night sweats, and unexplained body weight loss of 10% or more over the preceding 6 months. Another rather specific symptom is severe and unexplained pruritus.

However, the clinical presentation varies considerably, ranging from life-threatening airway compression to the coincidental detection of an enlarged node or mediastinal tumor during an otherwise routine physical examination. Furthermore, clinical presentation varies across different geographic regions (see Table 13-2) Approximately 80% of children present with disease in one or both sides of the upper or lower neck. Involvement of the lymphoid tissues of Waldeyer's ring is uncommon without associated cervical lymphadenopathy. Approximately 60% to 80% of children have intrathoracic disease, most commonly in the anterosuperior mediastinum, paratracheal, and tracheobronchial lymph node groups. Pulmo-

nary involvement is rarely observed in the absence of hilar disease. Pleural effusions are uncommon; they are usually an indication of lymphatic obstruction from bulky central disease rather than a sign of advanced-stage disease. Pericardial effusion may occur in cases with pericardial involvement and is also seen most often in the setting of bulky mediastinal disease.[116] Intrathoracic Hodgkin's lymphoma is often asymptomatic but may be associated with nonproductive cough and chest pain. However, intrathoracic Hodgkin's lymphoma may present as a life-threatening condition, with dyspnea and severe superior vena cava syndrome. In these patients, invasive diagnostic procedures such as biopsy under general anesthesia may carry a high risk for respiratory and cardiac failure because of impaired blood flow to the heart and severe airway constriction. Intubation is an important consideration in patients with tumor-related constriction of the trachea and bronchi.

Hodgkin's lymphoma has a strong tendency for contiguous spread along adjacent lymph node regions (Fig. 13-5). In about two thirds of children with cervical nodes, intrathoracic disease is present (Fig. 13-6). Thus, in patients with enlarged cervical nodes in whom lymphoma is considered and biopsy is planned, a chest x-ray should be obtained to determine the absence or presence of mediastinal involvement. The chest x-ray typically shows a mediastinal mass with tuberous margins (Fig. 13-7). In patients with mediastinal tumors, only a computed tomography (CT) scan is required, however, whether critical airway obstruction is preexisting or not (see later, "Non-Hodgkin's Lymphoma"; Fig. 13-8B). Although about 30% of patients have supradiaphragmatic and infradiaphragmatic disease, Hodgkin's lymphoma limited to infradiaphragmatic sites is rare.[29] Palpable, inguinal lymph nodes are common in children; however, fewer than 7% of patients with Hodgkin's lymphoma have involvement of the inguinal nodes.

In Western Europe and North America, most children have stage II disease at diagnosis, according to the Ann Arbor Staging System (see Table 13-2). Extranodal involvement is diagnosed in about 30% of cases.

Laboratory findings are often nonspecific, although scrutiny of the complete blood count, erythrocyte sedimentation rate (ESR), and other acute-phase reactants may provide clues about the extent of disease. When the ESR is elevated at the time of diagnosis, it may be useful later as a nonspecific marker for detecting relapse. Other nonspecific laboratory findings generally associated with advanced-stage disease include the following:

1. Hematologic—neutrophilic leukocytosis, monocytosis, lymphopenia, eosinophilia, normochromic normocytic anemia
2. Elevated C-reactive protein level
3. Increased serum copper level
4. Elevated levels of alkaline phosphatase, which may indicate bone involvement
5. Autoimmune disorders (paraneoplastic syndromes), including nephritic syndrome, polymyositis, autoimmune hemolytic anemia, neutropenia, and thrombocytopenia or combinations of these; observed in patients with Hodgkin's lymphoma (idiopathic thrombocytopenic purpura [ITP] is most frequent)[117]
6. Serious paraneoplastic disorder of Hodgkin's lymphoma—may be limbic encephalitis or subacute cerebellar degeneration[118]

Patients with Hodgkin's disease often exhibit altered immunity characterized by reduced cellular immunity, whereas humoral immunity is usually relatively intact.[119] The nature of the immune defect is unclear. The severity of the impairment increases with advanced-stage, disease progression, and recurrence and after treatment with radiotherapy and chemotherapy. T-cell deficits may persist for a prolonged period in successfully

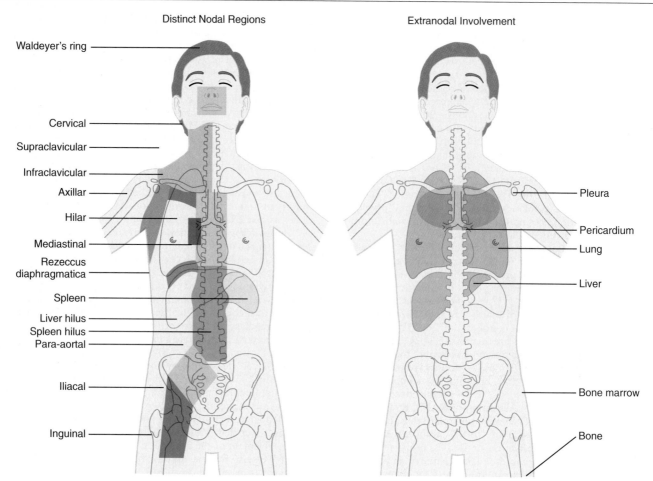

Figure 13-5. Distinct nodal regions according to the Ann Arbor staging classification for Hodgkin's lymphoma. (Adapted from Dörffel W, Schellong G. Morbus Hodgkins. In Gadner H, Gaedicke G, Niemeyer C, Ritter J (eds). Paediatrische Haematologie und Onkologie. Heidelberg, Germany, Springer, 2006, pp 770-776.)

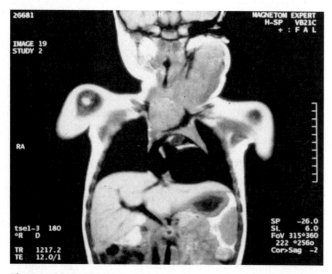

Figure 13-6. Magnetic resonance tomography of a child with Hodgkin's lymphoma. Shown is the nodal involvement of the neck, supraclavicular and infraclavicular regions, and nodes in the upper mediastinum. (Courtesy of Dr. W. Dörffel, Berlin.)

treated patients. As a result, patients with Hodgkin's lymphoma carry an increased risk of infection with opportunistic pathogens, fungi, tuberculosis, and viruses, as well as reactivation of viruses. The frequency and severity of the disturbed immune function increase not only with advanced-stage disease but also with unfavorable histologic subtypes of LDHL and MCHL.

Many systemic clinical features of Hodgkin's lymphoma may be the result of overexpression and an abnormal pattern of cytokines and chemokines, and their receptors, by Reed-Sternberg cells and the cells of the reactive background of the Hodgkin's lymphoma lesions. Table 13-4 summarizes correlations of abnormal cytokine and chemokine expression and related clinical and pathologic features of patients with Hodgkin's lymphoma.

Clinical features may differ among subtypes of Hodgkin's lymphoma. Thus, mediastinal involvement is present more often in adolescents with NSHL than in children younger than 10 years with MCHL.[120] The mixed cellularity subtype mainly affects younger children, has the strongest association with EBV, and often presents with widespread disease. In this subtype, uninvolved regions may interrupt the usual contiguous pattern of lymph node spread. With the rare LDHL subtype, involvement of bone and bone marrow is more frequently documented. NLPHL appears to have a less aggressive natural

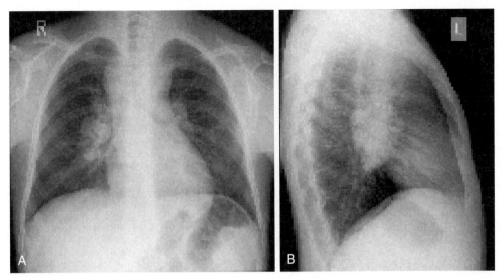

Figure 13-7. Chest roentgenogram of a patient with Hodgkin's lymphoma and involvement of the mediastinal nodes and hilum. The mediastinal mass has a typical tuberous appearance.

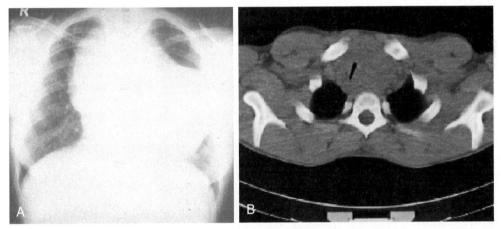

Figure 13-8. A, Chest roentgenogram showing a mediastinal tumor and left site pleural effusion in a child with T-cell lymphoblastic lymphoma. **B,** CT scan of the thorax of a child with T-cell lymphoblastic lymphoma demonstrating critical compression of the trachea by a mediastinal tumor ("scabbard trachea").

TABLE 13-4	Clinical Features and Abnormal Cytokine Production
Clinical Features	**Cytokines and Chemokines**
CONSTITUTIONAL (B) SYMPTOMS	TNF, LT-α, IL-1, IL-6
Polykaryon formation	IFN-γ, IL-4
Sclerosis	TGF-β, LIF, PDGF, IL-1, TNF
Acute phase reactions	IL-1, IL-6, IL-11, LIF
Eosinophilia	IL-5, GM-CSF, IL-2, IL-3
Plasmacytois	IL-6, IL-11
Mild thrombocytosis	IL-6, IL-11, LIF
T-cell and Hodgkin's and Reed-Sternberg cell interaction	IL-1, IL-2, IL-6, IL-7, IL-9, TNF, LT-α, CD30L, CD40L, B7 ligands (CD 80 and CD86)
IMMUNODEFICIENCY	TGF-β, IL-10
Autocrine growth factors (?)	IL-6, IL-9, TNF, LT-α, CD30L, GM-CSF
Increased alkaline phosphatase	GM-CSF
Neutrophil accumulation/activation	IL-8, TNF, TGF-β

IL-1, interleukin-1; IFN-γ, interferon gamma; LIF, leukemia-inhibiting factor; LT-α, lymphotoxin alpha; GM-CSF, granulocyte-macrophage colony-stimulating factor; PDGF, platelet-derived growth factor; TGF-β, transforming growth factor beta; TNF, tumor necrosis factor.
Adapted from Kadin ME, Liebowitz DM. Cytokines and cytokine receptors in Hodgkin's disease. In Mauch PM, Armitage JO, Diehl V, et al (eds). Hodgkin's Disease. Lippincott Williams & Wilkins, Philadelphia, 1999, pp 139-157.

course than CHL and usually presents as a localized disease involving only one peripheral lymph node region.

Diagnosis and Staging

The establishment of the diagnosis of Hodgkin's lymphoma is based on histopathology and immunohistochemistry of a lymph node biopsy. However, a complete characterization of the lymphoma cells would necessitate a more extended immunophenotypic examination. In individual cases, molecular genetic analysis of immunoglobulin gene and T-cell receptor gene rearrangements of the tumor cells can be of particular value in differentiating Hodgkin's lymphoma from ALCL or from reactive benign lymphoproliferative disorders. Major difficulties may arise in the separation of Hodgkin's lymphoma of the nodular sclerosis type from ALCL and of NLPHL from T-cell–rich large B-cell NHL and even reactive lymphoproliferative processes.

The differential diagnosis of Hodgkin's lymphoma includes other neoplastic conditions and infectious and inflammatory diseases associated with lymphadenopathy (see later, "Lymphadenopathy"). In many cases, only biopsy of a node may be able to exclude or prove malignant disease. Careful evaluation of the lymph node architecture is important, not only for accurate classification of Hodgkin's lymphoma but also to distinguish it from non-neoplastic adenopathy and NHL. Needle biopsy can be misleading, because it may not provide appropriate information about the lymph node architecture. Thus, needle biopsy is mostly restricted to situations in which surgery and general anesthesia may carry undue risks for the patient. If needle biopsy is performed, multiple biopsies should be taken to augment its diagnostic potential. As noted earlier, invasive diagnostic procedures in patients with mediastinal tumors, such as biopsy under general anesthesia, carry a high risk for respiratory and/or cardiac failure because of critical airway obstruction and/or impaired blood flow to the heart. Intubation in patients with tumor-related constriction of the trachea and bronchi can be problematic. Thus, needle biopsy should be considered in such cases. However, in patients with respiratory distress and/or severe upper vena cava syndrome caused by a mediastinal tumor, it is wise to avoid any form of invasive diagnostic procedure, but rather to start treatment immediately with corticosteroids and, if necessary, cyclophosphamide, allowing biopsy to be postponed until after stabilization of the patient's condition. An alternative is to start radiotherapy immediately to provide symptomatic relief and, when the patient has been stabilized, initiate invasive diagnostic procedures. A dramatic shrinkage of the tumor is usually achieved with doses of 10 to 15 Gy.

Staging

The Ann Arbor staging classification for Hodgkin's lymphoma was based on the recognized orderly spread of the disease, resulting from spread along contiguous lymph nodes, which predominates until late in the course of the disease. Clinical staging can be based on the history, physical examination, radiologic studies, and initial biopsy results (Table 13-5).[121] The distinct lymph node regions recognized by the Ann Arbor classification system are shown in Figure 13-5. The substage classifications A, B, and E amend each stage based on distinct features. Stage A designates asymptomatic disease, B indicates the presence of B symptoms, as defined in Table 13-5, and extralymphatic disease is designated as E, referring to limited extranodal extensions that easily can be encompassed within a radiotherapy portal. Extralymphatic disease is further designated as L (lung), P (pleura), and O (osseous) according to this

TABLE 13-5	Ann Arbor Staging Classification for Hodgkin Lymphoma
Stage	**Description**
I	Involvement of a single lymph node region (I) or a single extralymphatic organ or site (I$_E$)
II	Involvement of two or more lymph node regions on the same side of the diaphragm (II) or localized contiguous involvement of only one extralymphatic organ or site and its regional lymph node(s) on the same side of the diaphragm (II$_E$)
III	Involvement of lymph node regions on both sides of the diaphragm (III), which may also be accompanied by involvement of the spleen (III$_S$) or by localized contiguous involvement of an extralymphatic organ or site (III$_E$) or both (III$_{SE}$)
IV	Diffuse or disseminated involvement of one or more extralymphatic organs or tissues, with or without associated lymph node involvement
Designations applicable to any stage	
A	No B symptoms
B	B symptoms, defined as presence of fever (>38° C [100.4° F]) for 3 consecutive days, drenching night sweats, or unexplained loss of 10% or more of body weight in the preceding 6 mo
E	Involvement of a single extranodal site that is contiguous or proximal to the known nodal site

Adapted from Carbone PP, Kaplan HS, Musshoff K, et al. Report of the Committee on Hodgkin's Disease Staging Classification. Cancer Res. 1971;31:1860-1861.

system. The decision to classify extralymphatic disease either as substage E or as stage IV is based on the clinician's judgment, and often depends on whether the extralymphatic disease can be adequately covered in a radiotherapy treatment portal. Multiple E lesions are automatically considered to be stage IV. Although the Ann Arbor system assesses tumor extent, it does not adequately address tumor volume. Tumor volume and the number of involved nodal sites may have prognostic significance; however, this has not been shown in all studies (see later, "Prognostic Factors"). Thus, in an effort to account for prognostic factors not included in the Ann Arbor staging system and also the new imaging modalities of CT and magnetic resonance imaging (MRI), a revision to the Ann Arbor staging system called the Cotswolds revision was proposed in 1988.[122] It includes features not considered in the original Ann Arbor system, such as performance status, age, gender, assessments of mediastinal bulk, serum lactate dehydrogenase (LDH), albumin, ESR, total lymphocyte count, and number of nodal sites involved. In pediatrics, both systems are acknowledged, using the broadly accepted approach of adopting risk-adapted therapy based on specific factors shown in large retrospective series to separate patients into distinct prognostic groups for disease-free survival and overall survival.

Clinical Evaluation and Staging Procedures

The purpose of a staging evaluation is to identify all sites and characteristics of Hodgkin's disease in each patient to permit

TABLE 13-6	Recommended Staging Procedures in Children and Adolescents with Hodgkin Lymphoma
Stage	**Mandatory Procedure(s)**
1	History and physical examination by several investigators
2	Laboratory studies—complete blood count, with differential and platelet count; erythrocyte sedimentation rate, C-reactive protein; renal and liver function studies, including albumin, LDH, alkaline phosphatase, anti-EBV VCA, EBNA-1, 2 antibodies
3	Imaging studies Ultrasonography: peripheral lymph node regions, abdomen Chest roentgenography (posteroanterior and lateral views) Computed tomography (CT) of chest, abdomen, and pelvis (see text for discussion) Magnetic resonance imaging (MRI) or CT: abdomen, pelvis, head and neck Positron emission tomography
	Selected Indications
1	CT of head and neck in case of high neck adenopathy or/and suspicion of Waldeyer's ring involvement
2	Bone marrow biopsy, except stages IA, IIA
3	Bone scan in case of bone pain and elevated alkaline phosphatase level; all patients with stage IIB and higher Selective MRI or CT of suspicious lesions Bone biopsy of at least one suspicious lesion
4	Selective lymph node biopsy if involvement or noninvolvement is not unambiguous by physical examination and imaging studies, and if clarification is important for involved field irradiation
5	Selected laparoscopy or laparotomiy and biopsies (without splenectomy) if involvement or noninvolvement of abdominal sites is not unambiguous by imaging studies, and if clarification is important for involved field irradiation
6	Oophoropexy for any girl requiring pelvic irradiation
7	Fine-needle liver biopsy in case of suspected liver involvement

EBV VCA, Epstein-Barr virus viral capsid antigen; EBNA-1, 2, Epstein-Barr nuclear antigen 1, 2; LDH, lactate dehydrogenase.

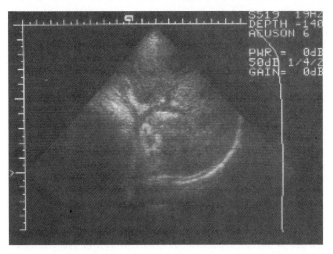

Figure 13-9. Splenic involvement in a child with Hodgkin's lymphoma. The nodal lesions of the spleen are depicted ultrasonographically as areas of reduced echogenicity.

accurate stratification of therapy based on risk, the definition of areas to be included in radiation fields, and follow-up imaging studies. Table 13-6 gives an overview of staging procedures, which are mandatory in all patients, and specific procedures for selected indications. The routine clinical evaluation of children with Hodgkin's lymphoma starts with a careful history and physical examination, with special attention to the lymphoid system. Several physicians representing the disciplines of oncology and radiotherapy should participate in the routine examination of every child. A biopsy should be performed on lymph nodes considered suspicious for involvement with Hodgkin's lymphoma or they should be treated as if they were involved with the disease. Although the growth rate of Hodgkin's lymphoma is variable, it is generally possible to complete thorough staging.

Knowledge of the recognized contiguity of spread of Hodgkin's lymphoma is important in the accuracy of clinical staging. Although lymph nodes in the upper half of the neck, in the anterior and posterior chains, and in the submandibular areas may often be associated with coexisting upper respiratory tract infections in children, firm lymph nodes in the lower half of the neck, including the supraclavicular fossa, are much more likely to indicate a more serious disease. Involvement of the lymphoid tissues of Waldeyer's ring is uncommon in Hodgkin's disease without associated high cervical lymphadenopathy. Asymmetrical tonsillar tissue in a patient with Hodgkin's lymphoma should be considered suspicious for disease involvement. Recommended imaging studies for children do not differ from those in adults, although their interpretation may be more difficult in young patients. Ultrasonography (US), chest x-ray, CT, and MRI are basic diagnostic imaging studies of value in Hodgkin's disease (see Fig. 13-6). These imaging methods have clear applications, depending on the suspected involvement of distinct topographic and anatomic regions. Thus, Doppler-pulsed US may be suitable to identify Hodgkin's lymphoma involvement of peripheral and abdominal nodes and to distinguish them from reactive adenopathy by determining whether the pattern of vascularization is hilar or capsular.[123] Moreover, US is superior to CT and MRI to detect nodal spleen involvement (Fig. 13-9).[124,125] A CT scan of the chest with contrast is particularly helpful for determining the extent of intrathoracic disease and has major value for detecting pulmonary involvement and subtle mediastinal adenopathy in the child with an apparently normal chest radiograph, as well as in the patient with obvious intrathoracic disease. MRI is less accurate for assessing the pulmonary parenchyma than thoracic CT scanning, but MRI is a superior method to detect pleural and pericardial involvement. Differentiating the normal thymus gland from thymic infiltration with Hodgkin's disease is a unique problem in the evaluation of the mediastinum in children.

CT scanning has become widely used as a noninvasive means of evaluating the retroperitoneum in patients with Hodgkin's disease. However, examination of children with Hodgkin's disease by CT scanning and lymphography has shown only an 82% correlation between the two studies, with negative results by both examinations for most patients.[126] The accuracy of CT scanning is hampered because of the following: (1) the nodal involvement of Hodgkin's disease is characteristically focal, with filling defects often too small to be imaged by CT; (2) the enlarged nodes of children that are abnormal on CT scans (larger than 1.5 cm) often represent reactive hyperplasia rather than Hodgkin's disease; (3) children characteristically lack retroperitoneal adipose tissue that provides an interface of nodal tissue against fat to differentiate tissue planes; and (4) children often cannot tolerate adequate amounts of oral contrast material, which makes accurate visualization of normal structures more difficult. MRI may provide better evaluation of retroperitoneal nodes compared with CT, but CT scanning and MRI have as yet not been compared for their value in detecting retroperitoneal adenopathy in children. Abdominal nodes smaller than 1 to 1.5 cm and pelvic nodes smaller than 2 to 2.5 cm are usually considered not to be involved in Hodgkin's disease. CT scanning has a low sensitivity of only 19% for detection of splenic involvement because of the small size of tumor deposits (generally smaller than 5.0 mm) and the absence of splenomegaly in most patients.[127] Similarly, hepatic involvement is rare in Hodgkin's disease.

Skeletal scintigraphy is sensitive to detect involvement of bone. Areas of increased activity in the skeletal scintigraphy should be further examined by CT or MRI. Skeletal scintigraphy as a screening procedure may not be mandatory, but may be confined to patients with symptoms of bone involvement, such as an elevated alkaline phosphatase level, and patients in an advanced stage. If bone lesions are detected by imaging studies, at least one lesion should be biopsied to verify lymphoma.

Bone marrow biopsy is indicated for any child with systemic symptoms at presentation and for those with clinical stage III or IV disease. It is rare to find marrow involvement in patients with clinical stage I or IIA disease.

Lymphoangiography and gallium scanning with gallium-67 are soon going to be replaced by positron emission tomography (PET) scanning.[128-130] PET scanning with ^{18}F-fluorodeoxyglucose (FDG) has become a widely used diagnostic tool for staging and restaging of malignant lymphomas (Fig. 13-10).[131] Increased ^{18}F-FDG uptake in lymphoma is based on elevated glycolysis and the longer residence time of ^{18}F-FDG in malignant cells compared with most normal tissues.[132] Numerous studies in adults with Hodgkin's lymphoma have demonstrated that PET is able to detect an

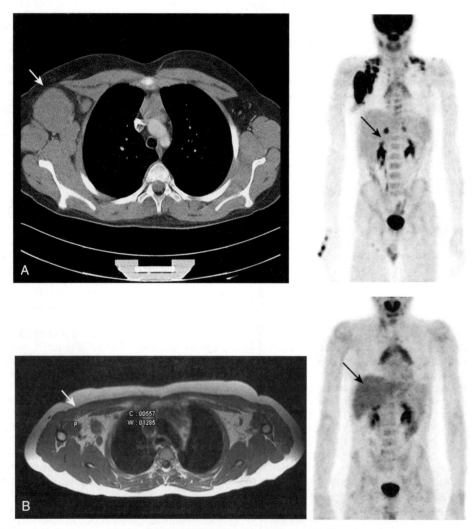

Figure 13-10. Positron emission tomography (PET) with ^{18}F-fluorodeoxyglucose (FDG) and magnetic resonance imaging (MRI) scans of an 11-year-old child with Hodgkin's lymphoma. **A,** At diagnosis, before therapy. Involvement of the right axillary nodes is depicted in this MRI scan (*arrow*). The whole-body FDG-PET scan depicts involvement of axillary and infra- and supraclavicular nodes (*right*) and supraclavicular nodes (*left*) as well as nodal involvement in the liver hilus (*arrow*). Nonspecific activity is seen in the thyroid, brain, kidney, pelvis, and bladder as well as at the site of FDG injection (*right*). **B,** Post-chemotherapy. In the MRI scan, residual nodes are visible in the right axillary region (*arrow*). The FDG-PET scan reveals no specific FDG uptake in the areas of initial disease involvement. (Courtesy of Dr. Mauz-Körholz, Halle, Germany.)

additional number of presumed Hodgkin's lymphoma lesions compared with conventional imaging studies, in particular CT and bone marrow biopsy, resulting in a modification of staging in 15% to 20% of patients, with an impact on disease management in 5% to 15% of cases.[133] Discordant findings occur in both directions, however. PET has demonstrated abnormalities not detectable by CT, resulting in altering staging in 15% to 20% of patients; CT shows abnormalities undetectable by PET with an impact on stage assignment in 10% to 20% of cases. Thus, from these studies, it appears that PET alone cannot replace CT for staging. Abnormal findings only detected by PET, affecting staging and disease management, include Hodgkin's lymphoma involvement of normal-sized lymph nodes, spleen and liver infiltration, and multifocal bone involvement. However, PET alone is unreliable to detect a limited degree of bone marrow (BM) involvement. Thus, PET cannot completely replace BM biopsy. In contrast to the extensive studies on the role of FDG-PET in the management of lymphomas in adults, there are only few studies evaluating the possible role of FDG-PET in childhood lymphoma. All reports have been retrospective studies comparing the results of FDG-PET with conventional imaging methods, such as MRI and/or CT.[130,134] In a retrospective single-center study, Hermann and colleagues[135] have compared FDG-PET with CT findings at initial staging; they evaluated 662 regions in 25 consecutive pediatric patients (17 with Hodgkin's lymphoma and 7 with NHL). Concordant findings were found in 92% of the analyzed regions (78% concordant negative, 14% concordant positive). In 7% of the analyzed regions, discordant findings were found; 4% were classified as PET+/CT–, whereas 3% were classified as PET–/CT+. Discordant findings were more frequent in extranodal regions compared with nodal regions. Staging based on PET findings resulted in a change of staging based on CT findings in 6 of the 25 patients. Increased uptake of FDG is not restricted to malignant cells, but can be observed in other non-malignant tissues with a high level of physiologic glucose metabolism, including the thymus gland and brown fat.[136,137] The limitations of both methods may be reduced by dual-modality PET-CT fusion images.[138,139] However, even in the case of concordant findings in PET and CT, differentiating between reactive hyperplasia (e.g., caused by inflammation) of lymph nodes and nodal tumor spread is not always possible.[135] A main limitation of most studies comparing findings of FDG-PET with findings of conventional imaging methods is the lack of histologic validation of lesions classified as tumor.[135,140] Furthermore, different histopathologic subtypes of Hodgkin's lymphoma show significantly different levels of FDG uptake.[141] Thus, prospective studies are required, not only to evaluate and verify the diagnostic role of FDG-PET in staging, but also to assess whether the different findings of FDG-PET compared with conventional imaging translate into modifications of therapy and whether this then results in improved outcome and/or reduction of treatment burden for patients.

The issue of surgical staging, including splenectomy previously, has been controversial in the management of children with Hodgkin's disease, largely because of concerns of morbidity related to operative staging. With the availability of high-resolution imaging techniques, routine staging laparotomy has now been largely abandoned for the management of pediatric Hodgkin's lymphoma patients.[142] Lymph nodes with a largest diameter of less than 1 cm can generally be considered uninvolved, whereas nodes with a diameter larger than 2 cm are most likely involved. In cases of lymph nodes more than 1 cm but less than 2 cm in size, however, further clarification is necessary. Considering the serious late risk of irradiation, whenever involvement or noninvolvement of a site would significantly influence staging or treatment, especially irradiation, and cannot be clarified unambiguously by physical examina-

tion and imaging studies, it is wise to carry out a biopsy to assess involvement. This applies also to abdominal sites. In the future, FDG-PET can be an alternative noninvasive method to clarify involvement or noninvolvement in such cases.[130] However, even if staging laparoscopy or laparotomy is performed, splenectomy should be avoided because of the late risks, especially in young children. In the German-Austrian experience of 1181 children with Hodgkin's lymphoma, the survival was poorer for children younger than 10 years because of episodes of infection and death caused by sepsis in splenectomized children.[142,143]

Treatment

The optimal setting is to enroll all children and adolescents diagnosed with Hodgkin's lymphoma in controlled clinical studies. Centers treating children with Hodgkin's lymphoma should have extended experience with a dedicated multidisciplinary team, including a pediatric surgeon, radiation oncologist, pediatric oncologist, pathologist, and diagnostic radiologist. If such a team is not available at the facility at which the child is initially seen, prompt referral to a comprehensive childhood cancer center is essential.

Hodgkin's lymphoma has become the malignancy of childhood and adolescence, with the highest cure rates of more than 90%. Because Hodgkin's lymphoma was also one of the first neoplasms with a high degree of curability, Hodgkin's lymphoma is also the prototype of a childhood malignancy winning the prize for successful therapy. Large numbers of former patients reach adult age and become subject to the recognition of late effects. Second cancers, infertility, endocrinologic dysfunction, and growth impairment are the most important. Thus, optimizing the balance of treatment efficacy and the late risks of therapy is the major challenge in the care of children and adolescents suffering from Hodgkin's lymphoma.[144,145]

Prognostic Factors—Stratification of Treatment

As with other malignancies, prognostic factors are useful as tools for defining risk groups for stratification of treatment intensity and treatment modalities. The stage of disease is a strong prognostic factor and widely used for stratification of treatment intensity.[28,142,146] Apart from the stage of disease, a number of variables have been reported to be associated with the risk of treatment failure (Table 13-7). However, there is a correlation between the predictive strength of prognostic factors and the treatment applied. Thus, weak prognostic factors may vanish with improved treatment whereas the impact of treatment on strong prognostic factors may be less pronounced. Furthermore, the prognostic impact of such features may depend on the number of patients investigated and the treatment applied. In a large series of unselected patients who achieved a high disease-free survival rate, the only factors with adverse prognostic impact in all three trials were B symptoms and nodular sclerosis type 2.[142] However, in this series, treatment intensity was already stratified according to presumed prognostic factors. Age at diagnosis and gender had no consistent influence on outcome in different larger studies as had laboratory findings such as subnormal hemoglobin level at diagnosis.[147] However, gender may be a criterion for stratification of treatment after the recognition that spermatogenesis of boys is more vulnerable to the gonadotoxic effect of procarbazine than the reproductive function of females.[148,149] Mediastinal bulky disease—defined as a mass larger than one third of the maximum chest diameter (as visualized on the initial upright

TABLE 13-7   **Risk Stratification of Treatment in Clinical Trials on Pediatric Hodgkin's Lymphoma**

| | STAGE | | |
Study Group	Low Risk	Intermediate Risk	High Risk
DAL-HD 90[142]	IA, IB, IE, IIA	IIEA, IIB, IIIA	IIEB, IIIEA, IIIB, IIIEB, IV
GPOH-HD 95[29]	IA, IB, IIA	IE, IIEA, IIB, IIIA	IIEB, IIIEA, IIIB, IV
CCG 5942[28]	I + IIA, without*	I + II with* IIB, III	IV
Stanford–St. Jude, Boston Consortium[170,663]	I, II, without†	"Unfavorable" I, II with† III, IV	
Pediatric Oncology Group[174,664]	I, IIA, IIIA1	"Unfavorable" IIB, IIIA$_2$, IIIB, IV	

*Adverse disease features (one or more of the following): hilar adenopathy, more than four nodal regions, mediastinal tumor $\geqq$ 33% of chest diameter, node or nodal aggregate with diameter > 10 cm.

†Presence of one or more of the following: bulky disease, peripheral nodal disease 6 cm or larger and/or mediastinal tumor one third of intrathoracic diameter or more, B symptoms.

chest radiograph)—was associated with increased risk for relapse in some studies but not in the German-Austrian trial DAL-HD 90.[150-153] However, differences in treatment details may hamper the comparability. Thus, in the DAL-HD 90 study, patients with a larger residual mass at the end of chemotherapy received a boost dose in addition to the involved field irradiation.[142,153] Similarly, male gender had an adverse impact on outcome in that trial. For boys, however, procarbazine was partially replaced by etoposide but girls received a full dose of procarbazine.

Thus, apart from stage of disease, there is considerable variation in the application of patient or disease-related factors for definition of risk groups and treatment stratification (see Table 13-7). This variability of definitions of risk groups hampers the comparability of results and conclusions from therapeutic studies confined to subgroups of Hodgkin's lymphoma patients. Patients with stage I or II disease are usually referred to as low-risk patients whereas those with stage III or IV are considered intermediate- or high-risk patients. B symptoms and contiguous extranodal involvement are other parameters more frequently used for the stratification of treatment. An interesting finding was that latent EBV infection of Reed-Sternberg cells in pediatric Hodgkin's lymphoma is an independent adverse prognostic factor for overall survival but not for failure-free survival to first-line therapy in the German-Austrian multicenter trials.[65] The kinetics of response to treatment has been elucidated to be the overriding prognostic parameter in many malignancies; for example, leukemia likely best reflecting sensitivity or resistance of the neoplasm. Functional imaging using FDG-PET may be a new tool to evaluate response kinetic (see later).

Treatment Options
Radiotherapy

Radiotherapy was used as the sole treatment modality for adolescents and young adults with limited disease in whom growth and development were not issues. Appropriate irradiation requires megavoltage treatment best administered by a well-collimated photon beam such as that generated by a linear accelerator, ideally of 4- to 8-MV energy. Scatter irradiation and depth dose inadequacies are significant limitations associated with cobalt-60 and orthovoltage and preclude their use. Electron fields may be useful for superficial ports, such as preauricular and femoral fields. Portal films should be obtained for all patients for simulation and verification. Opposed fields are generally used. For young patients who may move or have a risk of daily variation in fields, immobilization devices such as casts may be helpful for improving daily reproducibility. A well-

defined radiation dose-response curve has demonstrated that the risk of recurrence is 10% or less when radiation doses of 35 to 44 Gy are used as sole therapy.[154] When radiation is combined with chemotherapy, doses of 25 Gy or less appear to be adequate. Local control of 97% has been reported with the use of 15 to 25 Gy and six cycles of MOPP chemotherapy (**m**echlorethamine [nitrogen mustard], vincristine [**O**ncovin], **p**rocarbazine, and **p**rednisone).[155] The late sequelae of high-dose extended-volume radiotherapy in children soon became obvious, including musculoskeletal morbidities, growth inhibition, coronary heart disease, and second cancers.[156-159] The late risks of radiotherapy clearly correlate with the dose and volume of irradiation.[159]

Radiotherapy alone is only sufficient if also microscopically involved sites are included in the radiation field. Thus, radiotherapy alone generally requires surgical staging of disease and high-dose extended-field irradiation, or even total nodal irradiation (Fig. 13-11). Today, involved-field radiotherapy alone is not considered the optimal therapy for a child with Hodgkin's disease.[156] Combined-modality treatment combining radiotherapy with chemotherapy was introduced in the 1970s to reduce the late risks of radiotherapy. The introduction of effective chemotherapy made cure possible, even in advanced-stage disease. In addition to providing effective treatment of unrecognized microscopic disease, chemotherapy permitted a reduction in the dose and volume of irradiation to involved fields and made invasive staging procedures, such as laparotomy and splenectomy, unnecessary.[142,155,160-164] In current treatment protocols, radiation fields are reduced even further and individualized, taking into account the tolerance of involved or adjacent extranodal organs (see Fig. 13-11).[142,165] For optimal fractionation, 1.5 to 2 Gy/dose is recommended 5 days/week, with a reduction to 1.5 Gy/dose in case of large radiation volumes. The radiation dose to lung and liver should not exceed 12 to 15 Gy if larger parts of the organ are in the radiation field. Computer-based three-dimensional planning of irradiation provides further optimization of the balance of efficacy and site effects. General principles include the following: (1) avoid asymmetrical irradiation of the spine; (2) avoid irradiation of the tooth bud in case of Waldeyer's ring involvement; (3) block out the heart for doses above 16 to 20 Gy in case of mediastinal tumors; and (4) avoid irradiation of the spleen and testes. In females, irradiation of the breast should be avoided and, in case of pelvic irradiation, transposition of ovaries before pelvic irradiation is essential to preserve ovarian function. Whether the spleen should be routinely irradiated in the case of para-aortic but not overt splenic involvement is controversial. In the setting of controlled clinical trials, a review of staging imaging, recommendations for a radiotherapy plan, and review of radiation compliance can enhance substantially the quality of radiotherapy.[165,166]

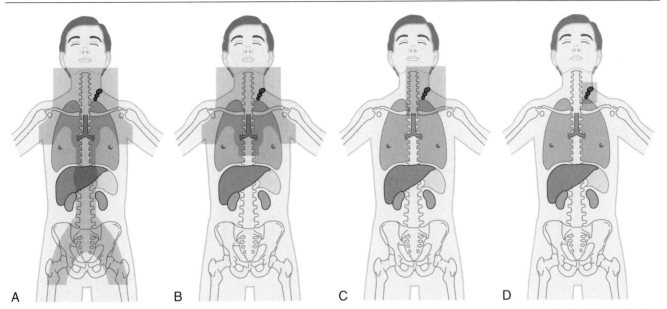

Figure 13-11. Radiation fields for treating Hodgkin's lymphoma. **A,** Total nodal irradiation. **B,** Mantle field. **C,** Involved field. **D,** Radiation field individualized to the patient's local disease, taking into account the tolerance of involved or adjacent extranodal organs. (Courtesy of Dr. W. Dörffel, Berlin.)

Combined-Modality Chemotherapy and Radiotherapy

Combined-modality therapy programs have emerged as the treatment of choice for children and adolescents who suffer from Hodgkin's lymphoma. The combined-modality approach allows the use of clinical staging, lower doses and volumes of radiation, and refined chemotherapy programs. The concept of involved-field radiotherapy combined with six cycles of MOPP chemotherapy was pioneered by the Stanford investigators in children with pathologically staged disease.[155] This pivotal study has served as the model for combined-modality treatment programs in children when therapy is designed to maximize cure and minimize late effects. The invention of the MOPP combination by Devita and coworkers[167] to treat patients with Hodgkin's lymphoma was fundamental for the development of combination chemotherapy. The basic rational was to combine single drugs with proven efficacy but different mechanisms of action and resistance, with few overlapping toxicities, to maximize antitumor effect and limit side effects with moderate doses of individual drugs. The second pivotal combination chemotherapy for the treatment of Hodgkin's lymphoma was ABVD (doxorubicin (*A*driamycin), *b*leomycin, *v*inblastine, *d*acarbazine) developed by Bandanna and coworkers.[168] Six to eight cycles of these two combinations given every 3 to 4 weeks and alternating combinations of both has become a standard of chemotherapy for Hodgkin's lymphoma in adults and children. However, significant but different late risks became obvious with both combinations. The main late risks of MOPP are second cancers, especially leukemia, associated with mechlorethamine, and male infertility associated with procarbazine. ABVD cardiomyopathy caused by doxorubicin and lung fibrosis as a sequelae of bleomycin are main late effects (see later, "Late Effects").

Because of the increased vulnerability of children, the development of combined-modality treatment programs for children and adolescents with Hodgkin's lymphoma since the 1980s has involved a sequence of attempts to provide maximum efficacy and minimize later risk. The main principles of this approach are to substitute drugs with increased risk for serious long-term effects with less dangerous drugs in both combinations, design hybrids of both, and reduce the cumulative dose of dangerous drugs. Table 13-8 gives an overview of chemotherapy combinations that are mainly derived from MOPP and ABVD or their hybrids. The most frequent substitutes are cyclophosphamide for mechlorethamine and etoposide to replace either procarbazine in MOPP or doxorubicin in ABVD. With most of these derivative combinations, comparable high disease-free survival rates could be achieved.[28,29,142,169-171] Some combinations avoided certain dangerous drugs, at least for the treatment of patients with limited-stage disease (Table 13-9). One example is the VAMP regimen of the Stanford-St. Jude-Boston consortium, with moderate cumulative doses of doxorubicin (see Table 13-8) and avoidance of alkylating agents, bleomycin, and etoposide.[169,170] Another example is the combination VBVP, used by a group in France that avoids alkylating agents, anthracyclines, and procarbazine.[171] One approach to limit and even reduce the cumulative doses of drugs that carry later risks is to increase the dose intensity over time, as in the Stanford V regimen for adults.[172]

A stringent strategy to balance efficacy and late risk of the combined-modality of chemotherapy and radiation therapy (RT) by the German-Austrian study group (Table 13-10) includes the following:

- Reduction of cumulative dose of alkylating agents and replacement of mechlorethamine of MOPP by doxorubicin (OPPA) and by cyclophosphamide (in reduced dose of 500 mg/m²) in COPP
- Reduction of radiotherapy (volume, dose, and number of patients who receive RT)
- Reduction of the risk of male infertility by partial replacement of procarbazine by etoposide for boys
- Reduction of invasive staging procedures by almost complete omission of laparotomy and splenectomy
- Refinement of treatment to include extranodal involvement adjacent to nodal disease and early response to therapy as stratification criteria as well as to stage and B symptoms

In two trials, the event-free survival (EFS) probability was comparable to that in the first two trials in the series. However,

TABLE 13-8   Combination Chemotherapy Courses for Treatment of Hodgkin's Lymphoma

Course	Drugs	Dosage and Route	Days
MOPP[155]	Mechlorethamine	6.0 mg/m², IV	1, 8
	Vincristine	1.4 mg/m², IV	1, 8
	Procarbazine	100 mg/m², PO	1-15
	Prednisone	40 mg/m², PO	1-15
MOPP DERIVATIVES			
COPP[160,665]	Cyclophosphamide	600 (500) mg/m², IV	1, 8
	Vincristine	1.4 mg/m², IV (max 2 mg)	1, 8
	Procarbazine	100 mg/m², PO	1-15
	Prednisone	40 mg/m², PO	1-15
COMP[173,665]	Cyclophosphamide	600 mg/m², IV	1, 8
	Vincristine	1.4 mg/m², IV (max 2 mg)	1, 8
	Methotrexate	40 mg/m², IV	1, 8
	Prednisone	40 mg/m², PO	1-15
COP[663]	Cyclophosphamide	600 mg/m², IV	1, 8
	Vincristine	1.4 mg/m², IV (max 2 mg)	1, 8
	Procarbazine	100 mg/m², PO	1-14
ABVD[168]	Doxorubicin	25 mg/m², IV	1, 15
	Bleomycin	10 U/m², IV	1, 15
	Vinblastine	6 mg/m², IV	1, 15
	Dacarbazine	375 mg/m², IV	1, 15
MOPP-ABVD HYBRIDS AND DERIVATIVES			
OPPA[160]	Vincristine	1.5 mg/m², IV (max 2 mg)	1, 8, 15
	Procarbazine	100 mg/m², PO	1-15
	Prednisone	60 mg/m², PO	1-15
	Doxorubicin	40 mg/m², IV	1, 15
OPA[173]	Vincristine	1.5 mg/m², IV (max 2 mg)	1, 8, 15
	Prednisone	60 mg/m², PO	1-15
	Doxorubicin	40 mg/m², IV	1, 15
OEPA[142]	Vincristine	1.5 mg/m², IV (max 2 mg)	1, 8, 15
	Etoposide	125 mg/m², IV	3-6
	Prednisone	60 mg/m², PO	1-15
	Doxorubicin	40 mg/m², IV	1, 15
ChIVPP[666]	Chlorambucil	6 mg/m², PO	1-14
	Vinblastine	6 mg/m², PO	1, 8
	Procarbazine	100 mg/m², PO	1-14
	Prednisone	40 mg/m², PO	1-14
VAMP[169]	Vinblastine	6 mg/m², IV	1, 15
	Doxorubicin	25 mg/m², IV	1, 15
	Methotrexate	20 mg/m², IV	1, 15
	Prednisone	40 mg/m², PO	1-14
VBVP[171]	Vinblastine	6 mg/m², IV	1, 8
	Bleomycin	10 mg/m², IV	1
	Etoposide	100 mg/m², IV	1-5
	Prednisolone	40 mg/m², PO	1-8
COPP-ABV[28]	Cyclophosphamide	600 mg/m², IV	0
	Vincristine	1.4 mg/m², IV	0
	Procarbazine	100 mg/m², PO	0-6
	Prednisolone	40 mg/m², PO	0-13
	Doxorubicin	35 mg/m², IV	7
	Bleomycin	10 U/m², IV	7
	Vinblastine	6 mg/m², IV	7
ABC[28]	A		
	Cytarabine	3 g/m², IV over 3 hr, q12h	0, 1
	Etoposide	200 mg/m², IV over 1 hr, q12h	0, 1
	G-CSF	5 µg/kg, SC	Starting on day 2
	B		
	COPP-ABVD	See COPP/ABVD	21-27
	G-CSF	5 µg/kg SC	Starting on day 28
	C		
	Vincristine	1.4 mg/m², IV	42
	Cyclophosphamide	1200 mg/m², IV	42-43
	Doxorubicin	25 mg/m²/day, continuous infusion	42-44
	Methylprednisolone	250 mg/m², IV q6h	42
	Prednisone	60 mg/m², PO	43-46
	G-CSF	5 µg/kg, SC	Starting on day 46

TABLE 13-8	Combination Chemotherapy Courses for Treatment of Hodgkin Lymphoma—cont'd		
Course	**Drugs**	**Dosage and Route**	**Days**
BEACOPP[667]	Bleomycin	10 U/m^2, IV	8
	Etoposide	200 mg/m^2, IV	1-3
	Doxorubicin	35 mg/m^2, IV	1
	Cyclophosphamide	1200 mg/m^2, IV	1
	Vincristine	2 mg/m^2 (max, 2 mg), IV	8
	Procarbazine	100 mg/m^2, PO	1-7
	Prednisone	40 mg/m^2, PO	1-14
DBVE[664]	Doxorubicin	25 mg/m^2, IV	1, 15
	Bleomycin	10 mg/m^2, SC	1, 15
	Vincristine	1.5 mg/m^2 (max, 2 mg), IV	1, 15
	Etoposide	100 mg/m^2, IV over 1 hr	1-5
Stanford V[172]	Mechlorethamine	6 mg/m^2, IV	1
	Vinblastine	6 mg/m^2, IV	1, 15
	Doxorubicin	25 mg/m^2, IV	1, 15
	Etoposide	60 mg/m^2, IV	15, 16
	Vincristine	1.4 mg/m^2 (max, 2 mg) IV	8, 22
	Bleomycin	5 U/m^2, IV	8, 22
	Prednisone	40 mg/m^2, PO	Every other day

G-CSF, granulocyte colony-stimulating factor.

the impact of distinct drugs became evident in the DAL-HD 85 study, when procarbazine was omitted without substitution for low-risk patients and low-dose methotrexate was substituted for intermediate- and high-risk patients to reduce gonadotoxicity. This study was stopped prematurely because of an excess of relapses compared with the previous study, DAL-HD 82. Subsequently, procarbazine has partially replaced etoposide for boys, whereas females receive full-dose procarbazine because of their lower risk of gonadal toxicity.[148,173]

In summary, when combining chemotherapy with radiotherapy, the balance of efficacy and later risk of standard MOPP-ABVD can be optimized by the following:

• Reducing cumulative doses of drugs with increased later risk
• Replacing drugs with increased later risk
• Reducing volume and dose of radiotherapy
• Stratifying treatment intensity and modality based on the patient's risk for relapse

A powerful tool for treatment optimization is prospective clinical trials, especially large multicenter trials that enroll random groups of patients. In several study groups of pediatric and adolescent Hodgkin's lymphoma, patients have been generally divided into low-, intermediate-, and high-risk groups. Many reports from these therapeutic studies are confined to a distinct risk group of patients. Table 13-11 summarizes treatment strategy and results of therapeutic studies confined to patient subgroups defined as low- or as intermediate- and high-risk patients, respectively (also see Table 13-9). The comparisons and conclusions from trials confined to patient subsets need to be interpreted with caution, however, because the definition of low risk and high risk and therefore the composition of subgroups vary considerably for each study. To remedy this shortcoming, the percentage of the respective risk group in the total group of Hodgkin's lymphoma patients and the treatment outcome for that group should be considered. Table 13-12 summarizes patient characteristics, stratification criteria, treatment strategy, and outcome from three large multicenter trials that enrolled children and adolescents newly diagnosed with Hodgkin's lymphoma in North America and Western Europe, respectively.[28,29,142] Clinical characteristics and the distribution of histologic subtypes can be compared. In all three studies, treatment intensity was stratified into three therapy groups. Although the Ann Arbor stage of the disease and presence of B symptoms were basic stratification criteria in all three studies, the composition of the three risk groups differed considerably because of the application of different criteria and the group allocation for risk stage. In the Children's Cancer Group (CCG) trial 5942, disease features deemed to be of adverse prognostic impact, such as hilar adenopathy, involvement of more than four nodal regions, presence of a mediastinal tumor more than one third of the chest diameter, or node aggregate with a diameter more than 10 cm, were used to group patients with stage I or II disease in the intermediate-risk group. In contrast, the German-Austrian-Scandinavian studies included extranodal tissue or organs adjacent to nodal disease as a criterion for grouping patients with limited stage disease into intermediate- and high-risk groups.

As a result, in the DAL-HD 90 and GPOH-HD 95 trials, the low-risk group contained 46% and 40%, respectively, of the total group of patients compared with 26% in the CCG trial. The high-risk group was twice as large in the DAL-HD 90 and GPOH-HD 95 trials compared with the CCG trial, in which the intermediate-risk group was the largest risk group. Although similar, comparing treatment outcome by risk groups may be invalid because of their difference in composition. However, the event-free and overall survival probability for the total group was similar in all three trials; the goal was to reduce later risks for the patients. There was, however, a different weighing of treatment components that carry special later risks. In the DAL-HD 90 and GPOH-HD 95 trials, no typical alkylating agent was given to the lowest risk group, which was comprised of about 40% of patients. Furthermore, boys in the low-risk group did not receive procarbazine to prevent testicular function but were given a moderate dose of etoposide as a substitute. In the high-risk group, comprised of one third of patients, rather high cumulative doses of the gonadotoxic procarbazine were included, whereas in the CCG trial, procarbazine was partially outweighed by slightly higher doses of other drugs. Both the CCG 5942 and GPOH-HD 95 trials focused on reducing the proportion of patients who receive radiotherapy based on their early responses to chemotherapy. Interestingly,

Text continues on p. 440

TABLE 13-9   Combined-Modality Treatment Strategy and Results for Selected Low-Risk Patients with Hodgkin's Lymphoma in Multicenter Trials

Group or Institution	No. of Patients	Stage	Chemotherapy*	Radiation (Gy), field	EFS or RFS Overall (%)	Survival (%)	Median Follow-up (Yr)	Adverse Prognostic Factors
Royal Marsden[666]	125	II	6-10 ChlVPP	35, IF	85	92	10	ng
DAL–HD 90[142]	267	I, IIA	Female: OPPA, ×2 Male: OEPA, ×2	IF, 25 Gy in TG 1, 2; IF, 20 Gy in TG 2; residual tumor, 30-35 Gy				ng
GPOH-HD 95[29]	281	I, IIA	Female: OPPA, ×2 Male: OEPA, ×2	CR‖: no RT (22%); non-CR: IF, 20 Gy; residual tumor, 30-35 Gy	94	NA	5	ng
French Society of Pediatric Oncology[171]	171 27	I, II I, II	4 VBVP, good responders; 4 VBVP + 1 or 2 OPPA, poor responders	20, IF 20, IF	91 78	97.5	5	Nodular sclerosis; Hb < 10.5 g/dL; B symptoms[†]
Stanford–St. Jude Boston Consortium[663]	15 62	I, II	3 VAMP, 3 COP 3 VAMP, 3 COP	15-25.5, IF 15-25.5, IF	100 78	NA NA	5.8	ng
Stanford–St. Jude Boston Consortium[170]	110	I, II§	4 VAMP	15-25.5, IF	93 (5 yr)	99	9.6	Two sites; non-CR end of chemotherapy[‡]
CCG 5942[28]		I + IIA without§	COPP-ABV × 4	CR,¶ random: IF-RT 21 Gy vs. no RT; PR, 21 Gy IF	95 (3 yr)	ng	ng	ng
POG 9226[664]	51	I, IIA, IIIA1	4 DBVE	25, IF	91(6 yr)	98	ng	ng

*For the composition of combination chemotherapy courses, see Table 13-8.
†Multivariate.
‡Univariate.
§Low risk is defined as stage I or II, peripheral nodal disease, <6 cm, mediastinal tumor smaller than one third of intrathoracic diameter, absence of extranodal involvement.
‖CR defined as reduction of tumor volume of >95% and residual mass < 2 mL.
¶CR defined as >70% reduction of initial tumor volume and gallium-negative if initially gallium-positive.
CR, complete remission; ng, not given in the report; Hb, hemoglobin; IF, involved field; IF-RT, involved field radiotherapy; PR, partial remission; RT, radiotherapy; TG 1, 2, therapy group 1, 2.

TABLE 13-10 Development of Treatment Strategy and Outcome for Children and Adolescents with Hodgkin's Lymphoma in Six Subsequent Trials of the German-Austrian Multicenter Study Group

Study	No. of Patients (EFS)*	THERAPY GROUP 1			THERAPY GROUP 2			THERAPY GROUP 3		
		Stages (% of patients) EFS†	Chemotherapy	Radiotherapy	Stages (% of patients) EFS†	Chemotherapy	Radiotherapy	Stages (% of patients) EFS*	Chemotherapy	Radiotherapy
DAL-HD 78[160]	170 (92%)	I, IIA (43%, 95%)	OPPA, ×2	EF, 36-40 Gy	>IIA (57%, 89%)	OPPA, ×2 COPP, ×4	EF, 36-40 Gy	Included in TG 2		
DAL-HD 82[163]	203 (96%)	I, IIA (49%, 99%)	OPPA, ×2	IF, 35 Gy	IIB, IIIA (26%, 96%)	OPPA, ×2 COPP, ×2	IF, 30 Gy§	IIIB, IV (25%, 87%)	OPPA, ×2 COPP, ×4	25 Gy§
DAL-HD 85[164]	103 (77%)	I, IIA 58% 59%	OPA, ×2	IF, 35 Gy	IIB, IIIA (20%, 62%)	OPA, ×2 COMP, ×2	IF, 30 Gy§	IIIB, IV (22%, 62%)	OPA, ×2 COMP, ×4	25 Gy§
DAL-HD 87[668]	204 (85%)	I, IIA (51%, 84%)	OPA, ×2	IF, 30 Gy§	IE, IIEA IIB, IIIA (17%, 82%)	OPPA, ×2 COPP, ×2	25 Gy§	IIIB, IV 28%, 89%	OPPA, ×2 COPP, ×4	25 Gy§
DAL-HD 90[142]	578 (91%)	I, IIA (46%) 94%	OPPA, ×2† OEPA ×2‡	IF, 25 Gy§	IE, IIEA IIB, IIIA (21%, 93%)	OPPA, ×2† COPP, ×2 OEPA, ×2‡ COPP, ×2	25 Gy§	IIEB, IIIEA IIIB, IV (31%, 86%)	OPPA, ×2† COPP, ×4 OEPA, ×2‡ COPP, ×4	20 Gy§
GPOH-HD 95[29]	1018 (88%)	I, IIA (40%, 94%)	OPPA, ×2† OEPA, ×2‡	CR: no RT (28%)‖; non-CR: IF, 20 Gy§	IE, IIEA IIB, IIIA (26%, 87%)	OPPA, ×2† COPP, ×2 OEPA, ×2‡ COPP, ×2	CR: no RT (19%)‖; non-CR: IF 20 Gy§	IIEB, IIIEA IIIB, IV (33%; 83%)	OPPA, ×2† COPP, ×4 OEPA, ×2‡ COPP, ×4	CR: no RT (17%)‖; non-CR: IF, 20 Gy§

For the composition of combination chemotherapy courses, see Table 13-8.
*EFS at 5 yr.
†Female.
‡Male.
§Boost to residual tumor to 30-35 Gy.
‖Percentage of patients in the treatment subgroup who did not receive radiotherapy.
EF, extended field; EFS, event-free survival; IF, involved field; TG 2, therapy group 2.

TABLE 13-11   Combined-Modality Treatment Strategy and Results for Selected Intermediate- and High-Risk Patients with Hodgkin's Lymphoma in Multicenter Trials

Group or Institution	No. of Patients	Stage	Chemotherapy	Radiation (Gy), Field	Survival (%; DFS, EFS, or RFS at 5 yr)	Overall Survival (%)	Follow-up Interval (yr)	Adverse Prognostic Factors
DAL-HD-90[142]	179	IIₑB, IIIₑA, B, IIIB, IVA, B	2 OEPA-OPPA + 4 COPP	IF, 25 Gy in TG 1, 2; IF, 20 Gy in TG 3, residual tumor 30-35 Gy	83, 91	98, 89	5	B symptoms; nodular sclerosis type 2*
GPOH-HD-95[29]	265	IIₑA, IIIₑA, B, IIIB, IVA, B	2 OPPA/OEPA + 4 COPP	CR‖: no RT (22%); non-CR: IF, 20 Gy; residual tumor, 30-35	90	90	5	ng
Stanford[155]	28	III-IV	6 MOPP	15-25.5, IF	84	78	7.5	ng
Stanford–St. Jude-Boston Consortium[663]	159	I-II unfavorable,‡ III, IV	3 VAMP/3 COP	15-25.5,§ IF	76	93		Hb < 11 g/dL; WBC > 13,500/μL
Pediatric Oncology Group[174]	80	IIB, IIIA₂, IIIB, IV	4 MOPP, 4 ABVD	21, EF	80	87	5	Non-CR after 3 cycles;† age > 13 yr
U.S. Children's Cancer Group[28]	394	I/IIB, IIB, III	6 COPP-ABV	21, IF	87	95	3	ng
U.S. Children's Cancer Group[28]	141	CS IV	COPP-ABV + CHOP + Ara-C	21, IF	90	100	3	ng

For the composition of combination chemotherapy courses, see Table 13-8.
*Multivariate.
†Univariate.
‡Defined as presence of one or more of the following: bulky disease: peripheral nodal disease 6 cm or larger or/and mediastinal tumor one third of intrathoracic diameter or larger, B symptoms.
§15 Gy for nonbulky sites and complete response after two cycles of chemotherapy.
‖CR defined as reduction of tumor volume of >95% and residual mass < 2 mL.
CR, complete remission; DFS, disease-free survival; EFS, event-free survival; Hb, hemoglobin; IF, involved field; ng, not given in report; RFS, relapse-free survival; TG 1, 2, 3 therapy group 1, 2, 3; WBC, white blood cell count.

TABLE 13-12 **Patient Characteristics, Treatment Strategy, and Results of Unselected Children and Adolescents with Hodgkin's Lymphoma**

Parameter	STUDY		
	CCG 5942[28]	DAL-HD-90[142]	GPOH-HD-95[29]
No. of patients	829	578	1018
Age, yr	0-21	2.7-17.9	2-18
Stage I	16%	15%	7%
Stage II	52%	51%	59%
Stage III	15%	19%	21%
Stage IV	17%	15%	12%
B symptoms	26%	32%	32%
	Rye Classification	Rye Classification	WHO Classification
HISTOLOGY			
NSHL	76.8%	65.2%	68.3%
MCHL	10.2%	24.2%	21.0%
LDHL	0.3%	0.5%	0.7%
Lymphocyte-predominant	9.4%	9.9%	LRHL, 0.7%; NLPHL: 9.3%
Unclassified	3.1%		
Stratification			
TG 1 (%)	I + IIA without* (26)	IA, IB, IE, IIA (46)	IA, IB, IIA (40)
TG 2 (%)	IIB, III, I + II with* (47)	IIEA, IIB, IIIA (21)	IE, IIEA, IIB, IIIA (26)
TG 3 (%)	IV (17)	IIEB, IIIEA, IIIB, IIIEB, IV (31)	IIEB, IIIEA, IIIB, IV (33)
CHEMOTHERAPY			
TG 1	COPP-ABV, ×4	F: OPPA, ×2 M: OEPA, ×2	F: OPPA, ×2 M: OEPA, ×2
TG 2	COPP-ABV, ×6	F: OPPA, ×2, COPP, ×2 M: OEPA ×2, COPP ×2	F: OPPA, ×2, COPP, ×2 M: OEPA, ×2, COPP, ×2
TG 3	ABC, ×2	F: OPPA, ×2, COPP, ×4 M: OEPA, ×2, COPP, ×4	F: OPPA, ×2, COPP, ×4 M: OEPA, ×2, COPP, ×4

	TG 1	TG 2	TG 3	TG 1	TG 2	TG 3	TG 1	TG 2	TG 3
Patients (%)	26	47	17	46	21	31	40	26	33
Cumulative dosage (mg/m²/TG)									
Cyclophosphamide	2400	3600	6000	0	2000	4000	0	2000	4000
Procarbazine	2800	4200	1400	F: 3000	6000	9000	F: 3000	6000	9000
				M: 0	3000	6000	M: 0	3000	6000
Doxorubicin	140	210	220	160	160	160	160	160	160
Bleomycin	40	60	20	0	0	0	0	0	0
Etoposide	0	0	1600	F: 0	0	0	F: 0	0	0
				M: 1000	1000	1000	M: 1000	1000	1000

Radiotherapy	CR†, random: 251 pts, IF-RT 21 Gy; 250 pts, no RT (30%) PR, 21 Gy IF	IF 25 Gy in TG 1, 2; IF 20 Gy in TG 2; residual tumor, 30-35 Gy	CR‡: no RT (22%); non-CR: IF, 20 Gy; residual tumor, 30-35 Gy
EFS (all)	87% (at 3 yr)	91% (at 5 yr)	88% (at 5 yr)
Survival	95% (at 3 yr)	98% (at 5 yr)	97% (at 5 yr)
EFS TG 1	95% (at 3 yr)	94% (at 5 yr)	94% (at 5 yr)
EFS TG 2	82% (at 3 yr)	93% (at 5 yr)	87% (at 5 yr)
EFS TG 3	83% (at 3 yr)	86% (at 5 yr)	83% (at 5 yr)
Prognostic factors (multivariate)	Not reported	B symptoms; nodular sclerosis type 2	Not reported

For the composition of combination chemotherapy courses, see Table 13-8.

*adverse disease features (one or more of the following): hilar adenopathy, more than four nodal regions, mediastinal tumor ≥33% of chest diameter, node or nodal aggregate with diameter >10 cm.

†Defined as presence of >70% reduction of initial tumor volume and gallium-negative if initially gallium-positive.

‡Defined as presence of reduction of tumor volume of >95% and residual mass <2 mL.

CR, complete remission; EFS, event-free survival; F, female; IF, involved field; IF-RT, involved-field radiotherapy; LRHL, lymphocyte- rich Hodgkin's lymphoma; M, male; NLPHL, nodular lymphocyte-predominant Hodgkin's lymphoma; PR, partial remission; pts, patients; RT, radiation therapy; TG 1, 2, 3, therapy group 1, 2, 3.

the percentage of patients who did not receive radiotherapy was comparable in both studies, as were the overall results.

Whether radiotherapy can be omitted from treatment for at least some children and adolescents with Hodgkin's lymphoma is one of the important questions in ongoing and future clinical trials. The results were inconsistent in the few clinical trials that addressed this question in randomized fashion. In the Pediatric Oncology Group (POG) trial 8725, patients with stages IIB, IIIA2, IIIB, and IV were randomized to receive eight alternating cycles of MOPP-ABVD chemotherapy, followed by total nodal irradiation (21 Gy) or no radiotherapy in cases of complete remission.[174] There was no difference in event-free survival (EFS) and a statistically nonsignificant higher overall survival of patients who received no radiotherapy in the beginning. However, it was difficult to determine the effect of radiotherapy in the combined-modality approach in this trial because there were more cycles of chemotherapy that included MOPP than in most of the concurrent studies. In the CCG 5942 trial (see Table 13-12), including all disease stages, patients received for their risk group four or six cycles of COPP-ABV or six cycles of ABC chemotherapy (see Table 13-8).[28] Patients with at least a 75% tumor volume reduction and negative gallium scan at the completion of chemotherapy were randomized to receive or not receive involved-field radiotherapy (IFRT) with 21 Gy. This randomized trial was stopped because of a significantly higher number of relapses, mostly at sites in the no-IFRT arm. However, patients who did not receive IFRT had a fairly high EFS probability at 3 years from the time of randomization of 85% ± 2.3% compared with 93% ± 2.2% of patients with IFRT. Furthermore, the overall survival probability was almost identical for patients of both randomization arms. Importantly, the probability of EFS (87%) and overall survival (95%) of that study's total population compared well with concurrent large multicenter trials with comparable late-risk potential of the chemotherapy applied (see Table 13-11).

Provided that longer follow-up will sustain these findings, especially the rather favorable outcome of nonirradiated patients, important conclusions can be drawn from the CCG 5942 study. There appears to be a significant proportion of children and adolescents with Hodgkin's lymphoma who can be cured with only chemotherapy, imparting moderate late-risk potential. Pediatric oncologists should keep the latter in mind. Chemotherapy alone may prove as effective as combined-modality treatment, but not at the expense of excessive doses, which increases the risk of late sequelae other than the late-risk potential of radiotherapy.

Furthermore, there is little room to accept a certain increase of the relapse rate when attempting to reduce the treatment burden, even given the fair chance that Hodgkin's lymphoma patients will survive with salvage therapy. Studies of long-term survivors have clearly indicated that salvage treatment for relapse significantly increases the risk for NHL mortality, especially as a result of second cancers.[159,175-178] The potential value of moderate-dose IFRT in a combined-modality treatment strategy is underlined by the fact, that across different studies, about 80% of all relapses occur at initially involved sites, whereas relapses at new sites are rare.[28,142,147] However, especially with respect to the risk of second cancers, there may be no real safe dose of radiotherapy. The increased risk of a second cancer appears to be equal to the dose of radiotherapy only in the very low dose range (between 2 to 5 and 10 Gy), and may increase only slightly with higher doses.[179,180]

Moderate chemotherapy alone without radiotherapy may be a successful treatment, especially in cases of tumors with high susceptibility to chemotherapy. The major task for the near-future may be to identify patients with a high predictive value. Patients with an early response to chemotherapy, indicating sensitivity to chemotherapy, may be promising candidates.

A favorable prognostic impact of complete response after two to four cycles of chemotherapy was observed in several studies.[170,174] In those trials, treatment response was mainly evaluated clinically with conventional imaging, including MRI and histologic examination of residual masses. However, a residual mass on imaging may not per se herald later relapse, because this mass often consists only of fibrosis and necrotic tissue. However, even biopsy may not preclude the ultimate prognostic meaning of a tumor remnant because of its heterogeneous composition. Functional imaging methods such as gallium scanning and PET are able to distinguish metabolic active tissue from necrosis. In the revised response criteria for malignant lymphoma, especially Hodgkin's lymphoma, PET is now the approved and preferred imaging method; gallium scanning is no longer considered state of the art.[181,182] The accuracy of PET to monitor treatment response in Hodgkin's lymphoma patients has been sustained in several studies. Moreover, the accuracy of PET to predict treatment outcome appears higher early in the course of treatment as compared with the end of chemotherapy.[183-185] In a prospective study including 77 adult Hodgkin's lymphoma patients receiving combined-modality treatment, early interim PET after two courses of chemotherapy was stronger than any other prognostic factor, including stage, in multivariate analysis.[183] Ten of 16 patients with positive PET after two cycles suffered from subsequent progress as compared with 3 of 61 patients with negative PET after two cycles. Most studies were performed in adults with Hodgkin's lymphoma. In the German-Austrian study GPOH-HD 2002, the predictive strength on outcome of early PET after two cycles and interim PET after four cycles was prospectively evaluated.[186] Published results are pending. However, evidence is accumulating that early PET, after one to three courses of chemotherapy, ideally in combination with a CT scan, appears to be a powerful tool to identify those patients with sufficient susceptibility for treatment with chemotherapy alone, with acceptable toxicity.

Treatment of Patients with Inherited or Acquired Immunodeficiency and Hodgkin's Lymphoma

A special challenge constitutes the treatment of children with inherited immunodeficiency syndrome suffering from Hodgkin's lymphoma, especially those with chromosomal breakage syndromes caused by their reduced tolerance to chemotherapy.[187] For these children, treatment needs to be adapted to their impaired therapy tolerance. However, patients with HIV-AIDS may tolerate standard therapy for Hodgkin's lymphoma.[188]

Relapsed Patients

Children and adolescents with Hodgkin's lymphoma have a fair chance to survive, even after failure of first therapy. Thus, in most series, overall survival probability is significantly higher than progression-free survival. However, in contrast to first-line therapy there is at present no established standard salvage therapy. There is some controversy about the role of high-dose chemotherapy with autologous hematopoietic stem cell transplantation (HDT-AHSCT) in the treatment of children and adolescents with recurrent disease. In a prospective randomized trial of the German Hodgkin's Lymphoma Study Group, adults with chemosensitive relapse had a significantly higher failure-free survival probability when treated with two cycles of dexamethasone, carmustine, etoposide, cytarabine, and melphalan (Dexa-BEAM) followed by HDT-AHSCT therapy as compared with patients receiving four cycles of Dexa-BEAM without HDT-AHSCT.[189] For childhood Hodgkin's lymphoma, there are very few prospective or even randomized trials. In a retrospective study of 51 pediatric patients with recurrent Hodgkin's lymphoma treated with different salvage regimens, there was a beneficial impact of HDT-AHSCT on survival only for patients with Hodgkin's lymphoma refractory or progressive to first-line therapy, but not for patients with later relapses.[190] The subgroup of patients receiving HDT-AHSCT was negatively selected, especially for the time point of failure to first-line therapy. Table 13-13 depicts the results of three larger studies of pediatric patients with progressive or recurrent Hodgkin's lymphoma. Whereas in the Nebraska and Stanford series all patients were to receive HDT-AHSCT, in the German-Austrian DAL-GPOH study HDT-AHSCT was performed in only 30% of the 176 patients. In that prospective study, overall, progression-free, and event-free survival probabilities of patients who failed first-line therapy compared well with those studies in which all patients received HDT-AHSCT.

In the DAL-GPOH study, there was a survival advantage only for patients who received HDT-AHSCT after second or subsequent relapse compared with patients not receiving HDT-AHSCT, but no advantage for those who had undergone HDT-AHSCT after first recurrence. Data from that study and a recent reported POG study have suggested that for many children and adolescents with recurrent Hodgkin's lymphoma, salvage chemotherapy combined with IFRT provides a fair chance for cure and avoidance of the late risks of HDT-AHSCT, among them pulmonary injury and second cancer (see later, "Late Effects").[178,191] The choice of salvage chemotherapy may depend on that used in first-line treatment and on the time to treatment failure. ABVD and COPP, if not used as first-line therapy, are salvage therapy options.[192,193] Combinations of ifosfamide, etoposide, and carboplatin (ICE) or ifosfamide, etoposide, and prednisone (IEP) have proved efficacious, especially in patients with early failure to front-line therapy.[178] Table 13-14 depicts chemotherapy courses for rescue, including

TABLE 13-13   Salvage Treatment and Outcome of Progressive and Recurrent Hodgkin's Lymphoma of Childhood and Adolescence

Parameter	STUDY			
	Nebraska[194]	Stanford[193]	DAL-GPOH[178]	POG[191]
No. of patients	53	41	176	31
First treatment failure	Not given	36	176	25
Subsequent failure	Not given	5	0	6
Initial presentation with:				
B symptoms	40%	56%	47%	Not given
Extranodal involvement	Not given	54%	36%	50%
Front-line therapy‡	Not given	MOPP, ABVD, COPP, VEPA, VAMP, Stanford V IF-RT	OPPA, OPA, OEPA, COPP, COMP; IF-RT, 20-35 Gy	MOPP-ABVD radiotherapy (n = 23)
Time to failure to front-line therapy	Not given	Initial remission, 23.5 mo (3-75)	Initiation of first therapy to recurrence, 1.1 yr (0.1-15.3)	First diagnosis to relapse, 19 mo (4-53)
Salvage				
Salvage chemotherapy‡	Not given	MOPP, DHAP, ICE	IEP, ABVD, COPP, 3-6 courses	APE, 8 cycles
Salvage radiotherapy	77% of patients	IF-RT, 4 patients	IF-RT, depending on radiation dose in first therapy, medium maximum dose, 25 Gy (0-44)	Optional
Autologous HSCT	53	41	53* (30%)	13 (42%)†
Median follow-up, yr	5.4 (0.5-11.9)	4.2 (0.7-11.9)	5.0 (0.1-17.1)	
Survival	43% (at 5 yr)	68% (at 5 yr)	75% (at 10 yr)	34% (at 8 yr)
EFS	Nd	53% (at 5 yr)	57% (at 10 yr)	23% (at 8 yr)
PFS	31% (at 5 yr)	63 (at 5 yr)	62% (at 10 yr)	Not given
Subsequent relapse	35	13	61	Not given
Death of HL	21	11	36	Not given
Toxic death	7	5	4	Not given
Second cancer	2	1	8 (4 deaths)	Not given
Death total	30	16	44	Not given
Adverse prognostic factors for survival (multivariate)	Chemorefractory disease; interval from diagnosis to HSCT ≤ 15 mo; increased LDH	Primary induction failure Initial extranodal disease; bulky mediastinal tumor at AHSCT	Primary progressive disease <3 mo after completion of front-line therapy Procarbazine-etoposide in front-line therapy; female gender	

*18 in 2; CR, 35 after recurrence subsequent to conventional salvage chemoradiotherapy.
†6 after subsequent relapse to APE therapy.
‡See Table 13-8.
AHSCT, autologous hematopoietic stem cell transplantation; CR, complete remission; HL, Hodgkin's lymphoma; HSCT, hematopoietic stem cell transplantation; IF-RT, involved-field radiotherapy; LDH, lactate dehydrogenase.

TABLE 13-14 Salvage Chemotherapy for Hodgkin's Lymphoma other than MOPP/ABVD-Derivatives

Study	Agent	Dosage	Days
DHAP[669]	Dexamethasone	40 mg IV (total, adults)	1-4
	Cisplatin	100 mg/m² 24-hr IV infusion	1
	Cytarabine	2 g/m² IV q12h	2
Dexa-BEAM[670]	Dexamethasone	12 mg/m² PO	1-10
	BCNU	60 mg/m² IV 1 hr	2
	Etoposide	150 mg/m² IV 2 hr	4-7
	Cytarabine	100 mg/m² IV 30 min, q12h	4-7
	Melphalan	20 mg/m² IV	3
IEP[178]	Ifosfamide	2,000 mg/m² continuous IV infusion, 24h	1-5
	Etoposide	125 mg/m², IV 2 hr	1-5
	Prednisone	100 mg/m², PO	1-5
APE[191]	Sequence of:		
	Cytarabine	375 mg/m² infusion, 10 min	Sequence repeated q12h for 3-4 per cycle and days 1, 2
	Cytarabine	125 mg/m² infusion, 60 min	
	Eoposide	20 mg/m² infusion, 20 min	
	Cytarabine	250 mg/m² infusion, 90 min	
	Cisplatin	15 mg/m² infusion, 20 min	
High-dose chemotherapy BEAM[189,671]	BCNU	300 mg/m² IV	-7
	Etoposide	150 mg/m² IV, q12h	-7 to -4
	Cytarabine	200 mg/m² IV, q12h	-7 to -4
	Melphalan	140 mg/m² IV	-3
CBV[194]	Cyclophosphamide	1,500 mg/m², ×4	Not given
	BCNU	300 mg/m² IV, ×1	
	Etoposide	125 mg/m² IV, ×6	
BEC[193]	BCNU	10-15 mg/kg, IV	-6
	Etoposide	60 mg/kg IV	-4
	Cyclophosphamide	100 mg/kg IV	-2

For the composition of combination chemotherapy courses, see Table 13-8.

HDT for AHSCT. The dosage of salvage IFRT ranges from 10 to 30 Gy, depending on the local radiation dose applied during front-line treatment.[178]

Despite the different uses of HDT-AHSCT in all three studies listed in Table 13-13, the time to first treatment failure was the most powerful prognostic factor for outcome in multivariate analyses. Patients with early progressive disease during or shortly after first-line therapy had significantly worse outcomes to salvage in terms of progression-free and overall survival.[178,193,194] Thus, for those patients and for patients with relapse subsequent to HDT-AHSCT, new treatment options are warranted in the future. Allogeneic HSCT after reduced intensity conditioning may be an option for these patients because there appears to be a graft–versus–Hodgkin's lymphoma effect.[195-200]

Nodular Lymphocyte–Predominant Hodgkin's Lymphoma

NLPHL, which corresponds to lymphocyte-predominant Hodgkin's disease of the Rye classification, is now considered a separate disease with distinct biologic and clinical features, such as male predominance, limited-stage disease, and a tendency for later relapses than CHL. Although Hodgkin's lymphoma patients with NLPHL are included in most therapeutic studies of childhood and adolescent Hodgkin's lymphoma, uncertainty exists as to whether these patients deserve identical treatment to patients with CHL, especially if they need further therapy after complete resection of localized disease. In some studies, these patients have better prognoses compared with patients with CHL, but not in others.[142,170,201-203] In a prospective trial of French investigators, 13 (stage I, 11; stage III, 2) of 27 patients with NLPHL received no further treatment after surgical resection whereas 14 (stage I, 11) patients received chemotherapy with or without (n = 1) IFRT.[204] Event-free survival was significantly higher for patients receiving complementary treatment as compared with those without further therapy. However, of the 9 patients with initial complete resection and no subsequent treatment, 6 remained free of relapse for follow-up times of 32 to 172 months, and 3 patients relapsed 5 to 24 months after resection; all 3 patients could be rescued. The French investigators concluded from their observations that a watchful waiting approach for patients with complete remission (CR) after initial surgery is appropriate. However, a careful postoperative staging is essential to exclude further manifestations. Patients with more extended disease require complementary treatment, which needs to be defined in prospective trials.

Late Effects

Given the high rate of curability of children and adolescents with Hodgkin's lymphoma, the late risks of their treatment become a major issue over the long term for these young people. In the scientific literature, the number of reports on late sequelae after successful treatment of pediatric Hodgkin's lymphoma patients presumably has exceeded that of reports on prospective therapeutic trials. These reports mainly visualized late sequelae connected with earlier treatment approaches of pediatric Hodgkin's lymphoma, as early as the 1960s. The treatment for pediatric Hodgkin's lymphoma since then has been a continuous process of outweighing efficacy and risks of therapy. Therefore, many of the reports may not necessarily indicate late risks of current treatment strategies.

TABLE 13-15	Late Effects of Treatment of Children and Adolescents with Hodgkin's Lymphoma		
Late Effect	**Radiotherapy**	**Chemotherapy**	**Staging Procedures**
Musculoskeletal growth impairment[156]	x		
Cardiomyopathy[205]		Anthracyclines	
Cardiovascular and conduction disorders[158,206]	x		
Stroke[207]	x		
Infections (overwhelming postsplenectomy infections)[143,175,208]			Splenectomy; spleen irradiation > 20 Gy
Thyroid dysfunction[213,214,224]	x		Lymphangiography(?)
Female gonadal dysfunction[215,156,672]	x		
Male infertility[148,149,216 218,221,673]	Inguinal, pelvic irradiation	Alkylating agents; procarbazine	
Lung dysfunction[193,674]	x	Bleomycin; BCNU; CCNU; busulfan	
Second cancer (hematologic)[159,224]		Alkylating agents; topoisomerase II inhibitors	
Solid tumors[159,224]	x		

In two large monocenter series of pediatric Hodgkin's lymphoma patients treated from 1960 to 1986 and 1995, respectively, the long-term cumulative risk of death from treatment-related sequelae, such as infections, cardiac disease, and second cancers, approached that of the risk of death from Hodgkin's lymphoma.[175,176] Table 13-15 lists other well-known nonfatal late effects that impair the quality of life for survivors. Some late effects of Hodgkin's lymphoma therapy can be attributed to a distinct treatment modality or a single drug; others may have a multifactorial pathogenesis with the impact of several modalities or drugs. Musculoskeletal growth impairment was one of the first sequelae, which was recognized early as a consequence of radiotherapy applying a standard dose of up to 40 Gy.[156] This complication is ameliorated by the low-dose IFRT now used that restricts the volume and dose of irradiation.

Cardiomyopathy can result from anthracycline therapy, and female gender appears to increase risk.[205] However, various cardiac disorders affecting the vessels, valves, and conduction system of the heart were attributed to Hodgkin's lymphoma treatment at a young age, especially radiotherapy that included the heart in the radiation volume.[158,206] Thus, death caused by cardiac disease was a major risk for pediatric Hodgkin's lymphoma patients after the Hodgkin's lymphoma itself and second cancers.[158,175] Recently, an increased risk for stroke has been described for pediatric Hodgkin's lymphoma patients who had received mantle field irradiation with "standard high" doses of 40 Gy.[207]

Death of overwhelming infections related to splenectomy was a major risk, which has been significant since splenectomy was abandoned from staging procedures.[143,175] Irradiation of the spleen may also induce functional impairment of the spleen, at least if doses of 20 Gy or more are applied.[208]

Chronic lung disease can result from irradiation of the lung and several drugs used for Hodgkin's lymphoma treatment may also contribute to lung injury, including bleomycin and the nitrosourea derivatives BCNU and CCNU. The cumulative dose of these drugs is certainly the most crucial determinant for chronic lung injury. However, in the case of bleomycin, a single dose may risk lung injury; 25 mg/m^2/dose appears to be a cut point.[209] Very young age may be an additional risk factor for possible fatal lung toxicity from BCNU and CCNU.[210] However, no significant increase of long-term lung toxicity was observed in children receiving up to a 300-mg/m^2 cumulative dose of BCNU, whereas there was clearly an increased risk with

a cumulative dose of 600 mg/m^2.[211] A preexisting history of atopy may increase the risk of chronic lung injury caused by these drugs.[212] It can reasonably be assumed that the combination of radiotherapy and drugs with lung toxicity may contribute to long-term lung disease. This might be of special concern in cases of salvage treatment for recurrent Hodgkin's lymphoma that includes high-dose chemotherapy.

Survivors of pediatric Hodgkin's lymphoma are at increased risk for thyroid malfunction, mainly hypothyroidism but also Graves' disease. The risk increases with the dose of cervical irradiation, age at treatment, and whether the patient is a white female.[213,214]

Gonadal toxicity of Hodgkin's lymphoma treatment requires separate considerations for females and males. Pelvic lymph node irradiation will ablate ovarian function; therefore, consideration of ovarian transposition before pelvic radiotherapy is essential. The likelihood of maintaining ovarian function is directly related to gonadal exposure and age at time of treatment. Among girls aged 13 to 18 years with Hodgkin's lymphoma, normal menses was maintained in 100% after oophoropexy and radiation.[156] For girls in whom chemotherapy was added to the treatment program, normal menses was maintained in 88%, whereas for women, normal menses was maintained in only 50% after pelvic irradiation and chemotherapy.[215] It is probable that the younger the patient, the greater the complement of oocytes at the time of treatment and the greater the likelihood of maintenance of ovarian function. Pregnancies have been observed in these women, with no increased risk of fetal wastage, spontaneous abortions, or birth defects.

The incidence of sterility in males is of much greater severity than that observed in females. High-dose pelvic radiation may be associated with transient oligospermia or azoospermia; however, recovery of function is common.[216] Dose-dependent testicular damage from germ cell depletion and Leydig cell dysfunction has also been documented in prepubertal and postpubertal boys after MOPP, ChlVPP (*chl*orambucil, *v*inblastine, *p*rocarbazine, and *p*rednisone), and OPPA-COPP chemotherapy.[217,218] However, rare cases of recovery have been reported 10 to 15 years after prolonged azoospermia.[219] The ABVD regimen appears to be less toxic to germ cells.[220] However, with hybrid MOPP-ABVD derivative chemotherapy such as COPP-ABV, which restricted the cumulative dose of cyclophosphamide to 2.4 to 4.8 g/m^2, a high rate of male infertility was observed.[221] Of 11 men treated for Hodgkin's lymphoma at a median age of 13 years, 9 were infertile based on semen analysis

TABLE 13-16 Pathologic Increased FSH Serum Concentration in Postpubertal Boys*

Therapy Group	Therapy Study	Chemotherapy	Cyclophosphamide (mg/m², cumulative)	Procarbazine (mg/m², cumulative)	Postpubertal Boys with Increased FSH (%)
TG 1	HD-78, HD-82	2 OPPA	0	3000	28.9
	HD-85	2 OPA	0	0	0
	HD-90	2 OEPA	0	0	0
TG 2	HD-78/82	2 OPPA, 2 COPP	2000	5800	45.5
	HD-85	2 OPA, 2 COMP	2000	0	0
	HD-90	2 OEPA, 2 COPP	2000	3000	37.5
TG 3	HD-78/82	2 OPPA, 4 COPP	4000	8,600-11,400	62.5
	HD-85	2 OPA, 4 COMP	4000	0	0
	HD-90	2 OEPA, 4 COPP	4000	6000	36.4

For the composition of combination chemotherapy courses, see Table 13-8.
*According to cumulative doses of cyclophosphamide and procarbazine of the German-Austrian trials of pediatric Hodgkin's lymphoma.[148,149,218]
FSH, follicle-stimulating hormone; TG, therapy group.

when examined 1.5 to 5 years after completion of therapy. Results from the German-Austrian studies on pediatric Hodgkin's lymphoma have shown clearly that with moderate doses of cyclophosphamide, male infertility correlates with the cumulative dose of procarbazine (Table 13-16). These investigators chose the serum concentration for follicle-stimulating hormone (FSH), basal and stimulated, as a surrogate parameter for impaired spermatogenesis. The percentage of postpubertal boys with pathologic increased FSH levels correlated with the replacement dose of procarbazine.[148,149,218] Patients receiving no procarbazine but a cumulative 4-g/m² dose of cyclophosphamide had no increased FSH levels. With only two cycles of COPP therapy, including a cumulative dose of procarbazine of 3000 mg/m², one third of postpubertal males had pathologic increased FSH levels. The percentage was similar with four COPP cycles but increased to two thirds of boys receiving cumulative doses of procarbazine of 8600 mg/m² or more. However, the parameter of pathologic increased FSH may underestimate the true rate of infertility. In the study of Hobbie and coworkers,[221] which used the gold standard spermatogram in addition to FSH level, all patients with increased FSH levels were infertile; however, some patients with azoospermia had normal FSH levels.[221] In both studies, there was no association of male infertility with pubertal status at the time of treatment for Hodgkin's lymphoma. Thus, from this observation, it became apparent that both the prepubertal and pubertal testes are vulnerable to cytotoxic drugs.[149,221]

In the U.S. Childhood Cancer Survivor Cohort consisting of more than 13,000 survivors of childhood cancers, former patients treated for Hodgkin's lymphoma were at the highest risk to develop a second malignant neoplasm (SMN).[222] An increasing rate of lost to follow-up cases with time may deviate the calculation of the true rate of SMNs.[223] Thus, the comparability of data on the risk of SMN from large series of pediatric Hodgkin's lymphomas may be hampered by different methodologies (e.g., inclusion or exclusion of SMN occurring within the first 5 years from completion of Hodgkin's lymphoma treatment), different proportions of lost to follow-up cases, and different follow-up time. Nevertheless, there is convincing evidence from several large cohorts of pediatric Hodgkin's lymphoma patients treated from the 1960s to the 1999s that have indicated a cumulative risk to develop SMN at 20 years of 7% to 10% (Table 13-17). Breast carcinoma is the most frequent SMN, followed by leukemias, including myelodysplastic syndromes, sarcomas, and thyroid tumors.[143,159,176,224-226] Other

SMNs are lung carcinoma, epithelial carcinoma of the intestinal tract, and NHL. Basal cell carcinoma is not included in most series of SMN after Hodgkin's lymphoma. With follow-up, an increasing number of patients develop third and subsequent neoplasms.[159]

The cumulative incidence of second leukemias ranges from 0.6% to 2.1% and reaches a plateau after 10 to 14 years.[143,159,176,177,224] In contrast, in the U.S. Late Effect Study Group (LESG) trial, the risk of solid tumor as SMN continued with extended follow-up, and approached 23.5% at 30 years from diagnosis of Hodgkin's lymphoma.[159] Considering risk factors for developing any SMN, salvage therapy for recurrent Hodgkin's lymphoma is a main risk factor across most studies whereas female gender is a risk factor in some studies at the expense of breast cancer.[159,176,177] The risk of second leukemias is associated with the cumulative dose of alkylating agents and is almost absent in patients treated with radiotherapy alone.[159,176] Data about whether splenectomy increases the risk to develop second leukemias are inconsistent.[176,227] For children younger than 5 years, treatment for Hodgkin's lymphoma and combined-modality chemotherapy-radiotherapy are risk factors for developing second solid tumors.[159,226] Most solid tumors arise in areas adjacent to or within the former irradiation fields.[143,159] Breast cancer as a SMN is almost absent in males. For females in the U.S. LESG group, the cumulative incidence of breast cancer at 20 years was approximately 5% to 6% and increased to 16.9% after 30 years.[143,159] In the LESG group, women had a 55.5-fold excess risk of breast cancer compared with the general population.[159] All patients who developed breast cancer had received 26 Gy or more irradiation to the mantle region. In some studies, the risk of developing breast cancer as a SMN was concentrated in girls 10 years or older at treatment for Hodgkin's lymphoma.[224-226] This was interpreted as an increased susceptibility of the proliferating breast tissue to the carcinogenic effect of radiotherapy. However, in the LESG group, age at diagnosis was no longer a statistically significant risk factor when the calculation of the relative risk to develop breast cancer was adjusted for normal changes in site- and gender-specific cancer risk that occurs in the general population.[159,222] The risk of developing thyroid cancer is clearly related to radiotherapy and is highest in children younger than 5 years at the time of Hodgkin's lymphoma therapy.[159,225,226] Almost all thyroid tumors arise within the radiation field.[159]

As shown in Table 13-17, most reports on SMNs after pediatric Hodgkin's lymphoma include patients treated with

TABLE 13-17   Second Cancers After Hodgkin's Lymphoma (HL) in Childhood and Adolescence

Period of Diagnosis of HL	No. of Patients	Median Follow-up (Yr)	Cumulative Incidence of SMN at 20 Yr (%)	SIR	Absolute Excess Risk/1000 Person-Yr of Follow-up	Risk Factor for SMN, Any Type	No. of SMNs	Leukemias	NHL	Solid Tumor	Breast Cancer
1970-1986[222]	1,815*	15.4	7.63	9.7	5.13	Female	111	9	7	95	35
1935-1994[226]	5,925	10.5†	6.5	7.7	ng		195	28	10	157	52
1943-1987[225]	1,641	10.4†	6.9	7.7			62	7	5	50	16
1960-1995[176]	694	12.3		15.4 F 10.6 M	8.68 F 4.38 M	Female gender, recurrent HL	59§	8	3	48	16
1955-1986[159]	1,380	17.0	10.6‡	18.5	6.5	Recurrent HL	143	27	7	109	30
1978-1999[177]	667	8.3	2.5 (15 yr)	ng	ng	Salvage therapy	10	5	0	5	0
1978-1995[143]	1245	11.1	11% (22 yr)	ng	ng	ng	46	6	4	36	4

*Patients who developed second cancer within 5 yr from diagnosis of HL are excluded.
†Average per patient.
§Without 25 nonmelanoma skin cancers and one carcinoma in situ of the cervix.
‡9.3% without basal cell carcinoma.

F, female; M, male; ng, not given in report; NHL, non-Hodgkin's lymphoma; SIR, standard incidence ratio (observed-to-expected number of cases); SMN, second malignant neoplasm.

early treatment regimens that included higher doses of alkylating agents and, most importantly, larger volumes and high doses of irradiation. The continuous optimization of the balance of treatment efficacy and risks since the 1980s has resulted in reduction of late sequelae resulting from tissue injury, such as musculoskeletal growth impairment and infertility. Whether it will also decrease the risk of developing second cancers is not yet known. However, only thoroughly designed and organized studies on late effects will be helpful. A recent report suggesting that dexrazoxane given as a cardioprotective agent in combination with anthracyclines may add to the risk of a second leukemia reminds us that well-meaning approaches may reveal unexpected results.[228]

Follow-up Treatment

Follow-up management includes follow-up studies to monitor remission status and studies aimed at identifying and monitoring late risks of treatment. With current combined-modality treatment regimens, about 90% of all relapses occur within 3 years from completion of therapy. In contrast, patients continue to be at increased risk for late effects, such as second cancers likely throughout life. Thus, studies to monitor remission status can be confined to the first 3 years after treatment whereas studies for monitoring late risks need to be performed for longer periods and lifelong for SMNs. Studies include accurate physical examination and imaging studies. Because the vast majority of relapses occur at the initial sites or adjacent areas, routine imaging studies can be confined and adapted to the initial sites, except when relapse is suspected elsewhere. It is most important to use imaging methods with the lowest risk for patients. During the 2 years after treatment, 3-month intervals to monitor the remission status may be appropriate, whereas in the third year, 6-month intervals may be enough. Thereafter, imaging may be indicated only in cases of suspected relapse. Most important is to alert patients to possible signs of relapse. Analyses of relapses have revealed that with longer follow-up, more relapses were detected by patients or guardians on their own than during their scheduled follow-up visits.[229,230]

Follow-up studies to monitor late risks of therapy should follow a structured plan as described in the COG Long-Term Follow-up Guidelines.[231] They should include studies of thyroid function, especially in case of cervical irradiation, heart function tests at least every 2 years, and tests of lung function after treatment with bleomycin, nitrosourea derivatives, or lung irradiation. With pelvic or inguinal irradiation and treatment with alkylating agents, it is important to determine whether it is appropriate for the patient's stage of pubertal development. Infertility, especially after procarbazine therapy, should be considered, especially in the follow-up care of young men. Follow-up studies to identify second cancers should take into account the specific risks described later (see "Late Effects"). For patients at risk for breast, thyroid, and intestinal tract cancers, inclusion in an early screening program should be considered. COG recommendations for monitoring patients at increased risk of breast cancer include clinical breast examinations annually until the age of 25 years, and then every 6 months, and annual mammograms beginning at age 25 years or 8 years following radiation, whichever comes last.[159] Most importantly, physicians should teach patients how to perform breast self-examination and encourage them to perform these every month, reporting any changes in the breast tissue promptly to the clinicians. For patients at high risk for colorectal malignancies, monitoring at 10 years following radiation or at age 25 years, whichever occurs last, is recommended by the American Cancer Society for people considered at the highest risk of developing these malignancies. An underestimated issue that needs to be monitored is the quality of life of survivors of Hodgkin's lymphoma.[232]

NON-HODGKIN'S LYMPHOMA

Definition

NHLs are a diverse collection of malignant neoplasms of lymphoid cell origin, including all the malignant lymphomas that are not classified as Hodgkin's disease. Until recently, the childhood NHLs represented a frustrating group of neoplasms for the clinician. NHLs are heterogeneous in their clinical behavior, and the histopathologic classification schemes used in the past were difficult to comprehend and were constantly changing. Moreover, the diseases followed an unpredictable aggressive course, therapies were unsatisfactory, and few children with NHL survived more than 1 year after diagnosis. Advances in the past 2 decades have brightened this gloomy picture. Laboratory investigations have improved our knowledge of the biology of NHLs, which has led in turn to the development of more rational classification schemes. In addition, improvements in understanding of the biology and management of NHL have translated into gratifying improvements in survival for affected children.

Histopathology and Classification

Whereas the Hodgkin's disease Reed-Sternberg cells define Hodgkin's lymphoma as a uniform entity, the NHL complementary group exhibits enormous morphologic and clinical heterogeneity. As a result, the classification of NHL has been and continues to be a topic of scientific discussion. Growth patterns (diffuse vs. nodular) and cytology (undifferentiated vs. differentiated) are the basic criteria used in Rappaport's classification system.[233] The Lukes Collins classification system is based primarily on splitting the lymphocytic system into T and B lymphocytes.[234] The Kiel classification system attempts to translate information about how the lymphatic system is organized into a classification system for NHL, in which the lymphoma cells are related morphologically and immunophenotypically to the cell categories of the immune system.[235,236] The National Cancer Institute Working Formulation (WF) for Clinical Usage, established in 1982, did not intend to constitute another classification of NHL; rather, it was to be a common language to translate between existing classifications.[237] The WF also took into consideration the clinical course of patients, which resulted in a grading of NHL into low-grade, intermediate-grade, and high-grade NHL. Therefore, the WF was widely used by clinicians in North America. In Europe and Asia, the Kiel classification was in broader use. The use of different classification systems hampered, or even made it impossible, to compare results of clinical trials. In the 1990s, the International Lymphoma Study Group (ILSG) undertook a major effort to overcome this confusion and to create a uniform classification of NHL based on biologic principles. The result was the *R*evised *E*uropean-*A*merican Classification of *L*ymphoid Neoplasms (REAL-Classification) which then became the World Health Organization (WHO) Classification of Tumors of the Hematopoietic and Lymphoid Tissues and was referred to as the WHO classification.[12,14] Its basic principles are as follows:

- Subdivision of neoplasms according to the lineage—B, T, or natural killer (NK) cell
- For each lineage, definition of distinct subtypes according to a combination of morphology, immunophenotype, genetic features, and clinical syndromes
- Postulation of a cell of origin for each subtype. The postulated cell of origin refers to the normal counterpart in the ontogenesis of B, T, and NK cells with respect to the phenotype of the malignant cell seen in the tumor. This implies that the malignant transformation event may have occurred in a more undifferentiated cell because the latter is still often unknown.
- Within the B-, T-, and NK-cell neoplasms, two major categories are recognized: neoplasms of precursor B and T cells of the foreign antigen–independent differentiation compartment and neoplasms of peripheral or mature B and T cells of the foreign antigen–dependent differentiation compartment.

Table 13-18 presents the main subtypes of NHL occurring in childhood and adolescence according to the WHO classification and their postulated cell of origin. The respective terms of the former WF are also listed.

The availability of more and newer methodologic tools, including cytogenetics, molecular genetics, and gene expression profiling, have greatly enhanced the accuracy of diagnostic classification of lymphomas and the determination of their relationship to non-neoplastic counterpart cells. However, these methodologies require the appropriate tumor material, such as fresh tumor cells, which may not be available in all cases. The increasing applicability of new methodologies such as immunophenotyping, fluorescence in situ hybridization (FISH), and comparative genomic hybridization (CGH) in paraffin-embedded tumor probes has significantly expanded diagnostic accuracy for a larger number of patients.

Neoplasms of Precursor B and T Cells (Lymphoblastic Lymphoma)

Neoplasms of the precursor B and T cells occur in two different clinical patterns, as acute lymphoblastic leukemia (ALL) or as lymphoblastic lymphoma (LBL; see Table 13-18). Regarding morphology and immunophenotype, both diseases are indistinguishable from each other. Conventionally, ALL and LBL are arbitrarily separated by the degree of bone marrow (BM) involvement. Cases with 25% lymphoblasts or more in the BM are diagnosed as ALL and cases with extramedullary manifestations and less than 25% BM lymphoblasts are referred to as LBL. The assumption is that ALL may primarily arise in the BM and subsequently spread to extra-BM lymphoid organs. Conversely, LBLs primarily arise in extra-BM sites, such as lymph nodes or the thymus, and subsequently spread to the BM. Thus, both conditions may primarily differ in the expression of certain homing factors such as adhesion molecules. About 80% of children with T-cell ALL and 90% of those with T-cell LBL have a mediastinal tumor at presentation. Thus, the thymus might be the site at which most of the precursor T-cell neoplasms arise and subsequently spread to other lymphoid organs and the BM. However, in a minority of cases, T-cell ALL occurs as BM disease alone and 10% of T-cell LBL cases have no thymus tumor. Whether ALL and LBL are biologically a uniform disease with different clinical manifestations or whether they represent two different, although related, disorders with overlapping clinical patterns is not clear. Recent observations of different gene expression profiles in childhood T-cell ALL as compared with T-cell LBL have provided a first hint that T-cell ALL and T-cell LBL may be biologically different diseases, although both arise from precursor T lymphocytes.[238] In North America and Western Europe, LBLs account for about 25% of childhood NHLs and most of them are of the precursor T-cell type.

Morphology

The neoplastic cells are uniform in size, with scanty or indistinct cytoplasm and nuclei larger than those of small lymphocytes with finely distributed chromatin and are referred to as the L1 and L2 types according to the French-American-British (FAB) Classification of Acute Leukemias (Table 13-19).[239] Nuclear membranes may possess subdivisions of varying prominence, giving rise to a distinction between convoluted and nonconvoluted variants of lymphoblastic lymphoma.[237] This distinction may be merely a histopathologic nuance, however,[240] and is not included in the WHO classification.

Immunophenotype

Most childhood LBL cases express the immunophenotype of precursor T cells and approximately 20% of cases have a precursor C-cell type. Table 13-20 depicts immunophenotypic features of precursor T-cell and B-cell LBL. Precursor T-cell

TABLE 13-18   Main Subtypes of Non-Hodgkin's Lymphoma of Childhood and Adolescence*

	LINEAGE	
Parameter	**B Lineage**	**T Lineage**
FOREIGN ANTIGEN–INDEPENDENT LYMPHOCYTE DIFFERENTIATION COMPARTMENT		
Basic biology	Precursor B cells; Ig gene recombination	Precursor T cells; TCR gene recombination
Topography	Bone marrow	BM → Thymus
Childhood neoplasms	Precursor B-cell LBL (<25% BM lymphoblasts); WF—lymphoblastic lymphoma (patients with ≥25% BM lymphoblasts are diagnosed as having precursor B-cell ALL)	Precursor-T cell LBL (<25% BM lymphoblasts) WF: lymphoblastic lymphoma (Patients with ≥25% BM lymphoblasts are diagnosed as precursor-T-cell ALL)
Childhood NHLs (%)	5	19
Basic morphology	Cytology: FAB-L1, L2; histology: lymphoblastic	Cytology: FAB-L1, L2 Histology: lymphoblastic
TdT	Positive	Positive
FOREIGN ANTIGEN-DEPENDENT LYMPHOCYTE DIFFERENTIATION COMPARTMENT		
Basic biology	Antigen-reactive mature B cells; germinal center reaction, IgH class switch	Antigen-reactive mature T cells (?)
Topography	Peripheral lymphoid tissue	Peripheral lymphoid tissue
Childhood neoplasms	• Burkitt's lymphoma or leukemia (B-ALL); WF: small noncleaved cell, Burkitt's type • Diffuse large B-cell lymphoma; WF: diffuse large cell, large cell immunoblastic, diffuse, mixed small and large cell • Primary mediastinal (thymic) large B-cell lymphoma; WF: diffuse large cell (juvenile) follicular lymphoma, follicular mixed small and large cell	• Anaplastic large cell lymphoma; WF: diffuse large cell immunoblastic, various other categories • Peripheral T-cell lymphoma; WF: various other categories
Childhood NHLs (%)	61	15
Basic morphology	Cytology: Burkitt's, FAB-L3; others not classifiable by FAB; nonlymphoblastic histology	Cytology not classifiable by FAB; nonlymphoblastic histology
TdT	Negative	Negative

*According to the WHO Classification of Tumors of Hematopoietic and Lymphoid Tissue and Postulated Cell of Origin.[12]
ALL, acute lymphoblastic leukemia; LBL, lymphoblastic lymphoma; TCR, T-cell receptor; TdT, terminal deoxyribonucleotide transferase; WF, respective terms of the National Cancer Institute Working Formulation.[237]
Data from German-Austrian-Switzerland multicenter studies NHL-BFM and German Co-ALL study enrolling all children with NHL in Germany and Austria.

LBLs are terminal deoxyribonucleotide transferase (TdT)–positive and variably express CD1a, CD2, CD3, CD4, CD5, CD7, and CD8, of which only CD3 is T-cell lineage–specific.[12] Most precursor B-cell LBLs express Pax5, TdT, cCD79a, and CD19. Surface immunoglobulin is characteristically absent from precursor LBL B cells.

Both precursor B-cell and precursor T-cell LBLs may coexpress myeloid CD13, CD33 and, rarely, CD117 antigens. A useful marker to distinguish LBL of precursor B and T cells from mature B-cell and T-cell neoplasms is TdT. The TdTs add single nucleotides to the end during the process of immunoglobulin (Ig) gene and TCR gene recombination, respectively, a process essential during precursor B-cell and T-cell differentiation.[241,242] TdT is only expressed during this process and thus is a specific marker for neoplasms of precursor B and T cells but not for mature T- and B-cell neoplasms.

ALL cases can be further subdivided according to the maturational stages of the leukemic cells, defined by the sequence of expression of antigens into pro-B, common ALL, and pre-B in the precursor B-cell ALL category and into pro-T, pre-T, thymus cortex type, and thymus medullary type in the precursor T-cell category.[243] Little data exist about whether the same subdivision is possible for LBL cases. In a series of 59 cases of childhood T-cell LBL subclassified according to the EGIL classification, 80% of cases expressed a thymus cortex type (TdT, sCD3, CD5, CD1a, and CD4-CD8 double-positive).[244]

Genetics

In contrast to ALL, few data are available on cytogenetic findings in lymphoblastic lymphoma, mainly because of the lack of fresh tumor tissue appropriate for cytogenetic research. In a recent study, chromosomal abnormalities were found in 11 of 13 cases investigated, including four translocations involving 14q11.2, the site of the α/δ T-cell receptor locus.[245]

Role of T-Cell Receptor Translocations. Classic recurring chromosomal rearrangements found in T-cell lymphoblastic leukemias and lymphomas (T-cell ALL) involve the *TCRB* locus (7q34) or the *TCRA/D* locus (14q11) and are generated from mistakes in the recombination process that generate functional T-cell antigen receptors during the development of normal thymocytes.[246-248] These translocations typically induce the aberrant expression of transcription factor oncogenes in T-cell progenitors, activating an irregular transcriptional program that interferes with normal T-cell development and contributes to leukemic transformation. Transcription factor oncogenes involved in these T-cell ALL–specific translocations include members of the basic helix-loop-helix (bHLH) family (*MYC, TAL1, TAL2, LYL1,* and *BHLHB1*),[249-254] the LIM-only domain protein genes (*LMO1* and *LMO2*),[255] homeodomain genes (*TLX1/HOX11, TLX3/HOX11L2,* and *HOXA9*),[256-259] *MYB*,[260,261] and *NOTCH1*.

TABLE 13-19   Morphology, Immunophenotype, and Specific Cytogenetics of Main Non-Hodgkin's Lymphoma Subtypes of Childhood and Adolescence

			SUBTYPE		
Parameter	**Lymphoblastic Lymphoma**	**Burkitt's Lymphoma, Leukemia**	**Diffuse Large B-Cell Lymphoma**	**Anaplastic Large Cell Lymphoma**	
Cytology					
Histology					
Immunophenotype	Precursor B-cell (~20%) Precursor T-cell (~80%)	Mature B-cell, sIg-pos light chain restriction κ or λ	Mature B-cell	T-cell	
TdT	Positive	Negative	Negative	Negative	
Cytogenetics	Only few data available so far	t(8;14)(q24;q32) t(2;8)(p11;q24) t(8;22)(q24;q11)		t(2;5)(p23;q35) t(1;2)(q21;p23) plus other less frequent translocations involving 2p23	

TdT, terminal deoxyribonucleotide transferase.

TABLE 13-20	Immunohistochemical Findings in Tumor Cells of Childhood and Adolescent Non-Hodgkin's Lymphoma Subtypes							
Marker	**T-cell LBL**	**PTCL**	**ALCL**	**NKCL nasal**	**pB-LBL**	**Burkitt's***	**DLBCL**	**PMLBL**
TdT	−	−	−	−	+		−	−
CD19	−	−	−	−	+	+	+	+
CD20	−	−	−	−	±	+	+	+
CD79a	±	−	−	−	+	+	+	+
Cyμ	−	−	−	−	±	±	±	−
sIg‡	−	−	−	−	−	+	±	−
Pax5	−	−	−	−	+	+	+	+
Bcl-6	−	−	−	−	−	+	±	−
CD1a	±	−	−	−	−	−	−	−
CD2	±	±		+	−	−	−	−
cμCD3	+	±	±	+	−	−	−	−
sCD3	±	±	±	−	−	−	−	−
CD4	±	±	±	±	−	−	−	−
CD5	±	±	±	±	−	−	±	−
CD7	±	±	±	±	−	−	−	−
CD8	±	±	±	±	−	−	−	−
CD56	−	±	±	+	−	−	−	−
CD10	±	−	−	−	±	+	±	−
Perforin-granzyme B	−	±	±	+	−	−	±	±
CD30	−	±	+	±	−	−	±	±
Alk	−	−	80%+	−	−	−	−†	−

*Including Burkitt's (FAB-L3) leukemia.

†In the rare plasmablastic variant only.

‡Light chain restriction κ or α.

ALCL, anaplastic large cell lymphoma; DLBCL, diffuse large B-cell lymphoma; NKCL nasal, extranodal natural killer T-cell lymphoma, nasal type; pB-LBL, precursor B-cell lymphoblastic lymphoma; PMLBL, primary mediastinal (thymic) large B-cell lymphoma; PTCL, peripheral T-cell lymphoma, unspecified; T-cell LBL, precursor T-cell lymphoblastic lymphoma.

Adapted from Jaffe ES, Harris NL, Stein H, Vardiman JW. WHO pathology and genetics of tumours of haematopoietic and lymphoid tissues. In Kleihues P, Sobin LH (eds). World Health Organization Classification of Tumours. Lyon, France, IARC Press, 2001.

Importantly, a number of chromosomal rearrangements that do not involve the TCR loci are also involved in the aberrant expression of some of these oncogenes. Thus, *MYB* can be activated by a t(6;7)(q23;q34) translocation,[260] or alternatively by a small intrachromosomal duplication selectively affecting the *MYB* locus in the long arm of chromosome 6.[261] The TAL1d rearrangement, a small intrachromosomal deletion that places the *TAL1* gene under the control of the promoter of the nearby *SIL* gene, is found in about 25% of T-cell ALL cases.[262] Similarly, *LMO2* can be activated by small intrachromosomal deletions in the short arm of chromosome 11.[263] Both *TAL1* and *LMO2* are frequently expressed biallelically in T-cell ALL cases without known alterations in their respective loci, suggesting that activation of upstream regulatory mechanisms controlling the expression of these genes may also participate in the pathogenesis of T-cell ALL.[264,265]

NOTCH1 Activation. The most characteristic molecular lesion associated with the pathogenesis of T-cell lymphoblastic leukemias and lymphomas is the aberrant activation of the NOTCH1 signaling pathway. The NOTCH signaling pathway plays a critical role in the hematopoietic system by participating at multiple stages of T-cell development.

During early hematopoiesis, NOTCH signaling is required for the commitment of multipotent hematopoietic progenitors to the T-cell lineage.[267-269] Thus, immunodeficient mice reconstituted with bone marrow progenitors expressing a constitutively active form of NOTCH1 show ectopic T-cell development in the bone marrow and fail to produce B lymphocytes.[268] Conversely, mice harboring a conditional deletion of *Notch1* in hematopoietic progenitors fail to develop T cells, and show ectopic B-cell development in the thymus.[269] In some systems, this occurs between CD4 and CD8 lineages.[270-273]

Mature NOTCH receptors (NOTCH1-4) are transmembrane heterodimeric proteins generated from a precursor polypeptide that is postranslationally cleaved by a furin protease in the trans-Golgi network. This first cleavage generates both N-terminal and C-terminal NOTCH fragments, which in the absence of a NOTCH signaling stimulus form a heterodimeric transmembrane protein. The N-terminal fragment of the receptor contains multiple EGF repeats involved in ligand interaction, followed by a series of LNR repeats that in the absence of ligand, stabilize the heterodimeric association between the N-terminal and C-terminal NOTCH fragments. The latter (membrane-bound) fragment of the receptor contains a transmembrane proximal RAM domain, followed by a series of ankyrin repeats, both of which participate in the interaction with the DNA binding factor CSL, and a carboxy-terminal PEST sequence responsible for the proteasomal degradation of the activated receptor in the nucleus.

The NOTCH signaling pathway is normally triggered by the interaction of a NOTCH receptor in one cell with a NOTCH DSL (Jagged 1,2 and Delta-like 1,3,4) ligand expressed in the surface of a neighboring cell. This ligand-receptor interaction induces two consecutive proteolytic cleavages at the cell surface that release the cytoplasmic domains of the receptor (ICN1) from the cell membrane.[274,275] The first of these ligand-induced cleavages is mediated by extracellular metalloproteases of the ADAM family. Two ADAM proteases (ADAM10 and ADAM17) have been implicated in the activation of the NOTCH signaling pathway in different organisms.[274,275] After S2 cleavage, the resultant activated membrane-bound form of NOTCH is further processed by the gamma-secretase complex, which catalyzes the final endomembrane cleavage step and releases the intracellular domains of NOTCH from the membrane.

After gamma-secretase cleavage, the consequent activated form of NOTCH rapidly translocates to the nucleus, where it interacts with the CSL DNA binding protein. In the absence of NOTCH signals, the CSL transcription factor binds to the DNA in NOTCH target promoters, where it recruits transcription inhibitory factors to form a multiprotein transcriptional corepressor complex.[275] Binding of ICN1 to CSL displaces these repressors and recruits the MAML1 coactivator to the complex, thereby switching the activity of CSL from repressor to activator and inducing the transcriptional activation of NOTCH CSL target genes.

The human *NOTCH1* receptor gene was originally identified as part of the t(7;9)(q34;q34.3), a rare chromosomal translocation that moves the *NOTCH1* gene next to the TCRB locus, leading to the aberrant expression of a truncated and constitutively active form of NOTCH1 in about 1% of human T-cell ALLs.[276] Despite evidence that NOTCH signaling plays a major role in the development of the T-cell lineage, and that aberrant NOTCH1 signaling can transform T-cell progenitors, the significance of activated NOTCH1 in human T-cell ALL seemed limited to rare human T-cell ALLs harboring the t(7;9). This perception was quickly revised after the identification of activating mutations in NOTCH1 in 50% of human primary T-cell ALL samples and more than 80% of human T-cell ALL cell lines.[277]

Activating mutations in *NOTCH1* in human T-cell ALL are concentrated in exons 26 and 27, which encode the homodimerization (HD) domain in the extracellular portion of the receptor, and in the 3′ end of exon 34, which encodes the PEST domain in the C-terminal region of the protein. *NOTCH1* HD mutations probably operate by inducing ligand-independent activation of NOTCH1, whereas *PEST* mutations are predicted to result in increased levels of intranuclear active NOTCH1 by impairing its degradation by the proteasome. Thus, both types of mutations result in increased NOTCH1 activity (5- to 10-fold over baseline). Importantly, double-mutant alleles harboring both HD and *PEST* mutations are often found in T-cell ALL samples and increase the activation of NOTCH1 10-fold more than HD or *PEST* mutations alone (50-fold over baseline).[277]

Aberrant activation of NOTCH1 signaling in hematopoietic progenitors drives commitment to the T-cell lineage and promotes malignant transformation by inducing deregulated cell growth, proliferation, and survival. Genomic studies on the identification of NOTCH1 direct target genes and pathways in T-cell ALL have uncovered a major role for oncogenic NOTCH1 as a critical regulator of cell growth and metabolism in T-cell lymphoblasts.[278] Thus, NOTCH1 directly binds the promoters of numerous genes involved in protein biosynthesis and anabolic pathways through CSL.[278] In addition, oncogenic NOTCH1 controls the expression of *MYC*, which further increases the expression of cell growth genes.[278-280]

The relevance of the NOTCH-MYC regulatory axis in T-cell transformation is further supported by the identification of mutations in *FBW7* in 15% of T-cell ALL cases.[281] This F box protein mediates the proteasomal degradation of activated NOTCH1, MYC, JUN, and cyclin E.[282] *FBW7* mutations found in T-cell ALL are clustered in three critical arginine residues involved in the interaction with its target proteins. Thus, mutant FBW7 works as a dominant negative factor to promote the stability of activated NOTCH1, mimicking the effect of NOTCH1 PEST mutations.[281] In addition mutant FBW7 also stabilizes MYC, which further enhances the

NOTCH-MYC axis (see earlier) and blocks the degradation of cyclin E, which may contribute to T-cell ALL transformation by promoting cell cycle progression.[282]

MYC. The *c-MYC* oncogene has been implicated in the pathogenesis of T-cell ALL by the t(8;14)(q24;q11) translocation that induces aberrantly high levels of *MYC* expression in T-cell progenitors.[283,284] Furthermore, the prominent role of MYC in T-cell transformation is reinforced by the identification of *MYC* as an important direct transcriptional target of NOTCH1[278-280] and by the identification of *FBW7* mutations that contribute to increased MYC levels by blocking the proteasomal degradation of the MYC protein.[281,282]

TAL1, TAL2, LYL1, and BHLHB1 bHLH Factors and LMO1 and LMO2 Transcriptional Oncoproteins. *TAL1* is a class II basic helix-loop-helix factor gene aberrantly expressed in more than 60% of T-cell ALL cases.[285] *TAL1* activation can occur by means of chromosomal translocation of the *TAL1* locus in the vicinity of *TCR* genes[286] or by a small intrachromosomal deletion that places the *TAL1* gene under the control of the nearby *SIL* locus, present in 25% of T-cell ALL cases.[251] In addition, sporadic cases of T-cell ALL harbor chromosomal rearrangements that place *TAL1*-related genes such as *TAL2*, *LYL1*, and *BHLHB1* in the vicinity of the *TCR* loci.[252-254] Class II bHLH factors heterodimerize with the class I bHLH proteins E12, E47, HEB, and E2-2 and modulate their transactivating activities.[287] T-cell tumors expressing TAL1 contain TAL1-E47 and TAL1-HEB heterodimers.[288] In addition, E2A-deficient mice develop T-cell lymphomas,[289,290] suggesting that TAL1 and related bHLH proteins TAL2, LYL1, and BHLHB1 may contribute to leukemia by interfering with E protein function.

Loss of function of E2A and HEB is also believed to be the mechanism of transformation in tumors with chromosomal translocations involving the LIM-only domain protein genes, *LMO1* and *LMO2*.[263] *LMO1* or *LMO2* are frequently coexpressed with TAL1[285] in T-cell ALL, and TAL1-LMO2-E2A complexes are detected in human T-cell ALL cells.[291,292] Furthermore, aberrant expression of *LMO2* accelerated the leukemogenic process in transgenic mice expressing *TAL1* in the thymus.[293]

HOX11(TLX1), HOX11L2(TLX3), and HOXA9 Homeobox Genes. Homeobox (*HOX*) genes constitute an evolutionarily conserved family of transcription factors that are expressed in specific patterns during embryogenesis and are responsible for the regulation of various developmental processes in vertebrates.[294] The *HOX11(TLX1)* family of *HOX* genes includes *HOX11L1 (TLX2)* and *HOX11L2(TLX3)*,[295] which are characterized by the presence of a threonine in the third helix of the homeodomain; this confers specific DNA-binding properties. Both *HOX11* and *HOX11L2* have been linked to the pathogenesis of T-cell ALL through the characterization of chromosomal translocations. In contrast, *HOX11L1* is normally expressed in T-cell progenitors and does not seem to play a role in the transformation of normal thymocytes.[285]

HOX11 was originally isolated from the recurrent t(10;14)(q24;q11) in T-cell ALL[256,257,296,297] and is aberrantly expressed in 5% of pediatric and up to 30% of adult T-cell ALL cases.[285,298-300] Like other *HOX* genes, *HOX11* plays an important role during embryonic development and acts as a master transcriptional regulator necessary for the genesis of the spleen.[301,302]

Several possible mechanisms through which aberrant *HOX11* expression might lead to malignant transformation have been proposed. In particular, the HOX11 protein is believed to function as a transcriptional regulator, a hypothesis supported by the presence of both a 61–amino acid, helix-turn-helix DNA-binding domain (or homeodomain) and by the localization of HOX11 in the cell nucleus.[295] In addition, HOX11 has been shown to bind to a protein serine-threonine phosphatase 2A catalytic subunit (PP2AC) and phosphatase 1 (PP1C). Both PP2A and PP1 are targets for oncogenic viruses and chemical tumor promoters. Thus, inactivation of PP2A by HOX11 could contribute to the transformation of T-cell progenitors.[303]

A second *HOX11* family member, *HOX11L2*, has been implicated in the pathogenesis of human T-cell ALL through characterization of the t(5;14)(q35;q32), a cryptic chromosomal translocation detectable only by FISH and chromosome painting techniques.[258] This translocation leads to the ectopic expression of *HOX11L2*, possibly by bringing it under the influence of regulatory elements in the *CTIP2/BCL11B* gene, which is highly expressed during T-lymphoid differentiation.[258,304] In contrast to the predominance of *HOX11* expression in adult T-cell ALL cases, both t(5;14) and *HOX11L2* expression are present in 20% to 25% of pediatric but in only 5% of adult T-cell ALL cases.[298,300,305,306] As is the case for HOX11, HOX11L2 plays an important role during embryonic development, when it is essential for the normal development of the ventral medullary respiratory center.[307]

The HOX11 and HOX11L2 proteins are closely related in structure and possess a high degree of sequence identity at the amino acid level, especially in the homeobox domain, where their sequences only differ in three amino acids. The high level of structural homology in their DNA binding domains supports the hypothesis that HOX11 and HOX11L2 may induce T-cell ALL through the regulation of the same transcriptional targets. Moreover, the identification of the *NUP214-ABL1* fusion oncogene[308] as an oncogenic event in T-cell ALL, with a very strong association with the presence of *HOX11* and *HOX11L2* overexpression adds further support to the hypothesis that these two transcription factor oncogenes share a common leukemogenic pathway. However, although the expression of *HOX11* is associated with a favorable prognosis in pediatric and adult T-cell ALL,[246,285,299] the aberrant expression of *HOX11L2* is associated with a higher incidence of relapse in children with T-cell ALL.[285,306,309,310] Thus, the aberrant expression of *HOX11* and *HOX11L2* in T-cell ALL is associated with clinically relevant differences that may reflect, at least in part, unidentified differences in the mechanisms of action of these two oncoproteins.

Major *HOX* genes involved in body patterning are organized in four paralog clusters that contain 9 to 11 *HOX* genes, with an evolutionary conserved organization and tightly regulated expression.[311] The rearrangement of the *HOXA* cluster in chromosome band 7p15 with the TCRB locus in T-cell ALL cases with inv(7)(p15q34) or t(7;7)(p15;q34) is associated with a global overexpression of the *HOXA* genes.[259] Importantly, overexpression of *HOXA* genes is a hallmark of *MLL*-rearranged and *CALM-AF10* leukemias (see later) and forced expression of *HOXA9* induces stem cell expansion[312] and leukemia in mice.[313]

MYB. The translocation t(6;7)(q23;q34) is a rare recurrent rearrangement that juxtaposes the *TCRB* and *MYB* loci in T-cell ALL cases characterized by an early onset (median age, 2.2 years).[260] The pathogenic role of *MYB* in T-cell ALL is further supported by the identification by molecular cytogenetic techniques of a short somatic duplication, which includes the *MYB* locus in 15% of T-cell ALL cases.[260,261] These abnormalities induce increased *MYB* expression, particularly in the case of the *TCRB-MYB*–rearranged leukemias. The Myb transcription factor is essential for primitive and adult hematopoiesis, includ-

ing in the T-cell lineage, and the *Myb* locus is a common site of retroviral insertional mutagenesis–induced leukemias; however, the specific mechanisms that mediate *MYB*-induced transformation in T-cell ALL remain to be elucidated. Notably, *MYB* is upregulated downstream of *HOXA9* and *MLL-ENL* T-cell oncogenes and is required for *HOXA9*- and *MLL-ENL*–induced leukemic transformation.[314]

Fusion Transcription Factor Oncogenes: *CALM-AF10* and *MLL-ENL*. The t(10;11)(p13;q14-21) is a recurrent chromosomal translocation found in patients with acute myeloid leukemia (AML) and T-ALL. The product of this translocation is a chimeric oncogene resulting from the fusion of *CALM* (clathrin assembly protein-like lymphoid-myeloid leukemia gene) and *AF10*.[315,316]

CALM is a ubiquitously expressed protein containing an epsin N-terminal homologous domain involved in the interaction with clathrin during endocytosis.[317] *AF10* is a ubiquitously expressed transcription factor originally identified as a partner of *MLL* in AML.[318,319] *CALM-AF10* rearrangements are present in 5% to 10% of T-cell ALL and seem to be particularly frequent in tumors, with a very early block in T-cell development or those expressing TCR-γ/δ.[320,321] Gene expression profiling studies have demonstrated that *CALM-AF10* expression is associated with high levels of *HOXA* genes, including *HOXA9*.[259,322]

Rearrangements of *MLL*, located on human chromosome 11q23, are frequent in infant and therapy-related leukemias and can occur in AML and ALL. These rearrangements typically generate a fusion oncogene containing the N-terminus part of MLL and various protein domains from more than 50 different fusion partners. The *MLL-ENL* fusion oncogene is found in rare cases of T-cell ALL and, in contrast with *MLL* rearrangements in other hematologic tumors, is associated with a favorable prognosis.[285] MLL is normally responsible for the maintenance of gene expression at the *HOX* paralog groups. *MLL* fusion oncogene products disrupt the normal function of MLL and result in aberrant expression of *HOX* genes.[323,324] *MLL*-rearranged T-cell ALL cases have high levels of expression of HOX genes, including *HOXA9* and *HOXA10*.[285,324]

Protein Kinases: *TEL-JAK2*, *LCK*, and *NUP214-ABL1*. The *TEL-JAK2* fusion oncogene is associated with rare cases of T-cell ALL harboring the t(9;12)(p24;p13).[103] This chimeric oncogene results in constitutively activated kinase with transforming activity.[325,326]

A rare translocation, the t(1;7)(p34;q34) involving the *TCRAD* loci, has been associated with overexpression of the *LCK* tyrosine kinase gene in T-cell ALL.[327] This translocation is thought to contribute to leukemogenesis by mimicking pre-TCR or TCR hyperstimulation, which normally controls the proliferation and survival of developing T-cell precursors.[328]

Cell Cycle Regulators: *p15^INK4B*, *p14^ARF*, and *p16^INK4A* Inactivation and Cyclin D2 Overexpression. Deletions of chromosome bands 9p21-229 involving the *p16^INK4A*, *p14^ARF*, and *p15^INK4B* tumor suppressor genes are the most common abnormality found in T-cell lymphoblastic tumors.[329,330] p15 and p16 are involved in cell cycle regulation by inhibiting cyclin-CDK complexes, whereas p14-ARF is a negative regulator of TP53. Thus, loss of these tumor suppressors affects both the control of cell proliferation and survival.

Chromosomal translocations targeting the cyclin D2 (*CCND2*) locus at chromosome band 12p13 and the *TCRB* or *TCRAD* loci result in high levels of cyclin D2 overexpression. *CCND2* expression is normally confined to early (double-

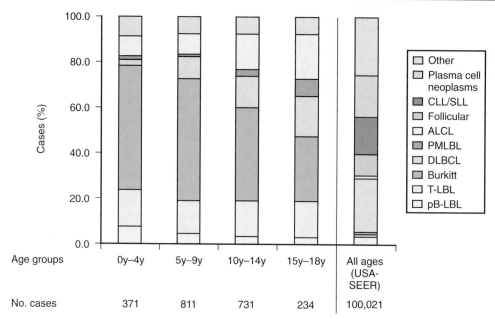

Figure 13-12. Distribution of non-Hodgkin's lymphoma subtypes in children and adolescents according to age groups. For comparison, the distribution of subtypes in all age groups, including adulthood, is depicted in the last column. Burkitt's lymphoma, lymphoblastic lymphoma, and anaplastic large cell lymphoma predominate in childhood but are the minority in adulthood. In contrast, plasma cell neoplasms, chronic lymphatic leukemia, and follicular lymphoma are rare or absent in children. The proportion of patients with diffuse large B-cell lymphoma increases constantly with increasing age. (Data for specific age groups from the German-Austrian-Switzerland NHL-BFM database, diagnosis 10/1986-2002. Data for USA-SEER adapted from Morton LM, Wang SS, Devesa SS, et al. Lymphoma incidence patterns by WHO subtype in the United States, 1992-2001. Blood. 2006;107:265-276., and include all age groups. Also, in the USA-SEER data precursor-B-cell and precursor-T-cell acute lymphoblastic leukemia cases are included in pB-LBL and T-LBL, respectively. See text for details.)

negative) stages of thymocyte differentiation and is replaced by *CCND3* in more mature (double-positive) cells, suggesting that sustained expression in *CCND2*-rearranged T-cell ALL cases may be oncogenic.[260]

Mature Peripheral B-cell Neoplasms

Only a limited number of the numerous subtypes of neoplasms of mature B cells occur during childhood and adolescence—Burkitt's lymphoma (BL), diffuse large B-cell lymphoma, and primary mediastinal (thymic) large B-cell lymphoma—and all others are rare in children (see Table 13-18).

Burkitt's Lymphoma

In 1958, Denis Burkitt described a "sarcoma involving the jaw in African children," which a short time later was shown by O'Connor to be a lymphoma. Burkitt also recognized the endemic nature of the disease.[331] This was substantiated by the isolation of the EBV infectious organism.[332] Most NHL cases in children in North America and Europe were morphologically indistinguishable from Burkitt's lymphoma. Because there was no geographic limitation and most cases were not associated with EBV infection, they were referred to as sporadic Burkitt's lymphomas, in contrast to the endemic Burkitt's lymphoma of central Africa.

According to the WHO classification, three clinical subtypes are recognized. These are morphologically indistinguishable but differ in clinical presentation and biology—endemic BL, sporadic BL, and immunodeficiency-associated BL[12]:

- Endemic BL occurs in equatorial Africa (lymphoma belt; see later, "Epidemiology and Causative Factors"), Papua New Guinea, and equatorial regions of South America. In up to 95% of endemic BL cases, the tumor cells carry the EBV genome and some express CD21, the receptor for C3d, which is also the receptor for EBV.[333]
- Sporadic BL occurs throughout the world in much lower incidence rates as compared with endemic BL. Nevertheless, in industrialized countries, BL lymphoma is the most frequent subtype of NHL in childhood and adolescence, and the most frequent of the mature B-cell neoplasms (Fig. 13-12). In contrast to areas with endemic BL in central Europe, only 10% to 15% of pediatric BL patients carry the EBV genome.[31,334]
- Immunodeficiency-associated BL occurs primarily in patients with HIV infection and may be the first defining condition of AIDS. In this BL type, the morphologic variant of BL with plasmocytic differentiation is observed more frequently. EBV is identified in up to 70% of pediatric HIV–associated BL cases.[335]

Morphology. Classic Burkitt's lymphoma is composed of monomorphic medium-sized cells with deep basophilic cytoplasm and round to ovoid nuclei, with granular dispersed chromatin and multiple nucleoli corresponding to L3 morphology according to the FAB classification (see Table 13-19).[239] Lipid vacuoles are frequently present in the cytoplasm and the nuclei, but are not mandatory. Numerous mitotic and apoptotic cells are usually seen. On histomorphology, a starry sky pattern is usually present, imparted by numerous macrophages that have ingested apoptotic cells. Using proliferation-associated markers such as Ki67, the growth fraction is high and can be up to 100%.[12]

Immunophenotype. BL cells invariably express the B-lineage antigens CD19, CD20, CD22, and CD79a and surface immunoglobulin, characterized by light chain restriction λ or κ, and are negative for CD5, CD23, and TdT.[12] The expression of the germinal center markers bcl-6 and CD10 points to a germinal center origin of BL cells.[336]

Genetics. BL cells carry one of the BL-specific chromosomal translocations t(8;14) (the majority) or, rarely, t(2;8) or t(8;22); all result in the juxtaposition of the proto-oncogene *c-myc* to the immunoglobulin heavy and light chain gene complex, respectively. This leads to aberrant regulation of *c-myc* function (see later, "Molecular and Cellular Biology").[337] The breakpoints on chromosomes 8 and 14 of the BL-specific translocation t(8;14) differ between endemic and sporadic BL.[338-340] In most endemic BL cases, the breakpoint on chromosome 8 lies outside the *myc* gene, but in up to 90% of sporadic BL cases, the breakpoint is located within the myc locus. On chromosome 14, the breakpoint more frequently involves the heavy chain–joining region in endemic BL, whereas in sporadic BL the Ig switch region is more often involved. The breakpoints of the translocation t(8;14) also differ between EBV-positive and EBV-negative cases, with breakpoints outside the *c-MYC* locus on chromosome 8 associated with EBV positivity and cases with breakpoints within the myc locus being more frequently EBV-negative.[339] Recent studies using immunoglobulin gene analysis have revealed two distinct cells of origin for EBV-positive and -negative cases, irrespective of the subtype (endemic, sporadic, or immunodeficiency-associated BL), suggesting that EBV status rather than the patient's geographic region determines the biology of the disease.[341]

BL exhibits a distinct gene expression profile characterized by the high-level expression of MYC target genes which allows accurate differentiation of BL from other NHL subtypes, such as diffuse large B-cell lymphomas (Fig. 13-13).[342,343]

Variants. Burkitt's-like lymphoma shows a greater pleomorphism in nuclear size and shape, and nucleoli are more prominent and fewer in number than in classic BL. However, there is low interinvestigator concordance for this variant and the proof of a c-MYC translocation is required for diagnosis.[12] In the variant type of BL with plasmacytoid differentiation, tumor cells often have eccentric basophilic cytoplasm with a single central nucleolus, and monotypic intracytoplasmic immunoglobulin can be demonstrated by immunohistochemistry. This variant is more common in immunodeficiency states.

Burkitt's lymphoma is universally characterized by the aberrant expression of *MYC*. This cellular oncogene encodes a helix-loop-helix transcription factor involved in the control of multiple cellular processes that contribute to cellular transformation, including cell growth, division, death, metabolism, adhesion, and motility. Chromosomal translocations characteristic of Burkitt's lymphoma juxtapose the *c-MYC* locus in chromosome band 8q24 with strong enhancers from the immunoglobulin genes and drive high levels of *MYC* expression.[344,345] In 80% of Burkitt's lymphoma cases, the t(8:14)(q24;q32) translocation places *MYC* in the vicinity of the *IGH* locus. In 15% of cases, the translocation partner is the *IGκ* locus at chromosome 2p11, whereas the remaining 5% of cases involve the *IGλ* locus at chromosome 22q11.

Tumors with the t(8;14) show differences in the location of the breakpoints relative to the *MYC* gene and the *IGH* genes, which are strongly associated with the geographic origin of the patient.[338-340,346,347] In endemic Burkitt's lymphoma, the chromosome 8 breakpoints are found up to 100 kb 5′ from the *c-MYC* exon 1, whereas the chromosome 14 breakpoints occur most frequently in the *IGH* joining regions (J_H). In contrast, in sporadic and AIDS-associated Burkitt's lymphoma, the chromosome 8 breakpoints are most frequently located between *c-MYC* exons 1 and 2, and those in chromosome 14 are found in the *IGH* Sμ switch region. In cases with *c-MYC* rearrangements involving the light-chain Ig genes, the breakpoints on chromosome 8 are located at variable distances from the 3′ of the *c-MYC* locus,[348,349] and the breakpoints on chromosomes 2 and 22 are located 5′ from the constant region of the *IGκ* and *IGλ* genes. These findings suggest that in sporadic and AIDS-associated Burkitt's lymphomas with the t(8;14), the chromosome 14 breakpoints are generated during Ig class switch recombination. This supports a germinal center B-cell origin for these tumors. In contrast, in endemic Burkitt's lymphoma, the breakpoints on chromosome 14 originate during RAG-mediated V(D)J recombination, suggesting that these tumors most probably derive from pre–B cells, which normally express RAG genes, or from germinal center B cells undergoing RAG gene re-expression.[350]

The first exon and first intron of c-MYC contain negative transcription regulatory sequences.[351,352] These negative regulators of *MYC* expression are removed in sporadic Burkitt's lymphoma, with t(8;14) breakpoints located in MYC intron 1. In contrast, in endemic Burkitt's lymphoma and sporadic Burkitt's lymphoma with light-chain gene translocations, the chromosomal breakpoints are located 5′ or 3′ to the *MYC* locus, respectively. However, in these tumors, the *MYC* exon 1 and intron 1 are frequently mutated and show loss of the negative transcriptional regulatory elements located in these regions.[353,354] Thus, even though the Ig enhancers drive high levels of *MYC* RNA expression, *MYC* levels are further increased in Burkitt's lymphoma by the deletion and/or mutation of negative regulatory sequences within the *MYC* locus.

Additionally, Burkitt's lymphoma tumors frequently show mutations of *MYC* at codon 58. These stabilize the MYC protein by disrupting a critical threonine phosphorylation site involved in the proteasomal degradation of this transcription factor.[355-358]

Other Recurrent Genetic Abnormalities

About 30% of Burkitt lymphomas have mutations in the *TP53* tumor suppressor gene at chromosome band 17p.[359,360] In addition, promoter hypermethylation and consequent transcriptional silencing of *TP73*, a functional homolog of *TP53*, is present in one third of cases.[361] MYC overexpression can induce apoptosis by TP53-dependent and TP53-independent mechanisms.[362-364] Thus, the loss of *TP73* and *TP53* genes, which have prominent roles in the control of programmed cell death, may enhance the transforming effects of MYC.

The *BCL6* oncogene (see earlier) is activated by mutations generated by aberrant somatic hypermutation in 30% to 50% of Burkitt lymphomas.[365,366]

Role of Epstein-Barr Virus

EBV infection is present in 90% of endemic Burkitt's lymphoma cases, 20% of sporadic Burkitt lymphoma cases, and about 40% of HIV-associated Burkitt lymphoma cases.[348] Although molecular data have indicated that EBV infection precedes or occurs concomitantly with B-cell transformation,[367] the specific mechanisms whereby EBV infection contributes to the pathogenesis of Burkitt's lymphoma have not been fully elucidated. However, the virally encoded *EBNA-1* gene may play an important role, because it can induce B-cell lymphomas in transgenic mice[368] and has been shown to be essential for EBV-induced B-cell transformation in vitro.[369,370]

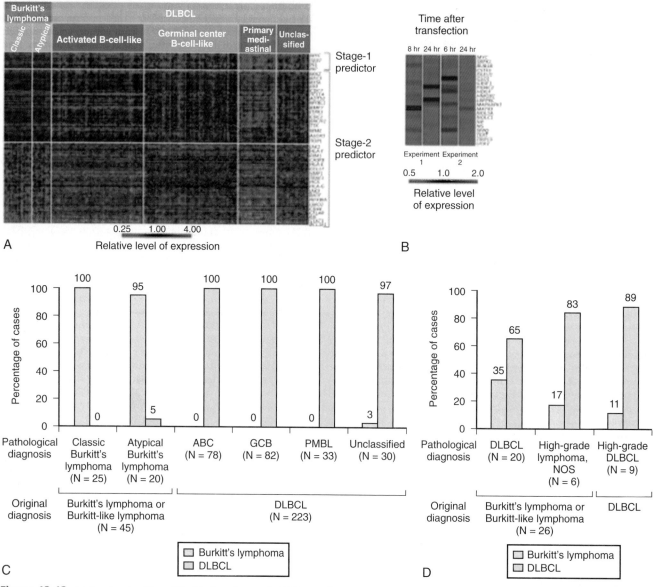

Figure 13-13. Molecular classifier of Burkitt lymphoma. **A,** Difference in gene expression between Burkitt's lymphoma and diffuse large B-cell lymphoma (DLBCL) derived from DNA microarray analysis. The relative levels of gene expression are depicted according to the color scale shown. The genes analyzed in stage 1 of constructing the classifier include *c-myc* and its target genes. The 196 genes analyzed in stage 2 of constructing the classifier include additional genes that distinguish Burkitt's lymphoma from the three subgroups of DLBCL. **B,** List of *c-myc* target genes identified with the use of RNA interference. The OCI-Ly10 DLBCL cell line was transfected with small interfering RNA targeting the *c-myc* gene. Gene expression of the transfected cells was compared with that of control cells by DNA microarray analysis at various hours after transfection in two separate experiments. The levels of gene expression relative to that of control cells are depicted according to the color scale shown; downregulation is depicted in shades of *green* and upregulation is shown in shades of *red.* **C,** The diagnostic performance of the molecular classifier based on gene expression—as compared with the original diagnosis and the pathologic diagnosis—according to leave-one-out cross-validation analysis. **D,** Molecular classification of the 26 specimens originally diagnosed as Burkitt's lymphoma or Burkitt's-like lymphoma that were diagnosed on pathology review as DLBCL or high-grade lymphoma not otherwise specified (NOS) and the 9 specimens that were originally diagnosed as high-grade DLBCL and were verified as such on pathology review. The molecular diagnosis sometimes disagreed with the pathologic diagnosis (*peach bars* in panel **D**). (Redrawn with permission from Dave SS, Fu K, Wright GW, et al. Molecular diagnosis of Burkitt's lymphoma. N Engl J Med. 2006;354:2431-2442.)

Diffuse Large B-Cell Lymphomas

Diffuse large B-cell lymphomas (DLBCLs) are composed of large, transformed lymphoid cells derived from germinal center and post–germinal center B cells.[12] Morphologically, DLBCLs are diverse and can be subdivided into distinct variants.

Centroblastic Variant. This variant is composed of medium-sized to large cells with basophilic cytoplasm, oval to round nuclei, and two to four membrane-bound nucleoli (see Table 13-19). The centroblastic variant is the most frequent DLBCL in children.

Immunoblastic Variant. More than 70% of cells are immunoblasts with deep basophilic cytoplasm and an oval nuclei with a single centrally located nucleolus.

Anaplastic Variant. Very large, round, oval, or polygonal cells with bizarre pleomorphic nuclei, which may resemble Reed-Sternberg cells, characterize this variant. Most of them express CD30. However, this variant is biologically unrelated to anaplastic large cell lymphoma (see later).

T-Cell and Histiocyte-rich Variant. Most cells of this type are non-neoplastic T cells, with or without histiocytes; less than 10% of the infiltrate are neoplastic B cells, which resemble immunoblasts, centroblasts, Hodgkin's cells, or L&H cells of NLPHL. Because of the predominance of reactive cells, this variant may be misdiagnosed as reactive lesions. Also, the distinction from NLPHL may be difficult and an overlap between both cannot be completely excluded.[12]

Immunophenotype

DLBCL cells consistently express pax5, CD79a, and CD20, whereas expression of all other B-lineage markers varies.

Genetics

Complex cytogenetic abnormalities are observed in DLBCL. So far, no entity-specific, nonrandom chromosomal translocations have been described for this subgroup, which may reflect its heterogeneity. In many cases, translocations, including the c-*MYC* locus 8q24, are observed, as well as abnormalities in 3q27, where the proto-oncogene *BCL6* is located.[371] Based on gene expression profiling, two main subtypes of DLBCL can be distinguished, germinal center B-cell–like (GCB) DLBCL and activated B-cell–like DLBCL.[372] The subdivision of DLBCL cases into GCB and non-GCB types by gene expression analysis could be reproduced by means of immunohistochemistry, applying the germinal center cell markers CD10 and BCL6, and the post–germinal center marker MUM1.[373] CD10 expression assigned cases to the GCB type independently of MUM1 expression, but in CD10-negative cases, BCL6 positivity and negativity for MUM1 were associated with GCB type. Although indistinguishable from adult DLBCL cases in terms of morphology, DLBCLs in children appear to comprise a biologically distinct subgroup of germinal center B-cell lymphomas.[374] In contrast to adult DLBCL, pediatric DLBCL is predominantly of germinal center origin but differs from adult DLBCL of the GCB type in that it invariably lacks t(14;18).

Plasmablastic B-Cell Lymphoma with Anaplastic Lymphoma Kinase Expression

In 1997, Delsol and coworkers[375] described an unusual subtype of large B-cell lymphoma with plasmablastic morphology, the cells of which contained cytoplasmic IgA and expressed a full-length ALK protein but not an ALK fusion protein. However, in a more recent report, two pediatric cases carrying the chromosomal translocation t(2;5) and expressing the NPM-Alk fusion transcript were described.[376] The translocation t(2;5) is discussed later (see "Anaplastic Large Cell Lymphoma").

Primary Mediastinal (Thymic) Large B-Cell Lymphoma

Primary mediastinal (thymic) large B-cell lymphoma (PMLBL) is characterized by its primary localization in the mediastinum and was first described as a B-cell lymphoma in 1986.[377] In most cases, a prominent compartmentalizing sclerosis dominates the histologic appearance. The malignant cells are of putative thymic B-cell origin and are large, often pleomorphic, lymphoid cells, with abundant pale cytoplasm. The neoplastic cells may express CD30 and in these cases distinction from NSHL may be crucial. In contrast to HL, the cells express CD45 and B-lineage markers such as CD19 and CD20, CD79a, but sIg is usually absent. Contrary to DLBCL, PMLBL cells do not express CD10 nor BCL6 and BCL2.[378] Overexpression of the *MAL* gene, which is involved in T-cell maturation, has been demonstrated in a high proportion of PMLBL patients.[379,380]

Juvenile Follicular Lymphoma

Follicular lymphoma (FL) accounts for about one third of NHL cases in adults but is rare in children and accounts for less than 2% of pediatric cases. FL has a predominantly follicular growth pattern, but diffuse areas may be present. Cytomorphologically, FLs are composed of two types of cells, small to medium-sized with twisted or cleaved nuclei and scant pale cytoplasm known as centrocytes or cleaved follicle center cells, and a variable number of large transformed cells with basophilic cytoplasm known as centroblasts or noncleaved follicular center cells. FL is graded by the number of centroblasts into three grades. From the few reported series, which included at least 20 patients each, it appears that FL occurring in childhood differs from FL in adulthood, primarily by the rarity or even absence of the translocation t(14;18) juxtaposing *BCL2* to the Ig heavy-chain locus on chromosome 14.[381,382]

Peripheral T-cell Neoplasms
Anaplastic Large Cell Lymphoma

ALCL was first described by Stein and colleagues[18] in 1985. It is characterized by large anaplastic cells with strong reactivity with the monoclonal antibody anti-CD30 and by activation markers such as the IL-2 receptor (CD25) and HLA-DR antigens.

Based on cytomorphologic criteria, several variants of ALCL have been described[12]:

- The common variant is characterized by sheets of large lymphoid cells, with chromatin-poor horseshoe-shaped nuclei containing multiple nucleoli (see Table 13-19). Cells with these cytologic features have been called hallmark cells because they are encountered in all ALCL variants, including the small cell and lymphohistiocytic variants.
- The lymphohistiocytic variant is characterized by a large number of reactive histiocytes, which may even mask the anaplastic tumor cell population and can therefore be misdiagnosed as reactive histiocytic disease or malignant histiocytosis.[383]
- The small cell variant is characterized by a predominant population of small to medium sized neoplastic cells with irregular nuclei. This variant was often misdiagnosed as peripheral T-cell lymphoma.[384-385]
- Other rare variants are the giant cell variant, sarcomatoid variant, and neutrophil-rich variant. In some cases, mixtures of histologic subtypes are observed in one lesion, whereas in other patients different subtypes can be seen in different lesions.

However, the relevance of such subclassification remains uncertain. Furthermore, relapses may reveal morphologic features different from those seen initially.

The clonal nature of ALCL has been confirmed by the detection of the nonrandom chromosomal translocation t(2;5)(p23;q35) in malignant cells.[386-388] This translocation causes the nucleophosmin (*NPM*) gene located at 5q35 to fuse with a gene at 2p23 encoding the receptor tyrosine kinase ALK.[389] The production of monoclonal antibodies directed against fixative-resistant epitopes of ALK allows its detection by immunohistochemistry.[390,391] Although the translocation t(2;5)(p23;q35) is the most frequent, more than 10 other chromosomal translocations juxtaposing the *ALK* gene at chromosome 2p23 to a partner gene have been detected (see Table 13-19). The partner gene of *ALK* determines the immunohistochemical Alk staining pattern. Only the NPM-ALK fusion protein is detectable in the cytoplasm and the nucleus because of the heterodimerization of the NPM portion with normal NPM, which functions in the nuclear shuttling of proteins.[392] All other fusion gene products lacking the NPM portion are detectable only in the cytoplasm. Conversely, the ALK staining pattern, cytoplasmic and nuclear versus extranuclear, distinguishes the NPM-ALK translocation from all others.[411] In children, more than 90% of ALCL cases are ALK-positive.[393]

The cellular origin of ALCL is still not completely clarified. The vast majority express T-lineage antigens, have clonally rearranged TCRγ and TCRβ genes, and express the cytotoxic molecules perforin, granzyme B, and T-cell-restricted intracellular antigen-1 (TIA-1; see Table 13-20).[394,395] However, findings of plasmablastic B-cell lymphoma carrying the translocation t(2 ;5) and expressing *NPM-ALK* transcripts have suggested that the ALK involving translocation may not be restricted to ALCLs of T-cell lineage.[396] In a minority of cases, the expression of the NK cell–associated marker CD56 and the lack of detectable TCR gene rearrangements suggest an origination from NK cells rather than cytotoxic T cells.[394,397]

In most cases, ALCL occurs as a de novo malignant lymphoma. On rare occasions, however, ALCL appears as a secondary lymphoma that evolves from a low-grade or high-grade malignant T-cell lymphoma, Hodgkin's lymphoma, or lymphomatoid papulosis.[398-401]

As mentioned above, the most characteristic molecular feature of ALCL is the presence of gene rearrangements involving the *ALK* locus in chromosome band 2p23. ALK is a transmembrane receptor tyrosine kinase of the insulin receptor superfamily normally expressed only in cells of neural origin. ALCL translocations lead to the aberrant expression and constitutive activation of ALK.[402] The most common of these translocations present in 80% of ALCL cases is the t(2;5)(p23;q35).[403,404] In this translocation, the 5′ region of the nucleophosmin gene (*NPM*) on chromosome 5q35 is fused to the *ALK* gene.[389,404-406] NPM is a ubiquitously expressed nucleolar phosphoprotein involved in the shuttling of ribonucleoproteins between the nucleus and cytoplasm.[407] The *NPM-ALK* fusion oncogene resulting from the t(2;5)(p23;q35) translocation encodes a constitutively active form of ALK,[404] which promotes cell transformation in vitro[392,408] and in vivo[409] by phosphorylating and activating important mediators in a number of critical signaling pathways, such as PLCG, PI3K-AKT-mTOR, JAK2, STAT3, STAT5, and MEK-ERK.[402,405,410]

As already mentioned, in addition to the t(2;5)(p23;q35) rearrangement, several other chromosomal translocations involving the *ALK* gene have been found in 20% of ALK-positive ALCL cases. All these rearrangements result in the fusion of the catalytic domain of ALK with different partners, such as tropomyosins 3 and 4, TGF, ATIC, clathrin heavy chain, moesin, AL017, and MYH9,[402,410] and result in constitutively active ALK phosphorylation and activation.[404]

The importance of the elucidation of constitutively active ALK as a major mechanism in the transformation of ALCL is highlighted by the development of specific ALK inhibitors.

These may provide a targeted therapeutic strategy for treatment of this disease.[412]

Primary Cutaneous Anaplastic Large Cell Lymphoma

The cytologic features of primary cutaneous anaplastic large cell lymphomas are similar to those of systemic ALCLs. In most cases, the tumor cells express CD30, CD3, TIA-1/GMP17, perforin, and/or granzyme B, but Alk expression is not yet described for this entity. Primary cutaneous ALCL may occur as de novo lymphoma or occur on the base of a preexisting lymphomatoid papulosis of the skin.[400,413]

Peripheral T-cell lymphomas other than ALCLs are rare in childhood and account for less than 1% of cases. They represent a heterogeneous group of neoplasms. In childhood, most of them are peripheral T-cell lymphomas, unspecified according to the WHO classification. Some cases express CD30, but Alk staining is consistently negative and an important parameter to distinguish these neoplasms from ALCLs. The cytologic spectrum is heterogeneous but most cases show a predominance of medium-sized cells, with irregular pleomorphic nuclei and a pale cytoplasm. The rare extranodal NK–T-cell lymphoma, nasal type, is characterized by a diffuse but angiocentric and angiodestructive growth pattern.

Epidemiology and Causative Factors

Differences of incidence rates according to geographic areas, gender, age, and ethnicity give clues to the cause and pathogenesis of childhood NHL because they reflect differences in exposure to environmental factors and genetic predisposition. The conceptual hypothesis includes disease-specific genetic alterations with significant impact on the pathogenesis that might be induced by environmental agents or infections. Host-dependent factors such as genetic polymorphisms or inherited genetic defects may modify metabolic and mutagenic effects of environmental factors, as well as immune responses to malignant transformed cells. The hormonal stages and aging processes of the host may be complementary factors, as well as interactions of environmental factors.

Incidence

The comparison of incidence rates of NHL in childhood and adolescence in different geographic areas is limited because of a paucity of true population-based registries, different degrees of completeness of their data, and differences in methodology. Table 13-21 lists age-standardized incidence rates for NHL in children aged 0 to 14 years from regional registries. The incidence rates range from 6.6/million in the United Kingdom to 12.5/million in Japan (Osaka). However, specific subtypes may occur with a much higher incidence in particular regions. Thus, endemic BL accounts for 74% of all childhood malignancies in equatorial Africa.[414-416] Burkitt's lymphoma also has a very high incidence in equatorial areas of South America.[417] Outside the endemic BL zone, the highest incidence of childhood NHL occurs in Mediterranean and Middle Eastern countries and in parts of South America.[418]

Time Trends in Incidence Rates

Data on time trends in the incidence of childhood NHL are inconsistent. In the Automated Childhood Cancer Information System (ACCIS) in Europe, incidence rates of NHL in childhood and adolescents increased from 1978 to 1997 by 0.9%/year on average, and the increase was highest in adolescents.[419]

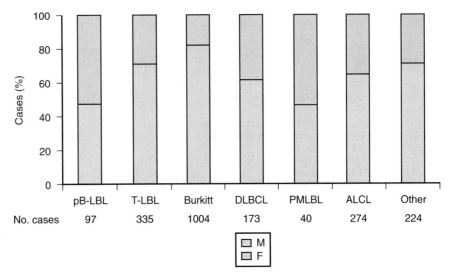

Figure 13-14. Distribution of gender according to main non-Hodgkin's lymphoma subtypes of childhood. See text for details. (Data from Burkhardt B, Zimmermann M, Oschlies I, et al. The impact of age and gender on biology, clinical features and treatment outcome of non-Hodgkin lymphoma in childhood and adolescence. Br J Haematol. 2005;131:39-49.)

TABLE 13-21	Age-Standardized Incidence Rate of Non-Hodgkin's Lymphoma in Children*									
	U.S. SEER		**Costa Rica**	**Australia**	**Europe**	**United Kingdom**	**Germany**	**Harare, Zimbabwe**	**Bombay, India**	**Osaka, Japan**
Parameter	**White**	**Black**								
Period	1980-1994	1980-1994	1980-1994	1980-1994	1978-1997	1980-1994	1980-1998	1980-1994	1980-1994	1980-1994
Incidence rate	9.0	6.3	11.1	9.1	9.4	6.6	8.0	9.3	6.4	12.5

*Aged 0-14 yr, by geographic region, per million.[418,419,423]

TABLE 13-22	Age-Specific Incidence Rates of Non-Hodgkin's Lymphoma in Europe.				
	AGE GROUP (YR) AND AGE-SPECIFIC INCIDENCE RATES PER MILLION				
Period	**0**	**1-4**	**5-9**	**10-14**	**15-19**
1988-1992	3.0	8.0	10.5	9.4	14.7
1993-1997	3.0	7.4	10.6	11.2	15.5

Data from Izarzugaza MI, Steliarova-Foucher E, Martos MC, Zivkovic S. Non-Hodgkin's lymphoma incidence and survival in European children and adolescents (1978-1997): report from the Automated Childhood Cancer Information System project. Eur J Cancer. 2006;42:2050-2063.

In contrast, there was little variation in the incidence rates of childhood NHL over the 20-year period from 1975 to 1995 in the U.S. SEER program.[1] Also, in single national and regional European registries, no increase was observed in the incidence rate of childhood NHL.[421-423] Thus, it is not clear what changes in specific diagnostics, classification, reporting, and methodology may contribute to changes in recognized incidence rates over time.

Age-Specific Incidence Rates

Across all registries, the age-specific incidence rate increases with increasing age (Table 13-22).[420-423] NHL is rare in infants and incidence rates increase consistently during childhood and adolescence.

Gender

In all registries, the incidence rates of NHL are higher in males than in females, usually by a factor of 2.[41,420-423] The male-to-female ratio varies considerably among different NHL subtypes (Fig. 13-14). Whether male predominance in most NHL subtypes reflects hormonal differences rather than loss of an X chromosome–linked tumor suppressor gene remains to be determined.

Ethnicity and Genetic Predisposition

In the U.S. SEER program, the incidence rate in white children is higher as compared with black children, which suggests variation in susceptibility by ethnic background.[41,418] A likely role for genetic susceptibility is sustained by the observation that the Israeli-born offspring of migrants to Israel from North Africa retain the high incidence rate of NHL observed in those countries.[424]

Familial Predisposition

In adults, an increased risk for NHL has been described in first-degree relatives of patients with hematopoietic malignancies.[76,425] So far, no larger studies are available about the familial risk for pediatric NHL, except for classic known hereditary syndromes predisposing for NHL.

Inherited immunodeficiency is a strong risk factor for developing NHL during childhood, and NHL is the most fre-

TABLE 13-23 Inherited Immunodeficiency and Bone Marrow Failure Syndromes Associated with Childhood Cancer

OMIM	Syndrome	Inheritance	Locus	Gene	Childhood Cancers
208900	Ataxia telangiectasia	AR	11q22	ATM	Lymphoma, leukemia
301000	Wiskott-Aldrich syndrome	X-linked	Xp11	WAS	NHL
210900	Bloom's syndrome	AR	15q26	BLM	NHL, Wilms' tumor, osteosarcoma
240500	Common variable immunodeficiency	Various	Various	Various	Lymphoma
300300	X-linked agammaglobulinemia	X-linked	Xq21-22	BTK	Lymphoma
137100	IgA deficiency	AD	6p21	IGAD1	Lymphoma
300400	Severe combined immunodeficiency	X-linked	Xq13	IL2RG	Lymphoma
308240	Duncan's disease	X-linked	Xq25	Various	Lymphoma
251260	Nijmegen's breakage syndrome	AR	8q21	NBS1	NHL

AD, autosomal dominant; AR, autosomal recessive; NHL, non-Hodgkin's lymphoma.
Adapted from Stiller CA. Epidemiology and genetics of childhood cancer. Oncogene. 2004;23:6429-6444.

quent cancer in children with those disorders, except for IgA deficiency.[426] Table 13-23 presents the main inherited immunodeficiencies associated with up to a 50-fold increased risk for lymphoma. The most important are ataxia telangiectasia (ATM), Nijmegen breakage syndrome (NBS), and Bloom's syndrome, which are all characterized by increased chromosomal instability, pointing to a possible defective regulation of immunoglobulin and T-cell receptor gene rearrangements in those patients.[427,428,675] Up to 15% of children affected by ATM develop NHL during childhood.[429] Although patients with inherited immunodeficiency syndromes account for only a small minority of children with NHL, studies have shown that heterozygous ATM gene alterations are prevalent in pediatric NHLs.[430-432] So far, little evidence exists that mutations of the NBS gene in heterozygotes may have a role in the pathogenesis of childhood NHL.[433,434]

Environmental Factors

There is increasing evidence that pesticides may be associated with an increased risk of NHL in adults, specifically NHL that carries the chromosomal translocation t(14;18) but not with t(14;18)–negative NHL.[435] However, similar evidence for an occupational risk for pediatric NHL is lacking. In a case-control study, the residential use of insecticides was associated with the risk of pediatric lymphoma.[436] In other studies, residential history, familial characteristics, birth order, and maternal and perinatal factors such as cesarean section were described as associated with the risk of NHL in children but seasonal variations were not.[437-441] However, despite an increasing number of studies on environmental factors, evidence in support of an association with the risk of childhood NHL is still limited because of the weakness of research methodology. Crucial issues are problems faced in exposure assessment, small numbers of exposed subjects, and difficulties in estimating critical windows of exposure.[442]

Based on our understanding today, NHL comprises an assembly of biologically different disorders, and the significant differences in gender ratios among subtypes may be a striking confirmation of this view. However, in most population-based registries, disease categories are registered based on the International Classification of Diseases for Oncology or the International Classification of Childhood Cancer.[443] Those categories are not directly transferable to the WHO classification of hematologic malignancies.[12] Moreover, there is considerable change in diagnostic practice, resulting in shifts of the proportions of distinct entities in the cohort of cases.[444] Therefore, comparisons about geographic differences in the distribution of NHL subtypes according to the WHO classification are limited. The distribution of NHL subtypes differs between childhood and adulthood.[445] This may have been substantiated in a large study on lymphoma incidence pattern by WHO subtype based on the U.S. SEER program, including more than 100,000 cases of all ages. The incidence in children younger than 15 years was higher than in older patients for lymphoblastic lymphomas of precursor B- and T-cell type.[41] In contrast, plasma cell neoplasms, follicular lymphoma, marginal zone lymphoma, mantle cell lymphoma, and chronic lymphocytic leukemia (CLL) are almost absent in childhood. Diffuse large B-cell lymphomas occur in childhood, but their incidence rate increases with age and is much higher in adults. Burkitt's lymphoma or leukemia shows a first peak in incidence in childhood, followed by a slightly decreased incidence in adolescence and young adults, and then gradually increases with age. Even in childhood, the distribution of NHL subtypes differs among specific age groups. Burkitt's lymphoma or leukemia is the predominant subtype in children younger than 10 years. The proportion of DLBCL, ALCL, and PMLBL cases is rare in the very young and increases with age (see Fig. 13-12).

The conclusion from these data is that the striking differences in incidence pattern and gender ratio strongly suggests causative heterogeneity among NHL entities and supports the pursuit of epidemiologic analysis by subtype rather than the whole spectrum of childhood NHLs. A strong correlation between a factor and a distinct NHL subtype may become blurred in the whole group. An example may be the correlation between the polymorphism of the methylenetetrahydrofolate reductase, resulting in altered folate metabolism with the risk of lymphoblastic lymphoma; however, no significant associations were determined for other biologic subtypes or for the entire group of pediatric NHL cases.[446] Similarly, polymorphism of the NAD(P)H–quinone oxidoreductase, an enzyme that protects cells against mutagenicity from free radicals and toxic oxygen, was found to be associated with an increased risk for BL but not for lymphoblastic neoplasms.[447]

Infections

Denis Burkitt not only recognized and described BL as a new disease entity but also established the epidemiologic basics for the current view of its association with EBV, malaria, and arbovirus infections.[331,416] Burkitt and coworkers[414] described the lymphoma belt of Africa, which stretches about 10 degrees north to 10 degrees south of the equator, with a tail extending south along the eastern coast of the continent (Fig. 13-15). In 1964, Epstein and associates[332] described viral particles—later

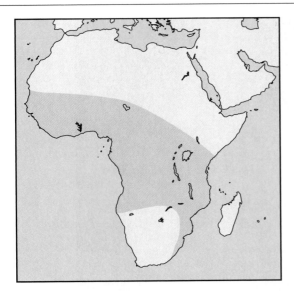

Figure 13-15. The lymphoma belt of Africa. Burkitt's lymphoma is endemic in regions with mean minimum temperatures that exceed 15.5° C and a yearly rainfall more than 50 mL, which stretch from about 10 degrees north to 10 degrees south of the equator. (Adapted from van den Bosch CA. Is endemic Burkitt's lymphoma an alliance between three infections and a tumour promoter? Lancet Oncol. 2004;5:738-746.)

referred to as EBV—in Burkitt's lymphoma probes that they received from Denis Burkitt from African patients. The EBV-positive BL cells express the EBV nuclear antigen 1 (EBNA1) with the absence of all other EBV proteins corresponding to the EBV latency type I.[19] The EBV genome is incorporated into 96% of endemic BL cases in the African lymphoma belt but in 80% of BL cases in Algeria, where BL has a lower incidence than in equatorial Africa but higher than in France, where only 10% to 15% of cases are EBV-positive.[334,448] Because malaria is holoendemic, where endemic BL was found it was postulated that EBV could be oncogenic in the presence of marked reactive lymphoid hyperplasia, which occurs in response to malaria infection, giving rise to malignant transformation.[449] However, Burkitt postulated for the first time that the higher vulnerability to the oncogenicity of EBV in those areas may be caused by suppression of immunity by malaria infection.[450] Later findings revealed that malaria infection expands the pool of EBV-positive cells in two ways: (1) by inducing polyclonal expansion of EBV-positive B lymphocytes; and (2) by inhibition of EBV-specific suppressor T cells.[451-453] From the gradient of the incidence rates of BL and the proportion of EBV-positive BL cases in equatorial Africa compared with North Africa and Europe, it was postulated that malaria infection (holoendemic in central Africa but not in North Africa and France) and EBV infection early in life (occurring more frequently in Africa than in France) may be crucial for the pathogenesis of EBV-positive BL.[334,454] In Germany, 11% of pediatric BL cases were found to be EBV-positive.[31] Interestingly, these children were significantly younger at time of diagnosis of BL as compared with their EBV-negative counterparts.

However, malaria and EBV alone cannot account for the occasional shifting foci and space-time clusters of endemic BL, and other environmental factors may play a role. Burkitt and his collaborators not only described the lymphoma belt. Their investigations revealed that BL was not found in places higher than 5000 feet above sea level and that altitude was only a limiting factor because it reflects temperature. Furthermore,

they found similarities between the altitude limitations of BL and mosquito-borne epidemics of o'nyong-nyong fever in the same region and raised the possibility of a mosquito-borne arbovirus as a common factor in Burkitt's lymphoma.[414,455,456] Arboviruses seem to be associated with case clusters of endemic BL and symptoms compatible with arbovirus infection have been observed immediately before onset of the tumor.[415,416,457] Also, arboviruses and EBV are promoted by extracts of a commonly used plant, *Euphorbia tirucalli*, whose distribution corresponds with the boundaries of the lymphoma belt.[458] Extracts from *E. tirucalli* are tumor promoters and can induce the translocation t(8;14) in EBV-infected cell lines and enhance EBV-mediated cell transformation.[416,459]

Thus, although BL was the first human malignancy for which a virus involvement in pathogenesis was described, the definitive role of EBV has still to be elucidated. In EBV-positive BL cases, the breakpoints on chromosome 8 of the BL-specific translocation t(8;14) is more frequently located outside the *MYC* locus, leaving the *MYC* gene intact, whereas in EBV-negative cases the breakpoint is predominantly within the myc locus.[338,339] This supports the hypothesis that EBV is required to contribute to the deregulation of *MYC* in the presence of some but not all types of *MYC* damage arising from the BL-specific translocations.[339] EBV is almost absent from other subtypes of childhood NHL, with the exception of the rare peripheral T-cell lymphomas other than ALCL.[31,460]

HIV-infected children are at a more than 150 times higher risk for developing NHL in comparison with general population rates.[461,462] NHLs are the most frequent neoplasms occurring in HIV-infected children and most are of B-cell lineage.[335,463] NHL may even be the first AIDS-defining condition and, in some children, the diagnosis of HIV infection may be established only when the tumor is diagnosed.[335,463] Many HIV-infected children did not show severe immunosuppression at the time of lymphoma diagnosis as measured by CD4+ cells. In an Italian series, 8 of 11 cases of HIV-associated NHL were EB-positive, and high loads of EBV DNA were measured during prolonged periods preceding onset of the tumor.[335] However, the ultimate role of EBV in AIDS-related NHL has still to be elucidated.

Little evidence exists about the role of other viruses in childhood NHL, including human T-cell lymphotropic virus type I, which is only rarely associated with T-cell lymphoma of childhood.[464,465]

Clinical Characteristics

NHL and HL of childhood and adolescence have many features in common. Thus, as in Hodgkin's lymphoma, the most frequent symptom of childhood NHL is painless lymphadenopathy. In contrast to Hodgkin's lymphoma, the nodes may enlarge more rapidly because of a much higher growth fraction of NHL. However, the variety of presenting features of childhood NHL is even larger than that for Hodgkin's lymphoma, ranging from a single painless enlarged lymph node, an asymptomatic asymmetrical enlarged tonsil, or a harmless looking skin papule to a life-threatening condition, which is more often the case as compared with Hodgkin's lymphoma. Almost any organ, tissue, and anatomic area can be involved. The most common disease sites are the cervical lymph nodes, abdomen (including the liver and spleen), mediastinum (see Fig. 13-8A), and head and neck region (Fig. 13-16). Lesions in the head and neck area may involve the tonsilla (usually one site), Waldeyer's ring, the paranasal sinuses, and any bone structure, including the skull and cranial base. Other sites are bone (Fig. 13-17), soft tissue, kidneys (enlarged kidneys caused by diffuse infiltration or tumors in the kidney parenchyma;

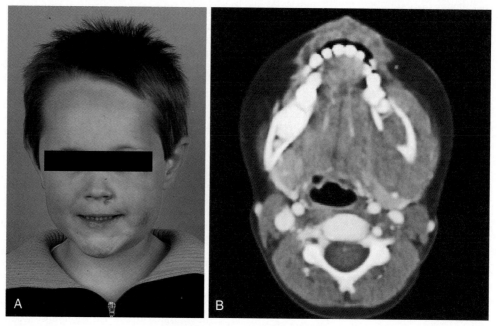

Figure 13-16. Osteolytic lesion of the left corpus mandibulae in a 4-year-old boy with Burkitt's lymphoma.

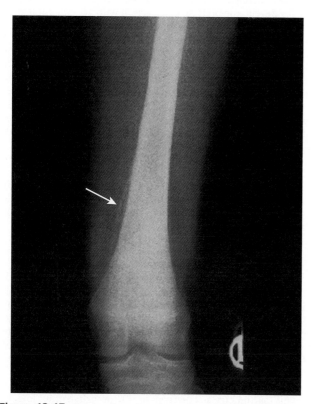

Figure 13-17. Primary bone lymphoma (*arrow*) in the distal metaphysis of the femur.

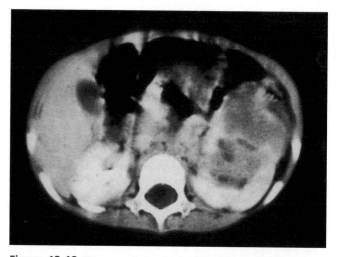

Figure 13-18. Timorous lesion in the left kidney in a patient diagnosed with primary mediastinal (thymic) large B-cell lymphoma.

Fig. 13-18), ovaries, and skin (Fig. 13-19). Testicular involvement occurs in less than 5% of boys and usually manifests as painless uni- or bilateral enlargement of the testicle. Involvement of ovaries is diagnosed in less than 5% of females. The pancreas, adrenal glands, thyroid gland, and salivary glands are rarely affected.

In industrial countries, general health status is not significantly compromised at the time of diagnosis in most children. Symptoms and signs depend on the localization of the tumor. They are more or less nonspecific and include fever, weight loss, nonspecific abdominal pain, bone pain, or retrosternal pain and chronic cough in the case of a mediastinal tumor. Headaches are a less common symptom (in cases of central nervous system [CNS] involvement). Impaired neurologic functions such as isolated cranial nerve palsy or discrete paraplegia may be presenting features in case of CNS disease or a paraspinal tumor (Fig. 13-20).

The presenting clinical features differ considerably, however, in patients suffering from different NHL subtypes. Figure 13-21 depicts key features of children and adolescents with different NHL subtypes. B symptoms are observed in about 30% of cases and are most frequent in ALCL patients. Abdominal disease is most frequent in BL with the intestinal

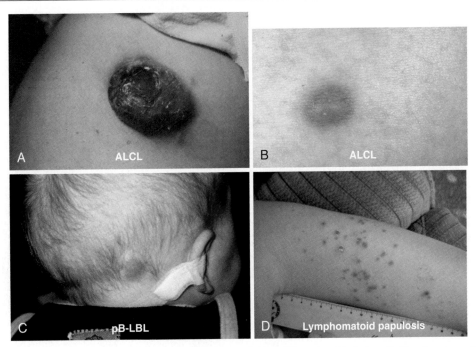

Figure 13-19. Skin involvement in anaplastic large cell lymphoma (ALCL). **A,** Ulcerative skin lesion. **B,** Papulomatous skin lesion. **C,** Lesion of precursor B-cell lymphoblastic lymphoma. **D,** Multiple skin lesions of lymphomatoid papulosis.

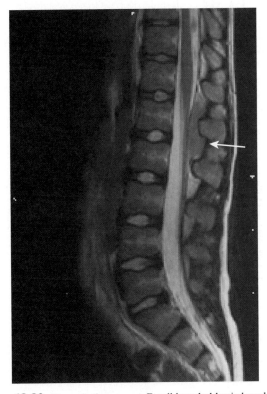

Figure 13-20. Paraspinal precursor B-cell lymphoblastic lymphoma.

tract, especially the ileocecal part, as the classic organ of involvement. The ileus and acute abdomen is a not infrequent presentation of children with abdominal NHL, with prognostically different underlying conditions. A small tumor adherent to the inner part of the intestinal wall may have been the perpendicu-

lum for intussusception (Fig. 13-22). Because of this "alarm clock," the tumor is discovered early, can be resected, and the patient cured with minimal chemotherapy. Other BL cases present with disseminated abdominal disease, massive ascites, and/or generalized infiltration of the intestinal wall, resulting in intestinal obstruction and ileus (Fig. 13-23). With abdominal NHL, life-threatening conditions mainly evolve from intestinal tract obstruction or even rupture and/or anuria. The latter can result for different reasons—obstruction of the uterus by retroperitoneal tumors, massive infiltration of the kidneys, spontaneous acute tumor lysis syndrome (ATLS), and any combination of these conditions. These patients require emergency management (see later, "Treatment and Outcome: Emergencies"). Both the abdomen and thorax can be affected in BL patients.

A mediastinal tumor is the typical manifestation of T-cell LBL but is not specific to it. In T-cell LBLs, the thymus and mediastinal mass usually do not show the tuberous margins typical for mediastinal nodal involvement in Hodgkin's lymphoma (compare Figs. 13-7 and 13-8). T-cell LBLs frequently spread to adjacent lymph node regions in the infra- and supraclavicular area as well as to subdiaphragmatic retroperitoneal nodes. In about 10% of T-cell LBL patients, a mediastinal mass is missing and the primary tumor arises from other sites. The rare PMLBL is by definition a mediastinal tumor, usually characterized by particularly aggressive invasive growth into adjacent structures and a tendency for focal involvement of the kidneys (see Fig. 13-18). A mediastinal mass is also observed in 40% of ALCL patients. A mediastinal tumor is frequently accompanied by large pleural and pericardial effusions, which may require rapid intervention. Patients with mediastinal NHL may go undetected for longer periods with slight retrosternal pain and chronic cough, sometimes misinterpreted as obstructive bronchitis or asthma. It may finally present as a life-threatening condition characterized by respiratory distress, superior vena cava syndrome caused by compression of mediastinal structures, and imminent low-output heart failure in case of

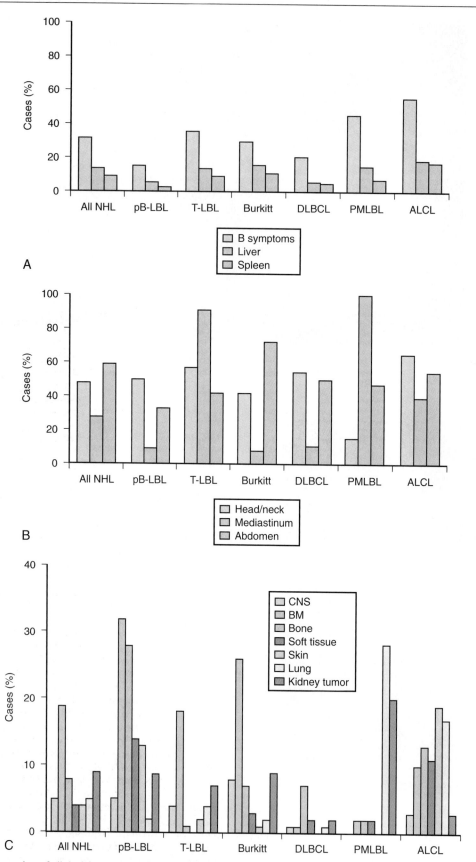

Figure 13-21. Presentation of clinical features by NHL subtypes (*N* = 2147). **A,** B symptoms and liver and/or spleen involvement. **B,** Involvement of anatomic areas—head and neck, mediastinum, and abdomen. **C,** Involvement of extranodal sites. See text for details. (Data derived from multicenter studies NHL BFM.)

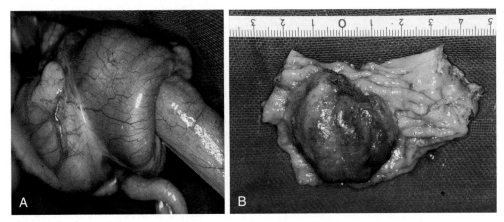

Figure 13-22. Ileocecal Burkitt lymphoma. The polypous tumor adherent to the inner intestine has been the perpendiculum for intussusception.

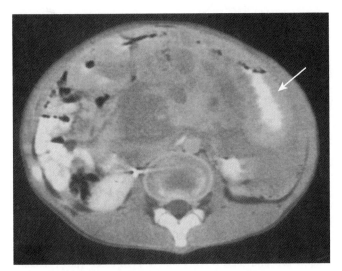

Figure 13-23. Disseminated abdominal disease in a child with Burkitt's lymphoma, including ascites, enlarged mesenteric nodes, and generalized infiltration of the intestinal wall (*arrow*).

massive pericardial effusion. Such patients are at high risk for death if not managed appropriately (see later, "Treatment and Outcome: Emergencies"). Intubation anesthesia is especially dangerous for patients with critical compression of the trachea and/or bronchi (see Fig. 13-8B).

The clinical pattern of precursor B-cell LBL differs significantly from that of T-cell LBL. There is a strong tendency for BM and bone involvement as well as for soft tissue and skin lesions. The skin lesions differ from those of ALCL in that the tendency for ulceration is lacking (see Fig. 13-19A,B). Precursor B-cell (pB) LBLs have a certain predilection for subcutaneous sites, such as the scalp and face.[466]

DLBCLs have a less characteristic clinical pattern compared with other subtypes. There is no clear predilection for a certain anatomic region or organ. The tendency for their dissemination to the BM or/and CNS is rather low and most patients present with localized disease (see Fig. 13-21).

The rare cases of pediatric follicular lymphoma also present most frequently with localized disease.[381] A peculiar feature of this entity is the presentation as primary testicular lymphoma in boys.[467]

ALCL may be the most intriguing subtype of childhood NHL; it is characterized by several distinctive features, including frequent extranodal disease of lung, skin, bone, and soft tissue and the presence of B symptoms (see Fig. 13-21).[393,398,399,468,469] Patients may have an indolent phase consisting of mild lymphadenopathy and a longer history of illness characterized by fever and, most intriguing, a waxing and waning course of lymph node adenopathy, until finally rapid progression takes place.[399,470] ALCL may mimic other diseases. Soft tissue involvement may occur as multiple tumors in the subcutaneous tissue and muscles, or as a single larger tumor resembling a soft tissue sarcoma. Bone manifestations vary from small osteolytic lesions to large tumors simulating bone tumors (see Fig. 13-17). Two types of skin lesions can be observed. There may be single or multiple bluish-colored cutaneous or subcutaneous nodules, large ulcerated lesions (see Fig. 13-19A), and multiple or disseminated papillomatous lesions of a red-yellow color. In contrast to adults, the disease in children and adolescents is rarely confined to the skin (see later). In rare cases, the neutrophil-rich ALCL may mimic inflammatory processes in bone, skin, and soft tissue. In such cases, fine-needle biopsy or needle aspiration may obtain, predominantly or even exclusively, neutrophils, which can lead to the misleading diagnosis of an abscess formation.[471-473] Compared with patients with BL or LBL, children with ALCL have microscopically detectable BM disease less frequently. The diagnosis of BM involvement may depend on the procedure applied (see later, "Diagnosis and Staging"). Not infrequently, marked hemophagocytosis by macrophages can be observed in the BM of ALCL patients. In rare cases, disseminated intravascular coagulation of yet unknown pathogenesis has been observed as a paraneoplastic syndrome.[474] Some of the distinctive clinical features of ALCL may be the result of cytokine production of tumor cells. ALCL cells have been shown to produce IL-6, which may be responsible for fever, bone lesions, and thrombocytosis, IL-9, IL-4, interferon-γ, and granulocyte-macrophage colony-stimulating factor (GM-CSF) and granulocyte-colony stimulating factor (G-CSF), which may induce leukocytosis.[475-478] Many ALCL patients have elevated serum concentrations of C-reactive protein (CRP) at diagnosis, which may correlate with disease activity.

Bone marrow and/or CNS involvement is observed in 15% to 30% and 5% to 8%, respectively, of patients with pB-LBL, T-cell LBL, and BL, but is rare in patients with DLBCL and PMLBL (see Fig. 13-21C). In the rare event of CNS involvement in DLBCL patients, an intraparenchymal mass is the predominant pattern, whereas in pB-LBL, T-LBL, and BL, most CNS-positive patients have meningeal disease with blasts in the cerebrospinal fluid (CSF).[479]

Of note, Burkitt's leukemia, often referred to as B-cell ALL, most often presents as a leukemic disease in combination with large tumors.[480] However, in some cases, the disease can be confined to the BM without any extramedullary involvement, except for the CNS.

Laboratory findings are unspecific except for increased serum LDH levels in advanced-stage disease, especially in BL and T-cell LBL cases. In children with Burkitt's leukemia, the peripheral blood (PB) may show the typical constellation of acute leukemia. However, in contrast to pediatric ALL, in Burkitt's leukemia the blast count in the PB rarely exceeds 30,000 to 50,000/µL. Also, the degree of anemia and thrombocytopenia is less in B-cell ALL patients as compared with pediatric ALL, reflecting a different degree of BM invasion.

Apart from these biologically well-defined NHL subtypes typical for childhood and adolescence, many other rare subtypes may be occasionally diagnosed in children, including those usually occurring only in adults. Peripheral T- and NK-cell neoplasms other than ALCL are probably the most frequent, although rare in terms of absolute number. They are an assemblage of heterogeneous disorders in terms of biology as well as clinical patterns. The rare extranodal T- and NK-cell lymphoma, nasal type, may be the only one with a repetitive characteristic clinical pattern, characterized by destructive lesions that arise from midline structures of the face and upper aerodigestive tract (previously termed *lethal midline granuloma*).

Non-Hodgkin's Lymphoma Confined to Extranodal Organs

In rare cases, NHL can occur in a single extranodal organ and may mimic other malignant or nonmalignant disorders.

Central Nervous System Lymphoma

Primary CNS NHL is a rare observation in children and adolescents but is more frequent in children affected by inherited or acquired immunodeficiency syndromes.[481] In a large cohort of 2170 patients of the NHL-BFM studies, only 10 patients were observed with primary CNS lymphoma.[479] The estimated incidence in North America is 15 to 20 cases/year.[482] Most cases present with uni- or multifocal intraparenchymal masses but some patients have meningeal disease only, or combinations of both. Diffuse large B-cell lymphoma is the most common subtype, followed by ALCL.[479,481] The clinical features resemble those of brain tumors characterized by signs of increased intracranial pressure, nerve palsies, personality changes, and endocrinologic disturbances.

Primary Cutaneous Non-Hodgkin's Lymphoma

Primary skin lymphoma is rare in childhood, although some cases may go unrecognized for longer periods.[483] In a series of 69 patients younger than 20 years, mycosis fungoides occurred most frequently, followed by CD30+ ALCL, lymphomatoid papillomatosis, marginal zone lymphoma, and precursor B-cell LBL (see Fig. 13-19).[484] Primary cutaneous CD30+ ALCLs differ biologically from systemic ALCLs (e.g., by the lack of Alk translocations).[483,485] Lymphomatoid papulosis is characterized by papulonodular eruptions of only a few millimeters of diameter in size (see Fig. 13-19) and spontaneous regressions. Some patients will develop CD30+ ALCL, and to differentiate between them may sometimes be difficult. In some of these patients, the first diagnosis can be ALCL, and only the course

of recurrent papulonodular skin eruptions or intensive questioning of the history will disclose the existence of lymphomatoid papulosis.[401,483]

Primary Bone Lymphoma

Although bone involvement is not infrequent in childhood NHL, only about 2% of pediatric NHL cases present as primary bone lymphoma without other manifestations, including missing BM involvement.[486,487] The most frequent histologic subtypes are LBL, DLBCL and ALCL.[487-489] Almost any bone can be the primary site and, in some cases, multiple bone lesions are present. Primary bone lymphoma can be localized at typical sites of primary bone tumors and can, on imaging, mimic osteosarcoma or Ewing's sarcoma (see Fig. 13-17). Thus, diagnostic errors may occur, especially between Ewing's sarcoma and primary lymphoblastic bone lymphoma, because both are small round blue cell tumors. Furthermore, both can express CD99, which was previously regarded as specific for Ewing's sarcoma.[490]

Diagnosis and Staging

Accurate classification is the prerequisite for allocation of the patients to the appropriate therapy strategy (see later, "Treatment and Outcome"). Table 13-24 shows the diagnostic program and the required preservation of appropriate material to establish the exact diagnosis.

If a malignant lymphoma is suspected, it is important to determine whether the diagnosis can be confirmed without an operation. Many children present with advanced-stage disease, including advanced BM invasion and/or malignant effusions. In most of these cases, correct diagnosis can be made by cytology, immunophenotyping by flow cytometry and, if necessary, cytogenetics. A diagnostic surgical procedure should only be performed if a definitive diagnosis cannot be achieved in this way. It is not helpful to perform surgery for an abdominal tumor first and then to diagnose Burkitt's leukemia during staging procedures. If surgery is to be performed, the procedure should be minimally invasive and should only be used to preserve enough biopsy material to characterize the disease fully. The role of initial surgery is discussed later. If biopsy is performed, ideally the pathologist and pediatric oncologist are present in the operating room and can process the tumor immediately after biopsy. One piece of the tumor should be subdivided for formalin fixation and for shock freezing so that the composition of the frozen piece can be determined from the formalin-fixated counterpart. Most cases can be correctly classified by cytology of tumor touch imprints, histomorphology, and immunohistochemistry with the available wide range of paraffin-resistant antibodies. Regarding the appropriate allocation of patients to therapy groups, there are some crucial diagnostic cutting sites that require additional selected diagnostic considerations. Typical interfaces are distinct between LBLs of precursor B-cell type and BL-BL variants or DLBCL, T-cell rich variant of DLBCL and NLPHL, PMLBL and NSHL, and the distinction of ALCL from other peripheral T-cell–NK-cell lymphomas or the anaplastic variant of DLBCL. In these cases, immunohistochemical staining for the expression of genes associated with differentiation compartments such as TdT (positive only in precursor B- and T-cell neoplasms) and the germinal center cell–associated marker bcl-6 can be helpful.[336] Finally, the identification of subtype-specific chromosomal translocations may be decisive.[491] However, appropriate material for cytogenetic evaluation is not always available in NHL patients. In such cases, FISH, which can be performed on the tumor touch preparations, or paraffin sections, is a valid method to

TABLE 13-24 **Procedures for Diagnosis and Classification of Non-Hodgkin's Lymphoma (NHL)**

Method	Appropriate Material
ESSENTIAL	
Cytomorphology	Tumor touch imprints, bone marrow smears; cytospin preparations of effusions
FAB classification	
Histopathology, immunohistochemistry, WHO classification	Tumor material, formalin-fixated
Immunophenotyping by flow cytometry (FACS analysis)	Vital cells of anticoagulated bone marrow malignant effusions
INDICATED IN SELECTED CASES	
Cytogenetics	Vital cells of anticoagulated bone marrow malignant effusions
FISH	Tumor touch imprints, bone marrow smears, cytospin preparations of effusions, fresh-frozen tumor tissue, paraffin-embedded tumor tissue
Detection of NHL subtype-specific fusion gene transcripts by RT-PCR	Vital cells, anticoagulated (EDTA or citrate) bone marrow malignant effusions
FUTURE PROCEDURES	
Matrix-comparative genomic hybridization	Vital cells of anticoagulated bone marrow effusions, fresh-frozen tumor tissue, paraffin-embedded tumor tissue
Gene expression profile	Vital cells of anticoagulated bone marrow effusions, fresh-frozen tumor tissue

FACS, fluorescence-activated cell sorting; FISH, fluorescence in situ hybridization; RT-PCR, reverse transcriptase-polymerase chain reaction.

visualize most of the known subtype-specific chromosomal translocations.[492,493] In selected cases, subtype-specific fusion genes or their transcripts can be detected by reverse transcriptase-polymerase chain reaction (RT-PCR) assay.[494] Gene expression profiling has enabled identification of distinct types of DLBCL.[372] It has been shown that BL has a reproducible gene expression profile that can be used to identify and distinguish molecular BL from morphologically and immunophenotypically indistinguishable cases of DLBCB (see Fig. 13-13).[342,343] Contrary to the case with adults, the distinction between molecular BL and DLBCL has little impact on treatment in children (however, see later, "Treatment and Outcome"). Genome-wide comparative genomic hybridization (matrix should be preserved) will become increasingly important to detect secondary chromosomal aberrations with possible impact on NHL pathogenesis and prognosis. After proper diagnostic classification of each patient, whenever possible, appropriate material for future research should be preserved (e.g., purified tumor cells or/and shock-frozen tumor tissue).[491]

With the currently available routine diagnostic tools, a needle aspiration or biopsy is generally not suitable for extracting appropriate material to classify the disease accurately and should therefore be reserved for exceptions, such as when a more invasive procedure would represent an undue risk for the patient (e.g., for patients with critically large mediastinal tumors; see later, "Emergencies"). However, with further refined molecular genetic methodologies, accurate classification by means of fine-needle aspiration may become applicable in a broader range of cases in the future.[495]

Staging Classification

The St. Jude staging system is widely accepted for the staging of childhood NHL (Table 13-25).[496] The distribution of stages varies greatly, depending on the NHL subtype (Fig. 13-24). The St. Jude staging system was primarily based on the clinicopathologic features of the main NHL subtypes of childhood, LBL and BL. It takes into account the different pattern of disease spread of these disorders as compared with Hodgkin's lymphoma, especially the more frequent extranodal involvement. The definition of stages is determined by the number and anatomic pattern of disease sites, their resectability, and the more frequent involvement of the BM and CNS in LBL

TABLE 13-25 **St. Jude Staging System for Pediatric Non-Hodgkin's Lymphoma**

Stage	Definition
I	A single tumor (extranodal) or involvement of a single anatomic area (nodal), with the exclusion of the mediastinum and abdomen
II	A single tumor (extranodal) with regional node involvement
	Two or more nodal areas on the same side of the diaphragm
	Two single (extranodal) tumors, with or without regional node involvement on the same side of the diaphragm
	A primary gastrointestinal tract tumor (usually in the ileocecal area), with or without involvement of associated mesenteric nodes, that is completely resectable
III	Two single tumors (extranodal) on opposite sides of the diaphragm
	Two or more nodal areas above and below the diaphragm
	Any primary intrathoracic tumor (mediastinal, pleural, or thymic)
	Extensive primary intra-abdominal disease
	Any paraspinal or epidural tumor, whether or not other sites are involved
IV	Any of the above findings with initial involvement of the central nervous system, bone marrow, or both

Adapted from Murphy SB. Classification, staging and end results of treatment of childhood non-Hodgkin's lymphomas: dissimilarities from lymphomas in adults. Semin Oncol. 1980;7:332-339.

and BL. Lymphoblastic neoplasms are considered acute lymphoblastic leukemia if there are 25% or more lymphoblasts in the BM. For BL, infiltration of the BM with more than 25% lymphoma cells is characterized as B-cell or Burkitt's cell leukemia, also referred to as B-ALL. The St. Jude staging system has proven useful for the stratification of therapy intensity for the treatment of these entities. For other entities, such as ALCL, its usefulness for treatment stratification is less well

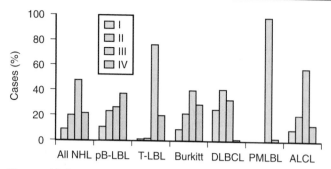

Figure 13-24. Distribution of stages according to non-Hodgkin's lymphoma subtypes (N = 2147). See text for details. (Data derived from multicenter studies NHL BFM.)

defined because of the different biologic behavior of this disorder as compared with LBL and BL. Its weakness is in the classification of patients with multifocal skin and with multifocal bone involvement for whom the bone marrow is not affected.

Furthermore, there is no specification of the imaging method to identify tumor sites because the St. Jude staging system was developed in the late 1970s based on imaging methods available at that time. Thus, with the imaging modalities now available, the recognition of involved sites may have changed. In addition, other criteria with important prognostic impact on outcome have been detected since then and are now used for stratification of treatment, such as tumor mass reflected by the surrogate parameter LDH.[497,498] However, in spite of these shortcomings, the St. Jude staging classification is useful because it provides physicians worldwide with a common basis for comparison of experience and treatment results in the care of children and adolescents with NHL.

Clinical Evaluation and Staging Procedures

The aim of staging procedures is to identify all disease manifestations as a basis for treatment and follow-up monitoring of treatment response. Principally, clinical evaluation and staging procedures of children and adolescents with NHL are similar to what has been described for patients with Hodgkin's lymphoma. However, in contrast to Hodgkin's lymphoma, local irradiation has little role in the treatment of childhood NHL. In addition, for many subtypes of childhood NHL, the anatomic and topographically defined stage of the disease is no longer the unique criterion for stratification of treatment intensity. Although accuracy is always demanded, there is less of a need for aggressive clarification of involvement or noninvolvement of single nodes or even certain extranodal sites, especially if invasive methods would be required. However, this may differ among different NHL subtypes (see later).

Because of the variety of clinical patterns of sites in childhood NHL, careful physical examination is essential. Also, a detailed interview of the patient and/or guardian is required to lend special attention to certain sites. As described in the section on clinical characteristics, almost any organ, tissue, and anatomic area can be involved. Concerning the examination of lymph node involvement, the considerations described for Hodgkin's lymphoma are also valid for NHL. Special attention should be drawn to signs of a critical space-occupying tumor, such as one that would cause respiratory distress and increased filling of the facial and cervical veins as a result of upper vena cava compression in case of a mediastinal tumor (see later, "Emergencies"). Because CNS involvement is not uncommon, careful neurologic examination is necessary, including cranial

nerve function, signs of paraparesis, and increased intracranial pressure.

Basic laboratory studies include peripheral blood counts, serum concentrations of LDH and CRP, basic coagulation parameters, liver function tests, and parameters to detect imminent ATLS, such as electrolyte levels and potassium, calcium, phosphorus, blood urea nitrogen (BUN), uric acid, and creatinine levels. Bone marrow aspiration is mandatory as well as a CSF examination (cell count and cytomorphology), except in an emergency situation.

Basic imaging studies include chest x-rays in two levels, abdominal ultrasound, and cranial cross-sectional imaging diagnostics. Chest radiography is routinely performed and is sufficient to detect a mediastinal mass and/or pleural effusions. In most cases, US is sufficient to detect involvement of abdominal and retroperitoneal tumors. Abdominal CT or MRI may be performed in some circumstances (e.g., suboptimal conditions for US). The need for routine cranial MRI or CT scan is debatable, because intracerebral involvement without the presence of CSF blasts and/or cranial nerve palsy is rare, but does occur.[479] Because of the adverse consequences for the patient if an intracerebral focus remains undetected at the time of diagnosis, a cranial MRI scan would seem to be justified. However, cranial imaging is mandatory in any case of neurologic impairment. The individual disease patterns will dictate whether other imaging studies need to be done. Appropriate imaging methods to examine specific anatomic areas were discussed for Hodgkin's lymphoma (see Table 13-6). For whole-body functional imaging to identify disease sites, gallium-67 scintigraphy was in use for staging studies in children with NHL but not in all countries, mainly because of the caveats around radiation exposure. Furthermore, gallium-67 uptake varies among different NHL subtypes; the radionuclide uptake is not specific for lymphoma tissue, but is also taken up by normal thymus and areas of inflammation.[499] As for children with Hodgkin's lymphoma, gallium-67 scintigraphy will be replaced by FDG-PET.[130]

The considerations discussed earlier ("Hodgkin's Lymphoma") on the possible role of FDG-PET in the staging of children and adolescents with lymphoma are relevant for NHL. However, the different avidity for FDG uptake of different NHL subtypes appears to be even more pronounced than for Hodgkin's lymphoma.[141,500] One aspect warrants careful consideration in children with NHL—namely, upstaging as far as disease stage is used to stratify treatment intensity. Children with St. Jude stage I or II disease have excellent outcomes with limited therapy. With few exceptions, this holds true for all NHL subtypes. The St. Jude staging was primarily based on clinical findings, x-ray results, and surgical resectability of abdominal tumors. Modern imaging methods, especially FDG-PET, most likely may alter stage allocation for patients when disease sites not detectable with the methods available when this staging system was developed are disclosed. For example, identification of a small lesion at the opposite side of diaphragm will change stage I to stage III according to the St. Jude staging classification. As a consequence, these patients may undergo more intense treatment, although their disease-free survival probability with limited therapy for stage I or II disease may be near 100%. Thus, prospective studies are required to evaluate and verify the diagnostic role of FDG-PET in staging and to assess whether different findings of FDG-PET compared with conventional imaging translate into different staging, and whether this will affect the outcome for patients demanding modification of therapy. However, functional imaging with FDG-PET may become a useful tool for evaluation of the kinetics of response to therapy, which in turn is probably a powerful prognostic parameter.[501] For that purpose, pretherapeutic (baseline) FDG-PET may be required, at least for distinct NHL subtypes with variable FDG uptake (see later).[133]

If the diagnosis of NHL is otherwise confirmed, the involvement of organs is usually based on clinical and imaging findings, and biopsy is restricted to uncertain cases if involvement or noninvolvement would alter treatment. Involvement of the testes is usually diagnosed in case of firm, painless, uni- or bilateral testes enlargement. Similarly, in females, involvement of the ovaries is usually based on imaging alone.

Skeletal scintigraphy can detect bone involvement. Because skeletal involvement was not an indication of negative significance for prognosis in several analyses, mandatory skeletal scintigraphy to detect clinically occult bone foci is unnecessary.[393,469,487,502] Specific imaging procedures may be confined to patients with symptoms of bone involvement, such as pain and swelling. Larger bone lesions are almost always symptomatic and can be depicted using simple x-ray diagnostics.

The involvement of BM and the CNS affects treatment of all subtypes of childhood NHL and therefore needs special attention. The diagnosis of BM involvement depends on the procedure used. BM aspiration and microscopic examination of stained smears are basic. If BM involvement alters treatment, further sites (at least two) should be examined in case the first BM aspirate does not contain blasts, because BM involvement may differ in different BM areas. Conventionally, BM involvement is diagnosed if more than 5% blasts are present in a representative BM aspiration smear. This applies especially for patients with LBL, because FAB L1 blasts are undistinguishable from immature hematopoietic cells when present in low numbers. However, because of the characteristic cytomorphology of BL and ALCL, their cells are microscopically identifiable at a much lower frequency in the BM (see Table 13-19). A generally agreed convention is lacking so far as to whether such patients are to be allocated as BM-positive or not. Compared with BM aspiration smears, BM biopsies may enable the detection of BM involvement in a higher proportion of patients, especially if disease-specific immunohistochemistry staining can be applied to identify lymphoma cells in the BM, as in the case of ALCL by means of Alk staining.[503] An even higher level of sensitivity may be achieved by using immunophenotyping for the detection of minimal numbers of malignant cells in the BM and blood.[504] Another option is PCR technology to detect disease-specific fusion gene products. Using this for pediatric ALCL patients, the frequency of patients with detectable lymphoma cells in the BM is even higher than 50%, whereas only about 5% of patients show microscopically identifiable ALCL cells in the BM smears.[469,505-507] Also in BL patients, lymphoma cells can be detected in the BM using PCR assay to identify the IgH *MYC* fusion of the BL-specific translocation t(8;14)(q24;q32) in microscopically negative patients.[508,509] Thus, the question arises as to whether the detection of lymphoma cells in the BM and PB below the microscopic sensitivity level has an additional effect on patient outcome. In other words, does minimally disseminated disease at the submicroscopic level simply reflect an increase of the total mass of tumor cells, or is it a biologically different and more aggressive disease with higher resistance to treatment? In children and adolescents with ALCL, the presence of minimally disseminated disease detected only by PCR-based identification of the NPM-ALK fusion gene transcript in the BM and PB is associated with a significantly increased risk of treatment failure.[506,507]

CNS involvement is usually diagnosed in the presence of an intracerebral mass and/or lymphoma cells in the CSF.[479,510-513] In patients with LBL, a CSF cell count more than 5/μL is also required.[479,514] In case of doubt, specific immunocytochemistry staining (e.g., Alk or TdT in case of ALCL and LBL, respectively, or FISH using disease-specific probes) may be useful for clarification.

However, there is no internationally standardized definition of CNS involvement in childhood NHL. Opinions differ on how cranial nerve paralysis and paraspinal involvement are considered as criteria for manifest CNS involvement without the concomitant presence of the hard criteria listed earlier. Cranial nerve paralysis alone is generally only considered a criterion for CNS involvement if extracerebral causes have been ruled out. Paraspinal involvement with no evidence of blasts in the CSF is considered to constitute CNS involvement in some study groups, but not in others.[244,498,502,510,511,513] In a recent report, 25 pediatric NHL patients with epidural tumors who were diagnosed and treated as CNS-negative had an EFS rate of 87%.[479]

Intracerebral lesions on cranial MRI in the absence of morphologically identifiable lymphoma cells in the CSF may create a diagnostic dilemma. If the diagnosis of NHL is established otherwise, an intracerebral mass on imaging is usually recognized as CNS involvement without biopsy proof, except that imaging suggests a different causality. In the rare cases of multiple intracerebral lesions, a genesis other than lymphoma may be acute disseminated myeloencephalitis or infection. In doubtful cases, guided stereotactic biopsy may be considered because of the importance of the differential diagnosis.

Clinical evaluations need to take into consideration special requirements of distinct subtypes. This applies especially for children who suffer from ALCL. In these cases, special attention should be directed to the examination of soft tissue and skin because of their relatively frequent involvement in ALCL patients. Because of the frequency and adverse prognostic impact of lung involvement, which may be missed on a routine chest x-ray, a CT scan of the thorax provides additional information regarding possible infiltration of the lungs and other thoracic organs. In case of skin lesions, a biopsy should be performed to prove or exclude skin involvement because this may alter treatment. If only skin lesions are present, careful evaluation of the patient is crucial to distinguish between primary cutaneous ALCL, ALCL evolving from lymphomatoid papillomatosis, and systemic ALCL with skin involvement. In the first case, a watchful waiting strategy may be appropriate, but skin involvement in systemic ALCL is a worse prognostic parameter.

Treatment and Outcome

Today, children and adolescents who suffer from NHL have more than an 80% survival rate but at the expense of very cumbersome treatment. Current treatment protocols are aggressive and carry a significant risk for the patient to die from treatment-related complications. Thus, these patients should only be treated in institutions with extensive experience in the treatment of children with cancer; they should have a dedicated multidisciplinary team and appropriate infrastructure to provide all the necessary support, including an intensive care unit and hemodialysis availability.

Emergencies

Children with NHL can be brought to emergency rooms with life-threatening emergency situations such as stridor, shortness of breath, and superior vena cava syndrome caused by a mediastinal tumor, ileus and acute abdomen in case of an abdominal tumor, oligoanuria, cranial nerve paralysis, amaurosis, paraplegia in the case of epidural involvement and, in rare cases, disseminated intravascular coagulation. Sometimes, invasive diagnostic measures create emergencies for previously compromised children. ATLS, one of the most challenging complications, can occur during the first days after initiation of chemotherapy or may already exist on admission.

Emergencies Caused by Mediastinal Tumor

A mediastinal tumor can cause respiratory distress or even failure and superior vena cava syndrome because of compression of the superior vena cava trachea, and main bronchi. Many of these patients have extensive pleural effusion and/or pericardial effusion, which can lead to cardiac tamponade and low-output heart failure. If there is considerable respiratory impairment, such as orthopnea, then all invasive diagnostic procedures, including BM aspiration and lumbar puncture, should be postponed. In case of a large pleural effusion, it should be carefully relieved under local anesthesia with an atraumatic device. For critical pericardial effusion, drainage is required. Cytoreductive therapy with prednisone, 60 mg/m^2/day, and cyclophosphamide, 100 to 200 mg/m^2/day, should be started immediately. An alternative is to start radiotherapy immediately. A dramatic shrinkage of tumor may be seen with doses of 10 to 15 Gy. Prevention or treatment of ATLS is essential (see later). After stabilization of the clinical condition, normally after 1 or 2 days, procedures to establish diagnosis may be undertaken.

In all cases of mediastinal tumor intubation, general anesthesia carries an increased risk to induce injury and/or swelling of the tracheal mucosa, which may lead to critical constriction during ventilation or after extubation. Therefore, a CT scan of the chest gives information on the degree to which the trachea and/or bronchi are constricted (see Fig. 13-8A,B). In case of significant constriction of the trachea, the procedure is as described earlier. If there is no significant impairment of airways, the next step is to try to establish a diagnosis by examining the bone marrow and any available pleural effusion. If surgery is necessary to establish the diagnosis, it is essential to know that life-threatening respiratory failure can occur because of tracheal edema and tracheal compression postoperatively. If intubation is performed on these patients, it is wise to continue ventilation after surgery, start cytoreductive therapy immediately, and postpone extubation until a significant shrinking of the tumor is achieved.

Incipient Paraplegia and Amaurosis

If the diagnosis of lymphoma can be established by other manifestations, cytoreductive therapy with cyclophosphamide, 200 mg/m^2/day, and prednisone, 60 mg/m^2/day, or dexamethasone, 10 mg/m^2/day, should be started immediately. If necessary, the dosage of both medications can be increased. Whether surgical decompression is mandatory depends on the degree and duration of paraplegia. Rapid surgical decompression may be advantageous in cases of higher degree and/or longer duration of paraplegia. In case of cranial nerve palsy caused by lymphoma localized at the epipharynx, paranasal sinus or skull base surgery should be restricted to biopsy if a decompressing resection would cause mutilation or a loss of function. In most cases, rapid tumor relief can be achieved by promptly beginning cytoreductive therapy, as described earlier. (**Caution:** Lumbar puncture may carry the risk of brainstem herniation.)

Oligoanuria and Acute Renal Failure

Oligoanuria can be caused by bilateral kidney infiltration or ureter compression by lymphomatous tumors, the consequences of spontaneous or chemotherapy-induced ATLS, or a combination of both. Oligoanuria is life-threatening for children because of the rapidly increasing hyperkalemia. Therefore,

equipment for hemodialysis should be available. Because of the rapid accumulation of potassium, the usual definition of oligoanuria may not be useful in this situation. Instead, oligoanuria may be diagnosed if urine excretion decreases significantly in spite of hydration with 130 to 200 mL/m^2/hr and full-dose medication with diuretics. The leading cause of oligoanuria needs to be determined using imaging diagnostics and laboratory studies. In the case of bilateral kidney infiltration and/or obstruction of the draining ureters by lymphoma masses, initiating cytoreductive therapy is a prerequisite for restoring kidney function. Intensive prophylaxis and therapy of ATLS is essential (see later). If ATLS is present without major infiltration of the kidneys and without urinary tract obstruction, ATLS should be treated first and the cytoreductive therapy postponed until kidney function has improved.

Prevention and Treatment of Acute Tumor Cell Lysis Syndrome

ATLS describes the metabolic derangements that occur with tumor cell breakdown, characterized by various combinations of hyperuricemia, hyperphosphatemia, hypocalcemia, hyperkalemia, and eventually acute renal failure, uremia, and death.[515-517] Clinical manifestations include nausea, vomiting, lethargy, tetany, seizures, cardiac dysrhythmias, fluid overload, congestive heart failure, and sudden death caused by asystole. The incidence of ATLS differs among tumor entities and depends primarily on the growth fraction, tumor mass, and chemotherapeutic sensitivity of the tumor. Patients with advanced-stage Burkitt's lymphoma or leukemia or LBL are at high risk to develop ATLS. ATLS may not only result in the early death of some patients, but the impaired renal function caused by ATLS may also increase the risk of death because of toxicity later in the course of treatment. The risk of ATLS is highest during the first few days after initiation of chemotherapy. Howver, some patients may present with ATLS before beginning antitumor therapy because of spontaneous tumor cell lysis, especially in BL. Hyperuricemia, hyperphosphatemia, and hyperkalemia result from the massive release of nucleic acid, phosphorus, and potassium from lysed tumor cells, whereas hypocalcemia and renal failure are the consequences that may lead to death from hyperkalemia. Purine nucleic acids released from dying tumor cells are metabolized to hypoxanthine and then to xanthine and uric acid. The latter two reactions are catabolized by the enzyme xanthine oxidase. Hyperuricemia occurs when uric acid production exceeds the excretion capacity of the kidneys. If the product exceeds its solubility, then uric acid can crystallize out which is enhanced by acidic pH. Crystallization of uric acid takes place in the renal tubules, collecting tubules and medullary vessels. The resulting oligoanuria aggravates hyperkalemia, which may lead to rapid death because of ventricular fibrillation or asystole.

Hyperhydration, alkalinization, and the administration of allopurinol, an inhibitor of xanthine oxidase, were mainstays of prevention and treatment of ATLS aimed at the reduction of uric acid production and prevention of its precipitation in the kidneys. Although effective, this approach has some limitations. Alkalinization favors the precipitation of phosphorus with calcium as calcium phosphate in both the kidney tubules and other tissues (e.g., pancreas), resulting in hypocalcemia, tissue necrosis, and anuria. Also, precipitation of hypoxanthine, the first metabolite of nucleic acids, is increased at a pH of 7.5 or higher.[518] Thus, overzealous alkalinization of the urine aimed at the prevention of crystallization of uric acid can favor the precipitation of other products of cell lysis, which leads to impaired renal function. Allopurinol as an inhibitor of xanthine oxidase only prevents further synthesis of uric acid but does not degrade the existing uric acid. Moreover, because of blocked catabolism of hypoxathine and xanthine to uric acid, the concentration of these metabolites increases, which in turn can cause precipitation in the renal tubules. An alternative is to catabolize uric acid to allantoin by urate oxidase, an enzyme not found in humans.[519,520] Allantoin has much higher solubility in urine than uric acid. Administration of rasburicase, a recombinant form of urate oxidase, was found to reduce uric acid concentration in children with hematologic malignancies rapidly and significantly as compared with allopurinol administration.[521,522] Thus, the accumulation of toxic precursor metabolites of uric acid can be avoided. Also, alkalinization and its adverse impact on the precipitation of calcium phosphate and hypoxathine in renal tubules can be decreased and even avoided. Although there are no prospective randomized trials comparing the incidence of renal failure and toxic death in pediatric NHL patients receiving allopurinol versus urate oxidase, there is some evidence for a beneficial impact of urate oxidase from large clinical trials. In a French study, the incidence of children with advanced-stage B-cell NHL undergoing dialysis during the first days of treament was only 2.6% compared with 16% and 23% in other cooperative studies using the same French protocol.[523] The difference was that a nonrecombinant form of urate oxidase was available and used in the French study, whereas in the other studies, patients received only allopurinol. Even more importantly, the incidence of toxic death was much lower in the French study.

The mainstay of successful management of ATLS is to maintain a high index of suspicion and a proactive prophylactic strategy to prevent or reduce the severity of ATLS. Therefore, patients with high risk for ATLS should be treated in an intensive care unit by those who are trained and experienced with the complications of ATLS and availability of hemodialysis. The most important measure is the initiation and maintenance of a high urine output (100 to 250 mL/m^2/hr). If this is working well, then metabolic imbalances that require intervention are rare. If the uric acid, potassium, phosphate, and/or creatinine levels are already increased before the start of cytoreductive therapy, then measures for controlling these substances should be started first, before active cytoreductive therapy is begun. However, in patients with rapidly growing advanced-stage BL or LBL, it is critical not to wait too long to start cytoreductive therapy. If, in spite of sufficient hydration and diuretics, it is not possible to initiate and maintain a satisfactory urine output, early hemodialysis should be instituted. This situation probably occurs because of direct infiltration of the kidneys, obstruction of the urinary tract caused by lymphomatous compression, established urate or calcium phosphate nephropathy, or a combination of these conditions (see earlier). Hyperkalemia is the most frequent, immediately life-threatening complication of ATLS. If potassium levels rise above normal or, in the case of existing hyperkalemia, do not fall quickly after starting therapeutic measures, a life-threatening hyperkalemia can evolve within a few hours.

Classification and strategies for prevention and treatment of ATLS were recently described in an excellent review.[517] Basic principles are as follows:

- Hydration: 3000 to 5000 mL/m^2/day (two to four times maintenance)
- Maintain urine output > 100 mL/m^2/hr
- Maintain specific gravity of the urine ≤ 1.010
- Fluid balancing: Output = input − insensible losses
- For insufficient output: Furosemide 0.5 to 6 (to 10) mg/kg/day
- Body weight measured twice daily
- Initially, no extra potassium in infusion; slight hypokalemia not a problem

Additional measures for patients at risk for ATLS are as follows.

Prevention or Treatment of Hyperuricemia

Low-Risk Patients

- Localized stage LBL and BL, other NHL subtypes regardless of stage, no kidney involvement, normal serum values for uric acid, potassium, phophorus, renal function; LDH < 2× normal
- Allopurinol, 10 mg/kg/day PO, divided q8h, for 3 to 5 days
- Alkalinization of urine is controversial (see earlier); avoid excessive alkalinization; optimal urine pH = 6.5 to 7.0

High-Risk Patients

- Advanced stage LBL, BL, Burkitt's leukemia, and/or LDH > 2× normal, kidney involvement, increased serum values for uric acid, potassium, phophorus, renal function
- Rasburicase, 0.05 to 0.2 mg/kg/day IV over 30 minutes, for 3 to 5 days, depending on tumor size; alkalinization of urine unnecessary, could be a disadvantage because it might enhance precipitation of calcium phosphate in kidney tubules and tissues (e.g., pancreas). Avoid rasburicase in patients with glucose-6-phosphate dehydrogenase deficiency.
- Laboratory controls: Na, K, Cl, Ca, phosphate, uric acid, creatinine every 6, 12, or 24 hours, depending on degree of disturbances. (**Note:** If rasburicase is administered, blood samples for measurement of uric acid need to be placed on ice immediately to avoid ex vivo enzymatic degradation of uric acid, resulting in false low values.)

Recommendations for the management of electrolyte disturbances and renal dysfunction are as follows.[517]

Hyperphosphatemia

- Moderate (≥2.1 mmol/L): Avoid IV phosphate administration
- Aluminum hydroxide, 50 to 150 mg/kg/24 hr PO, divided q6h
- Severe: Dialysis, hemofiltration

Hypocalcemia

- Defined as ≤1.75 mmol/L
- Asymptomatic: No therapy
- Symptomatic: Calcium gluconate, 50 to 100 mg/kg IV (**Note:** Use caution in case of hyperphosphatemia.)

Hyperkalemia

- Moderate and asymptomatic (≥6.0 mmol/L): Avoid IV and oral potassium; electrocardiography and cardiac rhythm monitoring; sodium polystyrene sulfonate (Kayexalate), 1 g/kg with 50% sorbitol PO or per rectum; consider/prepare for dialysis
- Severe (>7.0 mmol/L) and/or symptomatic: Same as earlier, plus calcium gluconate (100 to 200 mg/kg) IV and/or regular insulin (0.1 unit/kg IV) + dextrose 25% (2 mL/kg), IV, dialysis

Acute Renal Dysfunction and Uremia

- Acute renal dysfunction resulting in uremia may be multifactorial including uric acid crystal obstructive uropathy, calcium phosphate nephrocalcinosis, renal tumor infiltration, ureteral obstruction by the tumor, intravascular volume depletion, nephrotoxic drugs, or a combination of these factors.

- Careful monitoring of heart function, fluid intake and output, serum electrolytes, treatment or prevention of hyperuricemia, management of hypertension, modification of the dosage of renally excreted drugs are main principles of the management of these patients.
- The availability of the equipment for dialysis is essential since in some cases renal replacement therapy may be required.
- Indications for dialysis include one or more of the following uncontrolled by medical management: hyperkalemia, hyperphosphatemia, product of calcium x phosphate (mmol/L) > 6, hyperuricemia uncontrolled by rasburicase, volume overload, uncontrolled hypertension, severe acidosis, severe uremia with central nervous system toxicity.

General Principles of Treatment

Childhood NHLs tend to spread early, so effective combination chemotherapy is the cornerstone of successful treatment. The risk of relapse increases with advanced stages and growth of the tumor mass, so these are important criteria for modifying the intensity and duration of chemotherapy. However, prognostic parameters with an impact on outcome differ among different entities. After reducing systemic relapses by effective combination chemotherapy, the recurrence or progression of local manifestations is the most common treatment failure across all subtypes (see Fig. 13-15). Therefore, the question of the role of local therapeutic measures continues to be an important one. A key moment in the development of current treatment concepts was the recognition that different NHL subtypes require different chemotherapeutic strategies. Also, the role of extracompartmental therapy needs special considerations for different NHL subtypes because of different frequencies and patterns of extracompartmental involvement, especially the CNS. However, all subtypes have many aspects in common as to the role of local therapeutic modalities, surgery and radiotherapy, incomplete tumor regression during treatments and appropriate monitoring of treatment response. Therefore, these considerations are discussed here.

Initial Surgery

The role of initial surgery is mainly diagnostic to provide sufficient biopsy material for comprehensive diagnostic classification. A complete resection of a small localized lymphoma may be beneficial for patients with mature B-cell NHL and ALCL. These patients have an almost 100% chance of survival with only two or three short chemotherapy courses. For patients with ALCL confined to single skin lesions, complete resection can be the definitive therapy (see earlier). However, resections at the expense of functional deficits are not justified for children with NHL. With advanced disease stages, surgeries should always be limited to minimally diagnostic procedures for preserving enough biopsy material. Partial resections, including subtotal resection, have no therapeutic value.[524] Conversely, gross sectional surgery may delay chemotherapy and is therefore obsolete.

Strategic Therapeutic Groups Differentiated by Biologic Subtypes

Differentiating NHL into lymphoblastic and nonlymphoblastic lymphomas is the most important subdivision for determining therapeutic strategy, especially for patients with advanced-stage disease.[525] Therapeutic regimens used for ALL, which are based on the principle of continual exposure to cytostatic agents for a long period, are efficacious for treating children with lympho-

blastic lymphoma.[244,525-528] In contrast, a strategy of short, intensive chemotherapy courses with high-dose intensity using corticosteroids, cyclophosphamide, and methotrexate has been shown to be more effective for treating patients with nonlymphoblastic NHL, especially BL.[498,510,525,529-534] Although this pulse type of therapy has also proved to be effective for treating patients diagnosed with ALCL, this subtype of childhood NHL has emerged to become a separate strategic treatment group.[469,524] The main reasons for the emergence of this new group were the different prognostic parameters related to treatment stratification and a higher chance to survive after relapse as compared with the other main subgroups of nonlymphoblastic NHL, BL, and DLBCL.[393,469,524,535] Internationally, the subdivision of childhood NHL into three main therapeutic groups has prevailed:

- Lymphoblastic lymphomas of precursor B-cell and T-cell type
- Peripheral B-cell lymphomas (B-NHL), including BL, Burkitt's leukemia, and DLBCL
- Anaplastic large cell lymphomas

Other rarer and currently less accurately defined NHL subtypes in children, including the small but heterogeneous group of peripheral and NK cell lymphomas, are not included in these strategic treatment groups, so their optimal treatment strategy has not yet been defined.

Therapy of Lymphoblastic Lymphoma

Chemotherapy

In large multicenter treatment studies, patients with lymphoblastic lymphomas achieved a probability of long-term EFS from 60% to more than 80% (Table 13-26). The LSA$_2$-L$_2$ protocol developed by Wollner and coworkers[526] early in the 1970s became a worldwide standard protocol for treating children with lymphoblastic lymphomas and has been used in numerous modified forms (Table 13-27).[528,536] Concurrently, in the Berlin-Frankfurt-Münster (BFM) group,[537] the strategy developed by Riehm and colleagues[527] originally designed to treat children with ALL, proved to be highly efficacious for treatment of children with LBL (see Table 13-27). In particular, there was a favorable outcome with the BFM ALL-type strategy for children with advance stage T-cell LBL.[244] Most treatment protocols listed in Table 13-26 include corticosteroids, vincristine, anthracyclines, L-asparaginase, cyclophosphamide, and the antimetabolites methotrexate (MTX), cytarabine, 6-mercaptopurine, and 6-thioguanine, but epipodophyllotoxins were part of only a few strategies.

The dose and schedule of drug administration differ. The BFM protocol is the only one that includes high-dose (HD) MTX, 5 g/m^2, in the form of a continuous IV infusion over 24 hours. The contribution of single drugs to patient cure is largely unknown because of the paucity of randomized trials. Evidence for the efficacy of L-asparaginase in patients with T-cell LBL can be derived from a randomized study conducted by the former Pediatric Oncology Group (POG).[538] Patients with T-cell LBL receiving weekly L-asparaginase after induction had a higher EFS than controls (see Table 13-26). A study designed around the BFM strategy showed instead that the administration of HD cytarabine in combination with HD MTX in the consolidation phase had no effect.[539] Dexamethasone instead of prednisone in induction resulted in improved outcome of children suffering from ALL, but at the expense of higher toxicity.[540] Randomized BFM-based trials are ongoing as to whether dexamethasone in induction can also further improve EFS of T-cell LBL patients. Early-dose

				Duration						
Protocol	**Stages**	**No. of Patients**	**pEFS ± SE (3-5 Yr)**	**(mo), Pulses (P)**	**CPM (g/m²)**	**Dox (mg/m²)**	**Epipod (mg/m²)**	**HD-MTX (g/m²)**	**CRT**	**LRT**
Modified LSA₂-L₂[528]	I-IV T + pB	84	75% ± 2%	24, P+	5.4	435	0	3 × 10 inf 3 hr	0	ICTR
UKCCSG 8503[676]	III + IV T	59	65% (CI, 50%-80%)	24, P+	0	270	1000	0	18 Gy	0
Modified LSA₂-L₂[536]	I-IV T + pB	143	74%	18, P+	4.2	270	0	0	0	Bulky
R vs. ADCOMP		138	64%	18, P+	11.2	360	0	0	0	15 Gy
POG 8704[538]	III + IV	83	L-Asp– 64% ± 6%	24, P+	6.1	390	7.200	0	0	0
L-Asp + R vs. L-Asp–	T	84	L-Asp+ 78% ± 5%							0
NHL-BFM 90[244]	I-IV T	105	90% (5 yr)	24, P–	3	240	0	5 × 4 inf 24 hr	12	0
NHL-BFM 95[677]	I-IV T + pB	198	80 +3% (5 yr)	24, P–	3	240	0	5 × 4 inf 24 hr	0	0

TABLE 13-26 Treatment Protocols and Results in Recent Multicenter Studies of Childhood and Adolescent Lymphoblastic Lymphoma

L-Asp, L-asparaginase; CI, confidence interval; CPM, cyclophosphamide; CRT, prophylactic cranial radiotherapy; Dox, doxorubicin; Epipod, epipodophyllotoxin; HD-MTX, high-dose methotrexate; ICTR, radiotherapy in case of incomplete tumor regression after induction therapy; LRT, local radiotherapy; P+, P–, with or without intensification pulses during maintenance; pB, precursor B-cell; inf, infusion; pEFS ± SE, Kaplan-Meier estimate of event-free survival ± standard error; POG, Pediatric Oncology Group; R vs., randomized versus; T, T-cell; UKCCSG, United Kingdom Children's Cancer Study Group.

TABLE 13-27 Treatment Protocols for Lymphoblastic Lymphoma

Drug	**Dosage**	**Days Given**
LSA₂-L₂ PROTOCOL[536]		
Induction, days 0-30 (phase I)		
Prednisone (PO)	60 mg/m²	2-30
Cyclophosphamide (IV)	1200 mg/m²	0
Vincristine (IV)	2 mg/m² (max 2 mg)	2, 9, 16, 23
Daunorubicin (IV)	60 mg/m²	11, 12
Cytarabine (IT)	20 to 70 mg dep. on age	0
Methotrexate (IT)	6 to 12 mg dep. on age	16, 30 (+ days 9, 23 if CNS+)
Consolidation, days 30-58 (phase II)		
Prednisone (PO)	60 mg/m²	0-70, then taper until day 25
Cytarabine (IV, SC)	100 mg/m²	0-4, 7-11
6-Thioguanine (PO)	50 mg/m²	0-4, 7-11
L-Asparaginase (IM)	6000 U/m²	14-27
BCNU (IV)	30 mg/m²	28
Methotrexate (IT)	6 to 12 mg dep. on age	7, 14, 21, 28
Continuation (phase III), minimum of five courses of:		
Methotrexate (IT)	6 to 12 mg dep. on age	1
6-Thioguanine (PO)	300 mg/m²	1-4
Cyclophosphamide (IV)	600 mg/m²	4
Hydroxyurea (PO)	2400 mg/m²	15-18
Daunorubicin (IV)	30 mg/m²	18
Methotrexate (PO)	10 mg/m²	29-32
BCNU (IV)	30 mg/m²	32
Cytarabine (IV, SC)	150 mg/m²	43-46
Vincristine (IV)	2 mg/m² (max 2 mg)	46
BFM PROTOCOL[244,595]		
Induction Ia, weeks 1-5		
Prednisone (PO)	60 mg/m²	1-28, then taper over 3 × 3 days
Vincristine (IV)	1.5 mg/m² (max 2 mg)	8, 15, 22, 29
Daunorubicin (IV over 1 hr)	30 mg/m²	8, 15, 22, 29
L-Asparaginase (IV)	10,000 IU/m²	12, 15, 18, 21, 24, 27, 30, 33
Induction Ib, weeks 7-9		
Cyclophosphamide (IV over 1 hr)†	1000 mg/m²	36, 64
Cytarabine (IV)	75 mg/m²	38-41, 45-48, 52-55, 59-62
6-Mercaptopurine (PO)	60 mg/m²	36-63
Methotrexate (IT)‡	12 mg‡	1, 12, 33, 45, 59*

Continues

TABLE 13-27   **Treatment Protocols for Lymphoblastic Lymphoma—cont'd**

Drug	Dosage	Days Given
Protocol M, weeks 11-19		
6-Mercaptopurine (PO)	25 mg/m^2	1-56
Methotrexate[§]	5 g/m^2	8, 22, 36, 50
Methotrexate (IT)[‡]	12 mg[‡]	8, 22, 36, 50
Reinduction IIa, weeks 21-26		
Dexamethasone (PO)	10 mg/m^2	1-21, then taper over 3 × 3 days
Vincristine (IV)	1.5 mg/m^2 (max 2 mg)	8, 15, 22, 29
Doxorubicin (IV over 1 hr)	30 mg/m^2	8, 15, 22, 29
L-Asparaginase (IV)	10,000 IU/m^2	8, 11, 15, 18
Reinduction IIb, weeks 27-29		
Cyclophosphamide (IV over 1 hr)[†]	1000 mg/m^2	36
Cytarabine (IV)	75 mg/m^2	38-41, 45-48
6-Thioguanine (PO)	60 mg/m^2	36-49
Methotrexate (IT)[‡]	12 mg[‡]	38, 45
Maintenance, weeks 31-104		
6-Mercaptopurine (PO)	50 mg/m^2	daily
Methotrexate (PO)	20 mg/m^2	weekly

*Additional doses at days 18, 27 for CNS-positive patients.
[†]With mesna.
[‡]Doses were adjusted for children younger than 3 yr.
[§]10% of the dose over 30 minutes, 90% as a 23.5-hour continuous IV infusion; leucovorin rescue: 30 mg/m^2 IV at hour 42, 15 mg/m^2 IV at hours 48 and 54. Serum levels of MTX should be <3 μmol/L at hour 36 after the start of the MTX infusion, ≤1 μmol/L at hour 42, and ≤0.4 μmol/hour at hour 48.
    CNS+, central nervous system–positive; IT, intrathecal.

TABLE 13-28   **Incidence of Relapses and CNS Relapses in Therapeutic Studies in Advanced-Stage Childhood and Adolescent Lymphoblastic Lymphoma***

Prophylactive Cranial Radiation Therapy	Cumulative No. of Patients in Studies	Cumulative No. of Relapses	CNS Involved in Relapse
Yes[244,529,533,676]	357	52 (15%)	8 (2%)
No[528,536,538,595]	733	184 (25%)	27 (4%)

*With and without prophylactic cranial irradiation.
CNS, central nervous system.

intense treatment is considered important for the treatment of lymphoblastic neoplasias. However, in a French study, two dose-intense combination pulses including HD MTX, cyclophosphamide, and doxorubicin administered in front of a modified BFM strategy did not improve outcome of LBL patients as compared with studies that used the BFM protocol alone.[541]

Oral 6-mercaptopurine and MTX are basic elements of a maintenance therapy for remission; they are administered for the treatment duration for 18 to 24 months from the start of chemotherapy. With the exception of the BFM strategy, multiple intensification pulses of different composition are applied as an adjunct in many study protocols. When comparing overall results of studies, there is little evidence for a beneficial effect of those intensification pulses during maintenance. Most remaining relapses in T-cell LBL patients occur early during the first 12 months, whereas late relapses are rare.[244,542] Therefore, future trials may evaluate whether duration of maintenance can safely be reduced for these patients. Children with pB-LBL have a longer risk period.

Stratification of Treatment Intensity

In most reported therapeutic studies, treatment intensity was stratified according to stages I and II versus stages III and IV.

In the BFM strategy, only patients with stage III or VI received reintensification therapy, and those with stage I or II did not. Whether treatment for patients with localized LBL can be further reduced is difficult to determine. Children with stage I or II are rare. They achieved EFS rates more than 90% with reduced intensity and full-length maintenance therapy. In a POG trial, 24-week maintenance in addition to a 9-week induction was beneficial for patients with localized LBL, although their EFS rate was only 63%.[543] This suggests that their biologic similarity to ALL may be more important than their low tumor burden and that they might therefore benefit from an ALL-type treatment.

Extracompartmental Therapy

For patients with overt CNS disease, 18 to 24 Gy cranial radiation therapy (CRT), in addition to LSA$_2$-L$_2$ or BFM chemotherapy, is highly effective in preventing CNS recurrences.[244,479,536] In the BFM studies, CNS-positive LBL patients had event-free survival rates comparable to CNS-negative patients when receiving HD-MTX, 5 g/m^2 as IV infusion during 24 hours, intrathecal therapy and cranial irradiation with 18 Gy.[479] However, CRT is usually not applied in children younger than 1 year of age. With treatment that includes intrathecal MTX and systemic HD MTX (0.5 to 5 g/m^2), children with stage I

TABLE 13-29 **Treatment and Results in Recent Multicenter Studies on Childhood and Adolescent Mature B-Cell Neoplasms**

Study	Therapy Duration (No. Courses)	No. of Patients	Stage(s)	pEFS ± SE at 3-5 yr
NCI 89-C-41[497]	4 courses	41*	All, including B-cell ALL	92%
POG Total B[559]	8 (6) courses	59	IV	79% ± 9%
		74	B-ALL	65% ± 8%
SFOP/LMB 89[510]	2/5/8 courses	492	All, including B-cell ALL	92.5% (CI, 90-94%)
NHL-BFM 90[498]	2/4/6 courses	413	All, including B-cell ALL	89% ± 2%
NHL-BFM 95[564]	2/4/5/6 courses	505	All, including B-cell ALL	89% ± 1%
UKCCSG 9002[585]	8 courses	112	III, IV	84% (CI, 76%-89%)
CCG 5911 "Orange"[534]	6/9 courses	36	III, IV	77% ± 7%
AIEOP[556]	2/4/6 courses	144	I-IV	82% ± 6%

*20 adults and 21 children.
ALL, acute lymphoblastic leukemia; CCG, Children's Cancer Group; CI, confidence interval; pEFS ± SE: Kaplan-Meier estimate of event-free survival; POG, Pediatric Oncology Group; SFOP, Société Française d'Oncologie Pédiatrique; UKCCSG, United Kingdom Children's Cancer Study Group.

or II are sufficiently protected without CRT.[244,479,543] Whether CNS-directed chemotherapy alone without prophylactic cranial irradiation is sufficient CNS prevention for patients with advanced-stage LBL without overt CNS disease has not been proven in randomized fashion. However, cumulative data from several studies with and without prophylactic CRT have suggested that prophylactic cranial irradiation as an adjunct to high-dose MTX therapy can also be omitted for patients with stage III or IV who do not have apparent CNS involvement at diagnosis (Table 13-28; see Table 13-26). In the NHL BFM 95 study, including HD MTX (5 g/m^2 IV, four times daily) and 11 doses of intrathecal MTX but no CRT, disease-free and CNS relapse-free survival of patients were not significantly inferior to the historic control group of the preceding NHL BFM 86 and 90 trials, in which patients received prophylactic CRT.[595] HD MTX therapy also appears efficacious to prevent relapse in the testes.[244]

The therapy protocols for LBL have most complications in common with the protocols for the treatment of childhood ALL. Chemotherapy-induced neutropenia increasing the risk of infections is most frequently observed during induction consolidation and reintensification phases.[244,536,538] However, during maintenance therapy, patients also have increased risk for opportunistic infections. Other main complications are vincristine-induced peripheral neuritis and constipation syndrome, L-asparaginase–associated complications, thrombosis, hepatotoxicity, pancreatitis, neurotoxicity associated with HD MTX and intrathecal MTX, and osteonecrosis (see section on treatment of ALL). Death from infection is the most frequent reason for death unrelated to tumor; most of these events occur during the induction phase.[536,595]

Treatment of Mature (Peripheral) B-cell Neoplasms

Chemotherapy

The chemotherapy strategy for this group is tailored to the biologic particularities of BL, which dominates this group numerically. The strategy has also been proven effective for treating DLBCL of childhood. Chemotherapy for BL was pioneered in Africa, where Denis Burkitt achieved remissions in children with BL with single or few doses of cyclophosphamide, low-dose MTX, or vincristine.[544] He already recognized that children with a small tumor were more likely to achieve complete remission than those with large tumors, which suggests a relationship between tumor mass and response.[497] The next important step was the introduction of the combination che-

motherapy of cyclophosphamide, vincristine, methotrexate, and cytarabine, which was found to be non–cross-resistant and proved not only efficacious for African children with endemic BL but also for American patients with sporadic BL.[545,546] Also, the high incidence of CNS relapses and the failure of cranial irradiation to prevent them was described by this group, leading to the introduction of combined intrathecal chemotherapy.[545,547,548] Based on the African experience, Ziegler and colleagues first explored the principle of dose intensity and achieved complete remissions with high-dose chemotherapy in American BL patients immune to conventional therapy.[549]

In the 1980s, treatment strategies were further improved by the emerging information about the peculiar biologic features of BL. A most important characteristic regarding therapeutic strategy is its high proliferation activity and rapid generalization. Burkitt's lymphoma cells cycle extremely rapidly, with an estimated generation time of only 25 hours.[550] It can be estimated that within 48 to 72 hours, every Burkitt cell is likely to traverse the cell cycle, therefore encompassing a period of greatest sensitivity to cytotoxic treatment.[551-553] Based on this knowledge, combination chemotherapy courses were designed based on the principle of maintaining—by means of fractionated administration or continuous infusion—cytotoxically active drug concentrations for the length of time needed to affect as many lymphoma cells during the vulnerable active cell cycle as possible.[529-531,554] The combination of several cytostatic agents should take into account preexisting resistance mechanisms and prevent the development of new resistance. The objective is to have high dose intensity so that the maximum amount of tumor cell death occurs with each course. Considerable postchemotherapeutic bone marrow suppression is accepted with this strategy. Short intervals between therapy courses are supposed to lower the probability of tumor cell regrowth and the development of resistance. Therapeutic strategies that adhere to this principle of rapidly repeated cycles of 4 to 7 days of dose-intensive combination chemotherapy have resulted in a dramatic increase in the cure rate for this disease group. In large multicenter studies, EFS rates of 80% to 90% were achieved for the entire group (Table 13-29).

Corticosteroids, cyclophosphamide, ifosfamide, MTX, cytarabine, doxorubicin, vincristine, and etoposide were used in these protocols. The comparatively favorable results with regimens developed in multicenter studies by the French SFOP group and the German-Austrian-Switzerland BFM group were able to be reproduced by other large study groups and have led to their widespread use.[534,555,556]

Table 13-30 shows the therapy protocols of the French LMB and the BFM groups. Both strategies use similar drugs,

TABLE 13-30 Chemotherapy Courses for Treatment of B-Cell Non-Hodgkin's Lymphoma of Childhood and Adolescence

Study	Drug	Dosage and Route	Days Given
TOTAL B[559]			
Course A	Cyclophosphamide	300 mg/m^2 IV × 6, q12h	1-3
	Doxorubicin	50 mg/m^2 IV	4
	Vincristine	1.5 mg/m^2 IV (max 2 mg)	4, 11
	Cytarabine	50 mg/m^2 IT (max 50 mg)	1, 2, 3, 11
	MTX	12 mg/m^2 IT (max 12 mg)	4, 11
Course B	MTX	200 mg/m^2 IV	1
	MTX	800 mg/m^2 IV over 24 hr	1
	Cytarabine	3000 mg/m^2 IV over 3 hr × 4, q12h	2, 3
	Cytarabine	50 mg/m^2 IT (max 50 mg)	1
	MTX	12 mg/m^2 IT (max 12 mg)	1
NCI 89-C-41[568]			
Regimen A	Cyclophosphamide	800 mg/m^2 IV	1
	Cyclophosphamide	200 mg/m^2 IV	2-5
	Doxorubicin	40 mg/m^2 IV	1
	Vincristine	1.5 mg/m^2/m^2 IV	1, 8
	MTX	1200 mg/m^2 IV over 1 hr	10
	MTX	5520 mg/m^2 IV over 23 hr	10
	Cytarabine	70 mg IT*	1, 3
	MTX	12 mg IT*	15
Regimen B	Cytarabine	2000 mg/m^2 IV × 4, q12h	1, 2
	Ifosfamide	1500 mg/m^2 IV	1-5
	Etoposide	60 mg/m^2 IV	1-5
	MTX	12 mg IT*	5
POG-APO[571]			
Induction	Doxorubicin	75 mg/m^2 IV	1, 22
	Vincristine	1.5 mg/m^2 IV	1, 22
	Prednisone	40 mg/m^2	1-28
	MTX	IT*	1, 8, 22 (CNS+, additional 15, 29, 36
Maintenance every 21 days	Doxorubicin (cumulative 300 mg/m^2)	30 mg/m^2 IV	1
	Then MTX	60 mg/m^2 IV	1
15 cycles	Vincristine	1.5 mg/m^2 IV	1
	Prednisone	120 mg/m^2	1-5
	MTX	IT* cycles 1, 3, 5, CNS+: additional cycles 2, 4	1
	6-Mercaptopurine	225 mg/m^2	1-5
FAB/LMB-96[510, 513, 565,678]			
COP	Prednisone	60 mg/m^2 PO, IV	1-7
	Vincristine	1 mg/m^2 IV	1
	Cyclophosphamide	300 mg/m^2 IV	1
	MTX + HC	15 mg IT*	1
	Cytarabine (group C only)	30 mg IT*	1 (group C +3, 5)
COPADM1	Prednisone	60 mg/m^2 PO, IV	1-6
	Vincristine	2 mg/m^2 (max 2 mg) IV	1
	Cyclophosphamide	250 mg/m^2 IV × 6, q12h	2, 3, 4
	Doxorubicin	60 mg/m^2 IV over 6 hr	2
	Methotrexate	3 g/m^2 IV over 3 hr (group C, 8 g/m^2 IV 4 hr)	1
	MTX + HC	15 mg IT*	2, 6 (group C +4)
	Cytarabine (group C only)	30 mg IT*	2, 4, 6
COPADM2	Same as COPADM1, but with cyclophosphamide	500 mg/m^2 IV × 6, q12h	2, 3, 4
COPAD	Same as COPADM1, but no MTX, no IT therapy, additional vincristine	2 mg/m^2 (max 2 mg)	6
CYVE	Cytarabine	50 mg/m^2 IV over 12 hr	1-5
	Cytarabine	3 g/m^2 IV over 3 hr	2-5
	Etoposide	200 mg/m^2 IV	2-5
CYM	Methotrexate	3 g/m^2 IV 3h	1
	MTX + HC	15 mg IT*	2
	Cytarabine	100 mg/m^2 IV over 24 hr	2-6
	Cytarabine + HC	30, 15 mg IT*	6

TABLE 13-30 Chemotherapy Courses for Treatment of B-Cell Non-Hodgkin's Lymphoma of Childhood and Adolescence—cont'd

Study	Drug	Dosage and Route	Days Given
M1	Prednisone	60 mg/m² PO	1-5
	Vincristine	2 mg/m² (max 2 mg) IV	1
	Cyclophosphamide	500 mg/m² IV	1, 2
	Doxorubicin	60 mg/m² IV over 6 hr	2
	Methotrexate	3 g/m² IV over 3 hr (group C, 8 g/m² IV over 4 hr)	1
	MTX + HC	15 mg IT*	2
	Cytarabine (group C only)	30 mg IT*	2
M2, M4	Cytarabine	100 mg/m² SC (in 2 fractions)	1-5
	Etoposide	150 mg/m² IV	1-3
M3	Prednisone	60 mg/m² PO	1-5
	Vincristine	2 mg/m² (max 2 mg) IV	1
	Cyclophosphamide	500 mg/m² IV	1, 2
	Doxorubicin	60 mg/m² IV over 6 hr	2
NHL-BFM 95[564]			
Prephase V	Dexamethasone	5-10 mg/m² PO, IV	1-5
	Cyclophosphamide	200 mg/m² IV over 1 hr	1, 2
	MTX, cyt, Pred	12, 30, 10 mg IT*	1
Course A	Dexamethasone	10 mg/m² PO, IV	1-5
	Vincristine	1.5 mg/m² IV (max 2 mg)	1
	Ifosfamide	800 mg/m² IV over 1 hr	1-5
	Cytarabine	150 mg/m² IV q12h	4, 5
	Etoposide	100 mg/m² IV over 1 hr	4, 5
	Methotrexate	1 g/m² IV over 4 hr	1
	MTX, cyt, Pred	12, 30, 10 mg IT*	2
Course B	Dexamethasone	10 mg/m² PO, IV	1-5
	Vincristine	1.5 mg/m² IV (max 2 mg)	1
	Cyclophosphamide	200 mg/m² IV over 1 hr	1-5
	Doxorubicin	25 mg/m² IV over 1 hr	4, 5
	Methotrexate	1 g/m² IV over 4 hr	1
	MTX, cyt, Pred	12/30/10 mg IT*	2
Courses AA and BB[6]	Same as A, B, respectively, but with methotrexate	5 g/m² IV over 24 hr	1
	MTX, cyt, Pred	6, 15, 5 mg IT*	2, 5
Course CC	Dexamethasone	20 mg/m² PO, IV	1-5
	Vindesine	3 mg/m² IV (max 5 mg)	1
	Cytarabine	3 g/m² IV over 3 hr × 4, q12h	1, 2
	Etoposide	100 mg/m² IV over 3 hr × 5, q12h	3-5
	MTX, cyt, Pred	12, 30, 10 mg IT*	5

In all regimens, leucovorin rescue is given after IV MTX and mesna is given with cyclophosphamide and ifosfamide as prophylaxis for cystitis.
*IT doses were adjusted for children younger than 3 yr.
cyt, cytarabine; HC, hydrocortisone; IT, intrathecal; MTX, methotrexate; Pred, prednisone.

but partly at very different dose levels and different application forms. Although there are few randomized trials testing the impact of individual drugs of these combinations on the patient's cure, there is considerable evidence that cyclophosphamide and MTX may be key important drugs. Monotherapy with cyclophosphamide or combined with low-dose MTX and vincristine could induce durable remissions in African children with endemic BL.[544,546] Djerassi and Kim[557] have described remission induction in children with BL using higher doses of MTX monotherapy. The important role of MTX can be concluded from the effect of different dosages. In patients with stage III disease and high tumor mass (LDH ≥ 500 U/L, approximately twice or more the upper limit of normal for age), and in Burkitt's leukemia patients, a 10-fold increase of the dose of MTX from 0.5 to 5 g/m² resulted in significantly improved outcome.[480,498] Similarly, the elevation of the dose of MTX from 3 to 8 g/m² in the SFOP-LMB protocols resulted in an excellent outcome of patients with advanced-stage BL, including those with CNS involvement.[510,532,558] The efficacy of HD cytarabine has been shown in studies on newly diagnosed patients,[530,559] and the combination of HD cytarabine with etoposide was efficacious

to induce remissions in relapsed BL patients.[560] Comparatively little evidence exists as to the role of corticosteroids and anthracyclines. In a CCG study of the 1980s, addition of daunomycin to the combination of cyclophosphamide, vincristine, MTX, and prednisone (COMP) did not improve the outcome of patients with advanced-stage nonlymphoblastic lymphoma as compared with COMP alone.[561]

The antitumor effectiveness of these strategies correlates with a high degree of adverse effects, whereby oral intestinal mucositis is the clinically most significant acute toxicity. It is caused primarily, but not solely, by HD MTX. Together with the severe neutropenia that results from dose-intensive therapy courses, it promotes serious infections, primarily septicemia caused by intestinal bacteria. Patients with advanced disease stages are at the greatest risk. For these patients, the rate of toxicity-induced death is 4% to 5% even in the most recent treatment studies, and higher still for all B-cell ALL patients.[498,510] Postchemotherapeutic application of G-CSF had no effect on treatment-related toxicity, as demonstrated in a randomized trial.[562] Toxicity and the risk of toxic death is greatest during and after the first treatment course.

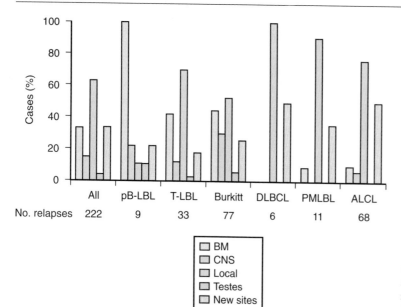

| No. relapses | 222 | 9 | 33 | 77 | 6 | 11 | 68 |

□ BM
□ CNS
□ Local
□ Testes
□ New sites

Figure 13-25. Site of relapse (isolated or combined) according to non-Hodgkin's lymphoma subtypes. BM, bone marrow; CNS, central nervous system. See text for details. (Data derived from multicenter studies NHL BFM.)

Risk-Adapted Stratification of Treatment Intensity and Duration

The most important prognostic criteria for stratifying therapeutic intensity are stage of disease, tumor mass, and involvement of the CNS. Patients with localized disease have excellent outcomes, almost 100% EFS across all studies, with the application of the basic drugs cyclophosphamide, vincristine, corticosteroid, and MTX at a low or intermediate dosage, with or without anthracycline.[195,498,510,543] However, stage alone may be less than optimal for stratification of treatment intensity. Descriptions of tumor burden as an important prognostic factor are in line with Goldie and Coldman's hypothesis[563] that the proportion of multiple resistant cells correlates with tumor mass.[497] The tumor mass and its surrogate parameter, the serum concentration of LDH, respectively, may vary largely in patients at the same stage, which is especially true for stage III BL patients (Fig. 13-26).

The use of LDH for stratification of treatment intensity was a major difference between the French LMB and the NHL BFM studies (Table 13-31). In both, patients with resected localized tumors are lowest risk patients, whereas patients with B-ALL and/or CNS disease belong to the highest risk group. Stratification concerns the number of drugs used, their dosage, and the number of treatment courses applied. Patients with localized, completely resectable lymphomas can be treated sufficiently with two 5-day therapy courses. Some of these patients may need even less therapy for cure. However, the very short therapy carries few late risks; therefore, overtreatment of some patients may be an acceptable price for an almost 100% chance to be cured. Patients with nonresectable localized lymphomas (stage I and II) and those with advanced disease stages (stage III, IV, and B-cell ALL) are given four, five, six, or eight therapy courses (see Table 13-31).[498,510,564] More treatment courses have little rationale because more than one third of relapses occur during therapy.[498,510,513,532,564,565] Other treatment protocols of short duration have been reported to result in high outcomes, especially for BL patients.[566,567] However, the numbers of patients included in these studies were too low to draw final conclusions. In the recent FAB LMB 96 trial,[565] based on the SFOP LMB 89 protocol, patients of the medium-risk group B in a randomized test had outcomes equal to four therapy courses as compared with those receiving a fifth therapy

course (see Table 13-31). In that trial, it was demonstrated that for the high-risk patients of group C, reduction of treatment intensity is crucial because it carries a high risk of increase of failure rate.[513] The shortness of latitude for reduction of treatment burden for high-risk patients became obvious in the randomized trial NHL BFM 95 aimed at the reduction of HD MTX-related toxicity by shortening the infusion time of MTX, 5 g/m², from the standard 24 hours to only 4 hours. The shorter infusion time resulted in an excess of tumor failures in patients with advanced disease.[564] Data from the NHL BFM 5 showed that toxicity and antitumor efficacy of MTX depends on duration of exposure to the drug. A 4-hour MTX infusion is less toxic than a 24-hour infusion, but is also less efficacious.[564] The required efficacy of MTX appears to be different according to the patient's risk for failure. For patients in the low- and intermediate-risk groups R1 and R2, 1 g/m² MTX for 4 hours was as efficient and less toxic than the 24-hour infusion (see Table 13-31). Mucositis grade III or IV and infection grade III or IV were observed after only 6% and 2%, respectively, of the treatment courses. Patients at high risk for failure benefit from higher MTX efficacy grades at the expense of higher toxicity. Patients with localized resected tumors may not need MTX because they had an excellent outcome in the SFOP-LMB 89 study with two courses of cyclophosphamide, vincristine, prednisone, and doxorubicin.[510]

Extracompartmental Therapy

Numerous studies have indicated that for patients without overt CNS involvement, intrathecal chemotherapy with MTX, cytarabine, and a corticosteroid, in combination with systemic MTX therapy, is sufficient protection to prevent CNS relapses.[479,498,510,513,532,533,565]

For patients with overt CNS disease at diagnosis, a favorable EFS of 78% was achieved in the LMB 89 study using HD MTX, 8 g/m² IV, over 4 hours combined with triple-drug intrathecal therapy, HD cytarabine (CYVE courses; see Table 13-31), and cranial irradiation after completion of chemotherapy.[510] The therapeutic role of cranial irradiation is difficult to determine because randomized trials are lacking.[568] In some CNS-positive patients, CNS relapse occurs before the end of chemotherapy, which means that scheduling cranial irradiation after chemotherapy is of questionable value.[510,529] Scheduling

TABLE 13-31 Treatment Stratification and Results in Two Large Multicenter Trials of Pediatric Mature B-Cell Neoplasms*

Group	Definition	Patients (%)	pEFS (%)	Chemotherapy Courses (Randomized Study Questions)	CUMULATIVE DOSAGES				
					MTX (g/m²)	CP (g/m²)	Ifo (g/m²)	Doxo (mg/m²)	Eto (mg/m²)
FAB/LMB 96[513,565,678] **(N = 1134)**									
A	Stage I, resected; stage II, abdominal	12	98	COPAD-COPAD	0	3	0	120	0
B	Stage I, not resected; stage II, nonabdominal; stages III, IV, bone marrow (BM) blasts ≦ 25%	67	90	COP-COPADM1-COPADM2-CYM-CYM-M1 (randomization for complete responders after COPADM1, half-dose CP and omission of M1; result: equally efficacious, less toxic)	3, ×4* 3, ×4 3, ×5 3, ×5	3.3* 4.3 4.8 5.8	0 0 0 0	120* 180 120 180	0 0 0 0
C	>25% BM blasts and/or CNS+ nonresponder to COP of group B	21	79	COP-COPADM1-COPADM2-CYVE1-CYVE2-M1-M2-M3-M4 (randomization for complete responders after COPADM1 + 2: reduced intensity "mini-CYVE" and omission of M2, M3, M4; result: inferior outcome)	8, ×3 (×4 for CNS+)	6.8, R 5.8	0 0	240, R180	2500, R800
NHL-BFM 95[564] **(N = 505)**									
R1	Stages I + II, resected	10	94	A-B (randomization: MTX IV over 24 hr vs. 4 hr; result: 4 hr less toxic, equally efficacious)	1, ×2	1.0	4	50	200
R2	Stages I + II, not resected; stage III, LDH < 500/U/L	46	94	p-A-B A-B (randomization: MTX IV over 24 hr vs. 4 hr; result: 4 hr less toxic, equally efficacious)	1, ×4	2.4	8	100	400
R3	Stage III, LDH 500-999 U/L; BM+ and LDH < 1000 U/L	16	85	p-AA-BB-CC-AA- BB (randomization: MTX in AA, BB IV over 24 hr vs. 4 hr; result: 4 hr less toxic, less effective)	5, ×4	2.4	8	100	900
R4	LDH ≥ 1000 U/L and/or CNS+	28	81	p-AA-BB-CC-AA-BB-CC (randomization: MTX in AA, BB IV over 24 hr vs. 4 hr; result: 4 hr less toxic, less effective)	5, ×4	2.4	8	100	1400

*For the composition of combination chemotherapy courses, see Table 13-30.
CP, cyclophosphamide; CNS+, central nervous system–positive; Doxo, doxorubicin; Eto, etoposide; Ifo, ifosfamide; LDH, lactate dehydrogenase; MTX, methotrexate; pEFS, Kaplan-Meier estimate of event-free survival; R, randomization.

TABLE 13-32 **Treatment and Results in Multicenter Studies of Childhood and Adolescent Anaplastic Large Cell Lymphoma**

Study, Protocol	No. of Patients	pEFS at 3-5 yr (%)	Therapy Duration	CUMULATIVE DOSAGE			Local Radiotherapy
				CPM/Ifo (g/m^2)	Dox (mg/m^2)	Epipod (mg/m^2)	
SFOP-M89/91, B-NHL-modified[393]	82	66	Six courses, 8 mo	10.3/-	360	1200	—
NHL-BFM 90, B-Cell NHL-type[469]	89	76	Stage I/II-r, 3 courses	1.4/8	50	200	—
			Stage II-nr, III, 6 courses*	3.4/12	150	600	—
			Stage IV, 6 courses 2-5 mo	2.4/8	100	1300	—
UKCCSG, B-Cell NHL type[502]	72	59	Five courses, 4 mo	5.8/-	240	2500	—
POG-APO[571]	86	72	17 courses,* 12 mo	0/-	300	0	Restricted to patients with vital residual tumor after induction
AIEOP LSA$_2$-L$_2$, modified[679]	34	65	24 mo	7.5/-	120	9450	Restricted to patients with residual tumor 5 cm or larger after consolidation

*For the composition of combination chemotherapy courses, see Table 13-29.

CPM, Cyclophosphamide; Ifo, Ifosfamide; Dox, Doxorubicin; Epipod, Epipodophyllotoxin; NHL, non-Hodgkin's lymphoma; pEFS, Kaplan-Meier estimate of event-free survival; SFOP, Société Française d'Oncologie Pédiatrique; UKCCSG, United Kingdom Children's Cancer Study Group.

it during the chemotherapy phase can delay chemotherapy, promoting systemic relapse.

Event-free survival rates of 65% to 70% for CNS-positive patients were achieved in several studies without applying cranial irradiation.[498,513,559,564] In those trials, CNS-positive B-cell NHL patients received therapy courses that included HD MTX in doses of 1.5, 5, and 8 g/m^2 and HD cytarabine, 2 to 3 g/m^2, in combination with intensive triple-drug intrathecal therapy. Nevertheless, treatment of CNS-positive B-cell NHL patients remains to be improved. Of note, not only are CNS relapses more frequent in initially CNS-positive patients as compared with CNS-negative patients, but also recurrent disease outside the CNS.[479]

Testicular relapse in boys is rare with therapy strategies that include HD MTX, even without specialized local treatment measures.[498,510]

Children and adolescents who suffer from mature B-cell neoplasms other than BL—namely, DLBCL, including rare variants such as T-cell–rich DLBCL and juvenile follicular lymphoma—appear to be efficaciously treated with therapies described for B-cell NHL.[382,569] However, the deviation of the prognosis of numerically smaller subgroups, such as PMLBL, may only become visible after examining the patient populations of several consecutive studies or large international collaborative trials.[570] In a POG study based on the APO regimen (doxorubicin, prednisone, vincristine), patients with DLBCL had an EFS at 4 years of 70%, suggesting an inferior prognosis for this patient subgroup.[571] However, in other large multicenter studies based on the LMB or BFM B-cell NHL strategies, EFS for children and adolescents with DLBCL was in the range of 90%.[498,510,564,565]

Therapy of Anaplastic Large Cell Lymphoma

ALCL has been accepted as a distinct clinicopathologic entity since the early 1990s.[399,468] Essential therapy-relevant characteristics distinguish ALCLs from other childhood NHLs—less

frequent CNS involvement initially and in relapse, frequent involvement of a new manifestation in relapse, and markedly better survival prognoses for patients in case of recurrent disease.

Chemotherapy

EFS rates in the range of 65% to 75% were reported from several therapeutic trials, including larger numbers of patients (Table 13-32). Comparable overall outcomes were achieved with different therapy protocols, including modified LSA$_2$-L$_2$ protocols and the short-pulse therapy strategy developed for B-cell NHL.

Steroids, vincristine, doxorubicin, MTX, and cyclophosphamide were common components in all regimens, except that cyclophosphamide was not part of the APO protocol. Other drugs, such as ifosfamide, cytarabine, epipodophyllotoxins, 6-mercaptopurine, thioguanine, and bleomycin, were included, with varying individual and cumulative doses in some but not all regimens. However, the number of drugs and individual doses differed among studies. In particular, the cumulative doses of drugs with special late risk potential differed considerably (see Table 13-32). Thus, the cumulative dose of doxorubicin ranged from 120 to 360 mg/m^2, whereas the cumulative dose of epipodophyllotoxins ranged from 0 to 9450 mg/m^2. Because of the heterogeneity of these regimens with respect to the use of individual drugs and drug dosages, only limited conclusions can be drawn about the role of individual components. Alkylating agents, high-dose MTX, and etoposide were main components of most regimens, but were absent in the APO regimen at the expense of rather high cumulative doses of doxorubicin, vincristine, and prednisone.[571] Thus, from this POG study (five-drug APO regimen), one might conclude that doxorubicin, vincristine, and steroids are key drugs. An intriguing observation was the efficacy of vinblastine in the management of recurrent ALCL.[535] The role of vinblastine in front-line therapy is currently under investigation in a large European intergroup randomized trial and a North American COG study.

These regimens also differed considerably in duration of treatment, although with rather short treatment duration of 2 to 5 months, patient outcome was not worse than with a treatment duration of 2 years (see Table 13-32). Most tumor failures occurred within the first 15 months from diagnosis. However, late recurrences were observed in all studies, regardless of the duration of therapy.

Stratification of Treatment Intensity

The criteria for stratifying the intensity of therapy are less well established than for other NHL entities, because the prognostic parameters are less well defined. Only in the BFM and UKCCSG studies was the treatment intensity stratified for presumed risk features, whereas in the other studies referenced in Table 13-32, all patients received the same treatment intensity. In the NHL BFM 90 study, treatment was stratified according to stage.[469] Patients with stage I or II disease and complete tumor resection had a 100% EFS with three 5-day courses of therapy, but all others received six courses. The dose of MTX was 0.5 g/m^2, except for patients with stage IV disease and/or multifocal bone involvement who received 5 g/m^2. Furthermore, the latter received high-dose cytarabine/etoposide. In an ongoing European intergroup trial, the presence of at least one of the risk factors—skin involvement, mediastinal mass, visceral involvement of the lung, liver, and/or spleen (defined as focal lesions and/or enlargement more than 5 cm below the costal margin)—is used to allocate patients to the high-risk group.[572]

Extracompartmental Therapy

The incidence of CNS relapse in patients who are initially CNS-negative is very low, with therapy protocols that involve corticosteroids and systemic MTX therapy with or without intrathecal therapy.[393,399,469,479] Prophylactic cranial irradiation is unnecessary. In the European intergroup trial ALCL99 based on the treatment strategy of the NHL BFM 90 study, including dexamethasone as a corticosteroid, it could be shown in randomized fashion that systemic MTX, 3 g/m^2, given as an IV infusion for 3 hours, is sufficient CNS protection for patients without overt CNS disease at diagnosis, and additional intrathecal chemotherapy is not necessary.[572]

Because of the small numbers of patients with overt CNS disease at diagnosis, no conclusions can currently be drawn about optimal treatment in this case. Therapeutic cranial irradiation with doses of 18 to 24 Gy, depending on age, may be efficacious in addition to HD MTX and HD cytarabine combined with triple-drug intrathecal therapy.[393,469]

Testicular involvement has not been observed, either initially or in relapse, in published study results.

Primary Cutaneous Anaplastic Large Cell Lymphoma

In childhood, ALCL confined to the skin is a rare observation. Although skin involvement in addition to nodal and/or extranodal disease has adverse prognostic impact (see later, "Prognostic Factors"), ALCL confined to the skin appears to have a good prognosis after complete resection, which is possible in most cases.[399,469] In some cases, primary skin ALCL may evolve from preexisting lymphomatoid papillomatosis. It is unclear whether these anaplastic large cell lymphomas limited to the skin require chemotherapy.[483] In the European intergroup study ALCL 99, these patients are put on a watchful waiting strategy after surgical resection and receive chemotherapy only in case of relapse.

Local Irradiation

There is little evidence for a beneficial role of local irradiation, although NHLs are certainly radiosensitive tumors. The incidence of tumor failure has been considerably reduced with modern combination chemotherapy, so the possible contribution to disease eradication of radiotherapy needs to be carefully balanced against its later risks (see earlier, "Hodgkin's Lymphoma"). Moreover, the therapeutic significance of radiation therapy needs to be viewed in relation to the efficacy of the chemotherapeutic modality used. In a randomized trial in children with lymphoblastic T-cell lymphomas, adjuvant mediastinal radiation (15 Gy) achieved a significantly better outcome than chemotherapy alone (probability of disease-free survival, 66% vs. 16%).[573] However, this result only proves that radiation therapy is an effective therapeutic element and the chemotherapy in the study has to be seen as not effective enough compared with modern protocols. Across all entities, patients with localized disease have excellent outcomes with chemotherapy alone. In a randomized trial, patients with localized stage I or II disease with involved field radiation had no advantage over patients without radiation, but they had a higher toxicity.[543,574] This applies also for patients with primary bone lymphoma or bone involvement in addition to other lesions. With histology-directed chemotherapy alone, these patients have superb outcomes without local irradiation of bone lesions.[486-489] Irradiation of bulky disease previously included in some treatment protocols for LBL and ALCL has been entirely abandoned because disease-free survival rates of more than 80% were attained with chemotherapy alone (see Tables 13-26 and 13-32). In patients with advanced disease, progression-free survival rates of 75% to 85% are also achieved with chemotherapy alone. Patients who relapse with current chemotherapy strategies usually have such extensive tumor involvement, particularly in the abdomen, that effective field radiation would be associated with high toxicity.[575] Especially in ALCL, the potential therapeutic value of local radiation is further challenged by the observation that frequently, in relapse, new regions are involved that were initially unaffected, and in some cases these new manifestations even represent the sole relapse localization (see Fig. 13-25). Nevertheless, because local sites are still the most frequent site of recurrence in childhood NHL, there might be selected patients who could benefit from local irradiation. The question is how these patients can be accurately identified to protect others from the late risks of irradiation.

Incomplete Tumor Regression, Second-Look Surgery, and Monitoring of Response

Incomplete regression of local lymphoma manifestations during induction chemotherapy is a frequent observation in the treatment of childhood and adolescent NHLs. The proportion of patients with tumor remnant varies according to the initial size and the NHL subtype. Also, the proportion may depend on the imaging method applied. Thus, although the chest x-ray may be normal, a significant residual mediastinal mass is still visible on a CT scan. Standardized response criteria, as defined for malignant lymphoma in adults, are therefore of limited value to assess the quality of treatment response in childhood NHL.[576] The challenge of incomplete tumor regression arises from the fact that the tumor remnant may be the result of resistant lymphoma or rather persistent fibrous or necrotic tissue, or a combination of both. Hence, the meaning of a residual tumor for the subsequent course of the patient may be different and require different treatment strategies. As a result, the role of local therapy modalities, such as surgical resection and/or local radiotherapy, is hard to evaluate and thus might be poorly

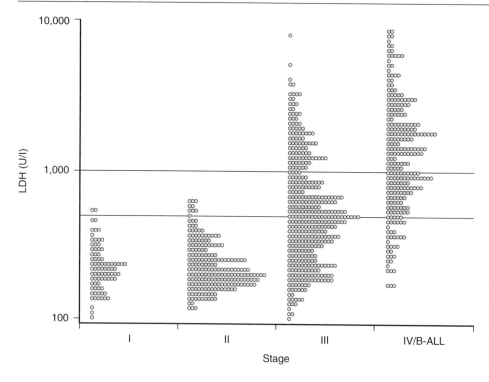

Figure 13-26. Distribution of pretherapeutic serum lactate dehydrogenase (LDH) concentrations in children and adolescents with Burkitt's lymphoma and leukemia according to St. Jude stage of disease. Each circle represents one patient. (Data derived from multicenter studies NHL BFM.)

determined. So far, there is no gold standard to distinguish the patient with a residual tumor that is prone to grow from those in whom the tumor remnant merely represents the fibrous or necrotic waste of the initial lymphoma, with no impact on outcome. The heterogeneity and complexity of initial manifestations in childhood NHL, and thus their remnants, hamper or even impede prospective evaluation of their prognostic significance in a reproducible manner with conventional imaging methods. Even second-look biopsy or resection has limited value because of difficulties in identifying or excluding residual lymphoma cells in the environment of fibrous or necrotic tissue. The only exception may be cases with clear viable tumor. Although there may be some differences according to NHL subtypes, general conclusions can be drawn from the findings of several treatment studies:

- Patients with delayed tumor regression during the first days and weeks of treatment are more likely to experience a subsequent progression than patients with rapid and complete tumor regression. This applies primarily to patients without recognizable tumor regression in the first days of therapy.[244,498,510,513,532,533,564,565]
- In most patients with rapid initial response but persisting tumor remnants detected with imaging techniques, only fibrotic or necrotic tissue without vital lymphoma is found with histologic testing of the resection material.*
- Patients with a vital residual tumor after the first 5 to 10 weeks of induction are at a high risk of suffering tumor progression subsequently.[244,399,513,533,565]

About two thirds of B-cell NHL patients with vital residual tumors after three to five therapy courses, for whom intensified chemotherapy or megadose chemotherapy was carried out with hematopoietic stem cell rescue, survived progression-free in more recent treatment studies.[498,510,565] However, the efficacy of this approach might differ for different NHL subtypes. Thus,

for patients with LBL or ALCL with vital residual tumor after the first weeks of treatment, a sufficient treatment approach is still to be determined.

As discussed earlier ("Hodgkin's Lymphoma"), functional imaging using FDG-PET can distinguish metabolic active tissue from necrosis. Functional imaging using FDG-PET is now included in the revised response criteria for malignant lymphoma.[181,182] A high accuracy of PET to monitor treatment response in adult Hodgkin's lymphoma patients was sustained in several studies.[183] So far, also for aggressive NHL, prospective studies to monitor treatment response by FDG-PET are only available from adult patients. In a meta-analysis of several studies, the specificity of FDG-PET at the end of chemotherapy for true identification of patients without later relapse was 100%, whereas the sensitivity for true identification of patients with later relapse was approximately 72%.[501] Evidence is accumulating that the accuracy of early FDG-PET after two cycles of chemotherapy to predict outcome appears higher as compared with FDG-PET at the end of chemotherapy.[577] Whether the findings from adult patients generalize to the typical NHL types of childhood and adolescents is unclear because the avidity of FDG-PET differs significantly among lymphoma subtypes.[500] So far, no data are available concerning the FDG-PET avidity of the predominant NHL types of childhood, LBL and BL.

Treatment of Children and Adolescents with Rare Non-Hodgkin's Lymphoma Subtypes

Children and adolescents diagnosed with the rare (juvenile) follicular lymphoma appear to have excellent outcomes when treated according to risk-adapted treatment regimens for mature B-cell lymphoma described earlier.[381,382]

Less than 2% of childhood NHLs are nonanaplastic peripheral T-cell lymphomas, which are a heterogeneous group of lymphomas. Differentiating them from the small cell variants of ALCL is sometimes difficult if a chromosome translocation typical of ALCL or ALK-1 positivity does not help make a differential diagnosis. The small case numbers and their clinical and biologic heterogeneity may be the main reason why the

---

*See references 244, 393, 399, 469, 498, 510, 513, 564, 565, and 570.

most appropriate therapy type has not yet been identified for these patients. In the NHL BFM treatment studies, peripheral T-cell lymphomas were treated using the strategy for lymphoblastic lymphomas, albeit with much less success.[479,533,578] For other even rarer entities, there are no proven specific therapeutic approaches. If typical adult NHL entities occur in children, one can try to treat them with the respective therapy protocols for adult patients.

Primary Central Nervous System Lymphoma

Because of its rarity and the lack of established treatment, children with primary CNS lymphoma represent a therapeutic challenge; radiotherapy is often considered necessary. However, most primary CNS NHLs of childhood are of the diffuse large B-cell subtype.[479,481] Their prognosis with the regular treatment for CNS-positive B-cell NHL as described earlier (without cranial irradiation) appears efficacious because only 1 of the 10 patients with primary CNS lymphoma suffered from relapse in the BFM series. Similarly, in another multi-institutional series of 12 patients, the 5-year event-free survival with chemotherapy alone was 70%, suggesting that radiotherapy may be avoidable for most children, at least as front-line therapy for those with the DLBCL subtype.[482]

Treatment of Non-Hodgkin's Lymphoma in Children with Inherited or Acquired Immunodeficiency Syndromes

Only few reports are available on treatment options and results for children with inherited or acquired immunodeficiency who develop NHL. In retrospective analyses, remission rates were estimated to be as low as 36%, with a median survival of only 10 months.[579,580] A more recent report from the BFM group has suggested that long-term remission is possible and adaptation of treatment to the reduced tolerance of these patients is crucial.[581] Of the 19 patients, 7 had chromosomal breakage syndromes, 6 patients were younger than 3 years at diagnosis, and most had advanced-stage disease. In 3 patients, NHL was the first diagnosis and immunodeficiency (ID) was only diagnosed at a young age and after unusually high treatment-related toxicity, which prompted the diagnosis for ID. Of the 19 patients, 17 were treated according to NHL BFM protocols stratified for their histology and stage.[430] Although the dosages of MTX, alkylators, and epipodophyllotoxins were reduced in most patients with known ID, toxicity was considerable and 3 patients died of toxicity. However, 12 of the 17 children achieved complete remission (CR) and only 1 patient suffered relapse. Thus, with reduced intensity treatment, such as a reduction in alkylator and topoisomerase II inhibitor dosages to 30% to 50% and MTX doses of a maximal 0.5 to 1 g/m^2, successful treatment of NHL appears possible for children with inherited ID, including chromosomal breakage syndromes. Radiotherapy should be avoided, especially in patients with chromosomal breakage syndromes. One might speculate whether the low incidence of tumor failure despite significant reduction of treatment intensity reflects a higher sensitivity of the malignant cells, especially in the patients with chromosomal breakage syndromes.

Similarly, little information exists on optimal treatment and outcome for HIV/AIDS-related NHL in children and adolescents. With varying treatments, event-free survival rates of 40% to 60% have been described.[335,463] From a larger Italian group, it was concluded that children with HIV/AIDS-related NHL should have access to the regular protocol treatment for NHL because 9 of 13 patients who received protocol treatment for B-cell NHL survived event-free.[335]

Treatment of Relapse

The chance of patients of relapsing after current front-line protocols is poor, although there are differences according to NHL subtypes. Relapses occur early in a considerable proportion of patients during front-line treatment. This reflects the lymphoma cell's high degree of resistance. Conversely, at the time of relapse, many patients have not recovered fully from the initial treatment and have a correspondingly lower tolerance for salvage therapy. Thus, a main challenge is to induce a stable second remission with a treatment tolerable for the patient. Established salvage treatment protocols with proven efficacy are widely lacking.

One of the most common treatments may be ICE (see Table 13-14).[192] In the CCG 5912 study with the DECAL protocol (dexamethasone, etoposide, cisplatin, high-dose cytarabine, and L-asparaginase), a complete remission was achieved in 40% of pediatric patients who experienced a first or subsequent relapse of NHL.[582] The 5-year survival was only 30%. In that study, outcome data were not broken down for distinct NHL entities.

In the German-Austrian-Switzerland BFM group, most patients with a relapse of LBL were treated according to therapy protocols for ALL relapse patients. The survival rate is below 30% for pB-LBL patients and even worse for T-cell LBL patients.[244,542,583] All relapsed T-cell LBL patients underwent allogeneic hematopoietic blood stem cell transplantation (HSCT).

For all patients with BL or B-cell ALL who failed to receive highly effective front-line treatment protocols, the survival rate is only 10% to 15%.[583-585] Therapy approaches have attempted to reinduce remission with high-intensity cytostatic combinations and then to secure the remission through a subsequent high-dose chemotherapy, along with autologous or allogeneic stem cell rescue.[585,586] We believe that the chances for survival of children with a relapse of a diffuse large cell B-cell NHL may probably be higher than BL patients. Prospective studies are needed to determine whether newer therapy options such as anti-B-cell-specific monoclonal antibodies[587,588] can play a role in the treatment of these patients.

The chance to survive after relapse appears to be higher for patients with ALCL than for patients with other NHL subtypes. Even after a second or third relapse, patients appear to survive for prolonged periods, which is unusual in other subtypes of childhood NHL. However, the course after relapse seems to be variable. The largest series has reported that the overall survival rate of 41 patients is 69% at 3 years.[335] Salvage chemotherapy was based on 3-week courses of CCNU, vinblastine, bleomycin, or cytarabine delivered every 6 weeks for 12 months, followed by autologous HSCT for some of the patients. An intriguing observation was that 10 of 11 patients achieved complete remission with weekly vinblastine, 6 mg/m^2, including 6 patients with follow-up relapse following autologous HSCT. This retrospective study included patients from as far back as the 1970s. For ALCL patients who failed current front-line protocols, less favorable survival rates were reported.[469,502] Early occurrence and high intensity of the front-line therapy seemed to confer a higher risk for failure of salvage therapy.[589] However, even in these high-risk patients, including patients with follow-up relapse after autologous HSCT, long-term remissions were observed after allogeneic HSCT.[589] Remarkably, even patients with active disease achieved long-term remissions after allogeneic HSCT. This may be a hint for a graft-versus-lymphoma effect. Prospective clinical trials are ongoing to test the feasibility and efficacy of new treatment strategies for children and adolescents with relapsed ALCL in the United States and Europe.

TABLE 13-33 **Prognostic Factors with Adverse Impact on Outcome of Children and Adolescents with Non-Hodgkin's Lymphoma (NHL) with Current Treatment Regimen**

| NHL Type | GROUP-SPECIFIC PROGNOSTIC FACTORS | | GENERAL PROGNOSTIC FACTORS | |
	Established	Candidate	Established	Candidate
LBL-pB, LBL-T	Female > 10 yr[677] Del 6q[594]	MRD monitoring[504]	Advanced stage	Cytogenetics, gene expression profiling, FDG-PET
Burkitt's	LDH > 2N > 500 > 1000 U/L[498,565] CNS disease[498,510,513,559] Age > 15 yr[510] Polymorphism of LTα-TNF[596] Nonresponse to prophase[510,565] Aber 13q;22, gain 7[593] Complex secondary aberrations[592]	MRD monitoring[508]		
DLBCL	Female > 14 yr of age[677]			
PMLBL	LDH > 2 N > 500 U/L[570]			
ALCL	Mediastinal mass, visceral involvement, skin[590] Lymphohistiocytic variant[591] MSD in BM, PB > 10 copies NPM-ALK/10,000 copies abl[507]	MRD monitoring[507,508]		

ALCL, anaplastic large cell lymphoma; BM, bone marrow; CNS, central nervous system; DLBCL, diffuse large B-cell lymphoma; FDG-PET, fluorodeoxyglucose–positron emission tomography; LBL-pB, lymphoblastic lymphoma–precursor B-cell; LBL-T, lymphoblastic lymphoma T-cell; LDH, lactate dehydrogenase; LTα, lymphotoxin alpha; MRD, minimal residual disease; MSD, minimal systemic disease; NPM-ALK, nucleophosmin–anaplastic lymphoma kinase; PB, peripheral blood; PMLBL, primary mediastinal (thymic) large B-cell lymphoma; TNF, tumor necrosis factor.

From Reiter A. Diagnosis and treatment of childhood non-Hodgkin lymphoma. Hematology Am Soc Hematol Educ Program. 2007;2007:285-296.

Prognostic Factors

The prognostic significance of individual parameters can only be analyzed in relation to the therapy applied and the overall outcome of the total group of patients. Hence, the adverse impact on outcome of any prognostic parameter may vanish with more efficacious treatment. Table 13-33 depicts prognostic factors with an adverse impact on patient outcome with current treatment regimens. Stage remains an important prognostic factor. Patients with localized stage I or II disease have a better chance of event-free survival than patients with advanced-stage disease. Increased serum concentration of LDH as a tumor mass parameter was described as having an adverse prognostic impact in addition to stage, especially in patients with B-cell NHL.[498,565,584] The prognostic impact of involvement of certain organs and sites may differ among NHL subtypes. CNS involvement was a negative prognostic factor for patients with B-cell NHL, especially BL, whereas CNS disease had no significant adverse impact on outcome in children with LBL.[479,498,510,513,530,531,555,559] CNS disease is rarely observed in ALCL patients, so information about its prognostic impact is not available. Bone involvement was not prognostically negative in any NHL subtype.[393,469,486-489] In contrast, the presence of a mediastinal mass, visceral involvement of lungs, liver, or spleen, and skin involvement had negative prognostic significance in ALCL.[590]

In contrast to adults with ALCL, the ALK-1 positivity or negativity had no significant impact on outcome for children and adolescents.[393,469] However, in ALCL patients, even minimal systemic disease, detectable only by PCR assay technology to amplify NMP-ALK fusion gene transcripts in BM and peripheral blood, was associated with a significantly increased risk of treatment failure.[506,507] Within the established treatment subgroups, the histologic subtype has no adverse prognostic impact, except for PMLBL and possibly the lymphohistiocytic variant of ALCL.[393,469,570,591]

Limited data on the prognostic impact of cytogenetic abnormalities of tumor cells are available from pediatric NHL patients. The main reason is a lack of fresh tumor cells appropriate for cytogenetic analysis. Preliminary data have suggested that complex secondary chromosomal aberrations and abnormalities of chromosomes 13q, 22, and 7 are associated with a high risk of failure in BL patients.[592,593] The prognostic significance of genetic aberrations in T-cell LBL could not be analyzed conclusively because of an insufficient number of investigated patients.[245] A recent study has revealed that deletions of the long arm of chromosome 6 were associated with a significantly worse outcome in children with T-cell LBL.[594]

A lack of response to the cytoreductive prophase was described as a strongly adverse prognostic factor in B-cell NHL patients.[510,565] The kinetics of treatment response is a strong prognostic parameter in many malignancies and has been underexplored in childhood NHL. The primary reason for this may be methodologic difficulties in evaluating the response kinetics because of their complex manifestations. Incomplete tumor regression during induction is a frequent observation. Its impact on the subsequent course may differ, because the tumor remnant may be a result of resistant lymphoma or persistent fibrous or necrotic tissue. Functional imaging using FDG-PET may provide a tool for the early assessment of treatment response (see earlier). In aggressive adult NHL, negative FDG-PET performed after the first two courses of chemotherapy was associated with a 2-year EFS of 82% compared with an EFS of 43% for patients with positive FDG-PET findings.[577] Whether these findings generalize to childhood NHL is unclear, because FDG-PET avidity differs significantly among lymphoma subtypes.[500] Furthermore, to determine treatment guidelines, prospective evaluation of prognostic accuracy will be necessary in the context of a given treatment. Monitoring residual clonal lymphoma cells in the blood and/or BM by means of aberrant immunophenotype- or PCR-based identification of specific fusion gene products may be an alternative tool for evaluating the kinetics of treatment response.[507,508] Host-related factors may also affect outcome. Age and gender were found to be associated with treatment results in some NHL subtypes but not in others.[595] Adolescent girls suffering from DLBCL and T-cell LBL had significantly worse outcomes as compared with boys. In patients with advanced-stage B-cell

NHL or B-cell ALL, genetic variations in the tumor necrosis factor (−308 [G-T]) and lymphotoxin alpha (+252 [a-G]) were significantly associated with an increased risk for events.[596] The polymorphism of the methylenetetrahydrofolate reductase, resulting in altered folate metabolism, was not associated with patient outcome.[597]

The availability of new methodologic tools will greatly enhance our ability to refine the definition of biologically distinct subtypes beyond histology and will enable application of subtype-specific therapies. However, the use of such methods (e.g., gene expression profiling) is often impeded by rather trivial factors, including a lack of appropriately preserved tumor material.

Late Effects

In contrast to pediatric Hodgkin's lymphoma, few reports are available on late effects in long-term survivors of childhood and adolescent NHL. The risk of second cancer for survivors of childhood and adolescent NHL appears to be much lower compared with patients with Hodgkin's lymphoma. In the Childhood Cancer Survivor Study, the excess risk for second cancers was among the lowest for children treated for NHL as compared with all other malignancies, with a cumulative risk for SMN of 1.9% after 20 years.[222,598] However, only events occurring 5 years or later from diagnosis of NHL were included in that analysis. Because AML as a second malignancy usually occurs earlier than 5 years from diagnosis of the first malignancy, the true risk for all SMNs may have been underestimated in that study. This assumption is supported by the lack of AML as a second cancer after childhood NHL in the report.[222] In a monocenter cohort of 497 former pediatric NHL patients, AML was reported to be the most frequent second malignancy.[599] In that study, the cumulative incidences of SMN at 10 and 20 years were 2.1% and 4.8%, respectively. Seven of 16 SMNs observed were AML, and exposure to epipodophyllotoxin was a risk factor to develop secondary AML. Few systematic studies on other late effects in long-term survivors of childhood NHL are available. In an analysis of 103 former patients, major late effects observed were cardiac toxicity and hepatitis C virus (HCV) infection, the latter presumably resulting from blood transfusions before HCV screening was introduced.[599a] Cardiotoxicity was observed in patients who received anthracycline doses of more than 400 mg/m², which is no longer in use today. Fertility was not greatly impaired. Irradiation was found to increase the likelihood of late effects. In long-term survivors of pediatric NHL, the risk for limitations on physical performance and daily activities was among the lowest compared with survivors of other childhood cancers, although higher compared with healthy siblings.[600] Furthermore, they are at increased risk for symptoms of depression and somatic distress compared with their siblings without cancer.[232]

Follow-up Care

After chemotherapy, the main risk period for relapses for patients with mature B-cell NHL is about 6 to 9 months, and risk is highest in the first 3 to 6 months after therapy ends. For patients with ALCL it is about 1 year. In children with lymphoblastic T-cell lymphomas, almost all relapses occur before maintenance therapy ends; with precursor B-cell lymphomas, they also occur later. During this period, patients should be closely monitored for remission. Appropriate testing includes blood count, serum LDH level, and clinical and imaging controls of the previous local manifestations. Bone marrow and cerebrospinal fluid studies are only indicated if

relapse is suspected. Over time, imaging, laboratory, and chemical studies are only necessary if there is a concrete suspicion of relapse. Nonetheless, clinical examinations should be performed at least annually to detect any possible late effects of the therapy.

Follow-up studies to monitor late risks of therapy should follow principles similar to those for patients with Hodgkin's lymphoma.

POST-TRANSPLANTATION LYMPHOPROLIFERATIVE DISEASE

Definition and Clinical Features

Lymphoproliferative disorders are the most frequent malignancies in children and adolescents with iatrogenic impaired immune function following solid organ transplantation (SOT) or allogeneic HSCT.[601] Post-transplantation lymphoproliferative disease (PTLD) represents a spectrum of clinically, morphologically, and biologically heterogeneous disorders. The initial clinical presentation is extraordinarily broad, ranging from a single, small, asymptomatic lymphomatous tumor, an infectious mononucleosis-like syndrome, and unexplained fever to a widespread disseminated disease with a rapid fatal course resulting in multiorgan failure. Any organ can be involved by interstitial infiltration of lymphocytes or tumorous lesions, including meninges and CNS. Occasional spontaneous regression is observed and may be a feature intrinsic to the nature of the disorder as a result of a disturbed balance of immune surveillance. Especially in HSCT patients, PTLD may even go unrecognized until autopsy because of the lack of localized tumors and may be clinically misdiagnosed for graft-versus-host disease (GVHD) or infection.[602] Laboratory findings are often nondefinitive, although an otherwise unexplained increase of LDH level may be a clue to suspect PTLD. Lymphocytosis may be present because of the broad spectrum of morphologic appearance, and diagnosis can rarely be based on the cytomorphologic features of blood, BM, or effusions.

Histopathology and Classification

According to the WHO classification of hematologic malignancies, PTLD is divided into three subtypes—early lesions, polymorphous lesions, and monomorphic lesions.[12] Disturbed nodal architecture and the presence of necrosis distinguish the latter two from early lesions. Monomorphic lesions are further subdivided into diffuse large B-cell lymphoma (most cases), Burkitt's and Burkitt's-like lymphoma, Hodgkin's-like lymphoma and, in rare cases, plasmacytoma. In the vast majority of cases, PTLD cells are of B-cell lineage, with a wide spectrum of phenotypes.[603] The B-lineage antigen CD20 is expressed in most cases, but not all.[604] In rare cases, a T-cell phenotype of PTLD is observed.[605] PTLD can be polyclonal, oligoclonal, or monoclonal, and polymorphous and homomorphous lesions could be observed in one patient.[606] Of post-SOT PTLD cases, 70% to 80% are associated with EBV, whereas almost all post-HSCT PTLD cases are EBV-positive.[12]

Post–Solid Organ Transplantation PTLD Versus Post-HSCT PTLD

Two main disparities exist between post-SOT PTLD and post-HSCT PTLD, reflecting fundamental differences of the transplantation biology of both procedures. In post-SOT PTLD, the malignant cells are almost invariably of recipient origin and PTLD cells are of donor origin in post-HSCT PTLD, because recipient hematopoietic cells are eradicated by the conditioning process.[607,608] However, with a reduced intensity nonmyeloablative conditioning regimen, PTLD of recipient origin has been described after allogeneic HSCT.[609] SOT recipients receive immunosuppressive therapy for a prolonged period or even lifelong to prevent graft rejection. In contrast, in HSCT recipients, the duration of immunosuppression to prevent GVHD is limited to a few months, allowing them to mount immunocompetence with time. Hence, the period of risk to develop PTLD is shorter in HSCT recipients as compared with SOT recipients who can develop PTLD several years after transplantation.[602,607,610]

Incidence and Risk Factors

Reported incidences of PTLD in pediatric SOT recipients range from 0.5% to 20%, and were lowest in kidney recipients and highest in intestinal transplant recipients.[607,611,612] The risk of PTLD strongly correlates with the degree of immunosuppression.[613] Thus, reported incidences of PTLD may differ because of different immunosuppression strategies. Recipient EBV seronegativity at the time of transplantation of an organ from an EBV-positive donor was identified as a risk factor for PTLD, suggesting that the lack of preexisting immunity impairs the capability of the immunosuppressed recipient to mount an effective cellular response to the primary EBV infection transmitted from the donor organ.[610] Recent studies have identified a strong risk of EBV seronegative recipients, regardless of the EBV status of the organ donor.[614,615] This may be at least partly why young children are at a much higher risk to develop PTLD than adults.[610,616]

In pediatric HSCT recipients, an incidence of PTLD of 1% and 1.6% has been reported.[602,617] Main determinants of the risk of PTLD are measured by the decreases or delay in T-cell function, including ex vivo T-cell depletion and antithymocyte globulin level, and the HLA disparity between donor and recipient.[608,618,619] Reduced intensity conditioning was also described to increase the risk of PTLD.[609] The risk of PTLD appears particularly high after selective ex vivo depletion of donor T-cells from the graft, corresponding to the observation that the PTLD cells are B cells of donor origin.[608] If both donor T cells and B cells are depleted, either ex vivo (e.g., by positive selection for CD34-positive cells) or in vivo (e.g., by infusion of anti-CD52 monoclonal antibodies), the risk of PTLD was not markedly increased.[620]

Preventive Strategies

PTLD is a serious complication of transplantation, with a high risk of death of 25% to almost 50% in cases of post-SOT PTLD, and even higher in cases of post-HSCT PTLD.[601,602,621] Because of the emerging knowledge concerning risk factors and the causative role of EBV, in most cases preventive strategies may be a realistic option to reduce the morbidity and mortality of transplant recipients from these disorders.

In contrast to cytomegalovirus (CMV), the prophylactic or preemptive use of antiviral drugs such as acyclovir or ganciclovir appears not to be efficacious to prevent EBV-related complications in transplant recipients.[622] In a randomized trial, a lower incidence of PTLD was observed in EBV-seronegative pediatric recipients of liver transplantation receiving IV immunoglobulin compared with controls, although the difference was statistically not significant.[615] Based on the recognition of the strong correlation of the risk of PTLD with the degree of immunosuppression and the role of EBV infection, modifications were made in management aimed at reduction of immu-

nosuppression and in monitoring patients for the actual risk of PTLD. Although randomized controlled clinical trials are lacking and may be difficult to perform, reduced incidences of PTLD compared with historical controls were reported with such a policy.[623-625] Because of the fundamental differences in the biologic determinants, these strategies require different considerations for SOT and HSCT recipients, respectively.

In SOT recipients, reducing immunosuppression was not only observed to reduce the risk of PTLD, but also could induce remissions in PTLD.[626] However, reduction of immunosuppression might increase the risk of graft rejection. Thus, there is a need for criteria to guide modification of immunosuppression.

Serial quantitative measurements of EBV DNA by real-time PCR in the blood of transplanted patients have revealed an increased load of EBV DNA in PTLD patients. This method facilitates the early recognition of PTLD in SOT and HSCT recipients[619,627-629] and could be an option to guide treatment decisions for preemptive alteration of immunosuppression. Although the sensitivity of the method to recognize PTLD appears to be high, the specificity seems to be less accurate. High levels of EBV load were observed in transplant recipients without development of PTLD.[628,630] In line with the recognition that T-cell immunity is important to control EBV infection, studies have revealed that combined testing for EBV viral load and the amount of EBV-specific T cells CD8- and/or CD4-positive in transplant recipients increases significantly the accuracy to predict the risk of PTLD.[631,632] However, further prospective studies and standardizing methodology appear warranted to establish these methodologies as guides for clinical decisions.

Treatment

There are currently no convincing published data on the efficacy of antiviral agents and IV immunoglobulins for PTLD. Reducing immunosuppression (RI) is an effective option to treat PTLD, and response rates of 60% were observed in pediatric cases of post-SOT PTLD.[607,621,626] There were inconsistent observations about the prognostic impact of factors such as histologic type, polymorphous versus monomorphous, increased LDH level, and dissemination of PTLD.[607,621] In nonresponders to RI, a response rate of 80% was observed with moderate pulses of chemotherapy with prednisone, 2 mg/kg for 5 days, and cyclophosphamide, 600 mg/m², at day 1.[633] However, chemotherapy may carry an increased risk for toxic death in these patients.[500] In most cases, PTLD cells express CD20; the monoclonal anti-CD20 antibody rituximab alone or in combination with moderate-dose chemotherapy has been described to induce responses in up to 60% of nonresponders to RI.[500,607,621,634] Thus, clinical trials are investigating response-triggered strategies starting with RI followed by rituximab in CD20-positive nonresponders to RI, followed by the addition of moderate chemotherapy in nonresponders to rituximab.

However, both rituximab and chemotherapy do not eliminate the ultimate cause of PTLD, impaired T-cell function, and EBV infection. Thus, recurrence of PTLD is frequently observed, especially in patients who do not mount an effective T-cell response to EBV.[635] The adoptive transfer of EBV-specific T-effector cells may be the more promising option to treat and prevent PTLD in the future.[628,636,637]

There are no published data on the efficacy of RI in post-HSCT PTLD cases, and only anecdotal reports on the efficacy of chemotherapy. In a prospective study of patients who underwent HSCT from unrelated or mismatched family donors, it was shown that a strategy of prompt intervention with EBV-specific CTL with or without rituximab in patients with increased EBV load accompanied by clinical signs of PTLD appears to be very efficacious[628]; all 8 (of 8) patients responded. The same study questioned the rationale for preemptive intervention in case of an increased EBV load because of its limited specificity of only 50%. Of 16 patients with repeatedly increased EBV load, 8 never developed signs of PTLD without any intervention.

Apart from the challenge for optimal management, PTLD also represents a unique opportunity for further investigation of the role of immune surveillance in the pathogenesis of lymphoma.

Outlook

Our insights into the pathogenesis and cellular biology of NHLs have dramatically improved over the last decade. Nevertheless, important issues need to be clarified until there is a complete understanding of the transformational process of malignant lymphoma. In contrast to the increasing perception of the molecular biologic features of the lymphomas, our knowledge of causative factors is still poor. Although lymphomas were among the first human malignancies for which an infectious cause was hypothesized, definitive clarification of the role of infectious agents in the pathogenesis of childhood lymphoma is still lacking. Disclosure of a possible causative role of a viral disease, such as EBV infection, could provide the basis for preventive strategies. Burkitt's lymphoma and Hodgkin's lymphoma, both suspected to be associated with EBV, account for a considerable proportion of childhood malignancies worldwide. Thus, the clarification of an interaction of genetic predisposition and infectious agents in their pathogenesis merits any efforts. Post-transplantation lymphoproliferative disease represents a broad spectrum of disorders, ranging from polymorphous and polyclonal early lesions to monoclonal lymphoid neoplasms. The risk of PTLD is associated with the degree of iatrogenic immunosuppression and, in most cases, PTLD is associated with EBV infection. Thus, PTLD may represent a unique opportunity for further investigation of the steps of lymphoma pathogenesis, the role of infectious agents, especially EBV, and the role of immune surveillance.

Despite striking successes in the treatment of childhood and adolescent lymphomas, the continued optimization of treatment remains a challenge. For many patients, obviously, more efficacious treatment is necessary to allow them to survive. For others, reduction of their treatment burden is warranted while maintaining efficacy. Therefore, both exploration of new treatment options and further refinement of the balance between the individual patient's treatment burden and the risk of failure are warranted. Identifying the parameters that predict a patient's outcome to current treatment with high accuracy is a major task. The kinetics of treatment response is a strong prognostic parameter in many malignancies and is underexplored in childhood NHL. Functional imaging using FDG-PET may provide a tool for early assessment of treatment response. Monitoring residual clonal lymphoma cells in the blood and/or BM by aberrant immunophenotype- or PCR-based identification of specific fusion gene products may be an additional or alternative option. The availability of new methodologies will greatly enhance our ability to identify biologically distinct subtypes beyond histology, which in turn will enable the application of subtype-specific therapies. Moreover, technologies such as genome-wide gene expression profiling may enable the identification of preexisting resistance to chemotherapy of the tumor cells and of host factors associated with the risk of toxicity; this will allow for therapy to be tailored for each patient.

However, any alteration of current therapy in terms of reduction of treatment intensity may be dangerous in the absence of a salvage strategy with proven efficacy. Therefore, the development of effective and tolerable therapeutic strategies for treating relapsed patients is a high-priority short-term goal.

For the future, it should be a realistic expectation that the enormous advances in the understanding of the biology of malignant lymphomas will afford not only the development of more efficacious treatment, but also more target-specific therapeutic interventions, which will increase a child's chances for survival.

Chimerical or humanized monoclonal antibodies (moAbs) directed against surface antigens of lymphoma cells are a new category of treatment options providing antitumor mechanisms beyond chemotherapy and radiotherapy. Because of the restricted expression of the target antigens, these antibodies can help eradicate antigen-positive lymphoma cells while allowing the regrowth of normal cells from antigen-negative precursor cells. The anti-CD20 moAb rituximab may currently be the most widely used agent for adult lymphoma patients. In contrast to adults, few data are available on the use of moAbs in children with malignant lymphoma. Their role in the treatment of childhood Hodgkin's lymphoma and NHL needs to be determined. As with any new category of drugs, this should occur in controlled clinical trials. It is questionable whether all findings from the use of moAbs in adults can be generalized to children with lymphoma for two reasons: (1) because of the different spectrum of biologic subtypes, especially for NHL; and (2) because of potential differences in the immunologic status of children compared with adults. Furthermore, the effect of these compounds on the tumor as well as on the host is unknown. Apart from activating immune effector mechanisms after binding with the target antigen on the surface of tumor cells, ligation of the target may induce intracellular signaling. Such effects may have a positive or negative impact on the ultimate aim to eradicate the target cell, but have not been completely explored yet. An example may be that binding of the humanized anti-CD30 antibody 5F11 with the antigen activates the NF-κB pathway and inhibits apoptosis in CD30-positive Hodgkin's lymphoma–derived cell lines.[638]

The increased incidence of cancer, especially lymphomas, in those with inherited or acquired immunodeficiency, strongly supports the concept of immune surveillance as an active process to control the emergence of malignant clones from transformed somatic cells.[639] The transfer of autologous EBV-specific T-effector cells has been shown to be successful treatment for PTLD.[636,637] Preliminary observations such as survival after allogeneic HSCT of children with relapsed ALCL or T-cell LBL refractory to chemotherapy suggest a graft-versus-lymphoma effect.[589,594] Thus, further research to disclose the mechanisms involved in the immune control of malignant clones and the escape mechanisms of tumor cells may help in the future development of successful immune antilymphoma strategies.

LYMPHADENOPATHY

The child with lymphadenopathy poses a relatively common diagnostic challenge for the pediatrician. In most patients, lymph node enlargement results from transient, self-limited disease processes that resolve without sequelae. However, serious, life-threatening benign and malignant diseases may present with lymphadenopathy as the primary manifestation and must be considered in the evaluation of the child with enlarged lymph nodes.

Enlargement of lymph nodes results from antigen-stimulated proliferation of lymphocytes and other cells intrinsic to the lymph node or from infiltration of the node by extrinsic cells, such as polymorphonuclear leukocytes or metastatic malignant cells. Most lymphadenopathy results from response to a local infection; thus, removal of the inciting antigen results in the regression of lymphadenopathy. Persistence of antigen (e.g., the presence of intracellular parasites) may result in chronically enlarged lymph nodes.[640]

Certain considerations narrow the diagnostic possibilities in evaluation of the child with lymphadenopathy. Not all masses that appear to be lymphadenopathy (particularly in the neck) represent enlarged lymph nodes; non–lymph node masses that may simulate cervical lymphadenopathy include thyroglossal duct cysts and branchial cleft cysts, but these rarely present a confusing clinical picture.[641] Evidence of recent or current upper respiratory infection and the presence of tender cervical adenopathy suggests inflammation as the cause. The presence of associated systemic symptoms, the chronicity of the adenopathy, and whether the adenopathy is generalized or regional are important considerations in the differential diagnosis. An abbreviated list of common causes of lymphadenopathy is presented in Box 13-2. More complete listings have been published elsewhere.[640,642,643]

Generalized adenopathy, which implies involvement of more than two contiguous lymph node regions, may include hepatosplenomegaly as well. The causes of generalized lymphadenopathy include disseminated bacterial, viral, fungal, and protozoan infections (notably, typhoid fever, tuberculosis,

---

| Box 13-2 | **Causes of Lymphadenopathy** |

INFECTION

Bacterial: Streptococcosis, staphylococcosis, mycobacteriosis
Brucellosis, tularemia, syphilis
Viral: Epstein-Barr virus, cytomegalovirus, human immunodeficiency virus, rubella
Fungal: Histoplasmosis, coccidioidomycosis
Protozoan: Toxoplasmosis, malaria

AUTOIMMUNE DISEASE

Rheumatoid arthritis, systemic lupus erythematosus, serum sickness, autoimmune hemolytic anemia

STORAGE DISEASE

Niemann-Pick disease, Gaucher's disease

DRUG REACTION

Phenytoin and others

MALIGNANCY

Lymphoma, leukemia, metastatic rhabdomyosarcoma, thyroid carcinoma, other carcinomas
Histiocytoses: Langerhans cell histiocytosis, malignant histiocytosis, sinus histiocytosis with massive lymphadenopathy

MISCELLANEOUS

Sarcoidosis, Kawasaki disease, cat-scratch fever

Data from Zuelzer WW, Kaplan J. The child with lymphadenopathy. Semin Hematol. 1975;12:323-334; Moussatos GH, Baffes TG. Cervical masses in infants and children. Pediatrics. 1963;33:351-376; and Bedros AA, Mann JP. Lymphadenopathy in children. Adv Pediatr. 1981;28: 341-376.

---

syphilis, brucellosis, mononucleosis, cytomegalovirus, histoplasmosis, coccidioidomycosis, toxoplasmosis, and malaria), autoimmune diseases, storage diseases, drug reactions, and disseminated neoplastic diseases such as leukemia, lymphoma, neuroblastoma, and the histiocytoses.

Regional lymphadenopathy is usually caused by lymphatic drainage of a local infection. The tender cervical adenopathy observed in children with upper respiratory infections and the axillary adenopathy observed in cat-scratch fever are typical examples. Mononucleosis characteristically presents with enlarged cervical lymph nodes (although generalized adenopathy and splenomegaly are common), as do the mononucleosis-like illnesses produced by cytomegalovirus, toxoplasmosis, brucellosis, and leptospirosis. In rare cases, lymphadenopathy caused by infectious mononucleosis may be difficult to distinguish from that caused by malignant lymphoma on clinical and histologic grounds.[644]

Bacterial lymphadenitis usually presents with fever and typical signs of inflammation with tender, enlarged nodes progressing to fluctuance and erythema of the overlying skin. The diagnosis and treatment of bacterial lymphadenitis are usually straightforward. Cervical lymphadenitis may also be caused by mycobacterial infections. Systemic disease usually accompanies cervical lymphadenitis caused by *Mycobacterium tuberculosis;* however, most occurrences of mycobacterial lymphadenitis are caused by atypical mycobacteria.[642] Nonsuppurative cervical adenitis may be caused by the mucocutaneous lymph node syndrome (Kawasaki's disease), a rare disease of infants and children with an obscure cause. The characteristic exanthem usually clarifies the diagnosis. Sarcoidosis is rare in children, but should be considered in African children with bilateral cervical adenopathy, hilar lymph node involvement, generalized lymph node involvement, peribronchial fibrosis, hepatosplenomegaly, and uveitis. Scalene nodes are almost always involved and are the preferred site for diagnostic biopsy.[642,645]

Finally, malignant neoplasms may present with regional adenopathy, and malignancy should be suspected, particularly if lymph nodes in the posterior triangle of the neck are involved.[641] Solid tumors in the head and neck region, especially rhabdomyosarcoma and nasopharyngeal carcinoma, may be associated with metastases to cervical lymph nodes and present clinically as cervical lymphadenopathy. The presence of epistaxis, nasal stuffiness, trismus, and signs of eustachian tube obstruction should suggest the possibility of a primary malignancy in the nasopharynx. Thyroid carcinomas often present with anterior cervical adenopathy, with or without a palpable thyroid nodule. The lymphomas have been discussed extensively in this chapter, and the histiocytoses are discussed in Chapter 24. An unusual benign form of histiocytosis that may be confused easily with malignant lymphoma results from sinus histiocytosis with massive lymphadenopathy.[646,647] The disease affects children (usually black Africans), and most patients are younger than 10 years. Massive, painless cervical lymphadenopathy associated with fever, weight loss, weakness, joint symptoms, and hypergammaglobulinemia are characteristic findings. Proptosis, bone lesions, and other systemic manifestations suggestive of malignancy may be present. The histologic picture is distinctive, demonstrating pericapsular fibrosis, dilation of the sinuses, and collections of plasma cells and macrophages containing phagocytosed lymphocytes.[646,647] The disease runs a protracted course, with spontaneous remissions and relapses.

Approach to the Patient

The management of the child with lymphadenopathy should be focused on obtaining clues to a diagnosis from the history, physical examination, and noninvasive testing, when possible, with the goals of ascertaining whether the lymphadenopathy is likely to be a manifestation of a serious illness and determining as early as possible in the workup whether the child should undergo lymph node biopsy. The history should include the duration of the adenopathy, associated symptoms, evidence of recent infection in the regions drained by the involved lymph node, exposure to illnesses, cats, or rodents, and current medications. The physical examination should be focused on ascertaining the location and number of enlarged nodes. Involvement of supraclavicular lymph nodes suggests mediastinal pathology and is usually associated with a serious disease mandating a prompt workup, including a chest radiograph. In contrast, the involvement of upper cervical lymph nodes is more likely to be the result of an upper respiratory tract infection. Signs of inflammation in the lymph nodes suggest an infectious cause; in particular, matted adenitis with nodes fixed to the skin in the upper anterior cervical and preauricular areas suggest atypical mycobacterial infection.[648]

A number of algorithms for the workup of the child with adenopathy have been proposed.[642] For the child with generalized lymphadenopathy, a complete blood count, blood culture, serologic testing for EBV, toxoplasmosis, cytomegalovirus (and, perhaps, HIV) and fungal disease, a tuberculin skin test, and chest radiograph will usually suggest a specific diagnosis. If no clues emerge, lymph node biopsy is probably indicated.

The workup of a child with regional lymphadenopathy must be tailored to the individual child. However, children with a high probability of serious disease can usually be selected for early lymph node biopsy. These include children with involvement of low cervical and supraclavicular nodes, because there is a high diagnostic yield from biopsies of such sites.[648] Children with constitutional complaints, including fevers for longer than 1 week, weight loss, weakness, or bone pain are likely to have a serious underlying disease and deserve prompt attention and early lymph node biopsy if less invasive tests prove unrevealing. In asymptomatic children, an appropriate strategy includes observation with careful measurement of lymph node size and possibly an empirical trial of antibiotic therapy. If the nodes increase in size over a 2-week period or fail to decrease to normal size after 4 to 6 weeks of observation, a lymph node biopsy is indicated.

In general, the largest possible node should be excised at biopsy, and specimens should be submitted for appropriate culture and supplemental studies, as well as for routine histopathologic examination. Great care is required in the biopsy procedure and in handling the specimen to maximize the yield of the procedure. Errors in technique are unquestionably the single most important cause of diagnostic difficulty in diseases of the lymph nodes.[643]

It is unfortunate that most lymph node biopsies fail to reveal a specific diagnosis. Nondiagnostic reactive hyperplasia is encountered in most patients.[648,649] However, in one large series, a specific cause of lymphadenopathy could be found in 41% of children undergoing lymph node biopsy.[648] It is noteworthy that a significant proportion (15% to 25%) of children with nondiagnostic lymph node biopsies ultimately prove to have a significant specific disease.[649,650] Therefore, if the initial workup and biopsy of the child with lymphadenopathy fail to confirm a specific diagnosis, close follow-up for persistent symptoms is essential, and another biopsy may be indicated.

MEDIASTINAL MASSES

Masses occurring in the mediastinum, whether the result of enlarged lymph nodes or involvement of extralymphatic tissues, represent urgent and challenging diagnostic problems. Most such masses in children are malignant neoplasms. Their proximity to vital structures and their propensity to cause life-threatening symptoms from vascular or airway compromise mandate an expeditious, systematic approach involving close cooperation among the surgeon, radiologist, oncologist, anesthesiologist, radiotherapist, and pathologist. The potential hazards associated with diagnostic procedures in children with malignant tumors of the mediastinum were discussed earlier. Selection of tissue for diagnostic biopsy should reflect an awareness of the potential dangers associated with biopsy in patients with vascular or airway compromise.

An appropriate differential diagnosis for a child with a mediastinal mass can usually be derived from examination of appropriate radiographs of the chest and determination of the anatomic location of the mass.[651,652] MRI and CT scanning may be extremely useful for selected patients. The mediastinum can be arbitrarily divided into three compartments—the anterior mediastinum, middle mediastinum, and posterior mediastinum. The anterior compartment contains the thymus, anterior pericardium, and heart and a few anterior mediastinal lymph nodes, as well as an occasional substernal extension of the thyroid gland. The bulk of the mediastinal lymph nodes, great vessels, and trachea are in the middle mediastinum. The posterior mediastinum includes the esophagus, thoracic duct, descending aorta, and sympathetic chain. Knowledge of the normal contents of each compartment, site of the mass, and age of the child are important considerations in planning the workup. A differential diagnosis of mediastinal masses according to location within the mediastinum is shown in Box 13-3.

Masses in the posterior mediastinum, particularly masses in the paravertebral sulcus, are likely to be neurogenic tumors arising from the nerve roots and sympathetic ganglia.[653] The presence of Horner's syndrome should suggest involvement of the superior cervical ganglion. Duplication cysts—embryonic abnormalities resulting from partial duplications of portions of the tracheobronchial or gastrointestinal system—should be suspected in the young infant with stridor, repeated episodes of respiratory distress, emphysema, or swallowing symptoms caused by compression. Older children may also be affected but are more likely to be asymptomatic or have mild symptoms. Surgical excision is curative, because these cysts are invariably benign. Sarcomas arising from the chest wall may also appear in the posterior mediastinum.[651,652,654,655]

Masses in the middle mediastinum most likely represent enlarged lymph nodes resulting from lymphoma or inflammatory conditions; malignant lymphomas are the most commonly observed masses in this location. In fact, malignant lymphoma was the most common mediastinal mass and the most common mediastinal tumor observed in one large series,[656] although neurogenic tumors were more common in other reports.[652,654,655] Inflammatory conditions of the mediastinal lymph nodes (e.g., tuberculosis and histoplasmosis) are usually associated with typical pulmonary parenchymal findings on radiographs and are rarely present as isolated mediastinal lymphadenopathy. Sarcoidosis almost always presents with striking bilateral involvement of cervical lymph nodes, from which a definitive diagnosis can usually be obtained.

In addition to malignant lymphomas, various benign and malignant tumors occur in the anterior mediastinum. Hyperplastic thymus glands account for a significant proportion of anterior mediastinal masses observed in infants and young children, but these masses rarely produce symptoms and usually undergo involutional atrophy.[150,652,655] Other neoplasms encountered in the anterior mediastinum include thymic cysts, benign teratomas, malignant germ cell tumors (seminomatous and nonseminomatous), and thymomas. Thymomas

Box 13-3	Differential Diagnosis of Mediastinal Masses

ANTERIOR MEDIASTINUM

Thymic cyst
Thymic "hyperplasia"
Benign teratoma
Malignant germ cell tumor
Lymphoma
Thymoma
Substernal thyroid
Pericardial cyst

MIDDLE MEDIASTINUM

Lymphoma
Tuberculosis
Histoplasmosis
Sarcoidosis
Anomalies of the great vessels

POSTERIOR MEDIASTINUM

Neuroblastoma
Ganglioneuroma
Neurofibroma
Sarcoma
Duplication cyst

Mediastinal meningocele. Adapted from Hope JW, Borns PF, Koop CE. Radiologic diagnosis of mediastinal masses in infants and children. Radiol Clin North Am. 1963;1:17; Haller JA, Mazur DO, Morgan WW. Diagnosis and management of mediastinal masses in children. J Thorac Cardiovasc Surg. 1969;58:385; and Bower RJ, Kiesewetter WB. Mediastinal masses in infants and children. Arch Surg. 1977;112:1003.

are rare malignant tumors involving the epithelial cells of the thymus. Such tumors may be encapsulated or invasive, factors that influence resectability and prognosis, and may be associated with myasthenia gravis, red cell aplasia, and hypogammaglobulinemia.

REFERENCES

1. Linet MS, Ries LA, Smith MA, et al. Cancer surveillance series: recent trends in childhood cancer incidence and mortality in the United States. J Natl Cancer Inst. 1999;91:1051-1058.
2. Kay NE, Ackerman SK, Douglas SD. Anatomy of the immune system. Semin Hematol. 1979;16:252-282.
3. Sklar J, Longtine J. The clinical significance of antigen receptor gene rearrangements in lymphoid neoplasia. Cancer. 1992;70:1710-1718.
4. Kuppers R, Klein U, Hansmann ML, Rajewsky K. Cellular origin of human B-cell lymphomas. N Engl J Med. 1999;341:1520-1529.
5. Kuppers R. Mechanisms of B-cell lymphoma pathogenesis. Nat Rev Cancer. 2005;5:251-262.
6. Hodgkin T. On some morbid appearances of the absorbent glands and spleen. Medico-Chirurgical Transactions. 1832;17:68.
7. Wilks S. Cases of enlargement of the lymphatic glands and spleen (Hodgkin's disease) with remarks. Guy's Hosp Rep. 1865;11:56.
8. Sternberg C. Über eine eigenartige, unter dem bilde der pseudo-leukaemie verlaufende tuberkulose des lymphatischen apparates. Z Heilk. 1989:19:21-90.
9. Reed DM. On the pathological changes in Hodgkin disease with special reference to its relation to tuberculosis. Bull Johns Hopkins Hosp. 1902;10:133-196.
10. Seif GS, Spriggs AI. Chromosome changes in Hodgkin's disease. J Natl Cancer Inst. 1967;39:557-570.
11. Kuppers R, Rajewsky K, Zhao M, et al. Hodgkin disease: Hodgkin and Reed-Sternberg cells picked from histological sections show clonal immunoglobulin gene rearrangements and appear to be derived from B cells at various stages of development. Proc Natl Acad Sci U S A. 1994;91:10962-10966.
12. Jaffe ES, Harris NL, Stein H, Vardiman JW (eds). World Health Organization Classification of Tumours. Pathology and Genetics of Tumours of Haematopoietic and Lymphoid Tissues. Lyon, France, IARC Press, 2001.
13. Lukes RJ, Butler JJ. The pathology and nomenclature of Hodgkin disease. Cancer Res. 1966;26:1063-1083.
14. Harris NL, Jaffe ES, Stein H, et al. A revised European-American classification of lymphoid neoplasms: a proposal from the International Lymphoma Study Group. Blood. 1994;84:1361-1392.
15. Seitz V, Hummel M, Marafioti T, et al. Detection of clonal T-cell receptor gamma-chain gene rearrangements in Reed-Sternberg cells of classic Hodgkin disease. Blood. 2000;95:3020-3024.
16. Stein H, Marafioti T, Foss HD, et al. Down-regulation of BOB.1/OBF.1 and Oct2 in classical Hodgkin disease but not in lymphocyte predominant Hodgkin disease correlates with immunoglobulin transcription. Blood. 2001;97:496-501.
17. Foss HD, Reusch R, Demel G, et al. Frequent expression of the B-cell-specific activator protein in Reed-Sternberg cells of classic Hodgkin's disease provides further evidence for its B-cell origin. Blood. 1999;94:3108-3113.
18. Stein H, Mason DY, Gerdes J, et al. The expression of the Hodgkin's disease–associated antigen Ki-1 in reactive and neoplastic lymphoid tissue: evidence that Reed-Sternberg cells and histiocytic malignancies are derived from activated lymphoid cells. Blood. 1985;66:848-858.
19. Rowe M, Rowe DT, Gregory CD, et al. Differences in B cell growth phenotype reflect novel patterns of Epstein-Barr virus latent gene expression in Burkitt's lymphoma cells. EMBO J. 1987;6:2743-2751.
20. Skinnider BF, Mak TW. The role of cytokines in classic Hodgkin lymphoma. Blood. 2002;99:4283-4297.
21. Maggio E, van den Berg A, Diepstra A, et al. Chemokines, cytokines and their receptors in Hodgkin's lymphoma cell lines and tissues. Ann Oncol. 2002;13(Suppl 1):52-56.
22. Kadin ME, Agnarsson BA, Ellingsworth LR, Newcom SR. Immunohistochemical evidence of a role for transforming growth factor beta in the pathogenesis of nodular sclerosing Hodgkin's disease. Am J Pathol. 1990;136:1209-1214.
23. Teruya-Feldstein J, Jaffe ES, Burd PR, et al. Differential chemokine expression in tissues involved by Hodgkin's disease: direct correlation of eotaxin expression and tissue eosinophilia. Blood. 1999;93:2463-2470.
24. MacLennan KA, Bennett MH, Vaughan HB, Vaughan HG. Diagnosis and grading of nodular sclerosing Hodgkin's disease: a study of 2190 patients. Int Rev Exp Pathol. 1992;33:27-51.
25. Anagnostopoulos I, Hansmann ML, Franssila K, et al. European Task Force on Lymphoma project on lymphocyte-predominant Hodgkin disease: histologic and immunohistologic analysis of submitted cases reveals 2 types of Hodgkin disease with a nodular growth pattern and abundant lymphocytes. Blood. 2000;96:1889-1899.

26. Diehl V, Sextro M, Franklin J, et al. Clinical presentation, course, and prognostic factors in lymphocyte-predominant Hodgkin's disease and lymphocyte-rich classical Hodgkin's disease: report from the European Task Force on Lymphoma Project on Lymphocyte-Predominant Hodgkin's Disease. J Clin Oncol. 1999;17:776-783.

27. Jackson H Jr, Parker F Jr. Hodgkin's Disease and Allied Disorders. New York, Oxford University Press, 1947, pp 17-34.

28. Nachman JB, Sposto R, Herzog P, et al. Randomized comparison of low-dose involved-field radiotherapy and no radiotherapy for children with Hodgkin's disease who achieve a complete response to chemotherapy. J Clin Oncol. 2002;20:3765-3771.

29. Dorffel W, Luders H, Ruhl U, et al. Preliminary results of the multicenter trial GPOH-HD 95 for the treatment of Hodgkin's disease in children and adolescents: analysis and outlook. Klin Padiatr. 2003;215:139-145.

30. Arya LS, Dinand V, Thavaraj V, et al. Hodgkin's disease in Indian children: outcome with chemotherapy alone. Pediatr Blood Cancer. 2006;46:26-34.

31. Karajannis MA, Hummel M, Oschlies I, et al. Epstein-Barr virus infection in Western European pediatric non-Hodgkin lymphomas. Blood. 2003;102:4244.

32. Savage KJ, Monti S, Kutok JL, et al. The molecular signature of mediastinal large B-cell lymphoma differs from that of other diffuse large B-cell lymphomas and shares features with classical Hodgkin lymphoma. Blood. 2003;102:3871-3879.

33. Copie-Bergman C, Plonquet A, Alonso MA, et al. MAL expression in lymphoid cells: further evidence for MAL as a distinct molecular marker of primary mediastinal large B-cell lymphomas. Mod Pathol. 2002;15:1172-1180.

34. Cartwright RA, Watkins G. Epidemiology of Hodgkin's disease: a review. Hematol Oncol. 2004;22:11-26.

35. International Agency for Research on Cancer. Cancer Incidence in Five Continents, vol VII (Publication No. 143). Lyon, France, IARC, 1997.

36. Macfarlane GJ, Evstifeeva T, Boyle P, Grufferman S. International patterns in the occurrence of Hodgkin's disease in children and young adult males. Int J Cancer. 1995;61:165-169.

37. Hjalgrim H, Askling J, Pukkala E, et al. Incidence of Hodgkin's disease in Nordic countries. Lancet. 2001;358:297-298.

38. Yeole BB, Jussawalla DJ. Descriptive epidemiology of lymphatic malignancies in Greater Bombay. Oncol Rep. 1998;5:771-777.

39. Chen YT, Zheng T, Chou MC, et al. The increase of Hodgkin's disease incidence among young adults. Experience in Connecticut, 1935-1992. Cancer. 1997;79:2209-2218.

40. Liu S, Semenciw R, Waters C, et al. Time trends and sex patterns in Hodgkin's disease incidence in Canada, 1970-1995. Can J Public Health. 2000;91:188-192.

41. Morton LM, Wang SS, Devesa SS, et al. Lymphoma incidence patterns by WHO subtype in the United States, 1992-2001. Blood. 2006;107:265-276.

42. Cartwright R, McNally R, Roman E, et al. Incidence and time trends in Hodgkin's disease: from parts of the United Kingdom (1984-1993). Leuk Lymphoma. 1998;31:367-377.

43. Kaatsch P, Spix C. Annual Report 2005: German Childhood Cancer Registry. Mainz, Germany, Institut für Medizinische Biometrie, Epidemiologie und Informatik, 2007, p 52.

44. Percy CL, Smith MA, Linet M, et al. Lymphomas and reticuloendothelial neoplasms. In Reis LAG, Smith MA, Gurney JG, et al (eds). Cancer Incidence and Survival Among Children and Adolescents: United States SEER Program 1975-1995 (NIH Publication No. 99-4649). Bethesda, Md, National Cancer Institute, SEER Program, 1999, pp 35-49.

45. Dörffel W, Schellong G. Morbus Hodgkin. In Gadner H, Gaedicke G, Niemeyer C, Ritter J (eds). Paediatrische Haematologie und Onkologie. Heidelberg, Germany, Springer, 2006, pp 770-776.

46. Dinshaw K, Pande S, Advani S, et al. Pediatric Hodgkin's disease in India. J Clin Oncol. 1985;3:1605-1612.

47. Vianna NJ, Polan AK. Epidemiologic evidence for transmission of Hodgkin's disease. N Engl J Med. 1973;289:499-502.

48. Glaser SL. Spatial clustering of Hodgkin's disease in the San Francisco Bay area. Am J Epidemiol. 1990;132:S167-S177.

49. Grufferman S, Cole P, Smith PG, Lukes RJ. Hodgkin's disease in siblings. N Engl J Med. 1977;296:248-250.

50. Alexander FE, Ricketts TJ, McKinney PA, Cartwright RA. Community lifestyle characteristics and incidence of Hodgkin's disease in young people. Int J Cancer. 1991;48:10-14.

51. Alexander FE, McKinney PA, Williams J, et al. Epidemiological evidence for the "two-disease hypothesis" in Hodgkin's disease. Int J Epidemiol. 1991;20:354-361.

52. Newell GR, Lynch HK, Gibeau JM, Spitz MR. Seasonal diagnosis of Hodgkin's disease among young adults. J Natl Cancer Inst. 1985;74:53-56.

53. Neilly IJ, Dawson AA, Bennett B, Douglas S. Evidence for a seasonal variation in the presentation of Hodgkin's disease. Leuk Lymphoma. 1995;18:325-328.

54. MacMahon B. Epidemiology of Hodgkin's disease. Cancer Res. 1966;26:1189-1201.

55. Rosdahl N, Larsen SO, Clemmesen J. Hodgkin's disease in patients with previous infectious mononucleosis: 30 years' experience. BMJ. 1974;2:253-256.

56. Evans AS, Comstock GW. Presence of elevated antibody titres to Epstein-Barr virus before Hodgkin's disease. Lancet. 1981;1:1183-1186.

57. Mueller N, Evans A, Harris NL, et al. Hodgkin's disease and Epstein-Barr virus. Altered antibody pattern before diagnosis. N Engl J Med. 1989;320:689-695.

58. Mueller N, Mohar A, Evans A, et al. Epstein-Barr virus antibody patterns preceding the diagnosis of non-Hodgkin's lymphoma. Int J Cancer. 1991;49:387-393.

59. Mueller N. Epidemiologic studies assessing the role of the Epstein-Barr virus in Hodgkin's disease. Yale J Biol Med. 1987;60:321-332.

60. Wagner HJ, Schlager F, Claviez A, Bucsky P. Detection of Epstein-Barr virus DNA in peripheral blood of paediatric patients with Hodgkin's disease by real-time polymerase chain reaction. Eur J Cancer. 2001;37:1853-1857.

61. Weiss LM, Strickler JG, Warnke RA, et al. Epstein-Barr viral DNA in tissues of Hodgkin's disease. Am J Pathol. 1987;129:86-91.

62. Weiss LM, Movahed LA, Warnke RA, Sklar J. Detection of Epstein-Barr viral genomes in Reed-Sternberg cells of Hodgkin's disease. N Engl J Med. 1989;320:502-506.

63. Gulley ML, Eagan PA, Quintanilla-Martinez L, et al. Epstein-Barr virus DNA is abundant and monoclonal in the Reed-Sternberg cells of Hodgkin's disease: association with mixed cellularity subtype and Hispanic American ethnicity. Blood. 1994;83:1595-1602.

64. Hjalgrim H, Askling J, Rostgaard K, et al. Characteristics of Hodgkin's lymphoma after infectious mononucleosis. N Engl J Med. 2003;349:1324-1332.

65. Claviez A, Tiemann M, Luders H, et al. Impact of latent Epstein-Barr virus infection on outcome in children and adolescents with Hodgkin's lymphoma. J Clin Oncol. 2005;23:4048-4056.

66. Salahuddin SZ, Ablashi DV, Markham PD, et al. Isolation of a new virus, HBLV, in patients with lymphoproliferative disorders. Science. 1986;234:596-601.

67. Schmidt CA, Oettle H, Peng R, et al. Presence of human beta- and gamma-herpesvirus DNA in Hodgkin's disease. Leuk Res. 2000;24:865-870.

68. Benharroch D, Shemer-Avni Y, Levy A, et al. New candidate virus in association with Hodgkin's disease. Leuk Lymphoma. 2003;44:605-610.

69. Chang ET, Zheng T, Weir EG, et al. Aspirin and the risk of Hodgkin's lymphoma in a population-based case-control study. J Natl Cancer Inst. 2004;96:305-315.

70. Bargou RC, Emmerich F, Krappmann D, et al. Constitutive nuclear factor-kappa B-RelA activation is required for proliferation and survival of Hodgkin's disease tumor cells. J Clin Invest. 1997;100:2961-2969.

71. Grulich AE, Wan X, Law MG, et al. Risk of cancer in people with AIDS. AIDS. 1999;13:839-843.

72. Biggar RJ, Jaffe ES, Goedert JJ, et al. Hodgkin lymphoma and immunodeficiency in persons with HIV/AIDS. Blood. 2006;108:3786-3791.

73. Razis DV, Diamond HD, Craver LF. Familial Hodgkin's disease: its significance and implications. Ann Intern Med. 1959;51:933-971.

74. Mack TM, Cozen W, Shibata DK, et al. Concordance for Hodgkin's disease in identical twins suggesting genetic susceptibility to the young-adult form of the disease. N Engl J Med. 1995;332:413-418.

75. Goldin LR, Pfeiffer RM, Gridley G, et al. Familial aggregation of Hodgkin lymphoma and related tumors. Cancer. 2004;100:1902-1908.

76. Chang ET, Smedby KE, Hjalgrim H, et al. Family history of hematopoietic malignancy and risk of lymphoma. J Natl Cancer Inst. 2005;97:1466-1474.

77. Kerber RA, O'Brien E. A cohort study of cancer risk in relation to family histories of cancer in the Utah population database. Cancer. 2005;103:1906-1915.

78. Altieri A, Hemminki K. The familial risk of Hodgkin's lymphoma ranks among the highest in the Swedish Family-Cancer Database. Leukemia. 2006;20:2062-2063.

79. Ferraris AM, Racchi O, Rapezzi D, et al. Familial Hodgkin's disease: a disease of young adulthood? Ann Hematol. 1997;74:131-134.

80. Altieri A, Castro F, Bermejo JL, Hemminki K. Number of siblings and the risk of lymphoma, leukemia, and myeloma by histopathology. Cancer Epidemiol Biomarkers Prev. 2006;15:1281-1286.

81. Robertson SJ, Lowman JT, Grufferman S, et al. Familial Hodgkin's disease. A clinical and laboratory investigation. Cancer. 1987;59:1314-1319.

82. Schlaifer D, Rigal-Huguet F, Robert A, et al. Epstein-Barr virus in familial Hodgkin's disease. Br J Haematol. 1994;88:636-638.

83. Landgren O, Bjorkholm M, Montgomery SM, et al. Personal and family history of autoimmune diabetes mellitus and susceptibility to young-adult-onset Hodgkin lymphoma. Int J Cancer. 2006;118:449-452.

84. Hjalgrim H, Rasmussen S, Rostgaard K, et al. Familial clustering of Hodgkin lymphoma and multiple sclerosis. J Natl Cancer Inst. 2004;96:780-784.

85. Straus SE, Jaffe ES, Puck JM, et al. The development of lymphomas in families with autoimmune lymphoproliferative syndrome with germline Fas mutations and defective lymphocyte apoptosis. Blood. 2001;98:194-200.

86. Hecht F, Hecht BK. Cancer in ataxia-telangiectasia patients. Cancer Genet Cytogenet. 1990;46:9-19.

87. Liberzon E, Avigad S, Yaniv I, et al. Molecular variants of the ATM gene in Hodgkin's disease in children. Br J Cancer. 2004;90:522-525.

88. Svejgaard A, Platz P, Ryder LP, et al. HL-A and disease associations—a survey. Transplant Rev. 1975;22:3-43.

89. Bodmer WF. Genetic factors in Hodgkin's disease: association with a disease-susceptibility locus (DSA) in the HL-A region. Natl Cancer Inst Monogr. 1973;36:127-134.

90. Hors J, Dausset J. HLA and susceptibility to Hodgkin's disease. Immunol Rev. 1983;70:167-192.

91. Chakravarti A, Halloran SL, Bale SJ, Tucker MA. Etiological heterogeneity in Hodgkin's disease: HLA linked and unlinked determinants of susceptibility independent of histological concordance. Genet Epidemiol. 1986;3:407-415.

92. Kamper PM, Kjeldsen E, Clausen N, et al. Epstein-Barr virus–associated familial Hodgkin lymphoma: paediatric onset in three of five siblings. Br J Haematol. 2005;129:615-617.

93. Pileri SA, Ascani S, Leoncini L, et al. Hodgkin's lymphoma: the pathologist's viewpoint. J Clin Pathol. 2002;55:162-176.

94. Kanzler H, Kuppers R, Hansmann ML, Rajewsky K. Hodgkin and Reed-Sternberg cells in Hodgkin's disease represent the outgrowth of a dominant tumor clone derived from (crippled) germinal center B cells. J Exp Med. 1996;184:1495-1505.

95. Marafioti T, Hummel M, Foss HD, et al. Hodgkin and Reed-Sternberg cells represent an expansion of a single clone originating from a germinal center B-cell with functional immunoglobulin gene rearrangements but defective immunoglobulin transcription. Blood. 2000;95:1443-1450.

96. Ohno T, Stribley JA, Wu G, et al. Clonality in nodular lymphocyte-predominant Hodgkin's disease. N Engl J Med. 1997;337:459-465.

97. Re D, Kuppers R, Diehl V. Molecular pathogenesis of Hodgkin's lymphoma. J Clin Oncol. 2005;23:6379-6386.

98. Martin-Subero JI, Gesk S, Harder L, et al. Recurrent involvement of the REL and BCL11A loci in classical Hodgkin lymphoma. Blood. 2002;99:1474-1477.

99. Cabannes E, Khan G, Aillet F, et al. Mutations in the IkBa gene in Hodgkin's disease suggest a tumour suppressor role for I kappa B alpha. Oncogene. 1999;18:3063-3070.

100. Emmerich F, Theurich S, Hummel M, et al. Inactivating I kappa B epsilon mutations in Hodgkin/Reed-Sternberg cells. J Pathol. 2003;201:413-420.

101. Joos S, Kupper M, Ohl S, et al. Genomic imbalances including amplification of the tyrosine kinase gene JAK2 in CD30+ Hodgkin cells. Cancer Res. 2000;60:549-552.

102. Kupper M, Joos S, von Bonin F, et al. MDM2 gene amplification and lack of p53 point mutations in Hodgkin and Reed-Sternberg cells: results from single-cell polymerase chain reaction and molecular cytogenetic studies. Br J Haematol. 2001;112:768-775.

103. Lacronique V, Boureux A, Valle VD, et al. A TEL-JAK2 fusion protein with constitutive kinase activity in human leukemia. Science. 1997;278:1309-1312.

104. De Keersmaecker K, Cools J. Chronic myeloproliferative disorders: a tyrosine kinase tale. Leukemia. 2006;20:200-205.

105. Woods DB, Vousden KH. Regulation of p53 function. Exp Cell Res. 2001;264:56-66.

106. Wlodarska I, Nooyen P, Maes B, et al. Frequent occurrence of BCL6 rearrangements in nodular lymphocyte predominance Hodgkin lymphoma but not in classical Hodgkin lymphoma. Blood. 2003;101:706-710.

107. Ye BH, Cattoretti G, Shen Q, et al. The BCL-6 proto-oncogene controls germinal-centre formation and Th2-type inflammation. Nat Genet. 1997;16:161-170.

108. Phan RT, Dalla-Favera R. The BCL6 proto-oncogene suppresses p53 expression in germinal-centre B cells. Nature. 2004;432:635-639.

109. Ranuncolo SM, Polo JM, Dierov J, et al. Bcl-6 mediates the germinal center B cell phenotype and lymphomagenesis through transcriptional repression of the DNA-damage sensor ATR. Nat Immunol. 2007;8:705-714.

110. Kapp U, Yeh WC, Patterson B, et al. Interleukin 13 is secreted by and stimulates the growth of Hodgkin and Reed-Sternberg cells. J Exp Med. 1999;189:1939-1946.

111. Trieu Y, Wen XY, Skinnider BF, et al. Soluble interleukin-13R alpha 2 decoy receptor inhibits Hodgkin's lymphoma growth in vitro and in vivo. Cancer Res. 2004;64:3271-3275.

112. Horie R, Watanabe T, Ito K, et al. Cytoplasmic aggregation of TRAF2 and TRAF5 proteins in the Hodgkin-Reed-Sternberg cells. Am J Pathol. 2002;160:1647-1654.

113. Gruss HJ, Hirschstein D, Wright B, et al. Expression and function of CD40 on Hodgkin and Reed-Sternberg cells and the possible relevance for Hodgkin's disease. Blood. 1994;84:2305-2314.

114. Carbone A, Gloghini A, Gruss HJ, Pinto A. CD40 ligand is constitutively expressed in a subset of T cell lymphomas and on the microenvironmental reactive T cells of follicular lymphomas and Hodgkin's disease. Am J Pathol. 1995;147:912-922.

115. Metkar SS, Naresh KN, Redkar AA, Nadkarni JJ. CD40-ligation-mediated protection from apoptosis of a Fas-sensitive Hodgkin's-disease-derived cell line. Cancer Immunol Immunother. 1998;47:104-112.

116. Bashir H, Hudson MM, Kaste SC, et al. Pericardial involvement at diagnosis in pediatric Hodgkin lymphoma patients. Pediatr Blood Cancer. 2007;49:666-671.

117. Sonnenblick M, Kramer R, Hershko C. Corticosteroid-responsive immune thrombocytopenia in Hodgkin's disease. Oncology. 1986;43:349-353.

118. Bierman PJ, Cavalli F, Armitage JO. Unusual syndromes in Hodgkin's disease. In Mauch PM, Armitage JO, Diehl V (eds). Hodgkin's Disease. Philadelphia, Lippincott Williams & Wilkins, 1999, pp 327-334.

119. Slivnick DJ, Ellis TM, Nawrocki JF, Fisher RI. The impact of Hodgkin's disease on the immune system. Semin Oncol. 1990;17:673-682.

120. Parker BR, Castellino RA, Kaplan HS. Pediatric Hodgkin's disease. I. Radiographic evaluation. Cancer. 1976;37:2430-2435.

121. Carbone PP, Kaplan HS, Musshoff K, et al. Report of the Committee on Hodgkin's Disease Staging Classification. Cancer Res. 1971;31:1860-1861.

122. Lister TA, Crowther D, Sutcliffe SB, et al. Report of a committee convened to discuss the evaluation and staging of patients with Hodgkin's disease: Cotswolds meeting. J Clin Oncol. 1989;7:1630-1636.

123. Mende U, Zierhut D, Ewerbeck V, et al. Ultrasound criteria for staging and follow-up of malignant lymphoma. Radiologe. 1997;37:19-26.

124. Siniluoto TM, Tikkakoski TA, Lahde ST, et al. Ultrasound or CT in splenic diseases? Acta Radiol. 1994;35:597-605.

125. Trauzeddel R, Dorffel W. The importance of spleen sonography in the initial staging of Hodgkin's disease in childhood and adolescents. (Personal communication.)

126. Daneman A, Martin DJ, Fitz CR, Chan HS. Computed tomography and lymphogram correlation in children with Hodgkin's disease. J Comput Tomogr. 1983;7:115-122.

127. Baker LL, Parker BR, Donaldson SS, Castellino RA. Staging of Hodgkin disease in children: comparison of CT and lymphography with laparotomy. AJR Am J Roentgenol. 1990;154:1251-1255.

128. Kostakoglu L, Leonard JP, Kuji I, et al. Comparison of fluorine-18 fluorodeoxyglucose positron emission tomography and Ga-67 scintigraphy in evaluation of lymphoma. Cancer. 2002;94:879-888.

129. Wirth A, Seymour JF, Hicks RJ, et al. Fluorine-18 fluorodeoxyglucose positron emission tomography, gallium-67 scintigraphy, and conventional staging for Hodgkin's disease and non-Hodgkin's lymphoma. Am J Med. 2002;112:262-268.

130. Hudson MM, Krasin MJ, Kaste SC. PET imaging in pediatric Hodgkin's lymphoma. Pediatr Radiol. 2004;34:190-198.

131. Reske SN, Kotzerke J. FDG-PET for clinical use. Results of the 3rd German Interdisciplinary Consensus Conference, "Onko-PET III," 21 July and 19 September 2000. Eur J Nucl Med. 2001;28:1707-1723.

132. Som P, Atkins HL, Bandoypadhyay D, et al. A fluorinated glucose analog, 2-fluoro-2-deoxy-D-glucose (F-18): nontoxic tracer for rapid tumor detection. J Nucl Med. 1980;21:670-675.

133. Juweid ME. Utility of positron emission tomography (PET) scanning in managing patients with Hodgkin lymphoma. Hematology Am Soc Hematol Educ Program. 2006;259-265.

134. Montravers F, McNamara D, Landman-Parker J, et al. [(18)F]FDG in childhood lymphoma: clinical utility and impact on management. Eur J Nucl Med Mol Imaging. 2002;29:1155-1165.

135. Hermann S, Wormanns D, Pixberg M, et al. Staging in childhood lymphoma: differences between FDG-PET and CT. Nuklearmedizin. 2005;44:1-7.

136. Brink I, Reinhardt MJ, Hoegerle S, et al. Increased metabolic activity in the thymus gland studied with 18F-FDG PET: age dependency and frequency after chemotherapy. J Nucl Med. 2001;42:591-595.

137. Yeung HW, Grewal RK, Gonen M, et al. Patterns of (18)F-FDG uptake in adipose tissue and muscle: a potential source of false-positives for PET. J Nucl Med. 2003;44:1789-1796.

138. Lardinois D, Weder W, Hany TF, et al. Staging of non-small-cell lung cancer with integrated positron-emission tomography and computed tomography. N Engl J Med. 2003;348:2500-2507.

139. Yeung HW, Schoder H, Smith A, et al. Clinical value of combined positron emission tomography/computed tomography imaging in the interpretation of 2-deoxy-2-[F-18]fluoro-D-glucose-positron emission tomography studies in cancer patients. Mol Imaging Biol. 2005;7:229-235.

140. Buchmann I, Reinhardt M, Elsner K, et al. 2-(Fluorine-18)-fluoro-2-deoxy-D-glucose positron emission tomography in the detection and staging of malignant lymphoma. A bicenter trial. Cancer. 2001;91:889-899.

141. Hutchings M, Loft A, Hansen M, et al. Different histopathological subtypes of Hodgkin lymphoma show significantly different levels of FDG uptake. Hematol Oncol. 2006;24:146-150.

142. Schellong G, Potter R, Bramswig J, et al. High cure rates and reduced long-term toxicity in pediatric Hodgkin's disease: the German-Austrian multicenter trial DAL-HD-90. The German-Austrian Pediatric Hodgkin's Disease Study Group. J Clin Oncol. 1999;17:3736-3744.

143. Schellong G, Riepenhausen M. Late effects after therapy of Hodgkin's disease: update 2003/04 on overwhelming post-splenectomy infections and secondary malignancies. Klin Padiatr. 2004;216:364-369.

144. Schellong G. The balance between cure and late effects in childhood Hodgkin's lymphoma: the experience of the German-Austrian Study-Group since 1978. German-Austrian Pediatric Hodgkin's Disease Study Group. Ann Oncol. 1996;7(Suppl 4):67-72.

145. Hudson MM. Pediatric Hodgkin's therapy: time for a paradigm shift. J Clin Oncol. 2002;20:3755-3757.

146. Henry-Amar M, Aeppli DM, et al. Workshop statistical report. In Somers, R, Henry-Amar M, Meerwald JK, London CP (eds). Treatment Strategy in Hodgkin's Disease. London, Inserm/John Libbey Eurotext, 1990.

147. Krasin MJ, Rai SN, Kun LE, et al. Patterns of treatment failure in pediatric and young adult patients with Hodgkin's disease: local disease control with combined-modality therapy. J Clin Oncol. 2005;23:8406-8413.

148. Bramswig JH, Heimes U, Heiermann E, et al. The effects of different cumulative doses of chemotherapy on testicular function. Results in 75 patients treated for Hodgkin's disease during childhood or adolescence. Cancer. 1990;65:1298-1302.

149. Gerres L, Bramswig JH, Schlegel W, et al. The effects of etoposide on testicular function in boys treated for Hodgkin's disease. Cancer. 1998;83:2217-2222.

150. Hoppe RT, Coleman CN, Cox RS, et al. The management of stage I-II Hodgkin's disease with irradiation alone or combined modality therapy: the Stanford experience. Blood. 1982;59:455-465.

151. Roskos RR, Evans RC, Gilchrist GS, et al. Prognostic significance of mediastinal mass in childhood Hodgkin's disease. Cancer Treat Rep. 1982;66:961-968.

152. Smith RS, Chen Q, Hudson MM, et al. Prognostic factors for children with Hodgkin's disease treated with combined-modality therapy. J Clin Oncol. 2003;21:2026-2033.

153. Dieckmann K, Potter R, Hofmann J, et al. Does bulky disease at diagnosis influence outcome in childhood Hodgkin's disease and require higher radiation doses? Results from the German-Austrian Pediatric Multicenter Trial DAL-HD-90. Int J Radiat Oncol Biol Phys. 2003;56:644-652.

154. Kaplan HS. Hodgkin's Disease, Cambridge, Mass, Harvard University Press, 1980.

155. Donaldson SS, Link MP. Combined modality treatment with low-dose radiation and MOPP chemotherapy for children with Hodgkin's disease. J Clin Oncol. 1987;5:742-749.

156. Donaldson SS, Kaplan HS. Complications of treatment of Hodgkin's disease in children. Cancer Treat Rep. 1982;66:977-989.

157. Donaldson SS, Link MP. Hodgkin's disease. Treatment of the young child. Pediatr Clin North Am. 1991;38:457-473.

158. Hancock SL, Donaldson SS, Hoppe RT. Cardiac disease following treatment of Hodgkin's disease in children and adolescents. J Clin Oncol. 1993;11:1208-1215.

159. Bhatia S, Yasui Y, Robison LL, et al. High risk of subsequent neoplasms continues with extended follow-up of childhood Hodgkin's disease: report from the Late Effects Study Group. J Clin Oncol. 2003;21:4386-4394.

160. Breu H, Schellong G, Grosch-Worner I, et al. Chemotherapy of different intensity and reduced radiotherapy of Hodgkin's disease in childhood—a report on 170 patients of the cooperative study HD 78. Klin Padiatr. 1982;194:233-241.

161. Oberlin O, Leverger G, Pacquement H, et al. Low-dose radiation therapy and reduced chemotherapy in childhood Hodgkin's disease: the experience of the French Society of Pediatric Oncology. J Clin Oncol. 1992;10:1602-1608.

162. Schellong G, Bramswig J, Ludwig R, et al. Combined treatment strategy in over 200 children with Hodgkin's disease: graduated chemotherapy, involved field irradiation with low dosage and selective splenectomy. A report of the cooperative therapy study DAL-HD-82. Klin Padiatr. 1986;198:137-146.

163. Schellong G, Waubke-Landwehr AK, Langermann HJ, et al. Prediction of splenic involvement in children with Hodgkin's disease. Significance of clinical and intraoperative findings. A retrospective statistical analysis of 154 patients in the German therapy study DAL-HD-78. Cancer. 1986;57:2049-2056.

164. Schellong G, Bramswig JH, Schwarze EW, Wannenmacher M. An approach to reduce treatment and invasive staging in childhood Hodgkin's disease: the sequence of the German DAL multicenter studies. Bull Cancer. 1988;75:41-51.

165. Dieckmann K, Potter R, Wagner W, et al. Up-front centralized data review and individualized treatment proposals in a multicenter pediatric Hodgkin's disease trial with 71 participating hospitals: the experience of the German-Austrian pediatric multicenter trial DAL-HD-90. Radiother Oncol. 2002;62:191-200.

166. Ruhl U, Albrecht M, Dieckmann K, et al. Response-adapted radiotherapy in the treatment of pediatric Hodgkin's disease: an interim report at 5 years of the German GPOH-HD 95 trial. Int J Radiat Oncol Biol Phys. 2001;51:1209-1218.

167. Devita VT Jr, Serpick AA, Carbone PP. Combination chemotherapy in the treatment of advanced Hodgkin's disease. Ann Intern Med. 1970;73:881-895.

168. Santoro A, Bonadonna G, Bonfante V, Valagussa P. Alternating drug combinations in the treatment of advanced Hodgkin's disease. N Engl J Med. 1982;306:770-775.

169. Donaldson SS, Hudson MM, Lamborn KR, et al. VAMP and low-dose, involved-field radiation for children and adolescents with favorable, early-stage Hodgkin's disease: results of a prospective clinical trial. J Clin Oncol. 2002;20:3081-3087.

170. Donaldson SS, Link MP, Weinstein HJ, et al. Final results of a prospective clinical trial with VAMP and low-dose involved-field radiation for children with low-risk Hodgkin's disease. J Clin Oncol. 2007;25:332-337.

171. Landman-Parker J, Pacquement H, Leblanc T, et al. Localized childhood Hodgkin's disease: response-adapted chemotherapy with etoposide, bleomycin, vinblastine, and prednisone before low-dose radiation therapy-results of the French Society of Pediatric Oncology Study MDH90. J Clin Oncol. 2000;18:1500-1507.

172. Horning SJ, Hoppe RT, Breslin S, et al. Stanford V and radiotherapy for locally extensive and advanced Hodgkin's disease: mature results of a prospective clinical trial. J Clin Oncol. 2002;20:630-637.

173. Schellong G, Hornig I, Bramswig J, et al. Significance of procarbazine in the chemotherapy of Hodgkin's disease—a report of the Cooperative Therapy Study DAL-HD-85. Klin Padiatr. 1988;200:205-213.

174. Weiner MA, Leventhal B, Brecher ML, et al. Randomized study of intensive MOPP-ABVD with or without low-dose total-nodal radiation therapy in the treatment of stages IIB, IIIA2, IIIB, and IV Hodgkin's disease in pediatric patients: a Pediatric Oncology Group study. J Clin Oncol. 1997;15:2769-2779.

175. Hudson MM, Poquette CA, Lee J, et al. Increased mortality after successful treatment for Hodgkin's disease. J Clin Oncol. 1998;16:3592-3600.

176. Wolden SL, Lamborn KR, Cleary SF, et al. Second cancers following pediatric Hodgkin's disease. J Clin Oncol. 1998;16:536-544.

177. Schellong G, Riepenhausen M, Creutzig U, et al. Low risk of secondary leukemias after chemotherapy without mechlorethamine in childhood Hodgkin's disease. German-Austrian Pediatric Hodgkin's Disease Group. J Clin Oncol. 1997;15:2247-2253.

178. Schellong G, Dorffel W, Claviez A, et al. Salvage therapy of progressive and recurrent Hodgkin's disease: results from a multicenter study of the pediatric DAL/GPOH-HD study group. J Clin Oncol. 2005;23:6181-6189.

179. Epstein R, Hanham I, Dale R. Radiotherapy-induced second cancers: are we doing enough to protect young patients? Eur J Cancer. 1997;33:526-530.

180. Prosnitz LR. Reducing treatment-related morbidity and mortality in early-stage Hodgkin's disease and why the recent Southwest Oncology Group Trial is not the way to go. J Clin Oncol. 2002;20:2225-2228.

181. Cheson BD, Pfistner B, Juweid ME, et al. Revised response criteria for malignant lymphoma. J Clin Oncol. 2007;25:579-586.

182. Juweid ME, Stroobants S, Hoekstra OS, et al. Use of positron emission tomography for response assessment of lymphoma: consensus of the Imaging Subcommittee of International Harmonization Project in Lymphoma. J Clin Oncol. 2007;25:571-578.

183. Hutchings M, Loft A, Hansen M, et al. FDG-PET after two cycles of chemotherapy predicts treatment failure and progression-free survival in Hodgkin lymphoma. Blood. 2006;107:52-59.

184. Kostakoglu L, Coleman M, Leonard JP, et al. PET predicts prognosis after 1 cycle of chemotherapy in aggressive lymphoma and Hodgkin's disease. J Nucl Med. 2002;43:1018-1027.

185. Hutchings M, Mikhaeel NG, Fields PA, et al. Prognostic value of interim FDG-PET after two or three cycles of chemotherapy in Hodgkin lymphoma. Ann Oncol. 2005;16:1160-1168.

186. Korholz D, Claviez A, Hasenclever D, et al. The concept of the GPOH-HD 2003 therapy study for pediatric Hodgkin's disease: evolution in the tradition of the DAL/GPOH studies. Klin Padiatr. 2004;216:150-156.

187. Niehues T, Schellong G, Dorffel W, et al. Immunodeficiency and Hodgkin's disease: treatment and outcome in the DAL HD78-90 and GPOH HD95 studies. Klin Padiatr. 2003;215:315-320.

188. Spina M, Gabarre J, Rossi G, et al. Stanford V regimen and concomitant HAART in 59 patients with Hodgkin disease and HIV infection. Blood. 2002;100:1984-1988.

189. Schmitz N, Pfistner B, Sextro M, et al. Aggressive conventional chemotherapy compared with high-dose chemotherapy with autologous haemopoietic stem-cell transplantation for relapsed chemosensitive Hodgkin's disease: a randomised trial. Lancet. 2002;359:2065-2071.

190. Stoneham S, Ashley S, Pinkerton CR, et al. Outcome after autologous hemopoietic stem cell transplantation in relapsed or refractory childhood Hodgkin disease. J Pediatr Hematol Oncol. 2004;26:740-745.

191. Wimmer RS, Chauvenet AR, London WB, et al. APE chemotherapy for children with relapsed Hodgkin disease: a Pediatric Oncology Group trial. Pediatr Blood Cancer. 2006;46:320-324.

192. Fields KK, Zorsky PE, Hiemenz JW, et al. Ifosfamide, carboplatin, and etoposide: a new regimen with a broad spectrum of activity. J Clin Oncol. 1994;12:544-552.

193. Lieskovsky YE, Donaldson SS, Torres MA, et al. High-dose therapy and autologous hematopoietic stem-cell transplantation for recurrent or refractory pediatric Hodgkin's disease: results and prognostic indices. J Clin Oncol. 2004;22:4532-4540.

194. Baker KS, Gordon BG, Gross TG, et al. Autologous hematopoietic stem-cell transplantation for relapsed or refractory Hodgkin's disease in children and adolescents. J Clin Oncol. 1999;17:825-831.

195. Anderson JE, Litzow MR, Appelbaum FR, et al. Allogeneic, syngeneic, and autologous marrow transplantation for Hodgkin's disease: the 21-year Seattle experience. J Clin Oncol. 1993;11:2342-2350.

196. Milpied N, Fielding AK, Pearce RM, et al. Allogeneic bone marrow transplant is not better than autologous transplant for patients with relapsed Hodgkin's disease. European Group for Blood and Bone Marrow Transplantation. J Clin Oncol. 1996;14:1291-1296.

197. Carella AM, Cavaliere M, Lerma E, et al. Autografting followed by nonmyeloablative immunosuppressive chemotherapy and allogeneic peripheral-blood hematopoietic stem-cell transplantation as treatment of resistant Hodgkin's disease and non-Hodgkin's lymphoma. J Clin Oncol. 2000;18:3918-3924.

198. Claviez A, Klingebiel T, Beyer J, et al. Allogeneic peripheral blood stem cell transplantation following fludarabine-based conditioning in six children with advanced Hodgkin's disease. Ann Hematol. 2004;83:237-241.

199. Claviez A, Glass B, Dreger P, Suttorp M. Elevated blood drug levels obtained from indwelling silicon catheters during oral cyclosporine A administration. Bone Marrow Transplant. 2002;29:535-536.

200. Peggs KS, Hunter A, Chopra R, et al. Clinical evidence of a graft-versus-Hodgkin's-lymphoma effect after reduced-intensity allogeneic transplantation. Lancet. 2005;365:1934-1941.

201. Sandoval C, Venkateswaran L, Billups C, et al. Lymphocyte-predominant Hodgkin disease in children. J Pediatr Hematol Oncol. 2002;24:269-273.

202. Karayalcin G, Behm FG, Gieser PW, et al. Lymphocyte predominant Hodgkin disease: clinico-pathologic features and results of treatment—the Pediatric Oncology Group experience. Med Pediatr Oncol. 1997;29:519-525.

203. Murphy SB, Morgan ER, Katzenstein HM, Kletzel M. Results of little or no treatment for lymphocyte-predominant Hodgkin disease in children and adolescents. J Pediatr Hematol Oncol. 2003;25:684-687.

204. Pellegrino B, Terrier-Lacombe MJ, Oberlin O, et al. Lymphocyte-predominant Hodgkin's lymphoma in children: therapeutic abstention after initial lymph node resection—a Study of the French Society of Pediatric Oncology. J Clin Oncol. 2003;21:2948-2952.

205. Lipshultz SE, Colan SD, Gelber RD, et al. Late cardiac effects of doxorubicin therapy for acute lymphoblastic leukemia in childhood. N Engl J Med. 1991;324:808-815.

206. Adams MJ, Lipsitz SR, Colan SD, et al. Cardiovascular status in long-term survivors of Hodgkin's disease treated with chest radiotherapy. J Clin Oncol. 2004;22:3139-3148.

207. Bowers DC, McNeil DE, Liu Y, et al. Stroke as a late treatment effect of Hodgkin's Disease: a report from the Childhood Cancer Survivor Study. J Clin Oncol. 2005;23:6508-6515.

208. Coleman CN, McDougall IR, Dailey MO, et al. Functional hyposplenia after splenic irradiation for Hodgkin's disease. Ann Intern Med. 1982;96:44-47.

209. Parvinen LM, Kilkku P, Makinen E, et al. Factors affecting the pulmonary toxicity of bleomycin. Acta Radiol Oncol. 1983;22:417-421.

210. O'Driscoll BR, Kalra S, Gattamaneni HR, Woodcock AA. Late carmustine lung fibrosis. Age at treatment may influence severity and survival. Chest. 1995;107:1355-1357.

211. Hartmann O, Benhamou E, Beaujean F, et al. Repeated high-dose chemotherapy followed by purged autologous bone marrow transplantation as consolidation therapy in metastatic neuroblastoma. J Clin Oncol. 1987;5:1205-1211.

212. Frankovich J, Donaldson SS, Lee Y, et al. High-dose therapy and autologous hematopoietic cell transplantation in children with primary refractory and relapsed Hodgkin's disease: atopy predicts idiopathic diffuse lung injury syndromes. Biol Blood Marrow Transplant. 2001;7:49-57.

213. Sklar C, Whitton J, Mertens A, et al. Abnormalities of the thyroid in survivors of Hodgkin's disease: data from the Childhood Cancer Survivor Study. J Clin Endocrinol Metab. 2000;85:3227-3232.

214. Metzger ML, Hudson MM, Somes GW, et al. White race as a risk factor for hypothyroidism after treatment for pediatric Hodgkin's lymphoma. J Clin Oncol. 2006;24:1516-1521.

215. Horning SJ, Hoppe RT, Kaplan HS, Rosenberg SA. Female reproductive potential after treatment for Hodgkin's disease. N Engl J Med. 1981;304:1377-1382.

216. Pedrick TJ, Hoppe RT. Recovery of spermatogenesis following pelvic irradiation for Hodgkin's disease. Int J Radiat Oncol Biol Phys. 1986;12:117-121.

217. da Cunha MF, Meistrich ML, Fuller LM, et al. Recovery of spermatogenesis after treatment for Hodgkin's disease: limiting dose of MOPP chemotherapy. J Clin Oncol. 1984;2:571-577.

218. Hassel JU, Bramswig JH, Schlegel W, Schellong G. Testicular function after OPA/COMP chemotherapy without procarbazine in boys with Hodgkin's disease. Results in 25 patients of the DAL-HD-85 study. Klin Padiatr. 1991;203:268-272.

219. Ortin TT, Shostak CA, Donaldson SS. Gonadal status and reproductive function following treatment for Hodgkin's disease in childhood: the Stanford experience. Int J Radiat Oncol Biol Phys. 1990;19:873-880.

220. Kulkarni SS, Sastry PS, Saikia TK, et al. Gonadal function following ABVD therapy for Hodgkin's disease. Am J Clin Oncol. 1997;20:354-357.

221. Hobbie WL, Ginsberg JP, Ogle SK, et al. Fertility in males treated for Hodgkins disease with COPP/ABV hybrid. Pediatr Blood Cancer. 2005;44:193-196.

222. Neglia JP, Friedman DL, Yasui Y, et al. Second malignant neoplasms in five-year survivors of childhood cancer: childhood cancer survivor study. J Natl Cancer Inst. 2001;93:618-629.

223. Donaldson SS, Hancock SL. Second cancers after Hodgkin's disease in childhood. N Engl J Med. 1996;334:792-794.

224. Bhatia S, Robison LL, Oberlin O, et al. Breast cancer and other second neoplasms after childhood Hodgkin's disease. N Engl J Med. 1996;334:745-751.

225. Sankila R, Garwicz S, Olsen JH, et al. Risk of subsequent malignant neoplasms among 1,641 Hodgkin's disease patients diagnosed in childhood and adolescence: a population-based cohort

study in the five Nordic countries. Association of the Nordic Cancer Registries and the Nordic Society of Pediatric Hematology and Oncology. J Clin Oncol. 1996;14:1442-1446.

226. Metayer C, Lynch CF, Clarke EA, et al. Second cancers among long-term survivors of Hodgkin's disease diagnosed in childhood and adolescence. J Clin Oncol. 2000;18:2435-2443.

227. Meadows AT. Risk factors for second malignant neoplasms: report from the Late Effects Study Group. Bull Cancer. 1988;75:125-130.

228. Tebbi CK, London WB, Friedman D, et al. Dexrazoxane-associated risk for acute myeloid leukemia/myelodysplastic syndrome and other secondary malignancies in pediatric Hodgkin's disease. J Clin Oncol. 2007;25:493-500.

229. Radford JA, Eardley A, Woodman C, Crowther D. Follow up policy after treatment for Hodgkin's disease: too many clinic visits and routine tests? A review of hospital records. BMJ. 1997; 314:343-346.

230. Dorffel W, Albrecht M, Luders H, et al. Multi-national therapy study for Hodgkin's disease in children and adolescents GPOH-DH 95. Interim report after $2\frac{1}{2}$ years. Klin Padiatr. 1998; 210:212-219.

231. Landier W, Bhatia S, Eshelman DA, et al. Development of risk-based guidelines for pediatric cancer survivors: the Children's Oncology Group Long-Term Follow-Up Guidelines from the Children's Oncology Group Late Effects Committee and Nursing Discipline. J Clin Oncol. 2004;22:4979-4990.

232. Zebrack BJ, Zeltzer LK, Whitton J, et al. Psychological outcomes in long-term survivors of childhood leukemia, Hodgkin's disease, and non-Hodgkin's lymphoma: a report from the Childhood Cancer Survivor Study. Pediatrics. 2002;110:42-52.

233. Rappaport H. Tumors of the hematopoetic system. In Atlas of Tumor Pathology, Section 3, Fascicles 8. Washington, DC, Armed Forces Institute of Pathology, 1966, pp 97-161.

234. Lukes RJ, Collins RD. Immunologic characterization of human malignant lymphomas. Cancer. 1974;34(Suppl):503.

235. Gerard-Marchant R, Hamlin I, Lennert K, et al. Classification of non-Hodgkin lymphomas [letter to the editor]. Lancet. 1974;ii: 406-408.

236. Stansfeld AG, Diebold J, Noel H, et al. Updated Kiel classification for lymphomas. Lancet. 1988;1:292-293.

237. National Cancer Institute sponsored study of classification on non-Hodgkin lymphomas: summary and description of a working formulation for clinical usage. The Non-Hodgkin's Lymphoma Pathology Classification Project. Cancer. 1982;49:2112-2135.

238. Raetz EA, Perkins SL, Bhojwani D, et al. Gene expression profiling reveals intrinsic differences between T-cell acute lymphoblastic leukemia and T-cell lymphoblastic lymphoma. Pediatr Blood Cancer. 2006;47:130-140.

239. Bennett JM, Catovsky D, Daniel MT, et al. Proposals for the classification of the acute leukaemias. French-American-British (FAB) co-operative group. Br J Haematol. 1976;33:451-458.

240. Griffith RC, Kelly DR, Nathwani BN, et al. A morphologic study of childhood lymphoma of the lymphoblastic type. The Pediatric Oncology Group experience. Cancer. 1987;59:1126-1131.

241. Desiderio SV, Yancopoulos GD, Paskind M, et al. Insertion of N regions into heavy-chain genes is correlated with expression of terminal deoxytransferase in B cells. Nature. 1984;311: 752-755.

242. Gilfillan S, Dierich A, Lemeur M, et al. Mice lacking TdT: mature animals with an immature lymphocyte repertoire. Science. 1993;261:1175-1178.

243. Bene MC, Castoldi G, Knapp W, et al. Proposals for the immunological classification of acute leukemias. European Group for the Immunological Characterization of Leukemias (EGIL). Leukemia. 1995;9:1783-1786.

244. Reiter A, Schrappe M, Ludwig WD, et al. Intensive ALL-type therapy without local radiotherapy provides a 90% event-free

245. Lones MA, Heerema NA, Le Beau MM, et al. Chromosome abnormalities in advanced stage lymphoblastic lymphoma of children and adolescents: a report from CCG-E08. Cancer Genet Cytogenet. 2007;172:1-11.

246. Ferrando AA, Look AT. Clinical implications of recurring chromosomal and associated molecular abnormalities in acute lymphoblastic leukemia. Semin Hematol. 2000;37:381-395.

247. Graux C, Cools J, Michaux L, et al. Cytogenetics and molecular genetics of T-cell acute lymphoblastic leukemia: from thymocyte to lymphoblast. Leukemia. 2006;20:1496-1510.

248. De Keersmaecker K, Marynen P, Cools J. Genetic insights in the pathogenesis of T-cell acute lymphoblastic leukemia. Haematologica. 2005;90:1116-1127.

249. Hayashi Y, Yamamoto K, Kojima S. T-cell acute lymphoblastic leukemias with a t(8;14) possibly involving a c-myc locus and T-cell-receptor alpha-chain genes. N Engl J Med. 1986;314: 650-651.

250. Bernard O, Guglielmi P, Jonveaux P, et al. Two distinct mechanisms for the SCL gene activation in the t(1;14) translocation of T-cell leukemias. Genes Chromosomes Cancer. 1990;1:194-208.

251. Brown L, Cheng JT, Chen Q, et al. Site-specific recombination of the tal-1 gene is a common occurrence in human T cell leukemia. EMBO J. 1990;9:3343-3351.

252. Mellentin JD, Smith SD, Cleary ML. lyl-1, a novel gene altered by chromosomal translocation in T cell leukemia, codes for a protein with a helix-loop-helix DNA binding motif. Cell. 1989;58:77-83.

253. Xia Y, Brown L, Yang CY, et al. TAL2, a helix-loop-helix gene activated by the (7;9)(q34;q32) translocation in human T-cell leukemia. Proc Natl Acad Sci U S A. 1991;88:11416-11420.

254. Wang J, Jani-Sait SN, Escalon EA, et al. The t(14;21)(q11.2;q22) chromosomal translocation associated with T-cell acute lymphoblastic leukemia activates the BHLHB1 gene. Proc Natl Acad Sci U S A. 2000;97:3497-3502.

255. Boehm T, Foroni L, Kaneko Y, et al. The rhombotin family of cysteine-rich LIM-domain oncogenes: distinct members are involved in T-cell translocations to human chromosomes 11p15 and 11p13. Proc Natl Acad Sci U S A. 1991;88:4367-4371.

256. Kennedy MA, Gonzalez-Sarmiento R, Kees UR, et al. HOX11, a homeobox-containing T-cell oncogene on human chromosome 10q24. Proc Natl Acad Sci U S A. 1991;88:8900-8904.

257. Hatano M, Roberts CW, Minden M, et al. Deregulation of a homeobox gene, HOX11, by the t(10;14) in T cell leukemia. Science. 1991;253:79-82.

258. Bernard OA, Busson-LeConiat M, Ballerini P, et al. A new recurrent and specific cryptic translocation, t(5;14)(q35;q32), is associated with expression of the Hox11L2 gene in T acute lymphoblastic leukemia. Leukemia. 2001;15:1495-1504.

259. Soulier J, Clappier E, Cayuela JM, et al. HOXA genes are included in genetic and biologic networks defining human acute T-cell leukemia (T-ALL). Blood. 2005;106:274-286.

260. Clappier E, Cuccuini W, Cayuela JM, et al. Cyclin D2 dysregulation by chromosomal translocations to TCR loci in T-cell acute lymphoblastic leukemias. Leukemia. 2006;20:82-86.

261. Lahortiga I, De Keersmaecker K, Van Vlierberghe P, et al. Duplication of the MYB oncogene in T cell acute lymphoblastic leukemia. Nat Genet. 2007;39:593-595.

262. Aplan PD, Lombardi DP, Ginsberg AM, et al. Disruption of the human SCL locus by "illegitimate" V-(D)-J recombinase activity. Science. 1990;250:1426-1429.

263. Van Vlierberghe P, van Grotel M, Beverloo HB, et al. The cryptic chromosomal deletion del(11)(p12p13) as a new activation mechanism of LMO2 in pediatric T-cell acute lymphoblastic leukemia. Blood. 2006;108:3520-3529.

264. Ferrando AA, Herblot S, Palomero T, et al. Biallelic transcriptional activation of oncogenic transcription factors in T-cell acute lymphoblastic leukemia. Blood. 2004;103:1909-1911.

265. Bash RO, Hall S, Timmons CF, et al. Does activation of the TAL1 gene occur in a majority of patients with T-cell acute lymphoblastic leukemia? A pediatric oncology group study. Blood. 1995;86:666-676.

266. Duncan AW, Rattis FM, DiMascio LN, et al. Integration of Notch and Wnt signaling in hematopoietic stem cell maintenance. Nat Immunol. 2005;6:314-322.

267. Jaleco AC, Neves H, Hooijberg E, et al. Differential effects of Notch ligands Delta-1 and Jagged-1 in human lymphoid differentiation. J Exp Med. 2001;194:991-1002.

268. Pui JC, Allman D, Xu L, et al. Notch1 expression in early lymphopoiesis influences B versus T lineage determination. Immunity. 1999;11:299-308.

269. Radtke F, Wilson A, Stark G, et al. Deficient T cell fate specification in mice with an induced inactivation of Notch1. Immunity. 1999;10:547-558.

270. Deftos ML, Huang E, Ojala EW, et al. Notch1 signaling promotes the maturation of CD4 and CD8 SP thymocytes. Immunity. 2000;13:73-84.

271. Fowlkes BJ, Robey EA. A reassessment of the effect of activated Notch1 on CD4 and CD8 T cell development. J Immunol. 2002;169:1817-1821.

272. Izon DJ, Punt JA, Xu L, et al. Notch1 regulates maturation of CD4+ and CD8+ thymocytes by modulating TCR signal strength. Immunity. 2001;14:253-264.

273. Robey E, Chang D, Itano A, et al. An activated form of Notch influences the choice between CD4 and CD8 T cell lineages. Cell. 1996;87:483-492.

274. Brou C, Logeat F, Gupta N, et al. A novel proteolytic cleavage involved in Notch signaling: the role of the disintegrin-metalloprotease TACE. Mol Cell. 2000;5:207-216.

275. Mumm JS, Schroeter EH, Saxena MT, et al. A ligand-induced extracellular cleavage regulates gamma-secretase-like proteolytic activation of Notch1. Mol Cell. 2000;5:197-206.

276. Ellisen LW, Bird J, West DC, et al. TAN-1, the human homolog of the Drosophila notch gene, is broken by chromosomal translocations in T lymphoblastic neoplasms. Cell. 1991;66:649-661.

277. Weng AP, Ferrando AA, Lee W, et al. Activating mutations of NOTCH1 in human T cell acute lymphoblastic leukemia. Science. 2004;306:269-271.

278. Palomero T, Lim WK, Odom DT, et al. NOTCH1 directly regulates c-MYC and activates a feed-forward-loop transcriptional network promoting leukemic cell growth. Proc Natl Acad Sci U S A. 2006;103:18261-18266.

279. Sharma VM, Calvo JA, Draheim KM, et al. Notch1 contributes to mouse T-cell leukemia by directly inducing the expression of c-myc. Mol Cell Biol. 2006;26:8022-8031.

280. Weng AP, Millholland JM, Yashiro-Ohtani Y, et al. c-Myc is an important direct target of Notch1 in T-cell acute lymphoblastic leukemia/lymphoma. Genes Dev. 2006;20:2096-2109.

281. Thompson BJ, Buonamici S, Sulis ML, et al. The SCFFBW7 ubiquitin ligase complex as a tumor suppressor in T cell leukemia. J Exp Med. 2007;204:1825-1835.

282. Minella AC, Clurman BE. Mechanisms of tumor suppression by the SCF(Fbw7). Cell Cycle. 2005;4:1356-1359.

283. Finger LR, Harvey RC, Moore RC, et al. A common mechanism of chromosomal translocation in T- and B-cell neoplasia. Science. 1986;234:982-985.

284. Shima EA, Le Beau MM, McKeithan TW, et al. Gene encoding the alpha chain of the T-cell receptor is moved immediately downstream of c-myc in a chromosomal 8;14 translocation in a cell line from a human T-cell leukemia. Proc Natl Acad Sci U S A. 1986;83:3439-3443.

285. Ferrando AA, Neuberg DS, Staunton J, et al. Gene expression signatures define novel oncogenic pathways in T cell acute lymphoblastic leukemia. Cancer Cell. 2002;1:75-87.

286. Chen Q, Cheng JT, Tasi LH, et al. The tal gene undergoes chromosome translocation in T cell leukemia and potentially encodes a helix-loop-helix protein. EMBO J. 1990;9:415-424.

287. Hsu HL, Cheng JT, Chen Q, Baer R. Enhancer-binding activity of the tal-1 oncoprotein in association with the E47/E12 helix-loop-helix proteins. Mol Cell Biol. 1991;11:3037-3042.

288. Hsu HL, Wadman I, Tsan JT, Baer R. Positive and negative transcriptional control by the TAL1 helix-loop-helix protein. Proc Natl Acad Sci U S A. 1994;91:5947-5951.

289. Bain G, Engel I, Robanus Maandag EC, et al. E2A deficiency leads to abnormalities in alphabeta T-cell development and to rapid development of T-cell lymphomas. Mol Cell Biol. 1997;17:4782-4791.

290. Yan W, Young AZ, Soares VC, et al. High incidence of T-cell tumors in E2A-null mice and E2A/Id1 double-knockout mice. Mol Cell Biol. 1997;17:7317-7327.

291. Ono Y, Fukuhara N, Yoshie O. Transcriptional activity of TAL1 in T cell acute lymphoblastic leukemia (T-ALL) requires RBTN1 or -2 and induces TALLA1, a highly specific tumor marker of T-ALL. J Biol Chem. 1997;272:4576-4581.

292. Ono Y, Fukuhara N, Yoshie O. TAL1 and LIM-only proteins synergistically induce retinaldehyde dehydrogenase 2 expression in T-cell acute lymphoblastic leukemia by acting as cofactors for GATA3. Mol Cell Biol. 1998;18:6939-6950.

293. Larson RC, Lavenir I, Larson TA, et al. Protein dimerization between Lmo2 (Rbtn2) and Tal1 alters thymocyte development and potentiates T cell tumorigenesis in transgenic mice. EMBO J. 1996;15:1021-1027.

294. Mark M, Rijli FM, Chambon P. Homeobox genes in embryogenesis and pathogenesis. Pediatr Res. 1997;42:421-429.

295. Dear TN, Sanchez-Garcia I, Rabbitts TH. The HOX11 gene encodes a DNA-binding nuclear transcription factor belonging to a distinct family of homeobox genes. Proc Natl Acad Sci U S A. 1993;90:4431-4435.

296. Dube ID, Kamel-Reid S, Yuan CC, et al. A novel human homeobox gene lies at the chromosome 10 breakpoint in lymphoid neoplasias with chromosomal translocation t(10;14). Blood. 1991;78:2996-3003.

297. Lu M, Gong ZY, Shen WF, Ho AD. The tcl-3 proto-oncogene altered by chromosomal translocation in T-cell leukemia codes for a homeobox protein. EMBO J. 1991;10:2905-2910.

298. Ferrando AA, Look AT. Gene expression profiling in T-cell acute lymphoblastic leukemia. Semin Hematol. 2003;40:274-280.

299. Kees UR, Heerema NA, Kumar R, et al. Expression of HOX11 in childhood T-lineage acute lymphoblastic leukaemia can occur in the absence of cytogenetic aberration at 10q24: a study from the Children's Cancer Group (CCG). Leukemia. 2003;17:887-893.

300. Berger R, Dastugue N, Busson M, et al. t(5;14)/HOX11L2-positive T-cell acute lymphoblastic leukemia. A collaborative study of the Groupe Francais de Cytogenetique Hematologique (GFCH). Leukemia. 2003;17:1851-1857.

301. Roberts CW, Shutter JR, Korsmeyer SJ. Hox11 controls the genesis of the spleen. Nature. 1994;368:747-749.

302. Dear TN, Colledge WH, Carlton MB, et al. The Hox11 gene is essential for cell survival during spleen development. Development. 1995;121:2909-2915.

303. Kawabe T, Muslin AJ, Korsmeyer SJ. HOX11 interacts with protein phosphatases PP2A and PP1 and disrupts a G2/M cell-cycle checkpoint. Nature. 1997;385:454-458.

304. MacLeod RA, Nagel S, Kaufmann M, et al. Activation of HOX11L2 by juxtaposition with 3'-BCL11B in an acute lymphoblastic leukemia cell line (HPB-ALL) with t(5;14)(q35;q32.2). Genes Chromosomes Cancer. 2003;37:84-91.

305. Mauvieux L, Leymarie V, Helias C, et al. High incidence of Hox11L2 expression in children with T-ALL. Leukemia. 2002;16:2417-2422.

306. Ballerini P, Blaise A, Busson-Le Coniat M, et al. HOX11L2 expression defines a clinical subtype of pediatric T-cell ALL associated with poor prognosis. Blood. 2002;100:991-997.

307. Shirasawa S, Arata A, Onimaru H, et al. Rnx deficiency results in congenital central hypoventilation. Nat Genet. 2000;24:287-290.

308. Graux C, Cools J, Melotte C, et al. Fusion of NUP214 to ABL1 on amplified episomes in T-cell acute lymphoblastic leukemia. Nat Genet. 2004;36:1084-1089.

309. Cave H, Suciu S, Preudhomme C, et al. Clinical significance of HOX11L2 expression linked to t(5;14)(q35;q32), of HOX11 expression, and of SIL-TAL fusion in childhood T-cell malignancies: results of EORTC studies 58881 and 58951. Blood. 2004;103:442-450.

310. Asnafi V, Buzyn A, Thomas X, et al. Impact of TCR status and genotype on outcome in adult T acute lymphoblastic leukemia: a LALA-94 study. Blood. 2005;105:3072-3078.

311. Krumlauf R. Hox genes in vertebrate development. Cell. 1994;78:191-201.

312. Thorsteinsdottir U, Mamo A, Kroon E, et al. Overexpression of the myeloid leukemia-associated Hoxa9 gene in bone marrow cells induces stem cell expansion. Blood. 2002;99:121-129.

313. Kroon E, Krosl J, Thorsteinsdottir U, et al. Hoxa9 transforms primary bone marrow cells through specific collaboration with Meis1a but not Pbx1b. EMBO J. 1998;17:3714-3725.

314. Hess JL, Bittner CB, Zeisig DT, et al. c-Myb is an essential downstream target for homeobox-mediated transformation of hematopoietic cells. Blood. 2006;108:297-304.

315. Dreyling MH, Martinez-Climent JA, Zheng M, et al. The t(10;11)(p13;q14) in the U937 cell line results in the fusion of the AF10 gene and CALM, encoding a new member of the AP-3 clathrin assembly protein family. Proc Natl Acad Sci U S A. 1996;93:4804-4809.

316. Dreyling MH, Schrader K, Fonatsch C, et al. MLL and CALM are fused to AF10 in morphologically distinct subsets of acute leukemia with translocation t(10;11): both rearrangements are associated with a poor prognosis. Blood. 1998;91:4662-4667.

317. Tebar F, Bohlander SK, Sorkin A. Clathrin assembly lymphoid myeloid leukemia (CALM) protein: localization in endocytic-coated pits, interactions with clathrin, and the impact of overexpression on clathrin-mediated traffic. Mol Biol Cell. 1999;10:2687-2702.

318. Chaplin T, Bernard O, Beverloo HB, et al. The t(10;11) translocation in acute myeloid leukemia (M5) consistently fuses the leucine zipper motif of AF10 onto the HRX gene. Blood. 1995;86:2073-2076.

319. Chaplin T, Ayton P, Bernard OA, et al. A novel class of zinc finger/leucine zipper genes identified from the molecular cloning of the t(10;11) translocation in acute leukemia. Blood. 1995;85:1435-1441.

320. Asnafi V, Radford-Weiss I, Dastugue N, et al. CALM-AF10 is a common fusion transcript in T-cell ALL and is specific to the TCRgammadelta lineage. Blood. 2003;102:1000-1006.

321. Asnafi V, Beldjord K, Libura M, et al. Age-related phenotypic and oncogenic differences in T-cell acute lymphoblastic leukemias may reflect thymic atrophy. Blood. 2004;104:4173-4180.

322. Dik WA, Brahim W, Braun C, et al. CALM-AF10+ T-cell ALL expression profiles are characterized by overexpression of HOXA and BMI1 oncogenes. Leukemia. 2005;19:1948-1957.

323. Armstrong SA, Staunton JE, Silverman LB, et al. MLL translocations specify a distinct gene expression profile that distinguishes a unique leukemia. Nat Genet. 2002;30:41-47.

324. Ferrando AA, Armstrong SA, Neuberg DS, et al. Gene expression signatures in MLL-rearranged T-lineage and B-precursor acute leukemias: dominance of HOX dysregulation. Blood. 2003; 102:262-268.

325. Lacronique V, Boureux A, Monni R, et al. Transforming properties of chimeric TEL-JAK proteins in Ba/F3 cells. Blood. 2000;95:2076-2083.

326. Carron C, Cormier F, Janin A, et al. TEL-JAK2 transgenic mice develop T-cell leukemia. Blood. 2000;95:3891-3899.

327. Tycko B, Smith SD, Sklar J. Chromosomal translocations joining LCK and TCRB loci in human T cell leukemia. J Exp Med. 1991;174:867-873.

328. Ciofani M, Zuniga-Pflucker JC. A survival guide to early T cell development. Immunol Res. 2006;34:117-132.

329. Nakao M, Yokota S, Kaneko H, et al. Alterations of CDKN2 gene structure in childhood acute lymphoblastic leukemia: mutations of CDKN2 are observed preferentially in T lineage. Leukemia. 1996;10:249-254.

330. Cayuela JM, Gardie B, Sigaux F. Disruption of the multiple tumor suppressor gene MTS1/p16(INK4a)/CDKN2 by illegitimate V(D)J recombinase activity in T-cell acute lymphoblastic leukemias. Blood. 1997;90:3720-3726.

331. Burkitt D. A sarcoma involving the jaws in African children. Br J Surg. 1958;46:218-223.

332. Epstein MA, Achong BG, Barr YM. Virus particles in cultured lymphoblasts from Burkitt's lymphoma. Lancet. 1964;15:702-703.

333. Tanner J, Weis J, Fearon D, et al. Epstein-Barr virus gp350/220 binding to the B lymphocyte C3d receptor mediates adsorption, capping, and endocytosis. Cell. 1987;50:203-213.

334. de-The G. Is Burkitt's lymphoma related to perinatal infection by Epstein-Barr virus? Lancet. 1977;1:335-338.

335. Caselli D, Klersy C, de Martino M, et al. Human immunodeficiency virus-related cancer in children: incidence and treatment outcome—report of the Italian Register. J Clin Oncol. 2000;18:3854-3861.

336. Cattoretti G, Chang CC, Cechova K, et al. BCL-6 protein is expressed in germinal-center B cells. Blood. 1995;86:45-53.

337. Berger R, Bernheim A. Cytogenetic studies on Burkitt's lymphoma-leukemia. Cancer Genet Cytogenet. 1982;7:231-244.

338. Pelicci PG, Knowles DM, Magrath I, la-Favera R. Chromosomal breakpoints and structural alterations of the c-myc locus differ in endemic and sporadic forms of Burkitt lymphoma. Proc Natl Acad Sci U S A. 1986;83:2984-2988.

339. Shiramizu B, Barriga F, Neequaye J, et al. Patterns of chromosomal breakpoint locations in Burkitt's lymphoma: relevance to geography and Epstein-Barr virus association. Blood. 1991;77:1516-1526.

340. Gutierrez MI, Bhatia K, Barriga F, et al. Molecular epidemiology of Burkitt's lymphoma from South America: differences in breakpoint location and Epstein-Barr virus association from tumors in other world regions. Blood. 1991;79:3261-3266.

341. Bellan C, Lazzi S, Hummel M, et al. Immunoglobulin gene analysis reveals 2 distinct cells of origin for EBV-positive and EBV-negative Burkitt lymphomas. Blood. 2005;106:1031-1036.

342. Dave SS, Fu K, Wright GW, et al. Molecular diagnosis of Burkitt's lymphoma. N Engl J Med. 2006;354:2431-2442.

343. Hummel M, Bentink S, Berger H, et al. A biologic definition of Burkitt's lymphoma from transcriptional and genomic profiling. N Engl J Med. 2006;354:2419-2430.

344. ar-Rushdi A, Nishikura K, Erikson J, et al. Differential expression of the translocated and the untranslocated c-myc oncogene in Burkitt lymphoma. Science. 1983;222:390-393.

345. Hayday AC, Gillies SD, Saito H, et al. Activation of a translocated human c-myc gene by an enhancer in the immunoglobulin heavy-chain locus. Nature. 1984;307:334-340.

346. Neri A, Barriga F, Knowles DM, et al. Different regions of the immunoglobulin heavy-chain locus are involved in chromosomal translocations in distinct pathogenetic forms of Burkitt lymphoma. Proc Natl Acad Sci U S A. 1988;85:2748-2752.

347. Joos S, Falk MH, Lichter P, et al. Variable breakpoints in Burkitt's lymphoma cells with chromosomal t(8;14) translocation separate c-myc and the IgH locus up to several hundred kb. Hum Mol Genet. 1992;1:625-632.

348. Magrath I. The pathogenesis of Burkitt's lymphoma. Adv Cancer Res. 1990;55:133-270.

349. Gerbitz A, Mautner J, Geltinger C, et al. Deregulation of the proto-oncogene c-myc through t(8;22) translocation in Burkitt's lymphoma. Oncogene. 1999;18:1745-1753.

350. Ohmori H, Hikida M. Expression and function of recombination activating genes in mature B cells. Crit Rev Immunol. 1998;18: 221-235.

351. Bentley DL, Groudine M. A block to elongation is largely responsible for decreased transcription of c-myc in differentiated HL60 cells. Nature. 1986;321:702-706.

352. Zajac-Kaye M, Levens D. Phosphorylation-dependent binding of a 138-kDa myc intron factor to a regulatory element in the first intron of the c-myc gene. J Biol Chem. 1990;265:4547-4551.

353. Cesarman E, Dalla-Favera R, Bentley D, Groudine M. Mutations in the first exon are associated with altered transcription of c-myc in Burkitt lymphoma. Science. 1987;238:1272-1275.

354. Zajac-Kaye M, Gelmann EP, Levens D. A point mutation in the c-myc locus of a Burkitt's lymphoma abolishes binding of a nuclear protein. Science. 1988;240:1776-1780.

355. Flinn EM, Busch CM, Wright AP. myc boxes, which are conserved in myc family proteins, are signals for protein degradation via the proteasome. Mol Cell Biol. 1998;18:5961-5969.

356. Salghetti SE, Kim SY, Tansey WP. Destruction of Myc by ubiquitin-mediated proteolysis: cancer-associated and transforming mutations stabilize Myc. EMBO J. 1999;18:717-726.

357. Bahram F, von der Lehr N, Cetinkaya C, Larsson LG. c-Myc hot spot mutations in lymphomas result in inefficient ubiquitination and decreased proteasome-mediated turnover. Blood. 2000;95:2104-2110.

358. Gregory MA, Hann SR. c-Myc proteolysis by the ubiquitin-proteasome pathway: stabilization of c-Myc in Burkitt's lymphoma cells. Mol Cell Biol. 2000;20:2423-2435.

359. Gaidano G, Ballerini P, Gong JZ, et al. p53 mutations in human lymphoid malignancies: association with Burkitt's lymphoma and chronic lymphocytic leukemia. Proc Natl Acad Sci U S A. 1991; 88:5413-5417.

360. Ichikawa A, Hotta T, Saito H. Mutations of the p53 gene in B-cell lymphoma. Leuk Lymphoma. 1993;11:21-25.

361. Corn PG, Kuerbitz SJ, van Noesel MM, et al. Transcriptional silencing of the p73 gene in acute lymphoblastic leukemia and Burkitt's lymphoma is associated with 5' CpG island methylation. Cancer Res. 1999;59:3352-3356.

362. Galaktionov K, Chen X, Beach D. Cdc25 cell-cycle phosphatase as a target of c-myc. Nature. 1996;382:511-517.

363. Hermeking H, Eick D. Mediation of c-Myc-induced apoptosis by p53. Science. 1994;265:2091-2093.

364. Shim H, Dolde C, Lewis BC, et al. c-Myc transactivation of LDH-A: implications for tumor metabolism and growth. Proc Natl Acad Sci U S A. 1997;94:6658-6663.

365. Capello D, Carbone A, Pastore C, et al. Point mutations of the BCL-6 gene in Burkitt's lymphoma. Br J Haematol. 1997;99: 168-170.

366. Capello D, Vitolo U, Pasqualucci L, et al. Distribution and pattern of BCL-6 mutations throughout the spectrum of B-cell neoplasia. Blood. 2000;95:651-659.

367. Raab-Traub N, Flynn K. The structure of the termini of the Epstein-Barr virus as a marker of clonal cellular proliferation. Cell. 1986;47:883-889.

368. Wilson JB, Bell JL, Levine AJ. Expression of Epstein-Barr virus nuclear antigen-1 induces B cell neoplasia in transgenic mice. EMBO J. 1996;15:3117-3126.

369. Swaminathan S, Tomkinson B, Kieff E. Recombinant Epstein-Barr virus with small RNA (EBER) genes deleted transforms

370. Fries KL, Sculley TB, Webster-Cyriaque J, et al. Identification of a novel protein encoded by the BamHI A region of the Epstein-Barr virus. J Virol. 1997;71:2765-2771.

371. Kramer MH, Hermans J, Wijburg E, et al. Clinical relevance of BCL2, BCL6, and MYC rearrangements in diffuse large B-cell lymphoma. Blood. 1998;92:3152-3162.

372. Alizadeh AA, Eisen MB, Davis RE, et al. Distinct types of diffuse large B-cell lymphoma identified by gene expression profiling. Nature. 2000;403:503-511.

373. Hans CP, Weisenburger DD, Greiner TC, et al. Confirmation of the molecular classification of diffuse large B-cell lymphoma by immunohistochemistry using a tissue microarray. Blood. 2004; 103:275-282.

374. Oschlies I, Klapper W, Zimmermann M, et al. Diffuse large B-cell lymphoma in pediatric patients belongs predominantly to the germinal-center type B-cell lymphomas: a clinicopathologic analysis of cases included in the German BFM (Berlin-Frankfurt-Munster) Multicenter Trial. Blood. 2006;107:4047-4052.

375. Delsol G, Lamant L, Mariame B, et al. A new subtype of large B-cell lymphoma expressing the ALK kinase and lacking the 2; 5 translocation. Blood. 1997;89:1483-1490.

376. Onciu M, Behm FG, Downing JR, et al. ALK-positive plasmablastic B-cell lymphoma with expression of the NPM-ALK fusion transcript: report of 2 cases. Blood. 2003;102:2642-2644.

377. Addis BJ, Isaacson PG. Large cell lymphoma of the mediastinum: a B-cell tumour of probable thymic origin. Histopathology. 1986;10:379-390.

378. Tsang P, Cesarman E, Chadburn A, et al. Molecular characterization of primary mediastinal B cell lymphoma. Am J Pathol. 1996;148:2017-2025.

379. Alonso MA, Weissman SM. cDNA cloning and sequence of MAL, a hydrophobic protein associated with human T-cell differentiation. Proc Natl Acad Sci U S A. 1987;84:1997-2001.

380. Copie-Bergman C, Gaulard P, Maouche-Chretien L, et al. The MAL gene is expressed in primary mediastinal large B-cell lymphoma. Blood. 1999;94:3567-3575.

381. Lorsbach RB, Shay-Seymore D, Moore J, et al. Clinicopathologic analysis of follicular lymphoma occurring in children. Blood. 2002;99:1959-1964.

382. Oschlies I, Burkhardt B, Krams M, et al. Pediatric follicular lymphoma: clinical, histopathological and genetic data of 20 cases and a comparison with pediatric diffuse large B-cell lymphoma. Pediatr Blood Cancer. 2007;46:842-843.

383. Pileri S, Falini B, Delsol G, et al. Lymphohistiocytic T-cell lymphoma (anaplastic large cell lymphoma CD30+/Ki-1 + with a high content of reactive histiocytes). Histopathology. 1990;16: 383-391.

384. Kinney MC, Collins RD, Greer JP, et al. A small-cell-predominant variant of primary Ki-1 (CD30)+ T-cell lymphoma. Am J Surg Pathol. 1993;17:859-868.

385. Benharroch D, Meguerian-Bedoyan Z, Lamant L, et al. ALK-positive lymphoma: a single disease with a broad spectrum of morphology. Blood. 1998;91:2076-2084.

386. Fischer P, Nacheva E, Mason DY, et al. A Ki-1 (CD30)-positive human cell line (Karpas 299) established from a high-grade non-Hodgkin's lymphoma, showing a 2;5 translocation and rearrangement of the T-cell receptor beta-chain gene. Blood. 1988;72: 234-240.

387. Kaneko Y, Frizzera G, Edamura S, et al. A novel translocation, t(2;5)(p23;q35), in childhood phagocytic large T-cell lymphoma mimicking malignant histiocytosis. Blood. 1989;73:806-813.

388. Le Beau MM, Bitter MA, Larson RA, et al. The t(2;5)(p23;q35): a recurring chromosomal abnormality in Ki-1-positive anaplastic large cell lymphoma. Leukemia. 1989;3:866-870.

lymphocytes and replicates in vitro. Proc Natl Acad Sci U S A. 1991;88:1546-1550.

389. Morris SW, Kirstein MN, Valentine MB, et al. Fusion of a kinase gene, ALK, to a nucleolar protein gene, NPM, in non-Hodgkin's lymphoma. Science. 1994;263:1281-1284.

390. Pulford K, Lamant L, Morris SW, et al. Detection of anaplastic lymphoma kinase (ALK) and nucleolar protein nucleophosmin (NPM)-ALK proteins in normal and neoplastic cells with the monoclonal antibody ALK1. Blood. 1997;89:1394-1404.

391. Pulford K, Falini B, Banham AH, et al. Immune response to the ALK oncogenic tyrosine kinase in patients with anaplastic large-cell lymphoma. Blood. 2000;96:1605-1607.

392. Bischof D, Pulford K, Mason DY, Morris SW. Role of the nucleophosmin (NPM) portion of the non-Hodgkin's lymphoma-associated NPM-anaplastic lymphoma kinase fusion protein in oncogenesis. Mol Cell Biol. 1997;17:2312-2325.

393. Brugieres L, Deley MC, Pacquement H, et al. CD30(+) anaplastic large-cell lymphoma in children: analysis of 82 patients enrolled in two consecutive studies of the French Society of Pediatric Oncology. Blood. 1998;92:3591-3598.

394. Foss HD, Anagnostopoulos I, Araujo I, et al. Anaplastic large-cell lymphomas of T-cell and null-cell phenotype express cytotoxic molecules. Blood. 1996;88:4005-4011.

395. Krenacs L, Wellmann A, Sorbara L, et al. Cytotoxic cell antigen expression in anaplastic large cell lymphomas of T- and null-cell type and Hodgkin's disease: evidence for distinct cellular origin. Blood. 1997;89:980-989.

396. Onciu M, Behm FG, Raimondi SC, et al. ALK-positive anaplastic large cell lymphoma with leukemic peripheral blood involvement is a clinicopathologic entity with an unfavorable prognosis. Report of three cases and review of the literature. Am J Clin Pathol. 2003;120:617-625.

397. Felgar RE, Salhany KE, Macon WR, et al. The expression of TIA-1+ cytolytic-type granules and other cytolytic lymphocyte-associated markers in CD30+ anaplastic large cell lymphomas (ALCL): correlation with morphology, immunophenotype, ultrastructure, and clinical features. Hum. Pathol. 1999;30:228-236.

398. Kadin ME, Sako D, Berliner N, et al. Childhood Ki-1 lymphoma presenting with skin lesions and peripheral lymphadenopathy. Blood. 1986;68:1042-1049.

399. Reiter A, Zimmermann W, Zimmermann M, et al. The role of initial laparotomy and second-look surgery in the treatment of abdominal B-cell non-Hodgkin's lymphoma of childhood. A report of the BFM Group. Eur J Pediatr Surg. 1994;4:74-81.

400. Davis TH, Morton CC, Miller-Cassman R, et al. Hodgkin's disease, lymphomatoid papulosis, and cutaneous T-cell lymphoma derived from a common T-cell clone. N Engl J Med. 1992;326:1115-1122.

401. Nijsten T, Curiel-Lewandrowski C, Kadin ME. Lymphomatoid papulosis in children: a retrospective cohort study of 35 cases. Arch.Dermatol. 2004;140:306-312.

402. Amin HM, Lai R. Pathobiology of ALK+ anaplastic large-cell lymphoma. Blood. 2007;110:2259-2267.

403. Pulford K, Morris SW, Turturro F. Anaplastic lymphoma kinase proteins in growth control and cancer. J Cell Physiol. 2004;199: 330-358.

404. Duyster J, Bai RY, Morris SW. Translocations involving anaplastic lymphoma kinase (ALK). Oncogene. 2001;20:5623-5637.

405. Wasik MA. Expression of anaplastic lymphoma kinase in non-Hodgkin's lymphomas and other malignant neoplasms. Biological, diagnostic, and clinical implications. Am J Clin Pathol. 2002;118(Suppl):S81-S92.

406. Bullrich F, Morris SW, Hummel M, et al. Nucleophosmin (NPM) gene rearrangements in Ki-1-positive lymphomas. Cancer Res. 1994;54:2873-2877.

407. Borer RA, Lehner CF, Eppenberger HM, Nigg EA. Major nucleolar proteins shuttle between nucleus and cytoplasm. Cell. 1989;56:379-390.

408. Fujimoto J, Shiota M, Iwahara T, et al. Characterization of the transforming activity of p80, a hyperphosphorylated protein in a Ki-1 lymphoma cell line with chromosomal translocation t(2;5). Proc Natl Acad Sci U S A. 1996;93(9):4181-4186.

409. Kuefer MU, Look AT, Pulford K, et al. Retrovirus-mediated gene transfer of NPM-ALK causes lymphoid malignancy in mice. Blood. 1997;90:2901-2910.

410. Medeiros LJ, Elenitoba-Johnson KS. Anaplastic large cell lymphoma. Am J Clin Pathol. 2007;127:707-722.

411. Falini B, Pulford K, Pucciarini A, et al. Lymphomas expressing ALK fusion protein(s) other than NPM-ALK. Blood. 1999;94:3509-3515.

412. Galkin AV, Melnick JS, Kim S, et al. Identification of NVP-TAE684, a potent, selective, and efficacious inhibitor of NPM-ALK. Proc Natl Acad Sci U S A. 2007;104:270-275.

413. Aoki M, Niimi Y, Takezaki S, Azuma A, et al. CD30+ lympho-proliferative disorder: primary cutaneous anaplastic large cell lymphoma followed by lymphomatoid papulosis. Br J Dermatol. 2001;145:123-126.

414. Burkitt D, O'Conor GT. Malignant lymphoma in African children. I. A clinical syndrome. Cancer. 1961;14:258-269.

415. van den Bosch CA, Hills M, Kazembe P, et al. Time-space case clusters of Burkitt's lymphoma in Malawi. Leukemia. 1993;7:1875-1878.

416. van den Bosch CA. Is endemic Burkitt's lymphoma an alliance between three infections and a tumour promoter? Lancet Oncol. 2004;5:738-746.

417. Sandlund JT, Fonseca T, Leimig T, et al. Predominance and characteristics of Burkitt's lymphoma among children with non-Hodgkin lymphoma in northeastern Brazil. Leukemia. 1997;11: 743-746.

418. Parkin DM. Epidemiology of cancer: global patterns and trends. Toxicol Lett. 1998;102-103, 227-234.

419. Izarzugaza MI, Steliarova-Foucher E, Martos MC, Zivkovic S. Non-Hodgkin's lymphoma incidence and survival in European children and adolescents (1978-1997): report from the Automated Childhood Cancer Information System project. Eur J Cancer. 2006;42:2050-2063.

420. Blair V, Birch JM. Patterns and temporal trends in the incidence of malignant disease in children: I. Leukaemia and lymphoma. Eur J Cancer. 1994;30A:1490-1498.

421. McNally RJ, Cairns DP, Eden OB, et al. Examination of temporal trends in the incidence of childhood leukaemias and lymphomas provides aetiological clues. Leukemia. 2001;15:1612-1618.

422. Clavel J, Goubin A, Auclerc MF, et al. Incidence of childhood leukaemia and non-Hodgkin's lymphoma in France: National Registry of Childhood Leukaemia and Lymphoma, 1990-1999. Eur J Cancer Prev. 2004;13:97-103.

423. Kaatsch P, Blettner M, Spix C, Jurgens H. Follow up of long-term survivors after childhood cancer in Germany. Klin Padiatr. 2005;217:169-175.

424. Iscovich J, Parkin DM. Risk of cancer in migrants and their descendants in Israel: I. Leukaemias and lymphomas. Int J Cancer. 1997;70:649-653.

425. Wang SS, Slager SL, Brennan P, et al. Family history of hematopoietic malignancies and risk of non-Hodgkin lymphoma (NHL): a pooled analysis of 10 211 cases and 11 905 controls from the International Lymphoma Epidemiology Consortium (InterLymph). Blood. 2007;109:3479-3488.

426. Filipovich AH, Mathur A, Kamat D, Shapiro RS. Primary immunodeficiencies: genetic risk factors for lymphoma. Cancer Res. 1992;52:5465s-5467s.

427. Swift M, Morrell D, Massey RB, Chase CL. Incidence of cancer in 161 families affected by ataxia-telangiectasia. N Engl J Med. 1991;325:1831-1836.

428. Peterson RD, Funkhouser JD. Speculations on ataxia-telangiectasia: defective regulation of the immunoglobulin gene superfamily. Immunol Today. 1989;10:313-314.

429. Taylor AM, Metcalfe JA, Thick J, Mak YF. Leukemia and lymphoma in ataxia telangiectasia. Blood. 1996;87:423-438.

430. Seidemann K, Henze G, Beck JD, et al. Non-Hodgkin's lymphoma in pediatric patients with chromosomal breakage syndromes (AT and NBS): experience from the BFM trials. Ann Oncol. 2000;11(Suppl 1):141-145.

431. Gumy-Pause F, Wacker P, Sappino AP. ATM gene and lymphoid malignancies. Leukemia. 2004;18:238-242.

432. Gumy-Pause F, Wacker P, Maillet P, et al. ATM alterations in childhood non-Hodgkin lymphoma. Cancer Genet Cytogenet. 2006;166:101-111.

433. Stanulla M, Stumm M, Dieckvoss BO, et al. No evidence for a major role of heterozygous deletion 657del5 within the NBS1 gene in the pathogenesis of non-Hodgkin's lymphoma of childhood and adolescence. Br J Haematol. 2000;109:117-120.

434. Stumm M, von Ruskowsky A, Siebert R, et al. No evidence for deletions of the NBS1 gene in lymphomas. Cancer Genet Cytogenet. 2001;126:60-62.

435. Chiu BC, Dave BJ, Blair A, et al. Agricultural pesticide use and risk of t(14;18)-defined subtypes of non-Hodgkin lymphoma. Blood. 2006;108:1363-1369.

436. Meinert R, Schuz J, Kaletsch U, et al. Leukemia and non-Hodgkin's lymphoma in childhood and exposure to pesticides: results of a register-based case-control study in Germany. Am J Epidemiol. 2000;151:639-646.

437. Bracci PM, Dalvi TB, Holly EA. Residential history, family characteristics and non-Hodgkin lymphoma, a population-based case-control study in the San Francisco Bay Area. Cancer Epidemiol Biomarkers Prev. 2006;15:1287-1294.

438. Grulich AE, Vajdic CM, Kaldor JM, et al. Birth order, atopy, and risk of non-Hodgkin lymphoma. J Natl Cancer Inst. 2005;97:587-594.

439. Grulich AE, Vajdic CM. The epidemiology of non-Hodgkin lymphoma. Pathology. 2005;37:409-419.

440. Adami J, Glimelius B, Cnattingius S, et al. Maternal and perinatal factors associated with non-Hodgkin's lymphoma among children. Int J Cancer. 1996;65:774-777.

441. Ross JA, Severson RK, Swensen AR, et al. Seasonal variations in the diagnosis of childhood cancer in the United States. Br J Cancer. 1999;81:549-553.

442. Jurewicz J, Hanke W. Exposure to pesticides and childhood cancer risk: has there been any progress in epidemiological studies? Int J Occup Med Environ Health. 2006;19:152-169.

443. Kramarova E, Stiller CA. The international classification of childhood cancer. Int J Cancer. 1996;68:759-765.

444. Clarke CA, Undurraga DM, Harasty PJ, et al. Changes in cancer registry coding for lymphoma subtypes: reliability over time and relevance for surveillance and study. Cancer Epidemiol Biomarkers Prev. 2006;15:630-638.

445. Sandlund JT, Downing JR, Crist WM. Non-Hodgkin's lymphoma in childhood. N Engl J Med. 1996;334:1238-1248.

446. Stanulla M, Seidemann K, Schnakenberg E, et al. Methylenetetrahydrofolate reductase (MTHFR) 677C>T polymorphism and risk of pediatric non-Hodgkin lymphoma in a German study population. Blood. 2005;105:906-907.

447. Kracht T, Schrappe M, Strehl S, et al. NQO1 C609T polymorphism in distinct entities of pediatric hematologic neoplasms. Haematologica. 2004;89:1492-1497.

448. Joab I. Epstein-Barr virus and Burkitt's lymphoma. Med Trop (Mars). 1999;59:499-502.

449. Dalldorf G, Barnhart FE. Childhood leukemia, malaria and Burkitt's lymphoma. N Engl J Med. 1972;286:1216.

450. Burkitt DP. Etiology of Burkitt's lymphoma—an alternative hypothesis to a vectored virus. J Natl Cancer Inst. 1969;42:19-28.

451. Greenwood BM, Oduloju AJ, Platts-Mills TA. Partial characterization of a malaria mitogen. Trans R Soc Trop Med Hyg. 1979;73:178-182.

452. Lam KM, Syed N, Whittle H, Crawford DH. Circulating Epstein-Barr virus-carrying B cells in acute malaria. Lancet. 1991;337:876-878.

453. Moss DJ, Burrows SR, Castelino DJ, et al. A comparison of Epstein-Barr virus-specific T-cell immunity in malaria-endemic and -nonendemic regions of Papua New Guinea. Int J Cancer. 1983;31:727-732.

454. deThé G. Epstein-Barr virus and associated diseases. Course of Medical Virology, Institut Pasteur, 1995/1996. Ann Med Interne (Paris). 1997;148:357-366.

455. Davies JN, Elmes S, Hutt MS, et al. Cancer in an African community, 1897-1956. An analysis of the records of Mengo Hospital, Kampala, Uganda. BMJ. 1964;1:259-264.

456. Haddow AJ. Age incidence in Burkitt's lymphoma syndrome. East Afr Med J. 1964;41:1-6.

457. Dean AG, Williams EH, Attobua G, et al. Clinical events suggesting Herpes-simplex infection before onset of Burkitt's lymphoma. A case-control study in West Nile, Uganda. Lancet. 1973;2:1225-1228.

458. Osato T, Mizuno F, Imai S, et al. African Burkitt's lymphoma and an Epstein-Barr virus-enhancing plant Euphorbia tirucalli. Lancet. 1987;1:1257-1258.

459. Aya T, Kinoshita T, Imai S, et al. Chromosome translocation and c-MYC activation by Epstein-Barr virus and Euphorbia tirucalli in B lymphocytes. Lancet. 1991;337:1190.

460. Lee SH, Su IJ, Chen RL, et al. A pathologic study of childhood lymphoma in Taiwan with special reference to peripheral T-cell lymphoma and the association with Epstein-Barr viral infection. Cancer. 1991;68:1954-1962.

461. Serraino D, Pezzotti P, Dorrucci M, et al. Cancer incidence in a cohort of human immunodeficiency virus seroconverters. HIV Italian Seroconversion Study Group. Cancer. 1997;79:1004-1008.

462. Newton R, Ziegler J, Beral V, et al. A case-control study of human immunodeficiency virus infection and cancer in adults and children residing in Kampala, Uganda. Int J Cancer. 2001;92:622-627.

463. Granovsky MO, Mueller BU, Nicholson HS, et al. Cancer in human immunodeficiency virus-infected children: a case series from the Children's Cancer Group and the National Cancer Institute. J Clin Oncol. 1998;16:1729-1735.

464. Lin KH, Su IJ, Chen RL, et al. Peripheral T-cell lymphoma in childhood: a report of five cases in Taiwan. Med Pediatr Oncol. 1994;23:26-35.

465. Bittencourt AL, Primo J, de Oliveira MF. Manifestations of the human T-cell lymphotropic virus type I infection in childhood and adolescence. J Pediatr (Rio J). 2006;82:411-420.

466. Neth O, Seidemann K, Jansen P, et al. Precursor B-cell lymphoblastic lymphoma in childhood and adolescence: clinical features, treatment, and results in trials NHL-BFM 86 and 90. Med Pediatr Oncol. 2000;35:20-27.

467. Finn LS, Viswanatha DS, Belasco JB, et al. Primary follicular lymphoma of the testis in childhood. Cancer. 1999;85:1626-1635.

468. Sandlund JT, Pui CH, Santana VM, et al. Clinical features and treatment outcome for children with CD30+ large-cell non-Hodgkin's lymphoma. J Clin Oncol. 1994;12:895-898.

469. Seidemann K, Tiemann M, Schrappe M, et al. Short-pulse B-non-Hodgkin lymphoma-type chemotherapy is efficacious treatment for pediatric anaplastic large cell lymphoma: a report of the Berlin-Frankfurt-Munster Group Trial NHL-BFM 90. Blood. 2001;97:3699-3706.

470. Greer JP, Kinney MC, Collins RD, et al. Clinical features of 31 patients with Ki-1 anaplastic large-cell lymphoma. J Clin Oncol. 1991;9:539-547.

471. Tamiolakis D, Georgiou G, Prassopoulos P, et al. Neutrophil-rich anaplastic large cell lymphoma (NR-ALCL) mimicking

lymphadenitis: a study by fine-needle aspiration biopsy. Leuk Lymphoma. 2004;45:1309-1310.

472. Mann KP, Hall B, Kamino H, et al. Neutrophil-rich, Ki-1-positive anaplastic large-cell malignant lymphoma. Am J Surg Pathol. 1995;19:407-416.

473. Mira JA, Fernandez-Alonso J, Macias J, et al. Bone involvement and abscess formation by neutrophil-rich CD30+ anaplastic large-cell lymphoma mimicking skeletal infection in an AIDS patient. J Infect. 2003;47:73-76.

474. Arber D, Bilbao J, Bassion S. Large-cell anaplastic (Ki-1-positive) lymphoma complicated by disseminated intravascular coagulation. Arch Pathol Lab Med. 1991;115:188-192.

475. Agematsu K, Takeuchi S, Ichikawa M, et al. Spontaneous production of interleukin-6 by Ki-1-positive large-cell anaplastic lymphoma with extensive bone destruction. Blood. 1991;77:2299-2301.

476. Merz H, Fliedner A, Orscheschek K, et al. Cytokine expression in T-cell lymphomas and Hodgkin's disease. Its possible implication in autocrine or paracrine production as a potential basis for neoplastic growth. Am J Pathol. 1991;139:1173-1180.

477. Merz H, Houssiau FA, Orscheschek K, et al. Interleukin-9 expression in human malignant lymphomas: unique association with Hodgkin's disease and large cell anaplastic lymphoma. Blood. 1991;78:1311-1317.

478. Nishihira H, Tanaka Y, Kigasawa H, et al. Ki-1 lymphoma producing G-CSF. Br J Haematol. 1992;80:556-557.

479. Salzburg J, Burkhardt B, Zimmermann M, et al. Prevalence, clinical pattern, and outcome of CNS-involvement in childhood and adolescent non-Hodgkin lymphoma differ according to NHL subtype—a BFM group report. J Clin Oncol. 2007;25:3915-3922.

480. Reiter A, Schrappe M, Ludwig WD, et al. Favorable outcome of B-cell acute lymphoblastic leukemia in childhood: a report of three consecutive studies of the BFM group. Blood. 1992;80:2471-2478.

481. Abla O, Weitzman S. Primary central nervous system lymphoma in children. Neurosurg Focus. 2006;21:E8.

482. Abla O, Sandlund JT, Sung L, et al. A case series of pediatric primary central nervous system lymphoma: favorable outcome without cranial irradiation. Pediatr Blood Cancer. 2006;47:880-885.

483. Bekkenk MW, Geelen FA, van Voorst Vader PC, et al. Primary and secondary cutaneous CD30(+) lymphoproliferative disorders: a report from the Dutch Cutaneous Lymphoma Group on the long-term follow-up data of 219 patients and guidelines for diagnosis and treatment. Blood. 2000;95:3653-3661.

484. Fink-Puches R, Chott A, Ardigó M, et al. The spectrum of cutaneous lymphomas in patients less than 20 years of age. Pediatr Dermatol. 2004;21:525-533.

485. Wood GS, Hardman DL, Boni R, et al. Lack of the t(2;5) or other mutations resulting in expression of anaplastic lymphoma kinase catalytic domain in CD30+ primary cutaneous lymphoproliferative disorders and Hodgkin's disease. Blood. 1996;88:1765-1770.

486. Furman WL, Fitch S, Hustu HO, et al. Primary lymphoma of bone in children. J Clin Oncol. 1989;7:1275-1280.

487. Lones MA, Perkins SL, Sposto R, et al. Non-Hodgkin's lymphoma arising in bone in children and adolescents is associated with an excellent outcome: a Children's Cancer Group report. J Clin Oncol. 2002;20:2293-2301.

488. Haddy TB, Keenan AM, Jaffe ES, Magrath IT. Bone involvement in young patients with non-Hodgkin's lymphoma: efficacy of chemotherapy without local radiotherapy. Blood. 1988;72:1141-1147.

489. Suryanarayan K, Shuster JJ, Donaldson SS, et al. Treatment of localized primary non-Hodgkin's lymphoma of bone in children: a Pediatric Oncology Group study. J Clin Oncol. 1999;17:456-459.

490. Peterson MR, Noskoviak KJ, Newbury R. CD5-positive B-cell acute lymphoblastic leukemia. Pediatr Dev Pathol. 2007;10:41-45.

491. Heerema NA, Bernheim A, Lim MS, et al. State of the Art and Future Needs in Cytogenetic/Molecular Genetics/Arrays in childhood lymphoma: summary report of workshop at the First International Symposium on childhood and adolescent non-Hodgkin lymphoma, April 9, 2003, New York City, NY. Pediatr Blood Cancer. 2005;45:616-622.

492. Siebert R, Matthiesen P, Harder S, et al. Application of interphase fluorescence in situ hybridization for the detection of the Burkitt translocation t(8;14)(q24;q32) in B-cell lymphomas. Blood. 1998;91:984-990.

493. Buno I, Nava P, varez-Doval A, et al. Lymphoma associated chromosomal abnormalities can easily be detected by FISH on tissue imprints. An underused diagnostic alternative. J Clin Pathol. 2005;58:629-633.

494. van Krieken JH, Langerak AW, Macintyre EA, et al. Improved reliability of lymphoma diagnostics via PCR-based clonality testing: report of the BIOMED-2 Concerted Action BHM4-CT98-3936. Leukemia. 2007;21:201-206.

495. Safley AM, Buckley PJ, Creager AJ, et al. The value of fluorescence in situ hybridization and polymerase chain reaction in the diagnosis of B-cell non-Hodgkin lymphoma by fine-needle aspiration. Arch Pathol Lab Med. 2004;128:1395-1403.

496. Murphy SB, Hustu HO. A randomized trial of combined modality therapy of childhood non-Hodgkin's lymphoma. Cancer. 1980;45:630-637.

497. Magrath I, Lee YJ, Anderson T, et al. Prognostic factors in Burkitt's lymphoma: importance of total tumor burden. Cancer. 1980;45:1507-1515.

498. Reiter A, Schrappe M, Tiemann M, et al. Improved treatment results in childhood B-cell neoplasms with tailored intensification of therapy: A report of the Berlin-Frankfurt-Munster Group Trial NHL-BFM 90. Blood. 1999;94:3294-3306.

499. Bekerman C, Port RB, Pang E, et al. Scintigraphic evaluation of childhood malignancies by 67Ga-citrate. Radiology. 1978;127:719-725.

500. Elstrom R, Guan L, Baker G, et al. Utility of FDG-PET scanning in lymphoma by WHO classification. Blood. 2003;101:3875-3876.

501. Zijlstra JM, Lindauer-van der WG, Hoekstra OS, et al. 18F-fluoro-deoxyglucose positron emission tomography for post-treatment evaluation of malignant lymphoma: a systematic review. Haematologica. 2006;91:522-529.

502. Williams DM, Hobson R, Imeson J, et al. Anaplastic large cell lymphoma in childhood: analysis of 72 patients treated on The United Kingdom Children's Cancer Study Group chemotherapy regimens. Br J Haematol. 2002;117:812-820.

503. Fraga M, Brousset P, Schlaifer D, et al. Bone marrow involvement in anaplastic large cell lymphoma. Immunohistochemical detection of minimal disease and its prognostic significance. Am J Clin Pathol. 1995;103:82-89.

504. Coustan-Smith E, Sancho J, Behm FG, et al. Prognostic importance of measuring early clearance of leukemic cells by flow cytometry in childhood acute lymphoblastic leukemia. Blood. 2002;100:52-58.

505. Downing JR, Shurtleff SA, Zielenska M, et al. Molecular detection of the (2;5) translocation of non-Hodgkin's lymphoma by reverse transcriptase-polymerase chain reaction. Blood. 1995;85:3416-3422.

506. Mussolin L, Pillon M, d'Amore ES, et al. Prevalence and clinical implications of bone marrow involvement in pediatric anaplastic large cell lymphoma. Leukemia. 2005;19:1643-1647.

507. Damm-Welk C, Busch K, Burkhardt B, et al. Prognostic significance of circulating tumor cells in bone marrow or peripheral blood as detected by qualitative and quantitative PCR in pediatric

NPM-ALK positive anaplastic large cell lymphoma. Blood. 2007;110:670-677.

508. Mussolin L, Basso K, Pillon M, et al. Prospective analysis of minimal bone marrow infiltration in pediatric Burkitt's lymphomas by long-distance polymerase chain reaction for t(8;14)(q24;q32). Leukemia. 2003;17:585-589.

509. Busch K, Borkhardt A, Wossmann W, et al. Combined polymerase chain reaction methods to detect c-myc/IgH rearrangement in childhood Burkitt's lymphoma for minimal residual disease analysis. Haematologica. 2004;89:818-825.

510. Patte C, Auperin A, Michon J, et al. The Société Française d'Oncologie Pédiatrique LMB89 protocol: highly effective multiagent chemotherapy tailored to the tumor burden and initial response in 561 unselected children with B-cell lymphomas and L3 leukemia. Blood. 2001;97:3370-3379.

511. Sandlund JT, Murphy SB, Santana VM, et al. CNS involvement in children with newly diagnosed non-Hodgkin's lymphoma. J Clin Oncol. 2000;18:3018-3024.

512. Gururangan S, Sposto R, Cairo MS, et al. Outcome of CNS disease at diagnosis in disseminated small noncleaved-cell lymphoma and B-cell leukemia: a Children's Cancer Group study. J Clin Oncol. 2000;18:2017-2025.

513. Cairo MS, Gerrard M, Sposto R, et al. Results of a randomized international study of high-risk central nervous system B non-Hodgkin lymphoma and B acute lymphoblastic leukemia in children and adolescents. Blood. 2007;109:2736-2743.

514. Burger B, Zimmermann M, Mann G, et al. Diagnostic cerebrospinal fluid examination in children with acute lymphoblastic leukemia: significance of low leukocyte counts with blasts or traumatic lumbar puncture. J Clin Oncol. 2003;21:184-188.

515. Frei E III, Bentzel CJ, Rieselbach R, Block JB. Renal complications of neoplastic disease. J Chronic Dis. 1963;16:757-776.

516. Bishop MR, Coccia PF. Tumor lysis syndrome. In Abeloff MD, Niederhuber JE, Armitage JO, Lichter AS (eds). Clinical Oncology. New York, Churchill Livingstone, 2000, pp 750-754.

517. Cairo MS, Bishop M. Tumour lysis syndrome: new therapeutic strategies and classification. Br J Haematol. 2004;127:3-11.

518. Jones DP, Mahmoud H, Chesney RW. Tumor lysis syndrome: pathogenesis and management. Pediatr Nephrol. 1995;9:206-212.

519. Brogard JM, Coumaros D, Franckhauser J, et al. Enzymatic uricolysis: a study of the effect of a fungal urate-oxidase. Rev Eur Etud Clin Biol. 1972;17:890-895.

520. Masera G, Jankovic M, Zurlo MG, et al. Urate-oxidase prophylaxis of uric acid-induced renal damage in childhood leukemia. J Pediatr. 1982;100:152-155.

521. Legoux R, Delpech B, Dumont X, et al. Cloning and expression in *Escherichia coli* of the gene encoding *Aspergillus flavus* urate oxidase. J Biol Chem. 1992;267:8565-8570.

522. Goldman SC, Holcenberg JS, Finklestein JZ, et al. A randomized comparison between rasburicase and allopurinol in children with lymphoma or leukemia at high risk for tumor lysis. Blood. 2001;97:2998-3003.

523. Patte C, Sakiroglu C, Ansoborlo S, et al. Urate-oxidase in the prevention and treatment of metabolic complications in patients with B-cell lymphoma and leukemia, treated in the Societe Francaise d'Oncologie Pediatrique LMB89 protocol. Ann Oncol. 2002;13:789-795.

524. Reiter A, Schrappe M, Tiemann M, et al. Successful treatment strategy for Ki-1 anaplastic large-cell lymphoma of childhood: a prospective analysis of 62 patients enrolled in three consecutive Berlin-Frankfurt-Munster group studies. J Clin Oncol. 1994;12:899-908.

525. Anderson JR, Wilson JF, Jenkin DT, et al. Childhood non-Hodgkin's lymphoma. The results of a randomized therapeutic trial comparing a 4-drug regimen (COMP) with a 10-drug regimen (LSA2-L2). N Engl J Med. 1983;308:559-565.

526. Wollner N, Lieberman P, Exelby P, et al. Non-Hodgkin's lymphoma in children: results of treatment with LSA2-L2 protocol. Br J Cancer Suppl. 1975;2:337-342.

527. Muller-Weihrich S, Henze G, Jobke A, et al. BFM study 1975/81 for treatment of non-Hodgkin lymphoma of high malignancy in children and adolescents. Klin Padiatr. 1982;194:219-225.

528. Patte C, Kalifa C, Flamant F, et al. Results of the LMT81 protocol, a modified LSA2L2 protocol with high dose methotrexate, on 84 children with non-B-cell (lymphoblastic) lymphoma. Med Pediatr Oncol. 1992;20:105-113.

529. Muller-Weihrich S, Henze G, Langermann HJ, et al. Childhood B-cell lymphomas and leukemias. Improvement of prognosis by a therapy developed for B-neoplasms by the BFM study group. Onkologie. 1984;7:205-208.

530. Murphy SB, Bowman WP, Abromowitch M, et al. Results of treatment of advanced-stage Burkitt's lymphoma and B cell (SIg+) acute lymphoblastic leukemia with high-dose fractionated cyclophosphamide and coordinated high-dose methotrexate and cytarabine. J Clin Oncol. 1986;4:1732-1739.

531. Patte C, Philip T, Rodary C, et al. Improved survival rate in children with stage III and IV B cell non-Hodgkin's lymphoma and leukemia using multi-agent chemotherapy: results of a study of 114 children from the French Pediatric Oncology Society. J Clin Oncol. 1986;4:1219-1226.

532. Patte C, Philip T, Rodary C, et al. High survival rate in advanced-stage B-cell lymphomas and leukemias without CNS involvement with a short intensive polychemotherapy: results from the French Pediatric Oncology Society of a randomized trial of 216 children. J Clin Oncol. 1991;9:123-132.

533. Reiter A, Schrappe M, Parwaresch R, et al. Non-Hodgkin's lymphomas of childhood and adolescence: results of a treatment stratified for biologic subtypes and stage—a report of the Berlin-Frankfurt-Munster Group. J Clin Oncol. 1995;13:359-372.

534. Cairo MS, Krailo MD, Morse M, et al. Long-term follow-up of short intensive multiagent chemotherapy without high-dose methotrexate ("Orange") in children with advanced non-lymphoblastic non-Hodgkin's lymphoma: a Children's Cancer Group report. Leukemia. 2002;16:594-600.

535. Brugieres L, Quartier P, Le Deley MC, et al. Relapses of childhood anaplastic large-cell lymphoma: treatment results in a series of 41 children—a report from the French Society of Pediatric Oncology. Ann Oncol. 2000;11:53-58.

536. Tubergen DG, Krailo MD, Meadows AT, et al. Comparison of treatment regimens for pediatric lymphoblastic non-Hodgkin's lymphoma: a Children's Cancer Group study. J Clin Oncol. 1995;13:1368-1376.

537. Riehm H, Gadner H, Welte K. The West Berlin therapy study of acute lymphoblastic leukemia in childhood—report after 6 years [author's translation]. Klin Padiatr. 1977;189:89-102.

538. Amylon MD, Shuster J, Pullen J, et al. Intensive high-dose asparaginase consolidation improves survival for pediatric patients with T cell acute lymphoblastic leukemia and advanced stage lymphoblastic lymphoma: a Pediatric Oncology Group study. Leukemia. 1999;13:335-342.

539. Millot F, Suciu S, Philippe N, et al. Value of high-dose cytarabine during interval therapy of a Berlin-Frankfurt-Münster-based protocol in increased-risk children with acute lymphoblastic leukemia and lymphoblastic lymphoma: results of the European Organization for Research and Treatment of Cancer 58881 randomized phase III trial. J Clin Oncol. 2001;19:1935-1942.

540. Bostrom BC, Sensel MR, Sather HN, et al. Dexamethasone versus prednisone and daily oral versus weekly intravenous mercaptopurine for patients with standard-risk acute lymphoblastic leukemia: a report from the Children's Cancer Group. Blood. 2003;101:3809-3817.

541. Bergeron C, Celine S, Pacquement H, et al. Childhood T-cell lymphoblastic lymphoma (TLL) Results of the SFOP LMT96 strategy. Pediatr Blood Cancer. 2006;46:967.

542. Burkhardt B, Reiter A, Lang PLL, et al. Relapse in pediatric patients with T-cell lymphoblastic lymphoma: clinical characteristics and outcome in the BFM group. Pediatr Blood Cancer. 2006;46:842.

543. Link MP, Shuster JJ, Donaldson SS, et al. Treatment of children and young adults with early-stage non-Hodgkin's lymphoma. N Engl J Med. 1997;337:1259-1266.

544. Burkitt D. Long-term remissions following one and two-dose chemotherapy for African lymphoma. Cancer. 1967;20:756-759.

545. Ziegler JL, Bluming AZ, Magrath IT, Carbone PP. Intensive chemotherapy in patients with generalized Burkitt's lymphoma. Int J Cancer. 1972;10:254-261.

546. Ziegler JL. Treatment results of 54 American patients with Burkitt's lymphoma are similar to the African experience. N Engl J Med. 1977;297:75-80.

547. Ziegler JL, Bluming AZ. Intrathecal chemotherapy in Burkitt's lymphoma. BMJ. 1971;3:508-512.

548. Olweny CL, Atine I, Kaddu-Mukasa A, et al. Cerebrospinal irradiation of Burkitt's lymphoma. Failure in preventing central nervous system relapse. Acta Radiol Ther Phys Biol. 1977;16:225-231.

549. Appelbaum FR, Deisseroth AB, Graw RG Jr, et al. Prolonged complete remission following high dose chemotherapy of Burkitt's lymphoma in relapse. Cancer. 1978;41:1059-1063.

550. Iversen OH, Iversen U, Ziegler JL, Bluming AZ. Cell kinetics in Burkitt lymphoma. Eur J Cancer. 1974;10:155-163.

551. Ziegler JL, Bluming AZ, Fass L, et al. Burkitt's lymphoma: cell kinetics, treatment and immunology. Bibl Haematol. 1973;39:1046-1052.

552. Murphy SB, Melvin SL, Mauer AM. Correlation of tumor cell kinetic studies with surface marker results in childhood non-Hodgkin's lymphoma. Cancer Res. 1979;39:1534-1538.

553. Murphy SB, Bowman WP, Hustu HO, Berard CW. Advanced stage (III-IV) Burkitt's lymphoma and B-cell acute lymphoblastic leukaemia in children: kinetic and pharmacologic rationale for treatment and recent results (1979-1983). IARC Sci Publ. 1985;405-418.

554. Brecher ML, Schwenn MR, Coppes MJ, et al. Fractionated cylophosphamide and back to back high-dose methotrexate and cytosine arabinoside improves outcome in patients with stage III high grade small non-cleaved cell lymphomas (SNCCL): a randomized trial of the Pediatric Oncology Group. Med Pediatr Oncol. 1997;29:526-533.

555. Atra A, Imeson JD, Hobson R, et al. Improved outcome in children with advanced stage B-cell non-Hodgkin's lymphoma (B-NHL): results of the United Kingdom Children Cancer Study Group (UKCCSG) 9002 protocol. Br J Cancer. 2000;82:1396-1402.

556. Pillon M, Di Tullio MT, Garaventa A, et al. Long-term results of the first Italian Association of Pediatric Hematology and Oncology protocol for the treatment of pediatric B-cell non-Hodgkin lymphoma (AIEOP LNH92). Cancer. 2004;101:385-394.

557. Djerassi I, Kim JS. Methotrexate and citrovorum factor rescue in the management of childhood lymphosarcoma and reticulum cell sarcoma (non-Hodgkin's lymphomas): prolonged unmaintained remissions. Cancer. 1976;38:1043-1051.

558. Patte C, Bernard A, Hartmann O, et al. High-dose methotrexate and continuous infusion Ara-C in children's non-Hodgkin's lymphoma: phase II studies and their use in further protocols. Pediatr Hematol Oncol. 1986;3:11-18.

559. Bowman WP, Shuster JJ, Cook B, et al. Improved survival for children with B-cell acute lymphoblastic leukemia and stage IV small noncleaved-cell lymphoma: a pediatric oncology group study. J Clin Oncol. 1996;14:1252-1261.

560. Gentet JC, Patte C, Quintana E, et al. Phase II study of cytarabine and etoposide in children with refractory or relapsed non-

561. Sposto R, Meadows AT, Chilcote RR, et al. Comparison of long-term outcome of children and adolescents with disseminated non-lymphoblastic non-Hodgkin lymphoma treated with COMP or daunomycin-COMP: A report from the Children's Cancer Group. Med Pediatr Oncol. 2001;37:432-441.

562. Patte C, Laplanche A, Bertozzi AI, et al. Granulocyte colony-stimulating factor in induction treatment of children with non-Hodgkin's lymphoma: a randomized study of the French Society of Pediatric Oncology. J Clin Oncol. 2002;20:441-448.

563. Goldie JH, Coldman AJ. The genetic origin of drug resistance in neoplasms: implications for systemic therapy. Cancer Res. 1984;44:3643-3653.

564. Woessmann W, Seidemann K, Mann G, et al. The impact of the methotrexate administration schedule and dose in the treatment of children and adolescents with B-cell neoplasms: a report of the BFM Group Study NHL-BFM95. Blood. 2005;105:948-958.

565. Patte C, Auperin A, Gerrard M, et al. Results of the randomized international FAB/LMB96 trial for intermediate risk B-cell non-Hodgkin lymphoma in children and adolescents: it is possible to reduce treatment for the early responding patients. Blood. 2007;109:2773-2780.

566. Schwenn MR, Blattner SR, Lynch E, Weinstein HJ. HiC-COM: a 2-month intensive chemotherapy regimen for children with stage III and IV Burkitt's lymphoma and B-cell acute lymphoblastic leukemia. J Clin Oncol. 1991;9:133-138.

567. Spreafico F, Massimino M, Luksch R, et al. Intensive, very short-term chemotherapy for advanced Burkitt's lymphoma in children. J Clin Oncol. 2002;20:2783-2788.

568. Magrath I, Adde M, Shad A, et al. Adults and children with small non-cleaved-cell lymphoma have a similar excellent outcome when treated with the same chemotherapy regimen. J Clin Oncol. 1996;14:925-934.

569. Tiemann M, Riener MO, Claviez A, et al. Proliferation rate and outcome in children with T-cell rich B-cell lymphoma: a clinico-pathologic study from the NHL-BFM-study group. Leuk Lymphoma. 2005;46:1295-1300.

570. Seidemann K, Tiemann M, Lauterbach I, et al. Primary mediastinal large B-cell lymphoma with sclerosis in pediatric and adolescent patients: treatment and results from three therapeutic studies of the Berlin-Frankfurt-Münster Group. J Clin Oncol. 2003;21:1782-1789.

571. Laver JH, Kraveka JM, Hutchison RE, et al. Advanced-stage large-cell lymphoma in children and adolescents: results of a randomized trial incorporating intermediate-dose methotrexate and high-dose cytarabine in the maintenance phase of the APO regimen: a Pediatric Oncology Group phase III trial. J Clin Oncol. 2005;23:541-547.

572. Brugieres L, Le Deley MC, Rosolen A, et al. Anaplastic large cell lymphoma (ALCL) in children: equal efficacy but greater toxicity of chemotherapy including methotrexate (MTX) 1g/m^2 in 24-hour infusion with intrathecal injection (IT) than chemotherapy with MTX 3g/m^2 in 3-hour infusion without IT: results of the ALCL99-R1 randomised trial. Blood. 2006;108:122a.

573. Mott MG, Chessells JM, Willoughby MI, et al. Adjuvant low dose radiation in childhood T cell leukaemia/lymphoma (report from the United Kingdom Children's Cancer Study Group—UKCCSG). Br J Cancer. 1984;50:457-462.

574. Link MP, Donaldson SS, Berard CW, et al. Results of treatment of childhood localized non-Hodgkin's lymphoma with combination chemotherapy with or without radiotherapy. N Engl J Med. 1990;322:1169-1174.

575. Murphy SB. Classification, staging and end results of treatment of childhood non-Hodgkin's lymphomas: dissimilarities from lymphomas in adults. Semin Oncol. 1980;7:332-339.

576. Cheson BD, Horning SJ, Coiffier B, et al. Report of an international workshop to standardize response criteria for non-

Hodgkin's lymphomas. NCI Sponsored International Working Group. J Clin Oncol. 1999;17:1244.

577. Haioun C, Itti E, Rahmouni A, et al. [18F]-Fluoro-2-deoxy-D-glucose positron emission tomography (FDG-PET) in aggressive lymphoma: an early prognostic tool for predicting patient outcome. Blood. 2005;106:1376-1381.

578. Bucsky P, Feller AC, Reiter A, et al. Low-grade malignant non-Hodgkin's lymphomas and peripheral pleomorphic T-cell lymphomas in childhood—a BFM study group report. Klin Padiatr. 1990;202:258-261.

579. Morrell D, Cromartie E, Swift M. Mortality and cancer incidence in 263 patients with ataxia-telangiectasia. J Natl Cancer Inst. 1986;77:89-92.

580. Filipovich AH, Mathur A, Kamat D, et al. Lymphoproliferative disorders and other tumors complicating immunodeficiencies. Immunodeficiency. 1994;5:91-112.

581. Seidemann K, Tiemann M, Henze G, et al. Therapy for non-Hodgkin lymphoma in children with primary immunodeficiency: analysis of 19 patients from the BFM trials. Med Pediatr Oncol. 1999;33:536-544.

582. Kobrinsky NL, Sposto R, Shah NR, et al. Outcomes of treatment of children and adolescents with recurrent non-Hodgkin's lymphoma and Hodgkin's disease with dexamethasone, etoposide, cisplatin, cytarabine, and L-asparaginase, maintenance chemotherapy, and transplantation: Children's Cancer Group Study CCG-5912. J Clin Oncol. 2001;19:2390-2396.

583. Attarbaschi A, Dworzak M, Steiner M, et al. Outcome of children with primary resistant or relapsed non-Hodgkin lymphoma and mature B-cell leukemia after intensive first-line treatment: a population-based analysis of the Austrian Cooperative Study Group. Pediatr Blood Cancer. 2005;44:70-76.

584. Cairo MS, Sposto R, Perkins SL, et al. Burkitt's and Burkitt-like lymphoma in children and adolescents: a review of the Children's Cancer Group experience. Br J Haematol. 2003;120:660-670.

585. Atra A, Gerrard M, Hobson R, et al. Outcome of relapsed or refractory childhood B-cell acute lymphoblastic leukaemia and B-cell non-Hodgkin's lymphoma treated with the UKCCSG 9003/9002 protocols. Br J Haematol. 2001;112:965-968.

586. Ladenstein R, Pearce R, Hartmann O, et al. High-dose chemotherapy with autologous bone marrow rescue in children with poor-risk Burkitt's lymphoma: a report from the European Lymphoma Bone Marrow Transplantation Registry. Blood. 1997;90:2921-2930.

587. Wossmann W, Schrappe M, Meyer U, et al. Incidence of tumor lysis syndrome in children with advanced stage Burkitt's lymphoma/leukemia before and after introduction of prophylactic use of urate oxidase. Ann Hematol. 2003;82:160-165.

588. Corbacioglu S, Eber S, Gungor T, et al. Induction of long-term remission of a relapsed childhood B-acute lymphoblastic leukemia with rituximab chimeric anti-CD20 monoclonal antibody and autologous stem cell transplantation. J Pediatr Hematol Oncol. 2003;25:327-329.

589. Woessmann W, Peters C, Lenhard M, et al. Allogeneic haematopoietic stem cell transplantation in relapsed or refractory anaplastic large cell lymphoma of children and adolescents—a Berlin-Frankfurt-Munster group report. Br J Haematol. 2006; 133:176-182.

590. Le Deley MC, Brugieres L, Williams DM, Reiter A. Prognostic factors in childhood anaplastic large cell lymphoma (ALCL): results of the European Intergroup Study. Blood. 2006; 108:581a.

591. Schmitt C, Delsol G, Brugieres L, et al. Lymphohistiocytic variant of anaplastic large cell lymphoma in children and adolescents: a long-term study by the French Society of Pediatric Cancer—Lymphoma Group. Pediatr Blood Cancer. 2006;46: 841-842.

592. Poirel HA, Heerema NA, Swansbury J, et al. Cytogenetic analysis of 238 pediatric mature B-cell non-Hodgkin lymphoma (NHL) cases from the randomized international FAB LMB96 trial identifies several patterns of chromosomal abnormality and new prognostic factors. Pediatr Blood Cancer. 2006;46:835.

593. Onciu M, Schlette E, Zhou Y, et al. Secondary chromosomal abnormalities predict outcome in pediatric and adult high-stage Burkitt lymphoma. Cancer. 2006;107:1084-1092.

594. Burkhardt B, Bruch J, Zimmermann M, et al. Loss of heterozygosity on chromosome 6q14-q24 is associated with poor outcome in children and adolescents with T-cell lymphoblastic lymphoma. Leukemia. 2006;20:1422-1429.

595. Burkhardt B, Woessmann W, Zimmermann M, et al. Impact of cranial radiotherapy on central nervous system prophylaxis in children and adolescents with central nervous system-negative stage III or IV lymphoblastic lymphoma. J Clin Oncol. 2006;24:491-499.

596. Seidemann K, Zimmermann M, Book M, et al. Tumor necrosis factor and lymphotoxin alfa genetic polymorphisms and outcome in pediatric patients with non-Hodgkin's lymphoma: results from Berlin-Frankfurt-Munster Trial NHL-BFM 95. J Clin Oncol. 2005;23:8414-8421.

597. Seidemann K, Book M, Zimmermann M, et al. MTHFR 677 (C→T) polymorphism is not relevant for prognosis or therapy-associated toxicity in pediatric NHL: results from 484 patients of multicenter trial NHL-BFM 95. Ann Hematol. 2006;85: 291-300.

598. Robison LL. The Childhood Cancer Survivor Study: a resource for research of long-term outcomes among adult survivors of childhood cancer. Minn Med. 2005;88:45-49.

599. Leung W, Sandlund JT, Hudson MM, et al. Second malignancy after treatment of childhood non-Hodgkin lymphoma. Cancer. 2001;92:1959-1966.

599a. Haddy TB, Adde MA, McCalla J, et al. Late effects in long-term survivors of high-grade non-Hodgkin's lymphomas. J Clin Oncol. 1998;16:2070-2079.

600. Ness KK, Mertens AC, Hudson MM, et al. Limitations on physical performance and daily activities among long-term survivors of childhood cancer. Ann Intern Med. 2005;143:639-647.

601. Buell JF, Gross TG, Woodle ES. Malignancy after transplantation. Transplantation. 2005;80(Suppl 2):S254-S264.

602. Baker KS, DeFor TE, Burns LJ, et al. New malignancies after blood or marrow stem-cell transplantation in children and adults: incidence and risk factors. J Clin Oncol. 2003;21:1352-1358.

603. Capello D, Cerri M, Muti G, et al. Analysis of immunoglobulin heavy and light chain variable genes in post-transplant lymphoproliferative disorders. Hematol Oncol. 2006;24:212-219.

604. Gulley ML, Swinnon LJ, Plaisance KT Jr, et al. Tumor origin and CD20 expression in posttransplant lymphoproliferative disorder occurring in solid organ transplant recipients: implications for immune-based therapy. Transplantation. 2003;76: 959-964.

605. Rajakariar R, Bhattacharyya M, Norton A, et al. Post transplant T-cell lymphoma: a case series of four patients from a single unit and review of the literature. Am J Transplant. 2004;4:1534-1538.

606. Chadburn A, Cesarman E, Liu YF, et al. Molecular genetic analysis demonstrates that multiple posttransplantation lymphoproliferative disorders occurring in one anatomic site in a single patient represent distinct primary lymphoid neoplasms. Cancer. 1995;75:2747-2756.

607. Hayashi RJ, Kraus MD, Patel AL, et al. Posttransplant lymphoproliferative disease in children: correlation of histology to clinical behavior. J Pediatr Hematol Oncol. 2001;23:14-18.

608. Micallef IN, Chhanabhai M, Gascoyne RD, et al. Lymphoproliferative disorders following allogeneic bone marrow transplantation: the Vancouver experience. Bone Marrow Transplant. 1998;22:981-987.

609. Cohen JL, Salomon BL. Therapeutic potential of CD4+ CD25+ regulatory T cells in allogeneic transplantation. Cytotherapy. 2005;7:166-170.

610. Ho M, Jaffe R, Miller G, et al. The frequency of Epstein-Barr virus infection and associated lymphoproliferative syndrome after transplantation and its manifestations in children. Transplantation. 1988;45:719-727.

611. Maecker B, Jack T, Zimmermann M, et al. CNS or bone marrow involvement as risk factors for poor survival in post-transplantation lymphoproliferative disorders in children after solid organ transplantation. J Clin Oncol. 2007;25:4902-4908.

612. Grant D. Intestinal transplantation: 1997 report of the international registry. Intestinal Transplant Registry. Transplantation. 1999;67:1061-1064.

613. Wilkinson AH, Smith JL, Hunsicker LG, et al. Increased frequency of posttransplant lymphomas in patients treated with cyclosporine, azathioprine, and prednisone. Transplantation. 1989;47:293-296.

614. Davis JE, Sherritt MA, Bharadwaj M, et al. Determining virological, serological and immunological parameters of EBV infection in the development of PTLD. Int Immunol. 2004;16:983-989.

615. Green M, Michaels MG, Katz BZ, et al. CMV-IVIG for prevention of Epstein Barr virus disease and posttransplant lymphoproliferative disease in pediatric liver transplant recipients. Am J Transplant. 2006;6:1906-1912.

616. Guthery SL, Heubi JE, Bucuvalas JC, et al. Determination of risk factors for Epstein-Barr virus-associated posttransplant lymphoproliferative disorder in pediatric liver transplant recipients using objective case ascertainment. Transplantation. 2003;75:987-993.

617. Gross TG, Steinbuch M, DeFor T, et al. B cell lymphoproliferative disorders following hematopoietic stem cell transplantation: risk factors, treatment and outcome. Bone Marrow Transplant. 1999;23:251-258.

618. Curtis RE, Travis LB, Rowlings PA, et al. Risk of lymphoproliferative disorders after bone marrow transplantation: a multiinstitutional study. Blood. 1999;94:2208-2216.

619. van Esser JW, van der Holt B, Meijer E, et al. Epstein-Barr virus (EBV) reactivation is a frequent event after alllogeneic stem cell transplantation (SCT) and quantitatively predicts EBV-lymphoproliferative disease following T-cell–depleted SCT. Blood. 2001;98:972-978.

620. Hale G, Waldmann H. Risks of developing Epstein-Barrr virus-related lymphoproliferative disorders after T-cell–depleted marrow transplants. CAMPATH Users. Blood. 1998;91:3079-3083.

621. Pinkerton CR, Hann I, Weston CL, et al. Immunodeficiency-related lymphoproliferative disorders: prospective data from the United Kingdom Children's Cancer Study Group Registry. Br J Haematol. 2002;118:456-461.

622. Green M, Reyes J, Webber S, Rowe D. The role of antiviral and immunoglobulin therapy in the prevention of Epstein-Barr virus infection and post-transplant lymphoproliferative disease following solid organ transplantation. Transpl Infect Dis. 2001;3:97-103.

623. McDiarmid SV, Jordan S, Kim GS, et al. Prevention and preemptive therapy of posttransplant lymphoproliferative disease in pediatric liver recipients. Transplantation. 1998;66:1604-1611.

624. Ganschow R, Schulz T, Meyer T, et al. Low-dose immunosuppression reduces the incidence of post-transplant lymphoproliferative disease in pediatric liver graft recipients. J Pediatr Gastroenterol Nutr. 2004;38:198-203.

625. Lee TC, Savoldo B, Rooney CM, et al. Quantitative EBV viral loads and immunosuppression alterations can decrease PTLD incidence in pediatric liver transplant recipients. Am J Transplant. 2005;5:2222-2228.

626. Rowe DT, Webber S, Schauer EM, et al. Epstein-Barr virus load monitoring: its role in the prevention and management of post-transplant lymphoproliferative disease. Transpl Infect Dis. 2001;3:79-87.

627. Rowe DT, Qu L, Reyes J, et al. Use of quantitative competitive PCR to measure Epstein-Barr virus genome load in the peripheral blood of pediatric transplant patients with lymphoproliferative disorders. J Clin Microbiol. 1997;35:1612-1615.

628. Wagner HJ, Cheng YC, Huls MH, et al. Prompt versus preemptive intervention for EBV lymphoproliferative disease. Blood. 2004;103:3979-3981.

629. Kullberg-Lindh C, Ascher H, Saalman R, et al. Epstein-Barr viremia levels after pediatric liver transplantation as measured by real-time polymerase chain reaction. Pediatr Transplant. 2006;10:83-89.

630. Benden C, Aurora P, Burch M, et al. Monitoring of Epstein-Barr viral load in pediatric heart and lung transplant recipients by real-time polymerase chain reaction. J Heart Lung Transplant. 2005;24:2103-2108.

631. Smets F, Latinne D, Bazin H, et al. Ratio between Epstein-Barr viral load and anti-Epstein-Barr virus specific T-cell response as a predictive marker of posttransplant lymphoproliferative disease. Transplantation. 2002;73:1603-1610.

632. Sebelin-Wulf K, Nguyen TD, Oertel S, et al. Quantitative analysis of EBV-specific CD4/CD8 T cell numbers, absolute CD4 solid organ transplant recipients with PLTD. Transpl Immunol. 2007;17:203-210.

633. Gross TG, Bucuvalas JC, Park JR, et al. Low-dose chemotherapy for Epstein-Barr virus–positive post-transplantation lymphoproliferative disease in children after solid organ transplantation. J Clin Oncol. 2005;23:6481-6488.

634. Messahel B, Taj MM, Hobson R, et al. Single agent efficacy of rituximab in childhood immunosuppression related lymphoproliferative disease: a United Kingdom Children's Cancer Study Group (UKCCSG) retrospective review. Leuk Lymphoma. 2006;47:2584-2589.

635. Savoldo B, Rooney CM, Quiros-Tejeira RE, et al. Cellular immunity to Epstein-Barr virus in liver transplant recipients treated with rituximab for post-transplant lymproliferative disese. Am J Transplant. 2005;5:566-572.

636. Heslop HE, Rooney CM. Adoptive cellular immunotherapy for EBV lymphoproliferative disease. Immunol Rev. 1997;157:217-222.

637. Savoldo B, Goss JA, Hammer MM, et al. Treatment of solid organ transplant recipients with autologous Epstein Barr virus-specific cytotoxic T lymphocytes (CTLs). Blood. 2006;108:2942-2949.

638. Böll B, Hansen H, Heuck F, et al. The fully human anti-CD30 antibody 5F11 activates NF-κB and sensitizes lymphoma cells to bortezomib-induced apoptosis. Blood. 2005;106:1839-1842.

639. Thomas L. Physiologic and pathologic alterations produced by the endotoxins of gram-negative bacteria. AMA Arch Intern Med. 1958;101:452-461.

640. Zuelzer WW, Kaplan J. The child with lymphadenopathy. Semin Hematol. 1975;12:323-334.

641. Moussatos GH, Baffes TG. Cervical masses in infants and children. Pediatrics. 1963;32:251-256.

642. Bedros AA, Mann JP. Lymphadenopathy in children. Adv Pediatr. 1981;28:341-376.

643. Dorfman RF, Warnke R. Lymphadenopathy simulating the malignant lymphomas. Hum Pathol. 1974;5:519-550.

644. Salvador AH, Harrison EG Jr, Kyle RA. Lymphadenopathy because of infectious mononucleosis: its confusion with malignant lymphoma. Cancer. 1971;27:1029-1040.

645. Kendig EL Jr. The clinical picture of sarcoidosis in children. Pediatrics. 1974;54:289-292.

646. Rosai J, Dorfman RF. Sinus histiocytosis with massive lymphadenopathy: a pseudolymphomatous benign disorder. Analysis of 34 cases. Cancer. 1972;30:1174-1188.

647. Foucar E, Rosai J, Dorfman R. Sinus histiocytosis with massive lymphadenopathy (Rosai-Dorfman disease): review of the entity. Semin Diagn Pathol. 1990;7:19-73.

648. Knight PJ, Mulne AF, Vassy LE. When is lymph node biopsy indicated in children with enlarged peripheral nodes? Pediatrics. 1982;69:391-396.

649. Lake AM, Oski FA. Peripheral lymphadenopathy in childhood. Ten-year experience with excisional biopsy. Am J Dis Child. 1978;132:357-359.

650. Kissane JM, Gephardt GN. Lymphadenopathy in childhood: long term follow-up in patients with nondiagnostic lymph node biopsies. Hum Pathol. 1974;5:431-439.

651. Hope JW, Borns PF, Koop CE. Radiologic diagnosis of mediastinal masses in infants and children. Radiol Clin North Am. 1963;1:17-50.

652. Haller JA Jr, Mazur DO, Morgan WW Jr. Diagnosis and management of mediastinal masses in children. J Thorac Cardiovasc Surg. 1969;58:385-393.

653. Saenz NC, Schnitzer JJ, Eraklis AE, et al. Posterior mediastinal masses. J Pediatr Surg. 1993;28:172-176.

654. Bower RJ, Kiesewetter WB. Mediastinal masses in infants and children. Arch Surg. 1977;112:1003-1009.

655. Pokorny WJ, Sherman JO. Mediastinal masses in infants and children. J Thorac Cardiovasc Surg. 1974;68:869-875.

656. King RM, Telander RL, Smithson WA, et al. Primary mediastinal tumors in children. J Pediatr Surg. 1982;17:512-520.

657. Weinreb M, Day PJ, Niggli F, et al. The consistent association between Epstein-Barr virus and Hodgkin's disease in children in Kenya. Blood. 1996;87:3828-3836.

658. Li PJ, Zhou XG, Liu SR. The association of Epstein-Barr virus with Hodgkin's lymphoma in childhood. Zhonghua Bing Li Xue Za Zhi. 1994;23:224-226.

659. Preciado MV, De ME, Diez B, et al. Presence of Epstein-Barr virus and strain type assignment in Argentine childhood Hodgkin's disease. Blood. 1995;86:3922-3929.

660. Jarrett AF, Armstrong AA, Alexander E. Epidemiology of EBV and Hodgkin's lymphoma. Ann Oncol. 1996;7(Suppl 4): 5-10.

661. Ambinder RF, Browning PJ, Lorenzana I, et al. Epstein-Barr virus and childhood Hodgkin's disease in Honduras and the United States. Blood. 1993;81:462-467.

662. Razzouk BI, Gan YJ, Mendonca C, et al. Epstein-Barr virus in pediatric Hodgkin disease: age and histiotype are more predictive than geographic region. Med Pediatr Oncol. 1997;28: 248-254.

663. Hudson MM, Krasin M, Link MP, et al. Risk-adapted, combined-modality therapy with VAMP/COP and response-based, involved-field radiation for unfavorable pediatric Hodgkin's disease. J Clin Oncol. 2004;22:4541-4550.

664. Tebbi CK, Mendenhall N, London WB, et al. Treatment of stage I, IIA, IIIA1 pediatric Hodgkin disease with doxorubicin, bleomycin, vincristine and etoposide (DBVE) and radiation: a Pediatric Oncology Group (POG) study. Pediatr Blood Cancer. 2006;46:198-202.

665. Morgenfeld MC, Pavlovsky A, Suarez A, et al. Combined cyclophosphamide vincristine, procarbazine, and prednisone (COPP) therapy of malignant lymphoma. Evaluation of 190 patients. Cancer. 1975;36:1241-1249.

666. Shankar AG, Ashley S, Radford M, et al. Does histology influence outcome in childhood Hodgkin's disease? Results from the United Kingdom Children's Cancer Study Group. J Clin Oncol. 1997;15:2622-2630.

667. Kelly KM, Hutchinson RJ, Sposto R, et al. Feasibility of upfront dose-intensive chemotherapy in children with advanced-stage Hodgkin's lymphoma: preliminary results from the Children's Cancer Group Study CCG-59704. Ann Oncol. 2002;13(Suppl 1):107-111.

668. Schellong G, Bramswig JH, Hornig-Franz I, et al. Hodgkin's disease in children: combined modality treatment for stages IA, IB, and IIA. Results in 356 patients of the German/Austrian Pediatric Study Group. Ann Oncol. 1994;5(Suppl 2):113-115.

669. Josting A, Rudolph C, Reiser M, et al. Time-intensified dexamethasone/cisplatin/cytarabine: an effective salvage therapy with low toxicity in patients with relapsed and refractory Hodgkin's disease. Ann Oncol. 2002;13:1628-1635.

670. Pfreundschuh MG, Rueffer U, Lathan B, et al. Dexa-BEAM in patients with Hodgkin's disease refractory to multidrug chemotherapy regimens: a trial of the German Hodgkin's Disease Study Group. J Clin Oncol. 1994;12:580-586.

671. Linch DC, Winfield D, Goldstone AH, et al. Dose intensification with autologous bone-marrow transplantation in relapsed and resistant Hodgkin's disease: results of a BNLI randomised trial. Lancet. 1993;341:1051-1054.

672. Byrne J. Infertility and premature menopause in childhood cancer survivors. Med Pediatr Oncol. 1999;33:24-28.

673. Ash P. The influence of radiation on fertility in man. Br J Radiol. 1980;53:271-278.

674. Cosset JM, Hoppe RT. Pulmonary late effects after treatment of Hodgkin's disease. In Mauch PM, Armitage JO, Diehl V (eds). Hodgkin's Disease. Philadelphia, Lippincott Williams & Wilkins, 1999, pp 633-645.

675. Stiller CA. Epidemiology and genetics of childhood cancer. Oncogene. 2004;23:6429-6444.

676. Eden OB, Hann I, Imeson J, et al. Treatment of advanced stage T cell lymphoblastic lymphoma: results of the United Kingdom Children's Cancer Study Group (UKCCSG) protocol 8503. Br J Haematol. 1992;82:310-316.

677. Burkhardt B, Zimmermann M, Oschlies I, et al. The impact of age and gender on biology, clinical features and treatment outcome of non-Hodgkin lymphoma in childhood and adolescence. Br J Haematol. 2005;131:39-49.

678. Gerrard M, Cairo MS, Weston C, et al. Results of the FAB LMB 96 international study in children and adolescents (C+A) with localised, resected B cell lymphoma (large cell [LCL], Burkitt's [BL] and Burkitt-like [BLL]). Proc Am Soc Clin Oncol. 2003;795.

679. Rosolen A, Pillon M, Garaventa A, et al. Anaplastic large cell lymphoma treated with a leukemia-like therapy: report of the Italian Association of Pediatric Hematology and Oncology (AIEOP) LNH-92 protocol. Cancer. 2005;104:2133-2140.

680. Reiter A. Diagnosis and treatment of childhood non-Hodgkin lymphoma. Hematology Am Soc Hematol Educ Program. 2007;2007:285-296.

IV Solid Tumors

Neuroblastoma

Pediatric Renal Tumors

Retinoblastoma

Tumors of the Brain and Spinal Cord

Hepatoblastomas and Other Liver Tumors

Rhabdomyosarcoma

Nonrhabdomyosarcomas and Other Soft Tissue Tumors

Ewing's Sarcoma

Osteosarcoma

Pediatric Germ Cell Tumors

Histocytoses

Rare Tumors of Childhood

14 Neuroblastoma

Suzanne Shusterman and Rani E. George

Neuroblastoma is an embryonal tumor of the sympathetic nervous system arising from the neural crest. It is a common solid tumor of childhood and is a disease distinguished by its clinical and biologic heterogeneity. The prognosis for neuroblastoma is variable and largely dependent on tumor biology. Although patients with localized disease and favorable tumor biology may be successfully treated with surgery alone or with minimal therapy, approximately half of all patients present with metastatic disease and/or adverse tumor-specific biologic features. For these children with high-risk disease features, cure rates remain poor. The development of resistance to chemotherapy and radiation is likely the cause of most treatment failures, and neuroblastoma accounts for 15% of all pediatric oncology deaths. This chapter summarizes our current understanding of neuroblastoma biology and pathogenesis, and how this rapidly evolving insight influences current and future treatment strategies.

EPIDEMIOLOGY

Neuroblastoma accounts for 7.5% of all cancer diagnoses in children younger than 15 years, with approximately 650 new cases diagnosed in the United States each year.[1] It is the most common extracranial solid tumor in childhood, affecting 1 in 7000 children younger than 5 years. It is the most commonly diagnosed cancer of infancy, with an incidence of 64/million, almost double the incidence of leukemia, the next most commonly diagnosed cancer of infancy.[1] The median age of diagnosis is 22 months, and neuroblastoma is rarely diagnosed after the age of 10 years. The incidence rate is 28.5/million in the 0- to 4-year-old age group, 3.0/million in the 5- to 9-year-old age group, and 0.8/million in the 10- to 14-year-old age group.[2] Historically, neuroblastoma has a reported slight male predominance, although recent data show a male-to-female ratio of 1.03:1.[3] There also is a small increased incidence in white infants compared with other races.[1,2]

The cause of neuroblastoma is largely unknown. The embryonal origin of the tumor cells as well as the young age of onset suggest that pre- and perinatal exposures may be important. Studies have investigated various prenatal exposures, including tobacco, alcohol, pesticides, and maternal medication or drug use, as well as birth characteristics, including small size for gestational age and maternal history of fetal loss.[4-8] The findings from these studies, however, have been inconsistent and none of these associations has been confirmed in large studies.

Because most neuroblastomas produce catecholamine metabolites that can be detected in the urine, infant screening programs have been conducted to see if it is possible to decrease the mortality from high-risk neuroblastoma by diagnosing cases earlier. In Japan, starting in 1985, a nationwide mass screening program for neuroblastoma was conducted in 6-month-old infants. Results showed that the incidence of neuroblastoma increased two- to threefold because of the screening, but that most patients had low-stage disease and biologically favorable features, and screening did not decrease overall neuroblastoma mortality,[9-14] implying that without screening many of these tumors would have regressed spontaneously and would not have been diagnosed clinically. The Quebec Neuroblastoma Screening Program screened infants at 3 weeks and 6 months and confirmed the Japanese results[15,16]; it also showed a significant complication rate in patients undergoing treatment for tumors found by screening.[17] The German Neuroblastoma Screening Study looked at postponing screening until 10 to 19 months of age.[18,19] They found less overdiagnosis of neuroblastoma and a greater frequency of patients with unfavorable clinical and biologic features. However, no decrease in the mortality of the patients with unfavorable features was documented. Because of these results, most mass screening efforts for neuroblastoma in infants have ended worldwide.

EMBRYOLOGY

Cell of Origin

The two predominant cell types comprising neuroblastoma are neuroblasts and Schwann cells. Neuroblasts are pluripotent cells that arise in the neural crest from where they migrate to the dorsal aorta and form various components of the sympathetic nervous system—the sympathetic ganglia, chromaffin cells of the adrenal medulla, and paraganglia, which are typical sites at which neuroblastic tumors can arise. What causes persistence of the embryonal cells that develop into peripheral neuroblastic tumors is unclear. Genes that dictate neural development are mutated, lost, or amplified, causing defects in the normal differentiation and programmed cell death pathways and leading to uncontrolled proliferation.[20,21]

The embryonal neuroblast can differentiate and mature into a ganglion cell or remain undifferentiated. On the other hand, the origin of Schwann cells, which form the stromal element of the tumor, is controversial. Originally, neuroblastic and Schwann cells were thought to arise from a common pluripotent tumor stem cell line. In an opposing view, based on the observation that Schwann cells are genetically normal, it has been suggested that these cells are a population of reactive cells arising from nonmalignant tissues that are recruited into the tumor during development.[22] However, in other studies, chromosomal and genetic abnormalities documented in neuroblastic cells are also seen in Schwann cells and this finding has led to the suggestion that both cell types are derived from the same progenitor cell.[23-25] In a recent study, identical X-inactivation profiles were noted in both Schwannian stromal cells and neuroblastic components. However, chromosomal imbalances were seen only in neuroblastic cells, leading to the conclusion that most stroma-rich tumors display polyclonal proliferation and that Schwann cells do not derive from neuroblasts, but that both cell types may arise from a common progenitor.[26]

Microscopic neuroblastic nodules have been reported in fetal adrenal glands during development, peaking at around 17 to 20 weeks' gestation and regressing by birth or within the first few months of postnatal life.[28] Beckwith and Perrin have termed these nodules, which were histologically identical to neuroblastoma, *neuroblastoma in situ*, which they noted during postmortem examinations of infants younger than 3 months who died of other causes.[29] These lesions were detected with a frequency 50-fold higher than the expected incidence of primary adrenal neuroblastoma and were initially thought to be neuroblastomas that regressed spontaneously. However, with new insights into the development of the adrenal gland, it is clear that these are remnants of normal fetal development.[5,29] The genetic profiles of normal developing neuroblasts and malignant neuroblastomas are similar in many respects, as shown by mRNA expression profiling of sympathetic neuroblasts from human fetal adrenal glands.[30]

Development of the Sympathetic Nervous System

The neural crest appears early in development and is composed of pluripotent cells that migrate from the neural tube ventrally

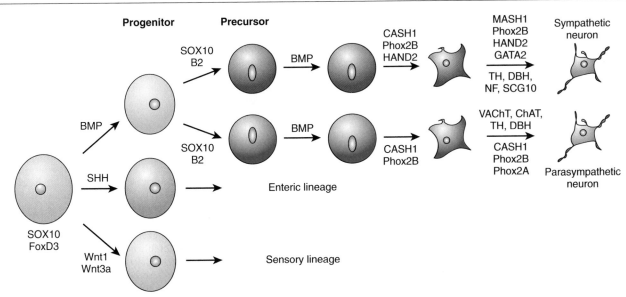

FIGURE 14-1. Schematic diagram summarizing the development of the autonomic nervous system. A series of growth factors and transcriptional regulators affect different stages of neurogenesis of neural crest–derived progenitor cells. Neural crest cells segregated from the neuroepithelium can be identified by the expression of FoxD3 and SOX10 (among other markers). Progenitor cells differentiate into sympathetic, parasympathetic, enteric, or sensory neurons, in part dependent on instructive signals encountered early at or near the time of egress from the neural tube. Additionally, extrinsic cues encountered during migration or at sites where neural crest–derived cells differentiate influence patterns of gene expression. *(Adapted from Howard MJ. Mechanisms and perspectives on differentiation of autonomic neurons. Dev Biol. 2005;277:271-286.)*

to the dorsal aorta and from there to sites where they differentiate into several lineages, including the sympathoadrenal lineage, which, when aberrant, can give rise to neuroblastoma. Development of the sympathetic phenotype is summarized in Figure 14-1.[31] In vivo studies have identified a series of transcriptional regulators and growth factors involved in neural crest cell migration, specification, and differentiation. Neural crest cells develop into sympathetic, parasympathetic, enteric, or sensory neurons, dependent in part on instructive signals encountered as they exit from the neural tube. In addition, these cells are influenced by extrinsic signals encountered during migration or at sites at which the neural crest–derived cells differentiate. Premigratory neural crest cells are characterized by the expression of several markers, including Foxd3 and SOX10. Foxd3 selectively specifies premigratory neural crest cells and is required for sublineage fate specification, migration, and survival. Zebrafish homozygous for Foxd3-inactivating mutations have near-complete loss of sympathetic neurons and their precursor populations.[32] Sox10 is responsible for the multipotency of neural crest–derived cells and is required for sympathetic nervous system and melanocyte development.[33] Bone morphogenetic proteins (BMPs) are produced in the dorsal aorta during development[34] and are a proximal signal in the transcription factor cascade required for differentiation of sympathetic neurons and acquisition of a noradrenergic phenotype. The importance of BMPs in supporting differentiation into sympathetic neurons is demonstrated by loss of expression of the noradrenergic markers of terminal differentiation, tyrosine hydroxylase (TH) and dopamine beta hydroxylase (DBH) when BMP expression is inhibited by its antagonist noggin.[35] Once neural crest cells have coalesced around the dorsal aorta, the first marker of their autonomic fate is expression of MASH1,[36] the vertebrate homologue of the *Drosophila* proneural gene achaete-scute, whose expression is maintained by BMPs.[35] In MASH1 null mice, all noradrenergic neurons are affected.[36,37] A group of transcription factors dictate the further differentiation of autonomic neurons once the neural progenitors localize at the sites where they will form ganglia—namely,

the sympathetic chain. These transcription factors include the homeodomain binding proteins PHOX2A and PHOX2B,[38,39] the bHLH DNA binding protein HAND2 (dHAND),[40,41] and the zinc finger protein GATA3 (Gata 2 in the chick).[42,43] The function of MASH1 is closely linked to PHOX2A and PHOX2B, which in turn regulate expression of the marker genes *TH* and *DBH*, whose encoded proteins are rate-limiting in catecholamine synthesis.[44,45] Loss-of-function studies have demonstrated that enteric and autonomic neuron precursors depend on PHOX2B for neuronal determination.[45,46] MASH1 in combination with HAND2 also induces expression of downstream differentiation markers.[40,41] Ectopic expression of HAND2 increases the amount of neural crest–derived cell differentiation into noradrenergic sympathetic ganglion neurons.[40] HAND2 is expressed during embryonic life, with undetectable postnatal expression. However, it is expressed in primary neuroblastoma tumors and cell lines, suggesting that many neuroblastoma tumors are blocked at an early stage of normal development when dHAND is expressed.[47] GATA2 in avian embryos functions as a cotranscriptional activator of DBH with HAND2 and PHOX2A. Abrogation of Gata2 expression also leads to decreased expression of TH in the sympathetic ganglia of the chick.

Neural crest cells from the cranial region migrate from the neural folds into the pharyngeal arches and heart, where they play essential roles in septation of the single outflow of the heart (the truncus arteriosus) and in the formation of the conotruncal portion of the ventricular septum.[48] It follows that coexistence of neuroblastoma with anomalies of other neural crest–derived structures is biologically plausible because of the shared roles of regulatory and developmental genes. Proper migration of neural crest cells is important, therefore, for the formation of neural crest–derived organs—for example, cardiogenesis; ablation of the cardiac neural crest results in congenital cardiovascular malformations in the chick embryo.[48] A significantly increased incidence of congenital cardiac malformations, especially those that are neural crest–derived, was noted in patients with neuroblastoma as compared with other malignancies, such as leukemia.[49] These cardiac anomalies were seen primarily in neuroblastoma patients younger than 1 year of age, and with lower stage tumors. Although the malignant transformation of neuroblasts and the disruption of normal cardiogenesis are likely to be multistep processes, it is possible that derangement of common genetic pathways contributes to both anomalies.

Congenital Anomalies Associated with Neuroblastoma

Neuroblastoma may occur rarely in association with chromosomal anomalies. In addition to the increased incidence of neuroblastoma in girls with Turner's syndrome,[50] neuroblastoma has also been noted to occur rarely in patients with Noonan's syndrome.[51] The protein phosphatase gene *PTPN11* is mutated in 50% of patients with Noonan's syndrome and is associated with an increased risk of leukemia[52] as well as neuroblastoma.[51] In a study of 89 primary neuroblastomas, three *PTPN11* mutations were identified, one of which was germline.[53] Mutations in the *NF1* gene have been detected in neuroblastoma cell lines[54,55] and there was a case report of a patient with a germline *NF1* mutation and neuroblastoma who had a homozygous deletion of *NF1* gene in the tumor.[56] However, germline inactivation of *NF1* does not predispose to neuroblastoma in the mouse.

PATHOGENESIS

Genetic and Molecular Pathology

Neuroblastoma Stem Cells

There is evidence to suggest that neuroblastoma, like other cancers, can arise in a stem cell compartment that is capable of self-renewal. β-Catenin signaling is thought to be involved in the maintenance and renewal of neural crest stem cells.[57,58] Neural stem cells promote resistance to cytokine and death receptor–mediated apoptosis, partly through developmentally downregulated caspase-8.[59] Most neuroblastomas do not express caspase-8 because of methylation of the caspase-8 promoter.[60] Thus, the absence of caspase-8 expression may reflect a block in the developmental program at a stage when neural crest stem cells have downregulated this gene. Recently, cells responsible for propagating neuroblastoma have been isolated and characterized from neuroblastoma tumors and bone marrow metastases.[61] These neuroblastoma stem cells have the ability to grow in conditions used to culture neural crest stem cells and are capable of self-renewal. Spheres generated from the tumors have been shown to differentiate under neurogenic conditions to form neurons. Neuroblastoma stem cells from high-risk tumors expressed markers of neural crest stem cells and clinical markers of neuroblastoma, renewed at a higher rate than those from low risk tumors, and formed metastatic tumors that could be serially passaged in xenograft models.[61]

Hereditary Predisposition

A family history has been identified in 1% to 2% of cases of neuroblastoma and is suggestive of autosomal dominant inheritance with incomplete penetrance.[62] In these children, as with hereditary retinoblastoma, neuroblastoma develops at an earlier age and frequently manifests as multiple tumors. However, there is clinical heterogeneity in the pedigrees, with affected individuals sharing the same predisposing genetic lesion, indicating that acquired secondary genetic alterations have a role

in determining the tumor phenotype. Knudson and colleagues[63] proposed that germline mutations may account for the initiation of tumors in 22% of cases of sporadic neuroblastoma. Thus, the timing and nature of the additional mutations appear to confer the ultimate phenotype, whether it is a spontaneously regressing tumor, a differentiated tumor, or one that is rapidly progressive.

Linkage analysis in studies of European families first identified a locus on chromosome 2p as being involved in hereditary neuroblastoma.[62] The aberrant gene at this locus has recently been identified as the ALK tyrosine kinase, germline mutations of which have been identified in a subset of hereditary neuroblastomas.[64] A genome-wide scan for linkage in five large neuroblastoma pedigrees and six "potential" pedigrees (sibling or cousin pairs) at approximately 6000 single-nucleotide polymorphisms has revealed a single region at 2p23-24 consistent with linkage. Four of the large pedigrees and one sibling pair showed single-base substitutions in highly conserved nucleotides within the region that encodes the *ALK* tyrosine kinase domain that segregated with the disease.[64] Activating mutations of the ALK kinase can also be acquired in somatic neural crest progenitors and *ALK* gene amplification has been documented in a substantial fraction of tumors with *MYCN* amplification, providing a target for the development of new drugs for the treatment of this disease.[65]

Mutations of the *PHOX2B* gene have been shown to occur in pedigrees and have led to cosegregation of neuroblastoma, ganglioneuroblastoma, congenital central hypoventilation syndrome (CCHS), and Hirschsprung's disease (HSCR).[20,66,67] Loss-of-function germline mutations have been identified in a small percentage of familial cases[20] and in 2.3% of children who develop sporadic neuroblastomas, usually in association with HSCR and/or CCHS.[68,69] Also, in several studies, the incidence of mutations in sporadic tumors was very low.[21,68,69]

PHOX2B plays a key role in the early differentiation of the sympathoadrenal lineage from neural crest cells. PHOX2B null mice fail to form sympathetic ganglia and cells expressing TH and DBH, key enzymes involved in terminal differentiation of sympathetic neurons, are largely absent in these animals.[39] On the other hand, overexpression of *PHOX2B* in the chick spinal cord promotes the differentiation of neural crest cells.[70] Moreover, forced expression of *PHOX2B* in human neuroblastoma cell lines has been shown to suppress cell proliferation and promote differentiation with retinoic acid.[21] *PHOX2B* mutations in neuroblastomas are missense alterations in highly conserved regions or nonsense mutations that lead to a truncated protein and absent second polyalanine motif.[20,66-68,71,72] Mutated PHOX2B also suppresses proliferation in vitro, but is not able to promote differentiation or activate expression of DBH, a downstream target of PHOX2B.[21] It is thought that mutant *PHOX2B* functions in a dominant negative role and that inhibition of *PHOX2B* affects terminal peripheral sympathetic neuron differentiation. This is also observed in vivo, in that abrogation of PHOX2B by morpholino knockdown in the zebrafish embryo leads to a block in terminal differentiation. This is evidenced by a decrease in the number of neurons in the cervical sympathetic ganglion expressing DBH and TH, while at the same time causing an excess of neurons expressing upstream markers, such as Zash1a.[73]

Traditional genetic analysis has also identified the short arms of chromosomes 16 (16p12-13) and 12 as likely predisposition loci, although mutant genes have not been identified.[62,74] Recently, a genome-wide association study from a large set of patients has revealed that common minor alleles of three consecutive single-nucleotide polymorphisms at chromosome 6p22 are associated with susceptibility to neuroblastoma.[75] Patients with neuroblastoma who were homozygous for the risk alleles were more likely to have metastatic disease, amplification of *MYCN*, and disease relapse.[75] However, the absolute risk conferred by the susceptibility allele is extremely small[75] and the risk that neuroblastoma may recur in families is estimated to be low.[76] This, plus the rarity of neuroblastoma, its variable natural history, and the high prevalence but low penetrance of neuroblastoma-associated chromosome 6p22 variants, preclude genetic screening at this time.[77]

DNA Ploidy

DNA ploidy is a way of assessing modal chromosomal content, and neuroblastoma tumors are classified into those with nuclear DNA content that is diploid (with a DNA index of 1) or hyperdiploid (DNA index greater than 1). Hyperdiploid tumors are often localized and have a good outlook, whereas diploid tumors not only tend to have a poor prognosis, but also are associated with other high-risk genetic aberrations, such as 17q gain and *MYCN* amplification. Originally, infants (those younger than 1 year of age) with a hyperdiploid modal chromosome number were found to respond well to conventional therapy, whereas those with advanced-stage disease with diploidy did not.[78,79] More recently, it has been reported that tumor cell ploidy predicts responsiveness to therapy in children younger than 18 months with advanced-stage neuroblastomas without *MYCN* amplification.[80] In an analysis of children 12 months and older with stage 4 disease, those 12 to 24 months old with nonamplified *MYCN* and hyperdiploidy had a survival rate of 72.7% compared with 26.7% for their older counterparts ($P = .0092$). This effect of ploidy was seen especially in the 12- to 18-month age group, in which the event-free survival (EFS) was 92.2% versus 37.5% for those 19 to 24 months of age ($P = .0037$).[80] Hyperdiploidy is detected because of whole chromosome losses or gains whereas diploidy is associated with chromosomal rearrangements and unbalanced translocations.

MYCN *Amplification*

MYCN was the first oncogene proven to be of clinical significance in neuroblastoma and has been noted in approximately 20% to 30% of primary tumors and 90% of cell lines.[81,82] Its presence is generally associated with a poor outcome and rapid tumor progression.[82,83] *MYCN* is a highly conserved nuclear transcription factor located on chromosome 2p24.3. Amplification manifests cytogenetically as double minutes (DMs) or homogeneously staining regions (HSRs), the latter occur mainly in tumors and the former in cell lines[84-86] (Fig. 14-2). However, there is no difference in clinical outcome whether *MYCN* amplification is manifested as DMs or HSRs in tumor samples

obtained at diagnosis.[87] Mice homozygous for disrupted *MYCN* die at about 10 days of gestation and have multiple organ defects, involving tissues of the central and peripheral nervous systems, mesonephros, lung, gut, and heart.[88,89]

MYCN is highly expressed in fetal and neonatal development but not in adult tissues; it is very high in newborn forebrain, hindbrain, kidney, and intestine.[90] *MYCN* is expressed in the fetal brain up to the onset of differentiation and is also present at high levels in neuroblasts migrating from the neural crest through the adrenal cortex.[91] Suppression of *MYCN* expression in neuroblastoma cell lines results in a more differentiated phenotype.[92] Downregulation of *MYCN* occurs in neuroblastoma cells induced to differentiate with chemical agents, and *MYCN* overexpression can block retinoic acid–induced differentiation.[93,94] Enhanced expression of *MYCN* and the mutant H-ras gene causes tumorigenic conversion of primary rat embryo fibroblasts, and these transformed cells elicit tumors in athymic mice and isogeneic rats.[95,96] Targeted expression of *MYCN* to the neuroectoderm of transgenic mice using a tyrosine hydroxylase promoter has resulted in the generation of neuroblastoma tumors, with cytogenetic abnormalities syntenic to those found in human tumors.[97,98]

MYCN amplification is noted in approximately 20% to 30% of all primary tumors and tends to be associated with advanced disease and a poor outcome.[83] It occurs in 5% to 10% of early-stage and stage 4S tumors and in 30% to 40% of tumors of patients with advanced-stage disease.[99,100] The detection of *MYCN* gene amplification in tumor cells at diagnosis is used by most cooperative groups to stratify patients to more intensive therapy. In 4S tumors, *MYCN* amplification predicts a poor outcome, although there is controversy as to whether this is also true in completely resected localized neuroblastoma.[101,102] *MYCN* copy number appears to be consistent throughout the natural course of the disease—that is, at diagnosis and relapse and between primary and metastatic tumors.[103] The Children's Oncology Group (COG) currently classifies *MYCN* amplification as more than 10 copies/diploid cell, but it is unclear whether lower levels of gain (i.e., *MYCN* copy number between 3 and 10) confers an adverse outcome. There is usually a correlation between amplification and increased *MYCN* expression, and tumors with *MYCN* amplification generally express higher levels of *MYCN* than nonamplified tumors; however, there is no link between high expression levels and a poor outcome.[104]

The genomic region amplified with *MYCN* is approximately 500 to 1000 kb and several genes have been shown to be coamplified with *MYCN* in neuroblastoma. These include *DDX1*,[105-107] *NAG*,[108,109] and *NCYM*[107,110,111] and these may contribute to the tumor phenotype.

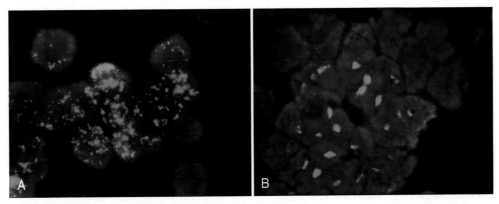

FIGURE 14-2. *MYCN* amplification in neuroblastoma. Fluorescence in situ hybridization image of neuroblastoma tumors depicting *MYCN* amplification manifested as double minutes **(A)** and homogeneously staining regions **(B)**. *(Courtesy L. Moreau, Dana-Farber Cancer Institute, Boston, MA.)*

ALK Amplification and Mutation in Neuroblastoma

ALK amplification has been detected in up to 15% of primary neuroblastomas with *MYCN* amplification.[65,112,113] Amplification has been associated with poor outcome.[64] ALK is a receptor tyrosine kinase of the insulin receptor superfamily. In human tumors, the most common mechanism of constitutive ALK activation involves chromosomal translocations that result in the generation of oncogenic *ALK* fusion genes, such as *NPM-ALK* in anaplastic large cell lymphoma[114] and *EML4-ALK* in non–small cell lung cancers,[115] among others.[116] However, translocations in human neuroblastoma tumors have not as yet been reported only in cell lines,[117] although the fusion partner has not been identified.

The ALK gene is also activated in neuroblastoma by mutations. Mutations have been identified in conserved positions in the tyrosine kinase domain in up to 8% of primary tumors,[65] of which the F1174L somatic mutation and the R1275Q germline mutation were found to be activating in Ba/F3 hematopoietic cells.[65] These mutations were associated with constitutive phosphorylation of ALK and that of downstream targets such as STAT3 and AKT. Ba/F3 cells and neuroblastoma cell lines expressing these mutations were found to be "addicted" to ALK and underwent apoptosis and cell cycle arrest after treatment with a small-molecule inhibitor of ALK. Thus, activating mutations of ALK provide a molecular rationale for targeted therapy of this disease.[65]

Allelic Loss of 1p

Deletion of the short arm of 1p has been described in neuroblastoma.[118] The common region of loss of heterozygosity is within 1p36.2-1p36.3.[119-121] However, this region may be much larger, extending from 1p35 to the terminal end.[122-124] This abnormality has also been reported in melanoma, pheochromocytoma, and medullary thyroid carcinoma, all of which are neural crest–derived tumors.[125-127]

Loss of heterozygosity (LOH) of 1p occurs in 30% to 40% of tumors[128] and is positively correlated with older age and advanced stage, *MYCN* amplification, and a poor outcome.[129] When *MYCN* amplification and 1p loss of heterozygosity are present together, they define a genetically distinct and very aggressive subset of neuroblastoma.[130] Because cases with *MYCN* amplification represent a subset of patients with 1p deletion (*MYCN* amplification is rarely found in the absence of 1p deletion), it is thought that 1p deletion may precede the development of *MYCN* amplification. Although in almost all samples with MYCN amplification 1p loss is also present, the latter is also seen in cases without *MYCN* amplification. 1p loss is strongly predictive of outcome, as documented in several studies, but a meta-analysis of several prognostic factors in neuroblastoma has revealed that *MYCN* amplification and ploidy are stronger predictors of outcome.[131] 1p loss thus may be used to identify patients with unfavorable outcome in patients without *MYCN* amplification.

There is evidence to suggest that loss or inactivation of a gene or genes on 1p is critical for the development or progression of neuroblastoma. This has been suggested by reports of constitutional 1p36 alterations in patients with neuroblastoma.[132] Transfection of chromosome 1p into a neuroblastoma cell line restores a differentiated phenotype and abrogates tumorigenicity.[133] In addition, cell fusion experiments between *MYCN*-amplified and single-copy cells have resulted in abrogation of *MYCN* expression, suggesting than *MYCN* expression is under the control of a suppressor gene located on 1p that is concomitantly deleted with *MYCN* amplification.[124] Several candidate tumor suppressor genes have been reported, including *CHD5*,[134-136] *KIF1B*,[137,138] *TP73*,[139] *CAMTA*,[140] and *CASTOR*.[141]

CHD5 (chromodomain helicase DNA binding domain 5), a member of the CHD family of proteins involved in chromatin remodeling, is preferentially expressed in the nervous system and maps to a small region of deletion on 1p36.3 in neuroblastomas.[136] Expression of CHD5 has been found to be low or absent in cell lines and tumors with 1p deletion. Low expression of CHD5 is also highly correlated with *MYCN* amplification, advanced stage, and unfavorable histology.[136,142] When CHD5 was expressed in neuroblastoma cell lines with low or absent expression, clonogenicity and tumor growth were abrogated.[135] Using chromosome engineering to generate mouse models with gain and loss of a region corresponding to human 1p36, CHD5 was identified as a tumor suppressor that controls proliferation, apoptosis, and senescence via the p19 (Arf)/p53 pathway.[134] CHD5 mutations are rare in neuroblastoma,[136] and the study by Bagchi and associates[134] has led to the suggestion that complete inactivation of the gene does not appear to be necessary for malignant transformation. Rather, gene dosage may be another mechanism that regulates tumor suppressor activity. In this study, increased dosage of CHD5 (as in wild-type or three copies) led to tumor suppressive properties. such as cellular senescence and apoptosis, whereas decreased dosage (as in heterozygous 1p deletion) enhances immortalization, spontaneous foci formation, and sensitivity to oncogenic transformation. Alternatively, it has been suggested that inactivation of the second allele may occur by an epigenetic phenomenon, because the CHD5 promoter was found to be highly methylated in two cell lines that lacked CHD5 expression.[135]

The kinesin KIF1B is located on 1p36.2 and is thought to function as a tumor suppressor gene in neuroblastoma and pheochromocytoma.[138] Germline loss-of-function mutations have been detected in neuroblastoma and the presence of these mutations causes abrogation of the apoptosis that is a requisite to normal neuronal developmental culling when NGF becomes limiting. Neuroblastoma cells have been shown to undergo apoptosis when NGF is withdrawn, which is mediated through the EglN3 prolyl hydroxylase. KIF1B acts downstream from EglN3. However, the one caveat is that in most cases with KIF1B mutations, the other allele is not deleted as predicted by the Knudson two-hit hypothesis.[143,144] Rather, it has been suggested that KIF1B haploinsufficiency may be sufficient for loss of its tumor suppressor activity, especially if combined with loss or abnormalities of other genes on 1p36, such as CHD5.[134] In support of this, when KIF1B levels were decreased to 50% using short hairpin RNA (shRNA) knockdown, apoptosis was blocked in these cells.[138]

The microRNA-34a (miRNA-34a) on 1p36.23 has been found to be expressed at lower levels in primary tumors and cell lines with 1p deletion and is also thought to function as a tumor suppressor gene.[145-147] Reintroduction of this miRNA into neuroblastoma cell lines with 1p deletion causes a dramatic reduction in cell proliferation through the induction of a caspase-dependent apoptotic pathway; this occurs by reducing levels of E2F3, a transcriptional inducer of cell cycle progression. miRNA-34a also increases during retinoic acid–induced differentiation of neuroblastoma cells.[145] In addition, miRNA-34a has also been found to be a direct target of *MYCN* and BCL2.[147] miRNA-34a causes significant suppression of cell growth through increased apoptosis and decreased DNA synthesis in neuroblastoma cell lines with *MYCN* amplification.[146]

Chromosome 17q Gain

Gain of chromosome 17q is the most common cytogenetic abnormality in neuroblastoma, occurring in more than 60% of tumors. It is associated with an unfavorable prognosis[148] and metastatic disease.[149] Gain usually takes the form of one to three extra copies. The breakpoints vary but, in general, gain of a region from 17q22–qter is observed. Partial gain often results from unbalanced translocation of 17q21-25 to another chromosome. Unbalanced 1;17 translocations occur in primary neuroblastoma and result in loss of distal 1p, with gain of 17q material.[150] Unbalanced 17q gain is associated with *MYCN* amplification and most likely harbors an oncogene that contributes to neuroblastoma tumorigenesis. However, 17q translocation breakpoints are not uniform and can involve other partner chromosomes, especially 11q.[151] The breakpoint positions on 11q were found to be variable, whereas all breakpoints on 17q appeared to cluster proximal to position 43.1 Mb on the DNA sequence map.[152]

Isogenic cell lines derived from *MYCN*-driven murine tumors in transgenic mice showed gains of regions syntenic with human 17q.[153] One of the candidate genes on 17q is survivin, whose expression is significantly associated with a poor prognosis.[154] Other candidate genes in the 17q region are nm23-H1 and nm23-H2, which are both strongly upregulated downstream targets of *MYCN*. Nm23-H1 binds to Cdc42, which is encoded on 1p36 and prevents induction of neuroblastoma cell differentiation. Overexpression of Nm23 caused by gain of 17q and the induction by *MYCN*, combined with decreased expression of Cdc42 caused by loss of 1p36, can block neuroblastoma tumor differentiation.[155]

Chromosome 11q Loss of Heterozygosity

Allelic loss of 11q occurs in 35% to 45% of primary tumors[156,157] but is rarely seen in tumors with *MYCN* amplification. Chromosome transfer experiments involving transfer of an intact chromosome 11 into a neuroblastoma cell line induces differentiation.[133] The common region of deletion has been mapped to 11q23, indicating that this could be a location for a neuroblastoma suppressor gene.[158] There have also been reports of constitutional rearrangements of 11q occurring in 4 patients.[159]

Chromosome 11q LOH is known to occur mainly in tumors without *MYCN* amplification but still identifies a high-risk subset of patients with advanced stage, older age, and unfavorable histology disease. Unbalanced deletion of 11q, which is deletion of the long arm with retention or gain of the short arm, occurs in 15% to 20% of cases and is associated with a poor event-free survival in patients with low- and intermediate-risk disease (Fig. 14-3).[160] Evaluation of 1p and 11q status and their effect on outcome is being prospectively evaluated in Children's Oncology Group (COG) studies and is now used for the risk stratification of intermediate-risk patients.

Chromosome 14q Loss of Heterozygosity

Deletion of 14q has also been reported in 25% of neuroblastomas,[161-163] with a common region of deletion within 14q23-qter.[164] LOH for 14q is inversely related to 1p36 LOH, *MYCN* amplification, and 11q LOH. It has been postulated that there may be two tumor suppressor genes on 14q, because there have been reports of two distinct regions of allelic loss on this chromosome arm.[165]

Other Rare Genetic and Molecular Aberrations

Other areas of gain noted especially in tumors with an aggressive clinical phenotype but not *MYCN* amplification include gain of 1q, 2p, 12q, and 17q.[166] Other chromosomal regions that have been deleted are 3p,[167] 4p,[168] 9p,[169] and 18q,[170] but these are all less common.

Mutations or deletions of p53 are rarely found in neuroblastoma[171-173] but may occasionally be associated with tumor progression[171] and in cell lines established at relapse.[174] Other mechanisms of involvement such as cytoplasmic sequestration, MDM2 amplification, or TWIST-mediated suppression have been proposed, although their contribution appears to be limited.[175-177] Although basal p53 expression in neuroblastoma cells is largely confined to the cytosol, p53 protein levels were found to increase mainly in the nucleus after radiation-induced DNA damage.[178] CDKN2 mutations and deletions also have rarely been found in neuroblastomas.[179,180] Although N-RAS was originally identified as the transforming gene in a neuroblastoma cell line no subsequent abnormalities in the RAS genes have been consistently reported. Targeting H-RAS to the neuroectoderm of mice leads to ganglioneuromas and, rarely, to neuroblastomas.[181] Rare examples of amplification of *CCND1*, *CDK4*, *MDM2*, and *MEIS1* have been reported in human neuroblastoma.[176,182-186] Microdeletions confined to the 5′ untranslated region (UTR) of the protein tyrosine phosphatase receptor D (PTPRD) gene have been detected in neuroblastomas.[186] It has also been shown that this 5′ UTR is also aberrantly spliced in more than 50% of primary tumors and cell lines. PTPRD is expressed at lower levels in high-stage neuroblastoma tumors, particularly those with amplification of *MYCN* relative to low-stage tumors or normal fetal adrenal neuroblasts. This is consistent with the possibility that loss of the 5′ UTR regions causes destabilization of the mRNA and is thus involved in neuroblastoma pathogenesis.[187]

Neurotrophin Expression in Neuroblastoma

The tyrosine kinase receptors TRKA, TRKB, and TRKC are receptors for the neurotrophic factors of the nerve growth factor family and are involved in normal neuronal development. The main ligand for TRKA is nerve growth factor (NGF), which promotes survival and induces differentiation in developing sympathetic neuroblasts. Neuroblastoma tumor cells with high levels of TRKA expression differentiate in the presence of NGF in vitro, but will undergo apoptosis in its absence.[188] Depending on the tumor microenvironment, therefore, TRKA signaling could induce differentiation or regression of favorable neuroblastomas. During normal development, depletion of NGF occurs in sympathetic neurons, causing TRKA signaling to activate predetermined apoptotic pathways. It has been postulated that spontaneous regression of neuroblastomas is only a delay in this normal developmental pattern.[189] A neurodevelopmentally regulated splice variant of TRKA, TrkAIII, has been identified that antagonizes the antioncogenic NGF/TRKA signaling and promotes neuroblastoma tumor growth.[190] High levels of TRKA expression are associated with a good prognosis in neuroblastoma and are strongly correlated with favorable tumor stage, younger age, and nonamplified *MYCN*. Patients with hyperdiploid tumors with favorable outcome identified by mass screening were also shown to have very high TRK-A expression.[188]

The TRKB transcript is expressed primarily in highly aggressive *MYCN*-amplified tumors.[191] The ligand for TRKB is BDNF, and activation by BDNF of TRKB leads to enhanced proliferation, migration, angiogenesis, and resistance to chemotherapy in neuroblastoma.[192] The full-length TRKB, which is expressed in about one third of tumors tested, is expressed primarily in those with *MYCN* amplification, whereas the truncated form resulting from alternative splicing, which lacks the tyrosine kinase domain, is expressed in ganglioneuromas and ganglioneuroblastoma.[191] The truncated TRKB is thought to sequester BDNF and thus prevent TRKB signaling.[193-195]

TRK-C, like TRKA, is involved in the biology of favorable neuroblastomas, and expression corresponds to lower stages.[196]

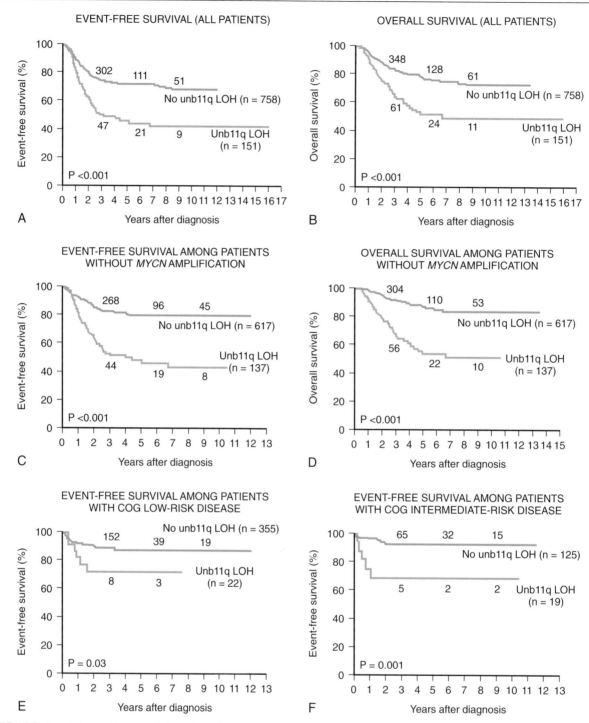

FIGURE 14-3. Survival according to unbalanced 11q loss of heterozygosity (unb11q LOH). The rates of event-free and overall survival are shown for all patients **(A, B)**, for those whose tumors did not have *MYCN* amplification **(C, D)**, and event-free survival for those with low-risk disease **(E)** and intermediate-risk disease **(F)** as defined by the Children's Oncology Group. The numbers of patients at risk for an event are shown along the curves. *(Adapted from Attiyeh EF, London WB, Mosse YP, et al. Chromosoe 1p and 11q deletions and outcome in neuroblastoma. N Engl J Med. 2005;353: 2243-2253.)*

It is expressed in 25% of primary neuroblastomas but does not have independent prognostic significance because all tumors with TRKC expression also have TRKA expression.

Apoptosis Pathways

Disruption of normal apoptotic pathways may be important in neuroblastoma. In contrast to most human tumor types, the

TP53 gene is rarely mutated in neuroblastoma. However, it has been found to be mutated in neuroblastoma cell lines established at relapse,[174] although the role that p53 plays in neuroblastoma apoptosis is unclear. BCl-2, an inhibitor of apoptosis, has been found to be associated with unfavorable histology and *MYCN* amplification.[197] Epigenetic modification of the proapoptotic gene caspase-8 has been observed in neuroblastomas.[60,198] Up to 70% of human neuroblastoma cell lines and 25% of primary tumors tested lack caspase-8 expression and fail to undergo apoptosis.[60,199,200] Loss of expression of both *CASP8* alleles is correlated with methylation of the caspase-8 gene,[60] and treatment with the demethylating agent, decitabine, restores caspase-8 expression[199,201] and increased susceptibility to doxorubicin-induced apoptosis.[60] In addition, methylation has been shown to be the mode of silencing of other genes involved in apoptosis—the four tumor necrosis factor–related apoptosis-inducing ligand (TRAIL) apoptosis receptors, the caspase-8 inhibitor FLIP (FLICE inhibitory protein), and other genes that function as tumor suppressors, such as *RASSF1A, p73, RB1, CD44, p14ARF,* and *p16INK4a*.[199,202] Because most of these genes may be involved in determining response to therapy, gene hypermethylation may be a mechanism of resistance to chemotherapeutic agents. Clinical trials of decitabine and other demethylating agents to determine the usefulness of exploiting this tumor specific aberration are ongoing.[203,204]

Drug Resistance

The multidrug resistance gene, P-glycoprotein, is thought to function by effecting enhanced drug efflux from the cell; its overexpression has been found to predict outcome of therapy for neuroblastoma.[205,206] The MRP gene located on chromosome 16p13.1 encodes a 190-kD membrane-bound glycoprotein that, like P-glycoprotein, mediates resistance to a number of drugs.[207,208] MRP is expressed by neuroblastoma tumors of all stages. Tumors with *MYCN* amplification have been shown to have significantly higher expression levels of MRP than those with normal *MYCN* copy numbers. Reduced MRP expression levels correlate with differentiation of neuroblastoma cells in vitro.[209] In addition, an association has been found between high levels of MRP expression and poor outcome, which is independent of *MYCN* amplification.[210] It is possible that both *MDR1* and *MRP* function together with several other factors that confer resistance to drug therapy in neuroblastoma such as *MYCN* amplification, TRKB signaling, or loss of p53 expression.[192,211]

Tumor Angiogenesis

Neuroblastoma is characterized by prominent angiogenesis, and neuroblastoma cells have been shown to induce angiogenesis in the chick embryo chorioallantoic membrane assay.[212] Increased tumor vascularity and microvascular proliferation are correlated with widely disseminated disease, *MYCN* amplification, unfavorable histology, and a poor outcome.[213-215] Such aggressive tumors are associated with high expression of vascular endothelial growth factor, basic fibroblastic growth factor, platelet-derived growth factor A,[213,216] and integrins, which are markers of active angiogenesis.[217] The presence of angiogenesis appears to be influenced by the cellular composition of the tumor in that in highly aggressive stroma-poor neuroblastoma, angiogenesis is present because of the secretion of angiogenic stimulators, whereas in stroma-rich tumors, numerous angiogenic inhibitors secreted by Schwann cells appear to maintain the inhibitory phenotype.[218] The Schwann cells in neuroblastoma tumors have been shown to have low tumor vascularity with production of angiogenesis inhibitors, such as tissue inhibitor of matrix metalloproteinase-2 (MMP-2), pigment epithelium–derived factor, and SPARC (secreted protein acidic and rich in cysteine), a calcium-binding matricellular glycoprotein.[213,219,220] SPARC expression has been found to be inversely correlated with the degree of malignant progression in neuroblastoma tumors, and neutralizing SPARC with antibodies reverses the antiangiogenic activity of Schwann cell–conditioned media.[219]

Metastasis

Little is known about the regulators of metastasis in neuroblastoma. Nevertheless, metalloproteinases such as MMP9, and CD44 and NM23-H1, which regulate tumor cell adhesion and migration, may play a role in metastasis.[221-223] Overexpression of MMP2 and MMP9 is associated with tumor invasion and metastasis in many types of cancer, whereas inhibitors of MMPs have been shown to suppress tumor invasion and angiogenesis. An association between increased levels of MMP-2 and -9 and advanced-stage tumors has been observed in neuroblastoma. Caspase-8 has also been shown to be a metastasis suppressor gene.[224] Decreased caspase-8 expression has been shown to occur during the establishment of neuroblastoma metastases in vivo, and induction of caspase-8 expression in deficient neuroblastoma cells suppresses these metastases. Caspase-8 selectively potentiates apoptosis in metastasizing cells, and loss of caspase-8 allows cellular survival in the stromal microenvironment and promotes metastases.

Histopathology

Neuroblastomas arise from primitive sympathetic precursors of the neural crest and belong to the family of small round blue cell tumors. The histopathology of the tumor cells correlates with stages of sympathetic nervous system development. Tumors are composed of small blue round cells, uniformly sized, containing dense hyperchromatic nuclei and scant cytoplasm. Surrounding the neuroblasts is stroma, known as Schwannian stroma. A typical feature of neuroblastoma is the presence of neuropil, which is made up of neuritic processes and is found in most neuroblastomas. One of the pathognomonic features of neuroblastoma is the Homer-Wright pseudorosette, a collection of neuroblasts surrounding areas of neuropil, which occurs in up to half of cases (1% to 50%; Fig. 14-4A).[225]

Neuroblastoma manifests as a spectrum of three histologic patterns, ranging from neuroblastoma to ganglioneuroblastoma to ganglioneuroma, based on the degree of tumor cell differentiation. Neuroblastomas are composed of mostly small immature blue round cells with scanty cytoplasm, little evidence of differentiation, and high mitotic activity. Ganglioneuroblastomas are tumors with differentiated ganglion cells admixed with neuroblastic tissue. These tumors may vary from predominantly neuroblastic, with rare ganglion cells, to predominantly maturing cells, with rare undifferentiated components such as neuroblastic cells. If there are less than 50% of maturing cells, the tumor is termed a *maturing neuroblastoma* and, if more than 50%, it is termed a *ganglioneuroblastoma*. Ganglioneuroblastomas can also be focal or diffuse and both types can exist in a single tumor. There are two forms of ganglioneuroblastoma: (1) the intermixed variety, in which cells in various stages of differentiation are interspersed with small nests of neuroblasts that predict a good outcome; and (2) the nodular type, in which there are hemorrhagic areas and macroscopic nodules, which is associated with a worse prognosis. Ganglioneuromas are fully differentiated tumors consisting entirely of maturing ganglion cells, neuropil Schwannian stroma, and nerve fibers.[226,227]

Primary histologic diagnosis may be enabled by hematoxylin and eosin (H&E) staining and light microscopy. Other techniques also help distinguish neuroblastomas from other small blue round cell tumors of childhood such as immunohistochemistry using antibodies for neural markers, such as neurofilament protein, synaptophysin, neuron-specific enolase, ganglioside GD2, chromogranin A, and tyrosine hydroxylase. Electron microscopy studies may exhibit dense core mem-

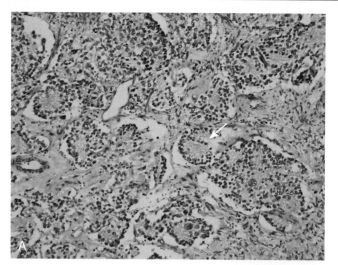

FIGURE 14-4. Neuroblastoma pathology. **A,** Neuroblastoma tumor showing aggregates of tumors, which are composed of small immature blue round cells, uniformly sized, containing dense hyperchromatic nuclei and scant cytoplasm. Homer-Wright pseudorosettes, which are rings of neuroblasts surrounding eosinophilic neuropil, are seen (*arrow*). **B,** Schematic representation of the International Neuroblastoma Pathology Classification. (*B from Park JR, Eggert A, Caron H. Neuroblastoma: biology, prognosis, and treatment. Pediatr Clin North Am. 2008;55: 97-120.*)

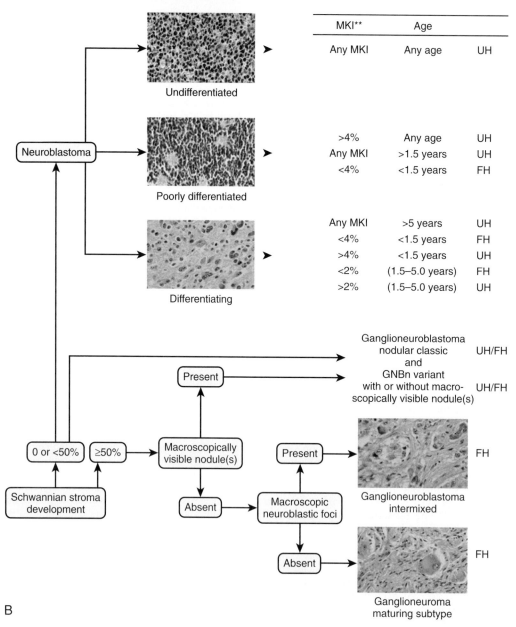

brane–bound neurosecretory granules, microfilaments and parallel arrays of microtubules within the neuropil.[228]

Tumor histology in neuroblastoma has traditionally been determined by the Shimada classification system.[229] Tumors are classified as favorable or unfavorable based on the three features of amount of stroma, degree of neuroblastic cell differentiation, and the mitosis-karyorrhexis index (MKI—the percentage of tumor cells in mitosis versus karyorrhexis). This, however, has one drawback in that it is age-linked, and age itself is a strong independent prognostic feature in neuroblastoma. The Joshi system is simpler in that it examines the presence of calcification and mitotic rate (≤10 mitoses/10 HPF [high-power fields]), and was designed to be independent of age and stage; however, it does not have the same prognostic power as the Shimada system.[230] Subsequently, a unified classification, the International Neuroblastoma Pathology Classification (INPC) was established in 1999[231] and revised in 2003.[232] This classification schema was formulated based on the natural history of neuroblastoma of involution and maturation, as described by Beckwith and Perrin.[29] In other words, it is based on the age-dependent normal ranges of morphologic features such as schwannian stroma, degree of neuroblastic differentiation, and MKI and seeks to divide neuroblastic tumors into those with favorable histology and those with unfavorable histology (see Fig. 14-4B).[233]

There are four main morphologic categories in the INPC system (Table 14-1):

1. Neuroblastoma (Schwannian stroma–poor). This is a tumor with nests of neuroblastic cells interspersed with little or minimal stroma. There are three subtypes, based on grade of differentiation: (1) undifferentiated; (2) poorly differentiated (some neuropil and less than 5% of cells exhibiting differentiation); and (3) differentiating (abundant neuropil and more than 5% of cells showing differentiation toward ganglion cells).
2. Ganglioneuroblastoma, intermixed (Schwannian stroma-rich). This tumor contains well-defined microscopic nests

of neuroblastic cells intermixed in ganglioneuromatous stroma. The nests are composed of neuroblastic cells in various stages of differentiation, but primarily composed of differentiating neuroblasts and maturing ganglion cells in a background of neuropil.
3. Ganglioneuroblastoma, nodular (composite Schwannian stroma-rich, stroma-dominant and stroma-poor). This tumor is composed of biologically different clones, an aggressive clone composed of grossly visible, hemorrhagic neuroblastic nodules (stroma-poor component), and a nonaggressive clone composed of ganglioneuroblastoma, intermixed (stroma-rich component) or ganglioneuroma (stroma-dominant component).
4. Ganglioneuroma (Schwannian stroma-dominant). There are two subtypes of these, maturing and mature. The maturing subtype is composed predominantly of ganglioneuromatous stroma with scattered differentiating neuroblasts or maturing ganglion cells, as well as fully mature ganglion cells. The mature subtype is composed of ganglion cells and Schwannian stroma.

In the new and revised International Neuroblastoma Risk Group (INRG) classification schema, tumor histology will be classified independent of age and will primarily be based on degree of differentiation and MKI.

CLINICAL PRESENTATION

Neuroblastomas are tumors of the sympathetic nervous system and can arise anywhere along the sympathetic chain or in any sympathetic ganglia. Most primary tumors occur in the abdomen (65%), and half of abdominal tumors occur in the adrenal gland. Other common sites of disease origin include the chest, neck, and pelvis although, rarely, a primary tumor cannot be found. Because the sites of origin of neuroblastoma

TABLE 14-1 International Neuroblastoma Pathology Classification

International Neuroblastoma Pathology Classification		Original Shimada Classification	Prognostic Group
Neuroblastoma Favorable	Schwannian stroma-poor*	Stroma-poor Favorable	Favorable
<1.5 yr	Poorly differentiated or differentiating and low or intermediate MKI tumor		
1.5-5 yr	Differentiating and low MKI tumor		
Unfavorable		Unfavorable	Unfavorable
<1.5 yr	1. Undifferentiated tumor† 2. High MKI tumor		
1.5-5 yr	1. Undifferentiated or poorly differentiated tumor 2. Intermediate or high MKI tumor		
≥5 yr	All tumors		
Ganglioneuroblastoma, nodular	Composite Schwannian stroma-rich/ stroma-dominant and stroma-poor	Stroma-rich nodular (Unfavorable)	Unfavorable‡
Ganglioneuroblastoma, intermixed	Schwannian stroma-rich	Stroma-rich intermixed (Favorable)	Favorable‡
Ganglioneuroma Maturing Mature	Schwannian stroma–dominant	Well-differentiated (favorable) Ganglioneuroma	Favorable‡

MKI, mitosis-karyorrhexis index.
*Subtypes of neuroblastoma are described in detail elsewhere (Shimada et al[390]).
†Rare subtype, especially diagnosed in this age group. Further investigation and analysis are required.
‡Prognostic grouping for these tumor categories is not related to patient age.
Adapted from Shimada H, Ambros IM, Dehner LP, et al. The International Neuroblastoma Pathology Classification (Shimada) System. Cancer. 1999;86:364-372.

are so diverse, the signs and symptoms of disease at presentation vary widely and depend on the location of the primary tumor and degree of disease dissemination.

Localized Disease

Approximately 40% of patients will present with localized disease.[234] Primary abdominal disease can present as an asymptomatic abdominal mass or with abdominal pain and fullness. Symptoms of obstruction can occasionally be seen, as well as renin-mediated hypertension caused by compression of the renal vasculature.[235] Abdominal or pelvic tumors can also occasionally cause compression of lower extremity venous and lymphatic drainage, leading to lower extremity and scrotal swelling. Rarely, abdominal tumors will spontaneously hemorrhage and patients will present with a sudden, dramatic enlargement of an abdominal mass, with increased distention and pain. Lower thoracic tumors are usually identified incidentally when a chest radiograph is obtained for unrelated reasons. Occasionally, large thoracic tumors are associated with mechanical obstruction and resultant superior vena cava syndrome. Upper thoracic or cervical tumors may cause Horner's syndrome.[236] Congenital tumors arising in this site can also cause heterochromia of the iris because of decreased pigmentation of the iris on the affected side.[237] Neuroblastoma arising from the paraspinal ganglia in the chest, abdomen, or pelvis can grow through the intervertebral foramina and compress the spinal cord. Patients may be asymptomatic or present with pain or neurologic deficits resulting from spinal cord compression. which requires emergent treatment (see later).

Metastatic Disease

Metastatic spread of neuroblastoma occurs through the lymphatics or hematogenously. Regional lymph node metastases are seen in one third of patients with apparently localized tumors, and half of patients present with hematogenous metastases.[234] Hematogenous spread occurs most frequently to the bone, bone marrow, and/or liver and rarely to the lungs and brain, usually at relapse rather than presentation. Classic signs of metastatic neuroblastoma include proptosis and periorbital ecchymoses (commonly referred to as raccoon eyes) caused by tumor infiltration of the periorbital bones. Patients also frequently present with limping and irritability caused by bone pain from bone and bone marrow disease as well as nonspecific symptoms, including fever and failure to thrive. The presence of fever is usually associated with extensive bone metastases. Signs and symptoms of bone marrow replacement are also sometimes seen, including most frequently pallor, which may also be caused by bleeding within the primary tumor, and bruising and increased risk infection caused by a low white blood cell count.[238]

Stage 4S (S, special) is a unique presentation of neuroblastoma seen in infants originally described by D'Angio and coworkers in 1971.[239] Infants with stage 4S neuroblastoma often present with massive hepatomegaly caused by diffuse liver metastases and nontender, bluish subcutaneous nodules caused by skin metastases. Stage 4S disease accounts for 7% to 12% of neuroblastoma diagnoses and is characterized by the presence of a small, localized primary tumor with metastases isolated to the liver, skin, and/or bone marrow.[240] This special neuroblastoma often spontaneously regresses, although infants younger than 2 months can present with respiratory compromise caused by a rapidly enlarging liver and may require cancer-directed treatment.[241]

Paraneoplastic Syndromes

Two paraneoplastic syndromes, opsoclonus-myoclonus syndrome and vasoactive intestinal peptide syndrome, are associated with neuroblastoma (see later). Patients with these syndromes usually have localized tumors with favorable biology. This may be because the syndrome causes early detection of tumor or, more likely, because of a correlation between the syndrome and the tumor biology.

Opsoclonus-myoclonus syndrome (OMS) is seen in 2% to 3% of children with neuroblastoma[242] and is usually diagnosed between the age of 1 and 3 years.[243] It is often referred to as dancing eyes, dancing feet syndrome and is characterized by the acute onset of rapid eye movements, ataxia, myoclonic jerking of the limbs and trunk, and behavioral disturbances.[243] Although children with neuroblastoma and opsoclonus-myoclonus generally have favorable tumor prognostic features and a high survival rate,[244-246] 70% to 80% suffer from long-term neurologic sequelae, which can include global developmental delay, speech and/or motor delay, behavioral disturbances, and cognitive deficits that can seriously affect quality of life.[242,245,247,248] OMS in children is associated with neuroblastoma more than half of the time.[243] After exclusion of central nervous system pathology, all children with OMS should be evaluated for neuroblastoma, with imaging of their abdomen, a ^{123}I-metaiodobenzylguanidine scan, and urine catecholamine analysis.[249]

OMS and its sequelae are thought to be immune-mediated, likely caused by the presence of an antineural antibody that cross-reacts with a common antigen on neuroblastoma and normal nervous system tissue.[243] Improvement in symptoms can be seen after tumor removal in some cases, but generally immunosuppression with glucocorticoids or adrenocorticotropic hormone is used to relieve acute symptoms.[243,245] However, over 80% of patients will have a relapse of symptoms with steroid weaning or in association with a viral syndrome,[249] and more than 50% of patients will need prolonged steroid treatment. Intravenous immune globulin has also been used in the treatment of OMS, with or without steroids, with varying success.[250,251] Case reports has shown efficacy of other immunomodulating strategies, including plasmapheresis and rituximab.[252-254] Although often effective in treating acute symptoms, none of these treatments has been consistently correlated with improved long-term outcome. Interestingly, a report from the Pediatric Oncology Group has suggested that patients who receive chemotherapy to treat their neuroblastoma have a more favorable neurologic outcome.[242] This benefit may be a result of the immunosuppressive effects of chemotherapy or of less severe activation of the immune system in patients with more advanced stages of tumor.[243] The same benefit was not observed in a similar review done by the Children's Cancer Group[245] and the benefit of chemotherapy for the treatment of OMS needs to be investigated further. COG is currently running a randomized trial for OMS in which patients with low-risk neuroblastoma who would not otherwise receive chemotherapy will receive cyclophosphamide in addition to steroids. Patients will also be randomized to intravenous immunoglobulin or not. Regardless of treatment, physicians caring for patients with OMS should anticipate long-term neurologic abnormalities and use early intervention strategies to help minimize these deficits.

Tumor secretion of vasoactive intestinal peptide can cause a syndrome of chronic water diarrhea and failure to thrive. Most tumors secreting vasoactive intestinal peptide are histologically mature. Surgical removal of the tumor usually results in complete resolution of symptoms.[255]

DIAGNOSIS AND EVALUATION

Diagnosis

The diagnosis of neuroblastoma is usually established from the histopathologic evaluation of primary tumor tissue.[256] In most cases, especially if features of neuronal differentiation are present, a tissue diagnosis of neuroblastoma can be made based on conventional H&E staining. However, in cases in which there is little differentiation and only small round blue cells are seen, immunohistochemical staining for neuron-specific enolase, chromogranin A, and/or synaptophysin, as well as cytogenetic and molecular analyses, can help differentiate neuroblastoma from other small round blue cell tumors of childhood.[252-254]

In addition to establishing the diagnosis, primary tumor material is essential for risk stratification and prognosis, particularly in children younger than 18 months with locoregional or metastatic spread. In cases in which primary tumor tissue cannot be obtained safely, the diagnosis of neuroblastoma can also be made by demonstrating unequivocal neuroblastoma cells in a bone marrow aspirate or biopsy in conjunction with increased urinary catecholamine levels. Urinary catecholamine metabolites are increased in 90% to 95% of neuroblastomas, as determined by sensitive detection techniques, such as high-performance liquid chromatography,[257,258] and can be helpful in establishing a diagnosis and in monitoring disease activity and response to therapy in patients known to excrete the metabolites. In sympathetic cells, the catecholamine precursor 3,4-dihydroxyphenylalanine (DOPA) is converted to dopamine by DOPA decarboxylase, which is converted to norepinephrine and then epinephrine by the enzyme phenylethanolamine *N*-methyltransferase, which is not present in neuroblastoma cells.[259] Instead, the enzymes catechol-O-methyl transferase and monoamine oxidase convert DOPA and dopamine to homovanillic acid (HVA) and norepinephrine and epinephrine to vanillylmandelic acid (VMA), inactive metabolites that are excreted in the urine. Both urinary HVA and VMA should be measured for diagnostic purposes. For undifferentiated tumors, urinary dopamine measurement may also be useful.[256] Despite this catecholamine production, symptoms of catecholamine excess such as hypertension, flushing, and sweating are rarely seen in neuroblastoma, likely because of the relatively low concentrations of active catecholamines in the circulation.

Clinical Disease Assessment

The primary tumor and the extent of disease should be evaluated using imaging techniques both at diagnosis and to evaluate response to treatment. Computed tomography (CT) or magnetic resonance imaging (MRI) should be used to evaluate the extent and origin of the primary tumor, as well as possible solid organ metastases. CT is generally the preferred method for evaluating tumors and metastases in the abdomen, pelvis, or mediastinum whereas MRI is superior for assessing paraspinal lesions, particularly those with possible intraspinal extension and spinal cord impingement. Although not as useful for assessing tumor volume and anatomy, abdominal ultrasonography may be useful as a noninvasive method for following tumor response or surveying for disease relapse. Brain imaging is only recommended if clinically indicated by symptoms or examination.

Bone and bone marrow disease can also be evaluated radiographically. Bone scan using ^{99m}Tc-diphosphonate scintigraphy is a relatively sensitive method to survey for occult bony metastases, although it is somewhat nonspecific. Metaiodo-benzylguanidine (MIBG) is a norepinephrine analogue that is selectively concentrated in more than 90% to 95% of neuroblastomas and can be combined with ^{131}I or ^{123}I isotopes for scanning purposes. MIBG scintigraphy provides enhanced sensitivity and specificity for detecting bony metastases over a traditional bone scan, and can also be used to assess the primary tumor and occult soft tissue disease (Fig. 14-5).[260] The ^{123}I isotope provides enhanced image resolution and is the isotope of choice, when available. Because not all neuroblastomas take up MIBG, it is common practice to obtain a bone scan and MIBG scan at diagnosis, particularly in patients with suspected metastatic disease. If the diagnostic bone scan does not provide independent information, it can be omitted in favor of the MIBG scan for further disease assessment.[234] Positron emission tomography (PET) can also be used to evaluate metastatic disease in neuroblastoma.[261-263] Its sensitivity and specificity in comparison to MIBG scintigraphy still need to be evaluated.

Bone marrow aspirates and biopsies from both iliac crests are recommended to assess for the presence of bone marrow disease using standard histologic analysis.[256,264] Both immunocytochemical and polymerase chain reaction (PCR)–based technologies can be used to increase the sensitivity of marrow detection. Immunocytochemical analysis of bone marrow aspirates with monoclonal antibodies directed against neural-specific antigens (e.g., GD2, NCAM) increases the sensitivity of detecting marrow involvement to 1 in 100,000 nucleated cells.[265] Reverse transcriptase PCR methodologies that target the expression of neuroblastoma-specific messages such as tyrosine hydroxylase, PGP 9.5, or GD2 synthase can enhance sensitivity further.[266-271] The clinical and prognostic significance of this enhanced detection, however, remains to be determined, and these studies are generally only recommended within the context of a clinical study.

Staging

The International Neuroblastoma Staging System (INSS) was established in the 1990s to replace three major staging systems used throughout the world in an effort to provide international uniformity so that clinical trials and biology studies done by different groups in different countries could be compared.[256,264] The INSS (Box 14-1) is based on clinical, radiographic, and surgical assessments of a patient at diagnosis and is currently in use nationally and internationally. However, one weakness of the current staging system is that surgical approaches are not uniform from one institution to another and the INSS stage for patients with locoregional disease can vary considerably, depending on the degree of initial tumor resection. To address this problem, an international presurgical staging system being considered will be largely based on imaging studies and bone marrow morphology. This new staging system will use an approach developed by the European International Society of Pediatric Oncology Neuroblastoma Group, which uses radiologic characteristics of the primary tumor to predict surgical risk and resectability.[272] Using this approach in the new staging system, locoregional disease will be staged according to whether or not the tumor is locally invasive.

Risk Stratification

Neuroblastoma is a tumor in which biologic factors are consistently used to influence disease risk stratification and treatment. The COG currently stratifies patients into low-, intermediate-, or high-risk categories based on prognostic features, including age at diagnosis, stage, tumor histology, DNA index (ploidy),

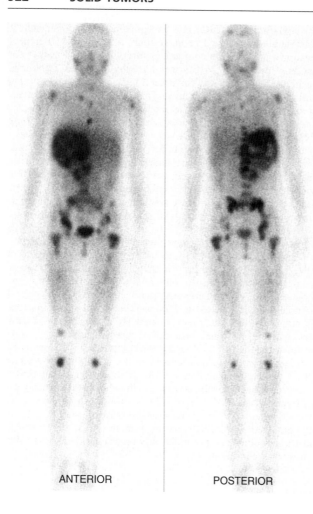

ANTERIOR   POSTERIOR

FIGURE 14-5. Metaiodobenzylguanidine (MIBG) scan. Primary tumor uptake (right adrenal gland) as well as bone and bone marrow metastases are visualized. *(Courtesy of Dr. F. Grant, Division of Nuclear Medicine, Children's Hospital, Boston.)*

Box 14-1 **International Neuroblastoma Staging System**

Stage 1: Localized tumor with complete gross excision, with or without microscopic residual disease; representative ipsilateral lymph nodes negative for tumor microscopically (nodes attached to and removed with the primary tumor may be positive).

Stage 2A: Localized tumor with incomplete gross excision; representative ipsilateral nonadherent lymph nodes negative for tumor microscopically.

Stage 2B: Localized tumor with or without complete gross excision, with ipsilateral nonadherent lymph nodes positive for tumor. Enlarged contralateral lymph nodes must be negative microscopically.

Stage 3: Unresectable unilateral tumor infiltrating across the midline,* with or without regional lymph node involvement;

or localized unilateral tumor with contralateral regional lymph node involvement;

or midline tumor with bilateral extension by infiltration (unresectable) or by lymph node involvement.

Stage 4: Any primary tumor with dissemination to distant lymph nodes, bone, bone marrow, liver, skin, and/or other organs (except as defined for stage 4S).

Stage 4S: Localized primary tumor (as defined for stage 1, 2A, or 2B), with dissemination limited to skin, liver, and/or bone marrow† (limited to infants younger than 1 year).

Note: Multifocal primary tumors (e.g., bilateral adrenal primary tumors) should be staged according to the greatest extent of disease, as defined earlier, followed by a subscript M (e.g., 3_M).

---

*The midline is defined as the vertebral column. Tumors originating on one side and crossing the midline must infiltrate to or beyond the opposite side of the vertebral column.

†Marrow involvement in stage 4S should be minimal—that is, less than 10% of total nucleated cells identified as malignant on bone marrow biopsy or aspirate. More extensive marrow involvement would be considered to be stage 4. The MIBG scan (if done) should be negative in the marrow.

From Brodeur GM, Pritchard J, Berthold F, et al. Revisions of the international criteria for neuroblastoma diagnosis, staging, and response to treatment. J Clin Oncol. 1993;11:1466-1477.

TABLE 14-2	**Current Children's Oncology Group Risk Group Classification**				
INSS	**Age (days)**	**MYCN***	**Ploidy**	**Shimada†**	**Risk Group**
1	Any	Any	Any	Any	Low
2	Any	Not amp	Any	Any	Low
2	Any	Amp	Any	Any	High
3	<547	Not amp	Any	Any	Intermediate
3	≥547	Not amp	Any	FH	Intermediate
3	≥547	Not amp	Any	UH	High
3	Any	Amp	Any	Any	High
4	<365	Amp	Any	Any	High
4	<365	Not amp	Any	Any	Intermediate
4	365–<547	Not amp	>1	FH	Intermediate
4	365–<547	Any	1	Any	High
4	365–<547	Any	Any	UH	High
4	365–<547	Amp	Any	Any	High
4	≥547	Any	Any	Any	High
4S	<365	Not amp	>1	FH	Low
4S	<365	Not amp	1	Any	Intermediate
4S	<365	Not amp	Any	UH	Intermediate
4S	<365	Amp	Any	Any	High

MYCN amplification status: Amp = amplified; Not amp = not amplified.
†International Neuroblastoma Pathology Classification: FH = favorable histology; UH = unfavorable histology.
INSS, International Neuroblastoma Staging System.
Adapted from Maris JM, Hogarty MD, Bagatell R, Cohn SL. Neuroblastoma. Lancet. 2007;369:2106-2120.

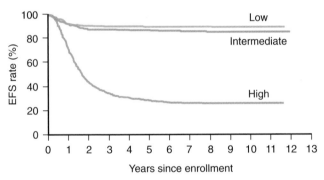

FIGURE 14-6. Event-free survival (EFS) of patients with neuroblastoma stratified according to risk group. *(Courtesy of Dr. W.B. London, Children's Oncology Group, Gainesville, FL.)*

and *MYCN* amplification status (Table 14-2). Treatment recommendations are based on this risk-grouping, as described in the next section, and prognosis is distinct for each risk group (Fig. 14-6).

In an effort to unify risk stratification internationally, the INRG classification system was formed by a working group composed of clinicians and researchers from all over the world, representing the major pediatric cooperative groups. Following a meeting in 2005 to review data obtained for 11,054 patients treated between 1974 and 2002, age (dichotomized at 18 months), stage at diagnosis, and *MYCN* status were selected for initial risk grouping. Other factors that are still being analyzed include histologic classification, ploidy, and 11q status. The significance of these risk factors is discussed later.

Clinical Variables

Age is an important prognostic factor in neuroblastoma. Traditionally, it was thought that infants (those younger than 1 year or 365 days old) had a more favorable outcome, whereas those older than 1 to 2 years had a more dismal outcome, especially those with metastatic disease at diagnosis.[273,274] Recent studies of a large series of cases have demonstrated, however, that age is a continuous prognostic variable in neuroblastoma and have identified 18 months as the age under which patients with stages 3 or 4 disease share the same favorable outlook as those younger than 1 year (Fig. 14-7).[80,275,276] Whether children between 12 and 18 months of age can be cured with less aggressive therapy is currently under investigation.

Stage has always been considered an important prognostic factor, with low-stage or localized disease having a better outcome than high-stage or metastatic disease; the overall prognosis for stages 1, 2 and 4S is 80% to 90%, whereas those between stages 3 and 4 have a 2-year survival rate of 20% to 40%.[259] Prior to 1990, various image-based and surgery-based staging systems were in place. In the 1990s, as noted, the INSS was developed in an effort to unify staging internationally.[256] However, because surgical approaches to locoregional disease can vary among countries, a presurgical staging system has been formulated that uses surgical risk factors to define extent of disease.[277] Surgical risk factors are those radiologic characteristics of the tumor that predict the resectability of the primary tumor and the risk of developing postoperative complications.[272] Therefore, in the proposed INRG staging system, extent of disease will be determined by imaging studies and bone marrow morphology. In this system, locoregional tumors that do not invade local structures (INRG stage L1) will be distinguished from locally invasive tumors (INRG stage L2) by radiologic features. Stages M and MS will categorize tumors that are widely metastatic or have an INSS stage 4S pattern of disease, respectively.[234] This risk grouping system is being prospectively validated in Europe and North America.

Pathologic features are also used to classify neuroblastomas. The Shimada classification divides tumors as having favorable and unfavorable histology by incorporating age with tumor differentiation, MKI, and schwannian stroma.[278] However, because age itself is a strong independent prognostic variable, new classification systems such as the INRG examine MKI and differentiation as independent variables, along with established clinical and biologic variables.

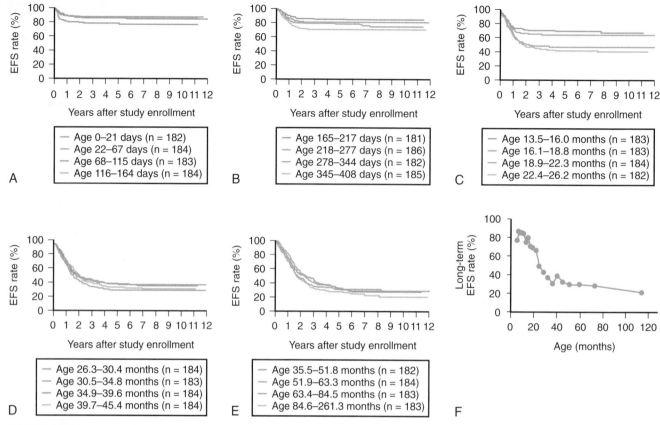

FIGURE 14-7. Kaplan-Meier event-free survival (EFS) curves by age group. **A,** 0 to 164 days. **B,** 165 to 408 days. **C,** 13.5 to 26.2 months. **D,** 26.3 to 45.4 months. **E,** 35.5 to 261.3 months. **F,** Long-term EFS rate by age group (not a Kaplan-Meier curve). *(Adapted from London WB, Castleberry RP, Matthay KK, et al. Evidence for an age cutoff greater than 365 days for neuroblastoma risk group stratification in the Children's Oncology Group. J Clin Oncol. 2005;23:6459-6465.)*

Biologic Variables

DNA index or ploidy is used in the current risk stratification system of neuroblastoma and is considered prognostic in children up to 18 months of age (see Table 14-2).[80] Neuroblastoma tumors are classified as diploid (DNA index [DI] = 1) and hyperdiploid (DI > 1). There are two situations in which a DI of 1 would automatically stratify a patient to the high-risk group:

1. 12 to 18 months of age, with stage 4 disease. In this age group, a DI of 1 stratifies patients to high risk regardless of *MYCN* amplification status or histology,
2. Similarly, presence of diploid DNA content in infants (younger than 12 months) with *MYCN* nonamplified, stage 4S disease will signify intermediate risk, regardless of tumor histology.

As described previously, *MYCN* amplification is found in 20% to 30% of neuroblastomas. It is strongly correlated with advanced-stage disease and a poor outcome. The presence of *MYCN* amplification automatically stratifies children into the high-risk category in most cases, except for completely resected INSS tumors, which remains controversial (see next section). Chromosome 1p loss occurs in older children with stage 3 or 4 disease. In addition, almost all cases of *MYCN* amplification occur with concomitant 1p loss, although isolated 1p loss has also been demonstrated.[128] Chromosome 1p LOH is a strong predictor of outcome,[128,279] and its greatest use may be to identify high-risk patients with *MYCN* single-copy tumors. Chromosome 11q loss is seen in 40% of patients and is inversely correlated with *MYCN* amplification[279]; it could potentially identify an additional high-risk subset of patients characterized by advanced stage, older age, and unfavorable histology. Unbalanced 11q loss, which occurs in a smaller number of cases (15% to 20%), is more clearly associated with high-risk biologic features.[160] Prospective evaluation of 1p and 11q status is ongoing in cooperative group trials and will be aimed at stratification of intermediate-risk patients.

APPROACH TO TREATMENT

The modalities used in the treatment of neuroblastoma include surgery, chemotherapy, radiotherapy, and biotherapy, as well as observation alone in a small subset of patients. The determination of treatment is largely based on prognostic factors and subsequent risk group assignment (see earlier). A major goal of ongoing neuroblastoma clinical trials is to validate the existing risk group assignments and evaluate newer prognostic markers for future refinement of risk stratification and treatment assignment. The general principles of therapy for each of the current risk groups are detailed here.

Risk Groups

Treatment of Low-Risk Disease

Surgical resection of the primary tumor is usually the only treatment required for patients with low-risk neuroblastoma. The COG currently recommends surgical resection followed by close observation for INSS 1 patients and INSS 2 patients with more than 50% tumor resected at diagnosis. A prospective CCG study for low-risk patients has reported a 93% 4-year EFS rate and a 99% 4-year overall survival (OS) rate for 141 Evans stage I patients.[280] This study also reported a 4-year EFS of 81% with surgery alone and a 4-year OS of 98% for 233 Evans stage II patients (56% INSS 2) with single-copy *MYCN*.[280] The extent of surgical resection had no effect on EFS or OS in the stage II patients. INSS 2 patients with less than 50% tumor resection at diagnosis are currently treated with two to four cycles of intermediate-risk chemotherapy, depending on biologic features (see later). Disease recurrence usually occurs within 1 year of diagnosis and most recurrences are local.[280-282] Local recurrences in low-risk patients can usually be managed with second surgeries. Metastatic recurrences are rare but often salvageable with more intensive systemic therapy.

Neuroblastoma is known to have one of the highest rates of spontaneous regression among malignant tumors, which has been well documented in stage 4S disease (see earlier). Data from mass screening studies in Japan show a two- to threefold higher incidence of neuroblastoma in areas with screening programs.[283] This increase in the rate of diagnosis supports the hypothesis that a subset of non–stage 4S neuroblastomas in young infants can undergo spontaneous regression as well. The German Society of Pediatric Oncology and Hematology recently reported a prospective trial supporting this hypothesis.[284] Ninety-three infants with localized neuroblastoma were observed without surgery or chemotherapy. Spontaneous regression was seen in 44 of 93 (47%) infants and 17 had a complete regression. The 3-year EFS (56% ± 5%) was low because approximately half of the infants required an intervention, but the OS remained excellent (99% ± 1%). The COG is currently running an observation study for perinatally detected adrenal tumors to explore the hypothesis of spontaneous regression in young infants with localized tumors further.[285]

The optimal treatment of the rare patient with *MYCN*-amplified localized neuroblastoma is controversial. Most studies have demonstrated a worse outcome for patients with localized tumors with *MYCN* amplification. A CCG prospective analysis of 374 patients with Evans stage I and II disease showed that 4 of 7 patients (4 with stage I disease and 3 with stage II disease) with *MYCN* amplification relapsed (3 metastatic) between 2 and 22 months from diagnosis and 3 of these patients died from disease progression.[280] Only patients with stage I disease were successfully treated with surgery alone. A Pediatric Oncology Group analysis of 329 stage A neuroblastoma patients showed that 4 of 11 patients with *MYCN* amplification remained disease-free 22 to 68 months after initial surgery and 4 of 7 patients with recurrent disease were successfully salvaged with additional treatment. Although these results clearly support a worse outcome for *MYCN*-amplified localized disease, they also show (based on a small sample size) that a subset of patients may achieve long-term remission with surgery alone.[281] A recent retrospective review of 600 patients (32 with *MYCN*-amplified tumors) with localized neuroblastoma enrolled in a COG neuroblastoma biology study from 1990 to 1999 suggests that ploidy might be useful for further risk stratification of these rare patients. In this study, ploidy was significantly correlated with outcome for patients with *MYCN*-amplified localized disease (7-year OS 87% ± 9% for patients with hyperdiploid tumors versus 38% ± 12% for patients with diploid or hypodiploid tumors).[102] Further prospective evaluation is needed to determine a consensus treatment strategy for these patients.

Cord compression from intraspinal tumor extension can occur in children who otherwise would be considered low risk and is an oncologic emergency requiring rapid intervention. The choice of emergent therapy is somewhat controversial, with pediatric oncologists favoring chemotherapy and neurosurgeons favoring laminectomy with spinal cord decompression.[286] Retrospective analyses have shown similar neurologic outcomes for patients treated with chemotherapy versus laminectomy.[287-289] Studies have also shown that because of the young age of most of these patients, laminectomy can result in significant long-term orthopedic problems.[290] For these reasons, intermediate-risk type chemotherapy is preferred in most cases for emergent treatment of spinal cord compression. Radiation therapy can also be used but is usually reserved for patients with progressive neurologic abnormalities despite chemotherapy and surgical decompression caused by the long-term morbidity of spinal irradiation in infants and young children.[286]

Most patients with INSS 4S disease have favorable biologic features (single-copy MYCN, hyperdiploid, and favorable Shimada histology) and are categorized as having low-risk disease. The Pediatric Oncology Group reviewed 110 patients with stage D(S) neuroblastoma diagnosed between 1987 and 1996 and found a 3-year OS rate of 85% ± 4%, with a significantly worse prognosis for infants younger than 2 months, or tumor cell diploidy, unfavorable histology, or *MYCN* amplification.[240] A report from the Children's Cancer Group has shown similar results for 80 infants, with a 5-year OS of 92%.[241] Patients with suspected INSS 4S neuroblastoma should undergo biopsy of the primary tumor or an accessible metastatic site (e.g., a subcutaneous nodule) to establish the diagnosis and determine biologic features of the tumor. Patients with favorable biologic features usually do not require therapy and should be observed closely.[291] Resection of the primary tumor is not necessary to achieve excellent outcome in these patients.[240] Patients with progressive or symptomatic disease and those who are too ill to undergo biopsy at diagnosis are generally treated with moderately intensive chemotherapy, such as that currently recommended for intermediate-risk disease.[240,241] Patients with hepatomegaly that progresses despite chemotherapy and causes respiratory compromise are treated with small doses of radiation, 450 to 600 cGy in 150-cGy fractions. The rare patient with INSS 4S disease with unfavorable ploidy and/or histology tumors should be treated with intermediate-risk type therapy. INSS 4S patients with *MYCN* amplification should be treated with high-risk type therapy.

Treatment of Intermediate-Risk Disease

The intermediate-risk classification group includes a wide spectrum of disease. The current approach to treatment uses a combination of moderate-dose multiagent chemotherapy and surgery with a goal of reduction of therapy in patients with favorable biologic features to maintain a 3-year OS of greater than 95%. The current COG intermediate-risk study is based largely on a study done in the CCG that was one of the first to stratify patients prospectively according to risk group and on the COG study that followed it. The CCG 3881 study treated Evans stage 3 patients with favorable biology (normal *MYCN*, favorable Shimada, and low serum ferritin level) with moderately dose-intensive chemotherapy (cyclophosphamide, doxorubicin, cisplatin, and etoposide) and local radiation for any gross residual disease following delayed surgery; it showed a 4-year EFS of more than 95%.[292] Following this study, the Children's Oncology Group A3961 study attempted to reduce acute and long-term toxicity of the CCG regimen by substituting carboplatin for cisplatin, decreasing total cumulative doses of chemotherapy while maintaining dose intensity, and eliminating radiation therapy in all patients, except those with unresectable primary tumors with unfavorable biologic features at the end of chemotherapy. Early reports have shown that despite the reduction of therapy, excellent overall survival was maintained.[293] The current COG intermediate-risk study is prospectively using 1p and 11q status to stratify patients further and reduce therapy for patients whose tumors lack loss of heterozygosity at 1p and 11q and who have other favorable biologic factors.[160]

Existing data suggest that adjuvant therapy could be further reduced, despite the presence of gross residual tumor in patients with locoregional tumors with favorable biology. Traditionally, patients receive chemotherapy with the goal of facilitating surgical resection. Experience from the Memorial Sloan-Kettering Cancer Center has shown that patients with non–stage 4, non–*MYCN*-amplified disease who had gross residual disease following initial surgery could be safely observed and maintain an excellent survival without cytotoxic therapy.[294] In this report, only 1 of 22 patients required chemotherapy and 4 of 13 patients with gross residual disease required a second surgery. This is also supported by the European experience. In the German NB 97 protocol, infants with stage 2 or 3 *MYCN* nonamplified tumors with incomplete resections were observed postoperatively without adjuvant chemotherapy. Regression without further treatment was seen in 32 of 55 patients and salvage therapy was effective for those who progressed or recurred, with a 3-year OS rate of 98%.[284] Based on this information, the current COG intermediate-risk study is using partial response as the treatment end point for patients with favorable biology INSS 2 or 3 disease.

Infants with INSS 4 neuroblastomas without *MYCN* amplification tend to have a much less aggressive clinical course than other INSS 4 patients and are treated with intermediate-risk type chemotherapy. As part of the CCG 3891 study described earlier, Schmidt and colleagues[295] have reported that infants with Evans stage IV disease without *MYCN* amplification had a 3-year EFS rate of 93% with the same treatment that the Evan stage III patients received. This is in contrast to the 3-year EFS of 10% for infants with *MYCN*-amplified tumors, many of whom were treated with more aggressive therapy. Children between the ages of 12 and 18 months may also have a less aggressive clinical course[80,276] (see earlier); the current COG intermediate-risk study is including patients in this age range who have all favorable biologic features.

Treatment of High-Risk Disease

Treatment of disseminated neuroblastoma remains one of the greatest challenges in pediatric oncology. High-risk neuroblastoma represents over half of all newly diagnosed neuroblastoma patients and is the cause of most of the mortality associated with the disease. Treatment approaches that use a combination of intensive induction therapy, myeloablative consolidation therapy with stem cell support, and biologic therapy for minimal residual disease have improved 5-year survival rates from less than 15% to 30% to 40%.[296,297] This modest improvement in survival, however, has come at the cost of increased doses of chemotherapy and radiotherapy, significantly increasing treatment-related morbidity in disease survivors.

Induction Therapy

The goal of induction therapy is to reduce the overall tumor burden maximally using a combination of chemotherapy, surgery, and radiation therapy. High-risk neuroblastoma is generally sensitive to initial chemotherapy, even in cases with *MYCN* amplification. A retrospective meta-analysis of 44 trials has shown that there is a correlation between dose intensity and treatment efficacy, including improved response and survival.[298] Induction chemotherapy for high-risk neuroblastoma generally consists of five to seven alkylator and platinum-based cycles using agents selected to reduce cross resistance. There are a number of combinations that have been used in the United States and Europe, including a regimen developed at Memorial Sloan-Kettering Cancer Center that was used in the last Children's Oncology Group phase 3 study. This regimen consists of cycles of cyclophosphamide, vincristine, and doxorubicin alternating with cycles of cisplatin and etoposide. In a single-institution study of this regimen, Kushner and associates[299] have reported a complete response rate of 63% and a complete plus very good partial response rate of 87% in 24 patients. More recently, however, the French Society of Pediatric Oncology Neuroblastoma Study Group used this induction regimen in a multi-institution study of 47 patients and found a complete response rate of only 45%.[300] Similar results were seen in a preliminary analysis of the Children's Oncology Group most recent phase III study, suggesting that chemotherapy resistance during induction remains an obstacle to cure.[301] One strategy to improve induction response is to decrease treatment intervals during induction to lead to more rapid cell death with less chance of drug resistance. Pearson and coworkers[302] have recently reported a European randomized clinical trial comparing treatment of 262 stage 4 neuroblastoma patients using rapid timing chemotherapy (cycle every 10 days) versus standard timing chemotherapy (cycle every 21 days); the same cumulative doses of five chemotherapeutic drugs given over 10 weeks or 18 weeks were used. The rapid regimen was feasible, without markedly increased toxicity. Complete or very good partial responses were achieved in 53% of patients assigned to conventional treatment versus 71% of patients assigned to rapid treatment ($P = .002$), although there was no significant difference in overall survival between the two regimens. The Children's Oncology Group is currently investigating an alternative strategy of using non–cross resistant chemotherapeutic agents to improve induction response rates further. Topotecan is a topoisomerase 1 inhibitor that has shown antineuroblastoma activity in phase I and II trials with a limited toxicity profile, including dose-limiting myelosuppression and mild to moderate nausea, vomiting, and mucositis.[303,304] The current COG phase 3 high-risk neuroblastoma trial incorporates high-dose topotecan into the Memorial Sloan-Kettering backbone and will compare the induction response rate to historical controls.[305]

There is a growing body of evidence that suggests that the quality of induction response correlates with outcome. Ladenstein and colleagues[306] have performed a multivariate analysis of 549 high-risk neuroblastoma patients registered on the European Bone Marrow Transplantation Solid Tumor Registry and showed that persistent cortical bone lesions ($P = .004$) and bone marrow involvement ($P = .03$) are the only independent adverse prognostic factors. More recent smaller retrospective studies have shown that MIBG response at the end of induction, as assessed by semiquantitative scoring methods, directly correlates with event-free survival following myeloablative therapy.[307-309] Efforts to improve survival further in high-risk disease may need to include response-based end of induction treatment stratification, although more prospective data are needed.

Local Control

Patients with high-risk disease usually have large and locally invasive primary tumors that chemotherapy alone is unlikely to eradicate. Local control is obtained using a combination of surgery and local radiation therapy. Definitive surgery on the primary tumor is usually performed near the end of induction therapy following four or five cycles of chemotherapy. Delaying surgical resection until after chemotherapy has been shown to improve resectability and may reduce the surgical complication rate.[310,311] However, the benefit of complete resection in the treatment of high-risk neuroblastoma remains controversial because it is unclear what impact aggressive treatment of the primary tumor site has on event-free survival in the face of metastatic disease. Several retrospective studies have shown contradictory results. La Quaglia and associates[312] reviewed 141 patients treated at Memorial Sloan-Kettering Cancer Center on sequential protocols between 1979 and 2002 and showed evidence of a significant improvement in survival with a gross total resection. Similarly, Adkins and coworkers[310] have reviewed 210 patients (out of 539 total patients) entered on the CCG 3891 study who achieved a complete response by resection and showed a trend to improved 5-year EFS and OS. However, a report from St. Jude Children's Research Hospital looking at the extent of resection compared with outcome in 107 children older than 1 year with stage 4 neuroblastoma treated on one of four consecutive protocols between 1984 and 2001 showed no evidence of association between survival and the extent of surgery.[313] In addition, von Allmen and colleagues[314] have reported on the local control of 76 patients treated at two institutions using the same treatment protocol with a consistent surgical approach. They found that aggressive surgery followed by local radiation provides excellent local tumor control, with no isolated local occurrences in patients who had more than 90% resection (60 of 76 patients). However, the completeness of resection was not correlated with a difference in EFS or OS. Further prospective evaluation of the role of surgery in high-risk neuroblastoma is needed. It is likely that resectability is a surrogate for tumor biology. Gross total resection with nodal resection should be the goal to provide adequate local control but should not be done if it is at the cost of vital organs or significant postoperative morbidity that would lead to a delay in further therapy.

Neuroblastoma is a highly radiosensitive tumor and local radiation given to the primary tumor site in high-risk disease has been shown to decrease the risk of local recurrence.[315-317] The total dose generally used in the United States is 2160 cGy in daily 180-cGy fractions. Local radiation is generally given at the end of induction or following recovery from consolidation chemotherapy. Patients whose radiation field includes their liver may be at higher risk of veno-occlusive disease if radiation is given prior to stem cell transplantation.[318]

Consolidation Therapy

The goal of the consolidation phase of therapy for high-risk neuroblastoma is to consolidate the response obtained during induction by eliminating any remaining tumor cells using myeloablative chemotherapy and stem cell rescue. The role of dose intensification to overcome tumor drug resistance mechanisms, followed by bone marrow or peripheral blood stem cell support, has been investigated for over 20 years. Early nonrandomized studies suggested a survival advantage compared with historical controls, but may have been influenced by selection bias.

The CCG conducted a randomized study from 1991 to 1996 testing the hypothesis that consolidation with myeloablative chemotherapy followed by purged autologous bone marrow rescue would improve EFS probability compared with nonmyeloablative consolidation chemotherapy.[297] A total of 539 eligible patients were enrolled in this clinical trial; 379 patients were randomly assigned to myeloablative therapy (consisting of carboplatin, etoposide, melphalan, and 1000 cGy of total body irradiation) with autologous marrow rescue (n = 189) or continuation chemotherapy (n = 190). An intent-to-treat analysis showed a significant improvement in 3-year EFS for the patients assigned to myeloablative therapy (34% ± 4% versus 22% ± 4%, P = .03; Fig. 14-8A). The German Society of Pediatric Oncology has shown similar results in a randomized study of

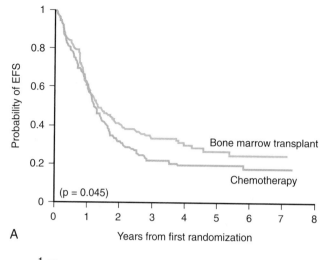

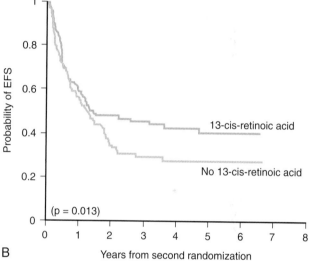

FIGURE 14-8. Children's Cancer Group study 3891 showing that autologous bone marrow transplantation (ABMT) and 13-cis-retinoic acid improve event-free survival (EFS) for high-risk neuroblastoma patients. Patients were treated with identical induction chemotherapy, randomized to ABMT or continuation chemotherapy, and then further randomized to receive 13-cis-retinoic acid or no further therapy. **A,** Event-free survival from time of randomization for patients randomized to ABMT (n = 189) or continuation chemotherapy (n = 180, P = .03). **B,** Event-free survival from time of randomization to 13-cis-retinoic acid (n = 130) or no further therapy (n = 128, P = .03). *(Adapted from Matthay KK, Villablanca JG, Seeger RC, et al. Treatment of high-risk neuroblastoma with intensive chemotherapy, radiotherapy, autologous bone marrow transplantation, and 13-cis-retinoic acid. Children's Cancer Group. N Engl J Med. 1999;341:1165-1173.)*

295 patients receiving myeloablative therapy with autologous stem cell rescue (n = 149) or consolidation with oral maintenance chemotherapy (n = 146). An intent to treat analysis again showed an improvement in 3-year EFS for patients assigned to myeloablative therapy (47%, 95% confidence interval [CI] = 38 to 55, vs. 31%, 95% CI = 23 to 39).[319]

Early myeloablative regimens for high-risk neuroblastoma used bone marrow as rescue, with allogeneic marrow showing no survival advantage compared with autologous marrow.[320,321] More recently, the use of peripheral blood stem cells has been shown to result in more rapid engraftment and less transplantation-related morbidity.[322,323] In addition, peripheral blood stem cells may be less likely to contain contaminating tumor cells.[324]

Peripheral blood stem cells are now the standard for myeloablative autotransplantation regimens and are typically harvested after two to four cycles of induction chemotherapy.

An important concern relating to autotransplantation is potential tumor cell contamination of the stem cell product, contributing to relapse. Strategies to purge tumor cells from harvested marrow or peripheral blood stem cells include ex vivo immunomagnetic purging based on neural specific antigens or CD34+ selection of hematopoietic progenitor cells.[323,325] A randomized clinical trial designed to test the efficacy of ex vivo purging of immunocytochemically negative peripheral blood stem cell products was recently completed by the COG. Preliminary analysis of this study did not show improvement in EFS or OS using purged stem cells.[326]

Given the improvement in event-free survival observed with single-transplant myeloablative strategies, tandem and even triple-transplant regimens have been evaluated in limited institution studies. The theoretic advantages to multiple transplants include exposure to multiple non–cross resistant therapies at maximal doses in a relatively rapid sequence and possible modulation of the tumor microenvironment during the first transplantation, potentiating cell kill with subsequent transplantation(s).[323] Between 1994 and 2002, Grupp and colleagues[323,327] treated 97 patients with high-risk neuroblastoma with tandem rapid sequence myeloablative consolidation regimens using peripheral blood stem cell support in a limited institution single-arm study. They showed that tandem transplantation was feasible, with rapid myeloid cell recovery and low treatment-related mortality (five treatment-related deaths, 82 patients completed two transplantations). The PFS rate at 5 years from diagnosis was 47% (95% CI, 36% to 56%) and the PFS at 7 years from diagnosis was 45% (95% CI, 24% to 55%) and the overall survival rate at 5 and 7 years, respectively, was 60% (95% CI, 42% to 64%) and 53% (95% CI, 40% to 64%; Fig. 14-9). In addition, Kletzel and associates[328] documented a 57% 3-year EFS in a cohort of 26 consecutive patients treated with a triple myeloablative consolidation regimen in a single-institution study. These studies suggest that further intensification of consolidation therapy may affect survival of high-risk neuroblastoma patients. The Children's Oncology Group is currently running a randomized trial of single versus tandem myeloablative consolidations to help evaluate the true impact of a tandem high-dose myeloablative consolidation strategy.

Treatment of Minimal Residual Disease

Even when a complete remission is obtained following myeloablative therapy and stem cell rescue, relapse remains a significant problem, suggesting the presence of highly chemotherapy-resistant minimal residual disease. Strategies targeting unique biologic features of neuroblastoma have therefore become an important part of current high-risk neuroblastoma treatment following consolidation therapy. Minimal residual disease therapy with the retinoid 13-cis-retinoic acid has become a standard for high-risk neuroblastoma care. Immunotherapy targeted against the GD2+ antigen is actively being investigated.

The retinoids have been shown to decrease proliferation, decrease expression of the *MYCN* oncogene, and induce differentiation in neuroblastoma cell lines, including those established from refractory tumors.[329,330] A phase 1 study of children with high-risk neuroblastoma showed that an intermittent schedule of high-dose 13-cis-retinoic acid following transplantation had minimal toxicity (primarily cheilitis, dry skin and hypertriglyceridemia) and resulted in the clearing of tumor cells in the bone marrow by morphologic assessment in 3 of 10 patients.[331] The efficacy of 13-cis-retinoic acid was tested in the

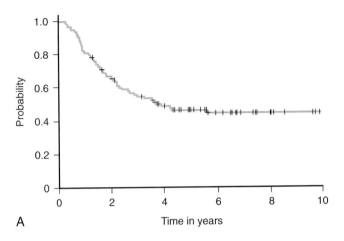

PROGRESSION-FREE SURVIVAL FROM DIAGNOSIS FOR ALL PATIENTS (n = 97)

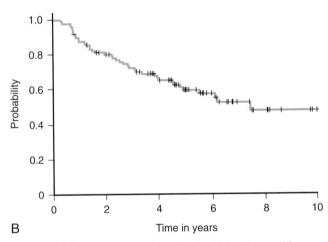

OVERALL SURVIVAL FROM DIAGNOSIS FOR ALL PATIENTS (n = 97)

FIGURE 14-9. Tandem transplantation for high-risk neuroblastoma. **A,** Progression-free survival. **B,** Overall survival from diagnosis of 97 patients. *(Adapted from George RE, Li S, Medeiros-Nancarrow C, et al. High-risk neuroblastoma treated with tandem autologous peripheral-blood stem cell-supported transplantation: long-term survival update. J Clin Oncol. 2006;24:2891-2896.)*

CCG randomized trial (see earlier) using a factorial design following randomization to myeloablative or continuation chemotherapy.[297] A total of 130 patients were randomized to receive six cycles of 13-cis-retinoic acid or no further therapy. The cohort of patients assigned to receive post-transplantation therapy with 13-cis-retinoic acid had a significantly improved EFS probability (46% ± 6% versus 29% ± 6% from second randomization, *P* = .03; see Fig. 14-8B).

Another biologic strategy that is being evaluated in the minimal residual disease phase of therapy is antibody therapy directed against the GD2 disialoganglioside that is highly expressed in neuroblastoma. Murine, chimeric, and humanized antibodies, either alone or with cytokines, have shown activity in preclinical models, particularly in the setting of minimal residual disease,[332-334] as well as in phase I and II clinical trials.[335-338] Because of low-level expression of GD2 on normal nervous tissue, neuropathic pain is a significant toxicity of antibody therapy and can be dose-limiting. COG is currently running a randomized clinical trial designed to test the efficacy

TABLE 14-3   **Definitions of Response to Treatment**

Response	Primary*	Metastases*	Markers*
CR	No tumor	No tumor (MIBG negative)	HVA, VMA normal
VGPR	Reduction 90%-100%	No tumor (MIBG negative)	HVA, VMA decreased >90%
PR	Reduction 50%-90%	No new lesions; 50%-90% reduction in measurable sites; no or one bone marrow sample with tumor; bone and marrow sites decreased by 50%	HVA, VMA decreased 50%-90%
MR	No new lesions; >50% reduction of any measurable lesion (primary or metastases) with <50% reduction in any other; <25% increase in any existing lesion[†]		
NR	No new lesions; <50% reduction but <25% increase in any existing lesion[†]		
PD	Any new lesion; increase of any measurable lesion by >25%; previous negative marrow positive for tumor		

*Evaluations of primary and metastatic disease as outlined in the text.

[†]Quantitative assessment does not apply to marrow disease.

CR, complete response; HVA, homovanillic acid; MR, mixed response; NR, no response; PD, progressive disease; PR, partial response; VGPR, very good partial response; VMA, vanillylmandelic acid.

From Brodeur GM, Pritchard J, Berthold F, et al. Revisions of the international criteria for neuroblastoma diagnosis, staging, and response to treatment. J Clin Oncol. 1993;11:1466-1477.

of ch14.18 with interleukin-2 (IL-2) and granulocyte-macrophage colony-stimulating factor (GM-CSF) and 13-cis-retinoic acid versus 13-cis-retinoic acid alone following myeloablative chemotherapy.

Assessment of Response to Treatment

Neuroblastoma response to treatment is assessed using the International Neuroblastoma Response Criteria (Table 14-3).[256] Determination of overall response requires assessment of primary and metastatic sites. This assessment should be made using the same modalities used at diagnosis. The timing of response assessments vary according to protocol and risk group but are generally done at the end of induction, before and after surgical procedures, and at the end of treatment. In addition to these response criteria, semiquantitative scoring systems for evaluating MIBG-positive disease have been developed.[307,339] The ability to quantify MIBG response objectively is particularly useful in clinical trials for relapsed disease. Relapsed patients often have only bone and/or bone marrow disease that can be seen by MIBG scan but that cannot be measured by CT or MRI using standard response criteria.

Late Effects of Therapy

Improvements in survival of high-risk neuroblastoma patients over the past 20 years has come at the cost of intensification of therapy, putting these patients at increased risk of experiencing late effects of treatment. Hearing loss caused by exposure to high cumulative doses of platinum chemotherapy at a young age is a particular problem that can put survivors at risk for learning problems and psychosocial difficulties.[340] Use of high doses of alkylating agents and topoisomerase inhibitors often results in sterility and puts patients at an increased risk of secondary leukemias.[341,342] Neuroblastoma survivors who received total body irradiation are also at risk for growth delay, cataracts, and thyroid insufficiency, as well as secondary cancers.[343] Survivors of high-risk neuroblastoma therapy should be followed regularly throughout their lives with anticipatory management for these potential problems.

Novel Therapies

Despite the intensive multimodality treatment described earlier, more than half of children with high-risk neuroblastoma still relapse. The prognosis for these children is poor, with the vast majority dying from progressive disease. There currently is no standard treatment regimen for these patients but there are several promising novel therapies that are currently in preclinical and clinical development. Some of these are highlighted below.

Targeted Radiotherapy

In addition to its use for staging and response evaluations, MIBG can be labeled with ^{131}I and used to deliver targeted radiotherapy. ^{131}I-MIBG has undergone extensive single-institution and, more recently, cooperative group clinical trials for the treatment of refractory neuroblastoma.[344,345] The results from a recently completed phase II study of 164 patients have shown that MIBG is active against refractory neuroblastoma, with an objective response rate of 36% and disease stabilization in 34% of patients with frequent palliation of pain.[346] Treatment-related toxicity, even at substantial doses, is usually minimal. The most significant reported toxicity is hematologic, with prolonged thrombocytopenia—most marked in patients with tumor in the bone marrow—and myelosuppression, both of which can be abrogated by autologous stem cell infusion.[346,347] Nonhematologic toxicities include brief nausea and vomiting, transient hepatic dysfunction, and chemical hypothyroidism. A phase I dose escalation study of ^{131}I-MIBG followed by myeloablative carboplatin, etoposide, and melphalan with stem cell rescue has shown a response rate of 27% in primary refractory patients. A phase II study at the maximal tolerated dose is currently underway to explore this approach further, with the consideration that ^{131}I-MIBG might be effective as part of up-front treatment of a subset of high-risk neuroblastoma patients.[348,349] Current clinical trials are also focusing on combining MIBG with radiosensitizing agents to enhance efficacy. In addition to MIBG, radiolabeled anti-GD2 antibodies are also under investigation to provide targeted radiotherapy.[350]

Immunotherapy

As discussed earlier, monoclonal antibody directed against the GD2 antigen in combination with cytokines is actively being investigated as part of the minimal residual disease phase of treatment in newly diagnosed high-risk patients and in relapsed patients. Preclinical studies have shown that the efficacy of antibody can be enhanced by creating a fusion protein consisting of antibody linked to a cytokine such as IL-2.[334,351] A phase II study of a humanized GD2 antibody fused to IL-2 (hu14.18–IL-2) has just been completed in a COG trial; preliminary results have shown a complete response in 5 of 24 patients with MIBG and/or bone marrow–only disease, with tolerable toxicity warranting further investigation.[352,353] Vaccine strategies and the use of engineered cytolytic T lymphocytes are also under development.[354-357]

Targeted Biologic Agents

Retinoids

It has already been established through a randomized trial that 13-cis-retinoic acid is efficacious in minimal residual disease.[297] Fenretinide (4-HPR) is a synthetic retinoid that is cytotoxic to neuroblastoma cells in vitro. Unlike 13-cis-retinoic acid, it does not induce tumor differentiation of cells, but is cytotoxic by inducing apoptosis.[358-360] Its mechanism of action is thought to be through de novo ceramide synthesis induction,[361-363] generation of reactive oxygen species,[364] angiogenesis inhibition,[365,366] and increased natural killer cell activity.[367] Fenretinide has been tested in preclinical and early phase clinical studies and shows promise in relapsed disease.

Tyrosine Kinase Inhibitors

Another promising area is tyrosine kinase inhibition. In animal models, CEP-701, a small-molecule inhibitor, has been shown to have activity against the TrkB tyrosine kinase.[368,369] Another druggable tyrosine kinase target is the epidermal growth factor receptor (EGFR) receptor.[370] EGFR overexpression has been observed in neuroblastomas.[371,372] In addition, the presence of ERBB2 positivity is a significant predictor of shorter median survival in patients with neuroblastoma.[373] Erlotinib, an oral inhibitor against EGFR with activity against ERBB2, has been tested in phase 1 trials of children with solid tumors and found to have tolerable toxicity.[374] Imatinib mesylate has also been studied in vitro because some neuroblastomas express vascular endothelial growth factor (VEGF).[375] Finally, the activating mutations that have been recently discovered in ALK may provide therapeutic targets. A dual MET/ALK inhibitor is currently in phase 1 trials in adult patients.[376] Efforts are ongoing to identify additional mutant proteins in neuroblastoma tumors that may also be targetable.

Targeting the Apoptosis Pathway

Another avenue of exploration is the regulation of apoptosis. In vitro studies using neuroblastoma cell lines have indicated that the expression of BCL-2 is associated with the inhibition of chemotherapy-induced apoptosis.[377] Higher expression has been associated with unfavorable histology, *MYCN* gene amplification, and a poor outcome.[378,379] A BCL-2 antisense compound, G3139, designed to bind to the first six codons of the human BCL-2 mRNA,[380,381] has been tested in phase 1 COG trials and was found to be well tolerated.[382] BCL-2 expression was seen to be reduced in peripheral blood mononuclear cells after exposure with this compound. It is now becoming clear, however, that apoptosis needs to be inhibited at multiple levels (e.g., at the level of BCL-2, reinduction of caspase-8 expression, and activation of TRAIL receptors).

Demethylating Agents

Other potential biologically targeted agents are demethylating agents. It is becoming increasingly clear that not only in other cancers but also in neuroblastoma, a large portion of the cancer genome is methylated—for example, methylation of caspase-8[60] and, more recently, that of the tumor suppressor gene, CHD5, on chromosome 1p.[135] Thus, epigenetic silencing of genes is a crucial mechanism for the silencing of genes that are important for programmed cell death; thus, demethylating agents such as decitabine are being studied and have shown some response in refractory tumors.[203,204]

Histone Deacetylase Inhibitors

Histone deacetylase (HDAC) agents have also shown preclinical activity against neuroblastoma[383,384] and are of potential therapeutic benefit because they cause apoptosis of human neuroblastoma cells, with an enhanced inhibitory effect when combined with retinoic acid.[384-386] Retinoids exert their effect via a nuclear receptor complex that has been recently found to contain histone deacetylase. It is hypothesized that HDAC inhibitors potentiate the derepression of retinoid responsive genes in the presence of ligand.[387] Depsipeptide, a histone deacetylase inhibitor, is currently in early phase trials. Others include suberoylanilide hydroxamic acid (SAHA) and valproic acid.

DNA demethylation and histone deacetylase inhibition have been found to act synergistically in the re-expression of genes silenced in cancer.[388,389] This finding has led to considerable interest in combining a histone deacetylase inhibitor and a demethylating agent (e.g., decitabine) to achieve synergistic activity in the treatment of recurrent neuroblastoma. In addition, HDAC inhibitors in combination with retinoids and DNA demethylating agents act synergistically in the re-expression of genes silenced in cancer, and also demonstrate synergistic activity in neuroblastoma cell lines and xenograft models.[384] These results suggest that HDAC inhibitors alone or in combination with retinoids or demethylating agents may prove to be useful in the treatment of neuroblastoma.

CONCLUSIONS AND FUTURE DIRECTIONS

The clinical heterogeneity of neuroblastoma is clearly correlated with tumor biology. The significant progress made to date in understanding neuroblastoma biology has led to the ability to stratify patients and adapt treatment according to prognostic variables, resulting in a significant reduction in therapy for low- and intermediate-risk patients and the intensification of treatment for high-risk patients. A remaining challenge for low- and intermediate-risk disease is to understand the biology of the small subset of patients better who have a poor outcome and tailor their therapy accordingly. High-risk disease remains a significant clinical problem. We have likely reached the limits of dose intensification and innovative approaches are needed to improve survival and decrease treatment-related morbidity. Future progress will likely be made by translating new discoveries about the underlying pathobiology of neuroblastoma into targeted therapies that can then be integrated into current treatment strategies for newly diagnosed patients.

REFERENCES

1. National Cancer Institute. Surveillance Epidemiology and End Results (SEER) Database, 2008. Available at http://seer.cancer.gov.
2. Gurney JG, Ross JA, Wall DA, et al. Infant cancer in the U.S.: histology-specific incidence and trends, 1973 to 1992. J Pediatr Hematol Oncol. 1997;19:428-432.

3. Li J, Thompson TD, Miller JW, et al. Cancer incidence among children and adolescents in the United States, 2001-2003. Pediatrics. 2008;121:e1470-e1477.

4. Yang Q, Olshan AF, Bondy ML, et al. Parental smoking and alcohol consumption and risk of neuroblastoma. Cancer Epidemiol Biomarkers Prev. 2000;9:967-972.

5. Kramer S, Ward E, Meadows AT, Malone KE. Medical and drug risk factors associated with neuroblastoma: a case-control study. J Natl Cancer Inst. 1987;78:797-804.

6. Schuz J, Kaatsch P, Kaletsch U, et al. Association of childhood cancer with factors related to pregnancy and birth. Int J Epidemiol. 1999;28:631-639.

7. Cook MN, Olshan AF, Guess HA, et al. Maternal medication use and neuroblastoma in offspring. Am J Epidemiol. 2004; 159:721-731.

8. Johnson KJ, Puumala SE, Soler JT, Spector LG. Perinatal characteristics and risk of neuroblastoma. Int J Cancer. 2008;123: 1166-1172.

9. Brodeur GM, Ambros PF, Favrot MC. Biological aspects of neuroblastoma screening. Med Pediatr Oncol. 1998;31:394-400.

10. Hayashi Y, Hanada R, Yamamoto K. Biology of neuroblastomas in Japan found by screening. Am J Pediatr Hematol Oncol. 1992;14:342-347.

11. Nakagawara A, Kadomatsu K, Sato S, et al. Inverse expression of Mycn and Mdr-1 in human neuroblastoma. Prog Clin Biol Res. 1991;366:11-19.

12. Sawada T, Matsumura T, Kawakatsu H, et al. Long-term effects of mass screening for neuroblastoma in infancy. Am J Pediatr Hematol Oncol. 1991;13:3-7.

13. Yamamoto K, Hanada R, Kikuchi A, et al. Spontaneous regression of localized neuroblastoma detected by mass screening. J Clin Oncol. 1998;16:1265-1269.

14. Suita S, Tajiri T, Higashi M, et al. Insights into infant neuroblastomas based on an analysis of neuroblastomas detected by mass screening at 6 months of age in Japan. Eur J Pediatr Surg. 2007;17:23-28.

15. Woods WG, Gao RN, Shuster JJ, et al. Screening of infants and mortality due to neuroblastoma. N Engl J Med. 2002;346: 1041-1046.

16. Woods WG, Tuchman M, Robison LL, et al. A population-based study of the usefulness of screening for neuroblastoma. Lancet. 1996;348:1682-1687.

17. Barrette S, Bernstein ML, Leclerc JM, et al. Treatment complications in children diagnosed with neuroblastoma during a screening program. J Clin Oncol. 2006;24:1542-1545.

18. Schilling FH, Spix C, Berthold F, et al. Neuroblastoma screening at one year of age. N Engl J Med. 2002;346:1047-1053.

19. Berthold F, Baillot A, Hero B, et al. Which cases are found and missed by neuroblastoma screening at 1 year? Results from the 1992 to 1995 study in three Federal States of Germany. J Clin Oncol. 1999;17:1200.

20. Trochet D, Bourdeaut F, Janoueix-Lerosey I, et al. Germline mutations of the paired-like homeobox 2B (PHOX2B) gene in neuroblastoma. Am J Hum Genet. 2004;74:761-764.

21. Raabe EH, Laudenslager M, Winter C, et al. Prevalence and functional consequence of PHOX2B mutations in neuroblastoma. Oncogene. 2008;27:469-476.

22. Ambros IM, Zellner A, Roald B, et al. Role of ploidy, chromosome 1p, and Schwann cells in the maturation of neuroblastoma. N Engl J Med. 1996;334:1505-1511.

23. Valent A, Benard J, Venuat AM, et al. Phenotypic and genotypic diversity of human neuroblastoma studied in three IGR cell line models derived from bone marrow metastases. Cancer Genet Cytogenet. 1999;112:124-129.

24. Mora J, Akram M, Cheung NK, et al. Laser-capture microdissected schwannian and neuroblastic cells in stage 4 neuroblastomas have the same genetic alterations. Med Pediatr Oncol. 2000;35:534-537.

25. Mora J, Cheung NK, Juan G, et al. Neuroblastic and schwannian stromal cells of neuroblastoma are derived from a tumoral progenitor cell. Cancer Res. 2001;61:6892-6898.

26. Bourdeaut F, Ribeiro A, Paris R, et al. In neuroblastic tumours, Schwann cells do not harbour the genetic alterations of neuroblasts but may nevertheless share the same clonal origin. Oncogene. 2008;27:3066-3071.

27. Unger MA, Rishi M, Clemmer VB, et al. Characterization of adjacent breast tumors using oligonucleotide microarrays. Breast Cancer Res. 2001;3:336-341.

28. Ikeda Y, Lister J, Bouton JM, Buyukpamukcu M. Congenital neuroblastoma, neuroblastoma in situ, and the normal fetal development of the adrenal. J Pediatr Surg. 1981;16:636-644.

29. Beckwith J, Perrin E. In situ neuroblastomas: a contribution to the natural history of neural crest tumors. Am J Pathol. 1963;43:1089-1104.

30. De Preter K, Vandesompele J, Heimann P, et al. Human fetal neuroblast and neuroblastoma transcriptome analysis confirms neuroblast origin and highlights neuroblastoma candidate genes. Genome Biol. 2006;7:R84.

31. Howard MJ. Mechanisms and perspectives on differentiation of autonomic neurons. Dev Biol. 2005;277:271-286.

32. Stewart RA, Arduini BL, Berghmans S, et al. Zebrafish foxd3 is selectively required for neural crest specification, migration and survival. Dev Biol. 2006;292:174-188.

33. Kim J, Lo L, Dormand E, Anderson DJ. SOX10 maintains multipotency and inhibits neuronal differentiation of neural crest stem cells. Neuron. 2003;38:17-31.

34. Shah NM, Groves AK, Anderson DJ. Alternative neural crest cell fates are instructively promoted by TGFbeta superfamily members. Cell. 1996;85:331-343.

35. Schneider C, Wicht H, Enderich J, et al. Bone morphogenetic proteins are required in vivo for the generation of sympathetic neurons. Neuron. 1999;24:861-870.

36. Guillemot F, Lo LC, Johnson JE, et al. Mammalian achaete-scute homolog 1 is required for the early development of olfactory and autonomic neurons. Cell. 1993;75:463-476.

37. Hirsch MR, Tiveron MC, Guillemot F, et al. Control of noradrenergic differentiation and Phox2a expression by MASH1 in the central and peripheral nervous system. Development. 1998; 125:599-608.

38. Pattyn A, Morin X, Cremer H, et al. Expression and interactions of the two closely related homeobox genes Phox2a and Phox2b during neurogenesis. Development. 1997;124:4065-4075.

39. Pattyn A, Morin X, Cremer H, et al. The homeobox gene Phox2b is essential for the development of autonomic neural crest derivatives. Nature. 1999;399:366-370.

40. Howard M, Foster DN, Cserjesi P. Expression of HAND gene products may be sufficient for the differentiation of avian neural crest-derived cells into catecholaminergic neurons in culture. Dev Biol. 1999;215:62-77.

41. Howard MJ, Stanke M, Schneider C, et al. The transcription factor dHAND is a downstream effector of BMPs in sympathetic neuron specification. Development. 2000;127:4073-4081.

42. Lim KC, Lakshmanan G, Crawford SE, et al. Gata3 loss leads to embryonic lethality due to noradrenaline deficiency of the sympathetic nervous system. Nat Genet. 2000;25:209-212.

43. Pandolfi PP, Roth ME, Karis A, et al. Targeted disruption of the GATA3 gene causes severe abnormalities in the nervous system and in fetal liver haematopoiesis. Nat Genet. 1995;11:40-44.

44. Goridis C, Brunet JF. Transcriptional control of neurotransmitter phenotype. Curr Opin Neurobiol. 1999;9:47-53.

45. Brunet JF, Pattyn A. Phox2 genes—from patterning to connectivity. Curr Opin Genet Dev. 2002;12:435-440.

46. Goridis C, Rohrer H. Specification of catecholaminergic and serotonergic neurons. Nat Rev Neurosci. 2002;3:531-541.

47. Gestblom C, Grynfeld A, Ora I, et al. The basic helix-loop-helix transcription factor dHAND, a marker gene for the developing human sympathetic nervous system, is expressed in both high- and low-stage neuroblastomas. Lab Invest. 1999;79:67-79.

48. Kirby ML, Waldo KL. Neural crest and cardiovascular patterning. Circ Res. 1995;77:211-215.

49. George RE, Lipshultz SE, Lipsitz SR, et al. Association between congenital cardiovascular malformations and neuroblastoma. J Pediatr. 2004;144:444-448.

50. Blatt J, Olshan AF, Lee PA, Ross JL. Neuroblastoma and related tumors in Turner's syndrome. J Pediatr. 1997;131:666-670.

51. Cotton JL, Williams RG. Noonan syndrome and neuroblastoma. Arch Pediatr Adolesc Med. 1995;149:1280-1281.

52. Tartaglia M, Niemeyer CM, Shannon KM, Loh ML. SHP-2 and myeloid malignancies. Curr Opin Hematol. 2004;11:44-50.

53. Bentires-Alj M, Paez JG, David FS, et al. Activating mutations of the noonan syndrome-associated SHP2/PTPN11 gene in human solid tumors and adult acute myelogenous leukemia. Cancer Res. 2004;64:8816-8820.

54. The I, Murthy AE, Hannigan GE, et al. Neurofibromatosis type 1 gene mutations in neuroblastoma. Nat Genet. 1993;3:62-66.

55. Johnson MR, Look AT, DeClue JE, et al. Inactivation of the NF1 gene in human melanoma and neuroblastoma cell lines without impaired regulation of GTP.Ras. Proc Natl Acad Sci U S A. 1993;90:5539-5543.

56. Martinsson T, Sjoberg RM, Hedborg F, Kogner P. Homozygous deletion of the neurofibromatosis-1 gene in the tumor of a patient with neuroblastoma. Cancer Genet Cytogenet. 1997;95:183-189.

57. Reya T, Clevers H. Wnt signalling in stem cells and cancer. Nature. 2005;434:843-850.

58. Chenn A, Walsh CA. Regulation of cerebral cortical size by control of cell cycle exit in neural precursors. Science. 2002;297:365-369.

59. Ricci-Vitiani L, Pedini F, Mollinari C, et al. Absence of caspase 8 and high expression of PED protect primitive neural cells from cell death. J Exp Med. 2004;200:1257-1266.

60. Teitz T, Wei T, Valentine MB, et al. Caspase 8 is deleted or silenced preferentially in childhood neuroblastomas with amplification of MYCN. Nat Med. 2000;6:529-535.

61. Hansford LM, McKee AE, Zhang L, et al. Neuroblastoma cells isolated from bone marrow metastases contain a naturally enriched tumor-initiating cell. Cancer Res. 2007;67:11234-11243.

62. Longo L, Panza E, Schena F, et al. Genetic predisposition to familial neuroblastoma: identification of two novel genomic regions at 2p and 12p. Hum Hered. 2007;63:205-211.

63. Knudson AG Jr, Strong LC, Anderson DE. Heredity and cancer in man. Prog Med Genet. 1973;9:113-158.

64. Mossé YP, Laudenslager M, Longo L, et al. Identification of ALK as a major familial neuroblastoma predisposition gene. Nature. 2008;455:930-935.

65. George RE, Sanda T, Hanna M, et al. Activating mutations in ALK provide a therapeutic target in neuroblastoma. Nature. 2008;455:975-978.

66. Amiel J, Laudier B, Attie-Bitach T, et al. Polyalanine expansion and frameshift mutations of the paired-like homeobox gene PHOX2B in congenital central hypoventilation syndrome. Nat Genet. 2003;33:459-461.

67. Mosse YP, Laudenslager M, Khazi D, et al. Germline PHOX2B mutation in hereditary neuroblastoma. Am J Hum Genet. 2004;75:727-730.

68. van Limpt V, Schramm A, van Lakeman A, et al. The Phox2B homeobox gene is mutated in sporadic neuroblastomas. Oncogene. 2004;23:9280-9288.

69. McConville C, Reid S, Baskcomb L, et al. PHOX2B analysis in non-syndromic neuroblastoma cases shows novel mutations and genotype-phenotype associations. Am J Med Genet A. 2006;140:1297-1301.

70. Dubreuil V, Hirsch MR, Pattyn A, et al. The Phox2b transcription factor coordinately regulates neuronal cell cycle exit and identity. Development. 2000;27:5191-5201.

71. Weese-Mayer DE, Berry-Kravis EM, Zhou L, et al. Idiopathic congenital central hypoventilation syndrome: analysis of genes pertinent to early autonomic nervous system embryologic development and identification of mutations in PHOX2b. Am J Med Genet. 2003;123A:267-278.

72. Matera I, Bachetti T, Puppo F, et al. PHOX2B mutations and polyalanine expansions correlate with the severity of the respiratory phenotype and associated symptoms in both congenital and late onset Central Hypoventilation syndrome. J Med Genet. 2004;41:373-380.

73. Luther W, Bayul T, Kanki J, et al. Phox2B in peripheral sympathetic nervous system development and neuroblastoma. Presented at the 8th International Conference on Zebrafish Development and Genetics. Madison, Wis, University of Wisconsin-Madison, June 2008.

74. Maris JM, Weiss MJ, Mosse Y, et al. Evidence for a hereditary neuroblastoma predisposition locus at chromosome 16p12-13. Cancer Res. 2002;62:6651-6658.

75. Maris JM, Mosse YP, Bradfield JP, et al. Chromosome 6p22 locus associated with clinically aggressive neuroblastoma. N Engl J Med. 2008;358:2585-2593.

76. Shojaei-Brosseau T, Chompret A, Abel A, et al. Genetic epidemiology of neuroblastoma: a study of 426 cases at the Institut Gustave-Roussy in France. Pediatr Blood Cancer. 2004;42:99-105.

77. Kushner BH, Cheung NK. Neuroblastoma—linking a common allele to a rare disease. N Engl J Med. 2008;358:2635-2637.

78. Look AT, Hayes FA, Nitschke R, et al. Cellular DNA content as a predictor of response to chemotherapy in infants with unresectable neuroblastoma. N Engl J Med. 1984;311:231-235.

79. Look AT, Hayes FA, Shuster JJ, et al. Clinical relevance of tumor cell ploidy and N-Myc gene amplification in childhood neuroblastoma: a Pediatric Oncology Group Study. J Clin Oncol. 1991;9:581-591.

80. George RE, London WB, Cohn SL, et al. Hyperdiploidy plus nonamplified MYCN confers a favorable prognosis in children 12 to 18 months old with disseminated neuroblastoma: a Pediatric Oncology Group study. J Clin Oncol. 2005;23:6466-6473.

81. Schwab M, Alitalo K, Klempnauer KH, et al. Amplified DNA with limited homology to myc cellular oncogene is shared by human neuroblastoma cell lines and a neuroblastoma tumour. Nature. 1983;305:245-248.

82. Brodeur G, Seeger RC, Schwab M, et al. Amplification of N-*myc* in untreated human neuroblastomas correlates with advanced disease stage. Science. 1984;224:1121-1124.

83. Seeger RC, Brodeur GM, Sather H, et al. Association of multiple copies of the N-myc oncogene with rapid progression of neuroblastomas. N Engl J Med. 1985;313:1111-1116.

84. Cox D, Yuncken C, Spriggs AI. Minute chromatin bodies in malignant tumours of childhood. Lancet. 1965;1:55-58.

85. Biedler JL, Spengler BA. A novel chromosome abnormality in human neuroblastoma and antifolate-resistant Chinese hamster cell lives in culture. J Natl Cancer Inst. 1976;57:683-695.

86. Balaban-Malenbaum G, Gilbert F. Relationship between homogeneously staining regions and double minute chromosomes in human neuroblastoma cell lines. Prog Cancer Res Ther. 1980;12:97-107.

87. Moreau LA, McGrady P, London WB, et al. Does MYCN amplification manifested as homogeneously staining regions at diagnosis predict a worse outcome in children with neuroblastoma? A Children's Oncology Group study. Clin Cancer Res. 2006;12:5693-5697.

88. Charron J, Malynn BA, Fisher P, et al. Embryonic lethality in mice homozygous for a targeted disruption of the N-myc gene. Genes Dev. 1992;6:2248-2257.

89. Stanton BR, Perkins AS, Tessarollo L, et al. Loss of N-myc function results in embryonic lethality and failure of the epithelial component of the embryo to develop. Genes Dev. 1992;6:2235-2247.

90. Zimmerman KA, Yancopoulos GD, Collum RG, et al. Differential expression of myc family genes during murine development. Nature. 1986;319:780-783.

91. Mugrauer G, Alt FW, Ekblom P. N-myc proto-oncogene expression during organogenesis in the developing mouse as revealed by in situ hybridization. J Cell Biol. 1988;107:1325-1335.

92. Negroni A, Scarpa S, Romeo A, et al. Decrease of proliferation rate and induction of differentiation by a mycn antisense DNA oligomer in a human neuroblastoma cell line. Cell Growth Differ. 1991;2:511-518.

93. Thiele CJ, Israel MA. Regulation of N-myc expression is a critical event controlling the ability of human neuroblasts to differentiate. Exp Cell Biol. 1988;56:321-333.

94. Thiele CJ, Reynolds CP, Israel M. Decreased expression of N-myc precedes retinoic acid-induced morphological differentiation of human neuroblastoma. Nature. 1986;313:404-406.

95. Yancopoulos GD, Nisen PD, Tesfaye A, et al. N-myc can cooperate with ras to transform normal cells in culture. Proc Natl Acad Sci U S A. 1985;82:5455-5459.

96. Schwab M, Varmus HE, Bishop JM. Human N-myc gene contributes to neoplastic transformation of mammalian cells in culture. Nature. 1985;316:160-162.

97. Weiss WA, Aldape K, Mohapatra G, et al. Targeted expression of MYCN causes neuroblastoma in transgenic mice. EMBO J. 1997;16:2985-2995.

98. Weiss WA, Godfrey T, Francisco C, Bishop JM. Genome-wide screen for allelic imbalance in a mouse model for neuroblastoma. Cancer Res. 2000;60:2483-2487.

99. Brodeur GM. Molecular basis for heterogeneity in human neuroblastomas. Eur J Cancer. 1995;31A:505-510.

100. Brodeur GM, Ambros PF. Genetic and biological markers of prognosis in neuroblastoma. In Brodeur GM, Sawada T, Tsuchida Y, Voute PA (eds). Neuroblastoma. Amsterdam, Elsevier Science, 2000, pp 355-369.

101. Cohn SL, Brodeur GM, Holbrook T, et al. N-myc gene amplification in localized neuroblastoma. A Pediatric Oncology Group Study. Cancer Res. 1995;55:721-726.

102. Schneiderman J, London WB, Brodeur GM, et al. Clinical significance of MYCN amplification and ploidy in favorable-stage neuroblastoma: a report from the Children's Oncology Group. J Clin Oncol. 2008;26:913-918.

103. Brodeur GM, Hayes FA, Green AA, et al. Consistent N-myc copy number in simultaneous or consecutive neuroblastoma samples from sixty individual patients. Cancer Res. 1987;47:4248-4253.

104. Cohn SL, London WB, Huang D, et al. MYCN expression is not prognostic of adverse outcome in advanced-stage neuroblastoma with nonamplified MYCN. J Clin Oncol. 2000;18:3604-3613.

105. Squire JA, Thorner PS, Weitzman S, et al. Co-amplification of MYCN and a DEAD box gene (DDX1) in primary neuroblastoma. Oncogene. 1995;10:1417-1422.

106. Manohar CF, Salwen HR, Brodeur GM, Cohn SL. Co-amplification and concomitant high levels of expression of a DEAD box gene with MYCN in human neuroblastoma. Genes Chromosomes Cancer. 1995;14:196-203.

107. George RE, Kenyon RM, McGuckin AG, et al. Investigation of co-amplification of the candidate genes ornithine decarboxylase, ribonucleotide reductase, syndecan-1 and a DEAD box gene, DDX1, with N-myc in neuroblastoma. United Kingdom Children's Cancer Study Group. Oncogene. 1996;12:1583-1587.

108. Wimmer K, Zhu XX, Lamb BJ, et al. Two-dimensional DNA electrophoresis identifies novel CpG islands frequently coamplified with MYCN in neuroblastoma. Med Pediatr Oncol. 2001;36:75-79.

109. Wimmer K, Zhu XX, Lamb BJ, et al. Co-amplification of a novel gene, NAG, with the N-myc gene in neuroblastoma. Oncogene. 1999;18:233-238.

110. George RE, Kenyon R, McGuckin AG, et al. Analysis of candidate gene co-amplification with MYCN in neuroblastoma. Eur J Cancer. 1997;33:2037-2042.

111. Chen QR, Bilke S, Wei JS, et al. cDNA array-CGH profiling identifies genomic alterations specific to stage and MYCN-amplification in neuroblastoma. BMC Genomics. 2004;5:70.

112. George RE, Attiyeh EF, Li S, et al. Genome-wide analysis of neuroblastomas using high-density single nucleotide polymorphism arrays. PLoS ONE. 2007;2:e255.

113. Miyake I, Hakomori Y, Shinohara A, et al. Activation of anaplastic lymphoma kinase is responsible for hyperphosphorylation of ShcC in neuroblastoma cell lines. Oncogene. 2002;21:5823-5834.

114. Morris SW, Kirstein MN, Valentine MB, et al. Fusion of a kinase gene, ALK, to a nucleolar protein gene, NPM, in non-Hodgkin's lymphoma. Science. 1994;263:1281-1284.

115. Soda M, Choi YL, Enomoto M, et al. Identification of the transforming EML4-ALK fusion gene in non-small-cell lung cancer. Nature. 2007;448:561-566.

116. Chiarle R, Voena C, Ambrogio C, et al. The anaplastic lymphoma kinase in the pathogenesis of cancer. Nat Rev Cancer. 2008;8:11-23.

117. McDermott U, Iafrate AJ, Gray NS, et al. Genomic alterations of anaplastic lymphoma kinase may sensitize tumors to anaplastic lymphoma kinase inhibitors. Cancer Res. 2008;68:3389-3395.

118. Brodeur GM, Sekhon GS, Goldstein MN. Chromosomal aberrations in human neuroblastomas. Cancer. 1977;40:2256-2263.

119. Fong CT, Dracopoli NC, White PS, et al. Loss of heterozygosity for the short arm of chromosome 1 in human neuroblastomas: Correlation with N-myc amplification. Proc Natl Acad Sci U S A. 1989;86:3753-3757.

120. Weith A, Martinsson T, Ciepluch C, et al. Neuroblastoma consensus deletion maps to 1p36.1-2. Genes Chromosomes Cancer. 1989;1:159-166.

121. White PS, Maris JM, Beltinger C, et al. A region of consistent deletion in neuroblastoma maps within human chromosome 1p36.2-36.3. Proc Natl Acad Sci U S A. 1995;92:5520-5524.

122. Schleiermacher G, Peter M, Michon J, et al. Two distinct deleted regions on the short arm of chromosome 1 in neuroblastoma. Genes Chromosomes Cancer. 1994;10:275-281.

123. Takeda O, Homma C, Maseki N, et al. There may be two tumor suppressor genes on chromosome arm 1p closely associated with biologically distinct subtypes of neuroblastoma. Genes Chromosomes Cancer. 1994;10:30-39.

124. Cheng NC, Van Roy N, Chan A, et al. Deletion mapping in neuroblastoma cell lines suggests two distinct tumor suppressor genes in the 1p35-36 region, only one of which is associated with N-myc amplification. Oncogene. 1995;10:291-297.

125. Dracopoli NC, Bruns GA, Brodeur GM, et al. Report and abstracts of the First International Workshop on Human Chromosome 1 Mapping 1994. Bethesda, Maryland, March 25-27, 1994. Cytogenet Cell Genet. 1994;67:144-165.

126. Dracopoli NC, Harnett P, Bale SJ, et al. Loss of alleles from the distal short arm of chromosome 1 occurs late in melanoma tumor progression. Proc Natl Acad Sci U S A. 1989;86:4614-4618.

127. Tsutsumi M, Yokota J, Kakizoe T, et al. Loss of heterozygosity on chromosomes 1p and 11p in sporadic pheochromocytoma. J Natl Cancer Inst. 1989;81:367-370.

128. Caron H, van Sluis P, de Kraker J, et al. Allelic loss of chromosome 1p as a predictor of unfavorable outcome in patients with neuroblastoma. N Engl J Med. 1996;334:225-230.

129. Caron H. Allelic loss of chromosome 1 and additional chromosome 17 material are both unfavourable prognostic markers in neuroblastoma. Med Pediatr Oncol. 1995;24:215-221.

130. Brodeur GM, Fong CT. Molecular biology and genetics of human neuroblastoma. Cancer Genet Cytogenet. 1989;41:153-174.

131. Riley RD, Heney D, Jones DR, et al. A systematic review of molecular and biological tumor markers in neuroblastoma. Clin Cancer Res. 2004;10(Pt 1):4-12.

132. Biegel JA, White PS, Marshall HN, et al. Constitutional 1p36 deletion in a child with neuroblastoma. Am J Hum Genet. 1993;52:176-182.

133. Bader SA, Fasching C, Brodeur GM, Stanbridge EJ. Dissociation of suppression of tumorigenicity and differentiation in vitro effected by transfer of single human chromosomes into human neuroblastoma cells. Cell Growth Differ. 1991;2:245-255.

134. Bagchi A, Papazoglu C, Wu Y, et al. CHD5 is a tumor suppressor at human 1p36. Cell. 2007;128:459-475.

135. Fujita T, Igarashi J, Okawa ER, et al. CHD5, a tumor suppressor gene deleted from 1p36.31 in neuroblastomas. J Natl Cancer Inst. 2008;100:940-949.

136. Thompson PM, Gotoh T, Kok M, et al. CHD5, a new member of the chromodomain gene family, is preferentially expressed in the nervous system. Oncogene. 2003;22:1002-1011.

137. Caren H, Ejeskar K, Fransson S, et al. A cluster of genes located in 1p36 are down-regulated in neuroblastomas with poor prognosis, but not due to CpG island methylation. Mol Cancer. 2005;4:10.

138. Schlisio S, Kenchappa RS, Vredeveld LC, et al. The kinesin KIF1Bbeta acts downstream from EglN3 to induce apoptosis and is a potential 1p36 tumor suppressor. Genes Dev. 2008;22:884-893.

139. Nakagawa T, Takahashi M, Ozaki T, et al. Negative autoregulation of p73 and p53 by DeltaNp73 in regulating differentiation and survival of human neuroblastoma cells. Cancer Lett. 2003;197:105-109.

140. Okawa ER, Gotoh T, Manne J, et al. Expression and sequence analysis of candidates for the 1p36.31 tumor suppressor gene deleted in neuroblastomas. Oncogene. 2008;27:803-810.

141. Liu Z, Yang X, Tan F, et al. Molecular cloning and characterization of human Castor, a novel human gene upregulated during cell differentiation. Biochem Biophys Res Commun. 2006;344:834-844.

142. White PS, Thompson PM, Gotoh T, et al. Definition and characterization of a region of 1p36.3 consistently deleted in neuroblastoma. Oncogene. 2005;24:2684-2694.

143. Knudson AG Jr, Strong LC. Mutation and cancer: neuroblastoma and pheochromocytoma. Am J Hum Genet. 1972;24:514-532.

144. Knudson AG Jr, Meadows AT. Developmental genetics of neuroblastoma. J Natl Cancer Inst. 1976;57:675-682.

145. Welch C, Chen Y, Stallings RL. MicroRNA-34a functions as a potential tumor suppressor by inducing apoptosis in neuroblastoma cells. Oncogene. 2007;26:5017-5022.

146. Wei JS, Song YK, Durinck S, et al. The MYCN oncogene is a direct target of miR-34a. Oncogene. 2008;27:5204-5213.

147. Cole KA, Attiyeh EF, Mosse YP, et al. A functional screen identifies miR-34a as a candidate neuroblastoma tumor suppressor gene. Mol Cancer Res. 2008;6:735-742.

148. Bown N, Cotterill S, Lastowska M, et al. Gain of chromosome arm 17q and adverse outcome in patients with neuroblastoma. N Engl J Med. 1999;340:1954-1961.

149. Scaruffi P, Coco S, Cifuentes F, et al. Identification and characterization of DNA imbalances in neuroblastoma by high-resolution oligonucleotide array comparative genomic hybridization. Cancer Genet Cytogenet. 2007;177:20-29.

150. Van Roy N, Laureys G, Van Gele M, et al. Analysis of 1;17 translocation breakpoints in neuroblastoma: implications for mapping of neuroblastoma genes. Eur J Cancer. 1997;33:1974-1978.

151. Lastowska M, Roberts P, Pearson AD, et al. Promiscuous translocations of chromosome arm 17q in human neuroblastomas. Genes Chromosomes Cancer. 1997;19:143-149.

152. Stallings RL, Carty P, McArdle L, et al. Molecular cytogenetic analysis of recurrent unbalanced t(11;17) in neuroblastoma. Cancer Genet Cytogenet. 2004;154:44-51.

153. Cheng AJ, Cheng NC, Ford J, et al. Cell lines from MYCN transgenic murine tumours reflect the molecular and biological characteristics of human neuroblastoma. Eur J Cancer. 2007;43:1467-1475.

154. Tajiri T, Tanaka S, Higashi M, et al. Biological diagnosis for neuroblastoma using the combination of highly sensitive analysis of prognostic factors. J Pediatr Surg. 2006;41:560-566.

155. Valentijn LJ, Koppen A, van Asperen R, et al. Inhibition of a new differentiation pathway in neuroblastoma by copy number defects of N-myc, Cdc42, and nm23 genes. Cancer Res. 2005;65:3136-3145.

156. Srivatsan ES, Ying KL, Seeger RC. Deletion of chromosome 11 and of 14q sequences in neuroblastoma. Genes Chromosomes Cancer. 1993;7:32-37.

157. Mertens F, Johansson B, Hoglund M, Mitelman F. Chromosomal imbalance maps of malignant solid tumors: a cytogenetic survey of 3185 neoplasms. Cancer Res. 1997;57:2765-2780.

158. Guo C, White PS, Weiss MJ, et al. Allelic deletion at 11q23 is common in MYCN single copy neuroblastomas. Oncogene. 1999;18:4948-4957.

159. Kaneko Y, Cohn SL. Ploidy and cytogenetics of neuroblastoma. In Brodeur GM, Sawada T, Tsuchida Y, Voute PA (eds). Neuroblastoma. Amsterdam, Elsevier Science, 2000, pp 41-56.

160. Attiyeh EF, London WB, Mosse YP, et al. Chromosome 1p and 11q deletions and outcome in neuroblastoma. N Engl J Med. 2005;353:2243-2253.

161. Takita J, Hayashi Y, Kohno T, et al. Allelotype of neuroblastoma. Oncogene. 1995;11:1829-1834.

162. Fong CT, White PS, Peterson K, et al. Loss of heterozygosity for chromosomes 1 or 14 defines subsets of advanced neuroblastomas. Cancer Res. 1992;52:1780-1785.

163. Takayama H, Suzuki T, Mugishima H, et al. Deletion mapping of chromosomes 14q and 1p in human neuroblastoma. Oncogene. 1992;7:1185-1189.

164. Thompson PM, Seifried BA, Kyemba SK, et al. Loss of heterozygosity for chromosome 14q in neuroblastoma. Med Pediatr Oncol. 2001;36:28-31.

165. Theobald M, Christiansen H, Schmidt A, et al. Sublocalization of putative tumor suppressor gene loci on chromosome arm 14q in neuroblastoma. Genes Chromosomes Cancer. 1999;26:40-46.

166. Mosse YP, Diskin SJ, Wasserman N, et al. Neuroblastomas have distinct genomic DNA profiles that predict clinical phenotype and regional gene expression. Genes Chromosomes Cancer. 2007;46:936-949.

167. Ejeskar K, Aburatani H, Abrahamsson J, et al. Loss of heterozygosity of 3p markers in neuroblastoma tumours implicate a tumour-suppressor locus distal to the FHIT gene. Br J Cancer. 1998;77:1787-1791.

168. Caron H, van Sluis P, Buschman R, et al. Allelic loss of the short arm of chromosome 4 in neuroblastoma suggests a novel tumour suppressor gene locus. Hum Genet. 1996;97:834-837.

169. Takita J, Hayashi Y, Kohno T, et al. Deletion map of chromosome 9 and p16 (CDKN2A) gene alterations in neuroblastoma. Cancer Res. 1997;57:907-912.

170. Reale MA, Reyes-Mugica M, Pierceall WE, et al. Loss of DCC expression in neuroblastoma is associated with disease dissemination. Clin Cancer Res. 1996;2:1097-1102.

171. Imamura J, Bartram CR, Berthold F, et al. Mutation of the p53 gene in neuroblastoma and its relationship with N-myc amplification. Cancer Res. 1993;53:4053-4058.

172. Vogan K, Bernstein M, Brisson L, et al. Absence of p53 gene mutations in primary neuroblastomas. Cancer Res. 1993;53: 5269-5273.

173. Komuro H, Hayashi Y, Kawamura M, et al. Mutations of the p53 gene are involved in Ewing's sarcomas but not in neuroblastomas. Cancer Res. 1993;53:5284-5288.

174. Tweddle DA, Malcolm AJ, Bown N, et al. Evidence for the development of p53 mutations after cytotoxic therapy in a neuroblastoma cell line. Cancer Res. 2001;61:8-13.

175. Moll UM, LaQuaglia M, Benard J, Riou G. Wild-type p53 protein undergoes cytoplasmic sequestration in undifferentiated neuroblastomas but not in differentiated tumors. Proc Natl Acad Sci U S A. 1995;92:4407-4411.

176. Corvi R, Savelyeva L, Breit S, et al. Non-syntenic amplification of *MDM2* and *MYCN* in human neuroblastoma. Oncogene. 1995;10:1081-1086.

177. Valsesia-Wittmann S, Magdeleine M, Dupasquier S, et al. Oncogenic cooperation between H-Twist and N-Myc overrides failsafe programs in cancer cells. Cancer Cell. 2004;6:625-630.

178. Goldman SC, Chen CY, Lansing TJ, et al. The p53 signal transduction pathway is intact in human neuroblastoma despite cytoplasmic localization. Am J Pathol. 1996;148:1381-1385.

179. Beltinger CP, White PS, Sulman EP, et al. No CDKN2 mutations in neuroblastomas. Cancer Res. 1995;55:2053-2055.

180. Thompson PM, Maris JM, Hogarty MD, et al. Homozygous deletion of CDKN2A (p16INK4a/p14ARF) but not within 1p36 or at other tumor suppressor loci in neuroblastoma. Cancer Res. 2001;61:679-686.

181. Sweetser DA, Kapur RP, Froelick GJ, et al. Oncogenesis and altered differentiation induced by activated Ras in neuroblasts of transgenic mice. Oncogene. 1997;15:2783-2794.

182. Van Roy N, Forus A, Myklebost O, et al. Identification of two distinct chromosome 12-derived amplification units in neuroblastoma cell line NGP. Cancer Genet Cytogenet. 1995;82: 151-154.

183. Jones TA, Flomen RH, Senger G, et al. The homeobox gene MEIS1 is amplified in IMR-32 and highly expressed in other neuroblastoma cell lines. Eur J Cancer. 2000;36:2368-2374.

184. Molenaar JJ, van Sluis P, Boon K, et al. Rearrangements and increased expression of cyclin D1 (CCND1) in neuroblastoma. Genes Chromosomes Cancer. 2003;36:242-249.

185. Spieker N, van Sluis P, Beitsma M, et al. The MEIS1 oncogene is highly expressed in neuroblastoma and amplified in cell line IMR32. Genomics. 2001;71:214-221.

186. Stallings RL, Nair P, Maris JM, et al. High-resolution analysis of chromosomal breakpoints and genomic instability identifies PTPRD as a candidate tumor suppressor gene in neuroblastoma. Cancer Res. 2006;66:3673-3680.

187. Nair P, DePreter K, Vandesompele J, et al. Aberrant splicing of the PTPRD gene mimics microdeletions identified at this locus in neuroblastomas. Genes Chromosomes Cancer. 2008;47:197-202.

188. Nakagawara A, Arima-Nakagawara M, Scavarda NJ, et al. Association between high levels of expression of the TRK gene and favorable outcome in human neuroblastoma. N Engl J Med. 1993;328:847-854.

189. van Limpt V, Chan A, Schramm A, et al. Phox2B mutations and the Delta-Notch pathway in neuroblastoma. Cancer Lett. 2005; 228:59-63.

190. Tacconelli A, Farina AR, Cappabianca L, et al. TrkA alternative splicing: a regulated tumor-promoting switch in human neuroblastoma. Cancer Cell. 2004;6:347-360.

191. Nakagawara A, Azar CG, Scavarda NJ, Brodeur GM. Expression and function of TRK-B and BDNF in human neuroblastomas. Mol Cell Biol. 1994;14:759-767.

192. Ho R, Eggert A, Hishiki T, et al. Resistance to chemotherapy mediated by TrkB in neuroblastomas. Cancer Res. 2002;62: 6462-6466.

193. Biffo S, Offenhauser N, Carter BD, Barde YA. Selective binding and internalisation by truncated receptors restrict the availability of BDNF during development. Development. 1995;121:2461-2470.

194. Haapasalo A, Koponen E, Hoppe E, et al. Truncated trkB.T1 is dominant negative inhibitor of trkB.TK+-mediated cell survival. Biochem Biophys Res Commun. 2001;280:1352-1358.

195. Eide FF, Vining ER, Eide BL, et al. Naturally occurring truncated trkB receptors have dominant inhibitory effects on brain-derived neurotrophic factor signaling. J Neurosci. 1996;16: 3123-3129.

196. Yamashiro DJ, Nakagawara A, Ikegaki N, et al. Expression of TrkC in favorable human neuroblastomas. Oncogene. 1996; 12:37-41.

197. Castle VP, Heidelberger KP, Bromberg J, et al. Expression of the apoptosis-suppressing protein bcl-2, in neuroblastoma is associated with unfavorable histology and N-myc amplification. Am J Pathol. 1993;143:1543-1550.

198. Teitz T, Lahti JM, Kidd VJ. Aggressive childhood neuroblastomas do not express caspase-8: an important component of programmed cell death. J Mol Med. 2001;79:428-436.

199. Eggert A, Grotzer MA, Zuzak TJ, et al. Resistance to tumor necrosis factor-related apoptosis-inducing ligand (TRAIL)-induced apoptosis in neuroblastoma cells correlates with a loss of caspase-8 expression. Cancer Res. 2001;61:1314-1319.

200. Hopkins-Donaldson S, Bodmer JL, Bourloud KB, et al. Loss of caspase-8 expression in highly malignant human neuroblastoma cells correlates with resistance to tumor necrosis factor-related apoptosis-inducing ligand-induced apoptosis. Cancer Res. 2000;60:4315-4319.

201. Fulda S, Kufer MU, Meyer E, et al. Sensitization for death receptor- or drug-induced apoptosis by re-expression of caspase-8 through demethylation or gene transfer. Oncogene. 2001;20: 5865-5877.

202. Eggert A, Grotzer MA, Zuzak TJ, et al. Resistance to TRAIL-induced apoptosis in neuroblastoma cells correlates with a loss of caspase-8 expression. Med Pediatr Oncol. 2000;35:603-607.

203. George RE, Medeiros-Nancarrow C, Adamson PC, et al. A phase I study of decitabine (DCT) in combination with doxorubicin (DOX) and cyclophosphamide (CTX) in the treatment of relapsed or refractory solid tumors: a Children's Oncology Group Study. J Clin Oncol. 2005 ASCO Annual Meeting Proceedings. 2005;23(Suppl):8530.

204. George R, Lahti J, Ingle M, Krailo M, et al. Decitabine (DAC) in combination with doxorubicin (DOX) and cyclophosphamide (CTX) in relapsed neuroblastoma (NBL): a Children's Oncology Group Study. J Clin Oncol. 2007 ASCO Annual Meeting Proceedings. 2007;25(Suppl):9565.

205. Chan HS, Haddad G, Thorner PS, et al. P-glycoprotein expression as a predictor of the outcome of therapy for neuroblastoma. N Engl J Med. 1991;325:1608-1614.

206. Goldstein LJ, Fojo AT, Ueda K, et al. Expression of the multidrug resistance, *MDR*1, gene in neuroblastomas. J Clin Oncol. 1990;8:128-136.

207. Cole SP, Bhardwaj G, Gerlach JH, et al. Overexpression of a transporter gene in a multidrug-resistant human lung cancer cell line. Science. 1992;258:1650-1654.

208. Zaman GJ, Flens MJ, van Leusden MR, et al. The human multidrug resistance-associated protein MRP is a plasma membrane drug-efflux pump. Proc Natl Acad Sci U S A. 1994;91:8822-8826.

209. Bordow SB, Haber M, Madafiglio J, et al. Expression of the multidrug resistance-associated protein (MRP) gene correlates with amplification and overexpression of the N-myc oncogene in childhood neuroblastoma. Cancer Res. 1994;54:5036-5040.

210. Norris MD, Bordow SB, Marshall GM, et al. Expression of the gene for multidrug-resistance-associated protein and outcome in

patients with neuroblastoma. N Engl J Med. 1996;334:231-238.

211. Jaboin J, Hong A, Kim CJ, Thiele CJ. Cisplatin-induced cytotoxicity is blocked by brain-derived neurotrophic factor activation of TrkB signal transduction path in neuroblastoma. Cancer Lett. 2003;193:109-114.

212. Ribatti D, Alessandri G, Vacca A, et al. Human neuroblastoma cells produce extracellular matrix-degrading enzymes, induce endothelial cell proliferation and are angiogenic in vivo. Int J Cancer. 1998;77:449-454.

213. Meitar D, Crawford SE, Rademaker AW, Cohn SL. Tumor angiogenesis correlates with metastatic disease, N-Myc amplification, and poor outcome in human neuroblastoma. J Clin Oncol. 1996;4:405-414.

214. Pavlakovic H, Von Schutz V, Rossler J, et al. Quantification of angiogenesis stimulators in children with solid malignancies. Int J Cancer. 2001;92:756-760.

215. Peddinti R, Zeine R, Luca D, et al. Prominent microvascular proliferation in clinically aggressive neuroblastoma. Clin Cancer Res. 2007;13:3499-3506.

216. Eggert A, Ikegaki N, Kwiatkowski J, et al. High-level expression of angiogenic factors is associated with advanced tumor stage in human neuroblastomas. Clin Cancer Res. 2000;6:1900-1908.

217. Erdreich-Epstein A, Shimada H, Groshen S, et al. Integrins alpha(v)beta3 and alpha(v)beta5 are expressed by endothelium of high-risk neuroblastoma and their inhibition is associated with increased endogenous ceramide. Cancer Res. 2000;60:712-721.

218. Chlenski A, Liu S, Cohn SL. The regulation of angiogenesis in neuroblastoma. Cancer Lett. 2003;197:47-52.

219. Chlenski A, Liu S, Crawford SE, et al. SPARC is a key Schwannian-derived inhibitor controlling neuroblastoma tumor angiogenesis. Cancer Res. 2002;62:7357-7363.

220. Huang D, Rutkowski JL, Brodeur GM, et al. Schwann cell-conditioned medium inhibits angiogenesis. Cancer Res. 2000;60:5966-5971.

221. Almgren MA, Henriksson KC, Fujimoto J, Chang CL. Nucleoside diphosphate kinase A/nm23-H1 promotes metastasis of NB69-derived human neuroblastoma. Mol Cancer Res. 2004;2:387-394.

222. Gross N, Balmas Bourloud K, Brognara CB. MYCN-related suppression of functional CD44 expression enhances tumorigenic properties of human neuroblastoma cells. Exp Cell Res. 2000;260:396-403.

223. Jodele S, Chantrain CF, Blavier L, et al. The contribution of bone marrow-derived cells to the tumor vasculature in neuroblastoma is matrix metalloproteinase-9 dependent. Cancer Res. 2005;65:3200-3208.

224. Stupack DG, Teitz T, Potter MD, et al. Potentiation of neuroblastoma metastasis by loss of caspase-8. Nature. 2006;439:95-99.

225. Russell DS, Rubenstein LJ. Tumors of peripheral neuroblasts and ganglion cells. In Pathology of Tumors of the Central Nervous System. Baltimore, Williams & Wilkins, 1989, pp 900-913.

226. Castleberry RP, Pritchard J, Ambros P, et al. The International Neuroblastoma Risk Groups (INRG): a preliminary report. Eur J Cancer. 1997;33:2113-2116.

227. Shimada H, Ambros IM, Dehner LP, et al. The International Neuroblastoma Pathology Classification (the Shimada system). Cancer. 1999;86:364-372.

228. Triche TJ, Askin FB, Kissane JM. Neuroblastoma, Ewing's sarcoma, and the differential diagnosis of small-, round-, blue-cell tumors. In Finegold M (ed). Pathology of Neoplasia in Children and Adolescents. Philadelphia, WB Saunders, 1986, pp 145-195.

229. Shimada H, Chatten J, Newton WA Jr, et al. Histopathologic prognostic factors in neuroblastic tumors: definition of subtypes of ganglioneuroblastoma and an age-linked classification of neuroblastomas. J Natl Cancer Inst. 1984;73:405-416.

230. Joshi VV, Cantor AB, Altshuler G, et al. Age-linked prognostic categorization based on a new histologic grading system of neuroblastomas. A clinicopathologic study of 211 cases from the Pediatric Oncology Group. Cancer. 1992;69:2197-2211.

231. Shimada H, Ambros IM, Dehner LP, et al. The International Neuroblastoma Pathology Classification (Shimada) System. Cancer. 1999;86:364-372.

232. Peuchmaur M, d'Amore ES, Joshi VV, et al. Revision of the International Neuroblastoma Pathology Classification: confirmation of favorable and unfavorable prognostic subsets in ganglioneuroblastoma, nodular. Cancer. 2003;98:2274-2281.

233. Park JR, Eggert A, Caron H. Neuroblastoma: biology, prognosis, and treatment. Pediatr Clin North Am. 2008;55:97-120.

234. Maris JM, Hogarty MD, Bagatell R, Cohn SL. Neuroblastoma. Lancet. 2007;369:2106-2120.

235. Weinblatt ME, Heisel MA, Siegel SE. Hypertension in children with neurogenic tumors. Pediatrics. 1983;71:947-957.

236. Musarella MA, Chan HS, DeBoer G, Gallie BL. Ocular involvement in neuroblastoma: prognostic implications. Ophthalmology. 1984;91:936-940.

237. Gesundheit B, Greenberg M. Images in clinical medicine. Medical mystery—one brown eye and one blue eye. N Engl J Med. 2005;353:1502.

238. Quinn JJ, Altman AJ. The multiple hematologic manifestations of neuroblastoma. Am J Pediatr Hematol Oncol. 1979;1:201-205.

239. D'Angio GJ, Evans AE, Koop CE. Special pattern of widespread neuroblastoma with a favorable prognosis. Lancet. 1971;1:1046-1049.

240. Katzenstein HM, Bowman LC, Brodeur GM, et al. Prognostic significance of age, MYCN oncogene amplification, tumor cell ploidy, and histology in 110 infants with stage D(S) neuroblastoma: the pediatric oncology group experience—a Pediatric Oncology Group study. J Clin Oncol. 1998;16:2007-2017.

241. Nickerson HJ, Matthay KK, Seeger RC, et al. Favorable biology and outcome of stage IV-S neuroblastoma with supportive care or minimal therapy: a Children's Cancer Group study. J Clin Oncol. 2000;18:477-486.

242. Russo C, Cohn SL, Petruzzi MJ, de Alarcon PA. Long-term neurologic outcome in children with opsoclonus-myoclonus associated with neuroblastoma: a report from the Pediatric Oncology Group. Med Pediatr Oncol. 1997;28:284-288.

243. Matthay KK, Blaes F, Hero B, et al. Opsoclonus myoclonus syndrome in neuroblastoma: a report from a workshop on the dancing eyes syndrome at the advances in neuroblastoma meeting in Genoa, Italy, 2004. Cancer Lett. 2005;228:275-282.

244. Cooper R, Khakoo Y, Matthay KK, et al. Opsoclonus-myoclonus-ataxia syndrome in neuroblastoma: histopathologic features—a report from the Children's Cancer Group. Med Pediatr Oncol. 2001;36:623-629.

245. Rudnick E, Khakoo Y, Antunes NL, et al. Opsoclonus-myoclonus-ataxia syndrome in neuroblastoma: clinical outcome and antineuronal antibodies-a report from the Children's Cancer Group Study. Med Pediatr Oncol. 2001;36:612-622.

246. Joshi VV, Cantor AB, Brodeur GM, et al. Correlation between morphologic and other prognostic markers of neuroblastoma. A study of histologic grade, DNA index, N-myc gene copy number, and lactic dehydrogenase in patients in the Pediatric Oncology Group. Cancer. 1993;71:3173-3181.

247. Hayward K, Jeremy RJ, Jenkins S, et al. Long-term neurobehavioral outcomes in children with neuroblastoma and opsoclonus-myoclonus-ataxia syndrome: relationship to MRI findings and anti-neuronal antibodies. J Pediatr. 2001;139:552-559.

248. Mitchell WG, Davalos-Gonzalez Y, Brumm VL, et al. Opsoclonus-ataxia caused by childhood neuroblastoma: developmental and neurologic sequelae. Pediatrics. 2002;109:86-98.

249. Swart JF, de Kraker J, van der Lely N. Metaiodobenzylguanidine total-body scintigraphy required for revealing occult neuroblas-

toma in opsoclonus-myoclonus syndrome. Eur J Pediatr. 2002; 161:255-258.

250. Veneselli E, Conte M, Biancheri R, et al. Effect of steroid and high-dose immunoglobulin therapy on opsoclonus-myoclonus syndrome occurring in neuroblastoma. Med Pediatr Oncol. 1998;30:15-17.

251. Petruzzi MJ, de Alarcon PA. Neuroblastoma-associated opsoclonus-myoclonus treated with intravenously administered immune globulin G. J Pediatr. 1995;127:328-329.

252. Bell J, Moran C, Blatt J. Response to rituximab in a child with neuroblastoma and opsoclonus-myoclonus. Pediatr Blood Cancer. 2008;50:370-371.

253. Pranzatelli MR, Tate ED, Travelstead AL, et al. Rituximab (anti-CD20) adjunctive therapy for opsoclonus-myoclonus syndrome. J Pediatr Hematol Oncol. 2006;28:585-593.

254. Yiu VW, Kovithavongs T, McGonigle LF, Ferreira P. Plasmapheresis as an effective treatment for opsoclonus-myoclonus syndrome. Pediatr Neurol. 2001;24:72-74.

255. Kaplan S, Holbrook C, McDaniel H, et al. Vasoactive intestinal peptide secreting tumors of childhood. Am J Dis Child. 1980; 134:21-24.

256. Brodeur GM, Pritchard J, Berthold F, et al. Revisions of the international criteria for neuroblastoma diagnosis, staging, and response to treatment. J Clin Oncol. 1993;11:1466-1477.

257. Graham-Pole J, Salmi T, Anton AH, et al. Tumor and urine catecholamines (CATS) in neurogenic tumors. Correlations with other prognostic factors and survival. Cancer. 1983;51: 834-839.

258. LaBrosse EH, Com-Nougue C, Zucker JM, et al. Urinary excretion of 3-methoxy-4-hydroxymandelic acid and 3-methoxy-4-hydroxyphenylacetic acid by 288 patients with neuroblastoma and related neural crest tumors. Cancer Res. 1980;40:1995-2001.

259. Brodeur GM, Maris JM. Neuroblastoma. In Pizzo PA, Poplack DG (eds). Principles and Practice of Pediatric Oncology. Philadelphia, JB Lippincott, 2002, pp 895-938.

260. Kushner BH, Yeh SD, Kramer K, et al. Impact of metaiodobenzylguanidine scintigraphy on assessing response of high-risk neuroblastoma to dose-intensive induction chemotherapy. J Clin Oncol. 2003;21:1082-1086.

261. Kushner BH, Yeung HW, Larson SM, et al. Extending positron emission tomography scan utility to high-risk neuroblastoma: fluorine-18 fluorodeoxyglucose positron emission tomography as sole imaging modality in follow-up of patients. J Clin Oncol. 2001;19:3397-3405.

262. Scanga DR, Martin WH, Delbeke D. Value of FDG PET imaging in the management of patients with thyroid, neuroendocrine, and neural crest tumors. Clin Nucl Med. 2004;29:86-90.

263. Shore RM. Positron emission tomography/computed tomography (PET/CT) in children. Pediatr Ann. 2008;37:404-412.

264. Brodeur GM, Seeger RC, Barrett A, et al. International criteria for diagnosis, staging and response to treatment in patients with neuroblastoma. J Clin Oncol. 1988;6:1874-1881.

265. Moss TJ, Reynolds CP, Sather HN, et al. Prognostic value of immunocytologic detection of bone marrow metastases in neuroblastoma. N Engl J Med. 1991;324:219-226.

266. Gilbert J, Haber M, Bordow SB, et al. Use of tumor-specific gene expression for the differential diagnosis of neuroblastoma from other pediatric small round-cell malignancies. Am J Pathol. 1999;155:17-21.

267. Cheung NK, Von Hoff DD, Strandjord SE, Coccia PF. Detection of neuroblastoma cells in bone marrow using GD2 specific monoclonal antibodies. J Clin Oncol. 1986;4:363-369.

268. Wang Y, Einhorn P, Triche TJ, et al. Expression of protein gene product 9.5 and tyrosine hydroxylase in childhood small round cell tumors. Clin Cancer Res. 2000;6:551-558.

269. Cheung IY, Cheung NK. Detection of microscopic disease: comparing histology, immunocytology, and RT-PCR of tyrosine

hydroxylase, GAGE, and MAGE. Med Pediatr Oncol. 2001;36: 210-212.

270. Lo Piccolo MS, Cheung NK, Cheung IY. GD2 synthase: a new molecular marker for detecting neuroblastoma. Cancer. 2001; 92:924-931.

271. Burchill SA, Lewis IJ, Abrams KR, et al. Circulating neuroblastoma cells detected by reverse transcriptase polymerase chain reaction for tyrosine hydroxylase mRNA are an independent poor prognostic indicator in stage 4 neuroblastoma in children over 1 year. J Clin Oncol. 2001;19:1795-1801.

272. Cecchetto G, Mosseri V, De Bernardi B, et al. Surgical risk factors in primary surgery for localized neuroblastoma: the LNESG1 study of the European International Society of Pediatric Oncology Neuroblastoma Group. J Clin Oncol. 2005;23: 8483-8489.

273. Breslow N, McCann B. Statistical estimation of prognosis for children with neuroblastoma. Cancer Res. 1971;31:2098-2103.

274. Evans AE. Natural history of neuroblastoma. In Evans AE (ed). Advances in Neuroblastoma Research. New York, Raven Press, 1980, pp 3-12.

275. London WB, Castleberry RP, Matthay KK, et al. Evidence for an age cutoff greater than 365 days for neuroblastoma risk group stratification in the Children's Oncology Group. J Clin Oncol. 2005;23:6459-6465.

276. Schmidt ML, Lal A, Seeger RC, et al. Favorable prognosis for patients 12 to 18 months of age with stage 4 nonamplified MYCN neuroblastoma: a Children's Cancer Group Study. J Clin Oncol. 2005;23:6474-6480.

277. Cohn SL LW, Monclair T, Matthay KK, et al. Update on the development of the international neuroblastoma risk group. Presented at the 43rd Annual Meeting of the American Society of Clinical Oncology, Chicago, June 2007.

278. Shimada H, Chatten J, Newton W Jr, et al. Histopathologic prognostic factors in neuroblastic tumors: definition of subtypes of ganglioneuroblastoma and an age-linked classification of neuroblastomas. J Natl Cancer Inst. 1984;73:405-416.

279. Maris JM. The biologic basis for neuroblastoma heterogeneity and risk stratification. Curr Opin Pediatr. 2005;17:7-13.

280. Perez CA, Matthay KK, Atkinson JB, et al. Biologic variables in the outcome of stages I and II neuroblastoma treated with surgery as primary therapy: a children's cancer group study. J Clin Oncol. 2000;18:18-26.

281. Alvarado CS, London WB, Look AT, et al. Natural history and biology of stage A neuroblastoma: a Pediatric Oncology Group study. J Pediatr Hematol Oncol. 2000;22:197-205.

282. Evans AE, Silber JH, Shpilsky A, D'Angio GJ. Successful management of low-stage neuroblastoma without adjuvant therapies: a comparison of two decades, 1972 through 1981 and 1982 through 1992, in a single institution. J Clin Oncol. 1996;14: 2504-2510.

283. Nishihira H, Toyoda Y, Tanaka Y, et al. Natural course of neuroblastoma detected by mass screening: s 5-year prospective study at a single institution. J Clin Oncol. 2000;18:3012-3017.

284. Hero B, Simon T, Spitz R, et al. Localized infant neuroblastomas often show spontaneous regression: results of the prospective trials NB95-S and NB97. J Clin Oncol. 2008;26:1504-1510.

285. Nuchtern JG. Perinatal neuroblastoma. Semin Pediatr Surg. 2006;15:10-16.

286. De Bernardi B, Balwierz W, Bejent J, et al. Epidural compression in neuroblastoma: Diagnostic and therapeutic aspects. Cancer Lett. 2005;228:283-299.

287. De Bernardi B, Pianca C, Pistamiglio P, et al. Neuroblastoma with symptomatic spinal cord compression at diagnosis: treatment and results with 76 cases. J Clin Oncol. 2001;19:183-190.

288. Katzenstein HM, Kent PM, London WB, Cohn SL. Treatment and outcome of 83 children with intraspinal neuroblastoma: the Pediatric Oncology Group experience. J Clin Oncol. 2001;19: 1047-1055.

289. Plantaz D, Rubie H, Michon J, et al. The treatment of neuroblastoma with intraspinal extension with chemotherapy followed by surgical removal of residual disease. A prospective study of 42 patients—results of the NBL 90 Study of the French Society of Pediatric Oncology. Cancer. 1996;78:311-319.

290. Hoover M, Bowman LC, Crawford SE, et al. Long-term outcome of patients with intraspinal neuroblastoma. Med Pediatr Oncol. 1999;32:353-359.

291. D'Angio GJ, Evans AE, Koop CE. Special pattern of widespread neuroblastoma with a favourable prognosis. Lancet. 1971;1:1046-1049.

292. Matthay KK, Perez C, Seeger RC, et al. Successful treatment of stage III neuroblastoma based on prospective biologic staging: a Children's Cancer Group study. J Clin Oncol. 1998;16:1256-1264.

293. Baker DL, Schmidt M, Cohn SL, et al. A phase III trial of biologically-based therapy reduction for intermediate risk neuroblastoma. J Clin Oncol. 2007 ASCO Annual Meeting Proceedings Part I. 2007;25(18S):9504.

294. Kushner BH, Cheung NK, LaQuaglia MP, et al. Survival from locally invasive or widespread neuroblastoma without cytotoxic therapy. J Clin Oncol. 1996;14:373-381.

295. Schmidt ML, Lukens JN, Seeger RC, et al. Biologic factors determine prognosis in infants with stage IV neuroblastoma: a prospective Children's Cancer Group study. J Clin Oncol. 2000;18:1260-1268.

296. Philip T, Ladenstein R, Lasset C, et al. 1070 myeloablative megatherapy procedures followed by stem cell rescue for neuroblastoma: 17 years of European experience and conclusions. European Group for Blood and Marrow Transplant Registry Solid Tumour Working Party. Eur J Cancer. 1997;33:2130-2135.

297. Matthay KK, Villablanca JG, Seeger RC, et al. Treatment of high-risk neuroblastoma with intensive chemotherapy, radiotherapy, autologous bone marrow transplantation, and 13-cis-retinoic acid. Children's Cancer Group. N Engl J Med. 1999;341(16):1165-1173.

298. Cheung NK, Heller G, Kushner BH, et al. Stage IV neuroblastoma more than 1 year of age at diagnosis: major response to chemotherapy and survival durations correlated strongly with dose intensity. Prog Clin Biol Res. 1991;366:567-573.

299. Kushner BH, LaQuaglia MP, Bonilla MA, et al. Highly effective induction therapy for stage 4 neuroblastoma in children over 1 year of age. J Clin Oncol. 1994;12:2607-2613.

300. Valteau-Couanet D, Michon J, Boneu A, et al. Results of induction chemotherapy in children older than 1 year with a stage 4 neuroblastoma treated with the NB 97 French Society of Pediatric Oncology (SFOP) protocol. J Clin Oncol. 2005;23:532-540.

301. Kreissman SG, Villablanca JG, Diller L, et al. Response and toxicity to a dose-intensive multi-agent chemotherapy induction regimen for high-risk neuroblastoma: a Children's Oncology Group (COG A3973) Study. J Clin Oncol. 2007 ASCO Annual Meeting Proceedings Part I. 2007;25(Suppl 18):9505.

302. Pearson AD, Pinkerton CR, Lewis IJ, et al. High-dose rapid and standard induction chemotherapy for patients aged over 1 year with stage 4 neuroblastoma: a randomised trial. Lancet Oncol. 2008;9:247-256.

303. Tubergen DG, Stewart CF, Pratt CB, et al. Phase I trial and pharmacokinetic (PK) and pharmacodynamics (PD) study of topotecan using a five-day course in children with refractory solid tumors: a Pediatric Oncology Group study. J Pediatr Hematol Oncol. 1996;18:352-361.

304. Kretschmar CS, Kletzel M, Murray K, et al. Response to paclitaxel, topotecan, and topotecan-cyclophosphamide in children with untreated disseminated neuroblastoma treated in an upfront phase II investigational window: a pediatric oncology group study. J Clin Oncol. 2004;22:4119-4126.

305. Park JR, Stewart CF, London WB, et al. A topotecan-containing induction regimen for treatment of high risk neuroblastoma. J Clin Oncol, 2006 ASCO Annual Meeting Proceedings Part I. 2006;24(Suppl 18):9013.

306. Ladenstein R, Philip T, Lasset C, et al. Multivariate analysis of risk factors in stage 4 neuroblastoma patients over the age of one year treated with megatherapy and stem-cell transplantation: a report from the European Bone Marrow Transplantation Solid Tumor Registry. J Clin Oncol. 1998;16:953-965.

307. Matthay KK, Edeline V, Lumbroso J, et al. Correlation of early metastatic response by 123I-metaiodobenzylguanidine scintigraphy with overall response and event-free survival in stage IV neuroblastoma. J Clin Oncol. 2003;21:2486-2491.

308. Katzenstein HM, Cohn SL, Shore RM, et al. Scintigraphic response by ^{123}I-metaiodobenzylguanidine scan correlates with event-free survival in high-risk neuroblastoma. J Clin Oncol. 2004;22:3909-3915.

309. Schmidt M, Simon T, Hero B, et al. The prognostic impact of functional imaging with (123)I-mIBG in patients with stage 4 neuroblastoma >1 year of age on a high-risk treatment protocol: results of the German Neuroblastoma Trial NB97. Eur J Cancer. 2008;44:1552-1558.

310. Adkins ES, Sawin R, Gerbing RB, et al. Efficacy of complete resection for high-risk neuroblastoma: a Children's Cancer Group study. J Pediatr Surg. 2004;39:931-936.

311. Shamberger RC, Allarde-Segundo A, Kozakewich HP, Grier HE. Surgical management of stage III and IV neuroblastoma: resection before or after chemotherapy? J Pediatr Surg. 1991;26:1113-1117.

312. La Quaglia MP, Kushner BH, Su W, et al. The impact of gross total resection on local control and survival in high-risk neuroblastoma. J Pediatr Surg. 2004;39:412-417.

313. McGregor LM, Rao BN, Davidoff AM, et al. The impact of early resection of primary neuroblastoma on the survival of children older than 1 year of age with stage 4 disease: the St. Jude Children's Research Hospital Experience. Cancer. 2005;104:2837-2846.

314. von Allmen D, Grupp S, Diller L, et al. Aggressive surgical therapy and radiotherapy for patients with high-risk neuroblastoma treated with rapid sequence tandem transplant. J Pediatr Surg. 2005;40:936-941.

315. Haas-Kogan DA, Swift PS, Selch M, et al. Impact of radiotherapy for high-risk neuroblastoma: a Children's Cancer Group study. Int J Radiat Oncol Biol Phys. 2003;56:28-39.

316. Kushner BH, Wolden S, LaQuaglia MP, et al. Hyperfractionated low-dose radiotherapy for high-risk neuroblastoma after intensive chemotherapy and surgery. J Clin Oncol. 2001;19:2821-2828.

317. Bradfield SM, Douglas JG, Hawkins DS, et al. Fractionated low-dose radiotherapy after myeloablative stem cell transplantation for local control in patients with high-risk neuroblastoma. Cancer. 2004;100:1268-1275.

318. Horn B, Reiss U, Matthay K, et al. Veno-occlusive disease of the liver in children with solid tumors undergoing autologous hematopoietic progenitor cell transplantation: a high incidence in patients with neuroblastoma. Bone Marrow Transplant. 2002;29:409-415.

319. Berthold F, Boos J, Burdach S, et al. Myeloablative megatherapy with autologous stem-cell rescue versus oral maintenance chemotherapy as consolidation treatment in patients with high-risk neuroblastoma: a randomised controlled trial. Lancet Oncol. 2005;6:649-658.

320. Matthay KK, Seeger RC, Reynolds CP, et al. Allogeneic versus autologous purged bone marrow transplantation for neuroblastoma: a report from the Childrens Cancer Group. J Clin Oncol. 1994;12:2382-2389.

321. Stram DO, Matthay KK, O'Leary M, et al. Consolidation chemoradiotherapy and autologous bone marrow transplantation versus continued chemotherapy for metastatic neuroblastoma: a report of two concurrent Children's Cancer Group studies. J Clin Oncol. 1996;14:2417-2426.

322. Cohn SL, Moss TJ, Hoover M, et al. Treatment of poor-risk neuroblastoma patients with high-dose chemotherapy and autologous peripheral stem cell rescue. Bone Marrow Transplant. 1997;20:543-551.

323. Grupp SA, Stern JW, Bunin N, et al. Tandem high-dose therapy in rapid sequence for children with high-risk neuroblastoma. J Clin Oncol. 2000;18:2567-2575.

324. Kletzel M, Longino R, Rademaker AW, et al. Peripheral blood stem cell transplantation in young children: experience with harvesting, mobilization and engraftment. Pediatr Transplant. 1998;2:191-196.

325. Reynolds CP, Seeger RC, Vo DD, et al. Model system for removing neuroblastoma cells from bone marrow using monoclonal antibodies and magnetic immunobeads. Cancer Res. 1986;46:5882-5886.

326. Kreissman SG, Villablanca JG, Seeger RC, et al. A randomized phase III trial of myeloablative autologous peripheral blood stem cell transplant for high-risk neuroblastoma (HR-NB) employing immunomagnetic purged (P) verging unpurged (UP) PBSC: A Children's Oncology Group Study. J Clin Oncol. 2008;26(Suppl):10011.

327. George RE, Li S, Medeiros-Nancarrow C, et al. High-risk neuroblastoma treated with tandem autologous peripheral-blood stem cell-supported transplantation: long-term survival update. J Clin Oncol. 2006;24:2891-2896.

328. Kletzel M, Katzenstein HM, Haut PR, et al. Treatment of high-risk neuroblastoma with triple-tandem high-dose therapy and stem-cell rescue: results of the Chicago Pilot II Study. J Clin Oncol. 2002;20:2284-2292.

329. Reynolds CP, Kane DJ, Einhorn PA, et al. Response of neuroblastoma to retinoic acid in vitro and in vivo. Prog Clin Biol Res. 1991;366:203-211.

330. Reynolds CP, Schindler PF, Jones DM, et al. Comparison of 13-cis-retinoic acid to trans-retinoic acid using human neuroblastoma cell lines. Prog Clin Biol Res. 1994;385:237-244.

331. Villablanca JG, Khan AA, Avramis VI, et al. Phase I trial of 13-cis-retinoic acid in children with neuroblastoma following bone marrow transplantation. J Clin Oncol. 1995;13:894-901.

332. Lode HN, Moehler T, Xiang R, et al. Synergy between an anti-angiogenic integrin alphav antagonist and an antibody-cytokine fusion protein eradicates spontaneous tumor metastases. Proc Natl Acad Sci U S A. 1999;96:1591-1596.

333. Kushner BH, Cheung NK. GM-CSF enhances 3F8 monoclonal antibody-dependent cellular cytotoxicity against human melanoma and neuroblastoma. Blood. 1989;73:1936-1941.

334. Neal ZC, Yang JC, Rakhmilevich AL, et al. Enhanced activity of hu14.18-IL2 immunocytokine against murine NXS2 neuroblastoma when combined with interleukin 2 therapy. Clin Cancer Res. 2004;10:4839-4847.

335. Cheung NK, Kushner BH, Cheung IY, et al. Anti-G(D2) antibody treatment of minimal residual stage 4 neuroblastoma diagnosed at more than 1 year of age. J Clin Oncol. 1998;16:3053-3060.

336. Cheung NK, Lazarus H, Miraldi FD, et al. Ganglioside GD2 specific monoclonal antibody 3F8: a phase I study in patients with neuroblastoma and malignant melanoma. J Clin Oncol. 1987;5:1430-1440.

337. Yu AL, Batova A, Alvarada C, et al. Usefulness of a chemeric anti-GD2 (ch 14.18) and GM-CSF for refractory neuroblastoma: a POG Phase II study. Proc Annu Meet Am Assoc Cancer Res. 1997;16:513a.

338. Kushner BH, Kramer K, Cheung NK. Phase II trial of the anti-GD2 monoclonal antibody 3F8 and granulocyte-macrophage colony-stimulating factor for neuroblastoma. J Clin Oncol. 2001;19:4189-4194.

339. Frappaz D, Bonneu A, Chauvot P, et al. Metaiodobenzylguanidine assessment of metastatic neuroblastoma: observer dependency and chemosensitivity evaluation. The SFOP Group. Med Pediatr Oncol. 2000;34:237-241.

340. Gurney JG, Tersak JM, Ness KK, et al. Hearing loss, quality of life, and academic problems in long-term neuroblastoma survivors: a report from the Children's Oncology Group. Pediatrics. 2007;120:e1229-e1236.

341. Kushner BH, Cheung NK, Kramer K, et al. Neuroblastoma and treatment-related myelodysplasia/leukemia: the Memorial Sloan-Kettering experience and a literature review. J Clin Oncol. 1998;16:3880-3889.

342. Meadows AT, Tsunematsu Y. Late effects of treatment for neuroblastoma. In Brodeur GM, Sawada T, Tsuchida Y, Voute PA (eds). Neuroblastoma. Amsterdam, Elsevier Science, 2000, pp 561-570.

343. Flandin I, Hartmann O, Michon J, et al. Impact of TBI on late effects in children treated by megatherapy for Stage IV neuroblastoma. A study of the French Society of Pediatric oncology. Int J Radiat Oncol Biol Phys. 2006;64:1424-1431.

344. Matthay KK, DeSantes K, Hasegawa B, et al. Phase I dose escalation of ^{131}I-metaiodobenzylguanidine with autologous bone marrow support in refractory neuroblastoma. J Clin Oncol. 1998;16:229-236.

345. Howard JP, Maris JM, Kersun LS, et al. Tumor response and toxicity with multiple infusions of high dose ^{131}I-MIBG for refractory neuroblastoma. Pediatr Blood Cancer. 2005;44:232-239.

346. Matthay KK, Yanik G, Messina J, et al. Phase II study on the effect of disease sites, age, and prior therapy on response to iodine-131-metaiodobenzylguanidine therapy in refractory neuroblastoma. J Clin Oncol. 2007;25:1054-1060.

347. DuBois SG, Messina J, Maris JM, et al. Hematologic toxicity of high-dose iodine-131-metaiodobenzylguanidine therapy for advanced neuroblastoma. J Clin Oncol. 2004;22:2452-2460.

348. Matthay KK, Tan JC, Villablanca JG, et al. Phase I dose escalation of iodine-131-metaiodobenzylguanidine with myeloablative chemotherapy and autologous stem-cell transplantation in refractory neuroblastoma: a New approach to Neuroblastoma Therapy Consortium Study. J Clin Oncol. 2006;24:500-506.

349. Yanik GA, Levine JE, Matthay KK, et al. Pilot study of iodine-131-metaiodobenzylguanidine in combination with myeloablative chemotherapy and autologous stem-cell support for the treatment of neuroblastoma. J Clin Oncol. 2002;20:2142-2149.

350. Kramer K, Humm JL, Souweidane MM, et al. Phase I study of targeted radioimmunotherapy for leptomeningeal cancers using intra-Ommaya 131-I-3F8. J Clin Oncol. 2007;25:5465-5470.

351. Lode HN, Xiang R, Varki NM, et al. Targeted interleukin-2 therapy for spontaneous neuroblastoma metastases to bone marrow. J Natl Cancer Inst. 1997;89:1586-1594.

352. Osenga KL, Hank JA, Albertini MR, et al. A phase I clinical trial of the hu14.18-IL2 (EMD 273063) as a treatment for children with refractory or recurrent neuroblastoma and melanoma: a study of the Children's Oncology Group. Clin Cancer Res. 2006;12:1750-1759.

353. Shusterman S, London WB, Gillies SD, et al. Anti-neuroblastoma activity of hu14.18-IL2 against minimal residual disease in a Children's Cancer Group phase II study. J Clin Oncol. 2008;26(Suppl):3002.

354. Bolesta E, Kowalczyk A, Wierzbicki A, et al. DNA vaccine expressing the mimotope of GD2 ganglioside induces protective GD2 cross-reactive antibody responses. Cancer Res. 2005;65:3410-3418.

355. Russell HV, Strother D, Mei Z, et al. Phase I trial of vaccination with autologous neuroblastoma tumor cells genetically modified to secrete IL-2 and lymphotactin. J Immunother. 2007;30:227-233.

356. Yu A, Batova A, Strother D, et al. Promising results of a pilot trial of a GD2 directed anti-idiotypic antibody as a vaccine for high risk neuroblastoma. Presented at the Eleventh Conference of Advances in Neuroblastoma Research 2004. Genoa, Italy, June 2004.

357. Gonzalez S, Naranjo A, Serrano LM, et al. Genetic engineering of cytolytic T lymphocytes for adoptive T-cell therapy of neuroblastoma. J Gene Med. 2004;6:704-711.

358. Reynolds CP, Wang Y, Melton LJ, et al. Retinoic-acid-resistant neuroblastoma cell lines show altered MYC regulation and high sensitivity to fenretinide. Med Pediatr Oncol. 2000;35:597-602.

359. Di Vinci A, Geido E, Infusini E, Giaretti W. Neuroblastoma cell apoptosis induced by the synthetic retinoid N-(4-hydroxyphenyl) retinamide. Int J Cancer. 1994;59:422-426.

360. Mariotti A, Marcora E, Bunone G, et al. N-(4-hydroxyphenyl) retinamide: a potent inducer of apoptosis in human neuroblastoma cells. J Natl Cancer Inst. 1994;6:1245-1247.

361. Maurer BJ, Metelitsa LS, Seeger RC, et al. Increase of ceramide and induction of mixed apoptosis/necrosis by N-(4-hydroxyphenyl)-retinamide in neuroblastoma cell lines. J Natl Cancer Inst. 1999;91:1138-1146.

362. Maurer BJ, Melton L, Billups C, et al. Synergistic cytotoxicity in solid tumor cell lines between N-(4-hydroxyphenyl)retinamide and modulators of ceramide metabolism. J Natl Cancer Inst. 2000;92:1897-1909.

363. Wang H, Maurer BJ, Reynolds CP, Cabot MC. N-(4-hydroxyphenyl)retinamide elevates ceramide in neuroblastoma cell lines by coordinate activation of serine palmitoyltransferase and ceramide synthase. Cancer Res. 2001;61:5102-5105.

364. Oridate N, Suzuki S, Higuchi M, et al. Involvement of reactive oxygen species in N-(4-hydroxyphenyl)retinamide-induced apoptosis in cervical carcinoma cells. J Natl Cancer Inst. 1997;89:1191-1198.

365. Ribatti D, Alessandri G, Baronio M, et al. Inhibition of neuroblastoma-induced angiogenesis by fenretinide. Int J Cancer. 2001;94:314-321.

366. Erdreich-Epstein A, Tran LB, Bowman NN, et al. Ceramide signaling in fenretinide-induced endothelial cell apoptosis. J Biol Chem. 2002;277:49531-49537.

367. Villa ML, Ferrario E, Trabattoni D, et al. Retinoids, breast cancer and NK cells. Br J Cancer. 1993;68:845-850.

368. Evans AE, Kisselbach KD, Yamashiro DJ, et al. The anti-tumor activity of CEP-751 (KT-6587) on human neuroblastoma and medulloblastoma xenografts. Clin Cancer Res. 1999;5:3594-3602.

369. Evans AE, Kisselbach KD, Liu X, et al. Effect of CEP-751 (KT-6587) on neuroblastoma xenografts expressing TrkB. Med Pediatr Oncol. 2001;36:181-184.

370. Ho R, Minturn JE, Hishiki T, et al. Proliferation of human neuroblastomas mediated by the epidermal growth factor receptor. Cancer Res. 2005;65(21):9868-9875.

371. Meyers MB, Shen WP, Spengler BA, et al. Increased epidermal growth factor receptor in multidrug-resistant human neuroblastoma cells. J Cell Biochem. 1988;38:87-97.

372. Zhang L, Jope RS. Muscarinic M3 and epidermal growth factor receptors activate mutually inhibitory signaling cascades in human neuroblastoma SH-SY5Y cells. Biochem Biophys Res Commun. 1999;255:774-777.

373. Layfield LJ, Thompson JK, Dodge RK, Kerns BJ. Prognostic indicators for neuroblastoma: stage, grade, DNA ploidy, MIB-1-proliferation index, p53, HER-2/neu and EGFr—a survival study. J Surg Oncol. 1995;59:21-27.

374. Jakacki RI, Hamilton M, Gilbertson RJ, et al. Pediatric phase I and pharmacokinetic study of erlotinib followed by the combination of erlotinib and temozolomide: a Children's Oncology Group Phase I Consortium Study. J Clin Oncol. 2008;Sep 15. [Epub ahead of print].

375. Beppu K, Jaboine J, Merchant MS, et al. Effect of imatinib mesylate on neuroblastoma tumorigenesis and vascular endothelial growth factor expression. J Natl Cancer Inst. 2004;96:46-55.

376. Christensen JG, Zou HY, Arango ME, et al. Cytoreductive antitumor activity of PF-2341066, a novel inhibitor of anaplastic lymphoma kinase and c-Met, in experimental models of anaplastic large-cell lymphoma. Mol Cancer Ther. 2007;6(Pt 1):3314-3322.

377. Dole M, Nunez G, Merchant AK, et al. Bcl-2 inhibits chemotherapy-induced apoptosis in neuroblastoma. Cancer Res. 1994;54:3253-3259.

378. Castle VP, Heidelberger KP, Bromberg J, et al. Expression of the apoptosis-suppressing protein bcl-2, in neuroblastoma is associated with unfavorable histology and N-myc amplification. Am J Pathol. 1993;143:1543-1550.

379. Mejia MC, Navarro S, Pellin A, et al. Study of bcl-2 protein expression and the apoptosis phenomenon in neuroblastoma. Anticancer Res. 1998;18:801-806.

380. Reed JC, Meister L, Tanaka S, et al. Differential expression of Bcl2 protooncogene in neuroblastoma and other human tumor cell lines of neural origin. Cancer Res. 1991;51:6529-6538.

381. Reed JC, Stein C, Subasinghe C, et al. Antisense-mediated inhibition of BCL2 protooncogene expression and leukemic cell growth and survival: comparisons of phosphodiester and phosphorothioate oligodeoxynucleotides. Cancer Res. 1990;50:6565-6570.

382. Rheingold SR, Hogarty MD, Blaney SM, et al. Phase I Trial of G3139, a bcl-2 antisense oligonucleotide, combined with doxorubicin and cyclophosphamide in children with relapsed solid tumors: a Children's Oncology Group Study. J Clin Oncol. 2007;25:1512-1518.

383. Jaboin J, Kim CJ, Kaplan DR, Thiele CJ. Brain-derived neurotrophic factor activation of TrkB protects neuroblastoma cells from chemotherapy-induced apoptosis via phosphatidylinositol 3'-kinase pathway. Cancer Res. 2002;62:6756-6763.

384. Coffey DC, Kutko MC, Glick RD, et al. The histone deacetylase inhibitor, CBHA, inhibits growth of human neuroblastoma xenografts in vivo, alone and synergistically with all-trans retinoic acid. Cancer Res. 2001;61:3591-3594.

385. Coffey DC, Kutko MC, Glick RD, et al. Histone deacetylase inhibitors and retinoic acids inhibit growth of human neuroblastoma in vitro. Med Pediatr Oncol. 2000;35:577-581.

386. Glick RD, Swendeman SL, Coffey DC, et al. Hybrid polar histone deacetylase inhibitor induces apoptosis and CD95/CD95 ligand expression in human neuroblastoma. Cancer Res. 1999;59:4392-4399.

387. Nagy L, Kao HY, Chakravarti D, et al. Nuclear receptor repression mediated by a complex containing SMRT, mSin3A, and histone deacetylase. Cell. 1997;89:373-380.

388. Cameron EE, Bachman KE, Myohanen S, et al. Synergy of demethylation and histone deacetylase inhibition in the re-expression of genes silenced in cancer. Nat Genet. 1999;21:103-107.

389. Zhu WG, Lakshmanan RR, Beal MD, Otterson GA. DNA methyltransferase inhibition enhances apoptosis induced by histone deacetylase inhibitors. Cancer Res. 2001;61:1327-1333.

390. Shimada H, Ambros IM, Dehner LP, et al. Terminology and morphologic criteria of neuroblastic tumors: recommendations by the International Neuroblastoma Pathology Committee. Cancer. 1999;86:349-363.

15 Pediatric Renal Tumors

Jeffrey S. Dome, Charles W. M. Roberts, and Pedram Argani

Pediatric renal tumors comprise approximately 5% of malignancies in children younger than 15 years and 3.6% of malignancies in children younger than 20 years.[1] Among 9731 patients registered with the National Wilms' Tumor Study Group (NWTSG; 1969-2002), Wilms' tumor comprised the vast majority of childhood renal tumors (92%), followed by clear cell sarcoma of the kidney (3.4%), congenital mesoblastic nephroma (1.7%), malignant rhabdoid tumor (1.6%), and rare miscellaneous neoplasms, including primitive neuroectodermal tumor (PNET), synovial sarcoma, neuroblastoma, and cystic nephroma (1.1%). Although not historically included on NWTSG studies, renal cell carcinoma accounted for 8% of renal tumors in children age 0 to 19 years according to data from the Surveillance, Epidemiology, and End Results (SEER) program.[1]

The study of pediatric renal tumors has had significant impact on the field of oncology. Wilms' tumor has provided a paradigm for multidisciplinary treatment approaches and the conduct of cooperative group studies. Wilms' tumor investigators took the lead in establishing one of the leading biologic sample banks, now containing several thousand annotated tumor, blood, and urine samples. Tenets of cancer biology, including Knudson's two-hit model and loss of imprinting in tumorigenesis, were demonstrated in Wilms' tumor. This chapter reviews the pathology, epidemiology, genetics and biology, and treatment of pediatric renal tumors.

PATHOLOGY OF PEDIATRIC RENAL TUMORS

Approximately 15% of renal neoplasms in children and adolescents are not Wilms' tumor. Because the clinical management of pediatric renal tumors varies greatly according to tumor type and stage, it is imperative for the pathologist to provide an accurate histologic diagnosis and staging designation.

Staging

Stage is the major determinant of prognosis and therapy for all pediatric renal neoplasms. Two staging systems are widely used (Table 15-1). The Children's Oncology Group (COG) staging system reflects tumor extent after surgery before chemotherapy is given. By contrast, the International Society of Pediatric Oncology (SIOP) system reflects tumor extent after 4 to 6 weeks of chemotherapy and surgery. The COG and SIOP staging systems are applied to all pediatric renal tumors except renal cell carcinoma, for which the TNM system is used.[2]

The COG staging schema is similar to that used in National Wilms' Tumor Study–5 (NWTS-5), although two changes distinguish the current COG staging criteria from the prior NWTS-5 criteria.[3,4] First, localized spillage or rupture, or any form of biopsy before removal of the kidney, is no longer considered stage II but instead is considered stage III. Second, several protocols that reduce therapy for stage I tumors require that regional nodes be examined microscopically. These protocols involve no adjuvant chemotherapy for young patients (younger than 2 years) with small (less than 550 g nephrectomy weight) stage I favorable histology Wilms' tumor, and no radiation therapy for stage I clear cell sarcoma of the kidney. If lymph nodes are not removed by the surgeon or identified by the pathologist, children who would otherwise qualify for these protocols will be ineligible.

The SIOP system was recently revised to classify tumors with local and regional lymph node involvement as stage III. Previously, lymph node involvement was considered stage II,

Stage	**Children's Oncology Group (COG) (Prechemotherapy)**	**International Society of Pediatric Oncology (SIOP) (Postchemotherapy)**
I	Tumor limited to kidney and completely resected: • Renal capsule intact, not penetrated by tumor • No tumor invasion of veins or lymphatics of renal sinus • No nodal or hematogenous metastases • No prior biopsy • Negative margins	Tumor limited to kidney and completely resected: • Renal capsule may be infiltrated by tumor, but tumor does not reach the outer surface • Tumor may protrude or bulge into the pelvic system or ureter, but does not infiltrate • Vessels of renal sinus not involved
II	Tumor extends beyond kidney but completely resected: • Tumor penetrates renal capsule • Tumor in lymphatics or veins of renal sinus • Tumor in renal vein with margin not involved • No nodal or hematogenous metastases • Negative margins	Tumor extends beyond kidney but completely resected: • Tumor penetrates the renal capsule into perirenal fat • Tumor infiltrates the renal sinus and/or invades blood and lymphatic vessels outside renal parenchyma but is completely resected • Tumor infiltrates adjacent organs or vena cava but is completely resected
III	Residual tumor or nonhematogenous metastases confined to abdomen: • Involved abdominal nodes • Peritoneal contamination or tumor implant • Tumor spillage of any degree occurring before or during surgery • Gross residual tumor in abdomen • Biopsy of tumor (including fine-needle aspiration) prior to removal of kidney • Resection margins involved by tumor	Incomplete excision of the tumor which extends beyond the resection margins (gross or microscopic residual): • Involved abdominal lymph nodes, including necrotic tumor or chemotherapy-induced changes • Tumor rupture before or intraoperatively • Tumor has penetrated the peritoneal surface • Tumor thrombi present at resection margins • Surgical biopsy prior to resection (does not include needle biopsy)
IV	Hematogenous metastases or spread beyond abdomen	Hematogenous metastases or spread beyond abdomen
V	Bilateral renal tumors: • Each side's tumor should be substaged separately according to the above criteria [e.g., stage V, substage II (right), substage I (left)]	Bilateral renal tumors: • Each side's tumor should be substaged separately according to the above criteria [e.g., stage V, substage II (right), substage I (left)]

TABLE 15-1   **Staging Systems for Pediatric Renal Tumors**

with separate designations for node-positive and node-negative disease.[5]

Overview

Wilms' Tumor (Nephroblastoma)

Gross Features

Wilms' tumor (WT) typically presents as a unicentric, spherical mass that is sharply demarcated from the renal parenchyma.[6] Approximately 10% of WTs are multicentric, a finding associated with an increased likelihood of WT formation in the contralateral kidney.

The cut surface of WT is most commonly pale gray and uniform, but hemorrhage, necrosis, and cyst formation are common. The texture is usually soft and friable, but stroma-rich neoplasms may have a dense, myomatous consistency. Calcification is relatively uncommon. Prominent septa frequently impart a multinodular appearance.

WT may arise anywhere in the cortex or medulla, frequently compressing and distorting renal parenchyma around its margin. Rarely, exophytic tumors connected to the renal surface by a narrow stalk may mimic extrarenal WT. Polyploid masses in the pelvicalyceal lumen may occur either as extensions from the primary intrarenal neoplasm or as separate neoplasms arising within the pelvic wall. The renal vein and its branches are not uncommonly filled by tumor thrombus that can extend via the inferior vena cava into the right atrium.

Cystic Variants of Wilms' Tumor

Scattered cysts are commonly encountered in conventional WT but, rarely, the encapsulated, well-delineated neoplasm is composed entirely of cystic spaces and delicate septa, without an expansile solid component. A neoplasm entirely composed of mature cells is termed *cystic nephroma* (CN). If the septa contain embryonal cell types, the designation cystic, partially differentiated nephroblastoma (CPDN) is appropriate. In contrast, cystic WT is distinguished by the presence of solid expansile regions that replace or distort the cystic spaces, rather than being passively molded by the cysts. This distinction is best made by careful examination of the gross specimen.[7]

CPDN may be a transitional stage in the development of pediatric CN, and these lesions seem to represent a cystic, highly favorable end of the WT spectrum. The epithelial cells lining the cysts of CN and CPDN range from flattened to columnar, and often are of the "hobnail" type, with prominent eosinophilic cytoplasm that is more abundant at the base than the apex. The cysts often have distinct walls composed of maturing spindle cells. The distinction of CN from CPDN has little clinical importance when the lesion has been completely resected, because both lesions are curable by resection alone. If resection is incomplete or associated with tumor spill, a slight potential for recurrence exists for each.

Microscopic Features

WTs are surpassed only by teratomas in their diversity of cell and tissue types and degrees of differentiation. Most WTs exhibit, at least focally, the so-called triphasic appearance, including cells of blastemal, stromal, and epithelial lineage (Fig. 15-1). However, monophasic and biphasic WTs are relatively common, consisting of only one or two of these cell lineages.

Each of the three major cell types can demonstrate a spectrum of patterns and degrees of differentiation, accounting for the remarkable diversity of appearances characterizing various WTs.

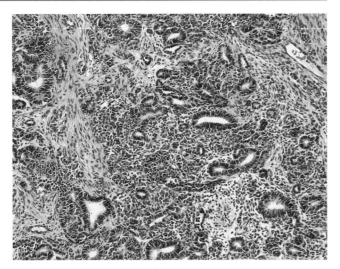

FIGURE 15-1. Wilms' tumor with favorable histology and triphasic pattern.

Blastemal Patterns. The blastemal cells of WT are small, tightly packed cells with a high nucleus-to-cytoplasm ratio, demonstrating little or no evidence of differentiation toward epithelial or stromal cell types at the light microscopic level. Their nuclei are usually round or oval, with moderately coarse chromatin, and mold to each other in the same fashion as the nuclei of small cell carcinoma of the lung. Nucleoli are relatively inconspicuous. Blastemal cells form several distinctive aggregation patterns that can be divided into two broad categories, diffuse and nested, based on their structure and degree of invasiveness.

Monomorphous, relatively dyscohesive sheets of blastemal cells with aggressively invasive margins characterize the diffuse blastemal pattern. This is the most consistently aggressive pattern of WT. Stage I WTs rarely show this pattern; most diffuse blastemal WTs present at an advanced stage, stage III or IV. Fortunately, most neoplasms with the diffuse blastemal pattern are highly responsive to modern therapeutic protocols, so this pattern remains in the favorable histology category.[8] The diffuse blastemal pattern can be readily confused with other small blue cell tumors of childhood, and ultrastructural or other special studies may be required to establish the correct diagnosis (Fig. 15-2).

Nested blastemal patterns are characterized by sharply outlined clusters of blastemal cells in a myxoid mesenchymal background. They usually lack the invasive behavior seen with the diffuse blastemal pattern, and these neoplasms have sharply defined margins at their advancing edge. Several nested patterns may be seen. The serpentine blastemal pattern features long, serpiginous, anastomosing cords of blastemal cells in a loose, stellate, spindled stroma. This is a highly distinctive pattern of WT, and helps distinguish WT from other small blue cell neoplasms of childhood. The nodular blastemal pattern resembles the serpentine pattern, but has rounded blastemal nests instead of long cell cords. The basaloid blastemal pattern resembles the serpentine or nodular patterns, except that the blastemal cell clusters are outlined by a palisaded layer of cuboidal or columnar cells, reminiscent of the architecture of cutaneous basal cell carcinoma.

Epithelial Patterns. Epithelial differentiation in WT produces various cell types and degrees of differentiation. Most of these recapitulate events in normal nephrogenesis (homologous differentiation). Others, such as squamous differentiation or

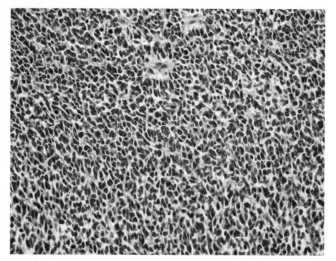

FIGURE 15-2. Wilms' tumor with favorable histology and a diffuse blastemal pattern.

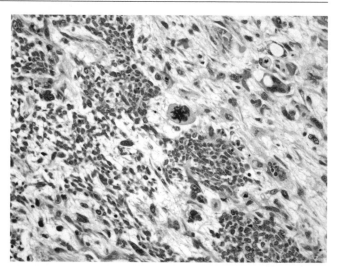

FIGURE 15-3. Wilms' tumor with anaplastic histology.

mucinous differentiation, do not occur in the normal kidney at any stage of development (heterologous differentiation).

Tubular differentiation is the most frequent epithelial pattern. This ranges from vague hints at tubular formation in blastemal foci, which may resemble rosettes, to highly differentiated tubules resembling those of the mature kidney. WTs in which tubular differentiation is predominant tend to be less aggressive, and most present at stage I. Although not usually invasive, tubular-predominant WTs often grow rapidly, and it is not uncommon to find huge tumors that remain confined to the kidney. Glomerular differentiation, present in many WTs, ranges from simple papillary formations barely suggesting glomerulogenesis to mature tumor glomeruli closely resembling those of normal developing kidneys.

Stromal Patterns. Immature myxoid and spindled mesenchymal cells are the most common stromal cell types seen in WTs. Skeletal muscle is the most common heterologous cell type. The presence of skeletal muscle (rhabdomyoblastic differentiation) in WT must not be confused with renal rhabdoid tumor (see later). In fact, the presence of skeletal muscle in a pediatric renal neoplasm is strong evidence supporting the diagnosis of WT.

Anaplasia: The Sign of Unfavorable Histology in Wilms' Tumor. Approximately 5% to 10% of WTs demonstrate anaplastic nuclear change, the only criterion of unfavorable histology.[9] All WTs lacking this feature are designated as having favorable histology. Anaplasia is almost never seen in WT diagnosed during the first year and is rare in the second year of life. The relative frequency of anaplasia increases after that age, and is found in approximately 10% of WTs diagnosed after the age of 5 years. Anaplastic nuclear change reflects extreme polyploidy and is usually apparent under low magnification (10× objective). The features of anaplasia include markedly enlarged tumor cell nuclei with increased chromatin content (hyperchromasia), and multipolar mitotic figures (Fig. 15-3). The former criteria reflect polyploidy, whereas the latter criterion helps exclude degenerative nuclear changes, as commonly seen in cells showing skeletal muscle differentiation, from the anaplastic category. Anaplasia is tightly correlated with the presence of *TP53* gene mutations.[10,11] Whereas favorable histology WTs almost never harbor *TP53* mutations, most anaplastic WTs do.

At a practical level, p53 protein overexpression by immunohistochemistry correlates well but not perfectly with morphologically defined anaplasia.[12,13]

Focal and Diffuse Anaplasia. Initially, the presence of anaplastic nuclear changes in any region of a WT was considered prognostically unfavorable. It subsequently has been hypothesized that anaplasia is an indicator of increased resistance to adjuvant chemotherapy and not necessarily a marker of increased tumor aggressiveness, so stage I anaplastic WT and WT with limited intrarenal foci of anaplasia (focal anaplasia) would be predicted to have an excellent prognosis. This concept implies that the prognosis for a patient with anaplastic WT is determined by the completeness of surgical removal of anaplastic cells.[14] However, recent data on patients with stage 1 anaplastic WT have challenged this concept.[15] Regardless, the definition of focal anaplasia (FA) includes only those WTs meeting all the following criteria:

1. Anaplasia confined to one or more discrete sites within the primary tumor and not present in extrarenal sites
2. Tumor cells outside anaplastic foci that show no "nuclear unrest" (nuclear or mitotic abnormalities that approach, but do not quite attain, the degree of severity required for a designation of anaplasia)

Any WT not meeting this definition of FA is designated as having diffuse anaplasia (DA). Any one of the following situations merits assignment to the DA category:

1. Nonlocalized anaplastic change
2. Anaplastic change or nuclear unrest in invasive sites, or any extrarenal deposits
3. Localized anaplastic change in a tumor that also has severe nuclear unrest elsewhere
4. Anaplasia in a random biopsy specimen
5. Anaplasia involving the edge of one or more sections, and the site(s) from which the sections were taken cannot be determined (with the latter emphasizing the importance of mapping the sections taken from a WT, best done on a photograph of a cut section of the tumor)

Anaplastic foci are usually clearly demarcated from adjacent nonanaplastic tumor. Most cases in the FA category have a single focus of anaplasia. Anaplastic foci are usually only a

	TABLE 15-2	Comparison of COG and SIOP Histologic Risk Classification Schemas

Children's Oncology Group (COG)	International Society of Pediatric Oncology (SIOP)
Favorable histology Wilms' tumor: • No evidence of anaplasia Focal anaplastic Wilms' tumor: • Anaplasia confined to one or more discrete sites within the primary tumor with no extrarenal involvement • No nuclear unrest outside anaplastic foci Diffuse anaplastic Wilms' tumor: • Nonlocalized anaplasia • Anaplasia in invasive sites or extrarenal deposits • Localized anaplasia with severe nuclear unrest elsewhere • Anaplasia in a random biopsy specimen. • Anaplasia involving the edge of one or more sections (non–Wilms' renal tumors not included in this classification schema)	Low risk: • Mesoblastic nephroma • Cystic partially differentiated nephroblastoma • Completely necrotic Wilms' tumor Intermediate risk: • Wilms' tumor of epithelial, stromal, mixed, or regressive types • Focal anaplastic Wilms' tumor High risk: • Blastemal-type Wilms' tumor • Diffuse anaplastic Wilms' tumor • Clear cell sarcoma of the kidney • Rhabdoid tumor of the kidney

few millimeters in diameter but can be larger if their localized nature can be convincingly documented.

International Society of Pediatric Oncology Postchemotherapy Histologic Classification System

Patients treated on SIOP protocols receive several weeks of chemotherapy before undergoing nephrectomy. Chemotherapy usually causes necrosis of immature and actively proliferating cell types in WT, whereas slowly replicating and differentiated cell types are usually unaffected. For example, tumors composed mostly of mature skeletal muscle or renal tubules show little clinical regression with chemotherapy, because few cells are proliferating.[16] The microscopic appearance of the tumor after chemotherapy has prognostic significance. Approximately 5% to 10% of WTs are completely necrotic after chemotherapy, a finding associated with a 98% 5-year relapse-free survival rate.[17] By contrast, WTs with a predominance of blastemal cells after chemotherapy, defined as viable cells in more than one third of the tumor mass and blastemal cells in at least two thirds of the viable component, have relapse rates of almost 40%.[5,18] Based on these observations, the SIOP histologic risk classification schema divides renal tumors into three risk categories—low risk, intermediate risk, and high risk. A comparison of the COG and SIOP histologic classification systems is summarized in Table 15-2.

Ultrastructural and Immunohistochemical Studies

Ultrastructural study is rarely necessary to establish a diagnosis of WT but can occasionally be helpful in distinguishing blastemal WT from other undifferentiated neoplasms.[19,20] The diversity of differentiation in WT creates a correspondingly varied profile of immunohistochemical results. Blastemal cells may or may not label for vimentin and cytokeratin, whereas various differentiating elements will label according to their patterns of

differentiation. For example, primitive rhabdomyoblasts within a tumor will label for the myogenic transcription factor myogenin and for cytoskeletal proteins such as actin and desmin. WT blastemal cells characteristically label for desmin but not for actin, myogenin, or other muscle markers.[21] Immunoreactivity for WT-1 protein is typically limited to the blastemal and epithelial components of WT, with the stroma being negative.[22] Hence, the absence of labeling for WT-1, particularly in a stroma-rich tumor, does not exclude the diagnosis of WT. Although WT-1 immunoreactivity may help distinguish WT from PNET, one should be aware that desmoplastic small round cell tumor typically labels for WT-1. Hence, although useful, WT-1 immunoreactivity cannot in and of itself establish or disprove a diagnosis of WT.

Nephrogenic Rests and Nephroblastomatosis

In more than 30% of kidneys resected for WT, the renal parenchyma contains one or more regions of persistent embryonal tissue, representing potential precursors of WT. These lesions have been given many names in the past; however, the term suggested by Dr. J. Bruce Beckwith, *nephrogenic rests* (NRs), is the currently accepted terminology.[23,24] The presence of multiple or diffusely distributed NRs is termed *nephroblastomatosis*. This term is most commonly applied when the rests are in an active state of cellular proliferation and are large enough to be apparent on imaging studies.

NRs have a dynamic life history that can yield various appearances. Beckwith's classification is based on the assumption that the structure of NRs reflects both the dynamic state and the history of an individual rest. A brief summary is provided here.

Two fundamental categories of NRs are recognized based on their topographic relation to the renal lobe. These are designated as perilobar nephrogenic rests (PLNRs) and intralobar nephrogenic rests (ILNRs). ILNRs may occur anywhere in the renal lobe, including the peripheral cortex. They may also occur in the renal sinus, including in the walls of the pelvicalyceal system. ILNRs have a more varied structure than PLNRs and typically intercalate between nephrons, whereas PLNRs usually are discrete structures that are well delineated from adjacent nephrons. Rests of either major category may be further classified based on their developmental fates. An individual NR may undergo any of the following fates, several of which often occur sequentially over time:

1. It may remain unchanged in size or composition, even for many years, as a tiny, microscopic blastemal focus (dormant NR).
2. It may undergo maturation, sclerosis, and eventual disappearance (sclerosing NRs and obsolescent NRs). This is the most common fate of NRs.
3. It may undergo hyperplasia, or coordinated proliferation of all susceptible cells of the rest, as distinguished from a clonal neoplastic process originating in a single cell of the rest. Hyperplastic NR may produce large, actively growing masses that have numerous mitotic figures, and a section from the interior of a hyperplastic NR may be indistinguishable from WT. Several features help make this distinction. First, diffuse hyperplastic growth, involving all or most cells of a rest, tends to preserve the original shape of the rest. When PLNRs form a continuous layer of embryonal cells at the lobar surface, hyperplastic proliferation will produce a thick "rind" of abnormal tissue at the renal surface. Ovoid and lenticular masses result from hyperplasia of NRs that originally had these shapes. An irregularly shaped, multinodular appearance will result if only some of the cells are capable

of proliferation. In contrast, WT, a neoplasm presumably arising from a single cell, tends to form spherical masses. The second important feature distinguishing actively hyperplastic NRs from WT is the usual absence of a pseudocapsule at the interface between hyperplastic NRs and the renal parenchyma.

4. Neoplastic induction is assumed to represent a clonal event originating in single cells of a rest, resulting in WT or benign adenomas. As noted, rapidly growing tumors originating at a single point (or cell) will tend to grow equally in all directions, forming spherical, expansile nodules with compressed rest remnants often present at the periphery.

5. Very rarely, anaplasia may develop in nephrogenic rests.[25]

An individual rest commonly progresses through several of these processes sequentially. For example, an incipient or dormant rest may undergo hyperplasia, followed by phases of growth arrest and maturation. This will result in a large but inactive-appearing lesion. Ultimately, one or more cells within the regressing rest may be induced to form WT.

ILNRs are most often found at the tumor-kidney interface, where they can be misinterpreted as infiltrating tumor cells or effaced by tumor compression. A helpful feature distinguishing ILNRs at the edge of a WT is the poorly defined, irregular outer border of the ILNR, which contrasts with the sharp pushing interface between the WT and the rest within which it arose. Also, ILNRs are usually less cellular than the adjacent WT that they surround.

The presence of NRs in a kidney removed for WT is correlated with an increased risk for subsequent WT formation in the remaining kidney. The type of rest and age of the patient modify this risk.[26] When a carefully sampled kidney is free of rests, the risk of contralateral WT is extremely low. The possibility of subsequent WT developing in the remaining kidney should be considered in planning the follow-up of patients whose nephrectomy specimen has revealed the presence of NRs in addition to WT.

Differential Diagnosis of Wilms' Tumor

Triphasic Wilms' Tumor. This pattern rarely presents a problem in diagnosis, except when small biopsies are obtained from large retroperitoneal masses of uncertain origin. In this setting, other mixed neoplasms might deserve consideration, including teratoma, hepatoblastoma, pancreatoblastoma, mesothelioma, synovial sarcoma, and intra-abdominal desmoplastic small round cell tumor. In the absence of nephrogenic differentiation or the distinctive nested blastemal patterns described earlier, ancillary studies such as immunohistochemistry, molecular biology, or electron microscopy may be required to distinguish some of these lesions from WT. WT with extensive heterologous differentiation (teratoid WT) is easily confused with immature teratoma. Renal teratomas are extremely rare, and some of the reported cases likely represent teratoid WT.

Blastemal Wilms' Tumor Versus Other Small Blue Cell Tumors of Childhood. This problem is most likely to arise when dealing with biopsies from metastatic sites or from large abdominal tumors of uncertain origin. The distinctive aggregation patterns of blastemal WT, the presence of nuclear molding, or the focal presence of tubular differentiation will often reveal the diagnosis. Early tubular differentiation in WT lacks lumens and therefore can sometimes be confused with rosettes of neuroblastoma or PNET. The presence of true lumens, even focally, confirms tubular differentiation, but neurofibrils are diagnostic of a neuroblastic pseudorosette. Neuroblastic rosettes rarely occur in WT, but usually only in teratoid WTs, which are not likely to

be confused with neuroblastomas or PNETs. Immunohistochemistry, electron microscopy, molecular diagnostic techniques, cytogenetics, circulating tumor markers, and other special studies are often required to confirm the nature of a small blue cell tumor.

Epithelial Predominant Wilms' Tumor Versus Papillary Renal Cell Carcinoma. This differential diagnosis is most often encountered in tumors from adolescents or adults. Papillary adenoma, the benign precursor of papillary renal cell carcinoma (PRCC), may resemble epithelial-predominant nephrogenic rests, and epithelial-predominant WTs can have a predominantly papillary architecture. Sometimes, PRCCs have a predominant tubular or solid component. Molecular or cytogenetic studies may be helpful, because PRCC characteristically contains increased copies of chromosomes 7 and 17 and, in tumors from male patients, deletion of Y.[27] Unequivocal glomerular differentiation, characteristic blastemal aggregation patterns, or the presence of heterologous cell types can confirm the diagnosis of WT. Immunoreactivity for cytokeratin 7 has been advocated as a useful marker for PRCC, but focal positive labeling for this marker occurs in many WTs. Only when diffusely positive is cytokeratin 7 labeling likely to be discriminatory. Nuclear labeling for WT1 protein may distinguish WT, nephrogenic rests, and metanephric adenoma from PRCC, because only the latter does not label.[28]

Clear Cell Sarcoma of the Kidney

Gross Appearance

Clear cell sarcoma of the kidney (CCSK) is always unicentric, with a distinct tumor-kidney junction. Tumors are usually relatively large, with a mean specimen diameter of approximately 11 cm.[29] The cut surface is often glistening and gelatinous. Cysts are almost always present and may be so prominent as to suggest cystic nephroma on gross examination or imaging studies.

Microscopic Appearance

Under low magnification, most CCSKs appear monomorphous, without the prominent lobulation usually seen in WT. CCSK usually has a scalloped border that appears fairly sharp under low power. Under higher magnification, the border appears less sharply defined because of the penetration of neoplastic cells a short distance into the surrounding kidney or the tumor capsule. This growth pattern tends to surround and isolate individual single nephrons, which is rarely if ever seen with WT. The entrapped tubules are usually confined to the peripheral 2 to 3 cm of a CCSK. Their epithelium commonly shows embryonal metaplastic changes similar to those entrapped in congenital mesoblastic nephroma, and the resultant basophilic epithelium creates confusion with WT. Dilation of these entrapped tubules produces intratumoral cysts that may mimic cystic nephroma. CCSK may show a wide variety of morphologic patterns (see later).[29-32]

Classic Pattern. The hallmark of this pattern is an evenly distributed network of vascular *septa*, which has a branching, chicken wire pattern similar to that seen in myxoid liposarcoma or oligodendroglioma.[33] These fibrovascular septa subdivide the tumor into a conspicuous pattern of cords and nests, averaging six to ten cells in width, and composed of polygonal cells that usually lack distinct cytoplasmic borders. Cells within the cords are less densely packed than those of blastemal WT, and overlapping nuclei are less frequent. Nuclear chromatin is usually finely granular, with inconspicuous nucleoli (Fig. 15-4). In well-fixed specimens, the fine nuclear chromatin pattern is

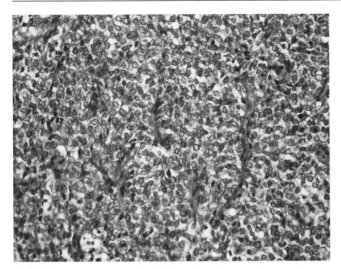

FIGURE 15-4. Clear cell sarcoma of the kidney.

the most helpful clue to the diagnosis. However, it is influenced markedly by the timing and type of fixation. Mitotic figures are variable in number but are usually less numerous than those in WT. The cytoplasm usually lacks distinct borders and is surrounded by extracellular mucopolysaccharides, which creates the illusion of clear cytoplasm.

CCSK is easily confused with other neoplasms because the classic pattern is often modified, presenting alterations that mimic other neoplasms to a sometimes striking degree. Fortunately, the classic pattern of CCSK predominates in most specimens and is present at least focally in over 90% of tumors. However, the pathologist unaware of these variant patterns is likely to diagnose CCSK as another neoplasm, with different therapeutic and prognostic implications. These variant patterns are described later.[29-31]

Epithelioid Patterns. Condensation of cord cells of the classic CCSK pattern creates striking epithelioid arrangements in approximately 15% of cases.[29] These condensations usually form trabeculae or rosettes. The epithelioid formations conform to the pattern of the original cell cords and can be straight or undulating in configuration. The epithelioid variants of CCSK are most likely to be mistaken for WT. In all the examples analyzed by immunohistochemistry, these epithelioid formations have been negative for epithelial markers, in contrast to the epithelial cells of WT.

Spindle Cell Patterns. Spindle cell patterns are seen in approximately 10% of cases and result from two mechanisms.[29] Proliferation of septal cells produces wide spindle cell septa that compress or obliterate the cell cords. Intersections of these hyperplastic septal cells often resemble the storiform patterns observed in fibrohistiocytic neoplasms. Spindled transformation of cord cells yields a spindled pattern, with preservation of thin fibrovascular septa.

Myxoid and Sclerosing Patterns. Most CCSKs contain abundant mucopolysaccharide, apparently produced by the cord cells.[29] This material separates cord cells and creates the appearance of clear cytoplasm. In approximately 30% of cases, mucopolysaccharide occupies more volume than the neoplastic cells themselves and forms large pools or cystic spaces.[29] As it accumulates, the tumor cells become progressively more isolated and eventually degenerate. In time, the mucoid material becomes denser, eosinophilic, and hyaline in appearance.

Hyaline sclerosis is found in 35% of CCSK. Complete replacement of cell cords by hyaline sclerosis preserves the original cord pattern with retention of the vascular septa, preserving the chicken wire appearance. More diffuse zones of dense stromal sclerosis surrounding individual tumor cells may create an osteosarcoma-like appearance. Dense stromal sclerosis is relatively uncommon in untreated WT, and this finding can be a clue to the diagnosis of CCSK or rhabdoid tumor in limited biopsy material.

Palisading (Verocay Body) Pattern. Nuclear palisading resembling schwannoma is focally prominent in approximately 10% of CCSK specimens.[29] Unlike schwannomas, these areas are not immunoreactive for S-100 protein.

Monstrocellular (Anaplastic) Pattern. Approximately 3% of CCSKs contain foci with enlarged, pleomorphic nuclei and bizarre mitotic figures, resembling the appearance of anaplastic WTs or pleomorphic sarcomas. This is the only pattern of CCSK that frequently overexpresses p53 protein.

Post-Therapy Patterns. Recurrences of CCSK after therapy may have a deceptively hypocellular and bland appearance, suggesting low-grade fibromatosis or myxoma. A lump appearing anywhere in a child with a history of CCSK should be viewed as a potential metastasis until proven otherwise.

Ultrastructure and Immunohistochemistry

Ultrastructural studies yield few clues about the putative cell of origin of CCSK.[34] The tumor cells are characterized by a high nuclear-to-cytoplasmic ratio, with nuclear shapes that are more irregular and variable than would be expected from light microscopy. The cytoplasm is usually tenuous, with elongated, irregular processes surrounding abundant intercellular matrix. This latter feature is responsible for the vacuoles often seen with the light microscope. The cytoplasm tends to be poor in organelles. Immunohistochemistry has afforded little new insight into the histogenesis of CCSK, except to exclude various potential lines of differentiation for this enigmatic neoplasm. Vimentin is positive in almost all specimens and bcl2 in some, but other markers are consistently negative. These include stains for epithelial markers (cytokeratins and EMA), neural markers (S-100 protein), neuroendocrine markers (chromogranin, synaptophysin), muscle markers (desmin), CD34, CD117 (c-kit), and CD99 (MIC2).[29]

Differential Diagnosis

The distinction of CCSK from other renal neoplasms can be extremely difficult, even for those with extensive experience in pediatric renal neoplasm pathology. The distinction of CCSK from rhabdoid tumor of the kidney is covered elsewhere in this chapter (see later). The following are the other major differential diagnostic concerns.

Clear Cell Sarcoma of the Kidney Versus Wilms' Tumor. Some blastemal WTs are richly vascular, and the vascular pattern may perfectly mimic that of CCSK. Several features help in this differential diagnosis. First, under low magnification, blastemal WTs often show distinctive nested patterns, whereas CCSKs are not typically nested. Second, blastemal WTs are more densely cellular than CCSKs. When cells are closely packed, most nuclei are overlapping, and nuclei mold to one another, WT is more likely than CCSK. Third, heterologous tissues such as skeletal muscle are never seen in CCSK. The presence of a focus resembling CCSK in an otherwise unequivocal WT can safely be ignored. Fourth, multicentricity is common in

WT, whereas multicentric and bilateral CCSKs have not been reported. Fifth, sclerotic, hyalinized stroma in an untreated tumor favors CCSK over WT. Finally, a fine nuclear chromatin pattern favors a diagnosis of CCSK over WT, although this feature is susceptible to fixation and processing artifacts.

Clear Cell Sarcoma of the Kidney Versus Congenital Mesoblastic Nephroma. Cellular congenital mesoblastic nephroma (CMN) may resemble spindled variants of CCSK, and the age ranges of these two entities overlap. Small foci resembling CCSK may occur in CMN, but CMN lacks the diversity of morphologic patterns that typifies CCSK. The absence of the t(12;15) chromosome translocation characteristic of cellular CMN in all CCSKs examined to date indicates that these two neoplasms are unrelated.

Congenital Mesoblastic Nephroma

Gross Appearance

CMN arises unicentrically and usually appears to have arisen deep within the medial parenchyma, near the renal sinus. The renal sinus and adjacent structures on the medial side of the kidney are major sites of extrarenal spread of CMN. Surgeons and pathologists must pay particular attention to the medial margin of the CMN resection specimen. However, because of the predominance of freely mobile fat in this location and retraction artifact, the medial specimen margin is notoriously difficult to evaluate, and it is rarely possible to be certain that it is free of involvement by CMN.

The appearance of the sectioned surface of CMN is variable and depends on the subtype. Classic CMNs have a tough whorled appearance resembling leiomyoma, but cellular CMNs may be soft friable tumors. Hemorrhage, necrosis, and cyst formation are present to some degree in most cellular CMNs.

Microscopic Appearance

CMN is a low-grade fibroblastic sarcoma of the infantile kidney. The classic type of CMN has a fibrous whorled gross appearance. Morphologically, classic CMN is identical to infantile fibromatosis; it is composed of bland fibroblastic-myofibroblastic cells, arranged in fascicles that dissect into the native kidney (Fig. 15-5).[35] Mitoses are usually rare, and necrosis is absent. The leading edge of the tumor characteristically

induces angiomatous vascular proliferation where it abuts perirenal fat. Entrapped renal tubules may acquire a primitive appearance (embryonal metaplasia); this may cause confusion with true neoplastic tubular differentiation, which would suggest a diagnosis of biphasic stromal-epithelial WT. In contrast, the cellular variant of CMN typically has a softer, fleshier, and hemorrhagic appearance, with necrosis and cystification. Microscopically, cellular CMN is identical to infantile fibrosarcoma (IFS).[36] Compared with the classic variant, cellular CMNs more often have a pushing border, demonstrate sheet-like growth patterns, are less often fascicular, are more cellular, and have a higher mitotic rate (Fig. 15-6). Tumor cells may be polygonal, with well-demarcated pink cytoplasm and nuclei with vesicular chromatin and prominent nucleoli; this raises the differential diagnosis of rhabdoid tumor of the kidney. Alternatively, the tumor cells may be thinner, primitive, and spindled, yielding a more embryonal blue cell appearance. Mixed CMNs have areas identical to cellular and classic CMN in varied proportions within the same tumor.

Immunohistochemistry and Ultrastructure

Immunohistochemistry is of limited value in the diagnosis of CMN. The cells of CMN label in a fashion consistent with fibroblasts or myofibroblasts.[37] Although actin may be focally positive, desmin and CD34 are typically negative (P. Argani, unpublished observations, 2000). INI1 protein is retained. Ultrastructural studies also reveal features consistent with fibroblasts or myofibroblasts.[38] Most CMN cells show abundant rough endoplasmic reticulum (RER) with branching and anastomosing profiles, and primitive cell junctions are often found.

Differential Diagnosis

The differential diagnosis for CMN includes stromal-predominant WT, CCSK, metanephric stromal tumor (MST), and malignant rhabdoid tumor (MRT). These distinctions are crucial, because most children with CMN do not require adjuvant chemotherapy whereas those with WT, CCSK, and MRT are treated on specific chemotherapy protocols. Features that distinguish CCSK and MRT from CMN are described elsewhere in this chapter, as are the features that distinguish CMN from WT and MST (see later).

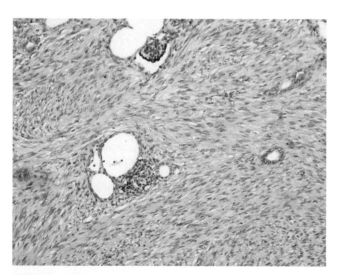

FIGURE 15-5. Congenital mesoblastic nephroma with classic histology.

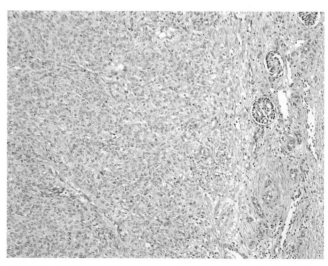

FIGURE 15-6. Congenital mesoblastic nephroma with cellular histology.

Congenital Mesoblastic Nephroma Versus Wilms' Tumor. As noted, embryonal metaplastic changes in nephrons surrounded by CMN cells are sometimes misinterpreted as tubular or papillary elements in a WT. Rarely, untreated WTs will be composed predominantly of stromal cells. In most of these, the presence of immature or mature skeletal muscle readily excludes the diagnosis of CMN. Specimens removed after chemotherapy are particularly challenging. Treatment often ablates the embryonal, proliferating elements of a WT but tends to spare stromal cells. The resulting appearances can readily be confused with CMN. The following features are helpful in the differential diagnosis:

1. A diagnosis of CMN should be considered suspect in a patient who has received prior therapy, unless the clinical and pathologic features are characteristic.
2. Most CMNs are diagnosed in the first 3 months of life, whereas WT is relatively uncommon at this age. Only 10% of CMNs are diagnosed after 1 year, and almost none after 2 years.
3. Most WTs express a diversity of cell types and tissue patterns. In contrast, blastemal foci do not occur in a CMN, and skeletal muscle is never seen. However, nodules of entrapped cartilage and squamous pearls may occur in CMN, likely reflecting coexisting renal dysplasia, and this should not be taken as evidence for WT.
4. The interdigitating irregular border of classic CMN distinguishes it from most WTs. However, cellular CMN often has a sharp pushing border, similar to that of most WTs.
5. Bilaterality, the presence of nephrogenic rests, or both strongly favor WT over CMN.

Congenital Mesoblastic Nephroma Versus Metanephric Stromal Tumor. Many tumors previously considered to be CMN in children older than 3 years are distinct from CMN, and represent the newly recognized entity, metanephric stromal tumor.[39] MST is identical to the stromal component of metanephric adenofibroma (MAF),[40] previously known as nephrogenic adenofibroma,[41] a biphasic tumor containing an epithelial component that is identical to metanephric adenoma (MA). MST is a benign lesion composed of spindled to stellate cells featuring thin hyperchromatic nuclei and thin indistinct cytoplasmic extensions. Several of the characteristic features of MST distinguish it from CMN. MST characteristically surrounds and entraps renal tubules and blood vessels to form concentric onionskin rings or collarettes around these structures. Most MSTs induce angiodysplasia of entrapped arterioles, consisting of epithelioid transformation of medial smooth muscle and myxoid changes. One fourth of MSTs feature juxtaglomerular cell hyperplasia within entrapped glomeruli, which may occasionally lead to hypertension associated with hyperreninism. Finally, unlike CMN, MSTs are typically immunoreactive for CD34, but labeling may be patchy.

Malignant Rhabdoid Tumor

Gross Appearance

Most MRTs are relatively small, because metastasis occurs early in the neoplasm's evolution. On gross examination, MRTs are typically fleshy or hemorrhagic neoplasms, with ill-defined borders and frequent satellite nodules that reflect the tumor's highly invasive nature.[42]

Microscopic Appearance

MRT was so-named because of the resemblance of the tumor cells to rhabdomyoblasts. However, this highly lethal infantile neoplasm does not demonstrate muscle differentiation. Micro-

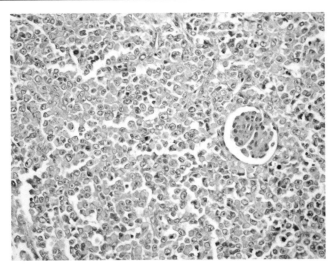

FIGURE 15-7. Rhabdoid tumor of the kidney (malignant rhabdoid tumor).

scopically, these neoplasms typically engulf native renal elements at their periphery and demonstrate extensive vascular invasion. MRT classically consists of sheets of monotonous cells featuring a characteristic cytologic triad—vesicular chromatin, prominent nucleoli, and hyaline cytoplasmic inclusions (Fig. 15-7). These features are variably well developed within a given tumor, so that one may need to examine multiple microscopic fields from many sections to find them.

Ultrastructure and Immunohistochemistry

Ultrastructurally, the cytoplasmic inclusions correspond to whorled intermediate filaments.[43] The whorled filaments may trap antibodies used for immunohistochemistry, yielding a nonspecific polyphenotypic pattern. With this caveat, strong vimentin and focal epithelial membrane antigen (EMA) labeling are characteristic immunohistochemical findings. An immunohistochemical assay for INI1 protein has become available. Loss of INI1 protein expression reflects *INI1* genetic status and is a sensitive and specific marker for MRT.[44]

Differential Diagnosis

The diagnosis of MRT is often challenging because a wide variety of renal and extrarenal tumors of adults and children may feature fully developed rhabdoid cytology, at least focally.[45,46] In the pediatric kidney, these include cellular CMN (of the plump cell type), CCSK, blastemal WT, PNET, renal medullary carcinoma, and rhabdomyosarcoma.[45] In general, thorough sampling of such tumors is most helpful, because it usually reveals specific differentiation that excludes MRT. Additionally, the age of the patient is helpful, because MRT is not seen outside of early childhood. Finally, loss of INI1 protein expression by immunohistochemistry is highly specific for MRT. Several specific differential diagnoses are covered later.

Malignant Rhabdoid Tumor Versus Wilms' Tumor. Both blastemal and myogenic elements of WT may contain cytoplasmic inclusions resembling those of MRT. A distinctive serpentine blastemal pattern, other distinctly nephrogenic features, or heterologous cells such as skeletal muscle supports the diagnosis of WT. The prominent nucleoli characteristic of MRT are not typically seen in WT, with the exception of some anaplastic specimens.

Malignant Rhabdoid Tumor Versus Cellular Congenital Mesoblastic Nephroma. The plump cell variant of cellular CMN often has vesicular nuclei with prominent nucleoli, and a rare CMN contains foci with hyaline cytoplasmic inclusions. A predominance of spindled patterns and a less invasive tumor periphery favors a cellular CMN over a rhabdoid tumor. Cytogenetic and/or molecular analysis may be invaluable in this setting; demonstration of chromosome 22q loss or loss of INI1 protein expression by immunohistochemistry supports MRT, whereas the presence of the ETV6-NTRK3 gene fusion supports cellular CMN.

Malignant Rhabdoid Tumor Versus Clear Cell Sarcoma of the Kidney. CCSK may rarely show prominent nucleoli, which can lead to difficulty in distinguishing CCSK from MRT. The presence of classic cytologic features of CCSK elsewhere and the presence of characteristic CCSK patterns are the major clues to the correct diagnosis in such cases. CCSKs lack the extreme invasiveness of MRTs and are generally more subtly invasive neoplasms.

Pediatric Renal Cell Carcinoma

All the common renal cell carcinomas (RCCs) of adulthood (clear cell, papillary, chromophobe, and collecting duct) may occasionally affect the pediatric kidney, but the clinical and differential diagnostic considerations differ in this setting. Children with von Hippel–Lindau syndrome are predisposed to develop conventional (clear cell) RCC. Children with tuberous sclerosis are at increased risk for developing either RCC or epithelioid angiomyolipoma,[47] and immunohistochemical analysis may be needed to distinguish these two. As discussed earlier, papillary renal cell carcinoma may overlap morphologically with epithelial-predominant Wilms' tumor or metanephric adenoma. However, most pediatric RCCs represent distinctive neoplastic entities. Four of these entities are described.

Xp11.2 Translocation Renal Cell Carcinomas

RCC with chromosome translocations involving Xp11.2 and resulting gene fusions involving the *TFE3* transcription factor gene were officially recognized in the 2004 World Health Organization (WHO) Renal Tumor Classification.[48] Although this subtype of RCC is relatively uncommon on a percentage basis in adults, it most likely comprises most pediatric RCCs. One distinctive subtype bears a t(X;17)(p11;q25), which results in the identical *ASPL-TFE3* gene fusion as was initially identified in alveolar soft part sarcoma (ASPS), and has been designated the *ASPL-TFE3* RCC.[49] Other subtypes are listed in Table 15-3.

Xp11.2 translocation RCCs closely resemble conventional (clear cell) renal carcinomas on gross examination, usually being tan-yellow, and often necrotic and hemorrhagic. A papillary carcinoma comprised of clear cells is the most distinctive histopathologic appearance (Fig. 15-8), because this combination is uncommon in other defined types of renal carcinomas. However, the Xp11.2-translocation RCCs often have nested architecture and often contain cells with granular eosinophilic cytoplasm. The histologies of Xp11.2-translocation RCC associated with different *TFE3* gene fusions differ. *ASPL-TFE3* RCCs feature cells with voluminous, clear to eosinophilic cytoplasm, discrete cell borders, vesicular nuclear chromatin, and prominent nucleoli. In contrast, *PRCC-TFE3* RCCs, characterized by a t(X;1)(p11.2;q21), typically have less abundant cytoplasm, fewer psammoma bodies, fewer hyaline nodules, and a more nested, compact architecture.[50]

Renal carcinomas with Xp11.2-associated translocations characteristically underexpress epithelial immunohistochemical markers such as cytokeratin and epithelial membrane antigen. Only approximately 50% of cases will be positive with these markers, and the labeling is often focal. Vimentin immunoreactivity is also often focal compared with the adjacent blood vessels; this also differs from conventional RCCs, which are diffusely positive. Rare Xp11.2-translocation carcinomas, specifically ones with variant gene fusions such as *PSF-TFE3* and *CLTC-TFE3*,[33] have labeled for melanocytic markers HMB45 and Melan A, creating confusion with epithelioid angiomyolipoma. The most distinctive immunohistochemical feature of these neoplasms is nuclear labeling for TFE3 protein using an antibody to the C-terminal portion of TFE3, which is retained in the gene fusions. Nuclear labeling for TFE3 is a common feature of all Xp11.2-translocation RCCs and ASPSs but does not occur in other RCCs (Fig. 15-9). Because native TFE3 is known to be ubiquitously expressed but is not detectable in normal tissues by immunohistochemistry, it is postulated that the different *TFE3* gene fusions consistently lead to overexpression of the fusion protein relative to native TFE3, so that the protein becomes detectable by this assay.[51]

When analyzed by electron microscopy, Xp11.2-associated carcinomas feature cell junctions, microvilli, intracytoplasmic fat, and glycogen, and thereby most closely resemble conventional renal carcinomas. However, a subset of cases demonstrates distinctive ultrastructural features. Most of the *ASPL-TFE3* RCCs contain membrane-bound cytoplasmic granules and a few have membrane-bound rhomboidal crystals that are identical to those seen in soft tissue ASPSs. Some *PRCC-TFE3* RCCs have had distinctive intracisternal microtu-

Gene Fusion	Chromosome Translocation	Age (yr)	Tumor
ASPL-TFE3	der(17)t(X;17)(p11.2;q25)	5-40	ASPS
ASPL-TFE3	t(X;17)(p11.2;q25)	2-68	RCC
PRCC-TFE3	t(X;1)(p11.2;q21)	2-70	RCC
PSF-TFE3	t(X;1)(p11.2;p34)	5-68	RCC
NoNo-TFE3	inv(X)(p11;q12)	39	RCC
CLTC-TFE3	t(X;17)(p11.2;q23)	14	RCC
Alpha-TFEB	t(6;11)(p21;q12)	6-53	RCC

TABLE 15-3   TFE Translocation Neoplasms

ASPS, alveolar soft part sarcoma; RCC, renal cell carcinoma.

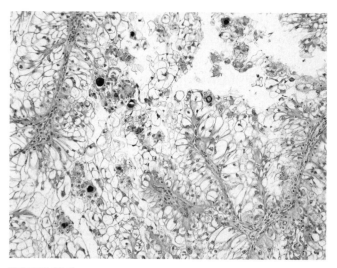

FIGURE 15-8. Renal cell carcinoma with the Xp11.2 translocation.

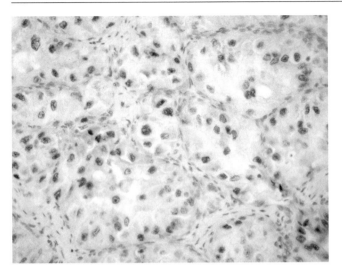

FIGURE 15-9. Renal cell carcinoma with the Xp11.2 translocation, showing TFE3 immunohistochemistry.

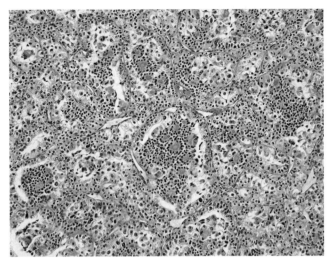

FIGURE 15-10. Renal cell carcinoma with the t(6;11)(p21;q12) translocation.

bules similar to those seen in malignant melanoma and extraskeletal myxoid chondrosarcoma.

t(6;11)(p21;q12) Renal Cell Carcinomas

Another distinctive type of RCC bears a t(6;11)(p21;q12). The distinctive clinicopathologic features of these neoplasms were not described until 2001.[52] On microscopic examination, these neoplasms usually feature nests and tubules of polygonal epithelioid cells, separated by thin capillaries. Some cases have had papillary formations. Most of the tumor cells have abundant clear to granular eosinophilic cytoplasm, well-defined cell borders, and round nuclei with small nucleoli. However, a second population of smaller epithelioid cells is also characteristic, typically (but not always) clustered around nodules of hyaline basement membrane material within larger acini (Fig. 15-10). The cases examined have generally been negative for cytokeratins by immunohistochemistry, but all have labeled at least focally for HMB45 and Melan A, again creating confusion with epithelioid angiomyolipoma.

The t(6;11)(p21;q12) has been shown to result in a fusion of the intronless, untranslated *Alpha* gene with *TFEB*, a gene belonging to the same transcription factor family as *TFE3*.[53,54] The consequence of the *Alpha-TFEB* fusion is dysregulated expression of the normal full-length TFEB protein. Along these lines, the t(6;11) RCC (also known as *Alpha-TFEB* RCC) demonstrates specific nuclear labeling for TFEB protein by immunohistochemistry, whereas other neoplasms and normal tissues do not (Fig. 15-11). Hence, nuclear labeling for TFEB is a sensitive and specific diagnostic marker for this neoplasm with a *TFEB* gene fusion, just as nuclear labeling for TFE3 is a sensitive and specific marker for neoplasms bearing *TFE3* gene fusions.[55]

Renal Medullary Carcinoma

Renal medullary carcinoma (RMC) was first described in 1995 by Davis and colleagues[56] as "the seventh sickle cell nephropathy." These tumors characteristically affect young patients (mean, 22 years) with sickle cell trait. Tumors are typically centered in the renal medulla, but demonstrate an aggressively infiltrative growth pattern, with frequent vascular permeation. The tumor cells feature vesicular chromatin and prominent nucleoli, frequently associated with hyaline intracytoplasmic

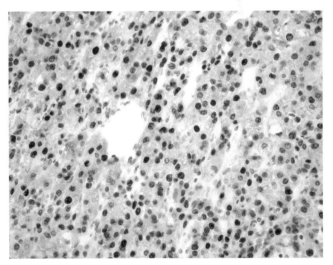

FIGURE 15-11. Renal cell carcinoma with the t(6;11)(p21:q12) translocation showing TFEB immunohistochemistry.

inclusions, thereby imparting a rhabdoid cytologic appearance. The tumor cells of RMC demonstrate diffuse (sheet-like), cribriform, gland-forming, microcystic or reticular growth patterns, the latter two simulating yolk sac tumor (Fig. 15-12). The stroma is typically desmoplastic and infiltrated by neutrophils, and close examination of extravasated red blood cells may reveal sickling. However, hemoglobin electrophoresis is more reliable than red blood cell morphology for determining that the patient has sickle cell trait. These tumors frequently present at a high stage and are highly lethal; Davis and associates reported a mean survival of 15 weeks. Given their medullary epicenter and high-grade cytology, RMCs are considered by some to be variants of collecting duct carcinoma, although the latter entity is a notoriously elusive one to define.

Oncocytic Renal Carcinomas in Neuroblastoma Patients

Medeiros and coworkers[57] have described oncocytic renal carcinomas arising in children who previously had neuroblastoma.

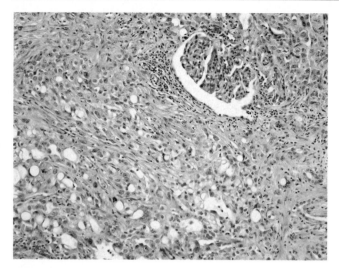

FIGURE 15-12. Renal medullary carcinoma.

The genetic alterations identified in these lesions did not match those of known renal carcinomas, suggesting that these are another distinctive entity.

Miscellaneous Renal Neoplasms

Primitive Neuroectodermal Tumor of Kidney

Primary renal PNET should be considered in the differential diagnosis of any undifferentiated blue cell tumor of the kidney. This neoplasm is encountered mainly in adolescent and young adult patients, and tends to present at an advanced stage.[38,58] Tumors consist of sheets of undifferentiated small blue cells, with frequent necrosis and occasional rosettes. Renal PNETs are frequently mistaken for blastemal WT of adolescent or adult patients and might account for some of the adverse prognosis attributed to adult WT. Compared with WT, tumor cell nuclei are less hyperchromatic and more evenly placed. Molecular detection of the *EWS-FLI1* gene fusion that results from the characteristic and specific t(11;22)(q24;q12) chromosome translocation is a useful way to confirm the diagnosis of PNET in suspected cases.[59] Also helpful is immunohistochemical labeling for CD99; the characteristic membrane staining pattern observed in PNETs is rarely, if ever, observed in WT blastemal cells or cellular CCSKs, which are the main differential diagnosis.[58]

Synovial Sarcoma of the Kidney

Like renal PNET, primary renal synovial sarcoma has been established as a distinctive neoplastic entity by demonstration of its specific chromosome translocation and gene fusion.[60,61] Genetically confirmed cases have affected young adults. Many were previously classified as adult blastemal WT, embryonal sarcoma of the kidney, adult cellular mesoblastic nephroma, or sarcoma arising in cystic nephroma. Renal synovial sarcomas are typically large, often cystic, and present at an advanced stage. The typical appearance is that of a monomorphic, highly cellular neoplasm composed of plump spindled cells growing in short fascicles. Tumor cells have ovoid nuclei and minimal cytoplasm, and may be associated with sclerosis. Grossly identified cysts are lined by mitotically inactive polygonal eosinophilic cells with apically oriented nuclei (hobnailed epithelium), and the cellularity of their walls may be deceptively low, creating confusion with cystic nephroma in limited biopsy samples.

Overall, the appearances are best conceptualized as monophasic spindle cell synovial sarcoma encircling native renal collecting ducts. True epithelial differentiation yielding a biphasic synovial sarcoma may occur, but is less common. Immunohistochemically, tumor cells label focally for epithelial markers (EMA more likely than cytokeratin), but many cases are completely negative for all epithelial markers. Many cases have labeled for CD99. The diagnosis can be confirmed in such cases by molecular demonstration of the *SYT-SSX* gene fusion that results from the t(X;18)(p11;q11) characteristic of this neoplastic entity. As with renal PNETs, renal synovial sarcoma is more aggressive than WT, and also may account for some of the adverse prognosis attributed to adult WT.

WILMS' TUMOR (NEPHROBLASTOMA)

Epidemiology

The age-adjusted incidence of pediatric renal tumors in the United States is 7.5/million children younger than 15 years and 6/million children younger than 19 years.[1] Although Wilms' tumor is the most common renal tumor overall, its relative frequency compared with other pediatric renal neoplasms varies according to patient age. Between 0 and 1 month of life, CMN is more common than Wilms' tumor[62] and, after age 14 years, RCC surpasses Wilms' tumor as the most prevalent renal cancer.[1] In North America, the average age of diagnosis for unilateral Wilms' tumor is 42 months for boys and 47 months for girls.[63] For bilateral Wilms' tumor, the average age of diagnosis is 30 months for boys and 33 months for girls.[63] The younger age of presentation for bilateral Wilms' tumor is caused by genetic predisposition, an observation that provided the basis for Knudson's two-hit model.[64] The reason for the later age of presentation in girls is more elusive. A recent analysis from the NWTSG has revealed that compared with boys, girls have a relative excess of PLNRs, Wilms' tumor precursor lesions associated with genetic alterations of the Beckwith-Wiedemann syndrome locus at chromosome 11p15.[65] Conversely, boys have a relative excess of ILNRs, distinct precursor lesions associated with mutations of the *WT1* gene at chromosome 11p13. ILNR-associated Wilms' tumors arise at an earlier age than PLNR-associated WTs, partially explaining the gender difference in age distribution. However, even in the absence of nephrogenic rests, girls present with Wilms' tumor a few months later, on average, than boys. In North America, there is a slight preponderance of Wilms' tumor in girls compared with boys, with a female-to-male ratio of 1.1 to 1.

There also are racial and ethnic differences in the predisposition to Wilms' tumor.[63] Most white populations have an age-adjusted incidence of 6 to 9 cases/million children/year. Black populations in North America and some parts of Africa exceed 10 cases/million children/year. In Japan, the Philippines, and China, the incidence is less than 4 cases/million children/year. Interestingly, in these East Asian populations, there is an excess of males with Wilms' tumor, the age at diagnosis is earlier than in North America, and PLNRs are rarely seen.[66]

Several studies have uncovered maternal and paternal environmental associations with Wilms' tumor. Maternal exposures that have been associated with Wilms' tumor include cigarettes, coffee or tea, oral contraceptives, hormonal pregnancy tests, hair coloring products, hypertension, household pesticide use, and vaginal infections.[67,68] However, none of these factors was confirmed by subsequent case-control studies conducted by the NWTSG.[69,70] A recent report from the COG has found that breast-feeding is associated with reduced risk of

Wilms' tumor, with the effect restricted to mothers with less than a college education.[71] On the paternal side, the occupations of machinist, welder, and other jobs involving exposure to hydrocarbons or lead were associated with increased risk of Wilms' tumor.[72-74] A subsequent case-control study found an association with the paternal occupations of vehicle mechanics, auto body repairmen, and welders, although no unifying exposure could be established.[75]

Molecular Biology and Genetics

Retinoblastoma and Wilms' tumor were the original tumors used by Knudson to establish the two-hit hypothesis of oncogenic transformation.[64] Unlike retinoblastoma, in which alterations of a single gene (*Rb*) account for the vast majority of tumors, several genes have been implicated in the genesis of Wilms' tumor, and a sizable proportion of WTs have an indeterminate genetic cause. Genes and loci that have been implicated in Wilms' tumor are summarized in Table 15-4.

WT1

WT1 was the first gene found to be specifically mutated in Wilms' tumor.[76-78] The gene was originally identified via a study of patients with the WAGR syndrome. Children with WAGR suffer from the constellation of *W*ilms' tumor, *a*niridia, *g*enitourinary abnormalities, and mental *r*etardation. Chromosomal analysis of these patients revealed heterozygous constitutional deletions at 11p13. Subsequent investigation of the genes contained within these deletions identified disruption of the *PAX6* gene as the basis of aniridia and *WT1* as the key tumor suppressor. The remaining allele of *WT1* is mutated in the WTs from these patients.

WT1 encodes an approximately 45-kD DNA-binding protein that contains domains rich in glutamine and proline in the amino terminus and four zinc fingers in the carboxyl terminus, collectively suggesting that it acts as a transcription factor. The *WT1* gene is complex because it encodes numerous distinct isoforms and contains an evolutionarily conserved cryptic splice site that can result in the insertion of three amino acids—lysine, threonine, and serine (KTS)—between zinc fingers 3 and 4. Notably, distinct functions have been identified for the different KTS isoforms. Patients with Frasier's syndrome, characterized by male pseudohermaphroditism, pro-gressive glomerulopathy, and an increased risk of Wilms' tumor, have a congenital donor splice site mutation in *WT1* that results in loss of the +KTS isoform.[79] Furthermore, mice that express only the +KTS or only the –KTS isoform have distinct phenotypes.[80]

Congenital point mutations in *WT1* are also the basis of the Denys-Drash syndrome.[81] Patients with this syndrome suffer from renal failure, pseudohermaphroditism, and a susceptibility to Wilms' tumor. Denys-Drash syndrome is caused by missense mutations in *WT1* that disrupt zinc finger binding to DNA. The phenotype of patients with Denys-Drash is severe and evidence has suggested that these mutations may lead to dominant negative protein that impairs function of the normal protein encoded by the remaining allele. Nonetheless, the remaining *WT1* allele is mutated in the WTs that arise in these patients, suggesting that mutation of both alleles is required for tumor formation. Notably, whereas mutations in *WT1* are the basis of several syndromes that predispose to the formation of Wilms' tumor, *WT1* is mutated in only 10% to 20% of sporadic tumors.[82]

Insight into the contributions of *WT1* to development and tumor suppression have come from mouse models. *WT1* is expressed at high levels in the developing kidney, gonads, spleen, and mesothelium and at lower levels in several other tissues. Mice deficient for *WT1* die midgestation with abnormalities of the metanephric blastema, gonads, mesothelium, heart, and lungs.[83] Cells from the metanephric blastema in these mice undergo apoptosis and consequently the metanephric kidney never develops. Based on these studies, it has been postulated that the WT1 protein regulates gene expression pathways required for morphogenesis of the kidney and that its disruption results in aberrant stimulation of tissue-specific growth. This role in differentiation may also explain why Wilms' tumor is largely a disease of early childhood because kidney morphogenesis is initiated in utero and is completed in early postnatal life. Indeed, the expression levels of *WT1* plummet within a few weeks following birth in mice.

β-Catenin and *WTX*

The Wnt signaling pathway regulates the cellular processes of proliferation, differentiation, motility, and survival. Central to the pathway is the transcriptional activator β-catenin, which is actively degraded in the absence of Wnt signaling.[84] Activating mutations in the *β-catenin (CTNNB1)* gene occur in approxi-

TABLE 15-4	**Genes and Loci Associated with Wilms' Tumor**		
Locus	**Gene**	**Gene Function**	**Associated Syndromes**
11p13	*WT1*	Transcription factor	WAGR; Denys-Drash; Frasier's
11p15	*WT2 (IGF2/ H19)*	Insulin-like growth factor pathway	Beckwith-Wiedemann
Xq11	*WTX*	Wnt signaling pathway	None
3p21	*CTNNB1 (β-Catenin)*	Wnt signaling pathway	None (in Wilms' tumor)
17q12-q21	*FWT1*	Unknown	Familial Wilms'
19q13	*FWT2*	Unknown	Familial Wilms'
17p13	*TP53*	Cell cycle checkpoint and apoptosis	Li-Fraumeni
13q12	*BRCA2 (FANCD1)*	DNA repair	Fanconi's anemia
16p12	*PALB2 (FANCN)*	DNA repair	Fanconi's anemia
15q26	*BLM*	DNA helicase	Bloom's syndrome
15q15	*BUB1B*	Mitotic spindle checkpoint	Mosaic variegated aneuploidy
Xq26	*GPC3*	Wnt signaling pathway	Simpson-Golabi-Behmel
7p14-15	*POU6F2*	Transcription factor	None
1q25	*CACNA1E*	Calcium channel	None
1q25-q32	*HRPT 2 (parafibromin)*	RNA processing; histone modification	Hyperparathyroid-jaw tumor
6q21	*HACE1*	Ubiquitin ligase	None

WAGR, *W*ilms' tumor, *a*niridia, *g*enitourinary abnormalities, and mental *r*etardation.

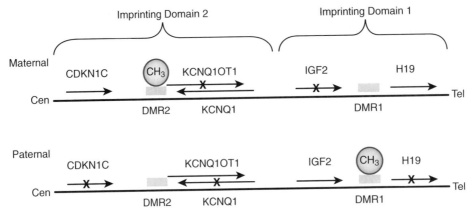

FIGURE 15-13. The Beckwith-Wiedemann syndrome (BWS) locus. The chromosome 11p15.5 locus contains several imprinted genes clustered in two imprinting domains, centromeric (Cen) and telomeric (Tel). Each domain has a differentially methylated region (DMR) that controls expression of surrounding genes. In normal individuals, the DMR of Domain 1 is methylated in the paternal allele, resulting in expression of *IGF2* and silencing of *H19*, whereas by contrast the DMR of Domain 2 is methylated in the maternal allele, resulting in expression of *CDKN1C (p57)* and *KCNQ1* and silencing of *KCNQ1OT(LIT1)*. BWS can arise from decreased methylation of Domain 2, increased methylation of Domain 1, duplication of the paternal 11p15 allele with no contribution of the maternal allele (uniparental isodisomy), or small deletions or rearrangements. Patients with increased methylation of Domain 1 and uniparental isodisomy have the greatest risk of developing Wilms' tumor.

mately 15% of Wilms' tumors.[85,86] Interestingly, mutations in β-*catenin* occur predominantly in tumors in which *WT1* is also mutated, suggesting that these two events cooperate in the genesis of Wilms' tumor.[86,87] In the developing kidney, *Wnt4* is an inducer of the mesenchymal to epithelial transition that underlies normal nephron development; disruption of normal renal development may be the means whereby β-*catenin* mutation contributes to the formation of Wilms' tumor.[88]

The recent discovery of the *WTX* gene has further implicated Wnt signaling in Wilms' tumor development.[89] *WTX* was discovered by an array comparative genomic hybridization screen that identified deletions of the Xq11.1 locus in male patients. Further investigation found deletions and mutations in girls. Intriguingly, *WTX* is inactivated by a single hit affecting either the sole *WTX* copy in males or the copy located on the active X chromosome in females. According to the initial report, *WTX* was deleted or mutated in approximately one third of WTs, although other groups have reported a lower mutation frequency.[89-91]

WTX encodes a protein that forms a complex with β-catenin, AXIN1, APC, and beta-TrCP2, ultimately promoting ubiquitination and degradation of β-catenin and thereby attenuating β-catenin–mediated transcription.[92] Downregulation of WTX leads to activation of Wnt signaling in human cell lines and zebrafish models.[92] Expression of *Wtx* during mouse development occurs at high levels in the lung, brain, kidney, and spleen, with expression in the kidney and brain declining rapidly during the first 3 postnatal weeks. Although *WT1* and β-catenin mutations are highly concordant, there is no clear relationship between *WT1* and *WTX* mutations.[90,93] The interactions between the WT1 and Wnt pathways remain to be unraveled.

WT2—The 11p15 Locus

Cytogenetic analyses have long suggested the presence of an additional Wilms' tumor gene at 11p15 distinct from the *WT1* locus at 11p13.[94] Loss of heterozygosity (LOH) at 11p15 occurs in some cases of sporadic Wilms' tumor. Additionally, this locus is linked to Beckwith-Wiedemann syndrome (BWS), an overgrowth disorder associated with macroglossia, umbilical hernia, gigantism, neonatal hypoglycemia, and predisposition to Wilms' tumor and other cancers. BWS arises from altera-

tions in several different genomically imprinted genes at the 11p15 locus.[95] Genomic imprinting is the preferential expression of a gene from the maternal or paternal allele. The molecular basis of genomic imprinting is epigenetic modification, most notably DNA methylation. The 11p15 locus has two imprinting domains (Fig. 15-13). The telomeric domain (Domain 1) includes the genes *insulin-like growth factor 2 (IGF2)* and *H19*. *IGF2* encodes a growth factor expressed at high levels in the developing kidney and Wilms' tumor.[96,97] *H19* encodes a biologically active untranslated RNA that may function as a tumor suppressor.[98] In normal cells, these genes are oppositely expressed so that *IGF2* is expressed only from the paternal allele and *H19* is expressed only from the maternal allele. The centromeric imprinting domain (Domain 2) contains several imprinted genes, including *KCNQ1 (KvLQT1)*, *KCNQ1OT (LIT1)*, and *CDKN1C (p57^{KIP2})*. *KCNQ1* encodes a subunit of a voltage-gated potassium channel that is implicated in several cardiac arrhythmia syndromes, including long-QT syndrome 1. *KCNQ1OT1* encodes a noncoding RNA with antisense transcription of *KCNQ1*. *CDKN1C* encodes a member of the cyclin-dependent kinase inhibitor family of proteins that negatively regulates cell proliferation and is a tumor suppressor. Molecular subgroups of BWS include those with the following: (1) loss of methylation in Domain 2, which is associated with decreased expression of *CDKN1C* (approximately 50%); (2) duplication of Domains 1 and 2 of the paternal allele with no maternal contribution (uniparental isodisomy; approximately 20%); (3) mutation of *CDKN1C* (approximately 10%); (4) gain of methylation of Domain 1, resulting in increased *IGF2* expression and decreased H19 expression (approximately 2% to 7%); (5) small duplications or chromosome rearrangements (less than 2%); and (5) unknown genetic cause (approximately 13% to 15%).[95] Interestingly, the Silver-Russell syndrome (SRS), associated with growth retardation, is caused by loss of methylation at Domain 1 and maternal 11p15 duplication (i.e., the opposite of BWS).[99,100]

In the past decade, correlations between BWS genotypes and cancer predisposition have emerged. Uniparental isodisomy and gain of methylation at Domain 1 carry the highest risk of Wilms' tumor. Loss of methylation at Domain 2 is associated with omphalocele, macrosomia, and a distinct lack of Wilms' tumor, although these individuals develop other tumor types.[101-103] A common thread in the patients most susceptible to Wilms' tumor is increased expression of *IGF2*.

GPC3

Mutations or deletions of the *GPC3* gene at chromosome Xq26 cause the Simpson-Golabi-Behmel syndrome, which is associated with overgrowth, coarse facial features, skeletal anomalies, accessory nipples, and renal dysplasia.[104] *GPC3* encodes a cell surface heparin sulfate proteoglycan that controls cell growth and interacts with the Wnt signaling pathway.[105] It is expressed at high levels in Wilms' tumor compared with adjacent normal kidney.[106] Of the 35 reported individuals with constitutional *GPC3* mutations, three developed Wilms' tumor.[107] *GPC3* mutations are infrequent in sporadic Wilms' tumor.[108,109]

BRCA2, PALB2, and BLM

Recently, inheritance of biallelic *BRCA2(FANCD1)* mutations was shown to predispose to Wilms' tumor and other childhood cancers.[110,111] BRCA2 is a member of a multiprotein complex that forms nuclear foci in response to DNA damage and participates in DNA repair.[112] Monoallelic *BRCA2* mutations predispose to breast and ovarian cancer, whereas biallelic mutations cause the D1 subgroup of Fanconi's anemia.[113] Five of 24 reported individuals with biallelic *BRCA2* mutations developed Wilms' tumor, including two brothers who developed both Wilms' tumor and brain tumors (glioblastoma and medulloblastoma).[111] Biallelic mutations of the *PALB2 (FANCN)* gene, which encodes a binding partner of BRCA2 that regulates its nuclear localization and stability, also predispose to Wilms' tumor and other childhood cancers.[114] Bloom's syndrome, characterized by short stature, skin photosensitivity, and alterations in pigmentation, immunodeficiency, and cancer predisposition, is caused by biallelic mutations of the *BLM* gene, which encodes a DNA helicase important in maintaining chromosomal stability. The estimated frequency of Wilms' tumor in those with Bloom's syndrome is approximately 3%.[107,115,116]

BUB1B

Mosaic variegated aneuploidy is an autosomal recessive condition characterized by multiple aneuploidies, notably trisomies and monosomies, involving a number of different chromosomes. Patients with MVA present with microcephaly, intrauterine growth retardation, various other anomalies, and a high risk of malignancies, including rhabdomyosarcoma, leukemia, and Wilms' tumor. Biallelic mutations in the *BUB1B* gene, which encodes one of the key proteins involved in the mitotic spindle checkpoint, was recently shown to cause MVA.[117] It is estimated that the risk of Wilms' tumor in those with biallelic *BUB1B* mutations is 25%, but *BUB1B* mutations are uncommon in sporadic Wilms' tumor.[107,118]

TP53

Constitutional mutations of the *TP53* gene are responsible for the Li-Fraumeni (cancer predisposition) syndrome (LFS).[119] *TP53*, one of the most commonly mutated genes in human cancer, encodes a transcription factor that is a master regulator of cell cycle arrest, apoptosis, and DNA repair in response to various stimuli. Although Wilms' tumor is not a defining criterion for LFS, several LFS families with Wilms' tumor have been identified.[120] Importantly, *TP53* mutations are associated with the anaplastic histology subtype of Wilms' tumor; approximately 75% of anaplastic WTs have detectable *TP53* mutations, whereas *TP53* mutations are uncommon in favorable histology tumors.[10,13,121] Several lines of evidence have suggested that anaplastic Wilms' tumor arises from the acquisition of a *TP53* mutation in a favorable histology Wilms' tumor. First, patients with bilateral Wilms' tumor often have discordant histologies between contralateral tumors.[15] Second, some WTs have favorable histologic features at diagnosis, but are found to have anaplastic histology at relapse.[13] Finally, microdissected Wilms' tumors were found to have *TP53* mutations restricted to areas of anaplasia within the tumor tissue.[11]

Nonsyndromic Familial Wilms' Tumor

Familial Wilms' tumor is a rare entity that accounts for less than 2% of all cases. The disorder appears to display autosomal dominant inheritance with incomplete penetrance. Mapping studies have excluded 11p13 and 11p15 in most cases, although rare Wilms' tumor pedigrees with *WT1* or 11p15 defects have been noted.[107] Linkage to chromosome 17q12-21 has been found in several pedigrees and the putative familial Wilms' tumor gene at this site has been named *FWT1*.[122,123] Other pedigrees show linkage to chromosome 19q13.3-q13.4, a locus now referred to as *FWT2*.[124] A specific Wilms' tumor gene has yet to be identified at the *FWT1* or *FWT2* loci. Comparative genomic hybridization studies have suggested the possibility of additional Wilms' tumor predisposition loci on chromosomes 1p, 3q, 4q, 7p, 9p, 16q, and 20p.[125]

Other Wilms' Tumor Loci

LOH studies have identified at least three regions at the 7p locus that may contain Wilms' tumor-related genes.[126,127] A candidate tumor suppressor gene at 7p14 called *POU6F2* has been identified.[128] *Pou6F2* is highly expressed in the developing kidney in mice and mirrors the expression of *WT1*.[129]

Analysis of the chromosome 6q21 breakpoint in a sporadic Wilms' tumor with a t(6;15)(q21;q21) rearrangement has led to the identification of the potential tumor suppressor *HACE1*.[130] *HACE1* encodes an E3 ubiquitin ligase protein that is widely expressed in human tissues, including mature and fetal kidney. *HACE1* has not been found to be deleted or mutated in Wilms' tumor, but is underexpressed in Wilms' tumor compared with normal kidney as a result of epigenetic modification.[131] Genetically engineered *Hace1*-null mice are prone to various cancers, including melanoma, mammary carcinoma, angiosarcoma, lung adenocarcinoma, and hepatocellular carcinoma, but not Wilms' tumor.[131]

Gain of chromosome 1q is a recurring abnormality seen in WTs, with a higher frequency in relapsing versus non-relapsing tumors.[132,133] The *HPRT2* gene at 1q25-31 causes the hyperparathyroidism-jaw-tumor syndrome, which is associated with parathyroid adenomas and renal abnormalities, including Wilms' tumor.[134] The *CACNA1E* gene at 1q25, which encodes a subunit of voltage-dependent calcium channels, was shown to be amplified in 8% of Wilms' tumors.[135] Overexpression of *CACNA1E* transcript in Wilms' tumor samples correlated with tumor relapse, as did nuclear localization of the protein, which is normally expressed on the apical membranes of distal tubules.

Clinical Presentation and Diagnostic Evaluation

The most common presenting signs and symptoms of Wilms' tumor are an abdominal mass (75%), abdominal pain (28%), hypertension (26%), gross hematuria (18%), microscopic hematuria (24%), and fever (22%).[136] The hypertension, which can be severe, may be caused by ectopic renin production by the tumor, compression of the renal artery by the tumor with resulting physiologic renin production, or ectopic ACTH production. Some patients have persistent hypertension after the tumor has been removed, suggesting underlying renal pathology. There are no tumor markers pathognomonic for Wilms' tumor, although associated laboratory findings include hematuria and anemia. An association between Wilms' tumor and acquired von Willebrand disease has been described.[137]

Wilms' tumor can spread locally or hematogenously. Locally, the tumor has the potential to spread into structures surrounding the kidney and can occasionally invade other organs such as the liver. If the tumor ruptures, peritoneal tumor deposits can be detected. Wilms' tumor also spreads to lymph nodes near the renal hilum and in the para-aortic chain. Six percent to 8% of Wilms' tumors spread through the renal vein and form a tumor thrombus in the inferior vena cava, which can propagate into the heart.[138,139] The most common sites of distant metastasis are the lung and liver. There are reports of Wilms' tumor spread to brain or bone, but this is uncommon. About 7% of patients have synchronous or metachronous bilateral tumors and 10% have unilateral multifocal tumors.[63]

The radiologic evaluation of Wilms' tumor focuses on the most prevalent sites of spread. A computed tomography (CT) scan of the abdomen and pelvis is recommended to visualize the primary tumor, contralateral kidney, lymph nodes, and intra-abdominal or pelvic tumor deposits. A Doppler ultrasound is recommended as a complementary test to evaluate for tumor thrombus in the renal vein and inferior vena cava. Chest x-rays have historically been used to assess patients for lung metastases, but CT scans are more sensitive for detecting nodules or effusions.[140,141] On NWTS-5, 129 patients had lung lesions detected on CT scan but not chest x-ray. Of these patients, 42 with CT-only nodules had lung biopsies and tumor was confirmed in 31 patients (73.8%).[142] Retrospective studies of the prognostic significance of CT-only lung nodules have yielded conflicting results.[140,143-146] The largest analysis to date included 186 patients with CT-only nodules from NWTS-4 and -5. These patients were treated heterogeneously (with or without doxorubicin and/or lung radiation) because the treatment decisions were left to the discretion of the local physicians. Outcome analysis has found that patients with CT-only nodules who were treated with doxorubicin have superior relapse-free survival compared with patients who did not receive doxorubicin. However, the use of lung radiation did not have a significant effect on outcome.[147] Based on these findings, the new COG studies recommend CT scans, but not chest x-rays, for the initial workup for Wilms' tumor. Lung nodules are considered to contain tumor unless proven negative by biopsy.

Bone scan and brain magnetic resonance imaging (MRI) are not routinely recommended in the evaluation of patients with newly diagnosed Wilms' tumor. Fluorodeoxyglucose (FDG) positron emission tomography (PET) scanning is not a routine part of the Wilms' tumor workup, although the initial experience with PET scans has indicated that most Wilms' tumors are FDG-avid.[148,149]

Treatment

The treatment approach to Wilms' tumor has evolved along two distinct pathways. The National Wilms' Tumor Study Group (NWTSG), which became the Renal Tumor Committee of the Children's Oncology Group (COG) in 2002, performs up-front nephrectomy followed by chemotherapy. This approach provides for accurate histologic diagnosis and staging information. By contrast, the International Society of Pediatric Oncology (SIOP) gives preoperative chemotherapy, which

shrinks the tumor, thereby reducing the risk of surgical complications such as intraoperative tumor spillage. It is difficult to compare the two approaches directly because of differences in the staging systems and treatment plans, but both approaches produce excellent outcomes. Regardless of the timing of initial surgery, the three pillars of Wilms' tumor treatment are surgery, radiation therapy, and chemotherapy.

Surgery

On the SIOP treatment protocols, patients 6 months of age or older receive chemotherapy before surgery unless there is evidence of tumor rupture. Open or needle biopsy is not routinely performed. Infants younger than 6 months old are treated with up-front nephrectomy because non-Wilms' renal tumors, such as mesoblastic nephroma or malignant rhabdoid tumor, are prevalent in this age group.

On the COG treatment protocols, all patients are considered candidates for immediate surgery, although there are several indications to give preoperative chemotherapy: (1) bilateral Wilms' tumor; (2) tumor thrombus in the IVC above the level of the hepatic veins; (3) tumors that invade adjacent organs such that resection of the tumor would involve resection of the other structure (except the adrenal gland); (4) tumors that, in the surgeon's judgment, would result in significant morbidity or mortality if resected before chemotherapy; and (5) respiratory distress from extensive pulmonary metastatic disease. If preoperative chemotherapy is given, it is recommended not to delay surgery beyond week 12 of treatment.

A generous transabdominal, transperitoneal, or thoracoabdominal incision is recommended for adequate exposure. Complete exploration of the abdomen should be performed, followed by a radical nephrectomy, dividing the ureter as distally as possible. Routine exploration of the contralateral kidney is not necessary if imaging is satisfactory and does not suggest a bilateral process. A recent study has shown that the chance of detecting a contralateral kidney tumor during surgery that is undetected with modern imaging techniques is less than 1%.[150] An important component of Wilms' tumor surgery is lymph node sampling, even if the nodes appear normal. NWTS-4 has shown that patients with positive lymph nodes have better outcomes than patients whose lymph nodes are not sampled, indicating that some patients who do not undergo lymph node sampling are understaged and undertreated.[151] Another important facet of surgery is to remove the tumor en bloc, avoiding tumor spillage. Intra-operative spillage was shown to increase the risk of tumor recurrence.[151]

Surgical resection or biopsy of lung nodules plays an important role in the diagnosis of metastatic Wilms' tumor. Current COG renal tumor studies consider circular lung nodules, regardless of size, to be metastatic disease unless proven benign by biopsy. The resection of lung metastases may also provide a therapeutic benefit. On the SIOP protocols, patients whose lung nodules are resected completely do not receive pulmonary radiation therapy (XRT). The current COG AREN0533 study is testing a new strategy for favorable histology Wilms' tumor with lung metastases. Lung nodules are assessed after 6 weeks of chemotherapy and XRT is omitted for patients with a complete response. With this approach, it is appropriate not to resect all lung nodules up front to assess chemosensitivity.

Radiation Therapy

Radiation therapy is a mainstay of Wilms' tumor treatment. Initially used in all patients with Wilms' tumor, successive studies from the NWTSG and SIOP have demonstrated that only patients with stage III or IV disease require radiation therapy (Table 15-5). Among these patients, radiation doses have been reduced over time, thereby decreasing the potential for late adverse effects.

The radiation guidelines for favorable histology Wilms' tumor that were used in NWTS-5 are commonly applied as standard practice in North America. Patients with positive lymph nodes, positive tumor margins after surgery, or tumor spillage receive 10.8 Gy to the flank. Patients with diffuse tumor spillage or peritoneal seeding receive 10.8 Gy to the whole abdomen. Sites of gross residual disease after surgery receive a boost of 10.8 Gy. Early reports from the NWTSG have demonstrated that XRT delay beyond 9 days from surgery

TABLE 15-5	Key Findings of National Wilms' Tumor and SIOP Studies		
National Wilms' Tumor Study (NWTS)	**Key Findings**	**International Society of Pediatric Oncology (SIOP) Study**	**Key Findings**
NWTS-1 (1969-1973)	Group I: XRT not beneficial for patients < 2 yr of age treated with AMD Groups II-III: VCR/AMD superior to either agent alone Anaplastic histology strongly predictive of adverse outcome	SIOP 1 (1971-1974)	Preoperative XRT reduces number of tumor ruptures and produces more low-stage tumors
		SIOP 2 (1974-1976)	9 mo of VCR/AMD equivalent to 15 mo of VCR/AMD; reduction of tumor ruptures in preoperative treatment group confirmed
NWTS-2 (1974-1978)	Group I: reduction of chemotherapy duration from 15 to 6 mo did not adversely affect RFS; XRT not needed for this group Group II: inferior outcome for those with lymph node involvement Group II-IV: addition of DOX to VCR/AMD improved outcome	SIOP 5 (1977-1979)	Preoperative chemotherapy equivalent to XRT in preventing tumor ruptures
NWTS-3 (1979-1986)	Stage I FH: RFS similar whether duration of VCR/AMD was 10 or 26 wk Stage II FH: addition of DOX to VCR/AMD did not improve RFS; XRT not necessary Stage III FH: 1. Without DOX, 20 Gy flank XRT superior to 10 Gy 2. Addition of DOX to 10 Gy flank XRT improved RFS 3. Addition of DOX to 20 Gy flank XRT did not improve RFS Stage IV FH: Addition of CYCLO did not improve RFS Stage II-IV diffuse anaplasia: addition of CYCLO appeared to improve RFS	SIOP 6 (1980-1987)	Stage I: 17 wk of VCR/AMD equal to 38 wk of VCR/AMD Stage IIN0: withholding XRT triggered stopping rule because of abdominal relapses; however, DFS and OS were not affected by withholding XRT Stage IIN+/III: doxorubicin improved DFS but not OS
		SIOP 9 (1987-1991)	4 wk of preoperative VCR/AMD equivalent to 8 wk in terms of percentage of stage I tumors, EFS, OS
		SIOP 93-01 (1993-1999)	Patients with stage I Wilms' tumor do just as well with 4 wk postoperative VCR/AMD as 38 wk VCR/AMD Postchemotherapy histology predictive of relapse: complete necrosis = low risk; blastemal predominance = high risk
NWTS-4 (1986-1994)	Stage I-IV FH: no difference in RFS when AMD given as single dose rather than as five doses; toxicity profile and cost better with single dose Stage III-IV FH: no difference in RFS when DOX given as a single dose rather than as three doses; toxicity profile and cost better with single dose Stage II-IV FH: no difference in RFS between 6 and 15 mo of therapy Stage II-IV diffuse anaplasia: improved RFS with addition of CYCLO confirmed		
NWTS-5 (1995-2002)	Stage I FH, age < 2 yr, tumor < 550 g: without chemotherapy, 2-year RFS was only 86% but OS was 100% Stage I-IV FH: LOH at 1p and 16q predict decreased RFS and OS Stage I anaplasia: RFS and OS inferior to stage I FH Stage II-IV diffuse anaplasia: best reported outcomes to date using VCR/DOX/CYCLO/ETOP		

AMD, dactinomycin; CYCLO, cyclophosphamide; DFS, disease-free survival; DOX, doxorubicin; EFS, event-free survival; ETOP, etoposide; FH, favorable histology; LOH, loss of heterozygosity; OS, overall survival; RFS, relapse-free survival; SIOP, International Society of Pediatric Oncology; VCR, vincristine; XRT, radiation therapy.

is an adverse prognostic factor.[152,153] Since then, NWTSG and COG studies have recommended that radiation commence by day 9 after surgery. However, a retrospective analysis of NWTS-3 and -4 did not detect a difference in local recurrence rate between patients who received radiation within 9 days and patients whose radiation was delayed beyond day 9, although few patients had XRT delayed much beyond day 10.[154] Patients whose tumors are initially unresectable have radiation therapy delayed until after definitive surgery.

The radiation doses that the SIOP treatment protocols use are higher than those on COG studies. Patients with lung metastases receive 15 Gy rather than 12 Gy. Patients with stage III intermediate-risk histology receive 14.4 Gy to the abdomen or flank rather than 10.8 Gy. Patients with stage II or III high-risk histology receive 25.2 Gy.

The radiation guidelines for patients with distant metastatic disease are evolving. The most common metastatic site is the lung. On the NWTSG studies, all patients with lung metastases received whole-lung radiation to a dose of 12 Gy at the beginning of treatment, yielding 16-year relapse-free survival rates of 80%.[155] On SIOP studies, patients whose lung nodules resolve with chemotherapy and surgery did not receive lung XRT. With this approach, the 4-year survival rate was 83%.[156] However, the United Kingdom Wilms' Tumor Study used the SIOP approach and observed a 6-year survival rate of only 65%.[157] This disparity may relate to differences in patient populations and treatment, but it raises the question of whether more stringent selection criteria should be used for withholding lung XRT. The current COG AREN0533 study is assessing whether XRT can be omitted for patients whose lung nodules disappear after 6 weeks of chemotherapy, thereby selecting a group of patients with highly chemosensitive disease. Patients who have metastatic disease in the bone, brain, and liver receive XRT to these respective sites.

Chemotherapy

In the mid-1950s, Farber and colleagues pioneered the use of dactinomycin (AMD) as an adjunct to surgery and radiation therapy for the treatment of Wilms' tumor. With the introduction of AMD, unprecedented survival rates were observed, particularly in patients with metastatic disease.[158] In the early 1960s, the Southwest Oncology Group found that vincristine (VCR) produced regression of metastatic Wilms' tumor and that the response to VCR plus XRT was similar to that reported for AMD.[159] In 1969, the first National Wilms' Tumor Study (NWTS-1) found the combination of VCR and AMD to be superior to either agent alone for group II and III tumors.[160] Since then, VCR/AMD has been the backbone of Wilms' tumor

therapy worldwide, although subsets of patients with stage I disease fare well with VCR alone or even surgery only, as discussed later. In the early 1970s, the third stalwart of Wilms' tumor chemotherapy regimens, doxorubicin (DOX), was introduced. NWTS-2 demonstrated the benefit of doxorubicin for patients with groups II-IV disease and NWTS-3 showed that radiation doses can be reduced when doxorubicin is used.[161,162] NWTS-4 refined how AMD and DOX are given. Both agents were as effective when delivered as a single dose rather than as separate doses over 5 (AMD) or 3 (DOX) days.[163] Not only was this pulse-intensive dosing more convenient and cost-effective, but it also was associated with less hematologic toxicity.[164,165] The key findings of the NWTSG studies are summarized in Table 15-5.

By the end of NWTS-4, the survival rate for patients with favorable histology Wilms' tumor was approximately 90%. Given this success, the priority for NWTS-5 was to identify novel prognostic markers to help stratify patients into risk-appropriate treatment groups. Pilot data from NWTS-3 and -4 have shown that LOH at chromosomes 1p and 16q is associated with adverse outcome in patients with Wilms' tumor.[166] Following this lead, NWTS-5 has prospectively evaluated the prognostic significance of LOH in more than 2000 patients.[167] There is no significant association between LOH and outcome in patients with anaplastic Wilms' tumor, CCSK, or MRT. However, LOH at 1p and 16q are each associated with increased risk of relapse and death in patients with favorable histology Wilms' tumor, with the greatest effect seen in tumors with LOH at both loci (Table 15-6).[167] Based on these findings, an aim of the current COG studies is to evaluate whether augmentation of chemotherapy improves outcomes in patients whose tumors contain LOH at both 1p and 16q.

A second objective of NWTS-5 was to determine whether therapy can be reduced in selected populations of patients with truly outstanding outcomes. Earlier studies have suggested that young patients with small stage I favorable histology tumors have excellent outcomes,[168] so NWTS-5 asked whether these patients could be treated with surgery alone without adjuvant chemotherapy and radiation therapy. Among 75 patients treated with surgery only, 8 patients relapsed and 3 patients developed metachronous tumors in the contralateral kidney.[169] The 2-year disease-free survival rate was only 86%, which triggered a stopping rule, and the study was discontinued. However, 74 of 75 patients survived, suggesting that the nephrectomy-only approach should be revisited. Although the standard treatment for stage I favorable histology Wilms' tumor in North America is 18 weeks of VCR/AMD, the United Kingdom Wilms' tumor group treated with 10 weeks of VCR only[170] and the SIOP 93-01 study has demonstrated that 4 weeks of postoperative

---

TABLE 15-6   Effect of Loss of Heterozygosity (LOH) on Patient Outcome (NWTS-5)

Stage	4-Year RFS (%)	RR	P	4-Year OS (%)	RR	P
Favorable histology stage I-II:						
No LOH	91.2	—		98.4	—	
LOH 1p only	80.4	2.19	0.02	91.2	4.03	0.02
LOH 16q only	82.5	1.91	0.01	98.1	1.40	0.6
LOH 1p and 16q	74.9	2.88	0.001	90.5	4.25	0.01
Favorable histology stage III-IV:						
No LOH	83.0	—		91.9	—	
LOH 1p only	89.0	0.69	0.37	97.6	0.52	0.36
LOH 16q only	85.3	0.89	0.67	92.0	0.88	0.76
LOH 1p and 16q	65.9	2.41	0.01	77.5	2.66	0.04

NWTS, National Wilms' Tumor Study; OS, overall survival; RFS, relapse-free survival; RR, relative risk, with group with no LOH as a baseline.

TABLE 15-7 **NWTS-5 Treatment Overview**

Tumor Histology and Stage	Chemotherapy Regimen	Radiation Therapy
Favorable histology Wilms' tumor		
Stage I-II	VCR/AMD × 18 wk	None
Stage III-IV	VCR/AMD/DOX × 24 wk	Flank or abdomen if local stage III, and to metastatic sites
Focal anaplastic Wilms' tumor		
Stage I	VCR/AMD × 18 wk	None
Stage II-IV	VCR/AMD/DOX × 24 wk	Flank or abdomen, and to metastatic sites
Diffuse anaplastic Wilms' tumor		
Stage I	VCR/AMD × 18 wk	None
Stage II-IV	VCR/DOX/CYCLO/ETOP × 24 wk	Flank or abdomen, and to metastatic sites
Clear cell sarcoma of the kidney		
Stage I-IV	VCR/DOX/CYCLO/ETOP × 24 wk	Flank or abdomen, and to metastatic sites
Malignant rhabdoid tumor		
Stage I-IV	CARBO/ETOP/CYCLO × 24 wk	Flank or abdomen, and to metastatic sites

AMD, dactinomycin; CARBO, carboplatin; CYCLO, cyclophosphamide; DOX, doxorubicin; ETOP, etoposide; NWTS, National Wilms' Tumor Study; VCR, vincristine.

treatment is equivalent to 18 weeks.[171] The treatment regimens from NWTS-5 are summarized in Table 15-7 and the corresponding outcomes are summarized in Table 15-8.

The current COG studies (started in 2006) are further refining the treatment of favorable histology Wilms' tumor. The AREN0532 study (very low- and standard-risk favorable histology Wilms' tumor) is reassessing the feasibility of surgery without adjuvant therapy for patients younger than 2 years old with stage I favorable histology Wilms' tumors less than 550 g. To be eligible to participate in this study arm, lymph nodes must be sampled and confirmed negative for tumor. AREN0532 also is assessing the benefit of therapy augmentation for patients with stage I or II FH with LOH at 1p and 16q. Instead of receiving the standard therapy with VCR/AMD, patients with LOH receive VCR/AMD/DOX. Similarly, the AREN0533 study (higher risk FH Wilms' tumor) is augmenting therapy for patients with stage III or IV FH with LOH at 1p and 16q. Instead of receiving VCR/AMD/DOX, these patients receive a new regimen that adds four cycles of cyclophosphamide (CYCLO) and etoposide (ETOP) to the standard treatment. AREN0533 also introduces a new approach to patients with lung metastases. Patients whose lung nodules respond completely after 6 weeks of VCR/AMD/DOX chemotherapy do not receive lung XRT. In contrast, patients whose lung nodules do not respond completely receive XRT and augmented chemotherapy with VCR/AMD/DOX/CYCLO/ETOP. The COG biology and classification study (AREN03B2) continues the NWTSG tradition of central pathology and surgery review and tumor banking. A new element of the central classification is central radiology review to assess for lung nodules, tumor thrombi, and evidence of bilateral renal tumors.

The current SIOP 2001 study aims to evaluate whether doxorubicin is needed for patients with stage II and III intermediate-risk tumors; patients are randomized to receive VCR/AMD with or without DOX. The study also adjusts chemotherapy based on histologic response to preoperative treatment. Patients with stage I blastemal predominance after 4 weeks of preoperative chemotherapy are treated with a regimen containing DOX instead of just VCR/AMD. Patients with stage II or III blastemal predominance receive a regimen of alternating CYCLO/DOX with CARBO/ETOP.

Anaplastic Wilms' Tumor

In 1978, Beckwith and Palmer published a detailed histopathologic review of the patients entered on the first National Wilms' Tumor Study.[172] Approximately 6% of the Wilms' tumor

TABLE 15-8 **Treatment Results: NWTS-5**

Stage	4-Year Relapse-Free Survival Rate (%)	4-Year Overall Survival Rate (%)
Favorable histology without LOH 1p		
I (<24 mo; tumor weight < 550 g)	95.6	100
I (≥24 mo; tumor weight ≥ 550 g)	94.2	98.4
II	86.2	97.7
III	86.5	94.4
IV	76.4	86.1
V	64.8	87.1
Focal anaplastic histology		
I	67.5	88.9
II	80.0	80.0
III	87.5	100
IV*	61.4	71.6
V	76.2	87.5
Diffuse anaplastic histology		
I	68.4	78.9
II	82.6	81.5
III	64.7	66.7
IV	33.3	33.3
V	25.1	41.6
Clear cell sarcoma†		
I	100	100
II	86.8	97.3
III	73.8	86.9
IV	35.6	45.0
Malignant rhabdoid tumor‡		
I	—	33.3
II	—	46.9
III	—	21.8
IV	—	8.4

*Results are for patients who received preoperative chemotherapy because very few patients in this group had up-front nephrectomy
†Results are reported as 5-year relapse-free and overall survival.
‡Results are combined results for NWTS 1-5.
LOH, loss of heterozygosity; NWTS, National Wilms' Tumor Study.

specimens contained anaplasia, as defined in the pathology section of this chapter. The presence of anaplasia was prognostically significant; 11 of 25 (44%) of patients with anaplasia died of tumor, whereas only 26 of 364 (7.1%) of patients without anaplasia died of tumor. Subsequent National Wilms' Tumor Studies, as well as the International Society of Pediatric Oncology (SIOP) and the United Kingdom Wilms' Tumor Study, have confirmed the adverse prognostic significance of anaplastic histology.[157,173,174]

The first NWTSG trial to stratify patients with anaplastic Wilms' tumor into a distinct treatment group was NWTS-3. On this study and on NWTS-4, patients received 15 months of VCR, AMD, and DOX, and were randomized to receive or not receive CYCLO. Patients with stages II to IV diffuse anaplastic Wilms' tumor had a 4-year relapse-free survival (RFS) estimate of 27.2% when treated without CYCLO, compared with 54.8% when treated with CYCLO ($P = .02$).[175] Patients with all stages of focal anaplastic histology and stage I diffuse anaplastic histology had excellent outcomes, regardless of treatment regimen.[162,175]

Based on these results, NWTS-5 incorporated CYCLO into the treatment plan for patients with stages II to IV diffuse anaplastic Wilms' tumor. Patients received a regimen consisting of VCR/DOX/CYCLO alternating with CYCLO/ETOP for 24 weeks of treatment and flank XRT to a dose of 10.8 Gy.[15] With this regimen, the 4-year RFS and OS compared favorably to historical data from NWTS-3 and -4 (see Table 15-8). Patients with stage I diffuse anaplastic histology were treated with VCR/AMD according to the regimen used for FH Wilms' tumor. With this approach, the 4-year event-free survival (EFS) was only 68.4%, significantly worse than that seen for stage I FH tumors.[15] Patients with stages II to IV focal anaplastic Wilms' tumor were treated with VCR/DOX/AMD/XRT and had outcomes intermediate between favorable histology and diffuse anaplasia (see Table 15-8).

AREN0321, the COG study for high-risk renal tumors, seeks to build on the NWTS-5 experience by adding carboplatin (CARBO) to the treatment regimen for diffuse anaplastic Wilms' tumor. Patients receive 31 weeks of alternating VCR/DOX/CYCLO and CYCLO/CARBO/ETOP with flank XRT. Based on the poorer than expected outcomes for stage I anaplastic Wilms' tumor, the AREN0321 study treats such patients with VCR/AMD/DOX/XRT instead of just VCR/AMD. Patients with stage IV diffuse anaplastic Wilms' tumor had a 4-year RFS estimate of only 33% on NWTS-5. For this group, the priority is to identify new chemotherapy combinations. The AREN0321 study includes a phase II window study to evaluate the antitumor activity of vincristine/irinotecan. This combination was selected based on preclinical and clinical data showing activity of the camptothecins (topotecan and irinotecan) against Wilms' tumor.[176]

Bilateral Wilms' Tumor

Of patients with Wilms' tumor, 4% to 6% have tumor involvement of both kidneys at initial presentation (synchronous bilateral Wilms' tumor).[63] These patients pose the dual challenge of eradicating the tumor cells while preserving renal function. Although renal failure occurs in less than 1% of patients with unilateral Wilms' tumor, the long-term incidence of renal failure in patients with bilateral Wilms' tumor is 11%.[177] Historically, synchronous bilateral Wilms' tumor was managed with surgical resection followed by chemotherapy. Typically, a unilateral nephrectomy of the more involved kidney was performed with biopsy or partial nephrectomy of the contralateral kidney, followed by adjuvant therapy. With the recognition that chemotherapy could decrease tumor volume and facilitate partial nephrectomy, preoperative chemotherapy has become the standard approach to treatment. Data from the NWTSG have shown no difference in outcome whether the tumor was resected at the time of diagnosis or after preoperative chemotherapy.[178-180] Despite the effectiveness of preoperative chemotherapy, approximately 60% of patients continue to undergo nephrectomy of at least one kidney. On NWTS-4, only 19% of patients underwent bilateral nephron-sparing procedures,[181] but recent data from St. Jude Children's Research Hospital have suggested that more patients are candidates for bilateral partial nephrectomies.[182] An aim of the current COG AREN0534 study for bilateral Wilms' tumor is to decrease the percentage of patients who require nephrectomy.

Chemotherapy regimens for bilateral Wilms' tumor use the same agents as for unilateral Wilms' tumor. On the NWTSG and SIOP studies, patients started treatment with VCR/AMD therapy and DOX was reserved for patients known to have distant metastatic disease, locally advanced disease, or poor response to therapy. With this treatment approach, long-term survival rates for patients with synchronous bilateral Wilms' tumors were approximately 70% to 80%.[178-180] The new COG AREN0534 study for bilateral Wilms' tumor will treat all patients with VCR/AMD/DOX prior to surgery to promote improved local control. Chemotherapy following surgery will be tailored according to histologic response, based on the postchemotherapy risk classification schema developed by the SIOP group.

Recurrent Wilms' Tumor

Approximately 10% of patients with favorable histology Wilms' tumor and 50% of patients with anaplastic Wilms' tumor develop recurrent disease. The survival rate after recurrence depends on several factors, including histology, time from diagnosis to recurrence, initial stage and treatment regimen, and site of recurrence.[183,184] The results of the NWTS-5 recurrent Wilms' tumor study were reported recently. Patients with favorable histology Wilms' tumor whose initial treatment consisted of VCR/AMD received VCR/DOX/CYCLO/ETOP and XRT as salvage therapy, resulting in 4-year EFS and overall survival (OS) estimates of 71.1% and 81.8%, respectively.[185] Patients whose initial treatment was VCR/AMD/DOX/XRT received a salvage regimen of alternating CYCLO/ETOP and CARBO/ETOP, resulting in 4-year EFS and OS of 42.3% and 48.0%.[186] Interestingly, females had better EFS and OS (54.7 and 58.7%) rates than males (28.6% and 38.0%). Other studies have demonstrated the efficacy of ifosfamide-carboplatin-etoposide (ICE) chemotherapy for the treatment of recurrent Wilms' tumor.[187,188] A phase II trial of topotecan has demonstrated a response rate of 48% in patients with multiply recurrent favorable histology Wilms' tumor.[176] The outcomes of patients with recurrent anaplastic Wilms' tumor are poor, with salvage rates on the order of 10%. Because up-front therapy for anaplastic Wilms' tumor involves the known active agents, patients with recurrent disease are candidates for phase I and II studies.

An unresolved question is whether high-dose chemotherapy (HDCT) with autologous stem cell rescue provides a benefit for patients with recurrent Wilms' tumor. Several series have reported survival rates of approximately 60% in patients with recurrent Wilms' tumor using single or tandem transplants.[189-191] However, similar results have been attained without high-dose therapy,[184] so the benefit of high-dose therapy remains undefined.

Late Effects of Wilms' Tumor Treatment

The excellent relapse-free survival rate for favorable histology Wilms' tumor heightens the importance of minimizing long-term effects of treatment. Follow-up of the NWTSG cohort has identified several treatment-related effects that current studies are aiming to minimize.

One of the most feared complications of Wilms' tumor therapy is cardiotoxicity. The cumulative frequency of congestive heart failure in patients treated on NWTS-1-4 was 4.4% at 20 years for patients treated initially with doxorubicin and 17.4% for patients treated with doxorubicin for recurrent disease.[192] The risk for congestive heart failure was strongly associated with female gender (relative risk [RR] = 4.5 compared with males), cumulative doxorubicin dose (RR = 3.3 for each 100 mg/m[2]); lung radiation (RR = 1.6), and left abdominal radiation (RR = 1.8).[193]

A second major complication of Wilms' tumor therapy is second malignant neoplasms (SMNs). The 15-year cumulative incidence of SMN in Wilms' tumor survivors treated on NWTSG studies between 1969 and 1991 was 1.6% and increasing steadily.[194] The second malignancies observed in this series were sarcomas, carcinomas, leukemias, lymphomas, and brain tumors. Whereas no cases of leukemia or lymphoma were seen after 8 years, the risk of developing a solid tumor continued to increase with time. Abdominal radiation increased the risk of SMNs, with doxorubicin potentiating the effect. Each 10 Gy of abdominal XRT was estimated to increase the SMN incidence by 22% without doxorubicin and by 66% with doxorubicin.

Renal failure is a concern for Wilms' tumor survivors because patients undergo nephrectomy or partial nephrectomy as part of their treatment. However, the cumulative incidence of end-stage renal disease (ESRD) at 20 years after Wilms' tumor diagnosis is only 0.6% in patients with nonsyndromic unilateral Wilms' tumor.[177] The cumulative incidence of ESRD is much higher for patients with unilateral Wilms' tumor and WAGR syndrome (36%), Denys-Drash syndrome (74%, but probably an underestimate because of inaccurate classification of the syndrome), and isolated genitourinary anomalies (7%).[177] The cumulative incidence of ESRD is also high in patients with nonsyndromic bilateral Wilms' tumor (12%). The high rate of renal failure in patients with bilateral Wilms' tumor is related mainly to bilateral nephrectomies performed for tumor control.[195] However, the renal failure seen with WAGR and Denys-Drash syndromes is caused by underlying renal pathology.[196]

A review of pregnancy outcomes in patients treated on NWTS-1-4 has revealed that fetal malposition and early or threatened labor are more frequent among women who received abdominal irradiation compared with unirradiated women.[197] There was an excess of infants born before 36 weeks of gestation to women who received flank radiation and an excess of infants with birth weight less than 2500 g. Most of the birth weights were appropriate for gestational age. Congenital malformations were more frequent among the offspring of women who received flank radiation compared with unirradiated women. Fertility was related to the dose and field of radiation therapy.[198] In general, fertility is preserved in Wilms' tumor survivors after upper abdominal radiation that does not include the pelvis.

Dental abnormalities (root stunting, enamel hypoplasia, and microdontia) in excess of the expected incidence in control patients were observed in Wilms' tumor survivors.[199] A small study of 49 Wilms' tumor survivors has revealed osteopenia in 27%.[200] Stature loss has been observed in Wilms' tumor survivors, with a predicted height deficit at age 18 years of 1.8 cm for children treated with 10 Gy to the flank at age 4 years.[201] Height deficits were negatively correlated with age (greater deficit with younger age of irradiation) and positively correlated with radiation dosage. Unlike cardiac effects or second malignancies, doxorubicin did not exacerbate reduction in stature.

CLEAR CELL SARCOMA OF THE KIDNEY

Epidemiology

The average age of onset of CCSK in the NWTSG experience was 36 months, with a range of 2 months to 14 years. In contrast to Wilms' tumor, a male predominance was noted, with a male-to-female ratio of 2:1. Among 351 cases of CCSK, no familial or bilateral CCSKs were described.[202]

Molecular Biology and Genetics

The genetic cause of CCSK is poorly understood. Most cases of CCSK have normal karyotypes, although a recurrent t(10;17) translocation has been identified in three cases of CCSK.[203-205] Although the *TP53* gene is located at the 17p13 breakpoint of these translocations, p53 is not thought to play a prominent role in the pathogenesis of CCSK because most CCSK tumors lack detectable p53 protein by immunostaining,[29,205,206] *TP53* mutations are infrequently detected by sequencing analysis,[206] and CCSK primary cell cultures have a functional p53 pathway in response to DNA damage.[207] Other recurrent abnormalities detected by conventional karyotyping or comparative genomic hybridization (CGH) include chromosome 14q deletion (two cases) and 1q gain (three cases).[205,208,209]

Gene expression analysis of CCSK tumors has revealed frequent upregulation of neural markers with activation of the sonic hedgehog and phosphoinositide-3-kinase–Akt pathways.[210] Among the upregulated members of the Akt signaling pathway was the epidermal growth factor receptor (*EGFR*) gene. A subsequent study found EGFR protein immunoreactivity in 12 of 12 CCSK samples, *EGFR* gene amplification in 1 of 12 samples, and a somatic *EGFR* mutation in 1 sample.[211] Two samples had mutations of *PTEN*, a negative regulator of the Akt pathway.[211] These results provide a rationale for evaluating EGFR inhibitors in patients with CCSK that is refractory to current treatment modalities.

Clinical Presentation and Diagnostic Evaluation

Although CCSK has been termed the *bone-metastasizing renal tumor of childhood*, metastatic disease at the time of initial presentation is distinctly uncommon. Only 4% of patients have distant metastatic disease at diagnosis, with bone, lung, and liver as the most common sites.[202] However, approximately 30% of patients who undergo local lymph node sampling are found to have tumor involvement in the renal hilar and periaortic lymph nodes.[202] The value of bone scan versus skeletal survey to detect bone metastases has been addressed. Most lesions are detectable by both modalities, but some lesions are seen by only one of the two modalities.[212] Despite the predilection of this tumor to bone, bone marrow involvement is uncommon and bone marrow aspiration is no longer recommended as part of the staging workup.

Treatment

Although considered one of the unfavorable histology renal tumors, significant progress has been made in the treatment of CCSK. Data from NWTS-1, -2, and -3 have suggested that the addition of DOX to the combination of VCR and AMD improves the 6-year RFS percentage.[213] The beneficial effect of

DOX was confirmed in a retrospective review of 351 cases, including 182 cases from NWTS-1 to 4.[202] NWTS-3 demonstrated no improvement in outcomes of patients with CCSK when CYCLO was added to the combination of VCR/AMD/DOX.[214] However, the CYCLO was delivered at a relatively low dosage and intensity. NWTS-4 asked whether the duration of therapy affects outcome for patients with CCSK. Compared with 6 months of VCR/AMD/DOX therapy, 15 months of therapy was associated with a trend toward improved 8-year RFS (87.8% vs. 60.6%, $P = .08$), although there was no difference in 8-year OS (87.5% vs. 85.9%).[215] NWTS-5 treated patients with 6 months of VCR/DOX/CYCLO alternating with CYCLO/ETOP. Preliminary analysis has shown 5-year event-free and overall survival estimates of 79% and 89%, respectively.[216] Interestingly, 14 patients had stage I disease and none of these patients relapsed. An aim of the current COG AREN0321 study is to assess whether the outstanding outcomes for stage I patients can be maintained without flank XRT.

An interesting observation on recent CCSK trials has been a shift in the site of recurrent disease. Although CCSK is associated with bone metastases, the brain has now surpassed the bone as the most common site of recurrence in North American and European studies.[216-218] The reason for this shift is unclear, but it is possible that improved disease control outside the central nervous system has uncovered the brain as a sanctuary site for tumor cells.

MALIGNANT RHABDOID TUMOR

Epidemiology

MRT occurs primarily in infants, with a mean age of diagnosis of 15 months.[219] However, older children and rare adults with MRT have been reported. MRT is associated with mutations of the *SNF5* gene at chromosome 22q11.1 and familial MRT has been described.[220] A recent report of three individuals with MRT whose parents shared a common site of employment raises the possibility of an environmental cause.[221]

Molecular Biology and Genetics

MRTs most frequently occur in the kidney, where they are referred to as rhabdoid tumor of the kidney and the central nervous system (CNS), where they are referred to as atypical teratoid-rhabdoid tumors, but they can also occur in soft tissues throughout the body, where they are generally referred to as extrarenal rhabdoid tumors. It had long been debated whether renal, CNS, and extrarenal rhabdoid tumors are distinct cancers that possess similar histologic appearances or whether they are the same cancer in different anatomic locations. This issue was largely resolved when most rhabdoid tumors from all anatomic sites were found to have specific biallelic inactivating mutations in *hSNF5* (also known as *INI1*, *BAF47*, and *SMARCB1*).[222,223] Inactivating mutations in both copies of *SNF5* occur in 70% of MRTs and an additional 20% to 25% of the tumors do not express SNF5 protein, even though a specific mutation cannot be identified.[224] Although loss of SNF5 occurs in most MRTs, mutation of another gene(s) may account for a minority of cases, a possibility supported by the report of two siblings with MRT in which loss of SNF5 function was convincingly excluded.[225]

Constitutional mutation in one allele of *SNF5* is the basis of familial MRT, a condition termed the *rhabdoid predisposition syndrome*.[226,227] Carriers have a markedly increased risk for MRT in all sites and can present with more than one primary tumor. Invariably, the second *SNF5* allele has been inactivated in these cancers. Constitutional mutation also accounts for the approximately 15% of patients who, following treatment for MRT, develop a second primary MRT. The frequency of germline mutations in patients presenting with new-onset rhabdoid tumor is somewhat unclear. It has been reported to be present in as many as 33% (16 of 49) of cases, although this number is likely inflated by selection bias.[224] Patients who carry a germline *SNF5* mutation typically present with early-onset RT. Most, but not all, of them are diagnosed before 1 year of age. Given the relatively high frequency of germline *SNF5* mutations, patients with new-onset MRT should have their brain and kidneys imaged to rule out additional tumors. Sequencing the *SNF5* gene from the peripheral blood of newly diagnosed patients should also be considered to rule out a constitutional mutation. If a constitutional mutation is identified, other family members should be screened for this mutation. Notably, although familial studies have identified cancer-free carriers, three families with multiple siblings affected by *SNF5* mutant MRT have been identified in which neither of the parents carried a *SNF5* mutation. This suggests that gonadal mosaicism in a parent can be the basis of familial cases. Consequently, the absence of a constitutional mutation in the parents of a patient with a germline *SNF5* mutation does not fully exclude the possibility that siblings may be affected.

SNF5 encodes a core member of the SWI-SNF chromatin remodeling complex. Tightly compacted chromatin provides an organizational structure for DNA but constitutes a significant barrier to gene expression. Nucleosomes, consisting of 147 base pairs of DNA wrapped around an octamer of histones, are a fundamental unit of chromatin. The SWI-SNF complex regulates the transcription of specific targets by using the energy of adenosine triphosphate (ATP) hydrolysis to mobilize nucleosomes and thereby control access of the transcriptional machinery to promoters. Mice heterozygous for *Snf5* are predisposed to the formation of rhabdoid tumors that display a histologic appearance essentially indistinguishable from human MRT.[228-230] Further, conditional inactivation of both Snf5 alleles leads to the extremely rapid formation of cancer with 100% of mice developing either lymphoma or MRT at a median onset of only 11 weeks. The contribution of *SNF5* to the activity of the SWI-SNF complex is unknown and thus the basis for its tumor suppressor activity is also not clear. However, accumulating evidence has suggested that the complex binds to the retinoblastoma protein (RB) and is required for appropriate regulation of the p16INK4A-RB-E2F pathway.[231-234] Perturbation of this activity may thus contribute to the oncogenesis that occurs following inactivation of *SNF5*.

Clinical Presentation and Diagnostic Evaluation

Children with MRT of the kidney present with signs and symptoms related to an intrarenal mass. Based on the young age at presentation, it is difficult to assess pain, yet most parents report fussiness. About 60% of patients have gross hematuria, which contrasts with Wilms' tumor, in which only 20% have hematuria.[235] Fever is a presenting feature in 50% of patients and hypertension is seen in up to 70%. Because MRT of the kidney can be associated with involvement of the central nervous system, patients may present with focal neurologic signs or signs of increased intracranial pressure.

The diagnosis of MRT must be made by histologic confirmation, although several laboratory features are suggestive of MRT. Approximately 25% of patients have hypercalcemia,

55% have hemoglobin levels less than 9 g/dL, and 75% have gross or microscopic hematuria. The most common sites of MRT metastasis are the lung, bone, and brain. Many of the CNS lesions likely represent second primary tumors rather than metastatic disease. The staging evaluation for MRT therefore includes a CT scan of the chest, abdomen, and pelvis, ultrasound of the abdomen to evaluate for tumor thrombus, bone scan, and MRI of the brain. Bone marrow aspirates and biopsies are not routinely required.

Treatment

MRT is one of the most lethal and aggressive pediatric cancers. Patients with rhabdoid tumor of the kidney historically were treated on NWTSG trials with VCR, AMD, DOX, with or without CYCLO.[162,236,236] The outcomes attained with these agents were poor (see Table 15-8).[219,237] SIOP has reported similarly unfavorable outcomes.[238] To try to improve on these results, NWTS-5 tested a treatment regimen consisting of CARBO/ETOP alternating with CYCLO, but this regimen did not yield improved survival compared with previous regimens.[219] Case reports have highlighted patients with metastatic rhabdoid tumor who had durable survival after treatment with various combinations of ifosfamide (IFOS), ETOP, CARBO, VCR, DOX, and CYCLO.[239-242] Survivors treated with high-dose therapy and autologous stem cell rescue have also been reported,[242] but it is unclear whether this provides a benefit compared with intensive regimens of standard-dose chemotherapy. Based on this limited experience, the current COG AREN0321 study is testing the efficacy of CYCLO/CARBO/ETOP, alternating with VCR/DOX/CYCLO.

The lack of treatment uniformity among reported patients makes it difficult to determine whether radiotherapy is effective for MRT. In NWTS-1-5, radiation therapy was given to the flank or abdomen at total dosages of 1080 to 3500 cGy, yet no relationship was observed between dose and outcome.[219] Radiation therapy is a cornerstone of treatment for central nervous system rhabdoid tumors, and some have suggested that the high doses delivered to the posterior fossa improve patients' outcomes.

RENAL CELL CARCINOMA

Epidemiology

Two European registries of childhood RCC have revealed that the median age of diagnosis in children and adolescents is 10 to 11 years, with a male-to-female ratio of 1 : 1.1.[243,244] In adults, clear cell RCC, associated with mutations of the von Hippel–Lindau (VHL) gene, is the predominant type of RCC. In children, the clear cell subtype is uncommon.[245,246] An association between oncocytoid RCC and a previous history of neuroblastoma has been described.[57,247] Translocation RCC, associated with translocations involving the *TFE3* (chromosome Xp11.1) or *TFEB* (chromosome) gene, has been associated with previous exposure to chemotherapy.[248]

Molecular Biology and Genetics

Little is known regarding the molecular pathogenesis of renal medullary carcinoma or the oncocytoid renal carcinomas in patients who survive neuroblastoma. However, the molecular pathogenesis of the Xp11.2 and t(6:11) translocation carcinomas is an area of active study.

The fusion partners of *TFE3* have variable functions. *PSF* and *NonO* are splicing factor genes. *PRCC* and *ASPL* are novel genes of unknown function, but the former may also be involved in splicing.[249-252] The clathrin heavy-chain gene (*CLTC*) trimerizes with a single light chain to form clathrin, the major protein constituent of the coat that surrounds organelles (cytoplasmic vesicles) to mediate selective protein transport.[253] All TFE3 fusion proteins retain the C-terminal portion of TFE3, including its leucine zipper dimerization domain, nuclear localization signal, and DNA-binding domain. It is likely that the genes fused 5′ to *TFE3* contribute strong promoters that cause overexpression of the chimeric protein, as suggested by results with TFE3 immunohistochemistry. Both PRCC-TFE3[254] and ASPL-TFE3 fusion proteins[255] localize to the nucleus and can act as aberrant transcription factors. PRCC-TFE3 may also interfere with splicing and mitotic checkpoint control via protein-protein interactions.[256]

Both alveolar soft part sarcoma (ASPS) and the t(X;17) renal carcinomas feature one of two types of *ASPL-TFE3* fusion transcript, in which the *ASPL* gene is fused to *TFE3* exon 4 (type 1 fusion) or *TFE3* exon 3 (type 2 fusion). Four types of *PRCC-TFE3* fusion transcripts have been described. Significant differences in clinicopathologic features between cases with different fusion types have yet to be established. Both *ASPL-TFE3* and *PRCC-TFE3* fusion transcripts are readily detected by conventional reverse transcriptase–polymerase chain reaction (RT-PCR) assay using appropriate primers, as described in detail elsewhere.[257,258]

A gene expression study has identified several novel genes that are differentially expressed between the Xp11 translocation carcinomas and conventional renal carcinomas, and has shown that Xp11 translocation carcinomas may be more similar to ASPS than to conventional renal carcinomas.[259] Additionally, gene expression profiling has identified potential therapeutic targets in the Xp11 translocation RCC. For example, the ASPL-TFE3 fusion protein transactivates the promoter of the MET receptor tyrosine kinase, leading to MET protein overexpression. Inhibition of the MET receptor tyrosine kinase may therefore be a potential avenue of targeted therapy for these RCC.[260]

The characteristic t(6;11)(p21;q12) translocation fuses the *Alpha* gene, an intronless gene of unknown function at 11q12, with the first intron of the *TFEB* transcription factor gene at 6p21. The breakpoint on *TFEB* is just upstream of the *TFEB* initiation ATG codon, which results in retention of the entire *TFEB* coding region in the fusion. Although the *Alpha* promoter drives expression of the fusion gene, the *Alpha* gene does not contribute to the open reading frame. Therefore, the consequence of the *Alpha-TFEB* fusion is dysregulated expression of the normal full-length TFEB protein. These findings explain why the t(6;11) renal carcinomas demonstrate specific nuclear labeling for TFEB protein by IHC whereas other neoplasms and normal tissues do not. The association of both the Xp11.2 and the t(6;11) renal translocation carcinomas with exposure of the child prior to chemotherapy raises the possibility that the *TFE3* and *TFEB* loci may be particularly susceptible to DNA damage that promotes chromosome translocations.[248]

It is now thought that the t(6;11) renal carcinomas are related to the Xp11-translocation carcinomas based on the following:

1. Their similar clinical predilection to affect young patients.
2. Their similar morphology. Both neoplasms are composed of nests of predominantly clear to eosinophilic epithelioid cells, typical of a conventional renal cell carcinoma on routine hematoxylin and eosin sections.
3. Their similar immunohistochemical profiles. Given their epithelioid morphology, both tumors underexpress epithe-

lial IHC markers (cytokeratins, EMA). Several Xp11-translocation carcinomas (specifically, those with PSF-TFE3 and CLTC-TFE3 fusions) have expressed melanocytic markers by IHC, just as the t(6;11) renal neoplasms characteristically do. Both tumors overexpress proteins in the MiTF/TFE transcription factor family (TFE3 fusion proteins or native TFEB) and, in each case, a routine IHC assay detects this overexpression in a highly sensitive and specific fashion.

4. Their related molecular pathology. TFEB, TFE3, TFEC, and Mitf comprise the members of the microphthalmia subfamily of basic helix-loop-helix transcription factors, which have homologous DNA binding domains and in fact bind to a common DNA sequence.[261] Members of the MiTF/TFE transcription factor family homodimerize and heterodimerize in all combinations to bind similar or identical DNA sequences. Therefore, it seems likely that the transcription factors overexpressed in these two tumors (TFE3 fusion proteins and native TFEB) have similar downstream targets. Most of these targets remain to be determined; however, genes normally expressed in melanocytic differentiation may be one such example. In cell line transfection assays, overexpression of TFE3 activates the promoter of the tyrosinase gene, whereas both TFEB and TFE3 activate the promoter of the tyrosinase related protein-1 gene.[262] The genes encoding tyrosinase and tyrosinase related-protein-1 are normally expressed in melanocyte differentiation, where they are regulated by another MiTF/TFE family member, MiTF. These results suggest that aberrant overexpression of TFEB may be responsible for the expression of melanocytic markers, a characteristic and distinctive feature of the t(6;11) renal carcinomas, and that some specific TFE3 fusion proteins may do so as well.

Mouse knockout studies have provided further evidence that MiTF family members may functionally overlap in certain cell types. In these studies, severe osteopetrosis occurs in mice with combined TFE3 and MiTF inactivation, but there is no effect of TFE3 or MiTF loss individually on osteoclasts.[263]

Therefore, based on these considerations, it has been suggested that one should classify the t(6;11) renal carcinomas and the Xp11.2 translocation carcinomas as members of the MiTF/TFE translocation carcinoma family.[264]

Clinical Presentation and Diagnostic Evaluation

The most common presenting signs and symptoms of pediatric RCC are flank or abdominal pain, hematuria, fever, nausea and vomiting, abdominal mass, anemia and pallor, and malaise.[243,244] It is unusual for children to present with the typical adult RCC triad of abdominal mass, hematuria, and hypertension. Approximately 20% of patients have locoregional lymph node metastases and up to 30% have distant metastatic disease at initial presentation. The lung, mediastinum, and liver are the most common sites of distant spread.[244,265] The imaging workup for pediatric RCC therefore includes CT of the chest, abdomen, and pelvis and bone scans. Some oncologists also perform a head MRI or CT scan because metastasis to the brain has been reported.

Treatment

Several series of pediatric RCC have demonstrated stage for stage outcomes that mirror outcomes seen in adult patients.[243,244,265] Survival rates for patients with stages I, II, III, and IV disease are about 92%, 85%, 73%, and 13%, respectively.[265] A difference between adult and pediatric RCC is the prognostic significance of local lymph node involvement in the absence of distant metastases.[265] Whereas the survival rate for adult patients with local lymph node involvement is in the 20% to 30% range, approximately 75% of children with local lymph node involvement survive.[244,265] This difference likely reflects the disparate histologies between adult and pediatric RCC. Given the good outcomes of children with localized RCC and the lack of agents with known efficacy, the current COG AREN0321 study is treating such patients without adjuvant therapy after surgical resection. Patients with metastatic RCC are treated according to physician choice.

Until recently, the only therapy with proven benefit for metastatic RCC was immunotherapy using interleukin-2, interferon alfa, or a combination of these agents. However, immunotherapy produces tumor responses in only 10% to 20% of patients, most of whom achieve a transient response and experience substantial toxicity.[266] After a dry spell in clinical progress for RCC, several molecularly targeted agents have demonstrated clinical benefit. Sunitinib, a tyrosine kinase inhibitor of vascular endothelial growth factor receptor (VEGFR)-1, -2, and -3, platelet-derived growth factor receptor (PDGFR)-α and -β, and other tyrosine kinases, has shown response rates of approximately 40% in phase II studies of patients with cytokine-refractory RCC.[267,268] A phase III trial comparing sunitinib with interferon alfa as first-line therapy for metastatic RCC has found higher response rates and improved progression-free survival in the sunitinib arm.[269] Sorafenib, another multitargeted tyrosine kinase inhibitor, has also demonstrated improved progression-free survival compared with placebo.[270,271] Both sunitinib and sorafenib have been approved by the U.S. Food and Drug Administration for the treatment of advanced RCC.[266] A randomized study comparing two doses of the anti-VEGF antibody bevacizumab with placebo has shown prolonged time to progression in the higher dose bevacizumab arm, but no improvement in survival.[272] The combination of bevacizumab and interferon alfa has improved progression-free survival when compared with interferon alfa alone.[273] Another pathway that has been targeted with success in RCC is the mammalian target of rapamycin (mTOR) pathway. The inhibitor temsirolimus was shown to prolong overall and progression-free survival compared with interferon alfa in patients with previously untreated advanced RCC.[274] The combination of interferon alfa and temsirolimus did not add benefit compared with temsirolimus alone. In the wake of these studies, molecularly targeted therapy has become the frontline treatment for advanced RCC in adult patients.

In considering treatment of pediatric RCC, it is important to recognize that childhood and adult RCC are distinct entities. Most of the patients enrolled in adult studies had the clear cell subtype of RCC, whereas most pediatric RCC patients have the translocation or papillary subtypes.[245,246] It therefore remains to be determined whether tyrosine kinase inhibition, mTOR inhibition, or immunotherapy are effective therapeutic modalities for childhood RCC.

A category of pediatric RCC with a distinctly poor outcome is renal medullary carcinoma, which is observed in patients with sickle cell trait.[275] Patients with renal medullary carcinoma almost always present with metastatic disease and have fatal outcomes. Transient responses have been observed after treatment with methotrexate-vinblastine-doxorubicin-cisplatin[276-278] or platinum-gemcitabine-taxane[279] chemotherapy. Agents that target the ABL tyrosine kinase may be considered for investigation in renal medullary carcinoma because these tumors have been reported to have ABL gene amplification and BCR-ABL rearrangements.[277,278] A patient with renal medullary carcinoma was shown to have a complete tumor response after treatment with the proteosome inhibitor bortezomib.[280]

CONGENITAL MESOBLASTIC NEPHROMA

Epidemiology

The average age of diagnosis of CMN is 3.4 months.[281] The vast majority of cases are diagnosed in infancy, but rare cases have been diagnosed in children up to 9 years of age. Of CMN cases, 14% were associated with congenital malformations, including genitourinary and gastrointestinal anomalies, polydactyly, and hydrocephalus.[281]

Molecular Biology and Genetics

Infantile fibrosarcoma (IFS) and cellular CMN have much in common. The two neoplasms have almost indistinguishable morphology and affect the same young age group. Both also are associated with a prognosis that is better than that expected given their ominous-appearing morphology; both IFS and cellular CMN only rarely metastasize. There had also been molecular hints of a relationship between IFS and cellular CMN, because both tumors are characterized by polysomies, particularly of chromosomes 11, 17, and 20.[282,283]

A major advance occurred in 1998, when it was discovered that IFS is characterized by a specific t(12;15)(p13;q25). The t(12;15) results in fusion of the *ETV6* gene on chromosome 12 with the *NTRK3* gene on chromosome 15.[284] The *ETV6 (TEL)* gene had previously been implicated in the t(12;21)(p13;q22) of pediatric precursor B cell acute lymphoblastic leukemia, and encodes a transcription factor with a helix-loop-helix protein dimerization domain. NTRK3 is a receptor tyrosine kinase that is activated by ligand-dependent dimerization, and is involved in neural development. The chimeric ETV6-NTRK3 protein is postulated to be constitutively dimerized, thereby activating tyrosine kinase growth pathway signaling. Importantly, neither infantile fibromatosis nor adult type fibrosarcomas, two entities in the histologic differential diagnosis of infantile fibrosarcoma, contain this gene fusion.

Given the clinicopathologic similarities of IFS and cellular CMN, the question arose as to whether cellular CMN bears the same chromosome translocation and gene fusion. Two studies have conclusively proven this to be true.[285,286] Ten of 11 cellular CMNs studied contained the fusion transcript, whereas all five classic CMNs (the renal counterpart of infantile fibromatosis) did not. Hence, one is tempted to consider cellular CMN to be essentially an IFS of the renal sinus, and there is no clinical, morphologic, histopathologic, or genetic reason to think otherwise. Also, these studies highlight the fact that classic and cellular CMN are molecularly distinctive neoplasms, not just two morphologic patterns of one neoplasm, as their names would suggest. An analogy between infantile fibroblastic tumors of the soft tissue and kidney may be drawn.[287]

Further studies have addressed the function of the *ETV6-NTRK3* fusion gene. Wai and colleagues[288] have shown that ETV6-NTRK3 chimeric tyrosine kinase is capable of transforming NIH3T3 cells. Tognon and associates[289] have subsequently shown that this requires activation of both the Ras-Raf1-Mek1-ERK1/2 mitogenic pathway and the phosphatidylinositol 3'-kinase (PI3K)-Akt cell survival pathway, so that inhibition of either pathway abolishes transformation. These findings raise the possibility that MEK or PI3K inhibitors could be potentially useful in treating the minority of patients who develop metastatic disease. Jin[290] has shown that the *ETVG-*

NTRK3 chimeric tyrosine kinase suppresses transforming growth factor-β (TGF-β) tumor suppressor activity by binding to the type II TGF-β receptor. Finally, the *ETV6-NTRK3* gene fusion has also been found to be consistently present in secretory carcinoma of the breast,[291] a rare epithelial cancer that tends to affect young people. Moreover, a rare case of acute myeloid leukemia has been shown to bear the same gene fusion.[292] Hence, the *ETV6-NTRK3* gene fusion is remarkable in that it may apparently transform cells of the mesenchymal, epithelial, and hematopoietic lineages.

Clinical Presentation and Diagnostic Evaluation

A palpable abdominal mass is the most common presenting symptom in infants with CMN. Other signs and symptoms at presentation include hematuria (18%), hypertension (4%), anemia (4%), and vomiting (6%).[281] Hypercalcemia has been reported as a presenting feature of CMN.[293] Patients with CMN generally do not present with metastatic disease, although the cellular histologic type has the potential to metastasize to the lung and, rarely, the brain later in the course of the disease. A baseline chest, abdomen, and pelvis CT scan are recommended.

Treatment

Outcomes for patients with congenital mesoblastic nephroma are generally excellent without adjuvant therapy, with overall survival rates of 95%.[281,294] The few tumors that recur are almost exclusively the cellular type of the CMN. In addition to cellular histologic subtype, age older than 3 months and stage III disease have been associated with relapse.

The standard therapy for all stages of classic CMN (noncellular) and stage I and II cellular CMN is surgical resection followed by observation with serial imaging studies. It remains to be established whether patients with stage III cellular CMN benefit from adjuvant chemotherapy. In a series published by the German Pediatric Oncology Group (GPOH), 2 of 5 patients with stage III cellular CMN developed recurrent disease, whereas only 1 of the remaining 45 patients had recurrence.[294] Experience with presurgical treatment of CMN shows that most of these tumors respond to VCR/AMD therapy.[294] Recurrent cellular CMN tumors are responsive to VCR/DOX/AMD, VCR/AMD/CYCLO, VCR/DOX/CYCLO, and IFOS/CARBO/ETOP.[295] There is no established role for radiation therapy in the treatment of CMN.

FUTURE DIRECTIONS

A broad view of the field of pediatric renal tumors provides cause for both celebration and trepidation. Treatment of favorable histology Wilms' tumor has been a terrific success, with cure rates in the 90% range. Remarkably, the success has been coupled with a reduction in treatment, thereby sparing patients of acute and long-term adverse effects. We also have a more complete understanding of renal tumor biology than ever before, with the discovery of several new genes (*WTX, BRCA2, INI1, TFE3,* and others) and increased understanding of the old genes (*WT1* and the *WT2* locus). Most importantly, the availability of a new pipeline of molecularly targeted agents provides opportunity to advance our therapies beyond the traditional cytotoxic agents.

On the other hand, challenges remain. Outcomes for children with anaplastic Wilms' tumor, bilateral Wilms' tumor, recurrent Wilms' tumor, renal cell carcinoma, and malignant rhabdoid tumor remain suboptimal (all less than 75% survival). For some of these tumor types, such as anaplastic Wilms' tumor and malignant rhabdoid tumor, we have increased the number of different agents, doses, and overall intensity of chemotherapy to the point that we are approaching the maximum level of patient tolerance without dramatic improvements in survival. Novel treatment approaches, such as molecularly targeted agents, differentiating agents, or immunotherapy, are required for these patients. A pitfall to the introduction of new agents is that the high-risk patient populations are small, so that clinical trials take years to execute. New initiatives for international collaboration between the COG and SIOP will facilitate the implementation of clinical research in these uncommon pediatric renal tumors. In addition, for tumor types such as pediatric renal cell carcinoma, we are only beginning to understand the tumor biology and natural clinical history. Broad support for basic and translational pediatric renal tumor research is essential for further progress.

REFERENCES

1. Ries LAG, Eisner MP, Kosary CL, et al. SEER Cancer Statistics Review, 1975-2000. Bethesda, Md, National Cancer Institute, 2004.
2. Guinan P, Sobin LH, Algaba F, et al. TNM staging of renal cell carcinoma: Workgroup No. 3. Union International Contre le Cancer (UICC) and the American Joint Committee on Cancer (AJCC). Cancer. 1997;80:992-993.
3. Beckwith JB. National Wilms Tumor Study: an update for pathologists. Pediatr Dev Pathol. 1998;1:79-84.
4. Perlman EJ. Pediatric renal tumors: practical updates for the pathologist. Pediatr Dev Pathol. 2005;8:320-338.
5. Vujanic GM, Sandstedt B, Harms D, et al. Revised International Society of Paediatric Oncology (SIOP) working classification of renal tumors of childhood. Med Pediatr Oncol. 2002;38:79-82.
6. Argani P, Beckwith JB. Renal neoplasms of childhood. In Mills SE, Carter D, Greenson JK, et al (eds). Sternberg's Diagnostic Surgical Pathology, 4th ed. Philadelphia, Lippincott Williams & Wilkins, 2004, pp 2001-2033.
7. Joshi VV, Beckwith JB. Multilocular cyst of the kidney (cystic nephroma) and cystic, partially differentiated nephroblastoma. Terminology and criteria for diagnosis. Cancer. 1989;64:466-479.
8. Beckwith JB, Zuppan CE, Browning NG, et al. Histologic analysis of aggressiveness and responsiveness in Wilms tumor. Med Pediatr Oncol. 1996;27:422-428.
9. Zuppan CW, Beckwith JB, Luckey DW. Anaplasia in unilateral Wilms' tumor: a report from the National Wilms' Tumor Study Pathology Center. Hum Pathol. 1988;19:1199-1209.
10. Bardeesy N, Falkoff D, Petruzzi MJ, et al. Anaplastic Wilms' tumour, a subtype displaying poor prognosis, harbours p53 gene mutations. Nat Genet. 1994;7:91-97.
11. Bardeesy N, Beckwith JB, Pelletier J. Clonal expansion and attenuated apoptosis in Wilms' tumors are associated with p53 gene mutations. Cancer Res. 1995;55:215-219.
12. Govender D, Harilal P, Hadley GP, Chetty R. p53 protein expression in nephroblastomas: a predictor of poor prognosis. Br J Cancer. 1998;77:314-318.
13. Hill DA, Shear TD, Liu T, et al. Clinical and biologic significance of nuclear unrest in Wilms tumor. Cancer. 2003;97:2318-2326.
14. Faria P, Beckwith B, Mishra K, et al. Focal versus diffuse anaplasia in Wilms tumor—new definitions with prognostic significance. Am J Surg Pathol. 1996;20:909-920.
15. Dome JS, Cotton CA, Perlman EJ, et al. Treatment of anaplastic histology Wilms' tumor: results from the fifth National Wilms' Tumor Study. J Clin Oncol. 2006;24:2352-2358.
16. Zuppan CW, Beckwith JB, Weeks DA, et al. The effect of preoperative therapy on the histologic features of Wilms' tumor. An analysis of cases from the Third National Wilms' Tumor Study. Cancer. 1991;68:385-394.
17. Boccon-Gibod L, Rey A, Sandstedt B, et al. Complete necrosis induced by preoperative chemotherapy in Wilms tumor as an indicator of low risk: report of the International Society of Paediatric Oncology (SIOP) nephroblastoma trial and study 9. Med Pediatr Oncol. 2000;34:183-190.
18. Weirich A, Leuschner I, Harms D, et al. Clinical impact of histologic subtypes in localized non-anaplastic nephroblastoma treated according to the trial and study SIOP-9/GPOH. Ann Oncol. 2001;12:311-319.
19. Mierau GW, Beckwith JB, Weeks DA. Ultrastructure and histogenesis of the renal tumors of childhood: an overview. Ultrastruct Pathol. 1987;11:313-333.
20. Weeks DA, Mierau GW, Malott RL, Beckwith JB. Practical electron microscopy of pediatric renal tumors. Ultrastruct Pathol. 1996;20:31-33.
21. Folpe AL, Patterson K, Gown AM. Antibodies to desmin identify the blastemal component of nephroblastoma. Mod Pathol. 1997;10:895-900.
22. Grubb GR, Yun K, Williams BR, et al. Expression of WT1 protein in fetal kidneys and Wilms tumors. Lab Invest. 1994;71:472-479.
23. Beckwith JB, Kiviat NB, Bonadio JF. Nephrogenic rests, nephroblastomatosis, and the pathogenesis of Wilms' tumor. Pediatr Pathol. 1990;10:1-36.
24. Beckwith JB. Precursor lesions of Wilms tumor: clinical and biologic implications. Med Pediatr Oncol. 1993;21:158-168.
25. Argani P, Collins MH. Anaplastic nephrogenic rest. Am J Surg Pathol. 2006;30:1339-1341.
26. Coppes MJ, Arnold M, Beckwith JB, et al. Factors affecting the risk of contralateral Wilms tumor development: a report from the National Wilms Tumor Study Group. Cancer. 1999;85:1616-1625.
27. Renshaw AA, Zhang H, Corless CL, et al. Solid variants of papillary (chromophil) renal cell carcinoma: clinicopathologic and genetic features. Am J Surg Pathol. 1997;21:1203-1209.
28. Muir TE, Cheville JC, Lager DJ. Metanephric adenoma, nephrogenic rests, and Wilms' tumor: a histologic and immunophenotypic comparison. Am J Surg Pathol. 2001;25:1290-1296.
29. Argani P, Perlman EJ, Breslow NE, et al. Clear cell sarcoma of the kidney: a review of 351 cases from the National Wilms Tumor Study Group Pathology Center. Am J Surg Pathol. 2000;24:4-18.
30. Sandstedt BE, Delemarre JF, Harms D, Tournade MF. Sarcomatous Wilms' tumour with clear cells and hyalinization. A study of 38 tumours in children from the SIOP nephroblastoma file. Histopathology. 1987;11:273-285.
31. Sotelo-Avila C, Gonzalez-Crussi F, Sadowinski S, et al. Clear cell sarcoma of the kidney: a clinicopathologic study of 21 patients with long-term follow-up evaluation. Hum Pathol. 1985;16:1219-1230.
32. Marsden HB, Lawler W. Bone-metastasizing renal tumour of childhood. Histopathologic and clinical review of 38 cases. Virchows Arch A Pathol Anat Histol. 1980;387:341-351.
33. Argani P, Lui MY, Couturier J, et al. A novel CLTC-TFE3 gene fusion in pediatric renal adenocarcinoma with t(X;17)(p11.2;q23). Oncogene. 2003;22:5374-5378.
34. Haas JE, Bonadio JF, Beckwith JB. Clear cell sarcoma of the kidney with emphasis on ultrastructural studies. Cancer. 1984;54:2978-2987.
35. Bolande RP. Congenital mesoblastic nephroma of infancy. Perspect Pediatr Pathol. 1973;1:227-250.

36. Pettinato G, Manivel JC, Wick MR, Dehner LP. Classical and cellular (atypical) congenital mesoblastic nephroma: a clinicopathologic, ultrastructural, immunohistochemical, and glow cytometric study. Hum Pathol. 1989;20:682-690.

37. Nadasdy T, Roth J, Johnson DL, et al. Congenital mesoblastic nephroma: an immunohistochemical and lectin study. Hum Pathol. 1993;24:413-419.

38. O'Malley DP, Mierau GW, Beckwith JB, Weeks DA. Ultrastructure of cellular congenital mesoblastic nephroma. Ultrastruct Pathol. 1996;20:417-427.

39. Argani P, Beckwith JB. Metanephric stromal tumor: report of 31 cases of a distinctive pediatric renal neoplasm. Am J Surg Pathol. 2000;24:917-926.

40. Arroyo MR, Green DM, Perlman EJ, et al. The spectrum of metanephric adenofibroma and related lesions: clinicopathologic study of 25 cases from the National Wilms Tumor Study Group Pathology Center. Am J Surg Pathol. 2001;25:433-444.

41. Hennigar RA, Beckwith JB. Nephrogenic adenofibroma. A novel kidney tumor of young people. Am J Surg Pathol. 1992;16:325-334.

42. Weeks DA, Beckwith JB, Mierau GW, Luckey DW. Rhabdoid tumor of kidney. A report of 111 cases from the National Wilms' Tumor Study Pathology Center. Am J Surg Pathol. 1989;13:439-458.

43. Haas JE, Palmer NF, Weinberg AG. Ultrastructure of malignant rhabdoid tumor of the kidney: a distinctive renal tumor of children. Hum Pathol. 1981;12:646.

44. Hoot AC, Russo P, Judkins AR, et al. Immunohistochemical analysis of hSNF5/INI1 distinguishes renal and extra-renal malignant rhabdoid tumors from other pediatric soft tissue tumors. Am J Surg Pathol. 2004;28:1485-1491.

45. Weeks DA, Beckwith B, Mierau GW, Zuppan CW. Renal neoplasms mimicking thabdoid tumor of kidney. Am J Surg Pathol. 1991;15:1042-1054.

46. Parham DM, Weeks DA, Beckwith JB. The clinicopathologic spectrum of putative extrarenal rhabdoid tumors. An analysis of 42 cases studied with immunohistochemistry or electron microscopy. Am J Surg Pathol. 1994;18:1010-1029.

47. Pea M, Bonetti F, Martignoni G, et al. Apparent renal cell carcinomas in tuberous sclerosis are heterogeneous. The identification of malignant epithelioid angiomyolipoma. Am J Surg Pathol. 1998;22:180-187.

48. Argani P, Ladanyi M. Renal carcinomas associated with Xp11.2 translocations/TFE3 gene fusions. In Eble JN, Sauter G, Epstein J, Sesterhenn I (eds). Pathology and Genetics: Tumours of the Urinary System and Male Genital Organs. Lyon, France, International Agency for Research on Cancer, 2003, pp 37-38.

49. Argani P, Antonescu CR, Illei PB, et al. Primary renal neoplasms with the ASPL-TFE3 gene fusion of alveolar soft part sarcoma: a distinctive tumor entity previously included among renal cell carcinomas of children and adolescents. Am J Pathol. 2001;159:179-192.

50. Argani P, Antonescu CR, Couturier J, et al. PRCC-TFE3 renal carcinomas: morphologic, immunohistochemical, ultrastructural, and molecular analysis of an entity associated with the t(X;1)(p11.2;q21). Am J Surg Pathol. 2002;26:1553-1566.

51. Argani P, Lal P, Hutchinson B, et al. Aberrant nuclear immunoreactivity for TFE3 in neoplasms with TFE3 gene fusions: a sensitive and specific immunohistochemical assay. Am J Surg Pathol. 2003;27:750-761.

52. Argani P, Hawkins A, Griffin CA, et al. A distinctive pediatric renal neoplasm characterized by epithelioid morphology, basement membrane production, focal HMB45 immunoreactivity, and t(6;11)(p21.1;q12) chromosome translocation. Am J Pathol. 2001;158:2089-2096.

53. Davis I, His B-L, Arroyo JD, et al. Cloning of a novel alpha-TFEB fusion in renal tumors harboring the t(6;11)(p21;q12)

54. chromosome translocation. Proc Natl Acad Sci U S A. 2003;6051-6056.

54. Kuiper RP, Schepens M, Thijssen J, et al. Upregulation of the transcription factor TFEB in t(6;11)(p21;q13)-positive renal cell carcinomas due to promoter substitution. Hum Mol Genet. 2003;12:1661-1669.

55. Argani P, Lae M, Hutchinson B, et al. Renal carcinomas with the t(6;11)(p21;q12): clinicopathologic features and demonstration of the specific alpha-TFEB gene fusion by immunohistochemistry, RT-PCR, and DNA PCR. Am J Surg Pathol. 2005;29:230-240.

56. Davis CJ Jr, Mostofi FK, Sesterhenn IA. Renal medullary carcinoma. The seventh sickle cell nephropathy. Am J Surg Pathol. 1995;19:1-11.

57. Medeiros LJ, Palmedo G, Krigman HR, et al. Oncocytoid renal cell carcinoma after neuroblastoma: a report of four cases of a distinct clinicopathologic entity. Am J Surg Pathol. 1999;23:772-780.

58. Jimenez RE, Folpe AL, Lapham RL, et al. Primary Ewing's sarcoma/primitive neuroectodermal tumor of the kidney: a clinicopathologic and immunohistochemical analysis of 11 cases. Am J Surg Pathol. 2002;26:320-327.

59. Quezado M, Benjamin DR, Tsokos M. EWS/FLI-1 fusion transcripts in three peripheral primitive neuroectodermal tumors of the kidney. Hum Pathol. 1997;28:767-771.

60. Argani P, Faria PA, Epstein JI, et al. Primary renal synovial sarcoma: molecular and morphologic delineation of an entity previously included among embryonal sarcomas of the kidney. Am J Surg Pathol. 2000;24:1087-1096.

61. Kim DH, Sohn JH, Lee MC, et al. Primary synovial sarcoma of the kidney. Am J Surg Pathol. 2000;24:1097-1104.

62. van den Heuvel-Eibrink MM, Grundy P, Graf N, et al. Characteristics and survival of 750 children diagnosed with a renal tumor in the first seven months of life: a collaborative study by the SIOP/GPOH/SFOP, NWTSG, and UKCCSG Wilms tumor study groups. Pediatr Blood Cancer. 2008;50:1130-1134.

63. Breslow N, Olshan A, Beckwith JB, Green DM. Epidemiology of Wilms tumor. Med Pediatr Oncol. 1993;21:172-181.

64. Knudson AG, Strong LC. Mutation and cancer: a model for Wilms' tumor of the kidney. J Nat Cancer Inst. 1972;48:313-324.

65. Breslow NE, Beckwith JB, Perlman EJ, Reeve AE. Age distributions, birth weights, nephrogenic rests, and heterogeneity in the pathogenesis of Wilms tumor. Pediatr Blood Cancer. 2006;47:260-267.

66. Fukuzawa R, Breslow NE, Morison IM, et al. Epigenetic differences between Wilms' tumours in white and east-Asian children. Lancet. 2004;363:446-451.

67. Stjernfeldt M, Berglund K, Lindsten J, Ludvigsson J. Maternal smoking during pregnancy and risk of childhood cancer. Lancet. 1986;1:1350-1352.

68. Bunin GR, Kramer S, Marrero O, Meadows AT. Gestational risk factors for Wilms' tumor: results of a case-control study. Cancer Res. 1987;47:2972-2977.

69. Olshan A, Breslow N, Faletta JM, et al. Risk factors for Wilms Tumor; Report from the National Wilms Tumor Study. Cancer. 1993;72:938-944.

70. Cooney MA, Daniels JL, Ross JA, et al. Household pesticides and the risk of Wilms' tumor. Environ Health Perspect. 2007;115:134-137.

71. Saddlemire S, Olshan AF, Daniels JL, et al. Breast-feeding and Wilms' tumor: a report from the Children's Oncology Group. Cancer Causes Control. 2006;17:687-693.

72. Kantor AF, Curnen MG, Meigs JW, Flannery JT. Occupations of fathers of patients with Wilms' tumour. J Epidemiol Community Health. 1979;33:253-256.

73. Wilkins JR III, Sinks TH Jr. Paternal occupation and Wilms' tumour in offspring. J Epidemiol Community Health. 1984;38:7-11.

74. Bunin GR, Nass CC, Kramer S, Meadows AT. Parental occupation and Wilms' tumor: results of a case-control study. Cancer Res. 1989;49:725-729.

75. Olshan A, Breslow N, Daling JR, et al. Wilms tumor and paternal occupation. Cancer Res. 1990;50:3212-3217.

76. Bonetta L, Kuehn SE, Huang A, et al. Wilms tumor locus on 11p13 defined by multiple CpG island-associated transcripts. Science. 1990;250:994-997.

77. Call KM, Glaser T, Ito CY, et al. Isolation and characterization of a zinc finger polypeptide gene at the human chromosome 11 Wilms' tumor locus. Cell. 1990;60:509-520.

78. Gessler M, Poustka A, Cavenee W, et al. Homozygous deletion in Wilms tumours of a zinc-finger gene identified by chromosome jumping. Nature. 1990;343:774-778.

79. Barbaux S, Niaudet P, Gubler MC, et al. Donor splice-site mutations in WT1 are responsible for Frasier syndrome. Nat Genet. 1997;17:467-470.

80. Hammes A, Guo JK, Lutsch G, et al. Two splice variants of the Wilms' tumor 1 gene have distinct functions during sex determination and nephron formation. Cell. 2001;106:319-329.

81. Pelletier J, Bruening W, Kashtan CE, et al. Germline mutations in the Wilms' tumor supressor gene are associated with abnormal urogenital development in Denys-Drash syndrome. Cell. 1991; 67:437-447.

82. Huff V. Wilms tumor genetics. Am J Med Genet. 1998;79: 260-267.

83. Kreidberg JA, Sariola H, Loring JM, et al. WT-1 is required for early kidney development. Cell. 1993;74:679-691.

84. Barker N, Clevers H. Mining the Wnt pathway for cancer therapeutics. Nat Rev Drug Discov. 2006;5:997-1014.

85. Koesters R, Ridder R, Kopp-Schneider A, et al. Mutational activation of the β-catenin proto-oncogene is a common event in the development of Wilms tumors. Cancer Res. 1999;59:3880-3882.

86. Maiti S, Alam R, Amos CI, Huff V. Frequent association of beta-catenin and WT1 mutations in Wilms tumors. Cancer Res. 2000; 60:6288-6292.

87. Li CM, Kim CE, Margolin AA, et al. CTNNB1 mutations and overexpression of Wnt/beta-catenin target genes in WT1-mutant Wilms' tumors. Am J Pathol. 2004;165:1943-1953.

88. Stark K, Vainio S, Vassileva G, McMahon AP. Epithelial transformation of metanephric mesenchyme in the developing kidney regulated by Wnt-4. Nature. 1994;372:679-683.

89. Rivera MN, Kim WJ, Wells J, et al. An X chromosome gene, WTX, is commonly inactivated in Wilms tumor. Science. 2007; 315:642-645.

90. Ruteshouser EC, Robinson SM, Huff V. Wilms tumor genetics: mutations in WT1, WTX, and CTNNB1 account for only about one-third of tumors. Genes Chromosomes Cancer. 2008;47: 461-470.

91. Perotti D, Gamba B, Sardella M, et al. Functional inactivation of the WTX gene is not a frequent event in Wilms' tumors. Oncogene. 2008 Apr 7. [Epub ahead of print].

92. Major MB, Camp ND, Berndt JD, et al. Wilms tumor suppressor WTX negatively regulates WNT/beta-catenin signaling. Science. 2007;316:1043-1046.

93. Rivera MN, Kim WJ, Wells J, et al. An X chromosome gene, WTX, is commonly inactivated in Wilms tumor. Science. 2007; 315:642-645.

94. Reeve AE, Sih SA, Raizis AM, Feinberg AP. Loss of allelic heterozygosity at a second locus on chromosome 11 in sporadic Wilms' tumor cells. Mol Cell Biol. 1989;9:1799-1803.

95. Weksberg R, Shuman C, Smith AC. Beckwith-Wiedemann syndrome. Am J Med Genet C Semin Med Genet. 2005;137C: 12-23.

96. Scott J, Cowell J, Robertson ME, et al. Insulin-like growth factor-II gene expression in Wilms' tumour and embryonic tissues. Nature. 1985;317:260-262.

97. Reeve AE, Eccles MR, Wilkins RJ, et al. Expression of insulin-like growth factor-II transcripts in Wilms' tumour. Nature. 1985;317:258-260.

98. Hao Y, Crenshaw T, Moulton T, et al. Tumour-suppressor activity of H19 RNA. Nature. 1993;365:764-767.

99. Gicquel C, Rossignol S, Cabrol S, et al. Epimutation of the telomeric imprinting center region on chromosome 11p15 in Silver-Russell syndrome. Nat Genet. 2005;37:1003-1007.

100. Eggermann T, Schonherr N, Meyer E, et al. Epigenetic mutations in 11p15 in Silver-Russell syndrome are restricted to the telomeric imprinting domain. J Med Genet. 2006;43:615-616.

101. Bliek J, Maas SM, Ruijter JM, et al. Increased tumour risk for BWS patients correlates with aberrant H19 and not KCNQ1OT1 methylation: occurrence of KCNQ1OT1 hypomethylation in familial cases of BWS. Hum Mol Genet. 2001;10:467-476.

102. DeBaun MR, Niemitz EL, McNeil DE, et al. Epigenetic alterations of H19 and LIT1 distinguish patients with Beckwith-Wiedemann syndrome with cancer and birth defects. Am J Hum Genet. 2002;70:604-611.

103. Weksberg R, Nishikawa J, Caluseriu O, et al. Tumor development in the Beckwith-Wiedemann syndrome is associated with various constitutional molecular 11p15 alterations including imprinting defects of KCNQ1OT1. Hum Mol Genet. 2001;10: 2989-3000.

104. Pilia G, Hughes-Benzie RM, MacKenzie A, et al. Mutations in GPC3, a glypican gene, cause the Simpson-Golabi-Behmel overgrowth syndrome. Nat Genet. 1996;12:241-247.

105. Song HH, Shi W, Xiang YY, Filmus J. The loss of glypican-3 induces alterations in Wnt signaling. J Biol Chem. 2005;280: 2116-2125.

106. Toretsky JA, Zitomersky NL, Eskenazi AE, et al. Glypican-3 expression in Wilms tumor and hepatoblastoma. J Pediatr Hematol Oncol. 2001;23:496-499.

107. Scott RH, Stiller CA, Walker L, Rahman N. Syndromes and constitutional chromosomal abnormalities associated with Wilms tumour. J Med Genet. 2006;43:705-715.

108. White GR, Kelsey AM, Varley JM, Birch JM. Somatic glypican 3 (GPC3) mutations in Wilms' tumour. Br J Cancer. 2002;86: 1920-1922.

109. Gillan TL, Hughes R, Godbout R, Grundy PE. The Simpson-Golabi-Behmel gene, GPC3, is not involved in sporadic Wilms tumorigenesis. Am J Med Genet. 2003;122A:30-36.

110. Hirsch B, Shimamura A, Moreau L, et al. Association of biallelic BRCA2/FANCD1 mutations with spontaneous chromosomal instability and solid tumors of childhood. Blood. 2004;103: 2554-2559.

111. Reid S, Renwick A, Seal S, et al. Biallelic BRCA2 mutations are associated with multiple malignancies in childhood including familial Wilms tumour. J Med Genet. 2005;42:147-151.

112. Wang W. Emergence of a DNA-damage response network consisting of Fanconi anaemia and BRCA proteins. Nat Rev Genet. 2007;8:735-748.

113. Howlett NG, Taniguchi T, Olson S, et al. Biallelic inactivation of BRCA2 in Fanconi anemia. Science. 2002;297:606-609.

114. Reid S, Schindler D, Hanenberg H, et al. Biallelic mutations in PALB2 cause Fanconi anemia subtype FA-N and predispose to childhood cancer. Nat Genet. 2007;39:162-164.

115. Cairney AEL, Andrews M, Greenberg M, et al. Wilms tumor in three patients with Bloom syndrome. J Pediatr. 1987;111:414-416.

116. German J. Bloom's syndrome. XX. The first 100 cancers. Cancer Genet Cytogenet. 1997;93:100-106.

117. Hanks S, Coleman K, Reid S, et al. Constitutional aneuploidy and cancer predisposition caused by biallelic mutations in BUB1B. Nat Genet. 2004;36:1159-1161.

118. Hanks S, Coleman K, Summersgill B, et al. Comparative genomic hybridization and BUB1B mutation analyses in childhood cancers

associated with mosaic variegated aneuploidy syndrome. Cancer Lett. 2006;239:234-238.

119. Malkin D, Li FP, Strong LC, et al. Germ line p53 mutations in a familial syndrome of breast cancer, sarcomas, and other neoplasms. Science. 1990;250:1233-1238.

120. Birch JM, Alston RD, McNally RJQ, et al. Relative frequency and morphology of cancers in carriers of germline TP53 mutations. Oncogene. 2001;20:4621-4628.

121. Malkin D, Sexsmith E, Yeger H, et al. Mutations of the p53 tumor suppressor gene occur infrequently in Wilms' tumor. Cancer Res. 1994;54:2077-2079.

122. Rahman N, Arbour L, Tonin P, et al. Evidence for a familial Wilms' tumour gene (FWT1) on chromosome 17q12-q21. Nat Genet. 1996;13:461-463.

123. Rahman N, Abidi F, Ford D, et al. Confirmation of *FWT1* as a Wilms' tumour susceptibility gene and phenotypic characteristics of Wilms" tumour attributable to *FWT1*. Hum Genet. 1998; 103:547-556.

124. McDonald JM, Douglass EC, Fisher R, et al. Linkage of familial Wilms' tumor predisposition to chromosome 19 and a two-locus model for the cause of familial tumors. Cancer Res. 1998;58: 1387-1390.

125. Altura RA, Valentine M, Li H, et al. Identification of novel regions of deletion in familial Wilms' tumor by comparative genomic hybridization. Cancer Res. 1996;56:3837-3841.

126. Grundy RG, Pritchard J, Scambler P, Cowell JK. Loss of heterozygosity for the short arm of chromosome 7 in sporadic Wilms tumour. Oncogene. 1998;17:395-400.

127. Perotti D, Testi MA, Mondini P, et al. Refinement within single yeast artificial chromosome clones of a minimal region commonly deleted on the short arm of chromosome 7 in Wilms tumours. Genes Chromosomes Cancer. 2001;31:42-47.

128. Perotti D, De VG, Testi MA, et al. Germline mutations of the POU6F2 gene in Wilms tumors with loss of heterozygosity on chromosome 7p14. Hum Mutat. 2004;24:400-407.

129. Di RF, Doneda L, Menegola E, et al. The murine Pou6f2 gene is temporally and spatially regulated during kidney embryogenesis and its human homolog is overexpressed in a subset of Wilms tumors. J Pediatr Hematol Oncol. 2006;28: 791-797.

130. Anglesio MS, Evdokimova V, Melnyk N, et al. Differential expression of a novel ankyrin-containing E3 ubiquitin-protein ligase, Hace1, in sporadic Wilms' tumor versus normal kidney. Hum Mol Genet. 2004;13:2061-2074.

131. Zhang L, Anglesio MS, O'Sullivan M, et al. The E3 ligase HACE1 is a critical chromosome 6q21 tumor suppressor involved in multiple cancers. Nat Med. 2007;13:1060-1069.

132. Hing S, Lu YJ, Summersgill B, et al. Gain of 1q is associated with adverse outcome in favorable histology Wilms' tumors. Am J Pathol. 2001;158:393-398.

133. Lu YJ, Hing S, Williams R, et al. Chromosome 1q expression profiling and relapse in Wilms' tumour. Lancet. 2002;360: 385-386.

134. Hobbs MR, Pole AR, Pidwirny GN, et al. Hyperparathyroidism-jaw tumor syndrome: the HRPT2 locus is within a 0.7-cM region on chromosome 1q. Am J Hum Genet. 1999;64:518-525.

135. Natrajan R, Little SE, Reis-Filho JS, et al. Amplification and overexpression of CACNA1E correlates with relapse in favorable histology Wilms' tumors. Clin Cancer Res. 2006;12:7284-7293.

136. Green DM. Diagnosis and Management of Malignant Solid Tumors in Infants and Children. Boston, Martinus Nijhoff, 1985, pp 129-186.

137. Coppes MJ, Zandvoort SW, Sparling CR, et al. Acquired von Willebrand disease in Wilms' tumor patients. J Clin Oncol. 1992;10:422-427.

138. Shamberger RC, Ritchey ML, Haase GM, et al. Intravascular extension of Wilms tumor. Ann Surg. 2001;234:116-121.

139. Lall A, Pritchard-Jones K, Walker J, et al. Wilms' tumor with intracaval thrombus in the UK Children's Cancer Study Group UKW3 trial. J Pediatr Surg. 2006;41:382-387.

140. Wilimas JA, Douglass EC, Magill HL, et al. Significance of pulmonary computed tomography at diagnosis in Wilms' tumor. J Clin Oncol. 1988;6:1144-1146.

141. Corey B, Yang CH, Wilimas JA, et al. Significance of pleural effusion at diagnosis of Wilms tumor. Pediatr Blood Cancer. 2004;42:145-148.

142. Ehrlich PF, Hamilton TE, Grundy P, et al. The value of surgery in directing therapy for patients with Wilms' tumor with pulmonary disease. A report from the National Wilms' Tumor Study Group (National Wilms' Tumor Study 5). J Pediatr Surg. 2006; 41:162-167.

143. Green DM, Fernbach DJ, Norkool P, et al. The treatment of Wilms' tumor patients with pulmonary metastases detected only with computed tomography: a report from the National Wilms' Tumor Study. J Clin Oncol. 1991;9:1776-1781.

144. Wilimas JA, Kaste SC, Kauffman WM, et al. Use of chest computed tomography in the staging of pediatric Wilms' tumor: interobserver variability and prognostic significance. J Clin Oncol. 1997;15:2631-2635.

145. Meisel JA, Guthrie KA, Breslow NE, et al. Significance and management of computed tomography detected pulmonary nodules: a report from the National Wilms Tumor Study Group. Int J Radiat Oncol Biol Phys. 1999;44:579-585.

146. Owens CM, Veys PA, Pritchard J, et al. Role of chest computed tomography at diagnosis in the management of Wilms' tumor: a study by the United Kingdom Children's Cancer Study Group. J Clin Oncol. 2002;20:2768-2773.

147. Dirks A, Li S, Breslow N, Grundy P. Outcome of patients with lung metastases on NWTS 4 and 5. Med Pediatr Oncol. 2003;41: 251-252.

148. Shulkin BL, Chang E, Strouse PJ, et al. PET FDG studies of Wilms tumors. J Pediatr Hematol Oncol. 1997;19:334-338.

149. Kaste SC, Dome JS. Wilms' tumor. In Charron M (ed). Practical Pediatric PET Imaging. New York, Springer, 2006, pp 256-266.

150. Ritchey ML, Shamberger RC, Hamilton T, et al. Fate of bilateral renal lesions missed on preoperative imaging: a report from the National Wilms Tumor Study Group. J Urol. 2005;174:1519-1521.

151. Shamberger RC, Guthrie KA, Ritchey ML, et al. Surgery-related factors and local recurrence of Wilms tumor in National Wilms Tumor Study-4. Ann Surg. 1999;229:292-297.

152. D'Angio GJ, Tefft M, Breslow N, Meyer JA. Radiation therapy of Wilms' tumor: results according to dose, field, post-operative timing and histology. Int J Radiat Oncol Biol Phys. 1978;4: 769-780.

153. Thomas PR, Tefft M, Farewell VT, et al. Abdominal relapses in irradiated second National Wilms' Tumor Study patients. J Clin Oncol. 1984;2:1098-1101.

154. Kalapurakal JA, Li SM, Breslow NE, et al. Influence of radiation therapy delay on abdominal tumor recurrence in patients with favorable histology Wilms' tumor treated on NWTS-3 and NWTS-4: a report from the National Wilms' Tumor Study Group. Int J Radiat Oncol Biol Phys. 2003;57:495-499.

155. Green DM. The treatment of stages I-IV favorable histology Wilms' tumor. J Clin Oncol. 2004;22:1366-1372.

156. de Kraker J, Lemerle J, Voute PA, et al. Wilms' tumor with pulmonary metastases at diagnosis: the significance of primary chemotherapy. International Society of Pediatric Oncology Nephroblastoma Trial and Study Committee. J Clin Oncol. 1990;8:1187-1190.

157. Pritchard J, Imeson J, Barnes J, et al. Results of the United Kingdom Children's Cancer Study Group first Wilms' tumor study. J Clin Oncol. 1995;13:124-133.

158. Farber S. Chemotherapy in the treatment of leukemia and Wilms' tumor. JAMA. 1966;198:826-836.

159. Vietti TJ, Sullivan MP, Haggard ME, et al. Vincristine sulfate and radiation therapy in metastatic Wilms' tumor. Cancer. 1970;25:12-20.

160. D'Angio GJ, Evans AE, Breslow N, et al. The treatment of Wilms' tumor: results of the national Wilms' tumor study. Cancer. 1976;38:633-646.

161. D'Angio GJ, Evans A, Breslow N, et al. The treatment of Wilms' tumor: results of the Second National Wilms' Tumor Study. Cancer. 1981;47:2302-2311.

162. D'Angio GJ, Breslow N, Beckwith JB, et al. Treatment of Wilms' tumor. Results of the Third National Wilms' Tumor Study. Cancer. 1989;64:349-360.

163. Green DM, Breslow NE, Beckwith JB, et al. Effect of duration of treatment on treatment outcome and cost of treatment for Wilms' tumor: a report from the National Wilms' Tumor Study Group. J Clin Oncol. 1998;16:3744-3751.

164. Green DM, Breslow NE, Evans I, et al. The effect of chemotherapy dose intensity on the hematologic toxicity of the treatment for Wilms' tumor. A report from the National Wilms' Tumor Study. Am J Pediatr Hematol Oncol. 1994;16:207-212.

165. Green DM, Breslow NE, Evans I, et al. Relationship between dose schedule and charges for treatment on National Wilms' Tumor Study-4. A report from the National Wilms' Tumor Study Group. J Natl Cancer Inst Monogr. 1995;(19):21-25.

166. Grundy PE, Telzerow PE, Breslow N, et al. Loss of heterozygosity for chromosomes 16q and 1p in Wilms' tumors predicts an adverse outcome. Cancer Res. 1994;54:2331-2333.

167. Grundy PE, Breslow NE, Li S, et al. Loss of heterozygosity for chromosomes 1p and 16q is an adverse prognostic factor in favorable-histology Wilms tumor: a report from the National Wilms Tumor Study Group. J Clin Oncol. 2005;23:7312-7321.

168. Larsen E, Perez-Atayde A, Green DM, et al. Surgery only for the treatment of patients with stage I (Cassady) Wilms' tumor. Cancer. 1990;66:264-266.

169. Green DM, Breslow NE, Beckwith JB, et al. Treatment with nephrectomy only for small, stage I/favorable histology Wilms' tumor: a report from the National Wilms' Tumor Study Group. J Clin Oncol. 2001;19:3719-3724.

170. Pritchard-Jones K, Kelsey A, Vujanic G, et al. Older age is an adverse prognostic factor in stage I, favorable histology Wilms' tumor treated with vincristine monochemotherapy: a study by the United Kingdom Children's Cancer Study Group, Wilms' Tumor Working Group. J Clin Oncol. 2003;21:3269-3275.

171. de Kraker J, Graf N, van TH, et al. Reduction of postoperative chemotherapy in children with stage I intermediate-risk and anaplastic Wilms' tumour (SIOP 93-01 trial): a randomised controlled trial. Lancet. 2004;364:1229-1235.

172. Beckwith JB, Palmer NF. Histopathology and prognosis of Wilms tumor. Cancer. 1978;41:1937-1948.

173. Tournade MF, Com-Nougue C, Voute PA, et al. Results of the sixth international society of pediatric oncology Wilms' tumor trial and study: a risk-adapted therapeutic approach in Wilms' tumor. J Clin Oncol. 1993;11:1014-1023.

174. Tournade MF, Com-Nougue C, de Kraker J, et al. Optimal duration of preoperative therapy in unilateral and nonmetastatic Wilms' tumor in children older than 6 months: results of the Ninth International Society of Pediatric Oncology Wilms' Tumor Trial and Study. J Clin Oncol. 2001;19:488-500.

175. Green DM, Beckwith JB, Breslow NE, et al. Treatment of children with stages II to IV anaplastic Wilms' tumor: a report from the National Wilms' Tumor Study Group. J Clin Oncol. 1994;12:2126-2131.

176. Metzger ML, Stewart CF, Freeman BB III, et al. Topotecan is active against Wilms tumor: results of a multi-institutional phase II study. J Clin Oncol. 2007;25:3130-3136.

177. Breslow NE, Collins AJ, Ritchey ML, et al. End stage renal disease in patients with Wilms tumor: results from the National Wilms Tumor Study Group and the United States Renal Data System. J Urol. 2005;174:1972-1975.

178. Bishop HC, Tefft M, Evans AE, D'Angio GJ. Survival in bilateral Wilms' tumor—review of 30 National Wilms Tumor Study cases. J Pediatr Surg. 1977;12:631-638.

179. Blute ML, Kelalis PP, Offord KP, et al. Bilateral Wilms' tumor. J Urol. 1987;138:968-973.

180. Montgomery BT, Kelalis PP, Blute ML, et al. Extended followup of bilateral Wilms tumor: results of the National Wilms Tumor Study. J Urol. 1991;146:514-518.

181. Horwitz JR, Ritchey ML, Moksness J, et al. Renal salvage procedures in patients with synchronous bilateral Wilms' tumors: a report from the National Wilms' Tumor Study Group. J Pediatr Surg. 1996;31:1020-1025.

182. Davidoff AM, Giel DW, Jones DP, et al. The feasibility and outcome of nephron-sparing surgery for children with bilateral Wilms tumor. The St. Jude Children's Research Hospital experience: 1999-2006. Cancer. 2008;112:2060-2070.

183. Grundy P, Breslow N, Green DM, et al. Prognostic factors for children with recurrent Wilms' tumor: results from the Second and Third National Wilms' Tumor Study. J Clin Oncol. 1989;7:638-647.

184. Dome JS, Liu T, Krasin M, et al. Improved survival for patients with recurrent Wilms tumor: the experience at St. Jude Children's Research Hospital. J Pediatr Hematol Oncol. 2002;24:192-198.

185. Green DM, Cotton CA, Malogolowkin M, et al. Treatment of Wilms tumor relapsing after initial treatment with vincristine and actinomycin D: a report from the National Wilms Tumor Study Group. Pediatr Blood Cancer. 2007;48:493-499.

186. Green DM, Cotton CA, Malogolowkin M, et al. Treatment of Wilms tumor relapsing after initial treatment with vincristine and actinomycin D: a report from the National Wilms Tumor Study Group. Pediatr Blood Cancer. 2007;48:493-499.

187. Kung FH, Desai SJ, Dockerman JD, et al. Ifosfamide/Carboplatin/Etoposide (ICE) for recurrent malignant solid tumors of childhood: a pediatric oncology group phase I/II study. J Pediatr Hematol Oncol. 1995;17:265-269.

188. Abu-Ghosh AM, Krailo MD, Goldman SC, et al. Ifosfamide, carboplatin and etoposide in children with poor-risk relapsed Wilms' tumor: a Children's Cancer Group report. Ann Oncol. 2002;13:460-469.

189. Pein F, Michon J, Valteau-Couanet D, et al. High-dose melphalan, etoposide, and carboplatin followed by autologous stem-cell rescue in pediatric high-risk recurrent Wilms' tumor: a French Society of Pediatric Oncology study. J Clin Oncol. 1998;16:3295-3301.

190. Kremens B, Gruhn B, Klingebiel T, et al. High-dose chemotherapy with autologous stem cell rescue in children with nephroblastoma. Bone Marrow Transplant. 2002;30:893-898.

191. Campbell AD, Cohn SL, Reynolds M, et al. Treatment of relpased Wilms' tumor with high-dose therapy and autologous hematopoietic stem-cell rescue: the experience at Children's Memorial Hospital. J Clin Oncol. 2004;22:2885-2890.

192. Green DM, Grigoriev YA, Nan B, et al. Congestive heart failure after treatment for Wilms' tumor: a report from the National Wilms' Tumor Study group. J Clin Oncol. 2001;19:1926-1934.

193. Green DM, Grigoriev YA, Nan B, et al. Correction to "Congestive heart failure after treatment for Wilms' tumor." J Clin Oncol. 2003;21:2447-2448.

194. Breslow NE, Takashima JR, Whitton JA, et al. Second malignant neoplasms following treatment for Wilms' tumor: A report from the national Wilms' tumor study group. J Clin Oncol. 1995;13:1851-1859.

195. Ritchey ML, Green DM, Thomas PR, et al. Renal failure in Wilms' tumor patients: a report from the National Wilms' Tumor Study Group. Med Pediatr Oncol. 1996;26:75-80.

196. Breslow NE, Takashima JR, Ritchey ML, et al. Renal failure in the Denys-Drash and Wilms' tumor-aniridia syndromes. Cancer Res. 2000;60:4030-4032.

197. Green DM, Peabody EM, Nan B, et al. Pregnancy outcome after treatment for Wilms tumor: a report from the National Wilms Tumor Study Group. J Clin Oncol. 2002;20:2506-2513.

198. Kalapurakal JA, Peterson S, Peabody EM, et al. Pregnancy outcomes after abdominal irradiation that included or excluded the pelvis in childhood Wilms tumor survivors: a report from the National Wilms Tumor Study. Int J Radiat Oncol Biol Phys. 2004;58:1364-1368.

199. Marec-Berard P, Azzi D, Chaux-Bodard AG, et al. Long-term effects of chemotherapy on dental status in children treated for nephroblastoma. Pediatr Hematol Oncol. 2005;22:581-588.

200. Othman F, Guo CY, Webber C, et al. Osteopenia in survivors of Wilms tumor. Int J Oncol. 2002;20:827-833.

201. Hogeboom CJ, Grosser SC, Guthrie KA, et al. Stature loss following treatment for Wilms tumor. Med Pediatr Oncol. 2001;36:295-304.

202. Argani P, Perlman EJ, Breslow NE, et al. Clear cell sarcoma of the kidney: a review of 351 cases from the National Wilms Tumor Study Group Pathology Center. Am J Surg Pathol. 2000;24:4-18.

203. Punnett HH, Halligan GE, Zaeri N, Karmazin N. Translocation 10;17 in clear cell sarcoma of the kidney. A first report. Cancer Genet Cytogenet. 1989;41:123-128.

204. Rakheja D, Weinberg AG, Tomlinson GE, et al. Translocation (10;17)(q22;p13): a recurring translocation in clear cell sarcoma of kidney. Cancer Genet Cytogenet. 2004;154:175-179.

205. Brownlee NA, Perkins LA, Stewart W, et al. Recurring translocation (10;17) and deletion (14q) in clear cell sarcoma of the kidney. Arch Pathol Lab Med. 2007;131:446-451.

206. Hsueh C, Wang H, Gonzalez-Crussi F, et al. Infrequent p53 gene mutations and lack of p53 protein expression in clear cell sarcoma of the kidney: immunohistochemical study and mutation analysis of p53 in renal tumors of unfavorable prognosis. Mod Pathol. 2002;15:606-610.

207. Brownlee NA, Hazen-Martin DJ, Garvin AJ, Re GG. Functional and gene expression analysis of the p53 signaling pathway in clear cell sarcoma of the kidney and congenital mesoblastic nephroma. Pediatr Dev Pathol. 2002;5:257-268.

208. Barnard M, Bayani J, Grant R, et al. Comparative genomic hybridization analysis of clear cell sarcoma of the kidney. Med Pediatr Oncol. 2000;34:113-116.

209. Schuster AE, Schneider DT, Fritsch MK, et al. Genetic and genetic expression analyses of clear cell sarcoma of the kidney. Lab Invest. 2003;83:1293-1299.

210. Cutcliffe C, Kersey D, Huang CC, et al. Clear cell sarcoma of the kidney: up-regulation of neural markers with activation of the sonic hedgehog and Akt pathways. Clin Cancer Res. 2005;11:7986-7994.

211. Little SE, Bax DA, Rodriguez-Pinilla M, et al. Multifaceted dysregulation of the epidermal growth factor receptor pathway in clear cell sarcoma of the kidney. Clin Cancer Res. 2007;13:4360-4364.

212. Feusner JH, Beckwith JB, D'Angio GJ. Clear cell sarcoma of the kidney: accuracy of imaging methods for detecting bone metastases. Report from the National Wilms' Tumor Study. Med Pediatr Oncol. 1990;18:225-227.

213. Green DM, Breslow NE, Beckwith JB, et al. Treatment of children with clear-cell sarcoma of the kidney: a report from the National Wilms' Tumor Study Group. J Clin Oncol. 1994;12:2132-2137.

214. Green DM, Breslow NE, Beckwith JB, et al. Treatment of children with clear-cell sarcoma of the kidney: a report from the National Wilms' Tumor Study Group. J Clin Oncol. 1994;12:2132-2137.

215. Seibel NL, Li S, Breslow NE, et al. Effect of duration of treatment on treatment outcome for patients with clear-cell sarcoma of the kidney: a report from the National Wilms' Tumor Study Group. J Clin Oncol. 2004;22:468-473.

216. Seibel NL, Sun J, Anderson JR, et al. Outcome of clear cell sarcoma of the kidney (CCSK) treated on the National Wilms Tumor Study-5 (NWTS). Proc Am Soc Clin Oncol. 2006;24:502S.

217. Furtwangler R, Reignhard H, Beier R, et al. Clear-cell sarcoma (CCSK) of the kidney—results of the SIOP 93-01/GPOH trial. Pediatr Blood Cancer. 2005;45:423.

218. Radulescu VC, Gerrard M, Moertel C, et al. Treatment of recurrent clear cell sarcoma of the kidney with brain metastasis. Pediatr Blood Cancer. 2008;50:246-249.

219. Tomlinson GE, Breslow NE, Dome J, et al. Rhabdoid tumor of the kidney in the National Wilms' Tumor Study: age at diagnosis as a prognostic factor. J Clin Oncol. 2005;23:7641-7645.

220. Janson K, Nedzi LA, David O, et al. Predisposition to atypical teratoid/rhabdoid tumor due to an inherited INI1 mutation. Pediatr Blood Cancer. 2006;47:279-284.

221. Swinney RM, Bowers DC, Chen TT, Tomlinson GE. Rhabdoid tumors in a shared parental environment. Pediatr Blood Cancer. 2006;47:343-344.

222. Versteege I, Sevenet N, Lange J, et al. Truncating mutations of hSNF5/INI1 in aggressive paediatric cancer. Nature. 1998;394:203-206.

223. Biegel JA, Zhou J-Y, Rorke LB, et al. Germ-line and acquired mutations of INI1 in atypical teratoid and rhabdoid tumors. Cancer Research. 1999;59:74-79.

224. Biegel JA. Molecular genetics of atypical teratoid/rhabdoid tumor. Neurosurg Focus. 2006;20:E11.

225. Fruhwald MC, Hasselblatt M, Wirth S, et al. Non-linkage of familial rhabdoid tumors to SMARCB1 implies a second locus for the rhabdoid tumor predisposition syndrome. Pediatr Blood Cancer. 2006;47:273-278.

226. Sevenet N, Sheridan E, Amram D, et al. Constitutional mutations of the hSNF5/INI1 gene predispose to various cancers. Am J Hum Genet. 1999;65:1342-1348.

227. Taylor MD, Gokgoz N, Andrulis IL, et al. Familial posterior fossa brain tumors of infancy secondary to germline mutation of the hSNF5 gene. Am J Hum Genet. 2000;66:1403-1406.

228. Roberts CW, Galusha SA, McMenamin ME, et al. Haploinsufficiency of Snf5 (integrase interactor 1) predisposes to malignant rhabdoid tumors in mice. Proc Natl Acad Sci U S A. 2000;97:13796-13800.

229. Klochendler-Yeivin A, Fiette L, Barra J, et al. The murine SNF5/INI1 chromatin remodeling factor is essential for embryonic development and tumor suppression. EMBO Rep. 2000;1:500-506.

230. Guidi CJ, Sands AT, Zambrowicz BP, et al. Disruption of Ini1 leads to peri-implantation lethality and tumorigenesis in mice. Mol Cell Biol. 2001;21:3598-3603.

231. Betz BL, Strobeck MW, Reisman DN, et al. Re-expression of hSNF5/INI1/BAF47 in pediatric tumor cells leads to G1 arrest associated with induction of p16ink4a and activation of RB. Oncogene. 2002;21:5193-5203.

232. Oruetxebarria I, Venturini F, Kekarainen T, et al. P16INK4a is required for hSNF5 chromatin remodeler-induced cellular senescence in malignant rhabdoid tumor cells. J Biol Chem. 2004;279:3807-3816.

233. Versteege I, Medjkane S, Rouillard D, Delattre O. A key role of the hSNF5/INI1 tumour suppressor in the control of the G1-S transition of the cell cycle. Oncogene. 2002;21:6403-6412.

234. Isakoff MS, Sansam CG, Tamayo P, et al. Inactivation of the Snf5 tumor suppressor stimulates cell cycle progression and cooperates with p53 loss in oncogenic transformation. Proc Natl Acad Sci U S A. 2005;102:17745-17750.

235. Amar AM, Tomlinson G, Green DM, et al. Clinical presentation of rhabdoid tumors of the kidney. J Pediatr Hematol Oncol. 2001;23:105-108.

236. Dome JS, Hill DA, McCarville M. Rhabdoid tumor of the kidney. eMedicine Journal. 2007. (http://www.emedicine.com/ped/topic3012.htm)

237. Weeks DA, Beckwith B, Mierau GW, Luckey DW. Rhabdoid tumor of kidney. Am J Surg Pathol. 1989;13:439-458.

238. Vujanic GM, Sandstedt B, Harms D, et al. Rhabdoid tumour of the kidney: a clinicopathologic study of 22 patients from the International Society of Paediatric Oncology (SIOP) nephroblastoma file. Histopathology. 1996;28:333-340.

239. Waldron PE, Rodgers BM, Kelly MD, Womer RB. Successful treatment of a patient with stage IV rhabdoid tumor of the kidney: Case report and review. J Pediatr Hematol Oncol. 1999;21:53-57.

240. Wagner L, Hill DA, Fuller C, et al. Treatment of metastatic rhabdoid tumor of the kidney. J Pediatr Hematol Oncol. 2002;24:385-388.

241. Yamamoto M, Suzuki N, Hatakeyama N, et al. Treatment of stage IV malignant rhabdoid tumor of the kidney (MRTK) with ICE and VDCy: a case report. J Pediatr Hematol Oncol. 2006;28:286-289.

242. Madigan CE, Armenian SH, Malogolowkin MH, Mascarenhas L. Extracranial malignant rhabdoid tumors in childhood: the Children's Hospital Los Angeles experience. Cancer. 2007;110:2061-2066.

243. Indolfi P, Terenziani M, Casale F, et al. Renal cell carcinoma in children: a clinicopathologic study. J Clin Oncol. 2003;21:530-535.

244. Selle B, Furtwangler R, Graf N, et al. Population-based study of renal cell carcinoma in children in Germany, 1980-2005: more frequently localized tumors and underlying disorders compared with adult counterparts. Cancer. 2006;107:2906-2914.

245. Bruder E, Passera O, Harms D, et al. Morphologic and molecular characterization of renal cell carcinoma in children and young adults. Am J Surg Pathol. 2004;28:1117-1132.

246. Geller JI, Argani P, Adeniran A, et al. Translocation renal cell carcinoma: lack of negative impact due to lymph node spread. Cancer. 2008;112:1607-1616.

247. Fleitz JM, Wootton-Gorges SL, Wyatt-Ashmead J, et al. Renal cell carcinoma in long-term survivors of advanced stage neuroblastoma in early childhood. Pediatr Radiol. 2003;33:540-545.

248. Argani P, Lae M, Ballard ET, et al. Translocation carcinomas of the kidney after chemotherapy in childhood. J Clin Oncol. 2006;24:1529-1534.

249. Weterman MA, Wilbrink M, Geurts van KA. Fusion of the transcription factor TFE3 gene to a novel gene, PRCC, in t(X;1)(p11;q21)-positive papillary renal cell carcinomas. Proc Natl Acad Sci U S A. 1996;93:15294-15298.

250. Sidhar SK, Clark J, Gill S, et al. The t(X;1)(p11.2;q21.2) translocation in papillary renal cell carcinoma fuses a novel gene PRCC to the TFE3 transcription factor gene. Hum Mol Genet. 1996;5:1333-1338.

251. Skalsky YM, Ajuh PM, Parker C, et al. PRCC, the commonest TFE3 fusion partner in papillary renal carcinoma, is associated with pre-mRNA splicing factors. Oncogene. 2001;20:178-187.

252. Ladanyi M, Lui MY, Antonescu CR, et al. The der(17)t(X;17)(p11;q25) of human alveolar soft part sarcoma fuses the TFE3 transcription factor gene to ASPL, a novel gene at 17q25. Oncogene. 2001;20:48-57.

253. Smith CJ, Pearse BM. Clathrin: anatomy of a coat protein. Trends Cell Biol. 1999;9:335-338.

254. Weterman MJ, van Groningen JJ, Jansen A, van Kessel AG. Nuclear localization and transactivating capacities of the papillary renal cell carcinoma-associated TFE3 and PRCC (fusion) proteins. Oncogene. 2000;19:69-74.

255. Nagai M, Tsuda M, Saito T, et al. Functional properties of ASPL-TFE3 and identification of CYP17A1 and UPP1 as direct transcriptional targets. Proc Am Assoc Cancer Res. 2005;4518.

256. Weterman MA, van Groningen JJ, Tertoolen L, van Kessel AG. Impairment of MAD2B-PRCC interaction in mitotic checkpoint defective t(X;1)-positive renal cell carcinomas. Proc Natl Acad Sci U S A. 2001;98:13808-13813.

257. Argani P, Antonescu CR, Illei PB, et al. Primary renal neoplasms with the ASPL-TFE3 gene fusion of alveolar soft part sarcoma: a distinctive tumor entity previously included among renal cell carcinomas of children and adolescents. Am J Pathol. 2001;159:179-192.

258. Argani P, Antonescu CR, Couturier J, et al. PRCC-TFE3 renal carcinomas: morphologic, immunohistochemical, ultrastructural, and molecular analysis of an entity associated with the t(X;1)(p11.2;q21). Am J Surg Pathol. 2002;26:1553-1566.

259. Lae M, Argani P, Olshen A, et al. Global gene expression profiles of renal carcinomas with Xp11 translocatiions (TFE3 gene fusions) suggest a closer relationshipto alveolar Soft Part Sarcoma tan to Adult Type Renal Cell Carcinomas. Mod Pathol. 2004;17(Supp 1):163A.

260. Tsuda M, Davis IJ, Argani P, et al. TFE3 fusions activate MET signaling by transcriptional up-regulation, defining another class of tumors as candidates for therapeutic MET inhibition. Cancer Res. 2007;67:919-929.

261. Hemesath TJ, Steingrimsson E, McGill G, et al. microphthalmia, a critical factor in melanocyte development, defines a discrete transcription factor family. Genes Dev. 1994;8:2770-2780.

262. Verastegui C, Bertolotto C, Bille K, et al. TFE3, a transcription factor homologous to microphthalmia, is a potential transcriptional activator of tyrosinase and TyrpI genes. Mol Endocrinol. 2000;14:449-456.

263. Steingrimsson E, Tessarollo L, Pathak B, et al. Mitf and Tfe3, two members of the Mitf-Tfe family of bHLH-Zip transcription factors, have important but functionally redundant roles in osteoclast development. Proc Natl Acad Sci U S A. 2002;99:4477-4482.

264. Argani P, Ladanyi M. Translocation carcinomas of the kidney. Clin Lab Med. 2005;25:363-378.

265. Geller JI, Dome JS. Local lymph node involvement does not predict poor outcome in pediatric renal cell carcinoma. Cancer. 2004;101:1575-1583.

266. Oudard S, George D, Medioni J, Motzer R. Treatment options in renal cell carcinoma: past, present and future. Ann Oncol. 2007;18(Suppl 10):25-31.

267. Motzer RJ, Rini BI, Bukowski RM, et al. Sunitinib in patients with metastatic renal cell carcinoma. JAMA. 2006;295:2516-2524.

268. Motzer RJ, Michaelson MD, Redman BG, et al. Activity of SU11248, a multitargeted inhibitor of vascular endothelial growth factor receptor and platelet-derived growth factor receptor, in patients with metastatic renal cell carcinoma. J Clin Oncol. 2006;24:16-24.

269. Motzer RJ, Hutson TE, Tomczak P, et al. Sunitinib versus interferon alfa in metastatic renal-cell carcinoma. N Engl J Med. 2007;356:115-124.

270. Ratain MJ, Eisen T, Stadler WM, et al. Phase II placebo-controlled randomized discontinuation trial of sorafenib in patients with metastatic renal cell carcinoma. J Clin Oncol. 2006;24:2505-2512.

271. Escudier B, Eisen T, Stadler WM, et al. Sorafenib in advanced clear-cell renal-cell carcinoma. N Engl J Med. 2007;356:125-134.

272. Yang JC, Haworth L, Sherry RM, et al. A randomized trial of bevacizumab, an anti-vascular endothelial growth factor antibody, for metastatic renal cancer. N Engl J Med. 2003;349:427-434.

273. Escudier B, Pluzanska A, Koralewski P, et al. Bevacizumab plus interferon alfa-2a for treatment of metastatic renal cell carcinoma:

a randomised, double-blind phase III trial. Lancet. 2007;370: 2103-2111.

274. Hudes G, Carducci M, Tomczak P, et al. Temsirolimus, interferon alfa, or both for advanced renal-cell carcinoma. N Engl J Med. 2007;356:2271-2281.

275. Davis CJ, Mostofi FK, Sesterhenn IA. Renal medullary carcinoma: the seventh sickle cell nephropathy. Am J Surg Pathol. 1995;19:1-11.

276. Pirich LM, Chou P, Walterhouse DO. Prolonged survival of a patient with sickle cell trait and metastatic renal medullary carcinoma. J Pediatr Hematol Oncol. 1999;21:67-69.

277. Stahlschmidt J, Cullinane C, Roberts P, Picton SV. Renal medullary carcinoma: prolonged remission with chemotherapy, immunohistochemical characterisation and evidence of bcr/abl rearrangement. Med Pediatr Oncol. 1999;33:551-557.

278. Simpson L, He X, Pins M, et al. Renal medullary carcinoma and ABL gene amplification. J Urol. 2005;173:1883-1888.

279. Strouse JJ, Spevak M, Mack AK, et al. Significant responses to platinum-based chemotherapy in renal medullary carcinoma. Pediatr Blood Cancer. 2005;44:407-411.

280. Ronnen EA, Kondagunta GV, Motzer RJ. Medullary renal cell carcinoma and response to therapy with bortezomib. J Clin Oncol. 2006;24:e14.

281. Howell CG, Othersen HB, Kiviat NE, et al. Therapy and outcome in 51 children with mesoblastic nephroma: A report of the National Wilms' Tumor Study. J Pediatr Surg. 1982;17:826-831.

282. Schofield DE, Yunis EJ, Fletcher JA. Chromosome aberrations in mesoblastic nephroma. Am J Pathol. 1993;143:714-724.

283. Mascarello JT, Cajulis TR, Krous HF, Carpenter PM. Presence or absence of trisomy 11 is correlated with histologic subtype in congenital mesoblastic nephroma. Cancer Genet Cytogenet. 1994;77:50-54.

284. Knezevich SR, McFadden DE, Tao W, et al. A novel ETV6-NTRK3 gene fusion in congenital fibrosarcoma. Nat Genet. 1998;18:184-187.

285. Knezevich SR, Garnett MJ, Pysher TJ, et al. ETV6-NTRK3 gene fusions and trisomy 11 establish a histogenetic link between mesoblastic nephroma and congenital fibrosarcoma. Cancer Res. 1998;58:5046-5048.

286. Rubin BP, Chen CJ, Morgan TW, et al. Congenital mesoblastic nephroma t(12;15) is associated with ETV6-NTRK3 gene fusion: cytogenetic and molecular relationship to congenital (infantile) fibrosarcoma. Am J Pathol. 1998;153:1451-1458.

287. Argani P, Fritsch M, Kadkol SS, et al. Detection of the ETV6-NTRK3 chimeric RNA of infantile fibrosarcoma/cellular congenital mesoblastic nephroma in paraffin-embedded tissue: application to challenging pediatric renal stromal tumors. Mod Pathol. 2000;13:29-36.

288. Wai DH, Knezevich SR, Lucas T, et al. The ETV6-NTRK3 gene fusion encodes a chimeric protein tyrosine kinase that transforms NIH3T3 cells. Oncogene. 2000;19:906-915.

289. Tognon C, Garnett M, Kenward E, et al. The chimeric protein tyrosine kinase ETV6-NTRK3 requires both Ras-Erk1/2 and PI3-kinase-Akt signaling for fibroblast transformation. Cancer Res. 2001;61:8909-8916.

290. Jin W, Kim BC, Tognon C, et al. The ETV6-NTRK3 chimeric tyrosine kinase suppresses TGF-beta signaling by inactivating the TGF-beta type II receptor. Proc Natl Acad Sci U S A. 2005;102:16239-16244.

291. Tognon C, Knezevich SR, Huntsman D, et al. Expression of the ETV6-NTRK3 gene fusion as a primary event in human secretory breast carcinoma. Cancer Cell. 2002;2:367-376.

292. Eguchi M, Eguchi-Ishimae M, Tojo A, et al. Fusion of ETV6 to neurotrophin-3 receptor TRKC in acute myeloid leukemia with t(12;15)(p13;q25). Blood. 1999;93:1355-1363.

293. Chan HS, Cheng MY, Mancer K, et al. Congenital mesoblastic nephroma: a clinicoradiologic study of 17 cases representing the pathologic spectrum of the disease. J Pediatr. 1987;111:64-70.

294. Furtwaengler R, Reinhard H, Leuschner I, et al. Mesoblastic nephroma—a report from the Gesellschaft fur Padiatrische Onkologie und Hamatologie (GPOH). Cancer. 2006;106:2275-2283.

295. Loeb DM, Hill DA, Dome JS. Complete response of recurrent cellular congenital mesoblastic nephroma to chemotherapy. J Pediatr Hematol Oncol. 2002;24:478-481.

16 Retinoblastoma

Shizuo Mukai, Eric F. Grabowski, Yannek I. Leiderman, and Szilárd Kiss

INTRODUCTION

Retinoblastoma (RB) is a malignant primary intraocular tumor that arises in the retina and is usually seen in children younger than 3 years of age. It is the most common pediatric primary intraocular cancer, occurring in one or both eyes in approximately 1 in 20,000 infants, and represents approximately 4% of all childhood malignancies.[1-4] The tumors form when retinal cells lose the protein product of the RB gene *(RB1)* in the eye; this usually results from inactivation of both copies of *RB1*. The gene inactivation can result from a combination of a germ-line mutation (either inherited or new) and a subsequent mutation (resulting in hereditary RB) or from two somatic mutations (seen in nonhereditary RB).[5,6] Because approximately 40% of RB is hereditary, it is the responsibility of the physician who diagnoses RB to inform the family that it could be hereditary.

Early diagnosis and improved therapy have dramatically improved the prognosis for the eye and for life in patients with RB who, only a century ago, would probably not have survived. In fact, the rate of decrease in mortality rates in patients with RB has been faster than in any other cancer in children or adults. By 2003, RB had the highest survival rate of any childhood cancer, and in developed countries, the survival rate is more than 99%.[2] In addition, 90% of survivors of RB will have normal vision in at least one eye, and most children have essentially normal visual function with only one eye.[2,3,7]

EPIDEMIOLOGY

The incidence of RB is one in 18,000 to 30,000 live births worldwide, and it is estimated that 5000 to 8000 new cases are diagnosed each year.[8] In the United States, approximately 250 to 350 new cases are diagnosed yearly.[9] The incidence of hereditary RB appears to be constant in the various populations of the world, and no gender, racial, environmental, or socioeconomic predilection has been observed.[10] In contrast, geographic differences seem to occur in nonhereditary RB, and there appears to be more frequent occurrence in the poorer, tropical, and subtropical regions. Viral infection (e.g., human papillomavirus; HPV) and a diet deficient in fruits and vegetables have been suggested as possible causes.[11,12] There is a fiftyfold difference in the incidence of RB worldwide; the African countries of Mali, Uganda, and Zimbabwe have the highest rates. Globally, there are differences even in ethnically similar populations, and although there is no clear pattern, environmental factors, including susceptibility to environmental factors, appear to play a role.[13]

New germ-line mutations in *RB1* are much more common (90%) in the copy of the gene inherited from the father, and they are thought to occur prior to conception.[14-18] Mechanisms such as exposure to mutagens and faulty DNA repair in the setting of the increasing number of cell divisions in spermatogenesis with age have been postulated. For example, the number of cell divisions from a germinal stem cell to a mature spermatocyte is estimated to be 197 at age 20 years and 772 at age 45 years.[19] Because of this, advanced paternal age was hypothesized to predispose to new germ-line *RB1* mutations, but the results of the studies are not convincing and show a difference of only approximately 1 year between the ages of fathers of RB patients and the general population.[20-23] This difference is significantly smaller than in the conditions such as achondroplasia in which advanced paternal age is an established risk factor, and a 4- to 10-year difference is seen. In general, epidemiologic studies that have looked at the putative risk factors are relatively few and are limited in scope. Metal manufacturing appears to

be one such risk, and there are possible associations with exposure to smoking, radiation, and welding fumes.[24]

The difference in parental origin of the *RB1* mutation is not seen in non–germ-line, nonhereditary cases.[14,15] The mutations that inactivate each of the *RB1* genes are somatic and occur after conception, either in utero or after birth. The search for risk factors has tried to focus on environmental exposures experienced by the pregnant mother and the child. The data, although not conclusive, suggest possible risks, including maternal exposure to insecticides and radiation, father in a metal-related field (welder, machinist), maternal diet and vitamin use, in vitro fertilization, and maternal infection with HPV.[25-33] One might wonder if HPV vaccination could prevent some cases of RB.

CLINICAL PRESENTATION

The average age of diagnosis of RB (in cases not being screened for hereditary RB) is 3 to 18 months for hereditary RB and 18 to 24 months for nonhereditary cases.[34] In general, the child has no symptoms because the intraocular tumor is usually painless, and unless central vision in both eyes is affected, the child functions normally with the vision in one eye. The diagnosis is most commonly made by the observation of leukocoria, strabismus, or both.

Leukocoria, or white pupil, is the most common presenting sign in children with RB (Fig. 16-1). Approximately 60% of cases present with leukocoria.[35] It can be first noted by the parents as a "funny reflex" or "cat's eye" that is often seen in dim light like a night light, or as a white reflex rather than a red (red eye) in a photograph. It can also be detected by the pediatrician on a screening eye examination. Leukocoria is seen when the white RB tumor is large or centrally located and reflects the light back to the observer. If there is a history of a white pupil appearing on a photograph, multiple photographs should be examined to confirm that there is true leukocoria. Occasionally, a photograph taken at a certain angle could show a white reflex caused by light reflecting back from the optic disc; because the optic disc is only 1.5 mm in diameter and not at the visual axis, this usually does not show up in multiple photographs. If there is any doubt as to the presence of leukocoria, the child should be evaluated by a pediatric ophthalmologist promptly. Looking at multiple photographs taken over time may provide an estimate of the duration of the leukocoria (and the tumor).

Strabismus (the observation that one of the eyes turns inward or outward) is the second most common presenting sign of RB and is seen in approximately 20% of patients (Fig. 16-2).[35] Any tumor, even those that are small, that reduces

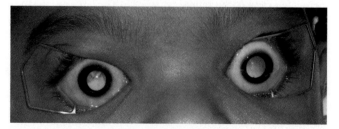

FIGURE 16-1. An 18-month-old child with bilateral leukocoria caused by advanced bilateral RB. The photograph was taken during an examination under anesthesia, with pupils pharmacologically dilated and lid specula in place.

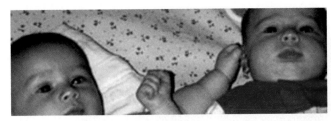

FIGURE 16-2. The infant on the left has strabismus and leukocoria in the left eye, whereas the right eye looks straight ahead and has a red reflex. The child on the right appears to have normal reflexes and alignment.

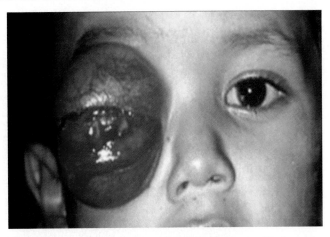

FIGURE 16-3. Child with large orbital RB. The tumor fills the entire orbit.

central vision, either directly by involving the fovea or indirectly by causing serous retinal detachment that involves the fovea or cells in the vitreous that obscure the fovea, can cause strabismus. Strabismus that is unusual, such as vertical deviations, usually indicates significant eye pathology, and the differential diagnosis includes RB, so one should consider prompt ophthalmologic evaluation.

Less commonly, cases of RB can present with a red, painful eye (e.g., from neovascular glaucoma), a cloudy cornea, poor vision, nystagmus, vitreous hemorrhage, or signs of orbital inflammation mimicking orbital cellulitis.[35] These cases are commonly associated with more advanced disease because these features are likely to represent secondary changes caused by advanced disease. There is also a small subset of cases of RB (less than 5%) that are diagnosed in older children, usually older than 5 years, and that often present with exudative retinal detachment mimicking Coats' disease or intraocular cells simulating uveitis.[36-39] The correct diagnosis of RB is often delayed in cases with atypical presentation.

Although it is still seen not infrequently in poorly developed areas, extraocular spread of intraocular tumor is rare in the United States. In such cases, the orbit can be filled with tumor, as seen in Figure 16-3.

DIAGNOSIS

A dilated retinal examination using indirect ophthalmoscopy by an ophthalmologist with expertise in RB is the most important step in the diagnosis of RB. A creamy-white appearance, unique vascular pattern, calcification, serous retinal detachment, and vitreous and subretinal seeding are characteristics of RB (Figs. 16-4 and 16-5A-D). Although often not essential for diagnosis, ultrasonography can demonstrate the shape of the mass, the size of the tumor, especially its height, the number of tumors, and the presence of calcification and retinal detachment (Fig. 16-6). Ultrasonography is extremely useful in cases in which there is no view of the retina, for example, because of vitreous hemorrhage, vitreous cells, or hazy cornea. Intraocular seeding into the vitreous and subretinal space reflects the friable nature of the tumor (see Fig. 16-5). Because of this characteristic, biopsy of RB can be extremely risky, and there is a high probability of extraocular spread as the result of such a procedure. In cases in which a biopsy or surgery is performed in an eye not originally suspected to contain RB, systemic chemotherapy, radiotherapy (RT) of the orbit, or both is required.[40] As a general rule, RB is treated without tissue confirmation, but in expert hands the accuracy of diagnosis is high, even with indirect ophthalmoscopy alone.

In the past, computed tomography (CT) was used routinely for diagnosis of RB. It was performed mainly to demon-

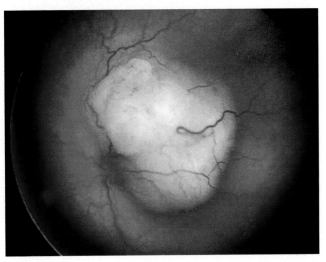

FIGURE 16-4. A fundus photograph of a characteristic large posterior RB involving the entire macula and overhanging the optic disc in the left eye. The tumor measured approximately 8 mm in diameter, and there was a cuff of subretinal fluid (retinal detachment) and subretinal seeding of the tumor.

strate calcification of the intraocular tumor. In addition, it was used as part of systemic workup for orbital and central nervous system (CNS) involvement by RB and to screen for pediatric neuroectodermal tumors (PNETs), especially pinealblastoma (Fig. 16-7).[41,42] Because of significant concern that the radiation exposure resulting from CT can contribute to nonocular malignancies in cases of hereditary RB, CT is now rarely used for the diagnosis of intraocular RB (calcification can be detected by ultrasonography), and neuroimaging for a CNS workup is usually performed by magnetic resonance imaging (MRI). Tests such as fluorescein angiography and optical coherence tomography may be more useful to differentiate entities that can simulate RB from cases of RB itself.

A family history of RB; of retinoma (a benign retinal tumor thought to be a precursor of RB or a regressed form of RB, and also known as retinocytoma; discussed later); or of nonocular malignancies associated with hereditary RB, such as osteosarcoma and PNET, may raise one's suspicion for hereditary RB. Examination of parents and siblings to look for RB or retinoma

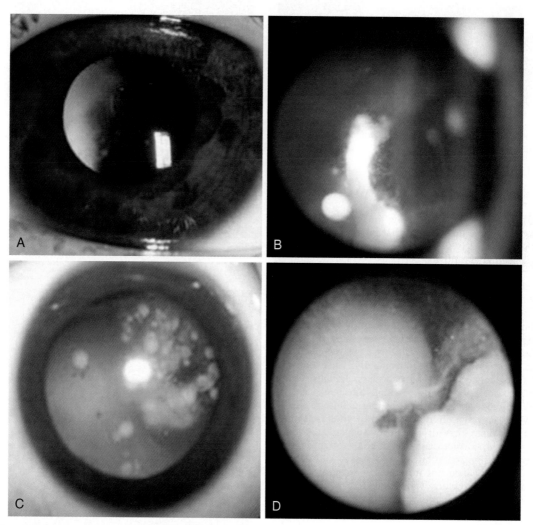

FIGURE 16-5. A-D, Examples of tumor seeding into the vitreous. The seeds can be subtle, mimicking uveitis, or can form clumps or larger balls (spherules).

is also helpful. There are occasional cases of RB that are diagnosed after the diagnosis of a nonocular malignancy associated with hereditary RB such as PNET.

DIFFERENTIAL DIAGNOSIS

The diseases that can simulate retinoblastoma include (1) ocular entities with whitish lesions in the retina, choroid, optic nerve, or vitreous; (2) exudative retinal lesions usually causing a retinal detachment and other forms of retinal detachment; and (3) cells in the vitreous. These are entities that also cause leukocoria and strabismus. Box 16-1 contains a representative list of pseudoretinoblastomas; the lesions that most commonly simulate RB, according to one large study, include persistent fetal vasculature (formerly known as persistent hyperplastic primary vitreous) (28%); Coats' disease (16%); and ocular toxocariasis (16%).[43] We feel that certain cases of Coats' disease are the most difficult to differentiate from RB (Fig. 16-8).[36]

SCREENING

As with many malignancies, early detection of RB leads to better prognosis for the eye and for survival. At a minimum, screening for RB should take place at two levels—by the parents and by the pediatrician to detect leukocoria and strabismus; and by the ophthalmologist to detect tumors in children at risk for RB such as those with positive family histories of RB.

Screening All Children

Although examination by the pediatrician of the eyes with dilation of the pupil is being tried in some areas, a penlight examination for red reflex in a darkened room is more universally used at this time. The timing of the test depends on the disorder for which one is screening. For RB, an early test may detect early tumors, but because a new retinoblastoma can appear until a child is 3 years old, three annual checks may be warranted. Unfortunately, a penlight test may pick up only the larger and more central tumors (the ones that usually cause

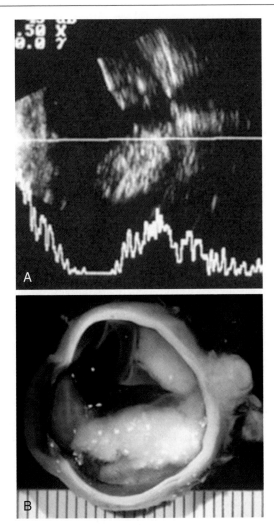

FIGURE 16-6. Ultrasound of an eye with multifocal RB (two distinct tumors are seen) and high internal reflectivity resulting from calcification. Gross pathology shows the two off-white tumors with flecks of white calcification, retinal detachment, and loose fragments of tumor.

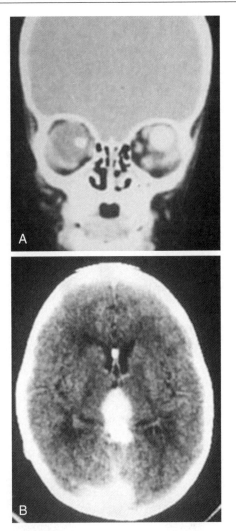

FIGURE 16-7. CT of a large pinealblastoma in a child with bilateral RB. The orbital scan shows a calcified mass nasally in the right eye and a prosthetic implant after enucleation on the left.

leukocoria and strabismus). Peripheral tumors are usually missed until they have enlarged significantly. In addition, the tumors that develop as the child gets older are more peripherally located in the retina, hence more difficult to detect early by using this test. It is to be hoped that a relatively simple test can be developed (perhaps something as basic as a flash digital photograph without the setting that eliminates red eye) so that the primary care physician can detect and document leukocoria and strabismus. The usefulness of such a test would depend on how easily and reliably it can be performed by the pediatrician.

Information that teaches parents how to be aware of the signs of RB is generally lacking. Specifically, there is very little in the lay literature available to parents that describes leukocoria, and some of the information available on the Internet is incorrect. Yet mechanisms that heighten awareness without inciting panic remain difficult to design. In addition, any system that is developed must not overwhelm the pediatrician or the pediatric ophthalmologist.

Screening Children with Increased Risk for Retinoblastoma

Children with family histories of RB are at higher risk for RB (unless they have been shown to be not at risk by genetic testing) and must be examined periodically by indirect ophthalmoscopy as often as every 3 months during the years when they are at risk, usually up to 3 years of age. The first examination should be made within the first few weeks of life; the subsequent one could be done in the office because infants are relatively easy to examine and because early tumors tend to be more centrally located in the retina. Later examinations usually require general anesthesia, although it can usually be delivered by mask. Dilated retinal examination by indirect ophthalmoscopy and peripheral retinal examination by scleral depression by an ophthalmologist experienced in RB diagnosis are the most reliable methods of diagnosis. Molecular genetic testing for detection of pathologic mutation in *RB1* can modify the risk in some families, and the frequency and type of examination

Box 16-1 **Differential Diagnosis of Intraocular Retinoblastoma**

White or whitish lesions in the posterior pole of the eye
  Persistent fetal vasculature/Persistent hyperplastic
    primary vitreous
  Coats' disease
  Retinopathy of prematurity
  Familial exudative vitreoretinopathy
  Astrocytic hamartoma (including tuberous sclerosis)
  Coloboma
  Myelinated nerve fibers
  Toxocariasis
  Toxoplasmosis
  Old vitreous hemorrhage
  Norrie disease
  Incontinentia pigmenti
Exudative retinal diseases and retinal detachment
  Coats' disease
  Familial exudative vitreoretinopathy
  Retinopathy of prematurity
  Toxocariasis
  X-linked retinoschisis
  Rhegmatogenous retinal detachment
Cells in the vitreous
  Toxocariasis
  Toxoplasmosis
  Pars planitis/intermediate uveitis
  Other uveitis
  Old vitreous hemorrhage

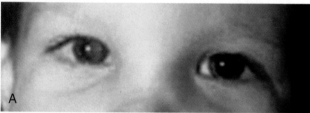

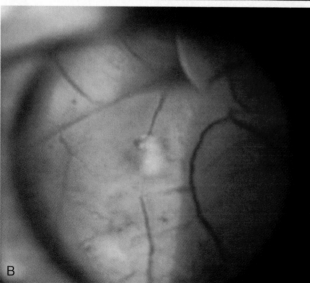

FIGURE 16-8. A boy with leukocoria and esotropia of the right eye with total serous retinal detachment caused by advanced Coats' disease.

(anesthesia versus office visit) can be customized according to the level of risk.[6,44]

PATHOLOGY

The pathology of the enucleated globe demonstrates many of the clinical characteristics of RB such as calcification, retinal detachment, vitreous and subretinal seeding, and multifocal tumors. In addition, histopathologic evaluation of the eye for characteristics that place it at higher risk for extraocular spread and metastasis is an essential part of the systemic workup in the patient who has RB.

Clinicopathologic Correlation

The gross pathology of a globe with RB, with calottes removed, is shown in Figure 16-6. This eye has two distinct tumor foci (multifocal disease), calcification, retinal detachment, and fragments of tumor floating in and out of the eye that are tumor clumps that have broken off during gross sectioning, demonstrating the discohesive nature of the tumor. All these features are clinically characteristic of RB. On histopathology with hematoxylin-eosin staining, one often sees clusters of densely packed, small, hyperchromatic cells with scant cytoplasm in a background of necrosis with a scattering of dense purplish-blue calcification.[45] The clusters commonly surround a blood vessel, and this complex has been termed a pseudorosette, in contradistinction to the Flexner-Wintersteiner and Homer Wright rosettes discussed later. Unfortunately, this terminology is confusing, but it continues to be used.

In advanced cases the tumors can fill the entire vitreous cavity, and histopathology shows areas of calcification and cell death (Fig. 16-9A). Higher power shows small cells with scant cytoplasm and hyperchromatic nuclei, mitotic figures or areas of presumed differentiation into rosettes or fleurettes (Fig. 16-9B). Rosettes with distinct lumina (thought to be analogous to the subretinal space) are called Flexner-Wintersteiner rosettes and are characteristic of RB. Those without lumina are called Homer Wright rosettes, and their cells surround a tangle of cytoplasmic filaments. Homer Wright rosettes also can be seen in neuroblastoma and other tumors. It is common to see areas of poorly differentiated and well-differentiated cells in the same tumor, which demonstrates phenotype heterogeneity within a given tumor.

Routes of Extraocular Spread

Advanced RB can fill the eye and extend out of the eye by invading the optic nerve, choroid, emissary canals (scleral channels for vessels and nerves), and trabecular meshwork (where intraocular fluid filters out of the eye into venous channels). This invasion eventually leads to hematogenous or lymphatic spread. Mortality and morbidity from RB increases dramatically with metastatic spread. It is therefore critical to identify features that predispose a patient to extraocular spread. Although, in general, clinical findings are not useful in predicting extraocular spread; histopathologic analysis appears to be a better predictor.

The most common route of extraocular spread of RB is the optic nerve.[45-50] The subarachnoid space extends anteriorly around the optic nerve to just posterior to the globe, so the tumor can access the CNS via this space. It is for this reason that lumbar puncture for cytology is performed in advanced cases of RB.

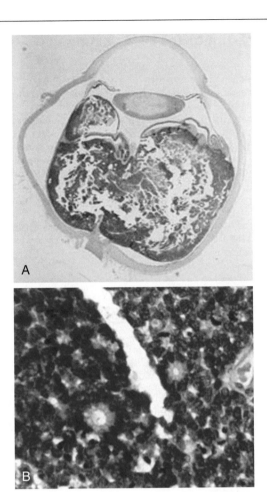

FIGURE 16-9. Histopathology of an eye with RB. **A,** Low power shows the tumor filling the vitreous cavity. There are clusters of blue cells in a background of pink necrosis, with flecks of purplish blue that are calcium. Retinal detachment is also seen. **B,** Higher magnification reveals densely packed hyperchromatic cells, scant cytoplasm, and Flexner-Wintersteiner rosettes (with lumina), Homer Wright rosettes (without lumina), and mitotic figures.

The next most common way RB spreads outside the eye is by massive invasion of the choroid.[48,50-54] The choroid has one of the highest perfusion rates of all tissues in the body, and significant tumor invasion is thought to lead to hematogenous spread. Hematogenous spread is also thought to happen after direct extension into other tissues such as orbital soft tissues that also receive high vascular supply.[55] One of the common targets of metastasis is bone, so bone marrow aspirate and biopsy are performed for this reason and in expectation of systemic chemotherapy in advanced RB.

Histopathologic Features That Predict Extraocular Spread

Based on the previous observations, it is possible to predict that: (1) invasion by the tumor of the optic nerve posterior to the lamina cribrosa, especially if the tumor also involves the subarachnoid space; (2) presence of the tumor at the surgical margin of the optic nerve; (3) massive extension by the tumor into the choroid; (4) extension by the tumor into the anterior segment; and (5) extrascleral spread of the tumor are signs of the increased probability of metastasis (Box 16-2).[46-51,56] When these features are seen in an enucleated eye, especially in combination, prophylactic systemic chemotherapy is usually recommended and, in some cases, the addition of intrathecal chemotherapy (see later discussion).

The degree of optic nerve involvement correlates with the likelihood of mortality. Although superficial involvement of the optic nerve head does not seem to increase the risk for spread, the risk goes up to 29% when the tumor is in the lamina cribrosa, to 42% when it is retrolaminar, and to 80% when the surgical margin is positive for tumor.[46-51,56,57] Because of this, the traditional method was to remove as long a piece as possible of the optic nerve with the globe at the time of enucleation to minimize the risk for having a positive surgical margin. Studies that compared the prognosis for globes with optic nerve lengths longer than 5 mm with the prognosis for those with nerve lengths shorter than 5 mm seemed to show poorer prognosis for the group with the shorter optic nerves. But another study showed no correlation between optic nerve length and prognosis.[52] In addition, the location of the tumor in the optic nerve (posterior tumors having poorer prognosis) and concurrent choroidal invasion appear to increase the risk.[46-52] A standardized pathologic protocol for sectioning and for reading the slides in conjunction with a prospective study of patient outcome would be useful in evaluating these factors. In addition, correlation of pre-enucleation imaging such as high resolution MRI with pathology may allow for pre-enucleation determination of factors predicting high risk.

The invasion by tumor into and through the sclera is a risk factor for metastatic RB.[51,58,59] Intrascleral spread without extrascleral tumor occurs in 1% to 8% of cases, and extrascleral extension occurs in 2% to 13% of cases.

A positive surgical margin can be caused by optic nerve involvement and by extrascleral spread, although the optic nerve margin appears to be clinically more important. Orbital seeding from the positive surgical margin leads to rapid tumor growth, most likely because of the excellent vascular supply in the orbit, and to invasion into the surrounding tissues. If metastasis occurs, the likelihood of mortality is extremely high, ranging from 68% to 100%.[60,61] Because of this, histopathologic identification of a positive surgical margin is critical so that appropriate therapy can be initiated. In addition, if extraocular extension is suspected by imaging prior to enucleation, chemotherapy can be administered to decrease the tumor burden and to decrease the chance of having a positive surgical margin, although the benefit of such an approach is not clear. These surgical scenarios highlight the importance of the care one should take in operating on eyes with RB or with conditions whose differential diagnosis includes RB.

Orbital recurrence of RB after enucleation is usually the result of the presence of tumor at the surgical margin. Orbital involvement that is not detected clinically or by histopathology can occur, but it is rare and can be confused with a second malignancy in germ-line cases of RB. In such a case, orbital biopsy might be indicated prior to therapy. The seeding of tumor can also occur iatrogenically. For example, we are aware of one case in which there was inadvertent scleral laceration during enucleation. Similarly, there are rare cases in which intraocular surgery has been performed on eyes in which RB was not suspected preoperatively.

Traditionally, choroidal tumor invasion has been classified qualitatively as absent, focal, or massive, without standardization. Despite the lack of a clear definition, massive choroidal involvement appears to increase the risk for extraocular spread via choroidal circulation or extrascleral extension.[46-51] In the literature, however, the risk for choroidal involvement by RB remains uncertain. The lack of standardization in the grading of choroidal tumor involvement confuses the results even more. Again, a standardized pathologic protocol evaluating prospectively the risk for extraocular spread would be helpful. If such a correlation is found, evaluation of the choroid before enucleation by high-resolution or functional imaging may permit in situ pathologic evaluation of this risk factor.

Involvement of the anterior segment is rare in RB, and there is a relative lack of reports describing it. Clinical examination is commonly more useful than pathology in evaluating for tumor in the anterior segment. Neovascularization of the iris (rubeosis iridis) and elevated intraocular pressure (usually neovascular glaucoma) correlate with optic nerve and choroidal involvement but do not necessarily indicate anterior segment tumor. Advanced disease in the posterior segment can cause anterior segment neovascularization without anterior segment tumor as the result of release of angiogenic factors by the tumor, retinal ischemia caused by retinal detachment, or both.

Although studies have attempted to evaluate these histopathologic risk factors' predictive power for metastasis, in general the studies have been limited by small sample size, differences in techniques used to evaluate the tissue specimens, differences in treatment strategies, and other variables. In addition, despite the association between the histopathologic risk factors and metastatic RB, there are reports of several cases in which metastases have developed without them. Until we have a better understanding of the cell and molecular biology of the metastasis of RB, both regionally and systemically, our ability to predict risk for metastasis is limited to methods based on histopathologic and clinical observations. With better understanding of the mechanisms involved in RB spread and invasion, the molecular pathways can be dissected and may serve as basis for future treatment strategies.

Tissue Handling and Processing

There is lack of agreement among eye pathologists about the optimal approach to the handling and processing of globes that have RB. The main questions are: (1) How many sections should be examined?; and (2) Which part of the globe should be evaluated for the risk factors discussed earlier? What is practical and feasible in a clinical pathology laboratory? Can representative sections that are strategically taken allow for efficient detection of the findings in question? If the entire globe must be sectioned and evaluated, is that practical? These questions have not been systematically addressed, and any discussion of risk factors such as choroidal invasion must consider them.

Use of Tumor for DNA Testing

The enucleated eye provides the opportunity of harvesting fresh tumor tissue for genetic analysis; the evaluation of tumor DNA increases the chances for obtaining useful information for molecular genetic diagnosis and subsequent genetic counseling. The surgeon and the pathologist must coordinate the process of obtaining fresh tumor tissue so that tissue for genetic testing can be obtained reliably, without jeopardizing the pathologic evaluation. A variety of techniques of collecting fresh tumor tissue have been described. They vary from making several incisions in the sclera of the intact enucleated eye to removing the tumor from the first calotte by the pathologist. The tumor and blood specimen must be sent properly and promptly to the genetics laboratory so that they reach the laboratory in a condition satisfactory for genetic testing.

RETINOMA (RETINOCYTOMA)

Retinoma (also known as retinocytoma) is a retinal tumor that appears to be the benign counterpart to RB.[62-65] Its clinical appearance closely resembles an RB tumor that has undergone regression from RT or chemotherapy. On histopathology, a retinoma contains cells that appear benign and well differentiated, and there is a relative lack of mitotic figures or areas of necrosis. The term *retinoma* was chosen to describe a benign retinal tumor. The alternative term, *retinocytoma*, was chosen because it is analogous to the use of *pinealocytoma* to describe a benign tumor of the pineal in contrast to *pinealblastoma*, a malignant tumor. *Retinoma* and *retinocytoma* are used interchangeably.

Although there was some belief that, because of its appearance, a retinoma was a spontaneously regressed form of RB, there is no definite evidence that this is so. The fact that some cases of retinoma undergo regression and that calcified vitreous seeds have been described in retinoma is intriguing. At this time, we are not able to determine whether retinoma represents a benign variant of RB, a spontaneously regressed form of RB, or both.

Relationship to Retinoblastoma

Retinoma is believed to be a more benign phenotype of a mutation in *RB1*.[62,64,66,67] In one hypothetical mechanism, the second of the two *RB1* mutations necessary for RB tumorigenesis occurs at a later stage than in the usual cases of RB in a cell that already has limited capacity to divide. The resultant tumor would be less malignant, resulting in a retinoma.[68]

There is evidence of a genetic relationship between retinoma and RB. Cases of retinoma and RB have been seen in the same family as well as in both eyes of a single patient.[62,63,69,70] In addition, retinoma appears to be more common in some families with low-penetrance RB (discussed later).[71-74] Low-penetrance RB can result from a partially functional RB protein (pRB) and cause a significantly lower number of tumors in carriers than in those with null mutations and no functional RB protein. One can postulate that the resultant tumors are less malignant and in some cases benign. On the other hand, there are also cases of malignant transformation of a retinoma.[75] It is possible that such an event accounts for the rare cases of retinoblastoma in adults.[76,77]

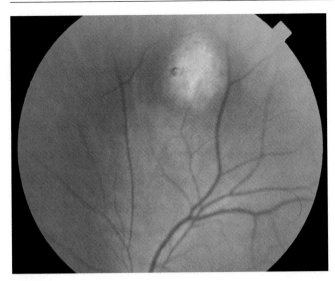

FIGURE 16-10. Retinoma discovered incidentally in one eye of the asymptomatic father of a child with bilateral RB. Note the translucent mass with calcification and pigmentary changes that resemble regressed RB after RT or chemotherapy.

Clinical Features

Although the incidence of retinoma in the general population is not known, its proportion in a population with RB is estimated to be 2% to 10%.[62,63] This would put the incidence at approximately 1 of 200,000 to 1,000,000 infants. Patients with retinoma are usually asymptomatic, and they are usually diagnosed incidentally on a routine dilated eye examination or on a screening examination when a family member is diagnosed with RB.[62,65] Retinoma is usually diagnosed in adults, and the signs of leukocoria and strabismus commonly seen in RB are rare. The ophthalmoscopic features of a translucent mass with calcification and areas of pigmentary and atrophic changes resemble RB tumors that have regressed after RT or systemic chemotherapy (Fig. 16-10).[62-65]

Management and Prognosis

A retinoma usually does not cause symptoms or progress, so no treatment is required. Annual ophthalmic examination is recommended to detect the rare case of malignant transformation into RB that would require treatment. Genetic counseling concerning the risk for RB and genetic testing for *RB1* mutations should be offered.

GENETICS AND MOLECULAR BIOLOGY

Molecular Basis of Retinoblastoma

Cancer results from the disruption of homeostatic signals that control cell division and differentiation. In normal cells, the interaction of multiple regulatory factors, both positive and negative, controls cellular homeostasis and growth. Genomic mutations that change the cumulative effects of these regulatory factors lead to cellular proliferation independent of intrinsic and extrinsic controls and result in unregulated cell growth and tumorigenesis.

Genes that are positive modulators of cell replication are called proto-oncogenes because their constitutive activation promotes uncontrolled cellular proliferation. Negative modulators, called tumor suppressors, act to inhibit cellular proliferation. A mutation need affect only a single allele of a diploid pair of a proto-oncogene to exert a biologic effect. In contrast, both alleles of a tumor suppressor must be functionally inactivated in a diploid cell to cause functional loss in a single tumor-suppressor gene.

In 1971 Knudson proposed the "two-hit" hypothesis of RB tumorigenesis based on empirical observations of the clinical genetics of RB and the principles of Mendelian genetics.[78] He proposed, "In the dominantly inherited form of [RB], one mutation is inherited via the germ line and the second occurs in somatic cells. In the nonhereditary form, both mutations occur in somatic cells." The two-hit hypothesis was validated when the team headed by Dryja and Weinberg cloned the RB susceptibility gene, *RB1*, the first tumor-suppressor gene to be identified.[5] Subsequent genotyping of RB tumors revealed that mutations in both alleles of *RB1* are necessary for RB tumor formation, exactly as predicted by Knudson's hypothesis.[5,79,80]

RB can occur as hereditary or nonhereditary disease.[2] Hereditary RB accounts for 40% of cases and is transmitted as an autosomal dominant trait with a high penetrance of approximately 90%. Nonhereditary RB accounts for the remaining 60%. Only 10% of patients have family histories of RB, and the remaining cases (composed of both the hereditary and nonhereditary genotypes) are the result of new mutations.

Patients with hereditary RB are heterozygous for an *RB1* mutation (the first hit) that: (1) is inherited from an affected or carrier parent; (2) occurs de novo in germ-line cells of a parent; or (3) occurs during embryonic development. *RB1* constitutional heterozygotes ($RB1^+/RB1^-$) require a single inactivating mutation (the second hit) in the functioning wild-type *RB1* allele of a retinal cell (a retinoblast) to confer biallelic loss of function and subsequent tumor formation. The presence of heterozygosity at the *RB1* locus in each retinoblast and the high probability of the second mutation underlies the epidemiologic observation that 90% of heterozygotes will develop RB. The existence in the developing retina of a large number of heterozygous retinoblasts that are susceptible to transformation by the inactivation of a single allele greatly increases the probability of transformation of at least one retinoblast. The frequency of such a somatic event is relatively high, and this is reflected in the occurrence of bilateral tumors in 90% of individuals with the $RB1^+/RB1^-$ genotype. Multiple (bilateral and unilateral multifocal) tumors arise by independent second inactivating mutations that yield distinct clonal populations of retinoblasts. Because of the near certainty of the second mutation in heterozygous carriers, hereditary RB is inherited as an autosomal dominant trait, although the mutation is recessive at the level of the gene.

Patients with nonhereditary RB, on the other hand, are constitutional wild-type homozygotes ($RB1^+/RB1^+$). They acquire somatic inactivating mutations in both *RB1* alleles in a clonal population of cells derived from a single retinoblast progenitor.[81-83] The probability of two distinct mutational events, each conferring loss of function at one of the *RB1* alleles of a single retinoblast, is very low in comparison with the case of the heterozygous carrier. Because of this, patients with nonhereditary RB nearly universally have unilateral, unifocal tumor.[81,82]

Gene and Protein Structure

RB1 is located at human chromosome 13q14 and contains 27 exons.[84] It encodes the RB polypeptide (pRB), a 110 kDa phosphoprotein[79] that shares homology with two other related proteins (paralogues), p130 and p107; they form the RB family of proteins.[85] They contain an N-terminal, a C-terminal, and intervening A/B domains.

The A/B region is conserved among the RB family members and mediates binding to most RB-associated proteins.[85] The A/B region codes for a polypeptide-pocket domain that is required for protein-protein interactions with endogenous proteins that mediate cell growth and differentiation and with exogenous viral proteins, such as adenovirus E1A, SV40 T antigen, and HPV E7.[86-88] Crystallographic analyses of the A/B region of pRB have revealed multiple protein-binding interface regions, suggesting its capacity to bind multiple polypeptides simultaneously.[89] This structure is consistent with the proposed role of pRB as a master regulator of subordinate proteins mediating cell growth.

The C-terminal region has not been as well characterized but also appears to be important in suppressing cell growth.[90] Sequence analysis demonstrates a nuclear-localization signal that regulates the transport of pRB from the cytoplasm into the nucleus and the concurrent transport of pRB-associated polypeptides lacking intrinsic nuclear-localization capability.[85] The C-terminal region also has intrinsic, nonspecific DNA-binding activity.[79,91] A mutation in this region has been described; it results in cases of hereditary RB with significantly lower penetrance[92] (low-penetrance RB; see later material for an additional discussion of the clinical and molecular genetics of this entity).

The N-terminal region binds the A/B pocket.[85] Mutations in this region can abolish the phosphorylation sites that mediate pRB function.[93]

pRB Function

pRB is a master regulator that controls a number of subordinate proteins that mediate cell replication. The best characterized interaction is that between pRB and the E2F family of transcription factors that help cells enter the S phase of the cell cycle.[94] pRB binds a number of polypeptides in the E2F family, sequesters them, and functionally inhibits the cell from entering the S phase.[94,95] It is the hypophosphorylated form of pRB that binds E2F, and this form therefore predominates in differentiating or quiescent cells. Hyperphosphorylation of pRB "inactivates" its tumor-suppressor function by releasing the bound E2F and allowing subsequent DNA synthesis.[96,97] pRB binds E2F at its transactivation domain, which controls the binding of E2F to DNA within promoters of genes that regulate the cell cycle.[98,99] pRB also has intrinsic transcriptional-repressor activity.[100,101] Higher-order suppression occurs where E2F places pRB near other transcription factors that are blocked from binding to the basal transcription complex directly by pRB. In this way, the pRB-E2F complex suppresses the transcription of genes containing enhancers proximal to the E2F sites.[100,102]

In addition, pRB inhibits the transcription of genes involved in cell proliferation by its interaction with histone deacetylases (HDACs).[103] DNA not actively undergoing transcription is bound to proteins that render the genes relatively inaccessible to the transcription machinery. HDACs remove acetyl groups from subsets of histones, enhancing the stability of the histone-DNA complex, and this diminishes the accessibility of chromatin to the transcription machinery. The prototype pRB-histone interaction is that with HDAC1, and pRB recruits HDACs to DNA-bound E2F, locally stabilizes the histone-DNA interaction, and represses gene transcription.[104-106]

Gene Mutations in *RB1*

Heterozygous carriers of an *RB1* mutation can exhibit variable phenotypic expression. The patients may develop one or more tumors in one or both eyes or may develop no tumor. Some may develop a retinoma. Such variability in phenotypic expression may be expected because a chance second inactivating mutation is required for tumor formation. Yet comparative studies of families in which RB appears have shown that differences in phenotypic expression among families harboring *RB1* mutations cannot be fully explained by stochastic distribution.[107] It is now recognized that specific mutations in *RB1* may confer variation in phenotypic expression, presumably in accordance with the extent of loss of function of pRB in vivo.

Mutations in *RB1* have been characterized in more than 1000 families with RB. Nonsense or frameshift mutations compose the majority of germ-line mutations.[108] These mutations are located within exons 2 through 25 and, with rare exceptions, cause bilateral RB. The exact location of a stop codon within the large gene will impact the phenotype accordingly. Yet this appears not to be the situation in *RB1*, because the site of the mutation within the gene usually does not modulate the phenotype.[107] This is perhaps caused, at least in part, by nonsense-mediated decay, a process in which transcripts of *RB1* alleles containing internal stop codons are detected by post-transcriptional surveillance mechanisms and cause the mutant transcripts to degrade.[107,109] The mutant transcripts, even with residual pRB function, would be degraded, leaving only the functional product of the wild-type allele. A loss-of-heterozygosity mutation of the remaining wild-type allele would similarly be subject to nonsense-mediated decay, which would result in the total absence of functional pRB.

Cases have been described of nonsense or frameshift mutations in individuals with isolated unilateral RB, and there is a case of two unaffected children who inherited different *RB1* alleles from a father with bilateral (therefore hereditary) RB.[81,110] This phenotype has been shown to result from somatic mosaicism, present in an estimated 10% of families with hereditary RB.

Point mutations in introns or exons that cause splice-site mutations constitute another important group of *RB1* mutations. Point mutations resulting in abnormal splicing commonly result in a premature stop codon. These mutations are usually associated with higher penetrance and with high expressivity because of the mechanism of nonsense-mediated decay described earlier.[107] Similar mutations that cause aberrant splicing and occur at less well-conserved splice sites, such as those within introns, commonly result in leaky mutations, in which a proportion of the total transcript is normal RNA, resulting in reduced production of functional protein.[111] The level of functional pRB may be greatly decreased, but it may be enough to cause some cases of decreased penetrance and decreased expressivity (unilateral disease) in germ-line carriers.[107,111] In a similar fashion, mutations in the *RB1* promoter could cause diminished, leaky transcription and reduced phenotypic expression, as in cases of splice-site mutations that yield diminished quantities of functional protein.[107]

Finally, in-frame and missense mutations occur in *RB1* and result in normal quantities of stable transcript. These mutations often result in amino acid insertion, deletion, or substitution within the A/B pocket and cause decreased penetrance and expressivity.[92,107,112]

The clinical observation of low-penetrance RB can be explained by another mechanism. There are reports of families with two isolated unilateral or uni- and bilateral cases of RB separated by four or more generations in the absence of other affected family members.[113-115] There have been a variety of attempts to explain this phenomenon, including mechanisms of epigenetic and epistatic modulation. One explanation is the presence of two independent genetic events in a moderately sized kindred.[71] The probability that a single family could harbor two independent cases of RB as a function of family size can be calculated by Poisson approximation. For example, in a large kindred of 300 individuals, this probability is 1.11×10^{-4}, implying that there could be 100 such families in the United States if enough individuals are assorted into family groups.[71]

Modifying Genetic Factors

Variability in phenotype can arise from protein dosage by distinct genetic alterations in *RB1*. In addition, epigenetic modulation of the dosage of functional pRB can also occur. Epigenetic modulation has been postulated to be the source of some degree of variation in phenotype within a given family. One study has identified two families with the identical base-pair substitution in intron 6 of *RB1*, resulting in a premature stop codon.[116] Although one would expect both families to have high penetrance and expressivity in the setting of nonsense-mediated decay, both families had incomplete penetrance. In addition, most individuals who inherited a mutant allele via the maternal germ-line were not affected, whereas of those who inherited the germ-line mutations from the father, nearly all had RB.[107,116] Further molecular analyses demonstrated that individuals with mutant alleles derived from the mother had a balanced ratio of mutant and wild-type RNA, whereas those with mutant alleles derived from the father had markedly reduced transcripts of mutant *RB1*, as predicted by nonsense-mediated decay.[116] How this differential silencing takes place is not known.

Mouse Models of Retinoblastoma

In the 1970s, adenovirus 12 injected into developing rodent and primate eyes caused them to develop RB.[117,118] We now know that adenovirus 12 E1A binds pRB and inactivates it.[88] E1A also binds p53. The first genetically engineered mouse model of hereditary RB (although it was not intentionally engineered to produce RB) was a transgenic mouse expressing SV40 T antigen in the retina.[119] T antigen inactivated pRB, thus causing retinal tumors, but because it also inhibited p107, p130, and p53, some considered this mouse model to be not a good model for human RB. In subsequent experiments, transgenic mice expressing HPV E7 (which inhibits pRB but not p53) did not develop RB until it was bred into p53-null mice.[120] In order to create a mouse model more similar to human hereditary RB, knock-out mice were created in which one copy of *RB1* was inactivated.[121-123] Unexpectedly, these mice did not develop RB although they did develop pituitary and other non-ocular tumors. It was later discovered that the pRB paralogue, p107, must be inactivated in addition to pRB for RB formation in mice[124] because p107 is upregulated to compensate for pRB inactivation in the mouse but not in humans,[125] elucidating the difference in RB tumorigenesis. Mice in which pRB and p107 have been inactivated do form RB that is of relatively low penetrance and aggressiveness, but when p53 is also inactivated, the mice form highly penetrant, aggressive RB.[120] It appears that in the mouse, p53 has to be inactivated for tumor formation that is similar to that in human RB. Recent studies show that although p53 is not mutated in human RB, the p53 pathway is suppressed by amplification of *MDMX* and *MDM2*.[126] The implication of this is discussed later.

Cell of Origin

Four possible cells of origin of RB have been postulated: retinal stem cell, retinal progenitor cell, newly postmitotic retinal cell, and differentiated retinal cell.[127] In the mouse models of RB, the retinal progenitor cell and the newly postmitotic cell appear to be the likely candidates for cell of origin of RB.[128] On one hand, conditional inactivation of pRB and p107 in retinal progenitor cells (but not in postmitotic cells) formed RB.[127,129-131] In addition, pRB inactivation in p107-inactivated retina showed increased cell division in retinal progenitor cells but not in postmitotic cells.[132] On the other hand, the retinas of mice deficient in pRB and p107 lack mitoses at the outer surface of the retina whereas S-phase cells are increased in the differentiating areas of the retina, suggesting that newly postmitotic cells are the cells of origin.[128] Additional studies are necessary to determine which of these cell types gives rise to RB in the mouse. Whether the candidate cells of origin seen in the mouse models are the possible cells of origin in human RB is yet to be elucidated.

In contrast to the idea of cell of origin is the possibility that there might be a cancer stem cell or a cancer initiating cell for RB. Such a cell is already committed to a cancer lineage and can self-renew or differentiate into a cancer cell.[133,134] This could account for the heterogeneity of RB cells observed on histopathology, even within a single tumor. Cancer stem cells have been found for other cancers such as brain tumors but as yet have not been identified in RB.

Postinitiation Events in Retinoblastoma

Although the initiating genetic events that inactivate both copies of *RB1* are well documented in RB, the events that must follow for the formation and progression of tumor are not well understood. For example, it is not clear why loss of pRB does not incite an apoptotic response that would stop clonal expansion of incipient RB. Most cancers escape apoptosis by acquiring mutations that block the p53 pathway. In fact, most tumors have inactivated both the pRB and the p53 pathways.[135-137] Yet studies have shown that p53 is not mutated in RB, and p53 can in fact be activated, implying that this protein is functional in human RB.[138,139] Because of these observations, it was postulated that RB may develop in cells that are inherently resistant to apoptosis and do not require inactivation of the p53 or a related pathway.[129]

Mouse models, on the other hand, showed that RB tumorigenesis is enhanced by inactivation of p53. Recent evidence shows that the p53 pathway is suppressed in human RB by amplification of the *MDMX* and *MDM2* genes and that the tumors do not arise in inherently apoptosis-resistant cells as postulated earlier.[126,129] It appears that the inactivation of the p53 pathway allows for the clonal expansion of the pRB-inactivated retinoblasts. If this is true, *MDMX* and *MDM2* can be potential targets for RB therapy. Early studies have shown that inhibition of *MDMX* and *MDM2* interaction with p53 by agents such as nutlin-3a may play a role in a new chemotherapeutic approach to RB.[126,140] The understanding of the pathways involved in RB tumorigenesis will allow for additional targeted treatment of RB in the near future.

GENETIC DIAGNOSIS

Prior to the cloning of the *RB1* gene and the availability of molecular genetic techniques for the genetic diagnosis of RB, the risk that a given individual is a carrier of the RB-predisposing mutation was calculated by statistical analysis based on clinical findings and family history.[2] Such factors as the number of tumors in the affected relative, the relationship of the individual to the affected relative, the number of affected relatives, and the number of unaffected siblings were considered in this calculation of risk.

Genetic diagnosis of a disease relies on methods that directly and indirectly detect the pathogenic mutations. In RB, prior to the cloning of *RB1*, direct detection of mutations was limited to a small number of cases in which high-resolution chromosome analyses such as karyotyping enabled detection of relatively large deletions involving the region of chromosome 13q14.[2] In approximately 15% of familial cases, the mutation can be detected indirectly by linkage analysis using polymorphic isoenzymes of esterase D, an enzyme marker linked to *RB1* on the long arm of chromosome 13, and this allowed for the prediction of the carrier or noncarrier state.[141-143]

Molecular genetic diagnosis of RB started in the early 1980s with the isolation of DNA probes on chromosome 13 that detected restriction fragment length polymorphisms.[144-146] DNA probes were used in indirect detection of disease-causing mutations by haplotype analyses and in direct detection of large deletions and reduction to homozygosity. As with any linked marker, the accuracy of these analyses depended on the distance between the marker and the mutation in the gene. The cloning of *RB1* in 1986[5,79,80] allowed for isolation of intragenic polymorphic markers for linkage and haplotype analyses; it also allowed for direct detection of the tumor-predisposing mutations by sequencing.[44,147-151]

The 25 exons, the flanking introns, and the promoter region of *RB1* can be sequenced to directly detect mutations.[147-151] The difficulty in this process stems from the large size of this gene and the fact that there is no hot spot for mutations. This makes the hunt for mutations expensive and time consuming. A variety of molecular screening techniques, such as single-strand conformation polymorphism, ribonuclease protection, and denaturing gel electrophoresis, have been used to screen for the area of the mutation prior to direct sequencing of the PCR-amplified DNA. Improved sequence-analysis technology, for example, with the use of DNA chip technology is starting to allow faster and less costly testing.

When a mutation is found, it is analyzed to see how it would affect the protein product to determine the probability that it is responsible for the disease. When the disease-causing mutation is found, the same mutation can be screened for in relatives easily and inexpensively by sequencing that specific area of the gene.

The identification of the pathogenic mutation is important in evaluating the carrier status of family members by means of presymptomatic diagnosis, including intrauterine testing by choriovillus sampling or amniocentesis, preimplantation testing of embryos for in vitro fertilization, or cord-blood testing. At present, the mutation can be found in as much as 90% of individuals known to be carriers. As the tests become more efficient, testing for unilateral cases without family history may become worthwhile. Recall that only about 15% of unilateral simplex cases are hereditary, and a negative result does not rule out carrier status.

Even if a mutation cannot be found, haplotype analysis of the individual, the family members, and the tumor, if available, can rule out risk in some instances and therefore can be important in genetic counseling for the family. This is reviewed in Wiggs and colleagues.[44]

It has been 38 years since Knudson proposed the two-hit hypothesis of the molecular tumorigenesis of RB[78] that established an elegant conceptual paradigm for oncogenesis that continues to be valid and useful today. During this time, a substantial body of work has elucidated the structure and function of the *RB1* gene and its protein product, pRB, including the complex regulation of transcription, translation, and post-translational tumor-suppressor activity. We are already able to detect the pathogenic mutations in *RB1* at a high rate and have used it clinically in genetic diagnosis of RB. Many categories of mutations have been characterized and correlated with phenotypic expression.[152] We are starting to characterize genotype-phenotype correlates in RB, and it is our hope that this will lead to prognostic predictors, improved genetic counseling and mutation-specific therapy.

GENETIC COUNSELING

Because RB is a genetic disease, it is critical that the family and the management team (see later) understand the implications.[6] The genetic counseling involves the family (at least the core family, the child and the parents), and the counseling is usually done by a genetic counselor, although in some instances it is provided by an ophthalmologist or oncologist with extensive background in RB genetics. Those providing the counseling must be able to: (1) explain the genetic nature of RB; (2) evaluate risk for RB of the individuals in the family; (3) discuss the availability and limitations of molecular testing, including prenatal and preimplantation testing; (4) help the family interpret the test results and their implications; and (5) make the family aware of other strategies of having children, including adoption.

Families with hereditary RB (bilateral disease, positive family history) are usually referred for genetic counseling, but those suspected to have nonhereditary RB because of unilateral disease and no family history often are not. We believe that every RB family should receive genetic counseling, and it is best to start it as soon as possible after diagnosis, even if the family is not planning additional children in the near future.

Genetic counseling in RB is much more complex than one might expect from a single-gene disease. This is in part because approximately 15% of unilateral simplex cases carry a germ-line mutation.[2] Those with cases of hereditary RB have significantly increased risks for second (third, fourth, and even fifth) nonocular tumors, and the nonocular tumors pose a much higher risk for mortality and morbidity than does the primary RB itself.[41,42] There are syndromes that include RB such as the 13q14 deletion syndrome in which mental retardation is common. Mental retardation can be seen in RB patients without 13q14 deletion, and other congenital anomalies such as those of the face and the ear are seen in higher than the expected 3% to 4% rate in the general population. In addition, there are cases of genetic mosaicism,[110,153] low-penetrance mutations,[112-115] and variable expressivity in RB[113] that make predictions of risk for RB difficult.

MANAGEMENT OF RETINOBLASTOMA

The management of RB patients and their families is usually very complex and is best performed by a team experienced in the care of patients who have RB. Ophthalmologist, ocular oncologist, pediatric oncologist, radiation oncologist, eye pathologist, pediatrician, genetic counselor, social worker, ocularist, and support groups all play a vital role in the care of patients with RB and their families. Expertise in caring for patients with RB and their families and in the optimal use of the resources available to the team is critical. The primary goal of treatment is to decrease the likelihood of mortality by: (1)

successful intraocular tumor control; (2) detection of risk factors for extraocular spread; (3) early detection of local recurrences, new tumors, metastases, and secondary malignancies; and (4) minimization of the life-threatening complications of therapy. The secondary goal is to save the tumor-bearing eye and to preserve as much vision as possible. The tertiary goal is to minimize morbidity resulting from treatment.

In general, the choice of treatment modality depends on the size and location (including seeding) of the tumors in the eye, the presence or absence of extraocular spread, the risk for metastasis, the risk for nonocular tumors, the expected visual prognosis, and the patient's response to treatment. The choice of the modalities also depends on the experience and expertise of the members of the treatment team as well as on the availability of the various modalities at a given institution. Many cases of RB require combination therapy given concurrently or in sequence. The treating physician must be able to identify the cases of inadequate response and plan subsequent management accordingly.

Communication with the Family

One of the most critical components of RB management, as is true in all pediatric cancers, is compassionate communication with the patient and the family concerning the findings, diagnosis, treatment options and plan, and prognosis. The news of the diagnosis of eye cancer in a young child, which includes not only the potential loss of the eye but also the loss of life, is a devastating blow to the family. It destroys the family's hope for a perfect child, especially because the eye is such a conspicuous part of the body. The entire clinical team must be knowledgeable, comfortable, and consistent in handling the difficult circumstances. The physicians must instill confidence and trust in the patient and the family concerning the soundness of both the diagnosis and the treatment plan. The team must make the family understand that it is acting in the best interest of the child and the family. The team initiates a conversation with the family members, allows them to voice their fears, anger, and sorrow freely, and gives them a chance to ask numerous questions.

The patient and family have tremendous needs during the initial phase of diagnosis and treatment.[154,155] Sit close to and at the eye level of the family, make eye contact (and be comfortable in doing so), and avoid being hurried. Everything takes a long time to sink in under these situations, so the team must remain patient, even if it requires answering the same question repeatedly. It is vital to speak clearly and use sentences that are easy to understand, avoid jargon, and pause frequently to allow the family to comprehend and digest the conversation and ask questions. We like to use models, drawings, and results of clinical tests such as fundus photography and ultrasonography to illustrate points. It is important to continue to monitor the status of the family and adjust the conversation accordingly. If some of the conversation can take place with other members of the team present, such as a pediatric ophthalmologist or oncology social worker, that person can serve as an important additional resource for the family. Spend as much time as possible with the family, and try to answer all of the immediate questions before setting up the next meeting which, in some cases, might be as early as later the same day. In situations in which there is some concern about the well-being of the family, the team should take the initiative in making the contact; sometimes this may mean a call every day for several days. In making telephone calls, we find that doing so when both parents can speak together (e.g., in the evening) works well.

Educating the family about RB and its management is of utmost importance, although the timing and schedule of doing so may differ according to the family. Descriptions of the tumors using fundus photography, ultrasonography, drawings, model eyes, and demonstration of leukocoria on photographs are useful in this process. Digital fundus photography and ultrasonography are especially useful in convincing the family of the existence of the tumor, especially when recommending procedures such as enucleation, chemotherapy, or RT that cast tremendous fear on the family. Literature and websites about RB, enucleation, and childhood blindness prepared for patients and their families are also helpful.[154-156] They address many of the questions that are commonly asked. We have also put together an enucleation book that displays actual orbital implant, temporary conformer, prosthetic eye, and photographs of children at various times after the enucleation. Similar educational materials addressing the details involved in the variety of treatment modalities for RB are also helpful. Give the family information that can be easily understood so that they can participate intelligently in the decision making. It is the responsibility of the ophthalmologist, as the leader of the team, to communicate continuously with the entire team to ensure that the information given to the patient and the family remains accurate, consistent, and complete, thereby minimizing doubt and anxiety while maintaining trust and confidence.

Although it is important to present options, it is also important to make a recommendation. Do not put the full burden of responsibility of the choice of treatment on the parents. Explain clearly the treatment options and the rationale for the recommendation. We usually offer to arrange for a second opinion so that the family can get a different perspective on the diagnosis and therapeutic recommendation. Usually a delay of few to several days to get another opinion will not change the clinical status. Yet one must always consider the confusion and stress resulting when significantly different recommendations are made. We have established a New England Retinoblastoma Group that includes many of the centers treating RB in New England; one of its roles is to function as a tumor board to consider difficult RB cases. Using e-mail, digital imaging, and teleconferencing, cases can be discussed even within a day or two and a recommendation made promptly. In addition, distant colleagues can be consulted by this system. We work to arrange contact with support groups, locally, nationally, and even internationally, although many of the families find chat lines and contacts via the Internet on their own. Finally, we must help the families to focus on what has to be done, especially when there are many distractions of guilt, blame, and shame.

Systemic Workup

All patients diagnosed with RB are referred for evaluation by a pediatric oncologist. This is done to determine whether there is any evidence of systemic spread of RB. We usually recommend at least an MRI of the head and orbits. The oncologist may consider a lumbar puncture or bone marrow aspiration and biopsy, depending on the severity of the case. There is frequent communication between the ophthalmologist and the oncologist about the clinical status. If enucleation is performed, the pathology report is reviewed promptly with the eye pathologist to determine whether there is histopathologic evidence of high-risk factors. In our practice, both the ophthalmologist and the oncologist review the pathology slides with the eye pathologist in high-risk cases.

The oncologist continues to monitor the patient for local or systemic tumor and for nonocular malignancies associated with the cancer syndrome that is hereditary RB. They include pinealoblastomas and other PNETs in early years to sarcomas later on. A partial list of second malignancies seen in hereditary RB is included in Table 16-1.[42] In addition, children who have received systemic chemotherapy may be predisposed to

TABLE 16-1	Second Nonocular Malignancies Seen in Hereditary Retinoblastoma	
Tumor Type	In Radiation Field (*n* = 59)	Out of Radiation Field (*n* = 34)
Osteosarcoma	24	13
Fibrosarcoma	6	
Soft tissue sarcoma	5	
Malignant melanoma		4
Squamous cell carcinoma	3	
Rhabdosarcoma	3	
Pinealblastoma		3
Fibrous histiocytoma	2	
Glioblastoma	2	
Papillary thyroid carcinoma		2
Ewing's sarcoma		2
Sarcoma	1	
Neuroblastoma	1	
Meningioma	1	
Angiosarcoma	1	
Mixed parotid	1	
Lymphoma	1	
Mesenchymoma	1	
Anaplastic tumor	1	
Papillary carcinoma	1	
Neurofibroma	1	
Testicular carcinoma		1
Liposarcoma		1
Hodgkin's disease		1
Leukemia		1
Astrocytoma		1
Wilms' tumor		1
Neuroepithelioma		1
Adenocarcinoma (Breast)		1
Unclassifiable	2	1
Insufficient data	2	1

Adapted from Abramson DH. Treatment of retinoblastoma. In Blodi FC (ed). Contemporary Issues in Ophthalmology, vol 2, Retinoblastoma. New York, Churchill Livingstone, 1985, p 89.

secondary cancers resulting from the treatment that are independent of hereditary RB.

General Principles in Treating Intraocular Retinoblastoma

Treatment of intraocular RB is determined by the size, number, location, and extent of spread of the tumor and on the genetic status of the child. In general, smaller tumors (<3 mm) are treated by the focal measures of laser treatment or cryotherapy.[157,158] These modalities are used to destroy the tumor cells directly; unfortunately, they usually destroy the normal tissues in the area of treatment, and in many instances the resultant scar, even though it may have initially spared critical structures such as the fovea, can expand into them with time (sometimes referred to as creep). Because of this, even small tumors (≤3 mm to foveola, ≤1.5 mm to the optic disc) that are close to or involve the fovea or the optic nerve are usually not treated by these techniques. RT or systemic chemotherapy with laser (either at the time of or subsequent to systemic chemotherapy)

is used in these instances to try to spare as much of the normal tissue as possible.[159-164] RT or systemic chemotherapy alone has the best chance of maintaining the best vision. The problem with chemotherapy is that by itself it has a relatively low cure rate[162-164]; RT, on the other hand, increases the rate of second malignancies in germ-line cases of RB.[41,42] The RT can be delivered by one of the external beam modalities, including stereotactic, intensity-modulated, and proton RT, or by brachytherapy with radioactive plaques.[160,161] Plaques are often difficult to apply to the back of the eye near the fovea and the optic nerve. RT is discussed in more detail later in the chapter.

Intraocular tumors of medium size cannot be treated by laser or cryotherapy alone. They require systemic chemotherapy or RT, and if chemotherapy is used, laser or cryotherapy is usually needed after the tumor has been reduced in size by the chemotherapy (referred to as chemoreduction).[162-164] Laser is sometimes used in conjunction with the chemotherapy, even before the tumor has been reduced in size (one form of this is chemothermotherapy).[165]

Large tumors also require systemic chemotherapy or RT. Again, after systemic chemotherapy, consolidation of a tumor that has been reduced in size is usually required, often by a form of RT, because, although smaller, the residual tumor is often still too large for cryotherapy or laser treatment. Studies have shown that a combination of laser treatment with each cycle of systemic chemotherapy can be effective in some cases of large tumors.[165]

When seeding of tumor cells is present, either in the vitreous or in the subretinal space, systemic chemotherapy and/or a form of external beam RT (EBRT) is used. An exception to this might occur when the seeding into the vitreous is minimal and can be included in the freeze of cryotherapy. The seeds are difficult to treat, perhaps because of slower cell proliferation resulting from being farther away from the blood supply of the tumor. Subconjunctival and sub-Tenon's chemotherapy (carboplatin) is also used with systemic chemotherapy in severe cases of seeding in an attempt to achieve higher levels of chemotherapy in the vitreous and subretinal space.[166,167]

In persistent or recurrent cases of RB after systemic chemotherapy, RT is usually used, but with the recent trials of subconjunctival and sub-Tenon's chemotherapy (carboplatin),[168] RT may not be necessary in some cases. Intraophthalmic artery chemotherapy[169,170] and even intravitreal chemotherapy[171,172] and gene therapy are being investigated.[173]

A number of classification schemes have been developed for the purpose of guiding the treatment of intraocular RB. The most commonly used was the Reese-Ellsworth (R-E) classification that was based on the response of intraocular tumors to EBRT (Table 16-2).[174] This classification was developed in 1963 and was well accepted and used universally. With the recent trend in treatment toward systemic chemotherapy and away from EBRT, the prognostic predictability of the R-E classification was questioned by some, and the new International Classification of Retinoblastoma (ICRB) has been developed on the basis of the response to systemic chemotherapy.[175] This is summarized in Table 16-3. The ICRB is being used clinically in various centers, including the clinical trials by the Children's Oncology Group (COG), which are being sponsored by the National Cancer Institute and the National Institutes of Health. In one retrospective study, the ICRB predicted treatment outcomes that involved diminishing possibilities of eye salvage with progressive groups: group A, 100%; group B, 93%; group C, 90%; group D, 47%; and group E, 0%.[176] Chemotherapy for intraocular RB is discussed later.

The application of a new classification system such as that of the ICRB introduces some concerns. First, it would be

TABLE 16-2	Reese-Ellsworth Classification of Intraocular Retinoblastoma		
Group	**Subgroup**	**Description**	**Prognosis**
I	Ia	Solitary tumor, <4 DD in size, at or posterior to the equator	Very favorable
	Ib	Multiple tumors, <4 DD in size, all at or posterior to the equator	
II	IIa	Solitary tumor, 4 to 10 DD in size, at or posterior to the equator	Favorable
	IIb	Multiple tumors, 4 to 10 DD in size, all at or posterior to the equator	
III	IIIa	Any tumor anterior to the equator	Doubtful
	IIIb	Solitary tumor >10 DD in size, posterior to the equator	
IV	IVa	Multiple tumors, some larger than 10 DD in size	Unfavorable
	IVb	Any tumor extending anterior to the ora serrata	
V	Va	Massive tumors involving more than half of the retina	Very unfavorable
	Vb	Vitreous seeding	

DD, disc diameter (approximately 1.5 mm).

TABLE 16-3	International Classification of Retinoblastoma (ICRB) Grouping System for Intraocular Retinoblastoma		
Group	**Subgroup**	**Quick Reference**	**Specific Features**
A	A	Small tumor	RB ≤3 mm in size, >3 mm from fovea, >1.5 mm from optic disc
B	B	Larger tumor	RB >3 mm in size or
		Macula	Macular RB location (≤3 mm to foveola)
		Juxtapapillary	Juxtapapillary RB (≤1.5 mm to optic stereotactic or disc)
		Subretinal fluid	Clear subretinal fluid ≤3 mm from margin
C		Focal seeds	RB with
	C1		Subretinal seeds ≤3 mm from RB
	C2		Vitreous seeds ≤3 mm from RB
	C3		Both subretinal and vitreous seeds ≤3 mm from RB
D		Diffuse seeds	RB with
	D1		Subretinal seeds >3 mm from RB
	D2		Vitreous seeds >3 mm from RB
	D3		Both subretinal and vitreous seeds >3 mm from RB
E	E	Extensive RB	Extensive RB occupying >50% globe or
			Neovascular glaucoma
			Opaque media from hemorrhage in anterior chamber, vitreous, or subretinal space
			Invasion of postlaminar optic nerve, choroid (>2 mm), sclera, orbit, anterior chamber

RB, retinoblastoma

difficult to compare the results of new studies using the ICRB with older ones that used the R-E classification. In addition, it is not always easy to reclassify cases originally described by the R-E classification into the ICRB groups. Because of this, many authors have used both the ICRB and the R-E classification when presenting their clinical data. In addition, because the ICRB is based on current treatment techniques, it may become a poorer predictor of outcome as treatment strategies change in the future. It is possible that the R-E classification may end up being as useful as the ICRB. It is to be hoped that with better understanding of the pathophysiology of RB, a classification scheme based on the biology of RB, rather than on response to a treatment modality, can be developed; it would allow for prognoses to be made even as treatment strategies change.

Cryotherapy

As a form of local treatment, trans-scleral cryotherapy has been effective in treating small RB tumors, usually in the range of up to 3 mm in diameter and 2 mm in thickness and confined to the retina (ICRB group A). The effectiveness correlates inversely with the size of the tumor; larger tumors are usually not successfully controlled by cryotherapy alone.[177] In rare instances, vitreous seeding that is present only very close to the tumor surface can be included in the freeze, but in general, vitreous seeding is a contraindication to cryotherapy, even if the tumor itself is small. In addition, cryotherapy can be useful in treating recurrent or persistent tumors after laser therapy, chemotherapy, or RT. It is thought to cause destruction of tumor cells because the freeze creates ice crystals that rupture cell membranes.

Cryotherapy is most commonly used in peripheral (anterior to the equator of the eye) tumors that can be reached by the cryoprobe without making an incision in the conjunctiva.[178] Using indirect ophthalmoscopy, the cryoprobe is applied outside the eye and the sclera is gently indented at the base of the tumor. The indentation is visualized and is verified to be centered at the base of the tumor. The entire tumor plus a margin of surrounding retina and overlying vitreous are frozen. The ice ball is allowed to thaw completely, and this cycle is usually repeated three times. The thaw should be complete before the probe is moved in order to avoid cracking the sclera and potentially seeding the orbit with tumor. The vessels on the surface of the tumor can break, causing small hemorrhages. Posterior tumors behind the equator of the globe can be treated by making a small incision in the conjunctiva that allows the cryoprobe to be advanced more posteriorly.

The goal of cryotherapy is to form a flat scar that can be seen a few weeks after treatment. Residual height (except for calcification) usually indicates persistent tumor and requires additional treatment. Repeat treatments are commonly necessary, and it is not unusual for a tumor to require two to three treatments. They are usually administered at 3- to 4-week intervals.

Complications are relatively rare but include vitreous hemorrhage and exudative retinal detachment soon after treatment; later, retinal thinning, retinal break, rhegmatogenous retinal detachment, dispersion of pigment into the vitreous, and scleral ectasia may be seen. Although rare, vitreous seeding of tumor cells can occur after cryotherapy.

Laser Treatment

Until the invention of indirect-ophthalmoscope and operating-microscope laser delivery systems in the 1980s, a xenon photocoagulator using a direct-ophthalmoscope delivery system was usually used to treat posterior, small RB tumors in the same range as those recommended for cryotherapy. This machine has been replaced by a variety of lasers; most are delivered using the indirect ophthalmoscope, which allows for the most versatile delivery of the laser.

In general, the laser is effective in destroying small tumors in the range of 3 mm in diameter and 2 mm in height that are confined to the retina (ICRB group A, similar to cryotherapy) with no seeding or retinal detachment. The laser cannot treat vitreous or subretinal seeding and does not work well when the retina is detached. Posterior tumors are usually treated by laser; more anterior tumors are usually treated by cryotherapy. The laser provides better control of the treatment area than cryotherapy, but by itself it does not work quite as well as cryotherapy. (In fact, the xenon photocoagulator that is no longer available worked better than some of the lasers available now.)

There is currently no standardization of laser therapy for RB. The lasers in use vary in wavelength from infrared (810 nm) to green (532 nm), and the technique varies from photocoagulation to hyperthermia and everything in between, including thermotherapy.

The traditional photocoagulation technique, originally described by Meyer-Schwickerath,[179] who used the xenon photocoagulator, surrounded the tumor with "hot burns" and provided light or no treatment of the tumor itself. The theory was to cut off the vascular supply to the tumor, but this approach was probably favored because vitreous seeding can be caused by direct vigorous photocoagulation of the tumor. We currently use green laser to photocoagulate tumors, either primarily or as part of consolidation after chemotherapy. Infrared diode laser is also effective when the retinal pigment epithelium beneath the tumor is intact. The tumor is treated directly, and photocoagulation is thought to heat the tissue to above 65° C, directly killing the tumor. In addition, the hyperthermia of the tumor around the coagulation spot may enhance the effect of chemotherapy or RT. Only enough power to achieve a moderately white reaction at the border of the tumor and normal retina (half the spot on the tumor) is used. Hemorrhage at the surface indicates that the power is too high. Once the appropriate level has been titrated, the tumor is surrounded by overlapping spots. Then the tumor itself is treated at the same setting and spacing. Friable RB tumors are fragile, and appropriate power settings with longer exposure times should be used to avoid explosive or other mechanical disruption and subsequent spread of the tumor. Finally, the green laser is the most versatile. Complications resulting from photocoagulation include vitreous seeding of the tumor, retinal fibrosis and traction, and retinal vascular occlusions (usually venous).

Hyperthermia and thermotherapy use an infrared diode laser, usually with a larger spot size and a longer duration at relatively low power, to directly kill tumor cells by raising the tumor's temperature to between 42° and 45° C in hyperthermia and between 60° and 65° C in thermotherapy.[180] They are used in primary treatment, for consolidation after systemic chemotherapy, and in cases of local recurrence. As in photocoagulation, these therapies are usually effective in small tumors up to 3 mm in diameter and 2 mm in height (ICRB group A) that are confined to the retina and there is no retinal detachment. At this wavelength the laser energy passes through the translucent tumor, and the laser uptake depends primarily on pigmentation. Therefore, initial treatments, when the retinal pigment epithelium is intact, appear to be most effective. Complications of thermotherapy include iris atrophy, focal cataract, tumor seeding into the vitreous, retinal scarring and traction, and retinal vascular occlusion (usually venous).

When hyperthermia is used in conjunction with systemic chemotherapy, the treatment is called thermochemotherapy or chemothermotherapy.[181] Hyperthermia (42° to 45° C) is applied using a diode laser and a long exposure (5 to 10 minutes) just prior to systemic chemotherapy and is thought to enhance the tumor-killing effects of the chemotherapy. Tumors with diameters up to 12 mm that are located posterior to the equator and have no seeding can be treated. The treatment is repeated with each cycle of chemotherapy.

In many instances the laser treatment used is not true photocoagulation or hyperthermia but involves a combination of the two. As with cryotherapy, the end point of successful laser treatment is a flat scar; residual elevation usually indicates persistent tumor. Repeated treatments are commonly required at several-week intervals, but in one series of photocoagulation, 76% of tumors were controlled by photocoagulation alone.[158] The remainder needed additional treatment by other modalities.

Radiotherapy for Retinoblastoma

In general, RB is radiosensitive and responds well to RT. Ionizing radiation causes DNA damage and cell death in the tumor cells. It is the high proportion of dividing cells in RB that makes it very radiosensitive.[159,182] Since the first report of using RT for intraocular RB in 1903, by Hilgartner, RT techniques have advanced greatly.[183] Preservation of the eye has been very good in R-E group I and group II; tumor control has been greater than 95% at 5 years.[184] Eyes that have tumors in group Vb were saved in approximately 53% of cases.[185] The effectiveness of RT must be balanced against the increased risk for second malignancies when patients with hereditary RB are exposed to radiation. Because of this, the recent advances in RB therapy have focused on modalities that avoid the use of RT and on RT modalities that allow more selective treatment of the tumor while minimizing the exposure of surrounding normal tissues.[160] Armstrong proposed that RT for RB should: (1) deliver adequate levels of uniform dose to the tumor target; (2) not expose the lens and surrounding tissues to radiation; (3) be able to be set up reproducibly and precisely; and (4) permit fast treatment.[186] None of the currently available approaches meets all of these criteria, although some are starting to approach it. Two forms of RT are currently being used: (1) brachytherapy, usually with radioactive episcleral plaques[161]; and (2) various forms of EBRT[160] (teletherapy).

Brachytherapy involves placement of radioactive material within or next to the tumor. In RB, a radioactive plaque is placed on the sclera covering the base of the tumor. The radioactive seeds, usually iodine-125 in the United States[187] and ruthenium-106 in Europe,[188] are placed in a gold carrier (plaque) that directs the radiation toward the center of the eye and shields it in other directions. The plaque is surgically placed on the scleral surface to cover the base of the tumor after dummy plaques are placed to verify size and location. The standard dose is in the range of 40 to 45 Gy delivered to the apex of the tumor; each plaque is calibrated to determine the duration of placement to achieve this dose.[189] There is a dose gradient in plaque brachytherapy, and in delivering the therapeutic dose to the apex, the base of the tumor is exposed to a very high dose. This can cause damage to all layers of the eye at the site of plaque placement, so many advocate not using plaques to treat tumors in the macula or around the optic nerve. In addition, there are anatomic difficulties in placing plaques in these areas. Surgical exposure of the back of the eye is difficult, especially in young children. The optic nerve's diameter is twice the diameter of the optic disc because of the optic nerve's sheath, and this makes treatment of peripapillary tumors difficult. The inferior oblique muscle, which is the largest of the extraocular muscles, inserts at the sclera behind the macula, and the plaque may not seat properly in this area. On the other hand, plaque brachytherapy is ideal for primary treatment of solitary midperipheral and anterior medium-sized tumors (ICRB group B). It is also useful for edge recurrences that are too large or extensive for laser treatment or cryotherapy.

In general, EBRT uses photons at a dose of approximately 40 to 45 Gy given in 1.8 to 2 Gy fractions. There is no controlled study that has tested the tumor control rate of RB when doses lower than 40 Gy are used. Fontanesi has reported on the single-institution experience at St. Jude Children's Research Hospital looking at doses of less than 36 Gy (the lowest dose was 21 Gy) in children younger than 1 year.[190] He found no difference in tumor control rate when the lower dose was used rather than a dose higher than 36 Gy, but most of the infants had R-E group I disease. Of the nine children who had group IV or V disease, one case was controlled by a dose greater than 36 Gy, but only three of eight cases that received doses less than 36 Gy were controlled. In terms of the daily fraction doses above 2 Gy, even in the range of 2.5 to 3.5 Gy, significantly increased risk for acute radiation-related eye complications was found.

A variety of irradiation techniques exist for photon EBRT. The traditional lateral approach uses a beam angled posteriorly or divided using a split-field to compensate for the divergent beam and to avoid irradiation of the anterior segment (especially the lens and the ciliary body) of the opposite eye. The anterior border of the beam was blocked at the equator of the eye, and the posterior volume went well into the orbit, irradiating most of the orbit and the optic nerve. These are the classic D-shaped fields.[191] Recurrent tumor growth after RT was seen more frequently in the anterior retina, and although they most likely included new tumors that arise more peripherally as a child becomes older, they were all considered to be treatment failures.[192,193] Because of this, techniques were developed to include the retina anterior to the equator in the treatment volume.[192,194] These techniques include eye-immobilization techniques using a suction contact lens that allows for accurate determination of the location of the eye, including the lens, so that the anterior border of the field can be brought forward to the posterior border of the lens or, in cases with very anterior disease, into the lens.[195-197] Other techniques use a split-beam with an additional anterior beam that has a central lens block, which allows for coverage of the anterior retina.[192] Despite the

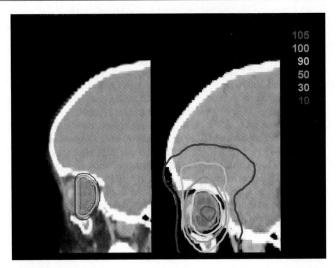

FIGURE 16-11. Dosimetry comparison of proton and photon RT plans demonstrating the significantly greater sparing of normal tissue and uniform dose distribution to the tumor target with proton RT (*left*) compared to standard EBRT (*right*). Numbers at upper right indicate percentage of prescribed target dose.

improvements, these techniques have continued to involve significant exposure of normal tissues, including the contralateral eye.

Recent advances in three-dimensional or stereotactic RT (confocal RT and intensity-modulated RT [IMRT])[198] and proton RT[160] have improved dramatically the specificity of irradiation of the target volume, although none is ideal. The photon modalities, in order of target specificity, are IMRT, three-dimensional confocal RT, and conventional two-dimensional RT. The increase in conformity in these techniques gives a sharper dose drop-off at the edge of the target volume, but this increases the volume of the normal tissue that receives the lowest doses. Any modality that might increase the volume of normal tissue irradiated, even at a low dose, is of concern in this radiation-sensitive cancer syndrome. In addition, even with the best IMRT plan, the orbit still receives a significant amount of the prescribed dose.

We have had the advantage of having a proton facility available to us for treatment of RB for the past 2 decades, first at the Harvard Cyclotron Laboratory and more recently at the Northeast Proton Treatment Center, now called the Burr Proton Center. When we compared the treatment plans for IMRT and proton RT on the same eye, the proton RT plans involved significantly less exposure of the surrounding tissues, even by a single lateral beam (Fig. 16-11). This is so because of two characteristics of the proton beam: the Bragg peak and the coherence of the beam. The Bragg peak allows deposition of essentially the entire dose in the tumor; it also allows us to stop the beam sharply downstream from the target. The coherence of the beam means that it produces almost no scatter. There is a higher entry dose with protons, and in a lateral field the lateral orbital bone is exposed.[199] With a combination of gantry angles and eye rotation, we have started to decrease this exposure significantly, and we are currently working on improving these techniques. Our technique approaches the target specificity we can already achieve in proton RT of uveal melanoma in adults.[200,201]

In improving the targeting of the tumor, the immobilization of both the eye and the head becomes critical in terms of knowing exactly where they are during treatment and making sure that they do not move significantly during the treatment. We use a combination of general anesthesia (usually

IV propofol), custom-molded plastic face masks, and a suction contact lens with a radio-opaque ring at the limbus. This allows for reproducible positioning and immobilization. A video camera monitors the child during treatment.

RT for RB should be administered by a radiation oncologist experienced in treating RB and in consultation with an ophthalmologist. The treatment plan and target volumes are determined by this collaboration. Historically, radiation oncologists have shown a bias toward treating the entire retina and in some cases the entire eye and anterior optic nerve in an attempt to "sterilize" these areas. On the other hand, ophthalmologists have tended to target the visible tumors in part because of the effectiveness of brachytherapy that targets the tumor and does not treat the entire retina. Close collaboration between these specialists is critical in the formulation of the treatment plan.

We use proton RT for tumors that require EBRT. Doses in the range of 44 Gy divided into 2-Gy fractions are used for primary treatment. Lower doses can be used for R-E group I and II disease, although we have not treated any patients with less than 40 Gy. In high-risk cases and in cases of chemotherapy failure, doses up to 48 Gy have been used. We recommend plaque RT for solitary, medium-sized, midperipheral to peripheral tumors, especially if they are nasally located. In addition, plaques are useful for edge recurrences after other modalities have been used.

Chemotherapy for Retinoblastoma

Although Kupfer first used intravenous nitrogen mustard with RT in 1953 for a case of advanced bilateral intraocular RB,[202] the role of systemic chemotherapy for RB has been traditionally reserved for cases of extraocular disease, often with suboptimal results. This changed dramatically in the early 1990s when several centers started administering primary systemic chemotherapy for intraocular RB, using the combination of carboplatin, etoposide, and vincristine that had been found to be effective against malignancies of the CNS such as neuroblastoma.[162,163] By that time, there had been dramatic movement away from EBRT because of the significant increase in second malignancies resulting from it in patients with hereditary RB. Combination therapy involving systemic chemotherapy and local modalities, including laser treatment, cryotherapy, and plaque RT, was especially effective.[164] The volume of the tumor was reduced by the chemotherapy (chemoreduction), which enabled treatment by the local measures described earlier. At present, the use of systemic chemotherapy for intraocular RB is widespread and is useful in avoiding EBRT in cases of hereditary RB. In addition to its recognized contribution to secondary nonocular malignancies in children with germ-line *RB1* mutations,[203] RT has been recognized to cause or contribute to radiation retinopathy and optic neuropathy, vitreous hemorrhage, neovascular glaucoma, dry eye caused by lacrimal gland injury, keratopathy, cataract, and impaired orbital bone growth.

Although systemic chemotherapy is now commonly used for intraocular RB, there is little agreement about how it should be administered. The chemotherapeutic agents, their doses, and the schedules of their delivery vary from center to center, although the most common regimen is the combination of carboplatin, etoposide, and vincristine (Table 16-4 shows standard doses). Systemic chemotherapy schedules have changed at many centers, and some centers have increased the number of agents in an attempt to achieve better tumor control. Some have started to include cyclosporin as a fourth agent in the hope of reducing multidrug resistance by inhibiting P-glycoprotein and decreasing transport of the drugs out of the cells.[17,204,205]

TABLE 16-4	Doses of Chemotherapy Used in Intraocular Retinoblastoma		
Drug	**Route**	**Dose**	**Days of Course**
Vincristine	IV push	0.05 mg/kg	1
Carboplatin	IV over 6 hr	8.35 mg/kg	1, 2
Etoposide	IV over 1 hr	5.0 mg/kg	1, 2

Criteria for starting carboplatin cycle: a. Absolute neutrophil count >1000/μL; b. Platelet count >100,000/μL; c. ALT <10 × the upper limit of normal; d. Normal glomerular filtration rate.

Others have decreased the number of drugs in an attempt to reduce toxicity, including the second malignancies associated with chemotherapeutic agents, especially etoposide.[206]

Systemic chemotherapy is usually used to shrink tumors (chemoreduction) so that they can be treated by focal modalities such as laser and cryotherapy. The optimal temporal schedule for this combination therapy has yet to be determined, and focal treatments may be given before, at the same time as, or after chemotherapy. To date, there has been no prospective, randomized clinical trial with adequate follow-up that compares the various chemotherapeutic and focal treatment regimens. Such studies are necessary to identify the optimal treatment modality and establish standardized care. Because RB is rare, multicenter trials are necessary to address these questions, and the COG protocols are starting to investigate some of them (Table 16-5).[168,207]

The increased role of systemic chemotherapy in the treatment of intraocular RB has made the role of pediatric oncologist critical in the management of the disease. In addition, chemotherapy is important for: (1) prophylaxis in children who, based upon globe and optic nerve pathology, may be at high risk for extraocular spread and may be candidates for chemoprophylaxis; (2) the treatment of localized bulky tumor (regional disease such as orbital recurrence or an optic nerve tumor at the margin of surgical section) or cerebrospinal fluid (CSF) tumor; and (3) treatment in combination with autologous stem-cell rescue of bone in bone marrow disease.

It was not clear whether the R-E classification of intraocular tumors that was developed to predict response to EBRT predicted outcomes for current treatment strategies that include chemotherapy and attempts to avoid EBRT. The new classification system, ICRB, was developed to test the new approaches and is gaining widespread acceptance, both internationally and by COG. For example, COG now uses the ICRB in its protocols (see Table 16-5).[168,207] For extraocular tumors, a staging system based on clinical presentation as well as globe and optic nerve pathology has been described previously,[208] and an updated version has been proposed (Table 16-6).[209]

It is important to keep in mind that the same stage of intraocular tumor may be treated differently depending on whether it is hereditary or nonhereditary. In particular, unilateral cases that lack positive family histories of RB and that are negative for mutation in the *RB1* gene (when molecular genetic test results are available) can be treated by radiation or enucleation. The use of radiation in these children does not increase the risk for second, nonocular tumors that is seen in hereditary cases. Enucleation of an eye containing advanced-stage tumor can be definitive therapy when there is no risk for developing RB in the other eye. Conversely, the increased risk for second, nonocular tumors seen in germ-line cases makes chemotherapy more attractive for this group. There is, however, likely to be some small effect even of chemotherapy in enhancing the inherent risk for a second tumor in germinal patients in addition to the risk for second malignancies caused by the chemotherapy itself. Consequently, chemotherapy for intraocular disease is generally offered primarily to children with bilateral or familial RB. In cases of extraocular tumor, children with germ-line and nongerm-line RB are both treated aggressively with chemotherapy and radiation.

The basic principles of chemotherapy for RB are as follows.

1. Treatment of intraocular tumor is directed toward saving the eye and vision, not life, and risks for fever, neutropenia, and other side effects of chemotherapy should be minimized. On the other hand, systemic chemotherapy has a special role in potentially enabling the avoidance of EBRT altogether in children harboring the germinal mutation. Such children are at high risk for second, nonocular tumors, a risk that is significantly higher in children who receive RT that includes the orbital bones in the radiation field.

2. Children with tumor invading the optic nerve but not at the surgical margin (when an eye is enucleated and globe and optic nerve pathology are evaluated) are at low to moderate risk (10% to 15%) for developing extraocular tumor weeks to months later. These children require systemic chemotherapy but not RT.

3. Children with tumor extending to or beyond the surgical margin require RT in addition to systemic chemotherapy.

4. Children with tumor extending regionally (into the orbit or preauricular lymph nodes) also require RT in addition to systemic chemotherapy. Ideally, bone marrow should be harvested from these children for possible future stem-cell transplantation (see later material), but they need not undergo stem-cell transplantation in the absence of distant hematogenous or CNS metastases.

5. Children with tumor extending to the CNS or bone and bone marrow should undergo remission induction by systemic chemotherapy followed by myeloablative chemotherapy and autologous stem-cell transplantation. In the absence of such an aggressive approach, long-term survival rates are limited to between 20% and 30% at most centers.[210-212]

Chemotherapy is administered to children with intraocular RB according to ICRB group.

Group A tumors are smaller than 3 mm and are generally managed by local measures carried out by the ophthalmologist (laser treatment, cryotherapy, or both). Note that group A does not include foveal and peripapillary tumors (Table 16-7; see also Table 16-3).

Group B tumors are larger than 3 mm or tumors of any size located less than 3 mm from the fovea or less than 1.5 mm from the optic disc. Friedman and colleagues used six cycles of vincristine, carboplatin, and etoposide to treat 39 eyes that were

Protocol ARET	Short Name	Full Name
TABLE 16-5	**The Children's Oncology Group* Protocols for Retinoblastoma**	
0331	Group B	Trial of Systemic Neoadjuvant Chemotherapy for Group B Intraocular Retinoblastoma
0231	Group C/D	A Single-Arm Trial of Systemic and Sub-Tenon's Chemotherapy for Groups C and D Intraocular Retinoblastoma
0332	Histopathologic risk	A Study of Unilateral Retinoblastoma with and without Histopathologic High-Risk Features and the Role of Adjuvant Chemotherapy
0321	Extraocular disease	A Trial of Intensive Multimodality Therapy for Extraocular Retinoblastoma

*www.childrensoncologygroup.org

TABLE 16-6 International Classification of Retinoblastoma Staging System for Retinoblastoma

Stage	Substage		Quick Reference	Specific Features
0			Intraocular RB	No evidence of extraocular RB Not necessary to have had an enucleation
I			RB completely removed by enucleation	High-risk characteristics can be present on pathology RB can be present in the other, nonenucleated eye
II			Residual orbital RB	RB is present at surgical margin of the optic nerve
III			Overt regional disease	
	Overt orbital RB			Orbital disease determined clinically or by neuroimaging
	LN extension (preauricular or cervical)			LN involvement determined clinically or by neuroimaging
IV	Hematogenous metastasis without CNS involvement	Single lesion	Metastatic disease	
		Multiple lesions		
	CNS disease	Prechiasmatic CNS mass Leptomeningeal disease		

CNS, central nervous system; LN, lymph node; RB, retinoblastoma.

TABLE 16-7   **Treatment Strategy for Intraocular Retinoblastoma Based on ICRB Grouping and Laterality**

ICRB Group	Unilateral	Bilateral, Based on the Most Advanced Tumor
A	Cryotherapy and/or laser	Cryotherapy and/or laser
B	Carboplatin and vincristine + laser and/or cryotherapy	Carboplatin and vincristine + laser and/or cryotherapy
	Plaque RT	Plaque RT
	Proton RT for macular and ON tumors	Proton RT for macular and ON tumors
C	Carboplatin, vincristine, and etoposide + laser and/or cryotherapy	Carboplatin, vincristine, and etoposide + laser and/or cryotherapy
	Proton RT for macular and ON tumors	Proton RT for macular and ON tumors
D	Enucleation	Carboplatin, vincristine, and etoposide + laser and/or cryotherapy with sub-Tenon's carboplatin
	Carboplatin, vincristine, and etoposide + laser and/or cryotherapy with sub-Tenon's carboplatin	
	Proton RT	
E	Enucleation	Enucleation
		If both eyes are equally advanced, carboplatin, vincristine, and etoposide + laser and/or cryotherapy with sub-Tenon's carboplatin followed by proton RT

ICRB, International Classification of Retinoblastoma; ON, optic nerve; RT, radiotherapy.

Chemotherapy is systemic unless otherwise noted.

chiefly in group B, and they avoided enucleation and EBRT in all.[164] Granulocyte colony-stimulating factor (G-CSF) was used to minimize episodes of prolonged neutropenia. Jubran and colleagues treated 11 eyes in this fashion and avoided enucleation and EBRT in nine.[213] Nonetheless, COG is now studying a two-agent protocol that uses six cycles of vincristine and carboplatin for patients in group B, with the same aim of avoiding radiation (COG protocol ARET 0331; see Tables 16-5 and 16-7).[207] We support this approach because the elimination of etoposide in one study still resulted in ocular preservation in 21 of 27 eyes in 16 patients,[214] while reducing the risk for hospitalization for fever and neutropenia and the risk for myelodysplasia and even acute myelogenous leukemia. In addition, the elimination of etoposide is unlikely to lead to undertreatment of intraocular tumors for several reasons. First, such tumors do respond to carboplatin alone.[215] Second, local treatment modalities remain in place to enhance the durability of responses to carboplatin and vincristine. Third, should these responses be considered insufficient, external beam or proton beam radiation can often still be used. Fourth, the importance of etoposide to chemotherapy responses in RB has not been well established. In children for whom a course of chemotherapy results in neutropenia, in subsequent courses we include daily G-CSF beginning 24 hours after completion of chemo-

therapy until the absolute neutrophil count is greater than 1000/μL.

We also recommend a two-agent regimen of carboplatin and vincristine for tumors that involve the macula or the peripapillary region, including consolidation by external beam radiation or proton beam radiation for tumors that do not fully respond. In some cases, we have administered primary treatment using proton RT without chemotherapy for macular tumors and have seen excellent preservation of macular function. Isolated group B tumors, especially if they are nasal and midperipheral in location, are excellent candidates for plaque RT, which can be used in both unilateral and bilateral tumors.

Group C and group D tumors are the most difficult to treat, except for the tumors in group E where the eyes are generally considered unsalvageable. Seeding of tumor cells into the vitreous or the subretinal space within a detached retina is the common and ominous feature of tumors in groups C and D; the difference between the two is the extent of seeding. These groups were determined by the border, which was arbitrarily chosen to be a distance of 3 mm from the tumor, but there appear to be similarities in the behavior of eyes with these tumors, and we are seeing many cases in which the two groups are considered together, as in one of the studies by COG ARET 0231.[168] It is interesting to note that the R-E classification had only one category for vitreous seeding (group Vb), which had the worst prognosis of all; the R-E classification did not consider subretinal seeding as a separate factor.

In general, three-drug chemotherapy using carboplatin, etoposide, and vincristine is the starting point for treating tumors in groups C and D. Local control using lasers, cryotherapy, or both is administered in an attempt to consolidate the treatment of retinal tumors. The variety of other measures that is used in addition to this treatment attests to the difficulty in controlling these tumors and seeds in these eyes. The measures include EBRT (including proton, IMRT, and stereotactic)[160,198,199] at full or reduced dose; sub-Tenon's or subconjunctival carboplatin[166,167]; systemic cyclosporin as part of a four-drug chemotherapy regimen[204,205]; and more experimental protocols that include selective ophthalmic artery infusion of melphalan,[169,170] intravitreal injection of chemotherapy,[171,172] and intravitreal gene therapy.[173]

Kaneko and colleagues in Japan developed a technique of ophthalmic arterial infusion of melphalan for intraocular RB.[169,170] They chose melphalan after evaluation by clonogenic assay of the chemosensitivity profiles of primary RB cell lines and comparison with various commonly used chemotherapeutic agents; they found melphalan to be the most effective agent.[170] Although they could perform "superselective catheterization" of the ophthalmic artery, they were concerned about intimal damage to the small vessel in young children. They chose instead to occlude temporarily the internal carotid with a balloon and infuse melphalan at the orifice of the ophthalmic artery.[169] They have treated more than 187 patients with this technique, but they have not published the tumor control and eye salvage rates of this series. The group at Memorial Sloan-Kettering are now directly catheterizing the ophthalmic artery for melphalan injections; their results too have not yet been published. We have referred one of our patients to the group at Children's Hospital in Boston for her first ophthalmic artery injection of melphalan.

Where proton beam radiation is available, our group believes that proton RT[160,199] preceded by a three-drug regimen of carboplatin, etoposide, and vincristine is an excellent strategy for tumors in groups C and D, although we have successfully treated some cases with proton RT alone.[160] Even though we are using a form of EBRT with protons, as discussed earlier, this radiotherapeutic modality limits the exposure of the orbital bones, including the growth plates.[199,216,217] Theoretically, this permits better growth and development of these structures while minimizing the risks for radiation-induced bone tumors.[203] We have had success with this approach, which included standard-dose proton RT (44 to 48 Gy). A combination of up-front systemic chemotherapy followed by proton beam radiation given at a lower dose than if offered alone may afford comparable eye salvage and useful vision as well as fewer and less severe side effects resulting from RT. We currently have a protocol that is investigating this approach. All smaller tumors that are 3 mm or more away from the macula or 1.5 mm or more away from the optic disc are treated by local measures, as are tumors in group A.

COG has a protocol that uses courses of carboplatin, etoposide, and vincristine that are given every 28 days for a total of six courses for tumors in group C, and for eight courses (with dose escalation) for tumors in group D (COG ARET 0231).[168] For each tumor in group C or D and for two of these courses, sub-Tenon's carboplatin is also given, at a dose of 1 mL of 10 mg/mL, at each of two sites in two quadrants (total dose of 20 mg) of each group C or D eye. G-CSF is used. Children with eyes that fail to respond to this chemotherapy regimen are considered "off study" and go on to either enucleation of a failed eye or RT to that eye. Of 22 eyes after 24 months or more of follow-up, 12 have not required enucleation or EBRT. We should point out, however, that a significant number (three to seven) of periocular injections of carboplatin have resulted in ischemic optic neuropathy.[218]

Enucleated eyes with high-risk features on histopathologic examination are found in children who have had one or both eyes enucleated and who have tumor involvement of the optic nerve beyond the lamina cribrosa, but not to the surgical margin; who have massive choroidal tumor, defined as posterior uveal invasion; and who have posterior uveal involvement with any optic nerve disease (optic nerve head, pre- and post-lamina cribrosa). Excluded from this category are those with extraocular tumors, including disease at the surgical margin and tumor in an emissary canal (intrascleral involvement) or on the scleral surface. The former children have an estimated 10% to 15% mortality rate resulting from recurrent tumor and therefore should receive chemotherapy that includes carboplatin, etoposide, and vincristine given every 28 days for six courses. COG protocol ARET 0332[220] addresses similarly high-risk eyes, but this study is limited to cases of unilateral retinoblastoma.

In view of our experience of having seen four cases of tumor involving the CSF only (each case had a repeat positive CSF cytology), we recommend a diagnostic lumbar puncture in cases of RB involving or obscuring the optic nerve. If the CSF cytology is positive (preferably confirmed by means of a repeat lumbar puncture for CSF cytology), we recommend including intrathecal chemotherapy with methotrexate and cytosine arabinoside at weeks 0, 1, 2, and 3, with age-related (and therefore, CSF-volume-related) dosing; doses for methotrexate are 6, 8, 10, and 12 mg for ages 4 to 11, 12 to 23, 24 to 36, and more than 37 months, respectively. Corresponding doses of cytosine arabinoside are 20, 30, 50, and 70 mg. For ages 0 to 3 months, we recommend half-doses of methotrexate and cytosine arabinoside of 3 and 10 mg, respectively. (In this situation, the extraocular tumor is technically no longer regional.) We consider RT to be unnecessary. Of 12 children we have treated in this manner, none developed extraocular tumor after 48 months or more of follow-up.

Regional extraocular tumors in children result in mortality rates in the range of 20%. These children have measurable or microscopic extraocular tumors that may include (1) orbital recurrence (orbital mass); (2) the presence of episcleral tumor

following enucleation; or (3) positive preauricular lymph nodes. Excluded are children with CNS or bone and bone marrow disease.

All patients should receive induction according to the new COG protocol for extraocular tumor (COG ARET 0321[219]), with four courses of vincristine, cisplatin, cyclophosphamide with mesna, and etoposide. G-CSF is given. Orbital RT (proton beam or stereotactic) should begin at week 6 to avoid orbital recurrence. More intensive (myeloablative) chemotherapy followed by stem-cell rescue is not warranted for regional extraocular tumors because children with such tumors have good prognoses with induction chemotherapy alone.

A good outcome in five of six patients following orbital recurrence has been reported by Goble and colleagues,[221] who used carboplatin, etoposide, and vincristine alternating with vincristine, doxorubicin, and ifosfamide for a total of three courses of each, with orbital radiation with or without intrathecal chemotherapy. G-CSF was used as noted earlier. Our group has had a similarly good outcome in two of two patients with orbital recurrence by using the same chemotherapy regimen combined with proton beam radiation.

Extraocular tumor with CNS and/or bone and bone marrow involvement places children in a category in which mortality in the absence of aggressive treatment approaches 100%. This category includes those with measurable extraocular tumor, which may include: (1) isolated meningeal disease with absence of disseminated meningeal tumor (two or more foci); (2) ectopic intracranial RB; and (3) bone and/or bone marrow tumor (bilateral bone marrow aspirates and biopsies). An exception appears to be the very rare case of a child with an isolated CSF tumor. We have treated such cases effectively by using the same treatments mentioned earlier for tumors with high-risk features.

Extraocular RB is usually very sensitive to chemotherapy,[208] but most centers report durable remission rates (at 3 to 5 years) in cases of bone and bone marrow disease of only 20% to 30%, indicating the need to offer myeloablative chemotherapy followed by stem-cell rescue to this subgroup. All patients should receive the same induction with four courses of vincristine, cisplatin, cyclophosphamide with mesna, and etoposide as is administered in cases of regional extraocular tumors. In addition, according to the same COG extraocular tumor protocol mentioned earlier (COG ARET 0321),[220] patients in this category should go on to consolidation with myeloablative chemotherapy with carboplatin, thiotepa, and etoposide, followed by autologous stem-cell rescue.[222,223] G-CSF is used. This approach can be taken if the child has adequate stem-cell yield upon collection of stem cells following induction chemotherapy and adequate remission status. EBRT (or proton RT) should be administered to the sites that initially harbored bulky disease on or about day 42 after stem-cell rescue. All patients should be followed by administering audiograms or brainstem auditory evolved response tests (BAERs) and echocardiograms.

Chemotherapy and RT options now exist that make possible the preservation of many more eyes for useful vision and the long-term survival of the overwhelming majority of children with RB, even those with high-risk features for micrometastases and regional extraocular tumor. Those who develop CNS or bone and bone marrow tumors, however, require intensive chemotherapy followed by autologous stem-cell rescue in order to have reasonable hope of long-term survival. Finally, 40% of all children with RB carry the germinal mutation in *RB1* and are at lifelong risk for second, nonocular malignancies. The recognition that one third to one half of these children will actually develop second tumors by the fourth decade of life makes vigilant follow-up care for these patients a necessity.

REFERENCES

1. Mahoney MC, Burnett WS, Majerovics A, Tanenbaum H. The epidemiology of ophthalmic malignancies in New York State. Ophthalmology. 1990;97:1143-1147.
2. Vogel F. Genetics of retinoblastoma. Hum Genet. 1979;52:1-54.
3. Abramson DH. Retinoblastoma in the 20th century: past success and future challenges: the Weisenfeld lecture. Invest Ophthalmol Vis Sci. 2005;46:2683-2691.
4. Balmer A, Zografos L, Munier F. Diagnosis and current management of retinoblastoma. Oncogene. 2006;25:5341-5349.
5. Friend SH, Bernards R, Rogelj S, et al. A human DNA segment with properties of the gene that predisposes to retinoblastoma and osteosarcoma. Nature. 1986;323:643-646.
6. Mukai S. Molecular genetic diagnosis of retinoblastoma. Semin Ophthalmol. 1993;8:292-299.
7. Abramson DH, Schefler AC. Update on retinoblastoma. Retina. 2004;24:828-848.
8. Seregard S, Lundell G, Svedberg H, Kivela T. Incidence of retinoblastoma from 1958 to 1998 in Northern Europe: advantages of birth cohort analysis. Ophthalmology. 2004;111:1228-1232.
9. Abramson DH. Retinoblastoma incidence in the United States. Arch Ophthalmol. 1990;108:1514.
10. Buckley JD. The aetiology of cancer in the very young. Br J Cancer Suppl. 1992;18:S8-S12.
11. Orjuela M, Castaneda VP, Ridaura C, et al. Presence of human papilloma virus in tumor tissue from children with retinoblastoma: an alternative mechanism for tumor development. Clin Cancer Res. 2000;6:4010-4016.
12. Orjuela MA, Titievsky L, Liu X, et al. Fruit and vegetable intake during pregnancy and risk for development of sporadic retinoblastoma. Cancer Epidemiol Biomarkers Prev. 2005;14:1433-1440.
13. Parkin DM, Kramarova E, Draper GJ, et al. International Incidence of Childhood Cancer. Lyon, France, International Agency for Research on Cancer, 1998.
14. Dryja TP, Morrow JF, Rapaport JM. Quantification of the paternal allele bias for new germline mutations in the retinoblastoma gene. Hum Genet. 1997;100:446-469.
15. Zhu XP, Dunn JM, Phillips RA, et al. Preferential germ-line mutation of the paternal allele in retinoblastoma. Nature. 1989;340:312-313.
16. Munier F, Spence MA, Pescia G, et al. Paternal selection favoring mutant alleles of the retinoblastoma susceptibility gene. Hum Genet. 1992;89:508-512.
17. Greger V, Debus N, Lohmann D, et al. Frequency and parental origin of hypermethylated *RB1* alleles in retinoblastoma. Hum Genet. 1994;94:491-496.
18. Kato MV, Ishizaki K, Shimizu T, et al. Parental origin of germ-line and somatic mutations in the retinoblastoma gene. Hum Genet. 1994;94:31-38.
19. Woodall AA, Ames BN. Nutritional prevention of DNA damage to sperm and consequent risk reduction in birth defects and cancer in offspring. In Bendich A, Deckelbaum RJ (eds), Preventive Nutrition: The Comprehensive Guide for Health Professionals. Totowa, NJ, Humana Press, 1997, pp 373-385.
20. Pellie C, Briard M-L, Feingold J, Freza J. Paternal age in retinoblastoma. Humangenetik. 1973;20:59-62.
21. Moll AC, Imhof SM, Kuik J, et al. High parental age is associated with sporadic hereditary retinoblastoma in Dutch Retinoblastoma Register 1862-1994. Hum Genet. 1996;98:109-112.
22. Matsunaga E, Minoda K, Sasaki MS. Parental age and seasonal variation in the births of children with sporadic retinoblastoma: a mutation-epidemiologic study. Hum Genet. 1990;84:155-158.
23. Czeizel A, Gardonyl J: Retinoblastoma in Hungary. Humangenetik. 1974;22:153-158.
24. Bunin G, Petrakova A, Meadows A, et al. Occupations of parents of children with retinoblastoma: a report from the Children's Cancer Study Group. Cancer Res. 1990;50:7129-7133.
25. Bunin GR, Meadows AT, Emanuel BS, et al. Pre- and post-conception factors associated with heritable and non-heritable retinoblastoma. Cancer Res. 1989;49:5730-5735.
26. Bunin GR, Nass CC, Kramer S, Meadows AT. Parental occupation and Wilms' tumor: results of a case-control study. Cancer Res. 1989;49:725-729.
27. Orjuela MA, Titievsky L, Liu X, et al. Fruit and vegetable intake during pregnancy and risk for development of sporadic retinoblastoma. Cancer Epidemiol Biomarkers Prev. 2005;14:1433-1440.
28. Bradbury BD, Jick H. In vitro fertilization and childhood retinoblastoma. Br J Clin Pharmacol. 2004;58:209-211.
29. Lidegaard O, Pinborg A, Anderson AN. Imprinting diseases and IVF: Danish National IVF cohort study. Hum Reprod. 2005;20:950-954.
30. Bruinsma F, Vern A, Lancaster P, et al. Incidence of cancer in children born after in vitro fertilization. Hum Reprod. 2000;15:604-607.
31. Orjuela M, Ponce Castaneda V, Ridaura C, et al. Presence of human papilloma virus in tumor tissue from children with retinoblastoma: an alternative mechanism for tumor development. Clin Cancer Res. 2000;6:4010-4016.
32. Montoya-Fuentes H, de la Paz Ramirez-Munoz M, Villar-Calvo V, et al. Identification of DNA sequences and viral proteins of 6 human papilloma virus types in retinoblastoma tissue. Anticancer Res. 2003;23:2853-2862.
33. Palazzi MA, Yunes JA, Cardinalli IA, et al. Detection of oncogenic human papilloma virus in sporadic retinoblastoma. Acta Ophthalmol Scand. 2003;81:396-398.
34. Shields CL, Shields JA. Basic understanding of current classification and management of retinoblastoma. Curr Opin Ophthalmol. 2006;17:228-234.
35. Abramson DH, Frank CM, Susman M, et al. Presenting signs of retinoblastoma. J Pediatr. 1998;132:505-508.
36. Walton DS, Mukai S, Grabowski EF, et al. Case records of the Massachusetts General Hospital. Case 5-2006. An 11-year-old girl with loss of vision in the right eye. N Engl J Med. 2006;354:741-748.
37. Shields CL, Shields JA, Shah P. Retinoblastoma in older children. Ophthalmology. 1991;98:395-399.
38. Bhatnagar R, Vine AK. Diffuse infiltrating retinoblastoma. Ophthalmology. 1991;98:1657-1661.
39. Foster BS, Mukai S. Intraocular retinoblastoma presenting as ocular and orbital inflammation. Int Ophthalmol Clin. 1997;37:153-160.
40. Shields CL, Honavar S, Shields JA, et al. Vitrectomy in eyes with unsuspected retinoblastoma. Ophthalmology. 2000;107:2250-2255.
41. Abramson DH. Second nonocular cancers in retinoblastoma: a unified hypothesis. The Franceschetti Lecture. Ophthalmic Genet. 1999;20:193-204.
42. Abramson DH. Treatment of retinoblastoma. In Blodi FC (ed). Contemporary Issues in Ophthalmology, vol 2, Retinoblastoma. New York, Churchill Livingstone, 1985, pp 88-93.
43. Shields JA, Parsons HM, Shields CL, Shah P. Lesions simulating retinoblastoma. J Pediatr Ophthalmol Strabismus. 1991;28:338-340.
44. Wiggs JL, Nordenskjöld M, Yandell DW, et al. Prediction of the risk of hereditary retinoblastoma using DNA polymorphisms within the retinoblastoma gene. New Engl J Med. 1988;318:151-157.
45. Sang DN, Albert DM. Retinoblastoma: clinical and histopathologic features. Hum Pathol. 1982;13:133-147.
46. Spencer WH. Optic nerve extension of intraocular neoplasms. Am J Ophthalmol. 1975;80:465-471.

47. Magramm I, Abramson DH, Ellsworth RM. Optic nerve involvement in retinoblastoma. Ophthalmology. 1989;96:217-222.

48. Stannard C, Lipper S, Sealy R, Sevel D. Retinoblastoma: correlation of invasion of the optic nerve and choroid with prognosis and metastasis. Br J Ophthalmol. 1979;63:560-570.

49. Shields CL, Shields JA, Baez K, et al. Optic nerve invasion of retinoblastoma: metastatic potential and clinical risk factors. Cancer. 1994;73:692-698.

50. Rubin CM, Robison LL, Camerson JD, et al. Intraocular retinoblastoma group V: an analysis of prognostic factors. J Clin Oncol. 1985;3:680-685.

51. Kheifaoui F, Validire P, Auperin A, et al. Histopathologic risk factors in retinoblastoma: a retrospective study of 172 patients treated in a single institution. Cancer. 1996;77:1206-1213.

52. Chantada GL, de Davila MT, Fandino A, et al. Retinoblastoma with low risk for extraocular disease. Ophthalmic Genet. 1999;20:133-140.

53. Erwenne CM, Franco EL. Age and lateness of referral as determinants of extraocular retinoblastoma. Ophthalmic Paediatr Genet. 1989;10:179-184.

54. Rootman J, Ellsworth RM, Hofbauer J, Kitchen D. Orbital extension of retinoblastoma: a clinicopathological study. Can J Ophthalmol. 1978;13:72-80.

55. MacKay CJ, Abramson DH, Ellsworth RM. Metastatic patterns of retinoblastoma. Arch Ophthalmol. 1984;102:391-396.

56. Karcioglu ZA, al-Mesfer SA, Abboud E, et al. Workup for metastatic retinoblastoma: a review of 261 patients. Ophthalmology. 1997;104:307-312.

57. Tosi P, Cintorino M, Toti P, et al. Histopathological evaluation of the prognosis of retinoblastoma. Ophthalmic Paediatr Genet. 1989;10:173-177.

58. Kopelman JE, McLean IW, Rosenberg SH. Multivariate analysis of risk factors for metastasis in retinoblastoma treated by enucleation. Ophthalmology. 1987;94:371-377.

59. Messmer EP, Heinrich T, Hopping W, et al. Risk factors in metastases in patients with retinoblastoma. Ophthalmology. 1991;98:136-141.

60. McLean IW, Burnier M, Zimmerman L, Jakobiec F. Tumors of the retina. In McLean IW, Burnier MN, Zimmerman LE, et al. (eds). Atlas of Tumor Pathology. Tumors of the Eye and Ocular Adnexa. Washington DC, Armed Forces Institute of Pathology, 1994, pp 100-135.

61. Hurwitz RL, Chévez-Barrios P, Chintagumpala M, et al. Retinoblastoma. In Pizzo PA, Poplack D (eds). Principles and Practice of Pediatric Oncology. 5th ed. Philadelphia, Lippincott-Raven, 2006, pp 825-846.

62. Gallie BL, Ellsworth RM, Abramson DH, Phillips RA. Retinoma: spontaneous regression of retinoblastoma or benign manifestation of the mutation? Br J Cancer. 1982;45:513-521.

63. Balmer A, Munier F, Gailloud C. Retinoma: case studies. Ophthalmic Paediatr Genet. 1991;12:131-137.

64. Balmer A, Munier F, Gailloud C. Retinoma and phthisis bulbi: benign expression of retinoblastoma. Klin Monatsbi Augenheilkd. 1992;200:436-439.

65. Singh AD, Santos CM, Shields CL, et al. Observations on 17 patients with retinocytoma. Arch Ophthalmol. 2000;118:199-205.

66. Abramson DH. Retinoma, retinocytoma, and the retinoblastoma gene. Arch Ophthalmol. 1983;101:1517-1518.

67. Gallie BL, Phillips RA, Ellsworth RM, Abramson DH. Significance of retinoma and phthisis bulbi for retinoblastoma. Ophthalmology. 1982;89:1393-1399.

68. Gallie BL, Dunn JM, Chen HS, et al. The genetics of retinoblastoma: relevance to the patient. Pediatr Clin North Am. 1991;38:299-315.

69. Lommatzsch PK, Zimmermann W, Lommatzsch R. Spontaneous growth inhibition in retinoblastoma. Klin Monatsbi Augenheilkd. 1993;202:218-223.

70. Lueder GT, Heon E, Gallie BL. Retinoma associated with vitreous seeding. Am J Ophthalmol. 1995;119:522-523.

71. Dryja TP, Rapaport J, McGee TL, et al. Molecular etiology of low-penetrance retinoblastoma in two pedigrees. Am J Hum Genet. 1993;52:1122-1128.

72. Kratzke RA, Otterson GA, Hogg A, et al. Partial inactivation of the RB product in a family with incomplete penetrance of familial retinoblastoma and benign retinal tumors. Oncogene. 1994;9:1321-1326.

73. Schubert EL, Strong LC, Hansen MF. A splicing mutation in RB1 in low penetrance retinoblastoma. Hum Genet. 1997;100:557-563.

74. Harbour JW. Molecular basis of low-penetrance retinoblastoma. Arch Ophthalmol. 2001;119:1699-1704.

75. Eagle RC Jr, Shields JA, Donoso L, Milner RS. Malignant transformation of spontaneously regressed retinoblastoma, retinoma/retinocytoma variant. Ophthalmology. 1989;96:1389-1396.

76. Rychener RO. Retinoblastoma in the adult. Trans Am Ophthalmol Soc. 1948;46:318-326.

77. Takahashi T, Tamura S, Inoue M, et al. Retinoblastoma in a 26-year-old adult. Ophthalmology. 1983;90:179-183.

78. Knudson AG Jr. Mutation and cancer: statistical study of retinoblastoma. Proc Natl Acad Sci U S A. 1971;68:820-823.

79. Lee WH, Bookstein R, Hong F, et al. Human retinoblastoma susceptibility gene: cloning, identification, and sequence. Science. 1987;235:1394-1399.

80. Fung YK, Murphree AL, T'Ang A, et al. Structural evidence for the authenticity of the human retinoblastoma gene. Science. 1987;236:1657-1661.

81. Lohmann DR, Gerick M, Brandt B, et al. Constitutional RB1-gene mutations in patients with isolated unilateral retinoblastoma. Am J Hum Genet. 1997;61:282-294.

82. Klutz M, Horsthemke B, Lohmann DR. RB1 gene mutations in peripheral blood DNA of patients with isolated unilateral retinoblastoma. Am J Hum Genet. 1999;64:667-668.

83. Shimizu T, Toguchida J, Kato MV, et al. Detection of mutations of the RB1 gene in retinoblastoma patients by using exon-by-exon PCR-SSCP analysis. Am J Hum Genet. 1994;54:793-800.

84. Toguchida J, McGee TL, Paterson JC, et al. Complete genomic sequence of the human retinoblastoma susceptibility gene. Genomics. 1993;17:535-543.

85. De Falco G, Giordano A. pRb2/p130: a new candidate for retinoblastoma tumor formation. Oncogene. 2006;25:5333-5340.

86. DeCaprio JA, Ludlow JW, Figge J, et al. SV40 large tumor antigen forms a specific complex with the product of the retinoblastoma susceptibility gene. Cell. 1988;54:275-283.

87. Dyson N, Howley PM, Munger K, Harlow E. The human papilloma virus-16 E7 oncoprotein is able to bind to the retinoblastoma gene product. Science. 1989;243:934-937.

88. Whyte P, Buchkovich KJ, Horowitz JM, et al. Association between an oncogene and an anti-oncogene: the adenovirus E1A proteins bind to the retinoblastoma gene product. Nature. 1988;334:124-129.

89. Lee JO, Russo AA, Pavletich NP. Structure of the retinoblastoma tumour-suppressor pocket domain bound to a peptide from HPV E7. Nature. 1998;391:859-865.

90. Whitaker LL, Su H, Baskaran R, et al. Growth suppression by an E2F-binding-defective retinoblastoma protein (RB): contribution from the RB C pocket. Mol Cell Biol. 1998;18:4032-4042.

91. Lee WH, Murphree AL, Benedict WF. Expression and amplification of the N-myc gene in primary retinoblastoma. Nature. 1984;309:458-460.

92. Bremner R, Du DC, Connolly-Wilson MJ, et al. Deletion of RB exons 24 and 25 causes low-penetrance retinoblastoma. Am J Hum Genet. 1997;61:556-570.

93. Shen WJ, Kim HS, Tsai SY. Stimulation of human insulin receptor gene expression by retinoblastoma gene product. J Biol Chem. 1995;270:20525-20529.

94. Dyson N. The regulation of E2F by pRB-family proteins. Genes Dev. 1998;12:2245-2262.

95. Harbour JW, Dean DC. Rb function in cell-cycle regulation and apoptosis. Nat Cell Biol. 2000;2:E65-E67.

96. Chen PL, Scully P, Shew JY, et al. Phosphorylation of the retinoblastoma gene product is modulated during the cell cycle and cellular differentiation. Cell. 1989;58:1193-1198.

97. Stein GH, Beeson M, Gordon L. Failure to phosphorylate the retinoblastoma gene product in senescent human fibroblasts. Science. 1990;249:666-669.

98. Flemington EK, Speck SH, Kaelin WG Jr. E2F-1-mediated transactivation is inhibited by complex formation with the retinoblastoma susceptibility gene product. Proc Natl Acad Sci U S A. 1993;90:6914-6918.

99. Helin K, Harlow E, Fattaey A. Inhibition of E2F-1 transactivation by direct binding of the retinoblastoma protein. Mol Cell Biol. 1993;13:6501-6508.

100. Chow KN, Dean DC. Domains A and B in the Rb pocket interact to form a transcriptional repressor motif. Mol Cell Biol. 1996;16:4862-4868.

101. Sellers WR, Rodgers JW, Kaelin WG Jr. A potent transrepression domain in the retinoblastoma protein induces a cell cycle arrest when bound to E2F sites. Proc Natl Acad Sci U S A. 1995;92: 11544-11548.

102. Weintraub SJ, Chow KN, Luo RX, et al. Mechanism of active transcriptional repression by the retinoblastoma protein. Nature. 1995;375:812-815.

103. Nielsen SJ, Schneider R, Bauer UM, et al. Rb targets histone H3 methylation and HP1 to promoters. Nature. 2001;412:561-565.

104. Brehm A, Miska EA, McCance DJ, et al. Retinoblastoma protein recruits histone deacetylase to repress transcription. Nature. 1998; 391:597-601.

105. Luo RX, Postigo AA, Dean DC. Rb interacts with histone deacetylase to repress transcription. Cell. 1998;92:463-673.

106. Magnaghi-Jaulin L, Groisman R, Naguibneva I, et al. Retinoblastoma protein represses transcription by recruiting a histone deacetylase. Nature. 1998;391:601-605.

107. Lohmann DR, Gallie BL. Retinoblastoma: revisiting the model prototype of inherited cancer. Am J Med Genet C Semin Med Genet. 2004;129:23-28.

108. Lohmann DR. RB1 gene mutations in retinoblastoma. Hum Mutat. 1999;14:283-288.

109. Frischmeyer PA, Dietz HC. Nonsense-mediated mRNA decay in health and disease. Hum Mol Genet. 1999;8:1893-1900.

110. Sippel KC, Fraioli RE, Smith GD, et al. Frequency of somatic and germ-line mosaicism in retinoblastoma: implications for genetic counseling. Am J Hum Genet. 1998;62:610-619.

111. Boerkoel CF, Exelbert R, Nicastri C, et al. Leaky splicing mutation in the acid maltase gene is associated with delayed onset of glycogenosis type II. Am J Hum Genet. 1995;56:887-897.

112. Otterson GA, Chen W, Coxon AB, et al. Incomplete penetrance of familial retinoblastoma linked to germ-line mutations that result in partial loss of RB function. Proc Natl Acad Sci U S A. 1997;94:12036-12040.

113. Connolly MJ, Payne RH, Johnson G, et al. Familial, EsD-linked, retinoblastoma with reduced penetrance and variable expressivity. Hum Genet. 1983;65:122-124.

114. Macklin MT. A study of retinoblastoma in Ohio. Am J Hum Genet. 1960;12:1-43.

115. Strong LC, Riccardi VM, Ferrell RE, Sparkes RS. Familial retinoblastoma and chromosome 13 deletion transmitted via an insertional translocation. Science. 1981;213:1501-1503.

116. Klutz M, Brockmann D, Lohmann DR. A parent-of-origin effect in two families with retinoblastoma is associated with a distinct splice mutation in the RB1 gene. Am J Hum Genet. 2002;71: 174-179.

117. Kobayashi S, Mukai N. Retinoblastoma-like tumors induced by human adenovirus 12 in rats. Cancer Res. 1974;34:1646-1651.

118. Mukai N, Kelter SS, Cummins LB, et al. Retinal tumor induced in baboon by human adenovirus 12. Science. 1980;210:1023-1025.

119. Windle JJ, Albert DA, O'Brien JM, et al. Retinoblastoma in transgenic mice. Nature. 1990;343:665-669.

120. Howes KA, Rensom N, Papermaster DS, et al. Apoptosis or retinoblastoma: alternative fates of photoreceptors expressing the HPV-16 E7 gene in the presence or absence of p53. Genes Dev. 1994;8:1300-1310.

121. Jacks T, Fazeli A, Schmitt EM, et al. Effects of an Rb mutation in the mouse. Nature. 1992;359:295-300.

122. Lee EY, Chang CY, Hu N, et al. Mice deficient for Rb are nonviable and show defects in neurogenesis and hematopoiesis. Nature. 1992;359:288-294.

123. Clarke AR, Maandag ER, van Roon M, et al. Requirement for a functional Rb-1 gene in murine develpment. Nature. 1992;359: 328-330.

124. Robanus-Maandag E, Dekker M, van der Valk M, et al. p107 is a suppressor of retinoblastoma development in pRb-deficient mice. Genes Dev. 1998;12:1599-1609.

125. Zhang J, Gray J, Wu L, et al. Rb regulates proliferation and rod photoreceptor development in the mouse retina. Nat Genet. 2004;36:351-360.

126. Laurie NA, Donovan SL, Shih C-S, et al. Inactivation of the p53 pathway in retinoblastoma. Nature. 2006;444:61-66.

127. Zhang J, Schweers B, Dyer MA. The first knockout mouse model of retinoblastoma. Cell Cycle. 2004;3:952-959.

128. Dyer MA, Bremner R. The search for the retinoblastoma cell of origin. Nat Rev Cancer. 2005;5:91-101.

129. Chen D, Livne-Bar I, Vanderluit JL, et al. Cell-specific effects of RB or RB/p107 loss on retinal development implicate an intrinsically death-resistant cell-of-origin in retinoblastoma. Cancer Cell. 2004;5:539-551.

130. MacPherson D, Sage J, Kim T, et al. Cell type-specific effects of Rb deletion in the murine retina. Genes Dev. 2004;18:1681-1694.

131. Vooijs M, te Riele H, van der Valk M, Berns A. Tumor formation in mice with somatic inactivation of the retinoblastoma gene in interphotorecptor retinol binding protein-expressing cells. Oncogene. 2002;21:4635-4645.

132. Donovan S, Schweeners B, Martins R, et al. Compensation by tumor suppressor genes during retinal development in mice and humans. BMC Biol. 2006;4:14.

133. Jordan CT, Guzman ML, Noble M. Cancer stem cells. N Engl J Med. 2006;355:1253-1261.

134. Wicha MS, Liu S, Dontu G. Cancer stem cells: an old idea—a paradigm shift. Cancer Res. 2006;66:1883-1890.

135. Sherr CJ, McCormick F. The RB and p53 pathways in cancer. Cancer Cell. 2002;2:103-112.

136. Hahn WC, Weinberg RA. Modeling the molecular circuitry of cancer. Nat Rev Cancer. 2002;2:331-341.

137. Vogelstein B, Kinzler KW. Cancer genes and the pathways they control. Nat Med. 2004;10:789-799.

138. Kato MV, Shimizu T, Ishizaki K, et al. Loss of heterozygosity on chromosome 17 and mutation of the p53 gene in retinoblastoma. Cancer Lett. 1996;106:75-82.

139. Nork TM, Poulsen GL, Millecchia LL, et al. p53 regulates apoptosis in human retinoblastoma. Arch Ophthalmol. 1997;115:213-219.

140. Elison JR, Cobrinik D, Claros N, et al. Small molecule inhibition of HDM2 leads to p53-mediated cell death in retinoblastoma cells. Arch Ophthalmol. 2006;124:1269-1275.

141. Sparkes RS, Murphree AL, Lingua RW, et al. Gene for hereditary retinoblastoma assigned to chromosome 13 by linkage analysis to esterase D. Science. 1983;219:971-973.

142. Mukai S, Rapaport JM, Shields JA, et al. Linkage of genes for human esterase D and hereditary retinoblastoma. Am J Ophthalmol. 1984;97:681-685.

143. Halloran SL, Boughman JA, Dryja TP, et al. Accuracy of detection of the retinoblastoma gene by esterase D linkage. Arch Ophthalmol. 1985;103:1329-1331.

144. Cavenee WK, Dryja TP, Phillips RA, et al. Expression of recessive alleles by chromosomal mechanisms in retinoblastoma. Nature. 1983;305:779-784.

145. Dryja TP, Cavenee W, White R, et al. Homozygosity of chromosome 13 in retinoblastoma. N Engl J Med. 1984;310:550-553.

146. Botstein D, White RL, Skolnick M, et al. Construction of genetic linkage map in man using restriction fragment length polymorphisms. Am J Hum Genet. 1980;32:314-331.

147. Bookstein R, Lee EYH, To H, et al. Human retinoblastoma susceptibility gene: genomic organization and analysis of heterozygous intragenic deletion mutants. Proc Natl Acad Sci U S A. 1988;85:2210-2214.

148. Yandell DW, Dryja TP. Detection of DNA sequence polymorphisms by enzymatic amplification and direct genomic sequencing. Am J Hum Genet. 1989;45:547-555.

149. Horsthemke B, Barnert HJ, Gregor V, et al. Early diagnosis in hereditary retinoblastoma by detection of molecular deletions at gene locus. Lancet. 1987;1:511-512.

150. Yandell DW, Campbell TA, Dayton SH, et al. Oncogenic point mutations in the human retinoblastoma gene: their application to genetic counseling. N Engl J Med. 1989;321:1689-1695.

151. Dunn JM, Phillips RA, Becker AJ, et al. Identification of germ line and somatic mutations affecting the retinoblastoma gene. Science. 1988;241:1797-1800.

152. Albrecht P, Ansperger-Rescher B, Schuler A, et al. Spectrum of gross deletions and insertions in the rb1 gene in patients with retinoblastoma and association with phenotypic expression. Hum Mutat. 2005;26:437-445.

153. Munier FL, Thonney F, Girardet A, et al. Evidence of somatic and germinal mosaicism in pseudo-low-penetrant hereditary retinoblastoma by constitutional and single-sperm mutation analysis. Am J Hum Genet. 1998;63:1903-1908.

154. Los Angeles Institute for Families of Blind Children. Breaking the News. 1991 (videotape).

155. Los Angeles Institute for Families of Blind Children. Diagnosis: retinoblastoma families in crisis. 1990 (videotape).

156. Chernus-Mansfield N, Horn M. My fake eye: the story of my prosthesis. Los Angeles, Los Angeles Institute for Blind Children, 1991.

157. Shields JA, Parsons H, Shields CL, et al. Role of cryotherapy on the management of retinoblastoma. Am J Ophthalmol. 1989;108: 260-264.

158. Shields JA, Shields CL, Parsons H, et al. Role of photocoagulation in the management of retinoblastoma. Arch Ophthalmol. 1990;108:205-208.

159. Abramson DH, Ellsworth RM, Tretter P, et al. Treatment of bilateral group I through III retinoblastoma with bilateral radiation. Arch Ophthalmol. 1981;99:1761-1762.

160. Mukai S, Munzenrider JE, Gragoudas ES. Proton beam treatment of retinoblastoma. Invest Ophthalmol Vis Sci. 1991; 32(suppl):981.

161. Shields CL, Shields JA, DePotter P, et al. Plaque radiotherapy in the management of retinoblastoma. Ophthalmology. 1993;100: 216-224.

162. White L. Chemotherapy in retinoblastoma: current status and future directions. Am J Pediatr Hematol Oncol. 1991;13:189-201.

163. Murphree AL, Villablanca JG, Deegan WF III, et al. Chemotherapy plus local treatment in the management of intraocular retinoblastoma. Arch Ophthalmol. 1996;114:1348-1356.

164. Friedman DL, Himelstein B, Shields CL, et al. Chemoreduction and local ophthalmic therapy for intraocular retinoblastoma. J Clinical Oncol. 2000;22:12-17.

165. Schefler AC, Ciccarelli N, Feuer W, et al. Macular retinoblastoma: evaluation of tumor control, local complications, and visual outcomes for eyes treated with chemotherapy and repetitive foveal laser ablation. Ophthalmology. 2007;114:162-169.

166. Abramson DH, Frank CM, Dunkel IJ. A phase I/II study of subconjunctival carboplatin for intraocular retinoblastoma. Ophthalmology. 1999;106:1947-1950.

167. Mulvill A, Budnig A, Jay V, et al. Ocular motility changes after sub-Tenon carboplatin for intraocular retinoblastoma. Arch Ophthalmol. 2003;121:1120-1124.

168. Children's Oncology Group protocol ARET 0231. Children's Oncology Group Website. Available at www.childrensoncologygroup.org. Accessed May 9, 2008.

169. Yamane T, Kaneko A, Mohri M. The technique of ophthalmic arterial infusion therapy for patients with intraocular retinoblastoma. Int J Clin Oncol. 2004;9:69-73.

170. Inomata M, Kaneko A. Chemosensitivity profiles of primary and cultured retinoblastoma cells in a human tumor clonogenic assay. Jpn J Cancer Res. 1987;78:858-868.

171. Seregard S, Koch B, af Trame E. Intravitreal chemotherapy for recurrent retinoblastoma in an only eye. Br J Ophthalmol. 1995;79:194-195.

172. Kaneko A, Suzuki S. Eye-preservation treatment of retinoblastoma with vitreous seeding. Jpn J Clin Oncol. 2003;33:601-607.

173. Chévez-Barrios P, Chintagumpala M, Mieler W, et al. Response of retinoblastoma with vitreous seeding to adenovirus-mediated delivery of thymidine kinase followed by ganciclovir. J Clin Oncol. 2005;23:7929-7935.

174. Reese AB, Ellsworth RM. The evaluation and current concept of retinoblastoma therapy. Trans Am Acad Ophthalmol Otolaryngol. 1963;67:164-172.

175. Murphree AL. Intraocular retinoblastoma: the case for a new group classification. Ophthalmol Clin North Am. 2005;18:41-53.

176. Shields CL, Shields JA. Basic understanding of current classification and management of retinoblastoma. Curr Opin Ophthalmol. 2006;17:228-234.

177. Abramson DH, Ellsworth RM, Rozakis GW. Cryotherapy for retinoblastoma. Arch Ophthalmol. 1982;100:1253-1256.

178. Lincoff H, McLean J, Long R. The cryosurgical treatment of intraocular tumors. Am J Ophthalmol. 1967;63:389-399.

179. Meyer Schwickerath G, Vogel MH. Malignant melanoma of the choroid treated with photocoagulation: a 10-year follow-up. Mod Probl Ophthalmol. 1974;12:544-549.

180. Oosterhuis JA, Journée-de Korver JG, Kakebeeke-Kemme HM, et al. Transpupillary thermotherapy in choroidal melanoma. Arch Ophthalmol. 1995;113:315-321.

181. Murphree AL, Villablanca JG, Deegan WF 3rd, et al. Chemotherapy plus local treatment in the management of intraocular retinoblastoma. Arch Ophthalmol. 1996;114:1348-1356.

182. Abramson DH, Ellsworth RM, Rosenblatt M, et al. Retreatment of retinoblastoma with external beam irradiation. Arch Ophthalmol. 1982;100:1257-1260.

183. Hilgartner H. Report of a case of double glioma treated by x-ray. Texas Med J. 1903;18:322-323.

184. Blach LE, McCormick B, Abramson DH. External beam radiation therapy and retinoblastoma: long-term results in the comparison of two techniques. Int J Radiat Oncol Biol Phys. 1996; 35:45-51.

185. Abramson DH, Beaverson KL, Chang ST, et al. Outcome following initial external beam radiotherapy in patients with Reese-Ellsworth group Vb retinoblastoma. Arch Ophthalmol. 2004;122: 1316-1323.

186. Armstrong DI. The use of 4-6 MeV electrons for the conservative treatment of retinoblastoma. Br J Radiol. 1974;47:326-331.

187. Sealy R, le Roux PLM, Rapley F, et al. The treatment of ophthalmic tumors with low-energy sources. Br J Radiol. 1976;49:551-554.

188. Lommatzsch PK. Treatment of choroidal melanoma with [106]Ru/[106]Rh beta-ray applications. Surv Ophthalmol. 1974;19:85-100.

189. Hernandez JC, Brady LW, Shields CL, et al. Conservative treatment of retinoblastoma. The use of plaque brachytherapy. Am J Clin Oncol. 1993;16:397-401.

190. Fontanesi J, Pratt CB, Kun LF, et al. Treatment outcomes and dose-response relationship in infants younger than 1 year treated for retinoblastoma with primary irradiation. Med Pediatr Oncol. 1996;26:297-304.

191. Cassadt JR, Sagerman RH, Tretter P, Ellsworth RM. Radiation therapy in retinoblastoma: an analysis of therapy in retinoblastoma: an analysis of 230 cases. Radiology. 1969;93:405-409.

192. Weiss DR, Cassady JR, Petersen R. Retinoblastoma: a modification in radiation therapy technique. Radiology. 1975;114:705-708.

193. Salmonsen PC, Ellsworth RM, Kitchin FD. The occurrence of new retinoblastomas after treatment. Ophthalmology. 1979;86:837-840.

194. Foote RL, Garretson BR, Schomberg PJ, et al. External beam irradiation for retinoblastoma: Patterns of failure and dose-dependent analysis. Int J Radiat Oncol Biol Phys. 1989;16:823-830.

195. Schipper J. An accurate and simple method for megavoltage radiation therapy of retinoblastoma. Radiother Oncol. 1983;1:31-41.

196. Schipper J, Tan KEWP, van Peperzeel HA. Treatment of retinoblastoma by precision megavoltage radiation therapy. Radiother Oncol. 1985;3:117-132.

197. Harnett AN, Hungerford JL, Lambert GD, et al. Improved external beam radiotherapy for the treatment of retinoblastoma. Br J Radiol. 1987;60:753-760.

198. Krasin MJ, Crawford BT, Zhu Y, et al. Intensity-modulated radiation therapy for children with intraocular retinoblastoma: potential sparing of the bony orbit. Clin Oncol (R Coll Radiol). 2004;16:215-222.

199. Krengli M, Hug EB, Adams JA, et al. Proton radiation therapy for retinoblastoma: comparison of various intraocular tumor locations and beam arrangements. Int J Radiat Oncol Biol Phys. 2006;61:583-593.

200. Gragoudas ES. Proton beam therapy of uveal melanomas. Arch Ophthalmol. 1986;104:349-351.

201. Goitein M, Miller T. Planning proton therapy of the eye. Med Phys. 1983;10:275-283.

202. Kupfer C. Retinoblastoma treated with intravenous nitrogen mustard. Am J Ophthalmol. 1953;36:1721-1723.

203. Wong FL, Boice JD Jr, Abramson DH, et al. Cancer incidence after retinoblastoma: radiation dose and sarcoma risk. JAMA. 1997;278:1262-1267.

204. Gallie BL, Budning A, DeBoer G, et al. Chemotherapy with local therapy can cure intraocular retinoblastoma without radiotherapy. Arch Ophthalmol. 1996;114:1321-1328.

205. Chan HS, DeBoer G, Thiessen JJ, et al. Combining cyclosporin with chemotherapy controls intraocular retinoblastoma without requiring radiation. Clin Cancer Res. 1996;2:1499-1508.

206. Rodriguez-Galindo C, Wilson MW, Haik BG, et al. Treatment of intraocular retinoblastoma with vincristine and carboplatin. J Clin Oncol. 2003;21:2019-2025.

207. Children's Oncology Group protocol ARET 0331. Children's Oncology Group Website. Available at www.childrensoncologygroup.org. Accessed May 9, 2008.

208. Grabowski E, Abramson DH. Intraocular and extraocular retinoblastoma. Hematol Oncol Clin North Am. 1987;1:721-735.

209. Chantada G, Doz F, Antonelli CB, et al. A proposal for an international retinoblastoma staging system. Pediatr Blood Cancer. 2006;47:801-805.

210. Chantada G, Fandino A, Cusak S, et al. Treatment of overt extraocular retinoblastoma. Med Pediatr Oncol. 2003;40:158-161.

211. Gündüz K, Müftüoglu O, Günalp I, et al. Metastatic retinoblastoma: clinical features, treatment, and prognosis. Ophthalmology. 2006;113:1558-1566.

212. Leal-Leal CA, Rivera-Luna R, Flores-Rojo M, et al. Survival in extra-orbital metastatic retinoblastoma: treatment results. Clin Transpl Oncol. 2006;8:39-44.

213. Jubran RF, Murphree AL, Villablanca JG. Low dose carboplatin/etoposide/vincristine and local therapy for intraocular retinoblastoma group II-IV eyes. Proceedings of the XIII Biannual Meeting of International Society of Genetic Eye Diseases and the X International Symposium on Retinoblastoma, May 4, 2001, Fort Lauderdale, Fla. USA.

214. Wilson MW, Haik BG, Liu T, et al. Effect on ocular survival of adding early intensive focal treatments to two-drug chemotherapy regimen in patients with retinoblastoma. Am J Ophthalmol. 2005;140:397-406.

215. Abramson DH, Lawrence SD, Beaverson KL, et al. Systemic carboplatin for retinoblastoma: change in tumour size over time. Br J Ophthalmol. 2005;89:1616-1619.

216. Imhof SM, Mouritis MP, Hofman P, et al. Quantification of orbital and mid-facial growth retardation after megavoltage external beam irradiation in children with retinoblastoma. Ophthalmology. 1996;103:263-268.

217. Kaste SC, Chen G, Fontanese J, et al. Orbital development in long-term survivors of retinoblastoma. J Clin Oncol. 1997;15:1183-1189.

218. Schmack I, Hubbard GB, Kang SJ, et al. Ischemic necrosis and atrophy of the optic nerve after periocular carboplatin injection for intraocular retinoblastoma. Am J Ophthalmol. 2006;142:310-315.

219. Children's Oncology Group protocol ARET 0332. Children's Oncology Group Website. Available at www.childrensoncologygroup.org. Accessed May 9, 2008.

220. Children's Oncology Group protocol ARET 0321. Children's Oncology Group Website. Available at www.childrensoncology.group.org. Accessed May 9, 2008.

221. Goble RR, McKenzie J, Kingston JE, et al. Orbital recurrence of retinoblastoma successfully treated by combined therapy. Br J Ophthalmol. 1990;74:97-98.

222. Dunkel IJ, Aledo A, Kernan NA, et al. Successful treatment of metastatic retinoblastoma. Cancer. 2000;89:2117-2121.

223. Matsubara H, Makimota A, Higa T, et al. A multidisciplinary treatment strategy that includes high-dose chemotherapy for metastatic retinoblastoma without CNS involvement. Bone Marrow Transplant. 2005;35:763-766.

17 Tumors of the Brain and Spinal Cord

Mark W. Kieran, Susan N. Chi, David Samuel, Mirna Lechpammer, Samuel Blackman, Sanjay P. Prabhu, Betsy Herrington, Christopher Turner, Karen J. Marcus, and Rosalind Segal

Tumors of the central nervous system (CNS) account for approximately 25% of pediatric cancer but are now the leading cause of cancer-related mortality in children. The complexities of tumors in this site are related to the large number of different histologies within the CNS and a historical nomenclature that is confusing, even to many in this field. With the need to modify therapies to spare important neurocognitive function in the youngest patients, and the presence of the blood-brain barrier, which restricts the delivery of effective therapies, improvement in outcome has lagged well behind that of many other cancers, especially childhood leukemia. The molecular revolution offers the chance to begin classifying tumors by the signals that drive their phenotype rather than their appearance under the microscope.[1] This chapter will discuss the different types of brain tumors in children and their diagnoses and treatments, and will incorporate the expanding knowledge of tumor biology.

Although clinical studies often focus on progression-free and overall survival, successful therapy incorporates much more. Accepting a lower overall cure rate, but preserving neurocognitive function is the norm for many tumors, especially those of infants and young children. Optimization of outcome requires expertise in multiple subspecialties that interact with these children. The skill of the neurosurgeon, the sophistication of the radiation planning, and the safe administration of chemotherapy are all important factors in improving the long-term outcome for these patients. In fact, many centers now employ neuro-oncologists who have completed additional training in this area. When combined with a large number of subspecialty services (e.g., endocrinology, neurology, neuropsychology, social work, back to school, physical and occupational therapy), truly optimal care is now possible for this patient population. Needs of the family continue to evolve as patients transition from diagnosis to treatment to post-therapy follow-up.[2] It is a comprehensive understanding of pediatric neuro-oncology and the delivery of comprehensive care to these patients and their families that will be the focus of this chapter.

To assist the reader, a number of important review articles summarizing different aspects of the care of children with CNS tumors are provided.[3-9]

EPIDEMIOLOGY

Primary CNS tumors rank second behind leukemia as the most common pediatric cancer diagnosed in the United States each year (Fig. 17-1). Brain tumors are the most common form of solid tumors in children and are the leading cause of death from solid tumors in children. The spectrum of adult brain tumors,[10] based on location, histology, and outcome, suggests that the causative events are different than that for pediatric brain tumors. No single standard system has been implemented, although attempts to develop a standardized platform for epidemiologic studies has been completed.[11] According to the most recent National Cancer Institute Surveillance Epidemiology and End Results (SEER) Cancer Statistics Report (CSR), published in 2007, the annual age-adjusted incidence rate of pediatric malignant brain and other nervous system tumors is 2.8 cases/100,000 children.[12] The 2007-2008 Central Brain Tumor Registry of the United States (CBTRUS) Statistical Report included primary nonmalignant as well as malignant pediatric brain and CNS tumors and increased the annual CNS tumor incidence to 4.5 cases/100,000 children. The rate is higher in males (4.7/100,000) compared with females (4.3/100,000). Approximately 3750 new cases of childhood primary CNS tumors will be diagnosed in the United States each year. Of these, an estimated 2820 will be in children younger than 15 years. The incidence for all brain tumors is

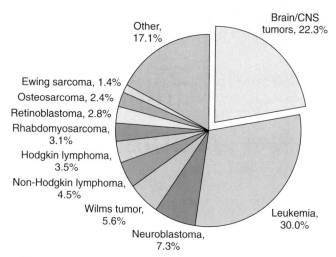

FIGURE 17-1. Incidence of pediatric cancer. *(Data from American Cancer Society. American Cancer Society Cancer Facts & Figures, 2007. Atlanta, American Cancer Society, 2007.)*

highest among 0- to 4-year-olds (5.2/100,000) and lowest among 10- to 14-year-olds (4.1/100,000). The 5-year survival rate following diagnosis of a primary CNS tumor is 66% for those aged 0 to 19 years. The prevalence rate for all malignant and benign pediatric CNS tumors (ages 0 to 19 years) is estimated at 9.5/100,000, with more than 26,000 children estimated to be living with this diagnosis in the United States in 2000. However, the prevalence rate for those with only malignant brain tumors was 7.9/100,000, with more than 21,000 children estimated to be living with a diagnosis of primary malignant CNS tumor in the United States in 2000.[13] The distribution of pediatric brain tumors by site is presented in Figure 17-2. Different brain tumor histologies have different age distributions (Fig. 17-3). The most common histologies in the younger age group (ages 0 to 14 years) include pilocytic astrocytomas and embryonal tumors (medulloblastoma), which account for 20% and 16% of cases, respectively. The broad category of glioma accounts for 56% of tumors in children younger than 15 years. The most common histologies in adolescents ages 15 to 19 years include pilocytic astrocytoma and pituitary tumors, which account for 15% and 14% of cases, respectively. The broad category of glioma accounts for 45% of tumors in adolescents ages 15 to 19 years. The rates among boys are slightly higher than those in girls and brain tumors are more common in whites (4.7/100,000) than in blacks (3/100,000).

The histologic-specific differences in brain and CNS tumor distribution by age and gender suggest that childhood tumors have different causes in which normal cells, possibly stem cells, are susceptible to mutation. Although certain histologic subtypes can also differ by race,[14,15] the overall concordance of tumor histologies among different ethnic groups would suggest that specific local environmental factors are not the cause of most cancers in children.[16-18] The incidence of common pediatric brain tumors such as medulloblastoma, malignant gliomas, and diffuse pontine glioma do not differ significantly in industrialized versus nonindustrialized countries, in vegetarian versus meat-eating societies, and in areas where smoking and drinking are permitted versus where they are not. Similarly, death rates for children with CNS tumors between different ethnic groups within the United States (Hispanics, Asians, blacks, whites) do not differ significantly for most tumor types.[19]

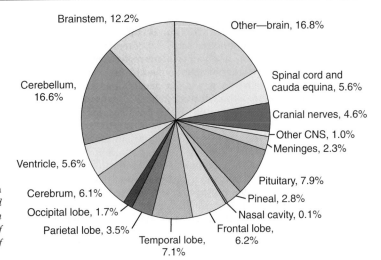

FIGURE 17-2. Incidence of pediatric CNS tumors by location (*N* = 5873). *(Data from Central Brain Tumor Registry of the United States [CBTRUS]. 2007-2008 Statistical Report: Primary Brain Tumors in the United States Statistical Report, 2000-2004 [Years of Data Collected]. Chicago, University of Illinois at Chicago School of Public Health, 2008.)*

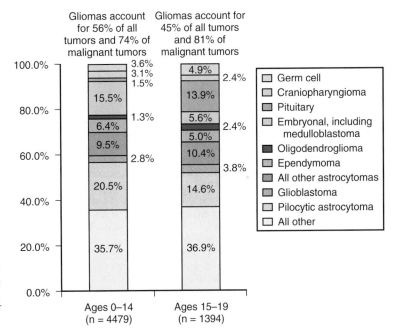

FIGURE 17-3. Incidence of pediatric brain tumors by histology. *(Data from Central Brain Tumor Registry of the United States [CBTRUS]. 2007-2008 Statistical Report: Primary Brain Tumors in the United States Statistical Report, 2000-2004 [Years of Data Collected]. Chicago, University of Illinois at Chicago School of Public Health, 2008.)*

In the mid-1990s, there appeared to be an increase in the incidence of childhood brain cancer compared with that in the previous 2 decades. This is now thought to reflect the introduction and widespread use of magnetic resonance imaging (MRI) technology in the mid-1980s, resulting in improved detection and reporting of pediatric brain tumors. More precise classification of brain tumors and diagnostic capabilities such as stereotactic biopsy may have also contributed to the increase in incidence. The rise in incidence was followed by the establishment of a new baseline that has remained stable. Mortality rates have not mirrored the increase in incidence.[20]

Primary CNS tumors develop from an accumulation of genetic changes. Such changes can result from inherited mutations or develop from exposure to chemical, physical, or biologic agents that damage DNA. Unlike adults, for whom lifetime exposure is significant, most pediatric tumors are believed to be the result of random genetic mutations that occur during normal cellular proliferation. Today, molecular biologic

techniques are being used to unravel the complex genetic errors that lead to the development of CNS tumors. Genetic polymorphisms in the glutathione S-transferase (GST) gene, which functions to metabolize and eliminate carcinogens, has been associated with an increased risk of malignant astrocytomas in pediatric-aged patients.[21]

The search for causative factors that place children at risk for developing CNS tumors has not yielded clear answers.[22] Numerous epidemiologic studies have evaluated potential risk factors. Like most pediatric cancers, no specific risk factor explains more than a small proportion of tumors.[23] Factors studied but not conclusively found to increase risk include tobacco and smoke exposure,[24] alcohol, traffic-related air pollution, electromagnetic field exposure, pesticides, occupational and industrial chemicals, diet, drugs and medications, infections and viruses, epilepsy, and consumption of cured meats during pregnancy.[25-34] The dramatic increase in the use of cellular telephones has generated concerns about the potential risk for developing brain tumors. A meta-analysis of nine case-control studies concluded that there is no overall increased risk of brain tumors in cellular phone users. The potential risk after long-term cellular phone use awaits confirmation by future studies.[35] A seasonal variation unique to medulloblastoma incidence by month of birth may provide evidence for an environmental exposure cause, although further studies are needed.[36] An association between atopic disease and a reduced risk of glioma has been observed in adult epidemiologic studies, with the implication that heightened immune surveillance decreases the risk of brain tumor development.[22,37] Prenatal multivitamin use has been associated with a protective effect in the development of pediatric brain tumors in a large meta-analysis.[38] Confirmation of this result in a prospective trial is needed.

The role of viruses in the pathogenesis of tumors has been documented in experimental animals and adenovirus serotypes have been shown to induce tumors in rodents. Adenoviral sequences were evaluated in over 500 tumors derived from 17 different pediatric cancer entities. Although most leukemias and solid tumors were negative for the presence of adenoviral sequences, tumor material from 25 of 30 glioblastomas, 22 of 30 oligodendrogliomas, and 20 of 30 ependymomas, as well as normal brain, were positive by polymerase chain reaction (PCR) assay for adenoviral gene sequences. This raises important questions about the contribution of this infectious agent to pediatric brain tumorigenesis.[39] In contrast, testing for polyoma-virus sequences in adult and pediatric CNS tumors were rarely positive.[40]

Ionizing radiation, immunosuppression, and certain hereditary genetic disorders are the only factors so far proven to increase a child's risk for CNS malignancy. Ionizing radiation exposure is a well-documented cause of brain tumors.[41] Children who undergo therapeutic irradiation to the CNS for the treatment of malignancy are at risk for developing a second tumor, specifically meningioma, high-grade glioma, or sarcoma. Since its introduction in the 1970s, computed tomography (CT) has become an essential tool in the diagnosis and treatment follow-up of disease. The growing use of CT scans has raised concerns about potential risks. Pediatric CT scans may result in a small but not negligible increased lifetime risk for cancer mortality.[42]

Immunocompromised children are at increased risk for primary CNS lymphoma. The risk for developing CNS lymphoma is 1% to 5% higher for adults and children undergoing transplantation and those with congenital immunodeficiencies. The risk is 2% to 6% higher for those with acquired immunodeficiency syndrome (AIDS). This risk will probably increase with longer survival because of improved AIDS treatment.

In summary, although a few environmental factors are associated with an increased risk of developing a pediatric CNS tumor, the vast majority of patients have no easily identifiable risk factors. For a small percentage (discussed later), inherited genetic mutations will be the cause of these tumors but for the remainder, their CNS tumors are likely the result of spontaneous mutations.

NEURODEVELOPMENT

Our understanding of the steps in hematopoietic development, together with the pathways and markers that distinguish precursors along each blood cell lineage, has been instrumental in allowing better classification and subsequently better treatment of leukemias. In the same way that leukemias can be viewed as deregulated expansion of hematopoietic precursor cell pools, pediatric brain tumors may similarly be considered as the proliferation of neuropoietic precursors. Thus, knowledge of the

steps and intermediates in neural development may help us understand and treat pediatric brain tumors. A current schema for neuropoiesis relies heavily on models for hematopoiesis, but introduces two additional aspects of developmental regulation. The first is the importance of regionalization. During neural development a rostral-caudal gradient delineates distinct zones for proliferation and differentiation, while the orientation of proliferating cells relative to the dorsal-ventral axis provides the basis for determining the progeny of each proliferative event.

The second aspect of neuropoiesis is the concept of mitogenic niches. Although hematopoietic stem cells can proliferate and give rise to the whole array of blood cell types when exposed to the environment of the immature or mature bone marrow, neural stem cells use a number of distinct niches, some of which are eliminated before birth, some that persist through early childhood, and some that remain extant into adult life. These niches provide important cues for proliferation and differentiation but may also provide an environment that fosters the growth of tumor cells.

Neural Tube

The nervous system develops as a specialized zone of the epithelium. In the third week after fertilization, the midline zone of the epithelium becomes specialized as the neural plate. This distinctive zone extends from the caudal to the rostral portion of the embryo. As the embryo turns, the neural plate grows and folds (Fig. 17-4). Subsequent fusion of the folds creates a

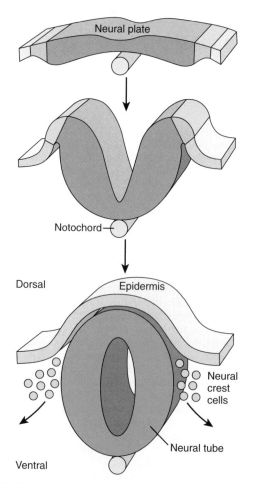

FIGURE 17-4. Growth and folding of the neural plate.

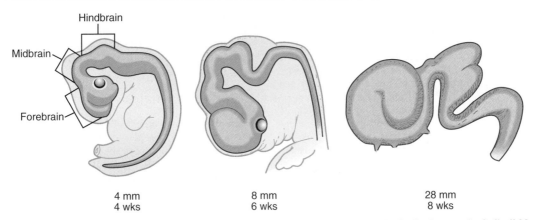

Hindbrain

Midbrain

Forebrain

| 4 mm | 8 mm | 28 mm |
| 4 wks | 6 wks | 8 wks |

FIGURE 17-5. Outpouching of the neural tube. *(Adapted from Diencephalon/telencephalon: Neural tube development. In Sodicoff M. Neuroanatomy Laboratory Assistant CD-ROM. Department of Anatomy and Cell Biology, Temple University School of Medicine, Philadelphia, 2004.)*

discrete neural tube that zips up from both the top and bottom. The two last places where the fold fuse are the hindbrain (the incipient cerebellum) and the lumbar spine. Cells at the crest of the developing neural tube are the neural crest cells, which give rise to the peripheral nervous system, including sympathetic ganglia, dorsal root ganglia, and Schwann cells as well as to melanocytes in the developing skin. The neural crest cells are the precursors to neuroblastomas,[43] neurofibromas,[44] and melanomas.[45]

After the neural tube fuses, rapid expansion of cell number continues but this occurs very differently along the rostral-caudal axis. The dramatic expansion of cell number in the rostral neural tube provides the building blocks for the brain, while the more caudal regions undergo more limited growth and engender the spinal cord.

Development of Brain Structures

Along the rostral-caudal axis of the neural tube, three outpouchings can be seen at the end of the fourth week after fertilization—the forebrain, midbrain, and hindbrain (Fig. 17-5). Subsequent branching of the forebrain forms two lateral protrusions that are destined to become the left and right cortex, and the midline portion of the forebrain gives rise to the thalamus. The midbrain does not undergo much expansion, but the hindbrain undergoes massive proliferation to give rise to the cerebellum and underlying pons, as well as the medulla. Cerebral cortical tumors, including supratentorial primitive neuroectodermal tumors (PNETs) and cortical and subependymal astrocytomas, all derive from the forebrain. Posterior fossa tumors, including the distinctive pontine gliomas, medulloblastomas, and cerebellar pilocytic astrocytomas, all derive from the hindbrain. Thus, the areas of the brain that undergo rapid expansion in early life engender most of the pediatric brain tumors. Along the dorsal-ventral plane of the neural tube, there is greater proliferation of neural tube precursors in the dorsal part of the tube than in the ventral tube. Proliferation of more dorsal precursors gives rise to the multilayer structures of the cerebral and cerebellar cortex; these areas are also the regions that give rise to most pediatric brain tumors.

Forebrain and Cerebral Cortex

In the forebrain, the open spaces within the lateral outpouchings of the neural tube become the lateral ventricles and proliferation continues adjacent to the ventricular zone. Early in development, these precursors divide in a symmetric manner, so that a proliferative cell divides and gives rise to two new precursor cells.[46,47] This symmetric phase of proliferation allows an exponential increase in cell number. As development proceeds, the precursors of the ventricular zone change the mode of cell division. In later cell divisions, one of the two cells generated continues to divide, although the other differentiates and migrates away from the ventricles into the incipient cortex. The early generated cells migrate to become the neurons of the innermost cortical layer (layer VI) and later mitoses give rise to neurons that occupy increasingly superficial layers. Thus, the cortex develops in an inside-out pattern. Toward the end of the prenatal neurogenic phase, the precursors of the ventricular zone generate glial cells, including astrocytes, oligodendrocytes, and ependymal cells.[48,49]

A small population of precursors remains in the subventricular zone, just above the ependymal cells, throughout life. These neural stem cells continue to generate glial cells and oligodendrocytes and also continue to give rise to a limited number of neuronal cells through adult neurogenesis. Thus, the neural stem cell represents a common precursor for glial and neuronal cells. Accumulating data suggest that many, if not most, brain tumors arise from such stem cells, or their early derivatives.

Cerebellar Cortex

The cerebellar cortex develops in a way that has some similarities to, but some differences from, the pattern in the cerebral cortex. The hindbrain is the site where the neural tube closes last. As closure occurs, the neural folds pucker to form the rhombic lips. These two protrusions will give rise to many cell types of the cerebellum and pons. Cells in the ventricular zone of the upper rhombic lip proliferate and then begin an unusual migration pattern. The precursor cells of the rhombic lip migrate over the top of the rhombic lip and disperse by moving from the caudal aspect of the pucker to cover the rhombic lip or incipient cerebellum. The rhombic lip–derived precursors settle in a zone that covers the developing cerebellum; this is called the external granule cell (external germinal cell [EGL]) layer. This layer constitutes a site of extensive postnatal proliferation and is a specialized mitogenic niche where precursors divide and give rise almost exclusively to cerebellar granule cells, the most numerous neuronal cells in the brain. This secondary proliferative zone may be necessary to generate this vast number of granule cells. To generate the 60 to 80 billion granule cell neurons, the granule cell precursors in the EGL undergo many rounds of cell divisions, beginning in the ninth week after fertilization and continuing through the first 18 months of life in humans.

A great deal of evidence has indicated that the granule cell precursors of the EGL are a cell of origin for medulloblastoma.[50] First, in very young children, medulloblastomas are often continuous with the EGL and an intermediate zone of dysplastic cells can sometimes be seen to join the EGL and tumor tissue. Second, the appearance and pattern of gene expression of the granule cell precursors resemble those of medulloblastoma cells. In particular, the expression of the zic family of transcription factors is characteristic of both populations. Finally, the growth factor–signaling pathways that normally regulate proliferation of granule cell precursors can, when constitutively active, cause medulloblastoma (see later).

As the rhombic lip begins the differentiation process, cells in the ventricular zone adjacent to the upper rhombic lip continue to proliferate. As these cells divide, they give rise to the Purkinje cells of the cerebellum, neurons of the deep cerebellar nuclei, and later to cerebellar interneurons and basket and stellate cells. These cells migrate dorsally; once they reach the white matter tracts of the incipient cerebellum, they can continue to divide postnatally to give rise to cerebellar interneurons and glia and may also have the potential to produce granule cells. It has been suggested that this less specialized cell can give rise to medulloblastomas. Indeed, molecular characterization of medulloblastomas suggests that there are genetically distinct tumor types; these may represent the oncogenic transformation of cerebellar precursor cells at different locations and stages.[51,52] This would be analogous to leukemias, in which oncogenic transformation of hematopoietic precursors at distinct developmental stages leads to distinct types of leukemias.

Cancer Stem Cells

Brain tumors have predominantly been classified as neuronal or glial in nature. The neuronal tumors include PNETs, pineoblastomas, and medulloblastomas, as well as ganglion cell tumors. Glial tumors include many different gliomas, such as juvenile pilocytic astrocytoma, subependymal giant cell astrocytoma, other low-grade astrocytomas, pontine glioma, malignant astrocytoma including glioblastoma multiforme, and tumors that resemble other glial cell types, oligodendroglioma and ependymoma. Although this classification schema remains useful, it appears that many brain tumors are generated by oncogenic mutations in neural stem–precursor cells, rather than more mature cell types. Furthermore, although cancers have traditionally been viewed as clonal, increasing evidence indicates that this is not the case. Instead, the concept has developed that there is a subpopulation of cancer stem cells, distinctive cells within the tumor that are uniquely capable of regenerating the cancer.[53] Recent studies on brain tumors have identified CD-133–positive cells as radioresistant, slowly proliferating cancer stem cells that are particularly prevalent in high-grade tumors, such as glioblastoma multiforme. The ability of these cancer stem cells to survive surgical resection, radiation, and cytotoxic chemotherapy is a major reason for the difficulty in curing high-grade brain tumors.

Genetic and Signaling Pathways Implicated in Development and in Pediatric Tumors

Inherited disorders that cause a familial propensity for brain tumors have provided an important method for identifying genetic pathways that contribute to these cancers.[54-56] Neurofibromatosis, tuberous sclerosis, Gorlin's syndrome, Turcot's syndrome, Cowden's syndrome, and the INI-1 mutation all represent heritable disorders associated with an increased risk of brain tumors[57] (Table 17-1).

Neurofibromatosis Type 1

Neurofibromatosis type 1 (NF-1) is an autosomal dominant neuroectodermal disorder characterized by café-au-lait spots and fibromatous tumors of the skin. Additional clinical features that can be seen in NF-1 (Box 17-1) include Lisch nodules in the iris, scoliosis, cognitive problems, and epilepsy.[58-60] Several tumors occur with greater frequency in this disorder, including pheochromocytoma, ependymoma, meningioma, and glioma. Among these, gliomas of the optic pathway are the most common tumors seen. The unique biology behind these tumors is slowly being elucidated with the development of NF-1 optic pathway animal models.[61] Neurofibromatosis is caused by heterozygous mutations in neurofibromin and the cancers seen in this disorder result from loss of heterozygosity at chromosome 17q11.2, leaving only the mutant NF-1 allele.[62] Although this disorder is inherited as an autosomal dominant disease, as many as 50% of patients represent new mutations and therefore do not have a family history of the disorder.

The neurofibromin protein is a 250-kD tumor suppressor that functions as a GTPase activator for the small G protein Ras.[63] In this way, active neurofibromin decreases the ratio of GTP-bound (active) to GDP-bound (inactive) Ras or Ras-like

TABLE 17-1	Common Chromosomal Abnormalities Associated with Pediatric Central Nervous System Tumors
Monosomy 22	Atypical teratoid-rhabdoid tumor
	Acoustic neuromas
	Meningioma
	Ependymoma
1p and/or 22q loss	Oligodendroglioma
Isochrome i17	Medulloblastoma
9q22 loss (PTCH gene)	Medulloblastoma
Loss of chromosome 10, 9p, 17p	Progression to high-grade glioma

Box 17-1	**Diagnostic Criteria of Neurofibromatosis Type 1 (NF-1)***

Six or more café-au-lait spots ≥1.5 cm in postpubescent or > 0.5 cm in prepubescent individuals
Two or more neurofibromas or one or more plexiform neurofibromas
Freckling in the axillae or groin
Optic glioma
Two or more Lisch nodules
Dysplasia of the sphenoid bone or dysplasia or thinning of the cortex of long bones
A first-degree relative with NF-1

*The diagnosis of NF-1 requires any two or more of these criteria.

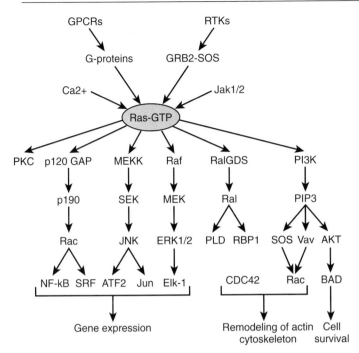

FIGURE 17-6. Ras and downstream pathway. GPCR, G protein coupled receptor; RTK, receptor tyrosine kinase. See text for other abbreviations.

protein. As activated Ras stimulates MAP kinases and PI3 kinases, the change in Ras activity leads to unregulated proliferation and survival (Fig. 17-6).[64] Although the incidence of brain tumors, particularly optic nerve gliomas, is significantly increased in NF-1 (approximately 5% to 15%), the tumors seen in these patients tend to be less aggressive than other gliomas. In fact, many stop growing spontaneously. These tumors are more susceptible to chemotherapeutic interventions, and thus can be treated differently than other gliomas. The unique developmental environment of the optic pathways may account for the differential occurrence of these tumors in patients with NF-1, as well as their increased responsiveness.[65] In addition to optic pathway gliomas, nonoptic pathway gliomas occur at frequencies 100 times greater than expected, with the most common sites being the brainstem (49%), cerebral hemispheres (21%), and basal ganglia (14%). Other MRI signal abnormalities within the brain are often observed in patients with NF-1.[66,67] The most characteristic is the unidentified bright object (UBO).[68] Unlike low-grade gliomas, these lesions are bright on T2-weighted imaging, do not demonstrate contrast enhancement, and usually produce neither mass effect nor symptoms. They often come and go and should not be biopsied or treated. The varied intracranial localization of lesions and variable need for neurosurgical intervention in a subset of children with NF-1 suggests that radiologic surveillance be based on careful and regular neurologic and ophthalmologic examinations.[69] NF-1 patients appear to be at increased risk of moyamoya syndrome[70,71] and this risk becomes especially high after cerebral radiation therapy. Patients with NF-1, even in the absence of a brain tumor, are also affected by a number of other problems as a result of their disease, in particular neurocognitive impairment, which can range from mild to severe.[64]

Neurofibromatosis Type 2 (Merlin)

Neurofibromatosis type 2 (NF-2) is characterized by familial, bilateral acoustic neuromas and is caused by mutations in the gene that encodes merlin, or schwannomin, at chromosome 22q12.2.[72,73] Merlin interacts with cytoskeletal components and appears to be important in adhesion-dependent growth control. Individuals with germline mutations also have skin tumors, with both peripheral schwannomas and neurofibromas, and a propensity to develop intracranial meningiomas or, more rarely, gliomas and spinal tumors.[74] The onset of symptomatic tumor growth is uncommon in childhood and most patients are identified in adulthood.

Tuberous Sclerosis

A third neurocutaneous disorder associated with an increased propensity for brain tumors is tuberous sclerosis (TS). This condition can be caused by mutations in either of two genes, *Tsc1* (hamartin, at chromosome 9q34)[75] or *Tsc2* (tuberin) and is characterized by hamartomata in multiple organs. The most common clinical manifestations include epilepsy, cognitive and behavioral problems, and characteristic skin lesions. The white leaf-shaped skin lesions can best be seen under a Wood's light; adenoma sebaceum (facial angiofibroma) can also be seen. Renal manifestations include angiomyolipomas, renal cysts and, more rarely, renal cell cancer. Between 5% and 14% of patients develop brain tumors, the most common being the subependymal giant cell astrocytoma (SEGA); other gliomas and ependymomas are also relatively frequent. Careful serial evaluations are required because of the possibility of additional tumor development in this patient population.[76] Cortical tubers can cause seizures and require specialized neurosurgical approaches in children.[77]

The similarity of Tsc1 and Tsc2 is explained by the finding that these two proteins interact directly with one another.[75] This complex acts as a GAP (GTPase activating protein) for Rheb. The decreased activity of Rheb inhibits the mammalian target of rapamycin (mTOR) and p70 ribosomal S6 kinase-1. As a result, there is diminished translation by eukaryotic translation initiation factor 4E-binding protein-1 (EIF4EBP1; 602223). The hamartin-tuberin complex thereby regulates growth and proliferation of subependymal and subventricular neural stem cells. The Tsc-mTOR pathways may normally be regulated by Wnt and IGF ligands during development. TS patients with SEGA or low-grade gliomas have demonstrated responses to mTOR inhibitors, confirming the clinical relevance of these findings.[78]

Gorlin's Syndrome

Gorlin's syndrome (basal cell nevus syndrome, nevoid basal cell carcinoma syndrome) is characterized by multiple basal cell carcinomas (BCCs) or basal cell nevi before the age of 30 years, odontogenic keratocysts or polyostotic bone cysts, and palmar and plantar pits. Other manifestations include rib or vertebral anomalies, large head circumference with frontal bossing, cardiac or ovarian fibroma, and lymphomesenteric cysts.[79] Gorlin's syndrome is caused by mutations in Ptc (chromosome 9q22.3), the receptor for the sonic hedgehog (Shh) ligand.[80-85] Approximately 4% to 10% of those with Gorlin's syndrome develop medulloblastoma. This syndrome also predisposes to other tumors, such as rhabdomyosarcoma.[86,87]

The Ptc1 gene product functions as both a receptor and negative regulator of signaling initiated by sonic hedgehog or the related ligands, Indian hedgehog and desert hedgehog. These ligands initiate an unusual and incompletely understood signaling pathway (Fig. 17-7). When a hedgehog ligand binds to Ptc, this alters the activation state of smoothened, or Smo, a seven-transmembrane protein. Normally, Ptc represses the activity of Smo; however, when a ligand binds to Ptc, this derepresses Smo activity. Active Smo initiates a cytoplasmic

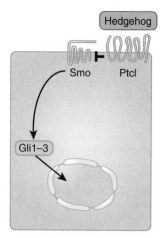

FIGURE 17-7. The Ptc1 gene product functions as both a receptor and negative regulator of signaling initiated by sonic hedgehog or the related ligands, Indian hedgehog and desert hedgehog. These ligands initiate an unusual and incompletely understood signaling pathway that culminates in Gli1-3 initiating transcription of cell cycle genes, including cyclin D1, D2.

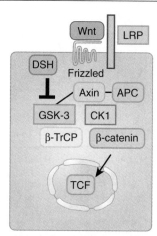

FIGURE 17-8. Wnts are a family of ligands that can act through two distinct signaling pathways. The canonical Wnt pathway is initiated when Wnt proteins bind to cell-surface receptors of the Frizzled family. This leads to activation of Dishevelled family proteins. When Dishevelled (DSH) becomes activated, it inhibits a protein complex that includes axin, GSK-3, and APC. The axin/GSK-3/APC complex usually promotes degradation of β-catenin. After this β-catenin destruction complex is inhibited, cytoplasmic β-catenin becomes stabilized so that it is able to enter the nucleus. Nuclear β-catenin interacts with the TCF family transcription factors to promote expression of a gene program that includes cyclin-D and thereby stimulates cell cycle progression.

signaling complex that includes a transcription factor of the Gli family (Gli1-3) and microtubule-associated components, such as suppressor of fused. This signaling complex results in the nuclear relocalization of Gli family members and increased expression of Gli family members, as well as the expression of N-myc, D-type cyclins, and the stem cell–associated chromatic complex component, Bmi-1. The active pathway thereby potentiates proliferation and inhibits apoptosis.

There is good evidence that constitutive activity of this pathway can cause medulloblastoma. Gorlin's syndrome is associated with increased incidence of medulloblastoma, as is the analogous mutation in mice. Activating mutations in Smo, or mutations in suppression of fused, can also lead to these brain tumors. Recent studies have suggested that specific inhibitors of Smo may provide valuable biologic therapies for medulloblastoma.

The value of understanding developmental pathways that normally regulate neural precursor proliferation to decipher the mechanisms that cause pediatric brain tumors is reinforced by data that Shh ligand stimulates and regulates proliferation of granule cell precursors and neural stem cells. Thus, it is perhaps not surprising that the Shh-responsive gene *Gli1-3* is expressed in gliomas and that inhibitors of Shh signaling may likewise play a role in treating gliomas.[88]

Turcot's Syndrome

Turcot's syndrome is characterized by familial polyposis of the colon, together with malignant brain tumors. This disorder can be caused by mutations in the adenomatous polyposis coli gene (*APC*, on chromosome 5q21) or in the mismatch repair genes *MLH1* (120436) or *PMS2* (600259). The distinction between the clinical entities that result from mutations in *APC* and mutations in repair genes[89] include the nature of the brain tumors seen; the characteristic brain tumors seen are medulloblastomas or astrocytomas, respectively. APC is a large protein whose activity is critical in the Wnt signaling pathway. Therefore, inactivating mutations of *APC* result in the aberrant accumulation of β-catenin and increased transcription of Tcf4-dependent genes, including *c-myc*. Mutations in β-catenin and in APC have also been reported in sporadic medulloblastoma,[89]

highlighting the importance of this pathway for this malignant cerebellar tumor.

Wnts constitute a family of ligands that can act through two distinct signaling pathways. The canonical Wnt pathway is initiated when Wnt proteins bind to cell-surface receptors of the Frizzled family. This leads to activation of Dishevelled family proteins. When Dishevelled (DSH) becomes activated, it inhibits a protein complex that includes axin, GSK-3, and APC (Fig. 17-8). The axin–GSK-3–APC complex promotes the proteolytic degradation of β-catenin. After this β-catenin destruction complex is inhibited, cytoplasmic β-catenin becomes stabilized and β-catenin is then able to enter the nucleus. Nuclear β-catenin interacts with TCF-LEF family transcription factors to promote the expression of a gene program that includes *c-myc*, *N-myc*, and *cyclin D1* and thereby stimulate cell cycle progression (Fig. 17-9). It is not clear whether the noncanonical Wnt pathway, which does not involve APC, also contributes to brain tumors.

As is the case for Shh signaling, the ability of deregulated Wnt pathway to cause medulloblastomas highlights the relevance of understanding neurodevelopment. In the absence of wnt1, the cerebellum does not form properly.[90] The Wnt and Shh pathways cooperate during normal development to generate normal cerebellar neurons. It is likely that these pathways also synergize in tumor formation, particularly during medulloblastoma oncogenesis.

Lhermitte-Duclos Disease, Cowden's Syndrome, and *PTEN* Mutation

Activation of PI3 kinase results in phosphorylation of phospholipids at the 3′ position; this phosphorylation is removed by the *PTEN* (phosphatase and tensin homologue) phosphatase. Therefore, mutations in *PTEN* result in excess and/or incorrectly localized activation of the PI3 kinase pathway. PI3 kinase is critical in several signaling pathways that regulate prolifera-

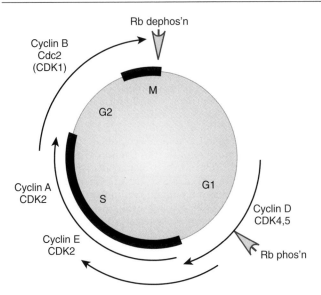

FIGURE 17-9. Cell cycle diagram. Oncogenic events can increase cyclin-D (i.e., hedgehog or Wnt signals) or alter other cell cycle regulators.

tion, survival, migration, and cell size. The multiplicity of functions explains the diverse spectrum of disorders seen in *PTEN* mutations, including neurologic, cutaneous, and oncologic syndromes.

Molecular studies on Lhermitte-Duclos disease tissue have revealed *PTEN* gene mutations in 83% of cases, with immunostaining showing lost or reduced *PTEN* expression in 78% of cases. As a consequence, there is increased Akt phosphorylation.[91] Initially, Cowden's syndrome was described as a familial predisposition for breast cancers, thyroid cancers, brain tumors, and other neoplasia. This syndrome was subsequently recognized as a spectrum of disorders that includes Lhermitte-Duclos disease and Bannayan-Ruvalcaba-Riley syndrome. The diagnosis of Lhermitte-Duclos disease depends on characteristic hamartomas of the cerebellum. These lesions in the cerebellar cortex exhibit thickened cerebellar folia, with misplaced cerebellar granule cells and enlarged size of the cerebellar neuronal cell bodies. In addition to cerebellar ataxia, these hamartomas can cause hydrocephalus and herniation. Another manifestation of the *PTEN* mutations is seen in Bannayan-Ruvalcaba-Riley syndrome, with macrocephaly, seizures, cognitive dysfunction, and autistic behaviors. Different manifestations of the mutation can be seen even within a family, so a careful consideration of family history is warranted.

Rb Mutations

The retinoblastoma gene was the first tumor suppressor gene identified. In addition to the retinal tumors seen in those with germline mutations in *Rb*, "trilateral" retinoblastoma has been described. In these individuals, bilateral retinoblastoma is accompanied by a pineal tumor (pineoblastoma) with similar characteristics to retinoblastoma. The other secondary tumors seen in patients with retinoblastoma are osteosarcomas. The Rb protein is required for the G1 checkpoint, and studies on this pathway have provided key insights into the mechanisms of growth regulation.

Atypical Teratoid Rhabdoid Tumor

Mutations in the SNF5/INI component of the SWI-SNF DNA remodeling complex cause rhabdoid tumors. These include renal and soft tissue tumors as well as brain tumors. In the CNS, these brain tumors, called atypical teratoid rhabdoid tumors, are characteristically found in the cerebellopontine angle or in supratentorial locations. Prior to the identification of their genetic mutation on chromosome 22, these tumors were historically grouped with medulloblastomas and primitive neuroectodermal tumors. However, their histology is distinct, with a mixture of atypical spindle cells, poorly differentiated small round blue cells, and rhabdoid cells with prominent cytoplasmic inclusions, large eccentric vesicular nuclei, and adjacent whorls of intermediate filaments. The cell of origin for these tumors, and why they predominantly arise in very young children, are as yet poorly understood.

CONCEPTUAL ORGANIZATION OF PEDIATRIC BRAIN TUMORS

Leukemias are considered in the context of their lineage and stage of development, whereas neuroblastoma is evaluated by the extent of spread, age of the child, and molecular phenotype. Neither of these approaches is well suited to CNS tumors. Although brain tumors share an anatomic site, there are a number of unique cell types, significant heterogeneity in distribution, and differences in the consequence of therapy that differ by age of the patient and location within the CNS. These factors, combined with a complicated historical nomenclature, require us to take a different approach to understanding these tumors.

The central nervous system is made up of three major elements and therefore three major groups of tumors are commonly observed:

1. Glial cells—responsible for structural support and maintenance of the CNS, and composed of three cell subtypes
   a. Astrocytes—structural support for the CNS → astrocytoma
   b. Ependycytes—help regulate homeostasis of the CNS → ependymoma
   c. Oligodendrocytes—myelination for the neural axons → oligodendroglioma
2. Neurons—electrical activity → medulloblastoma, pineoblastoma, CNS PNETs
3. Choroid plexus—production of cerebrospinal fluid (CSF) → choroid plexus carcinoma

Tumors arising from glia, neurons, or the choroid plexus account for approximately 90% of all pediatric CNS tumors. The remaining 10% of pediatric brain tumors arise from cells that are derived from extracranial sources but become entrapped in the developing CNS during embryogenesis (Fig. 17-10).

4. Germ cells, which arise in the primordial gonadal ridge and normally migrate down to their final resting place in the abdomen (ovaries) or scrotum (testes), can occasionally migrate upward and become enveloped in the developing brain → germinoma, nongerminomatous germ cell tumor (NGGCT).
5. Cells from Rathke's pouch, which normally gives rise to structures of the head and neck, can become trapped within the developing brain → craniopharyngioma.

Two additional tumor types that are rare in children but account for approximately 80% of CNS tumors in adults include metastatic carcinoma, especially breast, colon, lung, and prostate. Metastatic lesions to the brain in pediatric patients are exceptionally rare and, when they occur, are usually in the context of end-stage disease.[92-94] Meningiomas are the other common adult brain tumor that is rarely observed in children.

The five primary cell types of the brain are not evenly distributed in the central nervous system (Fig. 17-11):

1. Glia
   a. Astrocytes are found throughout the entire brain and spine.
   b. Ependycytes predominate in the posterior fossa.
   c. Oligodendrocytes are found around the junction of the gray-white matter.
2. Neural tumors are defined by location rather than histology.
   a. Medulloblastoma is found within the posterior fossa.
   b. Pineoblastoma is found within the pineal region.
   c. CNS PNETs can be found anywhere in the brain or spine.
3. Choroid plexus is predominantly located in the lateral ventricles.

4. Germ cell tumors are localized to the suprasellar region, the pineal area, or both.
5. Craniopharyngiomas are found within the suprasellar region.

Brain tumors tend to spread in one of two ways, by direct invasion into adjacent regions with focal expansion of the primary mass or by dissemination (seeding) of cells through the CSF, with resultant multifocal disease. Of the five tumor types listed, glial tumors and craniopharyngiomas tend to grow by direct extension and the other three tend to grow by seeding cells into the CSF. The workup of patients with newly diagnosed brain tumors will therefore require CT and MRI of the involved area for glial tumors and craniopharyngioma; craniospinal imaging and CSF cytology will be needed for seeding tumors (neural, choroid plexus, germ cell).

There are three major treatment strategies for all CNS tumors: (1) surgery, (2) radiotherapy, and (3) chemotherapy. Certain general principles can be applied to their use (Table 17-2):

1. Surgery is important for making the diagnosis, achieving rapid reduction in tumor size, and relieving elevated pressure from obstructive hydrocephalus.
2. Radiotherapy is effective for a wide range of tumors but has significant morbidity on the developing central nervous system, which frequently limits its applicability. In general, focal tumors (gliomas and craniopharyngiomas) are treated with focal radiation therapy, while seeding tumors (medulloblastoma, pineoblastoma, CNS PNETs, choroid plexus carcinoma, and germ cell tumors) are treated with craniospinal radiotherapy with a boost to the primary site and areas of metastatic disease, particularly in children 3 years and older.
3. Chemotherapy is effective for most seeding tumors and has become part of the initial therapy for these tumors (neural, choroid plexus and germ cell). By contrast, chemotherapy has had limited success for focal tumors (gliomas and craniopharyngiomas).

The classification of tumors based on their histologic characteristics is important in terms of providing prognostic information, although the unique environment of the brain makes the classification of benign versus malignant less important than for most other sites in the body. The brain and spine are critical for the control of basic autonomic response as well as higher

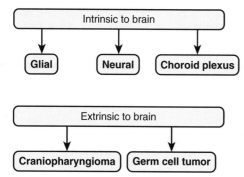

FIGURE 17-10. Most pediatric brain tumors can be classified into one of five different categories, based on cell of origin. Glial, neuronal, and choroid plexus tumors account for those that derive from cells within the central nervous system (CNS), although germ cell tumors and craniopharyngiomas arise from cells that are enclosed in the developing CNS in early development caused by abnormal migration.

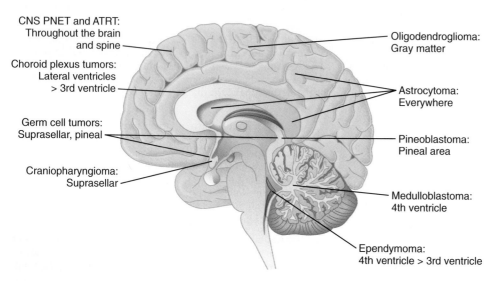

FIGURE 17-11. Common distributions of different pediatric central nervous system tumor histologies.

TABLE 17-2	Common Types of Treatment for Pediatric Central Nervous System Tumors*			
Type of Tumor	**Method of Spread**	**Attempted Surgery**	**Type of Radiation Therapy[†]**	**Chemotherapy**
Glial	Local	Yes	Focal	No[‡]
Neuronal	Seeding	Yes	CSI	Yes
Choroid	Seeding	Yes	CSI	Yes
Germ cell	Seeding	Yes	CSI	Yes
Cranio	Local	Yes	Focal	No

*Five major categories.
[†]Radiation therapy is often deferred in children younger than 3 years of age.
[‡]Certain low-grade gliomas are treated with chemotherapy to delay radiation therapy.
CSI, craniospinal irradiation.
Note: Tumors that exhibit focal growth receive attempted resection and focal radiation therapy. Tumors that are at high risk for early dissemination are treated with focal surgery, CSI, and chemotherapy.

order function and therefore limit the ability to obtain complete resection with a wide margin in most cases. Even benign tumors located in critical and inoperable structures may result in death if their growth cannot be stopped or slowed. Conversely, many highly malignant World Health Organization (WHO) grade IV brain tumors (defined histologically) that are responsive to radiation treatment (CNS germinoma) or radiation and chemotherapy (medulloblastoma) have an excellent prognosis. Because patients and their parents have preconceived notions about the importance of benign versus malignant, clarifying these terms early can be important.

The presenting symptoms for patients with CNS tumors can usually be categorized into one of two patterns, (1) direct compression of nerves or (2) obstructive hydrocephalus. The location of the tumor, histologic subtype, and age of the patient are major determinants in the length of clinical symptoms before the diagnosis is made.[95] Although dependent on the location and rapidity of growth, the time to diagnosis for many children may range from 3 to 8 months and multiple visits to primary care providers is not infrequent.[96] For younger children who cannot verbalize their symptoms and for whom fine motor coordination, speech, and gait are still developing, even greater delays may result.

Symptoms related to the direct compression of adjacent nerves by a tumor will cause a unique constellation of symptoms that can be localized to an area as a result of the highly organized structure of the CNS.

- The posterior fossa contains the brainstem, 12 cranial nerves, and the descending and ascending fibers connecting the upper and lower aspects of the CNS, in addition to the cerebellum, which is responsible for movement and balance. Tumors in this area result in cranial nerve dysfunction such as diplopia, choking, or facial asymmetry. Tumors of the brainstem can compress the descending motor tracts, resulting in lower motor deficits. Compression of the cerebellum will lead to ataxia or dysmetria.
- The thalamus is the major relay station of coordinated function from the motor strip and other areas of the cortex. Tumors in this area will often lead to significant hemiparesis.
- The frontal lobe regulates mood and behavior and contains the motor cortex. Patients with tumors in this area will often present with changes in behavior (more aggressive or more passive), worsening school performance, or specific motor deficits (except those controlled by the cranial nerves).[97,98] In some patients, more subtle signs of frontal lobe dysfunction such as fatigue, lack of interest, or decreased energy can be mistaken for the behaviors frequent in adolescence.
- The parietal lobe possesses the centers for sensory function. Tumors in this area can often compress a specific area of the

sensory cortex, resulting in a focal sensory deficit that does not follow classic dermatomal or peripheral nerve patterns.
- The hypothalamus and suprasellar regions contain the area that coordinates endocrine function (growth hormone, regulation of salts, pubertal development, and stress hormones). This area is near the optic nerves and chiasm. Tumors in this area often present as a change in growth (accelerated or delayed) or changes in vision.
- The occipital lobe organizes and interprets vision. Tumors in the occipital lobe will present with homonymous defects in vision.
- The pineal area sits adjacent to the centers of upward gaze (supranuclear tectal or pretectal areas). Lesions in this area can result in Parinaud's syndrome (paresis of upward gaze, enlarged pupils that are poorly reactive to light, and poor or limited convergence).
- The spinal cord possesses all the ascending and descending tracks for sensory and motor function to all areas innervated from that segment of the cord and below. Mass lesions in this area will reduce the motor and/or sensory activity of those areas below the lesion and can consist of motor, sensory, temperature, position, and vibration abnormalities.
- Gray matter is where neuron bodies are concentrated. Lesions in the gray matter of the frontal, parietal, temporal, and occipital lobes can result in seizure activity.[99] Although initially focal in nature, seizures can rapidly become generalized, obscuring the initial presenting focality.
- White matter tracts are the myelinated axons of neurons. Lesions in white matter tracts typically result in focal neurologic deficits that correspond to the tracts compressed.

Development of a differential diagnosis of a new tumor of the CNS can easily be developed using the preceding information. Symptoms will help localize the probable site of the tumor. In turn, the site will assist in developing a limited differential diagnosis of possible tumors at that site. Staging and treatment can then be considered in the context of focal versus seeding tumors. Although this exercise will not obviate the need for a definitive biopsy, it can help organize the large array of CNS tumors and ensure that appropriate presurgical planning and staging have been completed.

Obstructive Hydrocephalus and Raised Intracranial Pressure

The brain and spine float in the cranium and spinal canal, supported by CSF, which is largely localized to the subarachnoid space. CSF is initially made by the choroid plexus in the lateral ventricles and, to a lesser degree, in the third and fourth

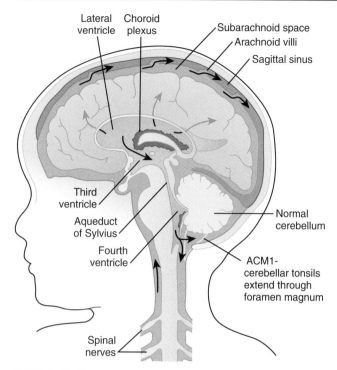

Lateral ventricle
Choroid plexus
Subarachnoid space
Arachnoid villi
Sagittal sinus
Third ventricle
Aqueduct of Sylvius
Fourth ventricle
Spinal nerves
Normal cerebellum
ACM1-cerebellar tonsils extend through foramen magnum

FIGURE 17-12. Normal flow of CSF. Blue arrows show compression of cortex due to obstructive hydrocephalus.

ventricles. The production of CSF is not linked to its passage from the lateral and third ventricles to the fourth ventricle and finally through the foramen of Magendie or foramen of Luschka, where it is eventually reabsorbed by the arachnoid villi (Fig. 17-12). The ventricles hold approximately 50 mL of CSF and, with approximately 500 mL of CSF produced each day, any failure to remove old CSF in the context of continued production will cause the fluid-filled ventricles to expand like water balloons in the closed cranium. Obstruction anywhere above the exit from the ventricles to the subarachnoid space (posterior fossa or above) will therefore result in obstructive hydrocephalus. The speed with which the accumulation of fluid occurs will in part determine the rapidity of the symptoms, as well as their severity. Obstructive hydrocephalus is considered a medical emergency because progressive expansion of the ventricular volume will force the brain to be compressed in all directions, including downward, resulting in tonsillar herniation.

The three common symptoms of obstructive hydrocephalus include headaches, often severe in nature, that are thought to arise as a result of stretching of vessels and the pial surfaces. These can often be worsened by changes in body position or head motion. They can be dull, aching, or stabbing in nature. Because of the prevalence of headaches in the general population, it is their persistence and worsening in the context of other symptoms (morning vomiting, focal neurologic deficits) that usually trigger further investigation. Patients will often have vomiting (often associated with a headache), especially early in the morning on wakening. Whether this results from hydrostatic pressure changes when first getting up, resulting in compression of the area postrema, or changes in CNS homeostasis on wakening, as a result of more rapid breathing and CO_2 release, is unknown. Unfortunately, the significance of this finding is often overlooked and thought to be related to school avoidance or the flu. Many patients present with prolonged histories of intermittent morning vomiting and headache, sug-

gesting that this process can be partial and relieved by the vomiting, which itself causes raised intra-abdominal pressure and equilibration of the CSF pressure gradient. A third common symptom in children with hydrocephalus is blurring of the optic discs, related to the increase in intracranial pressure. Patients will often complain of blurring or double vision, as well as difficulty in upward gaze. These symptoms likely result from a constellation of factors, including compression of the brainstem and cranial nerve, as well as edema and swelling of the optic discs and pathways leading to vision. The final common symptom of obstructive hydrocephalus is the presence of lower motor deficits, likely because of compression of motor tracts within the brainstem as well as difficulties with balance and gait, related to pressure on the cerebellum.

The symptoms of obstructive hydrocephalus differ in infants, in whom the presence of open sutures permits the head to expand. This relieves the buildup of pressure and thus the associated symptoms. As their head size expands, infants may begin to show some signs of delay in gaining milestones. Careful attention to head circumference changes will help identify these infants early, independent of the cause of the obstruction.

CT imaging of the brain is a rapid method for confirming the presence of obstructive hydrocephalus. Without the need for contrast, images will demonstrate enlargement of the ventricles above the area of obstruction. MR images will show large ventricles on T1- and T2-weighted images. Best seen on fluid-attenuated inversion recovery (FLAIR) sequences, the presence of a bright signal around the ventricles is suggestive of transependymal flow, which is thought to result from the backward transduction of pressure from the ventricle to the brain parenchyma (Fig. 17-13).[100] Obstructive hydrocephalus is a surgical emergency and requires urgent intervention. For posterior fossa tumors, such as medulloblastoma, ependymoma, or low-grade astrocytoma, relief from obstruction can be achieved with resection of the tumor in most patients, thus avoiding the need for a separate CSF diversion procedure.[101]

IMAGING STUDIES

Neuroimaging

Imaging of brain tumors entails determining the size and site of origin of the lesion, establishing primary diagnosis, and planning treatment. Neuroimaging is critical for the appropriate placement of catheters for stereotactic biopsy, resection, planning of radiation, guided application of experimental therapeutics, and delineation of tumor from functionally important neuronal tissue. After treatment, imaging is used to quantify treatment response and extent of residual tumor. At follow-up, imaging helps determine tumor progression and differentiate recurrent tumor growth from treatment-induced tissue changes, such as radiation necrosis.[102] Imaging brain tumors in children presents unique challenges not encountered in adult imaging, including the need for sedation and consideration of the long-term effects on a growing child. Cranial CT and MRI remain the main modalities for the primary diagnosis of brain tumors. However, several other techniques are being increasingly used in the evaluation of this patient population, including positron emission tomography (PET), MR perfusion and diffusion, and MR spectroscopy.

CT is a rapid and inexpensive modality to assess fluid, blood, and calcification in the central CNS. As such, it is the first imaging procedure in children with a presumed intracranial bleed or raised intracranial pressure that might need immediate neurosurgical intervention. Other than for lesions arising from the skull vault and to assess calcified tumors, CT scans are used

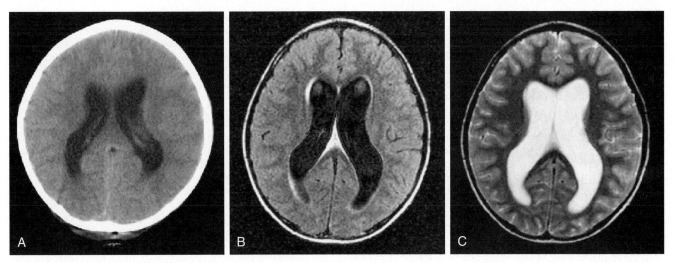

FIGURE 17-13. Hydrocephalus. **A,** Axial computed tomography (CT) noncontrast scan demonstrating significant enlargement caused by obstructive hydrocephalus. **B,** Axial fluid-attenuated inversion recovery (FLAIR) image demonstrates enlarged ventricles and transependymal flow suggestive of raised intracranial pressure. **C,** Axial T2-weighted image demonstrating enlarged ventricles.

less frequently for routine surveillance of pediatric patients because of an increase in long-term cancer risk caused by CT imaging.[42]

MRI is currently the modality of choice for localization and assessment of the size of brain tumors. MRI provides valuable information about secondary phenomena such as mass effect, edema, hemorrhage, necrosis, and signs of increased intracranial pressure. In addition, MRI provides excellent tissue contrast and high spatial resolution. Standard T1- and T2-weighted MRI sequences detect brain tumors with high sensitivity. Varying acquisition parameters, such as T1 or T2 weighting, techniques such as diffusion- and perfusion-weighted images, as well as FLAIR sequences, reveal a characteristic pattern of each tumor, depending on tumor type and grade. Susceptibility-weighted MRI is useful for detecting areas of hemorrhage, calcifications, and increased vascularity associated with brain tumors.[103] Recently, rapid-sequence MRI for the assessment of bleeds or hydrocephalus has been developed, which can avoid the radiation doses associated with CT scans and, like CT scans, can be performed without sedation, even in young children.[104]

Magnetic resonance spectroscopy (MRS) can also be helpful for the initial characterization of tumors[105,106]; it can also be used to differentiate tumor tissue from other tissue in children with CNS tumors in certain circumstances.[107] MRS has continued to evolve and the development of multivoxel and two-dimensional techniques has resulted in improved spatial resolution, thereby supplying additional information regarding tumor heterogeneity and intratumoral metabolite distribution. Although MRS is a sensitive technique, it still lacks specificity as a stand-alone technique in the clinical setting. In a recent study, brain proton MRS biomarkers were shown to predict survival of children with CNS tumors better than standard histopathology. More accurate prediction using this noninvasive technique represents an important advance and may suggest more appropriate therapy, especially when diagnostic biopsy is not feasible.[108] In general, decreased *N*-acetylaspartate (NAA) and creatine concentrations and increased choline concentrations correlate with tumor grade. Reduction of NAA is likely because of neuronal death or damage, although the reduction in creatine is likely to be a result of changes in cell energetics. The increase in choline is believed to reflect increased membrane synthesis. Increases in lipid and lactate concentra-

tions have been observed in some gliomas. Lactate accumulation is believed to be a result of central tumor necrosis.

Diffusion-weighted MR pulse sequences enable a quantitative and reproducible assessment of the diffusion changes, not only in areas exhibiting signal abnormality in conventional MR imaging but in areas of normal signal.[109] MR diffusion using predominantly echoplanar techniques has been useful in the characterization of tissue, tumor cellularity, tumor grading, tumor response to treatment, and distinction of tissue types.[110,111] Diffusion tensor imaging (DTI) provides visualization of fiber bundle direction and integrity, with in vivo characterization of the rate and direction of white matter diffusion. DTI is useful for presurgical planning or coregistration of tractography data with radiosurgical planning and functional MR imaging data.[112] Fractional anisotropy (FA) using DTI may prove helpful for the assessment of treatment-induced white matter changes in children.[113,114]

The usefulness of diffusion-weighted imaging (DWI) for characterizing intracranial cystic or cystlike lesions has been demonstrated in a number of studies.[115-118] DWI has long been used to differentiate between epidermoid and arachnoid cysts.[118,119] Arachnoid cysts are characterized by free diffusion, whereas epidermoids have an apparent diffusion coefficient similar to that of brain parenchyma, thereby demonstrating restricted diffusion.[116] The usefulness of DWI in the distinction between ring-enhancing cerebral lesions, such as brain abscesses, cystic or necrotic high-grade glioma, or metastasis, has been shown in multiple studies during the past decade, although this differentiation continues to be a challenge.[120] The ring enhancement of a brain abscess can be indistinguishable from that of a cystic or necrotic high-grade glioma or metastasis. Other lesions that may also have a similar appearance are subacute ischemic infarction, resorbing hematoma, and demyelinating disease.[109] Abscesses demonstrate high signal on DW images and a reduced apparent diffusion coefficient (ADC) in a cystic ring-enhancing cerebral lesion.[119,120] ADC values have been assessed for differentiation between tumor types; however, there can also be overlap between certain tumor types, requiring additional evaluation.[111,121] A retrospective study of ADC values of brain tumors in 275 patients in a pediatric and adult population has reported a significant negative correlation between ADC and WHO astrocytic tumor grades II through IV.[121] Other comparisons included higher ADC of dysembryoplastic neuroepithelial tumors (DNTs) than that of astrocytic grade II tumors (100% accuracy) or other glioneuronal tumors, lower ADC of malignant lymphomas compared with glioblastomas and metastatic tumors, lower ADC of PNETs compared with ependymomas, and lower ADC of meningiomas compared with schwannomas. The ADC of craniopharyngiomas was higher than that of pituitary adenomas, whereas the ADC of epidermoid tumors was lower than that of chordomas. In meningiomas, the ADC was not indicative of malignancy grade or histologic subtype. DWI has also been used to obtain additional information regarding tumor type and grade. The reduction in extracellular space, as well as high nuclear-to-cytoplasmic ratios of some cancer cells, causes a relative reduction in ADC values.[110,122] In some studies, however, there was overlap of ADC values of high- and low-grade gliomas.[111] The presence of glycosaminoglycans such as hyaluronin in the extracellular space of some high-grade gliomas may decrease water content and cause a reduction in ADC values.[123] In addition, one pitfall of DWI is in the case of high-grade tumors that may exhibit necrosis, which can lead to high ADC values.[124]

DWI and proton MRS have been evaluated as diagnostic tools in 17 children with posterior fossa lesions. Combining these approaches, MRI was successful in correctly identifying the histologic diagnosis in every case. Although this approach does not replace the pathologic diagnosis, it demonstrates the increasing accuracy of biologic-based imaging.[125,126] Similar results have been reported for ADC analysis.[127,128] DWI may also be helpful in differentiating postsurgical changes from tumor recurrence.[126] Diffusion-weighted images can also detect acute changes in white matter from methotrexate administration, which must be differentiated from progressive disease.[129]

Determination of the tumor margins is considered by many investigators to be extremely important for the management of brain tumors. Complete resection of tumors with minimal neurologic deficit is the ultimate goal of surgical resection. DWI has been shown in some studies to discriminate among tumor, infiltrating tumor, peritumoral edema, and normal brain parenchyma.[130,131] However, other studies have not found DWI to be helpful for evaluating tumor margins.[111,132]

MR diffusion imaging has also been assessed as a biomarker for early prediction of treatment response in patients with brain tumors. Recent studies have indicated the possibility of using functional diffusion map analysis as an early biomarker for treatment response preceding decrease in tumor size.[133,134] MR perfusion imaging is being increasingly used to evaluate cerebral perfusion dynamics by analysis of the hemodynamic parameters of relative cerebral blood volume (CBV), regional cerebral blood flow (rCBF), and mean transit time. CBV is the parameter most commonly quantified in brain tumors.[135] CBV is defined as the volume of blood in a region of brain tissue, commonly measured in mL/100 g of brain tissue. Cerebral blood flow (CBF) refers to the volume of blood/unit time passing through a given region of brain tissue, measured in mL/min/100 g of brain tissue. Mean transit time refers to the average time it takes blood to pass through a given region of brain tissue, commonly measured in seconds.[136] Perfusion imaging techniques include T2-weighted dynamic susceptibility techniques, arterial spin labeling (ASL) techniques, and T1-weighted dynamic contrast-enhanced perfusion techniques. These techniques use exogenous tracer agents, such as paramagnetic contrast material, or endogenous tracer agents, such as magnetically labeled blood (arterial water).[137] The most common method currently performed in the clinical setting is dynamic contrast-enhanced perfusion MR imaging with an exogenous tracer, such as gadopentetate dimeglumine (Gd-DTPA). It is assumed that the tracer is restricted to the intra-

vascular compartment and does not diffuse into the extracellular space. Imaging is performed dynamically (rapid imaging over time during a bolus injection) using echoplanar imaging–based spin echo or gradient echo sequences. It is thought that the spin echo sequences are more sensitive to capillary level blood vessels, whereas gradient echo techniques are more sensitive to the larger vessels.[138] Although gradient echo sequences are associated with more magnetic susceptibility artifacts, particularly in the posterior fossa, they are the more common of the two techniques. For young children and infants, there are challenges of intravenous access, smaller intravenous catheters, and limitations of contrast dose.

Dynamic T1-weighted contrast imaging can be used to assess microvascular permeability (Kps) in brain tumors.[139] Kinetic modeling of the dynamic signal changes can yield estimates of regional fractional blood volume (fBV) and Kps, which is an indicator of blood-brain barrier disruption and correlates with angiogenesis. This technique can be successfully performed in children, and applications of this technique may be useful for monitoring antiangiogenic therapies in pediatric patients with brain tumors.[140-142] ASL is an MR perfusion technique that does not use an IV contrast agent. The perfusion contrast in the image results from the subtraction of two successively acquired images, one with and one without proximal labeling of arterial water spins, with a magnetic gradient used to invert the magnetization of inflowing blood.[143] The signal-to-noise ratio, anatomic coverage, and shorter imaging time are currently better for the dynamic contrast perfusion techniques compared with ASL. However, ASL may have a future role in the imaging of pediatric brain tumors, particularly because it relies on a noninvasive endogenous contrast agent.[144]

A further advance in MRI imaging of brain tumors has come about with the availability of intraoperative scanners. These enable preoperative guidance for stereotactic biopsy and planning tumor resection, and review of the resection site for residual tumor prior to closure of the craniotomy.[145] Intraoperative DTI has been proposed to aid preservation of fiber tracts and minimize postoperative deficits.[146]

The use of PET and single-photon emission CT (SPECT) imaging continues to improve[147] and can be important in helping to differentiate treatment effect from tumor recurrence.[148-151] The usefulness of PET imaging is especially evident when a baseline evaluation is performed, so that postoperative changes can be evaluated in the context of the pretherapy PET avidity. This requires consideration of nuclear imaging early in the workup of these patients.[152,153]

Standardization of neuroimaging parameters for children with CNS tumors, and the testing of novel sequences that can be adapted to specific molecular inhibitors now being evaluated in this population, are being developed.[109,154]

Somatostatin receptor scintigraphy has been used to differentiate the presence of residual or recurrent tumor from scar and necrosis and is better than MRI scans for a number of pediatric tumor types.[155,156] Molecular imaging is likely to play an expanding role in neuro-oncology as more pathway specific inhibitors become available.

Posterior reversible leukoencephalopathy (PRES) is increasingly being identified in pediatric brain tumor patients, particularly in those with episodes of hypertension. Patients present with headaches, usually severe, mental and visual status changes, and seizures concurrent with hypertension and characteristic MRI findings, including T2 signal abnormalities.[157] MR imaging findings are those of vasogenic edema with T2 and FLAIR hyperintensities, involving predominantly the parietal and occipital regions bilaterally. The diffusion changes in PRES are traditionally thought to be represented by higher ADC values consistent with vasogenic edema. Focal areas of restricted diffusion (likely representing infarction–tissue injury with cytotoxic edema) are uncommon (11% to 26%) and may be associated with an adverse outcome.[158-162] Hemorrhage (focal hematoma, isolated sulcal-subarachnoid blood, or protein) is seen in approximately 15% of patients.[163,164] The parietal and occipital lobes are most commonly affected, followed by the frontal lobes, the inferior temporal-occipital junction, and the cerebellum.[163] Lesion confluence may develop as the extent of edema increases.

The mechanism of PRES remains controversial. Although the hypertension-hyperperfusion theory is favored because of the common presence of elevated blood pressure and perceived response to hypertension management. Key issues remain problematic, including PRES in normotensive patients with pressures rarely reaching autoregulatory limits, and brain edema lower in severe hypertensives. Hypertensive encephalopathy animal models do not reflect the systemic toxicity present, and hyperperfusion has not conclusively been demonstrated in patients.

Intracranial vasospasm has been seen with conventional and MR angiography, suggesting vasospasm as a possible pathophysiologic mechanism for the observed findings.[165] MR DWI was instrumental in establishing and consistently demonstrating that the areas of abnormality represent vasogenic edema. Prompt treatment with antihypertensive therapy or discontinuation of immunosuppressive agents can lead to complete recovery in some cases. However, if untreated, permanent neurologic deficits or even death may occur as a result of cerebral infarctions or hemorrhages[166] and 20% to 40% of patients with PRES can be normotensive.[167,168] PRES can be associated with a number of inciting events, including chemotherapy, radiation therapy, and antiangiogenic drugs.[169] This latter group of drugs may cause PRES as a result of their direct effect on vascular endothelial growth factor (VEGF) and raised blood pressure. Rapid recognition of this entity is critical to prevent permanent damage from occurring.

Surveillance Imaging

The role and usefulness of surveillance imaging for patients with a brain tumor remain controversial and depend on a number of factors, such as the age of the patient, histology of the tumor, time from diagnosis, and type of treatment. For example, in one study, only 9 of 318 imaging encounters identified an asymptomatic recurrence.[170] Other studies have demonstrated the cost-effectiveness of surveillance imaging,[171] recognizing that decisions are often made on the basis of insurance coverage. A common practice has been imaging every 3 months while on therapy (to assess continued response on therapy), and then every 3 months for the first year after completion of therapy. Beginning in year 2, scans are performed every 6 months for a year and then annually afterward. With time, the risk of tumor recurrence will go down, although the risks of radiation-induced vasculopathy and second tumors begin to increase. Modification of these guidelines for children with tumors at low risk of recurrence (completely resected craniopharyngioma or low-grade astrocytoma), or those who did not receive radiation therapy can be made on a case by case basis.

NEUROPATHOLOGY

The neuropathologic classification of pediatric brain tumors has evolved over the last century. Although multiple categorization systems have been developed, all suffer from an inherent problem—tumors are derived from a continuum of cell types and developmental stages whereas classification schema attempt to define criteria that put lesions into discrete categories. Categorizing tumors, however, can be helpful to guide therapy and estimate prognosis. A number of outstanding reviews on the classification of central nervous system tumors have been written.[172-180] When attempting to determine the treatment and/or prognosis of a tumor based on published reports or meeting abstracts, the classification schema used in those reports will become critical before applying this information to other patients.

Most current classification systems are based on the pioneering work of Cushing and Bailey almost 100 years ago. The major premise of this approach was to define tumors by their cell of origin, which continues today. This system was adapted by Kernohan when he proposed that certain tumors, especially those of glial origin, such as astrocytomas, ependymomas, and oligodendrogliomas, could be further classified by the degree of anaplasia. Most current systems now use these two criteria, cell of origin and degree of anaplasia, as the primary basis for classification of adult and pediatric CNS tumors. In spite of the usefulness of this classification schema, it is becoming progressively clear that brain tumors do not derive from a mature cell type, but rather from primitive precursors or stem cells that can differentiate down many different pathways, obscuring the cell of origin. Immunohistochemical analysis of tumor sections can help identify expression of cell type–specific markers, which are now used to support the presumed cell of origin of the tumor.

Significant advances have been made in the field of neuropathology. Less reliant on the appearance of cells under the microscope, neuropathology has embraced molecular classification for many tumors using highly specific immunohistochemical reagents.[173-176,181,182] In addition, the WHO classification of central nervous system tumors has recently been revised, with a number of important modifications.[183] A simplified WHO 2007 classification system is provided in Table 17-3. When combined with immunohistochemical analysis and the increasing use of cytogenetic classification and molecular profiling, the classification of tumors continues to become more defined. A simplified overview of the chromosomal abnormalities associated with pediatric brain tumors is presented in Table 17-1. For many large consortium-based studies in both Europe and North America, molecular profiling of tumors to ensure proper classification is now required, especially for medulloblastoma and atypical teratoid/rhabdoid tumors (ATRTs).

The immunohistochemical patterns used to classify CNS tumors require considerable experience on the part of the neuropathologist, as well as appropriate controls. Most markers lack specificity, can be identified in a wide array of histologies, and thus require interpretation by an experienced neuropathologist. Common markers used to classify pediatric CNS tumors are provided in Table 17-4. Three commonly used immunohistochemical markers are glial acidic fibrillary protein (GFAP), which stains glial cells (Fig. 17-14); synaptophysin, which stains neurons (Fig. 17-15); and Ki-67, which stains cells that have left G0 cell cycle and are at some stage of cellular division (Fig. 17-16).

TREATMENT STRATEGIES

Neurosurgery

The neurosurgeon is usually the first of the specialized team of caregivers called to see a child with a brain tumor, frequently from the emergency room or radiology department. The imme-

TABLE 17-3	Simplified World Health Organization Classification of Pediatric Central Nervous System Tumors		
Type	**Subtype**	**Example(s)**	**Grade**
Glial Tumors	Astrocytic tumors	Pilocytic astrocytoma	I
		Subependymal giant cell astrocytoma	I
		Pilomyxoid astrocytoma	II
		Pleomorphic xanthroastrocytoma	II
		Diffuse (fibrillary) astrocytoma	II
		Anaplastic astrocytoma	III
		Glioblastoma multiforme	IV
		Gliosarcoma	IV
		Gliomatosis cerebri	III-IV
	Oligodendroglial tumors	Oligodendroglioma	II
		Oligoastrocytoma	II
		Anaplastic oligodendroglioma	III
		Anaplastic oligoastrocytoma	III
	Ependymal tumors	Subependymoma	I
		Myxopapillary ependymoma	I
		Ependymoma	II
		Anaplastic ependymoma	III
Neural/Embryonal Tumors		Medulloblastoma	IV
		Pineocytoma	I
		Pineal parenchymal tumor of intermediate differentiation	II-III
		Papillary tumor of the pineal region	II-III
		Pineoblastoma	IV
		Primitive neuroectodermal tumor (PNET) (medulloepithelioma, ependymoblastoma)	IV
		Atypical teratoid-rhabdoid tumor	IV
Choroid Plexus Tumors		Choroid plexus papilloma	I
		Atypical choroid plexus papilloma	II
		Choroid plexus carcinoma	III
Germ Cell Tumors	Germinoma		III
	Non-germinoma	Embryonal carcinoma	III
		Yolk sac tumor	III
		Choriocarcinoma	III
		Mature teratoma	0
		Teratoma	I
		Immature teratoma	III
		Teratoma with malignant transformation	III
Craniopharyngioma	Craniopharyngioma	Adamantinomatous	I
		Papillary	I
Other	Mixed glial neuronal tumor	Ganglioglioma	I
		Gangliocytoma	I
		Anaplastic ganglioglioma	III
		Dysembryoplastic neuroepithelial tumor	I
		Desmoplastic infantile astrocytoma	I
		Central neurocytoma	II
		Extraventricular neurocytoma	II
	Neuroepithelial	Astroblastoma	—
	Nerve tumors	Schwannoma	I
		Neurofibroma	I
		Malignant peripheral nerve sheath tumor (MPNST)	II-IV
	Meningeal	Meningioma	I
		Atypical meningioma	II
		Anaplastic meningioma	III
		Hemangioblastoma	I

diate task of a neurosurgeon is to evaluate the patient, establish his or her stability and risk for rapid decompensation, and determine a plan that encompasses the ability to diagnose and/or treat the patient.[184-186] The most important function of neurosurgeons is to know their limitations and the circumstances that will influence the outcome of the patient.

Neurosurgery has seen remarkable advances in technology, from intraoperative microscopes, robotics, and computer-assisted navigation to intraoperative MR imaging.[187,188] Each of these has been instrumental in reducing the morbidity of neurosurgical procedures while ensuring that all of the ressectable disease is removed.

Acute Management Issues

The acute management of patients often starts with a CT scan to determine the degree of hydrocephalus. Because the severity of hydrocephalus is based on the amount of accumulated fluid,

TABLE 17-4	Immunohistochemical Markers of Pediatric Central Nervous System Tumors
Marker	**Tumor**
Glial fibrillary acidic protein (GFAP)	Astrocytoma, oligodendroglioma, ependymoma, choroid plexus papilloma, PNET, ATRT
Synaptophysin/NeuN	PNETs, ganglial tumor, neurocytoma
MIB-1/Ki-67	Measures all cells not in G0
Mitotic rate	Measures cells in mitosis
Neurofilament proteins (NFP):	Ganglial tumor, PNET, neurocytoma, subependymal giant cell tumor, ATRT
S-100 and neuron-specific enolase (NSE)	Normal and neoplastic glial and neuronal in origin
Retinal S-antigen	Pineal parenchymal tumor, PNET, retinoblastoma
Desmin	Muscle tumor, teratoma, PNET
Smooth muscle actin	Muscle tumor, ATRT
Cytokeratin	Chordoma, choroid plexus tumor, meningioma, some malignant gliomas, nongerminomatous germ cell tumor, PNET, ATRT
Epithelial membrane antigen (EMA)	Meningioma, ependymoma, teratoma, ATRT
Vimentin	Mesenchymal tumor, meningioma, sarcoma, melanoma, ependymoma, astrocytoma, chordoma, schwannoma, PNET, ATRT
Alpha-fetoprotein	Embryonal carcinoma, endodermal sinus (yolk sac) tumor
Human chorionic gonadotropin (β-HCG)	Germinoma, choriocarcinoma
Placental alkaline phosphatase	Germ cell tumor

ATRT, atypical teratoid/rhabdoid tumor; PNET, primary neuroectodermal tumor.

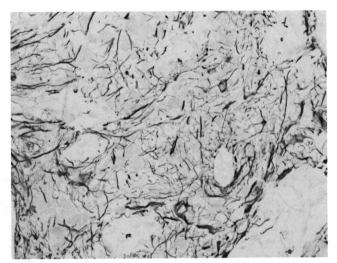

FIGURE 17-14. Glial acidic fibrillary protein (GFAP) staining of astrocytic cells in a child with glioblastoma multiforme (×400).

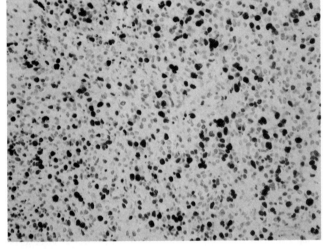

FIGURE 17-16. Ki-67 immunohistochemical staining in glioblastoma multiforme (×200).

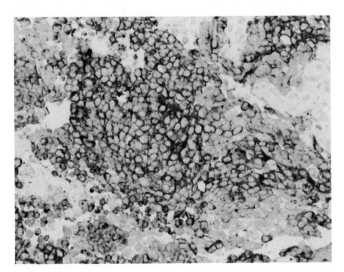

FIGURE 17-15. Synaptophysin immunohistochemical staining of medulloblastoma (×400).

but also the speed at which it has increased, experience in the assessment of the radiographic images and correlation with the patient's neurologic status is important. High-dose steroids will often produce significant relief in symptoms as peritumoral edema is suppressed. Intravenous mannitol is another rapid but transient method used to reduce intracerebral swelling and thus buy additional time before action is taken. Both of these are temporary approaches that can delay but usually not prevent the need for other aggressive intervention. Patients with suprasellar tumors can also have inadequate cortisol production or electrolyte disturbances, which need to be addressed as quickly as possible and often in concert with preparation for surgery.[189]

Because raised intracranial pressure resulting from the tumor is a medical emergency, relief of the pressure can be life-saving. Although this was previously achieved through the insertion of a ventricular-peritoneal catheter that shunts CSF around the obstruction, pediatric centers with sufficient expertise now routinely often use a third ventriculostomy to bypass the blockage.[190,191] This latter technique does not require the insertion of any artificial material or shunt that can become blocked, infected, or outgrown, but rather places a small communication between the third ventricle and subarachnoid space using an endoscope placed into the lateral ventricles and then guided to the correct location. A third ventriculostomy will not work with tumors filling the third ventricle, but for most pediatric patients, in whom fourth ventricular tumors predominate, this technique can save the patient a number of long-term morbidities. Like all complex procedures, there are rare but significant neurologic risks associated with this procedure in approximately 1% of cases.[192] The possibility of closure of a third ventriculostomy and resultant acute hydrocephalus requires careful consideration.

Certain tumors do not require routine biopsy or attempted resection at diagnosis (e.g., diffuse pontine gliomas, classic optic pathway tumors in children with NF-1, some suprasellar or pineal lesions with positive serum or CSF tumor markers). For tectal gliomas, biopsy or resection may only incur the potential morbidity of a surgical procedure and not affect the long-term survival rate. The leading factor in the outcome of a child with a brain tumor is not the presenting symptoms, age of the child, or the final pathology. Rather, it is the experience of the neurosurgeon performing the operation and the number of similar procedures performed over the prior few years.[193] With increasing cure rates in children with CNS tumors, careful consideration of the neurosurgical morbidity, which can often be lifelong, needs to be taken into account as a treatment plan is developed.

Endoscopic Procedures

Recent advances in image guided neurosurgical techniques have been considerable. Endoscopic procedures provide minimally invasive techniques to address not just obstructive hydrocephalus but also biopsy or resection of intracranial masses, with minimal morbidity in experienced hands.[194] New techniques using intraoperative ultrasound have been developed and are being used in pediatric patients.[195] Three-dimensional laser-guided maps can assist in the orientation and surrounding environment of the tumor during a procedure. More recently, intraoperative MRI facilities now allow surgeons to use MRI procedures with the same magnet strength as that used for diagnostic imaging while operating.[196] Real-time MRIs can assist the neurosurgeon in the detection of residual disease or hemorrhage before closure of the resection site.[197]

The surgical approach used by the neurosurgeon will depend on a number of factors that must balance the need for diagnosis with the potential risks of operating in a given area.[198] As the relative risks of general anesthesia and neurosurgical procedures continue to diminish with improving techniques, it is now common to perform staged operations in which a limited resection is done to confirm the diagnosis. Based on the pathologic results obtained, decisions about more complicated or risky surgery can be considered for those lesions in which complete resection is a critical component of improved outcome and deferred in those lesions in which additional resection would not significantly alter prognosis but could cause significant morbidity. Specialized techniques such as endonasal endoscopic approaches can allow a minimally invasive approach, with excellent outcome in centers with expertise in this approach.[199]

The need of neurosurgeons to be aware of the evolving treatment strategies for children reinforces the role of the multidisciplinary team. Over the last 5 years, this need has become even more important, because many pediatric brain tumors now require molecular classification to guide therapy. For example, in spite of their similar appearance, the treatment of posterior fossa medulloblastoma now differs significantly from posterior fossa ATRT. Treatment on national protocols therefore requires submission of fresh-frozen material obtained at the time of surgery for proper stratification on therapy protocols. As our molecular classification of pediatric brain tumors expands, and newer and better molecular inhibitors of specific pathways become available, the role of the neurosurgeon and neuropathologist in ensuring the proper processing of these samples will continue to expand.

A number of factors must be considered for the child having completed a tumor-based procedure. The rate of weaning steroids after an operation will depend on many factors, including the histology, degree of resection, post-tumor edema, and patient status. Although most patients can be weaned rapidly off steroids after an operation, it is important that the members of the team have a coordinated structure so that as children pass from neurosurgical care to the radiation therapist or oncologist, that overall management of these issues is seamless. A similar discussion holds true for anticonvulsants. Whereas many patients will receive preoperative or perioperative anticonvulsant therapy, most can be weaned rapidly, and will therefore require communication among team members.

Perioperative Issues

Hyponatremia is a common problem that can occur after neurosurgical intervention and requires immediate recognition.[200] Two common conditions, both resulting in hyponatremia but needing different interventions, can occur. Cerebral salt wasting (CSW) occurs because of excess renal loss of sodium with volume depletion and has been associated with abnormally high atrial natriuretic peptide (ANP) or brain natriuretic peptide (BNP) levels, which block all stimulators of zona glomerulosa steroidogenesis, resulting in mineralocorticoid deficiency.[201] CSW usually occurs 1 to 2 days after neurosurgical intervention and patients typically demonstrate polyuria, dehydration, serum sodium less than 130 mEq/L, and excess urine sodium or urine osmolarity. Duration of CSW was 1 to 9 days in a study of 12 pediatric patients.[202] CSW is generally treated with salt repletion, although fludrocortisone supplementation has also been successful.[203] Syndrome of inappropriate diuretic hormone (SIADH), by contrast, results when water is preferentially retained, causing dilution of serum sodium. Patients present with hyponatremia and an elevated urine sodium level.[204] The major clinical difference between CSW and SIADH is that in the former, dehydration is common, whereas in SIADH, symptoms of dehydration are lacking. SIADH is treated with water restriction. CSW was much more common than SIADH in one study of 30 patients.[205]

Posterior fossa syndrome (or cerebellar mutism syndrome) is a complex and heterogeneous disorder that tends to occur 24 to 48 hours after resection of a posterior fossa tumor,[206] usually medulloblastoma, ependymoma, or low-grade astrocytoma. Up to 25% of patients undergoing surgical resection in the posterior fossa will develop posterior fossa syndrome and, in most, it will be severe.[206] The incidence of posterior fossa syndrome appears greatest when the cerebellar vermis is cut vertically to expose the fourth ventricle at the time of the operation, although patients have had this difficulty even when horizontal cuts to preserve fibers have been performed. Also, patients in whom elevation of the cerebellar vermis without surgical disruption was performed have developed posterior fossa syndrome, suggesting that direct disruption of the vermis is not the cause. This is further supported by the onset of posterior fossa syndrome 24 to 48 hours postprocedure rather than immediately postoperatively. The exact clinical patterns of posterior fossa syndrome can vary among patients both in constellation and severity. Usually, the disorder includes loss of speech in patients who were capable of talking immediately postoperatively. Other symptoms include irritability, which may relate to difficulties in communication, emotional withdrawal, and motor difficulties with ataxia.[206] In a review of 450 children from two large Children's Cancer Group (CCG) protocols for high-risk and standard-risk medulloblastoma, 107 patients (24%) had posterior fossa syndrome. It was classified as severe in 43%, moderate in 49%, and mild in 8%. As with many neurologic insults, most patients demonstrated significant improvement, although neurologic abnormalities persisted in a large proportion of patients.[207] There are no uniform diagnostic criteria for posterior fossa syndrome, and radiologic imaging with SPECT has failed to define a specific controlling neurologic region.[208]

Venous thrombosis in adults with brain tumors is common, especially when compared with adults undergoing operations for non–brain tumor-related causes[209,210] and typically require therapy. A similar predilection to significant symptomatic thrombosis in children with CNS tumors has not been identified.[211] Because of the risks of spontaneous hemorrhage in patients on anticoagulants, their routine use is discouraged for pediatric patients.[212] When thromboses in this patient population are identified, other precipitating factors such as the presence of a central venous access device[211] are usually evident.[213] CNS hemorrhage is rare in pediatric patients undergoing tumor resection. Use of recombinant factor VIIa has been used successfully when bleeding was difficult to control.[214]

Radiotherapy

A detailed section on the fundamentals of radiation oncology is included elsewhere in this text (see Chapter 8). The primary goal of this brief discussion is to focus on radiation therapy issues that are specific to pediatric neuro-oncology.[215] An understanding of the basic principles of radiation therapy is critical, because this remains one of the most effective, albeit toxic, therapies for this patient population. Much of radiation therapy relates to understanding the terminology and acronyms used.

Like chemotherapy, radiation therapy targets dividing cells, one of the hallmarks of cancer. Unlike chemotherapy, however, delivery of radiation therapy is not limited by the blood-brain barrier. Radiation therapy works by causing damage to the DNA of tumor cells, which by their very nature have lost the regulation required to repair DNA damage before entering cell replication. By contrast, normal adjacent cells that receive radiation therapy will repair the damage between fractions. After weeks of continued radiation therapy, normal cells will have repaired themselves, although the repair process is not perfect and accounts for the toxicity to normal brain caused by radiation therapy. Tumor cells, on the other hand, will have accumulated significant damage, hopefully enough to lead to cell death. The concept of fractionation is the hallmark of radiation therapy.

Types of Radiation Therapy

There are a large number of techniques available to radiation therapists and many of these continue to evolve over time. The two forms of radiation therapy used for most patients with CNS tumors are photon radiotherapy and proton radiotherapy. Both these forms of irradiation provide the same treatment dose to the tumor tissue and therefore their differences are not related to efficacy. Rather, the differences in the therapeutic beams and the physical properties associated with them result in different dose distributions. The major clinical difference between the two techniques relates to potential toxicities to the normal brain.

Photon Therapy

Photons are packets of high energy that enter tissue, depositing their energy as they pass through both normal tissue and the tumor, eventually exiting the brain. The presence of an exit dose is one of the major differences between this modality and proton therapy. The generation of photon beams is easily achieved with a large array of commercially available machines and, with over 60 years of clinical experience, photon radiotherapy remains the most widely used form of radiation therapy. Significant advances in this modality have occurred through the development of more sophisticated planning algorithms that allow the radiation therapist to focus the beam to the area of interest more effectively.

Opposed Lateral Fields. Used largely before 1990, these are composed of two beam arrangements, one from the left and the other from the right, and at angles so that they do not overlap, except over the tumor volume (because the exit dose of one would add on to the entry dose of the other). These fields also irradiate a large area of normal tissue with a high dose. Although there are long-term survivors of pediatric brain tumors who have been treated with this approach, using opposed lateral fields is rarely done because of the significant morbidity associated with irradiating large areas of uninvolved brain.

Three-Dimensional Conformal Radiation Therapy. This has been a major advance in the treatment planning of children with CNS tumors and has been made possible through the development of sophisticated computers with CT, MRI, and coregistration software. This technique uses the principle of tumor volume definition through MRI scans, with the anatomic localization of the bony structures of the skull using CT scans. When fused together, radiation therapists can use landmarks on the skull to ensure correct planning of beam placement to maximize tumor coverage while avoiding normal brain. With the development of more rapid and powerful computers, the ability to generate a large number of different beam orientations has allowed for diffusion of the radiation dose over normal tissue, thus reducing long-term damage while ensuring complete coverage of the tumor volume.[216]

Stereotactic Radiotherapy. Stereotactic radiotherapy (SRT) is a further improvement on three-dimensional (3-D) conformal therapy by ensuring improved head immobility so that beam configuration may be further reduced without having to worry about head position and tumor location.[217] In the normal delivery of the radiation beam, some head movement may occur; therefore, the target volume must be expanded in all directions to ensure that at no time is part of the tumor outside the targeted area. To overcome this, a series of techniques have been developed that use head immobilization to ensure less head movement and consequently smaller target volumes. Options for such immobilization include frames bolted to the skull and then fixed to the radiation device; this is the standard procedure for stereotactic radiation surgery (see later). The major limitation of this, however, is that radiation therapy is delivered over approximately 6 weeks and bolting screws into the skull for this length of time is not practical. A second option is the use of a head mask made for each patient, which fits around the face and skull and can sometimes use the ear canals or palate to ensure exact and reproducible fits. A new development is the use of real-time CT scans that constantly re-evaluate the position of the skull, with computer software that corrects for changes in head position to reset the beams accordingly. In children, the additional dose of radiation therapy from CT scans is not trivial and needs to be considered in the choice of method.

Intensity-Modulated Radiation Therapy (IMRT).

Intensity-modulated radiation therapy (IMRT) gives radiation therapists the opportunity to modulate the intensity of a radiation beam so that instead of uniform dosing throughout a volume, areas of decreased intensity may spare critical structures.[218] For example, if a critical nerve runs through or adjacent to a tumor, IMRT allows the radiation therapist to spare the middle, like a doughnut, while still treating the entire surrounding tumor. IMRT is usually a device that fits onto the gantry of a radiation machine that moves small metal slots in and out of the beam path as it moves in arcs to deliver the required fields. Large metal (macroleaf) and small metal (microleaf) pieces are available. The microleaf collimators allow for a more refined shaping of the field. An important limitation of this technique is the development of hot spots in areas within the field. As a general rule, this technique can be added to 3-D conformal and stereotactic radiation therapy treatment plans.

Stereotactic Radiosurgery.

Stereotactic radiosurgery (SRS) techniques (e.g., gamma knife, cyber knife, or X knife) use a single fraction (or occasionally several fractions) rather than the prolonged treatment courses that are standard with radiation therapy. As the names imply in these techniques, all develop a focused beam of energy that covers a tight volume and causes the cells within the volume to die.[219] Unlike traditional radiation therapy, in which normal cells recover between successive doses while tumor cells do not, the principle for this technique is similar to focusing sunlight with a magnifying glass to burn a small area. Because of the significant toxicities possible with a technique designed to kill a targeted area, a specific volume that excludes normal adjacent structures is critical. To achieve this, the head is often bolted into a metal head frame, performed under general anesthesia, and then the metal frame is bolted to the radiation device. In this way, there can be no additional or unintended movement that would have the targeted beam miss part of the tumor and damage uninvolved adjacent normal brain. New methods that can avoid the need for fixed head localization are being developed.[220]

Radiation Toxicity.

Even with the significant advances in the highly precise delivery of radiation therapy, there are a number of circumstances that limit its usefulness for children. Humans achieve their maximum number of brain cells shortly after birth. From that time forward, there is a steady loss of cells that continues throughout life. As we age, our neurocognitive development is related to the development of new connections and interactions between cells, not the addition of cells. For reasons that are poorly understood, radiation can affect not only the proliferation of new cells in infancy, but also the ability of cells already present to form or maintain connections in children and adolescents.

Three major factors that determine the severity of the impairment after radiation therapy are the age of the patient, the volume of the brain to be irradiated, and the dose of radiation therapy required.

1. *Age.* Because the age of the patient at diagnosis is not mutable, simply withholding radiation therapy until a child has had an opportunity to grow older would reduce the long-term morbidity, but this approach may allow a tumor to recur. As such, the decision between accepting toxicity or foregoing efficacy is not uncommon in pediatric practice.
2. *Volume.* Although neurocognitive development is most active from birth until the age of 3 years, significant development occurs up to the age of 10 years and even into adulthood. This implies that radiation therapy to large parts of the brain can cause detrimental effects on cognition throughout life. Because the volume of brain to be irradiated is determined by the extent of tumor spread, radiation therapists must treat the required volumes with all the associated long-term morbidity or reduce the volume to be treated with a corresponding reduction in the efficacy that radiation provides.
3. *Dose.* The third factor related to radiation toxicity is the dose used. Because most brain tumors require the use of maximal tolerated doses to have a significant clinical impact on outcome, reducing the dose would again require a tradeoff between toxicity reduction and efficacy reduction.

Specific toxicities of radiation therapy are discussed later.

Proton Radiotherapy

The use of proton beam radiation therapy as an alternative to high-energy x-rays (photons) has the potential to limit some of the late effects of radiation therapy by reducing the exposure of normal tissue.[221,222] Physically, photon beams deliver their maximum radiation dose near the surface, followed by a continuously reducing dose with increasing depth. Tissues outside the target area receive an exit dose of the radiation beams. For example, when a single posterior field is used to treat the spinal axis, critical organs along the path, such as the heart, lung, bowel, and ovaries, may receive significant exposure. In contrast, in proton beam radiotherapy, as the charged particles—namely protons—move through tissue, they ionize particles and deposit their radiation dose along the path. The maximal dose, called the Bragg peak, occurs shortly before the point of greatest tissue penetration, which is dependent on the energy of the proton beam. Because the energy can be precisely controlled, the Bragg peak can be placed within the tumor targeted to receive the radiation dose. Because the protons are absorbed at this point, normal tissues beyond the target receive little irradiation (Fig. 17-17).[223] The cost of proton facilities has hampered their widespread use in pediatric radiation therapy. As more facilities become available, some of the limitations on availability will be resolved. The significantly greater cost of this approach without increased efficacy has raised some concerns regarding the use of health care resources. For patients likely to be long-term survivors of certain brain tumors (e.g., medulloblastoma, low-grade gliomas, completely resected ependymomas), techniques that reduce morbidity, including doses to the pituitary or auditory apparatus, may be very cost-effective over the long term (Fig. 17-18).

As with all technical advances, the use of highly focused radiation therapy must take into account the biology of the lesion being treated. Tumors with infiltrative margins may not be optimal candidates for highly focused radiation therapy. Similarly, patients who require craniospinal radiation therapy are less likely to benefit from all the advantages of focused methodologies. With the increasing complexity of radiation planning, a dedicated pediatric radiation oncology team is required to ensure appropriate care for the pediatric patient.[224]

Chemotherapy

The approach and use of chemotherapy, like radiation therapy, does not differ significantly for most children with brain tumors when compared with children with other cancers. Similarly, the effects of antiseizure medications on chemotherapy mirror those of other patient populations and agents susceptible to altered metabolism by enzyme-inducing anticonvulsants, such as irinotecan, require appropriate dose adjustments or switching to a nonenzyme anticonvulsant.[225,226] This has resulted in

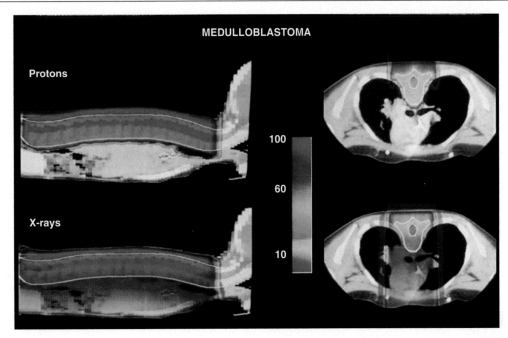

FIGURE 17-17. Different dose distribution between photon and proton therapy. Although efficacy between the two radiation techniques is the same (purple dose distribution covering the spinal cord and vertebral column), the ability to avoid radiation dose to areas uninvolved by tumor will reduce long-term morbidity (yellow dose areas anterior to the spine).

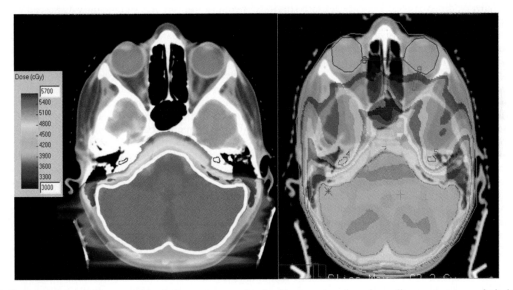

FIGURE 17-18. Proton therapy **(left)** can avoid exit dose to areas uninvolved by tumor, such as the auditory apparatus and pituitary fossa, which are commonly involved in photon field distribution **(right)**.

the development of many pediatric treatment regimens modified from adult studies. The increasing recognition of the unique nature of pediatric tumors in general and pediatric brain tumors in specific have led to the development of pediatric-specific preclinical models of cancer.[227] Incorporation of information from these models is likely to be slow as different combinations of chemotherapy, biologic therapies, and radiation therapy undergo evaluation.

Blood-Brain Barrier

The blood-brain barrier (BBB) results from the tight junctions of endothelial cells and astrocytic projections surrounding the brain that limit the penetration of substances, especially infections and inflammatory responses, from gaining access to the CNS. There is a slightly different barrier between the blood and CSF (called the blood-CSF barrier), although the primary role of the two systems remains the same—to isolate the brain from the entry of as many foreign chemicals and pathogens as possible.

As tumors develop, they grow and invade normal structures, which can disrupt the BBB. Tumors also need to secure a blood supply, and this can be achieved through the secretion of a large number of cytokines, the best characterized of which is VEGF. Before its discovery in stimulating angiogenesis, this molecule was initially discovered as vascular permeability factor

(VPF) because of its ability to open up endothelial junctions, allowing for changes in fluid shifts. The secretion of VEGF (VPF) by tumors is responsible for significant peritumoral edema and leakage of the BBB. For reasons that remain poorly understood at present, many tumors, or areas within tumors, do not demonstrate disruption of the BBB, making their detection on contrast-enhanced MRI scans more difficult.

General principles of chemotherapy administration in tumors of the central nervous system are similar to those of other tumors of the body. The CNS lacks a lymphatic system and, because of the presence of the BBB, extraneural metastases are uncommon. Thus, the goal of treatment remains focused on the brain and spine. Some agents may not fully penetrate through the BBB,[228,229] depending on the characteristics of the drug and local breakdown of the BBB. Although the chemical structure of compounds should be an important consideration in their predicted ability to penetrate the BBB, and thus have the potential for clinical activity, many hydrophilic drugs have demonstrated activity in brain tumors. However, some hydrophilic agents, which should easily traverse the BBB, do not. Even with extensive knowledge of the hydrophobicity of a drug, one cannot predict with certainty whether it will have activity in CNS tumors. The platinum drugs, for example, which would not be predicted to penetrate into the brain significantly, are active agents for various tumors in the brain and spine. This may in part relate to the breakdown of the blood-brain barrier around tumors, resulting in penetration of drugs into restricted areas. One important variable that can significantly affect BBB penetration is the degree of protein binding. To overcome this problem of drug delivery, direct application of drugs into surgical cavities or cysts is possible. Hydrostatic pressure gradients moving from tissue into an empty cavity draw most of the drugs away from the tumor and likely account for the limited activity of chemotherapeutic agent–impregnated wafers along the resection margin.

Intrathecal or Intraommaya Chemotherapy

Intrathecal administration of chemotherapy can overcome the blood-CSF barrier and is of importance in tumors with a predilection to seeding of the brain and spine. This technique is not safe in patients with obstructed CSF flow, but for those without this problem who also lack diversional shunts that would draw the drugs out of the CSF spaces, high concentrations can be delivered.[230] Because repeated access to the lumbar spine can be uncomfortable, insertion of an ommaya reservoir may reduce the difficulties of repeated administration. To assist in the delivery of chemotherapeutic agents into the CSF, insertion of reservoirs that sit on top of the skull or in the subcutaneous tissue of the abdomen or flank can make repeated administration more practical. Although a number of new agents have been investigated for intrathecal or intraommaya administration, including busulfan, etoposide, and mafosfamide,[231-233] overall there are a limited number of agents that may be safely administered to this compartment.

An important approach to increasing the penetration of chemotherapy into the brain has been the use of high-dose systemic therapy followed by stem cell rescue. The efficacy of this approach and management of the associated toxicities continue to be an area of significant study (see later).

Newer methods of targeting penetration of drugs into the CNS include blood-brain barrier disruption agents. These agents are in clinical trial and are designed to temporarily open up the tight junctions protecting the CNS.[234] They are typically administered just before the active anticancer agent is administered. Although promising and deserving of additional evaluation, a common problem to date has been the opening of the BBB in normal areas of the brain, resulting in greater toxicities to uninvolved areas. In a similar approach, new lipophilic carrier molecules have been designed to help transport drugs across the BBB, and further advances in these areas are expected.

Convection-Enhanced Delivery

With the movement of fluids away from areas of high interstitial pressure to areas of low interstitial pressure, passive diffusion of drugs deep into tumors is unlikely to occur in sufficient concentrations to be effective. To overcome this, developments in convection-enhanced delivery have been reported. These techniques require the implantation of small catheters that can be tunneled under the scalp, which then penetrate the solid tumor parenchyma or adjacent brain. By injecting drugs under high pressure, these agents move through the interstitial space between cells, allowing the drugs an opportunity to kill tumor cells. Because tumors usually penetrate along the pathway of least resistance, similar to fluids under pressure, this technique allows the drug to spread out in a fashion similar to that of the infiltrating tumor. A number of candidate molecules designed for convection-enhanced delivery are being developed. This technique should be equally well suited to small-molecule inhibitors, chemotherapeutic agents, biologic drugs, including large protein molecules, and gene vectors.

Novel Chemotherapeutic and Biologic Agents

The revolution in the molecular classification of adult and pediatric tumors has significantly advanced our understanding of pathways implicated in tumor initiation, progression, and metastases. These have also become important targets for new therapy approaches that are included in the realm of chemotherapy but differ in many fundamental ways. The unique mechanism of action of these inhibitors, and their lack of typical chemotherapy-related toxicity (myelosuppression) make them ideally suited for combination with traditional chemotherapy and radiation therapy.[3,235] In addition to classic cytotoxic agents, the use of agents that modulate the epigenome, such as histone deacetylases, which modify DNA methylation, a process critical in gene regulation, may allow apoptotic or differentiation genes to be reactivated while turning off proliferative pathways.[236]

The development of new formulations of old drugs also deserves comment. Many drugs that were tested in children with tumors of the CNS that did not demonstrate activity may have been the result of poor penetration or unknown pharmacokinetics. Modifications to older agents such as doxorubicin by pegylation and liposomal encapsulation will require additional clinical testing.[237] Even vincristine, which is commonly used in pediatric patients with CNS tumors despite a lack of clear data demonstrating its activity in these diseases, is being redeveloped to improve its potential activity.[238]

Numerous biologic targets are now available and each will require some early pediatric clinical experience regarding dosing and tolerability.[239] Unfortunately, most biologic agents are unlikely to possess significant single agent activity. Many of these drugs may be better at slowing tumor progression and will need combinations with other molecular inhibitors, radiation therapy, and/or chemotherapy. Many of these markers may also have important roles as prognostic markers as well as therapeutic targets.[240,241]

Small-Molecule Inhibitors

The sequencing of the human genome and the identification of a number of critical signaling pathways, especially the receptor tyrosine kinases, have provided the basis for a whole new class of anticancer agents.[242] Normal cells transmit signals from the external environment to the nucleus via receptor tyrosine kinases. These molecules sit on the cell surface and homo- or heterodimerize in the presence of ligand, which results in a conformational change in the intracellular domain of the receptor. This allows a phosphorylation event on the cytoplasmic component of the receptor that begins a complex cascade that results in the alteration of cell function. Many tumors use these receptors or their pathways to drive cell proliferation and migration as well as decouple cell repair and apoptosis.[243]

The activation of receptor tyrosine kinases results from the phosphorylation of a tyrosine residue in the intracellular domain of the receptor. This process can be blocked by the steric interference of small molecules designed to fit into the phosphorylation pocket. By carefully designing the shape of these molecules, the ability to define the specificity of these drugs to related receptors means that some inhibitors can disrupt only a single receptor or entire families of receptors. A number of experimental studies of these inhibitors have been tested in children with brain tumors, including those targeting the platelet-derived growth factor receptor (PDGFR)[244] and ras pathways.[245]

Immunotherapy

The brain and spine are considered immunologically privileged sites. In spite of this, the presence of lymphocytic infiltrates in many brain tumors suggests that activation of the immune system is possible. Significant attempts to activate the immune system against these tumors,[246] especially malignant gliomas, have followed two main approaches. Some groups have attempted to increase the immune activation of lymphocytes by cytokine stimulation of the innate immune system. In the second approach, a patient's own tumor is required to generate tumor-specific immune activated cells. As more is learned about how immune cells interact with and are activated by tumors, opportunities to develop immunotherapies will hopefully become more feasible[247]; some early encouraging results are already being reported.[248,249]

Gene Therapy

The use of gene vectors for the treatment of brain tumor allows for the expression of a large array of different molecules. Many experimental approaches have focused on modulators of the immune response.[250] An important component in the expansion of these approaches will be improvement in direct delivery of large molecules directly into the brain to bypass the blood-brain barrier.[251]

Antiangiogenic Agents

Over the last few decades, the role of angiogenesis in the development of cancer has gone from a novel hypothesis to a fundamental area of research and therapeutic intervention. Although not brain tumor–specific, the role of angiogenesis has been a hallmark of the progression of malignant gliomas. A large number of antiangiogenic inhibitors are now in clinical trials and have focused on targeting the cytokine vascular endothelial growth factor, although other inhibitors of the angiogenic cascade are being tested.[252,253] A developing area ideally suited for pediatric patients has been the use of antiangiogenic chemotherapy. The principle behind this approach is the use of very low-dose chemotherapy that targets dividing endothelial cells rather than tumor cells. A number of low-dose chemotherapy approaches are being tested and preliminary results are encouraging.[253-255]

Suppression of Tumor Resistance

The innate resistance of many tumors to cytotoxic agents, especially those of glial origin, is well documented by the near-complete and rapid progression of high-grade gliomas after up-front radiation and chemotherapy. There are a number of pathways that tumors can use to avoid cell death when confronted with DNA-damaging agents. Temozolomide has become widely used in conjunction with radiation therapy in adults and has demonstrated clear activity in these patients. Although this combination has demonstrated prolongation in time to progression, the vast majority of patients will eventually progress as resistance mechanisms are activated. In order to help overcome this, recent clinical trials have begun testing molecules that can bind and inactivate the enzymes responsible for resistance. One such example is O(6)-benzylguanine (O(6)-BG), a small molecular compound that can bind the enzyme O(6)-methyl DNA-methyltransferase (MGMT), which functions to remove the methyl group on the O(6) position of guanine after temozolomide treatment. By treating the patient in advance with O(6)-BG, all free MGMT can be consumed, at which point administration of temozolomide can damage the DNA. Although still early in pediatric testing, this approach offers considerable opportunity.[256,257] Additional resistance pathways have been identified in pediatric and adult brain tumors that may guide therapeutic approaches, as well as the development of new inhibitors of the resistance pathways.[258] For example, mutations within the PMS2 mismatch repair gene, which can lead to tumorigenesis and treatment resistance, may be influenced by the addition of retinoic acid.[259]

High-Dose Chemotherapy with Stem Cell Rescue

The principles of high-dose chemotherapy and stem cell rescue are similar to those for other malignant diseases. Many brain tumors, especially those of primitive neuroectodermal origin, such as medulloblastoma and PNETs, have demonstrated dose-dependent chemotherapy responses.[260-262] This technique has therefore been used extensively in children with relapsed disease after standard up-front therapy or in those with poor-prognosis diseases such as ATRT and PNET.[263,264] Although the conditioning regimens, disease histologies, and patient characteristics have differed significantly among patients, this approach has demonstrated positive results in those patients who were reinduced and could achieve minimal residual disease.[265,266] The evaluation of patients post-transplantation can be complicated by the presence of therapy-related signal changes on MRI scan, including heterogeneously enhancing lesions, often causing clinical symptoms related to their location. Although these lesions can appear consistent with disease progression early after transplantation, they do not progress and need to have long-term follow-up with regard to their clinical significance.[267]

PEDIATRIC BRAIN TUMORS

Gliomas

Glial tumors are composed of three main categories—astrocytomas, ependymomas, and oligodendrogliomas. Each is further divided by morphologic features, degree of invasiveness, and location and is assigned a grade ranging from I to IV as the features of malignancy increase. Grading of astrocytomas by WHO or St. Anne-Mayo criteria is predictive of patient survival.[268] In pediatrics, the modified WHO classification of CNS tumors[172] has become the standard classification system. Astrocytomas can be classified as low grade (WHO grades I and II) or high grade (WHO grades III and IV). Low-grade gliomas may consist of relatively pure tumors such as a juvenile pilocytic (grade I) or fibrillary (grade II) astrocytoma or mixed populations of both glial and neuronal lineages, such as ganglioglioma or glioneurocytoma. The classification of several other subtypes is still under debate. Although the differentiation of high-grade from low-grade glioma is universally used, with greater molecular definition of these tumors, the need to separate grade I from II and grade III from IV tumors regarding treatment and prognosis is increasing. Pediatric gliomas can also be discussed in the context of location, rather than grade. This approach recognizes some of the unique aspects of the environment in which tumors of similar histologies can grow and their effect on treatment and prognosis (Box 17-2).

Supratentorial, Cerebellar Pilocytic, and Other Low-Grade Astrocytomas

Pilocytic astrocytomas (PAs) are well-circumscribed tumors classified as WHO grade I.[269] These tumors were formally referred to as juvenile pilocytic astrocytomas (JPAs) but are now classified simply as pilocytic astrocytomas. Grade I tumors are the most common low-grade gliomas found in children, representing 20% to 30% of all childhood brain tumors. PAs typically appear in the first 2 decades, with no clear gender predominance. They are usually slow-growing, although their presentation can occur as acute deterioration as a result of obstructive hydrocephalus. NF-1 is the best example of a condition associated with an increased risk of PA.[270] The localization of PAs in the context of NF-1 and their improved long-term prognosis is well established, although the molecular basis for

this difference is unclear. Other predisposing factors such as common cytogenetic abnormalities are uncommon.[271] Low-grade astrocytomas typically lack epidermal growth factor receptor (EGFR) amplification,[272] although defects in the BRAF pathway have recently been reported.[273]

Clinical Presentation. Low-grade astrocytomas have a varied course, ranging from dissemination and persistent recurrence to spontaneous regression without therapy, and they behave differently from low-grade astrocytomas in adults.[274,275] The biologic factors that account for these differences remain investigational, although telomere length may play an important role.[276] Pilocytic astrocytomas commonly occur throughout the brain, including the optic pathways, optic chiasm–hypothalamus, thalamus and basal ganglia, cerebral hemispheres, cerebellum, and brainstem (dorsal exophytic brainstem glioma). Pilocytic astrocytomas of the spinal cord are less common.

The spectrum of clinical manifestations of a pilocytic astrocytoma depends on the site of origin, its size, age of the patient, and presence of raised intracranial pressure. Cerebellar pilocytic astrocytomas and dorsally exophytic brainstem PAs usually present with symptoms of increased intracranial pressure, such as headache, nausea, and vomiting. Children may also present with a relatively long history of progressive focal neurologic deficits, including gait disturbance; infants may present with progressive secondary macrocephaly. Signs of chronicity such as bone remodeling, scoliosis, or hemihypertrophy may be present, depending on the primary tumor location. The diencephalic syndrome is unique to low-grade astrocytomas, typically seen in infants whose tumors arise from the hypothalamus or optic pathways, and consists of emaciation, irritability, nystagmus, and normal linear growth.[277,278] Although many other deep-seated low-grade glial tumors are unresectable, patients with diencephalic syndrome appear to have a worse prognosis, suggesting that subtle biologic differences among these tumors and other PAs may exist.

Imaging and Histology. The typical MRI appearance of a grade I astrocytoma is an intensely homogeneous, well-circumscribed, contrast-enhancing lesion with minimal surrounding edema. Lesions are typically bright on both T1 and T2 images. Tumoral cysts are more prevalent in the cerebellum than in the cerebrum (Fig. 17-19) and often possess a contrast-enhancing mural nodule. Apparent diffusion coefficient imaging may be useful in differentiating PAs from higher grade astrocytomas.[279]

Histologic examination reveals a biphasic pattern, with a compacted component containing bipolar cells (Fig. 17-20) and Rosenthal fibers and a loose cellular array containing microcysts and eosinophilic granular bodies. Rosenthal fibers and eosinophilic granular bodies are pathologic hallmarks of pilocytic astrocytomas, although they can be observed in other diseases of the CNS. Rosenthal fibers are brightly eosinophilic, hyaline masses composed of alpha-B-crystalline and are best seen on tumor smear preparations (Fig. 17-21). Eosinophilic granular bodies are globular aggregates within astrocytic processes, also best visualized with smear preparations. Pilocytic astrocytomas stain intensely with the glial fibrillary acid protein (GFAP) immunoreagent. Invasion of the overlying meninges and adjacent brain parenchyma is commonly observed. Mitoses are rare and the MIB-1 labeling index is usually lower than 4%.[280] Although the pathologic criteria for anaplastic astrocytoma include the identification of mitoses, their presence in pilocytic astrocytomas does not indicate a higher grade. Inexperienced pathologists can often misinterpret these mitoses, resulting in a diagnosis of a malignant rather than low-grade glioma. Similarly, PAs can have vascular prolifera-

Box 17-2	**Histologic Classification of Low-Grade Gliomas**

Astrocytic tumors
  Pilocytic astrocytoma (PA)
  Pilomyxoid astrocytoma
  Diffuse astrocytomas (fibrillary, protoplasmic, gemistocytic)
  Pleomorphic xanthoastrocytoma (PXA)
  Subependymal giant cell astrocytoma (SEGA)
Oligodendroglial and mixed glial tumors
  Oligodendrocytoma
  Oligodendroglioma
  Oligoastrocytoma
Mixed glial-neuronal tumors
  Gangliocytoma
  Ganglioglioma
Dysembryoplastic infantile astrocytoma and dysembryoplastic infantile ganglioglioma (DIA, DIG)
Dysembryoplastic neuroepithelial tumor (DNT)
Special locations that are often not biopsied
  Optic pathway gliomas (OPGs)
  Tectal gliomas
  Cervicomedullary gliomas

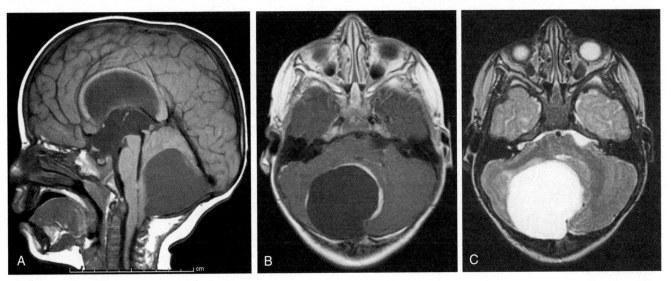

FIGURE 17-19. Posterior fossa pilocytic astrocytoma (juvenile pilocytic astrocytoma [JPA]). **A,** Sagittal T1 image without contrast. **B,** Axial T1 image with contrast. **C,** Axial T2 image.

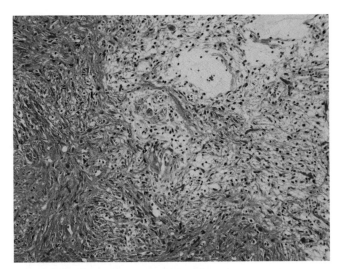

FIGURE 17-20. Pilocytic astrocytoma. Shown is a biphasic pattern of compact, fiber-rich tumor and hypocellular areas with microcysts (×200).

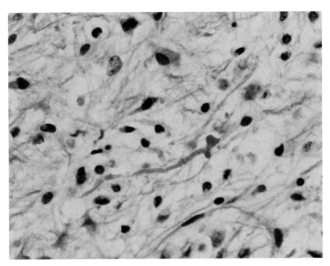

FIGURE 17-21. Rosenthal fiber in a pilocytic astrocytoma (H&E; ×1000).

tion, a hallmark of glioblastoma multiforme (grade IV astrocytoma) although, again, this does not indicate transformation to a more malignant phenotype. Rarely, pilocytic astrocytomas can present with diffuse leptomeningeal dissemination, especially in the variant of pilomyxoid astrocytoma.[281-284] Characteristic of the unique biology of PAs, each of the metastatic lesions continues to behave as a low-grade astrocytoma with a slow indolent course. These tumors are therefore not difficult to treat as a result of their aggressive metastatic phenotype, but rather as a result of their slow persistent recurrences.

Management. Surgery is the mainstay of therapy for pilocytic and other low-grade astrocytomas.[285] Gross total resection is often curative, even though residual microscopic disease may often be left behind. Radiation and chemotherapy are typically not required as part of up-front therapy after a complete resection.[286] PAs of the optic pathway in NF-1 patients do not

require surgical confirmation unless atypical features are present.[287] Patients with tectal gliomas require CSF diversion but do not benefit from biopsy; they can be diagnosed based on the presence of hydrocephalus and MRI appearance of the lesion alone.

Progressive or unresectable pilocytic astrocytomas, or those arising in infants or children causing alterations of vision or other neurologically relevant symptoms, may require adjuvant treatment.[320] Chemotherapy is assuming an increasingly important role in the management of unresectable and/or progressive low-grade gliomas, diencephalic low-grade gliomas in younger patients, or other unresectable tumors (Table 17-5). Various combination regimens, such as carboplatin and vincristine or thioguanine, procarbazine, lomustine (CCNU), and vincristine (TPCV) have produced consistent, durable responses,[306,307,313] reviewed in Perilongo.[319] Monthly carboplatin is more easily administered but may have less activity[288,321,322] and requires additional study.

TABLE 17-5   Chemotherapy for Pediatric Low-Grade Gliomas

Treatment	No. of Patients	Objective Response, % (CR + PR)	Overall Response, % (CR + PR + SD)	EFS or OS
Carboplatin[288]	80	2 CR, 17 PR	2 CR, 17 PR, 4 MR, 46 SD	72% 3-yr EFS in NF-1 patients; 62% 3-yr EFS in non–NF-1 patients
Carboplatin[289]	12 ND	4 PR	4 PR, 6 SD	
Carboplatin[290]	4 ND, 2 PD		6 SD	
Carboplatin[291]	13 ND/PD	1 CR/PR		
Iproplatin[291]	15 ND/PD	1 CR/PR	1 CR/PR, 9 SD	
Cyclophosphamide[292]	15 ND	1 CR	1 CR, 9 SD	
Cyclophosphamide[293]	1 PD, 3 ND with leptomeningeal dissemination		2 PR/MR, 2 SD	
Ifosfamide[294]	6	1 PR	1 PR, 3 SD	
Temozolomide[295]	21 PD	1 PR	1 PR, 20 SD	
Temozolomide[296]	13 PD	2 CR, 3 PR	2 CR, 3 PR, 3 MR, 4 SD	57% 3-yr EFS
Temozolomide[297]	10 ND, 20 PD	3 PR	3 PR, 1 MR, 25 SD	51% 2-yr PFS and 17% 4-yr PFS
Temozolomide[298]	2 PD		2 SD	
Methotrexate[299]	10 PD	2 PR	2 PR, 5 SD	
Topotecan[300]	2 PD	1 PR	1 PR, 1 SD	
Topotecan[301]	11 PD		5 SD	
Etoposide[302]	14 PD	1 CR, 4 PR	1 CR, 4 PR, 3 SD	
Etoposide[303]	12 ND		6 PR/SD	
Vincristine–actinomycin-D[304]	24 ND	3 PR	3 PR, 6 MR, 15 SD	
Vincristine-carboplatin[305]	123 ND		105/123 CR, PR or SD	61% 5-yr PFS
Vincristine-carboplatin[306]	78 ND	4 CR, 22 PR	4 CR, 22 PR, 18 MR, 29 SD	68% 3-yr PFS
Vincristine-carboplatin[307] (an additional 37 newly diagnosed patients are included in the report above[306])	24 PD	7 PR	7 PR, 5 MR, 5 SD	
Carboplatin-etoposide[308]	13 ND	1 CR	1 CR, 3 MR, 6 SD	69% patients alive at mean of 30 mo
Cisplatin-etoposide[309]	31 ND, 3 PD	1 CR, 11 PR	1 CR, 11 PR, 12 MR, 11 SD	3-year PFS 100% in patients older than 5 yr, 66% in patients younger than 5 yr
Vincristine-etoposide[310]	11 ND, 9 PD	1 PR	1 PR, 4 MR, 9 SD	
Tamoxifen-carboplatin[311]	12 ND, 1 PD	2/13 PR	2/13 PR, 9/13 SD	47% 3-year PFS, 69% 3-year OS
6-Thioguanine, vincristine, CCNU, dibromodulcitol, procarbazine (TPDCV)[312,313]	15 ND (4 patients were treated with other therapy and are not included), 42 ND	11 PR, 15 CR/PR	11/15 PR, 15 CR/PR + 25 SD	Median TTP not reached at 79 wk,[312] median TTP at 132 wk[313]
Procarbazine, carboplatin, vincristine, etoposide, cisplatin, cyclophosphamide[314]	85 ND	36/85	74/88; 36 CR or PR, 15 MR, 23 SD	34% 5-yr PFS, 89% 5-yr OS
Carboplatin, etoposide, cyclophosphamide, vincristine, CCNU, procarbazine[315]	7 ND, 3 PD	2/10	70% CR + PR + MR; 100%, including SD	70% PFS at 5.6 yr
5-Fluorouracil, vincristine, cyclophosphamide, etoposide[316]	13 (12 ND, 1 PD)	6/13, 1 CR, 5 PR	8/13, 1 CR, 5 PR, 2 SD	6-yr PFS 67%
Vinblastine[254]	9 (ND with carboplatin allergy; nonprogressive at time of therapy)	2/9	9/9; 1 CR, 1 PR, 5 MR, 2 SD	Median follow-up of patients, 10 mo
Thioguanine, procarbazine, CCNU, vincristine[317]	9 (5 ND with carbo allergy; nonprogressive at time of therapy, 4 PD)	0/9	7/9; 7 SD	78% at 13-mo progression-free
Cisplatin, etoposide, vinblastine[318]	16 ND	4/16 4 PR	9/16 4 PR, 5 SD	5-year PFS 56%

CR, complete remission; EFS, event-free survival; MR, minor response; ND, newly diagnosed; NF-1, neurofibromatosis type 1; OS, overall survival; PS, progression-free survival; PR, partial remission; SD, stable disease; TTP, time to progression.

Adapted from Perilongo G. Considerations on the role of chemotherapy and modern radiotherapy in the treatment of childhood low-grade glioma. J Neurooncol. 2005;75:301-307.

With these multiagent combinations, stabilization of tumors occurs in almost 50% of patients and radiographic response is observed in an additional 40%. Median time to progression is approximately 3 years, although up to 70% of patients will eventually demonstrate tumor growth. The ability to re-treat these patients with multiple regimens has allowed most patients to avoid radiation therapy, especially early in life when the long-term morbidity of this modality is greatest. Although the time to progression may appear short, and the overall progression rate of 70% appears high, these chemotherapy regimens are well tolerated, with few long-term complications. This is in contrast to radiation therapy (RT), which demonstrates a significantly improved response rate (95%) and duration of disease control (longer than 10 years), but radiotherapy also entails significant long-term morbidities, such as neurocognitive, vascular, hormonal, and second tumor risks. Because most children with low-grade gliomas will be long-term survivors, this is exactly the population that would benefit from the avoidance of the late effects of RT.

A recent randomized phase III clinical trial has been completed by the Children's Oncology Group, comparing the efficacies and morbidities of the regimens vincristine and carboplatin versus TPCV.[275] Although final results of this clinical trial have not yet been published, the results appear to confirm data from the prior reports regarding the overall usefulness of chemotherapy for the treatment of these tumors. The overall improved outcome for patients with NF-1 has also been confirmed, indicating that these tumors may have a unique biologic phenotype. Temozolomide, an orally active alkylating agent with a favorable side effect profile, has been shown to have some activity as monotherapy for adult low-grade gliomas.[323] Although it has not been widely studied, it appears to have a low response rate in low-grade gliomas in children, with a median time to progression of 6.7 months, although many patients appear to have prolonged stable disease.[296,324] Responses with temozolomide in disseminated low-grade astrocytomas have also been reported[281] although another alkylator, cyclophosphamide given every 3 weeks, lacked significant activity.[292] The role of temozolomide in combination with vincristine and carboplatin for pediatric low-grade gliomas is currently being investigated. Others have successfully used novel combinations, including 5-fluorouracil.[316] The metronomic application of vinblastine, a mitotic inhibitor, has resulted in some clinical responses or stable disease in children with low-grade gliomas unable to tolerate carboplatin.[254] Vinblastine is also being evaluated in combination with carboplatin in newly diagnosed patients. Although more information on the activity of these approaches is needed, responses in refractory low-grade gliomas have been reported with another metronomic-based chemotherapy approach,[253] suggesting that angiogenesis may be an important pathway in these tumors. This is also consistent with the presence of vascular proliferation observed in these tumors. Chemotherapy may also allow for improved surgical resection of previously unresectable lesions and should therefore be continuously re-evaluated as a therapeutic option.[325] Tumors treated with chemotherapy, even if not smaller, can be easier to resect because of less bleeding and a more firm texture at the time of the procedure.

Although most chemotherapy regimens for low-grade gliomas have been reserved for children younger than 10 years, older children seem to derive equal benefit with the use of these regimens, potentially avoiding radiation therapy and the risks of second tumors, vasculopathy, and hormonal dysfunction.[326] The use of dose-intensive chemotherapy has been piloted in a small series of children, with results similar to those observed using standard doses.[315]

Radiotherapy is considered contraindicated in children with NF-1 and is usually deferred in children with PAs and other low-grade gliomas, especially in diencephalic and optic pathway tumors. Even highly focused radiation therapy in these locations cannot avoid the potential cognitive, endocrine, or vascular risks associated with radiation therapy. In spite of this, highly focused radiation therapy is effective for low-grade gliomas and is without significant marginal failures, suggesting that these lesions are not deeply penetrated into surrounding brain.[327] Long-term concerns for second tumors, hormone dysfunction, and cognitive impact, however, still make this approach of concern for children. Additional late effects of RT when used in younger children with diencephalic gliomas may include strokes related to a moyamoya-like syndrome.[71,328,329]

Prognosis. The prognosis for surgically resectable tumors is excellent following gross total resection. For patients with PAs whose tumors can be completely surgically resected, depending on location, the 10-year progression-free survival approaches 90%.[283,330,331] Even in patients with incompletely resected lesions, treatment is not always required and, depending on the patient and clinical scenario, observation can be considered unless tumor or symptom progression is documented.[332] The most critical variable in the treatment of pilocytic astrocytomas is the anatomic location of the tumor. Complete resections are most difficult for tumors located in the brainstem, spinal cord, optic pathways, thalamus, and hypothalamus. As such, the progression-free survival of children with centrally located tumors (e.g., optic chiasm, thalamus, or hypothalamus) is less than 50%.[331] Given the favorable toxicity profile of chemotherapy versus radiation therapy in young children, chemotherapy is preferred as the first therapeutic modality in young patients with tumors not amenable to gross total resection.[306] The use of chemotherapy as initial treatment in patients with centrally located or unresectable lesions allows for the delay of radiation therapy until the child is less likely to incur the serious developmental and neuropsychological sequelae of radiation therapy. Patients demonstrating radiographic response to chemotherapy have progression-free survival similar to those whose tumors remained stable.[306,309] Ultimately, the quality of survival depends on multiple factors, including the tumor location, extent to which the tumor can be resected, timing of any radiotherapy, and side effects of surgery, chemotherapy, and radiotherapy.[333] Transformation of PAs into higher grade malignant gliomas is highly unusual.[334]

Optic Pathway Gliomas

Optic pathway gliomas (OPGs) represent approximately 4% to 6% of all primary pediatric brain tumors; the incidence is higher when asymptomatic lesions in NF-1 patients are also included.[335] OPGs are evenly distributed between boys and girls. These tumors may involve various parts of the optic pathway, such as the optic nerves, chiasm, optic tract, and optic radiations. They may also infiltrate the adjacent hypothalamus and temporal lobes. Optic nerve gliomas are strongly associated with NF-1, although sporadic lesions are not uncommon. OPGs in NF-1 patients have a more indolent course than those arising in patients without NF-1[336] and likely represent a different biology than sporadic tumors.[61] Although optic pathway gliomas may be considered a subset of pilocytic astrocytomas, their unique features and management necessitate a separate discussion.[337,338]

Clinical Presentation. Most optic pathway gliomas consist of pilocytic astrocytomas (WHO grade I).[339] The clinical course of OPGs can vary considerably, from an indolent mass in a child with NF-1 to a relatively aggressive, invasive, and expansile diencephalic tumor. Unilateral optic nerve gliomas often present with the classic triad of visual loss, proptosis, and optic atrophy. Optic nerve tortuosity, which can be present alone or in the context of optic pathway gliomas in children with NF-1, does not necessarily define the presence of disease nor the need for therapy.[340] Chiasmatic involvement may lead to unilateral or bilateral visual loss, a bitemporal visual field defect, and obstructive hydrocephalus as the tumor grows dorsally to obstruct CSF flow in the third ventricle. Further invasion into brain parenchyma may result in more pronounced visual field deficits as well as hemiparesis. Chiasmatic tumors in infants present as large suprasellar masses that may also extend into the hypothalamus and third ventricle, producing hydrocephalus and endocrine abnormalities. In cases of hypothalamic extension, in addition to nystagmus, visual loss, and hydrocephalus, the diencephalic syndrome may occasionally be seen. This syndrome consists of hyperkinesia, euphoria, and emaciation, with preserved normal linear growth.[278] Failure to thrive is a common presentation of this syndrome but in the context of a number of other conditions that may also cause failure to thrive during infancy, a delay in diagnosis of a brain tumor is not uncommon.[277] Endocrine deficiencies commonly accompany PAs in this location, and these tumors are more likely to have CSF dissemination in association with diencephalic syndrome, in spite of their histopathologic classification as benign.[341] Many patients with NF-1 will have long-standing, subtle ophthalmologic abnormalities, so regular visual evaluation is required. For these patients, routine surveillance MRI scans are not indicated because many asymptomatic and clinically irrelevant tumors will be diagnosed, creating a treatment dilemma.[342]

Imaging and Histology. The clinical diagnosis of an optic pathway glioma is suspected when a child presents with visual impairment, nystagmus, and/or optic atrophy. MRI of the brain or orbits typically shows a solid, cystic, or mixed type of tumor, with strong gadolinium enhancement. The imaging characteristics of low-grade gliomas of the optic pathway are similar to those of low-grade astrocytomas in other locations. The typical MRI appearance of a grade I astrocytoma is an intensely homogeneous, well-circumscribed, enhancing lesion with minimal surrounding edema (Fig. 17-22). Lesions are

typically bright on both T1- and T2-weighted images. MRI studies and clinical presentation may distinguish an OPG from other childhood tumors that arise in the suprasellar location, such as a germ cell tumor or craniopharyngioma. Histologically, optic pathway gliomas are usually grade I pilocytic astrocytomas or, less frequently, grade II fibrillary astrocytomas. Mixed low-grade gliomas have been reported in this region but the overall therapeutic approach is not altered, because most of these lesions are unresectable at diagnosis. Tumors with an elevated MIB-1 more than 1% and p53 expression were more likely to be WHO grade II and had a worse outcome compared with those with a MIB-1 and p53 labeling index less than 1%, all of which were pilocytic astrocytomas. Pilocytic astrocytomas with a more aggressive behavior had an MIB-1 labeling index of 2% to 3% but retained a low p53 labeling index of less than 1%.[339]

Management. The unpredictable clinical course of patients with optic pathway tumors has led to controversy regarding the optimal management of these tumors. The clinical course, age of onset, severity of symptoms, size and extent of the tumor, and presence of NF-1 may all affect management decisions. Treatment is frequently started promptly in younger patients, patients with progressive symptoms, and those with more extensive CNS involvement, with preservation of vision of paramount concern. The initial treatment of choice is chemotherapy (see Table 17-5),[319] which may cause stabilization or regression[343] and is not associated with the neurocognitive decline observed with radiation therapy.[344] Combination therapy with carboplatin and vincristine[305,306,345] or with thioguanine, procarbazine, CCNU, and vincristine (TPCV)[317] has been considered to have comparable beneficial effects. TPCV should not be used in children with NF-1 because of the increased risks of secondary tumors associated with alkylator-based treatment. After progression on vincristine and carboplatin, vincristine and actinomycin can be considered for patients with NF-1 to avoid further risks of alkylator therapy.[312,346] As for other low-grade gliomas, a number of new chemotherapy regimens are being developed (see earlier). Although delaying radiation therapy is paramount in young children, older patients

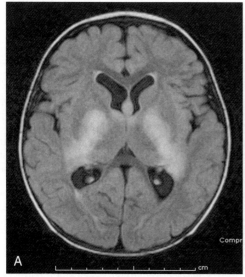
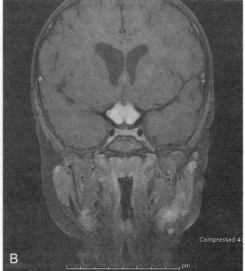

FIGURE 17-22. A large optic pathway glioma in a 2-year-old boy who does not have neurofibromatosis type 1 (NF-1). **A,** Axial T2 fluid-attenuated inversion recovery (FLAIR) image that demonstrates bilateral involvement of the optic tracts posterior to the chiasm. **B,** T1 gadolinium-enhanced coronal image demonstrating the enhancing tumor expanding the optic chiasm. The patient has no functional vision and is legally blind.

may also benefit from these chemotherapy approaches and delaying radiation therapy.[326]

A Children's Oncology Group (COG) study comparing a carboplatin-vincristine regimen with the TPCV regimen in the treatment of progressive low-grade astrocytoma in children younger than 10 years closed to accrual in 2005, and is awaiting publication. Preliminary results have suggested that both regimens are well tolerated and can delay or obviate the need for radiation therapy in most patients. Newer chemotherapy clinical trials for OPGs combine a number of agents such as temozolomide with vincristine and carboplatin and vinblastine and carboplatin. Although a definitive role for radiotherapy exists for the management of OPG,[347] current trends in treatment favor a delay in the initiation of radiotherapy in young patients.[348] Newer surgical techniques with direct administration of radiotherapy are also being explored and have demonstrated usefulness for selected patients.[349]

Prognosis. Although optic pathway tumors are almost always of low-grade histology, their location often results in serious morbidity. The growth rate of these tumors, however, often slows during late childhood so that by adulthood, tumors may become quiescent and do not require further therapy. Children with NF-1 have been shown to have a better progression-free survival, although an age of younger than 1 year is clearly associated with a higher risk of tumor progression.[350] NF-1 patients appear to be at high risk for the development of moyamoya[70] as well as radiation-induced second malignancies.[351] Patients with NF-1–associated optic nerve gliomas may remain stable for several years. Close observation and symptomatic management are recommended for these patients.

Low-Grade Astrocytomas of the Brainstem

Although most brainstem tumors are diffuse intrinsic pontine gliomas, approximately 20% of brainstem tumors are low-grade astrocytomas involving the medulla, midbrain, tectum, or cervicomedullary, pontomedullary, or midbrain-pontine junction. Although 20% of nonpontine tumors in these locations can be classified as grade III or IV malignant gliomas, 80% are low-grade glial lesions with a much better prognosis.[352] These lesions differ from diffuse pontine gliomas by their clinical presentation as well as their imaging characteristics. Early identification of the type of brainstem lesion is critical in the workup, consideration of neurosurgical intervention, treatment, and prognosis of these patients.[353]

Presentation. Patients with brainstem lesions can present with various clinical symptoms, depending on the location of the tumor. Medullary tumors are more common than midbrain tumors and the male-to-female ratio is approximately 1:1.[354] In spite of the eloquent function of the brainstem, most patients have an indolent course with subtle neurologic findings. Most commonly, patients present with cranial nerve dysfunction or head tilt. Lower motor weakness with subtle hemiparesis is also seen. Most parents have difficulty defining the start of the symptoms and refer to their child as having always been clumsy or weak. Rarely, these tumors can be multifocal in nature.[355]

Histology and Imaging. Most low-grade brainstem tumors are either grade I or II astrocytomas; less than 20% are malignant astrocytomas. Imaging characteristics are similar to those of other low-grade gliomas; pilocytic astrocytomas (grade I) tend to be bright on T1 and T2 images and enhance after contrast administration. Edema tends to be minimal. Fibrillary astrocytomas (grade II), by comparison, are less enhancing after contrast administration. The considerable overlap and variability in the imaging characteristics of grade I versus grade II astrocytomas, however, prevents accurate diagnosis based on MRI characteristics alone. The histologic features of brainstem low-grade astrocytomas are identical to grades I and II astrocytomas in other locations.

Management. Brainstem low-grade astrocytomas that remain focal can often be surgically resectable if they possess a plane between the brainstem and tumor.[356] If completely resected, these patients are unlikely to need additional therapy. Incompletely resected brainstem low-grade astrocytomas have a high recurrence rate and most of these patients will need additional therapy,[357] usually chemotherapy rather than radiation therapy, given the good long-term prognosis of these patients (see Table 17-5).[319] White matter tracts are often displaced by these tumors, and preoperative diffusion tensor imaging can assist the neurosurgeon regarding the optimal approach to maximize resection while minimizing morbidity in this patient population.[358] Although postsurgical morbidity such as problems with swallowing can be significant, many patients will eventually recover function, although this can take many months and extensive physical and occupational therapy.[359] The chemotherapy options for these tumors are identical to those for low-grade astrocytomas in other locations and include vincristine and carboplatin or TPCV chemotherapy. Recurrence and need for retreatment are common but most tumors will eventually stop growing as these patients enter adulthood.

Prognosis. Most low-grade brainstem glioma patients will be long-term survivors.[356] It is therefore important that the workup and treatment of these patients be adapted with this in mind. Differentiation from diffuse intrinsic pontine gliomas is usually easily made based on imaging and clinical criteria. Surgical intervention must be based on the expectation that minimal long-term morbidity will result, given the large number of other treatment options available for these patients.

Low-Grade Thalamic Astrocytomas

Thalamic tumors are rare in pediatric patients, accounting for less than 5% of intracranial tumors. Most thalamic tumors are unilateral and approximately 50% are low-grade astrocytomas.[360,361] Thalamic tumors occur at a slightly older age than many other low-grade gliomas of childhood. Low-grade thalamic tumors present as unilateral or bithalamic in location, which appears to have prognostic significance.

Clinical Presentation. Thalamic tumors can present with a number of different clinical findings.[362] Raised intracranial pressure, tremors, motor deficits, seizures, and mood changes are the most commonly observed presenting symptoms.[363] Unlike in adult tumors, dementia is a rare presenting symptom.[364]

Imaging and Histology. Imaging characteristics of thalamic tumors are similar to those of gliomas in other locations (Fig. 17-23). Low-grade and high-grade histologies are approximately equally distributed, although pathologic classification of these tumors can be influenced by sampling error from small biopsy specimens.[365] The use of PET or SPECT imaging can help identify areas to be biopsied.[366] Although astrocytic histologies predominate, oligodendroglial tumors have also been identified.[361]

Management. The presence of tumor in the thalamus presents a number of management difficulties. Because of their location, complete resection is difficult,[364] although surgery can result in symptom improvement in selected cases.[367] Even

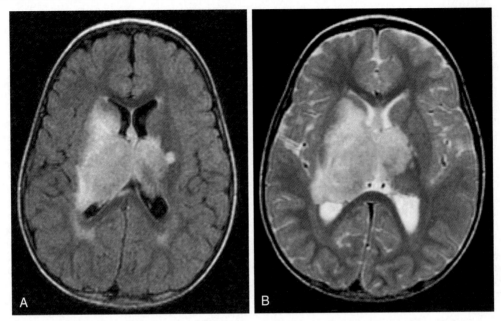

FIGURE 17-23. Bithalamic astrocytoma. **A,** Axial fluid-attenuated inversion recovery (FLAIR) image. **B,** Axial T2 image.

attempts at biopsy can result in significant morbidity. The small amount of surgical material often raises concerns of sampling error in attempting to determine the histopathologic grade of the tumor. Biopsy of the most malignant component of these deep-seated lesions can be guided with PET imaging.[366] This is particularly important for astrocytic tumors, for which samples of sufficient size and content are needed to define the elements of tumor grade. In the analysis of children with thalamic lesions, most tumors are unilateral in nature and approximately 50% to 60% are low-grade astrocytomas; the remaining 40% are high-grade lesions.[360] Some tumors are amenable to significant resection.[368,369] The response of low-grade thalamic tumors to chemotherapy and radiation is not known to be different from that of similar tumors in other locations. Thus, younger patients are often treated initially with chemotherapy used for other low-grade astrocytomas (see Table 17-5).[319] In those with rapid progression or histologic verification of high-grade features, radiotherapy can be used, although a significant portion of the brain will receive a substantial dose, resulting in long-term toxicity for survivors.

Prognosis. Contrary to some reports of poor outcome for bithalamic astrocytomas of any grade,[370] five of nine patients were long-term survivors in one retrospective series.[360] Part of the difficulty in assigning an accurate prognosis to these tumors is the limited biopsy material available for assessment. With a number of reports of survivors now available, even in the context of bilateral disease, all young patients should be given a trial of chemotherapy.

Low-Grade Diencephalic Astrocytomas

Diencephalic tumors remain a unique and poorly understood subtype of pediatric low-grade gliomas. They typically occur in young infants, although a few patients have presented late in the first or second decade of life.[371] A high incidence of dissemination throughout the neural axis has been recognized[355] and may relate to the increased frequency of the pilomyxoid variant in this location. The presence of failure to thrive in infants often leads to an extensive and prolonged workup for

gastrointestinal abnormalities before the correct cause is identified.[372] The presence of diencephalic tumors with early age of onset and the propensity to disseminate suggest that there may be unique biologic differences among these tumors and other low-grade astrocytomas, although no specific abnormalities have yet been documented.

Clinical Presentation. Diencephalic low-grade astrocytomas are differentiated from other low-grade gliomas in children by their presence around the hypothalamus–optic chiasm and a unique constellation of symptoms, including the three Es— emaciation, emesis, and euphoria. In spite of severe failure to thrive that is often seen, most infants retain normal growth rates and maintain normal pituitary secretion prior to surgical resection.[371] Although an accurate clinical picture for these patients continues to be defined, because many lack the typical constellation,[278] their management is difficult because of the deep-seated nature of these lesions and the frequent presence of leptomeningeal dissemination at diagnosis.[373] As such, these patients require full craniospinal imaging at diagnosis, along with CSF analysis. Any patient presenting with symptoms of spinal disease needs immediate restaging.

Imaging and Histology. The imaging characteristics of diencephalic low-grade gliomas do not differ from those of low-grade astrocytomas in other locations. Lesions are centered around the hypothalamus and chiasm, are bright on T2-weighted images, and usually show homogeneous enhancement after contrast administration.[374] The lesions are typically pilocytic or fibrillary astrocytomas, although the pilomyxoid variant can also be observed in this location.[365]

Management. The approach to therapy follows that for other low-grade astrocytomas. Because of the young age and deep location of these tumors, radiation therapy is usually contraindicated and will result in significant cognitive impairment over the long term.[328] Most patients undergo maximal safe surgery, followed by chemotherapy with vincristine and carboplatin or TPCV (see Table 17-5).[319] Radiographic response or stable disease accompanied by weight gain is common.[277,375,376]

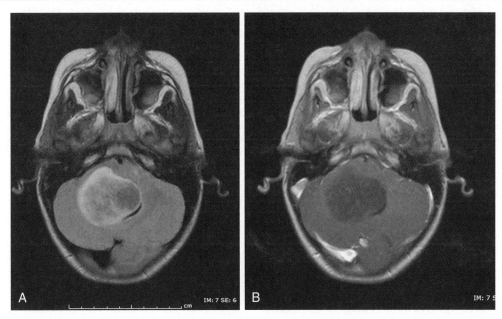

FIGURE 17-24. Grade II fibrillary astrocytoma. **A,** Axial T1 image with contrast. **B,** Axial fluid-attenuated inversion recovery (FLAIR) image.

High-dose chemotherapy has also been used successfully[377] as an investigational approach.

Prognosis. In spite of the low-grade nature of diencephalic tumors, these patients do less well than patients with similar tumors located in the optic pathway, brainstem, or cerebellum. In addition to the continued progression of these tumors compressing vital structures, patients are at high risk for surgery-induced hypothalamic damage resulting in obesity.

Fibrillary Astrocytomas

Fibrillary (WHO grade II) astrocytomas are low-grade astrocytomas (LGAs) and are distinct from PAs. Precise determination of the incidence of fibrillary astrocytomas is difficult because many tumors, particularly those in deep structures of the diencephalon or brainstem, cannot be resected sufficiently to provide the material required to classify the tumor accurately. Thus, the terms *fibrillary astrocytomas* and *low-grade astrocytoma* are often used interchangeably. Although all fibrillary astrocytomas are low-grade gliomas, most low-grade gliomas are pilocytic astrocytomas. Many tumors are classified as grade II astrocytoma with piloid features because a biopsy specimen may have been too small to identify all the elements required for classification as a pilocytic grade I astrocytoma. Similarly, the histologic term *pilocytic astrocytoma with fibrillary features* is used to indicate tumors that have all the components of grade I pilocytic astrocytomas but with areas of infiltration suggesting that they could be grade II. Other low-grade gliomas include pilomyxoid astrocytomas, oligodendrogliomas, and gangliogliomas. Fibrillary astrocytomas localized to the posterior fossa represent 3% to 15% of cerebellar tumors[378]; their incidence is lower in the remainder of the brain and spine. No gender predilection exists and the peak age at diagnosis is 6 to 10 years. Genetic abnormalities in low-grade gliomas are uncommon.[271] The reported incidence of low-grade gliomas has increased over the past several years. Although there is a purported association with paternal workplace exposure in the chemical and electrical industries, a more likely explanation is the increased use and availability of MRI and the diagnosis of presymptomatic lesions.[10,379]

Clinical Presentation. The initial symptoms of fibrillary astrocytomas vary, depending on the location of the tumor. Patients with medullary tumors may present with a long history of dysphagia, hoarseness, ataxia, and hemiparesis. Cervicomedullary tumors may cause medullary or upper cervical symptoms such as neck discomfort, weakness or numbness of the hands, and an asymmetrical quadriparesis. Patients with midbrain tumors such as a tectal glioma often present with signs and symptoms of raised intracranial pressure. Other symptoms include diplopia and hemiparesis. In children with dorsally exophytic brainstem glioma, a component of the tumor arises in the medulla and expands in a dorsal direction, resulting in noncommunicating hydrocephalus. Supratentorial fibrillary astrocytomas more commonly present with seizures, although thalamic lesions present with motor deficits. Hypothalamic lesions can present as diencephalic syndrome.[365] Low-grade astrocytomas in the brainstem are usually focal rather than diffuse. They tend to arise in the midbrain, cerebellar peduncles, medulla, or cervicomedullary region. Because of the slow rate of progression of these lesions, most patients have subtle neurologic changes that only become evident over a long period of time. Unlike adult fibrillary astrocytomas, in which degeneration to malignant gliomas is common, pediatric fibrillary astrocytomas remain low grade, even after multiple recurrences.[360,380] Symptoms may exist for months to years prior to the diagnosis of a low-grade astrocytoma.

Imaging and Histology. Most low-grade fibrillary astrocytomas appear isodense on CT without significant contrast enhancement. The tumors are hypointense on T1- and hyperintense on T2-weighted MRI, with minimal or no gadolinium enhancement (Fig. 17-24) except for dorsally exophytic brainstem tumors. This is in contrast to most pilocytic astrocytomas, in which homogeneous contrast enhancement is common. Pathologic examination may demonstrate some cellular pleomorphism but no mitoses, necrosis, or endothelial proliferation are present (i.e., no histologic features of malignancy). Although pilocytic astrocytomas are usually well-circumscribed lesions with a biphasic pattern of areas of bipolar cells and Rosenthal fibers and other areas with microcysts, fibrillary astrocytomas have greater cellularity and infiltrating boundaries.[381] In contrast to grade III or IV astrocytomas, fibrillary astrocytomas must lack features of malignancy, including significant atypia and pleomorphism, mitoses, vascular proliferation, and palisading necrosis. A number of other subtypes of grade II astrocytomas have been identified. These include the lipoastrocytic,[382] protoplasmic, gemistocytic,[383] and xanthomatous types.[381] These subtypes are much less common in pediatric patients compared with adults and may have a worse outcome compared with fibrillary and pilocytic astrocytomas. The rarity of these lesions prevents formal studies of these subtypes.

Management. Management of most fibrillary astrocytomas is similar to pilocytic astrocytomas and depends on the clinical prodrome, age, and location of the primary tumor.[384] Rapidly evolving clinical symptoms in the setting of an operable tumor usually warrant prompt neurosurgical intervention. On the other hand, a lesion with a long history of indolent and mild symptoms is often managed with close MRI and clinical surveillance.[332] Patients who subsequently show progressive neurologic symptoms and MRI studies suggesting tumor growth require therapeutic intervention.[385] Diffuse fibrillary astrocytomas in eloquent locations such as the thalamus or motor regions are often biopsied to confirm the diagnosis and exclude higher grade glial tumors. They do not lend themselves to radical resections, as is commonly done for PAs. However, in certain cases, such as a dorsally exophytic brainstem astrocytomas, radical resection can often confer a long symptom-free outcome. In cases in which resection is not feasible, chemotherapy or radiotherapy may be indicated.[320] As in the case of progressive or unresectable pilocytic astrocytomas, chemotherapy is the preferred first approach for younger patients (see Table 17-5).[317,319,386-388] Patients respond well to vincristine and carboplatin or TPCV chemotherapy. A recent randomized clinical trial of grades I and II astrocytomas has been completed comparing these two treatment regimens. Although recurrences occur in most patients, necessitating retreatment with other chemotherapeutic agents, the overall prognosis remains good. Limited experience with novel combinations of agents[309,316] or high-dose chemotherapy is available.[315] Radiotherapy is reserved for older children or younger patients whose tumors progress and are refractory to chemotherapy. Reduced radiation doses to adjacent normal tissue, with equivalent tumor control to that of standard photon therapy, can be achieved with conformal proton therapy.[347] Radiation therapy delivered at the time of initial diagnosis does not appear to provide additional benefit for event-free or overall survival.[286]

Prognosis. The long-term survival rate for completely resected pediatric supratentorial low-grade astrocytomas is excellent, especially when compared with similar tumors in adults.[275] Even partially or unresected fibrillary astrocytomas may remain stable for many years. An example of this is the focal midbrain or tectal glioma, which is rarely biopsied or resected.[389,390] Response to chemotherapy appears similar to that observed in pilocytic astrocytomas, although most patients will experience one or more episodes of progression, requiring retreatment with additional chemotherapy.[391,392] However, children with primary tumors arising in the pons or thalamus have a worse prognosis.[352,393] The presence of a gemistocytic component characterized by a predominance of large astrocytes, with thick processes and dramatic accumulation of GFAP, represents a histologic variant of low-grade fibrillary (grade II) astrocytoma. This variant may be associated with p53 mutations and may also convey a higher predisposition to malignant transformation.[394,395]

Although most patients with low-grade astrocytomas will survive, patients with fibrillary astrocytomas have a poorer outcome than patients with grade I astrocytomas.[396] Because pilocytic astrocytomas are more focal and easier to resect than fibrillary astrocytomas, prognosis may be related to the ease of resection rather than to biologic differences between these histologic variants. Overall survival after chemotherapy of children and adolescents with low-grade astrocytomas at 10 years is 70% to 80%.[286,305,326] The role of MIB-1 expression in the prognosis of low-grade astrocytomas was not established after age and degree of resection were excluded.[397] Survivors of low-grade astrocytomas still have a number of limitations.[333,398] Future treatment efforts for these tumors will therefore need to combine effective therapy with improved quality of survivorship in these patients.

Tectal Gliomas

Tectal gliomas are typically hamartomas or low-grade astrocytomas and patients present with acute hydrocephalus in most cases. These tumors appear to represent a unique variant of low-grade tumors, based on their positive long-term outcome, with relief of hydrocephalus as the sole therapeutic intervention. Because biopsy or surgical resection of these lesions is rarely required, little is known about the pathways that drive their activation. There are no known genetic syndromes that give rise to these tumors.

Presentation. Most patients with tectal gliomas present with the symptoms of obstructive hydrocephalus because of expansion of these lesions adjacent to the periaqueductal space. When picked up incidentally, many patients will demonstrate prolonged periods of stability and do not require treatment.

Imaging and Histology. The radiographic appearance of most tectal gliomas is similar to that of other low-grade gliomas. Most tumors lack contrast enhancement (Fig. 17-25). Based on their location and presenting symptoms, histologic verification is not required to make the diagnosis and can cause significant morbidity if attempted.

Management. Biopsy or resection of tectal gliomas is usually not required. Rather, most patients require immediate CSF diversion through a third ventriculostomy.[399,400] Failures of third ventriculostomies have been reported, even many years after the initial procedure, necessitating the proper education of families regarding symptoms that should precipitate immediate evaluation.[401] Rarely, tectal gliomas larger than 10 cm at presentation will continue to progress over time and may require surgical debulking and/or chemotherapy.[402] Tumors that have atypical radiographic features, rapid progression, or repeated recurrence may require a biopsy. Tumors with asymptomatic progression can often be observed carefully.[403] When treatment is required, approaches similar to those used for other low-grade astrocytomas are recommended. Patients are usually initiated on chemotherapy. Radiation therapy is not required for most patients and continued progression of these lesions into adulthood is rare.

Prognosis. The long-term outcome for patients with tectal gliomas remains excellent, which is surprising given the unresectable nature of the lesion and absence of therapy for most patients. Overall survival approaches 100% in this population[404] and thus avoidance of unnecessary surgical or radiation-related long-term morbidity is critical.

Pilomyxoid Astrocytomas

Pilomyxoid astrocytomas are a newly stratified group of grade II pediatric tumors in the 2007 WHO classification[183,269] that were previously grouped together with pilocytic astrocyto-

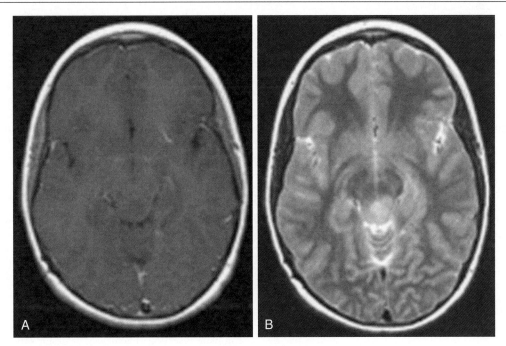

FIGURE 17-25. Tectal glioma. **A,** Axial T1 image with contrast. **B,** Axial T2 image.

mas.[405,406] Although no specific molecular pathway responsible for these tumors has yet been identified, the presence of defects in the *BCR* gene on chromosome 17[407] provides possible clues that will require further analysis. Other chromosomal aberrations have also been identified.[408] Pilomyxoid astrocytomas are found most commonly in the midline of the brain and spine.[409] These tumors are usually identified in infants, although their presence in adults has been reported.[410] At recurrence, tumors can appear as classic PAs, suggesting a developmental relationship between the two.[411]

Clinical Presentation. Although pilomyxoid astrocytomas present in a manner similar to that of other low-grade gliomas, the incidence of metastatic disease at presentation appears higher and requires a full workup, including spinal MRI and CSF for cytology. Patients with pilomyxoid astrocytomas may be at greater risk for spontaneous hemorrhage at the time of diagnosis or resection, or during follow-up.[412,413]

Imaging and Histology. On MRI, pilomyxoid astrocytomas appear similar to PAs, with well-circumscribed margins and little peritumoral edema.[414] They are usually found in the midline and can be solid or solid and cystic. They are usually bright on T1- or T2-weighted and FLAIR sequences, and they enhance with contrast administration.[415] In approximately 50% of cases, the contrast enhancement is heterogeneous.[416,417] Adjacent areas of brain can demonstrate elevated choline-to-creatinine ratios suggestive of an infiltrative margin.[417] Histologically, these lesions lack many features of PAs, including Rosenthal fibers and a biphasic pattern. Rather, there is a monophasic pattern and myxoid background, with strong GFAP and synaptophysin staining.[418] Like other glial tumors, mixed lineages may also be possible for pilomyxoid astrocytoma.[419] The variable histologic appearance compared with pilocytic astrocytomas,[420] MRS signal changes,[421] and higher incidence of progression and dissemination support their distinction from PAs.[405] There appears to be a predilection for younger age when localized to the pituitary-hypothalamic region.[422]

Management. Because of the more aggressive nature of these tumors compared with pilocytic astrocytomas, pilomyxoid astrocytomas are now classified as grade II gliomas. Treatments typically follow those of other low-grade gliomas, including vincristine and carboplatin or TPCV chemotherapy. Well-organized clinical trials for this rare subtype are not possible, however. Up-front chemoradiation therapy combinations have also been tried for these tumors.[423] Because of the young age and deep location of these tumors in many patients, radiation-based strategies will lead to significant long-term morbidity in most survivors. Many patients with pilomyxoid astrocytomas are infants and have diencephalic syndrome with dissemination, so complete surgical resection is not possible. Thus, most patients will start with low-grade glioma chemotherapy. The use of intrathecal therapy for those with disseminated disease unable to receive craniospinal radiation can be considered.

Prognosis. Without well-defined studies, the prognosis of pilomyxoid astrocytoma is difficult to assess with certainty. Confounding issues of deep-seated lesions, especially around the hypothalamic region, in which surgical options are limited, along with the young age of these patients and presence of metastatic disease, likely affect the overall poor prognosis. A mean overall survival of 60 months for patients with pilomyxoid astrocytoma versus 220 months for patients with grade I pilocytic astrocytomas has been reported.[422] Whether their unique biology affects survival is unknown, although these tumors can recur as typical grade I pilocytic astrocytomas.[411]

Ganglioglioma and Glial-Neuronal Tumors

Gangliogliomas are low-grade (WHO grade I) glioneuronal tumors. These tumors represent 4% to 8% of primary brain tumors in children, with 80% occurring before age 30 years and a mean age of younger than 10 years.[424] They are frequently associated with seizures and tend to be slow-growing tumors. Gangliogliomas can occur throughout the CNS[425,426] although most are localized to the temporal and parietal lobes.[424]

Clinical Presentation. Seizures are the first manifestation in 50% of cases of ganglioglioma and many have a prolonged history of seizures of longer than 2 years.[424] Complex partial seizures are common because gangliogliomas are frequently located in the temporal lobe, particularly the temporomesial region,[427] although they can occur anywhere in the brain or spine.

Imaging and Histology. Gangliogliomas are typically contrast-enhancing cystic lesions on CT scan. The MRI appearance of these tumors can be variable, but is frequently hypointense on T1-weighted sequences and hyperintense on T2-weighted images. Gadolinium enhancement varies in intensity from absent to significant and can be nodular, solid, or circumferential.[428] An infantile variant of ganglioglioma, desmoplastic infantile ganglioglioma (DIG), can occur (see later). Pathologic studies show synaptophysin and neuronal nuclear antigen (NeuN)–positive ganglion cells as well as a GFAP-positive astrocytic component.[429] Lesions associated with the ganglion cell but lacking the astrocytic component are called gangliocytomas. Gangliogliomas are frequently WHO grade I tumors, although some may show anaplastic features in the glial component. MIB-1 positive cells are usually localized to the astrocytic component.[430]

Management. Complete or near-total resection is the treatment of choice[427] and, in most cases, can eliminate or significantly improve seizure frequency in this patient population.[431,432] Recurrent or unresectable tumors may be treated with radiation therapy,[424,433] although these lesions may respond to low-grade glioma chemotherapy, and thus patients may avoid some of the long-term toxicity of radiation.[326] In the case of recurrent or unresectable ganglioglioma, response to low-grade glioma chemotherapy has been demonstrated.[424] Treatment of recurrent or unresectable gangliogliomas is included in current low-grade glioma chemotherapy trials. It should be noted that these tumors have been shown to undergo malignant transformation over time, usually involving the astrocytic component.

Prognosis. Gross total resection is often curative, making tumor location and extent of resection the most important prognostic factors.[427] Most patients are rendered seizure-free following gross total resection.[432] Gangliogliomas of the posterior fossa have also been reported and their outcomes appear similar to those for supratentorial lesions. Patients whose tumors can be fully resected to remove the enhancing components are likely to remain disease-free, although those with subtotal resected disease often require additional resection, chemotherapy, and/or radiation therapy.[425] The uncommon presentation of these tumors in the infratentorial location and the limited sample sizes in case reports limit the confidence on which therapeutic approaches can be recommended. Spinal cord ganglioglioma appear to have an indolent course. Those with a complete resection are often cured. Even patients with subtotal resection can remain stable for prolonged periods. Therefore, treatment should be deferred to those lesions that show clear evidence of progressive disease.[434]

Desmoplastic Infantile Gangliogliomas

DIGs are supratentorial tumors involving the leptomeningeal surface and are identified predominantly in children younger than 2 years.[435] These lesions are often very large, in part because of the presence of cysts, and they frequently involve the dura. Although precise estimates of their incidence are lacking, they make up less than 1% of pediatric brain tumors. No causative chromosomal aberrations have been identified.

Clinical Presentation. Most patients present with increasing head circumference, bulging fontanelle, and lethargy. Older patients present with focal motor deficits.

Imaging and Histology. DIGs are large cystic structures on CT scan, with contrast enhancement of the solid component. T1-weighted MRI sequences demonstrate an isointense tumor; T2 intensity of the tumor is variable. The tumors usually enhance after contrast administration. Peritumoral edema is uncommon. DIGs possess a desmoplastic stromal background, with neoplastic neurons and astrocytes. They often have areas with elevated MIB-1, although this does not represent transformation to a more malignant phenotype. Tumors lacking the neural component are called desmoplastic infantile astrocytoma (DIAs).

Management. Cure can be achieved with complete resection. Many patients have remained progression-free after total resection without additional treatment.[436] Chemotherapy with vincristine and carboplatin, as for other low-grade astrocytomas, can be considered for symptomatic or progressive cases for whom surgical removal is not feasible.[429,437]

Prognosis. Most patients will be long-term survivors if a complete resection is achieved.[436] Lesions that are more deep-seated may have a poorer outcome and initiation of chemotherapy may be considered at the first signs of progression in these unresectable tumors.[435] Metastatic lesions have been reported, suggesting that in rare cases, a more malignant phenotype can occur.[429]

Dysembryoplastic Neuroepithelial Tumors

Dysembryoplastic neuroepithelial tumors (DNETs) are recently described tumors that may comprise as much as 1% of all brain tumors in patients younger than 20 years.[438] Two thirds of all DNETs are located in the temporal lobe and DNETs are found in 5% to 15% of temporal lobe resections for intractable epilepsy. These lesions are classified as WHO grade I tumors.[439] Thought to be developmental in nature, they are treated with surgery. They are considered to have limited proliferative potential, suggesting that complete surgical resection is not required for long-term disease control.[440] In spite of this, however, recurrences can occur.[441]

Clinical Presentation. The diagnosis of DNET should be a consideration in children and young adults with new-onset seizures or a long history of epilepsy. Patients with these tumors typically present with a long history of complex partial seizures, with an average age of onset of 9 years. In many patients, the seizures are refractory to antiseizure medications. The superficial cortical location of DNETs may account for the high risk of seizures.

Imaging and Histology. Contrast-enhanced cranial MRI typically shows a temporal or frontal lobe lesion, absent peritumoral edema, and only minimal, if any, gadolinium enhancement. They are bright on T2-weighted sequences and hypointense on T1-weighted images (Fig. 17-26). Mass effect is minimal to absent. The pathologic findings include a specific glioneuronal element manifested by GFAP-negative oligodendroglia-like cells and neurons in a mucinous eosinophilic background that give the appearance of floating neurons.[442] Because oligodendrocytes, astrocytes, or both are found on histopathologic analysis, the pathologic differential diagnosis often includes oligodendroglioma, mixed oligoastrocytoma, and ganglioglioma. Differentiation of DNETs from other low-grade gliomas can be difficult.

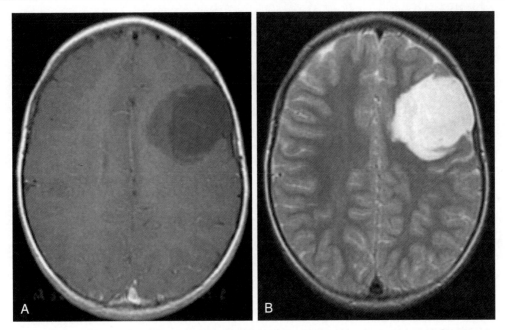

FIGURE 17-26. Left frontal dysembryoplastic neuroepithelial tumor (DNET). **A,** Axial T1 image with contrast. **B,** Axial T2 image.

Management. Although these tumors have a benign course, the associated seizures may be refractory to antiepileptic drugs because of the increased expression of multidrug transporters.[443] Gross total resection is often curative and typically alleviates the seizures, although some case series have shown a significant number of patients who continue to have residual seizures.[440,441] Adjuvant chemotherapy or radiation therapy is not recommended. Rare cases of malignant transformation of DNET following radiation and chemotherapy have been reported.[444]

Prognosis. The stable behavior of these tumors over time results in an excellent prognosis after gross total or partial resection.[440]

Pleomorphic Xanthoastrocytomas

Pleomorphic xanthoastrocytomas (PXAs) are uncommon grade II cortical tumors that mainly occur in children and adolescents and account for less than 1% of CNS tumors. The median age at the time of diagnosis is 14 years. The molecular pathogenesis of these tumors is poorly understood and no causative chromosomal abnormalities have been identified. A recent analysis of 50 PXAs by comparative genomic hybridization, however, has revealed loss of chromosome 9 to be the most common chromosomal lesion.[445] A few reports of PXA in conjunction with NF-1 may implicate the ras pathway in this disease.[446]

Clinical Presentation. PXAs are typically large and superficially located, especially in the temporal lobes. Seizures are the most common presenting feature. For tumors of the cerebellum or spine, direct nerve compression results in focal deficits. Rare cases of dissemination have been reported.[447]

Imaging and Histology. PXAs typically manifest enhancement on MRI, with occasional intratumoral cysts and calcification (Fig. 17-27). Peritumoral edema is uncommon. Tumors usually extend to the meninges. The typical histopathologic picture includes a pleomorphic appearance of the astrocytic component, with significant cellular atypia and bizarre multi-nucleated giant cells with intracellular lipid accumulation. The proliferative indices are usually low, although necrosis, endothelial proliferation, and mitoses have been described. PXA can be confused with glioblastoma multiforme[448] because of the presence of multinucleated cells and occasional foci of necrosis.[449] The expression of CD34 on most tumors may be useful in the histologic classification of difficult or atypical cases.[450] Prognosis appears to correlate with MIB-1 expression.[451] In lesions with mitoses, elevated MIB-1, and necrosis, the term *pleomorphic xanthoastrocytoma with anaplastic features* is used.

Management. The clinical diagnosis of PXA should be suspected in children who present with new-onset seizures, focal deficits, and a large, enhancing cortical mass on brain imaging. The goal of surgery is to achieve a gross total resection, which is usually curative.[452] Adjuvant therapy can be deferred, although the patient is followed expectantly. Tumors that recur and incompletely resected lesions with anaplastic features may be treated with chemotherapy[453] or radiotherapy,[454] although significant activity for these modalities has not been demonstrated. Formal clinical trials for this rare subtype are lacking.

Prognosis. Several series have reported a 5-year progression-free survival of more than 70%. However, the presence of mitoses, endothelial proliferation, or necrosis on the pathologic specimen, although rare, may significantly alter the clinical behavior and prognosis.[451] Cases of anaplastic PXA with subsequent malignant transformation have been reported.[455,456] Radiation therapy does not alter the poor outcome in these cases.

Subependymal Giant Cell Astrocytomas (SEGAs)

SEGAs usually originate in the ependymal walls of the lateral ventricles and are associated almost exclusively with tuberous sclerosis (TS), an autosomal dominant disorder.[457] TS patients have hamartomas and benign tumors of multiple organs, including the brain. The CNS manifestations include cortical

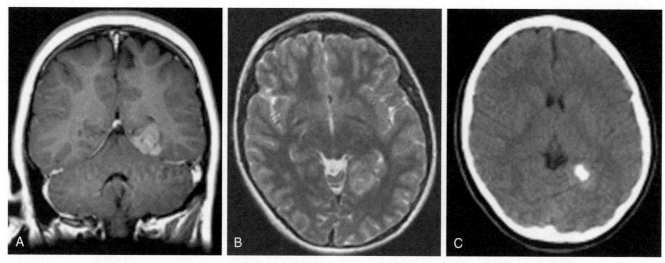

FIGURE 17-27. Pleomorphic xanthoastrocytoma (PXA). **A,** Coronal T1 image with contrast. **B,** Axial T2 image. **C,** Noncontrast computed tomography (CT) image.

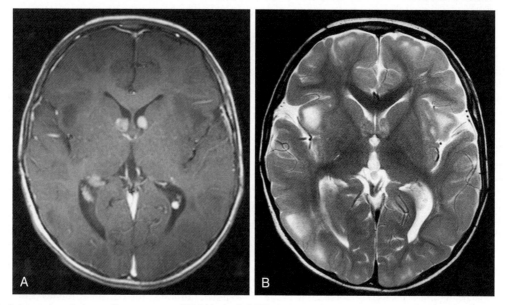

FIGURE 17-28. Subependymal giant cell astrocytoma (SEGA). **A,** Axial T1 image with contrast. **B,** Axial T2 image.

tubers (hamartomas), subcortical glioneuronal hamartomas, subependymal glial nodules, and subependymal giant cell astrocytomas.[458] Two genetic defects, one in the *TSC1* gene on 9q and the other in the *TSC2* gene in 16p, account for TS. Sporadic cases are rare.[459]

Clinical Manifestations. SEGA is sometimes the presenting feature of TS in patients without the typical physical stigmata of the syndrome. Because of the variable phenotype of TS, a consensus on diagnostic criteria has been developed. Presentation in older children and adolescents is common. Although patients with TS typically have multiple periventricular SEGAs, those that produce symptoms of hydrocephalus arise in close proximity to the foramen of Monro, although lesions around the pineal gland can also result in symptoms.[460] Most patients with known TS are followed with regular neuroimaging and the SEGAs are removed in anticipation of more serious neurologic syndromes, such as headaches, altered sensorium, or weak-

ness.[76] Of note, patients with TS may have other significant neurologic symptoms, such as seizures and cognitive deficiency related to cortical tubers.[461]

Imaging and Histology. CT and MRI are essential for early and accurate diagnosis. Although CT is better for detecting small calcified lesions, MRI is superior to CT for identifying areas of gliosis, heterotopia, and SEGA, which gives the typical radiographic appearance of candle dripping.[462] SEGAs typically show diffuse contrast enhancement on CT and MRI studies (Fig. 17-28).[76] SEGAs are considered grade I astrocytomas. They are well-circumscribed tumors that are positive for GFAP, neurofilament, neuron-specific enolase, and synaptophysin.[463,464] Mitoses can be identified but do not indicate a higher grade or more malignant phenotype.

Management. Total gross resection is the treatment of choice for SEGAs that are larger than 5 mm, progressive, and

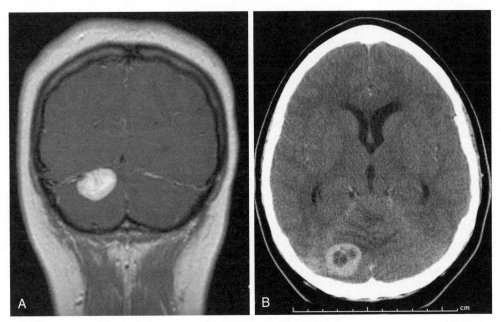

FIGURE 17-29. Cerebellar hemangioblastoma. **A,** Coronal T1 image with gadolinium. **B,** CT image.

cause obstructive hydrocephalus[465] or seizures.[466] The major risk of surgery is injury to the forniceal columns resulting in memory disturbance. The benign behavior of these tumors warrants reoperation in the case of recurrence or progression after subtotal resection. A recent report has documented tumor regression with the administration of rapamycin.[78]

Prognosis. SEGAs are essentially benign tumors and gross total resection is generally curative. However, multiple tumors may arise in some patients with TS, requiring ongoing radiologic surveillance.[76] The overall prognosis for patients with TS is good, despite increased susceptibility to other tumor types, including rhabdomyomas of the myocardium and angiomyomas of the kidney, liver, adrenals, and pancreas.[467]

Hemangioblastomas

Hemangioblastomas are WHO grade I lesions associated with von Hippel–Lindau syndrome (VHL). They occur primarily in adults and are centered in the cerebellum, brainstem and spinal cord.[468] Although sporadic tumors can arise, pediatric cases are usually associated with the inherited syndrome. Cases associated with VHL syndrome can be single or multifocal although most sporadic cases involve isolated nodules. Hemangioblastomas are highly vascularized lesions, although the genetic defect is localized to the stromal elements rather than the vasculature.[469] Tumor development appears to be related to the deregulation of VEGF. Patients with hemangioblastomas need to undergo complete genetic evaluation for VHL and, for those with the inherited disease, careful lifelong screening is necessary.[470]

Clinical Presentation. Obstruction of CSF flow is the primary reason for symptomatology in VHL patients diagnosed with hemangioblastomas. Headaches, morning vomiting, and long tract signs are therefore common. Ataxia and cranial nerve dysfunction can also be observed.[471]

Imaging and Histology. Hemangioblastomas are typically well-circumscribed cystic lesions with a solid tumor nodule.

The solid component tends to enhance brightly with contrast and is usually located peripherally within the cyst (Fig. 17-29). Flow voids are commonly observed on MR imaging and can be well delineated with angiography. Peritumoral edema is commonly observed. Tumors are usually composed of two elements—the stromal cells, which express vimentin and VEGF, and the endothelial cells, which express the VEGF receptor VEGFR2. Hemangioblastomas typically have low proliferative levels based on MIB-1 immunoreactivity and are considered grade I tumors.

Management. The management of these tumors requires specialized neurosurgical expertise because of the high risk of bleeding. The primary approach to these lesions, which tend to occur most commonly in the posterior fossa and cervicomedullary area, is maximal surgical resection.[470] This provides long-term control in most patients[472] although, because of the underlying genetic predisposition, new tumors may continue to develop throughout the life of the patient. Embolization can reduce the intraoperative risks of bleeding.[473] Radiosurgery can successfully treat the mural component of these tumors, although control is negatively influenced by the presence of the cysts.[474] Recently, VEGF inhibitors have been tested in this population, with encouraging results.[475]

Prognosis. Because of the genetic basis of these lesions, recurrences are common and likely represent new tumors rather than recurrences of previously resected ones. This indicates the importance of continued careful evaluation in this patient population.

Rare Low-Grade Gliomas

Tanycytic Astrocytomas. Tanycytic astrocytomas are rare and poorly characterized tumors, usually of the hypothalamic region.[476] Their malignant potential is not well defined, although recurrences after complete resection have been observed.

Lipoastrocytomas. Lipoastrocytomas are rare cortical tumors that, as the name suggests, possess fat droplets that give them the appearance of adipocytes in the context of a low-grade astrocytic lesion. These tumors express GFAP.[382] Recurrences can occur and are treated with resection. Malignant transformation has not been reported in this tumor type.

Dysplastic Cerebellar Gangliocytomas. Dysplastic cerebellar gangliocytomas are rare tumors of the cerebellum and fourth ventricle region that are of limited proliferative potential. They have a characteristic imaging pattern on MRI, with an abnormal laminated pattern in the cerebellum, although this is not pathognomonic and can be mimicked by medulloblastoma. As such, biopsy is recommended to differentiate the two entities.[477] Dysplastic cerebellar gangliocytoma do not typically require therapeutic intervention.

High-Grade Gliomas

High-grade gliomas are categorized in a similar manner as for low-grade gliomas. Although important differences in the time to progression for grade 3 versus grade 4 malignant gliomas is well recognized, most of these patients eventually succumb to their disease. As will be discussed later, a few notable exceptions occur. First, infants with malignant gliomas have a significant long-term survival rate (estimated around 25%), even without radiation therapy, while patients with diffuse intrinsic pontine gliomas typically suffer rapid progression and death, even when their histology suggests a lower grade lesion. The following sections will therefore discuss high-grade lesions in the context of location, and grade.

Supratentorial High-Grade Astrocytomas

High-grade astrocytomas (HGAs) are much less common in children than adults. Although over 30% of all pediatric brain tumors are low-grade gliomas, supratentorial high-grade astrocytomas represent only 6% to 12% of all primary pediatric brain tumors and diffuse brainstem gliomas represent another 10%. High-grade gliomas are anaplastic astrocytoma (WHO grade III) or glioblastoma multiforme (WHO grade IV). A number of genetic abnormalities have been implicated in high-grade gliomas in adult and pediatric patients, including the overexpression or mutation of EGFR,[478] alterations in phosphatidylinositol 3′-kinase (PI3K) signaling via mutations of the PTEN tumor suppressor,[479-481] topoisomerase II-alpha,[482] p14ARF,[483] and DNA repair enzyme alterations.[484] In the Children's Cancer Group CCG945 study of children with malignant high-grade gliomas, p53 status was an important independent prognostic variable, with a 5-year progression-free survival of 44% in low p53-expressing tumors versus 17% in those with overexpression of p53.[485] Similar results from other studies have supported these conclusions.[486,487] In addition to histopathologic differences, there are genetic differences between grades III and IV astrocytomas—notably, less frequent mutations of PTEN, amplification of EGFR, and loss of 10q in anaplastic astrocytomas compared with glioblastoma. However, mutation of TP53 has been shown to be more common in anaplastic astrocytoma.[488] It should be noted that most studies of genetic features of anaplastic astrocytoma and glioblastoma, and their association with prognosis, have been based on adult tumors.

It is becoming increasingly clear that the study of adult glioblastoma may be less informative regarding the molecular pathways involved in pediatric glioblastoma than previously thought.[489,490] Pediatric tumors have demonstrated abnormalities in the Ras and Akt pathways, as well as Y-box protein-1.[491] Microsatellite instability, which has been associated with a number of adult tumors, was not identified in an analysis of 71 pediatric gliomas, 41 of which were high-grade lesions.[492] An

analysis of 62 cases from the Children's Cancer Group study CCG945 identified only a single case of EGFR mutation, present in up to 50% of adult tumors, with 14 of 38 samples showing overexpression of EGFR. Only one case of PTEN mutation was identified, although an additional seven cases of PTEN loss were detected.[493] These results confirm that adult and pediatric tumors with identical histologies use different pathways or different mechanisms of activation of the same pathway. Similar results have been reported by others.[243] MIB-1 staining is usually elevated in HGAs and correlates with grade and prognosis. Patients with MIB-1 levels above 36% had a 5-year progression-free survival of 11% compared with 33% in those with MIB-1 levels less than 18%.[494]

High-grade gliomas occur more commonly in certain genetic syndromes. These include hereditary nonpolyposis colorectal carcinoma (HNPCC)[89] and Li-Fraumeni syndrome, a dominantly inherited mutation syndrome involving the p53 tumor suppressor gene.[495] *p53* mutations are rare in sporadic pediatric CNS tumors lacking a typical family history.[496] Cases of congenital glioblastoma multiforme (GBM) have also been observed at birth or within the first 3 months of life and appear genetically distinct from their childhood and adult counterparts. Long-term survival has been reported in these patients and supports the unique characteristics of these otherwise fatal tumors.[497-502]

Thalamic gliomas can occur as high-grade or low-grade lesions.[361] In a retrospective review of 69 thalamic tumors, 32 were identified as unilateral low-grade astrocytomas, 22 were unilateral high-grade gliomas, 6 were thalamoperduncular, and 9 were bithalamic. Most patients with unilateral low-grade astrocytomas were long-term survivors.[360] Poor prognostic factors in these patients included short interval of symptoms, high-grade histology, and inability to resect the lesion.[360]

Clinical Presentation. The clinical manifestations of HGA depend on the anatomic location as well as the age of the patient. The clinical prodrome is usually short and rapidly evolving. with signs and symptoms of elevated intracranial pressure and/or focal neurologic deficits. A protracted course may evolve in the context of malignant transformation of a low-grade fibrillary astrocytoma.[503] The presence of a malignant glioma within the volume of a previously irradiated field is difficult to differentiate from a radiation-induced malignant transformation of a low-grade astrocytoma, although preliminary studies have identified some differences between de novo and radiation-induced glioblastoma multiforme.[504] Dissemination of malignant gliomas into the cerebrospinal fluid is less common than for medulloblastoma and other neural tumors but is being recognized more frequently,[505] particularly as patients survive longer. Approximately 3% of pediatric patients with malignant gliomas will have metastatic disease at presentation.[506]

Imaging and Histology. Typical high-grade astrocytomas have an MRI appearance of heterogeneous enhancement or diffuse nonenhancing tumor with significant edema on the T1-weighted image, compressing or displacing adjacent ventricular structures and occasionally causing hydrocephalus. The T2 signal is often more diffuse, consistent with both infiltrative tumor and edema (Fig. 17-30). Magnetic resonance spectroscopy demonstrates a markedly elevated choline-to-NAA ratio. Lesions tend to be FDG-PET avid. ^{99m}Tc-sestamibi SPECT (MIBI SPECT) imaging can also detect malignant gliomas and can be used to follow for response or recurrence.[151] Areas of hemorrhage within pediatric GBMs at diagnosis are not uncommon.[507] Malignant features on histopathologic examination include nuclear pleomorphism, mitoses, palisading necrosis (Fig. 17-31), endothelial proliferation (Fig. 17-32), and a high Ki-67 or MIB-1 labeling index (see Fig. 17-16). Most pediatric

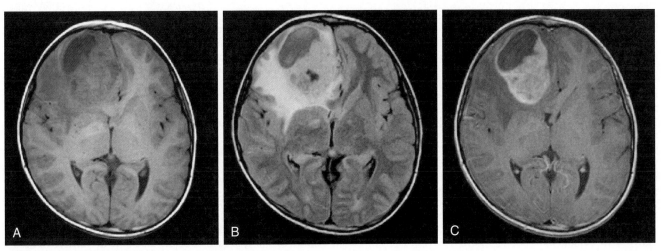

FIGURE 17-30. Right frontal glioblastoma multiforme. **A,** Axial T1 image without contrast. **B,** Axial fluid-attenuated inversion recovery (FLAIR) image. **C,** Axial T1 image with contrast.

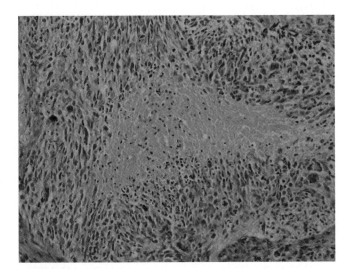

FIGURE 17-31. Palisading necrosis in a child with glioblastoma multiforme (H&E; ×400).

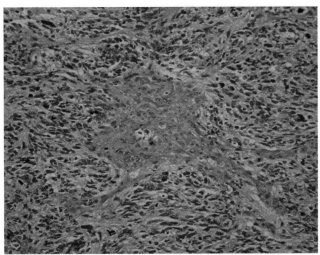

FIGURE 17-32. Vascular proliferation with glomeruloid tuft in a child with glioblastoma multiforme (H&E; ×400).

malignant gliomas are nestin-positive on immunohistochemistry.[508] Distinguishing between grade III and IV tumors relies on differences in histologic features, with grade III tumors having the first two of four features (nuclear atypia, mitoses, endothelial proliferation, necrosis) present, and grade IV tumors having three or four present. A rare subtype of pediatric glioblastoma called giant cell glioblastoma has been reported.[509] Although time to progression in this variant may be slightly longer, overall prognosis is not significantly better than other pediatric malignant gliomas.

Management. Most HGAs in children, similar to those in adults, arise in the cerebral hemispheres and treatment options are similar to those for adults.[503,510] The initial management following neuroimaging is to administer high-dose corticosteroids. The goals of neurosurgery include establishing a histologic diagnosis and, whenever possible, achieving radical resection.[511] Internal decompression or debulking makes subsequent radiotherapy more tolerable and probably more effective, given the lower tumor burden. Resection also diminishes

the duration of corticosteroid therapy[512] but complete resections are difficult to achieve as a result of the infiltrative properties of high-grade astrocytomas. The role of radiation therapy in the treatment of older children has been clearly established over the past 25 years.[513,514] The prognosis for children with HGA is poor but better than in adults. A report from the Children's Cancer Group[515] showed that the 5-year progression-free survival (PFS) rates for anaplastic astrocytoma were 44% ± 11% and 22% ± 6% for children who underwent radical resection versus other types of surgery, respectively. The 5-year PFS rates for glioblastoma multiforme were 26% ± 9% and 4% ± 3% for children who underwent radical resection versus other types of surgery, respectively. Radical resection and the absence of p53 immunostaining were favorable risk factors,[485] although O6-methylguanine DNA methyltransferase (MGMT) levels correlated with a worse prognosis.[516-518] PTEN deletions and EGFR amplification were not commonly identified.[493]

Chemotherapy currently has an emerging role, both alone and concomitantly with radiation therapy. Several studies have shown that chemotherapy with radiation therapy may have a clinically significant role in children with HGA.[519] The overall 5-year survival of children with supratentorial HGA treated with chemotherapy and radiation is approximately 43% versus 18% for radiation alone.[520] Building on the results of a large clinical trial for adults with high-grade gliomas that showed a survival benefit to combined radiotherapy and temozolomide,[521,522] the Children's Oncology Group conducted a pediatric clinical trial using a similar treatment regimen. Although the results of this trial are pending, this regimen appears well tolerated and equivalent to previous clinical trials combining radiation therapy and multiagent chemotherapy. Additional studies building on this temozolomide backbone are underway,[324] including one that uses lomustine (CCNU).[523] To overcome the resistance of MGMT, inhibitors of this resistance pathway are being combined with temozolomide.[256] This approach, however, includes significant increased risk for toxicity, because MGMT expression in normal tissue as well as in tumor tissue is targeted.

Preirradiation chemotherapy has been studied with the goal of delaying radiation. This approach is especially important for children younger than 3 years. Treatment with high-dose chemotherapy and autologous bone marrow or stem cell transplantation has been conducted in children with HGA.[524,525] The risk-benefit ratio is still under investigation,[526] with initial reports of 23% overall response but a mortality rate of 16%.[527]

Patients with diffuse thalamic and pontine high-grade tumors have the worst prognosis, in part because these tumors are unresectable.[370] Diffuse, infiltrating brainstem tumors have been treated with high-dose chemotherapy and stem cell rescue, with disappointing results.

The success of therapy for newly diagnosed high-grade glioma patients is limited, even with maximal resection, radiation therapy, and adjuvant chemotherapy. Not surprisingly, chemotherapy in the setting of relapsed disease has demonstrated little long-term success. Use of temozolomide as a single agent in recurrent disease has failed to demonstrate significant clinical activity, although occasional responses were observed.[528] Other novel approaches are clearly needed for this population.[489,513] A number of agents have been tested in recurrent disease, although no cytotoxic chemotherapy has been shown to have significant activity once tumors progress after radiation therapy. Blood-brain barrier disruption approaches have not demonstrated improved survival.[234] Immunologic recruitment approaches, including the use of oral cyclophosphamide and gamma interferon in combination or oral topotecan, have also not been successful in improving outcomes.[529,530]

Prognosis. The prognosis for children with HGA is poor but better than in adults.[484,500,531] The degree of surgical resection is associated with better progression-free survival.[515,532] Patients with anaplastic astrocytoma have a more favorable prognosis than those with glioblastoma multiforme.[494,533] A report from the Children's Cancer Group[515] showed that the 5-year PFS rates for anaplastic astrocytoma were 44% ± 11% and 22% ± 6% for children who underwent radical resection versus other types of surgery, respectively. The 5-year PFS rates for glioblastoma multiforme were 26% ± 9% and 4% ± 3% for children who underwent radical resection versus other types of surgery, respectively. Radical resection and the absence of p53 immunostaining are favorable risk factors.[485] The role of MGMT expression in pediatric tumors has confirmed the results reported in adults[521]; lack of MGMT expression, which repairs the damage done by certain chemotherapy, correlates with improved outcome when temozolomide is used.[516] MGMT expression in pediatric tumors also predicted poor outcome in patients who did not receive drugs targeting O6 methylation, suggesting that MGMT may be a prognostic marker.

Children younger than 5 years appear to have a better response rate and overall survival than older children.[531] Survivors of congenital glioblastoma multiforme have been reported, supporting the observation that infants with malignant glioma have a better prognosis than children or adults with the same disease.[534]

New treatment approaches include radiosurgical boost to the postoperative residual tumor following external beam radiotherapy, radiosensitizing agents such as gemcitabine[535] or gadolinium texaphyrin,[536] and new biologic agents that directly target aberrant signaling pathways. Multiple experimental agents are currently undergoing phase I and II evaluation in children, including various small-molecule inhibitors such as the EGFR antagonists erlotinib and gefitinib, the mTOR inhibitors sirolimus and everolimus, the farnesyltransferase inhibitors R115777 and SCH66336, and antiangiogenesis agents such as bevacizumab, AZD2171, and cilengitide.[537] Other experimental approaches include convection-enhanced delivery of potent cellular toxins, novel antimetabolites such as pemetrexed, immune-based therapy,[248] the ansamycin antibiotic 17-AAG, and platinum analogues such as oxaliplatin.[252,513]

Diffuse Intrinsic Pontine Gliomas

Tumors of the brainstem occur in approximately 10% to 20% of pediatric patients with central nervous system tumors. The median age at diagnosis is 7 to 9 years but these tumors may occur throughout childhood.[538] Various classification schemes have been developed to describe brainstem tumors,[539,540] looking at anatomic localization and imaging characteristics.[541,542] Anatomically, brainstem tumors can arise from the tectum, midbrain, pons, or cervicomedullary junction in either a focal or diffuse manner and, for this reason, the term *brainstem glioma* has generated considerable confusion. Intrinsic diffuse pontine gliomas (DPGs) are a unique subset of brainstem tumors with a dismal prognosis[543,544] and should be considered differently from other high-grade astrocytomas.[538]

In the past, patients with diffuse pontine gliomas were often not biopsied. Significant morbidities were previously observed and the information from the biopsy samples was limited. Many samples were from areas at the periphery of the tumor and included normal cells and reactive gliosis, which complicated the histopathologic classification of these tumors. It is from autopsy samples that newer information has been learned, such as the overexpression of Erb1.[545] With the revolution in neurosurgical techniques and the advent of new molecular analyses using minuscule quantities of tissue, the need to reconsider biopsy of these tumors is underway, especially now that many new specifically targeted drugs to these pathways are becoming available. In a recently reported series of 24 patients, biopsies were safely performed in all 24 patients, with only 2 suffering transient neurologic deficits.[546] The development of nonhuman primate models of direct drug delivery into the brainstem opens up another avenue for developing improved therapies for these tumors.[547,548]

Clinical Presentation. The clinical presentation of patients with brainstem tumors appears to fall into two groups. Patients with short presenting histories (i.e., less than 2 to 6 months), multiple cranial neuropathies (unilateral or bilateral), long tract signs (e.g., Babinski sign, hyperreflexia, weakness) and cerebellar signs (e.g., ataxia, dysmetria, dysarthria) are likely to have a diffuse pontine glioma. Patients with low-grade brainstem gliomas tend to demonstrate a more insidious history of isolated cranial nerve palsy or weakness. Hydrocephalus is observed in less than 10% of patients. Care must be taken to exclude children with an acute clinical history of obstructive hydrocephalus as the sole measure of rapid onset of symptoms. Although the

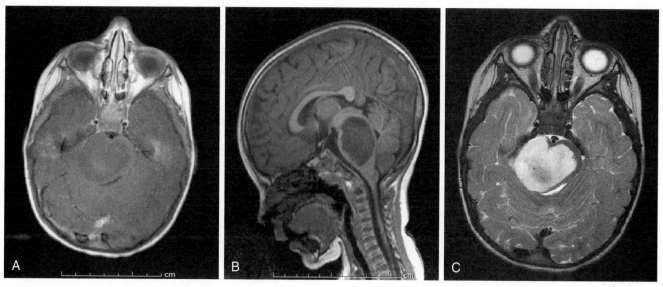

FIGURE 17-33. Diffuse intrinsic pontine glioma. **A,** Axial T1 image with contrast with minimal enhancement. Note the tumor encroachment around the basilar artery. **B,** Sagittal T1 image without contrast. This is a large, diffusely expanding, low T1-weighted lesion of the pons with little encroachment into the midbrain or medulla. **C,** Axial T2 image.

pons is not typically associated with behavior changes, pathologic laughter or separation anxiety have been symptoms noted in this population, either at diagnosis or at the time of progression.[549]

Imaging and Histology. The diagnosis of diffuse pontine gliomas may be made based on the classic MRI appearance of a diffusely expanded pons with encirclement of the basilar artery.[550] Most diffuse brainstem tumors appear to be hypointense on T1-weighted MRI imaging and hyperintense on T2-weighted imaging. A prominent edema signal is common. The ventral pons may appear swollen and infiltrated. Contrast enhancement can be variable, from homogeneous rim enhancement to patchy enhancement to complete absence of enhancement. Newer molecular imaging with magnetic resonance spectroscopy has identified a specific spectrum consistent with the malignant potential of DPGs. More importantly, this method can detect positive responses in patients after radiation therapy, as well as changes indicative of progression in advance of MRI changes.[551] Serial measurement and estimation of response may be best achieved with FLAIR imaging,[552] although no radiologic methodology is optimal for disease assessment or response. Time to progression or overall survival rather than radiographic response may therefore be the best determination of treatment activity in clinical trials for this population.[553] In contrast to DPGs, low-grade focal lesions of the brainstem present with a more circumscribed appearance and associated contrast enhancement that occupies less than 50% of the axial diameter of the brainstem. Tumors may be composed of cystic and solid components. Hydrocephalus may infrequently be present at diagnosis but is not typically associated with DPG.

Pathologically, brainstem tumors are a complex group of lesions and are predominantly of astrocytic origin. They can be low-grade or high-grade tumors.[354] A small percentage are found to be of neural origin (e.g., PNET, ATRT) or ganglioglioma[554,555] and treatment should be based on pathology rather than location. Therefore, careful clinical evaluation, detailed history, and assessment of imaging become critical in identifying patients who would benefit from a diagnostic biopsy, as well as those with probable low-grade lesions who may be treated

with less intensive therapy and may have a better prognosis. The histologic appearance of diffuse pontine gliomas is similar to that of other high-grade astrocytomas.[556] Most biopsy samples have shown evidence of atypia and mitoses and qualify as grade 3 anaplastic astrocytomas. Differentiation between WHO grades 3 and 4 histology in the pons is not relevant because these patients all appear to do equally poorly.

Management. Over the last 30 years, little progress has been made in the treatment of DPGs.[557] Radiation therapy has improved the median overall survival from weeks to months, but can at best be considered palliative therapy. Few patients survive more than a few years.[558] A number of adjuvant therapies such as radiation sensitizers, differentiation agents, and cytotoxic drugs have been studied but none has significantly affected the outcomes for these patients.[244,559-564]

Depending on location and radiographic appearance, the role of surgical resection and even biopsy is controversial and, because of the surgical morbidity risks in light of the overall outcomes, the option is not generally offered at the time of diagnosis for patients with diffusely infiltrating tumors. A meta-analysis by Hargrave and colleagues[565] has indicated that 26% of patients underwent a biopsy. There are certain circumstances whereby tissue sampling may be indicated, specifically when the diagnosis cannot be rendered by radiographic imaging alone.[566] As biologic-based therapies become available, a better understanding of the pathways involved in these tumors will require tissue at diagnosis, and the technical issues for doing this now appear feasible, at least in specialized centers.[546]

Radiation therapy remains the mainstay and standard treatment for diffuse pontine gliomas. Conventional focal doses to the brainstem range from 5400 to 5940 cGy. Multiple studies have attempted hyperfractionation techniques, ranging from 6600 to 7800 cGy.[567-573] However, all studies have been unsuccessful at improving the long-term cure rates for these tumors and this modality is still considered palliative. Radiation therapy can allow for relief of neurologic symptoms and reduction of steroid use. Infant brainstem gliomas appeared to do equally poorly[574] in one study, although other reports were able to demonstrate a less aggressive course.[575-577]

A number of phase I and II clinical trials have been performed using chemotherapeutic agents in various approaches.[543] These have included preirradiation multiagent chemotherapy,[564,578] topotecan as a radiosensitizer,[561,579] etanidazole as a radiosensitizer,[562] chemotherapy concurrent with radiation including thalidomide,[580] trofosfamide, and etoposide,[563] carboplatin,[581] carboplatin and etoposide,[582] radiation with temozolomide and cis-retinoic acid,[583] chemotherapy with blood-brain barrier disruption,[584] and a postradiation high-dose chemotherapy setting.[585] Unfortunately, the use of chemotherapy prior to, during, or after radiation therapy, whether conventional or hyperfractionated, has not shown any consistent survival advantage over radiation therapy alone. However, one large analysis of patients registered in multicenter studies over 18 years in Germany identified longer survival in patients who received adjuvant chemotherapy as compared with those who received radiation alone, although overall survival remained limited.[558] Direct administration of drugs into the tumor was also reported in one patient with a diffuse pontine glioma.[586]

The presence of intratumoral hemorrhage in diffuse pontine gliomas is not uncommon and may affect treatment options. In a retrospective study, the incidence of intratumoral hemorrhage was noted to be only approximately 6% at the time of diagnosis, although the cumulative incidences at 6 and at 12 months were 15% and 24%, respectively.[587] It should be noted that the rates of symptomatic intratumoral hemorrhage were somewhat lower—9% and 18% at 6 months and 12 months, respectively. In addition, this analysis did not identify any patient or treatment-related characteristics associated with intratumoral hemorrhage. Rather, it was thought that, because diffuse brainstem tumors are often higher grade lesions and associated with areas of necrosis, this phenomenon is seen because of the inherent biologic characteristics of this type of tumor.

Prognosis. The typical diffuse intrinsic pontine glioma tragically remains the most challenging of tumors to cure. Despite all approaches, most survival curves are superimposable with regard to overall survival.[565] On meta-analyses of numerous clinical reports, median progression-free survival ranges from 5 to 9 months, with a median overall survival at 6 to 16 months. One-year and 2-year survival ranged from 17% to 50% and 7% to 29%, respectively, with less than 10% survival at 3 years.[565,588] The prognosis for patients with focal brainstem lesions was more optimistic, with published results of 68% to 83%, depending on duration of symptoms (longer than 6 months), location (medulla or tectum), and absence of basilar artery engulfment.[555]

Although both high-grade gliomas and diffuse pontine gliomas are not stratified according to disease stage, nor is spinal imaging part of the routine workup at diagnosis, the incidence of neuraxis dissemination at the time of recurrence has been reported to be approximately 17%.[505,589,590] Patients with diffuse thalamic and pontine high-grade tumors have the worst prognosis, in part because their tumors are unresectable.[370]

Currently, there are a number of experimental clinical trials[513] investigating small-molecule inhibitors, such as farnesyltransferase inhibitors, epidermal growth factor receptor inhibitors, antiangiogenic therapies, blood-brain disruption techniques, enhanced delivery techniques, and radiosensitizers, in addition to other high-dose chemotherapy approaches. However, the one well-recognized limitation in progress for these tumors is that their biology is poorly understood. There are ongoing studies using cerebrospinal fluid analyses and autopsy materials to characterize these tumors better. In this new era, in which the biology has driven the direction of man-agement in other tumor types, surgical biopsy at the time of diagnosis is once again being reconsidered for brainstem tumors.

Gliomatosis Cerebri

Although much more common in adults, gliomatosis cerebri has also been identified in children.[591] Similar to adults, these lesions are often grade III astrocytomas that diffusely infiltrate the brain and appear to favor white matter tracts,[592] and can easily cross the corpus callosum. In spite of the widespread presence of disease, often involving both hemispheres and multiple lobes, a large primary focal mass is usually absent. All parts of the brain and spine can be involved. The overall prognosis is very poor by virtue of their diffuse nature and unresectability. Patients can be palliated for longer than would be expected for widely diffuse lesions, suggesting a different biology from that of typical grade III astrocytomas.[593] Genetic aberrations, including loss of 13q and 10q or gains of 7q, have been shown to be markers of poor outcome.[594] Some tumors demonstrate abnormalities in the p53 pathway.[595,596]

Clinical Presentation. The clinical presentation of children with gliomatosis cerebri is varied. Children present more frequently than adults with refractory seizures that can be palliated with surgical intervention.[597] Other presentations of this disease include raised intracranial pressure and cognitive impairment.[598] Tumors involving the brainstem can have cranial nerve deficits, although those in the optic pathway can present with visual or field deficits.

Imaging and Histology. Gliomatosis cerebri is diagnosed on MRI scan and demonstrates a characteristic diffuse infiltrative pattern.[599] T1-weighted sequences are usually isointense to hypointense and underestimate the extent of disease, although T2-weighted sequences are hyperintense and highlight the full extent of the disease (Fig. 17-34). Signal abnormality usually involves multiple lobes.[600] The presence of contrast enhancement is strongly correlated with a poorer prognosis in both adult and pediatric patients.[593,594] A solid area of tumor is usually not evident. Magnetic resonance spectroscopy demonstrates elevation of choline and decrease in NAA levels.[601] Although the hallmark of gliomatosis cerebri is an infiltrative astrocytic tumor, areas of oligodendroglial cells are not uncommon for adult and pediatric patients.[602,603] Most tumors are consistent with grade III histology and mitoses are often present. MIB-1 staining can vary considerably. The absence of mitoses is more likely because of sampling error. GFAP and S100 can be positive or negative. Nestin and vimentin can be positive.[604] Because of their infiltrative growth and co-opting of existing blood vessels, these tumors lack the abundant neovascularization observed in other malignant gliomas,[605] which suggests that they will not be effectively treated with antiangiogenic agents.

Management. Currently, patients with gliomatosis undergo biopsy to confirm the diagnosis. Given the diffuse nature of these tumors, complete resection is rarely feasible. The mainstay of therapy is irradiation to the involved region and, for the pediatric patient, this may require almost complete whole-brain therapy. In addition to significant morbidity, large-volume radiation therapy for gliomatosis cerebri has not been proven effective,[603] although it may delay the time to progression.[606] Objective responses to temozolomide have been documented[607,608] and, in oligodendrogliomas, correlate with chromosome 1p and/or 19q loss.[609] The impact of MGMT expression on response and outcome has not yet been determined.

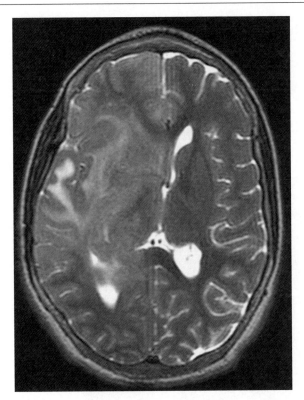

FIGURE 17-34. Gliomatosis cerebri. This axial T2 image demonstrates the diffuse infiltration. Note that a solid uniform mass is absent.

Prognosis. Pediatric patients with gliomatosis cerebri have a poor outcome.[593] In a large series of pediatric and adult patients, a median survival of 14.5 months was demonstrated. Younger age, lower grade histology, and chemoresponsiveness were associated with slightly longer survival times.[610] Although long-term survival is unlikely, adults whose tumors have chromosomal 1p and/or 19q loss can show more chemoresponsiveness to agents such as temozolomide.[594] Similar activity in pediatric patients has not been reported because of the rarity of these tumors in this population.

Ependymomas

Ependymomas are glial tumors that arise from ependymal cells that line the ventricles in the CNS. Ependymal cells play an essential role in the transport of cerebrospinal fluid. Recent experimental evidence has indicated that these cells may be derived from radial glia.[611,612] Ependymal tumors represent approximately 10% of all childhood intracranial neoplasms, constituting the third most common pediatric brain tumor, after astrocytomas and medulloblastoma. They are equally distributed between males and females and the median age at diagnosis is approximately 6 years old. They are significantly less common in blacks than whites.

Ninety percent of pediatric ependymomas are intracranial, with 66% to 75% arising from the posterior fossa.[613] Supratentorial ependymomas are often located in the brain parenchyma, away from the ependymal surface, in contrast to infratentorial ependymomas. Spinal cord ependymomas represent less than 10% of pediatric intramedullary spinal tumors. In contrast, ependymomas represent over 50% of intramedullary spinal tumors in adults.[614]

The WHO classification system recognizes three grades—subependymoma and myxopapillary ependymoma (WHO grade I), classic ependymoma (WHO grade II), and anaplastic ependymoma (WHO grade III). Subependymomas are benign, slow-growing, and often asymptomatic intraventricular neoplasms that are usually found incidentally in middle-aged and older adults, or at autopsy. Myxopapillary ependymomas (WHO grade I) are also slow-growing tumors of the conus medullaris, cauda equina, and filum terminale and manifest primarily in young adults. They account for approximately 10% of all ependymomas.

The most consistent genetic defects in ependymoma are monosomy 22 or structural abnormalities of 22q.[615] This raises the possibility that a tumor suppressor gene may be located on chromosome 22.[616-618] Comparative genomic hybridization has demonstrated significant differences between infant and childhood ependymoma, suggesting that the pathogenesis of this disease differs by age.[619] A number of other molecular defects have been described in ependymomas, including the abnormal expression of ERBB2 and ERBB4 receptors,[620] defects in the p53 homologue p73,[621] increased expression of the vascular endothelial growth factor protein,[622] amplification or overexpression of the p53 regulator MDM2,[623] overexpression of COX-2,[624] presence of telomerase activity,[625] and expression of protein 4.1.[626] Other molecules implicated in the pathogenesis of ependymoma have been reported using proteomic fractionation of tumor tissue. Future studies will be required to determine the significance of these molecules and their potential use as diagnostic markers and targets for therapy.[240]

Significant progress has also been made in the use of these markers in attempting to understand and characterize the putative ependymoma stem cell.[627] The role of telomerase may also be an important factor in the recurrence of ependymomas[628] and additional markers are being developed.[617,629] Finally, the presence of JC viral sequences identified in 5 of 18 ependymomas (but 0 of 32 medulloblastomas) raises the possibility that this agent is associated with ependymal tumorigenesis.[630] SV40 viral, large, T-antigen sequences have also been identified in ependymomas and choroid plexus papillomas[631] but are negative in adjacent normal brain.[632] Although these results have generated significant discussion, they have not been confirmed.[633,634] Further studies will be needed to validate these findings.

Individuals with NF-2 have an increased susceptibility to intramedullary spinal cord ependymomas.[635] Although the NF-2 gene is located at chromosome 22q12, mutations in NF-2 are rarely found in sporadic ependymomas.[636] A recent microarray analysis of pediatric ependymomas has identified a cluster of genes distinct from NF-2 that may be involved in ependymoma tumorigenesis.[617] Expression profiling has indicated that histologically similar ependymomas from different parts of the central nervous system are molecularly and clinically distinct disease subgroups.[611,637] Certain familial colon cancer syndromes may also be associated with an increased incidence of ependymoma in offspring.[638]

Clinical Presentation. The presenting symptoms of infratentorial ependymomas are a result of their origin from ependymal tissue lining the fourth ventricle. Hydrocephalus results when the tumor fills the fourth ventricle, causing headache, irritability, nausea, vomiting, and ataxia. Papilledema can often be found on physical examination. Tumors that extend out of the foramen of Luschka may compromise lower cranial nerve function and cause hearing impairment, hoarseness, and/or dysphagia. If the tumor extends through the foramen of Magendie, the patient may complain of neck discomfort or be noted to have torticollis. The most common signs of the tumor in infants are vomiting, ataxia, headache, lethargy, increased head

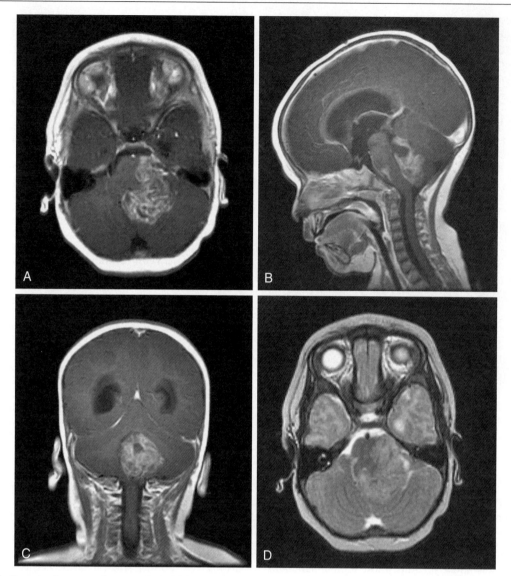

FIGURE 17-35. Posterior fossa ependymoma. **A,** Axial T1 image with contrast. **B,** Sagittal T1 image with contrast. **C,** Coronal T1 image with contrast. **D,** Axial T2 image.

circumference, and irritability.[639] Supratentorial ependymomas, which represent approximately one third of ependymomas, are more common in older children and adults. These patients present with focal neurologic deficits and seizures. Spinal ependymomas are typically located in the cervical region. The most common presenting symptom is pain or motor deficits localized to the level of the spinal cord lesion. The pain is typically described as being worse at night, presumably because of congestion of the spinal venous plexus that occurs when the patient is in the recumbent position. The second most common symptom is radicular dysesthesias, and a late manifestation of this symptom is progressive spastic quadriparesis. Thoracic ependymomas are associated with scoliosis. Myxopapillary ependymomas of the conus medullaris and filum terminale may cause low back pain, radicular pain, saddle anesthesia, and sphincter dysfunction.[640] When these tumors disseminate, they usually remain in the spine, although cranial metastases have been reported; therefore, craniospinal imaging at diagnosis should be undertaken.[641] Pediatric myxopapillary ependymoma may have a higher propensity to spread compared with adult tumors.[641]

Imaging and Histology. A typical MRI appearance of a fourth ventricular ependymoma is that of a homogeneously enhancing well-circumscribed solid mass, extending out one of the foramina of Luschka or Magendie with obstructive hydrocephalus. Hemorrhage and calcifications can be observed and are more common in supratentorial lesions (Fig. 17-35). Ependymomas may occasionally spread via CSF, seeding the leptomeninges or ventricles, either at diagnosis or at recurrence.[642] Careful attention to staging of patients is therefore important.

The characteristic microscopic feature of a classic ependymoma is that of dense cellularity, intermixed with perivascular pseudorosettes consisting of tumor cells and surrounding a neoplastic blood vessel (Fig. 17-36). True ependymal rosettes representing abortive canals are relatively uncommon.[643] Histologically, the anaplastic variant is recognized by the presence of mitoses, necrosis, and vascular proliferation. They tend to be more cellular than grade II ependymomas but usually remain well demarcated. MIB-1 rates above 5% in incompletely resected tumors or more than 15% in completely resected tumors correlate with more aggressive behavior.[644] GFAP and

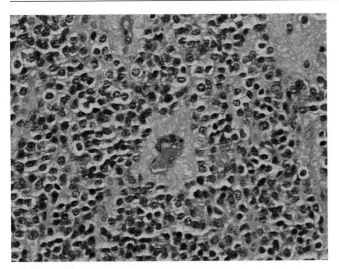

FIGURE 17-36. Ependymal pseudorosette (H&E; ×600).

S100 are positive in most ependymomas and epithelial membrane antigen (EMA) stains are positive in anaplastic variants. The presence of perivascular elastic fibers may also be a diagnostic feature of these tumors.[645] In patients in whom the diagnosis of ependymoma is indeterminate, electron microscopic analysis of cilia structure and junctional complexes, which are found in most ependymomas, can be used to confirm or exclude the diagnosis. Myxopapillary ependymomas have a mucinous appearance and arise almost exclusively in the cauda equine.[640] Their MIB-1 is typically low. Tanycytic ependymomas are a rare subtype of ependymoma that can occur throughout the brain or spine.[476,646] Other rare subtypes include cellular ependymoma, papillary ependymoma,[647] and clear cell ependymoma[648] variants.

Management. Evaluation of patients at diagnosis or recurrence should include an MRI of the brain and spinal cord, as well as cytologic evaluation of the CSF. The usefulness of CSF sampling in patients at relapse may not be particularly sensitive.[649] A number of factors have been associated with an unfavorable outcome, including younger age at diagnosis, subtotal resection, and a high MIB-1. Anaplastic histology remains controversial as a negative prognostic factor. Of these, the single most important factor in the determination of prognosis appears to be whether a complete resection can be accomplished.[650]

The first line of treatment is surgery with the goal of gross total resection. If a complete resection with clear margins of a grade II spinal cord or supratentorial ependymoma can be achieved, adjuvant therapy can be deferred in some patients. Technologic advances such as the operating microscope, Cavitron ultrasonic aspirator (CUSA), intraoperative ultrasound, and MRI, as well as electrophysiologic monitoring, have facilitated the safety of resections of intra-axial spinal cord tumors while reducing operative morbidity.[651] Overall, spinal cord ependymomas are more easily resectable than astrocytomas because of the presence of a better demarcated cleavage plane. Tumors with an infiltrative boundary, or those with anaplastic histology, require adjuvant therapy. All posterior fossa tumors, independent of grade and degree of resection, should also receive adjuvant treatment. Spinal myxopapillary ependymoma with a complete surgical resection have an excellent prognosis and do not usually require adjuvant therapy.[652]

Regarding radiation therapy, there is a long history of deferring radiation therapy for infants and young children with posterior fossa ependymomas, using various conventional chemotherapy regimens instead. Previous treatment recommendations included radiation therapy for patients in whom gross resection was not achieved or for patients with recurrent disease. However, partially resected tumors almost invariably recur, requiring further surgery, radiotherapy, and conventional chemotherapy. As such, the current strategy for ependymoma in the United States recommends deferral of adjuvant therapy in completely resected supratentorial ependymoma, involved field radiotherapy alone for completely resected posterior fossa ependymoma, and the use of multiagent chemotherapy for subtotally resected ependymoma, followed by second-look surgery and involved field RT.[653-655] A benefit to hyperfractionation has not been established.[656] Craniospinal radiation therapy does not appear to be superior to focal radiation therapy.[613] Several studies have suggested that radiotherapy prolongs progression-free survival after subtotal resection of an ependymoma. Deferral of radiation therapy after initial complete resection can result in reduced cure, even when complete resection is achieved a second time.[657] Proton radiation therapy appears to have equal efficacy when compared with photon therapy; it can reduce the potential long-term toxicity by decreasing the volume of normal brain tissue that is also targeted.[658]

Until recently, there was no clear role for chemotherapy in the management of ependymomas outside of clinical trials.[659] Several small series in newly diagnosed and recurrent disease have shown objective responses to the following drugs: carboplatin, cisplatin, ifosfamide, and etoposide.[660] Chemotherapy is more often used for infants and younger children with incompletely resected or disseminated disease.[661-663] Encouraging results have been reported from the most recent cooperative group clinical trial involving preirradiation chemotherapy, which showed a 40% complete response rate in patients who received preirradiation chemotherapy for residual postoperative tumor.[664] The two factors associated with a favorable outcome were the achievement of a complete resection and supratentorial disease. Chemotherapy should therefore be used to achieve a complete response or improve the chances of a complete surgical resection at second-look surgery. It is not highly effective as sole treatment for this disease, and recurrences occur relatively rapidly in a significant percentage of patients if radiotherapy is not administered early. The use of high-dose chemotherapy and stem cell rescue in infants with ependymoma has failed to demonstrate a significant advantage over standard modalities.[665] Although uncommon, up to 10% of patients can have leptomeningeal spread of ependymoma. Response to intrathecal liposomal cytarabine has been reported.[661]

Recurrences of intracranial ependymoma can occur throughout the first decade after initial therapy, although most recur within the first few years.[666] Surveillance scanning is important because it allows smaller asymptomatic tumors to be identified that may be more amenable to reresection. Most recurrences are within the original radiation field[667] and do not appear to be related to marginal failures.

Prognosis. The most important prognostic factors for intracranial and spinal cord ependymoma are age, tumor grade,[668] extent of surgical resection, and delivery of radiation therapy to doses of at least 5400 cGy.[669-672] Children younger than 3 years, those with WHO grade III disease, or those with less than a gross total resection have been shown to have lower survival.[673] The 5-year progression-free and overall survival for patients with subtotal versus total resection of posterior fossa ependymomas is 25% and 66%, respectively. The prognosis of patients with disseminated disease is worse.[384,670] Recently, a molecular assay for human telomerase reverse transcriptase expression has been shown to predict the likelihood of progression and survival of pediatric intracranial ependymoma.[628] Additional studies on the molecular profile of ependymomas will likely lead to improved stratification and prognostication of patients.[617,629] Patients with elevated MIB-1 more than 5% in incompletely resected or more than 15% in completely resected ependymomas were reported to have a worse prognosis in one study.[644] Patients with a deletion of 6q15.3 appear to have an improved outcome.[674]

Most patients with completely resected ependymoma followed by focal radiation therapy will be long-term survivors. Consideration of advanced radiation planning is critical to minimize long-term neurocognitive morbidity in this population.[675]

At the time of recurrence, no standard salvage regimen has been proven to be effective. Reoperation to achieve a complete resection has been curative in some patients and is typically the first modality considered[676]; this can be combined with reirradiation.[677] Patients with metastatic disease or infiltration into the brainstem or other critical structures have a poor salvage rate, presumably because of the lack of good therapies for recurrent disease and the inoperable nature of the lesions. Oral etoposide alone,[678] or in combination as a metronomic therapy combination, has demonstrated responses in this disease.[253]

Recurrence of myxopapillary ependymoma can occur after complete resection and can be associated with dissemination. Although cranial metastases have been reported, most cases result in regional metastases of the spine but not beyond the foramen magnum.[679] Many of these patients can be salvaged with radiation therapy. Consequently, frequent surveillance scanning of myxopapillary ependymoma patients is recommended to identify recurrent disease early.

Oligodendrogliomas

Oligodendrogliomas are rare cancers in children, representing less than 1% of all pediatric brain tumors.[680,681] The mean age at diagnosis is approximately 10 to 13 years old, with a male predominance.[682,683] The WHO grading system recognizes two grades for oligodendroglial tumors, well-differentiated grade II oligodendroglioma and grade III anaplastic oligodendroglioma.[684] As with other glial tumors, higher grade is a predictor of decreased overall survival. Other reported markers in oligodendrogliomas include deletions of the cyclin-dependent kinase inhibitor 2A (CDKN2A) gene on chromosome 9p, mutations in *p53* and *PTEN*, and amplification of the EGFR.[685,686] However, it is not known whether these factors are predictive of outcome in pediatric patients.

Clinical Presentation. Oligodendrogliomas are diffusely infiltrating tumors that tend to occur in the white matter of the cerebral hemispheres. Patients frequently present with seizures, although higher grade tumors may present with evidence of increased intracranial pressure because of more rapid growth.[687] Other symptoms at presentation can include headache, visual field defect, paresis, and cranial nerve palsy.[683] Although uncommon, oligodendrogliomas can also occur throughout other areas of the brain, including the posterior fossa and spine.[688-691]

Imaging and Histology. MRI evaluation of oligodendrogliomas typically reveals increased T2 signal and decreased T1 signal.[687] Gadolinium contrast enhancement is more common in tumors that grow as solid masses and less common in purely infiltrative tumors. Contrast enhancement is also more common in grade III than in grade II oligodendrogliomas.[692] Although oligodendrogliomas bear morphologic similarity to oligodendrocytes, the cellular origin of these tumors has remained difficult to prove. Histologic examination of fixed specimens of oligodendrogliomas reveals a monotonous pattern of cells with round nuclei and clear perinuclear halos (fried egg appearance). This appearance is an artifact of formalin fixation and is not seen in frozen sections or tumor smears. Higher grade anaplastic oligodendrogliomas (WHO grade III) are characterized by increased nuclear variability, increased mitotic activity, and/or microvascular proliferation. These features can occur diffusely throughout the tumor or in discrete foci. The differentiation between oligodendrogliomas and other diffuse gliomas such as astrocytomas and oligoastrocytomas is difficult because of a lack of reliable molecular markers that distinguish oligodendroglial tumors from astrocytic tumors. Mature oligodendrocyte-specific markers such as myelin basic protein, 2'3'-CNPase, and myelin-associated glycoprotein are not expressed in oligodendrogliomas, although astrocytic markers such as GFAP and S-100β are expressed in both astrocytomas and oligodendrogliomas.[684] More recently, the lineage markers OLIG1 and OLIG2 have been evaluated in the hope that they may enable specific identification of oligodendroglial tumors.[693] However, despite the restriction of OLIG2 expression to normal oligodendrocytes and their precursors, OLIG2 stains all diffuse gliomas and precludes specific immunohistochemical classification of these tumors.[694] The loss of chromosome 1p and/or 19q is commonly seen in adult oligodendrogliomas and correlates strongly with chemotherapy responsiveness and outcome.[695] Pediatric oligodendrogliomas have a much lower incidence of chromosome 1p and/or 19q deletions.[696,697] Even in children in whom these deletions are identified, the greater chemoresponsiveness observed in adults is less evident.

Management. Treatment of pediatric oligodendrogliomas, like other glial tumors, involves surgical resection, radiation therapy, and chemotherapy. The goal of surgery is to facilitate accurate diagnosis and remove as much of the tumor as is safely possible. In the adult literature, there is uncertainty as to whether extent of resection correlates with overall survival. Although some larger case series have shown no prognostic value in the extent of resection,[695] most evidence seems to indicate that the extent of resection may be associated with better prognosis.[698,699] In pediatric patients, it appears that the extent of resection is a sensitive predictor of outcome.[392] Fewer pediatric low-grade oligodendroglial tumors progress to high-grade tumors, so it is possible that patients with subtotally resected tumors may still have a good outcome. For example, in one series of 20 patients with oligodendrogliomas treated with surgery only, 70% remained progression-free at a median of 5 years.[700]

Despite the fact that oligodendroglial tumors are radiosensitive,[701] the use of adjuvant radiation therapy in asymptomatic children with incompletely resected oligodendrogliomas is not favored because of the well-described late effects of radiation therapy.[286] Children who are symptomatic, with tumors in critical locations such as the brainstem, or with progressive disease despite resection and/or chemotherapy may benefit from radiotherapy.[330] However, it is now clear that a subset of these children can be effectively treated with chemotherapy, allowing for a delay in, or avoidance of, radiation therapy.[702] The combination of carboplatin and vincristine chemotherapy has demonstrated activity in various low-grade astrocytomas, regardless of histologic subtype. This therapy should therefore be considered for patients with oligodendroglioma.[306] Older children may also benefit from chemotherapy.[326] Based on overlapping activity in children with low-grade astrocytomas, the combination of 6-thioguanine, procarbazine, lomustine, and vincristine (TPCV) might also be of use in patients who do not respond to or progress on vincristine and carboplatin. The combination of procarbazine, lomustine, and vincristine (PCV) or temozolomide monotherapy could also be considered based on the responses seen in adults, but these treatments have not yet been adequately tested in children.[312,703,704]

In patients with anaplastic oligodendroglioma or progressive disease, despite surgery and adjuvant chemotherapy, the risks of radiation therapy may be offset by the risk of further tumor growth. A recent survey of adult neuro-oncologists has found that the most commonly recommended treatment for anaplastic oligodendroglioma is the use of concurrent temozolomide and radiotherapy followed by adjuvant temozolomide.[705] In rare cases of dissemination, the overall prognosis for these patients is poor, although transient chemotherapy responsiveness can be achieved.[706] Patients with oligodendroglial gliomatosis cerebri have a very poor prognosis.

Prognosis. Overall, long-term survival from low-grade oligodendrogliomas appears comparable to other low-grade gliomas. It should be noted, however, that there are only limited numbers of case series, making comparisons among studies difficult. Bowers and coworkers[700] have reported an overall survival of at least 5.5 years in a series of 20 patients with low-grade oligodendrogliomas treated initially with surgical resection alone. Six of 20 patients in this series had disease progression at a median of 2.2 years following initial resection. Other studies have reported 5-year overall survival rates of 65% to 84.4%,[682,683] although the proportion of patients treated with radiation therapy and/or chemotherapy differed among these studies. The rarity of anaplastic oligodendroglioma in children makes specific estimates of survival in pediatric patients difficult. Oligodendrogliomas that are more centrally located do not appear to do as well as those located more peripherally in the cortex.[682]

A number of studies from adult patients have indicated that allelic losses at chromosomes 1p and 19q, typically involving the entire chromosomal arm at both sites, correlate with histologic classification, response to treatment, and prognosis.[707] Loss at chromosome 1p is a predictor of chemosensitivity, and combined 1p/19q loss is associated with both chemosensitivity and longer recurrence-free survival.[708] Recent evidence has indicated that 1p/19q loss is associated with MGMT promoter methylation and lower expression of MGMT.[709] Interestingly, these chromosomal features appear to be less common in pediatric oligodendrogliomas.[696,697] One study has reported the lack of allelic loss in children younger than 9 years, although a modest number of tumors from children older than 9 years had losses of chromosome 1p (45%) and/or 19q (27%).[697] Nevertheless, the incidence of chromosomal losses is significantly less than that seen in adults (50% to 90%). Taken together, these studies suggest that the oncogenesis of these tumors is distinct from their adult counterparts.

Oligoastrocytomas

Oligoastrocytomas (OAs) are tumors containing a mixture of two distinct neoplastic cell types that morphologically resemble the tumor cells of oligodendrogliomas and diffuse astrocytomas. These tumors correspond histologically to WHO grade II. The demography of oligoastrocytomas and anaplastic oligoastrocytomas (WHO grade III) is difficult to ascertain because of a high variability in the histopathologic criteria used for classification of these tumors. Clinically, these tumors present with signs and symptoms similar to those of astrocytomas and oligodendrogliomas. Tumors arise most frequently in the cerebral hemispheres and lack any neuroradiologic features that would facilitate distinguishing them from oligodendrocytomas. Histologic diagnosis requires the recognition of the two different glial

components, both of which must be neoplastic.[710] Anaplastic oligoastrocytomas (AOAs) are WHO grade III oligoastrocytomas with histologic features of malignancy, including high cellularity, high mitotic activity, and increased nuclear atypia and pleomorphism. Currently, treatment for OA and AOA is similar to that for other grade II and III glial lesions—surgical resection with adjuvant chemotherapy and/or radiation therapy for higher grade or progressive lesions.

Embryonal Tumors

Embryonal tumors represent a large and important fraction of pediatric brain tumors, both for their clinical impact as well as the importance of the scientific insights gained through their study. The most common embryonal tumors include medulloblastoma, pineoblastomas, and CNS PNETs. A number of other tumors are grouped into this category, such as ATRTs, ependymoblastomas, and medulloepitheliomas (Table 17-6). Recent advances in gene expression array technologies have facilitated a new understanding of the molecular features of tumors within this set of diseases.[711] The grouping of these tumors into the larger category of CNS PNETs will continue to evolve as a better understanding of their origin progresses. Currently, all these tumors share a common property: high risk of dissemination and therefore the need to treat the entire craniospinal axis. It is expected that new technologies will soon allow for a better understanding of the cell of origin of the different tumor types. These are no longer intellectual exercises. Gene-based classification systems may be the key to improved stratification and management and will likely augment, if not replace, the current histopathology-based classification system that underlies current treatment protocols.

TABLE 17-6 Classification of Embryonal Tumors

Tumor Location	Histologic Classification	Histologic Subtype
Fourth ventricle	Medulloblastoma	Classic or nondesmoplastic Desmoplastic Anaplastic Large cell Melanotic
	Cerebellar neuroblastoma*	
	Atypical teratoid-rhabdoid tumor (ATRT)	
Pineal	Pineocytoma	
	Pineoblastoma	
	ATRT	
Supratentorial or intratentorial	Primitive neuroectodermal tumor (PNET*)	
	Cerebral neuroblastoma	
	ATRT	
	Ependymoblastoma†	

*The nomenclature for neuroblastoma and PNET in the central nervous system results from the historical grouping of these tumors with other small round blue cell tumors of the body. Primary cerebral or cerebellar neuroblastoma are unrelated to similarly named tumors in the body, and do not possess the abnormalities in the N-Myc pathway. Similarly, CNS PNET is unrelated to Ewing's sarcoma PNET and does not possess the classic chromosome 11;22 translocation.
†Ependymoblastomas were previously grouped with ependymomas but are now differentiated from this group as a result of their embryologic development and patterns of spread.

The history of small round blue cell tumors is a fascinating story that spans the evolving approach to cancer over the last century. Histopathology was, and remains, the cornerstone of all classification schemas. Tumors from different sites that appeared the same under microscopic examination were assumed to be similar tumors arising from different organs. With the introduction of immunohistochemical techniques of pathologic specimens, pathologists began to define important differences among populations. Small round blue cell tumors within the body were now divided into unique categories based on cells of origin. Tumors such as lymphoma, neuroblastoma, Ewing's sarcoma, rhabdomyosarcoma, and others became easily differentiated. The classification of small round blue cell tumors of the brain by contrast took a different direction. Medulloblastoma, a small round blue cell tumor of the cerebellum, was previously differentiated from other similar-appearing tumors based on its location within the posterior fossa,[712] but some thought that this arbitrary separation was unwarranted. Hart and Earle's system[713] attempted to classify all embryonal tumors based on the expanding array of immunohistochemical markers and variations in the patterns of staining among these tumors. Rather than clarify the classification of embryonal tumors, further blurring of the understanding of these tumors resulted. One contributing factor involved differing definitions for the grouping of embryonal tumors. For some, medulloblastoma was considered a PNET and was lumped with pineoblastoma and supratentorial PNETs, whereas for others, medulloblastoma remained a separate category. Another factor was the considerable variability in the quality of the staining pattern and heterogeneity within different areas of a single tumor and within different tumors of the same type. With the advances in molecular pathology, there is movement away from the simple microscopic appearance of a tumor to one that incorporates the pathways active in the tumor. Molecular signatures for these different tumors have been demonstrated; these have shown that they arise from different cell populations and, as a result, these tumors will likely require different treatments. Many prior treatment protocols grouped all these heterogeneous tumors together, which has confounded the true efficacy of the therapy under consideration and the prognoses for this heterogeneous group of tumors.

Medulloblastomas

Medulloblastomas represent approximately 15% of all pediatric brain tumors and approximately one third of posterior fossa tumors.[714,715] In addition, medulloblastoma accounts for over 50% of pediatric embryonal intracranial tumors. The incidence in males is twice that of females and the median age at diagnosis is 5 to 7 years, with most cases being diagnosed in the first decade of life.[716] Recent data from the National Cancer Institute's Surveillance, Epidemiology and End Results (SEER) registry have indicated that the incidence of medulloblastoma appears to be increasing.[717] No specific single environmental factor has been demonstrated to be associated with the development of medulloblastoma, although the nonrandom occurrence of disease detected in children born in the fall raises the possibility that some environmental or infectious pathogen may be implicated.[36]

The association between the development of medulloblastoma and viruses remains controversial. Multiple reports implicating polyomaviruses, including JC[718] and SV40[719,720] virus in animal models, as a causative agent in medulloblastoma have been published. Human medulloblastoma samples have been found to possess JC and SV40 viral sequences.[632,721,722] However, independent conformation of JC and SV40 sequences in human tumors could not be duplicated.[40,634] Prematurity was identified as a significant risk factor in one study.[723] Whites are 42% more affected than blacks.[717] In contrast, several genetic syndromes (e.g., nevoid basal cell carcinoma syndrome or Gorlin's syndrome, Turcot's syndrome, Li-Fraumeni syndrome) are associated with a significantly increased risk for the development of medulloblastoma.[724-726] Gorlin's syndrome, although rare, is an important factor that must be considered in the treatment of these patients, because they are at high risk for the development of nevoid basal cell carcinoma, especially within the involved radiation fields. Children of African-American descent require especially careful skin evaluation for the early detection of these lesions.[727]

Medulloblastoma is the most common malignant CNS tumor of childhood and, as such, has been the most studied of the embryonal tumors. As a consequence, there are a number of new insights regarding the cell of origin and molecular biology of this tumor.[728,729] Original reports by Bailey and Cushing in 1925 suggested that these tumors originated from multipotential "medulloblasts" thought to be capable of generating both glial and neuronal cells.[712] Recent experimental evidence now indicates that there are two main histopathologic subtypes of medulloblastoma, desmoplastic and nondesmoplastic (formerly classic), that originate from two distinct germinal zones within the cerebellum—the external germinal layer (EGL) which contains committed granule cell precursors (GCPs), and the ventricular zone (VZ), which contains multipotent stem cells that give rise to most cerebellar neurons. Although desmoplastic medulloblastoma tends to express markers of granule cell lineage, suggesting an origin from GCPs, nondesmoplastic medulloblastoma more frequently expresses markers associated with nongranule neurons, suggesting an origin in the ventricular zone of the developing cerebellum.[730] Gene expression analysis supports these data by demonstrating separate expression profiles, with desmoplastic medulloblastoma cells expressing genes more closely associated with proliferating GCPs and nondesmoplastic medulloblastoma expressing a more heterogeneous set of markers not clearly associated with any particular cerebellar cell type.[711] Gene profiling of these tumors has also identified a number of other genes and chromosomal areas of interest in the possible pathogenesis of these tumors.[731-734] The association of medulloblastoma with Gorlin's syndrome has become particularly important. In addition to providing insight into the molecular pathways involved in certain cases of medulloblastoma, Gorlin's syndrome has also provided the basis for the development of the first potential target for therapy. Patients with Gorlin's syndrome have a mutation in a developmental gene called patch (*PTCH*) that is part of the Sonic hedgehog signaling cascade. One inhibitor of this pathway is cyclopamine, a plant derivative, which is currently being modified to improve its tolerability in humans.[735]

The origin of the more aggressive forms of nondesmoplastic medulloblastoma, specifically the anaplastic and large-cell variants,[736] remains unknown. These tumors might have origins from other unique cell populations within the cerebellum or have unique mutations or aberrations in pathways not shared by the desmoplastic and nondesmoplastic classic variants. They account for approximately 25% of medulloblastoma cases, and patients have a significantly worse outcome when compared with similarly staged patients with nonanaplastic medulloblastoma.[737] The knowledge gained from molecular genetic analyses of these tumors will hopefully lead to a better understanding of their basic biology, improved risk stratification, and subtype-specific management that minimizes toxicity while maximizing survival.[738]

Clinical Presentation. Many of the clinical manifestations of medulloblastoma are similar to those of other tumors that arise in the fourth ventricular region and are related to obstructive hydrocephalus. Headache, nausea, and vomiting, characteristically in the morning, are the most common initial symptoms and usually precede diagnosis by 4 to 8 weeks, although longer intervals are not uncommon, especially if the headaches and vomiting caused by obstructive hydrocephalus are intermittent. Interestingly, it appears that the duration of presenting symptoms may correlate inversely with disease state at the time of presentation; patients with low-stage disease were shown in one series to have a longer median duration of symptoms than patients with high-stage disease.[739,740] Personality changes (irritability) are an early feature but may be difficult to recognize as a sign of a brain tumor. Other features that can lead to diagnosis include lethargy, diplopia, head tilt, and truncal ataxia. The common signs found on physical examination are papilledema, ataxia, dysmetria, and cranial nerve involvement. Abducens nerve (cranial nerve VI) palsy secondary to raised intracranial pressure may cause diplopia and head tilt. Torticollis can be a sign of cerebellar tonsil herniation. Less commonly, intratumoral hemorrhage may lead to acute onset of confusion, headache, and loss of consciousness. The presentation in infants may include an abnormal rate of increase in head circumference. Other presenting symptoms can include loss of previously achieved milestones and failure to thrive. With regard to metastatic disease, at the time of diagnosis, although lumbar CSF analysis or MRI-visualized leptomeningeal metastases occur in 20% to 30% of children with medulloblastoma,[741,742] clinical manifestations of metastases are uncommon. Back pain and radicular pain may indicate the rare complication of spinal canal dissemination. Attention to the clinical manifestation of posterior fossa tumors is important because the presenting signs mimic many other common ailments in children, including viral infections and stress. With a significant propensity to metastasize early, careful evaluation of associated neurologic signs (e.g., papilledema, diplopia) can help identify children in need of referral for imaging sooner.

Imaging and Histology. Most medulloblastomas arise in the cerebellar vermis and extend into the fourth ventricle, resulting in obstructive hydrocephalus. The remainder are localized to the cerebellar hemisphere, especially in older patients and those with the desmoplastic subtype.[743] The signs and symptoms of obstructive hydrocephalus such as severe headache, morning vomiting, long tract signs, and papilledema can be a medical emergency and require immediate evaluation. CT scanning of the head is the immediate choice of imaging to rule out an obstructive mass. This rapid study provides good differentiation between the fluid cavities and brain and will be sufficient to allow the neurosurgeon to determine whether immediate action is required. Often, CSF diversion can be avoided if tumor resection is immediately possible. When required, third ventriculostomy is preferred to ventriculoperitoneal (VP) shunts. All patients will require high-quality MRI scans of the brain and spine, including the entire thecal sac at the base of the spine. Lumbar puncture for CSF cytologic examination in newly diagnosed patients should be deferred if there is any question of elevated intracranial pressure; it is usually performed better after the tumor has been resected and CSF flow has been restored.

The MRI findings may differentiate medulloblastoma from other cerebellar tumors, such as ependymoma and pilocytic astrocytoma, and may be helpful before surgical resection. However, atypical appearances of these three tumors can also occur, thus making a diagnosis based solely on imaging characteristics currently not feasible. The appearance of a vermian location, hypercellularity (often demonstrated as dark areas of tumor on T2), and intratumoral hemorrhage is more compatible with a cellular medulloblastoma or ependymoma. A tumor that fills the fourth ventricle and extends through the foramina

of Luschka and Magendie is more likely to be an ependymoma, although one with a large cyst and mural nodule (small area of solid tumor) is more consistent with a pilocytic astrocytoma. Pilocytic astrocytomas typically arise in the cerebellar hemisphere and are seen on T2-weighted MRI as areas of homogeneous high signal intensity, with the fluid collections defining the less intense tissue components of the tumor.

Medulloblastoma has T1-weighted MRI signal characteristics more similar to those of gray matter, reflecting hypercellularity and typically resulting in a relatively homogeneous image. On T2-weighted images, these tumors can appear to be hyperintense or, more frequently, can display mixed signal characteristics indicative of small intratumoral cysts, calcification, or small areas of hemorrhage.[744,745] The background signal intensity of medulloblastoma on T2-weighted images is characteristically lower than in other tumor types, indicating a dense packing of cells and a high nuclear-to-cytoplasmic ratio. Because medulloblastoma typically arises in the roof of the fourth ventricle, a cleft of CSF beneath the tumor in the fourth ventricle helps distinguish this tumor from ependymoma. Tumors are typically enhancing with gadolinium administration (Fig. 17-37). The presence of characteristic gyriform morphology and a well-circumscribed appearance on MRI scan suggests the presence of the nodular subtype of medulloblastoma.[746] Functional imaging with PET and SPECT are ideally suited for the improved diagnosis of medulloblastoma. A number of agents such as oxidronate (OctreoScan) can directly assess for the presence and activity of certain cellular constituents, which helps differentiate recurrent disease from scar.[747]

Histopathologic analysis of resected tumor specimens is essential for diagnosis and treatment planning. It should be noted that the histopathologic classification and nomenclature of medulloblastoma, within the broader context of embryonal tumors, has long been controversial and even today shows signs of continued evolution.[730] The most current WHO classification schema considers medulloblastoma to be an independent entity in the group of embryonal tumors,[724] separate from supratentorial PNET (now called CNS PNET in the revised WHO classification[183]). Within medulloblastoma, it is also clear that these tumors are not a homogeneous entity from a histopathologic viewpoint. At present, five main groups are recognized—classic, desmoplastic-nodular, anaplastic, large cell, and medulloblastoma with extensive nodularity. In addition, any of the above five variants of medulloblastoma can have areas of myogenic or melanotic differentiation. Classic (nondesmoplastic) medulloblastoma is the most common subtype, with approximately two thirds of tumors being classified as such, followed by the desmoplastic subtype (25%). This distribution is not uniform and is influenced by factors such as age and presence of Gorlin's syndrome. Individual tumors are often heterogeneous with regard to the extent of desmoplasia.[748,749]

Classic medulloblastoma consists of uniform sheets of densely packed small round blue cells with round to oval hyperchromatic nuclei and scant cytoplasm[724] (Fig. 17-38). Desmoplastic medulloblastoma is characterized by so-called pale islands, or reticulin-free nodules, that are surrounded by reticulin-producing proliferating cells. Desmoplastic medulloblastoma is linked to the nevoid basal cell carcinoma (Gorlin's) syndrome, caused by mutations in the PTCH1 gene and leading to dysregulation of Sonic hedgehog (Shh) signaling. Only recently have the large-cell and anaplastic variants of medulloblastoma been identified. These variants are defined by light microscopy findings of prominent nuclei with a high degree of pleomorphism, high mitotic indices, increased cytoplasm, and a higher rate of necrosis than in other variants.[750] These tumors are uniformly positive for synaptophysin and generally positive for chromogranin. Anaplastic and large-cell medulloblastomas tend to have higher rates of metastasis at presentation, loss of

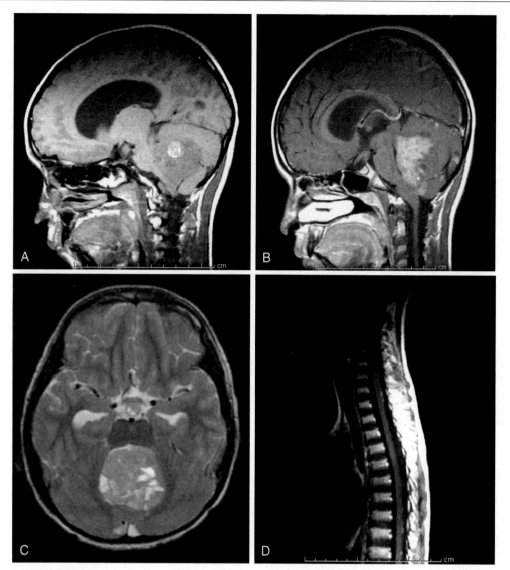

FIGURE 17-37. Medulloblastoma. **A,** Sagittal T1 image without contrast. An area of hemorrhage is present. **B,** Sagittal T1 image with contrast of medulloblastoma. **C,** Axial T2 image. The areas of low T2 signal suggest a cellular lesion. **D,** Saggital T1 with contrast. Thoracic-enhancing nodules represent metastatic disease.

17p13.3, and *MYC* amplification, and both have relatively poor prognoses.[751] These two variants can occur together and contain cells with markedly increased nuclear atypia and/or large nuclei with prominent nucleoli (Fig. 17-39).[737,751,752]

One of the cardinal features of medulloblastoma is its tendency to differentiate along one or more pathways, most commonly neuronal, astrocytic, and ependymal lineages. Synaptophysin expression, a characteristic feature of medulloblastomas, indicates neuronal lineage.[753] The expression of certain intermediate filament proteins, such as nestin, vimentin, and GFAP, can also be seen in medulloblastomas.[754] Medulloblastoma is divided into five variants:

1. Nondesmoplastic (classic) medulloblastoma may be strongly immunoreactive for vimentin. Although GFAP expression is typically restricted to developing and mature astrocytes, most classic medulloblastomas contain GFAP-positive cells, which could indicate astrocytic differentiation.[724]

2. Nodular-desmoplastic medulloblastoma has been shown to have an increased degree of reticulin staining,[755] with reticulin-free areas that can be identified throughout the lesion or only focally. The nodules represent regions of neuronal maturation.[724] This rare subtype makes up only 5% of medulloblastomas but accounts for 57% of medulloblastomas in infants[749] and accounts for the particularly good outcome in this age group.[756]

3. Anaplastic medulloblastoma has marked nuclear pleomorphism, a high mitotic rate, apoptotic cells, and significant atypia. If only small areas of anaplasia are identified, the tumor does not meet the diagnostic criteria for anaplastic subtype. Experienced pediatric neuropathologists are therefore required for difficult cases. Anaplasia may be related to abnormalities in *c-myc*.[757,758]

4. Large-cell medulloblastoma is a rare subtype with abundant mitoses and apoptotic bodies.[752] The name derives from the large nuclei present.[759] It often contains areas of anaplasia,

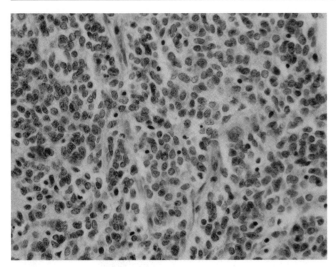

FIGURE 17-38. Nonanaplastic medulloblastoma. Lesions consist of sheets of homogeneous-appearing undifferentiated tumor cells (H&E; ×600).

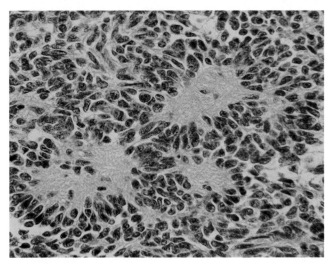

FIGURE 17-40. Homer-Wright rosettes (H&E; ×600).

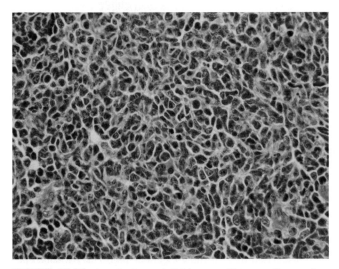

FIGURE 17-39. Anaplastic medulloblastoma. Tumor cells are pleomorphic with atypia, increased nuclear size, nuclear molding, and cell-cell wrapping (H&E; ×600).

possibly related to specific aberrant signaling pathways,[760] and thus many refer to these two variants as large-cell–anaplastic medulloblastoma.

5. Medulloblastoma with extensive nodularity, previously called cerebellar neuroblastoma, is typically identified in infants and has very large reticulin-free zones in comparison with desmoplastic medulloblastoma.[761]

Medulloblastoma with myogenic differentiation refers to the presence of rhabdomyoblastic elements[762,763] and can be seen with any of the five variants of medulloblastoma discussed earlier (classic, desmoplastic, anaplastic, large-cell, and medulloblastoma with extensive nodularity).[764] The historic term for medulloblastoma with rhabdomyoblastic elements was *medullomyoblastoma*,[765] although this latter term is no longer recommended. Similarly, medulloblastoma with melanotic differentiation refers to the presence of melanin and does not represent an additional unique variant of the disease.[766,767]

Rather, melanotic differentiation can occur with the other recognized variants discussed earlier. This tumor type was previously called melanocytic medulloblastoma.

Mitoses and other markers of proliferation such as MIB-1 are common features of these tumors and do not alter the prognosis.[768] A mitotic index of 0.5% to 2%, MIB-1 index higher than 20%, and the presence of Homer-Wright rosettes, cells arranged around a central lumen or hub (Fig. 17-40),[769] are often associated with increased atypia and mitotic activity and are seen in approximately one third of cases. Pseudorosettes, cells arranged around a central clearing with a vessel in the middle, are a common feature of medulloblastoma but are variable; they are not prognostic. Vascular proliferation and necrosis are uncommon (see Fig. 17-40).

Determining the cellular origin of medulloblastoma may be a key to the proper stratification and management of these tumors.[770] As noted earlier, current evidence indicates that patients with the desmoplastic variant, thought to originate from cerebellar granule cell precursors, have a better prognosis than those with the classic or anaplastic–large-cell variants.[771] Similarly, patients with the large-cell and anaplastic variants appear to have a worse prognosis, and our developing understanding of the unique pathways involved will likely allow better classification and therapy in future studies.

To date, the study of molecular prognostic markers of medulloblastoma has focused on amplification of *c-myc* as well as the presence of isochrome 17p (deletion of 17p and duplication of 17q), both of which have been associated with a worse prognosis. The presence of isochrome 17p is observed in a significant number of patients' samples (approximately 40% to 50%), although heterogeneity is observed within individual tumors.[772,773] Considerable data have evaluated the role of TrkC and its ligand neurotrophin-3. Tumors with paracrine or autocrine activation of this pathway appear to have a better prognosis.[768,774] In vitro data have suggested that TrkC activation induces tumor cell apoptosis; it is hypothesized that this may account for the improved outcome in this population.[775] The role of TrkC, however, has not been prospectively evaluated. A similar positive correlation of β-catenin and outcome has also been reported and awaits prospective analysis.[776] Activation of ErbB-2 and ErbB-4, by contrast, has been associated with a poorer prognosis in retrospective studies.[777,778]

Management. A high level of clinical suspicion is critical to make an early diagnosis of medulloblastoma. Neuroimaging

Stage M0: No evidence of subarachnoid or hematogenous metastases

Stage M1: Microscopic tumor cells found in the cerebrospinal fluid

Stage M2: Gross nodular metastatic seeding in the subarachnoid space or ventricular system distant from the primary site of disease

Stage M3a: Gross nodular seeding in the spine subarachnoid space without evidence of intracranial seeding

Stage M3b: Gross nodular seeding in the spinal subarachnoid space, as well as intracranial seeding

Stage M4: Extraneural metastases

is usually the first step, with CT scanning of the brain frequently performed in the acute setting. MRI of the brain and spine should be performed as soon as feasible. In children in whom the diagnosis of medulloblastoma is suspected, an MRI of the spine should be obtained because the incidence of CSF dissemination at diagnosis ranges between 20% and 30%.[741] Corticosteroids are usually used to control increased intracranial pressure. A lumbar puncture should be deferred until after intracranial hypertension has been relieved by surgery. Because extraneural spread of medulloblastoma is possible, bone marrow aspiration and biopsy should be considered for the complete evaluation of patients with medulloblastoma,[779] although these are no longer required for participation in cooperative clinical trials. Although the exact incidence of extraneural metastases is evolving, current estimates suggest that this occurs in less than 5% of patients. Because patients will require general anesthesia for insertion of a central line for the administration of chemotherapy, bone marrow samples and a baseline lumbar sample can be easily obtained with minimal trauma to the child or family. CSF obtained from the ventricular or cisternal fluid is not considered adequate to base staging decisions; thus, lumbar sampling is recommended for all patients in whom this is not contraindicated pretherapy.[780]

At present, risk stratification and treatment assignment are based primarily on clinical factors, although this will change with greater reliance on molecular profiling.[770] Recently, histology has been added in the risk assignment of medulloblastoma. The modified Chang criteria[781] are based on the extent of tumor and degree of metastasis (Box 17-3). Following the completion of the staging evaluation (MRI of brain and spine, CSF cytology, bone marrow studies), histology, and degree of resection, patients are stratified to the standard-risk, high-risk, or infant risk groups. The major determinants of clinical risk categorization are age at diagnosis (younger than 3 years versus 3 years or older),[717] metastasis or M stage (M0 versus higher than M0), volume of residual postoperative disease ($\leq$1.5 cm^3 residual versus >1.5 cm^3 residual),[782] and histology (anaplastic–large-cell versus other).[783]

Histology has just recently begun to be considered in risk stratification. Most prior published series of patients with medulloblastoma had incorporated those with anaplasia–large-cell medulloblastoma into standard-risk treatment if they met the other criteria for standard risk. The recognition that infants with the desmoplastic variant may do better than infants with the nondesmoplastic variant may provide an opportunity to

de-escalate therapy in this particular group. Newer protocols are now incorporating these variables. Tolerability of therapy has also recently come to light as more adult programs begin to treat older patients with regimens similar to those that have produced significant advances in pediatric patients. Older patients, including adolescents, do not tolerate therapy as well as younger children or infants, which argues for dose modifications in this group.[784]

Atypical teratoid rhabdoid tumors of the posterior fossa can easily resemble medulloblastoma. In prior cooperative group studies, up to 30% of patients with ATRT were misclassified as medulloblastoma.

Historical Perspective

Like most other treatments, the development of our current approaches to multimodality therapy for medulloblastoma is the result of a series of overlapping clinical trials. It is beyond the scope of this account to give a detailed recounting of the progression to our current understanding of medulloblastoma therapy. Rather, a few key events will provide some idea of why we do what we currently do and indicate some of the weaknesses on which our current assumptions are based.

For decades after the first description of medulloblastoma was published by Bail and Cushing in 1925, the prognosis for this highly malignant tumor was extremely poor. Cushing's development of neurosurgical techniques to remove tumors of the fourth ventricle, coupled with a dramatic decline in surgical morbidity, was critical to the development of effective therapies.[785] With the introduction of radiation therapy and further refinements in neurosurgical techniques between 1950 and 1970, significant improvements in survivorship were achieved. For the first time, patients with standard-risk disease had a 5-year event-free survival approaching 50%, whereas those with high-risk disease were estimated at approximately 20%. It was demonstrated that radiation therapy could cure a significant percentage of patients, thus securing its place in the standard approach for these tumors. The craniospinal dose for all patients was 3600 cGy (CSI), with a posterior fossa boost to an approximate total of 5400 cGy. The promising event-free survival was tempered, however, by the poor functioning levels seen in surviving patients.

Based on these outcomes and late effects, treatments were modified based on risk categories. For high-risk patients, chemotherapy was added to full-dose 3600 cGy craniospinal radiotherapy, and the resulting improvement in outcome was easily measured, with 3- and 5-year event-free survivals of approximately 60%. By contrast, the approach to patients with standard-risk disease was to reduce the dose of craniospinal radiotherapy from 3600 to 2400 cGy to spare neurocognitive function, while maintaining the boost to the posterior fossa of 5400 cGy. A national clinical trial was undertaken but, as the study progressed, there was concern that the number of recurrences in the 2400-cGy treatment arm was greater than that for the 3600-cGy treatment arm. Consequently, the study was terminated early. With further follow-up, however, the survival curves for the two treatment arms approached one another, such that no statistical difference in outcome was identified; the early termination of the trial hindered the determination of the statistical conclusion. The results from these treatment studies suggest that chemotherapy in combination with craniospinal radiation therapy could positively affect outcome. The strategy for standard-risk disease became the lower dose radiation therapy of 2400 cGy craniospinal irradiation (CSI) with the addition of chemotherapy. In follow-up studies of these combinations, progression-free survival of 86% and 79% at 3 and 5 years, respectively, was achieved for standard-risk patients.[786] The two approaches for high- and standard-risk disease have now become the basis of most North American treatment trials.

Treatment

Surgery

Treatment of medulloblastoma, as well as other embryonal tumors, is multimodal, consisting of surgery, radiation therapy, and chemotherapy, with current therapies guided primarily by age and stage at diagnosis. The initial goal of surgery is to control raised intracranial pressure, if present. Once the safety of the patient is ensured, consideration of tumor resection becomes the next objective. If metastatic tumor is already known to be present, immediate aggressive surgery within the posterior fossa will not reduce need for more intensive radiation and chemotherapy. Rather, the goal of surgical resection should be to achieve maximal tumor volume reduction without significant damage to adjacent areas. In balance, it is more important for the neurosurgeon to preserve function rather than maximize resection. Given the excellent prognosis for patients with medulloblastoma, even with metastatic disease, damage to the brain in a high percentage means a high percentage of survivors with permanent neurologic damage.[787] A third ventriculostomy (preferred) or VP shunt should be deferred prior to initial surgery but may be necessary if sufficient resection to reopen CSF flow is not achieved.

A number of surgical approaches are possible to optimize resection of posterior fossa and cerebellar tumors. Most fourth ventricular lesions will require interruption of the cerebellar vermis, although resections through the vermis using horizontal or vertical incisions have both been associated with posterior fossa syndrome. Even attempts at going under, rather than through the vermis, have been associated with this morbidity. The brainstem must also be protected while removing medulloblastomas within the fourth ventricle. Because these tumors can invade into the brainstem, intraoperative decisions regarding aggressiveness of resection must be made. Similarly, resection must protect the nearby cranial nerves. New neurosurgical techniques are now available that allow for greater guidance in resection as well as in physiologic monitoring so that damage to important anatomic structures can be avoided. The use of intraoperative MRIs has improved the neurosurgeon's ability to ensure adequate yet safe resection.[788,789]

Potential complications of surgery in this location, regardless of tumor type, include cerebellar mutism (also called posterior fossa syndrome) and aseptic meningitis. The posterior fossa, or cerebellar mutism, syndrome occurs in approximately 10% to 20% of cases, although it is being reported in an increasing percentage of patients as more attention is paid to the quality of survivorship. The characteristics are reduced speech output or mutism, personality changes, hypotonia, ataxia, and reduced oral intake. Symptoms typically appear one or two days after surgery, may range between mild to severe, and may last from days to months with varying degrees of recovery.[790]

Radiation Therapy

Radiotherapy has become an important modality in the long-term outcome of patients with medulloblastoma. Over the last 20 years, a great deal of effort has been focused on the reduction of craniospinal doses, as a result of significant long-term neurocognitive damage as well as secondary tumor risk and stroke. Radiotherapy is currently risk-adapted, and additional modifications to dose and volume continue.[791] For standard risk patients, 5400 to 5580 cGy are administered to the tumor bed. This volume continues to evolve, from inclusion of the entire posterior fossa, even when the tumor is small and focal, to more limited fields that encompass only structures in contact with the tumor and a small margin. Previous standard radiation therapy included craniospinal doses of 3600 cGy. A national clinical trial evaluating standard risk patients with a craniospinal dose of 2400 cGy demonstrated equal efficacy to historical reports, although this study did not randomize between the two CSI doses; 2400 cGy has been accepted as the new standard for this patient population.[792] An important conclusion from this study was the poor outcome of patients with high-risk disease treated with lower dose craniospinal radiotherapy, reinforcing the importance of proper staging and radiation planning in all patients. A Children's Oncology Group clinical trial for patients with standard risk medulloblastoma is ongoing, which randomizes children younger than 8 years to 2400 or 1800 cGy CSI and all children to full posterior fossa boost or involved field boost. This will help define the dose and field of radiation therapy required for this population. Because children younger than 8 years are most at risk for the neurocognitive damage caused by radiation therapy, this is the group most likely to benefit from dose reduction.

For patients with high-risk disease, either caused by the presence of bulk unresectable disease within the posterior fossa or by the presence of metastatic disease, treatment remains 3600 cGy to the craniospinal axis and a focal dose to the involved posterior fossa of 5400 to 5940 cGy. Although this dose to the entire brain and spine increases the morbidity of therapy, it is an important component of effective treatment. A number of cooperative group trials are currently evaluating drugs combined with radiotherapy (radiation sensitizers) to augment the activity of RT.

Infants with medulloblastoma (and other CNS PNETS) continue to pose the greatest therapeutic dilemma. Even in the presence of standard-risk disease, the contraindication for craniospinal radiation therapy limits the treatment options for this group and their long-term prognoses. The omission of craniospinal radiotherapy has required the acceptance of a lower cure rate, but a much higher functionality for those who do survive.[793] The use of treatment protocols that rely only on surgery and chemotherapy demonstrate a relatively poor outcome for this group in all but a select group (e.g., nodular desmoplastic medulloblastoma[756]), again supporting the importance of radiation therapy for the treatment of medulloblastoma. Because many relapses occur locally, many centers have piloted focal radiotherapy to the posterior fossa, forgoing the craniospinal component of therapy.[524,794] This approach attempts to improve local control to the cerebellum, which is thought to be an area less important for neurocognitive development than the cortex.

Hyperfractionation of radiotherapy—that is, twice-daily dosing of RT—has not demonstrated significant improvement in outcome,[795] although one pilot trial has reported such an improvement.[796] By contrast, significant delay in the completion of the radiation therapy appears to negatively affect survival.[797,798] Proton therapy is being increasingly used for children with medulloblastoma. Although efficacy is similar to that of conventional photon radiotherapy, the absence of an exit dose can reduce radiation exposure to areas uninvolved with tumor. The limited number of proton beam facilities currently open in the United States, however, restricts the wider application of this technique. Other more readily available radiation therapy options include intensity-modulated radiation therapy (IMRT). In particular, tighter margins within the posterior fossa and better three-dimensional conformal planning with IMRT-based techniques can help avoid the auditory apparatus and thus long-term hearing impairment.

The potential use of chemotherapy before craniospinal radiotherapy has been piloted.[798] Although the results were not statistically significant, delay in radiation therapy with chemotherapy trended to a reduction in event-free survival, although it also resulted in a decrease in some of the long-term side effects of the chemotherapy, particularly ototoxicity. A national clinical trial, randomizing between standard-dose radiation therapy (3600 cGy) compared with reduced dose (2340 cGy) craniospinal irradiation in low-stage (M0) patients not receiving adjuvant chemotherapy, resulted in an increased rate of recurrence outside of the posterior fossa.[799] However, it should be noted that no statistically significant difference was found between the two groups at 6 to 7 years following treatment.

Chemotherapy

The chemosensitivity of medulloblastoma and the benefits of adjuvant chemotherapy in treatment regimens have been demonstrated by a number of studies.[800-802] Over the past 20 years, studies have shown a nearly 20% to 30% improvement in event-free and overall survivals by using chemotherapy during and/or after radiation therapy. Most regimens have included vincristine, cisplatin, etoposide, and an alkylator (cyclophosphamide or CCNU). Chemotherapy is currently a standard adjuvant therapy in children. Similarly, infant studies with chemotherapy alone have shown the importance of chemotherapy as an effective strategy for patients with medulloblastoma. For most of these infant studies, the removal of CSI has negatively affected survival, although a significant proportion of survivors can achieve cure.[756] Recently, methotrexate has been added into multiagent chemotherapy for medulloblastomas and other PNETs with excellent tumor response. In one phase II study consisting of four cycles of carboplatin, etoposide, and methotrexate, complete response (CR) and partial response (PR) rates of 71% and 81% were achieved in patients younger than 3 years and older than 3 years, respectively.[803]

The concurrent use of craniospinal radiation therapy and multiagent chemotherapy for medulloblastoma can result in significant impairment of nutrition during therapy for these patients.[804] Patients who present with persistent vomiting likely initiate therapy in a negative nutritional state. A large proportion of patients will require nutritional support through a nasogastric tube or gastric tube. Constant surveillance of nutrition is important because this issue is often dismissed early and only recognized when severe weight loss has occurred.

Impairment in hearing function continues to be a major concern in survivors of medulloblastoma. The overlap between posterior fossa radiation therapy and the use of ototoxic drugs such as cisplatin has resulted in significant toxicity for this patient population. Conformal radiation planning with tighter margins, the use of IMRT, and the use of proton beam radiation therapy can all significantly reduce the damage to the auditory apparatus. Recent medulloblastoma treatment protocols have also reduced the cumulative doses of cisplatin. The use of amifostine continues to be controversial, with some studies showing efficacy at protecting hearing while others have not.[805,806] Concerns about protecting the tumor from the chemotherapy remain, and only a well-controlled randomized trial will resolve this question.

Standard-Risk Disease   The specific combination of chemotherapy used during and after CSI continues to evolve. A large national clinical trial, involving 2400 cGy CSI with a boost to 5400 cGy to the posterior fossa and randomizing between vincristine, cisplatin, and either CCNU or cyclophosphamide (COG A9961), have demonstrated that both treatment arms have approximately similar activity. The overall survival for both groups was approximately 90%, with only a slight difference in event-free survival between the two chemotherapy regimens (85% for patients who received CCNU versus 83% for those who received cyclophosphamide). The emphasis in the ongoing clinical study has been to reduce the CSI dose further in a randomized fashion for children younger than 8 years (i.e., those most at risk for the severe neurocognitive impact of radiation therapy) while combining the CCNU and cyclophosphamide agents to reduce the total exposure to each. The safety of 1800 cGy craniospinal radiotherapy was piloted in 10 patients with standard-risk medulloblastoma and, in this small cohort, outcome appeared equally effective to 2400 cGy therapy and with less neurocognitive impairment.[807] Radiation- and chemotherapy-adapted approaches are especially important for younger patients given the significant dose-dependent neurocognitive impact of radiation therapy in this population.[808]

High-Risk Disease.   Treatment strategies for this population have focused on the addition of new agents, including radiosensitizing agents and novel biologic inhibitors, targeting pathways important for these tumors in the hopes of further improving outcome.[809] It should be noted that the sequence of treatment has been shown to be of major importance, with the best survival rates being achieved if radiation therapy is not delayed.[810]

Infant Chemotherapy.   Patients younger than 3 years at diagnosis are considered to have higher risk disease at all stages and degrees of resection, related to the limitations of delivering craniospinal RT to this group. There is also an increased frequency of leptomeningeal dissemination at the time of diagnosis in young children (27% to 43%) versus older children (20% to 25%) with similar histologic diagnoses.[811] Following surgical resection, infants with medulloblastoma are often treated with chemotherapy alone or chemotherapy with involved field radiotherapy in an effort to reduce the high incidence of developmental and neuropsychological sequelae in young infants treated with craniospinal irradiation. It is clear that the risks of craniospinal radiation therapy in infants and young children are significantly greater than the benefits of therapeutic response in terms of neurocognitive development.[812] Currently, several chemotherapy regimens designed to delay or eliminate the need for whole-neuraxis radiation therapy are being investigated, including regimens using intraventricular chemotherapy.[756] In addition, high-dose regimens have been found to be feasible and effective for young children with disseminated, medulloblastoma.[813] The relative merits and risks of conventional multiagent chemotherapy compared with high-dose submyeloablative or myeloablative chemotherapy with stem cell support is under investigation.[264,525] An important finding in a recent study for infants with medulloblastoma is the particularly good outcome in infants with the desmoplastic variant, even without radiation therapy.[756] Ongoing studies to confirm this finding are underway but raise the possibility that desmoplastic medulloblastoma may form a new low-risk group that may extend to those older than 3 years.

Prognosis

Patients with standard-risk medulloblastoma have a 5-year survival of approximately 75% to 80%, whereas 5-year survival in high-risk medulloblastoma patients remains at between 40% and 60%.[792,814] Infants with metastatic disease or bulk unresectable disease continue to do poorly, with a 3-year event-free survival (EFS) of less than 40%, except in those with the desmoplastic variant. Patients with other rarer subtypes of medulloblastoma, including the large-cell, anaplastic, large-cell–anaplastic, and melanotic variants, continue to do poorly, even with maximal up-front therapy.[737] Various histologic features associated with improved prognosis have been evaluated, of which nodular appearance appears most important.[748] The presence of dissemination is the single most important factor that correlates with poor outcome.[815] Lifelong repeated surveillance imaging is required in anticipation of radiation-induced secondary malignancies, such as a meningioma or high-grade glioma.[816] Radiotherapy, particularly in young children, can also cause significant adverse late effects in cognitive development, growth, and endocrine function.[808,817,818] Molecular determinants such as p73 correlate with outcome and will need to await prospective validation.[819] These correlative findings can be of significant importance because if confirmed, they will not only permit better prognostication but potentially provide novel drug targets. Gene profiling of medulloblastoma was an accurate method of predicting outcome, even when evaluated in the context of clinical data. Variables such as age, M stage, and degree of resection did not significantly improve the predictive ability of this independent data set.[820]

Relapsed Medulloblastoma

Relapses occur as failures at the primary site, at distant sites, or both. Those occurring at the primary site within the posterior fossa may have a greater chance for salvage. Patients treated without up-front radiation therapy (infants, in particular) also have a good salvage rate.[821] Retrieval therapy is rarely curative but long-term disease control may occur with high-dose myeloablative chemotherapy in a small proportion of patients.[264,822] Past experience has shown that patients entering high-dose chemotherapy without chemotherapy-responsive disease, or with residual disease at the time of transplantation, are unlikely to benefit from this approach. There are a large number of new biologic and antiangiogenic agents being evaluated for relapsed medulloblastoma.[823] Although these agents are likely to be more effective when moved up early in the up-front setting, additional testing is still required.

Pineocytomas and Pineoblastomas

Tumors of the pineal region are often grouped together based on their location rather than their cellular origins and behavior. Embryonal tumors of the pineal region include pineocytoma, pineal parenchymal tumor of intermediate differentiation, pineoblastoma, and papillary tumor of the pineal region. Together, they account for less than 5% of all pediatric CNS tumors. Other pineal-based lesions include germ cell tumors and, less commonly, astrocytic tumors.[460] Germ cell tumors are discussed in a separate section.

Pineocytomas

These tumors arise from the pineocyte, whose primary function appears related to photoreceptor activity and neuroendocrine function.[824] They are classified as low-grade (grade I) neoplasms that are most common in adults and late adolescence, although they can be observed in young children. They account for approximately 50% of the tumors of pineal origin, although pineal region neoplasms account for only 1% to 5% of all pediatric CNS tumors.[825]

Clinical Presentation. Like other pineal region lesions, they often present with a constellation of symptoms related to their location. This includes obstructive hydrocephalus and Parinaud's syndrome,[826] a cluster of abnormalities of eye movements and papillary dysfunction characterized by paralyzed upgaze, pseudo–Argyll Robertson pupils, convergence-retraction nystagmus, eyelid retraction, and conjugate downgaze (setting-sun sign). Impairment of hypothalamic-pituitary, brainstem, and cerebellar function is also possible. Unlike malignant pineoblastomas, metastases are rare.

Imaging and Histology. On neuroimaging, pineocytomas are typically small focal lesions that can contain cysts and/or calcifications, best seen by CT. They are similar to other low-grade tumors on MRI, with strong contrast enhancement, hypointensity on T1-weighted sequences, and high signal on T2. Surgically, these tumors tend to be well-demarcated from surrounding tissue. Areas of hemorrhage are not uncommon. Microscopically, pineocytomas are made up of small, round, mature-looking cells that have maintained features of pineocytes, including rosettes.[827] These tumors demonstrate characteristic pineocytomatous rosettes that differentiate them from pineoblastoma. Mitoses are rare, as are other features of malignancy. Pineocytomas are usually strongly synaptophysin and neuron-specific enolase (NSE)-positive. If areas of pineoblastoma are identified with a pineocytoma, treatment is dictated by the most malignant element (i.e., pineoblastoma).

Management. Surgery remains the mainstay of the therapeutic approach for these lesions. Treatment directed at the hydrocephalus with third ventriculostomy may provide an opportunity to obtain a biopsy before aggressive and potentially morbid surgical resection is attempted.[828,829] Those with persistent growth can be irradiated although the benefit of this has not been clearly demonstrated. A role for chemotherapy has not been defined. Patients with incompletely resected tumors do not require therapy unless clear progression is demonstrated. Even patients with metastatic disease can remain untreated. The overall benign course observed with pineocytomas is in stark contrast to pineoblastomas.

Prognosis. The long-term prognosis remains excellent, even with incompletely resected disease. Conservative management should be followed with regard to attempted surgical resection and radiation therapy. Because almost all patients with pineocytomas will be long-term survivors, the need to avoid toxicity is paramount.

Pineal Parenchymal Tumor of Intermediate Differentiation

Pineal parenchymal tumors of intermediate differentiation (PPTIDs) are tumors of the pineal region that occur at all ages, although they are frequent in middle age, and are classified as grade II or III, depending on pathologic features. They account for 20% of pineal region tumors and were formally identified in 1993. Although reports are limited, there appears to be a slight female preponderance. Genetic evaluation has demonstrated a large number of abnormalities.[830]

Clinical Presentation. The presentation of patients with PPTID is similar to that of pineocytomas and includes obstructive hydrocephalus, as well as Parinaud's syndrome,[826] a cluster of abnormalities of eye movements, and papillary dysfunction characterized by paralyzed upgaze, pseudo–Argyll Robertson pupils, convergence-retraction nystagmus, eyelid retraction, and conjugate downgaze (setting-sun sign). Impairment of hypothalamic-pituitary, brainstem, and cerebellar function is also possible. Unlike pineocytomas, metastatic disease appears slightly more frequent.

Imaging and Histology. Imaging characteristics are similar to other lesions of pineal origin. They are cellular lesions with moderate nuclear atypia and a low mitotic index.[831] Because of sampling error, diagnosis can be difficult with tissue pieces, especially those obtained via third ventriculostomy.

Management. Because of the increasing degree of malignant potential when compared with pineocytomas, attempts at

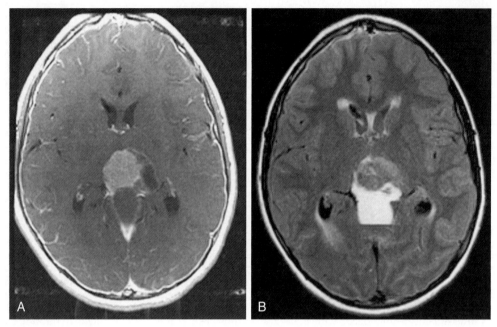

FIGURE 17-41. Large contrast-enhancing pineoblastoma. **A,** Axial T1 image with contrast. **B,** Axial fluid-attenuated inversion recovery (FLAIR) image demonstrating bright T2 signal.

surgical resection should be considered. Although formal pediatric studies are lacking, radiation therapy and chemotherapy should be considered. Intensity of treatment can be based on the localization of the tumor (focal, invasive, or disseminated) as well as the proportion of mitoses, necrosis, atypia, and possibly neurofilament protein expression.[832]

Prognosis. A definite prognosis for PPTID has not been clearly established. Grade is likely to play an important part in the long-term outcome of patients, as is the size and metastatic stage of patients.[833] Because these tumors span all age groups, large homogeneous studies are difficult.

Pineoblastoma

Unlike pineocytomas, pineoblastomas are highly malignant embryonal tumors. Like other small round blue cell tumors, these lesions are considered WHO grade IV and have a high propensity to metastasize. Typically, they are observed in children younger than those seen in pineocytomas, although there is considerable overlap. They can be associated with the genetic form of retinoblastoma and in such cases are often referred to as trilateral retinoblastomas.[834] An association with familial adenomatous polyposis has also been reported.[835] Little is known about the molecular classification of these tumors with respect to their genesis or association with other neural tumors of the CNS (PNET or medulloblastoma).[836] Defects in *TP53* have not been reported.

Clinical Presentation. Presenting symptoms of pineoblastoma are virtually identical to those for pineocytomas, although the duration of symptoms may be shorter than for other tumors in this location. They often present with a constellation of symptoms related to their location. This includes obstructive hydrocephalus in most patients,[837] as well as Parinaud's syndrome,[826] a cluster of abnormalities of eye movements and papillary dysfunction characterized by paralyzed upgaze, pseudo–Argyll Robertson pupils, convergence-retraction nystagmus, eyelid retraction, and conjugate downgaze (setting-sun

sign). Impairment of hypothalamic-pituitary, brainstem, and cerebellar function is also possible. Pineoblastomas have a much greater propensity to metastasize and thus may demonstrate symptoms beyond the pineal region.

Imaging and Histology. The neuroimaging characteristics of pineoblastomas are not pathognomonic for these tumors, but are differentiated from pineocytomas by significant increase in the volume of the tumor and the presence of much less distinct boundaries. MRI characteristics include low signal on T1-weighted sequences and heterogeneous areas of contrast enhancement (Fig. 17-41).[838] T2-weighted signals may be lower than in pineocytoma because of the higher nuclear-to-cytoplasmic ratio evident in these more malignant tumors.[839] On histologic analysis, these tumors are similar to other small round blue cell tumors, composed of sheets of cells but lacking the characteristic pineocytomatous rosettes of pineocytomas.[840] Pineoblastomas are typically synaptophysin- and NSE-positive and other markers, including those for photoreceptor pathways, can be present, consistent with the developmental role of the pineal gland.[832,841] Homer-Wright rosettes (cells with a central zone of cytoplasm; see Fig. 17-40) and Flexner-Wintersteiner rosettes (cells with a central zone of cytoplasm and a central space; Fig. 17-42) are common, but these can be seen in a large number of other embryonal tumors. These tumors often have significant atypia and mitotic activity can be high. When additional pathways of differentiation are present (e.g., melanin, cartilage, muscle), the tumors are called pineal anlage tumors. Regions of pineoblastoma can also be identified as part of a pineocytoma and are treated as a pineoblastoma. Although sporadic pineoblastoma has no clear genetic association, patients with hereditary (bilateral) retinoblastoma have a significant incidence of pineoblastoma (trilateral retinoblastoma). The clinical course of retinoblastoma-associated pineoblastoma can differ from that of sporadic pineoblastoma.[842]

Management. The therapeutic approaches for pineoblastoma have followed those of other embryonal seeding tumors

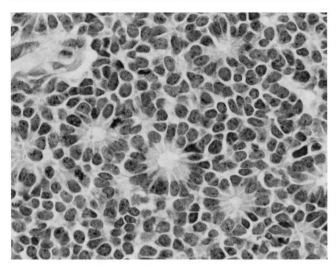

FIGURE 17-42. Flexner-Wintersteiner rosette in a patient with pineoblastoma (H&E; ×600).

of the CNS. The workup of patients with pineoblastoma includes immediate intervention for obstructive hydrocephalus and assessment of risk for herniation. A rapid CT scan, in conjunction with the examination and presenting history, will permit the neurosurgeon to assess these risks. If urgent CSF shunting is not required, then completion of the imaging baseline workup, including MRI of the brain and spine, can be performed and surgical resection planned. Unlike medulloblastoma, the location of pineoblastomas with adjacent vascular structures makes exploratory surgery much more risky and referral to a highly specialized center should be considered. A third ventriculostomy or VP shunt should be deferred prior to initial surgery but may be necessary if sufficient resection to reopen CSF flow is not achieved. In many patients, an endoscopic biopsy of the tumor to confirm the diagnosis and concurrent third ventriculostomy can be performed with a planned open craniotomy and resection once the patient is clinically stable, the pathology has been defined, and possible presurgical chemotherapy provided.[828] Patients with metastatic disease at diagnosis should not undergo up-front aggressive surgery because adjuvant therapy will be required. For patients with focal disease at diagnosis based on initial MR imaging and documentation of a negative lumbar puncture, complete removal of the tumor ultimately will be an important component of long-term prognosis,[843] but should not be undertaken at any costs. Consideration for staged surgeries (second- and even third-look approaches) may be equally effective without permanent neurologic damage).

Like other embryonal seeding tumors of the CNS, craniospinal radiotherapy is an important modality in treating microscopic metastatic disease at presentation. Unlike medulloblastoma, pineoblastomas do not have a standard risk category. All patients require aggressive therapy, including a craniospinal dose of 3600 cGy and a focal boost to the primary site of 5400 to 5940 cGy. Sites of metastatic disease require radiation boosts as well. Even with focal resectable disease, the prognosis for pineoblastoma falls significantly below that of medulloblastoma.[837] In those with disseminated disease, especially diffuse leptomeningeal spread, and infants, for whom craniospinal radiotherapy is contraindicated, the prognosis remains especially poor. The use of stereotactic radiosurgery (SRS) or other similar modalities to deliver single-fraction ablative radiation therapy may provide for added disease control

of unresectable tumor, although these approaches are limited to small areas of disease.

Chemotherapy is an important modality for patients with pineoblastoma, and significant responses to chemotherapy have been observed. Results from infant studies, which deferred radiotherapy, demonstrated that although chemotherapy can be effective at reducing bulk disease, few patients are long-term survivors with this modality alone.[844] Because of the rarity of this entity, most protocols have combined these patients with other embryonal tumors, including PNETs and, occasionally, medulloblastoma. Specific estimates of survival from different therapies have therefore been hard to determine. Current approaches continue to include initial craniospinal radiotherapy in combination with chemotherapy, followed by postradiation chemotherapy. Most regimens have used combinations of vincristine, cyclophosphamide, cisplatin, and etoposide.[843] Because of the chemoresponsiveness of these tumors, pilot clinical trials with high-dose chemotherapy with stem cell transplantation have also been undertaken.

The concurrent use of craniospinal radiation therapy and multiagent chemotherapy for pineoblastoma has resulted in a significant impairment of nutrition during therapy for these patients.[804] A large number will require nutritional support through a nasogastric tube or, more commonly, a gastric tube. Constant surveillance of nutrition is important because these issues are often dismissed early and are only recognized when severe weight loss has occurred. Patients with persistent vomiting usually initiate therapy in a negative nutritional state.

Prognosis. The outcome of patients with pineoblastoma remains poor. Those with focal disease that can be completely resected have 3- and 5-year event-free survivals of approximately 50%.[837,843] Infants, those with incompletely resected disease by the end of therapy, or those with metastatic disease continue to do poorly with 3- and 5-year EFS estimates of 20% or lower. Progression tends to occur early and can occur at the primary site, throughout the CNS, or both. Extracranial metastases are uncommon. There are, however, long-term survivors of patients with metastatic disease.[843] After recurrence, no standard therapy has been documented to be effective and most patients will succumb to their disease, usually within months.

Papillary Tumors of the Pineal Region

Papillary tumors of the pineal region (PTPRs) are rare tumors of children and adults that were separated from other pineal tumors in 2003.[183,845] As the name implies, these neuroepithelial lesions possess papillary structures and are thought to derive from specialized ependymal cells. Because of their varied appearance, they can be confused with ependymomas, choroid plexus tumors, and pineocytomas.[846] They appear to fall into the WHO grade II or III category.

Clinical Presentation. The clinical presentation of PTPRs is similar to other lesions of the pineal area. Hydrocephalus is present in almost all patients. Parinaud's syndrome,[826] a cluster of abnormalities of eye movements and papillary dysfunction characterized by paralyzed upgaze, pseudo–Argyll Robertson pupil, convergence-retraction nystagmus, eyelid retraction, and conjugate downgaze (setting-sun sign) is common. Impairment of hypothalamic-pituitary, brainstem, and cerebellar function is also possible. Metastatic disease does not appear as prevalent as in pineoblastomas.

Imaging and Histology. PTPRs are well-circumscribed, often cystic, lesions. They are hyperintense on T1-weighted sequences and hyperintense on T2 and are contrast-enhancing.[847,848] Histologically, these tumors stain strongly for keratins and are usually negative or weakly positive for GFAP (in contrast to ependymomas) and synaptophysin. Most of the tumor cells show strong expression of NSE, cytokeratins (particularly CK18), S-100 protein, and vimentin. The mitotic index and MIB-1 labeling index are intermediate but of unclear prognostic significance.[849]

Management. In spite of their differentiated appearance, PTPRs are aggressive tumors that are not highly responsive to therapy. In a recent report of 31 patients, 21 of whom achieved a gross total resection, adjuvant radiation therapy alone resulted in a progression-free survival rate of only 27%.[850] As for other malignant pineal-based tumors, maximal surgery, radiation therapy, and multiagent chemotherapy are therefore indicated.

Prognosis. In spite of complete resection and focal radiation therapy, local recurrences are common,[851] although patients with complete removal of these tumors may do better.[852]. Dissemination appears rare and craniospinal radiation therapy therefore does not appear to be required.

Supratentorial or Central Nervous System Primitive Neuroectodermal Tumors

PNETs are tumors of neuroepithelial origin.[853] The classification of supratentorial PNET (sPNET) as separate from medulloblastoma and other embryonal tumors, initially proposed in 1973,[713] has not been without controversy. Historically, these tumors have been called by various names, including cerebral medulloblastoma, cerebral neuroblastoma, and cerebral ganglioneuroblastoma. Rorke proposed that these tumors are the supratentorial equivalent of medulloblastoma, another common embryonal neoplasm.[854] Although these tumors are histologically similar to medulloblastoma, they respond poorly to medulloblastoma-specific therapy. Part of the confusion in the approach to CNS PNETs has been in the nomenclature—the overlap in the term *PNET* for tumors of the body as well. These tumors do not share the molecular pathways,[836] metastatic sites, or treatment responses of the extracranial PNET tumors. Even within the CNS, PNETs likely represent a heterogeneous group of tumors.[711] According to the WHO classification schema,[855] a number of subtypes of PNET are recognized—classic PNET, PNET with neuronal differentiation (called cerebral neuroblastoma) and, if ganglion cells are present as part of the tumor, cerebral ganglioneuroblastoma. Neither of the latter two entities is related to classic neuroblastoma, which is typically identified around the adrenal gland and shares a common name as a result of historical nomenclature only. New molecular determinants associated with PNETs of the brain have been identified using molecular and proteomic analysis and will hopefully be useful for better subclassification of the diseases that fall into this broad category of tumors.[240,856-858]

Supratentorial PNETs are relatively rare, occurring at a rate that is approximately 10% to 20% that of medulloblastoma.[859] Precise statistics regarding incidence are difficult to ascertain because of historically different views regarding classification and nosology. These tumors are more common in early childhood, with most diagnosed before the age of 10 years,[860] and whites make up most of the reported cases. Most cases are identified in early childhood, but they span all ages. Although they are classified as supratentorial in nature, these tumors have been identified in the infratentorial and spinal compartments. A better term has recently been adopted by WHO,[183] *CNS PNET.*

Clinical Presentation. Presenting features of CNS PNETs depend on the location of the lesion. Those adjacent to the ventricular flow path will usually include signs and symptoms of raised intracranial pressure as a result of obstructive hydrocephalus. Specific neurologic signs are dependent on the anatomic structures adjacent to the tumor and can include seizures, mood changes, or hemiparesis. Metastases are frequent in CNS PNETs and clinical symptoms unrelated to the primary site of disease require investigation.

Imaging and Histology. CNS PNETs appear similar, independently of location within the CNS. As in medulloblastoma and pineoblastoma, these tumors can have areas of cyst or necrosis evident on CT or MRI. Lesions are dark on T1-weighted sequences unless hemorrhage is present and dark on T2-weighted sequences, reflecting their high nuclear-to-cytoplasmic ratio.[861] They are usually contrast-enhancing after administration of gadolinium. Edema, as evident on T2-weighted or FLAIR sequences, is often prominent (Fig. 17-43). All CNS PNETs are considered WHO grade IV. The light microscopic features of CNS PNETs can be similar to those of medulloblastoma or pineoblastoma. Tumors are characterized by the presence of neuroepithelial cells. Many CNS PNETs have evidence of differentiation along glial, neuronal, ependymal, or oligodendroglial lines, although most (approximately 60%) appear undifferentiated.[862]

Immunohistochemical markers of CNS PNETs include synaptophysin, B-tubulin, and S-100. Occasionally, GFAP can be identified in these tumors and indicates their ability to undergo divergent differentiation. Mitotic rates are often high and, although variable, MIB-1 is usually abundant. Mutations of p53 are rare[863] and were identified in only 3 of 28 cases of CNS PNET in one study, although many tumors had overexpression of wild-type p53, which correlated with a poor prognosis.[864] Specific markers for supratentorial PNETs that distinguish them from medulloblastoma do not exist. Other features, such as Homer-Wright rosettes and perivascular pseudorosettes (cells around a central blood vessel) are observed in many different tumors (see Figs. 17-36 and 17-40). ATRTs may resemble PNETs but the presence of cells that stain positively for myosin but lack the protein produced of the *hSNF5/INI1* gene are diagnostic features.[865,866]

Medulloepitheliomas

CNS PNET tumors that have recreated features of the neural tube are called medulloepitheliomas, are typically found in very young children,[867] and have even been reported in newborns. They can occur throughout the brain, spine, and optic tract[868] and can also occur outside the CNS. Their imaging characteristics differ somewhat from other CNS PNETs, with bright appearance on T2.[869] They tend to be large on macroscopic appearance. Additional immunohistochemical markers include nestin and vimentin staining.[855] Like with other CNS PNETs, maximal surgical resection, chemotherapy, and radiation are the cornerstone of therapy. The predilection for young age in this subset of PNETs limits the use of craniospinal radiation.

Ependymoblastomas

PNET tumors with ependymoblastic rosettes are called ependymoblastomas. These tumors predominate in infants and young children[870] and can be found throughout the CNS, although most are associated with the ventricular system.[855] Dissemination throughout the CNS is common[871] and symptoms include obstructive hydrocephalus, enlarging head circumference in infants, and focal neurologic deficits. The MRI appearance is similar to other PNETs and edema is commonly

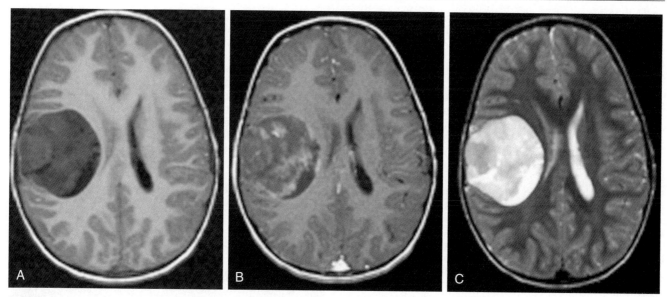

FIGURE 17-43. Primitive neuroectodermal tumor (PNET). **A,** Axial T1 image without contrast. **B,** Axial T1 image with contrast. **C,** Axial T2 image.

observed.[872] Treatment mirrors that of other CNS PNETs. Maximal resection is paramount, followed by multiagent chemotherapy. Although craniospinal radiation therapy is likely important for outcome, the prevalence of ependymoblastoma in infants precludes its use. Prognosis is poor, with rapid disease progression in most patients.

Cerebral Neuroblastomas

PNETs with neuronal differentiation are called cerebral neuroblastoma and are rare tumors of infancy and childhood. They are unrelated to the common form of neuroblastoma and predominate in young infants,[873] occurring in both the cerebrum[874] and posterior fossa.[875] Lack of immunohistochemical staining with IGF-II and IGFR-I, which is positive in many other infant CNS tumors, can help with the diagnosis.[855,876]

A related entity of cerebral neuroblastoma is termed *ganglioneuroblastoma*, which has the presence of ganglion cells in addition to the neuronal component.[855] These tumors cannot be differentiated from other malignant seeding tumors of infancy by MRI characteristics.[877] Unlike most other CNS PNETs, cerebral neuroblastoma and CNS ganglioneuroblastoma may have a better prognosis[878] with surgery and chemotherapy.

Embryonal Tumor

Embryonal tumor with abundant neuropil and true rosettes (ETANTR) is another rare CNS PNET tumor with a spectrum of histologic features and chromosomal abnormalities.[855] These lesions can be large, cystic, and calcified and come to clinical presentation as a result of mass effect.[879] Their rarity makes treatment recommendations difficult, although most are approached in a manner similar to that of other PNETs of the brain. The presence of isochrome 17[880] in only a few cases suggests that they are biologically distinct from medulloblastoma.[881] Various cytogenetic abnormalities have been defined but no one region or gene has yet been implicated.[882]

Treatment Strategies

A number of treatment protocols based on the successful therapeutic approaches of medulloblastoma have been applied to

CNS PNETs.[809] Repeated studies using maximal surgery, high-dose craniospinal radiotherapy to 3600 cGy with a boost to the primary site of at least 5400 cGy, and multiagent chemotherapy have not fared as well for CNS PNETs[883,884] as for high-risk medulloblastoma, with 4-year survival of approximately 40% in one retrospective series.[860] In one study of 55 patients treated with maximal surgery, craniospinal radiation therapy, and CCNU, vincristine, and prednisone versus 8-in-1 chemotherapy sandwiched in the middle, overall and event-free survival were comparable. The 3-year EFS was approximately 50% in the two groups and thus appeared similar to other studies. Poor prognostic variables included presence of metastases and age younger than 2 years. Patients with pineoblastoma did better, with an estimated 3-year PFS of 65%.[884] As compared with medulloblastoma, CNS PNETs often respond poorly to medulloblastoma-specific therapy, despite the fact that they are histologically similar.[885] The use of high-dose chemotherapy with stem cell rescue has been successful for some young children in eliminating the need for radiation therapy, with 5-year EFS of 39%.[886] The exact conditioning regimen and number of cycles of intensive chemotherapy remain under investigation.[887] Recurrences are often disseminated,[885,888] even when craniospinal radiation therapy is delivered up-front, and salvage for these patients is exceedingly poor. In spite of these overall poor results, there have been reports of survivors after surgery, especially gross total resection, and radiation therapy.[889]

The concurrent use of craniospinal radiation therapy and multiagent chemotherapy for CNS PNETs has resulted in a significant impairment of nutrition during therapy for these patients.[804] A large number will require nutritional support through a nasogastric tube or, more commonly, a gastric tube. Constant surveillance of nutrition is important because these issues are often dismissed early and are only recognized when severe weight loss has occurred. Patients with persistent vomiting may initiate therapy in a negative nutritional state.

Prognosis. Although the prognosis of CNS PNET is well below that of medulloblastoma, 40% of patients will be long-term survivors. The most important variable for prolonged survival is the ability to achieve a complete resection in patients with nonmetastatic disease, followed by craniospinal irradiation and multiagent chemotherapy. The ability to salvage relapsed patients is exceedingly poor, even with high-dose chemotherapy and stem cell rescue.[890]

Atypical Teratoid Rhabdoid Tumors

ATRTs are uncommon, highly malignant tumors seen primarily in infants and in young children,[891-893] with a peak incidence between birth and 3 years. Cases throughout childhood[894] and in adults, however, have been reported,[895] as have hereditary transmission of the susceptibility gene, resulting in congenital disease.[896] Although central nervous system ATRTs account for approximately 1% to 2% of childhood brain tumors, they represent almost 10% of CNS tumors in infants.[897,898] Rhabdoid tumors may arise anywhere in the body but are most common in the kidney and central nervous system. CNS ATRTs are most commonly identified in the posterior fossa (60%) at the cerebellopontine angle, although supratentorial ATRTs are also frequently seen.[899] Pineal, spine, and suprasellar area ATRTs have also been reported. ATRTs have a spectrum of morphologic and molecular variants,[900] although most have loss of the INI-1 gene product on chromosome 22; this has become a standard assessment tool for making the diagnosis of ATRT in atypical cases.[866] CNS tumors tend to have specific mutational hotspots in the INI-1 gene, although treatment response and outcome are not known to be influenced by specific mutations. There is a strong male preponderance and metastases at diagnosis are common.[899]

Clinical Presentation. Presenting symptoms are dependent on the age and location of the tumor. In those with posterior fossa tumors, obstructive hydrocephalus with headaches, morning vomiting, and long tract signs are common. Because most patients are young, irritability, lethargy, or failure to thrive may be evident. In those without closed fontanelles, rapidly enlarging head circumference is observed. Cranial nerve dysfunction is common, resulting in head tilt and diplopia. Patients with supratentorial tumors will often have obstructive hydrocephalus because of the rapid growth and concurrent cysts that obstruct CSF flow. Additional symptoms can be referred to direct compression of neural structures adjacent to the tumor and thus are dependent on location.[899,901] Although uncommon, spinal ATRT can occur and present with focal motor deficits. Because of the high incidence of metastatic disease, patients with symptoms related to a specific area away from the primary tumor site require thorough investigation. Although rare, constitutional loss of the *INI1* gene can occur,[897] resulting in intracranial and metachronous extraneural disease. Patients should therefore undergo CT evaluation of the chest, abdomen, and pelvis.

Imaging and Histology. Imaging characteristics are similar to other neuroectodermal tumors (medulloblastoma and PNET) of the CNS,[902] including isointense appearance on T1-weighted MR imaging and heterogeneity on FLAIR and T2 sequences.[903,904] Cystic areas are common. Tumors are usually heterogeneously enhancing with contrast administration. Because of their high cellular composition, restricted diffusion is often observed. The presence of hemorrhage and calcifications is not uncommon.[905]

ATRT has been recognized as a distinct pathologic entity, differentiated from medulloblastoma and other PNETs.[906] This has been supported by findings of deletions or loss at chromosome 22q11.2, the identification of the tumor suppressor gene *hSNF5/INI-1*, and the finding of germline and somatic mutations of INI-1 in approximately 75% of cases of CNS ATRTs,[907] although ATRTs based on morphologic criteria with normal expression of INI-1 have been identified.[908] Rhabdoid cells have

the characteristic appearance of an eccentric nucleus, prominent eosinophilic nucleoli, and abundant cytoplasm, with an eosinophilic globular cytoplasmic inclusion (Fig. 17-44).[909] These cells stain with EMA and vimentin. GFAP and synaptophysin can also be positive. INI-1 staining is routinely used to confirm the diagnosis. The expression of this nuclear protein, which remains expressed in endothelial cells, is characteristically lost in tumor cells (Fig. 17-45). Tumors without the presence of rhabdoid cells but with loss of INI-1 staining are still considered ATRTs.[908] Whether choroid plexus tumors can have loss of INI-1 expression or whether these represent actual ATRTs is controversial.[865,910] ATRTs are classified as WHO grade IV,[909] lesions with elevated MIB-1, and are composed of primitive neuroepithelial, epithelial, and mesenchymal components. Large areas of small round blue cells can predominate, resulting in the misdiagnosis of medulloblastoma or PNET. In

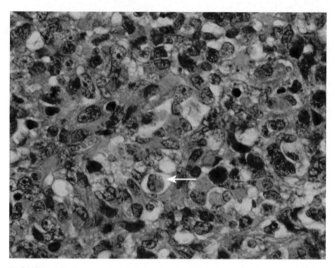

FIGURE 17-44. Atypical teratoid rhabdoid tumor (*arrow*) demonstrating prominent nucleoli and eosinophilic globular cytoplasmic inclusions (H&E; ×600).

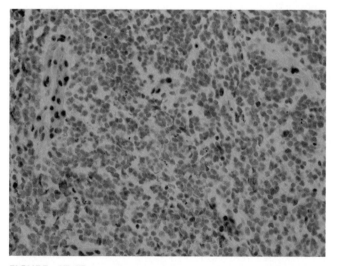

FIGURE 17-45. Atypical teratoid rhabdoid tumor (ATRT) with absence of INI-1 immunoreactivity in the tumor cells. Normal endothelial cells within the blood vessels have normal INI-1 expression (INI-1 immunostaining; ×400).

a review of 55 cases from the Pediatric Oncology Group (POG) study, the small cell component resembled medulloblastoma[911] and ATRT was misclassified as medulloblastoma in over 50% of cases.[891] These findings emphasize the need for confirmatory testing with INI-1 immunohistochemical staining or fluorescence in situ hybridization (FISH) to look for monosomy chromosome 22 to help confirm or exclude the diagnosis of ATRT.[911] Similarly, a central pathology review of 227 of 284 eligible infants with brain tumors from a CCG clinical trial for infant patients (CCG-9921) showed that ATRT is a significant component of the tumors in this population and that frequent misdiagnoses occur.[662] Since the original description of monosomy 22 in ATRTs, a tumor suppressor gene *INI-1* (integrase interactor 1, also known as *hSNF5*) has been cloned from this region[912] and functions as a chromatin remodeling complex.[913] Mutations and loss of *INI-1* gene and protein expression may not be confined to ATRTs alone as reports on choroid plexus carcinoma, supratentorial PNET, and medulloblastoma[891] have been published. It remains controversial whether these later reports represent other diseases with *INI-1* mutations or atypical cases of ATRT. Given the predominance of *INI-1* loss of expression in ATRT, it is now standard practice to evaluate *INI-1* expression for treatment stratification onto the appropriate disease-specific protocols.

Management. Multimodality protocols developed for the treatment of medulloblastoma have not been effective for ATRT. Some success has been achieved using treatment protocols based on therapy for children with rhabdomyosarcoma[901,914] and high-dose myeloablative chemotherapy.[899] The discovery of the function of the new tumor suppressor gene *hSNF5/INI-1* will hopefully lead to more specific targeted therapies. Currently, the optimal therapy for pediatric ATRT remains maximal surgical resection, multiagent chemotherapy, and radiation therapy.[894,915] Older patients appear to have a better prognosis and, with complete surgical resection, multiagent chemotherapy, and craniospinal radiotherapy, have 2-year EFS and OS of 78% and 89%, respectively. In contrast, children younger than 3 years have a dismal outcome with EFS and OS of 11% and 17%, respectively.[894] A recent risk-adapted treatment protocol in which patients received maximal surgery, multiagent chemotherapy, both systemic and intrathecal, and focal radiation therapy in children younger than 3 years and CSI in older patients has demonstrated encouraging results. The 2-year EFS and OS in this group of patients, most of whom were younger than 3 years, was 53% and 70%, respectively.[915] These results indicate that ATRT can be effectively treated and that even patients with metastatic disease can be long-term survivors. The need for radiation therapy in the treatment of ATRT remains controversial, especially for the youngest patients, although some centers have encouraged its use.[916] The overall positive outcomes seen in infants treated with three-dimensional conformal therapy, as well as those treated with the high-dose chemotherapy and a stem cell transplantation approach without RT, have suggested that craniospinal therapy is not needed in all patients. The identification of a radiation-resistant CD31 positive stem cell may explain some of the innate resistance of this tumor to current therapies.[917] Coupled with an improved understanding of the pathways aberrant in these tumors, newer targeted therapies will hopefully soon be available.[918]

Prognosis. Until recently, estimates of survival rates for ATRT ranged from 6 to 11 months.[662,911,919,920] Although tumors tend to be initially responsive to chemotherapy, rapidly recurrence occurs, both locally and with metastatic disease.[907] However, the prognosis for patients with ATRT may be improved dramatically with intensive multimodality treatment.[894,915] Although extremely uncommon, some survivors of relapsed disease have been reported.[901]

Neurocytomas

Central neurocytomas are rare tumors, comprising between 0.25% and 0.5% of all brain tumors.[921,922] First described in 1982 by Hassoun and colleagues, neurocytomas typically occur in adolescents and young adults. These tumors are of neural lineage based on the expression of neuronal markers such as βIII-tubulin, neural cell adhesion molecular (NCAM), neuron-specific enolase (NSE), and synaptophysin.[923,924] A gene expression profile comparison of central neurocytoma cells with normal adult ventricular zone progenitors has demonstrated significant overlap, indicating that central neurocytoma is most consistent with proneural cells and that these neurocytoma cells differ from progenitor cells by the increased expression of insulin-like growth factor 2 (IGF-2) and receptors, and effectors of the canonical Wnt signaling pathway and *PDGFD*.[925] Neurocytomas usually arise in the lateral ventricles, especially in proximity to the third ventricle and foramen of Monro, and are called central neurocytomas. Those localized to the brain parenchyma are called extraventricular neurocytomas. Historically, neurocytomas have been frequently described as benign lesions because of the positive outcome of patients with complete surgical resections, although aggressive behavior and poor outcome are not uncommon.[926,927] Furthermore, there have been numerous reports of tumors with MIB-1 labeling indices more than 3%, and/or atypical histologic features such as increased mitotic activity, vascular proliferation, and/or focal necrosis.[928] The mean age at presentation in adults is 28 to 29 years, with most patients between the ages of 20 and 40 years,[921] and a male-to-female ratio of 3:2.[929] A review of neurocytoma in 60 children younger than 18 years, compiled primarily from reports in the medical literature, has demonstrated a median age of 16 years, with a similar male predominance (61%).[930]

Clinical Presentation. Most neurocytomas are located in the ventricular system,[931] specifically the anterior portion of the lateral ventricles near the foramen of Monro, although extraventricular tumors have been described.[927,932] Symptoms of raised intracranial pressure are common as a result of tumor obstruction of CSF flow at the level of the foramen of Monro or cerebral aqueduct.[926] Patients with neurocytoma typically present with symptoms including headache, visual changes, nausea, and vomiting.[933] Focal neurologic deficits are less common presenting signs. Hemorrhage can result in acute symptoms, leading to the diagnosis. Primary disease in the fourth ventricle[934] or spinal cord has been reported in children.[935]

Imaging and Histology. The typical MRI appearance of central neurocytoma is that of a well-circumscribed lobulated mass in the anterior portion of the lateral ventricles, making it difficult to distinguish from other intraventricular neoplasms such as ependymomas, astrocytomas, and oligodendrogliomas. Tumors often have an isointense or slightly hypointense signal relative to the cerebral cortex on T1-weighted and hyperintense signal on T2-weighted MR images with enhancement on administration of gadolinium (Fig. 17-46).[936-938] Proton MRS has recently been described as a possible diagnostic tool in central neurocytoma. A characteristic MRS appearance of a high choline peak, a low NAA peak, and a glycine peak at 3.55 ppm is seen in a subset of patients.[939]

Histopathologic analysis of neurocytomas often reveals benign-appearing tissue composed of uniform round cells.

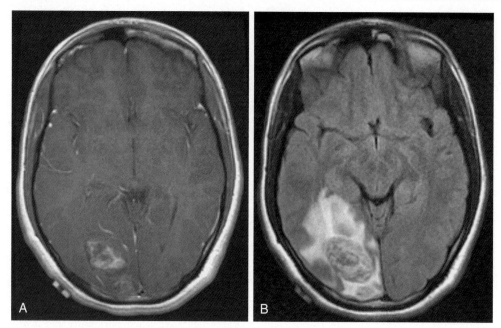

FIGURE 17-46. Right occipital extraventricular neurocytoma. **A,** Axial T1 image with contrast. **B,** Axial fluid-attenuated inversion recovery (FLAIR) image. This is an iso- to hyperintense extraventricular neurocytoma with surrounding edema.

Neurocytomas are classified as WHO grade II.[940] Features such as large fibrillary areas, calcifications, and perivascular pseudo-rosettes are commonly observed.[941] Routine hematoxylin and eosin (H&E) staining of a neurocytoma can reveal the presence of cells with perinuclear halos suggestive of oligodendroglioma. However, the reactivity with immunohistochemical staining for neuronal markers such as synaptophysin, βIII-tubulin, NCAM, and NSE helps establish the diagnosis of a neurocytoma.[942] As noted earlier, atypical forms with mitoses, necrosis, and endo-thelial proliferation have been reported.[943,944] In tumors lacking synaptophysin or Neu-N staining, electron microscopy can assist in confirming the diagnosis.[945] A MIB-1 labeling index is useful for prognostic purposes. Patients with a MIB-1 labeling index greater than 2% to 3% are referred to as having atypical neurocytoma and have a worse prognosis for local control and survival.[928,943,944] Subtotal resection, atypical histologic features, and older patient age have been associated with an increased risk of recurrence.[946]

Management. Gross total resection can be curative for central neurocytomas and is the treatment of choice for pedi-atric patients. A review of 73 children younger than 18 years pooled from multiple studies has shown an overall survival of 100% at 10 years for children who underwent a gross total resection.[947] Local failure was demonstrated in approximately 15% of patients who underwent complete resection alone versus 0% in patients who underwent complete resection with adjuvant radiation therapy. However, given the absence of sur-vival difference and the potential neurocognitive toxicities, adjuvant radiation therapy is not recommended as initial treat-ment.[930] Children with incomplete resections have a signifi-cantly higher risk of recurrence (mean, 100 months) and a lower overall survival (82%). Adjuvant radiation therapy has been shown to reduce the risk of recurrence but not the risk of death.[930] In the case of incomplete resection, radiotherapy may be beneficial at a dose of 5400 cGy,[948] although it should be noted that the number of patients available for evaluation in these studies is small. Radiotherapy should be more seriously considered for atypical neurocytomas, such as those with a high

MIB-1 labeling index (higher than 3%). A recent meta-analysis has shown that patients with lesions that have an MIB-1 less than 3% have less than a 15% risk of recurrence and a 95% 5-year overall survival, compared with 38% and 66%, respec-tively, for patients with tumors that have an MIB-1 index higher than 3%.[928] In a review of 85 adult and pediatric patients, Rades and colleagues[949] have demonstrated a marked difference in 5-year survival for incompletely resected atypical neurocytoma (43%). The addition of adjuvant radiation therapy increased 5-year survival rates to 78%. Complete resection was again found to be the best treatment, with 5-year survival rates of 93%. Adjuvant radiotherapy held no additional benefit in cases of completely resected atypical neurocytomas. Stereotactic radiosurgery has been explored as a potential first-line treat-ment for neurocytoma, but only in limited numbers of adult patients.[950] SRS is likely not the optimal initial treatment for pediatric patients. Historically, the use of chemotherapy for central neurocytoma has been limited, with only case reports and small case series being reported.[951] Brandes and associ-ates[952] have described three adult patients with progressive neurocytoma treated with etoposide, cisplatin, and cyclophos-phamide, which led to disease stabilization in two patients and complete remission in one.

Prognosis. Complete surgical resection and an MIB-1 rate of less than 2% are the most important prognostic markers. Even with extraventricular location and atypical features, most patients will be long-term survivors. Thus, judicious use of therapeutic modalities that can lead to significant long-term morbidity, such as radiation therapy, is indicated.

Choroid Plexus Tumors

Choroid plexus tumors usually arise from the epithelium of the choroid plexus in the lateral or fourth ventricles, where the choroid plexus is found. Although choroid plexus lesions rep-resent only 3% of pediatric brain tumors, they comprise 10% to 20% of tumors that develop in the first year of life and

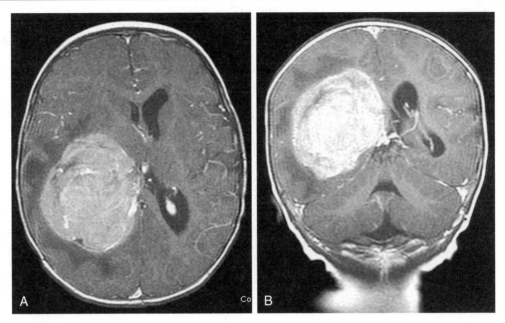

FIGURE 17-47. Choroid plexus carcinoma (CPC). **A,** Axial T1 image with contrast. **B,** Sagittal T1 image with contrast.

account for a considerable percentage of in utero diagnoses.[953] The median age at diagnosis for choroid plexus tumors is younger than 2 years.[954] Three histologic choroid plexus variants have been described—papillomas, atypical papillomas, and carcinomas.[955] Choroid plexus papillomas outnumber choroid plexus carcinomas by a ratio of at least 5:1. Both tumors typically arise in the lateral ventricles in 50% of cases and in the fourth ventricle in 40%. Tumors arising from multiple ventricles represent only 5% of cases. Because of their rarity, little is known about the molecular abnormalities that give rise to these tumors,[956] although their strong association with the Li-Fraumeni p53 cancer susceptibility gene is well established.[957] A significant percentage of choroid tumors will have abnormalities on array comparative genomic hybridization (CGH) analysis.[615] The presence of normal INI-1 staining in these tumors can be used to exclude ATRTs, which share many histologic features.[865]

Little is known at present about the developmental or molecular biology of choroid plexus tumors, although a number of markers have been identified using gene array analysis.[958] In rare cases, choroid plexus carcinomas have been found in Li-Fraumeni patients who have a germline mutation of p53.[957] DNA sequences from sporadic papillomas may harbor the human neurotropic John Cunningham virus.[630] The role of SV40 (another polyomavirus) in the development of pediatric CNS tumors, particularly ependymomas and choroid plexus, is an interesting one. SV40 sequences are found in the tumor tissue of up to 50% of patients but not in adjacent areas of normal brain. SV40 is known to induce brain tumors in preclinical models and SV40 can transform human cells in vitro. This may support a causative role for this polyomavirus in choroid plexus tumors.[631] Polio vaccines used in certain countries in the 1950s and 1960s were contaminated with SV40. In countries that have used uncontaminated vaccines, the identification of SV40 sequences in choroid plexus tumors is rare. However, the incidence of choroid plexus tumors is similar between the two populations and thus appears independent of both SV40 exposure and SV40 detection within the tumors.[633,959] Because of the strong association of Li-Fraumeni syndrome and p53 mutations with choroid plexus carcinoma, patients need a comprehensive family history to ascertain the incidence of asso-

ciated cancers and assist in the screening of family members. The presence of a p53 germline mutation may affect the choice of radiation therapy as a therapeutic option and would indicate the need for genetic counseling in other family members.[957] The presence of PDGFR expression in a high percentage of cases (87%) is a rationale for the use of targeted inhibitors of this pathway in the context of a clinical trial.[960]

Clinical Presentation. Initial symptoms are usually secondary to elevated intracranial pressure (ICP) and hydrocephalus and include headaches, nausea, and vomiting, with papilledema. Other possible manifestations include lethargy, seizures, and failure to thrive. Because these tumors tend to arise in infants who retain open sutures, the presentation may be relatively delayed and the tumors may reach an exceptional size. Infants typically demonstrate irritability, lethargy, vomiting, a tense fontanelle, and macrocephaly, with splayed sutures. Although most choroid plexus tumors arise in the lateral ventricles, predominantly in infants, fourth ventricular choroid plexus tumors occur in all ages, including adults. Metastatic disease can occur in choroid plexus papillomas (CPPs), although these patients still have a good prognosis and many of the tumors will not progress. Leptomeningeal dissemination is common with choroid plexus carcinomas (CPCs) and is a poor prognostic marker because of the limited use of craniospinal radiation therapy in this very young population. Dissemination through a VP shunt has been reported.[961]

Imaging and Histology. A choroid plexus tumor should be suspected when a large enhancing tumor in the lateral ventricle is visualized on gadolinium-enhanced MRI (Fig. 17-47). Multilobular, calcified, well-delineated contrast-enhancing intraventricular masses are characteristic of choroid plexus tumors. Tumors are usually isodense on T1-weighted images and bright on T2.[962] CPCs often have more heterogeneous enhancement and edema signal on FLAIR than is routinely seen in CPPs.[963] Unique characteristics of MRS can differentiate CPP from CPC at diagnosis although, for most patients, this will not obviate the need for surgery because of the high incidence of CSF flow obstruction in these patients necessitating neurosurgical intervention.[964]

CPPs (WHO grade I) have the lowest proliferative rate and are composed of fibrovascular fronds covered by a single layer of epithelial cells. They closely resemble the normal choroid plexus. Cytokeratin, S-100 protein, podoplanin, and vimentin are typically expressed on immunohistochemistry. GFAP, which is typically not seen in the normal choroid plexus, is found in approximately 25% to 50% of choroid plexus papillomas.[965] In contrast, CPCs (WHO grade III) manifest higher cell density, nuclear pleomorphism, frequent mitoses (more than 5/10 high-power fields [HPF]), high nuclear-to-cytoplasmic ratios, necrosis, and invasive appearance (i.e., blurring of the papillary structures). Up to 20% of CPCs can be positive for GFAP.[966] Atypical choroid plexus papillomas (WHO grade II) refer to cases in which the distinction between choroid plexus papilloma and carcinoma is not clear (e.g., only one or two histologic features of malignancy). Clear diagnostic criteria for these atypical tumors have not been established. These tumors can possess greater pleomorphism, increased cellularity, and areas of necrosis, but these elements are not required for diagnosis. However, it appears that the presence of mitotic activity (2 mitoses or more/10 HPF) is the sole atypical histologic feature independently associated with recurrence.[966] Atypical CPPs accounted for approximately 15% of all choroid plexus papillomas in one large series.[966]

Management. Following diagnostic neuroimaging studies, patients are often placed on high-dose corticosteroids when elevated ICP is suspected. Because the extent of surgical resection is the single most important factor that determines the prognosis in choroid plexus tumors, the goal of the neurosurgeon is to perform a gross total resection.[967] This may require more than one surgical procedure but appears to improve outcome.[968] One obstacle to the surgical removal of choroid plexus tumors is the rich vascular network that is often located within the tumor. The choroid plexus receives its blood supply from the anterior and posterior choroidal arteries, branches of the internal carotid artery, and the posterior cerebral artery. Achieving a gross total resection in cases of choroid plexus papilloma and atypical papilloma is often curative, and adjuvant therapy may be deferred following a normal restaging evaluation.

Because most children diagnosed with choroid plexus carcinoma are younger than 3 years, chemotherapy is the treatment of choice in those for whom a complete resection cannot be achieved.[844,954] Various multiagent chemotherapy regimens have been explored and preliminary evidence suggests that choroid plexus carcinomas are chemosensitive tumors. The role of radiotherapy is controversial and is usually reserved for children older than 3 years who have had a subtotal resection, malignant features within the tumor, or dissemination of the tumor along the neuraxis.

Prognosis. Gross total resection is often curative for choroid plexus papilloma. Even in patients with a subtotal resection, 50% of the residual tumor will not demonstrate progression.[969] The 5- and 10-year progression-free and overall survivals for patients with papillomas are 81% and 77%, respectively, versus 41% and 35%, respectively, for those with carcinomas.[954] Atypical CPP can recur and thus careful follow-up is needed. The long-term prognosis for this group of patients remains excellent.[966] Patients with dissemination at diagnosis do less well. Several adjuvant platinum-based chemotherapy regimens have been used, with some measure of success,[970] but at present there is no standard protocol established for choroid plexus carcinoma. An international protocol for the prospective treatment and outcome of choroid papilloma, atypical choroid plexus papilloma, and choroid plexus carcinoma is underway.

Germ Cell Tumors

Central nervous system germ cell tumors (GCTs) are the most prevalent tumors of the pineal region and represent approximately 3% to 5% of intracranial childhood malignances in the United States. These tumors are much more common in Asia, particularly in Japan.[971,972] The reason for this geographic variability is unknown. Most germ cell tumors occur in early adolescence and males are significantly more affected than females.[973] Males are much more likely to have both pineal and suprasellar germ cell tumors, with a reported male-to-female ratio of approximately 14:1.[974] Germinomas are much more common than nongerminomas.[975] Histologically, these tumors resemble the germ cell tumors that arise in the gonads.

Most (95%) germ cell tumors arise in midline sites such as the infundibular region (40%) and pineal region (50%), although 5% arise simultaneously in both regions without an apparent connection.[976] Occasionally, they are isolated to the basal ganglia[977] but can be approached in a similar fashion to those in the pineal or suprasellar area.[978] CNS GCTs are presumed to result from the abnormal migration of primitive germ cells early in embryogenesis within the gonadal ridge.[979,980] Occasionally, metachronous lesions at both sites are detected at the time of diagnosis.[979] CNS GCTs are divided into two clinical groups, which reflect sensitivity to cytotoxic therapies— pure germinomas (60%) and nongerminomatous germ cell tumors (40%).[971,981] Nongerminomatous germ cell tumors (NGGCTs) include yolk sac tumors (endodermal sinus tumors), embryonal carcinomas, choriocarcinomas, immature teratomas, teratomas with malignant transformation, and mixed germ cell tumors. Mixed germ cell tumors are defined as tumors that contain any two of the elements listed earlier and can include mixtures of germinoma and nongerminoma. Germinomas are the most common germ cell tumor of the pineal region,[974] although NGGCTs and germinomas arise with equal frequency in the suprasellar region. A male excess occurs in pineal region tumors, although both genders are equally affected by tumors in the suprasellar region. Mature teratomas of the brain causing significant mass effect have been reported.[982] Their peak age of occurrence is in the second and third decade of life.

No clear genetic predisposition to CNS germ cell tumors has been identified other than males with Klinefelter's syndrome (47XXY).[983] Of interest, a number of CNS germ cell tumors have an abnormal karyotype, including gain of chromosome X, and raises the possibility that Klinefelter's patients are uniquely at risk because of the presence of their additional X chromosome. A number of cases of germ cell tumors in patients with Down syndrome have also been reported.[984,985]

Clinical Presentation. The clinical presentation between suprasellar and pineal region germ cell tumors can differ. Patients diagnosed with suprasellar germ cell tumors often have a long prodrome, often several years in duration.[986] The earliest symptoms usually involve endocrine dysfunction, most frequently symptoms of diabetes insipidus.[987] This presenting symptom can also be observed in other lesions of the pituitary region, such as lymphocytic hypophysitis.[988] In some patients with diabetes insipidus, a mass is not identified on MRI scan but, over time, a mass becomes evident, leading to the diagnosis. Eventually, other endocrine manifestations may occur, such as growth impairment, delayed puberty, and hypothyroidism. Visual loss and symptoms of raised ICP are late manifestations when the tumor has reached appreciable size or spread in a periventricular distribution. Even in patients without MRI evidence of pituitary or hypothalamic involvement of tumor, endo-

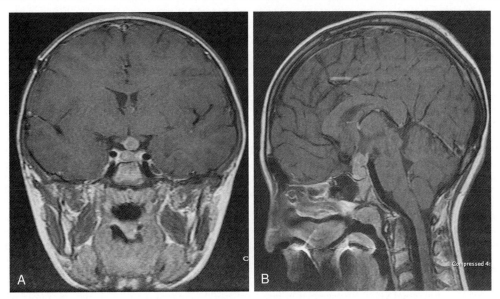

FIGURE 17-48. Pituitary germinoma. **A,** Coronal T1 fat-saturated image. **B,** Sagittal T1 fat-saturated image.

scopic evaluation can often detect subtle areas of tumor.[989] It is not yet clear whether endoscopically identified regional disease patients should be upstaged.

Tumors arising in the pineal region often produce headache, nausea, and vomiting because of obstructive hydrocephalus. Limitation of vertical gaze, convergence nystagmus, impaired pupillary reflexes, and double vision may occur because of tectal compression (Parinaud's syndrome). Atypical presentations occur when germ cell tumors arise in unusual locations such as the basal ganglia, when they present with widespread leptomeningeal metastases, or when they diffusely infiltrate deep white matter structures.

Germ cell tumors can cause precocious puberty because of release of β-human chorionic gonadotropin (β-HCG).[990,991] Atypical presentations, such as movement disorders or depression as the presenting symptom, can result in significant delays in diagnosis.[97,986]

Imaging and Histology. Germ cell tumors can have a heterogeneous appearance on CT and MR imaging and can differ between the pineal and suprasellar regions.[992] Most are contrast-enhancing solid lesions, with isointense signal on T1-weighted sequences and bright signal on T2 (Fig. 17-48).[993] Cysts are commonly observed, especially in nongerminomas.[994] These signal characteristics overlap with other common tumors of the pineal region and require biopsy or hormone marker analysis for accurate diagnosis.[981,995] An important exception is CNS teratoma. These lesions are composed of all three mature tissue elements and therefore will demonstrate calcified areas with adjacent cysts and low-density regions of fat. Areas of bright signal on T1, consistent with hemorrhage, are suggestive of choriocarcinoma.[994]

The nongerminomatous germ cell tumors are unique among central nervous system tumors in that they can be diagnosed solely on the basis of expression of tumor markers.[996,997] Either or both β-HCG, a normal product of syncytiotrophoblasts, and α-fetoprotein (AFP), a normal product of yolk sac endoderm, can be detected in the blood and CSF of patients with NGGCTs. β-HCG is associated with choriocarcinoma, although low levels can also be associated with germinomas. CSF levels tend to be higher than those in the serum.[998] AFP is expressed by yolk sac tumors, although low immunohistochemical expression can be observed in some teratomas.

Although placental alkaline phosphatase (PLAP) and lactate dehydrogenase (LDH) isoenzymes and CSF c-kit have been used as markers of germinoma,[996,999-1001] immunohistochemical staining for these markers is more commonly used for diagnosis. Because AFP is normally expressed in newborns, considerable attention must be given to interpretation of these levels in infants.[1002]

The histologic identification of CNS germ cell tumors is critical for proper therapeutic assignment and prognostic counseling. Seven major categories are recognized by the WHO.[1003] Clinically, mixed germ cell tumors are encountered in most patients, except those with pure germinomas or mature teratomas, and the most malignant component typically dictates the type and intensity of the therapy.

Germinoma is the most common CNS germ cell tumor encountered and is considered the equivalent of the testicular seminoma. The appearance of these large cells on H&E staining, frequent mitoses, and lymphocytic infiltrates is characteristic and can easily be observed on smear preparations. Cells stain brightly for both c-kit and octamer-4 (Oct-4).[1004,1005] Placental alkaline phosphatase has been less reliable. Even pure germinomas can possess syncytiotrophoblastic giant cells, resulting in low-level expression of β-HCG, which does not upstage their classification to the more malignant choriocarcinoma.[991]

NGGCT is typically used to refer to one of three different malignant germ cell tumor variants as well as teratomatous elements with atypical or malignant degeneration. The first, yolk sac tumor, is an epithelial tumor that can mimic the appearance of germinomas but highly expresses AFP throughout the cytoplasm. Embryonal carcinoma (endodermal sinus tumor) is an epithelial-derived tumor that has a characteristic appearance with abundant mitoses and diffuse presence of cytokeratin. This latter feature can help differentiate these tumors from germinomas because both can express PLAP and Oct-4. Lastly, choriocarcinoma is a trophoblastic tumor of extraembryonic origin. It requires the identification of cytotrophoblastic elements and syncytiotrophoblastic giant cells. Hemorrhagic necrosis is a common feature of this tumor and the giant cells stain brightly for β-HCG.

Teratoma refers to a group of three lesions that have evidence of differentiation along the three embryonic germ cell layers—ectoderm, endoderm, and mesoderm:

1. Mature teratoma possesses fully differentiated tissue elements of all three layers. The ectodermal components often contain skin, brain, and/or choroid plexus. The mesodermal component can frequently include cartilage, bone, fat, and/or muscle, although the endodermal component often contains respiratory or gastrointestinal cysts lined by epithelium. Teratomas usually have an absent or low mitotic index.
2. Immature teratoma is similar to mature teratoma but possesses some elements from one or more of the germ cell layers that are not fully differentiated. Most commonly seen are mitotically active stromal elements or neuroectodermal cells. These immature elements are at considerable risk for malignant degeneration and thus require additional therapy unless a complete resection has been performed.[1006]
3. Teratomas with malignant transformation are rare lesions in which an area of malignant cells of any histologic type is observed. Rhabdomyosarcoma or undifferentiated sarcoma is the most commonly seen, although almost any tumor can occur in the context of teratomas because teratomas already possess all three germ cell layers.[1007]

The diagnosis of an intracranial GCT is suspected in any patient with acquired diabetes insipidus (DI) or Parinaud's syndrome. Although location of the primary tumor on neuroimaging studies and certain features of the clinical presentation are supportive of the diagnosis of a CNS germ cell tumor, the diagnosis must be confirmed by histology or CSF tumor markers (Table 17-7). Histologic confirmation may not be necessary in patients with elevated serum and/or CSF concentrations of tumor markers (AFP or β-HCG) consistent with a NGGCT.[996,997]

The tumor markers β-HCG and AFP are useful in not only confirming the presence of a CNS germ cell tumor but also in monitoring response to therapy and in suspecting earlier recurrence. Elevation of AFP alone suggests yolk sac (endodermal sinus tumor), whereas a high level of β-HCG suggests choriocarcinoma. Pure germinomas may have modest elevations of CSF β-HCG, usually lower than 50 mIU/mL (100 mIU/mL at some institutions). LDH isoenzymes, the soluble c-kit oncogene product, and PLAP are also detectable in the CSF of germinoma patients.[996,1000,1001] Serum markers of β-HCG at diagnosis can be negative, even in the presence of significantly elevated CSF levels, demonstrating the importance of a comprehensive workup for this patient population, including MRI of the spine and CSF for markers and cytology.[996,1008] Proper prospective studies using ventricular CSF rather than lumbar CSF have not been completed and should therefore not be used for staging at present.[780]

Management. Preoperative evaluation should include contrast-enhanced brain and spine MRI, serum and CSF tumor markers (if lumbar puncture can be safely performed), CSF cytology, assessment of endocrine function and visual acuity, and visual field examinations for suprasellar disease. In the absence of elevated lumbar CSF tumor markers, a biopsy should be performed. Aggressive resection leading to morbidity is neither necessary nor advisable in cases of germinoma because of the tumor's exquisite sensitivity to cytotoxic and radiation therapies. Thus, less invasive neurosurgical procedures to obtain a tissue sample, such as an endoscopic or stereotactic biopsy, are used more frequently.[828,989] A third ventriculostomy is frequently performed at the same time as an endoscopic biopsy in patients with noncommunicating hydrocephalus and a pineal region tumor.[1009] Radical resections of a NGGCT may be easier to accomplish after several courses of chemotherapy.[1010]

Patients with germinomas have a number of nonsurgical treatment options.[1011,1012] With RT alone for pure germinoma, the 5-year overall survival (OS) has approached 90% to 95% in clinical series[1013]; however, RT alone is inadequate for NGGCT, with 5-year OS ranging from 30% to 0%.[1014,1015] Several new treatment strategies are under investigation in an attempt to minimize some of the late effects of RT, as seen in long-term survivors of CNS germinomas.[1016] Administering an intermediate radiation dose of approximately 4000 to 5000 cGy encompassing the brain and ventricles is curative treatment for most patients with localized intracranial germinomas. Craniospinal radiation therapy is no longer routinely used for this population. Although whole-brain radiation therapy has been used in the past, whole ventricular fields are now recommended to spare the outer margin of the cortex without increasing the risk of recurrence. Typically, 3000 cGy is administered to the whole ventricular region and the primary tumor receives an additional 1500 cGy. This therapy is effective, with 10-year event-free survival in excess of 90% and distant recurrences such as spinal metastases rarely occurring.[1017] Patients with concurrent pineal and pituitary location represent regional rather than metastatic disease and can also be adequately treated with whole ventricular radiation therapy.[1018] Like other brain tumor patients receiving radiation therapy, these children often suffer late consequences of RT, such as cognitive and endocrine deficiencies and RT-induced secondary tumors.[1016] This has led to the development of treatment regimens using adjuvant chemotherapy followed by response-based radiotherapy to permit a selective reduction in not only dose (from 4500 to 3000 cGy) but also volume (from whole ventricular to involved field) in patients whose tumors completely disappear after two to four courses of chemotherapy.[1019-1021] A similar

TABLE 17-7   Common Marker Analysis in Central Nervous System Germ Cell Tumors*

Type of Tumor	Placental Alkaline Phosphatase	Oct-4	c-kit	AFP	β-HCG	Cytokeratin	Cerebrospinal Fluid Marker Positivity
Germinoma	+	+	+	−	+	−	c-kit, low level of β-HCG[†]
Yolk sac tumor	−	−	−	+	−	+	AFP
Embryonal carcinoma	−	−	−	−	−	+	−
Choriocarcinoma	−	−	−	−	+	+	β-HCG
Mature teratoma	−	−	−	−	−	−	−
Immature teratoma	−	−	−	−	−	−	−
Teratoma with malignant transformation	−	−	−	−	−	−	−

*The common staining patterns provided do not include positive reactions in small subsets of cells.
†Germinomas can express low concentrations of β-HCG (50-100 mIU/mL), depending on institutional preference.
AFP, α-fetoprotein; β-HCG, β-human chorionic gonadotropin; Oct-4, octamer-4.

approach has been used with success by the Japanese cooperative group, including an intermediate risk group of germinomas with elevated β-HCG.[1022] Focal radiotherapy only to sites of disease may not be sufficient therapy because a number of failures have been noted with this approach.[1023] The optimal dose and field of radiation and the best combination of chemotherapy are still being investigated and will require further follow-up to confirm efficacy and decreased toxicity.

Attempts at treating patients with chemotherapy alone have demonstrated significant responses but a recurrence rate of approximately 50% in one study.[1024] Although these patients had an excellent salvage with radiation therapy, a higher craniospinal dose of 3600 cGy is then required. For this reason, chemotherapy alone is not used for germinomas outside of formal clinical trials. Recently, the identification of an intermediate risk group of CNS germinoma patients has been identified, specifically those with germinoma histology and elevated β-HCG. With treatment consisting of whole ventricular radiation therapy, this group of patients can achieve outcomes similar to those of other germinoma patients.[991]

For NGGCT, more aggressive chemotherapy, radical tumor resection, and high-dose and high-volume radiotherapy are required for survival.[1019,1025-1028] NGGCTs are highly chemotherapy-responsive, as seen in one study with 16 of 17 patients achieving a CR or PR with two cycles of cisplatin and cyclophosphamide-based therapy, one third of whom were long-term survivors.[1025] The use of consolidation with high-dose chemotherapy and stem cell rescue is being developed[264] and appeared to further improve outcome in a small pilot series.[1029] Many patients initially treated with chemotherapy with progressive disease can be salvaged with high-dose chemotherapy and craniospinal radiation therapy.[1030] Immature teratomas are classified as NGGCTs but can often be treated with a more conservative approach. A complete resection may be sufficient therapy and the prognosis is good. Those with incomplete resection likely require adjuvant therapy.[1006]

Germ cell tumors after treatment can demonstrate significant progressive growth on MRI scan with concurrent clinical decline in the setting of normal tumor markers (β-HCG and/or AFP). Although a nonsecreting germ cell recurrence cannot be excluded, most of these cases represent growing teratoma syndrome.[1031] These lesions are nonmalignant progression of the teratomatous component of lesions that when resected, will relieve the clinical symptoms.[1031] Patients with growing teratomatous syndrome are not considered to have progressive disease, in spite of the dramatic increase in the size of the lesion on MRI. These patients should discontinue neither their radiation therapy nor their chemotherapy.

Prognosis. Patients with germinoma have an excellent prognosis. because of the tumor's sensitivity to radiation and chemotherapy. For these patients, the major treatment challenge is maximizing the quality of life and limiting long-term sequelae of therapy. The Children's Oncology Group is currently conducting a randomized phase III study comparing standard RT alone versus chemotherapy followed by response-dependent reduced-intensity radiation therapy, in which the primary outcome measures are progression-free survival, overall survival, and quality of life. For germinoma patients who progress after radiation therapy, many can be salvaged with high-dose chemotherapy, with or without stem cell transplantation, followed by higher dose and volume radiation therapy.[1032,1033] Chemotherapy and radiation therapy for those not previously treated with radiation therapy can also lead to a high salvage rate.[1030]

Nongerminomas have a less favorable prognosis and thus clinical trials are evaluating conventional multiagent chemotherapy followed by dose-intensive myeloablative chemother-

apy and second-look surgery for poor responders, followed by high-dose craniospinal RT. A small fraction of these patients can be salvaged with high-dose chemotherapy and stem cell rescue.[1033] The response rate of recurrent NGGCT to second-line chemotherapy is poor. Poor prognostic factors in NGGCTs include degree of resection, presence of hemorrhage, and metastases.[1034] A rise in CSF β-HCG can be a sensitive marker of pending relapse and was identified well in advance of elevated levels in the serum.[998]

Craniopharyngiomas

Craniopharyngiomas are benign nonglial tumors in children and account for 3% to 5% of all pediatric brain tumors with a peak age ranging between 6 and 14 years. These tumors arise from Rathke's pouch epithelium and are classified as WHO grade I tumors.[1035] Craniopharyngiomas are slow-growing tumors that arise in the sella and parasellar regions, composed of both solid and cystic components, which often extend into the parasellar cisterns and occasionally invade adjacent cortical and vascular structures.[1036] Calcification is a common finding of these lesions,[1037] although this is not pathognomonic for these tumors. Compression of critical intracranial structures can lead to pituitary, hypothalamic, and optic dysfunction. As a result, these patients often have complicated medical courses and long-term sequelae. Nigerian and Japanese children appear to have a greater risk for these tumors.[972,1038] A strong association between β-catenin mutations and adamantinomatous craniopharyngioma has been identified.[1039,1040]

Clinical Presentation. The typical onset of craniopharyngioma is insidious and can extend over several years. It is often made in retrospect on recognizing one or more slowly evolving symptoms, such as progressive visual loss, delay in sexual maturation, growth failure, weight gain, and diabetes insipidus.[1041] Eventually, clinical recognition is heralded by a change in mental status as enlargement of the cystic component causes obstructive hydrocephalus. More than 70% of children have growth hormone deficiency, obstructive hydrocephalus, short-term memory deficits, and/or psychomotor slowing at the time of diagnosis. The presenting feature in young adults also includes other symptoms of hypopituitarism, such as galactorrhea or amenorrhea in females and impotence in males. The differential diagnosis of a suspected craniopharyngioma is limited because of the characteristic radiographic findings of these lesions.[1042] Congenital craniopharyngioma associated with a paraneoplastic expression of parathyroid hormone–related protein expression has been reported.[1043]

Imaging and Histology. MRI features (Fig. 17-49) usually include a multicystic and solid enhancing suprasellar mass.[1044] The T1-weighted signal is usually isointense. The chiasm is often stretched over the suprasellar mass and, if there is sufficient dorsal extension, hydrocephalus will be apparent.[1045] A classic neuroimaging distinction of craniopharyngiomas from other suprasellar tumors such as a diencephalic glioma or germ cell tumor is the presence of calcifications on a noncontrast CT scan. With contrast, the solid components of craniopharyngiomas are usually bright on CT. Transcranial Doppler can also be used in the diagnosis and surveillance of these tumors.[1046]

Histologically, craniopharyngiomas are divided into adamantinomatous and papillary subtypes. Adamantinomatous craniopharyngiomas are the more common variant in adults and children and typically consist of cystic and solid areas, with frequent calcifications. Papillary tumors, seen almost exclusively in adults, are predominantly solid, without calcification,

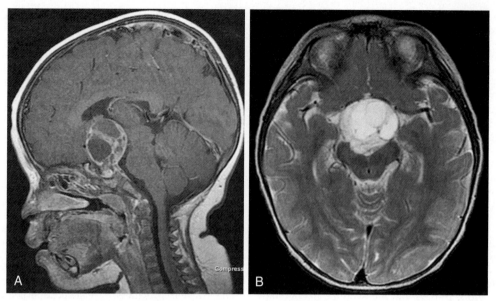

FIGURE 17-49. Craniopharyngioma with multiple cysts. **A,** Sagittal T1 image with contrast. **B,** Axial T2 image.

and are less infiltrative. The cysts seen in craniopharyngioma usually contain a dark liquid with the consistency of machine oil. The diagnosis of adamantinomatous craniopharyngioma requires the presence of squamous epithelium bordered by palisading columnar epithelium.[1035] Gliosis and Rosenthal fibers can be observed but rarely result in misdiagnosis because of the other characteristic features of craniopharyngioma. Palisading columnar cells can have a high MIB-1 rate, ranging from 0% to 15% but this does not correlate with a poorer outcome than for patients with a low MIB-1 index.[1047,1048]

Management. Surgical resection remains the standard approach for craniopharyngioma in many centers.[1042,1049] When the child presents with acute raised ICP, the initial management will relate to measures to alleviate this condition with high-dose corticosteroids and intensive care unit (ICU) monitoring. Because patients may have unappreciated panhypopituitarism, baseline hormonal and electrolyte levels should be obtained and the child empirically given stress-dose steroids.

Although somewhat controversial, a complete microsurgical resection of the entire tumor is the treatment of choice for newly diagnosed craniopharyngiomas.[1050] A multistaged operative approach may be planned, including a combination of trans-sphenoidal, pterional, and transcallosal approaches, depending on the extent and location of the tumor. Many tumors are adherent to adjacent structures, which will either limit the degree of resection or result in potentially significant postsurgical morbidity.[1036]

Despite the surgical accessibility of many of these tumors, radical resection does not guarantee recurrence-free survival and the 3-year EFS following a gross total resection (GTR) is 60%.[1051] Aggressive resection can result in more extensive hypothalamic deficiencies and visual complications.[1049] Careful management of diabetes insipidus can be required immediately after the surgical resection of these patients,[1052] which may lead to a permanent condition. Postoperative behavioral sequelae include altered regulation of appetite and weight control, impulsivity, hypersexuality, and changes in memory.

An alternative treatment strategy for the long-term control of craniopharyngiomas is subtotal resection followed by involved field high-dose radiotherapy.[1053-1055] Whether this approach is superior in terms of tumor control and preservation of quality of life remains to be established, but several studies have reported comparable PFS and OS statistics in retrospective, uncontrolled institutional series.[1051,1056,1057] Long-term complications of radiation include secondary malignancies, optic neuropathy, and vascular injury leading, rarely, to moyamoya disease.[71,1058-1060]

A temporizing approach to control the cystic components of the tumor is the intracystic instillation of sclerosing agents such as bleomycin or ^{32}P.[1061,1062] The use of intralesional bleomycin has also been shown to help delay the need for aggressive surgery or radiation therapy, although prospective clinical trials of this approach are needed.[1063] This procedure has the risk of leakage of the bleomycin from the cyst into adjacent brain and should be reserved for patients who have failed all other management approaches.[1064] However, the solid tumor usually continues to grow and make new cysts, thus making subsequent resections more difficult. In addition, subsequent external beam radiotherapy treatment planning may be difficult because of the unpredictable dosimetry of ^{32}P.[1062]

Recurrent or progressive craniopharyngiomas may be treated with reoperation, radiosurgery, fractionated radiotherapy or chemotherapy. Responses to chemotherapy have been reported with interferon, vinblastine, cisplatin, and other agents,[1057,1065-1070] although well-designed studies to test different agents for craniopharyngioma are lacking.[1071]

Prognosis. The most important factors that correlate with progression-free survival are the extent of resection and postoperative radiation therapy. Larger tumors and those with cysts are more likely to recur.[1072] In a surgical series, recurrence or progression occurred in 7% to 15% of cases after total resection and in 50% of cases after subtotal resection.[1073] The recurrence rate of 15% is observed when subtotal resection is followed by radiation therapy.[1074] The outcome between adult and pediatric patients does not appear to be different.[1075] Recurrences along the surgical tract have been reported but are thought to be related to the procedure rather than representing metastatic disease and are treated with surgery and focal irradiation, if needed.[1076] Unfortunately, many long-term survivors experience significant morbidity related to panhypopituitarism,[1077] cognitive impairment, sleep pattern disturbance, and obesity.[1075,1078,1079] Growth hormone deficiency is present in

100% of patients,[1080] but the early use of growth hormone in these patients is not thought to be contraindicated.[1081,1082] Although narcolepsy is uncommon,[1083] control of weight and regulation of sleep can be difficult. The use of stimulants has been investigated, with preliminary positive results,[1084] although clear efficacy for these interventions is lacking.[1085-1087] Finally, psychosocial problems can be significant in this patient population and require a comprehensive team approach.[1088]

Infant Tumors

Infants younger than 1 year and even children younger than 3 years with brain tumors have a poor outcome, especially with CNS PNETs and ependymoma. Five-year event-free and overall survival is as low as 19% and 25%, respectively, for those younger than 1 year.[1089] This poor prognosis can be related to unique characteristics of the tumors in this age group, as well as the significant limitations with regard to therapy. Evidence from numerous sources has suggested that neural development extends from the embryonic period through adolescence and is especially prominent during the first 3 years of life, making young children most susceptible to neurotoxic insults.[1090] These findings are in keeping with early observations that the most devastating consequences of radiotherapy in children, in terms of neuropsychological sequelae, were greatest in children younger than 3 years.[1091] Although early observations have led to the arbitrary age limit of 3 years as the cutoff for introduction of radiation therapy, numerous subsequent studies have shown that even older children can experience cognitive, endocrine, behavioral, and many other medical problems.[1092,1093] Consequently, several strategies have emerged to delay or eliminate radiotherapy through the use of chemotherapy in an attempt to preserve cognitive, neurologic, and endocrine function in the younger child.[1094,1095]

Data from the Childhood Brain Tumor Registry of the United States from 2000 to 2004 has shown that approximately 28% of childhood brain tumors occur in children younger than 4 years[1096] and 18% of brain tumors occur in children younger than 2 years.[1097] Tumor location in infants and young children is different from that in the older child, with a predominance of supratentorial tumors.[1097-1099] Seventy percent of tumors that present in the first week of life are also located supratentorially[1100] compared with 56% for the pediatric population.[1101] The male-to-female ratio in this age group is also different in that there is a lower male predominance in this age group[1098] when compared with childhood brain tumors overall. Histopathologic subtypes in infants and young children are also different from those in the older child but accurate determination of this has been difficult. This is because early epidemiologic data collected by the traditional data collection agencies such as the SEER registry and National Brain Tumor Registry did not have standardized histologic subtype information. For example, PNET was not previously recognized as a separate entity in the SEER Registry. In the large cooperative groups, brain tumors were categorized differently, so that the POG excluded medulloblastoma from PNET protocols, although the Children's Cancer Group (CCG) routinely included medulloblastoma into PNET protocols.[1094] The distribution of tumor types treated in the infant POG clinical trial (Baby POG) was medulloblastoma, followed by ependymoma, PNET, and malignant glioma.[1102] However, in a review of 1289 patients aged younger than 1 year reported in the literature, astrocytoma was the most common diagnosis, comprising 31% of cases (of which 75% were low-grade and 25% were reported as high-grade), followed by medulloblastoma at 12%, ependymoma at 11%, choroid plexus tumors at 11%, supratentorial PNET (sPNET) at 7%, and teratoma at 5%.[1098] Astrocytoma and

medulloblastoma remain the most common in the young age group, although there is a peak of ependymoma seen within the first 2 years of life and an increased incidence of PNET.[1089]

Two important histologic diagnoses in infants include teratomas and ATRTs, which account for 4.9% and 0.3%, respectively, of infant brain tumors.[1098] Briefly, ATRT is a rare tumor of childhood (see earlier), which has only recently been recognized as a separate entity; 75% of these tumors carry a unique 22q11.2 cytogenetic abnormality.[911] An initial description of malignant rhabdoid tumors of the kidney,[1103] followed by the description of the simultaneous appearance of renal and CNS tumors with similar histologic features,[1104] eventually resulted in the recognition that this unique histology represents a separate entity.[891,920] ATRT primarily affects young children at a mean age of 17 to 24.5 months, with 75% occurring in children younger than 3 years.

Clinical Presentation. The clinical presentation of brain tumors in infants and young children is most often associated with the symptoms of obstructive hydrocephalus, which in this age group manifests as persistent vomiting, irritability, lethargy, abnormal gait and coordination difficulties, failure to thrive, bulging and splayed fontanelles, seizures, and loss of developmental milestones. In a meta-analysis of 13 studies reported in the literature consisting of 332 children younger than 4 years presenting with intracranial tumors, increasing head circumference and macrocephaly was reported as the most common presentation (41%). Other presentations included focal motor weakness, head tilt, squint, abnormal eye movements, altered levels of consciousness, and hemiplegia.

Management. The historical approach to treating infants and young children with brain tumors had focused on the use of surgery and radiation. In the late 1960s, serious functional and neurocognitive sequelae that were incompatible with a normal productive life, especially for children younger than 2 years, were recognized.[1091] As a result, several different strategies to delay or exclude radiotherapy from the treatment of young children with brain tumors were developed and were centered on the use of chemotherapy.[1094,1095,1105] Van Eys and coworkers[1106] treated 12 young children with medulloblastoma using mechlorethamine, Oncovin [vincristine], procarbazine, prednisone (MOPP) chemotherapy without radiotherapy and found that 8 of 12 patients were long-term survivors. This strategy led to other clinical trials, including those investigated by POG, which worked on the premise of giving chemotherapy until the child achieved an age at which radiotherapy was accepted as less detrimental and its benefits could still be realized.[1094,1095] The Baby POG I protocol, initiated in 1986, enrolled 198 children, 132 of whom were younger than 24 months who were treated with chemotherapy for 2 years and an additional 66 children who were between the ages of 24 and 36 months who received chemotherapy for 1 year prior to receiving radiotherapy.[1102] Chemotherapy consisted of two 28-day cycles of cyclophosphamide plus vincristine followed by one 28-day cycle of cisplatin and etoposide; these cycles were given for 1 or 2 years, depending on the age of the child at diagnosis or until there was disease progression, following which radiotherapy was given. After two cycles of cyclophosphamide and vincristine, 39 of 109 evaluable patients showed a complete or partial response, although patients with brainstem glioma and PNET did poorly. The PFS at 1 year for children diagnosed between the ages of 24 to 36 months and PFS at 2 years in children diagnosed at younger than 24 months were 41% and 39%, respectively. The 5-year PFS was reported as 30% ± 5% and the 5-year OS was 39% ± 4%. The single most important predictor of survival was the degree of surgical resection, because children with a gross total resection had a

5-year OS of 62% ± 7% compared with those with a subtotal resection, whose 5-year survival was only 31% ± 5%. Of great importance in this landmark study was its demonstration that a small subset of children could achieve disease control without radiotherapy, and that even a delay of 1 or 2 years did not adversely affect outcome in all patients.[1094,1095,1105] Other study groups have adopted a similar approach of delaying radiotherapy using chemotherapy. The CCG 9921 clinical trial for infants with medulloblastoma, sPNET, and ependymoma used up-front chemotherapy for 1 year followed by focal radiotherapy to the involved site or craniospinal radiotherapy.[1107] This was an 8-drugs-in-1-day clinical trial that included 46 children with medulloblastoma who were younger than 18 months at the time of diagnosis, most of whom had gross total resections and were able to avoid radiotherapy; 22% were progression-free at 3 years.[1107] The German Pediatric Brain Tumor Study Group piloted an intensive chemotherapy regimen, consisting of procarbazine, ifosfamide, cisplatin, cytarabine, vincristine, and high-dose methotrexate for children to delay or avoid radiotherapy (HIT-SKK87). A direct comparison to the results of baby POG cannot be made because the results of HIT-SKK87 are not yet published. The United Kingdom Children's Cancer Study Group (UKCCSG) piloted a Baby Brain protocol in 1989 using weekly alternating cycles of myelosuppressive and nonmyelosuppressive chemotherapy consisting of vincristine and carboplatin, vincristine and methotrexate, vincristine and cyclophosphamide, and cisplatin to delay or avoid radiotherapy. Although only 28 children were treated on the protocol, the 4-year overall survival was 35%.[1108]

The overall results of these Baby chemotherapy protocols were thus somewhat disappointing, with event-free survivals of 20% to 40%, although the ability to defer radiation therapy in this patient population was an important advance. Given the high response rate for infants on these protocols, strategies centered on high-dose chemotherapy with autologous stem rescue were developed to improve the response rates already being observed further.[525] The French Society of Pediatric Oncology used this approach of high-dose chemotherapy with autologous bone marrow rescue in their BBSFOP protocol in an attempt to salvage young children with relapsed or progressive disease on conventional chemotherapy. Twenty children with medulloblastoma, median age of 23 months, who developed progressive disease while treated with conventional chemotherapy, were treated with high-dose busulfan and thiotepa followed by autologous stem cell rescue. Of these patients, 75% demonstrated a radiographic response to chemotherapy. For patients with initial local relapses only, an event-free survival of 50% and median survival of 39.5 months were achieved.[1109] A follow-up report of this study demonstrated a 69% 5-year overall survival in locally relapsed patients while eliminating the need for craniospinal radiotherapy in 30% to 50% of patients. The need for a complete resection limits this strategy for many patients, especially those with metastatic disease.[1105]

Another chemotherapy-based approach has been the "Head Start" protocols, in which conventional induction chemotherapy followed by high-dose chemotherapy with autologous stem cell transplantation is used in the newly diagnosed setting to delay or defer radiation therapy in infants and young children. Head Start I consisted of five induction cycles of cisplatin, vincristine, etoposide, and cyclophosphamide. Following this, patients with no radiologic evidence of disease, or following second-look surgery or reresection of tumor, underwent myeloablative therapy with carboplatin, thiotepa, and etoposide with autologous bone marrow rescue (ABMR). Radiotherapy was deferred in patients who achieved complete remission. Of 62 children enrolled, median age of 30 months,

37 patients proceeded to ABMR, of which 15 patients were free of disease and required no further treatment; this resulted in a 3-year EFS and OS of 40% and 25%, respectively. There were 7 deaths from treatment-related complications. These results are similar to those noted earlier and again demonstrate that a subset of patients can be effectively treated with chemotherapy and avoid radiotherapy.[1110] Head Start II further intensified the induction regimen with the addition of high-dose methotrexate. This chemotherapy-based protocol was primarily aimed at patients with high-risk tumors (nonmedulloblastoma) or those presenting with evidence of metastatic spread. A total of 21 patients with disseminated medulloblastoma were treated, 17 of whom had a complete response yielding a 3-year EFS and OS of 49% and 60%, respectively.[813] In this cohort of patients, 13 had a gross total resection and 10 patients received radiotherapy as part of their up-front or salvage therapy; 6 patients avoided radiotherapy altogether. For patients with sPNETs, this approach appears to confer an improved 5-year EFS and OS of 39% and 49%, respectively.[886] Nonpineal sPNET patients fared better than those with pineal-based tumors although metastatic disease at diagnosis, age, and extent of resection were not significant prognostic factors; 60% of survivors were able to avoid radiotherapy. In contrast, this approach has not demonstrated equivalent results for patients with ependymoma with an estimated 5-year EFS and OS of 12% and 38%, respectively, with younger age as the only significant prognostic factor.[665] In this cohort of 29 children, 22 were younger than 36 months and only 8% of patients were radiation-free at 5 years.

To further increase chemotherapy dose intensity, others have followed induction chemotherapy with tandem cycles of high-dose chemotherapy with stem cell rescue. In a small series of 15 infants between 4 and 38 months old, with varied histologies, including five medulloblastomas, four CNS sPNETs, five malignant gliomas, and one ependymoma, patients were treated with induction chemotherapy. This consisted of three cycles of cisplatin, cyclophosphamide, and etoposide followed by three cycles of tandem high-dose therapy with carboplatin and etoposide and autologous stem cell rescue.[1111] Although the follow-up period was short, the 2-year progression-free and overall survivals of 52% and 72%, respectively, is encouraging. Furthermore, of the 10 patients who were alive, only 5 received local radiotherapy and only 1 patient with M1 stage medulloblastoma received craniospinal radiotherapy.[1111] Similar results have also been reported by the French Society for Pediatric Oncology in a small series of seven patients with medulloblastoma and sPNET using high-dose therapy with busulfan and melphalan.[1112] Although three patients received additional thiotepa and two patients received additional topotecan, all patients were able to avoid radiotherapy. Their progression-free survival was 71% ± 17%, although longer follow-up will be needed.

With regard to the long-term benefits of adjuvant chemotherapy strategy of delaying or deferring radiotherapy, one infant study evaluated their neuropsychological outcomes in a follow-up report. Of the six children who did not receive radiotherapy, all had IQs within the normal range, with a mean of 101, although the five children who had received radiation therapy had lower IQs, with a mean of 85 at 5.8 years and a continued decline to a mean of 63 by 10 years.[1113]

Specific Management Issues in Infants and Young Children

A more detailed description of the diagnosis and management of individual disease categories has been given earlier, but management issues specific to infant tumors are described here.

Infant Medulloblastoma

Despite significant improvements in the treatment of standard-risk medulloblastoma in older children, the outcome of infants and young children with medulloblastoma remains poor, mainly because of limitations in the use of radiotherapy to the developing brain, increased risk of metastatic disease at presentation, and difficulty in achieving a complete surgical resection in infants.[1114] Although the strategies of delayed radiotherapy with chemotherapy and intensification of treatment with stem cell rescue have shown some promising results in infants and young children, the small number of patients, heterogeneous histologies, and varied staging limit their immediate widespread adaptation.[813,1111,1112] Salvage therapy in infants and young children has also been shown to be feasible in up to 50% of patients but requires the use of radiotherapy. Thus, some cognitive impact and compromise will be required in these patients if disease control is to be achieved with this modality.[1115] Attempts at reduction in radiotherapy dose to reduce neurodevelopmental damage can significantly compromise overall survival.[1116] Alternative therapeutic strategies are therefore needed in the treatment of medulloblastoma of the infant and young child.

The incorporation of high-dose methotrexate in chemotherapy regimens has been investigated. In the German HIT-SKK study, intrathecal methotrexate and systemic methotrexate were administered to 43 children with medulloblastoma younger than 3 years, including 26 patients with M+ disease. The 5-year OS for patients with completely resected tumors, residual tumor, and macroscopic metastases was 93% ± 6%, 56% ± 14%, and 38% ± 15%, respectively, an improvement as compared with historical controls.[756] Only 38% of survivors received radiotherapy. Of note, desmoplastic histology was highly predictive of good outcome, with an overall survival of 95% ± 4% versus an OS of 41% ± 11% for patients with classic histology; histology was found to be an independent prognostic marker, along with age younger than 2 years. High-dose methotrexate has also been investigated in the Head Start II protocol and was shown to be particularly effective for young patients with high-risk medulloblastoma.[813] The major concern, however, with the use of methotrexate is that this agent has been associated with white matter changes on MR imaging, especially when methotrexate is administered following radiation therapy.[1117,1118] In spite of this, the use of methotrexate continues to be investigated, given the overall poor prognoses for this subset of patients. Stratification of risk groups through better histologic diagnosis, together with an improved understanding of the biology of medulloblastoma, may help improve survival in this age group.[1114,1119]

Infant Central Nervous System Primitive Neuroectodermal Tumors and Pineoblastoma

Central nervous system PNET is a neuroepithelial tumor similar to medulloblastoma but with a significantly worse prognosis.[855] The most recent WHO classification clarifies the nomenclature of this heterogeneous group of tumors. It was traditionally referred to as sPNET and is now called CNS PNETs, not otherwise specified (NOS), and includes biologically similar tumors that can also be found in the brainstem and spinal cord.[183] Even though medulloblastoma and sPNET are classified together as embryonal tumors, there is cytogenetic[881,882] and molecular evidence from microarray analyses[711] to suggest that there are biologic differences between these tumors. Pineoblastomas are also tumors of embryonal origin with a clinically aggressive course.[840]

CNS PNETs are the fourth most common brain tumors of infants[1098] and account for approximately 10% of all brain tumors occurring in children younger than 3 years.[1120] It is also the most common malignant brain tumor in the first year of life[1097] and, from SEER data, has a dismal overall survival of 19% in this age group.[1089] POG 8633 treated 13 nonpineal CNS PNET patients younger than 3 years. These patients presented with large, well-demarcated tumors with limited edema. In this study, CNS PNET was the most common supratentorial tumor in this age group. Presenting symptoms included seizures, nausea, vomiting, lethargy, irritability, headache, focal motor weakness, and increased head circumference; 12 of 13 had symptoms for less than 1 month at the time of presentation.[1121] For reasons that are unknown, younger children with CNS PNETs and pineoblastomas present with more aggressive disease and a higher frequency of leptomeningeal disease.[1122,1123] Whether this is inherent to the biology of the disease, or related to clinical factors, remains controversial. In a retrospective review of 50 patients with CNS PNET, metastatic disease at diagnosis, extent of initial resection, and tumor site did not affect overall survival, although it was affected by age younger than 2 years and the use of radiotherapy and chemotherapy.[860] Similar findings were also reported in 46 patients with sPNET registered on the CCG-9921 study; treatment regimen, M stage, extent of resection, and age were not found to be significant prognostic factors.[662] In contrast, baby POG I treated 28 patients with supratentorial PNET, including 11 with pineoblastoma, all of whom received chemotherapy and delayed radiotherapy.[1094] In this study, there was a considerable difference in the 3-year survival between the 4 patients who achieved a gross total resection (100% survival) compared with the 9 patients with a subtotal resection (11% survival). This study also concluded a lack of benefit from chemotherapy.[1094] No benefit from chemotherapy was seen in the French BBSFOP protocol for 25 patients with supratentorial embryonal tumors, which included 17 patients with sPNET treated with chemotherapy to delay or omit radiotherapy. Of the 5 patients with sPNET who survived, 4 were salvaged with high-dose chemotherapy and/or surgery and radiotherapy.[1124] Results from the Head Start studies have also suggested a benefit from intensification of chemotherapy because 60% of this cohort of 43 patients with sPNET avoided radiotherapy and achieved an estimated 5-year EFS and OS of 39% and 49%, respectively.[886] Interestingly, metastasis at diagnosis, age, and extent of resection were not significant factors, although numbers were small and the interpretation of individual subgroups is limited.

Pineoblastoma in infants has been associated with a dismal outcome. The baby POG study treated 11 patients, 1 to 35 months (8 were younger than 12 months), and all patients had local recurrences, the majority with metastatic disease. All children died 4 to 13 months from the time of diagnosis, despite the use of radiotherapy in 6 patients.[844] Similar dismal results have been reported in the CCG 921 protocol in which eight infants with predominantly nonmetastatic, subtotally resected tumors all progressed within 3 to 14 months (median, 4 months) with a median time to death of 10 months.[1125] Similarly, five children younger than 3 years with pineoblastoma, treated on the German Pediatric Oncology Group HIT-SKK87 and HIT-SKK92 protocols, all progressed within 6 months and had a median overall survival of 0.9 year.[1122] Although there have been reports of better survival in pineal region PNETs, patients tended to be older and more often received radiotherapy.[843,1125]

A treatment strategy for infants and young children with CNS PNETs may involve intensification of treatment, as demonstrated by the Head Start I and II experience in which 5-year EFS and OS of 39% and 49%, respectively, were achieved.[886] High-dose chemotherapy and autologous stem cell rescue have also been reported to be successful in a series of newly diagnosed children and adults, which included two infants who avoided radiotherapy. The 4-year progression-free and overall survivals of 69% and 71%, respectively, were observed.[1126] In contrast, the German HIT-SKK87 and HIT-SKK92 studies had progression-free and overall survivals of only 15% and 17%, respectively, for 29 children between the ages of 3 and 37 months who were treated with chemotherapy to delay radiotherapy. A positive impact on survival was seen in patients who were able to achieve complete resection and those who received radiotherapy.[1127] The use of radiotherapy in some of these patients may improve survival, but RT diminishes the quality of survivorship.[1128] Findings from the CCG 921 study showed that all children with sPNET who received radiotherapy and were younger than 9 years were significantly developmentally delayed.[1125] The current recommendations for infants with CNS PNETs include maximal safe surgery, multiagent chemotherapy, consideration of high-dose chemotherapy with stem cell rescue, and focal three-dimensional conformal radiation therapy, if the field size and tumor location permits.

Infant Ependymoma

Ependymoma is the third most common tumor of infants and young children and the second most common CNS malignancy in children younger than 3 years referred for treatment.[1102] Approximately 43% of ependymomas occur in children younger than 2 years.[870,1089] Unlike adult ependymoma, most ependymomas in infants and young children occur intracranially and, unlike other infant brain tumors, are predominantly infratentorial.[1129] Negative prognostic factors from several studies have demonstrated the importance of extent of resection (less than gross total resection or biopsy) and young age (younger than 3 years at diagnosis).[673,1130,1131] Another prognostic factor that has been reported includes anaplastic histology. However, the heterogeneity of anaplasia seen in tumors and the differences in the diagnostic criteria for anaplastic histology by pathologists, which have ranged from 7% to 89%, have made a full prognostic assessment of this factor difficult.[650] An MIB-1 or Ki-67 index of 20 or higher[1132] may also be a negative prognostic marker.[1133] Although the 5-year overall survival for children with ependymoma has been estimated at 55% to 66%,[670,673] the 5-year survival for infants and young children remains around 25% and is worse if radiotherapy is delayed or a complete resection is not achieved.[663] The role of chemotherapy remains controversial in this population, even though cisplatin is an active agent against ependymoma.[1134] Several studies incorporating chemotherapy have shown lack of efficacy,[1134] including those with dose escalation such as in Head Start, as reported by Zacharoulis and coworkers.[665]

The importance of radiotherapy in the treatment of ependymoma has been clearly established and stereotactic RT administration has been demonstrated to be safe and effective.[327] A phase II study of conformal radiotherapy treating 88 young children, many of whom were younger than 18 months (after chemotherapy and maximal surgical resection were completed), yielded a PFS rate of 75% ± 6% and reduced early neurocognitive deficits, even though younger patients received 5400 cGy of conformal radiotherapy, supporting the use of the modality in these patients.[653] Although long-term neurocognitive follow-up of this younger population is not yet known, this study formed the basis for the COG cooperative group clinical trial of conformal radiotherapy, including short-duration chemotherapy in the subset of patients who achieved only subtotal resections. A previous CCG clinical trial (CCG 9942) of up-front chemotherapy before radiation therapy in children with incompletely resected ependymoma has also been completed.

Experience from the UKCCSG-SIOP (International Society for Pediatric Oncology) collaboration for patients with ependymoma has suggested some benefit from the administration of alternating courses of nonmyelosuppressive with myelosuppressive chemotherapy in nonmetastatic, incompletely resected patients.[1135] In this series of 89 children younger than 3 years, in which 9 patients had metastatic disease, preirradiation chemotherapy resulted in a 5-year EFS and OS of 42% and 63%, respectively. In addition, the 5-year cumulative incidence of freedom from radiotherapy was 42% in the nonmetastatic cohort. Also, patients who received the highest dose intensity had a 5-year overall survival of 76% compared with those with the lowest dose intensity, who had a 5-year overall survival of 52%.[1135] All patients with metastatic disease in this study relapsed and the 5-year overall survival in this group was approximately 25%.[1135] The outcome of patients with metastatic disease at presentation compared with those with localized disease has ranged from no difference in outcome[663,672] to relapse and death in all patients within 2 years of surgery.[1136] Fortunately, less than 10% of patients with ependymoma present with metastatic disease, although this is slightly higher in infants.[663,672] In a retrospective meta-analysis of prognostic factors of 40 patients with metastatic ependymoma, including 29 children younger than 3 years, those who achieved a gross total resection had the best 5-year EFS and OS of 35% ± 13% and 59% ± 13%, respectively, compared with the 5-year EFS and OS of 25% ± 9% and 32% ± 10%, respectively, for those who did not.[1137] The event-free survival for patients who received radiotherapy was 57% ± 19% and 40% ± 22% for those who received combined chemoradiotherapy. For patients treated with chemotherapy alone, the EFS was 20% ± 9%. Because there was no statistical difference in the 5-year overall survival between M1 and M3 patients (51% ± 16% and 40% ± 9%), even those with bulky disease can be treated if a gross total resection can be achieved.[1137]

Infant Glioma

Astrocytoma is the most common tumor in children younger than 3 years[1120] as well as in infants younger than 1 year, and constitutes 30% of the total, of which 75% are low-grade and 25% reported as high-grade tumors.[1098] Management of these tumors in infants and young children mirrors the approaches used in older children, including observation for patients with completely resected low-grade lesions, chemotherapy for patients with symptomatic progressive low-grade tumors, and chemotherapy and radiotherapy for patients with high-grade lesions. One major difference between young children and adults with high-grade gliomas is the improved prognosis observed in children. In the Baby POG series, 18 children younger than 3 years diagnosed with high-grade glioma (13 of whom were younger than 12 months) had 5-year progression-free and overall survivals of 43% ± 23% and 50% ± 14%, respectively.[501] Four survivors completed the 24 months of therapy but were not radiated because of parental refusal and remained without evidence of recurrence. Similar results have been reported in the French BBSFOP trial, in which 21 children younger than 5 years (13 with WHO grade III tumors and 8 with grade IV) received postoperative chemotherapy and had 5-year progression-free and overall survivals of 35% and 59%, respectively. Of the 12 survivors, 10 did not receive radiotherapy at the time of reporting.[531] Another retrospective review of 16 patients younger than 3 years showed similar results, with 5-year event-free and overall survivals of 29% (standard error [SE], 12%) and 66% (SE, 12%), respectively, although 6 patients received up-front radiation therapy and an additional 6 patients received radiation therapy at the time of progression.[1138]

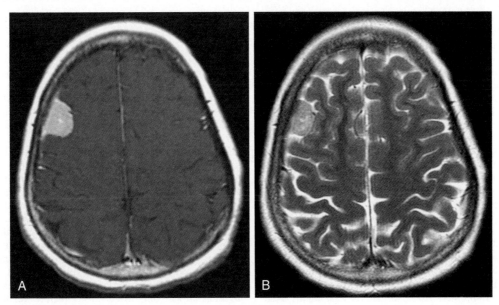

FIGURE 17-50. Peripheral contrast-enhancing meningioma. **A,** Axial T1 image with contrast. Note the dural tail. **B,** Axial T2 image—bright T2 signal of a right frontal meningioma.

Infant Choroid Plexus Carcinoma

Choroid plexus tumors account for 1% to 3% of childhood brain tumors and approximately 30% to 40% are choroid plexus carcinomas,[1139] with 70% occurring before the age of 2 years.[1140] Gross total resection has been shown to be prognostic,[1141] although technically difficult because of the highly vascular nature of these lesions.[1098] The role of radiotherapy for the treatment of this highly invasive tumor is controversial.[1142,1143] The Baby POG study reported eight patients with choroid plexus tumors, two of whom were alive without radiotherapy.[1141] Others have also reported long-term survival without radiotherapy in this group.[1144] Because the numbers of patients with this rare disease are so small, international collaboration is needed to determine the best treatment strategy for this group of patients. Currently, maximal safe surgery and adjuvant chemotherapy constitutes a reasonable approach to avoid or delay radiotherapy[1098] and salvage therapy is possible, not necessarily including craniospinal radiation therapy.[1145]

Other Tumors

Meningiomas

Meningiomas are rare pediatric tumors that are often seen in conjunction with either NF-2 or after radiation therapy[1146]; they account for 1% to 3% (range, 0.4% to 4.1%) of all childhood tumors of the central nervous system.[1147,1148] Familial meningiomas have been reported and thus a detailed family history is required.[1149] In one study of children who received radiation therapy to the CNS for childhood leukemia, 20% developed meningiomas on routine surveillance imaging.[1150] Although uncommon in pediatric patients, meningiomas are the second most common primary brain tumor in adults, after gliomas. Meningiomas are frequently identified as an incidental finding on autopsy, suggesting that many remain small and asymptomatic. Molecular differences between symptomatic lesions and those that remain asymptomatic suggest that they may be distinct entities.[1151] Meningiomas are known to express hormone receptors and a number of cell cycle pathways have been impli-

cated in their dysregulated growth.[1152] In a review of the literature, radiation-induced meningiomas were the second most common radiation-induced malignancy after malignant glioma in children treated for a primary malignant neoplasm, with a mean latency of 21.1 and 13.7 years for atypical and benign meningiomas, respectively.[1153] Similarly, in a cohort of children with acute lymphoblastic leukemia who received cranial radiotherapy (1800 to 2400 cGy) and were monitored by serial scans, meningiomas were the most common tumor, with a mean latency of 21 years.[1150]

Clinical Presentation. The most common clinical presentations in children are seizures (33%), headaches (13%), ataxia (10%), and hemiparesis (10%). Tumor locations are primarily supratentorial (64%), with the rest distributed infratentorially (16%), intraventricularly (12%), and in the spinal cord (8%).[1147] A few small series have indicated that the location and behavior of meningiomas in children may differ from those in adults, with a greater male preponderance, intraventricular location, and increased atypical or anaplastic subtypes (15% in childhood).[1148,1154]

Imaging and Histology. Meningiomas are usually well-circumscribed dural lesions on CT and MR imaging. Areas of calcification are common and are best seen on CT scans. Tumors tend to have low T1-weighted and bright T2 and FLAIR signals. They are usually brightly contrast-enhancing and can be associated with edema.[1155] A dural tail is a common finding on MRI scans in which there is dural thickening, tailing away from the lesion (Fig. 17-50). This finding does not indicate a greater propensity of the tumor to invade.[1156] Although most pediatric meningiomas are low-grade lesions (WHO grade I), a higher number of pediatric meningiomas have features of atypia or anaplasia (WHO grade II and III) as compared with adult patients, especially in spontaneously arising tumors. This can be more pronounced with younger age.[1146] In adult meningiomas, there is good correlation between histologic atypia, recurrence, and staining for the Ki-67 monoclonal antibody, a marker of proliferation. This is not seen in pediatric meningiomas, suggesting that the aggressiveness of pediatric meningioma is not related to proliferation alone.[1157] A number of histologic variants of meningioma can occur in children.[1158-1161] Most meningiomas stain for EMA and vimentin. Loss of chromosome 22 is commonly observed in grade I meningiomas. Additional chromosomal abnormalities can be observed in atypical and anaplastic meningioma. In patients without NF-2, a high incidence of mutations in this gene are still detected.[1162]

Management. The management of pediatric meningiomas is difficult to define as a result of their rare occurrence and association with other mitigating factors, such as prior radiation therapy or association with NF-2.[1146] Treatment guidelines from cooperative groups such as the British Children's Cancer and Leukemia Group are beginning to emerge.[1163]

Meningiomas that are asymptomatic are usually left untreated and followed carefully for the development of neurologic sequelae, radiologic progression, or radiologic evidence of transformation, at which point neurosurgical intervention should be considered. Gross total resection is usually curative, although the appearance of other lesions is not uncommon. In those with progressive or symptomatic lesions, radiotherapy can be delivered and can often stop tumor progression. For unresectable lesions, stereotactic radiosurgery is also being used with increasing frequency. Meningiomas that develop following radiotherapy in the pediatric population can take on a more malignant phenotype, and early surgical resection should therefore be considered. This may lead to a better outcome, especially if a gross total resection can be achieved.[1150] There is a limited role for chemotherapy in the treatment of meningiomas. Recurrent malignant and atypical meningiomas are difficult to treat successfully and chemotherapy has been unsuccessful. Brachytherapy has been proposed for the salvage of relapsed patients but with high accompanying morbidity.[1164] Partial responses to hydroxyurea[1165] and tamoxifen[1166] for refractory meningioma have been reported in the literature but need to be confirmed in larger clinical trials.[1167,1168] A number of new molecularly targeted therapies for meningiomas are now being developed and tested.[1169]

Prognosis. Because of the peripheral nature of many of these lesions, complete resection is achieved in a high percentage of cases. Surgery remains the primary modality of treatment of these tumors and is a major determinant of outcome.[1148] Histologic grade is a further determinant of event-free survival.[1147] Even though the overall survival of patients with meningioma has been reported to be close to 90%, length of follow-up is limited or unknown.[1170] One series extending between 1935 and 1984 has reported long-term survival of 35% in children, with a mean follow-up of 10 years following diagnosis.[1171] The true extent of the morbidity and mortality of this tumor in children is not accurately known[1170] and needs to be the subject of prospective study by national and international cooperative groups.

Pituitary Adenomas

Although infrequent in pediatric patients compared with adults, pituitary adenomas account for approximately 2.7% of pediatric brain tumors.[1172] The differential diagnosis of pituitary fossa tumors includes craniopharyngioma, germ cell tumors, and Langerhans cell histiocytosis (see elsewhere in this chapter) The vast majority of childhood pituitary adenomas are hormone-secreting or functional, meaning that they produce active hormones, including adrenocorticotropic hormone (ACTH), prolactin, growth hormone, thyroid-stimulating hormone (TSH), luteinizing hormone (LH), or follicle-stimulating hormone (FSH).[1173] Nonfunctioning adenomas account for only 3% to 6%.[1174,1175] Depending on the series, the two most commonly secreted hormones are prolactin and ACTH, fol-

lowed by growth hormone,[1174,1176-1179] and finally TSH, LH, and FSH.[1173,1180]

Clinical Presentation. The main clinical manifestations of pituitary adenomas are determined by their location and function and usually consist of headaches (with or without signs of raised ICP), visual field defects, endocrine dysfunction, and menstrual irregularities. Other endocrine-specific presentations can be related to hyperprolactinemia causing secondary amenorrhea and galactorrhea. Cushing's disease resulting from ACTH oversecretion presents with hypertension, weight gain, and occasionally diabetes, although gigantism and acromegaly are rarely observed as a result of growth hormone oversecretion. Hypopituitarism can manifest as hypogonadism with delayed or arrested puberty, amenorrhea, and hypoadrenalism, which can manifest as fatigue, hypoglycemia, and/or weight loss. Short stature or growth failure can result from growth hormone deficiency. Hypothyroidism with a low thyroxine (T_4) and low-normal TSH level can also be a manifestation, although hyperthyroidism from a thyrotropinoma is a rare finding in childhood.[1180] Nonfunctioning tumors can also have endocrine manifestations but these are typically related to pituitary insufficiency.[1181]

Imaging and Histology. The diagnostic workup and management of these tumors includes MR imaging of the pituitary region with and without contrast, although a CT scan can be useful in extensive disease or in an emergency to rule out local invasion or hemorrhage.[1182] Loss of the pituitary bright spot can indicate compression of the pituitary stalk.[1183] Microcystic and macrocystic structures are also easily identified on MRI (Fig. 17-51).[1183] A detailed biochemical workup in conjunction with an endocrinologist is vital to making a diagnosis and should include determination of serum prolactin, T_4 and TSH, LH, FSH, serum urea, electrolyte, and morning cortisol levels. Determination of growth hormone, IGF-1 and its binding partner IGF-BP3, and urine-free cortisol levels and a low-dose dexamethasone suppression test may be indicated if a growth hormone–secreting tumor or Cushing's disease is suspected. Occasionally, bilateral inferior petrosal sinus sampling for ACTH may be necessary for the diagnosis of Cushing's disease.[1184] Visual field testing should be done as part of a baseline assessment, and serum β-HCG and AFP should also be part of an initial assessment to rule out a germ cell tumor.

Management. Elevated secretion of prolactin can be associated with hyperplasia of TSH and prolactin-secreting cells but without the presence of a pituitary adenoma. Hypothyroidism should therefore be managed before surgical intervention in cases in which hyperplasia may be evident.[1185] In terms of managing patients with pituitary adenoma, medical management alone with agents such as bromocriptine or similar analogues may be all that is needed for prolactinoma.[1186] Trans-sphenoidal surgical resection is typically used for the treatment of growth hormone– and ACTH-secreting tumors,[1187] although a potential role for somatostatin analogues such as octreotide has been proposed for the medical treatment of acromegaly.[1188] Multimodal therapy with medication, surgery, or radiotherapy may be necessary where initial therapy has failed.[1179,1180] Fortunately, endocrinologic remission can be achieved in most patients with growth hormone– and ACTH-secreting tumors.[1178]

Multiple endocrine neoplasia type I (MEN1) is an autosomal dominant disorder characterized by hyperparathyroidism, enteropancreatic tumors, pituitary adenomas and, rarely, carcinoid, adrenal adenoma, and lipoma. Pituitary adenomas are observed at first presentation in 10% of cases.[1189] Although formal guidelines are lacking, because there is an increased

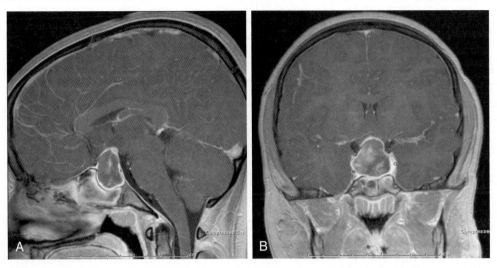

FIGURE 17-51. Large hemorrhagic pituitary adenoma. **A,** Sagittal T1 image with contrast. **B,** Coronal T1 fat-saturated image.

incidence of genetic disorders such as MEN1 in pituitary tumors in children compared with adults,[1190] the families of index cases of childhood pituitary adenoma should be referred for screening and long-term follow-up.

Prognosis. The long-term prognosis of children with pituitary adenomas is excellent. Remission from abnormal hormone secretion is common and, in one review, was achieved in 100% of those with Cushing's disease and 89% of those with growth hormone secretion.[1178] Although most patients can achieve disease control with surgery, 40% may require radiation therapy.[1191] Given the central location of these tumors, this patient population must be carefully followed for neurocognitive impact, radiation-induced tumors, and additional endocrinopathies because of pituitary dysfunction and radiation-mediated vascular damage.

Hamartomas

Hamartomas are an excessive but focal growth of cells and tissues native to the organs within which they occur. They have been described in the brain, eye, liver, lung, kidney, pancreas, heart, and gastrointestinal tract and in the lymphatic and vascular systems. Although they are benign lesions, hamartomas are regarded by pathologists as a link between developmental malformations and neoplasia. Because of the difficulty in distinguishing between these two entities, hamartomas can sometimes be tenuously and variously interpreted as benign neoplasms.[1192] However, despite their benign histology, their location and dysregulated growth in the brain can be the source of great morbidity, causing intractable seizures, obstructive hydrocephalus, and developmental delay.

Among the best-known conditions associated with hamartomas in the CNS are NF-1 and tuberous sclerosis (TS).[1193] NF-1–associated Lisch nodules are pigmented hamartomas in the iris and are found in more than 95% of affected adults and children older than 6 years; they are thought to be virtually pathognomonic for the condition.[1194] Although Lisch nodules remain asymptomatic and do not usually interfere with vision, they are important as a diagnostic criterion for NF-1. These lesions may be associated with unidentified bright spots (UBOs) seen in NF-1 patients[1195] and have been hypothesized ultimately to be related to neurofibromin levels.[1196] NF-2 results from loss of the tumor suppressor merlin and is characterized

by predisposition to developing multiple tumors, including schwannoma (particularly of the vestibular nerve), meningioma, and spinal cord glioma. Although not a commonly described association, combined pigment epithelial and retinal hamartoma have also been reported in NF-2 patients, although as a rare finding.[1197-1199] Their clinical significance is not clear. Tuberous sclerosis, like NF-1 and NF-2, results from the loss of the *TSC1* and *TSC2* tumor suppressor genes, which encode for hamartin and tuberin, respectively. These act by downregulating the Akt-mTOR pathway[1200] as well as by regulating transcription through cross-talk with the Wnt signaling pathway through the ability of TSC1 and TSC2 to form a β-catenin degradation complex.[1201] A pathologic feature of TS within the CNS is the formation of cortical tubers, which are hamartomatous growths, in addition to subependymal nodules and the propensity to develop subependymal giant cell astrocytomas (SEGAs). The clinical manifestation of this disorder is often seizures, cognitive disability, and other systemic manifestations, including dermatologic and visceral changes.[1193]

In considering other conditions that are associated with hamartomatous lesions in the brain, Cowden's disease (OMIM 158350) is important because it is characterized by the familial predisposition to multiple benign hamartomas. These patients are also at increased risk of malignant lesions in all three germ layers involving most major organs, including the brain, mucocutaneous tissue, breast, thyroid, and uterus,[1202] with multiple tricholemmomas or benign neoplasms of the hair follicle, which are considered pathognomonic.[1203] The gene responsible for Cowden's disease on chromosome 10 was cloned by linkage analysis and found to be a phospholipid phosphatase *PTEN* (*p*hosphatase *ten*ascin).[1204,1205] It is mutated in the germline in 80% of patients with Cowden's disease as well as in the Bannayan-Zonana syndrome, which is another familial hamartoma syndrome.[1206] The same gene is also mutated in 60% of patients with Bannayan-Riley-Ruvalcaba syndrome (OMIM 153480), which is manifested by macrocephaly, developmental delay, and intestinal hamartomas. Several authors have reported mutations in the *PTEN* gene in patients with Proteus or Proteus-like syndrome, both of which develop hamartomatous growths. Some authors have suggested that these syndromes are clustered with Cowden's disease and the Bannayan-Riley-Ruvalcaba syndrome into a new category called PTEN hamartoma tumor syndrome (PTHS), although controversy in this area remains.[1207] Although rare, Lhermitte-Duclos disease (LDD) is associated

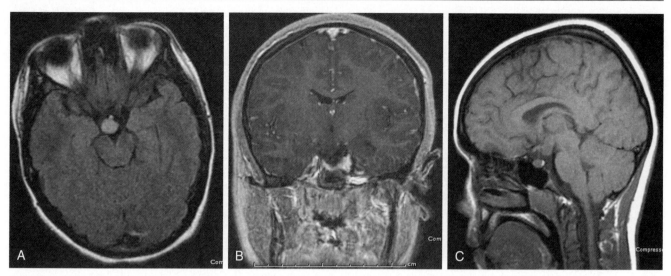

FIGURE 17-52. Hypothalamic hamartoma. **A,** Axial fluid-attenuated inversion recovery (FLAIR) image. **B,** Coronal T1 image with contrast demonstrates little contrast enhancement. **C,** Sagittal T1 image without contrast with hypo- to isointensity.

with hamartomas of the brain resulting in ataxia, increased ICP, and seizures. The underlying lesion is a dysplastic gangliocytoma of the cerebellum, which is thought to be a hamartomatous overgrowth of Cowden's disease.[1208,1209] In fact, adult onset of LDD is considered pathognomonic for Cowden's disease by the National Comprehensive Cancer Network Guidelines.[1193,1202]

Imaging and Histology. There is considerable variability in the imaging characteristics and pathologic appearance of hamartomas in the brain. Certain commonly observed features include areas of calcification on CT scan. On MRI scan, most lesions tend to be hypo- to isointense on T1-weighted sequences and bright on T2 and FLAIR (Fig. 17-52).[1210] Hamartomas of the brain are normally noncontrast-enhancing, which can help differentiate them from low-grade astrocytomas. The load of signal abnormality can be correlated with the severity of the symptoms and prognosis in many patients, such as those with TS.[1211] Using magnetoencephalography and concurrent SPECT imaging, precise tuber localization can be achieved and can assist in surgical planning.[1212,1213] Histologic features of hamartomas are highly dependent on their location.

Management. The detailed management of tumors arising from the hamartoma conditions of Lhermitte-Duclos and Cowden's disease, tuberous sclerosis, and neurofibromatosis is beyond the scope of this text. Multidisciplinary team management involving the input from the geneticist, neurologist, neuro-oncologist, neurosurgeon, and affiliated specialists such as the neuropsychologist is highly recommended to provide comprehensive care. Molecular testing of patients and tumor tissues is also mandatory as targeted therapies with new agents emerge. For example, rapamycin and its analogues and derivatives that specifically target mTOR, which is downstream from the PTEN/phosphoinositol-3-kinase/Akt pathway and is common to neurofibromatosis and tuberous sclerosis,[1200] are now being tested for treatment of low-grade astrocytomas in these patients.[78] Similar therapeutic agents are also available for targeting Ras through the inhibition of farnesyltransferase and are the subject of ongoing clinical trials for progressive plexiform neurofibroma.[1214] Pallister-Hall syndrome, which results in hypothalamic hamartomas, involves abnormalities in the Sonic hedgehog–Gli 3 pathway[1215] and a number of new

molecular inhibitors of this pathway are beginning clinical investigation.[1216]

Optimal management of hamartomatous lesions of the CNS is typically directed at the presenting symptoms.[1217] Seizures are a common presenting symptom and treatment with antiepileptic agents is the first approach. Hamartomatous lesions are often refractory to these medications, even when multiple drugs are coadministered. Complete resection of hamartomas is not always required to improve seizure control, because disconnection of the epileptiform focus without gross surgical resection has resulted in significant clinical improvement in hypothalamic hamartomas.[1218]

Prognosis. Although isolated hamartomatous lesions that can be resected have a good prognosis, patients usually present with a number of comorbid symptoms related to the hamartomas and to the underlying associated genetic syndrome. Mental retardation, autism, and behavioral issues can persist. Seizures are not always amenable to surgical intervention, especially in deep structures of the diencephalon. Even in successfully treated patients, their underlying genetic susceptibility places them at risk for the development of new lesions.

Astroblastomas

Astroblastoma is a rare glial tumor of the central nervous system that accounts for 0.45% to 2.8% of all primary brain gliomas[1219] and approximately 0.92% of all pediatric brain tumors.[1220] The tumor was first described by Bailey and Cushing in their 1924 classification of brain tumors,[712] but the term *astroblastoma* is argued by some as being confusing because the tumor is neither overtly astrocytic nor blastic in nature.[1221] The current widely accepted pathologic description of astroblastoma is that of a generally solid, well-circumscribed mass that is histologically defined by the presence of astroblastic pseudorosettes and perivascular hyalinization.[1222] Ependymoma is an important differential diagnosis because of the clinical and histopathologic similarity between these tumors, which includes perivascular orientation, pseudorosette formation, and immunohistochemical staining with GFAP and EMA. These histopathologic similarities have led to the suggestion that the tanycyte, or ependymal cell, may be a common precursor of ependymoma and astroblastoma.[1223] Even though astroblastoma does have some distinctive features, including broader tapering perivascular processes, lack of fibrillarity, and perivascular hyalinization, which is not seen in ependymoma, this rare tumor continues to be classified under "other neuroepithelial" tumors in the latest WHO classification of CNS tumors.[1224]

Clinical Presentation. The clinical presentation of astroblastoma is usually in children and young adults in the first 3 decades of life,[1221] with several reports in children 5 years or younger,[1220,1225-1228] as well as a congenital form.[1219] Several case series have shown a female preponderance.[1221,1229,1230] Presenting signs and symptoms are usually of headache and raised ICP because of mass effect or obstruction of CSF flow. The site of the tumor is most often supratentorial, peripherally located in the brain.

Imaging and Histology. Radiologically, astroblastomas appear as large, well-circumscribed, heterogeneous, lobulated, solid and cystic masses, with little vasogenic edema disproportional to their size. This lack of edema is a feature that can also help distinguish astroblastoma from ependymoma and high-grade gliomas. The solid component of the mass is described as bubbly and the MRI T2 signal is isointense with gray matter. Enhancement of the solid component is seen in 75% of cases and punctate calcification is occasionally seen.[1229,1230]

The histopathologic features of astroblastoma include strong immunoreactivity for S-100, GFAP, and vimentin, with focal staining with EMA.[1224] Histologic grade is considered as either well-differentiated, which correlates with the ability to achieve a gross total resection,[1221] or malignant, with features of anaplasia, which is a poor prognostic marker.[1228] MIB-1 immunoreactivity has been observed over a wide range (1% to 18%), although it is unclear whether increasing MIB-1 is related to a poorer outcome.[1221] A formal WHO grade has not yet been assigned.[1224]

Management. Treatment of these tumors includes maximal surgical resection followed by focal or whole-brain radiotherapy, especially when features of anaplasia are present. The role of temozolomide,[1231,1232] intensive chemotherapy in younger children,[1228] or other forms of chemotherapeutic agents[1220] has not been determined. The establishment of an international registry to gain more information on treatment responses and a detailed understanding of the biology of these tumors has been proposed to optimize treatment approaches for this rare tumor.[1233] To this end, studies of chromosomal abnormalities, such as gains of chromosome 20q and chromosome 19[1221] or loss of heterozygosity of chromosome 9p,[1234] are important and help distinguish this tumor from ependymoma. The description of variants of astroblastoma that have rhabdoid features and a better prognosis[1231,1235] warrants further study of this rare tumor.

Prognosis. The prognosis of astroblastoma is in part dependent on the histologic features. Anaplastic lesions do less well than those with low-grade features.[1222,1228] Complete resection is important for long-term survival and may be sufficient therapy for most patients, including some with more anaplastic-appearing lesions.[1221]

Primary Central Nervous System Lymphoma

CNS lymphoma is a rare group of tumors that can arise in the CNS. Although primarily associated with immunosuppression from HIV or other immunodeficiency states, CNS lymphoma has also been detected in patients lacking a prior infectious or immunocompromised history. These tumors are often very responsive to therapy, including radiation and/or chemotherapy.[1236]

Primary CNS (PCNS) lymphoma in childhood and young adults is an extremely rare tumor, accounting for about 1.2% to 1.5% of all brain tumors,[1237,1238] with an annual incidence rate of 0.02/100,000 based on data collected by the Childhood Brain Tumor Trust between 2000 and 2004. This would suggest approximately 16 new cases/year are expected in the United States.[714] Children with congenital immunodeficiency syndromes face an inherent 4% overall risk of developing cancer, which is 10,000 times higher than the expected rate, with the highest risk groups being ataxia-telangiectasia and common variable immunodeficiency.[1239] Data collected by the Immunodeficiency Cancer Registry have shown a median age of presentation in this group of children to be 10 years, and over 50% of the cases consist of non-Hodgkin's lymphoma, 30% of which were extranodal.[1240] Specific to PCNS lymphoma, which is more common than other inherited immunodeficiencies, Wiskott-Aldrich patients have the highest proportion of CNS lymphoma among the congenital immunodeficiencies, which is estimated at approximately 3%,[1241] followed by IgA deficiency, hyper-IgM syndrome, and severe combined immunodeficiency.[1242] Immunodeficiency following organ transplantation also carries a risk of between 1% and 5% for PCNS lymphoma and increasing rates are being observed in renal and cardiac, lung, and liver transplant recipients.[1243] Acquired immunodeficiency syndromes, particularly HIV-AIDS in adults, was responsible for a peak in CNS lymphoma in the mid-1990s, with 2% to 13% of adult AIDS patients affected.[1244] In one study of pediatric AIDS patients, the CDC has reported 18 of 6209 patients presenting with CNS lymphoma.[1245,1246] The overall risk of CNS lymphoma was estimated at 17% to 42% in pediatric AIDS patients.[1239,1247,1248] Subsequent reporting by the SEER program has not shown an increase in the rate of PCNS lymphoma in the 0- to 19-year-old age group, unlike in adults, whose rates have fallen dramatically since the peak in the 1990s.[1249] This is probably attributable to the introduction of multiantiretroviral therapies (i.e., highly active antiretroviral therapy [HAART]) and other therapeutic improvements.[1250]

Although patients with immunodeficiencies are at higher risk of developing PCNS lymphoma, most adult and pediatric patients who develop this malignancy are immunocompetent.[1236,1243,1251] The pathogenesis of PCNS lymphoma in the immunocompetent host is unknown. One hypothesis is that systemic inflammatory cells have become trapped in the brain and subsequently transform, isolated from the remainder of the immune system by virtue of the immunologic sanctuary status of the brain. This does not fully explain the fact that normally only T lymphocytes traffic through the CNS, although most PCNS lymphoma are of B-cell origin.[1252]

Clinical Presentation. Although the clinical presentation of PCNS lymphoma is in keeping with the diffuse infiltrative growth seen in adult patients and is dominated by cognitive dysfunction, psychomotor slowing, behavioral changes, raised ICP, and seizures,[1253,1254] most pediatric patients present with symptoms of increased intracranial pressure, hemiparesis, ataxia, and cranial nerve dysfunction.[1236,1237,1251]

Imaging and Histology. Radiologic features of PCNS lymphoma include enhancing unifocal or multifocal lesions, usually in the periventricular area, although cortical lesions are not uncommon. MRI is the best modality because these lesions are characteristically hypointense on T1-weighted sequences and T2 hyperintense tumor with edema.[1253] Most tumors are brightly enhancing on administration of contrast. PET and SPECT imaging can also help confirm the presence of lymphomas as well as identify metastases in the CNS and outside of the brain.[1255-1257] Using the Revised European American Lymphoma (REAL) classification system, the diffuse large B-cell phenotype accounts for most cases, followed by the small, noncleaved Burkitt's phenotype.[1258] Anaplastic large T-cell lymphoma is rare.[1251,1253] Pediatric AIDS patients, on the other hand, have been found to have small noncleaved B-cell tumors, both of the Burkitt's and non-Burkitt's types, and are more frequently associated with Epstein-Barr virus (EBV) infection.[1239,1259]

Management. The treatment of PCNS lymphoma has followed the adult practice because pediatric-based studies to define optimal therapy have not been conducted. Although PCNS lymphomas are aggressive tumors and require intensive treatment, they are responsive to radiation and chemotherapy. Historically, treatment for adults with CNS lymphoma had consisted of radiotherapy alone but also had high relapse rates, which led to the introduction of combination chemotherapy using high-dose methotrexate (1 g/m^2), a treatment that has proven to be effective.[1260] The role of whole-brain radiotherapy (WBRT) as part of consolidation therapy in adults is controversial given its toxicity, especially in older adults and when given in combination with high-dose methotrexate. Some consider it an essential part of therapy and should be excluded only in those of advanced age or with neurocognitive impairment.[1261] In contrast to the data with high-dose methotrexate, there is evidence to suggest that consolidation with WBRT and high-dose cytarabine or high-dose cytarabine alone does not improve survival in patients who achieve complete remission with high-dose methotrexate-based combination treatment.[1262] With effective salvage regimens such as retreatment with high-dose methotrexate or treatment options with temozolomide, rituximab, and other agents,[1260] there is a compelling argument to exclude WBRT as part of first-line treatment.

Although pediatric patients have been successfully treated with WBRT alone,[1236,1237] this is often too toxic, especially in younger children. In a multicenter retrospective review of 12 pediatric patients who had a 5-year event-free survival of 70% and overall survival of 75% (median follow-up of 79 months), only 2 patients received radiotherapy and 1 patient was treated with high-dose chemotherapy and autologous stem cell rescue, confirming that radiotherapy can be excluded from the up-front therapy of these patients.[1251] Most patients in this study received multiagent chemotherapy including high-dose methotrexate (8 g/m^2), high-dose cytarabine, and steroids, with patients having been treated on the French America British LMB-96 protocol (group C for those with CNS disease). All patients in this retrospective study had received intrathecal chemotherapy, with the exception of 1 immunocompromised patient who was treated with hydroxyurea only. Organ transplantation patients can be treated with multimodality therapy, as discussed earlier, in addition to a decrease in their immunosuppressive regimens,[1263] although care must be taken to protect their grafts.

Prognosis. Although the overall survival in pediatric patients with CNS lymphoma has been reported as 75%, which is better than the results observed in most adult studies with chemotherapy alone (50%),[1262] these results are based on a small cohort of mixed immunocompetent and immunocompromised patients. Further improvements in treatment outcome will require a large prospective multinational study that separates immunocompetent and immunocompromised patients with PCNS lymphomas to determine optimum therapy for this rare malignancy.

Dermoid, Epidermoid, and Arachnoid Cysts

A vast array of cysts can occur throughout the central nervous system[1264-1266] and, although not classified as tumors, these CNS lesions can cause significant morbidity and often require surgical intervention. If completely removed, recurrences are uncommon, although incompletely resected lesions can reaccumulate fluid, resulting in recurrence of symptoms and necessitating further resection[1267] or cyst drainage.[1268]

The benign cysts of the central nervous system are often divided into two main categories. The first are those that arise from tissue within the CNS and include porencephalic cysts, arachnoid cysts, ependymal cysts, hemangioblastomas, and those of infectious origin, such as cysticercosis or toxoplasmosis. The second group of cysts consists of those that arise from extracranial tissue and includes teratomas, dermoid and epidermoid cysts, craniopharyngioma, and endodermal, colloid, enterogenous, and Rathke's cleft cysts.[1264]

Arachnoid Cysts

Arachnoid cysts are CSF-filled cavities lined by arachnoid cells[1269,1270] that arise from the arachnoid layer of the meninges. They account for approximately 1% of all intracranial space-occupying lesions and are more common in boys.[1265] They are usually congenital and occur in early infancy[1271] but can also occur as a result of inflammation in older children. Arachnoid cysts usually occur in the supratentorial compartment, arising in areas that are rich in arachnoid tissue, with 50% occurring in the sylvian fissure,[1272] although they can occur anywhere in the CNS.[1273] These are often incidental findings on CT or MRI scans obtained for unrelated symptoms. Although usually isolated in their occurrence, multiple arachnoid cysts can be part of inherited syndromes such as the acrocallosal syndrome (a mutation in the *Gli3* gene, OMIM 200990) or the Chudley-McCullough syndrome (OMIM 604213), both of which are associated with agenesis of the corpus callosum. A familial pattern associated with cysts in multiple family members has been reported, one of which includes abnormalities on chromosome 16.[1274] Arachnoid cysts need to be distinguished from cysts associated with malignant primary or metastatic brain tumors, which are thought to develop as a result of a disrupted blood-brain barrier secondary to the malignant process.[1275]

Clinical Presentation. In infants and children, arachnoid cysts tend to present with increasing head circumference or hydrocephalus, seizures, headaches, and psychomotor retardation.[1265] In the suprasellar region, 90% of patients present with obstructive hydrocephalus,[1276] although precocious puberty has also been recognized.[1277] In this location, it may be necessary to distinguish arachnoid and Rathke's cleft cysts from craniopharyngioma, especially because the clinical management of craniopharyngioma differs significantly. Although differentiating these lesions can be difficult, arachnoid and Rathke's cleft cysts are usually uniformly cystic and lack a solid component. In contrast, craniopharyngiomas are solid in 10% of patients and solid and cystic in 43% of patients. Another distinguishing feature is the presence of calcification in approximately 90% of craniopharyngiomas, a finding that is rare in arachnoid cysts.[1278] Although the neurologic presentation of craniopharyngioma and arachnoid cysts can be similar, 95% of craniopharyngiomas have accompanying endocrine dysfunction, which is usually absent in patients with arachnoid cysts.

Imaging and Histology. The radiologic appearance of arachnoid cysts is usually nonenhancing, and they appear

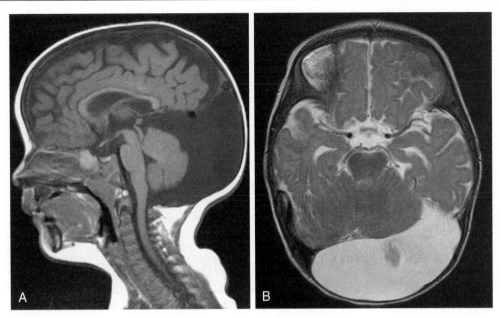

FIGURE 17-53. Arachnoid cyst. **A,** Sagittal T1 image without contrast. **B,** Axial T2 image.

hypodense on CT and isointense to CSF on MRI (Fig. 17-53).[1279] There have been several theories to explain the expansion of arachnoid cysts, which vary from the pulsatile movement of CSF into cyst cavities to osmotic gradients between cysts and CSF.[1265] Analysis of cyst fluid confirms that it is CSF, although the protein content tends to be elevated.[1280]

Management. The management of arachnoid cysts is usually conservative, especially if the patient is asymptomatic.[1281] A clearly expanding lesion or worsening signs and symptoms will necessitate surgical intervention with cyst fenestration[1277,1282] or cystoventricular shunting.[1268] Newer surgical approaches with endoscopic management have been developed and have been successful.[1276,1283] Most patients will have resolution of their presenting symptoms after surgical intervention, although approximately 20% will not.[1284,1285] Potential postsurgical complications include infections, subdural hygroma, and CSF leak.[192]

Prognosis. The long-term prognosis of children with arachnoid cysts is excellent. Because fluid reaccumulation can recur, repeat surgical procedures will be required in approximately 20% of patients.[1285] Those requiring shunting from the ventricles or cysts may require additional procedures as they grow.[192,1286,1287] Seizure control can require lifelong anticonvulsants, especially if complete surgical resection of the lesion is not feasible. Patients with a history of arachnoid cysts may be at increased risk of chronic subdural hematomas.[1288]

Dermoid and Epidermoid Cysts

Dermoid and epidermoid cysts account for 0.5% and 0.8%, respectively, of all intracranial space-occupying lesions[1289] and result from the intrusion of non-nervous tissue, mainly epithelia, into the neuraxis at the time of closure of the neural tube, between the weeks 3 and 5 of embryonic life.[1267,1290,1291] They are most often located in the major subarachnoid cisterns of the brain—namely the suprasellar cistern, pineal region, and cerebellopontine angle cistern.[1264] Although benign and slow-growing, these lesions can be problematic if they cause local mass effect or obstructive hydrocephalus, and they have a ten-

dency to recur if not completely resected or complicated by secondary infection. In general, dermoid cysts are primarily located in the midline in the suprasellar, frontobasal, and cisterna magna areas, although epidermoid cysts can also be found in the suprasellar area. Epidermoid cysts are more common in the lateral skull base around the cerebellopontine angle and are rare in the brain parenchyma or intraventricular region. Both dermoid and epidermoid cysts can occur in the brainstem and spinal cord.[1266,1267,1289,1292]

The presentation of intracranial dermoid cysts occurs in younger patients (10.5 years) as compared with epidermoid cysts, which present in adulthood with a mean age of 27 years.[1266] Although usually sporadic in their presentation, intracranial dermoid cysts can have a familial predisposition affecting several generations (OMIM 600679).[1293] Unlike arachnoid cysts, which have a more clearly defined association with intracranial syndromic malformations such as Aicardi's syndrome, dermoid and epidermoid cysts do not appear to follow the same pattern. However, patients with dermoid cysts can also have associated CNS malformations, such as agenesis of the corpus callosum (OMIM 600679).[1294,1295] In Goldenhar's syndrome, which is composed of oculoauricular dysmorphic features and hemifacial microsomia, associated epibulbar dermoid cysts have been reported (OMIM 164210) but do not have a link with cancer predisposition. In contrast, Gardner's syndrome, a variant of familial adenomatous polyposis with associated predisposition to colorectal carcinomas, includes hyperostosis of the skull and subcutaneous and intra-abdominal dermoid cysts (OMIM 175100). Turcot's syndrome is characterized by familial polyposis coli with a predisposition to the development of malignant neuroepithelial tumors[726] and is also associated with mutations in the adenomatous polyposis coli (APC) and mismatch repair genes.[1296,1297] The coexistence of Gardner's and Turcot's syndromes in a family,[1298,1299] coupled with the report of an intracranial epidermoid cyst in a patient with Gardner's syndrome,[1300] has suggested that dermoid and epidermoid cysts may share a common pathogenesis. Finally, epidermoid cysts can present as a late effect of a lumbar tap.[1301]

Clinical Presentation. Dermoid and epidermoid cysts can present with a wide array of symptoms, including recurrent fevers, headaches, signs of raised intracranial pressure, cerebel-

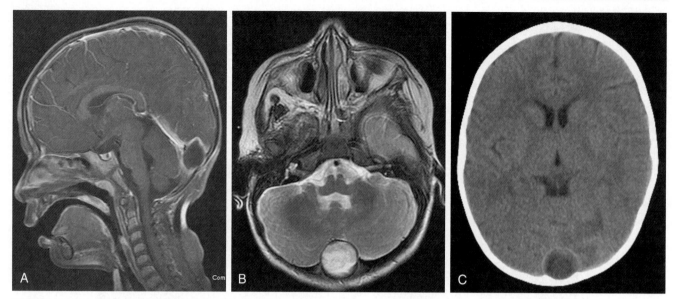

FIGURE 17-54. Occipital dermoid cyst. **A,** Sagittal T1 image with contrast. **B,** Axial T2 image. **C,** Computed tomography (CT) noncontrast image.

lar ataxia, behavioral changes, seizures, cranial nerve palsies, increased head circumference, Parinaud's syndrome, deafness, long tract signs, and cord compression.[1266,1267,1289]

Imaging and Histology. The MRI appearances of dermoid and epidermoid cysts are of well-circumscribed lesions with an accompanying sinus tract that is often visualized on imaging. They produce moderate mass effect but no perilesional edema. They are usually hypointense on T1-weighted imaging and hyperintense on T2, with enhancement of the solid component (Fig. 17-54).[1267] In a recent study of intraparenchymal epidermoid cysts, the imaging characteristics were similar to extracerebral epidermoid cysts with isointensity to CSF on both T1- and T2-weighted images, with additional diagnostic information from diffusion-weighted images.[1302] Histologically, dermoid and epidermoid cysts show overlap consistent with their ectodermal origin. Both are lined by squamous epithelium and some degree of keratin deposition and both lack features of invasion. In addition, dermoid cysts can have skin adnexa present in the cyst wall, including hair follicles, sebaceous glands with sebum, and keratin flakes in the cyst fluid.[1266,1303]

Management. The management of dermoid and epidermoid cysts is surgical when intervention is required. Maximal safe resection should be attempted but can be complicated by adherence of the cyst wall to vital structures, limiting the resection.[1267] Subtotal resection is associated with a high rate of recurrence, requiring repeated surgery.[1293] Potential complications include aseptic meningitis in cases of spillage of cyst contents and even malignant transformation.[1290]

Prognosis. Dermoid and epidermoid cysts can recur and continued surveillance is required, especially for lesions that are incompletely resected.

Spinal Cord Tumors

Spinal cord tumors of infants and children are rare and account for 1% to 10% of all tumors of the CNS. They can occur as extradural, intradural but extramedullary, or intramedullary.[1304]

Boys are affected more than girls and approximately 80% of tumors are low-grade neoplasms. Predominant histologies in the spine from one large series include ependymoma (19%), schwannoma (neurilemoma; 17%), and astrocytoma[409] (15%).[16] Benign cysts are also common in this location.[1305] Rare histologies identified in this region include neuroblastic tumors,[1306] oligodendroglioma,[688] gangliogliomas,[434] anaplastic ganglioglioma,[426] nongerminomatous germ cell tumor,[1307] teratoma,[1308] cavernous angioma,[1309] clear cell meningioma,[1310] lipoma,[1311] PNET,[1312] and ATRT.[1313] In a review of 164 patients with spinal cord tumors undergoing resection, the median age was 8.6 years.[1314]

Clinical Presentation. The clinical symptomatology of pediatric spinal cord tumors relates to neurologic impairment concordant with the level of the lesion. Because most spinal tumors grow along the cord, a number of segments are commonly involved. Each segment of the spinal cord (cervical, thoracic, lumbar, and sacral) can be involved by tumors and no histologic type is localized to a single area except myxopapillary ependymomas, which are predominantly found in the conus medullaris and filum terminale. Common symptoms of spinal cord tumors include pain (most common and identified in up to 80% of cases in most series), motor weakness, sensory loss, torticollis, and bladder and bowel incontinence.[1315-1317] Delay in diagnosis is common because of the nonspecific nature of the symptoms early in the disease process.[1318] Patients with evidence of a cerebral mass and spinal cord symptoms must undergo spinal imaging for metastatic disease.

Imaging and Histology. MR imaging is important in differentiating the location of tumors in the spine (extradural, intradural extramedullary, and intramedullary), as well as differentiating the possible histologies.[1319] As a general rule, the imaging characteristics of spinal cord lesion are similar to those of the same histology in the brain. Histologic evaluation of spinal cord tumors follows that of the same lesions in the brain.

Management. Complete or near-complete resection of intraspinal tumors can be achieved in a significant majority of

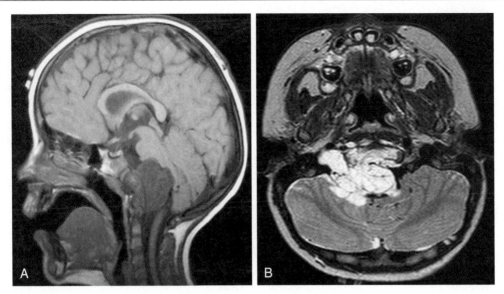

FIGURE 17-55. Large skull-based chordoma. **A,** Sagittal T1 image without contrast. **B,** Axial T1 image with contrast.

patients. In one large series of 164 patients, 76% (125 patients) obtained a greater than 95% resection.[1314] Because most spinal tumors are low-grade tumors and can be cured with complete resection, an experienced neurosurgeon is of utmost importance in achieving a complete resection. Other adjuvant therapies may be considered based on the histology of the tumor. Myxopapillary ependymoma are best managed with complete surgical resection, which is achievable in most patients. Radiation therapy is given to those with progressive disease.[652] Patients with spinal ependymoma may have better outcomes than those with similar tumors of the posterior fossa in that many children can be treated effectively with surgery alone, without the need for radiation therapy. In a group of 20 children, 14 were able to achieve a complete resection and 6 patients had subtotal resections. None of these 6 patients received radiation therapy and yet 3 remained without progressive disease.[1320] Children with high-grade astrocytomas of the spine treated with radiation therapy do as poorly as those with supratentorial tumors.[1321] Low-grade astrocytomas of the spine respond to vincristine and carboplatin[1322] or focal radiotherapy.[1323] Chemotherapy (irinotecan and cisplatin) has been used in infants with astrocytomas to delay the need for radiation therapy, with good results in 3 patients.[1324] Radiotherapy should be reserved for those in whom a complete resection cannot be obtained.[1325] Gangliogliomas are often cured with resection alone; those with incomplete resection or recurrence can be treated with low-grade glioma therapy or focal radiotherapy.[434]

Prognosis. The long-term outcomes for patients with spinal cord tumors are not significantly different from those with supratentorial tumors of the same histology and degree of resection. The morbidities of the tumor and therapies, however, may be significant. Direct neurologic consequences of spinal cord tumors include pain and motor and sensory deficits as well as urinary and bowel incontinence. Many patients will demonstrate significant improvement in these deficits after treatment. Negative predictive factors for prolonged or permanent motor deficits include older age, unilateral symptoms, preoperative urinary symptoms, and other preoperative deficits.[1326] High-grade astrocytic histology and a short history of symptomatology can also be poor prognostic markers.[1327] Patients who

present with sensory deficits do worse than those without this symptom at presentation.[1327] Those with symptoms related to cyst enlargement are most likely to regain function.[651] More than one fourth of patients (27%) develop long-term spinal deformity as a result of their initial laminectomy.[1328,1329] Chronic pain can be particularly difficult in this patient population and requires aggressive management.[1330]

Patients with radiation therapy to the cervical spine can experience paresthesias a few months after therapy that are often described as a feeling of electric shock in the spine. This phenomenon, called Lhermitte's sign, is related to transient demyelinization from radiation therapy.[1331] Patients are treated symptomatically and the sensations will typically resolve without the need for intervention.

Chordomas

Chordomas are rare tumors of the skull base that are thought to derive from remnants of the primitive notochord.[1332] Although most cases arise in adults, they can be observed at all ages, including infants.[1333] Whites appear to be more commonly affected than blacks and males are affected more than females.[1334,1335]

Clinical Presentation. Chordomas can present along the axial skeleton, including the skull base, spine, and sacral area. Skull-based lesions typically present with headaches and diplopia. Spinal lesions often result in pain, motor weakness, or sensory deficits. Although initially minor, these symptoms tend to progress and eventually result in referral for imaging. Rarely, metastatic disease identified on CSF cytology is detected and argues for complete staging of patients, particularly those with atypical or poorly differentiated disease.[1336]

Imaging and Histology. Chordomas are well-circumscribed lesions on CT imaging that can demonstrate areas of calcification. They are hypointense on MR T1-weighted images and bright on T2 and FLAIR sequences (Fig. 17-55). Chordomas can brightly enhance after gadolinium administration.[1334] The histologic appearance of chordomas can vary.[1337] Although conventional chordomas (58%) predominated in one pediatric series of 73 cases, 23% were chondroid chordomas and an additional 19% had high cellularity.[1338] Tumors stained positively for keratin, EMA, S-100, and vimentin. Mitoses and necrotic areas were also commonly observed.[1338]

Management. Radiation therapy can be effective in the treatment of chordomas. In addition to reducing the toxicity of radiation therapy to normal structures,[1339] proton beam radiation therapy in combination with IMRT can provide excellent delivery of a high dose to the lesion.[1340] In patients with more aggressive lesions, or those refractory to radiation therapy, chemotherapy is an option for therapy. Response to ifosfamide and doxorubicin was reported in one patient with metastatic disease in conjunction with triple intrathecal therapy (cytarabine, hydrocortisone, and methotrexate).[1341] The use of a combination of actinomycin D, cyclophosphamide, and methotrexate or cisplatin and 5-fluorouracil demonstrated no activity in this report.[1341]

The recent identification of PDGFR-alpha and PDGFR-beta in tumor cells and concurrent expression of the receptors in adjacent stromal cells suggest a possible role for therapeutic intervention with imatinib mesylate.[1342,1343] Another molecular target identified in these tumors includes EGFR; one patient with metastatic disease achieved a partial response with cetuximab and gifitinib.[1344] Modest activity in recurrent chordomas has also been observed with 9-nitrocamptothecin.[1345]

Prognosis. Patients with chordomas with poorly differentiated features have a worse prognosis than those with classic forms of the disease. Complete resection remains an important prognostic factor. In one large pediatric series, 81% of patients were alive at a median of 7 years after treatment with proton beam radiation therapy.[1338] Elevated MIB-1 has also been reported as an important predictor of recurrence and overall survival.[1346]

LATE EFFECTS OF TREATMENT

The long-term and late effects of therapy are a critical concern in pediatric neuro-oncology.[1347,1348] The developing nervous system is uniquely vulnerable to the long-term effects of radiation therapy and these effects can become apparent and progressive throughout the life span of the child into adulthood.[1349] Although much of the interest about late effects has refocused on the consequences of radiation therapy, there is increasing evidence that the presence of the tumor compressing the brain, the surgery needed to remove it, and the chemotherapy provided to treat it all add to the late effects' experience of survivors of pediatric brain tumors.[1350] The improving prognoses of patients with CNS tumors means that more children will be at risk for developing a wide range of late effects of therapy,[1351] including secondary malignancies.[1352] Of particular importance is the focus on the cognitive outcome of children treated for CNS tumors as we shift from number of survivors to the number of functioning survivors. This has required the development of specialized neurocognitive assessment tools.[1353-1355] It will also require the development of markers that will identify which patients are at risk for late effects from different therapies. Genetic constitution, pharmacogenomics, and individualized pharmacokinetics will need to be assessed when therapy is being planned and appropriate modifications will need to be made to adapt to the unique variables of each individual patient.[1356]

Not all late effects result solely from therapy. Many late effects are the direct result of the tumor or the raised ICP at presentation. Seizures, for example, can occur as a function of the location of the tumor, the therapy, or both. The occasional breakthrough seizure that is relatively well-controlled and not a major concern in childhood can become a significant problem with respect to work and driving as the survivor enters adulthood.[1357] The effect of having had a brain tumor on body image can also be significant. Facial asymmetry caused by tumor infiltration of the brainstem, visual impairment from tumors in the optic pathway, or gait abnormalities from involvement of the motor cortex provide daily reminders to patients that they continue to live with the effects of having had a brain tumor. Raised ICP can also lead to significant visual loss.[1358]

In considering the late effects in brain tumor survivors, we will focus on the major surgical, radiation, and chemotherapy-related factors.

Late Effects of Surgery

Although gross total resection is the goal of surgery for most types of brain tumors, the consequences of cerebellar or brainstem injury following resection of posterior fossa tumors or the behavioral and endocrine alterations following resection of suprasellar tumors may have a serious impact on the long-term quality of life for a patient. Many surgical morbidities may be acute and can improve over time but other deficits may persist, directly affecting the quality of life for survivors.[1359] The association between surgical dissection of the vermis for tumors involving the fourth ventricle and cerebellar mutism syndrome has been well documented, although a precise mechanism has yet to be elucidated. In a report from two large cooperative clinical trials for patients with medulloblastoma, up to 25% of patients were retrospectively identified as having cerebellar mutism syndrome and 92% of cases were deemed moderate or severe. More concerning, 1 year after surgery, a significant proportion of these patients were reported to have continued nonmotor speech, language, and neurocognitive deficits, and/or ataxia.[206] Changes in respiratory function related to cerebellar dysfunction can also persist.[1360] Long-term balance problems after posterior fossa surgery remains a major issue for patients and, although this may be improved with sparing of the deep cerebellar nuclei when resecting posterior fossa lesions, a significant proportion of children will still have residual deficits.[1361]

The increasing use of third ventriculostomies to treat hydrocephalus has helped reduce the need for prolonged VP shunt management. Those with VP shunts inserted will need long-term assessment of shunt function and, for patients who were very young at the time of VP shunt placement, reoperation to reposition and lengthen tubing may be required. Patients must be aware of the risks of shunt failure (both VP and third ventriculostomies) throughout their lives.

Pediatric brain tumor patients undergoing surgical resection as their sole treatment are often perceived to be the lucky ones. Many of these patients with benign histologies are expected to have few long-term effects from their tumor or treatment. However, with detailed neuropsychiatric and neurocognitive assessments, these patients are demonstrating significant abnormalities, including mood, behavioral, and academic difficulties.[1362] These results indicate that all brain tumor survivors, including those receiving minimal intervention, require long-term evaluation and support.

Late Effects of Radiation

Radiation therapy can produce acute, subacute, and late effects on the CNS.[1363] The subacute effects of radiation therapy typically become evident 2 to 6 months after treatment and include the radiation somnolence syndrome (RSS), Lhermitte's sign, and radiation necrosis.

Radiation somnolence syndrome typically follows within 1 to 2 months of large-volume cerebral irradiation. In a series of 19 adult patients treated with RT for their CNS tumors, 16 experienced RSS.[1364] Patients typically become lethargic and anorexic and may complain of fever and headaches. Drowsiness and inability to concentrate are also common.[1364] Many of the symptoms recapitulate those at presentation of the initial tumor and can be very distressing to patients and their parents. The syndrome spontaneously resolves within 1 month in most cases but occasionally low-dose corticosteroids are required.[1365]

Lhermitte's sign is described by patients as an electric shock sensation traveling down the spine on neck flexion, usually arising within several months of cervicothoracic spinal irradiation.[1331] Occurrence after administration of chemotherapy, especially cisplatin, has also been reported.[1366] It is estimated to occur in 3% to 13% of adults[1367] but has not been well studied in the pediatric population. It usually resolves spontaneously within 2 to 3 months, although a few rare cases of prolonged sensory symptoms have been reported.[1367]

Radiation necrosis frequently occurs within months of treatment, although it can be observed even years later; a median of 9 months for onset was reported in one retrospective series.[1368] The incidence can increase in association with chemotherapy.[1369] Common findings on MRI include an enlargement of the tumor region, with a central area of necrosis and strong edema signal best demonstrated on T2-weighted or FLAIR sequences. Because of the overlapping symptoms and MRI appearance of radiation necrosis with tumor progression, surgery is sometimes required to confirm the diagnosis as well as to relieve symptoms. A number of newer imaging modalities are being evaluated to differentiate tumor necrosis from tumor progression better; these include perfusion MRI,[1370] diffusion tensor imaging,[1371] and ^{11}C-methionine or ^{13}N-NH3-PET imaging.[1372,1373] On histopathologic examination, if biopsied, a significant lymphocytic infiltration can be observed.[1374] The occurrence of radiation necrosis is associated with increasing doses of radiation therapy and is most common with doses above 6000 cGy and fraction sizes greater than 180 cGy. It is commonly associated with stereotactic radiation surgery, especially in highly cellular tumors. Small round blue cell tumors of the CNS and glioblastoma multiforme are at particular risk. The treatment of radiation necrosis has historically relied on the use of high-dose steroids to suppress the inflammatory response and resulting edema. More recently, the use of antiangiogenic agents has demonstrated activity in this regard. VEGF (initially identified as vascular permeability factor, VPF) regulates endothelial cell integrity. Thus, agents that target VEGF signaling may become important therapeutic options in this regard.[1375,1376]

The late effects of radiation therapy can occur over a wide time range. It is unclear whether certain risks such as vasculopathy and second tumors have a plateau. On MR imaging, transient T2 signal abnormalities have been identified in patients approximately 1 year after radiation and chemotherapy. These lesions are smaller than 1 cm and patients are generally asymptomatic. They occur in the high-dose radiation volumes and typically resolve on subsequent MRIs.[1377] These MRI findings can be concerning for tumor recurrence but will usually resolve without therapy.

Late consequences of CNS radiotherapy include subtle or symptomatic, progressive, cognitive deficiencies in areas such as attention[1378] and memory impairment; learning disabilities become apparent[818] and are related to the dose and volume delivered.[1379] Younger age at the time of radiation therapy is a critical variable. Those younger than 3 years are at severe risk; those aged 3 to approximately 10 years can anticipate some

cognitive decline. Even older children and adults will demonstrate some cognitive deficits after large-volume, high-dose cranial irradiation. It is unclear whether this effect reaches a plateau. Abnormal patterning of the hippocampus in patients undergoing radiation therapy have been observed and may account for some of the memory difficulties in this group of survivors.[1380] Similarly, distinct patterns of volume loss in the posterior components of the corpus callosum in patients treated for medulloblastoma have also been reported and follow the radiation dosimetry in these regions.[1381] A detailed evaluation and assessment of the neurocognitive effects caused by therapy requires standardized and validated tools.[1382] Unfortunately, although a number of measures have been developed, all have certain weaknesses and none is currently being uniformly applied.

Leukoencephalopathy has been described in children with acute lymphoblastic leukemia who received intrathecal and intravenous methotrexate[1383] and whole-brain irradiation.[1384] Similar findings are reported in association with high-dose cytarabine. Leukoencephalopathy may manifest subtle but progressive cognitive decline as well as seizures. In its severe form, the child becomes demented and incapacitated. MR and CT imaging show diffuse periventricular leukomalacia, with patchy necrosis and calcification. The administration of high-dose IV methotrexate following cranial irradiation may lead to an especially high risk of leukoencephalopathy and this sequence of treatments should be avoided. Myelopathy may arise as a late consequence of spinal irradiation. Changes in white matter as a result of radiation therapy can have a dramatic impact on cognitive function later in life, and serial assessment of these changes may be used to guide survivorship issues and intervention.[1385,1386] Many patients with significant cognitive decline after radiation therapy, particularly of the temporal lobes, may not demonstrate specific white matter or vascular changes to explain the clinical deterioration.[1387]

Radiation injury to vascular endothelium may lead to ischemic strokes.[1388] If the process is slowly progressive, multiple small collateral vessels may arise consistent with a moyamoya pattern, as seen on angiography imaging. Patients with NF-1 are particularly at risk.[1363] This damage to vascular structures of the brain can result in long-term cerebrovascular problems, even decades later,[1389] ranging from acute hemorrhages and cavernous angiomas[1390] to slow and progressive loss of the vasculature and compensatory development of new vessels. The new vessels associated with moyamoya, however, are insufficient to replace the damaged ones.[71]

Secondary malignancies, including high-grade gliomas, atypical meningiomas,[1391] osteosarcomas,[1392] thyroid carcinoma,[1393] cavernous malformations, and schwannomas, have been observed within the treatment field several years after the completion of radiation therapy (Fig. 17-56). Most radiation-induced tumors are not observed before 5 years and can often occur in the marginal areas that received intermediate doses (Fig. 17-57). From a molecular basis, radiation-induced secondary tumors in children do not appear significantly different than those that arise de novo. The prognoses for secondary high-grade glioma (HGG), atypical meningiomas, and osteosarcomas remains exceedingly poor,[504] thus arguing for the judicious use of radiation therapy, especially for patients with low-grade tumors.[444] Patients with Turcot's syndrome, Gorlin's syndrome, and NF-1 are more likely to develop a secondary malignant glioma after radiation therapy compared with patients without these conditions.[1394]

Pediatric patients with central nervous system tumors are at high risk for various endocrinologic abnormalities as a result of their tumor,[1395] the surgery (especially for pituitary region tumors), or radiation therapy that hits the hypothalamus and/or pituitary region. Growth retardation is usually multifactorial.[1396]

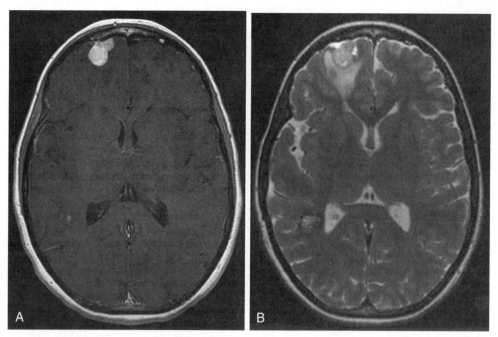

FIGURE 17-56. Radiation-induced meningioma and cavernous malformation. **A,** Axial T1 image with contrast. **B,** Axial T2 image.

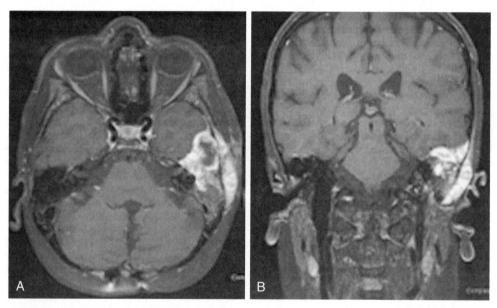

FIGURE 17-57. Radiation-induced left cranial osteosarcoma. **A,** Axial T1 image with contrast, with fat suppression. **B,** Coronal T1 image with contrast, with fat suppression.

Radiation to the pituitary gland may affect the production and release of growth hormone.[1397] Pituitary function may also be impaired by direct invasion of the gland by adjacent tumor. Obesity can be a direct result of radiation therapy on the hypothalamus.[1398] In addition, spinal radiation (as part of craniospinal treatment) affects the growth of the vertebral bones and overall bone density, within the radiation field and throughout the body.[1399] Ovarian function can be protected with laparoscopic oophoropexy preradiation therapy in prepubertal girls in whom the ovaries are likely to be near the midline.[1400] Growth failure after treatment requires active and continued participation by endocrinologists as the cause of growth failure changes from chemotherapy-induced cachexia to radiation-mediated growth hormone deficiency.[1401] Although many patients are discouraged from initiating growth hormone replacement because of concerns for reactivation of the primary tumor or a second malignancy, there is no evidence that this occurs.[1402,1403] In contrast, the morbidity of not replacing growth hormone for those that are deficient can be severe and lifelong.[1404] Although most centers start growth hormone 1 year after completion of therapy, there is no evidence to suggest that earlier treatment would increase the risk of tumor recurrence.

Late Effects of Chemotherapy

Although most chemotherapy-related toxicities occur acutely, a number of long-term side effects are well recognized. Many of the neurologic effects of chemotherapy become evident at the time of drug administration and will improve after cessation of drug. In some patients, however, these toxicities can become long-term issues. Peripheral neuropathy is a common late effect of several chemotherapy agents,[1405] particularly vincristine.[1405] Cisplatin and carboplatin mainly affect proprioception and spare pain and temperature sensation. The usual presenting symptoms are painful dysesthesias and tingling sensations in the toes and later in the fingers. Motor fibers are spared. In contrast, vincristine produces sensorimotor neuropathies. The first symptoms are usually tingling in the toes and fingers. Loss of ankle jerks is typically the first objective sign. Continued treatment with the drug leads to loss or decrease in reflexes and motor weakness involving the dorsiflexors of the feet. Patients with preexisting neuropathies may become quadriparetic after treatment with vincristine. Cerebellar syndromes of acute onset may be seen with high-dose cytarabine and occasionally with 5-fluorouracil. These complications are usually reversible within 2 weeks but severe irreversible damage to Purkinje cells may occur if the drug is given for several months or if the drug is reintroduced again at a later time.[1406] Transverse myelopathy is seen with prolonged treatments with intrathecal methotrexate or cytarabine. The risk is higher when combined with spinal irradiation.

Speech, language, and hearing are important components of daily functioning, and these can often be significantly impaired as a result of the brain tumor itself and its treatment.[1407] Many patients can be left with significant impairment that requires early and aggressive diagnosis and management.[1408] Radiation can cause long-term hearing impairment,[1409] but platinum agents such as cisplatin and, to a lesser extent, carboplatin, can cause significant sensorineural hearing loss in a dose-dependent manner. Although the higher frequencies of hearing, those above the normal hearing range, are usually affected initially, progressive loss can occur over time, including frequencies within the normal range. In one retrospective institutional study, 4% of patients treated with carboplatin and 57% of cisplatin-treated patients experienced significant hearing loss.[1410] Whether agents such as amifostine can reduce cisplatin-mediated hearing loss is controversial.[805,806] Patients at risk for hearing loss should therefore be followed regularly by audiologists so that early corrective action (e.g., dose reduction of platinum agents, hearing aids) can be instituted.[1411]

Renal dysfunction is a rare complication of cisplatin toxicity; it can lead to lifelong proteinuria and salt wasting.[1412] Various electrolytes can be lost with renal impairment and may require daily oral supplementation.

Secondary malignancies are a rare but significant late effect of chemotherapy. In children, acute myelogenous leukemia (AML) is the most common type of secondary malignancy induced by chemotherapy, most frequently caused by intravenous etoposide.[1413] The risk of AML appears dependent on the frequency and dose administered and is highest when etoposide is administered weekly, less when administered monthly, and very low when given daily in low-dose oral administration. These leukemias tend to occur 3 to 5 years after etoposide administration. Alkylating agents and platinum-based drugs are less commonly implicated. The transient genotoxic damage to chromosomes by chemotherapy may account for this risk.[1414]

A critical measure of the effectiveness of treatment of pediatric brain tumors is the patient's quality of life. Although this broad measure is difficult to define across all heterogeneous tumor types, age at presentation, and presenting morbidities, a greater emphasis on understanding how to optimize each child's potential has become the focus of many treatment protocols. The development of new assessment tools will also be important as new therapies are evaluated based on their efficacy and the quality of life.[1415]

Survivors have indicated the constant stress that they feel after the medical team, family, and friends have declared success in curing them and their brain tumors.[1416] They recognize their own impaired social functioning much of the time[1417] and yet can also be unaware of important psychosocial and behavioral issues evident to others.[1418] Depression is a frequent and often poorly recognized outcome in these patients.[1419] Even patients with excellent prognoses, such as those with a history of low-grade gliomas, demonstrate chronic medical problems, as evidenced in one report of 87 patients in which 100% of patients had such issues.[1420] Decline in attention and concentration in survivors of pediatric brain tumors are a major problem,[1421] even when compared with other populations that have received therapy directed toward the CNS, such as survivors of childhood acute lymphoblastic leukemia (ALL).[1422] Part of this likely reflects the dosimetry of radiation used for patients with brain tumors, which increases neurocognitive impairment.[1423] Verbal memory difficulties associated with the treatment of tumors in the third ventricular region are significantly greater than those seen in patients with posterior fossa tumors, in whom attention difficulties predominate.[1424] The development of models to assist in the risk assessment of having a poor outcome is needed.[1425] These issues become particularly acute for this population, especially when they reach adulthood, when they are often faced with insurance barriers preventing them from receiving much-needed therapy.[1426]

Given the broad issues faced by brain tumor survivors, it is hard to develop a single all-encompassing guideline for follow-up care. Multidisciplinary care in dedicated survivor programs can focus resources needed to identify and address issues in this patient population. From the imaging standpoint, many centers have adopted the standard of scanning patients who have completed therapy every 3 months for the first year, every 6 months for the second year, and then yearly thereafter. Routine surveillance of renal and audiologic assessments depends on the field and dose of radiation therapy, as well as the cumulative dose of platinum chemotherapy agents. The frequency of cardiac and pulmonary assessments also depends on particular agents previously used and their cumulative doses. Continued radiologic and blood chemistry surveillance is recommended for most patients as the risk of tumor recurrence decreases and is replaced by increased second tumor risk.

PALLIATIVE CARE

Although clinicians and caregivers focus a great deal of attention on attempts to eradicate disease, a significant proportion of patients with pediatric brain tumors will not survive and, in the process, many often suffer. The early introduction of palliative services, including discussions on the management of all symptoms[1427] and resuscitative measures (e.g., do not resuscitate [DNR] orders),[1428] can allow patients and families in the terminal phase of care a more peaceful and dignified death.[1429] Early and aggressive management of pain must be anticipated and the necessary expertise put in place.[1430] Children can often participate in discussion of end-of-life care.[1431] Decisions about where the child will die, either at home or in the hospital, as well as other aspects of terminal care must be addressed with the family and caregivers and require institutional support and resources.[1432] Finally, the discussion about the possibility of autopsy is never an easy one. The more time that patients, parents, and families have to consider an autopsy, separated in time from the actual death and grieving, the more likely they are to be able to make a decision that is right for themselves and their families. To understand the patient's disease better so that other children might be spared the same fate is comforting to families who consent to an autopsy.

Although limited by local governing policy, there is a low risk of transmission of cancer via transplanted organs from children with primary CNS tumors because of their infrequent spread outside the brain and spine. Given the severe shortage of organs, consideration of this option should be presented to the patient, family, and transplantation team.[1433]

Many families have expressed the importance of their relationship with the caregiving team. Actually, many feel abandoned after the child has died when communication and interaction with the medical team suddenly ends.[2] A number of palliative care programs and the expanding literature in this area are now available to help parents and caregivers through the grieving period.

REFERENCES

1. Tamber MS, Bansal K, Liang ML, et al. Current concepts in the molecular genetics of pediatric brain tumors: implications for emerging therapies. Childs Nerv Syst. 2006;22:1379-1394.
2. Jackson AC, Stewart H, O'Toole M, et al. Pediatric brain tumor patients: their parents' perceptions of the hospital experience. J Pediatr Oncol Nurs. 2007;24:95-105.
3. Partap S, Fisher PG. Update on new treatments and developments in childhood brain tumors. Curr Opin Pediatr. 2007;19:670-674.
4. Khatua S, Jalali R. Recent advances in the treatment of childhood brain tumors. Pediatr Hematol Oncol. 2005;22:361-371.
5. Walter AW, Hilden JM. Brain tumors in children. Curr Oncol Rep. 2004;6:438-444.
6. Rutka JT, Kuo JS, Carter M, et al. Advances in the treatment of pediatric brain tumors. Expert Rev Neurother. 2004;4:879-893.
7. Ullrich NJ, Pomeroy SL. Pediatric brain tumors. Neurol Clin. 2003;21:897-913.
8. Rashidi M, DaSilva VR, Minagar A, et al. Nonmalignant pediatric brain tumors. Curr Neurol Neurosci Rep. 2003;3:200-205.
9. MacDonald TJ, Rood BR, Santi MR, et al. Advances in the diagnosis, molecular genetics, and treatment of pediatric embryonal CNS tumors. Oncologist. 2003;8:174-186.
10. Wrensch M, Minn Y, Chew T, et al. Epidemiology of primary brain tumors: current concepts and review of the literature. Neuro Oncol. 2002;4:278-299.
11. Steliarova-Foucher E, Stiller C, Lacour B, et al. International Classification of Childhood Cancer, third edition. Cancer. 2005;103:1457-1467.
12. Ries LAG, Melbert D, Krapcho M, et al. SEER Statistics Review, 1975-2005. Bethesda, Md, National Cancer Institute, 2008. Available at http://www.cbtrus.org.
13. Davis FG, Kupelian V, Freels S, et al. Prevalence estimates for primary brain tumors in the United States by behavior and major histology groups. Neuro Oncol. 2001;3:152-158.
14. Suh YL, Koo H, Kim TS, et al. Tumors of the central nervous system in Korea: a multicenter study of 3221 cases. J Neurooncol. 2002;56:251-259.
15. Cho KT, Wang KC, Kim SK, et al. Pediatric brain tumors: statistics of SNUH, Korea (1959-2000). Childs Nerv Syst. 2002;18:30-37.
16. Zhou D, Zhang Y, Liu H, et al. Epidemiology of nervous system tumors in children: a survey of 1,485 cases in Beijing Tiantan Hospital from 2001 to 2005. Pediatr Neurosurg. 2008;44:97-103.
17. Rosemberg S, Fujiwara D. Epidemiology of pediatric tumors of the nervous system according to the WHO 2000 classification: a report of 1,195 cases from a single institution. Childs Nerv Syst. 2005;21:940-944.
18. Feltbower RG, Picton S, Bridges LR, et al. Epidemiology of central nervous system tumors in children and young adults (0-29 years), Yorkshire, United Kingdom. Pediatr Hematol Oncol. 2004;21:647-660.
19. Barnholtz-Sloan JS, Severson RK, Stanton B, et al. Pediatric brain tumors in non-Hispanics, Hispanics, African Americans and Asians: differences in survival after diagnosis. Cancer Causes Control. 2005;16:587-592.
20. Gurney JG. Topical topics: Brain cancer incidence in children: time to look beyond the trends. Med Pediatr Oncol. 1999;33:110-112.
21. Ezer R, Alonso M, Pereira E, et al. Identification of glutathione S-transferase (GST) polymorphisms in brain tumors and association with susceptibility to pediatric astrocytomas. J Neurooncol. 2002;59:123-134.
22. Connelly JM, Malkin MG. Environmental risk factors for brain tumors. Curr Neurol Neurosci Rep. 2007;7:208-214.
23. Baldwin RT, Preston-Martin S. Epidemiology of brain tumors in childhood—a review. Toxicol Appl Pharmacol. 2004;199:118-131.
24. Huncharek M, Kupelnick B, Klassen H. Maternal smoking during pregnancy and the risk of childhood brain tumors: a meta-analysis of 6566 subjects from twelve epidemiological studies. J Neurooncol. 2002;57:51-57.
25. Huncharek M, Kupelnick B. A meta-analysis of maternal cured meat consumption during pregnancy and the risk of childhood brain tumors. Neuroepidemiology. 2004;23:78-84.
26. Gurney JG, Chen M, Skluzacek MC, et al. Null association between frequency of cured meat consumption and methylvaline and ethylvaline hemoglobin adduct levels: the N-nitroso brain cancer hypothesis. Cancer Epidemiol Biomarkers Prev. 2002;11:421-422.
27. Raaschou-Nielsen O, Hertel O, Thomsen BL, et al. Air pollution from traffic at the residence of children with cancer. Am J Epidemiol. 2001;153:433-443.
28. Wrensch MR, Minn Y, Bondy ML. Epidemiology. New York, Thieme, 2000.
29. Boffetta P, Tredaniel J, Greco A. Risk of childhood cancer and adult lung cancer after childhood exposure to passive smoke: a meta-analysis. Environ Health Perspect. 2000;108:73-82.
30. Zahm SH. Childhood leukemia and pesticides. Epidemiology. 1999;10:473-475.
31. Blot WJ, Henderson BE, Boice JD Jr. Childhood cancer in relation to cured meat intake: review of the epidemiological evidence. Nutr Cancer. 1999;34:111-118.
32. Preston-Martin S, Mack W. Neoplasms of the nervous system. In Schottenfeld D, Fraumeni JF (eds). Cancer Epidemiology and Prevention. New York, Oxford University Press, 1996.
33. Wrensch M, Bondy ML, Wiencke J, et al. Environmental risk factors for primary malignant brain tumors: a review. J Neurooncol. 1993;17:47-64.

34. Thomas TL, Fontham ET, Norman SA, et al. Occupational risk factors for brain tumors. A case-referent death-certificate analysis. Scand J Work Environ Health. 1986;12:121-127.

35. Kan P, Simonsen SE, Lyon JL, et al. Cellular phone use and brain tumor: a meta-analysis. J Neurooncol. 2008;86:71-78.

36. Hoffman S, Schellinger KA, Propp JM, et al. Seasonal variation in incidence of pediatric medulloblastoma in the United States, 1995-2001. Neuroepidemiology. 2007;29:89-95.

37. Linos E, Raine T, Alonso A, et al. Atopy and risk of brain tumors: a meta-analysis. J Natl Cancer Inst. 2007;99:1544-1550.

38. Goh YI, Bollano E, Einarson TR, et al. Prenatal multivitamin supplementation and rates of pediatric cancers: a meta-analysis. Clin Pharmacol Ther. 2007;81:685-691.

39. Kosulin K, Haberler C, Hainfellner JA, et al. Investigation of adenovirus occurrence in pediatric tumor entities. J Virol. 2007;81:7629-7635.

40. Rollison DE, Utaipat U, Ryschkewitsch C, et al. Investigation of human brain tumors for the presence of polyomavirus genome sequences by two independent laboratories. Int J Cancer. 2005;113:769-774.

41. Ron E, Modan B, Boice JD Jr, et al. Tumors of the brain and nervous system after radiotherapy in childhood. N Engl J Med. 1988;319:1033-1039.

42. Chodick G, Ronckers CM, Shalev V, et al. Excess lifetime cancer mortality risk attributable to radiation exposure from computed tomography examinations in children. Isr Med Assoc J. 2007;9:584-587.

43. Schor NF. Neuroblastoma as a neurobiological disease. J Neurooncol. 1999;41:159-166.

44. Packer RJ, Gutmann DH, Rubenstein A, et al. Plexiform neurofibromas in NF1: toward biologic-based therapy. Neurology. 2002;58:1461-1470.

45. Rasheed S, Mao Z, Chan JM, et al. Is melanoma a stem cell tumor? Identification of neurogenic proteins in trans-differentiated cells. J Transl Med. 2005;3:14.

46. Sanada K, Tsai LH. G protein betagamma subunits and AGS3 control spindle orientation and asymmetric cell fate of cerebral cortical progenitors. Cell. 2005;122:119-131.

47. Chenn A, McConnell SK. Cleavage orientation and the asymmetric inheritance of Notch1 immunoreactivity in mammalian neurogenesis. Cell. 1995;82:631-641.

48. Gotz M, Barde YA. Radial glial cells defined and major intermediates between embryonic stem cells and CNS neurons. Neuron. 2005;46:369-372.

49. Gotz M, Huttner WB. The cell biology of neurogenesis. Nat Rev Mol Cell Biol. 2005;6:777-788.

50. Grimmer MR, Weiss WA. Childhood tumors of the nervous system as disorders of normal development. Curr Opin Pediatr. 2006;18:634-638.

51. Yang ZJ, Ellis T, Markant SL, et al. Medulloblastoma can be initiated by deletion of Patched in lineage-restricted progenitors or stem cells. Cancer Cell. 2008;14:135-145.

52. Schuller U, Heine VM, Mao J, et al. Acquisition of granule neuron precursor identity is a critical determinant of progenitor cell competence to form Shh-induced medulloblastoma. Cancer Cell. 2008;14:123-134.

53. Hemmati HD, Nakano I, Lazareff JA, et al. Cancerous stem cells can arise from pediatric brain tumors. Proc Natl Acad Sci U S A. 2003;100:15178-15183.

54. Rice JM. Inducible and transmissible genetic events and pediatric tumors of the nervous system. J Radiat Res (Tokyo). 2006;47(Suppl B):B1-B11.

55. Melean G, Sestini R, Ammannati F, et al. Genetic insights into familial tumors of the nervous system. Am J Med Genet C Semin Med Genet. 2004;129:74-84.

56. Taylor MD, Mainprize TG, Rutka JT. Molecular insight into medulloblastoma and central nervous system primitive neuroectodermal tumor biology from hereditary syndromes: a review. Neurosurgery. 2000;47:888-901.

57. Hottinger AF, Khakoo Y. Update on the management of familial central nervous system tumor syndromes. Curr Neurol Neurosci Rep. 2007;7:200-207.

58. McGaughran JM, Harris DI, Donnai D, et al. A clinical study of type 1 neurofibromatosis in northwest England. J Med Genet. 1999;36:197-203.

59. Gutmann DH. Learning disabilities in neurofibromatosis 1: sizing up the brain. Arch Neurol. 1999;56:1322-1323.

60. Friedman JM, Birch PH. Type 1 neurofibromatosis: a descriptive analysis of the disorder in 1,728 patients. Am J Med Genet. 1997;70:138-143.

61. Hegedus B, Banerjee D, Yeh TH, et al. Preclinical cancer therapy in a mouse model of neurofibromatosis-1 optic glioma. Cancer Res. 2008;68:1520-1528.

62. Sawada S, Florell S, Purandare SM, et al. Identification of NF1 mutations in both alleles of a dermal neurofibroma. Nat Genet. 1996;14:110-112.

63. Li Y, Bollag G, Clark R, et al. Somatic mutations in the neurofibromatosis 1 gene in human tumors. Cell. 1992;69:275-281.

64. Weeber EJ, Sweatt JD. Molecular neurobiology of human cognition. Neuron. 2002;33:845-848.

65. Warrington NM, Woerner BM, Daginakatte GC, et al. Spatiotemporal differences in CXCL12 expression and cyclic AMP underlie the unique pattern of optic glioma growth in neurofibromatosis type 1. Cancer Res. 2007;67:8588-8595.

66. Mentzel HJ, Seidel J, Fitzek C, et al. Pediatric brain MRI in neurofibromatosis type I. Eur Radiol. 2005;15:814-822.

67. Sheikh SF, Kubal WS, Anderson AW, et al. Longitudinal evaluation of apparent diffusion coefficient in children with neurofibromatosis type 1. J Comput Assist Tomogr. 2003;27:681-686.

68. Tognini G, Ferrozzi F, Garlaschi G, et al. Brain apparent diffusion coefficient evaluation in pediatric patients with neurofibromatosis type 1. J Comput Assist Tomogr. 2005;29:298-304.

69. Farmer JP, Khan S, Khan A, et al. Neurofibromatosis type 1 and the pediatric neurosurgeon: a 20-year institutional review. Pediatr Neurosurg. 2002;37:122-136.

70. Ullrich NJ, Robertson R, Kinnamon DD, et al. Moyamoya following cranial irradiation for primary brain tumors in children. Neurology. 2007;68:932-938.

71. Horn P, Pfister S, Bueltmann E, et al. Moyamoya-like vasculopathy (moyamoya syndrome) in children. Childs Nerv Syst. 2004;20:382-391.

72. Trofatter JA, MacCollin MM, Rutter JL, et al. A novel moesin-, ezrin-, radixin-like gene is a candidate for the neurofibromatosis 2 tumor suppressor. Cell. 1993;72:791-800.

73. Rouleau GA, Merel P, Lutchman M, et al. Alteration in a new gene encoding a putative membrane-organizing protein causes neuro-fibromatosis type 2. Nature. 1993;363:515-521.

74. Gold DR, Cohen BH. Brain tumors in neurofibromatosis. Curr Treat Options Neurol. 2003;5:199-206.

75. van Slegtenhorst M, de Hoogt R, Hermans C, et al. Identification of the tuberous sclerosis gene TSC1 on chromosome 9q34. Science. 1997;277:805-808.

76. Clarke MJ, Foy AB, Wetjen N, et al. Imaging characteristics and growth of subependymal giant cell astrocytomas. Neurosurg Focus. 2006;20:E5.

77. Weiner HL, Carlson C, Ridgway EB, et al. Epilepsy surgery in young children with tuberous sclerosis: results of a novel approach. Pediatrics. 2006;117:1494-1502.

78. Franz DN, Leonard J, Tudor C, et al. Rapamycin causes regression of astrocytomas in tuberous sclerosis complex. Ann Neurol. 2006;59:490-498.

79. Cowan R, Hoban P, Kelsey A, et al. The gene for the naevoid basal cell carcinoma syndrome acts as a tumour-suppressor gene in medulloblastoma. Br J Cancer. 1997;76:141-145.

80. Hahn H, Wojnowski L, Miller G, et al. The patched signaling pathway in tumorigenesis and development: lessons from animal models. J Mol Med. 1999;77:459-468.

81. Levanat S, Gorlin RJ, Fallet S, et al. A two-hit model for developmental defects in Gorlin syndrome. Nat Genet. 1996;12:85-87.

82. Gailani MR, Stahle-Backdahl M, Leffell DJ, et al. The role of the human homologue of Drosophila patched in sporadic basal cell carcinomas. Nat Genet. 1996;14:78-81.

83. Marigo V, Davey RA, Zuo Y, et al. Biochemical evidence that patched is the Hedgehog receptor. Nature. 1996;384:176-179.

84. Stone DM, Hynes M, Armanini M, et al. The tumour-suppressor gene patched encodes a candidate receptor for Sonic hedgehog. Nature. 1996;384:129-134.

85. Shimkets R, Gailani MR, Siu VM, et al. Molecular analysis of chromosome 9q deletions in two Gorlin syndrome patients. Am J Hum Genet. 1996;59:417-422.

86. Hahn H, Wojnowski L, Specht K, et al. Patched target Igf2 is indispensable for the formation of medulloblastoma and rhabdomyosarcoma. J Biol Chem. 2000;275:28341-28344.

87. Hahn H, Wojnowski L, Zimmer AM, et al. Rhabdomyosarcomas and radiation hypersensitivity in a mouse model of Gorlin syndrome. Nat Med. 1998;4:619-622.

88. Clement V, Sanchez P, de Tribolet N, et al. HEDGEHOG-GLI1 signaling regulates human glioma growth, cancer stem cell self-renewal, and tumorigenicity. Curr Biol. 2007;17:165-172.

89. Paraf F, Jothy S, Van Meir EG. Brain tumor-polyposis syndrome: two genetic diseases? J Clin Oncol. 1997;15:2744-2758.

90. McMahon AP, Bradley A. The Wnt-1 (int-1) proto-oncogene is required for development of a large region of the mouse brain. Cell. 1990;62:1073-1085.

91. Zhou XP, Marsh DJ, Morrison CD, et al. Germline inactivation of PTEN and dysregulation of the phosphoinositol-3-kinase/Akt pathway cause human Lhermitte-Duclos disease in adults. Am J Hum Genet. 2003;73:1191-1198.

92. Goldman S, Echevarria ME, Fangusaro J. Pediatric brain metastasis from extraneural malignancies: a review. Cancer Treat Res. 2007;136:143-168.

93. Kebudi R, Ayan I, Gorgun O, et al. Brain metastasis in pediatric extracranial solid tumors: survey and literature review. J Neurooncol. 2005;71:43-48.

94. Postovsky S, Ash S, Ramu IN, et al. Central nervous system involvement in children with sarcoma. Oncology. 2003;65:118-124.

95. Reulecke BC, Erker CG, Fiedler BJ, et al. Brain tumors in children: initial symptoms and their influence on the time span between symptom onset and diagnosis. J Child Neurol. 2008;23:178-183.

96. Mehta V, Chapman A, McNeely PD, et al. Latency between symptom onset and diagnosis of pediatric brain tumors: an Eastern Canadian geographic study. Neurosurgery. 2002;51:365-372.

97. Oreskovic NM, Strother CG, Zibners LM. An unusual case of a central nervous system tumor presenting as a chief complaint of depression. Pediatr Emerg Care. 2007;23:486-488.

98. Nakaji P, Meltzer HS, Singel SA, et al. Improvement of aggressive and antisocial behavior after resection of temporal lobe tumors. Pediatrics. 2003;112:e430.

99. Shuper A, Yaniv I, Michowitz S, et al. Epilepsy associated with pediatric brain tumors: the neuro-oncologic perspective. Pediatr Neurol. 2003;29:232-235.

100. Bradley WG Jr. Diagnostic tools in hydrocephalus. Neurosurg Clin N Am. 2001;12:661-684.

101. Morelli D, Pirotte B, Lubansu A, et al. Persistent hydrocephalus after early surgical management of posterior fossa tumors in children: is routine preoperative endoscopic third ventriculostomy justified? J Neurosurg. 2005;103:247-252.

102. Jacobs AH, Kracht LW, Gossmann A, et al. Imaging in neurooncology. NeuroRx. 2005;2:333-347.

103. Tong KA, Ashwal S, Obenaus A, et al. Susceptibility-weighted MR imaging: a review of clinical applications in children. AJNR Am J Neuroradiol. 2008;29:9-17.

104. Ashley WW Jr, McKinstry RC, Leonard JR, et al. Use of rapid-sequence magnetic resonance imaging for evaluation of hydrocephalus in children. J Neurosurg. 2005;103:124-130.

105. Panigrahy A, Krieger MD, Gonzalez-Gomez I, et al. Quantitative short echo time 1H-MR spectroscopy of untreated pediatric brain tumors: preoperative diagnosis and characterization. AJNR Am J Neuroradiol. 2006;27:560-572.

106. Warren KE. NMR spectroscopy and pediatric brain tumors. Oncologist. 2004;9:312-318.

107. Hourani R, Horska A, Albayram S, et al. Proton magnetic resonance spectroscopic imaging to differentiate between nonneoplastic lesions and brain tumors in children. J Magn Reson Imaging. 2006;23:99-107.

108. Marcus KJ, Astrakas LG, Zurakowski D, et al. Predicting survival of children with CNS tumors using proton magnetic resonance spectroscopic imaging biomarkers. Int J Oncol. 2007;30:651-657.

109. Poussaint TY, Rodriguez D. Advanced neuroimaging of pediatric brain tumors: MR diffusion, MR perfusion, and MR spectroscopy. Neuroimaging Clin N Am. 2006;16:169-192.

110. Gauvain KM, McKinstry RC, Mukherjee P, et al. Evaluating pediatric brain tumor cellularity with diffusion-tensor imaging. AJR Am J Roentgenol. 2001;177:449-454.

111. Kono K, Inoue Y, Nakayama K, et al. The role of diffusion-weighted imaging in patients with brain tumors. AJNR Am J Neuroradiol. 2001;22:1081-1088.

112. Witwer BP, Moftakhar R, Hasan KM, et al. Diffusion-tensor imaging of white matter tracts in patients with cerebral neoplasm. J Neurosurg. 2002;97:568-575.

113. Khong PL, Leung LH, Chan GC, et al. White matter anisotropy in childhood medulloblastoma survivors: association with neurotoxicity risk factors. Radiology. 2005;236:647-652.

114. Khong PL, Kwong DL, Chan GC, et al. Diffusion-tensor imaging for the detection and quantification of treatment-induced white matter injury in children with medulloblastoma: a pilot study. AJNR Am J Neuroradiol. 2003;24:734-740.

115. Lai PH, Hsu SS, Ding SW, et al. Proton magnetic resonance spectroscopy and diffusion-weighted imaging in intracranial cystic mass lesions. Surg Neurol. 2007;68(Suppl 1):S25-S36.

116. Bergui M, Zhong J, Bradac GB, et al. Diffusion-weighted images of intracranial cyst-like lesions. Neuroradiology. 2001;43:824-829.

117. Park SH, Chang KH, Song IC, et al. Diffusion-weighted MRI in cystic or necrotic intracranial lesions. Neuroradiology. 2000;42:716-721.

118. Tsuruda JS, Chew WM, Moseley ME, et al. Diffusion-weighted MR imaging of the brain: value of differentiating between extra-axial cysts and epidermoid tumors. AJNR Am J Neuroradiol. 1990;11:925-931.

119. Bukte Y, Paksoy Y, Genc E, et al. Role of diffusion-weighted MR in differential diagnosis of intracranial cystic lesions. Clin Radiol. 2005;60:375-383.

120. Chang SC, Lai PH, Chen WL, et al. Diffusion-weighted MRI features of brain abscess and cystic or necrotic brain tumors: comparison with conventional MRI. Clin Imaging. 2002;26:227-236.

121. Yamasaki F, Kurisu K, Satoh K, et al. Apparent diffusion coefficient of human brain tumors at MR imaging. Radiology. 2005;235:985-991.

122. Cha S. Update on brain tumor imaging: from anatomy to physiology. AJNR Am J Neuroradiol. 2006;27:475-487.

123. Sadeghi N, Camby I, Goldman S, et al. Effect of hydrophilic components of the extracellular matrix on quantifiable diffusion-

weighted imaging of human gliomas: preliminary results of correlating apparent diffusion coefficient values and hyaluronan expression level. AJR Am J Roentgenol. 2003;181:235-241.

124. Omuro AM, Leite CC, Mokhtari K, et al. Pitfalls in the diagnosis of brain tumours. Lancet Neurol. 2006;5:937-948.

125. Schneider JF, Viola A, Confort-Gouny S, et al. Infratentorial pediatric brain tumors: the value of new imaging modalities. J Neuroradiol. 2007;34:49-58.

126. Smith JS, Lin H, Mayo MC, et al. Diffusion-weighted MR imaging abnormalities in pediatric patients with surgically-treated intracranial mass lesions. J Neurooncol. 2006;79:203-209.

127. Rumboldt Z, Camacho DL, Lake D, et al. Apparent diffusion coefficients for differentiation of cerebellar tumors in children. AJNR Am J Neuroradiol. 2006;27:1362-1369.

128. Kan P, Liu JK, Hedlund G, et al. The role of diffusion-weighted magnetic resonance imaging in pediatric brain tumors. Childs Nerv Syst. 2006;22:1435-1439.

129. Rollins N, Winick N, Bash R, et al. Acute methotrexate neurotoxicity: findings on diffusion-weighted imaging and correlation with clinical outcome. AJNR Am J Neuroradiol. 2004;25:1688-1695.

130. Yoshiura T, Wu O, Zaheer A, et al. Highly diffusion-sensitized MRI of brain: dissociation of gray and white matter. Magn Reson Med. 2001;45:734-740.

131. Brunberg JA, Chenevert TL, McKeever PE, et al. In vivo MR determination of water diffusion coefficients and diffusion anisotropy: correlation with structural alteration in gliomas of the cerebral hemispheres. AJNR Am J Neuroradiol. 1995;16:361-371.

132. Stadnik TW, Chaskis C, Michotte A, et al. Diffusion-weighted MR imaging of intracerebral masses: comparison with conventional MR imaging and histologic findings. AJNR Am J Neuroradiol. 2001;22:969-976.

133. Moffat BA, Chenevert TL, Lawrence TS, et al. Functional diffusion map: a noninvasive MRI biomarker for early stratification of clinical brain tumor response. Proc Natl Acad Sci U S A. 2005;102:5524-5529.

134. Hamstra DA, Chenevert TL, Moffat BA, et al. Evaluation of the functional diffusion map as an early biomarker of time-to-progression and overall survival in high-grade glioma. Proc Natl Acad Sci U S A. 2005;102:16759-16764.

135. Covarrubias DJ, Rosen BR, Lev MH. Dynamic magnetic resonance perfusion imaging of brain tumors. Oncologist. 2004;9:528-537.

136. Vonken EJ, van Osch MJ, Bakker CJ, et al. Measurement of cerebral perfusion with dual-echo multi-slice quantitative dynamic susceptibility contrast MRI. J Magn Reson Imaging. 1999;10:109-117.

137. Tombach B, Benner T, Reimer P, et al. Do highly concentrated gadolinium chelates improve MR brain perfusion imaging? Intraindividually controlled randomized crossover concentration comparison study of 0.5 versus 1.0 mol/L gadobutrol. Radiology. 2003;226:880-888.

138. Rowley HA, Roberts TP. Clinical perspectives in perfusion: neuroradiologic applications. Top Magn Reson Imaging. 2004;15:28-40.

139. Wong JC, Provenzale JM, Petrella JR. Perfusion MR imaging of brain neoplasms. AJR Am J Roentgenol. 2000;174:1147-1157.

140. Cha S. Perfusion MR imaging: basic principles and clinical applications. Magn Reson Imaging Clin N Am. 2003;11:403-413.

141. Cha S, Knopp EA, Johnson G, et al. Intracranial mass lesions: dynamic contrast-enhanced susceptibility-weighted echo-planar perfusion MR imaging. Radiology. 2002;223:11-29.

142. Cha S, Lu S, Johnson G, et al. Dynamic susceptibility contrast MR imaging: correlation of signal intensity changes with cerebral blood volume measurements. J Magn Reson Imaging. 2000;11:114-119.

143. Wolf RL, Detre JA. Clinical neuroimaging using arterial spin-labeled perfusion magnetic resonance imaging. Neurotherapeutics. 2007;4:346-359.

144. Wang J, Licht DJ. Pediatric perfusion MR imaging using arterial spin labeling. Neuroimaging Clin N Am. 2006;16:149-167.

145. Bradley WG. Achieving gross total resection of brain tumors: intraoperative MR imaging can make a big difference. AJNR Am J Neuroradiol. 2002;23:348-349.

146. Jolesz FA, Talos IF, Schwartz RB, et al. Intraoperative magnetic resonance imaging and magnetic resonance imaging-guided therapy for brain tumors. Neuroimaging Clin N Am. 2002;12:665-683.

147. Connolly LP, Drubach LA, Ted Treves S. Applications of nuclear medicine in pediatric oncology. Clin Nucl Med. 2002;27:117-125.

148. Khanna G, O'Dorisio MS, Menda Y, et al. Somatostatin receptor scintigraphy in surveillance of pediatric brain malignancies. Pediatr Blood Cancer. 2008;50:561-566.

149. Patil S, Biassoni L, Borgwardt L. Nuclear medicine in pediatric neurology and neurosurgery: epilepsy and brain tumors. Semin Nucl Med. 2007;37:357-381.

150. Jadvar H, Connolly LP, Fahey FH, et al. PET and PET/CT in pediatric oncology. Semin Nucl Med. 2007;37:316-331.

151. Kirton A, Kloiber R, Rigel J, et al. Evaluation of pediatric CNS malignancies with (99m)Tc-methoxyisobutylisonitrile SPECT. J Nucl Med. 2002;43:1438-1443.

152. Pirotte B, Acerbi F, Lubansu A, et al. PET imaging in the surgical management of pediatric brain tumors. Childs Nerv Syst. 2007;23:739-751.

153. Pirotte B, Levivier M, Morelli D, et al. Positron emission tomography for the early postsurgical evaluation of pediatric brain tumors. Childs Nerv Syst. 2005;21:294-300.

154. Poussaint TY, Phillips PC, Vajapeyam S, et al. The Neuroimaging Center of the Pediatric Brain Tumor Consortium-collaborative neuroimaging in pediatric brain tumor research: a work in progress. AJNR Am J Neuroradiol. 2007;28:603-607.

155. Khanna G, O'Dorisio MS, Menda Y, et al. Somatostatin receptor scintigraphy in surveillance of pediatric brain malignancies. Pediatr Blood Cancer. 2008;50:561-566.

156. Fruhwald MC, Rickert CH, O'Dorisio MS, et al. Somatostatin receptor subtype 2 is expressed by supratentorial primitive neuroectodermal tumors of childhood and can be targeted for somatostatin receptor imaging. Clin Cancer Res. 2004;10:2997-3006.

157. Morris EB, Laningham FH, Sandlund JT, et al. Posterior reversible encephalopathy syndrome in children with cancer. Pediatr Blood Cancer. 2007;48:152-159.

158. Doelken M, Lanz S, Rennert J, et al. Differentiation of cytotoxic and vasogenic edema in a patient with reversible posterior leukoencephalopathy syndrome using diffusion-weighted MRI. Diagn Interv Radiol. 2007;13:125-128.

159. Lamy C, Oppenheim C, Meder JF, et al. Neuroimaging in posterior reversible encephalopathy syndrome. J Neuroimaging. 2004;14:89-96.

160. Ahn KJ, You WJ, Jeong SL, et al. Atypical manifestations of reversible posterior leukoencephalopathy syndrome: findings on diffusion imaging and ADC mapping. Neuroradiology. 2004;46:978-983.

161. Covarrubias DJ, Luetmer PH, Campeau NG. Posterior reversible encephalopathy syndrome: prognostic utility of quantitative diffusion-weighted MR images. AJNR Am J Neuroradiol. 2002;23:1038-1048.

162. Koch S, Rabinstein A, Falcone S, et al. Diffusion-weighted imaging shows cytotoxic and vasogenic edema in eclampsia. AJNR Am J Neuroradiol. 2001;22:1068-1070.

163. Bartynski WS, Boardman JF. Distinct imaging patterns and lesion distribution in posterior reversible encephalopathy syndrome. AJNR Am J Neuroradiol. 2007;28:1320-1327.

164. McKinney AM, Short J, Truwit CL, et al. Posterior reversible encephalopathy syndrome: incidence of atypical regions of involvement and imaging findings. AJR Am J Roentgenol. 2007; 189:904-912.

165. Bartynski WS. Posterior reversible encephalopathy syndrome, part 2: controversies surrounding pathophysiology of vasogenic edema. AJNR Am J Neuroradiol. 2008;29:1043-1049.

166. Stott VL, Hurrell MA, Anderson TJ. Reversible posterior leukoencephalopathy syndrome: a misnomer reviewed. Intern Med J. 2005;35:83-90.

167. Obeid T, Awada A. Posterior leukoencephalopathy without severe hypertension: utility of diffusion-weighted MRI. Neurology. 1999;53:1372-1373.

168. Ay H, Buonanno FS, Schaefer PW, et al. Posterior leukoencephalopathy without severe hypertension: utility of diffusion-weighted MRI. Neurology. 1998;51:1369-1376.

169. Ozyurek H, Oguz G, Ozen S, et al. Reversible posterior leukoencephalopathy syndrome: report of three cases. J Child Neurol. 2005;20:990-993.

170. de Graaf N, Hew JM, Fock JM, et al. Predictive value of clinical evaluation in the follow-up of children with a brain tumor. Med Pediatr Oncol. 2002;38:254-257.

171. Kovanlikaya A, Karabay N, Cakmakci H, et al. Surveillance imaging and cost effectivity in pediatric brain tumors. Eur J Radiol. 2003;47:188-192.

172. Louis DN, Ohgaki H, Wiestler OD, et al. WHO Classification of Tumours of the Central Nervous System, 4th ed. Lyon, France, World Health Organization, 2007.

173. Fuller CE, Perry A. Molecular diagnostics in central nervous system tumors. Adv Anat Pathol. 2005;12:180-194.

174. Rickert CH, Paulus W. Prognosis-related histomorphologic and immunohistochemical markers in central nervous system tumors of childhood and adolescence. Acta Neuropathol. 2005;109: 69-92.

175. Pietsch T, Taylor MD, Rutka JT. Molecular pathogenesis of childhood brain tumors. J Neurooncol. 2004;70:203-215.

176. Rickert CH. Prognosis-related molecular markers in pediatric central nervous system tumors. J Neuropathol Exp Neurol. 2004;63:1211-1224.

177. Zakrzewska M, Rieske P, Debiec-Rychter M, et al. Molecular abnormalities in pediatric embryonal brain tumors—analysis of loss of heterozygosity on chromosomes 1, 5, 9, 10, 11, 16, 17 and 22. Clin Neuropathol. 2004;23:209-217.

178. Rorke LB. The future of neuropathology in childhood. Childs Nerv Syst. 2000;16:805-808.

179. Kieran MW. Advances in pediatric neuro-oncology. Curr Opin Neurol. 2000;13:627-634.

180. Daumas-Duport C. The future of neuropathology. Clin Neurosurg. 2000;47:112-120.

181. Takei H, Bhattacharjee MB, Rivera A, et al. New immunohistochemical markers in the evaluation of central nervous system tumors: a review of 7 selected adult and pediatric brain tumors. Arch Pathol Lab Med. 2007;131:234-241.

182. Biegel JA, Pollack IF. Molecular analysis of pediatric brain tumors. Curr Oncol Rep. 2004;6:445-452.

183. Louis DN, Ohgaki H, Wiestler OD, et al. The 2007 WHO classification of tumours of the central nervous system. Acta Neuropathol. 2007;114:97-109.

184. Heuer GG, Jackson EM, Magge SN, et al. Surgical management of pediatric brain tumors. Expert Rev Anticancer Ther. 2007;7: S61-S68.

185. Rutka JT, Kuo JS. Pediatric surgical neuro-oncology: current best care practices and strategies. J Neurooncol. 2004;69: 139-150.

186. Maher CO, Raffel C. Neurosurgical treatment of brain tumors in children. Pediatr Clin North Am. 2004;51:327-357.

187. Albayrak B, Samdani AF, Black PM. Intra-operative magnetic resonance imaging in neurosurgery. Acta Neurochir (Wien). 2004;146:543-556.

188. Vitaz TW, Hushek S, Shields CB, et al. Intraoperative MRI for pediatric tumor management. Acta Neurochir Suppl. 2003;85: 73-78.

189. Matarazzo P, Genitori L, Lala R, et al. Endocrine function and water metabolism in children and adolescents with surgically treated intra/parasellar tumors. J Pediatr Endocrinol Metab. 2004;17:1487-1495.

190. Ray P, Jallo GI, Kim RY, et al. Endoscopic third ventriculostomy for tumor-related hydrocephalus in a pediatric population. Neurosurg Focus. 2005;19:E8.

191. Ruggiero C, Cinalli G, Spennato P, et al. Endoscopic third ventriculostomy in the treatment of hydrocephalus in posterior fossa tumors in children. Childs Nerv Syst. 2004;20:828-833.

192. Cinalli G, Spennato P, Ruggiero C, et al. Complications following endoscopic intracranial procedures in children. Childs Nerv Syst. 2007;23:633-644.

193. Smith ER, Butler WE, Barker FG 2nd. Craniotomy for resection of pediatric brain tumors in the United States, 1988 to 2000: effects of provider caseloads and progressive centralization and specialization of care. Neurosurgery. 2004;54:553-563.

194. Souweidane MM. Endoscopic management of pediatric brain tumors. Neurosurg Focus. 2005;18:E1.

195. Roth J, Biyani N, Beni-Adani L, et al. Real-time neuronavigation with high-quality 3D ultrasound SonoWand in pediatric neurosurgery. Pediatr Neurosurg. 2007;43:185-191.

196. Roth J, Beni-Adani L, Biyani N, et al. Classical and real-time neuronavigation in pediatric neurosurgery. Childs Nerv Syst. 2006;22:1065-1071.

197. McClain CD, Soriano SG, Goumnerova LC, et al. Detection of unanticipated intracranial hemorrhage during intraoperative magnetic resonance image-guided neurosurgery. Report of two cases. J Neurosurg. 2007;106:398-400.

198. Peretta P, Ragazzi P, Galarza M, et al. Complications and pitfalls of neuroendoscopic surgery in children. J Neurosurg. 2006;105:187-193.

199. Kassam A, Thomas AJ, Snyderman C, et al. Fully endoscopic expanded endonasal approach treating skull base lesions in pediatric patients. J Neurosurg. 2007;106:75-86.

200. Cole CD, Gottfried ON, Liu JK, et al. Hyponatremia in the neurosurgical patient: diagnosis and management. Neurosurg Focus. 2004;16:E9.

201. Papadimitriou DT, Spiteri A, Pagnier A, et al. Mineralocorticoid deficiency in post-operative cerebral salt wasting. J Pediatr Endocrinol Metab. 2007;20:1145-1150.

202. Jimenez R, Casado-Flores J, Nieto M, et al. Cerebral salt wasting syndrome in children with acute central nervous system injury. Pediatr Neurol. 2006;35:261-263.

203. Kinik ST, Kandemir N, Baykan A, et al. Fludrocortisone treatment in a child with severe cerebral salt wasting. Pediatr Neurosurg. 2001;35:216-219.

204. Hiranrat P, Katavetin P, Supornsilchai V, et al. Water and sodium disorders in children undergoing surgical treatment of brain tumors. J Med Assoc Thai. 2003;86(Suppl 2): S152-S159.

205. Cardoso AP, Dragosavac D, Araujo S, et al. Syndromes related to sodium and arginine vasopressin alterations in post-operative neurosurgery. Arq Neuropsiquiatr. 2007;65:745-751.

206. Turgut M. Cerebellar mutism. J Neurosurg Pediatrics. 2008;1:262.

207. Robertson PL, Muraszko KM, Holmes EJ, et al. Incidence and severity of postoperative cerebellar mutism syndrome in children with medulloblastoma: a prospective study by the Children's Oncology Group. J Neurosurg. 2006;105:444-451.

208. Ersahin Y, Yararbas U, Duman Y, et al. Single photon emission tomography following posterior fossa surgery in patients with and without mutism. Childs Nerv Syst. 2002;18:318-325.

209. Semrad TJ, O'Donnell R, Wun T, et al. Epidemiology of venous thromboembolism in 9489 patients with malignant glioma. J Neurosurg. 2007;106:601-608.

210. Blom JW, Vanderschoot JP, Oostindier MJ, et al. Incidence of venous thrombosis in a large cohort of 66,329 cancer patients: results of a record linkage study. J Thromb Haemost. 2006; 4:529-535.

211. Deitcher SR, Gajjar A, Kun L, et al. Clinically evident venous thromboembolic events in children with brain tumors. J Pediatr. 2004;145:848-850.

212. Tabori U, Beni-Adani L, Dvir R, et al. Risk of venous thromboembolism in pediatric patients with brain tumors. Pediatr Blood Cancer. 2004;43:633-666.

213. Levy ML, Granville RC, Hart D, et al. Deep venous thrombosis in children and adolescents. J Neurosurg. 2004;101:32-37.

214. Heisel M, Nagib M, Madsen L, et al. Use of recombinant factor VIIa (rFVIIa) to control intraoperative bleeding in pediatric brain tumor patients. Pediatr Blood Cancer. 2004;43:703-705.

215. Knab B, Connell PP. Radiotherapy for pediatric brain tumors: when and how. Expert Rev Anticancer Ther. 2007;7:S69-S77.

216. Kirsch DG, Tarbell NJ. Conformal radiation therapy for childhood CNS tumors. Oncologist. 2004;9:442-450.

217. Lo SS, Fakiris AJ, Abdulrahman R, et al. Role of stereotactic radiosurgery and fractionated stereotactic radiotherapy in pediatric brain tumors. Expert Rev Neurother. 2008;8:121-132.

218. Penagaricano JA, Papanikolaou N, Yan Y, et al. Application of intensity-modulated radiation therapy for pediatric malignancies. Med Dosim. 2004;29:247-253.

219. Suh JH, Barnett GH. Stereotactic radiosurgery for brain tumors in pediatric patients. Technol Cancer Res Treat. 2003;2:141-146.

220. Giller CA, Berger BD, Pistenmaa DA, et al. Robotically guided radiosurgery for children. Pediatr Blood Cancer. 2005;45:304-310.

221. Yock TI, Tarbell NJ. Technology insight: Proton beam radiotherapy for treatment in pediatric brain tumors. Nat Clin Pract Oncol. 2004;1:97-103.

222. Kirsch DG, Tarbell NJ. New technologies in radiation therapy for pediatric brain tumors: the rationale for proton radiation therapy. Pediatr Blood Cancer. 2004;42:461-464.

223. Levin WP, Kooy H, Loeffler JS, et al. Proton beam therapy. Br J Cancer. 2005;93:849-854.

224. Miralbell R, Fitzgerald TJ, Laurie F, et al. Radiotherapy in pediatric medulloblastoma: quality assessment of Pediatric Oncology Group Trial 9031. Int J Radiat Oncol Biol Phys. 2006;64:1325-1330.

225. Gajjar A, Chintagumpala MM, Bowers DC, et al. Effect of intrapatient dosage escalation of irinotecan on its pharmacokinetics in pediatric patients who have high-grade gliomas and receive enzyme-inducing anticonvulsant therapy. Cancer. 2003;97:2374-2380.

226. Crews KR, Stewart CF, Jones-Wallace D, et al. Altered irinotecan pharmacokinetics in pediatric high-grade glioma patients receiving enzyme-inducing anticonvulsant therapy. Clin Cancer Res. 2002;8:2202-2209.

227. Houghton PJ, Morton CL, Tucker C, et al. The pediatric preclinical testing program: description of models and early testing results. Pediatr Blood Cancer. 2007;49:928-940.

228. Gururangan S, Friedman HS. Innovations in design and delivery of chemotherapy for brain tumors. Neuroimaging Clin N Am. 2002;12:583-597.

229. Kellie SJ, Barbaric D, Koopmans P, et al. Cerebrospinal fluid concentrations of vincristine after bolus intravenous dosing: a surrogate marker of brain penetration. Cancer. 2002;94:1815-1820.

230. Stapleton S, Blaney S. New agents for intrathecal administration. Cancer Invest. 2006;24:528-534.

231. Gururangan S, Petros WP, Poussaint TY, et al. Phase I trial of intrathecal spartaject busulfan in children with neoplastic meningitis: a Pediatric Brain Tumor Consortium Study (PBTC-004). Clin Cancer Res. 2006;12:1540-1546.

232. Blaney SM, Boyett J, Friedman H, et al. Phase I clinical trial of mafosfamide in infants and children aged 3 years or younger with newly diagnosed embryonal tumors: a pediatric brain tumor consortium study (PBTC-001). J Clin Oncol. 2005;23:525-531.

233. Slavc I, Schuller E, Falger J, et al. Feasibility of long-term intraventricular therapy with mafosfamide (n = 26) and etoposide (n = 11): experience in 26 children with disseminated malignant brain tumors. J Neurooncol. 2003;64:239-247.

234. Warren K, Jakacki R, Widemann B, et al. Phase II trial of intravenous lobradimil and carboplatin in childhood brain tumors: a report from the Children's Oncology Group. Cancer Chemother Pharmacol. 2006;58:343-347.

235. Gururangan S, Friedman HS. Recent advances in the treatment of pediatric brain tumors. Oncology (Williston Park). 2004;18:1649-1661.

236. Furchert SE, Lanvers-Kaminsky C, Juurgens H, et al. Inhibitors of histone deacetylases as potential therapeutic tools for high-risk embryonal tumors of the nervous system of childhood. Int J Cancer. 2007;120:1787-1794.

237. Wagner S, Peters O, Fels C, et al. Pegylated-liposomal doxorubicin and oral topotecan in eight children with relapsed high-grade malignant brain tumors. J Neurooncol. 2008;86:175-181.

238. Kellie SJ, Koopmans P, Earl J, et al. Increasing the dosage of vincristine: a clinical and pharmacokinetic study of continuous-infusion vincristine in children with central nervous system tumors. Cancer. 2004;100:2637-2643.

239. Kieran MW, Packer RJ, Onar A, et al. Phase I and pharmacokinetic study of the oral farnesyltransferase inhibitor lonafarnib administered twice daily to pediatric patients with advanced central nervous system tumors using a modified continuous reassessment method: a Pediatric Brain Tumor Consortium Study. J Clin Oncol. 2007;25:3137-3143.

240. de Bont JM, den Boer ML, Kros JM, et al. Identification of novel biomarkers in pediatric primitive neuroectodermal tumors and ependymomas by proteome-wide analysis. J Neuropathol Exp Neurol. 2007;66:505-516.

241. de Bont JM, den Boer ML, Reddingius RE, et al. Identification of apolipoprotein A-II in cerebrospinal fluid of pediatric brain tumor patients by protein expression profiling. Clin Chem. 2006;52:1501-1509.

242. Warren K. Molecularly targeted therapy for pediatric brain tumors. J Neurooncol. 2005;75:335-343.

243. Nakamura M, Shimada K, Ishida E, et al. Molecular pathogenesis of pediatric astrocytic tumors. Neuro Oncol. 2007;9:113-123.

244. Pollack IF, Jakacki RI, Blaney SM, et al. Phase I trial of imatinib in children with newly diagnosed brainstem and recurrent malignant gliomas: a Pediatric Brain Tumor Consortium report. Neuro Oncol. 2007;9:145-160.

245. Widemann BC, Salzer WL, Arceci RJ, et al. Phase I trial and pharmacokinetic study of the farnesyltransferase inhibitor tipifarnib in children with refractory solid tumors or neurofibromatosis type I and plexiform neurofibromas. J Clin Oncol. 2006;24:507-516.

246. Worth LL, Jeha SS, Kleinerman ES. Biologic response modifiers in pediatric cancer. Hematol Oncol Clin North Am. 2001;15:723-740.

247. Raffaghello L, Nozza P, Morandi F, et al. Expression and functional analysis of human leukocyte antigen class I antigen-

processing machinery in medulloblastoma. Cancer Res. 2007; 67:5471-5478.

248. Rutkowski S, De Vleeschouwer S, Kaempgen E, et al. Surgery and adjuvant dendritic cell-based tumour vaccination for patients with relapsed malignant glioma, a feasibility study. Br J Cancer. 2004;91:1656-1662.

249. Caruso DA, Orme LM, Neale AM, et al. Results of a phase 1 study using monocyte-derived dendritic cells pulsed with tumor RNA in children and young adults with brain cancer. Neuro Oncol. 2004;6:236-246.

250. Kramm CM, Korholz D, Rainov NG, et al. Systemic activation of the immune system during ganciclovir treatment following intratumoral herpes simplex virus type 1 thymidine kinase gene transfer in an adolescent ependymoma patient. Neuropediatrics. 2002;33:6-9.

251. Pollack IF, Keating R. New delivery approaches for pediatric brain tumors. J Neurooncol. 2005;75:315-326.

252. Kieran MW. Anti-angiogenic therapy in pediatric neuro-oncology. J Neurooncol. 2005;75:327-334.

253. Kieran MW, Turner CD, Rubin JB, et al. A feasibility trial of antiangiogenic (metronomic) chemotherapy in pediatric patients with recurrent or progressive cancer. J Pediatr Hematol Oncol. 2005;27:573-581.

254. Lafay-Cousin L, Holm S, Qaddoumi I, et al. Weekly vinblastine in pediatric low-grade glioma patients with carboplatin allergic reaction. Cancer. 2005;103:2636-2642.

255. Sterba J, Pavelka Z, Slampa P. Concomitant radiotherapy and metronomic temozolomide in pediatric high-risk brain tumors. Neoplasma. 2002;49:117-120.

256. Broniscer A, Gururangan S, MacDonald TJ, et al. Phase I trial of single-dose temozolomide and continuous administration of o6-benzylguanine in children with brain tumors: a pediatric brain tumor consortium report. Clin Cancer Res. 2007; 13:6712-6718.

257. Neville K, Blaney S, Bernstein M, et al. Pharmacokinetics of O(6)-benzylguanine in pediatric patients with central nervous system tumors: a pediatric oncology group study. Clin Cancer Res. 2004;10:5072-5075.

258. Valera ET, Lucio-Eterovic AK, Neder L, et al. Quantitative PCR analysis of the expression profile of genes related to multiple drug resistance in tumors of the central nervous system. J Neurooncol. 2007;85:1-10.

259. Gottschling S, Reinhard H, Pagenstecher C, et al. Hypothesis: possible role of retinoic acid therapy in patients with biallelic mismatch repair gene defects. Eur J Pediatr. 2008;167: 225-229.

260. Ziegler DS, Cohn RJ, McCowage G, et al. Efficacy of vincristine and etoposide with escalating cyclophosphamide in poor-prognosis pediatric brain tumors. Neuro Oncol. 2006;8:53-59.

261. McCowage GB, Friedman HS, Moghrabi A, et al. Activity of high-dose cyclophosphamide in the treatment of childhood malignant gliomas. Med Pediatr Oncol. 1998;30:75-80.

262. Ashley DM, Longee D, Tien R, et al. Treatment of patients with pineoblastoma with high-dose cyclophosphamide. Med Pediatr Oncol. 1996;6:387-392.

263. Foreman NK, Schissel D, Le T, et al. A study of sequential high-dose cyclophosphamide and high dose carboplatin with peripheral stem-cell rescue in resistant or recurrent pediatric brain tumors. J Neurooncol. 2005;71:181-187.

264. Gardner SL. Application of stem cell transplant for brain tumors. Pediatr Transplant. 2004;8(Suppl 5):28-32.

265. Cheuk DK, Lee TL, Chiang AK, et al. Autologous hematopoietic stem cell transplantation for high-risk brain tumors in children. J Neurooncol. 2008;86:337-347.

266. Marachelian A, Butturini A, Finlay J. Myeloablative chemotherapy with autologous hematopoietic progenitor cell rescue for childhood central nervous system tumors. Bone Marrow Transplant. 2008;41:167-172.

267. Spreafico F, Gandola L, Marchiano A, et al. Brain magnetic resonance imaging after high-dose chemotherapy and radiotherapy for childhood brain tumors. Int J Radiat Oncol Biol Phys. 2008;70:1011-1019.

268. Daumas-Duport C, Beuvon F, Varlet P, et al. Gliomas: WHO and Sainte-Anne Hospital classifications. Ann Pathol. 2000; 20:413-428.

269. Scheithauer BW, Hawkins C, Tihan T, et al. Pilocytic astrocytoma. In Louis DN, Ohgaki H, Wiestler OD, et al (eds). WHO Classification of Tumours of the Central Nervous System, 4th ed. Geneva, World Health Organization Press, 2007, pp 14-21.

270. Rodriguez HA, Berthrong M. Multiple primary intracranial tumors in von Recklinghausen's neurofibromatosis. Arch Neurol. 1966;14:467-475.

271. Orr LC, Fleitz J, McGavran L, et al. Cytogenetics in pediatric low-grade astrocytomas. Med Pediatr Oncol. 2002;38:173-177.

272. Di Sapio A, Morra I, Pradotto L, et al. Molecular genetic changes in a series of neuroepithelial tumors of childhood. J Neurooncol. 2002;59:117-122.

273. Pfister S, Janzarik WG, Remke M, et al. BRAF gene duplication constitutes a mechanism of MAPK pathway activation in low-grade astrocytomas. J Clin Invest. 2008;118:1739-1749.

274. Stuer C, Vilz B, Majores M, et al. Frequent recurrence and progression in pilocytic astrocytoma in adults. Cancer. 2007; 110:2799-2808.

275. Shaw EG, Wisoff JH. Prospective clinical trials of intracranial low-grade glioma in adults and children. Neuro Oncol. 2003; 5:153-160.

276. Tabori U, Vukovic B, Zielenska M, et al. The role of telomere maintenance in the spontaneous growth arrest of pediatric low-grade gliomas. Neoplasia. 2006;8:136-142.

277. Huber J, Sovinz P, Lackner H, et al. Diencephalic syndrome: a frequently delayed diagnosis in failure to thrive. Klin Padiatr. 2007;219:91-94.

278. Fleischman A, Brue C, Poussaint TY, et al. Diencephalic syndrome: a cause of failure to thrive and a model of partial growth hormone resistance. Pediatrics. 2005;115:e742-e748.

279. Murakami R, Hirai T, Kitajima M, et al. Magnetic resonance imaging of pilocytic astrocytomas: usefulness of the minimum apparent diffusion coefficient (ADC) value for differentiation from high-grade gliomas. Acta Radiol. 2008;49:462-467.

280. Dirven CM, Koudstaal J, Mooij JJ, et al. The proliferative potential of the pilocytic astrocytoma: the relation between MIB-1 labeling and clinical and neuro-radiological follow-up. J Neurooncol. 1998;37:9-16.

281. Aryan HE, Meltzer HS, Lu DC, et al. Management of pilocytic astrocytoma with diffuse leptomeningeal spread: two cases and review of the literature. Childs Nerv Syst. 2005;21: 477-481.

282. Hukin J, Siffert J, Cohen H, et al. Leptomeningeal dissemination at diagnosis of pediatric low-grade neuroepithelial tumors. Neuro Oncol. 2003;5:188-196.

283. Fernandez C, Figarella-Branger D, Girard N, et al. Pilocytic astrocytomas in children: prognostic factors—a retrospective study of 80 cases. Neurosurgery. 2003;53:544-553.

284. Tihan T, Fisher PG, Kepner JL, et al. Pediatric astrocytomas with monomorphous pilomyxoid features and a less favorable outcome. J Neuropathol Exp Neurol. 1999;58:1061-1068.

285. Watson GA, Kadota RP, Wisoff JH. Multidisciplinary management of pediatric low-grade gliomas. Semin Radiat Oncol. 2001;11:152-162.

286. Mishra KK, Puri DR, Missett BT, et al. The role of up-front radiation therapy for incompletely resected pediatric WHO grade II low-grade gliomas. Neuro Oncol. 2006;8:166-174.

287. Wisoff JH. Management of optic pathway tumors of childhood. Neurosurg Clin N Am. 1992;3:791-802.

288. Gururangan S, Cavazos CM, Ashley D, et al. Phase II study of carboplatin in children with progressive low-grade gliomas. J Clin Oncol. 2002;20:2951-2958.

289. Aquino VM, Fort DW, Kamen BA. Carboplatin for the treatment of children with newly diagnosed optic chiasm gliomas: a phase II study. J Neurooncol. 1999;41:255-259.

290. Moghrabi A, Friedman HS, Burger PC, et al. Carboplatin treatment of progressive optic pathway gliomas to delay radiotherapy. J Neurosurg. 1993;79:223-227.

291. Friedman HS, Krischer JP, Burger P, et al. Treatment of children with progressive or recurrent brain tumors with carboplatin or iproplatin: a Pediatric Oncology Group randomized phase II study. J Clin Oncol. 1992;10:249-256.

292. Kadota RP, Kun LE, Langston JW, et al. Cyclophosphamide for the treatment of progressive low-grade astrocytoma: a Pediatric Oncology Group phase II Study. J Pediatr Hematol Oncol. 1999;21:198-202.

293. McCowage G, Tien R, McLendon R, et al. Successful treatment of childhood pilocytic astrocytomas metastatic to the leptomeninges with high-dose cyclophosphamide. Med Pediatr Oncol. 1996;27:32-39.

294. Heideman RL, Douglass EC, Langston JA, et al. A phase II study of every other day high-dose ifosamide in pediatric brain tumors: a Pediatric Oncology Group Study. J Neurooncol. 1995;25:77-84.

295. Nicholson HS, Kretschmar CS, Krailo M, et al. Phase 2 study of temozolomide in children and adolescents with recurrent central nervous system tumors: a report from the Children's Oncology Group. Cancer. 2007;110:1542-1550.

296. Khaw SL, Coleman LT, Downie PA, et al. Temozolomide in pediatric low-grade glioma. Pediatr Blood Cancer. 2007;49:808-811.

297. Gururangan S, Fisher MJ, Allen JC, et al. Temozolomide in children with progressive low-grade glioma. Neuro Oncol. 2007;9:161-168.

298. Chamoun RB, Alaraj AM, Al Kutoubi AO, et al. Role of temozolomide in spinal cord low grade astrocytomas: results in two paediatric patients. Acta Neurochir (Wien). 2006;148:175-179.

299. Mulne AF, Ducore JM, Elterman RD, et al. Oral methotrexate for recurrent brain tumors in children: a Pediatric Oncology Group study. J Pediatr Hematol Oncol. 2000;22:41-44.

300. Blaney SM, Phillips PC, Packer RJ, et al. Phase II evaluation of topotecan for pediatric central nervous system tumors. Cancer. 1996;78:527-531.

301. Kadota RP, Stewart CF, Horn M, et al. Topotecan for the treatment of recurrent or progressive central nervous system tumors—a pediatric oncology group phase II study. J Neurooncol. 1999;43:43-47.

302. Chamberlain MC. Recurrent cerebellar gliomas: salvage therapy with oral etoposide. J Child Neurol. 1997;12:200-204.

303. Chamberlain MC, Grafe MR. Recurrent chiasmatic-hypothalamic glioma treated with oral etoposide. J Clin Oncol. 1995;13:2072-2076.

304. Packer RJ, Sutton LN, Bilaniuk LT, et al. Treatment of chiasmatic/hypothalamic gliomas of childhood with chemotherapy: an update. Ann Neurol. 1988;23:79-85.

305. Gnekow AK, Kortmann RD, Pietsch T, et al. Low grade chiasmatic-hypothalamic glioma-carboplatin and vincristin chemotherapy effectively defers radiotherapy within a comprehensive treatment strategy—report from the multicenter treatment study for children and adolescents with a low grade glioma—HIT-LGG 1996—of the Society of Pediatric Oncology and Hematology (GPOH). Klin Padiatr. 2004;216:331-342.

306. Packer RJ, Ater J, Allen J, et al. Carboplatin and vincristine chemotherapy for children with newly diagnosed progressive low-grade gliomas. J Neurosurg. 1997;86:747-754.

307. Packer RJ, Lange B, Ater J, et al. Carboplatin and vincristine for recurrent and newly diagnosed low-grade gliomas of childhood. J Clin Oncol. 1993;11:850-856.

308. Castello MA, Schiavetti A, Padula A, et al. Does chemotherapy have a role in low-grade astrocytoma management? A report of 13 cases. Med Pediatr Oncol. 1995;25:102-108.

309. Massimino M, Spreafico F, Cefalo G, et al. High response rate to cisplatin/etoposide regimen in childhood low-grade glioma. J Clin Oncol. 2002;20:4209-4216.

310. Pons MA, Finlay JL, Walker RW, et al. Chemotherapy with vincristine (VCR) and etoposide (VP-16) in children with low-grade astrocytoma. J Neurooncol. 1992;14:151-158.

311. Walter AW, Gajjar A, Reardon DA, et al. Tamoxifen and carboplatin for children with low-grade gliomas: a pilot study at St. Jude Children's Research Hospital. J Pediatr Hematol Oncol. 2000;22:247-251.

312. Petronio J, Edwards MS, Prados M, et al. Management of chiasmal and hypothalamic gliomas of infancy and childhood with chemotherapy. J Neurosurg. 1991;74:701-708.

313. Prados MD, Edwards MS, Rabbitt J, et al. Treatment of pediatric low-grade gliomas with a nitrosourea-based multiagent chemotherapy regimen. J Neurooncol. 1997;32:235-241.

314. Laithier V, Grill J, Le Deley MC, et al. Progression-free survival in children with optic pathway tumors: dependence on age and the quality of the response to chemotherapy—results of the first French prospective study for the French Society of Pediatric Oncology. J Clin Oncol. 2003;21:4572-4578.

315. Bruggers CS, Greene D. A phase 2 feasibility study of sequential, dose intensive chemotherapy to treat progressive low-grade gliomas in children. J Pediatr Hematol Oncol. 2007;29:602-607.

316. Lee MJ, Ra YS, Park JB, et al. Effectiveness of novel combination chemotherapy, consisting of 5-fluorouracil, vincristine, cyclophosphamide and etoposide, in the treatment of low-grade gliomas in children. J Neurooncol. 2006;80:277-284.

317. Lancaster DL, Hoddes JA, Michalski A. Tolerance of nitrosourea-based multiagent chemotherapy regime for low-grade pediatric gliomas. J Neurooncol. 2003;63:289-294.

318. Hsu TR, Wong TT, Chang FC, et al. Responsiveness of progressive optic pathway tumors to cisplatin-based chemotherapy in children. Childs Nerv Syst. 2008;24:1457-1461.

319. Perilongo G. Considerations on the role of chemotherapy and modern radiotherapy in the treatment of childhood low grade glioma. J Neurooncol. 2005;75:301-307.

320. Zacharoulis S, Kieran MW. Treatment of low-grade gliomas in children: an update. Expert Rev Neurother. 2004;4:1005-1014.

321. Mahoney DH Jr, Cohen ME, Friedman HS, et al. Carboplatin is effective therapy for young children with progressive optic pathway tumors: a Pediatric Oncology Group phase II study. Neuro Oncol. 2000;2:213-220.

322. Moghrabi A, Friedman HS, Ashley DM, et al. Phase II study of carboplatin (CBDCA) in progressive low-grade gliomas. Neurosurg Focus. 1998;4:e3.

323. Quinn JA, Reardon DA, Friedman AH, et al. Phase II trial of temozolomide in patients with progressive low-grade glioma. J Clin Oncol. 2003;21:646-651.

324. Barone G, Maurizi P, Tamburrini G, et al. Role of temozolomide in pediatric brain tumors. Childs Nerv Syst. 2006;22:652-661.

325. Valera ET, Serafini LN, Machado HR, et al. Complete surgical resection in children with low-grade astrocytomas after neoadjuvant chemotherapy. Childs Nerv Syst. 2003;19:86-90.

326. Heath JA, Turner CD, Poussaint TY, et al. Chemotherapy for progressive low-grade gliomas in children older than ten years: the Dana-Farber experience. Pediatr Hematol Oncol. 2003;20:497-504.

327. Marcus KJ, Goumnerova L, Billett AL, et al. Stereotactic radiotherapy for localized low-grade gliomas in children: final results of a prospective trial. Int J Radiat Oncol Biol Phys. 2005;61: 374-379.

328. Arita K, Kurisu K, Sugiyama K, et al. Long-term results of conventional treatment of diencephalic pilocytic astrocytoma in infants. Childs Nerv Syst. 2003;19:145-151.

329. Serdaroglu A, Simsek F, Gucuyener K, et al. Moyamoya syndrome after radiation therapy for optic pathway glioma: case report. J Child Neurol. 2000;15:765-767.

330. Fisher BJ, Leighton CC, Vujovic O, et al. Results of a policy of surveillance alone after surgical management of pediatric low grade gliomas. Int J Radiat Oncol Biol Phys. 2001;51: 704-710.

331. Gajjar A, Sanford RA, Heideman R, et al. Low-grade astrocytoma: a decade of experience at St. Jude Children's Research Hospital. J Clin Oncol. 1997;15:2792-2799.

332. Benesch M, Eder HG, Sovinz P, et al. Residual or recurrent cerebellar low-grade glioma in children after tumor resection: is re-treatment needed? A single center experience from 1983 to 2003. Pediatr Neurosurg. 2006;42:159-164.

333. Aarsen FK, Paquier PF, Reddingius RE, et al. Functional outcome after low-grade astrocytoma treatment in childhood. Cancer. 2006;106:396-402.

334. Casadei GP, Arrigoni GL, D'Angelo V, et al. Late malignant recurrence of childhood cerebellar astrocytoma. Clin Neuropathol. 1990;9:295-298.

335. Shamji MF, Benoit BG. Syndromic and sporadic pediatric optic pathway gliomas: review of clinical and histopathological differences and treatment implications. Neurosurg Focus. 2007; 23:E3.

336. Deliganis AV, Geyer JR, Berger MS. Prognostic significance of type 1 neurofibromatosis (von Recklinghausen disease) in childhood optic glioma. Neurosurgery. 1996;38:1114-1118.

337. Binning MJ, Liu JK, Kestle JR, et al. Optic pathway gliomas: a review. Neurosurg Focus. 2007;23:E2.

338. Czyzyk E, Jozwiak S, Roszkowski M, et al. Optic pathway gliomas in children with and without neurofibromatosis 1. J Child Neurol. 2003;18:471-478.

339. Cummings TJ, Provenzale JM, Hunter SB, et al. Gliomas of the optic nerve: histological, immunohistochemical (MIB-1 and p53), and MRI analysis. Acta Neuropathol. 2000;99:563-570.

340. Armstrong GT, Localio AR, Feygin T, et al. Defining optic nerve tortuosity. AJNR Am J Neuroradiol. 2007;28:666-671.

341. Buschmann U, Gers B, Hildebrandt G. Pilocytic astrocytomas with leptomeningeal dissemination: biological behavior, clinical course, and therapeutical options. Childs Nerv Syst. 2003;19: 298-304.

342. King A, Listernick R, Charrow J, et al. Optic pathway gliomas in neurofibromatosis type 1: the effect of presenting symptoms on outcome. Am J Med Genet A. 2003;122A:95-99.

343. Silva MM, Goldman S, Keating G, et al. Optic pathway hypothalamic gliomas in children under three years : the role of chemotherapy. Pediatr Neurosurg. 2000;33:151-158.

344. Lacaze E, Kieffer V, Streri A, et al. Neuropsychologic outcome in children with optic pathway tumours when first-line treatment is chemotherapy. Br J Cancer. 2003;89:2038-2044.

345. Kato T, Sawamura Y, Tada M, et al. Cisplatin/vincristine chemotherapy for hypothalamic/visual pathway astrocytomas in young children. J Neurooncol. 1998;37:263-270.

346. Shuper A, Horev G, Kornreich L, et al. Visual pathway glioma: an erratic tumour with therapeutic dilemmas. Arch Dis Child. 1997;76:259-263.

347. Hug EB, Muenter MW, Archambeau JO, et al. Conformal proton radiation therapy for pediatric low-grade astrocytomas. Strahlenther Onkol. 2002;178:10-17.

348. Jahraus CD, Tarbell NJ. Optic pathway gliomas. Pediatr Blood Cancer. 2006;46:586-596.

349. Peraud A, Goetz C, Siefert A, et al. Interstitial iodine-125 radiosurgery alone or in combination with microsurgery for pediatric patients with eloquently located low-grade glioma: a pilot study. Childs Nerv Syst. 2007;23:39-46.

350. Opocher E, Kremer LC, Da Dalt L, et al. Prognostic factors for progression of childhood optic pathway glioma: a systematic review. Eur J Cancer. 2006;42:1807-1816.

351. Sharif S, Ferner R, Birch JM, et al. Second primary tumors in neurofibromatosis 1 patients treated for optic glioma: substantial risks after radiotherapy. J Clin Oncol. 2006;24:2570-2575.

352. Jallo GI, Biser-Rohrbaugh A, Freed D. Brainstem gliomas. Childs Nerv Syst. 2004;20:143-153.

353. Recinos PF, Sciubba DM, Jallo GI. Brainstem tumors: where are we today? Pediatr Neurosurg. 2007;43:192-201.

354. Badhe PB, Chauhan PP, Mehta NK. Brainstem gliomas—a clinicopathological study of 45 cases with p53 immunohistochemistry. Indian J Cancer. 2004;41:170-174.

355. Distelmaier F, Janssen G, Mayatepek E, et al. Disseminated pilocytic astrocytoma involving brain stem and diencephalon: a history of atypical eating disorder and diagnostic delay. J Neurooncol. 2006;79:197-201.

356. Lesniak MS, Klem JM, Weingart J, et al. Surgical outcome following resection of contrast-enhanced pediatric brainstem gliomas. Pediatr Neurosurg. 2003;39:314-322.

357. Kestle J, Townsend JJ, Brockmeyer DL, et al. Juvenile pilocytic astrocytoma of the brainstem in children. J Neurosurg. 2004; 101:1-6.

358. Phillips NS, Sanford RA, Helton KJ, et al. Diffusion tensor imaging of intraaxial tumors at the cervicomedullary and pontomedullary junctions. Report of two cases. J Neurosurg. 2005;103:557-562.

359. Jallo GI, Shiminski-Maher T, Velazquez L, et al. Recovery of lower cranial nerve function after surgery for medullary brainstem tumors. Neurosurgery. 2005;56:74-77.

360. Puget S, Crimmins DW, Garnett MR, et al. Thalamic tumors in children: a reappraisal. J Neurosurg. 2007;106:354-362.

361. Fernandez C, Maues de Paula A, Colin C, et al. Thalamic gliomas in children: an extensive clinical, neuroradiological and pathological study of 14 cases. Childs Nerv Syst. 2006;22: 1603-1610.

362. Colosimo C, di Lella GM, Tartaglione T, et al. Neuroimaging of thalamic tumors in children. Childs Nerv Syst. 2002;18: 426-439.

363. Martinez-Lage JF, Perez-Espejo MA, Esteban JA, et al. Thalamic tumors: clinical presentation. Childs Nerv Syst. 2002; 18:405-411.

364. Di Rocco C, Iannelli A. Bilateral thalamic tumors in children. Childs Nerv Syst. 2002;18:440-444.

365. Burger PC, Cohen KJ, Rosenblum MK, et al. Pathology of diencephalic astrocytomas. Pediatr Neurosurg. 2000;32: 214-219.

366. Messing-Junger AM, Floeth FW, Pauleit D, et al. Multimodal target point assessment for stereotactic biopsy in children with diffuse bithalamic astrocytomas. Childs Nerv Syst. 2002;18: 445-449.

367. Baroncini M, Vinchon M, Mineo JF, et al. Surgical resection of thalamic tumors in children: approaches and clinical results. Childs Nerv Syst. 2007;23:753-760.

368. Albright AL. Feasibility and advisability of resections of thalamic tumors in pediatric patients. J Neurosurg. 2004;100:468-472.

369. Tomita T, Cortes RF. Astrocytomas of the cerebral peduncle in children: surgical experience in seven patients. Childs Nerv Syst. 2002;18:225-230.

370. Reardon DA, Gajjar A, Sanford RA, et al. Bithalamic involvement predicts poor outcome among children with thalamic glial tumors. Pediatr Neurosurg. 1998;29:29-35.

371. Brauner R, Trivin C, Zerah M, et al. Diencephalic syndrome due to hypothalamic tumor: a model of the relationship between

weight and puberty onset. J Clin Endocrinol Metab. 2006; 91:2467-2473.

372. Dejkhamron P, Likasitwattankul S, Unachak K. Diencephalic syndrome: a rare and easily overlooked cause of failure to thrive. J Med Assoc Thai. 2004;87:984-987.

373. Perilongo G, Carollo C, Salviati L, et al. Diencephalic syndrome and disseminated juvenile pilocytic astrocytomas of the hypothalamic-optic chiasm region. Cancer. 1997;80: 142-146.

374. Poussaint TY, Barnes PD, Nichols K, et al. Diencephalic syndrome: clinical features and imaging findings. AJNR Am J Neuroradiol. 1997;18:1499-1505.

375. Gropman AL, Packer RJ, Nicholson HS, et al. Treatment of diencephalic syndrome with chemotherapy: growth, tumor response, and long term control. Cancer. 1998;83:166-172.

376. Shuper A, Bloch I, Kornreich L, et al. Successful chemotherapeutic treatment of diencephalic syndrome with continued tumor presence. Pediatr Hematol Oncol. 1996;13:443-449.

377. Kageji T, Nagahiro S, Horiguchi H, et al. Successful high-dose chemotherapy for widespread neuroaxis dissemination of an optico-hypothalamic juvenile pilocytic astrocytoma in an infant: a case report. J Neurooncol. 2003;62:281-287.

378. Akay KM, Izci Y, Baysefer A, et al. Surgical outcomes of cerebellar tumors in children. Pediatr Neurosurg. 2004;40: 220-225.

379. McKean-Cowdin R, Preston-Martin S, Pogoda JM, et al. Parental occupation and childhood brain tumors: astroglial and primitive neuroectodermal tumors. J Occup Environ Med. 1998;40:332-340.

380. Nishio S, Morioka T, Suzuki S, et al. Thalamic gliomas: a clinicopathologic analysis of 20 cases with reference to patient age. Acta Neurochir (Wien). 1997;139:336-342.

381. von Deirmling A, Burger PC, Nakazato Y, et al. Diffuse astrocytoma. In Louis DN, Ohgaki H, Wiestler OD, et al (eds). WHO Classification of Tumours of the Central Nervous System, 4th ed. Geneva, World Health Organization Press, 2007, pp 25-29.

382. Giangaspero F, Kaulich K, Cenacchi G, et al. Lipoastrocytoma: a rare low-grade astrocytoma variant of pediatric age. Acta Neuropathol. 2002;103:152-156.

383. Tomita T, Chou P, Reyes-Mugica M. IV ventricle astrocytomas in childhood: clinicopathological features in 21 cases. Childs Nerv Syst. 1998;14:537-546.

384. Ernestus RI, Schroder R, Stutzer H, et al. Prognostic relevance of localization and grading in intracranial ependymomas of childhood. Childs Nerv Syst. 1996;12:522-526.

385. Jallo GI, Danish S, Velasquez L, et al. Intramedullary low-grade astrocytomas: long-term outcome following radical surgery. J Neurooncol. 2001;53:61-66.

386. Schmandt SM, Packer RJ. Treatment of low-grade pediatric gliomas. Curr Opin Oncol. 2000;12:194-198.

387. Reddy AT, Packer RJ. Chemotherapy for low-grade gliomas. Childs Nerv Syst. 1999;15:506-513.

388. Allen JC, Siffert J. Contemporary chemotherapy issues for children with brainstem gliomas. Pediatr Neurosurg. 1996;24: 98-102.

389. Stark AM, Fritsch MJ, Claviez A, et al. Management of tectal glioma in childhood. Pediatr Neurol. 2005;33:33-38.

390. Hamilton MG, Lauryssen C, Hagen N. Focal midbrain glioma: long term survival in a cohort of 16 patients and the implications for management. Can J Neurol Sci. 1996;23:204-207.

391. Packer RJ. Brain tumors in children. Arch Neurol. 1999; 56:421-425.

392. Pollack IF, Claassen D, al-Shboul Q, et al. Low-grade gliomas of the cerebral hemispheres in children: an analysis of 71 cases. J Neurosurg. 1995;82:536-547.

393. Mauffrey C. Paediatric brainstem gliomas: prognostic factors and management. J Clin Neurosci. 2006;13:431-437.

394. Avninder S, Sharma MC, Deb P, et al. Gemistocytic astrocytomas: histomorphology, proliferative potential and genetic alterations—a study of 32 cases. J Neurooncol. 2006;78:123-127.

395. Reis RM, Hara A, Kleihues P, et al. Genetic evidence of the neoplastic nature of gemistocytes in astrocytomas. Acta Neuropathol. 2001;102:422-425.

396. Desai KI, Nadkarni TD, Muzumdar DP, et al. Prognostic factors for cerebellar astrocytomas in children: a study of 102 cases. Pediatr Neurosurg. 2001;35:311-317.

397. Fisher BJ, Naumova E, Leighton CC, et al. Ki-67: a prognostic factor for low-grade glioma? Int J Radiat Oncol Biol Phys. 2002;52:996-1001.

398. Beebe DW, Ris MD, Armstrong FD, et al. Cognitive and adaptive outcome in low-grade pediatric cerebellar astrocytomas: evidence of diminished cognitive and adaptive functioning in National Collaborative Research Studies (CCG 9891/POG 9130). J Clin Oncol. 2005;23:5198-5204.

399. Li KW, Roonprapunt C, Lawson HC, et al. Endoscopic third ventriculostomy for hydrocephalus associated with tectal gliomas. Neurosurg Focus. 2005;18:E2.

400. Wellons JC 3rd, Tubbs RS, Banks JT, et al. Long-term control of hydrocephalus via endoscopic third ventriculostomy in children with tectal plate gliomas. Neurosurgery. 2002;51:63-67.

401. Drake J, Chumas P, Kestle J, et al. Late rapid deterioration after endoscopic third ventriculostomy: additional cases and review of the literature. J Neurosurg. 2006;105:118-126.

402. Ternier J, Wray A, Puget S, et al. Tectal plate lesions in children. J Neurosurg. 2006;104:369-376.

403. Bowers DC, Georgiades C, Aronson LJ, et al. Tectal gliomas: natural history of an indolent lesion in pediatric patients. Pediatr Neurosurg. 2000;32:24-29.

404. Robertson PL, Muraszko KM, Brunberg JA, et al. Pediatric midbrain tumors: a benign subgroup of brainstem gliomas. Pediatr Neurosurg. 1995;22:65-73.

405. Komotar RJ, Mocco J, Jones JE, et al. Pilomyxoid astrocytoma: diagnosis, prognosis, and management. Neurosurg Focus. 2005;18:E7.

406. Komotar RJ, Mocco J, Carson BS, et al. Pilomyxoid astrocytoma: a review. MedGenMed. 2004;6:42.

407. Melendez B, Fiano C, Ruano Y, et al. BCR gene disruption in a pilomyxoid astrocytoma. Neuropathology. 2006;26:442-446.

408. Jeon YK, Cheon JE, Kim SK, et al. Clinicopathological features and global genomic copy number alterations of pilomyxoid astrocytoma in the hypothalamus/optic pathway: comparative analysis with pilocytic astrocytoma using array-based comparative genomic hybridization. Mod Pathol. 2008;21:1345-1356.

409. Mendiratta-Lala M, Kader Ellika S, Gutierrez JA, et al. Spinal cord pilomyxoid astrocytoma: an unusual tumor. J Neuroimaging. 2007;17:371-374.

410. Komotar RJ, Mocco J, Zacharia BE, et al. Astrocytoma with pilomyxoid features presenting in an adult. Neuropathology. 2006;26:89-93.

411. Chikai K, Ohnishi A, Kato T, et al. Clinico-pathological features of pilomyxoid astrocytoma of the optic pathway. Acta Neuropathol. 2004;108:109-114.

412. Hamada H, Kurimoto M, Hayashi N, et al. Pilomyxoid astrocytoma in a patient presenting with fatal hemorrhage. Case report. J Neurosurg Pediatrics. 2008;1:244-246.

413. Gottfried ON, Fults DW, Townsend JJ, et al. Spontaneous hemorrhage associated with a pilomyxoid astrocytoma. Case report. J Neurosurg. 2003;99:416-420.

414. Komakula ST, Fenton LZ, Kleinschmidt-DeMasters BK, et al. Pilomyxoid astrocytoma: neuroimaging with clinicopathologic correlates in 4 cases followed over time. J Pediatr Hematol Oncol. 2007;29:465-470.

415. Arslanoglu A, Cirak B, Horska A, et al. MR imaging characteristics of pilomyxoid astrocytomas. AJNR Am J Neuroradiol. 2003;24:1906-1908.

416. Komotar RJ, Zacharia BE, Sughrue ME, et al. Magnetic resonance imaging characteristics of pilomyxoid astrocytoma. Neurol Res. 2008;30:945-951.

417. Morales H, Kwock L, Castillo M. Magnetic resonance imaging and spectroscopy of pilomyxoid astrocytomas: case reports and comparison with pilocytic astrocytomas. J Comput Assist Tomogr. 2007;31:682-687.

418. Fuller CE, Frankel B, Smith M, et al. Suprasellar monomorphous pilomyxoid neoplasm: an ultastructural analysis. Clin Neuropathol. 2001;20:256-262.

419. de Chadarevian JP, Halligan GE, Reddy G, et al. Glioneuronal phenotype in a diencephalic pilomyxoid astrocytoma. Pediatr Dev Pathol. 2006;9:480-487.

420. Ceppa EP, Bouffet E, Griebel R, et al. The pilomyxoid astrocytoma and its relationship to pilocytic astrocytoma: report of a case and a critical review of the entity. J Neurooncol. 2007;81:191-196.

421. Cirak B, Horska A, Barker PB, et al. Proton magnetic resonance spectroscopic imaging in pediatric pilomyxoid astrocytoma. Childs Nerv Syst. 2005;21:404-409.

422. Komotar RJ, Burger PC, Carson BS, et al. Pilocytic and pilomyxoid hypothalamic/chiasmatic astrocytomas. Neurosurgery. 2004;54:72-79.

423. Enting RH, van der Graaf WT, Kros JM, et al. Radiotherapy plus concomitant and adjuvant temozolomide for leptomeningeal pilomyxoid astrocytoma: a case study. J Neurooncol. 2006;80:107-108.

424. Johnson JH Jr, Hariharan S, Berman J, et al. Clinical outcome of pediatric gangliogliomas: ninety-nine cases over 20 years. Pediatr Neurosurg. 1997;27:203-207.

425. Baussard B, Di Rocco F, Garnett MR, et al. Pediatric infratentorial gangliogliomas: a retrospective series. J Neurosurg. 2007;107:286-291.

426. Karabekir HS, Balci C, Tokyol C. Primary spinal anaplastic ganglioglioma. Pediatr Neurosurg. 2006;42:374-378.

427. Luyken C, Blumcke I, Fimmers R, et al. Supratentorial gangliogliomas: histopathologic grading and tumor recurrence in 184 patients with a median follow-up of 8 years. Cancer. 2004; 101:146-155.

428. Zentner J, Wolf HK, Ostertun B, et al. Gangliogliomas: clinical, radiological, and histopathological findings in 51 patients. J Neurol Neurosurg Psychiatry. 1994;57:1497-1502.

429. De Munnynck K, Van Gool S, Van Calenbergh F, et al. Desmoplastic infantile ganglioglioma: a potentially malignant tumor? Am J Surg Pathol. 2002;26:1515-1522.

430. Becker AJ, Wiestler OD, Figarella-Branger D, et al. Ganglioglioma and gangliocytoma. In Louis DN, Ohgaki H, Wiestler OD, et al (eds). WHO Classification of Tumours of the Central Nervous System, 4th ed. Geneva, World Health Organization Press, 2007, pp 103-105.

431. Cataltepe O, Turanli G, Yalnizoglu D, et al. Surgical management of temporal lobe tumor-related epilepsy in children. J Neurosurg. 2005;102:280-287.

432. Im SH, Chung CK, Cho BK, et al. Supratentorial ganglioglioma and epilepsy: postoperative seizure outcome. J Neurooncol. 2002;57:59-66.

433. Liauw SL, Byer JE, Yachnis AT, et al. Radiotherapy after subtotally resected or recurrent ganglioglioma. Int J Radiat Oncol Biol Phys. 2007;67:244-247.

434. Jallo GI, Freed D, Epstein FJ. Spinal cord gangliogliomas: a review of 56 patients. J Neurooncol. 2004;68:71-77.

435. Bachli H, Avoledo P, Gratzl O, et al. Therapeutic strategies and management of desmoplastic infantile ganglioglioma: two case reports and literature overview. Childs Nerv Syst. 2003;19: 359-366.

436. Sugiyama K, Arita K, Shima T, et al. Good clinical course in infants with desmoplastic cerebral neuroepithelial tumor treated by surgery alone. J Neurooncol. 2002;59:63-69.

437. Tamburrini G, Colosimo C Jr, Giangaspero F, et al. Desmoplastic infantile ganglioglioma. Childs Nerv Syst. 2003;19: 292-297.

438. Daumas-Duport C, Scheithauer BW, Chodkiewicz JP, et al. Dysembryoplastic neuroepithelial tumor: a surgically curable tumor of young patients with intractable partial seizures. Report of thirty-nine cases. Neurosurgery. 1988;23:545-556.

439. Daumas-Duport C, Pietsch T, Hawkins C, et al. Dysembryoplastic neuroepithelial tumour. In Louis DN, Ohgaki H, Wiestler OD, et al (eds). WHO Classification of Tumours of the Central Nervous System, 4th ed. Geneva, World Health Organization Press, 2007, pp 99-102.

440. Sandberg DI, Ragheb J, Dunoyer C, et al. Surgical outcomes and seizure control rates after resection of dysembryoplastic neuroepithelial tumors. Neurosurg Focus. 2005;18:E5.

441. Nolan MA, Sakuta R, Chuang N, et al. Dysembryoplastic neuroepithelial tumors in childhood: long-term outcome and prognostic features. Neurology. 2004;62:2270-2276.

442. Park JY, Suh YL, Han J. Dysembryoplastic neuroepithelial tumor. Features distinguishing it from oligodendroglioma on cytologic squash preparations. Acta Cytol. 2003;47:624-629.

443. Vogelgesang S, Kunert-Keil C, Cascorbi I, et al. Expression of multidrug transporters in dysembryoplastic neuroepithelial tumors causing intractable epilepsy. Clin Neuropathol. 2004;23:223-231.

444. Rushing EJ, Thompson LD, Mena H. Malignant transformation of a dysembryoplastic neuroepithelial tumor after radiation and chemotherapy. Ann Diagn Pathol. 2003;7:240-244.

445. Weber RG, Hoischen A, Ehrler M, et al. Frequent loss of chromosome 9, homozygous CDKN2A/p14(ARF)/CDKN2B deletion and low TSC1 mRNA expression in pleomorphic xanthoastrocytomas. Oncogene. 2007;26:1088-1097.

446. Saikali S, Le Strat A, Heckly A, et al. Multicentric pleomorphic xanthoastrocytoma in a patient with neurofibromatosis type 1. Case report and review of the literature. J Neurosurg. 2005; 102:376-381.

447. Passone E, Pizzolitto S, D'Agostini S, et al. Non-anaplastic pleomorphic xanthoastrocytoma with neuroradiological evidences of leptomeningeal dissemination. Childs Nerv Syst. 2006;22:614-618.

448. Hirose T, Ishizawa K, Sugiyama K, et al. Pleomorphic xanthoastrocytoma: a comparative pathological study between conventional and anaplastic types. Histopathology. 2008;52: 183-193.

449. Giannini C, Scheithauer BW, Burger PC, et al. Pleomorphic xanthoastrocytoma: what do we really know about it? Cancer. 1999;85:2033-2045.

450. Reifenberger G, Kaulich K, Wiestler OD, et al. Expression of the CD34 antigen in pleomorphic xanthoastrocytomas. Acta Neuropathol. 2003;105:358-364.

451. Sugita Y, Shigemori M, Okamoto K, et al. Clinicopathologic study of pleomorphic xanthoastrocytoma: correlation between histologic features and prognosis. Pathol Int. 2000;50:703-708.

452. Fouladi M, Jenkins J, Burger P, et al. Pleomorphic xanthoastrocytoma: favorable outcome after complete surgical resection. Neuro Oncol. 2001;3:184-192.

453. Cartmill M, Hewitt M, Walker D, et al. The use of chemotherapy to facilitate surgical resection in pleomorphic xanthoastrocytoma: experience in a single case. Childs Nerv Syst. 2001;17:563-566.

454. Bucciero A, De Caro M, De Stefano V, et al. Pleomorphic xanthoastrocytoma: clinical, imaging and pathologic features of four cases. Clin Neurol Neurosurg. 1997;99:40-45.

455. Marton E, Feletti A, Orvieto E, et al. Malignant progression in pleomorphic xanthoastrocytoma: personal experience and review of the literature. J Neurol Sci. 2007;52:144-153.

456. Tekkok IH, Sav A. Anaplastic pleomorphic xanthoastrocytomas. Review of the literature with reference to malignancy potential. Pediatr Neurosurg. 2004;40:171-181.

457. Kumar R, Singh V. Subependymal giant cell astrocytoma: a report of five cases. Neurosurg Rev. 2004;27:274-280.

458. Lopes MBS, Wiestler O, Stemmer-Rachamimov AO, et al. Tuberous sclerosis complex and subependymal giant cell astrocytoma. In Louis DN, Ohgaki H, Wiestler OD, et al (eds). WHO Classification of Tumours of the Central Nervous System, 4th ed. Geneva, World Health Organization Press, 2007, pp 218-221.

459. Stavrinou P, Spiliotopoulos A, Patsalas I, et al. Subependymal giant cell astrocytoma with intratumoral hemorrhage in the absence of tuberous sclerosis. J Clin Neurosci. 2008;15:704-706.

460. Dashti SR, Robinson S, Rodgers M, et al. Pineal region giant cell astrocytoma associated with tuberous sclerosis: case report. J Neurosurg. 2005;102:322-325.

461. DiMario FJ Jr. Brain abnormalities in tuberous sclerosis complex. J Child Neurol. 2004;19:650-657.

462. Nabbout R, Santos M, Rolland Y, et al. Early diagnosis of subependymal giant cell astrocytoma in children with tuberous sclerosis. J Neurol Neurosurg Psychiatry. 1999;66:370-375.

463. Buccoliero AM, Franchi A, Castiglione F, et al. Subependymal giant cell astrocytoma (SEGA): Is it an astrocytoma? Morphological, immunohistochemical and ultrastructural study. Neuropathology. 2009;29:25-30.

464. You H, Kim YI, Im SY, et al. Immunohistochemical study of central neurocytoma, subependymoma, and subependymal giant cell astrocytoma. J Neurooncol. 2005;74:1-8.

465. de Ribaupierre S, Dorfmuller G, Bulteau C, et al. Subependymal giant-cell astrocytomas in pediatric tuberous sclerosis disease: when should we operate? Neurosurgery. 2007;60:83-89.

466. Cuccia V, Zuccaro G, Sosa F, et al. Subependymal giant cell astrocytoma in children with tuberous sclerosis. Childs Nerv Syst. 2003;19:232-243.

467. Crino PB, Nathanson KL, Henske EP. The tuberous sclerosis complex. N Engl J Med. 2006;355:1345-1356.

468. Glasker S. Central nervous system manifestations in VHL: genetics, pathology and clinical phenotypic features. Fam Cancer. 2005;4:37-42.

469. Plate KH, Vortmeyer AO, Zagzag D, et al. Von Hippel-Lindau disease and haemangioblastoma. In Louis DN, Ohgaki H, Wiestler OD, et al (eds). WHO Classification of Tumours of the Central Nervous System, 4th ed. Geneva, World Health Organization Press, 2007, pp 215-217.

470. Winestone JS, Lin J, Sanford RA, et al. Subependymal hemangioblastomas of the cervicomedullary junction: lessons learned in the management of two cases. Childs Nerv Syst. 2007;23:761-764.

471. Jagannathan J, Lonser RR, Smith R, et al. Surgical management of cerebellar hemangioblastomas in patients with von Hippel-Lindau disease. J Neurosurg. 2008;108:210-222.

472. Vougioukas VI, Glasker S, Hubbe U, et al. Surgical treatment of hemangioblastomas of the central nervous system in pediatric patients. Childs Nerv Syst. 2006;22:1149-1153.

473. Montano N, Doglietto F, Pedicelli A, et al. Embolization of hemangioblastomas. J Neurosurg. 2008;108:1063-1064.

474. Matsunaga S, Shuto T, Inomori S, et al. Gamma knife radiosurgery for intracranial haemangioblastomas. Acta Neurochir (Wien). 2007;149:1007-1013.

475. Girmens JF, Erginay A, Massin P, et al. Treatment of von Hippel-Lindau retinal hemangioblastoma by the vascular endothelial growth factor receptor inhibitor SU5416 is more effective for associated macular edema than for hemangioblastomas. Am J Ophthalmol. 2003;136:194-196.

476. Lieberman KA, Wasenko JJ, Schelper R, et al. Tanycytomas: a newly characterized hypothalamic-suprasellar and ventricular tumor. AJNR Am J Neuroradiol. 2003;24:1999-2004.

477. Chen KS, Hung PC, Wang HS, et al. Medulloblastoma or cerebellar dysplastic gangliocytoma (Lhermitte-Duclos disease)? Pediatr Neurol. 2002;27:404-406.

478. Bredel M, Pollack IF, Hamilton RL, et al. Epidermal growth factor receptor expression and gene amplification in high-grade non-brainstem gliomas of childhood. Clin Cancer Res. 1999;5:1786-1792.

479. Gallia GL, Rand V, Siu IM, et al. PIK3CA gene mutations in pediatric and adult glioblastoma multiforme. Mol Cancer Res. 2006;4:709-714.

480. Korshunov A, Sycheva R, Gorelyshev S, et al. Clinical utility of fluorescence in situ hybridization (FISH) in nonbrainstem glioblastomas of childhood. Mod Pathol. 2005;18:1258-1263.

481. Raffel C, Frederick L, O'Fallon JR, et al. Analysis of oncogene and tumor suppressor gene alterations in pediatric malignant astrocytomas reveals reduced survival for patients with PTEN mutations. Clin Cancer Res. 1999;5:4085-4090.

482. Bredel M, Pollack IF, Hamilton RL, et al. DNA topoisomerase IIalpha predicts progression-free and overall survival in pediatric malignant nonbrainstem gliomas. Int J Cancer. 2002;99:817-820.

483. Newcomb EW, Alonso M, Sung T, et al. Incidence of p14ARF gene deletion in high-grade adult and pediatric astrocytomas. Hum Pathol. 2000;31:115-119.

484. Broniscer A, Gajjar A. Supratentorial high-grade astrocytoma and diffuse brainstem glioma: two challenges for the pediatric oncologist. Oncologist. 2004;9:197-206.

485. Pollack IF, Finkelstein SD, Woods J, et al. Expression of p53 and prognosis in children with malignant gliomas. N Engl J Med. 2002;346:420-427.

486. Ganigi PM, Santosh V, Anandh B, et al. Expression of p53, EGFR, pRb and bcl-2 proteins in pediatric glioblastoma multiforme: a study of 54 patients. Pediatr Neurosurg. 2005;41:292-299.

487. Sung T, Miller DC, Hayes RL, et al. Preferential inactivation of the p53 tumor suppressor pathway and lack of EGFR amplification distinguish de novo high grade pediatric astrocytomas from de novo adult astrocytomas. Brain Pathol. 2000;10:249-259.

488. Smith JS, Tachibana I, Passe SM, et al. PTEN mutation, EGFR amplification, and outcome in patients with anaplastic astrocytoma and glioblastoma multiforme. J Natl Cancer Inst. 2001;93:1246-1256.

489. Pytel P. Spectrum of pediatric gliomas: implications for the development of future therapies. Expert Rev Anticancer Ther. 2007;7:S51-S60.

490. Rickert CH, Strater R, Kaatsch P, et al. Pediatric high-grade astrocytomas show chromosomal imbalances distinct from adult cases. Am J Pathol. 2001;158:1525-1532.

491. Faury D, Nantel A, Dunn SE, et al. Molecular profiling identifies prognostic subgroups of pediatric glioblastoma and shows increased YB-1 expression in tumors. J Clin Oncol. 2007;25:1196-1208.

492. Eckert A, Kloor M, Giersch A, et al. Microsatellite instability in pediatric and adult high-grade gliomas. Brain Pathol. 2007;17:146-150.

493. Pollack IF, Hamilton RL, James CD, et al. Rarity of PTEN deletions and EGFR amplification in malignant gliomas of childhood: results from the Children's Cancer Group 945 cohort. J Neurosurg. 2006;105:418-424.

494. Pollack IF, Hamilton RL, Burnham J, et al. Impact of proliferation index on outcome in childhood malignant gliomas:

results in a multi-institutional cohort. Neurosurgery. 2002;50: 1238-1244.

495. Malkin D, Li FP, Strong LC, et al. Germ line p53 mutations in a familial syndrome of breast cancer, sarcomas, and other neoplasms. Science. 1990;250:1233-1238.

496. Portwine C, Chilton-MacNeill S, Brown C, et al. Absence of germline and somatic p53 alterations in children with sporadic brain tumors. J Neurooncol. 2001;52:227-235.

497. Hou LC, Bababeygy SR, Sarkissian V, et al. Congenital glioblastoma multiforme: case report and review of the literature. Pediatr Neurosurg. 2008;44:304-312.

498. Lasky JL, Choi EJ, Johnston S, et al. Congenital brain tumors: case series and review of the literature. J Pediatr Hematol Oncol. 2008;30:326-331.

499. Brat DJ, Shehata BM, Castellano-Sanchez AA, et al. Congenital glioblastoma: a clinicopathologic and genetic analysis. Brain Pathol. 2007;17:276-281.

500. Frappaz D. High-grade gliomas: babies are not small adults! Pediatr Blood Cancer. 2007;49:879-880.

501. Duffner PK, Krischer JP, Burger PC, et al. Treatment of infants with malignant gliomas: the Pediatric Oncology Group experience. J Neurooncol. 1996;28:245-256.

502. Geyer JR, Finlay JL, Boyett JM, et al. Survival of infants with malignant astrocytomas. A Report from the Childrens Cancer Group. Cancer. 1995;75:1045-1050.

503. Tamber MS, Rutka JT. Pediatric supratentorial high-grade gliomas. Neurosurg Focus. 2003;14:e1.

504. Donson AM, Erwin NS, Kleinschmidt-DeMasters BK, et al. Unique molecular characteristics of radiation-induced glioblastoma. J Neuropathol Exp Neurol. 2007;66:740-749.

505. Wagner S, Benesch M, Berthold F, et al. Secondary dissemination in children with high-grade malignant gliomas and diffuse intrinsic pontine gliomas. Br J Cancer. 2006;95:991-997.

506. Benesch M, Wagner S, Berthold F, et al. Primary dissemination of high-grade gliomas in children: experiences from four studies of the Pediatric Oncology and Hematology Society of the German Language Group (GPOH). J Neurooncol. 2005;72: 179-183.

507. Chang YW, Yoon HK, Shin HJ, et al. MR imaging of glioblastoma in children: usefulness of diffusion/perfusion-weighted MRI and MR spectroscopy. Pediatr Radiol. 2003;33:836-842.

508. Almqvist PM, Mah R, Lendahl U, et al. Immunohistochemical detection of nestin in pediatric brain tumors. J Histochem Cytochem. 2002;50:147-158.

509. De Prada I, Cordobes F, Azorin D, et al. Pediatric giant cell glioblastoma: a case report and review of the literature. Childs Nerv Syst. 2006;22:285-289.

510. Reddy AT, Wellons JC 3rd. Pediatric high-grade gliomas. Cancer J. 2003;9:107-112.

511. Pollack IF. The role of surgery in pediatric gliomas. J Neurooncol. 1999;42:271-288.

512. Kramm CM, Wagner S, Van Gool S, et al. Improved survival after gross total resection of malignant gliomas in pediatric patients from the HIT-GBM studies. Anticancer Res. 2006; 26:3773-3779.

513. Finlay JL, Zacharoulis S. The treatment of high grade gliomas and diffuse intrinsic pontine tumors of childhood and adolescence: a historical—and futuristic—perspective. J Neurooncol. 2005;75:253-266.

514. Walker MD, Alexander E, Jr, Hunt WE, et al. Evaluation of BCNU and/or radiotherapy in the treatment of anaplastic gliomas. A cooperative clinical trial. J Neurosurg. 1978;49: 333-343.

515. Wisoff JH, Boyett JM, Berger MS, et al. Current neurosurgical management and the impact of the extent of resection in the treatment of malignant gliomas of childhood: a report of the Children's Cancer Group trial no. CCG-945. J Neurosurg. 1998;89:52-59.

516. Donson AM, Addo-Yobo SO, Handler MH, et al. MGMT promoter methylation correlates with survival benefit and sensitivity to temozolomide in pediatric glioblastoma. Pediatr Blood Cancer. 2007;48:403-407.

517. Pollack IF, Hamilton RL, Sobol RW, et al. O6-methylguanine-DNA methyltransferase expression strongly correlates with outcome in childhood malignant gliomas: results from the CCG-945 Cohort. J Clin Oncol. 2006;24:3431-3437.

518. Chintagumpala MM, Friedman HS, Stewart CF, et al. A phase II window trial of procarbazine and topotecan in children with high-grade glioma: a report from the Children's Oncology Group. J Neurooncol. 2006;77:193-198.

519. Wolff JE, Wagner S, Sindichakis M, et al. Simultaneous radiochemotherapy in pediatric patients with high-grade glioma: a phase I study. Anticancer Res. 2002;22:3569-3572.

520. Lopez-Aguilar E, Sepulveda-Vildosola AC, Rivera-Marquez H, et al. Preirradiation ifosfamide, carboplatin and etoposide (ICE) for the treatment of high-grade astrocytomas in children. Childs Nerv Syst. 2003;19:818-823.

521. Stupp R, Mason WP, van den Bent MJ, et al. Radiotherapy plus concomitant and adjuvant temozolomide for glioblastoma. N Engl J Med. 2005;352:987-996.

522. Loh KC, Willert J, Meltzer H, et al. Temozolomide and radiation for aggressive pediatric central nervous system malignancies. J Pediatr Hematol Oncol. 2005;27:254-258.

523. Jakacki RI, Yates A, Blaney SM, et al. A phase I trial of temozolomide and lomustine in newly diagnosed high-grade gliomas of childhood. Neuro Oncol. 2008;10:569-576.

524. Massimino M, Gandola L, Luksch R, et al. Sequential chemotherapy, high-dose thiotepa, circulating progenitor cell rescue, and radiotherapy for childhood high-grade glioma. Neuro Oncol. 2005;7:41-48.

525. Dunkel IJ, Finlay JL. High-dose chemotherapy with autologous stem cell rescue for brain tumors. Crit Rev Oncol Hematol. 2002;41:197-204.

526. Massimino M, Biassoni V. Use of high-dose chemotherapy in front-line therapy of childhood malignant glioma. Expert Rev Anticancer Ther. 2006;6:709-717.

527. Finlay JL, Goldman S, Wong MC, et al. Pilot study of high-dose thiotepa and etoposide with autologous bone marrow rescue in children and young adults with recurrent CNS tumors. The Children's Cancer Group. J Clin Oncol. 1996;14:2495-2503.

528. Lashford LS, Thiesse P, Jouvet A, et al. Temozolomide in malignant gliomas of childhood: a United Kingdom Children's Cancer Study Group and French Society for Pediatric Oncology Intergroup Study. J Clin Oncol. 2002;20:4684-4691.

529. Wolff JE, Wagner S, Reinert C, et al. Maintenance treatment with interferon-gamma and low-dose cyclophosphamide for pediatric high-grade glioma. J Neurooncol. 2006;79:315-321.

530. Wagner S, Erdlenbruch B, Langler A, et al. Oral topotecan in children with recurrent or progressive high-grade glioma: a Phase I/II study by the German Society for Pediatric Oncology and Hematology. Cancer. 2004;100:1750-1757.

531. Dufour C, Grill J, Lellouch-Tubiana A, et al. High-grade glioma in children under 5 years : a chemotherapy only approach with the BBSFOP protocol. Eur J Cancer. 2006;42:2939-2945.

532. Bucci MK, Maity A, Janss AJ, et al. Near complete surgical resection predicts a favorable outcome in pediatric patients with nonbrainstem, malignant gliomas: results from a single center in the magnetic resonance imaging era. Cancer. 2004;101: 817-824.

533. Burger PC, Vogel FS, Green SB, et al. Glioblastoma multiforme and anaplastic astrocytoma. Pathologic criteria and prognostic implications. Cancer. 1985;56:1106-1111.

534. Winters JL, Wilson D, Davis DG. Congenital glioblastoma multiforme: a report of three cases and a review of the literature. J Neurol Sci. 2001;188:13-19.

535. Fabi A, Mirri A, Felici A, et al. Fixed dose-rate gemcitabine as radiosensitizer for newly diagnosed glioblastoma: a dose-finding study. J Neurooncol. 2008;87:79-84.

536. Ford JM, Seiferheld W, Alger JR, et al. Results of the phase I dose-escalating study of motexafin gadolinium with standard radiotherapy in patients with glioblastoma multiforme. Int J Radiat Oncol Biol Phys. 2007;69:831-838.

537. MacDonald TJ, Stewart CF, Kocak M, et al. Phase I clinical trial of cilengitide in children with refractory brain tumors: Pediatric Brain Tumor Consortium Study PBTC-012. J Clin Oncol. 2008;26:919-924.

538. Wolff JE, Classen CF, Wagner S, et al. Subpopulations of malignant gliomas in pediatric patients: analysis of the HIT-GBM database. J Neurooncol. 2008;87:155-164.

539. Barkovich AJ, Krischer J, Kun LE, et al. Brain stem gliomas: a classification system based on magnetic resonance imaging. Pediatr Neurosurg. 1990;16:73-83.

540. Epstein F. A staging system for brain stem gliomas. Cancer. 1985;56:1804-1806.

541. Sandri A, Sardi N, Genitori L, et al. Diffuse and focal brain stem tumors in childhood: prognostic factors and surgical outcome. Experience in a single institution. Childs Nerv Syst. 2006;22:1127-1135.

542. Fischbein NJ, Prados MD, Wara W, et al. Radiologic classification of brain stem tumors: correlation of magnetic resonance imaging appearance with clinical outcome. Pediatr Neurosurg. 1996;24:9-23.

543. Korones DN. Treatment of newly diagnosed diffuse brain stem gliomas in children: in search of the holy grail. Expert Rev Anticancer Ther. 2007;7:663-674.

544. Dunkel IJ, Souweidane MM. Brain stem tumors. Curr Treat Options Neurol. 2005;7:315-321.

545. Gilbertson RJ, Hill DA, Hernan R, et al. ERBB1 is amplified and overexpressed in high-grade diffusely infiltrative pediatric brain stem glioma. Clin Cancer Res. 2003;9:3620-3624.

546. Roujeau T, Machado G, Garnett MR, et al. Stereotactic biopsy of diffuse pontine lesions in children. J Neurosurg. 2007;107:1-4.

547. Sho A, Kondo S, Kamitani H, et al. Establishment of experimental glioma models at the intrinsic brainstem region of the rats. Neurol Res. 2007;29:36-42.

548. Jallo GI, Becker M, Liu YJ, et al. Local infusion therapy in the monkey brainstem: technical considerations. Surg Technol Int. 2006;15:311-316.

549. Hargrave DR, Mabbott DJ, Bouffet E. Pathological laughter and behavioural change in childhood pontine glioma. J Neurooncol. 2006;77:267-271.

550. Schumacher M, Schulte-Monting J, Stoeter P, et al. Magnetic resonance imaging compared with biopsy in the diagnosis of brainstem diseases of childhood: a multicenter review. J Neurosurg. 2007;106:111-119.

551. Laprie A, Pirzkall A, Haas-Kogan DA, et al. Longitudinal multivoxel MR spectroscopy study of pediatric diffuse brainstem gliomas treated with radiotherapy. Int J Radiat Oncol Biol Phys. 2005;62:20-31.

552. Hayward RM, Patronas N, Baker EH, et al. Inter-observer variability in the measurement of diffuse intrinsic pontine gliomas. J Neurooncol. 2008;90:57-61.

553. Hargrave D, Chuang N, Bouffet E. Conventional MRI cannot predict survival in childhood diffuse intrinsic pontine glioma. J Neurooncol. 2008;86:313-319.

554. Zagzag D, Miller DC, Knopp E, et al. Primitive neuroectodermal tumors of the brainstem: investigation of seven cases. Pediatrics. 2000;106:1045-1053.

555. Fisher PG, Breiter SN, Carson BS, et al. A clinicopathologic reappraisal of brain stem tumor classification. Identification of pilocystic astrocytoma and fibrillary astrocytoma as distinct entities. Cancer. 2000;89:1569-1576.

556. Kwon JW, Kim IO, Cheon JE, et al. Paediatric brain-stem gliomas: MRI, FDG-PET and histological grading correlation. Pediatr Radiol. 2006;36:959-964.

557. Massimino M, Spreafico F, Biassoni V, et al. Diffuse pontine gliomas in children: changing strategies, changing results? A mono-institutional 20-year experience. J Neurooncol. 2008; 87:355-361.

558. Wagner S, Warmuth-Metz M, Emser A, et al. Treatment options in childhood pontine gliomas. J Neurooncol. 2006;79: 281-287.

559. Korones DN, Fisher PG, Kretschmar C, et al. Treatment of children with diffuse intrinsic brain stem glioma with radiotherapy, vincristine and oral VP-16: a Children's Oncology Group phase II study. Pediatr Blood Cancer. 2008;50:227-230.

560. Greenberg ML, Fisher PG, Freeman C, et al. Etoposide, vincristine, and cyclosporin A with standard-dose radiation therapy in newly diagnosed diffuse intrinsic brainstem gliomas: a pediatric oncology group phase I study. Pediatr Blood Cancer. 2005;45:644-648.

561. Bernier-Chastagner V, Grill J, Doz F, et al. Topotecan as a radiosensitizer in the treatment of children with malignant diffuse brainstem gliomas: results of a French Society of Paediatric Oncology Phase II Study. Cancer. 2005;104:2792-2797.

562. Marcus KJ, Dutton SC, Barnes P, et al. A phase I trial of etanidazole and hyperfractionated radiotherapy in children with diffuse brainstem glioma. Int J Radiat Oncol Biol Phys. 2003;55:1182-1185.

563. Wolff JE, Westphal S, Molenkamp G, et al. Treatment of paediatric pontine glioma with oral trophosphamide and etoposide. Br J Cancer. 2002;87:945-949.

564. Jennings MT, Sposto R, Boyett JM, et al. Preradiation chemotherapy in primary high-risk brainstem tumors: phase II study CCG-9941 of the Children's Cancer Group. J Clin Oncol. 2002;20:3431-3437.

565. Hargrave D, Bartels U, Bouffet E. Diffuse brainstem glioma in children: critical review of clinical trials. Lancet Oncol. 2006;7:241-248.

566. Pincus DW, Richter EO, Yachnis AT, et al. Brainstem stereotactic biopsy sampling in children. J Neurosurg. 2006;104: 108-114.

567. Mandell LR, Kadota R, Freeman C, et al. There is no role for hyperfractionated radiotherapy in the management of children with newly diagnosed diffuse intrinsic brainstem tumors: results of a Pediatric Oncology Group phase III trial comparing conventional vs. hyperfractionated radiotherapy. Int J Radiat Oncol Biol Phys. 1999;43:959-964.

568. Packer RJ, Boyett JM, Zimmerman RA, et al. Outcome of children with brain stem gliomas after treatment with 7800 cGy of hyperfractionated radiotherapy. A Childrens Cancer Group Phase I/II Trial. Cancer. 1994;74:1827-1834.

569. Freeman CR, Krischer JP, Sanford RA, et al. Final results of a study of escalating doses of hyperfractionated radiotherapy in brain stem tumors in children: a Pediatric Oncology Group study. Int J Radiat Oncol Biol Phys. 1993;27:197-206.

570. Packer RJ, Boyett JM, Zimmerman RA, et al. Hyperfractionated radiation therapy (72 Gy) for children with brain stem gliomas. A Children's Cancer Group Phase I/II Trial. Cancer. 1993;72:1414-1421.

571. Freeman CR, Krischer J, Sanford RA, et al. Hyperfractionated radiation therapy in brain stem tumors. Results of treatment at the 7020 cGy dose level of Pediatric Oncology Group study #8495. Cancer. 1991;68:474-481.

572. Freeman CR, Krischer J, Sanford RA, et al. Hyperfractionated radiotherapy in brain stem tumors: results of a Pediatric Oncology Group study. Int J Radiat Oncol Biol Phys. 1988; 15:311-318.

573. Packer RJ, Littman PA, Sposto RM, et al. Results of a pilot study of hyperfractionated radiation therapy for children with

brain stem gliomas. Int J Radiat Oncol Biol Phys. 1987; 13:1647-1651.

574. Shah NC, Ray A, Bartels U, et al. Diffuse intrinsic brainstem tumors in neonates. Report of two cases. J Neurosurg Pediatrics. 2008;1:382-385.

575. Broniscer A, Laningham FH, Sanders RP, et al. Young age may predict a better outcome for children with diffuse pontine glioma. Cancer. 2008;113:566-572.

576. Schomerus L, Merkenschlager A, Kahn T, et al. Spontaneous remission of a diffuse brainstem lesion in a neonate. Pediatr Radiol. 2007;37:399-402.

577. Thompson WD Jr, Kosnik EJ. Spontaneous regression of a diffuse brainstem lesion in the neonate. Report of two cases and review of the literature. J Neurosurg. 2005;102:65-71.

578. Kretschmar CS, Tarbell NJ, Barnes PD, et al. Pre-irradiation chemotherapy and hyperfractionated radiation therapy 66 Gy for children with brain stem tumors. A phase II study of the Pediatric Oncology Group, Protocol 8833. Cancer. 1993;72: 1404-1413.

579. Sanghavi SN, Needle MN, Krailo MD, et al. A phase I study of topotecan as a radiosensitizer for brainstem glioma of childhood: first report of the Children's Cancer Group-0952. Neuro Oncol. 2003;5:8-13.

580. Turner CD, Chi S, Marcus KJ, et al. Phase II study of thalidomide and radiation in children with newly diagnosed brain stem gliomas and glioblastoma multiforme. J Neurooncol. 2007; 82:95-101.

581. Allen J, Siffert J, Donahue B, et al. A phase I/II study of carboplatin combined with hyperfractionated radiotherapy for brainstem gliomas. Cancer. 1999;86:1064-1069.

582. Walter AW, Gajjar A, Ochs JS, et al. Carboplatin and etoposide with hyperfractionated radiotherapy in children with newly diagnosed diffuse pontine gliomas: a phase I/II study. Med Pediatr Oncol. 1998;30:28-33.

583. Sirachainan N, Pakakasama S, Visudithbhan A, et al. Concurrent radiotherapy with temozolomide followed by adjuvant temozolomide and cis-retinoic acid in children with diffuse intrinsic pontine glioma. Neuro Oncol. 2008;10:577-582.

584. Hall WA, Doolittle ND, Daman M, et al. Osmotic blood-brain barrier disruption chemotherapy for diffuse pontine gliomas. J Neurooncol. 2006;77:279-284.

585. Bouffet E, Raquin M, Doz F, et al. Radiotherapy followed by high dose busulfan and thiotepa: a prospective assessment of high dose chemotherapy in children with diffuse pontine gliomas. Cancer. 2000;88:685-692.

586. Lonser RR, Warren KE, Butman JA, et al. Real-time image-guided direct convective perfusion of intrinsic brainstem lesions. Technical note. J Neurosurg. 2007;107:190-197.

587. Broniscer A, Laningham FH, Kocak M, et al. Intratumoral hemorrhage among children with newly diagnosed, diffuse brainstem glioma. Cancer. 2006;106:1364-1371.

588. Donaldson SS, Laningham F, Fisher PG. Advances toward an understanding of brainstem gliomas. J Clin Oncol. 2006; 24:1266-1272.

589. Singh S, Bhutani R, Jalali R. Leptomeninges as a site of relapse in locally controlled, diffuse pontine glioma with review of literature. Childs Nerv Syst. 2007;23:117-121.

590. Gururangan S, McLaughlin CA, Brashears J, et al. Incidence and patterns of neuraxis metastases in children with diffuse pontine glioma. J Neurooncol. 2006;77:207-212.

591. Caroli E, Orlando ER, Ferrante L. Gliomatosis cerebri in children. Case report and clinical considerations. Childs Nerv Syst. 2005;21:1000-1003.

592. Akimoto J, Nishioka H, Miki T, et al. Clinical diagnosis of gliomatosis cerebri: report of three cases. Brain Tumor Pathol. 2004;21:87-95.

593. Armstrong GT, Phillips PC, Rorke-Adams LB, et al. Gliomatosis cerebri: 20 years of experience at the Children's Hospital of Philadelphia. Cancer. 2006;107:1597-1606.

594. Ware ML, Hirose Y, Scheithauer BW, et al. Genetic aberrations in gliomatosis cerebri. Neurosurgery. 2007;60:150-158.

595. Mawrin C. Molecular genetic alterations in gliomatosis cerebri: what can we learn about the origin and course of the disease? Acta Neuropathol. 2005;110:527-536.

596. Mawrin C, Kirches E, Schneider-Stock R, et al. Analysis of TP53 and PTEN in gliomatosis cerebri. Acta Neuropathol. 2003;105:529-536.

597. Maton B, Resnick T, Jayakar P, et al. Epilepsy surgery in children with gliomatosis cerebri. Epilepsia. 2007;48:1485-1490.

598. Filley CM, Kleinschmidt-DeMasters BK, Lillehei KO, et al. Gliomatosis cerebri: neurobehavioral and neuropathological observations. Cogn Behav Neurol. 2003;16:149-159.

599. Vates GE, Chang S, Lamborn KR, et al. Gliomatosis cerebri: a review of 22 cases. Neurosurgery. 2003;53:261-271.

600. Yu A, Li K, Li H. Value of diagnosis and differential diagnosis of MRI and MR spectroscopy in gliomatosis cerebri. Eur J Radiol. 2006;59:216-221.

601. Guzman-de-Villoria JA, Sanchez-Gonzalez J, Munoz L, et al. 1H MR spectroscopy in the assessment of gliomatosis cerebri. AJR Am J Roentgenol. 2007;188:710-714.

602. Pal L, Behari S, Kumar S, et al. Gliomatosis cerebri—an uncommon neuroepithelial tumor in children with oligodendroglial phenotype. Pediatr Neurosurg. 2008;44:212-215.

603. Romeike BF, Mawrin C. Gliomatosis cerebri: growing evidence for diffuse gliomas with wide invasion. Expert Rev Neurother. 2008;8:587-597.

604. Hilbig A, Barbosa-Coutinho LM, Toscani N, et al. Expression of nestin and vimentin in gliomatosis cerebri. Arq Neuropsiquiatr. 2006;64:781-786.

605. Bernsen H, Van der Laak J, Kusters B, et al. Gliomatosis cerebri: quantitative proof of vessel recruitment by cooptation instead of angiogenesis. J Neurosurg. 2005;103:702-706.

606. Elshaikh MA, Stevens GH, Peereboom DM, et al. Gliomatosis cerebri: treatment results with radiotherapy alone. Cancer. 2002;95:2027-2031.

607. Levin N, Gomori JM, Siegal T. Chemotherapy as initial treatment in gliomatosis cerebri: results with temozolomide. Neurology. 2004;63:354-356.

608. Sanson M, Cartalat-Carel S, Taillibert S, et al. Initial chemotherapy in gliomatosis cerebri. Neurology. 2004;63:270-275.

609. Kaloshi G, Everhard S, Laigle-Donadey F, et al. Genetic markers predictive of chemosensitivity and outcome in gliomatosis cerebri. Neurology. 2008;70:590-595.

610. Taillibert S, Chodkiewicz C, Laigle-Donadey F, et al. Gliomatosis cerebri: a review of 296 cases from the ANOCEF database and the literature. J Neurooncol. 2006;76:201-205.

611. Taylor MD, Poppleton H, Fuller C, et al. Radial glia cells are candidate stem cells of ependymoma. Cancer Cell. 2005;8: 323-335.

612. Spassky N, Merkle FT, Flames N, et al. Adult ependymal cells are postmitotic and are derived from radial glial cells during embryogenesis. J Neurosci. 2005;25:10-18.

613. Paulino AC, Wen BC, Buatti JM, et al. Intracranial ependymomas: an analysis of prognostic factors and patterns of failure. Am J Clin Oncol. 2002;25:117-122.

614. Lee J, Parsa AT, Ames CP, et al. Clinical management of intramedullary spinal ependymomas in adults. Neurosurg Clin N Am. 2006;17:21-27.

615. Grill J, Avet-Loiseau H, Lellouch-Tubiana A, et al. Comparative genomic hybridization detects specific cytogenetic abnormalities in pediatric ependymomas and choroid plexus papillomas. Cancer Genet Cytogenet. 2002;136:121-125.

616. Karakoula K, Suarez-Merino B, Ward S, et al. Real-time quantitative PCR analysis of pediatric ependymomas identifies novel candidate genes including TPR at 1q25 and CHIBBY at 22q12-q13. Genes Chromosomes Cancer. 2008;47:1005-1022.

617. Suarez-Merino B, Hubank M, Revesz T, et al. Microarray analysis of pediatric ependymoma identifies a cluster of 112 candidate genes including four transcripts at 22q12.1-q13.3. Neuro Oncol. 2005;7:20-31.

618. Hulsebos TJ, Oskam NT, Bijleveld EH, et al. Evidence for an ependymoma tumour suppressor gene in chromosome region 22pter-22q11.2. Br J Cancer. 1999;81:1150-1154.

619. Dyer S, Prebble E, Davison V, et al. Genomic imbalances in pediatric intracranial ependymomas define clinically relevant groups. Am J Pathol. 2002;161:2133-2141.

620. Gilbertson RJ, Bentley L, Hernan R, et al. ERBB receptor signaling promotes ependymoma cell proliferation and represents a potential novel therapeutic target for this disease. Clin Cancer Res. 2002;8:3054-3064.

621. Kamiya M, Nakazato Y. The expression of p73, p21 and MDM2 proteins in gliomas. J Neurooncol. 2002;59:143-149.

622. Korshunov A, Golanov A, Timirgaz V. Immunohistochemical markers for prognosis of ependymal neoplasms. J Neurooncol. 2002;58:255-270.

623. Suzuki SO, Iwaki T. Amplification and overexpression of mdm2 gene in ependymomas. Mod Pathol. 2000;13:548-553.

624. Kim SK, Lim SY, Wang KC, et al. Overexpression of cyclooxygenase-2 in childhood ependymomas: role of COX-2 inhibitor in growth and multi-drug resistance in vitro. Oncol Rep. 2004;12:403-409.

625. Ridley L, Rahman R, Brundler MA, et al. Multifactorial analysis of predictors of outcome in pediatric intracranial ependymoma. Neuro Oncol. 2008;Aug 13. [Epub ahead of print].

626. Rajaram V, Gutmann DH, Prasad SK, et al. Alterations of protein 4.1 family members in ependymomas: a study of 84 cases. Mod Pathol. 2005;18:991-997.

627. Poppleton H, Gilbertson RJ. Stem cells of ependymoma. Br J Cancer. 2007;96:6-10.

628. Tabori U, Ma J, Carter M, et al. Human telomere reverse transcriptase expression predicts progression and survival in pediatric intracranial ependymoma. J Clin Oncol. 2006;24: 1522-1528.

629. Sowar K, Straessle J, Donson AM, et al. Predicting which children are at risk for ependymoma relapse. J Neurooncol. 2006; 78:41-46.

630. Okamoto H, Mineta T, Ueda S, et al. Detection of JC virus DNA sequences in brain tumors in pediatric patients. J Neurosurg. 2005;102:294-298.

631. Bergsagel DJ, Finegold MJ, Butel JS, et al. DNA sequences similar to those of simian virus 40 in ependymomas and choroid plexus tumors of childhood. N Engl J Med. 1992;326: 988-993.

632. Huang H, Reis R, Yonekawa Y, et al. Identification in human brain tumors of DNA sequences specific for SV40 large T antigen. Brain Pathol. 1999;9:33-42.

633. Sabatier J, Uro-Coste E, Benouaich A, et al. Immunodetection of SV40 large T antigen in human central nervous system tumours. J Clin Pathol. 2005;58:429-431.

634. Weggen S, Bayer TA, von Deimling A, et al. Low frequency of SV40, JC and BK polyomavirus sequences in human medulloblastomas, meningiomas and ependymomas. Brain Pathol. 2000;10:85-92.

635. Pollack IF, Mulvihill JJ. Neurofibromatosis 1 and 2. Brain Pathol. 1997;7:823-836.

636. Rubio MP, Correa KM, Ramesh V, et al. Analysis of the neurofibromatosis 2 gene in human ependymomas and astrocytomas. Cancer Res. 1994;54:45-47.

637. Ebert C, von Haken M, Meyer-Puttlitz B, et al. Molecular genetic analysis of ependymal tumors. NF2 mutations and chromosome 22q loss occur preferentially in intramedullary spinal ependymomas. Am J Pathol. 1999;155:627-632.

638. Hemminki K, Li X, Vaittinen P, et al. Cancers in the first-degree relatives of children with brain tumours. Br J Cancer. 2000; 83:407-411.

639. Comi AM, Backstrom JW, Burger PC, et al. Clinical and neuroradiologic findings in infants with intracranial ependymomas. Pediatric Oncology Group. Pediatr Neurol. 1998;18:23-29.

640. Nagib MG, O'Fallon MT. Myxopapillary ependymoma of the conus medullaris and filum terminale in the pediatric age group. Pediatr Neurosurg. 1997;26:2-7.

641. Fassett DR, Pingree J, Kestle JR. The high incidence of tumor dissemination in myxopapillary ependymoma in pediatric patients. Report of five cases and review of the literature. J Neurosurg. 2005;102:59-64.

642. West CR, Bruce DA, Duffner PK. Ependymomas. Factors in clinical and diagnostic staging. Cancer. 1985;56:1812-1816.

643. Wippold FJ 2nd, Perry A. Neuropathology for the neuroradiologist: rosettes and pseudorosettes. AJNR Am J Neuroradiol. 2006;27:488-492.

644. Zamecnik J, Snuderl M, Eckschlager T, et al. Pediatric intracranial ependymomas: prognostic relevance of histological, immunohistochemical, and flow cytometric factors. Mod Pathol. 2003;16:980-991.

645. Mierau GW, Goin L. Perivascular elastic fibers: a diagnostic feature of ependymoma. Ultrastruct Pathol. 2007;31:251-255.

646. Mohindra S, Bal A, Singla N. Pediatric tanycytic ependymoma of the cauda equina: case report and review of the literature. J Child Neurol. 2008;23:451-454.

647. Park SH, Park HR, Chi JG. Papillary ependymoma: its differential diagnosis from choroid plexus papilloma. J Korean Med Sci. 1996;11:415-421.

648. Kawano N, Yada K, Yagishita S. Clear cell ependymoma. A histological variant with diagnostic implications. Virchows Arch A Pathol Anat Histopathol. 1989;415:467-472.

649. Poltinnikov IM, Merchant TE. CSF cytology has limited value in the evaluation of patients with ependymoma who have MRI evidence of metastasis. Pediatr Blood Cancer. 2006;47: 169-173.

650. Bouffet E, Perilongo G, Canete A, et al. Intracranial ependymomas in children: a critical review of prognostic factors and a plea for cooperation. Med Pediatr Oncol. 1998;30:319-329.

651. McGirt MJ, Chaichana KL, Atiba A, et al. Neurological outcome after resection of intramedullary spinal cord tumors in children. Childs Nerv Syst. 2008;24:93-97.

652. Bagley CA, Kothbauer KF, Wilson S, et al. Resection of myxopapillary ependymomas in children. J Neurosurg. 2007;106: 261-267.

653. Merchant TE, Mulhern RK, Krasin MJ, et al. Preliminary results from a phase II trial of conformal radiation therapy and evaluation of radiation-related CNS effects for pediatric patients with localized ependymoma. J Clin Oncol. 2004;22:3156-3162.

654. Mansur DB, Drzymala RE, Rich KM, et al. The efficacy of stereotactic radiosurgery in the management of intracranial ependymoma. J Neurooncol. 2004;66:187-190.

655. Merchant TE, Zhu Y, Thompson SJ, et al. Preliminary results from a Phase II trail of conformal radiation therapy for pediatric patients with localised low-grade astrocytoma and ependymoma. Int J Radiat Oncol Biol Phys. 2002;52:325-332.

656. Massimino M, Gandola L, Giangaspero F, et al. Hyperfractionated radiotherapy and chemotherapy for childhood ependymoma: final results of the first prospective AIEOP (Associazione Italiana di Ematologia-Oncologia Pediatrica) study. Int J Radiat Oncol Biol Phys. 2004;58:1336-1345.

657. Massimino M, Giangaspero F, Garre ML, et al. Salvage treatment for childhood ependymoma after surgery only: Pitfalls of omitting "at once" adjuvant treatment. Int J Radiat Oncol Biol Phys. 2006;65:1440-1445.

658. MacDonald SM, Safai S, Trofimov A, et al. Proton radiotherapy for childhood ependymoma: initial clinical outcomes and dose comparisons. Int J Radiat Oncol Biol Phys. 2008;71:979-986.

659. Siffert J, Allen JC. Chemotherapy in recurrent ependymoma. Pediatr Neurosurg. 1998;28:314-319.

660. Valera ET, Machado HR, Santos AC, et al. The use of neoadjuvant chemotherapy to achieve complete surgical resection in recurring supratentorial anaplastic ependymoma. Childs Nerv Syst. 2005;21:230-233.

661. Lassaletta A, Perez-Olleros P, Scaglione C, et al. Successful treatment of intracranial ependymoma with leptomeningeal spread with systemic chemotherapy and intrathecal liposomal cytarabine in a two-year-old child. J Neurooncol. 2007;83:303-306.

662. Geyer JR, Sposto R, Jennings M, et al. Multiagent chemotherapy and deferred radiotherapy in infants with malignant brain tumors: a report from the Children's Cancer Group. J Clin Oncol. 2005;23:7621-7631.

663. Duffner PK, Krischer JP, Sanford RA, et al. Prognostic factors in infants and very young children with intracranial ependymomas. Pediatr Neurosurg. 1998;28:215-222.

664. Grill J, Le Deley MC, Gambarelli D, et al. Postoperative chemotherapy without irradiation for ependymoma in children under 5 years: a multicenter trial of the French Society of Pediatric Oncology. J Clin Oncol. 2001;19:1288-1296.

665. Zacharoulis S, Levy A, Chi SN, et al. Outcome for young children newly diagnosed with ependymoma, treated with intensive induction chemotherapy followed by myeloablative chemotherapy and autologous stem cell rescue. Pediatr Blood Cancer. 2007;49:34-40.

666. Agaoglu FY, Ayan I, Dizdar Y, et al. Ependymal tumors in childhood. Pediatr Blood Cancer. 2005;45:298-303.

667. Jaing TH, Wang HS, Tsay PK, et al. Multivariate analysis of clinical prognostic factors in children with intracranial ependymomas. J Neurooncol. 2004;68:255-261.

668. Merchant TE, Jenkins JJ, Burger PC, et al. Influence of tumor grade on time to progression after irradiation for localized ependymoma in children. Int J Radiat Oncol Biol Phys. 2002;53:52-57.

669. Tihan T, Zhou T, Holmes E, et al. The prognostic value of histological grading of posterior fossa ependymomas in children: a Children's Oncology Group study and a review of prognostic factors. Mod Pathol. 2008;21:165-177.

670. Shu HK, Sall WF, Maity A, et al. Childhood intracranial ependymoma: twenty-year experience from a single institution. Cancer. 2007;110:432-441.

671. Paulino AC. Radiotherapeutic management of intracranial ependymoma. Pediatr Hematol Oncol. 2002;19:295-308.

672. Pollack IF, Gerszten PC, Martinez AJ, et al. Intracranial ependymomas of childhood: long-term outcome and prognostic factors. Neurosurgery. 1995;37:655-666.

673. Horn B, Heideman R, Geyer R, et al. A multi-institutional retrospective study of intracranial ependymoma in children: identification of risk factors. J Pediatr Hematol Oncol. 1999;21:203-211.

674. Monoranu CM, Huang B, Zangen IL, et al. Correlation between 6q25.3 deletion status and survival in pediatric intracranial ependymomas. Cancer Genet Cytogenet. 2008;182:18-26.

675. Merchant TE, Kiehna EN, Li C, et al. Radiation dosimetry predicts IQ after conformal radiation therapy in pediatric patients with localized ependymoma. Int J Radiat Oncol Biol Phys. 2005;63:1546-1554.

676. Vinchon M, Leblond P, Noudel R, et al. Intracranial ependymomas in childhood: recurrence, reoperation, and outcome. Childs Nerv Syst. 2005;21:221-226.

677. Merchant TE, Boop FA, Kun LE, et al. A retrospective study of surgery and reirradiation for recurrent ependymoma. Int J Radiat Oncol Biol Phys. 2008;71:87-97.

678. Sandri A, Massimino M, Mastrodicasa L, et al. Treatment with oral etoposide for childhood recurrent ependymomas. J Pediatr Hematol Oncol. 2005;27:486-490.

679. Akyurek S, Chang EL, Yu TK, et al. Spinal myxopapillary ependymoma outcomes in patients treated with surgery and radiotherapy at M.D. Anderson Cancer Center. J Neurooncol. 2006;80:177-183.

680. Rizk T, Mottolese C, Bouffet E, et al. Pediatric oligodendrogliomas. Pediatr Neurosurg. 1999;30:166.

681. Rizk T, Mottolese C, Bouffet E, et al. Cerebral oligodendrogliomas in children: an analysis of 15 cases. Childs Nerv Syst. 1996;12:527-529.

682. Peters O, Gnekow AK, Rating D, et al. Impact of location on outcome in children with low-grade oligodendroglioma. Pediatr Blood Cancer. 2004;43:250-256.

683. Razack N, Baumgartner J, Bruner J. Pediatric oligodendrogliomas. Pediatr Neurosurg. 1998;28:121-129.

684. Reifenberger G, Kros J, Burger P. Oligodendrogliomas. In Kleihues P, Cavenee W (eds). Tumors of the Nervous System. Lyon, France, IARC Press, 2000, pp 56-61.

685. Nutt CL. Molecular genetics of oligodendrogliomas: a model for improved clinical management in the field of neurooncology. Neurosurg Focus. 2005;19:E2.

686. Ueki K, Nishikawa R, Nakazato Y, et al. Correlation of histology and molecular genetic analysis of 1p, 19q, 10q, TP53, EGFR, CDK4, and CDKN2A in 91 astrocytic and oligodendroglial tumors. Clin Cancer Res. 2002;8:196-201.

687. Tice H, Barnes PD, Goumnerova L, et al. Pediatric and adolescent oligodendrogliomas. AJNR Am J Neuroradiol. 1993;14:1293-1300.

688. Fountas KN, Karampelas I, Nikolakakos LG, et al. Primary spinal cord oligodendroglioma: case report and review of the literature. Childs Nerv Syst. 2005;21:171-175.

689. Baysefer A, Duz B, Erdogan E, et al. Pediatric cerebellar cystic oligodendroglioma: case report and literature review. Turk J Pediatr. 2004;46:95-97.

690. Gilmer-Hill HS, Ellis WG, Imbesi SG, et al. Spinal oligodendroglioma with gliomatosis in a child. Case report. J Neurosurg. 2000;92:109-113.

691. Nam DH, Cho BK, Kim YM, et al. Intramedullary anaplastic oligodendroglioma in a child. Childs Nerv Syst. 1998;14:127-130.

692. Jenkinson MD, du Plessis DG, Smith TS, et al. Histological growth patterns and genotype in oligodendroglial tumours: correlation with MRI features. Brain. 2006;129:1884-1891.

693. Lu QR, Park JK, Noll E, et al. Oligodendrocyte lineage genes (OLIG) as molecular markers for human glial brain tumors. Proc Natl Acad Sci U S A. 2001;98:10851-10856.

694. Ligon KL, Alberta JA, Kho AT, et al. The oligodendroglial lineage marker OLIG2 is universally expressed in diffuse gliomas. J Neuropathol Exp Neurol. 2004;63:499-509.

695. Hamlat A, Saikali S, Chaperon J, et al. Oligodendroglioma: clinical study and survival analysis correlated with chromosomal anomalies. Neurosurg Focus. 2005;19:E15.

696. Kreiger PA, Okada Y, Simon S, et al. Losses of chromosomes 1p and 19q are rare in pediatric oligodendrogliomas. Acta Neuropathol. 2005;109:387-392.

697. Raghavan R, Balani J, Perry A, et al. Pediatric oligodendrogliomas: a study of molecular alterations on 1p and 19q using fluorescence in situ hybridization. J Neuropathol Exp Neurol. 2003;62:530-537.

698. Dehghani F, Schachenmayr W, Laun A, et al. Prognostic implication of histopathological, immunohistochemical and clinical features of oligodendrogliomas: a study of 89 cases. Acta Neuropathol. 1998;95:493-504.

699. Scerrati M, Roselli R, Iacoangeli M, et al. Prognostic factors in low grade (WHO grade II) gliomas of the cerebral hemispheres: the role of surgery. J Neurol Neurosurg Psychiatry. 1996; 61:291-296.

700. Bowers DC, Mulne AF, Weprin B, et al. Prognostic factors in children and adolescents with low-grade oligodendrogliomas. Pediatr Neurosurg. 2002;37:57-63.

701. Fisher BJ, Bauman GS, Leighton CE, et al. Low-grade gliomas in children: tumor volume response to radiation. J Neurosurg. 1998;88:969-974.

702. Allison RR, Schulsinger A, Vongtama V, et al. Radiation and chemotherapy improve outcome in oligodendroglioma. Int J Radiat Oncol Biol Phys. 1997;37:399-403.

703. van den Bent MJ, Chinot O, Boogerd W, et al. Second-line chemotherapy with temozolomide in recurrent oligodendroglioma after PCV (procarbazine, lomustine and vincristine) chemotherapy: EORTC Brain Tumor Group phase II study 26972. Ann Oncol. 2003;14:599-602.

704. Cairncross G, Macdonald D, Ludwin S, et al. Chemotherapy for anaplastic oligodendroglioma. National Cancer Institute of Canada Clinical Trials Group. J Clin Oncol. 1994;12: 2013-2021.

705. Abrey LE, Louis DN, Paleologos N, et al. Survey of treatment recommendations for anaplastic oligodendroglioma. Neuro Oncol. 2007;9:314-318.

706. Bruggers C, White K, Zhou H, et al. Extracranial relapse of an anaplastic oligodendroglioma in an adolescent: case report and review of the literature. J Pediatr Hematol Oncol. 2007;29: 319-322.

707. Aldape K, Burger PC, Perry A. Clinicopathologic aspects of 1p/19q loss and the diagnosis of oligodendroglioma. Arch Pathol Lab Med. 2007;131:242-251.

708. Cairncross JG, Ueki K, Zlatescu MC, et al. Specific genetic predictors of chemotherapeutic response and survival in patients with anaplastic oligodendrogliomas. J Natl Cancer Inst. 1998; 90:1473-1479.

709. Brandes AA, Tosoni A, Cavallo G, et al. Correlations between O6-methylguanine DNA methyltransferase promoter methylation status, 1p and 19q deletions, and response to temozolomide in anaplastic and recurrent oligodendroglioma: a prospective GICNO study. J Clin Oncol. 2006;24:4746-4753.

710. Reifenberger G, Kros JM, Burger PC. Oligoastrocytomas. In Kleihues P, Cavenee WK (eds). Tumours of the Central Nervous System. Lyon, France, IARC Press, 2000, pp 65-67.

711. Pomeroy SL, Tamayo P, Gaasenbeek M, et al. Prediction of central nervous system embryonal tumour outcome based on gene expression. Nature. 2002;415:436-442.

712. Baily P, Cushing H. Medulloblastoma cerebelli: a common type of mid-cerebral glioma of childhood. Arch Neurol. Psychiatry. 1925;14:192-224.

713. Hart MN, Earle KM. Primitive neuroectodermal tumors of the brain in children. Cancer. 1973;32:890-897.

714. Central Brain Tumor Registry of the United States. Primary Brain Tumors in the United States, Statistical Report, 1997–2001, Years Data Collected. Chicago, Central Brain Tumor Registry of the United States, 2005.

715. Arseni C, Ciurea AV. Statistical survey of 276 cases of medulloblastoma (1935-1978). Acta Neurochir (Wien). 1981;57: 159-162.

716. Roberts RO, Lynch CF, Jones MP, et al. Medulloblastoma: a population-based study of 532 cases. J Neuropathol Exp Neurol. 1991;50:134-144.

717. McNeil DE, Cote TR, Clegg L, et al. Incidence and trends in pediatric malignancies medulloblastoma/primitive neuroecto-

718. Matsuda M, Yasui K, Nagashima K, et al. Origin of the medulloblastoma experimentally induced by human polyomavirus JC. J Natl Cancer Inst. 1987;79:585-591.

719. Fung KM, Trojanowski JQ. Animal models of medulloblastomas and related primitive neuroectodermal tumors. A review. J Neuropathol Exp Neurol. 1995;54:285-296.

720. Eibl RH, Kleihues P, Jat PS, et al. A model for primitive neuroectodermal tumors in transgenic neural transplants harboring the SV40 large T antigen. Am J Pathol. 1994;144:556-564.

721. Khalili K, Krynska B, Del Valle L, et al. Medulloblastomas and the human neurotropic polyomavirus JC virus. Lancet. 1999;353:1152-1153.

722. Krynska B, Del Valle L, Croul S, et al. Detection of human neurotropic JC virus DNA sequence and expression of the viral oncogenic protein in pediatric medulloblastomas. Proc Natl Acad Sci U S A. 1999;96:11519-11524.

723. Mellemkjaer L, Hasle H, Gridley G, et al. Risk of cancer in children with the diagnosis immaturity at birth. Paediatr Perinat Epidemiol. 2006;20:231-237.

724. Giangaspero F, Eberhart C, Haapasalo H, et al. Medulloblastoma. In Louis DN, Ohgaki H, Wiestler OD, et al (eds). WHO Classification of Tumours of the Central Nervous System, 4th ed. Geneva, World Health Organization Press, 2007, pp 132-140.

725. Gorlin RJ, Vickers RA, Kellen E, et al. Multiple basal-cell nevi syndrome. An analysis of a syndrome consisting of multiple nevoid basal-cell carcinoma, jaw cysts, skeletal anomalies, medulloblastoma, and hyporesponsiveness to parathormone. Cancer. 1965;18:89-104.

726. Turcot J, Despres JP, St Pierre F. Malignant tumors of the central nervous system associated with familial polyposis of the colon: report of two cases. Dis Colon Rectum. 1959;2: 465-468.

727. Smucker PS, Smith JL. Multifocal desmoplastic medulloblastoma in an African-American child with nevoid basal cell carcinoma (Gorlin) syndrome. Case report. J Neurosurg. 2006;105: 315-320.

728. Schuller U, Kho AT, Zhao Q, et al. Cerebellar "transcriptome" reveals cell-type and stage-specific expression during postnatal development and tumorigenesis. Mol Cell Neurosci. 2006;33: 247-259.

729. Rubin JB, Rowitch DH. Medulloblastoma: a problem of developmental biology. Cancer Cell. 2002;2:7-8.

730. Read TA, Hegedus B, Wechsler-Reya R, et al. The neurobiology of neurooncology. Ann Neurol. 2006;60:3-11.

731. Lo KC, Rossi MR, Burkhardt T, et al. Overlay analysis of the oligonucleotide array gene expression profiles and copy number abnormalities as determined by array comparative genomic hybridization in medulloblastomas. Genes Chromosomes Cancer. 2007;46:53-66.

732. Lo KC, Rossi MR, Eberhart CG, et al. Genome wide copy number abnormalities in pediatric medulloblastomas as assessed by array comparative genome hybridization. Brain Pathol. 2007;17:282-296.

733. Uziel T, Zindy F, Sherr CJ, et al. The CDK inhibitor p18Ink4c is a tumor suppressor in medulloblastoma. Cell Cycle. 2006;5:363-365.

734. Thompson MC, Fuller C, Hogg TL, et al. Genomics identifies medulloblastoma subgroups that are enriched for specific genetic alterations. J Clin Oncol. 2006;24:1924-1931.

735. Romer J, Curran T. Targeting medulloblastoma: small-molecule inhibitors of the Sonic Hedgehog pathway as potential cancer therapeutics. Cancer Res. 2005;65:4975-4978.

736. Perry A. Medulloblastomas with favorable versus unfavorable histology: how many small blue cell tumor types are there in the brain? Adv Anat Pathol. 2002;9:345-350.

737. Eberhart CG, Kepner JL, Goldthwaite PT, et al. Histopathologic grading of medulloblastomas: a Pediatric Oncology Group study. Cancer. 2002;94:552-560.

738. Gilbertson RJ. Medulloblastoma: signalling a change in treatment. Lancet Oncol. 2004;5:209-218.

739. Dorner L, Fritsch MJ, Stark AM, et al. Posterior fossa tumors in children: how long does it take to establish the diagnosis? Childs Nerv Syst. 2007;23:887-890.

740. Halperin EC, Watson DM, George SL. Duration of symptoms prior to diagnosis is related inversely to presenting disease stage in children with medulloblastoma. Cancer. 2001;91:1444-1450.

741. Meyers SP, Wildenhain SL, Chang JK, et al. Postoperative evaluation for disseminated medulloblastoma involving the spine: contrast-enhanced MR findings, CSF cytologic analysis, timing of disease occurrence, and patient outcomes. AJNR Am J Neuroradiol. 2000;21:1757-1765.

742. David KM, Casey AT, Hayward RD, et al. Medulloblastoma: is the 5-year survival rate improving? A review of 80 cases from a single institution. J Neurosurg. 1997;86:13-21.

743. Buhren J, Christoph AH, Buslei R, et al. Expression of the neurotrophin receptor p75NTR in medulloblastomas is correlated with distinct histological and clinical features: evidence for a medulloblastoma subtype derived from the external granule cell layer. J Neuropathol Exp Neurol. 2000;59:229-240.

744. Koeller KK, Rushing EJ. From the archives of the AFIP: medulloblastoma: a comprehensive review with radiologic-pathologic correlation. Radiographics. 2003;23:1613-1637.

745. Buhring U, Strayle-Batra M, Freudenstein D, et al. MRI features of primary, secondary and metastatic medulloblastoma. Eur Radiol. 2002;12:1342-1348.

746. Agrawal D, Singhal A, Hendson G, et al. Gyriform differentiation in medulloblastoma—a radiological predictor of histology. Pediatr Neurosurg. 2007;43:142-145.

747. O'Dorisio MS, Khanna G, Bushnell D. Combining anatomic and molecularly targeted imaging in the diagnosis and surveillance of embryonal tumors of the nervous and endocrine systems in children. Cancer Metastasis Rev. 2008;27:665-677.

748. Verma S, Tavare C, Gilles F. Histologic features and prognosis in pediatric medulloblastoma. Pediatr Dev Pathol. 2008;11:337-343.

749. McManamy CS, Pears J, Weston CL, et al. Nodule formation and desmoplasia in medulloblastomas-defining the nodular/desmoplastic variant and its biological behavior. Brain Pathol. 2007;17:151-164.

750. Lamont JM, McManamy CS, Pearson AD, et al. Combined histopathological and molecular cytogenetic stratification of medulloblastoma patients. Clin Cancer Res. 2004;10:5482-5493.

751. Brown HG, Kepner JL, Perlman EJ, et al. "Large cell/anaplastic" medulloblastomas: a Pediatric Oncology Group Study. J Neuropathol Exp Neurol. 2000;59:857-865.

752. Eberhart CG, Burger PC. Anaplasia and grading in medulloblastomas. Brain Pathol. 2003;13:376-385.

753. Smith TW, Nikulasson S, De Girolami U, et al. Immunohistochemistry of synapsin I and synaptophysin in human nervous system and neuroendocrine tumors. Applications in diagnostic neuro-oncology. Clin Neuropathol. 1993;12:335-342.

754. McLendon RE, Friedman HS, Fuchs HE, et al. Diagnostic markers in paediatric medulloblastoma: a Paediatric Oncology Group Study. Histopathology. 1999;34:154-162.

755. Giangaspero F, Chieco P, Ceccarelli C, et al. "Desmoplastic" versus "classic" medulloblastoma: comparison of DNA content, histopathology and differentiation. Virchows Arch A Pathol Anat Histopathol. 1991;418:207-214.

756. Rutkowski S, Bode U, Deinlein F, et al. Treatment of early childhood medulloblastoma by postoperative chemotherapy alone. N Engl J Med. 2005;352:978-986.

757. Stearns D, Chaudhry A, Abel TW, et al. c-myc overexpression causes anaplasia in medulloblastoma. Cancer Res. 2006;66:673-681.

758. Ellison D. Classifying the medulloblastoma: insights from morphology and molecular genetics. Neuropathol Appl Neurobiol. 2002;28:257-282.

759. Dagostino C, Clara E, Chio A, et al. Morphophenotype of medulloblastoma in children and adults. The size of nuclei. Clin Neuropathol. 2006;25:227-231.

760. Shakhova O, Leung C, van Montfort E, et al. Lack of Rb and p53 delays cerebellar development and predisposes to large cell anaplastic medulloblastoma through amplification of N-Myc and Ptch2. Cancer Res. 2006;66:5190-5200.

761. Suresh TN, Santosh V, Yasha TC, et al. Medulloblastoma with extensive nodularity: a variant occurring in the very young-clinicopathological and immunohistochemical study of four cases. Childs Nerv Syst. 2004;20:55-60.

762. Sachdeva MU, Vankalakunti M, Rangan A, et al. The role of immunohistochemistry in medullomyoblastoma—a case series highlighting divergent differentiation. Diagn Pathol. 2008;3:18.

763. Helton KJ, Fouladi M, Boop FA, et al. Medullomyoblastoma: a radiographic and clinicopathologic analysis of six cases and review of the literature. Cancer. 2004;101:1445-1454.

764. Polydorides AD, Perry A, Edgar MA. Large cell medulloblastoma with myogenic and melanotic differentiation: a case report with molecular analysis. J Neurooncol. 2008;88:193-197.

765. Er U, Yigitkanli K, Kazanci B, et al. Medullomyoblastoma: teratoid nature of a quite rare neoplasm. Surg Neurol. 2008;69:403-406.

766. Nozza P, Milanaccio C, Piatelli G, et al. Cerebellar medullomyoblastoma with melanotic tubular structures. Pediatr Blood Cancer. 2008;50:183-185.

767. Kubota KC, Itoh T, Yamada Y, et al. Melanocytic medulloblastoma with ganglioneurocytomatous differentiation: a case report. Neuropathology. 2009;29:72-77.

768. Ray A, Ho M, Ma J, et al. A clinicobiological model predicting survival in medulloblastoma. Clin Cancer Res. 2004;10:7613-7620.

769. Katsetos CD, Liu HM, Zacks SI. Immunohistochemical and ultrastructural observations on Homer Wright (neuroblastic) rosettes and the "pale islands" of human cerebellar medulloblastomas. Hum Pathol. 1988;19:1219-1227.

770. Gajjar A, Hernan R, Kocak M, et al. Clinical, histopathologic, and molecular markers of prognosis toward a new disease risk stratification system for medulloblastoma. J Clin Oncol. 2004;22:984-993.

771. Reardon DA, Jenkins JJ, Sublett JE, et al. Multiple genomic alterations including N-myc amplification in a primary large cell medulloblastoma. Pediatr Neurosurg. 2000;32:187-191.

772. Rossi MR, Conroy J, McQuaid D, et al. Array CGH analysis of pediatric medulloblastomas. Genes Chromosomes Cancer. 2006;45:290-303.

773. Giordana MT, Migheli A, Pavanelli E. Isochromosome 17q is a constant finding in medulloblastoma. An interphase cytogenetic study on tissue sections. Neuropathol Appl Neurobiol. 1998;24:233-238.

774. Grotzer MA, von Hoff K, von Bueren AO, et al. Which clinical and biological tumor markers proved predictive in the prospective multicenter trial HIT'91—implications for investigating childhood medulloblastoma. Klin Padiatr. 2007;219:312-317.

775. Kim JY, Sutton ME, Lu DJ, et al. Activation of neurotrophin-3 receptor TrkC induces apoptosis in medulloblastomas. Cancer Res. 1999;59:711-719.

776. Ellison DW, Onilude OE, Lindsey JC, et al. Beta-catenin status predicts a favorable outcome in childhood medulloblastoma: the United Kingdom Children's Cancer Study Group Brain Tumour Committee. J Clin Oncol. 2005;23:7951-7957.

777. Hernan R, Fasheh R, Calabrese C, et al. ERBB2 up-regulates S100A4 and several other prometastatic genes in medulloblastoma. Cancer Res. 2003;63:140-148.

778. Gilbertson RJ, Perry RH, Kelly PJ, et al. Prognostic significance of HER2 and HER4 coexpression in childhood medulloblastoma. Cancer Res. 1997;57:3272-3280.

779. Spencer CD, Weiss RB, Van Eys J, et al. Medulloblastoma metastatic to the marrow. Report of four cases and review of the literature. J Neurooncol. 1984;2:223-235.

780. Gajjar A, Fouladi M, Walter AW, et al. Comparison of lumbar and shunt cerebrospinal fluid specimens for cytologic detection of leptomeningeal disease in pediatric patients with brain tumors. J Clin Oncol. 1999;17:1825-1828.

781. Chang CH, Housepian EM, Herbert C Jr. An operative staging system and a megavoltage radiotherapeutic technic for cerebellar medulloblastomas. Radiology. 1969;93:1351-1359.

782. Albright AL, Wisoff JH, Zeltzer PM, et al. Effects of medulloblastoma resections on outcome in children: a report from the Children's Cancer Group. Neurosurgery. 1996;38:265-271.

783. Zeltzer PM, Boyett JM, Finlay JL, et al. Metastasis stage, adjuvant treatment, and residual tumor are prognostic factors for medulloblastoma in children: conclusions from the Children's Cancer Group 921 randomized phase III study. J Clin Oncol. 1999;17:832-845.

784. Tabori U, Sung L, Hukin J, et al. Medulloblastoma in the second decade of life: a specific group with respect to toxicity and management: a Canadian Pediatric Brain Tumor Consortium Study. Cancer. 2005;103:1874-1880.

785. Cohen-Gadol AA, Spencer DD. Inauguration of pediatric neurosurgery by Harvey W. Cushing: his contributions to the surgery of posterior fossa tumors in children. Historical vignette. J Neurosurg. 2004;100:225-231.

786. Packer RJ, Goldwein J, Nicholson HS, et al. Treatment of children with medulloblastomas with reduced-dose craniospinal radiation therapy and adjuvant chemotherapy: A Children's Cancer Group Study. J Clin Oncol. 1999;17:2127-2136.

787. Grill J, Viguier D, Kieffer V, et al. Critical risk factors for intellectual impairment in children with posterior fossa tumors: the role of cerebellar damage. J Neurosurg. 2004;101:152-158.

788. Kremer P, Tronnier V, Steiner HH, et al. Intraoperative MRI for interventional neurosurgical procedures and tumor resection control in children. Childs Nerv Syst. 2006;22:674-678.

789. Lam CH, Hall WA, Truwit CL, et al. Intra-operative MRI-guided approaches to the pediatric posterior fossa tumors. Pediatr Neurosurg. 2001;34:295-300.

790. Gelabert-Gonzalez M, Fernandez-Villa J. Mutism after posterior fossa surgery. Review of the literature. Clin Neurol Neurosurg. 2001;103:111-114.

791. Gajjar A, Chintagumpala M, Ashley D, et al. Risk-adapted craniospinal radiotherapy followed by high-dose chemotherapy and stem-cell rescue in children with newly diagnosed medulloblastoma (St. Jude Medulloblastoma-96): long-term results from a prospective, multicentre trial. Lancet Oncol. 2006;7:813-820.

792. Oyharcabal-Bourden V, Kalifa C, Gentet JC, et al. Standard-risk medulloblastoma treated by adjuvant chemotherapy followed by reduced-dose craniospinal radiation therapy: a French Society of Pediatric Oncology Study. J Clin Oncol. 2005;23:4726-4734.

793. Mabbott DJ, Barnes M, Laperriere N, et al. Neurocognitive function in same-sex twins following focal radiation for medulloblastoma. Neuro Oncol. 2007;9:460-464.

794. Grill J, Lellouch-Tubiana A, Elouahdani S, et al. Preoperative chemotherapy in children with high-risk medulloblastomas: a feasibility study. J Neurosurg. 2005;103:312-318.

795. Prados MD, Edwards MS, Chang SM, et al. Hyperfractionated craniospinal radiation therapy for primitive neuroectodermal tumors: results of a Phase II study. Int J Radiat Oncol Biol Phys. 1999;43:279-285.

796. Carrie C, Muracciole X, Gomez F, et al. Conformal radiotherapy, reduced boost volume, hyperfractionated radiotherapy, and online quality control in standard-risk medulloblastoma without chemotherapy: results of the French M-SFOP 98 protocol. Int J Radiat Oncol Biol Phys. 2005;63:711-716.

797. del Charco JO, Bolek TW, McCollough WM, et al. Medulloblastoma: time-dose relationship based on a 30-year review. Int J Radiat Oncol Biol Phys. 1998;42:147-154.

798. Hartsell WF, Gajjar A, Heideman RL, et al. Patterns of failure in children with medulloblastoma: effects of preirradiation chemotherapy. Int J Radiat Oncol Biol Phys. 1997;39:15-24.

799. Thomas PR, Deutsch M, Kepner JL, et al. Low-stage medulloblastoma: final analysis of trial comparing standard-dose with reduced-dose neuraxis irradiation. J Clin Oncol. 2000;18:3004-3011.

800. Krischer JP, Ragab AH, Kun L, et al. Nitrogen mustard, vincristine, procarbazine, and prednisone as adjuvant chemotherapy in the treatment of medulloblastoma. A Pediatric Oncology Group study. J Neurosurg. 1991;74:905-909.

801. Tait DM, Thornton-Jones H, Bloom HJ, et al. Adjuvant chemotherapy for medulloblastoma: the first multi-centre control trial of the International Society of Paediatric Oncology (SIOP I). Eur J Cancer. 1990;26:464-469.

802. Evans AE, Jenkin RD, Sposto R, et al. The treatment of medulloblastoma. Results of a prospective randomized trial of radiation therapy with and without CCNU, vincristine, and prednisone. J Neurosurg. 1990;72:572-582.

803. Kellie SJ, Wong CK, Pozza LD, et al. Activity of postoperative carboplatin, etoposide, and high-dose methotrexate in pediatric CNS embryonal tumors: results of a phase II study in newly diagnosed children. Med Pediatr Oncol. 2002;39:168-174.

804. Bakish J, Hargrave D, Tariq N, et al. Evaluation of dietetic intervention in children with medulloblastoma or supratentorial primitive neuroectodermal tumors. Cancer. 2003;98:1014-1020.

805. Fouladi M, Chintagumpala M, Ashley D, et al. Amifostine protects against cisplatin-induced ototoxicity in children with average-risk medulloblastoma. J Clin Oncol. 2008;26:3749-3755.

806. Gallegos-Castorena S, Martinez-Avalos A, Mohar-Betancourt A, et al. Toxicity prevention with amifostine in pediatric osteosarcoma patients treated with cisplatin and doxorubicin. Pediatr Hematol Oncol. 2007;24:403-408.

807. Goldwein JW, Radcliffe J, Johnson J, et al. Updated results of a pilot study of low dose craniospinal irradiation plus chemotherapy for children under five with cerebellar primitive neuroectodermal tumors (medulloblastoma). Int J Radiat Oncol Biol Phys. 1996;34:899-904.

808. Mulhern RK, Palmer SL, Merchant TE, et al. Neurocognitive consequences of risk-adapted therapy for childhood medulloblastoma. J Clin Oncol. 2005;23:5511-5519.

809. Jakacki RI. Treatment strategies for high-risk medulloblastoma and supratentorial primitive neuroectodermal tumors. Review of the literature. J Neurosurg. 2005;102:44-52.

810. Kortmann RD, Kuhl J, Timmermann B, et al. Postoperative neoadjuvant chemotherapy before radiotherapy as compared to immediate radiotherapy followed by maintenance chemotherapy in the treatment of medulloblastoma in childhood: results of the German prospective randomized trial HIT '91. Int J Radiat Oncol Biol Phys. 2000;46:269-279.

811. Heideman RL, Kuttesch J Jr, Gajjar AJ, et al. Supratentorial malignant gliomas in childhood: a single institution perspective. Cancer. 1997;80:497-504.

812. Silber JH, Radcliffe J, Peckham V, et al. Whole-brain irradiation and decline in intelligence: the influence of dose and age on IQ score. J Clin Oncol. 1992;10:1390-1396.

813. Chi SN, Gardner SL, Levy AS, et al. Feasibility and response to induction chemotherapy intensified with high-dose methotrexate for young children with newly diagnosed high-risk disseminated medulloblastoma. J Clin Oncol. 2004;22:4881-4887.

814. Packer RJ, Gajjar A, Vezina G, et al. Phase III study of craniospinal radiation therapy followed by adjuvant chemotherapy for newly diagnosed average-risk medulloblastoma. J Clin Oncol. 2006;24:4202-4208.

815. Helton KJ, Gajjar A, Hill DA, et al. Medulloblastoma metastatic to the suprasellar region at diagnosis: a report of six cases with clinicopathologic correlation. Pediatr Neurosurg. 2002;37:111-117.

816. Kantar M, Cetingul N, Kansoy S, et al. Radiotherapy-induced secondary cranial neoplasms in children. Childs Nerv Syst. 2004;20:46-49.

817. Nagel BJ, Delis DC, Palmer SL, et al. Early patterns of verbal memory impairment in children treated for medulloblastoma. Neuropsychology. 2006;20:105-112.

818. Mulhern RK, Reddick WE, Palmer SL, et al. Neurocognitive deficits in medulloblastoma survivors and white matter loss. Ann Neurol. 1999;46:834-841.

819. Zitterbart K, Zavrelova I, Kadlecova J, et al. p73 expression in medulloblastoma: TAp73/DeltaNp73 transcript detection and possible association of p73alpha/DeltaNp73 immunoreactivity with survival. Acta Neuropathol. 2007;114:641-650.

820. Fernandez-Teijeiro A, Betensky RA, Sturla LM, et al. Combining gene expression profiles and clinical parameters for risk stratification in medulloblastomas. J Clin Oncol. 2004;22:994-998.

821. Bowers DC, Gargan L, Weprin BE, et al. Impact of site of tumor recurrence on survival for children with recurrent or progressive medulloblastoma. J Neurosurg. 2007;107:5-10.

822. Dunkel IJ, Finlay JL. High dose chemotherapy with autologous stem cell rescue for patients with medulloblastoma. J Neurooncol. 1996;29:69-74.

823. Spiller SE, Ravanpay AC, Hahn AW, et al. Suberoylanilide hydroxamic acid is effective in preclinical studies of medulloblastoma. J Neurooncol. 2006;79:259-270.

824. Fevre-Montange M, Champier J, Szathmari A, et al. Microarray analysis reveals differential gene expression patterns in tumors of the pineal region. J Neuropathol Exp Neurol. 2006;65:675-684.

825. Cho BK, Wang KC, Nam DH, et al. Pineal tumors: experience with 48 cases over 10 years. Childs Nerv Syst. 1998;14:53-58.

826. Vogel R. Parinaud's syndrome and other related pretectal syndromes. Ophthalmic Semin. 1976;1:287-370.

827. Nakazato Y, Jouvet A, Scheithauer BW. Pineocytoma. In Louis DN, Ohgaki H, Wiestler OD, et al (eds). WHO Classification of Tumours of the Central Nervous System, 4th ed. Geneva, World Health Organization Press, 2007, pp 122-123.

828. Yamini B, Refai D, Rubin CM, et al. Initial endoscopic management of pineal region tumors and associated hydrocephalus: clinical series and literature review. J Neurosurg. 2004;100:437-441.

829. Yurtseven T, Ersahin Y, Demirtas E, et al. Neuroendoscopic biopsy for intraventricular tumors. Minim Invasive Neurosurg. 2003;46:293-299.

830. Rickert CH, Simon R, Bergmann M, et al. Comparative genomic hybridization in pineal parenchymal tumors. Genes Chromosomes Cancer. 2001;30:99-104.

831. Nakazato Y, Jouvet A, Scheithauer BW. Pineal parenchymal tumour of intermediate differentiation. In Louis DN, Ohgaki H, Wiestler OD, et al (eds). WHO Classification of Tumours of

the Central Nervous System, 4th ed. Geneva, World Health Organization Press, 2007, pp 124-125.

832. Jouvet A, Saint-Pierre G, Fauchon F, et al. Pineal parenchymal tumors: a correlation of histologic features with Prognosis. in 66 cases. Brain Pathol. 2000;10:49-60.

833. Fauchon F, Jouvet A, Paquis P, et al. Parenchymal pineal tumors: a clinicopathological study of 76 cases. Int J Radiat Oncol Biol Phys. 2000;46:959-968.

834. Popovic MB, Diezi M, Kuchler H, et al. Trilateral retinoblastoma with suprasellar tumor and associated pineal cyst. J Pediatr Hematol Oncol. 2007;29:53-56.

835. Gadish T, Tulchinsky H, Deutsch AA, et al. Pinealoblastoma in a patient with familial adenomatous polyposis: variant of Turcot syndrome type 2? Report of a case and review of the literature. Dis Colon Rectum. 2005;48:2343-2346.

836. Li MH, Bouffet E, Hawkins CE, et al. Molecular genetics of supratentorial primitive neuroectodermal tumors and pineoblastoma. Neurosurg Focus. 2005;19:E3.

837. Cuccia V, Rodriguez F, Palma F, et al. Pinealoblastomas in children. Childs Nerv Syst. 2006;22:577-585.

838. Chiechi MV, Smirniotopoulos JG, Mena H. Pineal parenchymal tumors: CT and MR features. J Comput Assist Tomogr. 1995;19:509-517.

839. Nakamura M, Saeki N, Iwadate Y, et al. Neuroradiological characteristics of pineocytoma and pineoblastoma. Neuroradiology. 2000;42:509-514.

840. Nakazato Y, Jouvet A, Scheithauer BW. Pineoblastoma. In Louis DN, Ohgaki H, Wiestler OD, et al (eds). WHO Classification of Tumours of the Central Nervous System, 4th ed. Geneva, World Health Organization Press, 2007, pp 126-127.

841. Yamane Y, Mena H, Nakazato Y. Immunohistochemical characterization of pineal parenchymal tumors using novel monoclonal antibodies to the pineal body. Neuropathology. 2002;22:66-76.

842. Finelli DA, Shurin SB, Bardenstein DS. Trilateral retinoblastoma: two variations. AJNR Am J Neuroradiol. 1995;16:166-170.

843. Gilheeney SW, Saad A, Chi S, et al. Outcome of pediatric pineoblastoma after surgery, radiation and chemotherapy. J Neurooncol. 2008;89:89-95.

844. Duffner PK, Cohen ME, Sanford RA, et al. Lack of efficacy of postoperative chemotherapy and delayed radiation in very young children with pineoblastoma. Pediatric Oncology Group. Med Pediatr Oncol. 1995;25:38-44.

845. Roncaroli F, Scheithauer BW. Papillary tumor of the pineal region and spindle cell oncocytoma of the pituitary: new tumor entities in the 2007 WHO Classification. Brain Pathol. 2007;17:314-318.

846. Hasselblatt M, Blumcke I, Jeibmann A, et al. Immunohistochemical profile and chromosomal imbalances in papillary tumours of the pineal region. Neuropathol Appl Neurobiol. 2006;32:278-283.

847. Chang AH, Fuller GN, Debnam JM, et al. MR imaging of papillary tumor of the pineal region. AJNR Am J Neuroradiol. 2008;29:187-189.

848. Amemiya S, Shibahara J, Aoki S, et al. Recently established entities of central nervous system tumors: review of radiological findings. J Comput Assist Tomogr. 2008;32:279-285.

849. Jouvet A, Nakazato Y, Scheithauer BW, et al. Papillary tumour of the pineal region. In Louis DN, Ohgaki H, Wiestler OD, et al (eds). WHO Classification of Tumours of the Central Nervous System, 4th ed. Geneva, World Health Organization Press, 2007, pp 128-129.

850. Fevre-Montange M, Hasselblatt M, Figarella-Branger D, et al. Prognosis and histopathologic features in papillary tumors of the pineal region: a retrospective multicenter study of 31 cases. J Neuropathol Exp Neurol. 2006;65:1004-1011.

851. Boco T, Aalaei S, Musacchio M, et al. Papillary tumor of the pineal region. Neuropathology. 2008;28:87-92.

852. Buffenoir K, Rigoard P, Wager M, et al. Papillary tumor of the pineal region in a child: case report and review of the literature. Childs Nerv Syst. 2008;24:379-384.

853. Burger PC. Supratentorial primitive neuroectodermal tumor (sPNET). Brain Pathol. 2006;16:86.

854. Rorke LB. The cerebellar medulloblastoma and its relationship to primitive neuroectodermal tumors. J Neuropathol Exp Neurol. 1983;42:1-15.

855. McLendon R, Judkins AR, Eberhart C, et al. Central nervous system primitive neuroectodermal tumours. In Louis DN, Ohgaki H, Wiestler OD, et al (eds). WHO Classification of Tumours of the Central Nervous System, 4th ed. Geneva, World Health Organization Press, 2007, pp 141-146.

856. Muhlisch J, Schwering A, Grotzer M, et al. Epigenetic repression of RASSF1A but not CASP8 in supratentorial PNET (sPNET) and atypical teratoid/rhabdoid tumors (ATRT) of childhood. Oncogene. 2006;25:1111-1117.

857. Inda MM, Munoz J, Coullin P, et al. High promoter hypermethylation frequency of p14/ARF in supratentorial PNET but not in medulloblastoma. Histopathology. 2006;48:579-587.

858. Inda MM, Perot C, Guillaud-Bataille M, et al. Genetic heterogeneity in supratentorial and infratentorial primitive neuroectodermal tumours of the central nervous system. Histopathology. 2005;47:631-637.

859. Yang HJ, Nam DH, Wang KC, et al. Supratentorial primitive neuroectodermal tumor in children: clinical features, treatment outcome and prognostic factors. Childs Nerv Syst. 1999;15: 377-383.

860. Johnston DL, Keene DL, Lafay-Cousin L, et al. Supratentorial primitive neuroectodermal tumors: a Canadian pediatric brain tumor consortium report. J Neurooncol. 2008;86:101-108.

861. Chawla A, Emmanuel JV, Seow WT, et al. Paediatric PNET: pre-surgical MRI features. Clin Radiol. 2007;62: 43-52.

862. Dirks PB, Harris L, Hoffman HJ, et al. Supratentorial primitive neuroectodermal tumors in children. J Neurooncol. 1996;29: 75-84.

863. Kraus JA, Felsberg J, Tonn JC, et al. Molecular genetic analysis of the TP53, PTEN, CDKN2A, EGFR, CDK4 and MDM2 tumour-associated genes in supratentorial primitive neuroectodermal tumours and glioblastomas of childhood. Neuropathol Appl Neurobiol. 2002;28:325-333.

864. Burns AS, Jaros E, Cole M, et al. The molecular pathology of p53 in primitive neuroectodermal tumours of the central nervous system. Br J Cancer. 2002;86:1117-1123.

865. Judkins AR, Burger PC, Hamilton RL, et al. INI1 protein expression distinguishes atypical teratoid/rhabdoid tumor from choroid plexus carcinoma. J Neuropathol Exp Neurol. 2005; 64:391-397.

866. Judkins AR, Mauger J, Ht A, et al. Immunohistochemical analysis of hSNF5/INI1 in pediatric CNS neoplasms. Am J Surg Pathol. 2004;28:644-650.

867. Molloy PT, Yachnis AT, Rorke LB, et al. Central nervous system medulloepithelioma: a series of eight cases including two arising in the pons. J Neurosurg. 1996;84:430-436.

868. Chavez M, Mafee MF, Castillo B, et al. Medulloepithelioma of the optic nerve. J Pediatr Ophthalmol Strabismus. 2004;41: 48-52.

869. Pang LM, Roebuck DJ, Ng HK, et al. Sellar and suprasellar medulloepithelioma. Pediatr Radiol. 2001;31:594-596.

870. Dohrmann GJ, Farwell JR, Flannery JT. Ependymomas and ependymoblastomas in children. J Neurosurg. 1976;45:273-283.

871. Mork SJ, Rubinstein LJ. Ependymoblastoma. A reappraisal of a rare embryonal tumor. Cancer. 1985;55:1536-1542.

872. Dorsay TA, Rovira MJ, Ho VB, et al. Ependymoblastoma: MR presentation. A case report and review of the literature. Pediatr Radiol. 1995;25:433-435.

873. Yaris N, Yavuz MN, Reis A, et al. Primary cerebral neuroblastoma: a case treated with adjuvant chemotherapy and radiotherapy. Turk J Pediatr. 2004;46:182-185.

874. Takahashi M, Ishihara T, Yokota T, et al. A case of cerebral composite ganglioneuroblastoma: an immunohistochemical and ultrastructural study. Acta Neuropathol. 1990;80:98-102.

875. Sohma T, Tuchita H, Kitami K, et al. Cerebellopontine angle ganglioneuroblastoma. Neuroradiology. 1992;34:334-336.

876. Ogino S, Kubo S, Abdul-Karim FW, et al. Comparative immunohistochemical study of insulin-like growth factor II and insulin-like growth factor receptor type 1 in pediatric brain tumors. Pediatr Dev Pathol. 2001;4:23-31.

877. Gasparetto EL, Rosemberg S, Matushita H, et al. Ganglioneuroblastoma of the cerebellum: neuroimaging and pathological features of a case. Arq Neuropsiquiatr. 2007;65:338-340.

878. Tanaka M, Shibui S, Nomura K, et al. Pineal ganglioneuroblastoma in an adult. J Neurooncol. 1999;44:169-173.

879. Dunham C, Sugo E, Tobias V, et al. Embryonal tumor with abundant neuropil and true rosettes (ETANTR): report of a case with prominent neurocytic differentiation. J Neurooncol. 2007;84:91-98.

880. Fuller C, Fouladi M, Gajjar A, et al. Chromosome 17 abnormalities in pediatric neuroblastic tumor with abundant neuropil and true rosettes. Am J Clin Pathol. 2006;126:277-283.

881. Burnett ME, White EC, Sih S, et al. Chromosome arm 17p deletion analysis reveals molecular genetic heterogeneity in supratentorial and infratentorial primitive neuroectodermal tumors of the central nervous system. Cancer Genet Cytogenet. 1997;97:25-31.

882. Russo C, Pellarin M, Tingby O, et al. Comparative genomic hybridization in patients with supratentorial and infratentorial primitive neuroectodermal tumors. Cancer. 1999;86:331-339.

883. Reddy AT, Janss AJ, Phillips PC, et al. Outcome for children with supratentorial primitive neuroectodermal tumors treated with surgery, radiation, and chemotherapy. Cancer. 2000;88: 2189-2193.

884. Cohen BH, Zeltzer PM, Boyett JM, et al. Prognostic factors and treatment results for supratentorial primitive neuroectodermal tumors in children using radiation and chemotherapy: a Childrens Cancer Group randomized trial. J Clin Oncol. 1995;13:1687-1696.

885. Hong TS, Mehta MP, Boyett JM, et al. Patterns of failure in supratentorial primitive neuroectodermal tumors treated in Children's Cancer Group Study 921, a phase III combined modality study. Int J Radiat Oncol Biol Phys. 2004;60: 204-213.

886. Fangusaro J, Finlay J, Sposto R, et al. Intensive chemotherapy followed by consolidative myeloablative chemotherapy with autologous hematopoietic cell rescue (AuHCR) in young children with newly diagnosed supratentorial primitive neuroectodermal tumors (sPNETs): report of the Head Start I and II experience. Pediatr Blood Cancer. 2008;50:312-318.

887. Sung KW, Yoo KH, Cho EJ, et al. High-dose chemotherapy and autologous stem cell rescue in children with newly diagnosed high-risk or relapsed medulloblastoma or supratentorial primitive neuroectodermal tumor. Pediatr Blood Cancer. 2007;48:408-415.

888. Paulino AC, Cha DT, Barker JL Jr, et al. Patterns of failure in relation to radiotherapy fields in supratentorial primitive neuroectodermal tumor. Int J Radiat Oncol Biol Phys. 2004;58: 1171-1176.

889. McBride SM, Daganzo SM, Banerjee A, et al. Radiation is an important component of multimodality therapy for pediatric non-pineal supratentorial primitive neuroectodermal tumors. Int

J Radiat Oncol Biol Phys. 2008;May 15. [Epub ahead of print].

890. Shih CS, Hale GA, Gronewold L, et al. High-dose chemotherapy with autologous stem cell rescue for children with recurrent malignant brain tumors. Cancer. 2008;112:1345-1353.

891. Strother D. Atypical teratoid rhabdoid tumors of childhood: diagnosis, treatment and challenges. Expert Rev Anticancer Ther. 2005;5:907-915.

892. Reddy AT. Atypical teratoid/rhabdoid tumors of the central nervous system. J Neurooncol. 2005;75:309-313.

893. Lee MC, Park SK, Lim JS, et al. Atypical teratoid/rhabdoid tumor of the central nervous system: clinico-pathological study. Neuropathology. 2002;22:252-260.

894. Tekautz TM, Fuller CE, Blaney S, et al. Atypical teratoid/rhabdoid tumors (ATRT): improved survival in children 3 years and older with radiation therapy and high-dose alkylator-based chemotherapy. J Clin Oncol. 2005;23:1491-1499.

895. Zarovnaya EL, Pallatroni HF, Hug EB, et al. Atypical teratoid/rhabdoid tumor of the spine in an adult: case report and review of the literature. J Neurooncol. 2007;84:49-55.

896. Jackson EM, Shaikh TH, Gururangan S, et al. High-density single nucleotide polymorphism array analysis in patients with germline deletions of 22q11.2 and malignant rhabdoid tumor. Hum Genet. 2007;122:117-127.

897. Biegel JA. Molecular genetics of atypical teratoid/rhabdoid tumor. Neurosurg Focus. 2006;20:E11.

898. Rickert CH, Paulus W. Epidemiology of central nervous system tumors in childhood and adolescence based on the new WHO classification. Childs Nerv Syst. 2001;17:503-511.

899. Hilden JM, Meerbaum S, Burger P, et al. Central nervous system atypical teratoid/rhabdoid tumor: results of therapy in children enrolled in a registry. J Clin Oncol. 2004;22:2877-2884.

900. Sasaki A, Kurihara H, Ishiuchi S, et al. Pediatric embryonal tumor of the cerebellum with rhabdoid cells and novel intracytoplasmic inclusions: distinction from atypical teratoid/rhabdoid tumor. Acta Neuropathol. 2005;110:69-76.

901. Zimmerman MA, Goumnerova LC, Proctor M, et al. Continuous remission of newly diagnosed and relapsed central nervous system atypical teratoid/rhabdoid tumor. J Neurooncol. 2005;72:77-84.

902. Koral K, Gargan L, Bowers DC, et al. Imaging characteristics of atypical teratoid-rhabdoid tumor in children compared with medulloblastoma. AJR Am J Roentgenol. 2008;190:809-814.

903. Warmuth-Metz M, Bison B, Dannemann-Stern E, et al. CT and MR imaging in atypical teratoid/rhabdoid tumors of the central nervous system. Neuroradiology. 2008;50:447-452.

904. Parmar H, Hawkins C, Bouffet E, et al. Imaging findings in primary intracranial atypical teratoid/rhabdoid tumors. Pediatr Radiol. 2006;36:126-132.

905. Meyers SP, Khademian ZP, Biegel JA, et al. Primary intracranial atypical teratoid/rhabdoid tumors of infancy and childhood: MRI features and patient outcomes. AJNR Am J Neuroradiol. 2006;27:962-971.

906. Rorke LB, Packer RJ, Biegel JA. Central nervous system atypical teratoid/rhabdoid tumors of infancy and childhood: definition of an entity. J Neurosurg. 1996;85:56-65.

907. Biegel JA, Kalpana G, Knudsen ES, et al. The role of INI1 and the SWI/SNF complex in the development of rhabdoid tumors: meeting summary from the workshop on childhood atypical teratoid/rhabdoid tumors. Cancer Res. 2002;62:323-328.

908. Haberler C, Laggner U, Slavc I, et al. Immunohistochemical analysis of INI1 protein in malignant pediatric CNS tumors: Lack of INI1 in atypical teratoid/rhabdoid tumors and in a fraction of primitive neuroectodermal tumors without rhabdoid phenotype. Am J Surg Pathol. 2006;30:1462-1468.

909. Judkins AR, Eberhart C, Wesseling P. Atypical teratoid/rhabdoid tumour. In Louis DN, Ohgaki H, Wiestler OD, et al (eds). WHO Classification of Tumours of the Central Nervous System, 4th ed. Geneva, World Health Organization Press, 2007, pp 147-149.

910. Gessi M, Giangaspero F, Pietsch T. Atypical teratoid/rhabdoid tumors and choroid plexus tumors: when genetics "surprise" pathology. Brain Pathol. 2003;13:409-414.

911. Burger PC, Yu IT, Tihan T, et al. Atypical teratoid/rhabdoid tumor of the central nervous system: a highly malignant tumor of infancy and childhood frequently mistaken for medulloblastoma: a Pediatric Oncology Group study. Am J Surg Pathol. 1998;22:1083-1092.

912. Versteege I, Sevenet N, Lange J, et al. Truncating mutations of hSNF5/INI1 in aggressive paediatric cancer. Nature. 1998;394:203-206.

913. Roberts CW, Orkin SH. The SWI/SNF complex—chromatin and cancer. Nat Rev Cancer. 2004;4:133-142.

914. Olson TA, Bayar E, Kosnik E, et al. Successful treatment of disseminated central nervous system malignant rhabdoid tumor. J Pediatr Hematol Oncol. 1995;17:71-75.

915. Chi S, Zimmerman MA, Yao X, et al. Intensive multimodality treatment for children with newly diagnosed CNS atypical teratoid rhabdoid tumor. J Clin Oncol. 2009;27:385-389.

916. Chen YW, Wong TT, Ho DM, et al. Impact of radiotherapy for pediatric CNS atypical teratoid/rhabdoid tumor (single institute experience). Int J Radiat Oncol Biol Phys. 2006;64:1038-1043.

917. Chiou SH, Kao CL, Chen YW, et al. Identification of CD133-positive radioresistant cells in atypical teratoid/rhabdoid tumor. PLoS ONE. 2008;3:e2090.

918. Fujisawa H, Misaki K, Takabatake Y, et al. Cyclin D1 is overexpressed in atypical teratoid/rhabdoid tumor with hSNF5/INI1 gene inactivation. J Neurooncol. 2005;3:117-124.

919. Packer RJ, Biegel JA, Blaney S, et al. Atypical teratoid/rhabdoid tumor of the central nervous system: report on workshop. J Pediatr Hematol Oncol. 2002;24:337-342.

920. Rorke LB, Packer R, Biegel J. Central nervous system atypical teratoid/rhabdoid tumors of infancy and childhood. J Neurooncol. 1995;24:21-28.

921. Hassoun J, Soylemezoglu F, Gambarelli D, et al. Central neurocytoma: a synopsis of clinical and histological features. Brain Pathol. 1993;3:297-306.

922. Hassoun J, Gambarelli D, Grisoli F, et al. Central neurocytoma. An electron-microscopic study of two cases. Acta Neuropathol. 1982;56:151-156.

923. Patt S, Schmidt H, Labrakakis C, et al. Human central neurocytoma cells show neuronal physiological properties in vitro. Acta Neuropathol. 1996;91:209-214.

924. Tsuchida T, Matsumoto M, Shirayama Y, et al. Neuronal and glial characteristics of central neurocytoma: electron microscopical analysis of two cases. Acta Neuropathol. 1996;91:573-577.

925. Sim FJ, Keyoung HM, Goldman JE, et al. Neurocytoma is a tumor of adult neuronal progenitor cells. J Neurosci. 2006;26:12544-12555.

926. Schmidt MH, Gottfried ON, von Koch CS, et al. Central neurocytoma: a review. J Neurooncol. 2004;66:377-384.

927. Ashkan K, Casey AT, D'Arrigo C, et al. Benign central neurocytoma. Cancer. 2000;89:1111-1120.

928. Rades D, Schild SE, Fehlauer F. Prognostic value of the MIB-1 labeling index for central neurocytomas. Neurology. 2004;62:987-989.

929. Leenstra JL, Rodriguez FJ, Frechette CM, et al. Central neurocytoma: management recommendations based on a 35-year experience. Int J Radiat Oncol Biol Phys. 2007;67:1145-1154.

930. Rades D, Schild SE, Fehlauer F. Defining the best available treatment for neurocytomas in children. Cancer. 2004;101:2629-2632.

931. Salvati M, Cervoni L, Caruso R, et al. Central neurocytoma: clinical features of 8 cases. Neurosurg Rev. 1997;20:39-43.

932. Tatter SB, Borges LF, Louis DN. Central neurocytomas of the cervical spinal cord. Report of two cases. J Neurosurg. 1994; 81:288-293.

933. Schild SE, Scheithauer BW, Haddock MG, et al. Central neurocytomas. Cancer. 1997;79:790-795.

934. Jouvet A, Lellouch-Tubiana A, Boddaert N, et al. Fourth ventricle neurocytoma with lipomatous and ependymal differentiation. Acta Neuropathol. 2005;109:346-351.

935. Singh A, Chand K, Singh H, et al. Atypical neurocytoma of the spinal cord in a young child. Childs Nerv Syst. 2007; 23:207-211.

936. Kerkovsky M, Zitterbart K, Svoboda K, et al. Central neurocytoma: the neuroradiological perspective. Childs Nerv Syst. 2008;24:1361-1369.

937. Sgouros S, Carey M, Aluwihare N, et al. Central neurocytoma: a correlative clinicopathologic and radiologic analysis. Surg Neurol. 1998;49:197-204.

938. Chang KH, Han MH, Kim DG, et al. MR appearance of central neurocytoma. Acta Radiol. 1993;34:520-526.

939. Yeh IB, Xu M, Ng WH, et al. Central neurocytoma: typical magnetic resonance spectroscopy findings and atypical ventricular dissemination. Magn Reson Imaging. 2008;26:59-64.

940. Figarella-Branger D, Soylemezoglu F, Burger P. Central neurocytoma and extraventricular neurocytoma. In Louis DN, Ohgaki H, Wiestler OD, et al (eds). WHO Classification of Tumours of the Central Nervous System, 4th ed. Geneva, World Health Organization Press, 2007, pp 106-109.

941. Zhang D, Wen L, Henning TD, et al. Central neurocytoma: clinical, pathological and neuroradiological findings. Clin Radiol. 2006;61:348-357.

942. Rajesh LS, Jain D, Radotra BD, et al. Central neurocytoma: a clinico-pathological study of eight cases. Indian J Pathol Microbiol. 2006;49:543-545.

943. Mackenzie IR. Central neurocytoma: histologic atypia, proliferation potential, and clinical outcome. Cancer. 1999;85: 1606-1610.

944. Soylemezoglu F, Scheithauer BW, Esteve J, et al. Atypical central neurocytoma. J Neuropathol Exp Neurol. 1997;56: 551-556.

945. Cenacchi G, Giangaspero F, Cerasoli S, et al. Ultrastructural characterization of oligodendroglial-like cells in central nervous system tumors. Ultrastruct Pathol. 1996;20:537-547.

946. Brat DJ, Scheithauer BW, Eberhart CG, et al. Extraventricular neurocytomas: pathologic features and clinical outcome. Am J Surg Pathol. 2001;25:1252-1260.

947. Rades D, Schild SE. Treatment recommendations for the various subgroups of neurocytomas. J Neurooncol. 2006;77: 305-309.

948. Rades D, Schild SE, Ikezaki K, et al. Defining the optimal dose of radiation after incomplete resection of central neurocytomas. Int J Radiat Oncol Biol Phys. 2003;55:373-377.

949. Rades D, Fehlauer F, Schild SE. Treatment of atypical neurocytomas. Cancer. 2004;100:814-847.

950. Yen CP, Sheehan J, Patterson G, et al. Gamma knife surgery for neurocytoma. J Neurosurg. 2007;107:7-12.

951. Amini E, Roffidal T, Lee A, et al. Central neurocytoma responsive to topotecan, ifosfamide, carboplatin. Pediatr Blood Cancer. 2008;51:137-140.

952. Brandes AA, Amista P, Gardiman M, et al. Chemotherapy in patients with recurrent and progressive central neurocytoma. Cancer. 2000;88:169-174.

953. Cavalheiro S, Moron AF, Hisaba W, et al. Fetal brain tumors. Childs Nerv Syst. 2003;19:529-536.

954. Wolff JE, Sajedi M, Brant R, et al. Choroid plexus tumours. Br J Cancer. 2002;87:1086-1091.

955. Pencalet P, Sainte-Rose C, Lellouch-Tubiana A, et al. Papillomas and carcinomas of the choroid plexus in children. J Neurosurg. 1998;88:521-528.

956. Losi-Guembarovski R, Kuasne H, Guembarovski AL, et al. DNA methylation patterns of the CDH1, RARB, and SFN genes in choroid plexus tumors. Cancer Genet Cytogenet. 2007;179:140-145.

957. Krutilkova V, Trkova M, Fleitz J, et al. Identification of five new families strengthens the link between childhood choroid plexus carcinoma and germline TP53 mutations. Eur J Cancer. 2005;41:1597-1603.

958. Hasselblatt M, Bohm C, Tatenhorst L, et al. Identification of novel diagnostic markers for choroid plexus tumors: a microarray-based approach. Am J Surg Pathol. 2006;30:66-74.

959. Ohgaki H, Huang H, Haltia M, et al. More about cell and molecular biology of simian virus 40: implications for human infections and disease. J Natl Cancer Inst. 2000;92:495-497.

960. Nupponen NN, Paulsson J, Jeibmann A, et al. Platelet-derived growth factor receptor expression and amplification in choroid plexus carcinomas. Mod Pathol. 2008;21:265-270.

961. Donovan DJ, Prauner RD. Shunt-related abdominal metastases in a child with choroid plexus carcinoma: case report. Neurosurgery. 2005;56:E412.

962. Guermazi A, De Kerviler E, Zagdanski AM, et al. Diagnostic imaging of choroid plexus disease. Clin Radiol. 2000;55: 503-516.

963. Meyers SP, Khademian ZP, Chuang SH, et al. Choroid plexus carcinomas in children: MRI features and patient outcomes. Neuroradiology. 2004;46:770-780.

964. Krieger MD, Panigrahy A, McComb JG, et al. Differentiation of choroid plexus tumors by advanced magnetic resonance spectroscopy. Neurosurg Focus. 2005;18:E4.

965. Jeibmann A, Wrede B, Peters O, et al. Malignant progression in choroid plexus papillomas. J Neurosurg. 2007;107:199-202.

966. Jeibmann A, Hasselblatt M, Gerss J, et al. Prognostic implications of atypical histologic features in choroid plexus papilloma. J Neuropathol Exp Neurol. 2006;65:1069-1073.

967. Gupta N. Choroid plexus tumors in children. Neurosurg Clin N Am. 2003;14:621-631.

968. Wrede B, Liu P, Ater J, et al. Second surgery and the prognosis of choroid plexus carcinoma—results of a meta-analysis of individual cases. Anticancer Res. 2005;25:4429-4433.

969. Krishnan S, Brown PD, Scheithauer BW, et al. Choroid plexus papillomas: a single institutional experience. J Neurooncol. 2004;68:49-55.

970. Greenberg ML. Chemotherapy of choroid plexus carcinoma. Childs Nerv Syst. 1999;15:571-577.

971. Packer RJ, Cohen BH, Cooney K. Intracranial germ cell tumors. Oncologist. 2000;5:312-320.

972. Mori K, Kurisaka M. Brain tumors in childhood: statistical analysis of cases from the Brain Tumor Registry of Japan. Childs Nerv Syst. 1986;2:233-237.

973. Villano JL, Propp JM, Porter KR, et al. Malignant pineal germ-cell tumors: an analysis of cases from three tumor registries. Neuro Oncol. 2008;10:121-130.

974. Cuccia V, Galarza M. Pure pineal germinomas: analysis of gender incidence. Acta Neurochir (Wien). 2006;148:865-871.

975. Keene D, Johnston D, Strother D, et al. Epidemiological survey of central nervous system germ cell tumors in Canadian children. J Neurooncol. 2007;82:289-295.

976. Jennings MT, Gelman R, Hochberg F. Intracranial germ-cell tumors: natural history and pathogenesis. J Neurosurg. 1985;63:155-167.

977. Okamoto K, Ito J, Ishikawa K, et al. Atrophy of the basal ganglia as the initial diagnostic sign of germinoma in the basal ganglia. Neuroradiology. 2002;44:389-394.

978. Wong TT, Chen YW, Guo WY, et al. Germinoma involving the basal ganglia in children. Childs Nerv Syst. 2008;24:71-78.

979. Hoffman HJ, Otsubo H, Hendrick EB, et al. Intracranial germ-cell tumors in children. J Neurosurg. 1991;74:545-551.

980. Sawamura Y, Ikeda J, Shirato H, et al. Germ cell tumours of the central nervous system: treatment consideration based on 111 cases and their long-term clinical outcomes. Eur J Cancer. 1998;34:104-110.

981. Echevarria ME, Fangusaro J, Goldman S. Pediatric central nervous system germ cell tumors: a review. Oncologist. 2008;13:690-699.

982. Bolat F, Kayaselcuk F, Tarim E, et al. Congenital intracranial teratoma with massive macrocephaly and skull rupture. Fetal Diagn Ther. 2008;23:1-4.

983. Kaido T, Sasaoka Y, Hashimoto H, et al. De novo germinoma in the brain in association with Klinefelter's syndrome: case report and review of the literature. Surg Neurol. 2003; 60:553-558.

984. Chik K, Li C, Shing MM, et al. Intracranial germ cell tumors in children with and without Down syndrome. J Pediatr Hematol Oncol. 1999;21:149-151.

985. Matsumura N, Kurimoto M, Endo S, et al. Intracranial germinoma associated with Down's syndrome. Report of 2 cases. Pediatr Neurosurg. 1998;29:199-202.

986. Crawford JR, Santi MR, Vezina G, et al. CNS germ cell tumor (CNSGCT) of childhood: presentation and delayed diagnosis. Neurology. 2007;68:1668-1673.

987. Ramelli GP, von der Weid N, Stanga Z, et al. Suprasellar germinomas in childhood and adolescence: diagnostic pitfalls. J Pediatr Endocrinol Metab. 1998;11:693-697.

988. Mikami-Terao Y, Akiyama M, Yanagisawa T, et al. Lymphocytic hypophysitis with central diabetes insipidus and subsequent hypopituitarism masking a suprasellar germinoma in a 13-year-old girl. Childs Nerv Syst. 2006;22:1338-1343.

989. Wellons JC 3rd, Reddy AT, Tubbs RS, et al. Neuroendoscopic findings in patients with intracranial germinomas correlating with diabetes insipidus. J Neurosurg. 2004;100:430-436.

990. Kuo HC, Sheen JM, Wu KS, et al. Precocious puberty due to human chorionic gonadotropin-secreting pineal tumor. Chang Gung Med J. 2006;29:198-202.

991. Ogino H, Shibamoto Y, Takanaka T, et al. CNS germinoma with elevated serum human chorionic gonadotropin level: clinical characteristics and treatment outcome. Int J Radiat Oncol Biol Phys. 2005;62:803-808.

992. Tomura N, Takahashi S, Kato K, et al. Germ cell tumors of the central nervous system originating from non-pineal regions: CT and MR features. Comput Med Imaging Graph. 2000;24:269-276.

993. Fujimaki T, Matsutani M, Funada N, et al. CT and MRI features of intracranial germ cell tumors. J Neurooncol. 1994;19:217-226.

994. Liang L, Korogi Y, Sugahara T, et al. MRI of intracranial germ-cell tumours. Neuroradiology. 2002;44:382-388.

995. Korogi Y, Takahashi M, Ushio Y. MRI of pineal region tumors. J Neurooncol. 2001;54:251-261.

996. Seregni E, Massimino M, Nerini Molteni S, et al. Serum and cerebrospinal fluid human chorionic gonadotropin (hCG) and alpha-fetoprotein (AFP) in intracranial germ cell tumors. Int J Biol Markers. 2002;17:112-118.

997. Sugiyama K, Arita K, Tominaga A, et al. Morphologic features of human chorionic gonadotropin- or alpha-fetoprotein-producing germ cell tumors of the central nervous system: histological heterogeneity and surgical meaning. Brain Tumor Pathol. 2001;18:115-122.

998. Fujimaki T, Mishima K, Asai A, et al. Levels of beta-human chorionic gonadotropin in cerebrospinal fluid of patients with malignant germ cell tumor can be used to detect early recurrence and monitor the response to treatment. Jpn J Clin Oncol. 2000;30:291-294.

999. Nakamura H, Takeshima H, Makino K, et al. C-kit expression in germinoma: an immunohistochemistry-based study. J Neurooncol. 2005;75:163-167.

1000. Takeshima H, Kuratsu J. A review of soluble c-kit (s-kit) as a novel tumor marker and possible molecular target for the treatment of CNS germinoma. Surg Neurol. 2003;60:321-324.

1001. Shinoda J, Yamada H, Sakai N, et al. Placental alkaline phosphatase as a tumor marker for primary intracranial germinoma. J Neurosurg. 1988;68:710-720.

1002. Ohama K, Nagase H, Ogino K, et al. Alpha-fetoprotein (AFP) levels in normal children. Eur J Pediatr Surg. 1997;7:267-269.

1003. Rosenblum M, Nakazato Y, Matsutani M. CNS germ cell tumours. In Louis DN, Ohgaki H, Wiestler OD, et al (eds). WHO Classification of Tumours of the Central Nervous System, 4th ed. Geneva, World Health Organization Press, 2007, pp 198-204.

1004. Ngan KW, Jung SM, Lee LY, et al. Immunohistochemical expression of OCT4 in primary central nervous system germ cell tumours. J Clin Neurosci. 2008;15:149-152.

1005. Takeshima H, Kaji M, Uchida H, et al. Expression and distribution of c-kit receptor and its ligand in human CNS germ cell tumors: a useful histological marker for the diagnosis of germinoma. Brain Tumor Pathol. 2004;21:13-16.

1006. Phi JH, Kim SK, Park SH, et al. Immature teratomas of the central nervous system: is adjuvant therapy mandatory? J Neurosurg. 2005;103:524-530.

1007. Freilich RJ, Thompson SJ, Walker RW, et al. Adenocarcinomatous transformation of intracranial germ cell tumors. Am J Surg Pathol. 1995;19:537-544.

1008. Fouladi M, Gajjar A, Boyett JM, et al. Comparison of CSF cytology and spinal magnetic resonance imaging in the detection of leptomeningeal disease in pediatric medulloblastoma or primitive neuroectodermal tumor. J Clin Oncol. 1999;17:3234-3237.

1009. Shono T, Natori Y, Morioka T, et al. Results of a long-term follow-up after neuroendoscopic biopsy procedure and third ventriculostomy in patients with intracranial germinomas. J Neurosurg. 2007;107:193-198.

1010. Weiner HL, Lichtenbaum RA, Wisoff JH, et al. Delayed surgical resection of central nervous system germ cell tumors. Neurosurgery. 2002;50:727-733.

1011. Finlay J, da Silva NS, Lavey R, et al. The management of patients with primary central nervous system (CNS) germinoma: current controversies requiring resolution. Pediatr Blood Cancer. 2008;51:313-316.

1012. Balmaceda C, Finlay J. Current advances in the diagnosis and management of intracranial germ cell tumors. Curr Neurol Neurosci Rep. 2004;4:253-262.

1013. Ogawa K, Shikama N, Toita T, et al. Long-term results of radiotherapy for intracranial germinoma: a multi-institutional retrospective review of 126 patients. Int J Radiat Oncol Biol Phys. 2004;58:705-713.

1014. Zissiadis Y, Dutton S, Kieran M, et al. Stereotactic radiotherapy for pediatric intracranial germ cell tumors. Int J Radiat Oncol Biol Phys. 2001;51:108-112.

1015. Dearnaley DP, A'Hern RP, Whittaker S, et al. Pineal and CNS germ cell tumors: Royal Marsden Hospital experience 1962-1987. Int J Radiat Oncol Biol Phys. 1990;18:773-781.

1016. Sands SA, Kellie SJ, Davidow AL, et al. Long-term quality of life and neuropsychologic functioning for patients with CNS germ-cell tumors: from the First International CNS Germ-Cell Tumor Study. Neuro Oncol. 2001;3:174-183.

1017. Rogers SJ, Mosleh-Shirazi MA, Saran FH. Radiotherapy of localised intracranial germinoma: time to sever historical ties? Lancet Oncol. 2005;6:509-519.

1018. Lafay-Cousin L, Millar BA, Mabbott D, et al. Limited-field radiation for bifocal germinoma. Int J Radiat Oncol Biol Phys. 2006;65:486-492.

1019. Robertson PL, DaRosso RC, Allen JC. Improved prognosis of intracranial non-germinoma germ cell tumors with multimodality therapy. J Neurooncol. 1997;32:71-80.

1020. Kretschmar C, Kleinberg L, Greenberg M, et al. Pre-radiation chemotherapy with response-based radiation therapy in children with central nervous system germ cell tumors: a report from the Children's Oncology Group. Pediatr Blood Cancer. 2007;48: 285-291.

1021. Douglas JG, Rockhill JK, Olson JM, et al. Cisplatin-based chemotherapy followed by focal, reduced-dose irradiation for pediatric primary central nervous system germinomas. J Pediatr Hematol Oncol. 2006;28:36-39.

1022. Matsutani M. Combined chemotherapy and radiation therapy for CNS germ cell tumors—the Japanese experience. J Neurooncol. 2001;54:311-316.

1023. Tseng CK, Tsang NM, Wei KC, et al. Radiotherapy to primary CNS germinoma: how large an irradiated volume is justified for tumor control? J Neurooncol. 2003;62:343-348.

1024. Kellie SJ, Boyce H, Dunkel IJ, et al. Intensive cisplatin and cyclophosphamide-based chemotherapy without radiotherapy for intracranial germinomas: failure of a primary chemotherapy approach. Pediatr Blood Cancer. 2004;43:126-133.

1025. Kellie SJ, Boyce H, Dunkel IJ, et al. Primary chemotherapy for intracranial nongerminomatous germ cell tumors: results of the Second International CNS Germ Cell Study Group protocol. J Clin Oncol. 2004;22:846-853.

1026. Calaminus G, Bamberg M, Jurgens H, et al. Impact of surgery, chemotherapy and irradiation on long term outcome of intracranial malignant non-germinomatous germ cell tumors: results of the German Cooperative Trial MAKEI 89. Klin Padiatr. 2004;216:141-149.

1027. Borg M. Germ cell tumours of the central nervous system in children—controversies in radiotherapy. Med Pediatr Oncol. 2003;40:367-374.

1028. Calaminus G, Andreussi L, Garre ML, et al. Secreting germ cell tumors of the central nervous system (CNS). First results of the cooperative German/Italian pilot study (CNS sGCT). Klin Padiatr. 1997;209:222-227.

1029. Tada T, Takizawa T, Nakazato F, et al. Treatment of intracranial nongerminomatous germ-cell tumor by high-dose chemotherapy and autologous stem-cell rescue. J Neurooncol. 1999;44:71-76.

1030. Merchant TE, Davis BJ, Sheldon JM, et al. Radiation therapy for relapsed CNS germinoma after primary chemotherapy. J Clin Oncol. 1998;16:204-209.

1031. Bi WL, Bannykh SI, Baehring J. The growing teratoma syndrome after subtotal resection of an intracranial nongerminomatous germ cell tumor in an adult: case report. Neurosurgery. 2005;56:188.

1032. Kamoshima Y, Sawamura Y, Ikeda J, et al. Late recurrence and salvage therapy of CNS germinomas. J Neurooncol. 2008;90: 205-211.

1033. Modak S, Gardner S, Dunkel IJ, et al. Thiotepa-based high-dose chemotherapy with autologous stem-cell rescue in patients with recurrent or progressive CNS germ cell tumors. J Clin Oncol. 2004;22:1934-1943.

1034. Shinoda J, Sakai N, Yano H, et al. Prognostic factors and therapeutic problems of primary intracranial choriocarcinoma/germ-cell tumors with high levels of HCG. J Neurooncol. 2004;66:225-240.

1035. Rushing EJ, Giangaspero F, Paulus W, et al. Craniopharyngioma. In Louis DN, Ohgaki H, Wiestler OD, et al (eds). WHO Classification of Tumours of the Central Nervous System, 4th ed. Geneva, World Health Organization Press, 2007, pp 238-240.

1036. Wang KC, Hong SH, Kim SK, et al. Origin of craniopharyngiomas: implication on the growth pattern. Childs Nerv Syst. 2005;21:628-634.

1037. Zhang YQ, Wang CC, Ma ZY. Pediatric craniopharyngiomas: clinicomorphological study of 189 cases. Pediatr Neurosurg. 2002;36:80-84.

1038. Aghadiuno PU, Adeloye A, Olumide AA, et al. Intracranial neoplasms in children in Ibadan, Nigeria. Childs Nerv Syst. 1985;1:39-44.

1039. Oikonomou E, Barreto DC, Soares B, et al. Beta-catenin mutations in craniopharyngiomas and pituitary adenomas. J Neurooncol. 2005;73:205-209.

1040. Buslei R, Nolde M, Hofmann B, et al. Common mutations of beta-catenin in adamantinomatous craniopharyngiomas but not in other tumours originating from the sellar region. Acta Neuropathol. 2005;109:589-597.

1041. Yasargil MG, Curcic M, Kis M, et al. Total removal of craniopharyngiomas. Approaches and long-term results in 144 patients. J Neurosurg. 1990;73:3-11.

1042. Jagannathan J, Dumont AS, Jane JA Jr, et al. Pediatric sellar tumors: diagnostic procedures and management. Neurosurg Focus. 2005;18:E6.

1043. Brown JL, Burton DW, Deftos LJ, et al. Congenital craniopharyngioma and hypercalcemia induced by parathyroid hormone-related protein. Endocr Pract. 2007;13:67-71.

1044. Rossi A, Cama A, Consales A, et al. Neuroimaging of pediatric craniopharyngiomas: a pictorial essay. J Pediatr Endocrinol Metab. 2006;19(Suppl 1):299-319.

1045. Brunel H, Raybaud C, Peretti-Viton P, et al. Craniopharyngioma in children: MRI study of 43 cases. Neurochirurgie. 2002;48:309-318.

1046. Lin KL, Wang HS, Lui TN. Diagnosis and follow-up of craniopharyngiomas with transcranial Doppler sonography. J Ultrasound Med. 2002;21:801-806.

1047. Agozzino L, Ferraraccio F, Accardo M, et al. Morphological and ultrastructural findings of prognostic impact in craniopharyngiomas. Ultrastruct Pathol. 2006;30:143-150.

1048. Raghavan R, Dickey WT Jr, Margraf LR, et al. Proliferative activity in craniopharyngiomas: clinicopathological correlations in adults and children. Surg Neurol. 2000;54:241-247.

1049. Muller HL. Childhood craniopharyngioma. Recent advances in diagnosis, treatment and follow-up. Horm Res. 2008;69: 193-202.

1050. Puget S, Grill J, Habrand JL, et al. Multimodal treatment of craniopharyngioma: defining a risk-adapted strategy. J Pediatr Endocrinol Metab. 2006;19(Suppl 1):367-370.

1051. Muller HL, Gebhardt U, Pohl F, et al. Relapse pattern after complete resection and early progression after incomplete resection of childhood craniopharyngioma. Klin Padiatr. 2006;218:315-320.

1052. Ghirardello S, Hopper N, Albanese A, et al. Diabetes insipidus in craniopharyngioma: postoperative management of water and electrolyte disorders. J Pediatr Endocrinol Metab. 2006;19(Suppl 1):413-421.

1053. Puget S, Garnett M, Wray A, et al. Pediatric craniopharyngiomas: classification and treatment according to the degree of hypothalamic involvement. J Neurosurg. 2007;106:3-12.

1054. Marchal JC, Klein O, Thouvenot P, et al. Individualized treatment of craniopharyngioma in children: ways and means. Childs Nerv Syst. 2005;21:655-659.

1055. Sainte-Rose C, Puget S, Wray A, et al. Craniopharyngioma: the pendulum of surgical management. Childs Nerv Syst. 2005;21: 691-695.

1056. Merchant TE, Kiehna EN, Kun LE, et al. Phase II trial of conformal radiation therapy for pediatric patients with craniopharyngioma and correlation of surgical factors and radiation dosimetry with change in cognitive function. J Neurosurg. 2006;104:94-102.

1057. Kalapurakal JA. Radiation therapy in the management of pediatric craniopharyngiomas—a review. Childs Nerv Syst. 2005;21: 808-816.

1058. Pereira AM, Schmid EM, Schutte PJ, et al. High prevalence of long-term cardiovascular, neurological and psychosocial morbidity after treatment for craniopharyngioma. Clin Endocrinol (Oxf). 2005;62:197-204.

1059. Rittinger O, Kranzinger M, Jones R, et al. Malignant astrocytoma arising 10 years after combined treatment of craniopharyngioma. J Pediatr Endocrinol Metab. 2003;16:97-101.

1060. Bitzer M, Topka H. Progressive cerebral occlusive disease after radiation therapy. Stroke. 1995;26:131-136.

1061. Kim SD, Park JY, Park J, et al. Radiological findings following postsurgical intratumoral bleomycin injection for cystic craniopharyngioma. Clin Neurol Neurosurg. 2007;109:236-241.

1062. Hasegawa T, Kondziolka D, Hadjipanayis CG, et al. Management of cystic craniopharyngiomas with phosphorus-32 intracavitary irradiation. Neurosurgery. 2004;54:813-820.

1063. Hukin J, Steinbok P, Lafay-Cousin L, et al. Intracystic bleomycin therapy for craniopharyngioma in children: the Canadian experience. Cancer. 2007;109:2124-2131.

1064. Lafay-Cousin L, Bartels U, Raybaud C, et al. Neuroradiological findings of bleomycin leakage in cystic craniopharyngioma. Report of three cases. J Neurosurg. 2007;107:318-323.

1065. Ierardi DF, Fernandes MJ, Silva IR, et al. Apoptosis in alpha interferon (IFN-alpha) intratumoral chemotherapy for cystic craniopharyngiomas. Childs Nerv Syst. 2007;23:1041-1046.

1066. Takahashi H, Yamaguchi F, Teramoto A. Long-term outcome and reconsideration of intracystic chemotherapy with bleomycin for craniopharyngioma in children. Childs Nerv Syst. 2005;21:701-704.

1067. Cavalheiro S, Dastoli PA, Silva NS, et al. Use of interferon alpha in intratumoral chemotherapy for cystic craniopharyngioma. Childs Nerv Syst. 2005;21:719-724.

1068. Plowman PN, Besser GM, Shipley J, et al. Dramatic response of malignant craniopharyngioma to cis-platin-based chemotherapy. Should craniopharyngioma be considered as a suprasellar "germ cell" tumour? Br J Neurosurg. 2004;18:500-505.

1069. Jakacki RI, Cohen BH, Jamison C, et al. Phase II evaluation of interferon-alpha-2a for progressive or recurrent craniopharyngiomas. J Neurosurg. 2000;92:255-260.

1070. Lippens RJ, Rotteveel JJ, Otten BJ, et al. Chemotherapy with Adriamycin (doxorubicin) and CCNU (lomustine) in four children with recurrent craniopharyngioma. Eur J Paediatr Neurol. 1998;2:263-268.

1071. Hargrave DR. Does chemotherapy have a role in the management of craniopharyngioma? J Pediatr Endocrinol Metab. 2006;19(Suppl 1):407-412.

1072. Gupta DK, Ojha BK, Sarkar C, et al. Recurrence in pediatric craniopharyngiomas: analysis of clinical and histological features. Childs Nerv Syst. 2006;22:50-55.

1073. Di Rocco C, Caldarelli M, Tamburrini G, et al. Surgical management of craniopharyngiomas—experience with a pediatric series. J Pediatr Endocrinol Metab. 2006;19(Suppl 1):355-366.

1074. Scott RM. Craniopharyngioma: a personal (Boston) experience. Childs Nerv Syst. 2005;21:773-777.

1075. Karavitaki N, Brufani C, Warner JT, et al. Craniopharyngiomas in children and adults: systematic analysis of 121 cases with long-term follow-up. Clin Endocrinol (Oxf). 2005;62:397-409.

1076. Novegno F, Di Rocco F, Colosimo C Jr, et al. Ectopic recurrences of craniopharyngioma. Childs Nerv Syst. 2002;18:468-473.

1077. Lee YY, Wong TT, Fang YT, et al. Comparison of hypothalamopituitary axis dysfunction of intrasellar and third ventricular craniopharyngiomas in children. Brain Dev. 2008;30:189-194.

1078. Pedreira CC, Stargatt R, Maroulis H, et al. Health related quality of life and psychological outcome in patients treated for craniopharyngioma in childhood. J Pediatr Endocrinol Metab. 2006;19:15-24.

1079. Kendall-Taylor P, Jonsson PJ, Abs R, et al. The clinical, metabolic and endocrine features and the quality of life in adults with childhood-onset craniopharyngioma compared with adult-onset craniopharyngioma. Eur J Endocrinol. 2005;152:557-567.

1080. Gonc EN, Yordam N, Ozon A, et al. Endocrinological outcome of different treatment options in children with craniopharyngioma: a retrospective analysis of 66 cases. Pediatr Neurosurg. 2004;40:112-119.

1081. Karavitaki N, Warner JT, Marland A, et al. GH replacement does not increase the risk of recurrence in patients with craniopharyngioma. Clin Endocrinol (Oxf). 2006;64:556-560.

1082. Maiter D, Abs R, Johannsson G, et al. Baseline characteristics and response to GH replacement of hypopituitary patients previously irradiated for pituitary adenoma or craniopharyngioma: data from the Pfizer International Metabolic Database. Eur J Endocrinol. 2006;155:253-260.

1083. Marcus CL, Trescher WH, Halbower AC, et al. Secondary narcolepsy in children with brain tumors. Sleep. 2002;25:435-439.

1084. Mason PW, Krawiecki N, Meacham LR: The use of dextroamphetamine to treat obesity and hyperphagia in children treated for craniopharyngioma. Arch Pediatr Adolesc Med. 2002;156:887-892.

1085. Muller HL, Handwerker G, Gebhardt U, et al. Melatonin treatment in obese patients with childhood craniopharyngioma and increased daytime sleepiness. Cancer Causes Control. 2006;17:583-589.

1086. Muller HL, Muller-Stover S, Gebhardt U, et al. Secondary narcolepsy may be a causative factor of increased daytime sleepiness in obese childhood craniopharyngioma patients. J Pediatr Endocrinol Metab. 2006;19(Suppl 1):423-429.

1087. Ismail D, O'Connell MA, Zacharin MR. Dexamphetamine use for management of obesity and hypersomnolence following hypothalamic injury. J Pediatr Endocrinol Metab. 2006;19:129-134.

1088. Jackson AC, Tsantefski M, Goodman H, et al. The psychosocial impacts on families of low-incidence, complex conditions in children: the case of craniopharyngioma. Soc Work Health Care. 2003;38:81-107.

1089. Gurney JG, Smith MA, Bunin G. CNS and miscellaneous intracranial and intraspinal neoplasms. In Ries LAG, Smith MA, Gurney JG, et al (eds). Cancer Incidence and Survival Among Children and Adolescents: United States SEER Program 1975 to 1995. Bethesda, Md, National Cancer Institute SEER Program, 1999.

1090. Rice D, Barone S Jr. Critical periods of vulnerability for the developing nervous system: evidence from humans and animal models. Environ Health Perspect. 2000;108(Suppl 3):511-533.

1091. Bloom HJ, Wallace EN, Henk JM. The treatment and prognosis of medulloblastoma in children. A study of 82 verified cases. Am J Roentgenol Radium Ther Nucl Med. 1969;105:43-62.

1092. Duffner PK. Long-term effects of radiation therapy on cognitive and endocrine function in children with leukemia and brain tumors. Neurologist. 2004;10:293-310.

1093. Anderson NE. Late complications in childhood central nervous system tumour survivors. Curr Opin Neurol. 2003;16:677-683.

1094. Duffner PK, Horowitz ME, Krischer JP, et al. The treatment of malignant brain tumors in infants and very young children: an update of the Pediatric Oncology Group experience. Neuro Oncol. 1999;1:152-161.

1095. Kellie SJ. Chemotherapy of central nervous system tumours in infants. Childs Nerv Syst. 1999;15:592-612.

1096. Central Brain Tumor Registry of the United States. Statistical report: Primary brain tumors in the United States, 2000-2004. Hinsdale, Ill, Central Brain Tumor Registry of the United States, 2008.

1097. Rickert CH, Probst-Cousin S, Gullotta F. Primary intracranial neoplasms of infancy and early childhood. Childs Nerv Syst. 1997;13:507-513.

1098. Larouche V, Huang A, Bartels U, et al. Tumors of the central nervous system in the first year of life. Pediatr Blood Cancer. 2007;49:1074-1082.

1099. Asai A, Hoffman HJ, Hendrick EB, et al. Primary intracranial neoplasms in the first year of life. Childs Nerv Syst. 1989;5: 230-233.

1100. Jellinger K, Sunder-Plassmann M. Connatal intracranial tumours. Neuropadiatrie. 1973;4:46-63.

1101. Wilne S, Collier J, Kennedy C, et al. Presentation of childhood CNS tumours: a systematic review and meta-analysis. Lancet Oncol. 2007;8:685-695.

1102. Duffner PK, Horowitz ME, Krischer JP, et al. Postoperative chemotherapy and delayed radiation in children less than three years with malignant brain tumors. N Engl J Med. 1993;328: 1725-1731.

1103. Beckwith JB, Palmer NF. Histopathology and prognosis of Wilms' tumors: results from the First National Wilms' Tumor Study. Cancer. 1978;41:1937-1948.

1104. Bonnin JM, Rubinstein LJ, Palmer NF, et al. The association of embryonal tumors originating in the kidney and in the brain. A report of seven cases. Cancer. 1984;54:2137-2146.

1105. Kalifa C, Grill J. The therapy of infantile malignant brain tumors: current status? J Neurooncol. 2005;75:279-285.

1106. van Eys J, Cangir A, Coody D, et al. MOPP regimen as primary chemotherapy for brain tumors in infants. J Neurooncol. 1985;3:237-243.

1107. Geyer JR, Zeltzer PM, Boyett JM, et al. Survival of infants with primitive neuroectodermal tumors or malignant ependymomas of the CNS treated with eight drugs in 1 day: a report from the Children's Cancer Group. J Clin Oncol. 1994;12:1607-1615.

1108. Lashford LS, Campbell RH, Gattamaneni HR, et al. An intensive multiagent chemotherapy regimen for brain tumours occurring in very young children. Arch Dis Child. 1996;74: 219-223.

1109. Dupuis-Girod S, Hartmann O, Benhamou E, et al. Will high dose chemotherapy followed by autologous bone marrow transplantation supplant cranio-spinal irradiation in young children treated for medulloblastoma? J Neurooncol. 1996;27:87-98.

1110. Mason WP, Grovas A, Halpern S, et al. Intensive chemotherapy and bone marrow rescue for young children with newly diagnosed malignant brain tumors. J Clin Oncol. 1998;16: 210-221.

1111. Thorarinsdottir HK, Rood B, Kamani N, et al. Outcome for children <4 years with malignant central nervous system tumors treated with high-dose chemotherapy and autologous stem cell rescue. Pediatr Blood Cancer. 2007;48:278-284.

1112. Perez-Martinez A, Quintero V, Vicent MG, et al. High-dose chemotherapy with autologous stem cell rescue as first line of treatment in young children with medulloblastoma and supratentorial primitive neuroectodermal tumors. J Neurooncol. 2004;67:101-106.

1113. Ater JL, van Eys J, Woo SY, et al. MOPP chemotherapy without irradiation as primary postsurgical therapy for brain tumors in infants and young children. J Neurooncol. 1997;32:243-252.

1114. Crawford JR, MacDonald TJ, Packer RJ. Medulloblastoma in childhood: new biological advances. Lancet Neurol. 2007;6: 1073-1085.

1115. Gajjar A, Mulhern RK, Heideman RL, et al. Medulloblastoma in very young children: outcome of definitive craniospinal irradiation following incomplete response to chemotherapy. J Clin Oncol. 1994;12:1212-1216.

1116. Saran FH, Driever PH, Thilmann C, et al. Survival of very young children with medulloblastoma (primitive neuroectodermal tumor of the posterior fossa) treated with craniospinal irradiation. Int J Radiat Oncol Biol Phys. 1998;42:959-967.

1117. Linnebank M, Pels H, Kleczar N, et al. MTX-induced white matter changes are associated with polymorphisms of methionine metabolism. Neurology. 2005;64:912-913.

1118. Surtees R, Clelland J, Hann I. Demyelination and single-carbon transfer pathway metabolites during the treatment of acute lymphoblastic leukemia: CSF studies. J Clin Oncol. 1998;16: 1505-1511.

1119. Gilbertson RJ, Langdon JA, Hollander A, et al. Mutational analysis of PDGFR-RAS/MAPK pathway activation in childhood medulloblastoma. Eur J Cancer. 2006;42:646-649.

1120. Rickert CH. Epidemiological features of brain tumors in the first 3 years of life. Childs Nerv Syst. 1998;14:547-550.

1121. Dai AI, Backstrom JW, Burger PC, et al. Supratentorial primitive neuroectodermal tumors of infancy: clinical and radiologic findings. Pediatr Neurol. 2003;29:430-434.

1122. Hinkes BG, von Hoff K, Deinlein F, et al. Childhood pineoblastoma: experiences from the prospective multicenter trials HIT-SKK87, HIT-SKK92 and HIT91. J Neurooncol. 2007;81: 217-223.

1123. Hong TS, Mehta MP, Boyett JM, et al. Patterns of treatment failure in infants with primitive neuroectodermal tumors who were treated on CCG-921: a phase III combined modality study. Pediatr Blood Cancer. 2005;45:676-682.

1124. Marec-Berard P, Jouvet A, Thiesse P, et al. Supratentorial embryonal tumors in children under 5 years : an SFOP study of treatment with postoperative chemotherapy alone. Med Pediatr Oncol. 2002;38:83-90.

1125. Jakacki RI, Zeltzer PM, Boyett JM, et al. Survival and prognostic factors following radiation and/or chemotherapy for primitive neuroectodermal tumors of the pineal region in infants and children: a report of the Childrens Cancer Group. J Clin Oncol. 1995;13:1377-1383.

1126. Gururangan S, McLaughlin C, Quinn J, et al. High-dose chemotherapy with autologous stem-cell rescue in children and adults with newly diagnosed pineoblastomas. J Clin Oncol. 2003;21:2187-2191.

1127. Timmermann B, Kortmann RD, Kuhl J, et al. Role of radiotherapy in supratentorial primitive neuroectodermal tumor in young children: results of the German HIT-SKK87 and HIT-SKK92 trials. J Clin Oncol. 2006;24:1554-1560.

1128. Larouche V, Capra M, Huang A, et al. Supratentorial primitive neuroectodermal tumors in young children. J Clin Oncol. 2006;24:5609-5610.

1129. Allen JC, Siffert J, Hukin J. Clinical manifestations of childhood ependymoma: a multitude of syndromes. Pediatr Neurosurg. 1998;28:49-55.

1130. Perilongo G, Massimino M, Sotti G, et al. Analyses of prognostic factors in a retrospective review of 92 children with ependymoma: Italian Pediatric Neuro-oncology Group. Med Pediatr Oncol. 1997;29:79-85.

1131. Healey EA, Barnes PD, Kupsky WJ, et al. The prognostic significance of postoperative residual tumor in ependymoma. Neurosurgery. 1991;28:666-671.

1132. Ritter AM, Hess KR, McLendon RE, et al. Ependymomas: MIB-1 proliferation index and survival. J Neurooncol. 1998; 40:51-57.

1133. Preusser M, Heinzl H, Gelpi E, et al. Ki67 index in intracranial ependymoma: a promising histopathological candidate biomarker. Histopathology. 2008;53:39-47.

1134. Bouffet E, Foreman N. Chemotherapy for intracranial ependymomas. Childs Nerv Syst. 1999;15:563-570.

1135. Grundy RG, Wilne SA, Weston CL, et al. Primary postoperative chemotherapy without radiotherapy for intracranial ependymoma in children: the UKCCSG/SIOP prospective study. Lancet Oncol. 2007;8:696-705.

1136. Rezai AR, Woo HH, Lee M, et al. Disseminated ependymomas of the central nervous system. J Neurosurg. 1996;85:618-624.

1137. Zacharoulis S, Ji L, Pollack IF, et al. Metastatic ependymoma: a multi-institutional retrospective analysis of prognostic factors. Pediatr Blood Cancer. 2008;50:231-235.

1138. Sanders RP, Kocak M, Burger PC, et al. High-grade astrocytoma in very young children. Pediatr Blood Cancer. 2007;49: 888-893.

1139. St Clair SK, Humphreys RP, Pillay PK, et al. Current management of choroid plexus carcinoma in children. Pediatr Neurosurg. 1991;17:225-233.

1140. Allen J, Wisoff J, Helson L, et al. Choroid plexus carcinoma—responses to chemotherapy alone in newly diagnosed young children. J Neurooncol. 1992;12:69-74.

1141. Duffner PK, Kun LE, Burger PC, et al. Postoperative chemotherapy and delayed radiation in infants and very young children with choroid plexus carcinomas. The Pediatric Oncology Group. Pediatr Neurosurg. 1995;22:189-196.

1142. Fitzpatrick LK, Aronson LJ, Cohen KJ. Is there a requirement for adjuvant therapy for choroid plexus carcinoma that has been completely resected? J Neurooncol. 2002;57:123-126.

1143. Wolff JE, Sajedi M, Coppes MJ, et al. Radiation therapy and survival in choroid plexus carcinoma. Lancet. 1999;353: 2126.

1144. Berger C, Thiesse P, Lellouch-Tubiana A, et al. Choroid plexus carcinomas in childhood: clinical features and prognostic factors. Neurosurgery. 1998;42:470-475.

1145. Chow E, Reardon DA, Shah AB, et al. Pediatric choroid plexus neoplasms. Int J Radiat Oncol Biol Phys. 1999;44:249-254.

1146. Greene S, Nair N, Ojemann JG, et al. Meningiomas in children. Pediatr Neurosurg. 2008;44:9-13.

1147. Rushing EJ, Olsen C, Mena H, et al. Central nervous system meningiomas in the first two decades of life: a clinicopathological analysis of 87 patients. J Neurosurg. 2005;103:489-495.

1148. Tufan K, Dogulu F, Kurt G, et al. Intracranial meningiomas of childhood and adolescence. Pediatr Neurosurg. 2005;41:1-7.

1149. Louis DN, Ramesh V, Gusella JF. Neuropathology and molecular genetics of neurofibromatosis 2 and related tumors. Brain Pathol. 1995;5:163-172.

1150. Goshen Y, Stark B, Kornreich L, et al. High incidence of meningioma in cranial irradiated survivors of childhood acute lymphoblastic leukemia. Pediatr Blood Cancer. 2007;49:294-297.

1151. Lusis EA, Chicoine MR, Perry A. High throughput screening of meningioma biomarkers using a tissue microarray. J Neurooncol. 2005;73:219-223.

1152. Simon M, Bostrom JP, Hartmann C. Molecular genetics of meningiomas: from basic research to potential clinical applications. Neurosurgery. 2007;60:787-798.

1153. Pettorini BL, Park YS, Caldarelli M, et al. Radiation-induced brain tumours after central nervous system irradiation in childhood: a review. Childs Nerv Syst. 2008;24:793-805.

1154. Arivazhagan A, Devi BI, Kolluri SV, et al. Pediatric intracranial meningiomas—do they differ from their counterparts in adults? Pediatr Neurosurg. 2008;44:43-48.

1155. Gasparetto EL, Leite Cda C, Lucato LT, et al. Intracranial meningiomas: magnetic resonance imaging findings in 78 cases. Arq Neuropsiquiatr. 2007;65:610-614.

1156. Rokni-Yazdi H, Azmoudeh Ardalan F, Asadzandi Z, et al. Pathologic significance of the "dural tail sign". Eur J Radiol. 2008;Feb 20. [Epub ahead of print].

1157. Sandberg DI, Edgar MA, Resch L, et al. MIB-1 staining index of pediatric meningiomas. Neurosurgery. 2001;48:590-595.

1158. Marhx-Bracho A, Rueda-Franco F, Ibarra-de la Torre A, et al. Chordoid meningioma of the foramen magnum in a child: a case report and review of the literature. Childs Nerv Syst. 2008; 24:623-627.

1159. Miyajima Y, Oka H, Utsuki S, et al. Tentorial papillary meningioma in a child: case report and review of the literature. Clin Neuropathol. 2007;26:17-20.

1160. Vural M, Arslantas A, Ciftci E, et al. An unusual case of cervical clear-cell meningioma in pediatric age. Childs Nerv Syst. 2007;23:225-229.

1161. Perry A, Louis DN, Scheithauer BW, et al. Meningiomas. In Louis DN, Ohgaki H, Wiestler OD, et al (eds). WHO Classification of Tumours of the Central Nervous System, 4th ed. Geneva, World Health Organization Press, 2007, pp 164-172.

1162. Wellenreuther R, Kraus JA, Lenartz D, et al. Analysis of the neurofibromatosis 2 gene reveals molecular variants of meningioma. Am J Pathol. 1995;146:827-832.

1163. Traunecker H, Mallucci C, Grundy R, et al. Children's Cancer and Leukaemia Group (CCLG): guidelines for the management of intracranial meningioma in children and young people. Br J Neurosurg. 2008;22:13-25.

1164. Ware ML, Cha S, Gupta N, et al. Radiation-induced atypical meningioma with rapid growth in a 13-year-old girl. Case report. J Neurosurg. 2004;100:488-491.

1165. Mason WP, Gentili F, Macdonald DR, et al. Stabilization of disease progression by hydroxyurea in patients with recurrent or unresectable meningioma. J Neurosurg. 2002;97:341-346.

1166. Goodwin JW, Crowley J, Eyre HJ, et al. A phase II evaluation of tamoxifen in unresectable or refractory meningiomas: a Southwest Oncology Group study. J Neurooncol. 1993;15: 75-77.

1167. Marosi C, Hassler M, Roessler K, et al. Meningioma. Crit Rev Oncol Hematol. 2008;67:153-171.

1168. Newton HB. Hydroxyurea chemotherapy in the treatment of meningiomas. Neurosurg Focus. 2007;23:E11.

1169. Wen PY, Drappatz J. Novel therapies for meningiomas. Expert Rev Neurother. 2006;6:1447-1464.

1170. Zwerdling T, Dothage J. Meningiomas in children and adolescents. J Pediatr Hematol Oncol. 2002;24:199-204.

1171. Rochat P, Johannesen HH, Gjerris F. Long-term follow up of children with meningiomas in Denmark: 1935 to 1984. J Neurosurg. 2004;100:179-182.

1172. Kane LA, Leinung MC, Scheithauer BW, et al. Pituitary adenomas in childhood and adolescence. J Clin Endocrinol Metab. 1994;79:1135-1140.

1173. Diamond FB Jr. Pituitary adenomas in childhood: development and diagnosis. Fetal Pediatr Pathol. 2006;25:339-356.

1174. Mindermann T, Wilson CB. Pediatric pituitary adenomas. Neurosurgery. 1995;36:259-268.

1175. Partington MD, Davis DH, Laws ER Jr, et al. Pituitary adenomas in childhood and adolescence. Results of transsphenoidal surgery. J Neurosurg. 1994;80:209-216.

1176. Webb C, Prayson RA. Pediatric pituitary adenomas. Arch Pathol Lab Med. 2008;132:77-80.

1177. Mehrazin M. Pituitary tumors in children: clinical analysis of 21 cases. Childs Nerv Syst. 2007;23:391-398.

1178. Pandey P, Ojha BK, Mahapatra AK. Pediatric pituitary adenoma: a series of 42 patients. J Clin Neurosci. 2005; 12:124-127.

1179. De Menis E, Visentin A, Billeci D, et al. Pituitary adenomas in childhood and adolescence. Clinical analysis of 10 cases. J Endocrinol Invest. 2001;24:92-97.

1180. Lafferty AR, Chrousos GP. Pituitary tumors in children and adolescents. J Clin Endocrinol Metab. 1999;84:4317-4323.

1181. Abe T, Ludecke DK, Saeger W. Clinically nonsecreting pituitary adenomas in childhood and adolescence. Neurosurgery. 1998;42:744-750.

1182. Rennert J, Doerfler A. Imaging of sellar and parasellar lesions. Clin Neurol Neurosurg. 2007;109:111-124.

1183. Delman BN, Fatterpekar GM, Law M, et al. Neuroimaging for the pediatric endocrinologist. Pediatr Endocrinol Rev. 2008;5(Suppl 2):708-719.

1184. Savage MO, Chan LF, Afshar F, et al. Advances in the management of paediatric Cushing's disease. Horm Res. 2008;69: 327-333.

1185. Alves C, Alves AC. Primary hypothyroidism in a child simulating a prolactin-secreting adenoma. Childs Nerv Syst. 2008;24: 1505-1508.

1186. Molitch ME. Medical management of prolactin-secreting pituitary adenomas. Pituitary. 2002;5:55-65.

1187. Jane JA Jr. Management of pediatric sellar tumors. Pediatr Endocrinol Rev. 2008;5(Suppl 2):720-726.

1188. Newman CB, Melmed S, George A, et al. Octreotide as primary therapy for acromegaly. J Clin Endocrinol Metab. 1998;83: 3034-3040.

1189. Trump D, Farren B, Wooding C, et al. Clinical studies of multiple endocrine neoplasia type 1 (MEN1). QJM. 1996;89: 653-669.

1190. Keil MF, Stratakis CA. Pituitary tumors in childhood: update of diagnosis, treatment and molecular genetics. Expert Rev Neurother. 2008;8:563-574.

1191. Joshi SM, Hewitt RJ, Storr HL, et al. Cushing's disease in children and adolescents: 20 years of experience in a single neurosurgical center. Neurosurgery. 2005;57:281-285.

1192. Maitra A, Kumar V. Diseases of infancy and childhood. In Kumar V, Abbas A, Fausto N (eds). Robbins and Cotran: Pathologic Basis of Disease, 7th ed. Philadelphia, Saunders, 2005.

1193. Farrell CJ, Plotkin SR. Genetic causes of brain tumors: neurofibromatosis, tuberous sclerosis, von Hippel-Lindau, and other syndromes. Neurol Clin. 2007;25:925-946.

1194. Huson S, Jones D, Beck L. Ophthalmic manifestations of neurofibromatosis. Br J Ophthalmol. 1987;71:235-238.

1195. Szudek J, Friedman JM. Unidentified bright objects associated with features of neurofibromatosis 1. Pediatr Neurol. 2002;27:123-127.

1196. Gutmann DH, Loehr A, Zhang Y, et al. Haploinsufficiency for the neurofibromatosis 1 (NF1) tumor suppressor results in increased astrocyte proliferation. Oncogene. 1999;18:4450-4459.

1197. Bosch MM, Boltshauser E, Harpes P, et al. Ophthalmologic findings and long-term course in patients with neurofibromatosis type 2. Am J Ophthalmol. 2006;141:1068-1077.

1198. Ragge NK, Baser ME, Riccardi VM, et al. The ocular presentation of neurofibromatosis 2. Eye. 1997;11(Pt 1):12-18.

1199. Meyers SM, Gutman FA, Kaye LD, et al. Retinal changes associated with neurofibromatosis 2. Trans Am Ophthalmol Soc. 1995;93:245-252.

1200. Houshmandi SS, Gutmann DH. All in the family: using inherited cancer syndromes to understand de-regulated cell signaling in brain tumors. J Cell Biochem. 2007;102:811-819.

1201. Jozwiak J, Wlodarski P. Hamartin and tuberin modulate gene transcription via beta-catenin. J Neurooncol. 2006;79:229-234.

1202. Pilarski R, Eng C. Will the real Cowden syndrome please stand up (again)? Expanding mutational and clinical spectra of the PTEN hamartoma tumour syndrome. J Med Genet. 2004; 41:323-326.

1203. Starink TM, Meijer CJ, Brownstein MH. The cutaneous pathology of Cowden's disease: new findings. J Cutan Pathol. 1985;12:83-93.

1204. Liaw D, Marsh DJ, Li J, et al. Germline mutations of the PTEN gene in Cowden disease, an inherited breast and thyroid cancer syndrome. Nat Genet. 1997;16:64-67.

1205. Nelen MR, van Staveren WC, Peeters EA, et al. Germline mutations in the PTEN/MMAC1 gene in patients with Cowden disease. Hum Mol Genet. 1997;6:1383-1387.

1206. Marsh DJ, Coulon V, Lunetta KL, et al. Mutation spectrum and genotype-phenotype analyses in Cowden disease and Bannayan-Zonana syndrome, two hamartoma syndromes with germline PTEN mutation. Hum Mol Genet. 1998;7:507-515.

1207. Lopiccolo J, Ballas MS, Dennis PA. PTEN hamartomatous tumor syndromes (PHTS): rare syndromes with great relevance to common cancers and targeted drug development. Crit Rev Oncol Hematol. 2007;63:203-214.

1208. Eng C, Murday V, Seal S, et al. Cowden syndrome and Lhermitte-Duclos disease in a family: a single genetic syndrome with pleiotropy? J Med Genet. 1994;31:458-461.

1209. Padberg GW, Schot JD, Vielvoye GJ, et al. Lhermitte-Duclos disease and Cowden disease: a single phakomatosis. Ann Neurol. 1991;29:517-523.

1210. Shepherd CW, Houser OW, Gomez MR. MR findings in tuberous sclerosis complex and correlation with seizure development and mental impairment. AJNR Am J Neuroradiol. 1995;16: 149-155.

1211. Chou IJ, Lin KL, Wong AM, et al. Neuroimaging correlation with neurological severity in tuberous sclerosis complex. Eur J Paediatr Neurol. 2008;12:108-112.

1212. Kamimura T, Tohyama J, Oishi M, et al. Magnetoencephalography in patients with tuberous sclerosis and localization-related epilepsy. Epilepsia. 2006;47:991-997.

1213. Wu JY, Sutherling WW, Koh S, et al. Magnetic source imaging localizes epileptogenic zone in children with tuberous sclerosis complex. Neurology. 2006;66:1270-1272.

1214. Dilworth JT, Kraniak JM, Wojtkowiak JW, et al. Molecular targets for emerging anti-tumor therapies for neurofibromatosis type 1. Biochem Pharmacol. 2006;72:1485-1492.

1215. Wallace RH, Freeman JL, Shouri MR, et al. Somatic mutations in GLI3 can cause hypothalamic hamartoma and gelastic seizures. Neurology. 2008;70:653-655.

1216. Fenoglio KA, Wu J, Kim do Y, et al. Hypothalamic hamartoma: basic mechanisms of intrinsic epileptogenesis. Semin Pediatr Neurol. 2007;14:51-59.

1217. Delande O, Rodriguez D, Chiron C, et al. Successful surgical relief of seizures associated with hamartoma of the floor of the fourth ventricle in children: report of two cases. Neurosurgery. 2001;49:726-730.

1218. Shim KW, Chang JH, Park YG, et al. Treatment modality for intractable epilepsy in hypothalamic hamartomatous lesions. Neurosurgery. 2008;62:847-856.

1219. Pizer BL, Moss T, Oakhill A, et al. Congenital astroblastoma: an immunohistochemical study. Case report. J Neurosurg. 1995;83:550-555.

1220. Navarro R, Reitman AJ, de Leon GA, et al. Astroblastoma in childhood: pathological and clinical analysis. Childs Nerv Syst. 2005;21:211-220.

1221. Brat DJ, Hirose Y, Cohen KJ, et al. Astroblastoma: clinicopathologic features and chromosomal abnormalities defined by comparative genomic hybridization. Brain Pathol. 2000;10: 342-352.

1222. Bonnin JM, Rubinstein LJ. Astroblastomas: a pathological study of 23 tumors, with a postoperative follow-up in 13 patients. Neurosurgery. 1989;25:6-13.

1223. Rubinstein LJ, Herman MM. The astroblastoma and its possible cytogenic relationship to the tanycyte. An electron microscopic, immunohistochemical, tissue- and organ-culture study. Acta Neuropathol. 1989;78:472-483.

1224. Aldape K, Rosenblum M. Astroblastoma. In Louis DN, Ohgaki H, Wiestler OD, et al (eds). WHO Classification of Tumours of the Central Nervous System, 4th ed. Geneva, World Health Organization Press, 2007, pp 88-89.

1225. Unal E, Koksal Y, Vajtai I, et al. Astroblastoma in a child. Childs Nerv Syst. 2008;24:165-168.

1226. Kim DS, Park SY, Lee SP. Astroblastoma: a case report. J Korean Med Sci. 2004;19:772-776.

1227. Mierau GW, Tyson RW, McGavran L, et al. Astroblastoma: ultrastructural observations on a case of high-grade type. Ultrastruct Pathol. 1999;23:325-332.

1228. Thiessen B, Finlay J, Kulkarni R, et al. Astroblastoma: does histology predict biologic behavior? J Neurooncol. 1998; 40:59-65.

1229. Bell JW, Osborn AG, Salzman KL, et al. Neuroradiologic characteristics of astroblastoma. Neuroradiology. 2007;49:203-209.

1230. Port JD, Brat DJ, Burger PC, et al. Astroblastoma: radiologic-pathologic correlation and distinction from ependymoma. AJNR Am J Neuroradiol. 2002;23:243-247.

1231. Fathi AR, Novoa E, El-Koussy M, et al. Astroblastoma with rhabdoid features and favorable long-term outcome: report of a case with a 12-year follow-up. Pathol Res Pract. 2008;204:345-351.

1232. Caroli E, Salvati M, Esposito V, et al. Cerebral astroblastoma. Acta Neurochir (Wien). 2004;146:629-633.

1233. Mangano FT, Bradford AC, Mittler MA, et al. Astroblastoma. Case report, review of the literature, and analysis of treatment strategies. J Neurosurg Sci. 2007;51:21-27.

1234. Hata N, Shono T, Yoshimoto K, et al. An astroblastoma case associated with loss of heterozygosity on chromosome 9p. J Neurooncol. 2006;80:69-73.

1235. Bannykh SI, Fan X, Black KL. Malignant astroblastoma with rhabdoid morphology. J Neurooncol. 2007;83:277-278.

1236. Makino K, Nakamura H, Yano S, et al. Pediatric primary CNS lymphoma: longterm survival after treatment with radiation monotherapy. Acta Neurochir (Wien). 2007;149:295-297.

1237. Kai Y, Kuratsu J, Ushio Y. Primary malignant lymphoma of the brain in childhood. Neurol Med Chir (Tokyo). 1998;38:232-237.

1238. Henry JM, Heffner RR Jr, Dillard SH, et al. Primary malignant lymphomas of the central nervous system. Cancer. 1974;34:1293-1302.

1239. Mueller BU, Pizzo PA. Cancer in children with primary or secondary immunodeficiencies. J Pediatr. 1995;126:1-10.

1240. Filipovich AH, Heinitz KJ, Robison LL, et al. The Immunodeficiency Cancer Registry. A research resource. Am J Pediatr Hematol Oncol. 1987;9:183-184.

1241. Perry GS 3rd, Spector BD, Schuman LM, et al. The Wiskott-Aldrich syndrome in the United States and Canada (1892-1979). J Pediatr. 1980;97:72-78.

1242. Filipovich AH, Mathur A, Kamat D, et al. Primary immunodeficiencies: genetic risk factors for lymphoma. Cancer Res. 1992;52:5465s-5467s.

1243. Schabet M. Epidemiology of primary CNS lymphoma. J Neurooncol. 1999;43:199-201.

1244. Forsyth PA, DeAngelis LM. Biology and management of AIDS-associated primary CNS lymphomas. Hematol Oncol Clin North Am. 1996;10:1125-1134.

1245. Mueller BU, Pizzo PA. Malignancies in pediatric AIDS. Curr Opin Pediatr. 1996;8:45-49.

1246. Centers for Disease Control and Prevention. U.S. HIV and AIDS cases reported through December 1994. HIV/AIDS Surveill Report. 1994;6:1-39.

1247. Arico M, Caselli D, D'Argenio P, et al. Malignancies in children with human immunodeficiency virus type 1 infection. The Italian Multicenter Study on Human Immunodeficiency Virus Infection in Children. Cancer. 1991;68:2473-2477.

1248. DiCarlo FJ Jr, Joshi VV, Oleske JM, et al. Neoplastic diseases in children with acquired immunodeficiency syndrome. Prog AIDS Pathol. 1990;2:163-185.

1249. Kadan-Lottick NS, Skluzacek MC, Gurney JG. Decreasing incidence rates of primary central nervous system lymphoma. Cancer. 2002;95:193-202.

1250. Newell ME, Hoy JF, Cooper SG, et al. Human immunodeficiency virus-related primary central nervous system lymphoma: factors influencing survival in 111 patients. Cancer. 2004;100:2627-2636.

1251. Abla O, Sandlund JT, Sung L, et al. A case series of pediatric primary central nervous system lymphoma: favorable outcome without cranial irradiation. Pediatr Blood Cancer. 2006;47:880-885.

1252. Lister A, Abrey LE, Sandlund JT. Central nervous system lymphoma. Hematology Am Soc Hematol Educ Program. 2002;283-296.

1253. Schlegel U, Schmidt-Wolf IG, Deckert M. Primary CNS lymphoma: clinical presentation, pathological classification, molecular pathogenesis and treatment. J Neurol Sci. 2000;181:1-12.

1254. Hochberg FH, Miller DC. Primary central nervous system lymphoma. J Neurosurg. 1988;68:835-853.

1255. Mohile NA, Deangelis LM, Abrey LE. The utility of body FDG PET in staging primary central nervous system lymphoma. Neuro Oncol. 2008;10:223-228.

1256. Nishiyama Y, Yamamoto Y, Monden T, et al. Diagnostic value of kinetic analysis using dynamic FDG PET in immunocompetent patients with primary CNS lymphoma. Eur J Nucl Med Mol Imaging. 2007;34:78-86.

1257. Kosuda S, Kusano S, Ishihara S, et al. Combined 201Tl and 67Ga brain SPECT in patients with suspected central nervous system lymphoma or germinoma: clinical and economic value. Ann Nucl Med. 2003;17:359-367.

1258. Deckert M, Paulus W. Malignant lymphomas. In Louis DN, Ohgaki H, Wiestler OD, et al (eds). WHO Classification of Tumours of the Central Nervous System, 4th ed. Geneva, World Health Organization Press, 2007, pp 188-192.

1259. McClain KL, Leach CT, Jenson HB, et al. Molecular and virologic characteristics of lymphoid malignancies in children with AIDS. J Acquir Immune Defic Syndr. 2000;23:152-159.

1260. Deangelis LM, Iwamoto FM. An update on therapy of primary central nervous system lymphoma. Hematology Am Soc Hematol Educ Program. 2006;311-316.

1261. Bessell EM, Hoang-Xuan K, Ferreri AJ, et al. Primary central nervous system lymphoma: biological aspects and controversies in management. Eur J Cancer. 2007;43:1141-1152.

1262. Ekenel M, Iwamoto FM, Ben-Porat LS, et al. Primary central nervous system lymphoma: The role of consolidation treatment after a complete response to high-dose methotrexate-based chemotherapy. Cancer. 2008;113:1025-1031.

1263. Traum AZ, Rodig NM, Pilichowska ME, et al. Central nervous system lymphoproliferative disorder in pediatric kidney transplant recipients. Pediatr Transplant. 2006;10:505-512.

1264. Hirano A, Hirano M. Benign cysts in the central nervous system: neuropathological observations of the cyst walls. Neuropathology. 2004;24:1-7.

1265. Gosalakkal JA. Intracranial arachnoid cysts in children: a review of pathogenesis, clinical features, and management. Pediatr Neurol. 2002;26:93-98.

1266. Sundaram C, Paul TR, Raju BV, et al. Cysts of the central nervous system : a clinicopathologic study of 145 cases. Neurol India. 2001;49:237-242.

1267. Caldarelli M, Massimi L, Kondageski C, et al. Intracranial midline dermoid and epidermoid cysts in children. J Neurosurg. 2004;100:473-480.

1268. McBride LA, Winston KR, Freeman JE. Cystoventricular shunting of intracranial arachnoid cysts. Pediatr Neurosurg. 2003;39:323-329.

1269. Hirano A, Hirano M. Benign cystic lesions in the central nervous system. Light and electron microscopic observations of cyst walls. Childs Nerv Syst. 1988;4:325-333.

1270. Rengachary SS, Watanabe I. Ultrastructure and pathogenesis of intracranial arachnoid cysts. J Neuropathol Exp Neurol. 1981;40:61-83.

1271. Jain F, Chaichana KL, McGirt MJ, et al. Neonatal anterior cervical arachnoid cyst: case report and review of the literature. Childs Nerv Syst. 2008;24:965-970.

1272. Rengachary SS, Watanabe I, Brackett CE. Pathogenesis of intracranial arachnoid cysts. Surg Neurol. 1978;9:139-144.

1273. Sharma A, Sayal P, Badhe P, et al. Spinal intramedullary arachnoid cyst. Indian J Pediatr. 2004;71:e65-e67.

1274. Arriola G, de Castro P, Verdu A. Familial arachnoid cysts. Pediatr Neurol. 2005;33:146-148.

1275. Lohle PN, Wurzer HA, Seelen PJ, et al. The pathogenesis of cysts accompanying intra-axial primary and metastatic tumors of the central nervous system. J Neurooncol. 1998;40:277-285.

1276. Ersahin Y, Kesikci H, Ruksen M, et al. Endoscopic treatment of suprasellar arachnoid cysts. Childs Nerv Syst. 2008;24:1013-1020.

1277. Starzyk J, Kwiatkowski S, Urbanowicz W, et al. Suprasellar arachnoidal cyst as a cause of precocious puberty—report of three patients and literature overview. J Pediatr Endocrinol Metab. 2003;16:447-455.

1278. Shin JL, Asa SL, Woodhouse LJ, et al. Cystic lesions of the pituitary: clinicopathological features distinguishing craniopharyngioma, Rathke's cleft cyst, and arachnoid cyst. J Clin Endocrinol Metab. 1999;84:3972-3982.

1279. Alkilic-Genauzeau I, Boukobza M, Lot G, et al. CT and MRI features of arachnoid cyst of the petrous apex: report of 3 cases. J Radiol. 2007;88:1179-1183.

1280. Sandberg DI, McComb JG, Krieger MD. Chemical analysis of fluid obtained from intracranial arachnoid cysts in pediatric patients. J Neurosurg. 2005;103:427-432.

1281. Tamburrini G, Del Fabbro M, Di Rocco C. Sylvian fissure arachnoid cysts: a survey on their diagnostic workout and practical management. Childs Nerv Syst. 2008;4:593-604.

1282. Sommer IE, Smit LM. Congenital supratentorial arachnoidal and giant cysts in children: a clinical study with arguments for a conservative approach. Childs Nerv Syst. 1997;13:8-12.

1283. Karabatsou K, Hayhurst C, Buxton N, et al. Endoscopic management of arachnoid cysts: an advancing technique. J Neurosurg. 2007;106:455-462.

1284. Tamburrini G, D'Angelo L, Paternoster G, et al. Endoscopic management of intra- and paraventricular CSF cysts. Childs Nerv Syst. 2007;23:645-651.

1285. Helland CA, Wester K. A population-based study of intracranial arachnoid cysts: clinical and neuroimaging outcomes following surgical cyst decompression in children. J Neurosurg. 2006;105:385-390.

1286. Zada G, Krieger MD, McNatt SA, et al. Pathogenesis and treatment of intracranial arachnoid cysts in pediatric patients younger than 2 years. Neurosurg Focus. 2007;22:E1.

1287. Kim SK, Cho BK, Chung YN, et al. Shunt dependency in shunted arachnoid cyst: a reason to avoid shunting. Pediatr Neurosurg. 2002;37:178-185.

1288. Mori K, Yamamoto T, Horinaka N, et al. Arachnoid cyst is a risk factor for chronic subdural hematoma in juveniles: twelve cases of chronic subdural hematoma associated with arachnoid cyst. J Neurotrauma. 2002;19:1017-1027.

1289. Guidetti B, Gagliardi FM. Epidermoid and dermoid cysts. Clinical evaluation and late surgical results. J Neurosurg. 1977;47:12-18.

1290. Abramson RC, Morawetz RB, Schlitt M. Multiple complications from an intracranial epidermoid cyst: case report and literature review. Neurosurgery. 1989;24:574-578.

1291. Baxter JW, Netsky MG. Epidermoid and dermoid tumors; pathology. In Wilkin RH, Rengachary SS (eds). Neurosurgery. New York, McGraw-Hill, 1985, pp 655-661.

1292. Caldarelli M, Colosimo C, Di Rocco C. Intra-axial dermoid/epidermoid tumors of the brainstem in children. Surg Neurol. 2001;56:97-105.

1293. Plewes JL, Jacobson I. Familial frontonasal dermoid cysts. Report of four cases. J Neurosurg. 1971;34:683-686.

1294. Barkovich AJ, Simon EM, Walsh CA. Callosal agenesis with cyst: a better understanding and new classification. Neurology. 2001;56:220-227.

1295. Jeeves MA, Temple CM. A further study of language function in callosal agenesis. Brain Lang. 1987;32:325-335.

1296. Attard TM, Giglio P, Koppula S, et al. Brain tumors in individuals with familial adenomatous polyposis: a cancer registry experience and pooled case report analysis. Cancer. 2007;109:761-766.

1297. Hamilton SR, Liu B, Parsons RE, et al. The molecular basis of Turcot's syndrome. N Engl J Med. 1995;332:839-847.

1298. Koot RW, Hulsebos TJ, van Overbeeke JJ. Polyposis coli, craniofacial exostosis and astrocytoma: the concomitant occurrence of the Gardner's and Turcot syndromes. Surg Neurol. 1996;45:213-218.

1299. Lasser DM, DeVivo DC, Garvin J, et al. Turcot's syndrome: evidence for linkage to the adenomatous polyposis coli (APC) locus. Neurology. 1994;44:1083-1086.

1300. Leblanc R. Familial adenomatous polyposis and benign intracranial tumors: a new variant of Gardner's syndrome. Can J Neurol Sci. 2000;27:341-346.

1301. Per H, Kumandas S, Gumus H, et al. Iatrogenic epidermoid tumor: late complication of lumbar puncture. J Child Neurol. 2007;22:332-336.

1302. Hu XY, Hu CH, Fang XM, et al. Intraparenchymal epidermoid cysts in the brain: diagnostic value of MR diffusion-weighted imaging. Clin Radiol. 2008;63:813-818.

1303. Harrison MJ, Morgello S, Post KD. Epithelial cystic lesions of the sellar and parasellar region: a continuum of ectodermal derivatives? J Neurosurg. 1994;80:1018-1025.

1304. Binning M, Klimo P Jr, Gluf W, et al. Spinal tumors in children. Neurosurg Clin N Am. 2007;18:631-658.

1305. Wilson PE, Oleszek JL, Clayton GH. Pediatric spinal cord tumors and masses. J Spinal Cord Med. 2007;30(Suppl 1):S15-S20.

1306. Duhem-Tonnelle V, Vinchon M, Defachelles AS, et al. Mature neuroblastic tumors with spinal cord compression: report of five pediatric cases. Childs Nerv Syst. 2006;22:500-505.

1307. Massimino M, Gandola L, Spreafico F, et al. Unusual primary secreting germ cell tumor of the spine. Case report. J Neurosurg Spine. 2006;5:65-67.

1308. Seol HJ, Wang KC, Kim SK, et al. Intramedullary immature teratoma in a young infant involving a long segment of the spinal cord. Childs Nerv Syst. 2001;17:758-761.

1309. Santoro A, Piccirilli M, Brunetto GM, et al. Intramedullary cavernous angioma of the spinal cord in a pediatric patient, with multiple cavernomas, familial occurrence and partial spontaneous regression: case report and review of the literature. Childs Nerv Syst. 2007;23:1319-1326.

1310. Jallo GI, Kothbauer KF, Silvera VM, et al. Intraspinal clear cell meningioma: diagnosis and management: report of two cases. Neurosurgery. 2001;48:218-221.

1311. Bulsara KR, Zomorodi AR, Villavicencio AT, et al. Clinical outcome differences for lipomyelomeningoceles, intraspinal lipomas, and lipomas of the filum terminale. Neurosurg Rev. 2001;24:192-194.

1312. Kwon OK, Wang KC, Kim CJ, et al. Primary intramedullary spinal cord primitive neuroectodermal tumor with intracranial seeding in an infant. Childs Nerv Syst. 1996;12:633-636.

1313. Yang CS, Jan YJ, Wang J, et al. Spinal atypical teratoid/rhabdoid tumor in a 7-year-old boy. Neuropathology. 2007;27:139-144.

1314. McGirt MJ, Chaichana KL, Atiba A, et al. Incidence of spinal deformity after resection of intramedullary spinal cord tumors in children who underwent laminectomy compared with laminoplasty. J Neurosurg Pediatrics. 2008;1:57-62.

1315. Baysefer A, Akay KM, Izci Y, et al. The clinical and surgical aspects of spinal tumors in children. Pediatr Neurol. 2004;31:261-266.

1316. Pollono D, Tomarchia S, Drut R, et al. Spinal cord compression: a review of 70 pediatric patients. Pediatr Hematol Oncol. 2003;20:457-466.

1317. Houten JK, Weiner HL. Pediatric intramedullary spinal cord tumors: special considerations. J Neurooncol. 2000;47:225-230.

1318. Parikh SN, Crawford AH. Orthopaedic implications in the management of pediatric vertebral and spinal cord tumors: a retrospective review. Spine. 2003;28:2390-2396.

1319. Rossi A, Gandolfo C, Morana G, et al. Tumors of the spine in children. Neuroimaging Clin N Am. 2007;17:17-35.

1320. Lonjon M, Goh KY, Epstein FJ. Intramedullary spinal cord ependymomas in children: treatment, results and follow-up. Pediatr Neurosurg. 1998;29:178-183.

1321. Merchant TE, Nguyen D, Thompson SJ, et al. High-grade pediatric spinal cord tumors. Pediatr Neurosurg. 1999; 30:1-5.

1322. Townsend N, Handler M, Fleitz J, et al. Intramedullary spinal cord astrocytomas in children. Pediatr Blood Cancer. 2004;43:629-632.

1323. Merchant TE, Kiehna EN, Thompson SJ, et al. Pediatric low-grade and ependymal spinal cord tumors. Pediatr Neurosurg. 2000;32:30-36.

1324. Mora J, Cruz O, Gala S, et al. Successful treatment of childhood intramedullary spinal cord astrocytomas with irinotecan and cisplatin. Neuro Oncol. 2007;9:39-46.

1325. Nadkarni TD, Rekate HL. Pediatric intramedullary spinal cord tumors. Critical review of the literature. Childs Nerv Syst. 1999;15:17-28.

1326. McGirt MJ, Chaichana KL, Atiba A, et al. Resection of intramedullary spinal cord tumors in children: assessment of long-term motor and sensory deficits. J Neurosurg Pediatrics. 2008;1:63-67.

1327. Bouffet E, Pierre-Kahn A, Marchal JC, et al. Prognostic factors in pediatric spinal cord astrocytoma. Cancer. 1998;83:2391-2399.

1328. Yao KC, McGirt MJ, Chaichana KL, et al. Risk factors for progressive spinal deformity following resection of intramedullary spinal cord tumors in children: an analysis of 161 consecutive cases. J Neurosurg. 2007;107:463-468.

1329. Fassett DR, Clark R, Brockmeyer DL, et al. Cervical spine deformity associated with resection of spinal cord tumors. Neurosurg Focus. 2006;20:E2.

1330. Klepstad P, Borchgrevink P, Hval B, et al. Long-term treatment with ketamine in a 12-year-old girl with severe neuropathic pain caused by a cervical spinal tumor. J Pediatr Hematol Oncol. 2001;23:616-619.

1331. Lewanski CR, Sinclair JA, Stewart JS. Lhermitte's sign following head and neck radiotherapy. Clin Oncol (R Coll Radiol). 2000;12:98-103.

1332. Pamir MN, Ozduman K. Tumor-biology and current treatment of skull-base chordomas. Adv Tech Stand Neurosurg. 2008; 33:35-129.

1333. Shinmura Y, Miura K, Yajima S, et al. Sacrococcygeal chordoma in infancy showing an aggressive clinical course: an autopsy case report. Pathol Int. 2003;53:473-477.

1334. Erdem E, Angtuaco EC, Van Hemert R, et al. Comprehensive review of intracranial chordoma. Radiographics. 2003;23:995-1009.

1335. McMaster ML, Goldstein AM, Bromley CM, et al. Chordoma: incidence and survival patterns in the United States, 1973-1995. Cancer Causes Control. 2001;12:1-11.

1336. Ali SZ, Semmelmeier SB, Urmacher C. Cytology of cervical chordoma in cerebrospinal fluid from a child. A case report. Acta Cytol. 1995;39:766-769.

1337. Paulus W, Scheithauer BW, Perry A. Mesenchymal, non-meningothelial tumours. In Louis DN, Ohgaki H, Wiestler OD, et al (eds). WHO Classification of Tumours of the Central Nervous System, 4th ed. Geneva, World Health Organization Press, 2007, pp 173-177.

1338. Hoch BL, Nielsen GP, Liebsch NJ, et al. Base of skull chordomas in children and adolescents: a clinicopathologic study of 73 cases. Am J Surg Pathol. 2006;30:811-818.

1339. Weber DC, Rutz HP, Bolsi A, et al. Spot scanning proton therapy in the curative treatment of adult patients with sarcoma: the Paul Scherrer institute experience. Int J Radiat Oncol Biol Phys. 2007;69:865-871.

1340. Timmermann B, Schuck A, Niggli F, et al. Spot-scanning proton therapy for malignant soft tissue tumors in childhood: first experiences at the Paul Scherrer Institute. Int J Radiat Oncol Biol Phys. 2007;67:497-504.

1341. Scimeca PG, James-Herry AG, Black KS, et al. Chemotherapeutic treatment of malignant chordoma in children. J Pediatr Hematol Oncol. 1996;18:237-240.

1342. Orzan F, Terreni MR, Longoni M, et al. Expression study of the target receptor tyrosine kinase of Imatinib mesylate in skull base chordomas. Oncol Rep. 2007;18:249-252.

1343. Casali PG, Messina A, Stacchiotti S, et al. Imatinib mesylate in chordoma. Cancer. 2004;101:2086-2097.

1344. Hof H, Welzel T, Debus J. Effectiveness of cetuximab/gefitinib in the therapy of a sacral chordoma. Onkologie. 2006; 29:572-574.

1345. Chugh R, Dunn R, Zalupski MM, et al. Phase II study of 9-nitro-camptothecin in patients with advanced chordoma or soft tissue sarcoma. J Clin Oncol. 2005;23:3597-3604.

1346. Saad AG, Collins MH. Prognostic value of MIB-1, E-cadherin, and CD44 in pediatric chordomas. Pediatr Dev Pathol. 2005; 8:362-368.

1347. Goldman S, Turner C. Late Effects of Treatment for Brain Tumors. Secaucus, NJ, Springer, 2008.

1348. Tao ML, Parsons SK. Quality-of-life assessment in pediatric brain tumor patients and survivors: lessons learned and challenges to face. J Clin Oncol. 2005;23:5424-5426.

1349. Sklar CA. Childhood brain tumors. J Pediatr Endocrinol Metab. 2002;15(Suppl 2):669-673.

1350. Perry A, Schmidt RE. Cancer therapy-associated CNS neuropathology: an update and review of the literature. Acta Neuropathol. 2006;111:197-212.

1351. Vinchon M, Dhellemmes P. The transition from child to adult in neurosurgery. Adv Tech Stand Neurosurg. 2007;32:3-24.

1352. Broniscer A, Ke W, Fuller CE, et al. Second neoplasms in pediatric patients with primary central nervous system tumors: the St. Jude Children's Research Hospital experience. Cancer. 2004;100:2246-2252.

1353. Lai JS, Cella D, Tomita T, et al. Developing a health-related quality of life instrument for childhood brain tumor survivors. Childs Nerv Syst. 2007;23:47-57.

1354. Nathan PC, Patel SK, Dilley K, et al. Guidelines for identification of, advocacy for, and intervention in neurocognitive problems in survivors of childhood cancer: a report from the Children's Oncology Group. Arch Pediatr Adolesc Med. 2007;161:798-806.

1355. Palmer SN, Meeske KA, Katz ER, et al. The PedsQL Brain Tumor Module: initial reliability and validity. Pediatr Blood Cancer. 2007;49:287-293.

1356. de Bont JM, Vanderstichele H, Reddingius RE, et al. Increased total-Tau levels in cerebrospinal fluid of pediatric hydrocephalus and brain tumor patients. Eur J Paediatr Neurol. 2008; 12:334-341.

1357. Macedoni-Luksic M, Jereb B, Todorovski L. Long-term sequelae in children treated for brain tumors: impairments, disability, and handicap. Pediatr Hematol Oncol. 2003;20:89-101.

1358. Arroyo HA, Jan JE, McCormick AQ, et al. Permanent visual loss after shunt malfunction. Neurology. 1985;35:25-29.

1359. Sonderkaer S, Schmiegelow M, Carstensen H, et al. Long-term neurological outcome of childhood brain tumors treated by surgery only. J Clin Oncol. 2003;21:1347-1351.

1360. Chen ML, Witmans MB, Tablizo MA, et al. Disordered respiratory control in children with partial cerebellar resections. Pediatr Pulmonol. 2005;40:88-91.

1361. Schoch B, Konczak J, Dimitrova A, et al. Impact of surgery and adjuvant therapy on balance function in children and adolescents with cerebellar tumors. Neuropediatrics. 2006;37:350-358.

1362. Meyer EA, Kieran MW. Psychological adjustment of "surgery-only" pediatric neuro-oncology patients: a retrospective analysis. Psychooncology. 2002;11:74-79.

1363. Kortmann RD, Timmermann B, Taylor RE, et al. Current and future strategies in radiotherapy of childhood low-grade glioma of the brain. Part II: Treatment-related late toxicity. Strahlenther Onkol. 2003;179:585-597.

1364. Faithfull S, Brada M. Somnolence syndrome in adults following cranial irradiation for primary brain tumours. Clin Oncol (R Coll Radiol). 1998;10:250-254.

1365. Ryan J. Radiation somnolence syndrome. J Pediatr Oncol Nurs. 2000;17:50-53.

1366. Ciucci G, De Giorgi U, Leoni M, et al. Lhermitte's sign following oxaliplatin-containing chemotherapy in a cisplatin-pretreated ovarian cancer patient. Eur J Neurol. 2003;10:328-329.

1367. Esik O, Csere T, Stefanits K, et al. A review on radiogenic Lhermitte's sign. Pathol Oncol Res. 2003;9:115-120.

1368. Chernov MF, Hayashi M, Izawa M, et al. Multivoxel proton MRS for differentiation of radiation-induced necrosis and tumor recurrence after gamma knife radiosurgery for brain metastases. Brain Tumor Pathol. 2006;23:19-27.

1369. Ruben JD, Dally M, Bailey M, et al. Cerebral radiation necrosis: incidence, outcomes, and risk factors with emphasis on radiation parameters and chemotherapy. Int J Radiat Oncol Biol Phys. 2006;65:499-508.

1370. Jain R, Scarpace L, Ellika S, et al. First-pass perfusion computed tomography: initial experience in differentiating recurrent brain tumors from radiation effects and radiation necrosis. Neurosurgery. 2007;61:778-786.

1371. Kashimura H, Inoue T, Beppu T, et al. Diffusion tensor imaging for differentiation of recurrent brain tumor and radiation necrosis after radiotherapy—three case reports. Clin Neurol Neurosurg. 2007;109:106-110.

1372. Terakawa Y, Tsuyuguchi N, Iwai Y, et al. Diagnostic accuracy of 11C-methionine PET for differentiation of recurrent brain tumors from radiation necrosis after radiotherapy. J Nucl Med. 2008;49:694-699.

1373. Xiangsong Z, Weian C. Differentiation of recurrent astrocytoma from radiation necrosis: a pilot study with 13N-NH3 PET. J Neurooncol. 2007;82:305-311.

1374. Chen CH, Shen CC, Sun MH, et al. Histopathology of radiation necrosis with severe peritumoral edema after gamma knife radiosurgery for parasagittal meningioma. A report of two cases. Stereotact Funct Neurosurg. 2007;85:292-295.

1375. Gonzalez J, Kumar AJ, Conrad CA, et al. Effect of bevacizumab on radiation necrosis of the brain. Int J Radiat Oncol Biol Phys. 2007;67:323-326.

1376. Batchelor TT, Sorensen AG, di Tomaso E, et al. AZD2171, a pan-VEGF receptor tyrosine kinase inhibitor, normalizes tumor vasculature and alleviates edema in glioblastoma patients. Cancer Cell. 2007;11:83-95.

1377. Helton KJ, Edwards M, Steen RG, et al. Neuroimaging-detected late transient treatment-induced lesions in pediatric patients with brain tumors. J Neurosurg. 2005;102:179-186.

1378. Kiehna EN, Mulhern RK, Li C, et al. Changes in attentional performance of children and young adults with localized primary brain tumors after conformal radiation therapy. J Clin Oncol. 2006;24:5283-5290.

1379. Ris MD, Ryan PM, Lamba M, et al. An improved methodology for modeling neurobehavioral late-effects of radiotherapy in pediatric brain tumors. Pediatr Blood Cancer. 2005;44:487-493.

1380. Nagel BJ, Palmer SL, Reddick WE, et al. Abnormal hippocampal development in children with medulloblastoma treated with risk-adapted irradiation. AJNR Am J Neuroradiol. 2004;25:1575-1582.

1381. Palmer SL, Reddick WE, Glass JO, et al. Decline in corpus callosum volume among pediatric patients with medulloblastoma: longitudinal MR imaging study. AJNR Am J Neuroradiol. 2002;23:1088-1094.

1382. Grill J, Kieffer V, Kalifa C. Measuring the neuro-cognitive side-effects of irradiation in children with brain tumors. Pediatr Blood Cancer. 2004;42:452-456.

1383. Lovblad K, Kelkar P, Ozdoba C, et al. Pure methotrexate encephalopathy presenting with seizures: CT and MRI features. Pediatr Radiol. 1998;28:86-91.

1384. Hertzberg H, Huk WJ, Ueberall MA, et al. CNS late effects after ALL therapy in childhood. Part I: Neuroradiological findings in long-term survivors of childhood ALL—an evaluation of the interferences between morphology and neuropsychological performance. The German Late Effects Working Group. Med Pediatr Oncol. 1997;28:387-400.

1385. Reddick WE, Glass JO, Palmer SL, et al. Atypical white matter volume development in children following craniospinal irradiation. Neuro Oncol. 2005;7:12-19.

1386. Reddick WE, White HA, Glass JO, et al. Developmental model relating white matter volume to neurocognitive deficits in pediatric brain tumor survivors. Cancer. 2003;97:2512-2519.

1387. Monje ML, Palmer T. Radiation injury and neurogenesis. Curr Opin Neurol. 2003;16:129-134.

1388. Kyrnetskiy EE, Kun LE, Boop FA, et al. Types, causes, and outcome of intracranial hemorrhage in children with cancer. J Neurosurg. 2005;102:31-35.

1389. Duhem R, Vinchon M, Leblond P, et al. Cavernous malformations after cerebral irradiation during childhood: report of nine cases. Childs Nerv Syst. 2005;21:922-925.

1390. Baumgartner JE, Ater JL, Ha CS, et al. Pathologically proven cavernous angiomas of the brain following radiation therapy for pediatric brain tumors. Pediatr Neurosurg. 2003;39:201-207.

1391. Santoro A, Minniti G, Paolini S, et al. Atypical tentorial meningioma 30 years after radiotherapy for a pituitary adenoma. Neurol Sci. 2002;22:463-467.

1392. Koshy M, Paulino AC, Mai WY, et al. Radiation-induced osteosarcomas in the pediatric population. Int J Radiat Oncol Biol Phys. 2005;63:1169-1174.

1393. Mazonakis M, Damilakis J, Varveris H, et al. Risk estimation of radiation-induced thyroid cancer from treatment of brain tumors in adults and children. Int J Oncol. 2003;22:221-225.

1394. Stavrou T, Bromley CM, Nicholson HS, et al. Prognostic factors and secondary malignancies in childhood medulloblastoma. J Pediatr Hematol Oncol. 2001;23:431-436.

1395. Merchant TE, Williams T, Smith JM, et al. Preirradiation endocrinopathies in pediatric brain tumor patients determined by dynamic tests of endocrine function. Int J Radiat Oncol Biol Phys. 2002;54:45-50.

1396. Lerner SE, Huang GJ, McMahon D, et al. Growth hormone therapy in children after cranial/craniospinal radiation therapy: sexually dimorphic outcomes. J Clin Endocrinol Metab. 2004;89:6100-6104.

1397. Muirhead SE, Hsu E, Grimard L, et al. Endocrine complications of pediatric brain tumors: case series and literature review. Pediatr Neurol. 2002;27:165-170.

1398. Lustig RH, Post SR, Srivannaboon K, et al. Risk factors for the development of obesity in children surviving brain tumors. J Clin Endocrinol Metab. 2003;88:611-616.

1399. Krishnamoorthy P, Freeman C, Bernstein ML, et al. Osteopenia in children who have undergone posterior fossa or craniospinal irradiation for brain tumors. Arch Pediatr Adolesc Med. 2004;158:491-496.

1400. Kuohung W, Ram K, Cheng DM, et al. Laparoscopic oophoropexy prior to radiation for pediatric brain tumor and subsequent ovarian function. Hum Reprod. 2008;23:117-121.

1401. Meacham LR, Mason PW, Sullivan KM. Auxologic and biochemical characterization of the three phases of growth failure in pediatric patients with brain tumors. J Pediatr Endocrinol Metab. 2004;17:711-717.

1402. Sklar CA, Mertens AC, Mitby P, et al. Risk of disease recurrence and second neoplasms in survivors of childhood cancer treated with growth hormone: a report from the Childhood Cancer Survivor Study. J Clin Endocrinol Metab. 2002;87:3136-3141.

1403. Packer RJ, Boyett JM, Janss AJ, et al. Growth hormone replacement therapy in children with medulloblastoma: use and effect on tumor control. J Clin Oncol. 2001;19:480-487.

1404. Shulman DI. Metabolic effects of growth hormone in the child and adolescent. Curr Opin Pediatr. 2002;14:432-436.

1405. Quasthoff S, Hartung HP. Chemotherapy-induced peripheral neuropathy. J Neurol. 2002;249:9-17.

1406. Friedman JH, Shetty N. Permanent cerebellar toxicity of cytosine arabinoside (Ara C) in a young woman. Mov Disord. 2001;16:575-577.

1407. Williams GB, Kun LE, Thompson JW, et al. Hearing loss as a late complication of radiotherapy in children with brain tumors. Ann Otol Rhinol Laryngol. 2005;114:328-331.

1408. Gonçalves MI, Radzinsky TC, da Silva NS, et al. Speech-language and hearing complaints of children and adolescents with brain tumors. Pediatr Blood Cancer. 2008;50:706-708.

1409. Merchant TE, Gould CJ, Xiong X, et al. Early neuro-otologic effects of three-dimensional irradiation in children with primary brain tumors. Int J Radiat Oncol Biol Phys. 2004;58:1194-1207.

1410. Dean JB, Hayashi SS, Albert CM, et al. Hearing loss in pediatric oncology patients receiving carboplatin-containing regimens. J Pediatr Hematol Oncol. 2008;30:130-134.

1411. Coradini PP, Cigana L, Selistre SG, et al. Ototoxicity from cisplatin therapy in childhood cancer. J Pediatr Hematol Oncol. 2007;29:355-360.

1412. Erdlenbruch B, Pekrum A, Roth C, et al. Cisplatin nephrotoxicity in children after continuous 72-h and 3x1-h infusions. Pediatr Nephrol. 2001;16:586-593.

1413. Le Deley MC, Vassal G, Taibi A, et al. High cumulative rate of secondary leukemia after continuous etoposide treatment for solid tumors in children and young adults. Pediatr Blood Cancer. 2005;45:25-31.

1414. Lopez de Mesa R, Lopez de Cerain Salsamendi A, Ariznabarreta LS, et al. Measurement and analysis of the chemotherapy-induced genetic instability in pediatric cancer patients. Mutagenesis. 2002;17:171-175.

1415. Wolff JE, Huttermann U, Askins MA. Quantifying health status outcomes in pediatric medulloblastoma patients. Anticancer Res. 2007;27:523-529.

1416. Gerhardt CA, Yopp JM, Leininger L, et al. Brief report: posttraumatic stress during emerging adulthood in survivors of pediatric cancer. J Pediatr Psychol. 2007;32:1018-1023.

1417. Zebrack BJ, Gurney JG, Oeffinger K, et al. Psychological outcomes in long-term survivors of childhood brain cancer: a report from the childhood cancer survivor study. J Clin Oncol. 2004;22:999-1006.

1418. Carpentieri SC, Meyer EA, Delaney BL, et al. Psychosocial and behavioral functioning among pediatric brain tumor survivors. J Neurooncol. 2003;63:279-287.

1419. Barrera M, Schulte F, Spiegler B. Factors influencing depressive symptoms of children treated for a brain tumor. J Psychosoc Oncol. 2008;26:1-16.

1420. Benesch M, Lackner H, Sovinz P, et al. Late sequela after treatment of childhood low-grade gliomas: a retrospective analysis of 69 long-term survivors treated between 1983 and 2003. J Neurooncol. 2006;78:199-205.

1421. Briere ME, Scott JG, McNall-Knapp RY, et al. Cognitive outcome in pediatric brain tumor survivors: delayed attention deficit at long-term follow-up. Pediatr Blood Cancer. 2008;50:337-340.

1422. Meeske K, Katz ER, Palmer SN, et al. Parent proxy-reported health-related quality of life and fatigue in pediatric patients diagnosed with brain tumors and acute lymphoblastic leukemia. Cancer. 2004;101:2116-2125.

1423. Merchant TE, Kiehna EN, Li C, et al. Modeling radiation dosimetry to predict cognitive outcomes in pediatric patients with CNS embryonal tumors including medulloblastoma. Int J Radiat Oncol Biol Phys. 2006;65:210-221.

1424. King TZ, Fennell EB, Williams L, et al. Verbal memory abilities of children with brain tumors. Child Neuropsychol. 2004;10:76-88.

1425. Micklewright JL, King TZ, Morris RD, Krawiecki N. Quantifying pediatric neuro-oncology risk factors: development of the neurological predictor scale. J Child Neurol. 2008;23:455-458.

1426. Taylor L, Simpson K, Bushardt R, et al. Insurance barriers for childhood survivors of pediatric brain tumors: the case for neurocognitive evaluations. Pediatr Neurosurg. 2006;42:223-227.

1427. Theunissen JM, Hoogerbrugge PM, van Achterberg T, et al. Symptoms in the palliative phase of children with cancer. Pediatr Blood Cancer. 2007;49:160-165.

1428. Postovsky S, Levenzon A, Ofir R, et al. "Do not resuscitate" orders among children with solid tumors at the end of life. Pediatr Hematol Oncol. 2004;21:661-668.

1429. Berg S. In their own voices: families discuss end-of-life decision making—part 2. Pediatr Nurs. 2006;32:238-242.

1430. Postovsky S, Moaed B, Krivoy E, et al. Practice of palliative sedation in children with brain tumors and sarcomas at the end of life. Pediatr Hematol Oncol. 2007;24:409-415.

1431. Hinds PS, Drew D, Oakes LL, et al. End-of-life care preferences of pediatric patients with cancer. J Clin Oncol. 2005;23:9146-9154.

1432. Bradshaw G, Hinds PS, Lensing S, et al. Cancer-related deaths in children and adolescents. J Palliat Med. 2005;8:86-95.

1433. Punnett AS, McCarthy LJ, Dirks PB, et al. Patients with primary brain tumors as organ donors: case report and review of the literature. Pediatr Blood Cancer. 2004;43:73-77.

18 Hepatoblastomas and Other Liver Tumors

Gail E. Tomlinson and Heung Bae Kim

INTRODUCTION AND EPIDEMIOLOGY

Liver tumors in children account for approximately 1.1% of all malignancies in children younger than 20 years of age, according to the SEER reports; approximately 100 to 150 new cases of liver cancer in children occur each year.[1] Liver malignancies in children can be divided into three broad classifications: hepatoblastomas, which make up two thirds of malignant liver cancers; hepatocellular carcinomas (HCCs); and other rare hepatic malignancies of childhood. In addition to malignant liver tumors, several benign tumors can occur in children, and that broadens the differential diagnosis of an infant or child with a liver mass.

In an early meta-analysis of 11 separate series totaling 1256 primary liver tumors in children, reported by Weinberg and Finegold, 43% were hepatoblastomas, 23% were HCCs, 13% were benign vascular tumors, 6% were mesenchymal hamartomas, 6% were sarcomas, 2% were adenomas, 2% were focal nodular hyperplasias, and 5% were other tumors.[2] Rare tumors of the liver also include rhabdoid tumors and hepatic germ cell tumors.

Hepatoblastomas are more common in males than in females. The male-to-female ratio in the cooperative group trials has ranged from 1.5:1 to 2:1; a combined analysis of five studies suggests that the male-to-female ratio of hepatoblastomas is 1.65:1.[3-7]

Hepatoblastomas have a unique age distribution (Fig. 18-1). Peaks occur at two ages: one at birth or within the first month of life and a second at age 16 to 18 months of age. Of the hepatoblastomas that occur, 90% appear when a child is younger than 4 years of age, and 97% of hepatoblastomas occur before a child has reached the age of 5. Hepatoblastomas have been seen in adults, although they are rare, as described in multiple reports of sporadic cases.[8-29] Hepatoblastomas in children older than 5 years is commonly more aggressive than typical hepatoblastomas, and they have the characteristics of HCCs. These tumors have also been termed transitional liver cell tumors.[30]

HCCs make up the bulk of liver tumors seen in children older than 10 years and throughout adolescence and adulthood. As with hepatoblastomas, HCCs are more common in males than in females.[31-33] The fibrolamellar variant of HCC is a notable exception; it occurs equally in males and females.[34,35]

The incidence of liver tumors has increased over recent decades. Although the rarity of liver tumors in children and the small numbers warrant caution in interpretation, SEER data comparing cancers occurring in infants between 1979 and 1981 to those occurring between 1989 and 1991 demonstrate that the incidence rate of hepatic tumors in infants under 1 year of age increased from 4 to 8 per million over a single decade.[36] The increase in rates was especially pronounced in female infants, in whom rates of hepatic cancer increased from 2 to 12 per million in 1 decade. Ross and Gurney have estimated that the average annual percentage of change in the incidence of hepatoblastoma between 1973 and 1992 has been 5.2% for males and 8.2% for females.[37] A recent updated study of trends in childhood cancer from 1992 through 2004 continues to demonstrate an annual increase of 4.3%.[38] The reasons for the increase in the incidence of hepatoblastomas are unknown, but one contributing factor is thought to be the increased survival rates of premature infants, who are at increased risk for hepatoblastomas (see subsequent material).

CAUSES OF MALIGNANT LIVER TUMOR DEVELOPMENT IN CHILDREN

As with other types of childhood cancers, the causes of most cases of hepatoblastoma remain largely unknown. Hepatoblastoma has long been thought to have prenatal origins,[39,40] and increasing evidence points to various contributing factors, including prematurity, prenatal exposures, and overgrowth in early infancy.

STEM CELL ORIGINS OF HEPATOBLASTOMA

It has long been presumed that embryonal tumors derive from primitive cells and that hepatoblastoma, an embryonal tumor of the liver, in which cells morphologically resemble cells in the developing embryonal and fetal liver, derives from a primitive hepatic cell. In rodents, immature oval cells, which proliferate

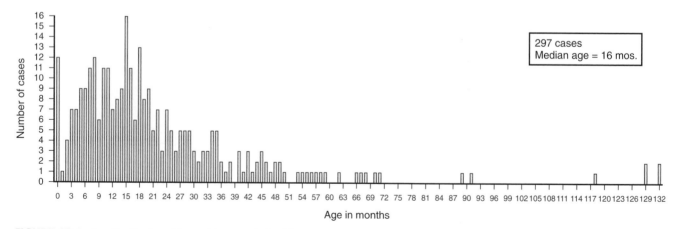

FIGURE 18-1. Age distribution of hepatoblastoma derived from 297 sequential cases representing all stages and histologies of hepatoblastoma enrolled in the Children's Oncology Group Hepatoblastoma Biology Study. An initial peak is seen at birth, reflecting tumors developing during gestation. The median age of all children with hepatoblastoma is 18 months, and the oldest age is 132 months. Of the cases, 97% were observed to occur by 5 years of age.

after exposure to hepatocarcinogens, express both biliary and hepatocytic markers.[41] These cells are characterized by staining with OV-1 and OV-6 markers. Ruck and colleagues have demonstrated the existence of a similar cell type in hepatoblastoma on the basis of marking with OV-1 and OV-6 in a small population of cells within the tumor.[42,43] These OV-1 and OV-6 staining cells are less than 1% of the cells within the tumor and argue for the existence of a population of stem cells in hepatoblastoma.

GENETIC PREDISPOSITION AND LIVER TUMORIGENESIS

In most cases of childhood liver malignancy, no apparent major genetic syndrome is associated. Familial cases of hepatoblastoma have been reported, as have numerous syndromes in association with hepatoblastoma or HCC. Of eight reported cases of hepatoblastoma in siblings, at least five are in families with familial adenomatous polyposis[44-47]; one pair of siblings was affected by type 1a glycogen storage disease,[48] and two pairs had no apparent familial syndrome.[49,50]

The genetic syndrome familial adenomatous polyposis (FAP) is best characterized by the presence of colonic polyps; without intervention their presence is associated with the virtual certainty of developing adenocarcinoma of the colon. FAP is caused by germ-line mutation in the adenomatous polyposis coli *(APC)* gene.[51] Numerous cases and small series report the occurrence of hepatoblastoma in FAP kindreds,[52-57] including reports of siblings with hepatoblastoma. Also reported in children from FAP kindreds, although less commonly, are liver tumors of other histologies.[58-60] Germ-line mutation of the *APC* gene is associated with a markedly increased risk for hepatoblastoma that is estimated to be 800-fold.[61] The risk that a parent with an *APC* mutation will have a child with hepatoblastoma is 0.4%.[62] Because FAP is an autosomal dominant disorder, genetic testing should demonstrate a predisposing mutation in 50% of offspring, such that the risk for hepatoblastoma in an infant who is a documented mutation carrier would be slightly less than 1%.

In a series of consecutive hepatoblastoma patients in the Pediatric Oncology Group Hepatoblastoma Biologic Study (POG 9346) in which family histories were obtained, approximately 8% of sequential cases of hepatoblastoma have family histories suggestive of FAP, and abnormalities of the *APC* gene were detectable in all cases.[63] It is conceivable, although not proven, that once a child has been diagnosed with hepatoblastoma in a family with FAP, the risk that a second child will develop hepatoblastoma is greater than the 1% chance in children in families that have FAP because of the presence of yet unknown genetic or environmental modifiers of risk.

Less clear is what percentage of the patients who have sporadic hepatoblastoma (those without obvious family histories) carry a germ-line mutation of the *APC* gene. One study has reported that in sporadic hepatoblastoma, germ-line mutations of the *APC* gene were identified in 10% of cases. It has been suggested both that children with hepatoblastoma be screened for germ-line *APC* mutations and that asymptomatic children in families known to have FAP be screened for hepatoblastoma.[64]

Within the *APC* gene, genotype-phenotype correlations suggest regions of the gene that predict both the severity of polyposis and the presence of extracolonic manifestations.[65] The literature suggests that in families with FAP that have children affected with hepatoblastoma, germ-line mutations

can occur throughout the gene (Fig. 18-2) and can also include whole gene deletions or chromosome rearrangements such that the site or type of the individual *APC* mutation cannot be used to predict the likelihood of occurrence of hepatoblastoma.[44,63,66] The functional role of the *APC* gene as a tumor suppressor in hepatoblastoma is further supported by the observation of biallelic inactivation of the *APC* gene in hepatoblastoma in a tumor specimen from a patient with a germ-line *APC* mutation.[67]

Beckwith-Wiedemann syndrome (BWS), an overgrowth disorder classically characterized by large birth weight, macroglossia, omphalocele, and visceromegaly,[68,69] is associated with a markedly increased risk for all embryonal tumors, including Wilms' tumor, hepatoblastoma, neuroblastoma, and adrenal cortical adenoma.[68,70,71] In a registry of children with BWS who were followed at the National Cancer Institute, it was determined that the relative risk for hepatoblastoma in children with BWS was 2280-fold and higher than the relative risk for any other type of cancer. Unlike hepatoblastoma and FAP, hepatoblastoma has not been seen in siblings with BWS despite the extraordinarily high relative individual risk. Presumably this is because of the low incidence of familial occurrence of BWS.

BWS maps to chromosome 11p15, a region known to show loss of alleles in hepatoblastoma[72,73] as well as parental-specific expression of genes (i.e., imprinting), including *IGF2* and *H19*. The extent to which loss of normal genomic imprinting at this locus contributes to hepatoblastoma pathogenesis is unclear.[74-77] Another gene at chromosome 11p15.5 is the *p57KIP2* gene, which has also been shown to be mutated in some but not all cases of BWS[78-81] but is not present in cases of BWS associated with Wilms' tumor.[81] Hartmann and colleagues demonstrated that although the *p57KIP2* gene is not mutated in hepatoblastoma, this gene was upregulated in hepatoblastomas as compared to matched liver samples.[82]

Clearly there is a role for tumor surveillance in BWS. Screening for embryonal tumors of the abdomen may be carried out by periodic sonography of the abdomen and may be effective in detecting Wilms' tumors at early stages.[83-85] It has been suggested that early detection of hepatoblastoma in children with BWS may be further enhanced by screening for serum α-fetoprotein.[86]

Although FAP and BWS are the genetic syndromes most commonly associated with hepatoblastoma, several occasional associations have also been reported (Table 18-1).

Simpson-Golabie-Behmel syndrome is X-linked, is characterized by overgrowth, and involves clinical features reminiscent of those in BWS, including increased risk for embryonal tumors. At least two cases of Simpson-Golabie-Behmel syndrome combined with hepatoblastoma have been reported.[87,88] The underlying gene for Simpson-Golabi-Behmel syndrome, *GPC3*, is highly expressed in hepatoblastoma compared to normal liver, suggesting that this gene may contribute to the tumorigenesis of hepatoblastoma.[89,90]

Li-Fraumeni syndrome predisposes to multiple tumor types in childhood and early adulthood.[91,92] Although liver tumors are not typically included in Li-Fraumeni syndrome, hepatoblastoma has been reported in two Asian kindreds who have Li-Fraumeni syndrome.[93,94] There is also the report of a kindred in which a child developed undifferentiated (embryonal) sarcoma of the liver.[95] Acquired mutations of the *TP53* gene in hepatoblastoma tumor specimens, however, are rare or absent, but they have been reported in undifferentiated embryonal sarcoma of the liver.[96-98]

Hepatoblastoma has also been reported to occur in children with primary biliary atresia as has childhood HCC.[99,100] It is unclear, however, whether liver tumor development in

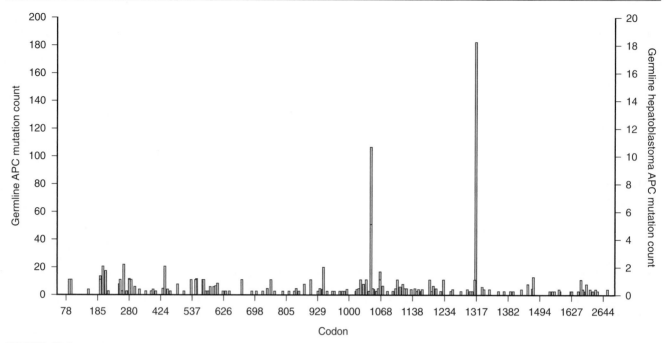

FIGURE 18-2. Frequency histogram of mutations in the adenomatous polyposis coli (APC) gene. Left axis and blue lines represent all known APC germ-line mutations. Right axis and orange lines represent APC germ-line mutations in children with hepatoblastoma. Germ-line mutations associated with hepatoblastoma are observed throughout the gene.[63]

TABLE 18-1	Genetic Syndromes That Cause Predisposition to Liver Tumors	
Disease	**Tumor Type**	**Gene**
Familial adenomatous polyposis	Hepatoblastoma, adenoma, HCC, biliary adenoma	APC
Beckwith-Wiedemann syndrome	Hepatoblastoma, hemangioendothelioma	Multiple candidates
Simpson-Golabi-Behmel syndrome	Hepatoblastoma	GPC3
Trisomy 18	Hepatoblastoma	No single gene
Li-Fraumeni syndrome	Hepatoblastoma, undifferentiated sarcoma	TP53
Glycogen storage disease types I-IV	Hepatocellular adenoma, HCC, hepatoblastoma	Glucose-6-phosphatase
Hereditary tyrosinemia	HCC	Fumarylacetoacetate hydrolase
Alagille's syndrome	HCC	JAGGED-1, NOTCH2
Other familial cholestatic syndromes	HCC	FIC1, *ABCB11*
Neurofibromatosis	HCC, malignant schwannoma, angiosarcoma	NF-1
Ataxia, telangiectasia	HCC	ATM
Fanconi's anemia	HCC, fibrolamellar cancer, adenoma	FAA, FAC others (20%)
Tuberous sclerosis	Angiomyolipoma	TSC1, TSC2

HCC, hepatocellular carcinoma.

children with biliary atresia is a complication resulting from liver disease, or whether a common predisposition to both biliary atresia and tumor development exists. It is worth noting that the same immature cells, thought to share similarities with stem cells, seen in hepatoblastoma are also seen in biliary atresia.[101]

Multiple cases of hepatoblastoma with trisomy 18 have been reported.[102-108] This is somewhat notable in that trisomy of chromosome 18 is not seen as an acquired event despite the observation of multiple other recurring trisomies.[109]

Hepatoblastoma has been reported in a female with monosomy 7 myelodysplasia, a predisposition syndrome not previously seen with hepatoblastoma.[110] Hepatoblastoma has also been reported in neurofibromatosis type 1, although it is not characteristic of this disorder.[111]

HCC, in contrast to hepatoblastoma, is seen in genetic syndromes that are characterized by hepatic cirrhosis. Progressive familial intrahepatic cholestasis, a condition marked by neonatal hepatic cirrhosis, is associated with liver tumor development in children. Both HCC and cholangiocarcinoma are known to occur in this disorder. The disorder, also known as Byler's disease, is a heterogeneous syndrome.[112] The underlying genetic cause is a germ-line mutation of the *ABCB11* gene, which encodes a bile acid export pump.[113] In a series of 11 cases of HCC in children under the age of 5 with neonatal hepatitis and clinical characteristics of familial intrahepatic cholestasis, 10 had immunohistochemical evidence of a deficiency in the bile acid transporter bile salt export pump.[114] In all patients in whom genotyping was possible, a germ-line mutation of the *ABCB11* gene encoding the bile salt export pump was detected.

Alagille's syndrome is an autosomal dominant disorder characterized by characteristic facies, congenital heart disease, and intrahepatic cholestasis, with resulting neonatal jaundice and a paucity of hepatic bile ducts that cause neonatal jaundice. The resulting liver pathology may progress to frank cirrhosis. HCC has been reported in children with Alagille's syndrome.[115-120] The vast majority of the HCCs associated with Alagille's syndrome occur in boys. In one family, three children were reported with HCC in the absence of any other type of liver disease except Alagille's syndrome.[116] Alagille's syndrome is associated with germ-line mutations in the *JAGGED1* gene, the endogenous ligand for *NOTCH2*, a developmental gene involved in the control of maturation of the heart and liver.[121] In a minority of cases of Alagille's syndrome, in which the *JAGGED1* gene is not found to be mutated, mutation of the *NOTCH2* gene itself is mutated.[93,122] It has been shown that the mechanism of liver disease in Alagille's syndrome may relate to an increased expression of hepatocyte growth factor in cells that carry *JAGGED1* mutations.[123]

The family of glycogen storage disorders has been associated with liver tumorigenesis. Glycogen storage disease type I has been reported in association with benign adenoma, HCC, and hepatoblastoma, although the last has been reported only in adolescents.[48,124,125] Similarly, glycogen storage disorder type III has been associated with HCC,[126] and type IV has been associated with hepatocellular adenoma.[127] HCC is known to occur in diseased liver, so with long-term follow-up HCC may be considered a complication of increased survival of glycogen storage disease patients.[125,128]

Hereditary tyrosinemia type 1, characterized by the deficiency of fumarylacetoacetate hydroxylase, is likewise associated with HCC in the setting of severe liver disease.[129]

Fanconi's anemia is associated with liver tumors, but the association has almost always been reported in association with androgenic steroid treatment.[130-137] In a review of 1301 reported cases of Fanconi's anemia, 2.8% were reported to have a liver tumor.[138] The most common type of liver tumor reported in Fanconi's anemia is HCC, but adenomas are also seen in these patients. The incidence appears to increase with age and does not appear to plateau. In multiple instances, liver malignancy was seen in patients with Fanconi's anemia who also had a diagnosis of leukemia. The extent of the associated androgen treatment and the development of hepatic malignancy as opposed to the effect of the underlying genetic defects in DNA repair as manifested by chromosome breakage in Fanconi's anemia is unclear, but a review of the association between androgens and liver tumors suggests that patients with Fanconi's anemia develop liver tumors after smaller and briefer androgen exposure than do individuals with non-Fanconi's anemia.[139] It is also unclear whether there is a difference among the genetic subtypes of Fanconi's anemia with regard to the predisposition to hepatic and other malignancies.[140]

In addition to syndromes predisposing to malignant liver tumors, several syndromes are associated with benign liver tumors. Tuberous sclerosis has been linked to the development of benign hepatic angiomyolipomas.[141,142] Although these hepatic growths are not as common as renal angiomyolipomas, which may develop in as much as 80% of patients with tuberous sclerosis, the hepatic lesions appear by imaging studies in approximately 13% of patients with tuberous sclerosis, accord-

ing to one study.[143] A complete summary of genetic syndromes and liver tumors in children is provided in Table 18-1.

PREMATURITY AS A RISK FACTOR

One of the most intriguing aspects of hepatoblastoma is its association with premature or low-birth-weight infants. This association was initially reported by Japanese investigators who analyzed patient diagnoses and birth weights in the Japan Children's Cancer Registry over the 9-year period between 1985 to 1993.[144] It was found that 3.9% of patients with hepatoblastoma were of very low birth weight. Moreover, it was observed, when subdividing data over 4-year periods, that the percentage of hepatoblastoma cases in infants with low birth weight rose from 0.7% in 1985 to 1989 to 8.6% in 1990 to 1993 and demonstrated a linearly increasing trend. The risk for hepatoblastoma has also been shown to be inversely proportional to birth weight.[145] The relative risk for an infant who weighs between 2000 and 2999 grams is 1.21, whereas the relative risk for an infant of less than 1000 grams is 15.64.

Data from the Children's Cancer Group survey confirm the excess numbers of formerly premature infants who developed hepatoblastoma in a series of 76 patients.[146] A second confirmation, this one in the United States, comes from the California population–based cancer registry, which also reported an elevated risk for hepatoblastoma in children of very low birth weight.[147] This study also pointed out that the age of diagnosis of hepatoblastoma in children of low birth weight was actually older than that of children of normal birth weight, which could in part be explained by gestational age.

It has been speculated that the increase in the percentage of low birth weights in children with hepatoblastoma may be caused in part by the increased survival rates of low-birth-weight infants. It is also believed that the increase in survival rates of premature infants at risk for hepatoblastoma may contribute to the overall increase in childhood liver tumors. Indeed, the rise in the occurrence rate of hepatoblastoma has been found to be consistent with the rise in the rate of low-birth-weight infants.[148] However, whether the pathways by which low-birth-weight infants develop hepatoblastoma involve key exposures in the newborn period, increased sensitivity of the liver in premature infants to potential carcinogens, disruption of the normal process of liver development resulting from premature birth, or a combination of these factors has yet to be determined. One small, single-institution study suggests that intensive long-term perinatal treatments may contribute to the development of hepatoblastoma; the study compared the treatment records of five infants who developed hepatoblastoma to those of infants of similar birth weights who did not develop hepatoblastoma.[149] A somewhat larger study of 12 cases of hepatoblastoma and 75 controls matched for birth weight suggests that the duration of oxygen therapy, the use of furosemide, and the length of time taken to regain body weight at birth were factors in predicting risk for development of hepatoblastoma in premature infants.[150] A study in the United Kingdom reports that when polyhydramnios and either eclampsia or pre-eclampsia have been present in the mother, the child is more likely to contract hepatoblastoma than is a child whose mother did not experience those difficulties. The report also notes that eclampsia or pre-eclampsia was also associated with low birth weight.[151]

A current case-control study of 600 patients with hepatoblastoma by the Children's Oncology Group (AEPI04C1) is examining exposures of low-birth-weight and other infants with hepatoblastoma and hopes to provide further insights into the precise risk factors associated with prematurity and hepatoblastoma.

ENVIRONMENTAL EXPOSURES AND HEPATOBLASTOMA

An epidemiologic case-control study of risk factors for hepatoblastoma by Buckley and colleagues that was based on parental interviews revealed an association between hepatoblastoma and maternal occupational exposure to metals when welding or soldering (OR = 8.0); to petroleum products, such as lubricating oils or greases (OR = 3.7; and to paints or pigments (OR = 3.7). There was also a significant association with paternal occupational exposure to metals (OR = 3.0, P = 0.01) and a marginally significant association with paternal occupational exposure to petroleum products (OR = 1.9).[152] Although the Buckley study did not find an association between parental smoking and hepatoblastoma, an association with parental smoking has been reported in several subsequent studies.[153-155] The risk for hepatoblastoma in children of parents who smoked was approximately double in all three studies.

VIRAL HEPATITIS AND LIVER TUMORS IN CHILDREN

Viral infection by hepatitis has historically accounted for a large percentage of cases of HCC. Prior to the introduction of the hepatitis B vaccine in Taiwan, HCC accounted for 80% of cases of liver tumors in children.[156] With the introduction of the hepatitis B vaccination in 1984, the rates of liver tumors in Taiwanese children over the age of 6 dropped significantly from 0.7 per 100,000 between 1981 and 1986 to 0.36 per 100,000 between 1990 and 1994.[157] The decrease in rate of HCC after the introduction of the vaccine was more pronounced in boys than in girls. The incidence of HCC decreased in boys but not in girls.[158] The male-to-female ratio of the incidence of HCC in Taiwan steadily decreased from 4.5 per 100,000 between 1981 and 1986 to 1.9 per 100,000 between 1990 and 1996, 6 to 12 years after the introduction of the vaccine. The reasons for these gender-related differences in response to the vaccine are not known.[159]

PRESENTATION AND EVALUATION

Aside from patients with the known genetic syndromes discussed earlier, most cases of hepatoblastoma occur in otherwise well children who present with abdominal masses, often with some degree of abdominal discomfort. Isosexual precocious puberty has been observed in some boys with hepatoblastoma, and it occurs secondary to tumor production of chorionic gonadotropin.[160-172] The incidence of precocious puberty in children with liver tumors in one study of 48 children was 6%.[173] To our knowledge, there are no known cases of precocious puberty associated with hepatoblastoma in girls.

Laboratory evaluation of a child with a liver mass should include a complete blood count and liver function tests as well as tests of α-fetoprotein (AFP) and β-human chorionic gonadotropin tumor marker levels. The platelet count is often high in cases of hepatoblastoma but is not diagnostic of hepatoblastoma in children with liver tumors.[174] This thrombophilia is associated with high serum levels of thrombopoietin, also

known as c-mpl ligand. Thrombopoietin is normally synthesized in the liver and has also been shown to be expressed in hepatoblastoma tumor tissues and is present at higher than normal levels in the serum of patients with hepatoblastoma.[175] In a large series of patients of various ages (13 to 84 years) who had hepatic tumors, thrombocytosis was noted in 2.7%. The high platelet count was correlated with higher serum levels of thrombopoietin.[176] Other components of the complete blood count are usually normal because bone marrow involvement with liver tumors has not been reported.

AFP is the primary serum marker used diagnostically, prognostically, and in surveillance, and its level should be obtained in the initial evaluation of any child with a liver mass. AFP levels are markedly elevated in more than 90% of hepatoblastomas and in more than 50% of HCCs. Care should be taken in interpreting AFP levels in a young infant because levels are normally high at birth and decline to below 10 ng/dL over the first year of life. It is worth noting that some liver malignancies, notably the small cell undifferentiated subtype of hepatoblastoma as well as the fibrolamellar variant of HCC, are not associated with elevation of AFP.[177,178] Likewise, sarcomas and rhabdoid tumors are not associated with elevated AFP. The International Society of Pediatric Oncology Liver Tumor Study Group (SIOPEL) has demonstrated that patients with hepatoblastomas and low AFP (less than 100 ng/mL) at diagnosis tend to present at a higher stage and are associated with poor outcomes.[177] The level of β-human chorionic gonadotropin is only occasionally elevated in hepatoblastoma, usually in cases that present with precocious puberty, as discussed earlier. β-human chorionic gonadotropin is also elevated in the rare choriocarcinoma of the liver as well as in the teratoma.

The evaluation of a child with a liver tumor should include a careful family history to document specifically cancers in relatives, and specific notation should be made of any early-onset colon cancers or colectomies, in addition to the presence of thyroid cancers or medulloblastomas, which can be part of the FAP syndrome. Testing for germ-line mutation of the APC gene may be indicated and, if done, should include appropriate genetic counseling. The patients with hepatoblastoma and germ-line APC mutations require long-term surveillance for colonic polyps and tumor development.

In addition, the medical history should note the birth weight, history of prematurity and presence or absence of stigmata of neonatal overgrowth, including omphalocele and hemihypertrophy, which would suggest BWS and a risk for other embryonal tumors.

STAGING

North American trials have traditionally used a postsurgical diagnostic staging group, as shown in Table 18-2. This staging is performed after the initial surgical procedure (biopsy or resection) and is similar to that used for other solid tumors.

The Europeans have developed a different system of staging pediatric liver tumors. The SIOPEL staging is based on the appearance on imaging prior to chemotherapy and surgical resection. Stages I through IV reflect how many sectors are involved with tumor. Other components of the staging system reflect extension into the vena cava, v; extension into the portal vein, p; extrahepatic abdominal disease, e; or distant metastases, m. The SIOPEL staging is shown schematically in Figure 18-3.

Figure 18-4 demonstrates a small hepatoblastoma tumor image that was diagnosed initially by surveillance ultrasound in a patient with BWS. This tumor involved two sectors and as

TABLE 18-2	North American Postsurgical Staging vs. European Presurgical Staging	
	North American Staging: Postsurgical Staging	**European Staging SIOPEL and PRETEXT: Presurgical Staging**
Stage I	No metastases; tumor completely resected	Tumor involving only one quadrant; three adjoining liver quadrants free of tumor
Stage II	No metastases; tumor grossly resected, with microscopic residual disease (i.e., positive margins, tumor rupture, or tumor spill at the time of surgery	Tumor involving two adjoining quadrants; two adjoining quadrants free of tumor
Stage III	No distant metastases; tumor unresectable or resected with gross residual tumor or positive nodes	Tumor involving three adjoining quadrants or two nonadjoining quadrants; one quadrant or two nonadjoining quadrants free of tumor
Stage IV	Distant metastases regardless of the extent of liver involvement	Tumor involving all four quadrants; no quadrant free of tumor

Adapted from National Cancer Institute, www.cancer.gov/cancertopics/pdq/treatment/childliver. Accessed May 3, 2008.

PRETEXT, pretreatment extent of disease; SIOPEL, International Society of Pediatric Oncology Liver Tumor Study Group.

such is classified as pretreatment extent of disease (PRETEXT) II but was completely excised surgically after diagnosis, so it is stage I in the North American staging system. Figure 18-5 demonstrates a multifocal hepatoblastoma that involves all four sectors, so it is PRETEXT IV. The patient had pulmonary metastases so was also stage IV in the North American staging system.

PATHOLOGY OF HEPATOBLASTOMA AND HEPATOCELLULAR CARCINOMA

Grossly, a hepatoblastoma occurs as a single expansile mass commonly located in the right lobe of the liver. A representative resected hepatoblastoma tumor is shown in Figure 18-6. Hepatoblastomas are composed primarily of epithelial cells that resemble various stages of the developing liver. Usually, a hepatoblastoma is a mixture of cells resembling fetal cells and cells resembling embryonal cells. A typical hepatoblastoma of fetal and embryonal histology is shown in Figure 18-7A. Because hepatoblastomas derive from immature cells that may retain the potential to differentiate, tumors often have foci of other types of more differentiated cells, including hematopoietic cells (Fig. 18-7B). A subset of hepatoblastomas is characterized by cholangiocyte-like cells, which suggests the differentiation of the neoplastic cells along the cholangiocyte lineage as opposed to the hepatocyte lineage.[179] When the epithelial cells are aligned in thick cordlike structures, the tumor is described as having macrotrabecular features. In approximately 5% of hepatoblas-

tomas, only fetal-type cells are seen histologically (Fig. 18-7C). As discussed in the treatment section, these pure fetal tumors are thought to have better prognoses.

The small cell, undifferentiated variant makes up approximately 5% of hepatoblastomas. Histologically, the cells are small and pleomorphic and show high mitotic rates (Fig. 18-7D). There are several reports of unique chromosome translocations involving chromosome 22q12, the region of the *SMARCB/INI1* gene, the gene most often associated with rhabdoid tumors and atypical teratoid tumors. Emerging evidence suggests that from histologic, cytogenetic, molecular genetic, and clinical perspectives these tumors resemble rhabdoid tumors. Mounting evidence suggests that the small cell variant is associated with a poor outcome.[177,180]

HCCs consist of cells that are well differentiated and resemble normal hepatocytes. A typical HCC is shown in Figure 18-8. The fibrolamellar variant of HCC is characterized by larger polygonal cells mixed with fibrous stroma, often eosinophilic cytoplasm, and occasionally cystic degeneration (Fig. 18-9A, B).[181,182] In contrast to hepatoblastoma, the adjacent liver tissue in a patient with HCC is commonly marked by cirrhosis. The fibrolamellar variant is an exception in which surrounding liver tissue is usually noncirrhotic.

ACQUIRED GENETIC CHANGES IN HEPATOBLASTOMA

Multiple studies have reported cases or small series of hepatoblastomas with abnormal cytogenetic findings. Karyotypic changes in hepatoblastomas can be classified into two broad categories: numerical changes and structural changes in individual chromosomes.[109]

Hepatoblastomas are characterized cytogenetically primarily by distinct patterns of numerical aberrations. Most result in the addition of whole chromosomes but occasionally result in the loss of chromosomes. The specific numerical changes are nonrandom. Trisomies of chromosome 2, 8, and 20 are the most common recurring numerical aberrations. The most commonly observed chromosomal losses occur in chromosomes 4 and 18. Although these whole-chromosome changes have been described previously by classical karyotype analysis, they can be better visualized by whole genome comparative genomic hybridization (Fig. 18-10).

The most common structural cytogenetic abnormality in hepatoblastoma involves unbalanced translocations involving the long arm of chromosome 1. The initial recurring translocation described was the translocation involving chromosomes 1 and 4, t(1;4)(q12;q34), which was reported by several groups.[183-185] It has since been reported in a large series that hepatoblastoma is characterized by a family of chromosome translocations with similar breakpoints on either chromosome 1q12 or 1q21.[109] Each such translocation observed is unbalanced, resulting in a gain in the long arm of chromosome 1, and is also commonly associated with numerous whole chromosomal gains. The clinical significance of these chromosomal abnormalities is not yet known.

HCC is characterized also by chromosomal gains and losses; loss of the Y chromosome is notable.[186] Duplication of chromosome 1q is also seen in HCC, with increased expression of numerous chromosome 1 genes.[187,188] Cytogenetic data on the fibrolamellar variant of HCC are sparse, but one childhood fibrolamellar carcinoma has been characterized by a hypertriploid karyotype with clonal evolution and multiple additional chromosomal gains as well as loss of the Y chromosome.[189]

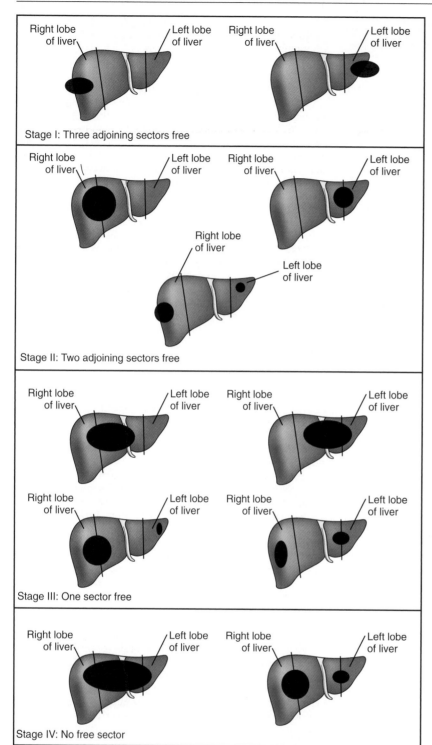

FIGURE 18-3. PRETEXT presurgical staging system used by SIOPEL and used to predict outcome. The liver image is divided into four sectors, and tumor stage is defined as the number of free sectors. In this system, stage is further defined by extension of tumor beyond the liver. v indicates extension into the vena cava and/or all three hepatic veins; p indicates extension into the main and/or both left and right branches of the portal vein; e indicates extrahepatic disease proven by biopsy; and m indicates the presence of distant metastases.[259]

TREATMENT: CHEMOTHERAPY

Although surgical resection, as discussed later, is essential for all malignant liver tumors, chemotherapy has been used extensively for hepatoblastoma to reduce tumor bulk prior to resection or to treat microscopic disease after resection. Much less success has been seen in the use of chemotherapy for HCC.

Effective use of vincristine as a single agent was documented in two early reports.[190,191] In one of these reports, com-

plete regression was noted in a 4-month-old child, and in the other report, a response was maintained for more than 20 months using vincristine alone. In an early multi-institutional phase II trial undertaken by the Acute Leukemia Group B, doxorubicin was shown to be effective in several pediatric solid tumors that had been refractory to other therapies. In the three cases of hepatoblastoma among these tumors, a complete response was observed in two of the three cases. The regimen of doxorubicin used was either a 4-day course of 15 to 20 mg/m^2/day or a 3-day course of 30 mg/m^2/day.[192]

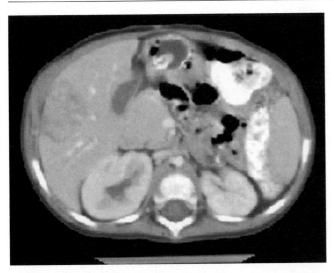

FIGURE 18-4. Computed tomography scan of a low-stage hepatoblastoma detected by periodic surveillance with ultrasound in a patient at high risk for hepatoblastoma because of Beckwith-Wiedemann syndrome. The tumor was fully resectable and classified as stage I. *(Image courtesy of Children's Medical Center, Dallas.)*

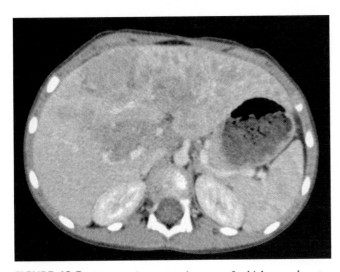

FIGURE 18-5. Computed tomography scan of a high-stage hepatoblastoma. The tumor occupies most of the left lobe and a portion of the right lobe. Preoperative chemotherapy rendered this tumor resectable. This tumor was also accompanied by pulmonary metastases (not shown) and therefore was classified as a stage IV. *(Image courtesy Children's Hospital Boston.)*

Subsequent studies in hepatoblastoma have been centered on platinum-based therapy. Douglass and colleagues of St. Jude Children's Research Hospital reported a response to *cis*-DDP (diamminedichloroplatinum) at a dose of 90 mg/m^2 in 9 of 11 patients with hepatoblastoma.[193] In five of these patients, DDP was used as a single agent in pretreated patients who had disease that was refractory to vincristine and doxorubicin, and only one of these five failed to have a significant response. In the remaining six patients, DDP was used initially as a single agent followed by a combination of cisplatin, vincristine, and doxorubicin. A subsequent study at MD Anderson Cancer Center in Houston used high-dose cisplatin at a dose of 150 mg/m^2 as a single dose in patients with unresectable hepatoblastoma and found a marked response in terms of primary tumor size as well as metastatic disease.[194]

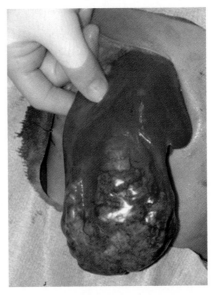

FIGURE 18-6. Gross pathology of resected hepatoblastoma tumor specimen. Tumor appears as a large expansile mass. The tumor has a whitish appearance compared to the darker adjacent liver in the background. The cut surface is shown at the bottom of the figure and has a variegated appearance. *(Picture courtesy Steve Meqisan, MD, Children's Medical Center, Dallas.)*

Platinum compounds have clearly emerged as the most effective means of treating hepatoblastoma, although it has been associated with considerable toxicity. Ototoxicity has been observed in 37% of children treated with platinum agents, according to a European study that included 120 children with cancer diagnosed at a median age of 2.6 years, including 11 patients with hepatoblastoma. The hearing loss was most severe in children younger than 3.6 years of age at diagnosis, and worsening of hearing loss was detected by prolonged follow-up.[195] Thus families of children with hepatoblastoma should be advised of the risks for hearing loss, and children should be monitored during post-treatment years.

The use of doxorubicin and cisplatin together in the treatment of hepatoblastoma has been shown to be effective as well. The first report of this combination in the literature concerned a 15-month-old girl with unresectable hepatoblastoma of mixed histology who received doxorubicin and cisplatin.[196] Quinn and colleagues reported on four patients with hepatoblastoma, three of whom had unresectable tumors, who were treated with cisplatin and doxorubicin.[196a]

The successful combination of cisplatin and doxorubicin was further studied in Toronto when 15 children, 13 of whom had unresectable disease, were treated with cisplatin 20 mg/m^2/day for 5 days together with doxorubicin 25 mg/m^2/day for 3 days.[7] Another report from Toronto documented success in administering similar doses of cisplatin and doxorubicin simultaneously as a continuous infusion in an attempt to further increase cell kill while minimizing toxicity.[197] Significant tumor reduction, allowing surgical resection, was attained in all of the six patients studied, with five of the six patients surviving long term and one child dying perioperatively of surgical complications. The Children's Cancer Study Group undertook a study administering cisplatin at a dose of 100 mg/m^2/day together with a continuous infusion of doxorubicin and reported efficacy in cases of initially unresectable hepatoblastoma.[198] Building on this observation of successful combination of doxorubicin and cisplatin, the two North American cooperative groups designed a study to determine the efficacy and safety of this

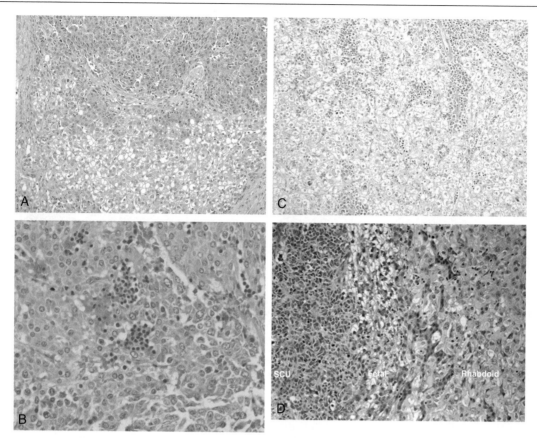

FIGURE 18-7. A, Mixed fetal and embryonal epithelial hepatoblastoma. This hepatoblastoma shows two different morphologic patterns. The fetal pattern, seen in the lower part of the image, is composed of uniform, small, cuboidal cells with distinct cell membranes, whereas the embryonal pattern, seen in upper part of the image, consists of smaller, angulated cells with hyperchromatic nuclei, higher nuclear/cytoplasmic ratios, and indistinct cell membranes. This is the most common histologic pattern of hepatoblastoma. **B,** Hepatoblastoma with extramedullary hematopoiesis. As is often observed in hepatoblastoma, islands of hematopoietic cells are observed as clusters of small dark cells with prominent nuclei within surrounding tumor tissue. **C,** Pure fetal epithelial hepatoblastoma. The pure fetal epithelial hepatoblastoma is composed of relatively uniform, small cuboidal cells. The cells have small round nuclei with inconspicuous nucleoli, abundant cytoplasm that may be clear or finely granular, and distinct cell membranes. The pure fetal variant composes approximately 5% of all hepatoblastomas and is associated with a favorable outcome. **D,** Small cell undifferentiated hepatoblastoma. The central portion shows cells resembling fetal hepatoblastoma. On the left, cells appear undifferentiated with round nuclei and minimal cytoplasm and fail to form tubules. At right, are more typical of rhabdoid-like histology. *(A and C, Images courtesy of Dinesh Rakeja, MD, Children's Medical Center, Dallas; B, Image courtesy of Victor Saldivar, MD, Santa Rosa Children's Hospital, San Antonio, Texas; D, Image courtesy Milton Finegold, Texas Children's Hospital, Houston, Texas.)*

regimen in a large number of patients. The doxorubicin and cisplatin regimen was found to be as effective as the cisplatin, 5-fluorouracil, vincristine (C5V) regimen; however, the toxicity level was greater, particularly in infants.[199]

The use of alternating the platinum analogues cisplatin and carboplatin without concomitant use of other agents was attempted in a randomized trial conducted by the Pediatric Oncology Group (POG 9645), but it resulted in the dismal outcome of a 37% event-free survival compared to a 57% event-free survival in patients receiving the C5V regimen. In addition, patients randomized to receive intensified platinum therapy only experienced more toxicity and a greater need for transfusions. Therefore the standard of care in North America has remained the C5V regimen administered either for four courses postresection in low-stage tumors or initially for two courses prior to resection and followed by additional courses postresection.

Early reviews of large series suggested that hepatoblastoma tumors that were purely of fetal histology had more favorable outcomes than those with predominantly embryonal histology or with macrotrabecular features.[200,201] The trend in cooperative group trials over the past 2 decades has therefore been to

decrease the extent of chemotherapy administered after full resection of hepatoblastomas of pure fetal histology. The first systematic attempt to reduce therapy in this subset of tumors was the Intergroup study (Pediatric Oncology Group 8945/Children's Cancer Study Group 8881. Patients with stage I tumors of purely fetal histology were treated with four courses of doxorubicin only, whereas other tumors were treated using multiagent therapy. The most recent trial by the Children's Oncology Group used an observation-only arm for stage I tumors of purely fetal histology. Although the final conclusions of this study are pending, the potential of eliminating adjuvant chemotherapy in some patients underscores the need for careful and thorough histologic analysis of the whole tumor specimen.

Compared to the successes in treating hepatoblastoma with chemotherapy, the progress in treating HCC has been for the most part disappointing in both children and adults. An early study indicated that doxorubicin induced remission of HCC in 14 of 44 patients (32%),[202] but subsequent studies have shown less success. Within the cooperative groups, because of the small numbers seen, HCC has previously been treated in the same way as hepatoblastoma, although it was acknowl-

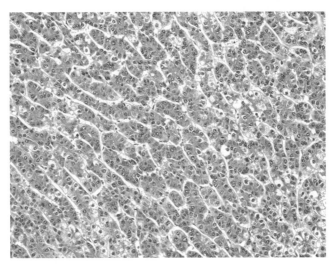

FIGURE 18-8. HCC. This well-differentiated HCC is composed of cords 2 to 4 layers thick or trabeculae of cells resembling normal hepatocytes. Sinusoidal-like spaces lined by endothelial cells are present between the trabeculae, further mimicking the architecture of normal liver. No portal tracts are present. *(Image courtesy Dinesh Rakeja, MD, Children's Medical Center, Dallas.)*

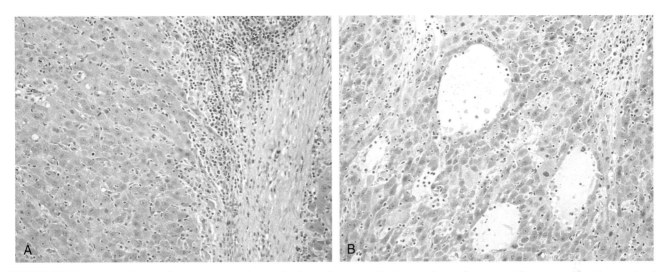

FIGURE 18-9. Fibrolamellar HCC, composed of sheets of polygonal tumor cells that are larger than normal hepatocytes and have a deeply eosinophilic cytoplasm, large nuclei, and prominent eosinophilic nucleoli. **A,** As shown prominently, the cells are embedded in collagenous stroma, and variably thick fibrous septa course through the tumor. Commonly there are focal infiltrates of mononuclear inflammatory cells. **B,** Foci of cystic degeneration (pseudogland formation). *(Image courtesy Dinesh Rakeja, MD, Children's Medical Center, Dallas.)*

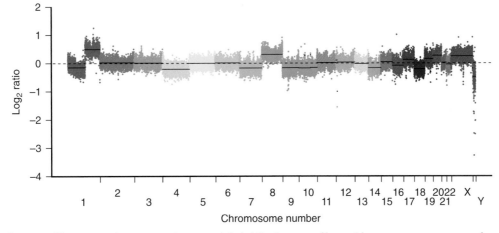

FIGURE 18-10. Genome-wide copy number comparative genomic hybridization scan of hepatoblastoma tumor as compared to a standard normal male control DNA. Hepatoblastoma is characterized by whole chromosome gains and losses as well as unbalanced translocations of chromosome 1, resulting in duplication of the long arm of chromosome 1q. This comparative genomic hybridization plot demonstrates increased copy number of chromosomes 8, 17, 19, and 20 as well as whole losses of chromosomes 4, 7, 9, 10, 14, and 18. In addition, a duplication of chromosome 1q and the loss of chromosome 1p is observed. Numerical aberrations of X and Y reflect the female sex of the child rather than tumor-specific changes.

edged as a distinct entity. Survival rates in cases of initially unresectable HCC have remained dismal. When patients treated with regimens of C5V were compared with those treated with continuous-infusion cisplatin and doxorubicin, using the same regimens shown to be effective in hepatoblastoma,[3] the results demonstrated that in patients with stage III and IV tumors, the survival rate was less than 20%.[33] However, of eight patients with HCC who underwent resection at diagnosis, the long-term survival rate was 88%. This is the largest treatment study of HCC in children, so it is clear that early resectability is an important factor in predicting survival rates; similar results have been observed in adults with HCC.

In 2007, the Food and Drug Administration approved the use of sorafenib, an oral tyrosine kinase inhibitor previously shown to be effective in treating advanced renal cell carcinoma, for the treatment of HCC. The decision was made after a trial of 602 adult patients demonstrated a median 10.7-month survival and a 5.5-month time to tumor progression in patients treated with 400 mg of sorafenib twice daily compared to a median 7.9 months of survival and 2.8 months to tumor progression in patients treated with placebo. The dose-limiting toxicity of sorafenib appears to be hand and foot skin reactions, diarrhea, and lipase or amylase elevation. A previous study at Memorial-Sloan Kettering demonstrated in a phase II, nonrandomized study that sorafenib was well tolerated, although it was only modestly efficacious, which would suggest an indication for future inclusion of sorafenib in multiagent trials of treatments of HCC.[203] This study also performed gene expression micro-array analysis of tumors treated with sorafenib and placebo and determined a pattern of gene expression that correlated with response to sorafenib. This information could conceivably serve as a means of treatment stratification in future trials. Table 18-3 shows a summary of recent cooperative group studies in Europe and North America.

SURGICAL ASPECTS OF LIVER TUMORS

Surgical resection is an important component in the management of both benign and malignant liver tumors. In the case of benign lesions, including adenoma, focal nodular hyperplasia, and mesenchymal hamartoma, complete resection of the tumor is usually curative. It can be performed by means of anatomic lobectomy when necessary, or by nonanatomic wedge resection, in cases of smaller peripheral lesions. In the case of hemangiomas and other vascular malformations of the liver, specific diagnosis is essential to avoid unnecessary surgical intervention or inappropriate use of steroids or chemotherapy agents.[204]

When assessing hepatoblastoma for resectability, a computed tomography scan or magnetic resonance image is essential.[205-207] Particular attention should be paid to the liver's vascular anatomy. A dual-phase computed tomography scan with both arterial and venous phases is the preferred modality for assessing vascular involvement and resectability. Although the PRETEXT staging system is a useful guide for deciding whether a lesion is resectable, the ultimate decision regarding surgical management should rest with the surgeon. If possible, primary resection should be undertaken for PRETEXT I or II tumors if there is no vascular involvement. Involvement of all three hepatic veins or both branches of the portal vein usually precludes surgical resection. However, a PRETEXT III or IV lesion that appears unresectable at the time of diagnosis may respond very well to chemotherapy, and repeat computed tomography following two or three cycles of chemotherapy might demonstrate adequate regression of the tumor away from vital vascular structures such that resection is possible. Very rarely will arterial or biliary involvement preclude tumor resection. In some cases of extensive tumor involving the bifurcation of the bile ducts, biliary reconstruction may be necessary. At the

TABLE 18-3	**A Summary of Cooperative Group Studies in Europe and North America**			
	Presurgical Chemotherapy	**Chemotherapy**	*n*	**Outcomes**
POG #869	No	C5V	73	3-year EFS Stage I(UH)/II: 91% Stage III: 67% Stage IV: 12.5%
COG #9645	Yes	C5V vs. intensified platinum*	33	5-year EFS Stage III: 73% Stage IV: 27%
INT 0098	Selected patients	C5V vs. cisplatin and doxorubicin	182	5-year EFS Stage I(UH)/II: >90% Stage III/IV: >50%
HB – 89	Yes	Ifosfamide, cisplatin, doxorubicin	72	3 year EFS Stage I: 100% Stage II: 50% Stage III: 74% Stage IV: 29%
HB – 9	Selected patients	Ifosfamide, cisplatin, doxorubicin	69	3-year EFS/OS Stage I: 96% Stage II: 100% Stage III: 76% Stage IV: 36%
SIOPEL 1	Yes	Cisplatin, doxorubicin	160	3-year OS 75%
SIOPEL 2	Yes	Cisplatin/carboplatin, doxorubicin; risk stratified	150	3-year OS[†] SR: 90% HR: 78%

*Only stage III and IV patients were enrolled.

[†]SR, Standard risk: hepatoblastoma confined to the liver and involving no more than three hepatic sectors; HR, High risk: hepatoblastoma extending into all four sectors and/or lung metastases and/or extrahepatic involvement.

C5V, cisplatin, fluorouracil, vincristine; COG, Children's Oncology Group, EFS, event-free survival; HB, hepatoblastoma; INT, intergroup study; OS, overall survival; POG, Pediatric Oncology Group; SIOPEL, International Society of Pediatric Oncology Liver Tumor Study Group; UH, unfavorable histology.

time of surgical resection, any suspicious porta hepatis, hepatic artery, celiac, or periaortic lymph nodes should be sampled. When complete tumor resection is not feasible despite adequate chemotherapy, liver transplantation should be performed.[208-211] Therefore, early referral of PRETEXT III or IV tumors to a center that performs liver transplantation is essential.

Surgery remains the mainstay treatment for HCC, given the poor response to chemotherapy and other modalities, including chemoembolization, radiofrequency ablation, and cryotherapy. When HCC develops with a background of cirrhosis, surgery may be limited by the lack of liver physiologic reserve. In these cases, transplantation may be the only safe option, even for early-stage disease.[212] In the fibrolamellar variant, the remaining liver is commonly normal, so resection is more likely to be possible, even with extensive disease, and this may be a factor contributing to the impression that fibrolamellar HCC has a better prognosis than standard HCC.[35] Other malignant tumors of the liver, including angiosarcomas, embryonal sarcomas, rhabdoid tumors, and rhabdomyosarcomas, require complete resection if there is to be any chance for cure.[213-223]

Transplantation has been used increasingly in the treatment of unresectable hepatoblastomas. In the majority of cases involving malignant liver tumors, complete surgical resection is a necessary component of therapy. Whether a tumor is benign or malignant, when complete surgical resection via partial hepatectomy is not possible because of the extent of disease or lack of hepatic reserve, liver transplantation is the only remaining option. Of children receiving liver transplants, approximately 2% are performed as treatment for hepatoblastoma.[224] Although liver transplantation for malignant disease was used during the early years of the development of liver transplantation, survival rates were poor because of complications resulting from transplantation and recurrent disease. More recent data demonstrate significantly improved survival rates in certain patients following transplantation for both hepatoblastoma and HCC.[225-230]

When planning therapy for patients with advanced hepatoblastomas that may require liver transplantation, early referral to a liver transplant center is mandatory. Options for transplantation include the traditional deceased-donor whole organ and the donor split-liver transplant and also, more recently, living-donor transplants.[224] Although there are no data to suggest an optimal timing for transplantation, most centers administer at least two rounds of chemotherapy prior to transplantation in an attempt to shrink the tumor and to determine whether resection without transplantation is an option. Given the small window of opportunity to perform a transplant between cycles, close communication between the oncology team and the transplant team is critical. Evaluation by an experienced transplant team should take place as soon after diagnosis as possible. The current United Network for Organ Sharing liver allocation policy provides high priority for children who require liver transplantation for hepatoblastoma (http:www.unos.org/). A child listed for transplantation who has a diagnosis of hepatoblastoma is automatically assigned 30 pediatric end-stage liver points and has the opportunity to be upgraded to status 1B after 30 days. This high-priority listing allows patients a reasonable chance of undergoing transplantation between cycles, when hematologic counts are not prohibitive. In the case of living-donor transplantation, the timing of the transplant can be scheduled electively. At the time of transplantation, an initial early abdominal exploration to rule out metastatic disease is required. If intra-abdominal metastatic disease is discovered and is not completely resectable, transplantation should be aborted. It is important to have a backup candidate available for such a circumstance so that a valuable liver graft is not wasted.

Liver transplantation for HCC has evolved significantly over the past several years. Most centers currently use the Milan criteria to determine patient selection for liver transplantation.[229] However, recent data from the group at University of California-San Francisco have demonstrated acceptable patient survival rates following transplantation in patients who exceed the Milan criteria.[231] The use of these criteria has not been validated for pediatric patients with HCC or for patients with the fibrolamellar variant of HCC.

LESS COMMON MALIGNANT TUMORS OF THE LIVER

Embryonal sarcoma of the liver, also termed undifferentiated embryonal sarcoma of the liver (UESL), is the third most common malignant liver tumor in children.[95] UESL was first recognized as a distinct entity in 1978. Histologically, these tumors are composed of mixtures of cells with histiocytoid, fibrohistiocytoid, myofibroblastic, and undifferentiated (primitive mesenchymal) morphologies.[232] They are thought to arise from a benign mesenchymal hamartoma.[220,233,234] A chromosome translocation similar to that seen in mesenchymal hamartomas has been reported.[235] UESL can be distinguished from biliary tract rhabdomyosarcoma by several immunohistochemical stains, including myogenin and MyoD1, which are negative in UESL and positive in rhabdomyosarcoma.[236] Unlike most other liver tumors, the male-to-female ration in UESL is 1 to 1. They are considered aggressive malignancies that should be treated with the multiagent regimens used for soft tissue sarcomas at other sites.[237] A European Cooperative Group study from Italy and Germany treated a series of 17 patients with UESL with chemotherapy, conservative surgery and, in two patients, radiotherapy. Of the 17 patients, 12 (70%) survived, and all 8 of those undergoing complete resection survived.[238] A recurring chromosomal translocation involving chromosome 19q13.4 has been reported in at least three cases.[220,239,240]

True rhabdomyosarcomas, when they are seen in the liver, occur in the biliary tract. These tumors histologically resemble rhabdomyosarcomas at other sites, with prominent myoblastic cells that stain for myogenin.[236] These tumors may have a botyroid appearance.[241,242] Embryonal sarcomas have historically been thought to have unfavorable prognoses.[238] They have been characterized by the same translocation seen in the benign mesenchymal hamartomas and may be the malignant counterpart. Like hepatoblastoma, UESL differs from rhabdomyosarcoma of the liver in that the median age of patients with UESL is 10.5 years compared to 3.6 years for rhabdomyosarcoma of the biliary tree, as reported by the Children's Oncology Group.[236]

Rhabdomyosarcoma of the biliary tract is also an embryonal tumor of mesenchymal origin. Obstructive jaundice, with or without abdominal distention, is the usual presenting sign.[242,243] Patients with rhabdomyosarcoma of the biliary tree should be treated with resection if possible and with multiagent therapy according to protocols for rhabdomyosarcomas in other sites. In a report from the Intergroup Rhabdomyosarcoma Study, 4 of 10 patients with biliary tract tumors survived.[243]

Primary germ-cell tumors of the liver are rare but have been reported.[244]

Angiosarcomas of the liver are rare but aggressive, high-grade malignancies derived from endothelial cells.[214,216,245] Angiosarcomas of the liver in children were previously known as infantile hemangioendothelioma type 2.[246] Fewer than 40 cases have been reported. Some cases have been preceded by

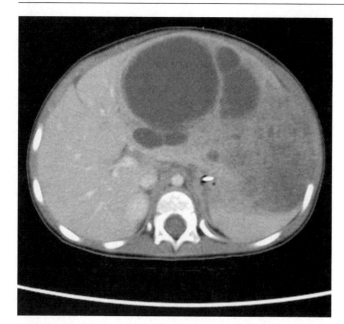

FIGURE 18-11. Computed tomography of a child with mesenchymal hamartoma. Note the multiple cysts with little solid component.

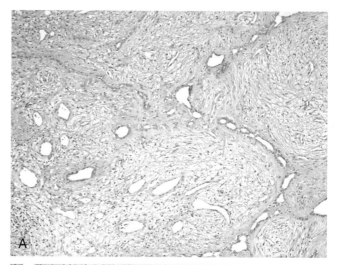

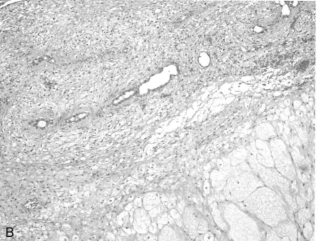

FIGURE 18-12. Mesenchymal hamartomas. Mesenchymal hamartomas are composed of haphazardly arranged and architecturally distorted elements that are normally found in the liver. **A,** Dilated and serpentine biliary ducts, each surrounded by a variably thick cuff of collagen. The bile ducts are lined with low cuboidal epithelial cells without cytologic atypia. **B,** Fluid-filled lymphatic-like cystic spaces. All these elements are embedded in a myxoid and edematous mesenchyme containing delicate fibroblasts. *(Image courtesy Dinesh Rakeja, MD, Children's Medical Center, Dallas.)*

a diagnosis of infantile hepatic hemangioendothelioma.[216,247,248] In contrast to other malignant liver tumors in children, angiosarcomas are more common in females than in males. Their pathology is distinct from that of angiosarcomas in adults in that kaposiform spindle cells are present. The overall prognosis is poor.[214]

Choriocarcinoma of the liver is also an extremely rare tumor. Most cases of infantile choriocarcinoma are actually metastases from gestational choriocarcinoma of the placenta that spreads to the child. However, primary tumors of the liver have been reported. They can be aggressive and devastating, and although the overall outcomes historically have been poor, there are now reports of cures through chemotherapy.[249-251]

BENIGN TUMORS OF THE LIVER

Hepatic mesenchymal hamartoma (HMH) is a benign tumor that parallels hepatoblastoma in terms of the age distribution of patients; almost all cases occur by the time a child is 5 years of age. A child with this tumor presents with an enlarged abdomen. Clinical presentation can be similar to that of hepatoblastoma, although α-fetoprotein levels are not elevated.[252] Like hepatoblastomas, the majority of mesenchymal hamartomas arise in the right side of the liver. Mesenchymal hamartomas are characterized by the presence of cysts, which are less characteristic of hepatoblastomas. Figure 18-11 demonstrates the cystic appearance on imaging. These benign tumors are characterized by massive growth and cause morbidity by compressing adjacent structures.[252] Occasionally these tumors are diagnosed prenatally and can be a cause of fetal demise.[252a] Microscopically, HMH consists of spindle cells in a myxoid background with occasional areas of extramedullary hematopoiesis similar to that seen in hepatoblastoma. Figure 18-12A, B shows the histologic pattern characteristic of mesenchymal hamartomas with fluid-filled cystic areas. Cytogenetically these tumors are characterized by translocations involving 19q13.4, which have been described in at least five cases.[220,239,253-255] The breakpoints involved in one such translocation have been char-

acterized.[256] An interstitial deletion at 19q13.4 has also been reported.[257] HMH can show malignant transformation into malignant mesenchymoma or embryonal sarcoma.[233,234] Treatment of HMH is usually surgical removal, although a more conservative approach of watchful waiting has been advocated in some cases. Intervention in the fetus in cases of intrauterine-detected HMH has been successfully carried out by aspiration of the cystic components of the mass.

Hemangioendothelioma is a term that has been used to denote a type of benign vascular tumor. Previously grouped together as infantile hepatic hemangioendothelioma, the pediatric benign hepatic vascular tumors have recently been shown to be at least two different lesions—hepatic infantile hemangioma and congenital hepatic vascular malformation with associated capillary proliferation. One type (infantile or juvenile hemangioma) often presents as multiple masses that usually involute and regress. The other type, which has been called a vascular malformation, is usually a large single mass that com-

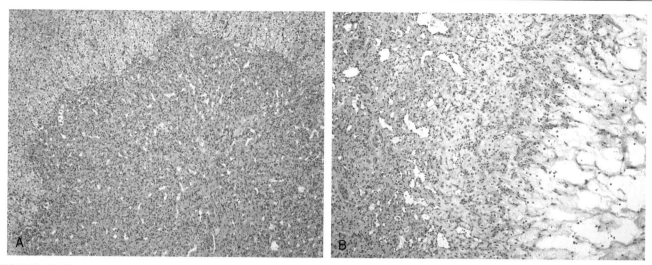

FIGURE 18-13. Benign hepatic vascular tumors. Previously clubbed together as infantile hepatic hemangioendotheliomas, the pediatric benign hepatic vascular tumors have recently been shown to be at least two different lesions. Hepatic infantile hemangioma can be distinguished from congenital hepatic vascular malformation with associated capillary proliferation by the presence or absence of GLUT1 staining. **A,** The infantile or juvenile hemangioma commonly presents as multiple masses that usually involute and regress. Microscopically, the lesions are sharply demarcated lobules composed of closely packed capillary-sized vessels that stain for the glucose transporter GLUT1. The other type, also known as hepatic vascular malformation, is usually a large single mass that often undergoes central infarction, does not regress, and may be associated with consumption coagulopathy. **B,** The area of infarct is surrounded by variably dilated thin-walled vessels with entrapped bile ducts and hepatocytes. The lesional vessels are negative for GLUT1. *(Image courtesy Dinesh Rakeja, MD, Children's Medical Center, Dallas.)*

monly undergoes central infarction, does not regress, and may be associated with consumption coagulopathy caused by platelet trapping in the abnormal vasculature. GLUT1 endothelial reactivity distinguishes the two entities histologically; hepatic infantile hemangiomas stains positively for GLUT1, whereas the hepatic vascular malformations do not exhibit GLUT1 immunoreactivity.[258] Figure 18-13A, B demonstrates these two benign hepatic vascular disorders. A patient with hepatic hemangioendothelioma usually presents with abdominal enlargement with or without congestive heart failure. Hemangioendothelioma has also been reported to occur in association with hydrops fetalis.[159]

FUTURE CHALLENGES

Although cure rates for liver tumors, particularly hepatoblastomas, have increased over past decades, multiple significant challenges remain. The rarity of these malignancies has been a contributing factor in the difficulty of design and implementation of clinical trials, and each clinical hypothesis proposed may take many years to test. Likewise, the testing of new agents for rare pediatric tumors is hampered by the relative rarity of cases. Agents of current interest for clinical testing to treat hepatoblastomas include irinotecan and oxaliplatin. Clinical trials for childhood HCC are likely to parallel those for adult HCC and use multikinase inhibitors.

The indications and consequences of administration of chemotherapeutic agents after liver transplantation have not been studied thoroughly, and challenges in collecting outcome data after transplantation remain significant. The need, if any, for dose reduction after liver transplantation remains unknown, as does the need for altering immunosuppression with concurrent chemotherapy.

There is a need for additional biologic markers for predicting prognosis and for risk stratification. Although several molecular pathways have been identified in pediatric liver tumors, additional therapies aimed at targeting relevant pathways are necessary.

REFERENCES

1. Bulterys M, Goodman M, Smith M, Buckley J. Hepatic tumors. In Ries L, Smith M, Gurney J (eds). Cancer Incidence and Survival Among Children and Adolescents: United States SEER Program 1975-1995. Bethesda, Md, National Cancer Institute, 1999, pp 91-97.
2. Weinberg A, Finegold M. Primary hepatic tumors of childhood. Hum Pathol. 1983;14:512-537.
3. Ortega J, Douglass E, Feusner J, et al. Randomized comparison of cisplatin/vincristine/fluorouracil and treatment of pediatric hepatoblastoma: a report from the Children's Cancer Group and the Pediatric Oncology Group. J Clin Oncol. 2000;18:2665-2675.
4. Perilongo G, Shafford E, Maibach R, et al. Risk-adapted treatment for childhood hepatoblastoma: final report of the second study of the International Paediatric Oncology—SIOPEL 2. Eur J Cancer. 2004;40:411-421.
5. Pritchard J, Brown J, Shafford E, et al. Cisplatin, doxorubicin and delayed surgery for childhood hepatoblastoma: a successful approach—results of the first prospective study of the International Society of Pediatric Oncology. J Clin Oncol. 2000;18: 3819-3828.
6. Weinblatt M, Siegel S, Siegel M, et al. Preoperative chemotherapy for unresectable primary hepatic malignancies in children. Cancer. 1982;50:1061-1064.
7. Filler R, Ehrlich, PF, Greenberg M, Babyn P. Preoperative chemotherapy in hepatoblastoma. Surgery. 1991;110:591-597.
8. Kasper HU, Longerich T, Stippel DL, et al. Mixed hepatoblastoma in an adult. Arch Pathol Lab Med. 2005;129:234-237.
9. Remes-Troche JM, Montano-Loza A, Meza-Junco J, et al. Hepatoblastoma in adult age: a case report and literature review. Ann Hepatol. 2006;5:179-181.

10. Zhang SH, Xu AM, Lin WH, Zhang XY. Mixed hepatoblastoma with teratoid features in an adult. Pathology. 2007;39:453-456.

11. Ke HY, Chen JH, Jen YM, et al. Ruptured hepatoblastoma with massive internal bleeding in an adult. World J Gastroenterol. 2005;11:6235-6237.

12. Yamazaki M, Ryu M, Okazumi S, et al. Hepatoblastoma in an adult: a case report and clinical review of literatures. Hepatol Res. 2004;30:182-188.

13. Inagaki M, Yagi T, Urushihara N, et al. Successfully resected hepatoblastoma in a young adult with chronic hepatitis B: report of a case. Eur J Gastroenterol Hepatol. 2001;13:981-984.

14. Ahn HJ, Kwon KW, Choi YJ, et al. Mixed hepatoblastoma in an adult—a case report and literature review. J Korean Med Sci. 1997;12:369-373.

15. Kacker LK, Khan EM, Gupta R, et al. Hepatoblastoma in an adult with biliary obstruction and associated portal venous thrombosis. HPB Surg. 1995;9:47-49.

16. Inoue S, Nagao T, Ishida Y, et al. Successful resection of a large hepatoblastoma in a young adult: report of a case. Surg Today. 1995;25:974-977.

17. Bortolasi L, Marchiori L, Dal Dosso I, et al. Hepatoblastoma in adult age: a report of two cases. Hepatogastroenterology. 1996;43:1073-1078.

18. Kuniyasu H, Yasui W, Shimamoto F, et al. Hepatoblastoma in an adult associated with c-met proto-oncogene imbalance. Pathol Int. 1996;46:1005-1010.

19. Bortolasi L, Marchiori L, Dal Dosso I, et al. Hepatoblastoma in adult age: a report of two cases. Hepatogastroenterology. 1996;43:1073-1078.

20. Harada T, Matsuo K, Kodama S, et al. Adult hepatoblastoma: case report and review of the literature. Aust N Z J Surg. 1995; 65:686-688.

21. Altmann HW. Epithelial and mixed hepatoblastoma in the adult: histological observations and general considerations. Pathol Res Pract. 1992;188:16-26.

22. Slugen I, Fiala P, Pauer M, et al. Mixed hepatoblastoma in the adult: morphological and immunohistochemical findings. Bratisl Lek Listy. 1990;91:507-515.

23. Green LK, Silva EG. Hepatoblastoma in an adult with metastasis to the ovaries. Am J Clin Pathol. 1989;92:110-115.

24. Sugino K, Dohi K, Matsuyama T, et al. A case of hepatoblastoma occurring in an adult. Jpn J Surg. 1989;19:489-493.

25. Seabrook GR, Collin JR, Britton BJ. Hepatoblastoma: successful resection in an adult. Br J Clin Pract. 1989;43:345-346.

26. Misra SC, Mansharamani GG. Hepatoblastoma of adulthood. Indian J Gastroenterol. 1988;7:58-59.

27. Bhatnagar A, Pathania OP, Champakam NS. Hepatoblastoma in an adult female. Indian J Gastroenterol. 1987;6:125-126.

28. Honan RP, Haqqani MT. Mixed hepatoblastoma in the adult: case report and review of the literature. J Clin Pathol. 1980;33:1058-1063.

29. Carter R. Hepatoblastoma in the adult. Cancer. 1969;23:191-197.

30. Prokurat A, Kluge P, Koscieza A, et al. Transitional liver cell tumors (TLCT) in older children and adolescents: a novel group of aggressive hepatic tumors expressing beta-catenin. Med Pediatr Oncol. 2002;39:510-518.

31. Lack E, Neave C, Vawter G. HCC: review of 32 cases in childhood and adolescence. Cancer. 1983;52:1510-1515.

32. Chen J-C, Chen C-C, Chen W-J, et al. HCC in children: clinical review and comparison with adult cancer. J Pediatr Surg. 1998;33:1350-1354.

33. Katzenstein H, Krailo M, Malogolowkin M, et al. HCC in children and adolescents: results from the Pediatric Oncology Group and the Chldren's Cancer Group intergroup study. J Clin Oncol. 2002;20:2789-2797.

34. Craig J, Peters R, Edmondson H, Omata M. Fibrolamellar carcinoma of the liver: a tumor of adolescents and young adults with distinctive clinco-pathologic features. Cancer. 1980;46:372-379.

35. Katzenstein H, Krailo M, Malogolowkin M, et al. Fibrolamellar hepatocellular carcinoma in children and adolescents. Cancer. 2003;97:2006-2012.

36. Kenney LB, Miller BA, Ries LAG, et al. Increased incidence of cancer in infants in the U.S.: 1980-1990. Cancer. 1998;82:1396-1400.

37. Ross JA, Gurney JG. Hepatoblastoma incidence in the United States from 1973 to 1992. Med Pediatr Oncol. 1998;30:141-142.

38. Linabery AM, Ross JA. Trends in childhood cancer incidence in the U.S. (1992-2004). Cancer. 2008;112:416-432.

39. Willis RA. Pathology of Tumors, 2nd ed. St. Louis, CV Mosby, 1953.

40. Ishak KG, Glunz PR. Hepatoblastoma and hepatocarcinoma in infancy and childhood. Report of 47 cases. Cancer. 1967;20:396-422.

41. Tsao M, Grisham J, Nelson K, Smith J. Phenotypic and karyotypic changes induced in cultured rat hepatic epithelial cells that express the "oval" cell phenotype by exposure to N-methyl-N'-nitro-N-nitrosoguanidine. Am J Pathol. 1985;118:306-315.

42. Ruck P, Xiao J-C, Kaiserling E. Small epithelial cells and the histogenesis of hepatoblastoma: electron microscopic, immuno-electron microscopic, and immunohistochemical findings. Am J Pathol. 1996;148:321-329.

43. Ruck P, Xiao J. Stem-like cells in hepatoblastoma. Med Pediatr Oncol. 2002;39:504-507.

44. deChadarevian JP, Dunn S, Malatack JJ, et al. Chromosome rearrangement with no apparent gene mutation in familial adenomatous polyposis and hepatocellular neoplasia. Pediatr Dev Pathol. 2002;5:69-75.

45. Thomas D, Pritchard J, Davidson R, et al. Familial hepatoblastoma and APC gene mutations: renewed call for molecular research. Eur J Cancer. 2003;39:2200-2204.

46. Ugarte N, Gonzalez-Crussi F. Hepatoma in siblings with progressive familial cholestatic cirrhosis of childhood. Am J Clin Pathol. 1981;76:172-177.

47. Sanders RP, Furman WL. Familial adenomatous polyposis in two brothers with hepatoblastoma: implications for diagnosis and screening. Pediatr Blood Cancer. 2006;47:851-854.

48. Ito E, Sato Y, Kawauchi K, et al. Type 1a glycogen storage disease with hepatoblastoma in siblings. Cancer. 1987;59:1776-1780.

49. Napoli V, Campell W. Hepatoblastoma in infant sister and brother. Cancer. 1977;39:2647-2650.

50. Fraumeni J, Rosen P, Hull E, et al. Hepatoblastoma in infant sisters. Cancer. 1969;24:1086-1090.

51. Groden J, Thliveris A, Samowitz W, et al. Identification and characterization of the familial adenomatous polyposis coli gene. Cell. 1991;66:589-600.

52. Kingston J, Draper G, Mann J. Hepatoblastoma and polyposis coli. Lancet. 1982;1:457.

53. Kingston JE, Herbert A, Draper GJ, Mann JR. Association between hepatoblastoma and polyposis coli. Arch Dis Child. 1983;58:959-962.

54. Li F, Thurber W, Seddon J, Holmes G. Hepatoblastoma in families with polyposis coli. JAMA. 1987;257:2475-2477.

55. Krush A, Traboulsi E, Offerhaus J, et al. Hepatoblastoma, pigmented ocular fundus lesions and jaw lesions in Gardner syndrome. Am J Med Genet. 1988;29:323-332.

56. Garber JE, Li FP, Kingston JE, et al. Hepatoblastoma and familial adenomatous polyposis. J Natl Cancer Inst. 1988;80:1626-1628.

57. Phillips M, Dicks-Mireaux C, Kingston J, et al. Hepatoblastoma and polyposis coli (familial adenomatous polyposis). Med Pediatr Oncol. 1989;17:441-447.

58. Gruner B, DeNapoli T, Andrews W, et al. Fibrolammelar HCC associated with Gardner's syndrome or familial adenomatous polyposis. Med Pediatr Onc. 1998;20:274-278.

59. Bala S, Wunsch P, Ballhausen W. Childhood hepatocellular adenoma in familial adenomatous polyposis: mutations in adenomatous polyposis coli gene and p53. Gastroenterology. 1997;112:919-922.

60. Cetta F, Mazzarella L, Bon G, et al. Genetic alterations in hepatoblastoma and HCC associated with familial adenomatous polyposis. Med Pediatr Oncol. 2003;41:496-497.

61. Giardiello F, Offerhaus G, Krush A, et al. Risk of hepatoblastoma in familial adenomatous polyposis. J Pediatr. 1991;119:766-768.

62. Hughes LJ, Michels VV. Risk of hepatoblastoma in familial adenomatous polyposis. Am J Med Genet. 1992;43:1023-1025.

63. Hirschman B, Pollock B, Tomlinson G. The spectrum of APC mutations in children with hepatoblastoma from familial adenomatous polyposis kindreds. J Pediatr. 2005;147:263-266.

64. Aretz S, Koch A, Uhlhaas S, et al. Should children at risk for familial adenomatous polyposis be screened for hepatoblastoma and children with apparently sporadic hepatoblastoma be screened for APC germ-line mutations? Pediatr Blood Cancer. 2006;47:811-818.

65. Wallis Y, Morton D, McKeown C, MacDonald F. Molecular analysis of the APC gene in 205 families: extended genotype-phenotype correlations in FAP and evidence for the role of the APC amino acid changes in colorectal cancer predisposition. J Med Genet. 1999;36:14-20.

66. Giardiello F, Petersen G, Brensinger J, et al. Hepatoblastoma and APC gene mutation in familial adenomatous polyposis. Gut. 1996;39:867-869.

67. Kurahashi H, Takami K, Oue T, et al. Biallelic inactivation of the APC gene in hepatoblastoma. Cancer Research. 1995;55:5007-5011.

68. Beckwith J. Macroglossia, omphalocele, adrenal cytomegaly, gigantism and hyperplastic visceromegaly. Birth Defects. 1969;5:188-196.

69. Wiedemann H. Complexe malformatif familial avec hernie ombilicale et macroglossie—"un syndrome nouveau"? J Genet Hum. 1964;13:223-232.

70. Sotelo-Avila C, Gonzalez-Crussi F, Fowler J. Complete and incomplete forms of Beckwith-Wiedemann syndrome: their oncogenic potential. J Pediatr. 1980;96:47-50.

71. Elliott M, Bayly R, Cole T, et al. Clinical features and natural history of Beckwith-Wiedemann syndrome: presentation of 74 new cases. Clin Genet. 1994;46:168-174.

72. Little M, Thomson D, Hayward N, Smith P. Loss of alleles on the short arm of chromosome 11 in a hepatoblastoma from a child with Beckwith-Wiedemann syndrome. Hum Genet. 1988;79:186-189.

73. Albrecht S, von Schweinitz D, Waha A, et al. Loss of maternal alleles on chromosome arm 11p in hepatoblastoma. Cancer Res. 1994;54:5041-5044.

74. Montagna M, Menin C, Chieco-Bianchi L, D'Andrea E. Occasional loss of constitutive heterozygosity at 11p15.5 and imprinting relaxation of the IGFII maternal allele in hepatoblastoma. J Cancer Res Clin Oncol. 1994;120:732-736.

75. Davies S. Maintenance of genomic imprinting at the IGF2 locus in hepatoblastoma. Cancer Res. 1993;53:4781-4783.

76. Rainer S, Dobry C, Feinberg A. Loss of imprinting in hepatoblastoma. Cancer Res. 1995;55:1836-1838.

77. Ross J, Radloff G, Davies S. H19 and IGF-2 allele-specific expression in hepatoblastoma. Br J Cancer. 2000;82:753-756.

78. Hatada I, Ohashi H, Fukushima Y, et al. An imprinted gene p57KIP2 is mutated in Beckwith-Wiedemann syndrome. Nat Genet. 1996;14:171-173.

79. O'Keefe D, Dao D, Zhao L, et al. Coding mutations in p57KIP2 are present in some cases of Beckwith-Wiedemann syndrome but are rare or absent in Wilms' tumors. Am J Hum Genet. 1997;61:295-303.

80. Lee M, DeBaun M, Randhawa G, et al. Low frequency of p57KIP2 mutations in Beckwith-Wiedemann syndrome. Am J Hum Gene. 1997;61:304-309.

81. Lam W, Hatada I, Ohishi S, et al. CDKN1C (p57KIP2) mutations in familial and sporadic Beckwith-Wiedemann syndrome (BSW) provides a novel genotype-phenotype correlation. J Med Genet. 1999;36:518-523.

82. Hartmann W, Waha A, Koch A, et al. p57(KIP2) is not mutated in hepatoblastoma but shows increased transcriptional activity in a comparative analysis of the three imprinted genes p57(KIP2), IFG2, and H19. Am J Pathol. 2000;157:1393-1403.

83. Craft A, Parker L, Stiller C, Cole M. Screening for Wilms' tumour in patients with aniridia, Beckwith syndrome, or hemihypertrophy. Med Pediatr Oncol. 1995;24:231-234.

84. Choyke P, Siegel M, Craft A, et al. Screening for Wilms' tumor in children with Beckwith-Wiedemann syndrome or idiopathic hemihypertrophy. Med Pediatr Oncol. 1999;32:196-200.

85. McNeil D, Brown M, Ching A, DeBaun M. Screening for Wilms' tumor and hepatoblastoma in children with Beckwith-Wiedemann syndromes: a cost-effective model. Med Pediatr Oncol. 2001;37:349-356.

86. Clericuzio C, Chen E, NcNeil E, et al. Serum alpha-fetoprotein screening for hepatoblastoma in children with Beckwith-Wiedemann syndrome or isolated hemihyperplasia. J Pediatr. 2003;143:270-272.

87. Li M, Shuman C, Fei Y, et al. GPC3 mutation analysis in a spectrum of patients with overgrowth expands the phenotypes of Simpson-Golabi-Behmel syndrome. Am J Med Genet. 2001;102;161-168.

88. Buonuomo P, Ruggiero A, Vasta I, et al. Second case of hepatoblastoma in a young patient with Simpson-Golabi-Behmel syndrome. Pediatr Hematol Oncol. 2005;22:623-628.

89. Toretsky J, Zitomersky M, Eskenazi A, et al. Glypican-3 expression in Wilms' tumor and hepatoblastoma. J Pediatr Hematol Oncol. 2001;23:496-499.

90. Zynger D, Gupta A, Luan C, et al. Expression of glypican 3 in hepatoblastoma: an immunohistochemical study of 65 cases. Hum Pathol. 2008;39:224-230.

91. Garber J, Goldstein A, Kantor A, et al. Follow-up study of twenty-four families with Li-Fraumeni syndrome. Cancer Res. 1991;51:6094-6097.

92. Nichols K, Malkin D, Garber J, Fraumeni J. Germ-line p53 mutations predispose to a wide spectrum of early-onset cancer. Cancer Epidemiol Biomarkers Prev. 2001;10:83-87.

93. Sameshima Y, Tsunematsu Y, Watanabe S, et al. Detection of novel germ-line p53 mutations in diverse cancer-prone families identified by selecting patients with childhood adrenocortical carcinoma. J Natl Cancer Inst. 1992;84:703-707.

94. Toguchida J, Yamaguchi T, Dayton S, et al. Prevalence and spectrum of germline mutations of the p53 gene among patients with sarcoma. N Engl J Med. 1992;326:1301-1308.

95. Lack EE, Schloo BL, Azumi N, et al. Undifferentiated (embryonal) sarcoma of the liver. Am J Surg Pathol. 1991;15:1-16.

96. Chen TC, Hsieh LL, Kuo TT. Absence of p53 gene mutation and infrequent overexpression of p53 protein in hepatoblastoma. J Pathol. 1995;176:243-247.

97. Kennedy S, Macgeogh C, Jaffe R, Spurr N. Overexpression of the oncoprotein p53 in primary hepatic tumors of childhood does not correlate with gene mutations. Hum Pathol. 1994;25:438-442.

98. Lepreux S, Rebouissou S, Le Bail B, et al. Mutation of TP53 gene is involved in carcinogenesis of hepatic undifferentiated (embryonal) sarcoma of the adult, in contrast with Wnt or telomerase pathways: an immunohistochemical study of three cases with genomic relation in two cases. J Hepatol. 2005;42:424-429.

99. Taat F, Bosman D, Aronson D. Hepatoblastoma in a girl with biliary atresia: coincidence or co-incidence? Pediatr Blood Cancer. 2004;43:603-605.

100. Tatekawa Y, Asonuma K, Uemoto S, et al. Liver transplantation for biliary atresia associated with malignant hepatic tumors. J Pediatr Surg. 2001;36:436-439.

101. Xiao JC, Ruck P, Kaiserling E. Small epithelial cells in extrahepatic biliary atresia: electron microscopic and immunoelectron microscopic findings suggest a close relationship to liver progenitor cells. Histopathology. 1999;35:454-460.

102. Dasouki M, Barr M. Trisomy 18 and hepatic neoplasia. Am J Med Genet. 1987;7:203-205.

103. Mamlok V, Nichols M, Lockhart L, Mamlok R. Trisomy 18 and hepatoblastoma. Am J Med Genet. 1989;33:125-126.

104. Teraguchi M, Nogi S, Ikemoto Y, et al. Multiple hepatoblastomas associated with trisomy 18 in a 3-year-old girl. Pediatr Hematol Oncol. 1997;14:463-467.

105. Bove K, Soukup S, Ballard E, Ryckman F. Hepatoblastoma in a child with trisomy 18: cytogenetics, liver anomalies and literature review. Pediatr Pathol Lab Med. 1996;16:253-262.

106. Tanaka K, Uemoto S, Asonuma K, et al. Hepatoblastoma in a 2-year-old girl with trisomy 18. Eur J Pediatr Surg. 1992;2:298-300.

107. Maruyama K, Ikeda H, Koizumi T. Hepatoblastoma associated with trisomy 18 syndrome: a case report and a review of the literature. Pediatr Int. 2001;43:302-305.

108. Takada K, Hamada Y, Sato M, et al. Cecal volvulus in children with mental disability. Pediatr Surg Int. 2007;23:1011-1014.

109. Tomlinson G, Douglass E, Pollock B, et al. Cytogenetic analysis of a large series of hepatoblastoma: numerical aberrations with recurring translocations involving 1q12-21. Genes Chromosome Cancer. 2005;44:177-184. (See also online supplement at http://www.interscience.wiley.com/jpages/1045-2257/suppmat/index.html.)

110. Neas K, Peters G, Jackson J, et al. Chromosome 7 aberrations in a young girl with myelodysplasia and hepatoblastoma: an unusual association. Clin Dysmorphol. 2006;15:1-8.

111. Ucar C, Caliskan U, Toy H, Gunel E. Hepatoblastoma in a child with neurofibromatosis type I. Pediatr Blood Cancer. 2007;49:357-359.

112. Bull LN, Carlton VE, Stricker NL, et al. Genetic and morphological findings in progressive familial intrahepatic cholestasis (Byler disease [PFIC-1] and Byler syndrome): evidence for heterogeneity. Hepatology. 1997;26:155-164.

113. Stautnieks S, Bull L, Knisely A, et al. A gene encoding a liver-specific ABC transporter is mutated in progressive familial intrahepatic cholestasis. Nat Genet. 1998;20:233-238.

114. Knisely A, Strautnieks S, Meier Y, et al. HCC in ten children under five years of age with bile salt export pump deficiency. Hepatology. 2006;44:478-486.

115. Kaufman S, Wood P, Shaw B, et al. Hepatocarcinoma in a child with the Alagille syndrome. Am J Dis Child. 1987;141:698-700.

116. Rabinovitz M, Imperial J, Schade R, Van Thiel D. HCC in Alagille's syndrome: a family study. J Pediatr Gastorenterol Nutr. 1989;8:26-30.

117. Castaneda C, Fragoso T, Gra B, et al. Alagille's syndrome in Cuba: a report of 9 cases. Genetics. 1992;46:341-346.

118. Chiaretti A, Zampino G, Botto L, Polidori G. Alagille syndrome and hepatocarcinoma: a case report. Acta Paediatr. 1992;81:937.

119. Kim B, Park S, Yang H, et al. HCC occuring in Alagille syndrome. Pathol Res Pract. 2005;201:55-60.

120. Bhadri V, Stormon M, Arbuckle S, et al. HCC in children with Alagille syndrome. J Pediatr Gastorenterol Nutr. 2005;8:26-30.

121. Oda T, Elkahloun A, Pike B, et al. Mutations in the human Jagged1 gene are responsible for Alagille syndrome. Nat Genet. 1997;16:235-242.

122. McDaniell R, Warthen DM, Sanchez-Lara PA, et al. NOTCH2 mutations cause Alagille syndrome, a heterogeneous disorder of the notch signaling pathway. Am J Hum Genet. 2006;79:169-173.

123. Yuan Z, Kobayashi N, Kohsaka T. Human Jagged1 mutants cause liver defect in Alagille syndrome by overexpression of hepatocyte growth factor. J Mol Biol. 2006;356:559-568.

124. Limmer J, Fleig W, Leupold D, et al. HCC in type 1 glycogen storage disease. Hepatology. 1988;8:531-537.

125. Franco LM, Krishnamurthy V, Bali D, et al. HCC in glycogen storage disease type Ia: a case series. J Inherit Metab Dis. 2005;28:153-162.

126. Haagsma E, Smit G, Niezen-Koning KE, et al. Type IIIb glycogen storage disease associated with end-stage cirrhosis and HCC. Hepatology. 1997;25:537-540.

127. Alshak N, Cocjin J, Podesta L, et al. Hepatocellular adenoma in glycogen storage disease type IV. Arch Pathol Lab Med. 1994;118:88-91.

128. Demo E, Frush D, Gottfried M, et al. Glycogen storage disease type III-HCC a long-term complication? J Hepatol. 2007;46:492-498.

129. Weinberg A, Mize C, Worthen H. The occurrence of hepatoma in the chronic form of hereditary tyrosinemia. J Pediatr. 1976;88:434-438.

130. Shapiro P, Ikeda RM, Ruebner BH, et al. Multiple hepatic tumors and peliosis hepatis in Fanconi's anemia treated with androgens. Am J Dis Child. 1977;131:1104-1106.

131. Holder L, Gnarra D, Lampkin B, et al. Hepatoma associated with anabolic steroid therapy. Am J Roentgenol Radium Ther Nucl Med. 1975;124:638-642.

132. Mulvihill J, Ridolfi R, Shultz F, et al. Hepatic adenoma in Fanconi anemia treated with oxymetholone. J Pediatr. 1975;87:122-124.

133. Obeid D, Hill F, Harnden D, et al. Fanconi anemia: oxymetholone hepatic tumors and chromosome aberrations associated with leukemic transition. Cancer. 1980;46:1401-1404.

134. Abbondanzo SL, Manz HJ, Klappenbach RS, Gootenberg JE. HCC in an 11-year-old girl with Fanconi's anemia: report of a case and review of the literature. Am J Pediatr Hematol Oncol. 1986;8:334-337.

135. LeBrun D, Silver M, Freedman M, Phillips J. Fibrolamellar carcinoma of the liver in a patient with Fanconi anemia. Human Path. 1991;22:396-398.

136. Moldvay J, Schaff Z, Lapis K. HCC in Fanconi's anemia treated with androgen and corticosteroid. Zentralblatt fur Pathologie. 1991;137:167-170.

137. Touraine R, Bertrand Y, Foray P, et al. Hepatic tumours during androgen therapy in Fanconi anaemia. Eur J Pediatr. 1993;152:691-693.

138. Alter B. Cancer in Fanconi anemia, 1927-2001. Cancer. 2003;97:425-440.

139. Velazquez I, Alter B. Androgens and liver tumors: Fanconi's Anemia and non-Fanconi's conditions. Am J Hematol. 2004;77:257-267.

140. Joenje H, Patel KJ. The emerging genetic and molecular basis of Fanconi anaemia. Nat Rev Genet. 2001;2:446-457.

141. Carmody E, Yeung E, McLoughlin M. Angiomyolipomas of the liver in tuberous sclerosis. Abdom Imaging. 1994;19:537-539.

142. Yeo W, Leong A, Ward SC, et al. Hepatic angiomyelolipoma and tuberous sclerosis. J Gastroenterol Hepatol. 1996;11:196-198.

143. Fricke B, Donnelly L, Casper K, Bissler J. Frequency and imaging appearance of hepatic angiomyolipomas in pediatric and adult patients with tuberous sclerosis. Am J Radiol. 2004;182:1027-1030.

144. Ikeda H, Matsuyama S, Tanimura M. Association between hepatoblastoma and very low birth weight: a trend or a chance? J Pediatr. 1997;130:557-560.

145. Tanimura M, Matsui I, Abe J, et al. Increased risk of hepatoblastoma among immature children with a lower birth weight. Cancer Res. 1998;58:3032-3035.

146. Feusner J, Plaschkes J. Hepatoblastoma and low birth weight: a trend or chance observation? Med Pediatr Oncol. 2002;39:508-509.

147. Reynolds P, Urayama K, von Behren J, Feusner J. Birth characteristics and hepatoblastoma risk in young children. Cancer. 2004;100:1070-1076.

148. Spector L, Feusner J, Ross J. Hepatoblastoma and low birth weight. Pediatr Blood Cancer. 2004;43:706.

149. Oue T, Kubota A, Okuyama H, et al. Hepatoblastoma in children of extremely low birth weight: a report from a single pernatal center. J Pediatr Surg. 2003;38:134-137.

150. Maruyama K, Ikeda H, Koizumi T, et al. Case-control study of perinatal factors and hepatoblastoma in children with an extremely low birth weight. Pediatr Int. 2000;42:492-498.

151. Ansell P, Mitchell C, Roman E, et al. Relationships between perinatal and maternal characteristics and hepatoblastoma: a report from the UKCCS. Eur J Cancer. 2005;41: 741-748.

152. Buckley J, Sather H, Ruccione K, et al. A case-control study of risk factors for hepatoblastoma: a report from the Chidren's Cancer Study Group. Br J Cancer. 1989;88:373-381.

153. Pang D, McNally R, Birch JM. Parental smoking and childhood cancer: results from the United Kingdom Childhood Cancer Study. Br J Cancer. 2003;88:373-381.

154. Sorahan T, Lancashire R. Parental cigarette smoking and childhood risks of hepatoblastoma: OSCC data. Br J Cancer. 2004;90: 1016-1018.

155. McLaughlin C, Baptiste M, Schymura M, et al. Maternal and infant birth characteristics and hepatoblastoma. Am J Epidemiol. 2006;163:818-828.

156. Chen W, Lee J, Hung W. Primary malignant tumors of liver in infants and children in Taiwan. J Pediatr Surg. 1988;23:457-461.

157. Chang M, Chen C, Lai M, et al. Hepatitis B vaccination in Taiwan and the incidence of HCC in children. Taiwan Childhood Hepatoma Study Group. N Engl J Med. 1997;336:1855-1859.

158. Chang M, Shau W, Chen C, et al. Hepatitis B vaccination and HCC rates in boys and girls. JAMA. 2000;284:3040-3042.

159. Skopec L, Lakatua D. Non-immune fetal hydrops with hepatic hemangioendothelioma and Kassabach-Merritt syndrome: a case report. Pediatr Pathol. 1989;9:87-93.

160. Braunstein GD, Bridson WE, Glass A, et al. In vivo and in vitro production of human chorionic gonadotropin and alpha-fetoprotein by a virilizing hepatoblastoma. J Clin Endocrinol Metab. 1972;35:857-862.

161. Behrle FC, Mantz FA Jr, Olson RL, Trombold JC. Virilization accompanying hepatoblastoma. Pediatrics. 1963;32:265-271.

162. McArthur JW, Toll GD, Russfield AB, et al. Sexual precocity attributable to ectopic gonadotropin secretion by hepatoblastoma. Am J Med. 1973;54:390-403.

163. Kumar EV, Kumar L, Pathak IC, et al. Clinical, hormonal and ultrastructure studies of a virilizing hepatoblastoma. Acta Paediatr Scand. 1978;67:389-392.

164. Flores F, Solano A, Rebeil R, et al. Isosexual precocious puberty in a male infant with hepatoblastoma. Rev Invest Clin. 1979;31: 251-255.

165. Butenandt O, Knorr D, Hecker WC, Lohrs U. Precocious puberty in a boy with HcG-producing hepatoma: case report. Helv Paediatr Acta. 1980;35:155-163.

166. Heinrich UE, Bolkenius M, Daum R, et al. Virilizing hepatoblastoma: significance of alpha-1-fetoprotein and human chorionic gonadotropin as tumor markers in diagnosis and follow-up. Eur J Pediatr. 1981;135:313-317.

167. Nakagawara A, Ikeda K, Hayashida Y, et al. Immunocytochemical identification of human chorionic gonadotropin- and alpha-fetoprotein-producing cells of hepatoblastoma associated with precocious puberty. Virchows Arch A Pathol Anat Histopathol. 1982;398:45-51.

168. Nakagawara A, Ikeda K, Tsuneyoshi M, et al. Hepatoblastoma producing both alpha-fetoprotein and human chorionic gonado-

169. tropin: clinicopathologic analysis of four cases and a review of the literature. Cancer. 1985;56:1636-1642.

169. Beach R, Betts P, Radford M, Millward-Sadler H. Production of human chorionic gonadotropin by a hepatoblastoma resulting in precocious puberty. J Clin Pathol. 1984;37:734-737.

170. Navarro C, Corretger JM, Sancho A, et al. Paraneoplasic precocious puberty: report of a new case with hepatoblastoma and review of the literature. Cancer. 1985;56:1725-1729.

171. Galifer RB, Sultan C, Margueritte G, Barneon G. Testosterone-producing hepatoblastoma in a 3-year-old boy with precocious puberty. J Pediatr Surg. 1985;20:713-714.

172. Heimann A, White PF, Riely CA, et al. Hepatoblastoma presenting as isosexual precocity: the clinical importance of histologic and serologic parameters. J Clin Gastroenterol. 1987;9:105-110.

173. Giacomantonio M, Ein SH, Mancer K, Stephens CA. Thirty years of experience with pediatric primary malignant liver tumors. J Pediatr Surg. 1984;19:523-526.

174. von Schweinitz D, Gluer S, Mildenberger H. Liver tumors in neonates and very young infants: diagnostic pitfalls and therapeutic problems. Eur J Pediatr Surg. 1995;5:72-76.

175. Komura E, Matsumura T, Kato T, et al. Thrombopoietin in patients with hepatoblastoma. Stem Cells. 1998;16:329-333.

176. Hwang SJ, Luo JC, Li CP, et al. Thrombocytosis: a paraneoplastic syndrome in patients with HCC. World J Gastroenterol. 2004;10:2472-2477.

177. De Ioris M, Brugieres L, Zimmermann A, et al. Hepatoblastoma with a low serum alpha-fetoprotein level at diagnosis: the SIOPEL group experience. Eur J Cancer. 2008;44:545-550.

178. Torbenson M. Review of the clinicopathologic features of fibrolamellar carcinoma. Adv Anat Pathol. 2007;14:217-223.

179. Zimmermann A. Hepatoblastoma with cholangioblastic features ("cholangioblastic hepatoblastoma") and other liver tumors with bimodal differentiation in young patients. Med Pediatr Oncol. 2002;39:487-491.

180. Haas JE, Feusner JH, Finegold MJ. Small cell undifferentiated histology in hepatoblastoma may be unfavorable. Cancer. 2001;92:3130-3134.

181. Edmondson HA. Differential diagnosis of tumors and tumor-like lesions of liver in infancy and childhood. AMA J Dis Child. 1956;91:168-186.

182. Farhi D, Shikes R, Murari P, Silverberg S. HCC in young people. Cancer. 1983;52:1516-1525.

183. Schneider N, Cooley L, Finegold M, et al. Report of the first recurring chromosome translocation: der(4)t(1;4)(q12;q34). Genes Chromosomes Cancer. 1997;19:291-294.

184. Sainati L, Leszl A, Stella M, et al. Cytogenetic analysis of hepatoblastoma: hypothesis of cytogenetic evolution in such tumors and results of a multicentric study. Cancer Genet Cytogenet. 1998;104:39-44.

185. Ma SK, Cheung AN, Choy C, et al. Cytogenetic characterization of childhood hepatoblastoma. Cancer Genet Cytogenet. 2000;119:32-36.

186. Bardi G, Johansson B, Pandis N, et al. Cytogenetic findings in three primary HCCs. Cancer Genet Cytogenet. 1992;58:191-195.

187. Park SJ, Jeong SY, Kim HJ. Y chromosome loss and other genomic alterations in HCC cell lines analyzed by CGH and CGH array. Cancer Genet Cytogenet. 2006;166:56-64.

188. Skawran B, Steinemann D, Weigmann A, et al. Gene expression profiling in HCC: upregulation of genes in amplified chromosome regions. Mod Pathol. 2008;21:505-516.

189. Lowichik A, Schneider NR, Tonk V, et al. Report of a complex karyotype in recurrent metastatic fibrolamellar HCC and a review of HCC cytogenetics. Cancer Genet Cytogenet. 1996;88:170-174.

190. Selawry OS, Holland JF, Wolman IJ. Effect of vincristine (NSC-67574) on malignant solid tumors in children. Cancer Chemother Rep. 1968;52:497-500.

191. Lascari A. Vincristine therapy in an infant with probable hepatoblastoma. Pediatrics. 1970;45:109-112.

192. Wang J, Holland J, Sinks L. Phase II study of adriamycin (NSC-123127) in childhood solid tumors. Cancer Chemother Rep 3. 1975;6:267-270.

193. Douglass E, Green A, Wrenn E, et al. Effective cisplatin (DDP) based chemotherapy in the treatment of hepatoblastoma. Med Pediatr Oncol. 1985;13:187-190.

194. Black C, Cangir A, Choroszy M, Andrassy R. Marked response to preoperative high-dose cis-platinum in children with unresectable hepatoblastoma. J Pediatr Surg. 1991;26:1070-1073.

195. Bertolini P, Lassalle M, Mercier G, et al. Platinum compound-related ototoxicity in children. J Pediatr Hematol Oncol. 2004;26:649-655.

196. Forouhar F, Quinn J, Cooke R, Foster J. The effect of chemotherapy on hepatoblastoma. Arch Pathol Lab Med. 1984;108:311-314.

196a. Quinn JJ, Attman AJ, Robinson HT, et al. Adriamycin and cisplatin for hepatoblastoma. Cancer. 1985;56:1926-1929.

197. Langevin A, Pierro A, Liu P, et al. Adriamycin and cis-platinum administered by continuous infusion preoperatively in hepatoblastoma unresectable at presentation. Med Pediatr Oncol. 1990;18:181-184.

198. Ortega JA, Krailo MD, Haas JE, et al. Effective treatment of unresectable or metastatic hepatoblastoma with cisplatin and continuous infusion doxorubicin chemotherapy: a report from the Children's Cancer Study Group. J Clin Oncol. 1991;9:2167-2176.

199. Ortega JA, Douglass EC, Feusner JH, et al. Randomized comparison of cisplatin/vincristine/fluorouracil and cisplatin/continuous infusion doxorubicin for treatment of pediatric hepatoblastoma: a report from the Children's Cancer Group and the Pediatric Oncology Group. J Clin Oncol. 2000;18:2665-2675.

200. Lack E, Naeve C, Vawter G. Hepatoblastoma: a clinical and pathological study of 54 cases. Am J Surg Pathol. 1982;6:693-705.

201. Weinberg A, Finegold M. Primary hepatic tumors of childhood. Hum Pathol. 1983;14:512-537.

202. Johnson PJ, Williams R, Thomas H, et al. Induction of remission in HCC with doxorubicin. Lancet. 1978;1:1006-1009.

203. Abou-Alfa G, Schwartz L, Ricci S, et al. Phase II study of sorafenib in patients with advanced hepatocellular. J Clin Oncol. 2006;24:4293-4300.

204. Christison-Lagay ER, Burrows PE, Alomari A, et al. Hepatic hemangiomas: subtype classification and development of a clinical practice algorithm and registry. J Pediatr Surg. 2007;42:62-67; discussion 7-8.

205. Dong Q, Xu W, Jiang B, et al. Clinical applications of computerized tomography 3-D reconstruction imaging for diagnosis and surgery in children with large liver tumors or tumors at the hepatic hilum. Pediatr Surg Int. 2007;23:1045-1050.

206. Lu M, Greer M. Hypervascular multifocal hepatoblastoma: dynamic gadolinium-enhanced MRI findings indistinguishable from infantile hemagioendothelioma. Pediatr Radiol. 2007;37:587-591.

207. Haliloglu M, Hoffer FA, Gronemeyer SA, et al. 3D gadolinium-enhanced MRA: evaluation of hepatic vasculature in children with hepatoblastoma. J Magn Reson Imaging. 2000;11:65-68.

208. Koneru B, Flye MW, Busuttil RW, et al. Liver transplantation for hepatoblastoma: the American experience. Ann Surg. 1991;213:118-121.

209. Al-Qabandi W, Jenkinson HC, Buckels JA, et al. Orthotopic liver transplantation for unresectable hepatoblastoma: a single center's experience. J Pediatr Surg. 1999;34:1261-1264.

210. Reyes JD, Carr B, Dvorchik I, et al. Liver transplantation and chemotherapy for hepatoblastoma and hepatocellular cancer in childhood and adolescence. J Pediatr. 2000;136:795-804.

211. Molmenti E, Wilkinson K, Molmenti H, et al. Treatment of unresectable hepatoblastoma with liver transplantation in the pediatric population. Am J Transplant. 2002;2:535-538.

212. Capussotti L, Ferrero A, Vigano L, et al. Liver resection for HCC with cirrhosis: surgical perspectives out of EASL/AASLD guidelines. Eur J Surg Oncol. 2007; (Aug 2; e-pub before print).

213. Premalata C, Kumar R, Appaji L, Prabhakaran P. Childhood hepatic angiosarcoma—a case report. Indian J Pathol Microbiol. 2005;48:487-489.

214. Dimashkieh H, Jum Q, Ashmead J. Pediatric hepatic angiosarcoma: case report and review of the literature. Pediatr Dev Pathol. 2004;7:527-532.

215. Gunawardena SW, Trautwein LM, Finegold MJ, Ogden AK. Hepatic angiosarcoma in a child: successful therapy with surgery and adjuvant chemotherapy. Med Pediatr Oncol. 1997;28:139-143.

216. Awan S, Davenport M, Portmann B, Howard E. Angiosarcoma of the liver in children. J Pediatr Surg. 1996;31:1729-1732.

217. Baron PW, Majlessipour F, Bedros AA, et al. Undifferentiated embryonal sarcoma of the liver successfully treated with chemotherapy and liver resection. J Gastrointest Surg. 2007;11:73-75.

218. Chowdhary SK, Trehan A, Das A, et al. Undifferentiated embryonal sarcoma in children: beware of the solitary liver cyst. J Pediatr Surg. 2004;39:E9-E12.

219. Kim DY, Kim KH, Jung SE, et al. Undifferentiated (embryonal) sarcoma of the liver: combination treatment by surgery and chemotherapy. J Pediatr Surg. 2002;37:1419-1423.

220. O'Sullivan M, Swanson P, Knoll J, et al. Undifferentiated embryonal sarcoma with unusual features arising within mesenchymal hamartoma of the liver: report of a case and review of the literature. Pediatr Dev Pathol. 2001;4:482-489.

221. Wagner LM, Garrett JK, Ballard ET, et al. Malignant rhabdoid tumor mimicking hepatoblastoma: a case report and literature review. Pediatr Dev Pathol. 2007;10:409-415.

222. Jayaram A, Finegold MJ, Parham DM, Jasty R. Successful management of rhabdoid tumor of the liver. J Pediatr Hematol Oncol. 2007;29:406-408.

223. Meyer-Pannwitt U, Kummerfeldt K, Broelsch CE. Primary pleomorphic rhabdomyosarcoma of the liver. Langenbecks Archiv fur Chirurgie. 1996;381:75-81.

224. Kasahara M, Ueda M, Haga H, et al. Living-donor liver transplantation for hepatoblastoma. Am J Transplant. 2005;5:2229-2235.

225. Otte JB. Paediatric liver transplantation—a review based on 20 years of personal experience. Transpl Int. 2004;17:562-573.

226. Otte JB, de Ville de Goyet J. The contribution of transplantation to the treatment of liver tumors in children. Semin Pediatr Surg. 2005;14:233-238.

227. Tiao G, Bobey N, Allen S, et al. The current management of hepatoblastoma: a combination of chemotherapy, conventional resection, and liver transplantation. J Pediatr. 2005;146:204-211.

228. Mazzaferro V, Chun YS, Poon RT, et al. Liver transplantation for HCC. Ann Surg Oncol. 2008;15:1001-1007.

229. Mazzaferro V, Regalia E, Doci R, et al. Liver transplantation for the treatment of small HCCs in patients with cirrhosis. N Engl J Med. 1996;334:693-699.

230. Yao FY. Expanded criteria for liver transplantation in patients with HCC. Hepatol Res. 2007;37(suppl 2):S267-S274.

231. Yao FY, Xiao L, Bass NM, et al. Liver transplantation for HCC: validation of the UCSF-expanded criteria based on preoperative imaging. Am J Transplant. 2007;7:2587-2596.

232. Aoyama C, Hachitanda Y, Sato J, et al. Undifferentiated (embryonal) sarcoma of the liver: a tumor of uncertain histogenesis showing divergent differentiation. Am J Surg Pathol. 1991;15:615-624.

233. Ramanujam T, Ramesh J, Goh D, et al. Malignant transformation of mesenchymal hamartoma of the liver: case report and review of the literature. J Pediatr Surg. 1999;34:1684-1686.

234. Begueret H, Trouette H, Vielh P, et al. Hepatic undifferentiated embryonal sarcoma: malignant evolution of mesenchymal hamartoma? Study of one case with immuno-histochemical and flow cytometric emphasis. J Hepatol. 2001;34:178-179.

235. Lauwers G, Grant L, Donnelly W, et al. Hepatic undifferentiated (embryonal) sarcoma arising in a mesenchymal hamartoma. Am J Surg Pathol. 1997;21:1248-1254.

236. Nicol K, Savell V, Moore J, et al. Distinguishing undifferentiated embryonal sarcoma of the liver from biliary tract rhabdomyosarcoma: a Children's Oncology Group study. Pediatr Dev Pathol. 2007;10:89-97.

237. Ninomiya T, Hayashi Y, Saijoh K, et al. Expression ratio of hepatocyte nuclear factor-1 to variant hepatocyte nuclear factor-1 in differentiation of HCC and hepatoblastoma. J Hepatol. 1996;25:445-453.

238. Bisogno G, Pilz T, Perilongo G, et al. Undifferentiated sarcoma of the liver in childhood: a curable disease. Cancer. 2002;94:252-257.

239. Bove K, Blough R, Soukup S. Third report of t(19q)(13.4) in mesenchymal hamartoma of liver with comments on link to embryonal sarcoma. Pediatr Dev Pathol. 1998;1:438-442.

240. Iliszko M, Czauderna P, Babinska M, et al. Cytogenetic findings in an embryonal sarcoma of the liver. Cancer Genet Cytogenet. 1998;102:142-144.

241. Taira Y, Nakayama I, Moriuchi A, et al. Sarcoma botryoides arising from the biliary tract of children: a case report with review of the literature. Acta Pathol Jpn. 1976;26:709-718.

242. Lack EE, Perez-Atayde AR, Schuster SR. Botryoid rhabdomyosarcoma of the biliary tract. Am J Surg Pathol. 1981;5:643-652.

243. Ruymann FB, Raney RB Jr, Crist WM, et al. Rhabdomyosarcoma of the biliary tree in childhood:a report from the Intergroup Rhabdomyosarcoma Study. Cancer. 1985;56:575-581.

244. Conrad RJ, Gribbin D, Walker NI, Ong TH. Combined cystic teratoma and hepatoblastoma of the liver: probable divergent differentiation of an uncommitted hepatic precursor cell. Cancer. 1993;72:2910-2913.

245. Nazir Z, Pervez S. Malignant vascular tumors of liver in neonates. J Pediatr Surg. 2006;41:e49-e51.

246. Ishak K, Goodman Z, Stocker J. Malignant mesenchymal tumors: tumors of the liver and intrahepatic bile ducts, Third Series, Fascicle 31. Washington, DC: American Registry of Pathology; 2001:301-306.

247. Kirchner S, Heller R, Kasselberg A, Greene H. Infantile hepatic hemangioendothelioma with subsequent malignant degeneration. Pediatr Radiol. 1981;11:42-45.

248. Strate S, Rutledge J, Weinberg A. Delayed development of angiosarcoma in multinodular infantile hepatic hemagioendothelioma. Arch Pathol Lab Med. 1984;108:934-944.

249. Szavay P, Wermes C, Fuchs J, et al. Effective treatment of infantile choriocarcinoma in the liver with chemotherapy and surgical resection: a case report. J Pediatr Surg. 2000;35:1134-1135.

250. Heath JA, Tiedemann K. Successful management of neonatal choriocarcinoma. Med Pediatr Oncol. 2001;36:497-499.

251. Yoon J, Burns R, Malogolowkin M, Mascarenhas L. Treatment of infantile choriocarcinoma of the liver. Pediatr Blood Cancer. 2007;49:99-102.

252. Yen J, Hong M, Lin J. Hepatic mesenchymal hamartoma. J Pediatr Child Health. 2003;39:632-634.

252a. Laberge JM, Patenaude Y, Desilets V, et al. Large hepatic mesenchymal hamartoma leading to mid-trimester fetal demise. Fetal Diagn Ther. 2005;20:141-145.

253. Speleman F, De Telder V, De Potter K, et al. Cytogenetic analysis of a mesenchymal hamartoma of the liver. Cancer Genet Cytogenet. 1989;40:29-32.

254. Mascarello J, Krous H. Second report of a translocation involving 19q13.4 in a mesenchymal hamartoma of the liver. Cancer Genet Cytogenet. 1992;58:141-142.

255. Rakheja D, Margraf L, Tomlinson G, Schneider N. Hepatic mesenchymal hamartoma with translocation involving chromosome band 19q13.4. Cancer Genet Cytogenet. 2004;153:60-63.

256. Rajaram V, Knezevich S, Bove K, et al. DNA sequence of the translocation breakpoints in undifferentiated embryonal sarcoma arising in mesenchymal hamartoma of the liver harboring the t(11;19)(q11;q13.4) translocation. Genes Chromosomes Cancer. 2007;46:508-513.

257. Talmon G, Cohen S. Mesenchymal hamartoma of the liver with an interstitial deletion involving chromosome band 19q14: a theory as to pathogeneisi. Arch Pathol Lab Med. 2006;130:1216-1218.

258. Mo JQ, Dimashkieh HH, Bove KE. GLUT1 endothelial reactivity distinguishes hepatic infantile hemangioma from congenital hepatic vascular malformation with associated capillary proliferation. Hum Pathol. 2004;35:200-209.

259. Abramson L, Arensman R. Liver tumors. eMedicine Website. Available at: www.emedicine.com/ped/topic3035.htm. Accessed May 4, 2008.

Rhabdomyosarcoma

Frederic G. Barr and Richard B. Womer

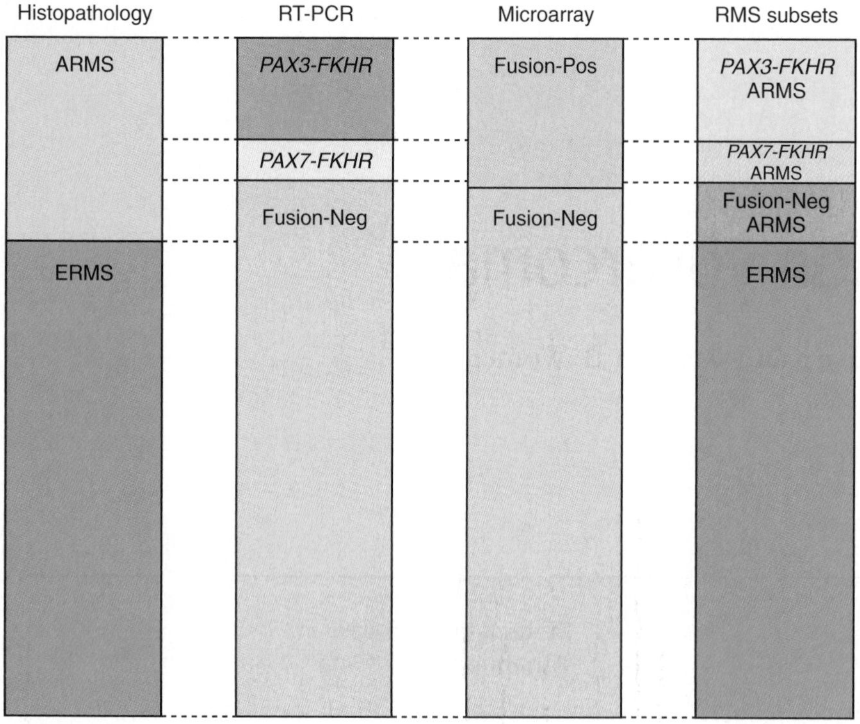

FIGURE 19-1. Categorization of rhabdomyosarcoma subsets by various methodologies. The columns represent the different subsets of RMS and how commonly they occur as defined by the methodologies of histopathologic analysis; RT-PCR detection of gene fusion status (*PAX3-FKHR* and *PAX7-FKHR*); and microarray-based gene expression profiling. The final column shows the subsets that have been established on the basis of a combination of histopathology and gene fusion analysis. It should be noted that there is a small difference in the size of the fusion-negative subset based on gene fusion analysis and microarray analysis because of the variant fusion cases that score as fusion-negative in the RT-PCR assay and fusion-positive in the microarray assay.

PATHOLOGIC CLASSIFICATION OF RHABDOMYOSARCOMA

The term *rhabdomyosarcoma* (RMS) comprises a heterogeneous family of tumors. These tumors are related in still poorly understood ways to the skeletal muscle lineage. Some of the tumors occur in the vicinity of skeletal muscle, but others occur in areas without obvious skeletal muscle; thus, these tumors cannot be defined solely as tumors of skeletal muscle. Instead, this tumor family is characterized by its derivation from mesenchymal precursors and the shared cellular program of skeletal myogenesis. However, this characterization does not rule out the possibility that some precursors intrinsically undergo myogenesis, whereas others may have developed this ability aberrantly.

Histopathologic classification has evolved over time, but two principal histopathologic subtypes have been recognized consistently: embryonal RMS (ERMS) and alveolar RMS (ARMS; Fig. 19-1). The criteria for these categories were refined over time as these subtypes were associated with clinically distinct phenotypes. As described in detail later, ERMS tends to occur in the head and neck, and genitourinary tract of younger patients and is associated with a favorable prognosis, whereas ARMS more often occurs in the extremities in older children and is associated with a less favorable prognosis. ERMS and ARMS account for 70% to 80% and 20% to 30% of RMS cases, respectively.

The diagnosis of RMS in general can be difficult because of the paucity of features of striated muscle differentiation. A variety of pediatric solid tumors, including RMS, neuroblastoma, Ewing's sarcoma, and non-Hodgkin's lymphoma, can present as collections of poorly differentiated cells (small round blue cell tumors). To detect more subtle evidence of myogenic differentiation, immunohistochemical reagents have been used to identify muscle-specific proteins, such as desmin, myoglobin, muscle-specific actin, and the myogenic transcription factors MyoD and myogenin. In addition, further evidence of the myogenic phenotype can be provided by electron microscopic examination and the detection of myofilaments.

ERMS is so named because of its histologic similarity to developing skeletal muscle (Fig. 19-2A). The tumor cells show varying degrees of differentiation along the myogenic spectrum, from small primitive round cells to larger oblong cells with eccentric oval nuclei and varying amounts of eosinophilic cytoplasm.[1] ERMS nuclei are often notable for a relatively bland chromatin pattern. These differentiated cells often elongate to assume a straplike appearance and occasionally show cross-striations and multinucleation. In addition to the characteristic cytology, ERMS tumors classically have variable cellularity, resulting in areas of hypercellularity alternating with areas of hypocellularity in a loose myxoid stroma.

Within the ERMS category, there are two variants that have superior outcomes. Botryoid RMS typically occurs in the lumen of a hollow viscus, such as the urinary bladder, vagina, or extrahepatic bile ducts, and grossly has multiple polypoid nodules.[1] At the microscopic level, this tumor typically has a dense cambium layer of tumor cells under an intact epithelial surface. Spindle-cell RMS has dense bundles or whorls of spindle-shaped cells that resemble smooth muscle cells. In children, these lesions commonly occur in the paratesticular region, but in adults, in whom the prognosis may not be as good, these lesions tend to occur in the head and neck. In both variants, the tumor cells can show marked rhabdomyoblastic differentiation.

In ARMS, the tumor cells are small blue round cells with only small amounts of cytoplasm (see Fig. 19-2B).[1,2] The prominent round nuclei generally have a monotonous, coarse chromatin pattern and often central nucleoli. These tumor cells form highly cellular aggregates that are separated by fibrovascular septae. Within these aggregates, there is a tendency to produce areas of discohesion, resulting in the formation of spaces or clefts lined by rhabdomyoblasts. This appearance of spaces within the fibrovascular septae results in the alveolar appearance for which this tumor is named. Other common features are the tendency of tumor cells to align along the septae in a picket-fence pattern and the appearance of tumor giant cells. In some cases (often associated with smaller biopsies),

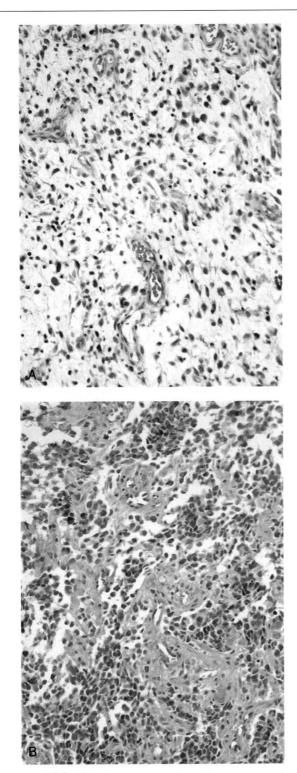

FIGURE 19-2. Histopathology of rhabdomyosarcoma subtypes. **A,** Embryonal rhabdomyosarcoma (hematoxylin-eosin; original magnification: 100×). **B,** Alveolar rhabdomyosarcoma (hematoxylin-eosin; original magnification: 100×). *(Photomicrographs provided by Dr. Bruce Pawel, Children's Hospital of Philadelphia.)*

there is a paucity of fibrovascular stroma, no evidence of alveolar-like spaces, and the predominance of a highly cellular small round cell population; the term *solid variant* applies to this situation.

There is also an RMS subset with features similar to those of anaplastic Wilms' tumors.[2] Although the anaplasia can be seen in both subtypes, it is more prevalent in ERMS. Anaplastic RMS tumors have large, lobated hyperchromatic nuclei and atypical mitoses. The anaplastic cells can be found either scattered throughout the tumor (focal anaplasia) or in clusters or sheets (diffuse anaplasia).

RHABDOMYOSARCOMA IN CANCER-PREDISPOSITION SYNDROMES

The majority of cases of RMS appear to arise as sporadic nonheritable tumors, but a small fraction are associated with heritable genetic syndromes (Table 19-1). In some cases, the proband with RMS inherited a mutant gene as part of an established familial syndrome, and in other cases a new germline mutation occurred in one germ cell that ultimately produced the proband. There are cancer-predisposition syndromes in which RMS is a common tumor (such as the Li-Fraumeni and Costello syndromes), and there are other syndromes in which RMS is a less common tumor (such as nevoid basal cell carcinoma syndrome; NBCCS). Finally, from a mechanistic standpoint, these syndromes can be divided into three groups: one involves the major p53 and retinoblastoma tumor suppressor pathways; the second involves the ras signaling pathway; and the third group involves other syndromes.

Germline Mutations Involving the p53 and Retinoblastoma Pathways

Li-Fraumeni Syndrome

Li-Fraumeni syndrome (LFS) is a familial cancer susceptibility syndrome characterized by a clustering of several different cancer types among first-degree relatives.[3] The most commonly involved tumors include RMSs and other soft tissue sarcomas, osteosarcomas, breast cancer, brain tumors, adrenal cortical carcinomas, and acute leukemia. The syndrome was first recognized by the finding of four patients who had a sibling or cousin with RMS among a group of 648 patients with RMS,[4] and additional studies delineated the associated feature of RMS occurrence at a young age (younger than 2 years of age).[5] Using a candidate gene approach, sequence analysis of the *TP53* gene identified germline alterations, usually point mutations in *TP53* exons 5 through 8, in as much as 70% of families in which LFS occurred.[6,7] Loss of the second wild-type *TP53* gene copy was shown in RMS tumors in individuals with germline *TP53* mutations[8,9] consistent with the second hit being a somatic event, as proposed in the "two-hit hypothesis" of tumor suppressor gene inactivation.[10] Furthermore, heightened tumor susceptibility was demonstrated by the finding of RMS accompanied by or followed by additional malignancies in individuals with confirmed *TP53* germline mutations.[11-14] Finally, an analysis of RMS patients without any family history of cancer predisposition identified germline *TP53* mutations in 3 of 33 sporadic RMS patients.[15] Of note, these mutations were found exclusively in patients younger than 3 years of age (3 of 13 patients), emphasizing the importance of early RMS onset as an important clue to a germline mutation, even without a family history of cancer susceptibility.

TABLE 19-1 Familial Cancer Predisposition Syndromes Associated with Rhabdomyosarcoma

Cancer Syndrome	Locus	Gene	Non-neoplastic Findings	Characteristic Tumors	RMS cases
Li-Fraumeni syndrome	17p13.1 22q12.1	TP53, CHEK2	None	Sarcomas, breast cancer, brain tumor, adrenocortical cancer, leukemia	0.1% to 9% of all cases
Hereditary retinoblastoma	13q14	RB1	None	Retinoblastoma, osteosarcoma	24 cases
Neurofibromatosis type 1	17q11.2	NF1	Café au lait spots, axillary freckling, Lisch nodules, learning deficits	Benign: Neurofibroma Malignant: Acute myelogenous leukemia, malignant peripheral nerve sheath tumor	0.5% to 6% of all cases
Costello syndrome	11p15.5	HRAS	Developmental delay, craniofacial defects, loose skin, palmar and plantar creases, cardiomyopathy	Benign: Skin papillomata Malignant: RMS, neuroblastoma, bladder cancer	13 cases
Beckwith-Wiedemann syndrome	11p15.5	Unknown	Macrosomia, macroglossia, hemihyperplasia, visceromegaly	Wilms' tumor, hepatoblastoma	8 cases
Nevoid basal cell carcinoma syndrome	9q22	PTCH	Macrocephaly, skin cysts, palmar and plantar pits, rib anomalies	Basal cell carcinoma, medulloblastoma	4 cases
Rubinstein-Taybi syndrome	16p13.3	CREBBP	Mental retardation, facial anomalies, broad thumbs	Leukemia, brain tumors	3 cases

There is also a subset of LFS families in which *TP53* germline mutations are not identified. In some of these families, including families with cases of RMS, germline mutations were identified in the *CHK2* gene.[16] This gene encodes a protein kinase that phosphorylates p53 in response to stimuli such as DNA damage, and thus both proteins contribute to a common signaling pathway that stops cell division at times of stress.

Hereditary Retinoblastoma

Hereditary retinoblastoma syndrome is characterized by the development of bilateral or multifocal retinal tumors at an early age and is caused by germline mutations in the *RB1* tumor suppressor gene. These tumors also develop following the occurrence of a somatic mutation in the second *RB1* allele in accord with the two-hit tumor suppressor hypothesis.[10] In addition to retinoblastoma, this syndrome is associated with the risk for other primary and treatment-related cancers, in particular osteosarcomas and other sarcomas,[17] including RMS. In a cohort of 963 survivors of hereditary retinoblastoma, with an average of 25 years of follow-up, 69 soft tissue sarcomas were diagnosed, including eight cases of RMS.[18] Seven of these RMS cases occurred in patients who had received radiation therapy, and all seven RMS tumors occurred within the radiation field. Four cases occurred 1 to 9 years following diagnosis of the first retinoblastoma tumor, and an additional three cases occurred 10 to 19 years after the first diagnosis. A second study described six RMS cases arising in the temporalis muscle in or near the radiation field after radiation therapy in patients with hereditary retinoblastoma.[19] Microscopic analysis of these tumors demonstrated an atypical small round cell appearance with perivascular pseudorosettes. The cytologic appearance was considered most consistent with a histologic diagnosis of ARMS, although characteristic gene fusion assays were negative in three tumors tested.

Germline Mutations of the ras Signaling Pathway

Neurofibromatosis Type 1

Neurofibromatosis type I is a common autosomal dominant disorder caused by mutations of the *NF1* gene. This gene encodes neurofibromin, a GTPase activating protein that negatively regulates the ras signaling pathway,[20,21] and thus *NF1* mutations serve to activate this pathway. Characteristic findings in this syndrome include café au lait spots, axillary freckling, neurofibromas, Lisch nodules, and developmental and learning deficits.[22] In addition to neurofibromas, other associated benign tumors include optic tract gliomas and pheochromocytomas. Malignant tumors associated with this syndrome include malignant peripheral nerve sheath tumors and acute myelogenous leukemia.[23] Multiple studies also indicate that neurofibromatosis type 1 is a contributing factor in the development of a subset of RMS cases. The percentage of RMS patients with neurofibromatosis type 1 ranged in various studies: 5 of 84 (6%); 5 of 249 (2%); 6 of 590 (1.0%); and 5 of 1025 (0.5%).[24-27] In general, the RMS tumors found in association with this syndrome were diagnosed as ERMS and occurred at urogenital sites.

Costello Syndrome

Costello syndrome is a rare genetic syndrome characterized by multiple developmental anomalies and tumor predisposition. The major developmental anomalies include postnatal growth retardation and developmental delay, coarse facies and other craniofacial abnormalities, loose skin and deep palmar and plantar creases, and cardiomyopathy.[28] The tumor predisposition includes the occurrence of benign skin papillomata in half of patients and an increased risk for malignant tumors, in particular RMS.[29] Among the estimated 200 known cases of this syndrome, there are 13 reported cases of RMS (11 of which were diagnosed as ERMS). Using a candidate gene approach, germline mutations were identified in the *HRAS* proto-oncogene in most patients with this syndrome,[30] thus indicating another mechanism of activating the ras signaling pathway. The mutations occur in *HRAS* codons 12 or 13, which are also commonly mutated in sporadic tumors and have transforming activity in standard cell culture assays. Therefore, in contrast to the germline mutations in tumor suppressor genes that result in loss of function, these germline *HRAS* mutations generate gain of function alleles. Of note, in one available case of RMS arising in the setting of Costello syndrome, the wild-type allele was lost, indicating that a second event related to the wild-type *HRAS* gene copy still occurs in a somatic cell in this gain-of-function mechanism.[31]

Costello syndrome demonstrates phenotypic overlap with Noonan syndrome and cardiofasciocutaneous (CFC) syndrome, which are all characterized by short stature, facial anomalies, heart defects, and other abnormalities.[32] Furthermore, the molecular basis of Noonan syndrome and CFC syndrome is germline mutations in genes encoding proteins within the ras signaling pathway. Mutations of *PTPN11* and *KRAS* occur in Noonan syndrome, whereas *KRAS*, *BRAF*, *MEK1*, and *MEK2* mutations occur in CFC syndrome. These results are particularly intriguing in light of the finding of RMS in patients with Noonan syndrome[33-35] and CFC syndrome.[36,37] It is noteworthy that Noonan syndrome has been linked to an increased risk for leukemia, but there is no clear evidence of cancer susceptibility in CFC syndrome.[32] Finally, RMS cases have also been found in patients with overlapping features of Noonan syndrome and neurofibromatosis type 1, which may be attributable to alterations in the *NF1* gene.[38,39] The overlap of these latter two genetic syndromes highlights the similarities in phenotype caused by all these various proteins, including neurofibromin, in the ras signaling pathway.

Other Syndromes

Beckwith-Wiedemann Syndrome

Beckwith-Wiedemann syndrome (BWS) is a rare heterogeneous overgrowth syndrome characterized by macrosomia, macroglossia, abdominal wall defects, hemihyperplasia, visceromegaly, and renal abnormalities.[40] Patients with this syndrome have an overall risk for tumor development of 7.5% and most commonly develop Wilms' tumor or hepatoblastoma or, less commonly, adrenocortical carcinoma, neuroblastoma, or RMS. The molecular basis for BWS is proposed to be dysregulation or alteration of one or more imprinted genes in the 11p15.5 chromosomal region, which includes genes encoding the growth factor IGF2 and tumor suppressors H19 and CDKN1C (p57/KIP2). There are eight reported cases of RMS associated with BWS.[41-46] These cases include four cases diagnosed as ERMS and three diagnosed as ARMS (although cytogenetics were negative for ARMS-associated translocations). The ages of patients diagnosed with RMS varied between 6 weeks and 13 years, and the sites included the orbit, abdomen, and bladder. In addition to complete BWS syndrome, ERMS was found in two patients in the setting of isolated hemihypertrophy, which may represent a mild BWS phenotype,[47,48] and in a third case orbital RMS was found in the setting of incomplete BWS.[49]

Nevoid Basal Cell Carcinoma Syndrome

NBCCS, or Gorlin's syndrome, is a rare autosomal dominant disorder associated with a predisposition for tumors and developmental abnormalities. NBCCS results from germline mutations in *PTCH*, a gene encoding a negative regulator of the sonic hedgehog signaling (SHH) pathway.[50] Developmental abnormalities in this syndrome include macrocephaly, skin cysts, palmar and plantar pits, odontogenic keratocysts, and rib anomalies.[51] This syndrome also commonly causes multiple basal cell carcinomas and less commonly medulloblastomas and ovarian fibrosarcomas. In addition, several cases of RMS[52-55] and benign fetal rhabdomyoma[51] have been reported as part of this syndrome.

Rubinstein-Taybi Syndrome

Rubinstein-Taybi syndrome is a malformation syndrome characterized by mental retardation, facial anomalies, and broad thumbs.[56] In the 724 documented cases of this syndrome, 17 malignant and 19 benign tumors have been reported,[57] including 3 cases of nasopharyngeal RMS.[47,58,59] This syndrome is caused by mutations of the *CREBBP* gene.[60-62] This gene encodes the ubiquitous protein CBP, which functions as a transcriptional coactivator and histone acetyltransferase.[63] CBP has been implicated as an important factor in the p53 pathway in the control of both p53 transcriptional activity as well as p53 protein stability.[64]

GENETICS OF SPORADIC RHABDOMYOSARCOMA

Classic Cytogenetic Analysis of Chromosomal Changes in Alveolar and Embryonal Rhabdomyosarcoma

In the Mitelman Database of Chromosome Aberrations in Cancer (http://cgap.nci.nih.gov/Chromosomes/Mitelman), there are karyotypes of 96 cases of ARMS and 68 cases of ERMS. These studies document significant differences between the two RMS subtypes detectable at the chromosomal level. Most important, several key references in this database first demonstrated that nonrandom chromosomal translocations distinguish the majority of ARMS tumors from ERMS tumors as well as from other pediatric solid tumors. The most prevalent finding in ARMS is a translocation, t(2;13)(q35;q14),[65-67] which was detected in 58% of cases of ARMS (Fig. 19-3). In addition, a variant translocation, t(1;13)(p36;q14), was identified in a small subset of approximately 6% of cases of ARMS.[68,69] As discussed later, this figure is an underestimate because the 1;13 translocation commonly is not visible because of a subsequent amplification event. In contrast to the high incidence of translocations in ARMS, among 69 cases of ERMS the 2;13 translocation was found in 2 cases (3%) and the 1;13 translocation was not found in any cases (0).[70,71] Such rare translocation-positive ERMS cases should be re-examined to determine whether they are ARMS tumors. No other structural chromosomal rearrangements were detected that further distinguish the two subtypes or are recurrent in either subtype. However, evidence of genomic amplification (double minute chromosomes or homogeneously staining regions) was detected in 18% of ARMS cases and 15% of ERMS cases.

A second set of karyotypic differences between ARMS and ERMS is the frequent occurrence of whole chromosome gains and losses (Fig. 19-4). ERMS generally shows a higher fraction of cases with gains and losses at most chromosomes than is found in ARMS. The most notable gains in ERMS were at chromosomes 2 (41%); 8 (50%); 11 (21%); 12 (31%); 13 (26%); and 20 (28%). The chromosomes most commonly lost in ERMS were chromosomes 4 (22%); 9 (22%); 13 (21%); 14 (21%); 15 (28%); and 17 (21%). Although the gains and losses in ARMS are usually lower, the chromosomes most commonly gained are 2 (19%); 12 (16%); and 20 (18%), and the chromosomes most commonly lost are 3 (19%); 10 (13%); 14 (13%); 16 (13%); and 21 (13%).

Comparative Genomic Hybridization Analyses of Copy Number Changes in Rhabdomyosarcoma

Comparative genomic hybridization (CGH) studies have provided insight into additional chromosomal changes in RMS and

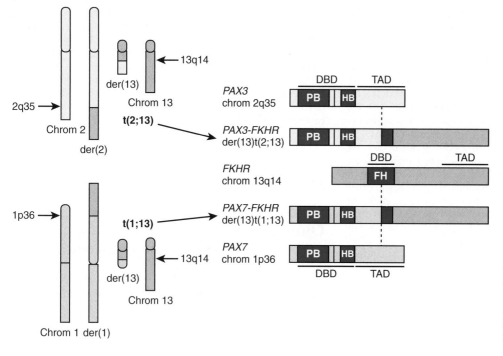

FIGURE 19-3. Diagrams of 2;13 and 1;13 chromosomal translocations and associated fusion products. A schematic representation of the normal and derivative chromosomes associated with t(2;13) and t(1;13) is shown on the left. The translocation breakpoints are indicated by *short horizontal arrows* indicating the location of the involved chromosomal region. The wild-type and fusion products associated with the 2;13 and 1;13 translocations are shown on the right. The paired box (PB), octapeptide, homeobox (HB), and forkhead (FH) domains are indicated as open boxes. Transcriptional domains (DNA-binding domain DBD and transcriptional activation domain TAD) are shown as solid bars. The vertical dashed line indicates the translocation fusion point.

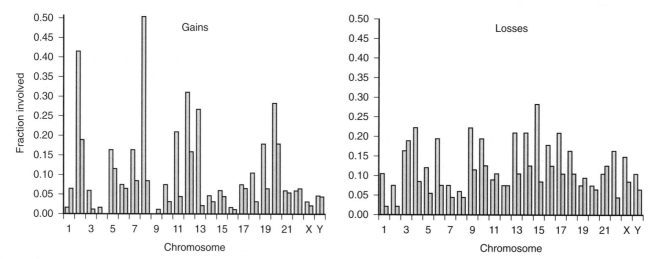

FIGURE 19-4. Chromosome gains and losses in embryonal and alveolar rhabdomyosarcomas. The fraction of ERMS (orange bar) and ARMS (blue bar) cases with each numeric change is calculated from the karyotypic data from 96 cases of ARMS and 68 cases of ERMS in the Mitelman Database of Chromosome Aberrations in Cancer (http://cgap.nci.nih.gov/Chromosomes/Mitelman).

have further highlighted genetic differences between ARMS and ERMS. CGH is a molecular cytogenetic method of screening a tumor for DNA gains and losses independent of prior knowledge of a gene or sequence from the affected region. In the original chromosomal CGH methodology, tumor and normal reference DNA preparations are differentially labeled with fluorescent dyes and cohybridized to normal metaphase chromosomes. Assessment of the ratio of tumor to normal DNA hybridization signals along each chromosome permits identification of regions in the tumor genome with copy number gains or losses. There have been three major CGH studies of cases of ERMS in which a total of 43 cases were analyzed.[72-74] These studies identified high frequency gain of chromosomes 2 or 2q (42%); 7 or 7q (49%); 8 (72%); 11 or 11p (35%); 12 (42%); 13 (30%); and 20 (30%), and loss of chromosomes 10

or 10p (21%). Finally, whereas two studies detected evidence of genomic amplification in only 1 of 10 or 1 of 11 ERMS tumors (each in the 12q13-15 region),[72,73] the other study detected amplification in 5 of 22 ERMS cases.[74] In the latter study, the incidence of amplification was further subdivided into 4 of 6 cases with anaplasia and 1 of 16 cases without anaplasia. In these anaplastic ERMS cases, amplification was found in various genomic regions, including 12q13-15 and 18q21.

In contrast to ERMS, the ARMS subtype was notable for the frequent occurrence of genomic amplification events (Table 19-2). Three CGH studies assessed the copy number status of 50, 23, and 11 ARMS cases and detected at least one amplification event in 66%, 26%, and 73% of the cases, respectively, for a combined incidence of 56%.[73-75] Therefore, the incidence of

TABLE 19-2	Commonly Amplified Chromosomal Regions in Alveolar Rhabdomyosarcoma		
		FREQUENCY OF OCCURRENCE	
Chromosome Region	**Genes Involved**	**CGH (%)**	**PCR (%)**
1p36	*PAX7*	6	70
2p24	*MYCN*	20	25
2q34-qter	*PAX3*	8	5
12q13-15	*CDK4*	18	11
	MDM2		12
13q14	*FKHR*	10	—
13q31	*GPC5*	10	16
	C13orf25		

CGH, comparative genomic hybridization; PCR, polymerase chain reaction.

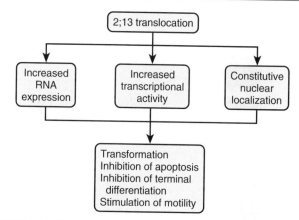

FIGURE 19-5. Multiple biologic effects of 2;13 translocation. The 2;13 translocation affects expression of the *PAX3-FKHR* gene product at multiple biologic levels (shown by boxes), resulting in multiple phenotypic changes in the target cell.

amplification appears similar in ARMS and anaplastic ERMS and is significantly higher than in nonanaplastic ERMS. In ARMS cases, the 12q13-15 and 2p24 chromosomal regions were the most commonly amplified, with evidence of amplification in 18% and 20% of cases, respectively. Amplified regions reported only in a subset of the studies include 13q14 (7-13%); 13q31 (10%); 2q34-qter (8%); and 1p36 (6%). In addition, the CGH studies of ARMS cases identified that the most common copy number gains involved chromosomes 1 or 1q (21%); 2 or 2p (20%); 5 or 5q (21%); 8 (20%); 12 or 12q (19%); and 20 or 20q (20%); and the most common copy number losses involved chromosomes 16 or 16q (15%); 17 or 17p (13%); and 22 (12%). These studies indicate that overall copy number gains and losses are generally lower in ARMS tumors than in ERMS tumors, supporting the view that different molecular mechanisms are involved in the development of these two RMS subtypes.

Molecular Genetics of Chromosomal Translocations in Alveolar Rhabdomyosarcoma

The 2;13 and 1;13 translocations break and rejoin portions of genes from the paired box and forkhead transcription factor families to generate fusion genes (see Fig. 19-3). The genes on chromosomes 2 and 1 rearranged by the 2;13 and 1;13 translocations are *PAX3* and *PAX7*, respectively.[76,77] These genes encode highly related members of the paired box family, which contain N-terminal DNA binding domains consisting of paired box and homeobox motifs and C-terminal transcriptional activation domains. The chromosome 13 locus involved in these translocations is *FKHR (FOX01)*, which encodes a member of the forkhead family with an N-terminal forkhead DNA binding domain and a C-terminal transcriptional activation domain.[77,78] The translocations break within intron 7 of *PAX3* or *PAX7*, respectively, and maintain the integrity of the N-terminal DNA binding domain but separate it from an essential part of the transactivation domain. Similarly, the translocations break within the first intron of *FKHR*, which disrupts the forkhead DNA binding domain and maintains the integrity of the transactivation domain. The 2;13 and 1;13 translocations result in the generation of fusion genes that are expressed as fusion transcripts, which are then translated into fusion pro-

teins. Although both reciprocal fusion genes resulting from a translocation, *PAX3-FKHR* and *FKHR-PAX3* (or *PAX7-FKHR* and *FKHR-PAX7*) are often present in the tumor cells, the higher and more consistent expression of *PAX3-FKHR* and *PAX7-FKHR* supports the premise that these products are involved in ARMS pathogenesis. In the chimeric transcripts, the 5′ *PAX3* (or 5′ *PAX7*) and 3′ *FKHR* coding sequences are fused in-frame to generate a 2508 or 2484 nt open reading frame encoding an 836 or 828 amino acid fusion protein, respectively. The distribution of translocation breakpoints within specific introns generates a functional protein that cannot be created by any other combination of *PAX3* and *FKHR* exons because of incompatible reading frames or loss of needed functional domains. These findings support the premise that rearrangements of *PAX3* or *PAX7* intron 7 and *FKHR* intron 2 are selected because of functional constraints related to the genomic organization of *PAX3*, *PAX7*, and *FKHR*.

The *PAX3-FKHR* and *PAX7-FKHR* fusion transcripts encode chimeric transcription factors containing the PAX3 or PAX7 DNA binding domain and the *FKHR* transcriptional activation domain (see Fig. 19-3). These fusion proteins activate transcription from PAX3/PAX7–binding sites but are more potent as transcriptional activators than the wild-type PAX3 and PAX7 proteins[79,80] (Fig. 19-5). In studies with model target genes, the wild-type PAX3 and PAX7 proteins induced low or undetectable levels of transcriptional activation, but the PAX3-FKHR and PAX7-FKHR fusion proteins induced as much as tenfold to 100-fold more activity. Rather than being directly attributable to simple differences between the transcriptional activation domains, this difference in transcriptional activity appears to be caused by a difference in sensitivity of the two activation domains to the inhibitory effects of N-terminal PAX3 and PAX7 domains.

In addition to changes in transcriptional function, the *PAX3-FKHR* or *PAX7-FKHR* gene fusion events affect the expression and subcellular localization of the corresponding fusion protein (see Fig. 19-5). In this way, the chromosomal changes in ARMS result in high levels of exclusively nuclear chimeric transcription factors that inappropriately activate transcription of genes with PAX3/PAX7 DNA binding sites. These biologic effects contribute to tumorigenesis by modulating myogenic differentiation, altering growth and apoptotic pathways, and stimulating motility and other metastatic pathways.

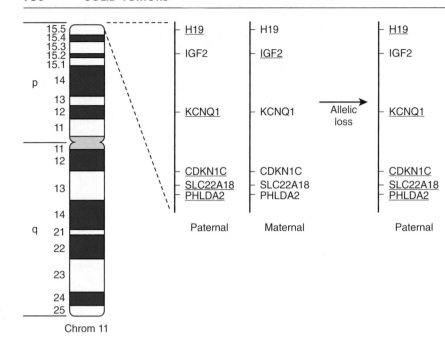

FIGURE 19-6. Allelic loss of imprinted region at 11p15.5 in rhabdomyosarcoma. In the 11p15.5 chromosomal region, there is parent-of-origin-specific expression (imprinting) of multiple genes. Expressed alleles are underscored; unexpressed alleles are not. In many cases of ERMS, a few cases of ARMS, and other tumors, the maternal alleles in the 11p15.5 region (and variable amounts of contiguous regions) are lost by one of a variety of genomic mechanisms in a process termed allelic loss, loss of heterozygosity, or conversion to homozygosity.

Molecular Genetics of Allelic Loss Events in Chromosomal Region 11p15.5 in Embryonal Rhabdomyosarcoma

Although recurrent chromosomal rearrangements have not been identified in ERMS, allelic loss has been detected commonly in ERMS tumors.[81] This process is defined by the absence of one of the two parental alleles at one or more contiguous chromosomal loci in the tumor cells. Allelic loss includes events such as chromosome loss and deletion, which can be detected with traditional and molecular cytogenetics, and also includes chromosome loss with duplication of the remaining chromosome or mitotic recombination, which do not produce an absolute loss of genetic material. Instead, these last two processes eliminate the contribution of one set of parental alleles and are detected by molecular strategies that use genetic polymorphisms to distinguish the two parental alleles.

Chromosome 11 is most commonly affected by allelic loss in ERMS.[82] The smallest chromosomal region of consistent allelic loss is 11p15.5.[83] Although 11p15.5 allelic loss is also detected in fusion-positive ARMS tumors, it is more common in ERMS tumors.[81,84] A recurrent region of allelic loss indicates the presence of a tumor suppressor gene that is inactivated in the associated malignancy. This premise is supported by the localization of the gene or genes responsible for BWS to this chromosomal region.[40] As discussed earlier, this syndrome predisposes to the development of several cancers, including RMS. Further support for a tumor suppressor gene relevant to ERMS tumorigenesis in chromosomal region 11p15 comes from studies in which the transfer of wild-type copies of chromosome 11 or fragments containing the 11p15 region into *RD* ERMS cells suppresses growth.[85,86] These findings suggest that a transferred wild-type gene restored a previously inactivated growth suppressive function.

Determination of the parent of origin of the two alleles revealed that ERMS tumors preferentially maintain the paternal allele and lose the maternal allele.[87] This preference suggests genomic imprinting, a normal epigenetic developmental process that selectively inactivates expression of alleles in a gamete-of-origin–dependent process. Studies of the human 11p15 chromosomal region and the corresponding mouse region revealed imprinting of several genes[40] (Fig. 19-6). For example, *IGF2*, which encodes an embryonic growth factor, is preferentially expressed from the paternally inherited allele, whereas *H19*, which produces a nontranslated RNA with tumor suppressor properties, is preferentially expressed from the maternally inherited allele. *CDKN1C* is also preferentially expressed from the maternally inherited allele and encodes a cyclin-dependent kinase inhibitor (p57/KIP2) that negatively regulates cell-cycle progression. These allelic loss studies suggest that ERMS tumorigenesis frequently involves inactivation of an imprinted tumor suppressor by allelic loss of the active maternal allele and retention of the inactive paternal allele.

Gene Amplification in Rhabdomyosarcoma

The CGH studies described earlier indicated that amplification events occur frequently in ARMS tumors, with the most common loci involved being 2p24 and 12q13-15 (see Table 19-2). Following the groundbreaking studies of *MYCN* amplification in neuroblastoma, there were multiple studies of amplification of the *MYCN* proto-oncogene situated in 2p24 in ARMS tumors. Initial studies evaluated small numbers of RMS cases using Southern blot or fluorescent in situ hybridization (FISH) assays, and evidence of amplification was found in 43% to 67% of ARMS cases, but in no ERMS cases.[88-90] In a more recent study, the *MYCN* copy number was quantified in a larger panel of RMS cases by quantitative polymerase chain reaction (qPCR).[91] Using a greater than fourfold increase as a cut-off for amplification, *MYCN* amplification was detected in 12 of 48 (25%) ARMS cases and 9 of 58 (16%) ERMS cases. The copy number was generally higher in the amplified ARMS cases than in the amplified ERMS cases. In addition, low copy number gains corresponding to a 1.5-fold to a fourfold increase were found in 54% of ARMS and 62% of ERMS cases. Finally, there was a correlation between expression and copy number for cases of ARMS but not for cases of ERMS, suggesting that

MYCN is a target of the copy number increase in ARMS but not in ERMS.

Amplification involving the 12q13-15 chromosomal region has been found in numerous cancers, including various soft tissue sarcomas, osteosarcoma, glial tumors, and several carcinomas.[92] The 12q13-15 region contains several genes encoding growth-related products, including the cell-cycle regulator CDK4 and the p53 regulator MDM2. In fact, detailed mapping of the 12q13-15 amplified regions in sarcomas demonstrated at least two distinct amplicons, one in the vicinity of *CDK4* and a second in the vicinity of *MDM2*.[93] In the largest published study to date of 12q13-15 amplification in RMS, qPCR analysis of *CDK4* copy number detected *CDK4* gene amplification in 1 of 9 cases of ARMS, 0 of 6 classic cases of ERMS, and 1 of 7 cases of anaplastic ERMS.[94] A qPCR assay of the *MDM2* copy number also detected amplification in a comparable distribution of cases, although the *MDM2*-amplified cases were different from the *CDK4*-amplified cases, indicating that the genes were located in distinct amplicons. Combining this study with two additional studies, the overall amplification frequency of *MDM2* in RMS is 12% (7/60).[95,96] Of note, immunostaining for CDK4 and MDM2 protein expression revealed that the two *CDK4*-amplified cases as well as additional nonamplified cases showed high CDK4 protein expression, whereas only one of the two *MDM2*-amplified cases and additional nonamplified cases showed high MDM2 expression. Therefore, although *MDM2* amplification may not result in high-level expression, there are additional mechanisms in these tumors that can lead to high levels of MDM2 or CDK4 protein.

The finding of frequent amplicons at 1p36 and 13q14 and infrequent amplicons at 2q35 corresponds to the chromosomal locations of the *PAX7*, *FKHR*, and *PAX3* genes. In particular, the *PAX7-FKHR* fusion gene is commonly amplified (70%), whereas the *PAX3-FKHR* fusion gene is much less commonly amplified (5%).[97] Despite this difference in the frequency of amplification, both fusion products are expressed in ARMS tumors at higher levels than the corresponding wild-type products.[98] This high level of expression is postulated to generate a level of fusion product above a critical threshold for oncogenic activity. Therefore, there is a common feature of fusion gene overexpression in the two ARMS fusion subtypes, but a striking difference in the mechanism of fusion gene overexpression. In *PAX7-FKHR*–expressing tumors, the fusion gene is overexpressed because of a copy number–dependent mechanism, in vivo amplification of the genomic region containing the fusion gene. In contrast, the *PAX3-FKHR* fusion gene is usually overexpressed because of a copy number–independent increase in transcriptional rate (see Fig. 19-5).

Another amplified region identified in the CGH studies is chromosomal region 13q31. A recent study of this amplicon in RMS further narrowed the minimal common region of amplification to a 2-megabase interval.[99] This interval contains two functional genes: *GPC5*, which encodes a cell surface proteoglycan, and *C13orf25*, which contains the mir-17-92 cluster of microRNAs. Assay of copy number of this region by qPCR for the *GPC5* gene demonstrated more than a 1.5–fold increase in copy number in 7 of 45 (16%) cases of ARMS and in 6 of 51 (12%) cases of ERMS. However, true amplification is present in only a subset of these cases, predominantly in ARMS, but the precise frequency is not reported. Comparison of copy number with gene expression as determined by quantitative reverse transcription (qRT)-PCR indicated a significant correlation for *GPC5* but not for *C13orf25*. However, if cases with true amplification are compared to cases without amplification, it appears that amplification is one possible mechanism for increasing the expression of either gene, although other copy number–independent mechanisms also exist.

Oncogene and Tumor Suppressor Gene Mutations in Rhabdomyosarcoma

The previously described analysis of RMS patients with cancer predisposition syndromes revealed genes that are mutated and corresponding pathways that are altered in the pathogenesis of rare RMS cases. In particular, RMS occurred in syndromes in which the *RB1* or *TP53* tumor suppressor genes were inactivated, and in syndromes in which the ras pathway was activated, either by activating a *RAS* family oncogene or inactivating the *NF1* tumor suppressor gene. The important next question is whether the corresponding pathways are also altered in sporadic tumors by mutating the same genes or different genes in these pathways (Fig. 19-7).

Although *RB1* gene alterations have not been found in sporadic RMS tumors,[100] changes have been found in genes encoding proteins that regulate RB1 function. As described earlier, *CDK4* amplification in a subset of ARMS and anaplastic ERMS cases results in overexpression of this protein that phosphorylates RB1 and thereby contributes to RB1 inactivation. In another subset of RMS cases, homozygous deletions occur in the locus including the *CDKN2A* and *CDKN2B* genes, and point mutations also occur in *CDKN2A*. These alterations occur in both ARMS and ERMS, with the frequency of homozygous deletion reported to be as high as 25% (3/12)[101] and the *CDKN2A* mutation frequency reported to be as high as 14% (6/44).[102] *CDKN2A* and *CDKN2B* encode inhibitors of both CDK4 and CDK6, and the loss of these inhibitors results in increased phosphorylation activity and resulting inactivation of the RB1 function.

In contrast to *RB1*, mutations have been identified in *TP53* in sporadic RMS tumors. Using PCR-based mutation screening assays, a total of 16 mutations has been detected in 91 RMS cases in multiple studies (18%).[95,96,103-107] Although most cases were not subclassifed for histopathologic subtype, mutations were found in both ARMS and ERMS. In addition to point mutations, Southern blot analysis demonstrated evidence of allelic loss of the 17p chromosomal region in 7 of 31 cases, and homozygous or hemizygous deletions involving *TP53* in 5 of 31 cases.[108] Finally, using an immunohistochemical assay to detect p53 overexpression as evidence of missense mutations that increase p53 protein half-life,

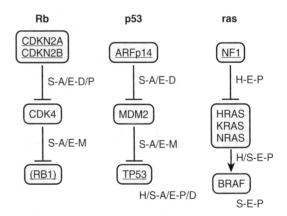

FIGURE 19-7. Gene pathways affected by mutations in rhabdomyosarcoma. The Rb, p53, and ras pathways are shown in three columns. Tumor suppressor products are underscored; oncogenes are not. A downstream activating step is shown by a vertical arrow, and a downstream inhibiting step is shown by a vertical inverted T. Adjacent to the name of each gene, a code is shown for the features of the mutation: A, occurs in ARMS; D, deletion; E, occurs in ERMS; H, inherited mutation; M, amplification, P, point mutation; S, sporadic mutation.

a recent study detected p53 overexpression in 22 of 72 cases (31%).[96] In addition to these direct changes in the *TP53* locus, changes in the p53 pathway may be caused by amplification of the *MDM2* gene (described earlier), which encodes a protein capable of binding and inactivating p53. Finally, deletion of the CDKN2A locus (described earlier) also eliminates expression of p14ARF, which is a protein that normally blocks MDM2 function and stabilizes the p53 protein.

Finally, the ras pathway can be activated in sporadic ERMS tumors by mutations in one of several genes. Analysis of the three members of the *RAS* gene family in 43 ERMS cases identified point mutations in 9 cases (21%; 3 × *HRAS*, 4 × *KRAS*, 2 × *NRAS*).[109-112] In contrast, *RAS* family gene mutations were not detected in 13 cases of ARMS. Furthermore, a *PTPN11* mutation was found in 1 of 20 ERMS and 0 of 11 ARMS cases,[112] and a *BRAF* mutation was detected in 2 of 6 unclassified RMS cases in one study and in 0 of 17 cases in a second study.[113,114] Finally, in a recent study of 50 RMS cases, a mutation in *BRAF* or a *RAS* family gene was found in 40% of ERMS cases and none of the ARMS cases.[115] Therefore, these findings indicate that one of several components involved in the ras pathway can be altered to activate this pathway specifically in sporadic ERMS, whereas there is no evidence of activation of this pathway in ARMS.

Hypermethylation as an Alternative Mechanism of Gene Inactivation in Rhabdomyosarcoma

In a final set of genomic changes in RMS, genetic loci are silenced by epigenetic events involving tumor-specific hypermethylation of CpG islands.[116] These CpG islands are DNA intervals of approximately 1 kb, which contain a high frequency of the dinucleotide CpG and are usually near the 5' end of genes. The cytosine residues in these dinucleotides are ordinarily unmethylated in normal cells but can become methylated during tumorigenesis, thereby altering the nearby chromatin structure and silencing the transcription of associated genes. This hypermethylation process thus provides an alternative nonmutagenic mechanism for inactivating tumor suppressor genes in cancer. Studies of small numbers of RMS cases have indicated that several genes often hypermethylated in other tumor types, such as *CDKN2A*, were not affected in a significant subset of RMS cases. However, a reasonable frequency of occurrence of hypermethylation was detected in *RASSF1A* (4 of 6 ARMS and 5 of 7 ERMS); *HIC1* (8 of 8 ARMS and 4 of 12 ERMS, $P < 0.005$); *CASP8* (4 of 6 ARMS and 9 of 10 ERMS); and *HIN1* (11 of 18 RMS, subtypes not distinguished).[117-120] Each methylatable gene encodes a known or putative tumor suppressor such as *CASP8*, which encodes caspase 8 and is involved in the apoptotic cascade. These hypermethylation events thereby result in loss of expression of the corresponding effector proteins and alteration of the associated pathways.

MOLECULAR AND CELLULAR BIOLOGY OF RHABDOMYOSARCOMA

Myogenic Pathways in the Tumorigenesis of Rhabdomyosarcoma

Based on the premise that RMS is related to the skeletal muscle lineage, the expression pattern of muscle-specific proteins has been extensively examined in RMS. In particular, many studies have focused on the family of myogenic transcription factors (MyoD, Myf5, myogenin, and MRF4) that are responsible in part for the determination of stem cells into myoblasts and then differentiation into myocytes. Assays of the corresponding genes detected RNA expression of *MYOD* and *MYF6* in all ARMS and ERMS tumors and RNA expression of *MYOG* (myogenin) and *MYF5* in all ARMS and most ERMS tumors.[121] Antibodies directed to MyoD and myogenin have proved to be suitable for immunohistochemistry on paraffin-embedded, formalin-fixed tissues.[122] Using these antibodies, the vast majority of RMS cases (about 97% in a recent study of 956 cases) showed positive nuclear immunostaining for each protein.[123] Because positive staining also occurred in multiple cases of pleuropulmonary blastoma, the specificity of these reagents was estimated to be approximately 90%. There are differences between ARMS and ERMS tumors in the myogenin staining patterns such that most cells within an ARMS tumor stain positive, whereas fewer cells within an ERMS tumor stain positive. This differential staining between ARMS and ERMS has also been shown for MyoD. There is a statistical difference in the extent of MyoD or myogenin expression between the RMS subtypes, but there is still overlap. Hence the immunohistochemical pattern of these myogenic proteins is not sufficient to classify cases but may be helpful in selecting cases for further testing.

Functional studies in RMS cell lines determined that MyoD is not an active transcription factor in the RMS environment[124] (Fig. 19-8). In particular, though MyoD is able to bind DNA at its specific binding sites in RMS cells, it is not capable of acting as a transcriptional activator on model genes with these DNA binding sites. These effects may contribute to the failure of RMS cells to undergo terminal differentiation. Various factors may contribute to this inhibition of transcriptional activation by MyoD. Experiments fusing RMS cell lines to a second normal cell line resulted in some instances in which the transcriptional activation block was overcome, suggesting that the RMS line was deficient in a transacting factor. In other instances, the block was not overcome by this cell fusion, suggesting a dominant acting inhibitory factor. As an example of the former recessive scenario, the p38 MAPK pathway is deficient in some RMS cell lines, resulting in the absence of an essential activator of MyoD during myogenic differentiation.[125] As an example of the latter dominant scenario, amplification of *MDM2* in an RMS cell line was found to be responsible for inhibition of MyoD activity by a mechanism involving competition for the transcription factor Sp1.[126,127] In addition, increased expression of the negative muscle growth regulator myostatin, which is found in cases of both ERMS and ARMS, is also capable of inhibiting MyoD-mediated transcriptional activity, possibly via Smad3 interactions.[128] Finally, in RMS associated with activation of the SHH pathway, expression of the transcription factor GLI1 or GLI2 inhibits MyoD-mediated transcriptional activation by reducing heterodimerization with its partner E12 and DNA binding.[129]

The identification of *PAX3-FKHR* and *PAX7-FKHR* gene fusions in ARMS also highlight PAX3 and PAX7 as important proteins in normal and aberrant myogenic transcriptional control. In murine systems, both Pax3 and Pax7 are involved in early embryonic development of cells giving rise to axial musculature, and Pax3 also has a necessary role in the early embryonic development of the limb musculature.[130-132] In the adult mouse, Pax7 has an important role in the development of the major population of myogenic satellite cells, and Pax3 is expressed in satellite cells in a subset of muscles.[133,134] This developmental biology of PAX3 and PAX7 is not relevant only to ARMS tumors, which express PAX3 or PAX7 as a fusion with FKHR,[135] but also to ERMS tumors, which express wild-type PAX3, PAX7, or both.[136]

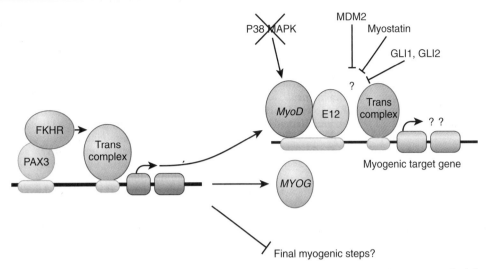

FIGURE 19-8. Influences on myogenic differentiation in ARMS. A model PAX3-FKHR target gene is shown on the left, with PAX3-FKHR binding to a positive-acting cis element and interacting with the transcriptional machinery at the promoter to upregulate the transcription of mRNA and ultimately increase production of the target protein. Two such targets are postulated to be MyoD and myogenin (*MYOG*). In turn, MyoD and its binding partner E12 bind to cis elements of myogenic target genes and stimulate the transcriptional machinery to upregulate transcription of the corresponding mRNAs. In ARMS (and ERMS), various upstream changes can influence the transcriptional activity of the MyoD protein and thereby inhibit myogenic differentiation.

The wild-type and fusion PAX proteins can variably affect the myogenic status of the cells expressing them. When wild-type Pax3 is introduced into explanted embryonic tissues, it can activate the myogenic program as shown by expression of MyoD, Myf5, and myogenin as well as myogenic differentiation products.[137] In contrast, *PAX3* could not induce this myogenic program in *NIH3T3* murine fibroblasts, suggesting that this murine fibroblast represents a less permissive environment.[138]

Studies of the PAX3-FKHR fusion protein have demonstrated a range of activities on the myogenic program (see Figs. 19-5 and 19-8). First, studies focusing on the *MYOD* and *MYOG* promoters provide evidence that both of these genes are transcriptional targets of PAX3-FKHR. Of two studies of NIH3T3 cells, one indicated that PAX3-FKHR induced the myogenic program, including the upstream products MyoD, myogenin, Six1, and Slug as well as downstream myogenic products, such as troponins and myosin light chain.[138] However, a second study of *NIH3T3* cells demonstrated induction of the upstream products MyoD, myogenin and desmin but no induction of the downstream product myosin heavy chain.[139] In contrast to these findings, transduction of *PAX3-FKHR* into two additional murine fibroblast lines (*10T1/2* and *Plus*) resulted in expression of both upstream and downstream myogenic products and fusion into multinucleated myotubes. In contrast, introduction of *PAX3* or *PAX3-FKHR* into two myogenic cell lines, *C2C12* myoblasts and MyoD-expressing *10T1/2* cells, inhibited terminal myogenic differentiation following stimulation of differentiation by growth factor withdrawal.[140] *PAX3-FKHR* was more potent than wild-type *PAX3* in this phenotypic activity. Finally, repression of *PAX3-FKHR* expression in an ARMS cell line with small interfering RNA (siRNA) resulted in expression of a series of genes related to normal myogenic differentiation, such as myosin light and heavy chain and troponins.[141] This finding indicates that PAX3-FKHR normally represses expression of this myogenic pathway in this cell type. The finding of both stimulatory and inhibitory effects of PAX proteins on myogenic events may be explained by the hypothesis that these wild-type or fusion PAX proteins facilitate entry into the myogenic pathway and variably inhibit the final steps of the pathway depending on the cellular environment.

Furthermore, the siRNA study in the ARMS cells suggests that PAX3-FKHR is inhibiting terminal differentiation in the ARMS environment.

Role of Insulin-like Growth Factors in Rhabdomyosarcoma

Insulin-like growth factor-II (IGF-II) is an important growth factor during the fetal period and is highly expressed in fetal skeletal muscle but not detectably expressed in adult skeletal muscle.[142] High-level IGF-II expression in murine myoblasts results in an increased proliferative rate, impaired myogenic differentiation, and anchorage independence, indicating a potential role of IGF-II in neoplasia of the myogenic lineage.[143] In accord with these findings, IGF-II is highly expressed by both ERMS and ARMS tumors as well as in derived RMS cell lines[144] (Fig. 19-9). In addition to the growth factor, both RMS subtypes express the IGF-I receptor, which is a cell surface receptor for IGF-II as well as IGF-I. This simultaneous expression of growth factor and receptor creates an autocrine loop that stimulates the growth and motility of RMS cells. No mutations have been detected in these genes, hence this autocrine situation may reflect the fetal muscle expression pattern that is maintained or induced by the other genetic alterations. The growth response is mediated through the IGF-I receptor, whereas the motility response is mediated through the distinct IGF-II/mannose-6-phosphate receptor.[145] Numerous studies have explored different strategies for interfering with the action of the IGF-I receptor. These strategies include an antibody directed to this receptor, a kinase-deficient mutant that acts as a dominant negative, and an antisense construct directed to this receptor.[146-148] Each of these strategies decreases the response of the cells to IGF-II stimulation, inhibits cell growth and anchorage independence in culture, and inhibits tumorigenicity in vivo.

As described earlier, the *IGF2* gene is located in the 11p15.5 chromosomal region, which is implicated in allelic loss events that occur in RMS tumors and in genetic alterations in the inherited disorder BWS, which predisposes to malignant

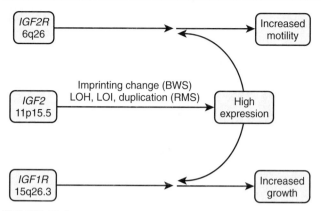

FIGURE 19-9. Changes in IGF pathway and associated phenotypic consequences in RMS. The three involved genes and their chromosomal locations are shown on the left. Genetic or epigenetic changes are indicated above the horizontal arrow. Changes in expression or phenotype are indicated on the right.

tumors, including RMS.[40,81,84] The *IGF2* gene is part of an imprinted region and is preferentially expressed from the paternally inherited alleles. The result of the allelic loss events and genetic changes in BWS is loss of the nonexpressed maternal allele and maintenance or gain of the expressed paternal allele. In addition to these genetic changes, other alterations of 11p15 involving the *IGF2* locus have been identified in both ARMS and ERMS tumors. In one study of 11 RMS tumors (including 4 ARMS and 6 ERMS), 1 ARMS and 3 ERMS cases demonstrated evidence of duplication of an *IGF2* allele.[149] Furthermore, although *IGF2* is normally expressed from only one allele, loss of imprinting can occur and result in a biallelic expression pattern. In RMS, loss of imprinting at the *IGF2* locus has been observed in 5 of 12 ERMS and 9 of 16 ARMS cases.[149-151] These duplication or imprinting changes increase the number of active *IGF2* alleles and may thereby contribute to the high expression of IGF2 mRNA and protein found in RMS tumors.

In mammalian cells, the subcellular localization of the wild-type FKHR (FOXO1) and related FOXO3 and FOXO4 proteins is regulated by a PI3K-AKT (PKB–dependent signaling pathway that is activated by survival- and growth-related signals such as IGF-II.[152] In this signaling pathway, AKT-mediated phosphorylation of FOXO proteins leads to protein transfer from the nucleus to the cytoplasm, and thus inactivates transcriptional function. Of the three AKT phosphorylation sites in FKHR, two are retained in PAX3-FKHR and PAX7-FKHR. If the fusion proteins are regulated by this pathway, the high level of IGF-II in ARMS cells would cause these proteins to be phosphorylated and sequestered in the cytoplasm. However, experiments show that PAX3-FKHR is retained in the nucleus and is transcriptionally active in cultured cells in the presence of active AKT and in ARMS cells.[153] Therefore, the fusion protein is resistant to upstream regulatory signals and shows exclusively nuclear localization (see Fig. 19-5).

Modulation of Growth and Apoptotic Pathways by Fusion Oncoproteins

Gene transfer experiments have investigated specific functions of the PAX3-FKHR and PAX7-FKHR fusion proteins and suggest that these proteins exert an oncogenic effect through multiple pathways (see Fig. 19-5). In initial studies of growth

control, transduction of *PAX3-FKHR* into murine *NIH3T3* or chicken embryo fibroblasts resulted in transforming activity, whereas wild-type *PAX3* did not transform these cells.[154,155] In a complementary study, a protein consisting of the N-terminal region of PAX3 fused to the KRAB transcriptional repression domain reverted the transforming activity of ARMS cells in culture and suppressed tumor formation of ARMS cells in mice.[156] In mutagenesis analyses, the homeodomain but not the paired box is needed by PAX3-FKHR for transformation, and thus target genes with paired box binding sites may not be required for cellular transformation. In addition, transforming activity is activated when the VP16 activation domain is substituted for the C-terminal domain of PAX3, suggesting that other activation domains can mimic the effect of the C-terminal FKHR domain.[157]

More recent studies indicate that there is an antagonistic balance between transforming activity and growth-suppressive or toxic activity in many cell types in which PAX3-FKHR is exogenously expressed.[158,159] Transforming activity is optimally exerted at low expression levels of exogenous fusion protein. In contrast, at higher expression levels, comparable to the levels in human ARMS tumors, PAX3-FKHR causes cell death or growth suppression in various nontransformed cell lines. Therefore, human ARMS cells can tolerate these high "physiologic" expression levels, whereas the non-ARMS cells do not tolerate these higher levels. The hypothesis proposed is that additional genetic alterations are necessary in ARMS to attenuate the toxic and growth-suppressive effects of the fusion protein. One such event may be inactivation of the *CDKN2A* tumor suppressor gene that collaborates with *PAX3-FKHR* to permit primary human skeletal muscle cell precursors to bypass the senescent growth arrest checkpoint.[160] It is noteworthy that mutation studies show that the growth suppressive and toxic activity is at least partly dependent on an intact paired box but does not require an intact homeodomain.[158] These findings suggest that there may be two separate sets of target genes mediating the transforming and toxic phenotypes as a result of the complex function of the PAX3-FKHR DNA binding domain.

Despite the ability of PAX3-FKHR to induce toxic effects when introduced into many cultured cells, an important function of the PAX3-FKHR oncoprotein in ARMS cells is maintenance of cell viability by inhibiting apoptosis (see Fig. 19-5). Treatment of ARMS cells with either an antisense oligonucleotide directed against the *PAX3* translational start site or with siRNAs directed against the 5′ *PAX3* region resulted in a decrease in PAX3-FKHR protein expression.[141,161] This expression change was associated with a significant decrease in cell number as well as with morphologic and biochemical characteristics of apoptosis. Similarly, expression of a tamoxifen-inducible *PAX3-KRAB* construct in ARMS cells demonstrated evidence of apoptosis when induced in low serum conditions or tumor xenografts.[162] One downstream transcriptional target of PAX3-FKHR that at least partially mediates this apoptotic function is the gene that encodes the transcription factor TFAP2B.[141] The functional role of TFAP2B is indicated by the induction of apoptosis in ARMS cells when this gene is downregulated by targeted siRNA and by the prevention of apoptosis mediated by siRNA directed against the 5′ *PAX3* region when a construct constitutively expressing TFAP2B is introduced into ARMS cells.

Metastatic Pathways in Rhabdomyosarcoma

Early studies of RMS metastasis examined subclones of the *RD* ERMS cell line. The metastatic capacity of different

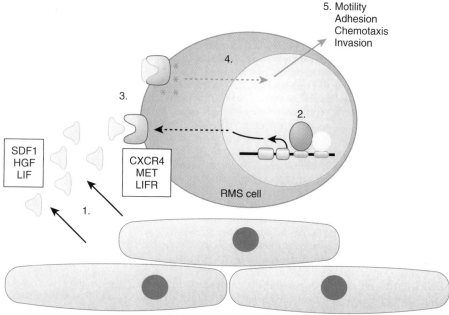

FIGURE 19-10. Role of secreted protein mediators in metastatic behavior of RMS cells. Bone marrow stromal cells secrete various protein mediators, including SDF1, HGF, and LIF (step 1). The RMS cells transcribe genes and then express cell surface receptors for these protein mediators (step 2). Binding of protein mediators to cognate receptors (step 3) activates various signaling pathways in the RMS cells (step 4). These signaling pathways ultimately modulate expression pathways in the nucleus that result in phenotypic changes (step 5).

subclones did not correlate with the tumorigenic or proliferative capability of the subclones.[163] After exposure to conditions that stimulate myogenic differentiation, some subclones showed increased differentiation manifested by an increased fraction of myosin-positive cells.[164] Although proliferative capability did not correlate with this in vitro differentiation, the metastatic efficiency was reduced in subclones demonstrating differentiation.

Additional studies with the *RD* line showed that its metastatic efficiency is affected by alterations of cell surface molecules. In the case of the cell surface glycoprotein NCAM, this protein is post-translationally modified by the addition of polysialic acid on its extracellular domain.[165] When the enzyme endoneuraminidase-N was injected intraperitoneally to cleave the polysialic acid from the surface of intraperitoneally implanted *RD* cells, there was a decrease in the frequency of lung and liver metastases. When the integrin VLA-2 (alpha2beta1), which is not normally expressed by *RD* cells, was introduced into these cells, there was increased adhesion to collagen and laminin in vitro, and more metastatic foci in mice following either intravenous or subcutaneous injection.[166]

Among the various RMS subtypes, there are differences in matrix metalloproteinase (MMP) expression that may contribute to differences in metastatic behavior. Immunohistochemical analysis of 5 MMPs in 33 RMS cases found higher expression of MMP1, MMP2, and MMP9 in ARMS than in ERMS cases.[167] After confirming the higher MMP2 expression in ARMS in a comparison of ARMS and ERMS cell lines, the high MMP2 expression was correlated with more invasive behavior in the ARMS cell lines.[168] In a human RMS cell line with spontaneous metastatic progression, there was upregulation of MMPs and downregulation of tissue inhibitors of metalloproteinases.[169] Finally, attachment of RMS cells to fibronectin results in increased MMP2 expression and in vitro invasive behavior along with increases in COX-2 expression and PGE2 production.[170] Treatment with exogenous *PGE2* can recapitulate this effect and increase MMP2 expression at the level of the *MMP2* promoter. In contrast, treatment of cells with COX-2 inhibitors can reverse the fibronectin effects on MMP expression and invasive behavior.

Three cell surface receptors, MET, CXCR4, and LIFR, are expressed in RMS and function in signaling pathways that impact metastatic behavior[171-173] (Fig. 19-10). Although *MET* and *CXCR4* genes are downstream targets of the PAX3-FKHR fusion protein (see Fig. 19-5), all three genes are expressed in both ARMS and ERMS tumors. CXCR4 is a G-protein–coupled chemokine receptor whose ligand is stromal derived factor-1 (SDF1), whereas MET is a member of the tyrosine kinase family of receptors whose ligand is hepatocyte growth factor/scatter factor (HGF/SF). Finally, leukemia inhibitory factor (LIF) binds to a heterodimeric membrane receptor composed of the LIF-specific LIFR and the gp130 receptor chain, which is also used as the receptor for interleukin-6, oncostatin M, and several other cytokines. All three ligands are secreted by the bone marrow, an important site of ARMS metastasis. The CXCR4-SDF1 signaling pathway is involved in the homing of normal cells to hematopoietic sites, and the MET-HGF/SF signaling pathway is involved in the proliferation and motility of various cell types. The LIF-LIFR signaling pathway has a variety of roles in multiple tissues, including proliferation of hematopoietic cells and muscle satellite cell production. For these reasons, usurpation of these signaling pathways has been proposed in the metastasis of various cancers.

Cell culture studies have explored the influence of CXCR4-SDF1, MET-HGF/SF, and LIFR-LIF signaling on the metastatic behavior of ARMS cells. SDF1, HGF, or LIF treatment of RMS cell lines induced cell culture changes in relevant properties, including motility, adhesion, chemotaxis, and invasion. In an in vivo experiment, more ARMS cells than ERMS cells are chemoattracted to and seed lethally irradiated bone marrow in association with the upregulation of HGF and SDF1 in irradiated bone marrow stroma. In addition, a selected ARMS subclone that preferentially responds to LIF demonstrates increased seeding of bone marrow, liver, and lymph nodes after intravenous injection, and increased cells in bone marrow and lung 6 weeks after intramuscular injection. Finally, as models of pathway-specific potential therapeutic strategies, a CXCR4-specific inhibitor blocked SDF1-directed adhesion and chemotaxis in ARMS cells, and an siRNA directed against LIFR inhibited in vivo metastasis of ARMS cells.

Studies of a metastatic RMS model system elucidated an important pathway involving the *Vil2* and *Six1* genes. In this model system, RMS tumors developed in transgenic mice that were deficient in *CDKN2A (Ink4/Arf)* and overexpressed *HGF/SF*.[174] In a comparison of gene expression profiles of highly and poorly metastatic cell lines derived from this system, 44 differentially expressed genes were identified (28 overexpressed and 16 underexpressed in highly metastatic cells), including the overexpressed genes, *Vil2* and *Six1*.[175] *Vil2* encodes ezrin, which is an adhesion molecule and member of the ERM family. Ezrin promotes cytoskeletal reorganization in pathways linked to survival, motility, invasion, and adherence. Six1 encodes a homeodomain-containing transcription factor involved in the development of several lineages, is a downstream target of PAX3-FKHR in NIH3T3 cells, and is expressed by ARMS cells.[138] Furthermore, the gene encoding ezrin is a direct transcriptional target of Six1.[176] These gene expression relationships were confirmed by RMS tumor studies in which both genes were generally expressed at higher levels in fusion-positive RMS tumors than in fusion-negative RMS tumors.

Expression of *Vil2* and *Six1* in RMS tumors was found to be correlated with clinical stage, which is consistent with a role in tumor progression and metastatic behavior.[175] There is direct proof of this role: transfer of either gene into to low metastatic RMS lines from the *HGF* transgenic system caused increased metastatic activity. Similarly, when expression of either gene was inhibited by shRNA, or the function of either gene product was repressed by a dominant-negative inhibitor, metastatic activity in the highly metastatic lines decreased. Finally, subsequent studies indicated that ezrin is needed for Six1 to exert its metastatic function, thus further confirming that ezrin acts downstream of Six1.[176] These studies provide the framework of a pathway that leads from the fusion proteins to Six1 to ezrin to metastatic activity.

ANIMAL MODELS OF RHABDOMYOSARCOMA

Inactivation of the *Trp53* Tumor Suppressor Gene

Mouse models of LFS, with homozygous and heterozygous inactivation of the *Trp53* tumor suppressor gene, have been noted to develop a variety of tumors, including RMS[177-179] (Table 19-3). An initial model was generated by developing a transgenic mouse with a mutant *Trp53* genomic fragment,[177] and then two knockout models were generated by gene targeting to replace exon 5[178] or exons 2 through 6 with a neomycin cassette.[179] In the knockout models, *Trp53*-null mice were viable, with no obvious fetal defects. *Trp53* heterozygotes developed fewer tumors than *Trp53*-null mice but they better mimic the p53 function and cancer susceptibility of the corresponding human genetic condition. No RMS tumors were detected in the exon 5 knockout model, but a low frequency of occurrence of RMS was detected in the other two models, both as an overall frequency (<5%) and as a fraction of the total number of tumors formed (2% to 7%).

Other studies crossed additional genetic features into these *Trp53* knockout mice to develop strains in which RMS occurs with higher incidence and with different phenotypic features. When crossed with a mutant *neu* oncogene expressed from the *MMTV-LTR*, 100% of male mice that were heterozygous for *Trp53* developed RMS in the genitourinary tract.[180] In particular, these tumors were pelvic masses located behind the urinary bladder, potentially arising from the sphincter of small striated muscle fibers in the periurethral region. When the *Trp53* knock-

out was crossed with a *Fos* knockout, more than 90% of the double-knockout homozygotes developed a highly proliferative and invasive form of RMS.[181] In contrast to the *neu* transgenic, the tumors developed in the facial and orbital regions of this mouse strain. Finally, a conditional mutant *Kras* allele was generated by targeting a mutant cDNA preceded by a stop codon flanked by *Lox* recombination sites into the first intron of the *Ryr2* gene.[182] This mutant gene was selectively expressed in postnatal skeletal muscle (right lower leg) by electroporation of a *Cre* expression construct. In *Trp53* homozygotes, activation of the mutant *Kras* gene resulted in a 100% incidence of RMS, with a microscopic appearance notable for pleomorphism and atypia.

Activation of the Shh Signaling Pathway

Two mouse models for *NBCCS* with engineered deletions in the *Ptch* locus have been described.[183,184] In contrast to *Trp53*-null mice, homozygous *Ptch* mutants are embryonic lethal as a result of profound neurodevelopmental defects. *Ptch* heterozygous mice are viable, with only subtle developmental abnormalities, similar to human *NBCCS* patients. In the two models, there was significant variation in incidence of medulloblastoma and RMS, depending on the genetic background. The incidence of medulloblastoma was increased when the *Ptch* mutation was crossed on a *Trp53* mutant background, but there was no change in the incidence or time of onset of soft tissue sarcomas in *Ptch+/−Trp53+/−* or *Ptch+/−Trp53−/−* mice.[185] The RMS tumors in *Ptch* mutant mice were commonly associated with skeletal muscle in the rear thigh, lumbar region, or abdominal wall.[184] These tumors demonstrate less aggressive growth and more differentiation than RMS tumors from p53+/− mice.[186] Finally, based on studies indicating that Shh promotes proliferation and inhibits myogenic differentiation of adult muscle satellite cells, these *Ptch*-associated RMS tumors are postulated to arise from satellite cells.[187]

The *Ptch*-associated tumors were found to have increased *Ptch* and *Gli1* expression, indicating activation of the Shh signaling pathway. The *Ptch* expression is derived from the mutant *Ptch* allele, whereas the wild-type allele is retained but reduced in expression.[188] Downstream expression consequences of the highly active Shh pathway in these tumors include increased expression of the growth factor Igf2, the transcription factor Foxf1, and the DNA damage-inducible gene Gadd45a.[186] There was no tumor formation when the *Ptch* mutation was crossed on a mutant *Igf2* background, indicating that *Igf2* expression is needed for RMS formation secondary to loss of *Ptch* function.[189]

Activation of Shh signaling by several additional strategies also leads to RMS. In a strategy comparable to the *Ptch* knockout, mice were derived with an inactivating mutation of the *Sufu* gene, which encodes a protein involved in the negative regulation of the Gli1 transcription factor. However, homozygotes were not viable and heterozygotes were indistinguishable from the wild type, with no evidence of tumor susceptibility. Further crosses with a *Trp53* mutant strain resulted in pronounced tumor susceptibility in the *Sufu+/−Trp53−/−* mice; this susceptibility was characterized by medulloblastomas and RMS similar to those in the *Ptch* knockout mice.[190] As an alternative strategy to activate the Shh pathway, a mutant *Smo* cDNA was targeted into the ubiquitously expressed *Rosa26* locus distal to a polyadenylation stop sequence cassette flanked by *Lox* recombination sites.[191] Mice with this allele were crossed with transgenic mice expressing Cre-ER, an inducible form of the *Cre* recombinase generated as a fusion with the estrogen receptor ligand binding domain and expressed from the ubiquitously active *CAGGS* promoter. Without any addition of an inducing

TABLE 19-3   Mouse Models of Rhabdomyosarcoma

Mouse Model	Genetic Alteration	Genetic Background	Overall Tumor Incidence	Predominant Tumors	RMS Incidence	RMS Sites
LFS model Mutant 53 transgenic	Mutant p53 genomic fragment	*C57BL/6*	22/112 (20%)	Lung adenocarcinoma Osteosarcoma Lymphoma	2/112 (2%)	N/A[1]
LFS model *Trp53+/−*	Replace *Trp53* exon 2 to intron 6 with neo[2]	*C57BL/6*	44/232 (19%)	Sarcoma	1/232 (0.4%)	N/A
Trp53−/−			56/70 (80%)	Lymphoma	3/70 (4%)	N/A
Mutant *neu* transgenic, *Trp53+/−*	Above *Trp53+/−* + MMTV–*neu*	*BALB/c*	10/10 (100%, male)	RMS	10/10 (100%, male)	Genitourinary
Fos−/−Trp53−/−	Above *Trp53+/−* + replace *Fos* exon 2 with neo	*129Sv×C57BL/6*	27/29 (93%)	RMS	27/29 (93%)	Facial and orbital regions
Conditional mutant *Kras* transgenic, *Trp53−/−* or *Trp53+/−*	Knock-in of floxed mutant *Kras* into *Ryr2* locus + *Trp53−/−* or +/− + *Cre* injection into right lower limb	*C57BL/6*	*Trp53−/−* 11/11 (100%) *Trp53+/−* 8/20 (40%)	RMS (pleomorphic)	11/11 (100%)	Right lower limb
NBCCS model *Ptch+/−*	Replace *Ptch* exons 1-2 with *lacZ*/neo	*129SV*	8/27 (30%)	Medulloblastoma	2/27 (7%)	"Soft tissue tumors"
	Replace *Ptch* exons 6-7 with neo	*CD1*	N/A	RMS	10/117 (9%)	Skeletal muscle in rear thigh, lumbar region, or abdominal wall
Sufu+/−Trp53−/−	Replace *Sufu* last exon with β-Geo[3] +*Trp53−/−*	*129Ola×C57BL/6*	15/46 (33%) 45/55 (82%)	Medulloblastoma	7/46 (15%) 5/55 (9%)	N/A
Conditional mutant *Smo* transgenic	Knock-in of floxed mutant *Smo* into R26 locus + CAGGS-CreER	Mixed (mostly *129/Sv* and Swiss Webster)	100%	RMS, basal cell carcinoma, medulloblastoma	100%	Thigh, abdominal wall, head and neck, paratesticular
HGF/SF Transgenic *Cdkn2a+/+*	MT1-HGF/SF	*FVB/N*	>24/69 (>35%)	Mammary cancer, melanoma	3/69 (4%)	Skin, peritoneum
Cdkn2a−/−	+ Replace *Cdkn2a* exons 2-3 with neo	Half *FVB/NCr* Half *C57BL/6*	35/36 (97%)	RMS	35/36 (97%)	Trunk Limb skeletal muscle
PAX3-FKHR conditional knock-in	Insert 3'*FKHR* (with *Lox* sites) after *PAX3* exon 7 + *Myf6-Cre*	*C57BL/6*	N/A	ARMS	1/228 (0.4%)	Extremities, trunk, head and neck
+ conditional *Trp53−/−*	+ Flank *Trp53* exons 2-10 with *Lox* sites				2/5 (40%)	
+ conditional *Cdkn2a−/−*	+ Flank *Cdkn2a* exons 2-3 with *Lox* sites				4/14 (29%)	
mdx mice	Spontaneous nonsense mutation in exon 23 of dystrophin (*Dmd*) gene	*C57BL/10*	6/94 (6%)	RMS	6/94 (6%)	Extremities

[1]N/A, not available.
[2]neo, neomycin.
[3]Geo, geomycin.

agent, there is sporadic low-level function of Cre that removes the polyadenylation stop sequence and activates expression of the mutant *Smo* gene in cells. This level of Cre activity was sufficient to cause RMS tumors in 100% of the mice (with an average of three tumors per mouse) and medulloblastomas in 27% of mice. Following a single intraperitoneal administration of the inducing agent tamoxifen at postnatal day 10, RMS tumors occurred in 100% of mice, with an average of seven tumors per mouse; basal cell carcinoma–like lesions also occurred in all animals, and medulloblastomas occurred in 40% of animals. The RMS tumors were similar to those occurring in *Ptch+/–* mice and consisted of a heterogeneous mixture of round undifferentiated cells and elongated spindle-shaped cells with evidence of myogenic differentiation in some tumor cells.

Abnormal Expression of HGF/SF

To investigate the consequences of abnormally expressing the HGF/SF growth factor in a broad range of tissues, an expression cassette consisting of the *HGF/SF* cDNA expressed from the mouse metallothionein 1 *(MT1)* promoter was used to develop a transgenic mouse.[192] In this mouse model, the ectopic production of HGF/SF resulted in the formation of ectopic skeletal muscle and the localization of melanocytes at aberrant sites. Along with these developmental abnormalities, the abnormal expression of HGF/SF in this mouse induced several cancers, including mammary gland tumors, melanomas, and RMS. Of note, RMS developed only in male transgenics (3 of 42, 7%). In most tumors, c-met mRNA was highly expressed, and was activated as indicated by phosphorylation status. The frequency of occurrence of RMS increased dramatically when this transgenic strain was crossed with a mouse strain in which the *Cdkn2a* locus (encoding the Ink4a and Arf tumor suppressor proteins) was inactivated by gene targeting.[174] In contrast to the *HGF/SF* transgenic with wild-type *Cdkn2a*, which developed a low frequency of occurrence of RMS, with an age of onset of approximately 8 months, the *HGF/SF* transgenic with homozygous inactivation of *Cdkn2a* developed multiple foci of RMS, with a mean age of onset of approximately 3.3 months, thus providing further evidence of synergism between the two genetic events in RMS development. The tumors in these mice often arose from the trunk and limb skeletal muscle but also arose from ectopic sites, such as the cerebellum, pituitary, stomach, pancreas, and esophagus. Based on the phenotype of the *HGF/SF* transgenic mouse, these tumors are hypothesized to arise from ectopic skeletal muscle forming at these sites.

Expression of the *PAX3-FKHR* Gene Product

Multiple approaches, ranging from standard transgenic to conditional knock-in, have been used to express *PAX3-FKHR* in a developing mouse.[193-196] These studies have resulted in a range of phenotypic changes involving neural- and neural-crest–derived or early myogenic lineages, and they appear to result from the loss or gain of *Pax3*-related functions. One major similarity among most of these systems is that the fusion protein exerted toxic effects, although the mechanism for this toxicity may differ among experiments and among cell types. Based on this toxicity, expression throughout a lineage may cause lineage-wide dysfunction and often severe consequences. The fact that tumors were not caused by the fusion protein in most systems undoubtedly resulted from early lethality and insufficient time for tumor development, if the fusion protein

was even expressed and functional in the appropriate susceptible lineage.

A mouse model of ARMS was developed using a conditional knock-in approach targeting expression mainly in differentiated skeletal muscle.[197] This approach used a knock-in allele consisting of a fragment of 3' *Fkhr* (flanked by *Lox* sites) inserted after *Pax3* exon 7. The Cre recombinase was introduced by crossing with a mouse expressing Cre from *Myf6* elements. *Pax3* is transcribed until Cre is activated by this promoter, resulting in generation of *Pax3-Fkhr*. Because *Myf6* is expressed predominantly in terminally differentiated skeletal muscle, *Pax3-Fkhr* is thus generated and expressed in this nondividing myogenic tissue (and possibly in other less abundant dividing *Myf6*-expressing populations). The viability and fertility of these mice indicate that *Pax3-Fkhr* is not toxic in this setting. The tumorigenicity of *Pax3-Fkhr* in these mice is low, and the latency is long (1 tumor/228 mice at 1 year of age). The tumor appeared to arise from muscle and had a microscopic appearance consistent with a solid variant of ARMS. Furthermore, immunohistochemistry revealed staining for myogenic markers, including myogenin, confirming the diagnosis of RMS. To evaluate other collaborating events, these mice were crossed with mice with conditional knockouts for *Cdkn2a* or *Trp53*. Based on the finding of highly increased tumor frequency in *Pax3-Fkhr* mice that were homozygous for either *Cdkn2a* or *Trp53*, there appears to be an important role for at least p53 pathway disruption in collaborating with *Pax3-Fkhr* in multistep ARMS tumorigenesis. Finally, homozygosity of *Pax3-Fkhr* was also necessary to achieve these enhanced effects, suggesting either the need for increased *Pax3-Fkhr* dosage or an inhibitory role for wild-type *Pax3* in this system.

Muscular Dystrophy in Mice

Recent studies have revealed that *mdx* mice, which have a spontaneous mutation of the dystrophin gene and provide a model for the human disease Duchenne's muscular dystrophy, have a propensity to develop RMS tumors as they age.[198] In particular, these tumors developed in the extremities of approximately 6% of *mdx* mice but did not occur in any wild-type mice. Unlike other tumors, this susceptibility is a feature of old mice, with an age of onset between 16.5 and 24 months. The lack of a corresponding notable increase in RMS development in human Duchenne's muscular dystrophy patients may be attributable to the significant decline in myofibers and satellite cells in the muscles of these human patients in contrast to those of the *mdx* mice, which maintain a more active regenerative capability.

Models in Other Species

In this exploration of animal models, brief consideration should be given to recent attempts to investigate the utility of using lower organisms to model aspects of RMS. For example, recent studies in *Drosophila* have revealed that, when the PAX7-FKHR fusion protein or wild-type PAX3 protein is expressed in differentiated muscle, mononucleated cells form and spread to distal sites such as the central nervous system.[199] Furthermore, this activity can be stimulated by the presence of an activated ras pathway. In zebrafish, embryos were injected with a construct consisting of a mutant *KRAS (KRASG12D)* expressed from a *rag2* promoter, which is expressed in the mononuclear skeletal muscle cells in addition to other cell types.[200] By 80 days post fertilization, 47% of mosaic transgenic fish developed invasive tumors, composed of a heterogeneous collection of differentiated (multinucleated) and undifferentiated (mononuclear) myogenic cells. These tumors express downstream myogenic markers (myod, myogenin, desmin) and satellite cell markers, confirming their diagnosis as RMS. To test for collaborating pathways, the transgene was injected into zebrafish embryos with a p53 loss of function mutation (Tu strain), resulting in significantly increased tumor incidence.

APPLICATIONS OF MOLECULAR GENETIC APPROACHES TO DIAGNOSIS AND PROGNOSIS

Detection of Recurrent Gene Fusions

As the genetics and biology of the recurrent *PAX3-FKHR* and *PAX7-FKHR* gene fusions in ARMS were elucidated, assays were developed to detect these fusions: Southern blot,[201,202] RT-PCR,[203,204] and fluorescent *in situ* hybridization (FISH)[205,206] methodologies have been used. To determine the frequency of occurrence of the PAX3-FKHR and PAX7-FKHR fusion transcripts in ARMS, multiple studies have applied RT-PCR assays to a large number of histopathologically diagnosed cases.[207-211] In particular, a large single study of RMS cases from the Intergroup Rhabdomyosarcoma Study (IRS)-IV protocol revealed that all 93 cases of RMS (or undifferentiated sarcoma) with a diagnosis other than ARMS were fusion-negative, whereas 77% of the 78 ARMS cases were fusion-positive.[212] Of these ARMS cases, 55% expressed *PAX3-FKHR*, 22% expressed *PAX7-FKHR*, and 23% were fusion-negative (see Fig. 19-1). It should be noted that the ratio of *PAX3-FKHR* to *PAX7-FKHR*–positive cases is an underestimate because the IRS-IV trial did not enroll patients older than 21 years of age and, as discussed later, fusion-positive ARMS tumors in young adults generally express the *PAX3-FKHR* fusion. Based on multiple smaller studies, this *PAX3-FKHR* to *PAX7-FKHR* ratio appears to be closer to 6 to 1.[207-211]

These molecular diagnostic studies clearly show that there is a significant subset of ARMS cases that do not express either gene fusion. Based on the findings of the IRS-IV study, with its pathology review and tissue banking processes,[212] these negative results cannot be explained by inaccurate or variable application of histopathologic diagnostic criteria or the suboptimal quality of the tissue samples. Further study of the *PAX3*, *PAX7*, and *FKHR* loci with additional RT-PCR and FISH approaches identified several subsets within this "fusion-negative" category. In several cases, variant fusions of *PAX3* or *PAX7* with other genes were detected, including fusion of *PAX3* with the *FKHR*-related locus *AFX1* (*FOXO4*)[213] and fusion of *PAX3* with *NCOA1*, a locus encoding a transcription factor unrelated to the forkhead family.[214] In another small subset of cases, the fusion is detectable at the DNA but not at the RNA level, suggesting that expression of the fusion gene may be extinguished.[213] Finally, the majority of cases are negative in all assays and thus appear to represent true fusion-negative cases with respect to these loci. Clinical correlative studies are needed to determine whether these fusion-negative ARMS subsets correspond to clinically distinct categories and whether these categories differ clinically from fusion-positive ARMS. It is worthy of note that two relatively rare and distinct presentations of RMS have been associated with fusion-negative ARMS tumors, BWS, and congenital ARMS.[46,215]

Aside from the well-established clinical differences between ARMS and ERMS, there is also evidence of clinical and pathologic differences among the ARMS fusion subtypes. Although no clinical differences were detected between fusion-negative ARMS cases and the two fusion-positive ARMS subsets in the IRS-IV study,[212] there was a histopathologic difference. Of the various histologic features compared, 7 of 16 fusion-negative cases lacked cystic foci and thus showed totally "solid alveolar" architecture, whereas these features were present in only 2 of 13 *PAX7-FKHR* cases and none of 36 *PAX3-FKHR* cases (*P* = 0.000136).[216] In contrast, there were no histopathologic differences between the two fusion-positive subsets, but there was a striking clinical difference: the fusion-positive ARMS tumors in younger patients tend to express *PAX7-FKHR*, whereas those in older patients tend to express *PAX3-FKHR*.[217] Differences in outcome were also found between these two fusion-positive subsets. In the IRS-IV study, the patients with localized *PAX3-FKHR*– and *PAX7-FKHR*–positive ARMS had comparable outcomes,[212] whereas in a recent study from Poland with small patient numbers, the patients with localized *PAX7-FKHR* tumors had better outcomes than those with localized *PAX3-FKHR* tumors (*P* = 0.04).[218] Among patients presenting with metastatic disease in the IRS-IV study, those with *PAX3-FKHR*–positive tumors had significantly poorer outcomes than those with *PAX7-FKHR*–positive tumors; the estimated 4-year overall survival rate was 75% for metastatic *PAX7-FKHR* compared to 8% for metastatic *PAX3-FKHR* (*P* = 0.0015).[212] An interesting feature of these metastatic cases was the high incidence of bone marrow involvement among *PAX3-FKHR*–positive metastatic tumors compared to no bone marrow involvement among *PAX7-FKHR* metastatic tumors (*P* = 0.044).

Gene Expression Profiling with Microarrays

Microarray-based analyses of genome-wide gene expression in RMS tumors have permitted the identification of patterns of gene expression that distinguish RMS subsets. In addition, these expression-profiling studies have been used to identify significant genes and pathways deregulated in RMS and to examine the role of the fusion proteins in these expression patterns and deregulated pathways. To date, four independent microarray studies of RMS cases have been published, three using oligonucleotide microarray platforms and one using a cDNA platform with probes derived primarily from muscle tissues.[214,219-221] The smallest study analyzed 10 RMS cases that included 5 *PAX3-FKHR*–positive and 5 fusion-negative ARMS cases; and the largest study analyzed 139 RMS cases that included 69 ERMS, 55 fusion-positive ARMS (39 *PAX3-FKHR*, 16 *PAX7-FKHR*), and 15 fusion-negative ARMS). In these various studies, unsupervised approaches were used to cluster the cases based on differences and similarities in gene expression patterns among the cases. In the studies that included both *PAX3-FKHR* and *PAX7-FKHR* cases, there were no clear expression differences between the two fusion-positive subsets, so these cases tended to cluster together (see Fig. 19-1). In contrast, there was a striking difference in expression pattern between the fusion-positive ARMS cases and the ERMS cases, confirming the biologic differences between these two entities. In addition, there was also a striking difference in expression pattern between the fusion-positive ARMS cases and the fusion-negative ARMS cases, except for the small subset of "fusion-negative" ARMS with variant fusions. The final comparison of the ERMS cases and the fusion-negative ARMS cases revealed relatively few, if any, detectable differences between these two groups of fusion-negative RMS cases. Therefore, based on expression pattern, the RMS cases could be divided into two major categories: the fusion-positive and the fusion-negative cases. Furthermore, when viewed as a multidimensional scaling plot, the fusion-positive group showed a dense cluster whereas the fusion-negative group showed a cluster with more heterogeneous spread.

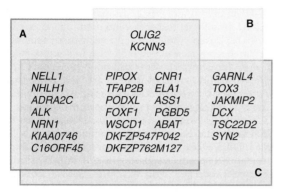

FIGURE 19-11. Genes that are differentially expressed between ARMS and ERMS tumors. In three independent studies, expression profiling was performed to determine genes differentially expressed between ARMS and ERMS tumors. The overlap among the top 50 entries in each study is shown. (**A,** *Wachtel M, Pettling M, Koscielniak E, et al.*[214]; **B,** *Lae M, Ahn EH, Mercado GE, et al.*[221]; **C,** *Davicioni E, Finckelstein FG, Shahbazian V, et al.*[220] *Adapted from Lae M, Ahn EH, Mercado GE, et al. Global gene expression profiling of* PAX-FKHR *fusion-positive alveolar and* PAX-FKHR *fusion-negative embryonal rhabdomyo-sarcomas. J Pathol. 2007;212:143-151.*)

To translate this information for prospective diagnostic purposes, gene expression lists were assembled using genes differentially expressed between the fusion-positive and fusion-negative RMS subsets. Using various statistical algorithms, the three published studies to date have generated signatures from 534 genes represented by 650 microarray entries (false discovery rate of 0.1%) to 121 genes corresponding to 136 microarray entries (Bonferroni-adjusted *P*-value <0.05).[214,220,221] Comparison of the top 50 entries ordered by statistical significance in each of these lists revealed 12 genes in common among the three lists and an additional 15 genes in common between any two of the lists (Fig. 19-11). In one study, four learning algorithms and cross-validation methodologies were used to identify a small and robust set of markers that distinguish fusion-negative ERMS and fusion-positive ARMS.[221] A 10-gene predictor was developed that was capable of distinguishing the two RMS subsets with about 95% accuracy (36/38) in the initial study. When applied to a previously published RMS dataset,[214] this predictor demonstrated a classification accuracy of 96% (25/26).

Many of the genes differentially expressed between fusion-positive and fusion-negative RMS tumors are postulated to be related to target genes of the fusion transcription factors. To explore this hypothesis, two complementary experimental systems were developed. In one system, constructs encoding each fusion protein were introduced into the *RD* ERMS cell line to express exogenously each protein in a myogenic tumor environment[220]; in the second system, a pair of siRNAs directed against *PAX3* sequences were introduced into an ARMS line to inhibit expression of the PAX3-FKHR protein.[141] Microarrays were used to identify genes with altered expression resulting from either upregulation of *PAX3-FKHR* (or *PAX7-FKHR*) in the ERMS cells or from downregulation of *PAX3-FKHR* in the ARMS cells. In the first system, comparison of *PAX3-FKHR*– and *PAX7-FKHR*–expressing *RD* cells to vector-transduced controls revealed 334 differentially expressed genes, 266 upregulated and 68 downregulated.[220] Further analysis showed that 24% of these genes (61 upregulated and 20 down-regulated) were differentially expressed between fusion-positive and fusion-negative RMS tumors. This group is enriched in genes involved in muscle development and function, neurogen-

esis, and cell proliferation, death, and adhesion. In the second system, 1834 genes were downregulated in anti-*PAX3* siRNA–treated ARMS cells 24 hours after treatment compared to scrambled siRNA-treated cells.[141] When compared to the 299-gene signature of genes differentially expressed between fusion-positive and fusion-negative tumors, 51 downregulated genes from the siRNA study overlapped this signature. This group is enriched for genes involved in signal transduction, enzymatic processes, and transcriptional regulation. As discussed previously, when the siRNA treatment continues for longer time periods, a group of repressed genes is induced, including a subset encoding myogenic differentiation products. Comparison of the 51 downregulated genes in the second study with the 61 upregulated genes in the first study revealed 9 genes in common, highlighting differences in the two experimental systems and the diverse range of downstream targets of these fusion transcription factors. In addition, these findings indicate that only a fraction of the expression differences between fusion-positive and fusion-negative tumors is directly attributable to the fusion protein; therefore, other expression differences must be attributable to additional genetic and environmental differences between these tumor subsets.

A hypothesis was proposed that the downstream target genes of these fusion oncoproteins would predict patient outcome. This hypothesis is based partially on the observations that the *PAX3-FKHR* and *PAX7-FKHR* expression levels vary over an eightyfold range in fusion-positive tumors, but this expression level does not correlate with patient survival. To explore this hypothesis, an investigation focused on the set of 81 target genes that were both modulated by the fusion proteins in *RD* cells and differentially expressed between the fusion-positive and fusion-negative subsets.[220] Cox regression modeling identified a subset of 28 genes corresponding to 33 microarray entries that had strong predictive power as a group. In particular, based on the expression of this group of genes, a score was calculated and used to divide the patients into three risk groups, which identify differences in outcome independent of known prognostic variables. This finding suggests that modulation of downstream target expression is associated with differences in the biologic aggressiveness of this malignancy.

Detection of Minimal Disseminated Rhabdomyocarcoma

Multiple studies with other cancers have used molecular markers and high-sensitivity detection methodologies to identify at diagnosis patients with disseminated disease that is not detected by conventional microscopic methods.[222-224] In the evaluation of solid tumors, bone marrow, peripheral blood, and lymph nodes are accessible and are commonly involved sites. In some cases, clinical correlative studies have demonstrated that the presence of minimal disseminated disease is predictive of a poor outcome.

Using several different methodologies, markers were developed to assay minimal disseminated disease in ARMS. An initial effort focused on the *PAX3-FKHR* and *PAX7-FKHR* gene fusions in ARMS and used RT-PCR methodology to detect the fusion transcripts.[225,226] Based on cell-mixing studies, standard RT-PCR assays for these gene fusions were reported to detect one tumor cell per 10^4 to 10^5 cells. Subsequent efforts focused on markers that would detect disseminated disease in fusion-negative ARMS and ERMS as well as fusion-positive ARMS, and would thereby provide a tool suitable for all RMS subtypes. As demonstrated in various other cancers, a common strategy is to assay for lineage-specific markers, which are generally expressed by the tumor and not by bone marrow or other sites assayed for disease spread. Therefore, for the RMS family of tumors, various myogenic markers of determination and differentiation have been investigated as minimal disease markers, including *MYOD*, myogenin *(MYOG)*, and the acetylcholine receptor genes *ACHRA* and *ACHRG*.[226,227] Using standard RT-PCR analysis, the sensitivity of assays for *MYOG* and *MYOD* were in the range of $1/10^4$ to $1/10^5$, and using qRT-PCR analysis, higher sensitivities for these and other markers were reported. Additional advantages of the quantitative assays include the ability to monitor changes in disease load over time and the ability to use these quantitative data to set an appropriate clinical threshold rather than allowing this threshold to be set by the inherent limits of the assay. Finally, antibodies were used to detect MyoD and myogenin protein in immunocytochemistry assays performed on mononuclear cell cytospins prepared from marrow aspirates.[228] In these assays, in which large numbers of cells were processed and multiple counts were performed on multiple cytospins, a high level of sensitivity, approximated to be $1/10^4$, was achieved.

These minimal disseminated disease assays were applied to clinical material from RMS patients in several different settings. Multiple studies of relatively small numbers of cases have addressed the feasibility of detecting occult disease in the bone marrow.[225-227] These studies have demonstrated that histologically positive bone marrows are consistently detected by these assays, regardless of the methodology or marker. For histologically negative marrows, various methodologies and markers detected submicroscopic disease, with the frequency tending to be higher in patients with ARMS than ERMS. In ARMS, which often metastasizes to the bone marrow, the frequency of a positive result in a histologically negative marrow ranges from 15% (2 of 13) to 60% (3 of 5). In ERMS, in which bone marrow is not a common site of metastasis, the frequency of a positive result in a histologically negative marrow ranges from 7% (1 of 15) to 33% (3 of 9). In an immunocytochemistry study of bone marrows from patients with nonmetastatic RMS, when the patients were grouped together, there was a clinically significant association between outcome and MyoD or myogenin staining in the bone marrow.[228] In particular, marrow involvement was associated with a significantly higher risk for recurrence (50% vs. 11%, $P = 0.011$) and poorer overall survival rates (47% vs. 92%, $P = 0.01$). In addition to these studies of bone marrows at the time of diagnosis, one study evaluated peripheral blood samples using qRT-PCR assays at diagnosis, during treatment, and following treatment.[227] Comparison of the positive results with outcome revealed that the finding of a positive at the end of treatment was associated with poor outcome, and the finding of persistent positive results preceded a metastatic relapse.

CLINICAL RESEARCH IN RHABDOMYOSARCOMA

RMS may be the most clinically complex tumor in pediatric oncology. In addition to its histologic and biologic diversity, RMS has a remarkable diversity of sites and clinical behaviors.

Much of our clinical knowledge of RMS has come from well-organized multi-institutional clinical trials in North America and Europe. In the United States and Canada (and later Australia, New Zealand, and Switzerland) the first Intergroup Rhabdomyosarcoma Study (IRS-I) opened in 1972 and closed in 1978, having recruited patients from the pediatric divisions of the Southwest Oncology Group (SWOG) and the Children's Cancer Study Group (CCSG). There were five further IRS studies (II, III, IV-pilot, IV, and V), during which the pediatric division of SWOG became the Pediatric Oncology

Group (POG), and the CCSG became the Children's Cancer Group (CCG). Finally, the IRS, POG, CCG, and National Wilms' Tumor Study merged to form the Children's Oncology Group (COG), and that group's Soft Tissue Sarcoma Committee completed the IRS-V studies before launching its own ARST (Rhabdomyosarcoma and Soft Tissue) series.

Meanwhile, in Europe, the International Society of Pediatric Oncology (SIOP) conducted a series of Malignant Mesenchymal Tumor (MMT) studies (SIOP 75 and MMT 84, 89, and 95). The German *Cooperative Weichteilsarkom Studie* (CWS) conducted four trials, CWS 81, 86, 91, and 96. The Italian Rhabdomyosarcoma Group had two clinical trials, RMS 79 and 88, before joining the CWS studies. Limited patient numbers made randomized controlled trials difficult, so the Europeans joined to form the European Paediatric Soft Tissue Sarcoma Study Group (EpSSG), which has launched a randomized controlled trial involving patients with localized RMS (RMS-2005). Unfortunately, the results of many of the European studies have never been published.

INCIDENCE AND EPIDEMIOLOGY

Clinical Epidemiology

RMSs account for about half of the soft tissue sarcomas in children and adolescents and constitute about 3% of childhood cancer cases. RMSs account for about 40% of soft tissue sarcomas in patients younger than 20 years of age overall, but this rate varies with age; RMSs are 60% of soft tissue sarcomas in patients younger than 5 years and 23% in the 15- to 19-year age group.[229] They occurred in 4.6 children per million children per year between 1996 and 2003, according to the Surveillance, Epidemiology and End Results database.[230] The highest incidence (8.4 per million children) occurs in children 1 to 4 years old, after which the incidence is stable at about 4 per million children per year. Most studies report a slight male preponderance (about 5:4).

Clinical Presentation

RMSs occur in virtually all parts of the body outside of the central nervous system (though they may involve that system). Embryonal tumors often occur in areas where there is very little skeletal muscle, such as the orbit, pharynx, sinuses, vaginal wall, and paratesticular tissues. Alveolar tumors have a greater tendency to occur where there is skeletal muscle, such as in the trunk and limbs (Fig. 19-12).

The clinical presentations of either histology are myriad and vary with the primary site. For example, tumors of the parameningeal region (such as the sinuses and pharynx) may have cranial nerve deficits as initial symptoms; orbital tumors often produce proptosis and diplopia; and tumors of the bladder base and prostate usually cause urinary retention. Often, however, the tumor is a painless mass without associated symptoms. Usually it is hard or firm, smooth, fixed to surrounding tissues, and not tender. There may be palpable regional lymphadenopathy, and occasionally (with alveolar histology tumors) distant involved nodes and metastases to the skeleton or marrow.

Clinical Evaluation

The initial evaluation of a patient with suspected RMS has three components: the evaluation of the extent and anatomic relationships of the primary tumor; the detection of metastases;

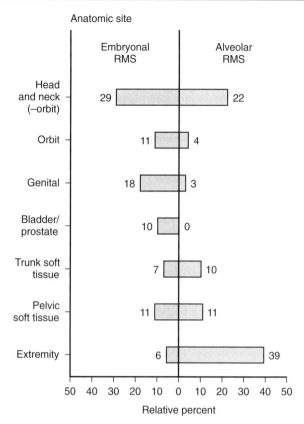

FIGURE 19-12. Primary sites of rhabdomyosarcoma, percent of distribution by histology. *(From Gurney JG, Young JL, Roffers SD, et al. Soft Tissue Sarcomas, SEER Pediatric Monograph, Bethesda, Md, National Cancer Institute, 1999, p 116.)*

TABLE 19-4	Clinical Features of Embryonal and Alveolar Rhabdomyosarcoma	
	Embryonal	**Alveolar**
Age	Younger	Older
Location	Central, not muscular	Peripheral, muscular
Invasiveness	Low/moderate	High
Metastases	Lung	Everywhere
Prognoses	40% to 90% + PFS	0 to 60% PFS

PFS, progression-free survival.

and the identification of other problems that may be related to the tumor (such as a cranial nerve palsy or urine retention) or that are unrelated but could affect therapy (such as neurofibromatosis type 1).

The most appropriate time for referral to a pediatric oncology center is upon the first suspicion of a possible malignancy. Imaging of the primary tumor is best performed by experienced radiologists before a biopsy has produced local hemorrhage and edema and using equipment that can share images with computerized radiation-therapy planning systems. If possible, the surgeon who will perform the definitive excision of the tumor should perform, or at least supervise, the diagnostic biopsy of a suspected sarcoma. Violation of tissue planes or neurovascular structures by inexpertly placed biopsy tracts, whether closed or open, may limit excision and reconstruction options, prevent limb salvage procedures, or increase the chances for local recurrence. Because sarcomas are often highly heterogeneous and contain large areas of necrosis, and because molecular techniques are helpful in the diagnosis of many sarcomas, generous fresh specimens are important. If closed techniques are used, many passes of the needle are usually required, with frozen-section confirmation of specimen adequacy. Fine-needle aspirates do not provide the tissue's architectural information currently necessary for diagnosis of pediatric sarcoma.

For evaluation of the primary tumor, the current standard of care is magnetic resonance imaging (MRI) with contrast enhancement, encompassing regional lymph nodes along with the primary tumor. For detection of pulmonary metastases, a spiral computed tomography (CT) scan without contrast is standard, although contrast is necessary to distinguish hilar adenopathy or mediastinal involvement and to distinguish a mass from a surrounding pleural effusion. A radionuclide bone scan is used to detect skeletal metastases, although a skeletal survey may be more sensitive in infants. Bilateral bone marrow aspirates and biopsies (by trephine) are performed to detect marrow involvement.

Other methods of staging are undergoing evaluation. The use of [18]fludeoxyglucose (FDG) positron emission tomography (PET) is particularly promising for the detection of involved regional nodes and distant metastases,[231,232] and its combination with CT scanning (PET-CT) can help to determine the extent of tumor versus peritumoral edema and whether a remote mass is tumor. Whole-body MRI scanning is currently the subject of a multi-institutional study; in a single-institution prospective study that included four patients with RMS, the findings on whole-body MRI matched those of conventional imaging by chest CT and bone scintigraphy.[233] A larger single-institution study compared the ability of whole-body MRI, FDG PET, and scintigraphy to detect skeletal metastases in 39 pediatric patients with a variety of tumors (including Ewing's sarcoma, RMS, osteosarcoma, lymphoma, melanoma, and Langerhans cell histiocytosis); all detected lesions were biopsied for histologic confirmation. PET had the highest sensitivity (90%), followed by whole-body MRI (82%) and skeletal scintigraphy (71%), although all three modalities had both false-positives and false-negatives, which varied with location (the high glucose uptake in the brain made PET relatively insensitive in the skull, for example). The greatest sensitivity (96%) was found in the combining of any two imaging modalities.[234]

Risk Group Classification

RMSs vary tremendously in prognosis, from almost 100% survival (for orbital embryonal tumors) to virtually no prospect of survival (for disseminated alveolar tumors). There has been a variety of schemes for classifying RMS to try to match treatment intensity to prognosis. Most of the schemes are prospective, in that they rely on tumor characteristics before therapy, but some are dynamic, subject to change based on response to surgery or chemotherapy. We consider individual prognostic variables and then discuss the ways in which they have been combined.

Histology

Patients with alveolar tumors are less likely to survive than patients with embryonal tumors, even if all other factors are equal. Alveolar tumors are also more likely to be regionally or metastatically disseminated at the time of diagnosis and are more likely to be invasive (Table 19-4). The difficulties in classifying tumors with alveolar histology that lack a *PAX-FKHR* gene fusion and the differences between alveolar tumors with fusions involving *PAX3* and *PAX7* have already been discussed. For the purposes of current clinical classification, the histology takes precedence over the fusion status.

Site

The clinical behavior and prognosis of RMS varies greatly with the site of the primary tumor. For example, an embryonal RMS of the orbit is almost always curable, whereas an embryonal tumor arising in the ethmoid sinus, just a few centimeters away, carries about a 25% mortality rate despite more intense therapy. The favorable sites for RMS are the orbit, superficial head and neck, biliary tree, vagina, and paratestis; all other sites are considered unfavorable. The biologic basis for this variability remains mysterious, with many different hypotheses (size at diagnosis, access to lymphatics, ploidy, and many others) having been explored and discarded.

Age

The prognosis for patients with RMS is best in preschool children and middle childhood and worse in infants and adolescents. An analysis of data from the IRSs III, IV pilot, and IV (spanning 1984 to 1997) revealed that when infants younger than 1 year of age are assigned a relative risk for treatment failure of 1, the relative risk for older children is 0.4 to 0.6 and that for adolescents (age 10 or older) is 0.8.[235] Although other prognostic variables, such as histology, nodal status, stage, site, and clinical group, differed among the three age groups, the impact of age remained when all other factors were controlled. Prognosis varies with age gradually, however, so the 1- and 10-year boundaries are somewhat arbitrary.

Invasiveness and Size (T status)

Invasive tumors, those that cross tissue planes or extend beyond the organ of origin (designated T2 in the TNM system), have worse prognoses that noninvasive tumors (T1). Similarly, patients with tumors 5 cm in diameter or larger (Tb) have worse prognoses than those with tumors smaller than 5 cm (Ta). The International Rhabdomyosarcoma Workshop pooled data from four studies conducted in the late 1970s and 1980s (the American IRS-II, the German CWS-81, the SIOP RMS 75, and the Italian Cooperative Group [ICG] study) to examine prognostic factors in 951 patients with localized disease. In multivariate analysis, site and invasiveness were the decisive factors.[236] Histology was not among the variables considered, but it is closely related to site and invasiveness. European studies have used invasiveness for risk classification but North American clinical trials have not, largely because of difficulty in arriving at a definition that would be usable in a large cooperative group.

Size is highly correlated with invasiveness in multivariate analyses[236] and is much simpler to measure. The current COG risk classification uses stage, which depends upon both site and size (Table 19-5).

Clinical Group

The extent of tumor when chemotherapy begins determines the clinical group (see Table 19-5). It is not a true staging system in that it is determined by the initial surgery; stage and group overlap only in patients with metastases (stage 4, group IV). IRS-I showed clinical group to be a powerful prognostic variable, but it is a complex one: site, invasiveness, the aggressiveness of the surgeon, the attitude of the family toward mutilating surgery, and the confidence of the treating team in chemotherapy and radiation therapy can all influence whether a tumor is

TABLE 19-5 Group (IRS) and Stage (COG)	
GROUP I: COMPLETE EXCISION No gross or microscopic residual disease	**STAGE 1: Favorable site** Orbit, superficial head and neck, biliary tree, paratestes, vagina
GROUP II: MICROSCOPIC RESIDUAL DISEASE IIa: Microscopically positive excision margins IIb: Excision margins negative; involved nodes but completely excised; most distant node negative IIc: Microscopically positive margins at primary site or grossly excised nodes; or most distant node positive	**STAGE 2: Unfavorable site, and** diameter ≤5 cm, and nodes clinically negative or unknown All sites except the favorable ones above are unfavorable.
GROUP III: GROSS RESIDUAL DISEASE Biopsy only or incomplete excision	**STAGE 3: Unfavorable site, and** diameter > 5 cm or clinically involved nodes
GROUP IV: DISTANT METASTASES	**STAGE 4: Distant metastases**

excised with negative margins at diagnosis (group I) or only biopsied (group III).

Lymph Node Involvement

Lymph node positivity is variably defined as clinical involvement on physical examination or imaging, or as histologic involvement at biopsy; some reports provide no definition. The International Rhabdomyosarcoma Workshop found lymph node involvement (undefined) to be a prognostic factor in univariate analysis, but not as strong as T status, size, or site.[236] Clinical involvement of local or regional lymph nodes was prognostically significant in IRS-III and IRS-IV patients with alveolar histology stage 3, group III tumors (5-year overall survival rate of 66% with negative nodes as opposed to 34% with positive nodes, $P = 0.01$) but not in patients with embryonal tumors.[237]

Metastases at Diagnosis

Patients with metastases at diagnosis fare poorly, and there has been little change over the years. Group IV patients had a 5-year overall survival rate of 20% in IRS-I, 23% in IRS-II, 20% in CWS-86, and 23% across a range of IRS studies beginning with IRS-III.[238-241] However, there are at least two populations of patients with metastatic RMS at diagnosis: those with embryonal tumors (usually metastatic to lung only), and those with alveolar tumors (whose metastases are often widespread). Patients younger than 10 years of age with metastatic embryonal RMS were classified as intermediate-risk (rather than high-risk) patients in the IRS-V series of studies because of a 51% failure-free survival rate in the previous three studies.[235,242] An analysis of patients with metastases at diagnosis in IRS-IV found that the number of metastatic sites and histology defined two risk groups. Patients with one or two metastatic sites, or three metastatic sites with embryonal histology, had a 3-year overall survival rate of 43% to 47%; but patients with three or more metastatic sites and alveolar histology had a 3-year survival rate of only 5%.[243]

Interactions

All of these variables interact, which complicates classification. For example, large primary tumors in the extremities commonly have alveolar histology, commonly have involved regional nodes, and commonly occur in teenagers; alveolar RMSs are usually invasive.

A recent analysis of 1164 CWS patients enrolled between 1980 and 2002 used multivariate analysis to identify as significant factors histology, age (10 years and younger vs. over 10), tumor size (5 cm cutoff), clinical group, site, and the use of radiation therapy in treatment. Further distillation produced three groups of patients: (1) those with embryonal tumors 5 cm or smaller whose 5-year event-free survival rate was 76%, whose relapses were only 19% systemic, and whose postrelapse survival rate was 46%; (2) those with embryonal tumors 5 cm or larger whose 5-year event-free survival rate was 64%, whose relapses were 32% systemic, and whose postrelapse survival rate was 18%; and (3) those with alveolar tumors whose 5-year event-free survival rate was 46%, whose elapses were 52% systemic, and whose postrelapse survival rate was 13%.[244]

Many different risk classification schemes exist for RMSs, and they change from one clinical trial to the next. In the system used by the COG for current studies, stage (which depends upon site and size), clinical group, and histology are combined to produce a three-way risk-classification (Table 19-6). The system used in the current European studies assigns patients to four risk groups (low, standard, high, and very high) on the basis of histology, clinical group (referred to as stage), site, nodal involvement, tumor size, and age; these four risk groups are then divided into eight subgroups (Table 19-7).

TREATMENT

Principles

Before the advent of chemotherapy for RMS, survival was rare; a retrospective review by the CCSG of 64 cases of RMS with "complete" surgical excisions revealed a survival rate of less than 8%.[245] The dramatic progress in the treatment and survival rates of patients with RMS over the past 40 years has flowed mostly from multidisciplinary care, in which surgeons, oncologists, radiologists, radiation oncologists, and pathologists approach treatment in a planned, coordinated fashion. Such care, which was pioneered in the late 1960s,[246] has been the foundation for clinical trials in RMS in the United States and Europe.

Chemotherapy

Systemic chemotherapy for all patients with RMS began with a CCSG randomized controlled trial that accrued patients from 1967 to 1971. Patients with complete excisions (group I) were randomly assigned to chemotherapy with vincristine and actinomycin D for 6 to 13 9-week cycles or to observation only; patients with microscopic residual disease (group II) were nonrandomly assigned to the chemotherapy arm. The relapse-free survival rate at 4 years was 82% in the chemotherapy group and 47% in the control group ($P = 0.03$); the relapse-free survival rate was 90% in group II.[245] This report established the role of chemotherapy in treating RMS and also established the feasibility and importance of coordinated multidisciplinary care on a national, multi-institutional scale.

Cyclophosphamide

Cyclophosphamide was part of combination chemotherapy for RMS in some of the earliest trials because of its efficacy as a single agent in patients with advanced RMS.[246,247] The combination of vincristine, actinomycin, and cyclophosphamide (VAC) has been in continuous use since IRS-I[239] and the first European cooperative group trials. The standard North American chemotherapy combination for patients with intermediate-risk tumors is still VAC. The exact composition of the VAC regimen has varied considerably over time (Table 19-8), but no randomized controlled trial has shown any particular combination to be more effective than others.

TABLE 19-6 **COG Risk Stratification for Rhabdomyosarcoma**

	Low Risk	Intermediate Risk	High Risk
Metastases	No	No	Yes
Histology	Embryonal	Any	Any
Stage	Any if group I or II; 1 if group III	1, 2, or 3 if alveolar histology; 2 or 3 if embryonal histology	4
Group	I, II, or III if stage 1; I or II if stage 2 or 3	III if stage 2 or 3; I, II, or III if alveolar histology	IV

TABLE 19-7 **EpSSG Risk Stratification for Rhabdomyosarcoma**

Risk Group	Subgroups	Pathology	Postsurgical Stage (IRS group)	Site	Node Stage	Size and Age
Low risk	A	Favorable	I	Any	N0	Favorable
Standard risk	B	Favorable	I	Any	N0	Unfavorable
	C	Favorable	II, III	Favorable	N0	Any
	D	Favorable	II, III	Unfavorable	N0	Favorable
High risk	E	Favorable	II, III	Unfavorable	N0	Unfavorable
	F	Favorable	II, III	Any	N1	Any
	G	Unfavorable	I, II, III	Any	N0	Any
Very high risk	H	Unfavorable	I, II, III	Any	N	Any

TABLE 19-8 Evolution of VAC Chemotherapy

	VCR Dose	VCR Schedule	AMD Dose	AMD Schedule[†]	CPM Dose	CPM Schedule	Duration	Total VCR	Total AMD	Total CPM
IRS-I	2 mg/m^2 max 2 mg	Weekly × 12	0.015 mg/kg/ d × 5 d, max 0.5 mg/dose	q12w	2.5 mg/kg	daily PO	2 y	12 doses	10 cycles	51.5 g/m^2
IRS-II*	2 mg/m^2 max 2 mg	Weekly × 12, then q4w	0.015 mg/kg/ d × 5 d, max 0.5 mg/dose	q4w	10 mg/kg/ d × 3	× 1, q3-4w	1 y for group II, 2 y for others	35 doses	24 cycles	27 doses, 24.3 g/m^2
IRS-III	1.5 mg/m^2 max 2 mg	Weekly × 12, then q3 to 4w	0.015 mg/kg/ d × 5 d, max 0.5 mg/dose	q3 to 4w	10 mg/kg/ d × 3	× 1, q3-4w	2 y	36 doses	21 cycles	27 doses, 24.3 g/m^2
IRS-IVP	1.5 mg/m^2 max 2 mg	Weekly × 12, then q3w with q1w intervals	1.35 mg/m^2 (1 dose)	q3w	3600 to 4500 mg/ m^2 (1st 4 cycles), then 2200 mg/ m^2 IV	× 1, q3w	38 weeks	32 doses	11 doses	13 doses, 34.2 to 37.8 g/m^2
IRS-IV	1.5 mg/m^2 max 2 mg	Weekly × 12, then q3w with q1w intervals	0.015 mg/kg/ d × 5 d, max 0.5 mg/ dose	q3w	2200 mg/ m^2 IV	× 1, q3w	44 weeks	32 doses	9 cycles	12 doses, 26.4 g/m^2
IRS-V	1.5 mg/m^2 max 2 mg	Weekly × 12, then q3w with q1w intervals	1.5 mg/m^2, max 2 mg	q3w	2200 mg/ m^2 IV	× 1, q3w	40 weeks	30 doses	12 doses	14 doses, 30.8 g/m^2
COG ARST[‡]	1.5 mg/m^2 max 2 mg	Weekly × 12, then q3w with q1w intervals	0.045 mg/kg (max 2.5 mg)[‡]	q3w	1200 mg/ m^2 IV	× 1, q3w	40 weeks	30 doses	12 doses	14 doses, 16.8 g/m^2

*Repetitive-pulse VAC;
[†]Except during radiation therapy;
[‡]Lower doses for infants.
AMD, actinomycin; ARST, Rhabdomyosarcoma and Soft Tissue; CPM, cyclophosphamide; VCR, vincristine.

In IRS-I, patients with group II tumors were randomized between 2-year regimens consisting of vincristine and actinomycin (with six doses of vincristine and 5 consecutive days of actinomycin per 9-week cycle) or VAC (12 weekly doses of vincristine at the start of therapy only, actinomycin every 12 weeks, and daily oral cyclophosphamide). There was no significant difference between the two arms,[239] but the design of the comparison allows one to conclude only that cyclophosphamide could substitute for 60 doses of vincristine and three cycles of actinomycin.

The IRS-II study addressed the role of cyclophosphamide in two randomizations. In group I patients, the VAC regimen from IRS-I (for 2 years) was compared to VA alone for 1 year, with the same 12 initial weekly doses of vincristine, and actinomycin every 12 weeks. VAC provided a statistically insignificant advantage in disease-free survival rates but no advantage in overall survival rates. For group II patients, there was a randomization between two 1-year regimens: VA with 9-week cycles incorporating 6 weekly doses of vincristine and one 5-day series of actinomycin doses per cycle; and a VAC modification with 4-week cycles each containing a single dose of vincristine, a single 5-day series of actinomycin injections, and intravenous cyclophosphamide. The contest was a draw,[240] and because the VA regimen had three times the vincristine and half the dactinomycin of the cyclophosphamide-containing regimen,

inferences regarding the role of cyclophosphamide are impossible.[248]

There is also no evidence of a relationship between the dosage of cyclophosphamide and its efficacy. For intermediate-risk patients receiving VAC, IRS-III prescribed the equivalent of 900 mg/m^2 per 3-week cycle in regimen 34[249]; IRS-IV used 2.2 g/m^2 per cycle in its VAC regimen[250]; and a pilot IRS study tried 3.6 g/m^2 of cyclophosphamide per cycle (a dosage of 4.5 g/m^2 proved too toxic).[251] However, there was no change in failure-free survival rates across these three trials despite a fourfold increase in cyclophosphamide dosage and dose intensity.[250,251]

Doxorubicin

Doxorubicin is probably the single most effective agent against sarcomas generally, but its role in RMS has been both unclear and controversial. It appears to be effective, but concerns about its cardiotoxicity (especially in young patients) have limited its use. The value of doxorubicin in treating RMS, and particularly its relative efficacy against embryonal and alveolar tumors, remain open questions despite 3 decades of study.

The IRSs have tried doxorubicin in a variety of ways. In IRS-I, patients with group III and IV tumors were randomized between VAC (with actinomycin every 12 weeks and continuous oral cyclophosphamide) and the same regimen with doxorubicin doses halfway between the actinomycin cycles. The addition of doxorubicin made no difference in either disease-free or overall survival rates.[239] The IRS-II study treated group III and IV patients with more modern, every-4-week intravenous regimens, randomizing between VAC and a regimen in which doxorubicin replaced actinomycin in alternating cycles. Again, there were no significant differences in disease-free or overall survival rates, although the results were much better than those of IRS-I.[240] Unfortunately, there was no analysis to see whether doxorubicin might have affected embryonal or alveolar histology differently.[248]

The third IRS used doxorubicin in two randomizations. For group II patients with favorable (embryonal) histology, vincristine-actinomycin-doxorubicin was superior to vincristine-actinomycin alone (89% vs. 54% 5-year survival rates, $P = 0.03$); however, the VA arm had worse results than in IRS-II, and when the IRS-II and -III results were combined, the statistical significance disappeared (89% vs. 73% for survival, $P = 0.14$).[249] Doxorubicin was also part of all three randomized regimens for clinical group III and IV patients but in complex ways that make its contribution to the results impossible to assess.[248]

The COG compared six phase II window regimens to IRS-III in 420 patients with group IV (metastatic) RMS. The doxorubicin-ifosfamide and ifosfamide-etoposide combinations and IRS-III did best in terms of failure-free survival rates, although there was no ultimate difference in overall survival rates.[238] Again, this analysis failed to shed any specific light on the role of doxorubicin.

In Europe, doxorubicin was part of the vincristine-actinomycin D-cyclophosphamide-Adriamycin (VACA) and vincristine-actinomycin D-ifosfamide-Adriamycin (VAIA) regimens of CWS-81 and CWS-86, respectively; it was part of the retrieval regimens for poor responders in MMT-84 and was widely used in the Italian RMS 79 and RMS 88 studies, but no randomized comparisons were made.[241,252] The addition of epirubicin, a doxorubicin analogue, along with carboplatin and etoposide proved to be no improvement over ifosfamide-vincristine-actinomycin (IVA) in the MMT-95 study.[253] We still do not know the value of doxorubicin (or other anthracyclines) in treating RMS.

Ifosfamide

DeKraker and Voute reported promising phase II results of the combination of vincristine and ifosfamide and went on to substitute ifosfamide for cyclophosphamide in the VAC combination in an 18-patient study of previously untreated patients.[254] The German CWS-86 study substituted ifosfamide for cyclophosphamide to change its VACA combination to VAIA, and the results were slightly better[241]; however, it was not a randomized controlled trial. A randomized controlled comparison of cyclophosphamide and ifosfamide had to await IRS-IV; 457 patients were randomly assigned to either VAC (with cyclophosphamide as a single 2.2 g/m^2 dose) or VAI (with ifosfamide as five daily doses of 1.8 g/m^2 each); the Kaplan-Meier plots of failure-free survival were superimposed.[250] Thus, although the IVA regimen has long been the European standard for intermediate-risk RMS, no data demonstrate its superiority to VAC; and ifosfamide has more urothelial, renal, and neurologic toxicity than cyclophosphamide.[255,256]

Etoposide

A phase II study of etoposide showed some activity in RMS.[257] The third IRS had a three-way randomization for intermediate-risk patients, which included a comparison of VAC with VAC plus cisplatin, plus or minus etoposide. Neither the cisplatin nor the cisplatin-etoposide combination added to the efficacy of VAC.[249]

In a comparison of phase II window regimens for patients with metastatic disease at diagnosis, in contrast, ifosfamide-etoposide was significantly superior to the IRS-III regimen of ifosfamide-doxorubicin, irinotecan, vincristine-melphalan, topotecan, or topotecan-cyclophosphamide in producing failure-free survival. The survival rates of the patients treated with ifosfamide-etoposide were also higher, although the proportion surviving at 5 years was no better.[238]

The combination of ifosfamide and etoposide produced complete or partial responses in 9 of 13 patients with recurrent or refractory RMS in a phase II National Cancer Institute study,[258] a remarkable level of activity. In the IRS-IV study, intermediate-risk patients were randomly assigned to chemotherapy with vincristine-ifosfamide-etoposide, VAC, or VAI; the three regimens had almost identical efficacy.[250] This showed not only that cyclophosphamide and ifosfamide are interchangeable (as given in the trial), but so are etoposide and actinomycin. Actinomycin can be given in a single dose rather than 3 to 5 daily doses, and all four patients who developed myeloid leukemia or myelodysplasia as a second malignancy in IRS-IV had received etoposide,[250] so VAC was carried forward as the control regimen for the IRS-V study.

Etoposide as a single agent, used daily by mouth for 21 days in every 28-day cycle, produced stable disease after two cycles in 3 of 11 patients with refractory or relapsed RMS or other soft tissue sarcoma in a British phase II trial.[259] Responses to oral etoposide appeared to be independent of previous etoposide exposure. A Turkish phase II study of a similar regimen included four patients with RMS; one had a durable complete response (more than 87 months), and another had a partial response lasting 10 months.[260] There have been no reports of regimens incorporating oral etoposide into initial therapy or of any combination regimens using it in RMS or other pediatric sarcomas.

Topotecan

Topotecan is a camptothecin analogue, and as such is a topoisomerase I poison that appeared to be active against a variety of pediatric solid tumors in preclinical trials. In a phase II POG study, the topotecan-cyclophosphamide combination produced complete or partial responses in 10 of 15 patients who had RMS.[261] The IRS and COG conducted a phase II window study of topotecan alone,[262] and then of topotecan with cyclophosphamide[263] in patients with group IV (metastatic-at-diagnosis) RMS, but neither distinguished itself in either event-free or overall survival rates.[238] More patients with alveolar histology responded to topotecan alone,[262] but the patients with embryonal and alveolar RMS responded similarly to topotecan-cyclophosphamide.[261,263]

The IRS-V intermediate-risk study randomized patients between VAC and VAC alternating with vincristine-topotecan-cyclophosphamide. Preliminary results showed no differences in disease-free or overall survival rates between the two arms, regardless of histology.[264]

Irinotecan

Irinotecan is another topoisomerase I poison with promising activity against pediatric solid tumors in preclinical models.[265] A British-French phase II study of irinotecan given as a single bolus dose every 3 weeks to patients with relapsed RMS produced only one complete response and three partial responses among 35 patients.[266] The results of a COG phase II study were similar, with one partial response among 18 RMS patients using a daily-times-five schedule (5 consecutive days of treatment every 3 weeks).[267] A daily-times-five-times-two schedule (5 days of treatment, 2 days off, then 5 more days of treatment, repeated every 3 weeks) was shown to be promising in both a xenograft model and in children with refractory solid tumors in a phase I study,[268] but in an Italian phase II study, only 2 of 12 patients with RMS had complete or partial responses.[269]

Vincristine and topotecan appeared to be synergistic in mouse xenografts,[270] inspiring a combination of vincristine and irinotecan in an IRS (later COG) study.[271] In the first part of the study, which enrolled patients with metastatic RMS at diagnosis, patients received 6 weeks (two cycles) of irinotecan using the daily-times-5-times-2 schedule, followed by VAC; in the second part, patients were treated with a combination of vincristine and irinotecan. The rate of response to the irinotecan window was 42%, but 32% had progressive disease; the rate of response to the combination vincristine-irinotecan window was 70%, with only 8% having progressive disease. Initial responses did not translate into improved survival rates, but patients who declined phase-II-window therapy received VAC alone and had response rates and failure-free survival rates (23%) similar to those of patients receiving vincristine-irinotecan.

A subsequent COG study randomized patients with relapsed or refractory RMS between the daily-times-5-times-2 schedule and a daily-times-5-times-1 schedule. The shorter regimen provided similar efficacy and toxicity.[271a] The current COG study of patients with intermediate-risk RMS randomizes patients between VAC and alternating 6-week blocks of vincristine-irinotecan and VAC.

Other Agents

Despite good results when the cisplatin-etoposide combination was tested in a phase II study,[272] cisplatin was shown not to add to the efficacy of VAC in intermediate-risk patients in IRS-III, either alone or in combination with etoposide (earlier). There has been no evaluation of carboplatin in a phase III study, but the addition of carboplatin to the ifosfamide-etoposide combination (the ICE regimen) in a phase II study produced a 51% rate of complete and partial responses in patients with a variety of relapsed sarcomas,[273] very similar to the rate of response to ifosfamide-etoposide and with greater toxicity. The SIOP MMT 98 study included a phase II window of carboplatin in 16 patients with RMS who had metastases at diagnosis.[274] Five patients had complete or partial responses after two cycles (31%), but four (25%) had progressive disease, limiting enthusiasm for this agent, especially in view of its prolonged myelotoxicity.

Melphalan with vincristine was a phase II window combination in an IRS-IV trial for patients with metastases at diagnosis; however, it produced an unimpressive response rate and more toxicity than ifosfamide-etoposide.[238,275]

Combinations

Two attempts to improve outcome for patients with intermediate-risk or high-risk RMS by administering intense combinations of several agents have failed in randomized controlled trials. IRS-III compared VAC with the same drugs plus doxorubicin and cisplatin, etoposide, or both; the outcomes were identical in the three arms.[249] The MMT 95 study randomly assigned similar patients to IVA or IVA plus carboplatin, epirubicin, and etoposide; the event-free and overall survival rates were the same at 3 years, although the toxicity of the intensified regimen was significantly greater.[253]

The success of alternating vincristine-doxorubicin-cyclophosphamide and ifosfamide-etoposide (VDC/IE) in Ewing's sarcoma inspired a limited-institution trial of that therapy in 46 patients with intermediate-risk RMS, and a comparison with the results in similar patients in IRS-IV. Failure-free survival rates with VDC/IE and IRS-IV were 82% and 72%, respectively ($P = 0.26$), and overall survival rates at 5 years was 76% for both. However, in a stratified analysis, a comparison of the patients administered VDC/IE with 346 patients in IRS-IV who were matched for site, histology, age, and clinical group showed a relative risk for failure of 0.5 with VDC/IE ($P = 0.06$).[276] The VDC/IE combination is currently under study, combined with vincristine and irinotecan, in high-risk patients in the COG.

Duration of Chemotherapy

The IRS-I, -II, and -III studies prescribed 2 years of treatment for most patients; in IRS-IV, the duration of treatment was trimmed to 44 weeks for patients with intermediate-risk tumors and 32 weeks for patients with low-risk tumors.[250] In contrast, the European MMT-84 and CWS-81 and CWS-86 studies used 30 to 56 weeks of therapy.[241,277] The current COG trials use only 22 weeks of therapy for patients with the lowest risk tumors and 42 and 51 weeks for patients with intermediate- and high-risk tumors, respectively. Although there have been no apparent adverse consequences of shorter durations of therapy, there have been no systematic controlled comparisons.

The current EpSSG study is testing the efficacy of "maintenance" therapy for 24 weeks using vinorelbine and oral cyclophosphamide after the completion of 26 weeks of intense cyclic chemotherapy for high-risk patients who achieve complete response.

Treatment Strategies

There have been three broad approaches to the treatment of RMSs. SIOP has used intense initial chemotherapy and then has tried to tailor primary tumor treatment according to responses to initial chemotherapy so as to minimize the use of surgery and radiation (with their accompanying late effects) in their MMT studies. The IRSs in North America have sought to maximize event-free survival through the use of chemotherapy, surgery, and radiotherapy in almost all patients (the IRS group is now the Soft Tissue Sarcoma Committee of the COG). The German-Italian CWS studies have taken an intermediate approach. The European groups established the EpSSG, which has launched a protocol for localized RMS (RMS-2005).

These various philosophies are illustrated in the groups' treatments for orbital RMSs. The MMT-84 and MMT-89 studies treated patients with intense multiagent chemotherapy and no radiation therapy for those achieving complete responses. The CWS studies modulated the radiation dose according to the response to intense multiagent chemotherapy: 40 or 50 Gy in CWS-81 and the ICG 88 study, and 32 or 54.4 Gy in CWS-86 for good and poor responders, respectively. The IRS gave all patients radiation therapy (45 to 55 Gy, depending upon the study), and evolving chemotherapy that was either relatively mild (vincristine and actinomycin) or intense (the IRS-IV randomization between VAC, VIE, and IVA). The three approaches led to very different event-free survival rates at 10 years (57% for MMT to 86% for IRS, $P < 0.001$), but the overall survival rates were almost identical (85% and 88%, $P = 0.67$). The incidence of radiation-associated late effects was higher in the IRS patients than in the MMT patients, although the total burden of therapy in the MMT studies includes the treatment of relapse in 37% of patients.[278]

A comparison of RMSs in all sites treated in MMT 89 and IRS-IV gave a considerable overall advantage to the IRS approach. Overall, IRS-IV had higher event-free and overall survival rates than MMT-89 (78% vs. 57% and 84% vs. 71%, respectively). For some sites (such as the genitourinary tract, not including bladder and prostate) there was no difference (IRS-IV vs. MMT 89, 83% vs. 82% event-free survival; 90% vs. 94% overall survival), but for others the difference was large (e.g., limbs, IRS-IV vs. MMT 89, 64% vs. 35% event-free survival; 71% vs. 46% overall survival). For patients with tumors of embryonal histology, the IRS approach showed a small advantage for overall survival rates (87% vs. 78%) but a large advantage for patients with tumors of alveolar histology (71% vs. 38%).[279] Another review found that the four major RMS clinical study groups enjoyed roughly equal success in preventing metastatic relapse, but there were considerable differences in local relapse, ranging from 13% for the IRS to 30% for the MMT; the CWS and Italian groups were in the middle, with 19% and 22%.[244]

More recent results call into question the CWS strategy of modifying treatment according to primary tumor response as assessed by conventional imaging (CT or MRI). A review of group III patients treated in IRS-IV demonstrated no relationship between response to the first 8 weeks of therapy (complete, partial, or none) and 5-year failure-free survival. This was true for patients who were initially treated with chemotherapy alone as well as for those with parameningeal tumors with intracranial extensions who received early radiation therapy. The only statistically significant difference was found in patients with alveolar tumors; those with no response had a better failure-free survival rate (81%) than did patients with complete (71%) or partial (39%) responses ($P = 0.04$).[232] Imaging using FDG-PET might prove to be useful because it can differentiate between viable tumor and a residual mass of necrosis or fibrosis,[280] but much work remains to determine the optimal timing and circumstances for such studies.

Current Practice and Protocols

Most patients with RMS in North America are enrolled in COG studies. Patients are classified as low, intermediate, or high risk on the basis of metastasis, stage, histology, and clinical group (Fig. 19-13 and see Table 19-6). Low-risk patients are currently treated with four cycles of VAC (using a single 1200 mg/m² dose of cyclophosphamide), followed by vincristine-actinomycin for a total of 6 months or 1 year of chemotherapy. Patients with group II or III tumors receive radiotherapy. Intermediate-risk patients are being randomized between the standard therapy of VAC for 1 year and a regimen in which blocks of vincristine-irinotecan therapy alternate with blocks of VAC. The results of treatment in high-risk patients are poor enough that it is difficult to designate any treatment as being standard; COG has a single-arm study using vincristine-irinotecan and interval-compressed (every-2-week) vincristine-doxorubicin-cyclophosphamide alternating with ifosfamide and etoposide.

The EpSSG is using a complex algorithm to classify patients without metastases into eight risk groups and subgroups, with further treatment subdivisions based on response to initial chemotherapy (see Table 19-7). Low-risk patients are being treated with eight cycles of vincristine-actinomycin. Standard-risk patients are receiving regimens including IVA and vincristine-actinomycin. High-risk patients are being enrolled in two randomized controlled trials, one evaluating the role of doxorubicin added to IVA and the other exploring maintenance chemotherapy with vinorelbine and cyclophosphamide. Very-high-risk patients (those with alveolar histology and involved nodes; EpSSG excludes patients with metastases) are being treated with IVA, doxorubicin, and maintenance vinorelbine-cyclophosphamide. All patients except those with group I embryonal tumors are also receiving radiation therapy.

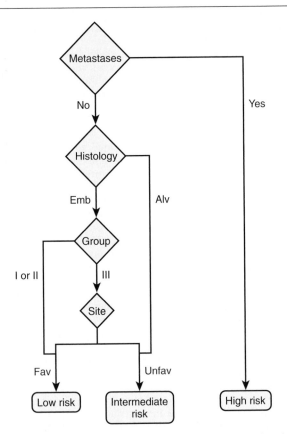

FIGURE 19-13. Algorithm for risk-group classification of patients with RMS. This represents the classification scheme in the current COG ARST series of protocols. Alv, alveolar; Emb, embryonal; Fav, favorable prognosis; Unfav, unfavorable prognosis.

Primary Tumor Treatment

Introduction

When only local therapy with surgery and radiation was available, the survival rate of patients with RMS was dismal. Chemotherapy has dramatically improved survival rates, and it has also changed the surgical and radiotherapeutic approaches; minimization of late effects has become a new priority. Optimal outcomes require multidisciplinary care.

Surgery

The surgeon is often involved with a patient with RMS from the time of initial biopsy. This is best done at the cancer center where treatment will occur and where a full complement of diagnostic tools (including molecular techniques) is available. The biopsy requires careful planning and execution because diagnosis, treatment, and late effects can all depend upon it. It is often possible to coordinate a biopsy and frozen section with the performance of marrow aspirates and biopsies for staging and the placement of a central venous catheter.

The earliest classification system for RMS, the IRS Clinical Grouping system, is based upon the amount of tumor remaining after the first surgical intervention, be it a complete excision with clear margins (group I) or only a biopsy with gross residual disease remaining (group III; see Table 19-5). The first IRS showed that clinical group is a powerful predictor of survival,[239] and it established the role of surgery in the treatment of RMS in the chemotherapy era. Although initial complete surgical excision can involve disfigurement or loss of function, it may have a smaller late-effects burden than primary tumor treatment by radiation in some patients, so multidisciplinary consultation is essential.

When a patient's initial excision leaves microscopically positive margins (group II), or when the initial excision was performed outside the pediatric cancer center, there may be value in a primary re-excision before chemotherapy begins. An analysis of patients with trunk or limb RMS in IRS-I and -II showed that group II patients converted to group I had the same survival rate as patients who were rendered group I in their initial procedure. Patients who were referred as group I patients and had primary re-excisions had superior outcomes to those who did not.[281]

Regional lymph node sampling is important in limb primary tumors, which commonly have alveolar histology and a predilection for nodal involvement. Patients 10 years old or older with paratesticular RMS also have an increased risk for paraspinal nodal relapse and should undergo node sampling. Otherwise, lymph node sampling may be limited to nodes that are suspicious by physical examination or imaging.[282,283]

Traditional surgical teaching holds that an attempt at excision is not valuable unless the patient can be left with, at most, microscopic residual disease (group I or II). Among patients with unresectable tumors (group III), debulking surgery may be beneficial even if the patients remain group III. In a retrospective study of IRS patients treated between 1984 and 1991 who had large (≥5 cm) group III or IV retroperitoneal tumors, patients with embryonal histology who underwent debulking surgery before chemotherapy fared better than those who did not (they had a failure-free survival rate of 72% vs. 39% at 4 years, $P = 0.03$); too few patients with alveolar histology tumors had debulking surgery to permit analysis.[284] It is not yet clear whether this principle applies only to retroperitoneal tumors or whether it is generally applicable. However, a retrospective analysis of the Italian RMS 79, 88, and 96 protocols that compared the fate of 323 patients with biopsy only and 71 patients with debulking surgery (defined as more than 50% excision, but still group III) found no overall benefit. One subgroup, patients 10 years old or older, appeared to benefit from debulking surgery (event-free survival rate of 73% vs. 50%, $P = 0.04$; overall survival rate of 83% vs. 62%, $P = 0.06$), but no other subgroup defined by site, size, histology, invasiveness, or response to initial chemotherapy did so.[285]

In patients with gross residual disease when chemotherapy begins (group III and IV), second-look operations and delayed excision of residual tumor masses, even after radiation therapy and chemotherapy, may improve the chances for survival. In a retrospective study of second-look operations in IRS-III, 12% of patients clinically thought to have had complete responses had residual viable tumor, and three quarters of patients clinically thought to have had partial responses or no response either had no viable tumor or were converted to the complete response group at surgery. These converted patients had the same 3-year survival rates as those whose complete responses were confirmed at second-look surgery (73% and 80%, respectively).[283] A single-institution study of 48 group III patients showed that those who had delayed complete surgical excision ($n = 22$) had relapse-free and overall survival rates superior to those who did not (approximately 90% vs. 60% relapse-free survival, $P = 0.013$).[286] Patient numbers were too small to permit a multivariate analysis, however, and histology and nodal status were also significant variables on univariate analysis.

Radiation Therapy

Because many RMSs occur in sites that are not amenable to surgery, radiation therapy plays a key role in primary tumor treatment. Advances in radiation therapy techniques are reducing the acute and late morbidities of treatment. However, there are large gaps in our knowledge of how best to use radiation to treat RMS.

The first knowledge gap is reflected by the question Who needs radiation therapy? A retrospective analysis of 439 group I patients in IRS-I, -II, and -III found no benefit of radiation in patients with embryonal tumors for overall survival (95% at 10 years for both groups, $P = 0.83$). For patients with alveolar and undifferentiated tumors, however, each of the IRS studies showed a benefit of radiation therapy, analyzing by treatment received.[287] A retrospective analysis of the CWS-81, 86, 91, and 96 studies showed that the use of radiation therapy roughly halved the risk of death in patients with embryonal tumors smaller than 5 cm ($P = 0.02$) and in patients with larger embryonal tumors ($P = 0.001$), but had a smaller effect in patients with alveolar tumors (risk for death ratio 0.7, $P = 0.09$).[244]

In patients with microscopic residual disease (group II), a retrospective analysis of 203 RMS patients in the four CWS studies (81, 86, 91, and 96) compared the 110 patients who received radiotherapy with the 93 who did not (for a variety of reasons). The two groups of patients differed significantly in histology (more irradiated patients had alveolar tumors); site (more irradiated patients had extremity and parameningeal tumors and fewer had vaginal-paratesticular tumors); and age (fewer irradiated patients were infants). All patients received combination chemotherapy following one of several regimens. Despite the greater number of unfavorable characteristics among the irradiated patients, local control was better (83% vs. 65%, $P < 0.04$), and event-free survival rates were better (76% vs. 58%, $P < 0.005$), although the overall survival rates of the irradiated and nonirradiated patients were similar (84% and 77%).[288] In the IRS studies I through IV, there were 37 patients with group II tumors who did not receive radiation; their failure-free survival rate was 69%, and their overall survival rate was 85%, very similar to the 73% and 78% for the entire cohort.[289] Thus, radiation therapy probably confers an advantage on group II patients, but it is far from indispensable for local control and survival.

Initially unresectable (group III) patients who subsequently undergo surgical excision are also a point of contention. The IRS and subsequent COG protocols have required radiation therapy for these patients, though European protocols have not. A single-institution study of 48 patients with group III RMSs identified 22 who had had complete excisions at second-look surgery, of whom 13 were treated with subsequent radiation and 9 were not. One patient in each group suffered relapse ($P = 0.67$), neither at the primary site.[286] In the MMT 89 study, 58% of the 289 survivors with "incomplete" initial surgery or biopsy only had either chemotherapy alone or chemotherapy plus conservative local therapy (defined as no functional deficits and no external beam radiation).[290] Unfortunately, these patients are not classified by stage or site, but radiation therapy was not indispensable for cure. Similarly, the CWS-86 study included 31 group III patients who did not receive radiation therapy (16 because they were younger than 3 years of age), again not classified by site or histology. All but one had complete responses to chemotherapy and surgery. The local relapse rate was 27%, versus 10% for patients receiving radiation ($P = 0.2$), and the overall relapse rate was 40%, versus 28% for irradiated patients ($P = 0.001$).[241] Thus, although radiation therapy seems to reduce the risk for local recurrence and improves the survival rate of patients with group III tumors, it is not indispensable.

Assuming the use of radiation therapy, the question becomes how much radiation the various presentations of RMS require to maximize the chances for cure. On the low side of the dose-response curve, it is unclear how much radiation is advisable. A single-institution study of 32 patients with IRS group II RMSs (all but two with embryonal histology) used chemotherapy (vincristine, doxorubicin, actinomycin, cyclophosphamide, with or without methotrexate, bleomycin, and carmustine) and between 30 and 60 Gy of radiation. Of the patients, 19 received 40 Gy or less, with only one local relapse; 14 received 36 Gy or less, with the same single local failure.[291] The CWS-86 study compared 67 group III patients who received 25 to 35 Gy (mean 31.6 Gy) with 49 patients who received 40 to 67 Gy (mean 52 Gy); 31% of the lower-dose group and 26% of the higher-dose group relapsed, although a higher proportion of the relapses in the higher-dose group were metastatic rather than local or regional.[241] In this study, the higher doses of radiation seem to have reduced the risk for local recurrence.

On the high side of the dose-response curve, IRS-IV randomized patients with group III tumors to between 50.4 Gy by conventional fractionation (180 cGy/day) and 59.4 Gy by hyperfractionation (110 cGy twice daily). The hyperfractionated regimen was designed to allow a higher dose without an increase in late effects. There was no difference in any outcome measure between the two regimens (failure-free survival, overall survival, local relapse, distant relapse) and no difference according to histology.[250] This indicates that 50.4 Gy is sufficient to control most gross residual RMSs; less radiation may be equally efficacious.

In an effort to spare normal tissues from radiation, some institutions have used brachytherapy at the time of second-look surgery.[292-295] This technique usually involves the placement of catheters in the tumor or tumor bed during surgery; the catheters are subsequently loaded with radioactive pellets and then removed when the dose is complete. The brachytherapy dose often has to be supplemented by external beam radiotherapy, and we have found that intensity-modulated radiation therapy (IMRT) has largely replaced brachytherapy.

Some institutions have also used intraoperative radiation therapy (IORT), which involves the delivery of a single large fraction of external beam radiation when the tumor or tumor bed is surgically exposed. Generally, larger radiation fractions decrease the therapeutic index, especially for late effects, and this may be the case in pediatric IORT. One series of children treated with IORT for neuroblastoma included seven long-term survivors (4 to 143 months); all seven had hypertension, five had vascular stenosis in the radiation field, and two patients died, one of mesenteric artery stenosis and bowel ischemia and the other of massive ascites.[296] Similarly, of eight surviving patients in another series treated for a variety of pediatric solid tumors, two patients required surgery for hydronephrosis and small bowel obstruction, a third developed severe renovascular hypertension and superior mesenteric artery stenosis, and two developed neuropathies.[297] In another series, 3 of 14 children treated with intraoperative radiotherapy for recurrent brain tumors developed radiation necrosis within 6 to 12 months.[298] However, the largest reported series of IORT-treated children (*n* = 59) who had a variety of malignancies recorded no long-term toxicities among the 14 long-term survivors.[299]

Proton therapy minimizes the irradiation of normal tissues surrounding the target, and its resulting potential to decrease late effects makes it particularly attractive for treating children. A study comparing conformal radiation, IMRT, and proton plans for a patient with parameningeal RMS calculated that protons reduced the risk for a second malignant neoplasm by a factor of two or more.[300] Proton therapy is currently available at only a few centers, and there have not been many systematic evaluations. One study compared the proton and three-dimensional conformal radiotherapy treatment plans of seven patients treated with protons for orbital RMS. Proton therapy reduced

the radiation dose to the hypothalamus, pituitary, temporal lobes, and optic chiasm by 82% to 94% and reduced the dose to the ipsilateral lens by 65%. One patient had a local relapse after radiotherapy, but all of the others were event-free survivors with a median follow-up of 6 years. None has any neuroendocrine abnormalities, and none has a cataract.[301] In another study 12 patients with RMS were among 16 children with soft tissue sarcomas reviewed. At a median of 18 months of follow-up, two patients with RMS had relapsed locally and died. Acute side-effects were mild, but the follow-up time was short for assessment of late effects.[302]

Special Situations

Infants and Toddlers

Treating small children with unresectable (group III) tumors while avoiding devastating late effects can be difficult because tissues irradiated to the doses used for RMS will not grow. Results in very young patients treated without radiation have challenged the dogma that radiotherapy is essential for cure of all but group I patients. In the CWS-86 study, 30 patients with stage III (equivalent to group III) tumors, about half of them younger than 3 years of age, were treated without radiation therapy, having achieved complete responses with chemotherapy and surgery. Of the 30, 12 (40%) relapsed, and 8 (27% of the 30 patients) had local recurrences, for a progression-free survival rate of about 60%.[241] This rate was similar to the event-free survival rate of stage III patients with complete responses to initial therapy in this study, but the patients are not classified according to other risk factors (such as site), and the numbers are too small for statistically meaningful comparison.

Infants and toddlers appear to tolerate aggressive chemotherapy less well than older children. In the IRS D9803 intermediate-risk study, which used VAC with a single dose of actinomycin and 2.2 g/m^2 of cyclophosphamide, there were 18 cases of hepatopathy resembling veno-occlusive disease, 4 of them fatal.[303] The total incidence of hepatopathy in 339 eligible patients was 6%, but it was 14% in patients younger than 36 months and only 4% in older patients. A modification of actinomycin and cyclophosphamide dosages for young patients ameliorated the problem. Cooperative group protocols have varying schemes for calculating infant chemotherapy dosages, including using weight as the basis, rather than surface area, reducing the dosages by 30% to 50%, or a combination; none has a foundation in data.

The effects of these compromises on outcome are unclear. A retrospective analysis of IRS-COG studies from 1984 to 1997 (IRS-III, IV pilot, and IV) found that patients younger than 1 year of age have much lower failure-free survival rates than patients aged 1 to 9 years and similar to those of adolescents (aged 10 years and older): 53% versus 72% versus 52%, *P* <0.001.[235] Infants were more likely than children aged 1 to 9 years to have embryonal or undifferentiated histology and to have bladder-prostate or head-and-neck primary sites. The study did not compare deviations from protocol therapy among the groups. In contrast, in the SIOP MMT-84 and -89 studies compared infants (less than 1 year of age) with localized RMS to children aged 1 to 9 years and to adolescents older than 10 years, and found identical event-free and overall survival rates between the infants and the older children, both of whom did better than the adolescents (event-free survival 57% vs. 58% vs. 42%; overall survival 72% vs. 72% vs. 59%, *P* <0.001 between adolescents and the other groups).[304] The infants had alveolar histology more commonly than older children and more commonly had bladder-prostate and limb primary sites. Again, there was no analysis of deviations from protocol therapy, leaving it unclear whether reduced therapy or biologic differences were responsible for the worse outcomes.

Bladder and Prostate Tumors

Because RMS can occur anywhere in the pelvis, and because pelvic tumors are often very large at the time of diagnosis, the exact primary site may be difficult to determine. One should not assume that a pelvic RMS is arising from the bladder or prostate without definitive imaging or cystoscopy. Bladder-prostate tumors usually produce urinary symptoms and are rarely of alveolar histology, so one should be especially suspicious that tumors without these characteristics are arising in nongenitourinary pelvic sites. This distinction can have important implications for the treatment of a primary tumor.

The evolution of approaches to bladder-prostate RMSs can be traced through the IRS trials. Early approaches included extensive surgery (often complete or partial pelvic exenteration) in addition to chemotherapy. In IRS-I, more than half the patients with bladder-prostate RMS underwent initial excisions (group I or group II), often involving anterior exenteration or cystectomy. The disease-free survival rate was 67%, and the overall survival rate was 76% at 5 years. The effectiveness of chemotherapy led to efforts to use initial chemotherapy and postpone and reduce surgery in favor of radiation therapy, in the hope of preserving genitourinary anatomy and function. When this approach was taken in IRS-II, the proportion of group I and II patients fell to 5%. However, the disease-free survival rate declined substantially (to 51%), although the overall survival rate was comparable (71%). The new approach had no effect on the proportions of patients alive and with intact bladders, however, which were 23% in IRS-I and 22% in IRS-II.[305] The IRS-III study used more intense chemotherapy (all patients receiving VAC plus doxorubicin, cisplatin, and etoposide), radiation therapy beginning at week 6, and second-look surgery at week 20. The percentage of patients retaining their bladders rose to 60%, with progression-free and overall survival rates improving to 74% and 83%, respectively.[249,306] IRS-IV used different chemotherapy, moved the radiation therapy from week 6 to week 9, and encouraged second surgical procedures short of complete cystectomy or prostatectomy unless there was biopsy-proven residual tumor or progression at the end of therapy. The overall survival rate of the 88 reviewed patients was 82%, and the failure-free survival rate was 77%; 63% retained their bladders.[307]

There have been two problems with these bladder-preserving strategies: often the bladders do not work very well, and the collateral side-effects can be considerable. Radiation therapy can cause fibrosis of the bladder and sphincters, leading to limited bladder capacity, dribbling, or incontinence. Radiation therapy to the pelvis limits bony growth, and even with modern IMRT techniques it can be difficult to avoid irradiation of the hip joints, leading to future orthopedic problems. A review of IRS-I and -II patients, which involved asking physicians whether their patients' urinary functions were normal, found normal urinary function in 73% of the 52 patients who had retained all or part of their bladders; the remaining 27% had incontinence, frequency, or nocturia. Radiation therapy and cyclophosphamide (before the availability of mesna) combined to produce hematuria after completion of treatment in 20% of patients. Outside the urinary tract, spontaneous reporting disclosed 4 patients with colostomies to repair fistulae or relieve strictures, and 6% with fecal incontinence, chronic diarrhea, or rectal stenosis; 8% had orthopedic problems, including slipped femoral epiphyses and pelvic fibrosis or hypoplasia.[308]

A more recent study of IRS-IV patients used routine follow-up forms and questionnaires that were sent to physicians. Of 55 patients with preserved bladders, two thirds were reported to have normal urinary function; the balance had late diversions, dribbling, incontinence, enuresis, hydronephrosis, or strictures. It is interesting that no differences in relapse rate or pattern could be found between patients who had protocol-specified radiation therapy and those who had major deviations in radiation therapy (including 9 who received none), although 2 irradiated patients developed second malignancies.[307]

The cooperative group data may underestimate the frequency and severity of late effects in this population, however. A single-institution study of 26 girls cured of pelvic RMS (including non–bladder-prostate sites) found that 23 (88%) had grade III or IV late effects at a median of 20 years' follow-up, and more than half required surgery for these complications. The most common problems were musculoskeletal hypoplasia, recurrent urinary tract infections, incontinence, urinary reflux, and short stature. There were three secondary solid tumors in radiation fields. Radiation therapy was associated with more late effects per patient ($P = 0.002$), and patients treated since 1984 had about twice as many late effects per patient than patients treated earlier (12.5 vs. 6.5, $P = 0.041$).[309]

None of these studies used urodynamics to measure bladder function objectively. One single-institution study that did so found 11 patients with pelvic RMS (7 of the bladder or prostate) and found that all 7 patients who had received radiation therapy had markedly reduced bladder capacity (11% to 48% of age norms) and abnormal voiding patterns; 4 had upper tract abnormalities and 2 had severe bilateral hydronephrosis.[310]

Bladder-prostate RMSs are unusual because they can be monitored easily by cystoscopy and biopsy. In view of the considerable late effects of radiation therapy in particular, some centers use cystoscopic and histologic monitoring to delay and minimize the use of radiation, moving in the direction of the SIOP MMT studies.[311] This requires expert pathologic interpretation, however, because distinguishing between viable RMS and harmless differentiated rhabdomyoblasts can be very difficult, especially in a field of previous surgery or radiation therapy.[311,312]

Parameningeal Tumors

The parameningeal sites include the nasal cavity and nasopharynx; the parapharyngeal space; the paranasal sinuses (ethmoid, maxillary, and sphenoid); the pterygopalatine and infratemporal fossae; and the middle ear and mastoid sinuses. Parameningeal RMSs have a tendency to invade the cranium and intracranial contents, either by eroding through the skull base or by extending through a foramen. It is curious that tumors arising in the orbits are much less aggressive. Complete excision of parameningeal tumors at diagnosis is almost never possible, so that they are at best stage 2, group III in the IRS-COG staging system. The large majority are of embryonal histology.

In the IRS-I study, the 5-year overall survival rate was only 47%[239]; it was identical in CWS-81.[313] The IRS-II study intensified therapy for patients with parameningeal tumors by means of craniospinal radiation and intrathecal chemotherapy (methotrexate, cytarabine, and hydrocortisone) beginning immediately after diagnosis, and overall survival improved to 67%.[240,314] IRS-III substituted whole-brain for craniospinal radiotherapy and began it early only in patients with cranial nerve palsies, intracranial extension or base-of-skull erosion on imaging; chemotherapy was also considerably more intense. Survival rates improved again, to 73%, but five patients (3.4%) developed ascending myelitis, which was fatal in three.[315] In IRS-IV, intrathecal chemotherapy was eliminated, and the radiation field was reduced to the involved area with a 5 cm margin, with no loss of efficacy found in a retrospective analysis of 611 IRS II-IV patients.[314]

A univariate analysis of parameningeal RMS patients in IRS-II through -IV identified as favorable features age between 1 and 9 years; site in the nasal cavity, nasopharynx, parapharynx, middle ear, or mastoid; and lack of bony erosion or intracranial extension.[314] Patients with entirely favorable features had a 92% overall survival rate at 5 years, compared to 57% for those with entirely unfavorable features. Size and histology were not statistically significant factors.

Results in Europe lagged far behind, with 5-year overall survival rates of 55% in SIOP, 47% in Germany, and 39% in Italy.[316] An international workshop in 1994 combining the American and European experiences recommended routine use of MRI to define the extent of tumor; treatment of all parameningeal RMS patients with radiation therapy (in the SIOP-84 study, 18 of 44 had not undergone radiotherapy, and only 5 survived); a minimum dose of 50 Gy with a 2 cm margin; and routine external quality control of radiation.[316]

Still controversial in the treatment of parameningeal RMS is the timing of radiotherapy. Early radiotherapy may increase the likelihood of survival, but delaying radiotherapy may permit the use of smaller fields, which could reduce late effects. In the IRS series, earlier radiotherapy was associated with better survival rates in IRS-II and -III, but there were so many other changes in treatment that its role cannot be isolated.[248] A retrospective study of radiation therapy variables in parameningeal cases in IRS-II through -IV compared 5-year local failure and failure-free survival rates of patients whose radiotherapy had begun within 2 weeks of entry into the study, as opposed to after 2 weeks of entry. Timely radiation therapy almost halved the local failure rates in patients with any meningeal impingement (33% vs. 18%, $P = 0.03$) or intracranial extension (37% vs. 16%, $P = 0.07$), but it had a much smaller and statistically insignificant effect on event-free survival rates.[317]

On the other hand, a single-institution study of 22 patients with parameningeal RMSs showed that the use of a shrinking-field technique reduced the mean treated area by half, from 99 cm² prechemotherapy to 48 cm² postchemotherapy, with no apparent effect on relapse-free survival rates.[318] A similar single-institution study was designed to begin radiotherapy at week 12 of treatment (it actually began at a median of 21 weeks), but used the prechemotherapy tumor volume as the target volume, with a 2 cm margin. Only 1 of 13 patients had an isolated local recurrence, and the 3-year event-free survival rate was 85%.[319] No patient in either study experienced local tumor progression during initial chemotherapy.

Megatherapy for Metastatic and Recurrent Rhabdomyosarcomas

A key question in the treatment of patients with metastases at diagnosis is the role of megatherapy: high-dose chemotherapy, with or without total body irradiation, with autologous (occasionally allogeneic) stem cell or marrow transplantation. There are vast differences among the various populations of patients with metastases; 3-year survival rates range from 5% to 47%. Similarly, an analysis of survival rates after relapse in IRS-III, -IV pilot, and -IV showed 5-year survival rates ranging from 3% (for patients with alveolar histology and originally group II, III, or IV tumors) to 72% (for patients with originally stage 1 or group I tumors and embryonal histology).[320]

There are also wide variations in the criteria for entry into megatherapy studies, ranging from having a complete response to initial salvage chemotherapy to failing to achieve a complete response to initial chemotherapy. Often, the entry criteria and key terms (e.g., high risk) remain undefined. For all these reasons, reports of the results of megatherapy in

RMS merit careful scrutiny (see Meyers[321] for an excellent review).

No randomized controlled trials examine the role of megatherapy in these patients. The IRS-COG has focused on "phase II window" designs for patients with metastases at diagnosis since the completion of IRS-III,[238] and it recently completed a study of patients with relapsed RMS that received intense multiagent chemotherapy but no megatherapy.[271] Until randomized controlled trials are performed, the role of megatherapy in RMS will remain undefined.

FOLLOW-UP AFTER TREATMENT

Surveillance and Patterns of Recurrence

Kaplan-Meier plots of many studies of newly diagnosed RMSs show that the vast majority of failures (progression or relapse) occur in the 3 years following diagnosis, although they can occur even 9 years after diagnosis. The complex nature of RMS persists in the complex patterns of failure, varying by primary site and histology, and in its ability to be local, regional (lymph nodes), metastatic, or any combination of these locales. In IRS-III, for example, local failures outnumbered distant failures by 7 to 1 in patients with orbital primary tumors; but among patients with primary sites in the extremities, distant and combined failures outnumbered local failures by almost 7 to 1. Among patients with embryonal histology tumors, local failures outnumbered combined and distant failures by about 2 to 1, but among patients with alveolar and other histologies, combined and distant failures were more common.[322]

In the same analysis of failure patterns in IRS-III, univariate analysis identified N1 (clinically positive) nodal status as the key risk factor for local or combined local and regional or distant failure; N1 nodal status was, in turn, associated with older age, alveolar histology, large (>5 cm) tumors, and unfavorable primary sites.[322] Distant failure was most likely in patients with N1 nodes and primary tumors in limbs.

Failure patterns appear to have changed across the first three IRS studies, but this may be the result of shifts in definitions and classifications. Attention to definitions is again necessary when assessing reports because, for example, failures in regional lymph nodes may be considered local (if they were within the radiation therapy field), regional, or distant.

The follow-up intervals prescribed in COG RMS protocols reflect the changes in risk over time. They include a history, physical examination, and chest imaging (radiograph or CT) every 3 months during the first year after therapy, every 4 months during the second and third years, and every 6 months during the fourth year, with primary site imaging depending upon the site and the primary tumor treatment used. During and annually after this follow-up for tumor recurrence, monitoring for late effects of treatment is also necessary.

Late Effects

The late effects of childhood cancer and its treatment are discussed thoroughly in Chapter 32. In patients treated for RMS, most observed late effects derive from the tumor itself (for example, cranial nerve palsies caused by parameningeal tumors), from surgery, or from radiation therapy. The sequelae of radiation therapy are particularly problematic because of the young ages of many of the patients and the locations of their tumors.

The late effects of chemotherapy are particularly relevant to RMS; they include late hemorrhagic cystitis resulting from cyclophosphamide and ifosfamide and secondary myelodysplasia or leukemia. Ifosfamide may cause nephropathy, which is occasionally progressive.[323] Relatively few patients treated according to current protocols receive anthracyclines (with the attendant risk that they will cause late heart disease) or cisplatin (with the risk that it will cause hearing loss and renal dysfunction). Sterility in males and early menopause in females may result from the high doses of alkylating agents used.

FUTURE DIRECTIONS

Among embryonal RMSs there is an enormous range of clinical behavior that varies with site and age. Fusion-bearing alveolar RMS is a highly aggressive tumor, with the *PAX7-FKHR*–bearing variant perhaps being less so. However, we remain far from having molecularly based classifications of RMS that correlate with, much less explain, the enormous heterogeneity we observe in clinical behavior. Techniques such as gene expression profiling and increasingly sophisticated analyses of combined clinical and laboratory data may allow us to discern the combinations of tumor and host variables that make, for example, a paratesticular embryonal RMS much more aggressive in a teenager than in a preschooler.

More sophisticated classifications allow for opportunities to tailor chemotherapy, but also present the challenge of smaller populations of patients for study. In the COG, it is already barely statistically feasible to carry out randomized controlled trials with intermediate-risk patients in 5 years. International collaboration has the benefit of providing larger patient numbers, but having fewer studies means that fewer ideas are tested. The bureaucratic and regulatory barriers are also formidable. The path through these obstacles is not clear.

Therapeutically, there are two challenges: identifying promising new agents and integrating them into existing therapy. One cannot predict which of the many newly discovered biochemical pathways and small-molecule inhibitors will lead to improvements in outcome in RMS patients. The numbers of patients are too small to provide an attractive market for the pharmaceutical industry, so an agent that would (for example) specifically block the action of the *PAX-FKHR* fusion protein is unlikely to become available. However, downstream from the fusion proteins lie potential pharmacologic targets that may well be commercially interesting.

The quest for new targets and agents is unlikely to lead to a magic bullet that makes current therapy obsolete, so we must further our efforts by using traditional chemotherapy, then carefully integrate new agents. Vast improvements in outcome have occurred in the leukemias in the past decade, through the use of a collection of drugs that are at least a quarter-century old; one of the advantages of that disease system is easy evaluation of response through marrow aspiration. Good early-response markers (perhaps PET) could extend some of the same advantages to RMS and other solid tumors.

REFERENCES

1. Parham DM, Ellison DA. Rhabdomyosarcomas in adults and children: an update. Arch Pathol Lab Med. 2006;130:1454-1465.
2. Qualman SJ, Coffin CM, Newton WA, et al. Intergroup Rhabdomyosarcoma Study: update for pathologists. Pediatr Dev Pathol. 1998;1:550-561.
3. Garber JE, Offit K. Hereditary cancer predisposition syndromes. J Clin Oncol. 2005;23:276-292.
4. Li FP, Fraumeni JF Jr, Rhabdomyosarcoma in children: epidemiologic study and identification of a familial cancer syndrome. J Natl Cancer Inst. 1969;43:1365-1373.
5. Birch JM, Hartley AL, Blair V, et al. Cancer in the families of children with soft tissue sarcoma. Cancer. 1990;66:2239-2248.
6. Malkin D, Li FP, Strong LC, et al. Germline p53 mutations in a familial syndrome of breast cancer, sarcomas, and other neoplasms. Science. 1990;250:1233-1238 (comment).
7. Varley JM, McGown G, Thorncroft M, et al. Germ-line mutations of *TP53* in Li-Fraumeni families: an extended study of 39 families. Cancer Res. 1997;57:3245-3252.
8. Sedlacek Z, Kodet R, Seemanova E, et al. Two Li-Fraumeni syndrome families with novel germline p53 mutations: loss of the wild-type p53 allele in only 50% of tumours. Br J Cancer. 1998;77:1034-1039.
9. Malkin D, Chilton-MacNeill S, Meister LA, et al. Tissue-specific expression of *SV40* in tumors associated with the Li-Fraumeni syndrome. Oncogene. 2001;20:4441-4449.
10. Knudson AJ. Mutation and cancer: statistical study of retinoblastoma. Proc Natl Acad Sci U S A. 1971;68:820-823.
11. Cornelis RS, van Vliet M, van de Vijver MJ, et al. Three germline mutations in the *TP53* gene. Hum Mutat. 1997;9:157-163.
12. Avigad S, Peleg D, Barel D, et al. Prenatal diagnosis in Li-Fraumeni syndrome. J Pediatr Hematol Oncol. 2004;26:541-545.
13. Khayat CM, Johnston DL. Rhabdomyosarcoma, osteosarcoma, and adrenocortical carcinoma in a child with a germline p53 mutation. Pediatr Blood Cancer. 2004;43:683-686.
14. Cavalier ME, Davis MM, Croop JM. Germline p53 mutation presenting as synchronous tumors. J Pediatr Hematol Oncol. 2005;27:441-443.
15. Diller L, Sexsmith E, Gottlieb A, et al. Germline p53 mutations are frequently detected in young children with rhabdomyosarcoma. J Clin Invest. 1995;95:1606-1611.
16. Bell DW, Varley JM, Szydlo TE, et al. Heterozygous germ line *hCHK2* mutations in Li-Fraumeni syndrome. Science. 1999;286:2528-2531.
17. Donaldson SS, Egbert PR, Newsham I, Cavenee WK. Retinoblastoma. In Pizzo PA, Poplack DG (eds). Principles and Practice of Pediatric Oncology, 3rd ed. Philadelphia, Lippincott-Raven, 1997, pp 699-715.
18. Kleinerman RA, Tucker MA, Abramson DH, et al. Risk of soft tissue sarcomas by individual subtype in survivors of hereditary retinoblastoma. J Natl Cancer Inst. 2007;99:24-31.
19. Hasegawa T, Matsuno Y, Niki T, et al. Second primary rhabdomyosarcomas in patients with bilateral retinoblastoma: a clinicopathologic and immunohistochemical study. Am J Surg Pathol. 1998;22:1351-1360.
20. Basu TN, Gutmann DH, Fletcher JA, et al. Aberrant regulation of *ras* proteins in malignant tumour cells from type 1 neurofibromatosis patients. Nature. 1992;356:713-715.
21. Xu GF, O'Connell P, Viskochil D, et al. The neurofibromatosis type 1 gene encodes a protein related to gap. Cell. 1990;62:599-608.
22. Rasmussen SA, Friedman JM. *NF1* gene and neurofibromatosis 1. Am J Epidemiol. 2000;151:33-40.
23. Plon SE, Peterson LE. Childhood cancer, heredity, and the environment. In Pizzo P, Poplack D (eds). Principles and Practice of Pediatric Oncology, 3rd ed. Philadelphia, Lippincott-Raven, 1997, pp 11-36.
24. McKeen EA, Bodurtha J, Meadows AT, et al. Rhabdomyosarcoma complicating multiple neurofibromatosis. J Pediatr. 1978;93:992-993.
25. Yang P, Grufferman S, Khoury MJ, et al. Association of childhood rhabdomyosarcoma with neurofibromatosis type I and birth defects. Genet Epidemiol. 1995;12:467-474.
26. Matsui I, Tanimura M, Kobayashi N, et al. Neurofibromatosis type 1 and childhood cancer. Cancer. 1993;72:2746-2754.

27. Sung L, Anderson JR, Arndt C, et al. Neurofibromatosis in children with rhabdomyosarcoma: a report from the Intergroup Rhabdomyosarcoma Study IV. J Pediatr. 2004;144:666-668.

28. Hennekam RC. Costello syndrome: an overview. Am J Med Genet. 2003;117C:42-48.

29. Gripp KW. Tumor predisposition in Costello syndrome. Am J Med Genet C Semin Med Genet. 2005;137:72-77.

30. Aoki Y, Niihori T, Kawame H, et al. Germline mutations in HRAS proto-oncogene cause Costello syndrome. Nat Genet. 2005;37:1038-1040.

31. Estep AL, Tidyman WE, Teitell MA, et al. *HRAS* mutations in Costello syndrome: detection of constitutional activating mutations in codon 12 and 13 and loss of wild-type allele in malignancy. Am J Med Genet A. 2006;140:8-16.

32. Schubbert S, Bollag G, Shannon K. Deregulated RAS signaling in developmental disorders: new tricks for an old dog. Curr Opin Genet Dev. 2007;17:15-22.

33. Khan S, McDowell H, Upadhyaya M, Fryer A. Vaginal rhabdomyosarcoma in a patient with Noonan syndrome. J Med Genet. 1995;32:743-745.

34. Jung A, Bechthold S, Pfluger T, et al. Orbital rhabdomyosarcoma in Noonan syndrome. J Pediatr Hematol Oncol. 2003;25:330-332.

35. Moschovi M, Vassiliki T, Anna P, et al. Rhabdomyosarcoma in a patient with Noonan syndrome phenotype and review of the literature. J Pediatr Hematol Oncol. 2007;29:341-344.

36. Bisogno G, Murgia A, Mammi I, et al. Rhabdomyosarcoma in a patient with cardio-fascio-cutaneous syndrome. J Pediatr Hematol Oncol. 1999;21:424-427.

37. Innes AM, Chudley AE. Rhabdomyosarcoma in a patient with cardio-fascio-cutaneous syndrome. J Pediatr Hematol Oncol. 2000;22:546-547.

38. Agras PI, Baskin E, Sakallioglu AE, et al. Neurofibromatosis: Noonan's syndrome with associated rhabdomyosarcoma of the urinary bladder in an infant: case report. J Child Neurol. 2003;18:68-72.

39. Oguzkan S, Terzi YK, Guler E, et al. Two neurofibromatosis type 1 cases associated with rhabdomyosarcoma of bladder, one with a large deletion in the *NF1* gene. Cancer Genet Cytogenet. 2006;164:159-163.

40. Weksberg R, Shuman C, Smith AC. Beckwith-Wiedemann syndrome. Am J Med Genet C Semin Med Genet. 2005;137:12-23.

41. Aideyan UO, Kao SC. Case report: urinary bladder rhabdomyosarcoma associated with Beckwith-Wiedemann syndrome. Clin Radiol. 1998;53:457-459.

42. Sotelo-Avila C, Gonzalez-Crussi F, Fowler JW. Complete and incomplete forms of Beckwith-Wiedemann syndrome: their oncogenic potential. J Pediatr. 1980;96:47-50.

43. Vaughan WG, Sanders DW, Grosfeld JL, et al. Favorable outcome in children with Beckwith-Wiedemann syndrome and intraabdominal malignant tumors. J Pediatr Surg. 1995;30:1042-1044.

44. Matsumoto T, Kinoshita E, Maeda H, et al. Molecular analysis of a patient with Beckwith-Wiedemann syndrome, rhabdomyosarcoma and renal cell carcinoma. Jpn J Hum Genet. 1994;39:225-234.

45. Rethy LL, Kalmanchey RR, Klujber VV, et al. Acid sphingomyelinase deficiency in Beckwith-Wiedemann syndrome. Pathol Oncol Res. 2000;6:295-297.

46. Smith AC, Squire JA, Thorner P, et al. Association of alveolar rhabdomyosarcoma with the Beckwith-Wiedemann syndrome. Pediatr Dev Pathol. 2001;4:550-558.

47. Ruymann FB, Maddux HR, Ragab A, et al. Congenital anomalies associated with rhabdomyosarcoma: an autopsy study of 115 cases. A report from the Intergroup Rhabdomyosarcoma Study Committee (representing the Children's Cancer Study Group, the Pediatric Oncology Group, the United Kingdom Children's Cancer Study Group, and the Pediatric Intergroup Statistical Center). Med Pediatr Oncol. 1988;16:33-39.

48. Samuel DP, Tsokos M, DeBaun MR. Hemihypertrophy and a poorly differentiated embryonal rhabdomyosarcoma of the pelvis. Med Pediatr Oncol. 1999;32:38-43.

49. Thavaraj V, Sethi A, Arya LS. Incomplete Beckwith-Wiedemann syndrome in a child with orbital rhabdomyosarcoma. Indian Pediatr. 2002;39:299-304.

50. Johnson RL, Rothman AL, Xie J, et al. Human homolog of patched, a candidate gene for the basal cell nevus syndrome. Science. 1996;272:1668-1671.

51. Gorlin RJ. Nevoid basal cell carcinoma syndrome. Dermatol Clin. 1995;13:113-125.

52. Beddis IR, Mott MG, Bullimore J. Case report: nasopharyngeal rhabdomyosarcoma and Gorlin's naevoid basal cell carcinoma syndrome. Med Pediatr Oncol. 1983;11:178-179.

53. Antley CA, Carney M, Smoller BR. Microcystic adnexal carcinoma arising in the setting of previous radiation therapy. J Cutan Pathol 1999;26:48-50.

54. Schweisguth O, Gerard-Marchant R, Lemerle J. Basal cell nevus syndrome: association with congenital rhabdomyosarcoma. Arch Fr Pediatr. 1968;25:1083-1093 (in French).

55. Cajaiba MM, Bale AE, Alvarez-Franco M, et al. Rhabdomyosarcoma, Wilms' tumor, and deletion of the patched gene in Gorlin syndrome. Nat Clin Pract Oncol. 2006;3:575-580.

56. Rubinstein JH, Taybi H. Broad thumbs and toes and facial abnormalities: a possible mental retardation syndrome. Am J Dis Child. 1963;105:588-608.

57. Miller RW, Rubinstein JH. Tumors in Rubinstein-Taybi syndrome. Am J Med Genet. 1995;56:112-115 (comments).

58. Siraganian PA, Rubinstein JH, Miller RW. Keloids and neoplasms in the Rubinstein-Taybi syndrome. Med Pediatr Oncol. 1989;17:485-491.

59. Sobel RA, Woerner S. Rubinstein-Taybi syndrome and nasopharyngeal rhabdomyosarcoma. J Pediatr. 1981;99:1000-1001 (letter).

60. Imaizumi K, Kuroki Y. Rubinstein-Taybi syndrome with de novo reciprocal translocation t(2;16)(p13.3;p13.3). Am J Med Genet. 1991;38:636-639.

61. Petrij F, Giles RH, Dauwerse HG, et al. Rubinstein-Taybi syndrome caused by mutations in the transcriptional co-activator CBP. Nature. 1995;376:348-351 (comments).

62. Tommerup NH, van der Hagen CB, Heiberg A. Tentative assignment of a locus for Rubinstein-Taybi syndrome gene to 16p13.3 by a de novo reciprocal translocation, t(7;16)(q34;p13.3). Am J Med Genet Genet. 1992;44:237-241.

63. Iyer NG, Ozdag H, Caldas C. p300/*CBP* and cancer. Oncogene. 2004;23:4225-4231.

64. Grossman SR. p300/*CBP/p53* interaction and regulation of the p53 response. Eur J Biochem. 2001;268:2773-2778.

65. Turc-Carel C, Lizard-Nacol S, Justrabo E, et al. Consistent chromosomal translocation in alveolar rhabdomyosarcoma. Cancer Genet Cytogenet. 1986;19:361-362.

66. Douglass EC, Valentine M, Etcubanas E, et al. A specific chromosomal abnormality in rhabdomyosarcoma. Cytogenet Cell Genet. 1987;45:148-155.

67. Wang-Wuu S, Soukup S, Ballard E, et al. Chromosomal analysis of sixteen human rhabdomyosarcomas. Cancer Res. 1988;48:983-987.

68. Biegel JA, Meek RS, Parmiter AH, et al. Chromosomal translocation t(1;13)(p36;q14) in a case of rhabdomyosarcoma. Genes Chromosomes Cancer. 1991;3:483-484.

69. Douglass EC, Rowe ST, Valentine M, et al. Variant translocations of chromosome 13 in alveolar rhabdomyosarcoma. Genes Chromosomes Cancer. 1991;3:480-482.

70. Mrozek K, Arthur DC, Karakousis CP, et al. Der(16)t(1;16) is a nonrandom secondary chromosome aberration in many types of human neoplasia, including myxoid liposarcoma, rhabdomyo-

sarcoma and Philadelphia chromosome-positive acute lymphoblastic leukemia. Int J Oncol. 1995;6:531-538.

71. Udayakumar AM, Sundareshan TS, Appaji L, et al. Rhabdomyosarcoma: cytogenetics of five cases using fine-needle aspiration samples and review of the literature. Ann Genet. 2002;45:33-37.

72. Weber-Hall S, Anderson J, McManus A, et al. Gains, losses, and amplification of genomic material in rhabdomyosarcoma analyzed by comparative genomic hybridization. Cancer Res. 1996;56:3220-3224.

73. Pandita A, Zielenska M, Thorner P, et al. Application of comparative genomic hybridization, spectral karyotyping, and microarray analysis in the identification of subtype-specific patterns of genomic changes in rhabdomyosarcoma. Neoplasia. 1999;1:262-275.

74. Bridge JA, Liu J, Qualman SJ, et al. Genomic gains and losses are similar in genetic and histologic subsets of rhabdomyosarcoma, whereas amplification predominates in embryonal with anaplasia and alveolar subtypes. Genes Chromosomes Cancer. 2002;33:310-321.

75. Gordon AT, Brinkschmidt C, Anderson J, et al. A novel and consistent amplicon at 13q31 associated with alveolar rhabdomyosarcoma. Genes Chromosomes Cancer. 2000;28:220-226.

76. Barr FG, Galili N, Holick J, et al. Rearrangement of the *PAX3* paired box gene in the paediatric solid tumour alveolar rhabdomyosarcoma. Nat Genet. 1993;3:113-117.

77. Davis RJ, D'Cruz CM, Lovell MA, et al. Fusion of *PAX7* to *FKHR* by the variant t(1;13)(p36;q14) translocation in alveolar rhabdomyosarcoma. Cancer Res. 1994;54:2869-2872.

78. Galili N, Davis RJ, Fredericks WJ, et al. Fusion of a forkhead domain gene to *PAX3* in the solid tumour alveolar rhabdomyosarcoma (published erratum appears in Nat Genet 1994;6:214). Nat Genet. 1993;5:230-235.

79. Bennicelli JL, Advani S, Schafer BW, Barr FG. PAX3 and PAX7 exhibit conserved *cis*-acting transcription repression domains and utilize a common gain of function mechanism in alveolar rhabdomyosarcoma. Oncogene. 1999;18:4348-4356.

80. Bennicelli JL, Edwards RH, Barr FG. Mechanism for transcriptional gain of function resulting from chromosomal translocation in alveolar rhabdomyosarcoma. Proc Natl Acad Sci U S A. 1996;93:5455-5459.

81. Visser M, Sijmons C, Bras J, et al. Allelotype of pediatric rhabdomyosarcoma. Oncogene. 1997;15:1309-1314.

82. Koufos A, Hansen MF, Copeland NG, et al. Loss of heterozygosity in three embryonal tumours suggests a common pathogenetic mechanism. Nature. 1985;316:330-334.

83. Scrable HJ, Witte DP, Lampkin BC, Cavenee WK. Chromosomal localization of the human rhabdomyosarcoma locus by mitotic recombination mapping. Nature. 1987;329:645-647.

84. Brinkschmidt C, Poremba C, Schafer KL, et al. Evidence of genetic alterations in chromosome 11 in embryonal and alveolar rhabdomyosarcoma. Verh Dtsch Ges Pathol. 1998;82:210-214 (in German).

85. Loh WE Jr, Scrable HJ, Livanos E, et al. Human chromosome 11 contains two different growth suppressor genes for embryonal rhabdomyosarcoma. Proc Natl Acad Sci U S A. 1992;89:1755-1759.

86. Koi M, Johnson LA, Kalikin LM, et al. Tumor cell growth arrest caused by subchromosomal transferable DNA fragments from chromosome 11. Science. 1993;260:361-364.

87. Scrable H, Witte D, Shimada H, et al. Molecular differential pathology of rhabdomyosarcoma. Genes Chromosomes Cancer. 1989;1:23-35.

88. Dias P, Kumar P, Marsden HB, et al. The N-*myc* gene is amplified in alveolar rhabdomyosarcomas (RMS) but not in embryonal rms. Int J Cancer. 1990;45:593-596.

89. Driman D, Thorner PS, Greenberg ML, et al. *MYCN* gene amplification in rhabdomyosarcoma. Cancer. 1994;73:2231-2237.

90. Hachitanda Y, Toyoshima S, Akazawa K, Tsuneyoshi M. N-*myc* gene amplification in rhabdomyosarcoma detected by fluorescence in situ hybridization: its correlation with histologic features. Mod Pathol. 1998;11:1222-1227.

91. Williamson D, Lu YJ, Gordon T, et al. Relationship between *MYCN* copy number and expression in rhabdomyosarcomas and correlation with adverse prognosis in the alveolar subtype. J Clin Oncol. 2005;23:880-888.

92. Knuutila S, Bjorkqvist AM, Autio K, et al. DNA copy number amplifications in human neoplasms: review of comparative genomic hybridization studies. Am J Pathol. 1998;152:1107-1123.

93. Berner JM, Forus A, Elkahloun A, et al. Separate amplified regions encompassing *CDK4* and *MDM2* in human sarcomas. Genes Chromosomes Cancer. 1996;17:254-259.

94. Ragazzini P, Gamberi G, Pazzaglia L, et al. Amplification of *CDK4, MDM2, SAS* and *GLI1* genes in leiomyosarcoma, alveolar and embryonal rhabdomyosarcoma. Histol Histopathol. 2004;19:401-411.

95. Taylor AC, Shu L, Danks MK, et al. *p53* Mutation and *MDM2* amplification frequency in pediatric rhabdomyosarcoma tumors and cell lines. Med Pediatr Oncol. 2000;35:96-103.

96. Takahashi Y, Oda Y, Kawaguchi K, et al. Altered expression and molecular abnormalities of cell-cycle-regulatory proteins in rhabdomyosarcoma. Mod Pathol. 2004;17:660-669.

97. Barr FG, Nauta LE, Davis RJ, et al. In vivo amplification of the *PAX3-FKHR* and *PAX7-FKHR* fusion genes in alveolar rhabdomyosarcoma. Hum Mol Genet. 1996;5:15-21.

98. Davis RJ, Barr FG. Fusion genes resulting from alternative chromosomal translocations are overexpressed by gene-specific mechanisms in alveolar rhabdomyosarcoma. Proc Natl Acad Sci U S A. 1997;94:8047-8051.

99. Williamson D, Selfe J, Gordon T, et al. Role for amplification and expression of glypican-5 in rhabdomyosarcoma. Cancer Res. 2007;67:57-65.

100. De Chiara A, T'Ang A, Triche TJ. Expression of the retinoblastoma susceptibility gene in childhood rhabdomyosarcomas. J Natl Cancer Inst. 1993;85:152-157.

101. Iolascon A, Faienza MF, Coppola B, et al. Analysis of cyclin-dependent kinase inhibitor genes (*CDKN2A, CDKN2B,* and *CDKN2C*) in childhood rhabdomyosarcoma. Genes Chromosomes Cancer. 1996;15:217-222.

102. Gao Z, Zhang S, Yang G. A study of p16 gene and its protein expression in rhabdomyosarcoma. Zhonghua Bing Li Xue Za Zhi. 1998;27:290-293.

103. Felix CA, Kappel CC, Mitsudomi T, et al. Frequency and diversity of *p53* mutations in childhood rhabdomyosarcoma. Cancer Res. 1992;52:2243-2247.

104. Stratton MR, Moss S, Warren W, et al. Mutation of the *p53* gene in human soft tissue sarcomas: association with abnormalities of the *RB1* gene. Oncogene. 1990;5:1297-1301.

105. Wurl P, Taubert H, Bache M, et al. Frequent occurrence of *p53* mutations in rhabdomyosarcoma and leiomyosarcoma, but not in fibrosarcoma and malignant neural tumors. Int J Cancer. 1996;69:317-323.

106. Mousses S, McAuley L, Bell RS, et al. Molecular and immunohistochemical identification of *p53* alterations in bone and soft tissue sarcomas. Mod Pathol. 1996;9:1-6.

107. Kusafuka T, Fukuzawa M, Oue T, et al. Mutation analysis of *p53* gene in childhood malignant solid tumors. J Pediatr Surg. 1997;32:1175-1180.

108. Mulligan LM, Matlashewski GJ, Scrable HJ, Cavenee WK. Mechanisms of *p53* loss in human sarcomas. Proc Natl Acad Sci U S A. 1990;87:5863-5867.

109. Stratton MR, Fisher C, Gusterson BA, Cooper CS. Detection of point mutations in *N-ras* and *K-ras* genes of human embryonal rhabdomyosarcomas using oligonucleotide probes and the polymerase chain reaction. Cancer Res. 1989;49:6324-6327.

110. Wilke W, Maillet M, Robinson R. *H-ras-1* point mutations in soft tissue sarcomas. Mod Pathol. 1993;6:129-132.

111. Kratz CP, Steinemann D, Niemeyer CM, et al. Uniparental disomy at chromosome 11p15.5 followed by *HRAS* mutations in embryonal rhabdomyosarcoma: lessons from Costello syndrome. Hum Mol Genet. 2007;16:374-379.

112. Chen Y, Takita J, Hiwatari M, et al. Mutations of the *PTPN11* and *RAS* genes in rhabdomyosarcoma and pediatric hematological malignancies. Genes Chromosomes Cancer. 2006;45:583-591.

113. Miao J, Kusafuka T, Fukuzawa M. Hotspot mutations of *BRAF* gene are not associated with pediatric solid neoplasms. Oncol Rep. 2004; 269-1272.

114. Seidel C, Bartel F, Rastetter M, et al. Alterations of cancer-related genes in soft tissue sarcomas: hypermethylation of *RASSF1a* is frequently detected in leiomyosarcoma and associated with poor prognosis in sarcoma. Int J Cancer. 2005;114:442-447.

115. Schaaf G, Hamdi M, Zwijnenburg D, et al. *SPRY1* functions as a collaborating oncogene in embryonal rhabdomyosarcoma cells expressing oncogenic *RAS* or *RAF*. Proc Annu Meet Am Assoc Cancer Res. 2007;48:5697.

116. Herman JG, Baylin SB. Gene silencing in cancer in association with promoter hypermethylation. N Engl J Med. 2003;349:2042-2054.

117. Harada K, Toyooka S, Maitra A, et al. Aberrant promoter methylation and silencing of the *RASSF1A* gene in pediatric tumors and cell lines. Oncogene. 2002;21:4345-4349.

118. Harada K, Toyooka S, Shivapurkar N, et al. Deregulation of caspase 8 and 10 expression in pediatric tumors and cell lines. Cancer Res. 2002;62:5897-5901.

119. Rathi A, Virmani AK, Harada K, et al. Aberrant methylation of the *HIC1* promoter is a frequent event in specific pediatric neoplasms. Clin Cancer Res. 2003;9:3674-3678.

120. Shigematsu H, Suzuki M, Takahashi T, et al. Aberrant methylation of *HIN-1* (high in normal-1) is a frequent event in many human malignancies. Int J Cancer. 2005;113:600-604.

121. Tonin PN, Scrable H, Shimada H, Cavenee WK. Muscle-specific gene expression in rhabdomyosarcomas and stages of human fetal skeletal muscle development. Cancer Res. 1991;51:5100-5106.

122. Sebire NJ, Malone M. Myogenin and *MyoD1* expression in paediatric rhabdomyosarcomas. J Clin Pathol. 2003;56:412-416.

123. Morotti RA, Nicol KK, Parham DM, et al. An immunohistochemical algorithm to facilitate diagnosis and subtyping of rhabdomyosarcoma: the Children's Oncology Group experience. Am J Surg Pathol. 2006;30:962-968.

124. Tapscott SJ, Thayer MJ, Weintraub H. Deficiency in rhabdomyosarcomas of a factor required for MyoD activity and myogenesis. Science. 1993;259:1450-1453.

125. Puri PL, Wu Z, Zhang P, et al. Induction of terminal differentiation by constitutive activation of p38 map kinase in human rhabdomyosarcoma cells. Genes Dev. 2000;14:574-584.

126. Fiddler TA, Smith L, Tapscott SJ, Thayer MJ. Amplification of *MDM2* inhibits MyoD-mediated myogenesis. Mol Cell Biol. 1996;16:5048-5057.

127. Guo CS, Degnin C, Fiddler TA, et al. Regulation of MyoD activity and muscle cell differentiation by MDM2, pRb, and Sp1. J Biol Chem. 2003;278:22615-22622.

128. Ricaud S, Vernus B, Duclos M, et al. Inhibition of autocrine secretion of myostatin enhances terminal differentiation in human rhabdomyosarcoma cells. Oncogene. 2003;22:8221-8232.

129. Gerber AN, Wilson CW, Li YJ, Chuang PT. The hedgehog-regulated oncogenes *Gli1* and *Gli2* block myoblast differentiation by inhibiting myod-mediated transcriptional activation. Oncogene. 2007;26:1122-1136.

130. Goulding MD, Chalepakis G, Deutsch U, et al. Pax-3, a novel murine DNA binding protein expressed during early neurogenesis. EMBO J. 1991;10:1135-1147.

131. Jostes B, Walther C, Gruss P. The murine paired box gene, Pax7, is expressed specifically during the development of the nervous and muscular system. Mech Dev. 1990;33:27-37.

132. Bober E, Franz T, Arnold HH, et al. Pax-3 is required for the development of limb muscles: a possible role for the migration of dermomyotomal muscle progenitor cells. Development. 1994;120:603-612.

133. Seale P, Sabourin LA, Girgis-Gabardo A, et al. Pax7 is required for the specification of myogenic satellite cells. Cell. 2000;102:777-786.

134. Relaix F, Montarras D, Zaffran S, et al. Pax3 and Pax7 have distinct and overlapping functions in adult muscle progenitor cells. J Cell Biol. 2006;172:91-102.

135. Barr FG. Gene fusions involving *FOX* and *PAX* family members in alveolar rhabdomyosarcoma. Oncogene. 2001;20:5736-5746.

136. Tiffin N, Williams RD, Shipley J, Pritchard-Jones K. *PAX7* expression in embryonal rhabdomyosarcoma suggests an origin in muscle satellite cells. Br J Cancer. 2003;89:327-332.

137. Maroto M, Reshef R, Munsterberg AE, et al. Ectopic Pax-3 activates MyoD and *Myf-5* expression in embryonic mesoderm and neural tissue. Cell. 1997;89:139-148.

138. Khan J, Bittner ML, Saal LH, et al. CDNA microarrays detect activation of a myogenic transcription program by the *PAX3-FKHR* fusion oncogene. Proc Natl Acad Sci U S A. 1999;96:13264-13269.

139. Scuoppo C, Riess I, Schmitt-Ney M, et al. The oncogenic transcription factor *PAX3-FKHR* can convert fibroblasts into contractile myotubes. Exp Cell Res. 2007;313:2308-2317.

140. Epstein JA, Lam P, Jepeal L, et al. Pax3 inhibits myogenic differentiation of cultured myoblast cells. J Biol Chem. 1995;270:11719-11722.

141. Ebauer M, Wachtel M, Niggli FK, Schafer BW. Comparative expression profiling identifies an in vivo target gene signature with TFAP2B as a mediator of the survival function of PAX3/FKHR. Oncogene. 2007;26:7267-7281.

142. Minniti CP, Helman LJ. *IGF-II* in the pathogenesis of rhabdomyosarcoma: a prototype of *IGF*'s involvement in human tumorigenesis. Adv Exp Med Biol. 1993;343:327-343.

143. Minniti CP, Luan D, O'Grady C, et al. Insulin-like growth factor II overexpression in myoblasts induces phenotypic changes typical of the malignant phenotype. Cell Growth Differ. 1995; 6:263-269.

144. El-Badry OM, Minniti C, Kohn EC, et al. Insulin-like growth factor II acts as an autocrine growth and motility factor in human rhabdomyosarcoma tumors. Cell Growth Differ. 1990;1:325-331.

145. Minniti CP, Kohn EC, Grubb JH, et al. The insulin-like growth factor II (IGF-II)/mannose 6-phosphate receptor mediates IGF-II–induced motility in human rhabdomyosarcoma cells. J Biol Chem. 1992;267:9000-9004.

146. Kalebic T, Tsokos M, Helman LJ. In vivo treatment with antibody against IGF-1 receptor suppresses growth of human rhabdomyosarcoma and down-regulates p34cdc2. Cancer Res. 1994;54:5531-5534.

147. Shapiro DN, Jones BG, Shapiro LH, et al. Antisense-mediated reduction in insulin-like growth factor-I receptor expression suppresses the malignant phenotype of a human alveolar rhabdomyosarcoma. J Clin Invest. 1994;94:1235-1242.

148. Kalebic T, Blakesley V, Slade C, et al. Expression of a kinase-deficient *IGF-I-R* suppresses tumorigenicity of rhabdomyosarcoma cells constitutively expressing a wild type *IGF-I-R*. Int J Cancer. 1998;76:223-227.

149. Pedone PV, Tirabosco R, Cavazzana AO, et al. Mono- and bi-allelic expression of insulin-like growth factor II gene in human muscle tumors. Hum Mol Genet. 1994;3:1117-1121.

150. Zhan S, Shapiro DN, Helman LJ. Activation of an imprinted allele of the insulin-like growth factor II gene implicated in rhabdomyosarcoma. J Clin Invest. 1994;94:445-448.

151. Anderson J, Gordon A, McManus A, et al. Disruption of imprinted genes at chromosome region 11p15.5 in paediatric rhabdomyosarcoma. Neoplasia. 1999;1:340-348.

152. Birkenkamp KU, Coffer PJ. Regulation of cell survival and proliferation by the Foxo (forkhead box, class o) subfamily of Forkhead transcription factors. Biochem Soc Trans. 2003;31:292-297.

153. del Peso L, Gonzalez VM, Hernandez R, et al. Regulation of the forkhead transcription factor FKHR, but not the PAX3-FKHR fusion protein, by the serine/threonine kinase AKT. Oncogene. 1999;18:7328-7333.

154. Scheidler S, Fredericks WJ, Rauscher FJ 3rd, et al. The hybrid PAX3-FKHR fusion protein of alveolar rhabdomyosarcoma transforms fibroblasts in culture. Proc Natl Acad Sci U S A. 1996; 93:9805-9809.

155. Lam PY, Sublett JE, Hollenbach AD, Roussel MF. The oncogenic potential of the PAX3-FKHR fusion protein requires the PAX3 homeodomain recognition helix but not the PAX3 paired-box DNA binding domain. Mol Cell Biol. 1999;19:594-601.

156. Fredericks WJ, Ayyanathan K, Herlyn M, et al. An engineered PAX3-KRAB transcriptional repressor inhibits the malignant phenotype of alveolar rhabdomyosarcoma cells harboring the endogenous PAX3-FKHR oncogene. Mol Cell Biol. 2000;20: 5019-5031.

157. Cao Y, Wang C. The *COOH*-terminal transactivation domain plays a key role in regulating the in vitro and in vivo function of Pax3 homeodomain. J Biol Chem. 2000;275:9854-9862.

158. Xia SJ, Barr FG. Analysis of the transforming and growth suppressive activities of the PAX3-FKHR oncoprotein. Oncogene. 2004;23:6864-6871.

159. Xia SJ, Rajput P, Strzelecki DM, Barr FG. Analysis of genetic events that modulate the oncogenic and growth suppressive activities of the PAX3-FKHR fusion oncoprotein. Lab Invest. 2007;87:318-325.

160. Linardic CM, Naini S, Herndon JE 2nd, et al. The *PAX3-FKHR* fusion gene of rhabdomyosarcoma cooperates with loss of p16INK4A to promote bypass of cellular senescence. Cancer Res. 2007;67:6691-6699.

161. Bernasconi M, Remppis A, Fredericks WJ, et al. Induction of apoptosis in rhabdomyosarcoma cells through down-regulation of PAX proteins. Proc Natl Acad Sci U S A. 1996;93:13164-13169.

162. Ayyanathan K, Fredericks WJ, Berking C, et al. Hormone-dependent tumor regression in vivo by an inducible transcriptional repressor directed at the *PAX3-FKHR* oncogene. Cancer Res. 2000;60:5803-5814.

163. Kalebic T, Judde JG, Velez-Yanguas M, et al. Metastatic human rhabdomyosarcoma: molecular, cellular and cytogenetic analysis of a novel cellular model. Invasion Metastasis. 1996;16:83-96.

164. Lollini PL, De Giovanni C, Landuzzi L, et al. Reduced metastatic ability of in vitro differentiated human rhabdomyosarcoma cells. Invasion Metastasis. 1991;11:116-124.

165. Daniel L, Durbec P, Gautherot E, et al. A nude mice model of human rhabdomyosarcoma lung metastases for evaluating the role of polysialic acids in the metastatic process. Oncogene. 2001;20:997-1004.

166. Chan BM, Matsuura N, Takada Y, et al. In vitro and in vivo consequences of *VLA-2* expression on rhabdomyosarcoma cells. Science. 1991;251:1600-1602.

167. Diomedi-Camassei F, Boldrini R, Rava L, et al. Different pattern of matrix metalloproteinase expression in alveolar versus embryonal rhabdomyosarcoma. J Pediatr Surg. 2004;39:1673-1679.

168. Onisto M, Slongo ML, Gregnanin L, et al. Expression and activity of vascular endothelial growth factor and metalloproteinases in alveolar and embryonal rhabdomyosarcoma cell lines. Int J Oncol. 2005;27:791-798.

169. Scholl FA, Betts DR, Niggli FK, Schafer BW. Molecular features of a human rhabdomyosarcoma cell line with spontaneous metastatic progression. Br J Cancer. 2000;82:1239-1245.

170. Ito H, Duxbury M, Benoit E, et al. Fibronectin-induced COX-2 mediates *MMP*-2 expression and invasiveness of rhabdomyosarcoma. Biochem Biophys Res Commun. 2004;318:594-600.

171. Libura J, Drukala J, Majka M, et al. CXCR4-SDF-1 signaling is active in rhabdomyosarcoma cells and regulates locomotion, chemotaxis, and adhesion. Blood. 2002;100:2597-2606.

172. Jankowski K, Kucia M, Wysoczynski M, et al. Both hepatocyte growth factor (HGF) and stromal-derived factor-1 regulate the metastatic behavior of human rhabdomyosarcoma cells, but only HGF enhances their resistance to radiochemotherapy. Cancer Res. 2003;63:7926-7935.

173. Wysoczynski M, Miekus K, Jankowski K, et al. Leukemia inhibitory factor: a newly identified metastatic factor in rhabdomyosarcomas. Cancer Res. 2007;67:2131-2140.

174. Sharp R, Recio JA, Jhappan C, et al. Synergism between INK4A/ARF inactivation and aberrant HGF/SF signaling in rhabdomyosarcomagenesis. Nat Med. 2002;8:1276-1280.

175. Yu Y, Khan J, Khanna C, et al. Expression profiling identifies the cytoskeletal organizer ezrin and the developmental homeoprotein Six-1 as key metastatic regulators. Nat Med. 2004;10:175-181.

176. Yu Y, Davicioni E, Triche TJ, Merlino G. The homeoprotein six1 transcriptionally activates multiple protumorigenic genes but requires ezrin to promote metastasis. Cancer Res. 2006;66:1982-1989.

177. Lavigueur A, Maltby V, Mock D, et al. High incidence of lung, bone, and lymphoid tumors in transgenic mice overexpressing mutant alleles of the p53 oncogene. Mol Cell Biol. 1989;9:3982-3991.

178. Donehower LA, Harvey M, Slagle BL, et al. Mice deficient for p53 are developmentally normal but susceptible to spontaneous tumours. Nature. 1992;356:215-221.

179. Jacks T, Remington L, Williams BO, et al. Tumor spectrum analysis in p53-mutant mice. Curr Biol. 1994;4:1-7.

180. Nanni P, Nicoletti G, De Giovanni C, et al. Development of rhabdomyosarcoma in *HER-2/neu* transgenic p53 mutant mice. Cancer Res. 2003;63:2728-2732.

181. Fleischmann A, Jochum W, Eferl R, et al. Rhabdomyosarcoma development in mice lacking *Trp53* and *Fos*: tumor suppression by the Fos proto-oncogene. Cancer Cell. 2003;4:477-482.

182. Tsumura H, Yoshida T, Saito H, et al. Cooperation of oncogenic *K-ras* and p53 deficiency in pleomorphic rhabdomyosarcoma development in adult mice. Oncogene. 2006;25:7673-7679.

183. Goodrich LV, Milenkovic L, Higgins KM, Scott MP. Altered neural cell fates and medulloblastoma in mouse patched mutants. Science. 1997;277:1109-1113.

184. Hahn H, Wojnowski L, Zimmer AM, et al. Rhabdomyosarcomas and radiation hypersensitivity in a mouse model of Gorlin syndrome. Nat Med. 1998;4:619-622.

185. Wetmore C, Eberhart DE, Curran T. Loss of p53 but not *ARF* accelerates medulloblastoma in mice heterozygous for patched. Cancer Res. 2001;61:513-516.

186. Kappler R, Bauer R, Calzada-Wack J, et al. Profiling the molecular difference between patched- and p53-dependent rhabdomyosarcoma. Oncogene. 2004;23:8785-8795.

187. Koleva M, Kappler R, Vogler M, et al. Pleiotropic effects of sonic hedgehog on muscle satellite cells. Cell Mol Life Sci. 2005;62:1863-1870.

188. Uhmann A, Ferch U, Bauer R, et al. A model for *PTCH1/Ptch1*-associated tumors comprising mutational inactivation and gene silencing. Int J Oncol. 2005;27:1567-1575.

189. Hahn H, Wojnowski L, Specht K, et al. Patched target *IgF2* is indispensable for the formation of medulloblastoma and rhabdomyosarcoma. J Biol Chem. 2000;275:28341-28344.

190. Lee Y, Kawagoe R, Sasai K, et al. Loss of suppressor-of-fused function promotes tumorigenesis. Oncogene. 2007;26:6442-6447.

191. Mao J, Ligon KL, Rakhlin EY, et al. A novel somatic mouse model to survey tumorigenic potential applied to the hedgehog pathway. Cancer Res. 2006;66:10171-10178.

192. Takayama H, LaRochelle WJ, Sharp R, et al. Diverse tumorigenesis associated with aberrant development in mice overexpressing hepatocyte growth factor/scatter factor. Proc Natl Acad Sci U S A. 1997;94:701-706.

193. Anderson MJ, Shelton GD, Cavenee WK, Arden KC. Embryonic expression of the tumor-associated PAX3-FKHR fusion protein interferes with the developmental functions of Pax3. Proc Natl Acad Sci U S A. 2001;98:1589-1594.

194. Lagutina I, Conway SJ, Sublett J, Grosveld GC. Pax3-FKHR knock-in mice show developmental aberrations but do not develop tumors. Mol Cell Biol. 2002;22:7204-7216.

195. Relaix F, Polimeni M, Rocancourt D, et al. The transcriptional activator *PAX3-FKHR* rescues the defects of *Pax3* mutant mice but induces a myogenic gain-of-function phenotype with ligand-independent activation of Met signaling in vivo. Genes Dev. 2003;17:2950-2965.

196. Keller C, Hansen MS, Coffin CM, Capecchi MR. Pax3-Fkhr interferes with embryonic Pax3 and Pax7 function: implications for alveolar rhabdomyosarcoma cell of origin. Genes Dev. 2004;18:2608-2613.

197. Keller C, Arenkiel BR, Coffin CM, et al. Alveolar rhabdomyosarcomas in conditional *Pax3-Fkhr* mice: cooperativity of *InK4A/arf* and *Trp53* loss of function. Genes Dev. 2004;18:2614-2626.

198. Chamberlain JS, Metzger J, Reyes M, et al. Dystrophin-deficient mdx mice display a reduced life span and are susceptible to spontaneous rhabdomyosarcoma. FASEB J. 2007;21:2195-2204.

199. Galindo RL, Allport JA, Olson EN. A drosophila model of the rhabdomyosarcoma initiator *PAX7-FKHR*. Proc Natl Acad Sci U S A. 2006;103:13439-13444.

200. Langenau DM, Keefe MD, Storer NY, et al. Effects of *RAS* on the genesis of embryonal rhabdomyosarcoma. Genes Dev. 2007;21:1382-1395.

201. Barr FG, Nauta LE, Hollows JC. Structural analysis of *PAX3* genomic rearrangements in alveolar rhabdomyosarcoma. Cancer Genet Cytogenet. 1998;102:32-39.

202. Fitzgerald JC, Scherr AM, Barr FG. Structural analysis of *PAX7* rearrangements in alveolar rhabdomyosarcoma. Cancer Genet Cytogenet. 2000;117:37-40.

203. Barr FG, Xiong QB, Kelly K. A consensus polymerase chain reaction-oligonucleotide hybridization approach for the detection of chromosomal translocations in pediatric bone and soft tissue sarcomas. Am J Clin Pathol. 1995;104:627-633.

204. Barr FG, Smith LM, Lynch JC, et al. Examination of gene fusion status in archival samples of alveolar rhabdomyosarcoma entered on the Intergroup Rhabdomyosarcoma Study-III trial: a report from the Children's Oncology Group. J Mol Diagn. 2006;8:202-208.

205. Biegel JA, Nycum LM, Valentine V, et al. Detection of the t(2;13)(q35;q14) and *PAX3-FKHR* fusion in alveolar rhabdomyosarcoma by fluorescence in situ hybridization. Genes Chromosomes Cancer. 1995;12:186-192.

206. Nishio J, Althof PA, Bailey JM, et al. Use of a novel FISH assay on paraffin-embedded tissues as an adjunct to diagnosis of alveolar rhabdomyosarcoma. Lab Invest. 2006;86:547-556.

207. Barr FG, Chatten J, D'Cruz CM, et al. Molecular assays for chromosomal translocations in the diagnosis of pediatric soft tissue sarcomas. JAMA. 1995;273:553-557.

208. de Alava E, Ladanyi M, Rosai J, Gerald WL. Detection of chimeric transcripts in desmoplastic small round cell tumor and related developmental tumors by reverse transcriptase polymerase

209. Arden KC, Anderson MJ, Finckenstein FG, et al. Detection of the t(2;13) chromosomal translocation in alveolar rhabdomyosarcoma using the reverse transcriptase-polymerase chain reaction. Genes Chromosomes Cancer. 1996;16:254-260.

210. Reichmuth C, Markus MA, Hillemanns M, et al. The diagnostic potential of the chromosome translocation t(2;13) in rhabdomyosarcoma: a PCR study of fresh-frozen and paraffin-embedded tumour samples. J Pathol. 1996;180:50-57.

211. Frascella E, Toffolatti L, Rosolen A. Normal and rearranged *PAX3* expression in human rhabdomyosarcoma. Cancer Genet Cytogenet. 1998;102:104-109.

212. Sorensen PH, Lynch JC, Qualman SJ, et al. *PAX3-FKHR* and *PAX7-FKHR* gene fusions are prognostic indicators in alveolar rhabdomyosarcoma: a report from the Children's Oncology Group. J Clin Oncol. 2002;20:2672-2679.

213. Barr FG, Qualman SJ, Macris MH, et al. Genetic heterogeneity in the alveolar rhabdomyosarcoma subset without typical gene fusions. Cancer Res. 2002;62:4704-4710.

214. Wachtel M, Dettling M, Koscielniak E, et al. Gene expression signatures identify rhabdomyosarcoma subtypes and detect a novel t(2;2)(q35;p23) translocation fusing *PAX3* to *NCOA1*. Cancer Res. 2004;64:5539-5545.

215. Grundy R, Anderson J, Gaze M, et al. Congenital alveolar rhabdomyosarcoma: clinical and molecular distinction from alveolar rhabdomyosarcoma in older children. Cancer. 2001;91:606-612.

216. Parham DM, Qualman SJ, Teot L, et al. Correlation between histology and *PAX/FKHR* fusion status in alveolar rhabdomyosarcoma: a report from the Children's Oncology Group. Am J Surg Pathol. 2007;31:895-901.

217. Kelly KM, Womer RB, Sorensen PH, et al. Common and variant gene fusions predict distinct clinical phenotypes in rhabdomyosarcoma. J Clin Oncol. 1997;15:1831-1836.

218. Kazanowska B, Reich A, Stegmaier S, et al. *PAX3-FKHR* and *PAX7-FKHR* fusion genes impact outcome of alveolar rhabdomyosarcoma in children. Fetal Pediatr Pathol. 2007;26:17-31.

219. De Pitta C, Tombolan L, Albiero G, et al. Gene expression profiling identifies potential relevant genes in alveolar rhabdomyosarcoma pathogenesis and discriminates *PAX3-FKHR* positive and negative tumors. Int J Cancer. 2006;118:2772-2781.

220. Davicioni E, Finckenstein FG, Shahbazian V, et al. Identification of a *PAX-FKHR* gene expression signature that defines molecular classes and determines the prognosis of alveolar rhabdomyosarcomas. Cancer Res. 2006;66:6936-6946.

221. Lae M, Ahn EH, Mercado GE, et al. Global gene expression profiling of *PAX-FKHR* fusion-positive alveolar and *PAX-FKHR* fusion-negative embryonal rhabdomyosarcomas. J Pathol. 2007;212:143-151.

222. Molnar B, Sipos F, Galamb O, Tulassay Z. Molecular detection of circulating cancer cells: role in diagnosis, prognosis and follow-up of colon cancer patients. Dig Dis. 2003;21:320-325.

223. Slade MJ, Coombes RC. The clinical significance of disseminated tumor cells in breast cancer. Nat Clin Pract Oncol. 2007;4:30-41.

224. Morgan TM, Lange PH, Vessella RL. Detection and characterization of circulating and disseminated prostate cancer cells. Front Biosci. 2007;12:3000-3009.

225. Kelly KM, Womer RB, Barr FG. Minimal disease detection in patients with alveolar rhabdomyosarcoma using a reverse transcriptase-polymerase chain reaction method. Cancer. 1996;78:1320-1327.

226. Sartori F, Alaggio R, Zanazzo G, et al. Results of a prospective minimal disseminated disease study in human rhabdomyosarcoma using three different molecular markers. Cancer. 2006;106:1766-1775.

227. Gallego S, Llort A, Roma J, et al. Detection of bone marrow micrometastasis and microcirculating disease in rhabdomyosarcoma by a real-time RT-PCR assay. J Cancer Res Clin Oncol. 2006;132:356-362.

228. McDowell HP, Donfrancesco A, Milano GM, et al. Detection and clinical significance of disseminated tumour cells at diagnosis in bone marrow of children with localised rhabdomyosarcoma. Eur J Cancer. 2005;41:2288-2296.

229. Gurney J, Young J, Roffers S, et al. Cancer incidence and survival among children and adolescents: United States SEER program 1975-1995. In Ries L, Smith MA, Gurney J, et al. (eds). SEER pediatric monograph. Bethesda, Md: National Cancer Institute, SEER Program; 1999:111-123.

230. Childhood cancer by the ICCC (CSR Section 29). In Ries LAG, Harkins D, Krapcho M, et al. (eds). SEER Cancer Statistics Review, 1975-2003. (Website): http://seer.cancer.gov/csr/1975_2003/results_merged/sect_29_childhood_cancer_iccc.pdf. Accessed June 1, 2008.

231. Klem ML, Grewal RK, Wexler LH, et al. PET for staging in rhabdomyosarcoma: an evaluation of PET as an adjunct to current staging tools. J Pediatr Hematol Oncol. 2007;29:9-14.

232. Volker T, Denecke T, Steffen I, et al. Positron emission tomography for staging of pediatric sarcoma patients: results of a prospective multicenter trial. J Clin Oncol. 2007;25:5435-5441.

233. Mazumdar A, Siegel M, Narra V, Lichtman-Jones L. Whole-body fast inversion recovery MR imaging of small cell neoplasms in pediatric patients. AJR Am J Roentgenol. 2002;179:1261-1266.

234. Daldrup-Link HE, Franzius C, Link TM, et al. Whole-body MR imaging for detection of bone metastases in children and young adults: comparison with skeletal scintigraphy and FDG pet. AJR Am J Roentgenol. 2001;177:229-236.

235. Joshi D, Anderson JR, Paidas C, et al. Age is an independent prognostic factor in rhabdomyosarcoma: a report from the soft tissue sarcoma committee of the Children's Oncology Group. Pediatr Blood Cancer. 2004;42:64-73.

236. Rodary C, Gehan EA, Flamant F, et al. Prognostic factors in 951 nonmetastatic rhabdomyosarcoma in children: a report from the International Rhabdomyosarcoma Workshop. Med Pediatr Oncol. 1991;19:89-95.

237. Meza J, Anderson J, Pappo AS, Meyer WH. Analysis of prognostic factors in patients with nonmetastatic rhabdomyosarcoma treated on Intergroup Rhabdomyosarcoma Studies III and IV: The Children's Oncology Group. J Clin Oncol. 2006;24:3844-3852.

238. Lager J, Lyden E, Anderson JR, et al. Pooled analysis of phase II window studies in children with contemporary high-risk metastatic rhabdomyosarcoma: a report from the Soft Tissue Sarcoma Committee of the Children's Oncology Group. J Clin Oncol. 2006;24:3415-3422.

239. Maurer H, Beltangady M, Gehan E, et al. The Intergroup Rhabdomyosarcoma Study-I: a final report. Cancer. 1988;61:209-220.

240. Maurer HM, Gehan EA, Beltangady M, et al. The Intergroup Rhabdomyosarcoma Study-II. Cancer. 1993;71:1904-1922.

241. Koscielniak E, Harms D, Henze G, et al. Results of treatment for soft tissue sarcoma in childhood and adolescence: a final report of the German Cooperative Soft Tissue Sarcoma Study CWS-86. J Clin Oncol. 1999;17:3706-3719.

242. Raney RB, Anderson JR, Barr FG, et al. Rhabdomyosarcoma and undifferentiated sarcoma in the first two decades of life: a selective review of Intergroup Rhabdomyosarcoma Study group experience and rationale for Intergroup Rhabdomyosarcoma Study-V. J Pediatr Hematol Oncol. 2001;23:215-220.

243. Breneman JC, Lyden E, Pappo AS, et al. Prognostic factors and clinical outcomes in children and adolescents with metastatic rhabdomyosarcoma: a report from the Intergroup Rhabdomyosarcoma Study-IV. J Clin Oncol. 2003;21:78-84.

244. Dantonello TM, Int-Veen C, Winkler P, et al. Initial patient characteristics can predict pattern and risk of relapse in localized rhabdomyosarcoma. J Clin Oncol. 2008;26:406-413.

245. Heyn RM, Holland R, Newton WA, et al. The role of combined chemotherapy in the treatment of rhabdomyosarcoma in children. Cancer. 1974;34:2128-2142.

246. Pratt C, Hustu H, Fleming I, Pinkel D. Coordinated treatment of childhood rhabdomyosarcoma with surgery, radiotherapy, and combination chemotherapy. Cancer Res. 1972;32:606-610.

247. Haddy T, Nora A, Sutow W, Vietti T. Cyclophosphamide treatment for metastatic soft tissue sarcoma. Am J Dis Child. 1967;114:301-308.

248. Womer RB. The Intergroup Rhabdomyosarcoma Studies come of age. Cancer. 1993;71:1719-1721.

249. Crist W, Gehan EA, Ragab AH, et al. The third Intergroup Rhabdomyosarcoma Study. J Clin Oncol. 1995;13:610-630.

250. Crist WM, Anderson JR, Meza JL, et al. Intergroup Rhabdomyosarcoma Study-IV: results for patients with nonmetastatic disease. J Clin Oncol. 2001;19:3091-3102.

251. Spunt SL, Smith LM, Ruymann FB, et al. Cyclophosphamide dose intensification during induction therapy for intermediate-risk pediatric rhabdomyosarcoma is feasible but does not improve outcome: a report from the soft tissue sarcoma committee of the Children's Oncology Group. Clin Cancer Res. 2004;10:6072-6079.

252. Flamant F, Rodary C, Rey A, et al. Treatment of non-metastatic rhabdomyosarcomas in childhood and adolescence: results of the second study of the International Society of Paediatric Oncology: *Mmt-84*. Eur J Cancer. 1998;34:1050-1062.

253. Stevens M, Rey A, Bouvet N, et al. Intensified (6-drug) versus standard (IVA) chemotherapy for high-risk non metastatic rhabdomyosarcoma (RMS) J Clin Oncol. 2004;22:802 (abstract).

254. de Kraker J, Voute PA. The role of ifosfamide in paediatric soft tissue sarcomas. Cancer Chemother Pharmacol. 1986;18(suppl 2):S23-S24.

255. Shaw PJ, Eden T. Ifosfamide in paediatric oncology: tried but not tested? Lancet. 1990;335:1022-1023.

256. Womer RB. Ifosfamide and paediatrics: should this marriage be saved? Eur J Cancer. 1996;32A:1100-1101.

257. Kung F, Hayes FA, Krischer J, et al. Clinical trial of etoposide (VP-16) in children with recurrent malignant solid tumors. A phase II study from the Pediatric Oncology Group. Investigational New Drugs. 1988;6:31-36.

258. Miser JS, Kinsella TJ, Triche TJ, et al. Ifosfamide with mesna uroprotection and etoposide: an effective regimen in the treatment of recurrent sarcomas and other tumors of children and young adults. J Clin Oncol. 1987;5:1191-1198.

259. Davidson A, Growing R, Lewis S, et al. Phase II study of 21-day-schedule of oral etoposide in children. Eur J Cancer. 1997;33:1816-1822.

260. Kebudi R, Gorgun O, Ayan I. Oral etoposide for recurrent/progressive sarcomas of childhood. Pediatr Blood Cancer. 2004;42:320-324.

261. Saylors RL, Stine SC, Sullivan J, et al. Cyclophosphamide plus topotecan in children with recurrent of refractory solid tumors: a Pediatric Oncology Group phase II study. J Clin Oncol. 2001;19:3463-3469.

262. Pappo AS, Lynden E, Breneman J, et al. Up-front window trial of topotecan in previously untreated children and adolescents with metastatic rhabdomyosarcoma: an Intergroup Rhabdomyosarcoma Study. J Clin Oncol. 2001;19:213-219.

263. Walterhouse D, Lyden E, Breitfeld P, et al. Efficacy of topotecan and cyclophosphamide given in a phase II window trial in children with newly diagnosed metastatic rhabdomyosarcoma: a Children's Oncology Group study. J Clin Oncol. 2004;22:1398-1403.

264. Arndt C, Hawkins D, Stoner J, et al. Randomized phase III trial comparing vincristine, actinomycin, cyclophosphamide (VAC)

with VAC/v topotecan/cyclophosphamide (tc) for intermediate-risk rhabdomyosarcoma (IRRMS). D9803, COG study. J Clin Oncol. 2007;25 (18 Suppl) No. 9509.

265. Houghton PJ, Santana VM. Clinical trials using irinotecan. J Pediatr Hematol Oncol. 2002;24:84-85 (comment).

266. Vassal G, Couanet D, Stockdale E, et al. Phase II trial of irinotecan in children with relapsed or refractory rhabdomyosarcoma: a joint study of the French Society of Pediatric Oncology and the United Kingdom Children's Cancer Study Group. J Clin Oncol. 2007;25:356-361.

267. Bomgaars LR, Bernstein M, Krailo M, et al. Phase II trial of irinotecan in children with refractory solid tumors: a Children's Oncology Group study. J Clin Oncol. 2007;25:4622-4627.

268. Furman WL, Stewart CF, Poquette CA, et al. Direct translation of a protracted irinotecan schedule from a xenograft model to a phase I trial in children. J Clin Oncol. 1999;17:1815-1824.

269. Bisogno G, Riccardi R, Ruggiero A, et al. Phase II study of a protracted irinotecan schedule in children with refractory or recurrent soft tissue sarcoma. Cancer. 2006;106:703-707.

270. Thompson J, George EO, Poquette CA, et al. Synergy of topotecan in combination with vincristine for treatment of pediatric solid tumor xenografts. Clin Cancer Res. 1999;5:3617-3631.

271. Pappo AS, Lyden E, Breitfeld P, et al. Two consecutive phase II window trials of irinotecan alone or in combination with vincristine for the treatment of metastatic rhabdomyosarcoma: the Children's Oncology Group. J Clin Oncol. 2007;25:362-369.

271a. Mascarenhas L, Lyden E, Breitfeld P, et al. Randomized phase II window study of two schedules of irinotecan (CPT-II) and vincristine (VCR) in rhabdomyosarcoma at first relapse/disease progression. J Clin Oncol. 2008;26:10013.

272. Carli M, Perilongo G, di Montezemolo LC, et al. Phase II trial of cisplatin and etoposide in children with advanced soft tissue sarcoma: a report from the Italian Cooperative Rhabdomyosarcoma Group. Cancer Treat Rep. 1987;71:525-527.

273. Van Winkle P, Angiolillo A, Krailo M, et al. Ifosfamide, carboplatin, and etoposide (ICE) reinduction chemotherapy in a large cohort of children and adolescents with recurrent/refractory sarcoma: the Children's Cancer Group (CCG) experience. Pediatr Blood Cancer. 2005;44:338-347.

274. Chisholm JC, Machin D, McDowell H, et al. Efficacy of carboplatin given in a phase II window study to children and adolescents with newly diagnosed metastatic soft tissue sarcoma. Eur J Cancer. 2007;43:2537-2544.

275. Breitfeld PP, Lyden E, Raney RB, et al. Ifosfamide and etoposide are superior to vincristine and melphalan for pediatric metastatic rhabdomyosarcoma when administered with irradiation and combination chemotherapy: a report from the Intergroup Rhabdomyosarcoma Study group. Pediatr Hematol Oncol. 2001;23:225-233.

276. Arndt CA, Hawkins DS, Meyer WH, et al. Comparison of results of a pilot study of alternating vincristine/doxorubicin/cyclophosphamide and etoposide/ifosfamide with IRS-IV in intermediate-risk rhabdomyosarcoma: a report from the Children's Oncology Group. Pediatr Blood Cancer. 2008;50:33-36.

277. Flamant F, Rodary C, Rey A, et al. Treatment of non-metastatic rhabdomyosarcoma in childhood and adolescence: results of the second study of the International Society of Paediatric Oncology: MMT84. Eur J Cancer. 1998;34:1050-1062.

278. Oberlin O, Rey A, Anderson J, et al. Treatment of orbital rhabdomyosarcoma: survival and late effects of treatment: results of an international workshop. J Clin Oncol. 2001;19:197-204.

279. Donaldson SS, Anderson JR. Rhabdomyosarcoma: many similarities, a few philosophical differences. J Clin Oncol. 2005;23:2586-2587 (comment).

280. Peng F, Rabkin G, Muzik O. Use of 2-deoxy-2-[f-18]-fluoro-d-glucose positron emission tomography to monitor therapeutic response by rhabdomyosarcoma in children: report of a retrospective case study. Clin Nucl Med. 2006;31:394-397.

281. Hays DM, Lawrence W Jr, Wharam M, et al. Primary reexcision for patients with microscopic residual tumor following initial excision of sarcomas of trunk and extremity sites. J Pediatr Surg. 1989;24:5-10.

282. Wiener ES, Anderson JR, Ojimba JI, et al. Controversies in the management of paratesticular rhabdomyosarcoma: is staging retroperitoneal lymph node dissection necessary for adolescents with resected paratesticular rhabdomyosarcoma? Semin Pediatr Surg. 2001;10:146-152.

283. Breneman JC, Wiener ES. Issues in the local control of rhabdomyosarcoma. Med Pediatr Oncol. 2000;35:104-109.

284. Blakely ML, Lobe TE, Anderson JR, et al. Does debulking improve survival rate in advanced-stage retroperitoneal embryonal rhabdomyosarcoma? J Pediatr Surg. 1999;34:736-742.

285. Cecchetto G, Bisogno G, De Corti F, et al. Biopsy or debulking surgery as initial surgery for locally advanced rhabdomyosarcomas in children?: the experience of the Italian Cooperative Group studies. Cancer. 2007;110:2561-2567.

286. Viswanathan A, Grier H, Litman H, et al. Outcome for children with group III rhabdomyosarcoma treated with or without radiotherapy. Int J Radiation Oncology Biol Phys. 2004;58:1208-1214.

287. Wolden SL, Anderson JR, Crist WM, et al. Indications for radiotherapy and chemotherapy after complete resection in rhabdomyosarcoma: a report from the Intergroup Rhabdomyosarcoma Studies I to III. J Clin Oncol. 1999;17:3468-3475.

288. Schuck A, Mattke AC, Schmidt B, et al. Group II rhabdomyosarcoma and rhabdomyosarcoma-like tumors: is radiotherapy necessary? J Clin Oncol. 2004;22:143-149.

289. Smith LM, Snderosn JR, Qualman SJ, et al. Which patients with microscopic disease and rhabdomyosarcoma experience relapse after therapy? A report from the Soft Tissue Sarcoma Committee of the Children's Oncology Group. J Clin Oncol. 2001;19:4058-4064.

290. Stevens MCG, Rey A, Bouvet N, et al. Treatment of nonmetastatic rhabdomyosarcoma in childhood and adolescence: third study of the International Society of Paediatric Oncology: SIOP malignant mesenchymal tumor 89. J Clin Oncol. 2005;23:2618-2628.

291. Mandell L, Ghavimi F, Peretz T, et al. Radiocurability of microscopic disease in childhood rhabdomyosarcoma with radiation doses less than 4,000 cGy. J Clin Oncol. 1990;8:1536-1542.

292. Nag S, Olson T, Ruymann F, et al. High-dose-rate brachytherapy in childhood sarcomas: a local control strategy preserving bone growth and function. Med Pediatr Oncol. 1995;25:463-469.

293. Nag S, Martinez-Monge R, Ruymann F, et al. Innovation in the management of soft tissue sarcomas in infants and young children: high-dose rate brachytherapy. J Clin Oncol. 1997;15:3075-3084.

294. Buwalda J, Schouwenburg P, Blank L, et al. A novel local treatment strategy for advanced-stage head and neck rhabdomyosarcomas in children: results of the Amore Protocol. Eur J Cancer. 2003;39:1594-1602.

295. Merchant TE, Zelefsky MJ, Sheldon JM, et al. High-dose rate intraoperative radiation therapy for pediatric solid tumors. Med Pediatr Oncol. 1998;30:34-39.

296. Gillis AM, Sutton E, Dewitt KD, et al. Long-term outcome and toxicities of intraoperative radiotherapy for high-risk neuroblastoma. Int J Radiat Oncol Biol Phys. 2007;69:858-864.

297. Schomberg PJ, Gunderson LL, Moir CR, et al. Intraoperative electron irradiation in the management of pediatric malignancies. Cancer. 1997;79:2251-2256.

298. Kalapurakal JA, Goldman S, Stellpflug W, et al. Phase I study of intraoperative radiotherapy with photon radiosurgery system in children with recurrent brain tumors: preliminary report of first dose level (10 Gy). Int J Radiat Oncol Biol Phys. 2006;65:800-808.

299. Haase GM, Meagher DP Jr, McNeely LK, et al. Electron beam intraoperative radiation therapy for pediatric neoplasms. Cancer. 1994;74:740-747.

300. Miralbell R, Lomax A, Cella L, Schneider U. Potential reduction of the incidence of radiation-induced second cancers by using proton beams in the treatment of pediatric tumors. Int J Radiat Oncol Biol Phys. 2002;54:824-829.

301. Yock T, Schneider R, Friedmann A, et al. Proton radiotherapy for orbital rhabdomyosarcoma: clinical outcome and a dosimetric comparison with photons. Int J Radiat Oncol Biol Phys. 2005;63:1161-1168.

302. Timmermann B, Schuck A, Niggli F, et al. Spot-scanning proton therapy for malignant soft tissue tumors in childhood: first experiences at the Paul Scherrer Institute. Int J Radiat Oncol Biol Phys. 2007;67:497-504.

303. Arndt C, Hawkins D, Anderson J, et al. Age is a risk factor for chemotherapy-induced hepatopathy with vincristine, dactinomycin, and cyclophosphamide. J Clin Oncol. 2004;22:1894-1901.

304. Orbach D, Rey A, Oberlin O, et al. Soft tissue sarcoma or malignant mesenchymal tumors in the first year of life: experience of the International Society of Pediatric Oncology (SIOP) malignant mesenchymal tumor committee. J Clin Oncol. 2005;23:4363-4371.

305. Raney RB, Gehan E, Hays DM, et al. Primary chemotherapy with or without radiation therapy and/or surgery for children with localized sarcoma of the bladder, prostate, vagina, uterus, and cervix: a comparison of the results in Intergroup Rhabdomyosarcoma Studies I and II. Cancer. 1990;66:2072-2081.

306. Lobe T, Wiener E, Andrassy R, et al. The argument for conservative, delayed surgery in the management of prostatic rhabdomyosarcoma. J Pediatr Surg. 1996;31:1084-1087.

307. Arndt C, Rodeberg D, Breitfeld PP, et al. Does bladder preservation (as a surgical principle) lead to retaining bladder function in bladder/prostate rhabdomyosarcoma? Results from Intergroup Rhabdomyosarcoma Study IV. J Urol. 2004;171:2396-2403 (comment).

308. Raney RB, Heyn R, Hays DM, et al. Sequelae of treatment in 109 patients followed 5 to 15 years after diagnosis of sarcoma of the bladder and prostate. Cancer. 1993;71:2387-2394.

309. Spunt SL, Sweeney TA, Hudson MM, et al. Late effects of pelvic rhabdomyosarcoma and its treatment in female survivors. J Clin Oncol. 2005;23:7143-7151.

310. Yeung C, Ward H, Ransley P, et al. Bladder and kidney function after cure of pelvic rhabdomyosarcoma in childhood. Br J Cancer. 1994;70:1000-1003.

311. Womer RB, Snyder HM. Bladder/prostate rhabdomyosarcoma: miles to go before we sleep. J Urol. 2006;176:1278-1279 (comment).

312. Arndt CA, Hammond S, Rodeberg D, Qualman S. Significance of persistent mature rhabdomyoblasts in bladder/prostate rhabdomyosarcoma: results from IRS IV. J Pediatr Hematol Oncol. 2006;28:563-567.

313. Koscielniak E, Jurgens H, Winkler K, et al. Treatment of soft tissue sarcoma in childhood and adolescence: a report of the German Cooperative Soft tissue Sarcoma study. Cancer. 1992;70:2557-2567.

314. Raney RB, Meza J, Anderson JR, et al. Treatment of children and adolescents with localized parameningeal sarcoma: experience of the Intergroup Rhabdomyosarcoma Study group protocols IRS-II through -IV, 1978-1997. Med Pediatr Oncol. 2002;38:22-32.

315. Raney B, Tefft M, Heyn R, et al. Ascending myelitis after intensive chemotherapy and radiation therapy in children with cranial parameningeal sarcoma. Cancer. 1992;69:1498-1506.

316. Benk V, Rodary C, Donaldson SS, et al. Parameningeal rhabdomyosarcoma: results of an international workshop. Int J Radiat Oncol Biol Phys. 1996;36:533-540.

317. Michalski JM, Meza J, Breneman JC, et al. Influence of radiation therapy parameters on outcome in children treated with radiation therapy for localized parameningeal rhabdomyosarcoma in Intergroup Rhabdomyosarcoma Study group trials II through IV. Int J Radiat Oncol Biol Phys. 2004;59:1027-1038.

318. Chen C, Shu HK, Goldwein JW, et al. Volumetric considerations in radiotherapy for pediatric parameningeal rhabdomyosarcomas. Int J Radiat Oncol Biol Phys. 2003;55:1294-1299.

319. Smith SC, Lindsley SK, Felgenhauer J, et al. Intensive induction chemotherapy and delayed irradiation in the management of parameningeal rhabdomyosarcoma. J Pediatr Hematol Oncol. 2003;25:774-779.

320. Pappo A, Anderson J, Crist W, et al. Survival after relapse in children and adolescents with rhabdomyosarcoma: a report from the Intergroup Rhabdomyosarcoma Study group. J Clin Oncol. 1999;17:3487-3493.

321. Meyers PA. High-dose therapy with autologous stem cell rescue for pediatric sarcomas. Curr Opin Oncol. 2004;16:120-125.

322. Wharam MD, Meza J, Anderson J, et al. Failure pattern and factors predictive of local failure in rhabdomyosarcoma: a report of group III patients in the third Intergroup Rhabdomyosarcoma Study. J Clin Oncol. 2004;22:1902-1908.

323. Skinner R, Sharkey IM, Pearson AD, Craft AW. Ifosfamide, mesna, and nephrotoxicity in children. J Clin Oncol. 1993;11:173-190 (review).

20 Nonrhabdomyosarcomas and Other Soft Tissue Tumors

Ian J. Davis, Antonio R. Perez-Atayde, and David E. Fisher

INTRODUCTION

Soft tissue sarcomas of childhood and adolescence constitute a heterogeneous group of tumors that exhibit features of mesenchymal differentiation (Tables 20-1 and 20-2). From a pediatric oncology perspective, the various types of rhabdomyosarcomas (RMSs), the most common soft tissue sarcomas in younger children, are grouped separately such that the remainder of these tumors is collectively termed nonrhabdomyosarcoma soft tissue sarcoma (NRSTS). It may seem odd to define a category of soft tissue sarcomas by exclusion and to group together various clinicopathologic entities distinguished by clinical features, molecular pathogenesis, and biologic behavior. However, the term *NRSTS* carries a unique value in pediatric oncology, enabling the study of significant cohorts of children with uncommon tumors. Sarcomas in children represent a some-

what distinct set of tumors that diverge in both incidence and histology from those in adults. The types of sarcomas that develop in adolescents and young adults are similar to those seen in older individuals; however, the relative incidence and response to therapy may differ. In addition, the term *NRSTS* permits the flexibility of including undifferentiated tumors and tumors that, based on treatment, are typically excluded from other groupings (e.g., desmoplastic small round cell tumors). Finally, by evoking those tumors prevalent in the pediatric population, the term *NRSTS* also permits consideration of the unique toxicities specific to children when one is evaluating treatment approaches.

NRSTSs are commonly characterized by distinct, consistent cytogenetic changes. Exploring the biology of these molecular alterations may offer insights into the biology of mesenchymal development and the pathogenesis of these

---

TABLE 20-1	**World Health Organization Classification of Soft Tissue Tumors: Intermediate (Rarely Metastasizing) and Malignant**	
	Intermediate (Rarely Metastasizing)	**Malignant**
Adipocytic		Dedifferentiated liposarcoma
		Myxoid liposarcoma
		Round cell liposarcoma
		Pleomorphic liposarcoma
		Mixed-type liposarcoma
		Liposarcoma, not otherwise specified
Fibroblastic/myofibroblastic	Solitary fibrous tumor	Adult fibrosarcoma
	Hemangiopericytoma	Myxofibrosarcoma
	Inflammatory myofibroblastic tumor	Low-grade fibromyxoid sarcoma, or hyalinizing spindle cell
	Low-grade myofibroblastic sarcoma	tumor
	Myxoinflammatory fibroblastic sarcoma	Sclerosing epithelioid fibrosarcoma
	Infantile fibrosarcoma	
So-called fibrohistiocytic	Plexiform fibrohistiocytic tumor	Undifferentiated pleomorphic sarcoma (pleomorphic MFH)
	Giant cell tumor of soft tissues	Undifferentiated pleomorphic sarcoma with giant cells (giant cell MFH)
		Undifferentiated pleomorphic sarcoma with prominent inflammation (inflammatory MFH)
Smooth muscle		Leiomyosarcoma
Pericytic (perivascular)		Malignant glomus tumor
		Glomangiosarcoma
Skeletal muscle		Embryonal rhabdomyosarcoma
		Alveolar rhabdomyosarcoma
		Pleomorphic rhabdomyosarcoma
Vascular tumors	Retiform hemangioendothelioma	Epithelioid hemangioendothelioma
	Papillary intralymphatic angioendothelioma	Angiosarcoma of soft tissue
	Composite hemangioendothelioma	
	Kaposi's sarcoma	
Chondro-osseous		Mesenchymal chondrosarcoma
		Extraskeletal osteosarcoma
Uncertain differentiation	Angiomatoid fibrous histiocytoma	Synovial sarcoma
	Ossifying fibromyxoid tumor	Epithelioid sarcoma
	Myoepithelioma	Alveolar soft part sarcoma
	Parachordoma	Clear cell sarcoma of soft tissue
		Extraskeletal myxoid chondrosarcoma
		Extraosseous Ewing's sarcoma/peripheral primitive neuroectodermal tumor
		Desmoplastic small round cell tumor
		Extrarenal rhabdoid tumor
		Malignant mesenchymoma
		Neoplasms with perivascular epithelioid differentiation (PEComa)
		Clear cell myomelanocytic tumor
		Intimal sarcoma

Adapted from Fletcher CD, Unni KK, Mertens F. World Health Organization Classification of Tumors. Pathology and Genetics. Tumors of Soft Tissue and Bone. Lyon, France, IARC Press; 2002.

TABLE 20-2   World Health Organization Classification of Soft Tissue Tumors: Benign and Intermediate (Locally Aggressive)

	Benign	Intermediate (Locally Aggressive)
Adipocytic	Lipoma Lipomatosis Lipomatosis of nerve Lipoblastoma/lipoblastomatosis Angiolipoma Chondroid lipoma Extrarenal angiomyolipoma Extra-adrenal myelolipoma Spindle cell/pleomorphic lipoma Hibernoma	Atypical lipomatous tumor/well-differentiated liposarcoma
Fibroblastic/myofibroblastic	Nodular fasciitis Proliferative fasciitis Proliferative myositis Myositis ossificans Fibro-osseous pseudotumor of digits Ischemic fasciitis Elastofibroma Fibrous hamartoma of infancy Myofibroma/myofibromatosis Fibromatosis coli Juvenile hyaline fibromatosis Inclusion body fibromatosis Fibroma of tendon sheath Desmoplastic fibroblastoma Mammary-type myofibroblastoma Calcifying aponeurotic fibroma Angiomyofibroblastoma Cellular angiofibroma Nuchal-type fibroma Gardner fibroma Calcifying fibrous tumor Giant cell angiofibroma	Superficial fibromatosis (palmar/plantar) Desmoid-type fibromatosis Lipofibromatosis
So-called fibrohistiocytic	Giant cell tumor of tendon sheath Diffuse-type giant cell tumor Deep benign fibrous histiocytoma	
Smooth muscle	Angioleiomyoma Deep leiomyoma Genital leiomyoma	
Pericytic (perivascular)	Glomus tumor (and variants) Myopericytoma	
Skeletal muscle	Rhabdomyoma	
Vascular	Hemangioma Epithelioid hemangioma Angiomatosis Lymphangioma	Kaposiform hemangioendothelioma
Chondro-osseous	Soft tissue chondroma	
Uncertain differentiation	Intramuscular myxoma Juxta-articular myxoma Deep ("aggressive") angiomyxoma Pleomorphic hyalinizing angiectatic tumor Ectopic hamartomatous thymoma	

Adapted from Fletcher CD, Unni KK, Mertens F. World Health Organization Classification of Tumors. Pathology and Genetics. Tumors of Soft Tissue and Bone. Lyon, France, IARC Press, 2002.

Epidemiology

In children younger than 5 years, RMS constitutes the most common type of soft tissue sarcoma (STS); however, by late school age and continuing into adolescence, the incidence of tumors and may lead to the development of new treatment strategies.

NRSTS rises to exceed that of RMS (Fig. 20-1). The total incidence of STS in children and adolescents younger than 20 years is approximately 11 per million, which represents 7.4% of cancer in this population.[1] NRSTS constitutes about one half of these cases, or about 3% to 4% of childhood malignancies. Within the class of NRSTS, specific tumor types demonstrate a strong age association. Although the median age at diagnosis is approximately 13 years, the NRSTSs prevalent in younger children include infantile fibrosarcoma and rhabdoid

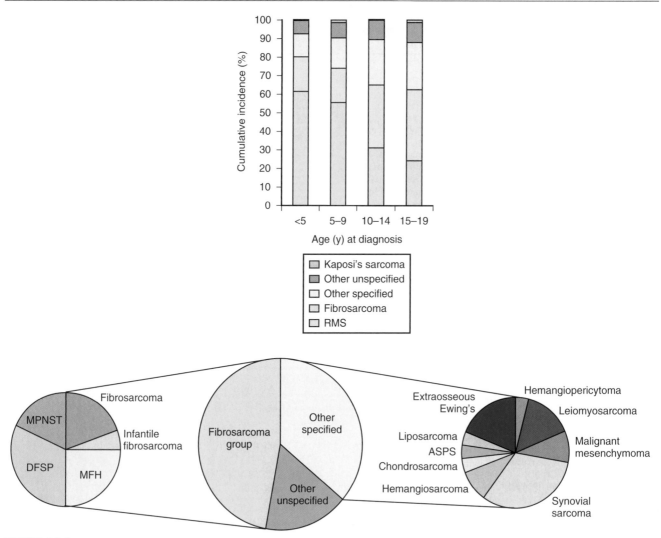

FIGURE 20-1. Incidence and distribution of pediatric soft tissue sarcomas. **A,** Age-adjusted incidence of soft tissue sarcomas of childhood are grouped according to the International Classification of Childhood Cancer.[601] Data extracted from the SEER data set.[1] **B,** Depiction of age-adjusted incidence of the specific tumors that compose the major classifications of NRSTS.[1] ASPS, alveolar soft part sarcoma; DFSP, dermatofibrosarcoma protuberans; MFH, malignant fibrous histiocytoma; MPNST, malignant peripheral nerve sheath tumor; RMS, rhabdomyosarcoma.

tumor, whereas synovial sarcoma and malignant peripheral nerve sheath tumor (MPNST) are more common in adolescents.[2-8]

Although the vast majority of cases of NRSTS occur spontaneously, several cancer predisposition syndromes are associated with the development of soft tissue sarcomas. Families that harbor mutations of the tumor suppressor p53 are prone to the development of many types of cancer.[9,10] Soft tissue sarcoma as well as osteosarcoma can be associated with germline p53 mutation.[11] The cell cycle regulatory protein RB has also been implicated in the development of STS. *RB* was originally identified as the locus deleted in hereditary and sporadic retinoblastoma.[12] However, retinoblastoma survivors are at risk for the development of STSs, including fibrosarcoma, malignant fibrous histiocytoma, and leiomyosarcoma, and molecular analysis of these tumors may demonstrate homozygous RB deletion.[13,14] In addition to other tumors, neurofibromatosis-1 (von Recklinghausen's disease) is associated with the development of MPNST and multifocal gastrointestinal stromal tumors.[15,16] Radiation therapy for optic nerve glioma in patients with neurofibromatosis type 1 (NF-1) increases the risk for subsequent development of MPNST.[17,18] Carney's triad is associated with multifocal gastrointestinal stromal tumor (as well as paragangliomas and pulmonary chondromas).[19,20] Individual Carney's triad tumors are associated with specific non–germline mutations, although a possible common association with chromosome 1 changes has been reported.[21] Gardner's syndrome, a phenotypic variant of familial adenomatous polyposis, results from mutation of the *APC* gene and is associated with an increased risk for abdominal desmoid tumor.[22-26] Werner's syndrome is caused by mutations of the DNA helicase gene *RECQL2* or the nuclear lamin gene *LMNA* and is associated with several cancers, including STSs in early and middle adulthood.[27-29] Typically resulting from mutations in *TSC1* or *TSC2*, dominantly inherited tuberous sclerosis is associated with spontaneously resolving cardiac rhabdomyomas in infants and renal angiomyolipoma, including the malignant epithelioid variant, as well as pulmonary lymphangiomyomatosis.[30-33]

In addition to cancer predisposition syndromes, environmental exposures have been linked to sarcoma development. Although osteosarcoma predominates, radiation exposure is associated with NRSTS, including fibrosarcoma and high-grade undifferentiated pleomorphic sarcoma.[34-36] Of the several environmental chemical exposures that have been linked to the development of sarcomas in adults, vinyl chloride exposure demonstrates the strongest association with the development of angiosarcoma.[37] Childhood cancer survivors also appear to be at a ninefold higher risk for the development of sarcomas (particularly NRSTS) in comparison with the general population, with a mean time from primary cancer diagnosis of 11 years.[38] Although an initial diagnosis of sarcoma was associated with the greatest risk, perhaps indicating an underlying predisposition, treatment by radiation or alkylating agents was also positively associated with sarcoma development.

Presentation and Evaluation

NRSTS typically presents as a persistent or enlarging, asymptomatic mass. Although NRSTS may arise in any location, extremities constitute the most common sites. However, within the first year of life, soft tissue tumors tend to develop in the trunk and the head and neck.[2] A significant fraction of tumors may be associated with pain that likely indicates invasion or compression of surrounding structures.[6]

The evaluation of NRSTS is typically initiated by appropriate imaging and followed by biopsy. For most tumors, a plain film and magnetic resonance (MR) imaging are justified. Technetium-99m–labeled methyldiphosphonate

(99 mTc MDP) nuclear scintigraphy (bone scan) can localize sites of bony metastatic disease. As a group these tumors tend to metastasize to the lungs, so computed tomography of the chest is commonly indicated for evaluation. Imaging may narrow the differential diagnosis and aid in assessing resectability by identifying tumor margins, involved tissue planes, and relationship to neurovascular structures. Combined positron emission tomography and computed tomography scans can identify primary tumors as well as metastatic spread and may detect metastatic lesions missed by bone scans.[39]

Accurate tissue diagnosis is critical for establishing a treatment plan and to predict prognosis.[4] The complexity of NRSTS diagnosis and grading requires the integration of histopathology with immunohistochemical, ultrastructural, cytogenetic, and molecular studies. In addition to standard histopathology and immunohistochemistry for appropriate markers, tumor material should be obtained for cytogenetic or molecular analysis (Table 20-3). The identification of cytogenetic abnormalities, many of which are highly specific for certain pediatric and young adult NRSTS, is helpful in arriving at or confirming a diagnosis (see Table 20-3). However, the same gene can be translocated in various tumor types. For example, the *EWS* gene is rearranged in desmoplastic small round cell tumor, clear cell sarcoma, and liposarcoma in addition to Ewing's sarcoma/primary neuroectodermal tumor. In contrast, the rearrangement of certain genes is highly restricted, such as that of *SS18*

TABLE 20-3   Diagnostic Studies in the Evaluation of NRSTS

Tumor	Immunohistochemical Markers	RECURRENT CYTOGENETIC CHANGES	
		Associated Karyotype	Genes Implicated
Alveolar soft part sarcoma	TFE3, MyoD1 (cytoplasmic), desmin (50%), S100 protein (25%), MSA (in some)	der(17)t(x;17)(p11;q25)	*ASPSCR1 (ASPL, TUG, RCC17), TFE3*
Angiomatoid fibrous histiocytoma	Vimentin, desmin (50%), CD68 (50%), CD99 (50%), epithelial membrane antigen (40%)	t(2;22)(q33;q12) t(12;16)(q13;p11) t(12;22)(q13;12)	*EWSR1, CREB1* *FUS, ATF1* *EWSR1, ATF1*
Angiosarcoma	Factor 8-associated (VWF), CD34, FLI1, CD31		
Congenital infantile fibrosarcoma	Vimentin, actins (30%), desmin (20%), cytokeratins (20%)	t(12;15)(p13;q25)	*ETV6, NTRK3 (TRKC)*
Clear cell sarcoma	MITF, HMB45, S100, Melan A	t(12;22)(q13;q12) t(12;2)(q13;q32)	*EWSR1, ATF1, CREB1*
Dermatofibrosarcoma protuberans	CD34, apolipoprotein D	t(17;22)(q22;q13)	*COL1A1, PDGFB*
Malignant desmoplastic round cell tumor	WT-1 (carboxy terminus), desmin (dotlike), EMA, cytokeratin, vimentin	t(11;12)(p13;q12)	*EWSR1, WT1*
Desmoid-type fibromatosis	Vimentin, actins, β-catenin (nuclear)	+8, +20	
Ectomesenchymoma	S100 protein, synaptophysin, GFAP, neurofilament protein, rhabdomyosarcoma markers (muscle-specific actin, desmin, myogenin, MyoD1)	+2, −6, +11, +20	
Epithelioid sarcoma	Cytokeratins, EMA, vimentin, CD34 (60%), CA-125		
Epithelioid hemangioendothelioma	VWF, CD31, CD34 cytokeratins (25% weak).		
Extraosseous Ewing's sarcoma	CD99 (membranous), NSE, vimentin, cytokeratins (25%), FLI1 (nuclear)	t(11;22)(q24;q12) t(21;22)(q21;q12) t(7;22)(p22;q12) t(17;22)(q12;q22) t(2;22)(q36;q12)	*EWSR1, FLI1* *EWSR1, ERG1* *EWSR1, ETV1* *EWSR1, ETV4 (E1AF)* *EWSR1, FEV*
Extrarenal rhabdoid tumor	Vimentin, cytokeratins, EMA, CD99, NSE, synaptophysin	Abnormalities of 22q11	*SMARCB1 (hSNF5, INI1, BAF47)*

Continues

TABLE 20-3   Diagnostic Studies in the Evaluation of NRSTS—cont'd

Tumor	Immunohistochemical Markers	RECURRENT CYTOGENETIC CHANGES	
		Associated Karyotype	Genes Implicated
	Vimentin, S100 protein (50%), cytokeratin (focal), EMA (30%) Neuroendocrine markers (chromogranin, NSE, synaptophysin) in t(9;17) tumors.	t(9;22)(q22;q12) t(9;17)(q22;q11) t(9;15)(q22;q21)	EWSR1, NR4A3 (TEC, CHN, CMSF, NOR1) TAF15 (RPB56, TAF2N), NR4A3 TCF12 (HTF4), NR4A3
Gastrointestinal stromal tumor	CD117 (KIT), CD34		
Extraskeletal myxoid chondrosarcoma	CD68, CD31, CD34		
Giant cell angioblastoma	Actins, vimentin		
Inflammatory myofibroblastic tumor	ALK, vimentin, actins, desmin (50%), cytokeratins (focal), CD68 (25%)	Multiple translocations involving 2p23	ALK, multiple partners
Kaposiform hemangioendothelioma	D2-40, CD31, CD34, FLI1, SMA, D2-40		
Kaposi's sarcoma	D2-40, CD31, CD34, FLI1, HHV-8 (in situ hybridization)		
Leiomyosarcoma	SMA, desmin, h-caldesmon	Complex	
Lipoblastoma	S100 protein, desmin	del(8)(q12;q24),r(8) t(7;8)(p22;q13)	HAS2, PLAG1 COL1A2, HAS2
Low grade fibromyxoid sarcoma	Vimentin, actins (focal)	t(7;16)(p33;p11)	FUS, CREB3L2 (BBF2H7)
Malignant peripheral nerve sheath tumor	S100 (50-90%), GFAP (50-90%), CD57 (50%), myelin basic protein (40%), p53	Numerical and structural abnormalities of chromosomes 1, 4, 7, 11, 12, 14, 16, 17 and 22	
Mesenchymal chondrosarcoma	S100 protein (cartilaginous component) NSE, CD57, CD99 (membranous) (undifferentiated component)	Complex cytogenetic alterations Robertsonian t(13;21)	
Myxoid liposarcoma	S100 protein	t(12;16)(q13;p11) t(12;22)(q13;q12)	FUS (TLS), DDIT3 (CHOP) EWSR1, DDIT3 (CHOP)
Plexiform fibrohistiocytic tumor	CD68, actins (70%), EMA (30%), BCL2 (30%)		
Solitary fibrous tumor	CD34, CD99 (cytoplasmic)		
Synovial sarcoma	EMA, cytokeratins, S100 protein (30%), CD99 (cytoplasmic), BCL2, TLE1	t(x;18)(p11;q11)	SS18 (SYT), SSX1 SS18 (SYT), SSX2
Undifferentiated pleomorphic sarcoma			

Note: These are the immunohistochemical markers and cytogenetic changes found in a large percent of tumors. The less common abnormalities are not listed.
EMA, epithelial membrane antigen; GFAP, glial fibrillary acidic protein; MITF, microphthalmia-associated transcription factor; MSA, muscle-specific actin; NSE, neuron-specific enolase; VWF, von Willebrand factor.

(SYT) in synovial sarcoma. Molecular studies, such as polymerase chain reaction (PCR) and interphase fluorescence in situ hybridization (FISH), may be required to evaluate for specific cytogenetic abnormalities, especially if there is a high index of suspicion and standard cytogenetics are unavailable or unremarkable.[40] Anticipating the rapid development of new strategies for diagnosis, including microarray-based gene expression profiling and biomarker identification, additional tumor material, if possible, should be preserved at −70° C for DNA or RNA analysis.

Staging and Grading

As with all cancers, appropriate recommendations for therapy depend on accurate predictions of clinical course and prognosis. Clinically informative classification schemes will accurately predict tumor outcome and will aid in the development and interpretation of the multicenter trials necessary to study these uncommon cancers. Studies of adult extremity STSs suggest that grade followed by tumor depth and size have independent prognostic value for the rates of distant metas-

tases and mortality resulting from the tumors.[41] However, the clinicopathologic classification of pediatric NRSTS poses unique challenges. The low incidence of these tumors results in the grouping of potentially disparate tumors in clinical trials. A patient's age may influence outcome. For some tumors, high grade does not predict clinically aggressive behavior, whereas other tumors behave aggressively regardless of histologic appearance. To address these issues, the Pediatric Oncology Group grading system incorporates histology, cytologic features, and age to classify NRSTS as low, intermediate, or high grade (Table 20-4).[42] Low grade is defined by histologic type, whereas intermediate grade takes into account necrosis and mitosis, with secondary consideration of nuclear atypia and tumor cellularity. High-grade tumors include those with specific histologies as well as tumors with more than 15% necrosis or five mitoses or more per 10 high-power fields. The National Cancer Institute and National Federation of French Cancer Centers (FNCLCC) grading specifications are alternative methodologies validated for sarcomas in adults.[43-46] Similar to the system used by the Pediatric Oncology Group, they take into consideration mitotic count, necrosis, and histologic type or tumor differentiation.

TABLE 20-4	Pediatric Oncology Group Histologic Grading System
Grade	
Grade 1—Low	Myxoid and well-differentiated liposarcoma
	Deep-seated dermatofibrosarcoma protuberans
	Well-differentiated or infantile (≤4 years old) fibrosarcoma
	Well-differentiated or infantile (≤4 years old) hemangiopericytoma
	Well-differentiated malignant peripheral nerve sheath tumor
	Extraskeletal myxoid chondrosarcoma
	Angiomatoid fibrous histiocytoma
Grade 2—Intermediate	Sarcomas not specifically included in grades 1 and 3, and in which: • <15% of the surface area shows necrosis • Mitotic count is ≤5 mitoses/10 high-power fields using a 40× objective • Absence of marked nuclear atypia* • Tumor is not markedly cellular*
Grade 3—High	Pleomorphic or round cell liposarcoma
	Mesenchymal chondrosarcoma
	Extraskeletal osteosarcoma
	Malignant triton tumor
	Alveolar soft part sarcoma
	Sarcomas not included in grade 1 with >15% of surface area with necrosis or ≥5 mitoses/10 high-power fields using a 40× objective

*Secondary criteria. Tumor diagnoses specified in grade 1 or 3 are excluded from grade 2.

Adapted from Parham DM, Webber BL, Jenkins JJ III, et al. Nonrhabdomyosarcomatous soft tissue sarcomas of childhood: formulation of a simplified system for grading. Mod Pathol. 1995;8:705-710.

TABLE 20-5		Surgical-Pathologic Grouping System of the Intergroup Rhabdomyosarcoma Study and the Children's Oncology Group
	Group	**Definition**
Low stage	I	Localized disease, completely resected
	II	Total gross resection with evidence of regional spread
	IIa	Grossly resected tumor with microscopic residual disease
	IIb	Regional disease with involved nodes, completely resected with no microscopic residual disease
	IIc	Regional disease with involved nodes, grossly resected but with evidence of microscopic residual disease and/or histologic involvement of the most distal regional lymph node from the primary site in the dissection.
High stage	III	Incomplete resection with gross residual disease
	IV	Distant metastatic disease present at onset

TABLE 20-6		SIOP-UICC TNM Soft Tissue Sarcoma Clinical Staging System
Stage	**Description**	
I	T1—Tumor confined to organ or tissue of origin	
	N0—No evidence of regional lymph node involvement	
	M0—No evidence of distant metastasis	
II	T2—Tumor involving one or more contiguous organs or tissues or with adjacent malignant effusion	
	N0	
	M0	
III	Any T	
	N1—Evidence of regional lymph node involvement	
	M0	
IV	Any T	
	Any N	
	M1—Evidence of distant metastases	

Adapted from Rodary C, Flamant F, Donaldson SS. An attempt to use a common staging system in rhabdomyosarcoma: a report of an international workshop initiated by the International Society of Pediatric Oncology (SIOP). Med Pediatr Oncol. 1989;17:210-215.

SIOP, International Society of Pediatric Oncology; UICC, International Union Against Cancer.

Pediatric multicenter studies also make use of the surgical-pathologic grouping system of the Intergroup Rhabdomyosarcoma Study (IRS; Table 20-5), which incorporates tumor spread and outcome of surgical resection, and of the International Society of Pediatric Oncology–International Union Against Cancer TNM classification system of pediatric tumors (Table 20-6).[47-49] STS may also be classified according to the American Joint Commission on Cancer staging system, which integrates tumor size, location relative to the superficial fascia, regional lymph node status, presence of distant metastases, and histologic grade (Table 20-7).[50]

NRSTS most commonly spreads locally and hematogenously but may exhibit regional lymph node metastases. The lung is the most common site of distant metastases, but less commonly, these tumors can metastasize to bone or brain. Metastatic spread at the time of diagnosis is likely to occur in alveolar soft part sarcoma, high-grade MPNST, clear cell sarcoma, high-grade angiosarcoma, and epithelioid sarcoma.[4]

Several factors have been shown to be prognostic for tumor associated mortality. In both univariate and multivariate analyses of patients with grossly resected tumors, tumor invasion into contiguous structures and size (>5 cm) are the most highly predictive of decreased 5-year event-free and overall survival. Other factors that correlate with poor outcome including female gender, older age, high-grade tumors, high-grade MPNST histology, and tumors in nonextremity locations.[4]

Treatment

Surgical resection constitutes the mainstay of treatment for localized tumors. Radiation therapy is typically reserved for tumors for which complete resection is not possible. However, the high radiation dose required for sarcoma therapy is associated with significant growth-associated side effects in children. Although surgery with or without radiation results in good outcome for localized and low-grade disease, high-grade disease is associated with significant morbidity and mortality rates. The role of conventional chemotherapy and biologically targeted therapies remains in evolution.

TABLE 20-7	American Joint Committee on Cancer Staging System			
	Primary Tumor (T)	Regional Lymph Nodes (N)	Distant Metastasis (M)	Histologic grade (G)
	1—Tumor ≤5 cm in maximum diameter 2—Tumor >5 cm in maximum diameter a—Superficial b—Deep	0—No metastasis 1—Regional lymph node metastasis	0—No distant metastasis 1—Distant metastasis	1—Well-differentiated 2—Moderately differentiated 3—Poorly differentiated 4—Poorly to undifferentiated
Stage I	Any	N0	M0	G1, G2
Stage II	T1a, T1b, T2a	N0	M0	G3, G4
Stage III	T2b	N0	M0	G3, G4
Stage IV	Any	N1	Any	Any
	Any	Any	M1	Any

Adapted from Greene FL, Page DL, Fleming ID, et al (eds). AJCC Cancer Staging Manual, 6th ed. Chicago, American Joint Committee on Cancer, 2002, pp 193-200.

Local Control

Surgical resection is typically the initial therapy for operable nonmetastatic NRSTS. Complete resection of NRSTS results in a 5-year overall survival rate in excess of 80%.[51-54] However, large, high-grade, and incompletely resected tumors have significant chances for local recurrence. Tumor location (e.g., abdomen vs. extremity) and invasion may limit the ability to perform the wide local excision necessary to achieve tumor-free margins. For these patients, external beam radiation therapy has been used to reduce the risk for local recurrence, based on adult studies.[55-57] Pediatric studies seem to confirm that radiotherapy reduces the risk for local recurrence associated with the inability to achieve a wide surgical margin (>1 cm) in high-grade disease.[58] The impact of postoperative radiation therapy may be most significant for IRS group II patients, although grade and size may mitigate this effect.[59] Radiation doses effective for NRSTS are associated with abnormalities of bone development, which complicates the delivery of this modality to growing children. Brachytherapy, interstitial, intercavitary, or surface placement of radioisotopes constitute alternative approaches to the delivery of radiotherapy.[60,61] Brachytherapy can precisely deliver high doses of radiation to the tumor or resection site while sparing normal tissue. Brachytherapy can also be administered concurrently with external beam radiation, and a study of adult STS suggests that the combination may result in increased rates of local control when surgical margins are positive.[62] Other techniques that augment local control include radiofrequency ablation, cryoablation, and embolization.[63-65] Strategies for local control that incorporate site-directed chemotherapy include intralesional chemotherapy followed by electroporation at accessible sites and intraperitoneal chemotherapy infusion.[66]

Chemotherapy

Complete resection of NRSTS is associated with a high rate of cure, so chemotherapy is employed principally when tumors are unresectable, incompletely resected, or metastatic. The uncommon appearance of each of the heterogeneous tumors that constitute the class of NRSTS makes clinical trials of chemotherapy particularly challenging. Even for multicenter groups to accrue sufficient subjects, the nonselective inclusion of NRSTS complicates the interpretation and extrapolation of most trials. Nonetheless, several consistent themes emerge. In contrast to the striking successes of chemotherapy for Ewing's

sarcoma and RMS, NRSTS tends to be relatively chemoresistant, although synovial sarcoma and extraosseous Ewing's sarcoma are exceptions.[4,53,67,68] For patients with fully resected tumors, the inclusion of chemotherapy fails to increase survival rates.[69,70] The impact of chemotherapy may be most significant in patients harboring tumors with the highest risk for metastatic spread. In high-grade, grossly resected tumors, chemotherapy was associated with a 5-year metastasis-free survival rate of 49.5%, compared to 0 in untreated patients.[71] Chemotherapy may also be beneficial for patients with unresectable tumors. For both chemotherapy-sensitive and -resistant tumors, neoadjuvant treatment may permit the subsequent surgical resection of initially nonresectable tumors.[67] Patients with unresected or metastatic tumors have poor outcomes, although 40% to 50% of patients with advanced disease demonstrate some response (partial or complete remission) to regimens containing ifosfamide and doxorubicin or cyclophosphamide and doxorubicin.[68,70,72] Treatment with doxorubicin, cyclophosphamide, and vincristine alternating with ifosfamide and etoposide together with aggressive local control of incompletely resected tumors or those metastatic at presentation, resulted in 80% of patients with a partial or complete remission.[72] Based on the principle that advanced sarcomas may respond to intensive therapies, the feasibility of dose-intensified neoadjuvant chemotherapy has been an end point of several trials using doxorubicin, ifosfamide, and dacarbazine in adults and using doxorubicin, cyclophosphamide, ifosfamide, etoposide, and vincristine in children.[68,73-76] The Children's Oncology Group has initiated a study of risk-based treatment for NRSTS (ARST 0332).

Regarding specific chemotherapeutic agents, topoisomerase 1 inhibitors may also have activity against these tumors. Topotecan with high-dose cyclophosphamide as well as irinotecan demonstrated limited efficacy against recurrent NRSTS, and the effect of irinotecan together with temozolomide is currently being studied.[77-80] The combination of vinorelbine with low-dose cyclophosphamide may also have activity against these tumors.[81] Gemcitabine and docetaxel, both of which have some activity against adult sarcomas, were more effective together than gemcitabine alone in adult patients with metastatic sarcoma.[82] In adults, advanced disease may also respond to the combination of gemcitabine and vinorelbine.[83] In children, however, the efficacy of gemcitabine or docetaxel administered individually in the setting of relapsed pediatric solid tumors seems small.[84-86] As previously mentioned, synovial sarcoma is considered an exception to the general chemoresistance of NRSTS. Children and adolescents exhibit a 5-year event-free survival of about 70%, with decreased event-free survival, progression-free survival, and overall survival associated with tumor size (>5 cm), local invasion, and IRS grouping (III and IV).[87-90] Another exception is extraosseous Ewing's sarcoma, which is generally grouped with bony Ewing's sarcoma for treatment purposes (see Chapter 21).

General Biologic Features

Soft tissue sarcomas can be classified into two groups based on cytogenetics. Tumors that occur in children and young adults tend to reveal relatively simple karyotypes that are commonly characterized by an easily recognizable and usually pathognomonic reciprocal chromosomal translocation. In contrast, STSs in adults typically demonstrate complex karyotypes without recurrent cytogenetic abnormalities. Cellular mechanisms for telomere maintenance may correlate with translocation status. Tumors harboring single translocations tend to have normal to short telomeres suggestive of active telomerase, whereas tumors with complex karyotypes have longer telomeres, suggesting the use of alternative mechanisms of telomere lengthening.[91-95] Although other cellular changes, in addition to translocations, are likely to be necessary for sarcoma development, the difference between sarcomas in children and young adults and those in older individuals may reflect divergent cellular origins. Experimentally, haploinsufficiency of the nonhomologous end-joining DNA repair pathway in the context of mice deficient in *Ink4a* and *Arf* leads to the development of sarcoma with varied histologies and karyotypes.[96] Although the tumors that develop in these mice demonstrate translocations, amplifications, and deletions, the translocated regions are not recognizably syntenic with known human translocations, suggesting that these sarcomas more closely reflect adult sarcomas. This finding also highlights the issue of whether complex cytogenetic abnormalities themselves result in oncogenesis or are a manifestation of the genomic instability associated with the loss of cell cycle checkpoints.

ADIPOCYTIC TUMORS

Liposarcoma is the most common soft tissue sarcoma in adults.[97] In children, however, approximately 95% of adipose tumors are benign lipomas and lipoblastomas; liposarcomas account for the remainder.[98] Lipoblastomas tend to occur in children younger than 3 years of age, whereas liposarcomas predominate in older children and adolescents. Liposarcomas are classified into five morphologic types: well-differentiated, dedifferentiated, myxoid, round cell, and pleomorphic.[99] Dedifferentiated and well-differentiated liposarcomas occur predominantly in the retroperitoneum, whereas myxoid and round cell liposarcomas tend to occur in the extremities. High-grade, dedifferentiated liposarcomas carry the highest risk for recurrence and metastasis.[100,101] In contrast to adults, most children present with the myxoid variant.[102,103] Myxoid liposarcoma is histopathologically characterized by proliferation of round to spindled primitive mesenchymal cells and scattered lipoblasts in an abundant, faintly eosinophilic, homogeneous myxoid matrix (Fig. 20-2). A network of delicate straight and curvilinear capillaries is distinctive. Complete resection is associated with prolonged tumor-free survival. When margins are microscopically positive, the addition of radiation therapy may increase the likelihood of disease-free survival. The histologic variants of liposarcoma are associated with differences in response to chemotherapy. Myxoid liposarcoma demonstrates the highest likelihood of response to a doxorubicin and ifosfamide regimen.[104] Myxoid liposarcoma also exhibits sensitivity

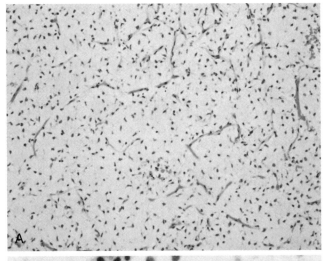

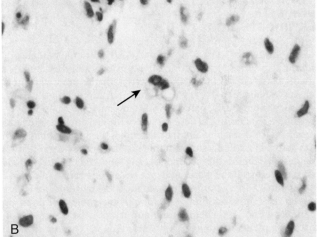

FIGURE 20-2. Myxoid liposarcoma. **A,** Uniform stellate and spindled cells in a prominent myxoid stroma; characteristic branching capillaries. **B,** Primitive tumor cells and scattered lipoblasts *(arrow)* in a myxoid background.

to trabectedin (ecteinascidin-743; ET-743), a DNA minor groove binding small molecule.[105]

Molecularly distinguished from other liposarcoma histologies, myxoid and round cell liposarcomas share recurrent chromosomal translocations. t(12;16)(q13;p11) results in fusion of the *FUS* (also known as *TLS*, an abbreviation for translocated in liposarcoma) with the transcription factor *DDIT3 (CHOP)*; and t(12;22)(q13;q11) fuses *EWS* with *DDIT3*.[106-108] *DDIT3* is a member of the b-ZIP family of transcriptional regulatory proteins and seems to function as a negative transcriptional regulator. Chimerism with both *EWS* and *FUS (TLS)* suggests that the retained domains of *EWS* and *FUS* confer similar activities to the DNA-binding domain of *DDIT3*. Ectopic expression of either *FUS-DDIT3* or *EWS-DDIT3* in NIH-3T3 cells resulted in characteristics of oncogenic transformation, including growth in soft agar and tumor formation in immunocompromised mice.[109] Furthermore, implantation of mice with primary murine mesenchymal progenitor cells transduced with *FUS-DDIT3* led to the development of tumors that morphologically and immunohistochemically resemble human myxoid liposarcoma.[110]

Well-differentiated liposarcomas are associated with complex karyotypes. However, a consistent finding is amplification of the *MDM2* locus. *MDM2* binds *p53* to inhibit its activity. In the context of wildtype *p53*, inhibition of *MDM2* by the small molecule nutlin3 results in increased apoptosis in liposarcoma cell lines.[111,112]

Chromosomal rearrangements of *8q12* are found in lipoblastoma, and their detection can aid in diagnosis. These rearrangements have implicated the zinc finger DNA-binding protein *PLAG1*. In lipoblastoma, translocation places the *PLAG1* coding exons under the transcriptional control of either the hyaluronan synthase 2 (*HAS2*) or the collagen, type I, alpha 2 (*COL1A2*) promoter.[113] *PLAG1* was originally identified based on its translocation in pleomorphic adenoma of the salivary gland.[114] In contrast to lipoblastoma, *PLAG1* is translocated downstream of the β-catenin promoter in pleomorphic adenoma.

FIBROBLASTIC AND MYOFIBROBLASTIC TUMORS

Desmoid Tumor

Desmoid tumor, also known as deep musculoaponeurotic fibromatosis, presents from infancy through adulthood, with a median age at diagnosis in the early thirties and a twofold higher incidence in women than in men. Although most tumors occur spontaneously, patients with familial adenomatous polyposis (FAP), and in particular those with Gardner's syndrome, have reported an incidence of desmoid tumors ranging from 3.5% to 32%.[23,115] Desmoid tumors in the pediatric population tend to occur in the second decade and are located in the extremities and the head and neck, in contrast to the adult population, in whom abdominal and truncal sites are common.[116,117] Abdominal desmoids are more common in patients with FAP, whereas limb and trunk locations predominate in patients without FAP.[118]

The tumors consist of an infiltrating, uniform, spindled cell proliferation lacking nuclear pleomorphism and mitotic activity (Fig. 20-3). Although desmoid tumors have a high potential for local invasion and recurrence, they never metastasize. Surgery is the primary treatment, but tumors have a significant chance for local recurrence, even if negative margins can be achieved.[117] Achieving negative margins without severe disfigurement or functional impairment may be impossible. In these circumstances, preoperative chemotherapy or partial resection and postoperative chemotherapy should be considered. Multiple drug regimens have been shown to shrink or stabilize desmoid tumor growth. They include methotrexate with vinblastine or tamoxifen with diclofenac.[119-122] Other active treatments include the combination of doxorubicin, vincristine, actinomycin D, and cyclophosphamide or the combination of doxorubicin and dacarbazine.[123-125] Response to imatinib has been demonstrated in about half of patients with desmoid tumors, possibly as the result of the inhibition of *PDGFRB*.[126]

Although most desmoid tumor cells are karyotypically diploid, abnormalities of the Y chromosome and 5q plus gains in chromosome 8 and 20 may be noted.[127-130] Abnormalities may be identified in a subset of tumor cells, and the finding of trisomy 8 may suggest an increased risk for recurrence.[128] Gardner's syndrome, which is associated with colonic polyposis and abdominal desmoid tumors, is a phenotypic variant of FAP. FAP is caused by mutation of the *APC* gene at 5q. *APC* regulates β-catenin, the downstream mediator of *WNT* signaling. Stabilized β-catenin forms a multiprotein complex with members of the T-cell factor/lymphoid enhancer factor family, resulting in transcriptional activation of T-cell factor/lymphoid enhancer factor target genes.[131-134] *APC* mutations resulting in

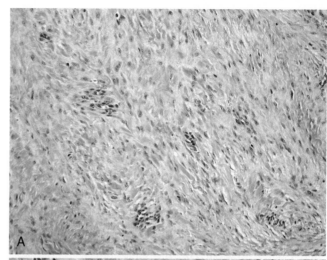

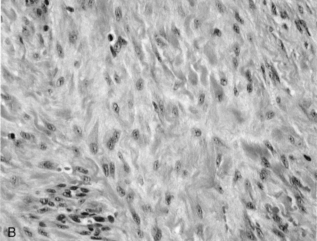

FIGURE 20-3. Desmoid tumor. **A,** Spindle cell neoplasm with prominent collagenization. **B,** Tumor cells are histopathologically bland, with ovoid uniform nuclei, open chromatin, and single small nucleoli. Some cells have abundant eosinophilic cytoplasm.

increased β-catenin or stabilizing mutations in β-catenin have been implicated in the proliferation of sporadic desmoid tumors.[135-137] Mice expressing either mutant *APC* or stabilized β-catenin develop aggressive fibromatoses.[138,139]

Infantile Myofibroma/Myofibromatosis and Hemangiopericytoma

In the most recent classification by the World Health Organization of soft tissue tumors, the term *hemangiopericytoma* is no longer used; instead, a majority of these tumors are currently regarded as solitary fibrous tumors.[140,141] Infantile hemangiopericytoma, recognized as a distinct category of benign hemangiopericytoma by Enzinger, is currently considered to be in the category of infantile myofibroma/myofibromatosis.[142] Infantile myofibromatosis is a benign proliferation of myofibroblastic cells affecting almost exclusively young children. Presentation in multiple siblings and across generations suggests an autosomal dominant pattern of inheritance.[143-145] The tumors are solitary or multicentric and may involve the skin, muscle, viscera, or bone. Approximately 60% are noted at birth, and 88% occur

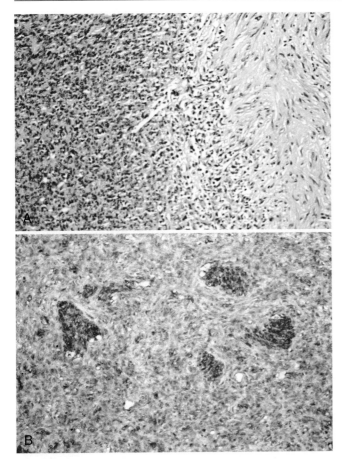

FIGURE 20-4. Infantile myofibromatoses. **A,** Biphasic tumor with an area of bland smooth muscle-like proliferation (to the right of the photograph) sharply demarcated from an area of cellular hemangiopericytoma-like tumor. **B,** Characteristic nests of strongly actin immunoreactive cells (in red) are scattered through a cellular hemangiopericytoma-like area.

before patients are 2 years old.[146] More commonly found in males, solitary lesions typically develop in the soft tissues of the head. neck, and trunk. In contrast, the multicentric form is more common in females and, in addition to affecting soft tissues, it can develop in bones and viscera. Histopathologically, infantile myofibroma and myofibromatosis have similar features. They are multinodular and biphasic, with alternating hemangiopericytoma-like, densely cellular areas and less cellular areas, and have smooth-muscle differentiation that is immunoreactive to actin (Fig. 20-4). Solitary lesions can recur, though rarely. Multicentric lesions undergo spontaneous regression, but multiple visceral lesions may increase in size and number before regression, thus compromising vital structures and, rarely, leading to death.[147] Optimal initial therapy involves complete surgical excision. Life-threatening multifocal disease has been treated successfully with low-dose vincristine and actinomycin-D or with low-dose vinblastine and methotrexate.[148] Urinary basic fibroblast growth factor has been shown to be elevated in an infant during the proliferative phase, and connective tissue growth factor is expressed in both tumor and stromal cells.[149,150]

Infantile myofibroma/myofibromatosis should be distinguished from t(7;12) pericytoma, a distinct tumor with the histologic, immunohistochemical, and ultrastructural features of pericytic differentiation and a translocation involving t(7;12)(p21-22;q13-15).[151] This translocation brings together the β-actin gene with the zinc finger transcription factor *GLI1*.[152] Originally identified on the basis of amplification in human glioma, *GLI1* is activated by sonic hedgehog signaling through the transmembrane receptor *PTCH*.[153-155] However, in t(7;12) pericytoma, the carboxyl terminus of *GLI1* is fused with the amino terminal domain of *ACTB*. It is intriguing that *GLI1* has also been found to be amplified in a subset of rhabdomyosarcoma and osteosarcoma that lacks typical markers of differentiation.[156]

Infantile Fibrosarcoma

Infantile (congenital) fibrosarcoma is one of the most common NRSTSs in young children.[157] In contrast to fibrosarcoma in adults, this low-grade tumor displays benign clinical behavior and is typically cured by surgical excision. However, large tumors for which surgical excision would result in significant morbidity may be treated with preoperative chemotherapy (Fig. 20-5A). Regimens with activity against these tumors include vincristine and actinomycin-D together with cyclophosphamide, ifosfamide, or doxorubicin.[158-164]

Histopathologically, the tumor is characterized by intersecting bundles with a herringbone pattern composed of cellular spindle to ovoid cells with a high proliferative rate, frequent mitoses, and areas of necrosis (see Fig. 20-5B, C). Some tumors may have a hemangiopericytoma-like pattern of growth. Scattered chronic inflammatory cells are commonly present. Tumor cells have a fibroblastic and myofibroblastic ultrastructure (see Fig. 20-5D) and immunophenotype with variable positivity for desmin and actin. Aberrant cytokeratin expression is observed in 15% to 20% of the tumors.

Infantile fibrosarcoma is characterized by t(12;15) (p13;q25).[165] This translocation fuses the amino terminal helix-loop-helix oligomerization domain of the *ETV6* transcription factor (also known as *TEL*) with the carboxyl terminal tyrosine kinase domain of the neurotrophin-3 receptor *NTRK3* (also known as *TRKC*). The detection of *ETV6-NTRK3* by RT-PCR is highly specific and can distinguish infantile fibrosarcoma from more aggressive spindle cell sarcomas.[166] It is intriguing that the same translocation also occurs in congenital mesoblastic nephroma and in secretory breast carcinoma.[167-169]

Chimerism results in constitutive activation by autophosphorylation of *NTRK3* tyrosine residues. Translocation also results in aberrant *NTRK3* expression. *ETV6* is widely expressed, whereas *NTRK3* is normally restricted to neuronal cells and fetal kidney.[170-172] *ETV6-NTRK3* transform *NIH3T3* cells as assayed by growth in soft agar and in xenografts in immunocompromised animals.[173] *ETV6-NTRK3* is associated with several signaling pathways that may be important in oncogenesis. *ETV6-NTRK3* activates both the mitogen-activated protein kinase and AKT pathways; AKT activation is mediated by direct interaction of *ETV6-NTRK3* with c-Src.[174,175] *ETV6-NTRK3*–mediated fibroblast transformation also requires the insulin-like growth factor receptor (IGFRI), possibly through direct interaction with the IGFRI substrate IRS-1.[176,177] The *ETV6-NTRK3* fusion may also act by suppressing transforming growth factor-β signaling through interaction with the type II transforming growth factor-β receptor.[178]

Specific Forms of Fibrosarcoma

Dermatofibrosarcoma protuberans (DFSP) is a rare cutaneous fibrohistiocytic tumor characterized by locally aggressive behavior. DFSP may begin as a plaquelike, raised, red-blue

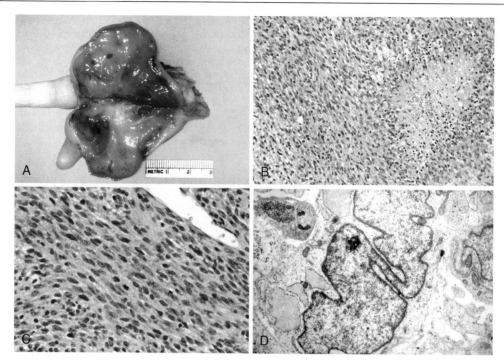

FIGURE 20-5. Infantile fibrosarcoma. **A,** Partial amputation of the hand in an infant with a rapidly growing soft tissue mass. On cut section the mass is fleshy and soft, with areas of hemorrhage and necrosis. **B,** Histopathology shows a cellular spindle cell sarcoma with frequent mitoses, apoptosis, and confluent areas of necrosis. **C,** At higher magnification, nuclei appear uniform and hyperchromatic, and cytoplasm is elongated and pink. Scattered inflammatory cells are also present. **D,** Ultrastructurally, tumor cells have the features of fibroblasts, with prominent secretory-type rough endoplasmic reticula.

lesion followed by a rapid growth phase that may be associated with the development of one or more nodules. DFSP appears as a cellular, spindle-cell proliferation, commonly with a distinct storiform pattern that infiltrates the surrounding dermis and subcutaneous fat (Fig. 20-6A). Tumor cells are typically immunoreactive for apolipoprotein A-III and CD34 (see Fig. 20-6B). The Bednár tumor refers to an uncommon DFSP variant with scattered dendritic cells containing melanin.[179] The majority of the tumors develop on the trunk and upper extremities and although typically diagnosed during the fourth or fifth decade, DFSP may occur in children and adolescents.[180] Inadequate resection of the tumor is associated with a significant risk for local recurrence.[181] Radiation therapy can be used effectively as an adjuvant for the treatment of resection sites with positive margins.[182-184] Rarely, DFSP can evolve into a high-grade fibrosarcoma often associated with a loss of CD34 staining and an increased risk for metastasis (Fig. 20-7A, B).[185]

Giant cell fibroblastoma, a rare tumor found predominantly in males less than 10 years of age, is in the spectrum of DFSP. Histopathologically, giant cell fibroblastoma is composed of variably cellular spindle or stellate cells often in a myxoid background containing pseudovascular spaces and multinucleated giant cells (see Fig. 20-7C).[186-188] Like DFSP, giant cell fibroblastoma is characteristically immunoreactive for CD34 and apolipoprotein A-III.[189]

DFSP and giant cell fibroblastoma harbor a pathognomonic translocation between the *collagen type 1 alpha1* gene and the *platelet derived growth factor β (PDGFB)* gene.[190-192] In contrast to the other sarcoma-associated translocations, the translocated *COL1A1-PDGFB* locus may be present as a low-level amplification on a ring chromosome. Detection of the resulting *COL1A1-PDGFB* transcript can provide confirmation of the diagnosis.[193] The fusion of *PDGFB* with *COL1A1* preserves the full coding region of *PDGFB*, and the resulting

chimeric polypeptide is subject to intracellular processing that results in the secretion of a native *PDGFB* molecule that is capable of activating its receptor, *PDGFR*.[194,195] Although the mechanisms of autocrine-activated *PDGFR* signaling are not known, they may function through *STAT3* and *ERK* activation.[196] Presumably, through the inhibition of autocrine *PDGFR* activation, the growth of xenografted primary human DFSP cells can be inhibited by the kinase inhibitor imatinib (Gleevec, STI571).[197] Treatment with imatinib has also been shown to be effective in patients with metastatic or unresectable disease.[198-202] Responses to vinblastine and methotrexate have also been reported.[203]

Low-Grade Fibromyxoid Sarcoma

Low-grade fibromyxoid sarcoma (LGFMS) typically develops in the lower extremities of young adults and occasionally in adolescents (Fig. 20-8). Described by Evans in 1987, it is characterized by bland, uniform spindle cells with a short fascicular or whorly pattern of growth in a dense collagenous or variably myxoid stroma (Fig. 20-9).[204,205] An abrupt transition between cellular myxoid and hypocellular collagenous areas is frequently present. Dense collagenous areas mimic desmoid tumor. Myxoid areas contain characteristic arcades of curvilinear vessels that may be sclerotic or be surrounded by more densely cellular spindle cells. The mitotic count is characteristically low. Occasionally, there are giant collagenous rosettes (hyalinizing spindle cell tumor with giant rosettes). Vimentin is the only constant marker present in tumor cells. Some tumors may be focally immunoreactive for actin, CD34, cytokeratins, or epithelial membrane antigen (EMA). Superficial locations are found more commonly in children.[206] Although primary resection typically results in disease control, local recurrence

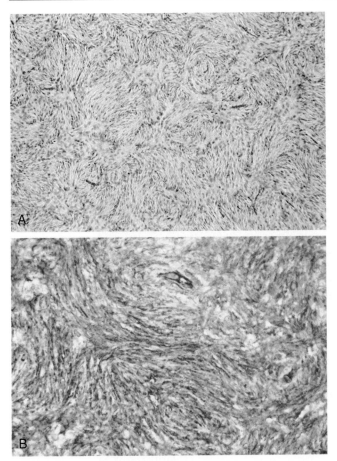

FIGURE 20-6. Dermatofibrosarcoma protuberans. **A,** Cellular spindle cell neoplasm with distinct storiform (cartwheel) pattern of growth. **B,** Tumor cells are diffusely immunoreactive with CD34.

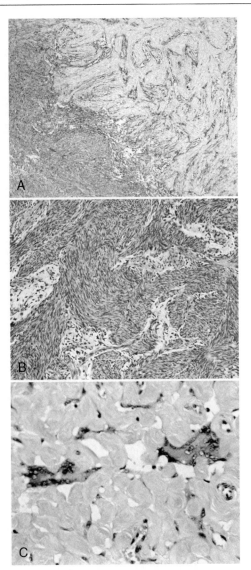

FIGURE 20-7. Fibrosarcoma in DFSP, giant cell fibroblastoma. **A,** Loss of CD34 immunoreactivity in the dedifferentiated fibrosarcoma area, which is sharply demarcated from adjacent CD34-positive DFSP (lower left corner). **B,** Highly cellular fibrosarcoma with fascicular pattern and numerous mitoses. **C,** Giant cell fibroblastoma with characteristic multinucleated giant cells and spindled cells with collagenization.

and pulmonary metastases can develop in 5% to 10% of patients after many years.[207] However, resection of recurrent disease can result in long-term remission. LGFMS seems to be chemoresistant.[208]

LGFMS is associated with t(7;16)(q34;p11), which results in the fusion of *FUS (TLS)* and *CREB3L2*.[209-211] One case of LGFMS was been reported with *FUS-CREB3L1* fusion.[212] Native *CREB3L2* (also known as *BBF2H7*) is a member of the *CREB* basic leucine zipper family of transcription factors and acts as a transducer of endoplasmic reticulum stress signals. Normally tethered through a transmembrane domain to the endoplasmic reticulum, metabolic stress on the endoplasmic reticulum results in cleavage of the cytoplasmic amino terminal b-ZIP domain, enabling it to translocate to the nucleus and to activate transcription from cyclic adenosine monophosphate–responsive elements.[213] Chimerism with *FUS*, a translocation partner with *CHOP* in myxoid liposarcoma, likely acts to deregulate *CREB3L2* transcriptional activity.[214] PCR-based identification of the fusion gene product from paraffin sections can be used to confirm the diagnosis.[215]

Myxofibrosarcoma

Myxofibrosarcoma (MFS) is one of the most common sarcomas of the elderly but has been reported in adolescents and young adults.[216,217] Typically developing during the sixth or seventh decade of life, MFS exhibits a predilection for the

dermal or subcutaneous tissues of the extremities.[218-220] MFS may alternatively be referred to as low-grade myxoid malignant fibrohistocytoma or as fibrosarcoma, myxoid type. Histopathologically, it is characterized by a multinodular growth of spindled or stellate cells in a myxoid stroma (Fig. 20-10). MFS grading has prognostic value and is based on cellularity, nuclear pleomorphism, and mitotic activity.[221] Resection is typically curative for low- or intermediate-grade tumors, but recurrent tumors may show morphologic and molecular multistep tumor progression.[222,223] Large tumor size, necrosis, and decreased myxoid stroma in low-grade tumors are associated with a significant risk for local and distant recurrence.[224] High-grade tumors have a significant risk for recurrence and metastasis. In a study of adults, 23% of patients with intermediate- or high-grade tumors developed metastases, most commonly to the lung and lymph nodes. A subset of intermediate- or high-grade

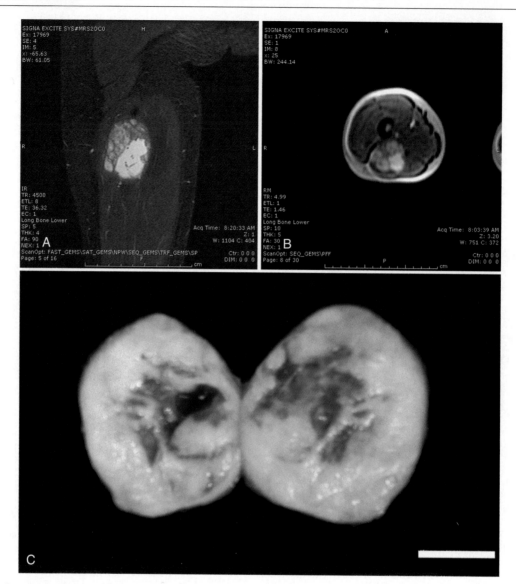

FIGURE 20-8. Low-grade fibromyxoid sarcoma. **A** and **B,** Enhancing well-delineated heterogeneous thigh mass seen on MR imaging. **C,** Grossly, the tumor is well circumscribed and shows a soft white-tan cut surface with areas of hemorrhage and cystification.

tumors exhibiting an epithelioid morphology seems to behave more aggressively than other high-grade histologies.[225] In addition to grade, an initial incomplete resection and infiltrative MR imaging T2 signal correlates with an increased risk for local recurrence.[226] Cytogenetically, MFS may be diploid but is typically complex. Numerous chromosomal gains and losses as well as ring chromosomes have been observed.[223,227] Isolated chromosomal translocations have been noted.[228,229]

Solitary Fibrous Tumor

A solitary fibrous tumor (SFT) is a fibroblastic tumor that was originally described in the pleura but can occur at other sites. Most of the tumors formerly classified as hemagiopericytomas are currently categorized as SFTs. Approximately 5% to 10% of soft tissue SFTs are malignant. SFTs may be associated with hypoglycemia as a result of synthesis by tumor cells of high-molecular-weight insulin-like growth factor II.[230,231] The histopathology is described as a patternless proliferation of spindle

cells with a hemangiopericytoma-like growth (Fig. 20-11). Areas of sclerosis and hyalinization are characteristic. The mitotic count is generally low. Although the behavior of SFTs cannot always be predicted by histopathology, the presence of frequent mitoses, hypercellularity, pleomorphism, or necrosis is generally associated with malignant behavior. Tumor cells are immunoreactive with CD34 and CD99 (see Fig. 20-11, inset). Some tumors also express EMA, actin, BCL2 APOD, or nuclear β-catenin.[232-234] Cytogenetically, SFTs are heterogeneous.

Inflammatory Myofibroblastic Tumor

Inflammatory myofibroblastic tumors (IMTs) occur primarily in the viscera and soft tissue (particularly lungs) of children and young adults; the mean age is 13.2 years.[235] Of intermediate biologic potential, these tumors often recur locally but rarely metastasize. They are characterized by a proliferation of myofibroblastic spindle cells and an inflammatory, predominantly

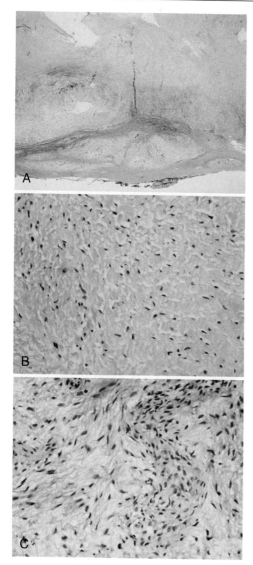

FIGURE 20-9. Low-grade fibromyxoid sarcoma. **A,** Multinodular, infiltrative growth at the tumor periphery and a variably myxoid stroma. **B,** Fibromatosis-like area with bland spindled cells immersed in a collagenous background. **C,** Characteristic curvilinear blood vessels, bland spindled cells, and a myxoid background.

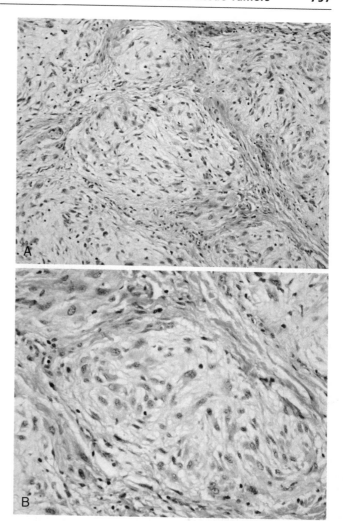

FIGURE 20-10. Myxofibrosarcoma. **A,** Multinodular growth pattern and prominent myxoid stroma. Numerous curvilinear vessels are present at the periphery of the nodules. **B,** Atypical myofibroblasts with large mildly pleomorphic nuclei and abundant cytoplasm.

lymphoplasmacytic infiltrate (Fig. 20-12A). Approximately half of IMTs show immunoreactivity for anaplastic lymphoma kinase (ALK; see Fig. 20-12B).

Clonal cytogenetic changes that activate ALK occur in 50% to 70% of IMTs.[236] The most common chromosomal translocation results in a fusion of the ALK receptor tyrosine kinase with the amino terminal coiled-coil domain of the tropomyosin 3 or tropomyosin 4 genes (*TPM3* and *TPM4*). ALK may also be fused to the amino terminal domains of clathrin heavy chain (*CTLC*), cysteinyl-tRNA synthetase, RAN-binding protein 2 (*RANBP-2*), or *SEC31L1*.[237-240] ALK rearrangements were first identified in anaplastic large cell lymphoma, in which the fusion of ALK with nucleophosmin is most common, although chimerism with *CTLC* has also been observed.[241,242] IMTs commonly demonstrate expression of *MYC*, cyclin D1, and *MCL1*, regardless of ALK status. ALK-positive IMTs are more common in younger patients and seem less likely to metastasize than ALK-negative disease, although local recurrence occurs with equal frequency.[235]

SO-CALLED FIBROHISTIOCYTIC TUMORS

Plexiform Fibrohistiocytic Tumor

A plexiform fibrohistiocytic tumor is a fibrohistiocytic neoplasm with a multinodular (plexiform) pattern of growth that occurs in the deep dermis and subcutaneous tissue, primarily in children, adolescents, and young adults.[243,244] Histopathologically, it is characterized by a plexiform growth of small nodules composed of mononuclear, histiocyte-like cells, fibroblasts and multinucleate giant cells (Fig. 20-13). Mitoses are infrequent and pleomorphism is minimal. This tumor has a tendency to recur locally and in about 5% of cases may metastasize, particularly to regional lymph nodes.[245] Cytogenetic abnormalities in the few cases reported are heterogeneous.

SMOOTH MUSCLE TUMORS

Sporadic Leiomyosarcoma

Leiomyosarcoma (LMS) is the most common soft tissue sarcoma in adults.[246] LMS can develop in uterus, bowel,

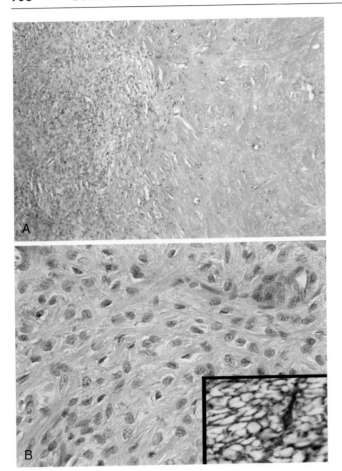

FIGURE 20-11. Solitary fibrous tumor. **A,** Spindle cell tumor with a prominent area of sclerosis. **B,** Patternless proliferation of spindled cells with uniform ovoid nuclei, inconspicuous nucleoli, and eosinophilic cytoplasm with poorly defined borders. Tumor cells are strongly immunoreactive with CD34 *(inset)*.

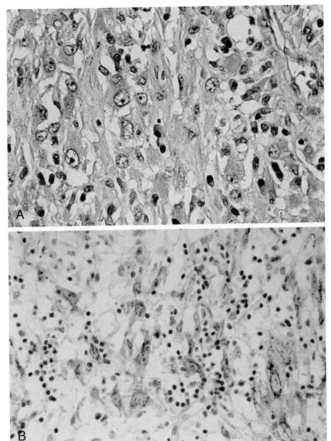

FIGURE 20-12. Inflammatory myofibroblastic tumor. **A,** Spindled and plump myofibroblasts with abundant eosinophilic cytoplasm, round to ovoid nuclei, and prominent single nucleolus. Intermingled are numerous lymphocytes and plasma cells. **B,** Neoplastic myofibroblasts show cytoplasmic immunoreactivity for ALK.

vascular structures, and skin as well as in soft tissue and bone.[247,248] In children, LMS most commonly develops in the gastrointestinal tract and skin. In infants, intestinal LMS can present with perforation and obstruction.[249,250] In the head/neck, trunk, and extremities, LMS has equal incidence and tends to exhibit a more low-grade morphology and a clinical behavior comparable to that in adults.[251,252] Secondary leiomyosarcoma may develop in the radiation field of childhood cancer survivors.[253] Histopathologically, LMS is characterized by intersecting fascicles of spindle cells with prominently eosinophilic cytoplasm and elongated cigar-shaped nuclei (Fig. 20-14). In some tumors, nuclear pleomorphism and hyperchromatism are present. Mitoses are usually easily found and their frequency is often uneven throughout the tumor. Tumor cells are immunoreactive for smooth muscle actin, desmin, and h-caldesmon. Ultrastructurally, tumor cells are invested by a continuous basal lamina and have subplasmalemmal densities; their cytoplasms contain abundant smooth-muscle-type myofilaments with evenly distributed dense bodies (Fig. 20-15). Because of the morphologic continuum of smooth muscle tumors, mitotic activity is the most reliable way to distinguish leiomyomas from leiomyosarcomas.

Patients with unresectable LMS treated with gemcitabine together with docetaxel demonstrated an overall response rate of 53%.[254] Treatment with bendamustine resulted in stable disease in 40% of patients with leiomyosarcoma refractory to other agents.[255] An overall response rate of 56% to ecteinascidin (ET-743) was found in pretreated leiomyosarcoma patients.[256]

Germline mutation of the fumarate hydratase gene resulting in *FH* deficiency is associated with a cancer predisposition syndrome and with an increased risk for renal cell carcinoma, benign leiomyoma of the skin and uterus, and uterine leiomyosarcoma.[257-259] Approximately half of LMSs demonstrate amplification of the 12q13-15 region that includes *CDK4* and *MDM2*.[260] Vascular endothelial growth factor overexpression detected by immunohistochemistry has been associated with a significantly shorter survival time.[261] Tissue and expression microarray based studies comparing uterine LMS with uterine leiomyoma have demonstrated increased expression of *p21*, *p53*, *PDGFR*, c-Kit, and *p16*.[262-267] Approximately 20% of transgenic mice expressing teratocarcinoma-derived growth factor 1 (also known as CRIPTO) from an *MMTV* promoter developed uterine LMS.[268,269] These tumors demonstrated activated Src, Akt, and GSK-3β as well as activated β-catenin. The majority of human uterine LMSs also demonstrate immunostaining for CR1. Conditional *Pten* inactivation in smooth muscle led to the development of abdominal LMS in mice.[270] Decreased tumor growth after treatment with the rapamycin derivative everolimus suggested the importance of *mTOR* activation in this model.

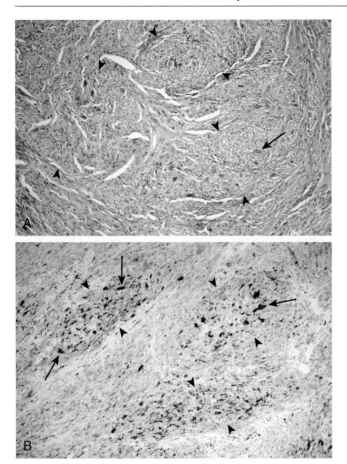

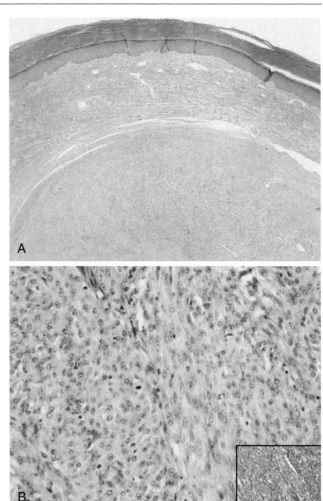

FIGURE 20-13. Plexiform fibrohistiocytic tumor. **A,** Multiple micronodules *(between arrowheads)* of fibrohistiocytic cells and multi-nucleated giant cells separated by collagenous stroma. **B,** Strong CD68 immunoreactivity of multinucleated giant cells *(arrows)* within micronodules *(between arrowheads)*.

FIGURE 20-14. Leiomyosarcoma. **A,** Large tumor nodule is centered in the deep dermis and subcutaneous tissue. **B,** Tumor cells are spindled, have brightly eosinophilic cytoplasm and prominent nuclei with distinct centrally located nucleoli. There is strong and diffuse immunoreactivity for smooth muscle actin *(inset)*.

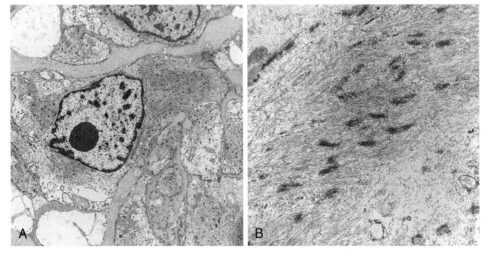

FIGURE 20-15. Leiomyosarcoma, electron microscopy. **A,** Tumor cells are individually invested by a continuous, well-developed basal lamina, and the abundant cytoplasm is filled with smooth-muscle–type filaments. **B,** Higher magnification shows actin-type filaments with uniformly distributed dense bodies, typical of smooth muscle.

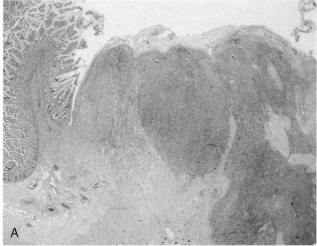

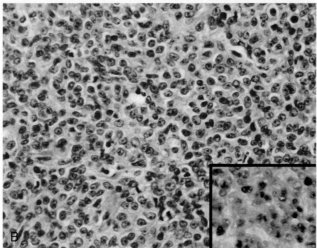

FIGURE 20-16. EBV-associated smooth muscle tumor. **A,** Small intestine with large ulcerating and infiltrative submucosal mass. **B,** The tumor is cellular, with spindled and round tumor cells that have uniform nuclei and distinct single nucleoli. Diffuse nuclear positivity for EBER is seen by in situ hybridization *(inset).*

Leiomyosarcoma Associated with the Epstein-Barr Virus

Immunosuppression associated with solid transplantation and HIV infection can result in LMS associated with the Epstein-Barr virus (EBV), particularly in children and young adults.[271] Multicentricity is common. The histopathologic, immunohistochemical, and ultrastructural features are similar to those in the sporadic LMSs (Fig. 20-16). In situ hybridization for Epstein Barr–encoded RNAs (EBER) shows nuclear positivity in nearly all tumor cells (see Fig. 20-16, inset). EBV can infect smooth muscle cells, resulting in expression of latent and replicative viral products and production of infectious viruses.[272] Reducing immunosuppression can lead to long-term remission.[273-275]

VASCULAR TUMORS

Epithelioid Hemangioendothelioma

Epithelioid hemangioendothelioma (EHE) is a vascular tumor that most commonly develops in the superficial or deep soft

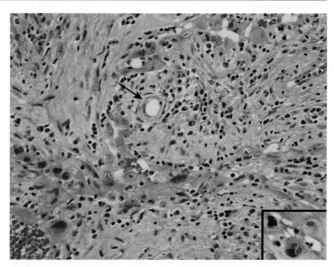

FIGURE 20-17. Epithelioid hemangioendothelioma. Poorly formed vascular channel lined by large epithelioid cells in an inflammatory stroma. Tumor cells have cytoplasmic vacuoles *(arrow).* Red blood cells within cytoplasmic vacuoles *(inset).*

tissue of the extremities.[276] Other sites include the liver, bone, lung, skin, lymph nodes, and central nervous system.[277-282] EHE often seems to arise from a medium to large vein. Unlike epithelioid hemangioma, vascular differentiation in EHE is primitive, with a solid growth pattern or in strands (Fig. 20-17). The stroma is usually myxoid. Tumor cells are large, with abundant eosinophilic cytoplasm. Intracellular vacuoles are characteristic and represent early lumen formation, sometimes containing erythrocytes. Occasionally there are associated eosinophils and lymphocytes. Focal cellular spindling, atypia, and necrosis are associated with a more aggressive course, but bland-appearing lesions may also metastasize.[283] The differential diagnosis includes metastatic carcinoma, melanoma, and various sarcomas with epithelioid appearances, in particular, epithelioid angiosarcoma and epithelioid sarcoma. Tumor cells are immunoreactive with vascular markers, such as CD31, factor VIII-related antigen, and CD34. Ultrastructurally, tumor cells reveal vascular differentiation, with prominent cytoskeletal intermediate filaments, Weibel-Palade granules, pinocytosis, and basal laminae. Although the genes involved are unknown, t(1;3)(p36.3q25) is thought to be a nonrandom translocation in EHE.[284] Extended periods of stable disease as well as partial spontaneous resolution have been noted.[285] Lower grade lesions can be conservatively resected, whereas malignant lesions are likely to justify radical surgical resection. Although surgical resection can result in cure, about one third of patients develop a local recurrence or distant metastasis, most commonly to the lung. Although EHE is considered to be chemoresistant, responses to carboplatin and etoposide for aggressive pulmonary disease and to interferon alfa-2b for multifocal or disseminated liver disease have been reported.[286-289]

Giant Cell Angioblastoma

Giant cell angioblastoma is a rare neonatal vascular tumor. Although the tumor grows slowly, it can be locally invasive and highly destructive.[290,291] Histopathologically it consists of nodular and plexiform aggregates of oval to spindle cells, mononuclear cells, and multinucleated giant cells in a perivascular distribution. Like epithelioid sarcoma, this tumor mimics granulomatous inflammation (Fig. 20-18). Based on previous

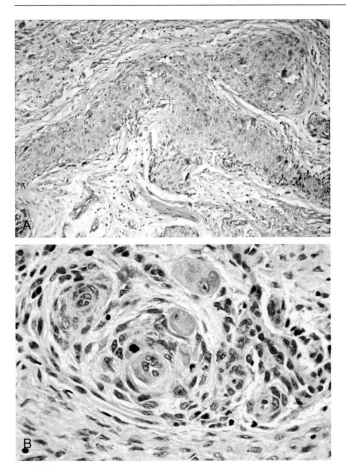

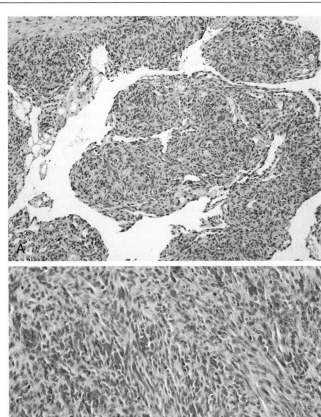

FIGURE 20-18. Giant cell angioblastoma. **A,** Nodular and plexiform aggregates of oval to spindle cells, mononuclear cells, and multinucleated giant cells in a perivascular distribution. **B,** Perivascular giant, spindled, and epithelioid cells.

FIGURE 20-19. Kaposiform hemangioendothelioma. **A,** Irregular nests of tumor with spindled cells and glomeruloid structures. **B,** Kaposi-like area with cellular spindled cell growth and erythrodiapedesis. Spindled cells are immunoreactive with D2-40, a marker associated with lymphatic differentiation *(inset)*.

success with hemangiomas, two patients have been effectively treated with interferon alfa-2b.[292]

Kaposiform Hemangioendothelioma

Kaposiform hemangioendothelioma (KHE), a vascular tumor of infancy and childhood, occurs in either superficial or deep soft tissue. Large lesions, particularly in the retroperitoneum, are aggressive and present with consumption coagulopathy and thrombocytopenia (Kasabach-Merritt syndrome).[293] The lesions usually develop postnatally; the mean age at diagnosis is 3 years 9 months. The lesions are multinodular, often with desmoplasia and vasoformative spindling of tumor cells resembling Kaposi sarcoma and glomeruloid structures (Fig. 20-19). Hyalin droplets, fragmentation of erythrocytes, hemosiderin granules, and fibrin thrombi are characteristic. A lymphatic component is usually present. A majority of tumor cells are immunoreactive to CD31, CD34, and D2-40.[294] In contrast to infantile hemangiomas, glut1 is negative.[295] Tumors can spread locally but do not metastasize distantly.[296]

The mortality rate associated with KHE approaches 30%, typically resulting from Kasabach-Merritt phenomenon, which presents with consumption coagulopathy characterized by moderate microangiopathic hemolytic anemia, severe thrombocytopenia, and hypofibrinogenemia.[297] Although Kasabach-Merritt phenomenon is thought to be a consistent association

with KHE, smaller lesions (<8 cm) may not result in sufficient platelet trapping to cause thrombocytopenia.[298] Surgical resection may be effective for superficial lesions. Unresectable tumors may respond to interferon alfa, corticosteroids, vincristine, and embolization.[299,300] For extensive disease, a combination therapy of vincristine, cyclophosphamide, and actinomycin D, with or without methotrexate, may result in long-term remission.[301,302]

Kaposi Sarcoma

Kaposi sarcoma (KS) is an endothelial cell malignancy that results from transformation by human herpesvirus 8 (HHV-8).[303-305] KS can be multifocal and represent clonal or oligoclonal disease.[306,307] Four clinical-epidemiologic variants of KS are recognized: African (endemic); classic; acquired immune deficiency syndrome (AIDS)–related (epidemic); and immunosuppression-associated. Immunosuppression-associated KS can develop after solid organ or bone marrow transplantation.[308] The incidence of AIDS-related KS has significantly decreased, probably because of improvements in anti-HIV therapies.[309] KS in immunosuppressed individuals tends to behave aggressively, presenting with multifocal skin lesions and involvement of mucosal surfaces, with spread to lymph nodes, brain, lung, gastrointestinal tract, and bones.[310-313]

The lymphadenopathic form of KS is most common in children; it is characterized by replacement of lymph nodes by a monotonous spindled cell proliferation, variable presence of slitlike vascular channels, and a lymphoplasmacytic infiltrate (Fig. 20-20A). Spindled cells show striking nuclear reactivity for HHV-8 by in situ hybridization (see Fig. 20-20B). HHV-8, like EBV, is a gammaherpesvirus, and similar to immunosuppression-related EBV-associated lymphoproliferative disorder, KS may respond to reduced immunosuppression. KS also responds to pegylated liposomal doxorubicin.[314-316]

Angiosarcoma

An angiosarcoma is a high-grade malignancy with endothelial differentiation that constitutes approximately 2% of vascular tumors in children.[317] Angiosarcomas typically develop in skin or soft tissues.[318] In young children angiosarcomas tend to occur in soft tissues and internal organs, including the liver, spleen, heart, and testes and may be associated with Aicardi and Klippel-Trénaunay-Weber syndromes.[319-322] In adults, angiosarcoma development is associated with chronic lymphedema and with exposure to radiation, vinyl chloride, arsenic, and thorium oxide.

Angiosarcomas are aggressive tumors with a 5-year survival rate of approximately 20%.[323-325] Complete surgical resection is associated with survival.[326] Angiosarcomas have a high rate of local and distant recurrence and can metastasize to the regional lymph nodes, lungs, soft tissues, bones, liver, and brain.[318] Although tumors are typically resistant to chemotherapy and radiation, a partial response by unresectable tumors to chemotherapy may facilitate resection.[327] Docetaxel with radiation, paclitaxel, liposomal doxorubicin, vinorelbine, and metronomic trofosfamide may be efficacacious in the treatment of these tumors.[328-331] Radiation therapy is associated with decreased incidence of local recurrence.[324] In contrast to hepatoblastoma, liver transplantation for angiosarcoma does not seem to result in increased survival rates, although long-term survival after transplantation has been reported for type II infantile hepatic hemangioendothelioma, which is considered a form of angiosarcoma.[332]

Angiosarcomas are vasoformative tumors with varying degrees of differentiation (Fig. 20-21). Tumor cells stain positive for factor 8, CD31, and CD34, supporting their endothelial nature.[333] The cellular target of the antiangiogenic compound angiostatin, annexin II, is expressed in angiosarcoma.[334] Although *p16INK4A* deletion seems uncommon, *p16INK4A* promoter methylation was detected commonly in hepatic angiosarcoma.[335]

CHONDRO-OSSEOUS TUMORS

Mesenchymal Chondrosarcoma

Mesenchymal chondrosarcoma is a rapidly growing, highly metastatic cartilaginous tumor. It usually develops in bone, but more than 30% can develop in extraskeletal sites.[336] In contrast to most chondrosarcomas, mesenchymal chondrosarcoma tends to occur in young adults and, infrequently, children. Histopathologically, mesenchymal chondrosarcoma has two components; one consists of well-differentiated

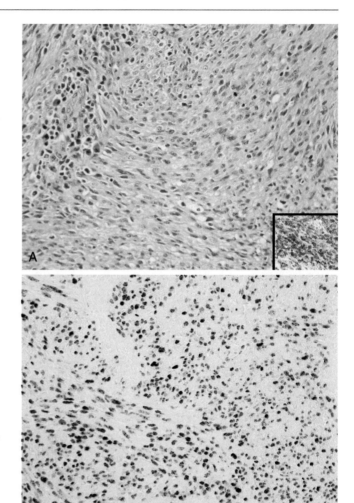

FIGURE 20-20. Kaposi sarcoma. **A,** Fascicles of monomorphic spindle cells and clusters of inflammatory cells, particularly lymphocytes and plasma cells. Spindled cells are strongly immunoreactive for D2-40, a lymphatic marker *(inset)*. **B,** The majority of tumor cells show nuclear staining for HHV-8 by in situ hybridization.

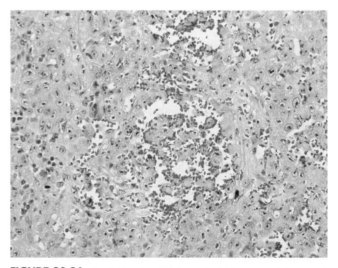

FIGURE 20-21. Angiosarcoma. High-grade angiosarcoma composed of large epithelioid cells with large pleomorphic nuclei, inclusion-like nucleoli, and abundant eosinophilic cytoplasm. There is vasoformation and hemorrhage.

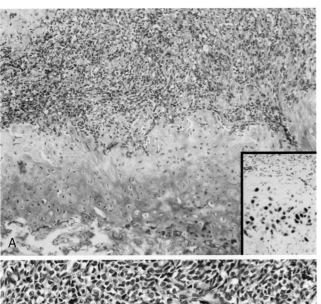

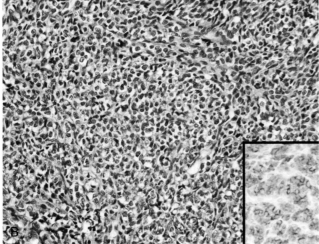

FIGURE 20-22. Mesenchymal chondrosarcoma. **A,** Biphasic tumor with a small cell Ewing's sarcoma–like component at the top of the photograph and well-differentiated cartilage at the bottom. The cartilage component is strongly immunoreactive to S100 protein *(bottom of inset)*. **B,** The small cell component at higher magnification shows undifferentiated small cells with membranous CD99 immunoreactivity *(inset)*.

cartilage and the other of small cells resembling Ewing's sarcoma (Fig. 20-22). Transition between these two components is usually abrupt. The small cell component commonly shows a hemangiopericytoma pattern of growth. The small cell component is immunoreactive with CD99 and the islands of cartilage with S100 protein. Given its malignant behavior, patients with this tumor have a 38-month median survival time and 5- and 10-year survival rates of 54.6% and 28%.[337,338] *SOX9* expression can distinguish mesenchymal chondrosarcoma from small round blue cell malignancies.[339]

Extraskeletal Myxoid Chondrosarcoma

Rare in children and adolescents, extraskeletal myxoid chondrosarcoma (EMC), also known as chordoid sarcoma, typically develops in older adults, with a peak incidence in the fifth or sixth decade.[340-342] EMC typically develops as a slowly growing, occasionally painful, deep mass, commonly in the extremities. Histopathologically, it exhibits a multinodular growth pattern

and a prominent chondroid appearance. Tumor cells are uniform, are arranged in cords or strands, and have an ovoid shape. The cytoplasm is usually eosinophilic and rarely has rhabdoid-type inclusions. Tumor cells are consistently immunoreactive to vimentin. About half the cells weakly express S100 protein; a lesser proportion are immunoreactive to cytokeratins, synaptophysin, and EMA.[343-346] Like other soft tissue sarcomas, EMC has a significant propensity for late recurrences and pulmonary metastases.[347,348]

EMC is characterized by several recurrent clonal translocations. The most common, t(9;22)(q22;q12), brings together the Ewing's sarcoma gene, *EWS*, with *NR4A3 (CHN, TEC, NOR-1, MINOR)*.[349,350] Other translocations fuse *TAF15 (TAF2N, TAFII-68, RBP56)* and *TCF12* with *NR4A3*.[351-353] In contrast to *EWS* and *TAF15*, which are ubiquitously expressed RNA-binding proteins and are translocated in many sarcomas, *TCF12* is a basic helix-loop-helix transcription factor that contributes its DNA-binding domain to the *NR4A3* fusion.[354,355] *NR4A3* is a member of a family of orphan nuclear receptors that includes *NUR77 (NR4A1)* and *NURR1 (NR4A2)*.[356-359] In contrast to typical nuclear receptors such as the estrogen receptors that require binding to a ligand for activity, the *NR4A* family of transcription factors regulate transcription in a ligand-independent fashion.[360] Their activity is controlled by regulated expression and post-translational modification by phosphorylation.[361-365] The *NR4A* family has been implicated in a variety of cellular processes, including T- and B-cell apoptosis and hepatic glucose metabolism.[366-368] Mice deficient for both *Nr4a1* and *Nr4a3* develop acute myeloid leukemia in the early postnatal period.[369] The fusion of *EWS* with *NR4A3* results in an increase in transactivation activity over the native *NRA3*.[370] The targets of the oncogenic fusion are not known, but expression profiling of EMC with differing histologies and translocations demonstrated a consistent RNA profile distinct from that of myxoid liposarcoma (which is characterized by an *EWS-CHOP* fusion).[371]

TUMORS OF UNCERTAIN DIFFERENTIATION

Synovial Sarcoma

Synovial sarcoma typically originates in proximity to major articular structures, bursae, and tendon sheaths, particularly those of the proximal lower extremity. In spite of its name, a true relationship with synovium is not longer believed to be the case, and intra-articular location is exceptional. Other sites for synovial sarcoma development include the trunk, head and neck, and mediastinum.[372-374] Synovial sarcoma is classified into two histologic subtypes: the more common monophasic spindle-cell morphology and the biphasic morphology (Fig. 20-23A-D). Both types exhibit an undifferentiated spindle-cell component. In addition, the biphasic type has a variable degree of epithelial differentiation in the form of glandular structures or clusters of poorly organized epithelial cells. A small proportion of cases are characterized by small round cells with an organoid, hemangiopericytomatous pattern that mimics Ewing's sarcoma (see Fig. 20-23C). This group is associated with a worse prognosis. Glandular structures, epithelial clusters and, focally, the spindle-cell component show intense immunoreactivity for keratin and EMA. Ultrastructurally, there is evidence of epithelial differentiation, with basal lamina, cell junctions, and microvilli in both glandular and spindle cell components (Fig. 20-24).

Cytogenetically, more than 95% of synovial sarcomas are characterized by t(X;18)(p11;q11), which results in the fusion of the *SS18* (also known as *SYT*) with *SSX1, SSX2,* or

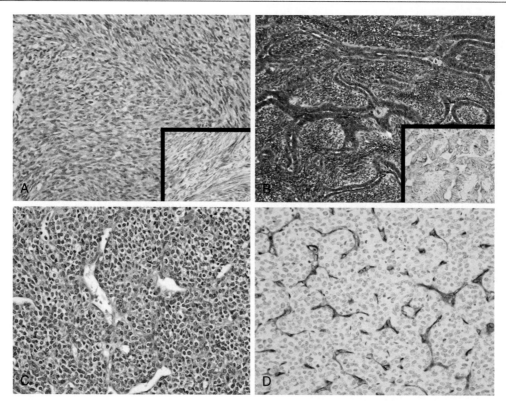

FIGURE 20-23. Synovial sarcoma. **A,** Monophasic synovial sarcoma composed of cellular undifferentiated spindled cells. Focal immunoreactivity for EMA *(inset)*. **B,** Biphasic synovial sarcoma with prominent slitlike glandular component and intervening undifferentiated spindled cells. The glandular component is strongly immunoreactive to cytokeratins *(inset)*. **C,** Small round cell synovial sarcoma with a hemangiopericytoma-like pattern mimicking a malignant primitive neuroectodermal tumor. **D,** Malignant primitive neuroectodermal tumor-like synovial sarcoma showing characteristic vessels highlighted by CD34 immunoreactive endothelium.

SSX4.[375-380] A variant fusion of the *SS18*-related gene *SS18L1* at 20.q13.3 with *SSX1* has also been reported.[381] Identification of the fusion by reverse transcriptase-polymerase chain reaction assay in paraffin-embedded tissue is an important diagnostic tool; it has a sensitivity of 95% and a specificity of 100%.[382-386] Nuclear immunostaining of *SYT* in paraffin-embedded tissue has a sensitivity of 85%.[387]

SSX1, -2, and *-4* are distinct genes that are located in proximity on the X chromosome.[388] *SSX1* and *-2* are highly conserved proteins characterized by acidic carboxyl termini and amino termini with homology to the Kruppel-associated box (*KRAB*) which, in the context of a DNA binding protein, has been implicated in transcriptional repression.[389] Whereas *SSX1* and *-2* demonstrate tissue specific expression, *SS18* is ubiquitously expressed, suggesting that the *SS18* fusion may function in part by the inappropriate expression of *SSX*.[390,391] The translocations found in synovial sarcoma encode nearly full-length *SS18* fused to the carboxyl two thirds of *SSX*.[380] *SS18* and the *SS18-SSX* chimeras demonstrate nuclear localization in a speckled distribution.[392] SS18 demonstrates transcriptional activity, and although the SSX KRAB homology domain is lost in the fusions, the SSX domain may attenuate *SS18* transcriptional activity.[393,394] Notably, neither *SS18* nor the *SSX* genes contains a DNA-binding domain. *SS18* and the *SSX* fusions may modulate transcription through interaction with the *SWI/SNF* chromatin remodeling complex.[395-397] SS18 was also found to interact with a nuclear coactivator (SIP/CoAA) that shares regional homology with EWS and TLS/FUS.[398,399] The SS18-SSX1 fusion can homo-oligomerize as well as hetero-oligomerize with native *SS18* to downregulate several genes.[400]

The *SS18-SSX1* fusion demonstrates transforming activity in a rat fibroblast cell line not shared by *SS18* or *SSX1* alone.[401] Tissue-specific activation of *SS18-SSX2* fusion controlled by the ubiquitous *ROSA26* promoter in a conditional knock-in system by myoblast *Myf5* activated *CRE* results in tumor development in 100% of surviving mice between 3 and 5 months of age (100% penetrance).[402] The mouse tumor demonstrates histopathology similar to that of human synovial sarcoma, having both monophasic and biphasic components, as well as limited shared gene expression. It is interesting that the timing of *SS18-SSX2* expression plays a critical role in the resulting phenotype. Expression of *SS18-SSX2* in early embryos was lethal, whereas expression in developing myocytes resulted in myopathy.

Several studies have attempted to identify pathologic and clinical differences among tumors harboring the most common fusions. Pathologically, tumors harboring the *SSX1* fusions demonstrate biphasic morphology and increased Ki67 staining, whereas those with the *SSX2* fusions are monophasic.[403,404] Although a large multicenter study comparing the outcomes of patients with tumors harboring the *SS18-SSX1* fusion with those having the *SS18-SSX2* fusion demonstrated that the *SSX1* fusion predicted a worse outcome,[405,406] a more recent multicenter study failed to confirm this finding but demonstrated that histologic grade was a strong predictor of survival.[407] An analysis of cell cycle–related proteins demonstrated that tumors with the *SS18-SSX1* fusion express higher levels of cyclin A and D1 than those with *SSX2* fusion.[408,409] There are biologic and epidemiologic differences between these fusions, but at this point it seems that the differences are likely to be subtle.

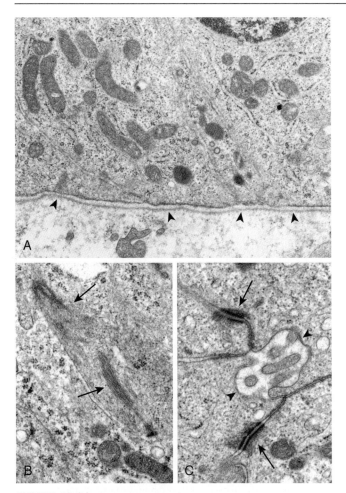

FIGURE 20-24. Synovial sarcoma, electron microscopy. **A,** Groups of tumor cells invested by a well-formed, continuous basal lamina *(arrowheads).* **B,** Well-developed cytoplasmic tonofilaments *(arrows).* **C,** Rudimentary intercellular lumen with microvilli *(arrowheads)* and well-developed desmosomes *(arrows).*

In addition to the *SSX* fusions, other genes have been associated with synovial sarcoma biology. The expression of insulin-like growth factor receptor-1 has been shown to correlate with a high incidence of lung metastases.[410] A significant fraction of synovial sarcoma also express hepatocyte growth factor and/or its receptor, MET.[411] Expression of human growth factor (HGF) or coexpression of MET and HGF were associated with large, high-grade and high-stage tumors and correlated with decreased survival rates.[412] mRNA microarray analysis has identified gene expression patterns that are specific to synovial sarcoma. Compared with malignant fibrous histiocytoma, synovial sarcoma shows increased expression of several growth factors and receptors, notably insulin-like growth factor binding protein 2 *(IGFBP2)*, the receptor tyrosine kinase HER2 *(ERBB2)*, insulin-like growth factor II *(IGF2)*, and fibroblast growth factor receptor 3 *(FGFR3)*.[413] Compared to other soft tissue sarcomas, it demonstrates increased expression of genes involved in the *WNT*, or notch signaling pathway, including *TLE1*, which was shown immunohistochemically to discriminate synovial sarcoma from other sarcomas.[414,415]

Alveolar Soft Part Sarcoma

Alveolar soft part sarcoma (ASPS) is a malignant tumor that usually presents in the thigh and trunk of young adults but can develop in the orbit or tongue in children.[416-418] Unusual primary locations include breast, heart, bladder, vagina, and uterine cervix.[419-423] The majority of patients present with metastatic disease. Because ASPS can metastasize to the brain in addition to the lung and bone, staging evaluation should include computed tomography of the head. Complete surgical resection is associated with long-term survival.[424,425] Although considered an indolent tumor, ASPS carries a poor prognosis because of its insidious propensity for late metastases. Nonmetastatic disease at presentation results in a 77% survival rate at 2 years, 60% at 5 years, 38% at 10 years, and 15% at 20 years.[427,428] Given the protracted course of ASPS, metastatic disease can be palliated by resection of metastatic disease to lung and brain.[429-431] ASPS is generally considered to be resistant to chemotherapy. Pulmonary metastases may demonstrate response to treatment with vincristine, but cyclophosphamide and doxorubicin alternating with etoposide and ifosfamide does not seem to extend survival.[426]

Histologically, ASPS is characterized by an organoid, pseudoalveolar proliferation of large polygonal cells that range from eosinophilic to clear (Fig. 20-25). Intravascular tumor growth is commonly present. A characteristic of these tumors is the presence of cytoplasmic periodic acid-Schiff–positive crystalline structures visible on light and electron microscopy. Ultrastructurally, these membrane-bound crystals consist of a latticework with distinctive periodicity (Fig. 20-26). The crystals are composed of monocarboxylate transporter protein MCT1 and its chaperone CD147.[432] The cell of origin for ASPS remains unclear; refuted evidence suggests a myogenic or neural crest derivation.[433,434] Tumor cells may show focal positivity for actin or desmin, but these markers are not muscle specific.

ASPS is characterized by a unique chromosomal translocation, t(X;17)(p11;q25).[435,436] The translocation is commonly unbalanced, consistently resulting in the fusion of *TFE3* with *ASPSCR1* (also known as *ASPL*).[437] *TFE3* is a member of the MiT basic helix-loop-helix leucine zipper transcription factor family.[438,439] *ASPSCR1* is not well characterized. However, amino acid sequence similarity suggests that *ASPSCR1* may be the human homologue of mouse *TUG*, a protein that regulates intracellular trafficking of the glucose transporter *GLUT4*.[440] The *ASPSCR1-TFE3* translocation may dysregulate *TFE3* expression by placing it under the control of the ubiquitous *ASPSCR1* promoter. Alterations in the *TFE3* locus can be detected cytogenetically, by FISH or PCR. In addition, nuclear immunoreactivity for *TFE3* provides a sensitive and possibly specific marker.[441] *ASPSCR1-TFE3* probably functions by altering target gene transcription. One potential target gene with therapeutic potential is the receptor tyrosine kinase *MET*.[442] *ASPCR1-TFE3* translocation can also be found in pediatric translocation-associated renal carcinoma.[443] The biologic importance of aberrant *TFE3* in ASPS classifies it together with a growing number of other MiT family-associated tumors, including clear cell sarcoma (see later material), translocation-associated renal carcinoma, and melanoma.

Clear Cell Sarcoma

Clear cell sarcoma (CCS) is a slowly growing soft tissue tumor that typically arises in the tendons, aponeuroses, and fascial structures of the extremities of adolescents and young

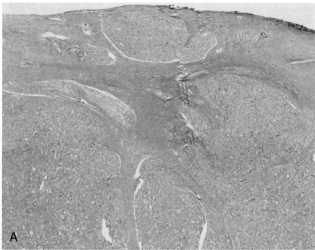

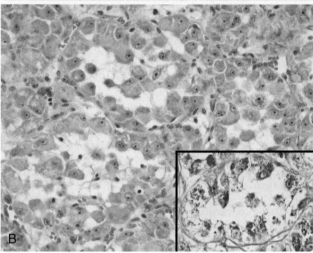

FIGURE 20-25. Alveolar soft part sarcoma. **A,** Multinodular growth with intervening fibrous septa. **B,** Large tumor cells with abundant eosinophilic cytoplasm, arranged with pseudoalveolar structures. Nuclei are large and round and contain single prominent nucleoli. Characteristic cytoplasmic periodic acid-Schiff–positive and diastase-resistant inclusions *(inset).*

adults.[444,445] It commonly presents as a small (<5 cm) painful nodule around the ankle or foot. CCS has a propensity for late metastasis, regionally to lymph nodes and distantly to lungs and bone. Overall, CCS is associated with a 5-year survival of 40% to 70%, with children faring somewhat better than adults.[446-449] Aggressive surgical management is critical to achieve disease control. In a pediatric population, fully resected and small tumors (<3 cm) are associated with a 5-year event-free survival rate of 90% to 100%, whereas larger tumors (>10 cm) result in a 20% 5-year event-free survival rate.[448] Postoperative radiotherapy is probably not necessary for fully resected CCS but may result in improved local control when negative margins cannot be achieved, a situation that commonly arises because complete surgical excision with wide margins at common locations is often not feasible without amputation. Unresectable, metastatic, relapsed CCS is refractory to conventional chemotherapy, but postoperative chemotherapy may be of benefit for localized resectable disease.[67,450]

CCS has an infiltrative, nesting, and fascicular pattern of growth (Fig. 20-27). The nesting pattern is highlighted by a reticulin framework. Tumor cells are usually ovoid or spindle-shaped with ovoid to elongated nuclei and distinct prominent eosinophilic nucleoli. CCS shares several histologic, immunophenotypic, and ultrastructural similarities with cutaneous melanoma, resulting in the alternative descriptor malignant melanoma of the soft parts.[445] Melanocytic differentiation of CCS is demonstrated by the expression of melanoma markers, including MITF, HMB45, S100, NSE, and melastatin.[451,452] Furthermore, about 70% of CCSs reveal melanin pigmentation by hematoxylin and eosin or Fontana stain and, ultrastructurally, they may contain premelanosomes and melanosomes.[452-454] By microarray expression analysis, CCS is segregated from other sarcomas by its melanocytic expression pattern.[455,456] However, clinically and cytogenetically, CCS and cutaneous melanoma are distinct. CCS presents as isolated masses in deep soft tissue, often originating from tendons and aponeuroses. CCS rarely shows the degree of anaplasia or microsatellite instability associated with melanoma, and unlike melanoma, CCS does not show *BRAF* mutation.[457-459] The vast majority of CCS tumors are distinguished by t(12;22)(q13;q12) that results in fusion of the Ewing's sarcoma gene *EWS* with the *CREB* transcription factor family member *ATF1.*[460] This translocation is not found in cutaneous mela-

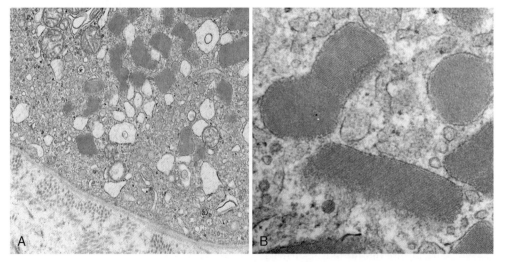

FIGURE 20-26. Alveolar soft part sarcoma, electron microscopy. **A,** Pseudoalveoli are invested by a well-developed basal lamina, and tumor cells contain prominent endoplasmic reticulum cisternae filled with dense proteinaceous material. **B,** At higher magnification, proteinaceous material shows a paracrystalline periodicity, which is typical of this tumor.

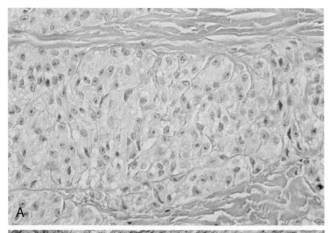

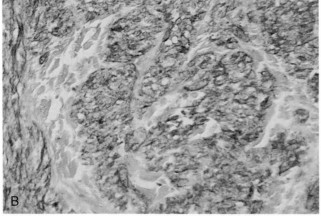

FIGURE 20-27. Clear cell sarcoma. **A,** Well-defined nest of tumor cells surrounded by fibrous septae. Tumor cells have abundant pale-staining cytoplasms and rounded vesicular nuclei with prominent single, centrally located nucleoli. **B,** Tumor cells are strongly immunoreactive for HMB45, a melanoma marker. Strong staining for S100 protein is also characteristic of clear cell sarcoma *(not shown)*.

noma. Native *ATF1* is regulated by serine phosphorylation in response to cAMP levels by protein kinase A.[461,462] In CCS, translocation dysregulates *ATF1* activity by replacing the kinase-inducible domain of *ATF1* with the carboxyl terminal region of *EWS*.[463]

Induction of *MITF* expression by EWS-ATF1 links the melanocytic phenotype of CCS with tumor proliferation and survival.[459] *MITF*, a member of the MiT basic helix-loop-helix leucine zipper transcription factor family, is the master regulatory factor of melanocyte differentiation and survival.[439,464] EWS-ATF1 co-opts the typically melanocyte-stimulating hormone-regulated cyclic adenosine monophosphate response element in the *MITF* promoter, aberrantly activating *MITF*. A critical transcriptional target, *MITF* mediates both the survival and proliferation and the melanocytic phenotype of CCS. *TFE3* and *TFEB*, other members of the *MiT* transcription factor family, can rescue the effect of inhibited *MITF* expression in CCS.[459] This functional redundancy places CCS among a family of tumors that share aberrant MiT transcription factor family expression, including cutaneous melanoma, alveolar soft part sarcoma, and translocation associated renal cell carcinoma. A gastrointestinal form of CCS is associated with a translocation that brings together *EWSR1* with *CREB1*.[465] Despite the related activity of *CREB1* and *ATF1*, this form of clear cell sarcoma does not express *MITF* or markers of melanocytic differentiation. Microarray expression profiling of the gastrointestinal CCS demonstrates a pattern that clusters more closely

with angiomatoid fibrous histiocytoma than with soft tissue CCS (see later material).[466]

Epidermal growth factor signaling may be important for CCS development. Clear sarcoma cell lines express ERBB3 and either ERBB2 or ERBB4.[455,467] Furthermore, ERBB3 is constitutively phosphorylated in cells expressing its ligand neuregulin (NRG1) and can be activated by exogenous neuregulin in cells that are not activated in an autocrine fashion. Treatment by the pan-ERBB inhibitor *CI-1033* decreases cell proliferation.[467]

Desmoplastic Small Round Cell Tumor

Desmoplastic small round cell tumor (DSRT) typically arises in intra-abdominal soft tissues and has a strong predilection for males. Although its most common site is the peritoneum, DSRT can arise in kidney, testes, ovaries, pleura, scalp, ethmoid sinuses, and pancreas.[468-472] DSRT usually presents with abdominal pain and weight loss and is commonly locally or distantly metastatic at the time of diagnosis. The diffuse paraserosal spread of DSRT may prevent resection with negative margins. A high tumor response rate in untreated DSRT and previously treated DSRT to high-dose cyclophosphamide, doxorubicin, and vincristine alternating with ifosfamide and etoposide may reduce bulky disease, permitting surgical resection and radiotherapy, if necessary.[473] Although the results are mixed, patients with high-risk disease may benefit from consolidation by high-dose chemotherapy and autologous stem cell rescue.[474,475] Relapsed disease may respond to irinotecan and temozolomide or low-dose cyclophosphamide and vinorelbine.[476,477] DSRT tends to develop and spread widely in the peritoneum, so based on its efficacy in peritoneal carcinomatosis, the use of continuous hyperthermic peritoneal infusion of chemotherapy is being studied, although initial results do not appear promising.[476,478] Multimodality therapy, consisting of aggressive surgical debulking, chemotherapy, and external beam radiotherapy, was associated with a 3-year survival rate of 55% compared to 27% when all three modalities were not used. Gross tumor resection was associated with a 58% 3-year survival rate compared to no survivors in the nonresected control group.[479] However, despite multimodality therapy, long-term survival rates remain very low.

As the name implies, DSRT appears histologically as malignant, undifferentiated, small round cells that are typically associated with a prominent desmoplastic reaction (Fig. 20-28).[480] Desmoplastic stroma, however, is not always present, and the location of the tumor may play a role in this regard. For example, desmoplastic small round cell tumor originating in the kidney characteristically lacks desmoplastic stroma.[468] Some tumors have glandular or rosette-like epithelial differentiation. Nuclei are usually hyperchromatic with little pleomorphism and with dispersed chromatin and small nucleoli. The scant cytoplasm is poorly outlined. A rhabdoid-type cytoplasmic inclusion can be observed focally in about half of cases. Areas of necrosis and frequent mitoses are common. Multiphenotypic differentiation is characteristic immunohistochemically. Most cases show immunoreactivity for cytokeratin, EMA, vimentin, and desmin. Desmin and vimentin commonly show a dotlike intracytoplasmic pattern corresponding to the rhabdoid-type inclusion. Nuclear WT1 expression with antibodies to the carboxy terminus is usually observed. Ultrastructurally, tumor cells are primitive and organelle-poor and may show paranuclear whorls of intermediate filaments (see Fig. 20-28C). Cell junctions including desmosomes may be observed focally.

Molecularly, DSRT is characterized by t(11;22)(p13;q12), which fuses the Ewing's sarcoma gene *EWS* with *WT1*.[481-484]

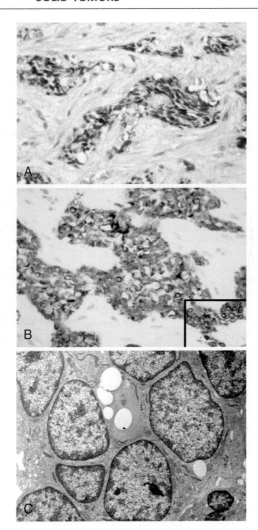

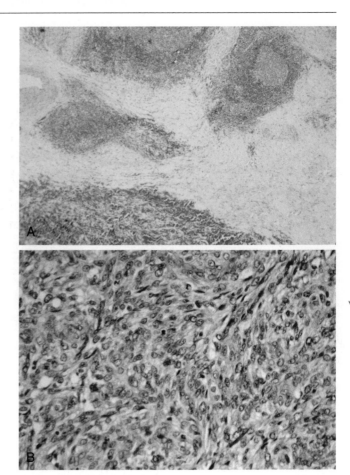

FIGURE 20-29. Angiomatoid fibrous histiocytoma. **A,** Nodular spindle cell proliferation with hemorrhage *(bottom)* and peripheral fibrous tissue with well-formed lymphoid follicles. **B,** Histiocyte-like cells and fibroblasts poorly arranged in short fascicles.

FIGURE 20-28. Malignant desmoplastic small round cell tumor. **A,** Infiltrative growth of elongated nests of variable sizes immersed in a densely collagenous stroma. Tumor cells are small, round, or ovoid, with hyperchromatic nuclei and poorly defined cytoplasmic borders. **B,** Tumor cells show strong diffuse and dotlike cytoplasmic immunoreactivity for desmin and diffuse cytoplasmic immunoreactivity for cytokeratin *(inset)*. **C,** Ultrastructurally, a cluster of undifferentiated small tumor cells with uniform round nuclei and occasional cytoplasmic whorls of intermediate filaments.

Although there is variability in the structure of the resulting chimera, the most common fusion includes *EWS* exons 1 through 7 and *WT1* exons 8 through 10.[484,485] *WT1* is a Cys_2-His_2 zinc finger DNA-binding protein that shares a high degree of homology and DNA recognition motif with the growth factor stimulated zinc finger DNA-binding protein *EGR1*.[486-489] The most common translocations result in *EWS-WT1* chimeras that preserve three of the four zinc finger motifs. However, because of molecular heterogeneity, chimeras may lack other *EWS* or *WT1* exons.[485] The *EWS-WT1* fusion has been detected in two intra-abdominal tumors that had histologic features of epithelioid leiomyosarcoma but lacked desmoplastic stroma, suggesting either a variant DSRT or another tumor type marked by *EWS-WT1*.[490] Based on the paradigm of the other transcription factors fused to the Ewing's sarcoma gene, *EWS-WT1* is thought to exert its oncogenic activity through transcriptional mechanisms, and several putative transcriptional targets have

been identified. The *EWS-WT1* fusion activates platelet-derived growth factor alpha *(PDGFA)*, T cell acute lymphoblastic leukemia-associated antigen 1 *(TALLA-1)*, and interleukin-2/15 receptor expression.[491-493] DSRTs stain positive for *PDGF* and for insulin-like growth factor II.[494] As a mitogen potentially acting on tumor-associated fibroblasts, *PDGF* seems to be a plausible cause for the desmoplastic reaction characteristic of these tumors. However, immunohistochemical analysis demonstrates an inverse correlation of *PDGF* expression with desmoplasia.[495] Although *PDGF* expression might suggest therapeutic *PDGFR* inhibition, imatinib mesylate demonstrates little to no activity as a single agent for DSRT.[496] About one third of DSRTs stain positive for androgen receptor, and androgen blockade may result in some response.[497]

Angiomatoid Fibrous Histiocytoma

Angiomatoid fibrous histiocytoma (AFH) was first described by Enzinger.[498] Histopathologically, it consists of a nodular fibrohistiocytic proliferation, usually surrounded by lymphoid follicles and a lymphoplasmacytic infiltrate (Fig. 20-29). The lesion commonly undergoes focal cystification and hemorrhage. In contrast to the more common (and similar sounding) adult tumor malignant fibrous histiocytoma (currently referred to as high-grade undifferentiated pleomorphic sarcoma; see later material), AFH is considered a low-grade malignancy that in children has not been reported to have the capacity to metastasize (grade I in the Pediatric Oncology Group's classification system), and surgery alone is considered curative treatment. However, incomplete resection is associated with a significant rate of local recurrence. Metastases to lung and brain have been reported in a single case of an adult with a large tumor.[499]

AFH is associated with a translocation of *EWSR1* or its related protein *FUS1* with *CREB1* or the related *CREB* family member *ATF1*.[466,500,501] These translocations are also characteristic of clear cell sarcoma (see earlier material). In contrast to typical CCS, these tumors do not express markers of melanocytic differentiation, including *MITF*. Because *SOX10* is required for *CREB1/ATF1*-mediated *MITF* activation, the differences in expression may reflect the absence of *SOX10* in AFH.[459]

Extrarenal Rhabdoid Tumor

A soft tissue rhabdoid tumor is a high-grade malignant tumor that occurs almost exclusively in infants and children. A subset is congenital, and may be disseminated at presentation.[502-504] Similar to its counterpart of renal origin, extrarenal rhabdoid tumor is an aggressive tumor with a very high rate of distant metastases, most commonly to the lung, lymph nodes, and liver.[505] Soft tissue rhabdoid tumors usually occur in the deep soft tissue, particularly in the paraspinal and neck regions. Some tumors arise adjacent to cutaneous benign mesenchymal lesions.[506,507] Tumor cells have little cohesiveness and grow in sheets or in a pseudoalveolar pattern, often mimicking alveolar rhabdomyosarcoma. Tumor cells are medium-sized and rounded and have large excentric nuclei and prominent eosinophilic nucleoli. Typically, the cytoplasm contains a paranuclear eosinophilic inclusion. Although extrarenal and renal rhabdoid tumors in children form a discrete entity, soft tissue rhabdoid tumors in adolescents and adults are a heterogeneous group without consistent cytogenetic aberrations.

A majority of tumor cells are immunoreactive for vimentin, EMA, and cam5.2. CD99, synaptophysin, and neuron-specific enolase are also commonly positive. Actin, S100 protein, desmin, myogenin, and CD34 are negative. Ultrastructurally, the rhabdoid inclusion corresponds to a paranuclear whorl of intermediate filaments.

Cytogenetic analysis of rhabdoid tumor consistently demonstrates abnormalities of 22q11.[508] The changes include deletions and translocations. Mapping the deleted region in a rhabdoid tumor cell line implicated the *SMARCB1 (hSNF5, INI1, BAF47)* gene, which was found to be mutated and truncated in other tumors.[509,510] *SMARCB1* is a component of the multiprotein *SWI/SNF* ATP-dependent chromatin remodeling complex. Loss of *SMARCB1* results in the polyploidization and chromosomal instability of rhabdoid cells. Expression of wild-type *SMARCB1* results in cell cycle arrest, possibly through restoration of DNA-damage–responsive cell cycle checkpoints or through replicative senescence, processes mediated by *p16INK4a* and *p21CIP/WAF1*.[511,512] For further discussion of rhabdoid tumor of the kidney and central nervous system, atypical teratoid/rhabdoid tumor, see Chapters 15 and 17.

Epithelioid Sarcoma

Epithelioid sarcoma is a distinctive high-grade soft tissue neoplasm that arises most commonly in the distal extremities of adolescents and young adults, particularly in the fingers, wrists, and hands. In young children, the tumor is more likely to arise in the head and neck as well as the pelvis.[513-516] The tumor can

present as a superficial ulcerated lesion or a deep painful mass. Dermis, subcutaneous tissue, fascia, and tendons can be involved, and upon recurrence the tumor has a propensity to spread locally along fascial planes and neurovascular bundles, resulting in the formation of proximal tumor satellites. Histologically, these tumors may resemble malignant peripheral nerve sheath tumors, synovial sarcomas, clear cell sarcomas, rhabdoid tumors, and melanomas.[517] Intravenous extension or lymph node involvement predicts a very high rate of pulmonary metastases.[518,519] In adults, epithelioid sarcoma demonstrates a 77% risk for local recurrence and a 45% risk for metastatic disease.[520] In children, epithelioid sarcoma is associated with a 5-year event-free survival of 61% and an overall survival rate that declines from 92.4% to 86.9% and 72% at 5, 10, and 15 years, indicating the propensity for late recurrence.[521] A small series of children with epithelioid sarcoma demonstrated that following lymphadenectomy with or without radiation, all patients were free of disease approximately 10 years after diagnosis.[5] Tumor size was the best predictor of prognosis; tumors larger than 5 cm were associated with a worse prognosis.[521,522] The more aggressive "proximal" type of variant exhibits a distinct rhabdoid phenotype, and the pattern of growth is more sheetlike than nodular.[523] The typical histology consists of nodular aggregates of medium size to large epithelioid and plump spindled cells with central necrosis and collagenization-simulating granulomas or metastatic carcinomas (Fig. 20-30A).[524] Immunohistochemically, tumor cells are commonly

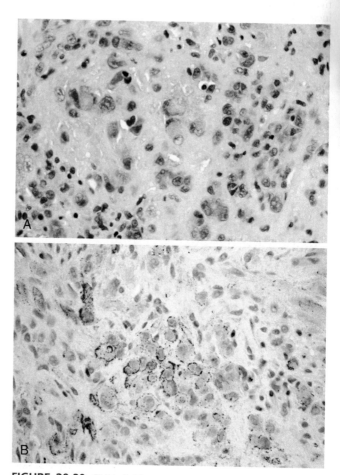

FIGURE 20-30. Epithelioid sarcoma. **A,** Granuloma-like cluster of large atypical cells, some with rhabdoid morphology, scattered inflammatory cells, and collagenization. **B,** Tumor cells are strongly immunoreactive for EMA (membranous pattern).

positive for keratin 8 and 19, EMA (see Fig. 20-30B), vimentin, and CD34.[525,526] Tumor cells are typically diploid, although deletions of the long arm of chromosomes 22 and 1, monosomy 21, and isochromosome 8q, as well as gains at 22q, have been noted.[527-532] t(8;22)(q22;q11) and t(6;8)(p25;q11.2) have been reported in isolated cases of epithelial sarcoma.[533,534] It is interesting to note that alterations in 22q11 in the proximal type of epithelioid sarcoma, which demonstrates a rhabdoid phenotype, have been associated with deletion of *SMARCB1*, the gene inactivated in malignant rhabdoid tumor.[535] Overexpression of epidermal growth factor receptor *(EGFR)* has been noted in epithelioid sarcoma, and one cell line derived from a recurrent malignant tumor demonstrates IL-6 secretion and IL-6 receptor expression, suggesting autocrine activation.[536-538] Autocrine MET activation by hepatocyte growth factor production has been speculated on the basis of detection of both proteins by immunohistochemistry.[411] Wide local excision with negative margins provides no advantage over primary amputation for patients with localized disease or regional metastases.[539] Treatment of epithelioid sarcoma cells in culture with retinoic acid and/or tumor necrosis factor-α results in inhibitory effects on growth.[540]

Extraosseous Ewing's Sarcoma

Although more commonly associated with an osseous origin, extraosseous Ewing's sarcoma (also known as peripheral primitive neuroectodermal tumor) can arise in many locations, including the small intestines, kidney, and spinal epidural space. Like its osseous counterpart, extraosseous Ewing's sarcoma consists of undifferentiated small round cells with minimal neuronal differentiation. It is characterized by membranous immunoreactivity for CD99 and harbors rearrangement of the *EWS* gene on chromosome 22 with a variety of partner genes, but most commonly with *FLI1* on chromosome 11. Other partner genes include *ERG, ETV1, EIAF,* and *FEV. EWSR1* break-apart FISH can be diagnostic. Extraosseous Ewing's sarcoma is treated much like the osseous form.[541,542] Given differences in treatment and prognosis, care should be taken to distinguish central nervous system Ewing's sarcoma from the CNS supratentorial primitive neuroectodermal tumors. For a more complete discussion of Ewing's sarcoma, see Chapter 21.

Gastrointestinal Stromal Tumor

Most commonly originating in the stomach or small intestine, gastrointestinal stromal tumors (GISTs) are mesenchymal neoplasms that can develop throughout the gastrointestinal tract. Typically GISTs occur in middle-aged to older adults, but approximately 3% of GISTs are identified in patients younger than 21 years of age.[543,544] Congenital GIST has been reported.[545,546] In children, the majority of tumors are identified in girls. Although isolated GIST predominates, multifocal epithelioid GIST is associated with Carney triad.[544] Pediatric GIST typically presents with gastrointestinal hemorrhage that can result in anemia. Although the majority of tumors identified in children are surgically resectable and are associated with good prognoses, GIST is commonly metastatic. The most common sites of metastases at the time of presentation or recurrence are the liver and omentum.[547]

The cell of origin of GIST is uncertain, but the observation that tumor cells have immunohistochemical[548] and ultrastructural[548,549] similarities to the interstitial cells of Cajal led to the proposition that GIST derives from these cells.[548,549] Histopathologically, most GISTs are composed of spindle cells with

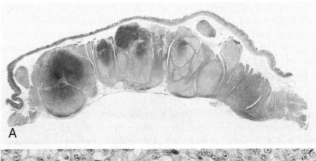

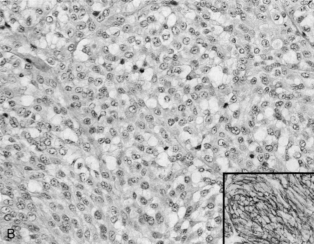

FIGURE 20-31. Gastrointestinal stromal tumor. **A,** Gastric antrum showing multifocal gastrointestinal stromal tumors centered within the muscularis propria. **B,** Nests of tumor are composed of spindled and epithelioid cells, diffusely immunoreactive for KIT *(CD117)*.

blunt-ended, elongated nuclei and moderately abundant cytoplasm (Fig. 20-31). They resemble smooth muscle or peripheral nerve sheath tumors. Unlike the immunohistochemistry in these tumors, however, the immunohistochemistry of GISTs in adults and children almost uniformly demonstrates the presence of the receptor tyrosine kinase *KIT (CD117);* see Fig. 20-31B, inset) and less commonly CD34.[550,551]

Several molecular features distinguish adult and pediatric GIST. Whereas GIST in adults is often associated with chromosomal losses of 1p, 14q, and 22q with additional chromosomal gains and losses in metastatic tumors, pediatric GIST typically lacks cytogenetic aberrancy.[552-554] GIST in adults is commonly associated with activating mutations identified in multiple regions of *KIT*.[555-557] Mutations include in-frame deletions and amino acid substitutions. In addition, a significant fraction of tumors that lack *KIT* mutations harbor activating mutations in platelet-derived growth factor receptor α *(PDGFRA)*.[558] However, in pediatric GIST, *KIT* and *PDGFRA* seem to be mutated only rarely.[544,559,560]

Historically, nonmetastatic GIST was managed surgically.[561] However, based on the growth-promoting properties of activated *KIT* and *PDGFR* in these tumors, treatment with the *KIT*- and *PDGFR*-targeted inhibitor imatinib has been examined.[562,563] In adults, a majority of GISTs demonstrated a significant and durable response to inhibitor treatment. Although a significant fraction of tumors progress because of acquired resistance to imatinib, they may respond to second-line treatment by sunitinib.[564,565] In children, the demonstration of *KIT* activation in the absence of mutation suggests that *KIT* inhibition may be effective.[554]

Ectomesenchymoma

Ectomesenchymoma is a rare tumor that affects primarily young children. Histopathologically, ectomesenchymomas are composed of a mixture of embryonal rhabdomyosarcomas, ganglioneuromas, and other neuroectodermal or mesenchymal components.[566-568] Treatment for these tumors typically involves surgical resection followed by chemotherapy based on sarcoma or rhabdomyosarcoma treatments.

NEUROECTODERMAL TUMORS

Malignant Peripheral Nerve Sheath Tumors

MPNSTs are sarcomas that ultrastructurally and immunohistochemically demonstrate nerve sheath differentiation.[569] Origin in a nerve or in a benign nerve sheath tumor or ganglioneuroma, as well as a history of NF-1, is also important in the diagnosis of these tumors. Previously referred to as malignant schwannomas and neurofibrosarcomas, the term *MPNST* is preferred, given the heterogeneity of tumor cell morphology. MPNSTs typically arise in the deep soft tissues of the extremities, head and neck, and trunk and may present with a mass or symptoms of nerve compression, including pain, dysesthesia,

or motor disturbance.[569,570] Between 50% and 80% of MPNSTs develop spontaneously; patients with NF-1 have lifetime incidences of MPNSTs of between 2% and 29%.[15,17,571-574] In a pediatric population with NF-1, MPNSTs tend to develop when children are older, and tumors tend to be larger, less likely to be resectable, and less likely to respond to chemotherapy than those that develop spontaneously.[570] MPNSTs are associated with a 5-year overall survival rate of 40% to 50% and a PFS of 35% to 37%.[570,575] However, the IRS grouping (see Table 20-5) strongly predicts both overall survival rate and progression-free survival (PFS) with complete surgical resection to be associated with an overall survival rate of 80% at 10 years. Histologically, MPNSTs are composed of fascicles of spindled cells with oval to wavy, slender nuclei with tapering poles, as well as pale cytoplasm with poorly defined borders (Fig. 20-32).[569] Perivascular hypercellularity and abrupt changes from dense cellular areas to zones containing abundant myxoid matrix are features that suggest nerve sheath differentiation. Pleomorphic, hyperchromatic nuclei are commonly present. Mitoses are usually frequent except in low-grade tumors arising in pre-existing neurofibromas in patients with neurofibromatosis (see Fig. 20-32A, B). High-grade MPNSTs are densely cellular with frequent mitoses and areas of necrosis (see Fig. 20-32C, D). MPNSTs with rhabdomyoblastic differentiation are referred to as malignant triton tumors, which have worse prognoses than typical MPNSTs. Osteosarcomatous or glandular differentiation may also occur. Immunohistochemically,

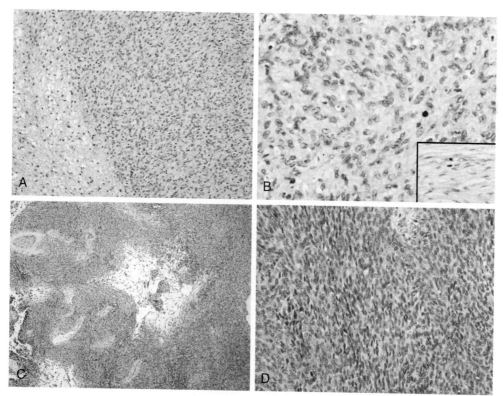

FIGURE 20-32. Malignant peripheral nerve sheath tumor. **A,** Low-grade MPNST showing a cellular area *(on right)* sharply demarcated from a less densely cellular component *(on left)*. **B,** At higher magnification, low-grade MPNST showing mild atypia and occasional mitoses. Low-grade MPNST showing focal strong nuclear and cytoplasmic immunoreactivity for S100 protein *(inset)*. **C,** High-grade MPNST showing densely cellular spindled cell tumor. **D.** At higher magnification, tumor cells in high-grade MPNST are densely arranged and have hyperchromatic nuclei and scattered mitoses and apoptosis.

MPNSTs may show focal positivity for S100 protein, EMA, and glial fibrillary acidic protein.

The development of MPNSTs is associated with loss of the tumor suppressor NF1 at *17q11.2,* which encodes neurofibromin. Neurofibromin is a guanosine triphosphatase (GTPase)-activating protein that modulates RAS signaling.[576-580] MPNSTs also frequently harbor mutations of *p53* and the *p16INK4a/p14ARF* locus, affecting both the *p53* and the RB pathways in 75% of tumors.[581] *p16INK4*a or *p14ARF* promoter inactivation by CpG island methylation may also downregulate expression.[582] Mice with homozygous *p53* and heterozygous NF1 deficiency develop sarcomas with histopathologic and immunohistochemical properties that resemble MPNSTs and malignant triton tumors. These tumors demonstrate loss of heterozygosity at the Nf1 locus.[583,584] EGFR may also play a role in the development of MPNST. EGFR seems to be consistently expressed in MPNSTs and MPNST-derived cell lines, and 26% of MPNSTs demonstrate amplification of the EGFR locus.[585,586] Enforced EGFR expression in transgenic mice results in Schwann cell hyperplasia with rare tumor development, whereas EGFR haploinsufficiency in NF-1+/-, *p53*+/- mice significantly reduces tumor formation.[587]

Melanotic Neuroectodermal Tumor of Infancy

A melanotic neuroectodermal tumor (retinal anlage tumor, melanotic progonoma) is a dysembryoplastic tumor that recapitulates embryonic retinal development. The majority of cases occur in the head and neck region, particularly in the maxilla, and it usually affects male children younger than 1 year of age. The tumor is a rapidly growing, locally invasive tumor and metastasizes in about 5% of cases.[588] Although complete surgical resection is required for cure, chemotherapy has been shown to decrease tumor mass, hence improving resectability.[589] The tumor is classified in the family of neuroblastic tumors, and rare cases are associated with elevated urinary vanillylmandelic acid. The histopathology is characteristically biphasic, with a component of neuroblast-like cells with neuropil arranged in nests and an epithelioid melanocyte-like component containing melanin (Fig. 20-33). The melanocyte-like cells are usually arranged at the periphery of the neuroblastic-like cells, forming pseudoglandular or pseudoalveolar structures in a densely fibrous stroma. Both cellular components are immunoreactive with neuroectodermal markers, such as synaptophysin, glial fibrillary acidic protein, and Leu7. Melanocyte-like cells are also immunoreactive with HMB45 and cytokeratins.

UNDIFFERENTIATED TUMORS

Undifferentiated Sarcoma/High-grade Undifferentiated Polymorphous Sarcoma

An undifferentiated sarcoma is a collection of tumors that lacks identifiable morphologic, immunohistochemical, or genetic changes permitting classification as a specific subtype of sarcoma (Fig. 20-34). For the purposes of therapeutic trials in childhood cancer, undifferentiated sarcoma had been grouped with rhabdomyosarcoma. However, the inclusion of MyoD1 and myogenin immunohistochemistry has permitted segregation of rhabdomyosarcoma from undifferentiated sarcoma, and the current Children's Oncology Group trial for NRSTS includes

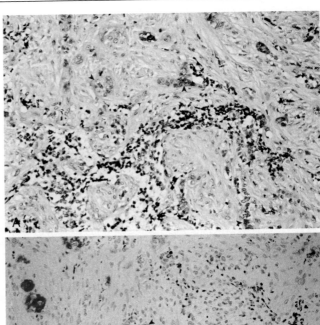
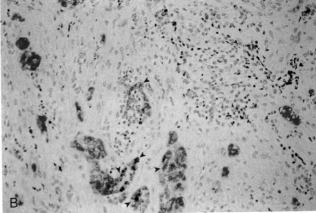

FIGURE 20-33. Retinal anlage tumor (progonoma). **A,** Biphasic tumor with a component of neuroblastic-like cells with neuropil arranged in nests and an epithelioid melanocyte-like cell component containing melanin *(arrowheads).* The melanocyte-like cells arranged at the periphery of the neuroblastic-like cells form pseudoglandular or pseudoalveolar structures in a densely fibrous stroma. **B,** Strong cytokeratin immunoreactivity in melanocyte-like cells *(in red).* The dark cytoplasmic granules represent melanin pigment *(arrowheads).*

undifferentiated sarcoma. A similar reclassification has also occurred for adult undifferentiated sarcoma. Many of the tumors previously labeled as the common soft tissue sarcoma malignant fibrous histiocytoma (MFH) have been reclassified to specific categories on the basis of immunohistochemistry, electron microscopy, and molecular genetics.[590-592] The remaining tumors are now referred to as high-grade undifferentiated polymorphous sarcoma (HGUPS).[140,593]

In infants, undifferentiated sarcoma constitutes the most common nonrhabdomyosarcoma malignant mesenchymal tumor. Surgery and chemotherapy result in a 10-year overall survival rate of 75%.[7] In contrast, HGUPS is a common soft tissue sarcoma of older adults that has peak incidence in the seventh decade and rarely occurs in children or adolescents.[594] A high-grade malignancy, HGUPS demonstrates a significant incidence of local and distant recurrence. Pulmonary and lymph node metastases are most common. The diversity in the histologic appearance of MFH, including both fibroblastic and histiocytic components, has led to controversy about whether the tumor evolves from histiocytic or mesenchymal origin. In a trial of docetaxel and gemcitabine compared to docetaxel alone in metastatic sarcoma, HGUPS was among the most responsive tumor types and demonstrated superior response to both agents in combination.[82]

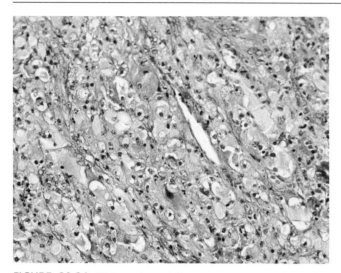

FIGURE 20-34. High-grade undifferentiated sarcoma. Undifferentiated, pleomorphic sarcoma composed of large, highly anaplastic tumor cells. Immunohistochemistry, electron microscopy, and cytogenetics defied further classification.

Although the classification of pediatric undifferentiated sarcomas based on the absence of lineage marker expression seems tenuous, common factors distinguish these tumors. Pediatric undifferentiated sarcomas often express vimentin, KIT and VEGF.[595] Hierarchical clustering of adult soft tissue sarcomas based on mRNA expression array profiling revealed an undifferentiated sarcoma class that is distinct from, among other tumors, fibrosarcoma and liposarcoma.[414] Expression analyses performed by other groups have also clustered HGUPS but with the intermingling of liposarcoma and leiomyosarcoma to varying degrees.[596,597] The similarity between liposarcoma and HGUPS is also suggested by cytogenetic studies demonstrating that a subset of undifferentiated sarcomas shares some features with liposarcomas.[598]

WNT signaling seems to play a central role in the development of undifferentiated sarcoma. DKK1, the secreted inhibitor of WNT signaling, is expressed in undifferentiated sarcoma, and it inhibits differentiation by blocking Wnt2/β-catenin signaling.[599] Conversely, treatment of an undifferentiated sarcoma cell line with either exogenous Wnt2 or Wnt5a induced markers of adipogenic or osteogenic differentiation. *JUN* deregulation may also play a role in undifferentiated sarcoma. *JUN* and *JNK* can be amplified in undifferentiated sarcoma, and *JUN* can block adipogenic differentiation.[600]

REFERENCES

1. Gurney JG, Young JL Jr, Roffers SD, et al. Soft tissue sarcomas. In Ries LAG, Smith MA, Gurney JG, et al (eds). Cancer Incidence and Survival among Children and Adolescents: United States SEER Program 1975-1995. Bethesda, Md, National Cancer Institute, SEER Program, NIH Pub. No. 99-4649, 1999, pp 111-124.
2. Coffin CM, Dehner LP. Soft tissue tumors in first year of life: a report of 190 cases. Pediatr Pathol. 1990;10:509-526.
3. Marcus KC, Grier HE, Shamberger RC, et al. Childhood soft tissue sarcoma: a 20-year experience. J Pediatr. 1997;131:603-607.
4. Ferrari A, Casanova M, Collini P, et al. Adult-type soft tissue sarcomas in pediatric-age patients: experience at the Istituto Nazionale Tumori in Milan. J Clin Oncol. 2005;23:4021-4030.
5. McGrory JE, Pritchard DJ, Arndt CA, et al. Nonrhabdomyosarcoma soft tissue sarcomas in children. The Mayo Clinic experience. Clin Orthop Relat Res. 2000:247-258.
6. Dillon P, Maurer H, Jenkins J, et al. A prospective study of nonrhabdomyosarcoma soft tissue sarcomas in the pediatric age group. J Pediatr Surg. 1992;27:241-244; discussion 244-245.
7. Orbach D, Rey A, Oberlin O, et al. Soft tissue sarcoma or malignant mesenchymal tumors in the first year of life: experience of the International Society of Pediatric Oncology (SIOP) Malignant Mesenchymal Tumor Committee. J Clin Oncol. 2005;23:4363-4371.
8. Dillon PW, Whalen TV, Azizkhan RG, et al. Neonatal soft tissue sarcomas: the influence of pathology on treatment and survival. Children's Cancer Group Surgical Committee. J Pediatr Surg. 1995;30:1038-1041.
9. Li FP, Fraumeni JF Jr. Rhabdomyosarcoma in children: epidemiologic study and identification of a familial cancer syndrome. J Natl Cancer Inst. 1969;43:1365-1373.
10. Li FP, Fraumeni JF Jr. Prospective study of a family cancer syndrome. JAMA. 1982;247:2692-2694.
11. Malkin D, Li FP, Strong LC, et al. Germ line *p53* mutations in a familial syndrome of breast cancer, sarcomas, and other neoplasms. Science. 1990;250:1233-1238.
12. Friend S, Bernards R, Rogelj S, et al. A human DNA segment with properties of the gene that predisposes to retinoblastoma and osteosarcoma. Nature. 1986;323:643-646.
13. Kleinerman RA, Tucker MA, Abramson DH, et al. Risk of soft tissue sarcomas by individual subtype in survivors of hereditary retinoblastoma. J Natl Cancer Inst. 2007;99:24-31.
14. Friend SH, Horowitz JM, Gerber MR, et al. Deletions of a DNA sequence in retinoblastomas and mesenchymal tumors: organization of the sequence and its encoded protein. Proc Natl Acad Sci U S A. 1987;84:9059-9063.
15. D'Agostino AN, Soule EH, Miller RH. Sarcomas of the peripheral nerves and somatic soft tissues associated with multiple neurofibromatosis (Von Recklinghausen's disease). Cancer. 1963;16:1015-1027.
16. Takazawa Y, Sakurai S, Sakuma Y, et al. Gastrointestinal stromal tumors of neurofibromatosis type I (von Recklinghausen's disease). Am J Surg Pathol. 2005;29:755-763.
17. Ducatman BS, Scheithauer BW, Piepgras DG, et al. Malignant peripheral nerve sheath tumors. A clinicopathologic study of 120 cases. Cancer. 1986;57:2006-2021.
18. Sharif S, Ferner R, Birch JM, et al. Second primary tumors in neurofibromatosis 1 patients treated for optic glioma: substantial risks after radiotherapy. J Clin Oncol. 2006;24:2570-2575.
19. Carney JA. Gastric stromal sarcoma, pulmonary chondroma, and extra-adrenal paraganglioma (Carney triad): natural history, adrenocortical component, and possible familial occurrence. Mayo Clin Proc. 1999;74:543-552.
20. Carney JA, Sheps SG, Go VL, Gordon H. The triad of gastric leiomyosarcoma, functioning extra-adrenal paraganglioma and pulmonary chondroma. N Engl J Med. 1977;296:1517-1518.
21. Matyakhina L, Bei TA, McWhinney SR, et al. Genetics of Carney triad: recurrent losses at chromosome 1 but lack of germline mutations in genes associated with paragangliomas and gastrointestinal stromal tumors. J Clin Endocrinol Metab. 2007;92(8):2938-2943.
22. Gardner EJ. Follow-up study of a family group exhibiting dominant inheritance for a syndrome including intestinal polyps, osteomas, fibromas and epidermal cysts. Am J Hum Genet. 1962;14:376-390.

23. Clark SK, Phillips RK. Desmoids in familial adenomatous polyposis. Br J Surg. 1996;83:1494-1504.

24. Eccles DM, van der Luijt R, Breukel C, et al. Hereditary desmoid disease due to a frameshift mutation at codon 1924 of the APC gene. Am J Hum Genet. 1996;59:1193-1201.

25. Kinzler KW, Nilbert MC, Su LK, et al. Identification of FAP locus genes from chromosome 5q21. Science. 1991;253:661-665.

26. Kinzler KW, Nilbert MC, Vogelstein B, et al. Identification of a gene located at chromosome 5q21 that is mutated in colorectal cancers. Science. 1991;251:1366-1370.

27. Yu CE, Oshima J, Fu YH, et al. Positional cloning of the Werner's syndrome gene. Science. 1996;272:258-262.

28. Chen L, Lee L, Kudlow BA, et al. LMNA mutations in atypical Werner's syndrome. Lancet. 2003;362:440-445.

29. Goto M, Miller RW, Ishikawa Y, Sugano H. Excess of rare cancers in Werner syndrome (adult progeria). Cancer Epidemiol Biomarkers Prev. 1996;5:239-246.

30. Anderson D, Tannen RL. Tuberous sclerosis and chronic renal failure: potential confusion with polycystic kidney disease. Am J Med. 1969;47:163-168.

31. van Baal JG, Fleury P, Brummelkamp WH. Tuberous sclerosis and the relation with renal angiomyolipoma: a genetic study on the clinical aspects. Clin Genet. 1989;35:167-173.

32. Cook JA, Oliver K, Mueller RF, Sampson J. A cross-sectional study of renal involvement in tuberous sclerosis. J Med Genet. 1996;33:480-484.

33. Harding CO, Pagon RA. Incidence of tuberous sclerosis in patients with cardiac rhabdomyoma. Am J Med Genet. 1990;37:443-446.

34. Weatherby RP, Dahlin DC, Ivins JC. Postradiation sarcoma of bone: review of 78 Mayo Clinic cases. Mayo Clin Proc. 1981;56:294-306.

35. Laskin WB, Silverman TA, Enzinger FM. Postradiation soft tissue sarcomas: an analysis of 53 cases. Cancer. 1988;62:2330-2340.

36. Kim JH, Chu FC, Woodard HQ, et al. Radiation-induced soft-tissue and bone sarcoma. Radiology. 1978;129:501-508.

37. Creech JL Jr, Johnson MN. Angiosarcoma of liver in the manufacture of polyvinyl chloride. J Occup Med. 1974;16:150-151.

38. Henderson TO, Whitton J, Stovall M, et al. Secondary sarcomas in childhood cancer survivors: a report from the Childhood Cancer Survivor Study. J Natl Cancer Inst. 2007;99:300-308.

39. McCarville MB, Christie R, Daw NC, et al. PET/CT in the evaluation of childhood sarcomas. AJR Am J Roentgenol. 2005;184:1293-1304.

40. Barr FG, Chatten J, D'Cruz CM, et al. Molecular assays for chromosomal translocations in the diagnosis of pediatric soft tissue sarcomas. JAMA. 1995;273:553-557.

41. Gaynor JJ, Tan CC, Casper ES, et al. Refinement of clinicopathologic staging for localized soft tissue sarcoma of the extremity: a study of 423 adults. J Clin Oncol. 1992;10:1317-1329.

42. Parham DM, Webber BL, Jenkins JJ 3rd, et al. Nonrhabdomyosarcomatous soft tissue sarcomas of childhood: formulation of a simplified system for grading. Mod Pathol. 1995;8:705-710.

43. Costa J, Wesley RA, Glatstein E, Rosenberg SA. The grading of soft tissue sarcomas. Results of a clinicohistopathologic correlation in a series of 163 cases. Cancer. 1984;53:530-541.

44. Trojani M, Contesso G, Coindre JM, et al. Soft-tissue sarcomas of adults; study of pathological prognostic variables and definition of a histopathological grading system. Int J Cancer. 1984;33:37-42.

45. Costa J. The grading and staging of soft tissue sarcoma. In Fletcher CDM, McKee PH (eds). Pathobiology of Soft Tissue Sarcoma. Edinburgh, UK: Churchill Livingstone, 1990, pp 221-238.

46. Guillou L, Coindre JM, Bonichon F, et al. Comparative study of the National Cancer Institute and French Federation of Cancer Centers Sarcoma Group grading systems in a population of 410 adult patients with soft tissue sarcoma. J Clin Oncol. 1997;15:350-362.

47. Meza JL, Anderson J, Pappo AS, Meyer WH. Analysis of prognostic factors in patients with nonmetastatic rhabdomyosarcoma treated on intergroup rhabdomyosarcoma studies III and IV: the Children's Oncology Group. J Clin Oncol. 2006;24:3844-3851.

48. Harmer MH. TNM classification of pediatric tumors. Geneva, Switzerland, UICC International Union Against Cancer, 1982, pp 23-38.

49. Rodary C, Flamant F, Donaldson SS. An attempt to use a common staging system in rhabdomyosarcoma: a report of an international workshop initiated by the International Society of Pediatric Oncology (SIOP). Med Pediatr Oncol. 1989;17:210-215.

50. American Joint Committee on Cancer. Soft tissue sarcoma. In Greene FL, Page DL, Fleming ID, et al (eds). AJCC Cancer Staging Manual. 6th ed. Chicago, AJCC, 2002, pp 193-200.

51. Spunt SL, Poquette CA, Hurt YS, et al. Prognostic factors for children and adolescents with surgically resected nonrhabdomyosarcoma soft tissue sarcoma: an analysis of 121 patients treated at St Jude Children's Research Hospital. J Clin Oncol. 1999;17:3697-3705.

52. Rao BN. Nonrhabdomyosarcoma in children: prognostic factors influencing survival. Semin Surg Oncol. 1993;9:524-531.

53. Pratt CB, Pappo AS, Gieser P, et al. Role of adjuvant chemotherapy in the treatment of surgically resected pediatric nonrhabdomyosarcomatous soft tissue sarcomas: a Pediatric Oncology Group Study. J Clin Oncol. 1999;17:1219-1226.

54. Horowitz ME, Pratt CB, Webber BL, et al. Therapy for childhood soft-tissue sarcomas other than rhabdomyosarcoma: a review of 62 cases treated at a single institution. J Clin Oncol. 1986;4:559-564.

55. Lindberg RD, Martin RG, Romsdahl MM, Barkley HT Jr. Conservative surgery and postoperative radiotherapy in 300 adults with soft-tissue sarcomas. Cancer. 1981;47:2391-2397.

56. Rosenberg SA, Tepper J, Glatstein E, et al. The treatment of soft-tissue sarcomas of the extremities: prospective randomized evaluations of (1) limb-sparing surgery plus radiation therapy compared with amputation and (2) the role of adjuvant chemotherapy. Ann Surg. 1982;196:305-315.

57. Yang JC, Chang AE, Baker AR, et al. Randomized prospective study of the benefit of adjuvant radiation therapy in the treatment of soft tissue sarcomas of the extremity. J Clin Oncol. 1998;16:197-203.

58. Blakely ML, Spurbeck WW, Pappo AS, et al. The impact of margin of resection on outcome in pediatric nonrhabdomyosarcoma soft tissue sarcoma. J Pediatr Surg. 1999;34:672-675.

59. Paulino AC, Ritchie J, Wen BC. The value of postoperative radiotherapy in childhood nonrhabdomyosarcoma soft tissue sarcoma. Pediatr Blood Cancer. 2004;43:587-593.

60. Fontanesi J, Rao BN, Fleming ID, et al. Pediatric brachytherapy. The St. Jude Children's Research Hospital experience. Cancer. 1994;74:733-739.

61. Merchant TE, Parsh N, del Valle PL, et al. Brachytherapy for pediatric soft-tissue sarcoma. Int J Radiat Oncol Biol Phys. 2000;46:427-432.

62. Alekhteyar KM, Leung DH, Brennan MF, Harrison LB. The effect of combined external beam radiotherapy and brachytherapy on local control and wound complications in patients with high-grade soft tissue sarcomas of the extremity with positive microscopic margin. Int J Radiat Oncol Biol Phys. 1996;36:321-324.

63. Yan TD, Esquivel J, Carmignani P, Sugarbaker PH. Cytoreduction and intraperitoneal chemotherapy for the management of non-gynecological peritoneal surface malignancy. J Exp Clin Cancer Res. 2003;22:109-117.

64. Imai Y, Habe K, Imada M, et al. A case of a large dermatofibrosarcoma protuberans successfully treated with radiofrequency ablation and transcatheter arterial embolization. J Dermatol. 2004;31:42-46.

65. Ahlmann ER, Falkinstein Y, Fedenko AN, Menendez LR. Cryoablation and resection influences patient survival for soft tissue sarcomas: impact on survivorship and local recurrence. Clin Orthop Relat Res. 2007;459:174-181.

66. de Bree R, Tijink BM, van Groeningen CJ, Leemans CR. Electroporation therapy in soft tissue sarcoma: a potentially effective novel treatment. Sarcoma. 2006;2006:85234.

67. Cecchetto G, Alaggio R, Dall'Igna P, et al. Localized unresectable non-rhabdo soft tissue sarcomas of the extremities in pediatric age: results from the Italian studies. Cancer. 2005;104:2006-2012.

68. Pappo AS, Devidas M, Jenkins J, et al. Phase II trial of neoadjuvant vincristine, ifosfamide, and doxorubicin with granulocyte colony-stimulating factor support in children and adolescents with advanced-stage nonrhabdomyosarcomatous soft tissue sarcomas: a Pediatric Oncology Group Study. J Clin Oncol. 2005;23:4031-4038.

69. Pappo AS, Rao BN, Jenkins JJ, et al. Metastatic nonrhabdomyosarcomatous soft-tissue sarcomas in children and adolescents: the St. Jude Children's Research Hospital experience. Med Pediatr Oncol. 1999;33:76-82.

70. Pratt CB, Maurer HM, Gieser P, et al. Treatment of unresectable or metastatic pediatric soft tissue sarcomas with surgery, irradiation, and chemotherapy: a Pediatric Oncology Group study. Med Pediatr Oncol. 1998;30:201-209.

71. Ferrari A, Brecht IB, Koscielniak E, et al. The role of adjuvant chemotherapy in children and adolescents with surgically resected, high-risk adult-type soft tissue sarcomas. Pediatr Blood Cancer. 2005;45:128-134.

72. Nathan PC, Tsokos M, Long L, et al. Adjuvant chemotherapy for the treatment of advanced pediatric nonrhabdomyosarcoma soft tissue sarcoma: the National Cancer Institute experience. Pediatr Blood Cancer. 2005;44:449-454.

73. Navid F, Santana VM, Billups CA, et al. Concomitant administration of vincristine, doxorubicin, cyclophosphamide, ifosfamide, and etoposide for high-risk sarcomas: the St. Jude Children's Research Hospital experience. Cancer. 2006;106:1846-1856.

74. Patel SR, Vadhan-Raj S, Burgess MA, et al. Results of two consecutive trials of dose-intensive chemotherapy with doxorubicin and ifosfamide in patients with sarcomas. Am J Clin Oncol. 1998;21:317-321.

75. Kraybill WG, Harris J, Spiro IJ, et al. Phase II study of neoadjuvant chemotherapy and radiation therapy in the management of high-risk, high-grade, soft tissue sarcomas of the extremities and body wall: Radiation Therapy Oncology Group Trial 9514. J Clin Oncol. 2006;24:619-625.

76. DeLaney TF, Spiro IJ, Suit HD, et al. Neoadjuvant chemotherapy and radiotherapy for large extremity soft-tissue sarcomas. Int J Radiat Oncol Biol Phys. 2003;56:1117-1127.

77. Saylors RL 3rd, Stine KC, Sullivan J, et al. Cyclophosphamide plus topotecan in children with recurrent or refractory solid tumors: a Pediatric Oncology Group phase II study. J Clin Oncol. 2001;19:3463-3469.

78. Kushner BH, Kramer K, Meyers PA, et al. Pilot study of topotecan and high-dose cyclophosphamide for resistant pediatric solid tumors. Med Pediatr Oncol. 2000;35:468-474.

79. Cosetti M, Wexler LH, Calleja E, et al. Irinotecan for pediatric solid tumors: the Memorial-Sloan Kettering experience. J Pediatr Hematol Oncol. 2002;24:101-105.

80. Bisogno G, Riccardi R, Ruggiero A, et al. Phase II study of a protracted irinotecan schedule in children with refractory or recurrent soft tissue sarcoma. Cancer. 2006;106:703-707.

81. Casanova M, Ferrari A, Bisogno G, et al. Vinorelbine and low-dose cyclophosphamide in the treatment of pediatric sarcomas: pilot study for the upcoming European Rhabdomyosarcoma Protocol. Cancer. 2004;101:1664-1671.

82. Maki RG, Wathen JK, Patel SR, et al. Randomized phase II study of gemcitabine and docetaxel compared with gemcitabine alone in patients with metastatic soft tissue sarcomas: results of sarcoma alliance for research through collaboration study 002 [corrected]. J Clin Oncol. 2007;25:2755-2763.

83. Dileo P, Morgan JA, Zahrieh D, et al. Gemcitabine and vinorelbine combination chemotherapy for patients with advanced soft tissue sarcomas: results of a phase II trial. Cancer. 2007;109:1863-1869.

84. Wagner-Bohn A, Paulussen M, Vieira Pinheiro JP, et al. Phase II study of gemcitabine in children with solid tumors of mesenchymal and embryonic origin. Anticancer Drugs. 2006;17:859-864.

85. Reid JM, Qu W, Safgren SL, et al. Phase I trial and pharmacokinetics of gemcitabine in children with advanced solid tumors. J Clin Oncol. 2004;22:2445-2451.

86. Zwerdling T, Krailo M, Monteleone P, et al. Phase II investigation of docetaxel in pediatric patients with recurrent solid tumors: a report from the Children's Oncology Group. Cancer. 2006;106:1821-1828.

87. Okcu MF, Despa S, Choroszy M, et al. Synovial sarcoma in children and adolescents: thirty-three years of experience with multimodal therapy. Med Pediatr Oncol. 2001;37:90-96.

88. Okcu MF, Munsell M, Treuner J, et al. Synovial sarcoma of childhood and adolescence: a multicenter, multivariate analysis of outcome. J Clin Oncol. 2003;21:1602-1611.

89. Ferrari A, Gronchi A, Casanova M, et al. Synovial sarcoma: a retrospective analysis of 271 patients of all ages treated at a single institution. Cancer. 2004;101:627-634.

90. Pappo AS, Fontanesi J, Luo X, et al. Synovial sarcoma in children and adolescents: the St Jude Children's Research Hospital experience. J Clin Oncol. 1994;12:2360-2366.

91. Montgomery E, Argani P, Hicks JL, et al. Telomere lengths of translocation-associated and nontranslocation-associated sarcomas differ dramatically. Am J Pathol. 2004;164:1523-1529.

92. Ulaner GA, Hoffman AR, Otero J, et al. Divergent patterns of telomere maintenance mechanisms among human sarcomas: sharply contrasting prevalence of the alternative lengthening of telomeres mechanism in Ewing's sarcomas and osteosarcomas. Genes Chromosomes Cancer. 2004;41:155-162.

93. Scheel C, Schaefer KL, Jauch A, et al. Alternative lengthening of telomeres is associated with chromosomal instability in osteosarcomas. Oncogene. 2001;20:3835-3844.

94. Henson JD, Hannay JA, McCarthy SW, et al. A robust assay for alternative lengthening of telomeres in tumors shows the significance of alternative lengthening of telomeres in sarcomas and astrocytomas. Clin Cancer Res. 2005;11:217-225.

95. Schneider-Stock R, Epplen C, Radig K, et al. On telomere shortening in soft-tissue tumors. J Cancer Res Clin Oncol. 1998;124:165-171.

96. Sharpless NE, Alson S, Chan S, et al. *p16(INK4a)* and *p53* deficiency cooperate in tumorigenesis. Cancer Res. 2002;62:2761-2765.

97. Dei Tos AP. Liposarcoma: new entities and evolving concepts. Ann Diagn Pathol. 2000;4:252-266.

98. Miller GG, Yanchar NL, Magee JF, Blair GK. Lipoblastoma and liposarcoma in children: an analysis of 9 cases and a review of the literature. Can J Surg. 1998;41:455-458.

99. Fletcher CD, Akerman M, Dal Cin P, et al. Correlation between clinicopathological features and karyotype in lipomatous tumors: a report of 178 cases from the Chromosomes and Morphology (CHAMP) Collaborative Study Group. Am J Pathol. 1996;148:623-630.

100. Henricks WH, Chu YC, Goldblum JR, Weiss SW. Dedifferentiated liposarcoma: a clinicopathological analysis of 155 cases

with a proposal for an expanded definition of dedifferentiation. Am J Surg Pathol. 1997;21:271-281.

101. Singer S, Antonescu CR, Riedel E, Brennan MF. Histologic subtype and margin of resection predict pattern of recurrence and survival for retroperitoneal liposarcoma. Ann Surg. 2003;238:358-370; discussion 370-371.

102. Shmookler BM, Enzinger FM. Liposarcoma occurring in children: an analysis of 17 cases and review of the literature. Cancer. 1983;52:567-574.

103. La Quaglia MP, Spiro SA, Ghavimi F, et al. Liposarcoma in patients younger than or equal to 22 years of age. Cancer. 1993; 72:3114-3119.

104. Jones RL, Fisher C, Al-Muderis O, Judson IR. Differential sensitivity of liposarcoma subtypes to chemotherapy. Eur J Cancer. 2005;41:2853-2860.

105. Grosso F, Jones RL, Demetri GD, et al. Efficacy of trabectedin (ecteinascidin-743) in advanced pretreated myxoid liposarcomas: a retrospective study. Lancet Oncol. 2007;8:595-602.

106. Crozat A, Aman P, Mandahl N, Ron D. Fusion of CHOP to a novel RNA-binding protein in human myxoid liposarcoma. Nature. 1993;363:640-644.

107. Rabbitts TH, Forster A, Larson R, Nathan P. Fusion of the dominant negative transcription regulator CHOP with a novel gene FUS by translocation t(12;16) in malignant liposarcoma. Nat Genet. 1993;4:175-180.

108. Panagopoulos I, Hoglund M, Mertens F, et al. Fusion of the EWS and CHOP genes in myxoid liposarcoma. Oncogene. 1996;12:489-494.

109. Zinszner H, Albalat R, Ron D. A novel effector domain from the RNA-binding protein TLS or EWS is required for oncogenic transformation by CHOP. Genes Dev. 1994;8:2513-2526.

110. Riggi N, Cironi L, Provero P, et al. Expression of the FUS-CHOP fusion protein in primary mesenchymal progenitor cells gives rise to a model of myxoid liposarcoma. Cancer Res. 2006;66: 7016-7023.

111. Muller CR, Paulsen EB, Noordhuis P, et al. Potential for treatment of liposarcomas with the MDM2 antagonist Nutlin-3A. Int J Cancer. 2007;121:199-205.

112. Singer S, Socci ND, Ambrosini G, et al. Gene expression profiling of liposarcoma identifies distinct biological types/subtypes and potential therapeutic targets in well-differentiated and dedifferentiated liposarcoma. Cancer Res. 2007;67:6626-6636.

113. Hibbard MK, Kozakewich HP, Dal Cin P, et al. PLAG1 fusion oncogenes in lipoblastoma. Cancer Res. 2000;60:4869-4872.

114. Kas K, Voz ML, Roijer E, et al. Promoter swapping between the genes for a novel zinc finger protein and beta-catenin in pleomorphic adenomas with t(3;8)(p21;q12) translocations. Nat Genet. 1997;15:170-174.

115. Griffioen G, Bus PJ, Vasen HF, et al. Extracolonic manifestations of familial adenomatous polyposis: desmoid tumours, and upper gastrointestinal adenomas and carcinomas. Scand J Gastroenterol Suppl. 1998;225:85-91.

116. Coffin CM, Dehner LP. Fibroblastic-myofibroblastic tumors in children and adolescents: a clinicopathologic study of 108 examples in 103 patients. Pediatr Pathol. 1991;11:569-588.

117. Faulkner LB, Hajdu SI, Kher U, et al. Pediatric desmoid tumor: retrospective analysis of 63 cases. J Clin Oncol. 1995;13:2813-2818.

118. Fallen T, Wilson M, Morlan B, Lindor NM. Desmoid tumors—a characterization of patients seen at Mayo Clinic 1976-1999. Fam Cancer. 2006;5:191-194.

119. Skapek SX, Ferguson WS, Granowetter L, et al. Vinblastine and methotrexate for desmoid fibromatosis in children: results of a Pediatric Oncology Group Phase II Trial. J Clin Oncol. 2007;25: 501-506.

120. Skapek SX, Hawk BJ, Hoffer FA, et al. Combination chemotherapy using vinblastine and methotrexate for the treatment of progressive desmoid tumor in children. J Clin Oncol. 1998;16: 3021-3027.

121. Lackner H, Urban C, Benesch M, et al. Multimodal treatment of children with unresectable or recurrent desmoid tumors: an 11-year longitudinal observational study. J Pediatr Hematol Oncol. 2004;26:518-522.

122. Weiss AJ, Lackman RD. Low-dose chemotherapy of desmoid tumors. Cancer. 1989;64:1192-1194.

123. Kinzbrunner B, Ritter S, Domingo J, Rosenthal CJ. Remission of rapidly growing desmoid tumors after tamoxifen therapy. Cancer. 1983;52:2201-2204.

124. Patel SR, Evans HL, Benjamin RS. Combination chemotherapy in adult desmoid tumors. Cancer. 1993;72:3244-3247.

125. Douglass HO Jr, Karakousis C. Alternating administration of adriamycin (NSC-123127) and vincristine (NSC-67574)-actinomycin D (NSC-3053) in advanced sarcomas. Cancer Chemother Rep. 1975;59:1045-1047.

126. Heinrich MC, McArthur GA, Demetri GD, et al. Clinical and molecular studies of the effect of imatinib on advanced aggressive fibromatosis (desmoid tumor). J Clin Oncol. 2006;24:1195-1203.

127. Bridge JA, Sreekantaiah C, Mouron B, et al. Clonal chromosomal abnormalities in desmoid tumors: implications for histopathogenesis. Cancer. 1992;69:430-436.

128. Fletcher JA, Naeem R, Xiao S, Corson JM. Chromosome aberrations in desmoid tumors: trisomy 8 may be a predictor of recurrence. Cancer Genet Cytogenet. 1995;79:139-143.

129. Dal Cin P, Sciot R, Aly MS, et al. Some desmoid tumors are characterized by trisomy 8. Genes Chromosomes Cancer. 1994; 10:131-135.

130. Mertens F, Willen H, Rydholm A, et al. Trisomy 20 is a primary chromosome aberration in desmoid tumors. Int J Cancer. 1995; 63:527-529.

131. Behrens J, von Kries JP, Kuhl M, et al. Functional interaction of beta-catenin with the transcription factor LEF-1. Nature. 1996;382:638-642.

132. Huber O, Korn R, McLaughlin J, et al. Nuclear localization of beta-catenin by interaction with transcription factor LEF-1. Mech Dev. 1996;59:3-10.

133. Molenaar M, van de Wetering M, Oosterwegel M, et al. XTcf-3 transcription factor mediates beta-catenin-induced axis formation in Xenopus embryos. Cell. 1996;86:391-399.

134. Roose J, Huls G, van Beest M, et al. Synergy between tumor suppressor APC and the beta-catenin-Tcf4 target Tcf1. Science. 1999;285:1923-1926.

135. Alman BA, Li C, Pajerski ME, et al. Increased beta-catenin protein and somatic APC mutations in sporadic aggressive fibromatoses (desmoid tumors). Am J Pathol. 1997;151: 329-334.

136. Li C, Bapat B, Alman BA. Adenomatous polyposis coli gene mutation alters proliferation through its beta-catenin-regulatory function in aggressive fibromatosis (desmoid tumor). Am J Pathol. 1998;153:709-714.

137. Tejpar S, Nollet F, Li C, et al. Predominance of beta-catenin mutations and beta-catenin dysregulation in sporadic aggressive fibromatosis (desmoid tumor). Oncogene. 1999;18:6615-6620.

138. Cheon SS, Cheah AY, Turley S, et al. Beta-Catenin stabilization dysregulates mesenchymal cell proliferation, motility, and invasiveness and causes aggressive fibromatosis and hyperplastic cutaneous wounds. Proc Natl Acad Sci U S A. 2002;99:6973-6978.

139. Smits R, van der Houven van Oordt W, Luz A, et al. Apc1638N: a mouse model for familial adenomatous polyposis-associated desmoid tumors and cutaneous cysts. Gastroenterology. 1998;114:275-283.

140. Fletcher CD. The evolving classification of soft tissue tumours: an update based on the new WHO classification. Histopathology. 2006;48:3-12.

141. Gengler C, Guillou L. Solitary fibrous tumour and haemangiopericytoma: evolution of a concept. Histopathology. 2006;48:63-74.

142. Enzinger FM, Smith BH. Hemangiopericytoma: an analysis of 106 cases. Hum Pathol. 1976;7:61-82.

143. Jennings TA, Duray PH, Collins FS, et al. Infantile myofibromatosis: evidence for an autosomal-dominant disorder. Am J Surg Pathol. 1984;8:529-538.

144. Ikediobi NI, Iyengar V, Hwang L, et al. Infantile myofibromatosis: support for autosomal dominant inheritance. J Am Acad Dermatol. 2003;49:S148-S150.

145. Zand DJ, Huff D, Everman D, et al. Autosomal dominant inheritance of infantile myofibromatosis. Am J Med Genet A. 2004;126:261-266.

146. Chung EB, Enzinger FM. Infantile myofibromatosis. Cancer. 1981;48:1807-1818.

147. Wiswell TE, Davis J, Cunningham BE, et al. Infantile myofibromatosis: the most common fibrous tumor of infancy. J Pediatr Surg. 1988;23:315-318.

148. Gandhi MM, Nathan PC, Weitzman S, Levitt GA. Successful treatment of life-threatening generalized infantile myofibromatosis using low-dose chemotherapy. J Pediatr Hematol Oncol. 2003;25:750-754.

149. Leaute-Labreze C, Labarthe MP, Blanc JF, et al. Self-healing generalized infantile myofibromatosis with elevated urinary bFGF. Pediatr Dermatol. 2001;18:305-307.

150. Kasaragod AB, Lucia MS, Cabirac G, et al. Connective tissue growth factor expression in pediatric myofibroblastic tumors. Pediatr Dev Pathol. 2001;4:37-45.

151. Perez-Atayde AR, Kozakewich HW, McGill T, Fletcher JA. Hemangiopericytoma of the tongue in a 12-year-old child: ultrastructural and cytogenetic observations. Hum Pathol. 1994;25:425-429.

152. Dahlen A, Fletcher CD, Mertens F, et al. Activation of the GLI oncogene through fusion with the beta-actin gene (ACTB) in a group of distinctive pericytic neoplasms: pericytoma with t(7;12). Am J Pathol. 2004;164:1645-1653.

153. Kinzler KW, Bigner SH, Bigner DD, et al. Identification of an amplified, highly expressed gene in a human glioma. Science. 1987;236:70-73.

154. Marigo V, Johnson RL, Vortkamp A, Tabin CJ. Sonic hedgehog differentially regulates expression of GLI and GLI3 during limb development. Dev Biol. 1996;180:273-283.

155. Lee J, Platt KA, Censullo P, Ruiz I, Altaba A. Gli1 is a target of sonic hedgehog that induces ventral neural tube development. Development. 1997;124:2537-2552.

156. Roberts WM, Douglass EC, Peiper SC, et al. Amplification of the gli gene in childhood sarcomas. Cancer Res. 1989;49:5407-5413.

157. Hayes-Jordan AA, Spunt SL, Poquette CA, et al. Nonrhabdomyosarcoma soft tissue sarcomas in children: is age at diagnosis an important variable? J Pediatr Surg. 2000;35:948-953; discussion 953-954.

158. Kynaston JA, Malcolm AJ, Craft AW, et al. Chemotherapy in the management of infantile fibrosarcoma. Med Pediatr Oncol. 1993;21:488-493.

159. Grier HE, Perez-Atayde AR, Weinstein HJ. Chemotherapy for inoperable infantile fibrosarcoma. Cancer. 1985;56:1507-1510.

160. Brock P, Renard M, Smet M, et al. Infantile fibrosarcoma. Med Pediatr Oncol. 1991;19:210.

161. Ninane J, Gosseye S, Panteon E, et al. Congenital fibrosarcoma: preoperative chemotherapy and conservative surgery. Cancer. 1986;58:1400-1406.

162. Hamm CM, Pyesmany A, Resch L. Case report: congenital retroperitoneal fibrosarcoma. Med Pediatr Oncol. 1997;28:65-68.

163. Shetty AK, Yu LC, Gardner RV, Warrier RP. Role of chemotherapy in the treatment of infantile fibrosarcoma. Med Pediatr Oncol. 1999;33:425-427.

164. McCahon E, Sorensen PH, Davis JH, et al. Non-resectable congenital tumors with the ETV6-NTRK3 gene fusion are highly responsive to chemotherapy. Med Pediatr Oncol. 2003;40:288-292.

165. Knezevich SR, McFadden DE, Tao W, et al. A novel ETV6-NTRK3 gene fusion in congenital fibrosarcoma. Nat Genet. 1998;18:184-187.

166. Bourgeois JM, Knezevich SR, Mathers JA, Sorensen PH. Molecular detection of the *ETV6-NTRK3* gene fusion differentiates congenital fibrosarcoma from other childhood spindle cell tumors. Am J Surg Pathol. 2000;24:937-946.

167. Knezevich SR, Garnett MJ, Pysher TJ, et al. *ETV6-NTRK3* gene fusions and trisomy 11 establish a histogenetic link between mesoblastic nephroma and congenital fibrosarcoma. Cancer Res. 1998;58:5046-5048.

168. Tognon C, Knezevich SR, Huntsman D, et al. Expression of the *ETV6-NTRK3* gene fusion as a primary event in human secretory breast carcinoma. Cancer Cell. 2002;2:367-376.

169. Rubin BP, Chen CJ, Morgan TW, et al. Congenital mesoblastic nephroma t(12;15) is associated with *ETV6-NTRK3* gene fusion: cytogenetic and molecular relationship to congenital (infantile) fibrosarcoma. Am J Pathol. 1998;153:1451-1458.

170. Golub TR, Barker GF, Lovett M, Gilliland DG. Fusion of PDGF receptor beta to a novel ets-like gene, tel, in chronic myelomonocytic leukemia with t(5;12) chromosomal translocation. Cell. 1994;77:307-316.

171. Lamballe F, Klein R, Barbacid M. trkC, a new member of the trk family of tyrosine protein kinases, is a receptor for neurotrophin-3. Cell. 1991;66:967-979.

172. Shelton DL, Sutherland J, Gripp J, et al. Human trks: molecular cloning, tissue distribution, and expression of extracellular domain immunoadhesions. J Neurosci. 1995;15:477-491.

173. Wai DH, Knezevich SR, Lucas T, et al. The *ETV6-NTRK3* gene fusion encodes a chimeric protein tyrosine kinase that transforms *NIH3T3* cells. Oncogene. 2000;19:906-915.

174. Tognon C, Garnett M, Kenward E, et al. The chimeric protein tyrosine kinase ETV6-NTRK3 requires both Ras-Erk1/2 and PI3-kinase-Akt signaling for fibroblast transformation. Cancer Res. 2001;61:8909-8916.

175. Jin W, Yun C, Hobbie A, et al. Cellular transformation and activation of the phosphoinositide-3-kinase-Akt cascade by the *ETV6-NTRK3* chimeric tyrosine kinase requires c-Src. Cancer Res. 2007;67:3192-3200.

176. Morrison KB, Tognon CE, Garnett MJ, et al. *ETV6*-NTRK3 transformation requires insulin-like growth factor 1 receptor signaling and is associated with constitutive IRS-1 tyrosine phosphorylation. Oncogene. 2002;21:5684-5695.

177. Lannon CL, Martin MJ, Tognon CE, et al. A highly conserved NTRK3 C-terminal sequence in the ETV6-NTRK3 oncoprotein binds the phosphotyrosine binding domain of insulin receptor substrate-1: an essential interaction for transformation. J Biol Chem. 2004;279:6225-6234.

178. Jin W, Kim BC, Tognon C, et al. The ETV6-NTRK3 chimeric tyrosine kinase suppresses TGF-beta signaling by inactivating the TGF-beta type II receptor. Proc Natl Acad Sci U S A. 2005;102:16239-16244.

179. Bednar B. Storiform neurofibromas of the skin, pigmented and nonpigmented. Cancer. 1957;10:368-376.

180. Criscione VD, Weinstock MA. Descriptive epidemiology of dermatofibrosarcoma protuberans in the United States, 1973 to 2002. J Am Acad Dermatol. 2007;56:968-973.

181. Khatri VP, Galante JM, Bold RJ, et al. Dermatofibrosarcoma protuberans: reappraisal of wide local excision and impact of inadequate initial treatment. Ann Surg Oncol. 2003;10:1118-1122.

182. Ballo MT, Zagars GK, Pisters P, Pollack A. The role of radiation therapy in the management of dermatofibrosarcoma protuberans. Int J Radiat Oncol Biol Phys. 1998;40:823-827.

183. Suit H, Spiro I, Mankin HJ, et al. Radiation in management of patients with dermatofibrosarcoma protuberans. J Clin Oncol. 1996;14:2365-2369.

184. Haas RL, Keus RB, Loftus BM, et al. The role of radiotherapy in the local management of dermatofibrosarcoma protuberans. Soft Tissue Tumours Working Group. Eur J Cancer. 1997;33:1055-1060.

185. Abbott JJ, Oliveira AM, Nascimento AG. The prognostic significance of fibrosarcomatous transformation in dermatofibrosarcoma protuberans. Am J Surg Pathol. 2006;30:436-443.

186. Dymock RB, Allen PW, Stirling JW, et al. Giant cell fibroblastoma: a distinctive, recurrent tumor of childhood. Am J Surg Pathol. 1987;11:263-271.

187. Jha P, Moosavi C, Fanburg-Smith JC. Giant cell fibroblastoma: an update and addition of 86 new cases from the Armed Forces Institute of Pathology, in honor of Dr. Franz M. Enzinger. Ann Diagn Pathol. 2007;11:81-88.

188. Shmookler BM, Enzinger FM, Weiss SW. Giant cell fibroblastoma. a juvenile form of dermatofibrosarcoma protuberans. Cancer. 1989;64:2154-2161.

189. West RB, Harvell J, Linn SC, et al. Apo D in soft tissue tumors: a novel marker for dermatofibrosarcoma protuberans. Am J Surg Pathol. 2004;28:1063-1069.

190. Simon MP, Pedeutour F, Sirvent N, et al. Deregulation of the platelet-derived growth factor B-chain gene via fusion with collagen gene COL1A1 in dermatofibrosarcoma protuberans and giant-cell fibroblastoma. Nat Genet. 1997;15:95-98.

191. Greco A, Fusetti L, Villa R, et al. Transforming activity of the chimeric sequence formed by the fusion of collagen gene COL1A1 and the platelet derived growth factor b-chain gene in dermatofibrosarcoma protuberans. Oncogene. 1998;17:1313-1319.

192. O'Brien KP, Seroussi E, Dal Cin P, et al. Various regions within the alpha-helical domain of the COL1A1 gene are fused to the second exon of the PDGFB gene in dermatofibrosarcomas and giant-cell fibroblastomas. Genes Chromosomes Cancer. 1998;23:187-193.

193. Wang J, Hisaoka M, Shimajiri S, et al. Detection of COL1A1-PDGFB fusion transcripts in dermatofibrosarcoma protuberans by reverse transcription-polymerase chain reaction using archival formalin-fixed, paraffin-embedded tissues. Diagn Mol Pathol. 1999;8:113-119.

194. Shimizu A, O'Brien KP, Sjoblom T, et al. The dermatofibrosarcoma protuberans-associated collagen type Ialpha1/platelet-derived growth factor (PDGF) B-chain fusion gene generates a transforming protein that is processed to functional PDGF-BB. Cancer Res. 1999;59:3719-3723.

195. Simon MP, Navarro M, Roux D, Pouyssegur J. Structural and functional analysis of a chimeric protein COL1A1-PDGFB generated by the translocation t(17;22)(q22;q13.1) in dermatofibrosarcoma protuberans (DP). Oncogene. 2001;20:2965-2975.

196. Lin N, Urabe K, Moroi Y, et al. Overexpression of phosphorylated-STAT3 and phosphorylated-ERK protein in dermatofibrosarcoma protuberans. Eur J Dermatol. 2006;16:262-265.

197. Sjoblom T, Shimizu A, O'Brien KP, et al. Growth inhibition of dermatofibrosarcoma protuberans tumors by the platelet-derived growth factor receptor antagonist STI571 through induction of apoptosis. Cancer Res. 2001;61:5778-5783.

198. Sawyers CL. Imatinib GIST keeps finding new indications: successful treatment of dermatofibrosarcoma protuberans by targeted inhibition of the platelet-derived growth factor receptor. J Clin Oncol. 2002;20:3568-3569.

199. Mizutani K, Tamada Y, Hara K, et al. Imatinib mesylate inhibits the growth of metastatic lung lesions in a patient with dermatofibrosarcoma protuberans. Br J Dermatol. 2004;151:235-237.

200. Savoia P, Ortoncelli M, Quaglino P, Bernengo MG. Imatinib mesylate in the treatment of a large unresectable dermatofibrosarcoma protuberans: a case study. Dermatol Surg. 2006;32:1097-1102.

201. Price VE, Fletcher JA, Zielenska M, et al. Imatinib mesylate: an attractive alternative in young children with large, surgically challenging dermatofibrosarcoma protuberans. Pediatr Blood Cancer. 2005;44:511-515.

202. McArthur GA, Demetri GD, van Oosterom A, et al. Molecular and clinical analysis of locally advanced dermatofibrosarcoma protuberans treated with imatinib: Imatinib Target Exploration Consortium Study B2225. J Clin Oncol. 2005;23:866-873.

203. Ng A, Nishikawa H, Lander A, Grundy R. Chemosensitivity in pediatric dermatofibrosarcoma protuberans. J Pediatr Hematol Oncol. 2005;27:100-102.

204. Evans HL. Low-grade fibromyxoid sarcoma: a report of two metastasizing neoplasms having a deceptively benign appearance. Am J Clin Pathol. 1987;88:615-619.

205. Evans HL. Low-grade fibromyxoid sarcoma: a report of 12 cases. Am J Surg Pathol. 1993;17:595-600.

206. Billings SD, Giblen G, Fanburg-Smith JC. Superficial low-grade fibromyxoid sarcoma (Evans' tumor): a clinicopathologic analysis of 19 cases with a unique observation in the pediatric population. Am J Surg Pathol. 2005;29:204-210.

207. Folpe AL, Lane KL, Paull G, Weiss SW. Low-grade fibromyxoid sarcoma and hyalinizing spindle cell tumor with giant rosettes: a clinicopathologic study of 73 cases supporting their identity and assessing the impact of high-grade areas. Am J Surg Pathol. 2000;24:1353-1360.

208. Canpolat C, Evans HL, Corpron C, et al. Fibromyxoid sarcoma in a four-year-old child: case report and review of the literature. Med Pediatr Oncol. 1996;27:561-564.

209. Panagopoulos I, Storlazzi CT, Fletcher CD, et al. The chimeric FUS/CREB3l2 gene is specific for low-grade fibromyxoid sarcoma. Genes Chromosomes Cancer. 2004;40:218-228.

210. Reid R, de Silva MV, Paterson L, et al. Low-grade fibromyxoid sarcoma and hyalinizing spindle cell tumor with giant rosettes share a common t(7;16)(q34;p11) translocation. Am J Surg Pathol. 2003;27:1229-1236.

211. Storlazzi CT, Mertens F, Nascimento A, et al. Fusion of the FUS and BBF2H7 genes in low grade fibromyxoid sarcoma. Hum Mol Genet. 2003;12:2349-2358.

212. Mertens F, Fletcher CD, Antonescu CR, et al. Clinicopathologic and molecular genetic characterization of low-grade fibromyxoid sarcoma, and cloning of a novel FUS/CREB3L1 fusion gene. Lab Invest. 2005;85:408-415.

213. Kondo S, Saito A, Hino S, et al. BBF2H7, a novel transmembrane bZIP transcription factor, is a new type of endoplasmic reticulum stress transducer. Mol Cell Biol. 2007;27:1716-1729.

214. Panagopoulos I, Moller E, Dahlen A, et al. Characterization of the native CREB3L2 transcription factor and the FUS/CREB3L2 chimera. Genes Chromosomes Cancer. 2007;46:181-191.

215. Guillou L, Benhattar J, Gengler C, et al. Translocation-positive low-grade fibromyxoid sarcoma: clinicopathologic and molecular analysis of a series expanding the morphologic spectrum and suggesting potential relationship to sclerosing epithelioid fibrosarcoma: a study from the French Sarcoma Group. Am J Surg Pathol. 2007;31:1387-1402.

216. Denschlag D, Kontny U, Tempfer C, et al. Low-grade myxofibrosarcoma of the vulva in a 15-year-old adolescent: a case report. Int J Surg Pathol. 2005;13:117-119.

217. Weiss SW, Enzinger FM. Myxoid variant of malignant fibrous histiocytoma. Cancer. 1977;39:1672-1685.

218. Merck C, Angervall L, Kindblom LG, Oden A. Myxofibrosarcoma: a malignant soft tissue tumor of fibroblastic-histiocytic origin. A clinicopathologic and prognostic study of 110 cases using multivariate analysis. Acta Pathol Microbiol Immunol Scand Suppl. 1983;282:1-40.

219. Mentzel T, Calonje E, Wadden C, et al. Myxofibrosarcoma. Clinicopathologic analysis of 75 cases with emphasis on the low-grade variant. Am J Surg Pathol. 1996;20:391-405.

220. Fujimura T, Okuyama R, Terui T, et al. Myxofibrosarcoma (myxoid malignant fibrous histiocytoma) showing cutaneous presentation: report of two cases. J Cutan Pathol. 2005;32:512-515.

221. Angervall L, Kindblom LG, Merck C. Myxofibrosarcoma: a study of 30 cases. Acta Pathol Microbiol Scand [A]. 1977;85A:127-140.

222. Fukunaga M, Fukunaga N. Low-grade myxofibrosarcoma: progression in recurrence. Pathol Int. 1997;47:161-165.

223. Willems SM, Debiec-Rychter M, Szuhai K, et al. Local recurrence of myxofibrosarcoma is associated with increase in tumour grade and cytogenetic aberrations, suggesting a multistep tumour progression model. Mod Pathol. 2006;19:407-416.

224. Huang HY, Lal P, Qin J, et al. Brennan MF, Antonescu CR. Low-grade myxofibrosarcoma: a clinicopathologic analysis of 49 cases treated at a single institution with simultaneous assessment of the efficacy of 3-tier and 4-tier grading systems. Hum Pathol. 2004;35:612-621.

225. Nascimento AF, Bertoni F, Fletcher CD. Epithelioid variant of myxofibrosarcoma: expanding the clinicomorphologic spectrum of myxofibrosarcoma in a series of 17 cases. Am J Surg Pathol. 2007;31:99-105.

226. Manoso MW, Pratt J, Healey JH, et al. Infiltrative MRI pattern and incomplete initial surgery compromise local control of myxofibrosarcoma. Clin Orthop Relat Res. 2006;450:89-94.

227. Meloni-Ehrig AM, Chen Z, Guan XY, et al. Identification of a ring chromosome in a myxoid malignant fibrous histiocytoma with chromosome microdissection and fluorescence in situ hybridization. Cancer Genet Cytogenet. 1999;109:81-85.

228. Sawyer JR, Binz RL, Gilliland JC, et al. A novel reciprocal (10;17)(p11.2;q23) in myxoid fibrosarcoma. Cancer Genet Cytogenet. 2001;124:144-146.

229. Clawson K, Donner LR, Dobin SM. Translocation (2;15)(p23;q21.2) and interstitial deletion of 7q in a case of low-grade myxofibrosarcoma. Cancer Genet Cytogenet. 2001;127:140-142.

230. Kishi K, Homma S, Tanimura S, et al. Hypoglycemia induced by secretion of high molecular weight insulin-like growth factor-II from a malignant solitary fibrous tumor of the pleura. Intern Med. 2001;40:341-344.

231. Tsuro K, Kojima H, Okamoto S, et al. Glucocorticoid therapy ameliorated hypoglycemia in insulin-like growth factor-II-producing solitary fibrous tumor. Intern Med. 2006;45:525-529.

232. West RB, Nuyten DS, Subramanian S, et al. Determination of stromal signatures in breast carcinoma. PLoS Biol. 2005;3:e187.

233. Ng TL, Gown AM, Barry TS, et al. Nuclear beta-catenin in mesenchymal tumors. Mod Pathol. 2005;18:68-74.

234. Morimitsu Y, Nakajima M, Hisaoka M, Hashimoto H. Extrapleural solitary fibrous tumor: clinicopathologic study of 17 cases and molecular analysis of the p53 pathway. Apmis. 2000;108:617-625.

235. Coffin CM, Hornick JL, Fletcher CD. Inflammatory myofibroblastic tumor: comparison of clinicopathologic, histologic, and immunohistochemical features including ALK expression in atypical and aggressive cases. Am J Surg Pathol. 2007;31:509-520.

236. Coffin CM, Patel A, Perkins S, et al. ALK1 and p80 expression and chromosomal rearrangements involving 2p23 in inflammatory myofibroblastic tumor. Mod Pathol. 2001;14:569-576.

237. Panagopoulos I, Nilsson T, Domanski HA, et al. Fusion of the SEC31L1 and ALK genes in an inflammatory myofibroblastic tumor. Int J Cancer. 2006;118:1181-1186.

238. Debelenko LV, Arthur DC, Pack SD, et al. Identification of CARS-ALK fusion in primary and metastatic lesions of an inflammatory myofibroblastic tumor. Lab Invest. 2003;83:1255-1265.

239. Ma Z, Hill DA, Collins MH, et al. Fusion of ALK to the Ran-binding protein 2 (RANBP2) gene in inflammatory myofibroblastic tumor. Genes Chromosomes Cancer. 2003;37:98-105.

240. Bridge JA, Kanamori M, Ma Z, et al. Fusion of the ALK gene to the clathrin heavy chain gene, CLTC, in inflammatory myofibroblastic tumor. Am J Pathol. 2001;159:411-415.

241. Morris SW, Kirstein MN, Valentine MB, et al. Fusion of a kinase gene, ALK, to a nucleolar protein gene, NPM, in non-Hodgkin's lymphoma. Science. 1994;263:1281-1284.

242. Touriol C, Greenland C, Lamant L, et al. Further demonstration of the diversity of chromosomal changes involving 2p23 in ALK-positive lymphoma: 2 cases expressing ALK kinase fused to CLTCL (clathrin chain polypeptide-like). Blood. 2000;95:3204-3207.

243. Enzinger FM, Zhang RY. Plexiform fibrohistiocytic tumor presenting in children and young adults: an analysis of 65 cases. Am J Surg Pathol. 1988;12:818-826.

244. Moosavi C, Jha P, Fanburg-Smith JC. An update on plexiform fibrohistiocytic tumor and addition of 66 new cases from the Armed Forces Institute of Pathology, in honor of Franz M. Enzinger, MD. Ann Diagn Pathol. 2007;11:313-319.

245. Remstein ED, Arndt CA, Nascimento AG. Plexiform fibrohistiocytic tumor: clinicopathologic analysis of 22 cases. Am J Surg Pathol. 1999;23:662-670.

246. Toro JR, Travis LB, Wu HJ, et al. Incidence patterns of soft tissue sarcomas, regardless of primary site, in the surveillance, epidemiology and end results program, 1978-2001: an analysis of 26,758 cases. Int J Cancer. 2006;119:2922-2930.

247. Mankin HJ, Casas-Ganem J, Kim JI, et al. Leiomyosarcoma of somatic soft tissues. Clin Orthop Relat Res. 2004:225-231.

248. Farshid G, Pradhan M, Goldblum J, Weiss SW. Leiomyosarcoma of somatic soft tissues: a tumor of vascular origin with multivariate analysis of outcome in 42 cases. Am J Surg Pathol. 2002;26:14-24.

249. Yamamoto H, Tsuchiya T, Ishimaru Y, et al. Infantile intestinal leiomyosarcoma is prognostically favorable despite histologic aggressiveness: case report and literature review. J Pediatr Surg. 2004;39:1257-1260.

250. Simpson BB, Reynolds EM, Kim SH, et al. Infantile intestinal leiomyosarcoma: surgical resection (without adjuvant therapy) for cure. J Pediatr Surg. 1996;31:1577-1580.

251. de Saint Aubain Somerhausen N, Fletcher CD. Leiomyosarcoma of soft tissue in children: clinicopathologic analysis of 20 cases. Am J Surg Pathol. 1999;23:755-763.

252. Swanson PE, Wick MR, Dehner LP. Leiomyosarcoma of somatic soft tissues in childhood: an immunohistochemical analysis of six cases with ultrastructural correlation. Hum Pathol. 1991;22:569-577.

253. Bisogno G, Spiller M, Scarzello G, et al. Secondary leiomyosarcomas: a report of 4 cases. Pediatr Hematol Oncol. 2005;22:181-187.

254. Hensley ML, Maki R, Venkatraman E, et al. Gemcitabine and docetaxel in patients with unresectable leiomyosarcoma: results of a phase II trial. J Clin Oncol. 2002;20:2824-2831.

255. Hartmann JT, Mayer F, Schleicher J, et al. Bendamustine hydrochloride in patients with refractory soft tissue sarcoma: a noncomparative multicenter phase 2 study of the German sarcoma group (AIO-001). Cancer. 2007;110:861-866.

256. Le Cesne A, Blay JY, Judson I, et al. Phase II study of ET-743 in advanced soft tissue sarcomas: a European Organisation for the Research and Treatment of Cancer (EORTC) soft tissue and bone sarcoma group trial. J Clin Oncol. 2005;23:576-584.

257. Lehtonen HJ, Kiuru M, Ylisaukko-Oja SK, et al. Increased risk of cancer in patients with fumarate hydratase germline mutation. J Med Genet. 2006;43:523-526.

258. Tomlinson IP, Alam NA, Rowan AJ, et al. Germline mutations in FH predispose to dominantly inherited uterine fibroids,

skin leiomyomata and papillary renal cell cancer. Nat Genet. 2002;30:406-410.

259. Alam NA, Rowan AJ, Wortham NC, et al. Genetic and functional analyses of FH mutations in multiple cutaneous and uterine leiomyomatosis, hereditary leiomyomatosis and renal cancer, and fumarate hydratase deficiency. Hum Mol Genet. 2003;12: 1241-1252.

260. Ragazzini P, Gamberi G, Pazzaglia L, et al. Amplification of *CDK4, MDM2, SAS* and *GLI* genes in leiomyosarcoma, alveolar and embryonal rhabdomyosarcoma. Histol Histopathol. 2004; 19:401-411.

261. Potti A, Ganti AK, Tendulkar K, et al. Determination of vascular endothelial growth factor (VEGF) overexpression in soft tissue sarcomas and the role of overexpression in leiomyosarcoma. J Cancer Res Clin Oncol. 2004;130:52-56.

262. Leiser AL, Anderson SE, Nonaka D, et al. Apoptotic and cell cycle regulatory markers in uterine leiomyosarcoma. Gynecol Oncol. 2006;101:86-91.

263. Anderson SE, Nonaka D, Chuai S, et al. *p53*, epidermal growth factor, and platelet-derived growth factor in uterine leiomyosarcoma and leiomyomas. Int J Gynecol Cancer. 2006;16:849-853.

264. O'Neill CJ, McBride HA, Connolly LE, McCluggage WG. Uterine leiomyosarcomas are characterized by high *p16*, p53 and *MIB1* expression in comparison with usual leiomyomas, leiomyoma variants and smooth muscle tumours of uncertain malignant potential. Histopathology. 2007;50:851-858.

265. Bodner-Adler B, Bodner K, Czerwenka K, et al. Expression of *p16* protein in patients with uterine smooth muscle tumors: an immunohistochemical analysis. Gynecol Oncol. 2005;96: 62-66.

266. Wang L, Felix JC, Lee JL, et al. The proto-oncogene c-kit is expressed in leiomyosarcomas of the uterus. Gynecol Oncol. 2003;90:402-406.

267. Hong T, Shimada Y, Uchida S, et al. Expression of angiogenic factors and apoptotic factors in leiomyosarcoma and leiomyoma. Int J Mol Med. 2001;8:141-148.

268. Strizzi L, Bianco C, Hirota M, et al. Development of leiomyosarcoma of the uterus in *MMTV-CR-1* transgenic mice. J Pathol. 2007;211:36-44.

269. Ciccodicola A, Dono R, Obici S, et al. Molecular characterization of a gene of the "EGF family" expressed in undifferentiated human *NTERA2* teratocarcinoma cells. EMBO J. 1989;8:1987-1991.

270. Hernando E, Charytonowicz E, Dudas ME, et al. The AKT-mTOR pathway plays a critical role in the development of leiomyosarcomas. Nat Med. 2007;13:748-753.

271. McClain KL, Leach CT, Jenson HB, et al. Association of Epstein-Barr virus with leiomyosarcomas in children with AIDS. N Engl J Med. 1995;332:12-18.

272. Jenson HB, Montalvo EA, McClain KL, et al. Characterization of natural Epstein-Barr virus infection and replication in smooth muscle cells from a leiomyosarcoma. J Med Virol. 1999;57: 36-46.

273. Brichard B, Smets F, Sokal E, et al. Unusual evolution of an Epstein-Barr virus-associated leiomyosarcoma occurring after liver transplantation. Pediatr Transplant. 2001;5:365-369.

274. Timmons CF, Dawson DB, Richards CS, et al. Epstein-Barr virus-associated leiomyosarcomas in liver transplantation recipients: origin from either donor or recipient tissue. Cancer. 1995;76:1481-1489.

275. Bonatti H, Hoefer D, Rogatsch H, et al. Successful management of recurrent Epstein-Barr virus-associated multilocular leiomyosarcoma after cardiac transplantation. Transplant Proc. 2005;37: 1839-1844.

276. Weiss SW, Enzinger FM. Epithelioid hemangioendothelioma: a vascular tumor often mistaken for a carcinoma. Cancer. 1982;50: 970-981.

277. Ishak KG, Sesterhenn IA, Goodman ZD, et al. Epithelioid hemangioendothelioma of the liver: a clinicopathologic and follow-up study of 32 cases. Hum Pathol. 1984;15:839-852.

278. Chan JK, Frizzera G, Fletcher CD, Rosai J. Primary vascular tumors of lymph nodes other than Kaposi's sarcoma: analysis of 39 cases and delineation of two new entities. Am J Surg Pathol. 1992;16:335-350.

279. Taratuto AL, Zurbriggen G, Sevlever G, Saccoliti M. Epithelioid hemangioendothelioma of the central nervous system: immunohistochemical and ultrastructural observations of a pediatric case. Pediatr Neurosci. 1988;14:11-14.

280. Dail DH, Liebow AA, Gmelich JT, et al. Intravascular, bronchiolar, and alveolar tumor of the lung (IVBAT): an analysis of twenty cases of a peculiar sclerosing endothelial tumor. Cancer. 1983;51:452-464.

281. Dail DH, Liebow AA. Intravascular bronchioloalveolar tumor. Am J Pathol. 1975;78:6a-7a.

282. Rock MJ, Kaufman RA, Lobe TE, et al. Epithelioid hemangioendothelioma of the lung (intravascular bronchioloalveolar tumor) in a young girl. Pediatr Pulmonol. 1991;11:181-186.

283. Mentzel T, Beham A, Calonje E, et al. Epithelioid hemangioendothelioma of skin and soft tissues: clinicopathologic and immunohistochemical study of 30 cases. Am J Surg Pathol. 1997; 21:363-374.

284. Mendlick MR, Nelson M, Pickering D, et al. Translocation t(1;3)(p36.3;q25) is a nonrandom aberration in epithelioid hemangioendothelioma. Am J Surg Pathol. 2001;25:684-687.

285. Kitaichi M, Nagai S, Nishimura K, et al. Pulmonary epithelioid haemangioendothelioma in 21 patients, including three with partial spontaneous regression. Eur Respir J. 1998;12:89-96.

286. Pinet C, Magnan A, Garbe L, et al. Aggressive form of pleural epithelioid haemangioendothelioma: complete response after chemotherapy. Eur Respir J. 1999;14:237-238.

287. Roudier-Pujol C, Enjolras O, Lacronique J, et al. Multifocal epithelioid hemangioendothelioma with partial remission after interferon alfa-2a treatment. Ann Dermatol Venereol. 1994;121: 898-904.

288. Kayler LK, Merion RM, Arenas JD, et al. Epithelioid hemangioendothelioma of the liver disseminated to the peritoneum treated with liver transplantation and interferon alpha-2B. Transplantation. 2002;74:128-130.

289. Galvao FH, Bakonyi-Neto A, Machado MA, et al. Interferon alpha-2B and liver resection to treat multifocal hepatic epithelioid hemangioendothelioma: a relevant approach to avoid liver transplantation. Transplant Proc. 2005;37:4354-4358.

290. Gonzalez-Crussi F, Chou P, Crawford SE. Congenital, infiltrating giant-cell angioblastoma. A new entity? Am J Surg Pathol. 1991;15:175-183.

291. Vargas SO, Perez-Atayde AR, Gonzalez-Crussi F, Kozakewich HP. Giant cell angioblastoma: three additional occurrences of a distinct pathologic entity. Am J Surg Pathol. 2001;25:185-196.

292. Marler JJ, Rubin JB, Trede NS, et al. Successful antiangiogenic therapy of giant cell angioblastoma with interferon alfa 2b: report of 2 cases. Pediatrics. 2002;109:E37.

293. Zukerberg LR, Nickoloff BJ, Weiss SW. Kaposiform hemangioendothelioma of infancy and childhood: an aggressive neoplasm associated with Kasabach-Merritt syndrome and lymphangiomatosis. Am J Surg Pathol. 1993;17:321-328.

294. Debelenko LV, Perez-Atayde AR, Mulliken JB, et al. D2-40 immunohistochemical analysis of pediatric vascular tumors reveals positivity in kaposiform hemangioendothelioma. Mod Pathol. 2005;18:1454-1460.

295. North PE, Waner M, Mizeracki A, Mihm MC Jr. GLUT1: a newly discovered immunohistochemical marker for juvenile hemangiomas. Hum Pathol. 2000;31:11-22.

296. Lyons LL, North PE, Mac-Moune Lai F, et al. Kaposiform hemangioendothelioma: a study of 33 cases emphasizing its

pathologic, immunophenotypic, and biologic uniqueness from juvenile hemangioma. Am J Surg Pathol. 2004;28:559-568.

297. Harper L, Michel JL, Enjolras O, et al. Successful management of a retroperitoneal kaposiform hemangioendothelioma with Kasabach-Merritt phenomenon using alpha-interferon. Eur J Pediatr Surg. 2006;16:369-372.

298. Gruman A, Liang MG, Mulliken JB, et al. Kaposiform hemangioendothelioma without Kasabach-Merritt phenomenon. J Am Acad Dermatol. 2005;52:616-622.

299. Blei F, Karp N, Rofsky N, et al. Successful multimodal therapy for kaposiform hemangioendothelioma complicated by Kasabach-Merritt phenomenon: case report and review of the literature. Pediatr Hematol Oncol. 1998;15:295-305.

300. Haisley-Royster C, Enjolras O, Frieden IJ, et al. Kasabach-Merritt phenomenon: a retrospective study of treatment with vincristine. J Pediatr Hematol Oncol. 2002;24:459-462.

301. Hu B, Lachman R, Phillips J, et al. Kasabach-Merritt syndrome-associated kaposiform hemangioendothelioma successfully treated with cyclophosphamide, vincristine, and actinomycin D. J Pediatr Hematol Oncol. 1998;20:567-569.

302. Hauer J, Graubner U, Konstantopoulos N, et al. Effective treatment of kaposiform hemangioendotheliomas associated with Kasabach-Merritt phenomenon using four-drug regimen. Pediatr Blood Cancer. 2007;49:852-854.

303. Chang Y, Cesarman E, Pessin MS, et al. Identification of herpes-virus-like DNA sequences in AIDS-associated Kaposi's sarcoma. Science. 1994;266:1865-1869.

304. Schalling M, Ekman M, Kaaya EE, et al. A role for a new herpes virus (KSHV) in different forms of Kaposi's sarcoma. Nat Med. 1995;1:707-708.

305. Moore PS, Chang Y. Detection of herpesvirus-like DNA sequences in Kaposi's sarcoma in patients with and without HIV infection. N Engl J Med. 1995;332:1181-1185.

306. Rabkin CS, Janz S, Lash A, et al. Monoclonal origin of multicentric Kaposi's sarcoma lesions. N Engl J Med. 1997;336:988-993.

307. Gill PS, Tsai YC, Rao AP, et al. Evidence for multiclonality in multicentric Kaposi's sarcoma. Proc Natl Acad Sci U S A. 1998;95:8257-8261.

308. Porta F, Bongiorno M, Locatelli F, et al. Kaposi's sarcoma in a child after autologous bone marrow transplantation for non-Hodgkin's lymphoma. Cancer. 1991;68:1361-1364.

309. Engels EA, Pfeiffer RM, Goedert JJ, et al. Trends in cancer risk among people with AIDS in the United States 1980-2002. AIDS. 2006;20:1645-1654.

310. Meduri GU, Stover DE, Lee M, et al. Pulmonary Kaposi's sarcoma in the acquired immune deficiency syndrome: clinical, radiographic, and pathologic manifestations. Am J Med. 1986; 81:11-18.

311. Friedman SL, Wright TL, Altman DF. Gastrointestinal Kaposi's sarcoma in patients with acquired immunodeficiency syndrome: endoscopic and autopsy findings. Gastroenterology. 1985;89: 102-108.

312. Caponetti G, Dezube BJ, Restrepo CS, Pantanowitz L. Kaposi sarcoma of the musculoskeletal system: a review of 66 patients. Cancer. 2007;109:1040-1052.

313. Rwomushana RJ, Bailey IC, Kyalwazi SK. Kaposi's sarcoma of the brain: a case report with necropsy findings. Cancer. 1975;36:1127-1131.

314. Money-Kyrle JF, Bates F, Ready J, et al. Liposomal daunorubicin in advanced Kaposi's sarcoma: a phase II study. Clin Oncol (R Coll Radiol). 1993;5:367-371.

315. Stewart S, Jablonowski H, Goebel FD, et al. Randomized comparative trial of pegylated liposomal doxorubicin versus bleomycin and vincristine in the treatment of AIDS-related Kaposi's sarcoma. International Pegylated Liposomal Doxorubicin Study Group. J Clin Oncol. 1998;16:683-691.

316. Gill PS, Wernz J, Scadden DT, et al. Randomized phase III trial of liposomal daunorubicin versus doxorubicin, bleomycin, and vincristine in AIDS-related Kaposi's sarcoma. J Clin Oncol. 1996;14:2353-2364.

317. Coffin CM, Dehner LP. Vascular tumors in children and adolescents: a clinicopathologic study of 228 tumors in 222 patients. Pathol Annu. 1993;28:97-120.

318. Meis-Kindblom JM, Kindblom LG. Angiosarcoma of soft tissue: a study of 80 cases. Am J Surg Pathol. 1998;22:683-697.

319. Tsao CY, Sommer A, Hamoudi AB. Aicardi syndrome, metastatic angiosarcoma of the leg, and scalp lipoma. Am J Med Genet. 1993;45:594-596.

320. McLaughlin ER, Brown LF, Weiss SW, et al. VEGF and its receptors are expressed in a pediatric angiosarcoma in a patient with Aicardi's syndrome. J Invest Dermatol. 2000;114:1209-1210.

321. Rossi NP, Kioschos JM, Aschenbrener CA, Ehrenhaft JL. Primary angiosarcoma of the heart. Cancer. 1976;37:891-894.

322. Lezama-del Valle P, Gerald WL, Tsai J, et al. Malignant vascular tumors in young patients. Cancer. 1998;83:1634-1639.

323. Mark RJ, Poen JC, Tran LM, et al. Angiosarcoma: a report of 67 patients and a review of the literature. Cancer. 1996;77: 2400-2406.

324. Ferrari A, Casanova M, Bisogno G, et al. Malignant vascular tumors in children and adolescents: a report from the Italian and German Soft Tissue Sarcoma Cooperative Group. Med Pediatr Oncol. 2002;39:109-114.

325. Maddox JC, Evans HL. Angiosarcoma of skin and soft tissue: a study of forty-four cases. Cancer. 1981;48:1907-1921.

326. Weitz J, Klimstra DS, Cymes K, et al. Management of primary liver sarcomas. Cancer. 2007;109:1391-1396.

327. Gunawardena SW, Trautwein LM, Finegold MJ, Ogden AK. Hepatic angiosarcoma in a child: successful therapy with surgery and adjuvant chemotherapy. Med Pediatr Oncol. 1997;28: 139-143.

328. Nagano T, Yamada Y, Ikeda T, et al. Docetaxel: a therapeutic option in the treatment of cutaneous angiosarcoma: report of 9 patients. Cancer. 2007;110:648-651.

329. Skubitz KM, Haddad PA. Paclitaxel and pegylated-liposomal doxorubicin are both active in angiosarcoma. Cancer. 2005; 104:361-366.

330. Anderson SE, Keohan ML, D'Adamo DR, Maki RG. A retrospective analysis of vinorelbine chemotherapy for patients with previously treated soft-tissue sarcomas. Sarcoma. 2006;2006: 15947.

331. Kopp HG, Kanz L, Hartmann JT. Complete remission of relapsing high-grade angiosarcoma with single-agent metronomic trofosfamide. Anticancer Drugs. 2006;17:997-998.

332. Walsh R, Harrington J, Beneck D, Ozkaynak MF. Congenital infantile hepatic hemangioendothelioma type II treated with orthotopic liver transplantation. J Pediatr Hematol Oncol. 2004;26:121-123.

333. Folpe AL, Chand EM, Goldblum JR, Weiss SW. Expression of Fli-1, a nuclear transcription factor, distinguishes vascular neoplasms from potential mimics. Am J Surg Pathol. 2001;25: 1061-1066.

334. Syed SP, Martin AM, Haupt HM, et al. Angiostatin receptor annexin II in vascular tumors including angiosarcoma. Hum Pathol. 2007;38:508-513.

335. Weihrauch M, Markwarth A, Lehnert G, et al. Abnormalities of the ARF-p53 pathway in primary angiosarcomas of the liver. Hum Pathol. 2002;33:884-892.

336. Nakashima Y, Unni KK, Shives TC, et al. Mesenchymal chondrosarcoma of bone and soft tissue: a review of 111 cases. Cancer. 1986;57:2444-2453.

337. Dabska M, Huvos AG. Mesenchymal chondrosarcoma in the young. Virchows Arch A Pathol Anat Histopathol. 1983;399: 89-104.

338. Huvos AG, Rosen G, Dabska M, Marcove RC. Mesenchymal chondrosarcoma: a clinicopathologic analysis of 35 patients with emphasis on treatment. Cancer. 1983;51:1230-1237.

339. Wehrli BM, Huang W, De Crombrugghe B, et al. Sox9, a master regulator of chondrogenesis, distinguishes mesenchymal chondrosarcoma from other small blue round cell tumors. Hum Pathol. 2003;34:263-269.

340. Greenspan A, Unni KK, Blake L, Rab G. Extraskeletal myxoid chondrosarcoma: an unusual tumour in a 6-year-old boy. Can Assoc Radiol J. 1994;45:62-65.

341. Hachitanda Y, Tsuneyoshi M, Daimaru Y, et al. Extraskeletal myxoid chondrosarcoma in young children. Cancer. 1988;61:2521-2526.

342. Enzinger FM, Shiraki M. Extraskeletal myxoid chondrosarcoma: an analysis of 34 cases. Hum Pathol. 1972;3:421-435.

343. Dei Tos AP, Wadden C, Fletcher CDM. Extraskeletal myxoid chondrosarcoma: an immunohistochemical reappraisal of 39 cases. Applied Immunohistochem. 1997;5:73-77.

344. Okamoto S, Hisaoka M, Ishida T, et al. Extraskeletal myxoid chondrosarcoma: a clinicopathologic, immunohistochemical, and molecular analysis of 18 cases. Hum Pathol. 2001;32:1116-1124.

345. Goh YW, Spagnolo DV, Platten M, et al. Extraskeletal myxoid chondrosarcoma: a light microscopic, immunohistochemical, ultrastructural and immuno-ultrastructural study indicating neuroendocrine differentiation. Histopathology. 2001;39:514-524.

346. Subramanian S, West RB, Marinelli RJ, et al. The gene expression profile of extraskeletal myxoid chondrosarcoma. J Pathol. 2005;206:433-444.

347. Saleh G, Evans HL, Ro JY, Ayala AG. Extraskeletal myxoid chondrosarcoma: a clinicopathologic study of ten patients with long-term follow-up. Cancer. 1992;70:2827-2830.

348. Meis-Kindblom JM, Bergh P, Gunterberg B, Kindblom LG. Extraskeletal myxoid chondrosarcoma: a reappraisal of its morphologic spectrum and prognostic factors based on 117 cases. Am J Surg Pathol. 1999;23:636-650.

349. Labelle Y, Zucman J, Stenman G, et al. Oncogenic conversion of a novel orphan nuclear receptor by chromosome translocation. Hum Mol Genet. 1995;4:2219-2226.

350. Clark J, Benjamin H, Gill S, et al. Fusion of the EWS gene to CHN, a member of the steroid/thyroid receptor gene superfamily, in a human myxoid chondrosarcoma. Oncogene. 1996;12:229-235.

351. Panagopoulos I, Mencinger M, Dietrich CU, et al. Fusion of the RBP56 and CHN genes in extraskeletal myxoid chondrosarcomas with translocation t(9;17)(q22;q11). Oncogene. 1999;18:7594-7598.

352. Attwooll C, Tariq M, Harris M, et al. Identification of a novel fusion gene involving hTAFII68 and CHN from a t(9;17)(q11.2) translocation in an extraskeletal myxoid chondrosarcoma. Oncogene. 1999;18:7599-7601.

353. Sjogren H, Wedell B, Meis-Kindblom JM, et al. Fusion of the NH2-terminal domain of the basic helix-loop-helix protein TCF12 to TEC in extraskeletal myxoid chondrosarcoma with translocation t(9;15)(q22;q21). Cancer Res. 2000;60:6832-6835.

354. Zhang Y, Babin J, Feldhaus AL, et al. HTF4: a new human helix-loop-helix protein. Nucleic Acids Res. 1991;19:4555.

355. Hu JS, Olson EN, Kingston RE. HEB, a helix-loop-helix protein related to E2A and ITF2 that can modulate the DNA-binding ability of myogenic regulatory factors. Mol Cell Biol. 1992;12:1031-1042.

356. Hazel TG, Nathans D, Lau LF. A gene inducible by serum growth factors encodes a member of the steroid and thyroid hormone receptor superfamily. Proc Natl Acad Sci U S A. 1988;85:8444-8448.

357. Law SW, Conneely OM, DeMayo FJ, O'Malley BW. Identification of a new brain-specific transcription factor, NURR1. Mol Endocrinol. 1992;6:2129-2135.

358. Milbrandt J. Nerve growth factor induces a gene homologous to the glucocorticoid receptor gene. Neuron. 1988;1:183-188.

359. Nakai A, Kartha S, Sakurai A, et al. A human early response gene homologous to murine nur77 and rat NGFI-B, and related to the nuclear receptor superfamily. Mol Endocrinol. 1990;4:1438-1443.

360. Wang Z, Benoit G, Liu J, et al. Structure and function of Nurr1 identifies a class of ligand-independent nuclear receptors. Nature. 2003;423:555-560.

361. Scearce LM, Laz TM, Hazel TG, et al. RNR-1, a nuclear receptor in the NGFI-B/Nur77 family that is rapidly induced in regenerating liver. J Biol Chem. 1993;268:8855-8861.

362. Fahrner TJ, Carroll SL, Milbrandt J. The NGFI-B protein, an inducible member of the thyroid/steroid receptor family, is rapidly modified posttranslationally. Mol Cell Biol. 1990;10:6454-6459.

363. Davis IJ, Hazel TG, Chen R-H, et al. Functional domains and phosphorylation of the orphan receptor Nur77. Mol Endocrinol. 1993;7:953-964.

364. Davis IJ, Hazel TG, Lau LF. Transcription activation by Nur77, a growth factor-inducible member of the steroid receptor superfamily. Mol Endocrinol. 1991;5:854-859.

365. Hazel TG, Misra R, Davis IJ, et al. Nur77 is differentially modified in PC12 cells upon membrane depolarization and growth factor treatment. Mol Cell Biol. 1991;11:3239-3246.

366. Liu ZG, Smith SW, McLaughlin KA, et al. Apoptotic signals delivered through the T-cell receptor of a T-cell hybrid require the immediate-early gene nur77. Nature. 1994;367:281-284.

367. Woronicz JD, Calnan B, Ngo V, Winoto A. Requirement for the orphan steroid receptor Nur77 in apoptosis of T-cell hybridomas. Nature. 1994;367:277-281.

368. Pei L, Waki H, Vaitheesvaran B, et al. NR4A orphan nuclear receptors are transcriptional regulators of hepatic glucose metabolism. Nat Med. 2006;12:1048-1055.

369. Mullican SE, Zhang S, Konopleva M, et al. Abrogation of nuclear receptors Nr4a3 and Nr4a1 leads to development of acute myeloid leukemia. Nat Med. 2007;13:730-735.

370. Labelle Y, Bussieres J, Courjal F, Goldring MB. The EWS/TEC fusion protein encoded by the t(9;22) chromosomal translocation in human chondrosarcomas is a highly potent transcriptional activator. Oncogene. 1999;18:3303-3308.

371. Sjogren H, Meis-Kindblom JM, Orndal C, et al. Studies on the molecular pathogenesis of extraskeletal myxoid chondrosarcoma-cytogenetic, molecular genetic, and cDNA microarray analyses. Am J Pathol. 2003;162:781-792.

372. Al-Rajhi N, Husain S, Coupland R, et al. Primary pericardial synovial sarcoma: a case report and literature review. J Surg Oncol. 1999;70:194-198.

373. Yano M, Toyooka S, Tsukuda K, et al. SYT-SSX fusion genes in synovial sarcoma of the thorax. Lung Cancer. 2004;44:391-397.

374. Miller DV, Deb A, Edwards WD, et al. Primary synovial sarcoma of the mitral valve. Cardiovasc Pathol. 2005;14:331-333.

375. Turc-Carel C, Dal Cin P, Limon J, et al. Involvement of chromosome X in primary cytogenetic change in human neoplasia: nonrandom translocation in synovial sarcoma. Proc Natl Acad Sci U S A. 1987;84:1981-1985.

376. Griffin CA, Emanuel BS. Translocation (X;18) in a synovial sarcoma. Cancer Genet Cytogenet. 1987;26:181-183.

377. Clark J, Rocques PJ, Crew AJ, et al. Identification of novel genes, SYT and SSX, involved in the t(X;18)(p11.2;q11.2) translocation found in human synovial sarcoma. Nat Genet. 1994;7:502-508.

378. de Leeuw B, Balemans M, Weghuis DO, et al. Molecular cloning of the synovial sarcoma-specific translocation (X;18)(p11.2;q11.2) breakpoint. Hum Mol Genet. 1994;3:745-749.

379. de Leeuw B, Balemans M, Olde Weghuis D, Geurts van Kessel A. Identification of two alternative fusion genes, SYT-SSX1 and

SYT-SSX2, in t(X;18)(p11.2;q11.2)-positive synovial sarcomas. Hum Mol Genet. 1995;4:1097-1099.

380. Crew AJ, Clark J, Fisher C, et al. Fusion of SYT to two genes, *SSX1* and *SSX2*, encoding proteins with homology to the Kruppel-associated box in human synovial sarcoma. EMBO J. 1995;14:2333-2340.

381. Storlazzi CT, Mertens F, Mandahl N, et al. A novel fusion gene, *SS18L1/SSX1*, in synovial sarcoma. Genes Chromosomes Cancer. 2003;37:195-200.

382. Argani P, Zakowski MF, Klimstra DS, et al. Detection of the *SYT-SSX* chimeric RNA of synovial sarcoma in paraffin-embedded tissue and its application in problematic cases. Mod Pathol. 1998;11:65-71.

383. Lasota J, Jasinski M, Debiec-Rychter M, et al. Detection of the SYT-SSX fusion transcripts in formaldehyde-fixed, paraffin-embedded tissue: a reverse transcription polymerase chain reaction amplification assay useful in the diagnosis of synovial sarcoma. Mod Pathol. 1998;11:626-633.

384. Hiraga H, Nojima T, Abe S, et al. Diagnosis of synovial sarcoma with the reverse transcriptase-polymerase chain reaction: analyses of 84 soft tissue and bone tumors. Diagn Mol Pathol. 1998;7: 102-110.

385. Guillou L, Coindre J, Gallagher G, et al. Detection of the synovial sarcoma translocation t(X;18) *(SYT;SSX)* in paraffin-embedded tissues using reverse transcriptase-polymerase chain reaction: a reliable and powerful diagnostic tool for pathologists: a molecular analysis of 221 mesenchymal tumors fixed in different fixatives. Hum Pathol. 2001;32:105-112.

386. van de Rijn M, Barr FG, Collins MH, et al. Absence of *SYT-SSX* fusion products in soft tissue tumors other than synovial sarcoma. Am J Clin Pathol. 1999;112:43-49.

387. He R, Patel RM, Alkan S, et al. Immunostaining for SYT protein discriminates synovial sarcoma from other soft tissue tumors: analysis of 146 cases. Mod Pathol. 2007;20:522-528.

388. Gure AO, Wei IJ, Old LJ, Chen YT. The *SSX* gene family: characterization of 9 complete genes. Int J Cancer. 2002;101: 448-453.

389. Witzgall R, O'Leary E, Leaf A, et al. The Kruppel-associated box-A (KRAB-A) domain of zinc finger proteins mediates transcriptional repression. Proc Natl Acad Sci U S A. 1994;91: 4514-4518.

390. de Bruijn DR, Baats E, Zechner U, et al. Isolation and characterization of the mouse homolog of *SYT*, a gene implicated in the development of human synovial sarcomas. Oncogene. 1996; 13:643-648.

391. de Bruijn DR, Kater-Baats E, Eleveld M, et al. Mapping and characterization of the mouse and human SS18 genes, two human SS18-like genes and a mouse Ss18 pseudogene. Cytogenet Cell Genet. 2001;92:310-319.

392. dos Santos NR, de Bruijn DR, Balemans M, et al. Nuclear localization of SYT, SSX and the synovial sarcoma-associated SYT-SSX fusion proteins. Hum Mol Genet. 1997;6:1549-1558.

393. Brett D, Whitehouse S, Antonson P, et al. The SYT protein involved in the t(X;18) synovial sarcoma translocation is a transcriptional activator localised in nuclear bodies. Hum Mol Genet. 1997;6:1559-1564.

394. Lim FL, Soulez M, Koczan D, et al. A KRAB-related domain and a novel transcription repression domain in proteins encoded by *SSX* genes that are disrupted in human sarcomas. Oncogene. 1998;17:2013-2018.

395. Thaete C, Brett D, Monaghan P, et al. Functional domains of the *SYT* and *SYT-SSX* synovial sarcoma translocation proteins and co-localization with the SNF protein BRM in the nucleus. Hum Mol Genet. 1999;8:585-591.

396. Soulez M, Saurin AJ, Freemont PS, Knight JC. *SSX* and the synovial-sarcoma-specific chimaeric protein *SYT-SSX* co-localize with the human Polycomb group complex. Oncogene. 1999;18: 2739-2746.

397. Perani M, Ingram CJ, Cooper CS, et al. Conserved SNH domain of the proto-oncoprotein *SYT* interacts with components of the human chromatin remodelling complexes, while the *QPGY* repeat domain forms homo-oligomers. Oncogene. 2003;22:8156-8167.

398. Perani M, Antonson P, Hamoudi R, et al. The proto-oncoprotein *SYT* interacts with *SYT*-interacting protein/co-activator activator (*SIP/CoAA*), a human nuclear receptor co-activator with similarity to *EWS* and *TLS/FUS* family of proteins. J Biol Chem. 2005;280:42863-42876.

399. Iwasaki T, Koibuchi N, Chin WW. Synovial sarcoma translocation (*SYT*) encodes a nuclear receptor coactivator. Endocrinology. 2005;146:3892-3899.

400. Ishida M, Miyamoto M, Naitoh S, et al. The *SYT-SSX* fusion protein downregulates the cell proliferation regulator *COM1* in t(x;18) synovial sarcoma. Mol Cell Biol. 2007;27:1348-1355.

401. Nagai M, Tanaka S, Tsuda M, et al. Analysis of transforming activity of human synovial sarcoma-associated chimeric protein *SYT-SSX1* bound to chromatin remodeling factor *hBRM/hSNF2* alpha. Proc Natl Acad Sci U S A. 2001;98:3843-3848.

402. Haldar M, Hancock JD, Coffin CM, et al. A conditional mouse model of synovial sarcoma: insights into a myogenic origin. Cancer Cell. 2007;11:375-388.

403. Skytting BT, Bauer HC, Perfekt R, et al. Ki-67 is strongly prognostic in synovial sarcoma: analysis based on 86 patients from the Scandinavian sarcoma group register. Br J Cancer. 1999;80:1809-1814.

404. Antonescu CR, Kawai A, Leung DH, et al. Strong association of *SYT-SSX* fusion type and morphologic epithelial differentiation in synovial sarcoma. Diagn Mol Pathol. 2000;9:1-8.

405. Kawai A, Woodruff J, Healey JH, et al. SYT-SSX gene fusion as a determinant of morphology and prognosis in synovial sarcoma. N Engl J Med. 1998;338:153-160.

406. Ladanyi M, Antonescu CR, Leung DH, et al. Impact of *SYT-SSX* fusion type on the clinical behavior of synovial sarcoma: a multi-institutional retrospective study of 243 patients. Cancer Res. 2002;62:135-140.

407. Guillou L, Benhattar J, Bonichon F, et al. Histologic grade, but not *SYT-SSX* fusion type, is an important prognostic factor in patients with synovial sarcoma: a multicenter, retrospective analysis. J Clin Oncol. 2004;22:4040-4050.

408. Xie Y, Skytting B, Nilsson G, et al. *SYT-SSX* is critical for cyclin D1 expression in synovial sarcoma cells: a gain of function of the t(X;18)(p11.2;q11.2) translocation. Cancer Res. 2002;62:3861-3867.

409. Xie Y, Skytting B, Nilsson G, et al. The *SYT-SSX1* fusion type of synovial sarcoma is associated with increased expression of cyclin A and D1: a link between t(X;18)(p11.2;q11.2) and the cell cycle machinery. Oncogene. 2002;21:5791-5796.

410. Xie Y, Skytting B, Nilsson G, et al. Expression of insulin-like growth factor-1 receptor in synovial sarcoma: association with an aggressive phenotype. Cancer Res. 1999;59:3588-3591.

411. Kuhnen C, Tolnay E, Steinau HU, et al. Expression of c-Met receptor and hepatocyte growth factor/scatter factor in synovial sarcoma and epithelioid sarcoma. Virchows Arch. 1998;432: 337-342.

412. Oda Y, Sakamoto A, Saito T, et al. Expression of hepatocyte growth factor (HGF)/scatter factor and its receptor c-MET correlates with poor prognosis in synovial sarcoma. Hum Pathol. 2000;31:185-192.

413. Allander SV, Illei PB, Chen Y, et al. Expression profiling of synovial sarcoma by cDNA microarrays: association of *ERBB2*, *IGFBP2*, and *ELF3* with epithelial differentiation. Am J Pathol. 2002;161:1587-1595.

414. Segal NH, Pavlidis P, Antonescu CR, et al. Classification and subtype prediction of adult soft tissue sarcoma by functional genomics. Am J Pathol. 2003;163:691-700.

415. Terry J, Saito T, Subramanian S, et al. *TLE1* as a diagnostic immunohistochemical marker for synovial sarcoma emerging

from gene expression profiling studies. Am J Surg Pathol. 2007;31:240-246.

416. Hunter BC, Devaney KO, Ferlito A, Rinaldo A. Alveolar soft part sarcoma of the head and neck region. Ann Otol Rhinol Laryngol. 1998;107:810-814.

417. Castle JT, Goode RK. Alveolar soft part sarcoma of the tongue: report of an unusual pattern in a child. Ann Diagn Pathol. 1999;3:315-317.

418. Font RL, Jurco S 3rd, Zimmerman LE. Alveolar soft-part sarcoma of the orbit: a clinicopathologic analysis of seventeen cases and a review of the literature. Hum Pathol. 1982;13:569-579.

419. Luo J, Melnick S, Rossi A, et al. Primary cardiac alveolar soft part sarcoma: a report of the first observed case with molecular diagnostics corroboration. Pediatr Dev Pathol. 2008;11:142-147.

420. Wu J, Brinker DA, Haas M, et al. Primary alveolar soft part sarcoma (ASPS) of the breast: report of a deceptive case with xanthomatous features confirmed by *TFE3* immunohistochemistry and electron microscopy. Int J Surg Pathol. 2005;13:81-85.

421. Amin MB, Patel RM, Oliveira P, et al. Alveolar soft-part sarcoma of the urinary bladder with urethral recurrence: a unique case with emphasis on differential diagnoses and diagnostic utility of an immunohistochemical panel including TFE3. Am J Surg Pathol. 2006;30:1322-1325.

422. Roma AA, Yang B, Senior ME, Goldblum JR. *TFE3* immunoreactivity in alveolar soft part sarcoma of the uterine cervix: case report. Int J Gynecol Pathol. 2005;24:131-135.

423. Chapman GW, Benda J, Williams T. Alveolar soft-part sarcoma of the vagina. Gynecol Oncol. 1984;18:125-129.

424. Pappo AS, Parham DM, Cain A, et al. Alveolar soft part sarcoma in children and adolescents: clinical features and outcome of 11 patients. Med Pediatr Oncol. 1996;26:81-84.

425. Kayton ML, Meyers P, Wexler LH, et al. Clinical presentation, treatment, and outcome of alveolar soft part sarcoma in children, adolescents, and young adults. J Pediatr Surg. 2006;41:187-193.

426. Nickerson HJ, Silberman T, Jacobsen FS, et al. Alveolar soft-part sarcoma responsive to intensive chemotherapy. J Pediatr Hematol Oncol. 2004;26:233-235.

427. Lieberman PH, Brennan MF, Kimmel M, et al. Alveolar soft-part sarcoma: a clinico-pathologic study of half a century. Cancer. 1989;63:1-13.

428. Portera CA Jr, Ho V, Patel SR, et al. Alveolar soft part sarcoma: clinical course and patterns of metastasis in 70 patients treated at a single institution. Cancer. 2001;91:585-591.

429. Ueda T, Uchida A, Kodama K, et al. Aggressive pulmonary metastasectomy for soft tissue sarcomas. Cancer. 1993;72:1919-1925.

430. Bindal RK, Sawaya RE, Leavens ME, et al. Sarcoma metastatic to the brain: results of surgical treatment. Neurosurgery. 1994;35:185-190; discussion 190-191.

431. Berman TM, Fuhrman SA, Johnson FE. Prolonged survival after bilateral thoracotomy for metastatic alveolar soft-part sarcoma. Minn Med. 1984;67:261-262.

432. Ladanyi M, Antonescu CR, Drobnjak M, et al. The precrystalline cytoplasmic granules of alveolar soft part sarcoma contain monocarboxylate transporter 1 and CD147. Am J Pathol. 2002;160:1215-1221.

433. Mathew T. Evidence supporting neural crest origin of an alveolar soft part sarcoma: an ultrastructural study. Cancer. 1982;50:507-514.

434. Miettinen M, Ekfors T. Alveolar soft-part sarcoma: immunohistochemical evidence for muscle cell differentiation. Am J Clin Pathol. 1990;93:32-38.

435. Heimann P, Devalck C, Debusscher C, et al. Alveolar soft-part sarcoma: further evidence by FISH for the involvement of chromosome band 17q25. Genes Chromosomes Cancer. 1998;23:194-197.

436. Joyama S, Ueda T, Shimizu K, et al. Chromosome rearrangement at 17q25 and xp11.2 in alveolar soft-part sarcoma: a case report and review of the literature. Cancer. 1999;86:1246-1250.

437. Ladanyi M, Lui MY, Antonescu CR, et al. The der(17)t(X;17)(p11;q25) of human alveolar soft part sarcoma fuses the *TFE3* transcription factor gene to *ASPL*, a novel gene at 17q25. Oncogene. 2001;20:48-57.

438. Henthorn PS, Stewart CC, Kadesch T, Puck JM. The gene encoding human *TFE3*, a transcription factor that binds the immunoglobulin heavy-chain enhancer, maps to Xp11.22. Genomics. 1991;11:374-378.

439. Hemesath TJ, Steingrimsson E, McGill G, et al. *microphthalmia*, a critical factor in melanocyte development, defines a discrete transcription factor family. Genes Dev. 1994;8:2770-2780.

440. Bogan JS, Hendon N, McKee AE, et al. Functional cloning of *TUG* as a regulator of *GLUT4* glucose transporter trafficking. Nature. 2003;425:727-733.

441. Argani P, Lal P, Hutchinson B, et al. Aberrant nuclear immunoreactivity for *TFE3* in neoplasms with *TFE3* gene fusions: a sensitive and specific immunohistochemical assay. Am J Surg Pathol. 2003;27:750-761.

442. Tsuda M, Davis IJ, Argani P, et al. *TFE3* fusions activate *MET* signaling by transcriptional up-regulation, defining another class of tumors as candidates for therapeutic *MET* inhibition. Cancer Res. 2007;67:919-929.

443. Argani P, Antonescu CR, Illei PB, et al. Primary renal neoplasms with the *ASPL-TFE3* gene fusion of alveolar soft part sarcoma: a distinctive tumor entity previously included among renal cell carcinomas of children and adolescents. Am J Pathol. 2001;159:179-192.

444. Enzinger FM. Clear-cell sarcoma of tendons and aponeuroses: an analysis of 21 cases. Cancer. 1965;18:1163-1174.

445. Chung EB, Enzinger FM. Malignant melanoma of soft parts. A reassessment of clear cell sarcoma. Am J Surg Pathol. 1983;7:405-413.

446. Deenik W, Mooi WJ, Rutgers EJ, et al. Clear cell sarcoma (malignant melanoma) of soft parts: a clinicopathologic study of 30 cases. Cancer. 1999;86:969-975.

447. Finley JW, Hanypsiak B, McGrath B, et al. Clear cell sarcoma: the Roswell Park experience. J Surg Oncol. 2001;77:16-20.

448. Ferrari A, Casanova M, Bisogno G, et al. Clear cell sarcoma of tendons and aponeuroses in pediatric patients: a report from the Italian and German Soft Tissue Sarcoma Cooperative Group. Cancer. 2002;94:3269-3276.

449. Lucas DR, Nascimento AG, Sim FH. Clear cell sarcoma of soft tissues: Mayo Clinic experience with 35 cases. Am J Surg Pathol. 1992;16:1197-1204.

450. Kawai A, Hosono A, Nakayama R, et al. Clear cell sarcoma of tendons and aponeuroses: a study of 75 patients. Cancer. 2007;109:109-116.

451. Granter SR, Weilbaecher MD, Quigley C, et al. Clear cell sarcoma shows immunoreactivity for microphthalmia transcription factor: further evidence for melanocytic differentiation. Mod Pathol. 2001;14:6-9.

452. Hasegawa T, Hirose T, Kudo E, Hizawa K. Clear cell sarcoma: an immunohistochemical and ultrastructural study. Acta Pathol Jpn. 1989;39:321-327.

453. Kindblom LG, Lodding P, Angervall L. Clear-cell sarcoma of tendons and aponeuroses: an immunohistochemical and electron microscopic analysis indicating neural crest origin. Virchows Arch A Pathol Anat Histopathol. 1983;401:109-128.

454. Benson JD, Kraemer BB, Mackay B. Malignant melanoma of soft parts: an ultrastructural study of four cases. Ultrastruct Pathol. 1985;8:57-70.

455. Schaefer KL, Brachwitz K, Wai DH, et al. Expression profiling of t(12;22) positive clear cell sarcoma of soft tissue cell lines

reveals characteristic up-regulation of potential new marker genes including *ERBB3*. Cancer Res. 2004;64:3395-3405.

456. Segal NH, Pavlidis P, Noble WS, et al. Classification of clear-cell sarcoma as a subtype of melanoma by genomic profiling. J Clin Oncol. 2003;21:1775-1781.

457. Garcia JJ, Kramer MJ, O'Donnell RJ, Horvai AE. Mismatch repair protein expression and microsatellite instability: a comparison of clear cell sarcoma of soft parts and metastatic melanoma. Mod Pathol. 2006;19:950-957.

458. Panagopoulos I, Mertens F, Isaksson M, Mandahl N. Absence of mutations of the *BRAF* gene in malignant melanoma of soft parts (clear cell sarcoma of tendons and aponeuroses). Cancer Genet Cytogenet. 2005;156:74-76.

459. Davis IJ, Kim JJ, Ozsolak F, et al. Oncogenic *MITF* dysregulation in clear cell sarcoma: defining the MiT family of human cancers. Cancer Cell. 2006;9:473-484.

460. Zucman J, Delattre O, Desmaze C, et al. *EWS* and *ATF-1* gene fusion induced by t(12:22) translocation in malignant melanoma of soft parts. Nat Genet. 1993;4:341-345.

461. Yamamoto KK, Gonzalez GA, Biggs WH 3rd, Montminy MR. Phosphorylation-induced binding and transcriptional efficacy of nuclear factor CREB. Nature. 1988;334:494-498.

462. Gonzalez GA, Yamamoto KK, Fischer WH, et al. A cluster of phosphorylation sites on the cyclic AMP-regulated nuclear factor CREB predicted by its sequence. Nature. 1989;337:749-752.

463. Brown AD, Lopez-Terrada D, Denny C, Lee KAW. Promoters containing ATF-binding sites are de-regulated in cells that express the *EWS/ATF1* oncogene. Oncogene. 1995;10:1749-1756.

464. Hodgkinson CA, Moore KJ, Nakayama A, et al. Mutations at the mouse microphthalmia locus are associated with defects in a gene encoding a novel basic-helix-loop-helix-zipper protein. Cell. 1993;74:395-404.

465. Antonescu CR, Nafa K, Segal NH, et al. *EWS-CREB1*: a recurrent variant fusion in clear cell sarcoma—association with gastrointestinal location and absence of melanocytic differentiation. Clin Cancer Res. 2006;12:5356-5362.

466. Antonescu CR, Dal Cin P, Nafa K, et al. *EWSR1-CREB1* is the predominant gene fusion in angiomatoid fibrous histiocytoma. Genes Chromosomes Cancer. 2007;46:1051-1060.

467. Schaefer KL, Brachwitz K, Braun Y, et al. Constitutive activation of neuregulin/ERBB3 signaling pathway in clear cell sarcoma of soft tissue. Neoplasia. 2006;8:613-622.

468. Wang LL, Perlman EJ, Vujanic GM, et al. Desmoplastic small round cell tumor of the kidney in childhood. Am J Surg Pathol. 2007;31:576-584.

469. Gerald WL, Ladanyi M, de Alava E, et al. Clinical, pathologic, and molecular spectrum of tumors associated with t(11;22)(p13;q12): desmoplastic small round-cell tumor and its variants. J Clin Oncol. 1998;16:3028-3036.

470. Lae ME, Roche PC, Jin L, et al. Desmoplastic small round cell tumor: a clinicopathologic, immunohistochemical, and molecular study of 32 tumors. Am J Surg Pathol. 2002;26:823-835.

471. Kretschmar CS, Colbach C, Bhan I, Crombleholme TM. Desmoplastic small cell tumor: a report of three cases and a review of the literature. J Pediatr Hematol Oncol. 1996;18:293-298.

472. Bismar TA, Basturk O, Gerald WL, et al. Desmoplastic small cell tumor in the pancreas. Am J Surg Pathol. 2004;28:808-812.

473. Kushner BH, LaQuaglia MP, Wollner N, et al. Desmoplastic small round-cell tumor: prolonged progression-free survival with aggressive multimodality therapy. J Clin Oncol. 1996;14:1526-1531.

474. Mazuryk M, Paterson AH, Temple W, et al. Benefit of aggressive multimodality therapy with autologous stem cell support for intra-abdominal desmoplastic small round cell tumor. Bone Marrow Transplant. 1998;21:961-963.

475. Fraser CJ, Weigel BJ, Perentesis JP, et al. Autologous stem cell transplantation for high-risk Ewing's sarcoma and other pediatric solid tumors. Bone Marrow Transplant. 2006;37:175-181.

476. Anderson PM, Pearson M. Novel therapeutic approaches in pediatric and young adult sarcomas. Curr Oncol Rep. 2006;8:310-315.

477. Ferrari A, Grosso F, Stacchiotti S, et al. Response to vinorelbine and low-dose cyclophosphamide chemotherapy in two patients with desmoplastic small round cell tumor. Pediatr Blood Cancer. 2007;49:864-866.

478. Gil A, Gomez Portilla A, Brun EA, Sugarbaker PH. Clinical perspective on desmoplastic small round-cell tumor. Oncology. 2004;67:231-242.

479. Lal DR, Su WT, Wolden SL, et al. Results of multimodal treatment for desmoplastic small round cell tumors. J Pediatr Surg. 2005;40:251-255.

480. Gerald WL, Miller HK, Battifora H, et al. Intra-abdominal desmoplastic small round-cell tumor: report of 19 cases of a distinctive type of high-grade polyphenotypic malignancy affecting young individuals. Am J Surg Pathol. 1991;15:499-513.

481. Biegel JA, Conard K, Brooks JJ. Translocation (11;22)(p13;q12): primary change in intra-abdominal desmoplastic small round cell tumor. Genes Chromosomes Cancer. 1993;7:119-121.

482. Ladanyi M, Gerald W. Fusion of the *EWS* and *WT1* genes in the desmoplastic small round cell tumor. Cancer Res. 1994;54:2837-2840.

483. Rodriguez E, Sreekantaiah C, Gerald W, et al. A recurring translocation, t(11;22)(p13;q11.2), characterizes intra-abdominal desmoplastic small round cell tumors. Cancer Genet Cytogenet. 1993;69:17-21.

484. Gerald WL, Rosai J, Ladanyi M. Characterization of the genomic breakpoint and chimeric transcripts in the *EWS-WT1* gene fusion of desmoplastic small round cell tumor. Proc Natl Acad Sci U S A. 1995;92:1028-1032.

485. Liu J, Nau MM, Yeh JC, et al. Molecular heterogeneity and function of *EWS-WT1* fusion transcripts in desmoplastic small round cell tumors. Clin Cancer Res. 2000;6:3522-3529.

486. Call KM, Glaser T, Ito CY, et al. Isolation and characterization of a zinc finger polypeptide gene at the human chromosome 11 Wilms' tumor locus. Cell. 1990;60:509-520.

487. Haber DA, Buckler AJ, Glaser T, et al. An internal deletion within an 11p13 zinc finger gene contributes to the development of Wilms' tumor. Cell. 1990;61:1257-1269.

488. Christy BA, Lau LF, Nathans D. A gene activated in mouse 3T3 cells by serum growth factors encodes a protein with "zinc finger" sequences. Proc Natl Acad Sci U S A. 1988;85:7857-7861.

489. Sukhatme VP, Cao XM, Chang LC, et al. A zinc finger-encoding gene coregulated with c-fos during growth and differentiation, and after cellular depolarization. Cell. 1988;53:37-43.

490. Alaggio R, Rosolen A, Sartori F, et al. Spindle cell tumor with *EWS-WT1* transcript and a favorable clinical course: a variant of DSCT, a variant of leiomyosarcoma, or a new entity? Report of 2 pediatric cases. Am J Surg Pathol. 2007;31:454-459.

491. Lee SB, Kolquist KA, Nichols K, et al. The *EWS-WT1* translocation product induces *PDGFA* in desmoplastic small round-cell tumour. Nat Genet. 1997;17:309-313.

492. Ito E, Honma R, Imai J, et al. A tetraspanin-family protein, T-cell acute lymphoblastic leukemia-associated antigen 1, is induced by the Ewing's sarcoma-Wilms' tumor 1 fusion protein of desmoplastic small round-cell tumor. Am J Pathol. 2003;163:2165-2172.

493. Wong JC, Lee SB, Bell MD, et al. Induction of the interleukin-2/15 receptor beta-chain by the *EWS-WT1* translocation product. Oncogene. 2002;21:2009-2019.

494. Froberg K, Brown RE, Gaylord H, Manivel C. Intra-abdominal desmoplastic small round cell tumor: immunohistochemical evidence for up-regulation of autocrine and paracrine growth factors. Ann Clin Lab Sci. 1998;28:386-393.

495. Zhang PJ, Goldblum JR, Pawel BR, et al. *PDGF-A, PDGF-Rbeta, TGFbeta3* and bone morphogenic protein-4 in desmoplastic small round cell tumors with *EWS-WT1* gene fusion product and their

role in stromal desmoplasia: an immunohistochemical study. Mod Pathol. 2005;18:382-387.

496. Bond M, Bernstein ML, Pappo A, et al. A phase II study of imatinib mesylate in children with refractory or relapsed solid tumors: a Children's Oncology Group study. Pediatr Blood Cancer. 2008;50:254-258.

497. Fine RL, Shah SS, Moulton TA, et al. Androgen and c-Kit receptors in desmoplastic small round cell tumors resistant to chemotherapy: novel targets for therapy. Cancer Chemother Pharmacol. 2007;59:429-437.

498. Enzinger FM. Angiomatoid malignant fibrous histiocytoma: a distinct fibrohistiocytic tumor of children and young adults simulating a vascular neoplasm. Cancer. 1979;44:2147-2157.

499. Costa MJ, Weiss SW. Angiomatoid malignant fibrous histiocytoma: a follow-up study of 108 cases with evaluation of possible histologic predictors of outcome. Am J Surg Pathol. 1990;14:1126-1132.

500. Waters BL, Panagopoulos I, Allen EF. Genetic characterization of angiomatoid fibrous histiocytoma identifies fusion of the *FUS* and *ATF-1* genes induced by a chromosomal translocation involving bands 12q13 and 16p11. Cancer Genet Cytogenet. 2000;121:109-116.

501. Hallor KH, Mertens F, Jin Y, et al. Fusion of the *EWSR1* and *ATF1* genes without expression of the *MITF-M* transcript in angiomatoid fibrous histiocytoma. Genes Chromosomes Cancer. 2005;44:97-102.

502. Hsueh C, Kuo TT. Congenital malignant rhabdoid tumor presenting as a cutaneous nodule: report of 2 cases with review of the literature. Arch Pathol Lab Med. 1998;122:1099-1102.

503. Hosli I, Holzgreve W, Danzer E, Tercanli S. Two case reports of rare fetal tumors: an indication for surface rendering? Ultrasound Obstet Gynecol. 2001;17:522-526.

504. Costes V, Medioni D, Durand L, et al. Undifferentiated soft tissue tumor with rhabdoid phenotype (extra-renal rhabdoid tumor): report of a congenital case associated with medulloblastoma in a brother. Ann Pathol. 1997;17:41-43.

505. Fanburg-Smith JC, Hengge M, Hengge UR, et al. Extrarenal rhabdoid tumors of soft tissue: a clinicopathologic and immunohistochemical study of 18 cases. Ann Diagn Pathol. 1998;2:351-362.

506. Garcia-Bustinduy M, Alvarez-Arguelles H, Guimera F, et al. Malignant rhabdoid tumor beside benign skin mesenchymal neoplasm with myofibromatous features. J Cutan Pathol. 1999;26:509-515.

507. Perez-Atayde AR, Newbury R, Fletcher JA, et al. Congenital neurovascular hamartoma of the skin: a possible marker of malignant rhabdoid tumor. Am J Surg Pathol. 1994;18:1030-1038.

508. White FV, Dehner LP, Belchis DA, et al. Congenital disseminated malignant rhabdoid tumor: a distinct clinicopathologic entity demonstrating abnormalities of chromosome 22q11. Am J Surg Pathol. 1999;23:249-256.

509. Versteege I, Sevenet N, Lange J, et al. Truncating mutations of *hSNF5/INI1* in aggressive paediatric cancer. Nature. 1998;394:203-206.

510. Biegel JA, Zhou JY, Rorke LB, et al. Germline and acquired mutations of *INI1* in atypical teratoid and rhabdoid tumors. Cancer Res. 1999;59:74-79.

511. Vries RG, Bezrookove V, Zuijderduijn LM, et al. Cancer-associated mutations in chromatin remodeler *hSNF5* promote chromosomal instability by compromising the mitotic checkpoint. Genes Dev. 2005;19:665-670.

512. Chai J, Charboneau AL, Betz BL, Weissman BE. Loss of the *hSNF5* gene concomitantly inactivates *p21CIP/WAF1* and *p16INK4a* activity associated with replicative senescence in *A204* rhabdoid tumor cells. Cancer Res. 2005;65:10192-10198.

513. Schmidt D, Harms D. Epithelioid sarcoma in children and adolescents: an immunohistochemical study. Virchows Arch A Pathol Anat Histopathol. 1987;410:423-431.

514. Kodet R, Smelhaus V, Newton WA Jr, et al. Epithelioid sarcoma in childhood: an immunohistochemical, electron microscopic, and clinicopathologic study of 11 cases under 15 years of age and review of the literature. Pediatr Pathol. 1994;14:433-451.

515. Gross E, Rao BN, Pappo A, et al. Epithelioid sarcoma in children. J Pediatr Surg. 1996;31:1663-1665.

516. Billings SD, Hood AF. Epithelioid sarcoma arising on the nose of a child: a case report and review of the literature. J Cutan Pathol. 2000;27:186-190.

517. Mukai M, Torikata C, Iri H, et al. Cellular differentiation of epithelioid sarcoma: an electron-microscopic, enzyme-histochemical, and immunohistochemical study. Am J Pathol. 1985;119:44-56.

518. Prat J, Woodruff JM, Marcove RC. Epithelioid sarcoma: an analysis of 22 cases indicating the prognostic significance of vascular invasion and regional lymph node metastasis. Cancer. 1978;41:1472-1487.

519. Ross HM, Lewis JJ, Woodruff JM, Brennan MF. Epithelioid sarcoma: clinical behavior and prognostic factors of survival. Ann Surg Oncol. 1997;4:491-495.

520. Chase DR, Enzinger FM. Epithelioid sarcoma: diagnosis, prognostic indicators, and treatment. Am J Surg Pathol. 1985;9:241-263.

521. Casanova M, Ferrari A, Collini P, et al. Epithelioid sarcoma in children and adolescents: a report from the Italian Soft Tissue Sarcoma Committee. Cancer. 2006;106:708-717.

522. Evans HL, Baer SC. Epithelioid sarcoma: a clinicopathologic and prognostic study of 26 cases. Semin Diagn Pathol. 1993;10:286-291.

523. Guillou L, Wadden C, Coindre JM, et al. Proximal-type epithelioid sarcoma, a distinctive aggressive neoplasm showing rhabdoid features: clinicopathologic, immunohistochemical, and ultrastructural study of a series. Am J Surg Pathol. 1997;21:130-146.

524. Enzinger FM. Epitheloid sarcoma: a sarcoma simulating a granuloma or a carcinoma. Cancer. 1970;26:1029-1041.

525. Arber DA, Kandalaft PL, Mehta P, Battifora H. Vimentin-negative epithelioid sarcoma: the value of an immunohistochemical panel that includes *CD34*. Am J Surg Pathol. 1993;17:302-307.

526. Miettinen M, Fanburg-Smith JC, Virolainen M, et al. Epithelioid sarcoma: an immunohistochemical analysis of 112 classical and variant cases and a discussion of the differential diagnosis. Hum Pathol. 1999;30:934-942.

527. Ishida T, Oka T, Matsushita H, Machinami R. Epithelioid sarcoma: an electron-microscopic, immunohistochemical and DNA flow cytometric analysis. Virchows Arch A Pathol Anat Histopathol. 1992;421:401-408.

528. Sonobe H, Ohtsuki Y, Sugimoto T, Shimizu K. Involvement of 8q, 22q, and monosomy 21 in an epithelioid sarcoma. Cancer Genet Cytogenet. 1997;96:178-180.

529. Dal Cin P, Van den Berghe H, Pauwels P. Epithelioid sarcoma of the proximal type with complex karyotype including i(8q). Cancer Genet Cytogenet. 1999;114:80-82.

530. Debiec-Rychter M, Sciot R, Hagemeijer A. Common chromosome aberrations in the proximal type of epithelioid sarcoma. Cancer Genet Cytogenet. 2000;123:133-136.

531. Lee MW, Jee KJ, Han SS, et al. Comparative genomic hybridization in epithelioid sarcoma. Br J Dermatol. 2004;151:1054-1059.

532. Lualdi E, Modena P, Debiec-Rychter M, et al. Molecular cytogenetic characterization of proximal-type epithelioid sarcoma. Genes Chromosomes Cancer. 2004;41:283-290.

533. Cordoba JC, Parham DM, Meyer WH, Douglass EC. A new cytogenetic finding in an epithelioid sarcoma, t(8;22)(q22;q11). Cancer Genet Cytogenet. 1994;72:151-154.

534. Feely MG, Fidler ME, Nelson M, et al. Cytogenetic findings in a case of epithelioid sarcoma and a review of the literature. Cancer Genet Cytogenet. 2000;119:155-157.

535. Modena P, Lualdi E, Facchinetti F, et al. *SMARCB1/INI1* tumor suppressor gene is frequently inactivated in epithelioid sarcomas. Cancer Res. 2005;65:4012-4019.

536. Kusakabe H, Sakatani S, Yonebayashi K, Kiyokane K. Establishment and characterization of an epithelioid sarcoma cell line with an autocrine response to interleukin-6. Arch Dermatol Res. 1997;289:224-233.

537. Gusterson B, Cowley G, McIlhinney J, et al. Evidence for increased epidermal growth factor receptors in human sarcomas. Int J Cancer. 1985;36:689-693.

538. Gerharz CD, Ramp U, Reinecke P, et al. Analysis of growth factor-dependent signalling in human epithelioid sarcoma cell lines. Clues to the role of autocrine, juxtacrine and paracrine interactions in epithelioid sarcoma. Eur J Cancer. 2000;36:1171-1179.

539. Whitworth PW, Pollock RE, Mansfield PF, et al. Extremity epithelioid sarcoma: amputation vs local resection. Arch Surg. 1991;126:1485-1489.

540. Engers R, van Roy F, Heymer T, et al. Growth inhibition in clonal subpopulations of a human epithelioid sarcoma cell line by retinoic acid and tumour necrosis factor alpha. Br J Cancer. 1996;73:491-498.

541. Castex MP, Rubie H, Stevens MC, et al. Extraosseous localized Ewing tumors: improved outcome with anthracyclines—the French society of pediatric oncology and international society of pediatric oncology. J Clin Oncol. 2007;25:1176-1182.

542. Gururangan S, Marina NM, Luo X, et al. Treatment of children with peripheral primitive neuroectodermal tumor or extraosseous Ewing's tumor with Ewing's-directed therapy. J Pediatr Hematol Oncol. 1998;20:55-61.

543. Hamazoe R, Shimizu N, Nishidoi H, et al. Gastric leiomyoblastoma in childhood. J Pediatr Surg. 1991;26:225-227.

544. Miettinen M, Lasota J, Sobin LH. Gastrointestinal stromal tumors of the stomach in children and young adults: a clinicopathologic, immunohistochemical, and molecular genetic study of 44 cases with long-term follow-up and review of the literature. Am J Surg Pathol. 2005;29:1373-1381.

545. Wu SS, Buchmiller TL, Close P, et al. Congenital gastrointestinal pacemaker cell tumor. Arch Pathol Lab Med. 1999;123:842-845.

546. Shenoy MU, Singh SJ, Robson K, Stewart RJ. Gastrointestinal stromal tumor: a rare cause of neonatal intestinal obstruction. Med Pediatr Oncol. 2000;34:70-71.

547. DeMatteo RP, Lewis JJ, Leung D, et al. Two hundred gastrointestinal stromal tumors: recurrence patterns and prognostic factors for survival. Ann Surg. 2000;231:51-58.

548. Perez-Atayde AR, Shamberger RC, Kozakewich HW. Neuroectodermal differentiation of the gastrointestinal tumors in the Carney triad: an ultrastructural and immunohistochemical study. Am J Surg Pathol. 1993;17:706-714.

549. Kindblom LG, Remotti HE, Aldenborg F, Meis-Kindblom JM. Gastrointestinal pacemaker cell tumor *(GIPACT)*: gastrointestinal stromal tumors show phenotypic characteristics of the interstitial cells of Cajal. Am J Pathol. 1998;152:1259-1269.

550. Sarlomo-Rikala M, Kovatich AJ, Barusevicius A, Miettinen M. *CD117*: a sensitive marker for gastrointestinal stromal tumors that is more specific than *CD34*. Mod Pathol. 1998;11:728-734.

551. Smithey BE, Pappo AS, Hill DA. C-kit expression in pediatric solid tumors: a comparative immunohistochemical study. Am J Surg Pathol. 2002;26:486-492.

552. Assamaki R, Sarlomo-Rikala M, Lopez-Guerrero JA, et al. Array comparative genomic hybridization analysis of chromosomal imbalances and their target genes in gastrointestinal stromal tumors. Genes Chromosomes Cancer. 2007;46:564-576.

553. El-Rifai W, Sarlomo-Rikala M, Andersson LC, et al. DNA sequence copy number changes in gastrointestinal stromal tumors: tumor progression and prognostic significance. Cancer Res. 2000;60:3899-3903.

554. Janeway KA, Liegl B, Harlow A, et al. Pediatric *KIT* wild-type and platelet-derived growth factor receptor alpha-wild-type gastrointestinal stromal tumors share *KIT* activation but not mechanisms of genetic progression with adult gastrointestinal stromal tumors. Cancer Res. 2007;67:9084-9088.

555. Hirota S, Isozaki K, Moriyama Y, et al. Gain-of-function mutations of c-kit in human gastrointestinal stromal tumors. Science. 1998;279:577-580.

556. Lux ML, Rubin BP, Biase TL, et al. *KIT* extracellular and kinase domain mutations in gastrointestinal stromal tumors. Am J Pathol. 2000;156:791-795.

557. Duensing A, Heinrich MC, Fletcher CD, Fletcher JA. Biology of gastrointestinal stromal tumors: *KIT* mutations and beyond. Cancer Invest. 2004;22:106-116.

558. Heinrich MC, Corless CL, Duensing A, et al. *PDGFRA*-activating mutations in gastrointestinal stromal tumors. Science. 2003;299:708-710.

559. Agaimy A, Pelz AF, Corless CL, et al. Epithelioid gastric stromal tumours of the antrum in young females with the Carney triad: a report of three new cases with mutational analysis and comparative genomic hybridization. Oncol Rep. 2007;18:9-15.

560. Prakash S, Sarran L, Socci N, et al. Gastrointestinal stromal tumors in children and young adults: a clinicopathologic, molecular, and genomic study of 15 cases and review of the literature. J Pediatr Hematol Oncol. 2005;27:179-187.

561. Ng EH, Pollock RE, Munsell MF, et al. Prognostic factors influencing survival in gastrointestinal leiomyosarcomas: implications for surgical management and staging. Ann Surg. 1992;215:68-77.

562. Demetri GD, von Mehren M, Blanke CD, et al. Efficacy and safety of imatinib mesylate in advanced gastrointestinal stromal tumors. N Engl J Med. 2002;347:472-480.

563. Joensuu H, Roberts PJ, Sarlomo-Rikala M, et al. Effect of the tyrosine kinase inhibitor *STI571* in a patient with a metastatic gastrointestinal stromal tumor. N Engl J Med. 2001;344:1052-1056.

564. Prenen H, Cools J, Mentens N, et al. Efficacy of the kinase inhibitor *SU11248* against gastrointestinal stromal tumor mutants refractory to imatinib mesylate. Clin Cancer Res. 2006;12:2622-2627.

565. Demetri GD, van Oosterom AT, Garrett CR, et al. Efficacy and safety of sunitinib in patients with advanced gastrointestinal stromal tumour after failure of imatinib: a randomised controlled trial. Lancet. 2006;368:1329-1338.

566. Karcioglu Z, Someren A, Mathes SJ. Ectomesenchymoma. A malignant tumor of migratory neural crest (ectomesenchyme) remnants showing ganglionic, schwannian, melanocytic and rhabdomyoblastic differentiation. Cancer. 1977;39:2486-2496.

567. Kawamoto EH, Weidner N, Agostini RM Jr, Jaffe R. Malignant ectomesenchymoma of soft tissue: report of two cases and review of the literature. Cancer. 1987;59:1791-1802.

568. Oppenheimer O, Athanasian E, Meyers P, et al. Malignant ectomesenchymoma in the wrist of a child: case report and review of the literature. Int J Surg Pathol. 2005;13:113-116.

569. Meis JM, Enzinger FM, Martz KL, Neal JA. Malignant peripheral nerve sheath tumors (malignant schwannomas) in children. Am J Surg Pathol. 1992;16:694-707.

570. Carli M, Ferrari A, Mattke A, et al. Pediatric malignant peripheral nerve sheath tumor: the Italian and German soft tissue sarcoma cooperative group. J Clin Oncol. 2005;23:8422-8430.

571. Preston FW, Walsh WS, Clarke TH. Cutaneous neurofibromatosis (Von Recklinghausen's disease); clinical manifestation and incidence of sarcoma in sixty-one male patients. AMA Arch Surg. 1952;64:813-827.

572. Brasfield RD, Das Gupta TK. Von Recklinghausen's disease: a clinicopathological study. Ann Surg. 1972;175:86-104.

573. King AA, Debaun MR, Riccardi VM, Gutmann DH. Malignant peripheral nerve sheath tumors in neurofibromatosis 1. Am J Med Genet. 2000;93:388-392.

574. Evans DG, Baser ME, McGaughran J, et al. Malignant peripheral nerve sheath tumours in neurofibromatosis 1. J Med Genet. 2002;39:311-314.

575. deCou JM, Rao BN, Parham DM, et al. Malignant peripheral nerve sheath tumors: the St. Jude Children's Research Hospital experience. Ann Surg Oncol. 1995;2:524-529.

576. Ballester R, Marchuk D, Boguski M, et al. The NF-1 locus encodes a protein functionally related to mammalian GAP and yeast IRA proteins. Cell. 1990;63:851-859.

577. Buchberg AM, Cleveland LS, Jenkins NA, Copeland NG. Sequence homology shared by neurofibromatosis type-1 gene and IRA-1 and IRA-2 negative regulators of the RAS cyclic AMP pathway. Nature. 1990;347:291-294.

578. Martin GA, Viskochil D, Bollag G, et al. The GAP-related domain of the neurofibromatosis type 1 gene product interacts with ras *p21*. Cell. 1990;63:843-849.

579. Xu GF, Lin B, Tanaka K, et al. The catalytic domain of the neurofibromatosis type 1 gene product stimulates ras GTPase and complements ira mutants of *S. cerevisiae*. Cell. 1990;63:835-841.

580. Xu GF, O'Connell P, Viskochil D, et al. The neurofibromatosis type 1 gene encodes a protein related to GAP. Cell. 1990;62:599-608.

581. Perrone F, Tabano S, Colombo F, et al. *p15INK4b, p14ARF,* and *p16INK4a* inactivation in sporadic and neurofibromatosis type 1-related malignant peripheral nerve sheath tumors. Clin Cancer Res. 2003;9:4132-4138.

582. Gonzalez-Gomez P, Bello MJ, Arjona D, et al. Aberrant CpG island methylation in neurofibromas and neurofibrosarcomas. Oncol Rep. 2003;10:1519-1523.

583. Vogel KS, Klesse LJ, Velasco-Miguel S, et al. Mouse tumor model for neurofibromatosis type 1. Science. 1999;286:2176-2179.

584. Cichowski K, Shih TS, Schmitt E, et al. Mouse models of tumor development in neurofibromatosis type 1. Science. 1999;286:2172-2176.

585. Perry A, Kunz SN, Fuller CE, et al. Differential NF-1, p16, and EGFR patterns by interphase cytogenetics (FISH) in malignant peripheral nerve sheath tumor (MPNST) and morphologically similar spindle cell neoplasms. J Neuropathol Exp Neurol. 2002;61:702-709.

586. DeClue JE, Heffelfinger S, Benvenuto G, et al. Epidermal growth factor receptor expression in neurofibromatosis type 1-related tumors and NF-1 animal models. J Clin Invest. 2000;105:1233-1241.

587. Ling BC, Wu J, Miller SJ, et al. Role for the epidermal growth factor receptor in neurofibromatosis-related peripheral nerve tumorigenesis. Cancer Cell. 2005;7:65-75.

588. Pettinato G, Manivel JC, d'Amore ES, et al. Melanotic neuroectodermal tumor of infancy: a reexamination of a histogenetic problem based on immunohistochemical, flow cytometric, and ultrastructural study of 10 cases. Am J Surg Pathol. 1991;15:233-245.

589. Mello RJ, Vidal AK, Fittipaldi HM Jr, et al. Melanotic neuroectodermal tumor of infancy: clinicopathologic study of a case, with emphasis on the chemotherapeutic effects. Int J Surg Pathol. 2000;8:247-251.

590. Fletcher CD, Gustafson P, Rydholm A, et al. Clinicopathologic re-evaluation of 100 malignant fibrous histiocytomas: prognostic relevance of subclassification. J Clin Oncol. 2001;19:3045-3050.

591. Nakayama R, Nemoto T, Takahashi H, et al. Gene expression analysis of soft tissue sarcomas: characterization and reclassification of malignant fibrous histiocytoma. Mod Pathol. 2007;20:749-759.

592. Coindre JM, Mariani O, Chibon F, et al. Most malignant fibrous histiocytomas developed in the retroperitoneum are dedifferentiated liposarcomas: a review of 25 cases initially diagnosed as malignant fibrous histiocytoma. Mod Pathol. 2003;16:256-262.

593. Fletcher CD. Pleomorphic malignant fibrous histiocytoma: fact or fiction? A critical reappraisal based on 159 tumors diagnosed as pleomorphic sarcoma. Am J Surg Pathol. 1992;16:213-228.

594. Weiss SW, Enzinger FM. Malignant fibrous histiocytoma: an analysis of 200 cases. Cancer. 1978;41:2250-2266.

595. Somers GR, Gupta AA, Doria AS, et al. Pediatric undifferentiated sarcoma of the soft tissues: a clinicopathologic study. Pediatr Dev Pathol. 2006;9:132-142.

596. Baird K, Davis S, Antonescu CR, et al. Gene expression profiling of human sarcomas: insights into sarcoma biology. Cancer Res. 2005;65:9226-9235.

597. Nielsen TO, West RB, Linn SC, et al. Molecular characterisation of soft tissue tumours: a gene expression study. Lancet. 2002;359:1301-1307.

598. Chibon F, Mariani O, Derre J, et al. A subgroup of malignant fibrous histiocytomas is associated with genetic changes similar to those of well-differentiated liposarcomas. Cancer Genet Cytogenet. 2002;139:24-29.

599. Matushansky I, Hernando E, Socci ND, et al. Derivation of sarcomas from mesenchymal stem cells via inactivation of the Wnt pathway. J Clin Invest. 2007;117:3248-3257.

600. Mariani O, Brennetot C, Coindre JM, et al. *JUN* oncogene amplification and overexpression block adipocytic differentiation in highly aggressive sarcomas. Cancer Cell. 2007;11:361-374.

601. Kramarova E, Stiller CA. The international classification of childhood cancer. Int J Cancer. 1996;68:759-765.

Ewing's Sarcoma

21

Steven G. DuBois, Holcombe E. Grier, and Stephen L. Lessnick

In 1921, James Ewing described the cancer that came to carry his name—a primary bone tumor comprised of small round blue cells and devoid of the malignant osteoid that characterizes osteosarcoma.[1] Subsequently, pathologists described other clinicopathologic entities each initially thought to be distinct, such as peripheral primitive neuroectodermal tumor (PNET) of bone or soft tissue or the Askin tumor of the chest wall.[2] However, biologic studies and clinical responses to chemotherapy have now linked these tumors into one entity or family of tumors, a grouping that also includes extraosseous Ewing's sarcoma. Commonly used terms for this tumor include *Ewing's sarcoma*, *Ewing tumors*, and *Ewing's sarcoma family of tumors*. Throughout the chapter, we will generally use the World Health Organization–approved term, *Ewing's sarcoma*. When appropriate, we will highlight specific characteristics that differentiate Ewing's sarcoma, PNET, and Askin tumors.

We begin this chapter with a discussion of the epidemiology of Ewing's sarcoma. We then discuss the current understanding of the cellular and molecular features of these tumors and present an overview of the clinical presentation and prognostic features of patients with this disease. This overview is followed by a discussion of the management of patients with Ewing's sarcoma. We conclude with a review of the late effects seen in patients treated for these tumors.

EPIDEMIOLOGY

Ewing's sarcoma is the second most common type of primary bone cancer in the United States and Europe, accounting for approximately 25% to 34% of malignant bone tumors.[3-5] Approximately 250 new cases of Ewing's sarcoma are diagnosed in the United States each year. In the United States, Ewing's sarcoma has had a relatively stable average incidence of 2.5 to 3 cases/million/year from 1975 to 2000.[4,6] A similar age-adjusted incidence has been noted in Europe. As shown in Figure 21-1, the peak incidence occurs during adolescence with an average incidence of 4.6 cases/million/year for the 15- to 19-year age range. Younger children are affected less frequently and the disease is distinctly uncommon in adults older than 35 years. A male predominance has been noted, with a male-to-

female ratio of approximately 1.25:1.[5,7] However, one study has reported a female predominance in patients younger than 3 years at initial diagnosis.[8] There is no seasonal variation in the appearance of this disease.[7,9]

The incidence of Ewing's sarcoma varies markedly among races and countries, with the highest frequency reported from Australia and Sao Paolo, Brazil.[10] People of African ancestry appear to have the lowest incidence of this disease. Figure 21-2 demonstrates the dramatically lower incidence of these tumors in U.S. blacks.[5] Diagnosis beyond 25 years of age is exceedingly uncommon in blacks.[4,11] A similar low incidence in sub-Saharan Africa has been reported and suggests a possible genetic difference in the risk of developing Ewing's sarcoma.[10,12] Ewing's sarcoma also appears to be uncommon in people of East Asian ancestry, based on data from China, Japan, and Thailand.[10,13,14] Data from the Middle East, North Africa, and the Indian subcontinent suggest that Ewing's sarcoma is at least as common in these populations as in people of European ancestry. In small studies from Kuwait and Bombay, for example, Ewing's sarcoma was identified as the most common primary malignant bone tumor.[10,15-17]

The cause of Ewing's sarcoma remains largely obscure. These tumors are not generally believed to be familial, although rare cases of sibling pairs with Ewing's sarcoma have been reported.[18-20] First- and second-degree relatives of patients with Ewing's sarcoma do not appear to have an increased overall risk of cancer, although an excess of stomach cancer, melanoma, and brain tumors has been reported.[21,22]

Patients with Ewing's sarcoma appear to have an increased incidence of specific congenital anomalies. The most consistent finding has been an association between Ewing's sarcoma and congenital hernias, particularly inguinal hernias.[23-25] A pooled analysis of the available literature has confirmed this association, with an odds ratio of developing Ewing's sarcoma of 2.8 for children with congenital hernias compared with children without congenital hernias.[26] Whether a common hormonal or environmental mechanism underlies the development of both congenital hernias and Ewing's sarcoma remains unclear. Patients with Ewing's sarcoma have also been noted to have an increased incidence of bone anomalies, particularly rib and vertebral anomalies; other congenital anomalies, including cataracts and genitourinary anomalies, have been reported in

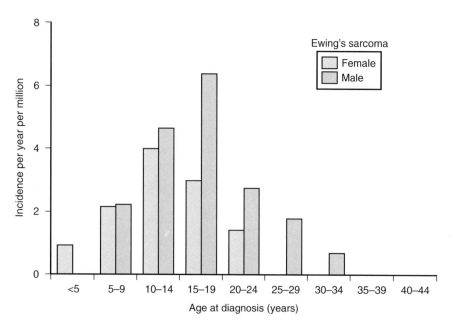

FIGURE 21-1. Incidence of Ewing's sarcoma for males and females according to age at initial diagnosis (SEER data, 1975-1999). *(Adapted from Mascarenhas L, Siegel S, Spector L, et al: Malignant bone tumors. In Bleyer A, O'Leary M, Barr R, et al (eds). Cancer Epidemiology in Older Adolescents and Young Adults 15 to 29 Years of Age, Including SEER Incidence and Survival 1975-2000. Bethesda, Md, National Cancer Institute, 2006, pp 98-109.)*

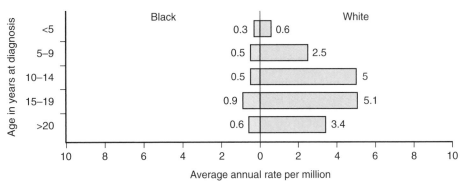

FIGURE 21-2. Incidence of Ewing's sarcoma by age according to race, demonstrating the marked rarity of the disease in U.S. blacks (SEER data, 1975-1995). *(Adapted from Gurney JG, Swensen AR, Bulterys M: Malignant bone tumors. In Ries L, Smith M, Gurney JG, et al (eds). Cancer Incidence and Survival among Children and Adolescents: United States SEER Program 1975-1995. Bethesda, Md, National Cancer Institute, 1999, pp 99-110.)*

patients with Ewing's sarcoma.[25,27-29] These anomalies occur at a low incidence in these patients and without a consistent pattern, suggesting that their occurrence together with Ewing's sarcoma may be coincidental.

Various parental exposures have been associated with the risk of developing Ewing's sarcoma. The most consistent finding has been an association between parental farm exposure around the time of conception through birth and the subsequent development of Ewing's sarcoma. This association has been reported in a series of case-control studies and affirmed in a meta-analysis, with an increased risk if either parent was involved in farming.[23,30-33] Specific exposures related to agricultural work that have been suggested as driving this increased risk include parental fertilizer, pesticide, solvent, and wood dust exposure.[31,32,34] Less consistently reported associations have included an increased risk of Ewing's sarcoma with parental cigarette smoking and parental occupation in manual labor. Family income does not appear to be associated with the risk of Ewing's sarcoma.

Additional attention has focused on features of physical growth and development that might distinguish patients with Ewing's sarcoma. Differences in birth weight between patients with Ewing's sarcoma and controls have not been observed.[35] Given its peak incidence during adolescence, some groups have investigated differences in the onset of puberty between patients with Ewing's sarcoma and controls. One group has reported that boys with Ewing's sarcoma began shaving earlier than boys without Ewing's sarcoma.[24] Other differences related to the development of secondary sex characteristics have not been observed. At the time of diagnosis, patients with Ewing's sarcoma do not seem to be taller than their peers.[35-37]

Several viruses have been suggested as playing a role in the pathogenesis of Ewing's sarcoma. One group has reported that the adenovirus *E1A* gene could specifically induce the chromosomal translocation characteristic of these tumors.[38] Follow-up studies have failed to corroborate this finding.[39-42] Based on increased Epstein-Barr virus (EBV) titers in patients with Ewing's sarcoma, other groups have evaluated Ewing's tumors for EBV infection and found no viral involvement.[43,44] Both BK and SV40 viral sequences have been variably identified in cases of Ewing's sarcoma, but the functional importance of these findings remains unknown.[45-47] The lack of a seasonal variation in the incidence of Ewing's sarcoma may also argue against a viral cause.

Ewing's sarcoma rarely develops as a second malignancy. Several case reports have described the development of Ewing's sarcoma years after the successful treatment of children with a range of hematologic malignancies and solid cancers.[48-53] More formal studies have indicated that Ewing's sarcoma as a second malignancy occurs only infrequently. In a large institutional

review, only 1.3% of second malignancies following treatment of pediatric cancer were Ewing's sarcoma or PNET.[54] Several large series of patients with secondary bone sarcomas have reported only a small number of patients with Ewing's sarcoma.[55-57] These secondary Ewing tumors do not appear to be radiation-related. In addition, the wide range of primary malignancies described in these patients suggests that these tumors do not arise as part of a specific cancer predisposition syndrome.

BIOLOGIC FEATURES

Chromosomal Rearrangements in Ewing's Sarcoma

In the mid-1980s, the presence of a recurrent reciprocal chromosomal translocation, t(11;22)(q24;q12), was reported in Ewing's sarcoma tumors and cell lines.[58,59] In addition to being found in Ewing's sarcoma of bone, the same translocation was also identified in PNET, supporting the hypothesis that these two tumors represent the same disease, which exhibits varying levels of differentiation along a neuronal pathway.[60] Subsequent studies have demonstrated that t(11;22)(q24;q12) is present in approximately 83% of Ewing's sarcomas.[61] A small percentage of tumors has demonstrated complex translocations involving chromosomes 11, 22, and a third chromosome. These cases probably represent additional examples of t(11;22)(q24;q12) existing in a complex background. Interestingly, 22q12 was rearranged in 92% of Ewing's sarcoma cases, whereas 11q24 was abnormal in only 88% of cases. This disparity would eventually be explained by the presence of an additional set of recurrent translocations involving chromosome 22 and other partner chromosomes (see later).

The early analysis of translocations in Ewing's sarcoma has demonstrated that the derivative chromosome 22 is always maintained as these tumors and cell lines undergo clonal evolution, whereas the derivative chromosome 11 could be lost.[59] This has demonstrated that the 22;11 derivative is the key chromosomal abnormality, and that the reciprocal 11;22 is unnecessary. Additionally, these are tumor-specific mutations, not constitutional, because they were not found in lymphoblasts or fibroblasts from analyzed patients.

In addition to the t(11;22)(q24;q12) rearrangement (and related translocations with similar molecular consequences; see later), other chromosomal abnormalities have also been reported in Ewing's sarcoma.[59,62-68] A careful analysis of these sometimes complex karyotypes has revealed a small group of recurrent, nonrandom chromosomal abnormalities. Gains (usually trisomies) of chromosome 8 may be observed in up to 50% of cases, and gains of chromosomes 12 and 1q are seen in approximately 25% of cases.[62,66,67,69,70] Gains in chromosome 20 have also been reported in 10% to 20% of cases.[71] Interestingly, a chromosomal translocation that is unrelated to the (11;22)(q24;q12) has been observed in approximately 20% of cases— der(16)t(1;16). This translocation is often found as an unbalanced rearrangement, and thus results in partial gains (trisomies and occasionally tetrasomies) of 1q and losses (monosomies) of 16q. The breakpoints of this translocation appear to be variable, and range from q11 through q32 on chromosome 1, and q11.1 through q24 on chromosome 16. This suggests that the translocation does not alter particular target genes at the breakpoint, but rather introduces gains of 1q and losses of 16q. Finally, losses at 1p36 have also been observed.[68] There has also been a report of genomic instability, as measured by microsatellite instability and loss of heterozygosity, in Ewing's sarcoma.[72] This finding, however, is somewhat controversial, because a second group was unable to replicate the microsatellite instability findings.[73]

Cloning of EWS/FLI

A major advance in the understanding of the pathogenesis of Ewing's sarcoma occurred when the breakpoint of the (11;22)(q24;q12) translocation was cloned in 1992.[74] The translocation breakpoint was localized roughly in the middle of two genes, *EWSR1* and *FLI1*. *EWSR1* had not been previously identified, and so was named on the basis of its involvement in the Ewing's sarcoma translocation breakpoint (*Ew*ing's *s*arcoma *r*earrangement domain *1*).[74,75] *FLI1* had previously identified in mice as the *F*riend *l*eukemia virus *i*ntegration site.[76] As a result of the translocation event, these two genes become fused and the expressed transcript encodes for the EWS/FLI fusion protein (Fig. 21-3).[74] It should be noted that the gene symbols used in this chapter are those designated by the Human Genome Organization (HUGO) Gene Nomenclature Committee, and are presented in italicized capital letters

(e.g., *EWSR1*). The symbols used for proteins and RNA transcripts in this chapter are those most commonly found in the literature, and are presented in nonitalicized capital letters (e.g., EWS).

Wild-type EWS Protein

EWSR1 encodes the EWS protein (see Fig. 21-3).[74] Wild-type EWS contains 656 amino acids, and appears to be ubiquitously expressed.[74,77,78] EWS is primarily localized to the nucleus,[79-81] although it has also been detected in the cytoplasm[82] and on the cell surface.[83] The amino terminus of EWS, sometimes referred to as NTD-EWS, contains 285 amino acids consisting of 31 pseudorepeats rich in tyrosine, glutamine, serine, threonine, glycine, alanine, and proline. This region bears some similarity to the carboxyl terminal domain (CTD) of RNA polymerase II. This similarity has suggested that the region could modulate RNA transcription. The carboxy terminus of EWS contains an RNA recognition motif (an RRM domain), as well as three arginine-glycine-glycine (RGG) domains often found in RNA binding proteins. It has been demonstrated in vitro that EWS can bind to RNA.[78,84] These findings suggest that wild-type EWS may be involved in RNA transcription or processing. The carboxy terminal region also contains a potential C_2C_2 zinc finger of uncertain significance.[85] There is evidence that EWS may undergo post-translational modifications, but the significance of these alterations is not well understood.[83,84,86,87]

EWS is highly related to two additional sarcoma-associated translocation partners, TLS (*t*ranslocated in *l*iposarcoma; also called FUS) and TAF15 (also known at TAF$_{II}$68, TAF2N, and RBP56), as well as to a *Drosophila melanogaster* protein named cabeza (also known as SARFH; originally called P19).[85,88-91] TLS was first identified in human myxoid liposarcoma in the context of the t(12;16)(q13;p11) translocation (Table 21-1). In this setting, the amino terminus of TLS is fused, in frame, to the carboxy terminus of the CHOP protein. TLS/CHOP appears to be the critical oncoprotein in myxoid liposarcoma. TLS and EWS have a high level of homology in their extreme

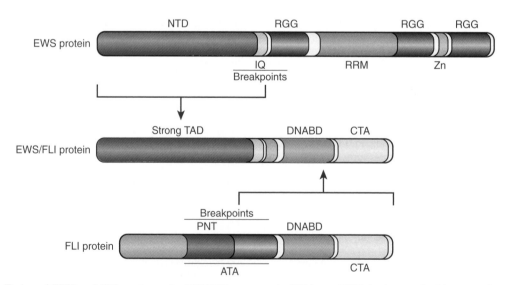

FIGURE 21-3. Fusion of EWS and FLI produces the EWS/FLI oncoprotein. Wild-type EWS is characterized by an amino-terminal domain (NTD), an IQ domain, three RGG regions, an RNA recognition motif (RRM), and a putative C2-C2 zinc finger domain (Zn). Wild-type FLI contains a pointed domain (PNT), amino- and carboxyl-terminal transcription activation domains (ATA and CTA, respectively), and an ETS DNA-binding domain (DNABD). The translocation breakpoint regions of each protein are shown. Following a translocation event, EWS/FLI is formed. EWS/FLI maintains the NTD of EWS, which functions as a strong transcriptional activation domain [TAD] in this context, and the DNA-binding and carboxyl-terminal activation domain of FLI.

TABLE 21-1 **Translocations Involving TET Family Members in Cancer***

Tumor Type	Translocation	Fusion Gene	Reference
Ewing's sarcoma	t(11;22)(q24;q12)	EWSR1/FLI1	74
	t(21;22)(q22;q12)	EWSR1/ERG	139
	t(7;22)(p22;q12)	EWSR1/ETV1	142
	t(17;22)(q12;q12)	EWSR1/ETV4	143
	t(2;22)(q35;q12)	EWSR1/FEV	144
	t(16;21)(p11;q22)	FUS/ERG	148
	t(2;16)(q35;p11)	FUS/FEV	147
Clear cell sarcoma	t(12;22)(q13;q12)	EWSR1/ATF1	378
Desmoplastic small round cell tumor	t(11;22)(p13;q12)	EWSR1/WT1	379
Extraskeletal myxoid chondrosarcoma	t(9;22)(q22;q12)	EWSR1/NR4A3	383
	t(9;17)(q22;q11)	TAF15/NR4A3	381
	t(9;15)(q22;q21)	TCF12/NR4A3	539
Myxoid liposarcoma	t(12;16)(q13;p11)	FUS/DDIT3	89
	t(12;22)(q13;q12)	EWSR1/DDIT3	384
Small round cell sarcoma	t(1;22)(p36.1;q12)	EWSR1/ZNF278	385
Undifferentiated bone sarcoma	t(6;22)(p21;q12)	EWSR1/POU5F1	540
Angiomatoid fibrous histiocytoma	t(12;16)(q13;p11)	FUS/ATF1	541
Low-grade fibromyxoid sarcoma	t(7;16)(q33;p11)	FUS/CREB3L2	542
Acute myelogenous leukemia	t(16;21)(p11;q22)	FUS/ERG	543
Acute myelogenous, lymphoblastic, or undifferentiated leukemia	t(12;22)(p13;q12)	EWSR1/ZNF384	93
	t(12;17)(p13;q11)	TAF15/ZNF384	93

*The genes are identified by their approved HUGO gene nomenclature, rather than by their corresponding protein names.

amino termini, as well as a significant homology in their carboxy termini. TAF15 is a member of the TFIID general transcription complex.[88] It is found fused to NR4A3, also called CHN, TEC, CSMF, or NOR1, in extraskeletal myxoid chondrosarcomas and to ZNF384, also called CIZ or NMP4, in acute leukemias (see Table 21-1).[92-94] TAF15 also has significant homology and domain organization to EWS and TLS. The three human proteins are sometimes described as the TET family of proteins (*T*LS, *E*WS, *T*AF15). Although the normal function of these proteins is not completely understood, there is evidence that they may be involved in RNA splicing and/or gene expression.[79,88,95-106]

Wild-type FLI Protein

FLI is a member of the ETS family of transcription factors.[107] This family is defined by the presence of an ETS type DNA-binding domain and consists of 27 different members in humans.[108] As with most transcription factors, ETS family members generally have a modular architecture with separate domains that contribute DNA binding and transcriptional functions.[109] The DNA-binding ETS domain of FLI is present in the carboxy-terminal portion of the protein (see Fig. 21-3).[107] Most ETS family members (including FLI) bind to sequences containing a GGAA or GGAT core sequence.[108,109] In addition to DNA binding function, FLI contains two separate transcriptional activation domains, one in the amino terminus and a second in the carboxy terminus (distal to the ETS DNA-binding domain; see Fig. 21-3).[110] Wild-type FLI also contains a PNT (pointed) domain in the amino-terminal portion of the protein.[111] In general, PNT domains are thought to mediate protein-protein interactions.[112]

The normal role of FLI appears to be primarily in the hematopoietic lineage. For example, FLI has been shown to regulate the expression of genes involved in megakaryocytic development, such as glycoproteins GPIX, GP1ba, and GPIIb[113] and the thrombopoietin receptor.[114] FLI is expressed in megakaryocytes and its forced expression in erythroleukemia cells results in megakaryocytic differentiation.[113,115] Knockout

of murine Fli-1 results in abnormal megakaryocytic differentiation and a loss in vascular integrity that results in embryonic lethality from central nervous system hemorrhage.[116,117] A role for FLI in human megakaryocytic development was shown by its hemizygous deletion in patients with Paris-Trousseau or Jacobson thrombocytopenia syndromes.[116,118,119] In addition to a role in megakaryocyte development, FLI appears to be important for vascular development in the mouse and zebrafish.[116,120] Finally, FLI may play a role in neural crest development. FLI is expressed in neural crest-derived mesenchyme in both the mouse and quail.[121,122] This finding is particularly interesting in light of the neural crest phenotype of Ewing's sarcoma.

FLI itself can function as an oncogene, at least in the hematopoietic context. Indeed, the murine *Fli* locus was first defined as a predominant *F*riend murine *l*eukemia virus (F-MuLV) *i*nsertion site. Thus, insertion of F-MuLV at the *Fli* locus results in upregulation of the *Fli* gene, and subsequent development of erythroleukemia.[76,107] The oncogenic activity of FLI appears to be limited to the hematopoietic system, although introduction of the protein into other models of oncogenesis, such as the NIH3T3 cell model, does not result in the transformed phenotype.[79]

EWS/FLI and Other TET/ETS Fusions in Ewing's Sarcoma

EWS/FLI consists of the amino terminus of EWS fused, in frame, to the carboxy terminus of FLI (see Fig. 21-3).[74] The EWS portion retained in the fusion contains the pseudorepeat domain that harbors a strong transcriptional activation function.[74,79,106] The RNA binding domain of EWS is lost in the fusion protein, and instead is replaced by the portion of FLI that contains its ETS DNA-binding domain.[74]

EWS/FLI functions as an oncoprotein. EWS/FLI can induce NIH3T3 cells (an immortalized mouse fibroblast cell line) to exhibit both anchorage-independent growth and growth as tumors when injected subcutaneously into immunodeficient mice.[123-125] Conversely, blockade of EWS/FLI expression or function (via antisense RNA, dominant-negative, blocking alleles, or RNA interference) causes Ewing's sarcoma cells to lose their transformed phenotype.[126-134] These data demonstrate that EWS/FLI expression is required for the oncogenic phenotype of Ewing's sarcoma. It has been reported that following therapy-induced neural differentiation of Ewing's sarcoma, EWS/FLI expression may also be lost.[135] Although these data support an important role for EWS/FLI expression in Ewing's sarcoma proliferation and/or transformation, they do not address whether EWS/FLI formation is the first step in Ewing's sarcoma development, or whether other oncogenic events occur first and are followed by EWS/FLI formation.

There are three main consequences of the t(11;22) (q24;q12) rearrangement. First, it places the transcriptional regulation of the EWS/FLI fusion under the control of the *EWSR1* promoter. This is important because the activity of the *FLI1* promoter is limited to hematopoietic (and perhaps neural crest) lineages, whereas the *EWSR1* promoter appears to be active in most, if not all, cell types (see previous sections). Second, the translocation results in a loss of one wild-type *EWSR1* allele and one wild-type *FLI1* allele. Loss of one *FLI1* allele is probably of no consequence, because wild-type *FLI1* is not expressed in Ewing's sarcoma.[134] Whether loss of one *EWSR1* allele is important in Ewing's sarcoma development is not known. The third consequence of the translocation is that it creates the EWS/FLI fusion protein. This is important because although EWS/FLI functions as an oncoprotein, neither wild-type EWS nor wild-type FLI could induce transformation of NIH3T3 cells, thus demonstrating a gain of function for the EWS/FLI fusion.[79] Initial structure-function analyses of EWS/FLI have demonstrated that both the amino-terminal EWS domain and the ETS DNA-binding domain of FLI are required for oncogenic transformation of NIH3T3 cells.[123] This result suggests that the fusion protein may be functioning as an aberrant transcription factor. Comparisons of EWS/FLI with wild-type FLI have demonstrated that the EWS domain included in the fusion protein could function as a much stronger transcriptional activation domain than the domain of FLI that was lost in the fusion.[79] These results suggest that EWS/FLI induced oncogenic transformation via binding to target genes through its ETS DNA-binding domain, and upregulating the expression of those genes through its EWS domain. Replacement of EWS sequences in EWS/FLI with other strong transcriptional activation domains resulted in a transforming oncoprotein, whereas replacement with weak activation domains did not.[106] Thus, transcriptional activation and DNA binding appear to be critical to the function of EWS/FLI.

The mechanisms whereby the EWS portion of the fusion functions as a transcriptional activation domain are only now beginning to be understood. Because wild-type EWS has been shown to interact with TFIID, RNA polymerase II, and/or the p300/CBP coactivators, it appears likely that these interactions are also important for EWS/FLI function.[96,98,103,104] This has been demonstrated in a limited number of studies.[136,137] RNA helicase A (RHA) has also been shown to be important for the transcriptional activity of EWS/FLI.[138] Thus, RHA may also function as a coactivator for gene expression mediated by the fusion protein.

The hypothesis that EWS/FLI functions as a transcriptional activator gained support when additional Ewing's sarcoma translocation breakpoints were cloned (see Table 21-1). As described, approximately 83% of Ewing's sarcoma tumors contain an (11;22)(q24;q12) translocation.[59-61] Approximately 10% of cases demonstrate an alternate translocation, t(21;22)(q22;q12).[139] Cloning of the breakpoint of this rearrangement has revealed that EWS is fused, in frame, to another

member of the ETS family, ERG. As in the case of EWS/FLI, the EWS/ERG fusion contains the amino terminus of EWS fused to the carboxy terminus of ERG, which harbors its ETS DNA-binding domain. Interestingly, the ETS DNA binding domains of FLI and ERG are 98% identical at the amino acid level.[139,140] Subsequent investigations have demonstrated that EWS/ERG also functions as an oncoprotein in the NIH3T3 cell model.[125,141] In subsequent years, additional translocations were identified in Ewing's sarcoma, including a t(7;22)(p22;q12), t(17;22)(q12;q12), and t(2;22)(q33;q12).[142-145] Cloning of transcripts from these translocations has demonstrated that in each case EWS is fused to another member of the ETS family. Currently, five EWS/ETS fusions have been described (see Table 21-1).[74,139,142-145]

It is assumed that all EWS/ETS fusion proteins bind similar (if not identical) target genes to induce oncogenic transformation. This has recently been experimentally evaluated, again using the NIH3T3 cell model.[146] A core group of target genes was shown to be dysregulated by all five of the EWS/ETS fusions. Although these results support the concept that all EWS/ETS proteins function similarly, they must be interpreted with caution, because they are based completely on the NIH3T3 model system. As discussed later, the NIH3T3 model may not be an accurate model for gene expression studies of EWS/ETS fusions.[134,146]

Overall, most cases of Ewing's sarcoma appear to harbor fusions between EWS and various ETS family members. On rare occasion, fusions between TLS and ETS family members may be present in Ewing's sarcoma instead, as shown by the identification of TLS/ERG fusions in four patients with Ewing's sarcoma, and the identification of a TLS/FEV fusion in another case (see Table 21-1).[147,148] These findings highlight the similarities across the TET family, and across the ETS family. Perhaps the most generic manner of describing the fusion proteins in Ewing's sarcoma would be as "TET/ETS" fusions. Because EWS/FLI is the most common fusion identified in Ewing's sarcoma, most experimental work has been performed using this fusion protein. Experimental findings based on EWS/FLI have only occasionally been confirmed using other Ewing's sarcoma fusion proteins.

In addition to the variability of fusion partners, there is also variability in the exonic structure of some of the fusion proteins (Fig. 21-4). The breakpoints found in Ewing's sarcoma translocations occur in the introns of *EWSR1* and *FLI1* (and presumably the other ETS factors as well, although in most cases this has not been experimentally confirmed).[74,75,149,150] The breakpoints in the *EWSR1* gene are found in one of two regions (3 and 1.2 kilobase [kb] in size) present in an approximately 6-kb region that includes 4 of the gene's 16 introns. The breakpoints in *FLI1* occur over an approximately 50-kb region, which includes 6 of 8 *FLI* introns. Splicing events join adjacent exons together in the fusion transcript. As a result of this variability in breakpoint and subsequent RNA splicing, at least 10 different EWS/FLI isoforms are generated (see Fig. 21-4).[74,75,123,149-151]

The most common Ewing's sarcoma translocation breakpoint pair fuses exon 7 of *EWSR1* to exon 6 of *FLI1*.[74,150] This 7/6 fusion is commonly referred to as a type 1 EWS/FLI fusion, and accounts for approximately 50% to 60% of EWS/FLI fusions.[150,152] A type 2 fusion joins exon 7 of *EWSR1* to exon 5 of *FLI1*, and is the second most common EWS/FLI fusion, accounting for approximately 20% to 30% of EWS/FLI fusions. Laboratory studies suggested that the type 1 EWS/FLI fusion was a weaker oncoprotein than the type 2 fusion, and this may have prognostic significance (see later).[153] In a limited evaluation, however, these functional differences were not reflected on changes in gene expression between types 1 and 2 fusions.[154]

GENOMIC STRUCTURES:

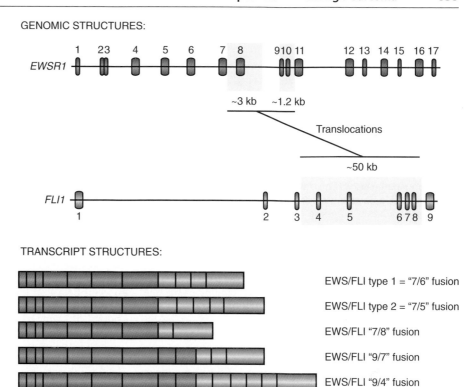

FIGURE 21-4. Translocation breakpoints may occur within one of two portions of a 6-kb region of the *EWSR1* gene and in a 50-kb region of the *FLI1* gene. This variety results in the observed heterogeneity of EWS/FLI fusion transcripts.

Although there is general agreement about the designation of types 1 and 2 fusions, there is no generalized nomenclature for the remaining fusions, and so these are best described in terms of which exons are fused to one another. In addition to variability in the EWS/FLI breakpoint, EWS/ERG has also been reported to demonstrate variability based on fusion points, with at least four fusions reported.[139,150] Because the other fusions are so rare, there is only minimal information as to whether they also show similar levels of breakpoint heterogeneity.

Ewing's Sarcoma Cell of Origin

The cell of origin of Ewing's sarcoma is unknown and has been an area of intense debate.[155] The original description by James Ewing in 1921 suggested that this round cell sarcoma was of endothelial origin, and hence properly referred to as a diffuse endothelioma of bone.[1] Dr. Ewing later suggested that it may arise from perivascular lymphatic endothelium.[156] A hematologic origin was proposed in the early 1970s following an in-depth evaluation of light and electron microscopic characteristics and cytochemistry of primary tumor and cell culture specimens.[157] In the early-1980s, a fibroblastic-mesenchymal derivation was proposed based on, among other things, the patterns of collagen expression of the tumor.[158,159] In the late 1980s, however, a neural crest derivation was proposed because of the occasional identification of certain neural features, such as the presence of Homer-Wright rosettes, neural processes, neurosecretory granules, and neural immunohistochemical markers.[160-165] Additionally, undifferentiated Ewing's sarcoma

cell lines can occasionally be induced to express markers of neural differentiation, including the expression of neurite-like elongated processes, neuron-specific enolase (NSE), cholinesterase, and neural filament triplet protein.[161,163,166-169] There are a few examples of neural differentiation of Ewing's sarcoma post-therapy, further supporting this theory.[135,170-172] Most recently, it was shown that introduction of EWS/FLI into mesenchymal stem cells could result in oncogenic transformation, suggesting that these may be the cell of origin.[173] This hypothesis has been further supported by microarray studies performed on Ewing's sarcoma cell lines in which EWS/FLI expression was reduced using RNA interference techniques.[174] In the absence of EWS/FLI expression, these cells had a gene expression pattern reminiscent of that of mesenchymal stem cells. Furthermore, these cells could be induced to differentiate into other mesenchymal cell types, such as fat and bone, a characteristic shared by mesenchymal stem cells.

Importantly, however, the phenotype of Ewing's sarcoma, at least the neural crest component, may be a *consequence* of the (11;22) translocation, rather than being related to the cell of origin of the tumor. Introduction of EWS/FLI into NIH3T3 murine fibroblasts induces a phenotype that is highly similar to Ewing's sarcoma, including the small, round, blue cell morphology and features of neural differentiation.[124,125] Similarly, expression of EWS/FLI in human rhabdomyosarcoma cells, neuroblastoma cells, or even normal human fibroblasts causes those cells to express genes similar to the genes expressed in Ewing's sarcoma.[175-177] This suggests that EWS/FLI may cause transdifferentiation of its target cells. Thus, the neural crest phenotype of Ewing's sarcoma may be induced by EWS/FLI.

Transcriptional profiling experiments, such as those using oligonucleotide or cDNA microarrays, in Ewing's sarcoma tumors and cell lines have allowed for a comprehensive analysis of the gene expression patterns associated with this disease. One of the earliest studies compared Ewing's sarcoma tumors and cell lines to other small round cell tumors of childhood, including neuroblastoma, non-Hodgkin's lymphoma, and rhabdomyosarcoma.[178] These studies have demonstrated that these histologically similar tumors could be distinguished from one another using gene expression data. A more recent analysis compared the expression of 180 sarcoma tumor samples, and again showed that tumors could be distinguished using gene expression patterns.[179] This latter study suggested a number of genes and pathways that may be associated with Ewing's sarcoma. Validation of these pathways remains to be completed. Additional studies in which the gene expression pattern of Ewing's sarcoma was compared with various normal tissues has supported the neural crest derivation, but has also suggested some similarity to endothelial cells.[180] As discussed earlier, analysis of some model systems has suggested a mesenchymal stem cell origin. A definitive understanding of the cell of origin of these tumors will require additional studies.

EWS/FLI Target Genes

Because most studies have suggested that EWS/FLI functions as a transcription factor, the two biggest questions in the field are the following: (1) which genes are dysregulated by EWS/FLI, and (2) what are the roles of these gene targets in oncogenic transformation? These questions are beginning to be answered. Because the cell of origin of Ewing's sarcoma is unknown, most laboratory-based studies of EWS/FLI have used heterologous cell types, with varying results. As noted, introduction of EWS/FLI into NIH3T3 immortalized mouse fibroblasts results in oncogenic transformation.[79,106,123] The earliest studies of EWS/FLI target genes therefore used the NIH3T3 model. A number of genes that are dysregulated by EWS/FLI were identified in this system, such as c-MYC, c-FOS, EAT-1, EAT-2, EAT-3, EAT-4, EAT-5, manic fringe (MFNG), stromelysin 1 (MMP3), cytokeratin 15, mE2-C, cytochrome P-450 F1, PDGFC, PIM3, and uridine phosphorylase.[181-187] Some of these have been shown to have a role in oncogenic transformation in the NIH3T3 transformation model, such as PDGFC, EAT2, MFNG, uridine phosphorylase, and PIM3.[184,185,187-189] Few of these have been validated in human Ewing's sarcoma. This latter point is particularly important, because recent evidence has suggested that NIH3T3 cells expressing EWS/FLI induce a gene expression pattern dissimilar to that of Ewing's sarcoma.[134,146] Thus, caution must be used when interpreting data derived from heterologous systems.

The most recent approaches toward the study of EWS/FLI have benefited from the use of RNA interference (RNAi).[131,133,134,190-193] The RNAi technique has allowed for the analysis of EWS/FLI in patient-derived Ewing's sarcoma cell lines themselves. This technique has avoided the concerns associated with the use of unvalidated heterologous cell types, such as NIH3T3 cells.

Gene expression analysis of Ewing's sarcoma cells in which EWS/FLI has been knocked down has allowed a comprehensive identification of genes that are modulated by the fusion protein.[131,134,190,192] The initial results of these studies have been somewhat surprising. It appears that EWS/FLI may downregulate at least as many, if not more, genes than it upregulates. This result is contrary to expectations based on early results demonstrating that EWS/FLI functions as a transcriptional activator, not a repressor.[79,106] There are at least two potential

explanations for these findings. First, EWS/FLI may have an undiscovered transcriptional repressive function, in addition to its activation function. Second, the downregulation of target genes may be an indirect function. That is, EWS/FLI may upregulate a second protein that serves as a transcriptional repressor. This latter hypothesis appears to be at least partially true. The gene expression studies have identified at least two likely transcriptional repressors or corepressors, NKX2.2 and NR0B1. Each of these targets has been shown to be required for the oncogenic phenotype of EWS/FLI in Ewing's sarcoma cells. The mechanisms whereby these proteins contribute to Ewing's sarcoma development are not yet known.

In addition to NKX2.2 and NR0B1, a number of additional EWS/FLI targets involved in the oncogenic phenotype of Ewing's sarcoma have been identified. For example, repression of transforming growth factor receptor 2 (TGFBR2, the receptor for TGF-β) is mediated by EWS/FLI.[194] It was shown that Ewing's sarcoma cells are resistant to the growth-suppressive effects of TGF-β, and reintroduction of TGFBR2 caused cells to become sensitive to this cytokine. Re-expression of TGFBR2 also blocked tumorigenicity. Thus, repression of TGF-β signaling appears to be critical for the oncogenic phenotype of Ewing's sarcoma.

Gene expression studies have demonstrated that EWS/FLI represses the expression of the insulin-like growth factor binding protein 3 (IGFBP-3).[131] IGFBP-3 appears to be involved in Ewing's sarcoma apoptosis, and thus decreased expression of this protein apparently prevents apoptosis. These data complement a growing body of literature that supports a critical role for IGF-1 signaling in Ewing's sarcoma development. For example, it has been shown that Ewing's sarcoma tumors and cell lines express IGF-1 and IGF receptors.[195,196] IGF-1 and its receptor appear to function in an autocrine-paracrine fashion in Ewing's sarcoma, and disruption of this signaling pathway blocks various functions that contribute to tumorigenesis.[195,197-202] This occurs in Ewing's sarcoma cell lines and in model systems.[195-205] Disruption of this pathway has been implicated as a potential molecularly targeted therapeutic approach for this disease.[202,206-209]

NPY1R was identified as an EWS/FLI target gene through microarray analysis.[134] Neuropeptide Y (NPY) is a small polypeptide neurotransmitter with diverse functions.[210,211] Engagement of NPY receptors by NPY in Ewing's sarcoma cell lines is growth inhibitory, suggesting a potential therapeutic role for these receptors.[211,212] This result was surprising, because Ewing's sarcoma cells also express the NPY ligand. It appears likely that Ewing's sarcomas are protected from the growth inhibitory effect of NPY/NPY1R interactions by the expression of dipeptidyl peptidase IV, which cleaves NPY into a form unable to bind NPY1R.[213] This cleaved form, NPY_{3-36}, functions as an angiogenic factor by binding to NPY2R receptors on endothelial cells, thus providing a likely explanation for the maintenance of this growth inhibitory autocrine pathway in Ewing's sarcoma cells.

Another protein that has been shown to be upregulated by EWS/FLI is vascular endothelial growth factor (VEGF).[176,214] VEGF levels are increased in Ewing's sarcoma cell lines and xenografts.[215] VEGF levels are also increased in the blood of patients with Ewing's sarcoma, and have been shown to be expressed in 55% of Ewing's sarcoma tumor samples by immunohistochemistry.[214,216,217] In the case of Ewing's sarcoma, VEGF may not only induce angiogenesis, but also vasculogenesis.[218,219] Blockade of VEGF function in Ewing's sarcoma model systems prevents tumor growth.[215,219-221] These preclinical studies have demonstrated the potential for VEGF inhibition as a therapeutic strategy for Ewing's sarcoma.

Most, but not all, studies of Ewing's sarcoma have shown that these tumors typically express telomerase activity.[222-225] It appears that hTERT, the catalytic subunit of the telomerase holoenzyme, is upregulated by EWS/ETS proteins.[137,214,226] This upregulation appears to be caused by specific binding of the ETS portion of the fusion to the *TERT* promoter.[214,226,227] These data suggest that EWS/ETS fusions regulate telomerase activity by direct activation of the *TERT* promoter.

One key protein whose expression may be regulated by EWS/FLI is CD99, also called MIC2.[176] In human fibroblasts engineered to express EWS/FLI, the expression of CD99 closely mimicked that of the fusion protein. In the early 1990s, it was found that CD99 is expressed at high levels in Ewing's sarcoma cells, but is uncommonly found on other tumor types.[228-230] The CD99 antigen is recognized by various monoclonal antibodies, including 12E7, HBA71, and O13, and these antibodies have an important role in the diagnosis of Ewing's sarcoma (see later).[228-237] The CD99 antigen is a membrane glycoprotein that plays a role in T-cell development and activation, and in migration of monocytes through endothelial junctions.[238-247] It is unclear whether it plays an active role in Ewing's sarcoma development or whether it is simply misregulated in this disease. Regardless of its normal role, there is emerging evidence to suggest that antibody-mediated engagement of CD99 may eventually be exploited as a new therapeutic approach to Ewing's sarcoma.[248,249] CD99 engagement in Ewing's sarcoma results in apoptosis of the tumor cells. This effect enhances tumor cell killing by chemotherapeutic agents.[248,250] Gene expression studies of CD99-mediated apoptosis have suggested a role for the cytoskeletal protein zyxin in this process, and this finding was confirmed through functional studies.[251] The identification of zyxin in this process was interesting in light of subsequent studies that demonstrated that zyxin acts as a tumor suppressor in Ewing's sarcoma.[252] Taken together, these studies suggest that CD99 may be an effective therapeutic target in Ewing's sarcoma by modulating cytoskeletal actin function.

DNA Binding Independent EWS/FLI Functions

Most of the early work on EWS/FLI suggested that it functions as an aberrant transcription factor by binding directly to DNA, and stimulating expression of target genes.[79,106,123,182] Some studies, however, have suggested that EWS/FLI does not need its DNA binding activity to mediate oncogenic function. For example, introduction of point mutations into the ETS domain that disrupt DNA binding in some cases causes the loss of target gene expression, but maintains the oncogenic function of the fusion protein.[253,254] Even more drastic alterations of the DNA binding domain, such as an almost complete deletion of the domain, also result in a protein with oncogenic function. These results were surprising and counterintuitive, based on previous work.

One possible explanation for these results is that EWS/FLI harbors nontranscription factor functions that also participate in the oncogenic function of the protein. The most frequently suggested of these is that EWS/FLI may alter normal splicing of nascent transcripts.[99,101,255,256] As noted, wild-type EWS may be involved in splice site selection. Similarly, it has been suggested that EWS/FLI can also alter splice site selection of model genes. It has also been shown that the splicing factor U1C can repress EWS/FLI–mediated transcriptional activity, suggesting that EWS/FLI interacts with components of the splicing machinery.[255] Whether this putative role in splicing is required for oncogenesis is unknown.

A role for DNA binding independent oncogenic functions of EWS/FLI must be interpreted with caution. These studies

were performed in the NIH3T3 model system, so their relevance to the human tumor has yet to be ascertained. Additionally, it is possible that EWS/FLI binds to critical target gene promoters or enhancers cooperatively.[186,257,258] In this case, protein-protein interactions may still allow for EWS/FLI to function as a transcription factor at key promoters, even without direct contact between the fusion protein and DNA. Additional work will be required to understand the relevance of these findings to Ewing's sarcoma development.

Pathways in Ewing's Sarcoma

Cooperative Pathways in Ewing's Sarcoma Oncogenesis

Multiple potentially cooperating mutations in addition to EWS/ETS fusions have been identified in Ewing's sarcoma. The most widely assessed are mutations in the p53 and RB pathways. The p53 pathway includes proteins such as p14^{ARF} and MDM2, and p53 itself.[259-263] When expressed in some heterologous systems, such as primary human fibroblasts, EWS/FLI induces the expression of p53.[176] This finding suggests that there is selective pressure to inhibit the p53 pathway, a hypothesis that appears to be at least partially true. Deletions in the *CDKN2A* locus, commonly called the *INK4a* locus encoding both p14^{ARF} and p16^{INK4a} proteins, have been identified in approximately 15% to 30% of primary Ewing's sarcoma tumors, and over 50% of Ewing's sarcoma cell lines.[264,265] Amplification or overexpression of *MDM2* is occasionally seen in Ewing's sarcoma.[266-269] Mutations in p53 are found in 5% to 20% of Ewing's sarcomas.[266,269-271] Taken together, mutations in the p53 pathway may be present in almost 70% of Ewing's sarcomas and these mutations may have prognostic significance in this disease (see later). Because there are likely additional components of the pathway yet to be identified and/or analyzed, the frequency of alterations in this pathway may be even higher.

The RB pathway regulates the cell cycle, and includes proteins such as CDK4, D-type cyclins, and p16^{INK4a}.[272-274] Mutations have been found in RB itself, and deletions of the *INK4a* locus have also been documented in Ewing's sarcoma.[264,265,275]

Mutations in the p53 and RB pathways are relatively common in Ewing's sarcoma, but mutations in other genes or pathways have only rarely been identified. For example, mutations in BRAF, which is also a member of the RAS/MAPK pathway, have been identified in 1 of 22 cell lines examined.[276] No mutations in other components of the pathway, including RAS or receptor tyrosine kinases, have been identified as of yet. This suggests that the RAS/MAPK pathway is only rarely activated via mutation in this disease.

Although the RAS/MAPK pathway does not appear to be frequently activated by mutation, there is some evidence for a requirement of pathway activation in Ewing's sarcoma tumor development. In the NIH3T3 model system, it was shown that expression of EWS/FLI induces phosphorylation of the ERK1 and ERK2 proteins (downstream members of the MAPK pathway).[277] This effect may be caused by autocrine stimulation of these transformed cells by platelet-derived growth factor C (PDGF-C), which was also shown to be induced by EWS/FLI expression in the NIH3T3 model and expressed in Ewing's sarcoma cell lines and tumor specimens.[187,278] There is some controversy as to whether PDGF-C plays a role in the human disease, because PDGFR-α, which is required for PDGF-C responsiveness, is not expressed in Ewing's sarcoma.[279] Although PDGF-C may not be involved in Ewing's sarcoma, inhibition of the MAPK pathway blocks oncogenic transformation mediated by EWS/FLI in the NIH3T3 model.[277] This finding was not replicated in Ewing's sarcoma cells, thus raising the question as to whether this is an NIH3T3-specific pathway.

Many members of the Wnt signaling pathway are expressed in Ewing's sarcoma, including soluble Wnt ligands, Wnt receptors (frizzled), and Wnt coreceptors (LRP5/6).[280] Additionally, microarray analysis of EWS/FLI target genes has demonstrated downregulation of the Wnt inhibitor DKK1 and upregulation of various Wnt signaling components.[134,175,192] These data suggest that Wnt signaling occurs in Ewing's sarcoma. In contrast, analysis of the pathway in Ewing's sarcoma cell lines in tissue culture has not demonstrated evidence of active Wnt autocrine signaling. If the pathway is involved in Ewing's sarcoma, it seems likely that it is important for processes such as migration and metastasis, rather than proliferation and transformation. Current studies have not addressed this possibility.

Gastrin-releasing peptide (GRP) has also been suggested to play a role in Ewing's sarcoma.[281] GRP was identified by differential display PCR comparing genes that were expressed in Ewing's sarcoma but not in other pediatric tumor types. The GRP receptor was also shown to be expressed in a subset of Ewing tumors. Importantly, activation of the receptor accelerated growth of a Ewing's sarcoma cell line, whereas blockade of the receptor with an antagonist inhibited cell growth. This result suggests that the GRP pathway plays a role in the proliferative capacity of at least some Ewing's sarcomas.

Apoptotic Pathways in Ewing's Sarcoma

As noted, mutations in the p53 pathway are relatively common in Ewing's sarcoma. These mutations likely confer resistance to the growth effects of TET/ETS fusions in the disease, and may also protect against apoptosis.[176,282,283] Although p53 is an important mediator of apoptosis, other signaling pathways are involved as well. These other pathways have been evaluated in Ewing's sarcoma in a number of studies.

Both Fas and the Fas ligand (FasL) are expressed in most Ewing's sarcomas.[284-286] There is some controversy as to the status of the FasL in Ewing's sarcoma; one study has reported soluble FasL in Ewing's sarcoma–conditioned media,[286] but another study reported that the FasL is only found intracellularly and thus is not accessible to cell surface receptors.[284] In terms of the receptor, Fas at the cell surface can be functional, but Ewing's sarcoma cells can be divided into Fas-sensitive, Fas-inducible, and Fas-resistant groups. Fas-sensitive lines are killed by coincubation with a FasL-expressing effector cell. Fas-inducible lines are only killed by this effector cell line following pretreatment with interferon-γ (IFN-γ) and/or cycloheximide. The Fas-resistant lines were resistant, regardless of pretreatment. The differences between sensitive and resistant cells is not completely known, but may involve differences in Fas expression, or expression of pro- or antiapoptotic mediators, such as BAD and BAR.[287] Strategies to improve Fas-mediated killing of Ewing's sarcoma cells have been investigated, such as allowing for accumulation of more FasL via the use of metalloproteinase inhibitors[288] and upregulation of Fas by administration of interleukin-12.[289,290]

In addition to Fas and FasL, evaluations of TRAIL and tumor necrosis factor-α (TNF-α) as inducers of Ewing's sarcoma apoptosis have also been conducted, in vitro and in vivo, alone and in combination with other agents.[291-302] Taken together, these data support a potential use of proapoptotic ligands in the treatment of Ewing's sarcoma. However, the variability of the effects seen demonstrate the need for an ongoing mechanistic evaluation of these pathways in this disease.

Summary

The identification of t(11;22)(q24;q12) and subsequent cloning of the EWS/FLI fusion protein represented a major advance in understanding the pathogenesis of Ewing's sarcoma. EWS/FLI appears to function primarily as an aberrant transcription factor to dysregulate gene targets involved in the development of this disease. Multiple gene targets and cooperating molecular pathways have been identified. These represent a wide array of functions, including growth factor signaling, survival and apoptosis pathways, angiogenesis, cellular immortalization, and cellular differentiation. Despite these myriad molecular functions, a unified mechanistic understanding of Ewing's sarcoma development has not yet been reached. Similarly, the cell of origin of the disease has not been clearly identified. Nonetheless, there is great hope that a detailed understanding of the molecular mechanisms involved in Ewing's sarcoma development will lead to new diagnostic, prognostic, and therapeutic approaches for this disease.

CLINICAL PRESENTATION AND DIAGNOSIS

Clinical Presentation

Patients with Ewing's sarcoma most commonly present with pain, a palpable mass, or both. In one series, 89% of patients with Ewing's sarcoma reported pain at the time of initial presentation.[303] Pain does not necessarily occur at night, with this pattern reported in only 19% of patients in one series. Patients may report that their pain began at the same time as a minor musculoskeletal injury. This presentation, reported in approximately 25% of patients, may delay the diagnosis. Unlike osteosarcoma, patients with Ewing's sarcoma may report constitutional symptoms such as fever and weight loss. Approximately 15% to 20% of patients have fever at presentation.[304-306] Other symptoms depend on the site of the disease. For example, 40% to 94% of patients with paraspinal tumors present with symptoms of spinal cord compression.[307-310] Patients with large pelvic tumors may complain of an alteration in voiding. Extensive bone marrow metastatic disease may cause symptoms related to anemia, thrombocytopenia, or neutropenia. Patients may have symptoms for many weeks or months prior to presenting for evaluation, with most studies reporting an average time from symptom onset to diagnosis of 3 to 5 months.[311-313]

Ewing's sarcoma can arise from any bone, but has a predilection for pelvic bones and long bones of the leg. Approximately 45% of Ewing's sarcomas develop in the axial skeleton, with more than half of these axial tumors arising from pelvic bones.[4,5] Up to 30% of Ewing's sarcomas arise from long bones in the leg, whereas up to 15% of tumors develop in long bones in the arm.[4,5] Tumors of the hands, feet, and head develop only rarely, accounting for 10% or less of all tumors.[4,5] The distribution of primary tumor site does not vary among ethnic and racial groups.[10] Soft tissue tumors may arise in any location, although axial sites seem to predominate.[314]

Laboratory studies in patients with newly diagnosed Ewing's sarcoma may reveal nonspecific abnormalities. More than a third of patients have an elevated erythrocyte sedimentation rate (ESR) at the time of diagnosis.[306,315] Similarly, serum lactate dehydrogenase (LDH) levels are elevated in approximately one third of patients.[305,315-317] Laboratory manifestations of tumor lysis syndrome are uncommon with these tumors. Unlike osteosarcoma, alkaline phosphatase is not typically elevated in patients with Ewing's sarcoma of the bone. Patients with advanced bone marrow metastatic disease may have anemia, thrombocytopenia, and neutropenia detected on a complete blood count. In one large series, 12% of patients had anemia, even in the absence of metastatic disease.[305]

Box 21-1 summarizes the differential diagnosis of Ewing's sarcoma. In most cases of Ewing's sarcoma of the bone, the main alternative diagnosis is osteosarcoma. Table 21-2 displays features that may aid in the differentiation of Ewing's sarcoma of the bone from osteosarcoma. Compared with osteosarcoma, Ewing's sarcoma is more likely to occur in the axial skeleton. Those Ewing's tumors that arise in long bones have a greater tendency to occur in the diaphysis, compared with the tendency of osteosarcoma to arise in the metaphysis of long bones.[318] Patients with Ewing's sarcoma are more likely to report constitutional symptoms than patients with osteosarcoma. Other malignant tumors in the differential diagnosis of Ewing's sarcoma of the bone include primary bone lymphoma, giant cell tumor of the bone, and bone metastasis of an extraosseous malignancy. The differential diagnosis of Ewing's sarcoma arising from the soft tissues is broader because the site of origin for these tumors is not restricted to the bone. The site of origin may help narrow the differential diagnosis. Paraspinal tumors may be confused with neuroblastoma, particularly in younger patients. Pelvic tumors may suggest rhabdomyosarcoma or malignant germ cell tumor. Lymphoma and other soft tissue sarcomas can arise at any site and should be included in the differential diagnosis.

Reports from several cooperative group studies have defined the metastatic behavior of Ewing's sarcoma. Approximately 25% of patients present with distant metastases.[319,320] Patients with pelvic primary tumors have an increased incidence of metastatic disease at initial diagnosis.[321] The lung is the most common metastatic site, with pulmonary dissemination reported in 50% to 60% of patients with metastatic disease.[322,323] Patients with isolated pulmonary metastasis represent 26% to 36% of cases of metastatic disease.[322,324] Patients most commonly have multiple lung nodules identified in both lungs.

The bone is the next most common metastatic site at presentation. A large cooperative group has reported cortical bone metastases in 43% of patients with metastatic disease and that the bone marrow is involved in approximately 19% of metastatic patients at initial diagnosis.[323] A smaller series has noted bone marrow involvement in 52% of patients with metastatic disease.[325] This group studied up to 10 bone marrow aspirates on patients at initial presentation, suggesting that routine sampling may underestimate the incidence of bone marrow involvement. Less than 10% of patients with metastatic disease have lymph node involvement at initial diagnosis, although the incidence of node involvement may be higher in patients with soft tissue rather than bone primary tumors.[323,326] Brain metastasis at initial diagnosis appears to be extremely uncommon. In two series of patients with brain metastasis from Ewing's sarcoma, all cases were reported at the time of disease recurrence and not at initial presentation.[327,328]

This metastatic pattern helps determine the appropriate staging evaluation for patients with Ewing's sarcoma (Box 21-2). In addition to computed tomography (CT) or magnetic resonance imaging (MRI) scans of the primary tumor, all newly diagnosed patients should be evaluated with a chest CT scan and a radiolabeled technetium bone scan. At least, bilateral bone marrow aspirates and biopsies should routinely be performed in newly diagnosed patients. Positron emission tomography (PET) scans may begin to play a role in the evaluation of newly diagnosed patients, but are not currently standard practice for the initial staging of Ewing's sarcoma (see later).

Box 21-1	Clinical Differential Diagnosis of Ewing's Sarcoma

EWING'S SARCOMA OF BONE

Osteosarcoma
Primary bone lymphoma
Langerhans cell histiocytosis
Osteomyelitis
Metastasis of an extraosseous malignancy
Benign bone tumor
Osteoblastoma
Chondrosarcoma
Giant cell tumor of the bone

EWING'S SARCOMA OF SOFT TISSUE

Rhabdomyosarcoma
Nonrhabdomyosarcoma soft tissue sarcoma
Lymphoma
Benign soft tissue tumor
Neuroblastoma
Malignant germ cell tumor

TABLE 21-2 Clinical Differentiation of Ewing's Sarcoma of Bone from Osteosarcoma

Parameter	Ewing's Sarcoma	Osteosarcoma
Age distribution	Peak in adolescence; occurs in young children; very rare in adults >40 yr	Peak in adolescence; very rare in children <5 yr; occurs in older adults
Racial distribution	Rare in patients of African or East Asian ancestry	No racial predilection
Predisposing factors	Not associated with radiation; no known familial predisposition	Radiation exposure; Li-Fraumeni syndrome; history of retinoblastoma
Constitutional symptoms	Yes	No
Involved bones	Both flat and long bones	Long bones more common
Location in long bones	Diaphyseal more common	Epiphyseal, metaphyseal more common
Type of periosteal reaction	Laminated, layered; onion-skin appearance	Spiculated, sunburst
Laboratory findings	Normal alkaline phosphatase; abnormal CBC if marrow disease	Elevated alkaline phosphatase; normal CBC
Histologic findings	Small round blue cells; no malignant osteoid	Malignant spindle cells; malignant osteoid

CBC = complete blood cell count.

These evaluations will indicate whether a patient has metastatic or nonmetastatic Ewing's sarcoma at initial diagnosis, a distinction that serves as the main staging classification in practice for these patients. Although a staging classification for musculoskeletal tumors has been devised by Enneking, this system is not routinely used in the clinical care of patients with Ewing's sarcoma.[329]

Imaging Features

Most patients presenting with Ewing's sarcoma of the bone are initially evaluated with a plain radiograph. Two representative radiographs are shown in Figure 21-5. These tumors typically appear as poorly circumscribed lesions arising from the bone, but with an associated soft tissue mass.[318] Both lytic and sclerotic areas may be seen within the bony component of the tumor. Given the aggressive nature of these tumors, periosteal reaction is commonly observed. A layered or laminated periosteal reaction is most typical, often giving an onion-skin appearance (see Fig. 21-5A).[318,330] A spiculated sunburst periosteal reaction is more commonly associated with osteosarcoma, but may be occasionally observed in Ewing's sarcoma (see Fig. 21-5B). Codman's triangle may also be seen in some cases. Cortical thickening is present in approximately 20% of tumors. Pathologic fractures occur in 15% of patients with Ewing's sarcoma of bone.[306,318,331]

CT and MRI scans are used to define the extent of local tumor in patients with both osseous and extraosseous tumors better. CT scans most commonly demonstrate a heterogeneous mass with heterogeneous contrast enhancement.[332-336] The soft tissue component generally has lower attenuation than muscle on nonenhanced CT scans.[332,334,337] MRI scans typically reveal a mass that is heterogeneous with respect to signal intensity and gadolinium contrast enhancement.[335,336,338] Typically T1- and T2-weighted MRI scans demonstrate areas of increased signal intensity of the soft tissue component compared with skeletal muscle. Although CT and MRI can delineate the soft tissue component of the tumor, MRI may be better able to determine the extent of bone marrow extension and the degree of growth plate involvement.[339]

Emerging evidence has suggested that fluorodeoxy glucose positron emission tomography (FDG-PET) may play an increasing role in the management of patients with Ewing's sarcoma. In one series, all 32 patients with Ewing's sarcoma evaluated by FDG-PET imaging prior to initiation of chemotherapy had FDG-avid tumors.[340] Figure 21-6 demonstrates an FDG-PET scan of a patient with widely metastatic Ewing's sarcoma at initial presentation. Several studies have evaluated the role of FDG-PET imaging in screening for metastatic disease and for disease recurrence. Two groups have demonstrated that FDG-PET imaging has superior sensitivity and specificity compared with conventional bone scans for detecting bone metastases in patients with Ewing's sarcoma.[341,342] In contrast, FDG-PET appears to be inferior to spiral CT scans in screening for pulmonary metastases in these patients.[343] In screening patients with Ewing's sarcoma for overall disease recurrence at any site, FDG-PET imaging may have lower sensitivity but higher specificity compared with conventional imaging.[344] Finally, one group has reported that a decrease in FDG avidity in response to neoadjuvant chemotherapy correlates with improved progression-free survival.[340]

Box 21-2	**Recommended Evaluations for Patients Newly Diagnosed with Ewing's Sarcoma**

ASSESSMENT OF PRIMARY TUMOR

Magnetic resonance imaging (MRI) scan
and/or
Computed tomography (CT) scan

EVALUATION FOR METASTATIC DISEASE

CT scan of the chest
Radiolabeled-technetium bone scan
Bone marrow aspirate and biopsy

EVALUATION PRIOR TO INITIATING CHEMOTHERAPY

Echocardiography
Serum creatinine (with formal creatinine clearance if renal function in question)

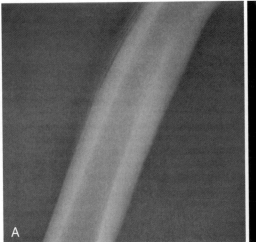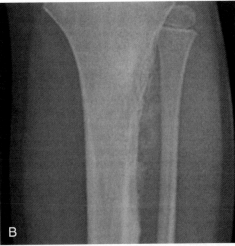

FIGURE 21-5. A, Plain radiograph of a femoral Ewing's sarcoma demonstrating a laminated periosteal reaction resulting in an onion-skin appearance. **B,** Plain radiograph of a tibial Ewing's sarcoma with a spiculated periosteal reaction. (*A courtesy of Dr. Stephan Voss, Department of Radiology, Children's Hospital, Boston.*)

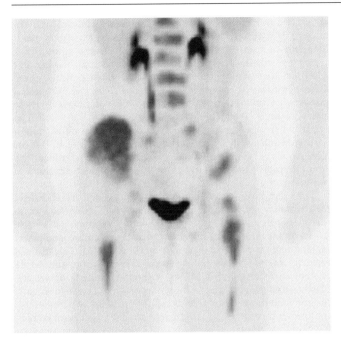

FIGURE 21-6. Whole-body FDG-PET scan of a patient with widely metastatic Ewing's sarcoma at initial diagnosis. FDG uptake is evident in bones, soft tissue, and bone marrow.

Pathologic Diagnosis

Once imaging studies have localized the tumor, diagnostic tissue must be obtained. The current pathologic diagnosis of Ewing's sarcoma depends on tumor morphology, immunohistochemistry findings, and demonstration of a Ewing's sarcoma–specific translocation by standard cytogenetics, fluorescence in situ hybridization (FISH), or reverse transcriptase–polymerase chain reaction (RT-PCR) assays.[345] In planning for biopsy, one must ensure that adequate tissue will be available to perform each of these tests. For example, one series has reported successful cytogenetic analysis in only 59% of fine-needle aspirations performed for Ewing's sarcoma.[346] Most centers use a core or open biopsy to ensure collection of adequate diagnostic material. The biopsy should be planned with an eye toward ultimate local control of the tumor. If surgical resection is ultimately planned, the biopsy tract should be included in the resected specimen.[347]

Ewing's sarcoma and PNET form a morphologic continuum, ranging from tumors with no apparent neural differentiation to tumors with evidence of early neural differentiation. Of note, the histologic classification of these tumors does not imply site of origin, because tumors with either histology may arise in the bone or soft tissue. Ewing's sarcoma appears as relatively monomorphic, small, round blue-staining cells with scant cytoplasm (Fig. 21-7).[348,349] The nuclei tend to be round without prominent nucleoli. These cells demonstrate positive periodic acid-Schiff staining because of cytoplasmic glycogen, and electron microscopy may reveal these glycogen stores.[345,349] The tumor cells grow in sheets without additional structure. A large cell or atypical Ewing's sarcoma has been described with large irregular nuclei and more conspicuous nucleoli.[348-350] Up to 30% of tumors with Ewing's sarcoma histology arise in soft tissues rather than bone. PNETs typically display primitive Homer-Wright pseudorosette formation. Electron microscopy may reveal additional features suggestive of neural differentiation, such as neurosecretory granules.[351] Tumors without pseu-

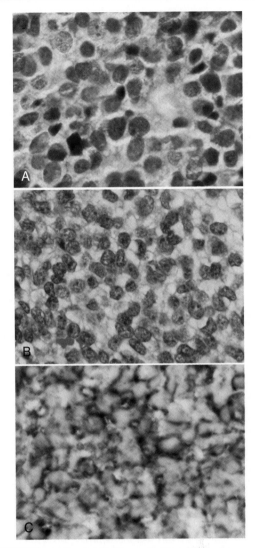

FIGURE 21-7. A, Characteristic morphology of Ewing's sarcoma with monomorphic, small, round blue cells without pseudorosette formation. **B,** Morphologic features of a primitive neuroectodermal tumor (PNET), including a pseudorosette formation in the center of the panel. **C,** Characteristic strong membranous CD99 immunohistochemical staining of Ewing's sarcoma. *(Courtesy of Dr. Antonio Perez-Atayde, Department of Pathology, Children's Hospital, Boston.)*

dorosette formation may also be classified as PNET if they express two or more neural markers (see later). Approximately 50% of tumors with PNET histology arise in bone. Despite these morphologic differences, Ewing's sarcoma and PNET are now viewed as the same biologic entity.

Immunohistochemistry plays a key role in differentiating Ewing's sarcoma and PNET from other small round cell tumors of children and young adults. The most useful antigen in the diagnosis of Ewing's sarcoma appears to be CD99. This protein product of the *MIC2* gene is expressed in a limited number of normal tissues, including strong staining of ependymal cells, pancreatic islet cells, anterior pituitary gland, testicular Sertoli cells, ovarian granulosa cells, and maturing T lymphocytes.[229,352] Less intense staining has been noted in scattered endothelial cells. Ewing's sarcoma and PNET both display prominent CD99 immunostaining in a membranous pattern (see Fig. 21-7). Multiple series have found strong CD99 immunostaining in more than 90% of cases of Ewing's sarcoma and

PNET.[229-231,236,237,352-355] Staining for neural markers, such as synaptophysin, S-100, NSE, and neurofilament, is variable and helps characterize tumors as Ewing's sarcoma or PNET.[345,348-350] These tumors also commonly stain with vimentin, whereas desmin staining is distinctly uncommon.[356] Approximately 30% of Ewing's sarcomas and PNETs demonstrate diffuse c-kit (CD117) staining.[357-359]

Several tumors also express CD99 and may confuse the diagnosis. Strong CD99 immunostaining has been observed in ependymoma, glioblastoma, and pancreatic islet cell tumors.[229,352] These tumors are not typically within the clinical differential diagnosis of Ewing's sarcoma or PNET. In contrast, lymphoblastic lymphoma (particularly T cell), neuroblastoma, alveolar rhabdomyosarcoma, synovial sarcoma, and desmoplastic small round cell tumor may demonstrate variable levels of CD99 staining and are frequently considered in the differential diagnosis of these tumors.[229,356,360-364] Whereas both Ewing's sarcoma and lymphoblastic lymphoma may demonstrate strong CD99 staining, Ewing's sarcoma and PNET should be negative for lymphocyte markers, particularly leukocyte common antigen (LCA) and terminal deoxynucleotidyl transferase (TdT).[350] Ewing's sarcoma and PNET are also more likely to demonstrate strong vimentin staining compared with lymphoblastic lymphoma. The immunohistochemical differentiation of Ewing's sarcoma and PNET from neuroblastoma is typically more straightforward, largely because CD99 staining in neuroblastoma, if present, is weak and patchy. Neuroblastomas commonly demonstrate strong staining with NSE, whereas Ewing's sarcoma and PNET occasionally will show weak to moderate NSE staining.[231,361] Poorly differentiated synovial sarcoma and desmoplastic small round cell tumor may both also demonstrate CD99 staining and morphologically be difficult to differentiate from Ewing's sarcoma and PNET. In both cases, strong membranous staining is more consistent with Ewing's sarcoma and PNET. In contrast, weak staining for CD99 and strong staining for cytokeratin and epithelial membrane antigen suggest synovial sarcoma. Desmoplastic small round cell tumors reliably demonstrate nuclear staining for WT1, but Ewing's sarcoma and PNET typically do not stain with WT1.[364] Nuclear staining for FLI1 may also help differentiate these tumors from other pediatric CD99 small round cell tumors. Most cases of Ewing's sarcoma and PNET demonstrate nuclear FLI1 staining, whereas synovial sarcoma, neuroblastoma, and rhabdomyosarcoma only rarely show positive nuclear FLI1 staining.[348,365,366] However, a high proportion of lymphoblastic lymphomas also exhibit nuclear FLI1 staining.

The combination of characteristic morphology and immunohistochemistry typically allows an experienced pathologist to render the diagnosis of Ewing's sarcoma or PNET. The identification of recurrent chromosomal translocations and their associated oncoproteins in these tumors has allowed for the incorporation of molecular testing into their diagnosis. These methods play a role as confirmatory tests in the setting of typical morphology and immunohistochemistry. In more unusual cases, these molecular tests may serve as the key feature on which the diagnosis is based. Although these molecular approaches have been effective, it is worth recognizing their strengths and weaknesses when interpreting diagnostic studies.

Karyotypic analysis is one approach toward confirming the diagnosis of Ewing's sarcoma. The presence of one characteristic translocation can be considered strong supportive evidence for the diagnosis.[59-61,367,368] It is important to recognize that false-negatives may occur from a number of sources, including overgrowth of nonmalignant elements during culture, complex translocations in which the characteristic Ewing-associated rearrangement is partially masked by the presence of an additional fusion partner,[61,369-371] and cryptic rearrangements in which the translocation cannot be identified via typical techniques.[370,372] FISH can be helpful as a complementary technique to demonstrate that the *EWSR1* locus is split, which suggests a translocation event.[373-377] FISH for the *FLI1* and/or *ERG* loci that demonstrates a split signal from either of these genes, or fusion between *EWSR1* and *FLI1* or *ERG* signals, provides additional strong evidence for involvement of these genes in the rearrangement. A false-negative FISH result may occur when the fusion involves a more rare translocation partner, such as TLS (in lieu of EWS), or ETV1, ETV4, or FEV (in lieu of FLI or ERG).[142-145,148] These rare translocations are not typically included in the molecular diagnostic evaluation of these tumors.

One important shortcoming in the use of *EWSR1* FISH for diagnostic purposes is the presence of *EWSR1* rearrangements in tumor types other than Ewing's sarcoma (see Table 21-1). For example, clear cell sarcoma, also called malignant melanoma of the soft parts, usually harbors a t(12;22)(q13;q12) rearrangement.[378] This translocation fuses EWS to the ATF1 protein to form the EWS/ATF1 protein. Similarly, a desmoplastic small round cell tumor harbors a t(11;22)(p13;q12) rearrangement, which fuses the EWS protein to the Wilms' tumor suppressor WT1 to form the EWS/WT1 protein.[379] EWS or TAF15 can join the NR4A3 orphan nuclear receptor to form EWS/NR4A3 and TAF15/NR4A3 fusion proteins in extraskeletal myxoid chondrosarcoma.[94,380-383] EWS is occasionally fused to DDIT3, also called CHOP, to form EWS/DDIT3 in t(12;22)(q13;q12)–positive myxoid liposarcoma.[384] An EWS/ZNF278 fusion was identified in a small round cell sarcoma as a result of a t(1;22)(p36;q12) rearrangement.[385] In some cases, there may be diagnostic confusion between some of these tumor types and Ewing's sarcoma, and thus the presence of a rearranged *EWSR1* locus may not be adequate for diagnostic purposes. In rare cases, tumors may show biphenotypic differentiation with neural and myogenic patterns. At least some of these express EWS rearrangements (EWS/FLI or EWS/ERG fusions), as well as the classic PAX3/FKHR fusion protein associated with alveolar rhabdomyosarcoma.[386-388]

The use of RT-PCR may provide greater specificity in the diagnosis of Ewing's sarcoma. RT-PCR is a useful method for the detection of EWS/ETS fusions.[377,389-391] As with any PCR-based method, false-positive results may occur from contamination. False-negative results may occur because of degradation of the RNA or alternate fusion partners, or because an RT-PCR primer pair may be designed to detect some EWS/FLI transcripts but not others. False-negative results may also occur when biopsies do not capture viable tissue or primarily include nonmalignant elements. Despite their shortcomings, molecular techniques have become an important addition to the diagnostic approach for Ewing's sarcoma.

PROGNOSTIC FACTORS

A number of clinical and molecular features have been identified as prognostic variables in patients with Ewing's sarcoma. The presence of metastatic disease at initial diagnosis is widely regarded as the most important adverse clinical prognostic feature. In the largest analysis of prognostic features in this disease, patients with metastatic disease at presentation had a 5-year relapse-free survival of 21% compared with 55% for nonmetastatic patients.[321] Patients in this analysis received therapy according to several sequential treatment protocols. Patients with metastatic disease treated in the North American study INT-0091 had a similar 5-year event-free survival of 22%, regardless of their chemotherapy regimen.[320] Patients with isolated lung metastases may have a better outcome than patients with dissemination to other sites or to lungs plus other sites.[319,321,324,392] Within this group of patients, patients with unilateral lung metastases may fare better than patients with bilateral lung metastases.

Tumor size has long been recognized as a predictor of outcome in patients with Ewing's sarcoma. Patients with larger tumors are at increased risk for having metastatic disease at initial diagnosis. For example, a pooled analysis of German patients treated in the EICESS/CESS studies indicated that tumor volume more than 100 mL was an independent predictor of metastatic disease at initial diagnosis.[393] The effect of tumor size on outcome does not depend entirely on this increased risk of metastatic disease, however. Tumor size appears to be prognostic, even among patients with initially nonmetastatic tumors. The CESS-81 study demonstrated that tumor volume more than 100 mL is a significant adverse prognostic factor for patients treated with surgery or radiation.[394] The follow-up CESS-86 study found that tumor volume more than 200 mL was a major adverse prognostic feature for patients with localized Ewing's sarcoma.[395,396] The North American INT-0091 study has reported that nonmetastatic patients with tumors more than 8 cm in maximal dimension have an inferior outcome compared with patients with smaller tumors.[320] The French EW88 study has reported that tumor size, using tumor volume or longest dimension, was prognostic only for patients who received radiotherapy alone as the mode of local control.[315] Although some smaller studies have not observed this effect of tumor size on outcome,[397] most investigators consider tumor size prognostic. A large pooled analyses of prognostic factors in Ewing's sarcoma has identified large tumor volume as an independent predictor of poor outcome.[321]

Tumor site is also widely considered a prognostic factor in Ewing's sarcoma, with axial tumors carrying a worse prognosis. The IESS-1 study established pelvic site as an unfavorable prognostic feature.[398] Several other cooperative group studies have confirmed this finding and indicated that patients with axial tumors generally have a worse outcome compared with patients with nonaxial tumors.[312,320,399,400] In many of these studies, patients with pelvic primary tumors have been shown to have a particularly poor outcome compared with patients with other axial locations. However, the inferior outcomes in patients with pelvic tumors may be confounded by a higher incidence of large tumor size and metastatic disease.[321,393] For example, in the CESS-86 trial, axial tumor location was a significant adverse prognostic feature on univariate analysis.[396] After controlling for tumor size and chemotherapy response, however, the prognostic impact of axial site became insignificant. Several groups evaluated only patients with nonmetastatic tumors and found that patients with pelvic tumors still have an inferior outcome compared with patients with nonpelvic tumors.[320,398,399] Two other groups used multivariate methods to evaluate the prognostic impact of axial tumor location in nonmetastatic patients.[305,321] Both groups reported that axial tumors have an inferior outcome compared with extremity tumors, even after controlling for potential confounders, but neither analysis controlled for tumor size. Therefore, whether axial tumor location portends a poor outcome independent of large tumor size remains unclear.

A number of groups have specifically evaluated histologic response to neoadjuvant chemotherapy as a predictor of outcome. Patients with a favorable chemotherapy response, typically 90% to 100% tumor necrosis depending on the grading scale used, at the time of surgery were found to have a decreased risk of disease recurrence compared with patients with less necrosis.[224,315,394,396,401-404] For patients with nonmetastatic tumors of the extremity, chemotherapy response is prognostic, independently of age and tumor size.[402] Despite these results,

grading of chemotherapy response in Ewing's sarcoma has not yet become routine practice, perhaps at least in part because this variable is not evaluable in those patients who receive definitive radiotherapy as their mode of local control. An alternative to histologic grading is radiographic grading of chemotherapy response. Two groups have reported that favorable radiographic response to chemotherapy is a predictor of favorable outcome.[400,401] Evaluation of radiographic response may also not be possible in all patients, particularly in patients with tumors confined to bone without an associated soft tissue mass.

Age at initial diagnosis has been increasingly recognized as an important prognostic feature in Ewing's sarcoma. Several studies have indicated that younger patients have an improved outcome compared with older patients.[305,316,320,321,397,398] Older patients have an increased risk of presenting with large tumors, but, interestingly, not a higher incidence of metastatic disease at initial diagnosis.[393] Even controlling for these potential confounders, age has been identified as an independent predictor of outcome in a number of studies.[399] Most studies have used a single cut point in the 12- to 15-year age range. One study divided patients into three groups (younger than 10 years, 10 to 17 years, and older than 18 years) and found that nonmetastatic patients older than 18 years of age at initial diagnosis had a particularly poor outcome (44% 5-year event-free survival).[320] A number of studies have focused on outcomes in older adolescents and adults with Ewing's sarcoma. These studies have typically identified the same adverse prognostic features (metastatic disease, large size, axial location, and poor chemotherapy response) in older patients that have been identified in larger studies in patients at a wide range of ages.[405-408] The mechanism underlying these differences in outcome with age remains unclear. Possible explanations include biologic differences in tumor and host as well as health care delivery differences in compliance and dose intensity.

Serum LDH levels at initial diagnosis also appear to be prognostic. Several early studies have reported that patients with elevated serum LDH levels at diagnosis had an increased risk of disease recurrence.[409-411] More recent studies have confirmed this finding and have found that the negative prognostic impact of an elevated LDH remains, even after controlling for other possible confounding variables.[305,316,412] A meta-analysis evaluating a range of tumor markers in Ewing's sarcoma has also concluded that elevated LDH at diagnosis is associated with inferior outcomes.[413] Presumably, elevated LDH levels indicate greater tumor cell turnover and therefore more aggressive clinical behavior.

Various other clinical and demographic features at diagnosis have been variably reported to be prognostic in Ewing's sarcoma. One group has reported that female gender is an independent predictor of favorable outcome.[305,316] Other groups have not corroborated this finding.[320,321,395] A greater degree of neural differentiation has been reported as an unfavorable marker by some groups, but not by others.[164,231,326,349,350,396,414-418] Fever, anemia, leukocytosis, elevated ESR, and hypoalbuminemia at initial diagnosis have also been suggested as unfavorable prognostic features, but their prognostic value has not yet been validated.[305,315,412,419]

The nature of the Ewing's sarcoma–specific translocation may provide prognostic information. One group has demonstrated that patients with any type of EWS/FLI1 translocation have similar outcomes to patients with any type of EWS/ERG translocation.[420] Another report has suggested that patients with nonmetastatic disease and a type 1 EWS/FLI translocation have a better relapse-free survival compared with all other types of EWS/FLI or EWS/ERG translocations.[152] A follow-up study has confirmed that the type 1 translocation is associated with more favorable overall survival than other types of EWS/FLI translocations, even after controlling for other known prognostic factors.[421]

Several studies have measured EWS/FLI fusion transcripts in the peripheral blood or bone marrow to predict outcome. These studies use PCR techniques to identify occult metastatic disease, with 25% of clinically nonmetastatic patients noted to have detectable EWS/FLI fusion transcripts in blood or bone marrow in one early study.[422] The results of studies correlating these findings to clinical outcome have been mixed. In one report, patients with clinically localized disease but positive peripheral blood EWS/FLI PCR at diagnosis had a higher risk of relapse compared with patients with negative peripheral blood EWS/FLI PCR.[423] A second study evaluating bone marrow EWS/FLI PCR at diagnosis was not able to confirm this finding.[424] Patients in this study had follow-up EWS/FLI PCR performed on blood and/or bone marrow. Patients with positive blood or bone marrow EWS/FLI PCR as their last evaluation had a significantly increased risk of clinical disease recurrence. The usefulness of this methodology for predicting outcome in patients with Ewing's sarcoma requires further prospective evaluation.

Chromosomal changes beyond the characteristic TET/ETS translocations may also provide prognostic information. Although it is the most common additional karyotypic abnormality in Ewing's sarcoma, at least two groups have reported that trisomy 8 does not appear to influence outcome.[425,426] A small series of 21 patients has reported that all three patients with gain of chromosome 1q died of disease.[427] A larger study of 124 patients with Ewing's sarcoma included 26 patients with gain of chromosome 1q.[425] This study confirmed that patients with gain of chromosome 1q have a worse outcome, independently of other clinical prognostic factors.

Several key regulators of cell cycle progression, senescence, and apoptosis have been correlated with outcome in patients with Ewing's sarcoma. The 10% to 15% of patients with mutations in the *TP53* gene, encoding the p53 protein, have consistently been shown to have a significantly worse outcome compared with patients with wild-type *TP53*, even after controlling for other prognostic factors.[428,429] Additional work has suggested that mutations or deletions of the *CDKN2A/INK4A* gene may also confer a poor outcome in these patients.[265,429,430] For example, aberrant *TP53* and/or *CDKN2A/INK4A* gene status in one study was shown to be an independent negative prognostic feature.[429] Other research has evaluated telomerase activity in the peripheral blood at diagnosis and during follow-up.[224] Although telomerase activity at diagnosis did not predict outcome, high telomerase activity during follow-up was strongly associated with disease recurrence. None of the patients in this study with low telomerase activity during follow-up had disease recurrence.

TREATMENT

Nonmetastatic Ewing's Sarcoma

Local Control

Patients with nonmetastatic Ewing's sarcoma require aggressive multimodality therapy to achieve long-term disease control. Local control of the primary tumor plays a key role in modern treatment for these patients. Historically, patients received radiation therapy alone as local control. Surgical local control was less commonly used because therapy was generally viewed as palliative. With improved outcomes with chemotherapy, however, the late effects of radiotherapy on long-term survivors of Ewing's sarcoma have become apparent. In addition, limb salvage surgical techniques have become more advanced. As a result, surgical local control of resectable tumors has become the standard of care. Radiotherapy for local control of the primary tumor is now generally reserved for unresectable tumors or tumors that have been resected with inadequate margins. This section reviews the principles of radiotherapy and surgical resection in the care of patients with Ewing's sarcoma.

Surgical resection is generally recommended for those tumors deemed completely resectable with wide or radical margins. For extremity tumors, surgical resection may take the form of an amputation or limb-sparing procedure. Rotationplasty is another option for patients with femoral tumors.[347] Technical advances, such as expandable implanted prostheses, have made limb-sparing procedures increasingly appealing.[431] However, the choice of a limb-sparing procedure over other surgical options must not compromise the adequacy of the resection. Tumor infiltration of surrounding neurovascular structures, muscle, or skin should raise concern that a limb-sparing procedure will not result in the desired wide resection. Often, neoadjuvant chemotherapy will produce sufficient response to allow for limb salvage when this option did not appear feasible at initial presentation.[347] However, two small reports from a single institution have suggested that neither the likelihood of an adequate margin nor the overall outcome does not differ between patients who had surgical resection at initial diagnosis compared with patients who had surgical resection after a period of neoadjuvant chemotherapy.[432,433] Nevertheless, the current standard approach is for patients to receive neoadjuvant chemotherapy.

Investigators from the CESS group and the Rizzoli Institute have evaluated the impact of surgical margins on outcome in Ewing's sarcoma in two retrospective case series.[434,435] These groups have both reported the rate of obtaining an adequate surgical margin as approximately 75% in those patients selected for planned definitive resection. Both groups observed that an adequate margin is more difficult to obtain in axial tumors. For example, the Rizzoli group reported that approximately 25% of the extremity tumors treated with a limb salvage procedure had inadequate margins. In contrast, none of the paraspinal or sacral tumors in their large series of surgically treated patients had an adequate margin.[434] The Rizzoli group observed that the 5-year event-free survival rate was higher for patients with an adequate surgical margin, although this finding may reflect improved outcome with smaller, more resectable tumors. In both series, a small group of patients with inadequate surgical margins did not receive postoperative radiotherapy. Only 14% to 21% of these patients experienced a local recurrence. However, the risk of local recurrence was diminished by the addition of postoperative radiotherapy, which is the current standard practice.

Radiation therapy alone can provide adequate local control for Ewing's sarcoma. In fact, the radiosensitivity of these tumors was one of the early characteristics that distinguished Ewing's sarcoma from osteosarcoma.[1] Local control rates with definitive radiation therapy in a large series have been reported to range from 53% to 86%.[436] For patients treated with radiation therapy alone, axial tumors (particularly pelvic tumors) have a higher rate of local failure than extremity tumors.[399,437-439] One group has reported that patients with metastatic disease treated with radiation alone or surgery plus radiation have a higher rate of local failure compared with patients with nonmetastatic disease.[440]

Several studies have evaluated the appropriate treatment volume, dose, timing, and schedule of radiotherapy in Ewing's sarcoma. The IESS-1 study group reported on their experience with radiotherapy.[438] All patients received radiotherapy as the mode of local control in this study. Across the range of doses administered (30 Gy to more than 60 Gy), no differences in local failure rates were observed, although few patients received less than 40 Gy. Although most patients received radiation to the whole bone involved with tumor, some patients were treated with more limited fields. Patients who received radiotherapy to the primary tumor plus a 5-cm margin had the same local failure rate as patients treated with whole-bone radiotherapy (8% for both groups). Patients treated with less than a 5-cm margin had an inferior local control rate.

The Pediatric Oncology Group conducted a study from 1983 and 1988 with the specific aim of determining the appropriate radiation dose for patients with Ewing's sarcoma of the bone.[437] Patients with tumors in expendable bones were recommended for surgical resection. Other patients were randomized to receive whole bone irradiation or involved field radiation. Patients treated with whole-bone irradiation received 39.6 Gy to the entire bone containing tumor plus a boost to 55.8 Gy to the tumor with a 2-cm margin. Patients treated with involved field radiation received 55.8 Gy to the tumor with a 2-cm margin. Because of enrollment issues, 20 patients were randomized to whole-bone radiation and 20 patients to involved field radiation. An additional 54 patients were nonrandomly assigned to involved field radiation. The 5-year event-free survival did not differ between patients randomized to whole-bone radiation and patients randomized to involved field radiation (37% and 39%, respectively). The local control rate was 53% in both treatment arms. Of note, patients who received radiotherapy according to protocol guidelines for dose and volume had a superior local control rate (80%) compared with patients with major deviations (16% local control rate) or minor deviations (48% local control rate). Deviations in treatment volume seemed to be more critical. These results indicate that involved field radiation is an acceptable mode of local control for these patients, but that treatment to the initial tumor volume plus an adequate margin is necessary.

Several retrospective single institution case series have evaluated the impact of radiation dose on local control in Ewing's sarcoma.[440-442] In one series, patients treated with less than 49 Gy had a 5-year local control rate of 37% compared with 89% for patients treated with 49 Gy or more.[441] In this study, higher doses seemed particularly important for larger tumors. In another series, patients with larger tumors had a uniform local failure rate regardless of radiation dose, whereas patients with smaller tumors treated with more than 40 Gy had a higher local control rate compared with patients with smaller tumors treated with less than 40 Gy.[442] A third case series reported no difference in outcome between patients treated with radiation doses above and below 54 Gy.[440] The CESS-81 trial randomized extremity tumors to receive 46 or 60 Gy. The local failure rate was similar in these two groups.[394]

Three studies have specifically commented on the use of lower dose radiotherapy.[419,443,444] The first study administered approximately 30 Gy in patients mainly in conjunction with some type of surgical resection, although 5 patients received radiotherapy only.[443] No local failures were noted in this group. The other two studies administered 30 to 36 Gy as definitive local control to patients with an objective response to neoadjuvant chemotherapy.[419,444] This strategy resulted in an unacceptably high local failure rate.

The timing of radiotherapy may be important for patients receiving definitive radiotherapy and not for patients receiving radiotherapy following surgery. A retrospective analysis of patients treated with surgery followed by radiation therapy in the CESS-86 and EICESS-92 trials has demonstrated that the interval between surgery and radiation does not affect local control rate or event-free survival, even up to intervals beyond 90 days.[445] In contrast, a retrospective analysis of patients with pelvic Ewing's sarcoma has suggested that initiating definitive

radiotherapy earlier may result in a lower local failure rate.[446] A pooled analysis has also suggested that longer periods of neoadjuvant chemotherapy before starting radiation therapy may negatively affect overall survival.[447]

Two retrospective case series have evaluated hyperfractionated radiotherapy in the management of Ewing's sarcoma.[440,448] Both series concluded that local control rates were not improved by hyperfraction. One group reported better functional results with the hyperfractionated schedule.[448] The CESS-86 trial randomized patients to conventional or hyperfractionated radiation schedules.[449,450] Patients on the conventional schedule had chemotherapy held during radiotherapy, whereas patients on the hyperfractionated schedule continued to receive chemotherapy during radiation. For patients treated with radiotherapy alone, the local control rate was 82% for patients on the conventional schedule and 86% for patients on the hyperfractionated schedule. The radiation schedule did not affect overall or relapse-free survival. The radiation schedule did not affect disease control in patients treated with surgery followed by radiation.[450]

Based on this experience with radiotherapy for Ewing's sarcoma, current practice is for patients with unresectable tumors to receive definitive radiotherapy after four to six cycles of chemotherapy. Most groups administer 54.4 to 60 Gy as definitive radiotherapy. Patients typically receive treatment as 45 Gy to the pretreatment volume plus a safety margin of at least 2 cm, followed by a boost to full-dose radiotherapy to the treatment volume remaining after neoadjuvant chemotherapy.[436] Tumors with soft tissue extension, but not infiltration, into the chest or pelvic cavities often receive treatment to the postchemotherapy volume plus a safety margin. Some centers advise full-dose preoperative radiotherapy to tumors that may become fully resectable with such therapy. Patients with inadequate surgical margins are recommended to receive postoperative radiation. The EURO-EWING group has also recommended postoperative radiotherapy for patients with adequate surgical margins and a poor histologic response to chemotherapy, although this practice is not standard in North America. The EURO-EWING group has recommended a hyperfractionated schedule of radiotherapy, whereas the standard in North America remains conventional fractionation.

Several groups have compared the three available modes of local control—surgery, definitive radiation, and surgery plus radiation. A number of studies have clearly documented that patients who undergo surgical resection have higher local control rates and/or improved overall outcomes compared with patients who receive definitive radiotherapy only.* These studies must be interpreted with caution because of the presence of confounding by indication. For example, because small extremity tumors are typically selected for surgery and large axial tumors are typically managed with radiotherapy alone, the outcome between these two groups might be expected to be different because of reasons other than the chosen mode of local control. Not all studies have concluded that surgery provides superior disease control compared with radiation. A retrospective single-institution study of 76 patients with nonmetastatic Ewing's sarcoma has concluded that overall survival and rate of local control is equivalent among patients who received local control as surgery, radiation, or surgery plus radiation, although the power to detect a difference may have been limited by the small size of this study.[452] A secondary analysis of data from the UKCCSG ET-2 trial reached the

---

*References 305, 312, 315, 316, 320, 434, 435, 437, 450, and 451.

same conclusion.[453] In addition, the overall rate of disease recurrence did not differ among local control groups. In the SE 91-CNR Italian cooperative group trial, the 3-year event-free survival did not differ between patients who received surgery alone or radiotherapy alone.[397]

Although a randomized trial might resolve the issue of optimal mode of local control, such a randomization would be untenable to patients. Several analyses have evaluated this issue by attempting to control for the known confounding factors influencing both outcome and choice of local control modality. An analysis from the Rizzoli Institute has shown that patients treated with definitive radiotherapy have inferior event-free survival compared with patients treated with surgery alone, even after controlling for age, tumor size, and serum LDH level.[434] This group did not control for tumor site in this analysis. Two similar previous analyses by this same group controlled for tumor site, among other factors.[305,316] In these analyses, patients treated with radiotherapy did not have an increased risk of relapse.

The EICESS/CESS experience with local control has also been retrospectively reviewed in several analyses.[435,450,451] On univariate analyses, these studies have demonstrated that patients treated surgically have improved local control compared with patients treated with definitive radiotherapy. Although this group has not reported a multivariate analysis of outcome based on local control, they have reported a subgroup analysis based on tumor size (above and below 100 cm^3) and site (axial vs. appendicular).[451] Patients treated with radiation alone had inferior local control for all combinations of tumor size and site, except small central tumors. However, patients treated with surgery appeared to have a higher rate of systemic failure compared with patients treated with radiation alone, such that the overall rate of disease recurrence was the same between groups.[435,451] This finding has not been reported by other groups.

Systemic Treatment with Chemotherapy

The use of chemotherapy for patients with Ewing's sarcoma has revolutionized the care of these patients. Prior to the 1970s, standard therapy for this disease consisted solely of local control directed at the primary tumor. Most patients treated in this manner ultimately died from local or systemic recurrent disease.[454-456] In one series, patients treated with local control alone had a median survival of 11 months.[455] In the 1960s and 1970s, evidence emerged that systemic chemotherapy could prevent recurrent disease in a substantial number of patients with Ewing's sarcoma. This section reviews the development of modern chemotherapy regimens for this disease. Table 21-3 lists major chemotherapy regimens evaluated for Ewing's sarcoma, along with abbreviations for these regimens. Table 21-4 provides a summary of the major cooperative group trials that have contributed to current treatment approaches to this disease.

Early Improvements with Vincristine, Actinomycin D, Doxorubicin, and Cyclophosphamide

Given the poor outcomes observed with local control alone, investigators began using single-agent chemotherapy for Ewing's sarcoma. Although single-agent therapy did not substantially improve the long-term outcomes for these patients, these studies did identify a group of drugs capable of inducing tumor regression. Some of the most effective agents included vincristine, actinomycin D, doxorubicin, and cyclophosphamide. Investigators soon began to evaluate the use of these drugs in combination for patients with Ewing's sarcoma.

One group evaluated two different combinations—vincristine with cyclophosphamide given in 8-week cycles for five cycles and vincristine, actinomycin D, doxorubicin, and cyclophosphamide (VACA) given in weekly components for 18 months.[455] Most patients received radiotherapy as the mode of local control. In both regimens, chemotherapy and radiotherapy started simultaneously at the initiation of treatment. Patients who received either regimen had a statistically significant improvement in outcome compared with historic controls who received only local control, with a suggestion that the VACA regimen results in better outcomes than the vincristine-cyclophosphamide regimen.

Another group reported on 30 patients with nonmetastatic Ewing's sarcoma treated with 18 months of vincristine, doxorubicin, cyclophosphamide, and procarbazine.[456] Chemotherapy and radiotherapy were given concurrently at the start of therapy. The 6-year disease-free survival rate was 49%, which was a substantial improvement on outcomes in historical controls treated with radiotherapy alone.

The Memorial Sloan-Kettering Cancer Center treated 20 patients with localized Ewing's sarcoma with 18 to 20 months of VACA as adjuvant therapy.[457] The cumulative dose of doxorubicin on this study typically exceeded 500 mg/m^2, higher than in most other studies. The 5-year disease-free survival was 75%, perhaps highlighting the sensitivity of Ewing's sarcoma to doxorubicin. The cardiotoxicity associated with these doses of doxorubicin resulted in a reduction in the cumulative doxorubicin exposure in subsequent studies by this group.[458]

The St. Jude Children's Research Hospital has evaluated the use of neoadjuvant therapy with cyclophosphamide and doxorubicin for five cycles. An early report on this regimen reported that 19 of 23 evaluable patients had a complete response to therapy.[459] After these five cycles of neoadjuvant therapy, patients received local control, most commonly with radiotherapy. With the start of local control, patients began adjuvant therapy with vincristine and actinomycin D for approximately 11 weeks, followed by an additional six cycles of cyclophosphamide and doxorubicin. At the time of a follow-up report of 50 evaluable patients with nonmetastatic disease treated in this manner, 17 patients had developed recurrent disease.[419] A larger cooperative group study evaluating radiotherapy in Ewing's sarcoma used a similar chemotherapy regimen and reported a 5-year event-free survival of 51% in patients with nonmetastatic disease.[437]

The Rizzoli Institute performed a series of trials evaluating adjuvant (after local control) and neoadjuvant (prior to local control) VACA regimens. In the first trial, patients received adjuvant therapy with vincristine, doxorubicin, and cyclophosphamide (VDC) for 2 years.[454] At the time of diagnosis, patients began chemotherapy together with local control of the

TABLE 21-3	Major Chemotherapy Regimens Evaluated for Ewing's Sarcoma
Abbreviation	**Regimen**
VAC	Vincristine, actinomycin D, and cyclophosphamide
VACA	Vincristine, actinomycin D, cyclophosphamide, and doxorubicin
VDC	Vincristine, doxorubicin, and cyclophosphamide
IE	Ifosfamide and etoposide
VAI	Vincristine, actinomycin D, and ifosfamide
VDI	Vincristine, doxorubicin, and ifosfamide
VAIA	Vincristine, actinomycin D, ifosfamide, and doxorubicin
VIDE	Vincristine, ifosfamide, doxorubicin, and etoposide

TABLE 21-4	Outcome for Patients with Localized Ewing's Sarcoma of Bone in Cooperative Group Trials			
Trial	**Years**	**Regimen(s)**	**5-yr EFS or RFS**	**Reference**
VACA TRIALS				
IESS-1	1973-1978	VACA	60%	398
		VAC + WLI	44%	
		VAC	24%	
IESS-2	1978-1982	High-dose VACA	73% nonpelvic	462
			55% pelvic	478
		Protracted VACA	56% nonpelvic	462
First French	1978-1984	VACA	52% (4 yr)	400
UKCCSG ET-1	1978-1986	VACA	41%	312
CESS-81	1981-1985	VACA	55%	394
French EW88	1988-1991	Protracted VACA	58%	315
VACA/IE TRIALS				
Second French	1984-1987	VAI/VDI	52%	304
CESS-86	1986-1991	VAIA for high risk	53% (10 yr)	396
		VACA for low risk	49% (10 yr)	
UKCCSG ET-2	1987-1993	VAI/VDI	62%	399
INT-0091	1988-1992	VACA/IE	69%	320
		VACA	54%	
SSG IX	1990-1996	VDI/PDI	58%	313
Italian SE 91-CNR	1991-1997	VACA/IE	69%	397
EICESS-92	1992-1999	VAIA or VACA	Pending	
		VAIA or VAIAE	Pending	
DOSE-INTENSIFIED VACA/IE TRIALS				
INT-0154	1995-1998	VACA/IE standard	76% (3 yr)	470
		VACA/IE intensified	74% (3 yr)	
AEWS0031	2001-2005	VACA/IE 3 wk	Pending	
		VACA/IE 2 wk	Pending	
EURO-EWING 99	Ongoing	VIDE	Ongoing	

EFS = event-free survival; PDI = cisplatin, doxorubicin, and ifosfamide; RFS = relapse-free survival; VAIAE = vincristine, actinomycin D, ifosfamide, doxorubicin, and etoposide; WLI = whole-lung irradiation. See also Table 21-3 for additional abbreviations.

primary tumor. In the 85 patients with localized disease treated in this manner, the 5-year event-free survival was 34%.[311] In contrast, only 5% of historical controls treated with local control only remained continuously disease-free.[454] The successor study treated 59 patients with localized disease with 18 months of VACA.[460] In this study, the 5-year event-free survival was 59%, suggesting a benefit to the addition of actinomycin D. The next study by this group evaluated VDC given as three neoadjuvant cycles followed by VACA chemotherapy after local control for a total of 15 months.[311,461] The 5-year event-free survival for the 108 patients with localized disease treated on this study was 49%. Compared with VACA given exclusively as adjuvant therapy, this result suggests that the change to neoadjuvant therapy did not improve outcomes for these patients.

Based on these promising results, several cooperative groups set out to evaluate vincristine, actinomycin D, and cyclophosphamide (VAC) and VACA regimens in large groups of uniformly treated patients. The first North American Intergroup Ewing's Sarcoma Study (IESS-1) was the first randomized study in patients with Ewing's sarcoma.[398] This study enrolled patients from 1973 to 1978. The 342 patients with nonmetastatic Ewing's sarcoma were randomized to one of three treatment arms. Patients in the first and second treatment arms received VAC, with patients in the second treatment arm also receiving prophylactic whole-lung irradiation. Patients in the third treatment arm received VAC plus doxorubicin. Patients in this arm received doxorubicin every 12 weeks and actinomycin D every 12 weeks, so that they received one of these agents every 6 weeks. Patients in the VAC arms received actinomycin D every 12 weeks. All patients received radiotherapy to the primary tumor. Patients who received doxoru-

bicin had a 5-year relapse-free survival of 60% compared with 24% for patients who received VAC only. Patients who received VAC with whole-lung irradiation had an intermediate 5-year relapse-free survival of 44%. These results indicated that the addition of doxorubicin to VAC significantly improves outcomes compared with VAC alone or VAC with whole-lung irradiation. The contribution of increased dose intensity in the doxorubicin arm to this improved outcome is not clear. Subgroup analysis has shown that outcomes are inferior for patients with pelvic primary tumors and do not differ by treatment arm for these patients. Doxorubicin performed as well as whole-lung irradiation in preventing lung metastasis. Based on these results, four-drug therapy with VACA has become the standard chemotherapy approach for patients with Ewing's sarcoma.

The IESS-2 study expanded on these results by randomizing patients with nonmetastatic disease not involving the pelvis to two different VACA dosing schedules.[462] Patients on one schedule received cycles of therapy every 3 weeks, and patients on the other schedule received more moderate doses of the same drugs at more frequent intervals. All patients received treatment for approximately 20 months. A total of 214 patients were enrolled on this study from 1978 to 1982. The 5-year relapse-free survival for patients with nonpelvic tumors who received higher dose intermittent VACA was 73% compared with 56% for patients who received more protracted VACA. Overall survival results have shown a similar pattern. These results indicate a significant survival advantage for the higher dose intermittent dosing schedule, at least for patients with tumors arising outside the pelvis.

The first German cooperative group trial for this disease (CESS-81) also used VACA given as 3-week cycles.[394] This trial enrolled 93 patients with nonmetastatic disease from 1981 to 1985. Treatment duration was only 10 months, which was shorter than treatment on the IESS protocols. The 5-year disease-free survival was 55%, including patients with pelvic tumors. This result is similar to the outcome of VACA-treated patients in IESS-1, which also included patients with pelvic tumors. This result suggested that a shorter treatment duration using higher dose every 3-week cycles of therapy does not compromise outcome.

The first Ewing's sarcoma study of the United Kingdom Children's Cancer Study Group (UKCCSG ET-1) sought to standardize the treatment of newly diagnosed Ewing's sarcoma using VACA-based chemotherapy.[312] This nonrandomized trial enrolled 142 patients from 1978 to 1986. Patients received one or two induction cycles of chemotherapy with VDC. Local therapy, with a preference for definitive radiotherapy, was administered next while patients received weekly cyclophosphamide and vincristine. Patients then received cycles of VDC alternating every 3 weeks with VAC, for a total of 1 year of therapy. The 5-year relapse-free survival was 41% and the 5-year overall survival was 44% for patients with nonmetastatic disease. The study authors have suggested that the inferior outcome in this trial compared with other VACA-based trials at the time may be partly the result of decreased early doxorubicin dose intensity.[312]

The first French cooperative group study of Ewing's sarcoma also used VACA-based chemotherapy as well as radiotherapy as the preferred mode of local control.[400] This study took place between 1978 and 1984. Patients received cycles of VDC alternating with VAC, for a total of 16 months of treatment. The 4-year disease-free survival for patients with nonmetastatic disease was 52%.

A follow-up French cooperative group study (EW88) enrolled 141 patients with nonmetastatic disease from 1988 to 1991.[315] This study administered cyclophosphamide in a more protracted manner, following a regimen piloted at St. Jude's Children's Research Hospital in the 1970s. Patients received initial chemotherapy with cyclophosphamide given daily for 7 days followed by doxorubicin on day 8. Patients received five cycles of this therapy before proceeding to local control. Surgery was recommended when possible. Radiotherapy was reserved for patients with unresectable tumors, incompletely resected tumors, or tumors with more than 5% viable tumor following initial chemotherapy. Following local control, patients received vincristine and actinomycin D for 12 weeks, followed by six additional cycles of cyclophosphamide and doxorubicin using the same schedule used neoadjuvantly. Using these standard four drugs in this manner resulted in a 5-year disease-free survival of 58%.

Addition of Ifosfamide and Ifosfamide plus Etoposide to VACA-Based Therapy

An initial report from the U.S. National Cancer Institute (NCI) has demonstrated a response rate of 45% in patients with recurrent Ewing's sarcoma treated with a 5-day course of ifosfamide.[463] A follow-up study by this group evaluated ifosfamide combined with etoposide (IE) for patients with recurrent pediatric tumors.[464] Of the 17 evaluable patients with recurrent Ewing's sarcoma included in the preliminary report, 16 patients had a partial response to therapy, for a response rate of 94%. A larger cooperative group study sponsored by the Pediatric Oncology Group included 55 patients with recurrent Ewing's sarcoma treated with ifosfamide and etoposide.[465] The response rate in this study was 25%. Based on these promising results in patients with recurrent disease, the St. Jude Children's Research Hospital has evaluated IE in patients with newly diagnosed high-risk disease.[466] This group gave three cycles of

IE as an initial window before proceeding with doxorubicin and cyclophosphamide chemotherapy. Only 1 of 26 patients failed to respond to IE, for a response rate of 95%.

A number of single-institution studies have incorporated ifosfamide and etoposide into the VACA backbone of therapy for newly diagnosed patients. One study from the NCI administered IE alternating with VDC or VAC for a total of 18 3-week cycles.[467] Ifosfamide was administered before and after local control. A total of 31 patients with nonmetastatic disease were treated and had a 5-year event-free survival of 64%. This outcome was significantly better than historical controls with nonmetastatic disease treated with VDC and whole-body irradiation with stem cell rescue. Two studies from the Rizzoli Institute introduced ifosfamide at different times and reached different conclusions. In the REN-2 study, patients with localized disease received ifosfamide for the first time after local control.[461] The cumulative ifosfamide dose was 54 g/m^2. The 5-year event-free survival for the 82 patients treated was 51%. This result was not different from historical controls treated with VACA-based therapy. In the REN-3 study, ifosfamide was introduced prior to local control, with the cumulative dose held constant at 54 g/m^2.[311] The 157 patients with nonmetastatic disease had a 5-year event-free survival of 71%, which was significantly better than any of the previous chemotherapy regimens evaluated at their center. These results suggest that early introduction of ifosfamide may improve outcome.

Several cooperative group studies have evaluated the efficacy of ifosfamide with and without etoposide. One of the first cooperative group studies incorporating ifosfamide was the second French cooperative group study of Ewing's sarcoma.[304] Patients were enrolled from 1984 to 1987 and received initial therapy with alternating 3-week cycles of vincristine, actinomycin D, and ifosfamide (VAI) and vincristine, doxorubicin, and ifosfamide (VDI) for a total of six cycles. Patients then underwent local control, with a preference for complete surgical resection. All patients were to receive radiotherapy, with the dose dependent on the extent of surgical resection. During radiotherapy, patients received two cycles of vincristine with doxorubicin and two cycles of vincristine with ifosfamide. Following local control, patients received alternating 3-week cycles of VAI and vincristine with doxorubicin to complete a total of 1 year of therapy. The 5-year disease-free survival was 52% for patients with nonmetastatic disease. This result prompted this group to conclude that substituting ifosfamide for cyclophosphamide does not improve outcomes. In addition, patients in this study had a higher than expected incidence of diminished cardiac function, prompting early closure of the study.

The CESS-86 trial was the first cooperative group attempt to risk-stratify patients and alter therapy based on risk.[396] Patients with small (less than 100-mL tumor volume) extremity tumors received VACA given as 3-week cycles for 36 weeks. Patients with large (larger than 100-mL) tumors or axial tumors received identical therapy, except ifosfamide was substituted for cyclophosphamide (VAIA). For the 301 nonmetastatic patients treated in this study, the 10-year event-free survival did not differ between patients who received VACA or VAIA (49% and 53%, respectively). However, multivariate analysis has demonstrated that, controlling for tumor size and site, VACA chemotherapy is less effective than VAIA.

The UKCCSG ET-2 study evaluated the substitution of ifosfamide for cyclophosphamide in newly diagnosed patients.[399] This nonrandomized trial enrolled 243 patients from 1987 to 1993. Patients received VDI for four 3-week cycles before undergoing local control. In contrast to ET-1, ET-2 suggested a preference for surgery as the mode of local control. Following local control, patients received VAI to complete 1 year of therapy. Patients received a cumulative doxorubicin dose of 420 mg/m^2 and a cumulative ifosfamide dose of 114 g/m^2. The

5-year relapse-free survival was 62% for patients with nonmetastatic disease. These results demonstrate a substantial improvement over the results of the UKCCSG ET-1 study. These improvements may be the result of increased doxorubicin dose intensity, use of ifosfamide, preference for surgery as local control, or a combination of these factors.

An Italian cooperative group study (SE 91-CNR) enrolled patients with nonmetastatic Ewing's sarcoma from 1991 to 1997.[397] Patients treated by this protocol received initial therapy with alternating 3-week cycles of VDC and VAI. After 24 weeks of therapy, patients received alternating 3-week cycles of IE and VAC to complete 36 total weeks of therapy. Surgery was the preferred mode of local control for resectable tumors. The 5-year event-free survival was 69.4%.

A Scandinavian Sarcoma Group trial (SSG IX) enrolled patients with metastatic and nonmetastatic Ewing's sarcoma from 1990 to 1996.[313] All patients received 35 weeks of chemotherapy given as 3-week cycles. Patients received cycles of VDI every 3 weeks, with cisplatin, doxorubicin, and ifosfamide substituted at cycles 2, 5, 8, and 11. Surgery was the preferred mode of local control. The 5-year metastasis-free survival was 58% for patients with initially nonmetastatic disease. The 5-year overall survival for these patients was 70%. The 5-year overall survival for patients presenting with metastatic disease was 28%. These results compare favorably to those of other contemporary trials.

Two randomized cooperative group trials have directly compared VACA-based chemotherapy to ifosfamide-containing chemotherapy. The North American intergroup study INT-0091 enrolled 518 patients with metastatic and nonmetastatic Ewing's sarcoma from 1988 to 1992.[320] The standard arm of this study consisted of 3-week cycles of VDC. The experimental arm consisted of 3-week cycles of VDC alternating with IE. In both treatment arms, actinomycin-D was substituted for doxorubicin after a cumulative doxorubicin dose of 375 mg/m^2. All patients received 17 cycles of therapy, for a total study duration of 49 weeks. Local control occurred at week 12 of the therapy, with the mode of local control determined on an individualized basis. The addition of IE significantly improved the outcome for patients with nonmetastatic disease, with a 5-year event-free survival of 69% compared with 54% for patients receiving VDC only. The incidence of local failure was also lower for patients who received IE, indicating that improved systemic therapy also improves local control. Based on these results, the combination of VDC and IE has become the standard therapy for patients with nonmetastatic Ewing's sarcoma treated in North America.

The EICESS-92 study represented a collaborative effort between the UKCCSG and German cooperative groups. This trial enrolled patients with localized and metastatic Ewing's sarcoma from 1992 to 1999. Patients with small (less than 100-mL tumor volume) localized tumors were deemed as standard risk. These patients received initial chemotherapy with VAIA given as 3-week cycles followed by a randomization between continued VAIA or VACA. All other patients were deemed high risk and were randomized to receive VAIA or VAIA plus etoposide. The final results of this trial have not yet been reported, although a preliminary report has demonstrated no difference in outcome for either randomization.[468]

Dose-Intensified VACA/IE Regimens

The next generation of chemotherapy regimens has focused on increasing the dose intensity of known active agents in this disease. The P6 protocol from the Memorial Sloan-Kettering Cancer Center used an augmented dose of cyclophosphamide given in combination with vincristine and standard-dose doxorubicin.[469] Patients received a total of seven cycles of alternating

VDC and IE together with local control of the primary tumor. The 4-year event-free survival for the 44 patients with localized disease was 82%, suggesting an improvement in outcome with higher dose cyclophosphamide.

Two North American cooperative group studies have investigated strategies for dose-intensifying therapy. The first trial, known as INT-0154, enrolled 492 patients with nonmetastatic Ewing's sarcoma from 1995 to 1998. Patients were randomized to receive alternating 3-week cycles of VDC and IE using a dose-intensified or standard-dose approach. The standard-dose arm emulated the therapy given to patients assigned to the experimental arm of INT-0091. Patients on the dose-intensified arm received higher individual doses of the alkylating agents than patients on the standard-dose arm, but cumulative drug doses were approximately equivalent between arms. Patients on the dose-intensified arm completed therapy in 30 weeks, whereas patients on the standard-dose arm completed therapy in 48 weeks. Although the final results of this study have not yet been reported, a preliminary analysis has reported a 3-year event-free survival of 74% for patients on the dose-intensified arm and 76% for patients on the standard-dose arm.[470]

In the Children's Oncology Group protocol AEWS0031, patients with nonmetastatic Ewing's sarcoma were randomized to receive cycles of VDC and IE alternating every 3 weeks or every 2 weeks. Individual and cumulative drug doses were equivalent between treatment arms. All patients received 14 cycles of therapy, requiring 42 weeks in the standard arm and 28 weeks in the interval compression arm. This trial enrolled patients from 2001 to 2005. Preliminary results of this trial indicate that patients assigned to the interval compression arm had a superior event-free survival compared with patients in the standard arm, and this approach has now become standard for North American patients with localized tumors, pending final publication of the results.

Several groups have evaluated chemotherapy regimens that combine multiple active agents given together during a cycle of therapy. In a protocol at St. Jude Children's Research Hospital, patients received ifosfamide, etoposide, cyclophosphamide, and doxorubicin given together for three cycles prior to local control.[471] Patients then received alternating cycles of IE and cyclophosphamide with doxorubicin, for a total of 41 weeks of therapy. The doses of ifosfamide, etoposide, and cyclophosphamide given after local control were higher than in previous studies. Patients were able to complete the planned neoadjuvant therapy, but myelosuppression limited the ability of patients to receive the planned adjuvant therapy on schedule. Specifically, only 66% of patients received all planned chemotherapy and only 25% of patients received all planned chemotherapy on schedule. Despite difficulties in achieving the desired degree of dose intensification, outcomes remained favorable. The 3-year event-free survival for patients with localized disease was 78%.

A British group has piloted the use of vincristine, ifosfamide, doxorubicin, and etoposide (VIDE) as neoadjuvant therapy for this disease.[472] Thirty patients with newly diagnosed Ewing's sarcoma were treated with six 3-week cycles of VIDE. Because of hematologic toxicity, etoposide was dose-reduced or omitted from 50% of the planned cycles. All attempts at collecting peripheral blood stem cells following a cycle of VIDE were successful. Of the 24 patients evaluable for radiographic response, only 1 patient had progressive disease. Patients in this pilot study received additional therapy following local control. The final results of this study are not yet available.

The European cooperative groups have initiated a combined trial known as EURO-EWING 99 that relies on VIDE as neoadjuvant therapy. All patients receive initial treatment with six 3-week cycles of VIDE. This trial then tailors therapy based on risk. Patients with small (less than 200-mL tumor volume) nonmetastatic tumors with good chemotherapy response are randomized to receive additional therapy with seven cycles of VAC or VAI. Patients with large tumors, pulmonary metastases, or poor chemotherapy response are randomized to receive additional therapy with seven cycles of VAI or high-dose therapy with stem cell rescue (see later).

Management of Tumors Arising at Special Sites

Pelvic Ewing's Sarcoma

Ewing's sarcoma frequently arises in the pelvis. These pelvic tumors tend be large and associated with crucial viscera, nerves, and bones (particularly of the acetabulum), making complete surgical resection difficult. The local failure rate for patients with pelvic primary tumors ranges from 15% to 27%, which is higher than the local failure rate typically reported for appendicular tumors.[473-477] In one large series, even after excluding patients with a local relapse, the outcome for patients with pelvic primary tumors was still inferior to outcomes at other sites.[474] This result suggests that systemic and local control are inadequate for these patients.

Recognizing the poor outcome of patients with pelvic primary tumors, the IESS-2 trial has nonrandomly assigned patients to the higher dose intermittent schedule VACA arm of that study.[478] In addition, an increased emphasis was placed on surgical control of pelvic tumors. With this strategy, patients with pelvic tumors had a 5-year relapse-free survival of 55% compared with only 23% on IESS-1. Because the higher dose VACA arm resulted in better outcomes in the randomized nonpelvic patients treated in IESS-2, the improvements in outcome seen in patients with pelvic tumors may have been the result of better systemic control, better local control, or both. Indeed, patients with pelvic tumors in IESS-2 were more likely to undergo complete surgical resection and had a lower local failure rate compared with patients with pelvic tumors in IESS-1. Compared with patients who did not have a complete resection, complete resection did not improve the overall or relapse-free survival in these patients in IESS-2.[478]

The optimal mode of local control for pelvic tumors has been difficult to determine with rigorous studies. A report from the Mayo Clinic has found that patients with pelvic Ewing's sarcoma treated with surgery have a statistically significant superior overall survival compared with patients treated without surgery.[479] In several other series of patients with pelvic primary tumors, the mode of local control has not clearly been shown to affect outcome,[474-476,480] although some trends have suggested improvements in survival in patients treated surgically. Some groups have also reported a trend toward a lower local recurrence rate in patients treated surgically,[446,474,475,479] although not all groups have reported this trend.[476] The results of these studies are often difficult to evaluate because patients treated with complete surgical resection typically have small resectable tumors. However, two groups have attempted to control for this and other confounding factors. The French cooperative group has reported on 53 patients with pelvic Ewing's sarcoma.[481] After controlling for size and other potentially confounding factors, patients treated with radiotherapy alone had an increased risk of recurrence and death compared with patients who received surgery or surgery with radiotherapy. The COG retrospectively analyzed 75 patients with pelvic primary tumors treated in INT-0091.[477] In contrast to the results of the French group, the mode of local control did not affect event-free survival or local failure after controlling for confounding factors such as size. As observed in the main analysis of all tumor sites, patients with pelvic tumors who were randomized

to receive VACA plus IE on this study had a lower risk of local failure compared with patients randomized to receive VACA alone.[477] Given this uncertainty and the risk of second tumors from radiotherapy, many groups have chosen to resect pelvic tumors that can be resected without functional consequences. For tumors that cannot be resected without functional consequences, options include definitive radiotherapy alone or preoperative radiotherapy, with the possible addition of wide resection.

Chest Wall Ewing's Sarcoma

Chest wall tumors also require specialized management, particularly because these tumors often invade the pleura or have associated pleural effusions. Some evidence has suggested that surgical resection of chest wall tumors provides superior local control, although these analyses do not account for differences in tumor size that influence resectability.[482,483] Other analyses have not shown a difference in outcome based on mode of local control for chest wall tumors.[484-486] Results from INT-0091 and INT-0154 have indicated that neoadjuvant chemotherapy prior to attempted resection of a chest wall tumor increases the likelihood of obtaining negative margins compared with results from attempted resection prior to chemotherapy. Delayed resection at this site therefore decreases the need for postoperative radiotherapy in these patients. Avoiding chest wall radiation is particularly appealing, given the added pulmonary and cardiac toxicities associated with this therapy.

Although several reports have suggested that an associated pleural effusion does not worsen outcome, patients with chest wall tumors and pleural effusions are often recommended to receive hemithorax irradiation on these studies.[483,484,487] A report from the French cooperative group has suggested that patients with rib primary tumors and an associated pleural effusion have an increased risk of local relapse without radiotherapy.[484] In the EICESS/CESS studies, patients who received hemithorax irradiation had more unfavorable features than patients who did not receive hemithorax irradiation.[488] Despite this difference, the rate of local relapse was the same in both groups, whereas the rate of systemic relapse was higher in the group of patients who did not receive hemithorax irradiation. This result may be interpreted as evidence of direct benefit of hemithorax irradiation in preventing dissemination of residual tumor cells from the pleural space. Alternatively, hemithorax irradiation may reduce the volume of lung at risk for subsequent relapse, because the IESS-1 trial noted that whole-lung irradiation can prevent lung metastasis in patients with initially nonmetastatic disease. Patients with chest wall primary tumors and positive pleural fluid cytology or pleural-based nodules treated by the most recent Children's Oncology Group protocol received hemithorax radiation.

Ewing's Sarcoma of the Spine

Management of patients with tumors arising along the spinal column require careful planning by a multidisciplinary team, including oncologists, radiation oncologists, orthopedic surgeons, general surgeons, and neurosurgeons. Small case series have suggested that local control and overall outcomes for patients with primary tumors at this site do not differ from outcomes for patients with tumors arising from other sites.[310,489] One group reported that sacral primary tumors fare less well than other vertebral tumors,[309] although this result was not replicated in other series.[307,308,310] The largest reported experience with vertebral Ewing's sarcoma comes from the EICESS/CESS studies.[490] A total of 116 patients had tumors arising from cervical, thoracic, or lumbar vertebrae. Given difficulties in obtaining a complete resection at this site, all but 4 patients received radiotherapy as part of local control of the tumor. The local failure rate for patients treated with radiotherapy alone did not differ from that of patients treated with surgery plus radiotherapy (22.6% and 18.7%, respectively). Local relapses typically occurred in the radiation field, suggesting that inadequate selection of radiotherapy fields was not to blame for these local relapses. Despite the fact that the spinal cord limits radiotherapy dosing at this site, the local failure rate for patients with vertebral tumors treated with radiotherapy alone was not higher than the local failure rate for patients with tumors of any location treated with radiotherapy alone.[451,490] This effect may be the result of the generally smaller size of paraspinal tumors compared with other tumors selected for local control with definitive radiotherapy. Of note, however, patients with a vertebral tumor treated with radiotherapy who recur locally often have few local control options, because additional radiotherapy may compromise the spinal cord.[490]

Outcomes

Patients with Ewing's sarcoma have shown great improvements in outcome over the past 4 decades. For patients with localized tumors, expected survival rates have increased to more than 70% with modern multimodality therapy. Figure 21-8 demonstrates these improvements graphically, using SEER data from 1975 to 2000. A similar pattern of steady improvement over time has also been reported using data from a large European registry.[491]

Metastatic Ewing's Sarcoma

Systemic Therapy

Despite a recognition that these patients have a poor prognosis, early studies often treated patients with metastatic disease with the same combined modality therapy used for nonmetastatic patients. Because the outcomes in these patients have not improved in concert with the gains seen in nonmetastatic patients, more aggressive strategies have been added to this backbone. These strategies are discussed here.

Attempts to improve outcomes for these patients through changes in chemotherapy regimens have been largely unsuccessful. The IESS-2 study attempted to improve on the 30%

5-year overall survival for metastatic patients treated in IESS-1.[323] This group added 5-fluorouracil to the VACA backbone of IESS-1. As in IESS-1, radiation to all metastatic sites was prescribed. The 5-year overall survival was 28%, despite the addition of 5-fluorouracil. Single-institution studies have suggested that the addition of IE to VACA does not improve the outcome for patients with initially metastatic disease.[467,469,471] The INT-0091 study has confirmed these disappointing results.[320,324] The Pediatric Oncology Group and Children's Cancer Group have conducted a phase II study alkylator-intensive chemotherapy for patients with newly diagnosed metastatic disease.[492] Patients in this study received topotecan or topotecan plus cyclophosphamide in an up-front window. Following the window phase, patients received IE alternating with VDC, using higher doses of ifosfamide and cyclophosphamide than were used in INT-0091. This strategy did not improve the outcomes for these patients. A regimen developed in Seattle has combined vincristine, doxorubicin, cyclophosphamide, ifosfamide, and etoposide given together each cycle.[493] All five patients with metastatic Ewing's sarcoma and evaluable disease obtained a complete radiographic response to this therapy. Only one of these patients remained disease-free 33 months from initial diagnosis. Results are not yet available for more recent studies attempting to improve outcomes for these patients by altering their chemotherapy regimens.

Patients with metastatic disease at initial diagnosis are candidates for novel approaches to the treatment of Ewing's sarcoma. The Children's Oncology Group has been evaluating the addition of metronomic chemotherapy with vinblastine and celecoxib to the VACA/IE backbone used in INT-0091. This approach uses an antiangiogenic approach together with known active cytotoxic chemotherapy in an attempt to improve the outcome for these patients. Patients with metastatic disease who do not respond to initial therapy may receive second-line chemotherapy (described below for patients with recurrent disease) and may also be candidates for other investigational therapies, including high-dose therapy with hematopoietic stem cell rescue (see later).

Role of Surgery and Radiation

Patients presenting with metastatic disease typically receive local control of their primary tumor. Because of their disseminated disease and poor prognosis, the local control strategy for these patients tends to be different from patients with nonmetastatic disease. In particular, patients with metastatic disease are more likely to receive definitive radiotherapy for local control because they often require radiotherapy to other sites of disease. Thus, surgical local control does not spare these patients from exposure to radiotherapy.

Whole-lung irradiation appears to be an effective therapy for patients with lung metastases. The St. Jude Children's Research Hospital has reported on patients at their center with lung metastases at initial diagnosis. Patients in this series received whole-lung irradiation if they had residual lung metastases following initial chemotherapy. Patients in this series who received whole-lung irradiation for residual lung metastases had an equivalent outcome to those patients whose lung metastases resolved with initial chemotherapy and who did not undergo whole-lung irradiation.[494] The authors argued that the patients with residual lung metastases after initial chemotherapy would have had an even worse outcome without the addition of whole-lung irradiation. Data from the CESS studies have suggested that a dose-response relationship may exist for whole-lung irradiation.[495] This group reported that patients with initial lung metastases who remained in clinical remission had received higher doses of whole-lung irradiation than patients who relapsed. The number of patients reported in this series was

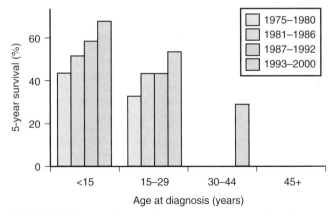

FIGURE 21-8. Overall survival rates at 5 years from initial diagnosis of Ewing's sarcoma according to age at initial diagnosis and treatment era (SEER data, 1975-2000). (*Adapted from Gurney JG, Swensen AR, Bulterys M: Malignant bone tumors. In Ries L, Smith M, Gurney JG, et al (eds). Cancer Incidence and Survival among Children and Adolescents: United States SEER Program 1975-1995. Bethesda, Md, National Cancer Institute, 1999, pp 99-110.*)

small, but the group reported that 4 of 10 patients who received 12 to 16 Gy remained in remission compared with 5 of 6 patients who received 18 to 21 Gy. Only 1 of 6 patients who did not receive whole-lung irradiation remained in clinical remission.[495]

The strongest evidence in favor of whole-lung irradiation for patients with lung metastases has come from the EICESS group. This group reported on 100 evaluable patients with isolated lung metastases, 75 of whom received 15- to 18-Gy whole-lung irradiation as part of their combined modality therapy.[319] The risk of pulmonary recurrence was significantly decreased with the addition of whole-lung irradiation. In addition, the overall risk of disease recurrence diminished with this intervention. The 5-year event-free survival for patients treated with whole-lung irradiation was 38% compared with 27% for patients who did not receive whole-lung irradiation. This result is even more striking when one notes that the indication for whole-lung irradiation in this trial was residual lung metastasis after chemotherapy. Although whole-lung irradiation was not prescribed in a randomized manner, potential confounding variables appeared to be balanced between patients who did and patients who did not receive whole-lung irradiation. In addition, a Cox regression model has indicated that whole-lung irradiation improves event-free survival after controlling for potential confounding variables.[319] An additional report from the EICESS group has indicated that whole-lung irradiation improves the outcome, even for patients with lung metastases combined with metastases at other sites.[322] Currently, whole-lung irradiation is commonly being used for patients with lung metastases at initial presentation, regardless of the radiographic response to initial chemotherapy. Patients with bone metastases also typically receive radiotherapy directed to these sites, although data supporting this strategy are lacking.

Pulmonary metastectomy plays little role in the management of patients with lung metastases at initial diagnosis. One small case series has suggested that pulmonary metastectomy might improve the outcome for these patients, although this result was confounded by the fact that only patients with resectable lung metastases underwent resection.[496] Surgical resection of pulmonary metastases was not shown to improve outcomes in patients treated by the EICESS group who had residual lung metastases after initial chemotherapy.[319]

Role of High-Dose Therapy with Hematopoietic Stem Cell Rescue

Patients with initially metastatic Ewing's sarcoma may be candidates for high-dose therapy with stem cell rescue. The role of high-dose therapy for these patients remains unclear. In most cases, patients have received autologous bone marrow or peripheral blood stem cells, although some groups have explored allogeneic transplantation for this disease. Numerous groups have demonstrated the feasibility of delivering myeloablative therapy as consolidation therapy after initial chemotherapy and local control in these high-risk patients. No completed studies have evaluated high-dose therapy in a randomized manner. As such, studies suggesting a benefit from this modality are subject to selection bias, in which only patients with good overall physical condition who attain a certain level of disease control are considered for high-dose therapy. Results from larger single-institution and multicenter studies are summarized here.

Two American groups carried out early studies of the use of 8-Gy whole-body irradiation with autologous bone marrow rescue as consolidation for patients with high-risk Ewing's sarcoma.[497,498] Patients received VDC with or without actinomycin D as initial chemotherapy, along with radiotherapy to their primary site. Patients who attained a complete response to this therapy proceeded to consolidation therapy. Despite selecting therapy-responsive patients, high-dose therapy did not improve the outcome for patients with metastatic disease. The 6-year overall survival for patients with metastatic disease in one study was only 14%.[498]

Two EICESS centers have evaluated 12-Gy whole-body irradiation combined with melphalan and etoposide as consolidation therapy in patients with bone metastases or early relapsed disease.[499,500] Patients in this series received either an autologous or allogeneic transplant if they had responded favorably to initial chemotherapy. Although an initial report has shown a relapse rate of only 52%, a follow-up report indicated that the event-free survival from the time of transplant for this cohort of patients was 24%. The outcome did not differ significantly between patients who received autologous or allogeneic stem cells, although patients who underwent allogeneic transplant had a higher rate of complications. A follow-up study from this same group has evaluated two consolidation courses of myeloablative melphalan and etoposide in 17 patients with bone metastases.[501] The 5-year event-free survival for these patients was 21%.

A later Children's Cancer Group study evaluated melphalan, etoposide, and 12-Gy whole-body irradiation for patients with newly diagnosed Ewing's sarcoma with bone or bone marrow metastases.[502] These patients received VDC alternating with IE for five cycles along with radiotherapy to their primary tumor and bone metastases. Patients with a complete response or a very good partial response to initial therapy received the planned myeloablative therapy. The 2-year event-free survival for all patients enrolled in this study was 20%. For the group of patients who were able to receive myeloablative therapy, the 2-year event-free survival was 24%. The outcome did not differ from a cohort of historical controls treated on protocol INT-0091. As such, the authors concluded that myeloablative therapy does not improve the outcome for patients with bone and bone marrow metastases.

A French multicenter trial prospectively has evaluated the role of high-dose therapy in patients with newly diagnosed metastatic disease.[392] Patients in this trial received initial chemotherapy with cyclophosphamide and doxorubicin alternating with IE. Of the 97 patients enrolled in the study, 75 patients had a favorable response to initial therapy and proceeded to consolidation therapy with busulfan and melphalan, followed by stem cell rescue. The 5-year event-free survival was 37% for all 97 patients and 47% for the 75 patients who received high-dose therapy. Much of the improvement from high-dose therapy appeared to be in patients with isolated lung metastases. These patients had a 5-year event-free survival of 52% compared with 24% of patients with metastases involving other sites.

A report of 171 patients treated by the EICESS group has indicated that high-dose therapy does not improve the outcome in patients with metastatic disease at initial diagnosis.[322] Further analysis has suggested that patients with multiple sites of metastases require some form of intensified therapy, either as high-dose therapy or whole-lung irradiation. The 4-year event-free survival for patients with multiple metastatic sites treated with high-dose therapy, whole-lung irradiation, or both modalities was 27% compared with 0% for patients who did not receive at least one form of intensified therapy.[322]

The only randomized study of high-dose therapy compared with other treatment for high-risk patients is ongoing. This trial, known as the EURO-EWING 99 study, has randomized newly diagnosed high-risk patients to receive consolidation therapy with busulfan and melphalan followed by stem cell rescue or continuation chemotherapy. Patients on this study with isolated pulmonary metastases are randomized to consolidation therapy with high-dose chemotherapy and stem cell rescue or to continuation chemotherapy followed by whole-lung irradiation. Patients with metastases beyond the lung are nonrandomly assigned to high-dose chemotherapy with stem cell rescue. Of note, patients with nonmetastatic disease with a poor response to neoadjuvant chemotherapy are also randomized to high-dose chemotherapy or to continuation chemotherapy. Results of this trial will not be available for several years.

The use of autologous stem cell infusion raises the concern of reinfusion of Ewing's cells contaminating the stem cell product. Several groups have investigated this issue using PCR techniques, with mixed results. The incidence of tumor cell contamination has ranged from 6% to 100% of pheresis products, depending on the study.[503-506] The largest and most recent evaluation of this issue studied 88 patients with high-risk Ewing's sarcoma treated with high-dose therapy with stem cell rescue.[506] Only seven patients had tumor cell contamination of their infused product. The outcome of these seven patients did not appear to differ from the outcome of patients without tumor cell contamination of their infused product.

Outcomes

Despite improvements in outcomes for patients with nonmetastatic disease over time, outcomes for patients with initially metastatic disease have not seen a similar improvement. Most reports have suggested that no more than 30% of patients with metastatic Ewing's sarcoma are long-term survivors, although this number may be slightly higher for patients with isolated lung metastases.[319,324] Even with combined modality therapy, many patients never attain a complete remission. One recent study has reported a complete response rate of only 43% after chemotherapy, surgery, and/or radiation for these patients.[492] As such, a number of these patients have treatment-refractory disease. For those patients who do attain a complete remission, disease recurrence remains a major barrier to durable cure.

Recurrent Ewing's Sarcoma

Location and Timing of Disease Recurrence

Among patients with disease recurrence, recurrence involving distant sites is more common than isolated local recurrence. Isolated distant relapse accounts for 48% to 71% of recurrences.[320,507-510] Another 10% to 29% of recurrences are combined local plus distant recurrences, but estimates of isolated local recurrence have varied widely among studies, ranging from 11% to 35%. Most initial distant relapses involve the lung and/or bones.[507,508]

Most episodes of disease recurrence occur once patients have completed their planned initial therapy. Disease recurrence within 2 years of initial diagnosis is more common than later recurrence. The median time to disease recurrence across several series has ranged from 17 to 27 months.[507-510] An analysis of data from the UKCCSG ET-1 and ET-2 studies has indicated that patients have a relatively stable rate of death during the first 2 years after diagnosis.[511] Between 2 and 5 years after diagnosis, the rate of death is lower but remains relatively constant during this interval. Only after 5 years from initial diagnosis does the risk of death plateau at an even lower rate that remains constant with extended follow-up. However, Ewing's sarcoma can recur very late. In one series, 5 of 31 patients who remained disease-free for 5 years from initial diagnosis later recurred.[512] Other series of patients with recurrent disease have included patients with disease recurrence beyond 10 years from initial diagnosis.[507,509] These results highlight the need for extended follow-up in patients with this disease.

General Approach

Patients with progressive or recurrent disease following initial therapy present a particular challenge to the clinical team. The time to disease recurrence provides an important indication of the likelihood of long-term survival for these patients (see later). More than 25% of patients with late recurrence (more than 2 years from initial diagnosis) may achieve long-term disease control with aggressive therapy.[507-510] Most clinicians initiate systemic chemotherapy for these patients to assess their sensitivity to the chosen chemotherapy regimen. For patients with chemotherapy-responsive disease, the use of surgery and/or radiation for sites of recurrence is often considered. For a local recurrence, a reattempt at local control may be undertaken with surgery, radiation, or both surgery and radiation. For patients with pulmonary recurrence, many clinicians will recommend whole-lung irradiation. Patients who respond well to second-line therapy may also be candidates for high-dose therapy with stem cell rescue. Patients with late recurrent disease that does not respond to initial chemotherapy are managed as for those with poor-risk recurrent disease according to the strategies outlined later.

For patients with an early recurrence (less than 2 years from initial diagnosis), the likelihood of long-term disease control is less than 10%.[507-510] Given these data, the appropriate treatment for these patients must be highly individualized, with a clear understanding of the patient's and family's goals for therapy. Various strategies are considered for these patients, ranging from palliative measures to aggressive multimodality therapy with curative intent. These patients often receive treatment with second-line chemotherapy regimens (see later) and are also candidates for investigational phase I and phase II clinical trials. For patients with chemotherapy-responsive disease, more aggressive measures can then be considered.

Systemic Chemotherapy

Historically, very few chemotherapy options existed for patients with recurrent Ewing's sarcoma. As such, patients with late relapse disease were often treated with agents that they had received at initial diagnosis. In one small series, a substantial number of patients who relapsed off-therapy responded again to the same agents that they received as initial therapy, and some of these patients had a durable second remission.[513] To avoid concerns of resistance to previously used agents, most clinicians now use newer chemotherapy regimens for patients at the time of relapse. However, for patients with late relapse, some clinicians will incorporate previously used active agents into an overall treatment plan that also includes newer second-line regimens. Some of these more common second-line regimens are reviewed here.

Camptothecin-containing regimens have demonstrated efficacy for patients with relapsed Ewing's sarcoma. Topotecan monotherapy appears to have limited activity against Ewing's sarcoma, with objective response rates of 0% to 10%.[514,515] In contrast, topotecan in combination with cyclophosphamide has a response rate of approximately 30% in patients with relapsed or refractory disease.[516,517] Patients with disease that was refractory to standard alkylator-containing therapy responded to this regimen, suggesting that this response rate is not solely because of cyclophosphamide but rather because of the combination of topotecan with cyclophosphamide. Patients with newly diagnosed metastatic disease treated in an up-front window study had a response rate of 57% to topotecan and cyclophosphamide.[492] This combination will be further evaluated in Children's Oncology Group trials for patients with both newly diagnosed and relapsed disease.

A second camptothecin-containing regimen has shown promise in patients with Ewing's sarcoma. An initial phase I study of irinotecan and temozolomide found that this well-tolerated regimen induced one complete response and one partial response among seven patients with Ewing's sarcoma treated in this study.[518] A follow-up report that included these seven patients plus seven additional evaluable patients reported an objective response in four patients (28%), although an additional four patients had a mixed response or stable disease.[519] Further evaluation of this combination is planned.

Two carboplatin-based regimens have benefited patients with relapsed or refractory Ewing's sarcoma. One group has reported a 26% response rate among 39 patients treated with carboplatin, cyclophosphamide, and etoposide.[520] A second group evaluated carboplatin, ifosfamide, and etoposide in patients with a range of relapsed or refractory sarcoma.[521] Of the 21 patients with Ewing's sarcoma, 48% had an objective response. The contribution of carboplatin to these responses is unclear, because both regimens contain first-line agents that are also effective in the treatment of this disease (ifosfamide, etoposide, and cyclophosphamide).

Role of Surgery and Radiation

Patients with recurrent Ewing's sarcoma typically must respond to systemic therapy for long-term disease control to be possible. However, surgery and radiation also play a role at the time of disease recurrence. One study has reported that patients who receive surgery for local recurrence have a superior outcome compared with patients who do not receive surgery, although this analysis did not control for the size of the recurrent tumor.[509] This same study reported that whole-lung irradiation may benefit patients with isolated pulmonary recurrence. Radiotherapy also plays an important role in controlling pain for patients with refractory Ewing's sarcoma.

Pulmonary metastectomy at relapse has a much more limited role in Ewing's sarcoma compared with other diseases, such as osteosarcoma. One group has reported that pulmonary metastectomy does not improve the outcome for patients with Ewing's sarcoma and isolated pulmonary relapse.[509] Two groups have compared patients who underwent pulmonary metastectomy to patients with lung metastases that were not resected.[496,522] Both groups have suggested that metastectomy improves the outcome for these patients. However, in both studies, patients were selected for resection only in the presence of resectable disease, so that the comparison group may have had a greater burden of disease. Another center has described 12 patients with isolated pulmonary relapse treated with surgery alone.[523] Five of these patients remained disease-free for at least 3 years. The authors noted that these 12 patients were selected for resection alone based on favorable characteristics, such as a small number of pulmonary nodules and a long period of time from diagnosis to relapse. Whether this strategy would benefit a less favorable group of patients remains to be demonstrated. Currently, pulmonary metastectomy at relapse is considered mainly for diagnostic purposes and only rarely for therapeutic purposes.

Role of High-Dose Therapy with Hematopoietic Stem Cell Rescue

Some clinicians recommend high-dose therapy as consolidation therapy for patients with recurrent Ewing's sarcoma who respond favorably to salvage therapy. Data supporting this approach are relatively limited, particularly because many of the reported studies have included patients with metastatic disease and patients with recurrent disease. Although most studies do not report specific outcomes for patients with recur-

rent disease, the EICESS group has reported that patients treated with high-dose therapy for early relapse have a 5-year event-free survival of approximately 45%.[501]

Two reports have retrospectively evaluated the impact of high-dose therapy on outcome in patients with recurrent disease. In one series of 64 patients with relapsed disease, 7 patients received high-dose therapy with stem cell rescue.[510] The outcomes for these 7 patients did not differ from outcomes for patients who received other types of relapse therapy. These results differ from a single-institution report of 55 patients with relapsed Ewing's sarcoma, of whom 13 received high-dose therapy with busulfan, melphalan, and thiotepa.[508] Patients who received high-dose therapy had a 5-year progression-free survival of 61% compared with 7% for other patients. Because high-dose therapy was only offered to patients who responded to second-line therapy, this report also compared outcomes between patients who received high-dose therapy and patients who had responsive disease but who did not receive high-dose therapy. In this analysis, high-dose therapy resulted in an improved 5-year progression-free survival over other therapy (61% vs. 21%). A multivariate analysis has confirmed that high-dose therapy is an independent predictor of favorable outcome.

Outcomes

The outcome for patients with recurrent disease is generally poor. In one large cooperative group analysis, the median overall survival from the time of recurrence was 14 months.[510] Estimates of 5-year overall survival from the time of disease recurrence range from 8% to 23%.[507-510] For patients with recurrent disease, the most widely recognized determinant of outcome is time to disease recurrence. An initial single-institution study has noted that 4 of 5 patients with relapse more than 5 years from diagnosis were salvaged, compared with only 2 of 44 patients with earlier relapses.[512] Follow-up studies have all confirmed this association. Estimates of 5-year progression-free survival for patients with recurrence more than 2 years from initial diagnosis have ranged from 19% to 49% compared with 5% to 8% for earlier relapses. Other clinical features, including type of relapse (distant or local) and metastatic site at recurrence, have not consistently been associated with outcome after relapse.

LATE EFFECTS IN PATIENTS TREATED FOR EWING'S SARCOMA

Given the nature of the therapy required to treat Ewing's sarcoma, patients treated for this disease have an increased risk of developing second cancers. In one large European cohort study, patients with Ewing's sarcoma had a 30-fold increased cumulative risk of developing a solid second cancer 25 years from initial diagnosis.[524] The relative risk of developing a second solid cancer or a bone cancer after Ewing's sarcoma was second only to patients with an initial primary cancer diagnosis of retinoblastoma.[55,524] A number of groups have reported that the risk of developing any second cancer continues to increase with increasing time from initial diagnosis of Ewing's sarcoma. Estimates of the cumulative incidence of developing any second malignancy from the time of initial diagnosis have ranged from 0.7% to 0.9% at 5 years, 2.9% to 6.5% at 10 years, 4.7% at 15 years, and 9.2% to 12.7% at 20 years.[525-528] Figure 21-9 demonstrates this trend in a representative report from the CESS group.[526]

Radiation-induced sarcomas and chemotherapy-induced acute leukemia constitute the majority of second malignancies

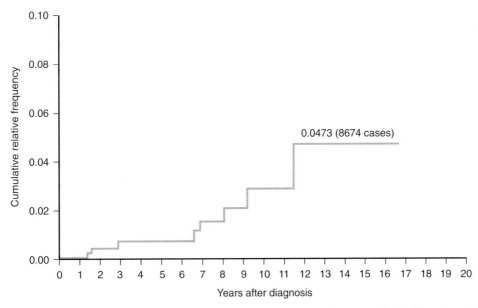

FIGURE 21-9. Cumulative incidence of second malignancies in patients treated for Ewing's sarcoma in the CESS-81 and CESS-86 studies. - *(Adapted from Dunst J, Ahrens S, Paulussen M, et al. Second malignancies after treatment for Ewing's sarcoma: a report of the CESS studies. Int J Radiat Oncol Biol Phys. 1998;42:379-84.)*

seen in these patients. Osteosarcoma accounts for approximately 25% of the secondary sarcomas, with various other bone and soft tissue sarcomas also observed.[525,527-529] Estimates of the incidence of secondary sarcomas in patients 20 years after treatment for Ewing's sarcoma have ranged from 6% to 22%.[55,526,527] This wide range is likely caused by variations in sample size, follow-up time, and second malignancy surveillance programs among studies. In almost all cases, these secondary sarcomas arise in the initial radiation field. One group has reported that the incidence of these secondary sarcomas increases with increasing radiation dose, with no cases of secondary sarcoma reported in patients who received less than 48 Gy.[527]

Secondary acute leukemia occurs significantly earlier than secondary sarcomas in these patients. Reported mean latency periods from initial diagnosis of Ewing's sarcoma to onset of acute leukemia have ranged from 2.3 to 4.8 years, although some patients have developed secondary acute leukemia while still receiving chemotherapy for Ewing's sarcoma.[525,529-531] Most of these cases of secondary acute leukemia are acute myeloid leukemia or myelodysplastic syndrome. In one large clinical trial, the cumulative incidence of secondary acute myeloid leukemia or myelodysplastic syndrome was approximately 2% 7 years from the initial diagnosis of Ewing's sarcoma, with no additional cases observed beyond that time point.[530] These cases are characterized by high frequencies of monosomy 5, monosomy 7, and abnormalities at 11q23.[530,531] These cytogenetic findings suggest a role for alkylating agents (cyclophosphamide and ifosfamide associated with monosomy 5 and monosomy 7) and topoisomerase II inhibitors (doxorubicin and etoposide associated with 11q23 abnormalities) in the pathogenesis of these cases. Interestingly, in protocol INT-0091, the incidence of secondary leukemia, including leukemias with the 11q23 abnormality, did not increase with the addition of ifosfamide and etoposide to the regimen of vincristine, doxorubicin, and cyclophosphamide.[530] Increased rates of secondary acute myeloid leukemia have been reported in patients with Ewing's sarcoma who received augmented doses of alkylating agents and anthracyclines compared with patients who received conventional doses. By way of contrast, in protocol INT-0154,

increasing the dose rate of alkylating agents while holding the cumulative dose constant did not increase the rate of secondary leukemias.[470]

Patients treated for Ewing's sarcoma are at risk for various late effects in addition to second cancers. Cardiac toxicity from anthracycline therapy can result in significant morbidity and mortality for these patients. In one small series, 6 of 30 Ewing's sarcoma survivors developed echocardiographic shortening fractions less than 20% compared with only 1 of 26 patients with soft tissue sarcomas treated with anthracyclines.[532] Both groups of patients received the same mean doxorubicin dose, but patients with Ewing's sarcoma received higher individual doses of doxorubicin at shorter intervals. The addition of ifosfamide to chemotherapy regimens for Ewing's sarcoma has resulted in the development of renal tubular dysfunction in some of these patients. A large European cohort of sarcoma survivors has reported an incidence of renal tubular dysfunction of 4.6% in patients treated with ifosfamide, with increasing risk with increasing cumulative ifosfamide dose.[533] Patients treated with radiation therapy to the bone are at risk for fractures in the radiation field, with an incidence of approximately 20% in one series of Ewing's sarcoma survivors.[534] Patients treated for Ewing's sarcoma may have hematologic changes following treatment, including mild thrombocytopenia and macrocytosis.[531]

Several studies have evaluated the psychosocial ramifications of treatment for bone sarcomas, including Ewing's sarcoma. A study from the Childhood Cancer Survivor Study has reported that survivors of lower extremity bone tumors overall have excellent self-reported orthopedic function and quality of life.[535] Approximately 5% of these patients reported severe or complete disability. Long-term function and quality of life did not appear to differ between patients who underwent amputation and patients who underwent limb salvage procedures.[535,536] In another report from the Childhood Cancer Survivor Study, survivors of lower extremity bone tumors were less likely to be married than siblings.[537] In addition, adolescents who underwent amputation were less likely to complete high school and were more likely to have difficulties with health insurance issues compared with sibling controls. Some of these findings were replicated in a single-institution study specific to Ewing's sarcoma survivors.[538] In this study, survivors had lower rates of employment and marriage than sibling controls, although educational attainment and insurance access did not differ between the two groups. All these studies highlight the importance of evaluation for late effects in survivors of Ewing's sarcoma. ·

FUTURE DIRECTIONS

This chapter has detailed the remarkable gains achieved in the treatment of patients with Ewing's sarcoma over the past 40 years. During this same period, our understanding of the biology of these tumors has also greatly progressed. Future improvements in the management of this disease will need to take advantage of this improved understanding of the events involved in Ewing's sarcoma tumorigenesis. Specific avenues of investigation will need to include therapies directed at key targets in Ewing's sarcoma, including IGF-1, CD99, angiogenesis pathways, and EWS/FLI itself. These therapies will likely be piloted first in those patients with the worst prognosis, patients with metastatic disease and patients with early relapse. Effective targeted therapies in these populations will then be applied to patients with lower risk disease. Targeted therapy holds promise not only for improving outcomes for patients with Ewing's sarcoma, but also for reducing exposure to conventional chemotherapy and the late effects of that therapy. For now, further studies of the clinical and molecular prognostic features of this disease are required so that current active agents may be applied in a more risk-adapted approach.

REFERENCES

1. Ewing J. Diffuse endothelioma of bone. Proc N Y Pathol Soc. 1921;21:17-24.
2. Askin FB, Rosai J, Sibley RK, et al. Malignant small cell tumor of the thoracopulmonary region in childhood: a distinctive clinicopathologic entity of uncertain histogenesis. Cancer. 1979;43:2438-51.
3. Stiller CA, Bielack SS, Jundt G, Steliarova-Foucher E. Bone tumours in European children and adolescents, 1978-1997. Report from the Automated Childhood Cancer Information System project. Eur J Cancer. 2006;42:2124-35.
4. Mascarenhas L, Siegel S, Spector L, et al: Malignant bone tumors. In Bleyer A, O'Leary M, Barr R, et al (eds). Cancer Epidemiology in Older Adolescents and Young Adults 15 to 29 Years of Age, Including SEER Incidence and Survival, 1975-2000. Bethesda, Md, National Cancer Institute, 2006, pp 98-109.
5. Gurney JG, Swensen AR, Bulterys M: Malignant bone tumors. In Ries L, Smith M, Gurney JG, et al (eds). Cancer Incidence and Survival Among Children and Adolescents: United States SEER Program 1975-1995. Bethesda, Md, National Cancer Institute, 1999, pp 99-110.
6. Ries L, Harkins D, Krapcho M, et al (eds). SEER Cancer Statistics Review, 1975-2003. Bethesda, Md, National Cancer Institute, 2006.
7. Glass AG, Fraumeni JF Jr. Epidemiology of bone cancer in children. J Natl Cancer Inst. 1970;44:187-99.
8. Maygarden SJ, Askin FB, Siegal GP, et al. Ewing sarcoma of bone in infants and toddlers. A clinicopathologic report from the Intergroup Ewing's Study. Cancer. 1993;71:2109-18.
9. Ross JA, Severson RK, Swensen AR, et al. Seasonal variations in the diagnosis of childhood cancer in the United States. Br J Cancer. 1999;81:549-53.
10. Parkin DM, Stiller CA, Nectoux J. International variations in the incidence of childhood bone tumours. Int J Cancer. 1993;53:371-6.
11. Polednak AP. Primary bone cancer incidence in black and white residents of New York State. Cancer. 1985;55:2883-8.
12. Bahebeck J, Atangana R, Eyenga V, et al. Bone tumours in Cameroon: incidence, demography and histopathology. Int Orthop. 2003;27:315-7.
13. Settakorn J, Lekawanvijit S, Arpornchayanon O, et al. Spectrum of bone tumors in Chiang Mai University Hospital, Thailand according to WHO classification 2002: a study of 1,001 cases. J Med Assoc Thai. 2006;89:780-7.
14. Guo W, Xu W, Huvos AG, et al. Comparative frequency of bone sarcomas among different racial groups. Chin Med J (Engl). 1999;112:1101-4.
15. Sarma NH, al-Fituri O, Visweswara RN, Saeed SO. Primary bone tumour in eastern Libya—a 10 year study. Cent Afr J Med. 1994;40:148-51.
16. Yeole BB, Jussawalla DJ. Descriptive epidemiology of bone cancer in greater Bombay. Indian J Cancer. 1998;35:101-6.
17. Katchy KC, Ziad F, Alexander S, et al. Malignant bone tumors in Kuwait: a 10-year clinicopathologic study. Int Orthop. 2005;29:406-11.
18. Zamora P, Garcia de Paredes ML, Gonzalez Baron M, et al. Ewing's tumor in brothers. An unusual observation. Am J Clin Oncol. 1986;9:358-60.
19. Hutter RV, Francis KC, Foote FW Jr. Ewing's sarcoma in siblings: Report of the second known occurrence. Am J Surg. 107:24:1964;20.
20. Joyce MJ, Harmon DC, Mankin HJ, et al. Ewing's sarcoma in female siblings. A clinical report and review of the literature. Cancer. 1984;53:1959-62.
21. Hartley AL, Birch JM, Blair V, et al. Cancer incidence in the families of children with Ewing's tumor. J Natl Cancer Inst. 1991;83:955-6.
22. Novakovic B, Goldstein AM, Wexler LH, Tucker MA. Increased risk of neuroectodermal tumors and stomach cancer in relatives of patients with Ewing's sarcoma family of tumors. J Natl Cancer Inst. 1994;86:1702-6.
23. Winn DM, Li FP, Robison LL, et al. A case-control study of the cause of Ewing's sarcoma. Cancer Epidemiol Biomarkers Prev. 1992;1:525-32.
24. Valery PC, McWhirter W, Sleigh A, et al. A national case-control study of Ewing's sarcoma family of tumours in Australia. Int J Cancer. 2003;105:825-30.
25. Cope JU, Tsokos M, Helman LJ, et al. Inguinal hernia in patients with Ewing sarcoma: a clue to cause. Med Pediatr Oncol. 2000;34:195-9.
26. Valery PC, Holly EA, Sleigh AC, et al. Hernias and Ewing's sarcoma family of tumours: a pooled analysis and meta-analysis. Lancet Oncol. 2005;6:485-90.
27. McKeen EA, Hanson MR, Mulvihill JJ, Glaubiger DL. Birth defects with Ewing's sarcoma. N Engl J Med. 1983;309:1522.
28. Schumacher R, Mai A, Gutjahr P. Association of rib anomalies and malignancy in childhood. Eur J Pediatr. 1992;151:432-4.
29. Narod SA, Hawkins MM, Robertson CM, Stiller CA. Congenital anomalies and childhood cancer in Great Britain. Am J Hum Genet. 1997;60:474-85.
30. Valery PC, Williams G, Sleigh AC, et al. Parental occupation and Ewing's sarcoma: pooled and meta-analysis. Int J Cancer. 2005;115:799-806.
31. Valery PC, McWhirter W, Sleigh A, et al. Farm exposures, parental occupation, and risk of Ewing's sarcoma in Australia: a national case-control study. Cancer Causes Control. 2002;13:263-70.

32. Holly EA, Aston DA, Ahn DK, Kristiansen JJ. Ewing's bone sarcoma, paternal occupational exposure, and other factors. Am J Epidemiol. 1992;135:122-9.

33. Hum L, Kreiger N, Finkelstein MM. The relationship between parental occupation and bone cancer risk in offspring. Int J Epidemiol. 1998;27:766-71.

34. Moore LE, Gold L, Stewart PA, et al. Parental occupational exposures and Ewing's sarcoma. Int J Cancer. 2005;114:472-8.

35. Buckley JD, Pendergrass TW, Buckley CM, et al. Epidemiology of osteosarcoma and Ewing's sarcoma in childhood: a study of 305 cases by the Children's Cancer Group. Cancer. 1998;83:1440-8.

36. Cotterill SJ, Wright CM, Pearce MS, Craft AW. Stature of young people with malignant bone tumors. Pediatr Blood Cancer. 2004;42:59-63.

37. Pendergrass TW, Foulkes MA, Robison LL, Nesbit ME. Stature and Ewing's sarcoma in childhood. Am J Pediatr Hematol Oncol. 1984;6:33-9.

38. Sanchez-Prieto R, de Alava E, Palomino T, et al. An association between viral genes and human oncogenic alterations: the adenovirus E1A induces the Ewing tumor fusion transcript EWS-FLI1. Nat Med. 1999;5:1076-9.

39. Kovar H, Fallaux FJ, Pribill I, et al. Adenovirus E1A does not induce the Ewing tumor-associated gene fusion EWS-FLI1. Cancer Res. 2000;60:1557-60.

40. Kovar H. E1A and the Ewing tumor translocation. Nat Med. 1999;5:1331.

41. Melot T, Delattre O. E1A and the Ewing tumor translocation. Nat Med. 1999;5:1331.

42. Meric F, Liao Y, Lee WP, et al. Adenovirus 5 early region 1A does not induce expression of the Ewing sarcoma fusion product EWS-FLI1 in breast and ovarian cancer cell lines. Clin Cancer Res. 2000;6:3832-6.

43. Kebudi R, Bilgic B, Gorgun O, et al. Is the Epstein Barr virus implicated in Ewing sarcoma? Med Pediatr Oncol. 2003;40:256-7.

44. Daugaard S, Hording U, Schiodt T. Ewing's sarcoma and Epstein-Barr virus. Eur J Cancer. 1991;27:1334.

45. De Mattei M, Martini F, Corallini A, et al. High incidence of BK virus large-T-antigen-coding sequences in normal human tissues and tumors of different histotypes. Int J Cancer. 1995;61:756-60.

46. Martini F, Lazzarin L, Iaccheri L, et al. Simian virus 40 footprints in normal human tissues, brain and bone tumours of different histotypes. Dev Biol Stand. 1998;94:55-66.

47. Negrini M, Rimessi P, Mantovani C, et al. Characterization of BK virus variants rescued from human tumours and tumour cell lines. J Gen Virol. 1990;71 (Pt 11):2731-6.

48. Aparicio J, Segura A, Montalar J, et al. Secondary cancers after Ewing sarcoma and Ewing sarcoma as second malignant neoplasm. Med Pediatr Oncol. 1998;30:259-60.

49. Anselmo AP, Cartoni C, Pacchiarotti A, et al. Peripheral neuroectodermal tumor of the chest (Askin tumor) as secondary neoplasm after Hodgkin's disease: a case report. Ann Hematol. 1994;68:311-3.

50. Fisher R, Kaste SC, Parham DM, et al. Ewing's sarcoma as a second malignant neoplasm in a child previously treated for Wilms' tumor. J Pediatr Hematol Oncol. 1995;17:76-80.

51. Helton KJ, Fletcher BD, Kun LE, et al. Bone tumors other than osteosarcoma after retinoblastoma. Cancer. 1993;71:2847-53.

52. Kim GE, Beach B, Gastier-Foster JM, et al. Ewing sarcoma as a second malignant neoplasm after acute lymphoblastic leukemia. Pediatr Blood Cancer. 2005;45:57-9.

53. Zoubek A, Simonitsch I, Panzer-Grumayer ER, et al. Ewing tumor after treatment of Ki-1+ anaplastic large cell lymphoma. Therapy-associated secondary neoplasm or unrelated coincidence? Cancer Genet Cytogenet. 1995;83:5-11.

54. Spunt SL, Rodriguez-Galindo C, Fuller CE, et al. Ewing sarcoma-family tumors that arise after treatment of primary childhood cancer. Cancer. 2006;107:201-6.

55. Tucker MA, D'Angio GJ, Boice JD Jr, et al. Bone sarcomas linked to radiotherapy and chemotherapy in children. N Engl J Med. 1987;317:588-93.

56. Newton WA Jr, Meadows AT, Shimada H, et al. Bone sarcomas as second malignant neoplasms following childhood cancer. Cancer. 1991;67:193-201.

57. Hawkins MM, Wilson LM, Burton HS, et al. Radiotherapy, alkylating agents, and risk of bone cancer after childhood cancer. J Natl Cancer Inst. 1996;88:270-8.

58. Aurias A, Rimbaut C, Buffe D, et al. Translocation involving chromosome 22 in Ewing's sarcoma. A cytogenetic study of four fresh tumors. Cancer Genet Cytogenet. 1984;12:21-5.

59. Turc-Carel C, Philip I, Berger MP, et al. Chromosome study of Ewing's sarcoma (ES) cell lines. Consistency of a reciprocal translocation t(11;22)(q24;q12). Cancer Genet Cytogenet. 1984;12:1-19.

60. Whang-Peng J, Triche TJ, Knutsen T, et al. Chromosome translocation in peripheral neuroepithelioma. New Engl J Med. 1984;311:584-585.

61. Turc-Carel C, Aurias A, Mugneret F, et al. Chromosomes in Ewing's sarcoma. I. An evaluation of 85 cases of remarkable consistency of t(11;22)(q24;q12). Cancer Genet Cytogenet. 1988;32:229-38.

62. Stark B, Mor C, Jeison M, et al. Additional chromosome 1q aberrations and der(16)t(1;16), correlation to the phenotypic expression and clinical behavior of the Ewing family of tumors. J Neurooncol. 1997;31:3-8.

63. Armengol G, Tarkkanen M, Virolainen M, et al. Recurrent gains of 1q, 8 and 12 in the Ewing family of tumours by comparative genomic hybridization. Br J Cancer. 1997;75:1403-9.

64. Betts DR, Avoledo P, von der Weid N, et al. Cytogenetic characterization of Ewing tumors with high-ploidy. Cancer Genet Cytogenet. 2005;159:160-3.

65. Douglass EC, Valentine M, Green AA, et al. t(11;22) and other chromosomal rearrangements in Ewing's sarcoma. J Natl Cancer Inst. 1986;77:1211-5.

66. Douglass EC, Rowe ST, Valentine M, et al. A second nonrandom translocation, der(16)t(1;16)(q21;q13), in Ewing sarcoma and peripheral neuroectodermal tumor. Cytogenet Cell Genet. 1990;53:87-90.

67. Hattinger CM, Rumpler S, Ambros IM, et al. Demonstration of the translocation der(16)t(1;16)(q12;q11.2) in interphase nuclei of Ewing tumors. Genes Chromosomes Cancer. 1996;17:141-50.

68. Hattinger CM, Rumpler S, Strehl S, et al. Prognostic impact of deletions at 1p36 and numerical aberrations in Ewing tumors. Genes Chromosomes Cancer. 1999;24:243-54.

69. Mugneret F, Lizard S, Aurias A, Turc-Carel C. Chromosomes in Ewing's sarcoma. II. Nonrandom additional changes, trisomy 8 and der(16)t(1;16). Cancer Genet Cytogenet. 1988;32:239-45.

70. Stark B, Zoubek A, Hattinger C, et al. Metastatic extraosseous Ewing tumor. Association of the additional translocation der(16)t(1;16) with the variant EWS/ERG rearrangement in a case of cytogenetically inconspicuous chromosome 22. Cancer Genet Cytogenet. 1996;87:161-6.

71. Ozaki T, Paulussen M, Poremba C, et al. Genetic imbalances revealed by comparative genomic hybridization in Ewing tumors. Genes Chromosomes Cancer. 2001;32:164-71.

72. Ohali A, Avigad S, Cohen IJ, et al. High frequency of genomic instability in Ewing family of tumors. Cancer Genet Cytogenet. 2004;150:50-6.

73. Ebinger M, Bock T, Kandolf R, et al. Standard mono- and dinucleotide repeats do not appear to be sensitive markers of

microsatellite instability in the Ewing family of tumors. Cancer Genet Cytogenet. 2005;157:189-90.

74. Delattre O, Zucman J, Plougastel B, et al. Gene fusion with an ETS DNA-binding domain caused by chromosome translocation in human tumours. Nature. 1992;359:162-5.

75. Zucman J, Delattre O, Desmaze C, et al. Cloning and characterization of the Ewing's sarcoma and peripheral neuroepithelioma t(11;22) translocation breakpoints. Genes Chromosomes Cancer. 1992;5:271-7.

76. Ben-David Y, Giddens EB, Bernstein A. Identification and mapping of a common proviral integration site Fli-1 in erythroleukemia cells induced by Friend murine leukemia virus. Proc Natl Acad Sci U S A. 1990;87:1332-6.

77. Aman P, Panagopoulos I, Lassen C, et al. Expression patterns of the human sarcoma-associated genes FUS and EWS and the genomic structure of FUS. Genomics. 1996;37:1-8.

78. Ohno T, Ouchida M, Lee L, et al. The EWS gene, involved in Ewing family of tumors, malignant melanoma of soft parts and desmoplastic small round cell tumors, codes for an RNA binding protein with novel regulatory domains. Oncogene. 1994;9:3087-97.

79. May WA, Lessnick SL, Braun BS, et al. The Ewing's sarcoma EWS/FLI-1 fusion gene encodes a more potent transcriptional activator and is a more powerful transforming gene than FLI-1. Mol Cell Biol. 1993;13:7393-8.

80. Sutherland HG, Mumford GK, Newton K, et al. Large-scale identification of mammalian proteins localized to nuclear subcompartments. Hum Mol Genet. 2001;10:1995-2011.

81. Zakaryan RP, Gehring H. Identification and characterization of the nuclear localization/retention Signal in the EWS proto-oncoprotein. J Mol Biol. 2006;363:27-38.

82. Felsch JS, Lane WS, Peralta EG. Tyrosine kinase Pyk2 mediates G-protein-coupled receptor regulation of the Ewing sarcoma RNA-binding protein EWS. Curr Biol. 1999;9:485-8.

83. Belyanskaya LL, Gehrig PM, Gehring H. Exposure on cell surface and extensive arginine methylation of Ewing sarcoma (EWS) protein. J Biol Chem. 2001;276:18681-7.

84. Deloulme JC, Prichard L, Delattre O, Storm DR. The prooncoprotein EWS binds calmodulin and is phosphorylated by protein kinase C through an IQ domain. J Biol Chem. 1997;272:27369-77.

85. Stolow DT, Haynes SR. Cabeza, a Drosophila gene encoding a novel RNA binding protein, shares homology with EWS and TLS, two genes involved in human sarcoma formation. Nucleic Acids Res. 1995;23:835-43.

86. Belyanskaya LL, Delattre O, Gehring H. Expression and subcellular localization of Ewing sarcoma (EWS) protein is affected by the methylation process. Exp Cell Res. 2003;288:374-81.

87. Guinamard R, Fougereau M, Seckinger P. The SH3 domain of Bruton's tyrosine kinase interacts with Vav, Sam68 and EWS. Scand J Immunol. 1997;45:587-95.

88. Bertolotti A, Lutz Y, Heard DJ, et al. hTAF(II)68, a novel RNA/ssDNA-binding protein with homology to the pro-oncoproteins TLS/FUS and EWS is associated with both TFIID and RNA polymerase II. EMBO J. 1996;15:5022-31.

89. Crozat A, Aman P, Mandahl N, Ron D. Fusion of CHOP to a novel RNA-binding protein in human myxoid liposarcoma. Nature. 1993;363:640-4.

90. Morohoshi F, Arai K, Takahashi EI, et al. Cloning and mapping of a human RBP56 gene encoding a putative RNA binding protein similar to FUS/TLS and EWS proteins. Genomics. 1996;38:51-7.

91. Rabbitts TH, Forster A, Larson R, Nathan P. Fusion of the dominant negative transcription regulator CHOP with a novel gene FUS by translocation t(12;16) in malignant liposarcoma. Nat Genet. 1993;4:175-80.

92. Attwooll C, Tariq M, Harris M, et al. Identification of a novel fusion gene involving hTAFII68 and CHN from a

t(9;17)(q22;q11.2) translocation in an extraskeletal myxoid chondrosarcoma. Oncogene. 1999;18:7599-601.

93. Martini A, La Starza R, Janssen H, et al. Recurrent rearrangement of the Ewing's sarcoma gene, EWSR1, or its homologue, TAF15, with the transcription factor CIZ/NMP4 in acute leukemia. Cancer Res. 2002;62:5408-12.

94. Sjogren H, Meis-Kindblom J, Kindblom LG, et al. Fusion of the EWS-related gene TAF2N to TEC in extraskeletal myxoid chondrosarcoma. Cancer Res. 1999;59:5064-7.

95. Meissner M, Lopato S, Gotzmann J, et al. Proto-oncoprotein TLS/FUS is associated to the nuclear matrix and complexed with splicing factors PTB, SRm160, and SR proteins. Exp Cell Res. 2003;283:184-95.

96. Araya N, Hirota K, Shimamoto Y, et al. Cooperative interaction of EWS with CREB-binding protein selectively activates hepatocyte nuclear factor 4-mediated transcription. J Biol Chem. 2003;278:5427-32.

97. Bertolotti A, Bell B, Tora L. The N-terminal domain of human TAFII68 displays transactivation and oncogenic properties. Oncogene. 1999;18:8000-10.

98. Bertolotti A, Melot T, Acker J, et al. EWS, but not EWS-FLI-1, is associated with both TFIID and RNA polymerase II: interactions between two members of the TET family, EWS and hTAFII68, and subunits of TFIID and RNA polymerase II complexes. Mol Cell Biol. 1998;18:1489-97.

99. Chansky HA, Hu M, Hickstein DD, Yang L. Oncogenic TLS/ERG and EWS/Fli-1 fusion proteins inhibit RNA splicing mediated by YB-1 protein. Cancer Res. 2001;61:3586-90.

100. Zinszner H, Albalat R, Ron D. A novel effector domain from the RNA-binding protein TLS or EWS is required for oncogenic transformation by CHOP. Genes Dev. 1994;8:2513-26.

101. Yang L, Chansky HA, Hickstein DD. EWS.Fli-1 fusion protein interacts with hyperphosphorylated RNA polymerase II and interferes with serine-arginine protein-mediated RNA splicing. J Biol Chem. 2000;275:37612-8.

102. Kasyapa CS, Kunapuli P, Cowell JK. Mass spectroscopy identifies the splicing-associated proteins, PSF, hnRNP H3, hnRNP A2/B1, and TLS/FUS as interacting partners of the ZNF198 protein associated with rearrangement in myeloproliferative disease. Exp Cell Res. 2005;309:78-85.

103. Petermann R, Mossier BM, Aryee DN, et al. Oncogenic EWS-Fli1 interacts with hsRPB7, a subunit of human RNA polymerase II. Oncogene. 1998;17:603-10.

104. Rossow KL, Janknecht R. The Ewing's sarcoma gene product functions as a transcriptional activator. Cancer Res. 2001;61:2690-5.

105. Thomas GR, Latchman DS. The pro-oncoprotein EWS (Ewing's Sarcoma protein) interacts with the Brn-3a POU transcription factor and inhibits its ability to activate transcription. Cancer Biol Ther. 2002;1:428-32.

106. Lessnick SL, Braun BS, Denny CT, May WA. Multiple domains mediate transformation by the Ewing's sarcoma EWS/FLI-1 fusion gene. Oncogene. 1995;10:423-31.

107. Ben-David Y, Giddens EB, Letwin K, Bernstein A. Erythroleukemia induction by Friend murine leukemia virus: insertional activation of a new member of the ets gene family, Fli-1, closely linked to c-ets-1. Genes Dev. 1991;5:908-18.

108. Seth A, Watson DK. ETS transcription factors and their emerging roles in human cancer. Eur J Cancer. 2005.

109. Sharrocks AD. The ETS-domain transcription factor family. Nat Rev Mol Cell Biol. 2001;2:827-37.

110. Rao VN, Ohno T, Prasad DD, et al. Analysis of the DNA-binding and transcriptional activation functions of human Fli-1 protein. Oncogene. 1993;8:2167-73.

111. Klambt C. The Drosophila gene pointed encodes two ETS-like proteins which are involved in the development of the midline glial cells. Development. 1993;117:163-76.

112. Mackereth CD, Scharpf M, Gentile LN, et al. Diversity in structure and function of the Ets family PNT domains. J Mol Biol. 2004;342:1249-64.

113. Bastian LS, Kwiatkowski BA, Breininger J, et al. Regulation of the megakaryocytic glycoprotein IX promoter by the oncogenic Ets transcription factor Fli-1. Blood. 1999;93:2637-44.

114. Deveaux S, Filipe A, Lemarchandel V, et al. Analysis of the thrombopoietin receptor (MPL) promoter implicates GATA and Ets proteins in the coregulation of megakaryocyte-specific genes. Blood. 1996;87:4678-85.

115. Athanasiou M, Clausen PA, Mavrothalassitis GJ, et al. Increased expression of the ETS-related transcription factor FLI-1/ERGB correlates with and can induce the megakaryocytic phenotype. Cell Growth Differ. 1996;7:1525-34.

116. Hart A, Melet F, Grossfeld P, et al. Fli-1 is required for murine vascular and megakaryocytic development and is hemizygously deleted in patients with thrombocytopenia. Immunity. 2000;13: 167-77.

117. Spyropoulos DD, Pharr PN, Lavenburg KR, et al. Hemorrhage, impaired hematopoiesis, and lethality in mouse embryos carrying a targeted disruption of the Fli1 transcription factor. Mol Cell Biol. 2000;20:5643-52.

118. Shivdasani RA. Lonely in Paris: when one gene copy isn't enough. J Clin Invest. 2004;114:17-9.

119. Raslova H, Komura E, Le Couedic JP, et al. FLI1 monoallelic expression combined with its hemizygous loss underlies Paris-Trousseau/Jacobsen thrombopenia. J Clin Invest. 2004;114:77-84.

120. Brown LA, Rodaway AR, Schilling TF, et al. Insights into early vasculogenesis revealed by expression of the ETS-domain transcription factor Fli-1 in wild-type and mutant zebrafish embryos. Mech Dev. 2000;90:237-52.

121. Mager AM, Grapin-Botton A, Ladjali K, et al. The avian fli gene is specifically expressed during embryogenesis in a subset of neural crest cells giving rise to mesenchyme. Int J Dev Biol. 1998;42:561-72.

122. Melet F, Motro B, Rossi DJ, et al. Generation of a novel Fli-1 protein by gene targeting leads to a defect in thymus development and a delay in Friend virus-induced erythroleukemia. Mol Cell Biol. 1996;16:2708-18.

123. May WA, Gishizky ML, Lessnick SL, et al. Ewing sarcoma 11;22 translocation produces a chimeric transcription factor that requires the DNA-binding domain encoded by FLI1 for transformation. Proc Natl Acad Sci U S A. 1993;90:5752-6.

124. Teitell MA, Thompson AD, Sorensen PH, et al. EWS/ETS fusion genes induce epithelial and neuroectodermal differentiation in NIH 3T3 fibroblasts. Lab Invest. 1999;79:1535-43.

125. Thompson AD, Teitell MA, Arvand A, Denny CT. Divergent Ewing's sarcoma EWS/ETS fusions confer a common tumorigenic phenotype on NIH3T3 cells. Oncogene. 1999;18:5506-5513.

126. Ouchida M, Ohno T, Fujimura Y, et al. Loss of tumorigenicity of Ewing's sarcoma cells expressing antisense RNA to EWS-fusion transcripts. Oncogene. 1995;11:1049-54.

127. Kovar H, Aryee DN, Jug G, et al. EWS/FLI-1 antagonists induce growth inhibition of Ewing tumor cells in vitro. Cell Growth Differ. 1996;7:429-37.

128. Tanaka K, Iwakuma T, Harimaya K, et al. EWS-Fli1 antisense oligodeoxynucleotide inhibits proliferation of human Ewing's sarcoma and primitive neuroectodermal tumor cells. J Clin Invest. 1997;99:239-47.

129. Toretsky JA, Connell Y, Neckers L, Bhat NK. Inhibition of EWS-FLI-1 fusion protein with antisense oligodeoxynucleotides. J Neurooncol. 1997;31:9-16.

130. Matsumoto Y, Tanaka K, Nakatani F, et al. Downregulation and forced expression of EWS-Fli1 fusion gene results in changes in the expression of G(1)regulatory genes. Br J Cancer. 2001;84: 768-75.

131. Prieur A, Tirode F, Cohen P, Delattre O. EWS/FLI-1 silencing and gene profiling of Ewing cells reveal downstream oncogenic pathways and a crucial role for repression of insulin-like growth factor binding protein 3. Mol Cell Biol. 2004;24:7275-83.

132. Chan D, Wilson TJ, Xu D, et al. Transformation induced by Ewing's sarcoma associated EWS/FLI-1 is suppressed by KRAB/FLI-1. Br J Cancer. 2003;88:137-45.

133. Chansky HA, Barahmand-Pour F, Mei Q, et al. Targeting of EWS/FLI-1 by RNA interference attenuates the tumor phenotype of Ewing's sarcoma cells in vitro. J Orthop Res. 2004;22:910-7.

134. Smith R, Owen LA, Trem DJ, et al. Expression profiling of EWS/FLI identifies NKX2.2 as a critical target gene in Ewing's sarcoma. Cancer Cell. 2006;9:405-16.

135. Knezevich SR, Hendson G, Mathers JA, et al. Absence of detectable EWS/FLI1 expression after therapy-induced neural differentiation in Ewing sarcoma. Hum Pathol. 1998;29:289-94.

136. Nakatani F, Tanaka K, Sakimura R, et al. Identification of p21WAF1/CIP1 as a direct target of EWS-Fli1 oncogenic fusion protein. J Biol Chem. 2003;278:15105-15.

137. Takahashi A, Higashino F, Aoyagi M, et al. EWS/ETS fusions activate telomerase in Ewing's tumors. Cancer Res. 2003;63: 8338-44.

138. Toretsky JA, Erkizan V, Levenson A, et al. Oncoprotein EWS-FLI1 activity is enhanced by RNA helicase A. Cancer Res. 2006;66:5574-81.

139. Sorensen PH, Lessnick SL, Lopez-Terrada D, et al. A second Ewing's sarcoma translocation, t(21;22), fuses the EWS gene to another ETS-family transcription factor, ERG. Nat Genet. 1994;6:146-51.

140. Prasad DD, Rao VN, Lee L, Reddy ES. Differentially spliced erg-3 product functions as a transcriptional activator. Oncogene. 1994;9:669-73.

141. Lessnick SL. Structural and Functional Requirements for Transformation Mediated by the Ewing's Sarcoma EWS/FLI-1 Fusion Protein [molecular biology dissertation]. Los Angeles, University of California, 1994.

142. Jeon IS, Davis JN, Braun BS, et al. A variant Ewing's sarcoma translocation (7;22) fuses the EWS gene to the ETS gene ETV1. Oncogene. 1995;10:1229-34.

143. Kaneko Y, Yoshida K, Handa M, et al. Fusion of an ETS-family gene, EIAF, to EWS by t(17;22)(q12;q12) chromosome translocation in an undifferentiated sarcoma of infancy. Genes Chromosomes Cancer. 1996;15:115-21.

144. Peter M, Couturier J, Pacquement H, et al. A new member of the ETS family fused to EWS in Ewing tumors. Oncogene. 1997;14:1159-64.

145. Urano F, Umezawa A, Hong W, et al. A novel chimera gene between EWS and E1A-F, encoding the adenovirus E1A enhancer-binding protein, in extraosseous Ewing's sarcoma. Biochem Biophys Res Commun. 1996;219:608-12.

146. Braunreiter CL, Hancock JD, Coffin CM, et al. Expression of EWS-ETS fusions in NIH3T3 cells reveals significant differences to Ewing's sarcoma. Cell Cycle. 2006;5:2753-9.

147. Ng TL, O'Sullivan MJ, Pallen CJ, et al. Ewing sarcoma with novel translocation t(2;16) producing an in-frame fusion of FUS and FEV. J Mol Diagn. 2007;9:459-63.

148. Shing DC, McMullan DJ, Roberts P, et al. FUS/ERG gene fusions in Ewing's tumors. Cancer Res. 2003;63:4568-76.

149. Zucman-Rossi J, Legoix P, Victor JM, et al. Chromosome translocation based on illegitimate recombination in human tumors. Proc Natl Acad Sci U S A. 1998;95:11786-91.

150. Zucman J, Melot T, Desmaze C, et al. Combinatorial generation of variable fusion proteins in the Ewing family of tumours. EMBO J. 1993;12:4481-7.

151. Kovar H, Jugovic D, Melot T, et al. Cryptic exons as a source of increased diversity of Ewing tumor-associated EWS-FLI1 chimeric products. Genomics. 1999;60:371-4.

152. Zoubek A, Dockhorn-Dworniczak B, Delattre O, et al. Does expression of different EWS chimeric transcripts define clinically distinct risk groups of Ewing tumor patients? J Clin Oncol. 1996;14:1245-51.

153. Lin PP, Brody RI, Hamelin AC, et al. Differential transactivation by alternative EWS-FLI1 fusion proteins correlates with clinical heterogeneity in Ewing's sarcoma. Cancer Res. 1999;59:1428-32.

154. Aryee DN, Sommergruber W, Muehlbacher K, et al. Variability in gene expression patterns of Ewing tumor cell lines differing in EWS-FLI1 fusion type. Lab Invest. 2000;80:1833-44.

155. Kovar H. Context matters: the hen or egg problem in Ewing's sarcoma. Semin Cancer Biol. 2005;15:189-96.

156. Ewing J. Further report on endothelial myeloma of bone. Proc N Y Pathol Soc. 1924;24:93-101.

157. Kadin ME, Bensch KG. On the origin of Ewing's tumor. Cancer. 1971;27:257-73.

158. Dickman PS, Liotta LA, Triche TJ. Ewing's sarcoma: Characterization in established cultures and evidence of its histogenesis. Lab Invest. 1982;47:375-382.

159. Navas-Palacios JJ, Aparicio-Duque R, Valdes MD. On the histogenesis of Ewing's sarcoma. An ultrastructural, immunohistochemical, and cytochemical study. Cancer. 1984;53:1882-901.

160. Lipinski M, Braham K, Philip I, et al. Neuroectoderm-associated antigens on Ewing's sarcoma cell lines. Cancer Res. 1987;47:183-7.

161. Cavazzana AO, Miser JS, Jefferson J, Triche TJ. Experimental evidence for a neural origin of Ewing's sarcoma of bone. Am J Pathol. 1987;127:507-18.

162. Henderson DW, Leppard PJ, Brennan JS, et al. Primitive neuroepithelial tumours of soft tissues and of bone: further ultrastructural and immunocytochemical clarification of 'Ewing's sarcoma', including freeze-fracture analysis. J Submicrosc Cytol Pathol. 1989;21:35-57.

163. Lizard-Nacol S, Volk C, Lizard G, Turc-Carel C. Abnormal expression of neurofilament proteins in Ewing's sarcoma cell cultures. Tumour Biol. 1992;13:36-43.

164. Ladanyi M, Heinemann FS, Huvos AG, et al. Neural differentiation in small round cell tumors of bone and soft tissue with the translocation t(11;22)(q24;q12): an immunohistochemical study of 11 cases. Hum Pathol. 1990;21:1245-51.

165. O'Regan S, Diebler MF, Meunier FM, Vyas S. A Ewing's sarcoma cell line showing some, but not all, of the traits of a cholinergic neuron. J Neurochem. 1995;64:69-76.

166. Cavazzana AO, Magnani JL, Ross RA, et al. Ewing's sarcoma is an undifferentiated neuroectodermal tumor. Prog Clin Biol Res. 1988;271:487-98.

167. Kodama K, Doi O, Higashiyama M, et al. Differentiation of a Ewing's sarcoma cell line towards neural and mesenchymal cell lineages. Jpn J Cancer Res. 1994;85:335-8.

168. Ohta S, Suzuki A, Shimada M, et al. Neuronal differentiation of Ewing's sarcoma induced by cholera toxin B and bromodeoxyuridine—establishment of Ewing's sarcoma cell line and histochemical study. Acta Paediatr Jpn. 1991;33:428-33.

169. Sugimoto T, Umezawa A, Hata J. Neurogenic potential of Ewing's sarcoma cells. Virchows Arch. 1997;430:41-6.

170. Collini P, Mezzelani A, Modena P, et al. Evidence of neural differentiation in a case of post-therapy primitive neuroectodermal tumor/Ewing sarcoma of bone. Am J Surg Pathol. 2003;27:1161-6.

171. Maeda G, Masui F, Yokoyama R, et al. Ganglion cells in Ewing's sarcoma following chemotherapy: a case report. Pathol Int. 1998;48:475-80.

172. Weissferdt A, Neuling K, English M, et al. Peripheral primitive neuroectodermal tumor with postchemotherapy neuroblastoma-like differentiation. Pediatr Dev Pathol. 2006;9:229-33.

173. Riggi N, Cironi L, Provero P, et al. Development of Ewing's sarcoma from primary bone marrow–derived mesenchymal progenitor cells. Cancer Res. 2005;65:11459-68.

174. Tirode F, Laud-Duval K, Prieur A, et al. Mesenchymal stem cell features of Ewing tumors. Cancer Cell. 2007;11:421-9.

175. Hu-Lieskovan S, Zhang J, Wu L, et al. EWS-FLI1 fusion protein up-regulates critical genes in neural crest development and is responsible for the observed phenotype of Ewing's family of tumors. Cancer Res. 2005;65:4633-44.

176. Lessnick SL, Dacwag CS, Golub TR. The Ewing's sarcoma oncoprotein EWS/FLI induces a p53-dependent growth arrest in primary human fibroblasts. Cancer Cell. 2002;1:393-401.

177. Rorie CJ, Thomas VD, Chen P, et al. The Ews/Fli-1 fusion gene switches the differentiation program of neuroblastomas to Ewing sarcoma/peripheral primitive neuroectodermal tumors. Cancer Res. 2004;64:1266-77.

178. Khan J, Wei JS, Ringner M, et al. Classification and diagnostic prediction of cancers using gene expression profiling and artificial neural networks. Nat Med. 2001;7:673-9.

179. Baird K, Davis S, Antonescu CR, et al. Gene expression profiling of human sarcomas: insights into sarcoma biology. Cancer Res. 2005;65:9226-35.

180. Staege MS, Hutter C, Neumann I, et al. DNA microarrays reveal relationship of Ewing family tumors to both endothelial and fetal neural crest-derived cells and define novel targets. Cancer Res. 2004;64:8213-21.

181. Arvand A, Bastians H, Welford SM, et al. EWS/FLI1 up regulates mE2-C, a cyclin-selective ubiquitin conjugating enzyme involved in cyclin B destruction. Oncogene. 1998;17:2039-2045.

182. Bailly RA, Bosselut R, Zucman J, et al. DNA-binding and transcriptional activation properties of the EWS-FLI-1 fusion protein resulting from the t(11;22) translocation in Ewing sarcoma. Mol Cell Biol. 1994;14:3230-41.

183. Braun BS, Frieden R, Lessnick SL, et al. Identification of target genes for the Ewing's sarcoma EWS/FLI fusion protein by representational difference analysis. Mol Cell Biol. 1995;15:4623-30.

184. Deneen B, Hamidi H, Denny CT. Functional analysis of the EWS/ETS target gene uridine phosphorylase. Cancer Res. 2003;63:4268-74.

185. Deneen B, Welford SM, Ho T, et al. PIM3 proto-oncogene kinase is a common transcriptional target of divergent EWS/ETS oncoproteins. Mol Cell Biol. 2003;23:3897-908.

186. Magnaghi-Jaulin L, Masutani H, Robin P, et al. SRE elements are binding sites for the fusion protein EWS-FLI-1. Nucleic Acids Res. 1996;24:1052-8.

187. Zwerner JP, May WA. PDGF-C is an EWS/FLI induced transforming growth factor in Ewing family tumors. Oncogene. 2001;20:626-33.

188. Thompson AD, Braun BS, Arvand A, et al. EAT-2 is a novel SH2 domain containing protein that is up regulated by Ewing's sarcoma EWS/FLI1 fusion gene. Oncogene. 1996;13:2649-58.

189. May WA, Arvand A, Thompson AD, et al. EWS/FLI1-induced manic fringe renders NIH 3T3 cells tumorigenic. Nat Genet. 1997;17:495-7.

190. Owen LA, Lessnick SL. Identification of target genes in their native cellular context: An analysis of EWS/FLI in Ewing's sarcoma. Cell Cycle. 2006;5.

191. Kovar H, Ban J, Pospisilova S. Potentials for RNAi in sarcoma research and therapy: Ewing's sarcoma as a model. Semin Cancer Biol. 2003;13:275-81.

192. Kinsey M, Smith R, Lessnick SL. NR0B1 Is required for the oncogenic phenotype mediated by EWS/FLI in Ewing's sarcoma. Mol Cancer Res. 2006;4:851-9.

193. Siligan C, Ban J, Bachmaier R, et al. EWS-FLI1 target genes recovered from Ewing sarcoma chromatin. Oncogene. 2005;24:2512-24.

194. Hahm KB, Cho K, Lee C, et al. Repression of the gene encoding the TGF-beta type II receptor is a major target of the EWS-FLI1 oncoprotein. Nat Genet. 1999;23:222-7.

195. Yee D, Favoni RE, Lebovic GS, et al. Insulin-like growth factor I expression by tumors of neuroectodermal origin with the t(11;22) chromosomal translocation. A potential autocrine growth factor. J Clin Invest. 1990;86:1806-14.

196. van Valen F, Winkelmann W, Jurgens H. Type I and type II insulin-like growth factor receptors and their function in human Ewing's sarcoma cells. J Cancer Res Clin Oncol. 1992;118:269-75.

197. Benini S, Zuntini M, Manara MC, et al. Insulin-like growth factor binding protein 3 as an anticancer molecule in Ewing's sarcoma. Int J Cancer. 2006;119:1039-46.

198. Scotlandi K, Maini C, Manara MC, et al. Effectiveness of insulin-like growth factor I receptor antisense strategy against Ewing's sarcoma cells. Cancer Gene Ther. 2002;9:296-307.

199. Scotlandi K, Avnet S, Benini S, et al. Expression of an IGF-I receptor dominant negative mutant induces apoptosis, inhibits tumorigenesis and enhances chemosensitivity in Ewing's sarcoma cells. Int J Cancer. 2002;101:11-6.

200. Scotlandi K, Benini S, Sarti M, et al. Insulin-like growth factor I receptor–mediated circuit in Ewing's sarcoma/peripheral neuroectodermal tumor: a possible therapeutic target. Cancer Res. 1996;56:4570-4.

201. Scotlandi K, Benini S, Nanni P, et al. Blockage of insulin-like growth factor-I receptor inhibits the growth of Ewing's sarcoma in athymic mice. Cancer Res. 1998;58:4127-31.

202. Scotlandi K, Manara MC, Nicoletti G, et al. Antitumor activity of the insulin-like growth factor-I receptor kinase inhibitor NVP-AEW541 in musculoskeletal tumors. Cancer Res. 2005;65:3868-76.

203. Toretsky JA, Kalebic T, Blakesley V, et al. The insulin-like growth factor-I receptor is required for EWS/FLI-1 transformation of fibroblasts. J Biol Chem. 1997;272:30822-7.

204. Strammiello R, Benini S, Manara MC, et al. Impact of IGF-I/IGF-IR circuit on the angiogenetic properties of Ewing's sarcoma cells. Horm Metab Res. 2003;35:675-84.

205. Hofbauer S, Hamilton G, Theyer G, et al. Insulin-like growth factor-I-dependent growth and in vitro chemosensitivity of Ewing's sarcoma and peripheral primitive neuroectodermal tumour cell lines. Eur J Cancer. 1993;29A:241-5.

206. Toretsky JA, Thakar M, Eskenazi AE, Frantz CN. Phosphoinositide 3-hydroxide kinase blockade enhances apoptosis in the Ewing's sarcoma family of tumors. Cancer Res. 1999;59:5745-50.

207. Mitsiades CS, Mitsiades NS, McMullan CJ, et al. Inhibition of the insulin-like growth factor receptor-1 tyrosine kinase activity as a therapeutic strategy for multiple myeloma, other hematologic malignancies, and solid tumors. Cancer Cell. 2004;5:221-30.

208. McAllister NR, Lessnick SL. The potential for molecular therapeutic targets in Ewing's sarcoma. Curr Treat Options Oncol. 2005;6:461-71.

209. Benini S, Manara MC, Cerisano V, et al. Contribution of MEK/MAPK and PI3-K signaling pathway to the malignant behavior of Ewing's sarcoma cells: therapeutic prospects. Int J Cancer. 2004;108:358-66.

210. Lin S, Boey D, Herzog H. NPY and Y receptors: lessons from transgenic and knockout models. Neuropeptides. 2004;38:189-200.

211. Kitlinska J. Neuropeptide Y in neural crest-derived tumors: Effect on growth and vascularization. Cancer Lett. 2006.

212. Kitlinska J, Abe K, Kuo L, et al. Differential effects of neuropeptide Y on the growth and vascularization of neural crest-derived tumors. Cancer Res. 2005;65:1719-28.

213. Kitlinska J, Kuo L, Abe K, et al. Role of neuropeptide Y and dipeptidyl peptidase IV in regulation of Ewing's sarcoma growth. Adv Exp Med Biol. 2006;575:223-9.

214. Fuchs B, Inwards CY, Janknecht R. Vascular endothelial growth factor expression is up-regulated by EWS-ETS oncoproteins and Sp1 and may represent an independent predictor of survival in Ewing's sarcoma. Clin Cancer Res. 2004;10:1344-53.

215. Zhou Z, Zhou RR, Guan H, et al. E1A gene therapy inhibits angiogenesis in a Ewing's sarcoma animal model. Mol Cancer Ther. 2003;2:1313-9.

216. Holzer G, Obermair A, Koschat M, et al. Concentration of vascular endothelial growth factor (VEGF) in the serum of patients with malignant bone tumors. Med Pediatr Oncol. 2001;36:601-4.

217. Pavlakovic H, Von Schutz V, Rossler J, et al. Quantification of angiogenesis stimulators in children with solid malignancies. Int J Cancer. 2001;92:756-60.

218. Bolontrade MF, Zhou RR, Kleinerman ES. Vasculogenesis plays a role in the growth of Ewing's sarcoma in vivo. Clin Cancer Res. 2002;8:3622-7.

219. Lee TH, Bolontrade MF, Worth LL, et al. Production of VEGF165 by Ewing's sarcoma cells induces vasculogenesis and the incorporation of CD34+ stem cells into the expanding tumor vasculature. Int J Cancer. 2006;119:839-46.

220. Dalal S, Berry AM, Cullinane CJ, et al. Vascular endothelial growth factor: a therapeutic target for tumors of the Ewing's sarcoma family. Clin Cancer Res. 2005;11:2364-78.

221. Guan H, Zhou Z, Wang H, et al. A small interfering RNA targeting vascular endothelial growth factor inhibits Ewing's sarcoma growth in a xenograft mouse model. Clin Cancer Res. 2005;11:2662-9.

222. Amiel A, Ohali A, Fejgin M, et al. Molecular cytogenetic parameters in Ewing sarcoma. Cancer Genet Cytogenet. 2003;140:107-12.

223. Sotillo-Pineiro E, Sierrasesumaga L, Patinno-Garcia A. Telomerase activity and telomere length in primary and metastatic tumors from pediatric bone cancer patients. Pediatr Res. 2004;55:231-5.

224. Ohali A, Avigad S, Cohen IJ, et al. Association between telomerase activity and outcome in patients with nonmetastatic Ewing family of tumors. J Clin Oncol. 2003;21:3836-43.

225. Ulaner GA, Hoffman AR, Otero J, et al. Divergent patterns of telomere maintenance mechanisms among human sarcomas: sharply contrasting prevalence of the alternative lengthening of telomeres mechanism in Ewing's sarcomas and osteosarcomas. Genes Chromosomes Cancer. 2004;41:155-62.

226. Shindoh M, Higashino F, Kohgo T. E1AF, an ets-oncogene family transcription factor. Cancer Lett. 2004;216:1-8.

227. Xiao X, Athanasiou M, Sidorov IA, et al. Role of Ets/Id proteins for telomerase regulation in human cancer cells. Exp Mol Pathol. 2003;75:238-47.

228. Kovar H, Dworzak M, Strehl S, et al. Overexpression of the pseudoautosomal gene MIC2 in Ewing's sarcoma and peripheral primitive neuroectodermal tumor. Oncogene. 1990;5:1067-70.

229. Ambros IM, Ambros PF, Strehl S, et al. MIC2 is a specific marker for Ewing's sarcoma and peripheral primitive neuroectodermal tumors. Evidence for a common histogenesis of Ewing's sarcoma and peripheral primitive neuroectodermal tumors from MIC2 expression and specific chromosome aberration. Cancer. 1991;67:1886-93.

230. Fellinger EJ, Garin-Chesa P, Triche TJ, et al. Immunohistochemical analysis of Ewing's sarcoma cell surface antigen p30/32MIC2. Am J Pathol. 1991;139:317-25.

231. Fellinger EJ, Garin-Chesa P, Glasser DB, et al. Comparison of cell surface antigen HBA71 (p30/32MIC2), neuron-specific enolase, and vimentin in the immunohistochemical analysis of Ewing's sarcoma of bone. Am J Surg Pathol. 1992;16:746-55.

232. Levy R, Dilley J, Fox RI, Warnke R. A human thymus-leukemia antigen defined by hybridoma monoclonal antibodies. Proc Natl Acad Sci U S A. 1979;76:6552-6.

233. Goodfellow P, Banting G, Sheer D, et al. Genetic evidence that a Y-linked gene in man is homologous to a gene on the X chromosome. Nature. 1983;302:346-9.

234. Dracopoli NC, Rettig WJ, Albino AP, et al. Genes controlling gp25/30 cell-surface molecules map to chromosomes X and Y and escape X-inactivation. Am J Hum Genet. 1985;37:199-207.

235. Ramani P, Rampling D, Link M. Immunocytochemical study of 12E7 in small round-cell tumours of childhood: an assessment of its sensitivity and specificity. Histopathology. 1993;23:557-61.

236. Perlman EJ, Dickman PS, Askin FB, et al. Ewing's sarcoma—routine diagnostic utilization of MIC2 analysis: a Pediatric Oncology Group/Children's Cancer Group Intergroup Study. Hum Pathol. 1994;25:304-7.

237. Devaney K, Abbondanzo SL, Shekitka KM, et al. MIC2 detection in tumors of bone and adjacent soft tissues. Clin Orthop Relat Res. 1995;176-87.

238. Banting GS, Pym B, Darling SM, Goodfellow PN. The MIC2 gene product: epitope mapping and structural prediction analysis define an integral membrane protein. Mol Immunol. 1989;26:181-8.

239. Banting GS, Pym B, Goodfellow PN. Biochemical analysis of an antigen produced by both human sex chromosomes. EMBO J. 1985;4:1967-72.

240. Bernard G, Zoccola D, Deckert M, et al. The E2 molecule (CD99) specifically triggers homotypic aggregation of CD4+ CD8+ thymocytes. J Immunol. 1995;154:26-32.

241. Bernard G, Breittmayer JP, de Matteis M, et al. Apoptosis of immature thymocytes mediated by E2/CD99. J Immunol. 1997;158:2543-50.

242. Choi EY, Park WS, Jung KC, et al. Engagement of CD99 induces up-regulation of TCR and MHC class I and II molecules on the surface of human thymocytes. J Immunol. 1998;161:749-54.

243. Hahn JH, Kim MK, Choi EY, et al. CD99 (MIC2) regulates the LFA-1/ICAM-1-mediated adhesion of lymphocytes, and its gene encodes both positive and negative regulators of cellular adhesion. J Immunol. 1997;159:2250-8.

244. Bernard G, Raimondi V, Alberti I, et al. CD99 (E2) up-regulates alpha4 beta1-dependent T cell adhesion to inflamed vascular endothelium under flow conditions. Eur J Immunol. 2000;30:3061-5.

245. Schenkel AR, Mamdouh Z, Chen X, et al. CD99 plays a major role in the migration of monocytes through endothelial junctions. Nat Immunol. 2002;3:143-50.

246. Waclavicek M, Majdic O, Stulnig T, et al. CD99 engagement on human peripheral blood T cells results in TCR/CD3-dependent cellular activation and allows for Th1-restricted cytokine production. J Immunol. 1998;161:4671-8.

247. Wingett D, Forcier K, Nielson CP. A role for CD99 in T cell activation. Cell Immunol. 1999;193:17-23.

248. Scotlandi K, Baldini N, Cerisano V, et al. CD99 engagement: an effective therapeutic strategy for Ewing tumors. Cancer Res. 2000;60:5134-42.

249. Sohn HW, Choi EY, Kim SH, et al. Engagement of CD99 induces apoptosis through a calcineurin-independent pathway in Ewing's sarcoma cells. Am J Pathol. 1998;153:1937-45.

250. Scotlandi K, Perdichizzi S, Bernard G, et al. Targeting CD99 in association with doxorubicin: an effective combined treatment for Ewing's sarcoma. Eur J Cancer. 2006;42:91-6.

251. Cerisano V, Aalto Y, Perdichizzi S, et al. Molecular mechanisms of CD99-induced caspase-independent cell death and cell-cell adhesion in Ewing's sarcoma cells: actin and zyxin as key intracellular mediators. Oncogene. 2004;23:5664-74.

252. Amsellem V, Kryszke MH, Hervy M, et al. The actin cytoskeleton-associated protein zyxin acts as a tumor suppressor in Ewing tumor cells. Exp Cell Res. 2005;304:443-56.

253. Jaishankar S, Zhang J, Roussel MF, Baker SJ. Transforming activity of EWS/FLI is not strictly dependent upon DNA-binding activity. Oncogene. 1999;18:5592-7.

254. Welford SM, Hebert SP, Deneen B, et al. DNA binding domain-independent pathways are involved in EWS/FLI1-mediated oncogenesis. J Biol Chem. 2001;276:41977-84.

255. Knoop LL, Baker SJ. The splicing factor U1C represses EWS/FLI-mediated transactivation. J Biol Chem. 2000;275:24865-71.

256. Knoop LL, Baker SJ. EWS/FLI alters 5′-splice site selection. J Biol Chem. 2001;276:22317-22.

257. Kim S, Denny CT, Wisdom R. Cooperative DNA binding with AP-1 proteins is required for transformation by EWS-Ets fusion proteins. Mol Cell Biol. 2006;26:2467-78.

258. Watson DK, Robinson L, Hodge DR, et al. FLI1 and EWS-FLI1 function as ternary complex factors and ELK1 and SAP1a function as ternary and quaternary complex factors on the Egr1 promoter serum response elements. Oncogene. 1997;14:213-21.

259. Crawford LV, Pim DC, Gurney EG, et al. Detection of a common feature in several human tumor cell lines—a 53,000-dalton protein. Proc Natl Acad Sci U S A. 1981;78:41-5.

260. Momand J, Zambetti GP, Olson DC, et al. The mdm-2 oncogene product forms a complex with the p53 protein and inhibits p53-mediated transactivation. Cell. 1992;69:1237-45.

261. Oliner JD, Kinzler KW, Meltzer PS, et al. Amplification of a gene encoding a p53-associated protein in human sarcomas. Nature. 1992;358:80-3.

262. Quelle DE, Zindy F, Ashmun RA, Sherr CJ. Alternative reading frames of the INK4a tumor suppressor gene encode two unrelated proteins capable of inducing cell cycle arrest. Cell. 1995;83:993-1000.

263. Stott FJ, Bates S, James MC, et al. The alternative product from the human CDKN2A locus, p14(ARF), participates in a regulatory feedback loop with p53 and MDM2. EMBO J. 1998;17:5001-14.

264. Kovar H, Jug G, Aryee DN, et al. Among genes involved in the RB dependent cell cycle regulatory cascade, the p16 tumor suppressor gene is frequently lost in the Ewing family of tumors. Oncogene. 1997;15:2225-32.

265. Tsuchiya T, Sekine K, Hinohara S, et al. Analysis of the p16INK4, p14ARF, p15, TP53, and MDM2 genes and their prognostic implications in osteosarcoma and Ewing sarcoma. Cancer Genet Cytogenet. 2000;120:91-8.

266. Kovar H, Auinger A, Jug G, et al. Narrow spectrum of infrequent p53 mutations and absence of MDM2 amplification in Ewing tumours. Oncogene. 1993;8:2683-2690.

267. Ladanyi M, Lewis R, Jhanwar SC, et al. MDM2 and CDK4 gene amplification in Ewing's sarcoma. J Pathol. 1995;175:211-217.

268. Miller CW, Aslo A, Won A, et al. Alterations of the p53, Rb and MDM2 genes in osteosarcoma. J Cancer Res Clin Oncol. 1996;122:559-65.

269. Radig K, Schneider-Stock R, Rose I, et al. p53 and ras mutations in Ewing's sarcoma. Pathology research and practice. 1998;194:157-162.

270. Komuro H, Hayashi Y, Kawamura M, et al. Mutations of the p53 gene are involved in Ewing's sarcomas but not in neuroblastomas. Cancer Res. 1993;53:5284-8.

271. Patino-Garcia A, Sierrasesumaga L. Analysis of the p16INK4 and TP53 tumor suppressor genes in bone sarcoma pediatric patients. Cancer Genet Cytogenet. 1997;98:50-55.

272. Serrano M, Hannon GJ, Beach D. A new regulatory motif in cell-cycle control causing specific inhibition of cyclin D/CDK4. Nature. 1993;366:704-7.

273. Weinberg RA. The retinoblastoma protein and cell cycle control. Cell. 1995;81:323-30.

274. Kamb A, Gruis NA, Weaver-Feldhaus J, et al. A cell cycle regulator potentially involved in genesis of many tumor types. Science. 1994;264:436-40.

275. Obana K, Yang HW, Piao HY, et al. Aberrations of p16INK4A, p14ARF and p15INK4B genes in pediatric solid tumors. Int J Oncol. 2003;23:1151-7.

276. Davies H, Bignell GR, Cox C, et al. Mutations of the BRAF gene in human cancer. Nature. 2002;417:949-54.

277. Silvany RE, Eliazer S, Wolff NC, Ilaria RL, Jr. Interference with the constitutive activation of ERK1 and ERK2 impairs EWS/FLI-1-dependent transformation. Oncogene. 2000;19:4523-30.

278. Zwerner JP, May WA. Dominant negative PDGF-C inhibits growth of Ewing family tumor cell lines. Oncogene. 2002;21:3847-54.

279. Uren A, Merchant MS, Sun CJ, et al. Beta-platelet-derived growth factor receptor mediates motility and growth of Ewing's sarcoma cells. Oncogene. 2003;22:2334-42.

280. Uren A, Wolf V, Sun YF, et al. Wnt/Frizzled signaling in Ewing sarcoma. Pediatr Blood Cancer. 2004;43:243-9.

281. Lawlor ER, Lim JF, Tao W, et al. The Ewing tumor family of peripheral primitive neuroectodermal tumors expresses human gastrin-releasing peptide. Cancer Res. 1998;58:2469-76.

282. Kovar H, Pospisilova S, Jug G, Printz D, Gadner H. Response of Ewing tumor cells to forced and activated p53 expression. Oncogene. 2003;22:3193-204.

283. Deneen B, Denny CT. Loss of p16 pathways stabilizes EWS/FLI1 expression and complements EWS/FLI1 mediated transformation. Oncogene. 2001;20:6731-41.

284. Kontny HU, Lehrnbecher TM, Chanock SJ, Mackall CL. Simultaneous expression of Fas and nonfunctional Fas ligand in Ewing's sarcoma. Cancer Res. 1998;58:5842-9.

285. Lee SH, Jang JJ, Lee JY, et al. Immunohistochemical analysis of Fas ligand expression in sarcomas. Sarcomas express high level of FasL in vivo. APMIS. 1998;106:1035-40.

286. Mitsiades N, Poulaki V, Kotoula V, et al. Fas ligand is present in tumors of the Ewing's sarcoma family and is cleaved into a soluble form by a metalloproteinase. Am J Pathol. 1998;153:1947-56.

287. Lee B, Galli S, Tsokos M. Sensitive Ewing sarcoma and neuroblastoma cell lines have increased levels of BAD expression and decreased levels of BAR expression compared with resistant cell lines. Cancer Lett. 2006;247:110-4.

288. Mitsiades N, Poulaki V, Leone A, Tsokos M. Fas-mediated apoptosis in Ewing's sarcoma cell lines by metalloproteinase inhibitors. J Natl Cancer Inst. 1999;91:1678-84.

289. Zhou Z, Lafleur EA, Koshkina NV, et al. Interleukin-12 up-regulates Fas expression in human osteosarcoma and Ewing's sarcoma cells by enhancing its promoter activity. Mol Cancer Res. 2005;3:685-91.

290. Jia SF, Duan X, Worth LL, et al. Intratumor murine interleukin-12 gene therapy suppressed the growth of local and distant Ewing's sarcoma. Cancer Gene Ther. 2006;13:948-57.

291. van Valen F, Winkelmann W, Burdach S, et al. Interferon gamma and tumour necrosis factor alpha induce a synergistic antiproliferative response in human Ewing's sarcoma cells in vitro. J Cancer Res Clin Oncol. 1993;119:615-21.

292. van Valen F, Kentrup-Lardong V, Truckenbrod B, et al. Regulation of the release of tumour necrosis factor (TNF) alpha and soluble TNF receptor by gamma irradiation and interferon gamma in Ewing's sarcoma/peripheral primitive neuroectodermal tumour cells. J Cancer Res Clin Oncol. 1997;123:245-52.

293. Van Valen F, Fulda S, Truckenbrod B, et al. Apoptotic responsiveness of the Ewing's sarcoma family of tumours to tumour necrosis factor-related apoptosis-inducing ligand (TRAIL). Int J Cancer. 2000;88:252-9.

294. Van Valen F, Fulda S, Schafer KL, et al. Selective and nonselective toxicity of TRAIL/Apo2L combined with chemotherapy in human bone tumour cells vs. normal human cells. Int J Cancer. 2003;107:929-40.

295. Abadie A, Besancon F, Wietzerbin J. Type I interferon and TNF alpha cooperate with type II interferon for TRAIL induction and triggering of apoptosis in SK-N-MC EWING tumor cells. Oncogene. 2004;23:4911-20.

296. Abadie A, Wietzerbin J. Involvement of TNF-related apoptosis-inducing ligand (TRAIL) induction in interferon gamma-mediated apoptosis in Ewing tumor cells. Ann N Y Acad Sci. 2003;1010:117-20.

297. Merchant MS, Yang X, Melchionda F, et al. Interferon gamma enhances the effectiveness of tumor necrosis factor-related apoptosis-inducing ligand receptor agonists in a xenograft model of Ewing's sarcoma. Cancer Res. 2004;64:8349-56.

298. Djavaheri-Mergny M, Wietzerbin J, et al. TNF alpha potentiates 2-methoxyestradiol-induced mitochondrial death pathway. Ann N Y Acad Sci. 2003;1010:159-62.

299. Mitsiades N, Poulaki V, Mitsiades C, Tsokos M. Ewing's sarcoma family tumors are sensitive to tumor necrosis factor-related apoptosis-inducing ligand and express death receptor 4 and death receptor 5. Cancer Res. 2001;61:2704-12.

300. Kumar A, Jasmin A, Eby MT, Chaudhary PM. Cytotoxicity of Tumor necrosis factor related apoptosis-inducing ligand towards Ewing's sarcoma cell lines. Oncogene. 2001;20:1010-4.

301. Kontny HU, Hammerle K, Klein R, et al. Sensitivity of Ewing's sarcoma to TRAIL-induced apoptosis. Cell Death Differ. 2001;8:506-14.

302. Javelaud D, Besancon F. NF-kappa B activation results in rapid inactivation of JNK in TNF alpha-treated Ewing sarcoma cells: a mechanism for the anti-apoptotic effect of NF-kappa B. Oncogene. 2001;20:4365-72.

303. Widhe B, Widhe T. Initial symptoms and clinical features in osteosarcoma and Ewing sarcoma. J Bone Joint Surg Am. 2000;82:667-74.

304. Oberlin O, Habrand JL, Zucker JM, et al. No benefit of ifosfamide in Ewing's sarcoma: a nonrandomized study of the French Society of Pediatric Oncology. J Clin Oncol. 1992;10:1407-12.

305. Bacci G, Ferrari S, Bertoni F, et al. Prognostic factors in nonmetastatic Ewing's sarcoma of bone treated with adjuvant chemotherapy: analysis of 359 patients at the Istituto Ortopedico Rizzoli. J Clin Oncol. 2000;18:4-11.

306. Wilkins RM, Pritchard DJ, Burgert EO Jr, Unni KK. Ewing's sarcoma of bone. Experience with 140 patients. Cancer. 1986;58:2551-5.

307. Ilaslan H, Sundaram M, Unni KK, Dekutoski MB. Primary Ewing's sarcoma of the vertebral column. Skeletal Radiol. 2004;33:506-13.

308. Grubb MR, Currier BL, Pritchard DJ, Ebersold MJ. Primary Ewing's sarcoma of the spine. Spine. 1994;19:309-13.

309. Pilepich MV, Vietti TJ, Nesbit ME, et al. Ewing's sarcoma of the vertebral column. Int J Radiat Oncol Biol Phys. 1981;7:27-31.

310. Venkateswaran L, Rodriguez-Galindo C, Merchant TE, et al. Primary Ewing tumor of the vertebrae: clinical characteristics, prognostic factors, and outcome. Med Pediatr Oncol. 2001;37:30-5.

311. Bacci G, Mercuri M, Longhi A, et al. Neoadjuvant chemotherapy for Ewing's tumour of bone: recent experience at the Rizzoli Orthopaedic Institute. Eur J Cancer. 2002;38:2243-51.

312. Craft AW, Cotterill SJ, Bullimore JA, Pearson D. Long-term results from the first UKCCSG Ewing's Tumour Study (ET-1). United Kingdom Children's Cancer Study Group (UKCCSG) and the Medical Research Council Bone Sarcoma Working Party. Eur J Cancer. 1997;33:1061-9.

313. Elomaa I, Blomqvist CP, Saeter G, et al. Five-year results in Ewing's sarcoma. The Scandinavian Sarcoma Group experience with the SSG IX protocol. Eur J Cancer. 2000;36:875-80.

314. Raney RB, Asmar L, Newton WA Jr, et al. Ewing's sarcoma of soft tissues in childhood: a report from the Intergroup Rhabdomyosarcoma Study, 1972 to 1991. J Clin Oncol. 1997;15:574-82.

315. Oberlin O, Deley MC, Bui BN, et al. Prognostic factors in localized Ewing's tumours and peripheral neuroectodermal tumours: the third study of the French Society of Paediatric Oncology (EW88 study). Br J Cancer. 2001;85:1646-54.

316. Bacci G, Forni C, Longhi A, et al. Long-term outcome for patients with non-metastatic Ewing's sarcoma treated with adjuvant and neoadjuvant chemotherapies. 402 patients treated at Rizzoli between 1972 and 1992. Eur J Cancer. 2004;40:73-83.

317. Farley FA, Healey JH, Caparros-Sison B, et al. Lactase dehydrogenase as a tumor marker for recurrent disease in Ewing's sarcoma. Cancer. 1987;59:1245-8.

318. Reinus WR, Gilula L. Radiology of Ewing's sarcoma: Intergroup Ewing's Sarcoma Study. Radiographics. 1984;4:929-944.

319. Paulussen M, Ahrens S, Craft AW, et al. Ewing's tumors with primary lung metastases: survival analysis of 114 (European Intergroup) Cooperative Ewing's Sarcoma Studies patients. J Clin Oncol. 1998;16:3044-52.

320. Grier HE, Krailo MD, Tarbell NJ, et al. Addition of ifosfamide and etoposide to standard chemotherapy for Ewing's sarcoma and primitive neuroectodermal tumor of bone. N Engl J Med. 2003;348:694-701.

321. Cotterill SJ, Ahrens S, Paulussen M, et al. Prognostic factors in Ewing's tumor of bone: analysis of 975 patients from the European Intergroup Cooperative Ewing's Sarcoma Study Group. J Clin Oncol. 2000;18:3108-14.

322. Paulussen M, Ahrens S, Burdach S, et al. Primary metastatic (stage IV) Ewing tumor: survival analysis of 171 patients from the EICESS studies. European Intergroup Cooperative Ewing sarcoma Studies. Ann Oncol. 1998;9:275-81.

323. Cangir A, Vietti TJ, Gehan EA, et al. Ewing's sarcoma metastatic at diagnosis. Results and comparisons of two intergroup Ewing's sarcoma studies. Cancer. 1990;66:887-93.

324. Miser JS, Krailo MD, Tarbell NJ, et al. Treatment of metastatic Ewing's sarcoma or primitive neuroectodermal tumor of bone: evaluation of combination ifosfamide and etoposide—a Children's Cancer Group and Pediatric Oncology Group study. J Clin Oncol. 2004;22:2873-6.

325. Oberlin O, Bayle C, Hartmann O, et al. Incidence of bone marrow involvement in Ewing's sarcoma: value of extensive investigation of the bone marrow. Med Pediatr Oncol. 1995;24:343-6.

326. Marina NM, Etcubanas E, Parham DM, et al. Peripheral primitive neuroectodermal tumor (peripheral neuroepithelioma) in children. A review of the St. Jude experience and controversies in diagnosis and management. Cancer. 1989;64:1952-60.

327. Parasuraman S, Langston J, Rao BN, et al. Brain metastases in pediatric Ewing sarcoma and rhabdomyosarcoma: the St. Jude Children's Research Hospital experience. J Pediatr Hematol Oncol. 1999;21:370-7.

328. Trigg ME, Glaubiger D, Nesbit ME Jr. The frequency of isolated CNS involvement in Ewing's sarcoma. Cancer. 1982;49:2404-9.

329. Enneking WF: Staging musculoskeletal tumors In Enneking WF (ed). Musculoskeletal Tumor Surgery. New York, Churchill Livingstone, 1983, pp 68-88.

330. Levine SM, Lambiase RE, Petchprapa CN. Cortical lesions of the tibia: characteristic appearances at conventional radiography. Radiographics. 2003;23:157-77.

331. Wagner LM, Neel MD, Pappo AS, et al. Fractures in pediatric Ewing sarcoma. J Pediatr Hematol Oncol. 2001;23:568-71.

332. Khong PL, Chan GC, Shek TW, et al. Imaging of peripheral PNET: common and uncommon locations. Clin Radiol. 2002;57:272-7.

333. Dick EA, McHugh K, Kimber C, Michalski A. Imaging of non-central nervous system primitive neuroectodermal tumours: diagnostic features and correlation with outcome. Clin Radiol. 2001;56:206-15.

334. Ibarburen C, Haberman JJ, Zerhouni EA. Peripheral primitive neuroectodermal tumors. CT and MRI evaluation. Eur J Radiol. 1996;21:225-32.

335. Sallustio G, Pirronti T, Lasorella A, et al. Diagnostic imaging of primitive neuroectodermal tumour of the chest wall (Askin tumour). Pediatr Radiol. 1998;28:697-702.

336. Winer-Muram HT, Kauffman WM, Gronemeyer SA, Jennings SG. Primitive neuroectodermal tumors of the chest wall (Askin tumors): CT and MR findings. AJR Am J Roentgenol. 1993;161:265-8.

337. O'Keeffe F, Lorigan JG, Wallace S. Radiologic features of extraskeletal Ewing sarcoma. Br J Radiol. 1990;63:456-60.

338. Gladish GW, Sabloff BM, Munden RF, et al. Primary thoracic sarcomas. Radiographics. 2002;22:621-37.

339. Frouge C, Vanel D, Coffre C, et al. The role of magnetic resonance imaging in the evaluation of Ewing sarcoma. A report of 27 cases. Skeletal Radiol. 1988;17:387-92.

340. Hawkins DS, Schuetze SM, Butrynski JE, et al. [18F]Fluorodeoxyglucose positron emission tomography predicts outcome for Ewing sarcoma family of tumors. J Clin Oncol. 2005;23:8828-34.

341. Gyorke T, Zajic T, Lange A, et al. Impact of FDG PET for staging of Ewing sarcomas and primitive neuroectodermal tumours. Nucl Med Commun. 2006;27:17-24.

342. Franzius C, Sciuk J, Daldrup-Link HE, et al. FDG-PET for detection of osseous metastases from malignant primary bone tumors: comparison with bone scintigraphy. Eur J Nucl Med. 2000;27:1305-11.

343. Franzius C, Daldrup-Link HE, Sciuk J, et al. FDG-PET for detection of pulmonary metastases from malignant primary bone tumors: comparison with spiral CT. Ann Oncol. 2001;12:479-86.

344. Franzius C, Daldrup-Link HE, Wagner-Bohn A, et al. FDG-PET for detection of recurrences from malignant primary bone tumors: comparison with conventional imaging. Ann Oncol. 2002;13:157-60.

345. Carpentieri DF, Qualman SJ, Bowen J, et al. Protocol for the examination of specimens from pediatric and adult patients with osseous and extraosseous Ewing sarcoma family of tumors, including peripheral primitive neuroectodermal tumor and Ewing sarcoma. Arch Pathol Lab Med. 2005;129:866-73.

346. Udayakumar AM, Sundareshan TS, Goud TM, et al. Cytogenetic characterization of Ewing tumors using fine needle aspiration samples. A 10-year experience and review of the literature. Cancer Genet Cytogenet. 2001;127:42-8.

347. Hosalkar HS, Dormans JP. Limb-sparing surgery for pediatric musculoskeletal tumors. Pediatr Blood Cancer. 2004;42:295-310.

348. Folpe AL, Goldblum JR, Rubin BP, et al. Morphologic and immunophenotypic diversity in Ewing family tumors: a study of 66 genetically confirmed cases. Am J Surg Pathol. 2005;29:1025-33.

349. Parham DM, Hijazi Y, Steinberg SM, et al. Neuroectodermal differentiation in Ewing's sarcoma family of tumors does not predict tumor behavior. Hum Pathol. 1999;30:911-8.

350. Schmidt D, Herrmann C, Jurgens H, Harms D. Malignant peripheral neuroectodermal tumor and its necessary distinction from Ewing's sarcoma. A report from the Kiel Pediatric Tumor Registry. Cancer. 1991;68:2251-9.

351. Ushigome S, Shimoda T, Takaki K, et al. Immunocytochemical and ultrastructural studies of the histogenesis of Ewing's sarcoma and putatively related tumors. Cancer. 1989;64:52-62.

352. Hamilton G, Fellinger EJ, Schratter I, Fritsch A. Characterization of a human endocrine tissue and tumor-associated Ewing's sarcoma antigen. Cancer Res. 1988;48:6127-31.

353. Lee CS, Southey MC, Waters K, et al. EWS/FLI-1 fusion transcript detection and MIC2 immunohistochemical staining

in the diagnosis of Ewing's sarcoma. Pediatr Pathol Lab Med. 1996;16:379-92.

354. Weidner N, Tjoe J. Immunohistochemical profile of monoclonal antibody O13: antibody that recognizes glycoprotein p30/32MIC2 and is useful in diagnosing Ewing's sarcoma and peripheral neuroepithelioma. Am J Surg Pathol. 1994;18:486-94.

355. Halliday BE, Slagel DD, Elsheikh TE, Silverman JF. Diagnostic utility of MIC-2 immunocytochemical staining in the differential diagnosis of small blue cell tumors. Diagn Cytopathol. 1998;19:410-6.

356. Lucas DR, Bentley G, Dan ME, et al. Ewing sarcoma vs lymphoblastic lymphoma. A comparative immunohistochemical study. Am J Clin Pathol. 2001;115:11-7.

357. Ahmed A, Gilbert-Barness E, Lacson A. Expression of c-kit in Ewing family of tumors: a comparison of different immunohistochemical protocols. Pediatr Dev Pathol. 2004;7:342-7.

358. Scotlandi K, Manara MC, Strammiello R, et al. C-kit receptor expression in Ewing's sarcoma: lack of prognostic value but therapeutic targeting opportunities in appropriate conditions. J Clin Oncol. 2003;21:1952-60.

359. Smithey BE, Pappo AS, Hill DA. C-kit expression in pediatric solid tumors: a comparative immunohistochemical study. Am J Surg Pathol. 2002;26:486-92.

360. Folpe AL, Schmidt RA, Chapman D, Gown AM. Poorly differentiated synovial sarcoma: immunohistochemical distinction from primitive neuroectodermal tumors and high-grade malignant peripheral nerve sheath tumors. Am J Surg Pathol. 1998;22:673-82.

361. Carter RL, al-Sams SZ, Corbett RP, Clinton S. A comparative study of immunohistochemical staining for neuron-specific enolase, protein gene product 9.5 and S-100 protein in neuroblastoma, Ewing's sarcoma and other round cell tumours in children. Histopathology. 1990;16:461-7.

362. Ozdemirli M, Fanburg-Smith JC, Hartmann DP, et al. Differentiating lymphoblastic lymphoma and Ewing's sarcoma: lymphocyte markers and gene rearrangement. Mod Pathol. 2001;14:1175-82.

363. Olsen SH, Thomas DG, Lucas DR. Cluster analysis of immunohistochemical profiles in synovial sarcoma, malignant peripheral nerve sheath tumor, and Ewing sarcoma. Mod Pathol. 2006;19:659-68.

364. Hill DA, Pfeifer JD, Marley EF, et al. WT1 staining reliably differentiates desmoplastic small round cell tumor from Ewing sarcoma/primitive neuroectodermal tumor. An immunohistochemical and molecular diagnostic study. Am J Clin Pathol. 2000;114:345-53.

365. Folpe AL, Hill CE, Parham DM, et al. Immunohistochemical detection of FLI-1 protein expression: a study of 132 round cell tumors with emphasis on CD99-positive mimics of Ewing's sarcoma/primitive neuroectodermal tumor. Am J Surg Pathol. 2000;24:1657-62.

366. Llombart-Bosch A, Navarro S. Immunohistochemical detection of EWS and FLI-1 proteinss in Ewing sarcoma and primitive neuroectodermal tumors: comparative analysis with CD99 (MIC-2) expression. Appl Immunohistochem Mol Morphol. 2001;9:255-60.

367. Dei Tos AP, Dal Cin P. The role of cytogenetics in the classification of soft tissue tumours. Virchows Arch. 1997;431:83-94.

368. Sorensen PHB, Triche TJ. Gene fusions encoding chimaeric transcription factors in solid tumors. Seminars in cancer biology. 1996;7:3-14.

369. Bonin G, Scamps C, Turc-Carel C, Lipinski M. Chimeric EWS-FLI1 transcript in a Ewing cell line with a complex t(11;22;14) translocation. Cancer Res. 1993;53:3655-7.

370. Desmaze C, Brizard F, Turc-Carel C, et al. Multiple chromosomal mechanisms generate an EWS/FLI1 or an EWS/ERG fusion gene in Ewing tumors. Cancer Genet Cytogenet. 1997;97:12-9.

371. Noguera R, Pellin A, Navarro S, et al. Translocation (10;11;22)(p14;q24;q12) characterized by fluorescence in situ hybridization in a case of Ewing's tumor. Diagn Mol Pathol. 2001;10:2-8.

372. Hattinger CM, Rumpler S, Kovar H, Ambros PF. Fine-mapping of cytogenetically undetectable EWS/ERG fusions on DNA fibers of Ewing tumors. Cytogenet Cell Genet. 2001;93:29-35.

373. McManus AP, Gusterson BA, Pinkerton CR, Shipley JM. Diagnosis of Ewing's sarcoma and related tumours by detection of chromosome 22q12 translocations using fluorescence in situ hybridization on tumour touch imprints. J Pathol. 1995;176:137-42.

374. Desmaze C, Zucman J, Delattre O, et al. Interphase molecular cytogenetics of Ewing's sarcoma and peripheral neuroepithelioma t(11;22) with flanking and overlapping cosmid probes. Cancer Genet Cytogenet. 1994;74:13-8.

375. Kaneko Y, Kobayashi H, Handa M, et al. EWS-ERG fusion transcript produced by chromosomal insertion in a Ewing sarcoma. Genes Chromosomes Cancer. 1997;18:228-31.

376. Hattinger CM, Zoubek A, Ambros PF. Molecular cytogenetics in ewing tumors: diagnostic and prognostic information. Onkologie. 2000;23:416-422.

377. Bridge RS, Rajaram V, Dehner LP, et al. Molecular diagnosis of Ewing sarcoma/primitive neuroectodermal tumor in routinely processed tissue: a comparison of two FISH strategies and RT-PCR in malignant round cell tumors. Mod Pathol. 2006;19:1-8.

378. Zucman J, Delattre O, Desmaze C, et al. EWS and ATF-1 gene fusion induced by t(12;22) translocation in malignant melanoma of soft parts. Nat Genet. 1993;4:341-5.

379. Ladanyi M, Gerald W. Fusion of the EWS and WT1 genes in the desmoplastic small round cell tumor. Cancer Res. 1994;54:2837-40.

380. Stenman G, Andersson H, Mandahl N, et al. Translocation t(9;22)(q22;q12) is a primary cytogenetic abnormality in extraskeletal myxoid chondrosarcoma. Int J Cancer. 1995;62:398-402.

381. Panagopoulos I, Mencinger M, Dietrich CU, et al. Fusion of the RBP56 and CHN genes in extraskeletal myxoid chondrosarcomas with translocation t(9;17)(q22;q11). Oncogene. 1999;18:7594-8.

382. Labelle Y, Zucman J, Stenman G, et al. Oncogenic conversion of a novel orphan nuclear receptor by chromosome translocation. Hum Mol Genet. 1995;4:2219-26.

383. Gill S, McManus AP, Crew AJ, et al. Fusion of the EWS gene to a DNA segment from 9q22-31 in a human myxoid chondrosarcoma. Genes Chromosomes Cancer. 1995;12:307-10.

384. Panagopoulos I, Hoglund M, Mertens F, et al. Fusion of the EWS and CHOP genes in myxoid liposarcoma. Oncogene. 1996;12:489-94.

385. Mastrangelo T, Modena P, Tornielli S, et al. A novel zinc finger gene is fused to EWS in small round cell tumor. Oncogene. 2000;19:3799-804.

386. Sorensen PH, Shimada H, Liu XF, et al. Biphenotypic sarcomas with myogenic and neural differentiation express the Ewing's sarcoma EWS/FLI1 fusion gene. Cancer Res. 1995;55:1385-92.

387. Tan SY, Burchill S, Brownhill SC, et al. Small round cell tumor with biphenotypic differentiation and variant of t(21;22)(q22;q12). Pediatr Dev Pathol. 2001;4:391-6.

388. de Alava E, Lozano MD, Sola I, et al. Molecular features in a biphenotypic small cell sarcoma with neuroectodermal and muscle differentiation. Hum Pathol. 1998;29:181-4.

389. Downing JR, Head DR, Parham DM, et al. Detection of the (11;22)(q24;q12) translocation of Ewing's sarcoma and peripheral neuroectodermal tumor by reverse transcription polymerase chain reaction. Am J Pathol. 1993;143:1294-300.

390. Giovannini M, Biegel JA, Serra M, et al. EWS-erg and EWS-Fli1 fusion transcripts in Ewing's sarcoma and primitive neuroecto-

dermal tumors with variant translocations. J Clin Invest. 1994;
94:489-96.

391. Sorensen PH, Liu XF, Delattre O, et al. Reverse transcriptase PCR amplification of EWS/FLI-1 fusion transcripts as a diagnostic test for peripheral primitive neuroectodermal tumors of childhood. Diagn Mol Pathol. 1993;2:147-57.

392. Oberlin O, Rey A, Desfachelles AS, et al. Impact of high-dose busulfan plus melphalan as consolidation in metastatic Ewing tumors: a study by the Société Française des Cancers de l'Enfant. J Clin Oncol. 2006;24:3997-4002.

393. Hense HW, Ahrens S, Paulussen M, et al. Factors associated with tumor volume and primary metastases in Ewing tumors: results from the (EI)CESS studies. Ann Oncol. 1999;10:1073-7.

394. Jurgens H, Exner U, Gadner H, et al. Multidisciplinary treatment of primary Ewing's sarcoma of bone. A 6-year experience of a European Cooperative Trial. Cancer. 1988;61:23-32.

395. Ahrens S, Hoffmann C, Jabar S, et al. Evaluation of prognostic factors in a tumor volume-adapted treatment strategy for localized Ewing sarcoma of bone: the CESS 86 experience. Cooperative Ewing sarcoma Study. Med Pediatr Oncol. 1999;32:186-95.

396. Paulussen M, Ahrens S, Dunst J, et al. Localized Ewing tumor of bone: final results of the cooperative Ewing's Sarcoma Study CESS 86. J Clin Oncol. 2001;19:1818-29.

397. Rosito P, Mancini AF, Rondelli R, et al. Italian Cooperative Study for the treatment of children and young adults with localized Ewing sarcoma of bone: a preliminary report of 6 years of experience. Cancer. 1999;86:421-8.

398. Nesbit ME Jr., Gehan EA, Burgert EO Jr., et al. Multimodal therapy for the management of primary, nonmetastatic Ewing's sarcoma of bone: a long-term follow-up of the First Intergroup study. J Clin Oncol. 1990;8:1664-74.

399. Craft A, Cotterill S, Malcolm A, et al. Ifosfamide-containing chemotherapy in Ewing's sarcoma: The Second United Kingdom Children's Cancer Study Group and the Medical Research Council Ewing's Tumor Study. J Clin Oncol. 1998;16:3628-33.

400. Oberlin O, Patte C, Demeocq F, et al. The response to initial chemotherapy as a prognostic factor in localized Ewing's sarcoma. Eur J Cancer Clin Oncol. 1985;21:463-7.

401. Lin PP, Jaffe N, Herzog CE, et al. Chemotherapy response is an important predictor of local recurrence in Ewing sarcoma. Cancer. 2006;34:27.

402. Picci P, Bohling T, Bacci G, et al. Chemotherapy-induced tumor necrosis as a prognostic factor in localized Ewing's sarcoma of the extremities. J Clin Oncol. 1997;15:1553-9.

403. Picci P, Rougraff BT, Bacci G, et al. Prognostic significance of histopathologic response to chemotherapy in nonmetastatic Ewing's sarcoma of the extremities. J Clin Oncol. 1993;11:1763-9.

404. Wunder JS, Paulian G, Huvos AG, et al. The histologic response to chemotherapy as a predictor of the oncologic outcome of operative treatment of Ewing sarcoma. J Bone Joint Surg Am. 1998;80:1020-33.

405. Fizazi K, Dohollou N, Blay JY, et al. Ewing's family of tumors in adults: multivariate analysis of survival and long-term results of multimodality therapy in 182 patients. J Clin Oncol. 1998;16:3736-43.

406. Baldini EH, Demetri GD, Fletcher CD, et al. Adults with Ewing's sarcoma/primitive neuroectodermal tumor: adverse effect of older age and primary extraosseous disease on outcome. Ann Surg. 1999;230:79-86.

407. Martin RC 2nd, Brennan MF. Adult soft tissue Ewing sarcoma or primitive neuroectodermal tumors: predictors of survival? Arch Surg. 2003;138:281-5.

408. Verrill MW, Judson IR, Harmer CL, et al. Ewing's sarcoma and primitive neuroectodermal tumor in adults: are they different from Ewing's sarcoma and primitive neuroectodermal tumor in children? J Clin Oncol. 1997;15:2611-21.

409. Brereton HD, Simon R, Pomeroy TC. Pretreatment serum lactate dehydrogenase predicting metastatic spread in Ewing's sarcoma. Ann Intern Med. 1975;83:352-4.

410. Bacci G, Avella M, McDonald D, et al. Serum lactate dehydrogenase (LDH) as a tumor marker in Ewing's sarcoma. Tumori. 1988;74:649-55.

411. Glaubiger DL, Makuch R, Schwarz J, et al. Determination of prognostic factors and their influence on therapeutic results in patients with Ewing's sarcoma. Cancer. 1980;45:2213-9.

412. Aparicio J, Munarriz B, Pastor M, et al. Long-term follow-up and prognostic factors in Ewing's sarcoma. A multivariate analysis of 116 patients from a single institution. Oncology. 1998;55:20-6.

413. Riley RD, Burchill SA, Abrams KR, et al. A systematic review of molecular and biologic markers in tumours of the Ewing's sarcoma family. Eur J Cancer. 2003;39:19-30.

414. Pinto A, Grant LH, Hayes FA, et al. Immunohistochemical expression of neuron-specific enolase and Leu 7 in Ewing's sarcoma of bone. Cancer. 1989;64:1266-73.

415. Llombart-Bosch A, Lacombe MJ, Peydro-Olaya A, et al. Malignant peripheral neuroectodermal tumours of bone other than Askin's neoplasm: characterization of 14 new cases with immunohistochemistry and electron microscopy. Virchows Arch A Pathol Anat Histopathol. 1988;412:421-30.

416. Daugaard S, Kamby C, Sunde LM, et al. Ewing's sarcoma. A retrospective study of histologic and immunohistochemical factors and their relation to prognosis. Virchows Arch A Pathol Anat Histopathol. 1989;414:243-51.

417. Hartman KR, Triche TJ, Kinsella TJ, Miser JS. Prognostic value of histopathology in Ewing's sarcoma. Long-term follow-up of distal extremity primary tumors. Cancer. 1991;67:163-71.

418. Terrier P, Henry-Amar M, Triche TJ, et al. Is neuro-ectodermal differentiation of Ewing's sarcoma of bone associated with an unfavourable prognosis? Eur J Cancer. 1995;31A:307-14.

419. Hayes FA, Thompson EI, Meyer WH, et al. Therapy for localized Ewing's sarcoma of bone. J Clin Oncol. 1989;7:208-13.

420. Ginsberg JP, de Alava E, Ladanyi M, et al. EWS-FLI1 and EWS-ERG gene fusions are associated with similar clinical phenotypes in Ewing's sarcoma. J Clin Oncol. 1999;17:1809-14.

421. de Alava E, Kawai A, Healey JH, et al. EWS-FLI1 fusion transcript structure is an independent determinant of prognosis in Ewing's sarcoma. J Clin Oncol. 1998;16:1248-55.

422. West DC, Grier HE, Swallow MM, et al. Detection of circulating tumor cells in patients with Ewing's sarcoma and peripheral primitive neuroectodermal tumor. J Clin Oncol. 1997;15:583-8.

423. Schleiermacher G, Peter M, Oberlin O, et al. Increased risk of systemic relapses associated with bone marrow micrometastasis and circulating tumor cells in localized ewing tumor. J Clin Oncol. 2003;21:85-91.

424. Avigad S, Cohen IJ, Zilberstein J, et al. The predictive potential of molecular detection in the nonmetastatic Ewing family of tumors. Cancer. 2004;100:1053-8.

425. Hattinger CM, Potschger U, Tarkkanen M, et al. Prognostic impact of chromosomal aberrations in Ewing tumours. Br J Cancer. 2002;86:1763-9.

426. Zielenska M, Zhang ZM, Ng K, et al. Acquisition of secondary structural chromosomal changes in pediatric Ewing sarcoma is a probable prognostic factor for tumor response and clinical outcome. Cancer. 2001;91:2156-64.

427. Kullendorff CM, Mertens F, Donner M, et al. Cytogenetic aberrations in Ewing sarcoma: are secondary changes associated with clinical outcome? Med Pediatr Oncol. 1999;32:79-83.

428. de Alava E, Antonescu CR, Panizo A, et al. Prognostic impact of P53 status in Ewing's sarcoma. Cancer. 2000;89:783-92.

429. Huang HY, Illei PB, Zhao Z, et al. Ewing sarcomas with p53 mutation or p16/p14ARF homozygous deletion: a highly lethal subset associated with poor chemoresponse. J Clin Oncol. 2005;23:548-58.

430. Wei G, Antonescu CR, de Alava E, et al. Prognostic impact of INK4A deletion in Ewing sarcoma. Cancer. 2000;89:793-9.

431. Baumgart R, Hinterwimmer S, Krammer M, et al. The bioexpandable prosthesis: a new perspective after resection of malignant bone tumors in children. J Pediatr Hematol Oncol. 2005;27:452-5.

432. Krasin MJ, Davidoff AM, Rodriguez-Galindo C, et al. Definitive surgery and multiagent systemic therapy for patients with localized Ewing sarcoma family of tumors: local outcome and prognostic factors. Cancer. 2005;104:367-73.

433. Krasin MJ, Rodriguez-Galindo C, Davidoff AM, et al. Efficacy of combined surgery and irradiation for localized Ewings sarcoma family of tumors. Pediatr Blood Cancer. 2004;43:229-36.

434. Bacci G, Longhi A, Briccoli A, et al. The role of surgical margins in treatment of Ewing's sarcoma family tumors: experience of a single institution with 512 patients treated with adjuvant and neoadjuvant chemotherapy. Int J Radiat Oncol Biol Phys. 2006; 65:766-72.

435. Ozaki T, Hillmann A, Hoffmann C, et al. Significance of surgical margin on the prognosis of patients with Ewing's sarcoma. A report from the Cooperative Ewing's Sarcoma Study. Cancer. 1996;78:892-900.

436. Donaldson SS. Ewing sarcoma: radiation dose and target volume. Pediatr Blood Cancer. 2004;42:471-6.

437. Donaldson SS, Torrey M, Link MP, et al. A multidisciplinary study investigating radiotherapy in Ewing's sarcoma: end results of POG #8346. Pediatric Oncology Group. Int J Radiat Oncol Biol Phys. 1998;42:125-35.

438. Razek A, Perez CA, Tefft M, et al. Intergroup Ewing's Sarcoma Study: local control related to radiation dose, volume, and site of primary lesion in Ewing's sarcoma. Cancer. 1980;46:516-21.

439. Tepper J, Glaubiger D, Lichter A, et al. Local control of Ewing's sarcoma of bone with radiotherapy and combination chemotherapy. Cancer. 1980;46:1969-73.

440. La TH, Meyers PA, Wexler LH, et al. Radiation therapy for Ewing's sarcoma: results from Memorial Sloan-Kettering in the modern era. Int J Radiat Oncol Biol Phys. 2006;64:544-50.

441. Paulino AC, Nguyen TX, Mai WY, et al. Dose response and local control using radiotherapy in non-metastatic Ewing sarcoma. Pediatr Blood Cancer. 2006.

442. Krasin MJ, Rodriguez-Galindo C, Billups CA, et al. Definitive irradiation in multidisciplinary management of localized Ewing sarcoma family of tumors in pediatric patients: outcome and prognostic factors. Int J Radiat Oncol Biol Phys. 2004;60: 830-8.

443. Merchant TE, Kushner BH, Sheldon JM, et al. Effect of low-dose radiation therapy when combined with surgical resection for Ewing sarcoma. Med Pediatr Oncol. 1999;33:65-70.

444. Arai Y, Kun LE, Brooks MT, et al. Ewing's sarcoma: local tumor control and patterns of failure following limited-volume radiation therapy. Int J Radiat Oncol Biol Phys. 1991;21:1501-8.

445. Schuck A, Rube C, Konemann S, et al. Postoperative radiotherapy in the treatment of Ewing tumors: influence of the interval between surgery and radiotherapy. Strahlenther Onkol. 2002;178: 25-31.

446. Burgers JM, Oldenburger F, de Kraker J, et al. Ewing's sarcoma of the pelvis: changes over 25 years in treatment and results. Eur J Cancer. 1997;33:2360-7.

447. Dunst J, Schuck A. Role of radiotherapy in Ewing tumors. Pediatr Blood Cancer. 2004;42:465-70.

448. Bolek TW, Marcus RB Jr, Mendenhall NP, et al. Local control and functional results after twice-daily radiotherapy for Ewing's sarcoma of the extremities. Int J Radiat Oncol Biol Phys. 1996;35:687-92.

449. Dunst J, Sauer R, Burgers JM, et al. Radiation therapy as local treatment in Ewing's sarcoma. Results of the Cooperative Ewing's Sarcoma Studies CESS 81 and CESS 86. Cancer. 1991;67: 2818-25.

450. Dunst J, Jurgens H, Sauer R, et al. Radiation therapy in Ewing's sarcoma: an update of the CESS 86 trial. Int J Radiat Oncol Biol Phys. 1995;32:919-30.

451. Schuck A, Ahrens S, Paulussen M, et al. Local therapy in localized Ewing tumors: results of 1058 patients treated in the CESS 81, CESS 86, and EICESS 92 trials. Int J Radiat Oncol Biol Phys. 2003;55:168-77.

452. Paulino AC, Nguyen TX, Mai WY. An analysis of primary site control and late effects according to local control modality in non-metastatic Ewing sarcoma. Pediatr Blood Cancer. 2006.

453. Shankar AG, Pinkerton CR, Atra A, et al. Local therapy and other factors influencing site of relapse in patients with localised Ewing's sarcoma. United Kingdom Children's Cancer Study Group (UKCCSG). Eur J Cancer. 1999;35:1698-704.

454. Bacci G, Picci P, Gitelis S, et al. The treatment of localized Ewing's sarcoma: the experience at the Istituto Ortopedico Rizzoli in 163 cases treated with and without adjuvant chemotherapy. Cancer. 1982;49:1561-70.

455. Chan RC, Sutow WW, Lindberg RD, et al. Management and results of localized Ewing's sarcoma. Cancer. 1979;43:1001-6.

456. Zucker JM, Henry-Amar M, Sarrazin D, et al. Intensive systemic chemotherapy in localized Ewing's sarcoma in childhood. A historical trial. Cancer. 1983;52:415-23.

457. Rosen G, Caparros B, Mosende C, et al. Curability of Ewing's sarcoma and considerations for future therapeutic trials. Cancer. 1978;41:888-99.

458. Rosen G, Caparros B, Nirenberg A, et al. Ewing's sarcoma: ten-year experience with adjuvant chemotherapy. Cancer. 1981; 47:2204-13.

459. Hayes FA, Thompson EI, Hustu HO, et al. The response of Ewing's sarcoma to sequential cyclophosphamide and adriamycin induction therapy. J Clin Oncol. 1983;1:45-51.

460. Bacci G, Toni A, Avella M, et al. Long-term results in 144 localized Ewing's sarcoma patients treated with combined therapy. Cancer. 1989;63:1477-86.

461. Bacci G, Picci P, Ferrari S, et al. Neoadjuvant chemotherapy for Ewing's sarcoma of bone: no benefit observed after adding ifosfamide and etoposide to vincristine, actinomycin, cyclophosphamide, and doxorubicin in the maintenance phase—results of two sequential studies. Cancer. 1998;82:1174-83.

462. Burgert EO Jr, Nesbit ME, Garnsey LA, et al. Multimodal therapy for the management of nonpelvic, localized Ewing's sarcoma of bone: intergroup study IESS-II. J Clin Oncol. 1990;8:1514-24.

463. Magrath I, Sandlund J, Raynor A, et al. A phase II study of ifosfamide in the treatment of recurrent sarcomas in young people. Cancer Chemother Pharmacol. 1986;18:S25-8.

464. Miser JS, Kinsella TJ, Triche TJ, et al. Ifosfamide with mesna uroprotection and etoposide: an effective regimen in the treatment of recurrent sarcomas and other tumors of children and young adults. J Clin Oncol. 1987;5:1191-8.

465. Kung FH, Pratt CB, Vega RA, et al. Ifosfamide/etoposide combination in the treatment of recurrent malignant solid tumors of childhood: A Pediatric Oncology Group Phase II study. Cancer. 1993;71:1898-903.

466. Meyer WH, Kun L, Marina N, et al. Ifosfamide plus etoposide in newly diagnosed Ewing's sarcoma of bone. J Clin Oncol. 1992;10:1737-42.

467. Wexler LH, DeLaney TF, Tsokos M, et al. Ifosfamide and etoposide plus vincristine, doxorubicin, and cyclophosphamide for newly diagnosed Ewing's sarcoma family of tumors. Cancer. 1996;78:901-11.

468. Paulussen M, Craft A, Lewis I, et al. Ewing tumor of bone—updated report of the European Intergroup Cooperative Ewing's Sarcoma Study EICESS 92 [abstract]. Am Soc Clin Oncol. 2002;21:1568.

469. Kolb EA, Kushner BH, Gorlick R, et al. Long-term event-free survival after intensive chemotherapy for Ewing's family of

tumors in children and young adults. J Clin Oncol. 2003;21: 3423-30.

470. Granowetter L, Womer R, Devidas M, et al. Comparison of dose-intensified and standard dose chemotherapy for the treatment of non-metastatic Ewing sarcoma and PNET of bone and soft tissue [abstract]. Med Pediatr Oncol. 2001;37:172.

471. Marina NM, Pappo AS, Parham DM, et al. Chemotherapy dose-intensification for pediatric patients with Ewing's family of tumors and desmoplastic small round-cell tumors: a feasibility study at St. Jude Children's Research Hospital. J Clin Oncol. 1999;17: 180-90.

472. Strauss SJ, McTiernan A, Driver D, et al. Single center experience of a new intensive induction therapy for ewing's family of tumors: feasibility, toxicity, and stem cell mobilization properties. J Clin Oncol. 2003;21:2974-81.

473. Evans R, Nesbit M, Askin F, et al. Local recurrence, rate and sites of metastases, and time to relapse as a function of treatment regimen, size of primary and surgical history in 62 patients presenting with non-metastatic Ewing's sarcoma of the pelvic bones. Int J Radiat Oncol Biol Phys. 1985;11:129-36.

474. Bacci G, Ferrari S, Mercuri M, et al. Multimodal therapy for the treatment of nonmetastatic Ewing sarcoma of pelvis. J Pediatr Hematol Oncol. 2003;25:118-24.

475. Hoffmann C, Ahrens S, Dunst J, et al. Pelvic Ewing sarcoma: a retrospective analysis of 241 cases. Cancer. 1999;85:869-77.

476. Scully SP, Temple HT, O'Keefe RJ, et al. Role of surgical resection in pelvic Ewing's sarcoma. J Clin Oncol. 1995;13: 2336-41.

477. Yock TI, Krailo M, Fryer CJ, et al. Local control in pelvic Ewing sarcoma: analysis from INT-0091—a report from the Children's Oncology Group. J Clin Oncol. 2006;24:3838-43.

478. Evans RG, Nesbit ME, Gehan EA, et al. Multimodal therapy for the management of localized Ewing's sarcoma of pelvic and sacral bones: a report from the second intergroup study. J Clin Oncol. 1991;9:1173-80.

479. Frassica FJ, Frassica DA, Pritchard DJ, et al. Ewing sarcoma of the pelvis. Clinicopathologic features and treatment. J Bone Joint Surg Am. 1993;75:1457-65.

480. Yang RS, Eckardt JJ, Eilber FR, et al. Surgical indications for Ewing's sarcoma of the pelvis. Cancer. 1995;76:1388-97.

481. Carrie C, Mascard E, Gomez F, et al. Nonmetastatic pelvic Ewing sarcoma: report of the French society of pediatric oncology. Med Pediatr Oncol. 1999;33:444-9.

482. Thomas PR, Foulkes MA, Gilula LA, et al. Primary Ewing's sarcoma of the ribs. A report from the intergroup Ewing's sarcoma study. Cancer. 1983;51:1021-7.

483. Schuck A, Hofmann J, Rube C, et al. Radiotherapy in Ewing's sarcoma and PNET of the chest wall: results of the trials CESS 81, CESS 86 and EICESS 92. Int J Radiat Oncol Biol Phys. 1998;42:1001-6.

484. Sirvent N, Kanold J, Levy C, et al. Non-metastatic Ewing's sarcoma of the ribs: the French Society of Pediatric Oncology Experience. Eur J Cancer. 2002;38:561-7.

485. Shamberger RC, LaQuaglia MP, Gebhardt MC, et al. Ewing sarcoma/primitive neuroectodermal tumor of the chest wall: impact of initial versus delayed resection on tumor margins, survival, and use of radiation therapy. Ann Surg. 2003;238: 563-7.

486. Shamberger RC, Laquaglia MP, Krailo MD, et al. Ewing sarcoma of the rib: results of an intergroup study with analysis of outcome by timing of resection. J Thorac Cardiovasc Surg. 2000;119: 1154-61.

487. Ozaki T, Lindner N, Hoffmann C, et al. Ewing's sarcoma of the ribs. A report from the cooperative Ewing's sarcoma study. Eur J Cancer. 1995;31A:2284-8.

488. Schuck A, Ahrens S, Konarzewska A, et al. Hemithorax irradiation for Ewing tumors of the chest wall. Int J Radiat Oncol Biol Phys. 2002;54:830-8.

489. Barbieri E, Chiaulon G, Bunkeila F, et al. Radiotherapy in vertebral tumors. Indications and limits: a report on 28 cases of Ewing's sarcoma of the spine. Chir Organi Mov. 1998;83: 105-11.

490. Schuck A, Ahrens S, von Schorlemer I, et al. Radiotherapy in Ewing tumors of the vertebrae: treatment results and local relapse analysis of the CESS 81/86 and EICESS 92 trials. Int J Radiat Oncol Biol Phys. 2005;63:1562-7.

491. Stiller CA, Craft AW, Corazziari I. Survival of children with bone sarcoma in Europe since 1978: results from the EUROCARE study. Eur J Cancer. 2001;37:760-6.

492. Bernstein ML, Devidas M, Lafreniere D, et al. Intensive therapy with growth factor support for patients with Ewing tumor metastatic at diagnosis: Pediatric Oncology Group/Children's Cancer Group Phase II Study 9457—a report from the Children's Oncology Group. J Clin Oncol. 2006;24:152-9.

493. Felgenhauer J, Hawkins D, Pendergrass T, et al. Very intensive, short-term chemotherapy for children and adolescents with metastatic sarcomas. Med Pediatr Oncol. 2000;34:29-38.

494. Spunt SL, McCarville MB, Kun LE, et al. Selective use of whole-lung irradiation for patients with Ewing sarcoma family tumors and pulmonary metastases at the time of diagnosis. J Pediatr Hematol Oncol. 2001;23:93-8.

495. Dunst J, Paulussen M, Jurgens H. Lung irradiation for Ewing's sarcoma with pulmonary metastases at diagnosis: results of the CESS-studies. Strahlenther Onkol. 1993;169:621-3.

496. Lanza LA, Miser JS, Pass HI, Roth JA. The role of resection in the treatment of pulmonary metastases from Ewing's sarcoma. J Thorac Cardiovasc Surg. 1987;94:181-7.

497. Miser JS, Kinsella TJ, Triche TJ, et al. Preliminary results of treatment of Ewing's sarcoma of bone in children and young adults: six months of intensive combined modality therapy without maintenance. J Clin Oncol. 1988;6:484-90.

498. Horowitz ME, Kinsella TJ, Wexler LH, et al. Total-body irradiation and autologous bone marrow transplant in the treatment of high-risk Ewing's sarcoma and rhabdomyosarcoma. J Clin Oncol. 1993;11:1911-8.

499. Burdach S, Jurgens H, Peters C, et al. Myeloablative radiochemotherapy and hematopoietic stem-cell rescue in poor-prognosis Ewing's sarcoma. J Clin Oncol. 1993;11:1482-8.

500. Burdach S, van Kaick B, Laws HJ, et al. Allogeneic and autologous stem-cell transplantation in advanced Ewing tumors. An update after long-term follow-up from two centers of the European Intergroup study EICESS. Stem-Cell Transplant Programs at Dusseldorf University Medical Center, Germany and St. Anna Kinderspital, Vienna, Austria. Ann Oncol. 2000; 11:1451-62.

501. Burdach S, Meyer-Bahlburg A, Laws HJ, et al. High-dose therapy for patients with primary multifocal and early relapsed Ewing's tumors: results of two consecutive regimens assessing the role of total-body irradiation. J Clin Oncol. 2003;21:3072-8.

502. Meyers PA, Krailo MD, Ladanyi M, et al. High-dose melphalan, etoposide, total-body irradiation, and autologous stem-cell reconstitution as consolidation therapy for high-risk Ewing's sarcoma does not improve prognosis. J Clin Oncol. 2001;19:2812-20.

503. Yaniv I, Cohen IJ, Stein J, et al. Tumor cells are present in stem cell harvests of Ewing's sarcoma patients and their persistence following transplantation is associated with relapse. Pediatr Blood Cancer. 2004;42:404-9.

504. Leung W, Chen AR, Klann RC, et al. Frequent detection of tumor cells in hematopoietic grafts in neuroblastoma and Ewing's sarcoma. Bone Marrow Transplant. 1998;22:971-9.

505. Fischmeister G, Zoubek A, Jugovic D, et al. Low incidence of molecular evidence for tumour in PBPC harvests from patients with high risk Ewing tumours. Bone Marrow Transplant. 1999;24:405-9.

506. Vermeulen J, Ballet S, Oberlin O, et al. Incidence and prognostic value of tumour cells detected by RT-PCR in peripheral blood

stem cell collections from patients with Ewing tumour. Br J Cancer. 2006;95:1326-33.

507. Bacci G, Ferrari S, Longhi A, et al. Therapy and survival after recurrence of Ewing's tumors: the Rizzoli experience in 195 patients treated with adjuvant and neoadjuvant chemotherapy from 1979 to 1997. Ann Oncol. 2003;14:1654-9.

508. Barker LM, Pendergrass TW, Sanders JE, Hawkins DS. Survival after recurrence of Ewing's sarcoma family of tumors. J Clin Oncol. 2005;23:4354-62.

509. Rodriguez-Galindo C, Billups CA, Kun LE, et al. Survival after recurrence of Ewing tumors: the St Jude Children's Research Hospital experience, 1979-1999. Cancer. 2002;94: 561-9.

510. Shankar AG, Ashley S, Craft AW, Pinkerton CR. Outcome after relapse in an unselected cohort of children and adolescents with Ewing sarcoma. Med Pediatr Oncol. 2003;40:141-7.

511. Weston CL, Douglas C, Craft AW, et al. Establishing long-term survival and cure in young patients with Ewing's sarcoma. Br J Cancer. 2004;91:225-32.

512. McLean TW, Hertel C, Young ML, et al. Late events in pediatric patients with Ewing sarcoma/primitive neuroectodermal tumor of bone: the Dana-Farber Cancer Institute/Children's Hospital experience. J Pediatr Hematol Oncol. 1999;21:486-93.

513. Hayes FA, Thompson EI, Kumar M, Hustu HO. Long-term survival in patients with Ewing's sarcoma relapsing after completing therapy. Med Pediatr Oncol. 1987;15:254-6.

514. Hawkins DS, Bradfield S, Whitlock JA, et al. Topotecan by 21-day continuous infusion in children with relapsed or refractory solid tumors: a Children's Oncology Group study. Pediatr Blood Cancer. 2006;47:790-4.

515. Pratt CB, Stewart C, Santana VM, et al. Phase I study of topotecan for pediatric patients with malignant solid tumors. J Clin Oncol. 1994;12:539-43.

516. Hunold A, Weddeling N, Paulussen M, et al. Topotecan and cyclophosphamide in patients with refractory or relapsed Ewing tumors. Pediatr Blood Cancer. 2006;47:795-800.

517. Kushner BH, Kramer K, Meyers PA, et al. Pilot study of topotecan and high-dose cyclophosphamide for resistant pediatric solid tumors. Med Pediatr Oncol. 2000;35:468-74.

518. Wagner LM, Crews KR, Iacono LC, et al. Phase I trial of temozolomide and protracted irinotecan in pediatric patients with refractory solid tumors. Clin Cancer Res. 2004;10: 840-8.

519. Wagner LM, McAllister N, Goldsby RE, et al. Temozolomide and intravenous irinotecan for treatment of advanced Ewing sarcoma. Pediatr Blood Cancer. 2007;48:132-9.

520. Whelan JS, McTiernan A, Kakouri E, Kilby A. Carboplatin-based chemotherapy for refractory and recurrent Ewing's tumours. Pediatr Blood Cancer. 2004;43:237-42.

521. Van Winkle P, Angiolillo A, Krailo M, et al. Ifosfamide, carboplatin, and etoposide (ICE) reinduction chemotherapy in a large cohort of children and adolescents with recurrent/refractory sarcoma: the Children's Cancer Group (CCG) experience. Pediatr Blood Cancer. 2005;44:338-47.

522. Briccoli A, Rocca M, Ferrari S, et al. Surgery for lung metastases in Ewing's sarcoma of bone. Eur J Surg Oncol. 2004;30:63-7.

523. Bacci G, Briccoli A, Picci P, Ferrari S. Metachronous pulmonary metastases resection in patients with Ewing's sarcoma initially treated with adjuvant or neoadjuvant chemotherapy. Eur J Cancer. 1995;31A:999-1001.

524. de Vathaire F, Hawkins M, Campbell S, et al. Second malignant neoplasms after a first cancer in childhood: temporal pattern of risk according to type of treatment. Br J Cancer. 1999;79: 1884-93.

525. Bacci G, Longhi A, Barbieri E, et al. Second malignancy in 597 patients with Ewing sarcoma of bone treated at a single institution

with adjuvant and neoadjuvant chemotherapy between 1972 and 1999. J Pediatr Hematol Oncol. 2005;27:517-20.

526. Dunst J, Ahrens S, Paulussen M, et al. Second malignancies after treatment for Ewing's sarcoma: a report of the CESS-studies. Int J Radiat Oncol Biol Phys. 1998;42:379-84.

527. Kuttesch JF Jr, Wexler LH, Marcus RB, et al. Second malignancies after Ewing's sarcoma: radiation dose-dependency of secondary sarcomas. J Clin Oncol. 1996;14:2818-25.

528. Paulussen M, Ahrens S, Lehnert M, et al. Second malignancies after ewing tumor treatment in 690 patients from a cooperative German/Austrian/Dutch study. Ann Oncol. 2001;12:1619-30.

529. Fuchs B, Valenzuela RG, Petersen IA, et al. Ewing's sarcoma and the development of secondary malignancies. Clin Orthop Relat Res. 2003;82-9.

530. Bhatia S, Krailo MD, Chen Z, et al. Therapy-related myelodysplasia and acute myeloid leukemia after Ewing sarcoma and primitive neuroectodermal tumor of bone: a report from the Children's Oncology Group. Blood. 2006;22:25.

531. Rodriguez-Galindo C, Poquette CA, Marina NM, et al. Hematologic abnormalities and acute myeloid leukemia in children and adolescents administered intensified chemotherapy for the Ewing sarcoma family of tumors. J Pediatr Hematol Oncol. 2000;22: 321-9.

532. Kakadekar AP, Sandor GG, Fryer C, et al. Differences in dose scheduling as a factor in the cause of anthracycline-induced cardiotoxicity in Ewing sarcoma patients. Med Pediatr Oncol. 1997;28:22-6.

533. Stohr W, Paulides M, Bielack S, et al. Ifosfamide-induced nephrotoxicity in 593 sarcoma patients: A report from the Late Effects Surveillance System. Pediatr Blood Cancer. 2006;58:54.

534. Fuchs B, Valenzuela RG, Inwards C, et al. Complications in long-term survivors of Ewing sarcoma. Cancer. 2003;98: 2687-92.

535. Nagarajan R, Clohisy DR, Neglia JP, et al. Function and quality-of-life of survivors of pelvic and lower extremity osteosarcoma and Ewing's sarcoma: the Childhood Cancer Survivor Study. Br J Cancer. 2004;91:1858-65.

536. Zahlten-Hinguranage A, Bernd L, Ewerbeck V, et al. Equal quality of life after limb-sparing or ablative surgery for lower extremity sarcomas. Br J Cancer. 2004;91:1012-4.

537. Nagarajan R, Neglia JP, Clohisy DR, et al. Education, employment, insurance, and marital status among 694 survivors of pediatric lower extremity bone tumors: a report from the childhood cancer survivor study. Cancer. 2003;97:2554-64.

538. Novakovic B, Fears TR, Horowitz ME, et al. Late effects of therapy in survivors of Ewing's sarcoma family tumors. J Pediatr Hematol Oncol. 1997;19:220-5.

539. Sjogren H, Wedell B, Meis-Kindblom JM, et al. Fusion of the NH2-terminal domain of the basic helix-loop-helix protein TCF12 to TEC in extraskeletal myxoid chondrosarcoma with translocation t(9;15)(q22;q21). Cancer Res. 2000;60:6832-35.

540. Yamaguchi S, Yamazaki Y, Tshikawa Y, et al. EWSR1 is fused to POU5F1 in a bone tumor with translocation t(6;22)(p21;q12). Genes Chromosomes Cancer. 2005;43:217-22.

541. Waters BL, Panagopoulos I, Allen EF: Genetic characterization of angiomatoid fibrous histiocytoma identifies fusion of the FUS and ATF-1 genes induced by a chromosomal translocation involving bands 12q13 and 16p11. Cancer Genet Cytogenet. 2000;121:109-16.

542. Storlazzi CT, Mertens F, Nascimento A, et al. Fusion of the FUS and BBF2H7 genes in low grade fibromyxoid sarcoma. Hum Mol Genet. 2003;12:2349-58.

543. Panagopoulos I, Aman P, Fioretos T, et al. Fusion of the FUS gene with ERG in acute myeloid leukemia with t(16;21)(p11;q22). Genes Chromosomes Cancer. 1994;11:256-62.

22

Osteosarcoma

Katherine A. Janeway, Richard Gorlick, and Mark L. Bernstein

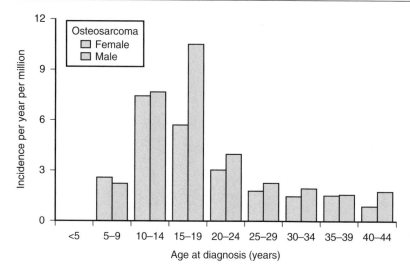

FIGURE 22-1. Age distribution of osteosarcoma based on U.S. cases between 1975 and 1999. *(Data from Bleyer A, O'Leary M, Barr R, Ries LAG [eds]. Cancer Epidemiology in Older Adolescents and Young Adults 15 to 29 Years of Age, Including SEER Incidence and Survival: 1975-2000 [NIH Publication No. 06-5767]. Bethesda, Md, National Cancer Institute, 2006.)*

Osteosarcoma is the most common primary bone tumor. There are approximately 600 cases/year in the United States.[1] The term *osteosarcoma* was first used in the early 1800s by Alexis Boyer,[2] the imperial family surgeon for Napoleon. Although low-grade forms of osteosarcoma do exist, over 90% of osteosarcomas are high-grade malignant lesions. Low-grade osteosarcomas will be discussed, but most of what follows pertains to high-grade osteosarcomas.

Osteosarcoma usually occurs in adolescents and young adults. Presenting symptoms can include tumor-related pain with or without a mass, painless mass, and pathologic fracture. The distal femur is the most frequent site of primary disease, followed by the proximal tibia and then the proximal femur, hip, and proximal humerus.[3] As early as 1818, it was recognized that untreated patients with osteosarcoma often developed metastatic disease.[2] The most common site of metastasis is the lungs, followed by bone. Metastatic disease is present in approximately 15% of patients at the time of diagnosis.[4]

Prior to the 1970s, when chemotherapy was first used to treat osteosarcoma, overall survival was approximately 20%. With modern chemotherapy and surgical control, the 10-year overall survival of patients with localized osteosarcoma is around 70%.[5] Overall survival is much worse for patients with metastases at diagnosis and for those with relapsed disease. In both groups, the 5-year overall survival rate is approximately 25%.[4,6,7] The most active chemotherapy agents in osteosarcoma are doxorubicin (Doxo), cisplatin (CP), and high-dose methotrexate (HDMTX). Ifosfamide and etoposide are also active against osteosarcoma and are typically used in addition to Doxo, CP, and HDMTX in patients with metastatic disease and in patients with recurrence.

In the past 3 decades, a number of discoveries have led to a better understanding of osteosarcoma biology. For example, the tumor suppressor genes *p53* and *retinoblastoma (Rb)* are altered in osteosarcoma. Oncogenes, including *MYC, MET,* and *FOS,* have also been implicated in osteosarcomagenesis. These tumor suppressors, oncogenes, and other biologic factors will be discussed in detail. Biomedical research tools with which to study osteosarcoma continue to improve. These advances will likely soon lead to basic discoveries that will have therapeutic applications.

EPIDEMIOLOGY

Osteosarcoma is the most common primary bone tumor in children.[1] The average annual incidence of osteosarcoma in children younger than 20 years in the United States is 4.8/million. Approximately 3% of all malignancies in this age group are osteosarcomas. In 2000, the most recent year for which data are available, there were 440 cases of osteosarcoma in children age 0 to 19 years in the United States. There were an additional 135 cases in young adults age 20 to 29.[1] Internationally, incidence rates approximate the U.S. rate, with the exception of a higher incidence in some African countries. In Sudan and Uganda, the osteosarcoma incidence in children younger than 14 years is 5.3 and 6.4/million respectively, compared with an incidence of between 2 and 3/million in this age group in the United States, Europe, and Asia.[8,9]

Osteosarcoma occurs rarely in children younger than 5 years. After age 5, the incidence increases steadily, reaching a peak at age 15 years.[10] After the adolescent peak, the rate of osteosarcoma steadily declines, leveling off at a rate of 1 to 2/million. A second peak in incidence, approximately half the magnitude of the adolescent peak, occurs in the sixth to seventh decade.[11,12] Osteosarcoma in older patients is associated with Paget's disease and prior radiation therapy, although approximately half of older patients with osteosarcoma have neither condition.[13] The adolescent peak occurs at age 13 years in girls and between ages 15 and 17 years in boys (Fig. 22-1). The age of peak incidence corresponds to the age of greatest growth velocity in each gender. This association contributes to the evidence supporting a role for growth in the cause of osteosarcoma (see later, "Cause"). Osteosarcoma is slightly more common in males, particularly in the 15- to 19-year-old age group.

In the United States, osteosarcoma is slightly more common in African Americans, Hispanics, and Asians–Pacific Islanders (Fig. 22-2). Several studies have reported that rates of osteosarcoma in black children younger than 14 years are about twice those in white children of the same age.[14,15] In the most recent report on osteosarcoma from the Surveillance, Epidemiology and End Results (SEER) Program of the National Cancer Institute, U.S. blacks younger than 20 years continue to have a slightly higher rate of osteosarcoma.[10] As shown in

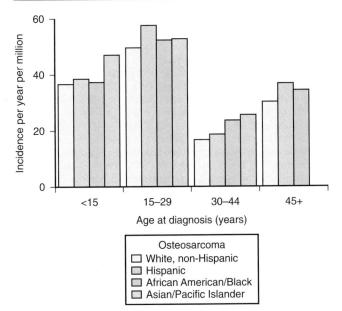

FIGURE 22-2. Incidence of osteosarcoma by racial group based on U.S. cases between 1990 and 1999. *(Data from Bleyer A, O'Leary M, Barr R, Ries LAG [eds]. Cancer Epidemiology in Older Adolescents and Young Adults 15 to 29 Years of Age, Including SEER Incidence and Survival: 1975-2000 [NIH Publication No. 06-5767]. Bethesda, Md, National Cancer Institute, 2006.)*

Figure 22-2, for the age group 15 to 29 years, the racial group with the highest rate of osteosarcoma is Hispanic. The relative risk of developing osteosarcoma for Hispanic children younger than 14 years of age, based on data collected between 1975 and 2003, is 1.3.[16] Asians–Pacific Islanders have the highest rate of osteosarcoma in the age groups younger than 15 years and 30 to 44 years. However, the reported incidence in Hispanics and Asians–Pacific Islanders is likely to be inaccurate given the small absolute number of affected individuals and uncertainty in the denominator (i.e., the number of Hispanics and Asians–Pacific Islanders within each age group living in the United States). In summary, there is evidence for a slightly increased incidence of osteosarcoma among U.S. blacks and Hispanics. Recent SEER data show an increased rate in Asians and Pacific Islanders younger than 15 years but this finding needs further investigation.

The most common anatomic sites of osteosarcoma at initial presentation are the long bones of the lower limbs. Fifty percent of osteosarcomas are located around the knee, in the distal femur, proximal tibia, or proximal fibula (Fig. 22-3). Approximately 10% of tumors occur in the mid- or proximal femur and 9% occur in the proximal humerus.[3,10] Of patients with osteosarcoma, 10% to 20% have metastatic disease at initial presentation. The most common site of metastasis is the lungs. Isolated pulmonary metastases are present in 61% of patients with metastatic disease at presentation. Isolated metastases to bone are present in 16% of patients, and 14% have both pulmonary and bone metastases. Seven percent of patients have metastases to other rare sites plus bone and/or pulmonary metastases, and 2% of patients have isolated metastases to rare sites. Rare sites of metastasis in patients with primary metastatic disease, as opposed to metastatic disease in patients with recurrent disease, are lymph nodes, central nervous system, liver, adrenal gland, and soft tissues.[4]

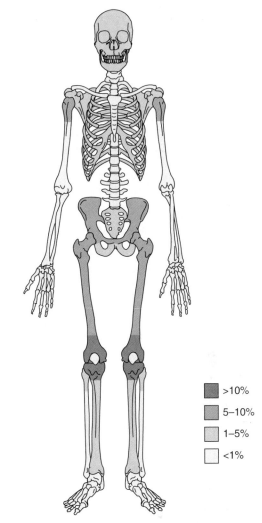

>10%

5–10%

1–5%

<1%

FIGURE 22-3. Anatomic sites of osteosarcoma at initial presentation. *(Adapted from Dahlin DC, Unni KK. Osteosarcoma of bone and its important recognizable varieties. Am J Surg Pathol. 1977;1:61-72.)*

CAUSE

When faced with a patient with osteosarcoma, it is often difficult to identify a cause. However, recognition of causative factors has led to the discovery of biologic mechanisms of transformation, as in the case of predisposition to osteosarcoma in Li-Fraumeni syndrome, or the identification of exposures to be avoided, as in the case of radiation-induced osteosarcoma. Inherited syndromes in which there is an increased occurrence of osteosarcoma are hereditary retinoblastoma and Li-Fraumeni, Rothmund-Thomson, Bloom, and Werner's syndromes. There is a clear association between the risk of osteosarcoma and prior radiation therapy or treatment with alkylating chemotherapy. Epidemiologic studies and clinical observation have suggested that increased height may be a risk factor for the development of osteosarcoma. Finally, environmental exposures to radium and beryllium likely increase the risk of osteosarcoma but exposure to high doses of these agents is rare.

As noted, peak rates of osteosarcoma coincide with the period of maximal linear growth during puberty. Most osteosarcomas occurring in the adolescent age group are in the long bones of the axial skeleton, the bones in which the most active growth occurs. These clinical observations have led to the hypothesis that the hormonal milieu during maximal linear growth encourages the development of osteosarcoma and that by extension, osteosarcoma would be more common in taller adolescents. Multiple epidemiologic studies have addressed this question[17-22] but results are contradictory. Approximately 50% of the studies have found that osteosarcoma patients are taller at diagnosis than age-matched controls or the normal population.[20-22] The remaining studies have not supported an association between height and the occurrence of osteosarcoma.[17-19] The larger studies[21] and those with more reliable sources of height data[20] have shown a positive association between tall stature and osteosarcoma. These data, in part, have led to the investigation of the insulin-like growth factor axis in osteosarcoma (see later, "Biology").

Approximately 1% of patients develop secondary bone tumors following treatment of a primary pediatric malignancy[23]; of these secondary bone tumors, 50% to 80% are osteosarcomas. On the other hand, secondary Ewing's sarcoma is rare.[23,24] The relative risk of secondary osteosarcoma increases greatly with radiation doses to the bone higher than 1000 cGy. In patients who received between 3000 and 5000 cGy to the bone during treatment of their primary pediatric malignancy, the relative risk of secondary osteosarcoma was variably reported, but may be as high as 100.[23,25] A study in patients with primary Ewing's sarcoma has concluded that only higher radiation doses increase the risk of secondary sarcomas, with no tumors developing in patients who had received less than 4800 cGy. The highest risk, 130 cases/10,000 person-years of observation, was observed among patients who had received 6000 cGy or more.[26] In the 92 published cases of secondary osteosarcoma for whom radiation dose was reported, the median radiation dose delivered was 4500 to 5400 cGy.[27] The average time between diagnosis of the primary malignancy and development of secondary osteosarcoma is 10 years.[24] Another factor that increases the likelihood that survivors of a primary cancer will develop secondary osteosarcoma is treatment with alkylating agents. This class of chemotherapy increases the relative risk of secondary osteosarcoma by a factor of 5.[23]

Data regarding an increased risk of cancer in people exposed to low levels of radiation from the atomic bombs in Hiroshima and Nagasaki have led to increased concern about the risk of diagnostic imaging with x-rays and computed tomography (CT) scans, particularly in pediatric patients.[28] However, current evidence does not suggest that osteosarcoma risk would be increased from commonly used imaging modalities.[29] In particular, the radiation dose of a CT scan is approximately 6 cGy and the risk of bone cancer in pediatric cancer survivors who received less than 1000 cGy to the bone is not increased.[23]

Osteosarcoma is seen in a number of inherited cancer predisposition syndromes. These syndromes have often illuminated mechanisms of transformation in sporadic osteosarcoma. Children with hereditary retinoblastoma have a germline heterozygous, inactivating deletion, and/or a frameshift or point mutation of the tumor suppressor gene *retinoblastoma 1*. Affected children develop retinoblastoma usually in one or both eyes. The cumulative incidence of a nonretinoblastoma malignancy in hereditary retinoblastoma is 51%, and approximately 40% of these second malignancies are osteosarcomas.[30] Both osteosarcomas and retinoblastomas in these patients have loss of heterozygosity of the *retinoblastoma 1* allele, resulting in a complete loss of Rb function. As discussed later (see "Biology"), loss of Rb function also occurs in sporadic osteosarcomas.[31,32]

In the Li-Fraumeni syndrome, patients carry a heterozygous inactivating mutation of the tumor suppressor gene *p53*. Affected individuals have a greatly increased cancer risk at a young age. The most common malignancies are breast cancer and bone and soft tissue sarcomas, brain tumors, and leukemia.[33] Slightly more than 10% of the malignancies in patients with Li-Fraumeni syndrome are osteosarcomas. Osteosarcomas and other cancers that develop in Li-Fraumeni syndrome patients have loss of the normal *p53* allele consistent with the tumor suppressor function of the p53 gene product. Loss of p53 function by *p53* mutation or amplification of *MDM2* or *COPS3* is also present in most sporadic osteosarcomas (see later, "Biology").[34]

Rothmund-Thomson, Bloom, and Werner's syndromes are members of a family of autosomal recessive disorders caused by mutations in one of the RECQ DNA helicases. Rothmund-Thomson syndrome, caused by mutations in the *RECQL4* gene, is characterized by skin rash, skeletal dysplasias, and sparse hair. Up to 30% of patients with Rothmund-Thomson syndrome develop osteosarcoma at a slightly younger age than in sporadic osteosarcoma.[35,36] Bloom syndrome, caused by mutations in the *BLM* or *RECQL2* gene, is characterized by short stature, telangiectasias, and an increased risk of developing a wide variety of cancers at a young age.[37] Unlike in Rothmund-Thomson syndrome, only a small percentage of cancers occurring in affected individuals are osteosarcomas. Werner's syndrome is caused by a mutation in the *WRN* or *RECQL3* gene. Patients have scleroderma-like skin changes, premature aging, and a typical body habitus with short stature, long spindly limbs, and a stocky trunk. Like Bloom syndrome, the risk of developing cancer at a young age is increased in Werner's syndrome. Also like Bloom syndrome, osteosarcoma constitutes fewer than 10% of the malignancies occurring in patients with Werner's syndrome.[38] For a further discussion of the role of RECQ DNA helicases in osteosarcoma, see later ("Biology").

The risk of developing osteosarcoma is increased in adults with Paget's disease. In Paget's disease, which affects up to 1% of adults over the age of 40 years, bone resorption by osteoclasts is increased. As a result, there is a compensatory increase in osteoblast activity and bone formation.[39] Osteosarcoma develops in less than 1% of patients with Paget's disease, but this represents a higher rate than that seen in the general population. The average age of Paget's disease–related osteosarcoma is 70 years.[13]

Previously, some believed that trauma may cause osteosarcoma. However, modern epidemiologic studies have not supported a relationship between trauma and osteosarcoma.[18] Prior observations linking trauma and osteosarcoma were likely the result of the fact that a traumatic event may result in a previously existing osteosarcoma being brought to medical attention.

Environmental exposures, other than ionizing radiation, for which there is evidence of an association between exposure and osteosarcoma risk, include exposure to radium and beryllium. Radium is a radioactive element that is variably present in well water. When ingested, radium retained in the body is deposited in bone. Studies of those exposed to high levels of radium while painting dials on clocks in the 1920s strongly indicated that exposure to high doses of radium causes osteosarcoma.[40] The risk of osteosarcoma from exposure to low levels of radium in drinking water is less clear. Two studies have shown a slight increase in risk of bone sarcoma or osteosarcoma in those born in areas with drinking water containing relatively high concentrations of radium.[41,42] Conversely, two studies have shown no link between mean levels of radium in water and osteosarcoma.[41,43] Beryllium is a metallic element with limited use in the production of aerospace structural material, x-ray tubes, and nuclear reactors. Although IV injection of beryllium salts causes osteosarcoma in rabbits, there is limited evidence of an increased risk of osteosarcoma caused by beryllium exposure in humans.[44] Case-control studies have failed to identify other environmental or occupational exposures that increase the risk of osteosarcoma.[22]

CLINICAL PRESENTATION AND EVALUATION

Clinical, laboratory, and radiologic findings are often highly suggestive of osteosarcoma but are not pathognomonic. Biopsy is always required for diagnosis. Atypical imaging characteristics, including a benign appearance in high-grade osteosarcoma, have been described.[45] The differential diagnosis of osteosarcoma includes benign and malignant bone tumors (Box 22-1; Fig. 22-4).

Clinical Features

Clinical symptoms of osteosarcoma are nonspecific; 25% of patients have pain and a palpable mass at presentation, and 70% of patients present with pain as their only complaint. Pain tends to be intermittent and exacerbated by activity. The remaining patients present with a painless mass.[46] The duration of symptoms before diagnosis ranges from 1 day to 5 years, with a median of $3\frac{1}{2}$ months. In approximately 10% of patients, symptom duration is longer than 6 months.[47] A pathologic fracture is present in 8% of patients at the time of diagnosis.[48]

Radiologic Evaluation

Radiologic evaluation in osteosarcoma informs the initial diagnostic impression, aids in the determination of the best approach for biopsy, facilitates surgical resection, and identifies sites of

Box 22-1	Differential Diagnosis of Osteosarcoma

OTHER MALIGNANT PRIMARY BONE TUMORS

Ewing's sarcoma
Chondrosarcoma
Fibrosarcoma
Langerhans cell histiocytosis

OTHER MALIGNANCIES PRESENTING WITH BONE TUMOR(S)

Lymphoma
Neuroblastoma
Metastatic rhabdomyosarcoma
Metastatic melanoma

BENIGN BONE TUMORS

Aneurysmal bone cyst
Osteoblastoma
Osteoid osteoma
Giant cell tumor of bone
Unicameral bone cyst

INFECTION

Osteomyelitis

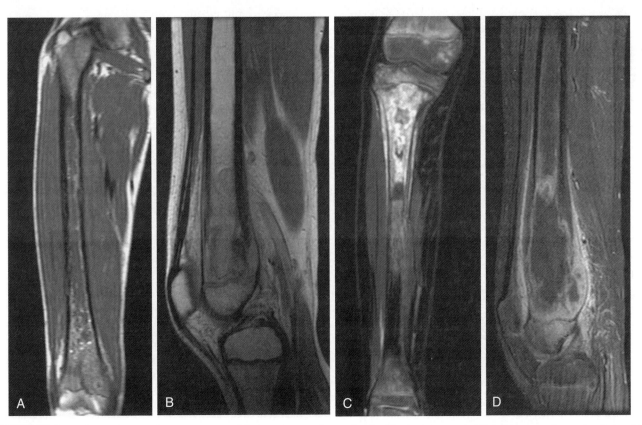

FIGURE 22-4. MRI appearance of osteosarcoma and lesions that can be confused with osteosarcoma in clinical presentation and radiographic appearance. **A,** Osteomyelitis of the femur. **B,** Lymphoma of the distal femur. **C,** Ewing's sarcoma of the proximal tibia. **D,** Osteosarcoma of the distal femur.

metastatic disease, if present. The recommended imaging studies for osteosarcoma at the time of diagnosis are a plain radiograph and magnetic resonance imaging (MRI) scan of the primary tumor site to evaluate the extent of local disease, a bone scan to screen for bony metastases, and a CT scan of the chest to determine whether pulmonary metastases are present. Whenever possible, these imaging studies should be performed prior to diagnostic biopsy because postsurgical atelectasis interferes with evaluation of the lung parenchyma. MRI of the primary tumor should include the entire bone from which the tumor arises and the closest adjacent joint to screen for skip metastases properly. An additional MRI scan should be obtained after neoadjuvant chemotherapy has been given but prior to definitive resection to determine the best plan for the surgical approach.

A plain radiograph of the primary tumor has usually been obtained prior to referral to an oncologist or orthopedist. Most appendicular osteosarcomas are located in the metaphyseal portion of the long bone. Both lytic destruction of bone and sclerotic irregular new bone formation can occur. Osteosarcoma usually has a mixed pattern of bone lysis and sclerosis, but one of these patterns can predominate. Regardless of the predominant pattern, the boundary between tumor and normal bone is usually irregular. The bone cortex is often disrupted by tumor growth into the surrounding soft tissue. Osteoid formation within the tumor results in areas of calcification visible in the bony and soft tissue components of the tumor. Periosteal new bone formation in osteosarcoma can be irregular or can

occur in a sunburst pattern. Sunburst refers to linear new bone growth that is perpendicular to the bony cortex and arranged in a fan-like pattern (Fig. 22-5).[49] In contrast, in Ewing's sarcoma, periosteal new bone growth typically occurs in an onionskin pattern in which linear new bone is oriented parallel to the bony cortex.[3] Periosteal new bone formation in osteosarcoma can also be present at the edge of the preserved cortex, resulting in Codman's triangle. Plain radiographs also assist in the diagnosis of pathologic fractures (Fig. 22-6).

Although plain radiographs of the primary tumor are informative, MRI is preferable for local staging, presurgical planning, and identification of skip metastases. CT is an acceptable alternative to MRI but most orthopedic surgeons and oncologists prefer MRI. In two studies directly comparing preoperative CT and MRI scans with pathologic findings in patients with osteosarcoma, MRI was found to be superior to CT in defining the longitudinal extent of intraosseous tumor,[50,51] extension into adjacent muscle compartments, and involvement of the neurovascular bundle. The two modalities were equivalent in their ability to define cortical bone and joint involvement. However, a more recent study in a larger patient population did not find a statistically significant difference between CT and MRI scans in their ability to predict the involvement of bone, muscle, joints, and the neurovascular bundle.[52] One possible explanation for the contradictory results is improvements in CT scan quality during the interval between the studies. In addition, the later study grouped all primary bone tumors together for analysis but, given that 60% of the

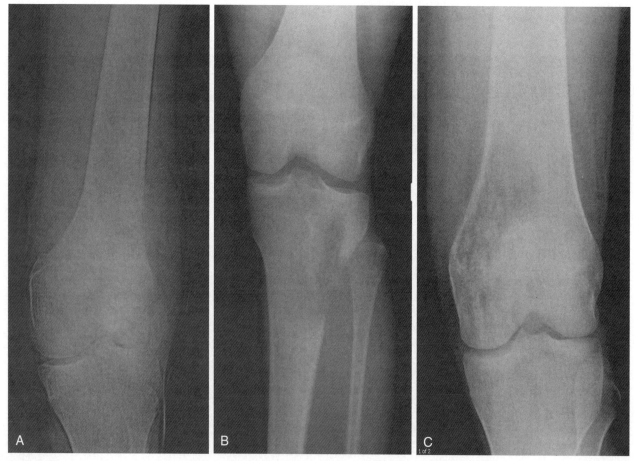

FIGURE 22-5. Three typical patterns observed in plain radiographs of osteosarcoma. **A,** Predominantly sclerotic pattern in an osteosarcoma of the distal femur with sunburst periosteal new bone formation. **B,** Predominantly lytic pattern in an osteosarcoma of the proximal tibia. **C,** Mixed lytic and sclerotic pattern in an osteosarcoma of the distal femur.

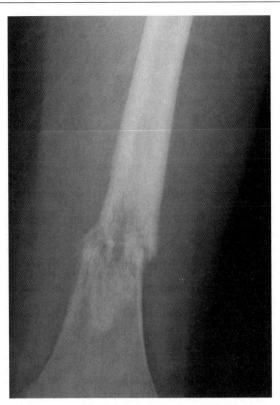

FIGURE 22-6. Pathologic fracture in an osteosarcoma of the distal femur.

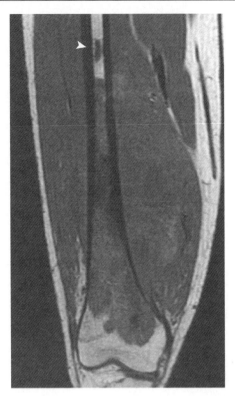

FIGURE 22-7. Skip metastasis (*arrowhead*) of an osteosarcoma of the distal femur as seen on T1-weighted MRI scan.

bone tumors were osteosarcoma, results would likely be similar for osteosarcomas alone. In comparison to CT and [99]technetium bone scanning, MRI more accurately predicts the intraosseous extent of osteosarcoma.[51] The presence of significant edema has been associated with inaccurate assessment of the margins of tumor on MRI. Because edema can resolve with chemotherapy, imaging performed for the purpose of surgical planning should be obtained after the administration of neoadjuvant chemotherapy.[53]

Skip metastasis is defined as a smaller distinct focus of osteosarcoma that is either within the same bone as the primary tumor or on the other side of the joint adjacent to the primary tumor.[54] There must be normal structures not involved with tumor present between the primary tumor and skip metastasis. Skip metastases are synchronous with the primary tumor and thus are present at initial presentation. Diagnosis of skip metastases is of critical importance for prognostication and because complete surgical remission in osteosarcoma with skip metastases requires complete resection of both the primary tumor and skip metastases. Over 80% of skip metastases are visible on MRI scans, as shown in Figure 22-7. In contrast, skip metastases are visible on bone scan, CT scans, and plain radiographs in only 46%, 45%, and 36% of cases, respectively.[55] Interestingly, a common reason for failure to identify skip metastases by bone scanning is merging of the signal from the primary tumor with the signal from the skip metastasis.[56] To ensure that skip metastases are identified, MRI of the primary tumor should include the entire bone and adjacent joint. Bony metastases that are not skip metastases are best identified with a [99]technetium bone scan (Fig. 22-8).[57] The usefulness of ^{18}F-fluorodeoxyglucose positron emission tomography (FDG-PET) in osteosarcoma has not yet been adequately evaluated. Results of preliminary studies have suggested that FDG-PET is more useful for assessing tumor response to chemotherapy and for post-therapy monitoring for recurrence than for assessing the initial tumor.[58] Because edema can resolve with chemotherapy, imaging performed for the purpose of surgical planning should be performed after the administration of neoadjuvant chemotherapy.[53]

CT scan of the chest is the most sensitive radiologic study for detection of pulmonary metastases. A generally accepted definition of definitive pulmonary metastatic disease is three or more lesions 5 mm or larger or one lesion 1 cm or larger.[59] The interpretation of very small lesions (less than 5 mm) and solitary lesions between 5 mm and 1 cm detected by high-resolution CT scanning can be difficult. In some cases, it is not possible to determine whether such CT findings represent metastatic disease or a nonmalignant lung process, and biopsy may be needed. Compared with a CT scan, a plain radiograph of the chest has a sensitivity of 57% and a [99]technetium bone scan has a sensitivity of 41%.[60] Although CT is highly sensitive, evaluation at the time of thoracotomy usually reveals more pulmonary metastases than are appreciated on the CT scan.[61] Importantly, chest CT scans should be obtained prior to biopsy of the primary tumor because postanesthesia atelectasis makes chest CT scans more difficult to interpret.

Biopsy

Traditionally, bone tumor tissue for pathologic examination was obtained by open biopsy. However, percutaneous core needle biopsies have become more common as the availability and sophistication of interventional radiology services have increased. A number of retrospective series have reported on the diagnostic yield and accuracy of core needle biopsies in

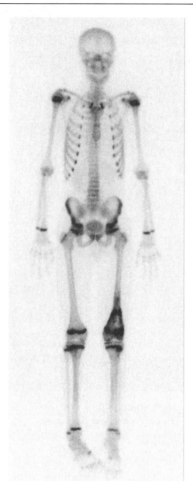

FIGURE 22-8. [99]Technetium bone scan showing an osteosarcoma of the distal femur without distant bony metastases.

osteosarcoma.[62-67] Although none specifically studies pediatric osteosarcoma, all series that provide patient age included children. In these published series, core needle biopsy resulted in a definitive, correct diagnosis in 78% to 94% of cases. The more recently published series have reported a diagnostic accuracy of 90% or greater.[63,67] It is important to note that even those percutaneous biopsies that yield sufficient tumor material for a diagnosis often do not yield sufficient tumor specimen for other biologic studies.

The outcome of percutaneous biopsy varies depending on the provider, technique, and patient population. In the published series reporting a high diagnostic yield, biopsies were performed by experienced interventional radiologists in consultation with orthopedic surgeons in tertiary or referral centers with considerable expertise in the diagnosis and management of bone tumors. In the more recent series, patients underwent conscious sedation or were given general anesthesia. Specific techniques included the use of fluoroscopic, CT, or ultrasound guidance, and use of at least a 14-gauge needle. The tumor component targeted for biopsy was the soft tissue mass, if present, followed by the lytic aspect of an intraosseous lesion.

The most common reason for failure to obtain diagnostic tissue by core needle biopsy is the presence of a highly sclerotic tumor.[64,65] Of the various types of osteosarcoma, telangiectatic osteosarcoma most often results in a nondiagnostic specimen or is misdiagnosed.[63,64] Development of osteosarcoma in a percutaneous biopsy tract has been reported.[68]

Therefore, it is important that the biopsy site be located so that it can be resected en bloc with the primary tumor. Because fine-needle aspiration has a diagnostic yield lower than core needle biopsy[62] and does not obviate the need for sedation in the pediatric population, it is not a recommended approach for diagnosis.

Surgical or open biopsy of bone tumors can be incisional or excisional. Excisional biopsy is almost never performed in osteosarcoma because neoadjuvant chemotherapy can decrease tumor edema and, in doing so, simplify resection. In addition, time is required for adequate surgical planning, especially for younger children in whom placement of a growing prosthesis is being considered. Complications of open biopsy include anesthesia-related events, infection, bleeding, and tumor seeding in the biopsy tract.[69] In addition, disruption of anatomic compartments and incorrect localization of the biopsy incision can lead to a more complex or more extensive tumor resection and can occasionally result in an amputation that would not have otherwise been necessary.[70] As with percutaneous biopsy, the incision for an open biopsy should be placed and oriented in a way that allows it to be excised en bloc with the primary tumor. Complications of open biopsy, including those that result in more extensive resections, are unusual when the biopsy is performed at a center specializing in the diagnosis and treatment of malignant bone tumors.[71]

In summary, the percutaneous and open biopsy routes are both acceptable. Given the implications for ultimate surgical resection of a poorly performed biopsy, biopsy should be performed or planned by an orthopedic surgeon with bone tumor expertise, ideally by the same orthopedic surgeon who will perform the ultimate resection. Percutaneous biopsies should only be performed by experienced interventional radiology staff working in conjunction with an experienced orthopedic surgeon. If the percutaneous route is recommended, it is important to counsel patients and families about the possible risks of core needle biopsy, including the potential for an inconclusive specimen. For a further discussion of the debate regarding the correct route for bone tumor biopsy, see Box 22-2.

Laboratory Evaluation

Laboratory test results are often normal in osteosarcoma. When laboratory abnormalities are present, they are nonspecific, having many other potential causes. Serum alkaline phosphatase is elevated in approximately 50% of patients presenting with osteosarcoma.[72,73] A higher percentage of patients with metastatic disease have a high alkaline phosphatase but this is not a reliable test of metastatic disease, because some patients with metastatic disease will have a normal result. As will be discussed later, alkaline phosphatase elevations are associated with a poorer prognosis. Lactate dehydrogenase (LDH) is elevated in approximately 30% of osteosarcoma patients.[74] The erythrocyte sedimentation rate is generally not elevated in osteosarcoma, whereas it is often elevated in Ewing's sarcoma.

PATHOLOGY AND STAGING

Pathology

On gross examination, osteosarcoma usually presents as a large mass located in the metaphysis (Fig. 22-9) arising in the medullary cavity and crossing the bony cortex, with invasion into the adjacent soft tissues. Microscopically, the malignant cells are pleomorphic but spindle cells typically predominate. Epithelioid, small round cells, multinucleated giant cells, and

| Box 22-2 | **Controversies in Osteosarcoma: Open Versus Core Needle Biopsy** |

There are two possible approaches to obtaining a diagnostic specimen in suspected osteosarcoma—open biopsy and core needle biopsy. Considerable controversy exists regarding which diagnostic approach is best. An open biopsy is performed in the operating room by an orthopedic surgeon. As discussed in more detail in the text, an open biopsy should be performed by an orthopedic surgeon with experience treating bone tumors and ideally by the same orthopedic surgeon who will ultimately perform the tumor resection. In a core needle biopsy, while imaging the tumor with CT, an interventional radiologist obtains several needle cores of tumor material. As with an open biopsy, a core needle biopsy should be performed by an interventional radiologist with expertise in the diagnostic evaluation of bone tumors. Planning for core needle biopsy should include a discussion with the orthopedic surgeon who will ultimately perform the resection. The relative merits of core needle and open biopsy as they relate to several core issues are as follows:

1. DEFINITIVE DIAGNOSIS

Because orthopedic surgeons directly visualize a tumor during an open biopsy and because pathologists often view frozen sections during open biopsies, nondiagnostic open biopsies are uncommon. In retrospective series,[62-67] core needle biopsy resulted in a definitive correct diagnosis in 78% to 94% of cases. The more recently published series have reported a diagnostic accuracy of 90% or greater.[63,67] It is important to note that the interventional radiology-guided core needle biopsies in these studies were performed in centers with considerable experience with the diagnosis of bone tumors, and similar diagnostic accuracy would not be expected in inexperienced centers. Less tumor material is obtained from core needle biopsies, which can compromise the pathologist's ability to perform additional testing, such as cytogenetics, in some cases.

2. POSTPROCEDURE RECOVERY

Both core needle and open biopsies require general anesthesia in children. In general, open biopsies are longer procedures, requiring a greater length of general anesthesia. Open biopsies are also more invasive and result in a longer postprocedure recovery.

3. IMPACT ON ULTIMATE RESECTION

Whether the biopsy approach is core needle or open, definitive surgical treatment of osteosarcoma, which is essential for cure, requires excision of the biopsy tract or site en bloc with the primary tumor. A poorly placed biopsy can convert a tumor amenable to limb-sparing surgery into one that requires amputation. This effect on ultimate resectability is one of the greatest potential negative aspects of core needle biopsy. Because interventional radiologists are less knowledgeable about surgical approaches for definitive tumor resection in osteosarcoma, the risk of a poorly placed biopsy is potentially higher with a core needle biopsy. However, supporters of core needle biopsy argue that this risk can be reduced through discussion of the biopsy with the patient's treating orthopedic surgeon.

4. IMPACT ON BIOLOGIC STUDIES OF OSTEOSARCOMA

Although the availability of tumor material for the study of osteosarcoma biology is not an important issue from the perspective of the individual patient with osteosarcoma, it is an important issue from the perspective of researchers and future patients who could benefit from research discoveries. Because tumor resection occurs after the administration of chemotherapy, osteosarcoma resection specimens are often not suitable for laboratory investigation. Following open biopsy there is usually sufficient prechemotherapy tumor material available for biologic studies after the diagnosis is made. This is not the case with core needle biopsies. Thus, progress in osteosarcoma research would likely be negatively affected if most centers were to perform core needle biopsies.

plasmacytoid cells may also be present and occasionally are the predominant morphology.[75] Osteoid, which can be plentiful or sparse, is currently essential for the diagnosis of osteosarcoma. Sometimes, it is not present in the initial biopsy sample, but is seen in the definitive resection specimen. If not present in either, the diagnosis of osteosarcoma cannot be made with certainty. The histologic appearance of osteoid is dense, pink, and amorphous. Classic or conventional osteosarcoma constitutes 70% to 80% of cases of osteosarcoma.[73] A number of other types of osteosarcoma are distinguished from classical osteosarcoma based on clinical or pathologic features (Table 22-1).

Classical osteosarcoma has a highly malignant appearance, with prominent anaplasia and frequent mitoses. There is vari-ability in the histologic appearance of conventional osteosarcoma. To facilitate pathologic diagnosis and best describe this variability in appearance, classical osteosarcoma is divided into three subtypes based on the predominant matrix produced by the malignant cells.[73] In the first, 50% of typical osteosarcoma is osteoblastic osteosarcoma, in which osteoid is the predominant matrix (Fig. 22-10). Next, 25% of typical osteosarcoma is chondroblastic osteosarcoma in which cartilaginous islands are the predominant matrix. This subtype is differentiated from chondrosarcoma by the presence of osteoid. Because osteoid can be sparse in chondroblastic osteosarcoma, distinguishing chondroblastic osteosarcoma from chondrosarcoma can require extensive biopsy material, which may necessitate rebiopsy. The remaining 25% of typical osteosarcoma is fibroblastic. In fibroblastic osteosarcoma, osteoid is minimal and spindle cells grow in a herringbone pattern.[3] Many osteosarcomas have a mixture of different histologies, but in mixed histology cases one histology usually predominates. Of note, the subtypes of typical osteosarcoma were originally designated for the purpose of diagnosis, and their prognostic significance is uncertain. A better histologic response to chemotherapy in fibroblastic osteosarcoma and a poorer histologic response to chemotherapy in chondroblastic osteosarcoma have been consistent findings in several studies.[74,76,77] Telangiectatic osteosarcoma also has a better histologic response to chemotherapy (see later). Whether these differences in histologic response to therapy are correlated with differences in overall survival is not entirely clear. In the largest study to evaluate this question, there was a slight, statistically significant 5-year overall survival advantage in patients with fibroblastic osteosarcoma. Unlike other types of osteosarcoma, histologic response to chemotherapy may not be correlated with outcome in chondroblastic osteosarcoma.[77]

The remaining 20% to 30% of osteosarcomas that are not classical osteosarcomas are divided into secondary (occurring in Paget's disease or postradiation), jaw, telangiectatic, small cell, parosteal, periosteal, and low-grade intramedullary osteosarcoma. Telangiectatic osteosarcoma accounts for 4% to 11% of all osteosarcoma cases.[73,78-80] The age and gender distribution are the same as in conventional osteosarcoma. Pathologic fracture is more common, occurring in 15% to 25% of cases.[73,79,80] Radiographically, a lytic pattern is present because of the presence of large or small cystic areas and minimal osteoid formation. Microscopically, cysts are divided by septa that are lined with malignant cells producing scant osteoid. Cysts are also lined by benign, multinucleated giant cells. The presence of cysts and multinucleated giant cells can lead to misdiagnosis as an aneurysmal bone cyst or giant cell tumor, both benign bone tumors.[73] Although case series published prior to the modern era of multiagent chemotherapy had reported that telangiectatic osteosarcoma has an adverse prognostic implication, more recent studies have reported a better histologic response to therapy and improved survival as compared with typical osteosarcoma.[77-79]

Small cell osteosarcoma is a rare but histologically distinct variant representing 1% to 4% of osteosarcomas.[81,82] The clinical and epidemiologic characteristics are the same as conven-

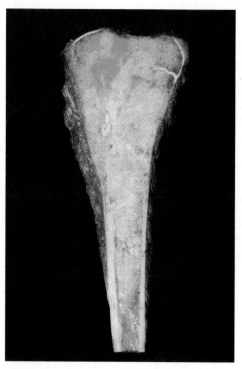

FIGURE 22-9. Osteosarcoma: gross pathology.

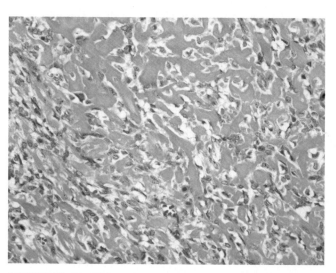

FIGURE 22-10. High-grade osteosarcoma composed of malignant-appearing tumor cells having a high nuclear-to-cytoplasmic ratio, hyperchromatism, and prominent nucleoli, and an abundant eosinophilic osteoid matrix.

TABLE 22-1	**Pathologic Features and Relative Frequency of Osteosarcoma Subtypes**	
Type	**Pathology**	**Approximate No. (%*)**
Classic	Anaplastic numerous mitoses	70-80
Osteoblastic	Predominant matrix osteoid	35
Chondroblastic	Predominant matrix chondroid	18
Fibroblastic	Spindle cells in herringbone pattern	18
Jaw	Similar to classic osteosarcoma	3-7
Secondary	Similar to classic osteosarcoma	7
Telangiectatic	Cysts and septa, scant osteoid, giant cells present	4-10
Small cell	Small round malignant cells, osteoid present but quantity variable	1-4
Low-grade intramedullary	Minimal atypia, few mitoses	1-2
Parosteal	Located on bone surface, low grade, matrix osteoid and, in 50%, cartilage	4
Periosteal	Located on bone surface, intermediate grade, predominant matrix cartilage	1-2

*Of all osteosarcomas.

tional osteosarcoma. Microscopically, tumors are composed of small round cells that produce variable amounts of osteoid. Differentiation from Ewing's sarcoma and lymphoma can be difficult.

Osteosarcomas of the jaw, located in the maxilla or mandible, deserve specific mention. Even when secondary osteosarcomas are excluded, the mean age of patients with osteosarcoma in this location is the mid-30s, older than in classical osteosarcoma.[73,83,84] These tumors are more often low grade; approximately 50% are low grade in most series.[84,85] Histologically, the appearance is similar to classical osteosarcoma but a larger proportion of tumors are chondroblastic. In concordance with the greater proportion of low-grade tumors, prognosis is better for osteosarcoma of the jaw. Although local recurrence does occur, especially when the initial resection is inadequate, metastasis is unusual.

Low-grade intramedullary osteosarcoma is relatively rare, making up approximately 1% to 2% of all osteosarcomas. Patients developing this form of osteosarcoma tend to be older than those with conventional osteosarcoma, with 30 years being the mean age at diagnosis. Microscopic examination reveals spindle cells permeating bony trabeculae, with minimal atypia and few mitoses. A variable amount of osteoid is present. Recurrence and metastasis are rare. With adequate resection, chemotherapy is generally not indicated.[86,87]

Parosteal osteosarcoma is another low-grade osteosarcoma distinguished from low-grade intramedullary osteosarcoma by its location on the cortical surface of the bone. It is generally a sclerotic tumor attached to the bone by a broad base. Microscopically, the stroma is sparsely populated by minimally atypical spindle cells. The matrix contains osteoid and, in 50% of cases, cartilage.[88] A limited degree of medullary involvement is seen in 25% of cases. Areas of dedifferentiation can be present at diagnosis or at the time of recurrence and portend a poorer prognosis. Of patients with dedifferentiation, 31% will die of disease, usually with pulmonary metastasis.[89] Parosteal osteosarcoma makes up approximately 4% of all osteosarcomas. Like intramedullary low-grade osteosarcoma, parosteal osteosarcoma occurs in slightly older patients than conventional osteosarcoma, and recurrence and metastasis are rare in adequately resected cases without dedifferentiation.[90]

Parosteal osteosarcoma must be distinguished from periosteal osteosarcoma, which also arises from the surface of the bone but is an intermediate- or high-grade lesion. Periosteal osteosarcoma has an age distribution similar to typical osteosarcoma but almost all tumors arise in the proximal tibia. The appearance on plain radiograph is highly characteristic and suggests the diagnosis. Histology is of a spindle cell neoplasm with osteoid and cartilaginous islands present, usually in large amounts. The prognosis is better than in conventional

osteosarcoma but probably not as good as in parosteal osteosarcoma without dedifferentiation or intermedullary low-grade osteosarcoma.[91]

Secondary osteosarcoma arises in previously irradiated bone or in patients with Paget's disease. In both cases, patients are older than those with conventional osteosarcoma. Pathology is similar to conventional osteosarcoma. Prognosis is poorer in Paget's disease than in conventional osteosarcoma.[75] There is some evidence that radiation-induced osteosarcomas have similar outcomes to de novo osteosarcoma if standard osteosarcoma chemotherapy is given.[92,93]

Staging

Staging of osteosarcoma follows the Enneking[94] or musculoskeletal society staging system (Table 22-2). The TNM system is not used for several reasons. The TNM system lacks biologic relevance in that osteosarcoma seldom metastasizes to lymph nodes. In addition, it is more complex than needed for predicting outcome, because patients in different TNM stages have overlapping prognoses.[94]

The Enneking staging system is based on tumor grade (G), site (T), and metastases (M). Low-grade (G1) tumors are well-differentiated and have few mitoses, corresponding to Broders' grades I and II.[95] Osteosarcoma is high grade (G2) if it is poorly differentiated and has numerous mitoses, corresponding to Broders' grades III and IV. As noted, most osteosarcomas are high grade (G2). Surgical site (T) is determined by whether the tumor is contained within its anatomic compartment of origin (T1) or extends beyond its compartment of origin (T2). For example, a typical osteosarcoma that arises in the medullary space and extends through the cortex into the soft tissue is T2. A parosteal osteosarcoma that does not extend from the bone surface, its site of origin, into the medullary space and does not invade the surrounding soft tissue is T1. Most classical osteosarcomas are T2. Metastases are absent (M1) or present (M2). Stages IA and IB are low-grade (G1) tumors. Stages IIA and IIB are high-grade tumors. Stage IA tumors are low-grade osteosarcomas that are T1, or lack extension beyond the compartment of origin. Stage IB tumors are low-grade osteosarcomas that are T2, or demonstrate extension beyond the compartment of origin. Similarly, stage IIA tumors do not have extracompartmental extension, whereas IIB tumors do. Stage III osteosarcomas are tumors of any grade and any site that have distant metastases.[94,96,97] The vast majority of osteosarcomas are stage IIB. The next most common stage for osteosarcoma at presentation is stage III. Stages IA, IB, and IIA are uncommon, with 3% to 5% of osteosarcomas falling into each of these categories.[98]

TABLE 22-2   Enneking Staging System for Osteosarcoma, Distribution of Osteosarcoma, and Indicated Treatment by Stage

Stage	Grade	Site	Metastasis	No. of Patients (%)[98]	Surgical Margin	Chemotherapy	Representative Subtype
IA	G1	T1	M0	5	Wide	No	Parosteal
IB	G1	T2	M0	3	Wide	No	
IIA	G2	T1	M0	5	Wide	Yes	Periosteal
IIB	G2	T2	M0	74	Wide	Yes	Classical
III	G1,2	T1,2	M1	13	Variable	Yes	Classical

G1, low grade, characterized by few mitoses and a relatively well-differentiated appearance; G2, high grade, characterized by higher mitotic rate and a less differentiated appearance; T1, tumor is intracompartmental or confined to anatomic compartment of origin; T2, tumor is extracompartmental or extends beyond anatomic compartment of origin; M0, no distant metastases present; M1, distant metastases present.

Adapted from Enneking WF, Spanier SS, Goodman MA. A system for the surgical staging of musculoskeletal sarcoma. Clin Orthop Relat Res. 1980;(153)106-120.

NATURAL HISTORY AND PROGNOSIS

The most significant predictor of survival in osteosarcoma is the presence of residual disease caused by incomplete resection of primary tumor in localized osteosarcoma, local recurrence, or the presence of metastases. Consequently, the natural history, prognosis, and prognostic factors of localized, relapsed, and metastatic osteosarcoma differ significantly.

Localized Disease

Natural History

Prior to the use of chemotherapy for osteosarcoma, the overall survival of patients with localized disease who had a complete resection was 20%. Death was almost always caused by complications of pulmonary metastases.[73,99] With wide or radical surgical margins, local recurrence was rare. The development of pulmonary metastases in 80% of patients treated with only complete resection of the primary tumor has been interpreted as evidence of the presence of micrometastatic foci in the lungs at the time of diagnosis[100] and was one rationale for adjuvant chemotherapy.

Five-year event-free survival and overall survival of localized osteosarcoma in the era of modern therapy are 65% to 75% and 70% to 80%, respectively.[101-104] Approximately 80% of relapses are pulmonary either alone or, in 25% of patients, with a second disease site, which is most often bone. Bone, distant from the initial resection, is the initial relapse site in 8% of patients; 1% to 2% of patients have recurrence isolated to unusual sites such as brain, kidneys, heart, or liver.[6,7,105] Local recurrence is seen in 2% to 8% of patients, despite having had adequate surgical margins.[48,106,107] Most relapses occur during the first 2 years after completion of chemotherapy. However, relapses occur as late as 10 years[106] and the event-free survival (EFS) decreases slowly between 2 and 10 years. In the few studies reporting long-term follow-up data, EFS decreases to 60% at 10 years from 65% at 5 years.[106,108]

Prognostic Factors

By multivariate analysis, the only factor that is a reproducible predictor of outcome in localized, fully resected osteosarcoma is the extent of tumor necrosis following neoadjuvant chemotherapy.[47,48,109-112] When investigators at the Memorial Sloan-Kettering Cancer Center first gave neoadjuvant, or preoperative, chemotherapy to facilitate surgical resection without amputation, they noted varying degrees of necrosis on pathologic examination of resected tumor specimens.[113] It was later observed that patients with significant necrosis had a better event-free and overall survival than those with lesser degrees of necrosis.[114]

The generally accepted grading system for tumor necrosis (Table 22-3) assigns higher grades to tumors with greater evidence of necrosis. In most studies, grades III and IV, in which more than 90% of the tumor is necrotic, define the group of patients whose tumors have a good response to chemotherapy. Patients whose tumors have a poor response have 10% or more viable tumor, corresponding to grades I and II. Patients with a poor response have disease-free survival (DFS) rates of 40% to 50%, whereas those with a good response have DFS rates of 70% to 80%[102,115-117] (Fig. 22-11). An improved outcome for poor responders is an objective of past and current trials (see later, "Chemotherapy for Localized Disease").

Tumor size has been identified as a significant prognostic factor by multivariate analysis in several studies.[47,48,104,111] However, other studies have not found this patient variable to

TABLE 22-3	Grading of Histologic Response to Neoadjuvant Chemotherapy	
Response	**Grade**	**Histology**
Poor	I	Necrosis minimal or absent
	II	Necrosis <90% of the tumor but greater than minimal
Good	III	Scattered areas of viable tumor but >90% of tumor necrotic
	IV	No viable tumor

Adapted from Rosen G, Caparros B, Huvos AG, et al. Preoperative chemotherapy for osteogenic sarcoma: selection of postoperative adjuvant chemotherapy based on the response of the primary tumor to preoperative chemotherapy. Cancer. 1982;49:1221-1230.

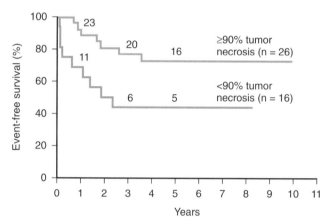

FIGURE 22-11. Representative event-free survival curve of patients with localized osteosarcoma ≥90% (blue line) or <90% (green line) tumor necrosis following neoadjuvant chemotherapy. *(Adapted from Goorin AM, Schwartzentruber DJ, Devidas M, et al. Presurgical chemotherapy compared with immediate surgery and adjuvant chemotherapy for nonmetastatic osteosarcoma: Pediatric Oncology Group Study POG-8651. J Clin Oncol. 2003;21:1574-1580.)*

be predictive of outcome.[109,118-120] One possible explanation for this conflict is variability in the definition of tumor size and measurement techniques. Some studies evaluate absolute tumor length, others use relative (to the entire bone) tumor length, and still others base analyses on tumor volume. Most studies showing size to be a significant predictor of outcome on multivariate analysis have measured tumor volume.[48,104,111] However, the volume that distinguishes small, low-risk tumors from large, high-risk tumors varies among studies. In summary, further studies using standard measurement techniques and risk criteria need to be conducted before tumor size can be used as a clinically significant predictor on which to counsel patients or base therapeutic decisions. The prognostic significance of tumor size might be caused by the influence of tumor size on resectability. In other words, larger tumors may confer a poorer prognosis because it is less likely that the tumor will be completely resected with wide margins.

Several studies have found an association between tumor site and outcome, with axial and proximal appendicular primary tumors having a worse prognosis than distal extremity tumors.[47,48,101,104,111,121-124] However, there are potential interactions between tumor site and other osteosarcoma prognostic factors. In particular, site and size are likely to be associated. A distal extremity osteosarcoma is likely to be noticed at a smaller size because of the relative lack of soft tissue. More importantly, the higher risk sites, such as axial skeleton, are also those for which a complete resection is less likely.

Elevated LDH and alkaline phosphatase at the time of diagnosis are associated with a poorer prognosis.[48,109,110] In one study,[109] the EFS of patients with a normal alkaline phosphatase at diagnosis was 88%, whereas it was 46% for patients with an elevated alkaline phosphatase. There are several issues that limit the usefulness of LDH and alkaline phosphatase as prognostic indicators. First, elevated levels are not consistently associated with a poorer prognosis in all studies. Second, elevations in LDH and alkaline phosphatase confer only a modestly increased relative risk (1.5 for LDH and 2 for alkaline phosphatase) of a poor outcome.[110]

Other prognostic factors that have been reported to be significant in a limited number of studies are age and gender.[47,48] Currently, there is insufficient evidence regarding the prognostic significance of these variables. As noted earlier, histologic subtype may be a prognostic factor. P-glycoprotein positivity, loss of heterozygosity at the *Rb* locus, and high ERBB2 and ezrin expression have all been identified as possible biology-based predictors of a poor outcome.[125-127] Further validation of these factors in large prospective populations is needed. These prognostic factors are discussed more extensively (see "Biology"). In summary, the extent of tumor necrosis is the most reliable prognostic indicator in localized, completely resected osteosarcoma. However, tumor response is not a true prognostic factor because it cannot be determined until after the initiation of chemotherapy.

Metastatic and Relapsed Disease

Overall survival for patients with relapsed disease is poor, with most series showing a 25% overall survival at 5 years.[6,7,105] As with primary osteosarcoma, the most significant prognostic factor for post-relapse survival is the ability to achieve complete resection of all disease sites. In one report of 162 patients with initially localized osteosarcoma who developed recurrent disease, the 5-year projected overall survival was 39% for those who had complete resection of all disease and 0% for those who did not.[6] With isolated pulmonary metastases, prognosis is significantly influenced by the number of pulmonary nodules and whether there is unilateral or bilateral pulmonary disease.[6,7,105] In particular, having more than one pulmonary nodule at relapse conveys a worse prognosis. An additional prognostic factor is the duration of remission. Patients relapsing less than 24 months after initial diagnosis have a worse outcome.[6,105] Finally, use of chemotherapy is associated with a slightly improved postrelapse prognosis,[7] particularly in patients with unresectable disease.[6]

Local recurrence warrants special mention because of its dismal prognosis. The 5-year disease-free survival is 0% to 15%.[106,107,128] Local recurrence is almost always associated with concurrent or delayed pulmonary metastasis.[106] In one series, the outcome of patients with local recurrence was strongly influenced by the presence or absence of systemic metastases at the time of local recurrence. The 5-year DFS was 25% for patients without systemic metastases at the time of local recurrence and it was 0% for those with systemic metastases.

The outcome and prognostic factors for metastatic disease present at diagnosis are similar to those for relapsed disease. The 5-year overall survival of patients presenting with primary metastatic disease is 20% to 30%.[4,129] One exception to the poor prognosis for patients with metastatic disease is skip metastases. In patients with skip metastases, overall survival is 50%, even when pulmonary metastases are also present.[55] Higher overall survival has been reported in some chemotherapy trials, possibly because of therapy efficacy or shorter periods

of follow-up.[130] An important predictor of a poor outcome is the inability to achieve complete surgical remission. Similarly, patients with metastases to more than one site or more than one organ are at increased risk of death from disease.[4,129] In one study, an alkaline phosphatase level higher than 500 IU/L was significantly associated with poor prognosis on multivariate analysis.[129]

BIOLOGY

Structural chromosomal alterations, loss of tumor suppressor function, and oncogene amplification have all been described in osteosarcoma. In addition, alterations in specific proteins contribute to chemotherapy resistance and metastatic behavior. A summary of genes altered in osteosarcoma is presented in Table 22-4.

Genetic Alterations

All osteosarcomas contain complex cytogenetic aberrations, which points to the involvement of multiple genes in osteosarcoma development. However, unlike Ewing's and synovial cell sarcoma, consistent translocations that can serve as starting points for biologic studies or therapeutic intervention have not been described. Copy number abnormalities, changes in ploidy, and structural rearrangements are seen in all high-grade osteosarcomas. Homogeneously staining regions and marker, double-minute, and ring chromosomes are seen in most tumors.[131,132] A representative karyotype is shown in Figure 22-12. Nonclonal changes, often superimposed on clonal aberrations, are present in many tumor specimens.[75] The nonclonal complex nature of the osteosarcoma genome makes the interpretation of karyotype, comparative genomic hybridization (CGH), and fluorescence in situ hybridization (FISH) data difficult and the identification of candidate genes implicated in a significant proportion of osteosarcomas challenging.[133]

Osteosarcoma DNA ploidy ranges from diploid to hexaploid.[131] Spectral karyotyping (SKY) of osteosarcomas reveals an average of 39 chromosomal rearrangements/tumor.[134] The chromosome regions most commonly affected by structural rearrangements have been reviewed by Sandberg and Bridge[133] and include the following regions, which are affected in 15% or more cases: 1p11-p13, 1q10-q12, 11p15, 12p13, 19q13, and 22q11-13. By karyotype analysis, loss of genetic material is more common than gain of genetic material. The most common losses involve chromosomes 9, 10, 13, and 17 and gains are commonly seen in chromosome 1. Because it is not possible to assign an origin to the homogeneous staining regions and marker, double-minute, and ring chromosomes seen in most tumors, classic cytogenetics do not fully characterize osteosarcomas. For example, chromosome 8 material is frequently present in marker chromosomes,[134] which can be determined by SKY but not by traditional karyotyping. Whereas karyotypes do not show a gain of 8q,[133] CGH analysis has identified 8q21.3-23 as a region with high-level amplification in almost 50% of cases.[135]

Multiple investigators have applied CGH analysis to identify genes of interest in osteosarcoma.[135-139] In almost all CGH analyses, gains are more common than losses. Amplified regions consistently seen in a significant proportion of tumors and across studies include 1q21-q24, 6p11.2-p12, 8q21.3-q24, 17p11.2-p12 (high-level amplification), 1p, 1q21, 5p14, and 6p12-21.3. Commonly seen deletions include 2q and 6q and chromosomes 9, 10, and 13q. Copy number alterations are also present in other regions but have been reported in a small pro-

TABLE 22-4   Genes Implicated in Osteosarcoma Pathogenesis and Biologic Progression

Gene	Alteration	Gene Function	Portion of Sporadic Osteosarcoma (%)
Rb	Deletion, inactivation	Cell cycle control	70
p53	Mutation, inactivation	Apoptosis; response to DNA damage; cell cycle control	50
MDM2	Gene amplification	p53 regulation	10-15
COPS3	Gene amplification	p53 regulation	25
INK4A	Deletion Promoter methylation	Cell cycle control through inhibition of cyclin-dependent kinase 4–cyclin D	15-20
MET	Increased expression	Motility Invasion	60
FOS	Increased expression	Proliferation Possibly, differentiation	60
MYC	Gene amplification	Proliferation	40
MDR1	Increased expression	Efflux of chemotherapeutic agents	25-45
DHFR	Increased expression	Folate metabolism; MTX target	60 relapsed tumors
erbB2	Increased expression	Growth factor receptor	40
Ezrin	Increased expression	Membrane cytoskeleton linker, facilitates metastasis	92
FAS	Decreased expression	Apoptosis	60 pulmonary metastases lack FAS
Reduced folate carrier	Decreased expression	MTX transport	65
IGF-IR	Increased expression	Growth factor receptor, proliferation	Unknown

MTX, methotrexate.

portion of cases or single studies only. Loss of 13q14[136] and gain of 8q (8q21.3-q22 or 8cen-q13)[135] have been associated with a worse prognosis, and 5q loss[136] has been associated with a better prognosis, although these findings have not been replicated. Higher detail analysis with FISH, quantitative polymerase chain reaction (PCR), or array CGH has revealed that amplification and deletion patterns are complex, in that individual genes in an amplified region may not be amplified.[140]

Some important candidate genes have been identified using genomic techniques. 12q13-14, which is amplified in 10%[135,137] of osteosarcomas, is important because it contains multiple potential oncogenes, including MDM2. In the commonly amplified region 17p11.2-p12, candidates PMP22, TOP3A, MAPK7, and COPS3 display high levels of amplification in more than 50% of cases using semiquantitative PCR and microsatellite markers.[141,142] The retinoblastoma gene is located at 13q14, a region that is lost in many osteosarcomas.[131,132] MDM2 and COPS3 amplifications and Rb loss are discussed further below.

The MYC gene, located at 8q24.1 is amplified in 7% to 10% of osteosarcomas when assessed by Southern blotting.[143,144] The more sensitive technique, CGH, detects MYC amplification in 44% of osteosarcomas.[139,143-145] c-Myc mRNA and protein levels are increased in a similar proportion of osteosarcomas and MYC expression might be correlated with metastasis. c-Myc, when complexed with MAX, activates the transcription of a number of genes, perhaps as many as 15% of all genes. Downstream effects of c-Myc transcriptional activation include proliferation, cell growth, inhibition of differentiation, and apoptosis. Exactly how c-Myc regulates these diverse cell processes and how MYC overexpression leads to cancer is an area of active investigation.[146,147]

Tumor Suppressors

Retinoblastoma

The retinoblastoma 1 gene, located at 13q14, was the first tumor suppressor gene identified and is one of the most frequently altered genes in osteosarcoma. As noted earlier (see "Cause"), the second most common tumor in patients with hereditary retinoblastoma who carry germline Rb mutations[31] is osteosarcoma. Rb abnormalities are also present in most sporadic osteosarcomas. Rb inactivation is thought to contribute to osteosarcoma tumorigenesis through its role in cell cycle control and possibly through its regulation of differentiation and apoptosis.

Hereditary retinoblastoma is a condition in which individuals with a heterozygous germline Rb mutation develop retinoblastoma, a malignant tumor of the embryonal neural retina, with 90% penetrance.[148] Germline Rb mutations can be sporadic or inherited. Rb germline mutations in patients who develop bilateral tumors are usually small deletions or frameshift mutations resulting in a null protein,[149] whereas 40% of Rb germline mutations in patients with unilateral tumors are in-frame point mutations.[149] The cumulative incidence of a second malignancy by 50 years after the initial retinoblastoma diagnosis is 51%. Approximately 50% of the second malignancies developing in patients with hereditary retinoblastoma are osteosarcomas.[30,150] Both osteosarcomas and retinoblastomas occurring in patients with hereditary retinoblastoma have somatic loss of the normal Rb allele, with resulting complete absence of a functional Rb protein.[31,151,152]

Somatic alterations in the Rb gene are seen in most sporadic osteosarcomas. Loss of heterozygosity (LOH) at the Rb locus is seen in 65%[32,127,153] of sporadic osteosarcomas. Structural changes, usually associated with LOH, are present in 30% to 40%[32,153,154] of tumors and homozygous deletions are seen in 23%[155] of tumors. Point mutations are rare and are present in only 6% of cases.[32] Overall, 70% of sporadic osteosarcomas have at least one Rb abnormality,[32] and many tumors have a combination of Rb alterations. Rb gene alterations are generally not seen in low-grade bone tumors.[32] There is some evidence that the initially mutated allele is usually of paternal origin and the allele that undergoes deletion is maternally derived.[156] Decreased Rb expression is seen in about 50% of osteosarcomas[157] but changes in Rb expression are not correlated with Rb gene alterations.[32] For example, in some tumors with Rb LOH, Rb protein levels are not reduced.

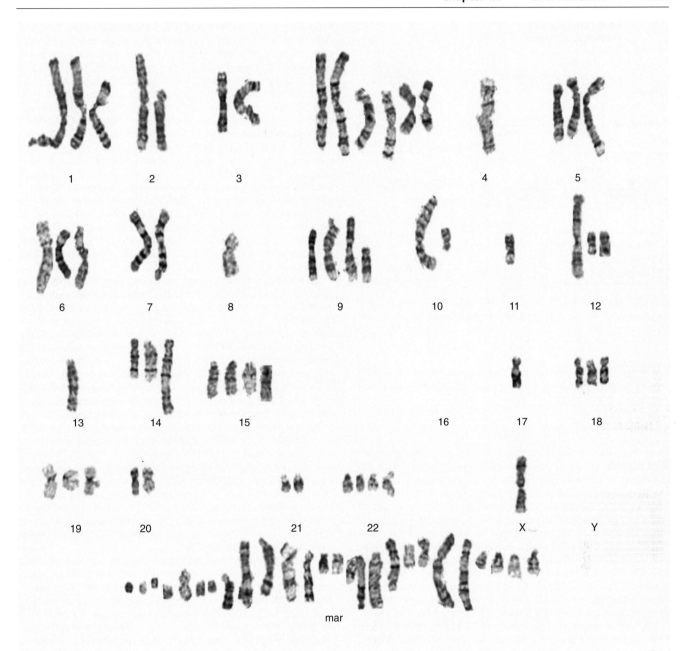

FIGURE 22-12. Representative osteosarcoma karyotype showing chromosome 16 loss, multiple marker chromosomes, monosomies, trisomies, and tetrasomies.

Some studies have found an association between *Rb* LOH and a poorer prognosis.[32,127] However, these studies were based on univariate analyses in relatively small populations and another study had contradictory results.[158] Theoretically, *Rb* inactivation could contribute to a poorer prognosis through increasing the expression of thymidylate synthase and dihydrofolate reductase, consequently increasing resistance to antimetabolites,[159] an important component of osteosarcoma therapy.

As reviewed by Classon and Harlow,[160] Rb is a key regulator of the G1 to S cell cycle transition. Rb, by binding and thereby inhibiting the E2F family of transcription factors, blocks the transition from the G1 to the S phase of the cell cycle. Rb is regulated by cyclin-dependent kinases (CDKs), particularly CDKs 4 and 6, which interact with cyclin D. These CDK-cyclin complexes phosphorylate Rb. Rb phosphorylation inhibits the Rb-E2F interaction, allowing transcriptional activa-

tion by E2F, which leads to progression from G1 to S (Fig. 22-13). Rb probably also controls cell cycle progression through chromatin remodeling, as reviewed by Khidr and Chen.[161] In particular, the Rb-E2F complex, by interacting with histone deacetylases, histone methyltransferases, and DNA methylases, contributes to the inactivation of E2F target genes during G0 and G1.

Genetically engineered *Rb* null mouse models have suggested that Rb regulates cellular differentiation and apoptosis. *Rb* deletion in mice results in embryonic lethality. The *Rb* null embryos have abnormalities in the development and differentiation of skeletal muscle, nervous system components, retina, adipocytes, and hematopoietic cells.[161,162] Some of these defects may be secondary to a placental defect in *Rb* null mice.[163] Through interaction with CBFA1, a key transcriptional regulator in osteoblasts, Rb induces osteogenic differentiation.[164] The

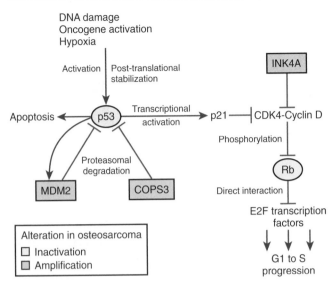

FIGURE 22-13. Selected regulators and effectors of *p53* and *Rb*. Alterations present in osteosarcoma are highlighted in yellow and blue.

significance of Rb differentiation and apoptosis roles in tumorigenesis in general and osteosarcomagenesis in particular is not clear.

p53

There is convincing evidence that abnormal p53 function is one of the central events in osteosarcomagenesis. Patients with Li-Fraumeni syndrome, who carry heterozygous germline *p53* mutations, are predisposed to osteosarcoma. Somatic alterations in the *p53* gene are found in a significant percentage of sporadic osteosarcomas. Furthermore, several different transgenic mouse models, with altered or absent p53 function, develop osteosarcoma. Finally, components of the p53 regulatory and effector pathways, MDM2 (murine double-minute 2), INK4A, also known as CDKN2A, cyclin-dependent kinase inhibitor 2A, and COPS 3 (COP9 constitutive photomorphogenic homolog subunit 3) are also frequently perturbed in osteosarcoma, particularly in tumors lacking *p53* mutations.

Of cancers arising in patients with Li-Fraumeni syndrome, 10% are osteosarcoma, making osteosarcoma the second most common tumor in Li-Fraumeni syndrome.[33] In addition to osteosarcoma, Li-Fraumeni patients are predisposed to breast cancer, various soft tissue sarcomas, brain tumors, and various carcinomas. *p53* germline mutations are present in 7% of osteosarcoma patients who have a personal history of multiple cancers but who do not meet Li-Fraumeni diagnostic criteria.[165] Individuals with Li-Fraumeni syndrome have germline mutations in *p53* located throughout the gene, although approximately 75% of the mutations are in exons 5 to 8,[166] which encode the DNA binding domain of the *p53* protein. Tumors arising in patients with Li-Fraumeni syndrome typically have loss of the normal *p53* allele.[167]

Somatic alterations of the *p53* gene are present in 20% to 50% of sporadic osteosarcomas.[34,126,168-175] Despite the prevalence of somatic *p53* mutations in sporadic osteosarcomas, germline *p53* mutations are rare in patients with sporadic osteosarcoma without a personal or family history of multiple cancers.[176,177] The wide range in the reported frequency of somatic *p53* alterations in sporadic osteosarcoma is the result of small study size, differences in techniques of ascertainment, and varying definitions of an abnormal result. *p53* point muta-

tions are present in 20% to 30% of osteosarcomas.[34,168,171-173] As with *p53* mutations in other cancer types, missense mutations constitute approximately 75% of osteosarcoma point mutations.[178] Point mutations are present throughout the *p53* coding sequence although, as with Li-Fraumeni syndrome germline mutations, approximately 73% occur in exons 5 to 8.[172] The initial *p53* abnormality to be recognized in osteosarcoma was gross rearrangements of the *p53* gene.[170] Gross rearrangements are present in 15% to 25% of cases.[168,169,171] Studies that evaluated *p53* for both point mutations and gross gene rearrangements have found that almost 50% of osteosarcomas examined have aberrant *p53*.[171,174] Because mutant p53 protein usually accumulates in cells because of an increased half-life,[179] p53 immunohistochemistry (IHC) has been used to screen for *p53* mutations in osteosarcoma. By IHC, 15% to 25% of osteosarcomas have p53 abnormalities,[126,175] reflecting the fact that IHC has a relatively low sensitivity for detecting *p53* mutations. Approximately 50% of osteosarcomas with *p53* point mutations have loss of the normal allele.[172]

Several genetically engineered mouse models with dysfunctional or absent *p53* develop osteosarcoma. In a genetically engineered mouse model in which *p53* and *Rb* deletion is restricted to osteoblasts, osteosarcoma develops with a high penetrance and short latency.[179a,179b] Mice homozygous for null *p53* develop a variety of tumors. Although lymphoma and hemangiosarcoma are the most common tumor types seen, 4% of the mice develop osteosarcoma.[180] Mice heterozygous for null *p53* develop tumors at 25% the rate and at an older age than homozygous null mice, but 25% of the tumors that develop are osteosarcomas.[181] Osteosarcomas are much more common in mice genetically engineered to be heterozygous for a common cancer-associated *p53* mutation, R172H. Almost 50% of these mice develop osteosarcoma, usually associated with hematogenous metastases.[182] Several other mouse models heterozygous for mutant *p53* develop osteosarcoma at a rate of 20% to 30%. Metastases are common in these models as well.[183,184] Transgenic mice expressing the SV40 T antigen from different promoters[185,186] develop osteosarcoma at a rate of approximately 70%. The mechanism of transformation in the SV40 T antigen expressing models probably involves the inactivation of p53 and Rb.

Other transgenic murine models that develop osteosarcoma include mice carrying a homozygous deletion of *WWOX*,[87] and conditional *MYC* overexpression from the EµSRa promoter.[188] The *WWOX* null mice develop osteosarcoma at a rate of 30% prior to premature death at 4 weeks postnatal age.[187] Only 1% of the *MYC* overexpressing mice develop osteosarcomas.[188] Rats receiving prolonged treatment with parathyroid hormone develop osteosarcoma at approximately $1\frac{1}{2}$ years of age.

In other cancers, *p53* mutation status has been associated with proliferation, response to chemotherapy, and outcome. In osteosarcoma, the response to chemotherapy is equivalent in *p53* mutant and *p53* wild-type osteosarcomas.[189] Several studies have examined the impact of *p53* mutation on survival in osteosarcoma. Only one study, in 30 patients, showed a worse survival in patients whose tumors had *p53* mutations.[174] The remainder of the studies did not show a relationship between *p53* mutation status and outcome.[126,171,189,190] Finally, *p53* mutations are not more common in metastatic disease than in localized disease.[172] Actually, the *p53* mutation status of primary and metastatic tumors tends to be concordant.[172]

As reviewed by Levine[179] and Vogelstein and colleagues,[191] *p53* mutations and structural alterations lead to transformation by interfering with p53 tumor suppressor functions and, possibly, by producing a p53 protein that has gained oncogenic function. p53 tumor suppressor activities include cell cycle control and induction of apoptosis. Several forms of cellular stress, including DNA damage, hypoxia, shortened telomeres, and oncogene activation lead to p53 post-translational stabilization and p53 activation. Following activation, p53 binds DNA and promotes the transcription of several genes, including *p21* and *MDM2*. As in other tumor types, the *p53* mutations seen in sporadic osteosarcomas and Li-Fraumeni syndrome are concentrated in the DNA-binding domain and interfere with the transcriptional activity of the protein.[178] p53 prevents progression from the G1 phase to the S phase of the cell cycle through the actions of one of its target genes, *p21*. p21 protein inhibits the cyclin-dependent kinase 4 (CDK4)–cyclin D complex, which in turn keeps Rb in an unphosphorylated state. Unphosphorylated Rb binds E2F transcription factors, preventing progression into the S phase (see Fig. 22-13).[191] p53 also plays a regulatory role in the G2 to M cell cycle checkpoint. Other inhibitors of CDK4–cyclin D are INK4A, also known as p16, and CDKN2A (cyclin-dependent kinase inhibitor 2A). INK4A abnormalities are also seen in osteosarcoma (see later).

As with p53-mediated cell cycle control, p53-mediated apoptosis is triggered by DNA damage. In addition, oncogene overexpression and *Rb* inactivation stimulate p53-mediated apoptosis. The pathways involved in p53-mediated apoptosis are not fully understood. However, they likely involve proapoptotic proteins whose genes are targets of p53 transcriptional activation, including BAX, NOXA, and P53AIP1.[191]

p53 inactivation allows cells to progress through the cell cycle and escape apoptosis, despite the presence of DNA damage. Consistent with this observation, the presence of a *p53* mutation in osteosarcoma is significantly correlated with a greater level of genomic instability.[34] Thus, promotion of genomic instability and the resultant accumulation of secondary mutations in oncogenes or tumor suppressors is yet another mechanism of transformation in *p53* mutant tumors.

p53 Regulators: MDM2 and COPS3

The regulators of p53 activity, MDM2 and COPS3, are amplified in a proportion of osteosarcomas. MDM2 inhibits p53 activity by direct interaction with the p53 DNA-binding domain and by transporting p53 to the cytoplasm.[192-194] In addition, MDM2 ubiquitinates p53, targeting it for proteasomal degradation. MDM2-mediated ubiquitination is enhanced by DNA damage.[195] The *MDM2* gene, located at 12q14, is amplified in 10% to 15% of osteosarcomas.[168,174,175,196-198] Usually, *MDM2* amplification occurs in tumors without p53 mutations, and thus *MDM2* amplification acts as an alternative mechanism of *p53* inactivation. There is limited evidence that *MDM2* amplification is more common in parosteal and other forms of low-grade osteosarcoma.[140,199,200]

COPS3, located at 17p11.2, a frequently amplified region in osteosarcoma, is a subunit of the COP9 signalosome. The COP9 signalosome interacts directly with p53 and, through phosphorylation, targets p53 for interaction with MDM2 and degradation by the 26S proteasome.[201] *COPS3* gene amplification is present in 25% to 30% of osteosarcomas.[202,203] Increased COPS3 expression through alternative mechanisms is present in some tumors lacking *COPS3* gene amplification.[202] Like *MDM2* amplification, *COPS3* overexpression may be an alternative mechanism of p53 inactivation. p53 mutations are present in a small proportion of COPS3-amplified osteosarcomas.[202,203]

INK4A and ARF

As described earlier, INK4A (also known as p16), like the p53-inducible protein p21, is an inhibitor of the CDK4–cyclin D complex. As with p21, inhibition of CDK4–cyclin D by INK4A prevents progression from the G1 to the S phase. Ten percent to 20% of osteosarcomas have *INK4A* homozygous deletion[168,173,174,204] and, in another 5% to 10%, the *INK4A* promoter is methylated. Similarly, by IHC, 16% of osteosar-

comas lack INK4A protein expression.[205] *INK4A* deletions appear to be more common in osteosarcomas grown in cell culture[206] but seem to be less common in osteosarcomas with *Rb* abnormalities, possibly because the two alterations have a similar effect on cell cycle control.[204] Few studies have evaluated the coexistence of *p53* mutations and *INK4A* deletions in osteosarcomas. There is limited evidence that the two abnormalities occur simultaneously.[174] ARF (also known as p19) is an alternatively spliced product of the gene encoding *INK4A*. ARF inhibits MDM2 by direct binding.[207] Thus, loss of ARF leads to increased MDM2-mediated p53 degradation. As a consequence of the gene structure, the 10% to 20% of osteosarcomas with *INK4A* homozygous deletion also lack functional ARF.

RECQ DNA Helicases

As noted earlier, osteosarcoma incidence is increased in three autosomal recessive cancer predisposition syndromes caused by RECQ DNA helicase mutations, Rothmund-Thomson syndrome (RTS), Werner's syndrome, and Bloom syndrome. The overlapping but distinct clinical features and specific nature of osteosarcoma predisposition in these syndromes has already been discussed (see "Cause"). Whereas germline *RECQL4* mutations predispose patients with these syndromes to osteosarcoma, somatic *RECQL4* mutations are not present in sporadic osteosarcomas.[208]

Patients with RTS caused by mutations in *RECQL4*[209] develop osteosarcoma with a prevalence of approximately 30% and probably do not have an increased susceptibility to other types of cancer.[210] Interestingly, osteosarcoma occurs only in the 60% of patients with RTS who have truncating or inactivating *RECQL4* mutations.[35] On the other hand, patients with Bloom and Werner's syndromes, caused by mutations in *RECQL2* and *RECQL3*, respectively,[211,212] are prone to a wide variety of cancers, and osteosarcoma represents less than 10% of the cancers occurring in these patients.[37,38] Why *RECQL4* mutations, in contrast to *RECQL2* and *RECQL3* mutations, specifically increase the risk of osteosarcoma is unknown.

The mechanism whereby loss of function of RECQ DNA helicases results in tumor development generally and in osteosarcoma in particular are not well understood. Proposed RECQ functions that could be related to tumor formation include participation in DNA recombination, maintenance of chromosome stability, recovery from DNA replication collapse, initiation of DNA replication, and telomere processing. The three RECQ DNA helicases mutated in cancer predisposition syndromes have overlapping but not identical functions. In vitro cell culture and mouse models of *RECQL4* mutant RTS display increased chromosomal instability with high rates of aneuploidy.[213] Bloom and Werner's syndrome models have abnormally high rates of homologous recombination events, with accumulation of recombination intermediates.[214] Studies with the *Xenopus RECQL4* homologue have suggested that RECQL4 participates in the initiation of DNA replication.[215] Several lines of evidence have indicated that the RECQ helicases likely play an essential role in reestablishing DNA replication following disruption of the replication fork.[214] Finally, WRN may be involved in telomerase-independent telomere maintenance.[214,216]

Oncogenes

MET

MET, a receptor tyrosine kinase, was first identified and noted to be oncogenic in a transformed human osteosarcoma cell line.

In the 1970s, Rhim and colleagues[217] treated a human osteosarcoma cell line with N-methyl-N′-nitronitrosoguanidine (MNNG), a chemical carcinogen. MNNG treatment resulted in a morphologic change and the acquisition of in vivo tumor-forming capacity. Subsequent studies have shown that the transforming event is formation of a fusion oncogene, TRP-MET, which leads to high levels of MET expression.[218,219]

MET is highly expressed in human osteosarcomas and osteosarcoma cell lines. The exact proportion of osteosarcomas that have high MET expression varies, depending on the detection method used. By Western blotting, 60% to 88% of osteosarcoma tumor specimens and 100% of osteosarcoma cell lines display high levels of MET protein.[220,221] Immunohistochemical analysis yields more variable results, with 35% to 75% of osteosarcomas highly expressing MET.[222,223] The quantitative PCR assay also demonstrates elevated MET expression in all osteosarcoma tumor specimens and cell lines studied.[224] Of note, the benign bone tumors osteoblastoma and nonossifying fibroma do not express MET but chondroblastoma and giant cell tumors do express MET.[220,221,223] When primary and metastatic tumors from the same patient are compared, metastatic tumors have higher MET expression than the primary tumors, suggesting a role for MET in osteosarcoma metastasis.[220,222,225] The mechanism of elevated MET expression in osteosarcoma is not known. When evaluated, MET gene amplification does not appear to be present in osteosarcoma.[220]

Functional studies in cell lines have contributed to the understanding of MET-transforming roles in osteosarcoma. Expression of MET carrying an activating mutation or overexpression of MET by lentiviral transfection transforms normal osteoblasts.[224] Despite a high level of MET expression, MET is not activated in the absence of its ligand, scatter factor (SF), also known as hepatocyte growth factor.[226] An autocrine-paracrine loop may cause MET activation in human osteosarcomas in vivo.[221] Addition of SF to MET-expressing osteosarcoma cell lines results in MET activation, activation of downstream signaling intermediates MAPK and AKT, and increased invasive growth.[226,227] MET-SF interaction in other model systems induces proliferation and enhances motility, cellular changes that frequently precede metastasis.[228]

As reviewed by Trusolino and Comoglio,[228] the MET receptor, its ligand HGF, and the related RON-macrophage–stimulating protein receptor-ligand pair turn on cellular programs that lead to invasive growth. Downstream mediators of MET activity include cadherins, integrins, and metalloproteinases, and the ultimate outcome of MET activation includes loss of cell-cell adhesion, increased cell motility, and extracellular matrix degradation. Physiologic requirements for invasive growth include organogenesis, tissue regeneration, and wound healing. Inappropriate activation in cancer cells leads to tissue invasion and metastasis.

FOS

FOS was initially identified as osteosarcomagenic through investigation of the FBJ murine virus. Mice inoculated with FBJ murine virus develop osteosarcomas that are pathologically similar to human tumors.[229] The viral protein responsible for transformation after infection with FBJ murine virus is v-fos, which, except for the last 49 amino acids, has almost complete homology with the murine c-fos protein.[230] v-fos was presumably derived from a recombination event, including the c-fos gene, between the murine and viral genomes. Transfection of a functional, highly expressed FOS gene transforms fibroblasts.[231]

Further evidence that c-fos overexpression can induce osteosarcomas has been provided by transgenic mouse models.

Transgenic mice in which c-fos is expressed from a major histocompatibility complex (MHC) class I promoter develop osteosarcoma with 100% penetrance.[232] In these mice, c-fos is highly expressed in both osteoblasts and osteosarcomas. Transgenic mice in which the gene is expressed from a different universally expressed promoter, human metallothionein, also develop osteosarcomas but at a much lower frequency,[233] suggesting that there is a dose-response relationship between the extent of FOS overexpression and the development of osteosarcoma.

FOS is overexpressed in human osteosarcoma tumor specimens. By immunohistochemical analysis, 50% to 60% of human osteosarcomas express high levels of FOS protein.[234,235] Only 20% of benign bone tumors have immunohistochemical positivity for FOS and the level of FOS immunohistochemical staining in benign tumors is not as high as in osteosarcomas.[234] When compared with normal tissues and nonosteosarcoma lesions, FOS expression, as assessed by IHC, is 150%.[235] FOS RNA levels are increased in 40% of osteosarcomas.[143] One study has found an association between FOS expression and the occurrence of metastasis or recurrence,[143] but another did not.[234]

Although it is known that FOS, a member of the AP1 transcription factor complex, is an important mediator between extracellular signaling and transcriptional activation in normal bone development, it is not known exactly how FOS overexpression contributes to osteosarcomagenesis. Induction of c-fos expression in osteoblasts alters cyclin levels and increases entry into the S phase.[236] Wagner[237] has noted that AP1 complex activity is regulated by vitamin D, transforming growth factor β, and parathyroid hormone, all of which are important factors influencing bone formation, growth, and healing. In particular, FOS appears to play an essential role in enchondral ossification. FOS null mice have significant osteopetrosis, suggesting that FOS activity is required for normal osteoclast function.[238,239]

Insulin-like Growth Factor

As noted earlier (see "Cause"), there is epidemiologic evidence for a link between normal bone growth and osteosarcoma, including the coincidence of osteosarcoma peak incidence with maximal linear growth in adolescence and the higher rate of osteosarcoma in larger dog breeds.[240] The observed epidemiologic links between osteosarcoma and bone growth could have alternate explanations. Osteosarcoma in large-breed dogs could be caused by the underlying genetics of breed founders rather than by rates of bone growth. Nevertheless, as central mediators of normal linear bone growth and cellular proliferation in general, insulin-like growth factor I (IGF-I) and its receptor, insulin-like growth factor I receptor (IGF-IR), have been investigated in osteosarcoma. In vitro and in vivo data have supported a possible role for IGF-I and IGF-IR in osteosarcoma proliferation and invasion.

IGF-I and IGF-IR are members of the family of insulin-like growth factors and insulin-like growth factor receptors. The other ligands in the IGF-I family are IGF-II and insulin. There are three tyrosine kinase receptors in the family, IGF-IR, IGF-IIR, and the insulin receptor. IGF-IR is the primary target of IGF-I and the most thoroughly studied insulin-like growth factor receptor in osteosarcoma. Other key modulators of IGF-IR activity are the insulin-like growth factor binding proteins (IGFBPs).[241] Growth hormone stimulates production of IGFs in the liver and other target tissues. IGFs, primarily IGF-I, mediate growth hormone–induced postnatal skeletal growth. Dog size is determined by IGF-I haplotype. In the haplotype present in larger dogs, a polymorphism in the IGF-I promoter results in higher IGF-I expression and serum levels.[242] Knockout mice lacking IGF-I or IGF-IR are approximately half the size of normal mice and have delayed formation of their ossification centers.[243] Several humans with intrauterine growth restriction and postnatal short stature were found to have mutations in IGF-IR.[244,245]

Competitive binding assays, affinity labeling experiments, and Northern and Western studies have demonstrated expression of IGF-IR by osteosarcoma cell lines.[246-248] IGF-I expression is variable across osteosarcoma cell lines.[249] Although less thoroughly studied than IGF-I, IGF-II appears to be expressed by osteosarcoma cells.[248,250] There has been limited investigation into IGFBPs in osteosarcoma, but one study has shown that IGFBP3 transcription is augmented in MG-63 osteosarcoma cells in response to IGF-I.[251]

In osteosarcoma cell lines, IGF-IR is not activated in the absence of its ligand.[247] Addition of IGF-I to osteosarcoma cells in culture results in IGF-IR activation,[252] activation of IGF-IR downstream signaling, including Akt and Erk activation,[252] and increased proliferation.[246,249,250] One study has shown that IGF-II is also mitogenic for osteosarcoma cell lines and that this effect is mediated by binding to IGF-IR.[250]

Multiple mechanisms of IGF-IR inhibition in vitro and in vivo suppress osteosarcoma growth and invasion. In a number of different osteosarcoma cell lines, antibodies to IGF-IR decrease osteosarcoma proliferation in a dose-dependent manner.[246,249,250,253] In some cases, antibody treatment causes 100% inhibition of IGF-I induced proliferation. Forced expression of IGFBP5 or IGFBP3 by genetic or chemical mechanisms results in decreased IGF-I expression, increased expression of differentiation markers, and decreased proliferation of osteosarcoma cells.[254,255] In vivo interruption of growth hormone by hypophysectomy or growth hormone–releasing hormone antagonism leads to a dramatic decrease in osteosarcoma xenograft tumor size and metastasis.[248,256]

IGF-I and IGFBP3 levels in patients with osteosarcoma are different than established age- and gender-matched normal values, with 68% of patients having low IGF-I levels. IGF-I and IGFBP3 levels are not correlated with clinical variables such as metastasis and outcome.[257] Phase I studies of octreotide pamoate, a growth hormone antagonist, in patients with osteosarcoma have shown a 50% decrease in serum IGF-I levels. However, there were no clinical responses to octreotide pamoate. There are several possible explanations that could reconcile these clinical findings, with evidence suggesting an important role for the IGF axis in osteosarcoma. The behavior of IGF-I and IGF-IR in osteosarcoma models may not accurately represent osteosarcoma in patients. More likely, IGF-I may act in a paracrine rather than endocrine manner, so that IGF-I serum levels are not representative of the tumor milieu. Alternatively, IGF-IR activation in osteosarcoma in vivo may be mediated by IGF-II or the extent of IGF-IR activation may not be determined by ligand concentration. Finally, osteosarcoma biology is likely to be heterogeneous, with the IGF axis being important in some tumors but not in others. IGF-IR antibodies and kinase inhibitors continue to be developed and are currently being tested in patients with osteosarcoma.

HER2/neu

The *c-erb* B-2 proto-oncogene (*erbB2*) encodes the human epidermal growth factor receptor 2 (HER2), a receptor tyrosine kinase in the epidermal growth factor receptor family. *erbB2* is amplified in 20% of breast cancers[258] and HER2 protein is expressed in a similar proportion of breast cancers.[259] In breast cancer, *erbB2* amplification or HER 2 expression is associated with a poorer prognosis. Trastuzumab, an anti-HER2 therapeutic antibody, improves survival in patients with *erbB2*-amplified tumors.[260]

HER2 protein levels are increased in 40% of osteosarcomas.[126,261,262] As with breast cancer, in osteosarcoma, expression of HER2 is associated with a worse prognosis, but this finding has been refuted by some other studies (see later). Some investigators have found evidence of erbB2 gene amplification in osteosarcoma[262] but others have not.[261,263,264] As discussed later (see "Treatment"), these findings led to a Children's Oncology Group study, AOST 0121, that evaluated the feasibility of adding trastuzumab to multiagent chemotherapy. Eligible patients were those with high-risk metastatic osteosarcoma whose tumors were HER2-positive.

Interestingly, some studies have contradicted the early research on erbB2/HER2 in osteosarcoma.[263,264] In one study, none of 21 pediatric osteosarcomas evaluated expressed HER2. In another study, HER2 expression was detected in 60% of tumors but, in the group of patients evaluated, HER2 expression was associated with an improved rather than worsened outcome.[265] In the recent Children's Oncology Group study, AOST 0121, 30% of the eligible patients had tumors expressing HER2.[266]

Determinants of Metastasis

One of the defining features of osteosarcoma is its tendency to metastasize early—hence, the need for systemic chemotherapy in all patients. Metastasis is a complicated process that involves motility, migration, degradation of extracellular matrix, extravasation, survival during transit through vasculature, invasion, and growth. Given the complicated nature of the process, many factors are likely to play a role in metastases, but it is difficult to decipher the specific contribution of each. Several of the factors that have been more extensively studied in the context of osteosarcoma will be discussed.

Chemokine stromal cell–derived factor 1 (SDF-1) is a cytokine-like protein expressed on the surface of vascular endothelial cells. Through binding to its chemokine receptor, CXCR4, it plays a role in cytoskeleton rearrangement, adhesion to endothelial cells, and chemotaxis.[267,268] Involvement of the CXCR4/SDF-1 pathway has been implicated in the metastatic potential of several cancers, including rhabdomyosarcoma and lymphoma.[269-271] CXCR4 mRNA has been shown to be expressed in osteosarcoma and associated with the presence of metastases at the time of diagnosis.[272,273] In vitro assays have shown that migration of osteosarcoma cells expressing CXCR4 follows an SDF-1 gradient and that their adhesion to endothelial and bone marrow stromal cells is promoted by SDF-1 treatment.[274] This study also provided a rationale for the propensity of osteosarcoma to metastasize to the lung, where SDF-1 concentration is high, and demonstrated prevention of pulmonary metastasis in a murine model by the administration of a CXCR4 inhibitor, suggesting molecular strategies inhibiting this axis as a therapeutic target.[274]

Ezrin is a membrane-cytoskeleton linker protein that allows direct cellular interactions with the microenvironment, facilitating signal transduction through growth factor receptors and adhesion molecules, thereby regulating cell migration and metastasis, among other processes.[125] In an orthotopic model of murine osteosarcoma, ezrin expression was threefold higher in the more aggressive K7M2 cell line, which correlated with its metastatic potential when compared with the less aggressive K12 cell line.[275,276] In follow-up experiments, ezrin expression was found to provide an early survival advantage for pulmonary metastatic osteosarcoma, which is in part mediated by AKT.[125] A significant correlation between high ezrin expression and poor outcome in osteosarcoma has been shown, with shorter DFS and higher risk of metastatic relapse, supporting the animal model data.[125]

Overexpression of the c-met proto-oncogene tyrosine kinase receptor (Met) and its ligand, hepatocyte growth factor (HGF) or scatter factor, in osteosarcoma cell lines suggests a role for the Met in its metastatic phenotype. Binding of HGF or scatter factor to the Met-HGF receptor stimulates both cell proliferation and motility, features associated with metastasis.[220,277] In a study of 17 osteosarcoma tumor samples, 60% expressed the HGF receptor at high levels.[220] When primary and metastatic tumors from the same patient are compared, metastatic tumors have higher Met expression than the primary tumors, indicating its role in potentiating the metastatic phenotype of osteosarcoma.[220-222]

FAS, also known as CD95, is a transmembrane receptor that activates the extrinsic cell death pathway on stimulation by its ligand, FASL (or CD95L). There is increasing evidence in a variety of tumor types that escape from apoptosis may enhance the ability of tumor cells to metastasize.[278] Studies in an osteosarcoma murine xenograft model with a high rate of pulmonary metastasis have suggested that decreased FAS expression enhances osteosarcoma metastasis. Therapies enhancing FAS expression inhibit the development of metastases in this model system. However, evidence that perturbations in FAS are a generalized mechanism of enhanced metastatic potential in osteosarcoma is limited.

The SAOS2 LM6 cell line was produced by serially passaging a human osteosarcoma cell line, SAOS2, through immunodeficient mice until pulmonary metastasis developed reliably and rapidly following tail vein injections. FAS protein and mRNA levels are lower in the SAOS2 LM6 metastasis–producing cell line compared with the seldom metastasizing parental cell line SAOS2.[279] Furthermore, when SAOS2 LM6 FAS expression is increased through transfection, the number and size of pulmonary metastases developing after tail vein injection decrease.[280] FAS expression can also be induced by interleukin-12 (IL-12).[279] Intrapulmonary aerosolized IL-12 gene therapy following SAOS2 LM6 tail vein injection increases FAS expression in metastatic tumors and inhibits the development of pulmonary metastases.[281-284] Interestingly, ifosfamide and IL-12 display a synergistic relationship when used together in this model system, possibly because of ifosfamide-induced expression of FASL.[281]

FAS expression has been evaluated in human osteosarcoma pulmonary metastases from 28 patients. FAS was not expressed in 60% of the tumors and the remaining 40% had only weak FAS expression.[285] Further study is needed to confirm that decreased FAS expression contributes to the metastatic potential of osteosarcoma occurring in humans and in osteosarcoma models other than the SAOS2 LM6 model.

Other factors that likely play a role in osteosarcoma metastases include expression of matrix metalloproteinases[286] and other degradative enzymes. The expression of these enzymes is necessary to degrade the extracellular matrix, permitting extravasation into the vasculature.

Biologic Markers of Response to Chemotherapy

Osteosarcoma's response to chemotherapy is evident in the change in patient survival resulting from its administration. Defining response is somewhat more difficult. Chemotherapy response in osteosarcoma is typically used to refer to the degree of necrosis in the definitive surgical resection specimen. The degree of necrosis seen in that specimen is a consistent predictor of patient survival across studies, as described elsewhere in this chapter. In the original description of the grading system,

a grade I response was considered indicative of no histologically visible response to chemotherapy. Subsequently, this was specified as being less than 50% necrosis, because untreated osteosarcomas could have as much as 25% spontaneous necrosis. It was therefore thought that necrosis more than double this amount would be attributable to a chemotherapy effect. Numerous biologic studies have been performed correlating a particular marker with the necrosis grading. In some of these studies, the necrosis grading was used as a surrogate for event-free survival, with the anticipation that these will correlate. The advantage of necrosis grading in this context is that the data are available much sooner than mature EFS data. In other contexts, the necrosis grading is used as a marker of chemotherapy response. Complicating these analyses, the standard of care in osteosarcoma is multiagent chemotherapy. Factors that only affect responsiveness to a single agent may not be predictive in the context of multiagent chemotherapy. Given these limitations, relating a genetic alteration to necrosis grading may provide a more robust relationship with chemotherapy response than survival, because survival may be influenced by many factors other than chemotherapy response. Similarly, necrosis grading may be a better marker of response than radiographic response in osteosarcoma, because the mineralized matrix of an osteosarcoma prevents radiographically visible shrinkage of the tumor.

Because chemotherapy has had a dramatic effect on the outcome of osteosarcoma, it is perhaps intuitive to assume that genetic alterations that produce drug resistance would be associated with inferior chemotherapy response and patient survival. Along these lines, perhaps the most extensively studied prognostic marker is the expression of P-glycoprotein (PGP). This is a transmembrane ATP-dependent efflux pump protein encoded by the multidrug resistance (MDR1) gene, which is responsible for the efflux of numerous chemotherapeutic agents from the malignant cell. In the context of osteosarcoma, the most important drug that can be effluxed by PGP is doxorubicin, although etoposide is also a substrate. Immunohistochemistry and reverse transcriptase (RT)–PCR quantification studies have explored PGP and MDR1 expression in osteosarcoma and demonstrated overexpression of PGP in 23% to 45% of tumors, with decreased survival reported for patients with PGP-positive tumors[287-292] in initial studies. Of interest, although many of these studies demonstrated a correlation with outcome, several key studies did not demonstrate a relationship with the necrosis grade. This suggests that use of necrosis grading as an early marker of outcome may not always be appropriate in the context of some biologic markers. A meta-analysis has proposed that PGP is associated with an increased risk of disease progression.[293] Although the early literature suggested that PGP may be a marker of drug resistance and aggressiveness in osteosarcoma, this finding has not been verified consistently across studies.[287-290,292] In addition, a prospective clinicopathologic cooperative group study has concluded that there is no correlation between PGP expression and percentage of osteosarcoma tumor necrosis after induction chemotherapy or event-free survival in localized osteosarcoma.[294] Overexpression of MDR1 has also been explored with regard to its prognostic relevance. Although a small pilot study has shown a trend toward a worse outcome in patients exhibiting high levels of MDR1 expression,[295] a larger prospective investigation did not identify a correlation between MDR1 mRNA expression and prognosis in osteosarcoma patients with patients with either very low or very high levels of MDR1 having a relatively poor outcome.[296]

High-dose methotrexate (MTX) with leucovorin rescue is a major component of current protocols for the treatment of osteosarcoma.[101,297] High-dose MTX is vastly more effective than conventional dose methotrexate in the treatment of osteosarcoma, a finding that is not observed in other malignancies treated with MTX, implying a mechanism of intrinsic MTX resistance within osteosarcoma tumor cells.[298] In experimental systems, resistance to methotrexate can occur through a variety of mechanisms, including impaired intracellular transport of the drug via the reduced folate carrier, upregulation of dihydrofolate reductase, and diminished intracellular retention caused by decreased polyglutamylation. Studies have demonstrated that impairment of drug influx as a result of decreased expression and mutations in the reduced folate carrier gene is the major basis of intrinsic resistance; 65% of osteosarcoma tumor samples were found to have decreased reduced folate carrier expression at the time of initial biopsy.[298] In contrast, dihydrofolate reductase overexpression was seen relatively infrequently at initial biopsy, in only 10% of tumor samples, compared with 62% of the tumors examined at the time of definitive surgery or relapse, suggesting dihydrofolate reductase overexpression as the major mechanism of acquired MTX resistance in osteosarcoma.[298]

Other potential mechanisms of drug resistance include alterations in multidrug resistance protein expression, topoisomerase II, glutathione *S*-transferases, DNA repair, DNA damage response, drug metabolism or inactivation, and reduced intracellular delivery. Few studies have been performed in osteosarcoma to indicate whether these processes play a role in defining chemotherapy response.

In other studies, necrosis following chemotherapy has been used as a marker of response, and investigators have attempted to identify genetic signatures predictive of response. In each of these studies, a large number of genes were required to define a profile of response. The studies reported using 60 genes,[299] 104 genes,[300] and 45 genes[301] to distinguish between responders and nonresponders. This may be related to the small sample sizes used in each of these studies. Alternatively, the lack of robust clustering may be caused by the heterogeneity of osteosarcoma itself. Lack of robust clustering on gene expression profiling appears to be a property of nontranslocation–associated sarcomas, a result of their high levels of genetic complexity.

TREATMENT

Local Control

Definitive surgical treatment of osteosarcoma, as discussed more extensively in Chapter 9, has two components, tumor resection and reconstruction. Tumor resection is essential for cure of osteosarcoma. Ten-year survival in patients with macroscopic residual tumor is less than 15%, even with multiagent chemotherapy.[47,302] Tissue margins on the resection specimen should be wide. Although the exact tissue margin required is not known, wide margins are generally defined as 2 to 5 mm for soft tissue and 2 to 3 cm for bone marrow. Marginal and intralesional margins are associated with a poor outcome and an increased risk of local recurrence.[48,303] As noted earlier (see "Natural History and Prognosis"), an additional factor increasing the risk of local recurrence and poor outcome is a poor histologic response to chemotherapy. In one study, inadequate margins and a poor histologic response to therapy were independent predictors of local recurrence.[304] In this study, having both a poor histologic response to therapy and inadequate margins dramatically increased the risk of local recurrence.[304]

Options for limb reconstruction include limb-sparing techniques that use allografts or fixed or expandable endoprostheses. Currently, 75% to 80% of patients with nonaxial tumors are treated with limb-sparing surgery.[101,106] As long as the resection margins are adequate, limb-sparing techniques do not change event-free or overall survival.[110,120] Because of the significant cosmetic impact, amputation and rotationplasty are often reserved for those patients whose tumors are not amenable to limb-sparing techniques. Occasionally, however, patients will opt for amputation or rotationplasty because of their advantages, which include a lower incidence of repeated surgical revisions and a greater ability to participate in high-impact activities.[305] Benefits of endoprostheses over allografts include a shorter postoperative recovery time and a lower incidence of perioperative complications. Allografts have the important advantage of allowing preservation of the growth plate. The relative strengths and weaknesses of the various surgical options are discussed further (see later, "Complications of Therapy") and in Chapter 9.

The optimal surgical approach should be determined by a multidisciplinary team that includes a radiologist, oncologist, and orthopedic surgeon with experience in the treatment of bone tumors. Adequate imaging, usually an MRI, is required to determine which surgical procedures will produce sufficient margins. Finally, a good understanding of the patient's and family's priorities is needed to provide appropriate counseling.

Chemotherapy for Localized Disease

The use of neoadjuvant and adjuvant chemotherapy has increased the overall survival of patients with localized high-grade osteosarcoma from 20% to 70% to 75%. The most active chemotherapeutic agents for localized osteosarcoma are HDMTX with leucovorin rescue, doxorubicin (Doxo), and cisplatin (CP). In addition, ifosfamide and etoposide have demonstrated efficacy in metastatic osteosarcoma. Institutional and cooperative group studies have attempted to identify the optimal combination of active agents, the most effective drug dosing, and the impact of dose intensity and schedule on outcome and toxicity (Tables 22-5 and 22-6). Much has been learned from these studies. However, important questions remain, including the ability to improve high-risk disease outcomes through chemotherapy intensification, the role of immune modulators in osteosarcoma therapy, and whether there is additional benefit of adding ifosfamide and etoposide to first-line therapy of localized disease.

Chemotherapy and Outcome

It has not always been clear that chemotherapy is effective in osteosarcoma. Successful treatment of osteosarcoma with chemotherapy was first reported in the literature in the early 1970s. Jaffe and colleagues[100] treated 20 patients with adjuvant HDMTX and vincristine (VCR). They noted one death in 20 patients compared with 14 expected deaths, based on historical controls. In 12 patients with completely resected primary tumors, there was one death, six fewer than predicted by historic controls.[100] Cortes and colleagues[306] saw similar dramatic improvements in overall survival (OAS) and EFS in 21 patients treated with surgery and Doxo. The Memorial Sloan-Kettering Cancer Center (MSKCC) has reported an OAS of 75% with neoadjuvant HDMTX containing multiagent chemotherapy.[114] Other groups reported improved survival compared with historic controls with adjuvant CP and Doxo[307] or adjuvant multiagent chemotherapy containing Doxo.[308] However, in other studies, chemotherapy did not appear to improve outcome. Lange and colleagues[309] treated 20 patients with completely resected nonmetastatic osteosarcoma with HDMTX, VCR, and Doxo and observed an OAS of only 26%, a rate similar to that of untreated historical controls.

TABLE 22-5 Randomized Controlled Trials of Chemotherapy for Nonmetastatic Osteosarcoma

Group	Year	Regimen(s)	No. of Patients	EFS (%)	Primary Objective(s)	Results and Conclusions
ADJUVANT CHEMOTHERAPY/XRT						
Mayo[122]	1984	HDMTX + VCR vs. observation	38	42	Demonstrate superior outcome with adjuvant chemotherapy.	1. EFS and OAS equivalent in chemo and observation arms. 2. EFS and OAS in observation arm better than historical controls. 3. Power inadequate to detect a difference. 4. Natural history may be improving.
POG[312]	1986	HDMTX + Doxo + BCD vs. observation	36	66 / 17	Demonstrate superior outcome with adjuvant chemotherapy.	1. Adjuvant chemotherapy improves outcome. 2. Natural history is not improving.
UCLA[313]	1987	HDMTX + VCR + Doxo + BCD vs. observation	59	55 / 20	Demonstrate superior outcome with adjuvant chemotherapy.	1. Adjuvant chemotherapy improves outcome. 2. Natural history is not improving.
CCG[118]	1987	HDMTX + VCR + Doxo vs. MDMTX + VCR + Doxo	166	38	Compare efficacy of HDMTX and MDMTX.	1. EFS equivalent in both arms.
EORTC-SIOP[368]	1988	HDMTX + Doxo + CTX vs. pulmonary XRT vs. HDMTX + Doxo + CTX + pulmonary XRT	205	40	Compare efficacy of adjuvant chemotherapy vs. adjuvant pulmonary XRT.	1. EFS and OAS equivalent in all arms. 2. Pulmonary XRT less toxic than chemotherapy.
NEOADJUVANT (NEOADJ.) CHEMOTHERAPY						
MSKCC (T10)[326]	1982	Neoadj.—HDMTX + BCD + Doxo; Good response—continue same; Poor response—HDMTX + CP; All groups—±VCR	57	93 / 96 / 91	Evaluate the effect of VCR on EFS.	1. Improved EFS compared with historical controls. 2. VCR has no impact on EFS.
COSS[115]	1984	Neoadj.—HDMTX + Doxo + BCD ± IFN vs. CP ± IFN-α	158	68	Compare efficacy of CP and BCD and evaluate IFN-α.	1. EFS equivalent in all arms.
COSS[116]	1988	Neoadj.—MTX + Doxo + CP; Good response—continue same; Poor response—ifosfamide + CP + BCD vs. Neoadj.—MTX + BCD; Good response—continue same; Poor response—Doxo + CP	141	58 / 49	Improve survival or decrease toxicity by altering chemotherapy intensity based on tumor response.	1. Lower intensity therapy results in a reduced EFS. 2. Higher intensity therapy for poor responders does not result in an increased EFS (compared with historical controls).
Rizzoli[109]	1990	Neoadj.—MTX + CP; Good response—continue same; Fair response—add Doxo; Poor response—add Doxo + BCD; All groups—HDMTX, 7500 mg/m² vs. MDMTX, 750 mg/m²	127	58 / 42	Compare efficacy of HDMTX and MDMTX.	1. EFS worse in patients receiving MDMTX, although result is not statistically significant. 2. Lower intensity therapy for good responders results in a reduced OAS.

Study	Year	Regimen	No.		Objective	Conclusions
EOI[117]	1992	HDMTX + Doxo + CP vs. Doxo + CP	198	41 / 57	Compare efficacy of multiagent regimen and two-agent regimen.	1. Two-drug regimen as efficacious as multiagent regimen.
EOI[333]	1997	HDMTX +VCR + BCD + Doxo + CP vs. Doxo + CP	407	44	Compare efficacy of multiagent, prolonged (44-wk) regimen and two-agent shorter (18-wk) regimen.	1. EFS and OAS equivalent in both arms. 2. Compliance better in shorter two-agent regimen.
MSKCC[103] (T12)	1998	Neoadj:—HDMTX + BCD Poor response—add Doxo + CP Good response— add Doxo vs. Neoadj:—HDMTX + BCD + Doxo + CP Poor or good response—continue	73	73 / 78	Improve outcome by intensifying preoperative chemotherapy.	1. Preoperative chemotherapy intensification increases percentage of good responders. 2. EFS is equivalent in both arms. 3. Intensifying preoperative chemotherapy does not increase DFS.
POG[102]	2003	Neoadj:—None Adj.— HDMTX + BCD + Doxo + CP vs. Neoadj:—HDMTX + Doxo + CP Adj.—+ BCD	106	65	Compare outcomes of patients treated with or without neoadjuvant chemotherapy.	1. Neoadjuvant chemotherapy does not improve or worsen EFS. 2. Limb salvage rates are similar in both arms.
COG[5,101]	2005	HDMTX + Doxo + CP ± MT-PPE ± ifosfamide	667	63	Improve outcome by intensifying chemotherapy with ifosfamide, MTP-PE, or both.	1. OAS and EFS were not statistically different between arms on initial analysis. 2. On follow-up analysis, OAS is slightly better in patients receiving MTP-PE.
EOI[334]	2007	Doxo + CP q3-wk cycles vs. Doxo + CP q2-wk cycles (with GCSF)	497	39 / 41	Improve survival by increasing dose intensity.	1. EFS and OAS equivalent in both arms. 2. Toxicity equivalent in both arms. 3. Outcome with two-agent shorter regimen (this study) significantly worse than with multiagent prolonged regimen (other studies).

Adj., adjuvant; BCD, bleomycin, cyclophosphamide, and dactinomycin; CP, cisplatin; DFS, disease-free survival; Doxo, doxorubicin; EFS, event-free survival; GCSF, granulocyte colony-stimulating factor; HDMTX, high-dose methotrexate; IFN-α, interferon-α; MDMTX, moderate-dose methotrexate; MTP-PE, muramyl tripeptide phosphatidylethanolamine; OAS, overall survival; VCR, vincristine; XRT, x-ray therapy.

TABLE 22-6   **Nonrandomized Uncontrolled Trials of Chemotherapy in Nonmetastatic Osteosarcoma**

Group	Date	Regimen(s)	No. of Patients	EFS (%)
CHOP[309]	1982	HDMTX + VCR + Doxo	20	26
CCG[120]	1997	Neoadjuvant—HDMTX + VCR + BCD +	268	53
		Good responders—Doxo		81
		Poor responders—Doxo + CP		46
COSS[121]	1998	Low risk—HDMTX + Doxo + CP	171	66
		High risk—HDMTX + Doxo + CP + I		
Rizzoli[106]	2000	Neoadj.—HDMTX + Doxo + CP	164	61
		Good response—continue same		
		Poor response—add IE		
St. Jude[321]	2001	HDMTX + Doxo + I	69	72
SSG[320]	2003	Neoadj.— HDMTX + Doxo + CP	113	63
		Good response—continue same		
		Poor response—add IE		
ISG-SSG[104]	2005	HDMTX + Doxo + CP + I	182	64

BCD, bleomycin, cyclophosphamide, and dactinomycin; CP, cisplatin; Doxo, doxorubicin; EFS, event-free survival; HDMTX, high-dose methotrexate; I, ifosfamide; IE, ifosfamide and etoposide; VCR, vincristine.

Randomized controlled trials comparing chemotherapy and observation have been conducted for several reasons, despite the positive results of some early chemotherapy studies. First, the improved outcome observed with chemotherapy could have been caused by an improved outcome for all patients unrelated to chemotherapy. Advances in diagnosis and surgical approach could have improved outcome, irrespective of other therapies provided. Results of a randomized controlled trial at the Mayo Clinic[122,310] in which the EFS was 42% in both treated and untreated patients, supported this theory. Second, because of the lack of a control group, the favorable results of these early chemotherapy trials could have been caused by patient selection.[311]

Two randomized controlled trials published in the mid-1980s confirmed the effectiveness of chemotherapy and an unchanged osteosarcoma natural history. In a multi-institutional study, 36 patients with nonmetastatic fully resected osteosarcoma were randomized to observation or treatment with HDMTX, Doxo, and bleomycin, cyclophosphamide, and dactinomycin (BCD).[312] The EFS was 66% in the group treated with chemotherapy but only 17% in the observed patients. Investigators at UCLA randomized 59 patients to a similar chemotherapy regimen or observation and obtained almost identical results.[313] Of treated patients, 55% were disease-free at 2 years whereas only 20% of observed patients remained disease-free.

Chemotherapeutic Agents

Cisplatin

In addition to the initially identified agents, HDMTX and Doxo, CP was identified as an active antiosteosarcoma drug in the late 1970s[314] and was rapidly incorporated into multiagent protocols. Adjuvant CP, in combination with Doxo, results in disease-free survival rates at least as high as those seen with adjuvant HDMTX and Doxo.[307] In the past, it was theorized that intra-arterial administration of cisplatin directly to the primary tumor might improve local control and survival. However, several randomized trials have failed to show survival gains from the intra-arterial administration route,[121,315] despite an increased proportion of tumors with a good histologic response in some studies. Thus, it is now generally accepted that intra-arterial administration of cisplatin is not of sufficient benefit to be worth the increased risk and inconvenience,

although countervailing opinions remain.[316] Carboplatin, which has successfully replaced cisplatin in some other cancers, has limited efficacy in osteosarcoma. In a Pediatric Oncology Group study, presurgical carboplatin produced pathologic tumor responses in only 1 of 37 chemotherapy-naive patients with metastatic osteosarcoma.[317]

A recently published trial conducted by the Société Française d'Oncologie Pédiatrique[318] has underscored the importance of cisplatin in osteosarcoma therapy. This study had two arms, with different preoperative chemotherapy regimens. In one arm, preoperative chemotherapy was HDMTX and Doxo, and patients in the other arm received HDMTX and ifosfamide and etoposide (IE). Patients with a poor histologic response to preoperative chemotherapy in the HDMTX-IE arm received postoperative CP-Doxo and had an EFS of 60%, whereas patients with a poor histologic response in the HDMTX-Doxo arm received postoperative IE without CP and had an EFS of 49%.

Ifosfamide and Etoposide

Following demonstration of antiosteosarcoma activity in unresectable or metastatic disease,[319] ifosfamide was incorporated into multiagent treatment protocols for localized disease with the goal of improving outcome[104,106,121,320] or minimizing toxicity.[321] In two separate nonrandomized studies, one conducted at the Rizzoli Institute (Italy) and one by the Scandinavian Sarcoma Group (SSG), patients with a poor histologic response were treated with the combination of ifosfamide and etoposide. In both studies, outcome was improved in patients with a poor response when compared with historical controls.[106,320] However, in a follow-up joint study by the SSG and the Italian Sarcoma Group (ISG), ifosfamide was given to all patients regardless of tumor response and outcome was similar to that of historical controls.[104] Because none of these trials was randomized, a definitive conclusion regarding the additional benefit gained by adding IE to first-line therapy of localized disease is not possible. In a randomized controlled Children's Oncology Group trial, the addition of ifosfamide to Doxo, CP, and HDMTX for patients with localized osteosarcoma did not increase survival.[101] Of note, in this trial, patients were treated with ifosfamide not in combination with etoposide, and ifosfamide was administered in a relatively low dosage (9 g/m²/course). An international, multigroup study, EURAMOS, is examining the efficacy of the addition of postoperative IE for improving EFS in patients whose tumors have a poor histologic response to chemotherapy.

Methotrexate

In early protocols, MTX was administered at dosages between 3 and 7.5 g/m^2.[100,114,119] However, methotrexate pharmacokinetics in children result in lower peak MTX levels for a given dosage/kg of body weight partly because of faster renal clearance.[322] Since this information became known, most regimens have used a MTX dosage of 12 g/m^2.[101,102] Several retrospective studies have shown a correlation between higher peak methotrexate levels (700 to 1000 μmol/L) and tumor necrosis[74] and disease-free survival.[323] At a methotrexate dosage of 12 g/m^2, more than 90% of patients achieve peak methotrexate levels above 1000 μmol/L.[323,324] However, the only study directly comparing 7.5 g/m^2 and 12 g/m^2 did not demonstrate improved survival with the higher dosage.[325] Moderate MTX dosages (600 to 750 mg/m^2) do not seem to be as effective as high MTX dosages.[109,118] Alkaline intravenous fluids and leucovorin are administered with HDMTX, and MTX levels should be monitored after MTX administration.

Vincristine

VCR was used in combination with MTX in the initial chemotherapy study by Jaffe and colleagues[100] because of preclinical data suggesting that VCR potentiated cellular MTX uptake. It is no longer used because a randomized controlled trial has shown no effect on EFS compared with MTX alone.[326]

Bleomycin, Cyclophosphamide, and Dactinomycin

The combination of bleomycin, cyclophosphamide, and dactinomycin (BCD) was initially used by investigators at MSKCC[114] in combination with other active agents. BCD was included in a number of other treatment regimens in a nonrandomized fashion. However, in a direct comparison of BCD and CP in combination with HDMTX, VCR, and Doxo conducted by the Cooperative Osteosarcoma Study Group (COSS), BCD was equivalent to CP.[115] In addition, BCD does not cause tumor regression in patients with previously treated metastatic disease.[327] Because of the equivalency with CP, lack of demonstrated efficacy in metastatic disease and potential pulmonary toxicity, BCD is no longer included in most osteosarcoma chemotherapy regimens.

Immune Modulators

In vitro, interferon-α (IFN-α) decreases the proliferation of osteosarcoma cell lines.[328] In vivo, growth of mouse osteosarcoma xenografts is inhibited by IFN-α.[329] Based on these preclinical data, investigators at the Karolinska Institute in Sweden gave IFN-α monotherapy to patients with localized fully resected osteosarcoma. The EFS was 53%.[330] Because of the impressive EFS in this study, further evaluation of IFN-α in combination with multiagent chemotherapy is ongoing in the international multigroup European and American Osteosarcoma Study Group EURAMOS 1 study.

Another immunomodulatory therapy that might have activity in osteosarcoma is muramyl tripeptide phosphatidylethanolamine (MTP-PE). MTP-PE is a liposomal encapsulated bacille Calmette-Guérin (BCG) cell wall component. It activates macrophages and, in mouse xenografts, induces tumoricidal activity.[331] Adjuvant treatment of osteosarcoma in dogs with MTP-PE alone led to a significantly increased DFS.[332] The addition of MTP-PE to HDMTX, Doxo, and CP was evaluated in a Children's Oncology Group (COG) randomized controlled trial.[101] In the initial analysis of this study, neither event-free nor overall survival were statistically significantly improved in patients treated with the addition of MTP-PE or MTP-PE and ifosfamide to standard three-drug HDMTX, CP, and Doxo when compared with those treated with the three-drug combination of HDMTX, CP, and Doxo alone. Interpretation of the study results remains controversial, especially in light of a recently published follow-up analysis of the study data. In this analysis, the addition of MTP-PE to the standard three-drug regimen of HDMTX, CP, and Doxo significantly improved 6-year overall survival from 70% to 78% but did not significantly improve event-free survival.[5] At present, the U.S. Food and Drug Administration (FDA) application for approval of MTP-PE is pending and MTP-PE is therefore not currently available.

Neoadjuvant Chemotherapy

Neoadjuvant chemotherapy is an approach in which some of the chemotherapy cycles are given prior to tumor resection and the remaining cycles are given postoperatively. Neoadjuvant chemotherapy in osteosarcoma has several potential benefits.[114] Theoretically, neoadjuvant chemotherapy could increase disease-free and overall survival through earlier treatment of microscopic metastatic foci.[114] From a practical perspective, neoadjuvant chemotherapy provides sufficient time for custom endoprosthesis preparation and other surgical planning. In addition, if sufficient tumor shrinkage occurs, neoadjuvant chemotherapy could make a patient who would have required amputation eligible for limb-sparing surgery. Postoperative healing could also be improved by neoadjuvant chemotherapy because there is less urgency to resume chemotherapy.

Theoretically, the greatest benefit of neoadjuvant chemotherapy is that it permits evaluation of tumor response to chemotherapy, the only clear predictor of outcome in osteosarcoma. Identifying patients with a poorer prognosis combined with subsequent therapeutic interventions could improve outcome. However, at present, there are no known therapeutic interventions that improve outcomes for patients with a poorer prognosis based on histologic response to chemotherapy. If therapeutic interventions that improve outcomes in patients with a poor tumor response to chemotherapy are not identified, the value of neoadjuvant chemotherapy will be diminished.

Neoadjuvant chemotherapy was initially used in MSKCC protocols.[114,326] OAS in patients treated with the MSKCC neoadjuvant protocols was 75% to 93%. Because an OAS of 93% was significantly better than outcomes reported with adjuvant chemotherapy, there was initial excitement that neoadjuvant therapy would improve survival. However, a COSS protocol using the neoadjuvant approach, COSS-80, had an EFS of 68%, similar to EFS in ongoing studies of adjuvant chemotherapy.[115] Nevertheless, essentially all protocols after 1980 included, in a nonrandomized fashion, neoadjuvant chemotherapy. In general, EFS in these neoadjuvant protocols was similar to EFS seen in protocols giving only adjuvant therapy.

In the only randomized controlled trial comparing adjuvant and neoadjuvant chemotherapy,[102] OAS and EFS were not significantly different for patients receiving adjuvant or neoadjuvant chemotherapy. Other than allowing the identification of a group of patients with a poorer prognosis, there did not appear to be significant additional benefits to neoadjuvant chemotherapy. The number of limb salvage procedures was the same in the adjuvant and neoadjuvant groups. Surgical complications were not reduced by neoadjuvant chemotherapy. Several patients had progression of the primary tumor during neoadjuvant chemotherapy, and a few of these patients developed pulmonary metastasis. Thus, patients with clearly documented tumor progression during neoadjuvant chemotherapy should proceed to resection without completing the planned course of neoadjuvant therapy. This is especially true in the case of proximal tumors at risk of becoming inoperable—for example, a proximal humeral lesion crossing the shoulder joint. On the other hand, chemotherapy-induced swelling of the tumor can sometimes be difficult to distinguish from progressive disease.

Response-Based Therapy

Multiple protocols have attempted to improve outcome in patients with a poorer prognosis by intensifying chemotherapy for this group of patients. In general, poor histologic tumor response after neoadjuvant chemotherapy has been used to stratify patients into an intensified treatment arm. Treatment intensification has generally been through the addition of one or two agents in the adjuvant phase not given during the neoadjuvant phase. For example, in CCG, Rizzoli Institute and COSS protocols using neoadjuvant therapy consisting of HDMTX and BCD adjuvant treatment was intensified by adding CP and Doxo.[109,116,120] Similarly, in the MSKCC T10 protocol, CP was administered to intensify therapy after neoadjuvant treatment with HDMTX, BCD, and Doxo.[326] With the exception of the T10 protocol, patients in the poor responder group had a similar outcome to historical controls (who did not get intensified chemotherapy), despite chemotherapy intensification.

In protocols in which both Doxo and CP are given neoadjuvantly, ifosfamide with or without etoposide has been used to intensify adjuvant chemotherapy for patients with a poor histologic response.[104,106,116,320] In the SSG protocol SSGVIII[320] and a recent Rizzoli protocol,[106] HDMTX, Doxo, and CP were given neoadjuvantly and IE was given adjuvantly to poor responders. In the Rizzoli trial, patients did not have a better outcome than historical controls (who did not receive IE intensification), whereas in the SSGVIII trial, outcome was better than historical controls, with an OAS of 70% in patients with a poor histologic response.

In a different approach to chemotherapy intensification, COSS divided patients into high-risk and low-risk groups based on tumor size, pathologic subtype, and clinical response to neoadjuvant chemotherapy, measured by bone scan. Patients in the high-risk group were treated with additional ifosfamide, added to the HDMTX, Doxo, and CP backbone. High-risk patients achieved the same outcome as low-risk patients. These results can be interpreted either as an indication than ifosfamide is effective at improving survival in high-risk patients or as indicating that the factors used to define the high-risk group do not actually convey a worse prognosis.[121] In summary, there is no convincing evidence that intensifying adjuvant chemotherapy for patients whose tumors have a poor histologic response results in an improved outcome. The lack of randomized studies addressing this question prevents a definitive conclusion about the usefulness of this approach.

On the other hand, there is fairly clear evidence that attempting to decrease toxicity for low-risk patients whose tumors have a good chemotherapy response by deintensifying chemotherapy results in a worse prognosis.[109,116] In one arm of COSS-82, neoadjuvant chemotherapy consisted of HDMTX and BCD and, during adjuvant therapy, a lower dose of Doxo (30 mg/m^2 × 2 days) was given than had been used in previous protocols. EFS was 41% in this arm, which was significantly less than in both the other study arms and in historical controls. In a trial at the Rizzoli Institute, after neoadjuvant therapy with HDMTX and CP, patients with a good response received only further HDMTX and CP. These patients had an EFS of only 27%.

The conclusion of a series of studies by the European Osteosarcoma Intergroup (EOI)[117,333,334] is that a two-drug

regimen of Doxo and CP is inferior to regimens that include three or more drugs. In the first and second randomized studies, outcomes in patients treated with CP and Doxo and those treated with regimens containing at least the three drugs were equivalent.[117] However, in these two studies and a third study, in which all patients were treated with Doxo and CP, EFS was approximately 40%, a lower rate than is seen in studies of multidrug regimens conducted by other groups.

Non–Risk-Based Chemotherapy Intensification

There are gains to be made in outcome for all osteosarcoma patients, not just those with high-risk disease. With this in mind, some groups have evaluated the impact of intensifying chemotherapy for all patients. The MSKCC T12 trial randomized patients to a more or less intensive neoadjuvant chemotherapy regimen. Patients randomized to the more intensive arm received HDMTX, BCD, Doxo, and CP neoadjuvantly and adjuvantly, whereas patients randomized to the less intensive arm received HDMTX and BCD neoadjuvantly, with adjuvant therapy based on tumor response. Doxo was continued for patients with a good response, with Doxo and CP used for poor responders. EFS was 73% for patients in the less intensive arm and 78% for those in the more intensive arm,[101] a difference that is neither clinically nor statistically significant.

The COG conducted a randomized trial to evaluate the impact of adding adjuvant ifosfamide and/or MTP-PE to a backbone of HDMTX, Doxo, and CP. As noted earlier, in the initial analysis of this trial, neither the addition of ifosfamide nor the addition of MTP-PE significantly improved survival.[101] However, in a follow-up analysis, MTP-PE was shown to improve 6-year overall survival significantly, by a small margin.[5] As noted, interpretation of these data remains uncertain. As with chemotherapy intensification for poor responders, randomized controlled trials are needed to determine whether additional benefit can be gained from adding ifosfamide, etoposide, or other active agents such as immunomodulators to the core antiosteosarcoma agents HDMTX, Doxo, and CP.

Dose Density

The most recent EOI study has evaluated the impact on toxicity and survival of shortening the interval between CP and Doxo courses from 3 to 2 weeks. In this randomized trial, patients on the every 2-week arm were supported with granulocyte colony-stimulating factor (GCSF) between chemotherapy cycles. The EOI found that the shortened interval dosing was equivalent in both toxicity and outcome to the longer interval dosing.[334]

Current Approach to Therapy

Most of the osteosarcoma research groups, COG, SSG, COSS, and the EOI, have collaborated on an international trial, EURAMOS 1. The chemotherapy backbone administered to all patients in the trial is neoadjuvant and adjuvant HDMTX, Doxo, and CP (Table 22-7). The objectives of this randomized trial are the following: (1) to determine whether the postoperative addition of IE improves EFS of patients with a poor response to neoadjuvant chemotherapy; and (2) to evaluate whether the postoperative addition of IFN-α following neoadjuvant chemotherapy improves outcome in patients with a good histologic response. All patients will receive a total of 10 weeks of neoadjuvant chemotherapy with HDMTX (four cycles), and Doxo and CP (two cycles). Patients with a poor response will be randomized to continue HDMTX, Doxo, and CP or to continue HDMTX, Doxo, and CP with the addition of IE. Patients with a good response will be randomized to continue

TABLE 22-7	Clinical Pearls: Schema of Typical Administration Schedules for Doxorubicin (A), Cisplatin (P), and High-Dose Methotrexate (M) Therapy of Osteosarcoma																	
Week*	1	4	5	6	9	10	11	12†	15	16	17	20	21	22	24	25	26	28	29
Chemo	A, P	M	M	A, P	M	M	Surgery	A, P	M	M	A, P	M	M	A	M	M	A	M	M

*Weeks 2, 3, 7, 8, 13, 14, 18, 19, 23, and 27 had no therapy scheduled.
†Week 12 chemotherapy is administered after adequate postoperative healing has occurred.

HDMTX, Doxo, and CP or to continue HDMTX, Doxo, and CP, with the addition of IFN-α. Results of this study, which might be available in 2012, will hopefully resolve several major questions about osteosarcoma therapy.

Treatment of Initially Metastatic Osteosarcoma

As noted earlier (see "Natural History and Prognosis"), the presence of metastatic disease at the time of initial diagnosis is the most unfavorable prognostic feature. Ten percent to 20% of patients have detectable metastases at the time of initial diagnosis. The largest study, a retrospective review of patients enrolled in COSS studies, has identified 202 patients with initially metastatic disease from a population of 1702 newly diagnosed patients.[4] The lung was involved in 164 patients (81%); in 124 patients, it was the only site of metastatic disease. Bones were the second most frequent site of metastasis, in 69 patients (34%), with lung and bone both involved in 28 patients. Seven others had lung, bone, or other sites of disease as well. Patients with multiple metastatic lesions had a more unfavorable outcome than those with solitary metastatic lesions. Importantly, those who did not achieve complete surgical remission had a significantly worse outcome than those who obtained complete surgical remission. Patients whose tumor showed a favorable histologic response to chemotherapy were more likely to achieve complete surgical remission (75% vs. 58%) and a more favorable outcome (51% vs. 24% overall survival at 5 years). Only a few patients (15) had isolated skip lesions. They had a relatively favorable outlook, a 5-year event-free survival of 47% ± 13%. This contrasts with the poor outcome of patients with other bone metastases, two thirds of whom had multiple sites of disease; 85% of these patients died at a median of 1 year from diagnosis.

In view of the unfavorable outlook of these patients, strategies that included higher toxicity regimens have been used in an effort to improve patient outcome. The Pediatric Oncology Group[317] administered carboplatin, 1 g/m^2 as a 48-hour continuous infusion, to patients with initially metastatic osteosarcoma as initial therapy. Only one patient had an overall partial response. Separately analyzing the primary and metastatic sites of disease, 3 patients had a partial response of their primary tumor (2 had histologic evaluation of the tumor at definitive surgery, showing between 50 and 90% necrosis), 3 had complete responses, and 1 had partial response of their pulmonary disease. However, 20 of 37 patients had unequivocal progressive disease while receiving carboplatin. Following induction, multiagent chemotherapy was administered with a combination of high-dose methotrexate, ifosfamide (2.4 g/m^2/day for 5 days, as a single agent), CP, and Doxo, for a total of 40 weeks. Overall outcome was poor, with an EFS of 24% and OAS of 40% at 3 years. Patients with isolated pulmonary metastasis had a more favorable outlook, as in the COSS series, with a 44% 3-year survival. Those with unresectable bony metastases had a particularly poor outcome, 6% survival at 3 years.

A subsequent Pediatric Oncology Group study began therapy with two cycles of high-dose ifosfamide (3.5 g/m^2/day for 5 days) and etoposide (100 mg/m^2/day, also for 5 days).[130] This was based on a prior phase I study of etoposide with escalating dosage of ifosfamide, in which 6 of 13 patients with recurrent osteosarcoma responded to therapy with higher dosage levels of ifosfamide.[335] Induction of ifosfamide and etoposide was followed by multiagent chemotherapy with high-dose methotrexate, CP, and Doxo, as well as three additional cycles of a slightly lower dosage of ifosfamide, 2.4 g/m^2/day for 5 days, and etoposide, 100 mg/m^2/day for 5 days. Surgery of the primary and resectable metastatic sites was encouraged. Of 41 evaluable patients, 2-year progression-free survival was 43%, with an overall survival probability of 55%. In the limited number of patients studied, survival was similar for patients with isolated pulmonary metastases, 52% at 2 years, as compared with patients with bone metastases, with or without lung metastases, 58% at 2 years. Toxicity was significant, however, with two toxic deaths, one from gram-negative sepsis and the second from congestive cardiac failure. Eighty-three percent of patients experienced severe neutropenia, with sepsis in 10% (including the septic death) and other bacterial infections in an additional 7%.

In view of the relatively favorable outcome of the regimen, however, it served as the model for the backbone for the next Children's Oncology Group study, AOST 0121. The ifosfamide dosage was one level lower, 2.8 g/m^2/day for 5 days, along with etoposide, 100 mg/m^2/day for 5 days, and the ordering of the cycles was slightly different. As noted earlier (see "Biology"), the presence of erbB-2 (HER2) in osteosarcoma confers an unfavorable prognosis. It may also represent a tumor target. Trastuzumab is a humanized antibody that binds specifically to the HER2 protein. Preclinically, it was found to antagonize the function of the growth-signaling properties of the HER2 system, signal immune cells to attack and kill tumor targets, and augment chemotherapy-induced cytotoxicity.[336-340] A pivotal randomized phase III trial in women with previously untreated HER2-positive metastatic breast cancer has shown a significantly improved response rate and survival for those who initially received trastuzumab along with chemotherapy.[260] Trastuzumab increased the risk of cardiotoxicity when given with anthracyclines. However, trastuzumab cardiotoxicity appears to be reversible on discontinuation of the drug.[341] In view of the possible increased risk of cardiac toxicity, entry into AOST 0121 was limited to the highest risk patients—those with bone metastases, bilateral lung metastases, or unilateral lung metastases with at least four nodules. In addition, dexrazoxane was administered as a cardioprotective agent prior to bolus doxorubicin. Approximately one third of patients had tumors that expressed HER2, and only these patients received trastuzumab. Toxicity data reported to the Children's Oncology Group showed only one patient who developed an asymptomatic and transient decrease in cardiac function. That patient was able to resume trastuzumab and complete therapy with no complications. Other toxicities, primarily febrile neutropenia, appeared similar in patients who received or did not receive trastuzumab. One patient died 12 days after the first dose of cisplatin-doxorubicin, having initially presented with fever, neutropenia, vomiting, diarrhea, severe dehydration, and renal failure. In preliminary outcome data, patients with HER2-positive tumors had a higher response rate (complete response plus partial response), 41% versus 27%, than patients with HER2-negative tumors, but this result was not statistically significant.[266]

The next Children's Oncology Group study for patients with initially metastatic osteosarcoma will incorporate zoledronate into the same background chemotherapy. Zoledronate is a nitrogen-containing bisphosphonate and the most potent of its class. It inhibits the development of osteolytic and osteoblastic bone lesions.[342] Preclinical models have shown cytotoxicity against osteosarcoma cell lines,[343,344] and in vivo models have shown prolonged survival in mice inoculated intravenously with the spontaneous murine osteosarcoma cell line POS-1 when treated with single-agent zoledronate.[345] Moreover, combination with ifosfamide has shown more activity than either agent alone in preventing tumor recurrence, improving tissue repair, and increasing bone formation.[346] Bisphosphonates may also improve bone integrity after limb salvage surgery.[347,348] The COG study will assess the feasibility and safety of adding zoledronate to the standard chemotherapy background being carried forward. The histologic response and EFS in patients with metastatic osteosarcoma treated with standard chemotherapy and zoledronic acid will also be compared with that of a similar cohort of patients treated by previous COG protocols.

Treatment of Recurrent Osteosarcoma

The recurrence of osteosarcoma is an unfavorable event, with subsequent outcome most influenced by the time to recurrence, burden of disease at the time of recurrence, and resectability of the recurrent disease. In a series from the COSS group,[7] 576 of an initial 1702 patients developed recurrent disease at a median time of 1.6 years (range, 0.1 to 14.3 years). Metastases occurred in 501 patients, 44 had local recurrence, and 31 had both. The most frequent metastatic site was the lungs, involved in 469 patients (81%). The lung was the only site of recurrence in 373 patients (65%). Bone metastases were found in 90 patients (16%); 45 of these also had other sites involved and 54 had sites other than lung or bone involved, but only 12 patients had other sites without lung or bone involved. There were 543 relapses (94%) within 5 years from biopsy; follow-up on the study was 4.5 to 23 years. Recurrence was solitary in 216 patients. Solitary recurrence was more frequent in those with initially localized disease and with recurrence more than 18 months from biopsy. The pleura was less likely to be involved than in those with multiple lesions. Event-free survival was 0.13 (standard error [SE], 0.01) at 5 years, 0.11 (SE, 0.02) at 10 years, with an overall survival of 0.23 (SE, 0.02) at 5 years, and 0.18 (SE, 0.02) at 10 years. The most important factor associated with survival was achievement of a second surgical complete remission. The ability to achieve second surgical complete remission was likely related to the number and bilaterality of pulmonary lesions, as well as pleural disruption by the pulmonary metastasis. Patients with multiple lesions, bilateral lesions, and lesions that disrupted the pleura fared less well. Chemotherapy was of limited benefit, with multiagent therapy probably more effective than single-agent therapy.

Similar results have been reported from the Rizzoli Institute[6] in a study of 175 patients. The median time to recurrence was slightly longer than in the COSS series, 23 months as compared with 19 months. As in the COSS series, 94% of recurrences were within 5 years of diagnosis. Again, achievement of a second surgical remission was key to survival and was more readily accomplished in patients with recurrence limited to the

lungs (97 of 125 [75%] of those with isolated pulmonary recurrence as compared with 21 of 37 [57%] of those with other than lung metastasis). Event-free survival was 16%, with postrelapse survival of 39% at 5 years for those who achieved a second complete surgical remission, but 0% among those who did not. A longer initial relapse-free interval (more than 24 months) and the presence of only one or two lung metastases were favorable prognostic indicators in patients with isolated pulmonary metastases who achieved a second complete surgical remission. Chemotherapy slightly prolonged survival in those who did not achieve a second surgical complete remission and possibly in those with three or more pulmonary nodules who underwent resection.

Other groups have reported comparable findings in smaller numbers of patients.[105,349,350] Aggressive and, if necessary, repeated thoracotomies have also been advocated by many.[351-355] A report from the Rizzoli group focusing on patients with recurrent osteosarcoma in bone has confirmed the inferior outcome of such patients.[128] Fifty-two patients were diagnosed with metastatic bone recurrence over a 27-year period (1972 to 1999), from a total patient population of 1148. Pain was the most common symptom at recurrence; 18 patients had recurrence in the extremities or the extremities and ribs. Their lesions were more amenable to resection than those of patients whose disease recurred in the pelvis or spine. Of the 6 patients who survived, 5 had only one lesion, which was resectable. They were the only patients to remain event-free at 5 years postrecurrence, yielding a rate of 11% (0% to 21% confidence interval). As compared with the more numerous patients (371) who first developed recurrent disease in the lungs, those with bone metastases were more likely to also have local recurrence, 36% as compared with 6%.

The Memorial-Sloan Kettering Cancer Center group analyzed their patients who had local recurrence.[356] The local recurrence rate was 4.2% among those whose primary disease was resectable (17 of 401), 3.7% for those with primary extremity disease, and 8.3% for those with primary axial disease. The presence of positive margins of resection was strongly correlated with subsequent local recurrence ($P < .0001$). A shorter time to recurrence (within 12 months from the primary resection), the presence of pulmonary metastases at recurrence, and failure to achieve complete surgical remission adversely affected outcome. Overall survival was 29% at 5 years and 10% at 10 years.

The development of pulmonary metastasis may be facilitated by the absence of FAS on the malignant cell surface. Tumor cells expressing FAS are eliminated by the lung endothelium, which constitutively expresses FAS ligand. The metastatic potential of osteosarcoma cells in model systems has been shown to be inversely related to FAS expression.[357,358] Blocking FAS signaling delays the clearance of osteosarcoma cells from the lung in an orthotopic mouse model.[285] In 38 patient samples, most were FAS-negative. Those that were weakly positive, and the one sample that was strongly positive, came from patients who had received salvage chemotherapy prior to lung resection. This suggests that chemotherapy may lead to a re-expression of FAS.[285] Gemcitabine administered by the inhalation route may be another way of activating FAS on the osteosarcoma cell surface.[359] An alternate means of enhancing FAS expression on osteosarcoma cells may be the administration of granulocyte-macrophage colony-stimulating factor (GM-CSF) by the inhalation route. A study at the Mayo Clinic in 40 patients with pulmonary metastases from a variety of malignancies has shown benefit in at least 50%.[360] Dose escalation in patients with melanoma has shown melanoma-specific T cells at the higher dosage levels of 1750 and 2000 µg administered by the inhalation route twice daily, 1 week on and 1 week off (S. Markovic, personal communication, 2008). An ongoing COG study (AOST 0221) is investigating the feasibility of such an approach in patients with recurrent osteosarcoma, with biologic end points including analysis of the FAS pathway and study of infiltrating dendritic cells. Dendritic cell therapy itself has shown antiosteosarcoma activity in a mouse model, particularly when pulsed in vitro with irradiated tumor and administered in a minimal residual disease setting.[361] Immune surveillance by T cells may delay or prevent the development of metastasis, as seen in a mouse model.[362] This suggests a role for the expansion of autologous T cells following the completion of immune-depleting chemotherapy.

Other possible targets include ezrin and the chemokine receptor CXCR4. Ezrin is a membrane-cytoskeleton linker that may be necessary as the malignant cell moves through its microenvironment, and may engage pathways important to successful metastasis.[125] There are currently no drugs that inhibit ezrin in clinical development. However, the mTOR pathway is activated downstream of ezrin. Rapamycin and temsirolimus (CI-779) inhibited the mTOR pathway and decreased lung metastasis in a mouse model of osteosarcoma.[363] Preclinical investigations in dogs with spontaneous osteosarcoma are ongoing. As noted earlier (see "Biology"), the chemokine receptor CXCR4 is involved in chemotaxis and endothelial cell binding and has been implicated in the development of metastasis. A CXCR4 inhibitor decreased the formation of pulmonary metastases in a mouse model of osteosarcoma.[274] In an orthotopic model of osteosarcoma, pigment epithelium–derived factor (PEDF), a potent antiangiogenic compound, inhibited the development of osteosarcoma metastases.[364,365] Novel antifolates such as pemetrexed may also hold promise, although single-agent in vitro studies have shown less activity than methotrexate.[366]

In summary, recurrent osteosarcoma carries a grave prognosis. Cure is most likely in the minority of patients who have a limited number of metastases that are completely resected, leading to a second complete surgical remission, especially if the first remission was of relatively long duration. The role of adjuvant therapy for patients with recurrent osteosarcoma is uncertain. Enrollment of such patients in clinical trials should be encouraged.

Radiotherapy

Radiotherapy is relatively ineffective against osteosarcoma, especially when compared with the combination of adequate surgery and multiagent chemotherapy. In vitro studies comparing osteosarcoma with other human cell lines have demonstrated that osteosarcoma cells are more resistant to irradiation.[367] In addition, those osteosarcomas with loss of p53 function would be expected to survive radiation-induced DNA damage.[179,191]

Adjuvant pulmonary radiation therapy has been compared in a randomized fashion with adjuvant vincristine plus high-dose methotrexate.[368] Although outcomes were the same in patients receiving chemotherapy and those receiving pulmonary irradiation, disease-free survival in both arms of the study was much lower (at 24%) than with the current standard approach of wide surgical resection and multiagent chemotherapy.[101] In addition, 14% of patients receiving adjuvant pulmonary irradiation experienced decreased pulmonary function. Thus, adjuvant pulmonary irradiation is not recommended.

Radiotherapy has been used for local control of osteosarcoma. When radiotherapy is the only local control measure (i.e., no operation is performed) the local recurrence rate is almost three times greater than is seen with surgical resection.[368] Nevertheless, when surgical resection of the primary lesion is not an option, there may be a role for radiotherapy. Machak and colleagues[369] have reported a 5-year overall survival of 60% in 31 patients who refused surgical resection of the primary tumor and were treated instead with local irradiation and multiagent chemotherapy. Similarly, patients with

osteosarcoma of the spine who had intralesional margins or no surgery tended to have a better outcome if they received local irradiation plus multiagent chemotherapy than chemotherapy alone, although the difference was not statistically significant.[370] Contrasting results have been presented by Hug and associates,[371] who saw local failures in 2 of 3 patients who did not undergo surgical resection of the primary tumor but were treated with local irradiation and multiagent chemotherapy.

Preoperative irradiation, in combination with neoadjuvant multiagent chemotherapy, has been given in an attempt to increase the rate of limb salvage surgery.[372] Although this approach has resulted in a higher percentage of limb salvage procedures compared with historical controls, local complications were also increased. Given the increased rate of local complications, this approach is not recommended.

Whether postoperative irradiation is useful when inadequate surgical margins are present is controversial. There are no randomized trials comparing postoperative irradiation with observation in patients whose tumor resection specimens had marginal or intralesional surgical margins. Studies that have compared such patients with similar historical controls show an improved local control rate and overall survival in patients treated with local postoperative irradiation.[370,373] However, a great diversity of tumor burden is present in patients with intralesional and marginal tumor margins, and chemotherapy regimens have changed over time. Thus, comparison with historic controls might not be valid.

Samarium 153 ethylenediaminetetramethylene phosphonate (^{153}Sm-EDTMP) is a pharmaceutical radioisotope that is efficiently and specifically taken up by bone. Patients with osteosarcoma bone metastases treated with ^{153}Sm-EDTMP experience a rapid decrease in pain symptoms.[374] At high doses of ^{153}Sm-EDTMP, peripheral blood stem cell rescue is required.

Complications of Therapy

Patients receiving osteosarcoma therapy can experience acute complications from chemotherapy and surgery. As noted, the usual osteosarcoma chemotherapy backbone is HDMTX, Doxo, and CP. Ifosfamide and etoposide are also given in many protocols. The acute toxicities of HDMTX, Doxo, and CP combination chemotherapy with and without ifosfamide have been well documented in numerous osteosarcoma treatment protocols.[102,104,121,320,333,334] The most common acute side effects, occurring in 75% of patients, are grades 3 or 4 leukopenia and neutropenia. Significant nausea and vomiting are also common and occur in 60% to 70% of patients, particularly during Doxo-CP cycles; 20% to 30% of patients experience mucositis. A similar percentage develops significant infections. Reversible transaminase elevations occur in about 15% of patients, usually because of HDMTX. Renal toxicity, which occurs in 1% to 2% of patients, presents as renal insufficiency or tubular dysfunction, with accompanying electrolyte abnormalities. Renal dysfunction can be acute or chronic. Neurologic toxicity presenting as seizures, headache, or radiologic changes is rare. The rate of therapy-related mortality varies from 0% to 4%, with most protocols reporting a 1% to 2% rate of therapy-related mortality, usually caused by infection and, less frequently, by cardiotoxicity.

A potential complication of HDMTX therapy in all disease settings is renal damage from insoluble MTX metabolites. Because MTX is primarily excreted by the kidneys, renal damage can lead to delayed MTX clearance, which in turn worsens renal dysfunction and further delays MTX clearance. Delayed MTX clearance, even in the setting of adequate leucovorin rescue, can lead to severe mucositis and prolonged myelosuppression. With adequate hydration, alkalinization, and monitoring of drug levels, the incidence of severely delayed MTX clearance is low. Delayed MTX clearance can be treated with increased hydration, adjustments in leucovorin dosing, hemodialysis, or carboxypeptidase (glucarpidase), an enzyme that converts MTX to inactive metabolites that are readily excreted in the urine.[375]

Acute complications of osteosarcoma primary resection surgeries are reviewed extensively in Chapter 9. Limb salvage procedures have a much higher rate of perioperative complications than amputations. In one study, 41% of limb-sparing procedures had wound complications compared with only 13% of amputations.[102] Acute complications of surgery include infection, flap necrosis, damage to the neurovascular bundle, and venous thrombosis.[102,376]

Chemotherapy late effects in osteosarcoma include cardiac dysfunction, hearing loss, secondary malignancy, and decreased fertility.[106] See Table 22-8 for guidelines regarding post-treatment monitoring for late effects and relapse. Many osteo-

TABLE 22-8 Clinical Pearls: Typical Monitoring After Completion of Therapy

ROUTINE MONITORING FOR TUMOR RECURRENCE (ALSO, IMAGING FOR SYMPTOMS, AS INDICATED)

First Year

Primary site	Plain film every 3 to 4 mo
Site(s) of bone metastases	Plain film every 3 to 4 mo
Chest	Chest CT every 3 mo

Second Year

Primary site	Plain film every 4 to 6 mo
Site(s) of bone metastases	Plain film every 4 to 6 mo
Chest	Chest CT every 4 to 6 mo

Third Year

Primary site	Plain film every 4 to 6 mo
Site(s) of bone metastases	Plain film every 4 to 6 mo
Chest	Chest radiography every 4 to 6 mo OR chest CT every 6 mo

Fourth and Fifth Years

Primary site	Plain film every 6 to 12 mo
Site(s) of bone metastases	Plain film every 12 mo
Chest	Chest radiography every 4 to 6 mo OR chest CT every 6 mo

Sixth to Tenth Years

Primary site	Plain film every 12 mo
Site(s) of bone metastases	Plain film every 12 mo
Chest	Chest radiography every 12 mo

MONITORING FOR CHEMOTHERAPY LATE EFFECTS

Cardiac	Echocardiography every 12 mo for 2-3 yr, then at time of pubertal growth spurt and pregnancy
Nephrotoxicity	Electrolytes, blood urea nitrogen, creatinine every 12 mo
Ototoxicity	Audiology at the end of therapy
Secondary malignancy	Complete blood count every 12 mo
Fertility	Semen analysis offered to postpubertal males
All	Physical examination every 3 mo × 1 yr, then every 3 to 6 mo until 4 yr postcompletion of therapy, every 6 mo until 5 years postcompletion of therapy, then yearly

Recommendations for post-treatment surveillance vary. For further reading see references 377a, 377b, and 377c.

sarcoma protocols use a cumulative doxorubicin dosage of 450 mg/m^2. Published rates of cardiac toxicity following treatment for osteosarcoma range from 0% to 5%.[102,111,320,334] Cardiac dysfunction caused by doxorubicin is irreversible and can be severe enough to cause death or require transplantation. Doxo-related cardiotoxicity is more common in women and is more likely with higher cumulative Doxo dosages.[377] Younger children treated with Doxo may develop delayed cardiac failure during rapid somatic growth in adolescence, and women may similarly develop cardiac failure as a result of the increased cardiac workload presented by pregnancy. The long-term cardiac outcome of patients treated with Doxo especially at a relatively high cumulative dosage remains to be defined. Administration of dexrazoxane in conjunction with Doxo in pediatric sarcoma patients has led to preservation of left ventricular function, without any change in outcome, compared with placebo control in an initial small clinical trial.[378] Recently, dexrazoxane administration in patients receiving therapy for Hodgkin's disease has been associated with an increased risk of subsequent acute myeloid leukemia and myelodysplastic syndrome.[379] It is uncertain whether these findings pertain to patients with other disease types.

Second malignancies occur at an increased rate in osteosarcoma survivors compared with the general population or patients with benign bone tumors.[380,381] The incidence of second malignancies ranges from 2% to 4%. Because a number of genetic cancer syndromes increase osteosarcoma risk, it is difficult to determine whether second malignancies are caused by an underlying genetic predisposition or a complication of osteosarcoma therapy. Certainly some of the osteosarcoma survivors who develop a second malignancy have no family history of cancer. No particular type of secondary malignancy predominates.

Ototoxicity as a result of osteosarcoma therapy is predominantly caused by cisplatin. In some patients, aminoglycoside treatment of infectious complications of chemotherapy may be a contributing factor. Mild ototoxicity, which does not involve the frequencies of audible speech, is relatively common. Significant ototoxicity involving the audible speech frequencies is rare, reported in 1% or fewer patients.[382] Amifostine, administered concurrently with cisplatin, has been tested in a small group of pediatric osteosarcoma patients. Compared with untreated controls, patients receiving amifostine had less severe myelosuppression, but the incidence of renal and ototoxicity was not decreased by amifostine therapy. Amifostine was emetogenic but was otherwise well tolerated.[383]

Azoospermia is known to be caused by alkylating agents and is common in osteosarcoma patients treated with ifosfamide. Azoospermia has also been seen in patients who were treated with HDMTX, Doxo, and CP and it is likely that this is chemotherapy-related.[384] Data on female infertility following osteosarcoma therapy are limited. In one study, 6% of female patients treated with HDMTX, Doxo, and CP plus ifosfamide had early menopause.[385]

Long-term orthopedic complications, which depend on the type of surgical resection performed, are discussed further in Chapter 9. Patients who have limb-sparing operations are more likely to have late orthopedic complications. Most late complications are caused by endoprosthesis or allograft failure, although late infections also occur.[376] Thirty percent of endoprostheses will require surgical revision or replacement by 10 years after the initial surgery.[386] Other problems that arise in patients undergoing limb-sparing surgery include poor joint mobility and leg length discrepancy, both of which can impair limb function. Although limb-sparing procedures have a higher complication rate, the functional outcome is superior when assessed by oxygen consumption during walking. Functionally, rotationplasty is equivalent to a below-knee amputation.[376] Data on quality of life following surgery for osteosarcoma are limited.

CONCLUSIONS AND FUTURE DIRECTIONS

Osteosarcoma treatment and prognosis have not changed significantly during the past 2 decades. The standard chemotherapy backbone for localized osteosarcoma—Doxo, CP, and HDMTX—has remained the same. Consequently, outcomes in patients with localized osteosarcoma are similar today to outcomes 20 years ago. New therapies, particularly ifosfamide and etoposide, have been used for patients with metastatic and recurrent disease, and there are early indications that this may result in a slight improvement in outcome. In contrast, surgical approaches have changed significantly over the past 20 years. Previously, amputations were common; currently, many patients have limb-sparing surgeries. In addition, there has been increasing recognition of the ability to increase survival via complete resection of pulmonary metastases.

This relatively slow rate of progress in treatment of osteosarcoma is partly the result of the biologic complexity of the disease. There have been a number of biologic insights over the past 2 decades, but none has revealed obvious drug targets that are of central relevance in a large proportion of osteosarcomas. An additional factor slowing the rate of progress in osteosarcoma is the small patient population available for clinical studies.

Several ongoing clinical studies should provide important clinical insights in the next 5 to 10 years. Results of the international cooperative study EURAMOS1 will hopefully determine whether the postoperative addition of ifosfamide and etoposide improves the EFS of patients with a poor response to neoadjuvant chemotherapy and whether the postoperative addition of interferon-α following neoadjuvant chemotherapy improves outcome in patients with a good histologic response. The proposed COG trial for patients with initially metastatic disease will determine whether it is feasible to administer zoledronate with multiagent chemotherapy and may give some indication as to whether zoledronate has possible efficacy in metastatic osteosarcoma. This question is also being addressed by an SFOP (Société Française d'Oncologie Pédiatrique) trial.

New therapeutic agents are likely to be evaluated in osteosarcoma in the next several years. A number of anti–IGF-IR antibody therapies have been developed and these are likely to be tested in osteosarcoma patients in phase I and II trials in the next few years. The Sarcoma Alliance for Research through Collaboration (SARC) is planning to study a src inhibitor in patients with metastatic osteosarcoma. Other existing agents that have preclinical data supporting use in osteosarcoma include mTOR and CXCR4 inhibitors. In addition to these newly developed agents, it is possible that there will be further evaluation of MTP-PE, given the continued debate about its impact on survival in prior trials.

Breakthroughs in the understanding of osteosarcoma biology are likely in the next 10 to 20 years as the number and sophistication of tools and techniques for biomedical research continue to increase. For example, improved transgenic mouse models of osteosarcoma are likely to be developed and these models will facilitate basic and applied studies. High-throughput genomic and proteomic techniques requiring minimal amounts of tumor tissue will facilitate the study of human osteosarcoma samples, which are in limited supply. The combination of these new techniques, with the proliferation of new drug compounds and the recently established international collaboration for clinical studies, will hopefully lead to significant advances in osteosarcoma in the near-future.

REFERENCES

1. Bleyer A, O'Leary M, Barr R, Ries LAG (eds). Cancer Epidemiology in Older Adolescents and Young Adults 15 to 29 Years of Age, Including SEER Incidence and Survival: 1975-2000 (NIH Publication No. 06-5767). Bethesda, Md, National Cancer Institute, 2006.
2. Peltier L. Tumors of bone and soft tissues. In Peltier L (ed). Orthopedics: A History and Iconography. Novato, Calif, Norman Publishing, 1993, pp 264-292.
3. Dahlin DC, Unni KK. Osteosarcoma of bone and its important recognizable varieties. Am J Surg Pathol. 1977;1:61-72.
4. Kager L, Zoubek A, Potschger U, et al. Primary metastatic osteosarcoma: presentation and outcome of patients treated on neoadjuvant Cooperative Osteosarcoma Study Group protocols. J Clin Oncol. 2003;21:2011-2018.
5. Meyers PA, Schwartz CL, Krailo MD, et al. Osteosarcoma: the addition of muramyl tripeptide to chemotherapy improves overall survival—a report from the Children's Oncology Group. J Clin Oncol. 2008;26:633-638.
6. Ferrari S, Briccoli A, Mercuri M, et al. Postrelapse survival in osteosarcoma of the extremities: prognostic factors for long-term survival. J Clin Oncol. 2003;21:710-715.
7. Kempf-Bielack B, Bielack SS, Jurgens H, et al. Osteosarcoma relapse after combined modality therapy: an analysis of unselected patients in the Cooperative Osteosarcoma Study Group (COSS). J Clin Oncol. 2005;23:559-568.
8. Parkin DM, Stiller CA, Draper GJ, Bieber CA. The international incidence of childhood cancer. Int J Cancer. 1988;42:511-520.
9. Stiller CA. International patterns of cancer incidence in adolescents. Cancer Treat Rev. 2007;33:631-645.
10. Ries LAG, Smith MA, Gurney JG, et al (eds). Cancer Incidence and Survival Among Children and Adolescents: United States SEER Program 1975-1995 (NIH Publication No. 99-4649). Bethesda, Md, National Cancer Institute, SEER Program, 1999.
11. Larsson SE, Lorentzon R. The incidence of malignant primary bone tumours in relation to age, sex and site. A study of osteogenic sarcoma, chondrosarcoma and Ewing's sarcoma diagnosed in Sweden from 1958 to 1968. J Bone Joint Surg Br. 1974;56:534-540.
12. Price CH. Osteogenic sarcoma; an analysis of the age and sex incidence. Br J Cancer. 1955;9:558-574.
13. Grimer RJ, Cannon SR, Taminiau AM, et al. Osteosarcoma over the age of forty. Eur J Cancer. 2003;39:157-163.
14. Kramer S, Meadows AT, Jarrett P, Evans AE. Incidence of childhood cancer: experience of a decade in a population-based registry. J Natl Cancer Inst. 1983;70:49-55.
15. Polednak AP. Primary bone cancer incidence in black and white residents of New York State. Cancer. 1985;55:2883-2888.
16. Howe HL, Wu X, Ries LA, et al. Annual report to the nation on the status of cancer, 1975-2003, featuring cancer among U.S. Hispanic/Latino populations. Cancer. 2006;107:1711-1742.
17. Buckley JD, Pendergrass TW, Buckley CM, et al. Epidemiology of osteosarcoma and Ewing's sarcoma in childhood: a study of 305 cases by the Children's Cancer Group. Cancer. 1998;83:1440-1448.
18. Operskalski EA, Preston-Martin S, Henderson BE, Visscher BR. A case-control study of osteosarcoma in young persons. Am J Epidemiol. 1987;126:118-126.
19. Brostrom LA, Adamson U, Filipsson R, Hall K. Longitudinal growth and dental development in osteosarcoma patients. Acta Orthop Scand. 1980;51:755-759.
20. Fraumeni JF Jr. Stature and malignant tumors of bone in childhood and adolescence. Cancer. 1967;20:967-973.
21. Longhi A, Pasini A, Cicognani A, et al. Height as a risk factor for osteosarcoma. J Pediatr Hematol Oncol. 2005;27:314-318.
22. Gelberg KH, Fitzgerald EF, Hwang S, Dubrow R. Growth and development and other risk factors for osteosarcoma in children and young adults. Int J Epidemiol. 1997;26:272-278.
23. Hawkins MM, Wilson LM, Burton HS, et al. Radiotherapy, alkylating agents, and risk of bone cancer after childhood cancer. J Natl Cancer Inst. 1996;88:270-278.

24. Newton WA Jr, Meadows AT, Shimada H, et al. Bone sarcomas as second malignant neoplasms following childhood cancer. Cancer. 1991;67:193-201.

25. Le VB, de VF, Shamsaldin A, et al. Radiation dose, chemotherapy and risk of osteosarcoma after solid tumours during childhood. Int J Cancer. 1998;77:370-377.

26. Kuttesch JF Jr, Wexler LH, Marcus RB, et al. Second malignancies after Ewing's sarcoma: radiation dose-dependency of secondary sarcomas. J Clin Oncol. 1996;14:2818-2825.

27. Koshy M, Paulino AC, Mai WY, Teh BS. Radiation-induced osteosarcomas in the pediatric population. Int J Radiat Oncol Biol Phys. 2005;63:1169-1174.

28. Pierce DA, Preston DL. Radiation-related cancer risks at low doses among atomic bomb survivors. Radiat Res. 2000;154:178-186.

29. Brenner D, Elliston C, Hall E, Berdon W. Estimated risks of radiation-induced fatal cancer from pediatric CT. AJR Am J Roentgenol. 2001;176:289-296.

30. Wong FL, Boice JD Jr, Abramson DH, et al. Cancer incidence after retinoblastoma. Radiation dose and sarcoma risk. JAMA. 1997;278:1262-1267.

31. Hansen MF, Koufos A, Gallie BL, et al. Osteosarcoma and retinoblastoma: a shared chromosomal mechanism revealing recessive predisposition. Proc Natl Acad Sci U S A. 1985;82:6216-6220.

32. Wadayama B, Toguchida J, Shimizu T, et al. Mutation spectrum of the retinoblastoma gene in osteosarcomas. Cancer Res. 1994;54:3042-3048.

33. Li FP, Fraumeni JF Jr, Mulvihill JJ, et al. A cancer family syndrome in twenty-four kindreds. Cancer Res. 1988;48:5358-5362.

34. Overholtzer M, Rao PH, Favis R, et al. The presence of p53 mutations in human osteosarcomas correlates with high levels of genomic instability. Proc Natl Acad Sci U S A. 2003;100:11547-11552.

35. Wang LL, Gannavarapu A, Kozinetz CA, et al. Association between osteosarcoma and deleterious mutations in the RECQL4 gene in Rothmund-Thomson syndrome. J Natl Cancer Inst. 2003;95:669-674.

36. Hicks MJ, Roth JR, Kozinetz CA, Wang LL. Clinicopathologic features of osteosarcoma in patients with Rothmund-Thomson syndrome. J Clin Oncol. 2007;25:370-375.

37. German J. Bloom's syndrome. XX. The first 100 cancers. Cancer Genet Cytogenet. 1997;93:100-106.

38. Goto M, Miller RW, Ishikawa Y, Sugano H. Excess of rare cancers in Werner syndrome (adult progeria). Cancer Epidemiol Biomarkers Prev. 1996;5:239-246.

39. Whyte MP. Clinical practice. Paget's disease of bone. N Engl J Med. 2006;355:593-600.

40. Rowland RE, Stehney AF, Lucas HF Jr. Dose-response relationships for female radium dial workers. Radiat Res. 1978;76:368-383.

41. Finkelstein MM, Kreiger N. Radium in drinking water and risk of bone cancer in Ontario youths: a second study and combined analysis. Occup Environ Med. 1996;53:305-311.

42. Finkelstein MM. Radium in drinking water and the risk of death from bone cancer among Ontario youths. CMAJ. 1994;151:565-571.

43. Guse CE, Marbella AM, George V, Layde PM. Radium in Wisconsin drinking water: an analysis of osteosarcoma risk. Arch Environ Health. 2002;57:294-303.

44. Vainio H, Kleihues P. IARC Working Group on Carcinogenicity of Beryllium. J Occup Med. 1994;36:1068-1070.

45. Rosenberg ZS, Lev S, Schmahmann S, et al. Osteosarcoma: subtle, rare, and misleading plain film features. AJR Am J Roentgenol. 1995;165:1209-1214.

46. Widhe B, Widhe T. Initial symptoms and clinical features in osteosarcoma and Ewing sarcoma. J Bone Joint Surg Am. 2000;82:667-674.

47. Bielack SS, Kempf-Bielack B, Delling G, et al. Prognostic factors in high-grade osteosarcoma of the extremities or trunk: an analysis of 1,702 patients treated on neoadjuvant cooperative osteosarcoma study group protocols. J Clin Oncol. 2002;20:776-790.

48. Bacci G, Longhi A, Versari M, et al. Prognostic factors for osteosarcoma of the extremity treated with neoadjuvant chemotherapy: 15-year experience in 789 patients treated at a single institution. Cancer. 2006;106:1154-1161.

49. Gross M, Stevens K. Sunburst periosteal reaction in osteogenic sarcoma. Pediatr Radiol. 2005;35:647-648.

50. Gillespy T III, Manfrini M, Ruggieri P, et al. Staging of intraosseous extent of osteosarcoma: correlation of preoperative CT and MR imaging with pathologic macroslides. Radiology. 1988;167:765-767.

51. Bloem JL, Taminiau AH, Eulderink F, et al. Radiologic staging of primary bone sarcoma: MR imaging, scintigraphy, angiography, and CT correlated with pathologic examination. Radiology. 1988;169:805-810.

52. Panicek DM, Gatsonis C, Rosenthal DI, et al. CT and MR imaging in the local staging of primary malignant musculoskeletal neoplasms: report of the Radiology Diagnostic Oncology Group. Radiology. 1997;202:237-246.

53. Pan G, Raymond AK, Carrasco CH, et al. Osteosarcoma: MR imaging after preoperative chemotherapy. Radiology. 1990;174:517-526.

54. Enneking WF, Kagan A. "Skip" metastases in osteosarcoma. Cancer. 1975;36:2192-2205.

55. Kager L, Zoubek A, Kastner U, et al. Skip metastases in osteosarcoma: experience of the Cooperative Osteosarcoma Study Group. J Clin Oncol. 2006;24:1535-1541.

56. Chew FS, Hudson TM. Radionuclide bone scanning of osteosarcoma: falsely extended uptake patterns. AJR Am J Roentgenol. 1982;139:49-54.

57. Franzius C, Sciuk J, Daldrup-Link HE, et al. FDG-PET for detection of osseous metastases from malignant primary bone tumours: comparison with bone scintigraphy. Eur J Nucl Med. 2000;27:1305-1311.

58. Brenner W, Bohuslavizki KH, Eary JF. PET imaging of osteosarcoma. J Nucl Med. 2003;44:930-942.

59. Picci P, Vanel D, Briccoli A, et al. Computed tomography of pulmonary metastases from osteosarcoma: the less poor technique. A study of 51 patients with histological correlation. Ann Oncol. 2001;12:1601-1604.

60. Vanel D, Henry-Amar M, Lumbroso J, et al. Pulmonary evaluation of patients with osteosarcoma: roles of standard radiography, tomography, CT, scintigraphy, and tomoscintigraphy. AJR Am J Roentgenol. 1984;143:519-523.

61. Kayton ML, Huvos AG, Casher J, et al. Computed tomographic scan of the chest underestimates the number of metastatic lesions in osteosarcoma. J Pediatr Surg. 2006;41:200-206.

62. White VA, Fanning CV, Ayala AG, et al. Osteosarcoma and the role of fine-needle aspiration. A study of 51 cases. Cancer. 1988;62:1238-1246.

63. Jelinek JS, Murphey MD, Welker JA, et al. Diagnosis of primary bone tumors with image-guided percutaneous biopsy: experience with 110 tumors. Radiology. 2002;223:731-737.

64. Ayala AG, Zornosa J. Primary bone tumors: percutaneous needle biopsy. Radiologic-pathologic study of 222 biopsies. Radiology. 1983;149:675-679.

65. Stoker DJ, Cobb JP, Pringle JA. Needle biopsy of musculoskeletal lesions. A review of 208 procedures. J Bone Joint Surg Br. 1991;73:498-500.

66. Yao L, Nelson SD, Seeger LL, et al. Primary musculoskeletal neoplasms: effectiveness of core-needle biopsy. Radiology. 1999;212:682-686.

67. Ahrar K, Himmerich JU, Herzog CE, et al. Percutaneous ultrasound-guided biopsy in the definitive diagnosis of osteosarcoma. J Vasc Interv Radiol. 2004;15:1329-1333.

68. Davies NM, Livesley PJ, Cannon SR. Recurrence of an osteosarcoma in a needle biopsy track. J Bone Joint Surg Br. 1993;75: 977-978.

69. Iemsawatdikul K, Gooding CA, Twomey EL, et al. Seeding of osteosarcoma in the biopsy tract of a patient with multifocal osteosarcoma. Pediatr Radiol. 2005;35:717-721.

70. Peabody TD, Simon MA. Making the diagnosis: keys to a successful biopsy in children with bone and soft-tissue tumors. Orthop Clin North Am. 1996;27:453-459.

71. Mankin HJ, Mankin CJ, Simon MA. The hazards of the biopsy, revisited. Members of the Musculoskeletal Tumor Society. J Bone Joint Surg Am. 1996;78:656-663.

72. Thorpe WP, Reilly JJ, Rosenberg SA. Prognostic significance of alkaline phosphatase measurements in patients with osteogenic sarcoma receiving chemotherapy. Cancer. 1979;43:2178-2181.

73. Dahlin DC, Unni KK (eds). Bone Tumors, 4th ed. Springfield, Ill, Charles C Thomas, 1986.

74. Bacci G, Ferrari S, Delepine N, et al. Predictive factors of histologic response to primary chemotherapy in osteosarcoma of the extremity: study of 272 patients preoperatively treated with high-dose methotrexate, doxorubicin, and cisplatin. J Clin Oncol. 1998;16:658-663.

75. Fletcher CDM, Unni KK, Mertens F (eds). World Health Organization Classification of Tumours. Pathology and Genetics, Tumours of Soft Tissue and Bone. Lyon, France, IARC Press, 2002.

76. Hauben EI, Weeden S, Pringle J, et al. Does the histological subtype of high-grade central osteosarcoma influence the response to treatment with chemotherapy and does it affect overall survival? A study on 570 patients of two consecutive trials of the European Osteosarcoma Intergroup. Eur J Cancer. 2002;38: 1218-1225.

77. Bacci G, Bertoni F, Longhi, A, et al. Neoadjuvant chemotherapy for high-grade central osteosarcoma of the extremity. Histologic response to preoperative chemotherapy correlates with histologic subtype of the tumor. Cancer. 2003;97:3068-3075.

78. Huvos AG, Rosen G, Bretsky SS, Butler A. Telangiectatic osteogenic sarcoma: a clinicopathologic study of 124 patients. Cancer. 1982;49:1679-1689.

79. Bacci G, Ferrari S, Ruggieri P, et al. Telangiectatic osteosarcoma of the extremity: neoadjuvant chemotherapy in 24 cases. Acta Orthop Scand. 2001;72:167-172.

80. Matsuno T, Unni KK, McLeod RA, Dahlin DC. Telangiectatic osteogenic sarcoma. Cancer. 1976;38:2538-2547.

81. Nakajima H, Sim FH, Bond JR, Unni KK. Small cell osteosarcoma of bone. Review of 72 cases. Cancer. 1997;79:2095-2106.

82. Ayala AG, Ro JY, Raymond AK, et al. Small cell osteosarcoma. A clinicopathologic study of 27 cases. Cancer. 1989;64:2162-2173.

83. Bertoni F, Dallera P, Bacchini P, et al. The Istituto Rizzoli-Beretta experience with osteosarcoma of the jaw. Cancer. 1991;68:1555-1563.

84. Clark JL, Unni KK, Dahlin DC, Devine KD. Osteosarcoma of the jaw. Cancer. 1983;51:2311-2316.

85. Gadwal SR, Gannon FH, Fanburg-Smith JC, et al. Primary osteosarcoma of the head and neck in pediatric patients: a clinicopathologic study of 22 cases with a review of the literature. Cancer. 2001;91:598-605.

86. Kurt AM, Unni KK, McLeod RA, Pritchard DJ. Low-grade intraosseous osteosarcoma. Cancer. 1990;65:1418-1428.

87. Bertoni F, Bacchini P, Fabbri N, et al. Osteosarcoma. Low-grade intraosseous-type osteosarcoma, histologically resembling parosteal osteosarcoma, fibrous dysplasia, and desmoplastic fibroma. Cancer. 1993;71:338-345.

88. Okada K, Frassica FJ, Sim FH, et al. Parosteal osteosarcoma. A clinicopathological study. J Bone Joint Surg Am. 1994;76:366-378.

89. Bertoni F, Bacchini P, Staals EL, Davidovitz P. Dedifferentiated parosteal osteosarcoma: the experience of the Rizzoli Institute. Cancer. 2005;103:2373-2382.

90. Agarwal M, Puri A, Anchan C, et al. Hemicortical excision for low-grade selected surface sarcomas of bone. Clin Orthop Relat Res. 2007;(459):161-166.

91. Unni KK, Dahlin DC, Beabout JW. Periosteal osteogenic sarcoma. Cancer. 1976;37:2476-2485.

92. Tabone MD, Terrier P, Pacquement H, et al. Outcome of radiation-related osteosarcoma after treatment of childhood and adolescent cancer: a study of 23 cases. J Clin Oncol. 1999;17: 2789-2795.

93. Shaheen M, Deheshi BM, Riad S, et al. Prognosis of radiation-induced bone sarcoma is similar to primary osteosarcoma. Clin Orthop Relat Res. 2006;(450):76-81.

94. Enneking WF, Spanier SS, Goodman MA. A system for the surgical staging of musculoskeletal sarcoma. Clin Orthop Relat Res. 1980;(153):106-120.

95. Broders AC. The microscopic grading of cancer. Surg Clin North Am. 1941;21:947-962.

96. Enneking WF, Spanier SS, Goodman MA. Current concepts review. The surgical staging of musculoskeletal sarcoma. J Bone Joint Surg Am. 1980;62:1027-1030.

97. Wolf RE, Enneking WF. The staging and surgery of musculoskeletal neoplasms. Orthop Clin North Am. 1996;27:473-481.

98. Mankin HJ, Hornicek FJ, Rosenberg AE, et al. Survival data for 648 patients with osteosarcoma treated at one institution. Clin Orthop Relat Res. 2004;(429):286-291.

99. Dahlin DC, Coventry MB. Osteogenic sarcoma. A study of six hundred cases. J Bone Joint Surg Am. 1967;49:101-110.

100. Jaffe N, Frei E III, Traggis D, Bishop Y. Adjuvant methotrexate and citrovorum-factor treatment of osteogenic sarcoma. N Engl J Med. 1974;291:994-997.

101. Meyers PA, Schwartz CL, Krailo M, et al. Osteosarcoma: a randomized, prospective trial of the addition of ifosfamide and/or muramyl tripeptide to cisplatin, doxorubicin, and high-dose methotrexate. J Clin Oncol. 2005;23:2004-2011.

102. Goorin AM, Schwartzentruber DJ, Devidas M, et al. Presurgical chemotherapy compared with immediate surgery and adjuvant chemotherapy for nonmetastatic osteosarcoma: Pediatric Oncology Group Study POG-8651. J Clin Oncol. 2003;21:1574-1580.

103. Meyers PA, Gorlick R, Heller G, et al. Intensification of preoperative chemotherapy for osteogenic sarcoma: results of the Memorial Sloan-Kettering (T12) protocol. J Clin Oncol. 1998;16: 2452-2458.

104. Ferrari S, Smeland S, Mercuri M, et al. Neoadjuvant chemotherapy with high-dose ifosfamide, high-dose methotrexate, cisplatin, and doxorubicin for patients with localized osteosarcoma of the extremity: a joint study by the Italian and Scandinavian Sarcoma Groups. J Clin Oncol. 2005;23:8845-8852.

105. Hawkins DS, Arndt CA. Pattern of disease recurrence and prognostic factors in patients with osteosarcoma treated with contemporary chemotherapy. Cancer. 2003;98:2447-2456.

106. Bacci G, Ferrari S, Bertoni F, et al. Long-term outcome for patients with nonmetastatic osteosarcoma of the extremity treated at the Istituto Ortopedico Rizzoli according to the Istituto Ortopedico Rizzoli/osteosarcoma-2 protocol: an updated report. J Clin Oncol. 2000;18:4016-4027.

107. Glasser DB, Lane JM, Huvos AG, et al. Survival, prognosis, and therapeutic response in osteogenic sarcoma. The Memorial Hospital experience. Cancer. 1992;69:698-708.

108. Eselgrim M, Grunert H, Kuhne T, et al. Dose intensity of chemotherapy for osteosarcoma and outcome in the Cooperative

Osteosarcoma Study Group (COSS) trials. Pediatr Blood Cancer. 2006;47:42-50.

109. Bacci G, Picci P, Ruggieri P, et al. Primary chemotherapy and delayed surgery (neoadjuvant chemotherapy) for osteosarcoma of the extremities. The Istituto Rizzoli Experience in 127 patients treated preoperatively with intravenous methotrexate (high versus moderate doses) and intraarterial cisplatin. Cancer. 1990;65:2539-2553.

110. Meyers PA, Heller G, Healey J, et al. Chemotherapy for non-metastatic osteogenic sarcoma: the Memorial Sloan-Kettering experience. J Clin Oncol. 1992;10:5-15.

111. Bieling P, Rehan N, Winkler P, et al. Tumor size and prognosis in aggressively treated osteosarcoma. J Clin Oncol. 1996;14:848-858.

112. Davis AM, Bell RS, Goodwin PJ. Prognostic factors in osteosarcoma: a critical review. J Clin Oncol. 1994;12:423-431.

113. Rosen G, Murphy ML, Huvos AG, et al. Chemotherapy, en bloc resection, and prosthetic bone replacement in the treatment of osteogenic sarcoma. Cancer. 1976;37:1-11.

114. Rosen G, Marcove RC, Caparros B, et al. Primary osteogenic sarcoma: the rationale for preoperative chemotherapy and delayed surgery. Cancer. 1979;43:2163-2177.

115. Winkler K, Beron G, Kotz R, et al. Neoadjuvant chemotherapy for osteogenic sarcoma: results of a Cooperative German/Austrian study. J Clin Oncol. 1984;2:617-624.

116. Winkler K, Beron G, Delling G, et al. Neoadjuvant chemotherapy of osteosarcoma: results of a randomized cooperative trial (COSS-82) with salvage chemotherapy based on histological tumor response. J Clin Oncol. 1988;6:329-337.

117. Bramwell VH, Burgers M, Sneath R, et al. A comparison of two short intensive adjuvant chemotherapy regimens in operable osteosarcoma of limbs in children and young adults: the first study of the European Osteosarcoma Intergroup. J Clin Oncol. 1992;10:1579-1591.

118. Krailo M, Ertel I, Makley J, et al. A randomized study comparing high-dose methotrexate with moderate-dose methotrexate as components of adjuvant chemotherapy in childhood nonmetastatic osteosarcoma: a report from the Childrens Cancer Study Group. Med Pediatr Oncol. 1987;15:69-77.

119. Goorin AM, Perez-Atayde A, Gebhardt M, et al. Weekly high-dose methotrexate and doxorubicin for osteosarcoma: the Dana-Farber Cancer Institute/the Children's Hospital—study III. J Clin Oncol. 1987;5:1178-1184.

120. Provisor AJ, Ettinger LJ, Nachman JB, et al. Treatment of non-metastatic osteosarcoma of the extremity with preoperative and postoperative chemotherapy: a report from the Children's Cancer Group. J Clin Oncol. 1997;15:76-84.

121. Fuchs N, Bielack SS, Epler D, et al. Long-term results of the co-operative German-Austrian-Swiss osteosarcoma study group's protocol COSS-86 of intensive multidrug chemotherapy and surgery for osteosarcoma of the limbs. Ann Oncol. 1998;9:893-899.

122. Edmonson JH, Green SJ, Ivins JC, et al. A controlled pilot study of high-dose methotrexate as postsurgical adjuvant treatment for primary osteosarcoma. J Clin Oncol. 1984;2:152-156.

123. Taylor WF, Ivins JC, Unni KK, et al. Prognostic variables in osteosarcoma: a multi-institutional study. J Natl Cancer Inst. 1989;81:21-30.

124. Hudson M, Jaffe MR, Jaffe N, et al. Pediatric osteosarcoma: therapeutic strategies, results, and prognostic factors derived from a 10-year experience. J Clin Oncol. 1990;8:1988-1997.

125. Khanna C, Wan X, Bose S, et al. The membrane-cytoskeleton linker ezrin is necessary for osteosarcoma metastasis. Nat Med. 2004;10:182-186.

126. Gorlick R, Huvos AG, Heller G, et al. Expression of HER2/erbB-2 correlates with survival in osteosarcoma. J Clin Oncol. 1999;17:2781-2788.

127. Feugeas O, Guriec N, Babin-Boilletot A, et al. Loss of heterozygosity of the RB gene is a poor prognostic factor in patients with osteosarcoma. J Clin Oncol. 1996;14:467-472.

128. Bacci G, Longhi A, Cesari M, et al. Influence of local recurrence on survival in patients with extremity osteosarcoma treated with neoadjuvant chemotherapy: the experience of a single institution with 44 patients. Cancer. 2006;106:2701-2706.

129. Mialou V, Philip T, Kalifa C, et al. Metastatic osteosarcoma at diagnosis: prognostic factors and long-term outcome—the French pediatric experience. Cancer. 2005;104:1100-1109.

130. Goorin AM, Harris MB, Bernstein M, et al. Phase II/III trial of etoposide and high-dose ifosfamide in newly diagnosed metastatic osteosarcoma: a pediatric oncology group trial. J Clin Oncol. 2002;20:426-433.

131. Bridge JA, Nelson M, McComb E, et al. Cytogenetic findings in 73 osteosarcoma specimens and a review of the literature. Cancer Genet Cytogenet. 1997;95:74-87.

132. Fletcher JA, Gebhardt MC, Kozakewich HP. Cytogenetic aberrations in osteosarcomas. Nonrandom deletions, rings, and double-minute chromosomes. Cancer Genet Cytogenet. 1994;77:81-88.

133. Sandberg AA, Bridge JA. Updates on the cytogenetics and molecular genetics of bone and soft tissue tumors: osteosarcoma and related tumors. Cancer Genet Cytogenet. 2003;145:1-30.

134. Bayani J, Zielenska M, Pandita A, et al. Spectral karyotyping identifies recurrent complex rearrangements of chromosomes 8, 17, and 20 in osteosarcomas. Genes Chromosomes Cancer. 2003;36:7-16.

135. Tarkkanen M, Elomaa I, Blomqvist C, et al. DNA sequence copy number increase at 8q: a potential new prognostic marker in high-grade osteosarcoma. Int J Cancer. 1999;84:114-121.

136. Ozaki T, Schaefer KL, Wai D, et al. Genetic imbalances revealed by comparative genomic hybridization in osteosarcomas. Int J Cancer. 2002;102:355-365.

137. Lau CC, Harris CP, Lu XY, et al. Frequent amplification and rearrangement of chromosomal bands 6p12-p21 and 17p11.2 in osteosarcoma. Genes Chromosomes Cancer. 2004;39:11-21.

138. Zielenska M, Bayani J, Pandita A, et al. Comparative genomic hybridization analysis identifies gains of 1p35 approximately p36 and chromosome 19 in osteosarcoma. Cancer Genet Cytogenet. 2001;130:14-21.

139. Stock C, Kager L, Fink FM, et al. Chromosomal regions involved in the pathogenesis of osteosarcomas. Genes Chromosomes Cancer. 2000;28:329-336.

140. Gisselsson D, Palsson E, Hoglund M, et al. Differentially amplified chromosome 12 sequences in low- and high-grade osteosarcoma. Genes Chromosomes Cancer. 2002;33:133-140.

141. van Dartel M, Cornelissen PW, Redeker S, et al. Amplification of 17p11.2 approximately p12, including PMP22, TOP3A, and MAPK7, in high-grade osteosarcoma. Cancer Genet Cytogenet. 2002;139:91-96.

142. Man TK, Lu XY, Jaeweon K, et al. Genome-wide array comparative genomic hybridization analysis reveals distinct amplifications in osteosarcoma. BMC Cancer. 2004;4:45.

143. Pompetti F, Rizzo P, Simon RM, et al. Oncogene alterations in primary, recurrent, and metastatic human bone tumors. J Cell Biochem. 1996;63:37-50.

144. Ladanyi M, Park CK, Lewis R, et al. Sporadic amplification of the MYC gene in human osteosarcomas. Diagn Mol Pathol. 1993;2:163-167.

145. Gamberi G, Benassi MS, Bohling T, et al. C-myc and c-fos in human osteosarcoma: prognostic value of mRNA and protein expression. Oncology. 1998;55:556-563.

146. Patel JH, Loboda AP, Showe MK, et al. Analysis of genomic targets reveals complex functions of MYC. Nat Rev Cancer. 2004;4:562-568.

147. Pelengaris S, Khan M, Evan G. c-MYC: more than just a matter of life and death. Nat Rev Cancer. 2002;2:764-776.

148. Corson TW, Gallie BL. One hit, two hits, three hits, more? Genomic changes in the development of retinoblastoma. Genes Chromosomes Cancer. 2007;46:617-634.

149. Richter S, Vandezande K, Chen N, et al. Sensitive and efficient detection of RB1 gene mutations enhances care for families with retinoblastoma. Am J Hum Genet. 2003;72:253-269.

150. Draper GJ, Sanders BM, Kingston JE. Second primary neoplasms in patients with retinoblastoma. Br J Cancer. 1986;53:661-671.

151. Cavenee WK, Hansen MF, Nordenskjold M, et al. Genetic origin of mutations predisposing to retinoblastoma. Science. 1985;228:501-503.

152. Cavenee WK, Dryja TP, Phillips RA, et al. Expression of recessive alleles by chromosomal mechanisms in retinoblastoma. Nature. 1983;305:779-784.

153. Toguchida J, Ishizaki K, Sasaki MS, et al. Chromosomal reorganization for the expression of recessive mutation of retinoblastoma susceptibility gene in the development of osteoblastoma. Cancer Res. 1988;48:3939-3943.

154. Wunder JS, Czitrom AA, Kandel R, Andrulis IL. Analysis of alterations in the retinoblastoma gene and tumor grade in bone and soft-tissue sarcomas. J Natl Cancer Inst. 1991;83:194-200.

155. Friend SH, Horowitz JM, Gerber MR, et al. Deletions of a DNA sequence in retinoblastomas and mesenchymal tumors: organization of the sequence and its encoded protein. Proc Natl Acad Sci U S A. 1987;84:9059-9063.

156. Toguchida J, Ishizaki K, Sasaki MS, et al. Preferential mutation of paternally derived RB gene as the initial event in sporadic osteosarcoma. Nature. 1989;338:156-158.

157. Benassi MS, Molendini L, Gamberi G, et al. Alteration of pRb/p16/cdk4 regulation in human osteosarcoma. Int J Cancer. 1999;84:489-493.

158. Heinsohn S, Evermann U, Zur SU, et al. Determination of the prognostic value of loss of heterozygosity at the retinoblastoma gene in osteosarcoma. Int J Oncol. 2007;30:1205-1214.

159. Li W, Fan J, Hochhauser D, et al. Lack of functional retinoblastoma protein mediates increased resistance to antimetabolites in human sarcoma cell lines. Proc Natl Acad Sci U S A. 1995;92:10436-10440.

160. Classon M, Harlow E. The retinoblastoma tumour suppressor in development and cancer. Nat Rev Cancer. 2002;2:910-917.

161. Khidr L, Chen PL. Rb, the conductor that orchestrates life, death and differentiation. Oncogene. 2006;25:5210-5219.

162. Nguyen DX, McCance DJ. Role of the retinoblastoma tumor suppressor protein in cellular differentiation. J Cell Biochem. 2005;94:870-879.

163. Wu L, de BA, Saavedra HI, et al. Extra-embryonic function of Rb is essential for embryonic development and viability. Nature. 2003;421:942-947.

164. Thomas DM, Carty SA, Piscopo DM, et al. The retinoblastoma protein acts as a transcriptional coactivator required for osteogenic differentiation. Mol Cell. 2001;8:303-316.

165. Malkin D, Jolly KW, Barbier N, et al. Germline mutations of the p53 tumor-suppressor gene in children and young adults with second malignant neoplasms. N Engl J Med. 1992;326:1309-1315.

166. Varley JM. Germline TP53 mutations and Li-Fraumeni syndrome. Hum Mutat. 2003;21:313-320.

167. Malkin D, Li FP, Strong LC, et al. Germ line p53 mutations in a familial syndrome of breast cancer, sarcomas, and other neoplasms. Science. 1990;250:1233-1238.

168. Miller CW, Aslo A, Won A, et al. Alterations of the p53, Rb and MDM2 genes in osteosarcoma. J Cancer Res Clin Oncol. 1996;122:559-565.

169. Miller CW, Aslo A, Tsay C, et al. Frequency and structure of p53 rearrangements in human osteosarcoma. Cancer Res. 1990;50:7950-7954.

170. Masuda H, Miller C, Koeffler HP, et al. Rearrangement of the p53 gene in human osteogenic sarcomas. Proc Natl Acad Sci U S A. 1987;84:7716-7719.

171. Toguchida J, Yamaguchi T, Ritchie B, et al. Mutation spectrum of the p53 gene in bone and soft tissue sarcomas. Cancer Res. 1992;52:6194-6199.

172. Gokgoz N, Wunder JS, Mousses S, et al. Comparison of p53 mutations in patients with localized osteosarcoma and metastatic osteosarcoma. Cancer. 2001;92:2181-2189.

173. Patino-Garcia A, Sierrasesumaga L. Analysis of the p16INK4 and TP53 tumor suppressor genes in bone sarcoma pediatric patients. Cancer Genet Cytogenet. 1997;98:50-55.

174. Tsuchiya T, Sekine K, Hinohara S, et al. Analysis of the p16INK4, p14ARF, p15, TP53, and MDM2 genes and their prognostic implications in osteosarcoma and Ewing sarcoma. Cancer Genet Cytogenet. 2000;120:91-98.

175. Lonardo F, Ueda T, Huvos AG, et al. p53 and MDM2 alterations in osteosarcomas: correlation with clinicopathologic features and proliferative rate. Cancer. 1997;79:1541-1547.

176. McIntyre JF, Smith-Sorensen B, Friend SH, et al. Germline mutations of the p53 tumor suppressor gene in children with osteosarcoma. J Clin Oncol. 1994;12:925-930.

177. Toguchida J, Yamaguchi T, Dayton SH, et al. Prevalence and spectrum of germline mutations of the p53 gene among patients with sarcoma. N Engl J Med. 1992;326:1301-1308.

178. Petitjean A, Achatz MI, Borresen-Dale AL, et al. TP53 mutations in human cancers: functional selection and impact on cancer prognosis and outcomes. Oncogene. 2007;26:2157-2165.

179. Levine AJ. p53, the cellular gatekeeper for growth and division. Cell. 1997;88:323-331.

179a. Walkley CR, Qudsi R, Sankaran VG, et al. Conditional mouse osteosarcoma, dependent on p53 loss and potentiated by loss of Rb, mimics the human disease. Genes Dev. 2008;22:1662-1676.

179b. Berman SD, Calo E, Landman AS, et al. Metastatic osteosarcoma induced by inactivation of Rb and p53 in the osteoblast lineage. PNAS. 2008;105:1851-1856.

180. Donehower LA, Harvey M, Slagle BL, et al. Mice deficient for p53 are developmentally normal but susceptible to spontaneous tumours. Nature. 1992;356:215-221.

181. Jacks T, Remington L, Williams BO, et al. Tumor spectrum analysis in p53-mutant mice. Curr Biol. 1994;4:1-7.

182. Olive KP, Tuveson DA, Ruhe ZC, et al. Mutant p53 gain of function in two mouse models of Li-Fraumeni syndrome. Cell. 2004;119:847-860.

183. Liu G, McDonnell TJ, Montes de Oca LR, et al. High metastatic potential in mice inheriting a targeted p53 missense mutation. Proc Natl Acad Sci U S A. 2000;97:4174-4179.

184. Lavigueur A, Maltby V, Mock D, et al. High incidence of lung, bone, and lymphoid tumors in transgenic mice overexpressing mutant alleles of the p53 oncogene. Mol Cell Biol. 1989;9:3982-3991.

185. Knowles BB, McCarrick J, Fox N, et al. Osteosarcomas in transgenic mice expressing an alpha-amylase-SV40 T-antigen hybrid gene. Am J Pathol. 1990;137:259-262.

186. Wilkie TM, Schmidt RA, Baetscher M, Messing A. Smooth muscle and bone neoplasms in transgenic mice expressing SV40 T antigen. Oncogene. 1994;9:2889-2895.

187. Aqeilan RI, Trapasso F, Hussain S, et al. Targeted deletion of Wwox reveals a tumor suppressor function. Proc Natl Acad Sci U S A. 2007;104:3949-3954.

188. Jain M, Arvanitis C, Chu K, et al. Sustained loss of a neoplastic phenotype by brief inactivation of MYC. Science. 2002;297:102-104.

189. Wunder JS, Gokgoz N, Parkes R, et al. TP53 mutations and outcome in osteosarcoma: a prospective, multicenter study. J Clin Oncol. 2005;23:1483-1490.

190. Pakos EE, Kyzas PA, Ioannidis JP. Prognostic significance of TP53 tumor suppressor gene expression and mutations in human

osteosarcoma: a meta-analysis. Clin Cancer Res. 2004;10:6208-6214.

191. Vogelstein B, Lane D, Levine AJ. Surfing the p53 network. Nature. 2000;408:307-310.

192. Haupt Y, Maya R, Kazaz A, Oren M. Mdm2 promotes the rapid degradation of p53. Nature. 1997;387:296-299.

193. Kubbutat MH, Jones SN, Vousden KH. Regulation of p53 stability by Mdm2. Nature. 1997;387:299-303.

194. Fuchs SY, Adler V, Buschmann T, et al. Mdm2 association with p53 targets its ubiquitination. Oncogene. 1998;17:2543-2547.

195. arcon-Vargas D, Ronai Z. p53-Mdm2—the affair that never ends. Carcinogenesis. 2002;23:541-547.

196. Oliner JD, Kinzler KW, Meltzer PS, et al. Amplification of a gene encoding a p53-associated protein in human sarcomas. Nature. 1992;358:80-83.

197. Ladanyi M, Cha C, Lewis R, et al. MDM2 gene amplification in metastatic osteosarcoma. Cancer Res. 1993;53:16-18.

198. Momand J, Jung D, Wilczynski S, Niland J. The MDM2 gene amplification database. Nucleic Acids Res. 1998;26:3453-3459.

199. Wunder JS, Eppert K, Burrow SR, et al. Co-amplification and overexpression of CDK4, SAS and MDM2 occurs frequently in human parosteal osteosarcomas. Oncogene. 1999;18:783-788.

200. Ragazzini P, Gamberi G, Benassi MS, et al. Analysis of SAS gene and CDK4 and MDM2 proteins in low-grade osteosarcoma. Cancer Detect Prev. 1999;23:129-136.

201. Bech-Otschir D, Kraft R, Huang X, et al. COP9 signalosome-specific phosphorylation targets p53 to degradation by the ubiquitin system. EMBO J. 2001;20:1630-1639.

202. Henriksen J, Aagesen TH, Maelandsmo GM, et al. Amplification and overexpression of COPS3 in osteosarcomas potentially target TP53 for proteasome-mediated degradation. Oncogene. 2003;22:5358-5361.

203. Yan T, Wunder JS, Gokgoz N, et al. COPS3 amplification and clinical outcome in osteosarcoma. Cancer. 2007;109:1870-1876.

204. Nielsen GP, Burns KL, Rosenberg AE, Louis DN. CDKN2A gene deletions and loss of p16 expression occur in osteosarcomas that lack RB alterations. Am J Pathol. 1998;153:159-163.

205. Maitra A, Roberts H, Weinberg AG, Geradts J. Loss of p16(INK4a) expression correlates with decreased survival in pediatric osteosarcomas. Int J Cancer. 2001;95:34-38.

206. Park YB, Park MJ, Kimura K, et al. Alterations in the INK4a/ARF locus and their effects on the growth of human osteosarcoma cell lines. Cancer Genet Cytogenet. 2002;133:105-111.

207. Sherr CJ. Divorcing ARF and p53: an unsettled case. Nat Rev Cancer. 2006;6:663-673.

208. Nishijo K, Nakayama T, Aoyama T, et al. Mutation analysis of the RECQL4 gene in sporadic osteosarcomas. Int J Cancer. 2004;111:367-372.

209. Kitao S, Shimamoto A, Goto M, et al. Mutations in RECQL4 cause a subset of cases of Rothmund-Thomson syndrome. Nat Genet. 1999;22:82-84.

210. Wang LL, Levy ML, Lewis RA, et al. Clinical manifestations in a cohort of 41 Rothmund-Thomson syndrome patients. Am J Med Genet. 2001;102:11-17.

211. Ellis NA, Groden J, Ye TZ, et al. The Bloom's syndrome gene product is homologous to RecQ helicases. Cell. 1995;83:655-666.

212. Yu CE, Oshima J, Fu YH, et al. Positional cloning of the Werner's syndrome gene. Science. 1996;272:258-262.

213. Mann MB, Hodges CA, Barnes E, et al. Defective sister-chromatid cohesion, aneuploidy and cancer predisposition in a mouse model of type II Rothmund-Thomson syndrome. Hum Mol Genet. 2005;14:813-825.

214. Hickson ID. RecQ helicases: caretakers of the genome. Nat Rev Cancer. 2003;3:169-178.

215. Sangrithi MN, Bernal JA, Madine M, et al. Initiation of DNA replication requires the RECQL4 protein mutated in Rothmund-Thomson syndrome. Cell. 2005;121:887-898.

216. Eller MS, Liao X, Liu S, et al. A role for WRN in telomere-based DNA damage responses. Proc Natl Acad Sci U S A. 2006;103:15073-15078.

217. Rhim JS, Park DK, Arnstein P, et al. Transformation of human cells in culture by N-methyl-N′-nitro-N-nitrosoguanidine. Nature. 1975;256:751-753.

218. Cooper CS, Park M, Blair DG, et al. Molecular cloning of a new transforming gene from a chemically transformed human cell line. Nature. 1984;311:29-33.

219. Park M, Dean M, Cooper CS, et al. Mechanism of met oncogene activation. Cell. 1986;45:895-904.

220. Scotlandi K, Baldini N, Oliviero M, et al. Expression of Met/hepatocyte growth factor receptor gene and malignant behavior of musculoskeletal tumors. Am J Pathol. 1996;149:1209-1219.

221. Ferracini R, Di Renzo MF, Scotlandi K, et al. The Met/HGF receptor is over-expressed in human osteosarcomas and is activated by either a paracrine or an autocrine circuit. Oncogene. 1995;10:739-749.

222. Oda Y, Naka T, Takeshita M, et al. Comparison of histological changes and changes in nm23 and c-MET expression between primary and metastatic sites in osteosarcoma: a clinicopathologic and immunohistochemical study. Hum Pathol. 2000;31:709-716.

223. Wallenius V, Hisaoka M, Helou K, et al. Overexpression of the hepatocyte growth factor (HGF) receptor (Met) and presence of a truncated and activated intracellular HGF receptor fragment in locally aggressive/malignant human musculoskeletal tumors. Am J Pathol. 2000;156:821-829.

224. Patane S, Avnet S, Coltella N, et al. MET overexpression turns human primary osteoblasts into osteosarcomas. Cancer Res. 2006;66:4750-4757.

225. Ferracini R, Angelini P, Cagliero E, et al. MET oncogene aberrant expression in canine osteosarcoma. J Orthop Res. 2000;18:253-256.

226. MacEwen EG, Kutzke J, Carew J, et al. c-Met tyrosine kinase receptor expression and function in human and canine osteosarcoma cells. Clin Exp Metastasis. 2003;20:421-430.

227. Coltella N, Manara MC, Cerisano V, et al. Role of the MET/HGF receptor in proliferation and invasive behavior of osteosarcoma. FASEB J. 2003;17:1162-1164.

228. Trusolino L, Comoglio PM. Scatter-factor and semaphorin receptors: cell signalling for invasive growth. Nat Rev Cancer. 2002;2:289-300.

229. Finkel MP, Biskis BO, Jinkins PB. Virus induction of osteosarcomas in mice. Science. 1966;151:698-701.

230. Van Beveren C, van Straaten F, Curran T, et al. Analysis of FBJ-MuSV provirus and c-fos (mouse) gene reveals that viral and cellular fos gene products have different carboxy termini. Cell. 1983;32:1241-1255.

231. Miller AD, Curran T, Verma IM. c-fos protein can induce cellular transformation: a novel mechanism of activation of a cellular oncogene. Cell. 1984;36:51-60.

232. Grigoriadis AE, Schellander K, Wang ZQ, Wagner EF. Osteoblasts are target cells for transformation in c-fos transgenic mice. J Cell Biol. 1993;122:685-701.

233. Ruther U, Komitowski D, Schubert FR, Wagner EF. c-fos expression induces bone tumors in transgenic mice. Oncogene. 1989;4:861-865.

234. Wu JX, Carpenter PM, Gresens C, et al. The proto-oncogene c-fos is over-expressed in the majority of human osteosarcomas. Oncogene. 1990;5:989-1000.

235. Franchi A, Calzolari A, Zampi G. Immunohistochemical detection of c-fos and c-jun expression in osseous and cartilaginous tumours of the skeleton. Virchows Arch. 1998;432:515-519.

236. Sunters A, Thomas DP, Yeudall WA, Grigoriadis AE. Accelerated cell cycle progression in osteoblasts overexpressing the c-fos proto-oncogene: induction of cyclin A and enhanced CDK2 activity. J Biol Chem. 2004;279:9882-9891.

237. Wagner EF. Functions of AP1 (Fos/Jun) in bone development. Ann Rheum Dis. 2002;61(suppl 2):ii40-ii42.

238. Johnson RS, Spiegelman BM, Papaioannou V. Pleiotropic effects of a null mutation in the c-fos proto-oncogene. Cell. 1992;71: 577-586.

239. Wang ZQ, Ovitt C, Grigoriadis AE, et al. Bone and haematopoietic defects in mice lacking c-fos. Nature. 1992;360:741-745.

240. Tjalma RA. Canine bone sarcoma: estimation of relative risk as a function of body size. J Natl Cancer Inst. 1966;36:1137-1150.

241. Larsson O, Girnita A, Girnita L. Role of insulin-like growth factor 1 receptor signalling in cancer. Br J Cancer. 2005;92:2097-2101.

242. Sutter NB, Bustamante CD, Chase K, et al. A single IGF1 allele is a major determinant of small size in dogs. Science. 2007; 316:112-115.

243. Liu JP, Baker J, Perkins AS, et al. Mice carrying null mutations of the genes encoding insulin-like growth factor I (Igf-1) and type 1 IGF receptor (Igf1r). Cell. 1993;75:59-72.

244. Abuzzahab MJ, Schneider A, Goddard A, et al. IGF-I receptor mutations resulting in intrauterine and postnatal growth retardation. N Engl J Med. 2003;349:2211-2222.

245. Kawashima Y, Kanzaki S, Yang F, et al. Mutation at cleavage site of insulin-like growth factor receptor in a short-stature child born with intrauterine growth retardation. J Clin Endocrinol Metab. 2005;90:4679-4687.

246. Pollak MN, Polychronakos C, Richard M. Insulin like growth factor I: a potent mitogen for human osteogenic sarcoma. J Natl Cancer Inst. 1990;82:301-305.

247. Scotlandi K, Manara MC, Nicoletti G, et al. Antitumor activity of the insulin-like growth factor-I receptor kinase inhibitor NVP-AEW541 in musculoskeletal tumors. Cancer Res. 2005;65: 3868-3876.

248. Braczkowski R, Schally AV, Plonowski A, et al. Inhibition of proliferation in human MNNG/HOS osteosarcoma and SK-ES-1 Ewing sarcoma cell lines in vitro and in vivo by antagonists of growth hormone-releasing hormone: effects on insulin-like growth factor II. Cancer. 2002;95:1735-1745.

249. Kappel CC, Velez-Yanguas MC, Hirschfeld S, Helman LJ. Human osteosarcoma cell lines are dependent on insulin-like growth factor I for in vitro growth. Cancer Res. 1994;54: 2803-2807.

250. Raile K, Hoflich A, Kessler U, et al. Human osteosarcoma (U-2 OS) cells express both insulin-like growth factor-I (IGF-I) receptors and insulin-like growth factor-II/mannose-6-phosphate (IGF-II/M6P) receptors and synthesize IGF-II: autocrine growth stimulation by IGF-II via the IGF-I receptor. J Cell Physiol. 1994;159:531-541.

251. Rosato R, Gerland K, Jammes H, et al. The IGFBP-3 mRNA and protein levels are IGF-I-dependent and GH-independent in MG-63 human osteosarcoma cells. Mol Cell Endocrinol. 2001;175:15-27.

252. Pasello M, Hattinger CM, Stoico G, et al. 4-Demethoxy-3′-deamino-3′-aziridinyl-4′-methylsulphonyl-daunorubicin (PNU-159548): a promising new candidate for chemotherapeutic treatment of osteosarcoma patients. Eur J Cancer. 2005;41: 2184-2195.

253. Maloney EK, McLaughlin JL, Dagdigian NE, et al. An anti-insulin-like growth factor I receptor antibody that is a potent inhibitor of cancer cell proliferation. Cancer Res. 2003;63: 5073-5083.

254. Velez-Yanguas MC, Kalebic T, Maggi M, et al. 1-alpha, 25-dihydroxy-16-ene-23-yne-26,27-hexafluorocholecalciferol (Ro24-5531) modulation of insulin-like growth factor-binding protein-3 and induction of differentiation and growth arrest in a human osteosarcoma cell line. J Clin Endocrinol Metab. 1996;81:93-99.

255. Schneider MR, Zhou R, Hoeflich A, et al. Insulin-like growth factor-binding protein-5 inhibits growth and induces differentia-

tion of mouse osteosarcoma cells. Biochem Biophys Res Commun. 2001;288:435-442.

256. Pollak M, Sem AW, Richard M, et al. Inhibition of metastatic behavior of murine osteosarcoma by hypophysectomy. J Natl Cancer Inst. 1992;84:966-971.

257. Rodriguez-Galindo C, Poquette CA, Daw NC, et al. Circulating concentrations of IGF-I and IGFBP-3 are not predictive of incidence or clinical behavior of pediatric osteosarcoma. Med Pediatr Oncol. 2001;36:605-611.

258. Seshadri R, Firgaira FA, Horsfall DJ, et al. Clinical significance of HER-2/neu oncogene amplification in primary breast cancer. The South Australian Breast Cancer Study Group. J Clin Oncol. 1993;11:1936-1942.

259. Muss HB, Thor AD, Berry DA, et al. c-erbB-2 expression and response to adjuvant therapy in women with node-positive early breast cancer. N Engl J Med. 1994;330:1260-1266.

260. Slamon DJ, Leyland-Jones B, Shak S, et al. Use of chemotherapy plus a monoclonal antibody against HER2 for metastatic breast cancer that overexpresses HER2. N Engl J Med. 2001;344: 783-792.

261. Onda M, Matsuda S, Higaki S, et al. ErbB-2 expression is correlated with poor prognosis for patients with osteosarcoma. Cancer. 1996;77:71-78.

262. Zhou H, Randall RL, Brothman AR, et al. Her-2/neu expression in osteosarcoma increases risk of lung metastasis and can be associated with gene amplification. J Pediatr Hematol Oncol. 2003;25:27-32.

263. Somers GR, Ho M, Zielenska M, et al. HER2 amplification and overexpression is not present in pediatric osteosarcoma: a tissue microarray study. Pediatr Dev Pathol. 2005;8:525-532.

264. Maitra A, Wanzer D, Weinberg AG, Ashfaq R. Amplification of the HER-2/neu oncogene is uncommon in pediatric osteosarcomas. Cancer. 2001;92:677-683.

265. Akatsuka T, Wada T, Kokai Y, et al. ErbB2 expression is correlated with increased survival of patients with osteosarcoma. Cancer. 2002;94:1397-1404.

266. Ebb D, Meyers P, Devidas M. Study Committee Progress Report AOST0121. Children's Oncology Group 10-1-2007.

267. Bleul CC, Fuhlbrigge RC, Casasnovas JM, et al. A highly efficacious lymphocyte chemoattractant, stromal cell-derived factor 1 (SDF-1). J Exp Med. 1996;184:1101-1109.

268. Gupta SK, Lysko PG, Pillarisetti K, et al. Chemokine receptors in human endothelial cells. Functional expression of CXCR4 and its transcriptional regulation by inflammatory cytokines. J Biol Chem. 1998;273:4282-4287.

269. Taichman RS, Cooper C, Keller ET, et al. Use of the stromal cell-derived factor-1/CXCR4 pathway in prostate cancer metastasis to bone. Cancer Res. 2002;62:1832-1837.

270. Libura J, Drukala J, Majka M, et al. CXCR4-SDF-1 signaling is active in rhabdomyosarcoma cells and regulates locomotion, chemotaxis, and adhesion. Blood. 2002;100:2597-2606.

271. Corcione A, Ottonello L, Tortolina G, et al. Stromal cell-derived factor-1 as a chemoattractant for follicular center lymphoma B cells. J Natl Cancer Inst. 2000;92:628-635.

272. Laverdiere C, Gorlick R. CXCR4 expression in osteosarcoma cell lines and tumor samples: evidence for expression by tumor cells. Clin Cancer Res. 2006;12:5254.

273. Laverdiere C, Hoang BH, Yang R, et al. Messenger RNA expression levels of CXCR4 correlate with metastatic behavior and outcome in patients with osteosarcoma. Clin Cancer Res. 2005;11:2561-2567.

274. Perissinotto E, Cavalloni G, Leone F, et al. Involvement of chemokine receptor 4/stromal cell-derived factor 1 system during osteosarcoma tumor progression. Clin Cancer Res. 2005;11:490-497.

275. Khanna C, Khan J, Nguyen P, et al. Metastasis-associated differences in gene expression in a murine model of osteosarcoma. Cancer Res. 2001;61:3750-3759.

276. Khanna C, Prehn J, Yeung C, et al. An orthotopic model of murine osteosarcoma with clonally related variants differing in pulmonary metastatic potential. Clin Exp Metastasis. 2000;18: 261-271.

277. Rong S, Jeffers M, Resau JH, et al. Met expression and sarcoma tumorigenicity. Cancer Res. 1993;53:5355-5360.

278. Mehlen P, Puisieux A. Metastasis: a question of life or death. Nat Rev Cancer. 2006;6:449-458.

279. Lafleur EA, Jia SF, Worth LL, et al. Interleukin (IL)-12 and IL-12 gene transfer up-regulate Fas expression in human osteosarcoma and breast cancer cells. Cancer Res. 2001;61:4066-4071.

280. Lafleur EA, Koshkina NV, Stewart J, et al. Increased Fas expression reduces the metastatic potential of human osteosarcoma cells. Clin Cancer Res. 2004;10:8114-8119.

281. Duan X, Jia SF, Koshkina N, Kleinerman ES. Intranasal interleukin-12 gene therapy enhanced the activity of ifosfamide against osteosarcoma lung metastases. Cancer. 2006;106:1382-1388.

282. Jia SF, Worth LL, Densmore CL, et al. Aerosol gene therapy with PEI: IL-12 eradicates osteosarcoma lung metastases. Clin Cancer Res. 2003;9:3462-3468.

283. Jia SF, Worth LL, Densmore CL, et al. Eradication of osteosarcoma lung metastases following intranasal interleukin-12 gene therapy using a nonviral polyethylenimine vector. Cancer Gene Ther. 2002;9:260-266.

284. Worth LL, Jia SF, Zhou Z, et al. Intranasal therapy with an adenoviral vector containing the murine interleukin-12 gene eradicates osteosarcoma lung metastases. Clin Cancer Res. 2000;6:3713-3718.

285. Gordon N, Arndt CA, Hawkins DS, et al. Fas expression in lung metastasis from osteosarcoma patients. J Pediatr Hematol Oncol. 2005;27:611-615.

286. Cho HJ, Lee TS, Park JB, et al. Disulfiram suppresses invasive ability of osteosarcoma cells via the inhibition of MMP-2 and MMP-9 expression. J Biochem Mol Biol. 2007;40:1069-1076.

287. Baldini N, Scotlandi K, Barbanti-Brodano G, et al. Expression of P-glycoprotein in high-grade osteosarcomas in relation to clinical outcome. N Engl J Med. 1995;333:1380-1385.

288. Serra M, Scotlandi K, Reverter-Branchat G, et al. Value of P-glycoprotein and clinicopathologic factors as the basis for new treatment strategies in high-grade osteosarcoma of the extremities. J Clin Oncol. 2003;21:536-542.

289. Chan HS, Grogan TM, Haddad G, et al. P-glycoprotein expression: critical determinant in the response to osteosarcoma chemotherapy. J Natl Cancer Inst. 1997;89:1706-1715.

290. Hornicek FJ, Gebhardt MC, Wolfe MW, et al. P-glycoprotein levels predict poor outcome in patients with osteosarcoma. Clin Orthop Relat Res. 2000;(373):11-17.

291. Park YB, Kim HS, Oh JH, Lee SH. The co-expression of p53 protein and P-glycoprotein is correlated to a poor prognosis in osteosarcoma. Int Orthop. 2001;24:307-310.

292. Yamamoto O, Wada T, Takahashi M, et al. Prognostic value of P-glycoprotein expression in bone and soft-tissue sarcoma. Int J Clin Oncol. 2000;5:164-170.

293. Pakos EE, Ioannidis JP. The association of P-glycoprotein with response to chemotherapy and clinical outcome in patients with osteosarcoma. A meta-analysis. Cancer. 2003;98:581-589.

294. Schwartz CL, Gorlick R, Teot L, et al. Multiple drug resistance in osteogenic sarcoma: INT0133 from the Children's Oncology Group. J Clin Oncol. 2007;25:2057-2062.

295. Wunder JS, Bell RS, Wold L, Andrulis IL. Expression of the multidrug resistance gene in osteosarcoma: a pilot study. J Orthop Res. 1993;11:396-403.

296. Wunder JS, Bull SB, Aneliunas V et al. MDR1 gene expression and outcome in osteosarcoma: a prospective, multicenter study. J Clin Oncol. 2000;18:2685-2694.

297. Meyers PA, Gorlick R. Osteosarcoma. Pediatr Clin North Am. 1997;44:973-989.

298. Guo W, Healey JH, Meyers PA, et al. Mechanisms of methotrexate resistance in osteosarcoma. Clin Cancer Res. 1999;5: 621-627.

299. Ochi K, Daigo Y, Katagiri T, et al. Prediction of response to neoadjuvant chemotherapy for osteosarcoma by gene-expression profiles. Int J Oncol. 2004;24:647-655.

300. Mintz MB, Sowers R, Brown KM, et al. An expression signature classifies chemotherapy-resistant pediatric osteosarcoma. Cancer Res. 2005;65:1748-1754.

301. Man TK, Chintagumpala M, Visvanathan J, et al. Expression profiles of osteosarcoma that can predict response to chemotherapy. Cancer Res. 2005;65:8142-8150.

302. Jaffe N, Carrasco H, Raymond K, et al. Can cure in patients with osteosarcoma be achieved exclusively with chemotherapy and abrogation of surgery? Cancer. 2002;95:2202-2210.

303. Grimer RJ, Taminiau AM, Cannon SR. Surgical outcomes in osteosarcoma. J Bone Joint Surg Br. 2002;84:395-400.

304. Picci P, Sangiorgi L, Rougraff BT, et al. Relationship of chemotherapy-induced necrosis and surgical margins to local recurrence in osteosarcoma. J Clin Oncol. 1994;12:2699-2705.

305. Grimer RJ. Surgical options for children with osteosarcoma. Lancet Oncol. 2005;6:85-92.

306. Cortes EP, Holland JF, Wang JJ, et al. Amputation and adriamycin in primary osteosarcoma. N Engl J Med. 1974;291:998-1000.

307. Ettinger LJ, Douglass HO Jr, Higby DJ, et al. Adjuvant adriamycin and cis-diamminedichloroplatinum (cis-platinum) in primary osteosarcoma. Cancer. 1981;47:248-254.

308. Sutow WW, Sullivan MP, Fernbach DJ, et al. Adjuvant chemotherapy in primary treatment of osteogenic sarcoma. A Southwest Oncology Group study. Cancer. 1975;36:1598-1602.

309. Lange B, Kramer S, Gregg JR, et al. High-dose methotrexate and adriamycin in osteogenic sarcoma: the children's hospital of Philadelphia study. Am J Clin Oncol. 1982;5:3-8.

310. Taylor WF, Ivins JC, Dahlin DC, et al. Trends and variability in survival from osteosarcoma. Mayo Clin Proc. 1978;53:695-700.

311. Lange B, Levine AS. Is it ethical not to conduct a prospectively controlled trial of adjuvant chemotherapy in osteosarcoma? Cancer Treat Rep. 1982;66:1699-1704.

312. Link MP, Goorin AM, Miser AW, et al. The effect of adjuvant chemotherapy on relapse-free survival in patients with osteosarcoma of the extremity. N Engl J Med. 1986;314:1600-1606.

313. Eilber F, Giuliano A, Eckardt J, et al. Adjuvant chemotherapy for osteosarcoma: a randomized prospective trial. J Clin Oncol. 1987;5:21-26.

314. Ochs JJ, Freeman AI, Douglass HO Jr, et al. cis-Dichlorodiammineplatinum (II) in advanced osteogenic sarcoma. Cancer Treat Rep. 1978;62:239-245.

315. Ferrari S, Mercuri M, Picci P, et al. Nonmetastatic osteosarcoma of the extremity: results of a neoadjuvant chemotherapy protocol (IOR/OS-3) with high-dose methotrexate, intraarterial or intravenous cisplatin, doxorubicin, and salvage chemotherapy based on histologic tumor response. Tumori. 1999;85:458-464.

316. Wilkins RM, Cullen JW, Odom L, et al. Superior survival in treatment of primary nonmetastatic pediatric osteosarcoma of the extremity. Ann Surg Oncol. 2003;10:498-507.

317. Ferguson WS, Harris MB, Goorin AM, et al. Presurgical window of carboplatin and surgery and multidrug chemotherapy for the treatment of newly diagnosed metastatic or unresectable osteosarcoma: Pediatric Oncology Group Trial. J Pediatr Hematol Oncol. 2001;23:340-348.

318. Le Deley MC, Guinebretiere JM, Gentet JC, et al. SFOP OS94: a randomised trial comparing preoperative high-dose methotrexate plus doxorubicin to high-dose methotrexate plus etoposide and ifosfamide in osteosarcoma patients. Eur J Cancer. 2007; 43:752-761.

319. Pratt CB, Horowitz ME, Meyer WH, et al. Phase II trial of ifosfamide in children with malignant solid tumors. Cancer Treat Rep. 1987;71:131-135.

320. Smeland S, Muller C, Alvegard TA, et al. Scandinavian Sarcoma Group Osteosarcoma Study SSG VIII: prognostic factors for outcome and the role of replacement salvage chemotherapy for poor histological responders. Eur J Cancer. 2003;39:488-494.

321. Meyer WH, Pratt CB, Poquette CA, et al. Carboplatin/ifosfamide window therapy for osteosarcoma: results of the St Jude Children's Research Hospital OS-91 trial. J Clin Oncol. 2001;19: 171-182.

322. Wang YM, Sutow WW, Romsdahl MM, Perez C. Age-related pharmacokinetics of high-dose methotrexate in patients with osteosarcoma. Cancer Treat Rep. 1979;63:405-410.

323. Graf N, Winkler K, Betlemovic M, et al. Methotrexate pharmacokinetics and prognosis in osteosarcoma. J Clin Oncol. 1994; 12:1443-1451.

324. Crews KR, Liu T, Rodriguez-Galindo C, et al. High-dose methotrexate pharmacokinetics and outcome of children and young adults with osteosarcoma. Cancer. 2004;100:1724-1733.

325. Jaffe N, Prudich J, Knapp J, et al. Treatment of primary osteosarcoma with intra-arterial and intravenous high-dose methotrexate. J Clin Oncol. 1983;1:428-431.

326. Rosen G, Caparros B, Huvos AG, et al. Preoperative chemotherapy for osteogenic sarcoma: selection of postoperative adjuvant chemotherapy based on the response of the primary tumor to preoperative chemotherapy. Cancer. 1982;49:1221-1230.

327. Pratt CB, Epelman S, Jaffe N. Bleomycin, cyclophosphamide, and dactinomycin in metastatic osteosarcoma: lack of tumor regression in previously treated patients. Cancer Treat Rep. 1987;71:421-423.

328. Strander H, Einhorn S. Effect of human leukocyte interferon on the growth of human osteosarcoma cells in tissue culture. Int J Cancer. 1977;19:468-473.

329. Masuda S, Fukuma H, Beppu Y. Antitumor effect of human leukocyte interferon on human osteosarcoma transplanted into nude mice. Eur J Cancer Clin Oncol. 1983;19:1521-1528.

330. Strander H, Bauer HC, Brosjo O, et al. Long-term adjuvant interferon treatment of human osteosarcoma. A pilot study. Acta Oncol. 1995;34:877-880.

331. Fidler IJ, Sone S, Fogler WE, Barnes ZL. Eradication of spontaneous metastases and activation of alveolar macrophages by intravenous injection of liposomes containing muramyl dipeptide. Proc Natl Acad Sci U S A. 1981;78:1680-1684.

332. MacEwen EG, Kurzman ID, Rosenthal RC, et al. Therapy for osteosarcoma in dogs with intravenous injection of liposome-encapsulated muramyl tripeptide. J Natl Cancer Inst. 1989;81: 935-938.

333. Souhami RL, Craft AW, Van der Eijken JW, et al. Randomised trial of two regimens of chemotherapy in operable osteosarcoma: a study of the European Osteosarcoma Intergroup. Lancet. 1997;350:911-917.

334. Lewis IJ, Nooij MA, Whelan J, et al. Improvement in histologic response but not survival in osteosarcoma patients treated with intensified chemotherapy: a randomized phase III trial of the European Osteosarcoma Intergroup. J Natl Cancer Inst. 2007;99:112-128.

335. Goorin A, Cantor A, Link MP. A phase I trial of etoposide and escalating doses of ifosfamide in recurrent pediatric sarcomas. Proc Am Soc Clin Oncol. 1994;13:A1458.

336. Pietras RJ, Fendly BM, Chazin VR, et al. Antibody to HER-2/neu receptor blocks DNA repair after cisplatin in human breast and ovarian cancer cells. Oncogene. 1994;9:1829-1838.

337. Arteaga CL, Winnier AR, Poirier MC, et al. p185c-erbB-2 signal enhances cisplatin-induced cytotoxicity in human breast carcinoma cells: association between an oncogenic receptor tyrosine kinase and drug-induced DNA repair. Cancer Res. 1994;54:3758-3765.

338. Hancock MC, Langton BC, Chan T, et al. A monoclonal antibody against the c-erbB-2 protein enhances the cytotoxicity of cis-diamminedichloroplatinum against human breast and ovarian tumor cell lines. Cancer Res. 1991;51:4575-4580.

339. Baselga J, Norton L, Albanell J, et al. Recombinant humanized anti-HER2 antibody (Herceptin) enhances the antitumor activity of paclitaxel and doxorubicin against HER2/neu overexpressing human breast cancer xenografts. Cancer Res. 1998;58:2825-2831.

340. Aboud-Pirak E, Hurwitz E, Pirak ME, et al. Efficacy of antibodies to epidermal growth factor receptor against KB carcinoma in vitro and in nude mice. J Natl Cancer Inst. 1988;80:1605-1611.

341. Hudis CA. Trastuzumab—mechanism of action and use in clinical practice. N Engl J Med. 2007;357:39-51.

342. Corey E, Brown LG, Quinn JE, et al. Zoledronic acid exhibits inhibitory effects on osteoblastic and osteolytic metastases of prostate cancer. Clin Cancer Res. 2003;9:295-306.

343. Evdokiou A, Labrinidis A, Bouralexis S, et al. Induction of cell death in human osteogenic sarcoma cells by zoledronic acid resembles anoikis. Bone. 2003;33:216-228.

344. Iguchi T, Miyakawa Y, Saito K, et al. Zoledronate-induced S phase arrest and apoptosis accompanied by DNA damage and activation of the ATM/Chk1/cdc25 pathway in human osteosarcoma cells. Int J Oncol. 2007;31:285-291.

345. Ory B, Heymann MF, Kamijo A, et al. Zoledronic acid suppresses lung metastases and prolongs overall survival of osteosarcoma-bearing mice. Cancer. 2005;104:2522-2529.

346. Heymann D, Ory B, Blanchard F, et al. Enhanced tumor regression and tissue repair when zoledronic acid is combined with ifosfamide in rat osteosarcoma. Bone. 2005;37:74-86.

347. Little DG, Smith NC, Williams PR, et al. Zoledronic acid prevents osteopenia and increases bone strength in a rabbit model of distraction osteogenesis. J Bone Miner Res. 2003;18:1300-1307.

348. Bobyn JD, Hacking SA, Krygier JJ, et al. Zoledronic acid causes enhancement of bone growth into porous implants. J Bone Joint Surg Br. 2005;87:416-420.

349. Duffaud F, Digue L, Mercier C, et al. Recurrences following primary osteosarcoma in adolescents and adults previously treated with chemotherapy. Eur J Cancer. 2003;39:2050-2057.

350. Saeter G, Hoie J, Stenwig AE, et al. Systemic relapse of patients with osteogenic sarcoma. Prognostic factors for long-term survival. Cancer. 1995;75:1084-1093.

351. Briccoli A, Rocca M, Salone M, et al. Resection of recurrent pulmonary metastases in patients with osteosarcoma. Cancer. 2005;104:1721-1725.

352. Antunes M, Bernardo J, Salete M, et al. Excision of pulmonary metastases of osteogenic sarcoma of the limbs. Eur J Cardiothorac Surg. 1999;15:592-596.

353. Harting MT, Blakely ML, Jaffe N, et al. Long-term survival after aggressive resection of pulmonary metastases among children and adolescents with osteosarcoma. J Pediatr Surg. 2006;41:194-199.

354. Pfannschmidt J, Klode J, Muley T, et al. Pulmonary resection for metastatic osteosarcomas: a retrospective analysis of 21 patients. Thorac Cardiovasc Surg. 2006;54:120-123.

355. Goorin AM, Delorey MJ, Lack EE, et al. Prognostic significance of complete surgical resection of pulmonary metastases in patients with osteogenic sarcoma: analysis of 32 patients. J Clin Oncol. 1984;2:425-431.

356. Nathan SS, Gorlick R, Bukata S, et al. Treatment algorithm for locally recurrent osteosarcoma based on local disease-free interval and the presence of lung metastasis. Cancer. 2006;107:1607-1616.

357. Jia SF, Worth LL, Kleinerman ES. A nude mouse model of human osteosarcoma lung metastases for evaluating new therapeutic strategies. Clin Exp Metastasis. 1999;17:501-506.

358. Worth LL, Lafleur EA, Jia SF, Kleinerman ES. Fas expression inversely correlates with metastatic potential in osteosarcoma cells. Oncol Rep. 2002;9:823-827.

359. Gordon N, Koshkina NV, Jia SF, et al. Corruption of the Fas pathway delays the pulmonary clearance of murine osteosarcoma cells, enhances their metastatic potential, and reduces the effect of aerosol gemcitabine. Clin Cancer Res. 2007;13:4503-4510.

360. Rao RD, Anderson PM, Arndt CA, et al. Aerosolized granulocyte macrophage colony-stimulating factor (GM-CSF) therapy in metastatic cancer. Am J Clin Oncol. 2003;26:493-498.

361. Joyama S, Naka N, Tsukamoto Y, et al. Dendritic cell immunotherapy is effective for lung metastasis from murine osteosarcoma. Clin Orthop Relat Res. 2006;(453):318-327.

362. Merchant MS, Melchionda F, Sinha M, et al. Immune reconstitution prevents metastatic recurrence of murine osteosarcoma. Cancer Immunol Immunother. 2007;56:1037-1046.

363. Wan X, Mendoza A, Khanna C, Helman LJ. Rapamycin inhibits ezrin-mediated metastatic behavior in a murine model of osteosarcoma. Cancer Res. 2005;65:2406-2411.

364. Ek ET, Dass CR, Contreras KG, Choong PF. Inhibition of orthotopic osteosarcoma growth and metastasis by multitargeted antitumor activities of pigment epithelium-derived factor. Clin Exp Metastasis. 2007;24:93-106.

365. Ek ET, Dass CR, Contreras KG, Choong PF. PEDF-derived synthetic peptides exhibit antitumor activity in an orthotopic model of human osteosarcoma. J Orthop Res. 2007.

366. Bodmer N, Walters DK, Fuchs B. Pemetrexed, a multitargeted antifolate drug, demonstrates lower efficacy in comparison to methotrexate against osteosarcoma cell lines. Pediatr Blood Cancer. 2007.

367. Weichselbaum R, Little JB, Nove J. Response of human osteosarcoma in vitro to irradiation: evidence for unusual cellular repair activity. Int J Radiat Biol Relat Stud Phys Chem Med. 1977;31:295-299.

368. Burgers JM, van Glabbeke M, Busson A, et al. Osteosarcoma of the limbs. Report of the EORTC-SIOP 03 trial 20781 investigating the value of adjuvant treatment with chemotherapy and/or prophylactic lung irradiation. Cancer. 1988;61:1024-1031.

369. Machak GN, Tkachev SI, Solovyev YN, et al. Neoadjuvant chemotherapy and local radiotherapy for high-grade osteosarcoma of the extremities. Mayo Clin Proc. 2003;78:147-155.

370. Ozaki T, Flege S, Liljenqvist U, et al. Osteosarcoma of the spine: experience of the Cooperative Osteosarcoma Study Group. Cancer. 2002;94:1069-1077.

371. Hug EB, Fitzek MM, Liebsch NJ, Munzenrider JE. Locally challenging osteo- and chondrogenic tumors of the axial skeleton: results of combined proton and photon radiation therapy using three-dimensional treatment planning. Int J Radiat Oncol Biol Phys. 1995;31:467-476.

372. Dincbas FO, Koca S, Mandel NM, et al. The role of preoperative radiotherapy in nonmetastatic high-grade osteosarcoma of the extremities for limb-sparing surgery. Int J Radiat Oncol Biol Phys. 2005;62:820-828.

373. DeLaney TF, Park L, Goldberg SI, et al. Radiotherapy for local control of osteosarcoma. Int J Radiat Oncol Biol Phys. 2005;61:492-498.

374. Anderson PM, Wiseman GA, Dispenzieri A, et al. High-dose samarium-153 ethylene diamine tetramethylene phosphonate: low toxicity of skeletal irradiation in patients with osteosarcoma and bone metastases. J Clin Oncol. 2002;20:189-196.

375. Buchen S, Ngampolo D, Melton RG, et al. Carboxypeptidase G2 rescue in patients with methotrexate intoxication and renal failure. Br J Cancer. 2005;92:480-487.

376. Nagarajan R, Neglia JP, Clohisy DR, Robison LL. Limb salvage and amputation in survivors of pediatric lower-extremity bone tumors: what are the long-term implications? J Clin Oncol. 2002;20:4493-4501.

377. Lipshultz SE, Lipsitz SR, Mone SM, et al. Female sex and drug dose as risk factors for late cardiotoxic effects of doxorubicin therapy for childhood cancer. N Engl J Med. 1995;332:1738-1743.

377a. Meyer JS, Nadel HR, Marina N, et al. Imaging guidelines for children with Ewing sarcoma and osteosarcoma: a report from the Children's Oncology Group Bone Tumor Committee. Pediatr Blood Cancer. 2008;51:163-170.

377b. Dauer LT, St. Germain J, Meyers PA. Let's image gently: reducing excessive reliance on CT scans. Pediatr Blood Cancer. 2008;51:838.

377c. Meyer JS, Nadel HR, Marina N, et al. Response to "Imaging guidelines for children with Ewing sarcoma and osteosarcoma. A report from the Children's Oncology Group Bone Tumor Committee." Pediatr Blood Cancer. 2008;51:839-840.

378. Wexler LH, Andrich MP, Venzon D, et al. Randomized trial of the cardioprotective agent ICRF-187 in pediatric sarcoma patients treated with doxorubicin. J Clin Oncol. 1996;14:362-372.

379. Tebbi CK, London WB, Friedman D, et al. Dexrazoxane-associated risk for acute myeloid leukemia/myelodysplastic syndrome and other secondary malignancies in pediatric Hodgkin's disease. J Clin Oncol. 2007;25:493-500.

380. Bacci G, Ferrari C, Longhi A, et al. Second malignant neoplasm in patients with osteosarcoma of the extremities treated with adjuvant and neoadjuvant chemotherapy. J Pediatr Hematol Oncol. 2006;28:774-780.

381. Aung L, Gorlick RG, Shi W, et al. Second malignant neoplasms in long-term survivors of osteosarcoma: Memorial Sloan-Kettering Cancer Center Experience. Cancer. 2002;95:1728-1734.

382. Stohr W, Langer T, Kremers A, et al. Cisplatin-induced ototoxicity in osteosarcoma patients: a report from the late effects surveillance system. Cancer Invest. 2005;23:201-207.

383. Petrilli AS, Oliveira DT, Ginani VC, et al. Use of amifostine in the therapy of osteosarcoma in children and adolescents. J Pediatr Hematol Oncol. 2002;24:188-191.

384. Longhi A, Macchiagodena M, Vitali G, Bacci G. Fertility in male patients treated with neoadjuvant chemotherapy for osteosarcoma. J Pediatr Hematol Oncol. 2003;25:292-296.

385. Longhi A, Pignotti E, Versari M, et al. Effect of oral contraceptive on ovarian function in young females undergoing neoadjuvant chemotherapy treatment for osteosarcoma. Oncol Rep. 2003;10:151-155.

386. Torbert JT, Fox EJ, Hosalkar HS, et al. Endoprosthetic reconstructions: results of long-term followup of 139 patients. Clin Orthop Relat Res. 2005;(438):51-59.

23 Pediatric Germ Cell Tumors

A. Lindsay Frazier and James F. Amatruda

Germ cell tumor is the designation given to neoplasms arising from the cells of the germline, the cells that are destined to become either the egg or the sperm. A number of unique features of these tumors, including their bimodal and wide age distribution, remarkable phenotypic diversity, and varying biologic behavior, make germ cell tumors a particular challenge for the pathologist and oncologist. However, the development of successful treatment regimens over the last several decades has focused current clinical research on ways to maintain efficacy and minimize toxicity for most patients and intensify treatment for patients who fail first-line therapy. Recent advances in understanding the underlying aberrations in germline development shed light on the genesis of these tumors, and may provide insight into new avenues for treatment.

DEVELOPMENT OF THE GERMLINE

The pathogenesis of germ cell tumors can best be understood through an analysis of the mechanisms of germline development.[1] The role of germ cells is to ensure the continuation of a species by producing the gametes, cells that will give rise to the next generation. Reflecting this unique role, germ cells are set aside from somatic cells early in development. In humans, germ cells arise in an extraembryonic position and must migrate to the site at which the gonads will form. The pluripotency of germ cells is reflected in the wide histopathologic diversity of germ cell tumors.

Specification of Primordial Germ Cells

Much of what is known about early molecular events in the mammalian germline comes from examination of germ cell development in the mouse.[2-5] Based on studies of human embryos and of human embryonic stem cells differentiating into germ cells in vitro,[6-10] it is a reasonable assumption that similar molecular mechanisms operate in humans. Development of the germline begins at the time of blastocyst implantation, when the extraembryonic ectoderm and the visceral endoderm send signals to cells in the proximal epiblast, also known as the embryonic ectoderm (Fig. 23-1). The major inductive signals are the bone morphogenetic proteins (BMPs), which are members of the transforming growth factor β (TGF-β) superfamily.[11-14] In response to BMPs, some of the epiblast cells begin to express the marker fragilis, signaling their competence to become germ cells.[2,15] Of these fragilis-expressing cells, a few will begin to express the transcriptional repressor *Blimp1/Prdm1*.[16] These cells, in which expression of somatic genes such as *hoxb1*, *T/Brachyury*, and *snail* is repressed, will become the primordial germ cells (PGCs). Unlike other epiblast-derived cells, PGCs regain or maintain expression of certain genes associated with pluripotency, such as *STELLA*, *OCT3/4*, and *NANOG*.[2,17-25] Certain pluripotency genes can be reactivated in germ cell tumors and may contribute to malignant potential; for example, *NANOG* and *OCT3/4* have been used as sensitive markers of malignant germ cells in studies of germ cell tumors.[26-30] In humans, PGCs can be identified in the wall of the yolk sac by their intrinsic alkaline phosphatase activity, beginning at about day 24. The PGCs begin to proliferate as they migrate out of the yolk sac into the embryo.[31]

Primordial Germ Cell Migration

In humans, as in many other organisms, PGCs arise in an extraembryonic location, distant from the eventual site at which

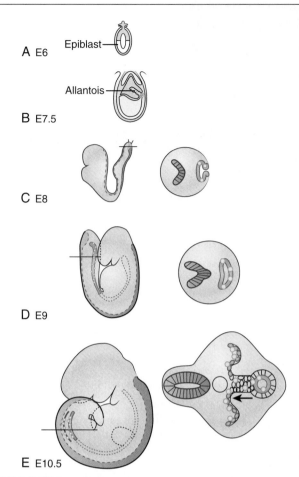

FIGURE 23-1. Development and migration of primordial germ cells. Stages of embryonic development and primordial germ cell (PGC) migration in the mouse. **A,** At E6, the epiblast (white) and extraembryonic tissue (gray) are discernible. **B,** By E7.5, the allantois has developed and the PGCs (yellow) appear. **C,** At E8, the neural tube (blue) and hindgut[71] are visible. In cross section (right side), the PGCs can be seen colonizing the hindgut. **D,** At E9, the embryo has turned and the posterior section is to the left; the PGCs are migrating through the hindgut. **E,** At E10.5, the PGCs begin exiting the hindgut and migrate through the dorsal mesentery (white cells) to enter the genital ridges (green). The equivalent stages of human embryonic development are weeks 1-2 (**A**), week 2.5 (**B**), week 3 (**C**), week 4 (**D**), and week 5 (**E**.) *(Adapted from Starz-Gaiano M, Lehmann R: Moving towards the next generation. Mech Dev. 2001;105:5-18.)*

the gonad will form. This physical separation may serve to insulate the germ cells from various proliferation and differentiation signals in the developing embryo, or to enforce a quality control by selecting for healthy PGCs capable of successfully navigating to the developing gonad. Proper PGC migration is critical to survival of the germ cells and formation of the gonad, and failure of this migration can result in ectopic germ cells. Persistence of these ectopic germ cells is one possible mechanism whereby extragonadal germ cell tumors are thought to arise.[32]

Toward the end of gastrulation, morphogenetic movements in the developing embryo bring the PGCs in proximity to the hindgut.[31] Invading the endoderm, the PGCs colonize the hindgut and begin vigorous, apparently random migratory movements, remaining confined to the gut. The receptor tyrosine kinase c-KIT, expressed in PGCs, and its ligand, Steel, expressed in somatic cells, are required for the colonization of the hindgut and for the survival and migration of PGCs within the gut.[33-36] Wylie and colleagues have shown that PGCs deficient in c-KIT signaling undergo apoptosis through the action of the p53-target gene, *Bax*.[36-39] At 5 to 6 weeks' postfertilization, the PGCs upregulate expression of the adhesion factor E-cadherin[40] and exit the hindgut on the dorsal side to begin colonization of the genital ridge primordial. The genital ridges are bilateral swellings of mesenchyme, covered by coelomic epithelium, situated on either side of the dorsal aorta on the posterior wall of the embryo in the lower thoracic and lumbar regions.[41] The genital ridges appear to attract the PGCs because of their expression of stromal-derived factor 1 (Sdf-1 or CXCL12), which is a ligand for the chemokine receptor CXCR4, expressed in the PGCs.[42,43] As the PGCs exit the hindgut, they divide into two lateral streams to colonize the genital ridges. PGCs that fail to colonize the ridges and remain in the midline are eliminated by apoptosis as the midline cells downregulate expression of Steel.[39] Once they have entered the genital ridges, PGCs become much less motile but continue through several more rounds of division. This proliferation is dependent on continued Steel–c-KIT signaling.[31,38,39,42,44]

Erasure of Imprinting

Imprinting refers to the epigenetic modification of certain genes, typically by cytosine methylation, so that only the maternal or paternal allele of the gene is expressed.[45-47] Lineage-specific patterns of imprinting are established in different tissues, including the germline, around the time of gastrulation.[46,48] On entering the gonadal ridges, however, PGCs actively erase these genomic methylation patterns. This erasure is necessary to allow the maternal and paternal imprinting patterns to be established in the oocytes and sperm, respectively. Imprinting is re-established in sex-specific patterns during gonadogenesis.[49-51] Germ cell tumors exhibit partial or total erasure of imprinting, implying their origin from early germ cells (reviewed by Oosterhuis and Looijenga[1]).

Gonadogenesis

Beginning shortly before the arrival of the PGCs in the genital ridges, the coelomic epithelium begins to proliferate and invade the underlying mesenchyme, forming the primitive sex cords. Migrating PGCs entering the gonad are surrounded by the cords. At this early stage, the appearance of the developing gonad is identical in males and females, and the tissue is referred to as the indifferent gonad. Subsequently, changes occur in the germ cells and gonadal somatic cells, according to the genetic gender of the embryo. In genetic males, gender determination occurs under the influence of the testis-determining *SRY* gene on the Y chromosome.[52-54] After the initial rounds of cell division, male germ cells enter a mitotic arrest that will persist until after birth.[14] In males, the primitive sex cords proliferate and penetrate deeper into the mesenchyme, forming the testis or medullary cords, which connect proximally to form the rete testis. By the fourth month of development, the cords consist of germ cells and the supporting Sertoli cells, which are derived from the surface epithelium of the genital ridge. The cords remain solid until puberty, when they form lumens to become seminiferous tubules. By the eighth week of development, the mesenchyme of the gonadal ridge gives rise in males to Leydig cells, which secrete testosterone. Secretion of antimüllerian hormone by the Sertoli cells and testosterone by the Leydig cells leads in males to degeneration of the paramesonephric ducts and the development of the mesonephric ducts into the vas deferens and epididymis. Testosterone is also necessary for male differentiation of the external genitalia.

Female gonadal development proceeds along different lines. In XX females in the absence of the Y chromosome, the sex cords initially degenerate and are replaced by a new set of cortical sex cords derived from the surface epithelium. By the fourth month, the cortical sex cords have become isolated clusters, with each cluster surrounding a single germ cell. In females, the primitive germ cells, called oogonia, continue rapid proliferation, reaching maximal numbers by the seventh month. After that point, most of the oogonia degenerate; the remaining cells, now called primary oocytes, enter meiosis and arrest at the diplotene stage of the first meiotic prophase. Granulosa cells (derived from the surface epithelium) and thecal cells (derived from the mesenchyme) together form the follicle cells that surround each primary oocyte. Beginning at adolescence, groups of oocytes periodically resume meiosis. In females, the paramesonephric (müllerian) ducts develop into the oviducts, uterus, cervix, and upper part of the vagina. The mesonephric ducts degenerate.

In summary, development of the germline requires the proper specification of primordial germ cells and their migration through the embryo to the gonadal ridges, where the gonads are formed through interactions of the germ cells with somatic cells. Concomitant with this process, the inherited pattern of genomic imprinting is erased, and a new, gender-specific pattern is formed. The complex process of gonadal organogenesis is subject to genetic and environmental influences. Abnormal development of the gonads during the embryonic and fetal periods leads to defects such as cryptorchidism and gonadal dysgenesis, which are strongly associated with the risk of developing germ cell tumors.

HISTOPATHOLOGY OF GERM CELL TUMORS

Germ cell tumors are a heterogeneous group of neoplasms with a wide variety of histopathologic features. This variety reflects the pluripotent nature of the primordial germ cells from which germ cell tumors arise.[1,55] Adding to the complexity of this tumor type, germ cell tumors with apparently similar histopathology can have different biologic behaviors when presenting at different ages or anatomic sites. The five major histologic subtypes of germ cell tumors are teratoma, yolk sac tumor, germinoma, embryonal carcinoma and choriocarcinoma. The World Health Organization (WHO) classification of germ cell tumors is presented in Boxes 23-1 and 23-2.

Overview

Testicular Germ Cell Tumors

In infants and children prior to puberty, teratoma and/or yolk sac tumors (YSTs) account for the vast majority of germ cell tumors.[56-58] Seminoma, embryonal carcinoma, and choriocarcinoma are rare in this age group. Germ cell tumors of the prepubertal testis differ from their adult counterparts, not only in the distribution of histologic subtypes, but also in their spectrum of cytogenetic abnormalities. Following the early peak of testicular YST and teratoma in the 0- to 4-year-old age group, testicular tumors are relatively rare until the onset of puberty. Between ages 15 and 40, there is a second peak in testicular tumor incidence, comprised of seminomas (the term used for a testicular germinoma) and nonseminomas (including embryonal carcinoma, teratoma, yolk sac tumor, and

Box 23-1	World Health Organization Classification of Germ Cell Tumors: Male

GERM CELL TUMORS

Intratubular germ cell neoplasia, unclassified
Other types
Tumors of one histologic type

SEMINOMA

Seminoma with syncytiotrophoblastic cells
Spermatocytic seminoma
Spermatocytic seminoma with sarcoma
Embryonal carcinoma

YOLK SAC TUMOR

Trophoblastic tumors
Choriocarcinoma
Trophoblastic neoplasms other than choriocarcinoma
Monophasic choriocarcinoma
Placental site trophoblastic tumor

TERATOMA

Dermoid cyst
Monodermal teratoma
Teratoma with somatic type malignancies

TUMORS OF MORE THAN ONE HISTOLOGIC TYPE

Mixed embryonal carcinoma and teratoma
Mixed teratoma and seminoma
Choriocarcinoma and teratoma/embryonal carcinoma
Others:
Sex cord–gonadal stromal tumors
Pure forms

LEYDIG CELL TUMOR

Malignant Leydig cell tumor

SERTOLI CELL TUMOR

Sertoli cell tumor, lipid-rich variant
Sclerosing Sertoli cell tumor
Large cell calcifying Sertoli cell tumor
Malignant Sertoli cell tumor

GRANULOSA CELL TUMOR

Adult-type granulosa cell tumor
Juvenile-type granulosa cell tumor

TUMORS OF THE THECOMA-FIBROMA GROUP

Thecoma
Fibroma
Sex cord–gonadal stromal tumor, incompletely differentiated
Sex cord–gonadal stromal tumor, mixed forms
Malignant sex cord–gonadal stromal tumor
Tumors containing both germ cell and sex cord–gonadal stromal elements
Gonadoblastoma
Germ cell-sex cord–gonadal stromal tumor, unclassified

Box 23-2	World Health Organization Classification of Germ Cell Tumors: Female

GERM CELL TUMORS

Dysgerminoma
Yolk sac tumor
Polyvesicular vitelline tumor
Glandular variant
Hepatoid variant
Embryonal carcinoma
Polyembryoma
Nongestational choriocarcinoma
Mixed germ cell tumor

TERATOMA

Biphasic or triphasic teratoma
Immature teratoma
Mature teratoma
Solid
Cystic
Dermoid cyst
Fetiform teratoma
Monodermal teratoma and somatic-type tumors associated with dermoid cysts

OTHERS

Thyroid (struma ovarii)
Carcinoid
Neuroectodermal
Carcinoma
Melanocytic
Sarcoma
Sebaceous tumors

GERM CELL-SEX CORD–STROMAL TUMORS

Gonadoblastoma
Variant with malignant germ cell tumor
Mixed germ cell sex cord–stromal tumor
Variant with malignant germ cell tumor
Sex cord-stromal tumors
Granulosa-stromal cell tumor

GRANULOSA CELL TUMOR

Adult-type granulosa cell tumor
Juvenile-type granulosa cell tumor

TUMORS OF THE THECOMA-FIBROMA GROUP

Thecoma
Fibroma

SERTOLI-STROMAL CELL TUMORS

Sertoli cell tumor
Stromal-Leydig cell tumor
Sex cord–stromal tumors of mixed or unclassified types

STEROID CELL TUMORS

Leydig cell tumor
Steroid cell tumor, not otherwise specified

choriocarcinoma). Postpubertal tumors demonstrate a wider array of histopathologic differentiation than germ cell tumors of the prepubertal testis. Moreover, adolescent and adult germ cell tumors share a common precursor cell of origin—the carcinoma in situ (CIS) or intratubular germ cell neoplasia, unclassified (IGCNU)—as well as characteristic cytogenetic abnormalities, including the near-universal presence of amplifications of chromosome 12p. These histopathologic and molecular cytogenetic differences have added support to the hypothesis that different pathogenic mechanisms underlie juvenile and adult testicular germ cell tumors.[59-61]

Ovarian Germ Cell Tumors

In neonates and infants, the most common ovarian lesions are ovarian cysts.[62] Cysts can occur at any time from late gestational stages onward, and occur with increased frequency in infants of mothers with diabetes, preeclampsia, and Rh immunization. Ovarian cysts in children often resolve spontaneously, without intervention.[63] Germ cell tumors account for 75% of ovarian tumors in the first 2 decades of life, and up to 90% of ovarian tumors in premenarchal girls. Most of these (95%) are benign mature teratomas,[64] but 5% of ovarian germ cell tumors are malignant; these include dysgerminomas, immature teratomas, mature teratomas with somatic malignancies, yolk sac tumors, choriocarcinomas, embryonal carcinomas, polyembryomas, and mixed germ cell tumors. Finally, gonadoblastoma is a mixed germ cell–sex cord stromal tumor occurring in cases of mixed gonadal dysgenesis with ambiguous genitalia, or 45,X Turner syndrome with Y chromosome material.[65-68] The histopathology of ovarian germ cell tumor types is similar to that of their testicular counterparts. After the third decade, ovarian germ cell tumors occur rarely, and carcinomas derived from the coelomic epithelial covering of the ovary are much more common.[69]

Intratubular Germ Cell Neoplasia, Unclassified

IGCNU,[70] also called testicular carcinoma in situ,[71] is considered the precursor for all invasive testicular germ cell tumors (TGCTs) of postpubertal males,[60,72-77] except spermatocytic seminoma.[78] Left untreated, IGCNU has up to a 50% probability of progressing to invasive TGCT, seminoma or nonseminoma, within 5 years.[75] Nonseminomas can be composed of embryonal carcinoma (the stem cell component), teratoma (somatic differentiation), and yolk sac tumor and choriocarcinoma (extraembryonic lineages). In IGCNU, germ cells with abundant vacuolated cytoplasm, large irregular nuclei, and prominent nucleoli are found within the seminiferous tubules, showing similarities to PGCs and early gonocytes.[70] IGCNU is found in 1% of cases of male infertility and in 2% to 4% of cryptorchid testes in adults.[70,74,77,79-82] In men with a TGCT, the prevalence of IGCNU is about 80% in the ipsilateral testis (range, 63% to 99%),[80,83] predominantly in men with nonseminomas,[84] and 5% in the contralateral testis.[72,85,86] Various markers, such as placental alkaline phosphatase (PLAP), c-KIT, transcription factor AP-2 gamma, OCT3/4 (POU5F1), and testis-specific protein Y-encoded (TSPY), have been extensively used for the immunohistochemical detection of IGCNU.[26,30,80,87-95] All these markers are also found in primordial germ cells and gonocytes, which supports the concept that IGCNU derives from primordial germ cells or gonocytes.[1,30,96,97]

Whether an identifiable precursor lesion exists for germ cell tumors of children is much less clear. In prepubertal children, the incidence of IGCNU appears to be low,[59,98,99] although several cases have been reported.[96,100-102] These data must be interpreted with caution, however, because of the difficulty of distinguishing IGCNU in the developing gonad, in which primitive germ cells normally express markers such as OCT3/4 and c-KIT.[97] The precursor lesion for the teratomas and yolk sac tumors of neonates and infants has yet to be identified. These pediatric tumors show partially erased imprinting, suggesting that the cell of origin is most likely a germ cell at an earlier development stage than that of IGCNU.[103-105]

IGCNU has been reported in a high percentage of gonadal biopsy specimens from children with disorders of sexual development (DSD), who are at risk for the development of germ cell malignancies.[106,107] These disorders include gonadal dysgenesis[108,109] and partial androgen insensitivity syndrome[110] and, less frequently, complete androgen insensitivity syndrome (AIS).[67,111-113] Development of these tumors in DSD patients in linked to the presence of a specific fragment of the Y chromosome, known as the GBY region.[29,94,95,114-117] For these patients, with an increased risk of germ cell malignancy, prophylactic gonadectomy is frequently indicated.[106,118] However, overdiagnosis of IGCNU is possible in this setting because of the frequent maturation delay of germ cells in DSD patients, resulting in the retained presence of c-KIT–positive germ cells.[21,119-121] Therefore, careful examination of the distribution pattern of OCT3/4-positive cells, and their position within the seminiferous tubule, are essential to making the diagnosis of IGCNU.[67,113,119]

Teratoma

Histopathology

Teratomas are tumors composed of multiple tissues that are normally foreign to, and able to proliferate in excess of, the site in which they occur.[122] In the usual definition of teratoma, tissue elements of all three germ layers (endoderm, mesoderm, and ectoderm) are present; however, teratomas also occur in which only one or two of the germ layers are present (referred to as monodermal or bidermal teratomas, respectively). The clinical and biologic behavior of teratomas vary significantly with differing anatomic location, degree of maturity of the tumor tissue, and age of onset. Grossly, teratomas are nodular and heterogeneous, with solid and cystic areas, depending on the types of differentiated tissue present. Cartilage, bone, hair, and pigmented areas may be recognizable (Fig. 23-2). At the

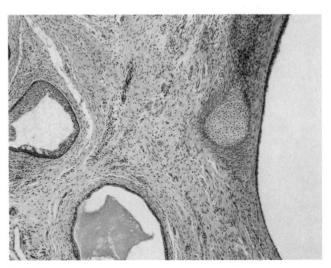

FIGURE 23-2. Mature teratoma. This low-power view shows a cystic tumor with areas of cartilaginous differentiation.

histopathologic level, ectodermal derivatives such as neuro-epithelium, skin, and hair are the most common tissues in teratomas of infants and children. However, almost any tissue type can be seen, including muscle, bone, cartilage, and well-differentiated glands (Fig. 23-3).

Mature teratomas are typically cystic and contain differentiated adult-type tissue from one or more of the germ layers. The term *dermoid cyst* refers to the frequent finding in mature teratomas of tissue resembling the adult epidermis and its appendages. Immature teratomas are those in which embryo-appearing tissue is present, typically in the form of neuroepithelial rosettes and tubules, and often mixed with mature tissue (Fig. 23-4). A loose myxoid stroma of immature mesenchyme, with focal differentiation into osteoid, fat, cartilage, and rhabdomyoblasts, may be present.[123] Hypercellularity, increased mitotic index, and nuclear atypia can be present. The prognostic significance of these findings is different for ovarian and testicular teratomas[57] (see later).

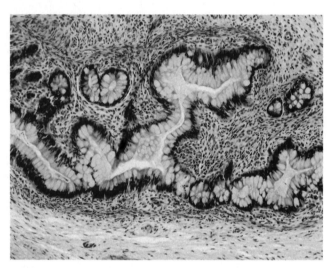

FIGURE 23-3. Mature teratoma with glandular differentiation.

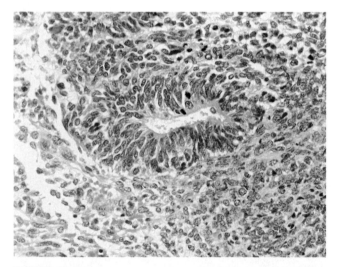

FIGURE 23-4. Immature teratoma. Immature teratomas are graded according to their content of primitive neuroepithelium. In this high-power view, the rosette formation characteristic of these tumors can be seen.

Testicular Teratoma

Testicular Teratoma in Infants and Children

In most series, testicular teratoma is the second most common germ cell tumor of the prepubertal testis, representing about 35% of germ cell tumors.[57,61,124-127] However, the actual incidence may be higher, because prepubertal testicular teratomas are uniformly benign, and thus may be underreported to tumor registries.[126-129] Histologically, 85% of prepubertal testicular teratomas are mature and 15% immature. Unlike what is found with ovarian teratomas, the degree of histologic immaturity of childhood testicular teratoma does not carry prognostic significance. In this age group, pure testicular teratomas lack metastatic potential and have not been found to recur following surgical removal of the tumor.[57,130-133] A review of cases of immature teratoma (IT) from Pediatric Oncology Group–Children's Cancer Group (POG-CCG) protocols has concluded that the presence of microscopic foci of YST, rather than the grade of IT, is the only valid predictor of recurrence in pediatric IT at any site.[134] The benign nature of these tumors has permitted the widespread use of testis-sparing enucleation surgery for prepubertal testicular teratomas.[59,128,135-137] In agreement with the benign clinical behavior of pure teratomas of the prepubertal testis, these tumors display normal karyotypes and normal results from comparative genomic hybridization.[127,138,139] Epidermoid cysts are rare tumors in the prepubertal testis and are most likely monodermal teratomas showing ectodermal differentiation.[64,128,140,141] These tumors have a characteristic ultrasonographic appearance, are hormonally inactive, and do not produce alpha-fetoprotein (AFP)[128]; as with other teratomas of the prepubertal testis, they are managed conservatively with testis-sparing surgery.[128,140,142] In the prepubertal testis, the seminiferous tubules surrounding the teratoma may contain germ cells with atypical features, such as enlarged nuclei. However, these features are distinct from the seminoma-like changes of IGCNU, and do not signify malignant transformation of the germ cells.[143,144]

Testicular Teratoma in Adolescents and Adults

Teratoma occurs as a component of 50% of mixed nonseminomas in the postpubertal testis. Pure teratoma is rare, accounting for only 2% to 3% of postpubertal TGCTs.[145,146] In contrast to testicular teratomas of infants and children, testicular teratomas in adolescents and adults are malignant tumors, even though they may appear to be well differentiated.[56,137] Indeed, these tumors may spread, giving rise to teratomatous and nonteratomatous metastases.[70] Furthermore, adult testicular teratomas typically are associated with IGCNU and exhibit characteristic cytogenetic abnormalities, such as isochromosome 12p, which are also found in seminomas and in other types of nonseminomatous TGCTs. Based on these findings, Ulbright[137,147] has proposed that teratomas in the adult testis arise from a germ cell that has already undergone malignant transformation; thus, the histogenesis of adult teratoma is distinct from that of teratomas arising in ovary or the prepubertal testis. Postpubertal teratomas may contain syncytiotrophoblastic giant cells, and patients with teratoma may present with gynecomastia[148] or with elevated serum β-human chorionic gonadotropin (β-hCG) or AFP.[149,150]

Ovarian Teratoma

Teratoma is the most common germ cell tumor (GCT) of the ovary, comprising more than 95% of all ovarian GCTs.[64] Ovarian teratomas differ in important ways from testicular teratomas. Teratomas in the prepubertal testis are uniformly benign. In adolescents and adults, testicular teratomas are almost always malignant, and occur as a component of mixed malignant germ cell tumors, with the exception being dermoid cysts of the testis. In the ovary, in contrast, the phenotype of teratomas does not vary as strikingly by age, and ovarian teratomas are usually pure tumors.[151,152] The great majority of ovarian tumors are mature benign tumors, often referred to as a dermoid cyst or mature cystic teratoma.[137,147,153,154] Less than 5% of ovarian teratomas are malignant; these are discussed separately later.

Benign, Mature Ovarian Teratoma

Mature ovarian teratomas are diploid, cytogenetically normal tumors.[127,155-158] This contrasts to postpubertal testicular teratomas, which are aneuploid and demonstrate cytogenetic abnormalities such as i12p. When polymorphic molecular markers are assayed, a high percentage of mature ovarian teratomas show a homozygous pattern, indicating that these tumors can arise from a germ cell that has completed meiosis I but not meiosis II.[110,138,155,159-164] Mature ovarian teratomas are usually cystic, although solid tumors can occur, especially in the first 2 decades.[165,166] Other characteristics of mature ovarian teratomas include a well-ordered, "organoid" appearance of the differentiated tissues within the teratoma and the absence of cytologic atypia.[167] Mature ovarian teratomas are uniformly benign, except in the rare case of post-teratomatous malignant degeneration of a dermoid cyst.[137,167,168]

Malignant Ovarian Teratoma

In children, immature teratoma is the most common type of malignant ovarian teratoma. Also in this category are other tumors that are rare in children, such as monodermal teratomas with malignant elements (e.g., papillary thyroid carcinoma in struma ovarii), dermoid cysts with malignant degeneration, and the rare case of mixed malignant ovarian germ cell tumor with a teratoma component.

Immature Teratoma. The term *immature teratoma* refers to teratomas containing immature-appearing tissues, principally neuroepithelium.[169] Additionally, foci of mitotically active glia may be present. A grading system has been developed for immature teratomas, based on the amount of neuroepithelial tissue present.[123,170] Mature teratomas containing only fully differentiated tissue are considered grade 0, and immature teratomas range from grade 1, comprised of less than 10% immature neuroepithelium, to grade 3, more than 50% immature neuroepithelium present. A two-component grading system (low and high grade) has also been proposed, and has been shown to have improved reproducibility.[171] In adult ovarian teratomas, the finding of grade 2 or 3 immature teratoma predicts the likelihood of metastasis and confers a worse prognosis.[123,165,171,172] In children, however, it is not clear that the same relationship of grade to outcome of immature teratomas holds true. A Pediatric Oncology Group study has concluded that surgery alone is curative in children and adolescents with Stage I immature teratomas of any grade, and that chemotherapy should be reserved for cases of relapse.[134,173,174]

Immature teratomas may be associated with implants of glial tissue on the peritoneum, known as gliomatosis peritonei.[175-177] If the implants are composed solely of mature tissues, the presence of gliomatosis peritonei confers a favorable prognosis, regardless of the degree of immaturity of the teratoma.[178,179] Recent evidence has suggested that the implants arise from metaplastic transformation of pluripotent müllerian stem cells in the peritoneum or underlying mesenchyme, rather than representing metastasis of the teratoma tissue.[180-182]

Monodermal Teratoma. Monodermal teratomas consist largely or exclusively of a single type of tissue, such as thyroid, carcinoid, or neuroectodermal tissue.[64,183-186] Monodermal teratomas with neuroectodermal differentiation include indolent types such as ependymoma and poorly differentiated forms such as primitive neuroectodermal tumor (PNET), as well as anaplastic tumors resembling glioblastoma.[127,187-191] These tumors are rare in children.

Teratoma with Malignant Transformation. Teratoma with malignant transformation makes up 0.2% to 1.4% of mature cystic tumors of the ovary.[137,168,192] In these tumors, more commonly seen in older women, somatic-type malignancies are seen among the individual tissues in the teratoma. Squamous cell carcinomas are the most common tumor type[193,194] but others, including melanoma, adenocarcinoma, small cell carcinoma, sarcomas (including PNET) and malignant glioma, may also occur.[137,167]

Yolk Sac Tumor

Histopathology

Yolk sac tumor is the most common malignant germ cell tumor in infancy and childhood.[57,58,122,126,195] The differentiation of the tumor cells is predominantly along endodermal lines and can take the form of intraembryonic endodermal derivatives, such as primitive gut and liver, and extraembryonic structures, such as allantois and yolk sac. There are many synonyms for yolk sac tumor, including orchioblastoma, Teilum's tumor, and clear cell adenocarcinoma. Although endodermal sinus tumor is commonly used as a synonym for yolk sac tumor, some consider the term problematic, because the endodermal sinus is not a component of normal human embryogenesis.[196] In macroscopic appearance, yolk sac tumors are yellowish, with multiple cysts and frequent areas of hemorrhage, necrosis, and liquefaction.[167] Microscopically, yolk sac tumors display a loose myxoid stroma containing a reticulated pattern of microcystic spaces (Fig. 23-5). The cysts are lined by a flattened, periodic acid–Schiff (PAS)-positive, diastase-resistant epithelium. About 20% of yolk sac tumors exhibit characteristic Schiller-Duval bodies, a clustering of cells around a small, central blood vessel

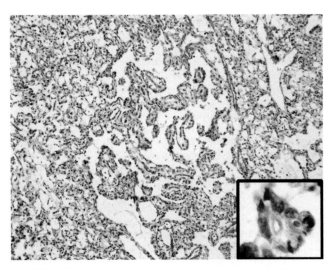

FIGURE 23-5. Yolk sac tumor. A loose myxoid stroma is filled with a labyrinthine network of cysts lined by clear, flattened epithelial cells. **Inset,** Schiller-Duval body.

(see Fig. 23-5, inset). In addition to the microcystic reticular pattern, several variant histologies of yolk sac tumor are described, including the solid, polyvesicular, and parietal types (corresponding to primitive endoderm and extraembryonic structures, such as allantois and yolk sac) and the glandular and hepatic types (corresponding to the intraembryonic endodermal derivatives, primitive lung, and liver).

Yolk sac tumors are typically cytokeratin-positive, which can help differentiate the solid YST variant from germinomas.[167] AFP expression is characteristic of these tumors, and AFP is a valuable tumor marker. Neonates and infants have high physiologic levels of AFP in serum, which can confound the use of serum AFP levels for the diagnosis of yolk sac tumor for monitoring therapy. Tables of normal serum AFP levels in neonates and infants have been published[197-199] (see Fig. 23-15). In addition, 70% to 100% of yolk sac tumors have detectable AFP expression by immunohistochemical assays.[200-204]

Testicular Yolk Sac Tumor

In Infants and Children

Yolk sac tumor[205] is the most common malignant germ cell tumor in infants and children, comprising approximately 65% of prepubertal testicular germ cell tumors.[125,206] YST is most common in male infants and boys aged 0 to 2 years, and can occur in pure form or as a malignant component of teratoma.[57] Histologically, prepubertal YSTs show the same spectrum of patterns as their adult counterparts—pseudopapillary, reticular, polyvesicular vitelline, and solid, with the pseudopapillary pattern being most common in children.[207] IGCNU is not a feature of childhood YST, and it is unlikely that p53 mutations play a role in pathogenesis.[98,99,139] Unlike childhood teratomas, yolk sac tumors in children are aneuploid, with characteristic, nonrandom chromosomal abnormalities, including gains at 3p and losses at 1p and 6q.[139,208,209] Immunohistochemistry detects AFP expression in more than 90% of YSTs and, in most cases, the serum AFP level is also elevated.[57,201,204,210-214]

In Adolescents and Adults

Yolk sac tumor in the adolescent and adult testis is extremely rare in the pure form, but occurs in approximately 40% of mixed TGCTs.[215] In one series of primary mediastinal germ cell tumors, yolk sac tumor was present in almost 50% of the tumors.[216] As in childhood yolk sac tumor, hematogenous metastases are common, especially to the liver. Most tumors stain positive for AFP, and serum AFP is commonly elevated.[217]

Ovarian Yolk Sac Tumor

Yolk sac tumor of the ovary is a clinically aggressive tumor that frequently presents at advanced stages, with metastasis to lymph nodes or peritoneal structures. The tumors are rarely bilateral.[122,202,218,219] The median age at diagnosis is 18 to 19 years.[62,220-222] In a series of 26 pediatric patients, the reticular type was the most common histology identified.[202]

Seminoma and Dysgerminoma

Histopathology

Seminomas represent a class of germ cell tumors in which the tumor cells resemble primitive, undifferentiated germ cells,

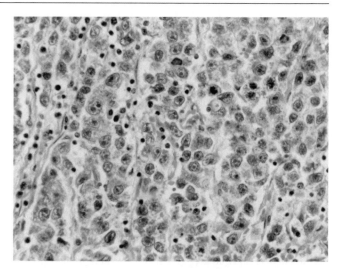

FIGURE 23-6. Dysgerminoma. Germinomas consist of sheets of large uniform cells with clear or granular cytoplasm, large central nuclei, and prominent nucleoli. A lymphocyte infiltrate is a typical feature of germinomas. The histologies of ovarian dysgerminoma, testicular seminoma, and extragonadal germinoma are identical.

both in morphology and in the expression of pluripotency genes such as *OCT3/4*, *NANOG*, and *STELLAR*.[28,30,91,92,223-225] These tumors are referred to as germinomas when they arise in extragonadal locations (e.g., the pineal gland, mediastinum, or retroperitoneum), dysgerminomas when in the ovary, and seminomas when in the testis. The histology of seminomas is identical, regardless of the site in which they occur. Grossly, these are rounded nodular tumors, separated into lobules by fibrous bands. Microscopically, seminomas are characterized by a monotonous proliferation of large uniform cells with large central nuclei and prominent nucleoli (Fig. 23-6). The cytoplasm is clear or granular, and frequently PAS-positive because of high glycogen content. A lymphocytic infiltrate is a typical feature of seminomas.

Seminoma

Seminoma is extremely rare in children. In the postpubertal testis, seminoma can occur in pure form or as a component of a mixed germ cell tumor.[70,147,226] The peak age of onset of seminoma is 34 to 45 years, slightly later than that of nonseminomatous tumors.[70,227] Several distinct variants of seminoma have been recognized. Up to 7% of classic seminomas contain syncytiotrophoblastic giant cells, and almost 25% of seminomas contain foci that stain positive for β-hCG.[228-231] These tumors may be accompanied by an elevation in serum β-hCG; however, the presence of syncytiotrophoblasts or elevated β-hCG does not worsen the prognosis.[232-234] Marked elevations of β-hCG, or persistently elevated β-hCG following orchiectomy, may indicate the presence of choriocarcinoma.[235] Anaplastic or atypical seminoma is the designation used for seminomas displaying increased mitotic activity, nuclear pleomorphism, and sparse lymphocytic infiltrate on histologic examination.[236-239] Whether these aggressive features portend a worse prognosis or a higher likelihood of metastasis remains controversial. Although some studies have suggested that anaplastic seminomas are clinically more aggressive tumors,[240,241] others have found no evidence of a worse prognosis when these features are present.[232,236,242]

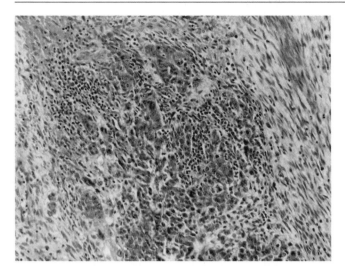

FIGURE 23-7. Embryonal carcinoma. Embryonal carcinomas consist of large, irregular epithelial-like cells with indistinct borders. The term *embryonal carcinoma* derives from the resemblance of the tumor cells to the early embryonic cells of the inner cell mass.

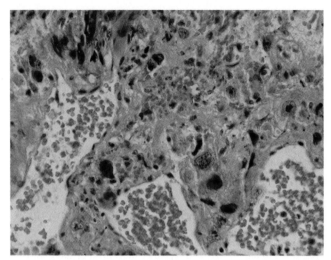

FIGURE 23-8. Choriocarcinoma. Choriocarcinomas are characterized by a mixture of syncytiotrophoblastic, cytotrophoblastic, and intermediate trophoblastic cells, with frequent areas of hemorrhage.

Dysgerminoma

Dysgerminoma is the most common malignant ovarian germ cell tumor of children and adolescents, and makes up one third of malignant ovarian GCTs.[243-245] Pathologically, dysgerminoma is the ovarian counterpart of the seminoma of the testis and the germinoma of extragonadal sites. Unlike seminomas of the testis, which are rare in the prepubertal period, dysgerminomas can occur at any age, although the peak incidence is 15 to 19 years.[245-248] Also unlike seminomas, which develop from IGCNU, dysgerminomas do not appear to arise from a precursor cell.[167] Dysgerminomas stain positive for octamer-4 (Oct4) on immunohistochemistry, which can be useful for distinguishing these tumors from nondysgerminomas.[249,250] As with seminomas, most dysgerminomas also stain positive for c-KIT,[251] and Hoei-Hansen and associates[252] have identified c-KIT mutations in a subset of ovarian dysgerminomas.

Embryonal Carcinoma

Histopathology

Embryonal carcinoma is rare in infants, but can occur in prepubertal females and adults of both genders. Embryonal carcinomas frequently have areas of hemorrhage and necrosis, and can be locally invasive into the epididymis and spermatic cord in males.[70,167] At the microscopic level, the tumors consist of large, epithelium-appearing cells that resemble the early embryonic cells of the inner cell mass (Fig. 23-7). The tumor cells may grow in solid, papillary, and reticular patterns, forming many clefts and gland-like structures. The tumors are typically cytokeratin- and CD30-positive, but negative for epithelial membrane antigen (EMA), carcinoembryonic antigen, and vimentin.[167,253] Syncytiotrophoblast cells, when present in the tumor, can produce β-hCG and cause precocious pseudopuberty in premenarchal girls or vaginal bleeding in older women.[200]

Testicular Embryonal Carcinoma in Adolescents and Adults

Embryonal carcinoma is the most common pure nonseminomatous TGCT in adults, representing about 2% to 10% of cases in this age group. Additionally, 80% of mixed malignant TGCTs contain embryonal carcinoma as one component.[254,255]

Ovarian Embryonal Carcinoma

Embryonal carcinoma occurs in the ovary less commonly than in the testis, accounting for 4% of malignant ovarian tumors.[200,202] The median age at diagnosis is 14 years, somewhat younger than for ovarian yolk sac tumor. Ovarian embryonal carcinoma is more frequently associated with β-hCG production and with hormonal manifestations such as precocious puberty, amenorrhea, and hirsutism.[200] Because of the totipotent nature of embryonal carcinoma cells, differentiation into various histologies may be seen, including teratomas and syncytiotrophoblastic giant cells resembling choriocarcinoma. Polyembryoma is a rare tumor in which multiple embryoid bodies resembling presomite-stage embryos are seen. Polyembryoma is considered by some to be an organoid variant of embryonal carcinoma,[167] although others have described it as one component of mixed germ cell tumors.[256,257]

Choriocarcinoma

Choriocarcinoma is a rare tumor composed of cytotrophoblast, syncytiotrophoblast, and extravillous trophoblast. Choriocarcinoma in infants can occur as a metastasis secondary to a placental choriocarcinoma, or as a primary tumor arising in the liver, lungs, brain, kidney, or skin.[258] The tumor can cause anemia and bleeding symptoms, as well as pseudoprecocious puberty because of expression of β-hCG by the tumor cells.[122] Choriocarcinomas are usually large tumors, with prominent foci of hemorrhage. The histopathology of choriocarcinoma is a mixture of syncytiotrophoblastic, cytotrophoblastic, and intermediate trophoblastic cells, often mixed in random fashion surrounding areas of hemorrhage and necrosis (Fig. 23-8).[70] Vascular invasion is a common feature of choriocarcinomas.

Testicular Choriocarcinoma in Adolescents and Adults

Choriocarcinoma, like yolk sac tumor, is very rare in pure form but occurs in approximately 8% of mixed TGCTs in adults.[254,259]

Ovarian Choriocarcinoma

Primary (nongestational) choriocarcinoma occurs rarely as a pure tumor but more often as a component of mixed ovarian germ cell tumor, usually in association with teratoma.[244] Choriocarcinoma in infants may arise as a primary tumor in the lung, liver, brain, kidney, or other location.[122,260,261] Gestational choriocarcinoma arises in the placenta and may metastasize widely in the mother; case reports have described metastasis of gestational choriocarcinoma to the infant.[262] In patients in their reproductive years, DNA analysis to detect the presence of paternal sequences can be helpful in determining the placental origin of gestational choriocarcinoma.[263,264]

Mixed Ovarian Germ Cell Tumor

Mixed ovarian germ cell tumors are composed of two or more of the malignant germ cell histologic subtypes. These tumors comprise 8% of malignant germ cell tumors of the ovary in children and adolescents and 20% of ovarian malignant germ cell tumors overall.[62,265,266] Mixed germ cell tumors thus represent only approximately 1% of all ovarian germ cell tumors, in contrast to the postpubertal testis, in which one third of germ cell tumors are of the mixed type.[64,70,147] Dysgerminoma, yolk sac tumor, or teratoma is the most frequent germ cell component, with embryonal carcinoma and choriocarcinoma present more rarely.[64,222]

Pathology of Mixed Germ Cell–Sex Cord Tumors

Gonadoblastoma

Gonadoblastomas contain mixtures of two cell types, large cells resembling primitive germ cells and smaller cells similar to immature Sertoli and granulosa cells (Fig. 23-9). It occurs most commonly in cases of mixed gonadal dysgenesis with ambiguous genitalia or 45,X Turner's syndrome with Y chromosome material.[65,66,68,113] Gonadoblastoma can occur as single or multiple nodules; foci of calcification are a characteristic finding.[122] Microscopically, nests of germ cells within basement membrane material are surrounded by supportive cells, such as Sertoli-granulosa cells. The stroma may have elements resembling Leydig or lutein-like cells.[267] The presence of gonadoblastoma substantially increases the risk that a malignant germ cell tumor will develop in a dysgenetic gonad. Several studies have found that the average incidence of germ cell tumors in gonadal biopsy specimens from patients with mixed gonadal dysgenesis is 12%.[67] Gonadoblastoma gives rise most frequently to dysgerminoma, and less frequently to embryonal carcinoma, teratoma, yolk sac tumor, and choriocarcinoma. The germ cells in dysgenetic gonads abnormally retain their embryonic characteristics, as demonstrated by their marker expression profile, including *OCT3/4* and *TSPY*. These cells give rise to gonadoblastoma in areas of undifferentiated gonadal tissue within the dysgenetic gonad, whereas IGCNU arises in regions with testicular differentiation.[21,26,29,30,67,113] Thus, just as IGCNU is the precursor lesion for invasive TGCTs, gonadoblastoma can be considered a precursor lesion for the invasive germ cell tumors of dysgenetic gonads.

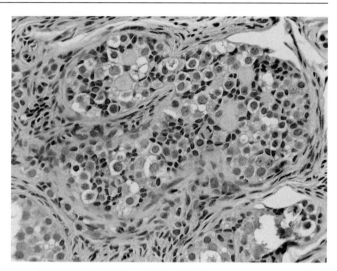

FIGURE 23-9. Gonadoblastoma. Gonadoblastomas are mixed germ cell–stromal tumors consisting of nests of primitive germ cells surrounded by immature-appearing Sertoli and Leydig cells.

Summary

The five major histologic subtypes of germ cell tumors are teratoma, yolk sac tumor, germinoma, embryonal carcinoma, and choriocarcinoma. In infants and children, teratoma and yolk sac tumor are the most common germ cell tumors. Yolk sac tumors occurring at any age are malignant tumors. Teratomas are benign in the prepubertal testis; in the postpubertal testis, teratomas occur as one component of nonseminomatous germ cell tumors and are uniformly malignant. Most ovarian teratomas are benign, but ovarian teratomas with a significant immature component are considered malignant. Germinomas in the ovary are known as dysgerminomas and may occur in children and adults. The testicular counterpart is known as seminoma and occurs exclusively in the postpubertal setting. Extragonadal germinomas can occur in both genders, typically in the midline of the retroperitoneum or mediastinum or in the pineal gland. The remaining tumor types, embryonal carcinoma, and choriocarcinoma, are very rare in children but can occur in the testis or ovary in adolescents and adults, either as pure tumors or as one component of a mixed germ cell tumor.

EPIDEMIOLOGY OF PEDIATRIC GERM CELL TUMORS

Incidence

Pediatric germ cell tumors account for only a small proportion of all cancers diagnosed in children younger than 20 years, but the incidence fluctuates dramatically with age. Teratomas are the most common neoplasm in the newborn, but malignant germ cell tumors are rarely diagnosed during the early childhood years; incidence begins to rise again at the onset of puberty (approximately age 8 in females and approximately age 11 in males; Fig. 23-10).[268] During adolescence, rates of GCT rise substantially for both males and females. In children younger than 15 years old, germ cell tumors represent only 3.5% of all cancer diagnoses but, during adolescence, between ages 15 and 19, germ cell tumors represent 16% of the total cancer burden.[268] The incidence of testicular germ cell tumors continues to rise

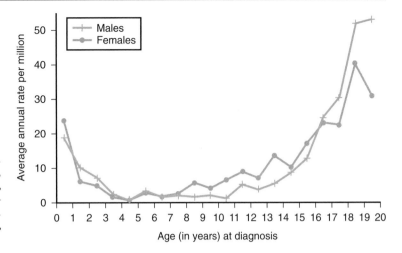

FIGURE 23-10. Age-specific incidence rates by gender and race for germ cell, trophoblastic, and other gonadal tumors, SEER, 1986-1994. *(Adapted from Bernstein L, Smith MA, Liu L, et al. Germ cell trophoblastic and other gonadal neoplasms, ICCC X. In Ries L, Melbert D, Krapcho M, et al (eds). SEER Cancer Statistics Review, 1975-2004. Bethesda, Md, National Cancer Institute, 2007, pp 125-137.)*

TABLE 23-1   **Average Annual Age-Adjusted* Incidence Rates (Per Million) for Germ Cell Trophoblastic and Other Gonadal Cancers[†]**

ICCC Group X	Description	Total	Males	Females
Xa-e	Germ cell, trophoblastic, and other gonadal tumors	11.6	12.0	11.1
Xa	Intracranial and intraspinal germ cell tumors	1.6	2.3	0.9
Xb	Other and unspecified nongonadal germ cell tumors. (this category includes the tumors of infants and young children that originate in the sacrococcygeal region, as well as mediastinal tumors primarily developing in older children.)	1.6	1.5	1.8
Xc	Gonadal germ cell tumors	6.7	8.0	5.3
	Testis	4.1	8.0	—
	Ovary	2.6	—	5.3
Xd	Gonadal carcinoma	1.4	0.1	2.9
	Ovary	1.3	—	2.6
	Other	0.1	0.1	0.3
Xe	Other and unspecified malignant gonadal tumors	0.2	0.1	0.3

ICCC, International Classification for Childhood Cancer.
*Adjusted to the 1970 U.S. standard population.
[†]By gender and subtype, age < 20 yr, all races, SEER, 1986-1995.
From Bernstein L, Smith MA, Liu L, et al. Germ cell trophoblastic and other gonadal neoplasms, ICCC X. In Ries L, Melbert D, Krapcho M, et al (eds). SEER Cancer Statistics Review, 1975-2004. Bethesda, Md, National Cancer Institute, 2007, pp 125-137.

in young adulthood, peaking in the third decade Testicular germ cell tumors are the most common solid tumor in men between the ages of 15 to 34 years.[269] In 2002, 7500 cases of testicular cancer were diagnosed in men.

Extrapolating from the SEER cancer registry of childhood cancer collected between 1986 and 1995, it was estimated that approximately 650 U.S. children and adolescents younger than 20 years are diagnosed with a gonadal or extragonadal germ cell tumor each year.[268] The incidence of GCT in childhood has a bimodal distribution; there is a peak in diagnosis at and during infancy and a second peak after the onset of puberty. Histology also varies dramatically with age. Yolk sac tumor is the predominant histology in newborns and younger children; tumors that arise in the peripubertal period contain a wider range of histologies, including YST, embryonal carcinoma, and choriocarcinoma, as well as germinomatous tumors (testicular seminoma and ovarian dysgerminoma).

The overall incidence for males is slightly higher than for females (12.0 vs. 11.1/million), but this varies by age (Table 23-1).[268] At birth, GCTs are more common in females than

males (because of the higher incidence of SCT in females) but, in early childhood, the overall incidence of GCT in boys exceeds that of girls. The relative incidence switches again in the peripubertal age range, with incidence in females higher than males but, beginning in midadolescence, around age 16, the incidence in males overtakes females because of the rapidly rising prevalence of testicular GCT in this age range (see Fig. 23-10).[268]

Examining incidence by site, gonadal tumors generally are more common than extragonadal tumors. Overall, approximately 15% of GCTs is extragonadal in males and approximately 33% of GCTs is extragonadal in females.[268] This ratio varies dramatically by age and gender. For example, prior to age 5, 42% of GCTs are sacrococcygeal teratomas.[57] Among males, in the first year of life, the rates of testicular and non–central nervous system (CNS) extragonadal tumors are approximately equal (Fig. 23-11A).[268] In contrast, among females, extragonadal GCTs (principally sacrococcygeal teratomas) are much more common than ovarian GCTs in the first year of life (see Fig. 23-11B). The incidence of all types of GCT remains

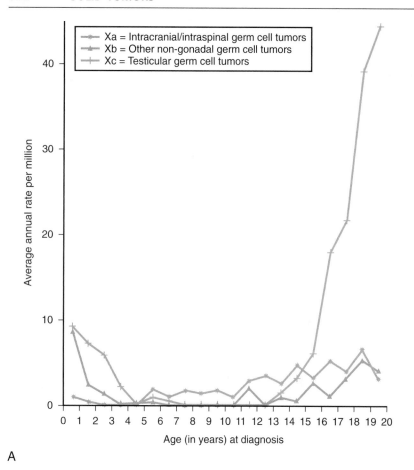

A

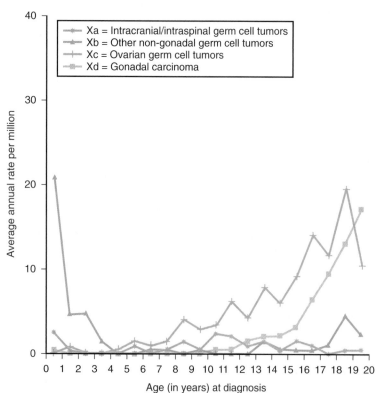

B

FIGURE 23-11. Age-specific incidence rates (all races) by selected International Classification for Childhood Cancer (ICCC) subgroups for germ cell, trophoblastic, and other gonadal tumors, SEER, 1986-1994. **A,** Males. **B,** Females. *(Adapted from Bernstein L, Smith MA, Liu L, et al. Germ cell trophoblastic and other gonadal neoplasms, ICCC X. In Ries L, Melbert D, Krapcho M, et al (eds). SEER Cancer Statistics Review, 1975-2004. Bethesda, Md, National Cancer Institute, 2007, pp 125-137.)*

TABLE 23-2 **Average Annual Age-Adjusted* Incidence Rates (Per Million) for Germ Cell Trophoblastic and Other Gonadal Cancers by Race and Gender[†]**

ICCC Group X	ICCC Germ Cell Tumor Category	White Male	Black Male	White Female	Black Female
Xa-e	All	12.3	3.2	9.0	10.8
Xc	Gonadal germ cell tumors	9.1	1.2	4.5	5.6
	Testis	9.1	1.2	—	—
	Ovary	—	—	4.5	5.6
Xa, b, d, e	Other than germ cell tumors	3.2	2.0	4.5	5.2

ICCC, International Classification for Childhood Cancer.

*Adjusted to the 1970 U.S. standard population.

[†]By race, gender, and subtype age < 20 yr, SEER, 1975-1995.

From Bernstein L, Smith MA, Liu L, et al. Germ cell trophoblastic and other gonadal neoplasms, ICCC X. In Ries L, Melbert D, Krapcho M, et al (eds). SEER Cancer Statistics Review, 1975-2004. Bethesda, Md, National Cancer Institute, 2007, pp 125-137.

low from about age 4 until age 11, when the incidence of testicular tumors begins to rise dramatically. The incidence of ovarian germ cell tumors decreases after the newborn period, and remains low until the onset of puberty (approximately age 8 years), when the incidence begins to rise as well, although not with the rate of increase seen in testicular GCT. The incidence of testicular GCT slightly exceeds the incidence of ovarian germ cell tumors at all ages, but this difference is most pronounced beginning in mid to late adolescence. In the German Cancer Registry, in children younger than 5 years, testicular germ cell tumors accounted for 29% of GCTs, whereas ovarian germ cell tumors accounted for only 5.6%.[248] At age 19, the rate of ovarian germ cell tumors is 10.4/million whereas the rate of testicular germ cell tumor is 44.5/million.[268] The incidence of extragonadal tumors also increases at onset of puberty in males, but at a much lower rate than testicular cancers. In females, the incidence of extragonadal tumors does not increase at puberty and extragonadal tumors are rare in females after the newborn period.

Incidence also varies by race (Table 23-2).[268] Among boys, testicular germ cell tumors are much more common in whites than blacks (9.1 vs. 1.2/million). This striking difference in the rate of diagnosis in young black males continues into adulthood; black men also have a low likelihood of being diagnosed with testicular cancer.[270] However, this may be changing; the incidence of seminoma and nonseminomatous germ cell tumors has increased in blacks by 50% to 100% since 1988, according to SEER data.[271] In contrast, ovarian germ cell tumors are slightly more common in black than white females (5.6 vs. 4.5/million).

The overall incidence of pediatric germ cell tumors in the United States has been increasing. In the period from 1975 to 1979, 3.7 million children younger than 15 years were diagnosed, whereas from 1990 to 1995, 5.4 million children were diagnosed with a GCT. In children younger than age 20, the incidence increased from 8.5 to 12.0/million in the same period.[268] In England and Wales, from 1962 to 1990, investigators examined trends in cancer registry data for testicular cancer in males younger than 15 years and reported that, on average, the incidence increased 1.3%/year over the interval studied.[272,273]

Delving deeper into the SEER data on trends in incidence, among younger prepubertal children, the increase is entirely caused by an increase in rates of intracranial and extragonadal germ cell tumors; rates of gonadal germ cell tumors did not increase. Almost all the increase in extragonadal germ cell tumors was caused by an increase in the reporting of malignant sacrococcygeal teratomas (SCTs) in the first year of life. This so-called increase must be interpreted with caution, because it may reflect surveillance bias. Even though only malignant

teratomas are reported to SEER; most SCTs in the first year of life are benign mature or immature teratomas. However, there has been increased recognition by pathologists that mature or immature teratomas may contain microscopic foci of yolk sac tumor, and therefore more careful scrutiny of these infant teratomas may have led to higher rates of malignant SCT being reported to SEER.

Among adolescents, an increase in the overall incidence of GCT has occurred in both males and females.[268] Both intracranial and gonadal germ cell tumors have increased in incidence, but most of the increase was attributable to gonadal germ cell tumors, both testicular and ovarian germ cell tumors. Among males aged 15 to 19 years, the incidence of testicular GCT increased from 22/million in 1975 to 1979 to 28/million in 1990 to 1995. In girls, the incidence of ovarian germ cell tumors increased from 8 to 13/million over the same 20-year interval.

An increase in testicular cancer has also been noted in men in the countries of the developed world since at least 1940. In the most recent analysis of U.S. data, the incidence of testicular germ cell tumors in men rose 44% between 1973 and 1998, with a more pronounced rise in seminoma (64%) than in nonseminoma (24%; Fig. 23-12).[274] In a study of 22 European countries, the incidence was noted to be increasing, from 1% (Norway) to 6% per year (Spain and Slovenia).[275] The fact that similar trends in incidence have been observed in both young children and adults strengthens the hypothesis that it is exposures that occur prenatally or in early childhood that are responsible for this increase in incidence.

Possible Environmental Causes

Given the worldwide increase in testicular cancer of almost 100% in the last 3 decades, and the concomitant rise in pediatric germ cell tumors, there has been significant interest in identifying potential environmental exposures that could be implicated. The parallel rise in children and young adults has pointed to early life exposure as likely being related to the development of germ cell tumors.

One of the primary hypotheses has been that induction of germ cell tumors occurs in the setting of prenatal exposure to high levels of maternal estrogens, which could affect gonadal development.[276] Several lines of evidence have suggested that this is a plausible hypothesis. When diethylstilbestrol (DES) is administered to pregnant mice, it causes maldescent of the testes and testicular hypoplasia. Male offspring of women who took DES during pregnancy have higher rates of cryptorchidism, a known risk factor for testicular GCTs in humans. Maternal use of DES has also been associated

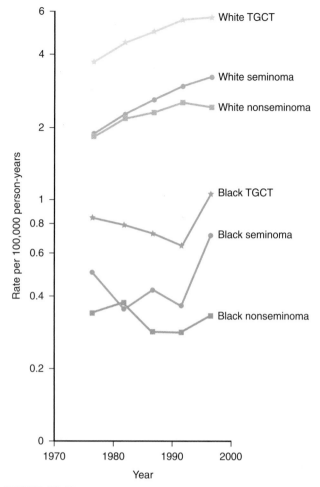

FIGURE 23-12. Incidence of testicular germ cell tumors (TGCTs) in the SEER program from 1973-1978 to 1994-1998. *(Adapted from McGlynn KA, Devesa SS, Sigurdson AJ, et al. Trends in the incidence of testicular germ cell tumors in the United States. Cancer. 2003;97:63-70.)*

with an increased risk of testicular cancer in some but not all studies.[277]

The fetus is also exposed to high levels of endogenous maternal estrogens during pregnancy (vs. exogenous sources, such as DES or oral contraceptives). Conditions of pregnancy, such as hyperemesis gravidum, are known to be associated with higher levels of serum estrogens and have also been linked to an increased risk of GCT. Testicular cancer is more common in first-born males, and twins, especially dizygotic twins; again, both conditions of pregnancy are known to be associated with higher levels of circulating estrogens.[276,278-281] Increased birth weight, which has been associated with a higher risk of testicular cancer, has been associated with higher estradiol and estriol levels in the first and third trimesters of pregnancy.[282] Increased maternal weight, also associated with an increased birth weight, is associated with higher insulin levels, leading to lower sex hormone–binding globulin levels, which thereby increases levels of bioavailable estrogens. Men born during World War II in Norway, Sweden, and Denmark have a decreased risk of testicular cancer compared with men born before or after the war. Maternal weight may explain in part this temporal association. Rationing during WWII in Norway resulted in a 15% to 20% energy restriction and a resultant decrease in maternal weight in the period from 1941 to 1945.[283] Height, determined

in part by childhood nutrition, has been found to be strongly associated with a risk of testicular cancer in two case-control studies.[284,285]

Because germ cell tumors are rare in children, the number of case-control studies conducted among children has been limited. The CCG conducted an epidemiologic study that included all children with cancer registered for treatment with CCG between 1982 and 1989.[286] Parents were asked to complete a 22-page self-administered questionnaire. Approximately 50% of eligible cancer cases completed the questionnaire; controls were obtained through a random digit dialing procedure. Among all the cases, there were 105 cases of children younger than 15 years with a malignant germ cell tumor and 639 controls. In this study, several factors were associated with a risk of germ cell tumor. Birth weight of more than 4000 g was related to a 2.4-fold increase in risk (95% confidence interval [CI] = 1.0 to 5.8) compared with a birth weight less than 3000 g, after adjustment for gestational age. Pregnancy conditions, such as nausea and vomiting and hypertension or eclampsia, were not associated with risk. An inverse association between maternal smoking and risk was noted; among mothers who smoked more than 15 cigarettes/day, the risk of germ cell tumor was reduced by 70%. Among mothers who ever reported being exposed to chemicals or solvents or to plastic and resin fumes, an increased risk was observed (odds ratio [OR], 4.6; CI = 1.9 to 11.3; OR, 12.0, CI = 1.9 to 75, respectively).

A more in-depth follow-up study that specifically focused on germ cell tumors in children was conducted under the auspices of the COG.[287] The study included 278 cases and 423 controls identified through random digit dialing. Subjects completed a self-administered questionnaire, telephone interview, and medical record review of the maternal records before and during the index pregnancy. The study did not confirm a relationship between maternal exposure to exogenous hormones (either DES or oral contraceptives) and risk of pediatric germ cell tumor. None of the pregnancy-related conditions, including birth weight, hyperemesis, preeclampsia, pregnancy-induced hypertension, or maternal weight gain, which can alter circulating levels of endogenous estrogen, was related to risk.[287] The study also failed to replicate the finding from the prior case-control study by the CCG that showed a relationship between maternal smoking and decreased risk of germ cell tumor[288]; neither environmental or occupational exposure to pesticides and other chemicals increased the risk of germ cell tumor in their offspring.[289]

Predisposing Syndromes

Certain syndromes affecting gonadal development and sex steroid production and regulation have clearly been implicated in the pathogenesis of pediatric GCT. These are detailed here.

Cryptorchidism and Testicular Cancer

Many studies have shown a definitive relationship between cryptorchidism and testicular cancer, with relative risks that range from 2.1% to 17.6.[290] Of note, cryptorchidism is three to four times more common in white than black males, which mirrors the difference in incidence by race. The cause of the relationship between cryptorchidism and testicular cancer remains unclear. It has been suggested that exposure of the testis to higher temperatures in the abdomen as compared with the scrotum in some way promotes cancer growth. In this case, orchiopexy should minimize risk, especially if it is done before the hormonal stimulation and proliferation of puberty. Others have suggested that the cause of the undescended testicle and the cancer is the same and, in this case, orchiopexy should not significantly decrease risk. It has been observed that there is an increased risk of testicular cancer in the descended contralateral testicle, which supports this hypothesis for a common cause. In a case-control study from Kaiser-Permanente of 183 cases of testicular cancer patients matched to 551 controls, there were 20 men who had had a cryptorchid testis.[291] Interestingly, if orchiopexy had been performed successfully by age 11, there was no increase in the risk of testicular cancer. However, in men whose cryptorchid testis were not treated until after their 11th birthday, had a failed orchiopexy, or had never had treatment, the odds of testicular cancer were increased 32-fold. Although the study was limited by small numbers, it would suggest that orchiopexy in early childhood prior to puberty may obviate the risk of subsequent testicular cancer. In the case in which an abdominal testes is discovered after the onset of puberty, an orchiectomy may be the most prudent procedure.

Turner's Syndrome and Gonadoblastoma

Turner's syndrome, the most common sex chromosome abnormality in girls (1 in 2000 live births), is caused by partial or total loss of an X chromosome, resulting in a 45,X karyotype. Most girls with Turner's syndrome have short stature and many have primary amenorrhea. Approximately two thirds of girls will have only the remnant of an ovary, or what is described as a streak gonad. Because of the increased risk of developing gonadoblastoma—a generally benign lesion that can undergo malignant degeneration—gonadectomy is recommended. A small subset of girls with Turner's syndrome actually has Y chromosome material. It had been estimated that the risk of gonadoblastoma was as high as 30% in this subset and gonadectomy was routinely suggested. However, a Danish study that examined 114 girls with Turner's syndrome documented the presence of the Y chromosome in 13 girls (12%).[292] In the 10 girls with Y chromosome material who subsequently underwent gonadectomy, gonadoblastoma was present in only one specimen. Therefore, the authors suggested that close ultrasound follow-up may be sufficient for monitoring rather than routine gonadectomy, but urged that more prospective follow-up was necessary.

Klinefelter's Syndrome

Klinefelter's syndrome, a condition present in between 1 in 500 to 1000 males, is caused by an extra X chromosome, resulting in the 47,XXY karyotype. Men with Klinefelter's syndrome have abnormal testicular development and are usually infertile. Men with Klinefelter's syndrome also have a substantially increased risk of developing mediastinal germ cell tumors, beginning in early adolescence.[293] The risk of testicular cancer, interestingly, does not appear to be increased.

Androgen Insensitivity Syndromes

Mutations either in the androgen receptor itself or its downstream effectors results in phenotypic females with an X,Y karyotype.[110] The prevalence of this disorder is estimated to be approximately 1 in 20,000 females. Often, these patients do not come to medical attention until presentation for evaluation of primary amenorrhea. Patients with complete androgen insensitivity often have little to no axillary or pubic hair, no uterus, and male serum testosterone levels. Testes are abdominal or inguinal but can also present on rare occasions as labial masses. These cryptorchid testes are at high risk for the development of gonadoblastoma or other more malignant germ cell tumors, and gonadectomy is advised.

MOLECULAR GENETICS OF GERM CELL TUMORS

The detection and analysis of genomic copy number imbalances (CNIs) in germ cell tumors provides some of the most important evidence supporting the contention that the pathogenesis for pediatric malignant germ cell tumors is distinct from that of adolescent and adult tumors.[61,158,208,294-296] In addition, the gain or loss of specific chromosomal regions may provide important clues about the molecular mechanisms of germ cell tumorigenesis.[1,70,96]

Adolescent and Adult Malignant Germ Cell Tumors

Adolescent and adult malignant testicular germ cell tumors are universally aneuploid, and polyploidization of germ cells has been emphasized as an early event in testicular germ cell tumorigenesis.[297,298] IGCNU and seminoma cells are hypertriploid, whereas nonseminomas of all histologic types are hypotriploid. TGCTs consistently exhibit biallelic expression of imprinted genes.[105,299-303] The erasure of parental imprinting occurs in mammalian embryonic germ cells,[304,305] implying the origin of TGCTs from an early germline cell.[1]

The most common cytogenetic aberrations in TGCTs are the relative loss of all or parts of chromosomes 4, 5, 11, 13, 18, and Y and gain of material from chromosomes 7, 8, 12, and X.[298,306-312] Of these, the most consistent chromosomal aberration in adolescent and adult malignant germ cell tumors is the overrepresentation of chromosome 12p, which is found in all histologic subtypes and primary sites (ovarian, testicular, and extragonadal).[313-322] A characteristic isochromosome 12p—i(12p)— can be detected cytogenetically in 80% of cases[60]; in other cases, an increased copy number of 12p sequences can be detected on derivative chromosomes.[323] Along with tumor markers such as β-hCG, the detection of i(12p) can identify a germ cell origin in cases of carcinoma of unknown primary.[324] Further analysis has identified a particular amplicon, 12p11-12p12.1, that is present in many TGCTs.[325,326] Candidate genes in the 12p region include the oncogenes *KRAS* and *CCND2*, as well as the stem cell–specific genes *NANOG* and *STELLAR*; however, the precise contribution of 12p amplification to the pathogenesis of GCTs remains unclear.[1,6,96,225,249,302,327-332] 12p amplification appears to be a late event in GCT pathogenesis, because it is not present in the precursor lesion, IGCNU.[333] Genome-wide association studies of cases of familial testicular GCT have so far not established a strong linkage of testicular cancer susceptibility to a specific locus.[334-337] An earlier report of linkage to Xq27[338] was not borne out by subsequent studies.[339] Other possible linked loci, including the gr/gr deletion region on the Y chromosome,[340,341] are undergoing further study. It is likely that inherited susceptibility to the adolescent and adult form of testicular GCT is caused by the effect of multiple genes, with each conferring a modest risk.[337]

Molecular genetic analysis of teratomas has further supported the hypothesis of different histogenetic origins of different types of teratomas.[137] The malignant teratoma component of mixed ovarian or testicular GCTs uniformly exhibits the same genomic aberrations as the other malignant components of the tumor, including i(12)p. In contrast, mature, cystic ovarian teratomas and dermoid and epidermoid cysts of the testis exhibit normal karyotypes.[127,155,156,189,209,319,322,342] Based on these observations, Ulbright[137] has proposed that mature ovarian teratomas develop directly from transformed germ cells, whereas postpubertal testicular teratomas develop through a malignant IGCNU stage, as do the other malignant postpubertal TGCTs.

Malignant Germ Cell Tumors of Infants and Children

The genomic aberrations seen in malignant GCTs of infants and children are generally distinct from those occurring in postpubertal tumors.[19,61,158,208,294] Pediatric germ cell tumors show only partial erasure of parental imprinting,[103,105,127,158,296,343,344] indicating that prepubertal GCTs likely arise from an earlier stage of embryonic germ cell development than postpubertal tumors. A similar pattern of imprinting is seen in gonadal and extragonadal pediatric GCTs, suggesting that gonadal and nongonadal tumors share a common pathogenesis and cell of origin.[103,105,158,296,344]

In analyses of chromosomal structure and copy number imbalances, differences between the pediatric and adolescent and adult GCTs are again consistently found. In the prepubertal period, pure teratomas of the testis or of extragonadal sites almost always exhibit a normal profile in genomic analyses, including classic cytogenetics, fluorescence in situ hybridization, loss of heterozygosity analysis, and array comparative genomic hybridization (CGH).[127,138,157,209,345-347] These data contrast sharply with the universally abnormal cytogenetic profile of postpubertal teratomas arising as a component of a mixed malignant germ cell tumor. In adolescents and adult germ cell tumors, only mature teratomas of the ovary and dermoid and epidermoid cysts of the testis exhibit normal cytogenetics, suggesting that these tumors may share a common pathogenesis with prepubertal teratomas.[127,137]

In children younger than 5 years, yolk sac tumor is the most common malignant germ cell tumor of the testis and of extragonadal sites. Unlike teratomas, cytogenetic and other genomic aberrations are consistently reported in analyses of yolk sac tumors in infants and children. The most common imbalances reported are gains at chromosomes 1p and 20q and losses at chromosome 1p and chromosome 6q.[103,138,139,158,294,295,346-350] More recently, the advent of higher resolution techniques, such as array-based CGH, has further defined chromosomal aberrations in this group of tumors. Veltman and coworkers[209] have reported the array-based CGH profiles of a series of 24 germ cell tumors from patients younger than 5 years, including 16 teratomas and 8 yolk sac tumors. Most of the teratomas had normal CGH profiles, with two teratomas exhibiting loss of chromosome 20p as the only recurrent change. In contrast, all the yolk sac tumors had abnormal profiles. The recurrent changes, seen in at least three of the eight yolk sac tumors, included gains of chromosomes 1q (1q32-1qter), 3p (3p21-pter), and 20q (20q13), and loss of chromosomes 1p (1p35-pter), 6q (6q24-qter), and 18q (18q21-qter). In their study, only one tumor from a child younger than 5 years exhibited gain of chromosome 12p, whereas five of seven cases from children older than 5 years showed gains at chromosome 12 p. Most of these tumors occurred in the ovary, supporting the hypothesis that ovarian and testicular malignant GCTs have a common pathogenesis, at least in older children and adults.[1,351] Recently, a larger study from the British Children's Cancer and Leukaemia Group examined the metaphase CGH profile of 34 malignant germ cell tumors in children younger than 16 years (Fig. 23-13).[352] This study supported the previous reports of an increased frequency of loss of chromosomes 1p and 6q and gain of chromosome 3p in yolk sac tumors. Intriguingly, 4 of 14 malignant GCTs from children younger than 5 years demonstrated gain of 12p, including gain of the 12p11 locus that is strongly associated with

adolescent and adult malignant GCTs in two cases. Therefore, childhood and adolescent and adult malignant GCTs may share more pathogenic mechanisms in common than was previously appreciated, based on the analysis of a relatively small number of cases.

Loss of chromosomes 1p and 6q correlates with loss of heterozygosity analysis, indicating true allelic loss in these regions in pediatric GCTs.[347,353] However, the most common chromosomal aberrations of pediatric GCTs—1p–, 1q+, 6q–, and 20q+—are not highly specific for GCTs, but are seen in other cancers of childhood, including neuroblastoma and Wilms' tumor, as well as carcinomas.[354,355] Deletion of chromosome 1p is associated with *MYCN* amplification and poor prognosis in neuroblastoma,[356,357] which has led to the speculation that one or more genes in this interval may act as a tumor suppressor in neuroblastoma.[358] Several candidate genes have been proposed, including *CHD5*, *TNFRSF25*, *CAMTA1*, and *AJAP1*.[359] *CHD5* was recently shown to act as a tumor suppressor in vivo.[71] Whether these or other genes in the 1p and 6q deleted regions play a pathogenic role in pediatric malignant GCTs is not currently known.

DIAGNOSIS AND STAGING OF PEDIATRIC GERM CELL TUMORS

In this section, the clinical presentation of germ cell tumors, evaluation of the patient for metastatic disease, and the use and interpretation of tumor markers in the diagnosis and staging of germ cell tumors will be discussed. The surgical approach, for diagnostic and staging purposes, will also be delineated.

Clinical Presentation

The clinical presentation of a pediatric germ cell tumor is determined by the site of origin, which varies by age. Gonadal tumors can present during infancy but are more common after the onset of puberty. The site of the extragonadal germ cell tumor also varies as a function of age at diagnosis. Sacrococcygeal tumors, much more common in females than males, present at birth or during the first 3 to 4 years of life. Mediastinal tumors are rare in infancy; the incidence begins to rise at onset of puberty, particularly in males. Site-specific features of the presentation are discussed in the sections that follow.

Testicular Germ Cell Tumors

Testicular germ cell tumors most often present with painless generalized swelling of the scrotum. Gynecomastia and infertility are rarely present,[226] although subfertile and infertile men appear to have an increased risk of developing TGCT.[360,361] Local extension to the spermatic cord and the epididymis may occur, and the presenting symptoms can be mistaken for those of epididymitis. Symptoms of metastasis, including back or abdominal pain, cough, or dyspnea, are present at diagnosis in about 10% of adult patients.[70] Choriocarcinoma is the most aggressive histologic subtype of testicular germ cell tumor, with a propensity to hematogenous metastasis. Patients may present with an occult primary tumor and few or no testicular complaints, but rather with symptoms caused by large-volume visceral metastases, such as hemoptysis, gastrointestinal hemorrhage, and neurologic disturbances. Extreme elevation of the serum β-hCG can be seen in choriocarcinoma, and occasional patients manifest thyrotoxicosis or gynecomastia because of the cross-reactivity of β-hCG with the thyroid and luteinizing hormone receptors.[226,362-366]

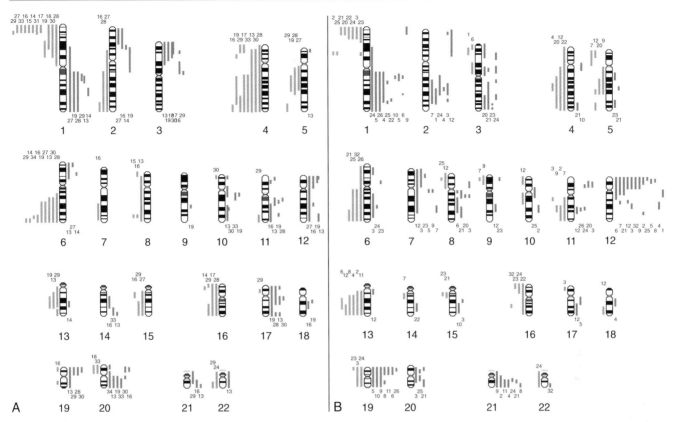

FIGURE 23-13. Comparative genomic hybridization of germ cell tumors in children and adolescents. In this technique, genomic DNA from tumor and control tissue is fluorescently labeled and hybridized to a metaphase chromosome spread or to a microarray representing the entire genome. Schematic views of human chromosomes 1 to 22 are shown; chromosomal gains in the tumor are shown as blue bars to the right of the chromosomes, and losses are shown as red bars to the left of the chromosomes. The numbers above the bars refer to individual cases. **A,** Summary karyograms for children younger than 5 years of age. Note the presence of frequent losses of chromosomes 1p, 4 and 6q and the occurrence of 4 tumors with amplification of chromosome 12p. **B,** Summary karyograms for children between 5 and 16 years of age. The predominant copy number imbalance is gain of chromosome 12p; also notable are gains at 1q and 19 and losses at chromosomes 1p, 6q, and 13. *(Adapted from Palmer RD, Foster NA, Vowler SL, et al. Malignant germ cell tumours of childhood: new associations of genomic imbalance. Br J Cancer. 2007;96: 667-676.)*

An ultrasound that shows the lesion to be intratesticular, with areas of microcalcification, is often helpful in clarifying the differential diagnosis which includes lymphoma and paratesticular rhabdomyosarcoma. Of children younger than 4 years, 85% will present with tumor confined to the testes (stage I), as compared with only 35% of adults.[367]

Ovarian Germ Cell Tumors

Ovarian GCTs typically present with abdominal pain and a palpable pelvic-abdominal mass (85%).[222,266,368] Symptoms of acute abdomen occur in about 10% to 25% of patients, usually caused by rupture, hemorrhage, or torsion of the ovarian tumor, which require immediate surgical exploration.[266] Other less common presenting symptoms include abdominal distention (35%), fever (10%), and vaginal bleeding (10%). Rarely, patients can present with precocious puberty because of the production of β-hCG by the tumor. Not uncommonly, a young girl with an abdominal-pelvic mass and an elevated β-hCG is assumed to be pregnant. This assumption is especially distressing for young females who are peripubertal and may not yet have initiated sexual intercourse.

If the diagnosis of dysgerminoma is made, it is important to recognize that 10% to 15% of cases are bilateral; therefore, the finding of dysgerminoma on frozen section during surgical exploration of an ovarian mass generally warrants close inspec-

tion and perhaps biopsy of the contralateral ovary.[369-372] Most dysgerminomas in the pediatric age group present as stage I (disease confined to the ovary),[369-372] but lymphatic metastasis of these tumors to pelvic, para-aortic, mediastinal, and supraclavicular lymph nodes can occur.[222,373,374] Five percent of dysgerminomas arise in dysgenetic gonads of girls with 46,XY (Swyer's syndrome, or testicular feminization) or who have 45,X–46,XY mosaicism.[375] Therefore, karyotyping should be considered for all girls with a prepubertal pelvic mass.[222] If dysgenetic gonads and the presence of Y chromosome material are detected, removal of the gonads is usually indicated because of the 25% to 50% risk of developing malignancy, such as gonadoblastoma or dysgerminoma.[67,113,376,377] (see earlier, "Epidemiology").

Sacrococcygeal Germ Cell Tumors

SCTs occur predominately in females. In Altman and colleagues' classic 1974 review[378] of 405 clinical cases, 74% occurred in females. However, even though SCTs are much more common in females, the rate of malignancy does not vary by gender. Of note, 18% of patients with SCTs had associated congenital anomalies. The most prevalent defects were in the musculoskeletal system, but other organ systems were involved, including renal, cardiovascular, CNS, and gastrointestinal. More than 50% of the patients were diagnosed on the first day of life but approximately 10% were diagnosed after 1 year of age.

Altman and associates[378] classified sacrococcygeal tumors by the degree of internalization versus externalization of the tumor (Fig. 23-14). An Altman type I SCT is a tumor that is entirely external; an Altman type IV SCT is entirely internal. This group was the first to note the correlation among rate of malignancy, age at diagnosis, and degree of internalization; 7% of girls and 10% of boys younger than 2 months had malignant tumors, whereas after 2 months of age, more than 50% of the tumors were malignant (48% of SCTs in girls and 67% of SCTs in boys).[378]

Most neonatal SCTs have a significant external component (Altman I or II) and can be completely excised in the neonatal period. Over 90% are benign lesions (mature or immature teratoma), which do not require further therapy. Recurrence rates after resection of neonatal mature or immature teratoma have been estimated to range from 4% to 21%, with a malignancy rate of 50% to 70%.[379,380] The reason why fraction of neonatal tumors do recur could be because of oversight of a malignant element during the initial pathologic review, such as a microscopic foci of yolk sac tumor, or because of malignant transformation of a small benign remnant left in situ after the initial procedure. Presacral tumors that are predominantly internal present later in infancy, through age 4. The usual presenting symptoms of an internal lesion are constipation or a gluteal or abdominal mass; the probability is high that these lesions are malignant.

Mediastinal Germ Cell Tumors

In a series of patients with mediastinal germ cell tumors registered in the German MAKEI protocols,[381] chest pain or respiratory symptoms, such as cough or dyspnea, were the most common presenting clinical symptoms. Others included the discovery of the mass as an incidental finding on fetal ultrasound or during a workup for pneumonia that did not resolve with standard antibiotics. In the MAKEI experience, all mediastinal tumors that presented at age younger than 1 year ($N = 9$) were mature or immature teratomas.[381] Mediastinal tumors presenting after infancy but prior to puberty were pure YST or had a predominant yolk sac component. Embryonal carcinoma was more prevalent after the age of 10. Mediastinal seminoma was not diagnosed before age 10.

Extragonadal Germ Cell Tumors at Other Sites

Extragonadal germ cell tumors are the most common fetal and neonatal neoplasms; perinatal teratomas present at a wide array of sites. In a review of all perinatal germ cell tumors reported in the literature from 1965 through 2004, 534 cases were identified.[57] The sacrococcygeal site is the most common (40%), but perinatal GCTs have also been reported in the cervical area (30%), oropharynx and nasopharynx (8%), and other sites, including cardiac (7.5%), gastric (2.6%), orbital (2.4%), facial (1.5%), mediastinal (2.6%), and placental (1.5%) locations. In addition, there were 17 teratomas reported in other sites, including the tongue, tonsil, liver, retroperitoneum, ileum, mesentery, vulva, and anorectal area. In addition, 25 cases of fetus in fetus were reported. The most common reasons for diagnosis included detection of a mass on prenatal ultrasound, polyhydramnios, or respiratory distress. Other symptoms were specific to site—for example, pericardial effusion and tamponade were the most common signs in neonates with intracardiac teratomas. The vast majority of perinatal germ cell tumors were benign, either mature or immature teratomas. Overall, the incidence of yolk sac tumor in the teratoma was 5.8%; the highest rate of yolk sac tumor (10%) was documented in sacrococcygeal teratomas. Teratomas detected antenatally had three times the mortality rates as those diagnosed postnatally. The fetal survival rate was 53% and the neonatal survival rate was 85%. The cause of death was most commonly caused by prematurity or hydrops. The survival rate was only 7% in patients whose tumors presented prior to 30 weeks of gestation.

Evaluation for Metastatic Disease

The current system for staging pediatric germ cell tumors in use by the Children's Oncology Group is shown in Box 23-3.[382] All patients suspected of having a germ cell tumor should have a radiologic evaluation of the extent of disease, including ultrasound, computed tomography (CT) or magnetic resonance

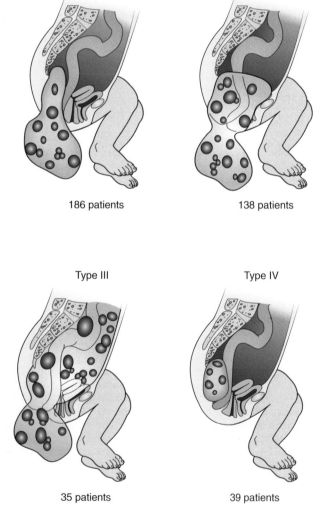

Type I

186 patients

Type II

138 patients

Type III

35 patients

Type IV

39 patients

FIGURE 23-14. Altman classification of sacrococcygeal germ cell tumors. Sacrococcygeal teratomas are classified according to their degree of internalization. Type I tumors are almost entirely external; in type II tumors, the mass extends equivalently into and external to the pelvis. Type III tumors have only a minimal external component and type IV tumors are entirely internalized. The numbers of patients with each type of tumor in this series of 398 patients is shown. - *(Adapted from Altman RP, Randolph JG, Lilly JR. Sacrococcygeal teratoma: American Academy of Pediatrics Surgical Section Survey—1973. J Pediatr Surg. 1974;9:389-398.)*

Box 23-3	Staging of Testicular, Ovarian, and Extragonadal Tumors

TESTICULAR

Stage I: Limited to testis, completely resected by high inguinal orchiectomy; no clinical, radiographic, or histologic evidence of disease beyond the testis; tumor markers normal after appropriate half-life decline; patients with normal or unknown markers at diagnosis must have negative ipsilateral retroperitoneal lymph node sampling to confirm stage I disease

Stage II: Transcrotal orchiectomy; microscopic disease in scrotum or high in spermatic cord (<5 cm from proximal end); retroperitoneal lymph node involvement (<2 cm) and/or increased tumor markers after appropriate half-life decline

Stage III: Tumor-positive retroperitoneal lymph node(s) >2 cm in diameter; no visceral or extra-abdominal involvement

Stage IV: Distant metastases that may include liver

OVARIAN

Stage I: Limited to ovary, peritoneal washings negative for malignant cells; no clinical, radiologic, or histologic evidence of disease beyond the ovaries (gliomatosis peritonei did not result in upstaging); tumor markers negative after appropriate half-life decline

Stage II: Microscopic residual or positive lymph nodes (<2 cm); peritoneal washings negative for malignant cells (gliomatosis peritonei did not result in upstaging); tumor markers positive or negative

Stage III: Gross residual or biopsy only, tumor-positive lymph node(s) >2 cm in diameter; contiguous visceral involvement (omentum, intestine, bladder); peritoneal washings positive for malignant cells

Stage IV: Distant metastases that may include liver

EXTRAGONADAL

Stage I: Complete resection at any site, coccygectomy included as management for sacrococcygeal site, negative tumor margins

Stage II: Microscopic residual; lymph nodes negative

Stage III: Gross residual or biopsy only; regional lymph nodes negative or positive

Stage IV: Distant metastases that may include liver

Data from Cushing B, Giller R, Cullen JW, et al. Randomized comparison of combination chemotherapy with etoposide, bleomycin, and either high-dose or standard-dose cisplatin in children and adolescents with high-risk malignant germ cell tumors: a pediatric intergroup study—Pediatric Oncology Group 9049 and Children's Cancer Group 8882. J Clin Oncol. 2004;22:2691-2700.

cell tumors can also metastasize to brain and bone. Although bone and brain metastases are generally considered rare, German investigators have reported that up to 10% of patients have bone metastasis and that the incidence was as high as 26% in stage IV patients.[383] In the last combined U.S. Intergroup GCT study, 6% of patients overall had bone metastases, but the frequency increased in stage IV patients, in whom 13% had bone metastases at diagnosis.[384] Brain metastases are present in about 4% of adults with GCTs. In a review of the St. Jude experience in 206 cases of pediatric GCT from 1962 to 2002, 16 patients in the series had brain metastases at some point during treatment.[385] Only 2 patients (1%) presented at diagnosis with brain metastases; 12 patients were diagnosed at relapse and 2 patients were discovered to have brain metastases at autopsy. Most patients with brain metastases had clinical symptoms (12 of 16) and also had other concurrent pulmonary metastases (14 of 16). The data likely overestimated the incidence of brain metastases, however, because 11 of 16 were diagnosed prior to 1982, before the use of cisplatinum-based chemotherapy. Risk factors for the development of brain metastases included extragonadal site ($P = .013$), advanced stage ($P = .02$) and choriocarcinoma ($P < .001$). In comparison, in a more recent cohort of patients treated from 1990 to 1996 in the U.S. Pediatric Intergroup study, only 3 of 299 patients were diagnosed with brain metastases; 2 were stage IV at diagnosis.[384] All patients had other sites of metastatic disease; the histology of all 3 patients included choriocarcinoma; 2 of these 3 are alive and well—1 was treated with standard-dose cisplatin (PEB) alone and 1 patient with PEB plus x-ray therapy. Therefore, a bone scan should be obtained in all patients with advanced stage disease (stage III or IV), but head CT or brain MRI is recommended only for stage IV patients (unless the patient has concerning clinical neurologic symptoms), particularly in patients who have choriocarcinoma.

The use of ^{18}F-fluorodeoxyglucose positron emission tomography (PET) has not been systematically evaluated in pediatrics, but its use is becoming more routine in adult patients with germ cell tumors in the setting of a residual mass post-chemotherapy. In a German study that compared the sensitivity and specificity of three different modalities for the evaluation of the residual mass, PET versus CT versus tumor markers (TMs), the results were as follows: PET, 59% sensitivity and 92% specificity; CT, 55% sensitivity and 86% specificity; and TMs, 42% sensitivity and 100% specificity.[386] The positive and negative predictive values for PET were 91% and 62%, respectively. Teratomas were not PET-avid. The authors concluded that PET does not add to the preoperative inference in the setting of a mass in which viable tumor was suspected by CT and TM, but it was a useful adjunct in the setting in which tumor markers had normalized and/or the patient had marker-negative disease at diagnosis. PET-negative masses still require resection because of the possibility of residual teratoma that is PET-negative.

Tumor Markers

Specific subtypes of germ cell tumors secrete proteins that can be used as markers of tumor presence. The pattern of these tumor markers and degree of elevation provide an indication of the likely histology (Table 23-3). AFP is a glycoprotein synthesized by fetal liver and yolk sac. AFP is elevated in patients with yolk sac tumor,[205] although low levels of AFP (less than 100 μg/L) can be observed in immature teratoma, perhaps because of occult microscopic foci of YST within the tumor. Low levels of AFP can also be secreted by a seminoma or dysgerminoma, or by an embryonal carcinoma. When an elevated AFP level is detected, one must consider other possible causes, including

imaging (MRI) of the primary site, abdominal-pelvic CT if the tumor is likely to drain to the lymph nodes of the retroperitoneum and abdomen, and chest CT. Radiologic staging is preferably obtained preoperatively so that the clinician does not have to differentiate between malignant involvement and postoperative changes (i.e., atelectasis on the chest CT or postoperative lymph node enlargement after surgery.) Germ

TABLE 23-3   Histologic Subtype and Tumor Marker Levels

Term	Synonym	Comments	Incidence: Prepuberty vs. Postpuberty	Tumor Marker
Seminoma	Dysgerminoma, germinoma	Seminoma-testes tumor; dysgerminoma-ovarian tumor; germinoma-extragonadal tumor	Postpuberty	Low levels of AFP; low levels of β-hCG in dysgerminoma because of presence of multinucleated syncytiotrophoblastic giant cells
Endodermal sinus tumor	Yolk sac tumor	Most common form prior to puberty, in addition to teratoma	Prepuberty	AFP +++
Embryonal carcinoma			Postpuberty	AFP+; β-hCG+
Choriocarcinoma		Pure forms rare; most commonly one component of mixed GCT	Postpuberty	β-hCG+++
Teratoma			Prepuberty and postpuberty	
Immature teratoma			Prepuberty and postpuberty	~33% of immature teratoma produce low levels of AFP
Polyembryoma				AFP+; β-hCG+
Mixed germ cell tumor (GCT)		Tumors with more than one component are categorized by most malignant component, not by most common component	Prepuberty and postpuberty	Depends on components

+, slightly elevated; +++, markedly elevated; AFP, α-fetoprotein; β-hCG, β-human chorionic gonadotropin.

synthesis by a liver tumor, such as a hepatoma or hepatoblastoma, or other disease states, such as hypothyroidism, folate deficiencies, autoimmune disorders, AIDS, congenital heart defects, cystic fibrosis, and platelet aggregation disorders. β-hCG is a peptide hormone produced in pregnancy that is synthesized by the embryo soon after conception and later by the syncytiotrophoblast (part of the placenta). Its role is to prevent disintegration of the corpus luteum of the ovary and thereby maintain progesterone production, which is critical for pregnancy in humans. In tumors that originate in extraembryonic tissues, such as choriocarcinoma, β-hCG can be significantly elevated. β-hCG is also sometimes mildly elevated in seminoma or dysgerminoma (less than 50 IU/L).

Interpretation of AFP levels must incorporate knowledge of age-related norms[197] (Fig. 23-15).[198] AFP is elevated in all infants at birth because of continued synthesis of AFP by the fetal liver. During the first 2 years of life, AFP declines in normal infants as the synthesis in the liver ceases. To establish normal values for infants, Blohm and coworkers[198] have analyzed data on 414 full-term infants, 90 preterm infants, and 259 children up to age 2 from the University Hospital Dusseldorf (Germany). Using regression analysis, the authors estimated that the half-life of AFP increases with age over the first 2 years of life. From birth to day 28, the half-life is estimated to be 5.1 days. The half-life of AFP increases thereafter to 14 days at 1 to 2 months of age, to 28 days at 2 to 4 months of age, and to 42 days at 4 to 6 months of age. The increase in the half-life of AFP with age also results in a shouldering of the AFP curve during the first 2 years of life. Not all children reach adult levels of AFP by 2 years of age. In the Blohm study, the mean AFP at age 2 was 8 ng/mL, but the 95% range extended between 0.8 and 87 ng/mL. Similar results were reported in an earlier and smaller study by Wu and colleagues.[197] It has been suggested that values of AFP obtained in children younger than

2 years be plotted on the nomogram developed by Blohm and associates[198] to determine whether the value falls within the normal range (see Fig. 23-15).

Tumor markers may also be prognostic, which is why it is important to obtain preoperative levels. In men with testicular cancer, the prognostic significance of tumor markers is well established. An international consortium pooled data on over 5000 men with testicular cancer and used multivariate analysis to investigate prognostic factors that could divide patients into good-, intermediate-, and poor-risk groups. The classification is known as the International Germ Cell Consensus Classification (IGCCC; see Fig. 23-4).[387] Elevated tumor markers is one of the primary variables that determines risk group assignment in adults. Evaluation of the prognostic significance of tumor markers in pediatrics has been limited. In men, the failure of tumor markers to decline appropriately in poor-risk patients has also been shown to be a poor prognostic feature. An elevated AFP of more than 10,000 IU/L has been found to indicate a poor prognosis in analysis of U.S., British, and French data from pediatric germ cell trials.[388-391] (See later, "Prognostic Factors at Diagnosis," for further discussion of the prognostic significance of tumor markers in pediatrics.)

Tumor markers are also used prospectively to differentiate between stage I and II tumors. For patients with gonadal germ cell tumors who have had all disease completely removed surgically, and in whom no evidence of further disease is noted on pathologic or radiologic staging evaluations, a watch and wait strategy is often recommended. However, if tumor markers fail to decline according to their expected half-life, the patient by definition has occult metastatic disease. The patient should be upstaged to stage II and therapy commenced.

There is one situation in which tumor markers may increase and not be cause for alarm. During the first cycle of chemotherapy, it has been observed that tumor markers can

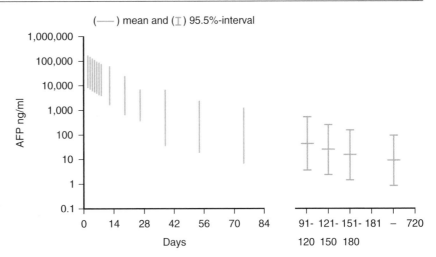

FIGURE 23-15. Serum α-fetoprotein (AFP) values in term babies. *(Adapted from Blohm ME, Vesturing-Horner D, Calaminus G, Gobel U. Alpha 1-fetoprotein (AFP) reference values in infants up to 2 years of age. Pediatr Hematol Oncol. 1998;15:135-142.)*

increase transiently. However, levels should have declined to the expected level by the start of the second cycle of chemotherapy.

Surgery for Diagnosis and Staging

Surgery is necessary to establish the diagnosis and for pathologic staging of the extent of tumor spread. The surgical approach is determined by the site of the disease. For gonadal tumors, a primary resection of the tumor is standard of care, but testicular germ cell tumors only undergo further pathologic staging if the involvement of regional lymph nodes is ambiguous radiographically. In contrast, patients with ovarian tumors are surgically staged, in part because resection of the tumor has already necessitated entry into the pelvis and abdomen. In contrast, for extragonadal tumors, the surgeon must decide whether to attempt a primary resection or to delay resection until after chemotherapy has been used to reduce the size of the mass. Evidence is mounting that delayed resection of extragonadal tumors does not just decrease morbidity but also, more importantly, may increase survival, because of the ability to achieve complete resection at the time of the delayed surgery.

An important factor in the outcome of the patient is the experience of the surgeon. There is accumulating evidence, at least in the case of men with testicular cancer, that the outcome is inferior in patients treated at institutions that do not have a large volume of testicular cancer patients.[392,393] The experience of the surgeon and oncologist should be taken into account in dealing with these relatively uncommon patients who require complicated surgeries.

Surgical Approach to Sacrococcygeal Tumors

Most neonatal tumors have a significant external component (Altman I or II; see Fig. 23-14) and can be completely excised in the neonatal period. Over 90% are benign lesions, either mature or immature teratoma, which do not require further therapy. Recurrence rates after resection of neonatal mature or immature teratoma have been estimated to range from 4% to 21%, with a malignancy rate of 50% to 70%.[379,380] A fraction of neonatal tumors recurs possibly because of an unrecognized malignant element during the initial pathologic review, such as a microscopic foci of yolk sac tumor, or malignant transformation of a small benign remnant left in situ after the initial procedure.

Children with an internal sacrococcygeal tumor should be evaluated for feasibility of resection. Significant functional morbidity has been reported in long-term follow-up of patients with sacrococcygeal tumors, including 46% who reported impaired bowel function and/or urinary incontinence (9% involuntary bowel movements, 13% soiling, 17% constipation), and 31% urinary incontinence. Therefore, a primary biopsy with a delayed resection must be seriously considered if morbidity is likely to be reduced.[394] In patients whose lesions involve the rectum or extend into the sacral bone, or in patients already shown to have metastatic disease, biopsy rather than resection is the more appropriate initial surgical approach. If a needle biopsy is used to obtain diagnostic material, multiple passes should be carried out because of the histologic heterogeneity of these tumors, and the possibility that the malignant foci will not be found in every sample. The histologic diagnosis should also be evaluated in the context of the information from tumor markers. A benign histologic diagnosis, in the setting of elevated tumor markers, should lead one to question whether there was a sampling error in the sample obtained or in the pathologic review.

Delayed resection of a sacrococcygeal teratoma has been definitively demonstrated not to affect survival adversely. German investigators have shown that patients with locally advanced or metastatic tumors actually have better overall survival when treated with chemotherapy prior to tumor resection. Overall survival for patients with delayed resection was 83%, whereas overall survival for patients who had an initial resection was only 45% (*P* = .01).[383] Preoperative chemotherapy allowed for more complete primary resection of the tumor; 19 of 31 patients had a complete resection after preoperative chemotherapy, versus only 11 of 35 patients who had a complete resection when definitive surgery was attempted prior to chemotherapy. Complete resection of the tumor, either at diagnosis or delayed until after chemotherapy, was the most significant predictor of EFS in the German series of sacrococcygeal tumors (Fig. 23-16).[383] Analysis of the data from the U.S. Pediatric Intergroup Trial (POG9049/CCG 8882) also has confirmed that delayed resection does not have an adverse effect on prognosis.[380]

Most presacral lesions will be initially approached through a posterior transsacral incision. Superior extension of the tumor into the pelvis usually requires a laparotomy. If laparotomy is performed, retroperitoneal lymph nodes should be examined and biopsied if enlarged. In all cases, the coccyx must be completely removed en bloc with the primary tumor. The importance of the resection of the coccyx was first noted by Gross

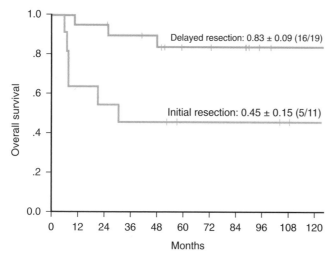

FIGURE 23-16. 5-year overall survival of 30 patients with locally advanced and metastatic malignant sacrococcygeal germ cell tumors (stage T2b M1) treated with initial resection versus delayed resection (*P* = .01; log-rank test). *(Adapted from Gobel U, Schneider DT, Calaminus G, et al. Multimodal treatment of malignant sacrococcygeal germ cell tumors: a prospective analysis of 66 patients of the German cooperative protocols MAKEI 83/86 and 89. J Clin Oncol. 2001;19:1943-1950.)*

and associates,[395] who reported a recurrence rate of 38% in those who had not had coccygectomy and 0% in those who had had a coccygectomy.

Surgical Approach to Testicular Tumors

Because the most frequent sites of metastasis of a testicular germ cell tumor are the retroperitoneal lymph nodes, a pelvic-abdominal CT scan should be obtained preoperatively. If the CT scan is delayed until after surgical exploration of the inguinal region, reactive retroperitoneal lymphadenopathy may be noted on CT scans and may be difficult to differentiate from metastatic disease. Similarly, evaluating the lungs for pulmonary metastases with chest CT prior to surgery is advisable, because postoperative atelectasis can make evaluation for malignant disease more difficult. Tumor markers should also be obtained preoperatively, because these levels are important to confirm the initial diagnosis and provide prognostic information. In addition, the rate of decline is important to be able to track postoperatively in patients, especially stage I patients who are being expectantly observed, reserving chemotherapy only for those patients who have demonstration of residual malignant disease.

The surgical approach for a scrotal tumor should be via an inguinal incision. Control of the testicular vessels and vas deferens is gained at the level of the inguinal ring. The testis is then mobilized out from the scrotum. Occasionally, a large testicular mass cannot be mobilized out of the scrotum into the inguinal region; in this case, the inguinal incision should be enlarged to the superior aspect of the scrotum to avoid tumor rupture during mobilization. A radical orchiectomy is then performed, with high ligation of all cord structures at the level of the internal inguinal ring. In a prepubertal boy, if a lesion appears to involve only a portion of the testicle, excision only of the involved portion of the testis is an appropriate procedure. If frozen section is consistent with teratoma, the testis can then be placed back in the scrotal position, because enucleation is adequate therapy for a testicular teratoma. In the postpubertal boy, however, the tumor is more likely to contain a malignant component and full orchiectomy should be undertaken.

Rates of adherence to surgical guidelines have been evaluated in 63 patients with stage I GCT of the testes who were treated with observation only in the last U.S. intergroup trial from 1990 to 1996.[396] Adherence to guidelines could be verified in only 69% of patients. The likelihood of adherence was directly related to having suspected tumor preoperatively. In patients in whom the preoperative diagnosis was malignant tumor, the surgical guidelines were followed in 80% of patients, whereas in patients in whom another preoperative diagnosis was suspected (e.g., hydrocele, hernia, torsion), the guidelines were followed in only 17%. However, there was no difference in recurrence rate in those patients in whom the surgical guidelines were followed and in those for whom the guidelines were not followed, with the exception of patients who had had scrotal violations. In the 4 patients with trans-scrotal violation, 3 had recurrence of disease.

The experience of the last pediatric intergroup study has led to revision of the recommendation in the case of scrotal violation. In cases in which a scrotal orchiectomy has been performed without violation of the tumor capsule, the patient may still remain a stage I, assuming negative margins; however, the proximal cord structures should be resected to the level of the internal ring. If the cord structures show evidence of tumor spread, the patient should be upstaged to stage II. If a scrotal biopsy was performed as the initial procedure, however, the scrotum is considered to be contaminated and the patient should be treated as a stage II, but hemiscrotectomy is no longer required. In addition, a completion orchiectomy, with removal of all cord structures to the level of the internal ring, should be performed.

Evaluation of Retroperitoneal Nodes in Pediatric Testicular Germ Cell Tumors. Lymphatic drainage of the testes is to the retroperitoneal nodes and to the nodes below the renal vessels. Right testicular tumors usually metastasize to the nodes between the aorta and inferior vena cava (interaortocaval nodes). Left testicular tumors metastasize to the nodes lateral to the aorta (para-aortic).[397] Left supraclavicular nodes and pulmonary nodules have been observed in the absence of retroperitoneal adenopathy. In adults, it is estimated that up to 30% of patients have false-negative CT scans. In the most recent U.S. intergroup study of stage I testicular cancer in boys younger than 10 years, 5% of patients had failure of normalization of tumor markers post-operatively (i.e., patients who had occult disease that was not detected on initial CT scan—false-negative initial CT scan). In total, 22% of patients with presumed stage I at diagnosis eventually relapsed, but all were salvaged with chemotherapy, with 100% survival.[367]

If the preoperative CT scan of the abdomen has identified enlarged (4 cm or larger) retroperitoneal lymph nodes, biopsy is not necessary and one may assume that this represents metastatic disease; the patient should be treated as having stage III disease. If retroperitoneal lymph nodes are 2 to 4 cm, a biopsy should be performed. If the retroperitoneal nodes are smaller than 2 cm, a biopsy is not required; however, the tumor markers (AFP and β-hCG) should be followed and returned to normal, with appropriate decline according to the half-life (see earlier). In men, 10% to 20% of nodes between 1 and 2 cm will contain metastatic disease.

If the decision is made to biopsy a suspected node of the prepubertal boy, the retroperitoneal procedure should simply be a lymph node excision, not a full retroperitoneal lymph node dissection. If no biopsy is performed and the nodes are enlarged (more than 2 cm), the patient should be treated as a stage III patient. However, in adolescents (as in adults), if a biopsy is being undertaken to evaluate nodal disease, a nerve-sparing modified template retroperitoneal lymph node dissection (RPLND) should be used, which some surgeons would expand to a full bilateral nerve-sparing RPLND if any of the initial nodes are positive on frozen section. RPLND is diagnostic and potentially therapeutic. (See later discussion of RPLND for the treatment of adolescent boys with stage I testicular cancer.)

Metachronous Testicular Cancer. In adults, 3% to 5% of men with testicular cancer will have a metachronous tumor in the other testicle at diagnosis and 2% of men will subsequently develop a tumor in the contralateral testicle. These risks have not been quantified for pediatric patients and no formal evaluation of the contralateral testis is recommended in addition to a thorough physical examination. Patients who have developed a testicular tumor in a cryptorchid testis are at increased risk of malignancy in the normally descended contralateral testis.

Surgical Approach to Ovarian Tumors

The goals of the initial exploration of a suspected ovarian tumor are to evaluate the extent of disease completely, maximize the completeness of the tumor resection, and spare uninvolved reproductive organs. AFP and β-hCG should be determined preoperatively if the diagnosis is suspected. If not done preoperatively, these markers should be determined as soon as possible, even in the operating room, once the diagnosis is apparent. A priori likelihood of malignancy in a girl presenting with an ovarian mass has been estimated to be as high as 80%, but a larger series (still only 66 cases) has estimated lower rates—the incidence of malignancy was 19% at 0 to 5, 14% at 6 to 10, and 33% at 11 to 15 years.[266]

Surgical guidelines for ovarian germ cell tumors were originally based on the experience with ovarian epithelial carcinoma, in which aggressive surgical resection was associated with a higher chance of survival. Application of those surgical guidelines to ovarian germ cell tumors, which have a different pattern of spread and are also highly chemosensitive, is not warranted. It is clear from studies in women with germ cell tumors that fertility-sparing surgery, such as performing a unilateral instead of bilateral salpingo-oophorectomy, has no adverse outcome on survival.[244] In the most recently completed U.S. Intergroup Trial for gonadal tumors (CCG 8892/POG 9048), surgeons adhered to the guidelines in only 2% of patients,[398] but event-free survival (EFS) and overall survival (OS) were nonetheless excellent.[399] Surgical omissions resulting in protocol noncompliance resulted from failure to biopsy bilateral nodes (97%), no omentectomy (36%), no peritoneal cytology (21%), or no contralateral ovary biopsy (59%). However, in patients in whom peritoneal cytology was examined, 25% of patients had malignant tumors found, but biopsies of normal-appearing lymph nodes, omentum, and/or contralateral ovary had a very low incidence of malignant results.

Based on the excellent overall survival, despite low adherence to the surgical guidelines in the Pediatric Intergroup Trial, the current surgical guidelines for pediatric ovarian GCTs have been substantially revised. Given the high rate of positivity in the examination of peritoneal fluid, all patients with ascites should have the fluid collected for cytology. In the absence of ascites, peritoneal washings should be carried out and sent for pathologic review. The pelvic viscera should be examined and pelvic and retroperitoneal lymph nodes should be palpated bilaterally. Only suspicious or enlarged lymph nodes should be biopsied. The omentum and peritoneal surfaces should also be palpated and visualized. If the omentum is adherent, or has nodules or implants, partial or complete omentectomy that includes the lesions should be done. If the omentum does not appear grossly involved, an omentectomy does not need to be performed. Any nodules studding the peritoneal surfaces should be biopsied.

If only one ovary is involved, the tumor should be removed by unilateral oophorectomy. Attempts to preserve completely uninvolved fallopian tubes and the uterus should be made in all patients. Lesions adherent to the uterus may be managed by separation of the adherence if feasible, or by biopsy only, with planned second-look surgery after chemotherapy, if necessary. The tumor capsule should not be aspirated. If the capsule is violated, either by the surgeon or rupture by the tumor, or if there is microscopic capsule penetration seen by the pathologist in an apparently intact tumor, the patient should be upgraded to stage II. (This is in contrast to adult staging guidelines, in which a patient with capsular involvement is stage IC.) The ovary must be delivered intact and not removed fragmentally. The contralateral ovary should only be biopsied if it appears involved with tumor; biopsy of a normal-appearing contralateral ovary is discouraged because of the adverse impact on future fertility. Bilateral ovarian lesions were present in only 6% of patients ($N = 10$) in the U.S. Pediatric Intergroup Study. Of these, four were benign teratomas and six were malignancies. If a patient has bilateral disease, preservation of as much normal ovarian parenchyma as possible should be the goal.

Surgical Approach to Mediastinal Germ Cell Tumors

Analogous to the experience with sacrococcygeal tumors, in the German MAKEI experience, with mediastinal germ cell tumors, delayed resection increased the probability that the patient would have a complete resection of the primary tumor (10 of 11 patients at delayed tumor resection vs. 6 of 12 patients at primary tumor resection),[381] and a complete resection was a strong predictor of more favorable outcome (EFS, 0.94 ± 0.06 vs. 0.42 ± 0.33). Therefore, the surgeon must decide whether it is more prudent to attempt a primary resection or to obtain a biopsy and plan for delayed resection.

The resection may be through a lateral thoracotomy or median sternotomy, as determined by the site of the lesion. The margin of resection should include contiguous nonvital structures, such as the thymus and pericardium. Regional lymph nodes should be evaluated and biopsied when possible in all patients.

Surgical Approach to Extragonadal Tumors at Other Sites

Yolk sac tumor, also referred to as endodermal sinus tumor, of the vagina is a rare tumor occurring exclusively in children younger than 3 years. The mass can be confused with sarcoma botryoides. Only small lesions that can be resected with vaginal preservation should be excised at initial presentation. In others, a careful vaginal examination and limited biopsy should be performed. After completion of chemotherapy, repeat evaluation and complete excision of residual disease should be done.

Malignant germ cell tumors found at other locations should be completely excised, if possible, without sacrifice of adjacent organs. Biopsy only may be appropriate at the initial operation, with planned secondary procedures for delayed excision after chemotherapy. Any enlarged regional lymph nodes in the area should be sampled.

Prognostic Factors at Diagnosis

Tumor markers have prognostic significance, which is why it is important to obtain preoperative levels. In men with testicular cancer, the prognostic significance of tumor markers is well established. An international consortium pooled data on over 5000 men with testicular cancer and used multivariate analysis to investigate prognostic factors that could divide patients into good-, intermediate-, and poor-risk groups (see Table 23-7). Elevated tumor markers is one of the primary variables that determines risk group assignment in adults. Other adverse prognostic factors include mediastinal primary site and presence of nonpulmonary visceral metastases. Lactate dehydrogenase (LDH) has been shown to be prognostic in men with testicular cancer, but has not been shown to have prognostic significance in pediatric patients, although analyses to date have been underpowered to examine this issue.

Several retrospective studies in men with testicular cancer have shown that slower than expected decline in tumor markers after the initiation of treatment predicts lower EFS and OS.[400-402] In an analysis of men with testicular cancer treated between 1986 and 1998 at Memorial Sloan-Kettering, those with satisfactory decline in their tumor markers had excellent 2-year results (EFS, 91%; OS, 95%) versus those with unsatisfactory decline (EFS, 69%; OS, 72%).[402] A recent randomized trial in poor-risk testicular cancer patients compared standard therapy, four cycles of BEP (bleomycin, etoposide, cisplatin), to two cycles of BEP followed by two cycles of high-dose carboplatin, etoposide, and cyclophosphamide (BEP + HDCT). Although the overall results of the trial did not show a difference in survival between the two arms, in the subgroup of 67 patients with unsatisfactory tumor marker decline, the 1-year durable complete response was 61% for the patients who received HDCT compared with 34% for those who received BEP alone.[403]

Evaluation of the prognostic significance of tumor markers in pediatrics has been limited by relatively small numbers enrolled on clinical trials. Nonetheless, in data from the last U.S. Pediatric Intergroup trial, British GC2 trial, and French TGM85 and TGM90 trials, an AFP of 10,000 IU/L or higher portends a worse prognosis for EFS.[382,388-391] In multivariate analysis of the British data, AFP of 10,000 IU/L or higher was a stronger predictor of relapse than site or stage; those with AFP higher than 10,000 IU/L had four times the risk of relapse. In two pediatric studies, AFP was not found to be prognostic, but both analyses were restricted only to patients with extragonadal primaries.[404,405] β-hCG and LDH were evaluated in the U.S. data and not shown to be of prognostic significance when using the cut points developed for men in the IGCCC data set.[382,388] The extragonadal tumor site was of prognostic significance in the U.S., British, and French studies, although it was defined slightly differently in each study. Common to each study was the inclusion of mediastinal site, which is clearly associated with reduced EFS in all studies. The relative impact of other sites of extragonadal disease will require examination in a larger dataset. The impact of satisfactory versus unsatisfactory tumor marker decline has not been evaluated in pediatric germ cell tumor patients.

TREATMENT

Overview

Survival has improved markedly since the 1979 report by Einhorn that testicular germ cell tumors are responsive to cisplatin-based regimens.[406] As it becomes more and more established, at least from long-term studies of men who have been successfully treated for testicular germ cell tumors, that treatment is associated with significant long-term morbidities and even increased chance of mortality, the need to minimize

toxicity is apparent. Many patients will require no treatment in addition to complete surgical resection; chemotherapy can be reserved to salvage only those patients who recur. On the other end of the spectrum, it is also apparent that for a subset of approximately 20% of patients, the standard cisplatin-based regimens are insufficient, and more intensive chemotherapeutic strategies must be devised. A key part of future treatment strategies will be the ability to identify those patients at high risk of relapse at the time of their initial presentation, and to design chemotherapeutic regimens that increase the odds of long-term survival, both by optimal first-line therapies and salvage therapies for those who fail to respond.

Explanation of the Nomenclature

Germ cell tumors are generally divided into several categories when treatment is being discussed: (1) teratoma; (2) immature teratoma; (3) seminoma-dysgerminoma; and (4) other malignant germ cell tumors, which includes the histologies of yolk sac tumor (or endodermal sinus), embryonal carcinoma, and choriocarcinoma. Germ cell tumors can present as a single histology, such as pure yolk sac tumor, or with a mixture of different histologies, including histologies from all four categories (teratoma, immature teratoma, seminoma-dysgerminoma, and other malignant germ cell tumors). The terminology is somewhat confusing in that a "malignant germ cell tumor" is shorthand for a germ cell tumor that contains at least one of the other malignant components, which means yolk sac, embryonal carcinoma, or choriocarcinoma. These histologies have a more aggressive nature; however, both immature teratoma and seminoma-dysgerminoma are also malignant forms of germ cell tumors, although generally more sensitive to chemotherapy and radiation than the other malignant forms. A mixed malignant germ cell tumor refers to a tumor that contains at least one of the malignant histologies (yolk sac, embryonal carcinoma, choriocarcinoma) but may also contain histologies from any of the other categories. The general proviso is that one must treat the most malignant form of the germ cell tumor. However, it is important to remember the other histologies that are present. For example, if there is a significant portion of the original tumor that is mature teratoma at diagnosis, this part of the tumor is not likely to respond to chemotherapy and it will likely be necessary to excise the remaining teratoma surgically at the end of the chemotherapeutic regimen.

Seminoma and Dysgerminoma

The nomenclature of this subtype of pediatric germ cell tumor can be confusing. It is important to recognize that a tumor with the same histologic appearance will have a different name, depending on the site in which it arose. Germinoma typically refers to an intracranial lesion, usually in the pineal gland. Dysgerminoma describes a lesion in the ovary. Seminoma describes a lesion that arises in the testis.

Seminomas and dysgerminomas are much more common histologies in young and middle-aged adults than in adolescents. Diagnosis of a seminoma or dysgerminoma is exceedingly rare prior to the onset of puberty. However, in men overall, seminomas account for approximately 50% of all testicular cancers, occurring most frequently in the fourth decade.[269]

Because these tumors are exquisitely sensitive to radiotherapy, radiation was an important component of the original treatment regimen. In patients with ovarian tumors, radiation resulted in sterilization of the remaining ovary. Therefore, since the 1980s, chemotherapy with cisplatin-based therapy has replaced radiotherapy in the treatment of ovarian GCT. With longer follow-up of patients treated with radiotherapy, it has become clear that there was reason for serious concerns about induction of secondary malignancies and cardiovascular disease in irradiated patients. The hazard ratio of cardiac death after infradiaphragmatic radiotherapy was 1.6 (95% CI, 1.2 to 2.4)[407] and, in a large prospective study, the risk of cardiac events after intradiaphragmatic radiotherapy was 2.4 (95% CI, 1.04 to 5.5).[408] The risk of a second malignant neoplasm was 2.0 (95% CI, 1.9 to 2.2).[409]

Therapy has evolved, so that the current standard for stage I disease is surveillance, with an expected 15% to 20% relapse rate. With seminomas, relapses can occur late; 5% occur after 5 years and there are anecdotal reports of relapses occurring after 10 years. Currently, most pediatric radiotherapists would refuse to use radiotherapy to treat a seminoma or dysgerminoma because of the risk of late effects; chemotherapy has replaced radiation as first-line therapy.

Current treatment recommendations parallel those for children with nonseminomatous malignant GCT. Patients with stage I seminoma or dysgerminoma are advised to undergo a watch and wait strategy, reserving chemotherapy for the 15% to 20% who are expected to relapse. Patients with higher stage disease are treated with three cycles of BEP, with an excellent prognosis.

However, these histologies are rare enough in pediatrics that treatment recommendations derive directly from the adult experience. The pediatric oncologist who is referred a patient with one of these diagnoses should consult with an adult oncologist, and refer to an organization such as the National Cancer Care Network (NCCN) that maintains updated clinical practice guidelines for these tumors (http://www.nccn.org).

MALIGNANT NONSEMINOMATOUS GERM CELL TUMORS
There are three treatment options that a physician should consider and discuss with a patient with a stage I malignant nonseminomatous germ cell tumor (MNSGCT). The first option is surgery, followed by observation. Pediatric patients with stage I testicular germ cell tumors, stage I ovarian and, even in some countries, stage I extragonadal GCT, are being observed after surgery, withholding chemotherapy for those who recur. Surveillance in this watch and wait strategy involves radiologic surveillance of the primary sites of recurrence every 3 months in the first year and every 6 months in the second year. Tumor markers should be monitored every month during the first year and every 2 to 3 months in the second year.

In patients with testicular cancer, two other options exist. The first, retroperitoneal lymph node dissection, can be diagnostic and therapeutic. The last option is to give adjuvant chemotherapy. Because the patient is presumed most likely to have minimal disease at most, the number of cycles of chemotherapy is reduced from three to two cycles of BEP. Experience with these three options is most extensive in men with testicular cancer and is reviewed here.

Stage I Disease in Men

Active Observation

The watch and wait strategy of active observation is based on a plethora of data from adult trials of men with stage I MGCT. Over 2000 adult patients have been enrolled in clinical trials of surveillance, with a median follow-up of at least 10 years.[410] Relapse rates have ranged from 27% to 35%; 95% of relapses occurred in the first 2 years postorchiectomy. Almost all patients who relapsed had good-risk disease, as defined by the International Germ Cell Cancer Collaborative Group (IGCCCG) criteria; overall survival with chemotherapy was 98% to 99%.

An increasing concern is that a patient who undergoes surveillance is obligated to have serial CT scans at frequent intervals, which exposes the patient to a dose of radiation that may subsequently be the cause of secondary malignancy. The COG currently recommends scans every 3 months for the first year and every 6 months for the second year postdiagnosis. However, a whole-trunk CT scan (chest, abdomen, and pelvis) will produce a radiation dose of 10 to 30 mSv.[411] Currently, it is recommended that exposure be limited to 100 mSv over 5 years.[412] Although it has been suggested that the risk related to low doses of radiation may have been overestimated, a retrospective cohort study using data from 15 countries has estimated that a cumulative exposure of 100 mSv would lead to a 9.7% increase in risk of all mortality from cancer, excluding leukemia, and a 19% increase in mortality from leukemia.[413] Rustin and colleagues[414] have postulated that five total body CT scans, therefore, could induce one second cancer in every 200 patients, which is the risk of death after stage I testis cancer. Therefore, they designed a trial in men with stage I testicular cancer comparing a surveillance policy of two CT scans over the first year (at 3 and 12 months) versus the standard surveillance policy of five CT scans over the first 2 years (3, 6, 9, 12, and 24 months). Patients continued to have frequent evaluations, which included measurement of tumor markers and chest x-ray (once per month in year 1, every 2 months in the second year, and every 3 months in the third year). There was no difference in overall relapse rate between the two surveillance groups, no increase in more advanced stage at relapse between the two groups, and no difference in overall survival. A major limitation of the study was that only 10% of the patients were at high risk for relapse, on the basis of the presence of lymphovascular invasion, so it is not clear whether this schedule is vigilant enough for this group of patients. Given the increased radiosensitivity of children to the low dose of ionizing radiation associated with CT scans, the schedule of surveillance in children with stage I germ cell tumors deserves serious scrutiny.

Factors that Predict Relapse. The first study to examine this issue was a retrospective study from the Medical Research Council in England,[415] in which 259 tumor specimens from clinical stage I patients on surveillance were reviewed without knowledge of subsequent clinical outcome. Four prognostic features were identified: invasion of the testicular veins, invasion of the testicular lymphatics, absence of yolk sac element, and presence of embryonal carcinoma. This resulted in a classification based on the number of risk factors—3% of patients had none of these factors and 100% were relapse-free at 2 years; 31% of patients had one factor and had 91% relapse-free survival; 34% had two factors and had a 75% relapse-free survival; and 21% of patients had three or more factors and had a 42% relapse-free survival. In a prospective study (N = 366) confirming this risk classification, 20% of patients were high risk (three or more factors) and had a 3-year relapse-free survival of 54%.[416] Because it is difficult to differentiate between invasion of the blood vessel and invasion of the lymphatics, a composite variable of lymphovascular invasion (LVI)[417] was agreed on. Subsequent studies have confirmed that the single most important prognostic factor is lymphovascular invasion[417] bifurcating risk into low-risk (15% to 20%) and high-risk (40% to 50%) relapse. Although embryonal carcinoma is a significant prognostic variable in univariate analyses, its importance in multivariate models is subsumed by the presence of lymphovascular invasion. No immunohistochemical markers, including MIB-1, p53, bcl-2, cathepsin D, or E-cadherin, have added to the prognostic significance of LVI alone.[418-420]

Retroperitoneal Lymph Node Dissection (RPLND)

There is no doubt that surgical removal of retroperitoneal lymph nodes known to comprise the landing zones for metastatic disease from the testes is the most accurate way to stage a patient, and potentially therapeutic as well. Relapse in the surgical field is less than 1% post-RPLND. The consensus of a series of clinical trials has shown that between 30% and 50% of men with testicular stage I nonseminoma will have occult metastases at RPLND that were not detected by radiologic scans.

A serious concern for any patient undergoing RPLND is nerve injury that interferes with the ability to ejaculate, causing retrograde ejaculation or ejaculatory failure. Because of refinements in surgical technique and the development of so-called nerve-sparing approaches, it is estimated that preservation of ejaculatory function is as high as 90% to 95%, especially if the surgery is done by a urologist who performs a high volume of these procedures annually (e.g., 10 to 20). The surgery can be the cause of infrequent but not negligible complications, such as bowel complications, lymphocele, and chylous ascites, although these may decrease as the laparoscopic approach becomes more widely used. Referral of the adolescent male who chooses RPLND as primary therapy to a cancer center with a urologist who specializes in RPLND should be strongly considered.

However, RPLND does not mean that chemotherapy will be avoided. Ten percent of pathologic stage (PS) I patients will relapse post-RPLND (primarily in the lungs), and approximately one third of patients with PS II disease who have evidence of more extensive disease (multiple nodes, any nodes larger than 2 cm, or any evidence of extranodal spread) require chemotherapy, usually at least two cycles of BEP. One advantage of a primary RPLND is that it may reduce the odds of having to perform RPLND after chemotherapy. After chemotherapy, the operation is more technically challenging because of the desmoplastic reaction to chemotherapy and cicatrization. Another advantage of primary RPLND is that it removes any concurrent teratoma, which is a chemoresistant form of germ cell tumors. The incidence of teratoma in men may be as high as 30%. Because 5% to 10% of teratomas can undergo malignant degeneration to non–germ cell malignancies that are more difficult to treat, it is beneficial to resect these components of germ cell tumor early in the course of treatment.

Adjuvant Chemotherapy

Another option used for men with clinical stage I NSGCT is adjuvant chemotherapy with one or two cycles of BEP. Although 11 studies have now shown that the risk of relapse can be reduced to less than 2%, the concern remains that most patients, conservatively at least 50%, have no further need for chemotherapy after the orchiectomy, and therefore treatment with BEP is overtreatment for a large percentage. Moreover, accumulating evidence of significant long-term side effects associated with three or four cycles of cisplatin-based therapy, including a marked increase in cardiovascular disease and risk of second malignancy (see later, "Late Effects"), should invoke caution about the administration of even two cycles of the same therapy, because the relationship between dose and late effect has not been quantified.

Stage I Disease in Pediatric Patients

Active Observation

In the U.S. Pediatric Intergroup study (POG09048/CCG8891), boys younger than 11 years with stage I testicular malignant germ cell tumors were observed after surgery (watch and wait strategy). They were only given chemotherapy if tumor markers did not normalize as expected or if imaging revealed recurrent disease. In the 63 patients enrolled in the protocol, 11 patients had progression of disease and received chemotherapy (four cycles of standard-dose BEP; see later); 80% of the recurrences occurred in the first year after surgery. The 6-year EFS of active observation was 78.5% ± 7%, but all patients were salvaged with subsequent chemotherapy (6-year OS, 100%).[396]

In the British Germ Cell Tumor Study II, conducted between 1989 and 1997, all gonadal stage I tumors (testicular and ovarian) were observed without chemotherapy. Of 51 testicular GCT patients, 40 (78%) were successfully treated with surgery alone, as were 6 of 9 (66%) patients with ovarian stage I GCT. All patients who recurred after observation were cured with carboplatin, etoposide, and bleomycin chemotherapy.[389]

The German study used separate protocols for treating testicular tumors (MAHO protocols) and nontesticular, extracranial, pediatric germ cell tumors (MAKEI protocols). In the latest update of the MAHO protocols, the authors reported on results from 1982 to 2001.[421] A watch and wait approach was taken for patients with stage I nonseminomatous testicular tumors, but only if the malignant histology was pure yolk sac, pure teratoma, pure immature teratoma, or pure seminoma. Boys with testicular tumors that included a malignant component other than yolk sac were treated with standard chemotherapy that consisted of PVB (cisplatin, vinoblastine, and etoposide). Of the 140 boys with stage I yolk sac tumor,[205] 16 (13%) progressed and required standard chemotherapy 6 to 60 weeks' postorchiectomy.[421] Of the 140 patients, 139 are alive and well. All boys with either mature teratoma ($n = 40$), immature teratoma ($n = 19$), or seminoma ($n = 2$) were cured with surgery alone.

On the MAKEI 96 protocol, the observational strategy was extended to include stage I ovarian and extragonadal GCT. Excluded from this surgery-only approach were extragonadal tumors that arose in the sacrococcygeal region. Children with sacrococcygeal primaries, regardless of stage, were treated with four cycles of PEI (cisplatin, etoposide, and ifosfamide), except for infants younger than 4 months, who were treated with four cycles of PE (cisplatin and etoposide; see later, "Treatment of Pediatric Germ Cell Tumors in Germany"). Results of this approach have not yet been published.

Chemotherapy for Pediatric Germ Cell Tumors Higher Than Stage I

Prechemotherapy Evaluation. Prior to initiating chemotherapy, studies should be done to establish a baseline for monitoring toxicity and procedures undertaken to minimize the risk of late effects. The postpubertal male patient should be encouraged to bank sperm, because a small percentage of male patients will be infertile postchemotherapy. Oocyte cryopreservation (egg freezing) is a rapidly advancing field and should be considered in postpubertal females due to an ill-defined but apparently increased risk of infertility. In addition, patients who are to receive standard chemotherapy with bleomycin, cisplatin, and etoposide (BEP) should have baseline measurements of their renal function by measuring the glomerular filtration rate (GFR), preferably with a chromium EDTA clearance, pulmonary function tests (PFTs), including DLCO (diffusing capacity of the lung for carbon monoxide), and baseline audiometry that includes accurate measurements of the high-frequency region, because this is the region affected first by cisplatin-induced hearing loss.

History of Use of Chemotherapy In Men with Testicular Cancer. Treatment of pediatric germ cell tumors derives in large part from knowledge gained in the treatment of men with testicular cancer. In 1979, Einhorn[406] reported that the combination of cisplatin, vinblastine, and bleomycin (subsequently referred to as the Einhorn regimen, or PVB), cured a substantial portion of men with widely disseminated testicular cancer. A follow-up study has shown that substitution of etoposide for vinblastine (BEP vs. PVB) is a superior regimen, both in terms of increased efficacy and reduced neuromuscular toxicity,[422] and BEP became the standard of care. Finally, it was shown that three cycles of BEP were equivalent to four cycles of BEP in good-prognosis patients, as defined by the IGCCC[423] (Table 23-4 provides a definition of a good-risk patient).[387] Based on experience in the treatment of adult testicular cancer, the pediatric trials reviewed later were developed.

Treatment of Pediatric Germ Cell Tumors in the United States

Prior to the use of chemotherapy, the outcome of children with germ cell tumors was dismal; 3-year survival rates did not reach 20%.[218,424] In the mid-1970s, the first reports of the effective chemotherapy regimens for pediatric germ cell tumors were published.[425,426] These regimens were based on VAC—vincristine, dactinomycin and cyclophosphamide—but also included radiation therapy. Although the survival for average-risk patients improved to approximately 60%, children with advanced-stage disease continued to have a poor prognosis.

TABLE 23-4	Definition of the Germ Cell Consensus Classification	
Nonseminoma	**Seminoma**
GOOD PROGNOSIS	
Testis–retroperitoneal primary *and* no nonpulmonary visceral metastases *and* good markers—all of the following: AFP < 1000 ng/mL *and* hCG < 5000 IU/L (1000 ng/mL) *and* LDH < 1.5 × upper limit of normal	Any primary site *and* no nonpulmonary visceral metastases *and* normal AFP, any hCG, and LDH
INTERMEDIATE PROGNOSIS	
Testis–retroperitoneal primary *and* no nonpulmonary visceral metastases *and* intermediate markers—any of the following: AFP = 1,000-10,000 ng/mL *or* hCG = 5,000-50,000 IU/L *or* LDH = 1.5-10 × normal	Any primary site *and* nonpulmonary visceral metastases *and* normal AFP, any hCG, and LDH
POOR PROGNOSIS	
Mediastinal primary *or* nonpulmonary visceral metastases *or* poor markers—any of the following: AFP > 10,000 ng/mL *or* hCG > 50,000 IU/L (10,000 ng/mL) *or* LDH > 10 × upper limit of normal	No patients classified as poor prognosis

AFP, α-fetoprotein; hCG, human chorionic gonadotropin; LDH, lactate dehydrogenase.
Data from International Germ Cell Consensus Classification: A prognostic factor-based staging system for metastatic germ cell cancers. International Germ Cell Cancer Collaborative Group. J Clin Oncol. 1997:15:594-603.

After the Einhorn regimen of cisplatin, vinblastine, and bleomycin (PVB) was published in the late 1970s, showing that a high rate of cure was possible for men with metastatic testicular cancer,[406] cisplatin-based regimens were quickly adopted in pediatrics, with marked improvement in outcome, even for patients with advanced-stage disease. Ablin and colleagues initiated a regimen in the Children's Cancer Study Group (CCG-861) that combined the Einhorn regimen (PVB), with the drugs that previously had been shown to have activity—cyclophosphamide, actinomycin and Adriamycin.[427] At 18 weeks, patients in partial remission received radiation therapy and maintenance chemotherapy until 2 years postdiagnosis. This protocol enrolled 93 pediatric germ cell patients, excluding patients with testicular germ cell tumors and including patients with ovarian ($n = 30$), sacrococcygeal ($n = 37$), and mediastinal ($n = 17$) tumors. Ovarian tumors had a 4-year OS of 67% and EFS of 63%, whereas extragonadal tumors had lower rates of survival (EFS, 48%; OS, 42%). Even though this protocol included cisplatin, it was given at a low dose (60 mg/m^2) and dose intensity (every 9 weeks), so that its effectiveness was likely compromised.

Subsequently, the Children's Cancer Group (CCG) and Pediatric Oncology Group (POG) initiated an intergroup study from 1990 to 1995. The study divided patients into two risk groups: the low- and intermediate-risk group included stages I and II gonadal MGCT patients (treated in POG 9048/CCG 8891)[399] and the high-risk group included stages III and IV gonadal MGCT and stages I to IV extragonadal MGCT (treated in POG 9049/CCG 8892).[382]

With the low- and intermediate-risk protocol for treatment of low-stage gonadal tumors, only boys younger than 11 years were enrolled. Older boys were to be treated according to adult standards. Boys with stage I disease were treated with active observation (see earlier); boys with stage II testicular MGCT (including stage II relapses of initially stage I testicular MGCT) and girls with stage I or II ovarian MGCT (patients younger than 21 years) received four cycles of standard-dose BEP (bleomycin, 15 U/m^2 on day 1; etoposide, 100 mg/m^2/day on days 1 to 5; cisplatin, 20 mg/m^2/day on days 1 to 5). In both the low- and intermediate-risk and high-risk arms of the intergroup study, bleomycin was reduced from a weekly dose used on adult protocols to once per cycle, or every 3 weeks, to reduce the incidence of pulmonary fibrosis. Of note, both the British and German investigators similarly reduced the dose of bleomycin, without apparent adverse results. It is important to realize, however, that this reduction in dosage has never been studied in a randomized trial that compares weekly dose, as bleomycin is administered in the adult trials, versus the once-every-3-week regimen introduced by pediatric oncologists.

Patients with either pure immature teratoma higher than stage I or pure dysgerminoma or seminoma were excluded from the U.S. Pediatric Intergroup Trials (see later, "Mature and Immature Teratomas"). Patients were reevaluated with tumor markers and radiologic scans after 4 cycles. If imaging or tumor markers suggested residual disease, patients underwent surgical exploration, and if viable tumor was found pathologically and/or if tumor markers did not normalize, the patient was to receive an additional two cycles of BEP.[399]

In the low- and intermediate-risk arm of the study, overall 6-year EFS was 94.5% and 6-year OS was 95.7%.[399] Six-year EFS and OS by primary site were as follows: testicular stage II (100% and 100%), ovarian stage I (95% and 95%), and ovarian stage II (87% and 94%). Two patients underwent second-look surgery; one patient had evidence of residual malignant disease. Although 23% of patients had grade 3 or 4 hematologic toxicity, no delay in therapy was reported. No patient had grade 3 or 4 ototoxicity, renal toxicity, or pulmonary toxicity. Two patients with ovarian primaries developed acute myelogenous leukemia (AML) at 5 and 32 months after the initiation of therapy, but neither patient had the topoisomerase-induced 11q23 cytogenetic abnormality.[399]

To follow on this trial, the COG protocol AGCT0132 was opened in 2002 for low-risk (gonadal stage I patients, both ovarian and testicular) and intermediate-risk (stages II to IV gonadal tumors and stage I or II extragonadal tumors) patients. The aims of this trial were to evaluate a watch and wait strategy for low-risk patients, reserving chemotherapy for those who failed observation after surgery. For patients judged to be of intermediate risk, the protocol is evaluating the efficacy of three courses of BEP, rather than the four courses that had been used in the previous protocol, and whether the drugs can be given in a compressed manner over 3 days, rather than 5. Enrollment continues in this protocol and preliminary results are not yet available.

The high-risk protocol of the prior Pediatric Intergroup Trial (POG9049/CCG8892) was a randomized clinical trial comparing standard-dose BEP (total cisplatin dose = 100 mg/m^2) versus high-dose BEP (total cisplatin dose = 200 mg/m^2).[382] The results of the intergroup high-dose clinical trial for stages III and IV gonadal tumors and stages I to IV extragonadal MGCTs did not show a significant difference in 6-year OS between high-dose cisplatin (HDPEB) and PEB (92% vs. 86%). However, there was evidence of an increase in 6-year EFS in patients receiving HDPEB (89.6% ± 3.6% vs. 80.5 ± 4.8%; $P = .03$).[382] Overall 6-year EFS and OS by site and stage are as follows (Table 23-5): testicular stage III (94%

and 100%); testicular stage IV (88% and 91%); ovarian stage III (97% and 98%); ovarian stage IV (87% and 93%); extragonadal stages I and II (89% and 93%); extragonadal stage III (75% and 80%); and extragonadal stage IV (78% and 81%). The study was not powered to be able to examine response by site and stage, but in each subgroup, there was a trend toward higher EFS and OS for patients treated with HDPEB. This difference was most pronounced in patients with extragonadal MGCTs, in which it achieved borderline statistical significance. Patients treated with HDPEB had a 2-year EFS of 84% compared with 74% for patients treated with standard-dose PEB ($P = .09$).

Toxicity was much greater in the HDPEB arm of the study. Fatal infections accounted for seven deaths, and six occurred in the HDPEB arm. Hearing aids were needed in 67% of patients treated with HDPEB. Three patients who initially had been diagnosed with a mediastinal MGCT developed hematologic malignancies post-treatment. Two patients developed AML; neither had the characteristic 11q23 abnormality usually associated with etoposide-induced leukemias. One patient developed erythrophagocytic syndrome.

Given the trend observed for better survival in high-stage extragonadal GCT patients in the HDPEB arm, a follow-up pilot study was designed incorporating amifostine (825 mg/m^2/ day × 5 days), with the goal of reducing the observed toxicities of the higher dose of cisplatin, particularly the ototoxicity.[428] In the 20 patients enrolled, 17 were females, median age was 1.6 years, and the primary site was sacrococcygeal in 15

TABLE 23-5   Event-Free Survival and Survival Rates by Patient Characteristics

Parameter	No. of Patients	6-YEAR EFS RATE %	6-YEAR EFS RATE SE	6-YEAR OS RATE %	6-YEAR OS RATE SE
TREATMENT					
High-dose cisplatin (HDPEB)	149	89.6	3.6	91.7	3.3
Standard-dose cisplatin (PEB)	150	90.5	4.8	96.0	4.1
TUMOR TYPE					
Testicular	60	89.8	5.3	93.3	4.4
Ovarian	74	94.5	3.7	97.3	2.6
Extragonadal	165	79.0	4.9	83.4	4.4
GENDER AND AGE (YR)					
Males					
<15	71	88.5	5.2	89.3	5.0
≥15	45	70.2	10.2	75.4	9.7
All ages	116	81.4	5.1	83.8	4.8
Females					
<10	130	82.9	5.1	89.7	5.0
≥10	53	98.1	2.7	98.1	2.7
All ages	183	87.2	3.7	92.1	3.0
TUMOR TYPE AND STAGE					
Testicular stage III	17	94.1	6.9	100	6.4
Testicular stage IV	43	88.3	7.1	90.6	2.5
Ovarian stage III	58	96.6	3.5	98.3	7.6
Ovarian stage IV	16	86.7	10.5	93.3	5.9
Extragonadal stage I-II	30	89.4	7.0	92.8	8.3
Extragonadal stage III	61	75.1	9.4	80.9	7.3
Extragonadal stage IV	74	78.0	8.0	81.5	
OVERALL	299	85.0	3.0	98.8	2.6

EFS, event-free survival; HDPEB, high-dose cisplatin; OS, overall survival; PEB, standard-dose cisplatin; SE, standard error.

Data from Cushing B, Giller R, Cullen JW, et al. Randomized comparison of combination chemotherapy with etoposide, bleomycin, and either high-dose or standard-dose cisplatin in children and adolescents with high-risk malignant germ cell tumors: a pediatric intergroup study—Pediatric Oncology Group 9049 and Children's Cancer Group 8882. J Clin Oncol. 2004;22:2691-2700.

patients. Although the EFS and OS were acceptable (83% and 85%), amifostine at this dose and schedule did not protect against ototoxicity; 75% of patients had significant hearing loss.

A second pilot study for high-risk advanced-stage extragonadal patients has been completed by the COG. In this trial, standard-dose BEP was combined with escalating doses of cyclophosphamide. The three dose levels of cyclophosphamide were 1.2, 1.8, and 2.4 g/m^2. The study has closed to accrual but the results have not yet been released.

Treatment of Pediatric Germ Cell Tumors in the United Kingdom

From 1977 to 1988, patients in the United Kingdom were treated in the United Kingdom Children's Cancer Study Group (UKCCG) Germ Cell Tumor Studies 1 (GC1).[429] This protocol compared five regimens used sequentially over the time interval: low-dose VAC, high-dose VAC, high-dose Adria-VAC (doxorubicin plus VAC), PVB (platinum, vinblastine, bleomycin), and BEP (bleomycin, etoposide, cisplatin). GCI enrolled 52 patients who received chemotherapy until a complete response was documented and then two more cycles after achieving CR (complete response; CR + 2). Outcome varied significantly by regimen; BEP was clearly the most effective.

In 1989, based on preliminary data showing the efficacy of carboplatin in pediatric malignant GCT, the UKCCG initiated their second germ cell tumor study (GC2), in which cisplatin was replaced by carboplatin.[389] JEB chemotherapy consisted of etoposide, 120 mg/m^2/day for days 1 to 3 (total dose, 360 mg/m^2), carboplatin on day 2, in a dose calculated either as 600 mg/m^2 or using the area under the curve (AUC) formula—6 × (uncorrected GFR + [15 × surface area])—and bleomycin, 15 mg/m^2 on day 3. Clinicians were urged to use the AUC formula to calculate the carboplatin dose, rather than the dosing based on surface area, but 75% of patients enrolled in the study were dosed according to the mg/m^2 dose. It is important to note that this is a higher dose and dose intensity of carboplatin than that used in the French study of carboplatin in pediatric germ cell tumors (TGM90), in which the results with carboplatin were inferior to those in a previous trial that had used cisplatin (TGM8589).[430,431] As was the practice in GC1, patients in GC2 received chemotherapy until a complete response was documented, and then two further cycles.

The UK investigators have published an interim analysis of the patients treated between 1989 and 1997.[389] During this period, 184 patients younger than 16 years with localized or metastatic extracranial germ cell tumors were enrolled in GC2 and eligible for analysis. In total, JEB chemotherapy was administered to 137 patients. GC2 remained open to recruitment after analysis in 1997 and an additional 84 patients received JEB in this period, resulting in a total of 221 patients who eventually received chemotherapy. Patients with gonadal stage I tumors were observed without chemotherapy (watch and wait strategy). Forty of 51 testicular GCT patients (78%) and 6 of 9 (66%) patients with ovarian stage I GCT were successfully treated with surgery alone. All patients who recurred after observation were cured with JEB chemotherapy. The OS for all 137 JEB-treated patients at 5 years was 90.9% (95% CI, 83.8% to 95%) and EFS at 5 years was 87.8% (95% CI, 81.1% to 92.4%). Outcomes by site, stage, histologic classification, and initial presurgical AFP level are summarized in Table 23-6.[76] EFS according to site was 100% for testis, 90.7% for ovary, 86.5% for sacrococcygeal, and 75% for thorax. EFS according to stage was 100% for stage I, 93.8% for stage II, 84.8% for stage III, and 78% for stage IV. Toxicity was minimal with JEB. In GC2, only one child had severe deafness, likely attributable

TABLE 23-6	Event-Free Survival (EFS) of JEB-Treated Patients		
Prognostic Factor	**EFS (%)**	**95% CI (%)**	***P***
SITE			
Testis	100	85.2-100	.11
Ovary	90.7	78.2-96.4	
Vagina, uterus	80.0	37-6-96-4	
Sacrococcygeal region	86.5	72.0-94.1	
Thorax	75.0	46.8-91.1	
Other	72.7	43-4-90.3	
STAGE			
I	100	84.6-100	.07
II	93.8	79.8-98.3	
III	84.8	69.1-93.4	
IV	78.0	63.2-88.0	
HISTOLOGIC CLASSIFICATION			
Germinoma	100	78.2-100	.32
Malignant teratoma	87.0	74.4-93.9	
Yolk sac tumor	85.6	75.4-92.0	
AFP LEVEL			
<10,000 kU/L	95.3	87.1-98.4	.014
10,000-100,000 kU/L	76.5	61.8-86.8	
100,000-1,000,000 kU/L	80.0	54.8-93.0	

AFP, α-fetoprotein; CI, confidence interval; JEB, etoposide, bleomycin, and carboplatin.

Data from Mann JR, Raafat F, Robinson K, et al. The United Kingdom Children's Cancer Study Group's second germ cell tumor study: carboplatin, etoposide, and bleomycin are effective treatment for children with malignant extracranial germ cell tumors, with acceptable toxicity. J Clin Oncol. 2000; 18:3809-3818.

to a middle ear hemorrhage while thrombocytopenic, and none had severe renal toxicity. However, carboplatin is more myelotoxic than cisplatin; 36% of the total number of courses was delayed more than 28 days. Second-look surgery was undertaken in 45 patients (33%) in GC2. Necrotic or fibrotic tissue was found in 24 patients (53%), mature or immature teratoma was found in 19 patients (42%), and only 2 patients were found to have viable tumor.[76]

The current UKCCLG protocol (GC3) opened in May 2005. This protocol continues to use JEB chemotherapy as first-line treatment. Low-risk patients (stage I gonadal tumors) are treated surgically with close surveillance. Other patients receive four or six courses of JEB according to risk group stratification, determined by site, stage, age, and AFP level. Accrual is ongoing.

The results are very similar to those reported by the U.S. POG-CCG intergroup study (see Table 23-5)[382] and raise the question whether it is necessary to continue treatment with cisplatin in pediatric patients, given the higher toxicity profile of cisplatin. The concern is that carboplatin has been shown to be inferior to cisplatin in randomized clinical trials in adults with metastatic good-risk testicular cancer.[432,433] Similarly, in pediatric germ cell tumors, the French study has shown that carboplatin is inferior to prior studies using cisplatin (TGM 90 vs. TGM 85); however, both the dose (400 mg/m^2) and dose intensity (once every 6 weeks) were low in the French trial.[430,431] Consideration of carboplatin as first-line therapy for low- and intermediate-risk pediatric germ cell patients is warranted.

Treatment of Pediatric Germ Cell Tumors in Germany

The German Society of Pediatric Oncology has used separate protocols for treating testicular tumors (MAHO protocols) and nontesticular, extracranial pediatric germ cell tumors (MAKEI protocols). In the latest update of the MAHO protocols, published in 2002, the authors reported on results from 1982 to 2001.[421] A watch and wait approach was taken for patients with stage I testicular yolk sac tumors. All patients with stage I tumors who had a malignant component other than yolk sac, as well as patients with higher than stage I testicular tumors, were treated with standard chemotherapy that consisted of PVB. Four cycles were given every 28 days. If there was no complete response after two cycles, however, patients underwent exploratory laparotomy and, if viable disease was discovered, patients received four cycles of salvage therapy that consisted of PEI (etoposide, 80 mg/m^2/day on days 1 to 3; ifosfamide 1500 mg/m^2/day on days 1 to 4; cisplatin, 20 mg/m^2/day on days 2 to 5). If there was no evidence of disease at laparotomy, the patient received two more cycles of the standard PVB, for a total of four courses. In total, 59 patients received chemotherapy, with an overall survival of 95%. Survival in stages I and II patients was excellent; 41 of 42 patients survived. In stage III testicular cancer patients, 5 of 17 patients died, despite the use of salvage chemotherapy.

The German MAKEI protocols (MAKEI 83/86, MAKEI 89, MAKEI 96) specifically included only patients with an ovarian or extragonadal primary, and excluded patients with a testicular primary (treated on MAHO, as earlier). In MAKEI 83/86, patients were stratified into either low risk or high risk. Low risk included only stage I ovarian tumors; these patients received four cycles of PVB. High-risk patients included stages II to IV ovarian and stages I to IIb extragonadal primaries. These patients received four cycles of PVB followed by four cycles of PEI (cisplatin, etoposide, and ifosfamide). Because of concerns about the pulmonary toxicity associated with bleomycin and the neurotoxicity associated with vinblastine in the original Einhorn regimen, a modified Einhorn regimen was developed. Bleomycin was given prior to cisplatin, because cisplatin had been shown to reduce the clearance of bleomycin, as a continuous infusion over 3 days at 15 mg/m^2/day for 3 days or 45 mg/m^2/cycle. The cumulative dose of bleomycin was limited to 180 mg/m^2. This is substantially higher than the total dose of bleomycin received in either the U.S. or UK protocol, in which the per cycle dose of bleomycin was only 15 U/m^2 and most patients received between three and six cycles, or a total cumulative dose of 45 to 90 U/m^2. The German dose of bleomycin was more analogous to the cumulative doses of bleomycin one would find in an adult protocol for treating germ cell tumors, in which 30 U of bleomycin was administered weekly for 9 weeks, for an average total cumulative dose of 270 U or 135 U/m^2 in an average adult with a body surface area (BSA) of 2 m^2. Vinblastine was administered at 50% the dose of the original Einhorn regimen to reduce the associated neurotoxicity.

In MAKEI 89, changes were made to risk stratification and the overall amount of chemotherapy administered was reduced. Risk was stratified into three groups. Low risk remained stage I ovarian, medium risk included ovarian stages II and III and extragonadal stages I and IIa, and high risk was comprised of extragonadal stage IIb, coccygeal stages I and IIB, and ovarian stage IV. Therapy was reduced for these low- and intermediate-risk groups by 25% compared with MAKEI 83/86. Low-risk patients received three cycles of PEB and medium-risk patients received three cycles of PEB followed by three cycles of PIV (cisplatin, ifosfamide, vinblastine).

Outcome of the earlier MAKEI trials are as follows. In MAKEI 83/86, the low-risk group achieved 94% EFS, whereas the high-risk group achieved 76% EFS. In MAKEI 89, EFS in the low-risk arm was 91%, medium-risk 86%, and high-risk 83%. In terms of site, sacrococcygeal tumors had the lowest EFS without much significant change over time (74%, 80%, 77% in MAKEI 83, 86, and 89, respectively), whereas ovarian tumors had the best outcome, with significant improvement over time (EFS 77%, 92%, 90% in MAKEI 83, 86, and 89, respectively).

In MAKEI 96, several changes were made to the risk stratification and recommended therapies. Chemotherapy was determined by site, stage, and degree of resection. Bleomycin was removed from all chemotherapy protocols. All ovarian and extragonadal stage I patients, except stage I sacrococcygeal patients, were initially treated with a watch and wait strategy. Children with sacrococcygeal primaries, regardless of stage, were treated with four cycles of PEI: cisplatin, 20 mg/m^2/day on days 1 to 5; etoposide, 100 mg/m^2/day on days 1 to 3; and ifosfamide, 1500 mg/m^2/day on days 1 to 5 as a continuous infusion. Infants younger than 4 months with sacrococcygeal primaries were treated with four cycles of PE, omitting the ifosfamide. Patients with ovarian primaries received two cycles of PE (completely resected) or PEI (incompletely resected), and patients with extragonadal primaries received three cycles of PE (completely resected) or PEI (incompletely resected). Poor-prognosis patients with advanced-stage ovarian and extragonadal primaries were treated with four cycles of PEI. If the tumor had not been completely excised at the onset of therapy, three cycles of PEI were given and then the patient was to undergo resection. Postoperatively, an additional one to four cycles of PEI were administered, depending on whether the tumor was completely or incompletely resected. In all MAKEI protocols diagnosis was based on imaging, tumor markers, and histology. In advanced or bulky disease, diagnosis could be based on markers and imaging and a preoperative chemotherapy applied for downstaging.

Dose of Bleomycin in Treatment of Pediatric Germ Cell Tumors

In adults, investigators have shown that bleomycin can likely be safely omitted in good-risk patients if the patient receives an additional (fourth) cycle of etoposide and cisplatin.[434] Four cycles of etoposide is the standard of care at Memorial Sloan-Kettering for good-risk men with testicular cancer. Several randomized trials have suggested that results with four cycles of etoposide may be inferior to three cycles of BEP, but the results do not reach statistical significance and therefore are not conclusive.[435]

Concern about the possibility of bleomycin-induced pulmonary fibrosis has caused pediatric oncologists to evaluate the same issue. The British and American collaborative groups have reduced the dose of bleomycin from once weekly to once per cycle (or once every three weeks).[382,389] This dose of bleomycin represents a 67% reduction in the total dose of bleomycin when compared with adult regimens. Since the institution of these changes (1989 in Britain and 1990 in the United States), there have been no reported cases of fatal pulmonary fibrosis in over 137 British JEB-treated cases and 373 U.S. PEB-treated patients. On MAKEI 89, after two deaths occurred in children younger than 2 years from pulmonary fibrosis, German investigators no longer treated children younger than 1 year with bleomycin (EP) and children ages 1 to 2 years received half the standard dose of bleomycin. However, the dose of bleomycin for older children on MAKEI 83/86 and 89 was significant: 15 mg/m^2/day for 3 days with each cycle (total,

45 mg/m²/cycle). In MAKEI 96, bleomycin was omitted entirely from the chemotherapeutic regimens for all patients. No decrement in survival has been observed since its deletion.

Other countries in addition to Germany have decided to delete bleomycin from use in pediatric patients. A Brazilian study has reported preliminary results using four cycles of EP with 5-year survival rates of 92.3% in low-risk patients and 80.6% in high-risk patients.[436] Italian researchers also did not use bleomycin in their cooperative study (TCG91), but their regimen, which alternated carboplatin and etoposide with vincristine, dactinomycin, and ifosfamide, produced suboptimal results, particularly in higher stage patients, compared with other pediatric germ cell trials.[437]

Mature and Immature Teratomas

Complete surgical excision is adequate therapy for pure mature teratomas. Mature teratomas are much more common than immature teratomas. It is estimated that mature teratomas of the ovary, also called cystic teratoma or dermoid cyst, account for 95% to 99% of all ovarian teratomas. Mature teratomas that contain an element of a malignant germ cell tumor (yolk sac, endodermal sinus, choriocarcinoma, embryonal carcinoma) should be treated according to the guidelines for the treatment of malignant nonseminomatous germ cell tumors discussed earlier.

Immature teratomas are made up elements from the three germ layers and graded from 0 to 3, depending on the amount of immature neuroepithelium present in the tumor. Grade has been shown to correlate with stage and prognosis. Treatment for immature teratoma is more controversial and evolving.

A classic study by Norris and cowrokers[123] has reviewed 58 women with ovarian immature teratomas who had been treated with surgical resection alone; they reported that 70% of women who had grade 3 tumors at diagnosis subsequently relapsed. The recommendation was thus made that stage I, grade 3 ovarian immature teratomas be treated with chemotherapy.

Concern that the biology and behavior of immature teratoma might be different in childhood than adulthood led the U.S. pediatric oncology groups to investigate whether surgical resection was sufficient for stage I tumors, even in patients who had grade 3 tumors. Between 1990 and 1995, as part of the U.S. Intergroup Pediatric Study (POG9048/CCG 8891), 73 patients with pure stage I immature teratoma were enrolled in the study.[174] Central review of grade showed that 31.5% were grade 1, 38.4% were grade 2, and 30.1% were grade 3. The primary site of disease included ovarian ($n = 44$), testicular ($n = 7$), sacrococcygeal ($n = 5$), retroperitoneal ($n = 7$), and head and neck ($n = 7$). All pathology was centrally reviewed; 50 patients were confirmed to have pure immature teratoma, whereas 21 had microscopic foci of YST and 2 had microscopic foci of PNET. Since significant time had elapsed between the initial surgery and the central review of the pathology, usually at least 6 months, it was decided to continue to observe patients discovered to have a malignant focus at central pathology review. Tumor markers were elevated in 25 patients at diagnosis (AFP alone = 18, β-hCG alone = 5, both = 2). Overall, only 50% of patients with microscopic foci of YST had an elevated AFP at diagnosis (9 of 20 patients). However, in ovarian tumors, there was a tighter correlation between an elevated AFP and presence of YST; 84% of patients with elevated AFP at diagnosis were shown to have microscopic foci of YST.[134] Elevation of AFP at diagnosis was also strongly correlated with stage and grade of the immature teratoma.[134]

With a median follow-up of 35 months of stage I patient treated with surgery and close observation, the overall 3-year EFS was 93%, with 3-year EFS of 97.8%, 100%, and 80% for ovarian, testicular, and extragonadal tumors respectively. Five patients relapsed, all within 7 months of the original diagnosis; one had an ovarian primary and four had extragonadal primaries. Three of the five patients had YST present at diagnosis; one patient had PNET. The patient with PNET who recurred was resistant to platinum-based therapy. All the other patients were salvaged with PEB or JEB. Although the numbers were too small to draw a definitive conclusion, it appears that patients with extragonadal immature teratomas and foci of malignancy are at higher risk of relapse and warrant especially close follow-up.[174] Grade at diagnosis did not appear to affect the risk of relapse.

How to treat higher than stage I pure immature teratoma lacks clinical consensus and published data. There is generally a belief in the pediatric oncology community that the diagnosis of immature teratoma has a different meaning and clinical significance in the newborn versus the peripubertal period. In the newborn period, patients with incompletely resected immature teratomas are usually closely observed, reserving treatment (usually reoperation) for those who recur. Immature teratoma in the peripubertal (older child and adult) is generally considered to be a malignant disease that warrants treatment with chemotherapy. Treatment with three or four cycles of standard-dose BEP is generally recommended for patients with higher than stage I pure immature teratoma.

In Germany, the German Society for Pediatric Oncology and Hematology (GPOH) has prospectively studied all extracranial testicular and nontesticular mature and immature teratomas since 1982 in successive MAHO and MAKEI protocols.[438] All pathology was centrally reviewed at a single institution and grade of immaturity was classified according to Gonzalez-Crussi.[170] AFP and β-hCG were measured in all patients and, by definition, had to be within normal limits for age to establish the diagnosis of teratoma. The treatment of immature teratoma varied over time. In MAKEI 83/86, patients with incompletely resected immature teratoma grade 2 or 3 were treated with three cycles of VAC chemotherapy. In MAKEI 89, chemotherapy (three cycles of BEP) was given to patients with incompletely resected immature teratomas, grade 3. In MAKEI 96, patients with incompletely resected immature teratomas grade 2 or 3 were stratified to a watch and wait approach or to two courses of adjuvant chemotherapy. The therapy was switched from PEB to PEI, substituting ifosfamide, 1500 mg/m²/day on days 1 to 5, for the bleomycin. However, because of low accrual, the randomization was stopped in 2000 and patients have since been treated according to physician preference.

Overall, the completeness of the original tumor resection was the chief predictor of relapse. EFS after complete resection was 96%, whereas EFS was only 55% in those with incomplete resection at diagnosis. The German group used a strict definition of a complete resection. Complete resection of a coccygeal tumor was defined as resection of the tumor with its pseudocapsule and the coccygeal bone in one piece.

In MAKEI 83/86/89, 274 patients with teratoma were registered; 230 were treated with surgery alone and 40 patients were treated with chemotherapy.[438] The relapse rate overall was 13.3%. Predictors of relapse were the completeness of initial resection (EFS complete, 0.96 ± 0.01 vs. incomplete, 0.55 ± 0.09) as well as site. Relapses occurred in 20% of patients with sacrococcygeal tumors compared with 7% in patients with tumors at other extragonadal sites and only 2% of patients with ovarian primaries. The relapse rate was similar in patients treated with surgery alone versus patients treated with chemotherapy on the basis of higher grade of immaturity. However, no malignant components were found at the time of relapse in the 7 patients who relapsed after initial chemotherapy, whereas 15 of 29 of patients who relapsed after surgery only as first treatment had a malignant component detectable in their recurrence. Immature teratomas were more likely to relapse than mature; higher grade of immature teratoma was more likely to relapse than lower grade (grade 0 [mature], 10%; grade 1, 14%; grade 2, 21%; grade 3, 31%).

In MAKEI 96, 261 evaluable patients were enrolled.[438] Because the criteria for complete versus incomplete resection were more highly scrutinized, the percentage of incompletely resected tumors rose from 10% to 34% in MAKEI 96. This change was not associated with a reduced relapse rate in the completely resected patients (4.2%). However, the overall relapse rate decreased from 13.3% to 9.5% over the same period. The authors were not certain whether this reflects better surgical procedures, or a change in the distribution of the primary site of the tumor. The rates are similar to those reported in other studies.[439] It is easier to achieve a complete resection for a gonadal teratoma. Extragonadal teratomas are often adjacent to or infiltrating vital structures, such as the sacral plexus in the case of the SCT or large vessels. The probability of relapse in MAKEI 96 was not linked to the histologic grade of immaturity, as it had been in MAKEI 83/86/89. Half of the relapses in MAKEI 83/86/89 had a malignant component, whereas two thirds of the relapses in MAKEI 96 had a malignant component, illustrating the malignant potential of the teratoma.

Growing Teratoma Syndrome

Growing teratoma syndrome describes the situation in which tumors are noted to enlarge postchemotherapy in a patient with normalized tumor markers. Pathologically, these tumors are comprised entirely of mature teratoma. The incidence of this phenomenon has been described in approximately 3% of men with testicular cancer[440] and as high as 12% of women with ovarian germ cell tumors, particularly in women originally diagnosed with immature teratoma.[441] It has been hypothesized that this occurs because the chemotherapy might induce differentiation of residual immature teratoma into a mature teratoma. The median interval between chemotherapy and first detection of growing teratoma syndrome was 9 months in a retrospective study from the Institut Gustave-Roussy of women with ovarian immature teratomas, but the range extended from 1 to 12 years post-treatment.[441] The disease usually occurs at the site of prior disease; for example, women known to have peritoneal deposits of tumor at diagnosis were noted to have a peritoneal location for the growing teratoma syndrome. In most cases, the recurrence is treated with surgery only. In cases in which total resection was not possible, patients require continued surveillance. Regrowth of the teratoma has been observed, as well as disease stabilization, but regression has not been reported.

Extragonadal Tumors

Mediastinal Tumors

The German group has reported on the outcome of mediastinal tumors as a separate entity.[381] The report included all patients treated between 1983 and 1999 in their protocols, including MAKEI 83/86, 89, and 96. The authors examined the outcome of mediastinal teratomas (mature and immature; n = 21) and malignant germ cell tumors of the mediastinum (n = 26). All the mediastinal germ cell tumors diagnosed in the first year of life were teratomas (Fig. 23-17). The incidence of teratoma

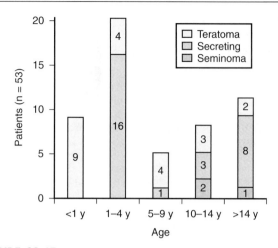

FIGURE 23-17. Age and histologic differentiation in all registered patients with mediastinal germ cell tumors (N = 53; 1 patient with insufficient histopathology was excluded). (Adapted from Schneider DT, Calaminus G, Reinhard H, et al. Primary mediastinal germ cell tumors in children and adolescents: results of the German cooperative protocols MAKEI 83/86, 89, and 96. J Clin Oncol. 2000;18:832-839.)

declined during infancy and adolescence; seminoma was not observed until after age 10.

Teratomas were surgically resected; no adjuvant chemotherapy or radiotherapy was given. Of the teratomas, 16 were mature and 5 were immature. All patients with teratoma underwent primary resection; surgery was microscopically complete in 17 of 21. All teratoma patients, regardless of the completeness of the tumor resection, were cured with surgery only.

Twelve of the 26 patients with malignant GCT had primary resection of the tumor, which was complete in 6 of 12. Four of the 6 patients with incomplete resections subsequently underwent second-look surgery and all achieved a complete resection of the residual tumor. Eleven patients underwent delayed resection of the primary tumor after preoperative chemotherapy and a complete resection was achieved in 10 of 11 patients. Three patients did not undergo resection of the tumor; 2 patients had a CR to first-line therapy and 1 had progressive disease on chemotherapy. Patients were treated with cisplatin-based regimens, for a total of three to eight courses[381] (Table 23-7). Excellent results in MAKEI 83/86 encouraged the German investigators to reduce the maximum number of courses from eight to four or five cycles, with no apparent detriment to overall survival. Overall 5-year EFS was 0.83 ± 0.05 at a median follow-up of 41 months. Complete resection of the tumor, either initially, at delayed resection, or at second-look surgery, was the strongest predictor of survival. Only 1 of 20 patients with complete resection relapsed, and that patient was cured with salvage therapy. The stage of tumor at diagnosis was not a significant predictor of outcome, although the analysis may have been limited by small sample size, in that EFS for patients without distant metastases was 0.93 ± 0.07 versus 0.65 ± 0.17 for those with distant metastases at diagnosis (P = .09). Histology at diagnosis and level of AFP at diagnosis were not prognostic.

Sacrococcygeal Tumors

The German investigators have reported on 71 patients with malignant sacrococcygeal tumors treated in MAKEI 83/86 and 89 from 1983 to 1995.[383] Of the 66 evaluable patients, there were 14 boys and 52 girls and the median age was 17.4

TABLE 23-7	Summary of Treatment of Nonseminomatous Malignant Germ Cell Tumors		
Tumor Type	**United States**	**Germany**	**United Kingdom**
TESTICULAR			
Stage I	W & W	W & W for pure yolk sac; other, two or three cycles PVB	W & W
Stage II	Three cycles of compressed BEP	Two or three cycles of PVB	JEB
Stage III or IV	Three cycles of compressed BEP	Two PVB, four PEI	JEB
OVARIAN			
Stage I	W & W	W & W	W & W
Stage II	Three cycles of compressed BEP	Two cycles of PE if completely resected; two cycles of PEI if incompletely resected	JEB
Stage III-IV	Three cycles of BEP	Four cycles of PEI	JEB
EXTRAGONADAL			
Stage I	Three cycles of compressed BEP	W & W except for sacrococcygeal tumors; stage I SCT; four cycles of PE or PEI*	W & W
Stage II	Three cycles of compressed BEP	Three cycles of PE if completely resected; three cycles of PEI if incompletely resected	JEB
Stage III or IV	High-risk protocol	Four or five cycles of PEI; poor responder: PEI, 1×; HDPEI, 3×	JEB
Relapse	TIC ± stem cell transplantation (SCT)	Local: 4× local deep hyperthermia + PEI; disseminated: PEI, 1×; HDPEI, 3×	

BEP, bleomycin, etoposide, cisplatin; HDPEI, high-dose cisplatin, etoposide, ifosfamide; JEB, carboplatin, etoposide, bleomycin, four to six cycles (number of cycles determined by risk group stratification); PE, cisplatin, etoposide; PEI, cisplatin, etoposide, ifosfamide; TIC, taxol, ifosfamide, carboplatin; W & W, watch and wait strategy—observation only after surgical excision of stage I tumor, with chemotherapy reserved for those who recur.

*Depending on age: <4 mo, PE; >4 mo, PEI.

months; 14 patients had stage T1 disease and 52 patients had T2 disease. Twelve patients had lymph node metastases and 30 patients had distant metastases (lungs, 21; liver, 8; bone, 8). On histologic examination, 45 patients had pure YSTs and 21 patients had mixed GCTs. Patients in MAKEI 83/86 received a total of eight cycles of cisplatin-based therapy, four cycles of PVB followed by four cycles of PEI. Patients in MAKEI 89 received a total of six cycles of cisplatin-based therapy, three cycles of PEB followed by three cycles of VIP. Event-free survival for the entire group was 0.76 ± 0.05 and overall survival was 0.81 ± 0.05. Overall survival did not differ by protocol (MAKEI 83/86 vs. 89) nor by stage (T1 vs. T2). The most significant predictor of favorable outcome was the completeness of tumor resection. The completeness of this resection could be established by tumor resection at initial diagnosis or at delayed resection after chemotherapy was given. In patients with advanced and metastatic disease (T2b M1), those who had a delayed resection fared better than patients with an initial resection (5-year OS, 0.83 ± 0.09 vs. 0.45 ± 0.15; $P = .01$). The presence of metastatic disease at diagnosis was only an adverse risk factor in those who had initial resection of their tumor at diagnosis. AFP levels at diagnosis were not prognostic, even when the analysis was restricted to children older than 1 year. The authors concluded that the therapeutic strategy of preoperative chemotherapy with delayed resection results in superior outcomes that abrogate prior reports that higher stage and higher pretherapy levels of AFP portend a worse prognosis.

An analysis of the prognostic factors in children with SCT treated in the U.S. intergroup study has confirmed the conclusions of the German report.[380] Of children with malignant SCT, 74 were randomized to receive standard-dose or high-dose BEP. Prognosis was excellent in this subgroup overall (4-year EFS, 84% ± 6%; 4-year OS, 90% ± 4%). Neither presence of metastatic disease nor delayed resection had an adverse effect on outcome. In this group of patients, AFP higher than 20,000 IU/L was associated with a higher than expected rate of failure.[439]

POSTCHEMOTHERAPY MANAGEMENT

At the end of chemotherapy, full restaging should be undertaken, including radiologic imaging of the primary site and most likely sites of nodal spread, chest CT, and assay of tumor markers (AFP and β-hCG). If tumor markers are elevated, and chest CT and pelvic-abdominal CT do not reveal the site of metastasis, a bone scan and brain MRI are indicated to look for other possible sites of metastatic disease. When tumor markers are elevated but no mass is detectable, a PET scan can sometimes be helpful in identifying occult disease.[386] The recommended surveillance postchemotherapy is similar to that recommended for stage I patients.

Retroperitoneal Lymph Node Dissection

If there is a residual mass detected or elevation of tumor markers, even in the case of no detectable mass radiographically, surgery is recommended to remove the mass or to explore and biopsy any potentially involved residual lymph nodes. There are limited data on findings from second-look surgeries in children with germ cell tumors. In England, after completion of JEB chemotherapy, 45 of 137 patients required surgery for residual mass seen on radiologic evaluation.[389] Of these patients, 53% had necrosis or fibrosis; 42% were found to have immature or mature teratoma. Only 2 patients had viable tumor; these patients received no further therapy after complete resection and both remain in complete remission.

Men with Testicular Cancer

In a retrospective review from Memorial Sloan-Kettering, 11% of men who underwent postchemotherapy (PC)–RPLND had viable residual germ cell tumor, 49% had fibrosis, and 40% were found to have teratoma in the PC surgical specimen.[442] In the subgroup of patients with teratoma, 85% had pure mature teratoma, 7% had immature teratoma, and 8% had teratoma with malignant transformation (to a non–germ cell tumor histology).[443] The median size of the node at PC-RPLND was 3.0 cm, but 18% of patients discovered to have teratoma had a node smaller than 2 cm and 11% had a node smaller than 1 cm. The 5- and 10-year probabilities of relapse-free survival were 83% and 80%, respectively. There is currently debate in the adult testicular cancer community as to the optimal surgical approach, a modified RPLND template versus bilateral infrahilar dissection. The complexity of these issues argues strongly for referral of the adolescent patient to a urologist well-versed in the data.[442,444]

Second-Look Surgery in Ovarian Malignancies

In women with epithelial ovarian carcinoma, second-look surgery postchemotherapy is performed on all patients to attain cytoreduction and has been found to improve prognosis. In women with malignant ovarian germ cell tumors, however, it has been shown that the yield of second-look surgery, in the setting of a negative radiologic evaluation and normal tumor markers, has a low probability of discovering occult residual malignant disease. Gershenson and colleagues[445] have noted that only 1 of 53 women with negative scans and tumor markers had a viable tumor at second-look surgery.

What should be the chemotherapeutic approach if tumor is found? The standard of care if viable tumor is found at PC lymph node resection has traditionally been two more cycles of the original chemotherapy. However, persistence of viable tumor after standard chemotherapy is used is increasingly viewed as evidence of resistant disease. Anecdotally, many adult oncologists are now treating patient with salvage-type therapy in this setting.

A higher than expected incidence of sarcoidosis has been noted in adult patients previously treated for germ cell tumors.[446] Sarcoidosis should be considered in the differential diagnosis of any adolescent patient with pulmonary nodules or infiltrates or mediastinal adenopathy in the setting of negative tumor markers.

RELAPSE AND SALVAGE THERAPY

In the German experience, more than 90% of relapses occurred locally.[447] In an analysis of 22 patients with recurrent sacrococcygeal tumors previously treated in the German MAKEI protocols, most patients (17 of 22) presented with local recurrence only; 2 patients presented with only distant metastases and 3 patients presented with combined local and distant recurrences.[344] Most relapses occurred within 6 months of completing primary therapy (median, 5.5 months; range, 0 to 21 months). Patients who achieved a second CR had a significantly better prognosis than patients who did not (5-year OS, second CR, 0.74 ± 0.13 vs. second PR, 0.1 ± 0.1). Complete surgical resection of the relapse was associated with a higher likelihood of continuous CR (5 of 7 patients in first relapse who had a microscopic CR of the relapsed tumor remained in CR). Only 1 of 5 patients who presented at relapse with distant metastases achieved a second continuous CR. Early versus late relapse (less than 1 year vs. more than 1 year postdiagnosis), AFP serum levels and tumor size at relapse were not prognostic. These data contrast with those from men with testicular GCT in whom favorable prognostic factors at relapse include testis primary site (vs. retroperitoneal or mediastinal), prior complete response to first-line therapy, low tumor markers at relapse, and low-volume disease.

Salvage Therapy

Surgery

Unlike many other forms of cancer, surgical excision can be curative for chemorefractory germ cell tumors in patients who have anatomically confined disease.[448] Most patients will also require chemotherapy to achieve a second remission.

Chemotherapy

Several different regimens have been used in men with relapsed or refractory GCT. VeIP (vinblastine, 0.11 mg/kg; cisplatin 25 mg/m^2 × 5; ifosfamide, 1.2 g/m^2 × 5) results in a complete response in 50% of patients but responses are durable in only 20% to 30%.[449] More recently, investigators from Memorial Sloan-Kettering have reported on a TIP regimen that substitutes paclitaxel for vinblastine (paclitaxel, 250 mg/m^2 on day 1; ifosfamide, 1.5 g/m^2 on days 2 to 5; cisplatin, 25 mg/m^2 on days 2 to 5) in which up to 70% of patients experience CR, with a durable CR rate of 63%.[450] These two regimens are currently being compared in a CALGB randomized trial in men with testicular cancer. Oxaliplatin and gemcitabine have both shown activity in phase II trials as single agents in men with relapsed testicular cancer.[451-453]

Two recent single-institution reports of treatment of relapsed patients with high-dose chemotherapy (HD-CT) have shown encouraging results. Kondagunta and associates[454] have reported on the treatment of 48 patients with a poor response to standard BEP therapy who were treated with two cycles of paclitaxel and ifosfamide followed by three cycles of carboplatin and etoposide with peripheral blood stem cell (PBSC) support administered at 14- to 21-day intervals. A CR was obtained in 55%, and 51% remained in remission at a median follow-up of 40 months. Einhorn and coworkers[455] have reported on the treatment of 184 patients with relapsed testicular cancer who were treated with two cycles of carboplatin and etoposide, with PBSC support. A CR was obtained in 63% of patients, with a median follow-up of 48 months. A high response rate was observed. even in the subset of patients who had cisplatin-refractory disease, or failed prior salvage regimens.

Limited data exist on optimal therapy for relapsed pediatric GCT patients. A trial of TIC (paclitaxel, 135 mg/m^2 on day 1; ifosfamide, 1.8 g/m^2 on days 1 to 5; carboplatin, use AUC formula to calculate dose—mg/m^2 = 6.5 × [0.93 × GFR + 15] on day 1) is currently under investigation by the COG. The decision was made to use carboplatin rather than cisplatin for two reasons. First, children are more sensitive to the ototoxicity of cisplatin and it is likely that many children would have a serious hearing impairment if further courses of cisplatin were administered after BEP. Second, carboplatin has been shown to be efficacious, potentially equal to cisplatin, in children with germ cell tumors in the GC2 study conducted in England.[389] The current study will evaluate response to two cycles of TIC. Additional therapy after two cycles of TIC—for example, to continue with TIC or proceed to HD-CT with SCT—is left to the physician's discretion.

Radiotherapy

Radiotherapy is not a standard part of salvage therapy in the United States, except as a palliative measure. However, in an analysis of outcome of patients with sacrococcygeal GCT tumors treated in Germany, Schneider and colleagues[344] have reported that 8 of 22 patients received local irradiation following relapse, mostly for an incompletely resected tumor. None of the patients who received less than 45 Gy achieved a stable second CR, whereas 3 of 5 patients who received more than 45 Gy achieved a stable continuous remission.

German investigators have also used local regional hyperthermia successfully in the control of local recurrence, especially if applied early in its course. Cisplatin is a thermosensitizer and thus this approach may be of use in overcoming cisplatin-resistant tumors.

Molecular Basis of Cisplatin Sensitivity and Resistance in Germ Cell Tumors

Compared with most other malignancies, germ cell tumors are unusually responsive to chemotherapy, especially to cisplatin-based regimens (with the exception of teratomas, which are chemoresistant). The reasons for this exquisite sensitivity are not fully known, precluding a complete understanding of the mechanisms of cisplatin resistance and hampering efforts to overcome chemoresistance in germ cell tumors. Several features of germ cell tumors are thought to contribute to their relative chemosensitivity.[456,457] In particular, germ cell tumors may differ from other malignancies in regard to uptake, efflux, and conjugation of cisplatin, as well as the cellular DNA repair and apoptotic response to cisplatin exposure. Uptake of cisplatin into germ cell tumors may occur by passive or facilitated diffusion. Recent work has highlighted the role of the copper transporter CTR1 in cisplatin uptake and the significance of altered CTR1 expression in cisplatin-resistant solid tumors.[458-460] However, it is unclear whether CTR1 significantly affects cisplatin uptake into germ cells. Similarly, overexpression of proteins capable of exporting cisplatin, such as LRP (lung resistance protein) and MRP2 (multidrug resistance-related protein) is not a consistent feature of cisplatin-resistant germ cell tumors.[456,457,461,462] Conjugation of cisplatin to glutathione can limit its cytotoxicity and facilitate export; in germ cells, this conjugation is mediated principally by the π isoform of glutathione-*S*-transferase (GST-π).[463-465] Strohmeyer and associates[457] have reported an overall low level of GST enzyme activity in germ cell tumors, and Mayer and coworkers[464] have found consistent GST-π expression in only 5 of 36 nonteratoma germ cell tumors. Thus, low levels of GST activity may contribute to the activity of cisplatin in germ cell tumors. However, in the study by Mayer and colleagues, the differences between cisplatin-responsive and refractory tumors were not significant.

In the absence of compelling evidence that import or export mechanisms predominantly determine cisplatin's effect on germ cell tumors, attention has focused on the role of DNA damage repair and apoptosis pathways in cisplatin-mediated cytotoxicity. Cisplatin causes bulky DNA adducts, which are removed via nucleotide excision repair (NER).[466] Most germ cell tumor cell lines exhibit low NER activity, which may be attributable to low expression levels of the NER proteins XPA, XPF, and ERCC1.[467-469] However, one study has found no difference in XPA expression between cisplatin-sensitive and cisplatin-resistant tumors,[470] and restoring XPA expression to a testicular tumor cell line did not increase cellular resistance to cisplatin,[471] calling into question whether NER is an important factor in germ cell tumor response to cisplatin. Another DNA damage repair pathway, mismatch repair (MMR), has also been investigated in relation to cisplatin treatment of GCTs. A hallmark of defects in the MMR pathway is the presence of microsatellite instability (MSI). Several studies have indicated a low level of MSI in germ cell tumors, implying that the MMR system is generally intact in these tumors.[472-474] In the presence of DNA damage, the MMR pathway can trigger p53-dependent apoptosis,[475,476] and this response may explain the sensitivity of most germ cell tumors to cisplatin. On the other hand, loss of MMR may confer chemoresistance. In one series, only 6% of unselected germ cell tumors displayed MSI, whereas 45% of chemoresistant tumors exhibited MSI or low levels of MMR proteins.[473] In another study of germ cell tumors, Velasco and associates[477] have found that low MMR expression and a high degree of MSI are associated with chemotherapy resistance, shorter time to recurrence, and poor survival. Loss of MMR function is associated with genomic instability and the acquisition of secondary mutations that may enhance tumor survival or aggressiveness.[478-480] Thus, the MMR system is an important determinant of cisplatin sensitivity in germ cell tumors, and loss of MMR may signal a worse prognosis.

As noted, the MMR pathway not only functions to maintain genome integrity, but is also one of the factors that triggers apoptosis in response to genotoxic damage, such as that caused by cisplatin. Apoptosis, or programmed cell death, is a key determinant of the death or survival of cancer cells and the effectiveness of chemotherapy.[481-486] The tumor suppressor protein p53 plays a central role in coordinating the apoptotic response to genotoxic damage,[487,488] and attention has focused on the role of the p53 pathway in the chemotherapy of germ cell tumors. Mutations in p53, which are commonly found in other tumor types, are rare in germ cell tumors.[456,489] The presence of high levels of wild-type p53 protein in germ cell tumors has been suggested to account for the unusual chemoresponsiveness of these tumors.[490,491]

However, p53 deficiency per se does not prevent an apoptotic response to cisplatin in germ cell tumor cell lines,[492] and the presence or absence of wild-type p53 correlates poorly with clinical response to chemotherapy.[489] Thus the importance of wild-type p53 expression in determining the cisplatin response of germ cell tumors is not clear. Also unclear is why germ cell tumors treated with cisplatin predominantly exhibit apoptosis, rather than undergoing cell cycle arrest, senescence, or other p53-mediated responses. Despite the absence of p53 mutations, other mechanisms exist in germ cell tumors to interfere with p53 function, including overexpression of the p53 inhibitor MDM2[493,494] and epigenetic silencing of p53 target genes.[495] Particularly interesting in this regard is the recent finding that the micro-RNA cluster miR-371-3 acts in germ cell tumors to neutralize the p53 response to oncogenic stress.[496] In summary, there is suggestive evidence that specific features of germ cell tumors—including their retention of a normal DNA damage repair, p53, and apoptosis pathways—may account for the unusual chemosensitivity of these cells. However, a simple loss of these mechanisms does not seem to account for most cases of chemoresistance. Recently, cGH analysis has revealed genomic copy number variation of specific chromosomal regions associated with acquired cisplatin resistance,[497,498] and further exploration of the genes involved in these regions may shed light on the mechanisms underlying resistance.

Prospects for Targeted Therapy of Germ Cell Tumors

Cisplatin-based chemotherapy of germ cell tumors has been highly effective and will continue to be a mainstay of treatment. However, the toxicity of these regimens, as well as the poor prognosis of cisplatin-resistant disease, indicate the need for more specific effective therapies. Such therapies will depend on advances in research focusing on the molecular mechanisms of germ cell tumorigenesis. To date, these mechanisms are only incompletely understood, but some case reports and small trials have raised intriguing prospects for targeted therapy of germ cell tumors. The receptor tyrosine kinase *c-KIT* oncogene is frequently overexpressed in seminomas, and activating mutations in *c-KIT* have been described in seminomas,[205,249,499] suggesting that germ cell tumors may be susceptible to treatment with the kinase inhibitor imatinib mesylate. Whereas case reports have documented the efficacy of imatinib in seminoma,[500] most of the described c-KIT mutations in seminomas are insensitive to imatinib,[501] and a phase II trial of imatinib in six patients with c-KIT–positive metastatic germ cell tumor has failed to show significant antitumor activity.[502] Although c-KIT remains a promising target in germ cell tumors and other malignancies, it is clear that not all c-KIT mutations will be susceptible to imatinib or other tyrosine kinase inhibitors (TKIs) currently in use.[503] Another potential TKI target, the epidermal growth factor receptor (EGFR), has also been investigated in relapsed or refractory germ cell tumors. Several studies have reported that EGFR is expressed in nonseminomas,[504-506] and a phase II study has been initiated to treat germ cell tumors with erlotinib, a small-molecule EGFR inhibitor. Early reports that germ cell tumors overexpress HER2/Neu, and might be susceptible to trastuzumab (a chimeric anti-HER2/Neu antibody),[507] have not been borne out by subsequent analyses.[508]

Differentiation therapy is another potential route to targeted therapy of germ cell tumors. Based on the differentiating effect of retinoic acid on germ cell tumor cell lines in vitro, 16 patients with chemoresistant germ cell tumors were treated with retinoic acid. However, no partial or complete responses occurred.[509]

Inhibition of tumor angiogenesis is a promising avenue currently under intense investigation for many tumor types. In germ cell tumors, increased expression of the proangiogenic vascular endothelial growth factor (VEGF) correlates with tumor metastasis.[510,511] Trials are now underway to evaluate the effect of inhibiting VEGF in patients with germ cell tumors using the small-molecule TKI sunitinib or the combination of oxaliplatin with the anti-VEGF antibody, bevacizumab.

It is important to note that most targeted therapy trials are based on preclinical models of adult germ cell tumors. Because the molecular pathogenesis of pediatric tumors likely differs from that of adults, targeted therapy developed for adult GCTs may not translate directly into clinical efficacy in children. More efforts will be required to define the targets for pediatric germ cell tumors and to develop animal models that accurately model human tumors. In children and young adults, germ cell tumors appear to arise from defects in early development.[1] Therefore, particular attention should be given to examining developmental and stem cell pathways, such as the Wnt/β-catenin, BMP, Notch, and Hedgehog pathways. Intriguingly, a recent report has described activation of the Wnt/β-catenin pathway in immature teratomas and yolk sac tumors, but not in germinomas, embryonal carcinomas, or choriocarcinomas.[512] The emerging role of micro-RNAs in human cancer is another area with potentially significant implications for understanding germ cell tumor pathogenesis.[513-515] Continued progress in molecular cytogenetics and pathway discovery in pediatric germ cell tumors will be critical to the development of improved therapies.

LATE EFFECTS

There are limited data on the short- and long-term side effects of treatment for germ cell tumors in children. Germ cell tumors are not included in the Childhood Cancer Survivor Study (CCSS), an invaluable source of information about late effects in children treated for other diagnoses. The only comprehensive survey of late effects of pediatric germ cell tumors is a single-institution St. Jude study of 73 patients treated from 1962 to 1988; two thirds of patients had at least one major complication.[516] However, this study is limited for several reasons, First,

the treatment of germ cell tumors has changed radically since 1962, even since 1988. In the era of the St. Jude study, most patients received radiotherapy as part of their treatment; radiotherapy is seldom used today. The chemotherapy for germ cell tumors during this era included VAC—vincristine, dactinomycin, and cyclophosphamide—either alone or in combination with a cisplatin-based regimen. The inclusion of an alkylator, cyclophosphamide, in the older regimens radically changed the profile of expected toxicities. Cumulative doses of drugs were also much higher in the older regimens because maintenance therapy often continued for 1 year, whereas the total duration of current regimens is generally only 9 to 12 weeks. For these reasons, the toxicities described in the St. Jude report, such as the high prevalence of delayed pubertal development and ovarian failure, are related to radiation or treatment with an alkylator; neither is part of standard care today.

Other pediatric studies have focused primarily on short-term toxicity, either occurring during the clinical trial or within the window of follow-up used to establish relapse rate. For example, in 33 children treated with BEP on GCI in the United Kingdom, 45% developed some degree of renal impairment and 10% developed auditory impairment (grades 1 to 3). One child developed acute myelogenous leukemia while receiving BEP. There were no deaths from bleomycin-induced pulmonary fibrosis after the dose of bleomycin was reduced to once per cycle every 3 weeks. There had been four deaths from pulmonary toxicity in children receiving weekly bleomycin. Of the 17 evaluable patients with SCT, 4 had neuropathic bladder and/or bowel and 1 had shortening of one leg.[389,429] In the 137 patients treated in GC2, which replaced carboplatin for cisplatin, only 1 patient had significant hearing loss, but this occurred after middle ear hemorrhages, and only 1 patient died of pulmonary failure (but had preexisting bronchopulmonary dysplasia).[449] All other renal and pulmonary toxicity noted on study was reversible. In the U.S. intergroup study, no patient treated with standard-dose PEB (total dose of cisplatin = 100 mg/m^2) developed hearing loss and no patients died of pulmonary toxicity.

In Men Treated for Testicular Cancer

Physicians who care for long-term survivors of pediatric germ cell tumors must be aware of and extrapolate from data emerging principally from follow-up studies of men treated for testicular cancer. Studies of men treated with testicular cancer are consistently demonstrating an increased risk of cardiovascular disease and second malignant neoplasm. However, the limitations of this approach are twofold. One is that age at treatment likely has an important bearing on the type and severity of toxicities. For example, adults are much more likely to develop tinnitus after cisplatinum therapy, or Raynaud's' phenomenon, than children. Younger age at treatment, however, increases the risk of development of a second malignant neoplasm. The other concern about extrapolating from the data on men who have been treated for testicular cancer is that one must assume that the experience of men can be applied without revision to the experience of women, an assumption proven to be false in other clinical situations.

Risk of Cardiovascular Disease

In a nationwide cohort in the Netherlands of 2707 5-year survivors of testicular cancer, the standardized incidence ratio of myocardial infarction, angina pectoris, or congestive heart failure was 1.4.[517] In another study of long-term survivors, the relative risk (RR) of cardiovascular disease was estimated to be 2.59 for patients treated with chemotherapy compared with patients on surveillance, with a median follow-up of 10 years.[214] A partial explanation for this excessive morbidity and mortality is the higher prevalence of cardiovascular risk factors in survivors, including hypertension, dyslipidemias, obesity, insulin resistance, and gonadal dysfunction,[518,519] as compared with patients treated with surgery and surveillance only or normal population controls. However, the reason that chemotherapy-treated patients have a higher prevalence of cardiovascular risk factors is not well understood. Another possible factor contributing to cardiovascular morbidity may be that chemotherapy induces vasospastic disease, as evidenced by the high post-chemotherapy incidence (up to 50%) of Raynaud's phenomenon in adult survivors of testicular cancer.[520-523] Another explanation for premature onset of cardiovascular events may be direct damage to the endothelial cell. Evidence of endothelial cell damage is the high prevalence (22%) of microalbuminuria observed in long-term survivors.[524] Other studies have noted an increase in plasma von Willebrand factor levels and in the intima-media thickness of the carotid artery post-treatment as further evidence of endothelial cell toxicity.[525]

Risk of Second Malignant Neoplasm

Several studies of the risk of second malignancy in men treated for testicular cancer have been conducted.[409,526,527] In the first two studies published ($n = 1025$; $n = 1909$), an increased risk of a second malignant neoplasm (SMN) was observed, principally gastrointestinal cancers, but secondary cancers occurred only in patients who had received radiotherapy.[526,527] A subsequent study that used population-based cancer registries identified almost 40,500 survivors of testicular cancer who had developed a total of 2,285 secondary solid cancers.[409,528] In this cohort, patients treated with chemotherapy alone exhibited a 1.8-fold excess risk of developing a second solid cancer, unlike prior studies, in which risk appeared to be restricted to those who had been treated with radiotherapy. Treatment with radiotherapy did incur a higher risk (RR, 2.0) than that observed with chemotherapy alone and a synergistic effect between chemotherapy and radiation therapy was also observed (RR, 2.9). This study was also the first to report an increased risk of supradiaphragmatic cancers (esophagus, pleura, and lung). Interestingly, cumulative risk at any given age increased with decreasing age at testicular cancer diagnosis. It was estimated that a patient diagnosed with seminoma at age 20 would have a cumulative risk of solid cancer of 47% by age 75, compared with 36% for a patient diagnosed at age 25 and 28% for a patient diagnosed at age 50. There was no plateau in the upward trend for risk throughout the 40-year period of follow-up, with serious implications for those diagnosed and treated at a young age.[409] A similar magnitude of increased risk of SMN was noted in the Dutch cohort of testicular cancer survivors (standardized incidence ratio [SIR], 2.1).[517]

Risk of Secondary Leukemia

The development of secondary leukemia or myelodysplastic syndrome after treatment with epipodophyllotoxins is a well-described clinical syndrome usually involving a translocation of the *MLL* gene. The risk of secondary leukemia in adult testicular patients has been estimated to be 0.6%.[529,530] An analysis of data that included children treated in the last U.S. Intergroup national protocol for pediatric germ cell tumors has estimated the risk to be almost identical (0.7%).[531] In a report of the German pediatric experience, 442 patients received chemotherapy and 174 patients received chemotherapy and radiotherapy.[532] Of these, 6 patients subsequently developed acute myelogenous leukemia; 4 of the 6 had the classic cytogenetic abnormalities associated with topoisomerase II inhibitor–

induced leukemias. The cumulative risk at 10 years for AML was 1% for children treated with chemotherapy alone and 4.2% for children treated with both chemotherapy and radiotherapy.

Other Significant Late Effects

Bleomycin and Pulmonary Toxicity. Bleomycin is known to cause fatal pulmonary fibrosis in 1% to 2% of patients, but all patients experience some measurable decrement in pulmonary function while on treatment. However, in adults, almost universally, pulmonary function tests recover to pretreatment values after completion of treatment.[533] Of more concern is the development of rapidly fatal adult respiratory distress syndrome (ARDS) in long-term survivors following general anesthesia. High concentrations of inspired oxygen have been implicated.[534,535] However, in a study reporting on the surgical management of patients who had been treated with bleomycin, the most significant predictor of postoperative oxygen saturation was the amount of blood transfused; intraoperative fractional oxygen was not significant in a multivariate analysis.[536] It was suggested that careful and conservative fluid management is at least as important as restriction of inspired oxygen during surgical procedures.

Most pediatric protocols have deleted or significantly reduced the amount of bleomycin used to avoid the complication of fatal pulmonary fibrosis completely (see earlier). It is not known how the reduction in dose will affect the development of ARDS during anesthesia post- treatment, and pediatric patients should be made aware of the risk.

Renal Toxicity. The glomerular filtration rate is decreased during treatment in almost all adult male patients but most studies have reported restoration of renal function to approximately 85% of pretreatment value by 4 years off therapy.[520,533,537-539] Persistent salt wasting (calcium, magnesium, phosphate) has been reported in 20% of patients.[520,538] Men have also been reported to have elevated renin and aldosterone levels after therapy.[540]

Gonadal Function. Abnormal sperm counts and motility and elevated levels of follicle-stimulating hormone (FSH) indicative of impaired spermatogenesis have been documented in two thirds of men after orchiectomy, prior to any adjuvant treatment.[541,542] One study has shown a similar clinical picture, even prior to the initial orchiectomy.[543] Despite these abnormalities in spermatogenesis at diagnosis, a significant proportion of men will recover sperm number and function after treatment.[541,544,545] In one study, 50% of men who were azoospermic at baseline recovered sperm counts to at least 10×10^6/mL, and 80% of patients who were oligospermic recovered normal sperm counts.[546] Elevated FSH (more than twice the upper limit of normal) was predictive of abnormal semen analysis at baseline and also after treatment.[546] Semen recovery usually occurs in the first 2 years following completion of treatment, but improvement has been observed as late as 4 years after treatment.[543] Encouragingly, paternity rates after treatment are high; most men (67% to 76%) who wished to be a parent have succeeded.[547]

Persistent endocrine dysfunction has been documented in men after treatment for testicular cancer, particularly in the pituitary-gonadal axis.[521] Several authors have noted elevations of FSH (up to 75% of men), luteinizing hormone (up to 50% of men)[214,521,537,548] and decreased testosterone (10% to 15%) in long-term survivors of testicular cancer.[521] One study has noted that the volume of the remaining testis is reduced in those men who received chemotherapy compared with those who underwent surgery only.[549] Moderate testosterone deficiency, as documented in some long-term survivors, may have a broader systemic impact. For example, testosterone deficiency has been correlated with higher levels of serum cholesterol[550] and lower testosterone levels are associated with lower levels of bone mineral density.[551] Site apparently was not related to endocrine dysfunction; patients with extragonadal primary tumors had the same profile of endocrine abnormalities.

CONCLUSIONS

Pediatric germ cell tumors are a highly curable form of cancer. Several challenges remain. One objective of current research is to elucidate a better understanding of the underlying biologic cause of these tumors. Work is also underway to improve on our current ability to predict who is likely to fail first-line therapy. Better prognostication will allow a more refined approach to treatment, reducing the amount of therapy for those likely to be cured. Given the seriousness of the emerging late effects of therapy on rates of cardiovascular disease and second malignant neoplasm in men treated for testicular cancer, physicians must reweigh the risks of adjuvant chemotherapy versus observation or primary RPLND. Conversely, the field is also challenged to find ways to intensify therapy for those for whom standard therapy is not sufficient. Finally, it is imperative that we catalogue the late effects of treatment for pediatric germ cell tumors so that we can adequately care for most pediatric patients who will be cured.

REFERENCES

1. Oosterhuis JW, Looijenga LH. Testicular germ-cell tumours in a broader perspective. Nat Rev Cancer. 2005;5:210-222.
2. Saitou M, Barton SC, Surani MA. A molecular programme for the specification of germ cell fate in mice. Nature. 2002;418:293-300.
3. Surani MA, Ancelin K, Hajkova P, et al. Mechanism of mouse germ cell specification: a genetic program regulating epigenetic reprogramming. Cold Spring Harb Symp Quant Biol. 2004;69:1-9.
4. Hayashi K, de Sousa Lopes SM, Surani MA. Germ cell specification in mice. Science. 2007;316:394-396.
5. Surani MA. Germ cells: the eternal link between generations. C R Biol. 2007;330:474-478.
6. Clark AT, Bodnar MS, Fox M, et al. Spontaneous differentiation of germ cells from human embryonic stem cells in vitro. Hum Mol Genet. 2004;13:727-739.
7. Geijsen N, Horoschak M, Kim K, et al. Derivation of embryonic germ cells and male gametes from embryonic stem cells. Nature. 2004;427:148-154.
8. Clark AT, Reijo Pera RA. Modeling human germ cell development with embryonic stem cells. Regen Med. 2006;1:85-93.
9. Kee K, Gonsalves JM, Clark AT, Pera RA. Bone morphogenetic proteins induce germ cell differentiation from human embryonic stem cells. Stem Cells Dev. 2006;15:831-837.
10. Clark AT. Establishment and differentiation of human embryonic stem cell derived germ cells. Soc Reprod Fertil Suppl. 2007;63:77-86.
11. Kierszenbaum AL, Tres LL. Primordial germ cell-somatic cell partnership: a balancing cell signaling act. Mol Reprod Dev. 2001;60:277-280.
12. Ying Y, Qi X, Zhao GQ. Induction of primordial germ cells from pluripotent epiblast. Scientific World Journal. 2002;2:801-810.
13. de Sousa Lopes SM, Roelen BA, Monteiro RM, et al. BMP signaling mediated by ALK2 in the visceral endoderm is necessary for the generation of primordial germ cells in the mouse embryo. Genes Dev. 2004;18:1838-1849.
14. Lacham-Kaplan O. In vivo and in vitro differentiation of male germ cells in the mouse. Reproduction. 2004;128:147-152.
15. Tanaka SS, Nagamatsu G, Tokitake Y, et al. Regulation of expression of mouse interferon-induced transmembrane protein-like gene-3, Ifitm3 (mil-1, fragilis), in germ cells. Dev Dyn. 2004;230:651-659.
16. Ohinata Y, Payer B, O'Carroll D, et al. Blimp1 is a critical determinant of the germ cell lineage in mice. Nature. 2005;436:207-213.
17. Scholer HR, Dressler GR, Balling R, et al. Oct-4: a germline-specific transcription factor mapping to the mouse t-complex. EMBO J. 1990;9:2185-2195.
18. Hansis C, Grifo JA, Krey LC. Oct-4 expression in inner cell mass and trophectoderm of human blastocysts. Mol Hum Reprod. 2000;6:999-1004.
19. Pesce M, Scholer HR. Oct-4: control of totipotency and germline determination. Mol Reprod Dev. 2000;55:452-457.
20. Pesce M, Scholer HR. Oct-4: gatekeeper in the beginnings of mammalian development. Stem Cells. 2001;19:271-278.
21. Rajpert-De Meyts E, Hanstein R, Jorgensen N, et al. Developmental expression of POU5F1 (OCT-3/4) in normal and dysgenetic human gonads. Hum Reprod. 2004;19:1338-1344.
22. Hatano SY, Tada M, Kimura H, et al. Pluripotential competence of cells associated with Nanog activity. Mech Dev. 2005;122:67-79.
23. Yamaguchi S, Kimura H, Tada M, et al. Nanog expression in mouse germ cell development. Gene Expr Patterns. 2005;5:639-646.
24. Payer B, Chuva de Sousa Lopes SM, Barton SC, et al. Generation of stella-GFP transgenic mice: a novel tool to study germ cell development. Genesis. 2006;44:75-83.
25. Buitrago W, DR. Oct-4: the almighty POUripotent regulator? J Invest Dermatol. 2007;127:260-262.
26. Looijenga LH, Stoop H, de Leeuw HP, et al. POU5F1 (OCT3/4) identifies cells with pluripotent potential in human germ cell tumors. Cancer Res. 2003;63:2244-2250.
27. de Jong J, Stoop H, Dohle GR, et al. Diagnostic value of OCT3/4 for pre-invasive and invasive testicular germ cell tumours. J Pathol. 2005;206:242-249.
28. Hart AH, Hartley L, Parker K, et al. The pluripotency homeobox gene NANOG is expressed in human germ cell tumors. Cancer. 2005;104:2092-2098.
29. Kersemaekers AM, Honecker F, Stoop H, et al. Identification of germ cells at risk for neoplastic transformation in gonadoblastoma: an immunohistochemical study for OCT3/4 and TSPY. Hum Pathol. 2005;36:512-521.
30. Cheng L, Sung MT, Cossu-Rocca P, et al. OCT4: biological functions and clinical applications as a marker of germ cell neoplasia. J Pathol. 2007;211:1-9.
31. McLaren A. Germ and somatic cell lineages in the developing gonad. Mol Cell Endocrinol. 2000;163:3-9.
32. Oosterhuis JW, Stoop H, Honecker F, Looijenga LH. Why human extragonadal germ cell tumours occur in the midline of the body: old concepts, new perspectives. Int J Androl. 2007;30:256-263.
33. Besmer P, Manova K, Duttlinger R, et al. The kit-ligand (steel factor) and its receptor c-kit/W: pleiotropic roles in gametogenesis and melanogenesis. Dev Suppl. 1993;125-137.
34. Buehr M, McLaren A, Bartley A, Darling S. Proliferation and migration of primordial germ cells in We/We mouse embryos. Dev Dyn. 1993;198:182-189.
35. Molyneaux KA, Stallock J, Schaible K, Wylie C. Time-lapse analysis of living mouse germ cell migration. Dev Biol. 2001;240:488-498.

36. Molyneaux K, Wylie C. Primordial germ cell migration. Int J Dev Biol. 2004;48:537-544.

37. Stallock J, Molyneaux K, Schaible K, et al. The pro-apoptotic gene Bax is required for the death of ectopic primordial germ cells during their migration in the mouse embryo. Development. 2003;130:6589-6597.

38. Molyneaux KA, Wang Y, Schaible K, Wylie C. Transcriptional profiling identifies genes differentially expressed during and after migration in murine primordial germ cells. Gene Expr Patterns. 2004;4:167-181.

39. Runyan C, Schaible K, Molyneaux K, et al. Steel factor controls midline cell death of primordial germ cells and is essential for their normal proliferation and migration. Development. 2006; 133:4861-4869.

40. Bendel-Stenzel MR, Gomperts M, Anderson R, et al. The role of cadherins during primordial germ cell migration and early gonad formation in the mouse. Mech Dev. 2000;91:143-152.

41. Johnson MH, Everitt BJ. Essential Reproduction, 5th ed. Malden, Mass, Blackwell, 2000.

42. Ara T, Nakamura Y, Egawa T, et al. Impaired colonization of the gonads by primordial germ cells in mice lacking a chemokine, stromal cell-derived factor-1 (SDF-1). Proc Natl Acad Sci U S A. 2003;100:5319-5323.

43. Molyneaux KA, Zinszner H, Kunwar PS, et al. The chemokine SDF1/CXCL12 and its receptor CXCR4 regulate mouse germ cell migration and survival. Development. 2003;130:4279-4286.

44. De Miguel MP, Cheng L, Holland EC, et al. Dissection of the c-Kit signaling pathway in mouse primordial germ cells by retro-viral-mediated gene transfer. Proc Natl Acad Sci U S A. 2002;99: 10458-10463.

45. da Rocha ST, Ferguson-Smith AC. Genomic imprinting. Curr Biol. 2004;14:R646-R649.

46. Wood AJ, Oakey RJ. Genomic imprinting in mammals: emerging themes and established theories. PLoS Genet. 2006;2:e147.

47. Munshi A, Duvvuri S. Genomic imprinting—the story of the other half and the conflicts of silencing. J Genet Genomics. 2007;34:93-103.

48. Barton SC, Surani MA, Norris ML. Role of paternal and maternal genomes in mouse development. Nature. 1984;311:374-376.

49. Allegrucci C, Thurston A, Lucas E, Young L. Epigenetics and the germline. Reproduction. 2005;129:137-149.

50. Trasler JM. Gamete imprinting: setting epigenetic patterns for the next generation. Reprod Fertil Dev. 2006;18:63-69.

51. Schaefer CB, Ooi SK, Bestor TH, Bourc'his D. Epigenetic decisions in mammalian germ cells. Science. 2007;316:398-399.

52. Gubbay J, Collignon J, Koopman P, et al. A gene mapping to the sex-determining region of the mouse Y chromosome is a member of a novel family of embryonically expressed genes. Nature. 1990;346:245-250.

53. Koopman P, Munsterberg A, Capel B, et al. Expression of a candidate sex-determining gene during mouse testis differentiation. Nature. 1990;348:450-452.

54. Wilhelm D, Palmer S, Koopman P. Sex determination and gonadal development in mammals. Physiol Rev. 2007;87:1-28.

55. Teilum G, Albrechtsen R, Norgaard-Pedersen B. The histogenetic-embryologic basis for reappearance of alpha-fetoprotein in endodermal sinus tumors (yolk sac tumors) and teratomas. Acta Pathol Microbiol Scand [A]. 1975;83:80-86.

56. Weissbach L, Altwein JE, Stiens R. Germinal testicular tumors in childhood. Report of observations and literature review. Eur Urol. 1984;10:73-85.

57. Isaacs H Jr. Perinatal (fetal and neonatal) germ cell tumors. J Pediatr Surg. 2004;39:1003-1013.

58. Walsh TJ, Grady RW, Porter MP, et al. Incidence of testicular germ cell cancers in U.S. children: SEER program experience 1973 to 2000. Urology. 2006;68:402-405.

59. Jorgensen N, Muller J, Giwercman A, et al. DNA content and expression of tumour markers in germ cells adjacent to germ cell tumours in childhood: probably a different origin for infantile and adolescent germ cell tumours. J Pathol. 1995;176:269-278.

60. van Echten J, Oosterhuis JW, Looijenga LH, et al. No recurrent structural abnormalities apart from i(12p) in primary germ cell tumors of the adult testis. Genes Chromosomes Cancer. 1995;14: 133-144.

61. Veltman IM, Schepens MT, Looijenga LH, et al. Germ cell tumours in neonates and infants: a distinct subgroup? APMIS. 2003;111:152-160.

62. Schultz KA, Sencer SF, Messinger Y, et al. Pediatric ovarian tumors: a review of 67 cases. Pediatr Blood Cancer. 2005;44: 167-173.

63. Strickland JL. Ovarian cysts in neonates, children and adolescents. Curr Opin Obstet Gynecol. 2002;14:459-465.

64. Ulbright TM. Germ cell tumors of the gonads: a selective review emphasizing problems in differential diagnosis, newly appreciated, and controversial issues. Mod Pathol. 2005;18(Suppl 2):S61-S79.

65. Hoepffner W, Horn LC, Simon E, et al. Gonadoblastomas in 5 patients with 46,XY gonadal dysgenesis. Exp Clin Endocrinol Diabetes. 2005;113:231-235.

66. Brant WO, Rajimwale A, Lovell MA, et al. Gonadoblastoma and Turner syndrome. J Urol. 2006;175:1858-1860.

67. Cools M, Stoop H, Kersemaekers AM, et al. Gonadoblastoma arising in undifferentiated gonadal tissue within dysgenetic gonads. J Clin Endocrinol Metab. 2006;91:2404-2413.

68. Talerman A, Roth LM. Recent advances in the pathology and classification of gonadal neoplasms composed of germ cells and sex cord derivatives. Int J Gynecol Pathol. 2007;26:313-321.

69. Quirk JT, Natarajan N. Ovarian cancer incidence in the United States, 1992-1999. Gynecol Oncol. 2005;97:519-523.

70. Woodward PJ, Heidenreich A, Looijenga LHJ, et al. Germ cell tumours. In Eble JN, Sauter G, Epstein JI, Sesterhenn IA (eds). World Health Organization Classification of Tumours: Tumours of the Urinary System and Male Genital Organs. Lyon, France, IARC Press, 2004, pp 221-250.

71. Bagchi A, Papazoglu C, Wu Y, et al. CHD5 is a tumor suppressor at human 1p36. Cell. 2007;128:459-475.

72. von der Maase H, Rorth M, Walbom-Jorgensen S, et al. Carcinoma in situ of contralateral testis in patients with testicular germ cell cancer: study of 27 cases in 500 patients. Br Med J (Clin Res Ed). 1986;293:1398-1401.

73. Skakkebaek NE, Berthelsen JG, Giwercman A, Muller J. Carcinoma-in-situ of the testis: possible origin from gonocytes and precursor of all types of germ cell tumours except spermatocytoma. Int J Androl. 1987;10:19-28.

74. Giwercman A, Bruun E, Frimodt-Moller C, Skakkebaek NE. Prevalence of carcinoma in situ and other histopathological abnormalities in testes of men with a history of cryptorchidism. J Urol. 1989;142:998-1001.

75. Dieckmann KP, Skakkebaek NE. Carcinoma in situ of the testis: review of biological and clinical features. Int J Cancer. 1999;83: 815-822.

76. Rorth M, Rajpert-De Meyts E, Andersson L, et al. Carcinoma in situ in the testis. Scand J Urol Nephrol Suppl. 2000;166:166-186.

77. Hoei-Hansen CE, Rajpert-De Meyts E, Daugaard G, Skakkebaek NE. Carcinoma in situ testis, the progenitor of testicular germ cell tumours: a clinical review. Ann Oncol. 2005;16:863-868.

78. Looijenga LH, Hersmus R, Gillis AJ, et al. Genomic and expression profiling of human spermatocytic seminomas: primary spermatocyte as tumorigenic precursor and DMRT1 as candidate chromosome 9 gene. Cancer Res. 2006;66:290-302.

79. Pedersen KV, Boiesen P, Zetterlund CG. Experience of screening for carcinoma-in-situ of the testis in young men with surgically corrected maldescended testes. Int J Androl. 1987;10:181-185.

80. Burke AP, Mostofi FK. Intratubular malignant germ cells in testicular biopsies: clinical course and identification by staining for placental alkaline phosphatase. Mod Pathol. 1988;1:475-479.

81. Bettocchi C, Coker CB, Deacon J, et al. A review of testicular intratubular germ cell neoplasia in infertile men. J Androl. 1994;15(Suppl):14S-16S.

82. Hoei-Hansen CE, Rajpert-De Meyts E, Carlsen E, et al. A sub-fertile patient diagnosed with testicular carcinoma in situ by immunocytological staining for AP-2gamma in semen samples: case report. Hum Reprod. 2005;20:579-582.

83. Giwercman A, Lindenberg S, Kimber SJ, et al. Monoclonal antibody 43-9F as a sensitive immunohistochemical marker of carcinoma in situ of human testis. Cancer. 1990;65:1135-1142.

84. Oosterhuis JW, Kersemaekers AM, Jacobsen GK, et al. Morphology of testicular parenchyma adjacent to germ cell tumours. An interim report. APMIS. 2003;111:32-40.

85. Berthelsen JG, Skakkebaek NE, von der Maase H, et al. Screening for carcinoma in situ of the contralateral testis in patients with germinal testicular cancer. Br Med J (Clin Res Ed). 1982;285:1683-1686.

86. Dieckmann KP, Loy V, Buttner P. Prevalence of bilateral testicular germ cell tumours and early detection based on contralateral testicular intra-epithelial neoplasia. Br J Urol. 1993;71:340-345.

87. Wahren B, Holmgren PA, Stigbrand T. Placental alkaline phosphatase, alphafetoprotein and carcinoembryonic antigen in testicular tumors. Tissue typing by means of cytologic smears. Int J Cancer. 1979;24:749-753.

88. Jacobsen GK, Norgaard-Pedersen B. Placental alkaline phosphatase in testicular germ cell tumours and in carcinoma-in-situ of the testis. An immunohistochemical study. Acta Pathol Microbiol Immunol Scand [A]. 1984;92:323-329.

89. Burke AP, Mostofi FK. Placental alkaline phosphatase immunohistochemistry of intratubular malignant germ cells and associated testicular germ cell tumors. Hum Pathol. 1988;19:663-670.

90. Hoei-Hansen CE, Nielsen JE, Almstrup K, et al. Transcription factor AP-2gamma is a developmentally regulated marker of testicular carcinoma in situ and germ cell tumors. Clin Cancer Res. 2004;10:8521-8530.

91. Jones TD, Ulbright TM, Eble JN, et al. OCT4 staining in testicular tumors: a sensitive and specific marker for seminoma and embryonal carcinoma. Am J Surg Pathol. 2004;28:935-940.

92. Jones TD, Ulbright TM, Eble JN, Cheng L. OCT4: a sensitive and specific biomarker for intratubular germ cell neoplasia of the testis. Clin Cancer Res. 2004;10:8544-8547.

93. Hoei-Hansen CE, Olesen IA, Jorgensen N, et al. Current approaches for detection of carcinoma in situ testis. Int J Androl. 2007;30:398-405.

94. Li Y, Tabatabai ZL, Lee TL, et al. The Y-encoded TSPY protein: a significant marker potentially plays a role in the pathogenesis of testicular germ cell tumors. Hum Pathol. 2007;38:1470-1481.

95. Li Y, Vilain E, Conte F, et al. Testis-specific protein Y-encoded gene is expressed in early and late stages of gonadoblastoma and testicular carcinoma in situ. Urol Oncol. 2007;25:141-146.

96. Honecker F, Oosterhuis JW, Mayer F, et al. New insights into the pathology and molecular biology of human germ cell tumors. World J Urol. 2004;22:15-24.

97. Honecker F, Stoop H, de Krijger RR, et al. Pathobiological implications of the expression of markers of testicular carcinoma in situ by fetal germ cells. J Pathol. 2004;203:849-857.

98. Manivel JC, Simonton S, Wold LE, Dehner LP. Absence of intratubular germ cell neoplasia in testicular yolk sac tumors in children. A histochemical and immunohistochemical study. Arch Pathol Lab Med. 1988;112:641-645.

99. Hawkins E, Heifetz SA, Giller R, Cushing B. The prepubertal testis (prenatal and postnatal): its relationship to intratubular germ cell neoplasia: a combined Pediatric Oncology Group and Children's Cancer Study Group. Hum Pathol. 1997;28:404-410.

100. Hu LM, Phillipson J, Barsky SH. Intratubular germ cell neoplasia in infantile yolk sac tumor. Verification by tandem repeat sequence in situ hybridization. Diagn Mol Pathol. 1992;1:118-128.

101. Stamp IM, Barlebo H, Rix M, Jacobsen GK. Intratubular germ cell neoplasia in an infantile testis with immature teratoma. Histopathology. 1993;22:69-72.

102. Renedo DE, Trainer TD. Intratubular germ cell neoplasia (ITGCN) with p53 and PCNA expression and adjacent mature teratoma in an infant testis. An immunohistochemical and morphologic study with a review of the literature. Am J Surg Pathol. 1994;18:947-952.

103. Schneider DT, Schuster AE, Fritsch MK, et al. Multipoint imprinting analysis indicates a common precursor cell for gonadal and nongonadal pediatric germ cell tumors. Cancer Res. 2001;61:7268-7276.

104. Schneider DT, Schuster AE, Fritsch MK, et al. Genetic analysis of mediastinal nonseminomatous germ cell tumors in children and adolescents. Genes Chromosomes Cancer. 2002;34:115-125.

105. Sievers S, Alemazkour K, Zahn S, et al. IGF2/H19 imprinting analysis of human germ cell tumors (GCTs) using the methylation-sensitive single-nucleotide primer extension method reflects the origin of GCTs in different stages of primordial germ cell development. Genes Chromosomes Cancer. 2005;44:256-264.

106. Lee PA, Houk CP, Ahmed SF, Hughes IA. Consensus statement on management of intersex disorders. International Consensus Conference on Intersex. Pediatrics. 2006;118:e488-e500.

107. Looijenga LH, Hersmus R, Oosterhuis JW, et al. Tumor risk in disorders of sex development (DSD). Best Pract Res Clin Endocrinol Metab. 2007;21:480-495.

108. Muller J, Skakkebaek NE, Ritzen M, et al. Carcinoma in situ of the testis in children with 45,X/46,XY gonadal dysgenesis. J Pediatr. 1985;106:431-436.

109. Muller J, Ritzen EM, Ivarsson SA, et al. Management of males with 45,X/46,XY gonadal dysgenesis. Horm Res. 1999;52:11-14.

110. Patil SR, Kaiser-McCaw B, Hecht F, et al. Human benign ovarian teratomas: chromosomal and electrophoretic enzyme studies. Birth Defects Orig Artic Ser. 1978;14:297-301.

111. Muller J, Skakkebaek NE. Testicular carcinoma in situ in children with the androgen insensitivity (testicular feminisation) syndrome. Br Med J (Clin Res Ed). 1984;288:1419-1420.

112. Cassio A, Cacciari E, D'Errico A, et al. Incidence of intratubular germ cell neoplasia in androgen insensitivity syndrome. Acta Endocrinol (Copenh). 1990;123:416-422.

113. Cools M, Drop SL, Wolffenbuttel KP, et al. Germ cell tumors in the intersex gonad: old paths, new directions, moving frontiers. Endocr Rev. 2006;27:468-484.

114. Tsuchiya K, Reijo R, Page DC, Disteche CM. Gonadoblastoma: molecular definition of the susceptibility region on the Y chromosome. Am J Hum Genet. 1995;57:1400-1407.

115. Schnieders F, Dork T, Arnemann J, et al. Testis-specific protein, Y-encoded (TSPY) expression in testicular tissues. Hum Mol Genet. 1996;5:1801-1807.

116. Hildenbrand R, Schroder W, Brude E, et al. Detection of TSPY protein in a unilateral microscopic gonadoblastoma of a Turner mosaic patient with a Y-derived marker chromosome. J Pathol. 1999;189:623-626.

117. Lau Y, Chou P, Iezzoni J, et al. Expression of a candidate gene for the gonadoblastoma locus in gonadoblastoma and testicular seminoma. Cytogenet Cell Genet. 2000;91:160-164.

118. Fallat ME, Donahoe PK. Intersex genetic anomalies with malignant potential. Curr Opin Pediatr. 2006;18:305-311.

119. Cools M, van Aerde K, Kersemaekers AM, et al. Morphological and immunohistochemical differences between gonadal matura-

tion delay and early germ cell neoplasia in patients with under-virilization syndromes. J Clin Endocrinol Metab. 2005;90:5295-5303.

120. Stoop H, Honecker F, Cools M, et al. Differentiation and development of human female germ cells during prenatal gonadogenesis: an immunohistochemical study. Hum Reprod. 2005;20:1466-1476.

121. Hannema SE, Scott IS, Rajpert-De Meyts E, et al. Testicular development in the complete androgen insensitivity syndrome. J Pathol. 2006;208:518-527.

122. Isaacs H Jr. Germ cell tumors. In Gilbert-Barness E, Kapur RJ, Oligny LL, Siebert JR (eds). Potter's Pathology of the Fetus, Infant and Child. St. Louis, Mosby, 2007, pp 1690-1709.

123. Norris HJ, Zirkin HJ, Benson WL. Immature (malignant) teratoma of the ovary: a clinical and pathologic study of 58 cases. Cancer. 1976;37:2359-2372.

124. Levy DA, Kay R, Elder JS. Neonatal testis tumors: a review of the Prepubertal Testis Tumor Registry. J Urol. 1994;151:715-717.

125. Ross JH, Rybicki L, Kay R. Clinical behavior and a contemporary management algorithm for prepubertal testis tumors: a summary of the Prepubertal Testis Tumor Registry. J Urol. 2002;168:1675-1678.

126. Pohl HG, Shukla AR, Metcalf PD, et al. Prepubertal testis tumors: actual prevalence rate of histological types. J Urol. 2004;172:2370-2372.

127. Harms D, Zahn S, Gobel U, Schneider DT. Pathology and molecular biology of teratomas in childhood and adolescence. Klin Padiatr. 2006;218:296-302.

128. Walsh C, Rushton HG. Diagnosis and management of teratomas and epidermoid cysts. Urol Clin North Am. 2000;27:509-518.

129. Wu HY, Snyder HM 3rd. Pediatric urologic oncology: bladder, prostate, testis. Urol Clin North Am. 2004;31:619-627, xi.

130. Carney JA, Thompson DP, Johnson CL, Lynn HB. Teratomas in children: clinical and pathologic aspects. J Pediatr Surg. 1972;7:271-282.

131. Tosi SE, Richardson JR Jr. Simple cyst of the testis: case report and review of the literature. J Urol. 1975;114:473-475.

132. Brown NJ. Teratomas and yolk-sac tumours. J Clin Pathol. 1976;29:1021-1025.

133. Brosman SA. Testicular tumors in prepubertal children. Urology. 1979;13:581-588.

134. Heifetz SA, Cushing B, Giller R, et al. Immature teratomas in children: pathologic considerations: a report from the combined Pediatric Oncology Group/Children's Cancer Group. Am J Surg Pathol. 1998;22:1115-1124.

135. Manivel JC, Reinberg Y, Niehans GA, Fraley EE. Intratubular germ cell neoplasia in testicular teratomas and epidermoid cysts. Correlation with prognosis and possible biologic significance. Cancer. 1989;64:715-720.

136. Rushton HG, Belman AB, Sesterhenn I, et al. Testicular sparing surgery for prepubertal teratoma of the testis: a clinical and pathological study. J Urol. 1990;144:726-730.

137. Ulbright TM. Gonadal teratomas: a review and speculation. Adv Anat Pathol. 2004;11:10-23.

138. Bussey KJ, Lawce HJ, Olson SB, et al. Chromosome abnormalities of eighty-one pediatric germ cell tumors: sex-, age-, site-, and histopathology-related differences—a Children's Cancer Group study. Genes Chromosomes Cancer. 1999;25:134-146.

139. Mostert M, Rosenberg C, Stoop H, et al. Comparative genomic and in situ hybridization of germ cell tumors of the infantile testis. Lab Invest. 2000;80:1055-1064.

140. Ross JH, Kay R, Elder J. Testis sparing surgery for pediatric epidermoid cysts of the testis. J Urol. 1993;149:353-356.

141. Garrett JE, Cartwright PC, Snow BW, Coffin CM. Cystic testicular lesions in the pediatric population. J Urol. 2000;163:928-936.

142. Eisenmenger M, Lang S, Donner G, et al. Epidermoid cysts of the testis: organ-preserving surgery following diagnosis by ultrasonography. Br J Urol. 1993;72:955-957.

143. Stamp IM, Jacobsen GK. Infant intratubular germ cell neoplasia. Am J Surg Pathol. 1995;19:489.

144. Hawkins E, Hicks MJ. Solid tumors and germ cell tumors induce nonneoplastic germ cell proliferations in testes of infants and young children. Hum Pathol. 1998;29:1547-1548.

145. von Hochstetter AR, Hedinger CE. The differential diagnosis of testicular germ cell tumors in theory and practice. A critical analysis of two major systems of classifiction and review of 389 cases. Virchows Arch A Pathol Anat Histol. 1982;396:247-277.

146. Mostofi FK, Sesterhenn IA, Davis CJ Jr. Immunopathology of germ cell tumors of the testis. Semin Diagn Pathol. 1987;4:320-341.

147. Ulbright TM. Germ cell neoplasms of the testis. Am J Surg Pathol. 1993;17:1075-1091.

148. Daly DW, Dossett JA, Jull JW. An oestrogen-secreting sex-chromatin-positive teratoma of the testis, associated with gynaecomastia. Br J Surg. 1963;50:816-819.

149. Javadpour N. The value of biologic markers in diagnosis and treatment of testicular cancer. Semin Oncol. 1979;6:37-47.

150. Javadpour N. Misconceptions and source of errors in interpretation of cellular and serum markers in testicular cancer. J Urol. 1986;135:879.

151. Kurman RJ, Norris HJ. Malignant mixed germ cell tumors of the ovary. A clinical and pathologic analysis of 30 cases. Obstet Gynecol. 1976;48:579-589.

152. Scully RE, Young RH, Clement PB. Tumors of the ovary, maldeveloped gonads, fallopian tube and broad ligament. In Atlas of Tumor Pathology, 3rd Series, Fascicle 23. Washington, DC, Armed Forces Institute of Pathology, 1998.

153. Katsube Y, Berg JW, Silverberg SG. Epidemiologic pathology of ovarian tumors: a histopathologic review of primary ovarian neoplasms diagnosed in the Denver Standard Metropolitan Statistical Area, 1 July-31 December 1969 and 1 July-31 December 1979. Int J Gynecol Pathol. 1982;1:3-16.

154. Koonings PP, Campbell K, Mishell DR Jr, Grimes DA. Relative frequency of primary ovarian neoplasms: a 10-year review. Obstet Gynecol. 1989;74:921-926.

155. Surti U, Hoffner L, Chakravarti A, Ferrell RE. Genetics and biology of human ovarian teratomas. I. Cytogenetic analysis and mechanism of origin. Am J Hum Genet. 1990;47:635-643.

156. Hoffner L, Shen-Schwarz S, Deka R, et al. Genetics and biology of human ovarian teratomas. III. Cytogenetics and origins of malignant ovarian germ cell tumors. Cancer Genet Cytogenet. 1992;62:58-65.

157. Stock C, Ambros IM, Lion T, et al. Detection of numerical and structural chromosome abnormalities in pediatric germ cell tumors by means of interphase cytogenetics. Genes Chromosomes Cancer. 1994;11:40-50.

158. Schneider DT, Schuster AE, Fritsch MK, et al. Genetic analysis of childhood germ cell tumors with comparative genomic hybridization. Klin Padiatr. 2001;213:204-211.

159. Linder D. Gene loss in human teratomas. Proc Natl Acad Sci U S A. 1969;63:699-704.

160. Ott J, Hecht F, Linder D, et al. Human centromere mapping using teratoma data. Birth Defects Orig Artic Ser. 1976;12:396-398.

161. Ott J, Linder D, McCaw BK, et al. Estimating distances from the centromere by means of benign ovarian teratomas in man. Ann Hum Genet. 1976;40:191-196.

162. Parrington JM, West LF, Povey S. The origin of ovarian teratomas. J Med Genet. 1984;21:4-12.

163. Dahl N, Gustavson KH, Rune C, et al. Benign ovarian teratomas. An analysis of their cellular origin. Cancer Genet Cytogenet. 1990;46:115-123.

164. Vortmeyer AO, Devouassoux-Shisheboran M, Li G, et al. Microdissection-based analysis of mature ovarian teratoma. Am J Pathol. 1999;154:987-991.

165. Thurlbeck WM, Scully RE. Solid teratoma of the ovary. A clinicopathological analysis of 9 cases. Cancer. 1960;13:804-811.

166. Beilby JO, Parkinson C. Features of prognostic significance in solid ovarian teratoma. Cancer. 1975;36:2147-2154.

167. Nogales F, Talerman A, Kubich-Huch RA, et al. Germ cell tumours. In Tavassoli FA, Devilee P (eds). World Health Organization Classification of Tumours: Tumours of the Breast and Female Genital Organs. Lyon, France, IARC Press, 2003, pp 163-179.

168. Comerci JT Jr, Licciardi F, Bergh PA, et al. Mature cystic teratoma: a clinicopathologic evaluation of 517 cases and review of the literature. Obstet Gynecol. 1994;84:22-28.

169. Gershenson DM, del Junco G, Silva EG, et al. Immature teratoma of the ovary. Obstet Gynecol. 1986;68:624-629.

170. Gonzalez-Crussi F. Extragonadal teratomas. In Atlas of Tumor Pathology, 2nd Series, Fascicle 18. Washington, DC, Armed Forces Institute of Pathology, 1982.

171. O'Connor DM, Norris HJ. The influence of grade on the outcome of stage I ovarian immature (malignant) teratomas and the reproducibility of grading. Int J Gynecol Pathol. 1994;13:283-289.

172. Kooijman CD. Immature teratomas in children. Histopathology. 1988;12:491-502.

173. Cushing B, Giller R, Ablin A, et al. Surgical resection alone is effective treatment for ovarian immature teratoma in children and adolescents: a report of the Pediatric Oncology Group and the Children's Cancer Group. Am J Obstet Gynecol. 1999;181:353-358.

174. Marina NM, Cushing B, Giller R, et al. Complete surgical excision is effective treatment for children with immature teratomas with or without malignant elements: a Pediatric Oncology Group/Children's Cancer Group Intergroup Study. J Clin Oncol. 1999;17:2137-2143.

175. El Shafie M, Furay RW, Chablani LV. Ovarian teratoma with peritoneal and lymph node metastases of mature glial tissue: a benign condition. J Surg Oncol. 1984;27:18-22.

176. Harms D, Janig U, Gobel U. Gliomatosis peritonei in childhood and adolescence. Clinicopathological study of 13 cases including immunohistochemical findings. Pathol Res Pract. 1989;184:422-430.

177. Muller AM, Sondgen D, Strunz R, Muller KM. Gliomatosis peritonei: a report of two cases and review of the literature. Eur J Obstet Gynecol Reprod Biol. 2002;100:213-222.

178. Robboy SJ, Scully RE. Ovarian teratoma with glial implants on the peritoneum. Hum Pathol. 1970;1:643-653.

179. Nielsen SN, Scheithauer BW, Gaffey TA. Gliomatosis peritonei. Cancer. 1985;56:2499-2503.

180. Ferguson AW, Katabuchi H, Ronnett BM, Cho KR. Glial implants in gliomatosis peritonei arise from normal tissue, not from the associated teratoma. Am J Pathol. 2001;159:51-55.

181. Best DH, Butz GM, Moller K, et al. Molecular analysis of an immature ovarian teratoma with gliomatosis peritonei and recurrence suggests genetic independence of multiple tumors. Int J Oncol. 2004;25:17-25.

182. Kwan MY, Kalle W, Lau GT, Chan JK. Is gliomatosis peritonei derived from the associated ovarian teratoma? Hum Pathol. 2004;35:685-688.

183. Robboy SJ, Scully RE. Strumal carcinoid of the ovary: an analysis of 50 cases of a distinctive tumor composed of thyroid tissue and carcinoid. Cancer. 1980;46:2019-2034.

184. Talerman A. Carcinoid tumors of the ovary. J Cancer Res Clin Oncol. 1984;107:125-135.

185. Soga J, Osaka M, Yakuwa Y. Carcinoids of the ovary: an analysis of 329 reported cases. J Exp Clin Cancer Res. 2000;19:271-280.

186. Roth LM, Talerman A. The enigma of struma ovarii. Pathology. 2007;39:139-146.

187. Shuangshoti S, Tharavej A. Neoplasms of neuroepithelial origin arising in a cystic teratoma of ovary. J Med Assoc Thai. 1980;63:284-290.

188. Aguirre P, Scully RE. Malignant neuroectodermal tumor of the ovary, a distinctive form of monodermal teratoma: report of five cases. Am J Surg Pathol. 1982;6:283-292.

189. Harms D, Janig U. Immature teratomas of childhood. Report of 21 cases. Pathol Res Pract. 1985;179:388-400.

190. Kleinman GM, Young RH, Scully RE. Primary neuroectodermal tumors of the ovary. A report of 25 cases. Am J Surg Pathol. 1993;17:764-778.

191. Nogales FF, Ruiz Avila I, Concha A, del Moral E. Immature endodermal teratoma of the ovary: embryologic correlations and immunohistochemistry. Hum Pathol. 1993;24:364-370.

192. Ayhan A, Bukulmez O, Genc C, et al. Mature cystic teratomas of the ovary: case series from one institution over 34 years. Eur J Obstet Gynecol Reprod Biol. 2000;88:153-157.

193. Peterson WF. Malignant degeneration of benign cystic teratomas of the ovary: collective review of the literature. Obstet Gynecol Surv. 1957;12:793-830.

194. Hirakawa T, Tsuneyoshi M, Enjoji M. Squamous cell carcinoma arising in mature cystic teratoma of the ovary. Clinicopathologic and topographic analysis. Am J Surg Pathol. 1989;13:397-405.

195. Ross JH, Kay R. Prepubertal testis tumors. Rev Urol. 2004;6:11-18.

196. Enders AC, King BF. Development of the human yolk sac, In Nogales F (ed). Yolk Sac and Yolk Sac Tumors. Berlin, Springer-Verlag, 1993, pp 33-47.

197. Wu JT, Book L, Sudar K. Serum alpha fetoprotein (AFP) levels in normal infants. Pediatr Res. 1981;15:50-52.

198. Blohm ME, Vesterling-Horner D, Calaminus G, Gobel U. Alpha 1-fetoprotein (AFP) reference values in infants up to 2 years of age. Pediatr Hematol Oncol. 1998;15:135-142.

199. Bader D, Riskin A, Vafsi O, et al. Alpha-fetoprotein in the early neonatal period—a large study and review of the literature. Clin Chim Acta. 2004;349:15-23.

200. Kurman RJ, Norris HJ. Embryonal carcinoma of the ovary: a clinicopathologic entity distinct from endodermal sinus tumor resembling embryonal carcinoma of the adult testis. Cancer. 1976;38:2420-2433.

201. Jacobsen GK, Jacobsen M. Alpha-fetoprotein (AFP) and human chorionic gonadotropin (HCG) in testicular germ cell tumours. A prospective immunohistochemical study. Acta Pathol Microbiol Immunol Scand [A]. 1983;91:165-176.

202. Morris HH, La Vecchia C, Draper GJ. Endodermal sinus tumor and embryonal carcinoma of the ovary in children. Gynecol Oncol. 1985;21:7-17.

203. Eglen DE, Ulbright TM. The differential diagnosis of yolk sac tumor and seminoma. Usefulness of cytokeratin, alpha-fetoprotein, and alpha-1-antitrypsin immunoperoxidase reactions. Am J Clin Pathol. 1987;88:328-332.

204. Chaudhary RK, Kher A, Bobhate SK, Grover S. Alpha-fetoprotein in germ cell tumors. An immunohistochemical study. Indian J Pathol Microbiol. 1989;32:167-173.

205. Tian Q, Frierson HF Jr, Krystal GW, Moskaluk CA. Activating c-kit gene mutations in human germ cell tumors. Am J Pathol. 1999;154:1643-1647.

206. Hawkins EP, Finegold MJ, Hawkins HK, et al. Nongerminomatous malignant germ cell tumors in children. A review of 89 cases from the Pediatric Oncology Group, 1971-1984. Cancer. 1986;58:2579-2584.

207. Grady RW. Current management of prepubertal yolk sac tumors of the testis. Urol Clin North Am. 2000;27:503-508, ix.

208. van Echten J, Timmer A, van der Veen AY, et al. Infantile and adult testicular germ cell tumors. a different pathogenesis? Cancer Genet Cytogenet. 2002;135:57-62.

209. Veltman I, Veltman J, Janssen I, et al. Identification of recurrent chromosomal aberrations in germ cell tumors of neonates and infants using genomewide array-based comparative genomic hybridization. Genes Chromosomes Cancer. 2005;43:367-376.

210. Teilum G, Albrechtsen R, Norgaard-Pedersen B. Immunofluorescent localization of alpha-fetoprotein synthesis in endodermal sinus tumor (yolk sac tumor). Acta Pathol Microbiol Scand [A]. 1974;82:586-588.

211. Norgaard-Pedersen B, Albrechtsen R, Teilum G. Serum alpha-foetoprotein as a marker for endodermal sinus tumour (yolk sac tumour) or a vitelline component of "teratocarcinoma." Acta Pathol Microbiol Scand [A]. 1975;83:573-589.

212. Fernandes ET, Etcubanas E, Rao BN, et al. Two decades of experience with testicular tumors in children at St Jude Children's Research Hospital. J Pediatr Surg. 1989;24:677-681.

213. Shebib S, Sabbah RS, Sackey K, et al. Endodermal sinus (yolk sac) tumor in infants and children. A clinical and pathologic study: an 11-year review. Am J Pediatr Hematol Oncol. 1989;11:36-39.

214. Huddart SN, Mann JR, Gornall P, et al. The UK Children's Cancer Study Group: testicular malignant germ cell tumours 1979-1988. J Pediatr Surg. 1990;25:406-410.

215. Talerman A. The incidence of yolk sac tumor (endodermal sinus tumor) elements in germ cell tumors of the testis in adults. Cancer. 1975;36:211-215.

216. Nichols CR, Saxman S, Williams SD, et al. Primary mediastinal nonseminomatous germ cell tumors. A modern single institution experience. Cancer. 1990;65:1641-1646.

217. Sesterhenn IA, Davis CJ Jr. Pathology of germ cell tumors of the testis. Cancer Control. 2004;11:374-387.

218. Kurman RJ, Norris HJ. Endodermal sinus tumor of the ovary: a clinical and pathologic analysis of 71 cases. Cancer. 1976;38:2404-2419.

219. Gershenson DM, Del Junco G, Herson J, Rutledge FN. Endodermal sinus tumor of the ovary: the M.D. Anderson experience. Obstet Gynecol. 1983;61:194-202.

220. Micha JP, Kucera PR, Berman ML, et al. Malignant ovarian germ cell tumors: a review of thirty-six cases. Am J Obstet Gynecol. 1985;152:842-846.

221. Chow SN, Yang JH, Lin YH, et al. Malignant ovarian germ cell tumors. Int J Gynaecol Obstet. 1996;53:151-158.

222. Zalel Y, Piura B, Elchalal U, et al. Diagnosis and management of malignant germ cell ovarian tumors in young females. Int J Gynaecol Obstet. 1996;55:1-10.

223. Palumbo C, van Roozendaal K, Gillis AJ, et al. Expression of the PDGF alpha-receptor 1.5 kb transcript, OCT-4, and c-KIT in human normal and malignant tissues. Implications for the early diagnosis of testicular germ cell tumours and for our understanding of regulatory mechanisms. J Pathol. 2002;196:467-477.

224. Almstrup K, Hoei-Hansen CE, Wirkner U, et al. Embryonic stem cell-like features of testicular carcinoma in situ revealed by genome-wide gene expression profiling. Cancer Res. 2004;64:4736-4743.

225. Ezeh UI, Turek PJ, Reijo RA, Clark AT. Human embryonic stem cell genes OCT4, NANOG, STELLAR, and GDF3 are expressed in both seminoma and breast carcinoma. Cancer. 2005;104:2255-2265.

226. Bahrami A, Ro JY, Ayala AG. An overview of testicular germ cell tumors. Arch Pathol Lab Med. 2007;131:1267-1280.

227. Spitz MR, Sider JG, Pollack ES, et al. Incidence and descriptive features of testicular cancer in United States whites, blacks, and Hispanics, 1973-1982. Cancer. 1986;58:1785-1790.

228. Fossa SD, Risberg T. beta-HCG producing seminoma. Prog Clin Biol Res. 1985;203:105-106.

229. Mostofi FK, Sesterhenn IA. Pathology of germ cell tumors of testes. Prog Clin Biol Res. 1985;203:1-34.

230. Fossa A, Fossa SD. Serum lactate dehydrogenase and human choriogonadotrophin in seminoma. Br J Urol. 1989;63:408-415.

231. Weissbach L, Bussar-Maatz R, Mann K. The value of tumor markers in testicular seminomas. Results of a prospective multicenter study. Eur Urol. 1997;32:16-22.

232. Hori K, Uematsu K, Yasoshima H, et al. Contribution of cell proliferative activity to malignancy potential in testicular seminoma. Pathol Int. 1997;47:282-287.

233. Fujikawa K, Matsui Y, Oka H, et al. Prognosis of primary testicular seminoma: a report on 57 new cases. Cancer Res. 2000;60:2152-2154.

234. Bruns F, Raub M, Schaefer U, Micke O. No predictive value of beta-hCG in patients with stage I seminoma—results of a long-term follow-up study after adjuvant radiotherapy. Anticancer Res. 2005;25:1543-1546.

235. Weissbach L, Bussar-Maatz R, Lohrs U, et al. Prognostic factors in seminomas with special respect to HCG: results of a prospective multicenter study. Seminoma Study Group. Eur Urol. 1999;36:601-608.

236. Johnson DE, Gomez JJ, Ayala AG. Anaplastic seminoma. J Urol. 1975;114:80-82.

237. Shulman Y, Ware S, Al-Askari S, Morales P. Anaplastic seminoma. Urology. 1983;21:379-381.

238. Ulbright TM, Roth LM. Recent developments in the pathology of germ cell tumors. Semin Diagn Pathol. 1987;4:304-319.

239. Suzuki T, Sasano H, Aoki H, et al. Immunohistochemical comparison between anaplastic seminoma and typical seminoma. Acta Pathol Jpn. 1993;43:751-757.

240. Mor Y, Leibovich I, Raviv G, et al. Testicular seminoma: clinical significance of nuclear deoxyribonucleic acid ploidy pattern as studied by flow cytometry. J Urol. 1995;154:1041-1043.

241. Warde P, Gospodarowicz MK, Banerjee D, et al. Prognostic factors for relapse in stage I testicular seminoma treated with surveillance. J Urol. 1997;157:1705-1709.

242. Zuckman MH, Williams G, Levin HS. Mitosis counting in seminoma: an exercise of questionable significance. Hum Pathol. 1988;19:329-335.

243. Abell MR, Johnson VJ, Holtz F. Ovarian neoplasms in childhood and adolescence. Am J Obstet Gynecol. 1965;92:1059-1081.

244. Kurman RJ, Norris HJ. Malignant germ cell tumors of the ovary. Hum Pathol. 1977;8:551-564.

245. Smith HO, Berwick M, Verschraegen CF, et al. Incidence and survival rates for female malignant germ cell tumors. Obstet Gynecol. 2006;107:1075-1085.

246. dos Santos Silva I, Swerdlow AJ. Ovarian germ cell malignancies in England: epidemiological parallels with testicular cancer. Br J Cancer. 1991;63:814-818.

247. Moller H, Evans H. Epidemiology of gonadal germ cell cancer in males and females. APMIS. 2003;111:43-46.

248. Schneider DT, Calaminus G, Koch S, et al. Epidemiologic analysis of 1,442 children and adolescents registered in the German germ cell tumor protocols. Pediatr Blood Cancer. 2004;42:169-175.

249. Looijenga LH, de Leeuw H, van Oorschot M, et al. Stem cell factor receptor (c-KIT) codon 816 mutations predict development of bilateral testicular germ-cell tumors. Cancer Res. 2003;63:7674-7678.

250. Cheng L, Thomas A, Roth LM, et al. OCT4: a novel biomarker for dysgerminoma of the ovary. Am J Surg Pathol. 2004;28:1341-1346.

251. Sever M, Jones TD, Roth LM, et al. Expression of CD117 (c-kit) receptor in dysgerminoma of the ovary: diagnostic and therapeutic implications. Mod Pathol. 2005;18:1411-1416.

252. Hoei-Hansen CE, Kraggerud SM, Abeler VM, et al. Ovarian dysgerminomas are characterised by frequent KIT mutations and

abundant expression of pluripotency markers. Mol Cancer. 2007; 6:12.

253. Niehans GA, Manivel JC, Copland GT, et al. Immunohisto-chemistry of germ cell and trophoblastic neoplasms. Cancer. 1988;62:1113-1123.

254. Krag Jacobsen G, Barlebo H, Olsen J, et al. Testicular germ cell tumours in Denmark 1976-1980. Pathology of 1058 consecutive cases. Acta Radiol Oncol. 1984;23:239-247.

255. Mostofi FK, Sesterhenn IA, Davis CJ Jr. Developments in histo-pathology of testicular germ cell tumors. Semin Urol. 1988;6: 171-188.

256. King ME, Hubbell MJ, Talerman A. Mixed germ cell tumor of the ovary with a prominent polyembryoma component. Int J Gynecol Pathol. 1991;10:88-95.

257. Jondle DM, Shahin MS, Sorosky J, Benda JA. Ovarian mixed germ cell tumor with predominance of polyembryoma: a case report with literature review. Int J Gynecol Pathol. 2002;21: 78-81.

258. Blohm ME, Gobel U. Unexplained anaemia and failure to thrive as initial symptoms of infantile choriocarcinoma: a review. Eur J Pediatr. 2004;163:1-6.

259. Fischer CG, Waechter W, Kraus S, et al. Urologic tumors in the Federal Republic of Germany: data on 56,013 cases from hospital cancer registries. Cancer. 1998;82:775-783.

260. Turner HB, Douglas WM, Gladding TC. Choriocarcinoma of the Ovary. Obstet Gynecol. 1964;24:918-920.

261. Shitara T, Oshima Y, Yugami S, et al. Choriocarcinoma in children. Am J Pediatr Hematol Oncol. 1993;15:268-269.

262. Sebire NJ, Lindsay I, Fisher RA, Seckl MJ. Intraplacental cho-riocarcinoma: experience from a tertiary referral center and rela-tionship with infantile choriocarcinoma. Fetal Pediatr Pathol. 2005;24:21-29.

263. Lorigan PC, Grierson AJ, Goepel JR, et al. Gestational chorio-carcinoma of the ovary diagnosed by analysis of tumour DNA. Cancer Lett. 1996;104:27-30.

264. Shigematsu T, Kamura T, Arima T, et al. DNA polymorphism analysis of a pure non-gestational choriocarcinoma of the ovary: case report. Eur J Gynaecol Oncol. 2000;21:153-154.

265. Gershenson DM, Del Junco G, Copeland LJ, Rutledge FN. Mixed germ cell tumors of the ovary. Obstet Gynecol. 1984;64:200-206.

266. De Backer A, Madern GC, Oosterhuis JW, et al. Ovarian germ cell tumors in children: a clinical study of 66 patients. Pediatr Blood Cancer. 2006;46:459-464.

267. Sesterhenn IA, Cheville J, Woodward PJ, et al. Sex card/gonadal stromal tumours. In Eble JN, Sauter G, Epstein JI, Sesterhenn IA (eds). World Health Organization Classification of Tumours: Tumours of the Urinary System and Male Genital Organs. Lyon, France, IARC Press, 2004, pp 250-258.

268. Bernstein L, Smith MA, Liu L, et al. Germ cell trophoblastic and other gonadal neoplasms ICCC X. In Ries L, Melbert D, Krapcho M, et al (eds). SEER Cancer Statistics Review, 1975-2004. Besthesda, Md, National Cancer Institute, 2007, pp 125-137.

269. Bosl GJ, Motzer RJ. Testicular germ-cell cancer. N Engl J Med. 1997;337:242-253.

270. Brown LM, Pottern LM, Hoover RN, et al. Testicular cancer in the United States: trends in incidence and mortality. Int J Epide-miol. 1986;15:164-170.

271. McGlynn KA, Devesa SS, Graubard BI, Castle PE. Increasing incidence of testicular germ cell tumors in black men in the United States. J Clin Oncol. 2005;23:5757-5761.

272. Mann JR, Stiller CA. Changing pattern of incidence and survival in children with germ cell tumors (GCTs). Adv Biosci. 1994; 91:59.

273. dos Santos Silva I, Swerdlow AJ, Stiller CA, Reid A. Incidence of testicular germ-cell malignancies in England and Wales: trends

274. McGlynn KA, Devesa SS, Sigurdson AJ, et al. Trends in the incidence of testicular germ cell tumors in the United States. Cancer. 2003;97:63-70.

275. Bray F, Richiardi L, Ekbom A, et al. Trends in testicular cancer incidence and mortality in 22 European countries: continuing increases in incidence and declines in mortality. Int J Cancer. 2006;118:3099-3111.

276. Henderson BE, Benton B, Jing J, et al. Risk factors for cancer of the testis in young men. Int J Cancer. 1979;23:598-602.

277. Strohsnitter WC, Noller KL, Hoover RN, et al. Cancer risk in men exposed in utero to diethylstilbestrol. J Natl Cancer Inst. 2001;93:545-551.

278. Walker AH, Ross RK, Haile RW, Henderson BE. Hormonal factors and risk of ovarian germ cell cancer in young women. Br J Cancer. 1988;57:418-422.

279. Brown LM, Pottern LM, Hoover RN. Prenatal and perinatal risk factors for testicular cancer. Cancer Res. 1986;46:4812-4816.

280. Depue RH, Pike MC, Henderson BE. Estrogen exposure during gestation and risk of testicular cancer. J Natl Cancer Inst. 1983;71:1151-1155.

281. Schottenfeld D, Warshauer ME, Sherlock S, et al. The epidemiol-ogy of testicular cancer in young adults. Am J Epidemiol. 1980;112:232-246.

282. Zhang Y, Graubard BI, Longnecker MP, et al. Maternal hormone levels and perinatal characteristics: implications for testicular cancer. Ann Epidemiol. 2007;17:85-92.

283. Aschim EL, Grotmol T, Tretli S, Haugen TB. Is there an associa-tion between maternal weight and the risk of testicular cancer? An epidemiologic study of Norwegian data with emphasis on World War II. Int J Cancer. 2005;116:327-330.

284. Rasmussen F, Gunnell D, Ekbom A, et al. Birth weight, adult height, and testicular cancer: cohort study of 337,249 Swedish young men. Cancer Causes Control. 2003;14:595-598.

285. Richiardi L, Askling J, Granath F, Akre O. Body size at birth and adulthood and the risk for germ-cell testicular cancer. Cancer Epidemiol Biomarkers Prev. 2003;12:669-673.

286. Shu XO, Nesbit ME, Buckley JD, et al. An exploratory analysis of risk factors for childhood malignant germ-cell tumors: report from the Childrens Cancer Group (Canada, United States). Cancer Causes Control. 1995;6:187-198.

287. Shankar S, Davies S, Giller R, et al. In utero exposure to female hormones and germ cell tumors in children. Cancer. 2006;106: 1169-1177.

288. Chen Z, Robison L, Giller R, et al. Risk of childhood germ cell tumors in association with parental smoking and drinking. Cancer. 2005;103:1064-1071.

289. Chen Z, Stewart PA, Davies S, et al. Parental occupational expo-sure to pesticides and childhood germ-cell tumors. Am J Epide-miol. 2005;162:858-867.

290. Buetow SA. Epidemiology of testicular cancer. Epidemiol Rev. 1995;17:433-449.

291. Herrinton LJ, Zhao W, Husson G. Management of cryptorchism and risk of testicular cancer. Am J Epidemiol. 2003;157:602-605.

292. Stochholm K, Juul S, Juel K, et al. Prevalence, incidence, diag-nostic delay, and mortality in Turner syndrome. J Clin Endocri-nol Metab. 2006;91:3897-3902.

293. Hasle H, Mellemgaard A, Nielsen J, Hansen J. Cancer incidence in men with Klinefelter syndrome. Br J Cancer. 1995;71: 416-420.

294. Perlman EJ, Valentine MB, Griffin CA, Look AT. Deletion of 1p36 in childhood endodermal sinus tumors by two-color fluo-rescence in situ hybridization: a pediatric oncology group study. Genes Chromosomes Cancer. 1996;16:15-20.

295. Perlman EJ, Hu J, Ho D, et al. Genetic analysis of childhood endodermal sinus tumors by comparative genomic hybridization. J Pediatr Hematol Oncol. 2000;22:100-105.

296. Schneider DT, Calaminus G, Gobel U. Diagnostic value of alpha 1-fetoprotein and beta-human chorionic gonadotropin in infancy and childhood. Pediatr Hematol Oncol. 2001;18:11-26.

297. Oosterhuis JW, Castedo SM, de Jong B, et al. Ploidy of primary germ cell tumors of the testis. Pathogenetic and clinical relevance. Lab Invest. 1989;60:14-21.

298. Oosterhuis JW, Castedo SM, de Jong B. Cytogenetics, ploidy and differentiation of human testicular, ovarian and extragonadal germ cell tumours. Cancer Surv. 1990;9:320-332.

299. van Gurp RJ, Oosterhuis JW, Kalscheuer V, et al. Biallelic expression of the H19 and IGF2 genes in human testicular germ cell tumors. J Natl Cancer Inst. 1994;86:1070-1075.

300. Looijenga LH, Verkerk AJ, De Groot N, et al. H19 in normal development and neoplasia. Mol Reprod Dev. 1997;46:419-439.

301. Looijenga LH, Verkerk AJ, Dekker MC, et al. Genomic imprinting in testicular germ cell tumours. APMIS. 1998;106:187-195.

302. Looijenga LH, Oosterhuis JW. Pathogenesis of testicular germ cell tumours. Rev Reprod. 1999;4:90-100.

303. Kraggerud SM, Lee MP, Skotheim RI, et al. Lack of parental origin specificity of altered alleles at 11p15 in testicular germ cell tumors. Cancer Genet Cytogenet. 2003;147:1-8.

304. Edwards RG. Genetics, epigenetics and gene silencing in differentiating mammalian embryos. Reprod Biomed Online. 2006;13:732-753.

305. Kerr CL, Gearhart JD, Elliott AM, Donovan PJ. Embryonic germ cells: when germ cells become stem cells. Semin Reprod Med. 2006;24:304-313.

306. Castedo SM, Oosterhuis JW, de Jong B. Cytogenetic studies of testicular germ cell tumors: pathogenetic relevance. Recent Results Cancer Res. 1991;123:101-106.

307. Rodriguez E, Mathew S, Reuter V, et al. Cytogenetic analysis of 124 prospectively ascertained male germ cell tumors. Cancer Res. 1992;52:2285-2291.

308. Korn WM, Oide Weghuis DE, Suijkerbuijk RF, et al. Detection of chromosomal DNA gains and losses in testicular germ cell tumors by comparative genomic hybridization. Genes Chromosomes Cancer. 1996;17:78-87.

309. Ottesen AM, Kirchhoff M, De-Meyts ER, et al. Detection of chromosomal aberrations in seminomatous germ cell tumours using comparative genomic hybridization. Genes Chromosomes Cancer. 1997;20:412-418.

310. Summersgill B, Goker H, Weber-Hall S, et al. Molecular cytogenetic analysis of adult testicular germ cell tumours and identification of regions of consensus copy number change. Br J Cancer. 1998;77:305-313.

311. Kraggerud SM, Skotheim RI, Szymanska J, et al. Genome profiles of familial/bilateral and sporadic testicular germ cell tumors. Genes Chromosomes Cancer. 2002;34:168-174.

312. Skotheim RI, Autio R, Lind GE, et al. Novel genomic aberrations in testicular germ cell tumors by array-CGH, and associated gene expression changes. Cell Oncol. 2006;28:315-326.

313. Atkin NB, Baker MC. Specific chromosome change, i(12p), in testicular tumours? Lancet. 1982;2:1349.

314. Atkin NB, Baker MC. i(12p): specific chromosomal marker in seminoma and malignant teratoma of the testis? Cancer Genet Cytogenet. 1983;10:199-204.

315. Bosl GJ, Dmitrovsky E, Reuter VE, et al. Isochromosome of the short arm of chromosome 12: clinically useful markers for male germ cell tumors. J Natl Cancer Inst. 1989;81:1874-1878.

316. Mukherjee AB, Murty VV, Rodriguez E, et al. Detection and analysis of origin of i(12p), a diagnostic marker of human male germ cell tumors, by fluorescence in situ hybridization. Genes Chromosomes Cancer. 1991;3:300-307.

317. Bosl GJ, Ilson DH, Rodriguez E, et al. Clinical relevance of the i(12p) marker chromosome in germ cell tumors. J Natl Cancer Inst. 1994;86:349-355.

318. Chaganti RS, Rodriguez E, Mathew S. Origin of adult male mediastinal germ-cell tumours. Lancet. 1994;343:1130-1132.

319. Rodriguez E, Melamed J, Reuter V, Chaganti RS. Chromosome 12 abnormalities in malignant ovarian germ cell tumors. Cancer Genet Cytogenet. 1995;82:62-66.

320. Chaganti RS, Houldsworth J. The cytogenetic theory of the pathogenesis of human adult male germ cell tumors. Review article. APMIS. 1998;106:80-83.

321. Reuter VE. Origins and molecular biology of testicular germ cell tumors. Mod Pathol. 2005;18(Suppl 2):S51-S60.

322. Poulos C, Cheng L, Zhang S, et al. Analysis of ovarian teratomas for isochromosome 12p: evidence supporting a dual histogenetic pathway for teratomatous elements. Mod Pathol. 2006;19:766-771.

323. Rodriguez E, Houldsworth J, Reuter VE, et al. Molecular cytogenetic analysis of i(12p)-negative human male germ cell tumors. Genes Chromosomes Cancer. 1993;8:230-236.

324. Motzer RJ, Rodriguez E, Reuter VE, et al. Molecular and cytogenetic studies in the diagnosis of patients with poorly differentiated carcinomas of unknown primary site. J Clin Oncol. 1995;13:274-282.

325. Suijkerbuijk RF, Sinke RJ, Weghuis DE, et al. Amplification of chromosome subregion 12p11.2-p12.1 in a metastasis of an i(12p)-negative seminoma: relationship to tumor progression? Cancer Genet Cytogenet. 1994;78:145-152.

326. Mostert MC, Verkerk AJ, van de Pol M, et al. Identification of the critical region of 12p over-representation in testicular germ cell tumors of adolescents and adults. Oncogene. 1998;16:2617-2627.

327. Houldsworth J, Reuter V, Bosl GJ, Chaganti RS. Aberrant expression of cyclin D2 is an early event in human male germ cell tumorigenesis. Cell Growth Differ. 1997;8:293-299.

328. Bartkova J, Rajpert-de Meyts E, Skakkebaek NE, Bartek J. D-type cyclins in adult human testis and testicular cancer: relation to cell type, proliferation, differentiation, and malignancy. J Pathol. 1999;187:573-581.

329. Looijenga LH, de Munnik H, Oosterhuis JW. A molecular model for the development of germ cell cancer. Int J Cancer. 1999;83:809-814.

330. Roelofs H, Mostert MC, Pompe K, et al. Restricted 12p amplification and RAS mutation in human germ cell tumors of the adult testis. Am J Pathol. 2000;157:1155-1166.

331. McIntyre A, Summersgill B, Spendlove HE, et al. Activating mutations and/or expression levels of tyrosine kinase receptors GRB7, RAS, and BRAF in testicular germ cell tumors. Neoplasia. 2005;7:1047-1052.

332. Goddard NC, McIntyre A, Summersgill B, et al. KIT and RAS signalling pathways in testicular germ cell tumours: new data and a review of the literature. Int J Androl. 2007;30:337-348.

333. Looijenga LH, Zafarana G, Grygalewicz B, et al. Role of gain of 12p in germ cell tumour development. APMIS. 2003;111:161-171.

334. Leahy MG, Tonks S, Moses JH, et al. Candidate regions for a testicular cancer susceptibility gene. Hum Mol Genet. 1995;4:1551-1555.

335. Rapley EA, Crockford GP, Easton DF, et al. Localisation of susceptibility genes for familial testicular germ cell tumour. APMIS. 2003;111:128-133.

336. Lutke Holzik MF, Rapley EA, Hoekstra HJ, et al. Genetic predisposition to testicular germ-cell tumours. Lancet Oncol. 2004;5:363-371.

337. Rapley E. Susceptibility alleles for testicular germ cell tumour: a review. Int J Androl. 2007;30:242-250.

338. Rapley EA, Crockford GP, Teare D, et al. Localization to Xq27 of a susceptibility gene for testicular germ-cell tumours. Nat Genet. 2000;24:197-200.

339. Crockford GP, Linger R, Hockley S, et al. Genome-wide linkage screen for testicular germ cell tumour susceptibility loci. Hum Mol Genet. 2006;15:443-451.

340. Nathanson KL, Kanetsky PA, Hawes R, et al. The Y deletion gr/gr and susceptibility to testicular germ cell tumor. Am J Hum Genet. 2005;77:1034-1043.

341. Linger R, Dudakia D, Huddart R, et al. A physical analysis of the Y chromosome shows no additional deletions, other than Gr/Gr, associated with testicular germ cell tumour. Br J Cancer. 2007;96:357-361.

342. Baker BA, Frickey L, Yu IT, et al. DNA content of ovarian immature teratomas and malignant germ cell tumors. Gynecol Oncol. 1998;71:14-18.

343. Ross JA, Schmidt PT, Perentesis JP, Davies SM. Genomic imprinting of H19 and insulin-like growth factor-2 in pediatric germ cell tumors. Cancer. 1999;85:1389-1394.

344. Schneider DT, Wessalowski R, Calaminus G, et al. Treatment of recurrent malignant sacrococcygeal germ cell tumors: analysis of 22 patients registered in the German protocols MAKEI 83/86, 89, and 96. J Clin Oncol. 2001;19:1951-1960.

345. Riopel MA, Spellerberg A, Griffin CA, Perlman EJ. Genetic analysis of ovarian germ cell tumors by comparative genomic hybridization. Cancer Res. 1998;58:3105-3110.

346. Schneider DT, Zahn S, Sievers S, et al. Molecular genetic analysis of central nervous system germ cell tumors with comparative genomic hybridization. Mod Pathol. 2006;19:864-873.

347. Zahn S, Sievers S, Alemazkour K, et al. Imbalances of chromosome arm 1p in pediatric and adult germ cell tumors are caused by true allelic loss: a combined comparative genomic hybridization and microsatellite analysis. Genes Chromosomes Cancer. 2006;45:995-1006.

348. Oosterhuis JW, Castedo SM, de Jong B, et al. Karyotyping and DNA flow cytometry of an orchidoblastoma. Cancer Genet Cytogenet. 1988;36:7-11.

349. Perlman EJ, Cushing B, Hawkins E, Griffin CA. Cytogenetic analysis of childhood endodermal sinus tumors: a Pediatric Oncology Group study. Pediatr Pathol. 1994;14:695-708.

350. Bussey KJ, Lawce HJ, Himoe E, et al. Chromosomes 1 and 12 abnormalities in pediatric germ cell tumors by interphase fluorescence in situ hybridization. Cancer Genet Cytogenet. 2001;125:112-118.

351. Veltman I, van Asseldonk M, Schepens M, et al. A novel case of infantile sacral teratoma and a constitutional t(12;15)(q13;q25) pat. Cancer Genet Cytogenet. 2002;136:17-22.

352. Palmer RD, Foster NA, Vowler SL, et al. Malignant germ cell tumours of childhood: new associations of genomic imbalance. Br J Cancer. 2007;96:667-676.

353. Hu J, Schuster AE, Fritsch MK, et al. Deletion mapping of 6q21-26 and frequency of 1p36 deletion in childhood endodermal sinus tumors by microsatellite analysis. Oncogene. 2001;20:8042-8044.

354. Praml C, Finke LH, Herfarth C, et al. Deletion mapping defines different regions in 1p34.2-pter that may harbor genetic information related to human colorectal cancer. Oncogene. 1995;11:1357-1362.

355. Schwab M, Praml C, Amler LC. Genomic instability in 1p and human malignancies. Genes Chromosomes Cancer. 1996;16:211-229.

356. Brodeur GM, Maris JM, Yamashiro DJ, et al. Biology and genetics of human neuroblastomas. J Pediatr Hematol Oncol. 1997;19:93-101.

357. Attiyeh EF, London WB, Mosse YP, et al. Chromosome 1p and 11q deletions and outcome in neuroblastoma. N Engl J Med. 2005;353:2243-2253.

358. White PS, Thompson PM, Gotoh T, et al. Definition and characterization of a region of 1p36.3 consistently deleted in neuroblastoma. Oncogene. 2005;24:2684-2694.

359. Okawa ER, Gotoh T, Manne J, et al. Expression and sequence analysis of candidates for the 1p36.31 tumor suppressor gene deleted in neuroblastomas. Oncogene. 2008;27:803-810.

360. Moller H, Skakkebaek NE. Risk of testicular cancer in subfertile men: case-control study. BMJ. 1999;318:559-562.

361. Jacobsen R, Bostofte E, Engholm G, et al. Risk of testicular cancer in men with abnormal semen characteristics: cohort study. BMJ. 2000;321:789-792.

362. Greenwood SM, Forman BH, Goodman JR, et al. Choriocarcinoma in a man. The relationship of gynecomastia to chorionic somatomammotropin and estrogens. Am J Med. 1971;51:416-422.

363. Morley JE, Jacobson RJ, Melamed J, Hershman JM. Choriocarcinoma as a cause of thyrotoxicosis. Am J Med. 1976;60:1036-1040.

364. Caron P, Salandini AM, Plantavid M, et al. Choriocarcinoma and endocrine paraneoplastic syndromes. Eur J Med. 1993;2:499-500.

365. O'Reilly S, Lyons DJ, Harrison M, et al. Thyrotoxicosis induced by choriocarcinoma: a report of two cases. Ir Med J. 1993;86:124.

366. Goodarzi MO, Van Herle AJ. Thyrotoxicosis in a male patient associated with excess human chorionic gonadotropin production by germ cell tumor. Thyroid. 2000;10:611-619.

367. Rescorla F, Billmire D, Vinocur C, et al. The effect of neoadjuvant chemotherapy and surgery in children with malignant germ cell tumors of the genital region: a pediatric intergroup trial. J Pediatr Surg. 2003;38:910-912.

368. Gershenson DM. Management of ovarian germ cell tumors. J Clin Oncol. 2007;25:2938-2943.

369. Asadourian LA, Taylor HB. Dysgerminoma. An analysis of 105 cases. Obstet Gynecol. 1969;33:370-379.

370. De Palo G, Lattuada A, Kenda R, et al. Germ cell tumors of the ovary: the experience of the National Cancer Institute of Milan. I. Dysgerminoma. Int J Radiat Oncol Biol Phys. 1987;13:853-860.

371. Mayordomo JI, Paz-Ares L, Rivera F, et al. Ovarian and extragonadal malignant germ-cell tumors in females: a single-institution experience with 43 patients. Ann Oncol. 1994;5:225-231.

372. Akyuz C, Varan A, Buyukpamukcu N, et al. Malignant ovarian tumors in children: 22 years of experience at a single institution. J Pediatr Hematol Oncol. 2000;22:422-427.

373. Krepart G, Smith JP, Rutledge F, Delclos L. The treatment for dysgerminoma of the ovary. Cancer. 1978;41:986-990.

374. Mandai M, Konishi I, Koshiyama M, et al. Ascitic positive cytology and intraperitoneal metastasis in ovarian dysgerminoma. J Obstet Gynaecol Res. 1996;22:89-94.

375. Andrews J. Streak gonads and the Y chromosome. J Obstet Gynaecol Br Commonw. 1971;78:448-457.

376. Verp MS, Simpson JL. Abnormal sexual differentiation and neoplasia. Cancer Genet Cytogenet. 1987;25:191-218.

377. Rutgers JL. Advances in the pathology of intersex conditions. Hum Pathol. 1991;22:884-891.

378. Altman RP, Randolph JG, Lilly JR. Sacrococcygeal teratoma: American Academy of Pediatrics Surgical Section Survey—1973. J Pediatr Surg. 1974;9:389-398.

379. Gobel U, Calaminus G, Engert J, et al. Teratomas in infancy and childhood. Med Pediatr Oncol. 1998;31:8-15.

380. Rescorla F, Billmire D, Stolar C, et al. The effect of cisplatin dose and surgical resection in children with malignant germ cell tumors at the sacrococcygeal region: a pediatric intergroup trial (POG 9049/CCG 8882). J Pediatr Surg. 2001;36:12-17.

381. Schneider DT, Calaminus G, Reinhard H, et al. Primary mediastinal germ cell tumors in children and adolescents: results of

the German cooperative protocols MAKEI 83/86, 89, and 96. J Clin Oncol. 2000;18:832-839.

382. Cushing B, Giller R, Cullen JW, et al. Randomized comparison of combination chemotherapy with etoposide, bleomycin, and either high-dose or standard-dose cisplatin in children and adolescents with high-risk malignant germ cell tumors: a pediatric intergroup study—Pediatric Oncology Group 9049 and Children's Cancer Group 8882. J Clin Oncol. 2004;22:2691-2700.

383. Gobel U, Schneider DT, Calaminus G, et al. Multimodal treatment of malignant sacrococcygeal germ cell tumors: a prospective analysis of 66 patients of the German cooperative protocols MAKEI 83/86 and 89. J Clin Oncol. 2001;19:1943-1950.

384. Malogolowkin MH, London WB, Cushing B, et al. Site of metastases does not influence the clinical outcome of children with metastatic germ cell tumors (GCT). A report from the Children's Oncology Group (COG). J Clin Oncol, American Society of Clinical Oncology Meeting Proceedings, Part I. 2006;24:9002.

385. Spunt SL, Walsh MF, Krasin MJ, et al. Brain metastases of malignant germ cell tumors in children and adolescents. Cancer. 2004;101:620-626.

386. Kollmannsberger C, Oechsle K, Dohmen BM, et al. Prospective comparison of [18F]-fluorodeoxyglucose positron emission tomography with conventional assessment by computed tomography scans and serum tumor markers for the evaluation of residual masses in patients with nonseminomatous germ cell carcinoma. Cancer. 2002;94:2353-2362.

387. International Germ Cell Cancer Collaborative Group. International Germ Cell Consensus Classification: a prognostic factor-based staging system for metastatic germ cell cancers. J Clin Oncol. 1997;15:594-603.

388. Frazier AL, Rumcheva P, Olson T, et al. Application of the adult international germ cell classification system to pediatric malignant nonseminomatous germ cell tumors: a report from the Children's Oncology Group. Pediatr Blood Cancer. 2008;50:746-751.

389. Mann JR, Raafat F, Robinson K, et al. The United Kingdom Children's Cancer Study Group's second germ cell tumor study: carboplatin, etoposide, and bleomycin are effective treatment for children with malignant extracranial germ cell tumors, with acceptable toxicity. J Clin Oncol. 2000;18:3809-3818.

390. Baranzelli MC, Bouffet E, Quintana E, et al. Nonseminomatous ovarian germ cell tumours in children. Eur J Cancer. 2000;36:376-383.

391. Baranzelli MC, Kramar A, Bouffet E, et al. Prognostic factors in children with localized malignant nonseminomatous germ cell tumors. J Clin Oncol. 1999;17:1212.

392. Harding MJ, Paul J, Gillis CR, Kaye SB. Management of malignant teratoma: does referral to a specialist unit matter? Lancet. 1993;341:999-1002.

393. Stiller CA. Non-specialist units, clinical trials and survival from testicular cancer. Eur J Cancer. 1995;31A:289-291.

394. Derikx JP, De Backer A, van de Schoot L, et al. Long-term functional sequelae of sacrococcygeal teratoma: a national study in The Netherlands. J Pediatr Surg. 2007;42:1122-1126.

395. Gross RW, Clatworthy HW Jr, Meeker IA Jr. Sacrococcygeal teratomas in infants and children; a report of 40 cases. Surg Gynecol Obstet. 1951;92:341-354.

396. Schlatter M, Rescorla F, Giller R, et al. Excellent outcome in patients with stage I germ cell tumors of the testes: a study of the Children's Cancer Group/Pediatric Oncology Group. J Pediatr Surg. 2003;38:319-324.

397. Donohue JP, Zachary JM, Maynard BR. Distribution of nodal metastases in nonseminomatous testis cancer. J Urol. 1982; 128:315-320.

398. Billmire D, Vinocur C, Rescorla F, et al. Outcome and staging evaluation in malignant germ cell tumors of the ovary in children and adolescents: an intergroup study. J Pediatr Surg. 2004;39: 424-429.

399. Rogers PC, Olson TA, Cullen JW, et al. Treatment of children and adolescents with stage II testicular and stages I and II ovarian malignant germ cell tumors: a Pediatric Intergroup Study—Pediatric Oncology Group 9048 and Children's Cancer Group 8891. J Clin Oncol. 2004;22:3563-3569.

400. Toner GC, Geller NL, Tan C, et al. Serum tumor marker half-life during chemotherapy allows early prediction of complete response and survival in nonseminomatous germ cell tumors. Cancer Res. 1990;50:5904-5910.

401. Murphy BA, Motzer RJ, Mazumdar M, et al. Serum tumor marker decline is an early predictor of treatment outcome in germ cell tumor patients treated with cisplatin and ifosfamide salvage chemotherapy. Cancer. 1994;73:2520-2526.

402. Mazumdar M, Bajorin DF, Bacik J, et al. Predicting outcome to chemotherapy in patients with germ cell tumors: the value of the rate of decline of human chorionic gonadotrophin and alpha-fetoprotein during therapy. J Clin Oncol. 2001;19:2534-2541.

403. Motzer RJ, Nichols CJ, Margolin KA, et al. Phase III randomized trial of conventional-dose chemotherapy with or without high-dose chemotherapy and autologous hematopoietic stem-cell rescue as first-line treatment for patients with poor-prognosis metastatic germ cell tumors. J Clin Oncol. 2007;25:247-256.

404. Marina N, London WB, Frazier AL, et al. Prognostic factors in children with extragonadal malignant germ cell tumors: a pediatric intergroup study. J Clin Oncol. 2006;24:2544-2548.

405. Calaminus G, Schneider DT, Bokkerink JP, et al. Prognostic value of tumor size, metastases, extension into bone, and increased tumor marker in children with malignant sacrococcygeal germ cell tumors: a prospective evaluation of 71 patients treated in the German cooperative protocols Maligne Keimzelltumoren (MAKEI) 83/86 and MAKEI 89. J Clin Oncol. 2003;21: 781-786.

406. Einhorn LH. Combination chemotherapy with cis-dichlorodiam mineplatinum(II) in disseminated testicular cancer. Cancer Treat Rep. 1979;63:1659-1662.

407. Fossa SD, Aass N, Kaalhus O. Long-term morbidity after infra-diaphragmatic radiotherapy in young men with testicular cancer. Cancer. 1989;64:404-408.

408. Aass N, Fossa SD, Host H. Acute and subacute side effects due to infra-diaphragmatic radiotherapy for testicular cancer: a prospective study. Int J Radiat Oncol Biol Phys. 1992;22:1057-1064.

409. Travis LB, Fossa SD, Schonfeld SJ, et al. Second cancers in 40,576 testicular cancer patients: focus on long-term survivors. J Natl Cancer Inst. 2005;97:1354-1365.

410. de Wit R, Fizazi K. Controversies in the management of clinical stage I testis cancer. J Clin Oncol. 2006;24:5482-5492.

411. Rehani MM, Berry M. Radiation doses in computed tomography. The increasing doses of radiation need to be controlled. BMJ. 2000;320:593-594.

412. International Commission on Radiological Protection (ICRP). Recommendations of the International Commission on Radiological Protection (ICRP Publication 60). Oxford, England, Pergamon Press, 1991.

413. Cardis E, Vrijheid M, Blettner M, et al. Risk of cancer after low doses of ionising radiation: retrospective cohort study in 15 countries. BMJ. 2005;331:77.

414. Rustin GJ, Mead GM, Stenning SP, et al. Randomized trial of two or five computed tomography scans in the surveillance of patients with stage I nonseminomatous germ cell tumors of the testis: Medical Research Council Trial TE08, ISRCTN56475197—the National Cancer Research Institute Testis Cancer Clinical Studies Group. J Clin Oncol. 2007;25:1310-1315.

415. Freedman LS, Parkinson MC, Jones WG, et al. Histopathology in the prediction of relapse of patients with stage I testicular teratoma treated by orchidectomy alone. Lancet. 1987;2:294-298.

416. Read G, Stenning SP, Cullen MH, et al. Medical Research Council prospective study of surveillance for stage I testicular teratoma. Medical Research Council Testicular Tumors Working Party. J Clin Oncol. 1992;10:1762-1768.

417. Fizazi K, Tjulandin S, Salvioni R, et al. Viable malignant cells after primary chemotherapy for disseminated nonseminomatous germ cell tumors: prognostic factors and role of postsurgery chemotherapy—results from an international study group. J Clin Oncol. 2001;19:2647-2657.

418. Vergouwe Y, Steyerberg EW, Eijkemans MJ, et al. Predictors of occult metastasis in clinical stage I nonseminoma: a systematic review. J Clin Oncol. 2003;21:4092-4099.

419. Heidenreich A, Sesterhenn IA, Mostofi FK, Moul JW. Prognostic risk factors that identify patients with clinical stage I nonseminomatous germ cell tumors at low-risk and high risk for metastasis. Cancer. 1998;83:1002-1011.

420. Spermon JR, Debruyne FM, Witjes JA. Important factors in the diagnosis and primary staging of testicular tumours. Curr Opin Urol. 2002;12:419-425.

421. Schmidt P, Haas RJ, Gobel U, Calaminus G. [Results of the German studies (MAHO) for treatment of testicular germ cell tumors in children—an update.] Klin Padiatr. 2002;214:167-172.

422. Williams SD, Birch R, Einhorn LH, et al. Treatment of disseminated germ-cell tumors with cisplatin, bleomycin, and either vinblastine or etoposide. N Engl J Med. 1987;316:1435-1440.

423. de Wit R, Roberts JT, Wilkinson PM, et al. Equivalence of three or four cycles of bleomycin, etoposide, and cisplatin chemotherapy and of a 3- or 5-day schedule in good-prognosis germ cell cancer: a randomized study of the European Organization for Research and Treatment of Cancer Genitourinary Tract Cancer Cooperative Group and the Medical Research Council. J Clin Oncol. 2001;19:1629-1640.

424. Chretien PB, Milam JD, Foote FW, Miller TR. Embryonal adenocarcinomas (a type of malignant teratoma) of the sacrococcygeal region. Clinical and pathologic aspects of 21 cases. Cancer. 1970;26:522-535.

425. Smith JP, Rutledge F. Advances in chemotherapy for gynecologic cancer. Cancer. 1975;36:669-674.

426. Wollner N, Exelby PR, Woodruff JM, et al. Malignant ovarian tumors in childhood: prognosis in relation to initial therapy. Cancer. 1976;37:1953-1964.

427. Ablin AR, Krailo MD, Ramsay NK, et al. Results of treatment of malignant germ cell tumors in 93 children: a report from the Children's Cancer Study Group. J Clin Oncol. 1991;9:1782-1792.

428. Marina N, Chang KW, Malogolowkin M, et al. Amifostine does not protect against the ototoxicity of high-dose cisplatin combined with etoposide and bleomycin in pediatric germ-cell tumors: a Children's Oncology Group study. Cancer. 2005;104:841-847.

429. Mann JR, Raafat F, Robinson K, et al. UKCCSG's germ cell tumour (GCT) studies: improving outcome for children with malignant extracranial non-gonadal tumours—carboplatin, etoposide, and bleomycin are effective and less toxic than previous regimens. United Kingdom Children's Cancer Study Group. Med Pediatr Oncol. 1998;30:217-227.

430. Baranzelli MC, Flamant F, De Lumley L, et al. Treatment of non-metastatic, nonseminomatous malignant germ-cell tumours in childhood: experience of the "Societe Francaise d'Oncologie Pediatrique" MGCT 1985-1989 study. Med Pediatr Oncol. 1993;21:395-401.

431. Baranzelli MC, Patte C. The French experience in paediatric malignant germ cell tumours. In: Jones WG, Appleyard I, Harnden P, eds. Germ Cell Tumours IV. London, John Libbey, 1998, pp 219-226.

432. Horwich A, Sleijfer DT, Fossa SD, et al. Randomized trial of bleomycin, etoposide, and cisplatin compared with bleomycin, etoposide, and carboplatin in good-prognosis metastatic nonseminomatous germ cell cancer: a Multi-institutional Medical Research Council/European Organization for Research and Treatment of Cancer Trial. J Clin Oncol. 1997;15:1844-1852.

433. Bokemeyer C, Kohrmann O, Tischler J, et al. A randomized trial of cisplatin, etoposide and bleomycin (PEB) versus carboplatin, etoposide and bleomycin (CEB) for patients with "good-risk" metastatic nonseminomatous germ cell tumors. Ann Oncol. 1996;7:1015-1021.

434. Kondagunta GV, Bacik J, Bajorin D, et al. Etoposide and cisplatin chemotherapy for metastatic good-risk germ cell tumors. J Clin Oncol. 2005;23:9290-9294.

435. Culine S, Kerbrat P, Kramar A, et al. Refining the optimal chemotherapy regimen for good-risk metastatic nonseminomatous germ-cell tumors: a randomized trial of the Genito-Urinary Group of the French Federation of Cancer Centers (GETUG T93BP). Ann Oncol. 2007;18:917-924.

436. Lopes LF, Sonaglio V, Ribeiro KC, et al. Improvement in the outcome of children with germ cell tumors. Pediatr Blood Cancer. 2008;50:250-253.

437. Lo Curto M, Lumia F, Alaggio R, et al. Malignant germ cell tumors in childhood: results of the first Italian cooperative study "TCG 91." Med Pediatr Oncol. 2003;41:417-425.

438. Gobel U, Calaminus G, Schneider DT, et al. The malignant potential of teratomas in infancy and childhood: the MAKEI experiences in non-testicular teratoma and implications for a new protocol. Klin Padiatr. 2006;218:309-314.

439. Rescorla FJ, Sawin RS, Coran AG, et al. Long-term outcome for infants and children with sacrococcygeal teratoma: a report from the Childrens Cancer Group. J Pediatr Surg. 1998;33:171-176.

440. Tonkin KS, Rustin GJ, Wignall B, et al. Successful treatment of patients in whom germ cell tumour masses enlarged on chemotherapy while their serum tumour markers decreased. Eur J Cancer Clin Oncol. 1989;25:1739-1743.

441. Zagame L, Pautier P, Duvillard P, et al. Growing teratoma syndrome after ovarian germ cell tumors. Obstet Gynecol. 2006;108:509-514.

442. Carver BS, Shayegan B, Eggener S, et al. Incidence of metastatic nonseminomatous germ cell tumor outside the boundaries of a modified postchemotherapy retroperitoneal lymph node dissection. J Clin Oncol. 2007;25:4365-4369.

443. Carver BS, Shayegan B, Serio A, et al. Long-term clinical outcome after postchemotherapy retroperitoneal lymph node dissection in men with residual teratoma. J Clin Oncol. 2007;25:1033-1037.

444. Garnick MB. Redefining the refined retroperitoneal lymph node dissection in testis cancer: a SWOT analysis of nonrandomized data. J Clin Oncol. 2007;25:4337-4338.

445. Gershenson DM, Copeland LJ, del Junco G, et al. Second-look laparotomy in the management of malignant germ cell tumors of the ovary. Obstet Gynecol. 1986;67:789-793.

446. Toner GC and Bosl GJ. Sarcoidosis, "Sarcoid-like lymphadenopathy," and testicular germ cell tumors. Am J Med. 1990;89:651-656.

447. Gobel U, Calaminus G, Schneider DT, et al. Management of germ cell tumors in children: approaches to cure. Onkologie. 2002;25:14-22.

448. Murphy BR, Breeden ES, Donohue JP, et al. Surgical salvage of chemorefractory germ cell tumors. J Clin Oncol. 1993;11:324-329.

449. Hartmann JT, Einhorn L, Nichols CR, et al. Second-line chemotherapy in patients with relapsed extragonadal nonseminomatous germ cell tumors: results of an international multicenter analysis. J Clin Oncol. 2001;19:1641-1648.

450. Kondagunta GV, Bacik J, Donadio A, et al. Combination of paclitaxel, ifosfamide, and cisplatin is an effective second-line therapy for patients with relapsed testicular germ cell tumors. J Clin Oncol. 2005;23:6549-6555.

451. Kollmannsberger C, Rick O, Derigs HG, et al. Activity of oxaliplatin in patients with relapsed or cisplatin-refractory germ cell cancer: a study of the German Testicular Cancer Study Group. J Clin Oncol. 2002;20:2031-2037.

452. Bokemeyer C, Gerl A, Schoffski P, et al. Gemcitabine in patients with relapsed or cisplatin-refractory testicular cancer. J Clin Oncol. 1999;17:512-516.

453. Einhorn LH, Stender MJ, Williams SD. Phase II trial of gemcitabine in refractory germ cell tumors. J Clin Oncol. 1999;17:509-511.

454. Kondagunta GV, Bacik J, Sheinfeld J, et al. Paclitaxel plus ifosfamide followed by high-dose carboplatin plus etoposide in previously treated germ cell tumors. J Clin Oncol. 2007;25:85-90.

455. Einhorn LH, Williams SD, Chamness A, et al. High-dose chemotherapy and stem-cell rescue for metastatic germ-cell tumors. N Engl J Med. 2007;357:340-348.

456. Mayer F, Honecker F, Looijenga LH, Bokemeyer C. Towards an understanding of the biological basis of response to cisplatin-based chemotherapy in germ-cell tumors. Ann Oncol. 2003;14:825-832.

457. Mayer F, Stoop H, Scheffer GL, et al. Molecular determinants of treatment response in human germ cell tumors. Clin Cancer Res. 2003;9:767-773.

458. Ishida S, Lee J, Thiele DJ, Herskowitz I. Uptake of the anticancer drug cisplatin mediated by the copper transporter Ctr1 in yeast and mammals. Proc Natl Acad Sci U S A. 2002;99:14298-4302.

459. Kuo MT, Chen HH, Song IS, et al. The roles of copper transporters in cisplatin resistance. Cancer Metastasis Rev. 2007;26:71-83.

460. Yoshizawa K, Nozaki S, Kitahara H, et al. Copper efflux transporter (ATP7B) contributes to the acquisition of cisplatin-resistance in human oral squamous cell lines. Oncol Rep. 2007;18:987-991.

461. Izquierdo MA, Scheffer GL, Flens MJ, et al. Broad distribution of the multidrug resistance-related vault lung resistance protein in normal human tissues and tumors. Am J Pathol. 1996;148:877-887.

462. Kool M, de Haas M, Scheffer GL, et al. Analysis of expression of cMOAT (MRP2), MRP3, MRP4, and MRP5, homologues of the multidrug resistance-associated protein gene (MRP1), in human cancer cell lines. Cancer Res. 1997;57:3537-3547.

463. Klys HS, Whillis D, Howard G, Harrison DJ. Glutathione S-transferase expression in the human testis and testicular germ cell neoplasia. Br J Cancer. 1992;66:589-593.

464. Strohmeyer T, Klone A, Wagner G, et al. Glutathione S-transferases in human testicular germ cell tumors: changes of expression and activity. J Urol. 1992;147:1424-1428.

465. Jansen BA, Brouwer J, Reedijk J. Glutathione induces cellular resistance against cationic dinuclear platinum anticancer drugs. J Inorg Biochem. 2002;89:197-202.

466. Reed E. Platinum-DNA adduct, nucleotide excision repair and platinum based anti-cancer chemotherapy. Cancer Treat Rev. 1998;24:331-344.

467. Koberle B, Masters JR, Hartley JA, Wood RD. Defective repair of cisplatin-induced DNA damage caused by reduced XPA protein in testicular germ cell tumours. Curr Biol. 1999;9:273-276.

468. Welsh C, Day R, McGurk C, et al. Reduced levels of XPA, ERCC1 and XPF DNA repair proteins in testis tumor cell lines. Int J Cancer. 2004;110:352-361.

469. Koberle B, Roginskaya V, Wood RD. XPA protein as a limiting factor for nucleotide excision repair and UV sensitivity in human cells. DNA Repair (Amst). 2006;5:641-648.

470. Honecker F, Mayer F, Stoop H, et al. Xeroderma pigmentosum group a protein and chemotherapy resistance in human germ cell tumors. Lab Invest. 2003;83:1489-1495.

471. Koberle B, Roginskaya V, Zima KS, et al. Elevation of XPA protein level in testis tumor cells without increasing resistance to cisplatin or UV radiation. Mol Carcinog. 2008;7:580-586.

472. Devouassoux-Shisheboran M, Mauduit C, Bouvier R, et al. Expression of hMLH1 and hMSH2 and assessment of microsatellite instability in testicular and mediastinal germ cell tumours. Mol Hum Reprod. 2001;7:1099-1105.

473. Mayer F, Gillis AJ, Dinjens W, et al. Microsatellite instability of germ cell tumors is associated with resistance to systemic treatment. Cancer Res. 2002;62:2758-2760.

474. Velasco A, Riquelme E, Schultz M, et al. Mismatch repair gene expression and genetic instability in testicular germ cell tumor. Cancer Biol Ther. 2004;3:977-982.

475. Li GM. The role of mismatch repair in DNA damage-induced apoptosis. Oncol Res. 1999;11:393-400.

476. Seifert M, Reichrath J. The role of the human DNA mismatch repair gene hMSH2 in DNA repair, cell cycle control and apoptosis: implications for pathogenesis, progression and therapy of cancer. J Mol Histol. 2006;37:301-307.

477. Velasco A, Corvalan A, Wistuba, II, et al. Mismatch repair expression in testicular cancer predicts recurrence and survival. Int J Cancer. 2008;122:1774-1777.

478. Charames GS, Bapat B. Genomic instability and cancer. Curr Mol Med. 2003;3:589-596.

479. Li GM. DNA mismatch repair and cancer. Front Biosci. 2003;8:d997-1017.

480. Bertholon J, Wang Q, Galmarini CM, Puisieux A. Mutational targets in colorectal cancer cells with microsatellite instability. Fam Cancer. 2006;5:29-34.

481. Thompson HJ, Strange R, Schedin PJ. Apoptosis in the genesis and prevention of cancer. Cancer Epidemiol Biomarkers Prev. 1992;1:597-602.

482. Martin SJ, Green DR. Apoptosis and cancer: the failure of controls on cell death and cell survival. Crit Rev Oncol Hematol. 1995;18:137-153.

483. Lowe SW, Lin AW. Apoptosis in cancer. Carcinogenesis. 2000;21:485-495.

484. Ehlert JE, Kubbutat MH. Apoptosis and its relevance in cancer therapy. Onkologie. 2001;24:433-440.

485. Yu J, Zhang L. Apoptosis in human cancer cells. Curr Opin Oncol. 2004;16:19-24.

486. Kim R, Emi M, Tanabe K. The role of apoptosis in cancer cell survival and therapeutic outcome. Cancer Biol Ther. 2006;5:1429-1442.

487. Hussain SP, Harris CC. p53 biological network: at the crossroads of the cellular-stress response pathway and molecular carcinogenesis. J Nippon Med Sch. 2006;73:54-64.

488. Vousden KH, Lane DP. p53 in health and disease. Nat Rev Mol Cell Biol. 2007;8:275-283.

489. Kersemaekers AM, Mayer F, Molier M, et al. Role of P53 and MDM2 in treatment response of human germ cell tumors. J Clin Oncol. 2002;20:1551-1561.

490. Chresta CM, Masters JR, Hickman JA. Hypersensitivity of human testicular tumors to etoposide-induced apoptosis is associated with functional p53 and a high Bax:Bcl-2 ratio. Cancer Res. 1996;56:1834-1841.

491. Lutzker SG, Mathew R, Taller DR. A p53 dose-response relationship for sensitivity to DNA damage in isogenic teratocarcinoma cells. Oncogene. 2001;20:2982-2986.

492. Burger H, Nooter K, Boersma AW, et al. Distinct p53-independent apoptotic cell death signalling pathways in testicular germ cell tumour cell lines. Int J Cancer. 1999;81:620-628.

493. Momand J, Jung D, Wilczynski S, Niland J. The MDM2 gene amplification database. Nucleic Acids Res. 1998;26:3453-3459.

494. Momand J, Wu HH, Dasgupta G. MDM2—master regulator of the p53 tumor suppressor protein. Gene. 2000;242:15-29.

495. Christoph F, Kempkensteffen C, Weikert S, et al. Frequent epigenetic inactivation of p53 target genes in seminomatous and

nonseminomatous germ cell tumors. Cancer Lett. 2007;247:137-142.

496. Voorhoeve PM, le Sage C, Schrier M, et al. A genetic screen implicates miRNA-372 and miRNA-373 as oncogenes in testicular germ cell tumors. Cell. 2006;124:1169-1181.

497. Wilson C, Yang J, Strefford JC, et al. Overexpression of genes on 16q associated with cisplatin resistance of testicular germ cell tumor cell lines. Genes Chromosomes Cancer. 2005;43:211-216.

498. Noel EE, Perry J, Chaplin T, et al. Identification of genomic changes associated with cisplatin resistance in testicular germ cell tumor cell lines. Genes Chromosomes Cancer. 2008;47:604-613.

499. Coffey J, Linger R, Pugh J, et al. Somatic KIT mutations occur predominantly in seminoma germ cell tumors and are not predictive of bilateral disease: report of 220 tumors and review of literature. Genes Chromosomes Cancer. 2008;47:34-42.

500. Pedersini R, Vattemi E, Mazzoleni G, Graiff C. Complete response after treatment with imatinib in pretreated disseminated testicular seminoma with overexpression of c-KIT. Lancet Oncol. 2007;8:1039-1040.

501. Kemmer K, Corless CL, Fletcher JA, et al. KIT mutations are common in testicular seminomas. Am J Pathol. 2004;164:305-313.

502. Einhorn LH, Brames MJ, Heinrich MC, et al. Phase II study of imatinib mesylate in chemotherapy refractory germ cell tumors expressing KIT. Am J Clin Oncol. 2006;29:12-13.

503. Longley BJ, Reguera MJ, Ma Y. Classes of c-KIT activating mutations: proposed mechanisms of action and implications for disease classification and therapy. Leuk Res. 2001;25:571-576.

504. Moroni M, Veronese S, Schiavo R, et al. Epidermal growth factor receptor expression and activation in nonseminomatous germ cell tumors. Clin Cancer Res. 2001;7:2770-2775.

505. Kollmannsberger C, Mayer F, Pressler H, et al. Absence of c-KIT and members of the epidermal growth factor receptor family in refractory germ cell cancer. Cancer. 2002;95:301-308.

506. Madani A, Kemmer K, Sweeney C, et al. Expression of KIT and epidermal growth factor receptor in chemotherapy refractory nonseminomatous germ-cell tumors. Ann Oncol. 2003;14:873-880.

507. Kollmannsberger C, Pressler H, Mayer F, et al. Cisplatin-refractory, HER2/neu-expressing germ-cell cancer: induction of remission by the monoclonal antibody Trastuzumab. Ann Oncol. 1999;10:1393-1394.

508. Soule S, Baldridge L, Kirkpatrick K, et al. HER-2/neu expression in germ cell tumours. J Clin Pathol. 2002;55:656-658.

509. Moasser MM, Motzer RJ, Khoo KS, et al. all-trans retinoic acid for treating germ cell tumors. In vitro activity and results of a phase II trial. Cancer. 1995;76:680-686.

510. Fukuda S, Shirahama T, Imazono Y, et al. Expression of vascular endothelial growth factor in patients with testicular germ cell tumors as an indicator of metastatic disease. Cancer. 1999;85:1323-1330.

511. Devouassoux-Shisheboran M, Mauduit C, Tabone E, et al. Growth regulatory factors and signalling proteins in testicular germ cell tumours. APMIS. 2003;111:212-224.

512. Fritsch MK, Schneider DT, Schuster AE, et al. Activation of Wnt/beta-catenin signaling in distinct histologic subtypes of human germ cell tumors. Pediatr Dev Pathol. 2006;9:115-131.

513. Calin GA, Dumitru CD, Shimizu M, et al. Frequent deletions and down-regulation of micro-RNA genes miR15 and miR16 at 13q14 in chronic lymphocytic leukemia. Proc Natl Acad Sci U S A. 2002;99:15524-15529.

514. Thomson JM, Newman M, Parker JS, et al. Extensive post-transcriptional regulation of microRNAs and its implications for cancer. Genes Dev. 2006;20:2202-2207.

515. Viswanathan SR, Daley GQ, Gregory RI. Selective blockade of microRNA processing by Lin28. Science. 2008;320:97-100.

516. Hale GA, Marina NM, Jones-Wallace D, et al. Late effects of treatment for germ cell tumors during childhood and adolescence. J Pediatr Hematol Oncol. 1999;21:115-122.

517. van den Belt-Dusebout AW, de Wit R, Gietema JA, et al. Treatment-specific risks of second malignancies and cardiovascular disease in 5-year survivors of testicular cancer. J Clin Oncol. 2007;25:4370-4378.

518. Gietema JA, Sleijfer DT, Willemse PH, et al. Long-term follow-up of cardiovascular risk factors in patients given chemotherapy for disseminated nonseminomatous testicular cancer. Ann Intern Med. 1992;116:709-715.

519. Bissett D, Kunkeler L, Zwanenburg L, et al. Long-term sequelae of treatment for testicular germ cell tumours. Br J Cancer. 1990;62:655-659.

520. Bokemeyer C, Berger CC, Kuczyk MA, Schmoll HJ. Evaluation of long-term toxicity after chemotherapy for testicular cancer. J Clin Oncol. 1996;14:2923-2932.

521. Berger CC, Bokemeyer C, Schuppert F, Schmoll HJ. Endocrinological late effects after chemotherapy for testicular cancer. Br J Cancer. 1996;73:1108-1114.

522. Teutsch C, Lipton A, Harvey HA. Raynaud's phenomenon as a side effect of chemotherapy with vinblastine and bleomycin for testicular carcinoma. Cancer Treat Rep. 1977;61:925-926.

523. Vogelzang NJ, Torkelson JL, Kennedy BJ. Hypomagnesemia, renal dysfunction, and Raynaud's phenomenon in patients treated with cisplatin, vinblastine, and bleomycin. Cancer. 1985;56:2765-2770.

524. Meinardi MT, Gietema JA, van der Graaf WT, et al. Cardiovascular morbidity in long-term survivors of metastatic testicular cancer. J Clin Oncol. 2000;18:1725-1732.

525. Nuver J, Smit AJ, van der Meer J, et al. Acute chemotherapy-induced cardiovascular changes in patients with testicular cancer. J Clin Oncol. 2005;23:9130-9137.

526. van Leeuwen FE, Stiggelbout AM, van den Belt-Dusebout AW, et al. Second cancer risk following testicular cancer: a follow-up study of 1,909 patients. J Clin Oncol. 1993;11:415-424.

527. Bokemeyer C, Schmoll HJ. Secondary neoplasms following treatment of malignant germ cell tumors. J Clin Oncol. 1993;11:1703-1709.

528. Travis LB, Curtis RE, Storm H, et al. Risk of second malignant neoplasms in long-term survivors of testicular cancer. J Natl Cancer Inst. 1997;89:1429-1439.

529. Bokemeyer C, Schmoll HJ, Kuczyk MA, et al. Risk of secondary leukemia following high cumulative doses of etoposide during chemotherapy for testicular cancer. J Natl Cancer Inst. 1995;87:58-60.

530. Nichols CR, Breeden ES, Loehrer PJ, et al. Secondary leukemia associated with a conventional dose of etoposide: review of serial germ cell tumor protocols. J Natl Cancer Inst. 1993;85:36-40.

531. Smith MA, Rubinstein L, Anderson JR, et al. Secondary leukemia or myelodysplastic syndrome after treatment with epipodophyllotoxins. J Clin Oncol. 1999;17:569-577.

532. Schneider DT, Hilgenfeld E, Schwabe D, et al. Acute myelogenous leukemia after treatment for malignant germ cell tumors in children. J Clin Oncol. 1999;17:3226-3233.

533. Osanto S, Bukman A, Van Hoek F, et al. Long-term effects of chemotherapy in patients with testicular cancer. J Clin Oncol. 1992;10:574-579.

534. Goldiner PL, Carlon GC, Cvitkovic E, et al. Factors influencing postoperative morbidity and mortality in patients treated with bleomycin. BMJ. 1978;1:1664-1667.

535. Jules-Elysee K, White DA. Bleomycin-induced pulmonary toxicity. Clin Chest Med. 1990;11:1-20.

536. Donat SM, Levy DA. Bleomycin associated pulmonary toxicity: is perioperative oxygen restriction necessary? J Urol. 1998;160:1347-1352.

537. Hansen SW, Groth S, Daugaard G, et al. Long-term effects on renal function and blood pressure of treatment with cisplatin,

vinblastine, and bleomycin in patients with germ cell cancer. J Clin Oncol. 1988;6:1728-1731.

538. Boyer M, Raghavan D, Harris PJ, et al. Lack of late toxicity in patients treated with cisplatin-containing combination chemotherapy for metastatic testicular cancer. J Clin Oncol. 1990;8: 21-26.

539. Petersen PM, Hansen SW. The course of long-term toxicity in patients treated with cisplatin-based chemotherapy for nonseminomatous germ-cell cancer. Ann Oncol. 1999;10:1475-1483.

540. Bosl GJ, Leitner SP, Atlas SA, et al. Increased plasma renin and aldosterone in patients treated with cisplatin-based chemotherapy for metastatic germ-cell tumors. J Clin Oncol. 1986;4:1684-1689.

541. Nijman JM, Schraffordt Koops H, Kremer J, et al. Fertility and hormonal function in patients with a nonseminomatous tumor of the testis. Arch Androl. 1985;14:239-246.

542. Fossa SD, Abyholm T, Aakvaag A. Spermatogenesis and hormonal status after orchiectomy for cancer and before supplementary treatment. Eur Urol. 1984;10:173-177.

543. Petersen PM, Skakkebaek NE, Rorth M, Giwercman A. Semen quality and reproductive hormones before and after orchiectomy in men with testicular cancer. J Urol. 1999;161:822-826.

544. Stephenson WT, Poirier SM, Rubin L, Einhorn LH. Evaluation of reproductive capacity in germ cell tumor patients following treatment with cisplatin, etoposide, and bleomycin. J Clin Oncol. 1995;13:2278-2280.

545. Lampe H, Horwich A, Norman A, et al. Fertility after chemotherapy for testicular germ cell cancers. J Clin Oncol. 1997;15: 239-245.

546. Fossa SD, Theodorsen L, Norman N, Aabyholm T. Recovery of impaired pretreatment spermatogenesis in testicular cancer. Fertil Steril. 1990;54:493-496.

547. Huyghe E, Matsuda T, Daudin M, et al. Fertility after testicular cancer treatments: results of a large multicenter study. Cancer. 2004;100:732-737.

548. Strumberg D, Brugge S, Korn MW, et al. Evaluation of long-term toxicity in patients after cisplatin-based chemotherapy for nonseminomatous testicular cancer. Ann Oncol. 2002;13: 229-236.

549. Hansen SW, Berthelsen JG, von der Maase H. Long-term fertility and Leydig cell function in patients treated for germ cell cancer with cisplatin, vinblastine, and bleomycin versus surveillance. J Clin Oncol. 1990;8:1695-1698.

550. Goldberg RB, Rabin D, Alexander AN, et al. Suppression of plasma testosterone leads to an increase in serum total and high density lipoprotein cholesterol and apoproteins A-I and B. J Clin Endocrinol Metab. 1985;60:203-207.

551. Holmes SJ, Whitehouse RW, Clark ST, et al. Reduced bone mineral density in men following chemotherapy for Hodgkin's disease. Br J Cancer. 1994;70:371-375.

24 Histiocytoses

Barbara A. Degar, Mark D. Fleming, and Barrett J. Rollins

Histiocytoses are a collection of rare hematologic diseases that resist easy classification. This is so at least in part because of the imprecise definition of the word *histiocyte*, which broadly refers both to cells of the macrophage lineage and to dendritic cells, only some types of which are macrophage-derived. The numerous descriptive and functional subsets of macrophages and dendritic cells only add to the confusion. Nonetheless, a degree of uniformity among these childhood diseases justifies their collective consideration: they present with infiltration of bone, secondary lymphoid organs, or liver, with or without concomitant involvement of visceral organs. At the same time, prognosis and treatment options are subtype-specific, so an appreciation of the individual varieties of histiocytoses is mandatory.

This chapter is divided into two main sections corresponding to the two most common clinical histiocytic disorders, Langerhans cell histiocytosis (LCH) and hemophagocytic lymphohistiocytosis (HLH). Also included is a relatively brief discussion of non-Langerhans cell histiocytoses and Rosai-Dorfman disease. Each section begins with a description of the normal counterparts of the relevant histiocytes and their ontogeny so as to provide a context for the description of how these cells are pathologically involved in the histiocytic disorders. Each section also includes a description of the clinical manifestations and current approaches to treatment.

LANGERHANS CELL HISTIOCYTOSIS

Dendritic Cells

Types of Dendritic Cells

The pathologic cells of LCH are derived from normal epidermal Langerhans cells (LCs), which are the primary antigen-presenting cells (APCs) of skin.[1] LCs are one type of the general class of APCs known as dendritic cells (DCs) because of the characteristic dendritelike morphology they assume when activated. DCs are, in turn, just one of several types of "professional" APCs, so called because they can, by themselves, fully activate naïve T lymphocytes by providing both the antigen/major histocompatibility complex ligand for T-cell receptor binding and the accessory signals required for full activation.[2,3]

Because DCs can render T cells tolerant to specific antigens as well as activate them,[4] DCs have become a major focus of basic immunologic research. This has revealed a surprising level of functional and phenotypic diversity among DCs, which will undoubtedly be relevant to the proliferative disorders affecting these cells. Several authors, including Shortman and Steinman, have provided helpful guides to thinking about and classifying DCs.[2,3] Overall, one can divide DCs into two types, conventional and inflammatory (Box 24-1). Conventional DCs are present in lymphoid and nonlymphoid organs in the basal state, and their primary function is to collect antigens for presentation to T cells to activate or tolerize them, depending on the antigen's source (i.e., nonself versus self). Inflammatory DCs arise in response to specific inflammatory or infectious signals and are ordinarily not present in the basal state. In addition to presenting antigen, these cells secrete cytokines and other mediators, including tumor necrosis factor, that enhance host defense.

Within the conventional DC category, one can distinguish between migratory DCs and lymphoid-tissue–resident DCs. Migratory DCs fulfill the sentinel role of this leukocyte class and include LCs, dermal DCs, and interstitial DCs of other organs. They shuttle between end-organs that interface with the external world (e.g., skin), in the case of LCs, and regional

---

Box 24-1	**Dendritic Cells**

CONVENTIONAL DENDRITIC CELLS

Migratory Dendritic Cells

Gather antigen in peripheral tissues, then migrate to regional lymph nodes to present antigen to T lymphocytes
Examples: Langerhans cells, dermal dendritic cells, interstitial dendritic cells

Lymphoid Tissue Dendritic Cells

Gather antigen within lymphoid tissue and present antigen to T lymphocytes within the same lymphoid tissue
Examples: thymic dendritic cells, splenic dendritic cells

INFLAMMATORY DENDRITIC CELLS

Arise in response to inflammatory signals; can gather antigen and present antigen to T lymphocytes; can secrete cytokines
Example: tumor necrosis factor- and iNOS-producing dendritic cells (TipDCs)

MUCOSAL DENDRITIC CELLS

Resident in mucosal surface tissues; can gather antigen and present antigen to T lymphocytes and help direct responses toward activation or tolerance

PREDENDRITIC CELLS

Cells that can develop dendritic cell function directly in response to inflammatory stimuli
Examples: plasmacytoid dendritic cells, monocytes

---

iNOS, inducible nitrous oxide synthase.
Adapted from Shortman K, Naik SH. Steady-state and inflammatory dendritic-cell development. Nat Rev Immunol. 2007;7:19-30.

---

lymph nodes. This trafficking occurs at a low level in the basal state but can be greatly enhanced in the presence of foreign antigen or inflammatory signals.[5-8] The migratory DC takes up antigen in the periphery and, once activated, travels to regional nodes either to present antigen itself or to transfer antigen to resident DCs in the node, which then perform the presentation function to T cells. Although the molecular signals that control this migratory behavior are not understood in detail, chemokines and their receptors play an important role.[9,10] In the case of LCs, resting cells express the chemokine receptor CCR6 whose ligand, CCL20, is secreted by cutaneous keratinocytes. Upon antigen uptake and activation, LCs downregulate CCR6 and in its place upregulate another chemokine receptor, CCR7, whose ligands, CCL19 and CCL21, are secreted by cells in regional lymph nodes. This receptor switch has the dual effect of removing the LCs' anchors to the skin and attracting them to regional lymph nodes.

In contrast, lymphoid-tissue–resident DCs are nonmigratory. They make up most of the DCs populating the thymus and spleen and about half of the DCs in lymph nodes.[6,11] Unlike migratory DCs, which are mature when they appear in lymph nodes, resident DCs are immature, which allows them to take up, process, and present local antigens. Surface markers can distinguish several subsets of resident DCs, which are presumed to have specialized functions. In the mouse, these include CD8+ and CD8– cells, and among the CD8– population are CD4+ and CD4– subpopulations.[12]

LCs bear distinctive intra- and extracellular markers that permit their distinction from lymphoid-tissue–resident DCs after the LCs migrate to lymph nodes. Most characteristic are Birbeck granules, which are pentilaminar tennis-racket–shaped cytoplasmic organelles that appear to be uniquely present in LCs.[13] Langerin, also known as CD207, is a characteristic cell surface marker for LCs that associates with Birbeck granules when internalized.[14] Langerin is a C-type lectin with specificity for mannose-containing sugars, suggesting that it may be involved in the processing and trafficking of antigens bearing these sugars. Dectin-2 is another C-type lectin restricted to DCs,[15] and DEC-205 (CD205) is yet another lectin that is often used to identify LCs, although its expression is not as restricted to LCs as is that of the other lectins.[16] In the appropriate histologic context, from a diagnostic standpoint, CD1a and langerin are the most reliable lineage-specific markers.[17]

Some authors also distinguish a group of so-called predendritic cells that do not ordinarily have DC functions or morphology.[18,19] However, these cells can develop directly into DCs upon stimulation, without the need for proliferation. One well-studied example is the plasmacytoid DC, which circulates as a nondescript mononuclear cell but acquires APC function and secretes large amounts of α-interferon when activated.[20] Technically, using this definition, monocytes would also be predendritic cells. After exposure to interleukin-4 and granulocyte-macrophage colony-stimulating factor, monocytes become functional DCs, although their phenotype is closer to that of inflammatory DCs than conventional DCs.[21]

Origins of Dendritic Cells

The availability of genetically modified mice that carry lineage-restricted markers has greatly expanded our understanding of the origins and development of DCs. The major insight these animals provide is that a salient characteristic of DC ontogeny is flexibility. For example, although DCs generally have myeloid characteristics, all DC subtypes in the mouse can arise from either committed lymphoid or committed myeloid precursors.[22-24] And even though half of thymic DCs show evidence of immunoglobulin rearrangements, suggesting a lymphoid phenotype, they also transcribe the granulocyte-macrophage colony-stimulating factor receptor gene, a myeloid characteristic.[25] Activation of *Flt3*, a growth factor receptor, is required for DC development and it has been suggested that committed myeloid or lymphoid precursors expressing *Flt3* can differentiate into DCs in the presence of the *Flt3* ligand.[26]

Splenic DCs have a relatively rapid turnover rate (every 3 days).[27] These cells are repopulated both by DC division and splenic precursors as well as by bone marrow precursors. In contrast, LCs are very long-lived.[27] After their migration from the skin, the population is replenished from a pool of LC precursors in the skin as well as by circulating monocytes.[28] The latter process is dependent on the action of the chemokine CCL2 acting on its receptor CCR2.[29,30] Thus the ontogeny of LCs is distinct from that of splenic DCs. Inflammatory DCs (iDCs) are more closely related to LCs but appear to be derived from noninflammatory monocytes (CCR2–).[31] Plasmacytoid DCs (pDCs) split off from conventional DCs early in development, consistent with their distinct functional characteristics.[32]

Langerhans Cell Histiocytosis

The hallmark of LCH is the proliferation and accumulation of bone-marrow–derived DCs in one or more tissues or organs. The clinical manifestations of LCH are highly diverse. They result both from the direct, local effects of the growth and accumulation of pathologic LCs and from the indirect, secondary effects these activated cells may have on other normal tissues, particularly cells of the immune system. The most commonly involved sites of disease are the bone and skin, but virtually any organ or system may be involved, and the pattern of involvement is not necessarily related to patterns of normal LC or DC migration.

The fact that pathologic LCs are related to immunomodulatory cells and that they elicit inflammatory infiltrates suggests that LCH is a reactive rather than a neoplastic disease. Indeed, there is ample precedent for this mechanism among the histiocytoses, including the secondary HLH syndromes that arise in response to viral infection.[33] However, there have been no reproducible reports of viral genomes recovered from LCH cells, and epidemiologic studies are not consistent with an infectious or environmental cause of LCH.[34-36] Rather, the preponderance of evidence indicates that LCH arises as a consequence of intrinsic genetic abnormalities. The most salient argument that LCH is a tumor and not a reactive phenomenon is that pathologic LCs are clonal, as demonstrated by nonrandom X chromosome inactivation both in whole LCH tissue (in a proportion corresponding to the proportion of CD1a+ cells in the lesion)[35] and in sorted CD1a+ cells.[37] To date, however, there is only a single report of cytogenetic abnormalities in LCH.[38] Although pathologic LCs are clonal, some have cited the high rate of spontaneous remission in LCH as evidence against their neoplastic nature. Nonetheless, other aspects of the disease suggest that it has some neoplastic characteristics. For example, LCH tends to be extremely responsive to chemotherapy and radiation therapy. This may be explained, in part, by the fact that pathologic LCs overexpress p53.[39]

Incidence and Etiology

The incidence of LCH is difficult to determine precisely because of the rarity and marked clinical variability of the disorder. Estimates are in the range of 2.6 to 8.9 cases per million per year for children younger than 15 years of age.[40-43] This corresponds to roughly one tenth the incidence of acute leukemia in childhood. LCH occurs in people of all races and all ages. The peak age of diagnosis is 2 years, but the disorder can present at any time from birth to old age. There is no evidence of seasonal variation in the time of presentation of LCH. Several studies have shown a slight male predominance.[44,45]

There is no identified cause of LCH and no known predisposing factors for the development of the disease in the vast majority of cases.[46] Studies have demonstrated concordance of the disorder in monozygotic twins, suggesting an inherited predisposition to LCH that might account for approximately 1% of cases.[47] However, a positive family histories is lacking in most cases. It has been proposed that certain viral infections may be associated with the development of LCH, although there has been no convincing, reproducible evidence to support this suggestion.[48] It is interesting that isolated pulmonary LCH in adults is closely linked to cigarette smoking, and it often resolves with smoking cessation.[49] However, exposure to cigarette smoke has not been linked to pediatric LCH.

There is an intriguing, although incompletely understood, association between malignancy and LCH. Children with a history of cancer appear to be at increased risk for the development of LCH. Conversely, children with a history of LCH appear to be at increased risk for the development of cancer. This suggests the possibility that underlying genetic abnormalities may place individual patients at increased risk for LCH.[50] Alternatively, the association between LCH and cancer may be more appropriately viewed as falling within the spectrum of secondary, post-therapy effects because irradiation and drugs such as etoposide, which is used to treat LCH, induce tumor-promoting genotoxic injury.

There is a unique association of LCH with hematologic malignancies. Multiple cases of LCH arising in the setting of T-cell acute lymphoblastic leukemia have been described, most typically when the leukemia is in remission while the patient is on therapy or in the early post-therapy period.[51] A clonal link between the initial leukemia and pathologic LCs of LCH has been established in several cases, suggesting that the LCH represents a manifestation of the malignant clone rather than a distinct reactive or neoplastic process related to the leukemia or to its therapy.[52,53]

Clinical Features

The clinical manifestations of LCH are protean. Although distinct patterns of clinical presentation have been described, the disease is appropriately viewed as a spectrum. LCH may involve a single site, multiple sites in a single organ system, or multiple organ systems. Limited disease commonly manifests as bone pain, soft tissue swelling, or skin rash. More extensive disease may present with symptoms of diabetes insipidus (DI), respiratory insufficiency, or signs of systemic illness consisting of fever, jaundice, lymphadenopathy, and organomegaly.

In the past, three distinct clinical syndromes were recognized based on the pattern of disease involvement: eosinophilic granuloma, Hand-Schuller-Christian disease, and Letterer-Siwe disease.[54] Eosinophilic granuloma, a term still commonly used by radiologists and orthopedists, refers to the presence of one or more lytic bone lesions. Hand-Schuller-Christian disease was composed of the triad of bone defects, exophthalmos, and polyuria. Letterer-Siwe disease was described as a fulminant disorder of the reticuloendothelial system, characterized by hepatosplenomegaly, lymphadenopathy, skin rash, bone lesions, anemia, and bleeding tendency. This classification has important historical significance, but it is of limited applicability in clinical decision making. Once it was recognized that the diverse clinical manifestations of the disease share common histopathologic features, the three syndromes were unified under the term histiocytosis X,[55] and late LCH. This led to the introduction of clinical staging of the disorder.[56] Stratification of patients based on the presence of single versus multiple sites of disease and the presence or absence of involvement of high-risk organs has proved to be useful in predicting prognosis and planning therapy.[57-60] Single-system disease (usually affecting bone, less frequently skin, and rarely lymph node) accounts for approximately two thirds of pediatric LCH cases. Multisystem disease, which tends to afflict younger children, accounts for the remainder. Roughly one half of children with multisystem disease manifest high-risk features, described later.[43,61]

Biopsy of lesional tissue is required to establish the diagnosis of LCH. The pathologic diagnosis is usually fairly straightforward, but because the disease is rare, varied, and may mimic many other conditions, a delay in diagnosis occurs commonly. The astute clinician should consider LCH in any patient who presents with skeletal lesions, persistent rash, chronically draining ears, DI, unexplained lymphadenopathy, respiratory insufficiency with a reticulonodular pattern on chest radiograph, hepatosplenomegaly, or cytopenias.

Once clinical suspicion has been raised, a directed workup should proceed to biopsy of the most accessible site of disease. Complete surgical excision of the lesion is generally unnecessary for the diagnosis or the treatment of LCH. Lesions at all sites share a common histopathology: a proliferation of large neoplastic LCs with a moderate amount of dense pink cytoplasm and plump, distinctive C-shaped, coffee-bean, or cleaved nuclei admixed with variable numbers of inflammatory cells, including T lymphocytes, macrophages, plasma cells, and eosinophils. The composition and architecture of the infiltrate characteristically differs according to the location. Osteolytic bone lesions commonly contain many non-neoplastic osteoclasts as well as multinucleated tumor giant cells and large numbers of eosinophils, the latter speaking to the origin of the term *eosinophilic granuloma*. Mature, burned-out bone lesions may be difficult to distinguish from chronic osteomyelitis, which is often included in the clinical and radiographic differential diagnosis. LCH infiltration of the skin typically involves the superficial dermis, with tumor cells infiltrating the epidermis—so-called epidermotropism or exocytosis—which alters epidermal barrier function, leading to superinfection and the characteristic appearance of some LCH rashes. In all cases, the neoplastic LCs express the LC markers CD1a[17] and langerin[62,63] as well as S100 protein[64] and fascin[65] (Fig. 24-1). Electron microscopy, historically used to demonstrate the presence of Birbeck granules indicative of an LC lineage, has little diagnostic utility at the present time. Similarly, there is no role for cytogenetics or other molecular studies other than to exclude other diseases with similar clinical presentations or histologies. Furthermore, there are no immunohistochemical or other laboratory methods that are useful in distinguishing clinically indolent from clinically aggressive forms of the disease.

Bone

Bone is the most commonly involved site in patients with LCH; bone involvement is present in approximately 75% of children with the disease.[45] Any bone may be affected, but the most commonly involved are the femur and the bones of the skull, and pelvis[44] (Fig. 24-2). Bone pain (often worse at night), swelling, and limp are typical presenting symptoms. Not uncommonly, a history of local trauma precedes or coincides with the onset of symptoms. The typical plain radiographic appearance is of a smooth-edged, punched-out hole in the bone. Lesions in the long bones most commonly involve the diaphysis, but metaphyseal and epiphyseal lesions occur. Involvement of a vertebral body may manifest as flattening or loss of height (vertebra plana) or as wedge deformity. Axial imaging (computed tomography or magnetic resonance imaging) may show an attendant soft tissue mass. The radiographic differential diagnosis of osseous LCH lesions includes malignancy, especially Ewing's sarcoma, and osteomyelitis (Fig. 24-3).

LCH of the bone may involve one site (mono-ostotic) or multiple sites (polyostotic), and it may present in association with disease in other organ systems. Among patients with bone involvement, mono-ostotic disease is the most common presentation, especially in older children, occurring in approximately 70% of cases.[61,66] Imaging of all bones with both skeletal survey and bone scan is recommended to obtain a comprehensive assessment of skeletal involvement.[67,68] These complementary imaging modalities detect lesions at various stages of evolution. Compared with plain radiographs, bone scintigraphy may detect smaller, evolving sites of disease based on the presence of abnormal local metabolic activity. It should be kept in mind that healed lesions take many months to resolve on imaging. Active lesions usually show increased radiotracer uptake, whereas older lesions may appear photopenic on bone scintigraphy. Experience with [18]fludeoxyglucose-positron emission tomography (PET) scanning is now accumulating for LCH. PET scan appears to be a very sensitive imaging modality for lesion detection in LCH and may be particularly useful in follow-up of patients.[69,70]

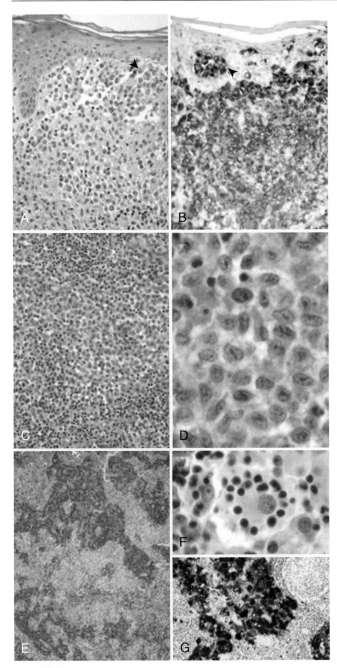

FIGURE 24-1. Histopathology of Langerhans cell histiocytosis (LCH) and sinus histiocytosis with massive lymphadenopathy (SHML). **A,** Hematoxylin-eosin (H&E), and **B,** CD1a immunostain of LCH involving the skin. Lesional cells infiltrate the upper dermis and focally *(arrowheads)* involve the epidermis. **C** and **D,** Low (200×) and high (1000×) magnification. Power views of an H&E-stained section of an LCH bone lesion. The low-power view (C) demonstrates tumor cells present in association with a mixed inflammatory infiltrate rich in eosinophils. The high-power view (D) illustrates the histologic features of the lesional Langerhans cells, including the characteristic C-shaped nuclei and abundant pink cytoplasm. **E** and **F,** Low-power (40×) magnification and high-power (1000×) magnification views of an H&E-stained section of SHML involving a lymph node. The pale areas in E are dilatated sinuses replaced by lesional histiocytes. A histiocyte (F) contains numerous lymphocytes typical of the emperipolesis characteristic of SHML. **G,** Lesional histiocytes are highlighted by an S100 immunostain.

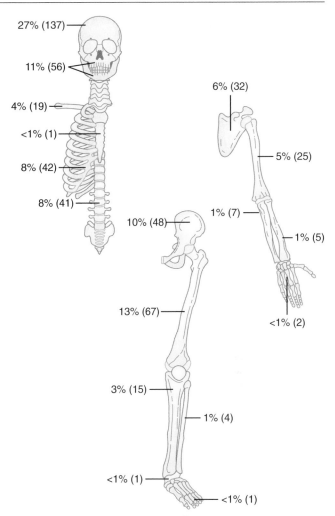

FIGURE 24-2. Anatomic distribution of 503 osseous lesions among 263 patients with LCH of bone. *(Redrawn from Kilpatrick SE, Wenger DE, Gilchrist GS, et al. Langerhans cell histiocytosis (histiocytosis X) of bone: a clinicopathologic analysis of 263 pediatric and adult cases. Cancer. 1995;76:2471-2484.)*

Skin

The skin is the second most commonly involved site of disease in LCH, occurring in about one third of patients.[42,43,57] Skin rash may be extremely variable, and misdiagnosis is common. Cutaneous LCH may present as single or multiple nodules, vesicles, or scaly, seborrhea-like patches or plaques. Although the rash may be located anywhere on the body, it is typically most intense in the flexural areas, such as the neck, axillary areas, and inguinal folds. Involvement of the scalp, the ear canals, and the posterior auricular areas is also characteristic. Ear canal involvement may lead to chronic ear drainage that may be malodorous. Diaper rash may be severe, persistent, and refractory to topical preparations. Cutaneous involvement may represent the only site of disease, but more commonly it occurs in association with other sites of disease.

Compared with older children and adults, infants appear to be at higher risk for manifesting cutaneous involvement. Some infants with isolated cutaneous LCH prove to have a benign, self-healing disorder known as Hashimoto-Pritzker disease.[71] However, a significant proportion of infants who initially present with apparently isolated cutaneous LCH go on to

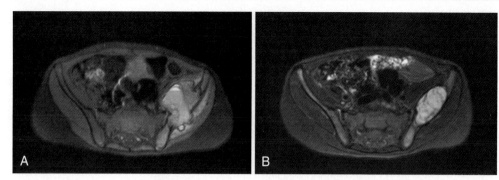

FIGURE 24-3. Magnetic resonance imaging scan of the pelvis of a 2-year-old male with unifocal LCH of the left ilium. **A,** An expansile, destructive iliac lesion and large soft tissue mass. **B,** The lesion and mass decreased dramatically in size within 3 months after intralesional glucocorticoid injection.

develop multisystem disease. Therefore, self-healing cutaneous LCH is a diagnosis that can be made accurately only in retrospect.[72,73] The differential diagnosis of cutaneous LCH may include superficial candidiasis, seborrheic dermatitis (cradle cap), contact dermatitis, and viral exanthems. Skin biopsy is required to confirm the diagnosis.

Central Nervous System

There are several different patterns of central nervous system (CNS) involvement in patients with LCH, including extra-axial extension of bone-based lesions, infiltration of the pituitary infundibulum resulting in pituitary dysfunction, and intraparenchymal soft tissue masses. Additionally, there is a rare and poorly defined neurodegenerative syndrome that may develop years after treatment for LCH.

Central DI is the most common and best-characterized CNS manifestation of LCH. It is thought to result from infiltration of the pituitary stalk by lesional cells, leading to deficiency in antidiuretic hormone secretion.[74] Although DI is the most common endocrinopathy in children with LCH and is usually the first to become clinically apparent, anterior pituitary dysfunction, especially growth hormone deficiency, or panhypopituitarism, may develop.[75] The diagnosis of DI may precede, coincide with, or occur years after the diagnosis of LCH. Estimates of the frequency of occurrence of DI in LCH vary considerably owing to variability in study populations. One large retrospective review reported a 12% incidence of DI, with 6% having DI present at the time of LCH diagnosis. In this analysis, the risk for DI correlated significantly with the location and extent of LCH involvement. Children with craniofacial lesions or multisystem disease are at significantly higher risk for the development of DI.[76]

DI may be a forme fruste of LCH or it may represent the initial clinical manifestation of evolving disease. Among children with new presentations of DI, LCH is the cause in a significant proportion—approximately 15% of cases.[77] In these patients, the absence of posterior pituitary hyperintensity (the pituitary "bright spot") or thickening of the pituitary infundibulum may be noted on brain imaging; however, these radiographic findings are neither sensitive nor specific. In the setting of DI, the differential diagnosis includes brain tumors, especially germinoma, and hypophysitis. Thorough investigation of other sites of LCH is worthwhile because it may spare the patient a pituitary biopsy.[78]

Screening for DI in children with LCH, including a careful history, is essential, and referral to an endocrinologist should be considered if symptoms of polyuria, polydipsia, nocturia, or dehydration are elicited. Urinary specific gravity greater than

1.015 weighs against a diagnosis of DI and can be determined easily by analysis of first morning–voided urine. Performing formal water-deprivation tests in asymptomatic children is generally not recommended because DI is usually clinically apparent. Furthermore, there is no firm evidence that rapid diagnosis and initiation of LCH-directed treatment, even in patients with incipient DI, influence the development of this complication. Although there are anecdotal reports of reversal of DI,[79,80] under most circumstances, it is a lifelong, irreversible condition once established.

Separate from, or in addition to, hypothalamic-pituitary involvement, tumorlike mass lesions and neurodegenerative lesions occur in patients with LCH. Parenchymal mass lesions composed of granulomatous accumulation of CD1a+ cells admixed with other inflammatory cells represent active LCH and can occur in isolation or in association with concomitant disease activity in other sites. Depending on the extent and location of the lesions, headaches, seizures, and focal neurologic symptoms may result. These lesions may be effectively managed surgically or by chemotherapy[81] or radiotherapy. Even more problematic is the late development of progressive neurodegeneration in some patients years after a diagnosis of LCH. In these cases, signal abnormality confined to the brainstem and cerebellum may be detected on magnetic resonance imaging. Posterior fossa symptoms or neurocognitive dysfunction may be clinically apparent. Biopsies show gliosis, neuronal cell loss, and lymphocytic infiltration without active CD1a+ cell infiltration.[74,82] The course of this manifestation of LCH is variable but it may be severe and progressive.

Risk Sites

Although the behavior of LCH is unpredictable, it has long been appreciated that children with disease involving the bone marrow, liver, or lungs have the potential to experience a serious, life-threatening course of illness.[58,59] Conventionally, organ involvement has been defined by the presence of organ dysfunction rather than on histopathologic grounds.[58] In children, single-system disease isolated to one risk organ is extremely uncommon. Typically, risk organ involvement is a component of disseminated disease involving multiple systems and is associated with overt constitutional symptoms, including persistent fever or failure to thrive. Involvement of one or more risk organs occurs in approximately one half of children with multisystem LCH. Risk organ involvement is usually present at diagnosis, but it can develop later. Risk organ involvement is clearly associated with young age; more than half of children diagnosed with LCH under the age of 2 years manifest risk organ involvement. The association between young age and aggressive disease accounts for the perception that young age is an adverse prognostic feature.[41] However, it has not been conclusively demonstrated that young age is an independent adverse prognostic factor.

Peripheral blood cytopenias are well-recognized manifestations of systemic LCH; they are associated with aggressive clinical behavior and adverse outcomes. The presence of peripheral blood cytopenias in patients with pathologically confirmed LCH is referred to as hematologic dysfunction, which is taken to be synonymous with bone marrow involvement. However, evidence of bone marrow infiltration by clusters of morphologically apparent LCs is not typically seen in these patients. Most often, the marrow contains a lymphohistiocytic infiltrate with hemophagocytosis that can be highly reminiscent of hemophagocytic syndromes (see later), perhaps further illustrating that the neoplastic LCs retain some of the immunomodulatory function of their normal counterparts.[83-85] Splenomegaly is commonly seen in association with hematologic dysfunction in children with disseminated LCH. The spleen may be enlarged because of disease infiltration, extramedullary hematopoiesis, or hemophagocytosis. Hypersplenism as a consequence of splenomegaly may contribute to cytopenias in these patients.

Hepatic dysfunction, like hematologic dysfunction, is associated with serious illness and a high risk for morbidity and mortality. *Hepatic dysfunction* is an inclusive term that comprises any of the following findings: hepatomegaly, ascites, hyperbilirubinemia, increased serum concentrations of hepatic transaminases (especially gamma glutamyl transferase), and impaired hepatic synthetic function (hypoalbuminemia, hypoproteinemia). As with bone marrow involvement, liver involvement is heterogeneous. In some cases, hepatomegaly and transaminitis are the consequence of macrophage activation in a sinusoidal pattern in the liver, which is associated with multisystem disease. In other cases, a cholestatic laboratory picture predominates, presumably resulting from the infiltration of hepatic bile ducts by CD1a+ LCs, although these cells may not be demonstrable on percutaneous liver biopsy.[86] In these patients, progressive hepatic dysfunction may lead over time to irreversible hepatic cirrhosis, requiring liver transplantation, even after resolution of active LCH.[87]

Pulmonary involvement occurs in a minority of children with LCH and almost always in the setting of multisystem disease. Involvement of the lung may be asymptomatic in up to one half of affected children, with radiographic evidence of diffuse micronodular interstitial disease or cyst formation on chest imaging. However, overt respiratory symptoms, including tachypnea, chronic cough, dyspnea, and pneumothorax, are seen in some patients. Some studies have suggested that pulmonary involvement is an adverse prognostic feature, warranting its classification as a risk organ in the Histiocyte Society stratification (see later material). However, pulmonary involvement in childhood LCH is usually seen in the context of multisystem disease along with hematologic or hepatic involvement. Recent retrospective studies have shown that in the absence of other risk organ involvement, pulmonary involvement does not appear to be an independent negative prognostic indicator in childhood LCH.[88-90]

In contrast, adults with LCH often present with disease limited to the lung. Pulmonary LCH in adults is closely linked to cigarette smoking. Cessation of smoking leads to resolution in the majority of patients.[49]

Other Sites

Lymphadenopathy occurs occasionally in children with LCH, usually in the setting of multisystem disease but sometimes in a single site of disease. The pathologic pattern of lymph node involvement is characteristically interfollicular and may be subtle.

The gastrointestinal tract is another uncommon site of disease in LCH, but its incidence may be underappreciated. When it does occur, it is usually in the context of multisystem involvement.[91] Clinical signs may include diarrhea, bloody stools, failure to thrive, and hypoalbuminemia.[91-93] Gastrointestinal biopsies typically demonstrate a sparse infiltrate of LCs in the lamina propria.

Therapeutic Considerations

A rational approach to therapy for LCH must account for the variability in its clinical behavior, which ranges from a benign, self-resolving process to a relentlessly aggressive and potentially fatal illness. This begs the question of whether LCH is fundamentally a reactive or a neoplastic disease,[94] as discussed earlier. On one hand, LCH is an uncontrolled proliferation of a clonal population of cells that have the capacity to behave extremely aggressively and the potential to involve multiple sites and organ systems. Additionally, it may be effectively treated with cytotoxic chemotherapy and radiotherapy. On the other hand, LCH is histologically benign, sometimes resolves spontaneously, and may respond to immunomodulatory or immunosuppressive agents. The broad range of therapies that have been used in LCH reflects the uncertainty about the fundamental nature of the disorder.

The fact that LCH may spontaneously remit without intervention is both fascinating and frustrating. In the absence of large, rigorously controlled trials, it is practically impossible to demonstrate that any intervention is effective in this disease. But controlled clinical trials are difficult to perform in LCH because of the rarity and the variability of the disorder. As a consequence, the LCH literature is often descriptive, anecdotal, and retrospective. Since the 1980s, several collaborative groups have carried out prospective clinical trials that have resulted in standardization and improvement in treatment.

Accumulated experience shows that the treatment of LCH must be matched with the clinical scenario. The risks of the therapy should not outweigh the risks of the disease. Patients with localized disease have an excellent prognosis with little or no intervention. In these children, the goal of therapy is to minimize symptoms and avoid long-term disability and potential late effects of therapy. On the other hand, children with multisystem disease are at risk for significant morbidity and mortality. In these children, systemic therapy, sometimes even to the point of hematopoietic cell transplantation (HCT), is justified.

Therapy of Single-System Disease

Children with LCH limited to a single bone have an excellent prognosis, regardless of the treatment administered. Various local and systemic therapies appear to be efficacious,[95] but retrospective trials have failed to demonstrate a comparative advantage for any specific intervention or modality, including: observation only, biopsy, curettage, simple excision, intralesional steroid instillation, local radiotherapy, and systemic therapy.[96,97]

The biopsy procedure performed to establish the diagnosis of LCH often appears to provide therapeutic benefit. In many cases, adequate tissue for diagnosis may be obtained via percutaneous needle biopsy under the guidance of ultrasound or computed tomography. Neurosurgeons tend to prefer open biopsy of orbital and skull base lesions and simple excision or curettage of calvarial lesions. Regardless of the surgical approach, most patients experience progressive healing after the procedure, even when complete excision of the lesion has not been attempted or achieved. In cases in which LCH is strongly suspected or has been confirmed intraoperatively on frozen section, methylprednisolone can be instilled directly into the site.[98,99] This intervention yields rapid relief of pain and it may hasten resolution of the lesion.[100] Intralesional steroid injection is not usually used in the management of cranial lesions.

In the past, radiotherapy was routinely used in the management of bone lesions. A relatively low dose, in the range of 600 to 1000 cGy, was commonly administered[44,101] because evidence of a dose-response relationship was lacking. However, the role of radiotherapy has waned in the past decade. Children with localized disease do well irrespective of therapy, so the long-term risks involved with radiotherapy, especially secondary malignant neoplasms, are rarely justified. In the setting of disseminated disease, local radiotherapy contributes little.[102]

Systemic chemotherapy may be offered to patients with mono-ostotic LCH who suffer from unrelenting pain or are at significant risk for pathologic fractures or permanent disability related to the location or size of their lesions. Some clinicians apply this principle to patients with lesions involving the craniofacial bones (CNS-risk lesions in the LCH-III trial) because these children appear to be at increased risk for the development of DI and other neurologic sequelae.[76] However, it has not been established that systemic therapy decreases the risk for neurologic complications in these patients.

Likewise, systemic therapy should be considered for all children with polyostotic LCH, especially when numerous bone lesions are present. In addition to controlling pain and reducing the risk for orthopedic complications, systemic therapy may mitigate the risk for future reactivation of disease in these patients.[57,61] Although the likelihood of survival of children with multifocal bone involvement is excellent, they are at significantly higher risk for disease reactivation than those with unifocal disease (4-year event-free survival rates are approximately 60% compared with 90%, respectively).[103] Reactivation can occur in the original site of bone disease or, more commonly, in distant bones or occasionally in another system (e.g., DI). Children with LCH of bone who require systemic therapy are treated using the same approach used for those with multisystem disease without risk organ involvement (see later material).

Within a 3-month interval of intervention, radiographic evidence of bone healing should be apparent. It is valuable to document evidence of improvement objectively. However, complete radiographic resolution may take many more months. In cases of vertebral collapse, reconstitution of vertebral height sometimes occurs in time.[104] In the absence of new symptoms, routine surveillance imaging is not usually recommended, at least in part because the risk for diagnostic radiation begins to mount. Close clinical follow-up, including careful history, physical examination, and prompt evaluation of signs or symptoms of disease for a minimum of 2 years from diagnosis is warranted.

When treatment for LCH involving the skin is required, topical medications often suffice. Topical corticosteroids in one form or another are the mainstay of therapy. In cases of severe cutaneous involvement, a solution of nitrogen mustard may be effective.[105] Occasionally, systemic therapy is required to control extensive or severe skin involvement, especially when it is associated with pain, disfigurement, or superinfection. Systemic chemotherapy approaches are described later. Alternatives such as psoralens and ultraviolet A light[106,107] or interferon[108] have been used with success in some patients who have had resistant cutaneous involvement.

Therapy of Multisystem Disease

In contrast to single-system LCH, multisystem LCH is a clear indication for systemic therapy. However, the optimal therapy for this diverse group of patients has not been established. Over the years, a wide variety of immunosuppressive and cytotoxic drugs have demonstrated activity. The first encouraging results were published in the early 1960s; they used corticosteroids[109] and vinblastine.[110] Then the list of potentially active agents expanded to include alkylating agents[111,112] and antimetabolites.[113] Among heterogeneous groups of patients with multisystem illness, response rates to a variety of single agents and combination regimens were in the range of 30% to 60%. No clearly superior treatment regimen emerged from the early studies, and small patient numbers and variations in evaluation criteria hampered comparison among them. In the 1980s, the epipodophyllotoxin etoposide was shown to have particular cytotoxicity for cells of the monocyte-macrophage lineage. This agent showed promising results in children with refractory LCH and was subsequently studied in newly diagnosed patients.[114-118] More recently, the nucleoside analogue 2-chlorodeoxyadenosine (2-CdA) has shown promise in the treatment of children with refractory LCH[119-122] and in adults.[123] A general principle that has emerged over many decades of clinical experience is that survival of low-risk patients is excellent, whereas a subset of high-risk patients experience refractory, relentlessly progressive, and ultimately fatal disease.[58,111,124,125]

To accrue sufficient numbers of patients with multisystem LCH for clinical trials, collaboration among pediatric oncology programs is a necessity. The Deutsche Arbeitsgemeinschaft fur Leukamieforschung und Behandlung im Kindersalter (German Working Group for Research and Treatment of Leukemia in Childhood) performed two consecutive multicenter studies (known as DAL-HX 83 and DAL-HX 90) in which children with multifocal bone or multisystem LCH were treated with a nonrandomized, risk-adapted, prospective, multidrug regimen. After initial therapy with prednisolone, vinblastine, and etoposide, children with multisystem disease went on to receive 1 year of continuation therapy with prednisolone, vinblastine, etoposide, and mercaptopurine. On DAL-HX 83, those with organ dysfunction also received methotrexate. In these trials, approximately 67% of the patients who had organ dysfunction responded to therapy; 42% of them experienced subsequent disease reactivation. In contrast, the multisystem patients without organ dysfunction and multifocal bone patients had a roughly 90% response rate and a 20% reactivation rate.[57,126] Although direct comparison with the less-intensive LCH I study (described later) is difficult, these response rates were relatively high, and reactivation rates were relatively low. Unfortunately, death resulting from refractory or progressive LCH occurred in about 20% of patients in the DAL-HX studies as well as in LCH I. Mortality was essentially restricted to children with disseminated disease, organ dysfunction, and unfavorable responses to initial therapy.

In 1991, The Histiocyte Society initiated LCH I, the first international, randomized clinical trial in LCH. This study compared the efficacy of 6 months of vinblastine (arm A) to etoposide (arm B) in children with multisystem disease.[114] The results showed that the two treatment arms were equivalent in all respects, including: response at week 6 (57% and 49%); toxicity (47% and 58%); probability of survival (76% and 83%); probability of disease reactivation (61% and 55%); and probability of developing permanent sequelae (39% and 51%), including DI (22% and 23%), in arms A and B, respectively. Of the 29 children in the study who died from disease, all had risk organ involvement. The probability of survival of children older than 2 years of age without risk organ involvement was

100%. One patient in the etoposide arm developed secondary acute myeloid leukemia. In light of the fact that etoposide was not shown to be superior to vinblastine, the study suggested that the added risk of etoposide may not be justified.

It is important to note that analysis of LCH I revealed that early response to therapy is an extremely powerful prognostic indicator in multisystem LCH. Children older than 2 years with multisystem involvement who failed to respond to 6 weeks of initial therapy had a dismal prognosis of 17%, compared with an 88% chance for survival in those who responded favorably to initial therapy (Fig. 24-4). The prognostic value of early response was confirmed in a retrospective analysis of the DAL-HX 83 and 90 studies.[127]

The Histiocyte Society's successor study, LCH II, intensified treatment for all patients and further explored the role of etoposide in high-risk LCH. All children received 6 weeks of initial therapy, which was composed of continuous oral prednisone and weekly vinblastine. Low-risk children (risk-organ-negative) went on to continuation therapy with pulse prednisone every 3 weeks and vinblastine for a total of 6 months. High-risk children (risk-organ–positive) received mercaptopurine in addition and were randomly assigned to receive (arm B) or not receive (arm A) etoposide during both the initial and the continuation phases. LCH II did not demonstrate a statistically significant benefit of the addition of etoposide in multisystem LCH; response at week 6 (63% vs. 71%); survival (74% vs. 79%); disease reactivation (46% in both arms); and permanent consequences (43% vs. 37%) were all similar in arms A and B, respectively. However, in comparison to the less intensive therapy studied in LCH I, the more intensive LCH II regimen did show a somewhat higher rapid response rate and a lower mortality rate in children with risk organ involvement.[128]

LCH III opened to enrollment in 2001. For the highest risk group of subjects in this study—children with multisystem disease and involvement of risk organs—methotrexate was added to the backbone of prednisone, vinblastine, and mercaptopurine in a randomized fashion. The total duration of therapy was lengthened to 12 months for all high-risk patients. Children without risk organ involvement were randomized to receive vinblastine and prednisone for 6 versus 12 months. The results of this trial have not been published at the time of this writing. Preliminarily, there appears to be no obvious benefit to the addition of methotrexate. Prolongation of therapy from 6 to 12 months does appear to be associated with a lower reactivation rate.

Reactivation of Langerhans Cell Histiocytosis

Children with LCH remain at risk for disease reactivation after initial improvement or resolution of the disease. Patients with multisystem disease are at higher risk for reactivation than are those with single-system disease. Most reactivations occur within 1 year of diagnosis, and almost all develop within 2 years.[61,129] Some children experience a single reactivation, but occasional patients experience a chronic relapsing and remitting course. Aggressive radiographic surveillance for reactivation is discouraged because the site of reactivation is unpredictable and the risks of imaging may exceed the risks of reactivation. However, monitoring by means of physical examination and observation of growth and development is advised, along with prompt evaluation of any new signs or symptoms. Elevation of the erythrocyte sedimentation rate and the platelet count can be a tip-off to disease reactivation.[130]

Bone is the most common site of disease reactivation in children with LCH. Fortunately, reactivation in risk organs is distinctly uncommon in children who did not have risk organ involvement at presentation.[131] Localized reactivations, such as a single bony site or recurrent rash, may be effectively managed by local therapy alone (surgery, radiotherapy, intralesional or topical corticosteroid). However, systemic therapy is often necessary in reactivated disease to control symptoms, prevent permanent sequelae, and decrease the severity and frequency of subsequent reactivations. In contrast to recurrent cancer, wherein acquired drug resistance limits the efficacy of cytotoxic drugs after previous exposure, in reactivated LCH, medications used successfully in the setting of newly diagnosed disease often remain effective in the treatment of reactivated disease. When standard systemic therapies such as corticosteroids, vinca alkaloids, and antimetabolites fail to provide durable disease control or when side effects are limiting, more intensive or less conventional options are worth exploring. In these relatively rare cases, therapy must be individualized, keeping in mind the specific sites, symptoms, and risks for reactivation as well as the specific side effects of the therapy.

Alternatives to conventional therapy that have been used in LCH reactivation, especially of bone, include nonsteroidal anti-inflammatory agents (e.g., indomethacin[107]) and bisphosphonates (e.g., pamidronate[132,133]). These agents may act to ameliorate pain and may not directly inhibit disease activity. Thalidomide has shown some efficacy in patients with low-risk LCH that is refractory to conventional therapy. The presumed mechanism of action is inhibition of tumor necrosis factor and other cytokines.[134] It should be kept in mind that many children who demonstrate a chronic relapsing course of illness develop permanent disabilities related to the LCH. Notwithstanding, their overall prognoses are good and the likelihood of their survival approaches 100%.[135]

Refractory Langerhans Cell Histiocytosis

Children who have multisystem LCH that does not respond promptly to vinblastine and prednisone have unfavorable prognoses; survival rates are in the range of 10% to 34%.[114,126] In the setting of refractory disease, other immunosuppressive and cytotoxic agents may be substituted or added. Unfortunately, LCH that is resistant to vinblastine and corticosteroids is relatively unlikely to respond to other conventional agents. Recently, cladribine (2CdA) has shown significant promise as "salvage" therapy in children with reactivated or refractory disease.[119,136] Also, dramatic responses have been achieved with the combina-

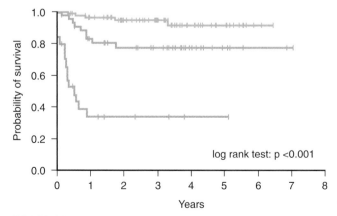

FIGURE 24-4. Results of the LCH I clinical trial for the treatment of multisystem LCH in children. Survival related to response to treatment at week 6. Blue line represents responders (*n* = 71/76); green line represents intermediate responders (*n* = 32/41); and orange line represents nonresponders (*n* = 10/25). (*Redrawn from Gadner H, Grois N, Arico M, et al. A randomized trial of treatment for multisystem Langerhans cell histiocytosis. J Pediatr. 2001;138:728-734.*)

tion of cladribine and cytarabine in children who have refractory LCH with hematologic dysfunction.[122] The Histiocyte Society is currently sponsoring a trial designed to investigate the efficacy of the cytarabine-cladribine combination followed by continuation therapy with standard agents in children with resistant disease involving risk organs.

HCT has been performed successfully in a relatively small number of children with refractory multisystem LCH.[137-140] It is not surprising that toxicity is a significant obstacle to success in these very ill patients. Of five patients who had refractory LCH with hematologic dysfunction and underwent allogeneic HCT, there were two deaths resulting from toxicity and three complete responses, two of which were durable. Of three children who received autologous transplants, all relapsed and two died of progressive disease.[141] Transplant regimens that incorporate reduced-intensity conditioning are especially appealing in refractory LCH; they are associated with lower transplant-related morbidity and mortality rates.[142]

Conclusions

Approach to Single-System Disease. Children with localized LCH have an excellent prognosis. Most may be safely observed without additional intervention after biopsy or resection. Local therapy may be added to accelerate the resolution of symptoms. In certain cases, systemic therapy using corticosteroids with or without vinblastine may be necessary to control symptoms and prevent long-term (especially orthopedic and neuroendocrine) sequelae.

Approach to Multisystem Low-Risk Disease. Children with disseminated LCH (i.e., multisystem or multifocal bone disease) who do not have involvement of risk organs also have an excellent prognosis. Their course of illness is generally favorable, so maximizing response while minimizing short- and long-term toxicities is the primary objective. When possible, enrollment in a clinical trial is encouraged. When this is not possible, the current standard of care in the United States is the combination of vinblastine and prednisone for a total duration of 6 to 12 months.

Approach to High-Risk Disease. Children with disseminated LCH and involvement of risk organs are at significant risk for morbidity and mortality. So far, up-front intensification of therapy has not been shown to improve outcome. Children with adverse prognostic features who respond favorably to standard chemotherapy have a good prognosis. However, those who do not respond rapidly to standard treatment are at high risk for death resulting from progressive disease. For this group of patients, intensive chemotherapy, investigational agents, and HCT should be considered.

The Long Term

Roughly one half of survivors of LCH experience irreversible long-term consequences of their illnesses and, to a lesser extent, of the therapies they received. The incidence and pattern of sequelae strongly correlate with the initial extent and pattern of disease involvement; patients who have multisystem disease and multiple reactivations of illness are at highest risk.[129,143,144] A considerable fraction of irreversible complications seen in survivors of LCH are present at the time of diagnosis. Therefore, not all long-term complications are preventable.

Orthopedic complications are the most commonly seen permanent sequelae in survivors of single-system LCH. Examples include spinal deformity leading to scoliosis or kyphosis, dental loss caused by involvement of the jaw, and facial asym-

metry or proptosis resulting from involvement of orbital or facial bones. Conductive hearing loss caused by chronic inflammation of the middle and external ear is reversible, whereas sensorineural hearing loss caused by involvement of osseous structures is usually permanent. Although permanent orthopedic and cosmetic consequences are relatively common, they do not necessarily adversely affect the quality of survival.[135]

DI is an irreversible condition in almost all cases in which it occurs, and a lifelong need for exogenous vasopressin is to be expected. Similarly, other endocrinopathies such as growth hormone deficiency and panhypopituitarism are not responsive to LCH-directed therapy but are managed by hormone supplementation. Awareness of and close attention to growth and development are very important in the follow-up care of these patients.[76]

Rarely, survivors of LCH experience progressive end organ damage in the absence of demonstrable activity of LCs. Progressive hepatic cirrhosis and liver failure requiring liver transplantation is a rare but well-recognized late event.[87] A somewhat analogous process may occur in the lungs, with pulmonary fibrosis, cystic changes, or spontaneous pneumothoraces resulting. Adult survivors of pediatric LCH should be counseled to avoid exposure to cigarette smoke because of their potentially increased risk for developing pulmonary abnormalities.[145]

Neurodegeneration is the most dreaded late event in survivors of LCH. This poorly understood entity is characterized by posterior fossa symptoms, including ataxia with cerebellar and brainstem signal abnormalities on magnetic resonance imaging. This process may progress unpredictably and may be associated with cognitive decline.[146] The risk factors for the development of neurodegeneration include multisystem disease, especially with craniofacial involvement.[147] There is no known effective therapy for this disorder. There is some suggestion that intravenous immunoglobulin may slow the progression of the disorder, but it has been tested in only a relatively small number of affected patients.[148]

NON-LANGERHANS CELL HISTIOCYTOSES

In addition to LCH, there is a spectrum of other, even rarer, histiocytic lesions that affect both children and adults. In general, they include a large number of clinically benign, not infrequently progressive dermatologic disorders that are pathologically characterized by proliferations of Langerhans-like cells, often with distinctive cytosolic features (see Fig. 24-1).[149,150] Rare non-LCHs, most notably Erdheim-Chester disease and the "true" malignancies such as LC sarcoma and histiocytic sarcoma,[151] may result in high mortality rates. With the exception of juvenile xanthogranuloma (JXG) and sinus histiocytosis with massive lymphadenopathy (SHML), because of their rarity, these disorders are not discussed further here; the reader is referred to several authoritative reviews of the subject.[149,150]

Juvenile Xanthogranuloma

JXG is a generally benign tumoral proliferation of histiocytes with the following immunophenotype: CD1a−, S100−, langerin−, CD68+, CD163+, fascin+. Like LCH, it is believed to be derived from dermal interstitial DCs. Lesions characteristically present as reddish to yellowish-brown cutaneous nodules in the head and neck region of children less than 1 year of age; the median age of onset is 5 months, and tumors may be congenital. Multifocality is not uncommon, particularly in male infants.[149,152] There is an association with neurofibromatosis 1, Noonan's syndrome, and juvenile myelomonocytic leukemia.[153] The natural history of most lesions is spontaneous regression; however, they are often diagnosed by excisional biopsy, leaving little or no residual tumor. Extranodal involvement of the deep soft tissues, liver, spleen, conjunctivae, and CNS—so-called systemic JXG—with or without cutaneous involvement occurs in nearly 5% of cases.[152,154] Although systemic lesions also typically regress, local disease, as in the eye and CNS, may lead to significant morbidity. Occasionally patients with systemic disease involving the CNS or liver have died of the disease.[152,154,155] In cases demanding treatment, single agents[156,157] or multiagent regimens similar to those used for LCH have been employed with success.[158]

Sinus Histiocytosis with Massive Lymphadenopathy

SHML, also known by the eponym Rosai-Dorfman disease,[159] is an enigmatic histiocytic disorder associated with a proliferation of CD1a–, langerin–, S100+, CD68+, CD163+, fascin+ histiocytes with abundant foamy cytoplasm.[149] Most characteristically, a subset of lesional histiocytic cells contains a large number of lymphocytes and other cells, but unlike in the hemophagocytic syndromes (see later), these cells are not contained within phagolysosomes. Rather, they are "just passing through" with invaginations of the cell membrane in a process termed emperipolesis (see Fig. 24-1).[160] In lymph nodes, these histiocytes preferentially involve the nodal sinuses and secondarily the interfollicular areas, leading to remarkably extensive lymphadenopathy, which gives the disease its name.

Because the literature concerning SHML, particularly since 1990 when a patient registry was last updated,[161] is largely retrospective, the reported patterns of clinical presentation and natural history of the disease are undoubtedly biased. Nevertheless, the prototypical clinical presentation is massive, painless cervical lymphadenopathy. In addition, as much as 40% of patients present with extranodal disease, most commonly in the skin, upper respiratory tract, and bone.[161] The orbit and meninges are also not uncommon extranodal sites.[162,163] Extensive nodal and extranodal disease—especially in the kidney, lower airway, and liver—and coexisting immunologic disorders tend to correlate with adverse prognoses, but it is apparent that many if not most cases remit spontaneously without therapy.[161,164,165] Constitutional symptoms, including fever associated with neutrophilia, increased erythrocyte sedimentation rate, and polyclonal hypergammaglobulinemia, are often associated with SHML and usually respond to systemic corticosteroids. In cases in which disease has compromised organ function, hence requiring therapy, there is no clearly preferred treatment modality; surgical debulking and radiation therapy generally result in some amelioration, but the response to systemic chemotherapy, often a combination of alkylators, vinca alkaloids, and steroids, is inconsistent.[161,166]

HEMOPHAGOCYTIC LYMPHOHISTIOCYTOSIS

Monocytes and Macrophages

Resident tissue macrophages play essential roles in host defense, especially when they populate tissues that face the external environment (e.g., alveolar macrophages in the lung). But macrophages also contribute to tissue homeostasis through their repair and clearance activities. The functional and morphologic heterogeneity of macrophages was recognized long ago, and identification of specific subsets has been aided by antibody-based identification of characteristic cell surface markers.[167] Some of these subsets may be involved in the histiocytoses of macrophage origin.

Among the macrophages active in host defense and inflammation, alveolar and gut macrophages are best understood. These cells express pattern recognition receptors and scavenger receptors that enhance recognition of microbial products,[168] they are highly phagocytic, and they are efficient antigen presenters. However, even within this category there is some degree of heterogeneity because gut macrophages tend to secrete smaller amounts of proinflammatory cytokines. Kupffer cells are macrophage derived and may also play a primarily defensive role in the host. In contrast, macrophages involved in homeostasis include osteoclasts and microglia.

Macrophages in secondary lymphoid organs show additional degrees of heterogeneity, with specific cell types occupying characteristic anatomic niches.[168,169] In the spleen, red pulp macrophages, which express high levels of the murine surface marker F4/80, are distinguishable from tingible macrophages in the white pulp. Also present in the white pulp are metallophilic macrophages, which align adjacent to the marginal sinus.[170] Within the marginal zone itself are functionally distinct macrophages that express pattern recognition and scavenger receptors, which they may use to clear pathogens from the bloodstream.[171-173] These macrophages express much lower levels of the F4/80 marker than do the red pulp macrophages. Similar subanatomic heterogeneity is observed in lymph nodes: macrophages in cortical regions express low levels of F4/80 whereas those in the medullary sinuses, paracortex, and subcapsular sinuses express high levels of F4/80.[174]

In the absence of specific stimuli, tissue macrophages remain in a low-functioning, resting state. Activation induces functions that are characteristic of their roles in host protection or homeostasis. Based on in vitro analyses, four distinct pathways of macrophage activation have been described.[175-177] (1) Classical activation via interferon-γ or lipopolysaccharide induces microbicidal activities and upregulation of expression of class II major histocompatibility complex. (2) Alternative activation by interleukin-4 or -13 induces the expression of genes that are involved in tissue repair or suppression of inflammation. (3) Innate activation via toll-like receptor ligands also, not surprisingly, induces microbicidal activities. (4) Deactivation by stimulation of interleukin-10 or transforming growth factor-β reduces class II expression and increases secretion of anti-inflammatory cytokines. As clearly defined as these pathways are in vitro, there is little evidence as yet that they are relevant in vivo. However, secretion of cytokines by activated macrophage-derived cells may be a major pathophysiologic factor in histiocytoses.[178]

Origins of Macrophages

For the most part, steady-state renewal of tissue macrophages appears to be accomplished by local proliferation of similar cell types. However, under conditions of rapid turnover such as inflammatory states, macrophages are replaced by bone marrow precursors, that is, circulating monocytes.[179] More recent findings have revealed substantial heterogeneity among circulating monocytes and the roles played by specific subsets in macrophage development.

Broadly defined, circulating monocytes can be separated into two categories: classic, or inflammatory, cells; and resident cells, which have a phenotype that closely resembles tissue macrophages.[167,180] Cell surface markers can distinguish these subsets: inflammatory monocytes are CD14hi CD16– in humans and Ly6C+ in mice; resident monocytes are CD14+ CD16+ in humans and Ly6C– in mice. Experiments in mice have tracked the fates of some of these cells.[181] For example, bone marrow–derived Ly6C+ cells, which express high levels of the chemokine receptor CCR2 and low levels of the chemokine receptor CX3CR1, enter the circulation. Ordinarily, these cells are very short-lived, but in inflammatory states, they are attracted to affected sites, where they can differentiate into macrophages or DCs. Meanwhile, the precise process whereby circulating monocytes replenish resident macrophages (which are *CCR2–* and *CX3CR1hiLy6C–*) is unknown. Nonetheless, some of the signals that dictate tissue-specific macrophage differentiation are understood. For example, circulating mononuclear precursors that home to bone become osteoclasts under the influence of M-CSF and RANK-L.[182] This may have pathophysiologic relevance in histiocytic disorders that attack bone.

Hemophagocytic Lymphohistiocytosis

HLH is not a single disease entity but rather a syndrome composed of clinical signs and laboratory abnormalities that result from the uncontrolled and ineffective proliferation and activation of cells of the monocyte-macrophage lineage. Normally, monocytes and macrophages are responsible for phagocytosis of antigen and activation of other immune cells through the production of cytokines and chemokines. By way of their interactions with natural killer (NK) cells, macrophages are an important feature of the innate immune response. Additionally, they participate in adaptive immunity via their complex interactions with T cells. When pathogens, especially viral pathogens, are not rapidly eliminated by the innate immune response, the chemokines and cytokines produced by activated macrophages stimulate and perpetuate the activation of T lymphocytes. Activated macrophages are themselves regulated by stimulatory and inhibitory factors that they and other immune cells produce. When this complex process escapes control, extremely potent and destructive inflammatory forces are unleashed. Uncontrolled macrophage activity is the hallmark of HLH. The pathogenetic mechanisms underlying the hyperinflammatory state in HLH are heterogeneous, but the clinical features are shared.

The earliest published reports of hemophagocytic syndrome by Farquhar described four siblings who were afflicted in early infancy with fever, irritability, hepatosplenomegaly, and pancytopenia. Autopsy demonstrated histiocytic proliferation throughout the reticuloendothelial system and prominent hemophagocytosis.[183,184] The disorder was dubbed familial haemophagocytic reticulosis and was recognized as being distinct from Letterer-Siwe disease (i.e., Langerhans cell histiocytosis).[185] An autosomal recessive pattern of inheritance was proposed. Subsequently, sporadic cases with similar clinical features were seen in association with viral infection and were termed viral-associated hemophagocytic syndrome (VAHS).[186] Upon recognition that bacterial infections[187] and a host of other infections could also precipitate the syndrome, the terminology expanded to infection-associated hemophagocytic syndrome (IAHS).[188] Concomitantly, it was observed that certain systemic illnesses, notably rheumatologic conditions and malignancies, were occasionally complicated by the development of clinical features of hemophagocytic syndrome. In 1987, the Histiocyte Society adopted the unifying term hemophagocytic lymphohistiocytosis (HLH) and defined a set of diagnostic criteria to assist clinicians and researchers. The criteria have

subsequently been refined to account for advances in our understanding of the syndrome (Box 24-2).[189,190]

Incidence and Etiology

For practical purposes, HLH is categorized into two main forms: familial and acquired. Undoubtedly, this stark delineation is an oversimplification because significant clinical and perhaps even genetic overlap exists between the two forms. In familial HLH (FHL), an ordinary immune stimulus such as a common viral exposure triggers an uncontrolled hyperinflammatory state because of the existence of an inherited, intrinsic defect in the patient's immune system. Affected individuals inevitably encounter the immunologic stimuli that trigger the syndrome, and HLH is invariably fatal. Replacement of the defective immune system via HCT is the only known curative option for these patients. In contrast, secondary HLH develops as a consequence of an intense immunologic stimulus in the form of an infection, malignancy, or autoimmune process in an individual with an apparently normal immune system or with an acquired immune deficiency. In these patients, effective management of the triggering process, often in combination with a period of immunosuppressive therapy to control the HLH, has the potential to reverse the process permanently. It is important to note that the familial and acquired forms of HLH may be clinically indistinguishable at presentation.

The incidence of HLH is very difficult to determine. FHL is estimated to affect approximately 1 in 50,000 live births.[191] There are no good estimates of the incidence of nonfamilial HLH, but it is certainly a rare condition. The male-to-female ratio is roughly equal. A slight preponderance of males may be attributable to the occurrence of HLH in association with X-linked lymphoproliferative disorder (XLP). HLH occurs in people of all races.

Familial Hemophagocytic Lymphohistiocytosis

FHL is a disease of early infancy. Although congenital cases do occur, most affected infants are born healthy and grow normally until the onset of symptoms in the first few months of life, often following a bout with an otherwise routine childhood infection. The peak age at diagnosis is 1 to 6 months, and it is estimated that approximately 70% are diagnosed within the first year of life. However, the age range at diagnosis is wide. FHL has been reported in patients as old as 27 years.[192,193]

As noted, familial inheritance was recognized in the earliest descriptions of the clinical phenotype, and an autosomal recessive pattern of inheritance was inferred in many cases.[194] It is now evident that the familial forms of HLH can be subdivided into nonsyndromic forms, in which the only or the predominant clinical phenotype is a predisposition to hemophagocytic syndrome; and syndromic forms, in which hemophagocytosis is only one, often inconstant, phenotype present in association with other, easily recognizable systemic abnormalities, particularly pigmentation defects and immune deficiency (Table 24-1).

Nonsyndromic Familial Hemophagocytic Lymphohistiocytosis

Early on, genetic linkage studies performed on large families with nonsyndromic FHL indicated substantial genetic heterogeneity and potential linkages to several different loci, which were systematically named FHL1 through FHL4. FHL1, which was among the first to be mapped, continues to defy molecular characterization.[195] However, the genes responsible for FHL2, FHL3, and FHL4 have been cloned and have led to remarkable

HLH: 1994 Diagnostic Guidelines and 2004 Revised Version

DIAGNOSTIC GUIDELINES (1994)*

Clinical Criteria

Fever

Splenomegaly

Laboratory Criteria

Cytopenias (hemoglobin <9 g/L; platelets <100 × 10^9/L; neutrophils (<1 × 10^9/L)

Hypertriglyceridemia +/− hypofibrinogenemia (fasting triglycerides ≥3 SD, fibrinogen ≤3 SD of normal for age)

Histopathologic Criteria

Hemophagocytosis in marrow, spleen, or lymph nodes and no evidence of malignancy

REVISED DIAGNOSTIC GUIDELINES (2004)

Molecular Diagnosis Consistent with HLH;

or five of the following eight clinical, laboratory, histopathologic criteria:

Clinical Criteria

Fever

Splenomegaly

Laboratory Criteria

Cytopenias (hemoglobin <9 g/L; platelets <100 × 10^9/L; neutrophils <1.0 × 10^9/L)

Hypertriglyceridemia and/or hypofibrinogenemia (fasting triglycerides ≥3 SD, fibrinogen ≤3 SD of normal for age)

Hyperferritinemia (>500 μg/L)

Elevated CD25 (≥2400 U/L)

Low or absent NK function

Histopathologic Criteria

Hemophagocytosis in marrow, spleen, or lymph nodes and no evidence of malignancy

*All criteria are required. If hemophagocytic activity is not proven at presentation, further search is encouraged.
Adapted from Henter JI, Elinder G, Ost A. Diagnostic guidelines for hemophagocytic lymphohistiocytosis. The FHL Study Group of the Histiocyte Society. Semin Oncol. 1991;18: 29-33; and Henter JI, Horne A, Arico M, et al. HLH-2004: diagnostic and therapeutic guidelines for hemophagocytic lymphohistiocytosis. Pediatr Blood Cancer. 2007;48:124-131.

branes.[198] FHL2-associated mutations may lead to a complete lack of protein or a defect in protein maturation and transport, resulting in varying degrees of perforin deficiency and lymphocyte-mediated cytotoxicity.[199]

FHL2 is caused primarily by defects in the effector of cell-mediated toxicity itself; FHL3 and FHL4 are caused primarily by mutations in the protein components of the trafficking machinery required for exocytosis of cytotoxic granules. Prior to exocytosis, vesicles must associate, or "dock," with the membrane, a process facilitated by SNAPs (soluble n-ethyl malemide sensitive attachment proteins) on the vesicular compartment surface and SNAREs (SNAP receptors) on the target membrane (Fig. 24-5). Mutations in the putative vesicular SNAP, syntaxin-11 (STX11), are responsible for FHL4.[200] A mammalian homologue of the Caenorhabditis elegans protein UNC13, UNC13D (also known as MUNC13-4) is mutated in patients with FHL3.[201,202] UNC13 family members are thought to participate in preparing vesicles docked at the cell surface for fusion with the membrane—a process called priming.[203,204] Thus, it would appear that STX11 and UNC13D are necessary to deliver PRF1 extracellularly.[205] In toto, then, the deficiency of NK cell function in patients with FHL can be ascribed to a defect in the primary cytotoxicity effector pathway, leading to poor clearance of target cells and a continued state of immune activation, which is characteristic of the hemophagocytic syndromes.

Whereas the absolute frequency of occurrence of disease-causing mutations in each of these genes varies greatly from publication to publication and population to population, it is evident that up to half of the molecularly defined cases of FHL are attributable to mutations in PRF1, with fewer due to STX11 or UNC13D.[202,206-208] Nonetheless, approximately half of presumptive FHL cases still evade genetic characterization.

Hemophagocytic Lymphohistiocytosis Associated with Other Genetic Syndromes

HLH may occur in association with other inherited anomalies, including Chédiak-Higashi syndrome,[209] Griscelli syndrome type 2,[210,211] lysinuric protein intolerance[212] and X-linked lymphoproliferative syndrome-1.[213] In these patients, hemophagocytosis is a variable feature and it is not the sole manifestation of the disease. These disorders are diverse, each resulting from defects in distinct genes (see Table 24-1).

Not coincidentally, the proteins encoded by the genes involved in several of these disorders play roles in the process of cellular cytotoxicity. The Griscelli syndrome type 2 protein, Rab27a, a small GTPase of the ras-associated family, directly associates with the FHL3 protein, UNC13, and is similarly thought to regulate exocytosis.[214] Chédiak-Higashi syndrome, like Griscelli syndrome type 2, gives rise to pigmentation defects and is also caused by mutations in a protein, LYST, involved in vesicular trafficking. Patients with X-linked lymphoproliferative syndrome caused by mutations in the Src homology 2 domain-containing gene 1A (SH2D1A), which functions as a lymphocyte-signaling adapter, have a multifactorial humoral and cellular immune deficiency most saliently characterized by susceptibility to infection by the Epstein-Barr virus (EBV), to lymphoproliferative disorders, and to dysgammaglobulinemia (see Chapter 13).[215] Defects in NK- and T-cell development and function, including cytotoxicity, appear to predispose patients with X-linked lymphoproliferative syndrome-1 to HLH, particularly in the setting of primary EBV infection. How abnormalities in dibasic amino acid transport[216] should result in HLH is completely obscure; however, several individuals with lysinuric protein imbalance have presented with HLH.[212]

insights into the pathogenesis of this group of disorders: each is a component required for the development or trafficking of a mature, fully capacitated cytotoxic lymphocyte or NK cell cytotoxic granule.

FHL2 is caused by mutations in the gene encoding perforin (PRF1).[196,197] Perforin is a component of T lymphocyte and NK cell cytotoxic granules that is homologous to the pore-forming complement component C9 and, like its homologue, it facilitates lysis of target cells by creating holes in cell mem-

TABLE 24-1   Genes Involved with Familial Hemophagocytic Lymphohistiocytosis

Disease	Locus	Gene	Gene Symbol	Syndromic Associations
FHL1	9q22.1-23	Unknown	Unknown	None
FHL2	10q22	Perforin	*PRF1*	None
FHL3	17q25	Mammalian homologue of *C. elegans* Unc13	*UNC13D*	None
FHL4	6q24	Syntaxin-11	*STX11*	None
Griscelli syndrome type 2	15q21	*ras*-associated protein Rab27a	*RAB27A*	Hypopigmentation +/− neurodegeneration
Lysinuric protein intolerance	14q11.2	Solute carrier family 7, member 7	*SLC7A7*	Protein intolerance, malabsorption, failure to thrive
Chédiak-Higashi syndrome	1q42.1-42.2	Lysosomal trafficking regulator	*LYST*	Partial albinism, giant lysosomes or melanosomes, neutropenia, susceptibility to infection
XLP1	Xq25	SLAM-associated protein (SAP)	*SHD2D1A*	Sensitivity to EBV infection, hypogammaglobulinemia, lymphoma
XLP2	Xq25	X-linked inhibitor of apoptosis	*XIAP*	Splenomegaly, hypogammaglobulinemia

EBV, Epstein-Barr virus; XLP, X-linked lymphoproliferative disorder.

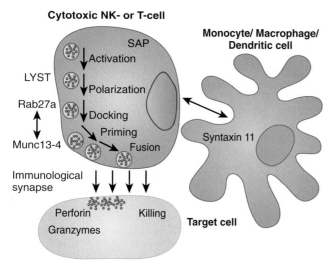

FIGURE 24-5. Molecular mechanisms based on the identification of genetic defects associated with the clinical picture of FHL, Griscelli syndrome, and Chédiak-Higashi syndrome. Cytotoxic granule processing involves a Rab27a/Munc13-4 complex and several other unknown proteins. Perforin and granzymes are secreted into the immunologic synapse and lead to apoptosis of the target cell. The exact functions of LYST and syntaxin 11 are not known. (*Redrawn from Janka GE. Hemophagocytic syndromes. Blood Rev. 2007;21:245-253.*)

Secondary Hemophagocytic Lymphohistiocytosis

Infection-Associated Hemophagocytic Lymphohistiocytosis

Virus-associated hemophagocytic syndrome was first described in a report of 19 adult patients, 14 of whom were immunocompromised.[186] Subsequently, it was shown that immunocompetent individuals may also develop this disorder. Although viruses, especially EBV and other members of the herpesvirus group, are the most commonly identified infectious triggers, a whole host of other infectious agents have been implicated, including bacteria,[187] fungi, and protozoa (e.g., leishmania).[217] In a review of the 219 cases of IAHS reported in the medical literature between 1979 and 1995, 55% were attributed to EBV.[218] The clinical features of infection-associated HLH are identical to those of familial HLH, although the median age of onset is higher: about 50% of cases occurred in children younger than 3 years and 18% in children younger than 1 year. An interesting but as yet unexplained fact is that about half of reported cases are people of Asian ancestry.

Malignancy-Associated Hemophagocytic Lymphohistiocytosis

In children, HLH occurs rarely in association with malignant neoplasms. The association presents in two uncommon but somewhat distinct forms: during treatment for a known cancer in clinical remission (e.g., acute lymphoblastic leukemia) or as a manifestation of an aggressive uncontrolled cancer that may be masked (e.g., T/NK cell leukemia/lymphoma). In the first case, the clinical features of HLH arise unexpectedly in patients undergoing cancer chemotherapy, presumably as the result of iatrogenic immune dysregulation. An infectious trigger may or may not be identified.[219] In the latter case, which occurs more commonly in adults, the hemophagocytic syndrome is a feature of the hematologic malignancy itself.[220,221] It is proposed that the malignant clone potentiates a state of hypercytokinemia that results in the clinical signs and symptoms of HLH. Some of these cancers are associated with infection by EBV. The majority of the reported cases are in individuals of Asian descent.

Macrophage Activation Syndrome

Macrophage activation syndrome (MAS) is a life-threatening complication of systemic inflammatory conditions that is characterized by all of the clinical symptoms and laboratory findings of HLH, leading to its classification as a form of secondary HLH. The syndrome was first described in 1985 in a report of seven children with systemic-onset juvenile idiopathic arthritis.[222] Rheumatologic conditions other than juvenile idiopathic arthritis such as systemic lupus erythematosus may also be associated with the syndrome in both children and adults.

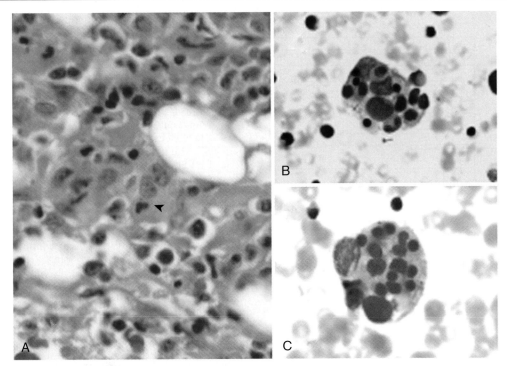

FIGURE 24-6. Histopathology of HLH. **A,** H&E-stained bone marrow biopsy section (400× magnification) showing marrow infiltration by benign-appearing macrophages. A macrophage containing a phagocytosed neutrophil is indicated by the *arrowhead*. **B** and **C,** Individual macrophages from a Wright-Giemsa–stained bone marrow aspirate smear (1000× magnification); B contains phagocytosed marrow elements, including mature eosinophils and erythroid precursors; C shows numerous erythroid precursors and a band neutrophil.

Typically the syndrome develops years after the diagnosis, but it may occur early or even concomitantly with the diagnosis of the rheumatologic disease.[223] With the onset of MAS, chronically ill children experience the acute and unexpected onset of unremitting fever, fall in blood counts, and organomegaly. The erythrocyte sedimentation rate may decrease concomitant with the development of MAS. Flare of the underlying disease, infection, and medication changes have been implicated as possible triggering events.[224,225]

It has been suggested that inherited defects in one or more of the genes associated with FHL might confer predisposition to the development of MAS in the setting of rheumatologic disease or, moreover, to the development of the rheumatologic condition itself.[226] A review of 133 children with systemic-onset juvenile idiopathic arthritis and 384 matched unrelated controls failed to demonstrate an increased incidence of detectable abnormalities in the genes encoding perforin, MUNC13D, granzyme B, or Rab27A.[227]

Clinical Features

The cardinal clinical features of HLH are persistent high fever, cytopenias, and splenomegaly, with or without hepatomegaly. Needless to say, this constellation of clinical signs and symptoms is neither rare nor specific. Further complicating the diagnostic picture is the fact that all of the clinical features of the disorder may not be initially or simultaneously present (Fig. 24-7).

Persistent and prolonged fever is essentially universal and it is usually the first sign of illness. Often, signs of a routine childhood upper respiratory or gastrointestinal illness accompany the fever. However, instead of resolving in the typical time course, or after a brief period of apparent improvement, constitutional symptoms rapidly progress. At presentation, affected

patients are usually acutely ill and require urgent evaluation and intervention.

Cytopenias affecting at least two cell lines are a key feature of HLH. Thrombocytopenia is almost always present. The platelet count may be only mildly depressed initially but it often falls precipitously as the disease progresses. Normocytic anemia with reticulocytopenia due to ineffective erythropoiesis is also common. In cytopenic patients, less than the expected increment may be seen in response to transfusions because of the shortened survival of transfused blood cells. Leukopenia and neutropenia are more variably present.

Abdominal distention and hepatosplenomegaly are usually present on physical examination. Jaundice and ascites may be noted. Biochemical evidence of liver dysfunction is typical, although it is not a universal feature of HLH. Hypertriglyceridemia,[228,229] increased transaminases, and hyperbilirubinemia may be present and may, in a very young child, raise the possibility of a metabolic disorder. Impaired hepatic synthetic function and clotting factor consumption may result in hypofibrinogenemia and prolongation of the prothrombin and partial thromboplastin times. When coagulopathy is combined with thrombocytopenia, a severe hemorrhagic tendency ensues.[230] Spontaneous hemorrhage, especially intracranially, may lead to acute decompensation and may raise an erroneous suspicion of child abuse.[231]

Typically, the serum ferritin level is markedly elevated in patients with active HLH.[232,233] Serum ferritin exceeding 10,000 μg/L is a highly sensitive and specific marker supporting the diagnosis of HLH.[234,235] However, although most patients with HLH have increased ferritin levels, not all demonstrate extreme hyperferritinemia. Furthermore, mild to moderate elevation of serum ferritin may be seen in disorders other than HLH, such as inflammatory conditions, infections, liver disease, hemochromatosis, and metabolic disorders. The precise mech-

Clinical features

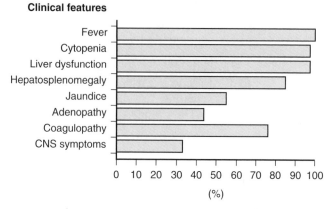

Laboratory findings

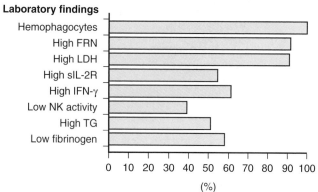

FIGURE 24-7. Incidence of clinical features and abnormal laboratory findings in 82 cases of HLH. (FRN, ferritin normal range 8 to 78 μg/L; IFN-γ, interferon gamma; LDH, lactate dehydrogenase, normal range 234 to 471 IU/L; sIL-2R, CD25, normal range <1090 U/mL); TG, triglycerides. *(Redrawn from Imashuku S, Hibi S, Todo S. Hemophagocytic lymphohistiocytosis in infancy and childhood. J Pediatr. 1997;130:352-357.)*

anism of ferritin elevation in HLH is unknown but it is probably related both to increased synthesis of ferritin mediated by high levels of cytokines[236] and to increased release of ferritin as the result of liver injury and hematopoietic cell turnover.

The term *hemophagocytosis* describes the pathologic finding of activated, histologically benign macrophages engulfing erythrocytes, leukocytes, platelets, and their precursor cells (Fig. 24-6). This process is often visible in the bone marrow, but it occurs throughout the reticuloendothelial system (i.e., in the liver, spleen, and lymph nodes) and sometimes in the CNS. Destruction of blood cells and their precursors leads to peripheral blood cytopenias despite bone marrow hypercellularity, often including erythroid hyperplasia. Analysis of the bone marrow is always recommended when a diagnosis of HLH is suspected, both to demonstrate hemophagocytosis and to rule out the presence of leukemia. The finding of hemophagocytosis in the bone marrow supports the diagnosis of HLH in the proper clinical context, but it is neither essential for the diagnosis nor pathognomonic of it. In a series of 122 children with HLH from the Histiocyte Society's International Registry, only 75% had evidence of hemophagocytosis at diagnosis.[237] In some cases, repeated bone marrow analyses may be necessary to document hemophagocytosis. Neither the pathophysiologic basis for hemophagocytosis nor its precise mechanism is well understood. In HLH, hemophagocytosis is a reactive process

that presumably results from the dysregulated and excessively exuberant immune response.

In keeping with a state of generalized, uncontrolled inflammation, the levels of various cytokines are increased in patients with active HLH, including interleukin-2, interleukin-2 receptor, interleukin-6, -8, and -10, interferon, and tumor necrosis factor.[238-240] Cytokine levels are not routinely measured in the clinical setting, but measurement of the soluble receptor for interleukin-2 (also known as CD25) is available on a clinical basis. CD25 elevation is a sensitive and reliable marker of HLH activity,[241] and it has been incorporated into the diagnostic criteria of HLH.[190] It must be borne in mind that CD25 levels are elevated in disorders other than HLH, notably lymphoid malignancies.

Despite the hyperactivity of the immune response in HLH and the presence of normal numbers of effector cells in many cases, the targeted killing function of the immune system is depressed or absent. In the laboratory, impairment in effector function may be demonstrated using a standard chromium release assay against K562 target cells. Successful performance of this test requires fresh blood cells from the patient and an experienced laboratory. In the setting of active HLH of any variety, the functional activity of NK cells is usually impaired.[242] Manipulation of the conditions of the NK cell functional assay by addition of mitogen, interleukin-2, or prolonged incubation times results in restoration of NK cell function in some samples from patients.[243] It appears that inability to reconstitute NK functional activity in vitro using modified assay conditions is associated with the familial form of the disease.[244] Along the same lines, patients in whom NK cell functional impairment persists despite treatment with immunosuppressive chemotherapy have a poor prognosis unless rescued by HCT.[245] Investigation has revealed some degree of correlation between the pattern of NK functional impairment and the molecular abnormality present in patients with FHL.[246,247]

Evaluation for infectious agents should be undertaken as part of the initial workup in patients with the clinical features of HLH. Bacterial cultures and tests for other pathogens, such as EBV, cytomegalovirus, herpes simplex virus, respiratory syncytial virus, adenovirus, fungi, and protozoa, should be performed based on patients' symptoms and exposure history. Identifying and treating (when possible) infection is a very important part of managing these critically ill patients. However, evidence of a bacterial, viral, or other infection in patients with HLH does not discriminate between the familial and acquired forms of the disease. In fact, patients with FHL commonly present after an identifiable infectious trigger.[237] Conversely, an infectious trigger is not always identified in patients who are found to have IAHS. Of course, the possibility of secondary infection must be assessed and managed conservatively in these patients, who are likely to be febrile and neutropenic and may be hemodynamically unstable.

A range of CNS symptoms, including irritability, lethargy, seizures, and focal deficits, may be seen. Analysis of the cerebrospinal fluid (CSF) may show pleocytosis (especially with activated monocytes present) or elevated CSF protein. Magnetic resonance imaging of the brain may demonstrate a range of abnormalities.[248] CNS manifestations, including neurologic symptoms, abnormal CSF, or both, have been reported in as much as 63% of children at diagnosis,[249] and they develop in most if not all children in whom disease cannot be controlled.[250,251] Occasionally, neurologic symptoms represent the most conspicuous manifestation of illness, obscuring and delaying the correct diagnosis of HLH.[252] Pathologically, CNS involvement is variable, with meningeal inflammation at the mild end and multifocal brain infiltration with necrosis at the severe end of the clinical spectrum.[253]

Therapeutic Considerations

The development of rational and effective therapy for HLH is challenged by the fact that affected patients demonstrate common clinical features despite variable underlying pathophysiology. Additionally, there is little time to wait for diagnostic clarity in affected patients because they may be desperately ill. Whether patients have the familial or the acquired form of the disease, the first objective of therapy is to cool down the overheated immune response. At the same time or later, the underlying cause of patients' disease processes must be addressed.

Without therapy, FHL is rapidly and invariably fatal, usually within a month or two of presentation. A comprehensive literature review performed prior to the discovery of effective chemotherapy showed that only 12% of children survived for 6 months, and only 3 of 101 children survived long term.[218] Acquired HLH is also a life-threatening condition, although it is much more variable. It is estimated that without therapy, the mortality rate of patients with EBV-associated HLH is approximately 50%.[33]

In 1980, Ambruso first reported the successful treatment of two infants with presumed FHL by etoposide (VP-16).[254] This was an enormous step forward because previously there had been no effective therapy for the disease.[255] However, disease control proved to be transient in these and subsequent patients, with the CNS being a major site of treatment failure. To address the problem of CNS disease, cranial irradiation and intrathecal methotrexate were added to the combination of VP-16 and corticosteroids.[256] Systemic and CNS relapses remained a significant problem and few, if any, patients survived long term. In the majority of the reported cases, patients maintained on etoposide eventually developed refractory disease that was fatal within 1 to 3 years.[256,257] Teniposide, also an epipodophyllotoxin, has been used in some patients with roughly equivalent results.[258]

In 1986, the first successful result of a matched sibling donor bone marrow transplant in a boy with FHL was published.[259] HCT was quickly recognized as the sole potentially curative modality for a group of patients for whom there had previously been no real possibility of cure. But allogeneic transplantation, which is always a high-risk procedure, is particularly toxic in children with HLH owing to their very young age, profound immune suppression, and underlying disease characteristics, such as liver dysfunction and hepatosplenomegaly. Control of the clinical signs of HLH prior to transplantation significantly improves the likelihood of successful outcomes.[260,261] Additionally, absence of CNS involvement and infection are favorable prognostic indicators for transplantation.[237] These factors drive the preference for early transplantation, as soon as possible after the achievement of disease control and prior to the onset of CNS manifestations or the acquisition of opportunistic infection. Unfortunately, a matched sibling donor exists for a minority of children with HLH, and identification of an alternative donor takes time.

Cyclosporine A, an inhibitor of T-cell activation, demonstrated efficacy in children with etoposide-refractory HLH who were awaiting transplantation.[262,263] Cyclosporine A is commonly given in the context of combination therapy to maintain disease control in children awaiting transplantation.

Initial Therapy

To standardize, improve, and study the treatment of this rare disease, the Histiocyte Society sponsored an international clinical trial, HLH-94.[264] This study, and its successor HLH-2004, defined a set of clear diagnostic criteria and laid out a nonrandomized treatment strategy combining chemotherapy (etoposide, glucocorticoids, and intrathecal methotrexate in select cases); immunotherapy (cyclosporine A); and HCT (when possible in familial, refractory, or relapsing cases). The HLH-94 study enrolled 113 children between 1994 and 1998. Because it is impossible to differentiate FHL from secondary HLH in many cases, confirmation of familial disease was not required, so both familial and secondary cases were included. Of the children studied, 25 had an affected sibling; 85% (90 patients) responded favorably to 8 weeks of initial therapy; 53% achieved resolution; and 32% improved without resolution. The remaining 15% died or did not improve within the first 2 months of treatment. Transplantation was performed in 65 patients, with a median time between onset of therapy and HCT of 187 days.

The combination of antithymocyte globulin (ATG), corticosteroids, and cyclosporine A may be an effective alternative to HLH-94 chemoimmunotherapy, although experience with it is much more limited. Among 38 children with confirmed FHL who received one or two courses of rabbit ATG, complete resolution was achieved in 73% and partial improvement in 24%. This includes favorable responses seen in 10 children who had received prior immunosuppressive treatment (including steroids, cyclosporine A, or chemotherapy). All of the patients were maintained on cyclosporine A. Of 19 patients, 16 who went on to receive allogeneic transplants after receiving ATG as first-line therapy are long-term survivors. All patients who did not receive transplants died. The therapy was relatively well tolerated, although infusional and infectious complications were not trivial.[265,266]

As stated previously, the CNS is not infrequently involved in children with HLH at diagnosis, and it is a major site of treatment failure in advanced FHL. Clearly, prompt and aggressive initiation of systemic chemoimmunotherapy, followed by allogeneic stem cell transplant (in familial, refractory, and relapsing cases) is the best strategy for minimizing the potential for CNS involvement.[251] The role of CNS-directed therapy is not well established. Intrathecal methotrexate and cranial irradiation have been routinely used in the context of systemic therapy. In HLH-94, intrathecal methotrexate was reserved for patients in whom neurologic symptoms progressed or CSF abnormalities did not resolve after 2 weeks of systemic treatment. It is worth noting that the same number of children (10 of 15) experienced normalization of neurologic symptoms by 2 months whether they had or had not received intrathecal therapy. Intrathecal methotrexate does not appear to prevent the development of CNS manifestations in patients who do not undergo transplantation. Furthermore, intensive intrathecal methotrexate is not sufficient to reverse CNS manifestations in children with advanced FHL.[251] Cranial irradiation is now rarely used because of the lack of established efficacy and the potential long-term toxicities in these very young patients.

Therapy of Secondary Hemophagocytic Lymphohistiocytosis

Infection-Associated Hemophagocytic Lymphohistiocytosis. HLH that is associated with EBV infection is the most common and best-studied type of IAHS and is the prototype of this disorder. Compared with children who have infectious mononucleosis, children with EBV-associated HLH have higher levels of the EBV genome copy number as measured by quantitative polymerase chain reaction. The EBV copy number quickly falls with the initiation of effective therapy and can be used as a marker of disease activity in these patients.[267] The role of antiviral agents (e.g., acyclovir) is not well established, but they are probably of some benefit during the phase of active viral replication. The need for immunosuppressive therapy has been well established in these patients. The efficacy of HLH-94–based immunochemotherapy has been clearly demonstrated and has yielded a survival rate of up to 90% in promptly treated patients.[268] Because of the potential short-term (myelosuppression) and long-term (secondary MDS/AML) toxicities linked to etoposide,[269] its role has been specifically evaluated. Mortality rates were 14 times higher in patients with EBV-associated HLH who did not receive etoposide within the first 4 weeks after diagnosis.[270] The risks associated with a relatively short course of etoposide appear to be acceptable when weighed against the high risks for morbidity and mortality in these patients and the knowledge that delayed treatment yields inferior outcomes. In a series of 78 patients with EBV-associated HLH, most of whom were treated according to HLH-94, 75% remained disease free, with a median follow-up of 43 months. Reactivations occurred in approximately 20% of cases, many of whom were eventually cured by HCT.[271]

An intriguing complementary therapeutic strategy for EBV-associated HLH is the use of B-cell–directed therapy with the goal of reducing the burden of EBV-infected B cells. Two young men known to have XLP and acute infectious mononucleosis who were treated with rituximab (anti-CD20 monoclonal antibody), in combination with corticosteroids, responded favorably.[272] There is a single case report of the successful use of rituximab in combination with immunosuppressive chemotherapy in a child with EBV-associated HLH.[273]

In patients with IAHS, identification of a potentially treatable precipitating infection is very important. When IAHS occurs in association with visceral leishmaniasis, a very uncommon infection in the United States, treatment of the underlying infection, perhaps by amphotericin B, is usually life-saving.[217]

Malignancy-Associated Hemophagocytic Lymphohistiocytosis. Treatment of reactive hemophagocytic syndrome, that is, malignancy-associated HLH and MAS, must be individualized. When an active malignancy is responsible for the hemophagocytic syndrome, administration of tumor-directed cancer chemotherapy is obviously the best treatment choice. The clinical features of HLH can be expected to resolve when or if the triggering cancer is controlled. The very rare patients who develop HLH while receiving immunosuppressive therapy for a cancer that is in remission may be very difficult to manage.[274] Discontinuation of immunosuppressive therapy is beneficial in some cases, but this is not always possible. Treatment by corticosteroids and etoposide may be indicated. When standard therapy for HLH fails, HCT should be considered.

Macrophage Activation Syndrome. MAS and rheumatologic disease-associated HLH fall into a clinical spectrum within which there are no generally accepted distinctions or definitions. *MAS* is a term that arose in the rheumatology literature and has become more or less synonymous with reactive HLH. It is likely that many patients in this disease spectrum do not come to the attention of pediatric hematologists and oncologists because pediatric or adult rheumatologists manage them. There are differences in approach between the two groups of specialists. High-dose, parenteral, pulsed corticosteroids are usually used in the initial management of MAS. Cyclosporine A may be effective when corticosteroids are not.[275] More recently, inhibitors of tumor necrosis factor, etanercept[276] and infliximab,[277] have been used successfully in patients with MAS that is refractory to steroids and cyclosporine.

In patients in whom HLH resolves completely and in whom a cause of the syndrome has not been determined (i.e., lack of a positive family history or identified genetic defect), HCT is not indicated. Very close monitoring in the period after cessation of therapy is warranted. Patients who remain well are presumed to have had secondary HLH. In the subset of patients who manifest signs of disease reactivation, chemoimmunotherapy should be promptly reinstituted to control the disease prior to HCT.

Supportive Care

It must be acknowledged that some of the progress in the management of HLH is attributable to advances in supportive care. Patients with new-onset and uncontrolled HLH are typically characterized by the presence of multiple organ-system dysfunction, including immunologic compromise, pancytopenia, hemorrhagic tendencies, and hepatic and neurologic dysfunction. Hemodynamic instability, respiratory insufficiency, renal dysfunction, and electrolyte imbalance may be present. Immunosuppressive and myelosuppressive chemotherapy in these critically ill patients magnifies their risk for serious infection. A significant fraction of children with HLH succumb to opportunistic infection. Empirical antibiotics for febrile neutropenia and *Pneumocystis jiroveci* pneumonia plus antifungal prophylaxis and intravenous immunoglobulin repletion are suggested. These interventions along with other supportive care measures, including aggressive blood-product support, certainly contribute substantially to the likelihood and quality of survival.

Hematopoietic Cell Transplantation

Multiple studies have demonstrated the necessity for allogeneic transplantation in the management of FHL. In the International Registry report of 122 children with HLH, HCT was performed in 29, for whom the 5-year survival rate after HCT was 66%. Most of the donors were fully matched or mismatched family donors; only three children received transplants from unrelated donors. Among those who did not receive transplantation, the 5-year survival rate was only 10%, with just three children surviving long term.[237] Only a minority of the patients received HCT, so the 5-year event-free survival rate for the entire cohort of 122 patients was just 21%.

The fact that only approximately 20% of children in need of allogeneic stem cell transplantation have an available matched family donor accounts in part for the poor overall survival rates of patients in the International Registry. Aside from availability, another limitation to the applicability of matched sibling donor transplantation in a genetic disorder such as HLH is the possibility that the sibling donor is at risk for developing the disease. Molecular tests are diagnostic in only about half of cases of FHL, so the identification of a potentially affected sibling may not be feasible. Most affected siblings develop clinical symptoms at approximately the same age as one another, although this is not always true.[237] There is at least one reported case in which a transplanted patient and matched sibling donor both developed HLH after transplantation. These factors, combined with the knowledge that FHL is invariably fatal without transplantation, has led to the increased use of alternative donors for HCT, and the results have been very encouraging.[261,278,279] The 3-year overall survival rate was 44% in 16 children who underwent transplantation for HLH from unrelated donors. Of 65 children in HLH-94 who underwent transplantation after immunochemotherapy, approximately half of whom were transplanted from an unrelated donor, the 3-year probability of survival was 62%. The impact of expanded access to HCT by increased use of alternative donors (among other factors) was borne out in the relatively high overall survival rate of 55% at 3 years in the HLH-94 study.

The most commonly employed conditioning regimen for HCT in patients with HLH is the combination of busulfan,

TABLE 24-2 **Characteristics, Laboratory Diagnosis, Treatment, and Prognosis of Langerhans Cell Histiocytosis (LCH) and Hemophagocytic Lymphohistiocytosis (HLH)**

	LCH		HLH	
	Single System	**Multisystem**	**Primary**	**Secondary**
Pathologic cell	Dendritic cell		Macrophage	
Histologic features	Clonal Langerhans cell proliferation (CD1a⁺, langerin⁺), mixed cellular infiltrate		Reactive macrophages (CD68⁺), hemophagocytosis	
Typical age at onset	Childhood	Infancy	Infancy	Childhood
Inheritance	Sporadic	Sporadic	Autosomal recessive	Sporadic
Clinical presentation	Bone pain, swelling, skin rash	Bone pain, swelling, skin rash, FTT, DI	Fever, hepatosplenomegaly, FTT, irritability, jaundice	
Laboratory and radiographic features	Lab results usually normal; lytic bone lesions	Cytopenias, $\uparrow\uparrow$ESR, $\uparrow\uparrow$bili, abnormal CXR, bone lesions	Cytopenias, $\uparrow\uparrow$ferritin, $\downarrow\downarrow$fibrinogen, $\uparrow\uparrow$triglycerides, $\downarrow\downarrow$NK cell function, $\uparrow\uparrow$soluble CD25, abnormal CSF	
Treatment	Observation, local, vinblastine and steroids	Vinblastine; steroids	Etoposide; steroids CSA HCT	Etoposide; steroids; CSA
Prognosis	Excellent	Variable Fatal in ~25%	Fatal without HCT Survival in ~50% with HCT	Variable Fatal in ~20%

DI, diabetes insipidus; bili, bilirubin; CSF, cerebrospinal fluid; ESR, erythrocyte sedimentation rate; HCT, hematopoietic cell transplantation; NK, natural killer.

cyclophosphamide, etoposide, and antithymocyte globulin. Transplant-related mortality rates are high. Roughly one third of recipients of unrelated donor transplants die within the first few months after transplantation as the result of infection, hepatopathy, pneumonitis, or uncontrolled disease. Disease remission at the time of transplantation is associated with a significantly better outcome than is found in active disease.[278] However, HCT should not be viewed as futile in children with active disease, even if it involves the CNS, because many children with active disease at the time of HCT have done well.[280] Despite high early mortality rates, late reactivation of disease is very uncommon in patients who have undergone allogeneic HCT for FHL.[280] Allogeneic transplantation with reduced intensity conditioning is an appealing concept in patients with HLH and has shown promise in a small number of patients.[281]

Conclusions

HLH is an acute, rapidly progressive, potentially life-threatening syndrome. The clinical features are attributable to immunologic dysregulation, but the underlying mechanisms are diverse. Prompt recognition and initiation of therapy is warranted, even when diagnostic certainty is elusive. Initial therapy using etoposide and corticosteroids, with or without cyclosporine A, is the standard of care in the United States. Analysis for defects in the genes known to be associated with the condition should be undertaken, although only about half of familial cases will have a confirmatory genetic test. Assessment for triggers of secondary HLH should be pursued, although identification of an infectious trigger does not reliably differentiate familial from secondary HLH. Children who have been determined to have FHL on the basis of a positive family history, the finding of a genetic abnormality, or refractory or relapsing course should be referred for allogeneic HST as soon as possible. Children not known to have FHL based on these criteria may be observed if they achieve disease resolution after 2 to 3 months of initial therapy (Table 24-2).

REFERENCES

1. Girolomoni G, Caux C, Lebecque S, et al. Langerhans cells: still a fundamental paradigm for studying the immunobiology of dendritic cells. Trends Immunol. 2002;23:6-8.
2. Shortman K, Naik SH. Steady-state and inflammatory dendritic-cell development. Nat Rev Immunol. 2007;7:19-30.
3. Steinman RM, Hemmi H. Dendritic cells: translating innate to adaptive immunity. Curr Top Microbiol Immunol. 2006;311: 17-58.
4. Yamazaki S, Inaba K, Tarbell KV, Steinman RM. Dendritic cells expand antigen-specific Foxp3+ CD25+ CD4+ regulatory T cells including suppressors of alloreactivity. Immunol Rev. 2006;212: 314-329.
5. Hemmi H, Yoshino M, Yamazaki H, et al. Skin antigens in the steady state are trafficked to regional lymph nodes by transforming growth factor-beta1-dependent cells. Int Immunol. 2001;13: 695-704.
6. Henri S, Vremec D, Kamath A, et al. The dendritic cell populations of mouse lymph nodes. J Immunol. 2001;167: 741-748.
7. Jakob T, Ring J, Udey MC. Multistep navigation of Langerhans/dendritic cells in and out of the skin. J Allergy Clin Immunol. 2001;108:688-696.
8. Kissenpfennig A, Henri S, Dubois B, et al. Dynamics and function of Langerhans cells in vivo: dermal dendritic cells colonize lymph node areas distinct from slower migrating Langerhans cells. Immunity. 2005;22:643-654.
9. Dieu MC, Vanbervliet B, Vicari A, et al. Selective recruitment of immature and mature dendritic cells by distinct chemokines expressed in different anatomic sites. J Exp Med. 1998;188:373-386.
10. Sallusto F, Schaerli P, Loetscher P, et al. Rapid and coordinated switch in chemokine receptor expression during dendritic cell maturation. Eur J Immunol. 1998;28:2760-2769.
11. Wilson NS, El-Sukkari D, Belz GT, et al. Most lymphoid organ dendritic cell types are phenotypically and functionally immature. Blood. 2003;102:2187-2194.

12. Vremec D, Pooley J, Hochrein H, et al. CD4 and CD8 expression by dendritic cell subtypes in mouse thymus and spleen. J Immunol. 2000;164:2978-2986.

13. Mierau GW, Favara BE, Brenman JM. Electron microscopy in histiocytosis X. Ultrastruct Pathol. 1982;3:137-142.

14. Valladeau J, Ravel O, Dezutter-Dambuyant C, et al. Langerin, a novel C-type lectin specific to Langerhans cells, is an endocytic receptor that induces the formation of Birbeck granules. Immunity. 2000;12:71-81.

15. Gavino AC, Chung JS, Sato K, et al. Identification and expression profiling of a human C-type lectin, structurally homologous to mouse dectin-2. Exp Dermatol. 2005;14:281-288.

16. Inaba K, Swiggard WJ, Inaba M, et al. Tissue distribution of the DEC-205 protein that is detected by the monoclonal antibody NLDC-145. I. Expression on dendritic cells and other subsets of mouse leukocytes. Cell Immunol. 1995;163:148-156.

17. Emile JF, Wechsler J, Brousse N, et al. Langerhans cell histiocytosis: definitive diagnosis with the use of monoclonal antibody O10 on routinely paraffin-embedded samples. Am J Surg Pathol. 1995;19:636-641.

18. Diao J, Winter E, Cantin C, et al. In situ replication of immediate dendritic cell (DC) precursors contributes to conventional DC homeostasis in lymphoid tissue. J Immunol. 2006;176:7196-7206.

19. Naik SH, Metcalf D, van Nieuwenhuijze A, et al. Intrasplenic steady-state dendritic cell precursors that are distinct from monocytes. Nat Immunol. 2006;7:663-671.

20. Colonna M, Trinchieri G, Liu YJ. Plasmacytoid dendritic cells in immunity. Nat Immunol. 2004;5:1219-1226.

21. Sallusto F, Lanzavecchia A. Efficient presentation of soluble antigen by cultured human dendritic cells is maintained by granulocyte/macrophage colony-stimulating factor plus interleukin 4 and downregulated by tumor necrosis factor alpha. J Exp Med. 1994;179:1109-1118.

22. Manz MG, Traver D, Miyamoto T, et al. Dendritic cell potentials of early lymphoid and myeloid progenitors. Blood. 2001;97:3333-3341.

23. Traver D, Akashi K, Manz M, et al. Development of CD8alpha-positive dendritic cells from a common myeloid progenitor. Science. 2000;290:2152-2154.

24. Wu L, D'Amico A, Hochrein H, et al. Development of thymic and splenic dendritic cell populations from different hemopoietic precursors. Blood. 2001;98:3376-3382.

25. MacDonald KP, Rowe V, Bofinger HM, et al. The colony-stimulating factor 1 receptor is expressed on dendritic cells during differentiation and regulates their expansion. J Immunol. 2005; 175:1399-1405.

26. Onai N, Obata-Onai A, Tussiwand R, et al. Activation of the *Flt3* signal transduction cascade rescues and enhances type I interferon-producing and dendritic cell development. J Exp Med. 2006;203:227-238.

27. Kamath AT, Pooley J, O'Keeffe MA, et al. The development, maturation, and turnover rate of mouse spleen dendritic cell populations. J Immunol. 2000;165:6762-6770.

28. Ginhoux F, Tacke F, Angeli V, et al. Langerhans cells arise from monocytes in vivo. Nat Immunol. 2006;7:265-273.

29. Mende I, Karsunky H, Weissman IL, et al. *Flk2+* myeloid progenitors are the main source of Langerhans cells. Blood. 2006;107:1383-1390.

30. Serbina NV, Pamer EG. Monocyte emigration from bone marrow during bacterial infection requires signals mediated by chemokine receptor CCR2. Nat Immunol. 2006;7:311-317.

31. Yrlid U, Jenkins CD, MacPherson GG. Relationships between distinct blood monocyte subsets and migrating intestinal lymph dendritic cells in vivo under steady-state conditions. J Immunol. 2006;176:4155-4162.

32. Fogg DK, Sibon C, Miled C, et al. A clonogenic bone marrow progenitor specific for macrophages and dendritic cells. Science. 2006;311:83-87.

33. Janka G, Imashuku S, Elinder G, et al. Infection- and malignancy-associated hemophagocytic syndromes: secondary hemophagocytic lymphohistiocytosis. Hematol Oncol Clin North Am. 1998;12:435-444.

34. Nichols KE, Egeler RM, Perry VH, Arceci R. Summary of the 12th Nikolas Symposium dendritic cell differentiation: signals, signaling and functional consequences as clues to possible therapy. J Pediatr Hematol Oncol. 2003;25:193-197.

35. Willman CL, Busque L, Griffith BB, et al. Langerhans-cell histiocytosis (histiocytosis X): a clonal proliferative disease. N Engl J Med. 1994;331:154-160.

36. Willman CL, McClain KL. An update on clonality, cytokines, and viral etiology in Langerhans cell histiocytosis. Hematol Oncol Clin North Am. 1998;12:407-416.

37. Yu RC, Chu C, Buluwela L, Chu AC. Clonal proliferation of Langerhans cells in Langerhans cell histiocytosis. Lancet. 1994;343:767-768.

38. Betts DR, Leibundgut KE, Feldges A, et al. Cytogenetic abnormalities in Langerhans cell histiocytosis. Br J Cancer. 1998;77:552-555.

39. Weintraub M, Bhatia KG, Chandra RS, et al. p53 expression in Langerhans cell histiocytosis. J Pediatr Hematol Oncol. 1998;20:12-17.

40. Alston RD, Tatevossian RG, McNally RJ, et al. Incidence and survival of childhood Langerhans cell histiocytosis in Northwest England from 1954 to 1998. Pediatr Blood Cancer. 2007;48:555-560.

41. A multicentre retrospective survey of Langerhans cell histiocytosis: 348 cases observed between 1983 and 1993. The French Langerhans Cell Histiocytosis Study Group. Arch Dis Child. 1996;75:17-24.

42. Guyot-Goubin A, Donadieu J, Barkaoui M, et al. Descriptive epidemiology of childhood Langerhans cell histiocytosis in France, 2000-2004. Pediatr Blood Cancer. 2008;51:71-75.

43. Stalemark H, Laurencikas E, Karis J, et al. Incidence of Langerhans cell histiocytosis in children: a population-based study. Pediatr Blood Cancer. 2008;51:76-81.

44. Kilpatrick SE, Wenger DE, Gilchrist GS, et al. Langerhans cell histiocytosis (histiocytosis X) of bone: a clinicopathologic analysis of 263 pediatric and adult cases. Cancer. 1995;76:2471-2484.

45. Hamre M, Hedberg J, Buckley J, et al. Langerhans cell histiocytosis: an exploratory epidemiologic study of 177 cases. Med Pediatr Oncol. 1997;28:92-97.

46. Bhatia S, Nesbit ME Jr, Egeler RM, et al. Epidemiologic study of Langerhans cell histiocytosis in children. J Pediatr. 1997;130:774-784.

47. Arico M, Nichols K, Whitlock JA, et al. Familial clustering of Langerhans cell histiocytosis. Br J Haematol. 1999;107:883-888.

48. McClain K, Jin H, Gresik V, Favara B. Langerhans cell histiocytosis: lack of a viral etiology. Am J Hematol. 1994;47:16-20.

49. Vassallo R, Ryu JH, Colby TV, et al. Pulmonary Langerhans-cell histiocytosis. N Engl J Med. 2000;342:1969-1978.

50. Egeler RM, Neglia JP, Arico M, et al. The relation of Langerhans cell histiocytosis to acute leukemia, lymphomas, and other solid tumors. The LCH-Malignancy Study Group of the Histiocyte Society. Hematol Oncol Clin North Am. 1998;12:369-378.

51. Trebo MM, Attarbaschi A, Mann G, et al. Histiocytosis following T-acute lymphoblastic leukemia: a BFM study. Leuk Lymphoma. 2005;46:1735-1741.

52. Feldman AL, Berthold F, Arceci RJ, et al. Clonal relationship between precursor T-lymphoblastic leukaemia/lymphoma and Langerhans-cell histiocytosis. Lancet Oncol. 2005;6:435-437.

53. Rodig SJ, Payne EG, Degar BA, et al. Aggressive Langerhans cell histiocytosis following T-ALL: clonally related neoplasms with persistent expression of constitutively active NOTCH1. Am J Hematol. 2008;83:116-121.

54. Broadbent V, Egeler RM, Nesbit ME Jr. Langerhans cell histiocytosis—clinical and epidemiological aspects. Br J Cancer Suppl. 1994;23:S11-S16.

55. Lichtenstein L. Histiocytosis X: integration of eosinophilic granuloma of bone, Letterer-Siwe disease, and Schuller-Christian disease as related manifestations of a single nosologic entity. AMA Arch Pathol. 1953;56:84-102.

56. Nezelof C, Frileux-Herbet F, Cronier-Sachot J. Disseminated histiocytosis X: analysis of prognostic factors based on a retrospective study of 50 cases. Cancer. 1979;44:1824-1838.

57. Gadner H, Heitger A, Grois N, et al. Treatment strategy for disseminated Langerhans cell histiocytosis. DAL HX-83 Study Group. Med Pediatr Oncol. 1994;23:72-80.

58. Lahey ME. Histiocytosis X: comparison of three treatment regimens. J Pediatr. 1975;87:179-183.

59. Komp DM, Herson J, Starling KA, et al. A staging system for histiocytosis X: a Southwest Oncology Group Study. Cancer. 1981;47:798-800.

60. Donadieu J, Piguet C, Bernard F, et al. A new clinical score for disease activity in Langerhans cell histiocytosis. Pediatr Blood Cancer. 2004;43:770-776.

61. Titgemeyer C, Grois N, Minkov M, et al. Pattern and course of single-system disease in Langerhans cell histiocytosis data from the DAL-HX 83 and -90 study. Med Pediatr Oncol. 2001; 37:108-114.

62. Lau SK, Chu PG, Weiss LM. Immunohistochemical expression of langerin in Langerhans cell histiocytosis and non-Langerhans cell histiocytic disorders. Am J Surg Pathol. 2008;32:615-619.

63. Chikwava K, Jaffe R. Langerin (CD207) staining in normal pediatric tissues, reactive lymph nodes, and childhood histiocytic disorders. Pediatr Dev Pathol. 2004;7:607-614.

64. Takahashi K, Isobe T, Ohtsuki Y, et al. Immunohistochemical study on the distribution of alpha and beta subunits of S-100 protein in human neoplasm and normal tissues. Virchows Arch B Cell Pathol Incl Mol Pathol. 1984;45:385-396.

65. Pinkus GS, Lones MA, Matsumura F, et al. Langerhans cell histiocytosis immunohistochemical expression of fascin, a dendritic cell marker. Am J Clin Pathol. 2002;118:335-343.

66. Bollini G, Jouve JL, Gentet JC, et al. Bone lesions in histiocytosis X. J Pediatr Orthop. 1991;11:469-477.

67. Azouz EM, Saigal G, Rodriguez MM, Podda A. Langerhans cell histiocytosis: pathology, imaging and treatment of skeletal involvement. Pediatr Radiol. 2005;35:103-115.

68. Hoover KB, Rosenthal DI, Mankin H. Langerhans cell histiocytosis. Skeletal Radiol. 2007;36:95-104.

69. Binkovitz LA, Olshefski RS, Adler BH. Coincidence FDG-PET in the evaluation of Langerhans cell histiocytosis: preliminary findings. Pediatr Radiol. 2003;33:598-602.

70. Blum R, Seymour JF, Hicks RJ. Role of 18FDG-positron emission tomography scanning in the management of histiocytosis. Leuk Lymphoma. 2002;43:2155-2157.

71. Walia M, Paul P, Mishra S, Mehta R. Congenital Langerhans cell histiocytosis: the self-healing variety. J Pediatr Hematol Oncol. 2004;26:398-402.

72. Minkov M, Prosch H, Steiner M, et al. Langerhans cell histiocytosis in neonates. Pediatr Blood Cancer. 2005;45:802-807.

73. Lau L, Krafchik B, Trebo MM, Weitzman S. Cutaneous Langerhans cell histiocytosis in children under one year. Pediatr Blood Cancer. 2006;46:66-71.

74. Grois N, Prayer D, Prosch H, Lassmann H. Neuropathology of CNS disease in Langerhans cell histiocytosis. Brain. 2005;128: 829-838.

75. Donadieu J, Rolon MA, Thomas C, et al. Endocrine involvement in pediatric-onset Langerhans cell histiocytosis: a population-based study. J Pediatr. 2004;144:344-350.

76. Grois N, Potschger U, Prosch H, et al. Risk factors for diabetes insipidus in Langerhans cell histiocytosis. Pediatr Blood Cancer. 2006;46:228-233.

77. Maghnie M, Cosi G, Genovese E, et al. Central diabetes insipidus in children and young adults. N Engl J Med. 2000;343:998-1007.

78. Prosch H, Grois N, Prayer D, et al. Central diabetes insipidus as presenting symptom of Langerhans cell histiocytosis. Pediatr Blood Cancer. 2004;43:594-599.

79. Ottaviano F, Finlay JL. Diabetes insipidus and Langerhans cell histiocytosis: a case report of reversibility with 2-chlorodeoxyadenosine. J Pediatr Hematol Oncol. 2003;25:575-577.

80. Rosenzweig KE, Arceci RJ, Tarbell NJ. Diabetes insipidus secondary to Langerhans cell histiocytosis: is radiation therapy indicated? Med Pediatr Oncol. 1997;29:36-40.

81. Dhall G, Finlay JL, Dunkel IJ, et al. Analysis of outcome for patients with mass lesions of the central nervous system due to Langerhans cell histiocytosis treated with 2-chlorodeoxyadenosine. Pediatr Blood Cancer. 2008;50:72-79.

82. Barthez MA, Araujo E, Donadieu J. Langerhans cell histiocytosis and the central nervous system in childhood: evolution and prognostic factors: results of a collaborative study. J Child Neurol. 2000;15:150-156.

83. Favara BE, Jaffe R, Egeler RM. Macrophage activation and hemophagocytic syndrome in Langerhans cell histiocytosis: report of 30 cases. Pediatr Dev Pathol. 2002;5:130-140.

84. McClain K, Ramsay NK, Robison L, et al. Bone marrow involvement in histiocytosis X. Med Pediatr Oncol. 1983;11:167-171.

85. Minkov M, Potschger U, Grois N, et al. Bone marrow assessment in Langerhans cell histiocytosis. Pediatr Blood Cancer. 2007;49: 694-698.

86. Jaffe R. Liver involvement in the histiocytic disorders of childhood. Pediatr Dev Pathol. 2004;7:214-225.

87. Braier J, Ciocca M, Latella A, et al. Cholestasis, sclerosing cholangitis, and liver transplantation in Langerhans cell Histiocytosis. Med Pediatr Oncol. 2002;38:178-182.

88. Ha SY, Helms P, Fletcher M, et al. Lung involvement in Langerhans cell histiocytosis: prevalence, clinical features, and outcome. Pediatrics. 1992;89:466-469.

89. Braier J, Latella A, Balancini B, et al. Outcome in children with pulmonary Langerhans cell Histiocytosis. Pediatr Blood Cancer. 2004;43:765-769.

90. Odame I, Li P, Lau L, et al. Pulmonary Langerhans cell histiocytosis: a variable disease in childhood. Pediatr Blood Cancer. 2006;47:889-893.

91. Hait E, Liang M, Degar B, et al. Gastrointestinal tract involvement in Langerhans cell histiocytosis: case report and literature review. Pediatrics. 2006;118:e1593-e1599.

92. Nanduri VR, Kelly K, Malone M, et al. Colon involvement in Langerhans cell histiocytosis. J Pediatr Gastroenterol Nutr. 1999;29:462-466.

93. Geissmann F, Thomas C, Emile JF, et al. Digestive tract involvement in Langerhans cell histiocytosis. The French Langerhans Cell Histiocytosis Study Group. J Pediatr. 1996;129:836-845.

94. Laman JD, Leenen PJ, Annels NE, et al. Langerhans-cell histiocytosis: insight into DC biology. Trends Immunol. 2003;24: 190-196.

95. Nauert C, Zornoza J, Ayala A, Harle TS. Eosinophilic granuloma of bone: diagnosis and management. Skeletal Radiol. 1983;10: 227-235.

96. Slater JM, Swarm OJ. Eosinophilic granuloma of bone. Med Pediatr Oncol. 1980;8:151-164.

97. Womer RB, Raney RB Jr, D'Angio GJ. Healing rates of treated and untreated bone lesions in histiocytosis X. Pediatrics. 1985;76:286-288.

98. Cohen M, Zornoza J, Cangir A, et al. Direct injection of methyl-prednisolone sodium succinate in the treatment of solitary eosinophilic granuloma of bone: a report of 9 cases. Radiology. 1980;136:289-293.

99. Capanna R, Springfield DS, Ruggieri P, et al. Direct cortisone injection in eosinophilic granuloma of bone: a preliminary report on 11 patients. J Pediatr Orthop. 1985;5:339-342.

100. Egeler RM, Thompson RC Jr, Voute PA, Nesbit ME Jr. Intralesional infiltration of corticosteroids in localized Langerhans cell histiocytosis. J Pediatr Orthop. 1992;12:811-814.

101. Richter MP, D'Angio GJ. The role of radiation therapy in the management of children with histiocytosis X. Am J Pediatr Hematol Oncol. 1981;3:161-163.

102. Gramatovici R, D'Angio GJ. Radiation therapy in soft-tissue lesions in histiocytosis X (Langerhans cell histiocytosis). Med Pediatr Oncol. 1988;16:259-262.

103. Jubran RF, Marachelian A, Dorey F, Malogolowkin M. Predictors of outcome in children with Langerhans cell histiocytosis. Pediatr Blood Cancer. 2005;45:37-42.

104. Levine SE, Dormans JP, Meyer JS, Corcoran TA. Langerhans cell histiocytosis of the spine in children. Clin Orthop Relat Res. 1996:288-293.

105. Sheehan MP, Atherton DJ, Broadbent V, Pritchard J. Topical nitrogen mustard: an effective treatment for cutaneous Langerhans cell histiocytosis. J Pediatr. 1991;119:317-321.

106. Kwon OS, Cho KH, Song KY. Primary cutaneous Langerhans cell histiocytosis treated with photochemotherapy. J Dermatol. 1997;24:54-56.

107. Munn S, Chu AC. Langerhans cell histiocytosis of the skin. Hematol Oncol Clin North Am. 1998;12:269-286.

108. Kwong YL, Chan AC, Chan TK. Widespread skin-limited Langerhans cell histiocytosis: complete remission with interferon alfa. J Am Acad Dermatol. 1997;36:628-629.

109. Avioli LV, Lasersohn JT, Lopresti JM. Histiocytosis X (Schuller-Christian disease): a clinico-pathological survey, review of ten patients and the results of prednisone therapy. Medicine (Baltimore). 1963;42:119-147.

110. Beier FR, Thatcher LG, Lahey ME. Treatment of Reticuloendotheliosis with vinblastine sulfate: preliminary report. J Pediatr. 1963;63:1087-1092.

111. Starling KA, Donaldson MH, Haggard ME, et al. Therapy of histiocytosis X with vincristine, vinblastine, and cyclophosphamide. The Southwest Cancer Chemotherapy Study Group. Am J Dis Child. 1972;123:105-110.

112. Lahey ME, Heyn RM, Newton WA Jr, et al. Histiocytosis X: clinical trial of chlorambucil: a report from Children's Cancer Study Group. Med Pediatr Oncol. 1979;7:197-203.

113. Jones B, Kung F, Chevalier L, et al. Chemotherapy of reticuloendotheliosis: comparison of methotrexate plus prednisone vs. vincristine plus prednisone. Cancer. 1974;34:1011-1017.

114. Gadner H, Grois N, Arico M, et al. A randomized trial of treatment for multisystem Langerhans cell histiocytosis. J Pediatr. 2001;138:728-734.

115. Ceci A, de Terlizzi M, Colella R, et al. Etoposide in recurrent childhood Langerhans cell histiocytosis: an Italian cooperative study. Cancer. 1988;62:2528-2531.

116. Broadbent V, Pritchard J, Yeomans E. Etoposide (VP16) in the treatment of multisystem Langerhans cell histiocytosis (histiocytosis X). Med Pediatr Oncol. 1989;17:97-100.

117. Viana MB, Oliveira BM, Silva CM, Rios Leite VH. Etoposide in the treatment of six children with Langerhans cell histiocytosis (histiocytosis X). Med Pediatr Oncol. 1991;19:289-294.

118. Ladisch S, Gadner H, Arico M, et al. LCH-I: a randomized trial of etoposide vs. vinblastine in disseminated Langerhans cell histiocytosis. The Histiocyte Society. Med Pediatr Oncol. 1994;23:107-110.

119. Stine KC, Saylors RL, Saccente S, et al. Efficacy of continuous infusion 2-CDA (cladribine) in pediatric patients with Langerhans cell histiocytosis. Pediatr Blood Cancer. 2004;43:81-84.

120. Stine KC, Saylors RL, Williams LL, Becton DL. 2-Chlorodeoxyadenosine (2-CDA) for the treatment of refractory or recurrent Langerhans cell histiocytosis (LCH) in pediatric patients. Med Pediatr Oncol. 1997;29:288-292.

121. Weitzman S, Wayne AS, Arceci R, et al. Nucleoside analogues in the therapy of Langerhans cell histiocytosis: a survey of members of the histiocyte society and review of the literature. Med Pediatr Oncol. 1999;33:476-481.

122. Bernard F, Thomas C, Bertrand Y, et al. Multi-centre pilot study of 2-chlorodeoxyadenosine and cytosine arabinoside combined chemotherapy in refractory Langerhans cell histiocytosis with haematological dysfunction. Eur J Cancer. 2005;41:2682-2689.

123. Saven A, Burian C. Cladribine activity in adult Langerhans-cell histiocytosis. Blood. 1999;93:4125-4130.

124. Komp DM, Silva-Sosa M, Miale T, et al. Evaluation of a MOPP-type regimen in histiocytosis X: a Southwest Oncology Group study. Cancer Treat Rep. 1977;61:855-859.

125. Egeler RM, de Kraker J, Voute PA. Cytosine-arabinoside, vincristine, and prednisolone in the treatment of children with disseminated Langerhans cell histiocytosis with organ dysfunction: experience at a single institution. Med Pediatr Oncol. 1993;21:265-270.

126. Minkov M, Grois N, Heitger A, et al. Treatment of multisystem Langerhans cell histiocytosis: results of the DAL-HX 83 and DAL-HX 90 studies. DAL-HX Study Group. Klin Padiatr. 2000;212:139-144.

127. Minkov M, Grois N, Heitger A, et al. Response to initial treatment of multisystem Langerhans cell histiocytosis: an important prognostic indicator. Med Pediatr Oncol. 2002;39:581-585.

128. Gadner H, Grois N, Potschger U, et al. Improved outcome in multisystem Langerhans cell histiocytosis is associated with therapy intensification. Blood. 2008;111:2556-2562.

129. Pollono D, Rey G, Latella A, et al. Reactivation and risk of sequelae in Langerhans cell histiocytosis. Pediatr Blood Cancer. 2007;48:696-699.

130. Calming U, Henter JI. Elevated erythrocyte sedimentation rate and thrombocytosis as possible indicators of active disease in Langerhans cell histiocytosis. Acta Paediatr. 1998;87:1085-1087.

131. Minkov M, Steiner M, Potschger U, et al. Reactivations in multisystem Langerhans cell histiocytosis: data of the International LCH Registry. J Pediatr. 2008; June 25 (E-pub ahead of print).

132. Farran RP, Zaretski E, Egeler RM. Treatment of Langerhans cell histiocytosis with pamidronate. J Pediatr Hematol Oncol. 2001;23:54-56.

133. Arzoo K, Sadeghi S, Pullarkat V. Pamidronate for bone pain from osteolytic lesions in Langerhans-cell histiocytosis. N Engl J Med. 2001;345:225.

134. McClain KL, Kozinetz CA. A phase II trial using thalidomide for Langerhans cell histiocytosis. Pediatr Blood Cancer. 2007;48:44-49.

135. Lau LM, Stuurman K, Weitzman S. Skeletal Langerhans cell histiocytosis in children: permanent consequences and health-related quality of life in long-term survivors. Pediatr Blood Cancer. 2008;50:607-612.

136. Mottl H, Stary J, Chanova M, et al. Treatment of recurrent Langerhans cell histiocytosis in children with 2-chlorodeoxyadenosine. Leuk Lymphoma. 2006;47:1881-1884.

137. Stoll M, Freund M, Schmid H, et al. Allogeneic bone marrow transplantation for Langerhans cell histiocytosis. Cancer. 1990;66:284-288.

138. Greinix HT, Storb R, Sanders JE, Petersen FB. Marrow transplantation for treatment of multisystem progressive Langerhans cell histiocytosis. Bone Marrow Transplant. 1992; 10:39-44.

139. Nagarajan R, Neglia J, Ramsay N, Baker KS. Successful treatment of refractory Langerhans cell histiocytosis with unrelated cord blood transplantation. J Pediatr Hematol Oncol. 2001;23: 629-632.

140. Suminoe A, Matsuzaki A, Hattori H, et al. Unrelated cord blood transplantation for an infant with chemotherapy-resistant progressive Langerhans cell histiocytosis. J Pediatr Hematol Oncol. 2001;23:633-636.

141. Akkari V, Donadieu J, Piguet C, et al. Hematopoietic stem cell transplantation in patients with severe Langerhans cell histiocytosis and hematological dysfunction: experience of the French Langerhans Cell Study Group. Bone Marrow Transplant. 2003;31:1097-1103.

142. Steiner M, Matthes-Martin S, Attarbaschi A, et al. Improved outcome of treatment-resistant high-risk Langerhans cell histiocytosis after allogeneic stem cell transplantation with reduced-intensity conditioning. Bone Marrow Transplant. 2005;36: 215-225.

143. Willis B, Ablin A, Weinberg V, et al. Disease course and late sequelae of Langerhans cell histiocytosis: 25-year experience at the University of California, San Francisco. J Clin Oncol. 1996;14:2073-2082.

144. Haupt R, Nanduri V, Calevo MG, et al. Permanent consequences in Langerhans cell histiocytosis patients: a pilot study from the Histiocyte Society-Late Effects Study Group. Pediatr Blood Cancer. 2004;42:438-444.

145. Bernstrand C, Cederlund K, Sandstedt B, et al. Pulmonary abnormalities at long-term follow-up of patients with Langerhans cell histiocytosis. Med Pediatr Oncol. 2001;36:459-468.

146. Nanduri VR, Lillywhite L, Chapman C, et al. Cognitive outcome of long-term survivors of multisystem Langerhans cell histiocytosis: a single-institution, cross-sectional study. J Clin Oncol. 2003;21:2961-2967.

147. Mittheisz E, Seidl R, Prayer D, et al. Central nervous system-related permanent consequences in patients with Langerhans cell histiocytosis. Pediatr Blood Cancer. 2007;48:50-56.

148. Imashuku S, Okazaki NA, Nakayama M, et al. Treatment of neurodegenerative CNS disease in Langerhans cell histiocytosis with a combination of intravenous immunoglobulin and chemotherapy. Pediatr Blood Cancer. 2008;50:308-311.

149. Weitzman S, Jaffe R. Uncommon histiocytic disorders: the non-Langerhans cell histiocytoses. Pediatr Blood Cancer. 2005;45: 256-264.

150. Caputo R, Marzano AV, Passoni E, Berti E. Unusual variants of non-Langerhans cell histiocytoses. J Am Acad Dermatol. 2007; 57:1031-1045.

151. Pileri SA, Grogan TM, Harris NL, et al. Tumours of histiocytes and accessory dendritic cells: an immunohistochemical approach to classification from the International Lymphoma Study Group based on 61 cases. Histopathology. 2002;41:1-29.

152. Janssen D, Harms D. Juvenile xanthogranuloma in childhood and adolescence: a clinicopathologic study of 129 patients from the Kiel pediatric tumor registry. Am J Surg Pathol. 2005;29: 21-28.

153. Burgdorf WH, Zelger B. JXG, NF1, and JMML: alphabet soup or a clinical issue? Pediatr Dermatol. 2004;21:174-176.

154. Dehner LP. Juvenile xanthogranulomas in the first two decades of life: a clinicopathologic study of 174 cases with cutaneous and extracutaneous manifestations. Am J Surg Pathol. 2003;27: 579-593.

155. Freyer DR, Kennedy R, Bostrom BC, et al. Juvenile xanthogranuloma: forms of systemic disease and their clinical implications. J Pediatr. 1996;129:227-237.

156. Auvin S, Cuvellier JC, Vinchon M, et al. Subdural effusion in a CNS involvement of systemic juvenile xanthogranuloma: a case report treated with vinblastin. Brain Dev. 2008;30:164-168.

157. Unuvar E, Devecioglu O, Akcay A, et al. Successful therapy of systemic xanthogranuloma in a child. J Pediatr Hematol Oncol. 2007;29:425-427.

158. Nakatani T, Morimoto A, Kato R, et al. Successful treatment of congenital systemic juvenile xanthogranuloma with Langerhans cell histiocytosis-based chemotherapy. J Pediatr Hematol Oncol. 2004;26:371-374.

159. Rosai J, Dorfman RF. Sinus histiocytosis with massive lymphadenopathy: a pseudolymphomatous benign disorder. Analysis of 34 cases. Cancer. 1972;30:1174-1188.

160. Sanchez R, Sibley RK, Rosai J, Dorfman RF. The electron microscopic features of sinus histiocytosis with massive lymphadenopathy: a study of 11 cases. Ultrastruct Pathol. 1981;2:101-119.

161. Foucar E, Rosai J, Dorfman R. Sinus histiocytosis with massive lymphadenopathy (Rosai-Dorfman disease): review of the entity. Semin Diagn Pathol. 1990;7:19-73.

162. Foucar E, Rosai J, Dorfman RF. The ophthalmologic manifestations of sinus histiocytosis with massive lymphadenopathy. Am J Ophthalmol. 1979;87:354-367.

163. Foucar E, Rosai J, Dorfman RF, Brynes RK. The neurologic manifestations of sinus histiocytosis with massive lymphadenopathy. Neurology. 1982;32:365-372.

164. Foucar E, Rosai J, Dorfman RF, Eyman JM. Immunologic abnormalities and their significance in sinus histiocytosis with massive lymphadenopathy. Am J Clin Pathol. 1984;82:515-525.

165. Foucar E, Rosai J, Dorfman RF. Sinus histiocytosis with massive lymphadenopathy. An analysis of 14 deaths occurring in a patient registry. Cancer. 1984;54:1834-1840.

166. Pulsoni A, Anghel G, Falcucci P, et al. Treatment of sinus histiocytosis with massive lymphadenopathy (Rosai-Dorfman disease): report of a case and literature review. Am J Hematol. 2002;69:67-71.

167. Gordon S, Taylor PR. Monocyte and macrophage heterogeneity. Nat Rev Immunol. 2005;5:953-964.

168. Taylor PR, Martinez-Pomares L, Stacey M, et al. Macrophage receptors and immune recognition. Annu Rev Immunol. 2005; 23:901-944.

169. Kraal G. Cells in the marginal zone of the spleen. Int Rev Cytol. 1992;132:31-74.

170. Taylor PR, Zamze S, Stillion RJ, et al. Development of a specific system for targeting protein to metallophilic macrophages. Proc Natl Acad Sci U S A. 2004;101:1963-1968.

171. Geijtenbeek TB, Groot PC, Nolte MA, et al. Marginal zone macrophages express a murine homologue of DC-SIGN that captures blood-borne antigens in vivo. Blood. 2002;100:2908-2916.

172. Kang YS, Yamazaki S, Iyoda T, et al. SIGN-R1, a novel C-type lectin expressed by marginal zone macrophages in spleen, mediates uptake of the polysaccharide dextran. Int Immunol. 2003;15:177-186.

173. van der Laan LJ, Dopp EA, Haworth R, et al. Regulation and functional involvement of macrophage scavenger receptor MARCO in clearance of bacteria in vivo. J Immunol. 1999;162: 939-947.

174. Hume DA, Robinson AP, MacPherson GG, Gordon S. The mononuclear phagocyte system of the mouse defined by immunohistochemical localization of antigen F4/80: relationship between macrophages, Langerhans cells, reticular cells, and dendritic cells in lymphoid and hematopoietic organs. J Exp Med. 1983;158:1522-1536.

175. Goerdt S, Orfanos CE. Other functions, other genes: alternative activation of antigen-presenting cells. Immunity. 1999;10:137-142.

176. Gordon S. Alternative activation of macrophages. Nat Rev Immunol. 2003;3:23-35.

177. Mosser DM. The many faces of macrophage activation. J Leukoc Biol. 2003;73:209-212.

178. Bechan GI, Egeler RM, Arceci RJ. Biology of Langerhans cells and Langerhans cell histiocytosis. Int Rev Cytol. 2006;254:1-43.

179. van oud Alblas AB, van Furth R. Origin, kinetics, and characteristics of pulmonary macrophages in the normal steady state. J Exp Med. 1979;149:1504-1518.

180. Grage-Griebenow E, Flad HD, Ernst M. Heterogeneity of human peripheral blood monocyte subsets. J Leukoc Biol. 2001;69:11-20.

181. Geissmann F, Jung S, Littman DR. Blood monocytes consist of two principal subsets with distinct migratory properties. Immunity. 2003;19:71-82.

182. Matsuzaki K, Udagawa N, Takahashi N, et al. Osteoclast differentiation factor (ODF) induces osteoclast-like cell formation in human peripheral blood mononuclear cell cultures. Biochem Biophys Res Commun. 1998;246:199-204.

183. Farquhar JW, Claireaux AE. Familial haemophagocytic reticulosis. Arch Dis Child. 1952;27:519-525.

184. Marrian VJ, Sanerkin NG. Familial histiocytic reticulosis (familial haemophagocytic reticulosis). J Clin Pathol. 1963;16:65-69.

185. Nelson P, Santamaria A, Olson RL, Nayak NC. Generalized lymphohistiocytic infiltration: a familial disease not previously described and different from Letterer-Siwe disease and Chediak-Higashi syndrome. Pediatrics. 1961;27:931-950.

186. Risdall RJ, McKenna RW, Nesbit ME, et al. Virus-associated hemophagocytic syndrome: a benign histiocytic proliferation distinct from malignant histiocytosis. Cancer. 1979;44:993-1002.

187. Risdall RJ, Brunning RD, Hernandez JI, Gordon DH. Bacteria-associated hemophagocytic syndrome. Cancer. 1984;54:2968-2972.

188. Reiner AP, Spivak JL. Hematophagic histiocytosis: a report of 23 new patients and a review of the literature. Medicine (Baltimore). 1988;67:369-388.

189. Writing Group of the Histiocyte Society. Histiocytosis syndromes in children. Lancet. 1987;1:208-209.

190. Henter JI, Horne A, Arico M, et al. HLH-2004: Diagnostic and therapeutic guidelines for hemophagocytic lymphohistiocytosis. Pediatr Blood Cancer. 2007;48:124-131.

191. Henter JI, Elinder G, Soder O, Ost A. Incidence in Sweden and clinical features of familial hemophagocytic lymphohistiocytosis. Acta Paediatr Scand. 1991;80:428-435.

192. Clementi R, Emmi L, Maccario R, et al. Adult onset and atypical presentation of hemophagocytic lymphohistiocytosis in siblings carrying PRF1 mutations. Blood. 2002;100:2266-2267.

193. Allen M, De Fusco C, Legrand F, et al. Familial hemophagocytic lymphohistiocytosis: how late can the onset be? Haematologica. 2001;86:499-503.

194. Gencik A, Signer E, Muller H. Genetic analysis of familial erythrophagocytic lymphohistiocytosis. Eur J Pediatr. 1984;142:248-252.

195. Ohadi M, Lalloz MR, Sham P, et al. Localization of a gene for familial hemophagocytic lymphohistiocytosis at chromosome 9q21.3-22 by homozygosity mapping. Am J Hum Genet. 1999;64:165-171.

196. Stepp SE, Dufourcq-Lagelouse R, Le Deist F, et al. Perforin gene defects in familial hemophagocytic lymphohistiocytosis. Science. 1999;286:1957-1959.

197. Trizzino A, zur Stadt U, Ueda I, et al. Genotype-phenotype study of familial haemophagocytic lymphohistiocytosis due to perforin mutations. J Med Genet. 2008;45:15-21.

198. Stepp SE, Mathew PA, Bennett M, et al. Perforin: more than just an effector molecule. Immunol Today. 2000;21:254-256.

199. Risma KA, Frayer RW, Filipovich AH, Sumegi J. Aberrant maturation of mutant perforin underlies the clinical diversity of hemophagocytic lymphohistiocytosis. J Clin Invest. 2006;116:182-192.

200. zur Stadt U, Schmidt S, Kasper B, et al. Linkage of familial hemophagocytic lymphohistiocytosis (FHL) type-4 to chromosome 6q24 and identification of mutations in syntaxin 11. Hum Mol Genet. 2005;14:827-834.

201. Feldmann J, Callebaut I, Raposo G, et al. Munc13-4 is essential for cytolytic granules fusion and is mutated in a form of familial hemophagocytic lymphohistiocytosis (FHL3). Cell. 2003;115:461-473.

202. Rudd E, Bryceson YT, Zheng C, et al. Spectrum, and clinical and functional implications of UNC13D mutations in familial haemophagocytic lymphohistiocytosis. J Med Genet. 2008;45:134-141.

203. Zikich D, Mezer A, Varoqueaux F, et al. Vesicle priming and recruitment by ubMunc13-2 are differentially regulated by calcium and calmodulin. J Neurosci. 2008;28:1949-1960.

204. Basu J, Betz A, Brose N, Rosenmund C. Munc13-1 C1 domain activation lowers the energy barrier for synaptic vesicle fusion. J Neurosci. 2007;27:1200-1210.

205. Bryceson YT, Rudd E, Zheng C, et al. Defective cytotoxic lymphocyte degranulation in syntaxin-11 deficient familial hemophagocytic lymphohistiocytosis 4 (FHL4) patients. Blood. 2007;110:1906-1915.

206. Zur Stadt U, Beutel K, Kolberg S, et al. Mutation spectrum in children with primary hemophagocytic lymphohistiocytosis: molecular and functional analyses of PRF1, UNC13D, STX11, and RAB27A. Hum Mutat. 2006;27:62-68.

207. Goransdotter Ericson K, Fadeel B, Nilsson-Ardnor S, et al. Spectrum of perforin gene mutations in familial hemophagocytic lymphohistiocytosis. Am J Hum Genet. 2001;68:590-597.

208. Rudd E, Goransdotter Ericson K, Zheng C, et al. Spectrum and clinical implications of syntaxin 11 gene mutations in familial haemophagocytic lymphohistiocytosis: association with disease-free remissions and haematopoietic malignancies. J Med Genet. 2006;43:e14.

209. Rubin CM, Burke BA, McKenna RW, et al. The accelerated phase of Chédiak-Higashi syndrome: an expression of the virus-associated hemophagocytic syndrome? Cancer. 1985;56:524-530.

210. Menasche G, Pastural E, Feldmann J, et al. Mutations in RAB27A cause Griscelli syndrome associated with haemophagocytic syndrome. Nat Genet. 2000;25:173-176.

211. Kumar M, Sackey K, Schmalstieg F, et al. Griscelli syndrome: rare neonatal syndrome of recurrent hemophagocytosis. J Pediatr Hematol Oncol. 2001;23:464-468.

212. Duval M, Fenneteau O, Doireau V, et al. Intermittent hemophagocytic lymphohistiocytosis is a regular feature of lysinuric protein intolerance. J Pediatr. 1999;134:236-239.

213. Arico M, Imashuku S, Clementi R, et al. Hemophagocytic lymphohistiocytosis due to germline mutations in SH2D1A, the X-linked lymphoproliferative disease gene. Blood. 2001;97:1131-1133.

214. Neeft M, Wieffer M, de Jong AS, et al. Munc13-4 is an effector of rab27a and controls secretion of lysosomes in hematopoietic cells. Mol Biol Cell. 2005;16:731-741.

215. Coffey AJ, Brooksbank RA, Brandau O, et al. Host response to EBV infection in X-linked lymphoproliferative disease results from mutations in an SH2-domain encoding gene. Nat Genet. 1998;20:129-135.

216. Torrents D, Mykkanen J, Pineda M, et al. Identification of SLC7A7, encoding y+LAT-1, as the lysinuric protein intolerance gene. Nat Genet. 1999;21:293-296.

217. Rajagopala S, Dutta U, Chandra KS, et al. Visceral leishmaniasis associated hemophagocytic Lymphohistiocytosis: case report and systematic review. J Infect. 2008;56:381-388.

218. Janka GE. Familial hemophagocytic lymphohistiocytosis. Eur J Pediatr. 1983;140:221-230.

219. Yin JA, Kumaran TO, Marsh GW, et al. Complete recovery of histiocytic medullary reticulosis-like syndrome in a child with acute lymphoblastic leukemia. Cancer. 1983;51:200-202.

220. Petterson TE, Bosco AA, Cohn RJ. Aggressive natural killer cell leukemia presenting with hemophagocytic lymphohistiocytosis. Pediatr Blood Cancer. 2008;50:654-657.

221. Tong H, Ren Y, Liu H, et al. Clinical characteristics of T-cell lymphoma associated with hemophagocytic syndrome: comparison of T-cell lymphoma with and without hemophagocytic syndrome. Leuk Lymphoma. 2008;49:81-87.

222. Hadchouel M, Prieur AM, Griscelli C. Acute hemorrhagic, hepatic, and neurologic manifestations in juvenile rheumatoid arthritis: possible relationship to drugs or infection. J Pediatr. 1985;106:561-566.

223. Avcin T, Tse SM, Schneider R, et al. Macrophage activation syndrome as the presenting manifestation of rheumatic diseases in childhood. J Pediatr. 2006;148:683-686.

224. Sawhney S, Woo P, Murray KJ. Macrophage activation syndrome: a potentially fatal complication of rheumatic disorders. Arch Dis Child. 2001;85:421-426.

225. Ravelli A. Macrophage activation syndrome. Curr Opin Rheumatol. 2002;14:548-552.

226. Hazen MM, Woodward AL, Hofmann I, et al. Mutations of the hemophagocytic lymphohistiocytosis-associated gene UNC13D in a patient with systemic juvenile idiopathic arthritis. Arthritis Rheum. 2008;58:567-570.

227. Donn R, Ellison S, Lamb R, et al. Genetic loci contributing to hemophagocytic lymphohistiocytosis do not confer susceptibility to systemic-onset juvenile idiopathic arthritis. Arthritis Rheum. 2008;58:869-874.

228. Ansbacher LE, Singsen BH, Hosler MW, et al. Familial erythrophagocytic lymphohistiocytosis: an association with serum lipid abnormalities. J Pediatr. 1983;102:270-273.

229. Brown RE, Bowman WP, D'Cruz CA, et al. Endoperoxidation, hyperprostaglandinemia, and hyperlipidemia in a case of erythrophagocytic lymphohistiocytosis: reversal with VP-16 and indomethacin. Cancer. 1987;60:2388-2393.

230. McClure PD, Strachan P, Saunders EF. Hypofibrinogenemia and thrombocytopenia in familial hemophagocytic reticulosis. J Pediatr. 1974;85:67-70.

231. Rooms L, Fitzgerald N, McClain KL. Hemophagocytic lymphohistiocytosis masquerading as child abuse: presentation of three cases and review of central nervous system findings in hemophagocytic lymphohistiocytosis. Pediatrics. 2003;111:e636-e640.

232. Esumi N, Ikushima S, Hibi S, et al. High serum ferritin level as a marker of malignant histiocytosis and virus-associated hemophagocytic syndrome. Cancer. 1988;61:2071-2076.

233. Esumi N, Ikushima S, Todo S, Imashuku S. Hyperferritinemia in malignant histiocytosis and virus-associated hemophagocytic syndrome. N Engl J Med. 1987;316:346-347.

234. Allen CE, Yu X, Kozinetz CA, McClain KL. Highly elevated ferritin levels and the diagnosis of hemophagocytic lymphohistiocytosis. Pediatr Blood Cancer. 2008;50:1227-1235.

235. Henter JI. Pronounced hyperferritinemia: expanding the field of hemophagocytic lymphohistiocytosis. Pediatr Blood Cancer. 2008;50:1127-1129.

236. Zandman-Goddard G, Shoenfeld Y. Ferritin in autoimmune diseases. Autoimmun Rev. 2007;6:457-463.

237. Arico M, Janka G, Fischer A, et al. Hemophagocytic Lymphohistiocytosis: report of 122 children from the International Registry, FHL Study Group of the Histiocyte Society. Leukemia. 1996;10:197-203.

238. Kataoka Y, Todo S, Morioka Y, et al. Impaired natural killer activity and expression of interleukin-2 receptor antigen in familial erythrophagocytic lymphohistiocytosis. Cancer. 1990;65:1937-1941.

239. Henter JI, Elinder G, Soder O, et al. Hypercytokinemia in familial hemophagocytic lymphohistiocytosis. Blood. 1991;78:2918-2922.

240. Imashuku S, Hibi S, Fujiwara F, Todo S. Hyper-interleukin (IL)-6-naemia in haemophagocytic lymphohistiocytosis. Br J Haematol. 1996;93:803-807.

241. Komp DM, McNamara J, Buckley P. Elevated soluble interleukin-2 receptor in childhood hemophagocytic histiocytic syndromes. Blood. 1989;73:2128-2132.

242. Perez N, Virelizier JL, Arenzana-Seisdedos F, et al. Impaired natural killer activity in lymphohistiocytosis syndrome. J Pediatr. 1984;104:569-573.

243. Schneider EM, Lorenz I, Muller-Rosenberger M, et al. Hemophagocytic lymphohistiocytosis is associated with deficiencies of cellular cytolysis but normal expression of transcripts relevant to killer-cell-induced apoptosis. Blood. 2002;100:2891-2898.

244. Horne A, Zheng C, Lorenz I, et al. Subtyping of natural killer cell cytotoxicity deficiencies in haemophagocytic lymphohistiocytosis provides therapeutic guidance. Br J Haematol. 2005;129:658-666.

245. Imashuku S, Hyakuna N, Funabiki T, et al. Low natural killer activity and central nervous system disease as a high-risk prognostic indicator in young patients with hemophagocytic lymphohistiocytosis. Cancer. 2002;94:3023-3031.

246. Ishii E, Ueda I, Shirakawa R, et al. Genetic subtypes of familial hemophagocytic lymphohistiocytosis: correlations with clinical features and cytotoxic T lymphocyte/natural killer cell functions. Blood. 2005;105:3442-3448.

247. Marcenaro S, Gallo F, Martini S, et al. Analysis of natural killer-cell function in familial hemophagocytic lymphohistiocytosis (FHL): defective CD107a surface expression heralds Munc13-4 defect and discriminates between genetic subtypes of the disease. Blood. 2006;108:2316-2323.

248. Goo HW, Weon YC. A spectrum of neuroradiological findings in children with haemophagocytic lymphohistiocytosis. Pediatr Radiol. 2007;37:1110-1117.

249. Horne A, Trottestam H, Arico M, et al. Frequency and spectrum of central nervous system involvement in 193 children with haemophagocytic lymphohistiocytosis. Br J Haematol. 2008;140:327-335.

250. Arico M, Caselli D, Burgio GR. Familial hemophagocytic lymphohistiocytosis: clinical features. Pediatr Hematol Oncol. 1989;6:247-251.

251. Haddad E, Sulis ML, Jabado N, et al. Frequency and severity of central nervous system lesions in hemophagocytic lymphohistiocytosis. Blood. 1997;89:794-800.

252. Rostasy K, Kolb R, Pohl D, et al. CNS disease as the main manifestation of hemophagocytic lymphohistiocytosis in two children. Neuropediatrics. 2004;35:45-49.

253. Henter JI, Nennesmo I. Neuropathologic findings and neurologic symptoms in twenty-three children with hemophagocytic lymphohistiocytosis. J Pediatr. 1997;130:358-365.

254. Ambruso DR, Hays T, Zwartjes WJ, et al. Successful treatment of lymphohistiocytic reticulosis with phagocytosis with epipodophyllotoxin VP 16-213. Cancer. 1980;45:2516-2520.

255. Perry MC, Harrison EG Jr, Burgert EO Jr, Gilchrist GS. Familial erythrophagocytic lymphohistiocytosis: report of two cases and clinicopathologic review. Cancer. 1976;38:209-218.

256. Fischer A, Virelizier JL, Arenzana-Seisdedos F, et al. Treatment of four patients with erythrophagocytic lymphohistiocytosis by a combination of epipodophyllotoxin, steroids, intrathecal methotrexate, and cranial irradiation. Pediatrics. 1985;76:263-268.

257. Alvarado CS, Buchanan GR, Kim TH, et al. Use of VP-16-213 in the treatment of familial erythrophagocytic lymphohistiocytosis. Cancer. 1986;57:1097-1100.

258. Henter JI, Elinder G, Finkel Y, Soder O. Successful induction with chemotherapy including teniposide in familial erythrophagocytic lymphohistiocytosis. Lancet. 1986;2:1402.

259. Fischer A, Cerf-Bensussan N, Blanche S, et al. Allogeneic bone marrow transplantation for erythrophagocytic lymphohistiocytosis. J Pediatr. 1986;108:267-270.

260. Blanche S, Caniglia M, Girault D, et al. Treatment of hemophagocytic lymphohistiocytosis with chemotherapy and bone marrow transplantation: a single-center study of 22 cases. Blood. 1991;78:51-54.

261. Baker KS, DeLaat CA, Steinbuch M, et al. Successful correction of hemophagocytic lymphohistiocytosis with related or unrelated bone marrow transplantation. Blood. 1997;89:3857-3863.

262. Loechelt BJ, Egeler M, Filipovich AH, et al. Immunosuppression: preliminary results of alternative maintenance therapy for familial hemophagocytic lymphohistocytosis (FHL). Med Pediatr Oncol. 1994;22:325-328.

263. Abella EM, Artrip J, Schultz K, Ravindranath Y. Treatment of familial erythrophagocytic lymphohistiocytosis with cyclosporine A. J Pediatr. 1997;130:467-470.

264. Henter JI, Samuelsson-Horne A, Arico M, et al. Treatment of hemophagocytic lymphohistiocytosis with HLH-94 immunochemotherapy and bone marrow transplantation. Blood. 2002;100: 2367-2373.

265. Stephan JL, Donadieu J, Ledeist F, et al. Treatment of familial hemophagocytic lymphohistiocytosis with antithymocyte globulins, steroids, and cyclosporin A. Blood. 1993;82:2319-2323.

266. Mahlaoui N, Ouachee-Chardin M, de Saint Basile G, et al. Immunotherapy of familial hemophagocytic lymphohistiocytosis with antithymocyte globulins: a single-center retrospective report of 38 patients. Pediatrics. 2007;120:e622-e628.

267. Teramura T, Tabata Y, Yagi T, et al. Quantitative analysis of cell-free Epstein-Barr virus genome copy number in patients with EBV-associated hemophagocytic lymphohistiocytosis. Leuk Lymphoma. 2002;43:173-179.

268. Imashuku S, Hibi S, Ohara T, et al. Effective control of Epstein-Barr virus-related hemophagocytic lymphohistiocytosis with immunochemotherapy. Histiocyte Society. Blood. 1999;93:1869-1874.

269. Imashuku S, Teramura T, Kuriyama K, et al. Risk of etoposide-related acute myeloid leukemia in the treatment of Epstein-Barr virus-associated hemophagocytic lymphohistiocytosis. Int J Hematol. 2002;75:174-177.

270. Imashuku S, Kuriyama K, Teramura T, et al. Requirement for etoposide in the treatment of Epstein-Barr virus-associated hemophagocytic lymphohistiocytosis. J Clin Oncol. 2001;19:2665-2673.

271. Imashuku S, Teramura T, Tauchi H, et al. Longitudinal follow-up of patients with Epstein-Barr virus-associated hemophagocytic lymphohistiocytosis. Haematologica. 2004;89:183-188.

272. Milone MC, Tsai DE, Hodinka RL, et al. Treatment of primary Epstein-Barr virus infection in patients with X-linked lymphoproliferative disease using B-cell-directed therapy. Blood. 2005; 105:994-996.

273. Balamuth NJ, Nichols KE, Paessler M, Teachey DT. Use of rituximab in conjunction with immunosuppressive chemotherapy as a novel therapy for Epstein-Barr virus-associated hemophagocytic lymphohistiocytosis. J Pediatr Hematol Oncol. 2007;29: 569-573.

274. Lackner H, Urban C, Sovinz P, et al. Hemophagocytic lymphohistiocytosis as severe adverse event of antineoplastic treatment in children. Haematologica. 2008;93:291-294.

275. Mouy R, Stephan JL, Pillet P, et al. Efficacy of cyclosporine A in the treatment of macrophage activation syndrome in juvenile arthritis: report of five cases. J Pediatr. 1996;129:750-754.

276. Prahalad S, Bove KE, Dickens D, et al. Etanercept in the treatment of macrophage activation syndrome. J Rheumatol. 2001;28:2120-2124.

277. Henzan T, Nagafuji K, Tsukamoto H, et al. Success with infliximab in treating refractory hemophagocytic lymphohistiocytosis. Am J Hematol. 2006;81:59-61.

278. Baker KS, Filipovich AH, Gross TG, et al. Unrelated donor hematopoietic cell transplantation for hemophagocytic lymphohistiocytosis. Bone Marrow Transplant. 2008;42:175-180.

279. Jabado N, de Graeff-Meeder ER, Cavazzana-Calvo M, et al. Treatment of familial hemophagocytic lymphohistiocytosis with bone marrow transplantation from HLA genetically nonidentical donors. Blood. 1997;90:4743-4748.

280. Horne A, Janka G, Maarten Egeler R, et al. Haematopoietic stem cell transplantation in haemophagocytic lymphohistiocytosis. Br J Haematol. 2005;129:622-630.

281. Cooper N, Rao K, Gilmour K, et al. Stem cell transplantation with reduced-intensity conditioning for hemophagocytic lymphohistiocytosis. Blood. 2006;107:1233-1236.

25 Rare Tumors of Childhood

Karen Albritton, John M. Goldberg, and Alberto Pappo

This chapter covers the rare tumors of childhood. No attempt has been made to consider the rarest of the rare tumors, and we will focus on the more common of the rare pediatric tumors that do not fall into other categories covered elsewhere in this text. The chapter is generally organized from top to bottom, with cancers of the head and neck at the beginning and cancers of the gastrointestinal tract following. The tumors discussed afflict mostly adults, and some are actually common cancers in older patients. Most are carcinomas, and will be more familiar to the oncologist who treats adults. These cancers tend to increase in incidence as children reach adolescence.

Evaluation of SEER data has shown that 9.2% of all childhood cancers are carcinoma, and 75% of these cases were diagnosed in children between the ages of 15 and 19 years.[1] Of these cases, 36% were thyroid carcinomas and 31% were melanomas. The next most common single carcinoma in children younger than 19 years was nasopharyngeal carcinoma, which comprised 4.5% of these cases. Thus, this chapter will emphasize a discussion of melanoma, thyroid carcinoma, and nasopharyngeal carcinoma, and reviews other rare tumors of childhood.

OROPHARYNGEAL CANCER

Squamous cell histology oropharyngeal cancer in children remains uncommon,[2] and most of the 1.3 children per year younger than 19 years of age per million who develop epithelial cancer of the nose, ears, and throat develop nasopharyngeal carcinoma. Nasopharyngeal carcinoma is the most prevalent form of head and neck cancer and is considered separately in this chapter. The increasing prevalence of smokeless tobacco and cigarette use in Western children raises the concern that the incidence of more adult types of squamous cell carcinoma of the oropharynx in children could change, because behavioral causes such as smokeless tobacco, cigarette smoking, and alcohol consumption are known risk factors for this disease in adults and seem to be difficult to eradicate in young people.[3] Although such habits ultimately lead to increased risk for a variety of cancers and early death from heart disease, it remains a theoretical concern that the use of smokeless tobacco by children, particularly by male adolescents, could increase the incidence of these tumors during adolescence and young adulthood.

Educational interventions have been shown to decrease the prevalence of cigarette and smokeless tobacco use in Massachusetts youth,[4] but restrictions on tobacco sales have a mixed record, because even a complete ban on sales of smokeless tobacco in Finland did not lead to a decrease in its use by adolescents.[5] Conversely, restrictions on smoking in public places have been demonstrated to decrease overall tobacco consumption (e.g., by up to 8% in Italy).[6] It is unlikely that many pediatric oncologists will be confronted by adult-type squamous cell carcinoma of the head and neck, but it is likely that pediatric oncologists will be confronted with tobacco use in young adult and adolescent survivors of pediatric cancer. A St. Jude Children's Research Hospital study has found that 29% of surviving children treated on an acute myelogenous leukemia (AML) protocol were found to be cigarette smokers on follow-up.[7] Although survivors of childhood cancer may not be seen frequently in the pediatric oncology clinic, tobacco use and prevention still merit mention during such visits.

Mucoepidermoid carcinoma of the salivary glands is still another type of head and neck carcinoma from which children suffer and is frequently associated with prior therapy for cancer, including radiation.[8] Most children are cured with surgery and sometimes surgery and radiation therapy. Any mass lesion or presenting complaint potentially related to a mass lesion in the salivary glands, particularly if found in a prior radiation field, should prompt a thorough evaluation, with suspicion for this tumor.

NASOPHARYNGEAL CARCINOMA

Nasopharyngeal carcinoma is a cancer of the epithelial lining of the nasopharynx. It shows varying degrees of differentiation, but is a type of squamous cell carcinoma. Most cases have undifferentiated histology; the undifferentiated type is associated with Epstein-Barr virus (EBV) infection of the nasopharyngeal epithelium, and virus is found in the tumor cells.[9] It is the most common type of epithelial tumor of the head and neck in children, accounting for up to 50% of head and neck tumors in children. Incidence varies widely among populations and in relationship to exposure to EBV, environmental exposures such as preserved or salted fish, and geographic location. Rates in China are particularly high, and ethnic Chinese born in China who move to the West have a higher incidence of the disease than ethnic Chinese who are born in Western countries.[9] In the United States, this cancer is more common in the South and more prevalent in African-American children, who have incidence rates of the disease that approach those of the Chinese.

Significant differences in survival by racial and ethnic background in the United States have not been described.[10,11]

Epidemiology

Nasopharyngeal carcinoma is more common in Asia and is strongly associated with Chinese ethnic origin within Asia, with some parts of China having incidence rates from 15 to 30 cases/100,000.[9] There is also a higher incidence of the cancer in Turkey.[12,13] The actual cancer cells are infected by EBV, suggesting a possible role for immunosuppression in the pathogenesis of the tumor, or at least that immune augmentation could help prevent recurrence of nasopharyngeal carcinoma.[9] In Greenland and other regions with similar native populations, high rates of nasopharyngeal carcinoma have been found. Additionally, high rates for other cancers associated with EBV infection, such as various forms of uterine cancer, are more common in families with EBV and nasopharyngeal carcinoma.[14,15] Population-based screening based on EBV serology in endemic areas can help detect nasopharyngeal carcinoma early. However, this would be impractical in nonendemic areas.

Presentation

The typical presenting signs and symptoms of nasopharyngeal carcinoma include evidence of tumor mass in the nasopharynx such as epistaxis, nasal obstruction, and discharge, Eustachian tube dysfunction, palsy of the fifth and sixth nerves relating to skull-based extension, and neck masses.[9] In children with epidemiologic factors making this disease more likely, clinicians must maintain a high index of suspicion for nasopharyngeal carcinoma and obtain imaging studies and consultation as necessary for these signs and symptoms. However, most children diagnosed with nasopharyngeal carcinoma in the United States are unlikely to have obvious epidemiologic associations for the cancer and, even in the United States, EBV infection in childhood is common enough that screening based on evidence of EBV infection would be impractical.

Staging and Evaluation

Proper evaluation of patients suspected of having nasopharyngeal carcinoma includes computed tomography (CT) scan and/or magnetic resonance imaging (MRI) of the head and biopsy of appropriate tissue for diagnosis. A clinical examination is key to evaluate for any apparent lymph node spread. Although systemic evaluation, including laboratory testing, positron emission tomography (PET) scanning, whole-body anatomic scanning, and bone marrow biopsy can be considered, they have not been shown to improve staging accuracy in patients with nasopharyngeal carcinoma.[9]

All nasopharyngeal carcinoma cases are considered squamous cell cancers, but the World Health Organization (WHO) classification of nasopharyngeal carcinoma defines type 1 histology as keratinizing squamous cell carcinoma, a form of cancer more common in adults, versus the type 2 histology, which does not show keratinization on light microscopy but does show some differentiation. Type 3 histology is nonkeratinized and nondifferentiated and is associated with endemic nasopharyngeal carcinoma.[9] Most children with nasopharyngeal carcinoma present with undifferentiated or WHO type III histology.

The American Joint Commission on Cancer (AJCC) TNM staging system (2002) is considered the most relevant for patients in the Western countries. The WHO staging system has fewer local (T) staging categories but seems to be adequate for patients in endemic areas.[9,16] The latest AJCC staging system is shown in Tables 25-1 and 25-2.

Treatment

Although nasopharyngeal carcinoma can be treated by radiation therapy only, it has been shown to be sensitive to chemotherapy in adults and children. Using chemotherapy may ultimately allow for curative radiotherapy at lower doses, with less risk for late effects from head and neck radiotherapy.[9,10,12,13,17] A Pediatric Oncology Group study has used four cycles of preirradiation chemotherapy with methotrexate with leucovorin, 5-fluorouracil (5-FU), and cisplatin to treat children with AJCC stage III or IV nasopharyngeal carcinoma. Children with stage I or II disease were treated with irradiation only. The 4-year event-free and overall survival were 77% ± 12% and 75% ± 12%, respectively.[10] Other agents used to treat nasopharyngeal carcinoma include bleomycin and doxorubicin.[13]

THYROID CARCINOMA

Thyroid nodules are extremely rare in children before puberty but the incidence of malignancy in these nodules is about 25%, which is significantly higher than the reported 5% incidence of malignancy in adults.[18,19] Thyroid carcinoma in children and adolescents accounts for 3% of all cancers in patients younger than 20 years, but 75% of cases occur in patients between the ages of 15 and 19 years (Fig. 25-1).[20]

Epidemiology

Radioactive exposure to the neck is a well-established risk factor for the development of thyroid carcinoma; the best recognized example is the post-Chernobyl nuclear power plant accident of April 1986.[21-25] Exposure to radioactive iodine and cesium isotopes after the accident resulted in a markedly increased rate of thyroid cancer in children; the estimated relative excess risk was calculated at 5.25/Gy of exposure.[24]

Long-term survivors of cancer who have been exposed to external radiation for treatment of their primary malignancy are at increased risk for developing thyroid carcinoma. This risk is higher in patients younger than 10 years of age and in those who received increasing radiation doses (highest risk from 20 to 29 Gy).[26] Other risk factors for the development of pediatric thyroid cancer include the presence of genetic syndromes, such as familial adenomatous polyposis, Cowden's disease, Carney's syndrome, and immune thyroid disorders, such as Hashimoto's thyroiditis.[18,27-30]

TABLE 25-1 **TNM Definitions for Nasopharyngeal Carcinoma**

Primary Tumor (T)	Regional Lymph Nodes (N)	Distant Metastasis (M)
TX: Primary tumor cannot be assessed	NX: Regional lymph nodes cannot be assessed	MX: Distant metastasis cannot be assessed
T0: No evidence of primary tumor	N0: No regional lymph node metastasis	M0: No distant metastasis
Tis: Carcinoma in situ	N1: Unilateral metastasis in lymph node(s), not more than 6 cm in greatest dimension, above the supraclavicular fossa†	M1: Distant metastasis
T1: Tumor confined to the nasopharynx		
T2: Tumor extends to soft tissues		
T2a: Tumor extends to the oropharynx and/or nasal cavity without parapharyngeal extension*	N2: Bilateral metastasis in lymph node(s), not more than 6 cm in greatest dimension, above the supraclavicular fossa†	
T2b: Any tumor with parapharyngeal extension*		
T3: Tumor invades bony structures and/or paranasal sinuses	N3: Metastasis in a lymph node(s)† larger than 6 cm and/or to supraclavicular fossa	
T4: Tumor with intracranial extension and/or involvement of cranial nerves, infratemporal fossa, hypopharynx, orbit, or masticator space	N3a: Larger than 6 cm	
	N3b: Extension to the supraclavicular fossa‡	

Note: The distribution and prognostic impact of regional lymph node spread from nasopharynx cancer, particularly of the undifferentiated type, are different from those of other head and neck mucosal cancers and justify the use of a different regional lymph node classification scheme.
*Parapharyngeal extension denotes posterolateral infiltration of tumor beyond the pharyngobasilar fascia.
†Midline nodes are considered ipsilateral nodes.
‡Supraclavicular zone or fossa is relevant to the staging of nasopharyngeal carcinoma and is the triangular region originally described in the Ho stage classification for nasopharyngeal cancer. It is defined by three points: (1) the superior margin of the sternal end of the clavicle; (2) the superior margin of the lateral end of the clavicle; and (3) the point where the neck meets the shoulder. Note that this would include caudal portions of levels IV and V. All cases with lymph nodes (whole or part) in the fossa are considered N3b.
From Greene FL, Page DL, Fleming ID, et al (eds). Pharynx (including base of tongue, soft palate and uvula). In AJCC Cancer Staging Manual, 6th ed. Chicago, American Joint Commission on Cancer, 2002, pp 33-46.

Pathology and Molecular Pathology

More than 90% of pediatric thyroid carcinomas have well-differentiated histology; papillary histology accounts for over 80% of cases and follicular histology for about 20% of cases.[31,32] Medullary thyroid cancer is seen in less than 10% of pediatric cases of thyroid cancer and can be found in association with multiple endocrine neoplasia (MEN) syndrome types 2A and 2B. The distribution of histologies is only slightly different in cases with known radiation carcinogenesis; in a study of 740 children with thyroid cancer, of whom 92% were exposed to radiation at Chernobyl, 90% of cases were papillary, about 5% were follicular, and 0.4% were medullary.[33]

RET-PTC rearrangements have been documented in 50% to 60% of pediatric cases of papillary thyroid carcinoma and in up to 70% of radiation-induced pediatric papillary thyroid carcinoma.[30,34] NTRK1 rearrangements and AKAP9-BRAF fusions have also been described in a small number of radiation-induced papillary tumors.[35-38] Unlike in adults, however, BRAF mutations are rarely seen in pediatric papillary tumors.[30,39,40] Follicular tumors are characterized by RAS mutations and peroxisome proliferator-activated receptor γ (PPARγ) rearrangements, whereas MEN-associated medullary thyroid carcinomas are characterized by germline-activating mutations of RET.[30,41]

Clinical Presentation and Staging

Most patients with thyroid carcinoma are older than 10 years. The most common clinical signs at presentation are palpable adenopathy and a thyroid nodule. Larger fixed nodules, prior history of radiation exposure, history of pheochromocytoma, hyperparathyroidism, Gardner's syndrome, familial adenomatous polyposis, Carney's complex, or Cowden's syndrome should raise suspicion for the presence of malignancy (more information is available at www.nccn.org/professionals/physician_gls/PDF/thyroid.pdf).

Ultrasound is a useful diagnostic technique and some prefer this method for evaluating thyroid nodules.[18] Scintigrams will detect the extent of intra- and extrathyroidal disease and identify functioning or nonfunctioning (cold) nodules. Approximately 5% of nonfunctioning nodules are malignant. Fine-needle aspiration is the most cost-effective and expeditious way to distinguish benign from malignant thyroid nodules, and a diagnosis of malignancy, when present, can be made in 90% of cases.[18] A simple cost-effective algorithm for the evaluation of thyroid nodules is shown in Figure 25-2.[42]

Patients with thyroid carcinoma are usually euthyroid. Measurement of serum calcitonin should be considered in patients with a family history of thyroid cancer, in those with findings suggestive of MEN, or in patients with solid thyroid nodules.[18] Baseline serum thyroglobulin and thyroperoxidase antibody levels can be helpful in identifying patients with autoimmune disorders such as Hashimoto's thyroiditis.[18]

TABLE 25-2	American Joint Committee on Cancer (AJCC) Stage Groupings for Nasopharyngeal Carcinoma*	
Stage	**Groupings**
0	Tis, N0, M0
I	T1, N0, M0
IIA	T2a, N0, M0
IIB	T1, N1, M0
	T2, N1, M0
	T2a, N1, M0
	T2b, N0, M0
	T2b, N1, M0
III	T1, N2, M0
	T2a, N2, M0
	T2b, N2, M0
	T3, N0, M0
	T3, N1, M0
	T3, N2, M0
IVA	T4, N0, M0
	T4, N1, M0
	T4, N2, M0
IVB	Any T, N3, M0
IVC	Any T, any N, M1

*Results of radiation therapy for nasopharyngeal carcinoma (locoregional control and survival) are usually reported by T stage and N stage separately or by specific T and N subgroupings, rather than by numerical stages I to IV. Outcome also depends on various biologic and technical factors related to treatment.

From Greene FL, Page DL, Fleming ID, et al (eds). Pharynx (including base of tongue, soft palate and uvula). In AJCC Cancer Staging Manual, 6th ed. Chicago, American Joint Commission on Cancer, 2002, pp 33-46.

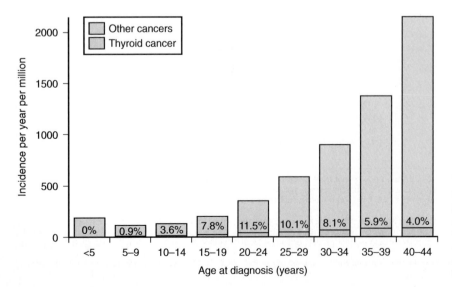

FIGURE 25-1. Incidence of thyroid carcinoma relative to all cancers, SEER 1975-2000. (*Data from Bleyer A, O'Leary M, Barr R, Ries LAG [eds]. Cancer Epidemiology in Older Adolescents and Young Adults 15 to 29 Years of Age, Including SEER Incidence and Survival: 1975-2000 [NIH Publication No. 06-5767]. Bethesda, Md, National Cancer Institute, 2006.*)

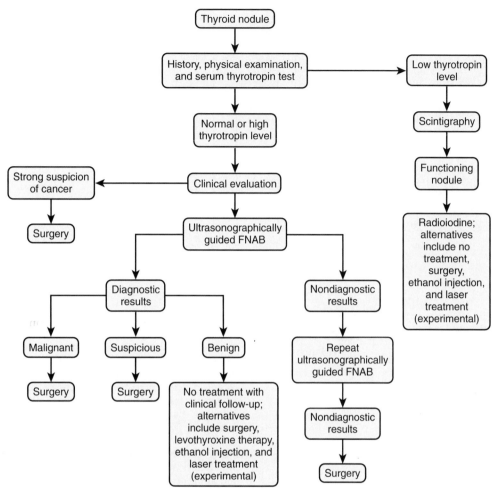

FIGURE 25-2. Algorithm for evaluating thyroid nodules. FNAB, fine-needle aspiration biopsy. *(Adapted from Hegedus L. Clinical practice. The thyroid nodule. N Engl J Med. 2004;351:1764-1771.)*

Extrathyroid disease, most commonly involving the lungs, is seen in at least 20% of patients. Follicular cancers most commonly spread to bones and lungs.

Treatment and Outcome

A recent evidence-based review of the treatment of differentiated thyroid carcinoma[43] has suggested the following treatment and follow-up guidelines for patients with thyroid carcinoma:

1. All patients with well-differentiated thyroid carcinoma should undergo total or near-total thyroidectomy with selective nodal dissection if nodes are involved, either during preoperative imaging or at the time of surgery.
2. Following surgery, all patients should undergo radioiodine remnant ablation within 4 to 6 weeks after thyroidectomy. Patients with low-risk disease, defined as those older than 10 years, with nodules less than 1.5 cm in size, no residual disease after surgery, and localized disease, should receive radioiodine at a dose of 100 mCi/1.73/m²; the remaining patients should receive a fixed dose of 100 mCi.
3. Thyroid replacement should include L-thyroxine at a dosage of 2 to 3 µg/kg/day to achieve thyroid-stimulating hormone (TSH) values less than 0.1 mU/L.

4. Lifelong follow-up is recommended. Scheduled evaluations should include whole-body scans, serum TSH, triiodothyronine (T_3), thyroxine (T_4), and thyroglobulin measurements, and neck ultrasound at 6, 12, 18, 24, 30, 36, 48, and 60 months after initial therapy. TSH stimulation-inducing hypothyroidism prior to diagnostic whole-body scans can be accomplished by withdrawing thyroid replacement or by administering recombinant human TSH.[43]

Despite a high incidence of metastases and recurrent disease, which in some series is as high as 40%,[44] the survival at 10 years is 98% or higher (Fig. 25-3).[31-33,44]

BREAST TUMORS

Breast masses are rare in young children. During puberty, benign fibroadenomas are the most common cause of a palpable breast lump (Table 25-3).[45] The estrogen stimulation during adolescence may cause exaggerated growth of the stroma and epithelium in a localized breast lobule that characterizes a fibroadenoma. They have been found in as many as 20% of women between the ages of 15 and 25 years on autopsy studies.[46] Fibroadenoma occurring in adolescence does not appear to be associated with concurrent or future

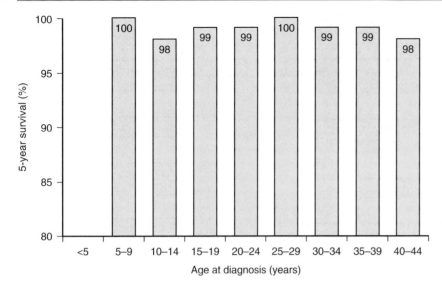

FIGURE 25-3. Five-year survival rates for thyroid carcinoma, SEER 1975-1999. *(Data from Bleyer A, O'Leary M, Barr R, Ries LAG [eds]. Cancer Epidemiology in Older Adolescents and Young Adults 15 to 29 Years of Age, Including SEER Incidence and Survival:1975-2000 [NIH Publication No. 06-5767]. Bethesda, Md, National Cancer Institute, 2006.)*

TABLE 25-3 **Breast Lesions in Adolescent Girls**	
Abnormality	**Incidence (%)**
Fibroadenoma	68
Miscellaneous	27
Juvenile hypertrophy	2
Giant fibroadenoma	1
Phyllodes tumor	<1
Cancer	<1
Metastatic	38
Adenocarcinoma (lobular or ductal)	31
Lymphoma	13

Data from Neinstein LS. Breast disease in adolescents and young women. Pediatr Clin North Am. 1999;46:607-629.

breast carcinoma. Any dominant discrete breast mass in an adolescent should be reexamined at midcycle after one or two menstrual cycles. Persistent masses should be imaged by ultrasound (not mammography) and referred to a surgeon. Lesions typical for fibroadenoma are sometimes followed clinically; fine-needle aspiration or core biopsy can also be performed to confirm the diagnosis.[47] Most fibroadenomas in adolescents self-resolve or shrink.[48]

Phyllodes tumors are stromal tumors that present as rapidly growing but clinically benign masses. Although the median age of presentation is 45 years, they can occur in adolescence.[49] Benign phyllodes tumors of the breast are pathologically similar to a large fibroadenoma, with more stromal cellularity. They are treated by resection, with at least 1-cm margins.[50] Malignant phyllodes tumors are sarcomas with nuclear pleomorphism and mitotic activity; treatment requires a multimodality sarcoma approach. Five-year disease-free survival has been reported to be 96%, 74%, and 66% for benign, borderline, and malignant phyllodes tumors, respectively, in adults[51]; it is thought that adolescents have a more favorable outcome.[52]

Breast masses can also represent primary or metastatic sites of pediatric cancers, such as rhabdomyosarcoma,[53] non-Hodgkin's lymphoma (NHL), Hodgkin's lymphoma, or neuroblastoma.[54]

Breast carcinoma under the age of 20 years is rare; five cases were seen at M. D. Anderson Cancer Center in a 10-year period compared with 180 between ages 20 and 30 and 1347 between ages 31 and 50 years.[55] The most common pathology is a juvenile secretory carcinoma, which secretes mucin and mucopolysaccharide-containing material. It is treated by excision and lymph node biopsy. No studies have evaluated outcomes in very young breast carcinoma patients (younger than 20 years) but multiple studies have shown that young age (younger than 30 or 35) is an independent predictor of poor response.[55] The two younger age groups at particular risk of breast cancer are women who have received radiation to the breast, usually for lymphoma, or who have a familial predisposition. These women should be taught breast self-examination and awareness at a young age.

PULMONARY TUMORS

Table 25-4 lists the most common pulmonary tumors in children.

Bronchial Adenomas

A large percentage of malignant pulmonary tumors in children are called bronchial adenomas and, although not benign, as the term implies, they are predominantly low grade in behavior. They include carcinoid tumor, mucoepidermoid carcinoma, and adenocystic carcinoma. Although pulmonary carcinoid tumors account for only 2% of all primary lung tumors in adults, nearly 40% to 80% of pediatric malignant lung lesions are carcinoids.[56-58] See later ("Carcinoid") for a more complete description of carcinoid and its management. Mucoepidermoid carcinomas (MECs)[59] and adenoid cystic carcinomas[60] are more often seen in the head and neck but can arise from mucous glands located in the respiratory submucosa.

Most bronchial adenomas are endobronchial; patients often have recurrent infections or obstructive pneumonitis before their diagnosis is determined (Fig. 25-4) and the most common presenting symptoms are cough, fever, or wheezing.[61,62] Although over 25% of adults with pulmonary carcinoid and MEC are asymptomatic, the figure is lower in children, who are less likely to have a radiographic study that would detect an incidental lesion.[63] Aggressive lesions can present with hemoptysis or chest pain. It is extremely rare for patients

TABLE 25-4	Pulmonary Tumors in Children
Malignant	**Benign**
Bronchial adenomas (40%-60%)	Hamartomas
Carcinoid	Hemangiomas
Mucoepidermoid carcinoma	Leiomyomas
Adenoid cystic carcinoma	Plasma cell granuloma
Pleuropulmonary blastoma (15%)	(inflammatory
Bronchogenic carcinoma (10%-15%)	pseudotumor)
Adenocarcinoma	Neurogenic tumors
Small cell carcinoma	
Bronchoalveolar carcinoma	
Squamous cell cancer	
Undifferentiated carcinoma	
Fetal lung adenocarcinoma	
Pulmonary mesothelioma	
Sarcomas (20%-25%)	
Rhabdomyosarcoma	
Synovial sarcoma	
Fibrosarcoma	
Hemangiopericytoma (solitary fibrous	
tumor)	

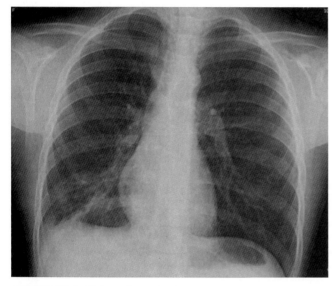

FIGURE 25-4. Plain radiograph of 9-year-old patient showing right lower lobe infiltrate persistent over 1 month. Further workup revealed a right lower lobe bronchus mucoepidermoid carcinoma.

with pulmonary carcinoid to present with carcinoid syndrome,[63] but a reported 4% of patients present with Cushing's syndrome.[62,64] A mass is usually detected by chest x-ray or chest CT, but endobronchial lesions may only be suspected by recurrent localized obstruction and volume loss (Fig. 25-5A and 5B). Octreotide scans have a sensitivity of 80% to 90% for carcinoids and can be useful at diagnosis to assess for metastatic disease.[65] Diagnostic biopsy is usually obtained by flexible fiberoptic bronchoscopy (see Fig. 25-5C). Lymph nodes can be involved, especially with higher grade tumors, but may also be enlarged as a reaction to obstructive pneumonitis rather than tumor.

The typical carcinoid tumor and low-grade MEC are pathologically bland and have a low rate of postresection recur-

rence or metastasis, even with local invasion.[56] The rarer atypical carcinoids and high-grade MEC have a higher mitotic rate and more necrosis and are more likely to behave aggressively.[66] The appropriate therapy is open resection of tumor and involved lymph node, the extent of which is determined by the centrality of the mass. Lobectomy or even pneumonectomy may be required for tumors of the main stem bronchus. Because adenoid cystic carcinomas can spread submucosally, the margin of resection should be determined intraoperatively by frozen sections of the bronchial margins. Local recurrences of bronchial adenomas can occur, especially for MECs, but metastases are rare. Estimates for metastases from bronchial carcinoid range from 5% to 27%.[62,67,68]

When surgery is not curative, other therapies can be used, but have shown limited success.[69] Octreotide, a somatostatin analogue used to treat the symptoms of carcinoid syndrome, has been known to stabilize carcinoid tumor growth but not result in regression; similarly, interferon has been used, with a modest response. Cytotoxic chemotherapy for carcinoid and MECs has been used but response rates, even with combination agents, are under 20%.[58,69] Novel molecular agents are being tested, including agents directed against vascular endothelial growth factor (VEGF), platelet-derived growth factor receptor (PDGFR), and mammalian target of rapamycin (mTor). Prognosis remains excellent for bronchial adenomas, even for locally invasive or high-grade tumors.

Pleuropulmonary Blastoma

This tumor in young children is distinct from pulmonary blastoma in adults; the pediatric tumor is composed of primitive blastema and neoplastic mesenchymal cells, without epithelial malignant cells.[70] There appears to be an increase in malformations and cancer in the afflicted child and family (Fig. 25-6).[71] The tumor is located peripherally and can be locally invasive. Most patients present with wheezing, respiratory distress or pneumothorax. Pathologically there are three subtypes: type 1 pleuropulmonary blastoma (PPB; exclusively cystic, without a macroscopically detectable solid component), type 2 PPB (with solid and true cystic areas), and type 3 PPB (a true solid tumor).[70]

Treatment involves resection. Adjuvant chemotherapy (doxorubicin, actinomycin, vincristine, and cyclophosphamide or ifosfamide), especially for types 2 and 3, may reduce the risk of recurrence[72] or can be used neoadjuvantly to improve the resectability of large lesions.[73] Radiation has been used adjuvantly or palliatively; its role is unclear. Event-free survival (EFS) for PPB is around 50%; overall survival is 50% to 70%. Prognosis correlates with subtype, with type 1 having the best and type 3 having the worst outcome.[74] Metastases can develop; the most common sites are the brain and spinal cord and bone.[72] An International PPB Registry (www.ppbregistry.org) has been established that collects clinical data on incident cases in an attempt to define the outcomes of patients with this rare disease.

Bronchogenic Carcinoma

Primary epithelial cancers of the lung are rarely seen in children; less than 100 cases have been reported in the literature. They are pathologically indistinguishable from the same tumors occurring in adults. Therapy should be planned after consultation with a medical oncologist experienced with lung cancers and, in general, should mimic the standard of care for adult tumors. When these histologies occur in children, they are often metastatic at diagnosis and have an aggressive

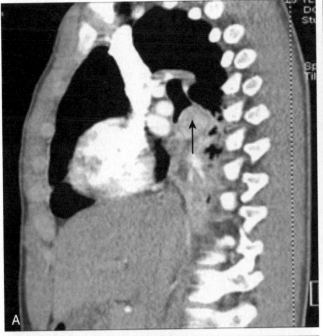

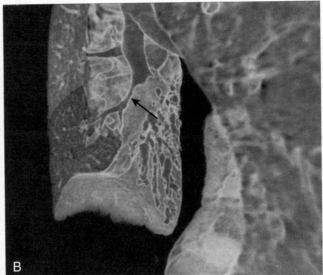

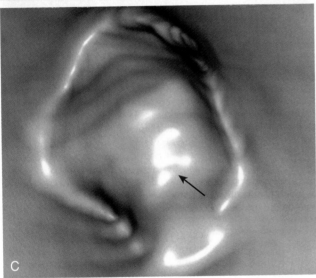

FIGURE 25-5. A, Carcinoid tumor (*arrow*) obstructing bronchus intermedius and causing peripheral consolidation of lung. **B,** Carcinoid tumor obstructing bronchus intermedius (*arrow*). **C,** Carcinoid tumor (*arrow*) obstructing bronchus intermedius.

course, and poor prognosis (Fig. 25-7).[58] Bronchioalveolar carcinoma (BAC) is a histology that accounts for less than 10% of lung malignancies in adults, with a mean age of presentation between the sixth and seventh decades. In children, mucinous BAC has been associated with congenital cystic-adenomatoid carcinoma malformation (CCAM) type 1.[75] Surgery is the primary treatment for BAC. Prognosis depends on nodal status and the resectability of the tumor; it appears to be slightly better for children than for adults with BAC or for children with other primary bronchogenic carcinomas.[76] Squamous cell carcinoma,[77] adenocarcinoma,[58] and small cell lung cancer[78,79] are occasionally seen in children.[61] There is no clear causative pathway or association with environmental exposure, and most patients have no family history to suggest a genetic component. A rare form of adenocarcinoma in children is well-differentiated fetal adenocarcinoma (WDFA), which histologically resembles fetal lung and has an excellent prognosis.[58,80,81]

Other Pulmonary Tumors

Sarcomas arise from mesenchymal cells and therefore can develop from connective tissue cells in the lung. The most common types seen are hemangiopericytoma, synovial sarcoma, fibrosarcoma, and rhabdomyosarcoma.[61] Ewing's sarcoma—peripheral primitive neuroectodermal tumor in the lung (Askin's tumor)—is often pleural-based. Given its marked chemosensitivity, it should be treated with chemotherapy prior to surgical resection, in contrast to almost all other lung tumors (see Chapter 21). Pleural mesothelioma is occasionally seen in children, with less than 100 cases in the literature and even fewer that have been confirmed by pathologic review.[82] Although there have been reports of assumed causation by asbestos exposure and chemotherapy and/or radiation for another malignancy, most cases appear in healthy children.[82,83] The tumor is similar to that in adult cases in its pathologic appearance and poor prognosis, with a median survival of approximately 10

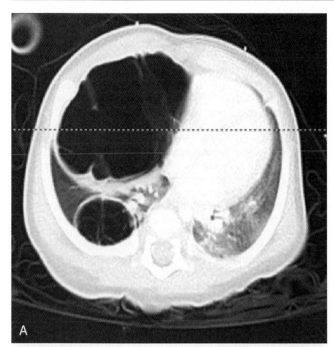

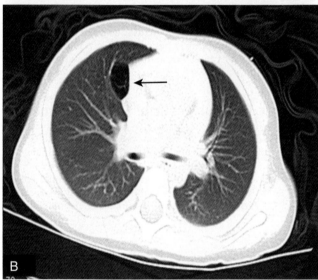

FIGURE 25-6. A, Two cystic lesons in 3-month-old infant, found to be pleuropulmonary blastoma (PPB) on resection. **B,** Brother of PPB patient in **A** with a benign cystic-adenomatoid carcinoma malformation (*arrow*).

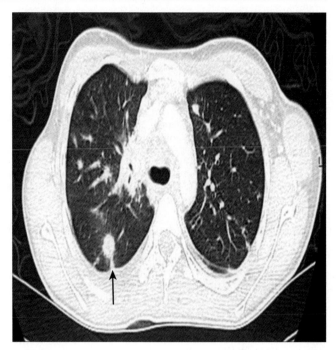

FIGURE 25-7. 14-year-old patient with primary pulmonary poorly differentiated carcinoma (*arrow*) and lung, bone, lymphatic, hepatic, and adrenal metastases.

months.[84,85] Most cases are treated with a multimodality approach, but tumors are often diffuse and unresectable, and are poorly responsive to chemotherapy and radiation. Current concepts in the therapeutic approach of adults with mesothelioma include the use of multitargeted antifolates[3] and aggressive surgery (extrapleural pneumonectomies).[86]

GASTROINTESTINAL TRACT MALIGNANCIES

Esophageal adenocarcinoma is rare in patients younger than 18 years, and the literature is mostly confined to case reports.[87] Some cases of esophageal carcinoma in children or young adults are associated with prior injury to the esophagus, including chemical burn[88] or repair of tracheoesophageal fistula as a child.[89,90] This could possibly be mediated by chronic inflammation.

Pancreatic tumors occur at an incidence of 0.1/million children younger than 19 years.[1] Pancreatic adenocarcinoma is rarely reported in children. Pseudopapillary tumor of the pancreas is a rare malignancy that usually can be cured by surgery alone.[91] Pancreatoblastoma is a rare tumor that can occur at any time of life but is usually considered a pediatric tumor. Surgery can be curative.[92]

Gastric adenocarcinoma is a rare tumor in childhood as well, and the published literature is confined to case reports. It can arise de novo, but many cases are associated with familial cancer syndromes, polyposis syndromes, or prior treatment for gastric lymphoma. Patients can present with abdominal pain, distention, anorexia, emesis or hematemesis, melena, hematochezia, and/or an abdominal mass.[93] Because this tumor is common in adults, treatment must be planned in consultation with medical oncologists familiar with the chemotherapy and radiation treatment plans used to augment surgical resection for this aggressive cancer.

Cholangiocarcinoma is also rare in children and the occasional case reports have been associated with congenital biliary dilation.[94] Liver tumors are covered elsewhere in this text (see Chapter 18).

GASTROINTESTINAL STROMAL TUMORS

Gastrointestinal Stromal Tumors in Adults

Gastrointestinal stromal tumors (GISTs) are the most common mesenchymal neoplasm of the gastrointestinal tract in adults, with an incidence of 14 cases/million, which translates into almost 5000 cases/year in the United States.[95-97] The cell of origin of GISTs appears to be related to the interstitial cells of Cajal, which function as a pacemaker-coordinating peristalsis.

The median age at diagnosis of GISTs is approximately 60 years and there is a slight male predominance. The most common presenting symptoms are a palpable mass, bloating, early satiety, and gastrointestinal bleeding. Not uncommonly, however, GISTs are detected incidentally during unrelated surgical procedures. Approximately 60% of GISTs arise in the stomach, 25% in the small intestine, and 10% in the large bowel, appendix, rectum, and esophagus. There are three major histologic subtypes of GIST:

1. Spindle cell type (70% of cases)
2. Epithelioid subtype (20% of cases)
3. Mixed (10% of cases)

Most GIST tumors in the stomach are of epithelioid or mixed histology, whereas spindle cell morphology predominates in other locations. Approximately 95% of GISTs stain with the immunohistochemical KIT (CD117) and up to 90% have activating mutations of *KIT*, most commonly involving exons 9, 11, 13, and 17.[97,98] A small proportion of adult GISTs (5%) lack *KIT* mutations but have mutually exclusive mutations of the activation loop or juxtamembrane domains of the *PDGFRA* gene.[99] Another small portion of GISTs (5% to 10%) lack mutations of *KIT* or *PDGFRA*.

Approximately 5% of GISTs occur within the context of three well-defined tumor-associated syndromes—neurofibromatosis type 1, Carney's triad, and familial GIST.[97,100] The occurrence of GISTs has been described in up to 6% of patients with neurofibromatosis type 1.[100] In this population, the tumors tend to involve the small intestine and are often multiple, and most tumors lack *KIT* and *PDGFR* mutations. GISTs in patients with Carney's triad (extra-adrenal paraganglioma, pulmonary chondroma, and GIST) more often affect women, are located in the stomach, have epithelioid histology, lack *KIT* and *PDGFR* mutations, and have an indolent clinical course.[97,101,102] Finally, there have been approximately 12 families reported to date with familial GIST, and the pattern of transmission appears to be autosomal dominant.[101] Molecular analyses of these families have revealed the presence of activating germline mutations of *KIT* and *PDFGR*, which are similar to those observed in sporadic GISTs.[101,103,104]

Treatment

Chemotherapy for unresectable or metastatic GISTs produces responses in less than 10% of patients, and the median survival for those with metastatic disease was historically approximately 20%.[105,106] The use of the tyrosine kinase inhibitor imatinib has revolutionized the treatment of GISTs. Administration of this drug to adults with unresectable or metastatic GISTs has been shown to produce responses in up to 85% of patients, and the median survival for this group of patients has increased to 58 months.[105-107] The likelihood of response to imatinib has been clearly correlated with tumor kinase mutational status; patients with *KIT* exon 11 mutations have a significantly higher response rate to imatinib than those with exon 9 mutations or no mutations.[97-99,108] A similar pattern has been documented for patients with *PDGFR* mutations; two thirds of patients with *PDGFR* lesions have the imatinib-resistant isoform D842V.[99] Administration of higher doses of imatinib has been associated with improved response rates in patients whose tumors harbor exon 9 mutations.[108] Patients whose tumors lack *PDGFR* or *KIT* mutations respond poorly to imatinib regardless of dose given. Table 25-5 summarizes the correlations among histopathologic features, primary tumor location, mutational status, and response to therapy.

Administration of sunitinib, a multitargeted tyrosine kinase inhibitor, has been recently reported to produce a fourfold improvement in the median time to progression in patients with imatinib-resistant GISTs.[109]

Pediatric Gastrointestinal Stromal Tumors

Pediatric GISTs account for less than 2.5% of all GISTs reported in the literature and their true U.S. incidence is unknown.[110] These tumors often affect females, arise in the stomach, tend to be multifocal, can affect locoregional lymph nodes, and have epithelioid or mixed histology (see Table 25-5).[111-117] Although one would assume a high incidence of

TABLE 25-5	Clinicopathologic Correlates in Gastrointestinal Stromal Tumors				
Mutation Type	**Approximate Frequency**	**Histologic Type**	**Anatomic Site**	**In Vitro Susceptibility to Imatinib**	**In Vivo Response to Imatinib**
KIT mutation	80%-85%	Predominantly spindle cell			
Exon 9	10%		Small bowel	Yes	Intermediate
Exon 11	60%-70%			Yes	Excellent
Exon 13	1%			Yes	Some responses*
Exon 17	1%			Yes	Some responses*
PDGFRA mutation	5%-10%	Epithelioid and mixed spindle and epithelioid	Stomach		
Exon 12	1%			Yes	Some responses*
Exon 14	<1%			Yes	Unknown
Exon 18	6%			Mixed† unknown/responsive	D842V not responsive; other mutations
Wild-type (no *KIT* or *PDGFR* mutation)	10%	Predominantly spindle cell		No	Poor

*Although there have been responses, there are very few patients that have been tested.
†Most isoforms with a substitution involving codon D842 (the most common mutation in exon 18) are resistant. However, other mutations in exon 18 are sensitive to imatinib.
From Rubin BP. Gastrointestinal stromal tumours: an update. Histopathology. 2006;48:83-96.

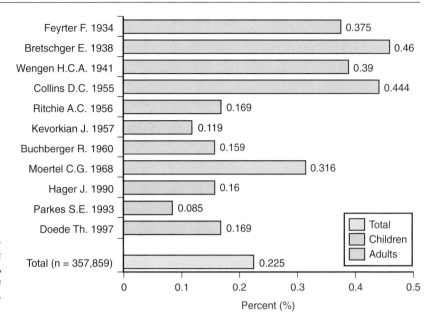

FIGURE 25-8. Percentage of appendectomy specimens found to have carcinoid tumor on pathologic examination. *(Adapted from Doede T, Foss HD, Waldschmidt J. Carcinoid tumors of the appendix in children—epidemiology, clinical aspects and procedure. Eur J Pediatr Surg. 2000;10:372-377.)*

well-defined genetic syndromes such as neurofibromatosis or Carney's triad, few reports have documented such an association.

The clinical course of pediatric GISTs is somewhat unpredictable, but studies have suggested that these tumors appear to behave more aggressively than their adult counterparts when prognostic criteria are applied.[110,111,114] However, pediatric GISTs have also been reported to have a more insidious and indolent course.

Most pediatric GISTs studied to date lack *KIT* and *PDGFR* mutations.[111,114,115,118] Expression profiling has revealed differences between pediatric and adult GISTs; neuroligin 4, ankyrin 3, frizzled 2, and insulin-like growth factor receptor appear to be preferentially upregulated in pediatric cases. The few reports addressing therapy with imatinib in pediatric GISTs have shown suboptimal responses to this agent.[111,114,119] A recent report has shown responses to sunitinib in three pediatric patients with imatinib-resistant GIST, suggesting that this therapeutic alternative should be studied further.[120]

CARCINOID

Carcinoid tumors are tumors of neuroendocrine cells that derive from embryonic divisions of the gut. The most common locations for carcinoid are in locations arising from the midgut—the appendix, small intestine, proximal colon, and rectum. Carcinoid tumor of the appendix is speculated to be the most common tumor of the gastrointestinal tract in children.[121] Tumors of the epithelial component of the bronchial mucosa arising from the foregut appear as carcinoids of the lung and bronchus. Biologically, carcinoid tumor cells contain membrane-bound neurosecretory granules that contain hormones and biogenic amines. When serotonin, 5-hydroxyindole acetic acid (5-HIAA), and other metabolites of the granules are released, a syndrome of flushing, diarrhea, and abdominal cramps can occur. The syndrome rarely occurs in children, because it is associated with large tumor mass, hepatic, or distant metastases.[122] Carcinoid tumors are one of the rarer tumors (less than 10%) seen in the autosomal dominant syndrome MEN type 1 (MEN1), caused by a mutation in the

tumor suppressor gene *MEN1* located at 11q13.[123,124] *MEN1* may be involved in sporadic carcinoid tumors as well, as evidenced by loss of heterozygosity (LOH) on chromosome 11 or inactivated copies of the *MEN1* gene.[125,126] Other possible contributors may be p53, K-ras-2, C-raf-1, and Bax/Bcl2.[124]

In a review over a 22-year period at St. Jude Children's Research Hospital, 0.08% of patients evaluated for malignancy had carcinoid tumors.[127] In that series, like others, the majority (approximately 60%) arose in the appendix. Pathologic examination of appendectomy specimens reveal carcinoid in 0.23%, with the figure slightly lower in children than adults (Fig. 25-8).[122] Most patients with appendiceal carcinoid present with symptoms of acute appendicitis; others have chronic abdominal pain, or an incidental appendectomy is done during another surgical procedure. The diagnosis is rarely made preoperatively.

Appendiceal carcinoid smaller than 1 cm rarely metastasize, and appendectomy alone is the appropriate therapy.[128] After a diagnosis of appendiceal carcinoid, it is reasonable to check levels of serum serotonin and chromogranin A and 24-hour urinary 5-HIAA, and abdominal imaging should be performed to look for metastases. Octreotide scans have a sensitivity of 80% to 90% for carcinoids and can be useful at diagnosis to assess for metastases[65,129] but, given the negligible incidence of distant disease in children, their use in pediatrics should probably be reserved for high-risk cases. For appendiceal tumors larger than 2 cm, right hemicolectomy is advocated in adults[130]; there is controversy regarding its use for tumors between 1 and 2 cm and for children, for whom cecal or ileocecal resection may suffice.[131-133]

No deaths from pediatric appendiceal carcinoid have been reported in several large recent series with extended follow-up.[121,132,133] In addition to increasing size, location at the base of the appendix and the presence of mucin-producing cells are thought to be poor prognostic indicators.[130] Given its rarity and benign behavior, recommended follow-up is controversial. Several authors have recommended a schedule of monitoring serotonin metabolites, with or without abdominal ultrasonography, in patients whose tumor diameter was more than 5 mm.[122,128] The findings that 14.6% of patients with appendiceal carcinoids in the Surveillance Epidemiology and End Results (SEER) registry had synchronous or metachronous noncarcinoid malignant tumors,[134] that the risk of offspring carcinoid (SIR 4.31) and secondary cancers (SIR 2.15-3.31) was elevated in a Swedish registry study,[135] and several case reports of patients with secondary adenocarcinoma of the colon[127,136,137] have raised other questions of appropriate counseling and follow-up for these patients.

For the rare metastatic carcinoid, octreotide, a somatostatin analogue, which has been used to treat the symptoms of carcinoid syndrome, has stabilized carcinoid tumor growth but not resulted in regression.[138] Similarly, interferon has been used, with a modest response.[139]

COLORECTAL CARCINOMA

In Western and developed countries, colorectal carcinoma is one of the most common malignant cancers and is responsible for significant morbidity and mortality. Conversely, colorectal carcinoma is rare in populations that do not have high rates of obesity and meat consumption. In the United States alone, approximately 153,000 patients/year are diagnosed with colorectal carcinoma and approximately 52,000 deaths/year are attributed to it.[140] However, colorectal carcinoma is rare in children, with fewer than 100 cases/year in the United States, as estimated by SEER data, and approximately one case/million in those younger than 20 years. The incidence of colorectal carcinoma relative to other cancers by age is shown in Figure 25-9, the 5-year survival rates of colorectal carcinoma by age are shown in Figure 25-10, and 5-year survival rates by age and stage are shown in Figure 25-11. Although case series offer suggestions about the biologic nature of this tumor in patients younger than 20 years, the rarity of this diagnosis in children means that comprehensive population-wide data are not available. Any case series from a large institution will be limited in number and by referral bias. Although many case series have suggested a higher stage at diagnosis for pediatric colorectal carcinoma and a prevalence of mucinous histology,[141,142] SEER data suggest that this disease in children more closely mirrors the adult presentation, and that referral bias could lead to the findings in the case series.

Most cases of colorectal carcinoma in adults occur sporadically and in association with lifestyle choices. Only approximately 10% of adults with colorectal carcinoma will have an

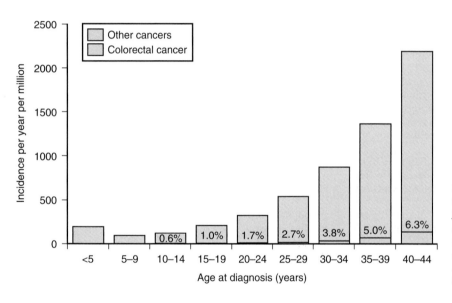

FIGURE 25-9. Incidence of colorectal cancer relative to all cancer, SEER 1975-2000. *(Data from Bleyer A, O'Leary M, Barr R, Ries LAG [eds]. Cancer Epidemiology in Older Adolescents and Young Adults 15 to 29 Years of Age, Including SEER Incidence and Survival: 1975-2000 [NIH Publication No. 06-5767]. Bethesda, Md, National Cancer Institute, 2006.)*

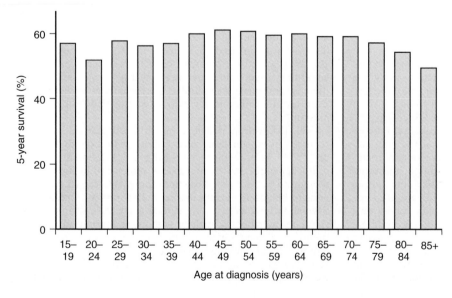

FIGURE 25-10. 5-year survival rate for colorectal carcinoma, SEER 1975-1999. *(Data from Bleyer A, O'Leary M, Barr R, Ries LAG [eds]. Cancer Epidemiology in Older Adolescents and Young Adults 15 to 29 Years of Age, Including SEER Incidence and Survival: 1975-2000 [NIH Publication No. 06-5767]. Bethesda, Md, National Cancer Institute, 2006.)*

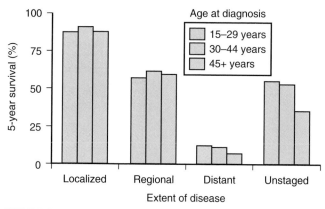

FIGURE 25-11. 5-year survival rate for colorectal cancer by extent of disease, SEER 1975-2000. *(Data from Bleyer A, O'Leary M, Barr R, Ries LAG [eds]. Cancer Epidemiology in Older Adolescents and Young Adults 15 to 29 Years of Age, Including SEER Incidence and Survival: 1975-2000 [NIH Publication No. 06-5767]. Bethesda, Md, National Cancer Institute, 2006.)*

identified inherited or acquired predisposition to it. These include patients with the dominantly inherited familial adenomatous polyposis (FAP) syndrome who have a mutation in the *FAP* tumor suppressor gene, patients with Lynch syndrome (also known as hereditary nonpolyposis colorectal cancer [HNPCC]), characterized by one of several defects in DNA mismatch repair genes, or patients with long-standing inflammatory bowel disease of more than 10 years' duration. It is not clear from the data whether children diagnosed with colorectal carcinoma are likely to have one of these common predispositions to the disease or if there is some other causative factor in these patients. Children with FAP, also known as Gardner's syndrome, are frequently found to have myriad polyps on colonoscopy and many ultimately undergo prophylactic total colectomy before the age of 21 years because of symptoms (e.g., continued blood loss) or because of a strong family history of colon cancer. The vast majority of patients with FAP syndrome develop colorectal cancer by the age of 40 years. Many of these children who do undergo prophylactic colectomy are found to have dysplasia that was not apparent on routine screening colonoscopy.[143] Other syndromes associated with colorectal carcinoma include Bloom, Peutz-Jeghers, Turcot's, Oldfield, and Rendu-Osler-Weber syndromes.[144-148]

Clinical Presentation

Colorectal carcinoma arises from the mucosal surface of the bowel, frequently growing from within a polyp. The tumor can cause intestinal obstruction through growth into the lumen of the bowel or can erode through the serosa and spread intraperitoneally. The early signs of colorectal carcinoma are difficult to separate from more common causes of abdominal complaints. Anemia, vague abdominal pain, bleeding, weight loss, and change in bowel habits have all been reported as the presenting complaint for children with colon cancer.[141] Many of these presenting complaints are common in pediatric care; it is possible that children who present with higher stages of colon cancer might be picked up if they were adults, because an older adult with these complaints would likely be referred for colonoscopy. In two relatively large series reporting on this rare tumor in children, 0 of 20 and 3 of 30 patients presented with modified Dukes stage B tumors.[141,142] All other patients were

stage C or D, and only 1 of 20 and 2 of 30 patients were alive without evidence of disease when these reports were published. In these two series, 16 of 20 and 25 of 30 patients had tumors with mucinous histology, a higher rate than that reported for adults with colorectal carcinoma. Again, these dire statistics likely reflect referral patterns, although they demonstrate that children with colorectal carcinoma can present with high-stage disease. Although vigilance for pediatric colorectal carcinoma remains important, in the absence of known risk factors for the disease, adult-oriented screening examinations, such as colonoscopy, routine testing of stool for occult blood, and sigmoidoscopy, are not indicated, because they would pick up many false-positives and would not be cost-effective.

Diagnosis and Staging

The diagnosis of colorectal carcinoma in children requires a high index of suspicion in patients presenting with the typical signs or symptoms, followed by tissue acquisition. The exact procedure required to obtain tissue for diagnosis is best determined in consultation with surgical colleagues and depends on the patient's clinical situation. For some patients, complete resection before chemotherapy may be appropriate, but for others, particularly those known to have metastatic disease, chemotherapy or radiotherapy may make resection possible in previously unresectable cases, so a less invasive approach to diagnosis is warranted after careful consultation with a multidisciplinary team. Any patient undergoing resection should have up to 12 lymph nodes sampled in an attempt to determine whether the cancer has spread.[149] An expert panel convened by the American Society of Clinical Oncology has not recommended adjuvant chemotherapy for those adult patients with stage II colorectal carcinoma that can be fully surgically resected. Children tend to present with more widespread disease; however, in the absence of data to support a contrary approach, for children with disease that can be fully resected at initial diagnosis, surgical intervention and subsequent observation seem to be indicated.[150]

For pediatric patients discovered to have colorectal carcinoma, full staging should involve functional and anatomic imaging (see later), as would be carried out in adult patients. In adults, linked PET and CT scans are increasingly becoming the norm, because this modality helps link fluorodeoxyglucose (FDG)-avid lesions with actual sites of disease more efficaciously than separate PET and CT scans, which cannot be linked because of bowel movement. Most large pediatric oncology centers now have access to linked PET and CT. Barium enema is sometimes used to help identify areas of concern prior to the diagnosis being made, and a bone scan can be used to identify bone metastases if there is concern that PET is not picking up lesions.[151] The American Joint Committee on Cancer staging for colorectal carcinoma is shown in Tables 25-6 and 25-7.

Treatment

Initial management of the patient is focused on the diagnostic and staging workup and on any surgical interventions that are urgently needed in the context of bowel-related emergencies, such as perforation or obstruction. Consultation with medical oncologists experienced in evaluating adult patients with colorectal carcinoma may help guide the workup. Because of the potential for anemia from bleeding and liver involvement, as well as the potential for peritoneal seeding, complete blood counts, liver function tests, and kidney function tests, with electrolyte levels should be obtained at diagnosis.[141]

TABLE 25-6   **TNM Definitions for Colorectal Carcinoma**

Primary Tumor (T)	Regional Lymph Nodes (N)[§]	Distant Metastasis (M)
TX: Primary tumor cannot be assessed T0: No evidence of primary tumor Tis: Carcinoma in situ—intraepithelial or invasion of the lamina propria* T1: Tumor invades submucosa T2: Tumor invades muscularis propria T3: Tumor invades through the muscularis propria into the subserosa or into nonperitonealized pericolic or perirectal tissues T4: Tumor directly invades other organs or structures and/or perforates visceral peritoneum[†,‡]	NX: Regional nodes cannot be assessed N0: No regional lymph node metastasis N1: Metastasis in one to three regional lymph nodes N2: Metastasis in four or more regional lymph nodes	MX: Distant metastasis cannot be assessed M0: No distant metastasis M1: Distant metastasis

*Tis includes cancer cells confined within the glandular basement membrane (intraepithelial) or lamina propria (intramucosal), with no extension through the muscularis mucosae into the submucosa.

[†]Direct invasion in T4 includes invasion of other segments of the colorectum by way of the serosa—for example, invasion of the sigmoid colon by a carcinoma of the cecum.

[‡]Tumor that is adherent macroscopically to other organs or structures is classified T4. If no tumor is present in the adhesion microscopically, however, the classification should be pT3. The V and L substaging should be used to identify the presence or absence of vascular or lymphatic invasion.

[§]A tumor nodule in the pericolorectal adipose tissue of a primary carcinoma without histologic evidence of residual lymph node in the nodule is classified in the pN category as a regional lymph node metastasis if the nodule has the form and smooth contour of a lymph node. If the nodule has an irregular contour, it should be classified in the T category and also coded as V1 (microscopic venous invasion) or as V2 (if it was grossly evident), because there is a strong likelihood that it represents venous invasion.

From Greene FL, Page DL, Fleming ID, et al (eds). Colon and rectum. In AJCC Cancer Staging Manual, 6th ed. Chicago, American Joint Commission on Cancer, 2002, pp 113-124.

TABLE 25-7   **AJCC Stage Groupings for Colorectal Carcinoma**

Stage	Groupings
0	Tis, N0, M0
I	T1, N0, M0
	T2, N0, M0
IIA	T3, N0, M0
IIB	T4, N0, M0
IIIA	T1, N1, M0
	T2, N1, M0
IIIB	T3, N1, M0
	T4, N1, M0
IIIC	Any T, N2, M0
IV	Any T, any N, M1

From Greene FL, Page DL, Fleming ID, et al (eds). Pharynx (including base of tongue, soft palate and uvula). In AJCC Cancer Staging Manual, 6th ed. Chicago, American Joint Commission on Cancer, 2002, pp 33-46.

Carcinoembryonic antigen (CEA) should also be determined, although most series have found that children tend not to have heightened CEA at diagnosis,[141,142] and subsequently followed to survey for occult recurrence. Many chemotherapeutic agents can increase CEA, so care should be taken when interpreting these values, especially when the patient is receiving oxaliplatin.[152] These patients should generally not have values checked until they have recovered from chemotherapy. If the patient did not have an elevated CEA level at diagnosis, the decision not to follow subsequent levels to screen for occult relapse is reasonable, but should be made in close consultation with medical oncology colleagues.

The treatment for children with colorectal carcinoma should be planned in conjunction with reports in the adult literature and with a medical oncologist experienced in treating gastrointestinal cancer in adults. Adult patients with stage II disease have not been shown to benefit from adjuvant chemotherapy if they have no evidence of disease after resection,[150]

and should undergo wide surgical resection with anastomosis, if possible. It is reasonable to recommend careful observation after surgical treatment for children in this scenario, in the absence of a clinical trial, because there is no standard of care therapy for these patients that has proven to reduce the risk for relapse. Although these patients should be considered for randomized controlled clinical trials, there are likely to be few trials available that include children younger than 18 years. If details of the case or of the surgical resection increase the concern that the patient could suffer a relapse, adjuvant therapy could be considered because the risk for recurrence could be from 51% to 73%.[153] The situation should include careful discussion between the oncologist and family. For stage III or higher patients, chemotherapy has demonstrated a survival benefit for adults with colorectal carcinoma, and children should be treated in a similar fashion.[154]

SEER data have suggested that the proportion of children presenting with colorectal carcinoma who have high-stage disease at diagnosis will mirror that of adults presenting with colorectal carcinoma. Thus, many children will have a higher stage disease at diagnosis that will not be fully resectable and that will require chemotherapy. These patients tend to have a poor prognosis. There are several regimens associated with prolonged survival for patients with metastatic colorectal carcinoma in adults based on the use of 5-FU, oxaliplatin, and irinotecan in a variety of combinations. Bevacizumab (Avastin) is also being used in conjunction with these regimens, often as second-line therapy in adults, with an improvement in survival benefit.[155] Children with high-stage colorectal carcinoma have a poor prognosis, and any child successfully cured may have years of life added, so it may be reasonable for pediatric oncologists to add bevacizumab to the established regimens as front line therapy. However, this will depend somewhat on the clinical scenario. A phase I trial of bevacizumab has been completed in children by the Children's Oncology Group, so there are pediatric oncologists available nationally who have experience administering this agent to children. Further information on chemotherapy regimens for patients with colorectal carcinoma can be found on the Internet (see http://www.cancer.gov/cancertopics/pdq/treatment/colon/HealthProfessional/page4).

Screening and Preventive Therapy for At-Risk Children

Children with a family history of FAP syndrome should generally begin undergoing colonoscopy at an early age, by the age of 10 or 12 years, and should be followed closely by geneticists and pediatric gastroenterologists.[156,157] For such patients, prophylactic colectomy is essential to prevent death from colorectal carcinoma later in life. The decision to undergo total colectomy must be made in conjunction with the family history and timing of cancer onset in the pedigree, the clinical situation, and the child's wishes. Patients with HNPCC are unlikely to develop colorectal carcinoma before the age of 18 years, but the accepted standard for such patients is to begin regular colonoscopy at 20 years of age or at least 10 years earlier than the earliest onset of colorectal carcinoma in their pedigree.[158] For patients with inflammatory bowel disease, care should be based on standard practices for pediatric gastroenterology. Cyclooxygenase-2 (COX-2) inhibitors have been shown to reduce the risk for developing colorectal carcinoma in adults, but are known to increase the risk for cardiovascular side effects, so are not universally recommended for adults at risk of developing colorectal carcinoma.[159] These agents have been used in the pediatric oncology setting, and may in the future be appropriate chemoprophylaxis for children at high risk for colorectal carcinoma.[160]

Follow-up

For the child with the sporadic occurrence of colorectal carcinoma who is cured by surgery or surgery and chemotherapy, careful observation must be recommended. However, there is little evidence available on the risk for such children to suffer recurrence or the risk for second malignancies later in life. Colorectal carcinoma is rare in children and often difficult to cure, so survivors are few. No large-scale randomized trials have documented the efficacy of a standard, postoperative monitoring program in adults to date. Therefore, given the long latency period for relapse for young children, they should probably be screened with regular colonoscopy and radiologic evaluation of the lungs, and perhaps PET scanning as well.[161,162] Because pediatric colorectal carcinoma is so rare, the child may suffer from a cancer predisposition syndrome and consideration should be given to such a diagnosis. The child may benefit from yearly colonoscopy and should be brought to medical attention with little delay for any blood in the stool or other symptoms of colon cancer. Screening for CEA at a reasonable interval could be considered, but is associated with a high rate of false-positives in adults. It should probably only be used for children who had high levels at presentation and are healthy enough to undergo risky surgery if any liver or lung metastases are found early by screening.[163] Although the 5-year survival rate for low-stage colon cancer is excellent (approximately 90%), patients with metastatic disease have less than a 10% 5-year survival rate. For those who survive metastatic pediatric colorectal cancer, it is unclear for how long surveillance against relapse should be done. The child should be followed in a clinic specializing in the long-term consequences of treatment for childhood cancer, regardless of what decisions are made about follow-up.

URINARY BLADDER CARCINOMA

Rhabdomyosarcoma is a relatively common tumor affecting the urinary tract and is discussed elsewhere in this text (see Chapter 19). Malignant epithelial tumors of the bladder are extremely rare in children in the Western world; the incidence of bladder cancer in general is higher in Africa because of the inflammation caused by chronic parasitic infection with bilharzial and other organisms.[164] Boys are more likely than girls to be diagnosed with this.[165] The presenting signs and symptoms of transitional cell tumors of the bladder in children include gross painless hematuria, urinary tract infections, voiding difficulties, and even hematospermia.

If a child is suspected of having a bladder tumor, the differential diagnosis must include malignancies such as epithelial bladder cancer and rhabdomyosarcoma, as well as benign lesions such as inflammatory masses. In the absence of obvious clinical signs of a mass, these patients will usually be seen first by the pediatric urologist. The initial workup should include urinalysis and culture, urine cytology, and imaging studies. CT or MRI can help define the lesion. Cystoscopy can help reveal the nature of the tumor and allow for biopsy of lesional tissue. Attempts at transurethral biopsy are a primary mode of obtaining a tissue diagnosis, with open procedures to be considered as a backup maneuver.[166] The outcome for children with bladder carcinoma seems to be better than for adults.

OVARIAN TUMORS

Approximately 50% of tumors occurring in the ovary in children are non-neoplastic. Furthermore, the minority of neoplastic lesions are malignant, so that only 10% to 20% of ovarian masses in children are cancerous (Box 25-1).[167,168] In children, and even in adolescents, surgical management plans should take into consideration the lower rate of malignancy than in adults, and minimize the risk of compromising hormonal function and fertility.[169] Ovarian masses usually present with abdominal pain, bloating, distention, or dysmenorrhea. The most appropriate and widely used initial evaluation tool for an ovarian mass is ultrasonography, which can distinguish the size, origin, and cystic nature of the tumor.[170] If cystic, unilateral, and presumed benign, a laparoscopic procedure is appropriate. Otherwise, further workup with chest, abdomen, and/or pelvic CT and tumor markers—beta-human chorionic gonadotropin (β-hCG), alpha-fetoprotein (AFP), cancer antigen-125 (CA-125), and CEA—is required, and open laparotomy should be the surgical approach.[170] Ovarian tumors are staged by the International Federation of Gynecology and Obstetrics (FIGO) system (Table 25-8).

Of the neoplastic tumors, germ cell tumors account for 65% to 70% (see Chapter 23). Epithelial carcinomas, the most common ovarian tumor in adults, account for 15% to 20% of pediatric ovarian tumors, with most occurring after menarche when the rate increases markedly (Fig. 25-12). Unlike in adults, most pediatric epithelial ovarian tumors are localized and pathologically most are of low malignant potential (borderline) or well differentiated.[171] Stage I low malignant potential tumors are appropriately treated by unilateral salpingo-oophorectomy alone, and have almost a 100% survival rate.[171] Surgery should include careful inspection of the peritoneum and contralateral ovary and lymph nodes.[172] For those rare children with invasive or advanced disease, platinum-based therapy developed for adult epithelial carcinomas has proven effective. Although a thorough family history should be obtained as a matter of course, studies suggest that Breast Cancer Gene 1 and 2 (BRCA1/2), breast and ovarian cancer syndrome and hereditary nonpolyposis colorectal cancer syndrome, account for few cases of epithelial cancer in young women (younger than 30 years).[173-175]

Box 25-1   **Ovarian Neoplasms**

MALIGNANT TUMORS

1. Germ cell (65%-70%)
2. Epithelial tumors (15%, including low malignant potential or borderline tumors)
   a. Adenocarcinoma
   b. Cystadenocarcinoma: mucinous, serous
   c. Endometroid
   d. Clear cell tumor
   e. Undifferentiated carcinoma
3. Stromal tumors (15%)
   a. Juvenile granulosa cell tumors (JGCTs)
   b. Sertoli-Leydig cell tumors
   c. Sclerosing stromal tumors
   d. Gynandroblastoma
4. Miscellaneous (<5%)
   a. Burkitt's
   b. Carcinosarcoma (malignant mixed müllerian tumor)

BENIGN TUMORS

1. Germ cell
   a. Cystic teratoma (dermoid)
2. Epithelial
   a. Cystadenomas
   b. Mucinous
   c. Papillary and nonpapillary serous
3. Stromal tumors
   a. Granulosa cell
   b. Theca cell
   c. Fibromas

Stromal Carcinomas

Tumors of the mesenchymal tissue of the ovary account for 15% of ovarian malignancies in pediatrics. Most present at an early stage and have a prognosis higher than 85%.[176] Sertoli-Leydig tumors often cause overproduction of androgen precursors, producing virilizing symptoms of amenorrhea, masculinization, and hirsutism. Juvenile granulosa cell tumors can overproduce estrogen and progesterone and present with precocious puberty. These tumors are sometimes classified with benign tumors, and many act in a benign fashion, but they have malignant potential and have been reported to metastasize and be fatal.[177] Nonlocalized tumors should be treated with adjuvant platinum-based chemotherapy with or without radiation.[178]

TUMORS OF THE CERVIX AND VAGINA

The most common nonovarian tumor of the female genital tract is rhabdomyosarcoma (82% in a registry series over 25 years in Great Britain)[179] and the appearance of a protruding cluster-of-grapes vaginal mass in a young child is classic for sarcoma botryoides. Cervical and vaginal carcinomas in children can be adenocarcinomas or squamous carcinomas; the ratio is skewed more toward adenocarcinoma in children than in adults. There is no known difference in causative factors, treatment, or prognosis between the two pathologies. Mesonephric adenocarci-

TABLE 25-8   **Carcinoma of the Ovary***

Stage	Extent of Growth
I	Growth limited to the ovaries
IA	Growth limited to one ovary; no ascites present containing malignant cells; no tumor on the external surface; capsule intact
IB	Growth limited to both ovaries; no ascites present containing malignant cells; no tumor on the external surface; capsules intact
IC*	Tumor either stage IA or IB, but with tumor on surface of one or both ovaries, or with capsule ruptured, ascites present containing malignant cells, or positive peritoneal washings
II	Growth involving one or both ovaries with pelvic extension
IIA	Extension and/or metastases to the uterus and/or tubes
IIB	Extension to other pelvic tissues
IIC[†]	Tumor either stage IIA or IIB, but with tumor on surface of one or both ovaries, or with capsule(s) ruptured, ascites present containing malignant cells, or positive peritoneal washings
III	Tumor involving one or both ovaries, with histologically confirmed peritoneal implants outside the pelvis and/or positive retroperitoneal or inguinal nodes; superficial live metastases equals stage III; tumor limited to the true pelvis, but with histologically proven malignant extension to small bowel or omentum
IIIA	Tumor grossly limited to the true pelvis, with negative nodes, but with histologically confirmed microscopic seeding of abdominal peritoneal surfaces or histologically proven extension to small bowel or mesentery
IIIB	Tumor of one or both ovaries with histologically confirmed implants, peritoneal metastasis of abdominal peritoneal surface, not exceeding 2 cm in diameter; nodes are negative
IIIC	Peritoneal metastasis beyond the pelvis >2 cm in diameter and/or positive retroperitoneal or inguinal nodes
IV	Growth involving one or both ovaries with distant metastases; if pleural effusion is present, there must be positive cytology to allot a case to stage IV; parenchymal liver metastasis equals stage IV

*International Federation of Gynecology and Obstetrics (FIGO) nomenclature, Rio de Janeiro, 1988.
[†]To evaluate the impact on prognosis of the different criteria for allotting cases to stage IC or IIC, it would be of value to know if rupture of the capsule was spontaneous, or caused by the surgeon; and if the source of malignant cells detected was peritoneal washings, or ascites.
From Heintz AP, Odicino F, Maisonneuve P, et al. Carcinoma of the ovary. FIGO 6th Annual Report on the Results of Treatment in Gynecological Cancer. Int J Gynaecol Obstet. 2006;95(Suppl 1):S161-S192.

noma is rare in adults but is a relatively more common subtype in children; it is thought to arise from mesonephric duct remnants and tends to arise deeply, without reaching the endocervical surface.[180]

Cervicovaginal clear cell adenocarcinomas are not associated with human papillomavirus (HPV) infection. Rather, a peak of incidence in children and adolescent girls was a historic phenomenon, caused by the maternal use of diethylstilbestrol (DES) therapy in pregnancy. Since its proscription, the tumor is again relatively uncommon in pediatrics. However, rates of non-DES cervical cancer in adolescents have been rising because of increasingly early sexual activity and higher rates of HPV infection.[181] HPV types 16 and 18 are the caus-

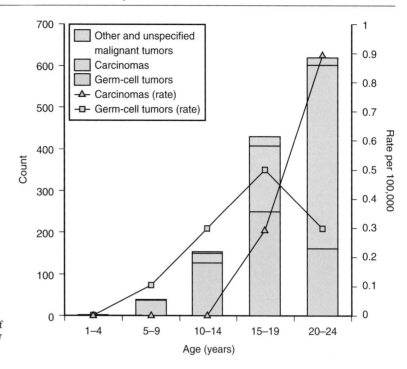

FIGURE 25-12. Incidence and rate per 100,000 cases of ovarian cancer in children and young adults, SEER-17 1998-2002.

ative agents in more than 70% of cervical cancer. The recent formulation of a vaccine against these viruses is being promoted for administration to 12-year-old girls.[182] Around puberty, the cervix has a particular biologic vulnerability to HPV infection, so that the sexually active adolescent has one of the highest risks of infection after exposure,[183] creating a risk for the development of squamous intraepithelial lesions that can progress over 10 to 15 years to invasive cervical cancer.[184] Recent data have shown that 29% of 9th-grade and 62% of 12th-grade girls report having had sexual intercourse.[185] These sexually active female adolescents have high rates of genital HPV infection (13% to 64%) and abnormal Pap smear results, as high as 38%.[183-185] The natural history of progression of cervical abnormalities (from squamous intraepithelial lesions to cervical intraepithelial neoplasia) appears similar in adolescents and adults.[186] Recommendations for adolescents with abnormal Pap smears are available on the American Society for Colposcopy and Cervical Pathology (ASCCP) website (www.asccp.org).

The most common clinical presentation of a cervical or vaginal tumor is vaginal bleeding, which may be difficult to distinguish from irregular menses in prepubescent and early pubescent girls. In one series evaluating causes of vaginal bleeding in children, tumors accounted for 11%.[187] These tumors often present at later stages in children and adolescents than adults because of the lack of screening Pap smears and hesitancy to perform pelvic examinations.[188]

Treatment includes surgical resection with lymph node exploration and adjuvant radiation for residual disease or lymph nodes. This preference of surgery over radiation differs from therapy for adults because of the need to avoid radiation toxicity in younger, growing children. Novel uterus-sparing techniques (e.g., radical vaginal trachelectomy) first adopted in adults have been used successfully in children.[189] In a retrospective study of women younger than 25 years, localized cervical cancer had a 5-year survival of 91% and regional disease had a 5-year survival of 46%.[190] A series of 37 pediatric cases of vaginal and cervical adenocarcinoma from St. Jude

Children's Research Hospital has found a 71% 3-year survival.[188]

Other rare tumors reported in the cervix and vagina are alveolar soft parts sarcoma,[94,191] endodermal sinus (yolk sac) tumor,[192] and Wilms' tumor.[193]

GESTATIONAL TROPHOBLASTIC TUMOR

Sexually active adolescents are at risk for these rare tumors, which arise as tumors of the products of conception. A hydatidiform mole, or molar pregnancy, is a uterine mass consisting only of placental-like tissue, without an intact fetus. Pregnancies in those younger than 15 years have a sixfold risk of being molar.[194] Hydatidiform moles are treated by dilation and curettage, with careful follow-up for resolution of elevated β-hCG levels.[195] Persistent or increasing β-hCG levels after a molar pregnancy, abortion, or term pregnancy indicate a malignant gestational trophoblastic tumor (GTT), the most aggressive of which is choriocarcinoma, a malignant tumor of the trophoblastic epithelium. The most common symptom is abnormal vaginal bleeding, but patients can also present with asymptomatic pulmonary metastases or neurologic symptoms, caused by brain metastases.[196] Patients with nonmetastatic or good-prognosis metastatic GTT are treated with single-agent chemotherapy (methotrexate, dactinomycin, or etoposide), and have an excellent prognosis.[197,198] Those with high-risk metastatic disease (high β-hCG, delay in start of chemotherapy, brain metastases, multiple sites of metastases) require multiagent cytotoxic chemotherapy.[199,200]

MELANOMA

Pediatric melanoma, which has been classified as an epithelial malignancy by the International Classification of Childhood

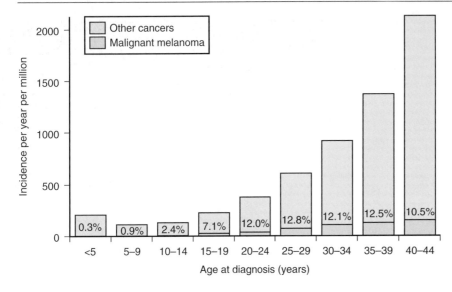

FIGURE 25-13. Incidence of malignant melanoma relative to all cancers, SEER 1975-2000. *(Data from Bleyer A, O'Leary M, Barr R, Ries LAG [eds]. Cancer Epidemiology in Older Adolescents and Young Adults 15 to 29 Years of Age, Including SEER Incidence and Survival: 1975-2000 [NIH Publication No. 06-5767]. Bethesda, Md, National Cancer Institute, 2006.)*

Cancer (ICCC), accounts for 30% of epithelial cancers in children and adolescents.[20,31] Although rare, particularly among prepubertal patients, it is estimated that nearly 450 cases of pediatric melanoma are diagnosed each year in the United States in patients younger than 20 years[31] and most cases affect 15- to 19-year olds, in whom this malignancy accounts for 7.1% of all cancers (Fig. 25-13).[31]

The incidence of melanoma in children younger than 20 years increased by 2.9%/year from 1973 to 2001, with the highest rates of increase in adolescents.[201] Most melanoma cases in pediatric patients affect white females, are localized superficial spreading melanoma, and involve the extremities and torso.[201] In children younger than 10 years, however, there is a higher preponderance of nonwhite patients, nodular histology, and disease that affects the face, head, and neck.

Risk Factors

Congenital and Infantile Melanoma

The most common transplacentally acquired malignancy, melanoma, is still rare,[201] with only six documented cases in the literature. The probability of developing fetal metastases as a consequence of placental involvement is about 20%. In the absence of metastases at birth, follow-up evaluations for the development of melanoma in infants should continue for 2 years after birth. These should include chest x-ray and liver enzyme and lactate dehydrogenase assays, performed at 6-month intervals.[202]

Most congenital or infantile melanomas arise from medium or large congenital nevi.[203] Giant congenital melanocytic nevi affects fewer than 1 in 20,000 newborns.[204] The risk of developing cutaneous melanoma in this patient population is about 3% and, although this number appears deceivingly small, this figure translates into a 465-fold increased risk for developing melanoma during childhood and adolescence.[204,205] Melanomas develop in patients with giant nevi, most often during the first decade of life, arise from preexisting nevi located on the trunk, although cases of unknown primary site and retroperitoneal and central nervous system melanoma have been reported, and occur in patients with increased numbers of satellite nevi and larger lesions (larger than 40 to 50 cm).[204-206] The role of surgical removal and its effect on preventing melanoma remain understudied.

Neurocutaneous melanosis is a rare disorder characterized by multiple congenital melanocytic nevi in association with melanocytic proliferations in the leptomeninges.[207] Asymptomatic neurocutaneous melanosis is seen in up to 25% of patients with large congenital nevi, and the vast majority of these patients have normal development and do not develop melanoma. The risk of developing symptomatic neurocutaneous melanosis, characterized by symptoms of increased intracranial pressure and developmental delay, in patients with giant melanocytic nevi ranges from 2.5% to 17%; the risk is increased in patients with large nevi (larger than 20 cm) in posterior axial locations with multiple satellites.[206,207] The risk of developing central nervous system melanoma in these patients ranges from 40% to 64%.

Several hereditary diseases predispose to pediatric melanoma. Xeroderma pigmentosum is a rare recessive nucleotide excision repair disease that affects approximately 1 in 250,000 individuals in the United States.[208-211] Patients with this condition have an increased risk (up to 1000-fold) of developing nonmelanoma skin cancer and melanoma. Up to 50% of patients with this condition develop cutaneous neoplasms by age 14 and 5% develop melanoma, with a median age at diagnosis of 19 years.[211] Patients with Werner's syndrome, a rare autosomal recessive disorder characterized by premature aging caused by mutations in the *WRN* gene, a member of the RecQ helicase gene family, are at increased risk of developing melanoma.[212,213] The distribution of melanoma in these patients is unusual, affecting areas such as the feet, nose, and esophagus. Survivors of hereditary retinoblastoma have a substantially increased risk (standardized incidence ratio of 28) of developing cutaneous melanoma. Administration of radiotherapy for the treatment of the primary retinoblastoma further increases the risk of melanoma in this patient population.[214]

Other Factors

Individuals who have received a renal or bone marrow transplant, or chemotherapy for primary tumors, are at increased risk of melanoma, suggesting a role for immunosuppression in pathogenesis. Melanoma in renal transplant recipients is most commonly seen within the first 5 years after transplantation and accounts for 15% of all post-transplantation de novo skin cancers in children.[215] Long-term survivors of childhood cancer are also at increased risk for developing melanoma; this risk appears most prominent in patients treated with spindle

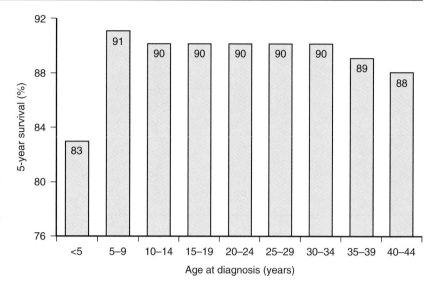

FIGURE 25-14. Overall 5-year survival rates for malignant melanoma, SEER 1975-1999. *(Data from Bleyer A, O'Leary M, Barr R, Ries LAG [eds]. Cancer Epidemiology in Older Adolescents and Young Adults 15 to 29 Years of Age, Including SEER Incidence and Survival: 1975-2000 [NIH Publication No. 06-5767]. Bethesda, Md, National Cancer Institute, 2006.)*

inhibitors, alkylating agents, or radiation doses exceeding 15 Gy.[216] Similarly, pediatric patients who have received a bone marrow transplant are at increased risk for developing melanoma.[217]

Lastly, in the absence of a known genetic syndrome, patients with an increased number of melanocytic nevi larger than 2 mm in diameter, fair complexion, inability to tan, facial freckling, and a family history of melanoma have an increased risk of developing melanoma.[218] The presence and number of dysplastic nevi confers a two- to 12-fold increased risk of developing melanoma. Inactivating mutations of the *CDKN2A* gene have been reported rarely in isolated cases of pediatric melanoma.[219-221]

Clinical and Pathologic Features

Pediatric melanoma resembles adult melanoma in its clinical presentation. The classic ABCDEs of melanoma (*a*symmetry, *b*order irregularity, *c*olor variegation, *d*iameter larger than 6 mm, and an *e*volving lesion) are commonly reported in childhood and adolescent cases.[220] Other signs and symptoms that have been documented in the literature that may suggest the diagnosis of pediatric melanoma include a mole that bleeds or itches or an obvious palpable mass secondary to lymph node metastases.[222] Because the diagnosis of melanoma is rarely suspected, it is estimated that up to 60% of pediatric patients with melanomas are initially misdiagnosed.[223]

The pathologic diagnosis of melanoma is often difficult and challenging. Increasing evidence has suggested that pediatric melanoma may have a significant variability in its pathologic spectrum. The term *melanocytic lesion with unknown metastatic potential* has gained popularity in recent years, adding to the uncertainty and confusion of diagnosing pediatric melanoma.[224]

Diagnosis and Staging

Guidelines for diagnosing and staging pediatric melanoma have been extrapolated from adult studies and are available on the Internet (see http://www.nccn.org/professionals/ physician_gls/ PDF/melanoma.pdf). We recommend following the current AJCC guidelines for staging all pediatric patients with melanoma. In one center's experience, the incidence of metastases

detected by routine imaging was significantly higher in pediatric patients when compared with adults.[225,226] This study was done prior to the use of sentinel node biopsies, so we recommend that appropriate staging procedures follow published adult guidelines and the use of additional baseline imaging studies be performed at the discretion of the treating physician. The use of sentinel node biopsy has gained popularity in recent years. Currently, it has become an accepted method for staging pediatric patients with melanomas at least 1 mm thick or in those with thinner lesions who have evidence of ulceration or are a Clark's level IV of invasion or higher.[224,227-230]

Treatment and Outcome

Surgery is the treatment of choice for pediatric melanoma, and guidelines for resection follow those outlined for adult patients with melanoma (http://www.nccn.org/professionals/ physician_gls/ PDF/melanoma.pdf). The administration of adjuvant high-dose interferon has been prospectively studied in two pediatric trials and appears to be better tolerated than in adults.[231,232] However, its role in improving outcome remains undetermined, given the small numbers of patients in these trials. Despite these limitations, we recommend considering the use of high-dose adjuvant interferon in patients with resected nodal disease.[233-235] The use of chemotherapy for disseminated disease has been poorly studied in pediatrics[236] and unfortunately vaccine trials are usually unavailable for this patient population. The overall survival of pediatric melanoma is excellent, exceeding 90% at 5 years (Fig. 25-14). However, patients younger than 10 years appear to have a worse prognosis (see Fig. 25-14) and, as in adults, stage is an important predictor of outcome (Fig. 25-15).[201,237,238]

A striking recent discovery in adult melanoma patients is the observation of activating mutations or amplifications in the *KIT* gene.[239] This molecular lesion was not previously observed at high frequency in melanomas, but was found to occur at a higher incidence in melanomas arising on mucosal surfaces, on acral surfaces (hairless palms, soles), and within chronically sun-damaged skin exhibiting histologic evidence of solar elastosis. Importantly, very early clinical experience has suggested major responsiveness of *c-Kit* mutant melanomas to targeted therapy using imatinib.[240] It remains to be seen whether other cases of unusual melanomas, such as those in pediatric populations, also exhibit *KIT* mutations, which may be amenable to

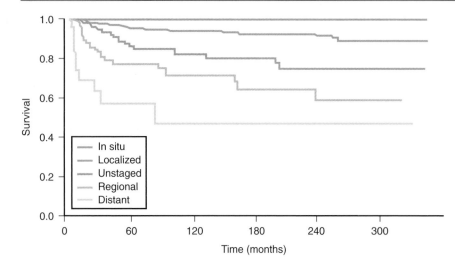

FIGURE 25-15. Survival of pediatric melanoma by stage, SEER 1973-2001. *(Adapted from Strouse JJ, Fears TR, Tucker MA, Wayne AS. Pediatric melanoma: risk factor and survival analysis of the surveillance, epidemiology and end results database. J Clin Oncol. 2005;23:4735-4741.)*

such kinase-targeted therapeutic strategies. It is also unclear whether the presence of KIT amplification (without gene mutation) may also portend responsiveness to KIT–targeted therapy; this is an important question in regard to an otherwise terribly challenging disease.

REFERENCES

1. Bernstein L, Gurney JG (eds). Carcinomas and Other Malignant Epithelial Neoplasms. SEER Pediatric Monograph. Bethesda, Md, National Cancer Institute, 2001. Available at http://seer.cancer.gov/publications/childhood/carcinomas.pdf.

2. Weir HK, Thun MJ, Hankey BF, et al. Annual report to the nation on the status of cancer, 1975-2000, featuring the uses of surveillance data for cancer prevention and control. J Natl Cancer Inst. 2003;95:1276-1299.

3. Ellis P, Davies AM, Evans WK, et al. The use of chemotherapy in patients with advanced malignant pleural mesothelioma: a systematic review and practice guideline. J Thorac Oncol. 2006;1:591-601.

4. Soldz S, Clark TW, Stewart E, et al. Decreased youth tobacco use in Massachusetts 1996 to 1999: evidence of tobacco control effectiveness. Tob Control 2002;11(Suppl 2):14-19.

5. Huhtala HS, Rainio SU, Rimpela AH. Adolescent snuff use in Finland in 1981-2003: trend, total sales ban and acquisition. Tob Control. 2006;15:392-397.

6. Gallus S, Zuccaro P, Colombo P, et al. Effects of new smoking regulations in Italy. Ann Oncol. 2006;17:346-347.

7. Leung W, Hudson MM, Strickland DK, et al. Late effects of treatment in survivors of childhood acute myeloid leukemia. J Clin Oncol. 2000;18:3273-3279.

8. Vedrine PO, Coffinet L, Temam S, et al. Mucoepidermoid carcinoma of salivary glands in the pediatric age group: 18 clinical cases, including 11 second malignant neoplasms. Head Neck. 2006;28:827-833.

9. Wei WI, Sham JS. Nasopharyngeal carcinoma. Lancet. 2005;365:2041-2054.

10. Rodriguez-Galindo C, Wofford M, Castleberry RP, et al. Preradiation chemotherapy with methotrexate, cisplatin, 5-fluorouracil, and leucovorin for pediatric nasopharyngeal carcinoma. Cancer. 2005;103:850-857.

11. Richey LM, Olshan AF, George J, et al. Incidence and survival rates for young blacks with nasopharyngeal carcinoma in the United States. Arch Otolaryngol Head Neck Surg. 2006;132:1035-1040.

12. Kupeli S, Varan A, Ozyar E, et al. Treatment results of 84 patients with nasopharyngeal carcinoma in childhood. Pediatr Blood Cancer. 2006;46:454-458.

13. Ozyar E, Selek U, Laskar S, et al. Treatment results of 165 pediatric patients with non-metastatic nasopharyngeal carcinoma: a Rare Cancer Network study. Radiother Oncol. 2006;81:39-46.

14. Friborg J, Wohlfahrt J, Koch A, et al. Cancer susceptibility in nasopharyngeal carcinoma families—a population-based cohort study. Cancer Res. 2005;65:8567-8572.

15. Albeck H, Bentzen J, Ockelmann HH, et al. Familial clusters of nasopharyngeal carcinoma and salivary gland carcinomas in Greenland natives. Cancer. 1993;72:196-200.

16. Ozyar E, Yildiz F, Akyol FH, Atahan IL. Comparison of AJCC 1988 and 1997 classifications for nasopharyngeal carcinoma. American Joint Committee on Cancer. Int J Radiat Oncol Biol Phys. 1999;44:1079-1087.

17. Kim TH, McLaren J, Alvarado CS, et al. Adjuvant chemotherapy for advanced nasopharyngeal carcinoma in childhood. Cancer. 1989;63:1922-1926.

18. Niedziela M. Pathogenesis, diagnosis and management of thyroid nodules in children. Endocr Relat Cancer. 2006;13:427-453.

19. Welker MJ, Orlov D. Thyroid nodules. Am Fam Physician. 2003;67:559-566.

20. Ries L, Smith M, Gurney J, et al (eds). Cancer Incidence and Survival Among Children and Adolescents: United States SEER Program 1975-1995 (NIH Publication No. 99.4649). Bethesda, Md, National Cancer Institute, 1999.

21. Cardis E, Howe G, Ron E, et al. Cancer consequences of the Chernobyl accident: 20 years on. J Radiol Prot. 2006;26:127-140.

22. Jacob P, Bogdanova TI, Buglova E, et al. Thyroid cancer among Ukrainians and Belarusians who were children or adolescents at the time of the Chernobyl accident. J Radiol Prot. 2006;26:51-67.

23. Jacob P, Bogdanova TI, Buglova E, et al. Thyroid cancer risk in areas of Ukraine and Belarus affected by the Chernobyl accident. Radiat Res. 2006;165:1-8.

24. Cardis E, Kesminiene A, Ivanov V, et al. Risk of thyroid cancer after exposure to ^{131}I in childhood. J Natl Cancer Inst. 2005;97:724-732.

25. Pacini F, Vorontsova T, Molinaro E, et al. Thyroid consequences of the Chernobyl nuclear accident. Acta Paediatr Suppl. 1999;88:23-27.

26. Sigurdson AJ, Ronckers CM, Mertens AC, et al. Primary thyroid cancer after a first tumour in childhood (the Childhood Cancer

Survivor Study): a nested case-control study. Lancet. 2005;365: 2014-2023.

27. Mauras N, Zimmerman D, Goellner JR. Hashimoto thyroiditis associated with thyroid cancer in adolescent patients. J Pediatr. 1985;106:895-898.

28. Belfiore A, Russo D, Vigneri R, Filetti S. Graves' disease, thyroid nodules and thyroid cancer. Clin Endocrinol (Oxf). 2001;55: 711-718.

29. Herraiz M, Barbesino G, Faquin W, et al. Prevalence of thyroid cancer in familial adenomatous polyposis syndrome and the role of screening ultrasound examinations. Clin Gastroenterol Hepatol. 2007;5:367-373.

30. DeLellis RA. Pathology and genetics of thyroid carcinoma. J Surg Oncol. 2006;94:662-669.

31. Bleyer A, O'Leary M, Barr R, Ries LAG (eds). Cancer Epidemiology in Older Adolescents and Young Adults 15 to 29 Years of Age, Including Seer Incidence and Survival: 1975-2000 (NIH Publication No. 06-5767). Bethesda, Md, National Cancer Institute, 2006.

32. Jarzab B, Handkiewicz-Junak D, Wloch J. Juvenile differentiated thyroid carcinoma and the role of radioiodine in its treatment: a qualitative review. Endocr Relat Cancer. 2005;12:773-803.

33. Demidchik YE, Demidchik EP, Reiners C, et al. Comprehensive clinical assessment of 740 cases of surgically treated thyroid cancer in children of Belarus. Ann Surg. 2006;243:525-532.

34. Klugbauer S, Lengfelder E, Demidchik EP, Rabes HM. High prevalence of RET rearrangement in thyroid tumors of children from Belarus after the Chernobyl reactor accident. Oncogene. 1995;11:2459-2467.

35. Brzezianska E, Karbownik M, Migdalska-Sek M, et al. Molecular analysis of the RET and NTRK1 gene rearrangements in papillary thyroid carcinoma in the Polish population. Mutat Res. 2006;599:26-35.

36. Ciampi R, Knauf JA, Kerler R, et al. Oncogenic AKAP9-BRAF fusion is a novel mechanism of MAPK pathway activation in thyroid cancer. J Clin Invest. 2005;115:94-101.

37. Alberti L, Carniti C, Miranda C, et al. RET and NTRK1 proto-oncogenes in human diseases. J Cell Physiol. 2003;195:168-186.

38. Musholt TJ, Musholt PB, Khaladj N, et al. Prognostic significance of RET and NTRK1 rearrangements in sporadic papillary thyroid carcinoma. Surgery. 2000;128:984-993.

39. Lima J, Trovisco V, Soares P, et al. BRAF mutations are not a major event in post-Chernobyl childhood thyroid carcinomas. J Clin Endocrinol Metab. 2004;89:4267-4271.

40. Nikiforova MN, Ciampi R, Salvatore G, et al. Low prevalence of BRAF mutations in radiation-induced thyroid tumors in contrast to sporadic papillary carcinomas. Cancer Lett. 2004;209: 1-6.

41. Castro P, Rebocho AP, Soares RJ, et al. PAX8-PPAR gamma rearrangement is frequently detected in the follicular variant of papillary thyroid carcinoma. J Clin Endocrinol Metab. 2006;91: 213-220.

42. Hegedus L. Clinical practice. The thyroid nodule. N Engl J Med. 2004;351:1764-1771.

43. Rachmiel M, Charron M, Gupta A, et al. Evidence-based review of treatment and follow up of pediatric patients with differentiated thyroid carcinoma. J Pediatr Endocrinol Metab. 2006;19:1377-1393.

44. Newman KD, Black T, Heller G, et al. Differentiated thyroid cancer: determinants of disease progression in patients <21 years of age at diagnosis: a report from the Surgical Discipline Committee of the Children's Cancer Group. Ann Surg. 1998;227: 533-541.

45. De Silva NK, Brandt ML. Disorders of the breast in children and adolescents, Part 2: Breast masses. J Pediatr Adolesc Gynecol. 2006;19:415-418.

46. Goehring C, Morabia A. Epidemiology of benign breast disease, with special attention to histologic types. Epidemiol Rev. 1997;19: 310-327.

47. Neinstein LS. Breast disease in adolescents and young women. Pediatr Clin North Am. 1999;46:607-629.

48. Cant PJ, Madden MV, Coleman MG, Dent DM. Non-operative management of breast masses diagnosed as fibroadenoma. Br J Surg. 1995;82:792-794.

49. Parker SJ, Harries SA. Phyllodes tumours. Postgrad Med J. 2001;77:428-435.

50. Mangi AA, Smith BL, Gadd MA, et al. Surgical management of phyllodes tumors. Arch Surg. 1999;134:487-493.

51. Reinfuss M, Mitus J, Duda K, et al. The treatment and prognosis of patients with phyllodes tumor of the breast: an analysis of 170 cases. Cancer. 1996;77:910-916.

52. Rajan PB, Cranor ML, Rosen PP. Cystosarcoma phyllodes in adolescent girls and young women: a study of 45 patients. Am J Surg Pathol. 1998;22:64-69.

53. Hays DM, Donaldson SS, Shimada H, et al. Primary and metastatic rhabdomyosarcoma in the breast: neoplasms of adolescent females, a report from the Intergroup Rhabdomyosarcoma Study. Med Pediatr Oncol. 1997;29:181-189.

54. Rogers DA, Lobe TE, Rao BN, et al. Breast malignancy in children. J Pediatr Surg. 1994;29:48-51.

55. Xiong Q, Valero V, Kau V, et al. Female patients with breast carcinoma age 30 years and younger have a poor prognosis: the M.D. Anderson Cancer Center experience. Cancer. 2001;92: 2523-2528.

56. Al-Qahtani AR, Di Lorenzo M, Yazbeck S. Endobronchial tumors in children: institutional experience and literature review. J Pediatr Surg. 2003;38:733-736.

57. Hartman GE, Shochat SJ. Primary pulmonary neoplasms of childhood: a review. Ann Thorac Surg. 1983;36:108-119.

58. Lal DR, Clark I, Shalkow J, et al. Primary epithelial lung malignancies in the pediatric population. Pediatr Blood Cancer. 2005;45:683-686.

59. Yousem SA, Hochholzer L. Mucoepidermoid tumors of the lung. Cancer. 1987;60:1346-1352.

60. Florentine BD, Fink T, Avidan S, et al. Extra-salivary gland presentations of adenoid cystic carcinoma: a report of three cases. Diagn Cytopathol. 2006;34:491-494.

61. Hancock BJ, Di Lorenzo M, Youssef S, et al. Childhood primary pulmonary neoplasms. J Pediatr Surg. 1993;28:1133-1136.

62. Wang LT, Wilkins EW Jr, Bode HH. Bronchial carcinoid tumors in pediatric patients. Chest. 1993;103:1426-1428.

63. Fauroux B, Aynie V, Larroquet M, et al. Carcinoid and mucoepidermoid bronchial tumours in children. Eur J Pediatr. 2005; 164:748-752.

64. Amer KM, Ibrahim NB, Forrester-Wood CP, et al. Lung carcinoid related Cushing's syndrome: report of three cases and review of the literature. Postgrad Med J. 2001;77:464-467.

65. Musi M, Carbone RG, Bertocchi C, et al. Bronchial carcinoid tumours: a study on clinicopathological features and role of octreotide scintigraphy. Lung Cancer. 1998;22:97-102.

66. Moraes TJ, Langer JC, Forte V, et al. Pediatric pulmonary carcinoid: a case report and review of the literature. Pediatr Pulmonol. 2003;35:318-322.

67. Lack EE, Harris GB, Eraklis AJ, Vawter GF. Primary bronchial tumors in childhood. A clinicopathologic study of six cases. Cancer. 1983;51:492-497.

68. Brandt B 3rd, Heintz SE, Rose EF, Ehrenhaft JL. Bronchial carcinoid tumors. Ann Thorac Surg. 1984;38:63-65.

69. Granberg D, Eriksson B, Wilander E, et al. Experience in treatment of metastatic pulmonary carcinoid tumors. Ann Oncol. 2001;12:1383-1391.

70. Dehner LP. Pleuropulmonary blastoma is THE pulmonary blastoma of childhood. Semin Diagn Pathol. 1994;11:144-151.

71. Priest JR, Watterson J, Strong L, et al. Pleuropulmonary blastoma: a marker for familial disease. J Pediatr. 1996;128:220-224.

72. Priest JR, Hill DA, Williams GM, et al. Type I pleuropulmonary blastoma: a report from the International Pleuropulmonary Blastoma Registry. J Clin Oncol. 2006;24:4492-4498.

73. Indolfi P, Casale F, Carli M, et al. Pleuropulmonary blastoma: management and prognosis of 11 cases. Cancer. 2000;89:1396-1401.

74. Indolfi P, Bisogno G, Casale F, et al. Prognostic factors in pleuropulmonary blastoma. Pediatr Blood Cancer. 2007;48:318-323.

75. Ramos SG, Barbosa GH, Tavora FR, et al. Bronchioloalveolar carcinoma arising in a congenital pulmonary airway malformation in a child: case report with an update of this association. J Pediatr Surg. 2007;42:E1-E4.

76. Ohye RG, Cohen DM, Caldwell S, Qualman SJ. Pediatric bronchioloalveolar carcinoma: a favorable pediatric malignancy? J Pediatr Surg. 1998;33:730-732.

77. La Salle AJ, Andrassy RJ, Stanford W. Bronchogenic squamous cell carcinoma in childhood; a case report. J Pediatr Surg. 1977;12:519-521.

78. Robinet G, Gouva S, Le Reste N, et al. Small cell bronchial cancer in a 17-year-old young man. Rev Mal Respir. 1994;11:607-609.

79. Yonemori K, Kunitoh H, Sekine I. Small-cell lung cancer with lymphadenopathy in an 18-year-old female nonsmoker. Nat Clin Pract Oncol. 2006;3:399-403.

80. Kantar M, Cetingul N, Veral A, et al. Rare tumors of the lung in children. Pediatr Hematol Oncol. 2002;19:421-428.

81. DiFurio MJ, Auerbach A, Kaplan KJ. Well-differentiated fetal adenocarcinoma: rare tumor in the pediatric population. Pediatr Dev Pathol. 2003;6:564-567.

82. Fraire AE, Cooper S, Greenberg SD, et al. Mesothelioma of childhood. Cancer. 1988;62:838-847.

83. Cooper SP, Fraire AE, Buffler PA, et al. Epidemiologic aspects of childhood mesothelioma. Pathol Immunopathol Res. 1989;8:276-286.

84. Coffin CM, Dehner LP. Mesothelial and related neoplasms in children and adolescents: a clinicopathologic and immunohistochemical analysis of eight cases. Pediatr Pathol. 1992;12:333-347.

85. Kelsey A. Mesothelioma in childhood. Pediatr Hematol Oncol. 1994;11:461-462.

86. Sugarbaker DJ. Macroscopic complete resection: the goal of primary surgery in multimodality therapy for pleural mesothelioma. J Thorac Oncol. 2006;1:175-176.

87. Sasaki H, Sasano H, Ohi R, et al. Adenocarcinoma at the esophageal gastric junction arising in an 11-year-old girl. Pathol Int. 1999;49:1109-1113.

88. Schettini ST, Ganc A, Saba L. Esophageal carcinoma secondary to a chemical injury in a child. Pediatr Surg Int. 1998;13:519-520.

89. Deurloo JA, Aronson DC. Possibility that esophageal atresia (EA) carries an increased risk for esophageal carcinoma. J Pediatr Surg. 2006;41:876-877; author reply 7.

90. Deurloo JA, van Lanschot JJ, Drillenburg P, Aronson DC. Esophageal squamous cell carcinoma 38 years after primary repair of esophageal atresia. J Pediatr Surg. 2001;36:629-630.

91. Choi SH, Kim SM, Oh JT, et al. Solid pseudopapillary tumor of the pancreas: a multicenter study of 23 pediatric cases. J Pediatr Surg. 2006;41:1992-1995.

92. Saif MW. Pancreatoblastoma. JOP. 2007;8:55-63.

93. Harting MT, Blakely ML, Herzog CE, et al. Treatment issues in pediatric gastric adenocarcinoma. J Pediatr Surg. 2004;39:e8-e10.

94. Morimitsu Y, Tanaka H, Iwanaga S, Kojiro M. Alveolar soft part sarcoma of the uterine cervix. Acta Pathol Jpn. 1993;43:204-208.

95. Demetri GD, Titton RL, Ryan DP, Fletcher CD. Case records of the Massachusetts General Hospital. Weekly clinicopathological exercises. Case 32-2004. A 68-year-old man with a large retroperitoneal mass. N Engl J Med. 2004;351:1779-1787.

96. Saund MS, Demetri GD, Ashley SW. Gastrointestinal stromal tumors (GISTs). Curr Opin Gastroenterol. 2004;20:89-94.

97. Corless CL, Fletcher JA, Heinrich MC. Biology of gastrointestinal stromal tumors. J Clin Oncol. 2004;22:3813-3825.

98. Heinrich MC, Corless CL, Demetri GD, et al. Kinase mutations and imatinib response in patients with metastatic gastrointestinal stromal tumor. J Clin Oncol. 2003;21:4342-4349.

99. Corless CL, Schroeder A, Griffith D, et al. PDGFRA mutations in gastrointestinal stromal tumors: frequency, spectrum and in vitro sensitivity to imatinib. J Clin Oncol. 2005;23:5357-5364.

100. Miettinen M, Fetsch JF, Sobin LH, Lasota J. Gastrointestinal stromal tumors in patients with neurofibromatosis 1: a clinicopathologic and molecular genetic study of 45 cases. Am J Surg Pathol. 2006;30:90-96.

101. Miettinen M, Lasota J. Gastrointestinal stromal tumors. Review of morphology, molecular pathology, prognosis and differential diagnosis. Arch Pathol Lab Med. 2006;130:1466-1478.

102. Rubin BP. Gastrointestinal stromal tumours: an update. Histopathology. 2006;48:83-96.

103. Lasota J, Miettinen M. A new familial GIST identified. Am J Surg Pathol. 2006;30:1342.

104. Li FP, Fletcher JA, Heinrich MC, et al. Familial gastrointestinal stromal tumor syndrome: phenotypic and molecular features in a kindred. J Clin Oncol. 2005;23:2735-2743.

105. Dematteo RP, Heinrich MC, El-Rifai WM, Demetri G. Clinical management of gastrointestinal stromal tumors: before and after STI-571. Hum Pathol. 2002;33:466-477.

106. Demetri GD, von Mehren M, Blanke CD, et al. Efficacy and safety of imatinib mesylate in advanced gastrointestinal stromal tumors. N Engl J Med. 2002;347:472-480.

107. Verweij J, van Oosterom A, Blay JY, et al. Imatinib mesylate (STI-571 Glivec, Gleevec) is an active agent for gastrointestinal stromal tumours, but does not yield responses in other soft-tissue sarcomas that are unselected for a molecular target. Results from an EORTC Soft Tissue and Bone Sarcoma Group phase II study. Eur J Cancer. 2003;39:2006-2011.

108. Debiec-Rychter M, Sciot R, Le Cesne A, et al. KIT mutations and dose selection for imatinib in patients with advanced gastrointestinal stromal tumours. Eur J Cancer. 2006;42:1093-1103.

109. Demetri GD, van Oosterom AT, Garrett CR, et al. Efficacy and safety of sunitinib in patients with advanced gastrointestinal stromal tumour after failure of imatinib: a randomised controlled trial. Lancet. 2006;368:1329-1338.

110. Miettinen M, Lasota J, Sobin LH. Gastrointestinal stromal tumors of the stomach in children and young adults: a clinicopathologic, immunohistochemical, and molecular genetic study of 44 cases with long-term follow-up and review of the literature. Am J Surg Pathol. 2005;29:1373-1381.

111. Prakash S, Sarran L, Socci N, et al. Gastrointestinal stromal tumors in children and young adults: a clinicopathologic, molecular, and genomic study of 15 cases and review of the literature. J Pediatr Hematol Oncol. 2005;27:179-187.

112. Hayashi Y, Okazaki T, Yamataka A, et al. Gastrointestinal stromal tumor in a child and review of the literature. Pediatr Surg Int. 2005;21:914-917.

113. Egloff A, Lee EY, Dillon JE. Gastrointestinal stromal tumor (GIST) of stomach in a pediatric patient. Pediatr Radiol. 2005;35:728-729.

114. Price VE, Zielenska M, Chilton-MacNeill S, et al. Clinical and molecular characteristics of pediatric gastrointestinal stromal tumors (GISTs). Pediatr Blood Cancer. 2005;45:20-24.

115. Kuroiwa M, Hiwatari M, Hirato J, et al. Advanced-stage gastrointestinal stromal tumor treated with imatinib in a 12-year-old

girl with a unique mutation of PDGFRA. J Pediatr Surg. 2005;40: 1798-1801.

116. Cypriano MS, Jenkins JJ, Pappo AS, et al. Pediatric gastrointestinal stromal tumors and leiomyosarcoma. Cancer. 2004;101: 39-50.

117. Price VE, Zielenska M, Chilton-MacNeill S, et al. Clinical and molecular characteristics of pediatric gastrointestinal tumors (GISTs). Pediatr Blood Cancer. 2005;45(1):20-24.

118. O'Sullivan MJ, McCabe A, Gillett P, et al. Multiple gastric stromal tumors in a child without syndromic association lacks common KIT or PDGFR-alpha mutations. Pediatr Dev Pathol. 2005;8:685-689.

119. Bond M, Bernstein ML, Pappo A, et al. A phase II study of imatinib mesylate in children with refractory or relapsed solid tumors: a Children's Oncology Group study. Pediatr Blood Cancer. 2008;50(2):254-258.

120. Janeway KA, Matthews DC, Butrynski JE, et al. Sunitinib treatment of pediatric metastatic GIST after failure of imatinib. J Clin Oncol. 2006;24(18S):9519.

121. Moertel CG, Dockerty MB, Judd ES. Carcinoid tumors of the vermiform appendix. Cancer. 1968;21:270-278.

122. Doede T, Foss HD, Waldschmidt J. Carcinoid tumors of the appendix in children—epidemiology, clinical aspects and procedure. Eur J Pediatr Surg. 2000;10:372-377.

123. Sachithanandan N, Harle RA, Burgess JR. Bronchopulmonary carcinoid in multiple endocrine neoplasia type 1. Cancer. 2005;103:509-515.

124. Schnirer, II, Yao JC, Ajani JA. Carcinoid—a comprehensive review. Acta Oncol. 2003;42:672-692.

125. Petzmann S, Ullmann R, Klemen H, et al. Loss of heterozygosity on chromosome arm 11q in lung carcinoids. Hum Pathol. 2001; 32:333-338.

126. Debelenko LV, Brambilla E, Agarwal SK, et al. Identification of MEN1 gene mutations in sporadic carcinoid tumors of the lung. Hum Mol Genet. 1997;6:2285-2290.

127. Spunt SL, Pratt CB, Rao BN, et al. Childhood carcinoid tumors: the St Jude Children's Research Hospital experience. J Pediatr Surg. 2000;35:1282-1286.

128. Prommegger R, Obrist P, Ensinger C, et al. Retrospective evaluation of carcinoid tumors of the appendix in children. World J Surg. 2002;26:1489-1492.

129. Kwekkeboom DJ, Krenning EP, Bakker WH, et al. Somatostatin analogue scintigraphy in carcinoid tumours. Eur J Nucl Med. 1993;20:283-292.

130. Gouzi JL, Laigneau P, Delalande JP, et al. Indications for right hemicolectomy in carcinoid tumors of the appendix. The French Associations for Surgical Research. Surg Gynecol Obstet. 1993;176:543-547.

131. Pelizzo G, La Riccia A, Bouvier R, et al. Carcinoid tumors of the appendix in children. Pediatr Surg Int. 2001;17:399-402.

132. Corpron CA, Black CT, Herzog CE, et al. A half-century of experience with carcinoid tumors in children. Am J Surg. 1995;170:606-608.

133. Parkes SE, Muir KR, al Sheyyab M, et al. Carcinoid tumours of the appendix in children 1957-1986: incidence, treatment and outcome. Br J Surg. 1993;80:502-504.

134. Sandor A, Modlin IM. A retrospective analysis of 1570 appendiceal carcinoids. Am J Gastroenterol. 1998;93:422-428.

135. Hemminki K, Li X. Familial carcinoid tumors and subsequent cancers: a nation-wide epidemiologic study from Sweden. Int J Cancer. 2001;94:444-448.

136. Zeitels J, Naunheim K, Kaplan EL, Straus F 2nd. Carcinoid tumors: a 37-year experience. Arch Surg. 1982;117:732-737.

137. Moertel CL, Weiland LH, Telander RL. Carcinoid tumor of the appendix in the first two decades of life. J Pediatr Surg. 1990;25:1073-1075.

138. Krenning EP, de Jong M, Kooij PP, et al. Radiolabelled somatostatin analogue(s) for peptide receptor scintigraphy and radionuclide therapy. Ann Oncol. 1999;10(Suppl 2):S23-S9.

139. Oberg K, Eriksson B. The role of interferons in the management of carcinoid tumors. Acta Oncol. 1991;30:519-522.

140. American Cancer Society: Cancer Facts and Figures 2007. Atlanta, American Cancer Society, 2007.

141. Rao BN, Pratt CB, Fleming ID, et al. Colon carcinoma in children and adolescents. A review of 30 cases. Cancer. 1985;55: 1322-1326.

142. Karnak I, Ciftci AO, Senocak ME, Buyukpamukcu N. Colorectal carcinoma in children. J Pediatr Surg. 1999;34:1499-1504.

143. Vasudevan SA, Patel JC, Wesson DE, et al. Severe dysplasia in children with familial adenomatous polyposis: rare or simply overlooked? J Pediatr Surg. 2006;41:658-661.

144. Pratt CB, Jane JA. Multiple colorectal carcinomas, polyposis coli, and neurofibromatosis, followed by multiple glioblastoma multiforme. J Natl Cancer Inst. 1991;83:880-881.

145. Houlston RS, Murday V, Harocopos C, et al. Screening and genetic counselling for relatives of patients with colorectal cancer in a family cancer clinic. BMJ. 1990;301:366-368.

146. Dean PA. Hereditary intestinal polyposis syndromes. Rev Gastroenterol Mex. 1996;61:100-111.

147. Jeghers H, McKusick KV, Katz KH. Generalized intestinal polyposis and melanin spots of the oral mucosa, lips and digits; a syndrome of diagnostic significance. N Engl J Med. 1949;241: 1031-1036.

148. Turcot J, Despres JP, St Pierre F. Malignant tumors of the central nervous system associated with familial polyposis of the colon: report of two cases. Dis Colon Rectum. 1959;2:465-468.

149. Compton C, Fenoglio-Preiser CM, Pettigrew N, Fielding LP. American Joint Committee on Cancer Prognostic Factors Consensus Conference: Colorectal Working Group. Cancer. 2000;88: 1739-1757.

150. Goetzl MA, Desai M, Mansukhani M, et al. Natural history and clinical outcome of sporadic renal cortical tumors diagnosed in the young adult. Urology. 2004;63:41-45.

151. Pratt C. Management of infrequent tumors of childhood. In Pizzo PA, Poplack DG (eds). Principles and Practice of Pediatric Oncology, 4th ed. Philadelphia, Lippincott Williams & Wilkins, 2002, pp 1149-1176.

152. Locker GY, Hamilton S, Harris J, et al. ASCO 2006 update of recommendations for the use of tumor markers in gastrointestinal cancer. J Clin Oncol. 2006;24:5313-5327.

153. Baddi L, Benson A 3rd. Adjuvant therapy in stage II colon cancer: current approaches. Oncologist. 2005;10:325-331.

154. NIH Consensus Conference. Adjuvant therapy for patients with colon and rectal cancer. JAMA. 1990;264:1444-1450.

155. Goldberg RM. Therapy for metastatic colorectal cancer. Oncologist. 2006;11:981-987.

156. Attard TM, Young RJ. Diagnosis and management of gastrointestinal polyps: pediatric considerations. Gastroenterol Nurs. 2006;29:16-22; quiz 3-4.

157. Lynch HT, Tinley ST, Shaw TG, et al. Challenging colonic polyposis pedigrees: differential diagnosis, surveillance, and management concerns. Cancer Genet Cytogenet. 2004;148:104-117.

158. Lindor NM, Petersen GM, Hadley DW, et al. Recommendations for the care of individuals with an inherited predisposition to Lynch syndrome: a systematic review. JAMA. 2006;296:1507-1517.

159. Bertagnolli MM, Eagle CJ, Zauber AG, et al. Celecoxib for the prevention of sporadic colorectal adenomas. N Engl J Med. 2006;355:873-884.

160. Gibbon DG, Schaar D, Kamen B. A call to action: cancer in adolescents and young adults: an unrecognized healthcare disparity. J Pediatr Hematol Oncol. 2006;28:549-551.

161. Bruinvels DJ, Stiggelbout AM, Kievit J, et al. Follow-up of patients with colorectal cancer. A meta-analysis. Ann Surg. 1994;219:174-182.

162. Martin EW Jr, James KK, Hurtubise PE, et al. The use of CEA as an early indicator for gastrointestinal tumor recurrence and second-look procedures. Cancer. 1977;39:440-446.

163. Dehner LP, Hill DA, Deschryver K. Pathology of the breast in children, adolescents, and young adults. Semin Diagn Pathol. 1999;16:235-247.

164. el-Mawla NG, el-Bolkainy MN, Khaled HM. Bladder cancer in Africa: update. Semin Oncol. 2001;28:174-178.

165. Snow B. Tumors of the lower urinary tract. In Kelalis P, King L, Belman A (eds). Clinical Pediatric Urology, 3rd ed. Philadelphia, WB Saunders, 1992, pp 1445-1455.

166. Defoor W, Minevich E, Sheldon C. Unusual bladder masses in children. Urology. 2002;60:911.

167. von Allmen D. Malignant lesions of the ovary in childhood. Semin Pediatr Surg. 2005;14:100-105.

168. Diamond MP, Baxter JW, Peerman CG Jr, Burnett LS. Occurrence of ovarian malignancy in childhood and adolescence: a community-wide evaluation. Obstet Gynecol. 1988;71:858-860.

169. Cass DL, Hawkins E, Brandt ML, et al. Surgery for ovarian masses in infants, children, and adolescents: 102 consecutive patients treated in a 15-year period. J Pediatr Surg. 2001;36:693-699.

170. Deligeoroglou E, Eleftheriades M, Shiadoes V, et al. Ovarian masses during adolescence: clinical, ultrasonographic and pathologic findings, serum tumor markers and endocrinological profile. Gynecol Endocrinol. 2004;19:1-8.

171. Tsai JY, Saigo PE, Brown C, La Quaglia MP. Diagnosis, pathology, staging, treatment, and outcome of epithelial ovarian neoplasia in patients age <21 years. Cancer. 2001;91:2065-2070.

172. Morowitz M, Huff D, von Allmen D. Epithelial ovarian tumors in children: a retrospective analysis. J Pediatr Surg. 2003;38:331-335.

173. Domanska K, Malander S, Masback A, Nilbert M. Ovarian cancer at young age: the contribution of mismatch-repair defects in a population-based series of epithelial ovarian cancer before age 40. Int J Gynecol Cancer. 2007;17:789-793.

174. Stratton JF, Thompson D, Bobrow L, et al. The genetic epidemiology of early-onset epithelial ovarian cancer: a population-based study. Am J Hum Genet. 1999;65:1725-1732.

175. Risch HA, McLaughlin JR, Cole DEC, et al. Population BRCA1 and BRCA2 mutation frequencies and cancer penetrances: a kin-cohort study in Ontario, Canada. J Natl Cancer Inst. 2006;98:1694-1706.

176. Schneider DT, Calaminus G, Harms D, Gobel U. Ovarian sex cord-stromal tumors in children and adolescents. J Reprod Med. 2005;50:439-446.

177. Calaminus G, Wessalowski R, Harms D, Gobel U. Juvenile granulosa cell tumors of the ovary in children and adolescents: results from 33 patients registered in a prospective cooperative study. Gynecol Oncol. 1997;65:447-452.

178. Schneider DT, Calaminus G, Wessalowski R, et al. Therapy of advanced ovarian juvenile granulosa cell tumors. Klin Padiatr. 2002;214:173-178.

179. La Vecchia C, Draper GJ, Franceschi S. Childhood nonovarian female genital tract cancers in Britain, 1962-1978. Descriptive epidemiology and long-term survival. Cancer. 1984;54:188-192.

180. Silverberg SG, Ioffe OB. Pathology of cervical cancer. Cancer J. 2003;9:335-347.

181. Crowther ME. Is the nature of cervical carcinoma changing in young women? Obstet Gynecol Surv. 1995;50:71-82.

182. Markowitz LE, Dunne EF, Saraiya M, et al. Quadrivalent human papillomavirus vaccine: recommendations of the Advisory Committee on Immunization Practices (ACIP). MMWR Recomm Rep. 2007;56:1-24.

183. Moscicki AB, Winkler B, Irwin CE Jr, Schachter J. Differences in biologic maturation, sexual behavior, and sexually transmitted disease between adolescents with and without cervical intraepithelial neoplasia. J Pediatr. 1989;115:487-493.

184. Mount SL, Papillo JL. A study of 10,296 pediatric and adolescent Papanicolaou smear diagnoses in northern New England. Pediatrics. 1999;103:539-545.

185. Tarkowski TA, Koumans EH, Sawyer M, et al. Epidemiology of human papillomavirus infection and abnormal cytologic test results in an urban adolescent population. J Infect Dis. 2004;189:46-50.

186. Wright JD, Davila RM, Pinto KR, et al. Cervical dysplasia in adolescents. Obstet Gynecol. 2005;106:115-120.

187. Hill NC, Oppenheimer LW, Morton KE. The aetiology of vaginal bleeding in children. A 20-year review. Br J Obstet Gynaecol. 1989;96:467-470.

188. McNall RY, Nowicki PD, Miller B, et al. Adenocarcinoma of the cervix and vagina in pediatric patients. Pediatr Blood Cancer. 2004;43:289-294.

189. Abu-Rustum NR, Su W, Levine DA, et al. Pediatric radical abdominal trachelectomy for cervical clear cell carcinoma: a novel surgical approach. Gynecol Oncol. 2005;97:296-300.

190. You W, Dainty LA, Rose GS, et al. Gynecologic malignancies in women aged less than 25 years. Obstet Gynecol. 2005;105:1405-1409.

191. Nielsen GP, Oliva E, Young RH, et al. Alveolar soft-part sarcoma of the female genital tract: a report of nine cases and review of the literature. Int J Gynecol Pathol. 1995;14:283-292.

192. Chen SJ, Li YW, Tsai WY. Endodermal sinus (yolk sac) tumor of vagina and cervix in an infant. Pediatr Radiol. 1993;23:57-58.

193. Babin EA, Davis JR, Hatch KD, Hallum AV 3rd. Wilms' tumor of the cervix: a case report and review of the literature. Gynecol Oncol. 2000;76:107-111.

194. Bagshawe KD, Dent J, Webb J. Hydatidiform mole in England and Wales 1973-83. Lancet. 1986;2:673-677.

195. Kohorn EI. The new FIGO 2000 staging and risk factor scoring system for gestational trophoblastic disease: description and critical assessment. Int J Gynecol Cancer. 2001;11:73-77.

196. Fisher PM, Hancock BW. Gestational trophoblastic diseases and their treatment. Cancer Treat Rev. 1997;23:1-16.

197. Lurain JR. Treatment of gestational trophoblastic tumors. Curr Treat Options Oncol. 2002;3:113-124.

198. McNeish IA, Strickland S, Holden L, et al. Low-risk persistent gestational trophoblastic disease: outcome after initial treatment with low-dose methotrexate and folinic acid from 1992 to 2000. J Clin Oncol. 2002;20:1838-1844.

199. Lurain JR, Singh DK, Schink JC. Primary treatment of metastatic high-risk gestational trophoblastic neoplasia with EMA-CO chemotherapy. J Reprod Med. 2006;51:767-772.

200. Soper JT, Mutch DG, Schink JC. Diagnosis and treatment of gestational trophoblastic disease: ACOG Practice Bulletin No. 53. Gynecol Oncol. 2004;93:575-585.

201. Strouse JJ, Fears TR, Tucker MA, Wayne AS. Pediatric melanoma: risk factor and survival analysis of the surveillance, epidemiology and end results database. J Clin Oncol. 2005;23:4735-4741.

202. Alexander A, Samlowski WE, Grossman D, et al. Metastatic melanoma in pregnancy: risk of transplacental metastases in the infant. J Clin Oncol. 2003;21:2179-2186.

203. Richardson SK, Tannous ZS, Mihm MC Jr. Congenital and infantile melanoma: review of the literature and report of an uncommon variant, pigment-synthesizing melanoma. J Am Acad Dermatol. 2002;47:77-90.

204. Bittencourt FV, Marghoob AA, Kopf AW, et al. Large congenital melanocytic nevi and the risk for development of malignant melanoma and neurocutaneous melanocytosis. Pediatrics. 2000;106:736-741.

205. Krengel S, Hauschild A, Schafer T. Melanoma risk in congenital melanocytic naevi: a systematic review. Br J Dermatol. 2006;155: 1-8.

206. Hale EK, Stein J, Ben-Porat L, et al. Association of melanoma and neurocutaneous melanocytosis with large congenital melanocytic naevi—results from the NYU-LCMN registry. Br J Dermatol. 2005;152:512-517.

207. Makkar HS, Frieden IJ. Neurocutaneous melanosis. Semin Cutan Med Surg. 2004;23:138-144.

208. Cleaver JE. Cancer in xeroderma pigmentosum and related disorders of DNA repair. Nat Rev Cancer. 2005;5:564-573.

209. Lindenbaum Y, Dickson D, Rosenbaum P, et al. Xeroderma pigmentosum/cockayne syndrome complex: first neuropathological study and review of eight other cases. Eur J Paediatr Neurol. 2001;5:225-242.

210. Lambert W, Kuo H, Lambert M. Xeroderma pigmentosum. Dermatol Clin. 1995;13:169-209.

211. Kraemer KH, Lee MM, Scotto J. Xeroderma pigmentosum. Cutaneous, ocular, and neurologic abnormalities in 830 published cases. Arch Dermatol. 1987;123:241-250.

212. van Brabant AJ, Stan R, Ellis NA. DNA helicases, genomic instability, and human genetic disease. Annu Rev Genomics Hum Genet. 2000;1:409-459.

213. Goto M, Miller RW, Ishikawa Y, Sugano H. Excess of rare cancers in Werner syndrome (adult progeria). Cancer Epidemiol Biomarkers Prev. 1996;5:239-246.

214. Kleinerman RA, Tucker MA, Tarone RE, et al. Risk of new cancers after radiotherapy in long-term survivors of retinoblastoma: an extended follow-up. J Clin Oncol. 2005;23:2272-2279.

215. Andres A. Cancer incidence after immunosuppressive treatment following kidney transplantation. Crit Rev Oncol Hematol. 2005;56:71-85.

216. Curtis RE, Freedman DM, Ron E, et al (eds). New Malignancies Among Cancer Survivors: SEER Cancer Registries 1973-2000 (NIH Publication No. 05-5302). Bethesda, Md, National Cancer Institute, 2006.

217. Ghelani D, Saliba R, Lima M. Secondary malignancies after hematopoietic stem cell transplantation. Crit Rev Oncol Hematol. 2005;56:115-126.

218. Youl P, Aitken J, Hayward N, et al. Melanoma in adolescents: a case-control study of risk factors in Queensland, Australia. Int J Cancer. 2002;98:92-98.

219. Tsao H, Zhang X, Kwitkiwski K, et al. Low prevalence of germline CDKN2A and CDK4 mutations in patients with early-onset melanoma. Arch Dermatol. 2000;136:1118-1122.

220. Pappo AS. Melanoma in children and adolescents. Eur J Cancer. 2003;39:2651-2661.

221. Whiteman DC, Milligan A, Welch J, et al. Germline CDKN2A mutations in childhood melanoma. J Natl Cancer Inst. 1997; 89:1460.

222. Boddie AW Jr, Smith JL Jr, McBride CM. Malignant melanoma in children and young adults: effect of diagnostic criteria on staging and end results. South Med J. 1978;71:1074-1078.

223. Saenz NC, Saenz-Badillos J, Busam K, et al. Childhood melanoma survival. Cancer. 1999;85:750-754.

224. Lohmann CM, Coit DG, Brady MS, et al. Sentinel lymph node biopsy in patients with diagnostically controversial spitzoid melanocytic tumors. Am J Surg Pathol. 2002;26:47-55.

225. Buzaid AC, Sandler AB, Mani S, et al. Role of computed tomography in the staging of primary melanoma. J Clin Oncol. 1993;11:638-643.

226. Kaste SC, Pappo AS, Jenkins JJ III, Pratt CB. Malignant melanoma in children: imaging spectrum. Pediatr Radiol. 1996;26: 800-805.

227. Su LD, Fullen DR, Sondak VK, et al. Sentinel lymph node biopsy for patients with problematic spitzoid melanocytic lesions: a report on 18 patients. Cancer. 2003;97:499-507.

228. Kogut KA, Fleming M, Pappo AS, Schropp KP. Sentinel lymph node biopsy for melanoma in young children. J Pediatr Surg. 2000;35:965-966.

229. Neville HL, Andrassy RJ, Lally KP, et al. Lymphatic mapping with sentinel node biopsy in pediatric patients. J Pediatr Surg. 2000;35:961-964.

230. Shah NC, Gerstle JT, Stuart M, et al. Use of sentinel lymph node biopsy and high-dose interferon in pediatric patients with high-risk melanoma: the Hospital for Sick Children experience. J Pediatr Hematol Oncol. 2006;28:496-500.

231. Chao MM, Schwartz JL, Wechsler DS, et al. High-risk surgically resected pediatric melanoma and adjuvant interferon therapy. Pediatr Blood Cancer. 2005;44:441-448.

232. Navid F, Furman WL, Fleming M, et al. The feasibility of adjuvant interferon alpha-2b in children with high-risk melanoma. Cancer. 2005;103:780-787.

233. Kirkwood JM, Ibrahim JG, Sosman JA, et al. High-dose interferon alfa-2b significantly prolongs relapse-free and overall survival compared with the GM2-KLH/QS-21 vaccine in patients with resected stage IIB-III melanoma: results of intergroup trial E1694/S9512/C509801. J Clin Oncol. 2001;19:2370-2380.

234. Kirkwood JM, Ibrahim JG, Sondak VK, et al. High- and low-dose interferon alfa-2b in high-risk melanoma: first analysis of intergroup trial E1690/S9111/C9190. J Clin Oncol. 2000;18:2444-2458.

235. Kirkwood JM, Strawderman MH, Ernstoff MS, et al. Interferon alfa-2b adjuvant therapy of high-risk resected cutaneous melanoma: the Eastern Cooperative Oncology Group Trial EST 1684. J Clin Oncol. 1996;14:7-17.

236. Hayes FA, Green AA. Malignant melanoma in childhood: clinical course and response to chemotherapy. J Clin Oncol. 1984;2: 1229-1234.

237. Hamre MR, Chuba P, Bakhshi S, et al. Cutaneous melanoma in childhood and adolescence. Pediatr Hematol Oncol. 2002;19: 309-317.

238. Rao BN, Hayes FA, Pratt CB, et al. Malignant melanoma in children: its management and prognosis. J Pediatr Surg. 1990;25: 198-203.

239. Curtin JA, Busam K, Pinkel D, Bastian BC. Somatic activation of KIT in distinct subtypes of melanoma. J Clin Oncol. 2006;24: 4340-4346.

240. Hodi FS, Friedlander P, Corless CL, et al. Major response to imatinib mesylate in KIT-mutated melanoma. J Clin Oncol. 2008;26:2046-2051.

V Supportive Care

26

Diagnostic Imaging in the Evaluation of Childhood Cancer

Stephan D. Voss

INITIAL IMAGING STUDIES AND STAGING

The imaging of children with suspected malignancy has evolved considerably over the past 2 decades. Nonetheless, the decision to perform an imaging study and the type of imaging that is selected still very much depends on the patient's clinical history and physical examination findings. In young children, presenting symptoms and complaints are frequently nonspecific. An easily performed, relatively inexpensive imaging assessment is therefore appropriate as a first step in the evaluation, and conventional radiography is still commonly used as the first imaging examination undertaken in children with suspected malignancy. These initial imaging studies provide valuable initial information and may help suggest a differential diagnosis and guide the subsequent imaging evaluation.

Although it is tempting to forego obtaining conventional radiography in favor of cross-sectional imaging modalities such as ultrasound and computed tomography (CT), radiographs of the abdomen, for example, still provide a sensitive and accurate method to assess for bowel obstruction or perforation. Chest radiographs are frequently adequate to identify primary intrathoracic or mediastinal tumors and pulmonary metastases. Chest radiographs are often critical in suggesting impending airway compromise, pneumothorax, or pneumomediastinum and are rapidly obtained, easy to perform, and can be interpreted fairly quickly. Oncologic emergencies are fortunately uncommon, but cardiorespiratory emergencies in a child, such as pneumothorax or pneumomediastinum, airway compression secondary to a large mediastinal mass (Fig. 26-1), and malignant pericardial or pleural effusions, can be effectively evaluated in the emergent setting by properly executed chest and abdominal radiographs. A CT scan may be contraindicated if radiographs indicate the presence of significant airway compromise in the setting of a large mediastinal mass, because supine positioning, with or without sedation, may lead to further

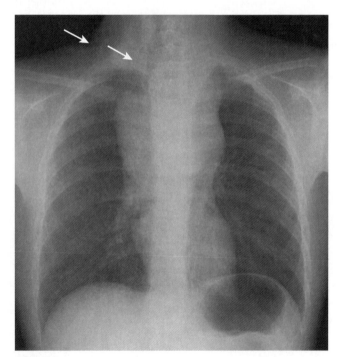

FIGURE 26-1. Chest x-ray showing marked tracheal deviation, pneumomediastinum, and subcutaneous emphysema along the right neck in a child with lymphoblastic lymphoma, emphasizing the severity of airway obstruction and potential for respiratory compromise. Arrows indicate pneumomediastinum and subcutaneous emphysema.

airway compression, impaired venous return, and acute cardiorespiratory collapse.[1]

Conventional radiography also still plays a role in specific conditions such as Langerhans cell histiocytosis, for which skeletal surveys are still used to detect the lytic lesions characteristic of this disease. Whether whole-body magnetic resonance imaging (MRI) or fluorodeoxyglucose–positron emission tomography (FDG-PET) scanning can be used to improve the sensitivity and specificity of detecting these lesions has been the subject of several investigations.[2-4]

The role of fluoroscopy in the primary evaluation of pediatric oncology patients is limited and has been largely replaced by CT. CT provides the advantage of visualizing endoluminal and surrounding mesenteric, intraperitoneal, and retroperitoneal processes, for which traditional fluoroscopic evaluations are limited.

Imaging Modalities

Ultrasound

The use of ultrasound in pediatric radiology is ubiquitous. Ultrasonography is relatively inexpensive, can be done portably, involves no radiation, and—in skilled hands—can be used to assess an anxious moving child accurately, for whom sedation may pose additional risk. Technically, ultrasound relies on the use of variable penetration and attenuation of sound waves by different tissue types. The routine ultrasound examination typically involves the combination of B-mode (brightness mode) scanning and color or pulsed wave–duplex Doppler sonography to assess flow within vascular structures. As an initial screening modality, ultrasound is sensitive at evaluating intra-abdominal solid organ viscera and is the initial imaging modality of choice in the evaluation of Wilms' tumor, neuroblastoma, and hepatoblastoma. Pelvic neoplasms, intraperitoneal free fluid, and musculoskeletal soft tissue tumors can all be effectively evaluated by ultrasound. Newer ultrasound imaging techniques rely on a large array of transducers, which afford high-resolution images independent of the size of the patient and depth of the lesion. Extended field of view image-processing algorithms offer the capability of visualizing large masses in their entirety, along with their relationships to normal structures. Although not in routine clinical use, three-dimensional ultrasound allows images to be displayed in multiple planes and may be useful in demonstrating relationships between solid organ malignancies and adjacent normal structures.[5] The use of ultrasound contrast agents, although in common use experimentally, has the potential to add to the diagnostic information obtained by conventional ultrasound but they are not yet being used routinely in clinical practice.[6-8]

Computed Tomography

After ultrasound, CT scanning is the primary imaging tool for evaluating most pediatric solid tumors. It is readily available and, in most institutions, can be performed rapidly and with newer generation scanners and provides high spatial resolution and multiplanar viewing capabilities. CT scanning involves the use of a fan-shaped or cone-shaped x-ray beam generated by the x-ray tube rotating 360 degrees around the body part being examined. At the same time that x-ray tube rotation is occurring, the patient is moving longitudinally through the scanner, allowing the sequential and almost simultaneous examination of multiple contiguous body parts. Once the x-rays pass through the patient, they strike an array of photodetectors that convert the x-ray energy into electrical signals; these are, in turn, used to reconstruct images from the region of the body through which the x-ray beam penetrated. The newest generation scanners are so-called multi-row detector helical CT scanners, and rely on multiple detector rows to acquire imaging information from larger segments of tissue simultaneously.[9,10] This allows for more rapid scanning and the reconstruction of imaging data in multiple planes with minimal artifact and image distortion. These multiplanar reconstructions also allow volumetric data to be evaluated, which may be important when assessing response to therapy.[11-13] In addition, the ability to view images in multiple planes serves as a convenient preoperative tool for the surgeon who is planning complicated cases.

For infants, it is usually still necessary for patients to be sedated to acquire high-quality imaging. In most patients, sedation can be performed safely and effectively with skilled nursing staff and monitoring equipment.[14,15] In particular, sedation is usually necessary prior to infusion of intravenous contrast agents, because the contrast infusion may be startling to an otherwise calm child and motion artifact will severely compromise the image quality.

The use of intravenous contrast agents, particularly for most pediatric solid tumors, is necessary to show relationships between primary neoplasms and adjacent structures properly. Although centers less experienced in the care of pediatric patients may consider performing scans without the use of intravenous contrast, in our institution, based on perceived increased risks of contrast reactions in children, a retrospective review of CT scanning results from over 12,000 contrast enhanced studies performed over a 5-year period has shown less than a 0.5% incidence of contrast reactions (57 reported adverse events), with the vast majority being minor reactions. No severe contrast reactions occurred in infants or very young children.[15a] Based on this, there are little data to support the omission of intravenous contrast in the evaluation of children suspected of malignancy and, in particular, the use of nonionic low-osmolar agents can be performed safely in most patients. Enteric contrast is also recommended to opacify the bowel lumen, allowing better discrimination between normal viscera and potential sites of mesenteric or retroperitoneal lymph node enlargement.

Although optimal imaging of the thorax for the purpose of evaluating the mediastinum and hilar structures requires the use of intravenous contrast, CT scanning of the chest to assess for pulmonary metastatic disease can generally be performed without the use of intravenous contrast. The use of multiplanar reconstructions and the ability to review slices in very thin sections improves the detection of pulmonary nodules.[16,17] In infants and small children who are asleep or in whom quiet breathing can be encouraged, the speed with which current generation scanners can acquire images may allow noncontrast examinations of the chest to be performed without sedation. In older children, for whom breath-holding is possible, image quality and sensitivity and specificity of pulmonary nodule detection is improved when images are obtained at the end of inspiration.

The use of intravenous contrast agents also requires skill on the part of the radiologist in interpreting the examination results, with awareness of potential causes of artifact. For example, the spleen has a variable pattern of enhancement that is well appreciated, but can be mistaken for splenic disease, particularly in the setting of lymphoma. Delayed scanning can usually help in discriminating artifact from disease.[18] In addition, acquisition of images at multiple phases following contrast infusion is often helpful in detecting subtle foci of disease which may only be seen at early arterial phases of enhancement, particularly in the liver (Fig. 26-2). Other lesions, in contrast, may only become evident after delayed enhancement, and knowledge of the typical patterns of enhancement for the particular disease that is being evaluated or suspected is impor-

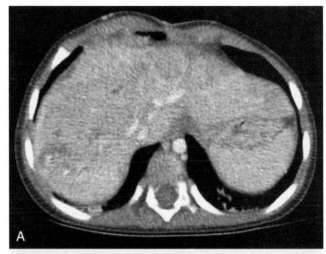

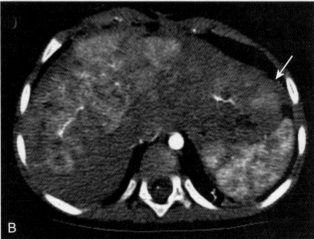

FIGURE 26-2. **A,** 20-month-old with unresectable hepatoblastoma, emphasizing the importance of multiphase scanning for optimal lesion detection. **B,** The presence of the left lateral segment lesion (*arrow*) was only seen on early arterial phase scanning. Its identification determined surgical unresectability in this patient.

tant in determining the scanning technique.[19] It is our practice to perform evaluations for hepatoblastoma in hepatic arterial and portal venous phases to maximize sensitivity of lesion detection and to provide optimal images to aid in surgical planning.

Discussions of radiation dose in the setting of diagnostic CT scanning have become widespread in the imaging and wider medical literature.[20-24] The data indicate measurable increases in incidence of malignancy attributable to radiation doses during diagnostic CT scanning, with cumulative increases in risk with increasing numbers of scans. Although these concerns are not to be underemphasized, particularly for otherwise well patients undergoing screening examinations, for patients with known malignancy or in whom malignancy is suspected, the relative benefit derived from the high-quality information obtained following diagnostic CT scanning almost always outweighs the modest incremental increase in risk associated with these techniques. Nonetheless, every effort should be made to limit the examination to involved regions of the body and to minimize the frequency of scanning in these heavily evaluated patients, using the ALARA (as low as reasonably achievable) principle as guidance.[23-26]

Magnetic Resonance Imaging

The physical principles of MR image formation are beyond the scope of this chapter and can be reviewed in articles devoted to this subject.[27,28] MRI imaging involves the use of an external magnetic field to orient protons—primarily contained in water molecules—in the body, after which radiofrequency pulses are applied in specific frequencies and orientations. These radiofrequency pulses force the protons aligned in the magnetic field to come out of alignment. After the radiofrequency energy is withdrawn, the protons gradually reassume their original alignment, or resonate, within the magnetic field. The process of relaxation is multidimensional and the rate with which longitudinal and transverse relaxation occurs (T1 and T2 relaxation times, respectively) is dependent on the properties of the specific tissue. The energy released during this realignment process can be measured much like the energy from a radio station transmitter is acquired by a standard radio receiver. This radiofrequency energy can be characterized in terms of its spatial location and frequency and this information, in turn, can be used to reconstruct images. The resultant magnetic resonance images provide very high-resolution images that reflect the tissue microenvironments within which the protons reside.

High– and low–field strength magnets are in common clinical use and, in general terms, with higher field strength, there is a higher signal-to-noise ratio.[27,29] Despite this, high–field strength magnets are susceptible to some image degradation and magnetic field artifact, and most imaging can be reliably performed at 1.5 T (tesla). With lower field strengths, signal to noise is considerably diminished. There are various radiofrequency coils that are used as receivers for the radiofrequency energy emitted during proton relaxation and reorientation. Newer coil designs allow for rapid scanning techniques and for very high-resolution imaging of specific body parts to be performed.[27,30]

Multiple magnetic resonance images of the same organ or tissue are typically generated, but the imaging technique chosen results in different patterns of tissue contrast, allowing the unique features that characterize distinct components of an organ or tissue to be depicted. The tissue contrast observed is the result of the interplay among the externally applied magnetic field, the inherent properties of the tissue (i.e., freely mobile water protons or highly ordered soft tissue protons), and the radiofrequency pulse sequence parameters chosen to acquire the image. The tissue properties that have the greatest influence on image contrast are the proton density (PD), and longitudinal (T1) and transverse (T2) proton relaxation times. Conventional MRI imaging techniques are acquired with so-called T1 and T2 weighting, in which the tissue contrast is weighted to reflect differences in the T1 and T2 relaxation times among the different tissues, respectively. This is accomplished by varying the interval between which the radiofrequency pulses are applied (the pulse repetition time, or TR) and the time that is allowed before the emitted signal is received (the so-called echo time, or TE). T1-weighted images typically have a short TR (300 to 600 milliseconds) and short TE (10 to 20 milliseconds) and emphasize T1 characteristics of tissues. On T1-weighted images, fat is typically bright, fluid has low signal intensity, and complex or proteinaceous fluid has intermediate to high signal intensity. Conventional contrast agents used in MRI result in T1 shortening and therefore produce increased signal on T1-weighted images. T2-weighted images have a longer TR (longer than 200 milliseconds) and longer TE (longer than 80 milliseconds). T2-weighted images typically display simple fluid such as cerebrospinal fluid (CSF) or urine as bright in signal intensity, whereas fat is low in signal intensity. Muscle and solid organs, depending on their tissue composition, have variable signal intensity on T2-weighted images. Beyond these simple T1- and T2-weighted images, specific pulse sequences can be created that eliminate fluid signal (fluid-attenuated inversion recovery [FLAIR]) or provide fat suppression, using chemically selective fat suppression techniques or so-called inversion recovery techniques, in which the echo time is selected to minimize signal from fat and maximize signal from non–fat-containing structures.

MRI angiography, diffusion weighted imaging, and MR spectroscopy are all standard imaging techniques in common practice in the evaluation of the central nervous system. MR angiography, in simplest terms, takes advantage of rapidly flowing blood moving in and out of the imaging slice. Alternatively, gadolinium (Gd)-enhanced MR angiography relies on the use of Gd-based contrast agents to display the vasculature. The use of dynamic enhanced MRI allows multiple acquisitions in a specific region, such as a tumor, to be obtained, and there is evidence to suggest that the relative rates of contrast uptake and perfusion in tumors may be a reflection of tumor cellularity and/or necrosis.[31,32] Diffusion-weighted imaging, which measures the free diffusion of water molecules in areas of cellular necrosis, as opposed to the more restricted movement of water in cellular regions of a tumor, has also been shown to correlate with tumor necrosis induced by treatment. This may be an important emerging technique for imaging neoplasms in the central nervous system and elsewhere in the body.[33,34]

MR spectroscopy is also used routinely in the evaluation of central nervous system (CNS) tumors, in which the metabolites *N*-acetylaspartate (NAA), creatine (Cr), and choline (Cho) have been defined and have specific and characteristic spectra. The use of spectroscopy, although not entirely diagnostic, adds additional information in evaluation of central nervous system (CNS) tumors.[35,36] For example, NAA is generally thought to correlate with neuronal density, whereas increases in choline levels usually signify increases in cell density and membrane turnover, reflecting the relatively rapid metabolic rate and division of actively dividing tumors. NAA peaks are typically decreased or absent in pediatric brain tumors and a decreased NAA/Cho ratio is a characteristic finding.[37,38] The presence of a prominent lactate peak, which is not typically present in the normal brain spectrum, signifies increases in cellular hypoxia and necrosis (Fig. 26-3), and has been described in more malignant CNS neoplasms.[36] Because obtaining good spectral data relies on relatively static body parts, proton spectroscopy has not been used routinely outside the brain. However, investigations are underway to develop a better understanding of the spectra observed in pediatric neoplasms outside the CNS.[39]

Nuclear Studies

Positron Emission Tomography

Positron emission tomography has emerged as an important imaging tool for the evaluation of patients with malignancy. A number of textbooks and recent reviews have been dedicated to this topic and should be consulted for a more in-depth discussion of this exciting technology.[40-49] The use of ^{18}F-fluorodeoxyglucose (^{18}F-FDG) is routine in adult practice and is becoming more commonplace in the evaluation of children with cancer.[50,51] FDG-PET scanning relies on the differential uptake of glucose by metabolically active tumor cells relative to surrounding tissues. The use of FDG-PET has been shown to be feasible for most pediatric tumors[51] and is likely to play an important role in monitoring responses to therapy, particularly with agents that do not produce immediate tumor shrinkage or cellular necrosis, but that do block specific metabolic pathways. Although ^{18}F-fluorine is the most common PET radionuclide

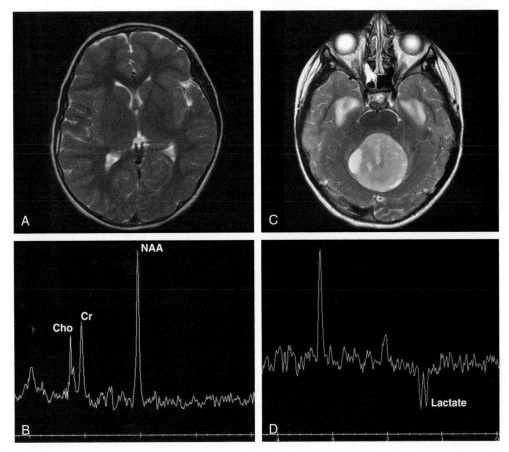

FIGURE 26-3. A, B, Normal MRI scan and MR spectrum demonstrating the increased choline peak, decreased or absent NAA peak, and lactate peak characteristically seen in malignant lesions. Compare this with the MRI scan and MR spectrum in a patient with medulloblastoma (**C, D**), NAA, *N*-acetylaspartate; Cho, choline; Cr, creatine.

used clinically, other agents are being developed and are in preclinical testing, including copper 64 (^{64}Cu)[52,53] and iodine 124 (^{124}I).[54] The use of biomarkers other than fluorodeoxyglucose is starting to emerge clinically, with compounds such as fluorinated thymidine (FLT) allowing DNA synthesis and cellular proliferation to be imaged directly.[55]

Multiple studies have shown that the use of PET imaging alone, without the simultaneous review of anatomic imaging data acquired by CT or MRI, results in a high sensitivity of lesion detection, but has an increased incidence of false-positives and an overall decreased specificity. The use of correlative cross-sectional imaging improves the specificity of lesions detected by PET scanning and also increases the sensitivity with which lesions are detected by conventional imaging techniques.[56-60] This has resulted in the development of PET CT scanners, in which the PET and CT scans are obtained on the instrument with the patient in the same position and orientation. This has revolutionized the use of PET scanning for the evaluation of oncology patients. In many institutions, it is considered standard of care for PET and CT scans to be reviewed simultaneously by skilled radiologists and nuclear medicine physicians, using the complementary information available from both imaging modalities to achieve greater confidence when rendering a diagnosis.[57,61] Postprocessing techniques, relying on newer software, also allow the functional data from PET scanners to be fused to MRI images acquired separately, much in the same way that PET images are fused to their correlative CT data. At least one major MRI manufacturer is also

in the process of developing a composite MRI-PET scanner to allow PET and MRI scanning to be performed during the same acquisition.[62] When this reaches the clinical arena, it is likely to have a significant impact on the imaging evaluation of pediatric oncology patients.

Other Nuclear Studies

In addition to PET scanning, conventional gamma emission planar and single-photon emission computed tomography (SPECT) imaging are still an important element of pediatric oncology imaging.[63-65] In particular, ^{123}I-metaiodobenzylguanidine (^{123}I-MIBG) and technetium 99m–methylenediphosphonate (^{99m}Tc-MDP) bone scintigraphy are commonly used in the evaluation of neuroblastoma patients.[66] Bone scintigraphy is also an important component of the sarcoma patient's evaluation.[65] As with PET scanning, SPECT images can be fused to anatomic data acquired by CT or MRI to provide correlative information, confirm sites of abnormality, and clarify areas of equivocal disease.[67]

Staging Considerations

A detailed discussion of the different staging classifications used in pediatric oncology is beyond the scope of this chapter. Specific staging considerations are discussed elsewhere in this text in the disease-specific chapters. It is important to note, however, that there are unique staging systems in pediatric oncology, such as the International Neuroblastoma Staging System (INSS), the Wilms' tumor staging system, Hodgkin's lymphoma staging system (Ann Arbor Staging), non-Hodgkin's lymphoma staging system (St. Jude Classification), and PRETEXT staging system for hepatoblastoma. Because these different staging systems do not simply rely on tumor size and nodal spread in determining disease stage, the imaging evaluation must be tailored to reflect the type of malignancy being evaluated, and the radiologist should work closely with the oncologist during the review of the initial imaging data to accurately determine the patient's disease stage and risk classification.

CENTRAL NERVOUS SYSTEM TUMORS

Primary CNS malignancies are the most common pediatric solid tumors, exceeded only by leukemia as a cause of pediatric cancer.[68,69] Although many pediatric CNS tumors are also seen in adults, there are several tumors that are unique to infancy and childhood and have characteristic imaging features and intracranial locations. The imaging evaluation should be directed at characterizing the location of the lesion (supratentorial or infratentorial) and whether it is intra- or extra-axial. CT is usually the first imaging study performed to investigate children with suspected CNS tumors. Although the role of CT has been diminished by the increased use of MRI for imaging the brain, CT is still widely available and readily accessible in almost all institutions. CT can effectively identify foci of hemorrhage or necrosis and critical abnormalities, such as brain edema or impending brain herniation. CT may also provide clues about the histologic nature of the tumor—for example showing a cystic or solid mass, or the presence of subtle calcifications. Bone invasion into the adjacent skull is typically depicted better by CT, and skull base lesions particularly should include evaluation by CT.

MRI of the brain, as with other parts of the body, provides enhanced spatial resolution and, with the variety of newly developed pulse sequences and imaging coils, can provide highly specific functional and anatomic information about the lesion in question and the condition of the surrounding brain.[36,70] MR angiography can be performed during the same imaging evaluation and allows assessment of arterial and venous systems. Obstruction to CSF flow can also be directly evaluated by MRI using specialized techniques aimed at monitoring CSF flow dynamics.

Newer techniques, beyond the scope of this general overview, include MR spectroscopy, functional MRI (fMRI), and diffusion tensor imaging.[36] These latter techniques allow biochemical and metabolic characterization of focal lesions, assessment of functional activity in the brain, and direct evaluation of the structural integrity of CNS white matter tracts, respectively. FDG-PET and PET scanning with newer radiotracers such as ^{18}F-thymidine may also be of additional value in delineating postsurgical margins from residual tumor and in predicting response to therapy.[71,72]

There are several classification systems for pediatric brain tumors. The most commonly used World Health Organization (WHO) classification of intracranial tumors is based on histopathologic characteristics and clinical course, with tumors further classified based on their intracranial location—specifically, whether lesions are supratentorial or infratentorial. This classification system allows a practical assignment of differential diagnoses to newly identified CNS tumors based on their location and provides prognostic information related to histologic subtype and grade when these additional data become available.

Supratentorial Tumors

Astrocytoma

The most common supratentorial brain tumor is the astrocytoma, representing from 55% to 65% of all primary pediatric brain tumors.[73] Astrocytomas are seen in all age groups; presenting symptoms are typically the result of increased intracranial pressure, with headache, nausea, and vomiting commonly seen. Astrocytomas can be reliably diagnosed by CT and MRI (Fig. 26-4). They range from benign to malignant in their histologic grade, with grade 1 lesions classified as benign, grade 2 as low-grade glioma, grade 3 as anaplastic glioma, and grade 4 as glioblastoma. The lesions are usually large with both solid and cystic components. Calcifications can occur, but are unusual. The parietal, frontal, and temporal lobes are common sites of astrocytoma. On fluid-sensitive sequences, the cystic component of the lesion may show characteristics of complex fluid, with decreased signal intensity relative to CSF on T2-weighted sequences. Following contrast infusion, homogeneous enhancement of the solid component of the lesion is typical. Higher grade, more malignant tumors often have less distinct margins, more heterogeneous enhancement, and increased peritumoral edema and mass effect.[73,74] Complete surgical resection is frequently not possible because of involvement of adjacent major neural structures. Five-year survival for low-grade astrocytomas is between 40% and 50%, with less than 5% survival for the higher grade malignancies. Because of a propensity to spread to the spine via the CSF, the staging evaluation must also include imaging of the entire spine.

Tumors of the midline deep gray matter, including the basal ganglia, thalamus, hypothalamus, and chiasmatic–optic pathway region, tend to be astrocytomas.[69,74] As with the cerebral hemispheric astrocytomas, tumor grades range from benign to highly anaplastic. The imaging features are similar to those of lesions located in the cerebral hemispheres, with decreased signal intensity on T1-weighted images, hyperintensity on T2-weighted images, and variable contrast enhancement. Because of their location, behavioral changes, emotional and memory changes, movement disorders, visual abnormalities, and hydrocephalus are all common symptoms associated with these deep gray matter tumors. Surgical resectability is often not possible, and the imaging evaluation is directed at identifying involvement of adjacent critical structures and monitoring post-therapy changes.[69]

The infratentorial-cerebellar form of astrocytoma, also known as juvenile pilocytic astrocytoma, is distinct from the diffuse supratentorial astrocytoma discussed here. It will be described in further detail later.

Oligodendroglioma

Oligodendroglioma, although common in adults, is relatively rare in children and adolescents.[74] The most common location is in the frontotemporal region, with less common involvement of the posterior fossa and spinal cord. Imaging evaluation shows a hypodense lesion on CT. Because most of these contain varying degrees of calcification, they are distinct as being the most common supratentorial tumor in childhood to calcify. The noncalcified solid component is typically isodense to the adjacent brain on CT. On MRI, the lesions are characterized by low signal intensity on T1-weighted images, hyperintensity on T2-weighted images, and minimal enhancement following infusion of gadolinium contrast (Fig. 26-5). Although these tend to be slow-growing lesions, depending on their size, there may be edema evident in the surrounding brain.

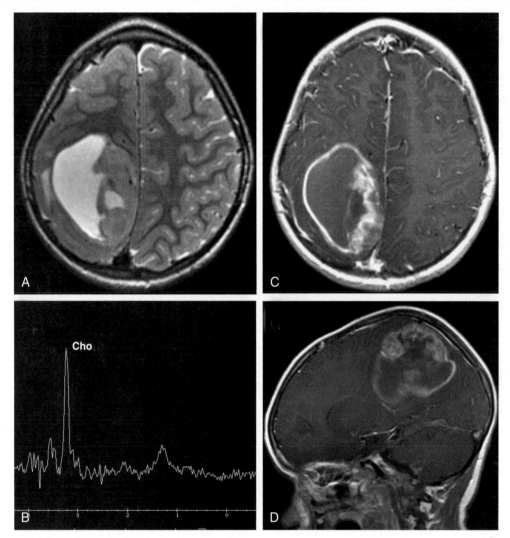

FIGURE 26-4. 4-year-old patient with hemispheric astrocytoma. **A,** T2-weighted and postgadolinium T1-weighted images (**C, D**) show cystic and solid masses with peripheral enhancement located in the frontoparietal region. **B,** MR spectroscopy of the solid component is notable for decreased NAA and elevated choline and lipid peaks, typical of a highly cellular tumor, NAA, *N*-acetylaspartate.

Ganglioglioma

Ganglioglioma and ganglioneuroma comprise about 5% of pediatric brain tumors.[73,74] As with their counterparts in the peripheral nervous system, calcification is seen in up to 40% of cases. The temporal lobes, frontoparietal lobes, and hypothalamic regions are the most common sites of involvement. The brainstem, posterior fossa, and spinal cord are less commonly involved. MRI demonstrates a low signal intensity lesion on T1-weighted images, with hyperintensity on T2-weighted images and hyperintense homogeneous enhancement following gadolinium infusion (Fig. 26-6).

Intraventricular Neoplasms

Intraventricular tumors include choroid plexus papilloma, neurocytoma, and dermoid-epidermoid tumors. Choroid plexus papilloma-carcinoma is relatively common, making up between 10% and 20% of the intraventricular tumors identified in the first year of life and comprising approximately 5% of all CNS neoplasms.[74] The imaging features are characteristic and typically reveal large lobulated intraventricular lesions (Fig. 26-7). These tumors are highly vascular, and are frequently associated with calcification and occasionally hemorrhage.[73,74] Depending on the size and location of the lesion, there may be obstructive hydrocephalus. MRI shows a low–signal intensity lesion on T1-weighted images, with variable hyperintensity on T2-weighted images. Magnetic susceptibility will be seen if hemorrhage is present and, following contrast infusion, these lesions typically show marked contrast enhancement. The combination of a lobulated, intensely enhancing intraventricular lesion is almost diagnostic of choroid plexus papilloma. Of these lesions, 5% to 10% will degenerate into choroid plexus carcinomas,[74] and this latter diagnosis is suggested by accompanying necrosis within the lesion and metastatic spread into the adjacent brain, either by direct extension into the adjacent brain or by CSF dissemination. Because of their intraventricular location, metastatic spread throughout the CNS via CSF dissemination is unfortunately common for choroid plexus carcinomas, resulting in a uniformly poor prognosis.[69]

Central Neurocytoma

Neurocytomas are rare in children and have imaging features that mimic those of oligodendroglioma, showing an intraventricular calcified mass with heterogeneous contrast enhancement. These tumors typically involve the lateral ventricle in the midline; however, surgical resection is necessary to distinguish

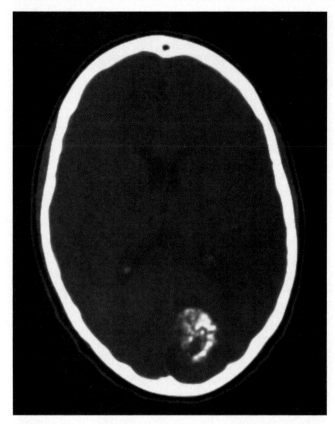

FIGURE 26-5. Oligodendroglioma. CT scan shows calcified low-attenuation lesion in the occipital cortex, with imaging features characteristic of oligodendroglioma.

this lesion from other intraventricular tumors, such as subependymal astrocytomas and ependymomas.

Midline Supratentorial Tumors

Tumors of the hypothalamic-suprasellar region include craniopharyngioma, hypothalamic hamartoma, and pineal region tumors.

Craniopharyngioma

Craniopharyngioma is the most common suprasellar tumor.[73,74] It has fairly characteristic imaging features, with lesions containing solid, cystic, and calcified elements. Symptoms usually result from increased intracranial pressure and local effects on the hypothalamic pituitary region and optic chiasm. Because these are relatively slow-growing lesions, they may be large at diagnosis. The presence of a calcified suprasellar mass at CT scan is usually suggestive of the diagnosis (Fig. 26-8); however, MRI is superior for evaluating the extent of involvement. Depending on the type of material present in the cystic component of the mass, variable signal intensity on T1- and T2-weighted images may be seen.[73] It is common, for example, for the complex proteinaceous, cholesterol-laden fluid to be variably hyperintense on both T1- and T2-weighted images (see Fig. 26-8). Following contrast infusion, the cyst wall frequently enhances. However, the solid components of the cyst often demonstrate inhomogeneous enhancement as well.

Pineal region masses are characterized by their location in the quadrigeminal plate cistern. These tumors typically arise

from primordial germ cells and include pineoblastoma, pineocytoma, and immature germ cell tumors.[69,73,74] It is important to distinguish these neoplastic lesions from benign pineal cysts, which are commonly seen within the pineal gland. Pineal cysts have a characteristic appearance on both CT and MRI, and do not distort or compress the adjacent ventricles. Simple pineal region cysts typically do not typically achieve sizes larger than 1 cm. Also of note is normal calcification within the pineal gland. Calcification is unusual before the age of 10 years, but is commonly seen in adolescents and older children.[75] Therefore, the presence of calcification in the pineal region in an infant or young child should raise suspicion for a pineal region mass or germ cell tumor and prompt further investigation.

Pineal gland tumors, including pineocytoma and pineoblastoma, are relatively rare. Pineocytoma is typically benign and nonaggressive, whereas pineoblastoma, representing an immature undifferentiated lesion, frequently metastasizes. Pineoblastoma is also a component of the so-called trilateral retinoblastoma and is seen with increased frequency in patients diagnosed with bilateral retinoblastoma. Pineocytomas are more frequently calcified than pineoblastomas. Pineoblastomas are typically larger, with low signal intensity on T1-weighted images, variable hyperintensity on T2-weighted images, and fairly homogeneous contrast enhancement.[74] Very large pineoblastomas may produce mass effect on the adjacent quadrigeminal cistern and, because of their large size, often show areas of necrosis (Fig. 26-9).

Germ Cell Tumors

The pineal region is the most common location for intracranial germ cell tumors.[74] Histopathologically, these are most often germinomas and usually associated with calcification. This is well demonstrated by CT. MRI is indicated for better delineation of the extent of the noncalcified solid portion of the mass, as well as heterogeneous cystic portions, which may also be present. On T2-weighted images, the solid portion is typically hyperintense with bright enhancement following contrast infusion. Other germ cell origin tumors are also seen, with choriocarcinomas more frequently showing hemorrhagic components and displaying more aggressive features. Benign teratomas, in contrast, display imaging features more in keeping with their well-differentiated dermoid or epidermoid components, including low attenuation fluid on CT, hyperdense fluid on T1-weighted sequences. and heterogeneous contrast enhancement (Fig. 26-10).

Hypothalamic Hamartoma

This is a rare congenital lesion, most often identified in infants younger than 2 years. Seizure disorders are common. The presence of precocious puberty or diabetes insipidus may provide clinical clues to suggest this diagnosis.

On imaging, CT scanning shows an isodense mass in the region of the hypothalamus. There is little to no contrast enhancement on CT or MRI scans.[74] On MRI, the lesion is usually isodense to brain on T1-weighted images, minimally hyperintense on T2-weighted images but, interestingly, may be hyperintense on fluid-attenuated inversion recovery (FLAIR) images (Fig. 26-11).

Infratentorial Tumors

The most common lesions of the posterior fossa and cerebellum are the juvenile pilocytic astrocytoma (JPA) and medulloblastoma.[69,73,74]

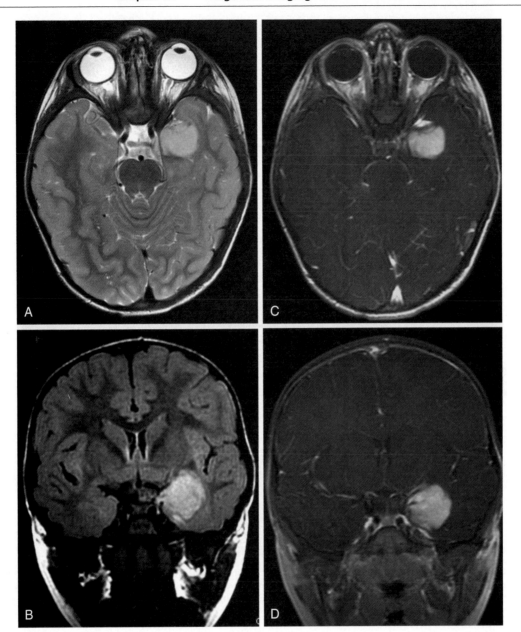

FIGURE 26-6. 4-year-old with left temporal lobe ganglioglioma, showing increased signal on T2-weighted images (**A**), and bright enhancement after gadolinium administration (**C, D**). Depending on their location, these lesions may be more conspicuous on fluid-attenuated inversion recovery (FLAIR) images (**B**).

Medulloblastoma

Medulloblastomas are slightly more common in incidence than cerebellar astrocytomas.[69] They typically occur in the first decade of life. Presenting symptoms usually relate to increased intracranial pressure secondary to obstructive hydrocephalus, typically on the fourth ventricle. Medulloblastomas are highly malignant and have a propensity to disseminate and seed the CNS via the CSF route.[73,74] Hematogenous spread to other sites may also occur in medulloblastoma.

CT scanning is usually the first imaging study performed to evaluate new-onset nausea, vomiting, headache, or seizures. CT scanning usually demonstrates a hyperintense solid lesion within the cerebellum, typically near the midline (Fig. 26-12). MRI is indicated to characterize the lesions better and to establish sites of local and metastatic spread. As with other highly

cellular CNS tumors, on T1-weighted images, medulloblastomas are usually hypointense relative to the adjacent cerebellum, with increased signal intensity on T2-weighted images (see Fig. 26-3) and homogeneous enhancement following gadolinium infusion.[73,74] Calcification and cystic areas are unusual in medulloblastoma. Because of the propensity to disseminate to other sites via the CNS, the staging evaluation must include a contrast-enhanced evaluation of the entire spine.

Cerebellar Astrocytoma

Astrocytomas are the next most common posterior fossa tumor.[69] As with their intracerebral counterpart, cerebellar astrocytomas range in histologic grade from benign to anaplastic. The characteristic juvenile pilocytic form makes up most of

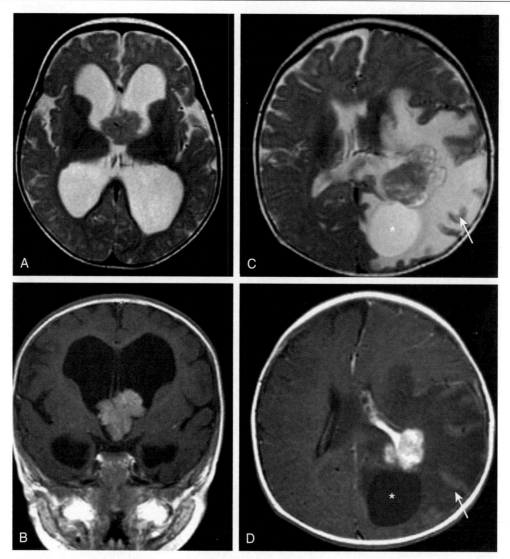

FIGURE 26-7. Choroid plexus papilloma in 8- and 10-month-old infants, both with large lobulated lesions causing obstructive hydrocephalus. **A, B,** In one patient, the tumor is centrally located, producing severe global hydrocephalus, whereas in the other **(C, D)**, the peripheral location is accompanied by extensive vasogenic edema (*arrow*) and left occipital horn hydrocephalus (*).

the cerebellar astrocytomas. Both the cystic and solid components are commonly seen in this type of astrocytoma (Fig. 26-13). Calcification is unusual.[73,74] Following resection, survival is excellent, with greater than 90% 10-year survival. As with medulloblastoma, CT scanning is usually the first imaging modality used to evaluate initial symptoms. CT shows a heterogeneous, predominantly cystic lesion in the posterior fossa, typically with a small mural nodule eccentrically along the margin of the tumor.[73,74] These lesions are frequently midline, near the vermis, but may also be eccentric in location. MRI is indicated to characterize the extent of cerebellar involvement better. Although the presence of a predominantly cystic component suggests a lower grade neoplasm, foci of local or metastatic spread may be present and will be manifest as a focus of increased enhancement following gadolinium infusion.[73] Therefore, the imaging evaluation should include conventional T1- and T2-weighted imaging as well as postcontrast enhanced scanning in all three imaging planes. Because higher grade neoplasms may also disseminate via the CSF, as with medulloblastoma, the initial staging evaluation should also include evaluation of the entire spine.

Brainstem Glioma

Brainstem gliomas make up most of the neoplasms involving the brainstem. These tumors are of astrocytoma origin and, because of their location, result in almost uniformly poor survival.[69] These predominantly cellular solid lesions are best evaluated by MRI, and typically appear as hypodense lesions on T1-weighted images, increased signal intensity on T2-weighted images, and heterogeneous enhancement.[73,74] Lower grade lesions, or lesions with larger cyst components, may only show very minimal contrast enhancement. As with the other tumors in these locations, spread is most often via the CSF to other portions of the brain.

Ependymoma

After medulloblastoma and juvenile pilocytic astrocytoma, the next most common posterior fossa tumor is the ependymoma. Most of these are benign and arise from the ependyma of the fourth ventricle. They typically present as a calcified intraventricular mass. Symptoms result from obstruction of CSF flow at the level of the fourth ventricle leading to obstructive

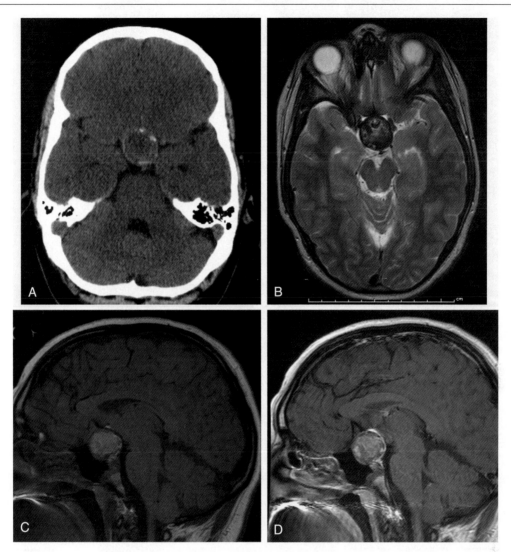

FIGURE 26-8. Craniopharyngioma. **A,** CT showing calcified suprasellar mass, with heterogeneous increased signal on both T2-weighted **(B)** and T1-weighted **(C)** images, with peripheral enhancement following gadolinium **(D).**

hydrocephalus. There are two histologic types, with the benign undifferentiated type being more common, and typically with less invasion locally and a lower likelihood of CSF dissemination. Malignant anaplastic ependymoma, in contrast, tends to spread via the CSF early on in the disease course to other sites within the CNS.[74] Because of their propensity to insinuate through neural foramina, resulting in a lobulated appearance, ependymomas have a fairly characteristic appearance on imaging (see Fig. 26-14). Depending on the degree of calcification, these lesions may be predominantly hypointense on T1- and T2-weighted images. In the absence of calcification, these are usually hyperintense lesions on T2-weighted images, with heterogeneous intense enhancement following gadolinium infusion.[74] Because of their propensity to seed throughout the CSF and ventricular system, the imaging evaluation must include examination of both the brain and spinal canal.

Hemangioblastoma

This is a benign vascular lesion that is more common in adults than children. However, the cerebellum is still the most common location in children, and multiple hemangioblastomas may be encountered in familial predisposition syndromes, such as the von Hippel–Lindau syndrome.[74] The imaging features demonstrate a predominantly cystic lesion, with an enhancing mural nodule that may be difficult to distinguish from the juvenile pilocytic astrocytoma. Similarly, these lesions show a cyst on MRI with low signal intensity on T1-weighted images and T2 hyperintensity and intense enhancement of the solid mural nodular component (Fig. 26-15). Depending on the size of the mural nodule, the degree of enhancement, and its location, these lesions may also be difficult to distinguish from a benign posterior fossa arachnoid cyst.

Other Central Nervous System Tumors

Metastatic Disease

A number of primary tumors are known to result in hematogenous spread to the CNS. The most common are rhabdomyosarcoma, Ewing's sarcoma, and osteogenic sarcoma.[74] A tumor with a particular propensity to metastasize to the brain is the rhabdoid tumor of the kidney, and imaging of the CNS is essential for children with this diagnosis. Metastatic disease to the CNS may also be seen in other common pediatric tumors,

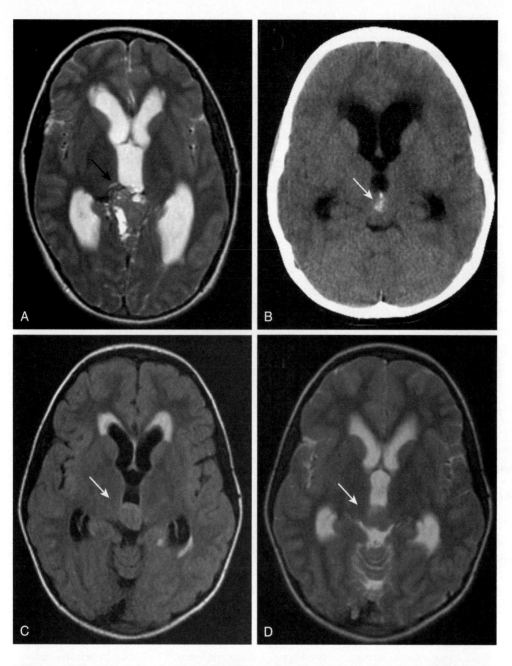

FIGURE 26-9. Two patients with pineoblastoma. **A,** The larger cystic/solid mass seen in one patient causes obstruction and hydrocephalus at the level of the quadrigeminal plate cistern. In the accompanying case, even the smaller calcified mass **(B)** causes hydrocephalus as a result of its central location abutting the ventricles. As noted in the text, the lesions are often hyperintense on fluid-attenuated inversion recovery **(C)** and isointense to cortex on T2-weighted images **(D)**. Arrows indicate the centrally located mass lesions.

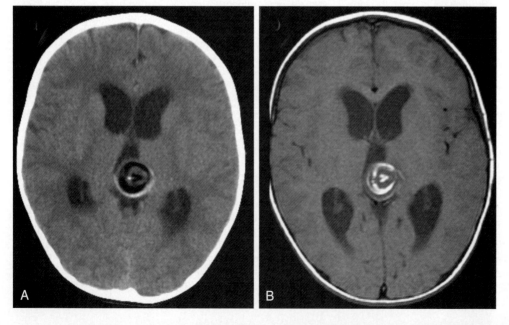

FIGURE 26-10. Pineal germ cell tumor. **A,** CT scan and T1-weighted axial MRI scan **(B)** show low-attenuation fluid on CT and hyperdense fluid on T1-weighted sequences, typical of a well-differentiated pineal germ cell tumor (teratoma).

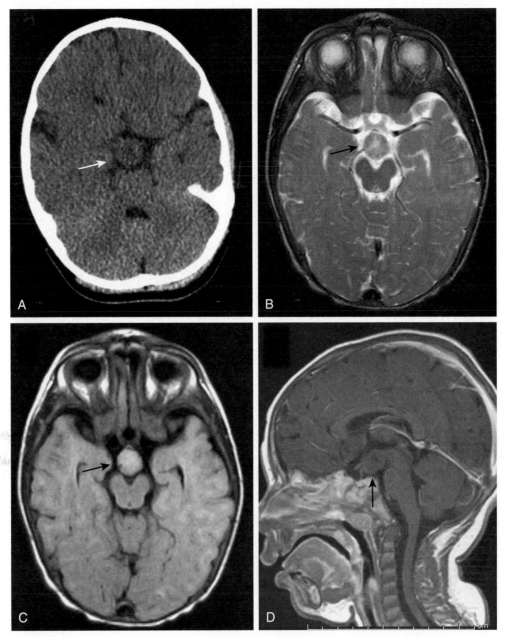

FIGURE 26-11. Hypothalamic hamartoma. **A,** CT scan shows a low-density suprasellar hypothalamic lesion (*arrow*). **B,** MRI scan shows the lesion to be isointense to brain on T2-weighted sequences, mildly hyperintense on fluid-attenuated inversion recovery (FLAIR) images **(C)**, with no significant enhancement following gadolinium infusion **(D)**.

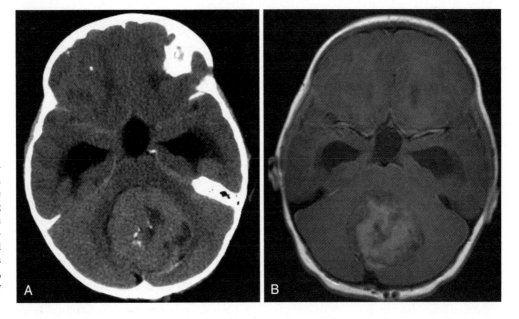

FIGURE 26-12. Medulloblastoma. **A,** Unenhanced CT scan shows a hyperdense mass in the posterior fossa, compressing the fourth ventricle with resultant obstructive hydrocephalus. **B,** Gadolinium-enhanced T1-weighted MRI scan shows enhancement of most of the mass, features consistent with a highly cellular medulloblastoma.

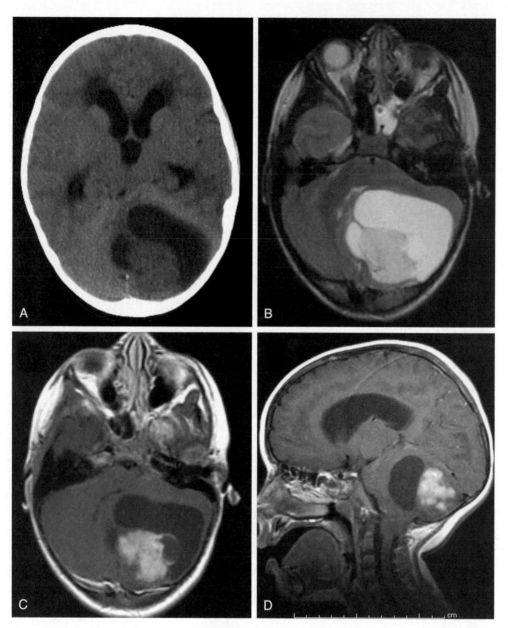

FIGURE 26-13. Cerebellar pilocytic astrocytoma. **A,** Unenhanced CT scan shows large, predominantly cystic mass, with a solid mural component in the posterior fossa with moderate hydrocephalus. **B,** T2-weighted MRI scan shows high signal intensity cystic fluid and intermediate signal mural nodule (**B**). **C, D,** Only the mural nodule enhances following gadolinium infusion.

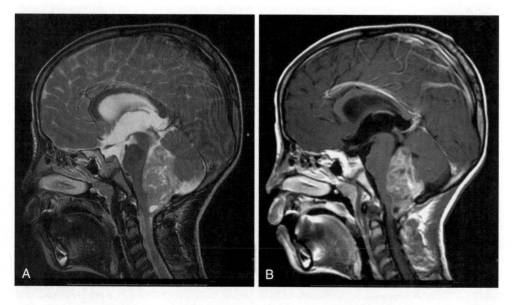

FIGURE 26-14. Ependymoma. 7-year-old with lethargy. **A,** T2-weighted and gadolinium-enhanced MRI (**B**) scans show a large heterogeneously enhancing posterior fossa mass compressing the brainstem and beginning to extend out through the foramen magnum.

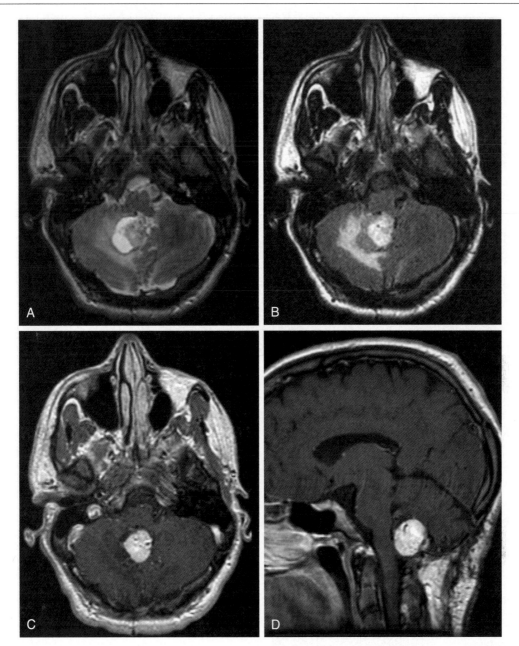

FIGURE 26-15. 28-year-old with history of von Hippel–Lindau syndrome and cerebellar hemangioblastoma, showing typical features on T2-weighted (**A**), fluid-attenuated inversion recovery (**B**), and post-gadolinium-enhanced images (**C, D**).

such as neuroblastoma and lymphoma. CNS involvement by leukemia is also common, although this is more frequently diagnosed by lumbar puncture and pathologic evaluation of the CSF rather than imaging. Although the imaging features may be variable, depending on the primary malignancy, the presence of any focal area of signal abnormality or enhancement with a known primary tumor should raise suspicion for metastatic spread of disease to the CNS.

Spinal Cord Tumors

In comparison to pediatric brain tumors, spinal cord tumors are relatively rare in children. Most of the intramedullary spinal tumors in children are low-grade astrocytomas, with the remainder being ependymomas.[74] The imaging features of these lesions mimic those of their intracranial counterparts. The imaging

assessment is usually prompted by neurologic symptoms and should include multiplanar T1, T2, and post–gadolinium-enhanced imaging. Because it may be difficult to distinguish a primary intraspinal tumor from metastatic disease, imaging of the brain must also be performed.

As in the brain, the imaging examination should be directed at identifying the site of origin of the tumor. It should be possible to make a distinction between primary intramedullary tumors, extramedullary intradural tumors, and extradural and epidural lesions. This is important because most spinal tumors in children are extramedullary. Intradural extramedullary lesions are, by definition, located within the subarachnoid space and are typically the result of dropped metastases or spread via the CSF from primary brain tumors (see earlier). Their appearance on imaging mimics that of their counterpart in the brain. Extradural extramedullary tumors may arise from local exten-

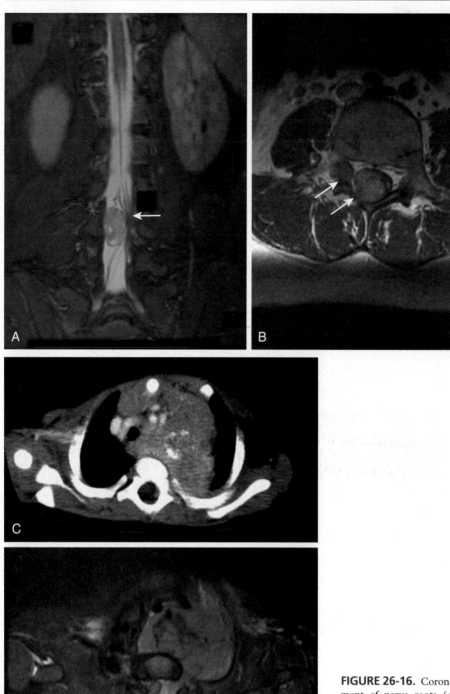

FIGURE 26-16. Coronal (**A**) and axial (**B**) MR images show displacement of nerve roots (*arrow*, **A**) and extension through the neural foramen (*arrows*, **B**) in a patient with extramedullary intraspinal Ewing's sarcoma. **C, D,** Patient with calcified left upper thoracic neuroblastoma initially detected on chest x-ray. MRI is superior in detecting the degree of intraspinal extension (**D**).

sion of other primary neoplasms, such as neuroblastoma, lymphoma, or Ewing's sarcoma (Fig. 26-16). When evaluating these other primary pediatric neoplasms, if their location is adjacent to the vertebral column, it is essential that a thorough imaging evaluation be undertaken to evaluate the presence and extent of intraspinal involvement. In particular, with neuroblastoma, this will influence staging and surgical resectability. The presence of intraspinal extension may be suggested by CT, but will usually be better delineated by MRI (Fig. 26-16C and D; Fig. 26-17).

PULMONARY AND INTRATHORACIC TUMORS

Thyroid and Parathyroid Tumors

Thyroid carcinoma in children is rare.[76] Three histologic subtypes are recognized in children, with most patients (approximately 80%) having papillary carcinoma; follicular (approximately 15%) and medullary (approximately 5%)

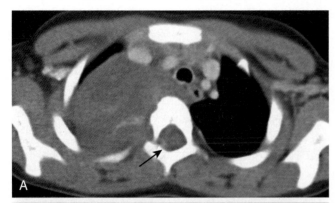

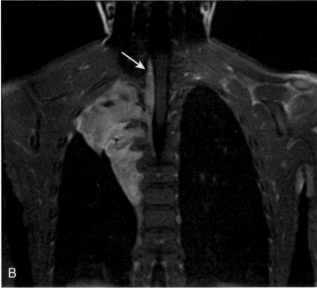

FIGURE 26-17. Upper thoracic paraspinal neuroblastoma in a 5-year-old with 2 weeks of upper respiratory infection symptoms. Chest x-ray revealed a right upper lobe opacity (not shown). This was found on CT to be a paraspinal mass. Intraspinal extension is evident on CT (**A,** *arrow*), but much better delineated by MRI (**B,** *arrow*).

thyroid cancers occur less frequently. The risk is increased in patients with prior history of neck radiation or with predisposing familial syndromes (multiple endocrine neoplasia [MEN]).[76] Presentation is typically a painless mass in the thyroid gland. Ultrasound is the imaging modality of choice for evaluating the thyroid gland and is usually sufficient to identify a palpable thyroid abnormality.[77] The goal of the ultrasound examination is to determine whether a cystic or solid mass is present (Fig. 26-18). The presence of increased blood flow and size of the mass is not reliable in distinguishing benign from malignant thyroid nodules. Malignant nodules are almost always cold on ^{123}I scintigraphy, relative to the surrounding thyroid gland.[77] Depending on the type of tumor, metastatic spread to adjacent lymph nodes and/or the lung may be present. In particular, papillary carcinoma of the thyroid often produces multiple small pulmonary nodules with a miliary distribution. These small pulmonary nodules may be challenging to detect by chest x-ray, and chest CT is indicated to provide increased sensitivity for lesion detection.[78] [123]I or ^{131}I scintigraphy may also detect lesions not seen by conventional imaging. Bone metastases and thoracic lymph node involvement are common sites of extrapulmonary metastatic spread.

Abnormalities of the parathyroid gland usually come to clinical attention during evaluation of hypercalcemic states. Functional parathyroid hyperplasia and parathyroid adenomas have a similar imaging appearance, and can be well characterized by ultrasound. There is usually no need for additional imaging by CT. Because of the variable anatomic locations of the parathyroid glands, it may be difficult to identify all potential sites of abnormality by conventional anatomic imaging techniques. ^{123}I-MIBG scintigraphy is very sensitive and specific at showing focal accumulation of radiotracer in sites of functional parathyroid activity and can be used to identify sites of otherwise occult disease (Fig. 26-19).

Mediastinal Masses and Tumors

The mediastinum is located in the center of the thorax, between the two thoracic cavities, diaphragm, and thoracic inlet. It is conventional to divide the mediastinum into anterior, middle, and posterior mediastinal compartments, based on their location as seen on the lateral chest radiograph. Although there are no distinct tissue planes that delineate these compartments, this system of classification is useful in characterizing diseases based on their tissue of origin. Classifying mediastinal masses within a single mediastinal compartment helps narrow the differential

FIGURE 26-18. Follicular thyroid carcinoma: palpable thyroid lesion, with typical ultrasound imaging characteristics. Longitudinal and transverse ultrasound images show hypoechoic well-circumscribed mass. The mass is too small (approximately 1 cm) to be characterized accurately by ^{123}I scintigraphy.

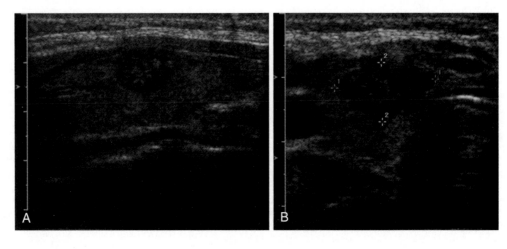

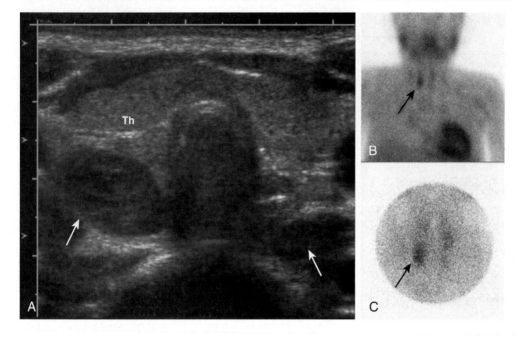

FIGURE 26-19. Parathyroid adenoma. Thyroid ultrasound **(A)** shows a large hypoechoic mass on the right and a smaller lesion on the left (*arrows*) at the expected location of the parathyroid glands in an 11-year-old patient with end-stage renal disease and secondary hyperparathyroidism. The dominant mass on the right (*arrows*) has corresponding increased uptake on ^{99m}Tc-metaiodobenzylguanidine (MIBG) scintigraphy **(B, C)**, consistent with parathyroid adenoma. Small lesions are optimally seen with a pinhole collimator **(C)**. The lower levels of uptake in the smaller lesions are more in keeping with hyperplastic parathyroid tissue. ^{99m}Tc-MIBG is also effective at locating ectopically located parathyroid tissue (e.g., substernal) not visualized on thyroid (Th) ultrasound.

diagnosis, calls attention to the potential effect of the mediastinal mass on adjacent compartmental structures, and thereby frequently guides clinical decision making.[79]

Anterior Mediastinal Masses

The anterior mediastinum is defined as the prevascular space situated between the sternum and the heart, pericardium, and great vessels. The anterior mediastinum extends superiorly from the thoracic to the level of the diaphragm. Organs located in the anterior mediastinum include the thymus, thyroid, and parathyroid glands and prevascular space lymphoid tissue. With respect to mediastinal mass formation, the thymus and anterior mediastinal lymph nodes are the two most important structures to be considered.

In infants, it is important to distinguish normal thymus from a mediastinal mass. The normal thymus usually has an undulating contour and, on chest radiographs, can be accurately identified based on subtle deformity by the costal cartilages of the adjacent anterior ribs. The normal thymus can be large and may extend posteriorly between the superior vena cava and aorta in the middle mediastinum, or superiorly into the lower neck, making the distinction from neoplasm difficult.[79,80] In the appropriate clinical setting, thymic hyperplasia may also be seen, characterized by a homogeneously enlarged thymus. The thymus also may rapidly involute in response to physiologic stress, which can also provide an indirect means of confirming its identity as normal thymus.

Lymphoma

Lymphoma is the most common tumor arising in the mediastinum, and most often arises in the anterior or middle mediastinum. Both Hodgkin's and non-Hodgkin's lymphomas can present as mediastinal masses. The imaging features of Hodgkin's lymphoma usually identify a bulky anterior mediastinal mass, with a nodular appearance. In addition, Hodgkin's disease is characterized by contiguous lymph node spread, which may aid in the distinction from other types of lymphoma. Approximately two thirds of pediatric patients with Hodgkin's lymphoma will present with lymphadenopathy involving the mediastinum. Non-Hodgkin's lymphomas include lymphoblastic lymphoma and other subtypes. Approximately one third of pediatric non-Hodgkin's lymphomas present with a mediastinal mass, and more than 50% of the lymphoblastic lymphomas have mediastinal involvement.[79] Although the distinction between non-Hodgkin's and Hodgkin's lymphoma may be difficult, acute T-lymphoblastic lymphomas frequently demonstrate a homogeneous infiltration and enlargement of the thymus gland, with encasement or compression of the vessels rather than displacement of the vessels (Fig. 26-20). All forms of lymphoma can result in significant tracheal compression or narrowing, vascular compression, and symptoms related to the superior mediastinal syndrome.[81] Pleural and pericardial effusions are seen in both non-Hodgkin's and Hodgkin's lymphomas of the mediastinum. Bone invasion by Hodgkin's lymphoma is unusual; non-Hodgkin's lymphomas often show more aggressive local involvement.

The imaging evaluation should always include chest radiography. Often, this is the most important imaging study to guide the subsequent care of the patient. The presence of significant tracheal narrowing or tracheal displacement in the context of a large anterior mediastinal mass, particularly if accompanied by respiratory symptoms (see Fig. 26-1), should raise immediate concern for impending respiratory or cardiopulmonary compromise and prompt intensive care unit (ICU) level monitoring.[81] Pneumomediastinum and pneumothorax may also be identified on these initial imaging studies (see Figs. 26-1 and 26-20). The placement of the patient in a recumbent position for CT scanning may further exacerbate the patient's already tenuous respiratory status, impair central venous return, and result in an acute cardiorespiratory event. In this setting, it may be necessary to delay CT imaging; the staging evaluation will have to follow stabilization of the patient's clinical status.

In the more stable patient, staging of anterior mediastinal lymphomas must include imaging of the neck to evaluate Waldeyer's ring of lymphoid tissue, and should also include the abdomen and pelvis. Intravenous contrast should be used to provide an accurate assessment of the mediastinal vascular structures. Oral contrast should be provided to opacify the bowel and aid in the distinction from mesenteric lymphadenopathy.

MRI, particularly with faster scanning techniques, may be effective in evaluating mediastinal masses, but currently has little value for the more acute stages of the evaluation. Gallium

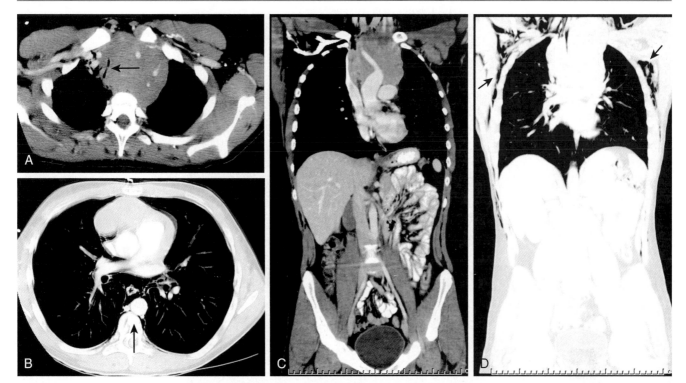

FIGURE 26-20. Lymphoblastic lymphoma and pneumomediastinum. This is the same patient whose chest x-ray is shown in Figure 26-1. On the admission CT, note the mediastinal mass (**A**, *arrow*) with mediastinal air (*arrow*) around the heart, pulmonary vessels, aorta, and esophagus (**B**). The trachea is markedly narrowed (**A**, *arrow*), likely the cause of the pneumomediastinum. Subcutaneous air is also evident in the anterior chest wall. Five days later, the findings had progressed considerably (**C, D**, *arrows*).

scintigraphy previously, and currently ^{18}F-FDG-PET imaging, are recognized as the standard of care for identifying sites of metabolically active lymphoma and identifying sites of disease otherwise undetected by conventional imaging techniques (Fig. 26-21). ^{18}F-FDG-PET scanning, in particular, has also been shown to play an important role in the post-treatment evaluation, helping stratify patients into early responder and non-responder groups to allow appropriate modulation of therapy based on their treatment response (Fig. 26-22).[62,82-85]

Following treatment, particularly in Hodgkin's disease, it is common for the mediastinal mass to regress slowly and for residual inflammatory tissue to persist, even months after therapy.[86] In contrast, lymphoblastic lymphomas usually respond rapidly to therapy, with very little residual soft tissue abnormality remaining in the anterior mediastinum, even after a relatively short duration of treatment. Increasingly, FDG-PET imaging is being used, with images being simultaneously acquired and coregistered as fused PET-CT images to distinguish persistent metabolically active disease from residual post-treatment inflammatory tissue.[87-89]

Germ Cell Tumor

Mediastinal germ cell tumors are primarily located in the anterior mediastinum, near the thymus gland, and make up about 10% to 20% of all childhood mediastinal tumors. Germ cell tumors are second only to lymphoma as the cause of a thymic/anterior mediastinal mass. When they present as predominantly solid masses they may be difficult to distinguish from lymphoma. Histologically, teratomas are the most common mediastinal germ cell tumor. At diagnosis, calcification of lymphoma is unusual, and the calcifications often present in teratoma may suggest the diagnosis. Germ cell tumors are frequently asymptomatic and may be identified incidentally as mediastinal

masses on chest radiographs obtained for other indications.[90] When symptoms are present, they are usually the result of compression of the tracheobronchial tree.

Either CT or MRI scanning is effective at further characterizing these masses. The presence of fluid attenuation, mixed attenuation fluids or gelatinous material, fat, and calcification all should suggest the diagnosis of mediastinal germ cell tumor (Fig. 26-23). Of the mediastinal germ cell tumors, 10% to 20% are malignant and will present with signs of local invasion into the pleura or pericardium. Malignant tumors include seminomatous and nonseminomatous histologic subtypes. Seminomas tend to be noncalcified bulky solid masses that remain localized or spread to local lymph nodes, whereas other malignant germ cell tumors display greater heterogeneity, with cystic and solid elements and more aggressive, locally invasive features.[91] Germ cell tumors may rupture into the pleural or pericardial spaces, the lung parenchyma, or the tracheobronchial tree. Imaging evaluation should be directed at determining the extent of rupture and sites of tissue involvement. Chemical pneumonitis can result from parenchymal rupture, whereas expectoration of blood, hair, and sebaceous material can result from rupture into the airways.[92]

Thymic Masses
Thymoma

Thymoma is rare in children, accounting for less than 4% of pediatric mediastinal tumors.[79] As with adults, thymoma may present with symptoms related to associated autoimmune disorders, including myasthenia gravis, diabetes, and Hashimoto's thyroiditis. Thymomas are typically solid lobulated masses arising in or around the thymus (Fig. 26-24). The imaging evaluation should be directed at assessing for aggressive features, such as invasion into adjacent pericardial or pleural

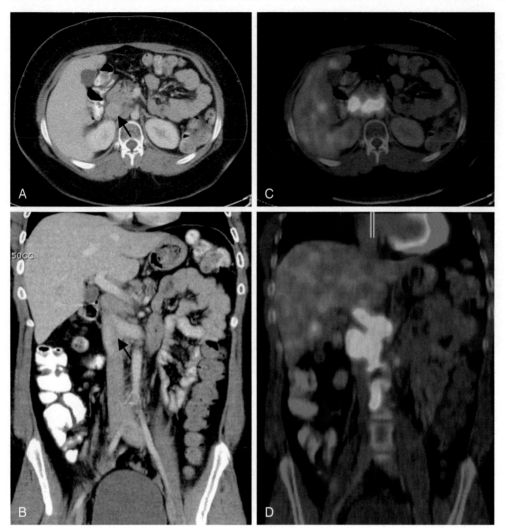

FIGURE 26-21. Axial **(A)** and coronal **(B)** CT and FDG-PET/CT **(C, D)** image fusion delineate equivocal areas of abnormality on CT (*arrows*), identifying foci of disease recurrence in a patient with Hodgkin's lymphoma.

structures. MRI and contrast-enhanced CT reveal a heterogeneously enhancing low-density mass that is isointense on T1-weighted images and mildly T2 hyperintense relative to muscle.[79] CT and MRI are excellent for delineating the relationship of these masses to the adjacent vascular structures. Nodular pleural or pericardial thickening should raise concern for invasive thymoma. Because complete surgical resection is the most effective treatment for ensuring long-term survival for patients with thymoma, postsurgical radiation therapy may be considered when invasive features are present.[93]

Thymolipoma

Thymolipoma, in contrast to thymoma, is relatively more common, making up about 5% to 10% of pediatric thymic tumors. These benign tumors are most often seen in older children, but can present in infancy. These heterogeneous masses may contain calcification and cystic areas, making distinction from germ cell tumors challenging. A predominantly fatty mass should, however, suggest the diagnosis of thymolipoma (Fig. 26-25). The fat characterization can be sensitively and specifically evaluated by MRI, showing a high-signal intensity mass on T1-weighted imaging, with loss of signal on fat-suppressed images. A low-attenuation mass on unenhanced or contrast-enhanced CT can also be seen, which suggests the presence of a fat-containing mass (see Fig. 26-25).

Middle Mediastinal Masses and Tumors
Tracheobronchial Tree Masses

The middle mediastinum is defined as the vascular space including the pericardium and heart, the great vessels, and trachea and proximal bronchi and associated lymph nodes. Although the most common middle mediastinal mass is lymphoma, lymphoma is rarely isolated to the middle mediastinum and usually occurs in conjunction with a large anterior mediastinal mass. The most common masses isolated to the middle mediastinum are benign bronchopulmonary foregut malformations, including bronchopulmonary sequestration, congenital cystic adenomatoid malformation, and foregut or bronchogenic cysts. These benign masses will not be discussed here except to emphasize that the distinction between congenital cystic adenomatoid malformation (CCAM) and pleuropulmonary blastoma cannot be made on the basis of imaging alone (Fig. 26-26), and surgical resection or histopathologic evaluation is required to distinguish the benign CCAM from its neoplastic counterpart.

Masses of the endobronchial tree are also exceedingly rare in children. The most common endobronchial neoplasm in children is the bronchial carcinoid tumor, making up about 50% of all bronchial neoplasms. Although these tumors may secrete neuroendocrine peptides, the classic carcinoid syndrome is relatively unusual in children with bronchial carcinoids, and these patients are more likely to present with

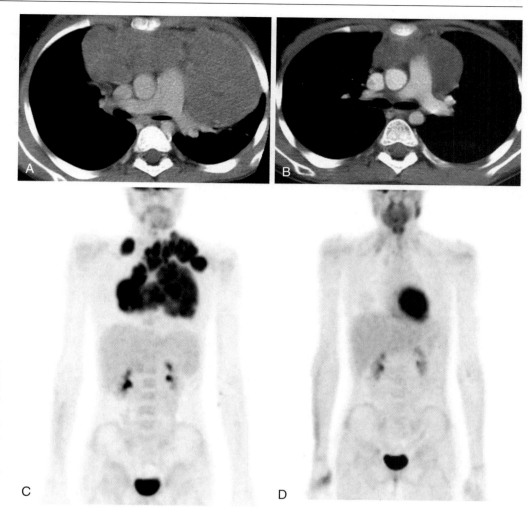

FIGURE 26-22. Hodgkin's lymphoma. CT scan **(A, B)** and FDG-PET scan **(C, D)** obtained at diagnosis **(A, C)** and after two cycles of chemotherapy **(B, D)** show excellent functional and anatomic response to therapy. Residual mediastinal mass on CT, with no residual FDG uptake, emphasizes the potential importance of functional imaging in response assessment.

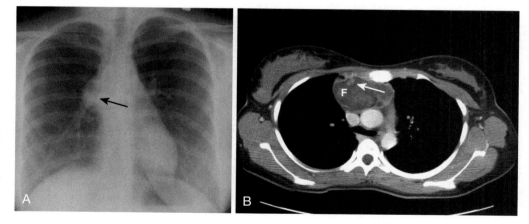

FIGURE 26-23. A, 15-year-old girl with mediastinal mass *(arrow)* seen incidentally on chest x-ray obtained as part of seizure evaluation. **B,** Note fat (F) and solid elements *(arrow)*, characteristic of germ cell tumor—in this case, mature teratoma.

respiratory symptoms such as hemoptysis or lobar atelectasis or partial collapse caused by the obstructing endobronchial lesion (Fig. 26-27). These lesions are frequently hilar in location and may be difficult to identify on chest radiographs. The presence of a persistent area of segmental or lobar collapse that does not resolve following appropriate therapy should prompt further investigation by CT scanning to directly assess the airways.

Newer or multidetector CT scans can provide exquisite three-dimensional re-formations of the airways and allow accurate detection of endobronchial abnormalities. Chest CT of patients with suspected endobronchial carcinoid tumor may be performed without intravenous contrast for the purpose of identifying the endobronchial lesion; however, contrast infusion typically shows prominent enhancement of these highly

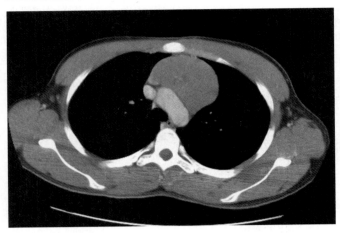

FIGURE 26-24. 15-year-old boy with myasthenia gravis. CT scan shows a lobular anterior mediastinal mass-like enlargement of the thymus. Surgery revealed thymoma.

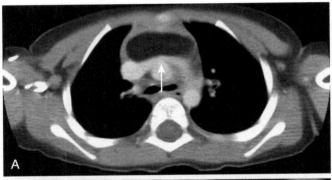

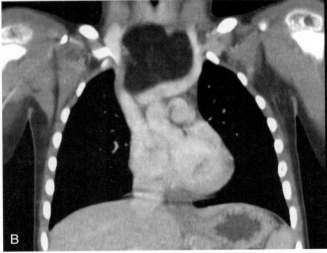

FIGURE 26-25. Thymolipoma in a child with incidentally detected mediastinal mass on chest x-ray. Axial and coronal CT images demonstrate a fat density mass (*arrow*) located within the thymus.

vascular lesions. There may be intraluminal, mural, and extraluminal components of these lesions, and the extraluminal extent of the lesion may exceed its intraluminal component. Although the presence of calcification in an endobronchial mass should suggest the diagnosis of carcinoid, calcification is still relatively rare in childhood bronchial carcinoid. Surgical resection is usually curative and, although the extent of local invasion around the primary lesion is variable, metastatic disease is relative rare (5% to 20%). Uptake of the neuroendocrine-specific radiotracer ^{111}In-octreotide provides highly specific scintigraphic imaging confirmation of the diagnosis (see Fig. 26-27C and D) and may aid in identifying occult sites of metastatic disease. ^{18}F-FDG PET imaging of metabolically active carcinoid tumors has also been carried out and, although not specific for neuroendocrine tumors, may prove to be a more sensitive means of identifying occult metastases.

Mucoepidermoid carcinoma is the second most common primary bronchial neoplasm. These patients also present primarily with respiratory symptoms caused by airway obstruction. Because primary airway neoplasia in children is rare and frequently characterized by nonspecific clinical symptoms, the diagnosis is often delayed and difficult to distinguish from infectious processes such as pneumonia. The most common finding on plain chest radiographs in patients with mucoepidermoid carcinoma is a central mass or nodule.[94,95] These tumors range from low to high grade, with high-grade neoplasms tending to invade the adjacent pulmonary parenchyma. As with carcinoid, multidetector CT with multiplanar and three-dimensional reformatting accurately identifies an airway abnormality.[95,96] However, in contrast to carcinoid, mucoepidermoid carcinoma is relatively hypovascular and shows minimal enhancement. Recent studies have also suggested that FDG-PET scanning may be used to advantage in staging patients with mucoepidermoid carcinoma,[95] with intense FDG uptake visualized (Fig. 26-28).

Tumors of the heart and pericardium are rare in children. Most of these are rhabdomyomas arising from the neoplastic transformation of cardiac myocytes. There is a well-known association between cardiac rhabdomyoma and tuberous sclerosis (Fig. 26-29), with approximately half of patients with this diagnosis having rhabdomyomas. Indeed, the presence of a cardiac rhabdomyoma should prompt further evaluation because rhabdomyomas may be the initial presenting sign of tuberous sclerosis.

When symptoms are present, they are usually the result of tumor protruding into the cardiac lumen resulting in outflow obstruction and congestive failure. Echocardiography is usually sufficient to suggest the diagnosis, but CT scanning and cardiac MRI are superior at defining the extent and attachments of these cardiac tumors and may be indicated for surgical planning. Cardiac fibromas and myxomas are much less common. It is more common to see secondary extension into the heart by other primary pediatric neoplasms such as neuroblastoma and Wilms' tumor, both of which have a propensity to extend into the heart via the inferior vena cava (IVC), hepatoblastoma, which may show direct intracardiac extension (Fig. 26-30), and mediastinal lymphoma, which may result in chest wall or pericardial involvement. Contrast-enhanced CT scanning usually allows an accurate delineation of sites of local extension in the thorax. Abdominal ultrasound or multiphase contrast-enhanced CT can be used to demonstrate intravascular or intracardiac extension from primary abdominal malignancies.

Posterior Mediastinal Masses

The posterior mediastinum is defined dorsally by the chest wall or vertebral column and ventrally by the pericardium and posterior wall of the great vessels, superiorly by the thoracic inlet,

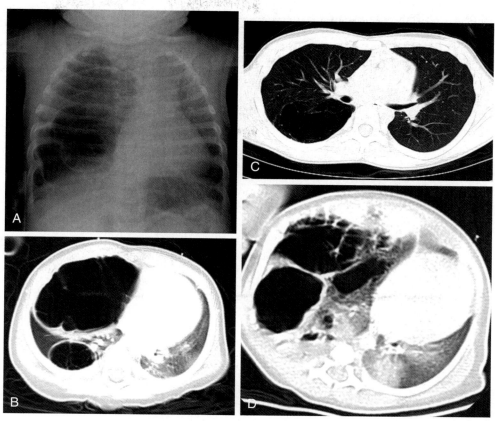

FIGURE 26-26. Pleuropulmonary blastoma **(A, B)**, emphasizing the difficulty in distinguishing this malignancy from congenital cystic adenomatoid malformation (CCAM) **(C, D)**.

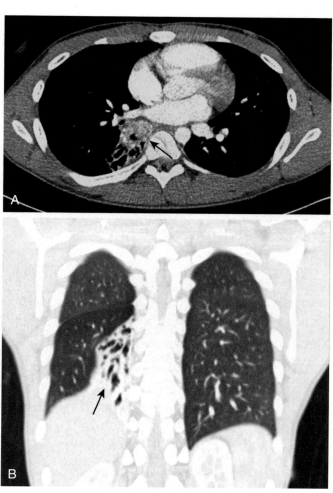

FIGURE 26-27. Bronchial carcinoid, with CT scans **(A, B)** showing hypervascular, enhancing endobronchial mass **(A,** *arrow)* causing post-obstructive collapse of the right lower lobe **(B,** *arrow).*
Continues on next page.

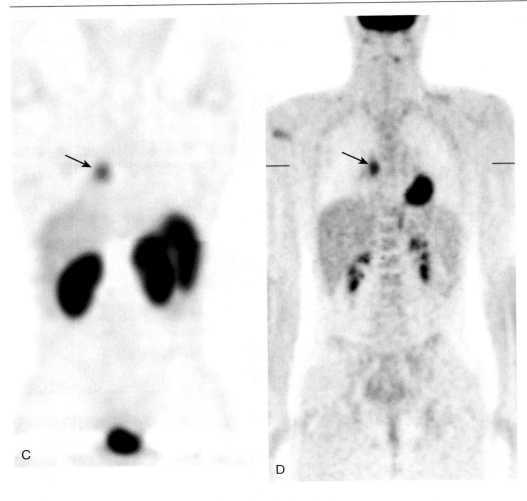

FIGURE 26-27, cont'd. ^{111}In-Octreotide scintigraphy (**C**) and ^{18}F-FDG-PET (**D**) both show accumulation in the mass, and were helpful in staging this patient.

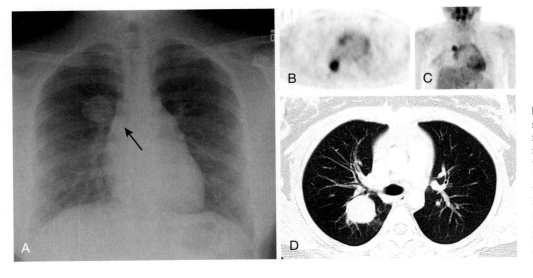

FIGURE 26-28. Mucoepidermoid carcinoma. This chest x-ray for nonspecific upper respiratory infection symptoms showed a right upper lobe mass (**A,** *arrow*). **B, C,** ^{18}F-FDG-PET showed intense uptake and was helpful for staging. **D,** CT scan shows a posterior segment upper lobe mass compressing the posterior segment bronchus, with mild associated air trapping.

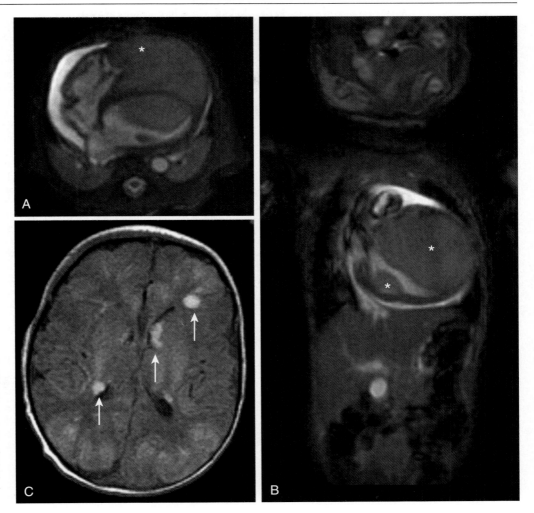

FIGURE 26-29. Cardiac rhabdomyoma in a 5-day-old infant with a large chest mass and tuberous sclerosis. **A, B,** Cardiac MRI scans show multiple rhabdomyomas (*), with the largest obliterating the right ventricle, and multiple smaller tumors in the left ventricle, both adherent to the septum and along the free wall. **C,** Brain MRI scan shows multiple subependymal and cortical tubers (*arrows*).

and inferiorly by the diaphragm. The primary components of the posterior mediastinum are the paravertebral sympathetic ganglia, azygos and hemiazygos veins, descending thoracic aorta, esophagus, and lymph nodes. Most posterior mediastinal masses in children are neurogenic in origin[79,97] and include ganglion cell tumors, nerve sheath tumors, and other nervous tissue neoplasms, such as paragangliomas. Ganglion cell tumors arise from sympathetic chain ganglia, and range from well-differentiated and benign ganglioneuromas to malignant neuroblastomas. Ganglioneuroblastomas contain elements of benign and malignant tissue types. The distinction between these different histologic subtypes cannot be made reliably based on imaging features.

Age at presentation is important in narrowing the differential diagnosis. Neuroblastoma, the most common non-CNS solid tumor in children, typically occurs in young children, with a median age at presentation of younger than 2 years and more than 95% of cases occurring by the age of 10 years. In contrast, the median age at presentation of ganglioneuroblastoma is approximately 5.5 years, whereas mature ganglioneuromas occur in later childhood or early adolescence, typically after the age of 10.[98]

It is important to emphasize that these lesions may be present in an otherwise asymptomatic child, and a thorough inspection of the chest radiograph using multiple windows and levels is necessary to identify small foci of disease. This is of particular importance, as shown in Figure 26-31, because a localized low-stage favorable histology neuroblastoma identi-

fied in a child younger than 1 year may make the difference between low stage disease and the child being treated on low-risk protocols, with higher likelihood of overall and disease-free survival, versus more advanced stages of disease, when the patient's risk of relapse and treatment failure increase.[99] Primary intra-abdominal neuroepithelial tumors may also have a significant posterior mediastinal extent, and often have an associated posterior mediastinal or paravertebral component near the thoracic inlet. Therefore, it may be prudent to include imaging of the chest, in addition to the abdomen and pelvis, in the staging evaluation of patients with suspected neuroblastoma.

Radiographically, ganglion cell tumors appear as paraspinal soft tissue masses. Calcifications may be present. The presence of chest wall invasion or destructive bony changes is more common with neuroblastoma, although benign ganglioneuromas can produce a considerable neural foraminal widening. As with primary adrenal neuroblastomas, staging should include ^{123}I-MIBG scintigraphy. ^{99m}Tc-MDP bone scintigraphy is also commonly performed to identify sites of cortical bone involvement.[66] Although the presence of a paraspinal mass can usually be adequately assessed by CT scanning, particularly with sagittal and coronal reconstructions, the extent of intraspinal extension is better depicted by MRI (Fig. 26-32).[79] MRI also provides a more accurate assessment of chest wall involvement, nerve root compression, and impingement on the spinal cord. The MR imaging of ganglion cell tumors typically reveals a low signal intensity lesion on T1-weighted images and intermediate to high signal intensity on T2-weighted and fast spin-echo

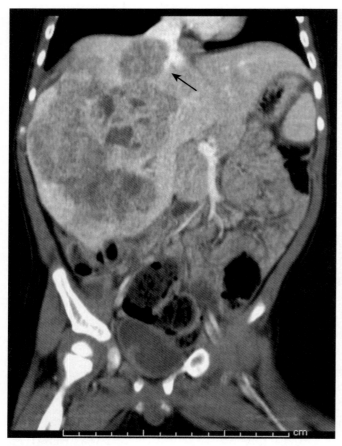

FIGURE 26-30. Coronal contrast-enhanced CT scan showing direct extension into the inferior vena cava (*arrow*) in a 15-month-old infant with hepatoblastoma.

inversion recovery (FSEIR) images, with variable patterns of enhancement. Bone marrow metastases are well demonstrated by MRI, with replacement of normal bone marrow signal by areas of low signal intensity on T1-weighted images and high signal intensity on T2-weighted images. Several studies have suggested MRI may be sufficient to identify sites of bone marrow involvement in neuroblastoma, although this has not yet become common clinical practice.[100,101] The use of FDG-PET in neuroblastoma has received attention as an alternative to conventional imaging techniques,[66,102] but has not yet been shown to offer a clear advantage over MIBG scintigraphy in the staging of patients with thoracic neuroblastoma.

Nerve sheath tumors, including schwannomas and neurofibromas, may be similar in appearance to mature ganglion cell tumors, presenting as relatively sharply marginated, lobulated paraspinal masses. The presence of rib erosions and neural foraminal widening is frequently seen with nerve sheath tumors, although intraspinal extension is less common. Paraspinal paragangliomas are catecholamine-secreting tumors arising from extra-adrenal chromaffin cells present in sympathetic chain ganglia and occur much less frequently than primary ganglion cell or nerve sheath neoplasms. Distinguishing between these tissue types is difficult on the basis of imaging, and surgical resection is the mainstay of therapy. Local recurrence can occur, however, and close imaging follow-up is necessary for these patients.

Chest Wall and Pleural-based Neoplasms

Most of these tumors are of mesenchymal origin and are primary neoplasms arising from the chest wall. They are relatively rare in infants and children, with a reported incidence of approximately 2% of all pediatric tumors.[103]

Ewing's Sarcoma

The most common chest wall neoplasms are the Ewing's sarcoma family of tumors and primitive neuroectodermal tumor

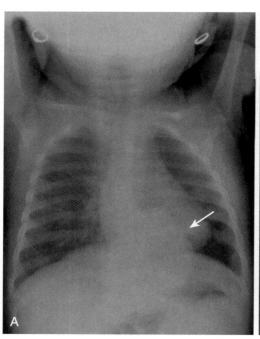

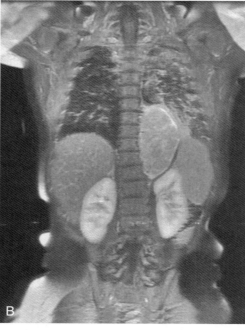

FIGURE 26-31. Posterior mediastinal neuroblastoma in a 5-month-old infant who presented with upper respiratory infection symptoms. A posterior mediastinal mass was identified by chest x-ray **(A)** and MRI **(B)**. Surgery revealed neuroblastoma. Subsequent staging confirmed low-stage disease.

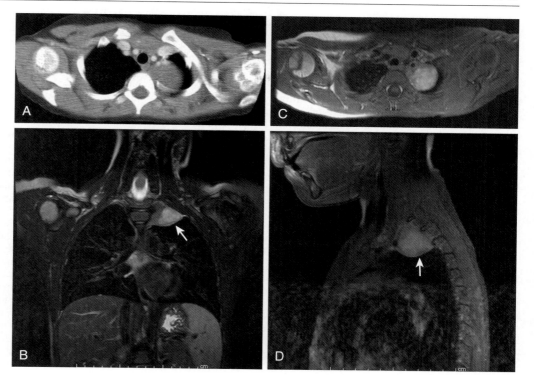

FIGURE 26-32. 7-year-old with cough had chest x-ray showing left upper lobe opacity. **A,** CT scan shows paraspinal mass. MRI scans show the mass to much better advantage (**B-D**). **B,** Coronal spin-echo inversion recovery and post–gadolinium-enhanced images (**C, D**) show the mass abutting the neural foramina and left subclavian vessels (*arrows*). MIBG scanning showed barely detectable uptake in the mature ganglioneuroma.

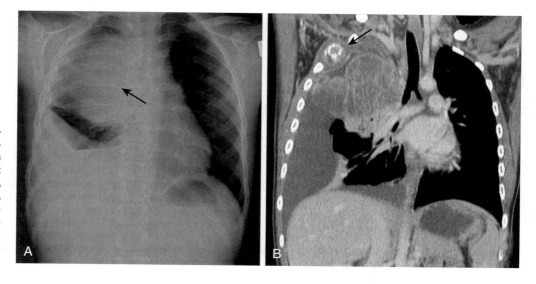

FIGURE 26-33. Ewing's sarcoma of the chest wall in a 6-year-old with fever and chest wall mass detected by chest x-ray. **A,** Chest x-ray shows pleural effusion, central chest wall mass (*arrow*), and partial lung collapse. **B,** Contrast-enhanced CT scan shows large locally invasive chest wall mass, with pleural involvement and rib destruction (*arrow*).

(PNET), collectively known as Askin tumors. These tumors have a peak incidence between 10 and 15 years of age and are more common in males. Because of their origin within the chest wall and propensity to invade the adjacent bone, symptoms are frequently of a palpable mass or pain secondary to local extension. Chest radiography should be the first imaging study in the evaluation of these patients, and is usually accurate at depicting sites of bone destruction, pleural effusion, and pleural thickening. CT scanning and/or MRI are almost always performed to delineate the extent of local disease better. CT scanning of the chest is essential to assess for the presence of pulmonary metastatic disease (Fig. 26-33). For paravertebral and intercostal masses, MRI may also be necessary to identify and accurately delineate the extent of intraspinal involvement. FDG uptake is usually seen with these tumors and, as with Ewing's sarcomas of the appendicular skeleton, FDG-PET scanning should be considered for identifying sites of occult disease that would otherwise go undetected and for monitoring responses to therapy when complete surgical resection cannot be achieved (see Fig. 26-33).[104]

Wide excision of the primary tumor is critical for local disease control, with variable response to radiation therapy and chemotherapy.[105,106] These chest wall neoplasms are extremely malignant and can be destructive, demonstrating extensive invasion into the airways, local vascular structures, and lung parenchyma. There is a high frequency of metastatic spread and local recurrence, and cure requires intensive therapy to control distant and local disease. The presence of disseminated disease invariably results in a poor long-term outcome in patients with these aggressive and poorly responsive tumors.[106]

Rhabdomyosarcoma

Rhabdomyosarcoma is the most common soft tissue sarcoma of childhood, and is the second most common malignancy of the chest wall in children.[105] Occurring in a younger population of children than thoracic Ewing's sarcoma and PNETs, approximately 7% of pediatric rhabdomyosarcomas involve the chest wall and should be included in the differential diagnosis for a chest wall mass in children younger than 10 years. Biopsy is necessary to make the diagnosis, and the imaging features are nonspecific, with considerable overlap between chest wall Ewing's sarcoma and rhabdomyosarcoma. Chest radiographs reveal a large, unilateral chest mass, often with accompanying pleural thickening or effusion. As with Ewing's sarcoma, there may be associated rib destruction changes. Cross-sectional imaging by CT or MRI better delineates the extent of local disease spread. These tumors are heterogeneous in density and attenuation on CT, with variably increased signal on both T1- and T2-weighted MRI scans. Contrast enhancement is heterogeneous, and these features likely reflect varying degrees of tumor necrosis. Tumor size, nodal status, and gross total tumor resection (upfront or delayed) have been significant predictors of event-free and overall survival. Tumors 5 cm or smaller have been shown to be amenable to up-front surgical resection. Tumor size and the ability to achieve gross total resection were the strongest predictors of overall survival, with local recurrence after resection resulting in poor overall outcome.[107,108] As with other malignant sarcomas, FDG-PET has been used effectively for staging and response assessment in patients with rhabdomyosarcoma,[109-111] and should be considered in the imaging evaluation of these patients.

Mesenchymal Hamartoma

Mesenchymal hamartomas of the chest wall are rare benign neoplasms occurring during infancy. The presence of a large chest wall mass, often containing calcifications with associated rib destruction and chest wall deformity, should prompt this diagnosis. Because these lesions may contain a significant necrotic or cystic component, the distinction between Langerhans cell histiocytosis, lymphoma, and metastatic neuroblastoma may be difficult to make. These masses frequently become large, and the radiographic findings are often sufficient to suggest the diagnosis, showing a large calcified extrapleural mass with expansion or destruction of multiple ribs. CT or MRI allows more accurate measure of size, characterization of the soft tissue component of the lesion, and mass effect on the lung and adjacent structures.[112] In particular, the presence of hemorrhagic cystic components has been described as charac-

teristic of these benign neoplasms.[112] There is some evidence to suggest that spontaneous resolution of these masses may also occur, although the extent of local invasion and tissue destruction may prompt surgical resection, which if complete, is usually curative. The importance of the imaging evaluation is to suggest this diagnosis to guide appropriate management of these benign lesions.

Pulmonary Metastases

Metastatic disease to the lung represents the most common pulmonary neoplasm encountered in childhood. The lung is a common site for metastatic disease spread, but is an uncommon site in childhood for primary malignancy.

Extrathoracic pediatric tumors that are frequently associated with pulmonary metastases include Wilms' tumor, rhabdomyosarcoma, hepatoblastoma, Ewing's sarcoma, and osteosarcoma. Neuroblastoma does not typically result in hematogenously spread pulmonary metastases, although in its disseminated form, pulmonary metastases may be seen.

The imaging evaluation in a patient with a known primary malignancy with a propensity to metastasize to the lung should include chest CT. CT is more sensitive than conventional radiography for detecting pulmonary metastatic disease, although the increased sensitivity of nodule detection has led to difficulty in distinguishing benign lesions from malignant pulmonary nodules (Fig. 26-34).[17,113] Once the staging evaluation has been completed and the absence of pulmonary metastatic disease and other sites of metastatic disease have been established, it may be reasonable to proceed with routine chest radiographs for subsequent follow-up, reserving CT for patients with suspected relapse or at high risk for relapse. In particular, in osteosarcoma, which has a high frequency of developing pulmonary metastases and for whom resection of these metastases may be curative, routine follow-up chest CT scanning is justifiable.

It is often difficult, particularly with small pulmonary nodules, to distinguish benign causes from malignancy.[17] Calcification within a pulmonary nodule is usually associated with benign causes (except in the case of osteosarcoma); however, there are no specific imaging findings that can be used to make this distinction reliably. Benign pulmonary nodules may result from postinflammatory change or represent small benign intrapulmonary lymph nodes. Short-interval follow-up and documentation of stability in areas of low suspicion are usually adequate to confirm the benign nature of these findings. For more suspicious or enlarging lesions, biopsy or surgical resection is necessary to arrive at a definitive diagnosis. The use of FDG-PET scanning has been advocated in an attempt to distinguish benign from malignant causes of pulmonary metastatic disease,[114] although CT scanning can accurately identify lesions

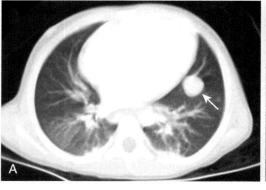
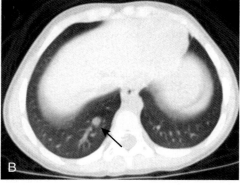

FIGURE 26-34. 2½-year-old child with metastatic Wilms' tumor. **A,** The nodule at the left lung base (*arrow*) at diagnosis was resected and found to be metastatic disease. **B,** The nodule at the right lung base (*arrow*) discovered 1 year later was resected and found to be a pulmonary hamartoma.

of only 1 to 2 mm in size, whereas even the newest generation PET scanners still have lower limits of resolution on the order of 5 mm to 1 cm.

Controversy still exists as to the significance of pulmonary nodules detected by chest CT in patients with Wilms' tumor.[115-117] There are still conflicting data about the importance of pulmonary nodules not visualized by chest radiography, but detectable by chest CT, in predicting relapse-free and overall survival in patients with Wilms' tumor. Nonetheless, it has been shown that the sensitivity of malignant nodule detection is enhanced by CT[115,116] and current treatment protocols routinely advocate the use of chest CT for staging these patients. In an effort to develop a better understanding of CT features that might distinguish benign from malignant pulmonary nodules,[115] current Children's Oncology Group Wilms' tumor protocols call for surgical resection or biopsy of persistent suspicious lung nodules detected by CT in intermediate- and high-risk patients.

CT scanning of the chest for identifying pulmonary metastatic disease need not include intravenous contrast, and the presence of hyperdense contrast material may confound the interpretation of a subtle parenchymal nodules. In addition, the newer generation multidetector row CT scanners allow the acquisition imaging data to be reviewed in 1-mm thick increments or less, as well as in sagittal and coronal planes. This allows the radiologist to make an accurate judgment about the presence or absence of a suspicious pulmonary nodule, and distinguish it from branching vessels. In addition, there is no evidence to suggest that additional high-resolution CT (HRCT) imaging, which is performed using a different image acquisition technique, provides any additional benefit or higher resolution over the approximately 1-mm thick slices obtained during the multidetector helical acquisition.[118]

Although the imaging features of small pulmonary nodules may be nonspecific and the difficulty in distinguishing benign from non-neoplastic causes may be frustrating, the presence and persistence of lung nodules in a child with a solid tumor that has a propensity to metastasize to the lung is usually indicative of metastatic disease. The use of CT for detecting these sites of disease spread is an essential component of the staging of most pediatric solid tumors.

GASTROINTESTINAL TUMORS

Tumors of the gastrointestinal tract, including the visceral abdominal organs, are relatively uncommon in childhood. In neonates, most intra-abdominal masses are nonmalignant. Children frequently present with nonspecific complaints such as abdominal pain, weight loss, or failure to thrive. The imaging evaluation should begin with abdominal radiography. These often provide valuable initial information, such as the presence of calcifications, mass effect on adjacent visceral organs, and the presence of bowel obstruction or perforation. Abdominal ultrasound is frequently used to gain further information about a suspicious mass. Doppler assessment may help distinguish cystic from solid masses and delineate patterns of blood flow in and around a tumor. These initial imaging studies are usually sufficient to narrow the initial differential diagnosis and to guide the subsequent imaging evaluation by CT, MRI, and/or PET.

Liver Tumors

Although rare in infants and young children, tumors of the hepatobiliary system are the most common of the gastrointes-

tinal tract tumors seen in childhood.[119-121] Usually, a combination of diagnostic studies is obtained, including imaging findings, clinical findings, and serum markers, to arrive at a definitive diagnosis. Benign and malignant tumors may be encountered.

Hepatoblastoma

Hepatoblastoma is the most common primary malignant tumor in children younger than 5 years.[121] Hepatoblastoma is usually encountered in infants and young children younger than 3 years, with an average age of presentation at 16 months. At diagnosis the mass is typically large (greater than 10 cm).

Metastatic disease is encountered in approximately 20% of patients, with pulmonary metastases most common. The imaging evaluation should be directed at determining surgical resectability, establishing sites of metastatic disease, and monitoring response to chemotherapy. More than 90% of children have elevated α-fetoprotein (AFP) levels at diagnosis; the presence of metastatic disease, high AFP levels, and high-stage pretreatment extent of liver involvement by tumor are all associated with poor outcome.[122-124] Surgical resection alone is insufficient to achieve cure in most cases, and the combination of surgery and chemotherapy has resulted in 5-year overall survival rates of over 70%.[124]

Abdominal radiographs typically show an abdominal mass. Calcifications may be present and pulmonary masses are often visible at the time of diagnosis at the lung bases (Fig. 26-35). Ultrasound should be the initial imaging test in a child with an abdominal mass, and reveals a large echogenic intrahepatic mass. It may be difficult with very large masses to define a margin between the hepatoblastoma and normal hepatic parenchyma (see Fig. 26-35). Hypoechoic areas may relate to necrosis or hemorrhage. Color Doppler imaging and pulsed wave Doppler should be used routinely to assess for intravascular extension of tumor,[121,123] IVC invasion, and portal vein thrombosis, which may affect eligibility for liver transplantation.[125]

CT and/or MRI are important for better definition of the relationship of the intrahepatic mass to adjacent vascular structures and adjacent organs, and to determine the extent of hepatic involvement and surgical respectability.[123] This is best accomplished with biphasic or angiographic techniques; imaging should include scanning after early arterial and portal venous phases of contrast of opacification, because small satellite lesions may only be visible on early arterial phase imaging (see Fig. 26-2).[126] Typically, hepatoblastomas show a heterogeneous pattern of enhancement. Multiplanar reconstructions are also crucial in aiding surgical planning and better delineating invasion into adjacent vascular structures (i.e., IVC invasion, portal venous thrombosis). MR imaging typically shows heterogeneously T2 hyperintense lesions with variable patterns of enhancement following gadolinium contrast administration (Fig. 26-36). MRI may be of particular value in delineating subtle lesions that are inconspicuous on contrast-enhanced CT scanning.

The pretreatment extent of disease (PRETEXT) staging system was developed by the International Liver Tumor Strategy Group (SIOPEL) in an effort to develop a pretreatment imaging-based measure of disease burden and surgical resectability as a basis for staging and risk stratification of children with hepatoblastoma.[123] In the PRETEXT system of staging, the liver is divided into sections, based in part on Couinaud's system of segmental anatomy. PRETEXT staging is based on the number of adjacent liver sections involved with tumor (Box 26-1) and has been shown to be effective in predicting resectability and overall survival in patients who complete neoadjuvant chemotherapy.[127] Because the PRETEXT staging system relies almost entirely on the pretreatment imaging assessment,

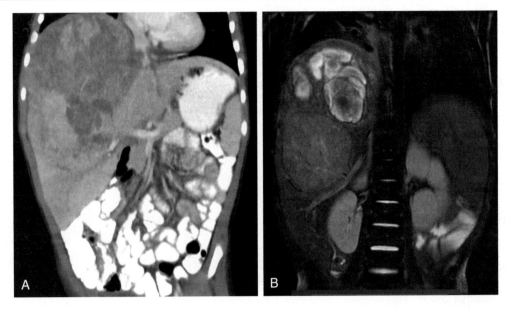

FIGURE 26-36. 3-year-old with hepatoblastoma, showing superiority of MRI scanning (**B**) for detecting the extent of liver involvement and relationship to adjacent structures, as compared with CT (**A**).

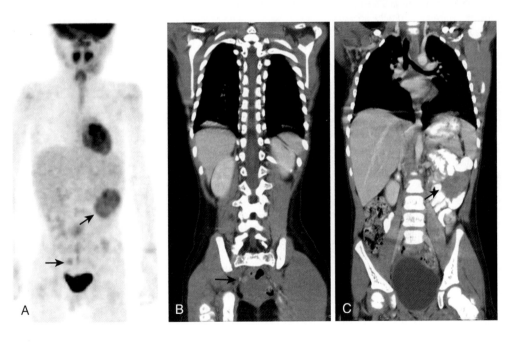

FIGURE 26-37. 5-year-old girl with metastatic hepatoblastoma, postresection, and in remission, with new rising α-fetoprotein levels. **A,** ^{18}F-FDG-PET scan shows two foci of uptake (*arrows*), corresponding to soft tissue masses on CT in the mesentery (**B**) and deep pelvis (**C**) (*arrows*). Surgery confirmed metastatic disease.

nation is often the first imaging study performed. Multiphase CT scanning with multiplanar reconstruction affords the greatest likelihood of detecting subtle lesions and in assessing relationships to adjacent structures and the vasculature.[120,126] The CT appearance of HCC depends on tumor size and phase of contrast administration. Lesions are typically isointense or mildly hypointense relative to liver and hyperattenuating on early arterial phase scanning, becoming isointense during later venous phases of imaging. Early arterial phase, portal venous phase, and delayed equilibration venous phase images have all been shown to contribute to enhancing lesion conspicuity, providing the greatest sensitivity and specificity for lesion detection.[130] MRI imaging may be of value in distinguishing hepatocellular carcinoma from benign liver lesions such as hepatic adenoma,[121] but biopsy is usually necessary to confirm the diagnosis (Fig. 26-38). Gadolinium-enhanced MRI, like CT, shows hyperenhancing lesions during early arterial phase imaging, with larger tumors showing variable signal intensity

and patterns of enhancement.[131] Superparamagnetic iron oxide particles, which are taken up by Kupffer cells present in normal liver and in focal nodular hyperplasia (FNH), have been used to help differentiate HCC, which contains few if any Kupffer cells, from benign liver masses and to enhance lesion conspicuity relative to the surrounding liver tissue.[131]

The fibrolamellar form of hepatocellular carcinoma occurs in adolescents and has distinctive imaging features, showing a central scar and often associated with calcification (Fig. 26-39). Fibrolamellar HCC is not associated with elevated AFP and overall survival is higher than hepatocellular carcinoma, in part because of its presentation as a solitary localized mass amenable to complete surgical resection.[132] Ultrasound reveals a hypoechoic mass, often with a focal central hyperechoic scar. After the initial characterization by ultrasound, CT or MRI is indicated for further staging. On CT, fibrolamellar HCC is usually a relatively low-attenuation, well-circumscribed mass with heterogeneous enhancement, initially becoming hyper-

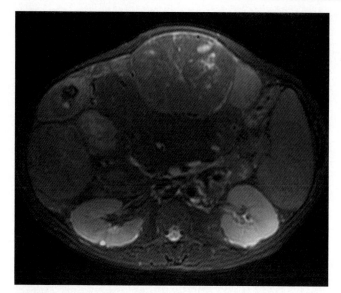

FIGURE 26-38. Hepatocellular carcinoma. Contrast-enhanced abdominal MRI scan in a teenage patient with type 1 glycogen storage disease, showing multiple adenomas and a large heterogeneously enhancing central mass that had enlarged since prior scans and was found on resection to be hepatocellular carcinoma.

intense relative to the surrounding liver parenchyma and ultimately becoming isointense to the liver during the equilibration phase of scanning. A nonenhancing central scar is seen in most cases (see Fig. 26-39)[133] on MRI lesions, are isointense to hypointense relative to the liver on T1-weighted images, and isointense to hyperintense on T2-weighted sequences. The pattern on gadolinium enhancement is similar to that observed by CT, with lesions becoming hyperintense early after contrast infusion and ultimately isointense to liver on delayed scanning. The distinction between fibrolamellar hepatocellular carcinoma and focal nodular hyperplasia, both of which have similar imaging characteristics and patterns of enhancement, may be difficult to make although, as shown in Figure 26-40, the uptake of iron oxide particles by the lesion is almost diagnostic of focal nodular hyperplasia.

Embryonal Sarcoma (Hepatic Mesenchymoma)

Embryonal sarcoma of the liver is the fourth most common hepatic neoplasm in children, after hepatoblastoma, hepatocellular carcinoma, and infantile hepatic hemangioma. These tumors are highly malignant, usually present in later childhood (between the ages of 6 and 10 years) and are typically accompanied by symptoms of abdominal pain and an abdominal mass. Embryonal sarcomas may be difficult to distinguish from mesenchymal hamartoma, although the latter tumors are more commonly diagnosed before the age of 2 years. At presentation, embryonal sarcomas are often large and contain cystic and solid areas, with areas of necrosis. Ultrasound reveals a heterogeneous echogenic mass, with many features overlapping with mesenchymal hamartoma and infantile hepatic hemangioma. Calcifications are rare. CT reveals a large hypodense mass, often with septations and areas of internal high attenuation. MRI shows a high signal intensity lesion on T2-weighted images (Fig. 26-41), with predominantly low signal on T1-weighted images. Following contrast enhancement, imaging by CT or MRI demonstrates peripheral enhancement and central areas of heterogeneous signal intensity that likely reflect solid tumor elements, cystic spaces, necrosis, and foci of hemorrhage.[134]

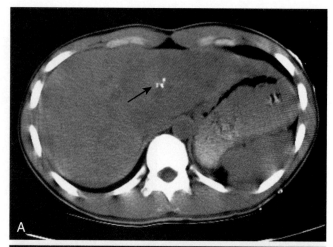

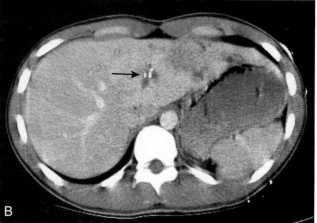

FIGURE 26-39. 16-year-old with fibrolamellar hepatocellular carcinoma. Unenhanced (A) and contrast-enhanced (B) CT scans show the calcifications and poorly enhancing central scar (*arrows*) typical of this form of hepatocellular carcinoma.

Despite their being highly malignant, complete surgical resection and adjuvant chemotherapy can be curative in most of these patients.[122,135]

Mesenchymal Hamartoma

Mesenchymal hamartoma, in contrast to hepatoblastoma, is a predominantly cystic mass most often occurring in infants younger than 2 years. It commonly presents as a painless, palpable abdominal mass comprised of mesenchymal tissue, bile ducts, hepatocytes, and hematopoietic cells. In contrast to hepatoblastoma, which is the primary differential consideration in an infant, the AFP levels are normal. On imaging, radiographs reveal a large right upper quadrant mass. Calcifications, which are seen in hepatoblastoma, are unusual in mesenchymal hamartoma.[121] Ultrasound examination typically shows a complex, predominantly cystic mass. MRI and CT may be of value in further characterizing the lesion and typically show large multilocular cystic masses with septations. Only minimal enhancement is seen. Some of the masses may have a predominantly solid component imparting a so-called Swiss cheese appearance to the mass and contributing to some difficulty in the differential diagnosis. MRI may also demonstrate the complex nature of the cystic fluid, with gelatinous, more complex fluids showing high signal on T1-weighted images

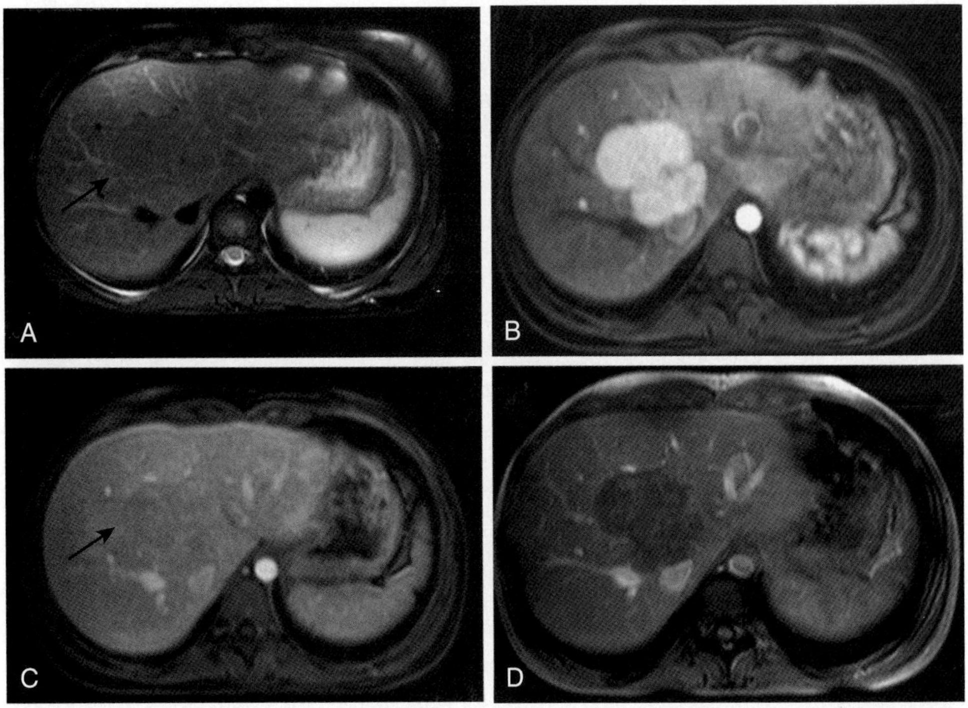

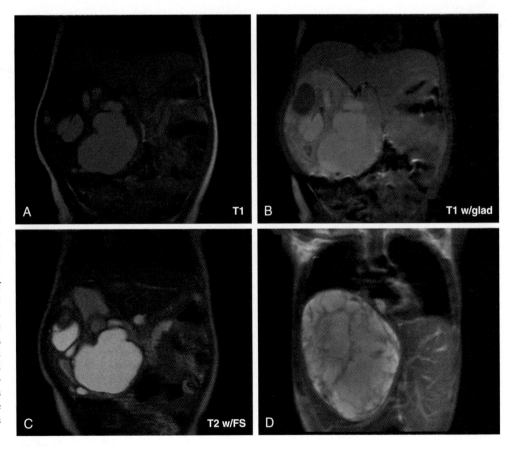

FIGURE 26-40. Patient with suspected focal nodular hyperplasia (FNH). **A,** T2-weighted MRI scan shows an almost inconspicuous lesion, with bright early enhancement following dynamic contrast administration **(B)**, becoming isointense to liver on delayed postcontrast imaging (*arrow,* **C**). **D,** The infusion of iron oxide nanoparticles (Reovist) shows signal loss in the lesion, compatible with iron uptake by reticuloendothelial cells in the lesion and highly suggestive of FNH, rather than hepatocellular carcinoma. (Images courtesy of Dr. Peter Ngo.)

FIGURE 26-41. Mesenchymal hamartoma. These MRI scans show the complex nature of the multiple cysts in a 13-month-old infant with mesenchymal hamartoma. Note the importance of obtaining T1-weighted images prior to contrast administration **(A)**, in addition to fluid-sensitive T2-weighted sequences **(C)**, because areas of complex fluid may be T1 bright **(A)** and should not be misinterpreted as enhancing solid components of the mass **(B)**. Note the similarity to the large embryonal sarcoma shown in **D**.

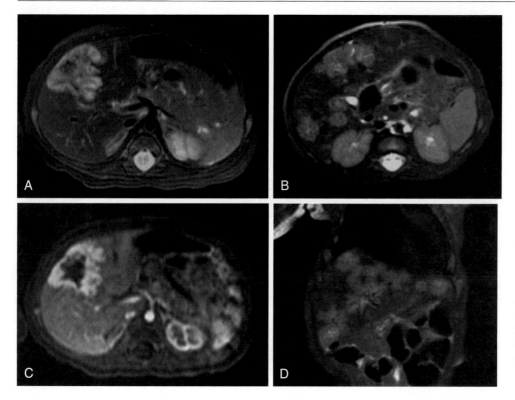

FIGURE 26-42. Involuting hepatic hemangioma and diffuse infantile hemangioma. Fat-suppressed T2-weighted **(A, B)** and post–gadolinium-enhanced **(C, D)** MRI scans showing large, solitary, peripherally enhancing lesion typical of involuting hepatic hemangioma **(A, C)** and the multifocal hepatic involvement in a patient with hypothyroidism and diffuse infantile hemangioma **(B, D)**.

versus the more common T2 bright or T1 dark serous fluid contained in most of the cysts (see Fig. 26-41). Treatment is surgical resection and recurrence is uncommon.[122]

Infantile Hepatic Hemangioma

Infantile hepatic hemangioma is a proliferative endothelial cell neoplasm that may be solitary or diffusely involve the liver. Infantile hepatic hemangiomas have characteristic phases of cellular proliferation followed by spontaneous involution. They are often referred to as hepatic hemangioendothelioma, creating some confusion in nomenclature, and must be distinguished from epithelioid hemangioendothelioma.[136] The latter is a proliferative tumor with malignant potential that does not involute, in contrast to the benign hepatic hemangioma. Infantile hepatic hemangiomas share the same growth characteristics as the more common cutaneous infantile hemangiomas. Most present by 6 months of age and about half are associated with cutaneous lesions. Most of the infantile hepatic hemangiomas involute spontaneously, and adverse outcomes are only observed when there is massive hepatic involvement and arteriovenous (AV) shunting, with accompanying high-output cardiac failure. The presence of extensive hepatic involvement and near-complete replacement of the liver parenchyma occurs in the diffuse infantile hemangioma variant, and is associated with profound hypothyroidism secondary to overproduction of type III iodothyronine deiodinase.[137]

Ultrasound is usually the first step in the evaluation and typically shows focal or multiple hepatic masses with heterogeneous echotexture. With large focal lesions it may be possible to identify a large draining varix or varices. Both arterial and venous waveforms are frequently detected and calcifications may be present. More characteristic findings are seen on CT and MRI. MRI typically shows homogeneously hypointense lesions on T1-weighted imaging, with heterogeneous hyperintense masses on T2-weighted images. Following contrast enhancement, imaging by CT or MRI reveals a typical pattern of peripheral contrast enhancement, with gradual filling in centrally (centripetal enhancement; Fig. 26-42).[138] Diffuse infantile hepatic hemangiomas may almost completely occupy the entire liver parenchyma (Fig. 26-43) and the associated hypothyroidism is caused by the elaboration of deiodinase enzymes affecting thyroid hormone synthesis, which can result in cardiac failure and neurologic impairment. These endocrinologic findings may be important in securing the diagnosis, because the multiple hepatic masses may share overlapping imaging features with malignant hepatic lesions, such as hepatoblastoma or metastatic neuroblastoma.

High-output cardiac failure associated with large varices and significant high-volume AV shunting can be effectively treated using interventional radiologic techniques, including coil and particle embolization. This may be essential for stabilizing the patient to initiate treatment to accelerate the involution of these benign proliferative lesions.[136]

Hepatic Adenoma

Other benign hepatic lesions include solitary hepatic adenoma. Hepatic adenomas are unusual in children in the absence of a predisposing condition, such as glycogen storage disease, galactosemia, or tyrosinemia. The imaging features of hepatic adenomas are not specific and imaging is usually directed at following these lesions for increases in size and number. Rapid increase in size is generally considered to be an indication of degeneration of benign adenoma to hepatocellular carcinoma, particularly in patients with glycogen storage disease.[139] Regular surveillance, typically by ultrasound, is indicated for these patients. MRI may be of additional value in distinguishing or characterizing new or multiple lesions.

Focal Nodular Hyperplasia

Focal nodular hyperplasia is rare in children, most commonly occurring in the teenage and adolescent years.[140] It is usually

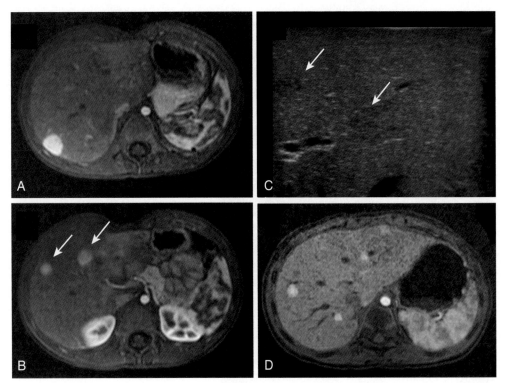

FIGURE 26-43. 19-month-old boy with history of treatment for stage 4 neuroblastoma. **A, B,** Follow-up MR imaging using dynamic contrast enhancement shows multiple brightly enhancing lesions throughout the liver. These rapidly become isointense to the liver during delayed scanning. They are not seen on any other sequences. The enhancement characteristics are typical of focal nodular hyperplasia (FNH). **C,** Intraoperative ultrasound localized lesions for biopsy, and confirmed as FNH. **D,** Similar lesions in a 2-year-old patient treated in infancy for stage 4 neuroblastoma.

found incidentally during imaging evaluation for other reasons. This benign lesion typically shows a central fibrous scar, with surrounding hyperplastic hepatocytes and small bile ducts. As noted earlier, these imaging features are also seen in the fibrolamellar variant of hepatocellular carcinoma, and the distinction between FNH and fibrolamellar carcinoma may be difficult. CT and MRI scans usually show rapid homogeneous early contrast enhancement during early arterial phase imaging (see Fig. 26-40). Lesions then typically become isodense to the liver during later phases of enhancement, with the central scar remaining hypodense, even during the delayed imaging period. This pattern of enhancement is considered diagnostic. Newer MR imaging techniques performed with iron oxide particle contrast agents, which accumulate in reticuloendothelial cells (Kupffer cells) present in the hyperplastic FNH lesions, show a characteristic pattern of decreased signal intensity on T2-weighted imaging (see Fig. 26-40). This, together with the early pattern of rapid gadolinium enhancement, is diagnostic of focal nodular hyperplasia.[140] These masses may be followed by ultrasound to ensure stability and do not typically require surgical resection unless they become symptomatic or undergo progressive enlargement. FNH has also been observed in patients who have completed therapy for nonhepatic primary tumors.[141,142] Although larger masses may be detected by ultrasound or CT, we have found that dynamic contrast-enhanced MRI is a highly sensitive technique for identifying these lesions. Occasionally, these lesions can be characterized by ultrasound using high-resolution high-frequency transducers, but they are unequivocally shown by contrast-enhanced MRI (see Fig. 26-43). These FNH lesions are typically isointense to the liver on conventional imaging sequences and display rapid early arterial enhancement, after which they become almost isointense to the liver and indistinguishable from the surrounding parenchyma. It is important to recognize this pattern of enhancement so as to not mistake this benign entity with recurrent disease or a new site of disease relapse.

Other lesions occurring in the liver include sarcomatous tumors, such as malignant angiosarcoma and rhabdomyosarcoma of the biliary tree, malignant vascular tumors, and metastatic disease. The most common metastatic lesions occurring in the liver include neuroblastoma, locally invasive and hematogenously disseminated Wilms' tumor, rhabdomyosarcoma, and Ewing's sarcoma.[121] The imaging characteristics of the metastatic hepatic lesions are typically nonspecific, with lesions characteristically hypoechoic on ultrasound relative to normal liver parenchyma, decreased attenuation on CT scan, low T1 and increased T2 signal intensity on T1- and T2-weighted MR images, respectively, and variable patterns of contrast enhancement with CT and MRI.

Spleen Tumors

Primary tumors of the spleen are exceedingly rare.[143] Angiosarcomas have been reported, but are not common in childhood. Involvement of the spleen by lymphoma and lymphoproliferative disease is the most common cause of malignant infiltration of the spleen.[144] Imaging evaluation by ultrasound will frequently demonstrate multiple or solitary hypoechoic masses (Fig. 26-44). CT scanning may be equivocal because of the variable phases of splenic parenchymal enhancement. MRI, in contrast, may be very sensitive at detecting focal lesions that are not detectable by CT and/or ultrasound. In the setting of lymphoma and lymphoproliferative disease, FDG-PET imaging has been shown to be an effective adjunctive imaging modality for detecting splenic involvement.[145] This is of importance for determining the patient's stage of disease at diagnosis and identifying sites of disease to be followed and assessed for response following treatment. In addition, the negative predictive value of FDG-PET in discriminating between benign and malignant lesions has been emphasized in patients with coexistent malignant disease and in those without a history of malignancy in

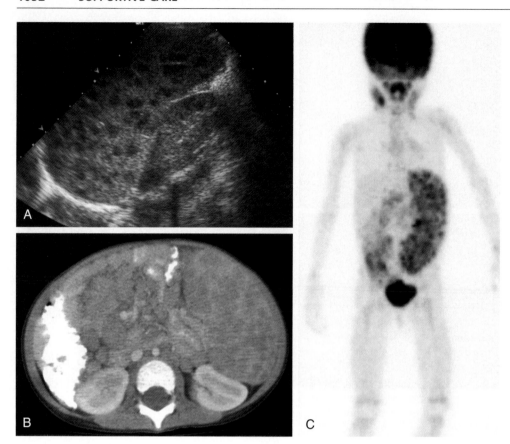

FIGURE 26-44. Lymphoproliferative disease. Ultrasound **(A)** and CT **(B)** demonstrate extensive splenic involvement and massive adenopathy in a patient with an unclassified lymphoproliferative disease. **C,** ^{18}F-FDG-PET shows multiple sites of disease and in particular confirms the extensive abnormalities in the spleen.

whom a solid splenic mass is identified by other imaging techniques.[146]

Biliary Tract Tumors

Tumors of the gallbladder and bile ducts are rare in children; these include biliary rhabdomyosarcoma and cholangiocarcinoma, with the latter occurring in the setting of chronic ulcerative colitis. The initial imaging evaluation is usually by ultrasound, frequently for symptoms of biliary tract obstruction, such as pain, jaundice, and weight loss. Ultrasound may show evidence of bile duct dilation and biliary tract obstruction, but identification of a focal mass usually requires additional evaluation by MRI or magnetic resonance cholangiopancreatography (MRCP), with diagnostic confirmation by endoscopic retrograde cholangiopancreatography (ERCP). Particularly in the setting of rhabdomyosarcoma, FDG-PET imaging may be of value in accurately determining the stage of disease. Biliary rhabdomyosarcoma can arise from the intrahepatic or extrahepatic biliary bile ducts, gallbladder, cystic duct, or ampulla of Vater. At the time of presentation with obstructive jaundice and abdominal pain, these neoplasms are usually large and, as a result, the distinction between biliary rhabdomyosarcoma, primary hepatic tumors arising in the hepatic hilum, pancreatic neoplasms, and renal/suprarenal masses may be challenging (Fig. 26-45).[147]

Pancreatic Tumors

Primary tumors of the pancreas are rare in children, in contrast to adults. In addition, the types of tumors found in children differ from the adult tumors, in which adenocarcinomas predominate. Pancreatic tumors can be classified into nonfunctional tumors of the exocrine pancreas and functional tumors of the endocrine pancreas, as well as secondary metastatic pancreatic neoplasia.

Malignant epithelial neoplasms arising from the exocrine pancreas include pancreatoblastoma and solid papillary epithelial neoplasms of the pancreas. Primary nonepithelial tumors of the pancreas are rare and include lymphoma, rhabdomyosarcoma, and primitive neuroectodermal tumors. Pancreatic endocrine neoplasms are rare in children and are usually associated with the MEN syndrome. These include hormonally active tumors such as insulinoma, gastrinoma, VIPoma, and glucagonoma.

Pancreatoblastoma

Pancreatoblastoma can occur at any age but is most common in children between the ages of 1 and 8 years. Pancreatoblastomas are reported as arising in or around the head of the pancreas in roughly half of cases. Because they are nonfunctional, they are typically large at the time of diagnosis. Presenting symptoms include abdominal pain, nausea, and weight loss. Obstructive symptoms, such as jaundice or pancreatitis, are less common, despite the large size of these masses, which has been attributed to their soft, gelatinous, and compliant consistency.[148] These tumors are usually well encapsulated and have heterogeneous patterns of echogenicity on ultrasound and variable patterns of contrast enhancement on CT (Fig. 26-46). Calcifications are commonly seen and are probably the sequelae of hemorrhage and necrosis known to occur within these tumors. MRI shows a similar pattern of heterogeneous signal intensity and enhancement, with masses usually hypointense on T1-weighted images and variably hyperintense on T2-weighted and post–gadolinium-enhanced images. As with hepatoblastoma,

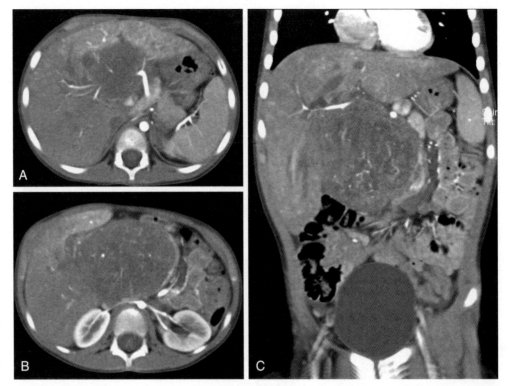

FIGURE 26-45. Biliary rhabdomyosarcoma. Dynamic contrast-enhanced CT scans with axial (**A, B**) and coronal (**C**) reconstructions reveal a large mass in the hepatic hilum, encasing the vessels and infiltrating adjacent structures. Note the lack of significant bile duct dilation, allowing the mass to become very large before producing symptoms of obstructive jaundice.

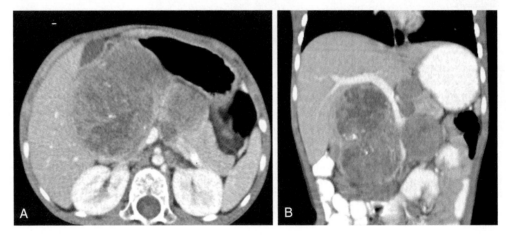

FIGURE 26-46. Pancreatoblastoma in a 4-year-old boy with a palpable abdominal mass. **A, B,** Contrast-enhanced axial (**A**) and coronal (**B**) CT shows large, calcified retroperitoneal mass centered in the pancreas. Both adrenal glands were normal. Lung metastases were also present (not shown). Biopsy showed pancreatoblastoma.

pulmonary metastatic disease is often present, and the staging evaluation must include CT of the chest. Because of their large size, the tissue of origin may be difficult to delineate clearly, and differential considerations will include exophytic hepatoblastoma, renal and suprarenal masses, and retroperitoneal neoplasms.[149]

Solid Pseudopapillary Neoplasm

Solid pseudopapillary neoplasm of the pancreas (also known, among other terms, as solid and papillary epithelial neoplasm[150]) is a rare primary pediatric pancreatic tumor. In contrast to other pancreatic tumors occurring in children, however, the prognosis after complete surgical resection is favorable.[151] Studies have reported up to a 90% survival rate following complete resection. In one small study, median age at presentation was 13 years, with abdominal pain, a palpable mass, dyspepsia, and pancreatitis being the most common presenting symp-

toms.[151] On imaging, usually by ultrasound and/or CT, solid pseudopapillary tumors appear as solid, well-demarcated masses. On ultrasound, there is heterogeneous echotexture, occasionally with fluid-filled cystic spaces (Fig. 26-47). CT shows a heterogeneous mass with peripheral contrast enhancement. Although these are slow-growing tumors with low-grade malignant behavior, FDG uptake on PET imaging has been shown in solid papillary tumors of the pancreas.[152] FDG-PET scanning may therefore be of value in follow-up imaging to assess for recurrence. Despite high rates of overall 5-year survival, if metastases are present and not resectable, survival is poor, with no clear beneficial role reported for adjuvant, chemo-, or radiation therapy.[150]

Pancreatic Sarcomas

Mesenchymal tumors of the pancreas include rare synovial cell sarcomas, myofibroblastic tumors, and metastatic rhabdomyo-

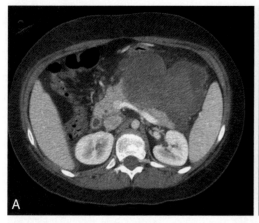

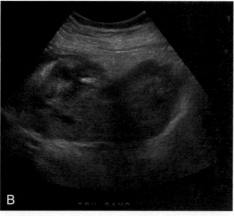

FIGURE 26-47. Pseudopapillary pancreatic tumor. 9-year-old with hypertension and increased abdominal girth. Ultrasound **(B)** shows a lobulated solid mass that could not be distinguished from the pancreas. CT **(A)** shows a low attenuation, heterogeneously enhancing lobulated mass arising from the pancreatic body and tail, abutting the greater curvature of the stomach (not shown).

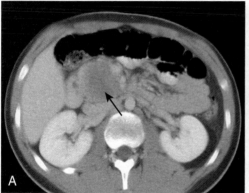

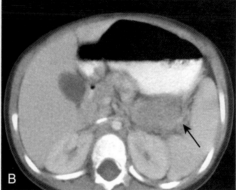

FIGURE 26-48. CT scanning shows rhabdomyosarcoma that metastasized to the pancreas (*arrows*) in two patients with extremity rhabdomyosarcoma. **A,** Patient had symptoms of pain. **B,** Patient had no abdominal symptoms and the lesion was detected by FDG-PET during routine surveillance.

sarcoma. Extremity rhabdomyosarcomas seem to have an unusual predilection for metastases to unusual sites such as the breast, ovary, testicle, and pancreas.[153] Two patients, shown in Figure 26-48, presented with metastatic rhabdomyosarcoma to the pancreas. Local presentation may include pancreatitis and abdominal pain, or may be incidental (see Fig. 26-48B). This emphasizes the importance of follow-up imaging in these patients and suggests an increasing role for FDG-PET scanning to identify unusual sites of metastatic spread in patients with rhabdomyosarcoma.

Pancreatic Lymphoma

Burkitt's lymphoma is well known to involve organs of the gastrointestinal tract, although isolated pancreatic involvement is unusual. Typically. pancreatic involvement will be accompanied by other sites of visceral and mesenteric disease. Diffuse pancreatic infiltration in the setting of Burkitt's lymphoma is shown in Figure 26-49 in a child who presented with symptoms of pancreatitis. On ultrasound, the pancreas was diffusely enlarged and heterogeneous in echogenicity. CT scan showed diffuse pancreatic enlargement, poor enhancement, and a homogeneous low attenuation. As is typical for the rapidly dividing Burkitt's lymphoma, a rapid response to chemotherapy was observed, with near-complete resolution of pancreatic abnormalities 10 days after onset of chemotherapy.

Pancreatic Islet Cell Tumor

Functioning islet cell tumors of the pancreas are rare but important clinically because of symptomatic endocrine abnor-

malities that result from constitutive secretion of hormones, which are normally tightly regulated by the endocrine pancreas. As shown in Figure 26-50, in which the patient presented with symptomatic hyperinsulinemic hypoglycemia, these tumors are often small and may be difficult to diagnose and characterize. As with other neuroendocrine neoplasms, optimal scanning techniques for detection of pancreatic islet cell tumors include early arterial phase scanning as part of a multiphase imaging technique. Thin sections (approximately 1 mm) are now routinely acquired by most multidetector row CT scanners and the evaluation should include a careful review of sagittal and coronal reconstructed images. Although there are no controlled studies comparing CT and MRI for evaluating these tumors, a well-administered MRI examination, with respiratory triggering or breath-holding, fast-gradient echo imaging, and dynamic contrast administration, is likely to yield comparable if not superior results to CT. These small lesions are often difficult to see by conventional ultrasound, but intraoperative ultrasound is invaluable in localizing small, nonpalpable lesions (see Fig. 26-50B).

Alimentary Tract Tumors

Tumors of the gastrointestinal tract, including esophagus, stomach, and large and small bowels are rare in children. In the stomach, lymphoma, leiomyoma, lyomyosarcoma and adenocarcinoma are all rare, as compared with adults. Gastrointestinal stromal tumors (GISTs) also have a low incidence in the pediatric population but, during the last decade, these tumors have attracted increased attention because of

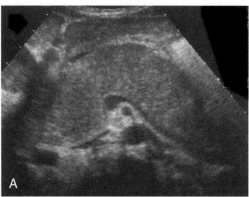

FIGURE 26-49. Burkitt's lymphoma of the pancreas in an 8-year-old patient who presented with pancreatitis. Ultrasound showed diffuse pancreatic infiltration (**A**), confirmed by CT (**B**), with disease limited to the pancreas. Ten days after initiating chemotherapy, the pancreas appeared normal (**C**), typical of the rapid responses observed with Burkitt's lymphoma.

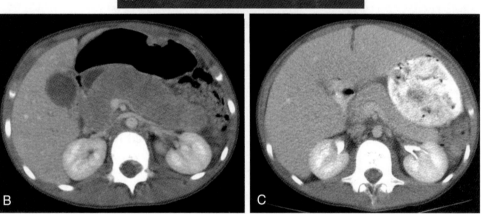

FIGURE 26-50. Pancreatic islet cell tumor. This patient had profound hypoglycemia. CT shows a small enhancing lesion in the pancreatic head, adjacent to the superior mesenteric vein, detected only during the early arterial phase of scanning (**A**, *arrow*) consistent with insulinoma. **B**, Intraoperative ultrasound was essential to localize this small nonpalpable lesion prior to resection.

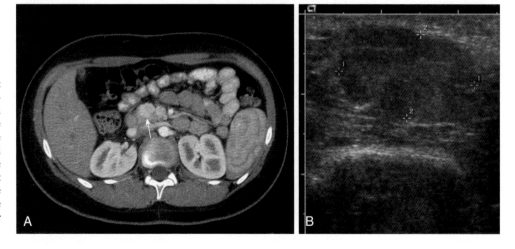

molecularly targeted therapies (e.g., imatinib [Gleevec]) specifically inhibiting cell surface receptors expressed on these cells. Although most pediatric GI stromal tumors apparently express a different cell surface receptor mutation (KIT or PDGFRA)[154] and thus do not respond to imatinib in the same way as adult GISTs, the radiographic features are similar, with patients presenting with a large mass closely apposed to the gastric wall. Depending on the size of the mass, it may be difficult to distinguish between a pancreatic tumor invading the posterior gastric wall and a primary gastric tumor. On CT, these tumors are frequently heterogeneous in attenuation, with modest enhancement relative to the adjacent pancreatic tissue. For patients with localized disease, complete surgical resection is still the mainstay of treatment for this tumor, with targeted therapies reserved for patients with advanced or metastatic

disease.[155] FDG-PET scanning has been shown to be important for staging and follow-up evaluation, both as a measure of metabolic response to molecularly targeted therapy[155] and for early detection of small, local sites of relapse within the gastric wall, which may be difficult to detect by conventional cross-sectional imaging techniques.

The most common primary bowel malignancy in childhood is lymphoma. The small bowel is more often involved than the large bowel, and this is most often non-Hodgkin's lymphoma. Presentation is typically with abdominal pain, weight loss, anemia, gastrointestinal bleeding, or constipation. Intussusception or a palpable abdominal mass may bring the patient to attention sooner. In an older child (older than 6 years) presenting with intussusception, lymphoma should be the leading diagnostic consideration (Fig. 26-51). Most

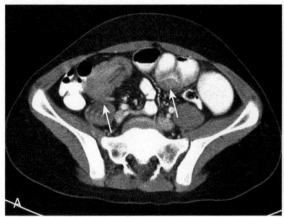
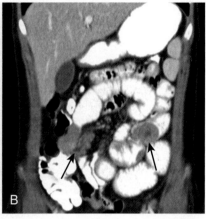

FIGURE 26-51. Burkitt's lymphoma of small bowel, presenting with abdominal pain, bowel wall thickening, intramural masses, and multiple small bowel intussusceptions (*arrows*), show on axial (**A**) and coronal CT scan (**B**).

small-bowel non-Hodgkin's lymphomas are Burkitt's lymphoma. These rapidly dividing tumors involve either the bowel or the small bowel or colonic mesentery and can become large and lead to intestinal obstruction. Burkitt's lymphoma responds rapidly to chemotherapy and can be effectively treated with no residual imaging abnormalities seen.

The imaging evaluation may initially involve fluoroscopic or barium studies to assess nonspecific symptoms of abdominal pain. In the setting of suspected intussusception, conventional radiography and ultrasound are usually sufficient to confirm the diagnosis. Attempts at hydrostatic or pneumatic enema reduction of intussusceptions occurring around pathologic lead points in the bowel caused by lymphomatous infiltration of the bowel or mesentery should be undertaken with caution, because of increased risk of perforation at the site of intussusception[156] and greater risk of failure at reducing the intussusception in these patients. Once the diagnosis of lymphoma has been made, a complete cross-sectional imaging (CT) staging examination, including the neck and chest, should be undertaken. Intravenous and oral contrast are necessary for this evaluation. CT reveals bowel wall thickening, mesenteric adenopathy, and often a large intraperitoneal/mesenteric mass. FDG-PET scanning has been shown to be effective in adult patients for staging and response assessment for non-Hodgkin's lymphoma and small case series have confirmed this finding in children. These data suggest FDG-PET should be included in the diagnostic staging and post-treatment assessment of these patients.[157-160]

Adenocarcinomas of the colon and rectum are fortunately rare in children. As in adults, colonoscopy may provide the best early diagnosis for a suspected carcinomatous lesion. The staging evaluation for metastatic spread should involve imaging of the chest, abdomen, and pelvis, again with both intravenous and oral contrast. There is no clear role established for routine use of FDG-PET scanning in the staging of children with adenocarcinomas of the GI tract.

Carcinoid tumors occurring in the gastrointestinal tract are rare, and are usually slow growing, but have malignant potential. The appendix is the most common location for carcinoid tumors. It is not uncommon for patients to present with symptoms of acute appendicitis, with carcinoid discovered at the time of appendectomy or incidentally during evaluation of the pathologic specimen.[161] When large, carcinoid tumors may also produce obstruction of the bowel or intussusception. Because of their propensity to metastasize to the liver, workup should include imaging of the entire abdomen and pelvis with intravenous and oral contrast. Somatostatin receptor analogues (octreotide) are useful for occult sites of metastatic disease spread. Hepatic metastases from carcinoid tumors are typically best demonstrated during the early arterial phase of contrast injection, which best delineates these hypervascular tumors

relative to the surrounding hepatic parenchyma. Complete surgical resection remains the mainstay of therapy for disease localized to the appendix and is usually curative.[161]

GENITOURINARY TUMORS

There are a number of different types of genitourinary tumors in the pediatric population, the majority of which include primary renal tumors, suprarenal and adrenal neoplasms, testicular and ovarian neoplasms, and tumors arising in or around the urinary bladder.

Renal Masses

Wilms' Tumor

Wilms' tumor is the most common renal malignancy in children, representing 6% to 10% of all pediatric malignancies and making up greater than 80% of pediatric renal masses. The peak age of incidence is between 3 and 4 years of age and bilateral disease is seen in between 5% and 10% of patients.[162,163] Wilms' tumor is often associated with syndromes and nephroblastomatosis, and typically presents as a painless, palpable abdominal mass. Occasionally, Wilms' tumor is an incidental finding during a radiologic assessment for other indications, such as trauma. Hypertension and hematuria only occur in about 25% of cases.[162]

Tumor staging, based on the National Wilms' Tumor Study Group classification, depends on surgical, pathologic and radiologic findings. The imaging evaluation should be directed at determining spread to adjacent organs such as the pancreas, spleen, and liver and for intravascular extension into the renal vein, IVC, and right atrium (Box 26-2).[164] In addition, the imaging examination should assess for the presence of distant metastatic disease (lung and liver) and contralateral kidney involvement.[163,165] Wilms' tumor is a rapidly growing malignancy, and intra-abdominal rupture—at diagnosis, during chemotherapy or at the time of surgical resection—is a well-appreciated complication and is a major risk factor for abdominal recurrence.[166] When tumor rupture is identified, these patients are upstaging and treated as having stage III disease.[163,165]

The initial examination is often a conventional abdominal x-ray obtained for symptoms of abdominal pain or a palpable mass. The typical findings include displacement of bowel and a masslike opacity in the abdomen. An ultrasound should serve as the initial evaluation and will usually confirm the renal origin

Box 26-2	**Childhood Wilms' Tumor: National Wilms' Tumor Study Group Staging**

STAGE I

Tumor is limited to the kidney and is completely resected.

The renal capsule is intact, and tumor is not ruptured or biopsied prior to removal.

There is no involvement of renal sinus vessels or evidence of the tumor at or beyond the margins of resection.

STAGE II

Tumor is completely resected, with no evidence of tumor at or beyond the margins of resection.

Tumor extends beyond the kidney, as evidenced by any one of the following:
1. Regional extension of the tumor (i.e., penetration of the renal sinus capsule, or extensive invasion of the soft tissue of the renal sinus).
2. Blood vessels within the nephrectomy specimen outside the renal parenchyma contain tumor.

STAGE III

Residual nonhematogenous intra-abdominal tumor following surgery.

Any one of the following may occur:
1. Lymph nodes within the abdomen or pelvis are involved by tumor.
2. Tumor implants are found on or penetrate through the peritoneal surface.
3. Gross or microscopic tumor remains.
4. Tumor is not completely resectable because of local infiltration.
5. Tumor spillage occurs before or during surgery, or tumor was biopsied before removal.
6. Tumor is removed in more than one piece (e.g., tumor thrombus within the renal vein is removed separately from the nephrectomy specimen).

STAGE IV

Hematogenous metastases (e.g., lung, liver, bone, brain), or lymph node metastases outside the abdominopelvic region are present.

STAGE V

Bilateral involvement by tumor is present at diagnosis.

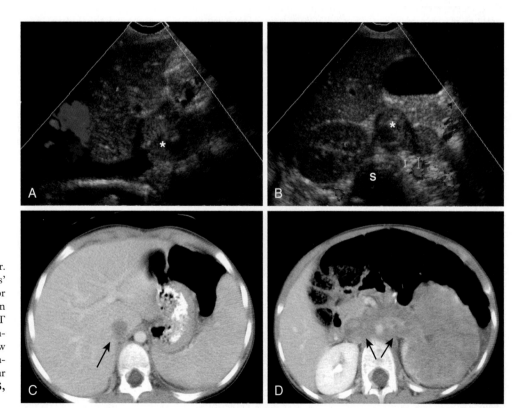

FIGURE 26-52. Wilms' tumor. 6-year-old with left renal Wilms' tumor and left renal vein–inferior vena cava (IVC) extension shown by ultrasound (★, **A, B**) and CT (**C, D,** *arrows*). Ultrasound confirms the complete absence of flow in the left renal vein (**B**) and documents the level of intravascular invasion into the IVC (**A, ★**). **S,** spine.

of the suspected mass. Sonographically, Wilms' tumors are often large, with relatively homogeneous echogenicity. There may be focal areas of hypoechogenicity or cystic change. Calcifications are uncommon. Ultrasound is also accurate and sensitive for detecting intravascular invasion; color and Doppler imaging are effective at establishing vascular patency (Fig. 26-52). Intravascular extension occurs in 4% to 10% of patients with Wilms' tumor, but is rare in neuroblastoma, helping to differentiate between these two tumors.[165] In addition, the ultrasound examination plays a crucial role in the pre-procedural management of these patients, because the presence of intravascular extension into the right atrium may increase the sedation or anesthesia risk for a child for whom subsequent CT or MRI is planned.

Once the diagnosis has been suggested by ultrasound, further imaging of suspected Wilms' tumor requires CT or MRI to stage the disease accurately. Multirow detector CT scanning allows for rapid scanning, and in some cases may allow sedation to be avoided. High-resolution imaging techniques, with multiplanar reconstructions, are essential for determining the extent of tumor spillage, local invasion, invasion into vascular structures, and presence of pulmonary metastatic disease. Early studies have suggested that pulmonary metastases detected only by CT should not result in upstaging of the patient, relying on chest x-ray for identifying pulmonary metastases.[165] Subsequent work by European investigators in SIOP and in North America with the National Wilms' Tumor Study Group has identified a small cohort of patients with pulmonary lesions visualized only by CT scanning, and in whom disease stage would be advanced based on the CT results.[165] One study has shown an increased risk of relapse in patients with positive CT findings,[167] with others reporting no difference in prognosis between patients with positive or negative chest CT scan.[116,168] These studies were limited by their retrospective nature, and it remains controversial whether these patients would have benefited from increased therapy.[163,165] Furthermore, other investigators have argued that chest x-ray and CT data are concordant in most cases,[117] and it has been shown that not all pulmonary lesions detected by CT represent metastases, even in the hands of experienced radiologists.[167] This suggests that surgical confirmation may be necessary to establish the malignant nature of suspicious lesions detected by CT in Wilms' tumor patients.[115] These considerations aside, it is now current practice to carry out chest CT for staging of all Wilms' tumor patients, with ongoing studies investigating the positive predictive value of this practice and its impact on overall clinical outcome.

Because of the need for chest CT in the staging evaluation, MRI is usually obtained for follow-up evaluation after resection or following chemotherapy. In addition, MRI is the imaging modality of choice for following nephrogenic rests that are seen in approximately 40% of unilateral Wilms' tumor patients and almost all bilateral Wilms' tumor patients (Fig. 26-53).[169,170] Nephrogenic rests are remnants of primitive blastomal tissue that persist after birth and have the potential to transform into Wilms' tumor. Nephroblastomatosis is the presence of multifocal or diffuse nephrogenic rests, and is prevalent in patients with hemihypertrophy.[162] The distinction between nephrogenic rests and Wilms' tumor may be difficult, but there are certain distinguishing MRI features that may help discriminate between the two. On T1-weighted MR images, Wilms' tumors appear as a well-defined heterogeneous mass, with slightly lower signal intensity as compared with the adjacent renal cortex. On T2-weighted images, Wilms' tumors appear isointense to slightly hyperintense relative to the normal renal cortex. Following intravenous gadolinium contrast administration, Wilms' tumors typically enhance heterogeneously, but less than the surrounding renal parenchyma. Nephrogenic rests also exhibit decreased signal intensity on T1-weighted images but, in contrast to Wilms' tumors, maintain a low signal on T2-weighted images.[171-173] Furthermore, nephrogenic rests show minimal enhancement following contrast infusion relative to the normal renal parenchyma, whereas foci of Wilms' tumors show heterogeneous enhancement.[171,172] A role for FDG-PET scanning in the routine management of Wilms' tumor patients has not been established. However, studies documenting increased FDG accumulation in metabolically active Wilms' tumors[174] have suggested that there may be a role for FDG-PET imaging in Wilms' tumor staging, post-therapy response evaluation, and possibly in helping discriminate benign nephrogenic rests from foci of transformed malignant tumor.

As discussed later, the major differential considerations in patients with suspected unilateral Wilms' tumor are clear cell sarcoma of the kidney and rhabdoid tumor of the kidney. However, there are no characteristic imaging features to make this distinction.

Clear Cell Sarcoma

Clear cell sarcoma of the kidney, also known as bone-metastasizing renal tumor of childhood, was previously thought to be a histologically aggressive variant of Wilms' tumor. It occurs less frequently than Wilms' tumor (4% to 5% of pediatric renal neoplasms), with an estimated 20 new cases diagnosed annually

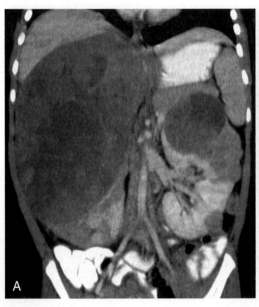
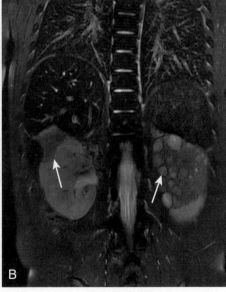

FIGURE 26-53. 3-year-old with bilateral Wilms' tumor, initially evaluated by CT (**A**). The patient underwent bilateral partial nephrectomies. MRI is now being used to follow nephrogenic rests on both kidneys (**B,** *arrows*), both for change in size and change in pattern of enhancement.

in the United States.[175] Although age at presentation ranges from infancy to the second decade, the peak incidence at about 2 to 3 years of age closely parallels that of Wilms' tumor, making differential diagnosis difficult. Bone metastases, which are unusual in Wilms' tumor, occur frequently in patients with clear cell sarcoma of the kidney, and can have osteolytic and osteoblastic activity.[162]

On imaging, there are no specific features that allow distinction to be made from Wilms' tumor. Ultrasound confirms the renal origin of the mass, showing a heterogeneous mass with areas of hypoechogenicity and isoechogenicity reflecting cystic and solid elements within the mass. CT scanning is usually performed to characterize the mass more completely and assess for regional invasion and metastatic disease. On CT, clear cell sarcomas of the kidney are typically heterogeneous in attenuation, with a variable pattern of contrast enhancement (Fig. 26-54). Vascular invasion is uncommon, and these tumors, in contrast to Wilms' tumors, do not have a pseudocapsule and commonly infiltrate the adjacent renal parenchyma and perinephric spaces.[162] The most common site of metastatic spread is to locoregional lymph nodes, followed by metastases to the lung and bone. Liver metastases also occur. As with Wilms' tumor, the management of clear cell carcinoma of the kidney involves a combination of nephrectomy and chemotherapy.

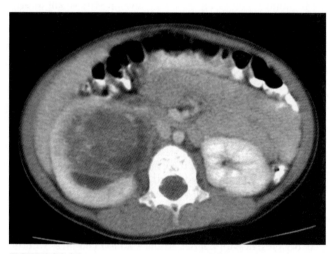

FIGURE 26-54. 2-year-old with clear cell sarcomas of the kidney. CT shows heterogeneous attenuation, ill-defined margins, cystic and solid areas, and a variable pattern of contrast enhancement.

Clear cell carcinomas are more aggressive than Wilms' tumor, with a higher relapse rate; the most common site of relapse is bone, and current recommendations include skeletal scintigraphy for follow-up screening examinations.

Rhabdoid Tumor of the Kidney

Rhabdoid tumor of the kidney is also extremely rare and is the most aggressive of the renal tumors in children. Previously thought to be a variant of Wilms' tumor histology, it is now recognized as a discrete entity and accounts for approximately 2% to 3% of pediatric renal tumors. Rhabdoid tumors tend to occur in young infants, with more than 80% occurring in patients younger than 2 years.[176]

CT, ultrasound, and MRI all show a large heterogeneous intrarenal mass that often involves the central renal hilum. There may be associated vascular invasion and calcifications may be seen. Although there are no distinctive imaging features to distinguish rhabdoid tumor of the kidney from Wilms' tumor (Fig. 26-55) reliably, the findings of calcification, subcapsular hematoma, and the presence of a lobular, centrally located heterogeneous renal mass have been reported as characteristic imaging findings in patients with rhabdoid tumors of the kidney.[177] In addition, the association between rhabdoid tumors of the kidney and the presence of primary brain tumors (posterior fossa tumors, including medulloblastoma, PNET, astrocytoma, and medulloblastoma) and synchronous or metachronous brain metastases are considered a unique and distinctive feature of this tumor.[176,178] Thus, once the diagnosis of rhabdoid tumor of the kidney has been established, subsequent staging and follow-up evaluations should always include imaging of the brain to assess for intracranial disease.

Renal Cell Carcinoma

As children enter their teenage years, the incidence of Wilms' tumor decreases and the incidence of renal cell carcinoma rises. Although there have been rare reports of renal cell carcinoma occurring in infancy, the vast majority occur in children in late adolescence.[162] Syndromes associated with renal cell carcinoma include von Hippel–Lindau syndrome, tuberous sclerosis, and Beckwith-Wiedemann syndrome. In contrast to adults, in whom hematuria and flank pain are common presenting complaints, children with renal cell carcinoma more often present with vague abdominal pain and an abdominal mass.

The imaging features of renal cell carcinoma and Wilms' tumor overlap, although renal cell carcinomas (RCCs) tend to show calcifications more often than Wilms' tumor. RCCs are

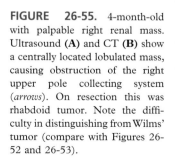

FIGURE 26-55. 4-month-old with palpable right renal mass. Ultrasound **(A)** and CT **(B)** show a centrally located lobulated mass, causing obstruction of the right upper pole collecting system (*arrows*). On resection this was rhabdoid tumor. Note the difficulty in distinguishing from Wilms' tumor (compare with Figures 26-52 and 26-53).

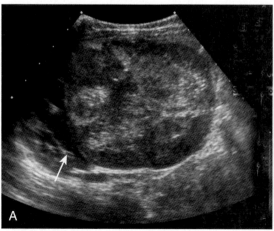
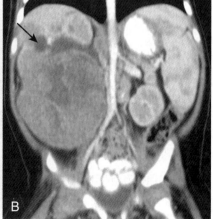

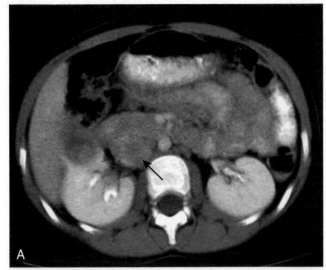

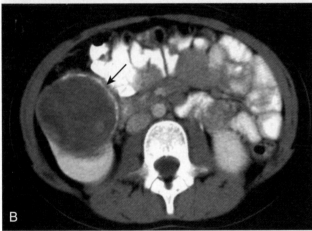

FIGURE 26-56. 9-year-old with right renal mass, found to be renal cell carcinoma. Note the rim calcification (**B,** arrow), heterogeneous attenuation and enhancement, and retroperitoneal lymph node spread (**A,** *arrow*).

more often bilateral and more commonly metastasize to bone than Wilms' tumors; however, it is primarily the older age at presentation that favors renal cell carcinoma over Wilms' tumor. CT, MRI, and ultrasound all reveal a heterogeneous-appearing intrarenal mass. Multiple bilateral renal cell carcinoma masses should suggest the diagnosis of von Hippel–Lindau syndrome.[176] Areas of cystic change are often seen, representing necrosis and hemorrhage, and calcifications are more common than in Wilms' tumor (Fig. 26-56). Following contrast infusion, a heterogeneous pattern of contrast enhancement is seen on both CT and MRI. Local invasion into retroperitoneal lymph nodes and vascular invasion, particularly into the IVC, are common with renal cell carcinoma and significantly influence the success of primary surgical resection and overall prognosis. Because of the increased incidence of bone metastases in renal cell carcinoma, the staging evaluation should also include bone scintigraphy in addition to CT scanning of the chest, abdomen, and pelvis.

Congenital Mesoblastic Nephroma

Congenital mesoblastic nephroma, although not the most common solid tumor in childhood, is the most common solid tumor of the neonatal period. It is a benign lesion with almost 75% of cases being identified within the first year of life. With the advent of prenatal ultrasound screening, the incidence of early diagnosis is expected to increase. Infants typically present with a large, palpable abdominal mass. The imaging evaluation typically begins with ultrasound, showing a large solid renal mass that frequently involves the renal hilum (Fig. 26-57).[176] Although not a distinguishing feature, cystic elements are less commonly seen in mesoblastic nephroma than Wilms' tumor. Congenital mesoblastic nephroma has been subdivided histologically into an aggressive high cell density variant and the classic variant, which has fewer active mitoses, less potential for local recurrence and metastasis, and overall better prognosis than the aggressive variant.[162,176] Hemorrhage, cysts, and necrosis, when present, are more often associated with the aggressive high cell density variant. Subsequent imaging by CT and/or MRI is usually performed to characterize the intrarenal lesion better and to assess for invasion into adjacent organs and structures. The imaging features alone do not allow distinction between mesoblastic nephroma and Wilms' tumor and surgical resection is indicated (see Fig. 26-57). Because there may be poorly defined margins and the lack of a definable capsule, a surgical resection with wide margins is usually performed. The conventional benign histologic variant of this tumor is composed primarily of benign connective tissue and mature mesenchymal cells, and prognosis is excellent if surgical resection is complete. Postoperative monitoring by ultrasound or MRI is still recommended, even with complete resection, for at least 1 year. With the aggressive cellular histologic variant, metastases and local spread of disease may require postoperative radiation and chemotherapy, and a more intensive follow-up imaging regimen should be directed at evaluating sites of local recurrence and typical metastatic spread (e.g., lungs, bone, brain).[176]

Multilocular Cystic Nephroma

Multilocular cystic nephroma is a benign renal tumor comprised almost entirely of coalescent cystic lesions with thin-walled septae.[179] Although the cystic appearance is distinctive, it is still not possible, based on imaging findings alone, to discriminate between the cystic variant of Wilms' tumor and the benign multilocular cystic nephroma. As with Wilms' tumor, the typical age of presentation is between 2 and 5 years, with a smaller percentage occurring in young adults. Typically, patients present with a large, painless abdominal mass with no systemic symptoms.[176]

Radiographs may show a large abdominal mass displacing loops of bowel. The use of ultrasound is particularly important to demonstrate the cystic characteristics of these lesions, because CT scanning may simply show a large, low-attenuation mass with septations, but may not clearly demonstrate the hypoechoic cystic spaces revealed by ultrasound (Fig. 26-58). MRI shows a characteristic fluid signal, with low signal intensity on T1-weighted images and high signal intensity on T2-weighted images. Following contrast enhancement by CT and MRI, enhancement of the thin-walled septae is seen, while most of the cystic mass remains unenhanced. Because the differentiation among cystic Wilms', clear cell sarcoma, and multilocular cystic renal tumor cannot be made on the basis of imaging features, surgical resection is required for diagnosis.[179] Long-term prognosis is excellent, but follow-up imaging is still necessary in the early stages postresection because a low incidence of local recurrence is still possible.

Rare Renal Tumors

Two additional very rare tumors of infancy are the ossifying renal tumor of infancy (Fig. 26-59) and desmoplastic small

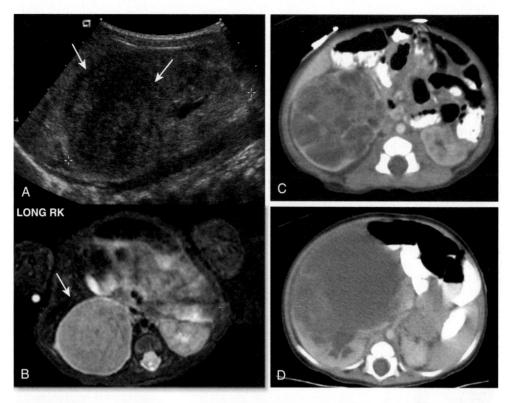

FIGURE 26-57. Congenital mesoblastic nephroma in 7-day-old infant with prenatally diagnosed solid right renal mass, confirmed by ultrasound (A) and MRI (B) after birth. The two other patients, newborn (C) and 5 months old (D), have large right renal masses showing both cystic and solid elements typical of congenital mesoblastic nephroma.

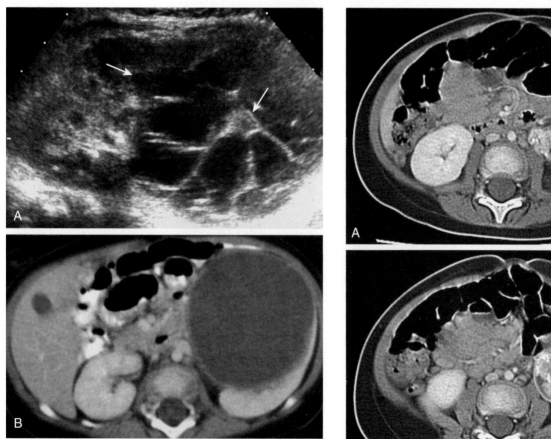

FIGURE 26-58. Multilocular cystic nephroma. A, Ultrasound shows a cystic left renal mass. Note how the cystic characteristics of these lesions and internal septations (A, *arrows*) are not well demonstrated by CT (B), which simply shows a large low-attenuation mass, perhaps with thin internal septations.

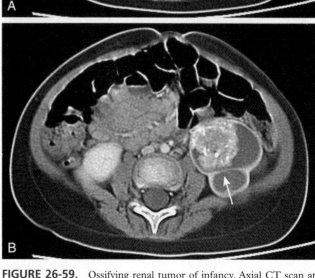

FIGURE 26-59. Ossifying renal tumor of infancy. Axial CT scan at the level of the left renal hilum (A) and lower pole (B). This lobular renal hilar mass has extensive calcification (*arrows*) that results from the ossifying renal tumors being composed of an osteoid core and osteoblastic tissue.

round cell tumors. Both tumors characteristically calcify. Figure 26-59 shows a renal hilar mass with extensive calcification that results from ossifying renal tumors being composed of an osteoid core and osteoblastic tissue. Surgical resection is usually curative.[176] Desmoplastic small round cell tumors are unusual as a primary renal neoplasm in children, but have been reported.[180] As in other locations, these should be included in a differential for a calcified renal mass in a young child. Finally, metastatic disease to the kidney is unusual, except in the setting of leukemia and lymphoma.[162] Leukemic involvement of the kidney typically manifests as diffuse nephromegaly. Lymphomatous involvement more often presents with discrete foci of lymphomatous infiltration, and occurs in both non-Hodgkin's and Hodgkin's lymphoma subtypes. Burkitt's lymphoma and T-lymphoblastic lymphoma are the non-Hodgkin's lymphoma types most frequently presenting with renal involvement. This is probably the result of hematogenous metastasis and, in the setting of Burkitt's lymphoma, is usually associated with extensive mesenteric and retroperitoneal lymphadenopathy.[176] In the case of leukemia, diffuse nephromegaly may also be accompanied by hepatosplenomegaly, but generalized adenopathy is less common. Ultrasound is usually sufficient to identify renal involvement by leukemia and lymphoma. Additional imaging by CT or MRI confirms the diagnosis, demonstrating low-density lesions with little enhancement relative to the surrounding renal parenchyma.

Bladder Neoplasms

In children, tumors involving the urinary bladder are uncommon, with rhabdomyosarcoma being the most common malignancy encountered. Adult-type tumors such as transitional cell carcinoma, fibroepithelial polyps, and adenomatous lesions are unusual.

Rhabdomyosarcomas

Pelvic rhabdomyosarcomas arise from the bladder wall, prostate, and vagina. Tumors arising in the bladder and prostate frequently result in obstruction of urinary flow, symptoms of dysuria and hematuria, and urinary retention. Vaginal rhabdomyosarcomas present as a pelvic mass, vaginal bleeding, and occasionally prolapse of tumor from the vaginal orifice onto the perineum.[181]

Imaging evaluation is initially by ultrasound, with rhabdomyosarcomas of the bladder presenting as diffuse bladder wall thickening or as polypoid or so-called botryoid soft tissue masses protruding from the bladder wall into the bladder lumen. Color and Doppler flow demonstrate increased vascularity of these lesions. Cystourethrography may be helpful to assess the degree of functional impairment and usually demonstrates filling defects in the bladder, diminished bladder volume and, depending on the size and location of the lesion, obstruction to the flow of urine.

Contrast-enhanced CT scanning, early after contrast infusion, prior to bladder filling, and after delayed bladder filling, is helpful to assess the degree of local invasion. MRI, however, is preferable to characterize the lesion in multiple planes and to evaluate spread into adjacent pelvic organs and neurovascular structures.[182] Rhabdomyosarcomas typically show intermediate signal intensity on T1-weighted images, with increased signal on T2-weighted images and heterogeneous or minimal enhancement on postcontrast images (Fig. 26-60). The imaging evaluation should be directed at assessing for local tumor extension into adjacent pelvic fat planes, adjacent lymph node enlargement, and involvement of the perivesical fat and adjacent musculature. Multiplanar T2-weighted images with fat suppression are well suited for detecting invasion of adjacent deep pelvic structures.

As with other rhabdomyosarcomas, metastases to the liver, bone, bone marrow, and lung occur, and the staging evaluation

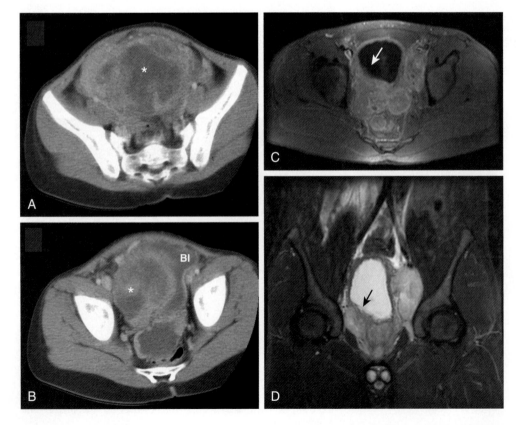

FIGURE 26-60. Rhabdomyosarcomas of the bladder and prostate. CT **(A, B)** shows large exophytic mass (⋆) arising from the bladder wall and compressing the bladder lumen (Bl). Contrast-enhanced **(C)** and fast spin-echo inversion recovery MR images **(D)** show invasion of the bladder wall by prostatic rhabdomyosarcoma (*arrows*); MRI is superior to CT at demonstrating extent of invasion in the pelvis.

should include chest CT and bone scintigraphy. The role of FDG-PET in imaging rhabdomyosarcoma has not been the focus of any controlled prospective trials, but it has been our experience and the experience of others that rhabdomyosarcomas are usually FDG-avid, and that FDG-PET imaging can play an important role in identifying sites of occult disease, monitoring responses to therapy, and evaluating equivocal foci of disease, locally or at metastatic sites, that are identified by CT or MRI.[110]

Adrenal and Suprarenal Tumors

Neuroblastoma

Neuroblastoma is the most common non-CNS pediatric solid tumor, and is the third most common pediatric malignancy, after leukemia and central nervous system tumors.[98,99] More than 90% of cases occur in children younger than 5 years. Patients with neuroblastoma often present with a painless abdominal mass. The most common site of origin is the retroperitoneum (adrenal gland), with other sites of origin in the posterior mediastinum, neck, and pelvis (at the level of the iliac bifurcation—organ of Zuckerkandl).[98] Symptoms at presentation may also result from compression of adjacent organs, extension into the spinal canal, vascular compression or invasion, and bone involvement. Hypertension is seen in about 10% of patients because of elevated catecholamine production. Paraneoplastic syndromes include the opsoclonus myoclonus syndrome and watery diarrhea. These symptoms frequently resolve after resection or chemotherapeutic treatment of the primary tumor.

The age and stage of disease remain the most important prognostic factors in neuroblastoma.[99] Infants younger than 1 year with localized disease have the highest rates of cure. Older patients with metastatic disease continue to be the most challenging population of patients to treat. The most widely used staging system for neuroblastoma is the International Neuroblastoma Staging System (INSS; Box 26-3).[183,184] This involves a combination of radiographic, scintigraphic, and surgical findings and bone marrow evaluation. Lower stage disease is characterized by localized tumor involvement, whereas infiltration across the midline and/or encasement of major blood vessels that results in surgical unresectability defines stage 3 disease. Widespread disease with cortical bone, bone marrow, or visceral organ involvement is defined as stage 4 disease. A unique feature of the staging of patients with neuroblastoma is the category stage 4S (special), which is defined as localized primary tumor with dissemination limited to liver and skin and less than 10% bone marrow involvement.[99]

The initial imaging modalities used for evaluating patients with neuroblastoma are directed at the presenting symptoms, and abdominal films, chest radiographs, and skeletal films are usually obtained to assess abdominal distention, suspected pneumonia, or limp/extremity pain (Fig. 26-61). Ultrasound is widely available and should be the first choice for evaluating a child with a suspected abdominal mass. Depending on the size of the mass, ultrasound can effectively demonstrate the presence of a retroperitoneal or suprarenal mass (Fig. 26-62), and is sensitive and specific for evaluating for the presence of hepatic metastatic disease and localized vascular invasion. Calcifications are common in neuroblastoma and are seen sonographically as areas of acoustic shadowing. Depending on the age and size of the patient, intraspinal extension can also be detected.

CT scanning is widely used for defining the extent of primary tumor involvement and, particularly with multiplanar reconstructions, has become critical in the staging and surgical

planning for patients with neuroblastoma (Fig. 26-63). The use of intravenous and oral contrast is essential in this evaluation, and scanning should include the chest, abdomen, and pelvis. The presence of intraspinal extension can often be detected by CT scanning, but MRI is considered superior to CT for characterizing epidural extension or leptomeningeal spread of disease.[66] MRI, particularly with the advent of faster,

---

Box 26-3 Childhood Neuroblastoma: International Neuroblastoma Staging System (INSS)

STAGE 1

Localized tumor with complete gross excision, with or without microscopic residual disease

Representative ipsilateral lymph nodes, separate from the primary tumor, are negative for tumor microscopically

STAGE 2A

Localized tumor with incomplete gross excision

Representative ipsilateral nonadherent lymph nodes are negative for tumor.

STAGE 2B

Localized tumor with or without complete gross excision

Ipsilateral nonadherent lymph nodes are positive for tumor.

Enlarged contralateral lymph nodes must be negative microscopically.

STAGE 3

Unresectable unilateral tumor infiltrating across the midline, with or without regional lymph node involvement; or

Localized unilateral tumor with contralateral regional lymph node involvement; or

Midline tumor with bilateral extension by infiltration (unresectable) or by lymph node involvement. The midline is defined as the vertebral column.

STAGE 4

Any primary tumor with dissemination to distant lymph nodes, bone, bone marrow, liver, skin, and/or other organs, except as defined for stage 4S.

STAGE 4S

Localized primary tumor, as defined for stage 1, 2A, or 2B, and

1. Dissemination limited to skin, liver, and/or bone marrow
2. Limited to infants younger than 1 year
3. Minimal marrow involvement (i.e., <10% of total nucleated cells in aspirate); more extensive bone marrow involvement is stage 4 disease.
4. Metaiodobenzylguanidine (MIBG) scan should be negative for disease in the bone marrow.

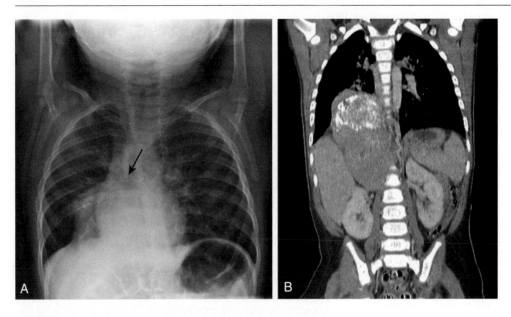

FIGURE 26-61. Neuroblastoma. **A,** This chest x-ray demonstrates calcified mass at the right lung base, seen on the lateral film to be posterior mediastinal (not shown). Coronal reconstructions from contrast-enhanced CT (**B**) reveal a large calcified right suprarenal mass with extension across the midline and into the thorax.

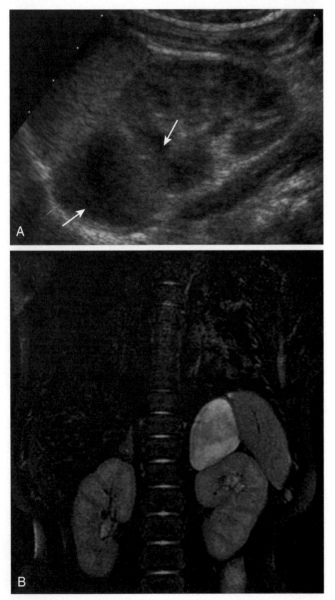

FIGURE 26-62. Neuroblastoma in 2-month-old infant being evaluated for vomiting. Ultrasound to assess for pyloric stenosis showed a well-defined left suprarenal mass (**A,** *arrows*) confirmed by MRI (**B**).

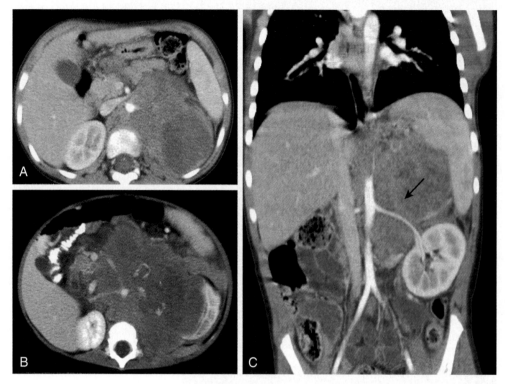

FIGURE 26-63. Neuroblastoma. **A, B,** Contrast-enhanced CT scans show bulky retroperitoneal masses in two patients, with encasement of vessels and extension across midline. **C,** Coronal reconstruction shows inferior displacement of the left kidney by the mass and demonstrates traction on the left renal artery (arrow), which often leads to hypertension in these patients.

whole-body scanning techniques, has also been advocated for use in determining extent of bone marrow involvement.[100,185] In addition, MRI is effective for evaluating unsuspected sites of bone marrow disease delineated by MIBG scintigraphy, and should also be used for monitoring infants and children with low-risk disease for whom treatment does not routinely involve radiotherapy and reduction in radiation exposure is desirable.

The staging and monitoring of patients with neuroblastoma also depend on the use of scintigraphic studies, including bone scanning and MIBG scintigraphy. ^{99m}Tc-MDP scintigraphy has historically been used to detect the presence of cortical bone metastases and has been shown to be superior to conventional radiography.[66] MIBG is a catecholamine analogue taken up by neuroblastoma cells. ^{123}I-MIBG has been used to localize neuroblastoma at primary sites (Fig. 26-64), as well as in bone, bone marrow, and lymph nodes, and is effective in identifying sites of disease in more than 90% of patients.[66,186] In particular, sites of previously unsuspected disease in the bone marrow are effectively detected by MIBG. Normal uptake by the liver, however, does limit the use of MIBG for detecting small foci of hepatic disease, and uptake by normal adrenal tissue following contralateral adrenalectomy may make postoperative follow-up challenging. Nonetheless, the relative sensitivity and specificity of MIBG for detecting disease not evident by other techniques has led many investigators to include routinely MIBG scintigraphy in the diagnostic and post-treatment evaluation of neuroblastoma patients.[187,188]

Although large controlled studies are lacking, a number of smaller consortium studies have shown that MIBG scanning at the time of staging has prognostic significance and that early response to therapy as detected by MIBG scintigraphy correlates with overall response and event-free survival.[189-193] As a result, MIBG scoring symptoms have been proposed to allow enumeration of the number and extent of MIBG disease foci and have been used for following responses to therapy, with good correlation with overall clinical response.[192,194]

FDG-PET scanning, although commonly used for many other tumor types, has not gained universal acceptance in the staging and follow-up evaluation of patients with neuroblastoma. PET scanning allows increased sensitivity and higher spatial resolution for disease detection,[51,102,195] but reports of false-positive FDG uptake and false-negative studies, combined with the general acceptance of MIBG scintigraphy and cross-sectional imaging, have resulted in the slow acceptance of FDG-PET scanning for the evaluation of patients with neuroblastoma.[66] Larger studies are needed to compare the sensitivity and specificity of FDG-PET with MIBG directly to determine the efficacy of FDG-PET imaging in the staging and post-treatment evaluation of patients with neuroblastoma.

Radiolabeled monoclonal antibodies, labeled with ^{131}I, ^{123}I, ^{99m}Tc, and ^{64}Cu, have all been used in animal and clinical models of neuroblastoma.[53,196,197] The antibodies on which these imaging agents are based are directed against the disialoganglioside GD2, which has increased expression in neuroblastoma, and these same antibodies have been used clinically to treat patients with advanced-stage disease.[198] However, the routine use of radioimmunodetection has still remained investigational in neuroblastoma patients.

Stage 4S neuroblastoma is unique among pediatric neoplasms. As earlier defined, stage 4S disease may have extensive hepatic and primary site involvement, but may also completely resolve with observation alone and no additional chemotherapy (Fig. 26-65). The importance of the prenatal detection of neuroblastoma has also been emphasized recently by Blackman and colleagues[198a]; in their study, a prenatal ultrasound and subsequent prenatal MRI delineated a large paraspinal mass. In this case, the detection of spinal cord compression by MRI, combined with decreased fetal movement, led to a rapid delivery, biopsy, further staging, and early initiation of treatment, which resulted in tumor response and preservation of lower extremity neurologic function.

The opsoclonus myoclonus ataxia (OMA) syndrome is a paraneoplastic neurologic syndrome that has been associated

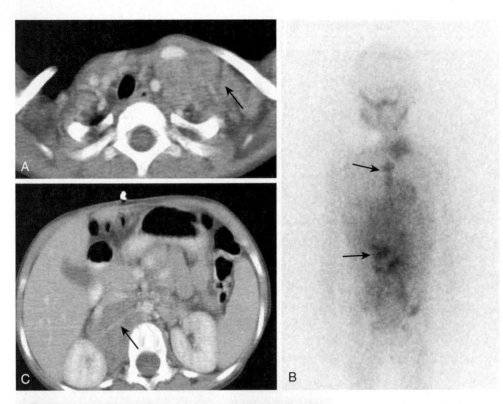

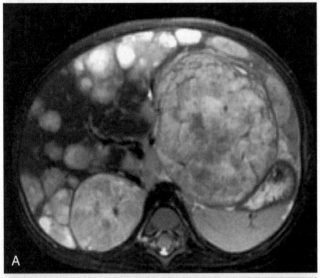

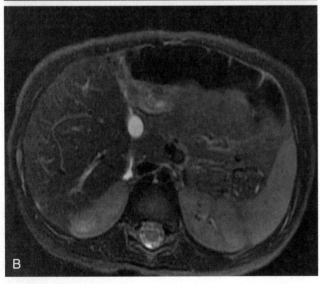

FIGURE 26-64. Neuroblastoma. Contrast-enhanced CT **(A, C)** and MIBG **(B)** in a 5-year-old showing intra-abdominal **(C)**, left supraclavicular **(A)**, and vertebral disease **(C)** (*arrows*). The thoracic vertebral disease is readily seen by MIBG, but was not evident on CT.

FIGURE 26-65. Neuroblastoma in a 6-month-old infant with abdominal mass and MRI showing extensive liver involvement **(A)**. He was shown to be stage 4S. **B,** After 7 months of observation only, and no chemotherapy, repeat MRI showed near-complete resolution of disease. This child continued on observation only.

with occult neuroblastoma. Frequently, the primary tumors associated with OMA syndrome are small, localized, and paraspinal or extra-abdominal. The identification of sites of disease is important, because symptoms often diminish or resolve on identification and treatment or resection of the neuroblastoma.[199,200] The imaging of patients with suspected OMA should include imaging of the chest, abdomen, and pelvis by MRI or CT, as well as MIBG scintigraphy.[66,201] MIBG scanning, in particular, has been shown to be sensitive and specific at revealing occult neuroblastoma in patients with the OMA syndrome.[202]

The distinction between neuroblastoma and its more differentiated counterparts, ganglioneuroblastoma and ganglioneuroma, cannot be made on the basis of imaging studies alone.[98] Ganglioneuroma, by definition, shows completely differentiated stromal and cellular elements, with neuroblastoma containing less than 50% differentiated elements and ganglioneuroblastoma intermediate between the two. Frequently, patients who have responded to therapy will have residual lesions that remain MIBG-avid and, on biopsy, are shown to be differentiated ganglioneuroma. In fact, novel treatment approaches are aimed at taking advantage of this potential for neuroblastoma to undergo differentiation, with *cis*-retinoic acid and its derivatives being used in an effort to accelerate the pathway toward differentiation.[203] Although biopsy and surgical resection are ultimately required to confirm the diagnosis, ganglioneuromas and ganglioneuroblastomas tend to be localized, with the most common sites of disease in the posterior mediastinum and retroperitoneum. The age at presentation is also typically older than that of patients with neuroblastoma. Ganglioneuroma, like ganglioneuroblastoma and neuroblastoma, may accumulate MIBG, and MIBG uptake cannot be used to discriminate between these distinct histopathologic entities effectively.[204] Calcifications are often seen by CT and conventional radiography, and similar MR imaging appearances are seen with all three histopathologic types, with low signal intensity on T1-weighted images, intermediate to high signal on T2-weighted images, and heterogeneous enhancement following gadolinium infusion. It is also important to recognize that sampling error can result following biopsy, and complete resection, if feasible, ensures a thorough sampling of the tumor specimen and a more confident diagnosis of ganglioneuroma.

Gonadal and Extragonadal Germ Cell Tumors

Gonadal and extragonadal germ cell tumors are relatively rare in children, representing only about 1% of tumors diagnosed in children younger than 15 years. The most common extragonadal sites of disease in older children are the mediastinum and brain; these tumors are discussed elsewhere in this chapter (see "Mediastinal Masses and Tumors"). Sacrococcygeal germ teratomas are the most common germ cell tumor occurring in infancy and account for approximately 40% of all teratomas identified in children.

Ovarian Germ Cell Tumors

Ovarian germ cell tumors include benign and malignant neoplasms.[181] Most ovarian tumors are benign, with the most common tumor being the mature cystic teratoma or dermoid cyst. Malignant ovarian tumors include neoplasms of stromal and germ cell origin, with the former including Sertoli-Leydig cell, granulosa thecal cell, and undifferentiated stromal tumors. Malignant ovarian tumors of germ cell origin include dysger-

minoma, immature teratoma, endodermal sinus tumor, embryonal carcinoma, and choriocarcinoma.

The imaging evaluation of malignant ovarian germ cell tumors should be directed at characterizing the primary lesion and identifying possible sites of metastatic spread of disease. Ultrasound is usually the first imaging study performed to identify and characterize a suspected primary ovarian or pelvic mass. Ultrasound reliably distinguishes between cystic and solid lesions and is helpful to assess blood flow to the lesion. The presence of associated ascites may also aid in the differential diagnosis. Additional evaluation by MRI and/or CT is typically performed, as needed, to characterize the primary lesion further and assess for locoregional and metastatic spread of disease.

Sonographically, the benign, mature cystic teratoma may be a homogeneous echogenic mass or a predominantly fluid-filled mass with an echogenic mural nodule. The presence of fat, calcification, or fat-fluid levels are all common findings in mature cystic teratoma (Fig. 26-66).[181] Large masses may be better characterized by CT and MRI, with CT scanning revealing low-Hounsfield Unit (HU) densities in fat-containing elements, with higher HU values and heterogeneous enhancement of the solid components. Calcifications, particularly microcalcifications, are effectively identified by CT.

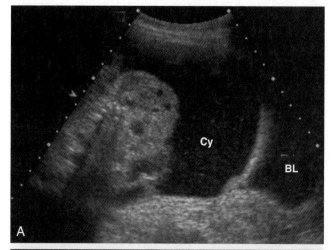

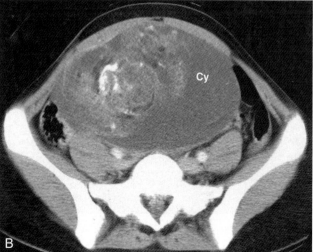

FIGURE 26-66. Mixed ovarian germ cell tumor. **A,** Ultrasound shows a complex cystic and solid mass, which on CT showed areas of calcification within the solid mass **(B)**, typical of germ cell tumors; BL, bladder; Cy, cystic component.

MRI findings are variable, depending on the characteristics and tissue composition of the teratomatous elements. Typically, mature teratomas have areas of high and low signal on T1- and T2-weighted images, with suppression of signal on fat-suppressed T1-weighted sequences. As shown in Figure 26-66, the presence of calcification, teeth, or hair may be useful in confirming the diagnosis. Even in the presence of mature elements, surgical resection is indicated, because the imaging features cannot clearly discriminate between malignant components of mixed germ cell tumors and the entirely benign mature counterparts. The presence of lymph node involvement, extension into contiguous organs/structures, hematogenous spread, and evidence of peritoneal or omental seeding all should suggest the presence of malignant disease.[181]

It is important to correlate the imaging findings with the age of the patient. Functional ovarian neoplasms such as granulosa thecal cell tumors may result in precocious puberty, and sonographic findings discordant with the patient's age (Fig. 26-67). Correlation with serum hormone, AFP, and β–human chorionic gonadotropin (HCG) levels are all important adjuncts to the imaging evaluation.

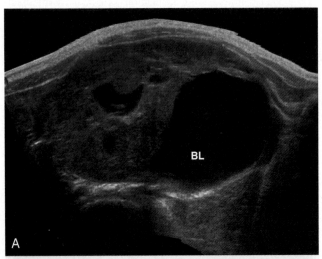

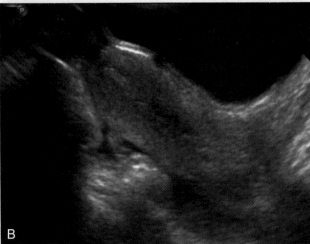

FIGURE 26-67. Granulosa cell tumor in 5½-year-old child with onset of menses. **A,** Abdominal ultrasound shows a mass adjacent to and above the mass, likely arising from the left ovary. **B,** Note the postpubertal appearance of the uterus, indicating a hormonally active mass. Luteinizing hormone–to–follicle-stimulating hormone ratio < 0.1, estradiol = 144.5 pg/mL (normal for a child of this age is 0-30 pg/mL). BL, bladder.

The distinction between neoplastic masses of the ovary and non-neoplastic cysts, particularly hemorrhagic cysts, may be difficult. Non-neoplastic cysts are the most common causes for ovarian masses in infants and adolescent girls.[181] These hormonally responsive lesions arise as a result of follicular stimulation and/or corpus luteal maturation. Serial imaging by ultrasound is helpful in documenting the stability and resolution of these benign processes and helps make the distinction from their malignant neoplastic counterparts. Complex cysts and hemorrhagic cysts may be challenging to distinguish from solid neoplasms and MRI, with inclusion of fat suppression and magnetic susceptibility weighted sequences, can be helpful in discriminating fat-containing solid masses from complex hemorrhagic cysts.

Testicular Germ Cell Tumors

Malignant testicular tumors are primarily of germ cell origin, with most of these being malignant. The most common malignant testicular germ cell tumor is the yolk sac, or endodermal sinus, tumor. Other malignant germ cell tumors include embryonal carcinoma and teratocarcinoma. The benign teratomas seen more frequently in the ovary are less commonly encountered in the testes. Adult type tumors such as seminomas and choriocarcinomas are less frequently encountered in infancy, and begin to emerge around the time of puberty.[181]

Most testicular masses present with nontender scrotal swelling. Elevated serum AFP levels are common and there is often spread to adjacent inguinal and retroperitoneal lymph nodes. The initial evaluation is usually by ultrasound to assess for the presence of a testicular mass and to distinguish between malignancy and non-neoplastic causes of scrotal swelling, such as epididymo-orchitis, inguinal hernia or hydrocele, and testicular torsion. Sonographic features include an intratesticular mass with increased or decreased echogenicity relative to the testicular parenchyma (Fig. 26-68). Color and Doppler assessment frequently reveal increased vascularity. The presence of an associated hydrocele, thickening of the spermatic cord, and extension of the mass through the tunica albuginea may indicate extratesticular spread of disease.[181] Once a mass has been confirmed, the staging evaluation should include imaging of the chest, abdomen, and pelvis to assess for regional lymph node spread and evidence of hematogenous disease spread, particularly to the liver and lungs.

FDG-PET scanning has been advocated for staging and follow-up evaluation of patients with malignant germ cell tumors, with several studies showing the effectiveness of FDG-PET in identifying sites of disease that would otherwise have escaped detection on conventional cross-sectional imaging alone.[205-207] One should be aware of the potential for false-negative findings on FDG-PET, particularly in the setting of mature differentiated teratoma.[207]

Non-germ cell tumors of the testes include Sertoli and Leydig cell tumors, both of stromal origin, as well as leukemia and lymphoma. Sertoli cell tumors are more common in infancy, with Leydig cell tumors occurring in early childhood, often accompanied by virilization or gynecomastia.

Sonographically, these testicular lesions are frequently heterogeneous and hypoechoic relative to the normal testicular parenchyma, and usually demonstrate increased blood flow. MRI is not usually required to characterize the local site of disease; however, the MRI features of these testicular lesions include decreased signal intensity on T1-weighted images relative to the normal testicular parenchyma, increased T2 signal intensity, and heterogeneous enhancement. As with testicular germ cell tumors, extension into the spermatic cord, as well as inguinal and retroperitoneal lymph node involvement, can be effectively demonstrated by MRI.

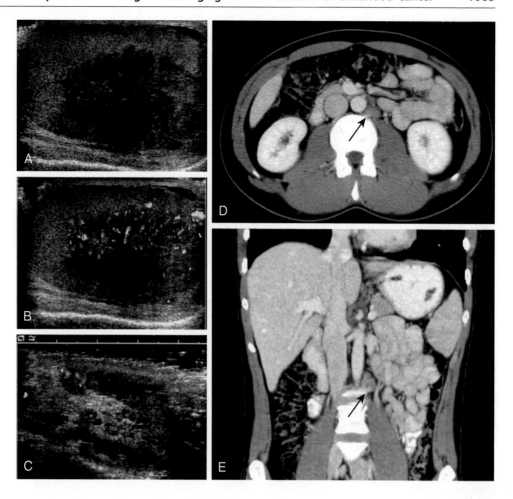

FIGURE 26-68. Testicular germ cell tumor (embryonal carcinoma) in an 18-year-old with palpable left testicular mass. **A,** Ultrasound shows hypoechoic mass with increased vascularity **(B)** and thickening of the epididymis and spermatic cord **(C).** A small hydrocele was also present. CT showed an enlarged left retroperitoneal lymph node, suspicious for extratesticular spread of disease **(D, E,** *arrows*).

In children with cryptorchid testes, the presence of an undescended testicle is considered a major factor leading to development of testicular tumors in childhood. Although the increased relative risk varies in published reports, there is little dispute that the risk of testicular cancer is increased in children and men with undistended testes.

Withdrawal of maternal estrogen at birth leads to a rise in testosterone and stimulation of testicular descent. Spontaneous descent of testes into the scrotum after 1 year of age is uncommon. The imaging evaluation of children with undescended testes should include a thorough ultrasound examination, with examination of the scrotum, inguinal canal regions, retroperitoneum, and kidneys. Frequently, undescended testes can be located in the inguinal canal and effectively relocated in the scrotum by orchidopexy. The retroperitoneal location of the undescended testes, although less common, is associated with a higher risk of malignancy as compared with those located in the inguinal canal. MRI may also be helpful for identifying undescended testes not detectable by ultrasound, particularly in older children, in whom the homogeneously T2 bright testes can often be located along the expected pathway of descent of the developing testes.

Sacrococcygeal Germ Cell Tumors

Sacrococcygeal germ cell tumors are the most common germ cell tumor in children. These germ cell tumors include mature and immature teratomas and endodermal sinus tumors. Both mature and immature teratomas are considered benign, whereas mixed malignant germ cell tumors indicate the presence of benign teratomatous elements and malignant yolk sac (endodermal sinus) tumor elements. Most sacrococcygeal teratomas are detected in the newborn period, whereas endodermal sinus tumors may be discovered later in childhood.[208] With the advent of prenatal sonography and prenatal MRI, an extensive prebirth evaluation of the tumor can be performed, facilitating a prompt surgical resection.

Sacrococcygeal teratomas are classified according to the system of Altman[209] as type I, predominantly external with a very small presacral component; type II, predominantly external with a significant intrapelvic component; type III, predominantly internal, with both pelvic and intraabdominal components; and type IV, entirely presacral, without significant intra-abdominal or external extension. The incidence of malignant elements is closely linked to the type of tumor, with almost 40% of type IV tumors having malignant components.[181]

In addition to the prenatal imaging evaluation, CT and MRI can be used to stage sacrococcygeal teratomas effectively.[208] MRI is often preferable for determining the extent of adjacent muscular, neurovascular, and intra-abdominal invasion. MRI findings typically reflect the heterogeneous nature of these tumors, with variable signal intensity on T1-weighted images, increased signal intensity on T2-weighted images, and heterogeneous enhancement following contrast administration (Fig. 26-69).[182] The presence of calcification, bone, and other more mature tissue elements may be better seen on CT. Metastatic disease to the lung, liver, and draining retroperitoneal lymph nodes can occur, and CT scanning of the chest and

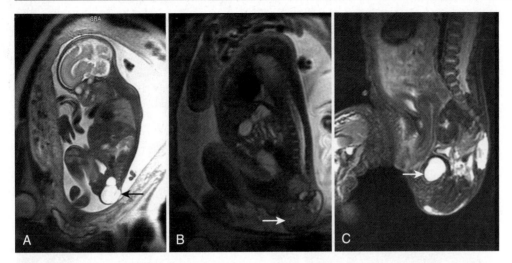

FIGURE 26-69. Sacrococcygeal germ cell tumor. Prenatal MR images show both cystic (**A**) and solid elements (**B**) within a large presacral mass. At birth, the solid elements predominated, although large cystic spaces were still present (**C**). Arrows indicate the presacral mass.

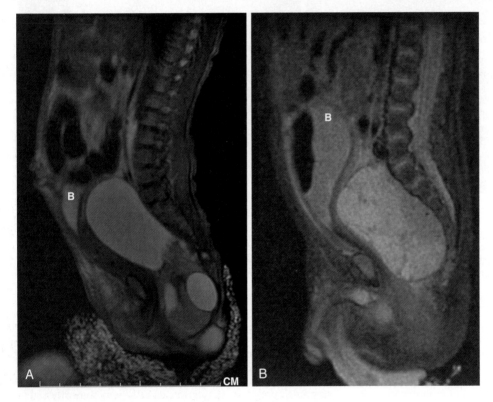

FIGURE 26-70. Sacrococcygeal germ cell tumor (**A**) and presacral cystic neuroblastoma (**B**) in two patients with prenatally diagnosed cystic presacral mass. Fluid-sensitive MRI showed similar-appearing complex cystic masses, both compressing the bladder *(B)*, with very similar imaging appearance, emphasizing the importance of including neuroblastoma in the differential for some sacrococcygeal teratomas.

abdomen is an important component of the staging evaluation. Approximately 20% of these patients have pulmonary metastases at the time of diagnosis.[181]

These tumors arise from coccygeal tissue elements, and surgical resection must include resection of the coccyx. When complete resection can be accomplished, survival rates are higher than 95% with tumors that have benign mature teratomatous elements. The presence of malignant elements results in much lower rates of long-term survival.[181]

In addition to sacrococcygeal teratomas, presacral solid masses that must also be included in the differential include neuroblastoma and lymphoma. In particular, the distinction between presacral cystic neuroblastoma and type IV germ cell tumor may be difficult on the basis of imaging alone (Fig. 26-70). The presence of intraspinal extension, which is commonly seen in neuroblastoma, is unusual in the setting of sacro-

coccygeal germ cell tumor, aiding in the differential diagnosis. Predominantly cystic germ cell tumors may also be difficult to distinguish from lumbosacral myelomeningoceles or the related fat-containing lipomyelomeningocele. Again the extent of intraspinal involvement, which is best demonstrated by MRI, may help in narrowing the differential diagnosis.

MUSCULOSKELETAL NEOPLASMS

Pediatric bone tumors are relatively rare, comprising less than 5% of the new cancer diagnoses in children younger than 9 years, and between 8% to 11% in children between the ages of 10 and 19 years. Osteosarcoma is the most common primary malignant bone tumor occurring in the first 2 decades of life.

The remaining bone malignancies include the Ewing's family of tumors (Ewing's sarcoma) and primary lymphoma of the bone. Because symptoms are frequently nonspecific, there is often a delay in diagnosis. The goal of the imaging evaluation is to establish a preliminary diagnosis,[210] because about 50% of bone lesions detected in children are benign. Based on these preliminary assessments, a more detailed imaging evaluation can then be undertaken. It is beyond the scope of this review to discuss the nonmalignant lesions that may mimic malignancy; however, chronic osteomyelitis, osteoid osteoma, bone cysts, and stress-related injury are all included in the differential considerations for primary bone lesions.[211]

Conventional radiography is essential as a first step in the evaluation.[212] Radiographs afford high spatial resolution, can be readily obtained, are relatively inexpensive, and do not require sedation. Most importantly, the radiographs are critical in guiding the next step in the evaluation, based on the pattern of bone reaction and involvement and surrounding soft tissue involvement. MRI is usually the imaging modality of choice to characterize primary bone lesions further.[210,211] MRI sequences should include, at a minimum, T1- and T2-weighted imaging in at least two orthogonal planes as well as post–gadolinium-enhanced imaging. Fat suppression sequences are almost always of value in distinguishing focal areas of enhancement from intramedullary fatty marrow or surrounding soft tissue fat. Fluid-sensitive sequences are highly sensitive, but lack specificity, and tumor, edema, hemorrhage, and focal fluid collections all may show increased signal on fluid-sensitive sequences. More importantly, the fluid-sensitive sequences allow the relationship of signal abnormalities in the bone and soft tissues to adjacent neurovascular structures to be closely assessed. It remains controversial whether post–gadolinium contrast-enhanced images, simple T1-weighted images, or fat-suppressed T2-weighted images allow the best discrimination between the true intraosseous tumor margins and surrounding peritumoral edema and bone reaction.

CT has a relatively limited role in assessing the primary bone lesions, given the increased use of MRI. However, for focal bone lesions such as osteoid osteoma, CT is helpful in characterizing the focal osseous abnormality. In addition, for primary bone tumors, particularly Ewing's sarcoma involving the chest wall and ribs, CT may be preferable. The staging evaluation of primary bone tumors must also include a CT of the chest to assess for pulmonary metastatic disease. The use of bone scintigraphy, using ^{99m}Tc or ^{18}F, is often useful for assessing multifocal sites of disease.[65] FDG-PET scanning, although not in common practice, has been shown in several studies to be effective in detecting sites of lymph node spread and metastatic disease outside of the primary site and for helping determine the margin of metabolically active tumor involvement.[111,213-215] In addition, FDG-PET scanning has been effective at showing early responses to chemotherapy; studies have shown that early responses to chemotherapy, manifest as decreased metabolic activity and decreased FDG uptake, correlate with improved outcome and overall survival.[104,111,216,217]

Osteosarcoma

Osteosarcomas are the most common primary bone tumor occurring in children older than 10 years, with Ewing's sarcoma being more common in younger children.[218-220] This may relate to the period of rapid bone growth occurring in early or mid-adolescence, corresponding to the peak incidence of osteosarcoma. Most osteosarcomas are of the classic high-grade histologic type, with telangiectatic and surface osteosarcomas occurring with less frequency; the latter two entities are divided into paraosteal and periosteal subtypes. Osteosarcomas most commonly occur in the metaphysis of the rapidly growing ends of the long bones, including distal femur, proximal tibia, proximal femur, and proximal humerus. Involvement of the axial skeleton and flat bones is much less common, except where osteosarcoma has developed secondary to radiation treatment or chemotherapy. At diagnosis, approximately 20% of patients will have pulmonary metastatic disease detectable by chest CT. Other sites of metastatic disease spread are unusual.

The radiographic appearance of osteosarcoma varies widely; however, the typical lesion is an aggressive destructive lesion centered in the metaphysis (Fig. 26-71). Smaller lesions may show periosteal reaction, most commonly a sunburst-type

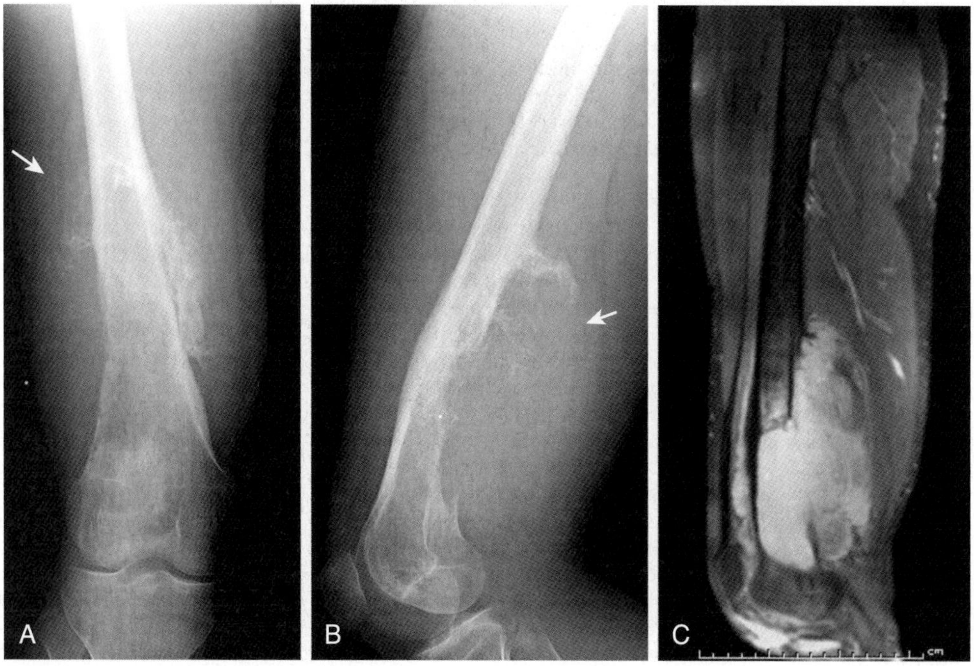

FIGURE 26-71. Osteosarcoma in 19-year-old young man with enlarging right leg mass. **A, B,** Radiographs show a large destructive lesion with extensive periosteal reaction. A large soft tissue mass is also evident on the radiographs (*arrows*). **C,** MRI shows better delineation of the associated soft tissue mass and the extent of osseous involvement.

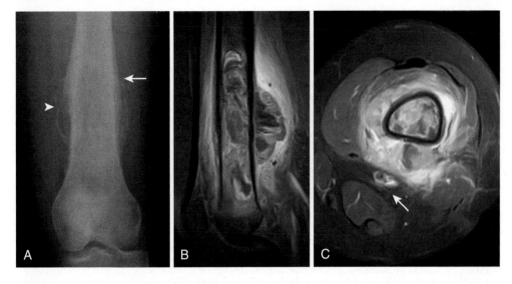

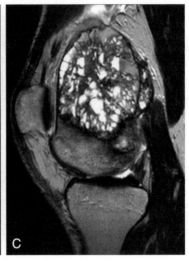

FIGURE 26-72. 14-year-old girl with osteosarcoma. **A,** Radiograph shows a large distal femoral destructive lesion with osteoblastic activity, lamellated periosteal reaction (*arrow*) and Codman's triangle (*arrowhead*). **B,** Contrast-enhanced MRI shows the associated soft tissue mass to better advantage, and the extent of bone involvement. **C,** Axial MR image shows mass abutting the neurovascular bundle (*arrow*), but not encompassing it.

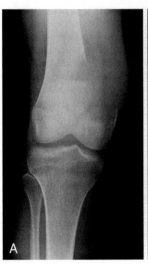

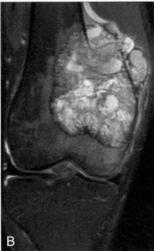

FIGURE 26-73. Osteosarcoma in 18-year-old man with leg pain and swelling. **A,** Radiograph shows a destructive lesion in the distal femur with an associated soft tissue mass. Gadolinium contrast-enhanced **(B)** and fluid-sensitive fast spin-echo inversion recovery **(C)** MR images demonstrate multiple fluid-fluid levels with heterogeneous contrast enhancement. The appearance is common in telangiectatic osteosarcoma, but in this patient, with high-grade metastatic osteosarcoma, it was caused by multiple solid and necrotic elements within the tumor.

reaction. Codman's triangle formation indicates periosteal new bone formation with the free edge of the periosteal new bone disrupted by growth of the tumor mass. A lamellated onion-skin-type periosteal reaction may also be seen in smaller lesions, but this is more typically associated with Ewing's sarcoma. Although the diagnosis of osteosarcoma is usually suggested by plain films, they are relatively insensitive at determining the extent of disease. As noted earlier, MRI is essential for determining the extent of long bone involvement and the degree of soft tissue involvement and invasion into adjacent neurovascular structures (Fig. 26-72).[219,221] Although we tend to think of epiphyseal involvement and crossing of the growth plate by osteosarcoma as unusual, reports have suggested that this may occur in as many as 80% of patients.

MRI is also helpful for characterizing the primary lesion. The presence of fluid-fluid levels, common to telangiectatic osteosarcoma, is best demonstrated by MRI (Fig. 26-73). The initial imaging evaluation should also assess for the presence of pathologic fracture, and must include the joint proximal and distal to the primary lesion to aid in surgical planning and decision making. Skeletal scintigraphy and chest CT are necessary for the staging evaluation to assess for locoregional and distant metastatic disease.[219] Follow-up imaging will usually be dic-tated by individual treatment protocols, but typically includes imaging of the primary site of disease and chest CT.

Ewing's Sarcoma

Ewing's sarcoma is usually a poorly differentiated tumor arising from the bone, although it may also arise from adjacent soft tissues. The neuroectodermal derivative of this tumor is known as the peripheral primitive neuroectodermal tumor (PPNET). Ewing's sarcomas arising in the chest wall comprise about 10% of the Ewing's family of tumors. Clinically, pain and a palpable mass are the most common presenting complaints. As with osteosarcoma, the imaging evaluation should be initially directed at characterizing the primary site of abnormality. Anatomically, Ewing's sarcomas occur with roughly equal distribution in the axial and appendicular skeleton, with about two thirds occurring in the pelvis and/or lower extremities. At the time of presentation, the size of the mass and extensive local invasion may make it difficult to determine whether the lesion has arisen primarily within the bone or surrounding soft tissue. Metastatic disease is also common at the time of diagnosis, with sites of metastatic disease reflecting hematogenous spread, including lung, bone, and bone marrow.

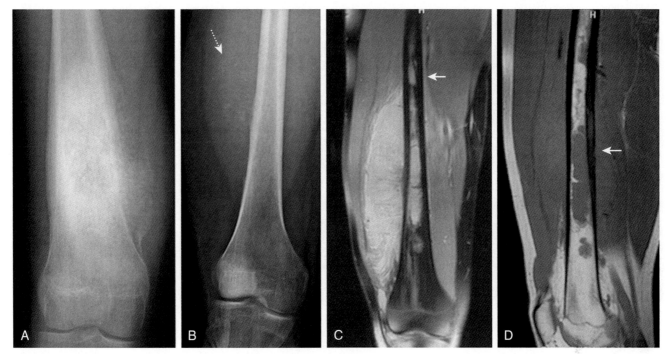

FIGURE 26-74. Ewing's sarcoma—radiographs from two patients with Ewing's sarcoma, showing the onionskin periosteal reaction characteristic of this tumor **(A)** and the sunburst periosteal reaction that is also frequently seen **(B,** *dashed arrow*). Fast spin-echo fat-suppressed T2-weighted (FSE T2/fs, **C**) and T1-weighted **(D)** MR images from the patient shown in **B** demonstrate intramedullary high signal on the FSE T2/fs images **(C)** and corresponding loss of normal intramedullary fat signal **(D)**, indicating more widely extensive tumor than suggested by the radiographic findings and highlighting the importance of MRI in evaluating the extent of disease in these patients.

Radiographically, Ewing's sarcoma of the bone is primarily a lytic lesion with a permeative destructive appearance.[222] The onionskin or lamellated periosteal reaction is characteristically described with Ewing's sarcoma, although it is not specific for this diagnosis, and other forms of periosteal reaction are also seen (Fig. 26-74), reflecting the variable degree of bone destruction and bone response to the tumor. There is usually a large accompanying soft tissue mass. Particularly in the axial skeleton (pelvis and ribs), the soft tissue component may predominate.

Plain radiographs should include imaging of the involved long bones, chest, and/or pelvis. MRI is indicated to further assess the appendicular skeleton and long bones and, as with osteosarcoma, the entire length of the bone, including the proximal and distal joints, should be included. The choice of MRI pulse sequence is similar to osteosarcoma, but should include at minimum T1-weighted and fat-suppressed T2-weighted images in orthogonal planes as well as post–gadolinium-enhanced images. The axial images, particularly proton density and T2-weighted, are useful for demonstrating the extent of subperiosteal and periosteal extension, and neurovascular invasion. Sagittal or coronal images are effective for defining the margin of bone marrow involvement and surrounding tissue edema.

Rib and chest wall lesions are best evaluated by CT and, particularly with multiplanar three-dimensional image reconstruction capabilities on modern CT scanners, the extent of osseous involvement and adjacent lung and pleural involvement can usually be adequately demonstrated by CT (Fig. 26-75). For paraspinal lesions, MRI may be necessary to delineate intraspinal invasion. MRI is also useful for characterizing subtle abnormalities and chest wall muscle involvement as well as

neurovascular involvement, particularly in the upper thorax and lung apices.

In contrast to osteogenic sarcoma, Ewing's sarcoma does not typically show the presence of soft tissue calcifications. Bone scintigraphy is effective for delineating sites of skeletal involvement; however, there is no clear evidence that skeletal scintigraphy is superior to MRI for characterizing local disease. FDG-PET scanning has recently been advocated for the staging evaluation of Ewing's sarcoma, particularly with respect to identifying sites of occult bone marrow metastatic disease. In addition, as with osteosarcoma, the use of FDG-PET has been advocated for monitoring response to therapy (Fig. 26-76).[58,104,214,216]

Other Bone Tumors

Primary lymphoma of the bone is a relatively unusual site of presentation in non-Hodgkin's lymphoma, but must be included in the differential diagnosis of a primary destructive lesion with intramedullary involvement. Radiographically, the evaluation is similar to that for Ewing's sarcoma, and biopsy is usually needed to confirm the diagnosis.

Although not primary bone neoplasms, leukemia and Langerhans cell histiocytosis (LCH) are both pediatric neoplastic conditions that may manifest as bone involvement. Leukemia, described later, often produces metaphyseal lucency and may result in an aggressive permeative, moth-eaten appearance to the bone, occasionally accompanied by periosteal reaction. Pain is also common at this stage of bone reaction to the leukemic involvement of the bone. Langerhans cell histiocytosis can manifest as localized disease or widespread osseous involve-

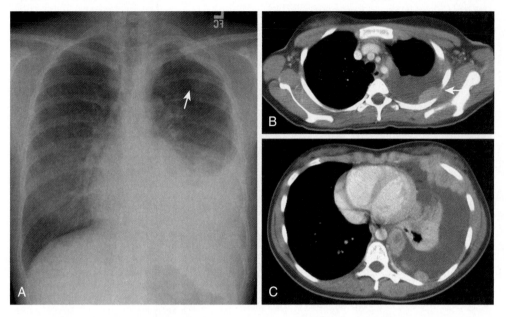

FIGURE 26-75. Ewing's sarcoma of the chest wall in a 14-year-old girl with chest pain. **A,** Chest x-ray shows a large left pleural effusion and multiple nodular densities (*arrow*), apparently arising from the chest wall and pleura. **B, C,** Contrast-enhanced CT scans show extensive soft tissue masses lining the chest cavity, with large effusion and left lower lobe collapse. Biopsy showed Ewing's sarcoma.

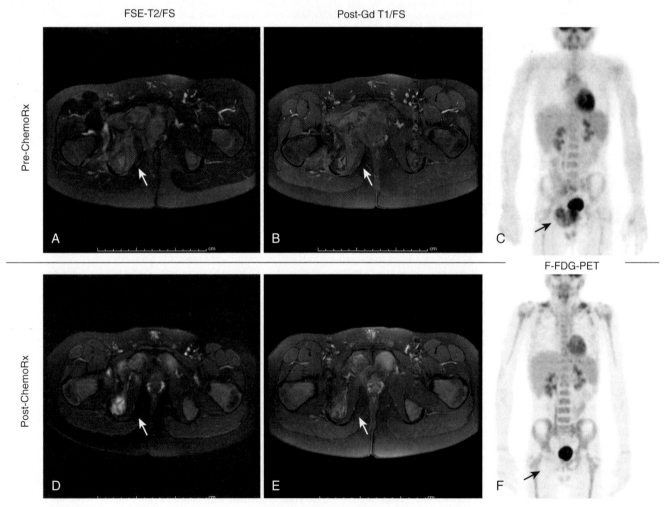

FIGURE 26-76. Ewing's sarcoma response assessment of 10-year-old child with nonmetastatic Ewing's sarcoma of the right pelvis. T2-weighted **(A, D)** and contrast-enhanced T1-weighted MR **(B, E)** images show ill-defined enhancing mass centered in the right ischium, with soft extension into the surrounding pelvis. Pretreatment ^{18}F-FDG-PET image **(C)** shows moderately intense uptake in the mass. **D, E,** Following chemotherapy, MRI shows persistent areas of increased T2 signal and enhancement; FDG-PET **(F)** shows no residual metabolic activity in the mass, demonstrating an excellent response to therapy and suggesting the MRI findings may relate to necrotic tumor and enhancing scar or granulation tissue rather than active disease.

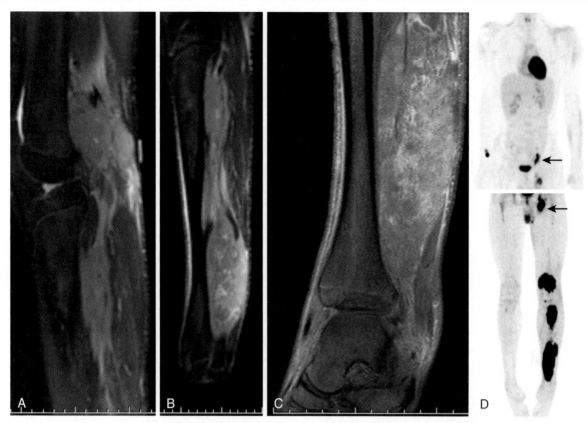

FIGURE 26-77. Rhabdomyosarcoma in 16-year-old with left leg mass and MRI findings showing T2 bright **(A, B)** enhancing **(C)** lesion localized in the deep soft tissues of the calf with extension proximally along fascial planes into the popliteal fossa **(A)**. **D,** FDG-PET showed multiple sites of disease, including left inguinal lymph node involvement that would not have been detected on the MRI. Biopsy showed alveolar rhabdomyosarcoma.

ment. Typical LCH osseous lesions are lytic on conventional radiographs. Because they are relatively slow-growing and do not elicit a significant response from the surrounding bone, these lesions may go undetected by bone scintigraphy, and a skeletal survey is still advocated to assess for the extent of osseous involvement in LCH. Recent studies have also suggested that FDG-PET scanning may be more sensitive for determining sites of intraosseous involvement and sites of soft tissue involvement that would go undetected by conventional scintigraphy or skeletal survey.[4]

Muscle and Soft Tissue Tumors

The nonosseous musculoskeletal malignancies of childhood are typically sarcomas that arise from immature mesenchymal tissue. Rhabdomyosarcomas, of skeletal muscle origin, comprise about half of pediatric soft tissue sarcomas.[220,223] The nonrhabdomyomatous soft tissue sarcomas include fibrosarcoma, synovial sarcoma, alveolar soft part sarcoma, malignant fibrous histiocytoma, and primitive peripheral neuroectodermal tumors. Ultimately, the distinction between these different histiologic subtypes is made pathologically. The imaging approach is directed at determining the size and extent of primary tumor involvement, relationship to critical adjacent structures such as nerves and blood vessels, and local involvement of bone or regional lymph nodes. All the soft tissue sarcomas have a propensity to metastasize to the lung, and a CT of the chest should be performed at the time of diagnosis. Bone scintigraphy is also indicated to assess for additional sites of skeletal involvement.

Rhabdomyosarcomas are the most common soft tissue sarcoma of childhood, making up more than half of all soft tissue sarcomas in children.[220] Although the head and neck and genitourinary tract are common sites of rhabdomyosarcoma presentation, about 25% of these tumors are also located in the extremities. These are typically of the alveolar or undifferentiated histologic type.[224] The imaging characteristics are not specific but typically a T2 bright lesion is seen localized in the deep soft tissues, with extension along fascial planes (Fig. 26-77). Following contrast infusion, these tend to be hypervascular tumors with bright enhancement. FDG-PET scanning has been shown in several studies to yield intense FDG uptake and may be of value for identifying sites of occult disease at the time of staging and assessing response to therapy.[111,225]

Synovial Sarcoma

Synovial sarcoma typically occurs in older patients in their teenage years. Synovial sarcomas are the most common nonrhabdomyosarcomatous soft tissues in children[223] and, despite their name, arise from undifferentiated mesenchymal cells, typically located in a para-articular location. They are more common in the lower extremities than in the upper extremities or axial skeleton. Conventional radiographs are indicated for extremity lesions and show calcifications in about 30% of cases. MRI shows a lobulated lesion that is usually isointense to muscle on T1-weighted images and isointense to slightly hyperintense on T2-weighted images, with a relatively homogeneous appearance.[226] Following contrast infusion, there is typically intense enhancement (Fig. 26-78). Although these findings are

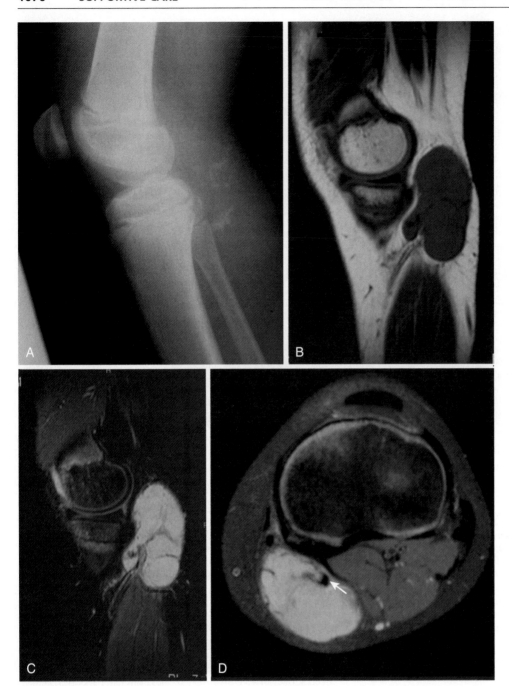

FIGURE 26-78. Synovial sarcoma in 11-year-old child with palpable leg mass showing a calcified mass behind the knee (**A**). MRI shows lobular mass in the medial compartment posterior to the knee, encasing the semimembranous tendon (**D**, *arrow*), characterized by low signal on T1-weighted images (**B**), high signal on T2-weighted images (**C**) and intense contrast enhancement (**D**). These features are all characteristic findings in synovial sarcoma.

not specific for synovial sarcoma, the presence of a lobulated calcified lesion with the earlier described MRI signal characteristics should suggest the diagnosis.

The clinical presentation is typically of a painless mass. The median duration of symptoms before presentation is approximately 14 months. The staging evaluation is important for predicting the overall survival of these patients. Patients with localized disease and/or with disease allowing gross total resection have an estimated 80% 5-year overall survival, as compared with patients with metastatic disease at diagnosis for whom the diagnosis is almost always fatal. These lesions most often occur in extremities and may mimic benign disease such as synovial or ganglion cysts. The MRI examination, therefore, must include contrast enhancement to discriminate between a

solid enhancing lesion and a predominantly fluid-containing cystic lesion. Because of the importance of local control, imaging is also essential for determining resectability and establishing the preoperative margins for surgical planning.

Tumor size has also been shown to be a key prognostic factor in synovial sarcoma, with lesions larger than 5 cm resulting in greater than 75% metastasis-free survival, in contrast to those with lesions larger than 5 cm in whom metastasis-free survival falls to less than 50%.[227]

Infantile (Desmoid-type) Fibromatosis

Infantile fibromatosis is a benign fibrous proliferation, although it can be locally aggressive and deforming.[228] Infantile desmoid-

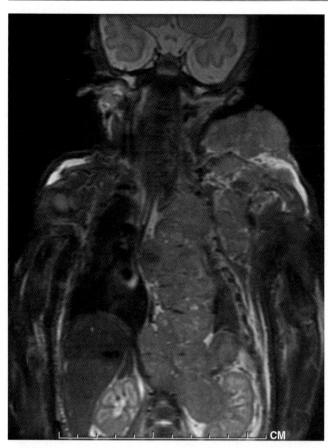

FIGURE 26-79. Infantile fibromatosis. MRI scan of 4-week-old infant shows extensive mediastinal, retroperitoneal, and intra-abdominal disease. Biopsy showed infantile fibromatosis.

type fibromatosis must be distinguished from congenital generalized fibromatosis, also known as infantile myofibromatosis.[229] This latter disorder is characterized by lesions consisting of smooth muscle and fibroblastic spindle cells in contrast to the more differentiated fibroblastic cells seen in desmoid-type fibromatosis. The presence of deep soft tissue involvement and visceral involvement of organs such as lung and liver has a worse prognosis than localized disease. The extent of involvement is optimally determined by MRI (Fig. 26-79), with lesions typically characterized by low signal on both T1- and T2-weighted sequences because of the relatively high collagen content in these tumors.[229]

It may be difficult based on imaging findings alone to distinguish between aggressive multifocal fibromatosis and congenital fibrosarcoma. The desmoid-type lesions, in contrast, tend to be localized and have a less aggressive appearance.

Other mesenchymal tumors, such as alveolar soft part sarcoma, epithelioid sarcoma, and malignancy fibrous histiosarcoma, are very rare in children and do not have distinctive imaging characteristics. As with the other mesenchymal tumors, lesions are typically isointense to slightly hyperintense on both T1- and T2-weighted images, with variable patterns of enhancement.

The distinction between liposarcoma and the benign lipoblastoma cannot be made on the basis of imaging alone, with both lesions showing high signal intensity on T1-weighted images, decreased signal intensity on T2-weighted images, and minimal enhancement. As with the other malignant sarcomas, metastatic disease to the chest must be excluded and the staging evaluation should include chest CT.

LYMPHOPROLIFERATIVE NEOPLASMS

Leukemia

Of the pediatric cancers, approximately one third are leukemias. Together with brain tumors, leukemia accounts for over half of childhood tumors.

More than 75% of pediatric leukemia is acute lymphoblastic leukemia (ALL),[230] and most patients have B-lineage ALL, with 15% to 20% having T-cell ALL and 1% to 2% with mature B-cell ALL. Acute myelogenous leukemia (AML) makes up 15% to 20% of pediatric leukemia cases; the remainder are leukemias that are uncommon in children, such as chronic myelogenous leukemia and juvenile myelomonocytic leukemia.

The most common presenting symptoms and physical examination findings are nonspecific and include fever, bleeding, bone pain, lymphadenopathy, and splenomegaly. In addition to fatigue, pallor, and anorexia, which are seen in almost all leukemic patients, hepatosplenomegaly and fever are seen in approximately two thirds of cases.

Because of the nonspecific nature of presenting symptoms and physical examination findings, radiologic imaging may be useful for confirmation and for directing the next step in the evaluation. Common imaging findings include pulmonary edema, secondary to high-output cardiac failure in the setting of peripheral leukemic blast crisis (related to anemia), organomegaly, including enlargement of the spleen, liver, kidneys, and heart, and pulmonary air space opacities, related to leukostasis or infection.[231] Skeletal changes can range from subtle metaphyseal lucent bands to frank bone destruction resulting from leukemic infiltration. CNS hemorrhage may be encountered as a result of leukostasis and thrombocytopenia in patients with very high peripheral leukemic cell counts.[232] Although such imaging findings alone do not make the diagnosis of leukemia, the initial imaging evaluation can be critical in assessing the overall physiologic burden of the patient's disease.

Acute Lymphoblastic Leukemia

Peripheral skeletal lesions may be detected on conventional radiographs in approximately 25% of patients newly diagnosed with ALL.[233] In the patient presenting with fatigue and poorly localized bone pain, metaphyseal lucent bands (also known as leukemic lines) may be seen (Fig. 26-80). This finding was initially thought to represent leukemic infiltration in the submetaphyseal bone, although the discovery of elevated parathyroid hormone levels in patients with leukemia has suggested paraneoplastic effects on bone resorption likely contribute to the observed radiographic changes.[234] Metaphyseal lucent lines are not unique to leukemia, and may also be seen in other marrow-infiltrative malignancies, such as neuroblastoma and lymphoma, and in response to physiologic stress, such as infection, systemic inflammatory reactions, and radiation.

Metaphyseal lucent lines may be difficult to distinguish from the diffuse metaphyseal lucency that represents a combination of direct leukemic infiltration of the bone and accompanying bone resorption. This pattern of infiltration typically results in a broad irregularity and more poorly demarcated pattern of metaphyseal lucency. It is also frequently associated with pain and localized tenderness and, depending on the degree of bone destruction, may also be accompanied by focal lytic lesions. Leukemic infiltration of the bone can also yield a moth-eaten appearance with a marked pattern of periosteal reaction.

More advanced imaging techniques such as MRI may be helpful for demonstrating the extent of leukemic infiltration by

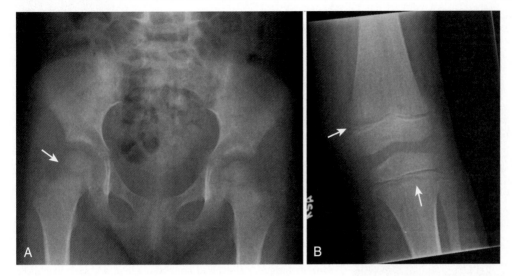

FIGURE 26-80. Leukemic lines in 4½-year-old child with limp and leg pain. **A, B,** Radiographs of the hips, pelvis, and knees show submetaphyseal lucency and loss of the normal trabecular architecture, particularly in the femoral necks **(A)**, distal femoral and proximal tibial metaphyses **(B)** (*arrows*). Bone marrow aspiration confirmed leukemia.

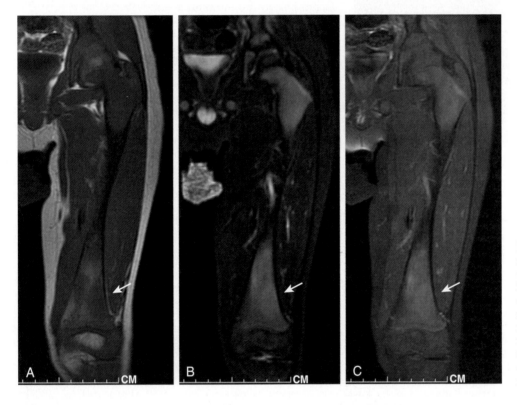

FIGURE 26-81. MRI of marrow infiltration in leukemia in 3-year-old child with persistent limp and lower extremity pain. MRI (*arrows*) showed patchy areas of marrow replacement **(A)**, heterogeneous increased signal **(B)** and enhancement **(C),** suggestive of diffuse marrow infiltration. Bone marrow aspiration confirmed acute B-lymphoblastic leukemia.

showing focal and diffuse replacement of normal fatty marrow signal (Fig. 26-81).[235] However, heterogeneous patterns of marrow signal are a normal finding in children, because hematopoietic marrow gradually converts to fatty marrow. Furthermore, therapeutic agents that stimulate bone marrow recovery following ablative chemotherapy (e.g., CSF) can mimic leukemic marrow replacement, and the extent of leukemic infiltration may be difficult to determine on the basis of MRI.[236,237]

In the setting of T-cell acute lymphoblastic leukemia (T-ALL), children and adolescents frequently present with wheezing caused by large mediastinal masses (Fig. 26-82). The diffuse thymic infiltration seen in T-ALL (and T-cell lymphoblastic lymphoma) typically produces a bland, homogeneous-appearing mediastinal mass (Fig. 26-83). Pericardial and pleural effusions are common, as is leukemic infiltration of the kidneys. Despite the bulky disease frequently encountered at the time of presentation, T-ALL and lymphoblastic lymphomas respond rapidly to chemotherapy. Within a short period of time, radiographic studies return to normal, although the significance of incomplete response of the mediastinal mass to therapy with respect to overall outcome is uncertain.[238]

Childhood Acute Myelogenous Leukemia

Acute myelogenous leukemia represents a heterogeneous group of leukemias encompassing the spectrum and extent of myeloid differentiation.[239] When patients with AML present with high peripheral blast counts (leukocyte counts higher than 100,000/mm³), clinical leukostasis may result, characterized by global CNS changes or respiratory distress caused by pulmonary vascular involvement. Imaging findings in the brain may suggest diffuse microvascular thrombi (Fig. 26-84), without focal neurologic signs. CNS changes secondary to leukostasis may be difficult to detect by CT and standard MRI sequences, but are readily demonstrated on paramagnetic susceptibility-sensitive gradient echo sequences, caused by the paramagnetic effects of

hemoglobin breakdown products (i.e., hemosiderin) accumulating at sites of microvascular thrombus formation.

Acute promyelocytic leukemia (APML) accounts for 5% to 10% of childhood AML and characteristically presents with a severe consumptive coagulopathy, which is further exacerbated by cytotoxic chemotherapy because of cell lysis and release of procoagulant intracellular contents. The resulting coagulopathy can result in clinically significant bleeding, necessitating emergent imaging studies to assess for cerebral hemorrhage, which can be profound and rapidly progressive (see Fig. 26-84).

Chloromas (also called granulocytic sarcomas) are seen in up to 10% of patients with AML, and are also encountered in chronic myelogenous leukemia (CML) and myelodysplasia.[240] They are frequently asymptomatic; however, CNS involvement can result in mental status changes and lead to focal neurologic deficits. CNS chloromas are typically extra-axial and contiguous with the meninges. They may be almost undetectable by CT, where they are isodense or occasionally hyperdense, to normal cortex. On MRI, these lesions are typically hypointense to isointense on T1-weighted images and heterogeneously isointense to hyperintense on T2-weighted images, with homogeneous contrast enhancement (Fig. 26-85).[240] Outside the CNS, chloromas commonly produce adjacent bone destruction and are often seen in the orbits, spine, paranasal sinuses, and adjacent soft tissues.[240] Chloromas are radiosensitive and chemosensitive, although they still have an approximately 25% recurrence rate.

Lymphoma

Pediatric lymphomas are classified as Hodgkin's or non-Hodgkin's lymphomas.[241,242] Because there is considerable overlap in the imaging features, age at presentation and sites of involve-

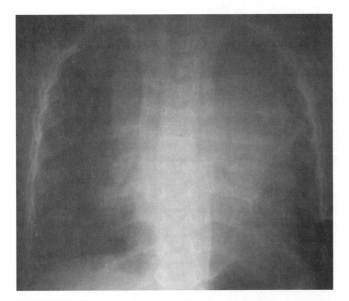

FIGURE 26-82. T-ALL in 4-year-old with first-time wheezing. This chest x-ray shows a large mediastinal mass and narrowing of the proximal bronchi and air bronchograms, suggesting airway compression.

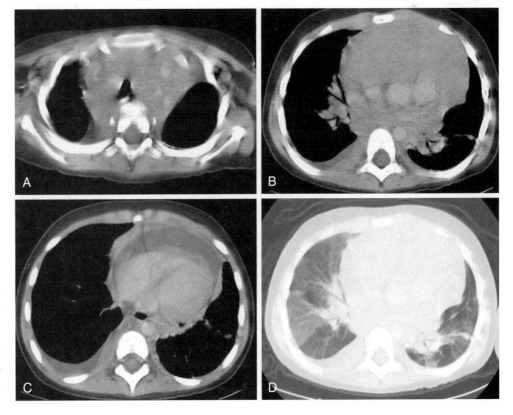

FIGURE 26-83. T-ALL leukemia in 4-year-old child (see chest x-ray in Fig. 26-82) with wheezing and mediastinal mass. Contrast-enhanced chest CT shows findings typical of T-lymphoblastic lymphoma, including mediastinal mass extending into the neck **(A)**, with homogeneous density infiltrating the thymus **(A, B)**. The mass causes marked airway compression and bronchial narrowing **(A, B)** and is associated with pericardial and pleural effusions **(C)** and mosaic lung attenuation **(D)** indicative of air trapping and airway obstruction. Based on bone marrow involvement of greater than 50% marrow, the patient was diagnosed with T-ALL.

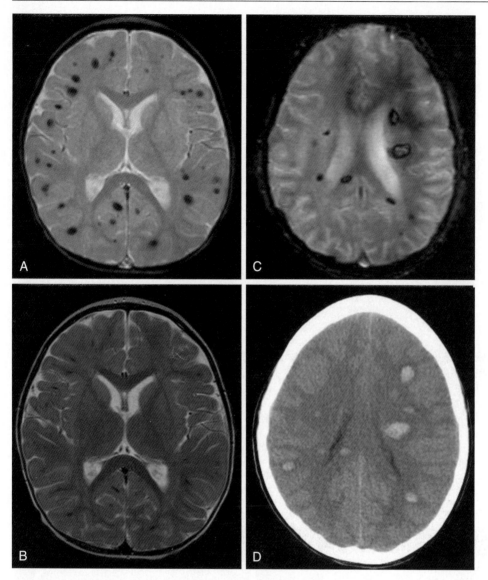

FIGURE 26-84. Acute myelocytic leukemia (AML) and acute promyelocytic leukemia (APML). Shown are gradient echo and fast spin-echo T2-weighted axial MR images through the brain of a 17-month-old girl with AML who presented with a white blood cell count >300,000/mm³. Brain MRI obtained after the patient was stabilized showed multiple areas of paramagnetic susceptibility throughout the brain (**A**), with no corresponding T2 signal abnormality (**B**); these were interpreted as foci of microthrombus formation secondary to leukostasis. A separate patient with APML presented with seizures, high WBC count, and CT showing multiple foci of acute hemorrhage (**D**). **C**, MRI showed multiple areas of paramagnetic susceptibility, likely caused by leukostasis, with acute hemorrhage caused by coagulopathy, reperfusion injury at sites of microthrombus formation, or both.

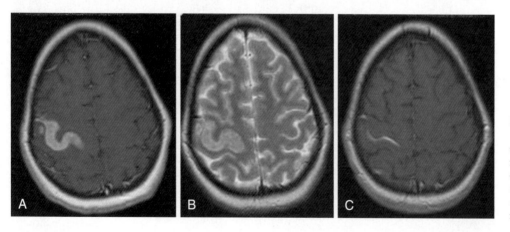

FIGURE 26-85. Chloroma in a 12-year-old with AML. Brain MRI shows typical findings of chloroma, including isointensity to cortex on T2-weighted images (**B**), homogeneous enhancement (**A**), and good response to radiation (**C**).

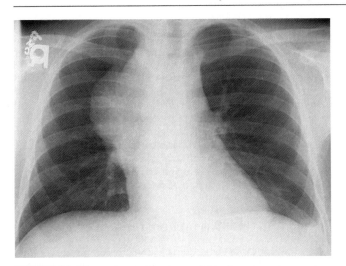

FIGURE 26-86. Hodgkin's lymphoma. This chest x-ray in a patient presenting with nonspecific upper respiratory infection symptoms shows anterior mediastinal and paratracheal masses.

ment are useful for helping distinguishing the types of disease.

Hodgkin's Disease

In Hodgkin's lymphoma, the bulky mediastinal mass characteristically seen radiographically (Fig. 26-86) is made up primarily of inflammatory cells, with the malignant Reed-Sternberg cell, from which the histologic diagnosis of Hodgkin's disease is made, comprising only 1% or less of the cells in the bulky lymph node mass.[243] Hodgkin's disease is typified by involvement of contiguous lymph node groups,[244] and is staged according to the number and extent of lymph node involvement in distinct nodal sites.

Staging

The most commonly used staging system is the Ann Arbor system (Box 26-4),[245,246] which involves determining the extent and pattern of lymph node involvement. One unique feature of Hodgkin's disease relates to splenic involvement. For the purpose of disease staging, the spleen is considered localized lymphoid tissue, and lymphomatous infiltration of the spleen in Hodgkin's disease is not classified as stage IV metastatic disease, but rather as stage III disease.

The initial diagnosis is often prompted by chest x-ray evaluation for upper respiratory symptoms and vague constitutional symptoms, such as fever and night sweats (see Fig. 26-86). At the time of diagnosis, a mediastinal mass is encountered in more than two thirds of patients with Hodgkin's disease.[233] CT scanning is most commonly used for staging these patients. In addition to determining the extent of lymph node involvement, pericardial and pleural effusions may be seen. Multiple sites of organ involvement may also be demonstrated, most commonly liver, spleen, and kidneys (Fig. 26-87). Children do not typically present with symptoms referable to intra-abdominal disease, so a thorough radiologic evaluation (IV and oral contrast-enhanced CT, FDG-PET, and/or gallium scan) is essential to stage these patients completely. The staging evaluation for Hodgkin's disease should always include scanning of the neck to the level of the skull base to evaluate the nasopharyngeal and tonsillar lymphoid tissues (Waldeyer's ring) for tumor involvement. Extensive involvement of the lymphoid tissue in Waldeyer's ring may produce complete obliteration of

Box 26-4 | **Childhood Hodgkin's Lymphoma: Ann Arbor Classification**

STAGE I

Involvement of a single lymph node region, or direct extension from that node to an adjacent extralymphatic region—stage I(E)

STAGE II

Involvement of two or more lymph node regions (number to be indicated) on the same side of the diaphragm, or direct extension from any one of these lymph nodes to an adjacent extralymphatic organ—stage II(E)

STAGE III

Involvement of lymph node regions on both sides of the diaphragm.

Stage III(E): May be accompanied by extension to an adjacent extralymphatic organ
Stage III(S): May be accompanied by involvement of the spleen
Stage III(E+S): Involvement of both an adjacent extralymphatic organ and the spleen

STAGE IV

Noncontiguous involvement of one or more extralymphatic organs or tissues, with or without associated lymph node involvement

the airway, requiring emergent intervention by a tracheostomy. As is true for all mediastinal lymphomas, the bulky anterior mediastinal mass common in Hodgkin's disease may produce tracheal, bronchial, and central vascular compression (the superior vena cava syndrome). This can result in acute airway compromise, particularly during procedures requiring general anesthesia and muscle relaxation. In addition, large anterior mediastinal masses can produce jugular vein thrombosis, venous sinus thrombosis, and CNS venous infarction (Fig. 26-88).

Pulmonary involvement in Hodgkin's disease is unusual (seen in less than 5% of children younger than 10 years and less than 15% of adolescents[233]), but its identification may distinguish stage II from stage IV disease, resulting in dramatically different treatment regimens. Although pulmonary involvement can be extensive (Fig. 26-89), pulmonary nodules or masses are usually associated with an ipsilateral hilar mass, and probably result in part from spread along peribronchial lymphatics.[244]

In addition to staging by CT, functional imaging by gallium and FDG-PET scanning is proving essential in both staging and monitoring response to therapy (Fig. 26-90; see Figs. 26-21 and 26-22). The time course to achieving gallium negativity has been correlated with event-free and overall survival.[247] Gallium has prolonged retention in the bowel, limiting its usefulness for evaluating intraperitoneal disease.[85] FDG-PET imaging has been shown to affect staging and response assessment in a significant number of patients,[83,84,87,157,248,249] and its use in lymphoma is the subject of several new clinical trials. The purpose is to provide earlier identification of sites of relapse, as well as to identify radiographically occult disease, particularly in the spleen (see Fig. 26-90).[145] In addition, there

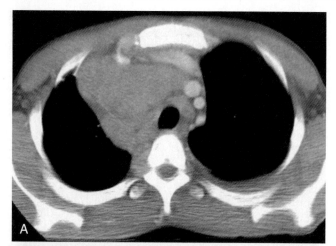

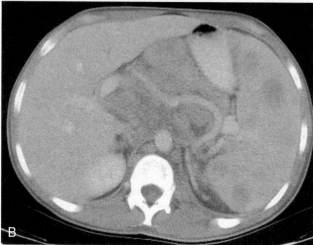

FIGURE 26-87. Hodgkin's lymphoma. This is a contrast-enhanced CT scan in a patient whose chest x-ray is shown in Figure 26-86. **A,** CT shows the mediastinal mass and left pleural effusion. **B,** The images in the abdomen show extensive splenic, mesenteric, and retroperitoneal lymphadenopathy.

is growing evidence to suggest that early response to therapy, defined as rapid early resolution of previously FDG-avid sites of disease, even in the presence of residual disease by CT or MRI, also correlates with improved overall outcome.[250] However, there have been no prospective trials in children testing whether relying solely on FDG-PET to determine early response to therapy can be used to reduce chemotherapy and radiation therapy in patients achieving a rapid early response, reserving intensified treatment regimens for patients not achieving an early response. In one adult trial, however, results have suggested that this approach may be overly simplistic; a higher rate of early relapses was observed in patients for whom involved field radiation was omitted, based on early resolution of FDG-avid disease.[251]

Non-Hodgkin's Lymphoma

The non-Hodgkin's lymphomas are a broad group of diseases.[242] Anaplastic large cell lymphoma frequently involves the soft tissues, skin, and bone, whereas Burkitt's lymphoma most commonly presents with intra-abdominal and mesenteric disease. Lymphoblastic lymphoma, particularly of the T-cell type, frequently presents with a mediastinal mass, although the appearance of the mass is characteristically distinct from the multilobulated bulky mass usually associated with Hodgkin's disease. The distinction between T-lymphoblastic lymphoma and its histologically identical leukemic counterpart is made on the basis of bone marrow aspirates—more than 25% marrow involvement results in a diagnosis of T-cell lymphoblastic leukemia.

Staging of non-Hodgkin's lymphoma in most centers is done according to the St. Jude classification (Box 26-5).[252] Although there is considerable overlap in the imaging features of the lymphomas, as shown in Figure 26-91, an anterior mediastinal mass that is not associated with other sites of significant contiguous lymph node enlargement is more likely to be non-Hodgkin's lymphoma (NHL). NHL is also more likely to be disseminated at the time of diagnosis. Chest wall and pericardial invasion are more common in the setting of NHL than in Hodgkin's lymphoma (see Fig. 26-91).[242] The mediastinal mass in acute T-lymphoblastic lymphoma characteristically responds rapidly to chemotherapy, whereas other non-Hodgkin's mediastinal lymphomas respond more slowly, with residual medias-

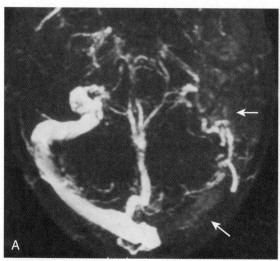

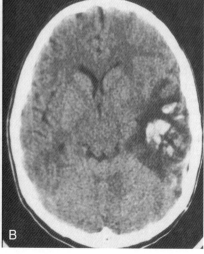

FIGURE 26-88. Hodgkin's lymphoma. **A,** MR angiogram and unenhanced head CT (**B**) in a patient with large mediastinal mass, brachiocephalic vein compression, and associated left jugular vein thrombosis, showing venous sinus thrombus involving the left transverse and sigmoid sinus (**A,** *arrows*) and associated hemorrhagic venous infarction (**B**). *(Courtesy of Dr. Laureen Sena.)*

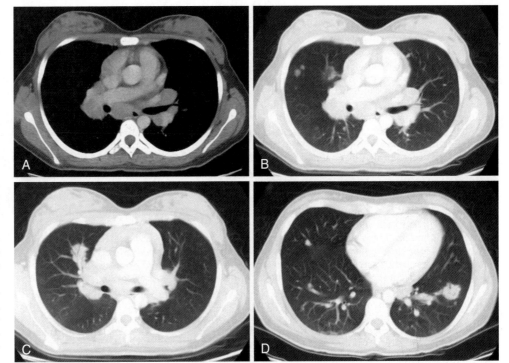

FIGURE 26-89. Hodgkin's lymphoma and pulmonary involvement. **A,** This patient has extensive mediastinal and bilateral hilar nodal disease. The presence of discrete pulmonary nodules **(B, D)** may be the result of hematogenously spread disease, although contiguous spread along peribronchovascular lymphatics **(C, D)** is more common in Hodgkin's lymphoma.

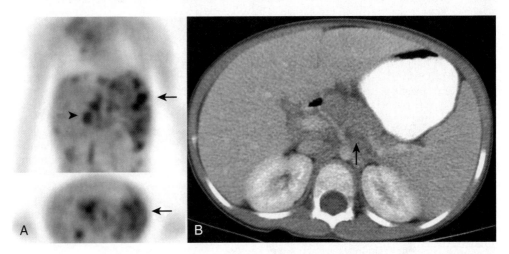

FIGURE 26-90. Hodgkin's lymphoma. Contrast-enhanced CT images of the abdomen **(B)** fail to demonstrate the multiple foci of splenic disease that are evident by ^{18}F-FDG-PET **(A,** *arrows*). Extensive retroperitoneal adenopathy is seen by CT **(B,** *arrow*) and PET (*arrowhead*) in this patient with stage III disease.

Box 26-5	Childhood Non-Hodgkin's Lymphoma: St. Jude (Murphy) Classification

STAGE I

A single tumor (extranodal) or nodal area is involved, excluding the abdomen and mediastinum.

STAGE II

Disease is limited to
  A single tumor (extranodal) with regional node involvement, or
  Two or more tumors or nodal areas involved on one side of the diaphragm, or
  A primary gastrointestinal tract tumor (completely resected), with or without regional node involvement.

STAGE III

Tumors or involved lymph node areas occur on both sides of the diaphragm; includes
  Any primary intrathoracic (mediastinal, pleural, or thymic) disease
  Extensive primary intra-abdominal disease
  Any paraspinal or epidural tumors

STAGE IV

Tumors involve bone marrow (<25%) and/or central nervous system (CNS) disease, regardless of other sites of involvement.

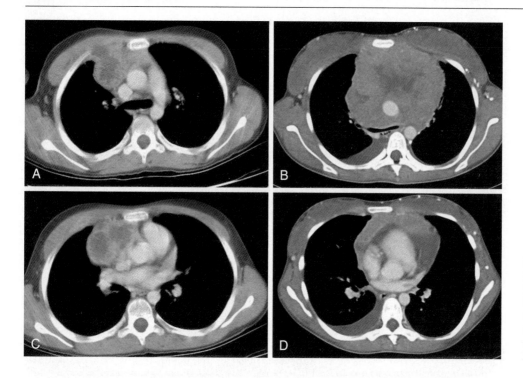

FIGURE 26-91. Non-Hodgkin's lymphoma. Diffuse large B-cell (**A, B**) and B-cell–rich (**C, D**) non-Hodgkin's lymphomas, showing chest wall and pericardial invasion that is more commonly seen in mediastinal non-Hodgkin's lymphoma.

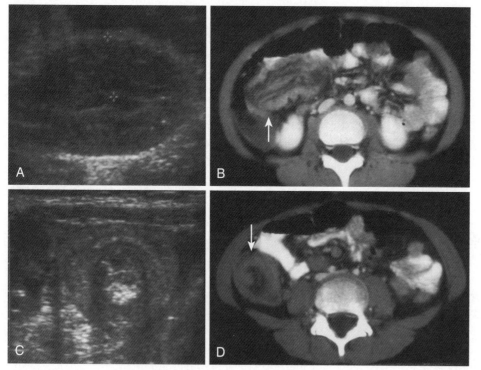

FIGURE 26-92. Non-Hodgkin's lymphoma and intussusception. **A, C,** Ultrasound imaging in a patient with Burkitt's lymphoma and CT in a patient with large cell lymphoma (**B, D**) showing typical features of intussusception, either small bowel–small bowel (**A, B**) or ileocolic (**C, D**).

tinal abnormalities frequently seen, even after multiple cycles of chemotherapy.

Non-Hodgkin's lymphomas of the bone can present primarily or in the setting of widespread metastatic disease. They often present with pathologic fractures and bone destruction.[243] MRI may be helpful for delineating the extent of marrow and adjacent soft tissue involvement. Staging of NHL includes bone scintigraphy, which can be useful for distinguishing between localized osseous involvement and more widespread disease,[65]

although it remains to be determined whether FDG-PET can replace bone scintigraphy for identifying sites of bone involvement in NHL.

Ileocecal involvement is common in NHL (see Fig. 26-91). In the abdomen, intussusception in an older child should raise concern for a pathologic lead point caused by lymphoma. This is commonly seen in the setting of Burkitt's lymphoma (Fig. 26-92; Fig. 26-51), but may also be seen in other forms of NHL.[242,243] The sporadic form of Burkitt's lymphoma, which

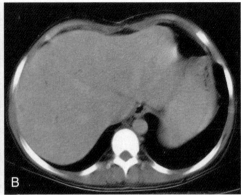

FIGURE 26-93. A, 22-year-old patient with renal transplant who develop extensive post-transplantation lymphoproliferative disease (PTLD) involving the liver. **B,** Four months after reducing the immunosuppressive therapy, the PTLD had almost completely resolved.

is more commonly encountered in Western and developed countries, is not causally linked to Epstein-Barr virus (EBV) infection. It frequently has a pattern of bulky mesenteric and pelvic adenopathy, as well as involvement of multiple visceral organs, including the liver, kidneys, and pancreas. Response of Burkitt's lymphoma to chemotherapy is often rapid, with bulky disease responding within weeks. In contrast, the endemic form of Burkitt's lymphoma, which is encountered in equatorial Africa, is usually associated with EBV infection (95%), and characteristically presents with jaw, orbit, paraspinal, and CNS involvement.[233]

Post-transplantation lymphoproliferative disease (PTLD) is seen in the setting of solid organ and bone marrow transplantation, and results directly from the immunosuppressive regimens used.[253] The lymphoproliferative disease, which is usually EBV-related, frequently responds to reduction in immunosuppression (Fig. 26-93). However, the lymphoproliferative disease may progress to an aggressive B-cell lymphoma, resulting in widespread malignant disease. PTLD can involve multiple organs and systems and responds variably to conventional lymphoma therapies. The use of FDG-PET imaging, although not routinely used for the management of PTLD, has been advocated by some to improve early disease detection and staging.[254]

Just as for Hodgkin's lymphoma, the role of FDG-PET scanning in non-Hodgkin's lymphoma is currently being validated. Several studies of small cohorts of patients have indicated that FDG-PET is valuable for staging and predicting response to therapy in patients with various forms of NHL.[84,86,158,255-258] As suggested by these studies, FDG-PET, particularly when combined with cross-sectional imaging by CT or MRI, is extremely sensitive at detecting sites of disease that might not have otherwise been identified. It seems obvious that identifying the extent of disease should affect staging and monitoring of treatment response, but prospective trials are needed to determine whether FDG-PET response alone can be used to direct response-based modulation in therapy.

Sites of Relapse

In the treatment of leukemia and lymphoma, radiologic evaluation plays an important role in monitoring for disease relapse. In addition to intramedullary (i.e., bone marrow) relapse, common sites of extramedullary leukemic relapse include kidneys, spleen, CNS, and bone. Although less common, relapse to "sanctuary sites" such as the testicle can occur, with diffuse organ infiltration and enlargement and with focal mass deposits (Fig. 26-94). Relapse to these sites may occur, even in the setting of bone marrow remission.

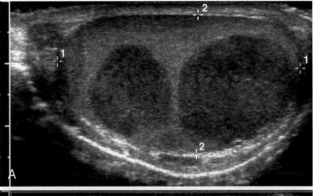
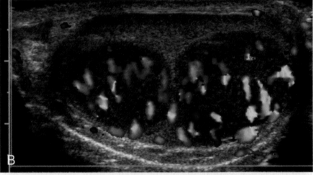
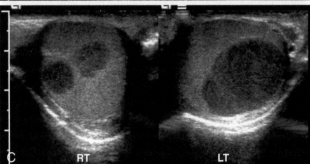

FIGURE 26-94. Scrotal relapse of leukemia in 17-year-old patient with high-risk acute lymphocytic leukemia, post–bone marrow transplantation. He presented with painless scrotal swelling and palpable abnormalities on examination. **A-C,** Scrotal ultrasound shows multiple bilateral hypoechoic masses (relative to testicular parenchyma), with increased blood flow to the masses, diagnostic of scrotal relapse.

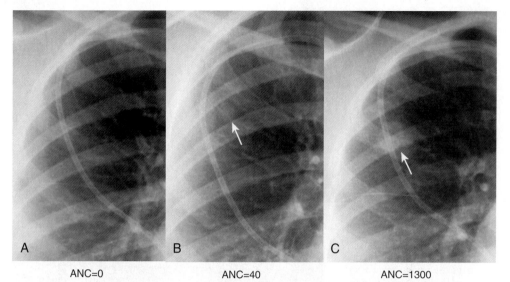

A   ANC=0   B   ANC=40   C   ANC=1300

FIGURE 26-95. Imaging the neutropenic patient. A 12-year-old patient with acute myelogenous leukemia. Note the appearance of focal lung nodule (*arrow*) (*Aspergillus*) as the patient's blood cell counts recover (**A-C**), suggesting the appearance of infectious lesions in neutropenic patients may be challenging to detect until the marrow has recovered after ablative chemotherapy. ANC, absolute neutrophil count.

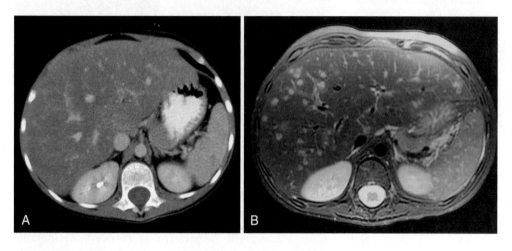

A   B

FIGURE 26-96. Imaging hepatosplenic fungal infection. MRI (**B**), using fluid-sensitive fast spin-echo inversion recovery (or similar) sequences, is sensitive for detecting lesions not seen by CT (**A**) or ultrasound.

IMAGING TREATMENT COMPLICATIONS

Complications resulting from the treatment of pediatric malignancies are myriad. It is important to note that the radiographic manifestations of fungal and other infectious diseases may not be manifest during periods of profound neutropenia (Fig. 26-95). Frequently, abnormalities on imaging studies emerge only after peripheral neutrophil counts recover and infection-fighting white blood cells become available to mount an inflammatory response. Infections complications include typical bacterial and viral infections, as well as localized and disseminated fungal infection. The extent of hepatic and splenic fungal involvement may be better detected by MRI (Fig. 26-96).

Cardiomyopathy results from cardiotoxic chemotherapy agents such as doxorubicin. Echocardiography has become the imaging modality of choice in monitoring these patients. Pulmonary toxicity can range from subtle ground glass opacity, often an early manifestation of bronchiolitis obliterans with organizing pneumonia (BOOP, also known as cryptogenic pneumonia), to frank interstitial pulmonary fibrosis.[259]

Children with cancer also have a poorly understood hypercoagulable state. Pulmonary emboli and other sites of venous thrombosis occur with increased frequency in these patients and may be detected incidentally (Fig. 26-97) or in response to specific clinical symptoms. Clinically, the probability of thromboembolic disease may be difficult to assess. The presence of multiple known risk factors, including indwelling catheters, concurrent infection, immobility, dehydration, and chemotherapy all increase the risk of thromboembolic events in these patients,[260] and the clinician and radiologist must be vigilant in their respective examinations to enable early detection and treatment of these potentially life-threatening complications.

GI complications occur during periods of neutropenia and can range from typhlitis, with localized inflammation of the cecum, to extensive pancolitis and bowel necrosis (Fig. 26-98).[261,262] Asparaginase, which is included in many chemotherapy regimens for ALL and lymphoblastic lymphoma, results in pancreatitis in approximately 5% to 10% of patients. The severity of pancreatitis can range from a mild chemical pancreatitis to frank pancreatic necrosis and subsequent pseudocyst formation (Fig. 26-99). This is best evaluated initially by ultrasound, with CT reserved for persistent or worsening clinical pancreatitis or to assess for complications such as pseudocyst.

Bony complications can arise after chronic treatment with corticosteroids and include osteopenia, fractures, bone marrow infarcts, and osteonecrosis (Fig. 26-100); osteonecrosis is most typically seen in the hips and knees.[263] Second tumors, particularly musculoskeletal tumors, may be seen following radiation therapy. Osteochondromas involving the clavicles and

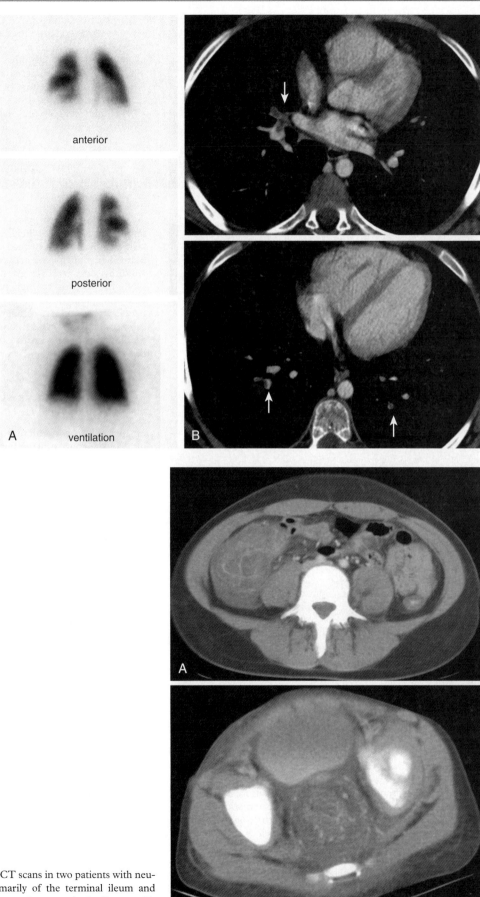

FIGURE 26-97. Pulmonary emboli in 6-year-old boy with T-cell acute lymphoblastic leukemia, fever, and neutropenia. CT scans of the chest identified multiple pulmonary emboli involving multiple lung segments **(B)**. CT findings were confirmed by ventilation-perfusion scanning **(A)**, which demonstrates multiple perfusion defects corresponding to involved segments identified by CT, but with no corresponding ventilation defects.

FIGURE 26-98. Contrast-enhanced CT scans in two patients with neutropenic colitis, showing disease primarily of the terminal ileum and cecum (i.e., typhlitis; **A**) and more extensive pancolonic disease with severe rectal necrosis **(B)** that required diverting ileostomy.

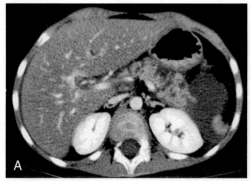

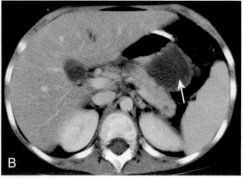

FIGURE 26-99. 11-year-old with acute lymphoblastic leukemia, on asparaginase, who developed severe pancreatitis **(A)** and subsequent pseudocyst formation (*arrow*), with the pseudocyst closely adherent to the posterior wall of the stomach **(B)**.

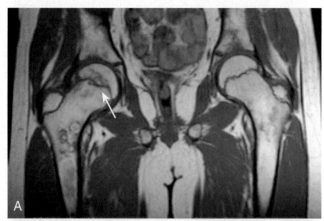

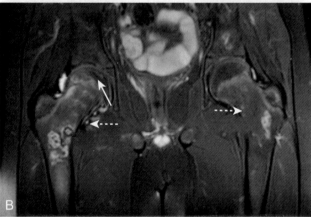

FIGURE 26-100. Osteonecrosis–avascular necrosis in 13-year-old with history of high-risk acute lymphoblastic leukemia on high-dose steroids, with right hip pain. Unenhanced T1-weighted **(A)** and gadolinium-enhanced **(B)** MRI scans of the hips and pelvis show osteonecrosis of the right femoral head (arrows) and evidence of bone infarcts in both femoral necks (dashed arrows).

sternoclavicular junction, for example, are common in patients with lymphoma who have received mantle radiation, particularly if radiation treatment occurred at an early age. Malignant degeneration of these lesions is rare.

Central nervous system changes can develop after radiation and chemotherapy. In one study, hemorrhagic events were seen in 4 of 120 children with ALL. All these children had been disease-free for more than 2 years and had been treated with prior chemotherapy and cranial radiation.[264] These events are most commonly related to treatment-induced vasculopathy,

and may be diffuse or localized vasculopathy. Asparaginase may also produce venous sinus thrombosis, leading to profound neurologic deficits and areas of venous infarction (Fig. 26-101). Methotrexate, which is given systemically and intrathecally for CNS prophylaxis to high-risk ALL patients, may produce a leukoencephalopathy characterized by symmetrical periventricular white matter signal abnormalities. These changes may be transient or permanent. They are not specific to methotrexate and can be seen with other chemotherapeutic agents that penetrate the CNS.

NEW IMAGING TECHNIQUES

Historically, the standard tools of radiology—CT, MRI, and ultrasound—have provided primarily anatomic information, with relatively little direct functional information being evident. Nuclear medicine imaging has provided useful functional information, but has been limited by the lack of accompanying anatomic detail offered by conventional planar, SPECT and, to a lesser extent, PET images. Of the three major cross-sectional imaging technologies, MRI has come closest to providing direct information about cellular function, for example by using diffusion-weighted imaging to assess regions of localized ischemia and using ^{1}H spectroscopy to derive metabolic information about specific regions being imaged. Functional MRI of the brain relies on relative changes in blood oxygen level in metabolically active tissues to yield exquisite information about cerebral activation in response to various stimuli. The relative success enjoyed by MRI in generating functional images derives mostly from the rich and varied information contained in the MR signal from different materials. Although most of the magnetic resonance information obtained routinely arises from the protons contained in hydrogen atoms from water molecules and lipids, a vast amount of metabolic information can also be derived from MR signals arising from molecules other than water.

The FDA, in its critical path initiative, has emphasized the need to increase the speed, efficiency, and cost-effectiveness of drug development for cancer and other diseases.[265] Molecular imaging and functional imaging probes have great potential to identify and characterize disease-specific targets and to provide target and treatment-specific imaging end points for therapy. In particular, as markers of biologic response, imaging end points that characterize cellular vitality or apoptosis, receptor downregulation or functional inactivation, and treatment-specific changes to cellular metabolism will be critical in determining the success or failure of newer classes of molecular-based therapies. As we have learned with imatinib (Gleevec) and GI stromal tumors, noncytolytic therapies that slowly extinguish tumor metabolic activity will not immediately result in tumor shrinkage, and imaging techniques that directly measure tumor

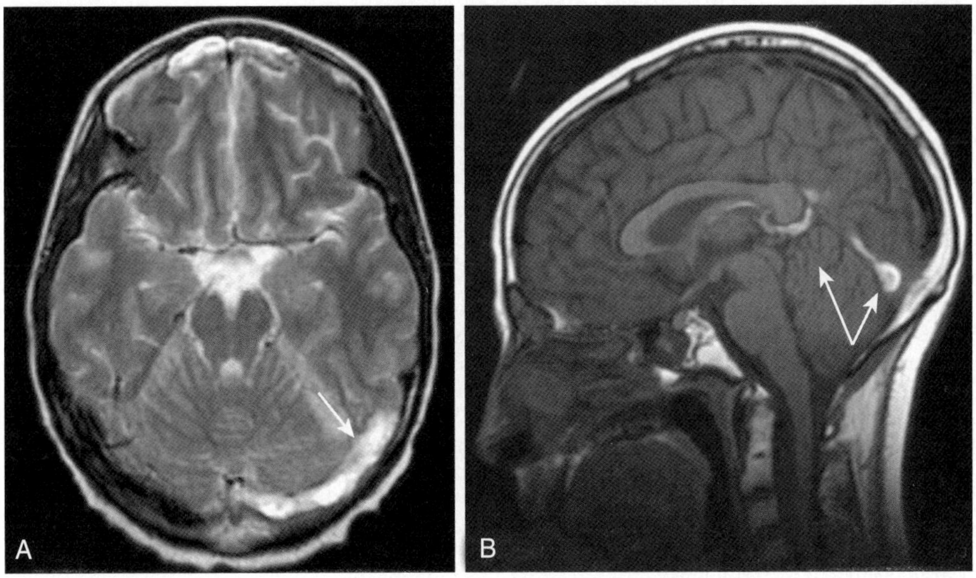

FIGURE 26-101. Cerebral sinus thrombosis. Shown are axial T2-weighted (**A**) and sagittal T1-weighted (**B**) MR images in a 15-year-old with acute lymphoblastic leukemia receiving asparaginase during induction therapy, showing high signal intensity abnormality in the left transverse sinus, straight sinus, and deep cerebral veins (*arrows*).

metabolism will be necessary to directly demonstrate a response to therapy.[266] In addition, for many molecularly targeted agents, such as antibodies, it is unclear whether the agents ever localize in tumor in vivo. For these compounds, it is critical to develop surrogate end points of response. The ability to image the distribution and targeting of such agents directly in vivo would significantly benefit this assessment, particularly when there is a poor overall clinical response to therapy.

Newer functional imaging approaches are also expected to affect treatment strategy and drug design, with an emphasis on response-based treatment regimens. This allows patients with a high likelihood of response to be treated less aggressively, whereas those not responding to therapy are identified early and redirected into more aggressive therapeutic regimens.

Molecular Imaging

Molecular imaging has been defined by the Commission on Molecular Imaging of the American College of Radiology as the "spatially localized and temporally resolved sensing of molecular and other processes in vivo."[267] Although molecular imaging techniques, particularly in nuclear medicine, have been in use for many years, this terminology has recently been applied to the rapidly growing area of radiologic investigation aimed at developing tools to allow direct imaging of cellular and molecular events. These investigations include development of optical imaging probes, imaging gene expression, imaging marker genes, tracking cells in vivo, and developing targeted biomolecular conjugates to allow visualization of specific cellular and molecular events in vivo.[268]

Most of these investigations are still in the early stages of development.[265,267,269] Perhaps the most fruitful area of research has been in the application of near-infrared fluorescent (NIRF) imaging for evaluation of malignant disease.[270-273] Fluorescence in the near-infrared range of the spectrum has been pursued because these wavelengths penetrate biologic tissue further than visible or infrared light. Light in the visible spectrum is largely absorbed by abundant biomolecules such as hemoglobin, which are present in most tissues, whereas light in the infrared range is almost completely absorbed by water.[274] The ability to image fluorescing tissues has long been in use in the laboratory setting, but has not yet found clinical usefulness. The development of

so-called "smart" NIRF imaging probes has allowed tumor-specific enzymatic activity to be imaged directly by fluorescence. These probes are synthesized so that the NIR fluorophore is attached to a peptide scaffold that, by virtue of its amino acid sequence, is selectively cleaved by tumor-specific proteases. Fluorescence of the NIR fluorophores is quenched because of their close proximity in the intact peptide scaffold. Upon enzymatic cleavage in the tumor, the fluorophores are released, and the resultant NIRF signal provides a specific signal that allows tumor visualization. This technique has been used successfully to detect tumor-specific cathepsin activity in colon and breast cancer models,[271] and more recently has been used to guide the endoscopic detection of colonic lesions in vivo.[275] Although the depth of penetration of NIR light still limits this technique to structures near the surface, there is potential for NIRF imaging to be used intraoperatively to provide guidance in determining tumor margins, sites of lymph node spread, and evaluation of cavities and tissue linings such as the peritoneum, which are poorly imaged by other techniques.

As novel cancer therapies evolve to include gene therapy approaches, the direct imaging of gene expression will be important to evaluate these techniques. Radiolabeling of viral and liposomal vectors has been used to monitor vector delivery. More importantly, the imaging of gene activity has been accomplished using various reporter gene strategies. One of the most elegant approaches has used a reporter gene and therapeutic gene driven by the same promoter, allowing the activity of the therapeutic gene to be inferred from reporter gene expression. Alternatively, some genes, such as the herpes simplex virus (HSV) thymidine kinase (TK) gene, can be used for imaging and therapy. The therapeutic effect results from enzymatic conversion of the prodrug ganciclovir to its toxic metabolite, and TK activity can be directly imaged using trace amounts of ^{18}F-ganciclovir analogues. This approach has been used in a clinical trial of HSV-tk gene therapy for gliomas, and the extent of HSV-tk expression determined by PET imaging was found to correlate with therapeutic response.[276]

Magnetic Resonance Spectroscopy

Whole-body MR imaging uses the aggregate signal characteristics of a given tissue to generate high-resolution images, which reveal information about the anatomy and state of health of the tissue, but give little direct information about the biochemical makeup of the tissue. In contrast, MR spectroscopy focuses on acquiring chemical information from small volumes of tissue, with the aim of characterizing the ongoing chemical processes unique to specific tissues. This is accomplished by separating the signals derived from specific tissue and cellular constituents into their different chemical forms. The protons contained within tissues will experience a molecular environment that is unique to the tissue. These variations in molecular environment produce alterations or chemical shifts in the resonant frequency of the constituent protons. In theory, when the nuclear magnetic resonance (NMR) signal is displayed as a function of resonant frequency the different chemical forms in the tissue should yield a unique spectroscopic fingerprint. In practice, large water and lipid peaks dominate the proton NMR spectra from biologic tissues, with the less abundant elements giving lower signal. Because of the need to reduce heterogeneity of tissue within the voxel being interrogated, the small volumes of tissue evaluated by MR spectroscopy generally produce low signal, and prolonged imaging times are needed to acquire useful spectra. With prolonged imaging times, degradation of spectra caused by motion artifact occurs; to date, most of the routine spectroscopic examinations have focused on applications in the brain, where the tissues being examined remain relatively static.[36]

With higher field strength magnets, faster scanning sequences, and advances in postprocessing techniques, [1]H-MR spectroscopy is increasingly being used for non-neurologic body applications. Some investigators have used [1]H-MR spectroscopy, together with dynamic contrast-enhanced MR imaging, to show that increases in vertebral marrow fat content and accompanying decreases in marrow perfusion correlate with varying states of osteopenia and osteoporosis.[277] Others have evaluated the usefulness of [1]H-MR spectroscopy to characterize and monitor response to therapy in some pediatric solid tumors, including neuroblastoma.[278] The response of neuroblastoma to chemotherapy has been shown to correlate with decreases in cellular choline peaks.[279] Whether this will turn out to be a better predictor of response to therapy than conventional imaging techniques will need to be evaluated prospectively in larger clinical trials.

[1]H-MR spectroscopy has also been used to characterize bone and soft tissue tumors, with elevated choline levels detected in lesions shown to have a malignant histology, but not in most benign lesions.[280] Preul and associates[281] have suggested that a pattern recognition analysis of the biochemical information obtained from [1]H-MR spectroscopy of brain tumors could reliably distinguish benign, low-grade, and high-grade tumors, and that specific tumor and nontumor fingerprints might ultimately provide an accurate noninvasive preoperative characterization of particular lesions. Although considerable progress has been made, much work will be needed to develop a similar library of characteristic spectra for other pediatric solid tumors.

Other nuclei that can be evaluated with MR scanners, particularly at higher field strengths, include ^{31}P, ^{13}C, and [23]Na. These nuclei all have lower gyromagnetic ratios than protons and resonate at lower frequencies than protons for a given field strength. The molecules and ions containing these nuclei are also much less abundant than water protons, so that the signal-to-noise ratios (SNRs) from these nuclei are low compared with those associated with proton NMR. As such, large voxels must be sampled from a given tissue to obtain sufficient SNRs with a reasonable scan time. ^{31}P-MR spectroscopy enables the observation of energy metabolism and intracellular compartmentation through the signals of phosphomonoesters (PMEs), phosphodiesters (PDEs), inorganic phosphate (Pi), and nucleo-tide triphosphates, mainly adenosine triphosphate (ATP). Depending on the tissue being studied, a peak from phosphocreatine may also be seen, such as brain and muscle. When compared with [1]H-MR spectroscopy in the evaluation of bone and soft tissue tumors, ^{31}P-MR spectroscopy was superior for identifying lesions shown to have a malignant histology.[280]

[31]P spectroscopy is also of interest with respect to molecularly directed therapies that affect cellular receptors and target intracellular tyrosine kinase activity. Agents such as imatinib and gefitinib (Iressa) inhibit receptor-associated tyrosine kinase activity.[282] Many of these agents will not result in immediate tumor shrinkage; it will be important to establish early surrogate end points that assess the effect of therapy before visible tumor shrinkage occurs. Whether ^{31}P spectroscopic measurement of intratumoral changes in phosphate metabolite profile will be feasible and valuable in response assessment remains to be validated.

Targeted Contrast Agents

One of the major obstacles facing the design of targeted MRI contrast agents is the necessity for producing detectable changes in the MR signal intensity of the target tissue or organ by altering its MR relaxation properties. Contrast agents typically affect both $1/T1$ and $1/T2$. In general, the major considerations governing the detectability of an MRI contrast agent are its local concentration and the magnitude of the perturbation produced by an individual agent on tissue water protons. Paramagnetic agents, such as chelates of the lanthanide metal gadolinium(III), increase $1/T1$ and $1/T2$ and are best detected using T1-weighted sequences. Ferromagnetic particles, on the other hand, produce relatively greater increases in $1/T2$ and are best detected using T2-weighted pulse sequences.

For paramagnetic agents, there must be a large number of paramagnetic centers selectively bound to the target tissue. It may also be desirable that these agents are of sufficiently high molecular weight to prolong vascular retention and thus slow tissue clearance. Over the past several years, various approaches have been used to address both these issues,[283] including the conjugation of paramagnetic chelates to macromolecules such as serum albumin and linear polymers. Polymeric paramagnetic liposomes and dendrimer-based metal chelates have also been used for tissue specific targeting. However, significant challenges remain with respect to pharmacokinetics and tissue-specific targeting. In addition, although gadolinium chelates bound to the cell surface may have prolonged tissue retention, there may be concern about endosomal degradation of surface-bound gadolinium chelates leading to toxicity from the release of unconjugated gadolinium.[284]

In an effort to improve sensitivity and specificity of MRI detection, monocrystalline iron oxide nanoparticle (MION)–based agents have been used to permit detection of as little as 100 nmol Fe/g of tissue.[285,286] These 10- to 20-nm superparamagnetic particles affect both $1/T1$ and $1/T2$ relaxivity, are sufficiently small to be coupled chemically to peptides, have rapid biodistribution, and have relatively long half-lives in vivo. Weissleder and coworkers[287] have discussed the factors governing the detectability of agents based on ferromagnetic particles, and have emphasized that the lower limit of detectability is determined by various factors, including spatial resolution, imaging field strength, size of the particle, and number of particles per cell. An important observation was that signal amplification could be achieved by cellular internalization of the contrast material. Targeting MIONs to various cell surface structures has been shown to result in internalization and formation of intracellular aggregates. Transferrin receptor targeting, HIV-Tat (transactivator of transcription) peptide-mediated cell binding, and annexin-targeted imaging of apoptosis have all been shown in in vivo model systems to yield enough cell-specific signal to generate an MR image.[288-290] Despite the technical feasibility of these approaches, however, the imaging data have been insufficiently compelling to lead to their widespread clinical use.

To overcome some of the disadvantages inherent in targeted MRI contrast agent development, PET-MRI has recently emerged as a hybrid technology that offers the possibility of combining the sensitive metabolic and molecular-targeted imaging feasible by PET with the high spatial resolution and soft tissue detail that can be achieved with MRI.[291] The use of newly developed ultrafast MRI scanners equipped with 32 receiver channels and up to 76 independent array coil elements connected simultaneously allows complete head-to-toe coverage in a single scan. The incorporation of integrated PET detectors into these scanners is currently entering clinical development and offers the potential to acquire whole-body MRI data and functional PET imaging data simultaneously during the same examination. This opens the way to correlating functional PET data with spectroscopic, diffusion, perfusion, and conventional dynamic MR angiographic techniques. Current hybrid PET-CT scanners allow fusion of PET images with concurrently acquired CT data. However, these CT images are acquired primarily for the purpose of providing attenuation correction for the PET images, and are frequently of suboptimal quality for assessing soft tissue structures and other anatomic regions outside the chest. PET-CT is usually not performed with intravenous or oral contrast. Despite these limitations, PET-CT has become the standard of care for many aspects of oncologic imaging.[48] Clearly, the opportunity to develop hybrid PET-MRI technology would overcome some of the limitations inherent in PET-CT. Furthermore, for pediatric applications, PET-MRI could be performed with a single sedation, would not be associated with additional radiation exposure, and would allow imaging with improved inherent soft tissue contrast relative to CT, without administration of exogenous intravenous or parenteral contrast agents.

CONCLUSION

The approach to imaging pediatric oncology patients is rapidly evolving. We have left the era when the radiologist played a peripheral role in the care of the child with cancer. Although the imaging features of many pediatric cancers are distinctive, as outlined in this chapter, the development of new imaging techniques and the incorporation of these techniques into new treatment designs based on imaging end points has led to exciting opportunities and challenges to detect, stage, and monitor malignant disease more effectively. The next decade of imaging will require close collaboration between the pediatric oncologist and pediatric imaging specialist to determine which of these imaging techniques is best suited to these patients.

REFERENCES

1. Choo SP, Lim DW, Lo CP, et al. Variable problems in lymphomas: CASE 1. Burkitt's lymphoma presenting with central airway obstruction. J Clin Oncol. 2005;23:8112-8113.
2. Binkovitz LA, Olshefski RS, Adler BH. Coincidence FDG-PET in the evaluation of Langerhans' cell histiocytosis: preliminary findings. Pediatr Radiol. 2003;33:598-602.
3. Daldrup-Link HE, Franzius C, Link TM, et al. Whole-body MR imaging for detection of bone metastases in children and young adults: comparison with skeletal scintigraphy and FDG PET. AJR Am J Roentgenol. 2001;177:229-236.
4. Kaste SC, Rodriguez-Galindo C, McCarville ME, Shulkin BL. PET-CT in pediatric Langerhans cell histiocytosis. Pediatr Radiol. 2007;3:615-622.
5. Minagawa M, Makuuchi M, Kubota K, Kondo Y. Intraoperative three-dimensional visualization of liver vasculature by ultrasonography. Hepatogastroenterology. 2004;51:1448-1450.
6. Atri M. New technologies and directed agents for applications of cancer imaging. J Clin Oncol. 2006;24:3299-3308.
7. Delorme S, Krix M. Contrast-enhanced ultrasound for examining tumor biology. Cancer Imaging. 2006;6:148-152.
8. Wilson SR, Burns PN. Microbubble contrast for radiological imaging: 2. Applications. Ultrasound Q. 2006;22:15-18.
9. Dalrymple NC, Prasad SR, El-Merhi FM, Chintapalli KN. Price of isotropy in multidetector CT. Radiographics. 2007;27:49-62.
10. Dalrymple NC, Prasad SR, Freckleton MW, Chintapalli KN. Informatics in radiology (infoRAD): introduction to the language of three-dimensional imaging with multidetector CT. Radiographics. 2005;25:1409-1428.
11. Sorensen AG, Patel S, Harmath C, et al. Comparison of diameter and perimeter methods for tumor volume calculation. J Clin Oncol. 2001;19:551-557.
12. Sohaib SA, Turner B, Hanson JA, et al. CT assessment of tumour response to treatment: comparison of linear, cross-sectional and volumetric measures of tumour size. Br J Radiol. 2000;73:1178-1184.
13. Barnacle AM, McHugh K. Limitations with the response evaluation criteria in solid tumors (RECIST) guidance in disseminated pediatric malignancy. Pediatr Blood Cancer. 2006;46:127-134.
14. Mason KP, Sanborn P, Zurakowski D, et al. Superiority of pentobarbital versus chloral hydrate for sedation in infants during imaging. Radiology. 2004;230:537-542.
15. Mason KP, Zgleszewski SE, Dearden JL, et al. Dexmedetomidine for pediatric sedation for computed tomography imaging studies. Anesth Analg. 2006;103:57-62.
15a. Callahan MJ, Poznauskis L, Zurakowski D, Taylor GA. Incidence of non-ionic iodinated intravenous contrast related reactions in a large urban Children's hospital: Retrospective analysis of 12,494 patients. Radiology. (In press.)
16. Iwano S, Makino N, Ikeda M, et al. Solitary pulmonary nodules: optimal slice thickness of high-resolution CT in differentiating malignant from benign. Clin Imaging. 2004;28:322-328.
17. McCarville MB, Lederman HM, Santana VM, et al. Distinguishing benign from malignant pulmonary nodules with helical chest CT in children with malignant solid tumors. Radiology. 2006;239:514-520.
18. Fenchel S, Boll DT, Fleiter TR, et al. Multislice helical CT of the pancreas and spleen. Eur J Radiol. 2003;45(Suppl 1):S59-S72.
19. Oto A, Tamm EP, Szklaruk J. Multidetector row CT of the liver. Radiol Clin North Am. 2005;43:827-848.
20. Brenner D, Elliston C, Hall E, Berdon W. Estimated risks of radiation-induced fatal cancer from pediatric CT. AJR Am J Roentgenol. 2001;176:289-296.
21. Brenner DJ, Doll R, Goodhead DT, et al. Cancer risks attributable to low doses of ionizing radiation: assessing what we really know. Proc Natl Acad Sci U S A. 2003;100:13761-13766.
22. Brenner DJ, Hall EJ. Computed tomography—an increasing source of radiation exposure. N Engl J Med. 2007;357:2277-2284.
23. Frush DP, Donnelly LF, Rosen NS. Computed tomography and radiation risks: what pediatric health care providers should know. Pediatrics. 2003;112:951-957.
24. Slovis TL. Children, computed tomography radiation dose, and the As Low As Reasonably Achievable (ALARA) concept. Pediatrics. 2003;112:971-972.

25. Donnelly LF, Emery KH, Brody AS, et al. Minimizing radiation dose for pediatric body applications of single-detector helical CT: strategies at a large Children's Hospital. AJR Am J Roentgenol. 2001;176:303-306.

26. Paterson A, Frush DP. Dose reduction in paediatric MDCT: general principles. Clin Radiol. 2007;62:507-517.

27. Jacobs MA, Ibrahim TS, Ouwerkerk R. AAPM/RSNA physics tutorials for residents: MR imaging: brief overview and emerging applications. Radiographics. 2007;27:1213-1229.

28. Pooley RA. AAPM/RSNA physics tutorial for residents: fundamental physics of MR imaging. Radiographics. 2005;25:1087-1099.

29. Tanenbaum LN. Clinical 3T MR imaging: mastering the challenges. Magn Reson Imaging Clin N Am. 2006;14:1-15.

30. Bammer R, Schoenberg SO. Current concepts and advances in clinical parallel magnetic resonance imaging. Top Magn Reson Imaging. 2004;15:129-158.

31. Choyke PL, Dwyer AJ, Knopp MV. Functional tumor imaging with dynamic contrast-enhanced magnetic resonance imaging. J Magn Reson Imaging. 2003;17:509-520.

32. O'Connor JP, Jackson A, Parker GJ, Jayson GC. DCE-MRI biomarkers in the clinical evaluation of antiangiogenic and vascular disrupting agents. Br J Cancer. 2007;96:189-195.

33. Hayashida Y, Yakushiji T, Awai K, et al. Monitoring therapeutic responses of primary bone tumors by diffusion-weighted image: Initial results. Eur Radiol. 2006;16:2637-2643.

34. Uhl M, Saueressig U, van Buiren M, et al. Osteosarcoma: preliminary results of in vivo assessment of tumor necrosis after chemotherapy with diffusion- and perfusion-weighted magnetic resonance imaging. Invest Radiol. 2006;41:618-623.

35. Tzika AA, Astrakas LG, Zarifi MK, et al. Multiparametric MR assessment of pediatric brain tumors. Neuroradiology. 2003;45:1-10.

36. Poussaint TY, Rodriguez D. Advanced neuroimaging of pediatric brain tumors: MR diffusion, MR perfusion, and MR spectroscopy. Neuroimaging Clin N Am. 2006;16:169-192.

37. Tzika AA, Astrakas LG, Zarifi MK, et al. Spectroscopic and perfusion magnetic resonance imaging predictors of progression in pediatric brain tumors. Cancer. 2004;100:1246-1256.

38. Tzika AA, Vajapeyam S, Barnes PD. Multivoxel proton MR spectroscopy and hemodynamic MR imaging of childhood brain tumors: preliminary observations. AJNR Am J Neuroradiol. 1997;18:203-218.

39. Margolis DJ, Hoffman JM, Herfkens RJ, et al. Molecular imaging techniques in body imaging. Radiology. 2007;245:333-356.

40. Oehr P, Biersack HJ, Coleman RE (eds). PET and PET-CT in Oncology. New York, Springer-Verlag, 2004.

41. Czernin J, Dahlbom M, Ratib O, Schiepers C (eds). Atlas of PET/CT Imaging in Oncology. New York, Springer-Verlag, 2004.

42. Phelps ME (ed). PET: Molecular Imaging and its Biological Applications. New York, Springer-Verlag, 2004.

43. Gambhir SS. Molecular imaging of cancer with positron emission tomography. Nat Rev Cancer. 2002;2:683-693.

44. Iyer M, Sato M, Johnson M, et al. Applications of molecular imaging in cancer gene therapy. Curr Gene Ther. 2005;5:607-618.

45. Jadvar H, Connolly LP, Fahey FH, Shulkin BL. PET and PET/CT in pediatric oncology. Semin Nucl Med. 2007;37:316-331.

46. Saleem A, Charnley N, Price P. Clinical molecular imaging with positron emission tomography. Eur J Cancer. 2006;42:1720-1727.

47. Schmidt GP, Kramer H, Reiser MF, Glaser C. Whole-body magnetic resonance imaging and positron emission tomography-computed tomography in oncology. Top Magn Reson Imaging. 2007;18:193-202.

48. von Schulthess GK, Steinert HC, Hany TF. Integrated PET/CT: current applications and future directions. Radiology. 2006;238:405-422.

49. Wong TZ, Paulson EK, Nelson RC, et al. Practical approach to diagnostic CT combined with PET. AJR Am J Roentgenol. 2007;188:622-629.

50. Jadvar H, Alavi A, Mavi A, Shulkin BL. PET in pediatric diseases. Radiol Clin North Am. 2005;43:135-152.

51. Shulkin BL. PET imaging in pediatric oncology. Pediatr Radiol. 2004;34:199-204.

52. Smith SV. Molecular imaging with copper-64. J Inorg Biochem. 2004;98:1874-1901.

53. Voss SD, Smith SV, DiBartolo N, et al. Positron emission tomography (PET) imaging of neuroblastoma and melanoma with 64 Cu-SarAr immunoconjugates. Proc Natl Acad Sci U S A. 2007;104:17489-17493.

54. Glaser M, Luthra SK, Brady F. Applications of positron-emitting halogens in PET oncology (review). Int J Oncol. 2003;22:253-267.

55. Salskov A, Tammisetti VS, Grierson J, Vesselle H. FLT: measuring tumor cell proliferation in vivo with positron emission tomography and 3'-deoxy-3'-[18F]fluorothymidine. Semin Nucl Med. 2007;37:429-439.

56. Blodgett TM, Meltzer CC, Townsend DW. PET/CT: form and function. Radiology. 2007;242:360-385.

57. Furth C, Denecke T, Steffen I, et al. Correlative imaging strategies implementing CT, MRI, and PET for staging of childhood Hodgkin disease. J Pediatr Hematol Oncol. 2006;28:501-512.

58. Gerth HU, Juergens KU, Dirksen U, et al. Significant benefit of multimodal imaging: PET/CT compared with PET alone in staging and follow-up of patients with Ewing tumors. J Nucl Med. 2007;48:1932-1939.

59. Pfannenberg AC, Aschoff P, Brechtel K, et al. Value of contrast-enhanced multiphase CT in combined PET/CT protocols for oncological imaging. Br J Radiol. 2007;80:437-445.

60. Wechalekar K, Sharma B, Cook G. PET/CT in oncology—a major advance. Clin Radiol. 2005;60:1143-1155.

61. Kaste SC. Issues specific to implementing PET-CT for pediatric oncology: what we have learned along the way. Pediatr Radiol. 2004;34:205-213.

62. Martinez MJ, Torres I, Ladebeck R, et al. Whole-body MR-PET: characterization of PET performance by Monte Carlo simulations. Program and Abstracts of the Society of Nuclear Medicine 54th Annual Meeting: June 3-6, 2007, Washington, DC. J Nucl Med. 2007;48(Suppl 2):46P.

63. Buscombe JR, Bombardieri E. Imaging cancer using single photon techniques. Q J Nucl Med Mol Imaging. 2005;49:121-131.

64. van Dalen JA, Vogel WV, Corstens FH, Oyen WJ. Multi-modality nuclear medicine imaging: artefacts, pitfalls and recommendations. Cancer Imaging. 2007;7:77-83.

65. Connolly LP, Drubach LA, Ted Treves S. Applications of nuclear medicine in pediatric oncology. Clin Nucl Med. 2002;27:117-125.

66. Kushner BH. Neuroblastoma: a disease requiring a multitude of imaging studies. J Nucl Med. 2004;45:1172-1188.

67. von Schulthess GK. Integrated modality imaging with PET-CT and SPECT-CT: CT issues. Eur Radiol. 2005;15(Suppl 4):D121-D126.

68. Pollack IF. Brain tumors in children. N Engl J Med. 1994;331:1500-1507.

69. Pollack IF. Pediatric brain tumors. Semin Surg Oncol. 1999;16:73-90.

70. Talos IF, Mian AZ, Zou KH, et al. Magnetic resonance and the human braIn anatomy, function and metabolism. Cell Mol Life Sci. 2006;63:1106-1124.

71. Chen W, Delaloye S, Silverman DH, et al. Predicting treatment response of malignant gliomas to bevacizumab and irinotecan by imaging proliferation with [18F] fluorothymidine positron emission tomography: a pilot study. J Clin Oncol. 2007;25:4714-4721.

72. Yamamoto Y, Wong TZ, Turkington TG, et al. 3′-Deoxy-3′-[F-18]fluorothymidine positron emission tomography in patients with recurrent glioblastoma multiforme: comparison with Gd-DTPA enhanced magnetic resonance imaging. Mol Imaging Biol. 2006;8:340-347.

73. Poussaint TY. Magnetic resonance imaging of pediatric brain tumors: state of the art. Top Magn Reson Imaging. 2001;12:411-433.

74. Faerber EN, Roman NV. Central nervous system tumors of childhood. Radiol Clin North Am. 1997;35:1301-1328.

75. Doyle AJ, Anderson GD. Physiologic calcification of the pineal gland in children on computed tomography: prevalence, observer reliability and association with choroid plexus calcification. Acad Radiol. 2006;13:822-826.

76. Dinauer C, Francis GL. Thyroid cancer in children. Endocrinol Metab Clin North Am. 2007;36:779-806.

77. Castellote A, Vazquez E, Vera J, et al. Cervicothoracic lesions in infants and children. Radiographics. 1999;19:583-600.

78. Bal CS, Kumar A, Chandra P, et al. Is chest x-ray or high-resolution computed tomography scan of the chest sufficient investigation to detect pulmonary metastasis in pediatric differentiated thyroid cancer? Thyroid. 2004;14:217-225.

79. Franco A, Mody NS, Meza MP. Imaging evaluation of pediatric mediastinal masses. Radiol Clin North Am. 2005;43:325-353.

80. Slovis TL, Meza M, Kuhn JP. Aberrant thymus—MR assessment. Pediatr Radiol. 1992;22:490-492.

81. Lam JC, Chui CH, Jacobsen AS, et al. When is a mediastinal mass critical in a child? An analysis of 29 patients. Pediatr Surg Int. 2004;20:180-184.

82. Gallamini A, Rigacci L, Merli F, et al. The predictive value of positron emission tomography scanning performed after two courses of standard therapy on treatment outcome in advanced stage Hodgkin's disease. Haematologica. 2006;91:475-481.

83. Hutchings M, Loft A, Hansen M, et al. FDG-PET after two cycles of chemotherapy predicts treatment failure and progression-free survival in Hodgkin lymphoma. Blood. 2006;107:52-59.

84. MacManus MP, Seymour JF, Hicks RJ. Overview of early response assessment in lymphoma with FDG-PET. Cancer Imaging. 2007;7:10-18.

85. Mody RJ, Bui C, Hutchinson RJ, et al. Comparison of (18)F Flurodeoxyglucose PET with Ga-67 scintigraphy and conventional imaging modalities in pediatric lymphoma. Leuk Lymphoma. 2007;48:699-707.

86. Rademaker J. Hodgkin's and non-Hodgkin's lymphomas. Radiol Clin North Am. 2007;45:69-83.

87. Hudson MM, Krasin MJ, Kaste SC. PET imaging in pediatric Hodgkin's lymphoma. Pediatr Radiol. 2004;34:190-198.

88. Kaste SC, Howard SC, McCarville EB, et al. 18F-FDG-avid sites mimicking active disease in pediatric Hodgkin's. Pediatr Radiol. 2005;35:141-154.

89. Kazama T, Faria SC, Varavithya V, et al. FDG-PET in the evaluation of treatment for lymphoma: clinical usefulness and pitfalls. Radiographics. 2005;25:191-207.

90. Dulmet EM, Macchiarini P, Suc B, Verley JM. Germ cell tumors of the mediastinum. A 30-year experience. Cancer. 1993;72:1894-1901.

91. Drevelegas A, Palladas P, Scordalaki A. Mediastinal germ cell tumors: a radiologic-pathologic review. Eur Radiol. 2001;11:1925-1932.

92. Choi SJ, Lee JS, Song KS, Lim TH. Mediastinal teratoma: CT differentiation of ruptured and unruptured tumors. AJR Am J Roentgenol. 1998;171:591-594.

93. Rothstein DH, Voss SD, Isakoff M, Puder M. Thymoma in a child: case report and review of the literature. Pediatr Surg Int. 2005;21:548-551.

94. Kim TS, Lee KS, Han J, et al. Mucoepidermoid carcinoma of the tracheobronchial tree: radiographic and CT findings in 12 patients. Radiology. 1999;212:643-648.

95. Lee EY, Vargas SO, Sawicki GS, et al. Mucoepidermoid carcinoma of bronchus in a pediatric patient: (18)F-FDG-PET findings. Pediatr Radiol. 2007;37:1278-1282.

96. Yikilmaz A, Lee EY. CT imaging of mass-like nonvascular pulmonary lesions in children. Pediatr Radiol. 2007;37:1253-1263.

97. Strollo DC, Rosado-de-Christenson ML, Jett JR. Primary mediastinal tumors: part II. Tumors of the middle and posterior mediastinum. Chest. 1997;112:1344-1357.

98. Lonergan GJ, Schwab CM, Suarez ES, Carlson CL. Neuroblastoma, ganglioneuroblastoma, and ganglioneuroma: radiologic-pathologic correlation. Radiographics. 2002;22:911-934.

99. Maris JM, Hogarty MD, Bagatell R, Cohn SL. Neuroblastoma. Lancet. 2007;369:2106-2120.

100. Kellenberger CJ, Epelman M, Miller SF, Babyn PS. Fast STIR whole-body MR imaging in children. Radiographics. 2004;24:1317-1330.

101. Meyer JS, Siegel MJ, Farooqui SO, et al. Which MRI sequence of the spine best reveals bone-marrow metastases of neuroblastoma? Pediatr Radiol. 2005;35:778-785.

102. Kushner BH, Yeung HW, Larson SM, et al. Extending positron emission tomography scan utility to high-risk neuroblastoma: fluorine-18 fluorodeoxyglucose positron emission tomography as sole imaging modality in follow-up of patients. J Clin Oncol. 2001;19:3397-3405.

103. Sallustio G, Pironti T, Lasorella A, et al. Diagnostic imaging of primitive neuroectodermal tumour of the chest wall (Askin tumour). Pediatr Radiol. 1998;28:697-702.

104. Hawkins DS, Schuetze SM, Butrynski JE, et al. [18F] Fluorodeoxyglucose positron emission tomography predicts outcome for Ewing sarcoma family of tumors. J Clin Oncol. 2005;23:8828-8834.

105. Shamberger RC, Grier HE. Ewing's sarcoma/primitive neuroectodermal tumor of the chest wall. Semin Pediatr Surg. 2001;10:153-160.

106. Shamberger RC, Tarbell NJ, Perez-Atayde AR, Grier HE. Malignant small round cell tumor (Ewing's-PNET) of the chest wall in children. J Pediatr Surg. 1994;29:179-184.

107. Andrassy RJ, Wiener ES, Raney RB, et al. Thoracic sarcomas in children. Ann Surg. 1998;227:170-173.

108. Chui CH, Billups CA, Pappo AS, et al. Predictors of outcome in children and adolescents with rhabdomyosarcoma of the trunk—the St Jude Children's Research Hospital experience. J Pediatr Surg. 2005;40:1691-1695.

109. Arush MW, Israel O, Postovsky S, et al. Positron emission tomography/computed tomography with 18fluoro-deoxyglucose in the detection of local recurrence and distant metastases of pediatric sarcoma. Pediatr Blood Cancer. 2007;49:901-905.

110. Klem ML, Grewal RK, Wexler LH, et al. PET for staging in rhabdomyosarcoma: an evaluation of PET as an adjunct to current staging tools. J Pediatr Hematol Oncol. 2007;29:9-14.

111. Volker T, Denecke T, Steffen I, et al. Positron emission tomography for staging of pediatric sarcoma patients: results of a prospective multicenter trial. J Clin Oncol. 2007;25:5435-5441.

112. Groom KR, Murphey MD, Howard LM, et al. Mesenchymal hamartoma of the chest wall: radiologic manifestations with emphasis on cross-sectional imaging and histopathologic comparison. Radiology. 2002;222:205-211.

113. Absalon MJ, McCarville MB, Liu T, et al. Pulmonary nodules discovered during the initial evaluation of pediatric patients with bone and soft-tissue sarcoma. Pediatr Blood Cancer. 2008;50:1147-1153.

114. O JH, Yoo Ie R, Kim SH, et al. Clinical significance of small pulmonary nodules with little or no 18F-FDG uptake on PET/CT images of patients with nonthoracic malignancies. J Nucl Med. 2007;48:15-21.

115. Ehrlich PF, Hamilton TE, Grundy P, et al. The value of surgery in directing therapy for patients with Wilms' tumor with pulmonary disease. A report from the National Wilms' Tumor Study

Group (National Wilms' Tumor Study 5). J Pediatr Surg. 2006;41:162-167.

116. Owens CM, Veys PA, Pritchard J, et al. Role of chest computed tomography at diagnosis in the management of Wilms' tumor: a study by the United Kingdom Children's Cancer Study Group. J Clin Oncol. 2002;20:2768-2773.

117. Wootton-Gorges SL, Albano EA, Riggs JM, et al. Chest radiography versus chest CT in the evaluation for pulmonary metastases in patients with Wilms' tumor: a retrospective review. Pediatr Radiol. 2000;30:533-537.

118. Studler U, Gluecker T, Bongartz G, et al. Image quality from high-resolution CT of the lung: comparison of axial scans and of sections reconstructed from volumetric data acquired using MDCT. AJR Am J Roentgenol. 2005;185:602-607.

119. Meyers RL. Tumors of the liver in children. Surg Oncol. 2007;16:195-203.

120. von Schweinitz D. Management of liver tumors in childhood. Semin Pediatr Surg. 2006;15:17-24.

121. Takano H, Smith WL. Gastrointestinal tumors of childhood. Radiol Clin North Am. 1997;35:1367-1389.

122. Emre S, McKenna GJ. Liver tumors in children. Pediatr Transplant. 2004;8:632-638.

123. Roebuck DJ, Olsen O, Pariente D. Radiological staging in children with hepatoblastoma. Pediatr Radiol. 2006;36:176-182.

124. Roebuck DJ, Perilongo G. Hepatoblastoma: an oncological review. Pediatr Radiol. 2006;36:183-186.

125. Czauderna P, Otte JB, Roebuck DJ, et al. Surgical treatment of hepatoblastoma in children. Pediatr Radiol. 2006;36:187-191.

126. McCarville MB, Kao SC. Imaging recommendations for malignant liver neoplasms in children. Pediatr Blood Cancer. 2006;46:2-7.

127. Aronson DC, Schnater JM, Staalman CR, et al. Predictive value of the pretreatment extent of disease system in hepatoblastoma: results from the International Society of Pediatric Oncology Liver Tumor Study Group SIOPEL-1 study. J Clin Oncol. 2005;23:1245-1252.

128. Mody RJ, Pohlen JA, Malde S, et al. FDG-PET for the study of primary hepatic malignancies in children. Pediatr Blood Cancer. 2006;47:51-55.

129. Philip I, Shun A, McCowage G, Howman-Giles R. Positron emission tomography in recurrent hepatoblastoma. Pediatr Surg Int. 2005;21:341-345.

130. Krishnamurthy G, Teo ELHJ. Liver tumours. In Carty H, Brunelle F, Stringer DA, Kao S (eds). Imaging Children. Edinburgh, Elsevier, 2004, pp 1579-1592.

131. Ward J. New MR techniques for the detection of liver metastases. Cancer Imaging. 2006;6:33-42.

132. Torbenson M. Review of the clinicopathologic features of fibrolamellar carcinoma. Adv Anat Pathol. 2007;14:217-223.

133. McLarney JK, Rucker PT, Bender GN, et al. Fibrolamellar carcinoma of the liver: radiologic-pathologic correlation. Radiographics. 1999;19:453-471.

134. Helmberger TK, Ros PR, Mergo PJ, et al. Pediatric liver neoplasms: a radiologic-pathologic correlation. Eur Radiol. 1999;9:1339-1347.

135. Nicol K, Savell V, Moore J, et al. Distinguishing undifferentiated embryonal sarcoma of the liver from biliary tract rhabdomyosarcoma: a Children's Oncology Group study. Pediatr Dev Pathol. 2007;10:89-97.

136. Kassarjian A, Zurakowski D, Dubois J, et al. Infantile hepatic hemangiomas: clinical and imaging findings and their correlation with therapy. AJR Am J Roentgenol. 2004;182:785-795.

137. Christison-Lagay ER, Burrows PE, Alomari A, et al. Hepatic hemangiomas: subtype classification and development of a clinical practice algorithm and registry. J Pediatr Surg. 2007;42:62-67.

138. Regier TS, Ramji FG. Pediatric hepatic hemangioma. Radiographics. 2004;24:1719-1724.

139. Bianchi L. Glycogen storage disease I and hepatocellular tumours. Eur J Pediatr. 1993;152(Suppl 1):S63-S70.

140. Okada T, Sasaki F, Kamiyama T, et al. Management and algorithm for focal nodular hyperplasia of the liver in children. Eur J Pediatr Surg. 2006;16:235-240.

141. Citak EC, Karadeniz C, Oguz A, et al. Nodular regenerative hyperplasia and focal nodular hyperplasia of the liver mimicking hepatic metastasis in children with solid tumors and a review of literature. Pediatr Hematol Oncol. 2007;24:281-289.

142. Joyner BL Jr, Levin TL, Goyal RK, Newman B. Focal nodular hyperplasia of the liver: a sequela of tumor therapy. Pediatr Radiol. 2005;35:1234-1239.

143. Abbott RM, Levy AD, Aguilera NS, et al. From the archives of the AFIP: primary vascular neoplasms of the spleen: radiologic-pathologic correlation. Radiographics. 2004;24:1137-1163.

144. Paterson A, Frush DP, Donnelly LF, et al. A pattern-oriented approach to splenic imaging in infants and children. Radiographics. 1999;19:1465-1485.

145. Rini JN, Leonidas JC, Tomas MB, Palestro CJ. 18F-FDG-PET versus CT for evaluating the spleen during initial staging of lymphoma. J Nucl Med. 2003;44:1072-1074.

146. Metser U, Miller E, Kessler A, et al. Solid splenic masses: evaluation with 18F-FDG PET/CT. J Nucl Med. 2005;46:52-59.

147. Kebudi R, Gorgun O, Ayan I, et al. Rhabdomyosarcoma of the biliary tree. Pediatr Int. 2003;45:469-471.

148. Montemarano H, Lonergan GJ, Bulas DI, Selby DM. Pancreatoblastoma: imaging findings in 10 patients and review of the literature. Radiology. 2000;214:476-482.

149. Roebuck DJ, Yuen MK, Wong YC, et al. Imaging features of pancreatoblastoma. Pediatr Radiol. 2001;31:501-506.

150. Moholkar S, Sebire NJ, Roebuck DJ. Solid-pseudopapillary neoplasm of the pancreas: radiological-pathological correlation. Pediatr Radiol. 2005;35:819-822.

151. Choi SH, Kim SM, Oh JT, et al. Solid pseudopapillary tumor of the pancreas: a multicenter study of 23 pediatric cases. J Pediatr Surg. 2006;41:1992-1995.

152. Sato M, Takasaka I, Okumura T, et al. High F-18 fluorodeoxyglucose accumulation in solid pseudo-papillary tumors of the pancreas. Ann Nucl Med. 2006;20:431-436.

153. Miller DV, Coffin CM, Zhou H. Rhabdomyosarcoma arising in the hand or foot: a clinicopathologic analysis. Pediatr Dev Pathol. 2004;7:361-369.

154. Janeway KA, Liegl B, Harlow A, et al. Pediatric KIT wild-type and platelet-derived growth factor receptor α wild-type gastrointestinal stromal tumors share KIT activation but not mechanisms of genetic progression with adult gastrointestinal stromal tumors. Cancer Res. 2007;67:9084-9088.

155. Judson I, Demetri G. Advances in the treatment of gastrointestinal stromal tumours. Ann Oncol. 2007;18(Suppl 10):20-24.

156. del-Pozo G, Albillos JC, Tejedor D, et al. Intussusception in children: current concepts in diagnosis and enema reduction. Radiographics. 1999;19:299-319.

157. Depas G, De Barsy C, Jerusalem G, et al. 18F-FDG-PET in children with lymphomas. Eur J Nucl Med Mol Imaging. 2005;32:31-38.

158. Querellou S, Valette F, Bodet-Milin C, et al. FDG-PET/CT predicts outcome in patients with aggressive non-Hodgkin's lymphoma and Hodgkin's disease. Ann Hematol. 2006;85:759-767.

159. Schaefer NG, Hany TF, Taverna C, et al. Non-Hodgkin lymphoma and Hodgkin disease: coregistered FDG-PET and CT at staging and restaging—do we need contrast-enhanced CT? Radiology. 2004;232:823-829.

160. Herrmann K, Wieder HA, Buck AK, et al. Early response assessment using 3′-deoxy-3′-[18F]fluorothymidine-positron emission tomography in high-grade non-Hodgkin's lymphoma. Clin Cancer Res. 2007;13:3552-3558.

161. Khanna G, O'Dorisio SM, Menda Y, et al. Gastroenteropancreatic neuroendocrine tumors in children and young adults. Pediatr Radiol. 2008;38:251-259.

162. Geller E, Smergel EM, Lowry PA. Renal neoplasms of childhood. Radiol Clin North Am. 1997;35:1391-1413.

163. Kaste SC, Dome JS, Babyn PS, et al. Wilms tumour: prognostic factors, staging, therapy and late effects. Pediatr Radiol. 2008;38:2-17.

164. D'Angio GJ, Breslow N, Beckwith JB, et al. Treatment of Wilms' tumor. Results of the Third National Wilms' Tumor Study. Cancer. 1989;64:349-360.

165. Brisse HJ, Smets AM, Kaste SC, Owens CM. Imaging in unilateral Wilms' tumour. Pediatr Radiol. 2008;38:18-29.

166. Shamberger RC, Guthrie KA, Ritchey ML, et al. Surgery-related factors and local recurrence of Wilms' tumor in National Wilms' tumor Study 4. Ann Surg. 1999;229:292-297.

167. Wilimas JA, Kaste SC, Kauffman WM, et al. Use of chest computed tomography in the staging of pediatric Wilms' tumor: interobserver variability and prognostic significance. J Clin Oncol. 1997;15:2631-2635.

168. Meisel JA, Guthrie KA, Breslow NE, et al. Significance and management of computed tomography detected pulmonary nodules: a report from the National Wilms' tumor Study Group. Int J Radiat Oncol Biol Phys. 1999;44:579-585.

169. Beckwith JB, Kiviat NB, Bonadio JF. Nephrogenic rests, nephroblastomatosis, and the pathogenesis of Wilms' tumor. Pediatr Pathol. 1990;10:1-36.

170. Lonergan GJ, Martinez-Leon MI, Agrons GA, et al. Nephrogenic rests, nephroblastomatosis, and associated lesions of the kidney. Radiographics. 1998;18:947-968.

171. Gylys-Morin V, Hoffer FA, Kozakewich H, Shamberger RC. Wilms' tumor and nephroblastomatosis: imaging characteristics at gadolinium-enhanced MR imaging. Radiology. 1993;188:517-521.

172. Munker R, Glass J, Griffeth LK, et al. Contribution of PET imaging to the initial staging and prognosis of patients with Hodgkin's disease. Ann Oncol. 2004;15:1699-1704.

173. Perlman EJ, Faria P, Soares A, et al. Hyperplastic perilobar nephroblastomatosis: long-term survival of 52 patients. Pediatr Blood Cancer. 2006;46:203-221.

174. Shulkin BL, Chang E, Strouse PJ, et al. PET FDG studies of Wilms' tumors. J Pediatr Hematol Oncol. 1997;19:334-338.

175. Argani P, Perlman EJ, Breslow NE, et al. Clear cell sarcoma of the kidney: a review of 351 cases from the National Wilms' tumor Study Group Pathology Center. Am J Surg Pathol. 2000;24:4-18.

176. Lowe LH, Isuani BH, Heller RM, et al. Pediatric renal masses: Wilms' tumor and beyond. Radiographics. 2000;20:1585-1603.

177. Chung CJ, Lorenzo R, Rayder S, et al. Rhabdoid tumors of the kidney in children: CT findings. AJR Am J Roentgenol. 1995;164:697-700.

178. Agrons GA, Kingsman KD, Wagner BJ, Sotelo-Avila C. Rhabdoid tumor of the kidney in children: a comparative study of 21 cases. AJR Am J Roentgenol. 1997;168:447-451.

179. Agrons GA, Wagner BJ, Davidson AJ, Suarez ES. Multilocular cystic renal tumor in children: radiologic-pathologic correlation. Radiographics. 1995;15:653-669.

180. Egloff AM, Lee EY, Dillon JE, Callahan MJ. Desmoplastic small round cell tumor of the kidney in a pediatric patient: sonographic and multiphase CT findings. AJR Am J Roentgenol. 2005;185:1347-1349.

181. Siegel MJ. Pelvic tumors in childhood. Radiol Clin North Am. 1997;35:1455-1475.

182. Siegel MJ, Hoffer FA. Magnetic resonance imaging of nongynecologic pelvic masses in children. Magn Reson Imaging Clin N Am. 2002;10:325-344.

183. Brodeur GM, Pritchard J, Berthold F, et al. Revisions of the international criteria for neuroblastoma diagnosis, staging, and response to treatment. J Clin Oncol. 1993;11:1466-1477.

184. Brodeur GM, Seeger RC, Barrett A, et al. International criteria for diagnosis, staging, and response to treatment in patients with neuroblastoma. J Clin Oncol. 1988;6:1874-1881.

185. Mazumdar A, Siegel MJ, Narra V, Luchtman-Jones L. Whole-body fast inversion recovery MR imaging of small cell neoplasms in pediatric patients: a pilot study. Am J Roentgenol. 2002;179:1261-1266.

186. Shulkin BL, Shapiro B. Current concepts on the diagnostic use of MIBG in children. J Nucl Med. 1998;39:679-688.

187. Kushner BH, Cheung NK. Exploiting the MIBG-avidity of neuroblastoma for staging and treatment. Pediatr Blood Cancer. 2006;47:863-864.

188. Kushner BH, Yeh SD, Kramer K, et al. Impact of metaiodobenzylguanidine scintigraphy on assessing response of high-risk neuroblastoma to dose-intensive induction chemotherapy. J Clin Oncol. 2003;21:1082-1086.

189. Katzenstein HM, Cohn SL, Shore RM, et al. Scintigraphic response by 123I-metaiodobenzylguanidine scan correlates with event-free survival in high-risk neuroblastoma. J Clin Oncol. 2004;22:3909-3915.

190. Matthay KK, Edeline V, Lumbroso J, et al. Correlation of early metastatic response by 123I-metaiodobenzylguanidine scintigraphy with overall response and event-free survival in stage IV neuroblastoma. J Clin Oncol. 2003;21:2486-2491.

191. Schmidt M, Simon T, Hero B, et al. The prognostic impact of functional imaging with (123)I-mIBG in patients with stage 4 neuroblastoma >1 year of age on a high-risk treatment protocol: results of the German Neuroblastoma Trial NB97. Eur J Cancer. 2008;44:1552-1558.

192. Suc A, Lumbroso J, Rubie H, et al. Metastatic neuroblastoma in children older than one year: prognostic significance of the initial metaiodobenzylguanidine scan and proposal for a scoring system. Cancer. 1996;77:805-811.

193. Ady N, Zucker JM, Asselain B, et al. A new 123I-MIBG whole body scan scoring method—application to the prediction of the response of metastases to induction chemotherapy in stage IV neuroblastoma. Eur J Cancer. 1995;31A:256-261.

194. Messina JA, Cheng SC, Franc BL, et al. Evaluation of semi-quantitative scoring system for metaiodobenzylguanidine (mIBG) scans in patients with relapsed neuroblastoma. Pediatr Blood Cancer. 2006;47:865-874.

195. Shulkin BL, Hutchinson RJ, Castle VP, et al. Neuroblastoma: positron emission tomography with 2-[fluorine-18]-fluoro-2-deoxy-D-glucose compared with metaiodobenzylguanidine scintigraphy. Radiology. 1996;199:743-750.

196. Fonti R, Cheung NK, Bridger GJ, et al. 99mTc-monoclonal antibody radiolabeled via hydrazino nicotinamide derivative for imaging disialoganglioside G(D2)-positive tumors. Nucl Med Biol. 1999;26:681-686.

197. Reuland P, Geiger L, Thelen MH, et al. Follow-up in neuroblastoma: comparison of metaiodobenzylguanidine and a chimeric anti-GD2 antibody for detection of tumor relapse and therapy response. J Pediatr Hematol Oncol. 2001;23:437-442.

198. Johnson E, Dean SM, Sondel PM. Antibody-based immunotherapy in high-risk neuroblastoma. Expert Rev Mol Med. 2007;9:1-21.

198a. Blackman SC, Evenson AR, Voss SD, et al. Prenatal diagnosis and subsequent treatment of an intermediate-risk paraspinal neuroblastoma: Case report and review of the literature. Fetal Diagn Ther. 2008;24:119-125.

199. Hayward K, Jeremy RJ, Jenkins S, et al. Long-term neurobehavioral outcomes in children with neuroblastoma and opsoclonus-myoclonus-ataxia syndrome: relationship to MRI findings and anti-neuronal antibodies. J Pediatr. 2001;139:552-559.

200. Rudnick E, Khakoo Y, Antunes NL, et al. Opsoclonus-myoclonus-ataxia syndrome in neuroblastoma: clinical outcome and antineuronal antibodies-a report from the Children's Cancer Group Study. Med Pediatr Oncol. 2001;36:612-622.

201. Parisi MT, Hattner RS, Matthay KK, et al. Optimized diagnostic strategy for neuroblastoma in opsoclonus-myoclonus. J Nucl Med. 1993;34:1922-1926.

202. Swart JF, de Kraker J, van der Lely N. Metaiodobenzylguanidine total-body scintigraphy required for revealing occult neuroblastoma in opsoclonus-myoclonus syndrome. Eur J Pediatr. 2002;161:255-258.

203. Reynolds CP, Matthay KK, Villablanca JG, Maurer BJ. Retinoid therapy of high-risk neuroblastoma. Cancer Lett. 2003;197:185-192.

204. Geoerger B, Hero B, Harms D, et al. Metabolic activity and clinical features of primary ganglioneuromas. Cancer. 2001;91:1905-1913.

205. Hain SF, O'Doherty MJ, Timothy AR, et al. Fluorodeoxyglucose positron emission tomography in the evaluation of germ cell tumours at relapse. Br J Cancer. 2000;83:863-869.

206. Hain SF, O'Doherty MJ, Timothy AR, et al. Fluorodeoxyglucose PET in the initial staging of germ cell tumours. Eur J Nucl Med. 2000;27:590-594.

207. Spermon JR, De Geus-Oei LF, Kiemeney LA, et al. The role of (18)fluoro-2-deoxyglucose positron emission tomography in initial staging and re-staging after chemotherapy for testicular germ cell tumours. BJU Int. 2002;89:549-556.

208. Keslar PJ, Buck JL, Suarez ES. Germ cell tumors of the sacrococcygeal region: radiologic-pathologic correlation. Radiographics. 1994;14:607-620.

209. Altman RP, Randolph JG, Lilly JR. Sacrococcygeal teratoma: American Academy of Pediatrics Surgical Section survey—1973. J Pediatr Surg. 1974;9:389-398.

210. Miller SL, Hoffer FA. Malignant and benign bone tumors. Radiol Clin North Am. 2001;39:673-699.

211. Fayad LM, Bluemke DA, Weber KL, Fishman EK. Characterization of pediatric skeletal tumors and tumor-like conditions: specific cross-sectional imaging signs. Skeletal Radiol. 2006;35:259-268.

212. Teo HE, Peh WC. The role of imaging in the staging and treatment planning of primary malignant bone tumors in children. Eur Radiol. 2004;14:465-475.

213. Brenner W, Bohuslavizki KH, Eary JF. PET imaging of osteosarcoma. J Nucl Med. 2003;44:930-942.

214. Gyorke T, Zajic T, Lange A, et al. Impact of FDG-PET for staging of Ewing sarcomas and primitive neuroectodermal tumours. Nucl Med Commun. 2006;27:17-24.

215. Kumar R, Chauhan A, Kesav Vellimana A, Chawla M. Role of PET/PET-CT in the management of sarcomas. Expert Rev Anticancer Ther. 2006;6:1241-1250.

216. Furth C, Amthauer H, Denecke T, et al. Impact of whole-body MRI and FDG-PET on staging and assessment of therapy response in a patient with Ewing sarcoma. Pediatr Blood Cancer. 2006;47:607-611.

217. Hawkins DS, Rajendran JG, Conrad EU 3rd, et al. Evaluation of chemotherapy response in pediatric bone sarcomas by [F-18]-fluorodeoxy-D-glucose positron emission tomography. Cancer. 2002;94:3277-3284.

218. Gorlick R, Anderson P, Andrulis I, et al. Biology of childhood osteogenic sarcoma and potential targets for therapeutic development: meeting summary. Clin Cancer Res. 2003;9:5442-5453.

219. Marina N, Gebhardt M, Teot L, Gorlick R. Biology and therapeutic advances for pediatric osteosarcoma. Oncologist. 2004;9:422-441.

220. Arndt CA, Crist WM. Common musculoskeletal tumors of childhood and adolescence. N Engl J Med. 1999;341:342-352.

221. Meyer JS, Dormans JP. Differential diagnosis of pediatric musculoskeletal masses. Magn Reson Imaging Clin North Am. 1998;6:561-577.

222. Mar WA, Taljanovic MS, Bagatell R, et al. Update on imaging and treatment of Ewing sarcoma family tumors: what the radiologist needs to know. J Comput Assist Tomogr. 2008;32:108-118.

223. Siegel MJ. Magnetic resonance imaging of musculoskeletal soft tissue masses. Radiol Clin North Am. 2001;39:701-720.

224. McCarville MB, Spunt SL, Pappo AS. Rhabdomyosarcoma in pediatric patients: the good, the bad, and the unusual. AJR Am J Roentgenol. 2001;176:1563-1569.

225. McCarville MB, Christie R, Daw NC, et al. PET/CT in the evaluation of childhood sarcomas. AJR Am J Roentgenol. 2005;184:1293-1304.

226. McCarville MB, Spunt SL, Skapek SX, Pappo AS. Synovial sarcoma in pediatric patients. AJR Am J Roentgenol. 2002;179:797-801.

227. Brecht IB, Ferrari A, Int-Veen C, et al. Grossly-resected synovial sarcoma treated by the German and Italian Pediatric Soft Tissue Sarcoma Cooperative Groups: discussion on the role of adjuvant therapies. Pediatr Blood Cancer. 2006;46:11-17.

228. Tolan S, Shanks JH, Loh MY, et al. Fibromatosis: benign by name but not necessarily by nature. Clin Oncol (R Coll Radiol). 2007;19:319-326.

229. Robbin MR, Murphey MD, Temple HT, et al. Imaging of musculoskeletal fibromatosis. Radiographics. 2001;21:585-600.

230. Margolin JF, Steuber CP, Poplack DG. Acute lymphoblastic leukemia. In Pizzo PA, Poplack DG (eds). Principles and Practice of Pediatric Oncology, 4th ed. Philadelphia, Lippincott Williams & Wilkins, 2002, pp 489-544.

231. Abbas AA, Baker DL, Felimban SK, Husain AH. Musculoskeletal and radiological manifestations of childhood acute leukaemia: a clinical review. Haematologica. 2004;7:448-455.

232. Vazquez E, Lucaya J, Castellote A, et al. Neuroimaging in pediatric leukemia and lymphoma: differential diagnosis. Radiographics. 2002;22:1411-1428.

233. Parker BR. Leukemia and lymphoma in childhood. Radiol Clin North Am. 1997;35:1495-1516.

234. Cohn SL, Morgan ER, Mallette LE. The spectrum of metabolic bone disease in lymphoblastic leukemia. Cancer. 1987;59:346-350.

235. Vande Berg BC, Lecouvet FE, Michaux L, et al. Magnetic resonance imaging of the bone marrow in hematological malignancies. Eur Radiol. 1998;8:1335-1344.

236. Fletcher BD, Wall JE, Hanna SL. Effect of hematopoietic growth factors on MR images of bone marrow in children undergoing chemotherapy. Radiology. 1993;189:745-751.

237. Kan JH, Hernanz-Schulman M, Frangoul HA, Connolly SA. MRI diagnosis of bone marrow relapse in children with ALL. Pediatr Radiol. 2008;38:76-81.

238. Attarbaschi A, Mann G, Dworzak M, et al. Mediastinal mass in childhood T-cell acute lymphoblastic leukemia: significance and therapy response. Med Pediatr Oncol. 2002;39:558-565.

239. Golub TR, Arceci RJ. Acute myelogenous leukemia. In Pizzo PA, Poplack DG (eds). Principles and Practice of Pediatric Oncology. Philadelphia, Lippincott Williams & Wilkins, 2002, pp 545-589.

240. Guermazi A, Feger C, Rousselot P, et al. Granulocytic sarcoma (chloroma): imaging findings in adults and children. AJR Am J Roentgenol. 2002;178:319-325.

241. Hudson MM, Donaldson SS. Hodgkin's disease. In Pizzo PA, Poplack DG (eds). Principles and Practice of Pediatric Oncology. Philadelphia, Lippincott Williams & Wilkins, 2002, pp 637-660.

242. McGrath IT. Malignant non-Hodgkin's lymphomas in children. In Pizzo PA, Poplack DG (eds). Principles and Practice of Pediatric Oncology. Philadelphia, Lippincott Williams & Wilkins, 2002, pp 661-705.

243. Guillerman RP, Parker BD (eds).Pediatric Lymphoma. Berlin, Springer-Verlag, 2004.

244. Roth SL, Sack H, Havemann K, et al. Contiguous pattern spreading in patients with Hodgkin's disease. Radiat Oncol. 1998;47:7-16.

245. Carbone PP, Kaplan HS, Musshoff K, et al. Report of the Committee on Hodgkin's Disease Staging Classification. Cancer Res. 1971;31:1860-1861.

246. Lister TA, Crowther D, Sutcliffe SB, et al. Report of a committee convened to discuss the evaluation and staging of patients with Hodgkin's disease: Cotswolds meeting. J Clin Oncol. 1989;7:1630-1636.

247. Front D, Ben-Haim S, Israel O, et al. Lymphoma: predictive value of Ga-67 scintigraphy after treatment. Radiology. 1992;182:359-363.

248. Dann EJ, Bar-Shalom R, Tamir A, et al. Risk-adapted BEACOPP regimen can reduce the cumulative dose of chemotherapy for standard and high-risk Hodgkin lymphoma with no impairment of outcome. Blood. 2007;109:905-909.

249. Kabickova E, Sumerauer D, Cumlivska E, et al. Comparison of 18F-FDG-PET and standard procedures for the pretreatment staging of children and adolescents with Hodgkin's disease. Eur J Nucl Med Mol Imaging. 2006;33:1025-1031.

250. Advani R, Maeda L, Lavori P, et al. Impact of positive positron emission tomography on prediction of freedom from progression after Stanford V chemotherapy in Hodgkin's disease. J Clin Oncol. 2007;25:3902-3907.

251. Picardi M, De Renzo A, Pane F, et al. Randomized comparison of consolidation radiation versus observation in bulky Hodgkin's lymphoma with post-chemotherapy negative positron emission tomography scans. Leuk Lymphoma. 2007;48:1721-1727.

252. Murphy SB, Fairclough DL, Hutchison RE, Berard CW. Non-Hodgkin's lymphomas of childhood: an analysis of the histology, staging, and response to treatment of 338 cases at a single institution. J Clin Oncol. 1989;7:186-193.

253. Scarsbrook AF, Warakaulle DR, Dattani M, Traill Z. Post-transplantation lymphoproliferative disorder: the spectrum of imaging appearances. Clin Radiol. 2005;60:47-55.

254. Bakker NA, van Imhoff GW, Verschuuren EA, van Son WJ. Presentation and early detection of post-transplant lymphoproliferative disorder after solid organ transplantation. Transpl Int. 2007;20:207-218.

255. Coleman M, Kostakoglu L. Early 18F-labeled fluoro-2-deoxy-D-glucose positron emission tomography scanning in the lymphomas: changing the paradigms of treatments? Cancer. 2006;107:1425-1428.

256. Hernandez-Maraver D, Hernandez-Navarro F, Gomez-Leon N, et al. Positron emission tomography/computed tomography: diagnostic accuracy in lymphoma. Br J Haematol. 2006;135:293-302.

257. Kostakoglu L, Goldsmith SJ, Leonard JP, et al. FDG-PET after 1 cycle of therapy predicts outcome in diffuse large cell lymphoma and classic Hodgkin disease. Cancer. 2006;107:2678-2687.

258. Amthauer H, Furth C, Denecke T, et al. FDG-PET in 10 children with Non-Hodgkin's lymphoma: initial experience in staging and follow-up. Klinische Pädiatrie. 2005;327-333.

259. Helton KJ, Kuhn JP, Fletcher BD, et al. Bronchiolitis obliterans–organizing pneumonia (BOOP) in children with malignant disease. Pediatr Radiol. 1992;22:270-274.

260. Babyn PS, Gahunia HK, Massicotte P. Pulmonary thromboembolism in children. Pediatr Radiol. 2005;35:258-274.

261. Kirkpatrick IDC, Greenberg HM. Gastrointestinal complications in the neutropenic patient: characterization and differentiation with abdominal CT. Radiology. 2003;226:668-674.

262. Parisi MT, Fahmy JL, Kaminsky CK, Malogolowkin MH. Complications of cancer therapy in children: a radiologist's guide. Radiographics. 1999;19:283-297.

263. Roebuck DJ. Skeletal complications in pediatric oncology patients. Radiographics. 1999;19:873-885.

264. Humpl T, Bruhl K, Bohl J, et al. Cerebral haemorrhage in long-term survivors of childhood acute lymphoblastic leukaemia. Eur J Pediatr. 1997;156:367-370.

265. Kelloff GJ, Krohn KA, Larson SM, et al. The progress and promise of molecular imaging probes in oncologic drug development. Clin Cancer Res. 2005;11:7967-7985.

266. Van den Abbeele AD, Badawi RD. Use of positron emission tomography in oncology and its potential role to assess response to imatinib mesylate therapy in gastrointestinal stromal tumors (GISTs). Eur J Cancer. 2002;38(Suppl 5):S60-S65.

267. Miller JC, Thrall JH. Clinical molecular imaging. J Am Coll Radiol. 2004;1:4-23.

268. Weissleder R, Mahmood U. Molecular imaging. Radiology. 2001;219:316-333.

269. Jaffer FA, Weissleder R. Molecular imaging in the clinical arena. JAMA. 2005;293:855-862.

270. Bremer C, Ntziachristos V, Weissleder R. Optical-based molecular imaging: contrast agents and potential medical applications. Eur Radiol. 2003;13:231-243.

271. Mahmood U, Weissleder R. Near-infrared optical imaging of proteases in cancer. Mol Cancer Ther. 2003;2:489-496.

272. Weissleder R, Ntziachristos V. Shedding light onto live molecular targets. Nat Med. 2003;9:123-128.

273. Frangioni JV. Translating in vivo diagnostics into clinical reality. Nat Biotechnol. 2006;24:909-913.

274. Frangioni JV. In vivo near-infrared fluorescence imaging. Curr Opin Chem Biol. 2003;7:626-634.

275. Marten K, Bremer C, Khazaie K, et al. Detection of dysplastic intestinal adenomas using enzyme-sensing molecular beacons in mice. Gastroenterology. 2002;122:406-414.

276. Jacobs A, Voges J, Reszka R, et al. Positron-emission tomography of vector-mediated gene expression in gene therapy for gliomas. Lancet. 2001;358:727-729.

277. Griffith JF, Yeung DK, Antonio GE, et al. Vertebral bone mineral density, marrow perfusion, and fat content in healthy men and men with osteoporosis: dynamic contrast-enhanced MR imaging and MR spectroscopy. Radiology. 2005;236:945-951.

278. Lindskog M, Spenger C, Klason T, et al. Proton magnetic resonance spectroscopy in neuroblastoma: current status, prospects and limitations. Cancer Lett. 2005;228:247-255.

279. Lindskog M, Spenger C, Jarvet J, et al. Predicting resistance or response to chemotherapy by proton magnetic resonance spectroscopy in neuroblastoma. J Natl Cancer Inst. 2004;96:1457-1466.

280. Negendank WG, Crowley MG, Ryan JR, et al. Bone and soft-tissue lesions: diagnosis with combined H-1 MR imaging and P-31 MR spectroscopy. Radiology. 1989;173:181-188.

281. Preul MC, Caramanos Z, Collins DL, et al. Accurate, noninvasive diagnosis of human brain tumors by using proton magnetic resonance spectroscopy. Nat Med. 1996;2:323-325.

282. Levitzki A. Tyrosine kinases as targets for cancer therapy. Eur J Cancer. 2002;38(Suppl 5):S11-S18.

283. Sosnovik DE, Weissleder R. Emerging concepts in molecular MRI. Curr Opin Biotechnol. 2007;18:4-10.

284. Caravan P, Ellison JJ, McMurry TJ, Lauffer RB. Gadolinium(III) chelates as MRI contrast agents: structure, dynamics, and applications. Chem Rev. 1999;99:2293-2352.

285. Hogemann D, Basilion JP. "Seeing inside the body": MR imaging of gene expression. Eur J Nucl Med Mol Imaging. 2002;29:400-408.

286. Weissleder R, Moore A, Mahmood U, et al. In vivo magnetic resonance imaging of transgene expression. Nat Med. 2000;6:351-355.

287. Weissleder R, Cheng HC, Bogdanova A, Bogdanov A Jr. Magnetically labeled cells can be detected by MR imaging. J Magn Reson Imaging. 1997;7:258-263.

288. Hogemann-Savellano D, Bos E, Blondet C, et al. The transferrin receptor: a potential molecular imaging marker for human cancer. Neoplasia. 2003;5:495-506.

289. Wunderbaldinger P, Josephson L, Weissleder R. Tat peptide directs enhanced clearance and hepatic permeability of magnetic nanoparticles. Bioconjug Chem. 2002;13:264-268.

290. Zhao M, Weissleder R. Intracellular cargo delivery using tat peptide and derivatives. Med Res Rev. 2004;24:1-12.

291. Gaa J, Rummeny EJ, Seemann MD. Whole-body imaging with PET/MRI. Eur J Med Res. 2004;9:309-312.

27

Infectious Diseases in Pediatric Cancer

Andrew Y. Koh and Philip A. Pizzo

INTRODUCTION

Children with cancer are predisposed to a variety of infectious complications as a consequence of perturbations of one or more components of their host defense systems; the most common cause of immune compromise is related to chemotherapy. The potential pathogens encountered in the compromised host are extensive and include bacteria, fungi, viruses, and protozoa.[1-3] The majority of organisms that cause infections in immunocompromised hosts can generally be found as components of the normal human endogenous microflora (i.e., gram-negative bacteria and *Candida albicans*). Other organisms, such as *Pseudomonas aeruginosa* and *Aspergillus* species, are usually acquired from exogenous sources and colonize the patient before infection. Still others, such as varicella-zoster virus and *Pneumocystis jiroveci* (formerly known as *Pneumocystis carinii*), may be present in a latent or subclinical stage for years before significant infection develops. Ultimately, the presence of an invasive infection is determined by the relative virulence of the resident or colonizing organism and the severity and type of the host's impairment.

MAJOR PATHOGENS RESPONSIBLE FOR INFECTIONS IN PEDIATRIC CANCER PATIENTS

Bacteria

Bacteria cause the majority of infections that are encountered in compromised patients and account for the greatest morbidity and mortality rates.[4] Of particular importance are the coagulase-positive and coagulase-negative staphylococci and the streptococci (including enterococci and α-hemolytic streptococci), which have replaced gram-negative isolates as the predominant organisms causing documented infections in cancer patients.[5-8] Although bacteremia caused by gram-positive organisms is generally associated with lower mortality rates than that associated with gram-negative organisms, the α-hemolytic viridans streptococci (*Streptococcus mitis* and *S. sanguis*), which are normal inhabitants of the oral cavity, are now well recognized as the cause of serious infectious complications, particularly in patients who have received high doses of cytarabine or who have significant oral mucositis.[9,10] Bacteremia caused by these organisms can lead to adult respiratory syndrome (3% to 33%); shock (7% to 18%); or endocarditis (8%); it is associated with a mortality rate of between 6% and 30%.[11,12] The emergence of penicillin resistance among these previously susceptible organisms is of significant concern.[8,13] Traditionally, methicillin-resistant *Staphylococcus aureus* (MRSA) has been classified as a health care–associated pathogen; however, community-acquired MRSA has emerged in pediatric cancer patients who are without established risk factors.[14,15] Community-acquired MRSA tends to cause localized skin and soft tissue infections, although more invasive disease does occur (e.g., sepsis,[16] necrotizing fasciitis,[17] and pneumonia[18]). Less common but still important gram-positive bacteria include *Corynebacterium* species, *Bacillus* species, and *Listeria monocytogenes*. The more common use of indwelling intravenous access devices such as Hickman-Broviac catheters has also contributed to the increase in gram-positive infections,[19] particularly with coagulase-negative staphylococci. The rise in the number of enterococcal infections, including the increased prevalence of vancomycin-resistant enterococci in some medical centers, has been related, in part, to the use of certain antibiotics, particularly the third-generation cephalosporins and the fluoroquinolones.[20]

The most common gram-negative bacterium associated with infection in compromised hosts is *Escherichia coli*. For still unexplained reasons, the incidence of infection by *Pseudomonas aeruginosa* has declined markedly in neutropenic cancer patients during the past 2 decades in the United States and Western Europe.[21] Less commonly encountered but still important gram-negative bacteria include *Klebsiella* species, *Citrobacter* species, *Enterobacter* species, *Serratia marcescens*, *Acinetobacter* species, non-*P. aeruginosa Pseudomonas* species, and *Legionella* species. The relative distribution of these organisms can vary from hospital to hospital and may be influenced by local environmental factors, antibiotic usage and resistance patterns, infection control practices, and the patient population being treated. Antibiotic resistance has also been observed with gram-negative bacteria, applying to essentially all the β-lactam agents (i.e., extended-spectrum penicillins and cephalosporins) as well as carbapenems, aminoglycosides, and quinolones. Of specific concern are *Enterobacter* and *Serratia* species, which are prone to rapid development of resistance because of extended-spectrum inducible β-lactamases. The pattern of antibiotic resistance as well as the relative distribution of predominant organisms varies by medical center and thus should be considered in the choice of antimicrobial therapy for cancer patients with documented bacterial infections.

Despite their predominance in the normal flora, anaerobic organisms are associated less commonly with bacteremia in febrile, neutropenic patients. The most commonly isolated anaerobic organisms are *Bacteroides* species and *Clostridium* species (both *C. perfringens* and nonperfringens clostridia).[22] These organisms have been associated with peritonitis, abdominal or pelvis abscesses, perianal cellulitis, and necrotizing gingivitis. *Clostridium septicum* can cause severe infections characterized by septic shock and rapidly progressive necrotizing fasciitis with myonecrosis, which can rarely occur without fever. In addition, a variety of other anaerobic organisms have been reported to cause systemic infections in immunocompromised hosts, including *Fusobacterium* species, *Peptococcus* species, and *Leptotrichia buccalis*.[23]

Mycobacterial infections are generally uncommon causes of infection in cancer patients. Patients with hairy cell leukemia appear to have an increased risk for infection with atypical mycobacteria (i.e., *Mycobacterium kansasii*, *M. fortuitum*, *M. chelonae*, and *M. avium-intracellulare*),[24] and certain "rapid growers" may cause significant infections around the exit sites of indwelling intravenous catheters. Infection by *Nocardia* species is uncommon, but pulmonary and disseminated disease have been observed in cancer patients.[25]

Fungi

The major fungal species that cause serious infections in compromised patients are *Candida* species, *Aspergillus* species, and *Cryptococcus neoformans*. Fungi that are encountered less often but that are still important pathogens include *Coccidioides immitis*, *Histoplasma capsulatum*, *Trichosporon beigelii*, *Fusarium* species, *Alternaria* species, *Malassezia furfur*, and the dematiaceous fungi.[1,26,27] As with bacterial infections, the predominant fungal pathogens vary according to the pattern of host impairment and the environmental setting. For example, infections by *Candida* or *Aspergillus* species are most common in patients with prolonged neutropenia, whereas infections by *C. neoformans*, *H. capsulatum*, or *C. immitis* are more common in patients with impaired cell-mediated immunity (CMI).

Candida species are the most common causes of fungal infections in children with cancer, with *C. albicans* accounting for most isolates.[28] In the past 20 years, other *Candida* species (*C. tropicalis*, *C. parapsilosis*, *C. krusei*, and *C. glabrata*) have become more common, and this changing pattern of infections may be caused in part by the use of oral antifungal agents such as fluconazole.[29] Although *Candida* species are often found as part of the endogenous microbial flora, patients receiving broad-spectrum antibiotics, requiring extensive hospitalization, or receiving immunosuppressive agents are more vulnerable to invasive disease because of the intercurrent mucosal disruption caused by surgery, tumor invasion, or chemotherapy.[30,31] The major risk factor for developing fungemia, however, is the presence of an intravascular catheter.[32,33]

Aspergillus species are the second most common cause of invasive fungal disease in children with cancer, with *A. fumigatus* and *A. flavus* being the most common species isolated.[34] *Aspergillus* species are most readily cultured from various sites in the hospital environment, including unfiltered air, ventilation systems, renovation or construction sites, food, and ornamental plants.[27] Air is the principal route of transmission in the hospital environment, and the respiratory tract is the most common portal of entry. Upper airway colonization by *Aspergillus* species probably precedes most occurrences of invasive infection, and nasal colonization may portend infection in certain high-risk settings.[35,36]

Another major fungal pathogen in children with cancer is *Pneumocystis jiroveci* (formerly referred to as *Pneumocystis carinii* and a protozoan, but recently found to be a genetically unique *Pneumocystis* organism that causes disease in the human host).[37] In patients with cancer, symptomatic infection caused by *P. jiroveci* is thought to be the result of reactivation of latent organisms, and it appears to be associated with a more rapidly progressive pneumonia than that seen in adults and older children infected with human immunodeficiency virus.[38] The risk for *Pneumocystis carinii* pneumonia (PCP) is related to the use of corticosteroids (particularly the tapering and discontinuation of steroids), which explains its occurrence in children with leukemia, lymphomas, and brain tumors.[39,40]

Viruses

The predominant viral infections that occur in children with cancer are caused by the herpes simplex virus (HSV), varicella-zoster virus (VZV), cytomegalovirus (CMV), Epstein-Barr virus (EBV), influenza and parainfluenza viruses, respiratory syncytial viruses, adenoviruses, and the enteroviruses. In a prospective study of children with leukemia, HSV and VZV were identified consistently as the most common viral pathogens, and the incidence of infection is higher in children undergoing induction or during relapse than during remission.[41]

Symptoms caused by HSV, VZV, EBV, or CMV may result from either primary infection or reactivation of latent infection. Both HSV-1 and HSV-2 may cause significant morbidity in the compromised host. Primary infection by HSV-1 occurs during childhood between the ages of 2 and 10 years and is most commonly transmitted by contact with oral secretions. In contrast, HSV-2 infection is spread by genital contact and is generally acquired after puberty. High titers of anti-HSV-1 have been correlated with the development of subsequent clinical infections in patients with aplastic anemia and in patients undergoing allogeneic bone marrow transplantation, as well as in patients with acute leukemias requiring aggressive chemotherapy.[42]

Primary VZV can cause serious morbidity in children with hematologic malignancies.[43] Secondary varicella infection, herpes zoster (also known as shingles), may occur in children after they receive chemotherapy, irradiation, or bone marrow transplantation.[1]

CMV may cause serious infections in patients undergoing allogeneic bone marrow or organ transplantation.[44] Most studies indicate a 60% to 70% prevalence of antibody to CMV by adulthood, although seropositivity varies with geography, socioeconomic status, and age.[45] Serious disease may occur either through reactivation of latent CMV infection as a result of immunosuppression or through primary infection.

EBV infection can cause lymphoproliferative disorders ranging from localized to disseminated lymphadenopathy to non-Hodgkin's lymphoma in immunocompromised patients[46,47] and has also been associated with a fatal hemophagocytic syndrome.[48] In addition, EBV infection has been found to play a role in the cause of smooth muscle tumors in immunocompromised patients.[49]

Protozoa

The protozoal pathogens most commonly encountered in children with cancer include *Toxoplasma gondii* and *Cryptosporidium* species. Although most of these parasites present as reactivation infections, *Cryptosporidium* species have been found in cases of person-to-person transmission (both in and out of the hospital) as well as in outbreaks caused by a water source.[50] *T. gondii* can cause fulminant disease but most commonly is localized to the central nervous system: stem cell transplant patients are at the highest risk for developing toxoplasmosis in the central nervous system.[51] *Cryptosporidium* species must always be considered in any pediatric cancer patient who exhibits severe or persistent diarrhea.[52]

ALTERATIONS IN HOST DEFENSE THAT CONTRIBUTE TO INFECTION

Physical Defense Barriers

The skin and mucosal surfaces represent the primary defense against both endogenous and exogenous sources of infection. Disruption of skin and mucosa may result from tumor invasion, the cytotoxic effects of chemotherapy or radiotherapy, the use of invasive diagnostic therapeutic procedures (e.g., intravenous catheters), and the effects of local infections.[53-55] Cytotoxic chemotherapy is a common cause for disruption of the gastrointestinal mucosal integrity in patients with malignancy, particularly cytarabine, the anthracyclines (daunarubicin, doxorubicin), methotrexate, 6-mercaptopurine, and 5-fluorouracil.[10] Stomatitis is usually the most easily recognizable clinical manifestation of gastrointestinal toxicity, but diffuse gastrointestinal involvement is common. A recent study demonstrated that recombinant human keratinocyte growth factor, palifermin, not only reduced the duration and severity of oral mucositis after intensive chemotherapy and radiotherapy for hematologic malignancies but was also associated with a lower incidence of blood-borne infections in the group treated with palifermin.[56]

In addition to mucosal breakdown, mechanical obstruction of body passages can also increase the risk for serious localized infection caused by stasis of local body fluids and resultant overgrowth of potentially pathogenic colonizing organisms. Common sites of secondary infections caused by obstruction include the lung, the urinary and biliary tracts, and the eustachian tube. Anatomic abnormalities can also contribute to the risk for infection.

Central venous catheters and peripherally inserted central catheters are devices that violate skin integrity and can lead to a significant increase in risk for infection. One study reports an estimated fourfold higher incidence of bacteremia in neutropenic patients who had catheters than in those who did not.[19] Foreign devices other than catheters have also been implicated in the risk for infectious complications in cancer patients (e.g., Ommaya intraventricular reservoirs). Finally, limb-sparing procedures in patients with osteosarcoma often use prosthetic bone-joint hardware that can be associated with infections. For instance, one retrospective study showed that in children and adolescents with bone malignancies who underwent limb-sparing surgery, focal bacterial infections occurred in 67% of patients and bacteremia in 21% of patients. Infections at the surgical site occurred in 26% of patients, and 21% of patients developed infections related to the orthopedic device.[57] It must be noted, however, that the relative risk for infection in children with limb prostheses is not known, and optimal management has not been standardized.

Phagocyte Defects

The polymorphonuclear leukocyte and the monocyte are the two most important components of cellular defense by a host against invasive bacteria and fungi. Both quantitative and qualitative defects affecting polymorphonuclear leukocytes and monocytes may occur in cancer patients.

Quantitative Abnormalities of Phagocytes

Granulocytopenia is among the most important risk factors for serious infections in the compromised host. The additional disruption of a mucosal barrier that accompanies cytotoxic therapy appears to increase the risk for infection by gram-negative bacteria, α-streptococci, or anaerobes in neutropenic cancer patients. In comparably granulocytopenic patients with aplastic anemia, the unbroken mucosal barrier appears to lower the risk for developing systemic bacterial infections.[58]

The relationship between granulocytopenia and serious infection was established unequivocally by the classic study of Bodey and associates in 1966 at the National Cancer Institute. The investigators concluded that the risk for infection was inversely proportional to the absolute neutrophil count, and the most severe infections were more prevalent when the absolute neutrophil count fell below 100 cells per mm^3. But not only was the depth of neutropenia an important risk factor; the duration of the neutropenia was the single most important risk factor for developing infection, with severe neutropenia that lasted longer than 3 weeks being associated with a 100% risk for infection and the highest mortality rates.[59] For practical purposes, granulocytopenia is usually defined as the presence of a neutrophil and band form count of 500 cells per mm^3 or fewer.

Granulocytopenia predisposes patients primarily to bacterial and fungal infections and does not, per se, appear to increase the incidence or severity of viral and parasitic infections.[1,2] Bacterial pathogens predominate during the early phase of neutropenia. The spectrum of bacteria involved is influenced not only by the patient's own colonizing flora but also by the prevalent organisms at a specific treatment center. Over the past 30 years, a shift from predominantly gram-negative to predominantly gram-positive bacterial organisms has occurred in neutropenic patients with cancer.[60,61] Fungal infections, although occasionally seen at the beginning of neutropenia, are more commonly associated with prolonged granulocytopenia, and the rates of mortality owing to infection by *Aspergillus* species, for example, are highly significant in patients with protracted granulocytopenia and in patients with severe aplastic anemia.[34]

Qualitative Abnormalities of Phagocytes

The microbicidal activity of granulocytes and monocytes involves complex interactions between the cells and the organisms at the inflammatory site. Some major functions important for microbicidal activity include migration of the cell to the inflammatory site (chemotaxis), cell activation, phagocytosis, and intracellular or extracellular killing through both oxygen-dependent and oxygen-independent pathways. Impaired phagocyte function commonly results in the formation of bacterial or fungal abscesses.

In children with cancer, the predominant defects affecting polymorphonuclear neutrophils are quantitative; however, qualitative abnormalities of phagocytes can result from pharmacologic agents used to treat the underlying cancer. The majority of cytotoxic drugs used for treatment of malignant and autoimmune diseases and transplantation (most notably methotrexate, 6-mercaptopurine, vincristine, vinblastine, cyclophosphamide, carmustine, and platinum compounds) have the potential ability to result in alterations in superoxide production, phagocytosis, chemotaxis, microbicidal activity, and hexose-monophosphate shunt activity.[62] Corticosteroids impair neutrophil chemotaxis; and, at high dosages, polymorphonuclear leukocyte phagocytosis, microbicidal activity, and antibody-dependent cytotoxicity also may be altered.[63] In addition, corticosteroids may cause monocytopenia as well as defects in monocyte chemotaxis, phagocytosis, and the killing of bacteria and fungi. Corticosteroids also may impair wound healing, increase skin fragility, and depress lymphocyte function and the production of cytokines and humoral immune response, making the host susceptible to a variety of infections. It is important to note that the signs and symptoms of even severe infections may be masked or greatly reduced in patients receiving corticosteroids.[64]

Defects in Cell-Mediated Immunity

Defective CMI may lead to infections caused by bacteria, fungi, viruses, and protozoa. The predominant pathogens are intracellular organisms, so they are less susceptible to alternative pathways of infection control, such as antibodies and complement.

Certain malignant disorders (especially Hodgkin's and non-Hodgkin's lymphomas) are associated with altered CMI that can persist even when the malignancy is in remission.[65] Nonmalignant hematologic disorders are only rarely associated with alterations in CMI, but some abnormalities have been described in patients with hemophilia who have received factor VIII concentrates, and patients with severe combined immunodeficiency (SCID) are anergic in association with zinc deficiency and decreased nucleoside phosphorylase activity.[66,67]

The treatment of hematologic disorders per se can lead to defective CMI response. Corticosteroids are the pharmacologic agents most often associated with CMI abnormalities, although they may also cause immune suppression because of effects on other host mechanisms.[64,68] Several cytotoxic drugs impair CMI, including methotrexate, 6-mercaptopurine, cyclophosphamide, and azathioprine. Children treated for acute lymphocytic leukemia, as well as patients receiving very intensive chemotherapy for solid tumors, are at an increased risk for developing *Pneumocystis* pneumonia or disseminated viral infections, presumably because of the combination of an underlying immune defect with iatrogenically induced immunosuppression. Although neutrophils, monocytes, and platelets recover to nearly normal numbers between cycles of intensive chemotherapy, CD4+ and CD8+ lymphocyte populations progressively decrease and remain deficient for several months after completion of chemotherapy; in fact, reduced lymphocyte subset populations were linked to the occurrence of opportunistic infections in a group of patients receiving dose-intensive chemotherapeutic regimens.[69] Allogeneic (and to a lesser degree autologous) bone marrow transplantation is associated with a high risk for infection by the herpesviruses because both humoral and cellular immune responses are impaired.[70]

Abnormalities of Humoral Defense Mechanisms

Humoral mechanisms of defense against infections include antibody- and complement-dependent mechanisms, such as opsonization of organisms, neutralization of toxins, inhibition of attachment of organisms to host cells, lysis by complement, and extracellular neutralization of viruses. Defects or deficiencies in immunoglobulin and complement can therefore be associated with serious infections that are caused mainly by encapsulated bacteria and, to a lesser extent, by the enteroviruses and *Giardia lamblia*. Primary humoral impairment is rare in children with cancer but has been described in adults with chronic lymphocytic leukemia or myeloma.

Splenectomy and Splenic Dysfunction

The spleen plays an adjunctive role in host defense by removing from the blood organisms that have been ineffectively opsonized by complement. In addition, the spleen participates in the primary immunoglobulin response and is involved in the regulation of the alternative complement pathway; low levels of immunoglobulins and properdin have been reported in patients after splenectomy. Alternative pathway and complement defects may be important in patients with severe combined immunodeficiency (SCID) and splenic dysfunction. Most asplenic patients are at increased risk for serious bacterial infections caused primarily by *S. pneumoniae* and *H. influenzae*, as well as *Neisseria* species.[71] Patients with SCID are predisposed to developing bacteremia or even splenic abscesses as the result of functional asplenia.[72,73]

PRACTICAL ISSUES IN THE EVALUATION, MANAGEMENT, AND PREVENTION OF INFECTIONS

Because bacteria account for the majority of infections in compromised patients, prophylactic strategies have focused on these pathogens, although the prevention of viral, fungal, and parasitic diseases has also been investigated. Simple measures include conscientious and careful hand washing before and after examining patients; vigilance concerning the detection of potentially transmissible diseases, such as respiratory virus infections and VZV; and knowledge of the specific susceptibilities of the immunocompromised host. Reverse isolation (placing the patient in a single room and the wearing of gowns, masks, and gloves by health care personnel) after the onset of neutropenia will not prevent infection because most of the organisms arise from the patient's endogenous flora.[74] The total protective environment, which includes a high-efficiency particulate air (HEPA)–filtered laminar airflow room together with an aggressive program of surface decontamination, including the sterilization of all objects that enter the room and an

intensive regimen to disinfect the patient's diet, can reduce infection in profoundly granulocytopenic individuals (e.g., after a stem cell transplant), but it is expensive and, because of the improvement in treating established infections, does not offer a current survival advantage to most patients.

The fluoroquinolones (norfloxacin, ciprofloxacin, and levofloxacin) have been used in recent years for prophylaxis in neutropenic patients. A meta-analysis of published randomized trials of prophylaxis by quinolone found that the incidence of gram-negative bacterial infections, microbiologically documented infections, total infections, and fevers was significantly reduced; but the incidence of gram-positive infections and infection-related deaths was not reduced.[75] Two studies investigating the use of prophylactic oral levofloxacin in patients receiving chemotherapy for solid tumors or lymphomas[76] or for hematologic malignancies[77] showed a reduction in the number of documented infections. It is interesting to note that a meta-analysis of all types of antibiotic prophylaxis in neutropenic cancer patients (95 trials performed between 1973 and 2004) concluded that prophylaxis by means of antibiotics significantly decreased the risk for death when compared with placebo or no treatment[78]; when trials that used only quinolones were selectively analyzed, a significant reduction in the risk for all-cause mortality, infection-related mortality, clinically documented infections, and microbiologically documented infections was noted. These results are very encouraging, but the increasing rates of antimicrobial resistance to quinolones was also reported in many of these studies.[77-79] For pediatric cancer patients, the use of prophylactic antibiotics is best guided by clinical protocols. Thus, if prophylaxis by quinolone is initiated, vigilant monitoring of the incidence of bacteremia (specifically gram-negative bacteremia) is mandatory to evaluate the loss of efficacy of quinolone prophylaxis.

The prophylactic use of fluconazole to prevent colonization and invasive infection by *Candida* species in bone marrow transplant recipients is becoming more common. Two randomized, prospective, placebo-controlled trials have shown that the administration of fluconazole to patients during neutropenia decreases both colonization and invasive infection by *Candida* species to below the levels seen in patients who received placebo.[80,81] The obvious concern is that widespread use of prophylactic fluconazole could result in a resistant *Candida* species. In fact, one retrospective review of patients undergoing stem cell transplantation who received prophylactic fluconazole noted that colonization by azole-resistant *Candida* species occurred, and that some invasive strains of *Candida* species were resistant to fluconazole.[82]

Fever and Neutropenia

Fever in a patient with neutropenia must always be treated as an emergency, and therapy has to be initiated promptly. Some of the current principles of the management of the febrile neutropenic child are outlined in Box 27-1. The overall management of neutropenic patients is based on the use of empirical antibiotics directed against a wide array of potential pathogens.[6] The rationale for this approach evolved from the observation that bacteremias in patients with neutropenia are rapidly lethal, especially if they are caused by gram-negative organisms and if antibiotic therapy has been delayed until an organism has been isolated or a site of infection identified. Although the goal of the initial evaluation of a febrile patient with neutropenia is to identify potential sources of infection, this will not be successful in the majority of patients.[83,84] Although it is uncommon, patients with neutropenia may present with serious infection in the absence of fever. Accordingly, should a patient with neutropenia develop localized symptoms (e.g., right lower

- Watch the patient closely if the neutrophil count is <500 cells per μL or is rapidly falling.
- Instruct the patient and caregiver to monitor the temperature at least three times daily. Seek medical help in the event of fever (single oral temperature above 38.5° C or three elevations above 38° C during a 24-hour period) or if patient complains of any new symptoms.
- In the event of fever, take a careful medical history; conduct a thorough physical examination, with attention to the skin, perirectal area, and other mucosal sites; obtain blood cultures from periphery and, if an indwelling catheter is present, from each lumen of the catheter. In patients with an Ommaya reservoir and fever, obtain cerebrospinal (ventricular fluid) for cultures as well.
- Initiate prompt therapy with broad-spectrum antibiotics. If the patient has an indwelling catheter, rotate the administration of antibiotics through each lumen.
- Monitor the patient closely for secondary infections requiring modification of initial therapy; obtain cultures daily, as long as the patient is febrile or if newly febrile. If the patient has a positive blood culture, monitoring cultures should be repeated daily until result is negative.
- Continue empirical therapy if the patient has prolonged (>1 week) neutropenia or no evidence of hematologic recovery.
- Add empirical antifungal therapy if the neutropenic patient remains or again becomes febrile after 4 to 7 days of broad-spectrum antibiotic therapy.
- Discontinue antibiotic therapy when the neutrophil count rises to above 500 cells per μL (high-risk patients), or is increasing (low-risk patients).
- Although 10 to 14 days of treatment is adequate for most patients with neutropenia, prolonged therapy is necessary for patients with residual foci of infection or invasive mycosis (e.g., chronic disseminated candidiasis).

quadrant abdominal pain) that are compatible with infection, empirical antibiotic therapy should be initiated even if the patient is afebrile.

The standard evaluation of a febrile patient with neutropenia should include a careful physical examination and history. Unfortunately, as stated previously, the physical examination will identify a potential site of serious infection in only a minority of patients. Visual inspection of common sites of infection (i.e., a catheter exit site, the oral cavity, and the perianal area) is important. At least two sets of blood cultures should be obtained, including a set from each lumen of an indwelling intravascular device. The utility of obtaining a chest radiograph at the time of initial evaluation has been challenged by several investigators[85-87]; one prospective pediatric study showed that the only children with abnormal chest radiographic findings were those who also had abnormal respiratory findings.[88] A chest radiograph, however, can serve as a valuable baseline, particularly in patients who are anticipated to have prolonged neutropenia (>7 to 10 days). Pulmonary infiltrates not present initially may become apparent with bone marrow recovery

because neutrophils are recruited to a site of previously silent infection. In addition, accessible sites of potential infection should be aspirated or sampled and appropriate material sent for Gram stain, culture, and histologic examination. Colonization by microorganisms often precedes development of significant infection. In spite of this, routine surveillance cultures are rarely helpful in a neutropenic patient, and multiple potential pathogens are usually isolated from any single site, making it difficult to ascertain the organisms responsible for infection.[83] Possible exceptions include cultures from the anterior nares to diagnose colonization by methicillin-resistant *S. aureus* or *Aspergillus* species and in patients at centers experiencing high rates of infections by resistant or highly virulent organisms, such as resistant *Enterococcus* or *Pseudomonas* species).

Efforts have focused on serologic measurements of both specific factors (e.g., *Candida* enolase, galactomannan) and nonspecific factors (e.g., computed tomography scan, acute-phase reactants such as C-reactive protein) to predict which patients are infected.[89,90] Although some of these tests are promising, they generally lack the sensitivity to make them clinically useful. Polymerase chain reaction–based diagnostic approaches to a variety of infectious diseases may provide more clinically useful rapid diagnostic tests in the near future.

Antibiotic Management of a Neutropenic Patient Who Becomes Febrile

The standard approach to the empirical management of a febrile patient with neutropenia has been a regimen of combined antibiotics.[6,91,92] An ideal empirical regimen should provide a broad spectrum of activity against a variety of pathogenic organisms, including but not limited to *Pseudomonas* species; should be bactericidal in the absence of neutrophils; and should have low potential to cause the adverse effects of the emergence of resistant organisms. Aminoglycoside/β-lactam combinations, the first empirical regimens with acceptable efficacy, are still widely used and represent a standard against which newer regimens are tested.[93] If an aminoglycoside-containing combination regimen is to be used, the choice of specific antibiotics should be based primarily on the institution's antibiotic-sensitivity pattern and secondarily on toxicity and cost differences.

Another successful approach is the combination of two β-lactam antibiotics, usually consisting of an expanded-spectrum carboxypenicillin or ureidopenicillin plus a third-generation cephalosporin (e.g., piperacillin and ceftazidime).[94] Coverage for *S. aureus* is less reliable, and the major drawback of these regimens is the potential for emergence of β–lactam-resistant gram-negative bacteria.

The advent of broad-spectrum β-lactam antibiotics with high serum bactericidal activity made monotherapy another option for the initial empirical therapy of a febrile neutropenic patient.[52] The third-generation cephalosporins (especially ceftazidime), cefepime,[95-97] and the carbapenems (i.e., imipenem-cilastin[84,98] and meropenem[99-101]) have superior activity against *P. aeruginosa* and are effective for the initial management of a febrile neutropenic patient, but modifications according to clinical and microbiologic data are necessary in about half of these patients.[84,93,102,103] In one randomized study, although imipenem-cilastin had a better anaerobic spectrum than ceftazidime, its use was associated with more side effects, especially nausea and *C. difficile*-associated diarrhea.[84] These side effects are, however, not shared by meropenem.

Because of the increasingly common occurrence of antibiotic-resistant α-hemolytic streptococci,[8,104,105] *S. aureus*, coagulase-negative staphylococci, *Corynebacterium jejuni*, and enterococci as causes of bacteremia in cancer patients, a number of centers have included vancomycin in empirical regimens.

However, although a reduction in gram-positive infections in patients receiving a vancomycin-containing regimen may be achieved, no significant differences in outcome or survival resulted when vancomycin was added in a pathogen-directed manner or when its administration was delayed while awaiting a microbiologic or a clinical indication.[60,106,107] However, in centers in which methicillin-resistant *S. aureus* or resistant α-hemolytic streptococci are a problem, vancomycin should be included in the initial regimen.[11]

The quinolones, a group of structurally distinct, synthetic antibiotics with a broad spectrum of activity and a unique mechanism of action, have activity against most gram-negative organisms encountered in a neutropenic host, but they have only moderate activity against many streptococcal species, including enterococci and *S. pneumoniae*. They are virtually devoid of activity against the clinically important anaerobic bacteria. Their role in the management of a neutropenic host is still undefined, but their excellent bioavailability, tolerability, and broad spectrum of activity have led to their increasing use in cancer patients, especially for prophylaxis.[75-77,79] However, it is worrisome that antibiotic resistance is emerging with more widespread use of quinolone prophylaxis.[11]

The monobactams (e.g., aztreonam) have a role in patients with neutropenia who have allergies to β-lactam antibiotics. However, they have a purely gram-negative spectrum of coverage and should not be given as a monotherapy to patients with neutropenia.[108] Also available are combinations of β-lactams with β-lactamase inhibitors (i.e., clavulanic acid and sulbactam). A number of studies have documented the efficacy of ticarcillin plus clavulanic acid combined with an aminoglycoside for initial empirical therapy of fever in a patient with neutropenia.

Management of Indwelling Intravenous Catheters

Several studies evaluating the use of central venous catheters in patients with cancer have confirmed that these devices increase the incidence of bacteremia, regardless of the level of bone marrow suppression.[19] Although gram-positive bacterial infections (especially staphylococci) are the most common cause of catheter-related infections, other bacterial and nonbacterial species can be encountered in an immunocompromised host.[55,109,110] It is therefore mandatory to culture all lumina of an intravascular device and to administer antibiotic therapy through all lumina as well. A prospective trial at the National Cancer Institute compared the complications involved with an externalized catheter (e.g., Hickman-Broviac) to those involved with a subcutaneously implanted device (e.g., Port-A-Cath) and did not show a difference in the incidence of documented infections between the two groups.[111]

The majority of simple catheter-related bacteremias and exit-site infections can be cleared by appropriate antibiotic therapy and do not necessitate catheter removal. However, if bacteremia persists after 48 hours of appropriate therapy, or if the patient shows signs of a tunnel infection, the catheter should be removed. Failures of therapy are most common when infections are caused by certain organisms, such as *Bacillus* species,[112] the rapidly growing mycobacteria (*Mycobacterium chelonae* and *M. fortuitum*),[113] *Candida* species,[114,115] and vancomycin-resistant enterococci. When these are isolated, the catheter should be removed a priori. One prospective study found that at the time of removal of implantable ports, 50% of children had deep venous thrombosis at the site (typically asymptomatic); thrombosis, however, did not appear to affect the risk for or outcome of bacteremia in these children.[116]

It is unresolved whether a non-neutropenic patient with an indwelling catheter who becomes newly febrile should receive antibiotics empirically. The safest policy is to begin antibiotics (using a third-generation cephalosporin, such as ceftriaxone or an aminoglycoside plus vancomycin) and continue them pending culture results and clinical response. If by 72 hours the cultures remain negative and the patient is stable, antibiotics can be discontinued.

Approach to a Patient with Prolonged Granulocytopenia

The prompt initiation of empirical therapy has become standard practice and has resulted in a significant reduction in early morbidity and mortality rates in febrile neutropenic patients.[1] However, the debate about the duration of therapy continues.[6,58,117]

At most centers, the majority of patients fall into a fever of undetermined origin. Their management is outlined in Figure 27-1. In an early study by the National Cancer Institute, patients with fever of unknown origin and persistent granulocytopenia were randomized to discontinue antibiotics on day 7 of therapy or to continue them until the resolution of neutropenia.[118] Nearly 40% of afebrile patients who stopped antibiotics developed recurrent fever, and 38% of febrile patients whose antibiotics were discontinued developed hypotensive episodes. It was concluded that day 7 was too early to discontinue antibiotics, especially in patients who remained both persistently febrile and neutropenic. Of the patients who became afebrile but remained neutropenic and whose antibiotic therapy was discontinued after a 14-day course (as if the patient had had an occult site of infection), nearly one third became febrile again but responded to reinstitution of the same antibiotics.

Patients with shorter periods of neutropenia and those who have evidence of hematologic recovery and who have become afebrile on antibiotics (even though their neutrophil counts are lower than 500 cells/mm³) appear to do well when antibiotics are discontinued and close monitoring is maintained.[119]

For persistently neutropenic patients with documented infections who have had clinical and microbiologic resolution of their infections and who are afebrile at day 14 (for a minimum of 7 days), antibiotics can be discontinued.[6,120] The ultimate decision about whether to continue or discontinue antibiotics rests on a number of clinical parameters, including the potential toxicity of the antibiotic, the predicted duration of neutropenia, the emergence of mononuclear phagocytes, the seriousness of the initial infection, and the continued presence or absence of an infection site and factors predisposing to subsequent infections.

Modification of Antibiotic Therapy During the Course of Granulocytopenia

The necessity of changing or modifying the initial empirical treatment is closely related to the duration of neutropenia and should be anticipated in a patient with prolonged neutropenia.[6] In a study performed at the National Cancer Institute, only 4% of patients with fever of unknown origin lasting fewer than 7 days needed a change in therapy, compared with 19% who had granulocytopenia for 7 to 14 days and 65% who had prolonged granulocytopenia that lasted for more than 2 weeks.[58,118,121] The reasons for modifying the initial regimen include lack of a clinical response (e.g., persistent or new fever after a week of empirical therapy or evidence that the patient's condition is deteriorating); the isolation of a pathogen that is not optimally

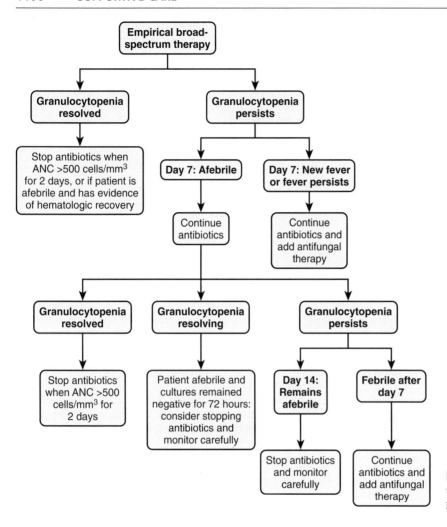

FIGURE 27-1. Treatment schema for fever of unknown origin in a febrile and neutropenic patient. ANC, absolute neutrophil count.

covered by the current regimen; the development of new specific findings on physical examination; or the emergence of a fungal, viral, or parasitic infection, particularly in a patient with prolonged neutropenia (Table 27-1).

The antibiotics that are most commonly added include (1) vancomycin for coagulase-negative staphylococci, methicillin-resistant *S. aureus*, enterococci, *Corynebacterium* species, or penicillin-resistant α-hemolytic streptococci; (2) aminoglycosides for *P. aeruginosa* or *Enterobacter*, *Serratia*, or *Citrobacter* species because these organisms are more likely to break through single-agent coverage as the result of inducible β-lactamases or mutations; and (3) clindamycin or metronidazole, when the initial regimen does not have adequate antianaerobic coverage and a site of presumably mixed infection is defined (e.g., necrotizing gingivitis, perianal tenderness).[58,84,122]

Empirical Antifungal or Antiviral Therapy During Prolonged Granulocytopenia

Fungi have emerged as an important cause of superinfections in cancer patients with prolonged neutropenia, and they may affect 9% to 31% of this population,[121,123] yet the diagnosis of a fungal infection, even when disseminated, is difficult in an immunocompromised patient.[33] The value of empirical antifungal therapy is supported by the results of two randomized clinical trials, one performed at the National Cancer Institute and the second from the European Organization for Research in the Treatment of Cancer.[121,124] Neutropenic patients who

remain persistently febrile despite a 4- to 7-day trial of broad-spectrum antibacterial therapy are particularly likely to have fungal infections.[26]

One quarter of all modifications to empirical antibiotic regimens investigated in a large multicenter trial involved the addition of systemic antifungal agents. In this trial, fungi were responsible for 7 bloodstream and 21 lung infections (causing 12 deaths) among 784 febrile episodes.[93] Traditionally, amphotericin B (at a dose of 0.5 mg/kg per day) has been the drug of choice for the empirical fungal treatment of a persistently febrile and neutropenic patient; however, higher doses, such as 1.0 to 1.5 mg/kg/day, may be necessary if infection by *Aspergillus* species constitutes a substantial risk, especially in patients with protracted neutropenia.[6,125]

The search for alternative antifungal agents has been prompted by the potential toxicity of amphotericin B (renal and infusion-related adverse events) and the emergence of fungi resistant to it. In general, the azoles represent a less toxic class of antifungal agents. Although fluconazole has been reported to be as effective as amphotericin in the treatment of candidemia in patients without neutropenia or other major immunodeficiency conditions,[126] the picture is less clear in febrile and neutropenic patients with cancer. Two prospective studies suggest that fluconazole is an equally effective but less toxic alternative to amphotericin B when given as empirical antifungal therapy to patients with cancer who have prolonged fever and neutropenia.[127,128] The azoles, however, may be less active than amphotericin B against some species. Fluconazole has no

TABLE 27-1	Modifications of Antibiotic Therapy During Neutropenia
Indication	**Modification**
Fever (persistent for >4 to 7 days or new in patient with persistent neutropenia)	Add empirical antifungal therapy
Positive blood cultures	
Gram-positive organisms	Add vancomycin pending results of sensitivity study
Pseudomonas aeruginosa, Enterobacter or *Citrobacter* species isolated during antibiotic therapy	Add aminoglycoside or an additional β-lactam antibiotic
Positive blood culture from central venous catheter	Attempt to treat; rotate administration of antibiotics through all lumina of catheter
	Exception: Positive cultures for *Bacillus* or *Candida* species: remove catheter; treat patient appropriately
Exit-site infections	Add vancomycin if gram-positive organisms are isolated
	Remove catheter and treat appropriately if rapidly growing mycobacteria (*M. chelonei, M. fortuitum*) or *Aspergillus* species are isolated
Tunnel infection	Remove catheter and treat patient appropriately
Sinus tenderness, nasal ulcerative lesions	Suspect fungal infection; try to establish diagnosis; treat with antifungal therapy
Mucositis with vesicular or ulcerative lesions	Test and culture for herpes simplex virus, and treat with acyclovir
Necrotizing gingivitis	Add antianaerobic antibiotic (clindamycin or metronidazole)
Painful swallowing	Suspect herpes simplex virus or *Candida* species infection; add antifungal therapy or acyclovir, or both
Abdominal pain, perianal tenderness	Optimize anaerobic coverage
Diarrhea	If positive for *C. difficile* toxin, treat with oral metronidazole (or oral vancomycin)
Pulmonary infiltrates	Send nasal secretions for testing and culturing of respiratory viruses (e.g., respiratory syncytial virus, influenza, parainfluenza)
Diffuse or interstitial pneumonitis	
Localized infiltrate	Consider adding coverage (macrolide or quinolone) for atypical microorganisms (e.g., *Mycoplasma* or *Legionella* species)
	If absolute neutrophil count is rising and patient is stable: continue antibiotics, observe carefully
	If persistent neutropenia or worsening clinical symptoms exist, consider performing biopsy or adding antifungal therapy, or both

useful activity against *Aspergillus* species and has less activity than amphotericin B against *C. tropicalis, C. krusei, C. lusitaniae,* and *C. glabrata.* In contrast, itraconazole and voriconazole have activity against *Candida* species, *Aspergillus* species, and some of the less common fungi. Voriconazole compared favorably with liposomal amphotericin B in adult cancer patients with fever and neutropenia.[129] Posaconazole, the most recently released oral azole, is notable for its broad spectrum of activity against a wide spectrum of fungal pathogens, including species of *Candida, Aspergillus, Zygomycetes,* and *Fusarium.*[130,131] Its efficacy as an empirical antifungal agent in febrile and neutropenic patients, however, has not been investigated.

Considerable focus has been placed on preparations of liposomal or lipid-associated amphotericin because of its lower documented toxicity in open-label phase 1 and phase 2 studies in patients with cancer and neutropenia.[132,133] In the only randomized, double-blind trial comparing liposomal amphotericin with conventional amphotericin B as empirical antifungal therapy, the outcomes were similar with respect to survival, resolution of fever, and discontinuation of the study drug because of toxic effects or lack of efficacy, but in patients treated with liposomal amphotericin B, there were fewer breakthrough fungal infections, less infusion-related toxicity, and less nephrotoxicity.[134] Finally, the higher therapeutic index of liposomal amphotericin B allows the use of substantially higher doses than those of conventional amphotericin. However, the only prospective randomized clinical trial comparing the efficacy of two doses of liposomal amphotericin (1 mg/kg/day versus 4 mg/kg/day) for treatment of invasive *Aspergillosis* species showed that the higher dosage was not more efficacious.[135]

The newest class of antifungal agents are the echinocandins (e.g., caspofungin, micafungin), large lipopeptide molecules that are inhibitors of β-(1,3)-glucan synthesis, which is essential for fungal cell wall synthesis. Both in vitro and in vivo, the echinocandins are rapidly fungicidal against most *Candida* species and are fungistatic against *Aspergillus* species, but they are not active against *Zygomycetes* species, *Cryptococcus neoformans,* or *Fusarium* species.[136] Adverse events are generally mild (e.g., for caspofungin: local phlebitis, fever, abnormal liver function tests, and mild hemolysis) because the drug target is not present in mammalian cells. Echinocandins can be administered only parenterally because of poor oral bioavailability. In a prospective randomized, double-blind trial comparing the efficacy and safety of caspofungin with that of liposomal amphotericin B, caspofungin was found to be as effective and generally better tolerated than liposomal amphotericin B when given as empirical antifungal therapy in patients with persistent fever and neutropenia.[137] Caspofungin was initially licensed for adult use, so the optimal dosing for pediatric patients is not yet known. One small prospective study investigated the pharmacokinetics and safety of caspofungin in pediatric patients and demonstrated that a caspofungin dose of 50 mg/m^2/day provided exposure comparable to that in adult patients treated with 50 mg/day without developing any serious drug-related adverse events or toxicity.[138] Finally, in the absence of potential mechanistic antagonism with other antifungal drugs and a mild adverse-event profile, combination antifungal therapy including echinocandins (particularly for invasion by *Aspergillosis* species) has been seriously considered.

Although viral infections result mainly from impaired cellular immunity, a child with prolonged granulocytopenia, especially after treatment with antineoplastic agents, may have symptoms of mucositis that can result from a viral infection. Empirical therapy with acyclovir is indicated in a child with suspected stomatitis or esophagitis caused by HSV infection or, less commonly, ganciclovir for suspected esophagitis caused by CMV infection.

Empirical Oral Antibiotic Therapy for Low-Risk Febrile Patients with Granulocytopenia

Outpatient management of low-risk febrile patients with neutropenia has also been actively investigated. Although no definitive consensus exists about the criteria used to distinguish high risk from low risk, several key factors that may increase the risk for infectious complications have been identified on the basis of a number of studies that have been conducted: anticipated duration of neutropenia[139]; significant medical comorbidity[139,140]; cancer status and cancer type; documented infection on presentation (i.e., pneumonia, intravenous catheter-site infection); evidence of bone marrow recovery (e.g., absolute monocyte count)[141,142]; and magnitude of fever.[5,141]

Oral antibiotic therapy has numerous advantages over parenteral therapy (potential cost reduction, outpatient administration, elimination of need for intravenous access devices). The benefits, however, must be balanced with the potential risks. Investigators have studied the use of many antibiotic regimens (pefloxacin,[143] ofloxacin,[144-148] ciprofloxacin,[149-151] cefixime,[152,153] and moxifloxacin[154]) for empirical coverage in low-risk febrile cancer patients with neutropenia. Although the results of these studies are encouraging, many clinical trials were statistically underpowered and were limited by methodologic issues. Two large, prospective, randomized studies of low-risk patients have evaluated the efficacy of oral ciprofloxacin plus oral amoxicillin-clavulanate with more conventional parenteral antibiotic therapies in an inpatient setting.[155,156] The relative efficacy of oral and intravenous regimens was comparable in both of these clinical studies; the authors of both studies, however, were quick to admonish that their findings should not be used to justify the use of empirical oral antibiotic therapy administered on an outpatient basis as the established standard for treating low-risk patients. The authors agreed that additional studies are needed to evaluate fully the use of oral regimens for fever and neutropenia in an outpatient setting. A analysis of the spectrum of infections in a very large cohort of low-risk febrile neutropenic patients (757 episodes of fever and neutropenia) at MD Anderson Cancer Center in Houston revealed that episodes of unexplained fever were predominant (58% of episodes), but both clinically documented and microbiologically documented infections were seen with equal frequency (21%).[157] Among the microbiologically documented infections, gram-positive (49%), gram-negative (36%), and polymicrobial (15%) infections were documented. This highlights the fact that although these patients were considered to be at low risk for developing infections, many developed serious infections necessitating broad-spectrum antibiotic therapy.

Use of Hematopoietic Growth Factors in Patients with Fever and Granulocytopenia

The hematopoeitic growth factors granulocyte-macrophage colony-stimulating factor (GM-CSF) and granulocyte colony-stimulating factor (G-CSF) have been evaluated as adjuncts to chemotherapy to assist in bone marrow reconstitution and to prevent neutropenia and reduce infectious complications in neutropenic patients with cancer. A recent meta-analysis of 16 randomized, controlled trials of prophylactic CSFs in pediatric patients receiving systemic chemotherapy revealed significant reductions in episodes of fever and neutropenia, in documented infection, and in length of hospitalization time.[158] It is interesting that when the subset of patients with acute lymphoblastic leukemia (ALL) was analyzed, it was found that the use of G-CSF resulted in minimal cost saving.[159] This insight coupled with the observation that the administration of G-CSF to children with ALL may increase the risk for developing therapy-associated myeloid leukemia or myelodysplastic syndrome[160] only emphasizes the importance of being cautious when making the decision about whether to use CSFs in pediatric patients with ALL. In terms of using CSFs as an adjunctive therapy for the treatment of febrile neutropenia, a study showed that the addition of CSFs to antibiotics resulted in only 1 less day of fever and 1 less day of hospitalization.[161]

Therefore, the most recent guidelines for the use of hematopoietic growth factors by the American Society of Clinical Oncology recommend that the use of CSFs is reasonable for the primary prophylaxis in pediatric patients with a likelihood of developing fever and neutropenia, although with the caveat that use of CSFs in children with ALL should always be considered with caution.[162] Ultimately, the use of CSFs in pediatric patients should be guided by clinical protocols.

MANAGEMENT OF FUNGAL INFECTIONS

Oropharyngeal Candidiasis (Thrush) and *Candida* Esophagitis

Patients with cell-mediated immune deficiencies are most prone to develop oropharyngeal or esophageal candidiasis.[27] Thrush rarely causes significant morbidity, except in a patient with HIV infection, whereas resistant *Candida* species can lead to significant symptoms.[163] Thorough mouth care, including topical clotrimazole, may be used as a prophylactic regimen in neutropenic patients. The presumptive diagnosis of oropharyngeal candidiasis is made by visual inspection. Creamy-white patches on the mucosal surfaces, which may be friable and bleed easily when scratched, are characteristic. However, it is often difficult to distinguish among mucositis caused by chemotherapy, *C. albicans*, and HSV, especially in granulocytopenic patients, and a combined therapeutic approach is often indicated.

- Esophageal candidiasis is a locally invasive infection, usually of the distal third of the esophagus, and symptoms may be mild or nonspecific.
- Retrosternal or epigastric burning, sometimes associated with local dysphagia, is the most commonly reported symptom in granulocytopenic patients, whereas HIV-infected children often have nonspecific symptoms, such as loss of appetite or failure to thrive.
- The absence of thrush does not rule out esophagitis caused by *Candida* species, because the distal esophagus may be the only focus of disease. In addition to *Candida* species, the differential diagnosis includes HSV, CMV, bacterial infections (often caused by *S. aureus*), and mixed infections, as well as noninfectious causes (e.g., chemotherapy, radiation therapy).[164-167]
- A barium swallow or upper gastrointestinal series may reveal mucosal irregularities suggestive of esophagitis caused by a *Candida* species ("cobblestoning"), but these radiographs are not helpful in definitively establishing the diagnosis.
- Only endoscopic biopsy with culture and histologic tissue examination is definitive, but it may not be feasible in a neutropenic host. Empirical initial therapy is therefore often

preferred, and endoscopic biopsy should be reserved for non-neutropenic patients (if relative risks and benefits allow) and patients with persistent symptoms despite adequate therapy.

The antifungal agents for the treatment of oropharyngeal candidiasis include oral nonabsorbable agents (e.g., nystatin or clotrimazole), oral systemically absorbed compounds (e.g., ketoconazole, fluconazole, and voriconazole[168]), and intravenously administered fluconazole, caspofungin,[169-171] or amphotericin B.[108] Although oropharyngeal candidiasis often responds to oral agents, a neutropenic child may not be able to swallow, and liposomal amphotericin B, intravenous fluconazole, or caspofungin then becomes the therapy of choice. A minimum of 5 days of therapy is recommended for neutropenic patients, and it is preferred that the therapy be continued until resolution of the granulocytopenia. In patients with esophagitis caused by *Candida* species, systemic therapy is required for effective treatment. A 14- to 21-day course of an azole compound (i.e., fluconazole, voriconazole, itraconazole); echinocandin (micafungin, caspofungin); or intravenous amphotericin B is recommended.[172]

Fungemia

Candida species are the most common fungi causing fungemia and are also the fourth leading cause of nosocomial bloodstream infections in the United States, with treatment costs estimated to be more than $1 billion annually.[173] The appropriate management of candidemia is important because it can be associated with high morbidity and mortality rates and may be a harbinger of disseminated *Candida* infection.[174] Neutropenic patients receiving broad-spectrum antibacterial agents, transplant recipients, postsurgical patients with indwelling catheters, and HIV-infected children with intravascular catheters are at increased risk.[31-33,175,176] The following factors should be considered.

- Fever might be the only sign of disseminated fungal infection. In some patients, embolic skin lesions (perhaps more commonly with *C. tropicalis*) or diffuse myalgias, indicative of *Candida* myositis, may be observed.[1,30,177]
- A positive blood culture should rarely be considered a "contaminant" in an immunocompromised host.
- It is important to evaluate all patients with documented candidemia for evidence of dissemination. The most common sites are the eye (endophthalmitis), skin, liver, and spleen.
- Clinical or radiographic evidence of organ involvement can be difficult to detect (in part because of the lack of an inflammatory response) when a patient is neutropenic.
- If a patient with documented candidemia has an intravenous catheter, the device must be removed because it can serve as a nidus for infection and source of dissemination.

Amphotericin B has long been the gold standard for the management of bloodstream infections caused by *Candida* species, but fluconazole,[126,178] caspofungin,[179] or the combination of fluconazole and amphotericin B (with the amphotericin B being administered for the first 5 to 6 days only)[172] have all been shown to have efficacy comparable to that of amphotericin B therapy for bloodstream infections caused by *Candida* species. Furthermore, because liposomal amphotericin B has efficacy comparable to that of amphotericin B but far fewer infusion-related and renal adverse effects, amphotericin B is now rarely used. The choice of therapy, however, should be individualized to consider the patient's clinical status as well as the particular species of *Candida* (particularly its antifungal

susceptibility). For example, in stable patients who have not recently received azole therapy or prophylaxis, fluconazole therapy could be initiated at 6 mg/kg/day or more.[180] *C. albicans*, *C. tropicalis*, and *C. parapsilosis* may be treated with either liposomal amphotericin B at 3 mg/kg/day, fluconazole at 6 mg/kg/day, or caspofungin.[172] Liposomal amphotericin or caspofungin is preferred in *C. krusei* infections. Likewise, many isolates of *C. lusitaniae* are resistant to amphotericin B; thus fluconazole is the treatment of choice. For uncomplicated candidemia, therapy should be continued for 2 weeks after the last positive blood culture and resolution of the signs and symptoms of infection. The evidence favoring removal of all existing central venous catheters is strongest in the non-neutropenic patient population, and in neutropenic patients, the role of the gut as a source of disseminated candidiasis has been supported by autopsy studies.[181] In an individual patient, however, it can be difficult to determine the relative contributions of the gut and a catheter as primary sources of candidemia. There are no randomized studies of this topic, but the consensus among experts in infectious diseases is that existing central venous catheters should be removed when feasible.[172] Persistent fever, localizing symptoms, or abnormal liver function tests (particularly alkaline phosphatase) should suggest the possibility of disseminated, invasive infection by *Candida* species.[2]

Chronic Disseminated (Hepatosplenic) Candidiasis

Chronic disseminated candidiasis, also known as hepatosplenic candidiasis, has emerged as a problematic intra-abdominal infection that affects cancer patients who have prolonged or recurrent episodes of neutropenia.[182,183] Typical findings in chronic disseminated candidiasis include the following:

- Persistent fever (unresponsive to standard antimicrobial therapy) after the recovery from neutropenia; "rebound leukocytosis"; an elevated serum alkaline phosphatase level; and abdominal pain may be noted.
- Ultrasonography, computed tomography, or magnetic resonance imaging can demonstrate evidence of the bull's-eye lesion that is suggestive of chronic disseminated candidiasis.[182] It is to be noted that these lesions are rarely detectable while the patient is still neutropenic.
- Biopsy may reveal granulomatous, disseminated 1-mm to 2-cm lesions, both deep-seated and localized on the surface of the liver.
- Cultures are almost always negative, even if yeast and pseudohyphae are visualized. Careful examination of the biopsy material is essential to confirm the diagnosis. Because treatment courses may be prolonged, it is important to establish the diagnosis before initiating therapy.

For treatment of hepatosplenic candidiasis, intravenous liposomal amphotericin B or fluconazole (oral or intravenous) is recommended. The administration of 5-flucytosine can be considered in combination with either amphotericin or fluconazole for more refractory infections.[172] Fluconazole at 6 mg/kg/day can be given to stable patients. Liposomal amphotericin B at 3 mg/kg/day may be used in acutely ill patients and in patients with refractory disease. Some clinicians recommend an initial 1- to 2-week course of liposomal amphotericin B for all patients, followed by a prolonged course of fluconazole.[184] Studies suggest that encapsulating amphotericin B into liposomes will allow for delivery of larger single and total doses with less toxicity and may both abbreviate and improve the treatment of hepatosplenic candidiasis.[185]

Infections Caused by *Aspergillus* Species

Infection by *Aspergillus* species is the second most commonly encountered fungal pathogen in compromised hosts. Serious invasive infections by *Aspergillus* species occur most commonly in patients with prolonged neutropenia (e.g., those with aplastic anemia or acute leukemia receiving cytotoxic therapy) and in patients receiving high doses of corticosteroids (particularly in association with other immunosuppressive regimens used for recipients of organ transplants).[34,186-188] The incidence of invasive infections by *Aspergillus* species has increased during the past 25 years in many centers.[189] Although there are hundreds of species, *A. fumigatus* and *A. flavus* account for the vast majority of human infections, with *A. niger* and other species reported less often.[188]

In compromised or noncompromised patients, *Aspergillus* species may cause saprophytic colonization of pulmonary cavities (primary or secondary aspergillomas). Primary aspergillomas tend to occur after granulocyte recovery in a patient who has had an episode of invasive pulmonary aspergillosis during a period of granulocytopenia (i.e., "walling off" the infection). Secondary aspergillomas occur most commonly in patients who have an underlying disease (e.g., sarcoidosis or tuberculosis) or other pulmonary lesions (e.g., cavitary neoplasms, bacterial abscess).

- The most common symptom of aspergilloma is hemoptysis, which occurs in 75% of patients and ranges from intermittent blood-tinged sputum to massive pulmonary hemorrhage with exsanguination.[190]
- Radiographically, a solitary rounded mass (of water density) within a spherical or ovoid cavity is sometimes overlain by a crescent of air (Monod's sign).[191]
- The first decision in the management of aspergilloma is whether therapy is required. Therapeutic options depend on the risk for life-threatening hemoptysis, which occurs in only a minority of patients.[191]
- Definitive treatment for aspergilloma is surgical resection; however, surgery has been associated with high morbidity and mortality rates.[191]

Infection by an *Aspergillus* species is acquired by inhalation of *Aspergillus* conidia. Invasive disease, therefore, usually involves the sinuses (5% to 10%) and lower respiratory tract (80% to 90%),[192] is often multifocal, and has a predilection for invading blood vessels and tissue parenchyma. Tissue infarction and subsequent necrosis commonly occur and may lead to rapidly progressive, extensive disease. In the absence of appropriate host defenses, the lesions respond poorly to available antimicrobial therapy. Invasive pulmonary infection by aspergillosis in granulocytopenic patients is associated with a mortality rate as high as 95%.

- The most common symptom of pulmonary aspergillosis is chest pain, which may develop before the appearance of pulmonary infiltrates (preceding it by an average of 6 days).[193]
- Sinus involvement manifests in the form of sinus pain and sometimes swelling, nasal ulceration or eschar, epistaxis, and nasal discharge. Infection of the maxillary sinuses may either invade into the roof of the hard palate or extend directly into the orbit or the central nervous system.[194]
- Radiographically, invasive pulmonary aspergillosis can range from discrete or multifocal nodular lesions through patchy densities to diffuse consolidation or even cavitation. Standard chest radiographs often underestimate the extent of pulmonary disease, especially if obtained during the early course of illness, but computed tomography scans may be more accurate in defining the extent of disease.[195,196] In patients with neutropenia, the most distinctive early lesions seen on computed tomography of the chest are small nodules, small pleural-based lesions with straight edges and surrounding low attenuation (the halo sign), or both.[192,197] The radiographic appearance of sinusitis caused by an *Aspergillus* species may range from minimal mucosal thickening to sinus obliteration and extensive bony erosion or destruction.[198]
- Blood cultures are rarely positive. Positive cultures derived from sputum or bronchoalveolar lavage are highly predictive of invasive disease in the symptomatic patient.[36,187]
- A number of tests for the diagnosis of invasive *Aspergillus* species have been developed: antibodies to *Aspergillus* species[199]; *Aspergillus* galactomannan in urine, sera, cerebrospinal fluid, and bronchoalveolar lavage specimens as determined by enzyme immunoassay and enzyme-linked immunosorbent assay[200-203]; and polymerase chain reaction assays.[204] The accuracy and reliability of these tests, however, still merits further investigation.
- Neither bronchoalveolar lavage, which indicates a recovery rate of approximately 50% in biopsy-proven *Aspergillus* pneumonia, nor transbronchial biopsy, which has a yield of about 20%, is highly sensitive for the diagnosis.[205] Furthermore, at present, the only definitive diagnosis of invasive infection by *Aspergillus* species is by histologic or microbiologic confirmation (via transbronchial biopsy, open lung biopsy, or sinus aspiration), which, however, may not be feasible in a thrombocytopenic and neutropenic host.[191]

For granulocytopenic patients with presumed or proven invasive aspergillosis, amphotericin B has historically been the treatment of choice, but recently liposomal amphotericin B or voriconazole has been used more frequently. Higher doses of liposomal amphotericin B (3 to 5 mg/kg/day) are often used in these clinical settings, although increased efficacy has not been definitely proven.[135] In a prospective, randomized, unblinded trial comparing the efficacy and safety of voriconazole with that of amphotericin B for the treatment of invasive aspergillosis, initial therapy using voriconazole led to better responses, improved survival rates, and fewer side effects.[206] Caspofungin, a member of the echinocandins that was initially approved for use in cases of refractory aspergillosis, was shown to provide a favorable response in 45% of patients with invasive aspergillosis that was refractory to amphotericin B, liposomal amphotericin B, and azole therapy.[207] Although successful use of caspofungin as first-line monotherapy for invasive aspergillosis has been reported,[208,209] no randomized controlled trials comparing its efficacy to other antifungal agents have yet been conducted. Given the decreased incidence of adverse effects and the theoretical lack of antagonism with other antifungal agents, combination therapy using voriconazole and caspofungin for invasive aspergillosis has been implemented and reported to be successful in isolated cases.[210-212] Randomized trials, however, are needed to determine whether this combination is truly better (from the standpoint of both efficacy and safety) than monotherapy or other combination-therapy regimens.

In general, surgical resection of lesions has a small role in severely immunocompromised patients because the disease is commonly multifocal and because other medical conditions frequently preclude even less invasive procedures. The response to therapy and the ultimate survival of patients who have invasive aspergillosis is most dependent on recovery from granulocytopenia. The use of granulocyte colony-stimulating factor or leukocyte transfusions (especially from granulocyte-colony-stimulating factor–stimulated donors) or interferon-γ[213,214] may be indicated in patients who do not show spontaneous rise in granulocytes. However, definitive data are lacking, and these modalities are not recommended for routine therapeutic use. In the only randomized multicenter trial evaluating the effectiveness of prophylactic inhalations of aerosolized amphotericin B to prevent invasive infections by *Aspergillus* species in patients after receiving chemotherapy or autologous bone marrow transplantation, there was no benefit from prophylactic amphotericin inhalations.[215] In a randomized multicenter study, patients with acute myelogenous leukemia or myelodysplastic syndrome who were treated with prophylactic posaconazole had lower incidences of proven or probable fungal disease (particularly invasive *Aspergillosis*) than did patients treated with fluconazole or itraconazole.[216]

Infections Caused by *Cryptococcus neoformans*

Cryptococcal infections range from mild or asymptomatic to life-threatening. Patients who have T-cell dysfunction as is associated with HIV infection, who have undergone organ transplantation or chronic corticosteroid therapy, as well as those with certain lymphoid malignancies (particularly Hodgkin's disease), are at increased risk for cryptococcal infections.[217,218] Children with these immunodeficiencies, however, have a lower incidence of cryptococcal disease than their adult counterparts—most likely a consequence of lack of exposure to sources *of Cryptococcus neoformans.*[219]

- Sites commonly involved (in descending order of occurrence) are the central nervous system, lungs, mediastinum, skin, bone, and prostate.[218,220]
- Symptoms of central nervous system involvement are commonly insidious and subtle, evolving over weeks to months. They include fevers, headaches, dizziness, somnolence, and signs of cognitive impairment as well as cranial nerve abnormalities (20%) and papilledema (30%).
- Symptoms of pulmonary and mediastinal involvement are commonly absent, and the diagnosis may be made incidentally on a routine chest radiograph. Solitary nodules caused by *Cryptococcus* species may be misdiagnosed as pulmonary metastasis.[217]
- Examination of cerebrospinal fluid may demonstrate elevated opening pressure, low glucose (in about 50% of cases), elevated protein levels, and mononuclear cell pleocytosis. However, patients with HIV infection and those on high dosages of corticosteroids may have little or no inflammatory response.
- The latex agglutination test for detection of cryptococcal polysaccharide antigen is sensitive and specific in more than 90% of cases and should be performed in both serum and cerebrospinal fluid.

The initial therapy for central nervous system cryptococcosis is amphotericin B, with or without 5-flucytosine. The combination of amphotericin B (0.7 to 1.0 mg/kg/day) plus 5-flucytosine (with serum concentrations between 50 and 100 µg/mL) for 6 to 10 weeks is generally considered to be the treatment of choice for cryptococcal meningitis in patients not infected with HIV.[220]

Other Fungi in Immunosuppressed Patients

Members of the Mucoraceae family, including the genera *Mucor, Rhizomucor, Rhizopus,* and *Absidia,* are the fourth most commonly encountered fungal pathogens that cause disease in immunocompromised patients.[221] Infections resulting from these organisms resemble those caused by *Aspergillus* species, both epidemiologically and clinically. In addition to granulocytopenia, diabetic ketoacidosis, and protein-calorie malnutrition, it has been recognized that iron overload is also a risk factor in these infections.[222] The two most common clinical presentations are rhinocerebral and pulmonary mucormycosis, which are seen mainly in patients with granulocytopenia. Treatment includes early and aggressive débridement (in rhinocerebral mucormycosis); antifungal antibiotics (intravenous amphotericin B [1 mg/kg/day] and possibly the newer drugs triazole or posaconazole); correction of underlying abnormalities or immunologic deficits is essential for the cure of mucormycosis.

Pseudallescheria boydii is a soil saprophyte and a cause of mycetoma. Disseminated pseudallescheriasis can follow a highly aggressive course, similar to that of aspergillosis. *P. boydii* is usually resistant to amphotericin B but is susceptible to miconazole.

Disseminated infection by *Fusarium* species may occur in patients who have prolonged neutropenia and is associated with high mortality rates. Infections in the granulocytopenic host are characterized by pulmonary infiltrates; prominent erythematous, maculopapular to nodular skin lesions; sinusitis; and positive blood cultures. Amphotericin B is the drug of choice for therapy, although resistance has been reported.

Disseminated disease caused by the yeast *T. beigelii* has been documented in severely immunosuppressed, often neutropenic, patients.[26] The lungs, kidneys, skin, and eyes are the main sites affected. Serum and cerebrospinal fluid results may be falsely positive for cryptococcal antigen. Early institution of amphotericin B and bone marrow recovery are important for a favorable outcome.

MANAGEMENT OF VIRAL INFECTIONS

Infection by the Herpes Simplex Virus

Primary or secondary HSV infection may lead to significant morbidity but rarely causes mortality in an immunocompromised host. Even in the most severely immunocompromised patients, HSV usually tends to remain localized and only rarely disseminates to distant sites. The most common sites are in or around the mouth, the nares and esophagus (HSV-1), and the perianal and perirectal area (HSV-2). Pain is the hallmark of lesions resulting from HSV infection. However, rapidly fatal pneumonitis, acute and subacute encephalitis, as well as infections caused by acyclovir-resistant viruses, are emerging, especially in patients who have undergone bone marrow transplantation and in those with HIV.[223]

Acyclovir and foscarnet (for acyclovir-resistant strains) are the drugs of choice for the treatment of HSV infections in immunocompromised patients.[108] The intravenous dose of acyclovir is 250 mg/m^2 (or 5 mg/kg) given every 8 hours, and 500 mg/m^2 is given every 8 hours for proven or suspected central nervous system or visceral involvement. Therapy should be continued for at least 1 week in uncomplicated cases and at least 10 days in patients with dissemination. Because of the emerging problems with resistant strains, prophylaxis of HSV infections by administering acyclovir should be restricted to specific indications (e.g., bone marrow transplantation). Oral valacyclovir or famciclovir can also be used for the treatment of recurrent HSV infection and also for the chronic suppression of HSV infections, but there is no evidence to suggest that these agents are more efficacious than acyclovir.

Infection by the Varicella-Zoster Virus

Primary varicella (chickenpox) may cause serious morbidity and mortality rates in patients with impaired CMI and low lymphocyte counts.[224,225] If a child with acute leukemia who is receiving immunosuppressive therapy is exposed to varicella and has not received either varicella-zoster immunoglobulin or early therapy with acyclovir, the likelihood of contracting pneumonitis is as high as 32% and the mortality rate is nearly one third.[226] Morbidity and mortality rates are lower in children with solid tumors or HIV disease but are still significant.

- The diagnosis of primary cutaneous chickenpox can usually be made on the appearance of the lesions; however, they may appear atypical in an immunosuppressed patient.
- The lung is the primary site of dissemination (occurring from 3 to 7 days after the onset of skin lesions); the central nervous system and liver are the two other most common sites. Some immunocompromised patients can have disseminated infections without having any visible skin lesions.[227,228]
- Polymerase chain reaction (vesicular fluid, CSF, or biopsy tissue) or direct fluorescent antibody (vesicle scraping) tests are the diagnostic methods of choice. Cultures of skin lesions often yield positive results but can take as long as 10 to 14 days.
- A chest radiograph and measurement of liver transaminases should be obtained if primary VZV infection is suspected.
- A child with suspected or proven varicella should be placed in strict isolation. All immunocompromised patients who have had contact with the patient during the infectious stage (beginning 48 hours before the appearance of the lesions and lasting until the crusting of all lesions) should be notified and, if susceptible, promptly be given varicella-zoster immunoglobulin.

Reactivation of latent VZV infection (herpes zoster, or shingles) is also more common in immunosuppressed populations, especially those with Hodgkin's disease (22% to 38%), those with non-Hodgkin's lymphoma (8%), and patients with solid tumors (2%).[229] As much as 50% to 75% of patients who have received bone marrow transplants show reactivation of VZV within the first 6 months after transplantation.[70] In cancer patients, zoster is usually unilateral and follows a dermatomal distribution. Visceral dissemination of herpes zoster is less common than it is after primary varicella infection.

Early institution of intravenous acyclovir (500 mg/m^2 (or 10 mg/kg) given every 8 hours) with adequate hydration can significantly reduce the incidence of visceral dissemination.[43,226,230] Therapy should be continued for a minimum of 7 days or until all lesions have crusted over. An increasing problem, especially in the HIV-infected population, is the emergence of acyclovir-resistant VZV strains, possibly associated with the use of oral acyclovir prophylaxis.[231] Intravenous foscarnet may offer an alternative treatment option. For mildly immunocompromised patients, oral valacyclovir or famciclovir (with careful observation of the patient) may provide another acceptable treatment alternative to intravenous therapy.[232]

Immunocompromised patients should not routinely be given the varicella vaccine.[232] The major risk to immunocompromised patients who are given the varicella vaccine is development of severe vaccine-strain varicella.[233-235]

Infection by the Cytomegalovirus

Infection by the CMV is associated with significant morbidity and mortality rates in immunosuppressed patients, especially those undergoing bone marrow transplantation and those infected by HIV.[236] Reactivation of endogenous virus occurs in as much as 80% of seropositive patients after transplantation.[70]

- Interstitial pneumonitis is the most common and most serious complication in non–HIV-infected patients. It is associated with a mortality rate of 80%.
- Retinitis, gastrointestinal infections (mouth ulcers, esophagitis, ileitis, colitis), pancreatitis, and cholecystitis, as well as hepatitis and central nervous system involvement, can occur in a child infected by HIV.
- CMV pneumonia is clinically and radiologically indistinguishable from other interstitial pneumonias and can occur in conjunction with other infectious agents.[197]
- Although positive cultures in blood, urine, or respiratory secretions should raise suspicion, they do not necessarily correlate with pulmonary infection.
- Diagnosis is made by culture, shell vial technique combined with specific antibodies, in situ hybridization, and polymerase chain reaction,[237] as well as classic histologic examination (showing typical intranuclear inclusion bodies).

Current therapeutic options include ganciclovir and foscarnet, either alone or in combination. The combination of ganciclovir with intravenous immunoglobulin (polyclonal or CMV-specific) may improve outcome in patients with CMV pneumonitis who have undergone allogeneic bone marrow transplantation. Ganciclovir administered prophylactically to patients undergoing allogeneic bone marrow transplantation results in a reduction in the incidence of interstitial pneumonitis.[238] Other measures that have reduced the incidence of CMV pneumonitis after bone marrow transplantation include the use of CMV-negative blood in patients who are CMV-antibody–negative and the prophylactic use of ganciclovir or high doses of acyclovir.[238-240]

Other Viral Infections

Viruses such as influenza and parainfluenza viruses, respiratory syncytial virus, and adenovirus tend to follow a more aggressive course in an immunosuppressed child, sometimes causing localized infiltrates, although a diffuse process is more common. In one series, respiratory tract viruses were documented in about 25% of episodes of fever in neutropenic patients, but the role of these organisms could not be predicted on the basis of presenting symptoms, radiographic findings, or degree or duration of neutropenia.[112] Patients with hematologic disease are prone to infection by several viruses, including blood-product–associated pathogens, such as hepatitis A virus, hepatitis B virus, hepatitis C virus, and HIV-1. Their diagnosis and treatment are usually not different from those used in patients without underlying hematologic disorder, but these infections add to the medical and psychological burden of patients and caregivers.

EBV-associated lymphoproliferative disorders can occur after organ or bone marrow transplantation or in association with HIV disease.[47,241-244] The incidence appears to be at least partly related to the choice of immunosuppression used to prevent graft rejection, and some lymphoproliferative disorders will respond to a decrease in immunosuppression.[245,246] Treatment or prophylaxis with acyclovir has not been successful.[247] There are some anecdotal and animal data that support the use of interferon-α[248,249] or immunoglobulins,[250,251] but the most promising immunomodulatory agents are anti-B-cell monoclonal antibodies (particularly anti-CD20 antibody, rituximab[252-255]) and EBV-specific cytotoxic T cells.[256,257] Recently a multicenter prospective phase 2 trial using rituximab as first-line therapy for post-transplant lymphoproliferative disorder in patients after solid organ transplantation showed that rituximab was not only effective (there was a 67% survival rate after 1 year) but was also safe.[258]

Infection of an immunocompetent host by the human herpes virus 6 (HHV-6) is a common self-limited febrile illness (e.g., roseola) that usually occurs in early childhood (90% of children younger than 2 years of age are seropositive).[259] As with all herpesviruses, HHV-6 is capable of reactivating from latency, particularly in an immunocompromised host. In immunocompromised hosts, HHV-6 infection may manifest as fever, leukopenia, rash, encephalitis, and interstitial pneumonitis.[260-263] Infection by HHV-6 may lead to reactivation of other herpesviruses, particularly CMV, and may increase HIV replication.[263] Diagnosis can be made by culture, serology, polymerase chain reaction, and immunohistochemistry, but the challenge lies in distinguishing active from latent infection. Because HHV-6 is similar to CMV, the therapeutic options are similar: in vitro, ganciclovir and foscarnet have shown good activity, whereas HHV-6 is relatively resistant to acyclovir.[264] But the role of antiviral therapy in HHV-6 must be further studied.

MANAGEMENT OF PROTOZOAL INFECTIONS

Infection by *Pneumocystis jiroveci*

Pulmonary infections by *P. jiroveci* (formerly known as *P. carinii*) have in the past been a major problem in children with hematologic malignancies.[265,266] Extrapulmonary infections can occasionally be seen in immunocompromised patients as well.[267,268]

- The most common presentation (often with acute onset and rapid progression) in patients without HIV infection includes fever; tachypnea, generally with intercostal retractions; and the absence of detectable rales. PCP in HIV-infected children can be more indolent, taking an insidious course for a prolonged period of time or rapidly progressing and including severe respiratory symptoms.
- In one review of oncology patients with confirmed PCP, 70% of patients became symptomatic while corticosteroid dosages were being tapered.[40]
- The chest radiographs in patients not infected with HIV may have a hazy (ground-glass) appearance, with bilateral alveolar infiltrates beginning at the hilus and spreading to the periphery. However, radiographic presentations can also be atypical and show, for example, lobar consolidation or nodular, unilateral infiltrates; they can even be normal.
- Diagnosis can generally be confirmed by using the induced sputum technique or bronchoalveolar lavage, and an open-lung biopsy is now rarely indicated.[269,270]

The therapy of choice is intravenous trimethoprim-sulfamethoxazole (20 mg/kg/day of trimethoprim) for 14 days (for cancer patients) to 21 days (for HIV-infected patients). In patients unable to tolerate this regimen, intravenous pentamidine, trimetrexate, atovaquone, and clindamycin plus primaquine or, potentially, the antifolate trimetrexate, can be used. It has been demonstrated that the addition of corticosteroids is beneficial in patients with severe hypoxemia (PaO₂ less than 75 mm Hg).[271] If the patient fails to improve after 4 to 7 days on the initial regimen, modifications (e.g., adding pentamidine to the sulfamethoxazole-trimethoprim regimen) and possibly an open lung biopsy to rule out other pathogens, may be indicated.

A clear benefit has been demonstrated in preventing PCP by administering trimethoprim-sulfamethoxazole to children with leukemia, to patients undergoing bone marrow transplantation, and to HIV-infected children. Alternative, but potentially less effective prophylactic regimens include dapsone, aerosolized or intravenous pentamidine, and atovaquone.[272,273]

Other Parasitic Infections

Cryptosporidial infection, manifested by watery diarrhea, can develop into a prolonged and devastating wasting syndrome in an immunocompromised host. One outbreak caused by a contaminated water supply in Milwaukee not only affected the general population but also led to often intractable diarrhea complicated by electrolyte imbalances and severe dehydration in HIV-infected children and adults.[50]

The prevalence of *Toxoplasma gondii* varies according to geographic region and, until recently, its major complication was vertical transmission and congenital infection. However, with the advent of AIDS, the number of adult patients with cerebral or ocular toxoplasmosis increased dramatically, although these numbers have decreased with the introduction of highly active antiretroviral therapy. Cerebral toxoplasmosis is usually manifested by diffuse meningoencephalitis (fever, headaches, focal neurologic signs, including seizures, cranial nerve palsy, or hemiparesis). Radiologic examination by computed tomography typically demonstrates single or multiple mass lesions, often ring-enhancing, which may be difficult to distinguish from malignancies.[274] The recommended treatment is the combination of pyrimethamine with sulfadiazine or clindamycin, but atovaquone has shown some promise as well.[265,274,275]

IMPROVING HOST DEFENSE

Immunization against bacterial and viral pathogens has played an extremely important role in decreasing the incidence and severity of many infectious diseases. It is unfortunate that active immunization is generally unsuccessful in immunocompromised hosts because these persons are unable to mount or to sustain an antibody response to most vaccines.[71] Live-virus vaccines are not recommended for use in immunocompromised children, with the notable exception of live-attenuated varicella vaccine for children with acute lymphocytic leukemia in remission.[276] For assistance in treating children who were not fully immunized before the diagnosis of a malignancy, the American Academy of Pediatrics has provided guidelines for the administration of immunizations in immunocompromised children.[277]

Pooled immunoglobulin preparations do not appear to offer a benefit to neutropenic patients but are clearly indicated in patients who have either congenital or acquired hypogammaglobulinemia, such as patients who have undergone stem cell tranplantation.

REFERENCES

1. Pizzo PA, Rubin M, Freifeld A, Walsh TJ. The child with cancer and infection. II. Nonbacterial infections. J Pediatr. 1991;119: 845-857.
2. Pizzo PA, Rubin M, Freifeld A, Walsh TJ. The child with cancer and infection. I. Empiric therapy for fever and neutropenia, and preventive strategies. J Pediatr. 1991;119:679-694.
3. Raaf JH. Results from use of 826 vascular access devices in cancer patients. Cancer. 1985;55:1312-1321.
4. Viscoli C, Castagnola E, Rogers D. Infections in the compromised child. Baillieres Clin Haematol. 1991;4:511-543.
5. Hann I, Viscoli C, Paesmans M, et al. A comparison of outcome from febrile neutropenic episodes in children compared with adults: results from four EORTC studies. International Antimicrobial Therapy Cooperative Group (IATCG) of the European

Organization for Research and Treatment of Cancer (EORTC). Br J Haematol. 1997;99:580-588.

6. Hughes WT, Armstrong D, Bodey GP, et al. 2002 guidelines for the use of antimicrobial agents in neutropenic patients with cancer. Clin Infect Dis. 2002;34:730-751.

7. Awada A, van der Auwera P, Meunier F, et al. Streptococcal and enterococcal bacteremia in patients with cancer. Clin Infect Dis. 1992;15:33-48.

8. Bruckner LB, Korones DN, Karnauchow T, et al. High incidence of penicillin resistance among alpha-hemolytic streptococci isolated from the blood of children with cancer. J Pediatr. 2002;140:20-26.

9. Bochud PY, Eggiman P, Calandra T, et al. Bacteremia due to viridans streptococcus in neutropenic patients with cancer: clinical spectrum and risk factors. Clin Infect Dis. 1994;18:25-31.

10. Dybedal I, Lamvik J. Respiratory insufficiency in acute leukemia following treatment with cytosine arabinoside and septicemia with streptococcus viridans. Eur J Haematol. 1989;42:405-406.

11. Bochud PY, Calandra T, Francioli P. Bacteremia due to viridans streptococci in neutropenic patients: a review. Am J Med. 1994;97:256-264.

12. Elting LS, Bodey GP, Keefe BH. Septicemia and shock syndrome due to viridans streptococci: a case-control study of predisposing factors. Clin Infect Dis. 1992;14:1201-1207.

13. Sotiropoulos SV, Jackson MA, Woods GM, et al. Alpha-streptococcal septicemia in leukemic children treated with continuous or large dosage intermittent cytosine arabinoside. Pediatr Infect Dis J. 1989;8:755-758.

14. Fridkin SK, Hageman JC, Morrison M, et al. Methicillin-resistant *Staphylococcus aureus* disease in three communities. N Engl J Med. 2005;352:1436-1444.

15. Buescher ES. Community-acquired methicillin-resistant *Staphylococcus aureus* in pediatrics. Curr Opin Pediatr. 2005;17:67-70.

16. Gonzalez BE, Martinez-Aguilar G, Hulten KG, et al. Severe staphylococcal sepsis in adolescents in the era of community-acquired methicillin-resistant *Staphylococcus aureus*. Pediatrics. 2005;115:642-648.

17. Miller LG, Perdreau-Remington F, Rieg G, et al. Necrotizing fasciitis caused by community-associated methicillin-resistant *Staphylococcus aureus* in Los Angeles. N Engl J Med. 2005;352:1445-1453.

18. Gonzalez BE, Hulten KG, Dishop MK, et al. Pulmonary manifestations in children with invasive community-acquired *Staphylococcus aureus* infection. Clin Infect Dis. 2005;41:583-590.

19. Hiemenz J, Skelton J, Pizzo PA. Perspective on the management of catheter-related infections in cancer patients. Pediatr Infect Dis. 1986;5:6-11.

20. Koll BS, Brown AE. Changing patterns of infections in the immunocompromised patient with cancer. Hematol Oncol Clin North Am. 1993;7:753-769.

21. Roilides E, Butler KM, Husson RN, et al. Pseudomonas infections in children with human immunodeficiency virus infection. Pediatr Infect Dis J. 1992;11:547-553.

22. Bodey GP, Rodriguez S, Fainstein V, Elting LS. Clostridial bacteremia in cancer patients: a 12-year experience. Cancer. 1991;67:1928-1942.

23. Weinberger M, Wu T, Rubin M, et al. *Leptotrichia buccalis* bacteremia in patients with cancer: report of four cases and review. Rev Infect Dis. 1991;13:201-206.

24. Golomb HM, Hanauer SB. Infectious complications associated with hairy cell leukemia. J Infect Dis. 1981;143:639-643.

25. Berkey P, Bodey GP. Nocardial infection in patients with neoplastic disease. Rev Infect Dis. 1989;11:407-412.

26. Walsh TJ, Melcher GP, Rinaldi MG, et al. Trichosporon beigelii, an emerging pathogen resistant to amphotericin B. J Clin Microbiol. 1990;28:1616-1622.

27. Walsh TJ, Pizzo PA. Nosocomial fungal infections: a classification for hospital-acquired fungal infections and mycoses arising from endogenous flora or reactivation. Annu Rev Microbiol. 1988;42:517-545.

28. Ridola V, Chachaty E, Raimondo G, et al. Candida infections in children treated with conventional chemotherapy for solid tumors (transplant recipients excluded): the Institut Gustave Roussy Pediatrics Department experience. Pediatr Blood Cancer. 2004;42:332-337.

29. Wingard JR, Merz WG, Rinaldi MG, et al. Increase in *Candida krusei* infection among patients with bone marrow transplantation and neutropenia treated prophylactically with fluconazole. N Engl J Med. 1991;325:1274-1277.

30. Flynn PM, Marina NM, Rivera GK, Hughes WT. *Candida tropicalis* infections in children with leukemia. Leuk Lymphoma. 1993;10:369-376.

31. Richet HM, Andremont A, Tancrede C, et al. Risk factors for candidemia in patients with acute lymphocytic leukemia. Rev Infect Dis. 1991;13:211-215.

32. Lecciones JA, Lee JW, Navarro EE, et al. Vascular catheter-associated fungemia in patients with cancer: analysis of 155 episodes. Clin Infect Dis. 1992;14:875-883.

33. Walsh TJ, Gonzalez C, Roilides E, et al. Fungemia in children infected with the human immunodeficiency virus: new epidemiologic patterns, emerging pathogens, and improved outcome with antifungal therapy. Clin Infect Dis. 1995;20:900-906.

34. Weinberger M, Elattar I, Marshall D, et al. Patterns of infection in patients with aplastic anemia and the emergence of *Aspergillus* as a major cause of death. Medicine (Baltimore). 1992;71:24-43.

35. Pursell KJ, Telzak EE, Armstrong D. *Aspergillus* species colonization and invasive disease in patients with AIDS. Clin Infect Dis. 1992;14:141-148.

36. Yu VL, Muder RR, Poorsattar A. Significance of isolation of *Aspergillus* from the respiratory tract in diagnosis of invasive pulmonary aspergillosis: results from a three-year prospective study. Am J Med. 1986;81:249-254.

37. Stringer JR, Beard CB, Miller RF, Wakefield AE. A new name (*Pneumocystis jiroveci*) for pneumocystis from humans. Emerg Infect Dis. 2002;8:891-896.

38. Kovacs JA, Hiemenz JW, Macher AM, et al. Pneumocystis carinii pneumonia: a comparison between patients with the acquired immunodeficiency syndrome and patients with other immunodeficiencies. Ann Intern Med. 1984;100:663-671.

39. Arend SM, Kroon FP, van't Wout JW. Pneumocystis carinii pneumonia in patients without AIDS, 1980 through 1993: an analysis of 78 cases. Arch Intern Med. 1995;155:2436-2441.

40. Sepkowitz KA, Brown AE, Telzak EE, et al. Pneumocystis carinii pneumonia among patients without AIDS at a cancer hospital. JAMA. 1992;267:832-837.

41. Wood DJ, Corbitt G. Viral infections in childhood leukemia. J Infect Dis. 1985;152:266-273.

42. Patrick CC. Infections in Immunocompromised Infants and Children. New York, Churchill Livingstone, 1992.

43. Ho CM, Khuzaiah R, Yasmin AM. Varicella in children with haematological malignancy—outcome of treatment and prevention. Med J Malaysia. 1994;49:29-35.

44. Rokicka-Milewska R, Pacholska J, Lukowska K, et al. Cytomegalovirus infection in children with blood diseases. Acta Haematol Pol. 1992;23:191-195.

45. White NH, Yow MD, Demmler GJ, et al. Prevalence of cytomegalovirus antibody in subjects between the ages of 6 and 22 years. J Infect Dis. 1989;159:1013-1017.

46. Giller RH, Grose C. Epstein-Barr virus: the hematologic and oncologic consequences of virus-host interaction. Crit Rev Oncol Hematol. 1989;9:149-195.

47. Purtilo DT, Sakamoto K, Saemundsen AK, et al. Documentation of Epstein-Barr virus infection in immunodeficient patients with life-threatening lymphoproliferative diseases by clinical, virological, and immunopathological studies. Cancer Res. 1981;41:4226-4236.

48. Kikuta H, Sakiyama Y, Matsumoto S, et al. Fatal Epstein-Barr virus-associated hemophagocytic syndrome. Blood. 1993;82:3259-3264.

49. McClain KL, Leach CT, Jenson HB, et al. Association of Epstein-Barr virus with leiomyosarcomas in children with AIDS. N Engl J Med. 1995;332:12-18.

50. Mac Kenzie WR, Hoxie NJ, Proctor ME, et al. A massive outbreak in Milwaukee of cryptosporidium infection transmitted through the public water supply. N Engl J Med. 1994;331:161-167.

51. Pagano L, Trape G, Putzulu R, et al. *Toxoplasma gondii* infection in patients with hematological malignancies. Ann Hematol. 2004;83:592-595.

52. Russell TS, Lynch J, Ottolini MG. Eradication of *Cryptosporidium* in a child undergoing maintenance chemotherapy for leukemia using high-dose azithromycin therapy. J Pediatr Hematol Oncol. 1998;20:83-85.

53. Chanock S. Evolving risk factors for infectious complications of cancer therapy. Hematol Oncol Clin North Am. 1993;7:771-793.

54. D'Antonio D, Pizzigallo E, Iacone A, et al. Occurrence of bacteremia in hematologic patients. Eur J Epidemiol. 1992;8:687-692.

55. Ingram J, Weitzman S, Greenberg ML, et al. Complications of indwelling venous access lines in the pediatric hematology patient: a prospective comparison of external venous catheters and subcutaneous ports. Am J Pediatr Hematol Oncol. 1991;13:130-136.

56. Spielberger R, Stiff P, Bensinger W, et al. Palifermin for oral mucositis after intensive therapy for hematologic cancers. N Engl J Med. 2004;351:2590-2598.

57. Gaur AH, Liu T, Knapp KM, et al. Infections in children and young adults with bone malignancies undergoing limb-sparing surgery. Cancer. 2005;104:602-610.

58. Pizzo PA. After empiric therapy: what to do until the granulocyte comes back. Rev Infect Dis. 1987;9:214-219.

59. Bodey GP, Buckley M, Sathe YS, Freireich EJ. Quantitative relationships between circulating leukocytes and infection in patients with acute leukemia. Ann Intern Med. 1966;64:328-340.

60. Gram-positive bacteraemia in granulocytopenic cancer patients, EORTC International Antimicrobial Therapy Cooperative Group. Eur J Cancer. 1990;26:569-574.

61. Rubio M, Palau L, Vivas JR, et al. Predominance of gram-positive microorganisms as a cause of septicemia in patients with hematological malignancies. Infect Control Hosp Epidemiol. 1994;15:101-104.

62. Pickering LK, Ericsson CD, Kohl S. Effect of chemotherapeutic agents on metabolic and bactericidal activity of polymorphonuclear leukocytes. Cancer. 1978;42:1741-1746.

63. Mukwaya G. Immunosuppressive effects and infections associated with corticosteroid therapy. Pediatr Infect Dis J. 1988;7:499-504.

64. Cupps TR, Fauci AS. Corticosteroid-mediated immunoregulation in man. Immunol Rev. 1982;65:133-155.

65. Slivnick DJ, Nawrocki JF, Fisher RI. Immunology and cellular biology of Hodgkin's disease. Hematol Oncol Clin North Am. 1989;3:205-220.

66. Jin ZW, Cleveland RP, Kaufman DB. Immunodeficiency in patients with hemophilia: an underlying deficiency and lack of correlation with factor replacement therapy or exposure to human immunodeficiency virus. J Allergy Clin Immunol. 1989;83:165-170.

67. Reed JD, Redding-Lallinger R, Orringer EP. Nutrition and sickle cell disease. Am J Hematol. 1987;24:441-455.

68. Ferdman RM, Church JA. Immunologic and virologic effects of glucocorticoids on human immunodeficiency virus infection in children: a preliminary study. Pediatr Infect Dis J. 1994;13:212-216.

69. Mackall CL, Fleisher TA, Brown MR, et al. Lymphocyte depletion during treatment with intensive chemotherapy for cancer. Blood. 1994;84:2221-2228.

70. Hiemenz JW, Greene JN. Special considerations for the patient undergoing allogeneic or autologous bone marrow transplantation. Hematol Oncol Clin North Am. 1993;7:961-1002.

71. Chilcote RR, Baehner RL, Hammond D. Septicemia and meningitis in children splenectomized for Hodgkin's disease. N Engl J Med. 1976;295:798-800.

72. Pegelow CH, Wilson B, Overturf GD, et al. Infection in splenectomized sickle cell disease patients. Clin Pediatr Med Surg (Philadelphia). 1980;19:102-105.

73. Cavenagh JD, Joseph AE, Dilly S, Bevan DH. Splenic sepsis in sickle cell disease. Br J Haematol. 1994;86:187-189.

74. Pizzo PA. Considerations for the prevention of infectious complications in patients with cancer. Rev Infect Dis. 1989;11(suppl 7):S1551-S1563.

75. Engels EA, Lau J, Barza M. Efficacy of quinolone prophylaxis in neutropenic cancer patients: a meta-analysis. J Clin Oncol. 1998;16:1179-1187.

76. Cullen M, Steven N, Billingham L, et al. Antibacterial prophylaxis after chemotherapy for solid tumors and lymphomas. N Engl J Med. 2005;353:988-998.

77. Reuter S, Kern WV, Sigge A, et al. Impact of fluoroquinolone prophylaxis on reduced infection-related mortality among patients with neutropenia and hematologic malignancies. Clin Infect Dis. 2005;40:1087-1093.

78. Gafter-Gvili A, Fraser A, Paul M, Leibovici L. Meta-analysis: antibiotic prophylaxis reduces mortality in neutropenic patients. Ann Intern Med. 2005;142:979-995.

79. Bucaneve G, Micozzi A, Menichetti F, et al. Levofloxacin to prevent bacterial infection in patients with cancer and neutropenia. N Engl J Med. 2005;353:977-987.

80. Goodman JL, Winston DJ, Greenfield RA, et al. A controlled trial of fluconazole to prevent fungal infections in patients undergoing bone marrow transplantation. N Engl J Med. 1992;326:845-851.

81. Slavin MA, Osborne B, Adams R, et al. Efficacy and safety of fluconazole prophylaxis for fungal infections after marrow transplantation: a prospective, randomized, double-blind study. J Infect Dis. 1995;171:1545-1552.

82. Marr KA, Seidel K, White TC, Bowden RA. Candidemia in allogeneic blood and marrow transplant recipients: evolution of risk factors after the adoption of prophylactic fluconazole. J Infect Dis. 2000;181:309-316.

83. Kramer BS, Pizzo PA, Robichaud KJ, et al. Role of serial microbiologic surveillance and clinical evaluation in the management of cancer patients with fever and granulocytopenia. Am J Med. 1982;72:561-568.

84. Freifeld AG, Walsh T, Marshall D, et al. Monotherapy for fever and neutropenia in cancer patients: a randomized comparison of ceftazidime versus imipenem. J Clin Oncol. 1995;13:165-176.

85. Feusner J, Cohen R, O'Leary M, Beach B. Use of routine chest radiography in the evaluation of fever in neutropenic pediatric oncology patients. J Clin Oncol. 1988;6:1699-1702.

86. Renoult E, Buteau C, Turgeon N, et al. Is routine chest radiography necessary for the initial evaluation of fever in neutropenic children with cancer? Pediatr Blood Cancer. 2004;43:224-228.

87. Katz JA, Bash R, Rollins N, et al. The yield of routine chest radiography in children with cancer hospitalized for fever and neutropenia. Cancer. 1991;68:940-943.

88. Korones DN, Hussong MR, Gullace MA. Routine chest radiography of children with cancer hospitalized for fever and neutropenia: is it really necessary? Cancer. 1997;80:1160-1164.

89. Walsh TJ, Hathorn JW, Sobel JD, et al. Detection of circulating *Candida* enolase by immunoassay in patients with cancer and invasive candidiasis. N Engl J Med. 1991;324:1026-1031.

90. de Repentigny L. Serodiagnosis of candidiasis, aspergillosis, and cryptococcosis. Clin Infect Dis. 1992;14(suppl 1):S11-S22.

91. Bodey GP. Empirical antibiotic therapy for fever in neutropenic patients. Clin Infect Dis. 1993;17(suppl 2):S378-S384.

92. Hughes WT, Armstrong D, Bodey GP, et al. From the Infectious Diseases Society of America: Guidelines for the use of antimicrobial agents in neutropenic patients with unexplained fever. J Infect Dis. 1990;161:381-396.

93. De Pauw BE, Deresinski SC, Feld R, et al. Ceftazidime compared with piperacillin and tobramycin for the empiric treatment of fever in neutropenic patients with cancer: a multicenter randomized trial. The Intercontinental Antimicrobial Study Group. Ann Intern Med. 1994;120:834-844.

94. Joshi JH, Newman KA, Brown BW, et al. Double beta-lactam regimen compared to an aminoglycoside/beta-lactam regimen as empiric antibiotic therapy for febrile granulocytopenic cancer patients. Support Care Cancer. 1993;1:186-194.

95. Kieft H, Hoepelman AI, Rozenberg-Arska M, et al. Cefepime compared with ceftazidime as initial therapy for serious bacterial infections and sepsis syndrome. Antimicrob Agents Chemother. 1994;38:415-421.

96. Eggimann P, Glauser MP, Aoun M, et al. Cefepime monotherapy for the empirical treatment of fever in granulocytopenic cancer patients. J Antimicrob Chemother. 1993;32(suppl B):151-163.

97. Corapcioglu F, Sarper N. Cefepime versus ceftazidime + amikacin as empirical therapy for febrile neutropenia in children with cancer: a prospective randomized trial of the treatment efficacy and cost. Pediatr Hematol Oncol. 2005;22:59-70.

98. Rolston KV, Berkey P, Bodey GP, et al. A comparison of imipenem to ceftazidime with or without amikacin as empiric therapy in febrile neutropenic patients. Arch Intern Med. 1992;152:283-291.

99. Vandercam B, Gerain J, Humblet Y, et al. Meropenem versus ceftazidime as empirical monotherapy for febrile neutropenic cancer patients. Ann Hematol. 2000;79:152-157.

100. Cometta A, Calandra T, Gaya H, et al. Monotherapy with meropenem versus combination therapy with ceftazidime plus amikacin as empiric therapy for fever in granulocytopenic patients with cancer. The International Antimicrobial Therapy Cooperative Group of the European Organization for Research and Treatment of Cancer and the Gruppo Italiano Malattie Ematologiche Maligne dell'Adulto Infection Program. Antimicrob Agents Chemother. 1996;40:1108-1115.

101. Muller J, Garami M, Constantin T, et al. Meropenem in the treatment of febrile neutropenic children. Pediatr Hematol Oncol. 2005;22:277-284.

102. Pizzo PA, Hathorn JW, Hiemenz J, et al. A randomized trial comparing ceftazidime alone with combination antibiotic therapy in cancer patients with fever and neutropenia. N Engl J Med. 1986;315:552-558.

103. Liang R, Yung R, Chiu E, et al. Ceftazidime versus imipenem-cilastatin as initial monotherapy for febrile neutropenic patients. Antimicrob Agents Chemother. 1990;34:1336-1341.

104. Haslam DB. Managing the child with fever and neutropenia in an era of increasing microbial resistance. J Pediatr. 2002;140:5-7.

105. Lyytikainen O, Rautio M, Carlson P, et al. Nosocomial bloodstream infections due to viridans streptococci in haematological and non-haematological patients: species distribution and antimicrobial resistance. J Antimicrob Chemother. 2004;53:631-634.

106. Rubin M, Hathorn JW, Marshall D, et al. Gram-positive infections and the use of vancomycin in 550 episodes of fever and neutropenia. Ann Intern Med. 1988;108:30-35.

107. Karp JE, Dick JD, Angelopulos C, et al. Empiric use of vancomycin during prolonged treatment-induced granulocytopenia: randomized, double-blind, placebo-controlled clinical trial in patients with acute leukemia. Am J Med. 1986;81:237-242.

108. Freifeld AG. Infectious complications in the immunocompromised host: the antimicrobial armamentarium. Hematol Oncol Clin North Am. 1993;7:813-839.

109. Flynn PM, Van Hooser B, Gigliotti F. Atypical mycobacterial infections of Hickman catheter exit sites. Pediatr Infect Dis J. 1988;7:510-513.

110. Riikonen P, Saarinen UM, Lahteenoja KM, Jalanko H. Management of indwelling central venous catheters in pediatric cancer patients with fever and neutropenia. Scand J Infect Dis. 1993;25:357-364.

111. Mueller BU, Skelton J, Callender DP, et al. A prospective randomized trial comparing the infectious and noninfectious complications of an externalized catheter versus a subcutaneously implanted device in cancer patients. J Clin Oncol. 1992;10:1943-1948.

112. Cotton DJ, Gill VJ, Marshall DJ, et al. Clinical features and therapeutic interventions in 17 cases of *Bacillus* bacteremia in an immunosuppressed patient population. J Clin Microbiol. 1987;25:672-674.

113. Hoy JF, Rolston KV, Hopfer RL, Bodey GP. *Mycobacterium fortuitum* bacteremia in patients with cancer and long-term venous catheters. Am J Med. 1987;83:213-217.

114. Anaissie EJ, Rex JH, Uzun O, Vartivarian S. Predictors of adverse outcome in cancer patients with candidemia. Am J Med. 1998;104:238-245.

115. Eppes SC, Troutman JL, Gutman LT. Outcome of treatment of candidemia in children whose central catheters were removed or retained. Pediatr Infect Dis J. 1989;8:99-104.

116. Glaser DW, Medeiros D, Rollins N, Buchanan GR. Catheter-related thrombosis in children with cancer. J Pediatr. 2001;138:255-259.

117. Bash RO, Katz JA, Cash JV, Buchanan GR. Safety and cost effectiveness of early hospital discharge of lower risk children with cancer admitted for fever and neutropenia. Cancer. 1994;74:189-196.

118. Pizzo PA, Robichaud KJ, Gill FA, et al. Duration of empiric antibiotic therapy in granulocytopenic patients with cancer. Am J Med. 1979;67:194-200.

119. Buchanan GR. Approach to treatment of the febrile cancer patient with low-risk neutropenia. Hematol Oncol Clin North Am. 1993;7:919-935.

120. Lee JW, Pizzo PA. Management of the cancer patient with fever and prolonged neutropenia. Hematol Oncol Clin North Am. 1993;7:937-960.

121. Pizzo PA, Robichaud KJ, Gill FA, Witebsky FG. Empiric antibiotic and antifungal therapy for cancer patients with prolonged fever and granulocytopenia. Am J Med. 1982;72:101-111.

122. Coullioud D, Van der Auwera P, Viot M, Lasset C. Prospective multicentric study of the etiology of 1051 bacteremic episodes in 782 cancer patients. CEMIC (French-Belgian Study Club of Infectious Diseases in Cancer). Support Care Cancer. 1993;1:34-46.

123. Wiley JM, Smith N, Leventhal BG, et al. Invasive fungal disease in pediatric acute leukemia patients with fever and neutropenia during induction chemotherapy: a multivariate analysis of risk factors. J Clin Oncol. 1990;8:280-286.

124. Empiric antifungal therapy in febrile granulocytopenic patients: EORTC International Antimicrobial Therapy Cooperative Group. Am J Med. 1989;86:668-672.

125. Denning DW, Stevens DA. Antifungal and surgical treatment of invasive aspergillosis: review of 2,121 published cases. Rev Infect Dis. 1990;12:1147-1201.

126. Rex JH, Bennett JE, Sugar AM, et al. A randomized trial comparing fluconazole with amphotericin B for the treatment of candidemia in patients without neutropenia: Candidemia Study Group and the National Institute. N Engl J Med. 1994;331:1325-1330.

127. Bodey GP, Anaissie EJ, Elting LS, et al. Antifungal prophylaxis during remission induction therapy for acute leukemia fluconazole versus intravenous amphotericin B. Cancer. 1994;73:2099-2106.

128. Malik IA, Moid I, Aziz Z, et al. A randomized comparison of fluconazole with amphotericin B as empiric anti-fungal agents in cancer patients with prolonged fever and neutropenia. Am J Med. 1998;105:478-483.

129. Walsh TJ, Pappas P, Winston DJ, et al. Voriconazole compared with liposomal amphotericin B for empirical antifungal therapy in patients with neutropenia and persistent fever. N Engl J Med. 2002;346:225-234.

130. Groll AH, Walsh TJ. Posaconazole: clinical pharmacology and potential for management of fungal infections. Expert Rev Anti Infect Ther. 2005;3:467-487.

131. Sabatelli F, Patel R, Mann PA, et al. In vitro activities of posaconazole, fluconazole, itraconazole, voriconazole, and amphotericin B against a large collection of clinically important molds and yeasts. Antimicrob Agents Chemother. 2006;50:2009-2015.

132. Meunier F, Prentice HG, Ringden O. Liposomal amphotericin B (AmBisome): safety data from a phase II/III clinical trial. J Antimicrob Chemother. 1991;28(suppl B):83-91.

133. Walsh TJ, Yeldandi V, McEvoy M, et al. Safety, tolerance, and pharmacokinetics of a small unilamellar liposomal formulation of amphotericin B (AmBisome) in neutropenic patients. Antimicrob Agents Chemother. 1998;42:2391-2398.

134. Walsh TJ, Finberg RW, Arndt C, et al. Liposomal amphotericin B for empirical therapy in patients with persistent fever and neutropenia. National Institute of Allergy and Infectious Diseases Mycoses Study Group. N Engl J Med. 1999;340:764-771.

135. Ellis M, Spence D, de Pauw B, et al. An EORTC international multicenter randomized trial (EORTC number 19923) comparing two dosages of liposomal amphotericin B for treatment of invasive aspergillosis. Clin Infect Dis. 1998;27:1406-1412.

136. Denning DW. Echinocandin antifungal drugs. Lancet. 2003;362:1142-1151.

137. Walsh TJ, Teppler H, Donowitz GR, et al. Caspofungin versus liposomal amphotericin B for empirical antifungal therapy in patients with persistent fever and neutropenia. N Engl J Med. 2004;351:1391-1402.

138. Walsh TJ, Adamson PC, Seibel NL, et al. Pharmacokinetics, safety, and tolerability of caspofungin in children and adolescents. Antimicrob Agents Chemother. 2005;49:4536-4545.

139. Talcott JA, Siegel RD, Finberg R, Goldman L. Risk assessment in cancer patients with fever and neutropenia: a prospective, two-center validation of a prediction rule. J Clin Oncol. 1992;10:316-322.

140. Talcott JA, Finberg R, Mayer RJ, Goldman L. The medical course of cancer patients with fever and neutropenia: clinical identification of a low-risk subgroup at presentation. Arch Intern Med. 1988;148:2561-2568.

141. Rackoff WR, Gonin R, Robinson C, et al. Predicting the risk of bacteremia in childen with fever and neutropenia. J Clin Oncol. 1996;14:919-924.

142. Klaassen RJ, Goodman TR, Pham B, Doyle JJ. "Low-risk" prediction rule for pediatric oncology patients presenting with fever and neutropenia. J Clin Oncol. 2000;18:1012-1019.

143. Gardembas-Pain M, Desablens B, Sensebe L, et al. Home treatment of febrile neutropenia: an empirical oral antibiotic regimen. Ann Oncol. 1991;2:485-487.

144. Malik IA, Abbas Z, Karim M. Randomised comparison of oral ofloxacin alone with combination of parenteral antibiotics in neutropenic febrile patients. Lancet. 1992;339:1092-1096.

145. Malik IA, Khan WA, Aziz Z, Karim M. Self-administered antibiotic therapy for chemotherapy-induced, low-risk febrile neutropenia in patients with nonhematologic neoplasms. Clin Infect Dis. 1994;19:522-527.

146. Malik IA, Khan WA, Karim M, et al. Feasibility of outpatient management of fever in cancer patients with low-risk neutropenia: results of a prospective randomized trial. Am J Med. 1995;98:224-231.

147. Papadimitris C, Dimopoulos MA, Kostis E, et al. Outpatient treatment of neutropenic fever with oral antibiotics and granulocyte colony-stimulating factor. Oncology. 1999;57:127-130.

148. Hidalgo M, Hornedo J, Lumbreras C, et al. Outpatient therapy with oral ofloxacin for patients with low-risk neutropenia and fever: a prospective, randomized clinical trial. Cancer. 1999;85:213-219.

149. Velasco E, Costa MA, Martins CA, Nucci M. Randomized trial comparing oral ciprofloxacin plus penicillin V with amikacin plus carbenicillin or ceftazidime for empirical treatment of febrile neutropenic cancer patients. Am J Clin Oncol. 1995;18:429-435.

150. Rubenstein EB, Rolston K, Benjamin RS, et al. Outpatient treatment of febrile episodes in low-risk neutropenic patients with cancer. Cancer. 1993;71:3640-3646.

151. Aquino VM, Herrera L, Sandler ES, Buchanan GR. Feasibility of oral ciprofloxacin for the outpatient management of febrile neutropenia in selected children with cancer. Cancer. 2000;88:1710-1714.

152. Paganini HR, Sarkis CM, De Martino MG, et al. Oral administration of cefixime to lower risk febrile neutropenic children with cancer. Cancer. 2000;88:2848-2852.

153. Shenep JL, Flynn PM, Baker DK, et al. Oral cefixime is similar to continued intravenous antibiotics in the empirical treatment of febrile neutropenic children with cancer. Clin Infect Dis. 2001;32:36-43.

154. Chamilos G, Bamias A, Efstathiou E, et al. Outpatient treatment of low-risk neutropenic fever in cancer patients using oral moxifloxacin. Cancer. 2005;103:2629-2635.

155. Freifeld A, Marchigiani D, Walsh T, et al. A double-blind comparison of empirical oral and intravenous antibiotic therapy for low-risk febrile patients with neutropenia during cancer chemotherapy. N Engl J Med. 1999;341:305-311.

156. Kern WV, Cometta A, De Bock R, et al. Oral versus intravenous empirical antimicrobial therapy for fever in patients with granulocytopenia who are receiving cancer chemotherapy. International Antimicrobial Therapy Cooperative Group of the European Organization for Research and Treatment of Cancer. N Engl J Med. 1999;341:312-318.

157. Kamana M, Escalante C, Mullen CA, et al. Bacterial infections in low-risk, febrile neutropenic patients. Cancer. 2005;104:422-426.

158. Sung L, Nathan PC, Lange B, et al. Prophylactic granulocyte colony-stimulating factor and granulocyte-macrophage colony-stimulating factor decrease febrile neutropenia after chemotherapy in children with cancer: a meta-analysis of randomized controlled trials. J Clin Oncol. 2004;22:3350-3356.

159. Bennett CL, Stinson TJ, Laver JH, et al. Cost analyses of adjunct colony stimulating factors for acute leukemia: can they improve clinical decision making. Leuk Lymphoma. 2000;37:65-70.

160. Relling MV, Boyett JM, Blanco JG, et al. Granulocyte colony-stimulating factor and the risk of secondary myeloid malignancy after etoposide treatment. Blood. 2003;101:3862-3867.

161. Ozkaynak MF, Krailo M, Chen Z, Feusner J. Randomized comparison of antibiotics with and without granulocyte colony-stimulating factor in children with chemotherapy-induced febrile neutropenia: a report from the Children's Oncology Group. Pediatr Blood Cancer. 2005;45:274-280.

162. Smith TJ, Khatcheressian J, Lyman GH, et al. 2006 update of recommendations for the use of white blood cell growth factors: an evidence-based clinical practice guideline. J Clin Oncol. 2006;24:3187-3205.

163. Morace G, Tamburrini E, Manzara S, et al. Epidemiological and clinical aspects of mycoses in patients with AIDS-related pathologies. Eur J Epidemiol. 1990;6:398-403.

164. Gupta KL, Ghosh AK, Kochhar R, et al. Esophageal candidiasis after renal transplantation: comparative study in patients on different immunosuppressive protocols. Am J Gastroenterol. 1994;89:1062-1065.

165. McBane RD, Gross JB Jr. Herpes esophagitis: clinical syndrome, endoscopic appearance, and diagnosis in 23 patients. Gastrointest Endosc. 1991;37:600-603.

166. Walsh TJ, Belitsos NJ, Hamilton SR. Bacterial esophagitis in immunocompromised patients. Arch Intern Med. 1986;146:1345-1348.

167. Wilcox CM, Diehl DL, Cello JP, et al. Cytomegalovirus esophagitis in patients with AIDS: a clinical, endoscopic, and pathologic correlation. Ann Intern Med. 1990;113:589-593.

168. Ally R, Schurmann D, Kreisel W, et al. A randomized, double-blind, double-dummy, multicenter trial of voriconazole and fluconazole in the treatment of esophageal candidiasis in immunocompromised patients. Clin Infect Dis. 2001;33:1447-1454.

169. Dinubile MJ, Lupinacci RJ, Berman RS, Sable CA. Response and relapse rates of candidal esophagitis in HIV-infected patients treated with caspofungin. AIDS Res Hum Retroviruses. 2002;18:903-908.

170. Villanueva A, Arathoon EG, Gotuzzo E, et al. A randomized double-blind study of caspofungin versus amphotericin for the treatment of candidal esophagitis. Clin Infect Dis. 2001;33:1529-1535.

171. Villanueva A, Gotuzzo E, Arathoon EG, et al. A randomized double-blind study of caspofungin versus fluconazole for the treatment of esophageal candidiasis. Am J Med. 2002;113:294-299.

172. Pappas PG, Rex JH, Sobel JD, et al. Guidelines for treatment of candidiasis. Clin Infect Dis. 2004;38:161-189.

173. Wisplinghoff H, Bischoff T, Tallent SM, et al. Nosocomial bloodstream infections in US hospitals: analysis of 24,179 cases from a prospective nationwide surveillance study. Clin Infect Dis. 2004;39:309-317.

174. Ashkenazi S, Leibovici L, Samra Z, et al. Risk factors for mortality due to bacteremia and fungemia in childhood. Clin Infect Dis. 1992;14:949-951.

175. Meunier F, Aoun M, Bitar N. Candidemia in immunocompromised patients. Clin Infect Dis. 1992;14(suppl 1):S120-S125.

176. Walsh TJ, Pizzo A. Treatment of systemic fungal infections: recent progress and current problems. Eur J Clin Microbiol Infect Dis. 1988;7:460-475.

177. Allen U, Smith CR, Prober CG. The value of skin biopsies in febrile, neutropenic, immunocompromised children. Am J Dis Child. 1986;140:459-461.

178. Phillips P, Shafran S, Garber G, et al. Multicenter randomized trial of fluconazole versus amphotericin B for treatment of candidemia in non-neutropenic patients: Canadian Candidemia Study Group. Eur J Clin Microbiol Infect Dis. 1997;16:337-345.

179. Mora-Duarte J, Betts R, Rotstein C, et al. Comparison of caspofungin and amphotericin B for invasive candidiasis. N Engl J Med. 2002;347:2020-2029.

180. Buchner T, Fegeler W, Bernhardt H, et al. Treatment of severe *Candida* infections in high-risk patients in Germany: consensus formed by a panel of interdisciplinary investigators. Eur J Clin Microbiol Infect Dis. 2002;21:337-352.

181. Nucci M, Anaissie E. Revisiting the source of candidemia: skin or gut? Clin Infect Dis. 2001;33:1959-1967.

182. Pastakia B, Shawker TH, Thaler M, et al. Hepatosplenic candidiasis: wheels within wheels. Radiology. 1988;166:417-421.

183. Thaler M, Pastakia B, Shawker TH, et al. Hepatic candidiasis in cancer patients: the evolving picture of the syndrome. Ann Intern Med. 1988;108:88-100.

184. Edwards JE Jr, Bodey GP, Bowden RA, et al. International Conference for the Development of a Consensus on the Management and Prevention of Severe Candidal Infections. Clin Infect Dis. 1997;25:43-59.

185. Walsh TJ, Whitcomb P, Piscitelli S, et al. Safety, tolerance, and pharmacokinetics of amphotericin B lipid complex in children with hepatosplenic candidiasis. Antimicrob Agents Chemother. 1997;41:1944-1948.

186. Walsh TJ. Invasive pulmonary aspergillosis in patients with neoplastic diseases. Semin Respir Infect. 1990;5:111-122.

187. Gerson SL, Talbot GH, Hurwitz S, et al. Prolonged granulocytopenia: the major risk factor for invasive pulmonary aspergillosis in patients with acute leukemia. Ann Intern Med. 1984;100:345-351.

188. Patterson TF, Kirkpatrick WR, White M, et al. Invasive aspergillosis. Disease spectrum, treatment practices, and outcomes. I3 Aspergillus Study Group. Medicine (Baltimore). 2000;79:250-260.

189. Anaissie E. Opportunistic mycoses in the immunocompromised host: experience at a cancer center and review. Clin Infect Dis. 1992;14 (suppl 1):S43-S53.

190. Albelda SM, Talbot GH, Gerson SL, et al. Pulmonary cavitation and massive hemoptysis in invasive pulmonary aspergillosis: influence of bone marrow recovery in patients with acute leukemia. Am Rev Respir Dis. 1985;131:115-120.

191. Stevens DA, Kan VL, Judson MA, et al. Practice guidelines for diseases caused by *Aspergillus*. Infectious Diseases Society of America. Clin Infect Dis. 2000;30:696-709.

192. Denning DW. Invasive aspergillosis. Clin Infect Dis. 1998;26:781-803.

193. Gerson SL, Talbot GH, Lusk E, et al. Invasive pulmonary aspergillosis in adult acute leukemia: clinical clues to its diagnosis. J Clin Oncol. 1985;3:1109-1116.

194. Drakos PE, Nagler A, Or R, et al. Invasive fungal sinusitis in patients undergoing bone marrow transplantation. Bone Marrow Transplant. 1993;12:203-208.

195. Walsh TJ, Aoki S, Mechinaud F, et al. Effects of preventive, early, and late antifungal chemotherapy with fluconazole in different granulocytopenic models of experimental disseminated candidiasis. J Infect Dis. 1990;161:755-760.

196. Blum U, Windfuhr M, Buitrago-Tellez C, et al. Invasive pulmonary aspergillosis: MRI, CT, and plain radiographic findings and their contribution for early diagnosis. Chest. 1994;106:1156-1161.

197. Leung AN, Gosselin MV, Napper CH, et al. Pulmonary infections after bone marrow transplantation: clinical and radiographic findings. Radiology. 1999;210:699-710.

198. Ashdown BC, Tien RD, Felsberg GJ. Aspergillosis of the brain and paranasal sinuses in immunocompromised patients: CT and MR imaging findings. AJR Am J Roentgenol. 1994;162:155-159.

199. Tomee JF, Mannes GP, van der Bij W, et al. Serodiagnosis and monitoring of *Aspergillus* infections after lung transplantation. Ann Intern Med. 1996;125:197-201.

200. Haynes KA, Latge JP, Rogers TR. Detection of *Aspergillus* antigens associated with invasive infection. J Clin Microbiol. 1990;28:2040-2044.

201. Patterson TF, Miniter P, Patterson JE, et al. *Aspergillus* antigen detection in the diagnosis of invasive aspergillosis. J Infect Dis. 1995;171:1553-1558.

202. Rogers TR, Haynes KA, Barnes RA. Value of antigen detection in predicting invasive pulmonary aspergillosis. Lancet. 1990;336:1210-1213.

203. Rohrlich P, Sarfati J, Mariani P, et al. Prospective sandwich enzyme-linked immunosorbent assay for serum galactomannan: early predictive value and clinical use in invasive aspergillosis. Pediatr Infect Dis J. 1996;15:232-237.

204. Hebart H, Loffler J, Meisner C, et al. Early detection of *Aspergillus* infection after allogeneic stem cell transplantation by polymerase chain reaction screening. J Infect Dis. 2000;181: 1713-1719.

205. Levine SJ. An approach to the diagnosis of pulmonary infections in immunosuppressed patients. Semin Respir Infect. 1992;7: 81-95.

206. Herbrecht R, Denning DW, Patterson TF, et al. Voriconazole versus amphotericin B for primary therapy of invasive aspergillosis. N Engl J Med. 2002;347:408-415.

207. Maertens J, Raad I, Petrikkos G, et al. Efficacy and safety of caspofungin for treatment of invasive aspergillosis in patients refractory to or intolerant of conventional antifungal therapy. Clin Infect Dis. 2004;39:1563-1571.

208. Betts R, Glasmacher A, Maertens J, et al. Efficacy of caspofungin against invasive *Candida* or invasive *Aspergillus* infections in neutropenic patients. Cancer. 2006;106:466-473.

209. Candoni A, Mestroni R, Damiani D, et al. Caspofungin as first-line therapy of pulmonary invasive fungal infections in 32 immunocompromised patients with hematologic malignancies. Eur J Haematol. 2005;75:227-233.

210. Damaj G, Ivanov V, Le Brigand B, et al. Rapid improvement of disseminated aspergillosis with caspofungin/voriconazole combination in an adult leukemic patient. Ann Hematol. 2004;83: 390-393.

211. Marr KA, Boeckh M, Carter RA, et al. Combination antifungal therapy for invasive aspergillosis. Clin Infect Dis. 2004;39: 797-802.

212. Schuster F, Moelter C, Schmid I, et al. Successful antifungal combination therapy with voriconazole and caspofungin. Pediatr Blood Cancer. 2005;44:682-685.

213. Bernhisel-Broadbent J, Camargo EE, Jaffe HS, Lederman HM. Recombinant human interferon-gamma as adjunct therapy for *Aspergillus* infection in a patient with chronic granulomatous disease. J Infect Dis. 1991;163:908-911.

214. Gaviria JM, van Burik JA, Dale DC, et al. Comparison of interferon-gamma, granulocyte colony-stimulating factor, and granulocyte-macrophage colony-stimulating factor for priming leukocyte-mediated hyphal damage of opportunistic fungal pathogens. J Infect Dis. 1999;179:1038-1041.

215. Schwartz S, Behre G, Heinemann V, et al. Aerosolized amphotericin B inhalations as prophylaxis of invasive *Aspergillus* infections during prolonged neutropenia: results of a prospective randomized multicenter trial. Blood. 1999;93:3654-3661.

216. Cornely OA, Maertens J, Winston DJ, et al. Posaconazole vs. fluconazole or itraconazole prophylaxis in patients with neutropenia. N Engl J Med. 2007;356:348-359.

217. Allende M, Pizzo PA, Horowitz M, et al. Pulmonary cryptococcosis presenting as metastases in children with sarcomas. Pediatr Infect Dis J. 1993;12:240-243.

218. Leggiadro RJ, Kline MW, Hughes WT. Extrapulmonary cryptococcosis in children with acquired immunodeficiency syndrome. Pediatr Infect Dis J. 1991;10:658-662.

219. Speed BR, Kaldor J. Rarity of cryptococcal infection in children. Pediatr Infect Dis J. 1997;16:536-537.

220. Saag MS, Graybill RJ, Larsen RA, et al. Practice guidelines for the management of cryptococcal disease. Infectious Diseases Society of America. Clin Infect Dis. 2000;30:710-718.

221. Vartivarian SE, Anaissie EJ, Bodey GP. Emerging fungal pathogens in immunocompromised patients: classification, diagnosis, and management. Clin Infect Dis. 1993;17(suppl 2): S487-S491.

222. Sugar AM. Mucormycosis. Clin Infect Dis. 1992;14(suppl 1): S126-S129.

223. Gateley A, Gander RM, Johnson PC, et al. Herpes simplex virus type 2 meningoencephalitis resistant to acyclovir in a patient with AIDS. J Infect Dis. 1990;161:711-715.

224. Morgan ER, Smalley LA. Varicella in immunocompromised children: incidence of abdominal pain and organ involvement. Am J Dis Child. 1983;137:883-885.

225. Srugo I, Israele V, Wittek AE, et al. Clinical manifestations of varicella-zoster virus infections in human immunodeficiency virus-infected children. Am J Dis Child. 1993;147:742-745.

226. Feldman S, Lott L. Varicella in children with cancer: impact of antiviral therapy and prophylaxis. Pediatrics. 1987;80:465-472.

227. Stemmer SM, Kinsman K, Tellschow S, Jones RB. Fatal noncutaneous visceral infection with varicella-zoster virus in a patient with lymphoma after autologous bone marrow transplantation. Clin Infect Dis. 1993;16:497-499.

228. Manian FA, Kindred M, Fulling KH. Chronic varicella-zoster virus myelitis without cutaneous eruption in a patient with AIDS: report of a fatal case. Clin Infect Dis. 1995;21:986-988.

229. Feldman S, Hughes WT, Kim HY. Herpes zoster in children with cancer. Am J Dis Child. 1973;126:178-184.

230. Prober CG, Kirk LE, Keeney RE. Acyclovir therapy of chickenpox in immunosuppressed children—a collaborative study. J Pediatr. 1982;101:622-625.

231. Jacobson MA, Berger TG, Fikrig S, et al. Acyclovir-resistant varicella zoster virus infection after chronic oral acyclovir therapy in patients with the acquired immunodeficiency syndrome (AIDS). Ann Intern Med. 1990;112:187-191.

232. Cohen JI, Brunell PA, Straus SE, Krause PR. Recent advances in varicella-zoster virus infection. Ann Intern Med. 1999;130: 922-932.

233. LaRussa P, Steinberg S, Gershon AA. Varicella vaccine for immunocompromised children: results of collaborative studies in the United States and Canada. J Infect Dis. 1996;174(suppl 3):S320-S323.

234. Brunell PA, Geiser CF, Novelli V, et al. Varicella-like illness caused by live varicella vaccine in children with acute lymphocytic leukemia. Pediatrics. 1987;79:922-927.

235. Wise RP, Salive ME, Braun MM, et al. Postlicensure safety surveillance for varicella vaccine. JAMA. 2000;284:1271-1279.

236. Skinhoj P. Herpesvirus infections in the immunocompromised patient. Scand J Infect Dis Suppl. 1985;47:121-127.

237. Zaia JA, Gallez-Hawkins GM, Tegtmeier BR, et al. Late cytomegalovirus disease in marrow transplantation is predicted by virus load in plasma. J Infect Dis. 1997;176:782-785.

238. Schmidt GM, Horak DA, Niland JC, et al. A randomized, controlled trial of prophylactic ganciclovir for cytomegalovirus pulmonary infection in recipients of allogeneic bone marrow transplants; The City of Hope-Stanford-Syntex CMV Study Group. N Engl J Med. 1991;324:1005-1011.

239. Goodrich JM, Boeckh M, Bowden R. Strategies for the prevention of cytomegalovirus disease after marrow transplantation. Clin Infect Dis. 1994;19:287-298.

240. Meyers JD, Reed EC, Shepp DH, et al. Acyclovir for prevention of cytomegalovirus infection and disease after allogeneic marrow transplantation. N Engl J Med. 1988;318:70-75.

241. Hanto DW, Frizzera G, Purtilo DT, et al. Clinical spectrum of lymphoproliferative disorders in renal transplant recipients and evidence for the role of Epstein-Barr virus. Cancer Res. 1981;41:4253-4261.

242. Sokal EM, Caragiozoglou T, Lamy M, et al. Epstein-Barr virus serology and Epstein-Barr virus-associated lymphoproliferative disorders in pediatric liver transplant recipients. Transplantation. 1993;56:1394-1398.

243. Reece ER, Gartner JG, Seemayer TA, et al. Epstein-Barr virus in a malignant lymphoproliferative disorder of B cells occurring after thymic epithelial transplantation for combined immunodeficiency. Cancer Res. 1981;41:4243-4247.

244. Cen H, Williams PA, McWilliams HP, et al. Evidence for restricted Epstein-Barr virus latent gene expression and anti-EBNA antibody response in solid organ transplant recipients with posttransplant lymphoproliferative disorders. Blood. 1993; 81:1393-1403.

245. Swinnen LJ, Costanzo-Nordin MR, Fisher SG, et al. Increased incidence of lymphoproliferative disorder after immunosuppression with the monoclonal antibody OKT3 in cardiac-transplant recipients. N Engl J Med. 1990;323:1723-1728.

246. Starzl TE, Nalesnik MA, Porter KA, et al. Reversibility of lymphomas and lymphoproliferative lesions developing under cyclosporin-steroid therapy. Lancet. 1984;1:583-587.

247. Yao QY, Ogan P, Rowe M, et al. Epstein-Barr virus-infected B cells persist in the circulation of acyclovir-treated virus carriers. Int J Cancer. 1989;43:67-71.

248. Davis CL, Wood BL, Sabath DE, et al. Interferon-alpha treatment of posttransplant lymphoproliferative disorder in recipients of solid organ transplants. Transplantation. 1998;66:1770-1779.

249. O'Brien S, Bernert RA, Logan JL, Lien YH. Remission of post-transplant lymphoproliferative disorder after interferon alfa therapy. J Am Soc Nephrol. 1997;8:1483-1489.

250. Abedi MR, Linde A, Christensson B, et al. Preventive effect of IgG from EBV-seropositive donors on the development of human lympho-proliferative disease in SCID mice. Int J Cancer. 1997; 71:624-629.

251. Nadal D, Guzman J, Frohlich S, Braun DG. Human immunoglobulin preparations suppress the occurrence of Epstein-Barr virus-associated lymphoproliferation. Exp Hematol. 1997;25: 223-231.

252. Faye A, Van Den Abeele T, Peuchmaur M, et al. Anti-CD20 monoclonal antibody for post-transplant lymphoproliferative disorders. Lancet. 1998;352:1285.

253. Cook RC, Connors JM, Gascoyne RD, et al. Treatment of post-transplant lymphoproliferative disease with rituximab monoclonal antibody after lung transplantation. Lancet. 1999;354:1698-1699.

254. Niedermeyer J, Hoffmeyer F, Hertenstein B, et al. Treatment of lympho-proliferative disease with rituximab. Lancet. 2000;355: 499.

255. Oertel SH, Anagnostopoulos I, Bechstein WO, et al. Treatment of posttransplant lymphoproliferative disorder with the anti-CD20 monoclonal antibody rituximab alone in an adult after liver transplantation: a new drug in therapy of patients with posttransplant lymphoproliferative disorder after solid organ transplantation? Transplantation. 2000;69:430-432.

256. Rooney CM, Smith CA, Ng CY, et al. Use of gene-modified virus-specific T lymphocytes to control Epstein-Barr-virus-related lymphoproliferation. Lancet. 1995;345:9-13.

257. Khanna R, Bell S, Sherritt M, et al. Activation and adoptive transfer of Epstein-Barr virus-specific cytotoxic T cells in solid organ transplant patients with posttransplant lymphoproliferative disease. Proc Natl Acad Sci U S A. 1999;96:10391-10396.

258. Choquet S, Leblond V, Herbrecht R, et al. Efficacy and safety of rituximab in B-cell post-transplantation lymphoproliferative disorders: results of a prospective multicenter phase 2 study. Blood. 2006;107:3053-3057.

259. Robinson WS. Human herpesvirus 6. Curr Clin Top Infect Dis. 1994;14:159-169.

260. Drobyski WR, Dunne WM, Burd EM, et al. Human herpesvirus-6 (HHV-6) infection in allogeneic bone marrow transplant recipients: evidence of a marrow-suppressive role for HHV-6 in vivo. J Infect Dis. 1993;167:735-739.

261. Singh N, Carrigan DR, Gayowski T, Marino IR. Human herpesvirus-6 infection in liver transplant recipients: documentation of pathogenicity. Transplantation. 1997;64:674-678.

262. Cone RW, Hackman RC, Huang ML, et al. Human herpesvirus 6 in lung tissue from patients with pneumonitis after bone marrow transplantation. N Engl J Med. 1993;329:156-161.

263. Dockrell DH, Smith TF, Paya CV. Human herpesvirus 6. Mayo Clin Proc. 1999;74:163-170.

264. Singh N, Carrigan DR. Human herpesvirus-6 in transplantation: an emerging pathogen. Ann Intern Med. 1996;124:1065-1071.

265. Kovacs JA. Efficacy of atovaquone in treatment of toxoplasmosis in patients with AIDS. The NIAID-Clinical Center Intramural AIDS Program. Lancet. 1992;340:637-638.

266. Leibovitz E, Rigaud M, Pollack H, et al. *Pneumocystis carinii* pneumonia in infants infected with the human immunodeficiency virus with more than 450 CD4 T lymphocytes per cubic millimeter. N Engl J Med. 1990;323:531-533.

267. Esolen LM, Fasano MB, Flynn J, et al. *Pneumocystis carinii* osteomyelitis in a patient with common variable immunodeficiency. N Engl J Med. 1992;326:999-1001.

268. Raviglione MC. Extrapulmonary pneumocystosis: the first 50 cases. Rev Infect Dis. 1990;12:1127-1138.

269. Ognibene FP, Gill VJ, Pizzo PA, et al. Induced sputum to diagnose *Pneumocystis carinii* pneumonia in immunosuppressed pediatric patients. J Pediatr. 1989;115:430-433.

270. Browne MJ, Potter D, Gress J, et al. A randomized trial of open lung biopsy versus empiric antimicrobial therapy in cancer patients with diffuse pulmonary infiltrates. J Clin Oncol. 1990;8: 222-229.

271. Bozzette SA, Sattler FR, Chiu J, et al. A controlled trial of early adjunctive treatment with corticosteroids for *Pneumocystis carinii* pneumonia in the acquired immunodeficiency syndrome. California Collaborative Treatment Group. N Engl J Med. 1990;323: 1451-1457.

272. El-Sadr WM, Murphy RL, Yurik TM, et al. Atovaquone compared with dapsone for the prevention of *Pneumocystis carinii* pneumonia in patients with HIV infection who cannot tolerate trimethoprim, sulfonamides, or both. Community Program for Clinical Research on AIDS and the AIDS Clinical Trials Group. N Engl J Med. 1998;339:1889-1895.

273. Chan C, Montaner J, Lefebvre EA, et al. Atovaquone suspension compared with aerosolized pentamidine for prevention of *Pneumocystis carinii* pneumonia in human immunodeficiency virus-infected subjects intolerant of trimethoprim or sulfonamides. J Infect Dis. 1999;180:369-376.

274. Luft BJ, Hafner R, Korzun AH, et al. Toxoplasmic encephalitis in patients with the acquired immunodeficiency syndrome. Members of the ACTG 077p/ANRS 009 Study Team. N Engl J Med. 1993;329:995-1000.

275. Dannemann B, McCutchan JA, Israelski D, et al. Treatment of toxoplasmic encephalitis in patients with AIDS: a randomized trial comparing pyrimethamine plus clindamycin to pyrimethamine plus sulfadiazine. The California Collaborative Treatment Group. Ann Intern Med. 1992;116:33-43.

276. American Academy of Pediatrics. Committee on Infectious Diseases. Varicella vaccine update. Pediatrics. 2000;105:136-141.

277. American Academy of Pediatrics. Committee on Infectious Diseases. Red book: report of the Committee on Infectious Diseases. Elk Grove Village, IL, American Academy of Pediatrics, 2000, v.

28 Oncologic Emergencies

Elizabeth Mullen, Jennifer Whangbo, and Lynda M. Vrooman

Expert management of emergent situations is crucial in the practice of pediatric oncology. Although many emergencies are common across the spectrum of general pediatric patients, such as seizure, respiratory arrest, and electrolyte abnormalities, others stem from the underlying cancer or cancer therapy and are unique to this population of patients. Emergencies related to space-occupying lesions, metabolic derangements caused by breakdown of tumor cells, and disruption of the hematopoietic system by invasion of cancer cells all in some way relate to the abnormal presence of cancer cells disrupting the normal function of a cell or organ. This disruption can be rapidly progressive and life-threatening—for example, as in cases of T-cell lymphoblastic leukemia presenting with mediastinal mass and respiratory compromise. The treatments directed toward cancers also carry significant toxicities and can result in uniquely emergent complications. Many chemotherapy agents impart a state of significant immunocompromise and put patients at risk for unusual or opportunistic infections as well as fulminant presentations of infection with more common organisms. All chemotherapy drugs carry extensive profiles of possible side effects; errors of administration or dosage can magnify toxicity and any available therapeutic interventions must be administered immediately. Appropriate management of an emergent pediatric oncologic situation requires a clear understanding of the specific underlying disease process and of the effects and consequences of cancer-directed therapies.

Symptoms in children presenting with new diagnoses of cancer or receiving cancer treatment are myriad. Therefore, recognition of an emergency is not always straightforward, particularly in the young pediatric population, in whom obtaining an accurate history can be challenging. A high level of vigilance should be maintained by the clinician for the presentation of potentially life-threatening situations. A child with cough and mild respiratory distress is most likely to have a viral infection; however, these symptoms might be consistent with a child presenting with a marked mediastinal mass, developing leukostasis syndrome, or the onset of *Pneumocystis* pneumonia. A complaint of lower back pain in a child may relate to new physical activity or could represent developing spinal cord compression from tumor. The pediatric oncologist needs to be familiar with all pediatric oncologic emergent situations to evaluate and manage these high-risk patients appropriately. Rapid and appropriate triage of patient complaints is critical, because overlooked diagnoses, as well as inaction or inappropriate action, can have severe consequences.

Grouping of some of the emergent pediatric oncologic conditions into disease- and treatment-related events is presented in Box 28-1. There is clear overlap among the conditions listed; for example, tumor lysis syndrome can occur on presentation with a new diagnosis of leukemia or high-grade lymphoma, but can be markedly worsened by initiation of chemotherapy. Similarly, superior vena cava syndrome can result from a new or recurrent presence of a mass lesion, or as a complication of an indwelling catheter placed to deliver antineoplastic therapy. This chapter will focus discussion on several of the emergent situations unique to the pediatric oncology patient, with review of available data and overviews of current management strategies. The topics addressed in the chapter are tumor lysis syndrome, hyperleukocytosis and leukostasis, anterior mediastinal mass, spinal cord compression, and selected chemotherapy toxicities. Several topics unique to the pediatric oncology patient are covered elsewhere in this text and will not be readdressed in this chapter (e.g., management of fever and neutropenia, transfusion medicine, and pain management). Situations that can occur in the pediatric oncology patient, but are not unique to this population, such as seizure, cerebral vascular injury, disseminated intravascular coagulation, and pancreatitis, will not be discussed here.

Box 28-1	**Commonly Encountered Pediatric Oncologic Emergencies**

DISEASE-RELATED

Tumor lysis syndrome
Anterior mediastinal mass
Spinal cord compression
Leukocytosis and leukostasis
Uncal herniation
Disseminated intravascular coagulation
Hypercalcemia

TREATMENT-RELATED

Fever and neutropenia, sepsis
Cerebrovascular accident, clot, stroke
Typhlitis
Pancreatitis
Vesicant infiltration
Methotrexate toxicity
All *trans*-retinoic acid (ATRA) syndrome
Veno-occlusive disease

Although optimal management of many of these emergent situations has been difficult to study, given the relatively small number of patients presenting to each institution, a literature is evolving on many of these topics. Many institutions have established clinical practice guidelines (CPGs) to help manage the most common pediatric oncologic emergencies. CPGs provide uniform standards for management but must allow for adaptations for each specific clinical scenario. Uniform use of clinical guidelines with collection and analysis of outcomes has the potential to guide improvements in clinical practice.

TUMOR LYSIS SYNDROME

Tumor lysis syndrome is the most commonly encountered pediatric oncologic emergency. Diagnosis and treatment strategies have been rapidly evolving over the last decade. Morbidity and mortality have improved as the entity is now recognized and treated earlier in presentation. New therapeutic interventions have become available and are more widely used.

Overview

Following the incorporation of cytotoxic chemotherapy into the treatment of hematologic malignancies and solid tumors, there were recurrent observations of severe metabolic abnormalities associated with the onset of therapy.[1,2] The consistent occurrence of these metabolic and electrolyte imbalances, particularly in the setting of lymphoma and leukemia, eventually became recognized as tumor lysis syndrome (TLS). TLS describes the metabolic derangements that occur as a result of spontaneous or treatment-related breakdown of tumor cells. The release of intracellular contents from the tumor cells into the bloodstream leads to the characteristic triad of hyperuricemia, hyperkalemia, and hyperphosphatemia. TLS is most commonly associated with initiation of therapy for cancers with massive tumor burden or high proliferative rates, such as acute lymphoblastic leukemia and Burkitt's lymphoma. Predictors of TLS include the presence of bulky disease, adenopathy,

PURINE CATABOLISM

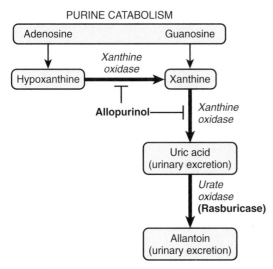

FIGURE 28-1. Pathophysiology of hyperuricemia in tumor lysis syndrome. Uric acid is a breakdown product of purine nucleotide catabolism. The current pharmacologic strategies for the management of hyperuricemia are allopurinol and rasburicase.

hepatosplenomegaly, and high leukocyte count. Additional risk factors for developing severe TLS include increased lactate dehydrogenase (LDH), uric acid, creatinine, and decreased urine output.[3-5] TLS can have high morbidity and mortality, with possible rapid progression to multiorgan failure. Thus, the prompt identification of patients at risk for this oncologic emergency and the institution of preventive measures are critical. Although the risk of developing TLS is highest at 12 to 72 hours after initiating chemotherapy, symptoms can also precede initiation of therapy or occur as long as 7 days later. The main principles of TLS prevention and treatment include hydration and diuresis, careful monitoring of electrolyte abnormalities, and management of hyperuricemia with allopurinol or rasburicase. In this section, we will discuss the pathophysiology, incidence, and recent advances in the management of TLS.

Pathophysiology

Although TLS can occur spontaneously prior to the administration of chemotherapy, it is most commonly observed following the initiation of therapy. In tumors with a high proliferative rate, large tumor burden, and high chemosensitivity, the exposure of the tumor cells to cytotoxic chemotherapy leads to massive cell lysis, with the release of intracellular anions, cations, and breakdown products of nucleic acids and proteins into the bloodstream. This rapid efflux of intracellular contents can exceed the renal capacity for clearance and consequently can lead to the metabolic derangements and electrolyte imbalances observed in TLS. Hyperuricemia is the most common finding in TLS; it results from the release of intracellular nucleic acids and the subsequent catabolism of the purine nucleotides, adenosine and guanosine. Uric acid, the final product of both endogenous and dietary purine nucleotide catabolism, is normally generated in the liver by oxidation of xanthine to uric acid by xanthine oxidase (Fig. 28-1). Uric acid is a weak acid, with a pK_a of 5.4 to 5.7. At normal concentrations and at physiologic pH, 98% of uric acid is in the ionized form as urate, which is soluble in urine.[6] However, when uric acid is present in high concentrations in acidic urine, it can crystallize in the

renal parenchyma, distal tubules, and collecting ducts, leading to intraluminal tubular obstruction and oliguria.

Hyperkalemia poses the greatest immediate threat of mortality because the rapid rise in serum potassium can result in severe arrhythmia and death. This life-threatening consequence of TLS is caused in part by the kidney's inability to excrete the massive quantities of intracellular potassium released from dying tumor cells. The kidney's inability to handle the excessive load of potassium can be amplified by renal dysfunction caused by precipitants such as uric acid. Hyperkalemia in the setting of TLS can be further exacerbated by concurrent metabolic acidosis or iatrogenic administration of potassium with intravenous fluids.

Hyperphosphatemia results from the rapid release of intracellular phosphorus from tumor cells, which can contain three to four times the amount of phosphorus in normal cells.[7,8] The development of hyperphosphatemia can also worsen in the setting of concurrent acute renal insufficiency secondary to uric acid precipitation. In TLS, the renal tubular capacity to reabsorb phosphorus can be exceeded and lead to hyperphosphaturia. A cyclic process commences, in which the acute hyperphosphatemia and hyperphosphaturia can then lead to acute nephrocalcinosis and renal failure via precipitation of calcium phosphate crystals, further impairing the renal tubular reabsorption of phosphorus. The normal calcium × phosphorus product ranges between 30 and 55 mg^2/dL^2. When this exceeds 70 mg^2/dL^2, there is a significant risk of calcium phosphate deposition in the kidney and other tissues.[9] Metastatic calcification caused by calcium phosphate crystals in other soft tissues is rarely seen in TLS, but has been described.[10] In addition, the precipitation of calcium phosphate can lead secondarily to asymptomatic or symptomatic hypocalcemia.

Incidence

The highest incidence of TLS occurs in acute lymphoblastic leukemia and high-grade non-Hodgkin's lymphoma (NHL). A retrospective study of 102 patients with high-grade NHL has revealed the incidence of TLS to be 42% based on laboratory evidence, although only 6% of the patients had clinically significant TLS.[11] Similarly, a pan-European retrospective chart review has reported TLS in 5.2% and 6.1% of patients with acute lymphoblastic leukemia and NHL, respectively.[12] This study also demonstrated a high incidence of mortality in those patients with clinical TLS. Of the patients with TLS in this study, 17.5% died from TLS-related causes.

The incidence of TLS appears to be similar in the pediatric population. A retrospective study of 1192 pediatric patients with any form of NHL has identified 63 patients (5.3%) with clinically significant TLS.[13] Among these 63 patients, two patients (3.2%) died within 48 hours of therapy because of electrolyte imbalances. However, another retrospective pediatric study has indicated that the incidence of TLS is significantly higher in patients with B-cell acute lymphoblastic leukemia or Burkitt's lymphoma stage III or IV, with LDH ≥ 500 U/L. Of the 218 patients who met these criteria initially (prior to the prophylactic use of urate oxidase), 35 (16.1%) developed TLS and 20 (9.2%) became anuric.[14]

Other hematologic malignancies that have been less commonly associated with TLS include acute myeloid leukemia, chronic lymphocytic leukemia, and multiple myeloma. Only isolated case reports of TLS have been described in other hematologic malignancies, such as chronic myeloid leukemia in blast crisis, myeloproliferative disorders and Hodgkin's disease. TLS is also uncommon in solid tumors, which generally have a longer doubling time and slow response to chemotherapy in comparison to lymphoproliferative malignancies. However,

TLS can be seen in solid tumors that are highly chemosensitive or that have high tumor burden, as in bulky, metastatic disease or in tumors that present with renal compromise. In the context of newly diagnosed solid tumors, renal compromise may occur from mass effect and compression. A literature review has identified 45 reported cases of TLS in solid tumors from 1977 to 2002.[15] Most of these cases occurred in tumors with a high response rate to cytotoxic therapy, such as small cell lung carcinoma, germ cell tumors, and breast carcinoma. Among the 45 reported cases, 16 (35.5%) died as a result of TLS. Risk factors for the development of TLS in solid tumors were similar to those in hematologic malignancies—increased LDH, hyperuricemia, and pretreatment renal impairment. However, the mortality rate caused by complications from TLS in these patients with solid tumors was higher than reported mortality rates in those with hematologic malignancies. This may be the result of better implementation of prophylactic measures in patients with hematologic malignancies resulting from a greater awareness of TLS in this population.

Diagnosis

As noted, TLS should be anticipated in patients presenting with large tumor burden and concurrent laboratory abnormalities. Although there are many general criteria for TLS, a uniform, widely accepted definition for TLS is lacking. A standardized definition would enable a more exact determination of TLS incidence and would also improve the ability to evaluate and compare therapies for the prevention of TLS. Two classification systems for TLS have been developed, but have not yet been incorporated into common clinical practice, the Hande-Garrow (Boxes 28-2 and 28-3) in 1993 and Cairo-Bishop in 2004. The Hande-Garrow classification system makes a distinction between laboratory and clinical TLS based on the observation that only a fraction of patients with TLS by laboratory criteria develop clinically significant TLS.[11] Laboratory TLS (LTLS) designates patients who have laboratory evidence of metabolic changes secondary to tumor cell breakdown, but who do not require any therapeutic intervention. Patients with any of the following metabolic changes occurring within the first 4 days of treatment are defined as having LTLS: (1) a 25% increase over pretreatment values in serum phosphate, potassium, uric acid, or urea nitrogen levels; or (2) a 25% decline in the serum calcium level. Clinical TLS (CTLS) is designated in any patient with LTLS who also experiences one of the following: (1) a rise in the serum creatinine level greater than 2.5 mg/dL; (2) a serum potassium level greater than 6.0 mmol/L; (3) a decline in the serum calcium to less than 6 mg/dL; (4) the development of a life-threatening arrhythmia; or sudden death. In practice, this classification system has several limitations. First, in requiring a 25% increase in the baseline laboratory value, the definition of laboratory TLS does not account for patients who have preexisting abnormal laboratory values at presentation. In addition, the definition requires that the laboratory changes occur within 4 days of starting therapy, which excludes patients with clinical evidence of TLS at presentation or patients who develop TLS beyond 4 days of therapy.

The Cairo-Bishop classification system is a modified version of the Hande-Garrow system that aims to be more clinically relevant (Table 28-1).[16] For example, the definition of LTLS has been extended to include a window of 3 days before and 7 days after the initiation of therapy. Similar to the Hande-Garrow system, the definition of CTLS requires the presence of LTLS, plus one or more of the three most significant clinical complications associated with TLS: renal insufficiency, cardiac arrhythmias or sudden death, and seizures. Cairo and Bishop also introduced a grading system for TLS that incorporates their definitions of no TLS, laboratory TLS, and clinical TLS. This grading system is currently being evaluated as part of a Children's Oncology Group (COG) study of chemoimmunotherapy and rasburicase in newly diagnosed non-Hodgkin's lymphoma (COG ANHL01P1). One of the specific aims of this study is to determine the incidences of TLS, consequent renal complications, and the requirement for assisted renal support (dialysis, hemofiltration) during the reduction phase and first induction phase of therapy in children with newly diagnosed advanced-stage leukemia or lymphoma.

Clinical Manifestations and Treatment

Clinical manifestations of acute TLS include nausea, anorexia, cardiac arrhythmias, seizures, muscle cramps, tetany, oliguria or anuria, and alterations in consciousness. These symptoms primarily result from the electrolyte disturbances seen in TLS (see earlier). The most important objectives for the successful management of acute TLS are the prompt identification of patients at high risk for developing TLS and aggressive institution of appropriate prophylactic measures to prevent and/or reduce the severity of the clinical manifestations of acute TLS (Box 28-4). Initial studies that can predict TLS and guide preventive management include serum electrolyte, calcium, phosphate, blood urea nitrogen, creatinine, and uric acid levels. This panel of laboratory assessments should be done promptly for any patient presenting with new diagnosis of malignancy. The main preventive measures are hydration and optimization of urine output, along with prevention of uric acid synthesis by allopurinol or rasburicase. In addition to the specific treatment recommendations discussed later, patients at risk for TLS should be carefully observed on cardiovascular and respiratory monitors. Frequent vital signs and strict fluid assessments including intake and output should be recorded. Laboratory tests should be performed at minimum every 6 to 8 hours initially and the results evaluated immediately (see Box 28-1).

Box 28-2	**Hande-Garrow Definition of Laboratory Tumor Lysis Syndrome (LTLS)***

25% increase over pretreatment values in serum phosphate, potassium, uric acid, or urea nitrogen

or

25% decline in serum calcium

---

*Any two of the above metabolic changes must occur within 4 days of treatment.

Box 28-3	**Hande-Garrow Definition of Clinical Tumor Lysis Syndrome (CTLS)***

Rise in serum creatinine >2.5 mg/dL
Serum potassium level >6.0 mmol/L
Decline in serum calcium to <6 mg/dL
Development of life-threatening arrhythmia or death

---

*CLTS is defined as the presence of laboratory tumor lysis syndrome (LTLS) and any one of the above-mentioned criteria.

TABLE 28-1		Cairo-Bishop Grading Classification of Tumor Lysis Syndrome		
Grade	LTLS	Creatinine Level	Cardiac Arrhythmia	Seizure
0	–	≤1.5 × ULN	None	None
I	+	1.5 × ULN	Intervention not indicated	None
II	+	>1.5-3.0 × ULN	Nonurgent medical intervention indicated	One brief generalized seizure, seizure(s) well controlled by anticonvulsants, infrequent focal motor seizures not interfering with ADLs
III	+	>3.0-6.0 × ULN	Symptomatic and incompletely controlled medically or controlled with device (e.g., defibrillator)	Seizure in which consciousness is altered, poorly controlled seizure disorder, breakthrough generalized seizures despite medical intervention
IV	+	>6.0 × ULN	Life-threatening (e.g., arrhythmia associated with CHF, hypotension, syncope, shock)	Seizures of any type that are prolonged, repetitive, or difficult to control (e.g., status epilepticus, intractable epilepsy)
V	+	Death	Death	Death

ADLs, activities of daily living; CHF, congestive heart failure; LTLS, laboratory tumor lysis syndrome; ULN, upper limit of normal.
Adapted from Cairo MS, Bishop M. Tumour lysis syndrome: new therapeutic strategies and classification. Br J Haematol. 2004;127:3-11.

Box 28-4 | Management of Patients at Risk for Tumor Lysis Syndrome

HYDRATION

D_5 (dextrose 5%) in half-normal saline with 40 mEq/L $NaHCO_3$ (without K+)
Recommended rate: 2 times maintenance (125 mL/m²/hr)

ALKALINIZATION

Modify $NaHCO_3$ as needed to maintain urine pH 7.0-8.0
Stop $NaHCO_3$ if serum bicarbonate level ≥ 30 mEq/L and/or urine pH > 8.0

DIURESIS

Maintain urine output at >100 mL/m²/hr and urine specific gravity at <1.010
Consider furosemide (0.5-1.0 mg/kg) or mannitol (0.5 g/kg) for low urine output in absence of hypovolemia

URIC ACID REDUCTION

Start allopurinol or urate oxidase (rasburicase):
Allopurinol: PO, 100 mg/ m² three times daily, or 10 mg/kg/day divided in three doses
Rasburicase: IV, 0.2 mg/kg once daily for up to 5 days
    Indicated when serum creatinine is >1.5 times upper limit or normal, or when uric acid > 7.0 mg/dL
    Contraindicated in glucose-6-phosphate deficiency patients
    Discontinue allopurinol if using rasburicase
    No bicarbonate necessary in IV fluid

METABOLIC ABNORMALITIES

Monitor serum electrolytes every 4 to 8 hr

HYPERKALEMIA

Moderate (≥6.0 mmol/L)
    Avoid IV and oral potassium
    Electrocardiogram and cardiorespiratory monitor
    Kayexalate (1 g/kg orally with 25% sorbitol every 6 hours)
Severe (>7.0 mmol/L and/or symptomatic)—same as above, plus:
    Albuterol nebulization treatment
    Insulin (0.1 units/kg) with concurrent 25% dextrose (2 mL/kg)
    Calcium gluconate (100-200 mg/kg)
    Dialysis

HYPERPHOSPHATEMIA

Moderate (≥5.0 mg/dL)—aluminum hydroxide (15-30 mL PO, every 6 hr)
Severe (with symptomatic hypocalcemia)—dialysis, continuous venovenous hemofiltration (CVVH), continuous venoarterial hemofiltration (CVAH)

HYPOCALCEMIA

Asymptomatic—no therapy
Symptomatic—calcium gluconate (50-100 mg/kg/dose)

Fluids and Alkalinization

Unless the patient presents with signs of acute renal failure or oliguria, aggressive hydration is the most important intervention. Intravenous fluids should be administered at a rate of 3000 mL/m²/day and brisk urine output should be maintained (more than 100 mL/m²/hr) with a urine specific gravity goal ≤ 1.010. This increased hydration and increase in urine flow promotes urinary excretion of uric acid and phosphate by enhancing renal blood flow and glomerular filtration. Potassium, calcium, and phosphate should not be added to initial hydration fluids to avoid iatrogenic aggravation of hyperkale-

mia, hyperphosphatemia, or calcium phosphate precipitation. If urine output remains low despite aggressive hydration (usually caused by third spacing), diuretics may be used as long as there is no evidence of acute obstructive uropathy and/or hypovolemia. Commonly used diuretics are mannitol (0.5 g/kg) or furosemide (0.5 to 1.0 mg/kg).

Urine alkalinization remains controversial, although historically it has been a general recommendation for prevention and treatment of TLS. An alkaline urine (urine pH ≥6.5) promotes urinary excretion of urate with maximal solubility of urate occurring at a pH of 7.5.[17] However, the solubility of its precursors, xanthine and hypoxanthine, significantly decreases at pH ≥ 6.5. Thus, excessive systemic and urinary alkalinization may lead to metabolic alkalosis and obstructive uropathies from xanthine and hypoxanthine crystallization. In addition, alkalinization of urine favors precipitation of calcium phosphate crystals in the renal tubules, a risk that can be further exacerbated by concomitant hyperphosphatemia. Metabolic alkalosis can also worsen the neurologic manifestations of hypocalcemia. Thus, sodium bicarbonate should be used judiciously, with checks of urine pH with every void. Its use should be discontinued once serum uric acid normalizes or its dose should be decreased for urine pH > 8.

Hyperkalemia

In the setting of TLS, hyperkalemia results from the massive efflux of intracellular potassium from dying tumor cells. Clinical manifestations include neuromuscular signs and symptoms such as muscle weakness, cramps, and paresthesias. Cardiac manifestations may include peaked T-waves on an electrocardiogram, malignant arrhythmias, and conduction disturbances. Hyperkalemia is usually defined by a serum potassium level ≥ 6.0 mmol/L. However, in the clinical setting of ongoing tumor lysis, a serum potassium level > 5.0 mmol/L and/or a trend of increasing values also merit intervention. Treatment of hyperkalemia is based on three approaches—driving extracellular potassium into cells, removing excess potassium from the body, and antagonizing the membrane effects of potassium. In asymptomatic patients, it is reasonable to begin simply with increased hydration with alkalinized fluids and diuresis with furosemide. The treatment of choice after alkalinization and optimization of urine output often is a potassium-binding cation exchange resin, sodium polystyrene sulfonate (1 g/kg/dose orally every 6 hours). This resin can also be given as a retention enema, but oral administration is more efficacious. Each gram of resin may bind as much as 1 mEq of potassium and release 1 to 2 mEq of sodium. For symptomatic patients, more rapidly acting treatments are required such as insulin and β_2-adrenergic agonists, which drive potassium into cells by enhancing the activity of the Na^+,K^+-ATPase pump in skeletal muscle. Insulin is usually given as a bolus (0.1 unit/kg) with concurrent glucose infusion (25% dextrose, 2 mL/kg). Commonly used β_2-adrenergic agonists in the treatment of hyperkalemia are albuterol nebulizer treatments and intravenous epinephrine. Interventions commonly used in the fluid management of TLS, such as alkalinization and diuretics, can also help in the reduction of serum potassium. The increase in systemic pH with sodium bicarbonate results in hydrogen ion release from the cells as part of the buffering reaction; this change results in the movement of potassium into the cells to maintain electroneutrality. Loop and thiazide diuretics can lead to a transient lowering of serum potassium. Calcium directly antagonizes the inactivation of sodium channels and decreased membrane excitability caused by hyperkalemia. Thus, calcium gluconate (100 to 200 mg/kg) can be given to stabilize myocardial conduction in cases of severe hyperkalemia or the presence of electrocardiographic abnormalities. Because concomitant hyperphosphatemia and alkalinization in the setting of TLS can increase the risk of calcium phosphate or calcium carbonate precipitation, calcium infusions should be given only when absolutely necessary. Finally, dialysis can be used if the conservative measures listed earlier are ineffective, or if the hyperkalemia is severe.

Hyperphosphatemia

Clinical manifestations of severe hyperphosphatemia include nausea, vomiting, diarrhea, lethargy, and seizures. Physiologically, hyperphosphatemia increases the risk of tissue precipitation of calcium phosphate, which can subsequently lead to intrarenal calcification, acute obstructive uropathy, or symptomatic hypocalcemia. Hyperphosphatemia is usually defined by a phosphorus level ≥ 5.0 mg/dL in children. Initial treatment for significant hyperphosphatemia consists of administration of oral forms of phosphate binders, such as aluminum hydroxide at a dosage of 50 to 150 mg/kg/day divided into equal doses every 6 hours. Acute severe hyperphosphatemia with symptomatic hypocalcemia can be life-threatening. However, given the real risk of worsening precipitation of calcium phosphate complexes, patients with hyperphosphatemia should not receive calcium infusions unless clinically symptomatic of hypocalcemia. Patients with impaired renal function may require more aggressive therapy, such as peritoneal dialysis, hemodialysis, or continuous venovenous hemofiltration (CVVH). Of these modalities, hemodialysis appears to be the most efficacious at clearing phosphorus.[18]

Hypocalcemia

During acute TLS, hypocalcemia commonly occurs because of precipitation of calcium phosphate, which in turn is a consequence of hyperphosphatemia. Many patients develop symptoms when their serum ionized calcium concentration is ≤0.7 mmol/L or their serum total calcium concentration is ≤7 mg/dL. Muscular manifestations of hypocalcemia include muscle cramps and spasms, paresthesias, and tetany. Cardiac abnormalities include ventricular arrhythmias, heart block, and hypotension. Neurologic complications include confusion, delirium, and seizures. Treatment of asymptomatic hypocalcemia is generally not recommended, particularly in the setting of hyperphosphatemia. In patients with severe hypocalcemia, intravenous calcium gluconate (50 to 100 mg/kg/dose) may be administered to correct marked or life-threatening clinical symptoms. However, this may increase the risk of calcium phosphate deposition.

Hyperuricemia

Hyperuricemia is defined as serum uric acid ≥ 8.0 mg/dL or a 25% increase from baseline 3 days before or 7 days after the initiation of chemotherapy. The major route of urate clearance is through the proximal renal tubule, and thus hyperuricemia develops when the excretory capacity of the renal tubule is exceeded. In combination with an acidic pH, hyperuricemia can lead to the formation of uric acid crystals in the renal tubule, resulting in intraluminal renal tubular obstruction and the development of acute renal dysfunction. The current pharmacologic strategies for the management of hyperuricemia are allopurinol and rasburicase.

Allopurinol was first approved for clinical use by the U.S. Food and Drug Administration (FDA) in 1966 to treat patients with gout.[19] An isomer of hypoxanthine, allopurinol is rapidly converted in vivo to oxypurinol, which functions as a competitive inhibitor of xanthine oxidase. This irreversible inhibition of xanthine oxidase prevents the metabolism of xanthine and hypoxanthine to uric acid (see Fig. 28-1). In 1965, one of the first studies to examine the use of allopurinol in TLS reported that 15 patients with leukemia or lymphoma had lowering of serum and urine uric acid levels following daily administration of allopurinol during the initiation of therapy.[20] A similar study was published in 1966, in which 33 patients with chronic leukemia, acute leukemia, or lymphoma had a dose-related reduction in uric acid after treatment with allopurinol.[21] It has since formed the backbone of both TLS prevention and treatment.

Allopurinol is available in two preparations, oral (PO) and IV, which have similar efficacies. However, the IV formulation is considerably more costly and should be reserved for patients who are unable to take oral drugs. Allopurinol is administered at a dosage of 100 mg/m^2 every 8 hours PO (maximum, 800 mg/day) or 200 to 400 mg/m^2/day in one to three divided doses IV (maximum, 600 mg/day). A significant limitation of allopurinol is that it cannot reduce uric acid produced prior to its initiation. Patients with hyperuricemia at presentation will not have a reduction in uric acid levels for 2 to 3 days after the initiation of allopurinol because the removal of existing uric acid is dependent on renal clearance.[22] Another concern is that treatment with allopurinol can lead to increased levels of the uric acid precursors hypoxanthine and xanthine via inhibition of xanthine oxidase. Because xanthine is less soluble than uric acid, it is possible that high levels of xanthine may lead to xanthine nephropathy or xanthine renal stones. The clinical significance of this hypothesis is not clear because xanthine nephropathy has been rarely reported. In a study of 19 children with acute lymphoblastic leukemia who received allopurinol for tumor lysis syndrome, precipitated xanthine was significantly more likely to be found in the urine sediment of patients with high urine xanthine levels (>350 mg/dL). However, there was no difference in the incidence of precipitated xanthine in patients who developed acute renal failure versus those who did not.[17]

Urate oxidase provides an alternate approach for treating hyperuricemia by promoting the catabolism of uric acid to allantoin. In comparison with uric acid, allantoin is five to ten times more water-soluble and is easily excreted in urine.[23] Urate oxidase is an endogenous enzyme found in many mammalian species, but not in humans. A nonrecombinant form of urate oxidase purified from the mold *Aspergillus flavus* has been demonstrated to reduce uric acid levels in patients at risk for TLS and has been available in Europe for more than 20 years. In the United States, a pediatric trial of this nonrecombinant urate oxidase was conducted in 126 children with newly diagnosed non–B-cell acute lymphoblastic leukemia. When compared with historical controls treated with allopurinol, patients treated with urate oxidase had significantly greater decreases in their blood uric acid levels (median maximal level during treatment, 2.3 vs. 3.9 mg/dL; $P < .001$).[24] However, the nonrecombinant urate oxidase was also associated with significant acute hypersensitivity reactions, including anaphylaxis, in 4.5% of patients receiving the drug.

More recently, a recombinant form of urate oxidase (rasburicase) produced by a genetically modified *Saccharomyces cerevisiae* strain has become available and appears to have a lower incidence of hypersensitivity reactions. Rasburicase offers potential advantage over allopurinol by affecting the direct breakdown of uric acid and consequently leading to a more rapid lowering of serum uric acid levels. Faster normalization of uric acid levels also allows for earlier discontinuation of alkalinized fluids. This likely results in better excretion of other metabolites, and avoids the increased risk of precipitation of calcium phosphate stones in the setting of overalkalinization. It should be noted that blood samples for uric acid measurement in patients receiving rasburicase therapy require special handling because of ex vivo degradation of uric acid by rasburicase at room temperature. To avoid falsely low uric acid levels, blood samples must be kept on ice and processed at 4° C within 4 hours of collection.

Pui and colleagues[25] initially administered rasburicase at a dose of 0.15 to 0.20 mg/kg IV for 5 to 7 days to 131 children with newly diagnosed leukemia or lymphoma. This study has demonstrated a significant reduction of the median uric acid level by 4 hours after treatment, from 9.7 to 1 mg/dL in the 65

patients who presented with hyperuricemia and from 4.3 to 0.5 mg/dL in the remaining 66 patients. Rasburicase was very well tolerated in this study, with 1 of 131 children developing bronchospasm. In addition, an open-label, multicenter, intent to treat, randomized, controlled trial was conducted to compare allopurinol with rasburicase in 52 pediatric patients with leukemia or lymphoma at high risk for TLS.[26] This study has shown that patients randomized to rasburicase compared with allopurinol achieve an 86% versus 12% reduction of initial serum uric acid levels 4 hours after the first dose. In addition, no hypersensitivity reactions were observed in this study. Limitations of this study included its open-label design and the difficulty of generalizing these results to an adult population, although children up to age 17 years were included. Randomized controlled trials of allopurinol versus rasburicase have not been performed in the adult population.

Rasburicase is contraindicated in patients known to have glucose-6-phosphate-dehydrogenase (G6PD) deficiency because the hydrogen peroxide generated in the breakdown of uric acid cannot be cleared by these patients.[23] The peroxide causes oxidative damage, resulting in hemolytic anemia and methemoglobinemia. The hemolytic anemia caused by rasburicase can be severe and can exacerbate renal damage in the setting of TLS. It is recommended that G6PD screening be performed before rasburicase administration whenever possible.[27] Screening should be performed prior to transfusion with packed red blood cells to avoid false-negatives. If screening cannot be performed in a timely manner, the use of rasburicase should be avoided in patients who by ethnic background or family history have a significant risk of G6PD deficiency. Other adverse reactions associated with rasburicase include rare occurrences of hypersensitivity reactions, rash, increased liver enzyme levels, headache, vomiting, and nausea.[28] Because of the high incidence of hypersensitivity reactions associated with the nonrecombinant urate oxidase, several studies have measured antibody formation to rasburicase. In one study, no patients experienced hypersensitivity reactions and none of the 23 of 27 patient samples tested contained detectable levels of antibodies to rasburicase.[26] In another study, 14% of patients developed antibodies, but none of these patients had hypersensitivity reactions.[25] It remains uncertain whether patients with detection of antibodies to rasburicase are at greater risk of hypersensitivity reactions with repeat courses. It has been suggested that patients with asthma and those with a high risk of hypersensitivity reactions based on allergy history should be monitored closely when receiving rasburicase.

Because of the high cost of rasburicase compared with allopurinol, it has been recommended that the use of rasburicase be reserved for those patients with significant hyperuricemia at presentation, or those at high risk of developing severe TLS. The significant cost of rasburicase therapy has led several groups to evaluate the efficacy of single-dose therapy. Several published reports have demonstrated rapid reduction of uric acid levels with a single dose of rasburicase, with persistent effects for up to 7 days.[29,30] Thus, single-dose therapy appears to be effective for both treatment and prophylaxis of hyperuricemia. However, when considering the use of rasburicase based on cost, it must be recognized that there are also significant costs associated with complications of hyperuricemia and TLS, such as acute renal failure and dialysis. For example, a European study that examined the economic consequences of TLS management found that the main cost drivers in TLS are interventions requiring intensive care.[31] Thus, studies aiming to analyze the cost difference between allopurinol and rasburicase should take into account the outcomes of acute renal failure and/or dialysis. Unfortunately, there have been no prospective randomized studies as yet comparing the incidence of renal failure or need for dialysis in patients at risk for TLS receiving allopurinol versus rasburicase.

Uremia and Acute Renal Failure

Causes for renal dysfunction, azotemia, and rising creatinine levels can be multifactorial during acute TLS. For example, any of the following conditions can result in renal injury: uric acid crystal obstructive uropathy, renal precipitation of calcium phosphate, renal tumor infiltration, xanthinuria, nephrotoxic drugs, or intravascular volume depletion. Despite appropriate medical management, some patients with increasing renal dysfunction and acute TLS require more aggressive measures, such as dialysis or hemofiltration. Indications for these therapies include metabolic derangements (e.g., hyperkalemia, hyperphosphatemia, hyperuricemia, hypocalcemia, uremia) or volume overload that cannot be adequately controlled by medical management. Hemodialysis, peritoneal dialysis, and continuous hemofiltration (arteriovenous and venovenous) have been used in pediatric and adult populations for the treatment of TLS.[32-34] Peritoneal dialysis, although commonly used in many forms of acute renal failure, cannot be safely used in patients with intra-abdominal tumors (e.g., Burkitt's lymphoma) and is not recommended in the oncologic setting because of risk of infection in immunocompromised hosts.[18] The major advantage of hemodialysis over the other modalities is the rapidity with which electrolyte abnormalities can be corrected. However, hemodialysis can lead to large swings in plasma electrolyte levels and also impose significant hemodynamic challenges. Continuous hemofiltration provides a more gradual method of correcting fluid and electrolyte disturbances, and may serve as a safer alternative to hemodialysis in some cases. Unfortunately, there is little evidence comparing the various dialysis modalities. Consultation with a nephrologist or an intensivist is recommended when weighing the options of hemofiltration and dialysis.

Conclusions

Tumor lysis syndrome is a constellation of metabolic derangements resulting from massive release of intracellular ions and nucleotides. Purine catabolism in the setting of TLS is particularly problematic for humans because of the lack of endogenous urate oxidase that can convert uric acid to the more soluble allantoin. The introduction of rasburicase has great promise for reducing the incidence and severity of complications from hyperuricemia in patients at high risk for TLS. Although rasburicase appears to have great potential, many questions remain unanswered:

Which dose and schedule of rasburicase is most effective?
Which patients only require allopurinol for prophylaxis or treatment?
Does rasburicase reduce morbidity and mortality from TLS in addition to lowering uric acid levels?

Future prospective studies will be required to resolve these concerns.

HYPERLEUKOCYTOSIS AND LEUKOSTASIS

Hyperleukocytosis is a clear, life-threatening pediatric oncologic emergency that requires immediate initiation of appropriate therapy. Marked metabolic abnormalities and mild to severe pulmonary and neurologic symptoms can accompany the initial finding of hyperleukocytosis, or can develop shortly

TABLE 28-2	Factors Associated with Occurrence of Hyperleukocytic Leukemias in Childhood	
Acute Lymphoblastic Leukemia	**Acute Myelogenous Leukemia**
Age < 1 yr	Age < 1 yr
11q23	11q23
T cell with mediastinal mass	FAB M4/M5
CNS involvement	FAB M3v
Hypodiploid	Inv 16
Philadelphia chromosome	FLT3 ITD*

*FLT3 internal tandem duplication, shown in young adults.[28]

after presentation. Stasis of leukemic cells within blood vessels and migration of blast cells into tissues can lead to the clinical entity of leukostasis. Morbidity and mortality are high; mortality can be 20% to 40%.[35-37] Despite the relative frequency of this true oncologic emergency, and several varied therapeutic options, there are no data-driven management guidelines because of overall small numbers of patients, variability of clinical presentation, molecular differences in the underlying disease, and the difficulty of conducting randomized clinical trials with these constraints.

Definition

Hyperleukocytosis is generally accepted as a white blood cell (WBC) count higher than 100×10^9/L, although some studies have included patients with WBC higher than 50×10^9/L. It is estimated to occur in 5% to 20% of childhood leukemias and is seen most frequently in infant acute lymphoblastic leukemia (ALL) and T-cell ALL. Hyperleukocytosis is more associated with certain subtypes of ALL and acute myelogenous leukemia (AML), and is seen in almost all cases of childhood CML (Table 28-2). It has long been observed that the occurrence of leukostasis does not correlate directly with degree of hyperleukocytosis. Although hyperleukocytosis is seen more frequently in childhood ALL, clinical leukostasis is seen more frequently in AML, particularly in M4-M5 subtypes. Clinical symptoms from hyperleukocytosis generally occur at WBC higher than 200 to 300×10^9/L in patients with AML,[38] and higher than 400 to 500×10^9/L in patients with ALL. However, symptoms of leukostasis have also been observed in patients with WBC lower than 100×10^9/L.[36,39,40]

Clinical symptoms of leukostasis are dependent on the system affected. Any small vessels, and therefore any organs, appear at risk. Although pulmonary and neurologic symptoms are most often observed, involvement of many other systems has also been reported. Hyperleukocytosis has been reported to result in leukostasis, causing renal failure, papilledema, dactylitis, priapism and clitorism, acute myocardial infarction, and cardiac failure.[3,41,42] Histopathologic studies have demonstrated aggregates of blast cells and thrombi leading to occlusion of small vessels in multiple organs of patients with hyperleukocytosis.[43] Corresponding to observed clinical symptoms, postmortem examinations have shown profound infiltration of multiple organs, including brain (including retinal vessels), liver, spleen, adrenals, and pulmonary vasculature, and in the alveoli and connective tissue of the lungs. A striking image of infiltration of a coronary artery was obtained by Thornton and Levis (Fig. 28-2).[41]

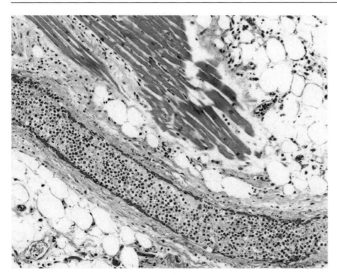

FIGURE 28-2. Small vessels throughout the body are at risk of occlusion in a patient with hyperleukocytosis. This image shows a coronary artery filled with FLT3 ITD acute myelogenous leukemia blasts. *(From Thornton K, Levis M. Images in clinical medicine. FLT3 mutation and acute myelogenous leukemia with leukostasis. N Engl J Med. 2007;357:1639.)*

The observance of the clinical expression of leukostasis and the accompanying related comorbidities has evolved to a description of a leukostasis syndrome. This has been defined as a critical condition with severe metabolic abnormalities, tumor lysis syndrome, severe coagulopathy, and multiorgan failure, which occurs in patients presenting with hyperleukocytic leukemia.[44,45]

Pathogenesis

The pathogenesis of leukostasis is under continued investigation as researchers have realized the importance and potential clinical relevance of understanding the pathophysiology involved. Increased blood viscosity is often postulated to contribute to the development of leukostasis. At high flow rates (in larger vessels), bulk viscosity of the blood is a function of the deformability of the blood cells and the fraction of blood represented by these cells.[40] The overall viscosity of the blood has been found generally not to increase, even with the marked increase in leukocytic cells, in part because of the corresponding decrease in erythrocrit with increasing leukocrit. In patients with associated moderate to severe anemia, observed leukocrits over 20% to 25% are needed to demonstrate an objective increase in blood viscosity. Transfusion of red blood cells prior to reduction of the leukocyte count will increase the erythrocrit and can therefore result in hyperviscosity. This can be extremely deleterious to the patient, causing clinical manifestations of hyperviscosity.

Blood viscosity in the microcirculation can increase, however, because the viscosity there is a function of the plasma viscosity and the deformability of the individual cells in the capillaries. Leukemic blasts are larger and less deformable than erythrocytes or normal leukocytes. Flow in microvessels will slow if the diameter of the poorly deformable blast cell approaches that of the channel. Lymphoblasts range in size from 250 to 350 mm³ and myeloblasts from 350 to 450 mm³. It has been suggested that the larger size of myeloblasts compared with lymphoblasts helps account for the greater

incidence of intracerebral hemorrhage that has been observed in patients with acute nonlymphoblastic leukemia (ANLL) over ALL.[38] Histopathologic studies have revealed leukocyte thrombi and aggregates in the cerebral vasculature of patients with ANLL.

There is increasing appreciation of the role of adhesion molecules and the endothelial lining of the blood vessels. Laboratory observations have shown that expression of intracellular adhesion molecule 1 (ICAM-1,) vascular cell adhesion molecule 1 (VCAM-1), and E-selectin can be induced in endothelial cells exposed to supernatants of blast cell cultures.[46] This effect was regulated by blast cell production of tumor necrosis factor-α and interleukin-1β. It is suggested that through this self-perpetuating interaction, leukemic blasts can promote their own adhesion to inactivated vascular endothelium. Alternate mechanisms of leukostasis have also been proposed and are under further study, including molecular interactions directly between leukemic blast cells, leading to clumping and intravascular aggregates.

The molecular origin and subsequent cell phenotype is likely important to the role in developing leukostasis. The expression of CD56 NCAM (neural cell adhesion molecule) on leukemic blasts in a study of adult patients with AML was correlated with the development of severe clinical leukostatic syndrome.[45] In another study of adult patients with acute promyelocytic leukemia (APML),[47] expression of CD13 (aminopeptidase N), a cell surface enzyme previously linked to tumor cell invasion, was highly associated with elevated leukocyte count and the development of all trans-retinoic acid (ATRA) syndrome. Further study in these intriguing areas of research is needed to confirm these findings and to test the applicability to pediatric patients. Better understanding of the underlying pathophysiology will hopefully lead to methods for early detection of patients at highest risk for severe leukostasis and eventually provide pharmacologic targets for disruption of the interaction of adhesion molecules, resulting in clinical improvements.

Clinical Presentation

Clinical manifestations can be myriad. Many patients with hyperleukocytosis are relatively asymptomatic. Clinical leukostasis can present subtly, and evolve rapidly. Most commonly, pulmonary symptoms are observed. Tachypnea, oxygen desaturation, and dyspnea can occur, and can progress rapidly to acute respiratory disease syndrome (ARDS) and respiratory failure. Neurologic symptoms can include headache, tinnitus, ataxia, behavioral changes, seizures, and stroke. Hemorrhagic stroke is a highly morbid complication of hyperleukocytosis, and is seen most often in the microgranular variant of M3 AML (M3v). Often, these patient have associated disseminated intravascular coagulation (DIC) and thrombocytopenia, increasing their risk for hemorrhage.

Symptoms can clearly worsen after initiation of therapy. It has been postulated that this may be caused by release of intracellular components of blast cells after lysis, including enzymes that can lead to injury in surrounding tissue, such as alveolar damage and interstitial edema.[48]

A number of studies have looked at the factors associated with more severe clinical events in patients with hyperleukocytic leukemias, with mixed conclusions. A clinical grading system has been proposed by Novotny and associates (Table 28-3).[44] The grading system groups patients into four categories—not present (0), possible (1), probable (2), and highly probable (3). The grading is based on the assumption that the severity of presenting symptoms may indicate the probability of leukostasis, provided other causes of the symptoms are not

TABLE 28-3 Grading of Symptoms in Hyperleukocytic Leukemia*

Group	Probability of Leukostasis Syndrome	Severity of Symptoms	Pulmonary Symptoms	Neurologic Symptoms	Other Organ Systems
0	Not present	No limitations	No symptoms and no limitations in ordinary activities	No neurologic symptoms	No symptoms
1	Possible	Slight limitations	Mild symptoms and slight limitation during ordinary activity, comfortable at rest	Mild tinnitus, headache, dizziness	Moderate fatigue
2	Probable	Marked limitations	Marked limitation in activity because of symptoms, even during less than ordinary activity, comfortable only at rest	Slight visual disturbances, severe tinnitus, headache, dizziness	Severe fatigue
3	Highly probable	Severe limitations	Dyspnea at rest, oxygen or respirator required	Severe visual disturbances (acute inability to read), confusion, delirium, somnolence, intracranial hemorrhage	Myocardial infarction, priapism, ischemic necrosis

*Probability of leukostasis deduced from the severity of symptoms attributable to leukostasis (no obvious other cause).
From Novotny JR, Müller-Beissenhirtz H, Herget-Rosenthal S, et al. Grading of symptoms in hyperleukocytic leukaemia: a clinical model for the role of different blast types and promyelocytes in the development of leukostasis syndrome. Eur J Haematol. 2005;74:501-510.

found. This assumption is supported by the knowledge that patients with respiratory distress or severe neurologic symptoms have a much increased mortality rate.[49] Novotny and coworkers used this clinical scoring system in conjunction with initial flow cytometry data to show that the detection of CD56 expression at baseline in patients with ANNL M4-M5 may identify patients at highest risk for fatal leukostasis. This has clear clinical relevance, but requires further validation prior to clinical application.

Treatment

Definitive treatment for hyperleukocytosis is the initiation of appropriate induction chemotherapy once a diagnosis is established. Prior to this, the initiation of intravenous hydration, urinary alkalinization, and allopurinol has been the clinical standard for the immediate initial treatment of acute hyperleukocytic leukemias for many years. In 1995, Basade and colleagues[50] reported that in a cohort of pediatric patients with ALL, an 81.5% reduction in WBC was achieved within a median of 36 hours with the use of IV hydration, urinary alkalinization, and allopurinol. No treatment-related complications occurred in their patient cohort. Although studies have not yet been published, the availability of urate oxalate is likely to modify this practice, because many of these patients clearly meet criteria for high risk of tumor lysis syndrome. Early therapy with urate oxalate has the potential to decrease the risk for TLS markedly in patients with acute hyperleukocytic leukemias, which could decrease the number of patients who develop the leukostasis syndrome, thereby positively affecting overall morbidity and mortality.

Additional measures to reduce the elevated WBC and associated morbidities have been studied. Cranial radiation has been proposed to decrease the chance of intracerebral hemorrhage. Based on a study of adult patients with ANLL and WBC higher than 200×10^9/L, Wiernik and Serpick[51] have proposed the prophylactic use of 400 to 600 rad of cranial x-ray therapy

to prevent intracranial hemorrhage. Several small series that used emergency cranial x-ray therapy in pediatric patients with ALL and hyperleukocytosis were then reported, with a low incidence of intracranial hemorrhage.[52] Subsequent experience, however, has not consistently shown a beneficial effect. Additionally, there are concerns with acute and chronic neuropsychiatric complications associated with cranial x-ray therapy in pediatric patients, so it is rarely used for this indication in current practice.[53-55]

The use of low-dose prednisone as initial treatment for patients with ALL and hyperleukocytosis has been proposed, with the rationale of inducing a gradual blast cell lysis, in an attempt to decrease the severity of metabolic derangements. Along with several other interventions, the use of low-dose prednisone was reviewed in a group of 124 patients followed by the Children's Cancer Study Group from 1981 to 1983 with newly diagnosed ALL and WBC higher than 200×10^9/L.[53] All patients received IV hydration, urinary alkalinization, and allopurinol. Some patients received additional measures (low-dose prednisone, cranial radiation, exchange transfusion, leukapheresis) in an attempt to decrease complications. It was concluded that pretreatment with low-dose prednisone does not correlate with fewer electrolyte abnormalities. However, many of the patients in this study received more than one additional treatment, complicating the analysis in this relatively small group of patients.

Leukapheresis and exchange transfusion have both been shown to be effective in reducing the total WBC and blast count. Patients weighing less than 12 kg usually are unable to undergo leukapheresis but may safely undergo exchange transfusion. Studies in pediatric patients have shown a mean reduction of 50% to 60% in WBC with exchange transfusion and leukapheresis.[54,56] However, the overall benefit of this cytoreduction is unclear.

In patients with ALL, the use of leukapheresis may decrease the risk of severe TLS. Patients with ALL and hyperleukocytosis in the Children's Cancer Study Group cohort[53] who received leukapheresis or exchange transfusion appeared to show some benefit of the procedures, with a lower incidence of severe electrolyte abnormalities and renal dysfunction. The same conclusion was reached by Bunin and Pui in a series of 161 patients with ALL and hyperleukocytosis.[38]

The three largest studies in patients with AML that examined the role of leukapheresis reached differing conclusions. In a group of 22 patients with newly diagnosed AML (ages 12 to 74 years),[57] it was found that decreasing the total WBC through leukapheresis by at least 30% correlates with improved outcome in those patients. In contrast, in a study by Porcu and colleagues,[49] 48 patients with AML or chronic myelocytic leukemia (CML) in blast crisis, ages 8 to 79 years, underwent immediate cytoreduction with leukapheresis, and no correlation between the degree of cytoreduction and early mortality rate was found. In the largest study, Giles and associates[58] reviewed outcomes of 146 patients (ages 16 to 86 years) with AML, 71 of whom underwent leukapheresis. An association with decreased early mortality rate was found; however, there was no improvement in the overall survival rate.

The use of leukapheresis in patients with APML is greatly discouraged because increased rates of mortality have been observed in these patients, largely caused by the increased incidence of hemorrhage. Vahdat and coworkers[47] have reported fatal or near-fatal hemorrhage in 9 of 11 patients with APML who underwent leukapheresis.

Hydroxyurea is known to be effective in reducing overall WBC and blast counts.[59] Preliminary results of a randomized study presented at the American Society of Hematology 2006 annual meeting on the use of hydroxyurea versus leukapheresis in patients presenting with AML noted equivalent outcome at 8 and 28 days, with no difference in death rate.[60]

The possible benefits from rapid reduction in WBC and blast count that can be achieved with leukapheresis or exchange transfusion need to be weighed against the risks of these procedures, which include placement of adequate venous access and anticoagulation. The decision to initiate leukapheresis must also take into account the time to arrange these procedures, including mobilization of specialized blood bank personnel and possible transfer to tertiary centers where such specialized procedures are available. Institution of these procedures can be particularly deleterious if they delay initiation of definitive chemotherapy treatments. With increased use of urate oxalate, the benefit of leukapheresis in ALL may need to be reassessed.

Conclusions

Acute hyperleukocytic leukemias present immediate clinical challenges to the treating pediatric oncologist and must be addressed rapidly and appropriately. Although many components of treatment of hyperleukocytosis are generally accepted, much ambiguity still exists about the appropriateness of many possible interventions. Although further study is appropriate, carrying out such studies poses many challenges. Box 28-5 groups treatment guidelines into those that have been shown to be clearly beneficial, those that have been shown to be harmful, and those of less certain benefit. Hopefully, translational research into the underlying pathophysiology of the leukostasis syndrome will lead to novel therapeutic modalities and pharmacologic interventions.

ANTERIOR MEDIASTINAL MASSES

Another commonly encountered oncologic emergency is the entity of anterior mediastinal mass. A clinician should always

---

Box 28-5 Clinical Guidelines for Patients with WBC > 50 × 10⁹ and Diagnosis of Acute Leukemia

RECOMMENDED FOR ALL

Careful clinical observation, neurologic examination, frequent laboratory evaluation per tumor lysis protocol, evaluation of renal function, chest x-ray, oxygen saturation monitoring, supplemental O_2 as needed

Treatment for TLS, with IVF, alkalinization and allopurinol **OR** rasburicase and no alkalinization; strong bias toward use of rasburicase if any parameters are met for high risk of TLS—increased uric acid, creatinine, LDH, potassium (see preceding section on TLS)

Correction of coagulopathy as appropriate with cryoprecipitate, FFP, vitamin K; special consideration to DIC and risk of intracerebral hemorrhage in M4/M5 AML, and even greater risk in M3v AML

Transfusion for platelet count <25 K or any clinical bleeding

Institution of appropriate chemotherapy as soon as diagnosis is made

RECOMMENDED IN SOME CLINICAL CIRCUMSTANCES

Consider exchange transfusion/leukopheresis in patients with ALL and WBC > 300-500 × 10⁹, or AML and WBC > 100-200 × 10⁹, particularly if any pulmonary or neurologic symptoms exist

Consider prednisone prophase prior to induction chemotherapy in patients with ALL and WBC > 300-500 × 10⁹—may decrease chance of TLS

CONTRAINDICATED

Avoid leukopheresis in APML—confers increased risk of hemorrhage

Avoid use of diuretics or transfusion of PRBC in patients with ALL and WBC > 300-500 × 10⁹, or AML and WBC > 100-200 × 10⁹—confers risk of increased viscosity

---

AML, acute myelogenous leukemia; APML, acute promyelocytic leukemia; DIC, disseminated intravascular coagulation; FFP, fresh-frozen plasma; IVF, intravenous fluid; LDH, lactate dehydrogenase; PRBC, packed red blood cells; TLS, tumor lysis syndrome; WBC, white blood cell count.

---

consider this in the differential diagnosis of a pediatric patient with new respiratory distress and must consider evaluation, even in the asymptomatic patient presenting with any of the variety of cancers known to be associated with the occurrence of anterior mediastinal masses.

Space-occupying lesions occurring in the anterior mediastinum can impinge on vital structures, causing significant cardiac or airway compromise. The anterior mediastinum is defined as the anatomic compartment bounded by the sternum, thoracic inlet, and anterior border of the heart.[61] The presence of a mass in this region can cause superior vena cava syndrome (SVCS), tracheobronchial compression, or compression of the heart or pulmonary vessels. The term *superior mediastinal syndrome* (SMS) has been used to denote the combination of great vessel and tracheobronchial tree compression. However, because these may be overlapping phenomena, particularly in the pediatric population, SVCS and SMS are often used interchangeably.

Neoplasms causing anterior mediastinal masses in the pediatric population and associated with SVCS and/or tracheal compression include NHL, ALL, and Hodgkin's disease (HD),[47] as well as neuroblastoma, germ cell tumors, sarcoma, thymoma, and thyroid cancer.[62,63] In a retrospective review of children with mediastinal masses treated at the Mayo Clinic, NHL and HD represented the majority of malignant causes of anterior mediastinal masses, although this review did not include patients with leukemia.[62] In a report on 3721 children with cancer treated at St. Jude Children's Research Hospital over a 15-year period, 24 children had SVC obstruction at initial presentation or with disease recurrence. Those presenting with SVC obstruction at initial presentation included 8 children with NHL, 4 with ALL, 2 with HD, 1 with neuroblastoma, and 1 with yolk sac tumor.[63] In contrast, in the adult population, small cell bronchogenic carcinoma is the most common underlying diagnosis associated with SVCS.[64]

SVCS was first described in a patient with a syphilitic aneurysm of the aorta in 1757.[65] The SVC is a thin-walled vessel with blood flowing under low pressure, and is easily compressible by the enlargement of surrounding structures in the thorax. In SVCS, compression and obstruction of the SVC cause restriction of blood return to the right atrium and impaired venous drainage from the upper extremities, head, and neck. Occlusion of the SVC by thrombus—for example, as a complication of a central venous line—can also result in SVCS. Just as the SVC can be compressed by an anterior mediastinal mass, the trachea and main stem bronchi in children are relatively compressible and have smaller intraluminal diameters compared with these structures in adults, making the pediatric patient with an enlarging mass susceptible to respiratory compromise (Fig. 28-3).[62]

Children with SVCS (SMS) can present with a constellation of signs and symptoms related to SVC and airway obstruction, including swelling, plethora, venous engorgement of the face, neck, and upper extremities, and cough, hoarseness, orthopnea, cyanosis, anxiety, syncope, and altered mental status.[66,67] The child can present in extremis, with shock caused by cardiac compromise or with respiratory failure. Conversely, patients with more indolent tumors, such as Hodgkin's lymphoma, can present with impressively large masses and surprisingly little symptomatology (Fig. 28-4). Symptoms are often more profound with the patient in the supine position, and may improve in the upright or prone position. In the supine position, thoracic volume is decreased because of decreased rib cage dimension and diaphragm position. In addition, blood flow to the mass itself can increase causing further expansion of the mass.[61] Therefore, pursuing testing such as computed tomography (CT) scanning in the supine position should be carefully considered.

An anterior mediastinal mass may be suspected based on medical history and physical examination, and can be identified on chest x-ray. To initiate tumor-specific therapy, a definitive diagnosis is needed. The least invasive diagnostic methods should be pursued. If the peripheral blood smear is abnormal, a bone marrow biopsy with local anesthetic may prove diagnostic. Biopsy of a peripheral lymph node, if present, may prove diagnostic. If a pleural effusion is present, pleural fluid aspiration may be possible with local anesthesia and may provide fluid for pathologic review and immunocytogenetic evaluation (Fig. 28-5).[68]

Identifying those at greatest risk for anesthetic complications is important in planning the diagnostic evaluation. Procedural sedation and anesthesia pose particular risks for the patient with an anterior mediastinal mass, with the potential for cardiopulmonary collapse and death.[66,67,69] A patient with

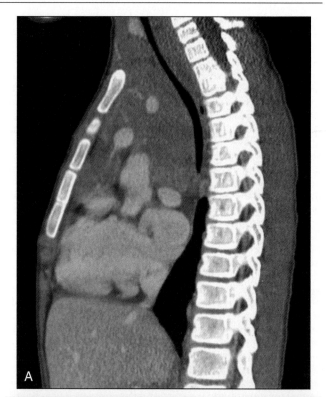

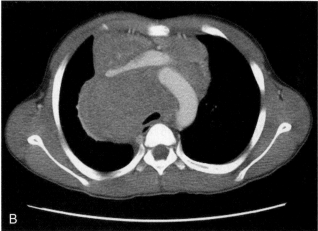

FIGURE 28-3. Chest CT scan of a patient with Hodgkin's disease. **A,** Sagittal and axial **(B)** images show the significant effects of the mass on structures within the mediastinum, with marked narrowing of the trachea and superior vena cava. Remarkably, the patient was symptomatic only with exercise.

stable respiratory status while awake, with spontaneous respirations, may develop significant obstruction under anesthesia. General anesthesia alters ventilatory mechanics, decreasing inspiratory muscle tone and functional residual capacity of the lung.[70] Chest wall tone is decreased by neuromuscular blockade. Airways are more compressible because of bronchial smooth muscle relaxation.[66] Positive pressure ventilation may further restrict an already narrowed airway.[71] In addition, general anesthetics can have negative inotropic effects and can contribute to decreasing cardiac output, precipitating hypoxemia, hypotension, or even cardiac arrest in the patient with compression of the great vessels.[72]

Respiratory symptoms occur in 40% to 60% of children with anterior mediastinal masses, but correlation of symptoms

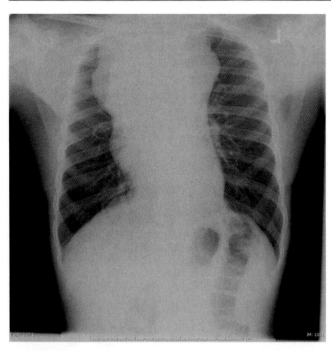

FIGURE 28-4. Chest x-ray of a patient with Hodgkin's disease showing a markedly enlarged mediastinum. The patient had a several-month history of intermittent cough and had only mild respiratory symptoms at presentation.

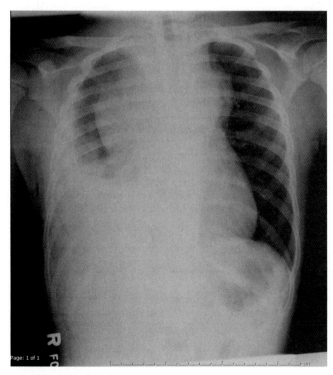

FIGURE 28-5. Chest x-ray of a patient who presented in near extremis, with facial swelling, plethora, and significant respiratory distress. The patient had large anterior mediastinal mass and marked pleural effusion. T-cell lymphoblastic lymphoma was diagnosed from the pleural fluid.

with anesthetic risk can be challenging.[66,73] Orthopnea has been associated with increased anesthetic risk.[73,74] Posterior anterior and lateral chest radiographs can demonstrate tracheal compression, but may not detect all cases.[73,75] CT can provide additional anatomic information and patients with less than 50% of expected tracheal cross-sectional area on CT have been shown to be a high-risk group.[66,73] However, obstruction distal to the trachea may be more difficult to appreciate. A prospective study assessing tracheal area and pulmonary function testing has found that general anesthesia can be used safely in children meeting the minimum criteria of tracheal area of larger than 50% and predicted peak expiratory flow rate (PEFR) more than 50%. Thirty-one children with mediastinal masses underwent pulmonary function testing in the sitting and supine positions as well as CT prior to undergoing 34 surgical procedures. Children with less than 50% of predicted cross-sectional tracheal area (or with less than 50% of PEFR) received only local rather than general anesthesia. Five patients had tracheal areas larger than 50% predicted but had low PEFR, and received local anesthesia. There were no intraoperative complications in those receiving anesthetics using these criteria.[76]

An accurate tissue diagnosis allows for initiation of the optimal treatment regimen. Patients in extremis or those with rapidly evolving respiratory compromise who would require sedation or general anesthesia are particularly challenging. If proceeding with general anesthesia, some have argued for preserving spontaneous respiration when at all possible, avoiding muscle relaxants, being prepared to change the patient's position and having an expert bronchoscopist and emergency cardiopulmonary bypass available.[69] Use of extracorporeal membrane oxygenation (ECMO) in individuals with anterior mediastinal masses with cardiopulmonary failure has been reported.[77] Use of inhaled heliox, a helium-oxygen mixture, has been advocated in case reports, to decrease resistance to airflow in obstructed airways, although its use in the setting of anterior mediastinal masses has not been studied.[78]

In some clinical situations, the risk of proceeding with diagnostic procedures is considered too great and empirical therapy aimed at reducing the mass must be initiated. Emergent treatment modalities include radiation, intravenous steroids, and combination chemotherapy. Radiation has traditionally been used in emergency management of anterior mediastinal masses, because most lymphomas such as NHL and HD will be radiosensitive. Daily radiation doses are based on those used for the presumed diagnosis that best fits the clinical data. Depending on the radioresponsiveness of the mass, prebiopsy radiation treatment can obscure the tissue diagnosis, even with low dose radiation therapy. Loeffler and colleagues[79] have reported that in 8 of 10 patients younger than 30 years who underwent emergent prebiopsy radiation for a mediastinal mass, a tissue diagnosis could not be established because of uninterruptible pathologic specimens.[79] Also of concern in the pediatric population is a risk of postirradiation respiratory deterioration caused by swelling of the trachea after radiation. Concurrent administration of steroid (e.g., dexamethasone at a dosage for airway edema, 0.5 to 2 mg/kg/day in divided doses every 6 hours) can be considered with the goal of preventing this complication, but may also contribute to obscuring the diagnosis.

The emergent use of empirical chemotherapy includes the use of intravenous steroids or combination chemotherapy. Steroid therapy should be considered in the emergent management of proven or presumed ALL or acute lymphoblastic lymphoma. Careful attention must be paid to fluid management given concerns for TLS in the patient with the potential for cardiovascular compromise. Consideration of the use of rasburicase may be warranted. Steroid dosing based on ALL treatment protocols can be used (e.g., methylprednisolone, 32 mg/m²/day IV, divided every 8 hours). Steroid therapy may also be effective in the setting of other NHL, as well as HD. Other chemotherapeutic agents for consideration in the emergent management of anterior mediastinal mass include cyclophosphamide, vincristine, and an anthracycline. Just as radiation may eliminate the ability to determine a definitive diagnosis, steroid therapy has also been reported to confound the ultimate diagnosis.[67] Without a definitive pathologic diagnosis, continued treatment of the patient for the presumed diagnosis that best fits the clinical data has been advocated. Masses found not to be responsive to treatment, such as germ cell tumors or benign tumors, may require surgical intervention.

The evaluation of a child with a suspected anterior mediastinal mass or SVCS should be initiated rapidly once the diagnosis is considered. Great variability in the course of evaluation and treatment may be encountered, depending on the specifics of each clinical situation, including clinical stability of the patient and underlying diagnosis. Figure 28-6 outlines a suggested evaluation and treatment algorithm. The clinician must adapt his or her care to the particular circumstances of the individual patient.

SPINAL CORD COMPRESSION

Spinal cord compression is overall a rare event in children, but several studies have shown an incidence of up to 5% in children with cancer.[80] Most frequently (67% of the time), in pediatric oncology patients, spinal cord compression occurs as the initial presentation of the malignant process.[81] Although such a presentation is usually associated with widely disseminated disease, spinal cord compression can also occur with a singular lesion as the initial presentation of a new diagnosis of cancer. In this scenario, along with preservation or restoration of lost neurologic functioning, proper diagnosis of the cancer through adequate tissue sampling is a management priority. Procurement of sufficient tissue for specialized testing and possible study enrollment is a lesser priority, but still should be thoughtfully considered in the overall management plan. Spinal cord compression is also encountered in relapsed and refractory disease, again as a single metastatic lesion but more commonly in the setting of widespread metastatic disease. In such situations, management strategies must take into account the likelihood of cure, effect of interventions on the patient, the role of palliation, and quality of life.

Most (71%) of tumors that cause spinal cord compression are extradural.[81] More than 50% of tumors causing spinal cord compression are found to be neuroblastoma or soft tissue sarcomas, most often Ewing's sarcoma, followed by rhabdomyosarcoma. A wide array of other tumors has also been reported as causes of spinal cord compression and must be considered in the differential diagnosis. Tumors reported include neuroblastoma, Ewing's sarcoma, medulloblastoma, rhabdomyosarcoma, osteosarcoma, Wilms' tumor, metastatic central nervous system tumors, acute myelogenous leukemia, and lymphoma.

Clinical Presentation

Back pain is the most common presenting sign of spinal cord compression. This complaint was present in 94% of patients characterized in a series of 70 pediatric patients with solid tumors presenting with spinal cord compression.[81] Because back pain in children is a fairly uncommon complaint, spinal lesions and spinal cord compression should always be considered in the differential diagnosis of this complaint—even in the absence of neurologic findings. In the known pediatric oncology patient, the index of suspicion must be particularly high. Any delay of diagnosis may contribute significantly to morbidity. A thorough physical examination should accompany a complete history. The history should include characterization of pain, including onset and duration. Neurologic findings, if present, will vary, depending on the spinal level of the lesion and the degree of compression. In their series of children with systemic cancer and spinal cord disease, Lewis and coworkers[80] noted that localized spine tenderness is the most reliable clinical finding. A spectrum of ataxia, gait disturbance, and paraplegia can be observed. Sphincter dysfunction is most commonly seen as urinary retention or constipation. Localization of the level of epidural cord compression along the spine is suggested by the specific effects on strength, tendon reflexes, sensory level, Babinski reflex, sphincter abnormalities, and rate of progression (Table 28-4).[80,82]

Evaluation and Imaging

When the possibility of spinal cord compression is considered, immediate evaluation should be undertaken. Spinal radiography is often the first-choice modality, because this is quickly and easily carried out. Plain films may be able to provide valuable clinical information rapidly, but one must be aware that they are positive in only approximately 30% of patients with spinal cord compression.[80] The presence of a compressive spinal lesion may be seen on a radiograph as a paraspinal soft tissue mass. In cases of neuroblastoma, calcifications are often present within the paraspinal mass. Classically, neuroblastoma

TABLE 28-4	**Epidural Cord Compression: Clinical Localization**		
	LOCATION		
SIGN	**Spinal Cord**	**Conus Medullaris**	**Cauda Equina**
Weakness	Symmetrical; profound	Symmetrical; variable	Asymmetrical; may be mild
Tendon reflexes	Increased or absent	Increased knee; decreased ankle	Decreased; asymmetrical
Babinski	Extensor	Extensor	Plantar
Sensory	Symmetrical; sensory level	Symmetrical; saddle	Asymmetrical; radicular
Sphincter abnormality	Spared until late	Early involvement	May be spared
Progression	Rapid	Variable; may be rapid	Variable; may be slow

From Lewis DW, Packer RJ, Raney B, et al. Incidence, presentation, and outcome of spinal cord disease in children with systemic cancer. Pediatrics. 1986;78:438-443.

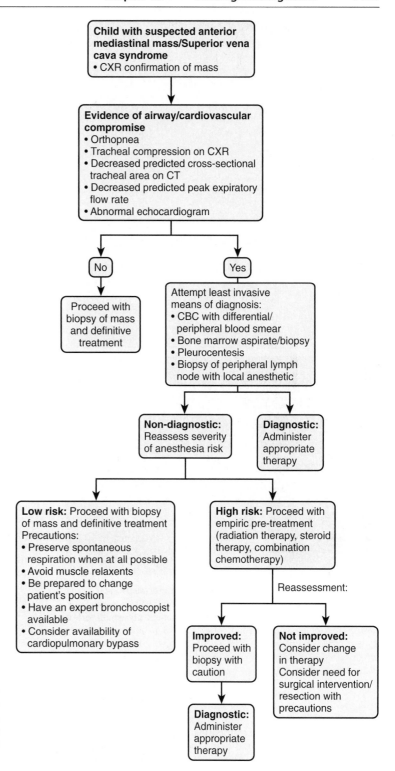

FIGURE 28-6. Suggested evaluation and treatment algorithm for a patient with an anterior mediastinal mass or superior vena cava syndrome. CT, computed tomography; CXR, chest x-ray. *(Adapted from Robie DK, Gursoy MH, Pokorny WJ. Mediastinal tumors—airway obstruction and management. Semin Pediatr Surg. 1994;3:259-266.)*

invading the spinal canal and intervertebral foramina classically may be visualized as a dumbbell-shaped lesion surrounding the spine. Other tumors, however, can have this appearance, emphasizing the importance of obtaining adequate tissue for diagnosis (Fig. 28-7). In many spinal lesions, lytic or sclerotic changes in adjacent bone are often observed on x-ray. Diagnostic widening of interpeduncular distances and enlargement of the neural foramina can sometimes also be observed on radiographs.

Magnetic resonance imaging (MRI) is valuable when plain radiographs are negative and clinical suspicion still exists. MRI is also now commonly used for further delineation of lesions observed on plain radiographs. It has become widely accessible, so MRI has replaced previously used techniques of radionucleotide bone scanning, spinal CT with intrathecal contrast, and lumbar myelography. MRI offers the advantage of increased accuracy and a less invasive nature than previously used modalities. Careful comparison of axial, coronal,

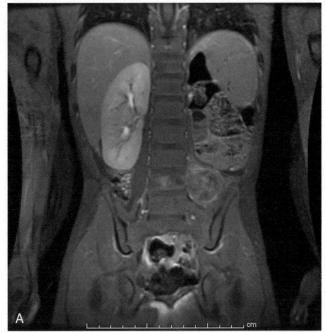

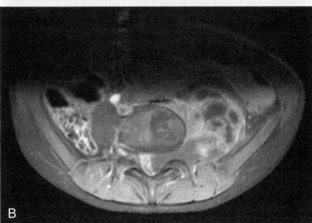

FIGURE 28-7. MRI scan, postcontrast, demonstrating a soft tissue retroperitoneal mass at the level of L4 with dumbbell appearance on both coronal **(A)** and axial **(B)** views. The patient presented with a short history of leg pain and limp, progressing to inability to ambulate, 2 years after completion of therapy for favorable histology Wilms' tumor.

and sagittal images can help categorize spinal tumors as extradural, intradural-extramedullary, or intramedullary, thereby aiding in differential diagnosis.[83] MRI sequences with and without gadolinium should be obtained for patients being evaluated for spinal cord compression. Contrast enhancement is less helpful for extradural tumors than intradural-extramedullary or intramedullary lesions. Fat suppression techniques are most helpful for evaluating extradural lesions. It should also be remembered that it is important to image the whole spine to identify the possibility of involvement at several levels, even if the physical examination has localized the most likely area of compression.

MRI can also accurately detect compression and dislocation of the spinal cord. Coronal images can elucidate the degree of cranial and caudal extension on the intraspinal component of a mass lesion. Because of increased cellularity and high nuclear-to-cytoplasmic ratio, lesions are usually iso- to hypodense on T2-weighted images.[84] Cord edema can be seen as a hyperintense signal in T2-weighted images. Contrast enhancement is generally marked in the presence of intraspinal lesions.

If the clinical situation allows time for further radiologic evaluation, CT with bone windows can provide complementary information to MRI findings. Detailed information on bone architecture and cortical appearance is better obtained by CT.

Treatment

Treatment options for a patient presenting with spinal cord compression include surgery (laminectomy or laminotomy), chemotherapy, steroid therapy, and radiation therapy. The best choice of initial therapy will vary, depending on the clinical situation. There are many clinical situations in which more than one choice of a modality may be appropriate, and situations in which more than one modality can appropriately be used at once. The complexity of the choice of the best initial therapy stems largely from simultaneously competing goals—the desire to prevent further loss of neurologic function, the need to make an accurate diagnosis with sufficient histologic and biologic information for assignment of appropriate treatment, the hope of regaining any lost function present at presentation, and the concern regarding the late effects of the available treatment modalities. After a brief overview of the basic treatment options, the conclusions of several clinical studies will be presented.

Surgery

Laminectomy is the most common surgical approach to relieve spinal cord compression caused by solid tumor. Laminectomy involves removal of the bony arch, or lamina, of a vertebra. This is often combined with biopsy and/or debulking of the tumor. The advantage of laminectomy is the rapid decompression of the spinal cord. Laminectomy is generally accepted as the most likely modality to stabilize or improve lost neurologic function. Another significant advantage of laminectomy is the procurement of tumor tissue for proper histologic diagnosis, and the option of obtaining tissue for relevant biology studies or possible protocol enrollment. The disadvantage of laminectomy is the high risk for late effects, with a significant percentage of patients developing kyphosis or scoliosis. Depending on the degree of spinal cord injury and how long symptoms have been present, laminectomy may not provide an advantage over treatment with chemotherapy only, and may expose the child to risks of the surgical procedure and greater risks of long-term orthopedic sequelae.

The technique of osteoplastic laminotomy involves removal of part of the lamina above and below an affected nerve, with subsequent bracing for a period of 6 to 8 weeks. Although historically not commonly used, this technique may offer a decreased incidence of long-term sequelae and may be considered by the surgeon.

Chemotherapy

It has been shown that chemotherapy can be used successfully to reduce some neoplastic masses causing spinal cord compression. This has been most studied in cases of neuroblastoma or Ewing's sarcoma that present with spinal cord compression. In the more rare cases of leukemic infiltrates, chemotherapy is a clear standard of initial therapy once the diagnosis has been established.

Advantages of up-front chemotherapy for lesions causing spinal cord compression are that it is noninvasive and long-term surgical consequences may be avoided. In addition, patients may proceed with tumor-specific therapy without the need for delay from postsurgical healing. However, the use of chemotherapy depends on first being able to make an adequate pathologic diagnosis of the type of cancer. In cases of metastatic tumor, it may be possible to make a diagnosis by biopsy of other primary or metastatic lesions. Isolated paraspinal masses can be more diagnostically difficult. If surgery is avoided completely, and chemotherapy started presumptively, the possibility of incorrect diagnosis will exist. Also, if no tissue is obtained, even though an isolated paraspinal mass may eventually be diagnosed as neuroblastoma by elevated urine catecholamine levels or positive metaiodobenzylguanidine (MIBG) activity, the opportunity to obtain valuable biologic information, such as histology and *N-myc* status, could be lost.

In patients who develop spinal cord compression in the setting of relapsed disease, the choice of using chemotherapy over surgery or radiation therapy can become more complex, because the rate and overall likelihood of response can be substantially decreased in pretreated patients. Radiation therapy or surgeries may have been used previously, complicating these options. Such clinical situations must be carefully weighed individually. Initiation of chemotherapy over surgery or radiation therapy or comfort palliation must involve the specifics of the patient's overall chance of long-term cure, the history of treatment and response and, importantly, the patient's and family's goals of treatment and desired level of intensity of therapy.

In the patient with a new presentation of cancer, the choice of a chemotherapy regimen must be based on clear identification of the malignant process. Once a diagnosis is known and a decision has been made to avoid surgery or radiation and commence with chemotherapy, standard induction therapy for the malignancy identified is accepted as the best initial chemotherapy in patients with spinal cord compression.

Dexamethasone

Dexamethasone is routinely recommended throughout the literature on treatment of pediatric spinal cord compression. It is theorized that decreased swelling of the cord will help minimize neurologic damage through minimizing the effect of vasogenic edema and venous congestion. In a review of the adult literature compiled to create an evidence-based guideline for the emergency treatment of extradural spinal cord compression in adult patients, Loblaw and Laperriere have reviewed the available studies on the use of dexamethasone.[85] They found strong evidence to support the use of high-dose dexamethasone with radiation therapy, with improved outcome, but significant associated toxicity.[86] They also reported evidence judged to be fair that dexamethasone does not need to be given to asymptomatic ambulatory patients with spinal cord compression receiving x-ray therapy.[87] Although there is no corresponding evidence to support the role of dexamethasone in improving outcome in spinal cord compression caused by solid tumors in pediatric patients, little substantial detrimental effect has been observed with the routine use of dexamethasone in the setting of acute spinal cord compression. Increased infection and delayed wound healing are possible concerns. The use of gastric protectants is advised with dexamethasone, and these can include H2 blockers and proton pump inhibitors. Blood pressure should be monitored and any increase above age norms treated appropriately.

In the case of a child presenting with a high index of suspicion of spinal cord compression caused by tumor and *any* neurologic compromise, rapid administration of dexamethasone at 1 to 2 mg/kg IV to be administered over 30 minutes is suggested. This should be administered prior to imaging. If no neurologic symptoms are present, lower oral dosing, 0.25 to 0.5 mg every 6 hours, may be initiated while imaging is arranged. If the child is found to have a spinal lesion, and radiation therapy is chosen as the modality for treatment of cord compression, moderate-dose dexamethasone is sometimes continued to decrease the effects of radiation-induced swelling and vasogenic edema.

Radiotherapy

Most tumors causing spinal cord compression in the pediatric population will respond to radiotherapy, so this modality can often be used emergently to relieve symptoms of spinal cord compression effectively. The benefits of its use include possible rapid response, reasonable tolerance, and avoidance of more invasive procedures. Drawbacks include possible long-term effects on the spinal column, including stunted growth, cord damage, scoliosis, thyroid dysfunction, and the risk of second tumors. Additionally, young pediatric patients may require anesthesia for planning and delivery of x-ray therapy fractions. For safety and accuracy, adequate imaging, usually through MRI, is required to define the length, depth, and width of the planned treatment field.

Several approaches can be used to deliver a therapeutic treatment dose.[88] Midline lesions, as well as lesions in the lumbar spine, may be treated through a parallel opposed anteroposterior-posteroanterior beam arrangement. A posterior field alone can be used for lesions in the thoracic spine. The cervical spine may be treated with opposed lateral fields in an effort to avoid the oral cavity. Current techniques can allow for more precise localization of the radiation therapy to the tumor volume; however, these methods require more elaborate planning, and may delay the initiation of therapy. The potential benefit of a more conformal field must be weighed against the additional time and planning required.

Radiotherapy dose and schedule are determined by the pathologic diagnosis, extent of spinal involvement, possible coadministration of chemotherapy, and patient's clinical situation (e.g., previously ambulatory or nonambulatory, overall life expectancy, likelihood of response to systemic therapy, previous history of radiation therapy.) A dosing range of 18 to 40 Gy can be used. Typical schedules include 30 Gy delivered in 10 fractions, 20 Gy given in 5 fractions, or up to 35 to 40 Gy spread over a more protracted course of 3 to 4 weeks.

The concomitant use of dexamethasone is often recommended with radiation therapy. Dexamethasone is usually begun at a high dose prior to starting XRT, continued at a lesser dose during the procedure, and tapered off after completion. The use of dexamethasone with a taper is thought to decrease some of the edema that can occur as a result of the radiotherapy.

Clinical Studies

Although much laudable investigation has been done on the question of the best choice of initial therapy for children with spinal cord compression, no consensus has been reached. The available data are most limited by relatively small sample size, given the rarity of occurrence. Larger series tend to group multiple histologic diagnoses, which may respond differently to the interventions of chemotherapy, radiation, and surgery. Many of the studies also span long intervals and cannot necessarily take into account modernization of practice, improved imaging modalities, and improved therapeutic options.

Pollono and colleagues[81] have reported on a review of 70 pediatric patients with spinal cord compression treated at a single institution from 1984 to 2001; 71% were extradural tumors and 54% were soft tissue sarcomas and neuroblastoma.

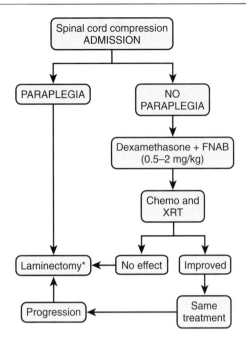

FIGURE 28-8. Algorithm for diagnosis and treatment of spinal cord compression. *With tumor resection, paraplegia of less than 96-hour evolution in patients less than 1 year and of less than 24 hours in older patients. Ch, chemotherapy; FNAB, fine-needle aspiration biopsy for diagnosis; Rdt, radiotherapy; XRT, x-ray therapy. *(Adapted from Pollono D, Tomarchia S, Drut R, et al. Spinal cord compression: a review of 70 pediatric patients. Pediatr Hematol Oncol. 2003;20:457-466.)*

Figure 28-8 presents the algorithm by which these patients were diagnosed and treated. Patients with paraplegia of less than 96 hours' duration underwent laminectomy, as did patients with primary spinal cord tumor or isolated recurrence of main tumor, progression of symptoms after radiation or chemotherapy or, if known, a radiation- and chemotherapy-resistant tumor. Surgery was avoided when the prognosis of primary tumor was poor or risks were thought to outweigh benefits. Of patients with paraplegia, 57% became ambulatory after laminectomy, whereas only 14% improved after chemotherapy and radiation; of patients who presented without paraplegia and received medical treatment without surgery, 87% remained ambulatory. Overall survival was related to the original malignancy. It was concluded that patients with chemotherapy- and radiotherapy-sensitive tumors without evidence of progressive neurologic damage may be treated with chemotherapy and/or radiation therapy, but that any indication of neurologic progression is a strong indication for laminectomy without delay.

The question of up-front chemotherapy versus surgery or radiation therapy for spinal cord compression has been most studied in pediatric patients with neuroblastoma, because rapid improvement with initial chemotherapy has been demonstrated. The first reports on the use of chemotherapy as front line therapy in children presenting with dumbbell neuroblastoma was published in 1984 by Hayes and associates[89]; 11 children with presenting neurologic symptoms were treated, and 9 had complete recovery and 2 demonstrated sustained paraplegia. In 1989, Sanderson and coworkers[90] also reported encouraging results of two children with paraplegia and two with paraparesis who both demonstrated full neurologic recovery after treatment with vincristine, cisplatin, etoposide, and cyclophosphamide (OPEC) therapy. Since then, more investigation has been done

on the use of front-line chemotherapy over neurosurgical intervention. Prospective and retrospective studies have attempted to elucidate whether chemotherapy or surgery is the best initial choice of therapy but the results yielded conflicting conclusions. The variability in outcome likely reflects the difficulty of appropriately grouping patients based on initial presenting signs and extent of disease, as well as institutional practice variations and availability of resources.

A series of these studies has been well summarized.[84] Studies from several major international cooperative groups (Italy, Germany, Poland, United Kingdom, and United States) were reviewed. The Italian Cooperative Group for Neuroblastoma has reported a prospective study in which 26 patients with neuroblastoma and spinal cord compression were preferentially given chemotherapy over surgery or radiation therapy. Prior to this study, patients followed between 1979 and 1998 by this group had been analyzed.[91] The retrospective analysis showed that radiotherapy, laminectomy, and chemotherapy have comparable ability to improve spinal cord compression. The following prospective study also concluded that chemotherapy adequately relieves neurologic symptoms in most patients. Neurologic and orthopedic sequelae were seen in a large number of patients, including those who received chemotherapy only.

In another prospective study carried out by the French Society of Paediatric Oncology,[92] 78 patients with intraspinal extension of neuroblastoma were treated, beginning in 1990. Of these, 86% were initially treated with chemotherapy; 63% had a complete neurologic recovery and 21% had a partial neurologic recovery. Also, 13% failed to improve with chemotherapy, 1 patient progressed, 14% underwent primary surgery, 23% of initially symptomatic patients (10 of 43) had severe neurologic sequelae, 16% had mild sequelae, and 23% were reported to have severe orthopedic sequelae.

One of the largest series reviewed was of 83 patients registered on the Pediatric Oncology Group (POG) NB Biology Protocol 9047[93]; 66 patients received up-front chemotherapy, 23 underwent primary laminectomy, 8 received initial radiotherapy, and 31 underwent initial surgical resection without laminectomy. From this series of retrospectively collected data, it was concluded that patients with neurologic symptoms can be managed without laminectomy, and that laminectomy should be reserved for patients who demonstrate progressive neurologic deterioration after initial chemotherapy. The likelihood of neurologic sequelae was found to be inversely related to the length of symptoms prior to initiation of treatment, and more severe sequelae were seen in patients presenting with more severe symptoms. Twenty-nine percent of patients had orthopedic sequelae; the incidence was significantly lower in patients managed with chemotherapy compared with those who underwent laminectomy.

After a review of multiple studies, the primary conclusion of the neuroblastoma workshop was that there exists a need for the creation of an international spinal registry.[84] It specified the need to standardize language and criteria to group patients with comparable degrees of neurologic compromise at presentation accurately and to characterize the late effects uniformly. A functional grading system proposed by Gilber and colleagues[93a] was used in some studies to aid in outcome analysis, but has not been universally adopted (Table 28-5). This grading system notably does not take into account sphincter dysfunction, an important neurologic finding.

It was also concluded that chemotherapy is a reasonable initial approach, but laminectomy should be used for patients who demonstrate progressive neurologic symptoms after presentation or no restoration in the short term.[84] Patients with symptoms occurring within 96 hours of presentation may also be considered as candidates for surgical intervention. There

TABLE 28-5	Functional Grading Scale of Spinal Cord Compression
Grade	**Patient Function**
1	Ambulatory, with or without weakness of lower extremities or ataxia
2	Not ambulatory, but able to lift legs against gravity when supine
3	Paraplegic and unable to move legs against gravity

From Lewis DW, Packer RJ, Raney B, et al. Incidence, presentation, and outcome of spinal cord disease in children with systemic cancer. Pediatrics. 1986;78:438-443.

was also a proposal that radiotherapy may be underused in spinal cord compression caused by neuroblastoma.

The findings of this group cannot be generalized for other types of malignancy. Smaller series of outcomes of patients with Ewing's sarcoma and intraspinal lesions have also described mixed use of up-front therapies, with variable outcomes. In a report of a series of seven patients with primary Ewing's sarcoma of the spine, as well as a review of the literature, Sharafuddin and colleagues[94] noted the importance of the location (sacral or nonsacral) of the presenting lesion in the response to treatment. Differences in response in adult and pediatric patients were also noted. Figure 28-9 shows the algorithm that they proposed for the management of primary Ewing's sarcoma of the spine. Initial chemotherapy or limited surgical decompression is recommended for all pediatric patients; surgical intervention is clearly indicated for patients who demonstrate progressive findings with medical treatment.

The rare cases of leukemia and lymphoma that present with spinal cord compression should be treated with initial chemotherapy. Radiotherapy can be considered for some special cases.

Late Effects

The long-term consequences of spinal cord compression and its management include neurologic compromise and orthopedic effects, and the choice of initial management takes heavily into account an attempt to minimize those late effects. A number of reports have supported the observation that neurologic sequelae are most related to the degree of presenting neurologic compromise; the more severe the neurologic compromise at presentation, the more likely long-term sequelae will be seen. Other studies have also shown that the duration of time between the development of neurologic symptoms and initiation of therapy is inversely correlated with the degree of neurologic recovery.[93] Although laminectomy may be the most likely method to correct or prevent neurologic sequelae, it is clearly not necessary in all cases of spinal cord compression, particularly in neuroblastoma, and carries the greatest risk of orthopedic sequelae. Orthopedic sequelae include scoliosis, growth impairment, and spinal instability. Orthopedic sequelae are related to the spinal level of the lesion and the age of the patient at treatment. The most severe sequelae are seen in patients with thoracic versus lumbar lesions and age younger than 12 months. Although a wide range of rates of sequelae has been reported, almost all studies have supported the observation of significantly greater orthopedic sequelae in patients who undergo surgery. A study by Hoover and associates[95] has found a scoliosis incidence of 67% in patients who underwent laminectomy compared with an incidence of 36% in patients who

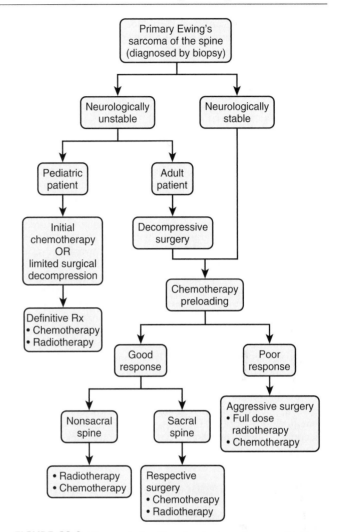

FIGURE 28-9. Proposed algorithm for the management of primary Ewing's sarcoma of the spine. *(Adapted from Sharafuddin MJA, Haddad FS, Hitchon PW, et al. Treatment options in primary Ewing's sarcoma of the spine: report of seven cases and review of the literature. Neurosurgery. 1992;30:610-618.)*

did not. Correlation between late effects, including differences in health-related quality of life and initial treatment, remain at the center of investigations into the optimal choice of initial therapy.

COMPLICATIONS OF CHEMOTHERAPY

The use of chemotherapeutic agents carries risks for multiple acute and chronic toxicities and potential complications. Here several oncologic emergencies related to the use of particular chemotherapeutic agents are summarized. These must be recognized and managed effectively to prevent patient morbidity and mortality.

Vesicant Extravasation

Extravasation of vesicant chemotherapeutic agents can result in severe patient morbidity, with the development of extensive tissue damage. Vesicant agents include anthracyclines, vinca alkaloids, mechlorethamine, and taxanes. Extravasation of anthracycline agents such as doxorubicin and daunorubicin can result in particularly severe and progressive tissue necrosis.[96] Importantly, the use of a central venous access device does not preclude the possibility of extravasation. Blood return or other evidence of patency, such as a dye study, is needed before a vesicant is administered in a central venous line. Once extravasation is suspected, usually because of swelling, redness, and pain at the injection site, administration of the agent should be stopped and assessment and treatment initiated.

Anthracycline extravasation has traditionally been managed by the application of ice packs, although many other local measures have been attempted, with undocumented success (e.g., injection of steroid, bicarbonate solution, or dimethylsulfoxide). Surgical débridement of affected areas may be required.[97] In 2007, the FDA approved dexrazoxane hydrochloride (Totect) for injection for the treatment of extravasation resulting from intravenous anthracycline chemotherapy.[98] In two studies, 57 evaluable patients underwent biopsy-proven extravasation of anthracycline from peripheral vein or central venous access sites. Totect was administered within 6 hours of extravasation for three doses, repeated 24 and 48 hours after the first dose. One patient required surgical intervention and the remaining patients had mild or no sequelae.[99] The use of Totect in the pediatric population has not been separately reported.

Mechlorethamine extravasation can also result in tissue necrosis. The manufacturer recommends the local injection of sodium thiosulfate into the extravasation area, followed by topical application of ice. Vinca alkaloid extravasation management includes application of warm compresses and local injections of hyaluronidase.[100] Cooling the area has been recommended for taxane extravasation.[97]

Methotrexate-Induced Renal Dysfunction

Nephrotoxicity associated with high-dose methotrexate administration can be considered a true oncologic emergency. Although the strategies of hydration, alkalinization, and leucovorin rescue with close monitoring of methotrexate concentration and serum creatinine usually allow for safe administration of high-dose methotrexate, nephrotoxicity still occurs in some patients. Renal dysfunction was found to occur in approximately 1.8% of patients with osteosarcoma treated in clinical trials.[101] Renal dysfunction can result in persistently elevated methotrexate levels. Delayed clearance of the drug amplifies methotrexate's other toxic effects, such as mucositis and myelosuppression.[102] In the patient with methotrexate-induced renal dysfunction, increasing leucovorin administration based on plasma methotrexate concentration remains a key intervention. Hemodialysis, hemoperfusion, and peritoneal dialysis have had inconsistent or limited success in this setting.[101] Carboxypeptidase-G2 (CPDG2), a recombinant bacterial enzyme, offers another emergency treatment option.[103,104] CPDG2 provides a route of elimination other than renal clearance by metabolizing methotrexate to the inactive metabolite, 2,4-diamino-N10-methylpteroic acid (DAMPA).[105] Within minutes of administration, CPDG2 results in an approximately 97% reduction in plasma methotrexate concentration, allowing for continued management with leucovorin.

Intrathecal Chemotherapy Overdose

Measures to prevent errors and overdose in the administration of intrathecal chemotherapeutic agents are key to avoiding this potentially devastating complication, fortunately making them rare events in clinical practice. Such errors, however, have been reported, underscoring the importance of having plans for treatment and management in place in case such an adverse event occurs. Immediate response is crucial; case reports and small series highlight potential strategies.

Intrathecal overdose of methotrexate can result in coma and death. Treatment options for intrathecal methotrexate overdoses have traditionally included cerebrospinal fluid (CSF) drainage, ventriculolumbar CSF perfusion, and systemic steroids and systemic leucovorin.[106] Immediate removal of CSF has been advocated. The intrathecal use of leucovorin has not been advocated.[107] The intrathecal use of carboxypeptidase G2 has also been reported.[108] In a 2004 report, Widemann and coworkers[106] presented results of a collaborative protocol assessing the intrathecal administration of carboxypeptidase G2 in seven cancer patients who had received accidental overdoses of intrathecal methotrexate, defined as a dose over 100 mg. They found that methotrexate concentrations in the CSF declined by more than 98% in all patients and that all patients recovered completely from the overdose, except for two patients of 61 and 77 years with memory impairment. Four of the cases were pediatric cases, with ages ranging from 5 to 9 years. Three of these cases received a 600-mg dose of methotrexate, two underwent CSF exchange, and all were reported to have a complete recovery. It was concluded that carboxypeptidase G2 should be considered for intrathecal methotrexate overdose.

One case report of an intrathecal overdose of cytarabine in a 4-year-old was managed with CSF exchange, and the patient survived.[109] At any dose, intrathecal vincristine is usually fatal.[110] Clearly, preventive measures in prescribing, preparing, and delivering intrathecal chemotherapy remain essential.

REFERENCES

1. Kravitz SC, Diamond HD, Craver LF. Uremia complicating leukemia chemotherapy; report of a case treated with triethylene melamine. JAMA. 1951;146:1595-1597.
2. Zusman J, Brown DM, Nesbit ME. Hyperphosphatemia, hyperphosphaturia and hypocalcemia in acute lymphoblastic leukemia. N Engl J Med. 1973;289:1335-1340.
3. Nicolin G. Emergencies and their management. Eur J Cancer. 2002;38:1365-1377.
4. Pession A, Barbieri E. Treatment and prevention of tumor lysis syndrome in children. Experience of Associazione Italiana Ematologia Oncologia Pediatrica. Contrib Nephrol. 2005;147:80-92.
5. Tiu RV, Mountantonakis SE, Dunbar AJ, Schreiber MJ Jr. Tumor lysis syndrome. Semin Thromb Hemost. 2007;33:397-407.
6. Klinenberg JR, Goldfinger SE, Seegmiller JE. The effectiveness of the xanthine oxidase inhibitor allopurinol in the treatment of gout. Ann Intern Med. 1965;62:639-647.
7. Frei E 3rd, Bentzel CJ, Rieselbach R, Block JB. Renal complications of neoplastic disease. J Chronic Dis. 1963;16:757-776.
8. Cohen LF, Balow JE, Magrath IT, et al. Acute tumor lysis syndrome. A review of 37 patients with Burkitt's lymphoma. Am J Med. 1980;68:486-491.
9. Hebert LA, Lemann J Jr, Petersen JR, Lennon EJ. Studies of the mechanism by which phosphate infusion lowers serum calcium concentration. J Clin Invest. 1966;45:1886-1894.
10. Avci Z, Alioglu B, Canan O, et al. Calcification of the gastric mucosa associated with tumor lysis syndrome in a child with non-Hodgkin lymphoma. J Pediatr Hematol Oncol. 2006;28:307-310.

11. Hande KR, Garrow GC. Acute tumor lysis syndrome in patients with high-grade non-Hodgkin's lymphoma. Am J Med. 1993;94: 133-139.

12. Annemans L, Moeremans K, Lamotte M, et al. Pan-European multicentre economic evaluation of recombinant urate oxidase (rasburicase) in prevention and treatment of hyperuricaemia and tumour lysis syndrome in haematologic cancer patients. Support Care Cancer. 2003;11:249-257.

13. Seidemann K, Meyer U, Jansen P, et al. Impaired renal function and tumor lysis syndrome in pediatric patients with non-Hodgkin's lymphoma and B-ALL. Observations from the BFM-trials. Klin Padiatr. 1998;210:279-284.

14. Wossmann W, Schrappe M, Meyer U, et al. Incidence of tumor lysis syndrome in children with advanced stage Burkitt's lymphoma/leukemia before and after introduction of prophylactic use of urate oxidase. Ann Hematol. 2003;82:160-165.

15. Baeksgaard L, Sorensen JB. Acute tumor lysis syndrome in solid tumors—a case report and review of the literature. Cancer Chemother Pharmacol. 2003;51:187-192.

16. Cairo MS, Bishop M. Tumour lysis syndrome: new therapeutic strategies and classification. Br J Haematol. 2004;127:3-11.

17. Andreoli SP, Clark JH, McGuire WA, Bergstein JM. Purine excretion during tumor lysis in children with acute lymphocytic leukemia receiving allopurinol: relationship to acute renal failure. J Pediatr. 1986;109:292-298.

18. Jones DP, Mahmoud H, Chesney RW. Tumor lysis syndrome: pathogenesis and management. Pediatr Nephrol. 1995;9:206-212.

19. Watts RW, Watts JE, Seegmiller JE. Xanthine oxidase activity in human tissues and its inhibition by allopurinol (4-hydroxypyrazolo[3,4-d] pyrimidine). J Lab Clin Med. 1965;66:688-697.

20. Krakoff IH, Meyer RL. Prevention of hyperuricemia in leukemia and lymphoma: use of alopurinol, a xanthine oxidase inhibitor. JAMA. 1965;193:1-6.

21. DeConti RC, Calabresi P. Use of allopurinol for prevention and control of hyperuricemia in patients with neoplastic disease. N Engl J Med. 1966;274:481-486.

22. Davidson MB, Thakkar S, Hix JK, et al. Pathophysiology, clinical consequences, and treatment of tumor lysis syndrome. Am J Med. 2004;116:546-554.

23. Yim BT, Sims-McCallum RP, Chong PH. Rasburicase for the treatment and prevention of hyperuricemia. Ann Pharmacother. 2003;37:1047-1054.

24. Pui CH, Relling MV, Lascombes F, et al. Urate oxidase in prevention and treatment of hyperuricemia associated with lymphoid malignancies. Leukemia. 1997;11:1813-1816.

25. Pui CH, Mahmoud HH, Wiley JM, et al. Recombinant urate oxidase for the prophylaxis or treatment of hyperuricemia in patients with leukemia or lymphoma. J Clin Oncol. 2001;19: 697-704.

26. Goldman SC, Holcenberg JS, Finklestein JZ, et al. A randomized comparison between rasburicase and allopurinol in children with lymphoma or leukemia at high risk for tumor lysis. Blood. 2001;97:2998-3003.

27. Browning LA, Kruse JA. Hemolysis and methemoglobinemia secondary to rasburicase administration. Ann Pharmacother. 2005;39:1932-1935.

28. Jeha S, Kantarjian H, Irwin D, et al. Efficacy and safety of rasburicase, a recombinant urate oxidase (Elitek), in the management of malignancy-associated hyperuricemia in pediatric and adult patients: final results of a multicenter compassionate use trial. Leukemia. 2005;19:34-38.

29. McDonnell AM, Lenz KL, Frei-Lahr DA, et al. Single-dose rasburicase 6 mg in the management of tumor lysis syndrome in adults. Pharmacotherapy. 2006;26:806-812.

30. Hutcherson DA, Gammon DC, Bhatt MS, Faneuf M. Reduced-dose rasburicase in the treatment of adults with hyperuricemia associated with malignancy. Pharmacotherapy. 2006;26:242-247.

31. Annemans L, Moeremans K, Lamotte M, et al. Incidence, medical resource utilisation and costs of hyperuricemia and tumour lysis syndrome in patients with acute leukaemia and non-Hodgkin's lymphoma in four European countries. Leuk Lymphoma. 2003;44:77-83.

32. Deger GE, Wagoner RD. Peritoneal dialysis in acute uric acid nephropathy. Mayo Clin Proc. 1972;47:189-192.

33. Heney D, Essex-Cater A, Brocklebank JT, et al. Continuous arteriovenous haemofiltration in the treatment of tumour lysis syndrome. Pediatr Nephrol. 1990;4:245-247.

34. Saccente SL, Kohaut EC, Berkow RL. Prevention of tumor lysis syndrome using continuous veno-venous hemofiltration. Pediatr Nephrol. 1995;9:569-573.

35. Cortes JE, Kantarjian HM. Acute lymphoblastic leukemia. A comprehensive review with emphasis on biology and therapy. Cancer. 1995;76:2393-2417.

36. Porcu P, Cripe LD, Ng EW, et al. Hyperleukocytic leukemias and leukostasis: a review of pathophysiology, clinical presentation and management. Leuk Lymphoma. 2000;39:1-18.

37. Creutzig U, Ritter J, Budde M, et al. Early deaths caused by hemorrhage and leukostasis in childhood acute myelogenous leukemia. Associations with hyperleukocytosis and acute monocytic leukemia. Cancer. 1987;60:3071-3079.

38. Bunin NJ, Pui CH. Differing complications of hyperleukocytosis in children with acute lymphoblastic or acute nonlymphoblastic leukemia. J Clin Oncol. 1985;3:1590-1595.

39. Wurthner JU, Kohler G, Behringer D, et al. Leukostasis followed by hemorrhage complicating the initiation of chemotherapy in patients with acute myeloid leukemia and hyperleukocytosis: a clinicopathologic report of four cases. Cancer. 1999;85:368-374.

40. Lichtman MA, Rowe JM. Hyperleukocytic leukemias: rheological, clinical, and therapeutic considerations. Blood. 1982;60: 279-283.

41. Thornton KA, Levis M. Images in clinical medicine. FLT3 Mutation and acute myelogenous leukemia with leukostasis. N Engl J Med. 2007;357:1639.

42. Williams DL, Bell BA, Ragab AH. Clitorism at presentation of acute nonlymphocytic leukemia. J Pediatr. 1985;107:754-755.

43. Dearth JC, Fountain KS, Smithson WA, et al. Extreme leukemic leukocytosis (blast crisis) in childhood. Mayo Clin Proc. 1978;53: 207-211.

44. Novotny JR, Muller-Beissenhirtz H, Herget-Rosenthal S, et al. Grading of symptoms in hyperleukocytic leukaemia: a clinical model for the role of different blast types and promyelocytes in the development of leukostasis syndrome. Eur J Haematol. 2005;74:501-510.

45. Novotny JR, Nuckel H, Duhrsen U. Correlation between expression of CD56/NCAM and severe leukostasis in hyperleukocytic acute myelomonocytic leukaemia. Eur J Haematol. 2006;76: 299-308.

46. Stucki A, Rivier AS, Gikic M, et al. Endothelial cell activation by myeloblasts: molecular mechanisms of leukostasis and leukemic cell dissemination. Blood. 2001;97:2121-2129.

47. Vahdat L, Maslak P, Miller WH Jr, et al. Early mortality and the retinoic acid syndrome in acute promyelocytic leukemia: impact of leukocytosis, low-dose chemotherapy, PMN/RAR-alpha isoform, and CD13 expression in patients treated with all-trans retinoic acid. Blood. 1994;84:3843-3849.

48. Myers TJ, Cole SR, Klatsky AU, Hild DH. Respiratory failure due to pulmonary leukostasis following chemotherapy of acute nonlymphocytic leukemia. Cancer. 1983;51:1808-1813.

49. Porcu P, Danielson CF, Orazi A, et al. Therapeutic leukapheresis in hyperleucocytic leukaemias: lack of correlation between degree of cytoreduction and early mortality rate. Br J Haematol. 1997;98: 433-436.

50. Basade M, Dhar AK, Kulkarni SS, et al. Rapid cytoreduction in childhood leukemic hyperleukocytosis by conservative therapy. Med Pediatr Oncol. 1995;25:204-207.

51. Wiernik PH, Serpick AA. Factors effecting remission and survival in adult acute nonlymphocytic leukemia (ANLL). Medicine (Baltimore). 1970;49:505-513.

52. Wald BR, Heisel MA, Ortega JA. Frequency of early death in children with acute leukemia presenting with hyperleukocytosis. Cancer. 1982;50:150-153.

53. Maurer HS, Steinherz PG, Gaynon PS, et al. The effect of initial management of hyperleukocytosis on early complications and outcome of children with acute lymphoblastic leukemia. J Clin Oncol. 1988;6:1425-1432.

54. Nelson SC, Bruggers CS, Kurtzberg J, Friedman HS. Management of leukemic hyperleukocytosis with hydration, urinary alkalinization, and allopurinol. Are cranial irradiation and invasive cytoreduction necessary? Am J Pediatr Hematol Oncol. 1993;15:351-355.

55. Butler RW, Hill JM, Steinherz PG, et al. Neuropsychologic effects of cranial irradiation, intrathecal methotrexate, and systemic methotrexate in childhood cancer. J Clin Oncol. 1994;12:2621-2629.

56. Eguiguren JM, Schell MJ, Crist WM, et al. Complications and outcome in childhood acute lymphoblastic leukemia with hyperleukocytosis. Blood. 1992;79:871-875.

57. Cuttner J, Holland JF, Norton L, et al. Therapeutic leukapheresis for hyperleukocytosis in acute myelocytic leukemia. Med Pediatr Oncol. 1983;11:76-78.

58. Giles FJ, Shen Y, Kantarjian HM, et al. Leukapheresis reduces early mortality in patients with acute myeloid leukemia with high white cell counts but does not improve long-term survival. Leuk Lymphoma. 2001;42:67-73.

59. Grund FM, Armitage JO, Burns P. Hydroxyurea in the prevention of the effects of leukostasis in acute leukemia. Arch Intern Med. 1977;137:1246-1247.

60. Kuo A, Terrault NA. Management of hepatitis C in liver transplant recipients. Am J Transplant. 2006;6:449-458.

61. Robie DK, Gursoy MH, Pokorny WJ. Mediastinal tumors—airway obstruction and management. Semin Pediatr Surg. 1994;3:259-266.

62. King RM, Telander RL, Smithson WA, et al. Primary mediastinal tumors in children. J Pediatr Surg. 1982;17:512-520.

63. Ingram L, Rivera GK, Shapiro DN. Superior vena cava syndrome associated with childhood malignancy: analysis of 24 cases. Med Pediatr Oncol. 1990;18:476-481.

64. Yellin A, Rosen A, Reichert N, Lieberman Y. Superior vena cava syndrome. The myth—the facts. Am Rev Respir Dis. 1990;141:1114-1118.

65. Hunter W. The history of an aneurysm of the aorta, with some remarks on aneurysms in general. Med Obser Inq. 1757;1:323.

66. Azizkhan RG, Dudgeon DL, Buck JR, et al. Life-threatening airway obstruction as a complication to the management of mediastinal masses in children. J Pediatr Surg. 1985;20:816-822.

67. Halpern S, Chatten J, Meadows AT, et al. Anterior mediastinal masses: anesthesia hazards and other problems. J Pediatr. 1983;102:407-410.

68. Chaignaud BE, Bonsack TA, Kozakewich HP, Shamberger RC. Pleural effusions in lymphoblastic lymphoma: a diagnostic alternative. J Pediatr Surg. 1998;33:1355-1357.

69. Ferrari LR, Bedford RF. General anesthesia prior to treatment of anterior mediastinal masses in pediatric cancer patients. Anesthesiology. 1990;72:991-995.

70. Bergman NA. Reduction in resting end-expiratory position of the respiratory system with induction of anesthesia and neuromuscular paralysis. Anesthesiology. 1982;57:14-17.

71. Shamberger RC. Preanesthetic evaluation of children with anterior mediastinal masses. Semin Pediatr Surg. 1999;8:61-68.

72. Pullerits J, Holzman R. Anaesthesia for patients with mediastinal masses. Can J Anaesth. 1989;36:681-688.

73. Shamberger RC, Holzman RS, Griscom NT, et al. CT quantitation of tracheal cross-sectional area as a guide to the surgical and anesthetic management of children with anterior mediastinal masses. J Pediatr Surg. 1991;26:138-142.

74. Anghelescu DL, Burgoyne LL, Liu T, et al. Clinical and diagnostic imaging findings predict anesthetic complications in children presenting with malignant mediastinal masses. Paediatr Anaesth. 2007;17:1090-1098.

75. Kirks DR, Fram EK, Vock P, Effmann EL. Tracheal compression by mediastinal masses in children: CT evaluation. AJR Am J Roentgenol. 1983;141:647-651.

76. Shamberger RC, Holzman RS, Griscom NT, et al. Prospective evaluation by computed tomography and pulmonary function tests of children with mediastinal masses. Surgery. 1995;118:468-471.

77. Frey TK, Chopra A, Lin RJ, et al. A child with anterior mediastinal mass supported with veno-arterial extracorporeal membrane oxygenation. Pediatr Crit Care Med. 2006;7:479-481.

78. Polaner DM. The use of heliox and the laryngeal mask airway in a child with an anterior mediastinal mass. Anesth Analg. 1996;82:208-210.

79. Loeffler JS, Leopold KA, Recht A, et al. Emergency prebiopsy radiation for mediastinal masses: impact on subsequent pathologic diagnosis and outcome. J Clin Oncol. 1986;4:716-721.

80. Lewis DW, Packer RJ, Raney B, et al. Incidence, presentation, and outcome of spinal cord disease in children with systemic cancer. Pediatrics. 1986;78:438-443.

81. Pollono D, Tomarchia S, Drut R, et al. Spinal cord compression: a review of 70 pediatric patients. Pediatr Hematol Oncol. 2003;20:457-466.

82. Rheingold SR, Lange BJ. Oncologic emergencies. In Pizzo PA, Poplack DG (eds). Principles and Practice of Pediatric Oncology, 5th ed. Philadelphia, Lippincott Williams & Wilkins, 2005, pp 1202-1230.

83. Khanna AJ, Shindle MK, Wasserman BA, et al. Use of magnetic resonance imaging in differentiating compartmental location of spinal tumors. Am J Orthop. 2005;34:472-476.

84. De Bernardi B, Balwierz W, Bejent J, et al. Epidural compression in neuroblastoma: diagnostic and therapeutic aspects. Cancer Lett. 2005;228:283-299.

85. Loblaw DA, Laperriere NJ. Emergency treatment of malignant extradural spinal cord compression: an evidence-based guideline. J Clin Oncol. 1998;16:1613-1624.

86. Sorensen S, Helweg-Larsen S, Mouridsen H, Hansen HH. Effect of high-dose dexamethasone in carcinomatous metastatic spinal cord compression treated with radiotherapy: a randomised trial. Eur J Cancer. 1994;30A:22-27.

87. Maranzano E, Latini P, Beneventi S, et al. Radiotherapy without steroids in selected metastatic spinal cord compression patients. A phase II trial. Am J Clin Oncol. 1996;19:179-183.

88. Porter AT, David M. Palliation of metastases: bone, spinal cord, brain, liver. In Gunderson LL, Tepper JE (eds). Clinical Radiation Oncology, 2nd ed. Philadelphia, Churchill-Livingstone, 2007, pp 449-455.

89. Hayes FA, Thompson EI, Hvizdala E, et al. Chemotherapy as an alternative to laminectomy and radiation in the management of epidural tumor. J Pediatr. 1984;104:221-224.

90. Sanderson IR, Pritchard J, Marsh HT. Chemotherapy as the initial treatment of spinal cord compression due to disseminated neuroblastoma. J Neurosurg. 1989;70:688-690.

91. De Bernardi B, Pianca C, Pistamiglio P, et al. Neuroblastoma with symptomatic spinal cord compression at diagnosis: treatment and results with 76 cases. J Clin Oncol. 2001;19:183-190.

92. Plantaz D, Rubie H, Michon J, et al. The treatment of neuroblastoma with intraspinal extension with chemotherapy followed by surgical removal of residual disease. A prospective study of 42

patients—results of the NBL 90 Study of the French Society of Pediatric Oncology. Cancer. 1996;78:311-319.

93. Katzenstein HM, Kent PM, London WB, Cohn SL. Treatment and outcome of 83 children with intraspinal neuroblastoma: the Pediatric Oncology Group experience. J Clin Oncol. 2001;19:1047-1055.

93a. Gilber RW, Kim J, Posner JB. Epidural spinal cord compression from metastatic tumor: diagnosis and treatment. Ann Neurol. 1978;3:40-51.

94. Sharafuddin MJ, Haddad FS, Hitchon PW, et al. Treatment options in primary Ewing's sarcoma of the spine: report of seven cases and review of the literature. Neurosurgery. 1992;30:610-618.

95. Hoover M, Bowman LC, Crawford SE, et al. Long-term outcome of patients with intraspinal neuroblastoma. Med Pediatr Oncol. 1999;32:353-359.

96. Linder RM, Upton J, Osteen R. Management of extensive doxorubicin hydrochloride extravasation injuries. J Hand Surg [Am]. 1983;8:32-38.

97. Schulmeister L. Managing vesicant extravasations. Oncologist. 2008;13:284-288.

98. Kane RC, McGuinn WD Jr, Dagher R, et al. Dexrazoxane (Totect): FDA review and approval for the treatment of accidental extravasation following intravenous anthracycline chemotherapy. Oncologist. 2008;13:445-450.

99. Mouridsen HT, Langer SW, Buter J, et al. Treatment of anthracycline extravasation with Savene (dexrazoxane): results from two prospective clinical multicentre studies. Ann Oncol. 2007;18:546-550.

100. Ener RA, Meglathery SB, Styler M. Extravasation of systemic hemato-oncologic therapies. Ann Oncol. 2004;15:858-862.

101. Widemann BC, Balis FM, Kempf-Bielack B, et al. High-dose methotrexate-induced nephrotoxicity in patients with osteosarcoma. Cancer. 2004;100:2222-2232.

102. Abelson HT, Fosburg MT, Beardsley GP, et al. Methotrexate-induced renal impairment: clinical studies and rescue from systemic toxicity with high-dose leucovorin and thymidine. J Clin Oncol. 1983;1:208-216.

103. Widemann BC, Balis FM, Murphy RF, et al. Carboxypeptidase-G2, thymidine, and leucovorin rescue in cancer patients with methotrexate-induced renal dysfunction. J Clin Oncol. 1997;15:2125-2134.

104. Buchen S, Ngampolo D, Melton RG, et al. Carboxypeptidase G2 rescue in patients with methotrexate intoxication and renal failure. Br J Cancer. 2005;92:480-487.

105. Widemann BC, Sung E, Anderson L, et al. Pharmacokinetics and metabolism of the methotrexate metabolite 2, 4-diamino-N(10)-methylpteroic acid. J Pharmacol Exp Ther. 2000;294:894-901.

106. Widemann BC, Balis FM, Shalabi A, et al. Treatment of accidental intrathecal methotrexate overdose with intrathecal carboxypeptidase G2. J Natl Cancer Inst. 2004;96:1557-1559.

107. Jardine LF, Ingram LC, Bleyer WA. Intrathecal leucovorin after intrathecal methotrexate overdose. J Pediatr Hematol Oncol. 1996;18:302-304.

108. O'Marcaigh AS, Johnson CM, Smithson WA, et al. Successful treatment of intrathecal methotrexate overdose by using ventriculolumbar perfusion and intrathecal instillation of carboxypeptidase G2. Mayo Clin Proc. 1996;71:161-165.

109. Lafolie P, Liliemark J, Bjork O, et al. Exchange of cerebrospinal fluid in accidental intrathecal overdose of cytarabine. Med Toxicol Adverse Drug Exp. 1988;3:248-252.

110. Trinkle R, Wu JK. Errors involving pediatric patients receiving chemotherapy: a literature review. Med Pediatr Oncol. 1996;26:344-351.

29 # Nursing Care of Patients with Childhood Cancer

Patricia A. Branowicki, Kathleen E. Houlahan, and Susanne B. Conley

HISTORY OF PEDIATRIC ONCOLOGY NURSING

Nursing is the largest health care occupation in the United States, representing 2.5 million jobs—a number that is expected to grow at a rate of 27% or more before 2014.[1,2] Because its roots are embedded in daily life and the caretaking role women traditionally assumed throughout history, nursing was not recognized as a profession until the mid-1800s, when Florence Nightingale identified the need for specialized education and training and developed the underpinnings of modern-day nursing practice.[1]

The first nurses were considered generalists and cared for patients of all ages. Pediatric nursing emerged as a specialty in the early 20th century, when free-standing children's hospitals became more common.[1] During this time, pediatric oncology patients were often cared for by pediatric nurses (sometimes called tumor therapy nurses) who learned to care for oncology patients through experience and self-directed, on-the-job training.[3-5]

The subspecialty of pediatric oncology nursing first appeared in the late 1940s and early 1950s, when courses specific to cancer nursing were introduced by the American Cancer Society, the University of Washington and the University of Minnesota School of Public Health.[1,4,6] It was formally recognized as a subspecialty practice in the mid-1970s, when more nursing schools began offering education specific to pediatric oncology, and a small cohort of nurses formed the Association of Pediatric Oncology Nurses (APON).[4,7,8] APON changed its name in 2006 to the Association of Pediatric Hematology/Oncology Nurses (APHON) and is considered the leading professional organization for registered nurses caring for children and adolescents with cancer and blood disorders.[9,10]

Over the years, the role of pediatric oncology nurses has evolved to match advances in cancer treatment. During the 1880s and early 1900s, the predominant treatment modality for cancer was surgery, and nursing care was focused primarily on relieving pain and meeting other postsurgical needs of patients.[6] Until the latter half of the 1900s, cancer was a metaphor for death, and nurses had few resources available to care for the patients it affected. Children diagnosed with cancer commonly died, diagnostic techniques and treatment were often not available, and care was typically palliative in nature.[4,5] The general attitude among health care professionals was that there was little to offer the person with cancer except a cheerful manner and a few comfort measures.[11]

After World War II, single-agent chemotherapy was introduced. This new therapy was administered only by physicians until the 1960s, when it was proposed that nurses assume this responsibility.[6] Today, chemotherapy is almost always administered by nurses, who as a discipline have been instrumental in developing standards for safe practice and education related to chemotherapy administration and symptom management.[7,12-14] Pediatric oncology nurses are also leaders in patient and family education, pain management, and palliative care. A 2006 survey of APON members highlights how nurses are integrally involved in caring for patients with all types of cancer. The top five practice areas noted in the survey were the specialties of leukemia/lymphoma (55%), solid tumor (38%), hematology (24%), hematopoietic stem cell transplantation (19%), and brain tumor (16%).[9]

Over the past few decades, a number of advanced-practice nursing roles have gained prominence. The term *advanced practice nurse* applies to nurses in specialized roles, including clinical nurse specialists, nurse practitioners, certified nurse midwives, and nurse anesthetists, who have completed additional formal education and training. In pediatric oncology settings, it is the clinical nurse specialist and the pediatric nurse practitioner who are most commonly employed. Although their responsibilities vary among institutions, the clinical nurse specialist generally focuses on the education of the staff and of patients and families, whereas the pediatric nurse practitioner usually provides direct patient care in consultation with the patient's oncologist. As a primary oncology provider, the pediatric nurse practitioner follows patients and families over time and helps to formulate, implement, and evaluate the patient's plan of care. Depending on institutional, state, and federal regulations, a pediatric nurse practitioner may also prescribe medications and perform procedures, such as bone marrow biopsies and lumbar punctures. Standards and guidelines regarding professional behaviors and scope of practice developed by APHON and the American Nurses Association also guide the practice of advanced practice nurses.[15]

Pediatric oncology nurses at all levels will continue to play critical roles in the care of children with cancer as new diagnostic and treatment techniques become available. Through persistence, vigilance, and dedication, nurses will shape the development and modification of practice standards that promote safe and effective pediatric cancer care.[16,7]

Nursing Education and Professional Certification

When nursing first emerged as a profession, nursing education was typically provided by hospital-based diploma programs.[17] Today, most of the diploma programs have closed and have been replaced by college- and university-based schools of nursing. Nurses specializing in pediatric oncology usually receive advanced training in all aspects of cancer and cancer treatment, including chemotherapy, the management of complications related to therapy, pediatric oncology protocols, and the protection of human subjects.[18-20] In addition to this specialized training, APHON and most health care organizations recommend that pediatric oncology nurses obtain professional certification, although it is not a requirement for practice. Certification was first introduced in 1999, and since then more than 1650 registered nurses have become certified pediatric oncology nurses.[10,21-23]

OVERVIEW OF THE PEDIATRIC ONCOLOGY NURSE'S ROLE

Historically, nurses were viewed as skillful technicians who provided physical care, advocated for patients, collected data, and served physicians.[5,24] Over time, the profile of nurses evolved, and today's nurses are respected for their professional expertise and unique contributions to patient care. Although still guided by medical orders and institutional policies, pediatric oncology nurses rely on their intellect, critical thinking abilities, expert communication skills, technical expertise, and up-to-date knowledge when caring for their patients.[20,24,25] These skills, when combined with intuition and caring, position pediatric oncology nurses to actively participate in and influence decisions concerning patient care and support, promote novel approaches to care, and optimize patient outcomes.[24-26]

When caring for patients, pediatric oncology nurses integrate information about the treatment modality with obser-

TABLE 29-1   The Nursing Process and Standards of Pediatric Oncology Nursing Care

Nursing Process	Standards of Care	Application: Case Study*
Assessment	The pediatric oncology nurse collects and documents data regarding the child and family.	• Obtained a patient history of severe chemotherapy-related nausea and vomiting during first treatment regimen
Diagnosis	The nurse uses assessment data from nursing and other disciplines to identify problems and determine nursing diagnoses.	• Severe chemotherapy-related nausea despite antiemetics • New protocol regimen is highly emetogenic.
Outcomes Identification	The nurse identifies expected and desired outcomes specific to the patient and family and related to their physical and emotional health, education, growth and development, and effects of disease and treatment.	Expected outcomes: • Patient will experience little or no nausea during chemotherapy and postchemotherapy period. • Patient and family will communicate effectiveness of antiemetic and patient satisfaction with the regimen.
Planning	The nurse develops an individualized plan that prescribes interventions to attain expected outcomes.	• Resume previous antiemetics (ondansetron, corticosteroids, and scopolamine). Add new antiemetic, aprepitant. • Have patient maintain a diary describing nausea and individual drug effectiveness.
Implementation	The nurse implements the plan of care to achieve the expected outcomes for the child and family.	• Administer first antiemetic doses in clinic to monitor effectiveness, and review timing of doses.
Coordination of Care	The nurse coordinates the delivery of care to support transition across the continuum of care.	• College student describes past use of dronabinol and lorazepam to control nausea. Patient states that these agents made him feel "loopy," which impeded his ability to attend class and keep up with studies.
Health Teaching and Health Promotion	The nurse employs strategies to educate families about maintaining health and providing a safe environment of care.	• Provided a detailed calendar outlining scheduled chemotherapy, predicted times of nausea, medication schedule, and escalation plan for unresolved nausea • Reviewed teaching sheets on all antiemetic drugs • Reviewed prn use of additional antiemetics
Evaluation	Working with other members of the care team, the nurse evaluates outcomes that have been achieved and follows the nursing process to adjust the plan of care as needed.	• Patient returned for cycle 2. Reviewed the drug diary with the patient to understand the duration of nausea and the patient's perspective on the effectiveness of the antiemetic regimen. • Patient reported no nausea, did not require supplemental antiemetics, and reported increased satisfaction with plan, noting that he had previously found the inability to control nausea extremely distressing.

*Applying the nursing process to the management of postchemotherapy nausea in a 19-year-old college student with relapsed Ewing's sarcoma. Case study of a patient at Dana-Farber/Children's Hospital Cancer Care managed by primary nurse A. Carnes, BSN, RN, CPON.

From Association of Pediatric Oncology Nurses, American Nurses Association. Scope and Standards of Pediatric Oncology Nursing Practice. Silver Spring, Md, Nurses Books, 2000.

vations of how the patient and family are responding to treatment and whether additional education and support are needed. Much of a pediatric oncology nurse's practice is grounded in standards of care and professional performance defined by APHON. These standards apply to clinical settings across the continuum of care and serve as a guide for nurses practicing in all aspects of care, from prevention, early detection, ongoing physical and psychosocial care, and long-term survival. These standards of care also define activities associated with each step of the nursing process—a process that includes assessing the patient, identifying problems requiring nursing intervention, specifying expected outcomes, planning and implementing a nursing plan of care, and evaluating the child's progress (Table 29-1).[15] This process is iterative, resulting in a plan of care that is continually adjusted in response to changes in the patient's condition and treatment plan.

As discussed in this chapter and highlighted in Box 29-1, pediatric oncology nurses are critical members of the oncology team, collaborating with colleagues and using an evidence-based approach to reduce the burden of cancer and meet the needs of patients and families.

The Nurse's Relationship with Patients, Families, and Other Providers

Meeting the varied needs of pediatric oncology patients and their families requires a broad range of professionals. For this reason, most pediatric cancer centers draw on an interdisciplinary team of providers, which may include physicians, nurses, social workers, psychologists, psychiatrists, pharmacists, child-life specialists, nutritionists, physical therapists, and others. The team approach has generally replaced the physician-centered model that was more common in the early years of cancer care, in which physicians worked alone to determine treatment and served as the sole source of information for patients and families.[3] Today, members of the care team rely on one another's observations, knowledge, and skills, with physicians and nurses working as interdependent partners toward the care and cure of children with cancer.[5,27,28]

Partnering with other members of the care team is fundamental to pediatric cancer care and pediatric oncology nursing. Equally important is coordinated and ongoing interaction between the child, the family and the members of the interdisciplinary team.

Box 29-1	The Role of the Pediatric Oncology Nurse in Reducing the Burden of Cancer: Ensuring Families' Needs Are Met

CARING

Provides compassionate, developmentally appropriate care

Considers cultural differences when developing and implementing a plan of care

Minimizes pain and suffering

Partners with patients and families to individualize approaches to care

Develops and coordinates all aspects of patients' experiences across the continuum

Collaborates with other disciplines to ensure optimal patient care

Demonstrates caring practices toward all patients, families, and members of the health care system

COMMUNICATION

Serves as an advocate for the needs of the patients and families

Exchanges ideas with other members of the clinical team to advance clinical practice and patient care

Facilitates communication:

With the community

With the patients and families

Between the patients and physicians

Between the patients and other members of the health care team

EDUCATION

Teaches patients and families about the cancer diagnosis and its treatment

Prepares patients and families to manage home care needs and transition back into the community

Encourages techniques supporting compassionate clinical and emotional care

Educates other members of the clinical team

Creates educational materials for patients, families, and other health care providers

Influences nursing practice at a local and national level

CLINICAL INQUIRY AND RESEARCH

Uses clinical judgment and reasoning to care for patients effectively

Guides pediatric oncology nursing practice by identifying key research areas

Advances nursing science using evidence as the basis for changes in practice

Masters the skills and competencies necessary to enhance patient outcomes

Serves as a change agent

Identifies patient care improvement opportunities

Box 29-2	Patient- and Family-Centered Care: Guidelines for Providers

- Consider how the core concepts of family-centered care can be incorporated into all aspects of professional practice.
- Convey respect for parents' or guardians' unique insights into and understanding of a child's behaviors and needs. Actively seek out their observations and incorporate family preferences into the care plan.
- Take into account the older child's and young adult's capacity for independent decision making and right to privacy and confidentiality.
- Offer parents and guardians the option of being present with their child during medical procedures, and offer them support before, during, and after the procedure.
- Promote the active participation of each child in the management and direction of his or her own health care, beginning at an early age and continuing into adulthood.
- In every health care encounter, share information with child and family in ways that are useful and affirming. Ensure that there are systems in place to facilitate access to consumer health information and support by children and families.
- Collaborate with the family and other health care professionals to examine systems of care, individual interactions with each patient and family, and patient flow, and modify them as needed to improve the patient's and family's experiences of care.
- Create ways for the child and family to serve as advisors, as participants in quality-improvement initiatives, as educators of staff and professionals in training; and as leaders or coleaders of peer support programs.
- Educate and train students, residents, and staff about family-centered care.

Adapted from American Academy of Pediatrics Committee on Hospital Care, Institute for Family-Centered Care. Family-centered care and the pediatrician's role. Pediatrics. 2003;112:691-696 [policy statement]; http://aappolicy. aappublications.org/cgi/content/full/.

Patient- and Family-Centered Care

Partnering with patients and families is the cornerstone of patient- and family-centered care. A model of care delivery commonly practiced in pediatric oncology settings, it is based on the understanding that the family is the child's primary source of strength and support, that the perspectives and information provided by the family, the child or the young adult are important to clinical decision making, and that the psychosocial and cultural needs of the family as well as the patient must be considered throughout the care process.[16,29-31] Guidelines developed by the American Academy of Pediatrics for clinicians interested in adopting a patient- and family-centered care model (Box 29-2) emphasize the importance of partnering with the patient and family throughout the course of treatment. Respecting the insights and perspectives of the parents regarding their child's needs, empowering the patient and family by providing them with information, and engaging the child in his or her own care are key aspects of the model. Organizations are also urged to involve patients and families in defining and improving institutional policies and care delivery systems.[29]

Although patient- and family-centered care is now widely embraced by pediatric health care professionals, there was a time when parental visitation was permitted only on a limited basis, information related to a child's diagnosis was often withheld from the patient and the family for fear of increasing anxiety, and decisions surrounding care were made within a paternalistic framework.[16,32] Nurses were often caught in the middle when a patient did not know the diagnosis or the family was not involved in shared decision making.[6,16] The cultural shift to a family-centered focus, along with improvements in survival rates, have helped members of the health care team develop a keener understanding of the long-term effects of diagnosis and treatment and an appreciation for how physiologic and psychological sequelae impact both the patient and the family members.[16] The patient- and family-centered approach has also helped parents to gain confidence in their ability to care for their child throughout the course of illness, and it has helped children and young adults to develop competence in helping to manage their own health care.[29]

Nurses routinely partner with patients and families during all aspects of the care trajectory, from diagnosis to end of life. This commitment to partnership is reflected in their efforts to involve patients and families in establishing short- and long-term goals, something that is particularly important for children because it gives them a feeling of control and enhances their sense of autonomy.[33] Although the ability of the child to participate in goal setting and decision making depends in part on their maturity and cognitive capacities, approaches and techniques usually can be tailored to match their capabilities.

Meeting the Emotional and Developmental Needs of Patients and Families

For pediatric oncology nurses, caring for patients often means spending long stretches of time with patients and families, particularly when the patients are hospitalized or receiving outpatient chemotherapy. Because of their frequent interactions with patients and families, nurses are often the first to recognize practical issues faced by families. Over time, many families view their nurses as advocates and welcome the nurses' efforts to communicate concerns that might otherwise go unnoticed by the health care team. The nurses' role, however, is not to provide all of the support families need, but rather to nurture support systems that are already established as well as identify other members of the team and available resources that might be of help.

Developing trusting relationships with patients and families is essential to effective oncology nursing practice.[33] Nurses often gain this trust simply through the care provided, the hours spent at the patients' bedsides, and the efforts undertaken to meet the needs of patients and families while facilitating communication with other providers. Among children and adolescents, trust is often more readily gained when the actions of the nurse reflect an appreciation for developmental needs and when nurses are forthright, honest, and maintain developmentally appropriate boundaries regarding the behavior of the child or adolescent.[34-36]

Children being treated for cancer are at risk for significant delays in growth and development, which are often functions of the length and type of treatment and the side effects that children experience.[37] Therefore, nurses caring for children with cancer incorporate developmentally supportive care into all phases of treatment. Such care requires knowledge of normal growth and development as well as an appreciation for the variations and abnormalities that may be encountered among children who are ill.

Using standard developmental assessment tools, as well as the parents' perspectives on past and current developmental concerns and accomplishments, nurses routinely evaluate key developmental milestones during each encounter with the patient, gauge the patient's progress by comparing findings with normal ranges, and tailor clinical interventions based on those findings. Physiologic parameters, including height and weight, are also evaluated during each hospital admission and clinic visit. In a child younger than 3 years of age, head circumference is also assessed. Deviations from expected findings typically trigger further evaluation.

Nurses use a variety of approaches to support a patient's growth and development and to help them reach their personal potential. Providing age-appropriate care that is individualized to each patient, encouraging parental involvement, and fostering normalcy whenever possible by maintaining routines and usual activities are just a few of the strategies nurses use. Nurses often consult child-life specialists to determine age-appropriate toys and diversional activities for children who are hospitalized or in treatment.[38,39]

Educating Patients and Families

A hallmark of comprehensive pediatric oncology care is educating patients and families about the diagnosis and treatment, empowering them to make informed decisions and become active partners in the treatment process.[40-43] Because the care process typically spans multiple settings, patients and families are likely to receive information and instruction from a variety of clinicians and care providers.

Nurses play a key role in the education of patients and families, routinely incorporating teaching into most patient encounters. Teaching sessions usually include information relative to medical care and are intended to help patients and families build skills and gain the self-confidence necessary to participate actively in ongoing care processes. When teaching patients and families, nurses use a variety of approaches and alter their teaching methods to meet the educational needs of individual patients and families. Nurses supplement verbal instructions with written materials that augment material covered in teaching sessions. Frequent opportunities to observe and practice the skills needed to manage care at home are typically offered.

Efforts to teach patients and families can be compromised by poor communication and language barriers, by a family's lack of trust in the information source, and by the absence of one parent when information is being provided.[34,44,45] Strategies to mitigate these barriers include matching the teaching method to the individuals' learning styles and using medical interpreters when English is not the learners' first language. In addition, listening carefully in order to identify questions and concerns as well as provide information in a simple and straightforward manner can maximize learning. To reduce inconsistencies in the instructions and information that is shared, it is imperative that all members of the clinical team document and communicate what has been taught.

Nurses have been instrumental on local, national, and international levels in developing educational materials for parents and age-appropriate materials for patients. In many hospitals and other care-delivery settings, nurses coordinate efforts to develop and evaluate educational materials on a wide range of topics, have the materials translated into various languages, and make them accessible to patients and families. A number of nursing organizations have also developed education resources. For example, APHON has developed a wide range of disease-specific pamphlets and education programs for patients and families that outline treatment options, side effects, and how to care for children at home.[46] The Children's Oncology Group also offers an informative website, a handbook, and numerous networking opportunities for parents.[47]

CARING FOR PATIENTS AND FAMILIES DURING THE DIAGNOSTIC PHASE

Receiving a diagnosis of childhood cancer is devastating and life altering.[48] For parents, the diagnostic phase is marked by extreme emotional, physical, and spiritual distress, with many describing the period of waiting and not knowing as one of the most difficult times in the journey.[49-51] It is during this wait that parents often are acutely aware that cancer is the probable diagnosis, but the type of cancer, the expected treatment, and the likely outcome have yet to be determined.[51] As a result, many of their fears stem from the unknown and surround questions the clinical team may not yet be ready to answer. Questions typically plaguing the parents during this phase include: Will our child survive? What will the future hold? Will our child suffer? Will we be able to comfort and protect our child from pain?[43,50]

The nurse caring for a child suspected of having cancer is in a unique position to offer support and guidance.[41,49] To do this, however, the nurse must have a thorough understanding of the various measures, tests, and procedures that are used to diagnose pediatric malignancies.[49]

The Diagnostic Workup

Establishing a cancer diagnosis can be a long process because many of the initial symptoms imitate normal childhood illnesses.[49] The diagnostic workup includes obtaining a complete history of the current illness, the incidence and duration of symptoms, and the existence of any predisposing factors.[52] It is during this phase that the nurse completes a comprehensive assessment that includes a physical examination, developmental assessment, and measurement of vital signs, height, and weight. The height and weight are used to calculate the body surface area, a key measure if cancer is confirmed because it is used to determine chemotherapy doses in patients 1 year of age and older (weight in kilograms, rather than body surface area, is typically used to calculate doses for children younger than 1 year). Accurate measurement of body surface area is critical; therefore, two nurses independently measure the initial height and weight and verify the calculations of body surface area.

Because the diagnostic phase involves numerous tests to determine the extent of disease, the nurse's role is focused on collecting specimens, coordinating the scheduling of the diagnostic workup, and preparing the patient and family.[52] The nurse is responsible not only for ensuring that preparative regimens for specific tests are observed, but must also facilitate the sequencing of various tests to ensure that preparative procedures do not conflict with one another, that sufficient time is allotted for traveling from one department to another, and that tests are scheduled in a manner that permits judicious use of sedation.[52] Before each test, the nurse speaks with the family, explaining the test and how long it will take, discussing whether contrast or sedation will be used, and answering any questions they may have about the procedure.

The diagnostic process is both emotionally and physically difficult because some of the necessary diagnostic tests, such as bone marrow aspirations, biopsies, and lumbar punctures, can be quite painful. Studies suggest that the invasive procedures needed for diagnostic purposes are painful and anxiety provoking, with some patients reporting that the pain associated with treatment and procedures was greater than the pain associated with the disease itself.[53,54]

Fortunately, there is much that can be done to prevent and manage procedure-related pain and anxiety. When possible, parents should be allowed to remain with the patient during the procedures. The use of a treatment room should also be considered for a hospitalized patient undergoing painful procedures in an effort to preserve the bed as a safe place. Because blood samples are commonly part of the diagnostic workup and are usually obtained via a venipuncture until a central venous access device is placed, they can be a source of discomfort and significant stress for pediatric patients. Limiting the number of attempts at venipuncture by a single health care provider is one technique used to minimize discomfort. It is recommended that a provider seek the assistance of another provider after three unsuccessful attempts. Additional techniques for managing procedure-related pain are discussed in the treatment section of this chapter.

Informing Patients and Families of the Diagnosis

Once the diagnostic workup is complete and the type and extent of the cancer is known, news of the diagnosis is usually shared with the parents or guardian during a meeting with the physician and nurse. In some centers, this meeting is called the Day One Talk. The purpose of this meeting is to review the extent of the disease, discuss the proposed treatment, and consider whether alternatives to that treatment are available. A consent form confirming the parents' or guardian's agreement to proceed with the proposed treatment is usually introduced during this meeting. If the proposed treatment is a research protocol, all issues related to the protocol, including the intent of the research, must be clearly explained to ensure informed decision making by parents.[51] Studies regarding informed consent have found that parents of pediatric cancer patients often do not understand some of the issues related to participating in clinical trials,[55] particularly that the purpose of research may be to benefit future patients rather than their own child.

The Day One Talk typically represents the first step toward developing the patient-provider relationship forming the basis for future care. Determining who should be present during the meeting is not always simple, and parents often ask the physician or nurse for advice about whether the patient should be in attendance. In cases involving younger children, a separate discussion tailored to the developmental level of the child is often suggested.[51] Many providers believe that teenagers should be invited to attend the meeting. If they are not included, they may assume that information later received is not completely true and that the diagnosis and treatment are worse than those stated in the information they have been given.[51] Including teenagers from the beginning may also help in later efforts to engage them in their own care. In rare circumstances, an adolescent's stage of development may make it difficult for him or her to participate in the family meeting concerning the diagnosis.

Receiving the news that a child has cancer and hearing the complex treatment plan is devastating for parents, who may be overwhelmed with feelings of anger, fear, guilt, sadness, and self-blame. The role of the nurse during the Day One Talk is to hear first-hand the information that is provided because parents may have difficulty retaining, processing, and understanding the information. Nurses are important sources of information and support for patients and parents as they process what they have been told. The signed consent form detailing the aspects of treatment and chemotherapy information sheets also serve as useful references for parents after the meeting.[51]

If the patient is an adolescent, consideration must be given to the potential impact the treatment may have on fertility, as well as possible fertility-preservation options. It is generally recommended that this conversation take place as early as possible before beginning treatment. Some physicians choose to discuss fertility-related issues during the Day One Talk with a follow-up referral to reproductive specialists.[56]

Supporting Patients and Families After Diagnosis

After the Day One Talk, nurses provide ongoing support as patients and parents express their fears and concerns. The reassurance and emotional support provided by nurses during this time are essential.[50] One survey found that mothers of children with cancer who felt they had received inadequate emotional support were more dissatisfied with the care given at the time of diagnosis and were at increased risk for distress.[57]

Once the diagnosis is made, patients and families are suddenly thrust into a complex plan of treatment that involves hospitals, ambulatory clinics, and home care agencies. Nurses help to arrange and coordinate appointments and other aspects of treatment and they facilitate collaboration and communication among care providers in various locations. During the weeks and months following the diagnosis, nurses also monitor patients and families carefully for signs that suggest they may be having difficulty coping.

All parents experience significant stress during this time, and some can even develop post-traumatic stress disorder. Missing appointments, avoiding contact with providers, failing to administer the child's medication, and other avoidance behaviors that can compromise a child's care may actually be symptoms of distress. Appearing unfeeling, uninvolved, or irritable[43] or exhibiting signs of substance abuse are other indications that may signify parental distress. Nurses also monitor parents for signs of fatigue because prolonged or excessive fatigue can interfere with physical and emotional stamina and can affect the parents' ability to think critically or to make sound judgments about their child's care.[41,43] If any signs of distress are observed, nurses work with colleagues on the care team to formulate a plan to help parents manage their stress and enhance the family's chances for the best possible outcomes.[43] Some parents may benefit from working with psychosocial clinicians, attending family support groups, or having regularly scheduled family meetings, whereas others may require more intensive interventions.

NURSING IMPLICATIONS OF PEDIATRIC CANCER TREATMENT

The treatment of childhood cancer has evolved into an increasingly complex set of treatment modalities and methods. Although advances in treatment are responsible for marked improvements in survival rates, they have resulted in a broad range of side effects that require diligent monitoring and supportive therapy. Knowledgeable and well-trained pediatric oncology nurses are critical to the safe and effective implementation of surgical, radiologic, and pharmacologic approaches to cancer treatment as well as to the management and oversight of clinical trials.

Nurses interact with patients during each treatment phase and in every care setting, making critical assessments and observations that guide decisions regarding the patients' care. Administering care specified by the treatment protocol, nurses continually monitor patients for complications and unexpected developments, offer emotional support to the patients and their families, and teach them what to expect during each treatment phase. Throughout the weeks, months, and years of care, nurses often develop a strong rapport with patients and families, becoming trusted sources of support and information.

Nursing Care Associated with Various Modes of Treatment

The care nurses provide varies with the mode of treatment. In this section, the specialized nursing care associated with the primary forms of pediatric oncology treatment—surgery, chemotherapy, radiation therapy, biotherapy, and hematopoietic stem cell transplant—are discussed. Complementary and integrative therapies and the nurse's role in clinical trials are also examined.

Surgery

Surgery is a major treatment modality for many pediatric solid tumors. Nurses play a central role in the preoperative and postoperative care of children and adolescents undergoing surgery. Preoperative nursing care involves preparing patients and their families for surgery and recovery by reviewing the plan and answering questions. In an effort to demystify the surgical experience, as well as to help children and adolescents understand the surgery and recovery period, many hospitals offer programs that allow patients to visit the inpatient surgical unit, meet nurses and other members of the staff, and see much of the equipment that will be used in their care.[58]

During the postoperative period, nurses oversee the recovery process by closely monitoring the patient's vital signs and overall clinical status. Coughing and deep breathing, frequent position changes, and early ambulation are just a few of the nursing interventions introduced following surgery to prevent complications. Ongoing assessment of fluid and electrolyte balance by tracking intake and output and watching for signs and symptoms of fluid shifts are a major priority. Wound and drain care is also important and involves taking precautions to maintain the integrity of drains and dressings; routinely recording the characteristics, amount, and texture of any drainage that might occur; and monitoring for signs and symptoms of infection. Fever is a common postoperative complication that can lead to significant complications in pediatric oncology patients, warranting careful monitoring and prompt treatment.[59]

Managing pain is a primary focus during the postoperative period. Pain can have a profound effect on physical and emotional well-being, as well as discourage children from engaging in activities that promote recovery. Medicines to control pain are typically initiated intraoperatively and are commonly continued for at least 72 hours after surgery.[60-62] During the postoperative period, nurses regularly assess for the presence of pain and the effectiveness of prescribed analgesics by watching for signs of discomfort using age-appropriate pain-rating scales.

Analgesics may be administered prior to activities such as walking or dressing changes to promote comfort and reduce the anxiety associated with procedures or activities that may cause pain.

Preparing patients and their families for discharge from the hospital following surgery typically begins prior to or at the time of admission. Discharge teaching involves reviewing the care regimen of the patients and coaching parents on how to perform aspects of physical care at home. Emphasis is placed on ensuring an understanding of the signs and symptoms of potential complications, when they should contact a provider and how to reach someone in the case of an emergency. Follow-up appointments with the surgical team and pediatric oncology providers are usually scheduled before children leave the hospital.

Chemotherapy

Chemotherapeutic agents are considered high-risk medications because of their narrow therapeutic indexes and the complexity of the treatment regimens in which they are used. If administered inappropriately, there is the potential for serious harm and even death.[63] Unlike other medications, many chemotherapeutic agents have broad arrays of doses and schedules, widely differing protocols, and weight-based dosing, making the administration of these highly toxic drugs challenging.[13,14,64,65]

Administering chemotherapy is the primary responsibility of pediatric oncology nurses, who are often viewed as the patient's last line of defense against medication errors. To minimize the risk for errors, nurses complete specialized training and follow standards of practice for chemotherapy administration developed by APHON. In addition, they receive ongoing education relative to new agents and protocols before any new agents are introduced.[63,66]

Before administering chemotherapy to a patient, the nurse reviews the patient's medical record and interviews the patient and family to determine past experience with chemotherapy, level of tolerance, and antiemetics used. During the interview, the nurse explains the current treatment plan, discusses how each agent works, reviews potential side effects, and completes a medication reconciliation process. The medication reconciliation process includes a review of chemotherapeutic agents, antiemetics, over-the-counter preparations, and herbal and nutritional supplements taken since the last visit. Querying the patient and family about medications at each visit helps to ensure an understanding of the treatment plan and medication doses and provides an opportunity to evaluate compliance with the prescribed plan. The nurse also assesses the patient for any drug-specific issues (e.g., constipation) to determine whether the chemotherapy can be taken as prescribed.[65,67]

Statistics revealing the incidence of medication errors have triggered widespread changes in all aspects of the medication process, from prescribing and dispensing to administering. The majority of medication errors have been noted to occur at the time an order is written, making prescribing errors the most common cause of medication errors.[68,69] Because prescribing errors related to chemotherapy agents can have serious and even lethal consequences, nurses in most institutions follow a special process to verify each chemotherapy order before the agent is administered. Each step of the verification process is designed to ensure chemotherapy is administered safely, the treatment protocol is observed, required pretreatment test results are within acceptable ranges, and that the correct chemotherapy agent and dose are administered.[70]

During the time a patient is receiving a dose of chemotherapy, the nurse monitors parameters specific to the par-

ticular agent. In addition to monitoring temperature, blood pressure, and heart rate, the nurse observes the patient for signs of an allergic reaction and watches the access site for signs of possible extravasation or leakage of intravenous fluid into the tissues. Special precautions must be taken to prevent extravasation when the agent being administered is a vesicant because these agents can cause blistering, severe tissue injury, or tissue necrosis if they extravasate.[71] If extravasation does occur, institutional polices and guidelines typically determine the appropriate actions to take.

After the chemotherapy has been administered, the nurse continues to evaluate the effectiveness of the antiemetic regimen and monitors the patient for signs of toxicity and adverse effects. Detecting adverse effects early and taking quick action can help to minimize their severity. The nurse records the patient's response to treatment carefully because these observations are used by the care team to evaluate the patient's tolerance to treatment and to determine whether changes need to be made in the overall plan of care.

For many families, the chemotherapy treatment phase is particularly difficult because they must cope with their own fears and anxieties while supporting the child or adolescent through treatment. Families often turn to the nurse for support and reassurance and find it comforting to work with a familiar and trusted team of nurses and providers. In some cases, families are asked to administer chemotherapy at home. Nurses work closely with these families to help them establish administration schedules, learn how to prepare and administer each medication safely, and understand which side effects to watch for and report (Box 29-3). They also teach the family about special considerations related to administering some agents. For example, if the child is taking a pill and has difficulty swal-

---

Box 29-3 | **General Guidelines for Administering Nonparenteral Chemotherapy by Family Members in the Home: What Families Need to Know**[63,72]

1. Treatment goals and plan, including the length of treatment, number of cycles and days of treatment
2. A schema or calendar that shows the general treatment plan
3. Names of all medications (brand and generic)
4. Indications for all medications
5. Doses of all medications, including the strengths
6. How to administer the medications
   a. Safe handling (e.g., disposal of waste products and management of chemotherapeutic exposure or spill)
   b. How to measure the medications, especially liquids
   c. What foods or drinks the medications can be mixed with or taken with
   d. What foods or drinks to avoid when taking the medications
7. How and when to take the medications (e.g., before or after meals, at bedtime)
8. The start and stop date or criteria for stopping
9. Expected and potential side effects and preventive measures for side effects
10. When to report side effects and whom to call

lowing it, the nurse instructs the family about how to safely crush and mix the pill, and teaches them what to do if the patient spits it out or vomits. (Most protocols and manufacturers now include specific instructions for these situations.) The nurse also helps the family arrange for routine blood work to monitor for myelosuppression between cycles. To make it more convenient for families, the nurse may arrange to have the blood drawn by a home care agency or a laboratory closer to home. School nurses and other caregivers may also need information on aspects of the child's care. The nurse may share this information after obtaining parental consent.

Because many chemotherapeutic agents are highly toxic, the National Institute of Occupational Safety and Health has developed standards to protect health care workers when handling or administering chemotherapy and caring for patients who have received chemotherapy.[72] The standards identify personal protective equipment, such as gowns, gloves, and eye shields, that must be used by those handling chemotherapeutic agents. In addition, standards recommend the use of closed systems, as well as the use of locking mechanisms on all syringes and tubing to prevent accidental disconnection and exposure. Research has shown that complying with these standards ensures adequate protection.[73] Although some patients and families may be frightened when they first see nurses and other clinicians using protective equipment and procedures, most are quickly accepting once they understand the rationale for such measures.

The safety concerns and precautions related to chemotherapy administration also apply to the patient's family, who must learn how to handle chemotherapeutic agents and the patient's body fluids. Body fluids can be a source of cytotoxic drugs and may pose a threat to the environment. As a result, special precautions for their disposal must be observed for 48 hours after chemotherapy administration, and family members should be given appropriate personal protective equipment and written instructions on how to handle the fluids safely. Family members who are of child-bearing age or who are pregnant should not be asked to prepare or administer cytotoxic drugs in the home; if they must handle the agent, they should minimize their risk by wearing appropriate protective equipment.[72]

Radiation Therapy

Radiation therapy is usually administered daily in an outpatient setting for a number of consecutive weeks until the radiation dose has been completed. Radiation therapy is often effective in controlling cancer, but can have significant side effects in children. During the weeks of treatment, nurses meet regularly with the patient and family to discuss the treatment plan and evaluate the patient's tolerance.

As part of the treatment planning process, most patients undergo radiation simulation to determine the radiation field. Simulation requires the use of markings, blocks, and immobilizing devices to ensure that the radiation will be delivered consistently to the same location during each radiation session. Children younger than 4 years of age usually require sedation and central venous access for their simulation and radiation treatments.[74,75] Children between 4 and 6 years of age may be able to tolerate the sessions without sedation if distraction techniques and nursing support are made available. Children older than 7 years of age usually tolerate the treatments well and are able to cooperate during the sessions.[75]

Nursing care for a child undergoing radiation therapy includes discussing the treatment plan with the patient and family, describing what the simulation process involves, assessing the patient for side effects, and teaching the patient and family how to prevent and manage side effects. Because the side effects of radiation therapy are related to the site that is irradiated, interventions to alleviate them vary accordingly. The mouth and skin are commonly affected, and all patients and families are taught proper mouth and skin care techniques before they begin treatment. Patients receiving radiation therapy in combination with chemotherapy or biotherapy are monitored closely because certain agents can produce an exacerbated effect known as radiation recall, a severe skin rash that requires special precautions and treatment.[74,75]

Biotherapy

In recent years, biotherapy has emerged as a treatment modality. Biotherapy agents interact with the child's immune system, often causing significant toxicities that can be acute or chronic but are generally not cumulative. Toxicities that occur are often influenced by the dose, route, and schedule of administration. The most common side effect of biotherapy is a flulike syndrome characterized by fever, chills, rigors, myalgias, headache, and fatigue.[76] Capillary leak syndrome, hypersensitivity reactions, infusion-related monoclonal reactions, first-dose phenomenon, and cognitive changes are among the more unusual side effects of biotherapy.

All patients receiving biotherapy are monitored closely for side effects. Before a biotherapy agent is administered, nurses obtain baseline vital signs and administer any prescribed premedications. During and after administration, the nurse observes the patient for tachycardia, hypotension, fever, chills, anaphylaxis, and signs of a local reaction. Nurses also teach the patient and family about potential side effects that might occur at home, when such side effects should be reported, and techniques for coping with them.[76]

Hematopoietic Stem Cell Transplant

In hematopoietic stem cell transplant (HSCT), healthy hematopoietic stem cells are administered to replace those that are diseased, damaged, or missing. In general, allogeneic transplants are used when the hematopoietic stem cells are diseased (as in leukemia), damaged (as in sickle cell disease), or absent (as in severe combined immunodeficiency disease), whereas autologous transplants are used to replace stem cells that have been destroyed by high doses of chemotherapy or radiation therapy.[77]

Patients receiving HSCT require the care of an experienced, multidisciplinary team. Specially trained nurses who are familiar with the immune and hematopoietic systems, stem cell transplant concepts, and complex treatment protocols are key members of the team and play critical roles during each phase of the treatment process.[78]

Preprocedure Phase

Only a limited number of institutions are capable of performing HSCT. As a result, many patients change providers and transfer their care to one of these institutions for the duration of HSCT treatment. Nurses may help to facilitate patient transfer by coordinating aspects of the referral process, clinical evaluation, or preprocedure education and counseling. The period before HSCT is one of great anxiety for patients and families. Good communication between the referring institution and the transplant center helps to ensure a smooth transfer process and fosters trust between the families and the new provider. Poor communication and delays only serve to increase fears and frustrations.

Preprocedure processes vary with the institution. For example, at one cancer center the patient and family meet with an HSCT nurse educator 1 to 2 weeks before admission. The patient's psychologist or social worker may also attend. During the meeting, the patient and family learn about the HSCT procedure, the roles they will play during the transplant process, are given an opportunity to tour the inpatient unit and hear about the resources the hospital offers to help them cope with the treatment and hospitalization. After the meeting, the HSCT nurse meets with the cancer center's oncology providers to exchange information about the patient's medical, emotional, and psychosocial behavior (C. Costello, oral communication, October 2008).

Inpatient Care

The length of time a patient is hospitalized can vary from as little as 2 weeks to as long as several months. Once a patient is admitted, a core team of nurses is usually assigned. This team is responsible for developing a nursing care plan and overseeing the patient's nursing care. With time, the team of nurses develops a comprehensive understanding of the patient's medical status and psychosocial needs and works with other members of the HSCT team to evaluate and revise the plan of care as needed.

Inpatient nursing care for a patient undergoing HSCT involves administering chemotherapy, helping to coordinate total body irradiation treatments, and monitoring the patient closely for adverse effects and complications. These include, but are not limited to, bone marrow suppression, diarrhea, nausea, vomiting, veno-occlusive disease, acute graft-versus-host disease, infection, graft failure, and disease recurrence. Other priorities include providing emotional support and teaching the patient and family about the care that will be required as they transition back into the community.

Planning for discharge should begin early in the hospitalization, and becomes a higher priority as engraftment approaches. Engraftment is indicated by an absolute neutrophil count greater than 500 per mm^3 for 3 consecutive days.[77] Discharge teaching should include instructions concerning medications that must be taken after discharge, the ambulatory treatment plan, the care that must be administered in the home, and arrangement of appropriate services. Careful discharge planning and efforts to help families anticipate how care will change can reduce the anxiety many families experience as they transition back to ambulatory care.

In general, patients are required to remain in close proximity to the transplant center for the first 100 days after allogeneic transplant. Autologous transplant patients may be referred back to their primary physician once engraftment occurs and HSCT complications have been resolved.[77]

Ambulatory Care and Acute Outpatient Follow-up

After discharge from the hospital, HSCT patients continue to require treatment and close observation and may need to visit the oncology clinic as often as 5 days a week for the first few weeks. Outpatient nurses regularly assess the patient's physical status while administering prescribed treatment and managing symptoms, particularly those associated with graft-versus-host disease and toxicities. They also monitor nutritional status, administer immunoglobulin, viral, and fungal prophylaxis, perform central-line care and blood drawing.[78]

The patient and family usually require a combination of outpatient and home care services. Some institutions provide housing close to the main hospital to improve the quality of life of the patient and family and ensure close supervision of the patient's status. Maintaining a consistent team of caregivers and good communication with the patient and family helps promote post-transplant recovery and minimizes toxicities and complications.

Clinical Trials

Clinical trials are crucial to the treatment of children with cancer. Access to trials and treatment at pediatric tertiary care centers have been correlated with a significant survival advantage.[79] Most children receiving treatment today are either in a trial or are receiving therapy based on the findings of a previous clinical trial.

Permission to participate in a clinical trial must be obtained. If the patient is under the age of 18, permission must be granted by the patient's parents or guardians[80]; however, many health care providers involved in treating young people believe that the child or adolescent should play a role in the decision to enter a research study, and they urge investigators to share information about the study with the child and obtain his or her assent or agreement to participate.[81] The National Commission for Protection of Human Subjects of Biomedical and Behavioral Research established age 7 as a reasonable minimum age for involving children in some kind of assent process.[80]

After consenting to participate in a clinical trial, the child and family may have lingering questions about the study and turn to their nurse for clarification and more information. The nurse may arrange for them to meet again with the consenting physician to ensure that all questions have been addressed and that their decision to participate is truly informed.[81]

After a patient has been enrolled in a trial, the trial's research coordinator, in partnership with the primary team, ensures that all required studies have been completed and that consent forms have been signed. Throughout the course of a trial, nurses help to oversee and maintain compliance with the study's protocol, provide ongoing staff education, and are primary collectors of the data used for dose adjustments and analyses. Nurses also administer investigational drugs; monitor the patient's responses; assess patients for adverse side effects in accordance with protocol criteria; collect timed specimens according to the protocol schedule; and carefully document the start and stop times of drug administration.[82] Nurses also provide essential patient and family education and support, checking in with them frequently and bringing unresolved concerns to the attention of the team.[79,82]

Complementary and Integrative Therapies

It is not uncommon for a family whose child has been diagnosed with cancer to turn to complementary and alternative medicine (CAM) at some point during the treatment process. CAM, also referred to as integrative therapies, includes practices and therapies that lie outside the realm of traditional medicine. They encompass a wide variety of approaches, including acupuncture, massage, imagery, energy healing, and prayer, as well as herbal, homeopathic, nutritional, and biologic therapies.[83] Although evidence that CAM improves immunity or promotes recovery is not well documented,[84] the use of integrative therapies among children and adolescents with cancer reportedly ranges between 46% and 85%.[85,86]

Even though integrative therapies are not a replacement for standard pediatric oncology treatment, many patients and families view them as a form of adjunctive therapy that may be used to help relieve symptoms, cope with life-threatening illness, and improve well-being.[87] While working with a patient and family, pediatric oncology nurses and other providers should routinely assess whether the patient has used CAM and evaluate understanding of the therapies tried. During all medication reviews, the patient and family should be asked to list any herbs and supplements the patient is taking. Although obtaining this information is an important part of the medication review process, many families report never having been asked about such practices.[87]

Patients often turn to nurses for information and insight about available therapies that might be useful to them. When trying to determine the best therapy for the patient, consideration should be given to the family's culture, spiritual beliefs, and practices and the patient's developmental level, education, and preferences.[83,88] Nurses' observations and documentation of a patient's response to CAM treatments are essential because they help providers gauge the impact of the treatments, as well as their potential interactions with individual therapies, and provide insight into the patient's coping strategies.

Symptom Management and Supportive Nursing Care

The advanced, complex treatment regimens designed to cure childhood cancer commonly produce multiple distressing side effects. Each treatment modality carries the potential for side effects that can occur during treatment or days, weeks, or years later. Side effects such as hair loss and low blood counts may be transient, whereas others, such as hearing loss and learning disabilities, can be permanent.[67,89] The most commonly reported side effects in children and adolescents with cancer include infection, bleeding, anemia, nutritional problems, nausea, vomiting, mucositis, fatigue, and pain.[53] Recent studies have found that children report nausea, fatigue, and pain as the most distressing.[90,91] Although many side effects can be effectively managed, some families believe suffering is to be expected among children with cancer. As a result, side effects may go unreported for a time and children may suffer unnecessary distress.[92,93]

Nurses help manage the side effects of cancer treatment by using strategies that have been tested and proven effective through research and evidence.[89] The nurse continually evaluates the effectiveness of symptom management strategies and, when necessary, collaborates with the interdisciplinary team to revise the plan so that it matches the needs and experiences of the individual patient. The following section summarizes specific nursing interventions associated with some of the most common and troubling side effects encountered in children with cancer.

Myelosuppression

The most common toxicity associated with radiation and many chemotherapeutic agents is myelosuppression.[89] Myelosuppression can also occur with certain malignancies, such as leukemia, sarcoma, neuroblastoma, and lymphoma.[53] Patients receiving myelosuppressive agents commonly experience a nadir between 10 and 14 days after the end of treatment. With subsequent courses of myelosuppressive agents, the nadir and recovery from the nadir can be affected by the number and type of agents given and the timing of their administration.[89,94] Pediatric oncology nurses play important roles in monitoring patients' response to treatment over time and anticipating complications of myelosuppression, such as infection, bleeding, and fatigue. Educating families to be aware of the signs and symptoms associated with complications related to myelosuppression, as well as when to report these symptoms, is an important part of the overall care of patients receiving cancer treatment.

The nursing care of patients with neutropenia, anemia, or thrombocytopenia due to myelosuppression is as follows:

Neutropenia

Neutropenia is characterized by an absolute neutrophil count of 1000 per mm[3] or less.[94a] It is the most severe consequence of bone marrow suppression, increasing a patient's risk for potentially life-threatening infections, a risk that is higher when neutropenia is prolonged for more than 7 days. The neutropenic patient often does not present with the routine signs of infection. In many cases, fever may be the only presenting symptom.[95,96]

Hand washing before and after contact with each patient minimizes the risk for microbial transmission and is the single most important method of preventing nosocomial infection.[97-99] The pediatric oncology nurse plays a critical role in managing and preventing infection in the neutropenic patient by teaching and practicing correct hand-washing techniques.

Biologic response modifiers can also help lower a patient's risk for infection by shortening the period of myelosuppression. These agents are usually given 24 hours after chemotherapy administration as a one-time subcutaneous injection or daily by the nurse, patient, or family member until the white blood cell count recovers.[100,100a] Many children associate subcutaneous injections with pain and fear, so nurses use creative techniques and special devices to ameliorate the discomfort associated with these injections. One device consists of a small infusion catheter that is inserted into the subcutaneous tissue. This catheter can be left in place for 5 to 7 days and is used to administer subcutaneous medications.[101] Ice or local anesthetic creams can also be used to help make subcutaneous injections more tolerable.

The administration of prophylactic antibiotics to prevent *Pneumocystis carinii* pneumonia is also a standard practice in many cancer treatment protocols.[102,103] These antibiotics are usually administered in an oral form and are commonly given throughout treatment. Getting children to take daily oral medications can be very distressing for parents of young children and adolescents. Teaching parents techniques that will help them to administer medications successfully and emphasizing the importance of the medications enhances the parents' ability to cope and has the potential to increase overall compliance with prescribed medication regimens.

Frequent blood draws are used to gauge the level of neutropenia with nurses closely monitoring results. Abnormal findings are reported to the clinical team and are used to determine the need for possible interventions. If a change in the plan of care is deemed necessary, the parents and patient should be notified.

Educating the patient and family about neutropenia is critically important. Elements of this education must include the meaning of blood counts, signs and symptoms of infection, an understanding that the time of greatest risk for infection occurs during nadir, and strategies to minimize the risk of infection (Box 29-4). Because the family plays an important role in monitoring a patient for signs of infection, nurses also focus on teaching them when to contact the child's provider. Family members are taught how to take a temperature and that the presence of a fever may signal an emergency; they are instructed to call the provider whenever the child's temperature is higher than 38° C on two occasions within 24 hours and to call immediately whenever it is higher than 38.5° C (or per institutional guidelines). They are also taught to report any respiratory symptoms, shaking chills, changes in the child's level of consciousness, and are instructed not to administer acetaminophen unless directed to do so by the provider. In addition to reviewing these instructions regularly, nurses make sure family members have emergency contact information. Families must be taught the critical nature of fever and neutropenia and the importance of initiating antibiotics rapidly.

Early assessment and intervention are key to successfully managing a febrile neutropenic patient.[89] Nurses help to ensure prompt and appropriate treatment by noting and reporting the patient's symptoms, as well as initiating and carrying out treat-

Neutropenic Precautions: Guidelines for Patients and Families[104,105]

- Notify the physician if the child exhibits any of the following:
     Oral or axillary temperature is ≥38.5°C or is 38°C two times within 24 hours
     Oral lesions
     Erythema at central venous access site
     Open skin lesions
     Perirectal laceration or irritation
     Cough
     Rhinorrhea
     Tachypnea
     Complaints of ear or throat pain
     Diarrhea
     Lethargy
- Perform meticulous hand washing.
- Do not take rectal temperatures or give suppositories.
- Avoid crowds and people who are sick.
- Do not share utensils with others.
- Do not let the child provide direct care to pets (e.g., they should not change kitty litter).
- Do not keep reptiles or birds as pets.
- The child and siblings should not receive live-virus vaccines.
- Avoid exposure to mold (e.g., digging in soil).
- Practice good mouth care.

ment orders. Whenever a fever is present, blood cultures are obtained from central venous access devices and peripheral sources. Broad-spectrum antibiotics are usually started within 60 minutes of the diagnosis of fever and neutropenia.[106] Treatment may be modified once the results of the culture and sensitivity are available and the specific organism has been identified. Antifungal therapy is often added if the patient's fever persists despite antibiotic treatment.

Most patients with fever and neutropenia are admitted to the hospital for treatment. During this time, nurses observe patients closely for signs and symptoms of septic shock by monitoring vital signs, peripheral perfusion, and intake and output. The patient's neurologic status is also monitored closely because lethargy, irritability, or a change in consciousness can indicate sepsis. Mouth care and perianal hygiene are performed on a routine basis. Rectal temperatures and suppositories are avoided in all neutropenic patients based on the risk for tearing the anal mucosa and introducing bacteria.

Anemia

Anemia can occur secondary to myelosuppression after chemotherapy or radiation therapy, most commonly appearing 7 to 10 days after treatment. It can also occur as a result of blood loss, metastasis to the bone marrow, or viral suppression.[89] Nurses routinely monitor all patients for symptoms of anemia, watching for pallor (particularly of the lips and conjunctiva), fatigue, tachycardia, gallop rhythm, headache, dizziness, dyspnea on exertion, and irritability.

Many children exhibit a high tolerance for low hemoglobin levels. Transfusions, however, are commonly necessary when the patient is symptomatic, hemoglobin is less than 7 g/dL, and

the hematocrit is less than 21%. Recombinant human erythropoietin may be used to increase red cell recovery and decrease the need for transfusions, especially when the patient and family object to blood transfusions on the basis of religious beliefs. It takes erythropoietin 2 to 4 weeks to stimulate red cell precursors, whereas the effects of a transfusion are immediate.[100] Transfusion amounts are generally in the range of 10 to 20 mL/kg. Red blood cells should be leukoreduced to decrease alloimmunization and irradiated to inactivate T cells and reduce the risk of graft-versus-host reactions.[107]

Because the patient and family are often the first to note symptoms of anemia, the nurse focuses patient and family education on anemia, its symptoms, when it is most likely to occur, and how to manage symptoms at home, such as providing frequent rest periods.

If a transfusion is ordered, nurses follow a standardized protocol to ensure that the blood product is administered safely and monitor the patient frequently for fever, chills, body aches, urticaria, pruritus, wheezing, respiratory distress, and other signs of reaction to transfusion.[89,108,109] Prior to the transfusion, a patient may require premedications to prevent transfusion reactions. Once the transfusion is complete, the nurse documents the patient's tolerance of the transfusion and whether premedications were administered; this information is important to guide future transfusions. Because a patient and family may be fearful of transfusions, nurses help them prepare for potential transfusions by reviewing how they are administered before they are needed.

Thrombocytopenia

Thrombocytopenia, or a platelet count of less than 100,000 per μL, can be caused by myelosuppressive therapy, disease, or coagulopathy.[109] Thrombocytopenic patients are at risk for internal bleeding when the platelet count falls below 20,000 per μL.[109,110] Education of the patient and family is an essential part of nursing care when a patient is at risk for bleeding. Nurses instruct the patient and family in strategies for preventing injury, hence minimizing the chances that bleeding will occur (Box 29-5). Nurses regularly assess a thrombocytopenic patient's risk for bleeding and communicate any pertinent laboratory findings or symptoms to the clinical team. Platelets are commonly administered when patients are symptomatic or in accordance with institutional or protocol guidelines. Patients receiving platelets are monitored carefully during and after the transfusion for signs of transfusion reaction.[107,109,110]

Fatigue

Fatigue is a major side effect of cancer treatment in children and adolescents.[91,112-114] Although defining fatigue in children undergoing cancer treatment has been challenging, research indicates that children and adolescents can reliably describe the physical and mental symptoms associated with fatigue. Fatigue can occur as the result of treatment, low blood counts, fever, too much activity, a change in the quality of sleep, and worry and fear. Parents also identify long waiting times and inadequate nutrition as contributing factors.

Nurses routinely assess children and adolescents for fatigue throughout the course of treatment. In addition to evaluating physical status, the nurse conducts a thorough assessment to determine possible factors that may contribute to fatigue, such as nutritional problems, pain, dehydration, and patterns of activity.[112,113] While caring for patients, nurses try to incorporate interventions designed to minimize fatigue. For example, with hospitalized children, incorporating adequate sleep time into the plan for the day and minimizing noise during sleep hours can sometimes be effective. In outpatient settings, nurses

Box 29-5	**Bleeding Precautions (Platelet Count Less than 20,000/mm³): Guidelines for Patients and Families**[111]

- Notify the physician if the child exhibits any of the following:
  - Increased bruising
  - Evidence of bleeding
    - If a nosebleed occurs, pinch the nostrils together for at least 10 minutes. (Use gauze to pinch the nostrils, holding it between your thumb and forefinger.) Go to the emergency room if the bleeding persists after this time.
  - Change in level of consciousness
- Whenever the platelet level drops below 50,000/mm³, avoid skateboarding, trampolines, contact sports, and other activities that can cause bleeding.
- Always wear a helmet when riding a bicycle.
- Shave only with an electric razor.
- Clean teeth with a soft toothbrush or gauze. Do not use dental floss.
- Avoid sharp foods such as tortillas that can cause gum injury and bleeding.
- Avoid aspirin, aspirin products, and ibuprofen.
- To prevent straining, keep stools soft using prescribed laxatives and stool softeners.
- Avoid taking rectal temperature, enemas, and suppositories.
- Oral contraceptives may be prescribed to prevent excess bleeding during menses.
- Avoid sexual intercourse.

work with other members of the care team to avoid long waiting times to conserve and maximize energy, ensure adequate time for rest, and work with patients and families to optimize the patient's nutritional status.

Other interventions and treatments that may decrease fatigue include pharmacologic assistance, physical activity, and distraction techniques. Integrative therapies that promote well-being and relaxation, such as massage and Reiki therapy, are increasingly employed in symptom management and show promise for relieving fatigue and promoting well-being.[83,87,88]

Nausea and Vomiting

Nausea and vomiting are common side effects of cancer treatment and are described by patients as the second most distressing symptom, after fatigue, of chemotherapy treatment.[90] Uncontrolled vomiting can produce its own complications because it may quickly lead to dehydration and electrolyte imbalance as well as to severe emotional distress. In some cases, nausea and vomiting can become dose-limiting side effects of chemotherapy if resolution requires a delay in treatment or a reduction in the chemotherapy dose.[67,89]

Nurses play central roles in managing a patient's nausea and vomiting by working to prevent or alleviate symptoms, thus enhancing a patient's quality of life. Efforts to establish an effective treatment plan require ongoing evaluation of a patient's symptoms and the effects of the antiemetic regimen.

For a patient just beginning chemotherapy, the first cycle offers predictors of the chemotherapy's emetogenic potential.

Antiemetics are typically ordered on the basis of symptoms observed during and after the cycle and adjusted according to the patient's response to subsequent cycles. The antiemetic regimen can also be adjusted to accommodate escalating doses of chemotherapy, as well as to manage breakthrough nausea and vomiting. Other interventions that may benefit some patients include antispasmodic therapy, relaxation techniques, acupuncture, and guided imagery.

Nurses routinely assess patients for nausea and vomiting during each chemotherapy cycle, obtaining information that helps in establishing and evaluating the effectiveness of the antiemetic regimen. They often encourage patients and families to maintain a diary describing the response to the antiemetic treatment and to list management strategies that the patient finds effective. Such information can help providers fine-tune the antiemetic regimen to the individual patient. When teaching patients and families about the regimen, nurses stress the importance of continuing antiemetics for the prescribed length of time.

Mucositis

Mucositis, or damage to the gastrointestinal cells and ulcerations of the mucosa, can develop as a result of chemotherapy or radiation therapy.[115] Ulcers that occur in the mouth are a dose-limiting toxicity that affects quality of life. Painful mouth ulcers make it difficult to eat and drink and can compromise a patient's nutritional status.[116,117]

Before treatment begins, patients are instructed to obtain dental care to ensure good oral hygiene and integrity. They are usually asked to have their braces removed to decrease the potential for infection and gum irritation. Once treatment starts, nurses work closely with patients and families to ensure adequate oral hygiene and decrease the risk for mucositis. Upon meeting with patients and their families, nurses assess baseline oral hygiene habits and instruct them in the techniques of good oral care, including rinsing the mouth frequently with water using a saline solution and a soft toothbrush or gauze to clean the teeth and gums three to four times a day.[89,118,119] Nurses also assess patients for mouth pain and discomfort and work with the care team to alleviate pain and promote adequate nutrition.

A wide variety of agents are marketed for the treatment and prevention of mucositis. Recent studies have shown that cold substances administered to the oral mucosa during chemotherapy administration (e.g., having patients suck on flavored ice pops) can help prevent mucosal cell damage.[115]

Pain

Pain is a common and distressing side effect of pediatric cancer and cancer treatment. Although techniques for managing pain effectively in children and adolescents are widely available, patients with cancer still experience unnecessary suffering. Inadequate pain assessment and poor communication between patients and providers are just two of the barriers to successful pain management. Other obstacles include lack of knowledge by health care providers about the manifestations of pain in pediatric patients and about how it is best managed. Taking the time to assess patients regularly to determine the type and cause of pain will assist in developing an individualized management plan to relieve pain and optimize quality of life.

Over the past decade, providers have become more aware of and concerned about pain in children, and efforts to understand and manage all aspects of pain have resulted in an overall improvement in pain management.[61,120] The creation of dedicated teams of clinicians who specialize in the treatment of pain has also contributed to the introduction of new drug

Box 29-6	**Common Myths and Barriers to Effective Pain Management in Children**

ASSESSMENT

A child reports pain to the nurse or doctor.

If a child does not complain of pain, the child is not suffering.

It is always possible to determine whether a child is faking pain or truly suffering.

Active or sleeping children cannot be in pain.

Pain must have an evident stimulus; without one, a child cannot be feeling pain.

If a child is in pain, the parent would know it.

DIAGNOSIS

Infants have immature nervous systems and therefore feel less pain.

Children do not remember painful events.

Children become accustomed to pain and no longer feel it.

Children cannot communicate the location and intensity of pain.

Neurologically impaired children do not feel pain.

Adolescents are drug seekers.

PAIN MANAGEMENT

It is unsafe to administer opioids to children because of respiratory depression and addiction.

The best way to give an analgesic is intramuscularly.

It is unsafe to give narcotics through a central line.

Administering morphine means the patient is dying.

Adapted from Jodarski K, Wilson K. Pain. In Kline NE, Brace-O'Neill J, Hooke MC, et al (eds). Essentials of Pediatric Oncology Nursing: A Core Curriculum, 2nd ed. Glenview, Ill. Association of Pediatric Oncology Nurses, 2004, pp 155.

combinations and techniques for the treatment and control of pain.[121]

Assessing Pain and Developing a Pain Management Plan

For pain to be effectively managed, dispelling the myths that exist regarding pain in children is important (Box 29-6) because believing any one of them can markedly compromise efforts to manage a patient's pain.[60,122] Although the most accurate and reliable indicator of pain remains the patient's report, many children cannot or do not consistently and independently report pain. Therefore, health care providers must consider the physiologic and psychological components of pain and develop techniques for routine assessment.[60,61]

Finding the most effective pain management strategy begins with assessment. Nurses conduct routine pain assessments, incorporating an understanding of the common types of pain and an appreciation of how pain is manifested by children at varying developmental stages. Because pain can affect patients differently, a comprehensive assessment typically includes the patient's pain threshold, fears related to particular drugs, cultural beliefs, anxiety level concerning pain control and, in adolescents and young adults, past use of alcohol or illicit drugs. A key component of the assessment also involves measuring the intensity of pain with an appropriate instrument. The most common scales use faces or numbers to gauge a patient's pain level. Scales that incorporate faces are particularly helpful in pediatrics because they can be understood by a variety of age groups and by patients who do not speak English.[123] Numerical scales, which generally ask the patient to rate pain on a scale of 1 to 10, are appropriate for children 5 years of age and older.[60,122,124]

Managing Pain and Stress during Invasive Procedures

Cancer treatment often involves numerous invasive procedures, such as bone marrow aspirations and lumbar punctures. Children with cancer perceive these procedures as extremely painful[125] and often report years later that the procedures were the most frightening and traumatic part of their cancer care.[116,126,127] Studies have demonstrated that children do not adapt to procedure-related pain; instead, the trauma and anxiety associated with procedures increases with repeated painful experiences.[53,125,128]

The pain and stress involved in procedures is commonly underestimated. Providers who believe that a procedure is brief and that sedation is time consuming may fail to manage procedural pain and anxiety with adequate attention. Offering support and preventing pain during procedures is the responsibility of nurses and physicians. A preprocedure assessment is usually conducted to determine the approach that is best suited to each particular patient.

Properly preparing a child to prevent trauma during the first procedure has been shown to have a direct impact on the ability of the child or adolescent to tolerate and cope with subsequent procedures.[116] A patient optimally managed through a combination of pain medication, careful timing, and parental support seems to be less anxious about and fearful of successive procedures.[124] A child who has had traumatic experiences during procedures in the past may demonstrate such symptoms as insomnia, anxiety, regression, and depression as the time for another procedure approaches.[53,122,127,128] If these symptoms do appear, providers should question whether past efforts to prevent or control pain have been adequate.

Researchers continue to build evidence for the best way to prepare a child for invasive procedures. Studies support general anesthesia as a safe and effective method of pain control and psychological support because procedural anesthesia does not require intubation and is accomplished quickly and effectively through the use of short-acting intravenous anesthetic agents.[125,129] If anesthesia services are not available, procedural conscious sedation is recommended. Conscious sedation uses various pharmacologic combinations, most commonly an opioid analgesic such as fentanyl and a benzodiazepine such as Versed, for anxiolysis and sedation.[54,126] Used in combination, these agents depress the level of consciousness while still allowing the child to maintain his or her airway independently and to respond to physical stimulation or verbal command. Carefully administering agents prior to and during the procedure can ensure a pain-free experience for children and adolescents.

A patient scheduled to receive general anesthesia or conscious sedation during a procedure is ordered to have nothing to eat or drink for 6 to 8 hours before the scheduled procedure. An infant may have clear liquids or breast milk for up to 2 hours before sedation. Ideally, the withholding of food and fluids begins at night and the procedure is performed early the following day to limit the child's distress. The nurse assisting with the procedure prepares the procedure room, ensuring that all necessary equipment such as oxygen saturation and cardiac monitor is available. For procedures performed under general anesthesia, the anesthesiologist ascertains that all the necessary anesthesia and emergency equipment is available, administers anesthetic agents, and monitors the patient. When procedural conscious sedation is used, the patient's physician or nurse practitioner usually determines the time of the procedure and prescribes the sedative agents to be used. The nurse assisting with the procedure administers the prescribed sedative agents and may also administer antiemetics if intrathecal chemotherapy is being given. During a procedure, the nurse carefully monitors vital signs and oxygenation. A pulse and oxygen saturation monitor is generally used throughout the procedure and for at least 30 minutes during the recovery period or until the patient's values return to baseline.[61,126]

For less invasive procedures, the application of a local anesthetic cream to the procedure site several hours before the procedure has been found to reduce pain. Applied in a thick layer (2 mm) and covered by an occlusive dressing that is left undisturbed for an hour, the anesthetic cream penetrates the skin and provides local anesthesia up to a depth of 5 mm for 2 to 3 hours. Anesthetic creams have been found to reduce the pain associated with a range of procedures, including venipuncture, lumbar puncture, injection, and accessing indwelling central venous lines.[120,130] In an ambulatory setting, a nurse may teach the parents to apply the cream before leaving home so it is at peak effectiveness upon arrival at the hospital. The cream's effectiveness may be decreased by poor hydration and dark skin pigmentation and offers limited effectiveness in controlling the pain of bone marrow aspiration, which requires the addition of locally injected lidocaine and procedural sedation or anesthesia.

Stress Reduction Techniques

Many times, a child benefits from having parents with them during a procedure. This is particularly true for toddlers and preschoolers for whom separation anxiety is a developmental issue. During the procedure, the parents should be positioned close to the child so they can offer reassurance and comfort and help the child use stress reduction and coping techniques. A parent who is uncomfortable staying with the child should be supported in that decision and given reassurance that the child will be well cared for and that a member of the team, such as a child life specialist or a member of the psychosocial staff, will be available to offer the child support.

A variety of behavioral techniques, such as music therapy, distraction, and relaxation methods, can be useful in reducing anxiety and managing the pain associated with cancer treatment and invasive procedures. Nurses routinely work with other members of the care team to identify techniques appropriate for the patient and to help the patient and family learn and use the techniques during treatment.[131]

The appropriate stress-reduction techniques for a particular child are determined in part by the child's developmental age and individual preferences. An infant, for example, may benefit from sucking on a pacifier or sucrose nipple, whereas a toddler may be distracted by a book, a tactile toy, or music. Guided imagery often works well with a child of school age or older; an adolescent may prefer being distracted by a CD player with headphones or a video game.

Medical play may also be used to help relieve a child's anxiety. Introduced before a procedure is performed, it allows the child to perform the procedure on a doll and to ask questions and examine equipment that will be used. Such play allows a child to gain insight into and understanding of the procedure and the sensations he or she will experience.[39,122]

Despite the advances in pain management that have been realized, there is still the potential for undertreatment of pain. Introducing strategies to control the pain and suffering of pediatric oncology patients through the use of medication or stress-reduction strategies is an important component of clinical practice.

Central Venous Access Devices

The introduction of central venous access devices (CVADs) is one of the most important advances in the treatment and supportive care of children with cancer. Prior to the introduction of these devices, gaining intravenous access to draw blood or administer blood products, chemotherapy, and other medications was a constant challenge and resulted in repeated and significant discomfort for patients. Today, a CVAD is considered integral to managing patients' care, and a line is usually inserted as one of the first steps in the treatment process.

The most commonly used CVADs are peripherally inserted central venous catheters, tunneled central venous catheters, and implanted vascular access devices consisting of a subcutaneous reservoir or port. Each of these devices can be used to administer chemotherapy, intravenous fluids, antibiotics and antifungal medications, and parenteral nutrition. They can also be used to obtain blood samples, administer blood products, and perform infusions in the patient's home.[132]

Once inserted, a CVAD can remain in a child for the duration of treatment. Barring any complications, the CVAD is not removed until after the completion of the treatment protocol or post-treatment scans. Complications associated with CVADs include local and systemic infections, catheter-related bloodstream infections, septic thrombophlebitis, and endocarditis.[97] Other potential complications include bleeding, thrombus formation, and catheter damage or dislodgment. The complications can be significant, but the benefits of using CVADs generally outweigh the risks. Among the most notable benefits is significant patient and family satisfaction.[132]

In order to minimize and prevent complications, meticulous care of the CVAD is required. During an inpatient stay, the line is cared for and maintained by the nurse. External devices, such as peripherally inserted central venous catheters and tunneled central venous catheters, are accessed by needleless systems, whereas implanted devices are accessed by puncturing the skin over the port using a noncoring, curved (Huber) needle. All external devices must be carefully secured in a manner appropriate to the patient's age to prevent tugging, irritation to the site, and accidental dislodgment.

One aspect of CVAD care is maintaining the patency of the line by flushing it as prescribed, typically daily when not infusing fluids. Confirmation of a patent line is required prior to the administration of all chemotherapy, especially agents that are considered vesicants. Patency is confirmed by aspirating the line and checking for a blood return. If blood cannot be aspirated, repositioning the patient is one technique that may achieve patency. After the patient has been repositioned, the nurse attempts again to flush and aspirate the line. If patency still cannot be confirmed, a thrombolytic agent may be required and is instilled by the nurse. If the occlusion persists, radiographic studies may be necessary to determine the cause.

To minimize the risk of infection and prevent the possibility of a nosocomial infection, caring for a patient with a CVAD requires particular attention to proper aseptic technique and good hand washing. Together, they have been shown to provide protection against infection.[97,98] Special care must be taken when cleansing the line's access port before it is used. Alcohol is commonly used to clean the access port, and some institutions have found that a 10-second wipe is the minimum necessary to remove bacteria. Extensive staff, patient, and family education must be conducted to ensure consistent and effective care of the CVAD. Guidelines developed by the manufacturer or institution-specific policies and procedures are designed to minimize the risk of infection and should be followed whenever a CVAD is accessed.[103,133]

One of the most common complications in a CVAD is a line-related or bloodstream infection. If a line-related infection is suspected, blood cultures are drawn immediately and antibiotic therapy is started. The administration of antibiotics for treatment of the infection should be alternated between the catheter's lumens, so that each lumen of a double- or triple-lumen catheter is used, and the risk for colonizing an unused lumen is minimized. Depending on the institution's guidelines, the CVAD may be removed, particularly if the patient has positive blood cultures 72 hours after antibiotics are initiated, evidence of tunnel infection, catheter-related septic shock, or occlusion of catheter that cannot be cleared by thrombolytic or chemical treatments.[106] If the CVAD is not removed, parenteral antibiotic therapy usually continues for 7 to 10 days after a first negative blood culture is obtained in a patient who is not immunocompromised, and for 10 to 14 days in an immunocompromised patient.[134,135]

Although a CVAD is typically cared for by the nurse while a patient is in the hospital, the patient and family assume that responsibility upon discharge from the hospital. Patient and family education related to using and caring for the line at home is an important part of nursing care. Teaching begins before the line is inserted and covers a range of topics, such as proper technique for CVAD dressing changes and how to flush the line with saline and heparin safely and recognize the signs and symptoms of complications. Education of the patient and family consists of a series of demonstrations by the nurse of all procedures necessary to care for the CVAD, followed by return demonstrations by the parents. During the return demonstration the nurse is able to evaluate technique and identify areas that need additional review. Other teaching materials, such as books and teaching dolls, may also be used. In addition to the management of the CVAD, the patient and family are taught to identify the signs and symptoms of infection and to report untoward findings to the physician immediately. Family members are instructed to avoid giving antipyretics unless directed by the provider.

A patient with a CVAD is also referred to a home care nursing service that provides nursing support and instruction in the child's home. The child's inpatient or clinic nurse works in collaboration with the home care agency to ensure that the supplies needed to care for the CVAD and any prescribed medications are delivered to the patient's home.

Caring for Patients Across Multiple Treatment Locations

For many pediatric cancer patients, treatment spans months or years and takes place in multiple settings. Much of a patient's care is delivered through an ambulatory clinic, but many patients are hospitalized from time to time and also receive care from home care providers. Coordinating care across multiple sites and providers presents a complex challenge for the pediatric oncology care team as well as for the patient and family. Nurses play a critical role in ensuring communication and coordination across settings.

Good communication, clear documentation, and careful planning are essential to safe and seamless care. Before a patient leaves a setting, the care team must develop a transition plan to ensure that the patient and family, as well as the team receiving the patient, are well informed about the patient's needs and treatment. In addition, nurses or social workers serving as case managers or care coordinators work with the primary care team to arrange for community services and obtain insurance approval for services and equipment the patient will need.[41,44]

Nursing agencies and other organizations in the community are often called on to help with a patient's care in the home. Some pediatric oncology patients may require home care nursing to assist with central line care, hyperalimentation, chemotherapy or antibiotic therapy, pain management, and psychological support. A home infusion company may also be involved to provide line care, infusion supplies, and pumps.

Although most patients receive the majority of their chemotherapy in an ambulatory clinic, some patients and families choose to administer chemotherapy at home, with the support of a home chemotherapy and infusion service. Research has shown that such home treatment programs are associated with lower total costs and yield no significant differences in patient outcomes.[136-138] Patients and families have noted that these programs not only help to decrease disruptions to their daily lives but also help reduce psychological distress.[139]

Whenever home care nurses or other community-based services are brought into a patient's home, the primary nurse from the inpatient or ambulatory setting should speak with the home care provider to provide a detailed patient history and outline specific home care needs. Written communication detailing specific flushing orders, cap changes, protocols, and blood sampling should also be provided. Once the patient is home, communication between the home care agency and the patient's providers must continue to ensure that the treatment plan is carried out appropriately and that the home care nurses know when and whom to call if they have questions or concerns.

SUPPORTING PATIENTS AND FAMILIES AT THE END OF TREATMENT

Usually, the patient and family eagerly await the completion of treatment. Its arrival, however, may be accompanied by uncertainty and fear. For some patients and families, ending treatment means a departure from the relative security of routine visits to the oncologist and signals a return to their precancer world. This transition is typically accompanied by a whole host of worries about their child's future and the potential for recurrence. Some of the anxieties troubling a patient and family stem from the fear that once the cancer is no longer actively battled, the child will become more vulnerable to illness or disease. This anxiety is often heightened by the gradual loss of contact with the health care team as providers pay more attention to "sick families," and by the loss of the psychosocial support that the team has long provided.[16,140-142]

Helping the patient and family transition from active treatment is an important part of comprehensive cancer care. The primary oncologist and nurse or nurse practitioner play key roles in this process because they provide much of the guidance and information that the patient and family need to transition from treatment successfully.[140,143]

The Emotional Impact of Transitioning from Treatment

For the patient and family, leaving the safety net provided by the health care team means they must adapt to living with the uncertainties of surviving cancer while re-establishing the life they had before cancer was diagnosed.[141-143] Many times, a patient finds it difficult to reassume the role of a well person and to integrate back into the contexts of family, school, and community.[141,142] Although the literature suggests that most childhood cancer survivors do relatively well from an emotional perspective, studies indicate that some survivors and their parents can exhibit trauma-related symptomatology and experience ongoing worry and alienation. For many survivors and families, the impact of the cancer experience stays with them long after treatment is over.[144-146]

The context of post-traumatic stress can help clinicians understand the long-term psychological reactions of the survivor and family.[146] The end of treatment may signal a return to normalcy from the providers' perspective, but it can hold a very different meaning for the patient and family. The psychological sequelae that result from prolonged uncertainty; the emotions, ranging from joy to unspeakable sadness; the restrictions the patient and family must still observe; and the extra work and overall loss associated with the cancer experience can impact an individual's ability to reintegrate into the community and adjust to a "new normal" as a cancer survivor.[142,145]

Supporting the Transition

Patients' descriptions of their experiences following cancer treatment suggest that they and their families often need help in accepting and dealing with their new situations and circumstances.[140,141] Before providers can help patients and families, however, they must first understand the psychosocial impact of childhood cancer, as well as the heightened fears and the intense need for reassurance that families experience once treatment is over. These needs and fears may be especially evident when the child experiences common illnesses or during follow-up procedures and appointments.[16,143,144]

Nurses, physicians, and other providers can help to alleviate the fears of patients and families by validating the psychological distress that may surface at the end of treatment, by answering all questions, providing honest feedback, and helping them to begin to trust their ability to adjust to life after treatment.[33,142] Additional strategies include providing patients and families with ample opportunity to discuss concerns, acknowledging that fears of recurrence are normal, and preventing additional anxiety by ensuring that all post-treatment test results are reported to patients and families in as timely a manner as possible.[141]

The oncology team can also help to prepare patients and families for the challenges that lie ahead by teaching them about what to expect once treatment is over and by connecting them to programs that support the reintegration process. Support groups, programs that help with school re-entry, camps that allow patients to socialize with other cancer survivors, and clinics that focus on cancer survival can all be instrumental in helping patients and families adjust to life after treatment.[16,57,140-142] Efforts to educate the patient and family and to support their transition from treatment will not only facilitate psychosocial adaptation, they can also improve the quality of life for cancer survivors.[143,147]

Because nurses are a primary source of support and information for patients and families, they play a critical role in ensuring a successful transition. Nurses should provide materials and information about resources that patients can draw on once they leave the oncology setting. Information about programs and support groups for cancer survivors and written materials that outline follow-up care and potential side effects of treatment can be invaluable resources for patients and families as they leave the structure and security of the hospital and transition to other care settings.[140]

NURSING CARE OF CHILDHOOD CANCER SURVIVORS

The treatment of childhood cancer is one of the great medical success stories of the past 30 years. During this time, the cure rate for all childhood cancers has risen to 78%, resulting in a dramatic increase in the population of childhood cancer survivors.[148] Today, approximately 1 in 640 adults between the ages of 20 and 39 have a history of childhood cancer.[149] One unfortunate consequence of this success is that late effects of childhood cancer treatment are now more commonly seen, effects that can occur during childhood or many years afterward, sometimes with devastating consequences. As many as two thirds of survivors experience late effects, and as many as a quarter experience an effect that is life-threatening.[149] Among the late effects that pose risks to cancer survivors are learning disabilities, infertility, heart problems, secondary tumors, and genetic issues.[140,150]

Although systematic and consistent follow-up of childhood cancer survivors is recommended, there is no consensus about where this care should be provided, who should provide it, or the detailed components that such care should entail.[149] The appropriate time to transfer care is also controversial and is dependent on the provider, although many suggest transitioning to long-term follow-up once a child has been off therapy for 2 years.

The primary pediatric oncology team, which typically has an intense investment in the childhood cancer survivor, may be reluctant to transition care to the primary provider; however, planning for the transition is essential and should begin well before follow-up care is needed. Developing a plan that includes detailed written information about the patient's specific cancer and treatment protocol ensures that the primary provider will have the necessary information to provide appropriate follow-up care. Other necessary information includes the medications the patient received (including dosages); the radiation therapy administered (including dosages); the surgical procedures performed; and any complications of therapy that the patient experienced. The oncology team should also equip the patient with documentation describing the cancer, its treatment, and possible long-term effects. Such a document in the form of a medical passport, notebook, or other transferable records is an important reference for the patient and for follow-up providers alike.

The patient and family should begin learning about late effects and follow-up care long before the end of treatment to ensure that they have a good understanding of the information presented and have a chance to ask questions and discuss concerns. Research on survivors of childhood cancer has shown that most survivors are unfamiliar with specific details of their diseases and treatments and are unaware of their risks for late effects.[151] One study found that only 30% of childhood and adolescent cancer survivors could provide adequate histories of their diseases and treatments.[152,153]

Providing a patient and family with information not only empowers them to advocate for adequate follow-up care, but also prepares them to navigate the health care system and play an active role in monitoring and managing late effects once the cancer treatment ends.[154] Pediatric oncology nurses play a critical role in preparing the patient and family for the transition to follow-up care by teaching them about the disease, its treatment, and possible physical or psychological late effects. While being careful not to overwhelm the patient and family with too much information,[153] nurses should also address risks specific to that patient's treatment and offer guidance about how to self-monitor for late effects.[149] Information about organizations that offer resources for childhood cancer survivors, such as the

Candlelighters Childhood Cancer Foundation and the National Children's Cancer Society,[155] is also helpful, as are books and other written materials that provide additional practical information.[152]

Follow-up Care and Care Settings

Over the past 10 years, many oncology centers have developed childhood cancer survivor clinics that monitor patients for late effects and provide treatment to improve survival rates and quality of life.[149] Centers that belong to the Children's Oncology Group are required to offer such a service. Care in these clinics is often provided by advanced practice nurses in collaboration with one or more pediatric oncologists. The nurses are trained in oncology and have extensive knowledge about survivorship issues and follow-up guidelines. During visits, nurses evaluate the patient's growth and development and conduct comprehensive screenings for late effects associated with the patient's particular cancer or treatment.[53] They also monitor the patient for systemic toxicities resulting from the cancer drugs and therapies they received. Some follow-up clinics are multidisciplinary in structure and offer the support of specialists, such as cardiologists, endocrinologists, fertility and genetic counselors, and social workers.

Although the number of specialized follow-up clinics is growing, most pediatric cancer survivors are followed by adult primary care providers. Childhood cancer survivors can also be encountered in a variety of other practice settings, such as primary pediatric settings and adult specialty clinics. Nurses and other providers in nononcology settings often have little experience working with survivors of childhood cancer and may not know about the possible consequences of cancer treatment or what to watch for. In addition, they often have little incentive to learn about the complex care required by childhood cancer survivors because many practices see very few such patients.[147]

Goals for the follow-up care of pediatric cancer survivors include identifying, preventing, treating, and curing late effects and bridging primary and special care services through education and outreach. To help support nononcology clinicians who are caring for pediatric oncology survivors, the Children's Oncology Group has developed a comprehensive set of guidelines for detecting and managing the late effects of childhood, adolescent, and young-adult cancers.[156] These guidelines were developed in a collaborative effort between the Nursing Discipline Committee of the Children's Oncology Group and the Late Effects Committee and are designed to enhance providers' awareness of potential late effects and to standardize the follow-up care of childhood cancer survivors.[154] The guidelines are risk based and exposure related and provide specific clinical recommendations for screening and managing late effects, beginning 2 years after cancer therapy has been completed. These guidelines can be obtained at no cost, and because they are on the Internet, they are readily accessible to primary care physicians, nurses, and the public.[156] Education materials developed by nursing experts are also available and can be used along with the guidelines to enhance the process of educating patients and empower patients to become proactive participants in their long-term follow-up care.[154,156]

The care of patients followed in nononcology settings can also be augmented by regular communication with the patients' pediatric oncology providers. Documentation of the cancers and the treatments given to patients (such as the medical notebook and other transferable records described earlier) is also an important reference for follow-up providers. Such communication, along with continuing education for community primary care providers, helps to ensure that survivors of childhood cancer receive comprehensive care and ongoing monitoring and treatment of late effects.[140]

Nurses in nononcology settings may not be aware of the guidelines for follow-up care and may not be knowledgeable about the late effects of childhood cancer. Although the guidelines of the Children's Oncology Group are helpful, additional methods of training nurses about specific interventions required by the survivor population are needed.[157,158]

Follow-up Nursing Care

Much of the care required by pediatric cancer survivors is the same as that required by other patients. For example, studies have indicated that survivors are at risk for establishing unhealthy lifestyle behaviors.[158] Because of this, nurses should use appropriate health promotion strategies and encourage survivors to exercise and maintain a healthy weight and balanced diet, avoid smoking, protect themselves from excessive sun exposure, and keep their consumption of alcohol to acceptable limits. Nurses working with adolescents, in particular, need to clarify the risks of unhealthy behaviors and encourage them to participate actively in decisions related to their health and follow-up care. Preventive screening techniques recommended for the general population (e.g., for colon, breast, and cervical cancer) should also be observed as minimum recommended follow-up.[149]

In addition to employing standard prevention and screening measures, nurses caring for pediatric cancer survivors must also help to monitor patients for late effects of cancer treatment. One of the most disturbing late effects for children and families is neurocognitive deficits. Childhood cancer survivors who received intrathecal chemotherapy or cranial irradiation or who were treated for tumors in the central nervous system are at particular risk for this late effect and should be routinely assessed for its symptoms. Patients with neurocognitive deficits may experience psychosocial problems and may have difficulties with school performance and academic achievement.[150] Memory loss and impaired intellectual or motor function can also occur and are more common in children, particularly girls, who received treatment when they were younger than 6 to 8 years of age.[159]

Survivors who have neurocognitive deficits are often placed in special education programs or programs for the learning-disabled and tend to have lower self-esteem than their siblings.[149] Families often describe the difficulties they encounter when dealing with learning issues, cognitive deficits, attention disorders, behavior disorders, and other problems associated with late effects relating to neurocognition. It is common for these families to need preparation for and assistance in working with school systems and help in obtaining referrals to and resources for neurocognitive testing. Nurses can play key roles in helping patients and families to obtain the support they need and should educate the survivors and families about three federal laws that ensure equal access to education. The Individuals with Disabilities Education Act requires states to provide free and appropriate education to all children between the ages of 3 and 21 years. The Americans with Disabilities Act prohibits discrimination against people with actual and perceived disabilities or histories of disability; the Rehabilitation Act prohibits schools that receive federal funding from discriminating against qualified students who have a history of cancer.[149] Nurses caring for pediatric cancer survivors should also become familiar with school re-entry programs and advocate for continued identification of appropriate cognitive programs to promote the success of these children.

Nurses also play roles in identifying late effects related to hormones and fertility. The potential fertility issues and options for their treatment, including sperm or egg banking, should be discussed with patients and families at the time of diagnosis. Once patients enter long-term follow-up, nurses should routinely assess and document patients' sexual development, including their histories of menses, sexual function, and Tanner scale staging, and should provide education and support to patients pursuing fertility options.

SUPPORTING PATIENTS AND FAMILIES DURING RELAPSE AND RECURRENCE

Although the cure rate for pediatric cancers has improved significantly over the past few decades, recurrence of the disease is still possible and is a source of great anxiety for patients and families. Identifying and diagnosing recurrence at an early stage is among the goals of post-treatment surveillance programs because early detection may enhance the chances of successful treatment by means of a second-line protocol.[160]

Some patients and families liken the possibility of relapse to having the sword of Damocles hanging over their heads. Many begin to express fears of relapse as the end of cancer therapy draws near or soon after treatment is over. For patients and families who experience actual relapse, the news can be more devastating than receiving the initial diagnosis of cancer. Nurses, physicians, and other providers working with cancer patients and their families must be aware of the fear surrounding relapse and be prepared to help patients and families manage their anxiety and cope with relapse should it occur.

Helping Patients and Families Cope with Fear of Relapse

In infants and very young children, the onus of fear related to relapse is generally carried by the parents. Once children reach school age, however, they too can experience fear of relapse and require the support of the oncology team. Some patients and families begin to raise the possibility of relapse during conversations with providers as they approach the end of treatment, whereas others do not address it until treatment is over. The fear may persist even after children or adolescents experience 5 cancer-free years, a time limit that is generally recognized as indicating recovery. In many cases the fear of relapse is brought on or is heightened by trigger events, such as when children catch colds or have other minor illnesses or experiences such as an increase in bruising.

The very fear of recurrence can be as burdensome to some patients and families as an actual recurrence. Patients and their families deal with their fears in various ways, according to their personal experiences, personalities, coping mechanisms, and prior psychological defenses.[161] Nurses and other members of the team should continually assess patients and families for signs that they are concerned about relapse: behaviors such as frequent questioning about the need for blood work, complaints of symptoms that suggest relapse, and statements by parents that they have "a feeling" their child's cancer has returned. Other signs signaling that a patient or family is concerned about relapse might include a decrease in appetite, changes in sleeping patterns, increased agitation, and indications that the patients or parents are growing frustrated with the staff.

Nurses monitor patients for signs and symptoms of distress throughout treatment. When such symptoms occur, nurses speak with the patients and families to explore what might be causing the distress, meeting with the patients and families

separately so that all can express their anxieties, thoughts, and feelings without the fear of alarming others. In addition to providing emotional support, nurses also answer the patients' and families' questions about relapse and provide accurate information about what it means. For many patients and families, openly discussing the possibility of relapse and exploring what they think might happen if a relapse were to occur helps them to lower their apprehension to manageable levels.

Because outpatient nurses encounter patients and families frequently and are commonly primary sources of support, they may be the first to notice signs suggesting that patients or families are worried about relapse, and they may be the first of the oncology team to whom the patients and families speak about their concerns. In addition to sharing their observations with other members of the team, nurses may recommend that patients and families meet with the oncology team's psychologist or social worker, who can help them identify ways of coping with fears and anxieties.

While encouraging patients and family members to verbalize their fears, nurses also emphasize the importance of maintaining a positive attitude because this benefits patients and families alike. Nurses also try to assess patients' siblings because they too can harbor fears of relapse and must be encouraged to verbalize these fears. In many centers, nurses or other providers have developed support groups for siblings that help them to express their feelings while engaging them in various activities, such as outings, discussion groups, or arts and crafts projects that allow them to spend time with others who have shared the same experience.

Recurrence

More upsetting than the fear of relapse is the experience of an actual relapse. The fear of recurrence can have a profound effect on patients and families, but experiencing actual relapse can be devastating. How families respond to the news of relapse has marked effects on the patients' responses to the illness and on the psychosocial environments in which they must continue to grow and develop.[50] Once parents are informed of a relapse, nurses and other members of the care team must help them manage their immediate emotional reactions so they can take necessary and curative actions on their children's behalf.[162] The behaviors of the nurses and the rest of the care team are critical in helping the patients and families cope and adapt as they endure what may be the greatest challenge of their lives.

Immediately after patients and families are told of recurrence, they are thrust once again into a state of waiting and not knowing.[50] During these difficult times, nurses focus on supporting the patients and the families by listening and providing them with opportunities to express their feelings. Patients and families may be confused about some of the information they have received and may ask nurses to go over it again. They may also feel helpless and overwhelmed as they contemplate decisions about additional treatment and realize they must once again take on the immense challenge of making decisions about their children's care. Collaborating with the health care team, coordinating the day-to-day care of siblings and work responsibilities may also add to parental distress. At this early stage, parents are especially dependent on physicians, nurses, and other health care professionals to communicate clearly and to share information about the illness and treatment that will help them plan and carry out their lives over the next weeks and months.[50]

Many cancer patients and families who experience recurrence express dissatisfaction with the initial treatment choice and may blame themselves for the treatment's ineffectiveness, calling themselves failures.[163] Parents often vacillate between hope for another remission and anticipatory grief while they struggle to determine whether they need to fight for cure or prepare for loss. These conflicting feelings are a part of coming to terms with the relapse, a process that involves limiting immediate emotional responses so they can take appropriate action.[162]

Along with providing support, information, and physical care, nurses also help to coordinate communication among providers and across treatment settings, which may include the clinic, the hospital, and the home. As treatment begins, patients and parents may become extremely vigilant about many of the details of therapy, such as the time a medication should be administered and the results of laboratory tests. Nurses and other providers must understand that such selective and watchful awareness is normal at this time and that it reflects the patients' and parents' need to gain control of the situation. During this time, parents often benefit from having predictable care routines and periods of time, however brief, in which they are free of any immediate worries. Such periods, parents say, help them to rest and recover from the burden of recurrence.[162] Patients, too, may require extra support. It is critical that patients' needs for support not be overlooked or minimized in the mistaken belief that the children are too young to understand the implications of recurrence. Research has shown that nurses who realize that school-age children may be aware of the uncertainty associated with relapse support patients more appropriately than do nurses who believe the patients are unaware of the status of their disease.[164]

Studies show that parents who have experienced relapse note the value of being kept apprised of treatment options and of how their children are responding to treatment.[162] Nurses address this need by speaking with family members during each encounter, reviewing what the families have been told, verifying information, answering questions, and helping them put new information into perspective.[50] Parents who have experienced the relapse of their children's illness also note the comfort they felt whenever providers demonstrated personal knowledge of or fondness for their children. Such actions, they said, told them that regardless of the treatment's outcome, their children would never be forgotten.[162]

NURSING CARE OF CHILDREN AT THE END OF LIFE

When efforts to treat patients' cancers are unsuccessful, end-of-life and bereavement care become critical aspects of the cancer journey.[165] As noted in a landmark report by the Institute of Medicine, the goal for children and families who face life-threatening diseases like cancer should be a health care system that provides "competent, consistent, and compassionate care that families can count on for support and solace as they experience a loved one's grave illness or death."[166] Unfortunately, most children who die of progressive illness in the United States do not receive state-of-the-art care at the end of life.[167] Clinicians' efforts to provide good end-of-life care are often compromised by current methods of organizing and financing palliative, end-of-life, and bereavement care services. Better data and scientific knowledge are also needed to support efforts to deliver more effective end-of-life care, educate professionals, and design supportive public services.[166] In spite of these challenges, many nurses and other health care providers have found that participating in end-of-life and bereavement care is a richly rewarding experience.

Nurses play critical roles in ensuring good end-of-life care because they provide much of the physical care while the patients are in the hospital and are key sources of support for patients and families while they are at home. Because of their ongoing and close contact with the patients and families, nurses have a unique appreciation of the patients' clinical conditions, the patients' and families' emotional needs, and the families' dynamics. Their observations and assessments are key to the care team's efforts to keep patients comfortable and enhance patients' quality of life. Nurses are also a vital source of information and support for patients and families, who often have many questions, worries, and concerns during patients' final months and days and need the continued support of the health care team.

In this section, some of the principles guiding end-of-life care and nurses' roles in the end-of-life and bereavement processes are examined more closely.

End-of-Life and Palliative Care

When discussing terminal illness, the words *end of life* refer not just to the last few hours before patients die, but also to the months and weeks that lead to death, the death itself, and the grieving or bereavement process that follows. Many of the challenges encountered when caring for patients and families at the end of life begin before patients enter the terminal phase. Managing pain and the side effects of treatment and coping with anxieties and fears are issues for all patients with cancer and their families and must be addressed throughout the treatment process. Palliative care, a specialized area of practice that focuses on preventing and relieving suffering and ensuring the best possible quality of life, is appropriate for all patients with cancer or any other life-threatening or debilitating illness and is particularly important for patients at the end of life.[167,168]

Palliative care is both a philosophy of care and an organized, highly structured system of delivering care.[169,170] Palliative care seeks to enhance patients' quality of life in the face of ultimately terminal conditions and to ensure that bereaved families remain functional and intact. Palliative treatments focus on relieving symptoms (e.g., pain and dyspnea) and conditions (e.g., loneliness) that cause distress and detract from children's enjoyment of life. Palliative care should begin as soon as children or adolescents receive diagnoses of life-threatening conditions and should continue throughout treatment until death, should it occur. The term *hospice care* refers to a package of palliative care services (including diagnostic and therapeutic interventions as well as medical equipment) that are generally provided at a limited per diem rate by a multidisciplinary group of physicians, nurses, and other personnel, such as chaplains, health aides, and bereavement counselors.[171]

An increasing number of hospitals and other health care organizations have specially trained palliative care teams that consult with patients' primary care teams and provide guidance about how to best meet patients' and families' physical, emotional, developmental, spiritual, and practical needs. These teams usually include clinicians from the medical, nursing, social work, chaplaincy, and other disciplines; such clinicians are knowledgeable about pain and symptom management and are trained in helping patients and families with the decisions and emotions that accompany life-threatening illnesses.

One of the most difficult decisions a family can face is deciding when to shift the focus from finding a cure to managing the end of a child's life. Historically, the conclusion that no curative options remain was arrived at solely by the treating physician. More recently, however, the parents or guardians have been routinely included in making end-of-life decisions, and the dying child is sometimes included as well.[172] In some cases, the family's decision about whether to shift the focus to end-of-life care may be complicated by an offer to participate in a clinical trial or to receive some form of innovative care. For the patient and the family these opportunities are usually unexpected, and deciding whether to participate in a trial or try a new treatment can be very difficult. Deciding what is right can also be difficult for health care providers who are also clinical investigators. They may experience discordance between their desire to advance science and improve the care of other children and their desire to protect the dying child by doing all that is in the child's best interest. This discordance may be lessened by the certainty that the dying child (when possible) and the family have been given all of the available information about the study and are making a well-informed decision.[172]

When discussing further treatment options or end-of-life care with a patient and family, clinicians must take the time to communicate clearly. How they approach the discussion should reflect appreciation of the child's developmental stage, how the child understands death, and awareness of the family's culture. The nurses who are caring for the child should be involved in the discussions because a family often calls on nurses to interpret what they have been told and looks to them for information and support when considering decisions and processing feelings. A recent qualitative study examining parental perceptions of the end-of-life experience identified six priorities for improving pediatric end-of-life care.[173] These priorities include honest and complete information, ready access to staff, communication and care coordination, emotional expression, support by staff, preservation of the integrity of the parent-child relationship, and faith.

Nurses' primary goal when caring for a child or adolescent dying of cancer is to maximize the patient's quality of life. Nursing interventions are based on the patient's needs and on the patient's and family's style, values, spirituality, culture, and ways of relating to and interfacing with others. To identify and support the unique needs of each patient and family, nurses assess the family's structure, dynamics, coping mechanisms, cognitive and emotional functioning, previous history with loss, family support system, and spiritual and religious beliefs on a continual basis, and they develop and revise the nursing plan of care accordingly.[168]

Aspects of nursing care in the hospital and home settings that are unique to patients at the end of life are discussed subsequently.

Nursing Care in the Inpatient Setting

As a profession, nursing focuses on preventing illness, alleviating suffering, and protecting, promoting, and restoring health. However, when the restoration of health is no longer possible, nursing care shifts to ensuring a comfortable, dignified death and the highest possible quality of remaining life. When a patient is facing the end of life in the hospital, keeping the patient comfortable by managing pain and other symptoms and helping the patient and family cope are major priorities. In some cases, nurses may spend as many as 12 hours at a patient's bedside, caring for the child and providing information and support to the family. Often nurses provide all of the child's clinical and physical care so that parents and other family members are free to meet the emotional needs of the child.

During the hospital stay, nurses try to normalize the patient's daily activities. Depending on the patient's age and developmental stage, this might mean encouraging parents to go for a walk with the child, read the child a story, or give the child a bath. Working with the other members of the care team, nurses might also introduce play therapy with puppets and storytelling or other techniques that help the child to express and cope with fears and anxieties. They may also work with the family to identify tangible ways of remembering the child or adolescent. Parents are often grateful when they are offered memory-making ideas, such as creating footprints and handprints, cutting a lock of the child's hair, or putting special mementos in a memory box.[165]

Throughout a child's hospitalization, nurses try to maintain consistent caregivers and routines because doing so helps to promote trust between the nurses and the patient and family and decreases a child's anxiety or irritability. They also encourage the family to observe age-appropriate limit setting. Although this may be difficult at times for both parents and nurses, it often enhances the child's and the family's ability to cope.

Outpatient, Home, and Hospice Care

Many children with progressive cancer die at home. Helping a child or adolescent to die peacefully at home presents a multitude of challenges to the care team, but it is critically important because the support of providers can enhance a family's ability to cope with the dying process and help them to adjust after the child's death. In the United States, much of the palliative and hospice care outside the hospital is currently provided by specially trained community nursing agencies; however, palliative care is a rapidly growing specialty in medicine and nursing, and many new services are being developed by hospitals, skilled nursing facilities, and other groups and providers.

Nurses in hospital and clinic settings play central roles in helping to arrange for home-based services and to ensure good communication between home care providers and clinicians in the hospital and clinic. When a patient is hospitalized, an inpatient case manager (often a nurse or social worker) is usually charged with identifying and arranging the community resources, including home heath and hospice care, that are needed by the patient and family. Once the patient is discharged, the outpatient pediatric oncology nurse usually coordinates communication between the clinic and the care providers in the community regarding new orders, the patient's status, or outstanding issues. If home care services are not available or are not covered by health insurance, outpatient nurses may play a more central role in coordinating care among the provider, patient, and family.[44]

Hospice is a philosophy of care that is rooted in the centuries-old idea of offering a place of shelter and rest, or "hospitality," to weary and sick travelers on long journeys. The term was first used in 1967 by Dame Cicely Saunders of St. Christopher's Hospice in London to describe specialized care for dying patients.[175] The hospice philosophy recognizes death as the final stage of life and seeks to enable patients to continue alert, pain-free lives and to manage other symptoms so that they may spend their last days with dignity and surrounded by their loved ones. Hospice affirms life and neither hastens nor postpones death. It treats the person rather than the disease and emphasizes the quality rather than the length of the person's life. Hospice care is considered appropriate when patients can no longer benefit from curative treatment, and life expectancy is, at most, no longer than 6 months. If patients' conditions improve or the disease goes into remission, they can be discharged from the hospice program and return to active treatment if they so desire. Hospice care can then be resumed at a later time.[175]

Hospice services provide family-centered care 24 hours a day, 7 days a week. Although it can be given in a hospital, nursing home, or private hospice facility, most hospice care in the United States is given in the home, with a family member serving as the primary caregiver, and the hospice staff offering ongoing consultation, guidance, and support. The hospice team usually encompasses an interdisciplinary group of providers made up of physicians, nurses, social workers, counselors, home health aides, clergy members, therapists, and trained volunteers. Care is focused on relieving pain and other symptoms and providing social, emotional, and spiritual support. Many hospices also provide respite and bereavement care.[176]

Choosing a hospice service can be a difficult decision for patients and families, and nurses and other providers often help by assisting them in gathering information and helping them to choose a hospice service that will meet their needs. Many providers are unfamiliar with the programs and hospice options that are available, so The Joint Commission has created a list of questions that patients, families, and providers can use to guide their selection of a home care or hospice program.[177]

Unfortunately, pediatric hospice services are not as widely available as services for adults. Often, the nursing agency that provides home care during treatment also provides palliative care at the end of life. Because round-the-clock, home-based pediatric nursing care is available only sporadically, most of the burden of care is placed on the parents. In some cases, enlisting the help of a surrogate caregiver to maintain daily routines and provide respite for the parents may be helpful.

Nurses are integral members of the hospice care team focusing on meeting the physical, emotional, and spiritual needs of patients and families. Hospice nurses work independently providing care in settings that are removed from many of the resources available in hospitals. Although the limits, functions, and titles of nurses involved in hospice care may vary from state to state, all hospice nurses are guided by the same holistic hospice philosophy and by a position statement from the American Nurses Association regarding the care of the dying patient that reinforces the obligation to promote comfort and ensure aggressive efforts to relieve pain and suffering.

The primary role of hospice nurses is to coordinate the care of a patient at the end of life while maintaining a focus on comfort, not cure. In the course of providing care within the patient's home, hospice nurses observe, assess, and record symptoms and work with the patient's physician or nurse practitioner to develop and help the family implement a plan that ensures optimal end-of-life care. Family members caring for the patient rely on hospice nurses for guidance in identifying and treating symptoms such as pain, agitation, and dyspnea and for instruction about when and who to call for assistance.

One of the major concerns of a dying patient and their family is the fear of intractable pain during the dying process. Overwhelming pain and other distressing symptoms can lead to serious problems, such as sleeplessness, loss of morale, fatigue, irritability, restlessness, and withdrawal.[179] Because nurses often have the most frequent and continuous contact with patients, they play central roles in assessing and managing a patient's pain and other distressing symptoms.

Bereavement Care

Grief and the bereavement experience are highly individualized and are strongly influenced by a family's culture, community, faith, and support system. For many grieving families, abruptly ending contact with health care providers can feel like abandonment.[165] This kind of family may find it helpful to stay connected with physicians, nurses, social workers, and hospice staff during the days, months, and years following a child's death. Some organizations have developed bereavement care programs through which professionals, volunteers, other families, and community agencies work together to meet the needs of a family.

Nurses, physicians, and other care providers often experience grief when a patient dies. Some may identify with the family and feel sad about the death, whereas others may experience awkwardness and not know how to respond.[180] The needs of health care providers working with dying children vary according to their personal and professional needs and experiences. Contrary to popular belief, nurses and other clinicians do not "get used to" working with dying children[181]; however, caregivers who have developed wide repertoires of coping skills through exposure to previous personal life stressors are probably better equipped to deal with the care of a dying child.[182]

Nurses and other providers who cope effectively tend to recognize their own feelings, take advantage of support groups provided by the health care institution, have an established support network outside of the hospital, understand their own limitations as health care providers, and feel their contributions to the patient's care have been positive. Those who detach themselves as the child's death approaches or who become overly involved and focus on the dying child and the child's family to the exclusion of their own personal needs tend to have a more difficult time coping with a child's death.[181] Although occasionally providers become overly involved with a patient or family, frequent overinvolvement is considered a danger signal because it often leads to burnout.

Nursing Education about End-of-Life Care

The care of dying patients is enhanced when it is provided by nurses who are experienced in and knowledgeable about end-of-life care.[167,183] Among the barriers to providing good pediatric palliative care are lack of formal courses in palliative care, high reliance on trial-and-error learning, lack of strong role models, and limited access to services focusing on pain management and palliative care.[175] Recognizing these barriers, many groups in the nursing community have made educating nurses about palliative and end-of-life care a priority.

In 1998, the American Association of Critical Care Nurses published a document specifying competencies that nursing students should acquire related to end-of-life care.[184] Since then, APHON has developed a curriculum and standards related to end-of-life care for use by cancer centers when training nursing staff, and the End-of-Life Nursing Education Consortium, which is composed of nationally recognized palliative care experts, has created a curriculum to train nurse educators in palliative and end-of-life care and prepare them for teaching nursing students and practicing nurses.[184] Other initiatives are under way to include palliative care content in licensing examinations of nurses and to revise nursing textbooks to include content concerning palliative care.[185]

In addition to training staff nurses in end-of-life care, there is also a growing need for nurses who have advanced knowledge and skills in palliative care.[185] Nurse practitioners and nurses at patients' bedsides who have such expertise can play vital roles in caring for patients across the life span and in shaping and leading organizations and programs that care for patients at the end of life.

ETHICAL NURSING PRACTICE

Complex patient care problems present themselves daily in pediatric oncology practices. Because of the interdisciplinary nature of pediatric oncology, many problems that involve ethical implications are foreseen, and anticipatory ethics is practiced (E. Tracey, oral communication, January 2007). Nurses dealing with ethical issues are guided by the Code of Ethics outlined by the American Nurses Association[186] (Box 29-7) and by the ethical standards for Pediatric Oncology Nursing Practice defined by APHON (Box 29-8).[187] These documents highlight fundamental principles of ethical practice—including respect for persons, beneficence, and justice[188]—that are considered basic to nursing and that underpin how

Box 29-7	**The American Nurses Association Code of Ethics for Nurses**

1. The nurse, in all professional relationships, practices with compassion and respect for the inherent dignity, worth, and uniqueness of every individual, unrestricted by considerations of social or economic status, personal attributes, or the nature of health problems.

2. The nurse's primary commitment is to the patient, whether an individual, family group, or community.

3. The nurse promotes, advocates for, and strives to protect the health, safety, and rights of the patient.

4. The nurse is responsible and accountable for individual nursing practice and determines the appropriate delegation of tasks consistent with the nurse's obligation to provide optimum patient care.

5. The nurse owes the same duties to self as to others, including the responsibility to preserve integrity and safety, to maintain competence, and to continue personal and professional growth.

6. The nurse participates in establishing, maintaining, and improving health care environments and conditions of employment conducive to the provision of quality health care and consistent with the values of the profession through individual and collective action.

7. The nurse participates in the advancement of the profession through contributions to practice, education, administration, and knowledge development.

8. The nurse collaborates with other health professionals and the public in promoting community, national, and international efforts to meet health needs.

9. The profession of nursing, as represented by associations and their members, is responsible for articulating nursing values, for maintaining the integrity of the profession and its practice, and for shaping social policy.

Reprinted with permission from American Nurses Association, Code of Ethics for Nurses with Interpretive Statements. © 2001 Nursesbooks.org, Silver Spring, Md.[186]

nurses think when confronted by problems involving ethical tensions (E. Tracey, oral communication, January 2007; A. Hamric, written communication, September 2006).

Several factors must be present for high-quality, ethical nursing care to occur. Perhaps the most important factor is that the nurses themselves must be moral individuals, possessing integrity, courage, honesty, and a sense of justice.[189] Further, they must be willing to use these virtues to protect patients' rights to self-determination and to ensure that an individual's wishes, goals, and viewpoints are considered when managing care.[189-191]

Nurses who frequently confront ethical issues benefit from forums that facilitate moral and ethical discussions, communication, and inquiry and that promote the exploration of options for patients. Guided sessions that focus on sorting through choices and their implications help nurses to gain a deeper understanding of nursing ethics and encourage them to embrace their role as patient advocate. The education provided by such forums not only helps nurses to develop skills needed to work through options when difficult situations arise, but it also helps

to cultivate the field of nursing ethics (E. Tracey, oral communication, January 2006).

The ways in which nurses approach ethical practice are somewhat different from the approaches used by other disciplines.[192] The differences may have their origins in the very core of each profession. Nursing and medicine, for example, often play complementary and virtually inseparable roles but have functionally different foci: nursing, a health-oriented profession, is focused predominantly on the care of patients and families while preserving and restoring health; medicine traditionally has been oriented toward the treatment, prevention, and cure of illness.[193] Because of these differences, the relationship that develops between patients and nurses can be very different from that which develops between patients and physicians.[192] Although both nurses and physicians serve as patients' advocates, the nurses' perspectives are informed by their proximity to the bedside, a proximity that allows nurses to develop unique relationships with patients and to witness directly the converging influences that surround care versus cure[190,193,194] (A. Hamric, written communication, September 2006).

During the course of pediatric oncology care, the varied and often complementary perspectives of each discipline have legitimate places in supporting the needs of patients and families. Nurses and physicians share responsibility for ensuring high-quality patient care and for achieving the best possible outcomes (A. Hamric, written communication, September 2006). Further, because the uncertain nature of cancer renders the children and their families vulnerable, the practices of both disciplines must possess the moral virtues of honesty, courage, and justice and must reflect commitment to ethical principles.[189,194]

Ethical dilemmas related to care are often unavoidable. Nurses and physicians alike have the responsibility to manage with care the trust shown them by their patients. And when the right or good thing to do is not clear, they must have the moral courage to analyze critically and, if necessary, to challenge practices and health policies so as to ensure the best possible outcomes[189,195,196] (A. Hamric, written communication, September 2006).

FUTURE TRENDS IN ONCOLOGY NURSING

Change is intrinsic to the nursing profession and to pediatric oncology nursing, which remains a dynamic subspecialty that is subject to constant advances in technology and science and the introduction of new treatment regimens.[3,197,198] Faced with a nursing shortage, direct and deliberate strategies to integrate these changes into nursing education, practice, and research are required to ensure that pediatric oncology nurses are positioned to continue providing high-quality care.[197] In the coming years, as new treatments are introduced and more aspects of care shift to the outpatient setting and the home, it is expected that the role of the pediatric oncology nurse will continue to expand and assume greater importance. Remaining current with new developments in the field will make it possible for nurses to influence pediatric nursing practice effectively and to develop innovative strategies for managing the care of patients and families.[17,197,199]

No single discipline can accomplish all that is necessary for a patient; therefore collaboration is critical.[13] Research has shown that interdisciplinary collaboration is associated with improved outcomes, suggesting that intensifying nurse-physician partnerships based on mutual trust, respect, teamwork, and open communication is a priority.[16,17,27,200] Even though both nurses and physicians recognize the importance

---

| Box 29-8 | Association of Pediatric Hematology and Oncology Nurses: Ethical Standards of Pediatric Oncology Nursing Practice |

Standard: The pediatric oncology nurse respects the rights of all children and families and makes decisions and designs interventions that are in agreement with ethical principles.

Rationale: Advances in technology and genetics, along with scarce resources in health care, have created an environment in which ethical issues frequently arise. The pediatric oncology nurse should advocate for the rights of children with cancer as well as identify and help resolve ethical conflicts.

Measurement Criteria:

The pediatric oncology nurse

- Understands and applies the basic ethical principles of autonomy (right to self-determination), beneficence (do what is in the best interest of the patient), nonmaleficence (do minimal harm), justice, and veracity (truth telling).
- Examines own beliefs relating to autonomy, rights of a minor, quality of life, death, suffering, truth telling, equality, and access to care.
- Identifies available resources, including the *Code of Ethics for Nurses with Interpretive Statements* (ANA, 2001) when formulating ethical decisions.
- Maintains confidentiality.
- Provides quality care to all children, regardless of race, culture, educational background, religious beliefs, socioeconomic status, or the ability to pay.

- Delivers care in a manner that preserves and protects patient autonomy, dignity, and rights.
- Acts as a patient advocate and assists children and families in developing skills so they can advocate for themselves.
- Identifies ethical conflicts and seeks to resolve them through multidisciplinary team discussions, including the child and family as appropriate.
- Addresses advance directives with young adults 18 years of age and older.
- Seeks to include minors in decision making as appropriate.
- Ensures that all children and families receive truthful information regarding diagnosis and treatment.
- Participates in the informed consent process by witnessing the signing of consent documents, obtaining ongoing education about research trials, answering the child and family's questions regarding their participation in research, and ensuring the child and family's continued desire to participate in the research trial.
- Reports illegal, incompetent, impaired, or unethical practices.
- Maintains therapeutic professional nurse-patient relationship with appropriate boundaries.

From Association of Pediatric Hematology/Oncology Nurses. Scope and Standards of Pediatric Oncology Nursing Practice. Silver Spring, Md, Nursesbooks.org, 2007. Reprinted with permission.

---

of collaboration, developing such partnerships may be a challenge.[201]

The primary focus of pediatric oncology nurses is healing rather than curing, but nurses will continue to play strategic roles in supporting the pursuit of a cure whenever possible.[17,25,202] As the consistent provider at the bedside, nurses have a distinct advantage to support translational research efforts. Leveraging this position by combining theory, research, science, and practice allows nurses to bring knowledge from the bench to the bedside and from the bedside to the bench.[203,204]

A 2006 survey of APHON members underscores the wide-ranging interests of pediatric oncology nurses and highlights some of the issues that cause them concern. These concerns include problems with care delivery systems, worries about meeting the needs of individual patients and families, and worries about national and global issues that impede clinicians' efforts to provide the best possible care to children with cancer.[205]

Factors that are critical to the future of pediatric oncology nursing are outlined in greater detail in the following section.

Cancer Treatment and the Roles of Nurses

Current trends toward shorter hospital stays and more outpatient therapy demand that pediatric oncology providers change their focus and pay more attention to evaluating the burden of care that is placed on families and to supporting patients and families through the treatment process.[3,8,139,206] Helping patients

and families to strengthen their personal support networks, learn about the disease, understand treatment options, and become knowledgeable about managing symptoms and side effects must continue to be a major focus for nursing and the entire health care team.[42,93,207]

Helping patients adjust to the diagnosis of cancer has become an increasingly important part of pediatric oncology nurses' roles. Research has shown that hope has a powerful influence on a patient's psychological and physiologic defenses.[208] These findings have significant implications for nurses, who work with patients and families to capitalize on their determination, courage, and optimism, helping them to develop a vision of hope, regardless of the child's age or the extent of disease.[208]

In the coming years, nursing's paradigm of professional practice will continue to shift toward a more holistic approach that requires knowledge of integrative therapies.[16,209] Therapies and interventions that strengthen the ability of the body and mind to influence healing are increasingly popular among pediatric oncology patients and families. As noted earlier, studies have found that as much as 85% of children and adolescents have used some form of integrative therapy.[85,86] These figures highlight the idea that developing an understanding of the risks and benefits of combining integrative therapies with traditional medicine is an important consideration for pediatric oncology nurses, now and in the future.[88,210] A committee formed by the Children's Oncology Group has highlighted the role of pediatric oncology nurses in CAM research and has noted that nurses are critical to the success of research in this area.[83]

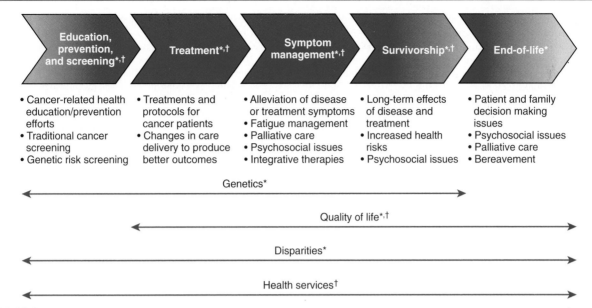

FIGURE 29-1. A continuum of oncology nursing research. *Research emphasis area of the National Institute of Nursing Research; †Priority area of the Oncology Nursing Society. *(From Bauer-Wu S, Epshtein A. Dana-Farber Cancer Institute, 2007.)*

Patient Safety

In 1979, NASA's Aerospace Human Factors Research Division linked inadequate communication, leadership, coordination, and decision-making skills, rather than pilot error, to most aviation accidents.[211] Since then, many health care organizations have translated this work into training courses designed to maximize teamwork among health care workers.[211] Clinicians participating in these courses have found that learning to communicate effectively and developing an understanding of one another's roles, responsibilities, and skills yields valuable insights and can positively influence the quality of patient care.[28] Such training programs will become increasingly important as organizations search for ways to minimize medical errors and improve the safety of the care environment.

Systems issues and other factors make many of the actions of nurses and physicians especially vulnerable to error. Nurses and physicians routinely make high-consequence decisions based on their knowledge and experience and an understanding of the relationship between patient-specific variables and environmental factors, such as work-flow patterns and the activities and norms of the patient care unit.[212] At times, these decisions are made in the context of factors—such as conflicting goals, obstacles, unpredictability, poorly designed technology, constant change, hazards, and missing data—that contribute to medical errors or near misses.[212] Maintaining vigilance in analyzing systems of care, identifying factors that contribute to errors or omissions, and introducing sustainable practice changes to promote safe patient care will continue to be a critical part of patient safety efforts.[213-215]

In many organizations, the growing focus on patient safety has impacted the culture of the work environment, shifting it from one that condones silence and blame to one that encourages open disclosure and promotes a team approach to problem solving.[216] Nurses in direct care roles confront patient safety directly and are important members of these problem-solving teams. They will continue to play critical roles in preventing medical errors and promoting safety in the health care environment.[216]

Self-Care

Nurses and physicians alike must find ways to preserve their interest in and passion for the work of caring for others. Although working to save, improve, or prolong the lives of others is rewarding, health care professionals often find that such work entails significant stress. This is particularly true in subspecialty practices like pediatric oncology, where patients are incredibly challenged by their diseases and often face uncertain futures. In addition to the emotional stress that stems from the focus on healing and helping, pediatric oncology providers often encounter workload and system constraints that contribute to chronic secondary stress and may lead to burnout or compassion fatigue.[217]

Understanding the concept of self-care and self-management is a pragmatic consideration for pediatric oncology nurses. Knowing how to renew oneself is critical to maximizing professional effectiveness and satisfaction.[16,17]

Nursing Research

The research training, methods, and rigor of nurse scientists are consistent with those of any other scientific discipline. Through the lens of professional nurses, research questions spanning the continuum of the cancer trajectory guide oncology nursing care (Fig. 29-1). Based on a holistic model, the needs of the patient and family are addressed using evidence-based strategies that help them cope with the physical and emotional sequelae of the cancer experience (S. Bauer Wu, PhD, written communication, April 2007).

Nurse scientists practicing in academic medical centers—at the juncture of clinical practice and clinical or patient-oriented research—have made noteworthy strides in the past decade as nurses have sought to change clinical practice on the basis of existing evidence. This trend toward evidence-based practice is widespread in the nursing community. The past decade has also witnessed a trend toward clinically based nurse-scientists who can bridge the knowledge gap between academia and clinical practice. More doctorally prepared nurses contributing to science will help to support a shift in the research paradigm to one that is multidisciplinary in nature, with nurse-scientists contributing to large multisite studies. This shift means more nurse scientists will have to be trained as members of larger multidisciplinary research teams.

A review of studies conducted by nurse researchers and of surveys among oncology nurses suggests that future nursing research will continue to focus on understanding the full scope of the patient experience and on identifying nursing interventions that ease the hardship of disease for patients and families alike.[205,218,219] Some of the high-priority areas for future nursing research include:

- Understanding issues related to long-term survivorship.
- Enhancing patients' quality of life, with a focus on the management of pain and symptoms.
- Evaluating and improving care at the end of life.
- Evaluating and promoting safe and effective nursing practice in all care settings, including the home.
- Understanding families' perspectives to find ways to support patients and families.
- Developing new ways to incorporate nursing research into practice and to promote and support interdisciplinary research.

These priorities reflect pediatric oncology nurses' appreciation for the ways in which cancer impacts patients and families and the toll it takes on their physical, psychological, and social well-being. The priorities also reflect nursing's continued commitment to preventing illness; to alleviating suffering; to protecting, promoting, and restoring health; and to ensuring a comfortable and dignified death and the highest possible quality of life when the restoration of health is no longer possible.

The advances in pediatric oncology that have occurred over the past half century are responsible for a remarkable increase in the number of patients who are cured; however, many patients still face uncertain futures and require ongoing care and support by health care professionals. Although the benefits to patients and families of an interdisciplinary approach to care cannot be underestimated, it is widely acknowledged that pediatric oncology nurses play a vital role in the care of patients and families. The knowledge, skills, and caring practices demonstrated by expert pediatric oncology nurses not only enhance the abilities of patients and families to cope with diagnoses of cancer but also help to reduce the overall burden of the disease.

REFERENCES

1. Wilson K. The evolution of the role of nurses: the history of nurse practitioners in pediatric oncology. J Pediatr Oncol Nurs. 2005; 22:250-253.
2. US Department of Labor, Bureau of Labor Statistics. Occupational Outlook Handbook, Registered Nurses. www.stats.bls.gov/oco/ocos083.htm. Accessed October 6, 2008.
3. Morra M. New opportunities for nurses as patient advocates. Semin Oncol Nurs. 2000;16:57-64.
4. Gibson F. Evidence in action: fostering growth of research-based practice in children's cancer nursing. Eur J Oncol Nurs. 2005;9: 8-20.
5. Ruccione K, Perin G. A living legend in pediatric oncology nursing: Gail Perin. J Pediatr Oncol Nurs. 2002;19:133-144.
6. Hilkemeyer R. A historical perspective in cancer nursing. Oncol Nurs Forum. 1982;9:47-56.
7. Loescher L. The influence of technology on cancer nursing. Semin Oncol Nurs. 2000;16:3-11.
8. Forte K. Pediatric oncology nursing: providing care through decades of change. J Pediatr Oncol Nurs. 2001;18:154-163.
9. Nelson M. APON becomes APHON to begin its second 30 years. APHON Counts. Glenview, Ill, Association of Pediatric Hematology/Oncology Nurses, 2006 (www.apon.org).
10. Association of Pediatric Hematology/Oncology Nurses Website. http://www.apon.org/i4a/pages/index.cfm?pageid=1. Accessed March 23, 2008.
11. Craytor J. Highlights in education for cancer nursing. Oncol Nurs Forum. 1982;9:51-59.
12. Marino B, Branowicki P, Bennett J, et al. Evaluating process changes in a pediatric hospital medication system. Outcomes Manag. 2002;6:10-15.
13. Branowicki P, Brace O'Neill J, Dwyer J, et al. Process improvement: improving complex medication systems—an interdisciplinary approach. J Nurs Adm. 2003;33:199-200.
14. Dinning C, Branowicki P, Brace O'Neill J, et al. Chemotherapy error reduction: a multidisciplinary approach to create templated order sets. J Pediatr Oncol Nurs. 2005;22:20-30.
15. Association of Pediatric Oncology Nurses, American Nurses Association. Scope and Standards of Pediatric Oncology Nursing Practice. Silver Spring, Md, Nurses Books, 2000.
16. Hicks MD, Lavender R. Psychosocial practice trends in pediatric oncology. J Pediatr Oncol Nurs. 2001;18:143-153.
17. Ruccione K, Fergusson J. A living legend in pediatric oncology nursing: Jean Ferguson. J Pediatr Oncol Nurs. 2001;18:229-238.
18. Joshi T, Ehrenberger H. Cancer clinical trials in the new millennium: novel challenges and opportunities for oncology nursing. Clin J Oncol Nurs. 2001;5:147-152.
19. Corrigan JJ, Feig SA, American Academy of Pediatrics. Guidelines for pediatric cancer centers. Pediatrics. 2004;113:1833-1835 (policy statement).
20. Sorokin P. New agents and future directions in biotherapy. Clin J Oncol Nurs. 2001;6:19-24.
21. Oncology Nursing Certification Corporation. ONCC Fact Sheet. www.oncc.org/about/docs/factsheet.pdf. Accessed October 6, 2008.
22. Heiney S, Wiley F. Historical beginnings of a professional nursing organization dedicated to the care of children and adolescents with cancer and their families: the Association of Pediatric Oncology Nursing from 1974 to 1993. J Pediatr Oncol Nurs. 1996;13: 196-203.
23. Lally R. Caring for kids with cancer takes passion, conviction, and commitment. ONS News. 2006;21:1-16.
24. Payne J. The nursing interventions classification: a language to define nursing. Oncol Nurs Forum. 2000;27:99-103.
25. Johnson M. Oncology nursing and integrative care: a new way of being. Integr Cancer Ther. 2003;2:353-357.
26. Miaskowski C, Eilers J, Dodd M. Introduction: shaping oncology nursing care for the future. Oncol Nurs Forum. 2004;31:3-4.
27. Anderson R, Marshall N. The importance of the pediatric oncologist–nurse partnership in the delivery of total care in pediatric oncology. Med Pediatr Oncol. 2000;34:263-264 (editorial).
28. Goldszer R. My day shadowing a nurse: learning about teamwork in health care. J Clin Outcomes Manag. 2004;11:165-166.
29. American Academy of Pediatrics Committee on Hospital Care, Institute for Family-Centered Care. Family-centered care and the pediatrician's role. Pediatrics. 2003;112:691-696 (policy statement). Also available at: http://aappolicy.aappublications.org/cgi/content/full/pediatrics;112/3/691. Accessed March 23, 2008.
30. Reid Ponte P, Conlin G, Conway J, et al. Making patient-centered care come alive. J Nurs Adm. 2003;33:82-90.
31. Frequently Asked Questions. Institute for Family-Centered Care. (Website): www.familycenteredcare.org/faq.html. Accessed March 23, 2008.

32. Barkley V. The best of times and worst of times: historical reflections from an American Cancer Society national nursing consultant. Oncol Nurs Forum. 1982;9:54-56.

33. Ritchie M. Psychosocial nursing care for adolescents with cancer. Issues Compr Pediatr Nurs. 2001;24:165-175.

34. Moore JB, Kordick MF. Sources of conflict between families and health care professionals. J Pediatr Oncol Nurs. 2006;23:82-91.

35. Decker C, Phillips C, Haase JE. Information needs of adolescents with cancer. J Pediatr Oncol Nurs. 2004;21:327-334.

36. Miller SA. Promoting self-esteem in the hospitalized adolescent: clinical interventions. Issues Compr Pediatr Nurs. 1987;10: 187-194.

37. Briseno-Toomey D. Side effects in treatment: growth and development. In Kline NE, Brace-O'Neill J, Hooke MC, et al (eds). Essentials of Pediatric Oncology Nursing: A Core Curriculum, 2nd ed. Glenview, IL, Association of Pediatric Oncology Nurses, 2004, pp 153-155.

38. Hooke M. Psychosocial issues. In Kline NE, Brace-O'Neill J, Hooke M, et al (eds). Essentials of Pediatric Oncology Nursing: A Core Curriculum, 2nd ed. Glenview, IL, Association of Pediatric Oncology Nurses, 2004, pp 196-227.

39. Beale KL, Bradlyn AS, Kato PM. Psychoeducational interventions with pediatric cancer patients. Part II. Effects of information and skills training on health-related outcomes. J Child Fam Stud. 2003;12:385-397.

40. Baggot C, Beale IL, Dodd MJ, Kato PM. A survey of self-care and dependent-care advice given by pediatric oncology nurses. J Pediatr Oncol Nurs. 2004;21:214-222.

41. Holm KE, Patterson JM, Gurney JG. Parental involvement and family-centered care in the diagnostic and treatment phases of childhood cancer: results from a qualitative study. J Pediatr Oncol Nurs. 2003;20:301-313.

42. Patterson K, Porock D. A survey of pediatric oncology nurses' perceptions of parent educational needs. J Pediatr Oncol Nurs. 2005;22:58-66.

43. Santacroce S. Uncertainty, anxiety, and symptoms of posttraumatic stress in parents of children recently diagnosed with cancer. J Pediatr Oncol Nurs. 2002;19:104-111.

44. Sobo EJ. Good communication in pediatric cancer care: a culturally-informed research agenda. J Pediatr Oncol Nurs. 2004;21: 150-154.

45. Clarke-Steffen L. Reconstructing reality: family strategies for managing childhood cancer. J Pediatr Nurs. 1997;12:278-287.

46. Association of Pediatric Hematology/Oncology Nurses. (Publications): www.association-office.com/APHON/etools/products/products.cfm. Accessed March 23, 2008.

47. CureSearch: for parents and families. National Childhood Cancer Foundation Children's Oncology Group. (Website): www.curesearch.org/for_parents_and_families. Accessed March 23, 2008.

48. Jacob E. Continuing care of the newly diagnosed child with cancer from hospital to home. Part 1. Home Health Care Consultant. 2000;7:1A-11A.

49. Leonard M. Diagnostic evaluations and staging procedure. In Baggott CR, Kelly KP, Fochtman D, Foley GV (eds). Nursing Care of Children and Adolescents with Cancer, 3rd ed. Philadelphia, Saunders, 2002, pp 66-89.

50. Clarke-Steffen L. Waiting and not knowing: the diagnosis of cancer in a child. J Pediatr Oncol Nurs. 1993;10:146-153.

51. Mack J, Grier H. The day one talk. J Clin Oncol. 2004;22:563-566.

52. Rubino P, Harley J. Diagnostic and staging procedures. In Kline NE, Brace-O'Neill J, Hooke MC, et al. Essentials of Pediatric Oncology Nursing, 2nd ed. Glenview, IL, Association of Pediatric Oncology Nurses, 2004, pp 74-78.

53. Hockenberry MJ, Kline NE. Nursing support of the child with cancer. In Pizzo PA, Poplack DG. Principles and Practice of Pediatric Oncology, 5th ed. Philadelphia, Lippincott Williams & Wilkins, 2006, pp 1380-1398.

54. Ljungman G, Gordh T, Sörensen S, Kreuger A. Lumbar puncture in pediatric oncology: conscious sedation vs. general anesthesia. Med Pediatr Oncol. 2001;36:372-379.

55. Joffe S, Cook EF, Cleary PD, et al. Quality of informed consent in cancer clinical trials: a cross-sectional survey. Lancet. 2001; 358:1772-1777.

56. American Society of Clinical Oncology. (Website): www.asco.org/portal/site. Accessed March 23, 2008.

57. Hoekstra-Weebers J, Jaspers J, Kamps W, Klip E. Psychological adaptation and social support of parents of pediatric cancer patients: a prospective longitudinal study. J Pediatr Psychol. 2001;26:225-235.

58. Bernier MJ, Samares DC, Owen SV, Newhouse PL. Preoperative teaching received and valued in a day surgery setting. AORN J. 2003;77:563-585.

59. Chang A, Hendershot E, Colapinto K. Minimizing the complications related to fever in the postoperative pediatric oncology patient. J Pediatr Oncol Nurs. 23;2006:75-81.

60. Sentivany-Collins S. Treatment of pain. In Baggott CR, Kelly KP, Fochtman D, Foley GV (eds). Nursing Care of Children and Adolescents with Cancer, 3rd ed. Philadelphia, WB Saunders, 2002:319-333.

61. American Academy of Pediatrics. The assessment and management of acute pain in infants, children, and adolescents. Pediatrics. 2001;108:793-796.

62. Oakes LL. Assessment and management of pain in the critically ill patient. Crit Care Nurs Clin North Am. 2001;13:281-295.

63. Ettinger A, Bond D, Sievers T. Chemotherapy. In Baggot CR, Kelly KP, Fochtman D, Foley GV (eds). Nursing Care of Children and Adolescents with Cancer, 3rd ed. Philadelphia, WB Saunders, 2002:133-176.

64. Ettinger A. Classification of chemotherapeutic agents. In Kline NE, Brace-O'Neill J, Hooke MC, et al. Essentials of Pediatric Oncology Nursing, 2nd ed. Glenview, IL Association of Pediatric Oncology Nurses, 2004: pp 37-65.

65. Sievers TD, Andam R. Chemotherapy administration and immediate postadministration issues. In Kline NE, Ecktencamp D, Norville R, et al (eds). The Pediatric Chemotherapy and Biotherapy Curriculum. Glenview, IL, Association of Pediatric Oncology Nurses, 2004, pp 76-98.

66. Kline NE, Echtencamp D, Norville R, et al (eds). The Pediatric Chemotherapy and Biotherapy Curriculum. Glenview IL, Association of Pediatric Oncology Nurses, 2004.

67. Herring RA, Hesselgrave J, Norville R. Toxicity and symptom management: In Kline NE, Ecktencamp D, Norville R, et al (eds). The Pediatric Chemotherapy and Biotherapy Curriculum. Glenview, IL, Association of Pediatric Oncology Nurses, 2004, pp 89-128.

68. Kaushal R, Bates D, Landrigan C, et al. Medication errors and adverse drug events in pediatric inpatients. JAMA. 2001;285: 2114-2120.

69. Marino BL, Reinhardt K, Eichelberger WJ, Steingard R. Prevalence of errors in a pediatric hospital medication system: implications for error proofing. Outcomes Manag. 2000;4:129-136.

70. Roll L. Preadministration considerations. In Kline NE, Brace-O'Neill J, Hooke MC, et al. Essentials of Pediatric Oncology Nursing, 2nd ed. Glenview, IL, Association of Pediatric Oncology Nurses; 2004: pp 73-125.

71. Anderson KN (ed). Mosby's Medical, Nursing and Allied Health Dictionary, 6th ed. St. Louis, Mosby, 2002.

72. Conley SB. Safe handling of chemotherapeutic agents. In Kline NE, Ecktencamp D, Norville R, et al (eds). The Pediatric Chemotherapy and Biotherapy Curriculum. Glenview, IL, Association of Pediatric Oncology Nurses, 2004, pp 67-72.

73. Ritchie M, McAdams C, Fritz N. Exposure risk in the handling and administration of chemotherapy agents: a review and syn-

thesis of the literature. Online J Knowl Synth Nurs. 2000;7 (www.stt.iupui.edu/library/ojksn).

74. Ruble K, Kelly KP. Radiation therapy in childhood cancer. Semin Oncol Nurs. 1999;15:292-302.

75. Cullen PM, Derrickson JD, Potter JA. Radiation Therapy. In Baggot CR, Kelly KP, Fochtman D, Foley GV (eds). Nursing Care of Children and Adolescents with Cancer, 3rd ed. Philadelphia, WB Saunders, 2002, pp 133-176.

76. Burks C. Principles of biotherapy. In Kline NE, Ecktencamp D, Norville R, et al (eds). The Pediatric Chemotherapy and Biotherapy Curriculum. Glenview, IL, Association of Pediatric Oncology Nurses; 2004, pp 31-36.

77. Norville R, Monroe R, Forte K. Hematopoietic stem cell transplantation. In Kline NE, Brace-O'Neill J, Hooke MC, et al. Essentials of Pediatric Oncology Nursing, 2nd ed. Glenview, IL, Association of Pediatric Oncology Nurses, 2004, pp 104-114.

78. Ryan LG, Kristovich K, Haugen MS, Hubbell MM. Hemapoietic stem cell transplantation. In Baggott CR, Kelly KP, Fochtman D, Foley GV (eds). Nursing Care of Children and Adolescents with Cancer, 3rd ed. Philadelphia, WB Saunders, 2002, pp 212-255.

79. Carlson C, Reilly M, Hitchens A. An innovative approach to the care of patients on phase I and phase II clinical trials: the role of the experimental therapeutics nurse. J Pediatr Oncol Nurs. 2005;22:353-364.

80. National Cancer Institute. Children's Assent to Clinical Trial Participation. National Cancer Institute. (Website): www.cancer.gov/clinicaltrials/understanding/childrensassent0101. Accessed March 23, 2008.

81. Bradlyn AS, Kato PM, Beale IL, Cole S. Pediatric oncology professionals' perceptions of information needs of adolescent patients with cancer. J Pediatr Oncol Nurs. 2004;21:335-342.

82. Silva M. Cancer research. In Kline NE, Ecktencamp D, Norville R, et al (eds). The Pediatric Chemotherapy and Biotherapy Curriculum. Glenview, IL, Association of Pediatric Oncology Nurses, 2004, pp 25-26.

83. Hawks R. Complementary and alternative medicine research initiative in the Children's Oncology Group and the role of the pediatric oncology nurse. J Pediatr Oncol Nurs. 2006;23:261-264.

84. Post-White J. Complementary and alternative treatments. In Kline NE, Brace-O'Neill J, Hooke MC, et al (eds). Essentials of Pediatric Oncology Nursing: A Core Curriculum, 2nd ed. Glenview, IL, Association of Pediatric Oncology Nurses, 2004, pp 120-127.

85. Gagnon EM, Recklitis CJ. Parents' decision-making preferences in pediatric oncology: the relationship to health care involvement and complementary therapy use. Psychooncology. 2003;12:442-452.

86. Post-White J, Sencer SF, Fitzgerald MA. Complementary and alternative treatments. In Baggott CR, Kelly KP, Fochtman D, Foley GV (eds). Nursing Care of Children and Adolescents with Cancer, 3rd ed. Philadelphia, WB Saunders, 2002, pp 256-265.

87. Post-White J, Hawks RG. Complementary and alternative medicine in pediatric oncology. Semin Oncol Nurs. 2005;21:107-114.

88. Ott MJ. Mind-body therapies for the pediatric oncology patient: matching the right therapy with the right patient. J Pediatr Oncol Nurs. 2006;23:254-257.

89. Panzarella C, Baggot CR, Comeau M, et al. Management of disease and treatment related complications. In Baggott CR, Kelly KP, Fochtman D, Foley GV. Nursing Care of Children and Adolescents with Cancer, 3rd ed. Philadelphia, WB Saunders 2002, pp 279-318.

90. Hedstrom M, Haglund K, Skolin I, Von Essen I. Distressing events for children and adolescents with cancer: child, parent, and nurse perceptions. J Pediatr Oncol Nurs. 2003;20:120-132.

91. Mooney-Doyle K. An examination of fatigue in advanced childhood cancer. J Pediatr Oncol Nurs. 2006;23:305-310.

92. Fochtman D. The concept of suffering in children and adolescents with cancer. J Pediatr Oncol Nurs. 2006;23:92-102.

93. Woodgate R, Degner L. Expectations and beliefs about children's cancer symptoms: perspectives of children with cancer and their families. Oncol Nurs Forum. 2003;30:479-491.

94. Hockenberry MJ. Symptom management research in children with cancer. J Pediatr Oncol Nurs. 2004;21:132-136.

94a. Herring RA, Hesslegrave J, Norille R, Madsen L. Toxicity and Symptom Management. In Kline NE, et al (eds.). The Pediatric Chemotherapy and Biotherapy Curriculum, 2nd ed., Glenview, IL: Association of Pediatric Hematology Oncology Nurses, 2007, pp 89-128.

95. Bryant R. Managing side-effects of childhood cancer treatment. J Pediatr Nurs. 2003;18:113-125.

96. Collins JJ, Byrnes ME, Dunkel IJ, et al. The measurement of symptoms in children with cancer. J Pain Symptom Manage. 2000;19:363-373.

97. O'Grady NP, Alexander M, Dellinger E, et al. Guidelines for the prevention of intravascular catheter-related infections. Pediatrics. 2002;110:51-75.

98. Centers for Disease Control and Prevention, Hospital Infections Program. National nosocomial infections surveillance (NNIS) system report, data summary from January 1990-May 1999, issued June 1999. Am J Infect Control. 1999;27:520-532.

99. Shulster I, Chinn RY. Guidelines for environmental infection control in health-care facilities. Recommendations of the CDC and Health care Infection Control Practices Advisory Committee (HICPAC). MMWR Recomm Rep. 2003;52:1-42.

100. Levine JE, Boxer LA. Clinical application of hematopoetic growth factors in pediatric oncology. Curr Opin Hematol. 2002;9:222-227.

100a. How can Neulasta help; When your start chemotherapy, start strong and support your natural defenses with Neulasta (www.neulasta.com/patient/howcanhelp/how_canhelp.jsp). Accessed October 11, 2008.

101. Dyer SL, Collins CT, Baghurst P, et al. Insuflon versus subcutaneous injection for cytokine administration in children and adolescents: a randomized crossover study. J Pediatr Oncol Nurs. 2004;21:79-86.

102. Clarke E, Glaser AW, Picton SV. *Pneumocystis carinii* pneumonia: a late presentation following treatment for stage IV neuroblastoma. Pediatr Hematol Oncol. 2003;20:467-471.

103. Kline N. Prevention and treatment of infection. In Baggott CR, Kelly KP, Fochtman D, Foley GV (eds). Nursing Care of Children and Adolescents with Cancer, 3rd ed. Philadelphia, WB Saunders, 2002, pp 266-278.

104. Wilson K. Bone marrow suppression. In Kline NE, Brace-O'Neill J, Hooke MC, et al (eds). Essentials of Pediatric Oncology Nursing: A Core Curriculum, 2nd ed. Glenview, IL, Association of Pediatric Oncology Nurses, 2004, pp 128-129.

105. Scott T. Neutropenia. In Kline NE, Brace-O'Neill J, Hooke MC, et al (eds). Essentials of Pediatric Oncology Nursing: A Core Curriculum, 2nd ed. Glenview, IL, Association of Pediatric Oncology Nurses, 2004, pp 64-66.

106. Barton SJ, Chase T, Latham B, Rayens MK. Comparing two methods to obtain blood specimens from pediatric central venous catheters. J Pediatr Oncol Nurs. 2004;21:320-326.

107. Pruss A, Kalus AL, Radtke H, et al. Universal leukodepletion of blood components results in a significant reduction of febrile non-hemolytic but not allergic transfusion reactions. Transfus Apher Sci. 2004;30:41-46.

108. Grass JA, Wafa T, Reames A, et al. Prevention of transfusion-associated graft-versus-host disease by photochemical treatment. Blood. 1999;93;3140-3147.

109. Herberg A. Blood product administration. In Bowden VR, Greenberg CS (eds). Pediatric Nursing Procedures. Philadelphia, Lippincott Williams & Wilkins, 2003, pp 113-125.

110. Enright H, Davis K, Gernsheimer T, et al. Factors influencing moderate to severe reactions to platelet transfusions: experience of TRAP multi-center clinical trial. Transfusion. 2003;43:1545-1552.

111. Elliott S. Thrombocytopenia. In Kline NE, Brace-O'Neill J, Hooke MC, et al (eds). Essentials of Pediatric Oncology Nursing: A Core Curriculum, 2nd ed. Glenview, IL, Association of Pediatric Oncology Nurses, 2004, pp 69-70.

112. Hockenberry M, Hinds PS, Barrera P, et al. Three instruments to assess fatigue in children with cancer: the child, parent, and staff perspectives. J Pain Symptom Manage. 2003;25:319-328.

113. Varni JW, Burwinkle TM, Katz ER, et al. The PedsQl in pediatric cancer: reliability and validity of the Pediatric Quality of Life Inventory Generic Core Scales, Multidimensional Fatigue Scale, and Cancer Module. Cancer. 2002;94:2090-2106.

114. Davies B, Whitsett SF, Bruce A, McCarthy P. A typology of fatigue in children and adolescents with cancer. J Pediatr Oncol Nurs. 2002;19:12-21.

115. Wohlschlaeger A. Prevention and treatment of mucositis: a guide for nurses. J Pediatr Oncol Nurs. 2004;21:281-287.

116. Chen CF, Wang RH, Cheng SN, Chang YC. Assessment of chemotherapy-induced oral complications in children with cancer. J Pediatr Oncol Nurs. 2004;21:33-39.

117. Bradlyn AS. Health-related quality of life in pediatric oncology: current status and future challenges. J Pediatr Oncol Nurs. 2004;21:137-140.

118. Rubenstein EB, Peterson DE, Schubert M, et al. Mucositis study section of the multinational association for supportive care in cancer: international society for oral oncology. Clinical practice guidelines for the prevention and treatment of cancer therapy-induced oral and gastrointestinal mucositis. Cancer. 2004;100:2026-2046.

119. Miller M, Kearney N. Oral care for patients with cancer: a review of the nursing literature. Cancer Nurs. 2001;24:241-254.

120. Vincent C, Denyes MJ. Relieving children's pain: nurses' abilities and analgesic administration practices. J Pediatr Nurs. 2004;53:1-10.

121. Jodarski K, Wilson K. Pain. In Kline NE, Brace-O'Neill J, Hooke MC, et al (eds). Essentials of Pediatric Oncology Nursing: A Core Curriculum, 2nd ed. Glenview, IL, Association of Pediatric Oncology Nurses, 2004, pp 155-159.

122. Broome ME, Rehwaldt M, Fogg L. Relationship between cognitive behavioral techniques, temperament, observed distress, and pain reports in children and adolescents during lumbar punctures. J Pediatr Nurs. 1998;13:48-54.

123. Chambers CR, Hardial J, Craig KD, et al. Faces scales for the measurement of postoperative pain intensity in children following minor surgery. Clin J Pain. 2005;21:277-285.

124. Ljungman G, Gordh T, Sörensen S, Kreuger A. Pain in paediatric oncology: interviews with children, adolescents and their parents. Acta Paediatr. 1999;88:623-630.

125. Crock C, Olsson C, Phillips R, et al. General anesthesia or conscious sedation for painful procedures in childhood cancer: the family's perspective. Arch Dis Child. 2003;88:253-257.

126. McPherson CF, Lundblad LA. Conscious sedation of pediatric oncology patients for painful procedures: development and implementation of a clinical practice protocol. J Pediatr Oncol Nurs. 1997;4:33-42.

127. Van Cleve L, Bossert E, Beecroft P, et al. The pain experience of children with leukemia during the first year after diagnosis. Nurs Res. 2004;19:40-50.

128. Weisman SJ, Bernstien B, Schechter NJ. Consequences of inadequate analgesia during painful procedures in children. Arch Pediatr Adolesc Med. 1998;152:147-149.

129. Jayabose S, Levendoglu-Tugal O, Giamelli J, et al. Intravenous anesthesia with propofol for painful procedures in children with cancer. Pediatr Hematol Oncol. 2001;23:290-293.

130. Luhman J, Hurt S, Shootman M, Kennedy R. A comparison of buffered lidocaine versus Ela-Max before peripheral intravenous catheter insertions in children. Pediatrics. 2004;113:217-220.

131. Christensen J, Fatchett D. Promoting parental use of distraction and relaxation in pediatric oncology patients during invasive procedures. J Pediatr Oncol Nurs. 2002;19:127-132.

132. Callahan C, De La Cruz J. Central line placement for the pediatric oncology patient: a model of advanced practice nurse collaboration. J Pediatr Oncol Nurs. 2004;21:16-21.

133. Shulster I, Chinn RY. Guidelines for environmental infection control in health-care facilities. Recommendations of the CDC and Health care Infection Control Practices Advisory Committee (HICPAC). MMWR Recomm Rep. 2003;52:1-42.

134. McInally W. Whose line is it anyway? Management of central venous catheters in children. Paediatr Nurs. 2005;17:14-18.

135. Peterson KK. Central line sepsis. Clin J Oncol Nurs. 2003;7:218-221; 241.

136. Clarke JN, Fletcher PC, Schneider MA. Mothers' home care work when their children have cancer. J Pediatr Oncol Nurs. 2005;22:365-373.

137. Raich DW, Holdsworth MT, Winters SS, et al. Economic comparison of home-care based versus hospital based treatment of chemotherapy-induced febrile neutropenia in children. Value Health. 2003;6:158-167.

138. Holdsworth MT, Raisch DW, Winter SS, et al. Pain and distress from bone marrow aspiration and lumbar punctures. Ann Pharmacother. 2003;37:17-22.

139. Stevens B, McKeever P, Law MP, et al. Children receiving chemotherapy at home: perceptions of children and parents. J Pediatr Oncol Nurs. 2006;23:276-285.

140. Duffy-Lind E, O'Holleran E, Healey M, et al. Transitioning to survivorship: a pilot study. J Pediatr Oncol Nurs. 2006;23:335-343.

141. Haase J, Rostad M. Experiences of completing cancer therapy: children's perspectives. Oncol Nurs Forum. 1994;21:1483-1494.

142. Labay L, Mayans S, Harris M. Integrating the child into home and community following the completion of cancer treatment. J Pediatr Oncol Nurs. 2004;21:165-169.

143. Arnold EM. The cessation of cancer treatment as a crisis. Soc Work Health Care. 1999;29:21-38.

144. Bruce M. A systematic and conceptual review of posttraumatic stress in childhood cancer survivors and their parents. Clin Psychol Rev. 2006;26:233-256.

145. Woodgate R, Faith Degner L. A substantive theory of keeping the spirit alive: the spirit within children with cancer and their families. J Pediatr Oncol Nurs. 2003;20:103-119.

146. Kazak A, Barakat L. Parenting stress and quality of life during treatment for childhood leukemia predicts child and parent adjustment after treatment ends. J Pediatr Psychol. 1997;22:749-758 (brief report).

147. Hudson M, Hester A, Sweeney T, et al. A model of care for childhood cancer survivors that facilitates research. J Pediatr Oncol Nurs. 2004;21:170-174.

148. Reis LAG, Eisner MP, Kosary CL, et al. SEER Cancer Statistics Review 1975-2000. Bethesda, Md, National Cancer Institute, 2003.

149. Institute of Medicine National Research Council. Hewitt M, Weiner SL, Simone J (eds). Childhood Cancer Survivorship: Improving Care and Quality of Life. Washington, DC, The National Academies Press, 2003.

150. Spencer J. The role of cognitive remediation in childhood cancer survivors experiencing neurocognitive late effects. J Pediatr Oncol Nurs. 2006;23:321-325.

151. Kadan-Lottick N, Robison L, Gurney J, et al. Childhood cancer survivors' knowledge about their past diagnosis and treatment. JAMA. 2002;287:1832-1839.

152. Keene N, Hobbie W, Ruccione K. Childhood Cancer Survivors: A Practical Guide to Your Future. Sebastopol, CA, O'Reilly and Associates, 2000.

153. Bashore L. Childhood and adolescent cancer survivors' knowledge of their disease and effects of treatment. J Pediatr Oncol Nurs. 2004;21:98-102.

154. Eshelman D, Landier W, Sweeney T, et al. Facilitating care for childhood cancer survivors: integrating Children's Oncology Group long-term follow-up guidelines and health links in clinical practice. J Pediatr Oncol Nurs. 2004;21:271-280.

155. Bottomly S. Late effects of childhood cancer: psychosocial effects, educational issues. In Kline NE, Brace-O'Neill J, Hooke MC, et al (eds). Essentials of Pediatric Oncology Nursing: A Core Curriculum, 2nd ed. Glenview, IL, Association of Pediatric Oncology Nurses, 2004, pp 260-267.

156. CureSearch. Long Term Follow-up Guidelines for Survivors of Childhood, Adolescent, and Young Adult Cancers. Children's Oncology Group. (Website). www.survivorshipguidelines.org. Accessed March 24, 2008.

157. Smith M, Hare ML. An overview of progress in childhood cancer survival. J Pediatr Oncol Nurs. 2004;21:160-164.

158. Smith AB, Bashore L. The effect of clinic-based health promotion education on perceived health status and health promotion behaviors of adolescent and young adult cancer survivors. J Pediatr Oncol Nurs. 2006;23:326-334.

159. Nelson MB. Late effects of chemotherapy. In Kline NE, Ecktencamp D, Norville R, et al (eds). The Pediatric Chemotherapy and Biotherapy Curriculum. Glenview, IL, Association of Pediatric Oncology Nurses 2004, pp 143-150.

160. Biasotti S, Garavanta A, Padovani P, et al. Role of active follow-up for early diagnosis of relapse after elective end of therapies. Pediatr Blood Cancer. 2005;45:781-786.

161. Lee-Jones C, Humphris G, Dixon R, Hatcher MB. Fear of cancer recurrence—a literature review and proposed cognitive formulation to explain exacerbation of recurrence fears. Psychooncology. 1997;6:95-105.

162. Hinds PS, Birenbaum LK, Clarke-Steffen L, et al. Coming to terms: a parent's response to first cancer recurrence in their child. Nurs Res. 1996;45:148-153.

163. Mahon SM, Cella DF, Donavan MI. Psychological adjustment to recurrent cancer. Oncol Nurs Forum. 1990;17(suppl 3):47-52.

164. Hockenberry-Eaton M, Dilorio C, Kemp V. The relationship of illness longevity and relapse with self-perception, cancer stressors, anxiety and coping strategies in children with cancer. J Pediatr Oncol Nurs. 1995;12:71-79.

165. Independent Lens. Pediatric Cancer. Independent Lens. (Website). www.pbs.org/independentlens/lioninthehouse/03_index.htm. Accessed March 25, 2008. (Based on information from film A Lion in the House, Bognar S, Reichert J, producers/directors.)

166. Institute of Medicine. Field M, Behrman RE (eds). When Children Die: Improving Palliative and End of Life Care for Children and Their Families. Washington, DC, The National Academies Press, 2002.

167. Dunn K, Otten C, Stephens E. Nursing experience and the care of the dying patients. Oncol Nurs Forum. 2005;32:97-104.

168. Kline N. Care of the terminally ill child and the family. In Kline NE, Brace-O'Neill J, Hooke MC, et al (eds). Essentials of Pediatric Oncology Nursing: A Core Curriculum, 2nd ed. Glenview, IL, Association of Pediatric Oncology Nurses, 2004: pp 243-244.

169. American Academy of Hospice and Palliative Medicine. College of Palliative Care. (Website): www.aahpm.org/about/college.html. Accessed: March 25, 2008.

170. National Coalition for Cancer Survivorship. (Website): www.canceradvocacy.org/about. Accessed March 25, 2008.

171. American Academy of Pediatrics. Committee on Bioethics and Committee on Hospital Care. Palliative care for children. Pediatrics. 2000;106:351-357.

172. Burghen E, Haluska H, Steen B, Hinds P. Children and adolescents participating in research and clinical care decisions at end of life. J Hospice Pall Nurs. 2004;6:176-186.

173. Meyer E, Ritholz M, Burns J, Troug R. Improving the quality of end-of-life care in the pediatric intensive care unit: parents' priorities and recommendations. Pediatrics. 2006;117:649-657.

175. Houlahan KE, Branowicki PA, Mack JW, et al. Can end-of-life care for the pediatric patient suffering with escalating and intractable symptoms be improved? J Pediatr Oncol Nurs. 2006;23:45-51.

176. American Cancer Society. What is Hospice Care? (Website): www.cancer.org/docroot/ETO/content/ETO_2_5X_What_Is_Hospice_Care.asp?sitearea=ETO. Accessed March 25, 2008.

177. The Joint Commission. Making better health care choices: helping you choose quality home care and hospice services. The Joint Commission. (Website): www.jointcommission.org/GeneralPublic/Choices/hc_ome.htm. Accessed March 25, 2008.

179. Ferrell BR, Coyle N. Palliative Nursing. New York, Oxford Press, 2001.

180. Saunders JM, Valente SM. Nurses' grief. Cancer Nurs. 1994;17:318-325.

181. Fochtman D. Palliative care. In Baggott CR, Kelly KP, Fochtman D, Foley GV (eds). Nursing Care of Children and Adolescents with Cancer, 3rd ed. Philadelphia, WB Saunders, 2002, pp 66-89.

182. Vachon MLS. Staff stress in the care of the critically ill and dying child. Issues Compr Pediatr Nurs. 1985;8:151-182.

183. Carper B. Fundamental patterns of knowing in nursing. In Nicoll LH (ed). Perspectives on Nursing Theory. Philadelphia, Lippincott Raven, 1978, pp 247-256.

184. American Association of Colleges of Nursing. The End-of-Life Nursing Education Consortium (ELNEC). (Website): www.aacn.nche.edu/elnec/pdf/FactSheet.pdf. Accessed March 25, 2008.

185. Hospice and Palliative Nurses Association. Scope and Standards of Hospice and Palliative Nursing Practice. Silver Spring, Md, American Nurses Association, 2002.

186. American Nurses Association. Code of Ethics for Nurses, with Interpretive Statements. (Website): nursingworld.org/MainMenuCategories/ThePracticeofProfessionalNursing/EthicsStandards/CodeofEthics.aspx. Accessed March 25, 2008.

187. Association of Pediatric Oncology Nurses. Scope and Standards of Pediatric Oncology Nursing Practice. Silver Spring, Md, American Nurses Association, 2000, pp 22-23.

188. Baker L, Marquis B. Nursing Administration Review and Resource Manual. Washington, DC, Institute of Research, Education and Consultation at the American Nurses Credentialing Center, 2003.

189. Gallagher A, Wainwright P. The ethical divide. Nurs Stand. 2005;20:22-25.

190. Hailstorm I, Leander G. Decision-making during hospitalization: parents' and children's involvement. J Clin Nurs. 2004;13:367-375.

191. Toiviainen L. Can practical nursing ethics be taught? Nurs Ethics. 2005;12:335-336.

192. Holm S. What should other health care professions learn from nursing ethics? Nurs Philos. 2006;7:165-174.

193. Breier-Mackie S. Medical ethics and nursing ethics: is there really any difference? Gastroenterol Nurs. 2006;29:182-183 (Ethics Connection).

194. Hallstrom I, Runeson I, Elander G. An observational study of the level at which parents participate in decisions during their child's hospitalization. Nurs Ethics. 2002;9:202-214.

195. Sorlie V, Kihlgren A, Kihlgren M. Meeting ethical challenges in acute nursing care as narrated by registered nurses. Nurs Ethics. 2005;12:133-142.

196. Gordon E, Hamric A. (2006). The courage to stand up: the cultural politics of nurses' access to ethics consultation. J Clin Ethics. 2006;17:231-244.

197. Loescher L. The influence of technology on cancer nursing. Semin Oncol Nurs. 2000;16:3-11.

198. Gibson F. Evidence in action: fostering growth of research-based practice in children's cancer nursing. Eur J Oncol Nurs. 2005; 9:8-20.

199. Sorokin P. New agents and future directions in biotherapy. Clin J Oncol Nurs. 2001;6:19-24.

200. Schmalenberg C, Kramer M, King C, et al. Excellence through evidence, securing collegial/collaborative nurse-physician relationships. Part 1. J Nurs Adm. 2005;35:450-466.

201. Ferrand E, Lemaire F, Regnier B. Discrepancies between perceptions by physicians and nursing staff of intensive care unit end-of-life decisions. Am J Respir Crit Care Med. 2003;67:1310-1315.

202. Pritchard M, Davies B. End of life in pediatric oncology: how clinical practice leads to research. J Pediatr Oncol Nurs. 2002; 19:191-197.

203. Freireich E. The future of clinical cancer research in the next millennium. Clin Cancer Res. 1997;3:2563-2570.

204. McGuire D, Ropka M. Research and oncology nursing practice. Semin Oncol Nurs. 2000;16:35-46.

205. Nelson M. What keeps APON nurses awake at night? Association of Pediatric Hematology/Oncology Nurses Association. (Website): www.apon.org/files/public/APHON06FALLarticles.pdf. Accessed March 25, 2008.

206. Buckley M. Childhood cancer: meeting the information needs of families. Paediatr Nurs. 2000;12:22-23.

207. Grant M, Golant M, Rivera L, et al. Developing a community program on cancer pain and fatigue. Cancer Pract. 2000;8:187-194.

208. Herth K. Development and implementation of a hope intervention program. Oncol Nurs Forum. 2001;28:1009-1017.

209. Krasuska M, Stanislawek A, Mazurkiewicz M. Complementary and alternative care within cancer care. Ann Univ Mariae Curie Sklodowska (Med). 2003;58:418-424.

210. Post-White J, Hawks R, O'Mara A. Ott M. Future directions of CAM research in pediatric oncology. J Pediatr Oncol Nurs. 2006;32:265-268.

211. David Oriol M. Crew resource management. J Nurs Adm. 2006;36:402-406.

212. Ebright P, Urden L, Patterson E, Chalko B. Themes surrounding novice nurse near-miss and adverse-event situations. J Nurs Adm. 2004;34:531-538.

213. Newhouse R. Selecting measures for safety and quality improvement initiatives. J Nurs Adm. 2006;36:109-113.

214. Allen D, Bockenhauer B, Egan C, Kinnaird L. Relating outcomes to excellent nursing practice. J Nurs Adm. 2006;36: 140-146

215. Potter P, Wolf L, Boxerman S, et al. Understanding the cognitive work of nursing in the acute care environment. J Nurs Adm. 2005;35:327-335.

216. Spears P. Managing patient care error: nurse leaders' perspective. J Nurs Adm. 2005;35:223-224.

217. Wicks R. Overcoming Secondary Stress in Medical and Nursing Practice. New York, Oxford University Press, 2006.

218. Ropka M, Guterbock T, Krebs L, et al. Year 2000 oncology nursing society research priorities survey. Oncol Nurs Forum. 2002;29:481-491.

219. Fochtman D, Hinds P. Identifying nursing research priorities in a pediatric clinical trials cooperative group: the pediatric oncology group experience. J Pediatr Oncol Nurs. 2000;17:83-87.

30 Palliative Care in Pediatric Oncology

Jennifer W. Mack, Elana E. Evan, Janet Duncan, and Joanne Wolfe

INTRODUCTION

More than 2000 children in the United States die each year of cancer-related causes,[1] and many thousands more are living with advanced cancer. In children with cancer, it is not always possible to determine whether the disease will be responsive to cancer-directed therapy, nor is it possible to determine which type of trajectory the dying process will take. Some children may die suddenly and unexpectedly—for example, children undergoing bone marrow transplantation who experience treatment-related complications. Others may experience steady and fairly predictable declines, such as children with progressive brainstem glioma after radiation therapy. Most children with progressive cancer experience varying periods of chronic illness punctuated by crises, one of which may prove fatal. One example of this type of trajectory occurs in children with relapsed metastatic neuroblastoma who may be palliated on a long-term basis before experiencing a life-ending event.

Although intensive, interdisciplinary supportive care—that is, palliative care—is essential for all children with cancer, it is especially critical for children living with more advanced stages of cancer. Palliative care, as defined by the World Health Organization,[2] is an approach to care that improves the quality of life of patients with life-threatening illness and their families through the prevention and relief of suffering by means of early identification of and impeccable assessment and treatment of pain and other problems, physical, psychosocial, and spiritual. The World Health Organization's definition of palliative care appropriate for children and their families is as follows:

- Palliative care for children is the active total care of the child's body, mind and spirit, and it also involves giving support to the family.
- Palliative care begins when illness is diagnosed and continues regardless of whether a child receives disease-directed treatment.
- Health providers must evaluate and alleviate a child's physical, psychological, and social distress.
- Effective palliative care requires a broad multidisciplinary approach that includes the family and makes use of available community resources; it can be successfully implemented even if resources are limited.
- Palliative care may be provided in tertiary care facilities, community health centers or the home.

Both data[3,4] and clinical experience favor a blended approach to care that includes disease-directed treatments *together with* palliative, or comfort, care. This approach is the one that is most commonly favored by parents who hope for life prolongation while also desiring maximal comfort and minimal pain and suffering for their children (Fig. 30-1). Pediatric palliative care should not involve a choice between life-prolonging treatments (such as chemotherapy) and comfort care. Rather, pediatric palliative care should be integrated into an overall care plan that is individualized and adaptable to changing circumstances.

INTEGRATING PALLIATIVE CARE AT THE TIME OF DIAGNOSIS

Although palliative care and end-of-life care are often considered to be a single entity, it is important to note that palliative care can be initiated at any time, not just in the end-of-life period. Rather than being restricted to the last phase of life, palliation may include attention to symptoms from the time of diagnosis. Palliative care may also allow for discussion of goals and preferences for care, long before death occurs.

In addition, rather than precluding intensive life-prolonging care, palliative care can be complementary to therapy with curative intent. With the inclusion of palliative care early in the course of disease, children can benefit from attention to symptoms and to quality of life concurrent with efforts to control disease. Parents often have goals for their children's care that go beyond cure and prolongation of life. Parents of children who have died of cancer, for example, recall holding the simultaneous goals of extending life and minimizing suffering during their children's treatments.[4,5] Concurrent disease-directed therapy and attention to the physical, psychosocial, and spiritual needs of children and families may be the optimal approach to meeting these seemingly conflicting goals.

In some pediatric cancer patients, such as children with pontine gliomas, the pattern of progression is relatively predictable, making planning for the end of life a logical part of care starting at diagnosis. Patients with other cancers, however, may have long periods during which the disease is controlled and there is relative clinical stability. Although ultimately these children may be expected to die of the disease, the particular relapse or acute decompensation that will result in death can be difficult to predict because early relapses may be responsive to intensive treatment.

In children with relapsed neuroblastoma, for instance, many years may elapse between the first recurrence and death. At any moment, the use of intensive chemotherapy may seem reasonable and may offer significant hope of life prolongation and remediation of symptoms. However, death after repeated intensive therapies, including chemotherapy-related toxicity, may not coincide with families' wishes for the end of the children's lives and may be associated with unnecessary suffering for the children. Even when families choose life-extending measures, they should have the opportunity to do so in the context of understanding the expected trajectory of illness.

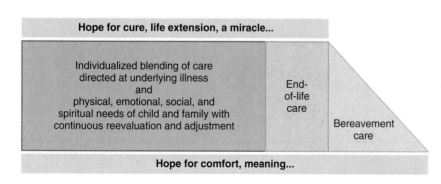

Hope for cure, life extension, a miracle...

Individualized blending of care directed at underlying illness and physical, emotional, social, and spiritual needs of child and family with continuous reevaluation and adjustment

End-of-life care

Bereavement care

Hope for comfort, meaning...

FIGURE 30-1. Pediatric palliative care includes individualized integration of palliative care principles to ensure combined hopes of varying degrees related to life extension and comfort, both of which can last throughout the children's lives. End-of-life care is an important component of palliative care, when the focus of care is almost entirely on comfort, although hope for a miracle can persist. The requirements of bereavement care can be intense and long lasting, gradually lessening over time.

Advantages of Early Integration of Palliative Care

Before patients are clearly in the last phase of life, physicians may find it difficult to initiate conversations about poor prognoses.[6] But the majority of parents of children with cancer say they want prognostic information, even when the news is upsetting.[7] Patients and families who are poorly prepared for death tend to choose more aggressive care at the end of life.[5,8] Without realistic information, they may not have the opportunity to make choices for care that are consistent with their values.

Although physicians may find the initiation of discussions about a poor prognosis difficult, families may find earlier integration of palliative care to be helpful. A study of bereaved family members of adult cancer patients, for example, found that half felt that palliative care was provided too late in the disease course, whereas less than 5% thought palliative care referrals occurred too early.[9] Clear communication by physicians was found to be an important contributing factor; families who felt that their physicians had communicated effectively about patients' prognosis and end-of-life care were less likely to feel that palliative care was introduced too late.

Early initiation of palliative care may also facilitate attention to symptoms and quality of life. Adults with advanced cancer, for example, tend to experience improvement in symptoms, including pain, anorexia, nausea, vomiting, sleeplessness, and constipation, after referral to palliative care services. In addition, patients who receive palliative care commonly experience improvements in overall quality of life and well-being.[10]

It is also possible that early discussions about palliative care can help parents to cope with death. Mothers who experience the sudden death of children tend to have more intense grief than mothers whose children die of chronic conditions.[11] These findings raise the possibility that emotional and psychological adjustment prior to death can help parents to cope with the loss of their children over time.

Perhaps most important, parents value preparation for the end-of-life period. In a study of bereaved parents of children with cancer, physicians' communication about what to expect in the end-of-life care period was a component of high-quality care.[12] Parents who felt prepared for the circumstances surrounding children's deaths were also more likely to consider care to be of high quality overall. Communication with parents in advance of children's deaths may allow them to process and be prepared for death before it happens and to make choices about end-of-life care that are right for them and their children.

Box 30-1 provides some general guidance for discussing end-of-life preferences.[13,14] Even if patients' outcomes are

---

Box 30-1	**Communicating with Children and Families About Integrating Palliative Care**

BEGINNING THE CONVERSATION

"What is your understanding of what is ahead for your child?"

"Would it be helpful to talk about how his or her disease may affect him or her in the months and years ahead?"

"As you think about what is ahead for your child, what would you like to talk about with me? What information can I give you that would be helpful to you?"

INTRODUCING THE POSSIBILITY OF DEATH

"I am hoping that we will be able to control the disease, but I am worried that this time we may not be successful."

"Although we do not know for certain what will happen for your child, I do not expect that your child will live a long and healthy life; most children with this disease eventually die because of the disease."

"I have been noticing that your child seems to be sick more and more often. I have been hoping that we would be able to make him or her better, but I am worried that his or her illness has become more difficult to control, and that soon we will not be able to help him or her to get over these illnesses. If that is the case, he or she could die of his or her disease."

ELICITING GOALS OF CARE

"As you think about your child's illness, what are your hopes?"

"As you think about your child's illness, what are your worries?"

"As you think about your child's illness, what is most important to you right now?"

"You mentioned that what is most important to you is that your child be cured of his or her disease. I am hoping for that too. But I would also like to know more about your hopes and goals for your child's care if the time comes when a cure isn't possible."

INTRODUCING PALLIATION

"Although I hope that we can control your child's disease as long as possible, at the same time I am hoping that he or she feels as good as possible each day."

"Although it is unlikely that this treatment will cure your child's disease, it may help him or her to feel better, and possibly to live longer."

TALKING ABOUT WHAT TO EXPECT

"Would it be helpful to talk about what to expect as your child's illness gets worse?"

"Although we cannot predict exactly what will happen to your child, most children with this disease eventually have [difficulty breathing]. If that happens to your child, our goal will be to help him or her feel as comfortable as possible. We can use medications to help control his or her discomfort."

TALKING TO CHILDREN

"What are you looking forward to most of all?"

"Is there anything that is worrying you or making you feel afraid?"

"Is there anything about how you are feeling that is making you feel worried or afraid?"

From Mack JW, Wolfe J. Early integration of pediatric palliative care: for some children, palliative care starts at diagnosis. Curr Opin Pediatr. 2006;18:10-14.

uncertain, death can be discussed as a possibility so that the patients have opportunities to express the desired goals of care.

MAKING THE TRANSITION TO PALLIATIVE CARE

Although integration of palliative care at the time of diagnosis is ideal, sometimes a clinical event such as relapse or a severe complication makes it necessary to discuss a poor prognosis for the first time. The transition from care intended to cure their children can be experienced by families as terrible loss. However, as with discussions about care at the time of diagnosis, honest communication about children's prognoses can help families make reasonable decisions about care on the basis of their own values.[15]

Delays in parental understanding of poor prognoses can affect the care they choose for their children. In a study of parents of children who died of cancer, parents recalled understanding that the children were likely to die about 3.5 months after the physician realized it. Earlier parental realization of the small likelihood of cure was associated with increased hospice use and decreased cancer-directed therapy during the end-of-life period.[5] Although parents sometimes have difficulty accepting poor prognoses, the difficulty physicians have in communicating poor prognoses also contributes to parents' overly optimistic expectations of cure.[16]

Discussing a Change in Prognosis

One statement physicians can use when introducing a discussion with parents about change in prognosis is, "Although I had hoped that your child would be cured and live a long life, I am now worried that this is no longer possible."[14] Acknowledging the sadness of the situation, responding to the parents' emotions, and allowing for silence can also be helpful. Parents may ask about treatment options, but such discussions should not obscure the fact that their children are unlikely to be cured. Physicians might respond to such requests by saying, for instance, "It is possible that treatment might help your child to feel better during the time she is here, but there is no treatment that will cure her." Although these conversations are difficult for families and for medical providers, such honesty can help parents to make the best possible decisions for their children. In addition, although honest provision of information is important, physicians may be able to clarify the goals of care without necessarily requiring parents to openly acknowledge that cure is not likely; this approach may be preferable to some parents.

DISCUSSING THE GOALS OF CARE

An important aspect of providing care for children with cancer is understanding the goals of care. It is common for these goals to be identified by the parents, but adolescents and even younger children are often able to define priorities for their care as well.[17] Understanding the goals of care allows the medical team to make recommendations for care that fit with patients' and families' values. In addition, the goals of care and conversations about these goals provide another window into parents' perceptions of what lies ahead.

A discussion about the goals of care can be started by simply asking parents what is most important to them as they think about what is ahead for their children.[14] Specific questions about hopes for the future and worries about what is to come can also be useful. Often, parents verbalize general goals, such as maintaining a good quality of life for as long as possible, minimizing suffering, prolonging life, or curing the cancer. It is common for parents to hold more than one goal, and they may have separate goals for cancer-directed and symptom-directed therapies; for example, the goal of cancer-directed therapy may be to cure the disease or to prolong life, whereas the goals of symptom-directed therapy may be to lessen suffering and maximize quality of life.[5,4] Although such goals may appear to be conflicting, holding more than one goal for care is normal, and physicians can make plans for care with both sets of goals in mind.

Acceptance of the parents' goals is an important aspect of acknowledging the parents' values, even when the goals are not in concert with the physicians' goals. At times, however, parents will continue to articulate the goal of cure when the medical team believes that such an outcome is not possible. Understanding what the parents would want if children cannot be cured can help the medical team to make plans for care. Back and colleagues[18] have recommended that physicians ask what the families would want if cure is not possible, a strategy described as hoping for the best but preparing for the worst. This strategy allows the medical team to have a conversation about what particular families would prefer in such a situation.

Even when parents hold the goal of cure, physicians should have clear discussions with them about the goals of treatment, especially cancer-directed treatment. Depending on the circumstances, oncologists may want to express the goal of controlling the disease for as long as possible, for example. When the purpose of treatment is to help cancer research, with little hope of benefit, that goal should be stated also.

Eliciting Children's Goals

Children and adolescents may express goals in general terms, like their parents, or they may have very specific wishes, such as staying at home, spending time with siblings, or minimizing invasive procedures.[17,19] Knowing about these goals, which can be elicited by asking children for their hopes and worries, and knowing what is most important to them when they think about what is ahead can allow the medical team to work toward meeting any specific hopes or needs.

Creating a Plan for Care Based on Goals

Once the goals of care have been elicited, a plan of care can be made. It is important to acknowledge that this plan is flexible and may change frequently and to acknowledge that each family is unique and even with similar goals, there may be very different plans of care. As previously mentioned, pediatric palliative care may be provided at the same time a family is seeking a life-prolonging or potentially curative therapy. Therefore, a plan of care may include preventive therapies, the search for life-prolonging or curative therapies, rehabilitation, and intensive quality-of-life and symptom management.[20] Having parents consider the following questions may help them to make decisions.

- How will this treatment affect my child's quality of life?
- What is likely to happen without this treatment?
- How will the treatment change my child's prognosis?
- What will it be like for my child (and family) to go through this treatment?

- Are there other options we should consider that might have the same outcome but use a different approach?

Particularly as cure becomes less likely, assisting parents to think deeply about what brings their children joy or what experiences provide good quality of life may help them in their decision making. Ideally, the children are included in these decisions and plans of care. In one study it was found that children between the ages of 8 to 17 years wanted to be told whether they were dying, and adolescents in particular wanted to participate in decisions concerning palliative care.[21]

Appointing a Health Care Proxy

For patients older than 18 years of age, the decision about whom to appoint as health care proxies may provide an opportunity for the discussion of care preferences. This document, usually completed upon admission to the hospital, allows patients to designate someone to make medical decisions if the patients are unable to do so. Ideally, the proxies make decisions based on knowledge of what the patients would want in various situations, and not on what the proxies would want or believe to be appropriate. Most hospitals have standard forms that are completed by patients and an admissions staff person. This could be an opportunity to explore the true wishes of young adult patients and can lead to rich discussion and meaningful decision making.

Resuscitation Status and Other Aspects of Advance Care Planning

Advance care planning involves choosing proxies for those over 18 years of age but encompasses a much broader scope. Planning may include (1) the designation of a decision maker; (2) discussion of the illness and prognosis; (3) the establishment of goals of care; (4) discussion of preferences for resuscitation, artificial nutrition and hydration, and palliative sedation; (5) the primary location of care and death; and (6) discussion of organ or tissue donation, including autopsy, and preferences for funeral arrangements.[22] Needless to say, advance care planning is a process that requires time and often occurs through multiple conversations and at different phases of children's illnesses. For example, Wolfe and colleagues showed that discussions about hospice care occurred approximately 2 months prior to death, but do-not-resuscitate (DNR) orders were written about 1 month before death.[3] Several resources are available to assist in these discussions. *Five Wishes*, for those older than 18 years of age (available at www.agingwithdignity.org) is a legal document in 37 states. This document presents information and questions in a way that enhances communication about these difficult subjects, and it addresses the kinds of nonmedical interventions that would be wanted, such as music, prayer, presence of family, and so on. Recently developed, *My Wishes*, which is for those younger than 18 years of age (www.agingwithdignity.org), is not a legal document, but with simple questions and the opportunity to write and draw, it affords children and adolescents the opportunity to communicate their wishes.

Other techniques may be helpful too, such as asking adolescents simply to list their wishes, realistic or not. Providers may also ask questions such as, "What is your understanding of your illness now?" Another technique is to suggest that adolescents write down, with a trusted person such as a child life specialist, psychosocial clinician, or parent, the questions they would like to ask of the health care team. In a study asking

parents whether they had talked to their children about death, none of those who had done so regretted it.[23] The parents had rich anecdotes concerning references their children had brought up about death (personal communication, U. Kreichbergs, 2006).

Making Recommendations

Even when curative therapies are no longer sought, families report wanting recommendations regarding available interventions. Most do not want the burden of making decisions completely on their own. Providers may feel that, especially when there are treatments with uncertain or marginal benefits, plans for care should be the parents' choice. However, parents can often be best supported by providers who clearly discuss the positives and negatives of each treatment or therapy and then recommend treatment in the context of the families' goals and values. This can apply to a wide spectrum of situations, such as participating in a phase I or II clinical treatment trial, putting in a chest tube for pleural effusions, using intravenous antibiotics to treat an infection, or instituting a DNR order. Clinicians who make recommendations can alleviate this burden on the parents and help to minimize parents' sense of regret and responsibility for choices that ultimately allow death to occur.

COMMUNICATING PLANS FOR CARE

The plan of care must be communicated to all involved in children's care. Consistency and honesty are among what bereaved parents tell us is most important.[24] Written documentation of team meetings, family meetings, and the care plan is essential. Documentation can also help to communicate plans of care to other providers, such as the home care team and those providing emergency services. Along with a home DNR or comfort care form, for instance, a letter that documents the children's situations and plans for care can be carried by the parents to help ensure that any care providers they encounter know their goals for care. By partnering with the children and families, the health care team in the hospital or home has the opportunity to enhance quality of life while the child is living and to affect the grieving and bereavement that will follow for the family.

Talking with Children About Palliative Care

To tell or not to tell? This is the question that typically arises when parents of and health care providers for children with life-threatening illnesses face the issue of discussing palliative care with children. Health care providers have reported a wide range (10% to 80%, with a median of a 45% prevalence) of types of open discussions among parents and children regarding the children's impending death.[25] Of a sample of 429 parents in Sweden, 34% discussed death with their children, and none of those parents regretted having that discussion. When children were given the information that their illnesses were terminal, most (63%) received it from the parents and physicians together.[23] In addition, several studies have shown that children as young as 6 to 10 years of age are willing to participate in end-of-life decision making.[17,26] Parents' and health care providers' distress in navigating these communication processes (especially regarding death) may prevent children and families from accessing appropriate and timely pediatric palliative care.[27]

Parents may be reluctant to discuss death with their children because of the understandable worry that such a conversation may be upsetting for the child. However, children may have some understanding that death is likely, but because they sense the parents' distress, they may feel unable to discuss this topic with parents. This choice often stems from concern for the parents' well-being. Providing children with the opportunity to talk, however, can be therapeutic for them. Therefore, we encourage parents to allow for such an opportunity. By describing to parents a nonthreatening mode of communication centered on exploring what the children know and what the children may be worrying about and hoping for in the time ahead, we can often reassure parents that this conversation will be sensitive and will be guided by the needs of the children.

The needs and wishes of individual children should guide the way in which communication takes place and its content. Children's ages and levels of cognitive development as well as their changing comprehension of death can help to shape appropriate conversations regarding their prognoses, treatment choices, and end-of-life decisions; however, all this information cannot necessarily predict what a child understands about death.[28] Thus, careful assessment of children's maturity, levels of comprehension, and coping abilities rests on the family and the health care team. Himelstein[22] explains appropriate communication interventions (i.e., language, details, expression, participation) based on age (Table 30-1). Chesler and colleagues found that the age at which children were diagnosed with cancer was strongly and significantly related to the amount of information the parents provided about the illness; the older the child, the more information was given.[29] Hurwitz and colleagues provide questions and statements children raise about dying when they are at various ages, thoughts that guide the behaviors, their underlying developmental understanding of death, and strategies and responses that can help children in these situations (Table 30-2).

Assessing children's level of autonomy, perceptions of threat and safety, and individual coping styles can help clinicians determine how to communicate with children regarding palliative care. Independence and individuation vary. For example, some adolescents, especially those who have close relationships with their parents, may not make a lot of the day-to-day decisions on their own and may depend on their parents' authority and life experience for critical decision making. Other adolescents may be accustomed to being head of the household and to making many of the daily decisions for their families.

Understanding children's family histories with regard to illness and experience with death is an important component to consider when broaching sensitive issues during palliative care. Children who have previously witnessed a relative die or suffer from a serious illness and have observed their families' grief may have unique needs related to this experience. Children who are accustomed to making decisions along with their

---

TABLE 30-1	Development of Death Concepts and Spirituality in Children			
Age Range	Characteristics	Predominant Concepts of Death	Spiritual Development	Interventions
0-2	Has sensory and motor relationship with environment Has limited language skills Achieves object permanence May sense that something is wrong	None	Faith reflects trust and hope in others.	Provide maximal physical comfort, familiar persons, transitional objects (favorite toys), and consistency. Use simple physical communication.
>2-6	Uses magical and animistic thinking Is egocentric Has thinking that is irreversible Engages in symbolic play Is developing language skills	Believes death is temporary and reversible, like sleep Does not personalize death Believes death can be caused by thoughts	Faith is magical and imaginative. Participation in ritual becomes important. The need for courage is important.	Minimize separation from parents. Correct perceptions of illness as punishment. Evaluate for sense of guilt and assuage if present. Use precise language (dying, dead).
>6-12	Has concrete thoughts	Develops adult concepts of death Understands that death can be personal Is interested in physiology and details of death	Faith concerns right and wrong. Eternal interpretations may be accepted as the truth. Ritual is connected with personal identity.	Evaluate child's fears of abandonment. Be truthful. Provide concrete details if requested. Support child's efforts to achieve control and mastery. Maintain access to peers. Allow child to participate in decision making.
>12-18	Has generality of thinking Sees reality as objective Is capable of self-reflection Sees body image and self-esteem as paramount	Explores nonphysical explanations of death	Internal interpretations start to be accepted as the truth. Relationship with God or higher power evolves. Meaning, purpose, hope, and the value of life are sought.	Reinforce child's self-esteem. Allow child privacy. Promote child's independence. Promote access to peers. Be truthful. Allow child to participate in decision making.

From Himmelstein BP, Hilden JM, Boldt AM, Weissman D. Pediatric palliative care. N Engl J Med. 2004;350:1752-1762.

TABLE 30-2   Statements About Dying at Various Stages of Development

Examples of Questions and Statements About Dying at Approximate Ages	Things That Guide Behavior	Developmental Understanding of Dying	Strategies and Responses to Questions and Statements About Dying
1-3 "Mommy, after I die, how long will it be before I'm alive again?" "Daddy, will you still tickle me while I'm dead?"	Limited understanding of accidental events, of future and past time, and of the difference between living and not living.	Death is often viewed as continuous with life. Life and death are often considered alternate states, like being awake and being asleep, or coming and going.	Maximize physical comfort, familiar persons, and favorite toys. Be consistent. Use simple physical contact and communication to satisfy the child's need for sense of self worth and love. "I will always love you." "You are my wonderful child and I will always find a way to tickle you."
3-5 "I have been a bad boy, so I have to die." "I hope the food is good in heaven."	Concepts are crude and irreversible. The child may not distinguish between reality and fantasy. Perceptions dominate judgment.	The child sees death as temporary and reversible and not necessarily universal (only old people die). Because of their egocentricity, the child often believes that he or she has somehow caused the death or views it as a punishment. Death is like an external force that can get you and may be personified (e.g., the bogeyman).	Correct the child's perception of illness as punishment. Maximize the child's time with his or her parents. A child of this age may be concerned about how the family will function without him or her. Help parents accept and appreciate the openness of these discussions. Reassure the child and help parents lessen guilt that the child may feel about leaving by using honest and precise language. "When you die, we will always miss you, but we will know that you are with us and that you are in a safe, wonderful place" (perhaps with another loved one who has died).
5-10 "How will I die? Will it hurt? Is dying scary?"	The child begins to demonstrate organized, logical thought. Thinking becomes less egocentric. The child begins to problem-solve concretely, reason logically, and organize thoughts coherently. However, he or she has limited abstract reasoning.	The child begins to understand death as real and permanent. Death means that your heart stops, your blood does not circulate, and you do not breathe. It may be viewed as a violent event. The child may not accept that death could happen to himself or herself or to anyone he or she knows but starts to realize that people he or she knows will die.	Be honest and provide specific details if they are requested. Help and support the child's need for control. Permit and encourage the child's participation in decision making: "We will work together to help you feel comfortable. It is very important that you let us know how you are feeling and what you need. We will always be with you, so you do not need to feel afraid."
Adolescent, 10-13 "I'm afraid if I die my mom will just break down. I'm worried that when I die, I'll miss my family, or forget them or something."	Thinking becomes more abstract, incorporating the principles of formal logic. The ability to generate abstract propositions, multiple hypotheses, and their possible outcomes becomes apparent.	The child begins to understand death as real, final, and universal. It could happen to him or her or family members. The biologic aspects of illness and death and details of the funeral may begin to interest the child. The child may see death as a punishment for poor behavior. The child may worry about who will care for him or her if a parent or caregiver dies. He or she needs reassurance that he or she will continue to be cared for and loved.	Help reinforce the adolescent's self-esteem, sense of worth, and self-respect. Allow and respect the adolescent's need for privacy, but maintain his or her access to friends and peers. Tolerate the teenager's need to express strong emotions and feelings. Support the need for independence, and permit and encourage participation in decision making. "Though I will miss you, you will always be with me and I will rely on your presence in me to give me strength."
Adolescent, 14-18 "This is so unfair!" "I cannot believe how awful this cancer has made me look." "I just need to be alone!" "I can't believe I'm dying....What did I do wrong?"	Thinking becomes more abstract. Adolescence is marked by risk-taking behavior that seems to deny the teenager's own mortality. At this stage, the teenager needs someone to use as a sounding board for his or her emotions.	A more mature and adult understanding of death develops. Death may be viewed as an enemy that can be fought against. Thus, dying may be viewed by the teenager as a failure, as giving up.	"I can't imagine how you must be feeling. You need to know that despite it all, you are doing an incredible job of handling all of this. I'd like to hear more about what you are hoping for and what you are worrying about."

From Hurwitz CA, Duncan J, Wolfe J. Caring for the child with cancer at the close of life: "There are people who make it, and I'm hoping I'm one of them." JAMA. 2004;292:2141-2149.

siblings may request to have siblings present during important decision making events.

Within the framework of American culture is the diversity of the various ethnic and religious cultural subgroups that use a range of guiding principles in regard to illness and truth telling. It is critical to assess families' identification with their particular cultures and inquire about their beliefs in regard to communication with children about issues pertaining to palliative care[30] because they may vary from the protective approach (shielding young patients and siblings from full knowledge of the disease) to a more open approach.[29]

Techniques of Communication

In many instances, communication with children regarding palliative care issues is best received when health care professionals are aware of the children's levels of desired information and concurrently reinforce the primary role of the parents.[31] Children between the ages of 8 and 17 who were interviewed about disclosure regarding their diagnoses and prognoses reported a range of views concerning the form of disclosure they preferred: a few thought it was better to hear the news at the same time as their parents, some thought it was more appropriate for their parents to be told first, and others reported no strong feelings either way.[32] Patients reported the roles their parents performed in facilitating communication with their health care teams: asking questions for them, being the source of information, and reframing the information from the health care team so they could understand it better. Some children reported feeling protected by the parents' executive role in screening the communication with doctors and marginalized by their nonparticipant status.[31]

The range of views reported by pediatric patients highlights the necessity of tailoring the approach of communication to individual children. The best way to determine the most appropriate way to communicate with particular children is by spending time with them. Providers who know the children well may be best suited for this conversation. Prior to the delivery of information, it is helpful to uncover what the children already know. This can be done through direct conversation or through nonverbal communication (drawing, symbolic play). Ensuring privacy, confidentiality, and support can facilitate the trust that is needed for children to disclose what it is that they already know. The next step is finding out what children want to know. Then clinicians can provide information in small chunks, responding to the children's reactions and feelings and reminding the children that there will be additional opportunities to discuss the issues at hand.[28]

Listening

Listening to children cannot be praised too highly or done too often. Children confronting life-threatening illnesses are at their most vulnerable, so listening to them can be a powerful tool that places some of the control back into the hands of the children. Allowing moments for silence in the discussion only reinforces the acknowledgment that clinicians are listening.[33] Providing children with tape recorders can be another method of empowering them. It allows children to record the questions they have for upcoming appointments with clinicians and allows them to record the clinicians' answers so they can be reviewed if necessary.[34] "Asking about and listening to children's priorities and providing choices when possible may allow children to participate in life-enhancing experiences, even at the close of life."[35]

SPIRITUALITY

Spirituality can be regarded as a multidimensional (mind, body, spirit) and unique expression that brings individuals hope, meaning, and purpose.[36] Spirituality is related to but different from religion such that "spirituality is a dynamic state of being in which the individual seeks connectedness, whereas religion represents the beliefs, values, practices, and rituals that are the observable aspect of a person's spirituality."[37] Spirituality is often inexpressible whereas religion is marked by greater structure.[36] Children can have a "highly developed awareness of spiritual concepts without ever having been part of a formal religious group."[38]

Spirituality in Children

In the same way they develop cognitive abilities, children display developing awareness of spiritual needs, meaning, or purpose within their lives at various ages. During infancy, children find meaning in their daily lives through unconditional love and trust. Toddlers desire self-assertion, worthiness, and success when performing new skills. Preschoolers and school-age children tend to derive their satisfaction from learning the concepts of right versus wrong, impulse control, and the benefits of peer socialization. Adolescents find purpose in their developing independence and individuality and sometimes in a deeper relationship with a higher being.[38] For children with life-threatening illnesses, spiritual concerns often include the need for unconditional love, forgiveness, hope, safety and security, and the development of a legacy. Children also experience loneliness and the loss of wholeness.[39] It can be helpful for children of all ages to be assured that they bring meaning to their families' lives and that when they are no longer alive, they will be remembered by their families.[36]

Children in general, more than adults, tend to attribute an illness to internal (personal) factors, as opposed to external (environmental) factors. Children younger than 7 years of age who have yet to develop the ability to think abstractly commonly see illness as a form of punishment for something they have done wrong (immanent justice belief).[37] Some older children may attribute illness to internal causes so as to maintain control, but others are able to attribute illness to external causes while continuing to seek the meaning and purpose of the illness—a task that may well be spiritual.[37]

The Spiritual Assessment

Children tend to reflect the religious and spiritual values of their parents and families, so a family-centered assessment of spirituality is often helpful. Providing spiritual care for parents can prepare them for the questions children ask, such as "Why is God doing this?" or "What is heaven like?" Parents need assurance that there is no specific right answer.[40]

One method of conducting a spiritual assessment is the use of the BELIEF questions[41]:

Belief system (e.g., Does your family take part in religious events or rituals? Have you discussed the idea of afterlife with your child? Do you believe in a higher power that influences your life?)

Ethics or values (e.g., What are the values you feel are most central to your family?)

Lifestyle (e.g., Are there rituals or dietary practices that you and your family follow?)

Involvement in a spiritual community (e.g., Are you involved with a spiritual community?)

Education (e.g., Do you and your family receive or have you received religious education?)

Future events (e.g., In the near future, are there any religious rites of passage set to occur for you or your family members? What role would you like the members of your faith community to play in the spiritual care of your child?)

However, most spiritual counselors and chaplains discourage the use of a checklist format in assessing spirituality. Instead, questions could be posed to families and children in a conversational format, depending on the situation.[38] Clinically effective pediatric spiritual assessments are conducted in narrative form and may use words, pictures, music, and play—inviting children to explain their sources of strength and areas of fear. Discussions with children and their families regarding spirituality early on in the disease course can help bring meaning to what the family is enduring and can provide hope and comfort at the end of life.[39]

Facing obstacles, challenges, and adversity in life often engenders spiritual thoughts and prompts adults and children alike to ask questions of a higher power such as Why me? Why my child? It is natural that spirituality is a significant issue for families of children with cancer.[36,42] Pastoral care providers at children's hospitals estimate that more than half of the children who are patients can benefit from spiritual care to deal with fear, anxiety, and coping with pain and familial difficulties.[43] Providers in this study identified three major barriers to providing spiritual care: "inadequate training of health care providers to detect patients' spiritual needs, inadequate staffing of the pastoral care office, and being called to visit with patients and families too late to provide all the spiritual care that could have been provided."[44] When the focus of clinical care is on cure for children, discussions about treatment involve medical facts and issues centered on resolving the "problem" by means of medications and therapies. In palliative care, by contrast, discussions are more about journeys of meaning, where there may be no clear solution.[36] Providing spiritual care to dying children and their families requires professionals to face their own issues with spirituality—something not all individuals have done or are ready to do.[36] Children's spirituality tends to be overlooked and, as a result, children may be more likely to feel unheard, invalidated, and alone in the end-of-life period.[45] Because a focus on spiritual beliefs during the end-of-life period is not only critical to the dying patient but also can have implications for bereavement outcomes, people who profess stronger spiritual beliefs may experience a more rapid and complete sense of closure after the death of a loved one.[46]

SCHOOL

Going to school is the job of school-age children. School provides them with their peer group and with the opportunity for discovery, mastery, and socialization.[47] Most children want to continue with their class unless they have not been well supported or unless they feel unable to participate. With families' and children's permission, creative solutions to problems involving participation can allow children to remain in school often until just days before death. Preparation of school staff and classmates is important, as is willingness on the families' part to provide candid information about their children's illnesses and treatment courses.

Ideally, this information is shared soon after children are diagnosed. Often hospital or clinic staff will travel to children's schools and provide information through a Back-to-School program, a program designed to offer information to the other children at school. A question that frequently arises during these sessions is whether the children/friends/peers will survive. Most school-age children have known an adult who has had cancer; some have survived and some have not. It is essential to address this subject in a hopeful way while acknowledging the uncertainty. In all instances, it is important that schools and communities have plans for sensitive communication of the death of children, plans that support classmates' questions, fears, and feelings.

To make it possible for sick children to attend school, the staff and the medical providers may have to find unusual solutions to obstacles. Perhaps the children are allowed to attend for half days, or just for lunch, or only on days when there are special activities. This can be rewarding for the children and their peers. Individualized education plans tailored to the needs of these children can allow resources to be mobilized. In addition, all children should be able to receive home or hospital schooling, and some may be able to complete computer courses or stay in touch with the classroom via teleconferencing.

One possibly disturbing aspect of school attendance by ill children is the change in the children's physical conditions. Reassuring classmates of the children's unchanging personhood may be necessary. Explaining absences, altered appearances, and altered abilities to participate in regular class activities may also be helpful.

Advance Care Planning and the School System

As disease progresses, children's families and medical teams may decide together that a DNR order should be put into effect. Challenges may arise in determining how to honor this choice within the children's communities. Many states have adopted "comfort care orders" to be followed outside of hospital settings as a form of protection for the children.[48] This ensures that when emergency personnel answer a 911 call, comfort care, not intubation or cardiac resuscitation, will be offered in the face of a life-ending event. However, most school districts do not have guidelines or policies to deal with this kind of situation, and those that do typically prohibit school staff from honoring such an order.[48] Nonetheless, ethical principles of beneficence, nonmaleficence, and autonomy have been offered as justification for honoring DNR orders for students.[48,49] At this point the children, families, and schools must come to a clear agreement about whether a DNR order would be observed if the children were at school during a life-ending event.[50,51]

Grief and Bereavement in the School

The grief and bereavement needs of classmates and school staff must be anticipated. Resources are available but affording the training and the opportunities for staff members to integrate this knowledge and experience may be a challenge.[52] As children with life-threatening illness are living longer, however, the goal of enhancing the quality of their lives must be honored whenever possible.

INTERDISCIPLINARY CARE

An interdisciplinary team is an essential aspect of palliative care for children.[20] How else would it be possible to address the physical, social, emotional, and spiritual needs of children with life-threatening illnesses and those of their families as well?[53]

Ideally, the team provides care from the time of diagnosis through death and bereavement.[14,20,54,55] Care may occur in the hospital, home, or community, so children commonly have primary teams whose members take the lead in day-to-day management. The team usually consists of a physician or nurse practitioner and a nurse. Other core team members include a psychologist or social worker, a chaplain, and a child life specialist, among many others. An entire team is necessary to provide children and families with the holistic care that is synonymous with palliative care.

Interdisciplinary care includes the children and their families as partners in the caretaking. Families' priorities are established, and their values, faiths, and cultures are included in decision-making processes. Family meetings, especially those used to address goals of care, include the parents, the children, if appropriate, and the interdisciplinary team members, so that information, emotional cues, and nonverbal language may be appreciated from different perspectives. This format also allows for responses that address the issues holistically. In addition to those already mentioned, at times an interpreter, physical therapist, teacher, respiratory therapist, nutritionist, or pharmacist may be present at family meetings. Research has shown that when physicians are working with psychosocial clinicians, there is closer agreement between the physicians and parents in the understanding of the children's prognoses.[5]

Interdisciplinary care is essential for addressing not only the children's and parents' needs but also those of the grandparents, siblings, school staff, classmates, and hospital, clinic, and home care staffs. Particularly when making a home visit, it is helpful to have several team members present so that the physical and emotional needs of the patients, parents, and siblings may receive attention. Team members also carry the responsibility to inform, teach, and reach out to their colleagues. Depending on the clinical setting, there inevitably will be times when different team members are called upon to take the lead.

Pediatric palliative care is particularly challenging. Providers have "an obligation to nurture relationships that can hold within their embrace both vulnerability and suffering: that which is experienced by our child patients and their families, and that which we experience within ourselves."[56] This kind of care touches practitioners at the core. All need the expertise, support, and companionship that interdisciplinary care can provide.

COORDINATION OF CARE

The coordination of care for children with life-threatening illnesses who move among hospital, home, clinic, and perhaps a rehabilitation facility is daunting. Despite the efforts of many providers, parents often report feeling overwhelmed by the responsibility of care and the coordination of services, particularly in the home. There are many barriers to the coordination of pediatric palliative care services, including lack of available staff to provide home-based services; lack of training of staff in pediatric palliative and hospice care; lack of funding for services; lack of a single agency that provides comprehensive services; and lack of information systems to support communication among sites of care.[22] Ideally, each hospital, clinic, community, and home care agency has designated personnel to perform coordination tasks for the children and families and has protocols specifying standards of practice.[20] Too often, however, care is fragmented. Palliative care programs that provide bridges to hospice do exist, but often the staffs are different, just as they are in hospitals and clinics. This is another clear challenge to providing consistent care and trusting relationships. As pediatric palliative care programs have developed, families seeking curative therapies for their children can often receive palliative

care at home simultaneously. Unfortunately, however, when the children require extended nursing hours, it often means that hospice services cannot be initiated in the home because of restrictions in insurance coverage.

LOCATION OF DEATH

It is generally assumed that children would prefer to die at home, although approximately half of children with progressive cancer die in hospitals,[57] as do the majority of infants and children who die of any illlness in the United States.[58] In a recent study in the United Kingdom,[59] research showed that of children dying in hospitals, 85.7% died in intensive care units, and this trend increased between 1997 and 2004. Parents may be reluctant to talk about withholding life-sustaining treatments until such therapies have been tried. Parents and clinicians alike may have greater difficulty making these decisions when long remissions have been enjoyed. For example, parents may hope that a new treatment is just over the horizon so think that no decisions should be made that might jeopardize their children's chances to survive until it is available. In addition, at times technologic advances in pain and symptom management also mean that children and families feel safer in the hospital so that new problems can be dealt with swiftly. Taking the opportunity to explore with parents what they would want for themselves may allow them to think about this difficult subject in a new way. Asking children where they would most like to spend time, even if they are very sick, and what they would hope to do in that time is often very instructive.

Preparation for Home Care

Preparing parents for events that may occur at home is essential. If they do not want to talk about it, they can be given written materials. Thinking ahead about the most likely symptoms, ways of managing the symptoms, the resources that will best match their needs, and who will be available on call are necessary parts of making care at home successful.

Children's primary providers must work closely with discharge planners, case managers, and social workers who know the intricacies of insurance benefits, home care nursing, and vendors of durable medical equipment so they can determine what each can and will provide. Even the most experienced families still need maximum physical and emotional supports in the home to care for children who are facing the end of life. The goal is to have enough support in place so that parents can simply be mom and dad, and so that family interactions and events may become experiences worth remembering.

Hospice Services

For families and children who know they want to be at home, hospice services can be invaluable. Many hospice agencies now have palliative care programs that offer greater flexibility and broaden the scope of care. There are many barriers, however, to the provision of hospice services to children.[53] Many fewer children than adults die, so maintaining a staff that is willing and able to provide care to children can be challenging. Families and practitioners often see hospice care as "giving up," and it has been difficult to change this assumption. Financially, provision of hospice care may also be a struggle because a hospice provides all the personnel, medications, equipment, and supplies that children need, and this is capped at a per diem rate ($120 per day in 2004).[60] There may be requirements, such as a life expectancy of no more than 6 months and the absence of life-sustaining treatments. The last requirement may be particularly challenging, because even families who understand that their children are likely to die often want to pursue therapies that might prolong life, such as chemotherapy, parenteral nutrition, or transfusions.

The first inpatient pediatric hospice in the United States, the George Mark Children's House in San Leandro, California, opened in 2004, and other pediatric hospice houses are being considered. Some adult inpatient hospice facilities are willing to accept children, but it is unusual, and the facility may need special dispensation to do so. In addition to hospice care, many families are in desperate need of respite care for their children, who may have prolonged palliative care trajectories.

Despite these barriers, palliative care, respite care, and hospice care for all children with life-threatening conditions is the recommendation of the Committee on Bioethics and the Committee on Hospital Care.[55] Hospice teams are ideally suited to provide comprehensive services to children, siblings, parents, and the members of the extended families. Hospice programs commonly have physicians, nurses, social workers, chaplains, and bereavement staff as well as volunteers, art therapists, music therapists, pet therapists, and complementary therapists who can provide massage and Reiki.[61]

CANCER-DIRECTED THERAPY

Parents often wish to continue some form of cancer-directed therapy in the end-of-life care period. The choice of cancer-directed therapy should be considered in the context of the goals of care. For example, if parents' primary goal is to minimize their children's suffering, an option that causes few distressing side effects and that necessitates few interventions may be a reasonable choice when parents wish to continue to provide cancer-directed therapy.

Some regimens with limited toxicity have established efficacy in relapsed or refractory tumors. For example, daily oral etoposide has been used in children with refractory solid tumors, with limited resulting toxicity and with the possibility of tumor response.[62-66] Oral temozolomide has had similar results in children with neuroblastoma.[67] In refractory acute lymphoblastic leukemia, maintenance-type regimens of 6-mercaptopurine, low-dose methotrexate, vincristine, and prednisone may be effective without causing significant side effects. Antibody therapies such as rituximab for children with B-cell malignancies, and molecular agents such as imatinib in potentially responsive cancers may also offer palliation with limited toxicity. Other examples of therapies with limited toxicity can be found in the literature.

Some parents may wish to continue more intensive regimens of chemotherapy. Physicians should ensure that such regimens offer reasonable hope of meeting the parents' and children's goals of care. Parents may also wish to pursue experimental options such as those provided in phase I clinical trials. In general, the likelihood of receiving significant benefit from agents offered in phase I trials is limited, typically, to less than 8%, even in children.[68] Misconceptions about the purpose of phase I trials are common; as with other clinical trials, many subjects believe that the purpose of such trials is to benefit them personally, rather than to benefit future patients.[69] When clinical trials are offered, clarity concerning the purpose of the trial is important so that parents and children can make informed decisions about whether such therapy will help to meet their goals. In addition, such therapies do not preclude concurrent attention to symptoms and quality of life. In fact, attention to life prolongation and symptoms simultaneously may best

meet the needs of children with advanced cancer and their families.[70,71]

Other cancer-directed options to be considered include local radiation or surgery. If a single lesion is causing significant pain or other symptoms, localized radiation therapy may offer palliation with few systemic side effects. Radiation therapy directed at an isolated painful bony metastasis is one such example. Surgery can be similarly beneficial, but a frank team discussion with the surgeon about the trajectory of recovery and the likelihood of recurrence can help when considering whether children will benefit from surgery. Debulking a rapidly growing abdominal tumor, for example, may provide little benefit, in contrast to controlling a single painful metastasis by radiation or surgery. Recommendations agreed on by the oncologist and surgeon or radiation oncologist should be provided to families.

Physicians sometimes feel the obligation to describe cancer-directed therapy as being either curative or palliative. Such a distinction may be difficult to make, however, because at times cancer-directed therapy may offer some chance of cure, even if the chance is small, as well as some possibility of symptom palliation and life extension. In addition, this distinction may be difficult for families, who may hold more than one goal for care. We recommend, rather than using the label *curative* or *palliative*, that cancer-directed therapy be discussed in terms of the goals for care. For example, parents might be told that the goals of a particular therapy are to control the disease for as long as possible, that there is a very small possibility of cure, and that there is a greater likelihood of decreasing symptoms for a period of time. If cure is clearly not a goal of therapy, that should be stated also.

Families who have been accustomed to using cancer-directed therapy at every recurrence may continue to pursue such options even when the medical team believes that the likelihood of benefit is extremely low. In such situations, the team should nonetheless reach consistent recommendations about cancer-directed therapy and should not offer therapies that have no chance for benefit and a high risk for harm. However, patients and families have different preferences for end-of-life care, and for some families, continuing to battle cancer until the time of death may hold personal meaning. In such situations, the team should follow the same standards for communication that were described earlier: assess the families' understanding of prognoses, allow for further communication about the prognoses if needed, elicit the goals of care, come to a team consensus about plans for care that fit with the goals, and make recommendations for care based on the families' and patients' goals and the teams' consensus. Aggressive interventions may be chosen by families who have inappropriately optimistic perceptions of prognoses[5,8]; ongoing communication about children's prognoses may allow families to readjust goals and to choose interventions that offer realistic chances for benefit. The team should never be obligated to provide care that they consider to be inappropriately harmful, and in such cases should work with hospital ethics teams to define appropriate responses to families' requests. But beyond the reaches of harm, families who make thoughtful decisions about care for their children should be allowed to do so, even when those plans for care do not match the ideals of staff members.

SYMPTOM-DIRECTED THERAPY

Managing symptoms in children with life-threatening conditions is of the utmost importance. Parents and children are partners in care and are the experts regarding the symptoms and treatments that make the most sense on the basis of their goals and values. Managing symptoms can be complicated and difficult. In research done by Wolfe and colleagues, 89% of children who died of cancer suffered a lot or a great deal from at least one symptom in the last month of life, according to parents' reports.[3] In a nationwide study in Sweden, parents of children who died of malignancies reported that pain, in particular, had a profound impact on their children.[72]

Many of the symptoms we describe are addressed in detail in the chapter on symptom management (see Chapter 31). We have therefore limited our discussion to management of common symptoms in the setting of palliative care. Medications used to manage common symptoms are listed in Table 30-3.

Pain

Pain is a critical symptom to treat; more than 80% of children with advanced cancer experience pain.[3,73] Pain should be considered a medical emergency. In addition, not only do the children suffer, the parents suffer as well. Pain affects not only the physical being but also the emotional and spiritual being. Pain, anxiety, and spiritual distress accompany one another, and separating them may not be possible. However, it is important to address coexisting or contributing factors.

Children's reports of pain are essential aspects of assessment.[74] Reliable scales that are consistent in the hospital and home are available, but assessment can be challenging, particularly with nonverbal children. Knowledge of children's usual behaviors and previous experience with pain management and with children who have had similar diagnoses can be helpful.[75] Tailored assessment tools can allow parents to equate behaviors with comfort or pain on individualized rating scales.[76]

Treatment of pain should be followed by assessment for effective relief. The World Health Organization provides the basis for a stepwise approach to treating pain.[77] This approach suggests moving from weak analgesics to strong analgesics although, depending on the presenting pain, strong analgesics may be initiated at the outset. Plans for treatment should be based on the type of pain, the children's history of use of pain medicine, and the parents' understanding of the pain and the possible treatment options.

Children and parents should be educated about the basic principles of self-report, around-the-clock dosing, and the need for frequent reevaluation. Providers should work to allay concerns and dispel common myths when necessary. Particularly when families are facing the end of children's lives, the meaning of a recommendation for morphine sulfate cannot be underestimated.[78-81] Often a thorough explanation is needed, and at times it may be helpful to suggest another opioid that is not as tightly associated with dying. Using opioids also necessitates the prophylactic treatment of common side effects.

In addition to analgesic agents, there are a variety of adjuvant therapies that may be used to alleviate pain (see Chapter 31). Increasingly, families are also being encouraged to use nonpharmacologic strategies such as distraction, heat, cold, positioning, and touch. Children may also benefit from acupuncture, hypnosis, Reiki, and guided imagery.[82-87]

Occasionally, children suffer from severe pain caused by malignancy and need massive infusions of opioids. Collins and colleagues found that 6% of children with terminal malignancies were in the category of needing more than 3 mg/kg of morphine dose equivalent per hour. Of 12, 8 required epidural or subarachnoid infusion, sedation, or both.[88] Children may also experience rapidly escalating symptoms of pain, dyspnea, and agitation. In these situations, it has been beneficial to have templated orders created by a multidisciplinary group of clinicians so that sound principles and standard management can be executed at the bedside.[89]

Transitioning children from the hospital to home with adequate symptom management may pose challenges to the home care system. Strategies such as using concentrated elixirs that can be administered buccally, by mouth, or by gastrointestinal tube, or using transdermal medications such as fentanyl patches[90,91] may be of benefit. Long-acting agents like methadone and transdermal fentanyl may be given in conjunction with shorter acting agents administered intravenously or orally. Compounding pharmacies can assist with multiple drug combinations for ease of administration in a variety of preparations. Many home care agencies, including hospice care, are able to provide intravenous patient-controlled analgesia in the home setting as well. Finally, exploring the potential use of midazolam or propofol infusions with the home care or hospice agency[92] may help to determine what can realistically be provided for children in extreme circumstances at home.

Dyspnea

Like pain, dyspnea is subjective and can be caused by a multitude of factors. Having children report the degree of distress

TABLE 30-3	**Medication Guidelines for Symptom Management**		
Symptom	**Medications**	**Dosage**	**Comment**
Anorexia	Megestrol acetate	100 mg PO, BID; if no effect in 2 weeks, double dose to 200 mg BID	Use only in children >10 years of age
	Dronabinol	2.5-5 mg/m²/dose every 4 hr	Use only in children >6 years of age;
	Dexamethasone	0.3 mg/kg/day PO/IV	contraindicated in depression
Agitation	Haloperidol	0.01 mg/kg PO TID prn	
		For acute onset: 0.025-.05 mg/kg PO; may repeat 0.025 mg/kg in 1 hr prn	
Anxiety	*Acute:* Lorazepam	0.025-0.1 mg/kg PO Q 4 to 6 hr	Always start with 0.025 mg/kg; increase dose by 20%-30% for effect
	Chronic: Fluvoxamine	25 mg/day; may increase by 25 mg every 4-7 days up to 200 mg/day	Rarely can worsen depression or cause suicidal thoughts
Constipation	Glycerin suppository	One suppository PR QD	
	Lactulose	5-10 mL Q 2 hr until stools	
	Polyethylene glycol (MiraLax)	0.8 g/kg/day PO; maximum dose 17 g/day PO	Always dissolve dose in 4-8 oz of liquid
	Children's Senokot liquid	2-6 yrs: 2.5-3.75 mL QD 6-12 yrs: 5-7.5 mL QD	
	Pediatric Fleet enema	One PR QD prn	

TABLE 30-3	Medication Guidelines for Symptom Management—cont'd		
Symptom	**Medications**	**Dosage**	**Comment**
Depression	Fluvoxamine	25 mg/day; may increase by 25 mg every 4-7 days up to 200 mg/day	Rarely can worsen depression or cause suicidal thoughts
	Methylphenidate	5 mg orally in the morning and at noon	Not recommended for children <6 years of age
Dyspnea	Morphine sulfate immediate release (MSIR)	0.1 mg/kg PO Q 1-4 hr	Starting dose, no ceiling
	Lorazepam	Starting dose 0.025-0.1mg/kg PO/IV Q 4 hr Maximum dose: 0.5 mg/kg	
Fatigue	Methylphenidate	5 mg orally in the morning and at noon	Not recommended for children <6 years of age
Fever	Acetaminophen	15 mg/kg PO Q 4 hr	
	Ibuprofen	10 mg/kg PO Q 6-8 hr	
Insomnia	Trazodone	0.75-1 mg/kg PO Q HS	
	Nortriptyline	0.1 mg/kg PO Q HS	Not recommended for children <10 years of age
Nausea and Vomiting	*Mild-moderate:* Diphenhydramine	1 mg/kg PO Q 6-8 hr, prn	
	Metoclopramide	0.25 mg/kg PO Q 8 hr, prn	
	Severe: Ondansetron	0.15 mg/kg PO Q 8 hr, prn	
	Dexamethasone	0.3 mg/kg/day PO/IV	
	Lorazepam	0.025-0.1 mg/kg Q 8 hr prn	Maximum dose: 3 mg/24hours
Pruritus	Diphenyhydramine	1 mg/kg PO/IV Q 4 hr, prn	
	Hydroxyzine	0.5 mg/kg PO Q 8 hr, prn	
	Hydrocortisone 1% cream	Q 6-8 hours	
Pain	*Mild pain:* Acetaminophen	15 mg/kg PO Q 4 hr, prn or ATC	Available in 160 mg/5 mL susp. or 80 mg/mL
	Moderate pain: Hydrocodone 7.5 mg w/ acetaminophen 500 mg	2 mg/kg PO Q 4-6 hr prn or ATC	
	Methadone	0.1 mg/kg PO/IV Q BID or TID	No dose adjustments for 72 hr (long half-life of drug); available in liquid
	Severe pain: Morphine sulfate immediate release (MSIR)	Infants <6 months: 0.1 mg/kg PO Q 3-4 hours >6 months: 50 kg: 0.3 mg/kg PO Q 3-4 hours for opioid-naïve patient; titrate by 50%-100%/dose; prescribe breakthrough dose of 0.15 mg/kg PO Q 15-30 min	
	Time-release morphine (MS Contin, Oramorph, Kadian) or OxyContin	Total daily dose of MSIR divided by 2 determines Q 12-hr dose (approximately 1 mg/kg PO Q 8 or 12 hr) Breakthrough dose approximately 10% of the 24-hr total given Q 1-2 hr	
	Oxycodone	0.1 mg/kg Q 3-4 hr PO	
	Hydromorphone	0.03-0.08 mg/kg Q 4 hr PO	
	Fentanyl patch	Children 2-12 years: do not exceed 15 µg/kg Q 72 hr	
Adjuvant Analgesics	*Bony metastases:* Ibuprofen	10 mg/kg PO Q 6 hr	
	Choline	25 mg/kg PO TID	
	Magnesium trisilicate	0.5 mg/kg Q HS	
	Neuropathic pain: Nortriptyline		
	Gabapentin	Initial dose: 10-15 mg/kg/day divided Q 8 hr; titrate if needed to 50 mg/kg/day; not to exceed 2400 mg/day	Maximum dose: 150 mg/day
	Severe visceral distention or bony disease: Prednisone	Oral solution: 1 mg/kg Q day or BID with food	
Secretions	Scopolamine	1.5 mg patch, apply topically Q 72 hr	
	Glycopyrrolate	0.04-0.1 mg/kg PO Q 4-8 hr	
	Hyoscyamine sulfate	Children < 2 years: 4 gtts PO Q 4 hr, prn (0.125 mg/mL solution) Children 2-12 years: 8 gtts PO Q 4 hr, prn (0.125 mg/mL solution)	Maximum dose: 24 gtts/24 hr
Seizures	Lorazepam	0.1 mg/kg PO/SL/PR; may repeat Q 15 min × 3 doses 4 mg single dose	Parents should be advised to contact physician if used
	Diazepam rectal gel (Diastat)	2-5 years: 0.2 mg/kg Q 15 min × 3 doses 6-11 years: 0.3 mg/kg Q 15 min × 3 doses >11 years: 0.2 mg/kg Q 15 min × 3 doses	Parents should be advised to contact physician if used

associated with dyspnea by using a scale similar to the visual analogue scale for pain may be helpful.[93] Recommended interventions should be congruent with the children's and families' goals, whether for extending life, relieving suffering, being in the hospital, or remaining at home. For instance, if pneumonia is diagnosed, some families may choose parenteral antibiotics, others enteral antibiotics, and others strictly comfort measures, including attentive management of associated symptoms. Diuretics may be given for situations involving fluid overload, and thoracentesis can be considered for pleural effusions, although such interventions may not provide effective palliation in patients with extensive parenchymal disease.[94] Transfusion can be considered if red blood cells are low with the hope of increasing oxygenation potential.

Oxygen is often considered for dyspnea.[95] In a recent study in adult patients with advanced cancer, Philip and colleagues found that patients reported relief with either room air or oxygen by nasal prongs.[96] They also found poor correlation between dyspnea complaints and measured oxygen saturation levels. In the hospital it may be easy to provide oxygen, whereas at home opening a window or providing a fan, in addition to positioning and relaxation techniques, may be useful.

Finally, opioid medications given intravenously or by mouth can provide relief[97,98] and can be used without hastening death or suppressing respirations. Dyspnea can often be relieved by an opioid dose lower than that used for pain; a starting dose that is 25% to 30% of the opioid dose used for pain is often effective, although the dose should then be titrated to symptom relief. Nebulized opioids have been used, although studies have not confirmed efficacy of this route.[99] In addition, anxiety often precedes or follows episodes of dyspnea and may be relieved by benzodiazepines,[100,101] hypnosis, or other relaxation techniques.

Airway Obstruction

Airway obstruction and the resulting noisy breathing caused by excessive secretions and the relaxation of oropharyngeal muscles can be very distressing to families. They must be educated to understand that deep suctioning may not be warranted (depending on the phase of illness and the families' goals) and, in fact, may cause discomfort. It may also be helpful to let parents know that an increase in the sounds of breathing is an expected part of children's decline, and that limited suffering is typically associated with it. Anticholinergics may be helpful to decrease secretions[102,103] as may a decrease in parenteral or enteral fluids, if they are being given. However, overly thickened secretions can lead to airway obstruction and greater distress, so careful titration of interventions is warranted.

A somewhat different situation occurs when tumor progression causes airway obstruction. In our experience, the respiratory distress that occurs in this situation can be quite difficult to control, even with massive opioid doses. If the child appears to be gasping and uncomfortable despite opioid therapy, palliative sedation may be warranted. In this case, it must be clear that the goal is to sedate the child and relieve the symptoms, not to hasten death.

Gastrointestinal Symptoms

Nausea and Vomiting

Slightly more than half of the parents of children who have died of cancer report that nausea and vomiting were present at the end of life, often with significant associated suffering.[3,104,105]

Such symptoms sometimes go unrecognized and untreated by physicians,[3,105,106] and even when treatment is offered, efficacy may be limited. Physicians should therefore assess for nausea and vomiting carefully, attend to symptoms promptly, and pay close attention to the efficacy of treatment.

Vomiting is stimulated by the gastrointestinal tract after local receptor stimulation by obstruction, stasis, or toxins; by the pharynx, as the result of mucus or mucosal breakdown; by the medullary vomiting center, in response to cortical, gastrointestinal, or chemoreceptor trigger zone stimulation; or by the cortex, in response to elevated intracranial pressure or emotional and sensory stimuli. Chapter 31 provides further detail about causes of nausea and vomiting in cancer patients. Because the cause may determine the most effective therapy, the most likely cause should be considered when evaluating and treating patients.[107]

In the end-of-life period, chemoreceptor trigger zone stimulation by toxins such as medications (chemotherapeutic agents, antibiotics, and opioids) and metabolic byproducts of uremia or hepatic failure in the blood and cerebral spinal fluid is a particularly common cause of nausea. In addition to effects on the chemoreceptor trigger zone, opioids induce nausea by decreasing gut motility and thereby causing gastroparesis and constipation. Patients may particularly experience nausea and vomiting after dose escalation, but this typically resolves after 3 to 4 days at a stable dose.[108] Opioid-induced nausea and vomiting are usually responsive to antiemetic therapy, especially with 5-hydroxytryptamine antagonists.[108-110]

Another important cause of nausea and vomiting in the end-of-life period is bowel obstruction, which deserves particular consideration in patients with abdominal tumors. Management of obstruction is discussed separately later.

Refractory nausea and vomiting in the end-of-life setting have been treated effectively with antipsychotics such as olanzapine[111] and haloperidol. It is also worth noting that dexamethasone may have limited efficacy against nausea and vomiting in the end-of-life setting[112] in contrast to its efficacy in chemotherapy-induced nausea, unless specific steroid-responsive causes, such as increased intracranial pressure or bowel obstruction, are present. Finally, because sights, smells, and children's emotional states can contribute to nausea, management of distress and of environmental triggers should be considered. Nonpharmacologic therapies like hypnosis and acupuncture may also be effective.

Constipation

Constipation is a common cause of pain and distress at the end of life,[3,104,105] particularly because it can be caused by the use of opioids to control pain. Opioids cause constipation by decreasing colonic motility and secretions and by increasing fluid absorption in the colon. Preventive measures should always be considered at the time of initiation of opioids by prescribing an osmotic or motility agent at initiation. Although many opioid-related side effects tend to decrease over time, constipation tends to remain a problem throughout the period of opioid use.[108]

Other important causes of constipation in the end-of-life care period are decreased patient mobility and decreased oral fluid and nutrition intake.[113] In addition, cord compression and bowel obstruction caused by intra-abdominal tumors should be considered as possible causes.

Unless evaluation reveals an underlying cause, such as bowel obstruction[114] or cord compression, therapy should be similar to that used for any children with cancer, regardless of phase of life. Because fluid intake is commonly limited at the end of life, however, fiber supplementation is not generally useful and can sometimes increase constipation. Similarly, stool softeners alone may be inadequate and should be replaced by or combined with osmotic agents or stimulants.

For severe opioid-related constipation, some authors have described the use of oral opioid antagonists such as naloxone.[115,116] Because of first-pass hepatic metabolism, most patients can tolerate oral naloxone without systemic opioid withdrawal. However, even small amounts of absorbed naloxone can precipitate withdrawal and pain.[117] Therefore we do not recommend the use of oral naloxone for constipation despite the fact that it may be tolerated in many circumstances.

Bowel Obstruction

Intestinal obstruction such as that caused by an abdominal tumor is a common cause of refractory nausea and vomiting in the end-of-life care period.[107] The goals of care and the patients' quality of life may guide the choice of treatment. Therapeutic surgical options include bypass of the intestinal obstruction or placement of a venting gastrostomy tube. However, nonsurgical alternatives exist for patients who wish to avoid surgery or who have limited abilities to tolerate invasive measures.[118] Options for medical management include corticosteroids, which can be useful in relieving obstruction,[119] and octreotide, which can markedly decrease nausea and vomiting by reducing gastrointestinal secretions.[120] Octreotide can be administered subcutaneously and can be used in the outpatient setting if desired. The combination of morphine, scopolamine, and haloperidol has also been used to relieve cramping, nausea, and vomiting.

Anorexia and Cachexia

Cachexia is a common finding in patients who have advanced cancer. Poor nutrition intake and the increased metabolic demands related to cancer appear to be its primary underlying causes. Mechanisms of increased catabolism, including lipolysis and proteolysis, are complex and are probably mediated in part by cytokines.[121-123]

Anorexia compounds the problem. It too is mediated by a number of factors, including gastrointestinal elements (nausea, constipation, mucositis, dysphagia); other physical elements (pain); medication-related elements (impaired ability to taste, decreased hunger); and psychological elements (depression). Commonly, multiple factors contribute to anorexia, and treatment should be directed to the specific causes when such causes can be discerned.[122,123]

Plans for care should include assessment of the meaning of this syndrome to individual patients and families. Some children and families are not significantly bothered by anorexia and cachexia, but other children and families find wasting to be extremely distressing, conjuring up the concern that the child is starving to death. Although severe cancer-related wasting is associated with poor outcomes in adult cancer patients,[124] increased nutrition is not enough to reverse this process.[125,126] Physicians may be able to address concerns about starvation by explaining that the cancer itself may be responsible for the condition and that increased nutritional intake often cannot halt the process. Goals for management should instead focus on symptoms such as the nausea and constipation that are associated with this process. Another important goal is the maintenance of children's levels of function.[127]

Treating any underlying causes, including associated psychological and spiritual issues, should be one of the first steps in management. Additional options such as enteral or parenteral[128] nutrition can be considered in light of the overall goals of care and the efficacy of treatment of underlying causes. If the family wishes to institute artificial nutrition, it can be helpful to discuss the fact that as children's cancers progress, there may be some point at which supplemental nutrition is no longer providing significant benefits relative to its actual or potential harms. Families and their physicians may wish to reassess the degree to which supplemental nutrition is meeting the goals of care, with the thought that at some point, discontinuation of supplemental nutrition may make the most sense for the children. Discussion of this issue with families at the time of instituting supplemental nutrition may make reconsideration of this intervention less distressing for families as the children's illnesses progress.

Pharmacologic therapeutic options include corticosteroids, which can increase appetite and nutrition intake. Their effect tends to wane after 4 weeks. Cannabinoids such as dronabinol can also increase appetite, as can megestrol acetate.[129] Because megestrol acetate is associated with severe adrenal suppression in children with cancer,[130] it should be used with caution; some have recommended routine steroid replacement for children on megestrol.[130]

Nutrition and Hydration

Near the end of life, fluid and nutrition needs diminish. Because parents commonly identify providing nutrition as one of their important roles, physicians should prepare parents for the expected decrease in fluid and nutrition needs as the end of life approaches. Preparation for decreased urine output as a manifestation of waning perfusion rather than of dehydration can also be helpful.

Most studies suggest that nutrition and hydration can be withheld or limited in the end-of-life period without causing suffering.[131-133] In fact, continued feeding via gastrostomy or nasogastric tube may be associated with abdominal discomfort or nausea when children are in the last stages of life. One study of terminally ill adult cancer patients, however, suggests that some degree of parenteral hydration may improve symptoms associated with dehydration.[134] Even in this study, limited volumes of parenteral fluid were sufficient to improve symptoms. Parenteral hydration also has the potential to affect other choices about care, such as the location in which families feel most comfortable receiving care, the need for medical services at the end of life, and the need for intravenous or subcutaneous access.

When the choice is made not to provide supplemental hydration or nutrition at the end of life, it is helpful to pay close attention to symptoms of dehydration, hunger, or thirst, with the goal of treating any symptoms that arise. Often, noninvasive measures such as moistening the lips or providing small tastes of food or fluid are enough to provide comfort.

Fatigue

Fatigue shapes the types of activities that children with life-limiting illnesses choose to participate in and has the potential to diminish children's quality of life significantly.[135] Parents consider fatigue to be the most common symptom in the last month of life and the cause of greatest distress for dying children.[3,136] Unfortunately, this symptom is also the least likely to be treated.[3]

In general, fatigue is a multidimensional symptom that has both physical elements (muscle weakness, decreased energy) and cognitive or affective elements (difficulty in concentrating and maintaining attention, lack of motivation and interest).[137] Younger children and adolescents with cancer define fatigue differently; younger children emphasize the physical aspects of the symptom, whereas adolescents describe multiple dimensions and distinguish between mental and physical fatigue.[138]

Parents of children with cancer note that physical and emotional dimensions of fatigue create significant disruptions for the entire family.[139] Parents describe mood changes in children and also report delays in household and family activities because of the need to accommodate fatigued children.[139] Fatigue also tends to limit children who wish to attend school until the very end of the illness rather than receive private tutoring from teachers in the hospital.[135]

Opioid analgesics contribute to diminished levels of energy as well as to decreased abilities to concentrate in children with advanced disease.[135] Coexisting or contributing factors include anemia, infection, pain, depression, and anxiety.[137,140] Assessment instruments commonly used to assess fatigue in cancer patients measure severity, onset, course, duration, and distress and concurrently assess other correlated symptoms.

Fatigue can seriously affect the quality of children's lives.[135] Multimodal approaches to treatment may be most effective; treatment of anxiety, depression, and sleep disturbance can also mitigate fatigue. Psychostimulants such as methylphenidate can be used to increase wakefulness, particularly when patients have opioid-related somnolence,[141] although their use has not been formally evaluated in children. Because methylphenidate has a short duration of action, patients can control the timing of doses to coincide with important events during the day, such as time with family and friends. Blood transfusions, exercise programs (including physiotherapy), psychosocial interventions, acupuncture, rest and relaxation (including playing and socializing), and nutrition and hydration counseling can also help to alleviate fatigue.[137,139,142] A qualitative study conducted by Hinds and colleagues[138] reported differing views of patients, parents, and staff regarding successful fatigue interventions: parents and staff considered themselves the primary responders to the children's fatigue and the source of its alleviation, whereas patients stated that rest and distraction were their first choices for alleviating symptoms of fatigue.

Psychological Symptoms

Among the most common psychological symptoms experienced by children with cancer are worry, sadness, nervousness, and irritability.[143,144] Some authors have reported that children as young as 7 who have cancer "can report clinically relevant and consistent information about their symptom experience," including psychological symptoms.[143] Through interviews with children who have life-threatening illnesses, Woodgate and colleagues[145] identified a symptom experience described by children as "I am hurting . . . my heart is sad." Children may have difficulty distinguishing among such symptoms, instead experiencing them more as an overall state, such as "experiences that cause . . . mental distress or suffering . . . from feeling sick to being scared." This phenomenon of a cluster of symptoms is also noted in quantitative studies in which children reporting high levels of symptom distress suggest an "interplay between psychological and physical symptoms," especially between psychological symptoms and the physical symptom of pain.[144] Additionally, when disease advances, it may be challenging for children to discuss with their loved ones and with the health care team some of the emotional issues that arise.

Depression

Children with life-threatening illnesses have been reported to experience symptoms of depression and may also meet diagnostic criteria for clinical depression. Gothelf found that 16 of 63 adolescents with cancer (25.4%) met the Diagnostic and Statistical Manual of Mental Disorders (DSM-IV) criteria for major depressive disorder.[146] Children older than 12 who had diagnoses of acute lymphoblastic leukemia, were receiving opiate analgesics, or were undergoing radiotherapy were significantly more likely to be receiving antidepressant medication.[147] Adolescents with higher levels of self-reported depression and lower levels of self-esteem had higher rates of nonadherence to medication; these same teens had lower rates of survival at a 6-year follow-up.[148] Collins and colleagues found that roughly 36% of 159 children with cancer between the ages of 10 and 18 reported feeling sad. Of this group, 17.5% rated the frequency of feeling sad as being "a lot to almost always"; 59.6% rated the intensity of the sadness as "moderate to very severe"; and 39.5% rated the distress it caused as "quite a bit to very much."[144]

In a younger cohort of children (ages 7 to 12) with cancer, Collins and colleagues[143] determined that 10.1% of the children surveyed reported feeling sad. Of this group, 53% reported feeling sad "a medium amount to almost all the time" on a scale of frequency; 60% reported feeling sad "a medium amount to a lot" on a scale of intensity; and 50% reported their sadness causing "a medium amount to very much" distress.[143] A slightly different story unfolded when Dejong and colleagues conducted a review of studies of depression in pediatric cancer patients published between 1980 and 2004. The majority of the studies reviewed were cross-sectional and had been conducted, at most, 5 years post diagnosis. Almost all found either no significant differences between depression rates in children with cancer and normal controls or significantly lower depression scores in the patients who had cancer when the scores were compared to those of the control group.[149]

There is mixed evidence that rates of sadness in children with cancer increase as disease advances. Parents have reported that a significant portion of their children (as much as 65%) experience sadness during the terminal phase,[104,150] and that sadness was the psychological symptom their children experienced most commonly during physical decline.[150] The well-being of children who died between the ages of 9 and 15 was moderately or severely affected by depression, although similar results were not found among children who died before the age of 4.[104]

Risk factors for depression in children with cancer include parental depression and perceived stress and social support; age and severity of illness are not consistently associated with depression.[149] However, variations in findings across studies may be attributed to factors such as having multiple informants concerning the children's symptoms. Another confounder in conducting accurate assessments of depression relates to the presence of other cancer symptoms or the medications being taken to alleviate those symptoms, which may exacerbate or mask the symptoms of depression.[151]

Anxiety

Anxiety appears to be quite common in children with life-threatening illnesses.[143,144] In a sample of 149 children between the ages of 7 and 12, 20.1% reported feeling "worry."[143] Of those children, 43% experienced it "a medium amount to a lot" (intensity); 43% experienced it "a medium amount to almost all the time" (frequency); and 30% reported that it caused them "a medium amount to very much" distress. Among 160 older children with cancer,[144] 35.4% reported feeling "worry." Of these children, 66.1% reported that worry was "moderate to very severe"; 28.6% reported a frequency between "a lot and almost always"; and 27.2% reported the worry caused "quite a bit to very much" distress.

In children with advanced disease, levels of anxiety have been described by parents and health care providers. Researchers studied the medical records of 28 children who died of cancer to understand their end-of-life experiences; 53.6% of the children were documented as experiencing anxiety.[105] In a separate study of 164 symptom assessments collected in the last month of life, 50.0% of children reported "no problem" with anxiety or depression; 27.4% reported a "minor" problem"; and 17.7% reported a "major problem."[152] Anxiety was found to influence significantly the prevalence of pain.[152] In documenting the experience of symptoms of 30 children who died of cancer, worrying and nervousness were found to be two of three symptoms "for which the proportion of children suffering a high level of distress (quite a bit to very much) was more than 50%."[136]

Parents of children who died of cancer were surveyed about their children's experiences of symptoms during the last month of life and reported that among other symptoms, their children's sense of well-being was moderately or severely affected by anxiety.[104] Children older than 9 years of age were reported to be more troubled by anxiety than were younger children.[104]

Qualitatively, children have described anxiety and fear together: "I am scared. . . . I don't know what is going to happen to me"[153]; often, children and families experienced fear so strong that they "could not focus their thoughts on anything but the cancer and [it paralyzed] children and families from participating in life."[153] In children undergoing cancer treatment, anxiety has been commonly linked to the experience of nausea, vomiting, insomnia, nightmares, and skin rashes. Younger children may act out behaviorally (kicking, fighting).[154] In children with advanced disease, those who identified themselves as feeling scared explained that the feeling was often the result of "painful treatments or procedures, experiencing unexpected and new symptoms, and experiencing feelings that there was a greater chance for relapse or death, . . . Sometimes the fear experienced by children would be so great this led them to not to talk about the symptoms or events that caused them to experience such intense fear and anxiety."[153]

Treatment for Depression and Anxiety

Pain, anxiety, distress, and suffering in children with advanced disease are interrelated, so providing relief for all of these symptoms is important. Given this reality, depression and anxiety, especially as they relate to other symptoms such as pain, should be treated simultaneously.

When treating depression and depressive symptoms in children in palliative care, the combination of medications and psychosocial therapies is optimal. Fluvoxamine and other types of serotonin reuptake inhibitors may be effective in children with cancer who also exhibit symptoms of depression and anxiety. In one study of adolescents receiving chemotherapy for advanced cancer, 25.4% of those given fluvoxamine experienced a significant decrease in the somatic and nonsomatic symptoms of major depressive disorder and experienced few side effects.[146] Methylphenidate also has antidepressant properties and may have a more rapid onset of antidepressant effects than other agents.[155] Other antidepressants may also be effective, as may counseling or psychotherapy or, ideally, a combination of medications and psychotherapy when indicated. In contrast, the administration of benzodiazepines alone is thought to be overused in cases of chronic anxiety.

Medications can be effective in palliative care, but therapeutic interventions that address children's anxieties must be tailored to their conditions, ages, and temperaments.[156] In children undergoing cancer treatment as well as at the terminal phases of the disease, supportive therapies such as hypnosis appear to be beneficial.[157,158] Pretend play has been suggested for younger children undergoing cancer treatment.[87]

Sleep Disturbance

Sleep disturbances in children who are critically ill typically take the form of insomnia (difficulty in falling asleep, trouble staying asleep, early-morning awakening, complaints of nonrestorative sleep) or periods of too much sleep or both. When Goldman and colleagues surveyed the records of children with terminal cancer, the number of children who reported that too much sleep was a problem almost doubled between the point of entry into the study (the palliative phase) and the last month of life.[152]

Data concerning the quality of sleep in children with critical illnesses (a study of children with HIV) compared to that in healthy controls showed that sick children slept approximately 1 hour less than healthy children, had more nightmares, and had more general sleep problems.[159] Children with serious illnesses also slept significantly less during nights when they were experiencing pain than during nights when they were pain free[160] and "reported poor sleep on an average of 43% of days with pain and 3% of days without pain."[161]

Predictors of sleep disturbances in cancer patients include pain, breathing difficulties, headaches, hot flashes, limb movements, frequent urination, nausea, and vomiting.[162] Patients who received greater amounts of radiation had poorer sleep.[163] In a study of adolescents with chronic pain, the investigators found a correlation between frequent pain and daytime sleepiness and between longer lasting pain and later bedtimes. Furthermore, sleep/wake problems (irregular sleeping habits, having a hard time falling asleep or waking up) were associated with reduced social and emotional well-being.[164]

The psychological consequences of impaired sleep include feelings of fatigue, impaired daytime functioning, mood disturbances,[165] and negative impact on the quality of life, the ability to cope, and the perception of the severity of the illness.[162] Cancer patients with sleep disturbances also reported high correlations between difficulty in falling asleep and fatigue, early awakening and fatigue, and difficulty in falling asleep and anxiety. Study results also support the idea that depression, anxiety, and sleep disturbances are related, as are cancer-related pain, fatigue, and sleep disturbances.[166]

Treatments of problems with sleep include various approaches, including pharmacologic and nonpharmacologic modalities. Pharmacologic treatments include benzodiazepines, antidepressants such as tricyclic antidepressants,[165] and antipsychotics (especially for cancer patients with delirium).[162] Psychological and behavioral interventions for sleep disturbance include stimulus control, sleep restriction, sleep education, relaxation training, and combinations of the aforementioned therapies.[165]

In cases in which sleep problems are linked to symptoms or correlated with a disorder, treatment of the underlying condition may improve the sleep problems.

Anemia and Bleeding

Decisions about treatment of anemia should center on children's quality of life and the expectations of the family and providers. In children whose major complaint is fatigue and who want to be active, a red blood cell transfusion may improve the quality of life.[167] Similarly, in children who are experiencing significant dizziness, tachycardia, or dyspnea, a red blood cell transfusion may be considered. For some children and families, however, the need for medical care associated with provision of transfusions may make transfusions less desirable.

Fear of profuse bleeding in the setting of thrombocytopenia at the end of life is worrisome for providers and family members. Most often, platelet transfusions are not possible in the home setting; therefore, careful planning and consideration are necessary so as not to disrupt the children's last days. Families may tolerate treating only symptomatic bleeding or may choose prophylactic scheduling of transfusions at a clinic or nearby hospital.[168] When children are at high risk for bleeding at home, parents and providers may want to develop a plan that minimizes distress for the children if bleeding should occur. For example, dark-colored sheets and towels on which blood is less apparent are often recommended in this situation.

Mucosal bleeding can sometimes be controlled by less invasive measures.[169] For example, aminocaproic acid can be used orally or intravenously to inhibit fibrinolysis.[170] Nausea is a common side effect, and aminocaproic acid should be avoided in patients who have hematuria. Topical options include fibrin sealants.[170] The tannins present in black teas can also help to stop bleeding. At home, patients can wet a tea bag with cool water and press it onto bleeding gums.

Fever and Infection

Parents of children with cancer are well aware of the consequences of fever and neutropenia during the children's treatment course. In palliative and end-of-life care, it may be appropriate to think about the role of antibiotics in a different way. Fevers may be caused by infection; however, they also may be caused by the underlying disease. If fevers and associated symptoms can be ameliorated by acetaminophen and other simple measures, that approach may be most beneficial to children. Other families may feel more comfortable with a course of antibiotics, oral or parenteral, on an inpatient or outpatient basis. If this is the case, it may be helpful to plan for a time-limited course, after which antibiotics may be discontinued if no infection has been detected. Over time, parents who prefer antibiotic therapy may become more comfortable with only antipyretic treatment if they see that their children can tolerate this management strategy. Meeting with parents and children to determine which investigative measures and treatments fit with their family goals will help to determine the most effective recommendations.[171]

Central Nervous System Symptoms

Seizures

Although seizures tend to be associated with limited suffering for the patient, parents may find seizures to be highly distressing at the end of life. Anticipating and planning for this possibility can therefore be an important aspect of preparing the family for the end-of-life care period. Seizures may occur near the end of life as a result of central nervous system disease, electrolyte abnormalities, fever, or hypoxia. When any patients under home care are deemed to be at risk for seizures, we recommend that rectal diazepam be available in the home setting. Parents should be educated in its use. At times, seizure prophylaxis may also be desirable, especially if patients are at high risk. Benzodiazepines can be highly effective in preventing seizures.

Increased Intracranial Pressure

Children with intracranial tumors are at risk for experiencing symptoms of increased intracranial pressure as the disease progresses. Common signs and symptoms include headache, vomiting, and somnolence. Although invasive therapies, such as surgical debulking or ventricular shunting, can be considered, the efficacy of such treatments may not be enduring in the end-

of-life setting; tumor growth can quickly block a shunt or lead to recurrence of elevated pressure. Administration of dexamethasone can be effective in alleviating symptoms, and the dosing can be titrated as new symptoms arise and if initial symptoms wane. Dexamethasone-associated side effects, including mood changes and a cushingoid appearance, can be a source of distress to patients, and such side effects should therefore be part of ongoing discussion about dose titration.

Spinal Cord Compression

Spinal cord compression is relatively uncommon at the end of life in children with cancer, but if present, it has the potential to impact quality of life severely. Early diagnosis and management maximize the chances of preserving function.[172] Presenting symptoms include sensory and motor changes as well as bowel and bladder function abnormalities. Prompt imaging, typically by magnetic resonance imaging, should be provided when cord compression is suspected. Dexamethasone can be used to decrease edema at the site of compression, thereby reducing symptoms and preserving neurologic function.[173] Local intervention, such as neurosurgery or radiation therapy, is the mainstay of treatment. Decompressive surgery plus radiotherapy increases the chances of recovery to ambulation,[174] but the specific intervention recommended should take into consideration the patients' overall functional status and goals of care.

Swallowing Impairment

Patients with brainstem involvement by a central nervous system tumor may develop swallowing impairment as one manifestation of disease progression. Such impairment has important implications for nutrition and hydration and may place patients at risk for aspiration pneumonia. Symptoms of coughing or choking when eating or drinking should be regarded as signs of aspiration and evaluated carefully. A swallowing study can establish which consistencies of liquids and solids patients can tolerate without aspirating. If thin liquids cannot be tolerated, additives can be used to thicken liquids until they are of tolerable consistency. Over time, swallowing should be reassessed because patients may develop progressive swallowing dysfunction.

Some patients are unable to tolerate adequate nutrition and hydration without a significant risk for aspiration. Placement of a gastrostomy tube to provide nutrition can be considered as an option; it can allow long-term sustenance while minimizing risks for food-related aspiration. This choice may be most appropriate in patients who are expected to live and to have a reasonable quality of life for some time. Even with gastrostomy tubes, patients remain at risk for aspiration of oropharyngeal secretions. Pharmacologic drying of secretions can offer some help, but most patients remain at risk for aspiration pneumonia. Chemical pneumonitis is also a risk in patients with reflux, and so acid control may also be beneficial.

For some families, placement and use of a gastrostomy tube may not fit with goals of care. Such families may choose to limit nutrition and hydration or to continue to provide oral nutrition and hydration despite the inherent risks. When eating provides significant pleasure to the patient, choosing to maintain oral feeding may positively impact quality of life. Some families may choose to use a gastrostomy tube for most nutrition but to give tastes by mouth so that the pleasure of eating is combined with a robust nutritional strategy. Such decisions should be made with sensitivity to the important nature of feeding in the parent-child relationship. As the end-of-life care period nears and needs for nutrition and hydration wane, nutritional strategies can be reassessed.

WHEN DEATH IS IMMINENT

Escalating Symptoms

For children with chronic conditions and progressive disease, escalating symptoms may occur over days, hours, or minutes. Ideally, family goals are known so that recommended interventions are consistent with them.[54] Meetings between families and their medical teams before rapid escalation of symptoms occurs allows for trust to be further established between the families and providers. The medical teams can then work to anticipate and proactively manage physical and emotional symptoms.

If home care or hospice is involved, escalating symptoms may be managed at home or perhaps by a day visit to the clinic. However, sometimes children have to be admitted for acute management. Whether children are at home or in the hospital, providers must respond to symptoms in a timely manner.

A palliative care team often can assist the primary provider by anticipating which interventions are likely to be the most helpful and to cause the least suffering, and by strategizing the means of carrying out plans for care. Care in a hospital differs from care at home in terms of what is readily available, possible to do, and timely to get. Home care services vary widely among regions and countries.[61,175,176] Palliative care teams may be able to assist with equi-analgesic opioid dosing, adjunctive medications, and best delivery methods as well as with engaging home care services and thinking through the benefits and challenges of end-of-life care at home.

In a hospital, one strategy is to have in place algorithms or templated orders that include starting doses and resources to be accessed. Such an escalating situation for a child at our institution prompted nurses, physicians, and pharmacists to develop a set of orders for the management of escalating pain, dyspnea, or agitation, using morphine, fentanyl, or Dilaudid to improve care in these relatively rare but highly demanding cases.[89] Some general recommendations for handling rapid escalation include:

- Bedside titration when symptoms arise, with bolus dosing every 10 to 15 minutes until pain is relieved.
- Initial bolus dose of 10% of the 24-hour morphine dose for patients already on opioids.
- Increase of bolus dose by 30% to 50% every third dose for unrelieved pain.
- Initiation of continuous infusion once pain is relieved, with additional dosing approximately equivalent to hourly rate for breakthrough pain.
- Increase of hourly rate and bolus by 30% to 50% when pain is unrelieved by existing regimen.[89]

At some institutions, a 24-hour on-call palliative care consultation service or pain treatment service is available to assist. Allowing children who are facing the end of life to be admitted directly to their usual inpatient unit where there are staff members who know them lessens the anxiety of families and children and allows for faster, more individualized care.

Palliative Sedation

Palliative sedation may be considered in rare circumstances. Sedation for refractory symptoms requires expertise in pain alleviation and palliative care and a trusting relationship with the children and their parents. It must be made clear that it is not euthanasia and is not intended to hasten death, although parents who are desperate to see their children at peace may ask for that. When children's refractory or unendurable symptoms cannot be managed by best standards, using opioids, benzodiazepines, and all other adjuncts, then palliative sedation may be warranted.[177,178]

Palliative sedation has the express outcome of relieving suffering and is considered only when physical and psychological symptoms are refractory to all other reasonable medical and complementary therapies.[179,180] The sedation is most commonly started by means of continuous infusion and titrated to achieve the effect the patients, parents, and medical teams have agreed on. The most common agents used are anxiolytic sedatives, sedating antipsychotics, barbiturates, or general anesthetics.[92,179,181,182] Suggested dosing may be found in *Fast Facts*,[183] which is available at www.eperc.mcw.edu, or in the National Hospice and Palliative Care Compendium.[184]

Before commencing palliative sedation, frank discussions should take place between the families and healthcare teams so that any questions, concerns, or misgivings may be addressed.[185] Staff and family members may express ethical concerns that can be addressed by the pain or palliative care team, the chaplaincy, or the ethics consultation service. Ethical principles, including the principle of double effect and the principle of proportionality, justify the use of such measures when the benefits outweigh the possible and unintended but foreseeable consequences. Allowing for a full discussion of ethical concerns as well as acknowledging the consistent intent to relieve suffering[185] may be helpful. Patients, families, and staff should agree on the symptoms, the levels of distress, and the reasonable outcomes of interventions. Being certain that patients and families have had the opportunity to express any final thoughts or feelings while the loved one is still awake and conversant may be important to reducing the potential for subsequent regrets.

Talking with Parents About What to Expect

Throughout this painful time, parents usually want to know what to expect as their children near death.[12] In particular, parents want to know how to achieve comfort for their children through the use of medications and nonpharmacologic interventions. Once it is clear that there is very little likelihood of the children's clinical situations remaining stable or improving, families might want to know when their children will die. Using parameters of prognosis such as hours to days, days to weeks, or weeks to months can be helpful because more specific prognostication can so easily be wrong.

Families often want to know what death will look like. Parents may especially want to know what to look for, so that they may be ready and be present at the moment of death. Some may wish to keep cardiac and respiratory monitors turned on to help them be prepared and know when it is "safe" to leave the bedside, if only momentarily. However, it may be helpful to describe possible physical changes such as decreased mobility, weakness, loss of interest in eating and drinking, and decreased interest in interacting.[57] Being frank about decreased urine output, cold and mottled extremities, vital sign and breathing changes, respiratory congestion, and decreased level of consciousness in the final days can allow the parents to recognize the situation when it occurs. At this time, it is also important to help families focus on being with their children in whatever ways are helpful to the children and families.

Despite our best efforts, not every death is peaceful. We assure families that we will do everything possible to alleviate suffering and allow for a peaceful death, but we cannot make promises. During such conversations, it is important to reaffirm the positive roles of the parents, siblings, and grandparents in the children's lives.

Talking About Autopsy

The discussion of autopsy is often dreaded by physicians, and sometimes it is avoided altogether. But the option of autopsy ideally is discussed by trusted caregivers before death occurs. Such a discussion may be prefaced by suggesting to families that in addition to thinking about location of death and how their children might die, it can be helpful to discuss ahead of time the options for organ or tissue donation and for autopsy. Some families may feel that the child has been through enough; however, some feel that this is a way to advance science and help other children who may suffer from the same condition. Autopsy may answer questions about the disease, the cause of death, or the side effects of treatments. Tissue or organ donation, including donation to science through autopsy, may be a part of children's legacies. Studies have shown that adults and children are altruistic even when facing death,[186] so autopsy may be offered as a kind of gift to future affected children, to medical science, and to the training of physicians who are seeking cures for diseases. In addition to inviting families to meet for a bereavement visit, inviting them to review the autopsy results with trusted providers may allow for a review and for the answering of lingering questions or concerns that may be causing parental distress.[187]

Care of Children's Bodies After Death

After death, whether it occurs at home or in the hospital, a family may value the opportunity to take time for memory-making activities, family rituals, and the sharing of stories and to have staff members visit to say good-bye. The family may also want to participate in routines such as cleaning or dressing the body. In the hospital, one of the most difficult moments occurs when a family leaves the hospital without the child. Having one staff member stay with the body while another accompanies the family to the lobby can be comforting. At home, this moment occurs when the staff of the funeral home arrives, puts the body on a stretcher, takes the body from the home, and puts it into the hearse. Again, having a caretaker present at this time may assist the family in an unspoken way. Ensuring bereavement follow-up may relieve the family by letting the members know that continued contact will occur and that they are not alone.

AFTER DEATH

Bereavement Care for Families

Bereavement is the term used to describe the overall experiences of family members and friends in the periods before, during, and after the death of loved ones.[188] It includes the unique grief that family members and loved ones feel (the emotional, internal processes experienced as a result of the loss) as well as the mourning process for the loss of the children (the more external process related to changing the environment as a result of the loss).[189]

Bereavement begins upon the diagnosis of any pediatric life-limiting condition because the diagnosis, in itself, signifies the loss of normal life and the beginning of significant emotional and physical adaptations on the part of families. Health care providers can begin to support families before the death of children by helping the families to stay connected with the children, communicate effectively with the children, process the concept of appropriate death, and develop memories. In addi-

tion, health care providers may help families to negotiate the medical system, obtain respite care, and assist with "prethinking" about the funeral.[190] Having this type of system in place before children's death can help families begin to adapt to life without their children.[191]

The grieving process of families who have just lost children is typically fraught with the ache of coming to the realization that they will no longer see or be with their children. This process is often layered with a sense of guilt as well—guilt that stems from questioning their treatment decisions, thinking that they caused the illnesses, and worrying that they perhaps gave more attention to the ill children than to the children's siblings.[190] The Two-Track Model of Bereavement described by Rubin[192,193] can guide interventions in dealing with the grief of family members by first assessing the individuals' functioning (for example their feelings of anxiety, depression, and guilt and their desire to return to work [track one] and then assessing the relationships of the individuals to the deceased person, even as they continue to evolve and change in meaning over the course of the surviving relatives' life spans [track two]). Similarly, in a review of recent literature concerning parents' grief, Davies rejects certain notions stating that bonds with the deceased individual must be broken for grief to be resolved and for closure to be attained. Instead, she concludes that "exploring the significance of their children's lives, as well as the continuing influence they have through continuing bonds, may be regarded as a positive means [of] dealing with bereavement."[194]

Spinetta and colleagues measured the postdeath (up to 3 years after the death) adaptation of parents whose children had died of cancer. Of 23 sets of parents interviewed, most had "adequately mastered" the return to normal activities, become active and zestful again, become able to confront physical reminders of their children, and had no regrets about the past. Other tasks, such as resolving remaining questions and healing relationships with siblings, were found to be more difficult for the bereaved parents.

Between 4 and 6 years after the deaths of children because of cancer, bereaved parents were more likely to report depression, low to moderate psychological well-being, and anxiety than were nonbereaved parents. Overall, self-reports of continued grief were associated with greater anxiety and depression. The risk for depression and anxiety in bereaved parents resembled that of nonbereaved parents 7 to 9 years after the deaths of the children; however, parents were at increased risk if their children were 9 years of age or older at the time of death.[195]

Immediate supportive bereavement interventions can take place during end-of-life care. In-depth qualitative interviews with 10 mothers of children who died of a variety of life-limiting illnesses revealed four main needs of mothers during the end of their children's lives: time with their dying children, space and privacy to be with their dying children, time to be with their children's bodies after death, and space and privacy to be with their children's bodies after death. Mothers who did not have time, quiet space, and dignity expressed distress and anguish about the unavailability of these elements.[196]

Shortly after their children's deaths, many parents said that attendance by members of the health care team at their children's memorial or funeral service tended to be helpful in coping with the loss. Parents also found that formal support groups where they could speak with other parents who had had similar experiences, follow-up contact with the health care team to discuss results of the autopsy, contact with the health care team on significant days (i.e., anniversaries of the death, Mother's or Father's Day), and guidance in helping siblings cope with the loss of a brother or sister proved to be beneficial while they mourned their loss.[197] Other, more long-term types of supportive care for bereaved families included individual grief counseling for one or both parents, couples counseling, family counseling, and social support groups.[190]

Care of Siblings

Siblings of children with cancer are deeply affected by their experiences of the sibling's illness and its effects within the family.[198] Siblings experience profound life changes as a result of the illness, and they experience intense positive and negative feelings.[199] In addition, the family dynamics and their roles within their families are often altered by the illness.[199]

The experiences of bereaved siblings are particularly intense. Their bereavement is often marked by feelings of anger, guilt, jealousy, and sadness.[200] A particular area of distress reported by siblings is a lack of involvement in the dying process.[200] Parents may choose not to involve siblings closely in the end-of-life period so as to protect them.[201] However, it is possible that limited involvement is an even greater problem for some siblings than being closely involved in the end-of-life period. Care providers should encourage open communication and allow involvement in care to the extent that siblings wish. Helping parents to understand that such involvement can be healing may be useful.

Care of Staff

Providing care to children with life-limiting illnesses and their families can be one of the most worthwhile acts a human being can offer. At the same time, providing pediatric palliative care services can place unique physical and emotional demands on the members of the health care team. Pediatric oncologists should be aware of the impact of these stressors on themselves and on colleagues and should take the appropriate steps to maintain physical and emotional well-being.

Stressors identified by hospice nurses and physicians include the care of patients with intractable symptoms, difficult communication issues, administrative concerns and paperwork, too many patients dying at the same time, the expectation (by family members, other staff, or self) that all patients' problems can be fixed, and becoming overly involved in the care of their patients.[202,203] When pediatric residents were asked to rate their personal experiences regarding death, similar emotional stressors were prevalent: guilt and feelings of responsibility for the children's deaths.[204]

Self-care can take the form of staff support sessions, educational seminars, and mechanisms in the medical system that allow for relief from patient service time to restore physical and emotional well-being. Methods of staff support can include regular, confidential debriefing sessions consisting of time for reflection and opportunities for staff to share challenges as well as effective ways of coping with these challenges.[205] These debriefing sessions can have a specific focus (e.g., processing the death of an individual child) or can have a more general focus that might take into account the day-to-day issues that arise when providing pediatric oncology and palliative care services.[206] Other types of staff support sessions can take the form of annual or semiannual memorial services to give health care teams a designated day to remember those children they cared for throughout the year.[202]

A combination approach, in which educational seminars regarding palliative care also include time to discuss and process emotions, can be quite effective in gathering a larger crowd of professionals, especially those who would not necessarily attend one type or the other. For example, a combination approach could include a 1-day or several-day death and bereavement retreat for residents to help them achieve the following goals: to gain experience in talking about children's deaths with parents; to practice being in emotional situations; to provide information about autopsy, organ donation, and ministry; to provide resources for supporting families; to gain insight into the impact of death on themselves so as to prevent burnout resulting from stress; and to provide resources for better understanding of parents' perspectives.[207-209]

Sumner suggests opportunities for professional growth for the seasoned professional as well as for new providers of pediatric oncology and palliative care services through mentorship programs. This type of program would encourage, for example, a new physician or pediatric oncology provider be partnered with an expert colleague.[202] The mentor, in turn, may experience a sense of satisfaction and self-efficacy by training new members of the team to provide pediatric palliative care.

ONGOING CHALLENGES

High-quality palliative care is now an expected standard,[20,55] and hospice and palliative medicine has been recognized as a formal medical subspecialty.[210] The American Academy of Pediatrics set the following as a minimum standard for pediatric palliative care: "Excellence in pediatric palliative care is essential for hospitals and other facilities caring for children. Program development in pediatric palliative care, along with community outreach and public education, must be a priority of tertiary care centers serving children."[55]

Although the principles of pediatric palliative care have been defined and refined over the past 2 decades, notable challenges remain in all domains of care, including communication, symptom management, coordination of care, and bereavement. The emerging field of pediatric palliative care is in need of rigorous research efforts, and these efforts should be integrated into curricula across disciplines and at all levels. Further, advocacy aimed at creating greater opportunity for children to receive palliative care across care settings is essential.[20]

REFERENCES

1. Hamilton BE, Minino AM, Martin JA, et al. Annual summary of vital statistics: 2005. Pediatrics. 2007;119:345-360.
2. Parker SL, Tong T, Bolden S, Wingo PA. Cancer statistics, 1996. CA Cancer J Clin. 1996;46:5-27.
3. Wolfe J, Grier HE, Klar N, et al. Symptoms and suffering at the end of life in children with cancer. N Engl J Med. 2000;342:326-333.
4. Bluebond-Langner M, Belasco JB, Goldman A, Belasco C. Understanding parents' approaches to care and treatment of children with cancer when standard therapy has failed. J Clin Oncol. 2007;25:2414-2419.
5. Wolfe J, Klar N, Grier HE, et al. Understanding of prognosis among parents of children who died of cancer: impact on treatment goals and integration of palliative care. JAMA. 2000;284:2469-2475.
6. Murray SA, Kendall M, Boyd K, Sheikh A. Illness trajectories and palliative care. BMJ. 2005;330:1007-1011.
7. Mack JW, Wolfe J, Grier HE, et al. Communication about prognosis between parents and physicians of children with cancer: parent preferences and the impact of prognostic information. J Clin Oncol. 2006;24:5265-5270.
8. Weeks JC, Cook EF, O'Day SJ, et al. Relationship between cancer patients' predictions of prognosis and their treatment preferences. JAMA. 1998;279:1709-1714.

9. Morita T, Akechi T, Ikenaga M, et al. Late referrals to specialized palliative care service in Japan J Clin Oncol. 2005;23:2637-2644.

10. Stromgren AS, Sjogren P, Goldschmidt D, et al. A longitudinal study of palliative care: patient-evaluated outcome and impact of attrition. Cancer. 2005;103:1747-1755.

11. Seecharan GA, Andresen EM, Norris K, Toce SS. Parents' assessment of quality of care and grief following a child's death. Arch Pediatr Adolesc Med. 2004;158:515-520.

12. Mack JW, Hilden JM, Watterson J, et al. Parent and physician perspectives on quality of care at the end of life in children with cancer. J Clin Oncol. 2005;23:9155-9161.

13. Hurwitz CA, Duncan J, Wolfe J. Caring for the child with cancer at the close of life: "there are people who make it, and I'm hoping I'm one of them." JAMA. 2004;292:2141-2149.

14. Mack JW, Wolfe J. Early integration of pediatric palliative care: for some children, palliative care starts at diagnosis. Curr Opin Pediatr. 2006;18:10-14.

15. Lamont EB, Christakis NA. Complexities in prognostication in advanced cancer: "to help them live their lives the way they want to." JAMA. 2003;290:98-104.

16. Mack JW, Cook EF, Wolfe J, et al. Understanding of prognosis among parents of children with cancer: parent optimism and the parent-physician interaction. J Clin Oncol. 2007;25:1357-1362.

17. Hinds P, Drew D, Oakes LL, et al. End-of-life care preferences of pediatric patients with cancer. J Clin Oncol. 2005;23:9055-9057.

18. Back AL, Arnold RM, Quill TE. Hope for the best, and prepare for the worst. Ann Intern Med. 2003;138:439-443 (comment).

19. Hinds PS, Gattuso JS, Fletcher A, et al. Quality of life as conveyed by pediatric patients with cancer. Qual Life Res. 2004;13:761-772.

20. Field MJ, Behrman RE, Institute of Medicine (U.S.). Committee on Palliative and End-of-Life Care for Children and Their Families. When Children Die: Improving Palliative and End-of-Life Care for Children and Their Families. Washington, DC, National Academy Press, 2003.

21. Ellis R, Leventhal B. Information needs and decision-making preferences of children with cancer. Psychooncology. 1993;2:277-284.

22. Himelstein BP, Hilden JM, Boldt AM, Weissman D. Pediatric palliative care. N Engl J Med. 2004;350:1752-1762.

23. Kreicbergs U, Valdimarsdottir U, Onelov E, et al. Talking about death with children who have severe malignant disease. N Engl J Med. 2004;351:1175-1186.

24. Contro NA, Larson J, Scofield S, et al. Hospital staff and family perspectives regarding quality of pediatric palliative care. Pediatrics. 2004;114:1248-1252.

25. Goldman A, Christie D. Children with cancer talk about their own death with their families. Pediatr Hematol Oncol. 1993;10:223-231.

26. Nitschke R, Humphrey GB, Sexauer CL, et al. Therapeutic choices made by patients with end-stage cancer. J Pediatr. 1982;101:471-476.

27. Himelstein BP. Palliative care in pediatrics. Anesthesiol Clin North Am. 2005;23:837-856.

28. Faulkner KW. Children's understanding of death. In Armstrong-Dailey A, Zarbock S (eds). Hospice Care for Children. New York, Oxford University Press, 2001, pp 9-21.

29. Chesler MA, Paris J, Barbarin OA. "Telling" the child with cancer: parental choices to share information with ill children. J Pediatr Psychol. 1986;11:497-516.

30. Diez B, Lascar E, Alizade A. Talking to a child with cancer: a valuable experience. Ann N Y Acad Sci. 1997;809:142-151.

31. Young B, Dixon-Woods M, Windridge KC, Heney D. Managing communication with young people who have a potentially life-threatening chronic illness: qualitative study of patients and parents. BMJ. 2003;326:305B-308B.

32. Bryce J, Boschi-Pinto C, Shibuya K, Black RE, Group WHOCHER. WHO estimates of the causes of death in children. Lancet. 2005;365:1147-1152.

33. Himelstein BP, Jackson NL, Pegram L. The power of silence. J Clin Oncol. 2003;21(suppl):41.

34. Orloff S, Quance K, Perszyk S, et al. Psychosocial and spiritual needs of the child and family. In Palliative Care for Infants, Children, and Adolescents. Baltimore, The Johns Hopkins University Press, 2004, pp 147-162.

35. Duncan J, Joselow M, Hilden JM. Program interventions for children at the end of life and their siblings. Child Adolesc Psychiatr Clin North Am. 2006;15:739-758.

36. Davies B, Brenner P, Orloff S, et al. Addressing spirituality in pediatric hospice and palliative care. J Palliat Care. 2002;18:59-67.

37. Pehler S. Children's spiritual response: validation of the nursing diagnosis Spiritual Distress. Nurs Diagn. 1997;8:55-65.

38. Heilferty CM. Spiritual development and the dying child: the pediatric nurse practitioner's role. J Pediatr Health Care. 2004;18:271-275.

39. Thayer P. Spiritual care of children and parents. In Armstrong-Dailey A, Zarbock S (eds). Hospice Care for Children. New York, Oxford University Press, 2001, pp 172-189.

40. Gibbons MB. Psychosocial aspects of serious illness in childhood and adolescence: curse or challenge? In Armstrong-Dailey A, Zarbock S (eds). Hospice Care for Children, 2nd ed. New York, Oxford University Press, 2001, pp 49-67.

41. McEvoy M. An added dimension to the pediatric health maintenance visit: the spiritual history. J Pediatr Health Care. 2000;14:216-220.

42. Donnelly JP, Huff SM, Lindsey ML, et al. The needs of children with life-limiting conditions: a healthcare-provider-based model. Am J Hosp Palliat Care. 2005;22:259-267.

43. Feudtner C, Haney J, Dimmers MA. Spiritual care needs of hospitalized children and their families: a national survey of pastoral care providers' perceptions. Pediatrics. 2003;111:67-72.

44. Feudtner C, Christakis DA, Connell FA. Pediatric deaths attributable to complex chronic conditions: a population-based study of Washington State, 1980-1997. Pediatrics. 2000;106:205-209.

45. Hufton E. Parting gifts: the spiritual needs of children. J Child Health Care. 2006;10:240-250.

46. Walsh K, King M, Jones L, et al. Spiritual beliefs may affect outcome of bereavement: prospective study. BMJ. 2002;324:1551.

47. Sourkes B, Frankel L, Brown MJ, et al. Food, toys, and love: pediatric palliative care. Curr Probl Pediatr Adolesc Health Care. 2005;35:347-386.

48. Kimberly M, Forte A, Carroll J, Feudtner C. Pediatric do-not-attempt-resuscitation orders and public schools: a national assessment of policies and laws. Am J Bioeth. 2005;5:59-65.

49. Ramer-Chrastek J. Hospice care for a terminally ill child in the school setting. J Sch Nurs. 2000;16:52-56.

50. Do not resuscitate orders in schools. Committee on School Health and Committee on Bioethics. American Academy of Pediatrics. Pediatrics. 2000;105:878-879.

51. Weise K. The spectrum of our obligations: DNR in public schools. Am J Bioeth. 2005;5:81-83.

52. Reid J, Dixon W. Teacher attitudes on coping with grief in the public school classroom. Psychol Sch. 1999;36:219-229.

53. Carter BS, Levetown M (eds). Palliative Care for Infants, Children, and Adolescents. Baltimore, The Johns Hopkins University Press, 2004.

54. Mack JW, Wolfe J. Early integration of pediatric palliative are: for some children, palliative care starts at diagnosis. Curr Opin Pediatr. 2006;18:10-14.

55. American Academy of Pediatrics, Committee on Bioethics and Committee on Hospital Care. Palliative care for children. Pediatrics. 2000;106:351-357.

56. Browning D. To show our humanness—relational and communicative competence in pediatric palliative care. Bioethics Forum. 2002;18:23-28.

57. Wolfe J, Friebert S, Hilden J. Caring for children with advanced cancer integrating palliative care. Pediatr Clin North Am. 2002; 49:1043-1062.

58. Feudtner C, Christakis DA, Zimmerman FJ, et al. Characteristics of deaths occurring in children's hospitals: implications for supportive care services. Pediatrics. 2002;109:887-893.

59. Ramnarayan P, Craig F, Petros A, Pierce C. Characteristics of deaths occurring in hospitalised children: changing trends. J Med Ethics. 2007;33:255-260.

60. Hellsten M, Hockenberry-Eaton M, Lamb D, et al. End-of-Life Care for Children. Austin, TX, The Texas Cancer Council, 2000.

61. Zwerdling T, Davies S, Lazar L, et al. Unique aspects of caring for dying children and their families. Am J Hosp Palliat Care. 2000;17:305-311.

62. Kebudi R, Gorgun O, Ayan I. Oral etoposide for recurrent/progressive sarcomas of childhood. Pediatr Blood Cancer. 2004; 42:320-324.

63. Schiavetti A, Varrasso G, Maurizi P, et al. Ten-day schedule oral etoposide therapy in advanced childhood malignancies. J Pediatr Hematol Oncol. 2000;22:119-124.

64. Mathew P, Ribeiro RC, Sonnichsen D, et al. Phase I study of oral etoposide in children with refractory solid tumors. J Clin Oncol. 1994;12:1452-1457.

65. Sandri A, Massimino M, Mastrodicasa L, et al. Treatment with oral etoposide for childhood recurrent ependymomas. J Pediatr Hematol Oncol. 2005;27:486-490.

66. Ashley DM, Meier L, Kerby T, et al. Response of recurrent medulloblastoma to low-dose oral etoposide. J Clin Oncol. 1996; 14:1922-1927.

67. Donfrancesco A, Jenkner A, Castellano A, et al. Ifosfamide/carboplatin/etoposide (ICE) as front-line, topotecan/cyclophosphamide as second-line and oral temozolomide as third-line treatment for advanced neuroblastoma over one year of age. Acta Paediatr Suppl. 2004;93:6-11.

68. Shah S, Weitman S, Langevin AM, et al. Phase I therapy trials in children with cancer. J Pediatr Hematol Oncol. 1998;20: 431-438.

69. Daugherty C, Ratain MJ, Grochowski E, et al. Perceptions of cancer patients and their physicians involved in phase I trials. J Clin Oncol. 1995;13:1062-1072.

70. Meyers FJ, Linder J, Beckett L, et al. Simultaneous care: a model approach to the perceived conflict between investigational therapy and palliative care. J Pain Symptom Manage. 2004;28: 548-556.

71. Ulrich CM, Grady C, Wendler D. Palliative care: a supportive adjunct to pediatric phase I clinical trials for anticancer agents? Pediatrics. 2004;114:852-855.

72. Jalmsell L, Kreichbergs U, Onelov E, et al. Symptoms affecting children with malignancies during the last month of life: a nationwide follow-up. Pediatrics. 2006;117:1314-1320.

73. Sirkia K, Hovi L, Pouttu J, Saarinen-Pihkala UM. Pain medication during terminal care of children with cancer. J Pain Symptom Manage. 1998;15:220-226.

74. Franck LS, Greenberg CS, Stevens B. Pain assessment in infants and children. Pediatr Clin North Am. 2000;47:487-512.

75. Hunt A, Mastroyannopoulou K, Goldman A, Seers K. Not knowing—the problem of pain in children with severe neurological impairment. Int J Nurs Stud. 2003;40:171-183.

76. Solodiuk J, Curley M. Pain assessment in nonverbal children with severe cognitive impairments: the individualized numeric rating scale (INRS). J Pediatr Nurs. 2003;18:295-299.

77. World Health Organization. Cancer Pain Relief and Palliative Care in Children. Geneva, World Health Organization, 1998.

78. Portenoy RK, Coyle N. Controversies in the long-term management of analgesic therapy in patients with advanced cancer. J Palliat Care. 1991;7:13-24.

79. Von Roenn JH, Cleeland CS, Gonin R, et al. Physician attitudes and practice in cancer pain management: a survey from the Eastern Cooperative Oncology Group. Ann Intern Med. 1993;119:121-126.

80. Field MJ, Cassel CK, Institute of Medicine (U.S.), Committee on Care at the End of Life. Approaching Death: Improving Care at the End of Life. Washington, DC, National Academy Press, 1997.

81. Potter VT, Wiseman CE, Dunn SM, Boyle FM. Patient barriers to optimal cancer pain control. Psychooncology. 2003;12: 153-160.

82. Rusy LM, Weisman SJ. Complementary therapies for acute pediatric pain management. Pediatr Clin North Am. 2000;47: 589-599.

83. Zeltzer LK, Tsao JC, Stelling C, et al. A phase I study on the feasibility and acceptability of an acupuncture/hypnosis intervention for chronic pediatric pain. J Pain Symptom Manage. 2002;24:437-446.

84. Snyder JR. Therapeutic touch and the terminally ill: healing power through the hands. Am J Hosp Palliat Care. 1997;14:83-87.

85. Giasson M, Bouchard L. Effect of therapeutic touch on the well-being of persons with terminal cancer. J Holist Nurs. 1998;16:383-398.

86. Olson K, Hanson J, Michaud M. A phase II trial of Reiki for the management of pain in advanced cancer patients. J Pain Symptom Manage. 2003;26:990-997.

87. Moore M, Russ S. Pretend play as a resource for children: implications for pediatricians and health professionals. J Dev Behav Pediatr. 2006;27:237-248.

88. Collins JJ, Grier HE, Kinney HC, Berde CB. Control of severe pain in children with terminal malignancy. J Pediatr. 1995;126: 653-657.

89. Houlahan KE, Branowicki PA, Mack JW, et al. Can end of life care for the pediatric patient suffering with escalating and intractable symptoms be improved? J Pediatr Oncol Nurs. 2006;23:45-51.

90. Noyes M, Irving H. The use of transdermal fentanyl in pediatric oncology palliative care. Am J Hosp Palliat Care. 2001;18: 411-416.

91. Hunt A, Goldman A, Devine TD, Phillips M. Transdermal fentanyl for pain relief in a paediatric palliative care population. Palliat Med. 2001;15:405-412.

92. Hooke M, Grund E, Quammen H, et al. Propofol use in pediatric patients with severe cancer pain at the end of life. J Pediatr Oncol Nurs. 2007;24:29-34.

93. Mancini I, Body JJ. Assessment of dyspnea in advanced cancer patients. Support Care Cancer. 1999;7:229-232.

94. Ripamonti C. Management of dyspnea in advanced cancer patients. Support Care Cancer. 1999;7:233-243.

95. Bruera E, Schoeller T, MacEachern T. Symptomatic benefit of supplemental oxygen in hypoxemic patients with terminal cancer: the use of the N of 1 randomized controlled trial. J Pain Symptom Manage. 1992;7:365-368.

96. Philip J, Gold M, Di Iulio J, et al. A randomized, double-blind, crossover trial of the effect of oxygen on dyspnea in patients with advanced cancer. J Pain Symptom Manage. 2006;32: 541-550.

97. Bruera E, MacEachern T, Ripamonti C, Hanson J. Subcutaneous morphine for dyspnea in cancer patients. Ann Intern Med. 1993;119:906-907.

98. Allard P, Lamontagne C, Bernard P, Tremblay C. How effective are supplementary doses of opioids for dyspnea in terminally ill cancer patients? A randomized continuous sequential clinical trial. J Pain Symptom Manage. 1999;17:256-265.

99. Noseda A, Carpiaux JP, Markstein C, et al. Disabling dyspnoea in patients with advanced disease: lack of effect of nebulized morphine. Eur Respir J. 1997;10:1079-1083.

100. Davis CL. ABC of palliative care: breathlessness, cough, and other respiratory problems. BMJ. 1997;315:931-934.

101. Abrahm JL. A Physician's Guide to Pain and Symptom Management in Cancer Patients, 1st ed. Baltimore, The Johns Hopkins University Press, 2000.

102. Bennett M, Lucas V, Brennan M, et al. Using anti-muscarinic drugs in the management of death rattle: evidence-based guidelines for palliative care. Palliat Med. 2002;16:369-374.

103. Bennett MI. Death rattle: an audit of hyoscine (scopolamine) use and review of management. J Pain Symptom Manage. 1996;12:229-233.

104. Jalmsell L, Kreicbergs U, Onelov E, et al. Symptoms affecting children with malignancies during the last month of life: a nationwide follow-up. Pediatrics. 2006;117:1314-1320.

105. Hongo T, Watanabe C, Okada S, et al. Analysis of the circumstances at the end of life in children with cancer: symptoms, suffering and acceptance. Pediatr Int. 2003;45:60-64.

106. Carter BS, Howenstein M, Gilmer MJ, et al. Circumstances surrounding the deaths of hospitalized children: opportunities for pediatric palliative care. Pediatrics. 2004;114:e361-e366.

107. Baines MJ. ABC of palliative care: nausea, vomiting, and intestinal obstruction. BMJ. 1997;315:1148-1150.

108. Abrahm J. A Physician's Guide to Pain and Symptom Management in Cancer Patients, 1st ed. Baltimore, Johns Hopkins University Press, 2000.

109. Mystakidou K, Befon S, Liossi C, Vlachos L. Comparison of the efficacy and safety of tropisetron, metoclopramide, and chlorpromazine in the treatment of emesis associated with far advanced cancer. Cancer. 1998;83:1214-1223.

110. Currow DC, Coughlan M, Fardell B, Cooney NJ. Use of ondansetron in palliative medicine. J Pain Symptom Manage. 1997;13:302-307.

111. Srivastava M, Brito-Dellan N, Davis MP, et al. Olanzapine as an antiemetic in refractory nausea and vomiting in advanced cancer. J Pain Symptom Manage. 2003;25:578-582.

112. Bruera E, Moyano JR, Sala R, et al. Dexamethasone in addition to metoclopramide for chronic nausea in patients with advanced cancer: a randomized controlled trial. J Pain Symptom Manage. 2004;28:381-388.

113. Fallon M, O'Neill B. ABC of palliative care: constipation and diarrhoea. BMJ. 1997;315:1293-1296.

114. Mancini I, Bruera E. Constipation in advanced cancer patients. Support Care Cancer. 1998;6:356-364.

115. Liu M, Wittbrodt E. Low-dose oral naloxone reverses opioid-induced constipation and analgesia. J Pain Symptom Manage. 2002;23:48-53.

116. Sykes NP. An investigation of the ability of oral naloxone to correct opioid-related constipation in patients with advanced cancer. Palliat Med. 1996;10:135-144.

117. Choi YS, Billings JA. Opioid antagonists: a review of their role in palliative care, focusing on use in opioid-related constipation. J Pain Symptom Manage. 2002;24:71-90.

118. Ripamonti C, Bruera E. Palliative management of malignant bowel obstruction. Int J Gynecol Cancer. 2002;12:135-143.

119. Laval G, Girardier J, Lassauniere JM, et al. The use of steroids in the management of inoperable intestinal obstruction in terminal cancer patients: do they remove the obstruction? Palliat Med. 2000;14:3-10.

120. Ripamonti C, Mercadante S, Groff L, et al. Role of octreotide, scopolamine butylbromide, and hydration in symptom control of patients with inoperable bowel obstruction and nasogastric tubes: a prospective randomized trial. J Pain Symptom Manage. 2000;19:23-34.

121. Bruera E, Sweeney C. Cachexia and asthenia in cancer patients. Lancet Oncol. 2000;1:138-147.

122. Bruera E. ABC of palliative care: anorexia, cachexia, and nutrition. BMJ. 1997;315:1219-1222.

123. Ross DD, Alexander CS. Management of common symptoms in terminally ill patients: Part II. Constipation, delirium and dyspnea. Am Fam Physician. 2001;64:1019-1026.

124. Dewys WD, Begg C, Lavin PT, et al. Prognostic effect of weight loss prior to chemotherapy in cancer patients. Eastern Cooperative Oncology Group. Am J Med. 1980;69:491-497.

125. Koretz RL. Parental nutrition: is it oncologically logical? J Clin Oncol. 1984;2:534-538.

126. Klein S, Koretz RL. Nutrition support in patients with cancer: what do the data really show? Nutr Clin Pract. 1994;9:91-100.

127. Bachmann P, Marti-Massoud C, Blanc-Vincent MP, et al. Summary version of the standards, options and recommendations for palliative or terminal nutrition in adults with progressive cancer (2001). Br J Cancer. 2003;89(suppl 1):S107-S110.

128. Torelli GF, Campos AC, Meguid MM. Use of TPN in terminally ill cancer patients. Nutrition. 1999;15:665-667.

129. De Conno F, Martini C, Zecca E, et al. Megestrol acetate for anorexia in patients with far-advanced cancer: a double-blind controlled clinical trial. Eur J Cancer. 1998;34:1705-1709.

130. Orme LM, Bond JD, Humphrey MS, et al. Megestrol acetate in pediatric oncology patients may lead to severe, symptomatic adrenal suppression. Cancer. 2003;98:397-405.

131. McCann RM, Hall WJ, Groth-Juncker A. Comfort care for terminally ill patients: the appropriate use of nutrition and hydration. JAMA. 1994;272:1263-1266.

132. Meares CJ. Terminal dehydration: a review. Am J Hosp Palliat Care. 1994;11:10-14.

133. Vullo-Navich K, Smith S, Andrews M, et al. Comfort and incidence of abnormal serum sodium, BUN, creatinine and osmolality in dehydration of terminal illness. Am J Hosp Palliat Care. 1998;15:77-84.

134. Bruera E, Sala R, Rico MA, et al. Effects of parenteral hydration in terminally ill cancer patients: a preliminary study. J Clin Oncol. 2005;23:2366-2371.

135. Bouffet E, Zucchinelli V, Costanzo P, Blanchard P. Schooling as a part of palliative care in paediatric oncology. Palliat Med. 1997;11:133-139.

136. Drake R, Frost J, Collins JJ. The symptoms of dying children. J Pain Symptom Manage. 2003;26:594-603.

137. Del Fabbro E, Dalal S, Bruera E. Symptom control in palliative care. Part II: cachexia/anorexia and fatigue. J Palliat Med. 2006;9:409-421.

138. Hinds PS, Hockenberry-Eaton M, Gilger E, et al. Comparing patient, parent, and staff descriptions of fatigue in pediatric oncology patients. Cancer Nurs. 1999;22:277-289.

139. Gibson F, Garnett M, Richardson A, et al. Heavy to carry: a survey of parents' and healthcare professionals' perceptions of cancer-related fatigue in children and young people. Cancer Nurs. 2005;28:27-35.

140. Greenberg DB. Fatigue. In Holland JC (ed). Management of Specific Symptoms. New York, Oxford University Press, 1998, pp 485-493.

141. Bruera E, Driver L, Barnes EA, et al. Patient-controlled methylphenidate for the management of fatigue in patients with advanced cancer: a preliminary report. J Clin Oncol. 2003;21:4439-4443.

142. Kohara H, Miyauchi T, Suehiro Y, et al. Combined modality treatment of aromatherapy, footsoak, and reflexology relieves fatigue in patients with cancer. J Palliat Med. 2004;7:791-796.

143. Collins JJ, Devine TD, Dick GS, et al. The measurement of symptoms in young children with cancer: the validation of the Memorial Symptom Assessment Scale in children aged 7-12. J Pain Symptom Manage. 2002;23:10-16.

144. Collins JJ, Byrnes ME, Dunkel IJ, et al. The measurement of symptoms in children with cancer. J Pain Symptom Manage. 2000;19:363-377.

145. Woodgate RL, Degner LF, Yanofsky R. A different perspective to approaching cancer symptoms in children. J Pain Symptom Manage. 2003;26:800-817.

146. Gotheif D, Rubinstein M, Shemesh E, et al. Pilot study: fluvoxamine treatment for depression and anxiety disorders in children and adolescents with cancer. J Am Acad Child Adolesc Psychiatry. 2005;44:1258-1262.

147. Portteus A, Ahmad N, Tobey D, Leavey P. The prevalence and use of antidepressant medication in pediatric cancer patients. J Child Adolesc Psychopharmacol. 2006;16:467-473.

148. Kennard BD, Stewart SM, Olvera R, et al. Nonadherence in adolescent oncology patients: preliminary data on psychological risk factors and relationships to outcome. J Clin Psychol Med Settings. 2004;11:31-39.

149. Dejong M, Fombonne E. Depression in paediatric cancer: an overview. Psychooncology. 2006;15:553-566.

150. Theunissen JM, Hoogerbrugge PM, van Achterberg T, et al. Symptoms in the palliative phase of children with cancer. Pediatr Blood Cancer. 2007;49:160-165.

151. Bennett DS. Depression among children with chronic medical problems: a metaanalysis. J Pediatr Psychol. 1994;19:149-169.

152. Goldman A, Hewitt M, Collins GS, et al. Symptoms in children/ young people with progressive malignant disease: United Kingdom Children's Cancer Study Group/Paediatric Oncology Nurses Forum survey. Pediatrics. 2006;117:e1179-e1186.

153. Woodgate RL, Degner LF. Expectations and beliefs about children's cancer symptoms: perspectives of children with cancer and their families. Oncol Nurs Forum. 2003;30:479-491.

154. Katz ER, Jay S. Psychological aspects of cancer in children, adolescents, and their families. Clin Psychol Rev. 1984;4:525-542.

155. Homsi J, Walsh D, Nelson KA, et al. Methylphenidate for depression in hospice practice: a case series. Am J Hosp Palliat Care. 2000;17:393-398.

156. Berde C, Wolfe J. Pain, anxiety, distress, and suffering: interrelated, but not interchangeable. J Pediatr. 2003;142:361-363.

157. Goodenough B, Hardy J, Jarratt R. "Riding my manta ray with Uncle Fester": hypnosis for managing pain and distress in a dying child. Aust J Clin Exp Hypn. 2003;31:95-102.

158. Katz ER, Jay SM. Psychological aspects of cancer in children, adolescents, and their families. Clin Psychol Rev. 1984;4:525-542.

159. Franck LS, Johnson LM, Lee K, et al. Sleep disturbances in children with human immunodeficiency virus infection. Pediatrics. 1999;104:e62.

160. Rees DC, Olujohungbe AD, Parker NE, et al. Guidelines for the management of the acute painful crisis in sickle cell disease. Br J Haematol. 2003;120:744-752.

161. Shapiro BS, Dinges DF, Orne EC, et al. Home management of sickle cell-related pain in children and adolescents: natural history and impact on school attendance. Pain. 1995;61:139-144.

162. Kvale EA, Shuster JL. Sleep disturbance in supportive care of cancer: a review. J Palliat Med. 2006;9:437-450.

163. Miaskowski C, Lee KA. Pain, fatigue, and sleep disturbances in oncology outpatients receiving radiation therapy for bone metastasis: a pilot study. J Pain Symptom Manage. 1999;17:320-332.

164. Palermo TM, Kiska R. Subjective sleep disturbances in adolescents with chronic pain: relationship to daily functioning and quality of life. J Pain. 2005;6:201-207.

165. Savard J, Morin CM. Insomnia in the context of cancer: a review of a neglected problem. J Clin Oncol. 2001;19:895-908.

166. Sela RA, Watanabe S, Nekolaichuk CL. Sleep disturbances in palliative cancer patients attending a pain and symptom control clinic. Palliat Support Care. 2005;3:23-31.

167. Monti M, Castellani L, Berlusconi A, Cunietti E. Use of red blood cell transfusions in terminally ill cancer patients admitted to a palliative care unit. J Pain Symptom Manage. 1996;12:18-22.

168. Gagnon B, Mancini I, Pereira J, Bruera E. Palliative management of bleeding events in advanced cancer patients. J Palliat Care. 1998;14:50-54.

169. Pereira J, Mancini I, Bruera E. The management of bleeding in patients with advanced cancer. In Portenoy RK, Bruera E (eds). Topics in Palliative Care. vol 4. New York, Oxford University Press, 2000, pp 163-183.

170. Pereira J, Phan T. Management of bleeding in patients with advanced cancer. Oncologist. 2004;9:561-570.

171. Pereira J, Watanabe S, Wolch G. A retrospective review of the frequency of infections and patterns of antibiotic utilization on a palliative care unit. J Pain Symptom Manage. 1998;16:374-381.

172. Loblaw DA, Laperriere NJ. Emergency treatment of malignant extradural spinal cord compression: an evidence-based guideline. J Clin Oncol. 1998;16:1613-1624.

173. Abrahm JL. Management of pain and spinal cord compression in patients with advanced cancer. ACP-ASIM End-of-life Care Consensus Panel, American College of Physicians-American Society of Internal Medicine. Ann Intern Med. 1999;131:37-46.

174. Patchell RA, Tibbs PA, Regine WF, et al. Direct decompressive surgical resection in the treatment of spinal cord compression caused by metastatic cancer: a randomised trial. Lancet. 2005;366:643-648.

175. Brook L, Vickers J, Pizer B. Home platelet transfusion in pediatric oncology terminal care. Med Pediatr Oncol. 2003;40:249-251.

176. Dangel T, Fowler-Kerry S, Karwacki M, Bereda J. An evaluation of a home palliative care programme for children. Ambulatory Child Health. 2000;6:101-114.

177. American Academy of Hospice and Palliative Medicine Statement on Palliative Sedation, 2006.

178. Krakauer E, Penson RT, Truog RD, et al. Sedation for intractable distress of a dying patient: acute palliative care and the principle of double effect. Oncologist. 2000;5:53-62.

179. De Graeff A, Dean M. Palliative sedation therapy in the last weeks of life: a literature review and recommendations for standards. J Palliat Med. 2007;10:67-85.

180. Postovsky S, Ben Arush MW. Care of a child dying of cancer: the role of the palliative care team in pediatric oncology. Pediatr Hematol Oncol. 2004;21:67-76.

181. Tobias JD. Propofol sedation for terminal care in a pediatric patient. Clin Pediatr (Phila). 1997;36:291-293.

182. Frager G. Palliative care and terminal care of children. Child Adolesc Psychiatr Clin North Am. 1997;6:889-909.

183. Salacz M, Weissman D. Controlled sedation for refractory suffering: part ii. Fast Facts and Concepts #107. End of Life/Palliative Education Resource Center. (Website): www.mywhatever.com/cifwriter/library/eperc/fastfact/ff107.html. Accessed May 5, 2008.

184. National Hospice and Palliative Care Organization. Compendium of Pediatric Palliative Care. Alexandria, VA, National Hospice and Palliative Care Organization, 2000.

185. Lo B, Rubenfeld G. Palliative sedation in dying patients. JAMA. 2005;294:1810-1816.

186. Hinds PS, Oakes L, Furman W, et al. End-of-life decision making by adolescents, parents, and healthcare providers in pediatric oncology: research to evidence-based practice guidelines. Cancer Nurs. 2001;24:122-134; quiz 135-136.

187. Pizzo PA, Poplack DG (eds). Principles and Practice of Pediatric Oncology, 4th ed. Philadelphia, Lippincott Williams & Wilkins, 2002.

188. Parkes CM, Weiss RS. Recovery From Bereavement. New York, Basic Books, 1983.

189. Christ GH, Bonnano G, Malkinson R, Rubin S. Bereavement experiences after the death of a child. In Field M, Behrman RE (eds). When Children Die: Improving Palliative and End-of-Life Care for Children and Their Families. Washington, DC, National Academies Press, 2002, pp 553-579.

190. Worden JW, Monahan JR. Caring for bereaved parents. In Armstrong-Dailey A, Zarbock S (eds). Hospice Care for Children. 2nd ed. New York, Oxford University Press, 2001, pp 137-156.

191. Spinetta JJ, Swarner JA, Sheposh JP. Effective parental coping following the death of a child from cancer. J Pediatr Psychol. 1981;6:251-263.

192. Rubin S. The two-track model of bereavement: overview, retrospect, and prospect. Death Studies. 1999;23:681-714.

193. Rubin S. A two-track model of bereavement: theory and research. Am J Orthopsychiatry. 1981;51:101-109.

194. Davies R. New understandings of parental grief: literature review. J Adv Nurs. 2004;46:506-513.

195. Kreicbergs U, Valdimarsdottir U, Onelov E, et al. Anxiety and depression in parents 4-9 years after the loss of a child owing to a malignancy: a population-based follow-up. Psychol Med. 2004;34:1431-1441.

196. Davies R. Mothers' stories of loss: their need to be with their dying child and their child's body after death. J Child Health Care. 2005;9:288-300.

197. Widger KA, Wilkins K. What are the key components of quality perinatal and pediatric end-of-life care? A literature review. J Palliat Care. 2004;20:105-112.

198. Wilkins KL, Woodgate RL. A review of qualitative research on the childhood cancer experience from the perspective of siblings: a need to give them a voice. J Pediatr Oncol Nurs. 2005;22:305-319.

199. Woodgate RL. Siblings' experiences with childhood cancer: a different way of being in the family. Cancer Nurs. 2006;29:406-414.

200. Nolbris M, Hellstrom AL. Siblings' needs and issues when a brother or sister dies of cancer. J Pediatr Oncol Nurs. 2005;22:227-233.

201. Giovanola J. Sibling involvement at the end of life. J Pediatr Oncol Nurs. 2005;22:222-226.

202. Sumner LH. Staff support in pediatric hospice care In Armstrong-Dailey A, Zarbock S (eds). Hospice Care for Children, 2nd ed. New York, Oxford University Press, 2001, pp 190-212.

203. Amery J, Lapwood S. A study into the educational needs of children's hospice doctors: a descriptive quantitative and qualitative survey. Palliat Med. 2004;18:727-733.

204. Serwint JR, Rutherford LE, Hutton N. Personal and professional experiences of pediatric residents concerning death. J Palliat Med. 2006;9:70-81.

205. Le Blanc PM, Hox JJ, Schaufeli WB, et al. Take care! The evaluation of a team-based burnout intervention program for oncology care providers. J Appl Psychol. 2007;92:213-227.

206. Rushton CH, Reder E, Hall B, et al. Interdisciplinary interventions to improve pediatric palliative care and reduce health care professional suffering. J Palliat Med. 2006;9:922-933.

207. Serwint JR, Rutherford LE, Hutton N, et al. "I learned that no death is routine": description of a death and bereavement seminar for pediatrics residents. Acad Med. 2002;77:278-284.

208. Bagatell R, Meyer R, Herron S, et al. When children die: a seminar series for pediatric residents. Pediatrics. 2002;110:348-353.

209. Kolarik RC, Walker G, Arnold RM. Pediatric resident education in palliative care: a needs assessment. Pediatrics. 2006;117:1949-1954.

210. Lauer ME, Mulhern RK, Schell MJ, Camitta BM. Long-term follow-up of parental adjustment following a child's death at home or hospital. Cancer. 1989;63:988-994.

Symptom Management in Children with Cancer

Christina K. Ullrich, Charles B. Berde, and Amy Louise Billett

Progress in understanding the causes of pediatric cancer, as well as advances in cancer-directed therapies, hold great promise in curing and extending the lives of many children diagnosed with cancer. However, as advances in medicine and technology improve the survival of children with life-threatening illness, attention to health-related quality of life and progress in symptom management has not kept pace with advances in disease-directed therapies. This phenomenon has created a population of children who are living with cancer but have suboptimally controlled symptoms.

Ameliorating symptoms experienced by a child with cancer does more than reduce a child's suffering from a troublesome symptom. Control of physical symptoms may allow attention to be focused on other issues that a family living with a child's cancer must face, such as psychosocial concerns and existential distress. In some cases, improved control of symptoms may also enhance the delivery of optimal cancer-directed therapy. Finally, optimal symptom control throughout the illness trajectory may also shape the child's and family's long-lasting impressions of their experience with cancer.

Relief from distressing symptoms is often possible with the myriad of therapeutic modalities available today. Pediatric oncologists play a key role in managing symptoms in their patients. This requires actively partnering with families to assess not only for the presence of symptoms but for the impact of uncontrolled symptoms on their daily lives, using appropriate interventions to ameliorate symptoms. Ideally, such attention to symptoms occurs in the context of attention to the child's overall condition so that the impact of symptoms on the child's overall quality of life is appreciated.

The vast majority of children with cancer suffer from multiple symptoms that could be ameliorated, but are not.[1-5] For example, Collins and colleagues have asked 10- to 18-year-old children and adolescents about the symptoms they experienced over the previous week. Symptoms included lack of energy (49%), pain (49%), nausea (45%), lack of appetite (40%), and itching (33%).[1] The prevalence of uncontrolled symptoms in children with cancer is likely to stem from various system-wide causes, including inadequate formal training dedicated to symptom management, a focus on cancer-directed treatment, and time constraints.

In addition, a lack of systematic research in the pediatric population, particularly with regard to nonpain symptoms, has led to a lack of evidence or standards on which to base interventions. Many symptom-directed interventions for children are currently based on extrapolation from adult studies or even individual or anecdotal experiences. Encouragingly, there are some guidelines that are strongly evidence-based, such as the National Comprehensive Care Network (NCCN) Guidelines for Pediatric Cancer Pain.[6] As advances in pediatric oncology extend into the realm of symptom management, additional guidelines for nonpain symptoms will assist pediatric oncologists in attending to their patient's symptoms.

As discoveries in pediatric oncology have led to promising survival rates, there is increasing attention to health-related quality of life and the human costs of cancer care.[7] With such a shift, efforts to understand and ameliorate the myriad of symptoms experienced by children with cancer are likely to be increasingly supported in the coming years.

PAIN

Pain is defined as "an unpleasant sensory and emotional experience associated with actual or potential tissue damage or described in terms of such damage."[8] This symptom is the most studied and best understood of all cancer symptoms in adults and children. Despite such attention, pain is often suboptimally controlled. For example, a recent large meta-analysis of studies aimed at evaluating the prevalence of pain in adults with cancer has found that 59% of those undergoing curative treatment and 64% of those with advanced illness experience pain.[9] In addition, of those with pain, more than one third rated their pain as moderate or severe.

Families and children confronting cancer often worry about potential pain caused by the disease as well as its treatment. Pain is the most feared problem for children with cancer.[10] To some extent, their concern is justified. For example, Collins and colleagues have demonstrated that children with cancer suffer from multiple symptoms, including pain.[1] Among 160 children and adolescents aged 10 to 18 years with cancer, pain was the second most common symptom, with a prevalence of 49.1%. In addition, 61.6% reported pain that was moderate to very severe in the 48 hours prior to completing the questionnaire and 40.9% reported pain that occurred "a lot" to "almost always." Moreover, the pain experienced by children was distressing, "quite a bit" to "very much" in 39.1%.

Pain control provides various benefits beyond the amelioration of suffering. Prompt pain relief is needed to prevent central sensitization, a centrally mediated hyperexcitability response that may result in escalating pain. Uncontrolled pain also leads to a physiologic stress response with various effects, such as altered metabolism and immune function. Control of pain with appropriate analgesia in the perioperative period can reduce some of these effects and prevent complications.[11]

Epidemiology

In general, pain experienced by children with cancer may be caused by various entities, including the disease itself (e.g., tumor invasion of bone, viscera, peripheral or central nervous system, or compression of the spinal cord), treatment (e.g., mucositis, radiation-induced dermatitis, drug-induced neuropathy), or procedures (e.g., venipuncture, lumbar puncture, bone marrow aspiration or biopsy, postoperative pain). A cross-sectional analysis of pain in inpatient children with cancer has found that the most frequent cause of pain is side effects of antitumor therapy.[12] There is also evidence that children with solid tumors outside the central nervous system have more pain and higher opioid requirements.[13]

Because most pediatric cancers respond at least initially to treatment, most pain that children experience early in the disease trajectory is procedure- and treatment-related. Later, if the cancer progresses, pain is more likely to be caused by tumor extension. In a series of structured interview surveys conducted by Ljungman and colleagues,[14] 49% of children with cancer experienced pain at diagnosis. Procedure- and treatment-related pain were the most significant types of pain at the start and, although procedure-related pain improved, treatment-related pain did not. In addition, pain intensity measurement was rarely performed.

A significant barrier to pain management in children is that research and development of evidence-based practice guidelines in pediatrics lags behind that in adults. The NCCN and World Health Organization (WHO) have developed comprehensive guidelines for managing pain in children with cancer[15] but, in many cases, pain management in children relies on extrapolation from adult data, anecdotal reports, and personal experience.

Children may also experience incidental, noncancer-related pain. Other pain-inducing disorders such as migraines, recurrent abdominal pain or injuries seen in the general pediatric population can occur in children with cancer. These types of disorders unrelated to the cancer diagnosis should always be included in the differential diagnosis of pain.

Pathophysiology

Nociception is a complex process whereby actual (or potential) tissue damage is perceived as pain by an individual. In many cases pain is a protective mechanism that alerts an individual to tissue injury. Nociception may be thought to occur on three levels, peripheral, spinal, and supraspinal (Fig. 31-1). Through transduction, the primary afferent nociceptors, thinly myelinated A-delta and unmyelinated C fibers, transmit biochemical changes at the sensory nerve endings generated by painful (chemical, thermal, or mechanical) stimuli into electrical

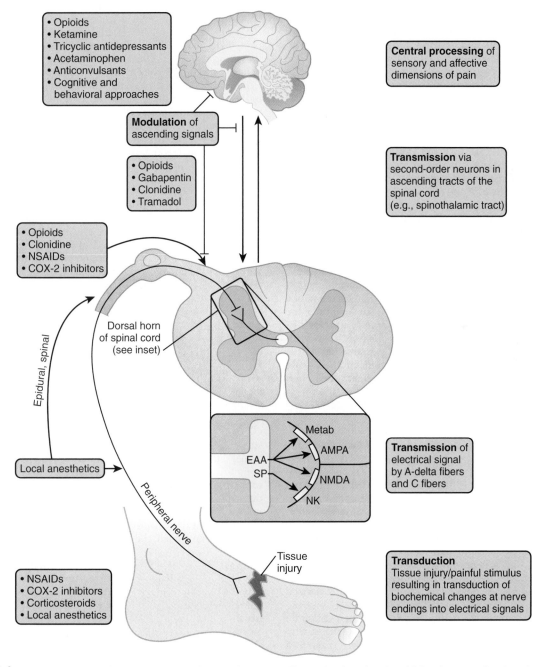

FIGURE 31-1. Anatomic scheme of the nociceptive pathway and corresponding analgesic action sites. Major elements of nociception are indicated in blue boxes. Analgesics are indicated in green boxes. *Inset*: Neurotransmission and neuromodulation in the dorsal horn of the spinal cord. Analgesics: COX-2, cyclooxygenase-2; NSAIDs, nonsteroidal anti-inflammatory drugs. Neurotransmitters: EAA, excitatory amino acids; SP, substance P. Receptors: Metab, metabotropic; AMPA, alpha-amino-3-hydroxy-5-methyl-4-isoxazolepropionic; NMDA, *N*-methyl-D-aspartate; NK, neurokinin.

signals. Stimulation of such nerve endings in the periphery may be increased or decreased by molecules such as prostaglandins, leukotrienes, bradykinin, and histamine. For example, bradykinin and histamine accompanying tissue inflammation can directly activate nociceptors in addition to reducing their threshold and increasing their response to suprathreshold stimulation.[16] The analgesic effect of nonsteroidal anti-inflammatory drugs (NSAIDs) is caused by their ability to inhibit prostaglandin synthesis and thus desensitize nociceptors.[17]

The electrical signals generated are propagated, or transmitted, to second-order neurons that synapse with sensory nociceptors in the dorsal horn of the spinal cord. Second-order neurons convey signals via ascending tracts in the spinal cord, including the anterolateral spinothalamic tracts, to supraspinal sites, including the brainstem, thalamus, and cortical areas involved in the sensory and affective dimensions of pain.

For example, descending inhibitory pathways from the thalamus and brainstem modulate excitatory transmission through such inhibitory neurotransmitters as serotonin, norepinephrine, and endogenous opioids. Several pharmacologic interventions, such as opioids and tricyclic antidepressants, exert their analgesic effects through such inhibitory processes at the spinal and supraspinal levels.

Pain is a complex sensory and emotional experience that involves nociception, but is modified by a range of contextual and psychological factors. Because the experience of pain is subjective, the degree of tissue injury and therefore nociceptive input do not necessarily correlate with the intensity of pain experienced. Interventions that may reduce the perception of pain include hypnosis and relaxation techniques.

Pain resulting from stimulation of intact neurons by impulses reflecting tissue injury or inflammation is called nociceptive pain. Conversely, pain resulting from abnormal excitability of neurons (e.g., caused by neuronal damage) is called neuropathic pain. Even if tissue damage initially accompanied neuropathic pain, neuropathic pain may persist long after the damage has resolved. Nociceptive pain may frequently be distinguished from neuropathic pain by its characteristics. Neuropathic pain is often described as burning or shooting and is often associated with paresthesias or allodynia (elicitation of pain by normally nonpainful stimuli, such as light touch).

Factors Influencing a Child's Experience of Pain

As a subjective experience, many factors affect a child's experience of pain. Recognizing such factors can facilitate an understanding of the pain as experienced by the child and in developing an effective pain treatment plan. Factors influencing the perception and meaning of pain are individual and contextual and include developmental and cognitive factors (e.g., understanding, control, expectation, relevance), behavioral and emotional factors (e.g., anxiety, fear, frustration, anger, guilt, isolation), and familiar and cultural factors.[18-20] Other factors, including age, gender, pain acceptance, and pain tolerance, have been hypothesized to influence pain perception in the pediatric population and have been summarized elsewhere.[21]

Importantly, previous painful experiences may heighten the experience of subsequent ones. For example, children who had inadequate procedural analgesia when newly diagnosed with cancer and were undergoing a first bone marrow aspirate or lumbar puncture had more severe distress during subsequent procedures, even when efficacious pain relief was subsequently provided.[22] This highlights the need to provide effective analgesia to prevent present and future painful experiences.

Assessment

Pain assessment and measurement provide the foundation for effectively addressing pain. Regular assessment of pain may improve pain management[23,24] and should be conducted in a developmentally appropriate manner. When permitted by the child's developmental status, self-report is considered the gold standard in pain assessment. Because there are bias and error in self-report, behavioral observations, physiologic changes, and clinician and/or parental report may be incorporated into the pain assessment. However, these methods also have inherent limitations. For example, tachycardia may reflect fever or intravascular volume depletion rather than pain.

Physiologic and behavioral signs and symptoms can indicate pain but lack of these signs does not indicate absence of pain, particularly in chronically or very ill children in whom these indicators are unreliable. In one study comparing a behavioral pain measure with two self-report measures, many children who reported severe pain showed few behavioral pain indicators.[25] In addition, these signs are not necessarily specific for pain itself and may reflect distress, which might or might not be pain-related. Parental and clinician estimates of the child's pain also have limitations, with clinicians and parents frequently underestimating pain.[26,27]

Examples of symptom assessment tools for children of various ages and developmental capacities are demonstrated in Figure 31-2. These tools may be helpful when assessing for symptoms and in measuring severity before and after interventions. They are not, however, all validated specifically for the population of children with cancer.[28] A particular tool should be used consistently with a particular child. When the assessment reveals the presence of pain, further inquiry regarding the nature (e.g., character of the pain, aggravating and alleviating factors), as well as the meaning that the pain holds for the child and family, should be undertaken.

Self-Report Instruments

Many children 3 years of age or older can self-report their symptoms. Because some young children, particularly those who are chronically ill, may be more mature than their chronologic age, their responses should be heeded, even those of young children. Self-report scales for children include the faces scale, color analogue scale, visual analogue scale (VAS),[29] Poker Chip Tool,[30] and numerical rating scales. With the faces scales, such as the Wong-Baker Faces Scale[31] and the Bieri Faces Pain Scale,[32] the child is asked to match how he or she feels with one of the faces. Color analogue scales and faces scales can be used by most children aged 4 years and older. Faces scales differ psychometrically—for example, in use of a smiling face for the no pain anchor, as in the Wong-Baker Faces Scale, versus a neutral face for the no pain anchor in the Bieri Faces Pain Scale. Although children often report that they like using the Wong-Baker Scale, some researchers regard the use of a neutral face for the no pain anchor, as in the Bieri Faces Scale, as psychometrically more specific. With the VAS, a child selects a point on a line that represents the intensity of their pain. These scales have been extensively studied and are appropriate for children 8 years of age and older.

Numerical rating scales do not require any equipment, are simple to use, and are already in frequent use with adults. These scales do require numeracy and the ability to think and express oneself in quantitative terms, and are therefore most appropriately used for children who are at least 8 years of age.[33] Children younger than this may provide an unreliable numerical response because, although they can count, they do not have an understanding of the quantitative meaning of numbers.[33] All

FLACC Behavioral Scale: Recommended for Children < 3 Years of Age

Categories*	Scoring*		
	0	1	2
Face	No particular expression or smile	Occasional grimace or frown, withdrawn, disinterested	Frequent to constant quivering chin, clenched jaw
Legs	Normal position or relaxed	Uneasy, restless, tense	Kicking, or legs drawn up
Activity	Lying quietly, normal position, moves easily	Squirming, shifting back and forth, tense	Arched, rigid, or jerking
Cry	No cry (awake or asleep)	Moans or whimpers; occasional complaint	Crying steadily, screams or sobs, frequent complaints
Consolability	Content, relaxed	Reassured by occasional touching, hugging, or being talked to, distractable	Difficulty to console or comfort

A

Wong-Baker FACES Pain Rating Scale: Recommended for Children ≥ 3 Years of Age

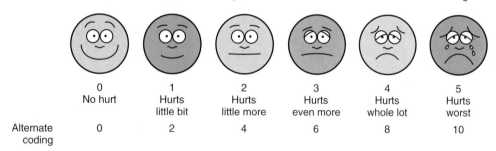

0	1	2	3	4	5
No hurt	Hurts little bit	Hurts little more	Hurts even more	Hurts whole lot	Hurts worst

Alternate coding   0   2   4   6   8   10

Brief word instructions: Point to each face using the words to describe the pain intensity. Ask the child
B to choose face that best describes own pain and record the appropriate number.

Numerical Rating Scale: Recommended for Children ≥ 8 Years of Age

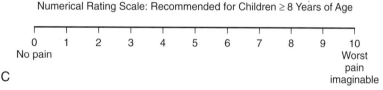

C

FIGURE 31-2. Pain assessment instruments. **A,** FLACC Scale, recommended for use in children younger than 3 years. Each of the five categories is scored from 0 to 2, which results in a total score between 0 and 10. **B,** Wong-Baker FACES Pain Rating Scale, recommended for children 3 years of age and older. **C,** Numerical Pain Rating Scale, recommended for children 8 years and older. (*A, from Merkel SI, Voepel-Lewis T, Shayevitz JR, Malviya S. The FLACC: A behavioral scale for scoring postoperative pain in young children. Pediatr Nurs. 1997;23:293-297; used with permission,* © *2002, The Regents of the University of Michigan.* **B, C,** *adapted from Hockenberry MJ, Wilson D, Winkelstein ML. Wong's Essentials of Pediatric Nursing, 7th ed. St. Louis, Mosby, 2005, p 1259, used with permission.*)

quantitative scales are based on the concept of counting, a universal concept for children who have this developmental capacity. It is therefore possible to develop quantitative tools for pain measurement that are appropriate for children of almost all cultures.[15]

Behavioral Observation Scales

Behavioral and physiologic cues are particularly useful for pre-verbal children and children who are not able to verbalize their symptoms because of cognitive impairment, developmental capacity, or sedation. Such scales may rely on facial expressions,[34] motor or verbal responses, or combinations of behavioral and autonomic responses.[35] Behavioral scales may actually rate distress, including fear and anxiety, rather than specifically assessing pain per se.

When behavior is used to assess pain, it is important to partner with parents or other caretakers who are particularly familiar with the child, because knowing the child, having familiarity with children with the same or similar conditions, and thoroughly grasping the science of symptom management are all important components of effective pain relief.[36] For example, the Paediatric Pain Profile was created to be a usable document for parents to assess and record their child's pain behavior. It is a well-validated instrument that uses behavioral cues, including changes in facial expression, vocal sounds, posture and movements, sleeping, eating, and mood, to assess pain.[37] The Individualized Numeric Rating Scale is an individualized scale for nonverbal children.[38] This scale is an adaptation of the numerical rating scale that allows parents or other clinicians who know the child well to identify the child's typical pain behavior and rank that behavior on a standard scale from 0 to 10.

The Face, Legs, Activity, Cry, Consolability (FLACC) tool was originally designed to score postoperative pain in children aged 2 to 7 years[39] but has also been validated for postoperative use in children with cognitive impairment.[40] This instrument may be advantageous because it uses various types of measures, such as activity and facial expression. Further work in the area of pain assessment in children with developmental or cognitive impairment is needed because children of this vulnerable population are less likely to be assessed for pain and to receive less analgesic medication.[41]

These assessment scales mainly simplify pain assessment as assessment of the intensity of pain. Although an oversimplification, the scales permit rapid evaluation of pain and help determine interventions aimed at ameliorating pain. Such scales are also key outcome measures in evaluations of pain-relieving interventions. Findings from one study, however, have highlighted the fact that such a simple screen for pain intensity fails to identify many individuals with significant functional interference from pain or pain significant enough to trigger a physician visit.[42] Regardless of the scale used, if clinical pain indicators are unclear, a trial of measures to ameliorate pain may clarify the cause of the distress or pain.

Beyond Assessment Instruments

Beyond using formal assessment tools, key elements in the history include alleviating and exacerbating factors, quality, location, onset, severity, and degree of impact on the child's function and well-being. Understanding the child's previous experiences with pain and strategies that have successfully been used in the past to address pain are also key components of the history and may inform the treatment plan. To this end, a multidimensional indicator of pain can help the clinician understand the existence, intensity, location, and pain that a child is experiencing. Techniques using more than one measure (self-report, behavioral, physiologic) will allow for a more accurate pain assessment.

In addition, understanding the holistic nature of pain, rather than pain as merely a physiologic phenomenon, is needed. For example, the meaning of the pain, the degree of distress it causes, and the impact of pain and pain treatment on the child's functional capacity and quality of life are crucial elements of the history. Exploring these issues may elicit exacerbating and potentially modifiable factors related to the pain experience. Finally, it is important to gain a clear understanding of the child's and family's beliefs about pain, as well as their treatment goals in terms of pain control.

Approach to the Child with Pain

Anticipation and prevention of pain constitutes the most effective treatment approach. Just as children and parents need information regarding their cancer treatment so that they know what to expect, informing them in a sensitive manner about the symptoms they may expect and strategies available for reducing the symptoms can reduce anxiety about the unknown. Often, without open conversations during which expectations can be addressed, the imagined reality that is substituted is worse than the true reality. By helping children understand what will happen and what will help, their fear and anxiety may be allayed, thereby reducing the symptoms that they may actually experience.

When a child reports pain, careful assessment by history and physical examination is imperative to generate a complete differential diagnosis. Determination of the underlying cause of pain may inform consideration of which modalities are likely to be most effective. Pharmacologic and nonpharmacologic approaches (e.g., cognitive-behavioral, physical, supportive) should be considered, including addressing factors that are likely to affect the child's experience of pain. Once a pain treatment plan is implemented, pain should be regularly reassessed. The goal of pain management should be to achieve the degree of comfort that the child finds satisfactory.

Pain of a moderate to severe rating should be treated with 24-hour analgesics, with rescue doses of the same or alternative analgesic available. Families often find it helpful to understand that preemptive analgesia is far more effective than catch-up analgesia administered for established pain.

The dosing interval, as determined by the pharmacokinetics of the agents being considered, and the feasibility of their administration by caregivers should also be taken into account. Behavioral, physical, and cognitive supports should be provided throughout treatment.

World Health Organization Guidelines

The WHO guidelines provide a stepwise approach to cancer pain. For mild pain in a child not on any analgesics, an NSAID or acetaminophen may be appropriate. Depending on the nature of the pain, it might also be appropriate to consider a short-acting opioid. For moderate pain, a short-acting opioid should be given, along with a bowel regimen to prevent constipation in most cases. For severe pain, a short-acting opioid should be rapidly titrated. In addition, adjuvant medications should be considered, regardless of pain severity.

The WHO guidelines, widely publicized for cancer pain, also provide pain control for many adults, with published success rates of 69% to 100%.[43-45] The WHO guidelines, which provide an effective, systematic approach to pain that includes strong opioids, have facilitated other WHO initiatives, such as increasing access to essential medicines for children with painful conditions worldwide.

The WHO approach, however, may inadequately emphasize an initial multidisciplinary approach. In this way, opportunities to use adjuvant medications (e.g., steroids, local anesthetics) and cognitive or behavioral interventions to reduce pain and pathologic responses to pain may be missed. In addition, the three-step ladder consisting of nonopioids, weak opioids, and strong opioids, may not be appropriate for some cancer patients, particularly those with advanced cancer. Studies have shown that a two-step ladder, in which treatment passes directly from step I (nonopioids) to step III (strong opioids) for mild to moderate pain, provides superior pain relief.[46,47] In addition, some medications historically used in step II (e.g., codeine, mixed agonist-antagonists) may be less useful for moderate pain compared with the continuation of acetaminophen and NSAIDs (unless contraindicated), along with titrated doses of other opioids.

Analgesic Medications and Interventions

Nonopioid Analgesics

This category of analgesics is appropriate for mild pain in a child not already receiving analgesics. Nonopioid analgesics include acetaminophen, NSAIDs, salicylates, and selective cyclooxygenase (COX-2) inhibitors.

Nonopioid analgesics are frequently used as monotherapy for mild pain and together with opioids for more severe pain. Unlike opioids, they do not cause sedation, tolerance, and respiratory depression. When given as an adjuvant to opioids, they enhance analgesia.[48,49] To this end, they may decrease the amount of opioid required for adequate analgesia,[50] thereby also limiting opioid-associated side effects. Combinations of nonopioids and opioids are available, although dosing of such combinations is often limited by the maximum dose of the nonopioid.

Salicylates and Nonsteroidal Anti-inflammatory Drugs

Salicylates and NSAIDs nonspecifically inhibit COX enzymes, thereby blocking production of various prostaglandins that mediate pain, inflammation, fever, and platelet function, protect gastric mucosa, and maintain a physiologic distribution of blood flow in the liver and kidneys. Aspirin's permanent effects on platelet function via permanent acetylation of cyclooxygenase are of particular concern in thrombocytopenic cancer patients because the antiplatelet effect lasts even after the drug has been metabolized. Trilisate is a salicylate that provides many of the same benefits as those provided by salicylates or NSAIDs, without known antiplatelet activity. Salicylates, however, have been associated with Reye's syndrome in children younger than 2 years.

No particular NSAID or route of administration has been found to be superior over another. Even ketorolac, the only parenteral NSAID widely used in the United States, is no more effective than orally administered NSAIDs, especially if doses are compared in an equivalent range. A single NSAID dose is roughly equivalent to 5 to 10 mg of intramuscular morphine in adults and has fewer side effects.[51] NSAIDs are commonly regarded as having a ceiling effect, with no added benefit at supramaximal doses, although the doses commonly recommended (based on safety concerns) generally remain well below the ceiling. NSAIDs can cause nephropathy, gastritis, and bleeding from reversible platelet dysfunction, a characteristic that may limit their use in the thrombocytopenic cancer patient. COX-2 inhibitors (e.g., celecoxib) selectively block production of prostaglandins that mediate inflammation and pain without impairing platelet function and with fewer effects on gastric mucosal integrity compared with traditional NSAIDs, particularly with short-term use.[52,53] Although concerns have been raised regarding the effects of COX-2 inhibitors on the risk of cardiovascular events in adults, there is little evidence that these concerns are relevant for children with neoplasms, except perhaps for the small pediatric subgroup of tumors or vascular anomalies with an increased risk for thrombotic events.

Acetaminophen

Acetaminophen is a nonopioid analgesic that reduces pain and fever. It may act in part by inhibiting prostaglandin synthesis in the central nervous system. Unlike salicylates and NSAIDs, which inhibit peripheral cyclo-oxygenases, it does not have peripheral anti-inflammatory properties. Acetaminophen is available in various oral formulations and as a rectal suppository, although its rectal administration should be avoided in neutropenic patients. When not contraindicated, rectal administration is helpful for children unwilling or unable to take oral medications, although its absorption is slow and variable, peaking at 70 minutes.[54] Because rectal absorption is less efficient, single dosing of 30 to 40 mg/kg can be given.[54] Subsequent doses should be smaller (20 mg/kg), and the interval between rectal doses should be 6 to 8 hours.[54,55] Dosing of oral acetaminophen is limited to 75 mg/kg/day, or a maximum of 3 g/day (whichever is smaller) because of the risk of hepatic toxicity.

Opioid Analgesics

General Considerations

Guidelines for initial opioid dosages are presented in Table 31-1 and are discussed in more detail later. Ultimately, the correct dose of opioid is the dose that provides the desired analgesia, with acceptable side effects. In general, intolerable side effects are usually the dose-limiting factor, as opposed to opioids having a ceiling effect. This should be explained to parents, as well as the fact that children with cancer who receive opioids for pain control do not become addicted to opioids. Addiction is an aberrant psychiatric condition in which the person exhibits maladapted, drug-seeking behavior. True addiction is comparatively rare in patients with cancer-related pain. If a child exhibits exaggerated pain behaviors (e.g., demanding pain medication, manipulative behaviors) they are far more likely to be demonstrating pseudoaddiction, in which case their behavior is a reflection of poorly controlled pain.

Addiction should be distinguished from dependence, which is a physiologic response to opioids such that if they are abruptly discontinued, the patient experiences symptoms of withdrawal. It may be helpful to draw a parallel to blood pressure medication, the abrupt cessation of which causes an undesired rebound hypertensive effect, because the body has adjusted to the presence of the antihypertensive. Addiction should also be distinguished from tolerance, which is another physiologic response of the body to the presence of opioids that requires increasing doses to achieve the same analgesic effect. The need to adjust dosing to account for tolerance is not an indication of addiction.

Opioids do not need to be saved for cases of extreme pain, because increasing pain can often be managed by increasing the opioid dose. When escalating doses provide marginal benefit, alternative opioids may be tried. It may be helpful to explain to parents that good initial pain control may improve pain control overall and actually minimize the amount of opioid needed, because large doses required to catch up to relieve uncontrolled pain may be avoided.

Some children with cancer, particularly those with advanced cancer, require extremely high doses of opioids. For example, Collins and colleagues have found that, in a sample of children with advanced cancer, in some patients the opioid infusions increased by more than 100-fold, from 3.8 to 518 mg/hr of morphine equivalent.[56]

Studies conducted in vitro and in animal models have demonstrated that opioids at physiologically relevant concentrations promote tumor angiogenesis.[57,58] In addition, the opioid receptor antagonist naloxone and the COX-2 inhibitor celecoxib inhibit angiogenesis, tumor growth, and metastasis in rodents.[58,59] There is no evidence to date that opioids promote tumor growth in humans. These preliminary in vitro and animal findings should not, by themselves, be used to conclude that the use of opioids to relieve cancer pain should be avoided. The data accumulated to date regarding the potential risks of opioids and the benefits of adequate analgesia are insufficient to recommend limiting opioid use for analgesia.

Developmental Pharmacology

Elements of renal clearance, such as glomerular filtration and tubular secretion, increase in the first few weeks of life, so that renal clearance commensurate with adult clearance is achieved by 8 months of age. When compared with infants, children, and adults, neonates and infants have reduced hepatic clearance because of hepatic enzyme immaturity. In addition, children 2 to 6 years of age have higher hepatic clearance than

TABLE 31-1   Guidelines for Initial Dosages for Opioid Analgesics*

| Drug | EQUIANALGESIC DOSES | | USUAL STARTING IV OR SUBCUTANEOUS DOSES AND INTERVALS | | Ratio of Parenteral to Oral Dose | USUAL STARTING ORAL DOSES AND INTERVALS | |
	Parenteral	Oral	Child <50 kg	Child ≥50 kg		Child <50 kg	Child ≥50 kg
Codeine	120 mg	200 mg	NR	NR	1:2	0.5-1.0 mg/kg every 3-4 hr	30-60 mg every 3-4 hr
Morphine	10 mg	30 mg (long term) 60 mg (single dose)	Bolus: 0.1 mg/kg every 2-4 hr Infusion: 0.03 mg/kg/hr Infusion:	Bolus: 5-8 mg/kg every 2-4 hr Infusion: 1.5 mg/hr	1:3 (long term) 1:6 (single dose)	Immediate release: 0.3 mg/kg every 3-4 hr Sustained release: 20-35 kg—10-15 mg every 8-12 hr 35-50 kg—15-30 mg every 8-12 hr	Immediate release: 15-20 mg every 3-4 hr Sustained release: 30-45 mg every 8-12 hr
Oxycodone	NA	15-20 mg	NA	NA	NA	0.1-0.2 mg/kg every 3-4 hr	5-10 mg every 3-4 hr
Methadone†	10 mg	10-20 mg	0.1 mg/kg every 4-8 hr	5-8 mg/kg every 4-8 hr	1:2	0.1-0.2 mg/kg every 4-8 hr	5-10 mg every 4-8 hr
Fentanyl	100 µg (0.1 mg)	NA	Bolus: 0.5-1.0 µg/kg every 1-2 hr Infusion: 0.5-2.0 µg/kg/hr	Bolus: 25-50 µg every 1-2 hr Infusion: 25-100 µg/hr	NA	NA	NA
Hydromorphone	1.5-2 mg	6-8 mg	Bolus: 0.02 mg every 2-4 hr Infusion: 0.006 mg/kg/hr	Bolus: 1 mg every 2-4 hr Infusion: 0.03 mg/hr	1:4	0.04-0.08 mg/kg every 3-4 hr	2-4 mg every 3-4 hr
Meperidine (pethidine)‡	75-100 mg	300 mg	Bolus: 0.8-1.0 mg/kg every 2-3 hr	Bolus: 50-75 mg every 2-3 hr	1:4	2-3 mg/kg every 3-4 hr	100-150 mg every 3-4 hr

*Doses are for patients older than 6 months of age. In infants younger than 6 months, initial per-kilogram doses should begin at roughly 25% of the per-kilogram doses recommended here. Higher doses are often required for patients receiving mechanical ventilation. All doses are approximate and should be adjusted according to clinical circumstances. Recommendations are adapted from previous summary tables, including those of a consensus statement from the World Health Organization and the International Association for the Study of Pain.

†Methadone requires additional vigilance because it can accumulate and produce delayed sedation. If sedation occurs, doses should be withheld until sedation resolves. Thereafter, doses should be substantially reduced; the interval between doses should be extended to 8 to 12 hours, or both.

‡The use of meperidine should generally be avoided if other opioids are available, especially with long-term use, because its metabolites can cause seizures.

NA, not applicable; NR, not recommended.

From Berde CB, Sethna N. Analgesics for the treatment of pain in children. N Engl J Med. 2002;347:1094-1103. Copyright © 2002 Massachusetts Medical Society. All rights reserved.

adults because of a larger liver mass to body weight ratio.[60] Therefore, drug doses may need to be given more frequently to children than to adults. Other age-related differences, such as changes in body composition and plasma concentrations of drug-binding proteins, can also influence pharmacokinetics.

Choice of Opioid

The usual starting opioid is morphine because of its low cost, wide availability, multiple routes of administration, and familiarity to clinicians. Because of its long history of use in children, it should be considered the first-line opioid in this population unless there are specific reasons to consider alternatives. Alternative opioids, including oxycodone and hydromorphone, and semisynthetic and synthetic compounds, such as fentanyl and methadone, can also be used in children. Use of alternative opioids may be predicated on availability, route of administra-

tion, presence of organ impairment, and the patient's prior experience with particular opioids.

Renal Failure. Metabolites of morphine, oxycodone, and hydromorphone (see later) may accumulate in renal failure. Some metabolites have analgesic activity, which may lead to delayed opioid toxicity (see later, "Opioid-induced Neurotoxicity"). For this reason, dosing intervals may need to be increased in patients with renal dysfunction. The pharmacokinetics of alternative opioids such as fentanyl and methadone are not changed with renal impairment, making these opioids better choices in this setting.

Hepatic Failure. Because glucuronidation is relatively well preserved in liver failure, opioids metabolized by glucuronidation (morphine, hydromorphone, buprenorphine) are generally better choices than those metabolized by oxidation via liver cytochromes (oxycodone, fentanyl, methadone) in this setting.[61] However, because of shunting in liver cirrhosis, the bioavailability of glucuronidated opioids may be increased. For this reason, initial opioid doses should be lower in those with hepatic impairment.

Weak Opioids. Tramadol is an atypical analgesic, with some direct noradrenergic and serotonergic agonist action and with an active metabolite that is a weak opioid. Tramadol does have numerous drug-drug interactions that should be considered. For example, it can produce seizures by itself, but this risk is greatly increased when tramadol is administered in combination with several classes of antidepressants. It is available as oral immediate and extended-release preparations and in combination formulations with acetaminophen.

Although codeine has historically been recommended as a weak opioid for mild to moderate pain, it has several limitations. Its gastrointestinal and neurologic side effects may make it intolerable. In addition, codeine is variably metabolized to its active form, morphine, providing unreliable analgesia. In fact, a study of 96 children has found that neither morphine nor its metabolites are detected in 36% of children given codeine.[62]

In various painful conditions in children, provision of codeine provides no benefit above that of NSAIDs. When codeine, ibuprofen, and acetaminophen monotherapy were compared in children presenting to an emergency room with musculoskeletal trauma, ibuprofen provided superior analgesia.[63] In the post-tonsillectomy setting, codeine in combination with acetaminophen caused more nausea, with no difference in pain or postoperative bleeding.[64] A meta-analysis has also found that weak opioids (e.g., codeine) in combination with NSAIDs fail to provide superior analgesia to that provided by NSAIDs alone,[51] but do have significantly more side effects. Based on these findings, we believe that there are very few cases in which codeine is a preferred choice among opioids.

Some opioids exhibit partial mu opioid receptor agonist activity (e.g., buprenorphine), kappa agonist activity (nalbuphine), or mixed agonist activity (butorphanol, pentazocine). Although these opioids have predominantly agonist activity, some also have significant antagonist activity. They may therefore reduce the effect of pure mu opioid receptor agonists given concurrently. In general, they do not provide superior analgesia, although they may have fewer gastrointestinal or respiratory side effects.

Strong Opioids. Meperidine is a strong opioid that should be avoided in most cases because of its side effect profile and lack of superiority to the strong opioids described later. For example, repeated doses of meperidine lead to accumulation of its metabolite, normeperidine, which in turn causes neuroexcitatory symptoms, including agitation, tremors, myoclonus, and seizures.[65] A double-blind trial comparing morphine with meperidine administered via patient-controlled analgesia (PCA) has found that morphine results in better analgesia and no more side effects than meperidine.[66] In low doses, meperidine does reduce postoperative shivering or rigors associated with amphotericin infusion.

Morphine. Morphine is the most frequently prescribed opioid in children and is the best studied opioid in this population. It has flexibility in terms of routes of administration. It is also available in a controlled-release formulation, and multiple randomized controlled trials have shown that this formulation can effectively control cancer pain when administered every 12 hours.[67] Morphine is extensively metabolized by glucuronidation in the liver to morphine 3-glucuronide (M3G) and morphine 6-glucuronide (M6G). M3G does not bind mu receptors

and has no analgesic activity, but may contribute to some of the neuroexcitatory side effects of morphine.[68] Conversely, M6G does bind mu receptors and is a potent analgesic.[69,70]

Oxycodone. Oxycodone is a semisynthetic derivative of morphine. It is frequently categorized as a weak opioid appropriate for mild to moderate pain (frequently administered in combination with acetaminophen [Percocet]), but this categorization is a reflection of its use at low doses. Oxycodone was shown to be as efficacious an analgesic as morphine or hydromorphone in one meta-analysis.[71] This meta-analysis has also shown no difference between oxycodone and morphine in terms of adverse effects, such as dry mouth, sedation, or nausea. Oxycodone itself has no ceiling effect or dose limit, although dosing may be limited when it is administered in combination with nonopioid agents, such as acetaminophen. Although it is available in parenteral formulations in other countries, it is only available in an oral formulation in the United States. It is available as an extended-release preparation.

Hydromorphone. Hydromorphone may be administered orally, intravenously, or subcutaneously. Although hydromorphone had previously been thought to have less neurotoxicity, hydromorphone metabolites have recently been shown to convey neuroexcitatory side effects. One advantage that hydromorphone does have over morphine is that its higher potency allows for smaller subcutaneous volumes to be delivered when this route of administration is used.

Fentanyl. Fentanyl may be given intravenously, with a rapid onset and short duration of action (20 to 30 minutes). For this reason, fentanyl is frequently used as an analgesic for brief painful procedures. Rapid administration of fentanyl may cause chest wall rigidity, requiring reversal with naloxone or even neuromuscular blockade and positive pressure ventilation.[72] In occasional patients, fentanyl may be better tolerated than other opioids, in part because it is associated with less histamine release[73] and creates no metabolites that may produce neurotoxicity.

Fentanyl transdermal patches last 72 hours and are a convenient parenteral mode of drug delivery preferred by many adults.[74,75] They have also been used successfully in children with chronic pain.[76] Although there is individual variation in fentanyl absorption, intraindividual absorption is stable.[77,78] In addition, hyperhidrosis, hypertrichosis, and the localization of patches on the skin do not appear to affect fentanyl absorption.[77] Because the onset of action is at least 12 hours, and because some fentanyl remains in the system for 72 hours after patch removal, transdermal fentanyl lacks flexibility for close titration for rapidly changing pain severity. The smallest patch size (25 μg/hr) may be too large a dose for some children. The reservoir design of the patch prevents the patch from being cut to adjust the dose delivered. For children previously on opioids who have developed some degree of tolerance, transdermal fentanyl was found to be a safe and well-tolerated alternative to oral opioid treatment in children as young as 2 years.[76] Transdermal fentanyl should not be used in opioid-naïve patients, because this may result in respiratory depression.

In addition to rapid onset of action and transdermal application, fentanyl provides several other benefits. When renal function is impaired, fentanyl does not accumulate to the same extent as morphine.[79] Some studies have demonstrated that transdermal fentanyl appears to cause less constipation than oral morphine, but it is unknown whether this is a route-related or drug-related observation.[80-82]

In adults or children already receiving 60 mg/day of morphine, oral transmucosal fentanyl (OTFC; Actiq) provides extremely rapid control of incident pain, with an onset of action of 5 to 10 minutes. This rapid onset of action is caused by its lipophilic nature and because this route bypasses first-pass hepatic metabolism. Because of its rapidity of onset of action, OTFC has been used to provide analgesia for brief painful procedures without the requirement for IV access.[83] OTFC is also useful for patients with breakthrough pain. A double-blind, double-dummy, randomized, crossover study of adult cancer patients with incident (breakthrough) pain found that OTFC reduces pain intensity more effectively than immediate-release oral morphine, and OTFC was favored over morphine sulfate immediate release (MSIR) by more patients after the study.[84] There is no conversion ratio for OTFC, and careful titration is needed to determine the correct dose. There is no correlation between the effective OTFC dose and the around-the-clock dose of an opioid.[85] Thus, the lowest strength (200 μg) should be tried first. If adequate pain relief is not achieved in 20 minutes, this dose may be repeated.

The fentanyl buccal tablet is another preparation of fentanyl that is rapidly absorbed via effervescent action through the oral mucosa. Patients should be on at least 60 mg/day of oral morphine in order to receive either OTFC or fentanyl buccal tablets. This way, they will have opioid tolerance so that they can safely receive a fixed dose of fentanyl, with such rapid onset of action, through the oral mucosa. The need for this degree of tolerance is highlighted by recent experiences with buccal and sublingual fentanyl, which when (inappropriately) administered to opioid-naïve patients may result in life-threatening respiratory depression.

Methadone. Methadone may be given orally, available as a tablet or liquid, or intravenously. One advantage to methadone in the pediatric population is that it is the only long-acting opioid widely available in liquid formulation. In addition, it is relatively inexpensive to manufacture, costing 90% less than extended-release morphine.[86] Methadone also exhibits unique receptor-binding properties in that the L-isomer binds mu opioid receptors and the D-isomer binds the *N*-methyl-D-aspartate (NMDA) receptor. Because the NMDA receptor is involved in opioid tolerance, opioid hyperalgesia, and neuropathic pain, it may be a useful opioid in these clinical situations (see later). Therefore, administration of methadone for analgesic purposes has become more popular in recent years.

Methadone's variable pharmacologic half-life, ranging from 12 to 150 hours, may result in delayed toxicity (sedation, hypoventilation) occurring many days after initiation of the drug.[87] Methadone's analgesic half life is commonly cited as 4 to 6 hours,[88] although some patients can require minimal rescue analgesia, with dosing at 8- or 12-hour intervals. Also, equianalgesic dose conversion from other opioids is variable and depends in part on the dose of the previous opioid. Its potency relative to morphine is highly dependent on the previous morphine dose.[89,90] Assistance in dose conversion can be found on the Internet at http://www.globalrph.com/narcoticonv.htm. Even with these calculations, there is enormous individual variability, and close follow-up is required to avoid delayed oversedation.

Methadone is metabolized through several cytochromes and therefore interacts with various other medications. Individual variation in cytochrome expression may account in part for significant blood concentration variability in patients.[91,92] Methadone, in conjunction with other medications, may prolong the QTc interval.[93] It is unclear whether this phenomenon explains the otherwise unexplained increased incidence of sudden cardiac arrest in adults on methadone therapy.[94] Until the potential for methadone to cause cardiotoxicity is better understood, it should be used cautiously in children with underlying cardiac conditions or those at risk for prolonged

QTc. Although methadone has several advantages, it does have some unique features that require familiarity with this agent for safe and effective use.

Oxymorphone. Oxymorphone is the active metabolite of oxycodone and is available as a rectal suppository. An extended-release oral formulation has been approved.

Opioid Starting Doses

For the opioid-naïve patient, recommended starting doses are listed in Table 31-1. For infants younger than 6 months, the starting dose should be roughly 25% the weight-scaled dose suggested in the table and titrated to effect. Opioids should be administered with caution in patients with disordered control of respiration, altered mental status, or altered drug metabolism. This is not to say that opioids should be withheld from these patients. Opioids can be safely delivered and adequate analgesia achieved, with careful titration to effect.

Routes and Methods of Administration

Medication should be given by the simplest, most effective, and least distressing route. Other considerations that should guide the choice of route include the severity and type of pain, ability of the child to tolerate a given route because of developmental or personal factors, and the ability of caregivers to administer medication via certain routes.

Oral Route. When possible, the oral route of administration should be attempted first. In general, the time for opioids to reach peak effect is about 60 minutes for the oral route. Most extended-release preparations are available in tablets or capsules. For children who cannot swallow tablets or capsules but who would benefit from an extended-release preparation or agent, liquid methadone can be used. If the child has a gastrostomy tube, ultra–extended-release morphine (given every 24 hours) may be suspended (but not crushed) and administered via gastrostomy tube. Ultra–extended-release morphine allows once-daily oral dosing, but unintended chewing or crushing may lead to overdose from immediate release of the morphine.[95,96] Opening the capsules and sprinkling onto applesauce may be an appropriate administration technique for adults,[95] but should be avoided in young children. Ultra–extended-release morphine may be considered for adolescents, but in younger children who may be at risk for accidentally chewing the capsules, these preparations should generally be avoided.

For intermittent dosing, oral opioids prepared as concentrated drops may provide analgesia without the requirement of swallowing larger volumes of liquid. Some children may not be able to take oral opioids reliably because of neurodevelopmental capacity or nausea and vomiting.

Rectal Route. Suppositories containing hydromorphone and morphine may be administered rectally. In addition, controlled-release morphine tablets may be given rectally.[97] Although the published potency of rectal opioids approximates that of oral opioids,[98] the pharmacokinetic properties of morphine—that is, first-pass metabolism to the active metabolite M6G by the portal circulation—should be noted when considering rectal administration. For example, Wilkinson and associates have determined that the areas under concentration-time curves for morphine metabolites are approximately twice those achieved after rectal administration. The maximal concentration of morphine and its metabolites was lower and time to achieve peak levels was longer for rectal administration. In this study, the variation in morphine kinetics did not correspond with altered pain ratings.[97] Although it is reasonable to start with 1:1 (oral to rectal) equianalgesic dosing of morphine, adjustments in dose or dosing interval should be anticipated.

Transdermal Route. Fentanyl is the only opioid manufactured in a transdermal formulation. Although other opioids such as morphine may be compounded to be delivered through this route, absorption of other opioids via this route is unreliable and alternative means of opioid administration should be sought.

Intravenous Route. This route, when appropriate, may provide rapid and reliable administration. In general, the time for morphine to reach peak effect is about 15 minutes via this route. It is frequently used when children are unable to take oral medications, such as children who are in the final stages of life.[13]

Subcutaneous Route. All intravenous opioids may be administered subcutaneously, although methadone may cause local irritation if infused continuously.[99] Delivery of opioids by this route adds approximately 30 minutes to the time of peak effect obtained by IV administration. This route is simple to use and requires only a portable syringe driver to administer the medication through a butterfly needle. In addition, it confers consistent delivery and easy titration without the requirement for IV access. Needles are changed every week, or more often if skin irritation occurs, and family members can often learn to administer medications via this route. Most patients can absorb 2 to 5 mL/hr subcutaneously.

Patient-controlled Analgesia. This mode of opioid delivery can provide a continuous IV or subcutaneous infusion of opioid to provide basal control of pain as well as a bolus, which provides relief from breakthrough pain. The PCA delivery system allows patients to manage their pain themselves, and there is no lag time between the request for and delivery of a bolus dose for uncontrolled pain, increasing their sense of control over their pain. One study comparing continuous infusion morphine with PCA has found that PCA requires less total opioid and provides equivalent control of the pain of bone marrow transplantation (BMT)–associated mucositis.[100]

Because opioid-induced sedation generally occurs before respiratory depression, it is rare for a patient to bolus himself or herself to the point of respiratory depression. PCA delivery has been used in the pediatric population with safety and efficacy. PCA does not increase the incidence of opioid-related complications, including sedation.[101] Clinical protocols for calculating the initial PCA opioid dose and subsequent opioid dose escalation can facilitate safe and efficacious implementation.[102] Thorough assessment of PCA use includes the total daily dose, ratio between continuous and bolus opioid, amount of baseline and breakthrough pain, and response to the bolus dose. A common recommendation is to adjust the continuous (basal) rate to supply roughly two thirds of the patient's daily opioid requirement. Although this is a reasonable starting point for most oncology patients with persistent disease-related pain, there are individual circumstances in which the parameters should be modified. For example, in the setting of brief, severe, episodic pain, it may be reasonable to use a lower basal rate and give more generous boluses. In postoperative care, there is considerable variation in the use of basal infusions. Our practice is to use them for operations expected to be more severely painful and/or in patients who are likely to underdose themselves. Conversely, we tend to avoid basal infusions or use very low basal rates for patients having less painful surgery, those who have received other nonopioid methods of analgesia (e.g., peripheral nerve blocks or plexus blocks), or those who have factors that increase respiratory risks.

PCA has been used successfully in children as young as 4 years.[103] PCA may also be administered by surrogates, commonly as nurse-controlled analgesia (NCA) or parent-controlled analgesia, or collectively as PCA by proxy. In theory, the safety of PCA is maximized when patients self-administer, because when they fall asleep, they stop pushing the button. Adverse events have been reported with PCA by proxy. Overall, the safety of NCA is well-established, and widely used for opioid-tolerant and opioid-naïve infants and children. Greater controversy persists with parent-controlled PCA. Our general practice is to limit its use greatly for routine care of opioid-naïve postoperative infants and children, but to use it widely for opioid-tolerant infants and children in palliative care, especially at home. Guidelines to increase the safety of PCA by proxy have been proposed.

Because the nurse assesses the child's pain and provides the bolus dose via NCA, the safety feature inherent in PCA to prevent respiratory depression is overridden. When used appropriately, NCA is associated only rarely with respiratory or neurologic complications.[104]

Intrathecal Route. Opioids may be administered intrathecally (see later, "Invasive Approaches to Pain Management").

Regardless of the route, if the patient has continuous pain, a regimen providing continuous pain control should be devised. To establish a patient's true analgesic needs, short-acting opioids, which can be easily titrated, may be given for the first 24 to 48 hours. Based on the amount of opioid required during the initial interval, longer acting opioid may then be substituted, with the provision of an as-needed short-acting opioid for incident or breakthrough pain.

Whatever regimen is devised, ensuring proper follow-up assessment is critical to ensure appropriate analgesia and to evaluate for potential opioid-associated side effects. Because constipation is a predicted and preventable side effect of opioids, a bowel regimen to prevent this side effect should always be instituted and adjusted as necessary whenever opioids are started or escalated.

Breakthrough Pain

Breakthrough pain is a transitory exacerbation of pain that occurs when pain is otherwise relatively controlled or stable at baseline. Cancer patients with chronic pain and superimposed breakthrough pain have worse overall pain, more impaired functioning, and higher psychological distress than those with chronic cancer pain alone.[105] It may occur as a result of incident pain (pain caused by a stimulus, such as movement or coughing) or end of dose failure, or may be spontaneous (e.g., lancinating pain attacks in postherpetic neuralgia).

A prospective study of pediatric inpatients with cancer has found that 57% of patients experience one or more episodes of breakthrough pain during the preceding 24 hours, with each episode lasting seconds to minutes. The pain was most commonly characterized as sharp and shooting by the children.[106]

Breakthrough pain may be challenging in that its onset may be unpredictable and rapid, and it may be more severe than pain typically experienced at baseline. Consequently, use of a pain diary may be particularly important in detecting patterns and factors associated with breakthrough pain. If end-of-dose breakthrough pain occurs, the total daily around-the-clock dose may be increased by 25%. Alternatively, the dosing interval may be shortened.

Breakthrough pain should be approached in the same manner as other types of pain, with the following caveats: (1) consideration of the underlying triggers and interventions aimed at the underlying problem; (2) optimization of the scheduled analgesic regimen; and (3) use of adequate analgesics for episodic pain (i.e., rescue medication). The rescue dose to treat such breakthrough pain should be the equivalent of the dose used every 4 hours, or 5% to 10% of the total daily opioid dose. For predictable incident pain, a short-acting opioid given just prior to the activity may be helpful. If the breakthrough pain has neuropathic features, consideration should be given to adjunctive use of analgesics with specificity for these types of pain (anticonvulsants or antidepressants), as will be discussed later.

OTFC may safely provide rapid pain relief in patients receiving the equivalent of 60 mg/day of oral morphine, as noted earlier. It may be especially useful when breakthrough pain is unpredictable and short-lived. Other hydrophilic agents such as morphine are often administered sublingually for breakthrough pain, but have a longer onset of action. A small study has indicated that methadone's rapid onset of action may make it a useful agent for treatment of breakthrough pain.[107]

Dose Escalation

For severe pain in a patient already on oral or IV opioids that persists despite a dose of breakthrough opioid medication, the dose should be increased by 50% to 100% and repeated. Once adequate analgesia is reached, the total amount given over 4 hours should be calculated to determine the effective dose for every 4 hours.[6] If more than two rescue doses are used in a 24-hour period, the total standing dose should be increased.

For patients on continuous IV opioids, a rescue dose for breakthrough pain consisting of 50% to 200% of the hourly infusion should be provided every 15 minutes as needed. For simplicity, the use of multiple different short-acting opioids is discouraged.

Opioid Tolerance

The response to acquired tolerance to an opioid is usually to increase the opioid dose. When this approach is not feasible because of opioid side effects such as neurotoxicity, rotating to a different opioid may be an option. Because the NMDA receptor plays a role in opioid tolerance, methadone, with its attendant NMDA antagonist properties, may control pain that is otherwise opioid-refractory.[108] Addition of adjuvant NMDA receptor antagonists such as ketamine may also reverse opioid tolerance. In animals, and in some patients, chronic administration of opioids can generate a condition of generalized hyperalgesia, meaning that new painful stimuli produce greater intensity of pain than that which would have occurred with the same stimulus for that subject in an opioid-naïve state. Opioid-induced hyperalgesia is discussed in greater detail later.

Opioid Rotation

Opioid rotation, or switching, may also be indicated because of intolerable side effects or route of administration. Equianalgesic tables are useful for conversion from one opioid to another and are widely available. Although no evidence exists demonstrating the superiority of one opioid over another in such a switch, changing opioids may be a successful strategy for alleviating dose-limiting side effects or opioid tolerance in children. For example, Drake and coworkers[109] have found that opioid rotation resolves adverse effects in 90% of children, without loss of analgesia or the need to increase morphine equivalents. Because of the phenomenon of incomplete tolerance, the equianalgesic dose of the second opioid should be decreased by 20% when a patient is transitioned from one opioid to another. The phenomenon of incomplete tolerance is particularly pronounced when converting to methadone,[89,90] probably because of the

ability of the D isomer of methadone to act as an NMDA receptor antagonist.[110]

Opioid Withdrawal and Opioid Tapering

Opioid withdrawal is a physiologic response. Sudden discontinuation of opioids in a patient who has been on long-standing opioids may prompt a withdrawal syndrome characterized by irritability, restlessness, dysphoria, anxiety, muscle aches, sweating, piloerection, diarrhea, nausea, vomiting, yawning, and sneezing. Withdrawal may be prevented by tapering opioids. Opioid doses may be safely cut in half without precipitating withdrawal. Continued tapering may be achieved by halving the dose every 3 days. An alternative strategy is to reduce the total daily dose by 10%/day. Maintaining the rescue dose at its original dose during the taper allows for effective treatment of breakthrough pain that may occur during the taper.

Opioid Side Effects

Nonrespiratory side effects from opioids include constipation, nausea, pruritus, somnolence or sedation and, particularly at high doses, neurotoxicity. A prospective study of pediatric oncology patients has found that in children receiving morphine, 38% had vomiting, 32% had nausea, and 24% had constipation postoperatively.[111] The high incidence of nausea and vomiting in this population is likely confounded by postoperative nausea and vomiting.

Opioid-associated sedation typically self-resolves within a few days of instituting opioids. In some cases, the sedation observed with instituting opioids is not a side effect of opioids per se, but rather a result of an exhausted patient finally able to sleep once pain is controlled. Nausea experienced by some patients on starting opioids similarly self-resolves within a few days and is often relieved with antiemetics. Switching to a different opioid because of nausea within the first 3 days of opioid therapy may be premature. Opioid-associated urinary retention is an uncomfortable symptom that may respond to use of an alternative opioid. Management of opioid-associated sedation and fatigue, constipation, pruritus, and nausea are discussed later in this chapter.

If side effects persist despite appropriate interventions, rotation to a different opioid may be helpful. Overall, there is no clear evidence at this point that one particular opioid has a different side effect profile than another. Individuals may exhibit different sensitivities to different opioids because of individual variability in opioid receptors, pharmacokinetics, and metabolism. Inroads have recently been made in understanding which genetic variants may influence an individual's response to opioids. For example, certain variants of the multidrug resistance-1 gene (MDR-1) or the gene encoding catechol-O-methyltransferase (COMT) are associated with central side effects, such as drowsiness or confusion.[112]

Opioid-associated side effects may also be improved with a reduction in opioid dose, which may be achieved without loss of analgesic effect if a coanalgesic medication is added. For example, gabapentin and morphine combined provide better analgesia from neuropathic pain at lower doses of each drug than either as a single agent.[113]

Opioid-induced Neurotoxicity

Opioid-induced neurotoxicity is typically encountered when opioid doses are rapidly increased, at high doses of opioid, or in the setting of renal failure. The patient may describe increased sensitivity to pain (hyperalgesia), pain in response to nonpainful stimuli (allodynia), worsening pain despite increasing opioids, or pain that appears to spread. Other findings of neurologic hyperexcitability such as myoclonus, delirium, or seizures may also be present. Opioid-induced hyperalgesia is likely caused by the accumulation of neurotoxic opioid metabolites such as M3G or hydromorphone 3-glucuronide (H3G). Such metabolites activate presynaptic calcium channels that release glutamate, which in turn activates NMDA receptors and depolarizes postsynaptic neurons in the central nervous system.[114]

If signs or symptoms of opioid neurotoxicity develop, the opioid should be decreased or changed to one with potentially less neurotoxic effects, such as fentanyl or methadone. Addition of a nonopioid analgesic may lessen the amount of opioid required. An alternative mode of analgesia, such as intrathecal, regional, or local analgesia, may be used in place of systemic opioids. If needed, parenteral ketamine, an NMDA receptor antagonist, may also be started to reduce NMDA receptor–mediated neurotoxicity.[115]

Myoclonus is frequently relieved by a benzodiazepine such as diazepam. Opioids may also play a role in the development of delirium (see later, "Mood Disorders and Mental Status Changes").

Management of Opioid Overdose

Respiratory depression occurs as a result of opioid receptor blockade of CO_2 chemoreceptors in the medulla. The risk of respiratory depression from opioids is small when opioids are dosed and titrated judiciously. Situations in which opioids may cause respiratory depression include the development of renal failure and a sudden decrease in pain, such as after a neurolytic block if opioid doses are not adjusted.

Respiratory depression characterized by hypopnea alone is not an indication for opioid reversal with naloxone. The administration of oxygen and reduction of the subsequent dose may be all that is needed. For a true respiratory emergency, naloxone should be administered by diluting the 0.4-mg/mL ampule in 10 mL of saline and administering 1 mL IV or subcutaneously every 3 minutes until respiratory depression is improved. If the patient is on long-acting opioids, repeated doses of naloxone or a naloxone infusion may be needed, with the hourly dose being the dose that was required initially to overcome respiratory depression. Overadministration of naloxone will block opioid receptors, resulting in withdrawal, which may be characterized by severe pain and sympathetic instability.

Adjuvant Treatments for Pain

Radiotherapy. Radiotherapy is commonly used to relieve pain, such as that from localized bone metastases. A review of 13 randomized trials in adults with painful bone metastases who received either radiotherapy or radioisotope injection for pain has found that 27% achieved total pain relief and 42% attained 50% pain relief. The largest trial found that the median duration of complete pain relief was 12 weeks. Various fractionation schedules were used, and there was no clear difference between schedules.[116]

Tricyclic Antidepressants. Tricyclic antidepressants (TCAs) often relieve neuropathic pain more quickly and at lower doses than those required to treat depression. They reduce neuropathic pain by inhibiting serotonin and norepinephrine uptake, which increases the transmission of inhibitory signals in the spinal cord. For children suffering from disturbed sleep, amitriptyline, which is a more sedating TCA, may be a good choice. However, amitriptyline also has more anticholinergic effects, such as xerostomia and constipation, in which case nortriptyline is an alternative TCA to consider.

Steroids. Pain attributable to swelling, such as headache from increased intracranial pressure, bone pain, nerve pain from compression by tumor, and hepatic capsular pain, may be responsive to steroids. A common starting dose is 10 mg followed by 4 mg four times daily in larger patients. Dosages of 10 mg/m² followed by 4 mg/m² four times daily can be used in smaller patients. If the response is favorable, the steroid dose should gradually be reduced to the lowest effective dose. An agent to provide concurrent gastric protection should also be prescribed.

Anticonvulsants. These agents control neuropathic pain by preventing peripheral nerve excitation. Carbamazepine has been widely studied for neuropathic pain such as trigeminal neuralgia. Carbamazepine, however, interacts with many other drugs and may suppress bone marrow function, limiting its usefulness for oncology patients. Gabapentin and pregabalin are newer anticonvulsants that lack such interactions and bone marrow toxicity. They target excitatory and inhibitory neurotransmitters through inhibition of sodium and voltage-gated calcium channels. Gabapentin may be sedating, requiring gradual initiation (i.e., 5 to 7 mg/kg/dose orally three times daily, gradually increased every 3 days) and titration to effect.

Clonidine. Clonidine is an alpha agonist that has historically been used to treat hypertension or opioid withdrawal. It may also be used for neuropathic pain or to enhance analgesia from opioids. Clonidine may be administered orally or transdermally, an additional benefit in the pediatric population. Clonidine has also been used in children for hyperactivity or steroid-associated psychiatric symptoms.

Ketamine. Ketamine is an effective adjuvant analgesic useful for its opioid-sparing and opioid-sensitizing capabilities. For example, it has been used successfully to supplement opioids for postoperative pain in children.[117]

Invasive Approaches to Pain Management

There is a small subgroup of patients for whom aggressive titration of analgesics and adjuvants still results in a circumstance of inadequate analgesia and/or intolerable side effects, including intolerable sedation. In some situations, it may be appropriate to consider regional anesthetic approaches; the most common are infusions of analgesics and local anesthetics via indwelling intrathecal, epidural, or plexus catheters. A number of considerations influence the choice of these methods, including patient's and surrogates' wishes in terms of balancing analgesia, alertness, and the risks and inconveniences of a technologic approach, availability of experts for catheter placement and ongoing management, and consideration of the nature of the pain, expected course of disease, and disease-related symptoms. There are a number of technical and management issues that cannot be readily extrapolated from similar infusions in adults or from perioperative infusions in children, so consultation with clinicians with past experience in these techniques should be encouraged.

In adults, there is a track record of using implantable programmable pumps that can be refilled infrequently—that is, at a frequency ranging from weekly to every several months. One study has indicated benefit of these systems for the relief of pain, quality of life scores, and even longevity.[118]

In children with cancer, it is generally necessary to combine small amounts of local anesthetic along with opioids in the spinal infusion. Because of the relatively low potency and low solubility of existing local anesthetics, this requirement makes it impractical to use the programmable pumps commonly used for adults. Therefore, in most of these cases, our preference has been to use implanted intrathecal ports rather than implanted pumps. These ports are placed in the operating room under general anesthesia in a lateral position. The intrathecal catheters are advanced cephalad from spinal entry near L3-4 under fluoroscopic guidance to position the tips near the spinal dorsal horn levels (rather than the exiting nerve root levels) relevant to the sites of greatest pain. An illustration of spinal dorsal horn levels can be found in Clemente's text.[119]

For example, for refractory pain caused by pelvic or lower extremity tumors predominantly involving lumbosacral dermatomes, we advance the catheter tips to a level around T11. Catheters are tunneled subcutaneously and connected to a port positioned over the lower ribs, near the anterior axillary line.

In the setting of refractory pain caused by advanced cancer, we think that coagulopathy should not generally be regarded as a major contraindication to this procedure. If necessary, platelets and/or fresh-frozen plasma are infused immediately before and during the procedure, as guided by coagulation parameters.

Use of indwelling ports is preferable for the sake of sterility and skin care. Ports are accessed with Huber needles similar to those used for IV ports. Although dilute local anesthetics are generally required for adequate analgesia, particularly with movement, these can generally be titrated in a manner that preserves reasonable lower body motor functioning. Depending on the side effect profile seen with opioids and local anesthetics, other spinal analgesics may be included in the mixture, including clonidine and ketamine.

The epidural route can be used, but we have found that the intrathecal route is more reliable over a longer period because of several factors, including the development of adhesions or fibrosis in the epidural space over periods of months with high-concentration infusions and because of the phenomenon of tolerance to local anesthetics. This can be overcome with intrathecal dosing but with much greater difficulty with prolonged epidural dosing. Clinicians' estimates of prognosis and longevity are often imprecise. If initially considering an invasive approach, we generally recommend first placing the type of implanted system that is most versatile and most likely to work successfully over the short term (i.e., a few weeks) and longer term (i.e., months to a year), and least likely to require a repeat procedure. One potential early complication of this procedure is cerebrosinal fluid (CSF) leak, leading to headache in the days following placement. In two cases, we have returned to the operating room several days later to resolve this problem with a fluoroscopically guided epidural blood patch. The introduction of spinal analgesic medication and the corresponding adjustment of systemic analgesics require careful attention, with the potential for oversedation and narcotization. Because the intensity of afferent nociceptive transmission is diminished by spinal medications, the stimulating effect of this nociceptive activity on alertness and respiratory drive is also diminished.

For occasional patients with tumor involving a single peripheral nerve or nerve plexus, indwelling tunneled catheters can be placed percutaneously along the nerve or in the plexus sheath. We prefer to use a combination of ultrasound and nerve stimulation guidance. These peripheral and plexus catheters can be extremely helpful if the pain remains highly localized. In most cases, however, tumor spreads beyond these more limited distributions, and we have therefore generally favored intraspinal infusions because of their greater versatility in covering pain arising from a broader area. For similar reasons, our general preference is to choose intraspinal drug infusions over neurolytic nerve blocks, except in very restricted circumstances, (e.g., the use of neurolytic celiac plexus blockade for tumor that is almost entirely restricted to upper abdominal solid viscera). Celiac plexus blockade has a good track record for treatment of refractory pain caused by pancreatic cancer in adults. It affects visceral innervation only, and produces no somatic sensory or motor deficits. Side effects such as diarrhea or orthostatic hypotension tend to be relatively short-lived and tolerable. For children and adolescents, we prefer to perform this procedure under general anesthesia with the patient in the prone position, using alcohol as the neurolytic agent, via a posterior approach using computed tomography (CT) guidance and in collaboration with an interventional radiologist.

Psychological and Nonpharmacologic Approaches to Pain

Because of the multifactorial nature of the experience of pain, a multidisciplinary approach is often helpful for optimizing pain management. Psychosocial assessment may be able to identify and address factors that contribute to pain that analgesic interventions alone cannot.

Depending on the developmental capacity of the child, interventions such as preparatory play, distraction, imagery, relaxation, deep breathing, hypnosis, and behavioral management can reduce anxiety and fear associated with pain. A child life specialist, psychologist, complementary medicine practitioner, or other specialist may provide some of these interventions.

Various cognitive and behavioral approaches to pain and invasive procedures may be helpful to reduce pain and distress. In a study of 56 children aged 3 to 13 years, a cognitive-behavioral package was compared with preprocedure diazepam or cartoon watching prior to bone marrow aspiration.[120] The cognitive-behavioral package consisted of breathing exercises, positive reinforcement, imagery, or distraction to provide the child with imaginative and cognitive tools to cope with procedural stress. Children who received the cognitive-behavioral package had overall lower pulse rates, distress, and pain scores when compared with diazepam or cartoon watching. However, during the actual aspiration procedure, there was no difference between groups, suggesting that it did not ameliorate distress associated with the intense experience of the actual procedure.[121] Cognitive-behavioral therapy (CBT) provides the child with mechanisms for coping with distressing procedures, and may explain why children who receive CBT display less distress following the procedure when compared with children who receive mask anesthesia alone.[122]

Hypnotherapy can be performed in children as young as 4 years.[123] Hypnosis can reduce procedural pain (e.g., bone marrow aspiration) and postoperative pain in children, as well as anticipatory nausea and dyspnea. In a randomized controlled trial of 30 children aged 5 to 15 years with cancer undergoing bone marrow aspiration, children who received hypnosis or CBT reported less pain and anxiety compared with their baseline symptoms or controls who did not receive either intervention. Children who underwent hypnosis also demonstrated less procedure-related distress than those in the other two groups.[124]

Music, art, and play therapy may also be helpful in reducing anxiety associated with procedures. For example, soft lullaby music reduces heart rates in children undergoing cast application or removal.[125] Even when specific nonpharmacologic techniques are not used, behavioral strategies that should always be used include appropriately preparing the child, giving them choices when possible, and providing developmentally appropriate and honest explanations and positive reinforcement. Patient education is also an important component of addressing pain.

Many patients find that therapies complementary to traditional medical approaches are of benefit in coping with stress, reducing the effects of treatment and illness, providing a sense of control, and enhancing quality of life.[126] In a survey of adults participating in cancer clinical trials, 63% used at least one type of complementary therapy, with an average use of two therapies per patient.[126] Many clinicians are unaware of these practices, and should therefore routinely inquire about them.

Although many practices such as acupuncture, massage, and healing touch seem promising in reducing cancer pain, the evidence base supporting the effectiveness of complementary therapies is weak. Barriers to the publication of such trials include issues of study quality and design, such as small study size, high attrition rates, and lack of a comparison arm, particularly in fields in which the placebo effect may be high.[127] Studies with adequate power, duration, and sham control are needed to evaluate the efficacy of these interventions for cancer pain.

Pediatric Cancer Pain Syndromes

Although pain should be approached with a systematic approach and use of analgesics, including opioids and adjuvants, certain cancer-related pain syndromes may respond to particular treatments.

Tumor-Mediated Pain

Gastrointestinal (GI) obstruction due to tumor may cause pain. Its treatment is discussed later ("Other Gastrointestinal Symptoms"). Visceromegaly, or invasion of organs, which often presents as a poorly localized, dull pain, is best treated with opioids, radiation, nerve blockade, or epidural or intrathecal techniques. Involvement of nerve or bone may result in neuropathic or bone pain (see later). Liver capsular pain may be alleviated by steroids.[128] Elevated intracranial pressure may present as headache and vomiting, and may respond to steroids or surgical decompression. In situations in which inflammation is thought to contribute to pain, pain may respond to steroids or NSAIDs.

Antineoplastic Therapy Administration–Related Pain

Antineoplastic therapy may produce various pain syndromes. Injection of chemotherapy into a peripheral vein may cause local transient pain or phlebitis. Extravasation of a vesicant such as vincristine or anthracycline may cause local pain, burning, swelling, and/or redness, as well as tissue necrosis. This is most likely to occur when the agent is injected peripherally. Dexrazoxane is a reversible topoisomerase II catalytic inhibitor that in preclinical studies was found to reduce the number, severity, and duration of wounds that developed in a dose-dependent manner after extravasation.[129] In a single-arm, open-label study of 53 patients with anthracycline extravasation, dexrazoxane was well tolerated. In this uncontrolled trial, 1 patient required surgical resection (1.8%).[130]

Intrathecal chemotherapy may cause arachnoiditis, which is associated with fever, headache, nuchal rigidity, nausea, and vomiting. A new liposomal formulation of cytarabine appears to have an increased risk of arachnoiditis in children, which can be mitigated with systemic dexamethasone.[131]

Prolonged steroid administration may result in avascular necrosis, which occurs most often in the hip.[132] NSAIDs may be helpful for this painful condition although, if pain is severe, opioid therapy may be indicated.

Bone Pain

Infiltration of bone is often experienced as a constant aching that may be relieved by steroids, NSAIDs, or opioid analgesics. Isolated bone metastases may be treated locally, such as with external beam radiation, or surgical techniques, such as vertebral body or long bone stabilization, or other more invasive treatments for pain (see later). Bisphosphonates, which reduce osteoclastic bone resorption, may be helpful when analgesics or radiotherapy are inadequate for the management of painful bone metastases.[133] Diffuse bone metastases may also be treated with radioisotopes, but these may cause myelosuppression.

Bone pain may also be caused by filgrastim or pegfilgrastim.[134] Although the mechanism underlying such pain has not been clearly established, it is frequently attributed to filgrastim-stimulated marrow expansion. In a study of 100 adults receiving care in a community oncology practice, 79% experienced moderate or severe bone pain caused by pegfilgrastim. Pain was commonly diffuse or located in the lower extremities, hips, or back. For those with the most severe pain, the mean duration of pain was 2.8 days after the injection. NSAIDs provided relief for 74% of those with moderate pain. Some with severe pain received opioids, with opioids providing relief in only 45% of patients. Interestingly, patients with lymphoma receiving concurrent steroids as lymphoma-directed therapy did not have significantly less bone pain.

Filgrastim-induced bone pain has not been well-studied in children, although anecdotally it appears to occur less frequently in children compared with adults. In a relatively small study of 28 children with cancer receiving pegfilgrastim after myelosuppressive chemotherapy (pegfilgrastim, 100 µg/kg, maximum dose 6 mg, for a total of 126 doses), 4 children reported bone pain.

Although the use of antihistamines to treat filgrastim-associated bone pain has been reported,[135] no clinical trials have evaluated this practice. Until there is evidence that antihistamines reduce this type of bone pain, antihistamines should not be used at the exclusion of established analgesic practices.

Mucositis

Mucositis is a common problem for children following chemotherapy, radiation, or bone marrow transplantation. It is particularly problematic in children undergoing high-dose chemotherapy or head and neck radiotherapy. Mucositis is associated with increased risk of infection and may impair the intake of adequate nutrition. It usually self-resolves within 14 days, or on recovery of the bone marrow. WHO has developed a mucositis rating scale that ranges from 0 (no visible evidence of mucositis, no pain, able to eat solids and drink) to 4 (erythema, ulceration present, significant pain, inability to eat or drink). Prophylactic antiviral or antifungal therapy does not decrease the incidence of mucositis. Superinfection, however, should be considered and cultures obtained when mucositis appears to be more severe or prolonged than anticipated.

The mainstay of pain control for mucositis has historically been parenteral opioid therapy, usually via PCA. This mechanism of analgesia delivery is safe and effective for this purpose.[102] An adjuvant mouthwash containing diphenhydramine, 2% viscous lidocaine, and liquid antacid (e.g., Maalox) in a 1:1:1 formulation may be tried for children older than 2 years who can spit out the medication rather than swallowing it. Topical application of straight viscous lidocaine carries with it the risk of systemic absorption if mucositis is widespread. Although the true risk of aspiration caused by local anesthesia of glottic structures is unclear, some centers avoid this strategy because of this concern. Severe mucositis can also cause abdominal pain, which is best treated with opioids. Perineal pain caused by mucositis may also be addressed with a topical barrier cream to soothe and protect the area.

Other measures may be used, such as regular administration of oral sucralfate during chemotherapy, low-dose laser therapy, and gum chewing.[136-138] Results of studies evaluating the efficacy of the free radical scavenger amifostine for reducing mucositis have been inconsistent.[139]

Recent advances in the understanding of the pathogenesis of mucositis have led to the development of targeted therapies. For example, palifermin is a keratinocyte growth factor that mediates epithelial cell growth and reduces epithelial cell apoptosis, factors that appear to be important processes in the evolution of mucositis. Palifermin was found to reduce mucosal injury, as manifested by decreased mucositis duration and severity and a reduced need for analgesics and parenteral nutrition in adults undergoing high-dose chemotherapy and radiotherapy requiring peripheral blood stem cell rescue. In one study of adults undergoing high-dose therapy with autologous stem cell rescue, the incidence of WHO grade 4 mucositis was reduced from 62% to 20% ($P < .001$).[140]

The role of L-glutamine in mucositis has also been investigated. Depletion of L-glutamine is associated with epithelial damage, and increased levels are associated with healing. The role of uptake-enhanced L-glutamine suspension (AES-14) in reducing mucositis has recently been studied. In a placebo controlled crossover study of 326 women undergoing chemotherapy for breast cancer, AES-14 reduced mucositis incidence and severity.[141] In addition, AES-14 demonstrated a carryover effect, with patients receiving AES-14 before placebo having a lower risk of mucositis.

Neuropathic Pain

Neuropathic pain may occur from infiltration or compression of nerves, nerve damage from surgery, herpes zoster, or side effects from antineoplastic therapies such as vinca alkaloids, cisplatin, oxaliplatin, or bortezomib. Children often describe it as burning or shooting pain that may be accompanied by dysesthesia or hyperalgesia.

Neuropathic pain may be related to chronic pain states in which chronic afferent input into the dorsal horn of the spinal cord leads to a hyperactive state. Mediators of this condition are excitatory amino acids, such as glutamate, which bind to the NMDA receptor. The NMDA-glutamate receptor is a calcium channel involved in opioid-resistant pain, neuropathic pain, allodynia, and hyperalgesia. NMDA receptor binding may lead to lasting increases in neuronal excitability, leading to the persistence of neuronal hyperactivity. The end result of such a phenomenon is hyperalgesia, allodynia, spontaneous pain, and phantom limb pain, even after the painful stimulus has resolved. Methadone, with its NMDA receptor antagonist properties, may be the most appropriate opioid for neuropathic pain. There is no clear evidence from human studies, however, that methadone is superior to other opioids in treating neuropathic pain.[142] In addition, other approaches, such as nerve blocks or adjuvant NMDA receptor antagonists, may disrupt ongoing nociceptive input and neuronal hyperexcitability.

Most therapies for neuropathic pain have been evaluated for noncancer-related neuropathic pain syndromes, such as diabetic neuropathy. Medications for neuropathic pain include TCAs and the newer atypical antidepressants venlafaxine and duloxetine. Duloxetine is the first antidepressant to be approved by the U.S. Food and Drug Administration (FDA) for the treatment of neuropathic pain. Neuroleptics such as topiramate, pregabalin, or gabapentin may also be effective.[113,143,144] In the cancer population, gabapentin effectively reduced tumor-related neuropathic pain in a randomized controlled study of

adults already receiving opioids, with lower average pain intensity scores and less dysesthesia in the gabapentin group.[145] In some cases, when tumor incites pain by spinal cord compression, dexamethasone may reduce pain.[146] Other interventions such as topical lidocaine or capsaicin, transcutaneous electrical nerve stimulation, surgical decompression, or nerve blocks may also relieve neuropathic pain.

Phantom Limb Pain

Phantom limb pain is a common phenomenon in children who undergo amputation of an extremity. It may be experienced as stump pain or the type of pain experienced preoperatively, and appears to improve over time.[147,148] It appears to be associated with preoperative limb pain. Therefore, it is best approached with preemptive regional anesthesia. Additional measures to treat this type of pain include anticonvulsants, TCAs, and topical agents such as lidocaine (Lidoderm). Some small series have reported success with gabapentin[149] or topiramate for phantom limb pain.[150] A preliminary observational study has found that use of a prosthesis to support limb use is associated with reduced phantom limb pain when compared with cosmetic prosthesis use.[151]

Pain Related to Graft-Versus-Host Disease

Graft-versus-host disease (GVHD) may cause various pain syndromes. It is a common cause of abdominal pain in children undergoing bone marrow transplantation.[152] Along with diarrhea, nausea and vomiting, weight loss, dysphagia, and early satiety, abdominal pain and cramping may occur in gut GVHD.[153] Gut GVHD may be so severe as to require opioids for analgesia.[103]

Oral GVHD usually does not cause pain. Development of oral pain is associated with ulceration or involvement of the soft palate.[154,155] Evaluation of pain in the setting of oral GVHD should also consider concomitant infection such as herpes simplex virus (HSV) infection or candidiasis. Oral GVH pain is usually reduced with GVH-directed treatment such as topical steroids or topical FK506 rinses. Pain associated with vulvovaginal GVHD may also respond to topical steroids or topical cyclosporine.[156,157] Other types of GVHD, such as myositis or fasciitis, may require systemic analgesia.

Postoperative Pain

A broader discussion of treatment of postoperative pain in children and adolescents can be found elsewhere.[158,159]

Cancer surgery is often distressing and anxiety-provoking to children and their parents. Unless specifically contraindicated, anxiolytic premedication with benzodiazepines should be considered as routine, using an oral or IV route as appropriate. For patients receiving opioids on a regular basis preoperatively, it is necessary to increase postoperative analgesic dosing accordingly. It is a common mistake to select routine parameters for opioid infusions or PCA for these patients; this invariably results in underdosing and inadequate analgesia. For major tumor resections in the lower extremities, pelvis, abdomen, and thorax, we make extensive use of epidural infusions for postoperative analgesia. Epidural analgesia in children requires specific training about the technical aspects, as well as pediatric-specific management protocols and a level of acute pain service coverage that permits optimal dose adjustment. For patients receiving epidural infusions who are opioid-tolerant preoperatively, it may be necessary to provide a systemic opioid along with an epidural opioid postoperatively, despite widespread disapproval of this combination, or it may be necessary to use larger than usual dosing of epidural opioids, addition of epidural clonidine, or other approaches to account for the patient's preexisting opioid tolerance, which may be accompanied by hyperalgesia.

Procedure-Related Pain

Brief needle procedures, including venipuncture, intravenous cannulation, lumbar puncture, and bone marrow biopsy and aspiration, are a major aspect of cancer treatment and a major source of distress for patients. Approaches to management of these interventions should be individualized, based on consideration of the child's age, temperament, coping style, and past pain experiences, as well as on the intensity of the procedure (e.g., bone marrow biopsy is more painful than simple venipuncture).

Explanations prior to procedures should be tailored according to the child's age, developmental status, and coping style. Parental presence can be helpful, especially when there is some coaching of parents to help them with facilitating positive coping. Parents should be there to provide support, not to hold the child or assist clinicians.

Various products are available for providing needle-free skin analgesia. These include local anesthetic creams, such as lidocaine and prilocaine (EMLA), liposome-encapsulated lidocaine (ELA-Max, or LMX4), tetracaine gel (Ametop), lidocaine and tetracaine patches (Synera), needleless injection systems (lidocaine [Zingo]), and lidocaine iontophoresis. These products differ in their onset time, propensity for vasodilation or vasoconstriction, cost, and availability in different countries. In a busy clinic, use of these topical anesthetic techniques is facilitated by standing order policies, so that they can be applied at an appropriate time before the planned procedure.

Several cognitive-behavioral approaches have been shown to be effective in reducing the distress of pediatric oncology procedures, including hypnosis, guided imagery, and related approaches to achieving a relaxed or dissociated state. These approaches have the virtue of safety and generalizability. A patient who learns these techniques for one setting can apply them to other situations.

Conscious sedation, deep sedation, or brief general anesthesia can be effective in alleviating the pain and distress of lumbar punctures and bone marrow biopsy and aspiration. Choice of approach will depend in part on the individual patient, intensity of pain involved in the procedure, degree of immobility required (e.g., for radiation therapy or magnetic resonance imaging [MRI]), and available resources.

There is considerable variation in the choices of drugs and depth of sedation, and about which staff members are involved in the various aspects of sedation. In some hospitals, a two-tiered approach is taken, with lower risk patients receiving sedation by oncologists and nurses and higher risk patients cared for by pediatric anesthesiologists.

Other hospitals use a different two-tiered approach, with low- to intermediate-risk patients receiving sedation by a sedation service involving nurses and pediatric subspecialists with specific expertise (e.g., pediatric intensivists or pediatric emergency physicians), with pediatric anesthesiologists caring for higher risk patients or those having more extensive procedures or requiring higher degrees of immobility. For example, for a cooperative, relatively healthy 12-year-old undergoing a lumbar puncture, a regimen that involves conscious sedation with midazolam and fentanyl, topical local anesthesia, followed by local anesthetic infiltration, is likely to be safe and effective. Conversely, a 2-year-old with a history of a difficult airway and cardiomyopathy, who is undergoing bone marrow aspiration, biopsy, lumbar puncture, and central line removal, would be

at higher risk and might therefore be referred for management by a pediatric anesthesiologist.

Regardless of local decisions about which specialists are involved in various procedures, we think that pediatric oncologists need to advocate for sufficient institutional resources to ensure that effective and safe approaches to conscious sedation and general anesthesia are available for all children with cancer. Some general recommendations for sedation programs are listed in Box 31-1. More detailed discussions of individual drugs and outcomes of pediatric sedation may be found elsewhere.[160,161]

Box 31-1 Recommendations for Pediatric Oncology Sedation Programs

1. A standardized preprocedure history and physical should be performed to identify factors that might modify risk (e.g., airway anomalies, respiratory difficulties, cardiac compromise).
2. Procedure checklists should be encouraged.
3. NPO guidelines should be consistent with those recommended for children undergoing general anesthesia.
4. Clinicians who are performing the procedure should have undivided attention during the procedure (e.g., their beeper and phone should be carried by someone else), and they should ensure that all necessary supplies (including kits, sterile supplies, chemotherapy, tubes) are already in the room before bringing the child into the room or initiating sedation.
5. Children receiving sedation should receive continuous monitoring, including a dedicated observer, continuous use of pulse oximetry, and regular recording of vital signs.
6. All procedure locations should have at least the following supplies, equipment, or systems at hand:
   a. Wall or tank oxygen supplies
   b. Wall or portable suction devices
   c. Monitoring equipment
   d. Airway equipment, including bags and suitably sized masks, laryngoscopes, endotracheal tubes, oral airways, and laryngeal mask airways
   e. An emergency cart, such as a code cart
   f. Communication protocols (often assisted by a code button or phone system)
7. Following the procedure, children require observation until they meet standardized recovery criteria, and often for a period of time thereafter. During recovery, and especially when they no longer appear sedated, children remain at significant risk for injuries caused by falling, hitting their head on bed rails, and so forth.
8. Observation and administration of medications should be performed by a clinician with no additional responsibilities—that is, not by the clinician performing the procedure. These clinicians should have training and competency in pediatric acute care and pediatric airway management.
9. Clinics and hospitals performing pediatric sedation should track outcomes related to efficacy (from a child-centered viewpoint) as well as safety to facilitate system-based improvements in quality of care.

Reassessing Interventions for Pain

Careful reassessment to determine response to therapy is a key component in effectively addressing pain. Interventions to reduce pain seek not only to reduce pain, but also to reduce distress and functional impairment and enhance quality of life. Pain relief measures do not necessarily achieve all these goals. For example, in one survey of adults with noncancer pain, those on opioid therapy did not experience improved quality of life or function, even when degree of pain was controlled for.[162] Therefore, evaluation of whether pain relief is attained and whether increased functional capacity and increased quality of life are achieved is crucial for symptom management.

Barriers to Effective Pain Management

Increasing interest in pain and pain treatment in recent years has resulted in a better understanding of pathophysiologic mechanisms of pain, better treatment options, and greater availability of pain treatment. These advances, however, have not necessarily resulted in a reduced prevalence of pain in cancer patients.[9]

This paradox is caused in part by the many barriers to effective pain management. Clinician-related barriers include a focus on cure at the exclusion of attention to symptoms, lack of optimal familiarity with pain management strategies, fear of regulatory repercussions for prescribing opioids or diversion to individuals for whom the opioid is not prescribed, and underappreciation of the multifactorial nature of the experience of pain. Patient-related factors may include fear of addiction, fear of side effects, including respiratory depression, fear that treating pain with opioids is equivalent to giving up, and the misperception that opioids should be saved for severe pain.

Educational strategies for clinicians and families alike are likely to surmount many of these problems with pain management. In addition, partnership with the child and family may increase attention to this important issue and provide added opportunities for addressing barriers to treating pain adequately. For example, a randomized clinical trial that tested the effectiveness of the PRO-SELF Pain Control Program, which actively involves adult patients and families in the pain management plan, has shown decreased pain intensity scores, increased appropriate analgesic prescriptions, and increased analgesic intake in oncology outpatients with pain from bone metastasis when compared with standard care.[163] Such an approach is endorsed by the American Pain Society and is likely to contribute greatly to overcoming barriers to successful pain management.

NAUSEA AND VOMITING

Pathophysiology

Vomiting may be caused by a wide variety of triggers, including motion, insults to the GI tract, hormonal changes, medications, and emotions. It is a complex process that involves the central and peripheral nervous systems, with biologic and psychological mechanisms playing a role.

Strides have been made over the past 3 decades in understanding the pathophysiologic components of nausea and vomiting and in the development of agents aimed at these factors. Investigations have focused primarily on chemotherapy-induced nausea and vomiting (CINV). Prior to the 1990s, dopamine was the major neurotransmitter recognized as important in mediating CINV, and dopamine blockade was the mainstay of therapy for CINV.

Vomiting is mediated by the vomiting center in the medullary lateral reticular formation. This center is not a discrete entity but is a group of loosely organized neurons in the medulla that are activated in a sequential manner during emetogenesis.[164,165] Sources of afferent input to the nucleus tractus solitarius in the vomiting center include the chemoreceptor trigger zone (CTZ), viscera (via vagal and sympathetic afferents), midbrain, vestibular system, and cerebral cortex (Fig. 31-3). To induce vomiting, the vomiting center causes the emission of coordinated efferent impulses to several targets, including the diaphragm, abdominal wall musculature, esophagus, and stomach, otherwise known as the vomiting reflex.

Chemotherapy-Induced Nausea and Vomiting

Chemotherapy can lead to nausea and vomiting through several mechanisms. One is by stimulation of the CTZ, which lies in the area postrema in the floor of the fourth ventricle. Although the CTZ is part of the central nervous system, it contains chemoreceptors outside the blood-brain barrier that can detect emetogenic agents present in the circulation and in the spinal fluid. Evidence suggests, however, that chemotherapy stimulates the CTZ indirectly because of the following: (1) it is unlikely that the CTZ has specific receptors that are activated by each type of chemotherapy agent; (2) the latency time to the onset of emesis is not compatible with direct action of the drugs on the CTZ; and (3) vagotomy and sympathectomy prevent cisplatin-induced emesis in the ferret, indicating that these inputs are needed for chemotherapy-induced vomiting to occur.[166,167]

Chemotherapy can also stimulate the vomiting center directly.[164] In addition, chemotherapeutic agents can stimulate the gut, leading to release of serotonin. This in turn stimulates the vagus nerve, which activates the vomiting center, either directly or via impulses to the CTZ.[168] The central cortex may also be involved in CINV by mediating feelings of anxiety that play a role in the genesis of nausea.

Several neurotransmitter pathways are known to play a role in nausea and vomiting. Although histamine and muscarinic receptors are prominent in vomiting associated with motion sickness,[169] serotonin, dopamine, and substance P appear to be particularly important in CINV.[170] Central blockade of the D2 subtype of dopamine receptors in the area postrema and vomiting center is the mechanism of action of antidopaminergic antiemetics such as metoclopramide. It was later found that in addition to dopamine receptor antagonism, metoclopramide is an antagonist of the 5-hydroxytryptamine-3 (5-HT$_3$) receptor,[171,172] prompting interest in the role of this receptor in nausea and vomiting.[164]

Serotonin is produced by enterochromaffin cells in the gut and is also found in a number of locations in the CNS. Several studies in animals and humans have confirmed that serotonin plays a major role in acute CINV. Cisplatin- and cyclophosphamide-induced vomiting in the ferret was drastically reduced with the administration of intravenous, intraperitoneal, or intracerebral injection of serotonin S3 receptor antagonists.[173] Serotonin receptor blockers and serotonin receptor blockade inhibited chemotherapy-induced vomiting in ferrets[166,174-177] and in other animal systems.[178,179] Depletion of serotonin stores was shown to also prevent cisplatin-induced vomiting.[180]

In humans, studies by Cubeddu and colleagues[181] have demonstrated that strongly emetogenic regimens containing cisplatin or dacarbazine result in a marked increase in serotonin

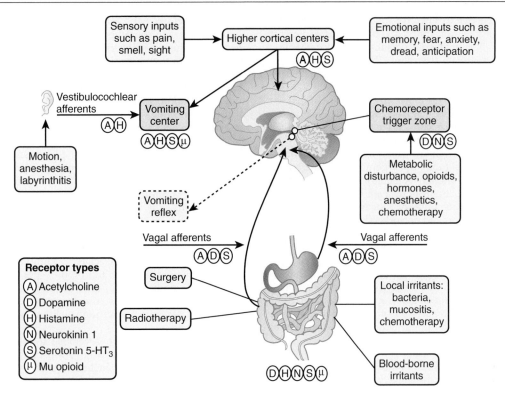

FIGURE 31-3. Pathogenesis of chemotherapy-induced nausea and vomiting.

metabolites in plasma and urine and have a time course similar to that of the vomiting experienced by patients receiving these agents. In addition, treatment with a serotonin synthesis inhibitor inhibits cisplatin-induced vomiting and increases in serotonin metabolites. The relationship between other chemotherapeutic agents and markers of serotonin metabolism has been further explored, with more emetogenic regimens resulting in higher serotonin metabolite levels.[181] Chemotherapeutic agents appear to be toxic to the enterochromaffin cells lining the upper small intestine, resulting in the generation of free radicals and release of serotonin.[167]

5-HT$_3$ receptors are present in the GI tract and in vagal afferents. They are also found throughout the human brainstem, including a high concentration in the CTZ.[182] Serotonin antagonists injected into the area postrema inhibit cisplatin-induced emesis in the ferret[173] but it appears that 5-HT$_3$ receptor antagonists also exert their antiemetic effect at the level of the peripheral nervous system by serotonin blockade in the vagal nerve.[183,184]

Substance P, which binds to the tachykinin neurokinin NK1 receptor, has been implicated more recently in mediating vomiting. Substance P is a neuropeptide found in the central nervous system and GI tract. Because of its localization pattern and its ability to induce vomiting when administered intravenously, it was suspected to play a role in the genesis of vomiting.[185] NK1 receptor antagonists appeared promising in that they inhibited vomiting induced by a range of agents known to produce vomiting by central and peripheral mechanisms in the ferret.[186,187] The site of antiemetic action of NK1 receptor antagonists has not yet been clearly defined. It may be peripheral, at the level of vagal motor neurons that control relaxation of the gastric fundus.[165] Investigation of the time course of the antiemetic effects of a 5-HT$_3$ antagonist and the NK1 receptor antagonist "aprepitant" has indicated that serotonin may mediate the early vomiting process (within the first 8 to 12

hours of cisplatin administration) although later vomiting may be mediated by substance P binding to NK1 receptors.[183]

Classification

Acute and Delayed Chemotherapy-Induced Nausea and Vomiting

Acute CINV, also known as post-treatment CINV, is traditionally defined as nausea and vomiting that occurs within the first 24 hours after the administration of chemotherapy. Delayed CINV occurs 24 hours after chemotherapy and may last up to 5 days. Delayed CINV is typically associated with certain chemotherapeutic agents such as cisplatin, which causes a peak of nausea and vomiting 48 to 72 hours after its administration.[188] The incidence of delayed CINV is as high as 89% in patients receiving cisplatin-based chemotherapy without antiemetic prophylaxis.[189] In patients receiving antiemetic prophylaxis with cisplatin-containing regimens, the incidence is variable, but has been reported to be as high as 73%.[190]

Delayed nausea may be more severe than acute nausea because it is often less responsive to standard antiemetic therapy. The recent introduction of the NK1 receptor antagonist aprepitant has provided new options for controlling delayed CINV. However, it remains clear that the single best predictor of delayed CINV is acute CINV and that control of acute CINV is a key factor in preventing delayed CINV.[188,191,192] For example, in a cohort of 705 patients receiving chemotherapy for the first time, when acute CINV was completely controlled with ondansetron plus dexamethasone, 92% had complete control of delayed CINV. However, of those who did have acute CINV, only 41% had complete control of delayed CINV.[192]

Although some pharmacologic agents have been developed to control delayed CINV, lack of recognition of this problem remains a major barrier to effective management. Grunberg and associates[193] have demonstrated that in a cohort of patients receiving moderately emetogenic chemotherapy for the first time, clinicians overestimate control of CINV, and this discrepancy is particularly notable for delayed CINV, in which case-control of symptoms was overestimated by 21% to 28%. More that 75% of clinicians underestimated the incidence of delayed CINV. This misperception may in part explain the observation that less than 50% of those who suffer from delayed CINV receive adequate prophylaxis that conforms to established guidelines.[194] Given the extent to which delayed CINV negatively affects the lives of those undergoing chemotherapy,[195] improved practice, in conjunction with pharmacologic advances, is needed to reduce suffering from delayed CINV.

Relatively little has been published regarding delayed vomiting in children. Pinkerton and coworkers[196] found that of 27 children who received cisplatin, cyclophosphamide, or carboplatin and ondansetron, 9 (33%) developed delayed emesis. In a larger prospective study of pediatric patients who did not receive antiemetics during the delayed phase following chemotherapy, 2 of 6 (33%) children who received high-risk antineoplastics (cyclophosphamide, cisplatin, or carboplatin) and 12 of 110 (11%) of those who received other chemotherapeutic agents developed delayed vomiting, although the accuracy of the incidence of delayed vomiting in the high-risk group was limited by the small number of children in that group.[197] As has been appreciated in adult patients, children who vomited in the acute phase were significantly more likely to have delayed vomiting (45%) compared with those who did not experience significant acute vomiting (13%). In addition, chemotherapy lasting 2 or more consecutive days was associated with a significantly higher rate of delayed vomiting (39%) compared with single-day chemotherapy (13%). In our experience, many children experience delayed CINV.

Anticipatory Nausea

Anticipatory nausea and vomiting is a conditioned response that occurs in anticipation of planned chemotherapy when vomiting has been poorly controlled in previous cycles. In adults, anticipatory nausea and vomiting occurs in 25% of adults undergoing chemotherapy.[198] It is associated with higher anxiety, more severe postchemotherapy nausea and vomiting, delayed onset of previous CINV, and a history of motion sickness.[198-201]

A similar pattern is seen in the pediatric population; the severity of distress from nausea and vomiting, greater expectation for severe nausea and vomiting, and the severity of nausea and vomiting actually sustained all correspond with a higher likelihood of anticipatory CINV.[202-204] Anticipatory nausea and vomiting is most likely to develop within the first 4 months of therapy, usually occurs hours before treatment, and is most severe at the actual time of chemotherapy administration.[202] Anticipatory nausea and vomiting in children appears to have features consistent with a conditioned response. These features suggest that this type of nausea and vomiting is a learned response, which accounts for its refractoriness to typical antiemetics.

Measurement and Assessment

Measurement

Although nausea and vomiting are often lumped together, as in the term *CINV*, they may be regarded as two distinct phenomena. Nausea, although it may be accompanied by physiologic changes such as pallor, sweating, or feeling hot or cold, is essentially a subjective experience that is measured by patient report. Therefore, nausea cannot be studied in models other than humans. On the other hand, vomiting can be objectively measured. Thus, it is invariably used as the outcome of choice when evaluating interventions for nausea and vomiting. Complete control of CINV is a frequently used outcome and is defined as the absence of any vomiting for a defined period of time after administration of chemotherapy. However, nausea may exist without vomiting, and changes in vomiting do not necessarily reflect a concomitant change in nausea.

Although they can occur together, nausea occurs more frequently than vomiting.[190,193,205] Much attention has been focused on the prevention of vomiting. This is an important goal because previous uncontrolled vomiting may stimulate anticipatory vomiting in subsequent cycles of chemotherapy. However, nausea is also an important symptom to assess and control, because it also impairs functioning and quality of life, even in the absence of vomiting.[195,206-209] Finally, although advances such as the 5-HT$_3$ receptor antagonists may have relieved chemotherapy-associated vomiting, related post-treatment nausea has not improved.[210] For all these reasons, attention to both nausea and vomiting is needed. Studies reporting only vomiting as an outcome are limited and interpretation of assessments relying solely on vomiting should be made with care.

Instruments have been developed to measure the subjective phenomenon of nausea in adults.[211,212] Instruments to assess nausea in children, including those who are preverbal, have been described but are not in widespread use.[213,214] One strategy for assessing nausea in children is a simple analogue or numerical scale on which children rate the severity of their nausea. Although application of such an instrument for children reporting their own nausea has not yet been studied, children as young as 5 years have reliably used a numerical scale to assess nausea experienced by characters in a vignette.[215] It is known that children 5 years or older can reliably use a color analogue scale to report severity of their pain[216] and children 7 years or older can report pain with a visual analogue scale[29] or numerical scale, so it is likely that they can report their nausea with similar reliability.

Hinds and associates[217] have shown that a symptom distress instrument that includes nausea assessment, designed for adults, is reliable and valid for adolescents with cancer. Other symptom distress scales that include nausea assessment, most notably the Memorial Symptom Assessment Scale, are also reliable and valid for children.[1,2]

Within the pediatric population, parental report is also an important source of information when assessing nausea and vomiting. In a small study of CINV, parent-child dyads were found to have a moderate to strong association when reporting symptoms of nausea and vomiting.[218] Studies by Zeltzer and coworkers[219,220] have also shown a high degree of correlation between parental and child reports of nausea, although Tyc and colleagues[221] have found that parents tend to underestimate their child's nausea.

Assessment

When nausea and vomiting in patients with cancer are considered, attention is often focused on CINV. When evaluating a patient with nausea and vomiting, however, it is imperative that other causes be considered in the differential diagnosis.

A full assessment of a patient with nausea and vomiting, extending beyond quantification of the severity of the symptom, permits the generation of a complete differential diagnosis. Only in this way can all possible mechanisms and therefore all potentially efficacious interventions be entertained.

Features such as whether nausea and vomiting is acute or chronic, intermittent or constant, and associated with any

Box 31-2	Patient-Related Risk Factors for Developing Chemotherapy-Induced Nausea and Vomiting

History of previous chemotherapy-induced emesis
Prechemotherapy nausea
Female gender
Emesis during past pregnancy
History of motion sickness
Low performance status
Low social functioning

TABLE 31-2	Schematic Approach to Chemotherapy-Induced Nausea and Vomiting (CINV)*		
Type of CINV		**Prophylaxis**	**Breakthrough**
Acute CINV			
	High risk	5-HT$_3$ receptor antagonist Dexamethasone Lorazepam ± aprepitant, scopolamine patch, metoclopramide, or cannabinoid if needed	Same as prophylaxis, initially as needed, then scheduled
	Moderate or low risk	5-HT$_3$ receptor antagonist Dexamethasone ± lorazepam, scopolamine patch, metoclopramide, or cannabinoid if needed	
Delayed CINV		Ondansetron Aprepitant Dexamethasone ± metoclopramide, cannabinoid, as needed	Same as prophylaxis, initially as needed, then scheduled
Anticipatory CINV		Prevention of CINV Lorazepam Nonpharmacologic approaches	Lorazepam

*Points to consider:
• Choose appropriate prophylactic antiemetics based on emesis risk, determined by patient-related risk factors, emetogenicity of chemotherapeutic agent(s).
• Assess effect of antiemetic regimen regularly.
• If breakthrough CINV occurs, augment prophylaxis regimen for subsequent chemotherapy cycles.

particular factors are important to consider. Other elements of the history, such as whether vomiting is projectile, bowel patterns, current medications, and prior history of nausea and vomiting can also be helpful in delineating the cause and therefore potentially effective interventions. For example, obtaining a history suggesting constipation as the cause of nausea and vomiting will lead to a workup and treatment plan entirely different than if the cause were suspected to be chemotherapy or labyrinthitis.

Another important component of the history is an assessment of the impact of the symptom on the patient's daily functioning and quality of life. Specific instruments to address these aspects have been developed, such as the Morrow Assessment of Nausea and Emesis, which is a self-report form that allows adults to assess their experience with acute, delayed, and anticipatory CINV.[222]

Predictors

The likelihood of CINV development and CINV severity is determined by treatment-related and patient-related factors. The particular agent used is the primary treatment-related risk factor for CINV (Table 31-2), but higher dosages of the agent, shorter infusion rates, combinations with other agents, and repeated cycles of chemotherapy can also increase the risk of CINV.[184,223,224] When combination chemotherapy is given, antiemetics should be prescribed according to the most emetogenic, and with the consideration that some combinations might act synergistically in creating CINV.

Patient-related factors, as determined in the adult population, also appear to affect risk for developing CINV (Box 31-2).[206,225,226] In one multivariate analysis, low social functioning, prechemotherapy nausea, and female gender were predictive of more severe CINV.[206] Patients with a history of vomiting in a previous cycle are at greater risk of vomiting with the subsequent cycle,[227] in part perhaps because of anticipatory vomiting. An assessment of the intended treatment and the patient's individual risk factors may help determine which patients are more at risk for developing CINV, and therefore in need of more intensive prophylaxis or rescue therapy.

Principles of Pharmacologic Therapy

Because prevention of acute CINV is a key element for reducing delayed CINV, the learned component of anticipatory CINV is based on prior experience, and there is inadequacy of rescue therapy once nausea and vomiting have developed, the optimal approach is to prevent these symptoms from occurring in the first place. Although a targeted approach based on the inciting cause and the suspected underlying pathophysiology, and/or on evidence demonstrating superiority of certain agents

or classes in different situations, is most effective, it is not always possible to know which is the optimal agent for an individual and should be chosen first. Guidelines for the initial choice of antiemetic, as well as dosing, are provided in Tables 31-2 and 31-3. Use of one (or two) agents, with titration of the dose and addition of other agents if necessary, might be the best strategy. For CINV, which is thought to be mediated through several pathways, a combination of antiemetics is usually warranted. This is particularly true with highly emetogenic chemotherapy, a case in which monotherapy is almost always insufficient.

Drugs used to manage CINV include true antiemetics and adjuvants. Adjuvant medications may be used to allay anxiety, induce amnesia, or induce sleep. Although many of these agents have been investigated in adults, evidence regarding their use in children, including optimal dosing and potential adverse effects, is frequently more limited. Where evidence in the pediatric population is available, it is included. However, we must often rely on evidence from adult studies and extrapolate appropriate dosing. Furthermore, guidelines and standard practices in adults may involve formulations of medications that cannot be adjusted (e.g., capsules or patches) for pediatric patients. Medications that are only available as tablets or capsules may also not be feasible for developmental or psychological reasons.

TABLE 31-3   Classes of Antiemetics, Dosing, and Routes of Administration

Class	Dose and Route	Indication	Notes
5-HT₃ RECEPTOR ANTAGONISTS			
Ondansetron	0.45 mg/kg/day every 24 hr IV or PO	First-line therapy for high-, moderate-, or low-risk CINV	May cause constipation, headache; available as an oral disintegrating tablet
Granisetron	≥2 yr: 20-40 µg/kg/day divided once or twice daily; maximum = 3 mg	First-line prophylaxis or breakthrough CINV	Granisetron available as oral solution
Dolasetron	≥2 yr: 1.8 mg/kg IV or PO as a single dose; maximum = 100 mg		Ondansetron, dolasetron may be extemporaneously prepared
DOPAMINE ANTAGONIST			
Metoclopramide	0.5 mg/kg IV or PO daily (for prophylaxis) 0.5 mg/kg IV or PO every 6 hr (for breakthrough CINV) 1 mg/kg IV or PO every 6 hr (for severe breakthrough CINV or if lower dose ineffective)	High-risk prophylaxis, breakthrough	Prescribe with diphenhydramine to prevent EPS; treat EPS with diphenhydramine or benztropine
CORTICOSTEROID			
Dexamethasone	BSA <1 m²: 10 mg/m² IV or PO daily BSA ≥1 m²: 10-12 mg IV or PO daily; may use 20 mg as a single dose on day 1	High-risk prophylaxis for acute or delayed CINV; breakthrough	Contraindicated in pulmonary radiation therapy Consider lower dose if given with aprepitant.
NK-1 ANTAGONIST			
Aprepitant	125 mg PO × 1 on day 1, then 80 mg PO daily on days 2, 3	Acute or delayed prophylaxis	Use only if ≥45 kg (limited data in pediatrics)
ANTICHOLINERGIC			
Scopolamine	1.5-mg patch applied transdermally; change every 72 hr	High-risk prophylaxis, breakthrough	Use only if ≥40 kg (cannot cut patch); may cause dry mouth, blurred vision
CANNABINOID			
Dronabinol	2.5-5 mg/m²/dose PO every 6 hr (10 mg/dose maximum)	High-risk prophylaxis; breakthrough	Do not use in children <6 yr; use with caution if 6-12 yr; may cause confusion, ataxia; no IV form
ANXIOLYTIC			
Lorazepam	<20 kg: 0.025 mg/kg IV or PO every 6 hr 20-40 kg: 0.0125 mg/kg IV or PO every 6 hr >40 kg: 0.5-2 mg IV or PO every 6 hr	High-risk prophylaxis; breakthrough; anticipatory CINV	May cause confusion, sedation, hallucinations, or memory impairment; avoid use of dose greater than 0.5 mg unless proven tolerance of 0.5 mg

CINV, chemotherapy-induced nausea and vomiting; EPS, extrapyramidal side effects; IV, intravenous; PO, by mouth.

Dopamine Receptor Antagonists

This category of antiemetics includes the butyrophenones (e.g., droperidol), phenothiazines (e.g., prochlorperazine), and substituted benzamides (e.g., metoclopramide; see later). Until the advent of 5-HT₃ receptor antagonists and other antiemetics in the 1990s, dopamine blocking agents were widely used. Use and efficacy of these agents are limited by their adverse effects, which include sedation and extrapyramidal symptoms. Extrapyramidal effects can be prevented by concomitant administration of an anticholinergic agent such as diphenhydramine.

Metopimazine, a phenothiazine derivative, is used as an adjunct to 5-HT₃ antagonists for CINV. Although it is not marketed in North America, it is used in children in Europe and a recent small study has demonstrated improved emetic control when combined with ondansetron, as compared with ondansetron monotherapy.[227a] Olanzapine, an atypical antipsychotic, has fewer extrapyramidal effects than older agents. In small studies in which it is combined with other antiemetics for CINV prophylaxis, it shows promise in preventing acute and delayed CINV. Chlorpromazine and droperidol may both cause prolongation of the QT interval, and droperidol has been associated with serious cardiac adverse events. Extreme caution, including electrocardiographic monitoring, should be taken if these agents are used, particularly in patients at risk for arrhythmias. Use of droperidol is now usually limited to the operative period in patients who do not respond to other agents.

5-Hydroxytryptamine-3 Receptor Antagonists

These agents have become the mainstay of therapy in the prevention and treatment of acute CINV since their introduction in the 1990s, when they were shown to be superior to most preexisting antiemetics such as prochlorperazine[228] and metoclopramide,[229-234] even when highly emetogenic chemotherapy such as cisplatin was administered.[230-232]

The superiority of these agents over others for preventing acute CINV in children has also been confirmed.[235-239] The efficacy of these agents appears to be further enhanced by the addition of a corticosteroid.[240-242] In one study of 33 children, ondansetron plus dexamethasone provided a complete response in 61% of patients, although ondansetron alone provided a complete response in only 21%.[241] Ondansetron has also been shown to reduce acute CINV, as compared with placebo, when chemotherapy is delivered intrathecally.[243]

First-generation agents in this class include ondansetron, dolasetron, and granisetron. Taken together, the data on these agents indicate that these agents are equally effective when given at equivalent doses.[244-251] They also appear to be equivalent in children, including cases involving high-dose therapy, such as preparative regimens for hematopoietic stem cell transplantation.[252-254] One small study has found that ondansetron controlled acute CINV caused by moderately emetogenic agents better than tropisetron. There was no difference between the two, however, in controlling acute CINV caused by highly emetogenic agents.

5-HT₃ antagonists are well tolerated by children,[242] with the most common side effects reported as mild headache and constipation.[243] For reasons of efficacy and tolerability, 5-HT₃ inhibitors in conjunction with a corticosteroid are now recommended as first-line therapy for children receiving moderately to highly emetogenic chemotherapy.[226,255]

Efficacy and tolerability of daily administration of high-dose oral ondansetron (24 or 32 mg daily) has been compared with a smaller dose (8 mg) given twice daily to adults. A large dose given daily is well-tolerated in adults.[256] In a large multicentered, randomized trial, the 24-mg daily dose provided the highest complete control of nausea and vomiting.[257] The superiority of more intensive dosing has been confirmed by others.[258-261] The efficacy of 24 over 32 mg has also been confirmed by Tsavaris and colleagues.[262]

Oral and intravenous routes of administration have been shown to be equally effective in adults and children.[263-266] Ondansetron, dolasetron, and granisetron are all available in intravenous formulations as well as an oral tablet. Ondansetron is available as an oral dissolving tablet and oral liquid, two preparations that are especially attractive in the pediatric population. Granisetron may be extemporaneously compounded by an apothecary. Successful administration of 16 mg of ondansetron daily as a suppository has been described in adults,[267] but not in children.

A second-generation 5-HT₃ receptor antagonist, palonosetron, differs from its predecessors in its stronger affinity for the 5-HT₃ receptor and its prolonged plasma half-life (four times that of the other 5-HT₃ antagonists), qualities that may enhance its duration of activity.[268,269] In randomized trials in adults, single doses of palonosetron appeared to be at least as good in the prevention of acute CINV as single doses of first-generation antagonists delivered 30 minutes before moderately emetogenic chemotherapy. Furthermore, the single dose of long-lasting palonosetron provided better protection from delayed CINV.[270-272] Palonosetron may prove to be a useful agent in pediatric patients for the prevention of acute CINV in multiple-day therapy when acute CINV is repeatedly induced and the prevention of delayed CINV, but at this time there are no data on its use in this population.

Corticosteroids

Corticosteroids have been frequently used as antiemetics, although their mechanism of action is unclear. Different corticosteroids are effective, but dexamethasone is the most widely used and is available in several different formulations. Disadvantages of corticosteroids include metabolic effects, gastritis, insomnia, hypertension, immune dysregulation, impaired wound healing, adverse psychiatric effects such as emotional lability, and, more rarely, psychosis. In general, short courses of corticosteroids do not usually produce significant side effects and are often well accepted and tolerated by patients.[273] Potentially beneficial side effects of corticosteroids are preservation of appetite and promotion of energy. The use of steroids may be prohibited when they are already part of a patient's chemotherapeutic regimen.

Dexamethasone is the best-studied corticosteroid and is currently the most commonly used although success with methylprednisolone has been described. The typical dexamethasone dose used for adults is 10 to 20 mg/day. Our starting dose for children is 10 mg/m², to a maximum of 10 mg/day. For persistent vomiting, this dose may be doubled to a maximum of 10 mg given twice daily.

Dexamethasone provides moderate protection from CINV, including delayed CINV, when used alone.[273-275] When first introduced, it provided an improvement over current agents such as prochlorperazine.[276] Dexamethasone has been shown to be as effective as metoclopramide for acute CINV in adults receiving moderately and highly emetogenic chemotherapy, and without the extrapyramidal effects of metoclopramide.[277,278]

Dexamethasone is especially useful in preventing delayed CINV from cisplatin, cyclophosphamide, and doxorubicin,[279-284] and may be even more effective for this purpose when combined with metoclopramide.[189] Dexamethasone is also very effective in potentiating the action of other antiemetics, including 5-HT₃ inhibitors[285] and metoclopramide.[281,283,284,286-289] In the pediatric population, dexamethasone combined with ondansetron was significantly more protective for acute CINV from highly emetogenic agents than ondansetron monotherapy, with 77% of children on ondansetron monotherapy having at least one episode of vomiting compared with 39% on ondansetron with dexamethasone.[241]

The benefit of improved protection from CINV must be weighed against the risks of corticosteroids. The potential short-term side effects of corticosteroids have been mentioned. Other potential risks include a decrease in action of a biologic response modifier and induction of radiation pneumonitis when steroid is withdrawn from patients who have received lung irradiation.[290,291] Caution is advised if using corticosteroids as antiemetics in conjunction with a treatment regimen associated with a high risk of infection or GI toxicity, such as induction regimens for acute myelogenous leukemia. Concomitant corticosteroids may further increase these risks. Concerns about the impact of steroids on the blood-brain barrier have led to a desire to avoid steroids as an antiemetic in patients with brain tumors, although chemotherapy-specific data are lacking.[292]

Metoclopramide

Metoclopramide, a procainamide derivative, exerts antiemetic effects via a central mechanism, dopamine receptor blockade in the CTZ, and a peripheral mechanism, promotion of gastric emptying.[293] It has been known to be an effective antiemetic in adults for the past 2 decades[294] as monotherapy or in conjunction with dexamethasone,[295] lorazepam,[296] or both.[297] Low-dose metoclopramide (i.e., 0.2 mg/kg) is effective in treating postoperative nausea and in promoting gastric emptying.

At high doses, metoclopramide also serves as a serotonin receptor antagonist[171,172] and provides better protection from CINV.[227] For these reasons, metoclopramide is usually given at high doses for CINV but at these higher doses, there is a greater risk for extrapyramidal side effects such as dystonia and akathisia, especially in children. In a dose-related toxicity study in children, significant extrapyramidal toxicity was observed at doses of 2 mg/kg or higher,[298] so high-dose metoclopramide is given with diphenhydramine to provide better protection from extrapyramidal side effects.[227] Extrapyramidal side effects can occur up to 24 hours later in patients who receive multiple daily doses of metoclopramide. Thus, diphenhydramine administration should continue until 24 hours after the last dose of metoclopramide. We have had personal experience using transdermal scopolamine as an anticholinergic in patients receiving once-daily dosing of metoclopramide.

Cannabinoids

Delta-9-tetrahydrocannabinol (THC) is the active ingredient in cannabis, or marijuana. THC was approved by the FDA in 1985 for the treatment of emesis. Synthetic THC, dronabinol (Marinol), has since become available. It is formulated in sesame oil and available as a 2.5- or 5-mg gelatin capsule. A homologue of THC, nabilone, has been recently approved by the FDA but was available in Canada and Europe for many years.

THC binds to the CB1 receptor found in the central and peripheral nervous systems, as well as the CB2 receptor, found in non-neural tissues. THC also interacts with dopaminergic, serotonin, monoaminergic, noradrenergic, and opioid systems, pathways that mediate both emesis and pain.

Sallan and associates have demonstrated that in patients who failed standard antiemetic therapy, THC provides better complete protection from CINV (36 of 79) than prochlorperazine (16/78).[298a] Interestingly, patients younger than 20 years had a higher proportion of complete responses than older patients. Those in the THC group also had significantly higher food intake.

An advantage of cannabinoids is their usefulness in treating pain. They are known to bind to kappa and delta receptors and act synergistically with opioids, a feature that may be useful when treating children with nausea and pain.[299] In addition, they are frequently used to stimulate appetite in patients who are not suffering from nausea or vomiting per se.

NK1 Receptor Antagonists

Aprepitant is the only approved agent in this category. Cisplatin-naïve patients receiving granisetron plus dexamethasone on day 1, and aprepitant (then called L-754,030) on day 1, aprepitant on days 1 to 5, or placebo on days 1 to 5 were compared. Of subjects in the aprepitant arms, 93% and 94%, respectively, had no acute vomiting compared with 67% in the placebo arm who had no vomiting. The aprepitant arms also had significantly better complete protection from delayed vomiting (82% and 78%) compared with placebo (33%). In addition, minimal or no nausea was noted in 49%, 48%, and 25%, respectively.[300]

Other studies have replicated these impressive findings in terms of control of delayed CINV, a historically difficult symptom to prevent, but they have not demonstrated improved protection from acute CINV seen in the aforementioned study.[301,302] For example, in a double-blind multicentered trial of 351 patients, aprepitant with dexamethasone provided no benefit in preventing acute emesis when compared with granisetron with dexamethasone. However, the addition of aprepitant to granisetron and dexamethasone more than doubled the efficacy of this regimen in preventing delayed vomiting.[301]

Aprepitant is generally well tolerated and easily administered by mouth daily for 3 consecutive days. In addition, it appears to decrease delayed cisplatin-induced CINV established to be refractory to the combination of 5-HT$_3$ antagonists and dexamethasone.[303] The efficacy of aprepitant appears to be sustained over multiple cycles of chemotherapy.[303,304] Use of aprepitant in adolescents has been reported, but studies are needed to determine the optimal dosing, safety, and efficacy in children.[305]

Aprepitant is a cytochrome P450 3A4 (CYP3A4) enzyme pathway substrate and therefore may interact with drugs that use or inhibit this pathway. For example, fentanyl and dexamethasone use the same pathway, and concomitant administration with aprepitant may increase the level of drugs such as dexamethasone, cyclophosphamide, thiotepa, or fentanyl.[306,307] Thus, it has been suggested that when coadministered together for CINV prophylaxis, the dexamethasone dose be decreased by 50%.[308] Aprepitant does not appear to alter the pharmacokinetics of ondansetron or granisetron.[309] Aprepitant should be used with caution in patients receiving warfarin.[310]

Other Agents

Lorazepam is often used as an adjuvant to true antiemetics because of its anxiolytic and amnestic properties. Early studies evaluating the addition of lorazepam have found that patients report less anxiety and prefer regimens that contain this additional agent, although it causes more sedation.[311-313] The acute antiemetic effect of several agents is enhanced when lorazepam is given concomitantly.[314-316] The addition of lorazepam to regimens that contain dexamethasone as prophylaxis against delayed CINV from cisplatin also appears to decrease delayed CINV.[280,314]

Scopolamine is a muscarinic antagonist known to reduce motion sickness. It is inadequate as monotherapy for CINV[317] but, in conjunction with other antiemetics such as metoclopramide and dexamethasone, it reduces cisplatin-induced CINV.[318] Scopolamine is administered as a 1.5-mg transdermal patch applied behind the ear, which releases 0.5 mg/day and must be changed every 3 days. Because the patch is only available in the 1.5-mg size and cannot be cut, we normally reserve it for children weighing 40 kg or more. Side effects from scopolamine include dry mouth, blurry vision, and mydriasis from systemic effects. Mydriasis on the side ipsilateral to the patch from unintentional touching of the patch, followed by rubbing the eyes, can also occur.[319]

Antihistamines such as dimenhydramine, hydroxyzine, and diphenhydramine are effective in reducing nausea associated with vertigo and motion sickness. For CINV management, diphenhydramine is often given in regimens containing high-dose metoclopramide to prevent extrapyramidal effects. Diphenhydramine does not, however, enhance the antiemetic effect of metoclopramide.[320,321]

Olanzapine is an atypical antipsychotic that binds to several receptors, including dopamine, serotonin and, to a lesser extent, histamine and muscarinic receptors. Because of its action at multiple receptor sites implicated in CINV, it may hold promise as therapy for CINV. In a small study of 10 adult patients receiving moderately to highly emetogenic chemotherapy with olanzapine, palonosetron, and dexamethasone as antiemetic prophylaxis, 100% had complete protection from nausea and vomiting in the first 24 hours after chemotherapy, with 50% and 75% of patients protected from nausea and vomiting, respectively, on days 2 to 5.[322] Olanzapine is consequently included in some guidelines for adults with CINV. No studies evaluating olanzapine for children with CINV have been published.

Gabapentin has also been evaluated for CINV in adults.[323] One study has shown a decrease in peak nausea scores for acute and delayed CINV, indicating that this agent may also hold promise as therapy for CINV.

Special Cases

Delayed Vomiting

Until rather recently, steroids and metoclopramide were the primary agents used to control delayed vomiting,[189,282,297] with modest protection from delayed CINV in 48% to 57% of adult patients. Some studies have demonstrated efficacy of 5-HT$_3$ antagonists in preventing delayed CINV[324,325] and providing

TABLE 31-4   Emetogenicity of Pediatric Chemotherapeutic Agents and Radiotherapy Fields

Modality	RISK OF EMESIS			
	High	**Moderate**	**Low**	**Minimal**
Chemotherapy	Carmustine (BCNU) Cisplatin Cyclophosphamide (>1500 mg/m^2) Dacarbazine (DTIC) Dactinomycin Ifosfamide ($\geq$500 mg/m^2) Lomustine (CCNU) Mechlorethamine (nitrogen mustard)	Carboplatin Cyclophosphamide (750-1500 mg/m^2) Cytarabine (>1000 mg/m^2) Cytarabine (intrathecal) Daunorubicin Doxorubicin Epirubicin Idarubicin Ifosfamide ($<$500 mg/m^2) Irinotecan Methotrexate (>1000 mg/m^2)	Cyclophosphamide ($\leq$750 mg/m^2) Cytarabine (<1000 mg/m^2) Etoposide (VP-16) Fluorouracil Gemcitabine Imatinib Methotrexate (50-1000 mg/m^2) Mitomycin Mitoxantrone Topotecan Vinblastine	2-Chloroxydeadenosine (cladribine) Asparaginase Bleomycin Busulfan Fludarabine Hydroxyurea Melphalan Mercaptopurine Methotrexate ($<$50 mg/m^2) Monoclonal antibodies (e.g., rituximab) Thioguanine Vincristine Vinorelbine
Radiotherapy	Total-body irradiation Upper abdomen (moderate to high risk)	Abdominal-pelvic Craniospinal Hemibody irradiation	Cranium Lower thorax Mantle	Other (e.g., extremity)

better protection when compared with existing drugs such as prochlorperazine.[326] However, most studies have demonstrated that the addition of a 5-HT$_3$ receptor antagonist to the standard, dexamethasone, does not confer greater protection from delayed CINV.[191,192,327-330] In a meta-analysis of the efficacy of 5-HT$_3$ antagonists, these antagonists did not confer protection from delayed CINV significantly beyond that provided by dexamethasone monotherapy. When ondansetron plus dexamethasone was compared with metoclopramide plus dexamethasone in randomized controlled trials, 5-HT$_3$ was equivocal at best.[331-333]

In one pediatric study evaluating ondansetron in acute and delayed CINV after treatment with carboplatin, cisplatin, or doxorubicin (Adriamycin) with cyclophosphamide or ifosfamide, ondansetron prevented acute CINV in 87% of children. Its efficacy in preventing delayed CINV was not nearly as high, preventing only 20% of children from experiencing nausea and 50% of children from vomiting after cisplatin or ifosfamide. Because of the significantly higher cost of 5-HT$_3$ receptor antagonists when compared with metoclopramide, it may be reasonable to start with dexamethasone and metoclopramide. In children who do not tolerate or who fail metoclopramide, a 5-HT$_3$ antagonist such as ondansetron may then be tried as an alternative.

In adults, some of the best protection from delayed CINV is conferred by the combination of a single dose of palonosetron, with three doses of aprepitant and concurrent dexamethasone. In one study, this regimen provided a complete response (no emesis and no rescue medication) for 88% of patients in the acute period and 78% during the delayed period.[334] Evidence for the efficacy of palonosetron in preventing delayed CINV is limited to regimens limited to single-day administration. There has been interest in consecutive daily dosing of palonosetron to cover multiday chemotherapy. Multiple dosing of palonosetron has recently been approved for adults.

A number of studies in adults have demonstrated the effectiveness of aprepitant for delayed CINV, as noted. Because most studies of aprepitant have been in the setting of single-day emetogenic treatment, it can be hard to deermine how to best use this drug in the setting of the multiday regimens common

in pediatrics. It is our practice to give aprepitant for up to 5 days, which may or may not continue beyond the end of the emetogenic treatment.

Anticipatory Nausea

Because anticipatory CINV is a learned response, typical antiemetics are generally ineffective. The best strategy for preventing CINV is the prevention of CINV in previous courses of chemotherapy.[193] Anxiety plays a key role in anticipatory nausea, so an anxiolytic such as lorazepam may be effective.

Breakthrough Emesis

Breakthrough emesis is defined as vomiting that occurs in spite of optimal preventive therapy. Although there are no studies or widely accepted standards for breakthrough emesis, a reasonable approach includes the following: (1) ensuring that the patient is receiving maximal doses of current antiemetics; and (2) adding a rescue agent from a category different from what the patient is already receiving. Although breakthrough agents may be started on an as-needed basis, scheduled administration may be needed during current or future cycles.

Radiation-Induced Nausea and Vomiting

Radiation-induced nausea and vomiting occur acutely in more than 90% of adult patients receiving total body irradiation for bone marrow transplantation and within 30 to 60 minutes in 80% of adults receiving single high-dose, large-field hemibody irradiation. Radiation-induced nausea and vomiting may also occur in 2 to 3 weeks in about 50% of adults receiving fractionated radiotherapy to the abdomen.[335] The incidence and severity of radiotherapy-induced nausea and vomiting are largely related to the location of the radiation field, as indicated in Table 31-4. In a prospective study of adults undergoing radiotherapy, the two radiotherapy-related risk factors for nausea and vomiting were the site of irradiation and field size, with significantly more vomiting in those who received radiation to the upper abdomen and in those with a radiation field size larger than 400 cm^2.[336] The only patient-related factor was previous experience with cancer chemotherapy. Because radiation to the upper or midhemibody results in an increase in circulating serotonin metabolites and because of the efficacy of 5-HT$_3$ receptor antagonists in this setting, it has been proposed that serotonin mediates radiation-induced emesis.[337]

In single-dose radiation to the upper abdomen, ondansetron has been demonstrated to be superior to metoclopramide in reducing vomiting and nausea.[338] In a randomized controlled trial comparing ondansetron with prochlorperazine in adults receiving fractionated radiotherapy to the abdomen, 43 (61%) of patients in the ondansetron arm and 23 (35%) of those in the prochlorperazine arm had a complete response—complete protection from emesis throughout the entire treatment course ($P = .002$). However, there was no difference in the incidence or severity of nausea in the two groups.[339] Although no controlled trials have been done in the pediatric population, studies have demonstrated its efficacy and tolerability during radiotherapy.[340] Dolasetron has also been used successfully to prevent nausea after a single high-dose fraction of radiotherapy to the upper abdomen.[341]

The addition of dexamethasone to ondansetron also appears to confer a slight benefit to ondansetron, even in multiply fractionated radiation to the upper abdomen.[342] Current adult guidelines recommend prophylaxis with a 5-HT$_3$ receptor antagonist for patients at high or moderate risk of radiation-induced vomiting (i.e., total body irradiation, upper abdomen), prophylaxis or rescue with a 5-HT$_3$ receptor antagonist in the low-risk group (lower thorax, pelvis, cranium), and rescue with a dopamine or 5-HT$_3$ antagonist in the minimal-risk group (head and neck, extremities, breast).[343] One study has evaluated ondansetron in children undergoing radiotherapy.[340] This study found that ondansetron provides 60% protection in children undergoing x-ray therapy for brain tumor, although no controls were used for comparison.

Postoperative Vomiting

Postoperative nausea and vomiting (PONV) is a common problem in all pediatric patients. Studies have demonstrated that dexamethasone is effective in preventing acute and late PONV.[344-346] Droperidol is also an effective agent but, given the high level of sedation, risk of extrapyramidal symptoms, and concerns about cardiotoxicity, this agent is no longer considered first-line prophylaxis.[347] There have also been a significant number of studies evaluating ondansetron in preventing PONV in children and it is considered the drug of choice for this situation.[347,348] In pooled analyses, however, the efficacy lies primarily in an antiemetic effect rather than an antinausea effect.[348]

A recent controlled study of adults undergoing surgery has also shown that scopolamine may be a promising agent in preventing PONV in adults, although it causes considerable dry mouth.[349] Two large adult studies have recently shown that one dose of aprepitant is superior to ondansetron in preventing postoperative vomiting, but only one study found a significant reduction in postoperative nausea.[350,351]

Vomiting from Other Causes

Opioid-Induced Nausea and Vomiting

Although frequently, and incorrectly, labeled as an allergy, opioids can cause nausea and vomiting. Such effects are mediated through direct effects of opioids on the CTZ, effects on the vestibular apparatus, and signals from the gut as a result of constipation. Except when caused by constipation, opioid-related nausea and vomiting tend to improve with repeated dosing of the opioid. Therefore, a reasonable strategy is to provide an antiemetic with the first few doses of opioid, particularly if the patient is at risk for nausea and vomiting. This prevents the problem of the patient being labeled as allergic to the opioid.

Although there is no evidence to indicate that one opioid is more emetogenic than another, it is commonly believed that morphine and codeine are the most likely to cause nausea and vomiting. If nausea and vomiting in response to an opioid persist despite antiemetics, it may be reasonable to consider changing the opioid or route of administration. Because tolerance to the emetogenic effect of the initial opioid usually develops in a few days, it is often difficult to know whether it was tolerance or the change in opioid that improved symptoms.

Evidence comparing antiemetics for opioid-induced nausea and vomiting is limited. One study compared 24 mg of daily ondansetron with either metoclopramide 10 mg orally three times daily or placebo. There were no differences detected in the three arms, although the study was terminated prematurely because of accrual difficulties.[352] In another study of adults with postsurgical pain, single doses of 8 or 16 mg ondansetron provided better emetic control than a single 10-mg dose of metoclopramide. One report also indicates that ondansetron may be effective for nausea and vomiting caused by spinal morphine.[353] Recent studies have also demonstrated that the addition of a low-dose naloxone infusion may reduce opioid-related side effects, including nausea, without effecting analgesia in adults and children.[354,355]

Disease-Related Vomiting

In addition to direct treatment-related nausea and vomiting, disease processes themselves may cause nausea and vomiting through various mechanisms, including increased intracranial pressure, gastrointestinal obstruction, altered gut motility, organ capsule distention, and GVHD. For example, altered gut motility appears to contribute to nausea and vomiting in patients recovering from bone marrow transplantation.[356-358] Reports of mirtazapine, a new serotonin-norepinephrine reuptake inhibitor (SNRI), to improve nausea and vomiting in patients with gastroparesis from various causes, have recently been published, but mirtazapine has not been studied for this purpose in bone marrow transplantation patients or children.[359-362]

In addition, other processes that might be related to the disease process or its treatment, such as GI infection, may be present. The mnemonic VOMIT may be used to review the possible underlying causes of nausea and vomiting so that a targeted approach to the situation may be used.[363] VOMIT indicates that nausea and vomiting may be caused by *v*estibular problems, *o*bstruction of the bowel (including constipation), gut dys*m*otility, *i*nfection and inflammation, and *t*oxins. Remarkably little is known about the effectiveness of antiemetics for these causes, and treatment of the underlying problem may be the best strategy. Ondansetron has a modest effect for controlling vomiting from acute gastroenteritis.[364]

Nonpharmacologic Interventions

Acupuncture and behavioral therapies are some of the best-studied nonpharmacologic interventions for CINV. Electroacupuncture has been found to reduce vomiting but not nausea in women undergoing myeloablative chemotherapy when compared with controls.[365] In children, P6 acupoint injections are as effective as droperidol in preventing postoperative nausea and vomiting.[366]

Acupressure and acustimulation have also been studied as interventions to mitigate CINV. In one relatively large study of

739 patients who were randomized to acupressure bands, an acustimulation band, or no band, those who received acupressure had less nausea on the day of treatment but there were no differences in delayed nausea.[367] In pooled analyses of trials evaluating acupuncture point stimulation, these interventions reduced the proportion of acute vomiting but not the severity of nausea. When broken down by modality, stimulation with needles and electroacupuncture reduced vomiting but not nausea. Acupressure reduced nausea but not vomiting, but these studies were uncontrolled.[368]

In children receiving chemotherapy, behavioral interventions such as hypnosis and cognitive distraction reduced nausea, vomiting, and the extent to which these symptoms bothered the children. These effects were maintained even after the interventions were discontinued and chemotherapy continued.[219] Behavioral interventions such as hypnosis and systemic desensitization also appear to be useful in treating anticipatory nausea, a phenomenon with a strong learned component.[369,370] Progressive muscle relaxation has been shown to reduce the duration of CINV in women with breast cancer but not the intensity or frequency of nausea or vomiting episodes.[371]

Role of the Patient and Family

Because patients who expect to experience CINV are significantly more likely to actually do so, discussing the role of interventions to prevent or mitigate CINV may enhance the efficacy of these interventions. Patients and families should also be encouraged to notify their medical team about uncontrolled symptoms when they occur, particularly because uncontrolled acute nausea is associated with an increased incidence of delayed nausea and anticipatory nausea with future chemotherapy. The phenomenon of delayed nausea should specifically be addressed, because children and their parents are usually at home and cannot be observed when the child may experience these symptoms.

Strategies to enhance a patient's sense of control over their treatment may also improve the experience. In one small study of adults with CINV controlled with IV antiemetics via pump, those who could control the pump themselves used less antiemetic.[372] More recent studies in adults and children have indicated that a continuous infusion, patient-controlled pump is well tolerated, safe, and effective in controlling CINV.[373,374] Patients should be encouraged to explore options for nonpharmacologic management, because they appear to have few adverse side effects and can also add to the patient's sense of control over the experience.

Future Directions

Significant advances have been made in the past few decades in managing nausea and vomiting, particularly CINV, but more remains to be done to improve the management of these symptoms in children. More information is needed regarding the assessment of nausea, as opposed just to measuring the number of vomiting episodes, and in predicting a child's risk for developing these symptoms. Pharmacogenomics may play a role in finding candidate genes that may predict emetic sensitivity and responsiveness to antiemetic therapy and help clinicians identify patients unlikely to respond to conventional therapies. Optimal regimens for multiple-day and high-dose chemotherapy or bone marrow transplantation, as well as new strategies for control of delayed and refractory symptoms, are needed as well. Exploratory studies using new drugs, such as the atypical antipsychotic medications or small molecules, may be useful.

For children in particular, more evidence of efficacy and side effects are needed, as are evidence-based guidelines for CINV management to address wide variations in practice that may exist. Finally, knowledge of nausea and vomiting in children has historically been based on CINV or postoperative situations. Much remains to be learned regarding nonchemotherapy-related nausea and vomiting.

OTHER GASTROINTESTINAL SYMPTOMS

Constipation

Constipation is the passage of hard feces that typically occurs with difficulty and decreased frequency. Most children who develop constipation have no history of bowel dysfunction prior to their cancer diagnosis. Children with cancer are predisposed to developing constipation when compared with healthy children because of their decreased fluid intake, variable diet, and decreased mobility, in addition to specific cancer and treatment-related causes. Constipation may be caused by direct effects of the cancer, such as tumor obstructing the intestinal lumen, infiltrating enteric nerves and muscles, or causing spinal cord compression or cauda equina syndrome. Cancer-directed therapy, particularly neurotoxic agents such as vinca alkaloids, may also cause constipation. In addition, the use of opioids may be one of the most important causes of constipation in this population.

Constipation may lead to painful bowel movements, which some children respond to by withholding stool, further exacerbating the problem. Constipation may lead to significant distress, discomfort (pain, nausea, bloating) and embarrassment for some children. Medical complications may include gastrointestinal obstruction, urinary obstruction, or infection.

Constipation is usually caused by altered gastrointestinal motility and/or altered fluid handling. Intestinal motility is controlled by neuronal, endocrine, and luminal factors. Acetylcholine is the chief neurotransmitter mediating peristalsis. Serotonin also plays an important role in mediating the gut's response to luminal contents. Opioids lead to constipation by reducing intestinal motility and secretions and increasing fluid absorption and blood flow,[375] as well as by decreasing sensitivity to luminal contents. The effects of opioids on the gut do not appear to be strongly dose-related.

Evaluation of the patient with constipation includes a thorough history and physical examination. If not contraindicated by a condition such as neutropenia or mucositis, a rectal examination may facilitate the distinction of lower (rectosigmoid) constipation from colonic inertia, or high obstruction, and may also allow assessment of anal sphincter tone and examination for fissures or hemorrhoids. When the diagnosis of constipation is unclear, a plain film of the abdomen (KUB) may facilitate the diagnosis.

In addition to medical interventions, the treatment of constipation includes strategies such as provision of a comfortable, easily accessible toilet or commode and addressing issues such as lack of privacy and the need for caregivers to help the patient with toileting. Although physical activity is associated with colonic peristalsis, increasing exercise does not necessarily reduce constipation.[376] In addition, the child's medications should be reviewed, and constipating medications such as opioids, tricyclic antidepressants, antihistamines, and 5-HT$_3$ receptor antagonists such as ondansetron and neuroleptics altered, if possible. For example, transdermal fentanyl may be less constipating than oral morphine.[377] Patients on methadone have less of a laxative requirement than those on morphine or hydromorphone, perhaps because methadone

indicator of more rapid mortality in adults with advanced cancer.[396]

Pathophysiology

The respiratory center that processes input from the respiratory system and coordinates respiratory activity is located in the medulla and pons. Afferent input arises from peripheral mechanoreceptors in respiratory muscles, chest wall, lungs, and upper airway, as well as central and peripheral chemoreceptors and pulmonary vagal afferents (Fig. 31-4). Chemoreceptors detect low pO_2 and high pCO_2 in the blood and send this input to the respiratory center. Pulmonary vagal afferents are activated by inputs from stretch receptors and irritant receptors, and they also trigger activity in tracts that project to the cerebral cortex. Based on this sensory input, the respiratory center coordinates the respiratory apparatus, consisting of the diaphragm, intercostal muscles, and accessory muscles. The cerebral cortex integrates sensory input, motor output, and cognitive and emotional input to create the sensation of breathing.[397]

The phenomenon of dyspnea occurs when the afferent sensory input to the brain—for example, input from mechanoreceptors in the chest wall—fails to match the outgoing motor signal emanating from the brain.[398] Situations in which such mismatch may occur include the following: (1) increased work of breathing, such as when breathing against increased resistance or with weakened muscles; (2) chemical changes, such as hypercapnia and hypoxemia; and (3) neuromechanical dissociation, such as when sensory input from a given inspiratory effort does not match the input anticipated by the brain.[397] The interpretation of this mismatch by the cerebral cortex, or perceived dyspnea, is affected by the individual's expectations, experiences, and beliefs, making the sensation of dyspnea highly subjective and individualized.

Diagnosis and Assessment

Neither clinical signs such as respiratory rate or oxygen saturation nor laboratory data such as arterial blood gases and hemoglobin concentration are reliable predictors of dyspnea. Because objective data correlate poorly with dyspnea, the gold standard for measuring and assessing dyspnea is the patient's self-report. The visual analogue scale[399] and Borg scale[400] are among the most widely used in adults. The Borg scale is a 10-point scale, with descriptive anchors at the ends. A numerical rating scale has also been evaluated in adult oncology patients, with score of 0 or 1 out of 10 having a 98% sensitivity and a 54% specificity. A score higher than 1 is predictive of dyspnea that may impair daily function and is recommended as a threshold score that needs further evaluation.[401] The Dalhousie dyspnea scale was developed to meet the need for a pediatric dyspnea assessment instrument.[402] This visual instrument actually contains three scales depicting three subconstructs of dyspnea, including throat closing, chest tightness, and effort. This instrument has been tested in children with asthma or cystic fibrosis and in healthy children. Children 8 years of age or older used the instrument reliably. Our review of the literature did not find any instruments that have been specifically developed for the measurement of dyspnea in the younger pediatric population.

Further assessment of dyspnea necessitates a history that should include triggers or exacerbating factors, alleviating factors, severity, and description of degree of functional impairment. Indications of complications such as infection, GVHD, and cardiac compromise should be sought, as should potential treatment-related causes such as chemotherapy and radiotherapy. Potential causes of dyspnea unrelated to malignancy such as asthma should also be considered. Finally, contributing psychosocial factors such as anxiety should be explored because

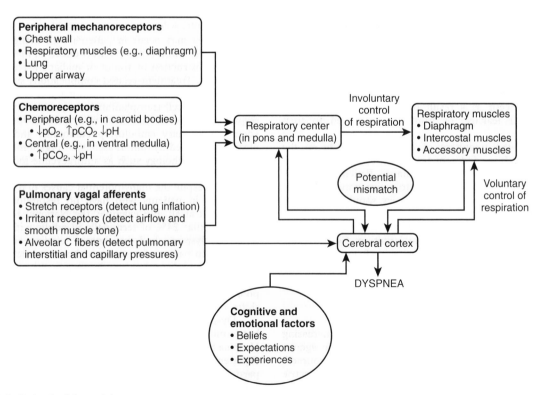

FIGURE 31-4. Pathophysiology of dyspnea.

emotional and cognitive factors may influence how someone interprets dyspnea as a symptom.

Evaluation beyond a thorough physical examination depends on the suspected cause of the dyspnea. Studies that may provide useful information include a complete blood count (CBC), noninvasive measures including pulse oximetry and capnometry, selective assessment of venous or arterial blood gases, and chest x-ray. Additional tests that may also be considered include pulmonary function testing, axial chest CT, echocardiography, electrocardiography, and spiral CT or ventilation-perfusion scan to assess for pulmonary embolus.

Treatment

Targeted approaches to treat dyspnea depend on the underlying cause and may include medical therapies such as chemotherapy, antibiotics, and diuretics. Procedural interventions may include pleurocentesis and stenting of the airways to relieve obstruction or surgical removal of obstruction. Consideration of such interventions should weigh the likely benefits and burdens for the child in view of the medical condition.

Symptomatic Treatment

Rapid and effective strategies for symptomatic management of dyspnea are available and applicable to patients who are candidates for targeted approaches and for those in whom such interventions are not appropriate. The mainstays of symptomatic management include opioids and oxygen. Other agents such as anxiolytics, steroids, and bronchodilators may also be of benefit, particularly if an inflammatory or bronchospastic component is suspected.

Opioids

Several studies in adult cancer patients have supported the use of opioids as an effective intervention for dyspnea.[403-406] Bruera and colleagues[403] and Mazzocato and associates[405] have conducted randomized placebo-controlled crossover studies demonstrating that opioids relieve dyspnea and do not cause clinically important respiratory depression. No studies demonstrating the efficacy of opioids for dyspnea in children have been published although, based on clinical experience, they appear as effective and safe in children.

The mechanism(s) whereby opioids relieve dyspnea has not yet been clearly elucidated. Opioid receptors present in the peripheral and central nervous system may play a role in relieving dyspnea. Opioids may alleviate dyspnea by blunting the effect of hypercapnia or hypoxia on ventilation, relieving anxiety, or modifying the sensation of dyspnea, related to their ability to modify the sensation of pain.

The dose required to relieve dyspnea is often relatively small, even when a patient is not opioid-naïve. For example, Allard and coworkers have shown that a 25% increase in the baseline dose controlled breakthrough dyspnea for up to 4 hours.[406] Our standard practice for opioid-naïve patients is to start by giving 0.025 mg/kg of morphine IV (25% of 0.1 mg/kg, the typical starting dose for pain) and titrating as indicated. In addition to short-acting preparations, long-acting preparations such as sustained-relief morphine are effective treatments for dyspnea.[407]

Because opioid receptors are present in the lower respiratory tract, it has been postulated that nebulized opioids might alleviate dyspnea. Case reports of inhaled morphine and fentanyl in adolescents with cystic fibrosis[408,409] and a small uncontrolled study in cancer patients using inhaled morphine fentanyl for reducing dyspnea have shown promise in this regard.[410] A crossover study conducted by Bruera and colleagues[411] comparing subcutaneous and nebulized morphine has suggested that both routes of administration may reduce dyspnea. However, perhaps because of small sample size or a placebo effect, a difference between the two routes could not be excluded. In addition, several other studies have not demonstrated the efficacy of nebulized opioids. Until larger studies using standardized doses of opioid and consistent delivery methods are carried out, there is insufficient evidence to support this method of delivery for dyspnea.[412]

Oxygen

When hypoxemia is suspected to be the cause of dyspnea, administration of oxygen to reverse hypoxemia may relieve this symptom. However, most patients with dyspnea are likely not to be hypoxemic or not to have dyspnea from hypoxemia alone. For example, in a study of adults with advanced cancer and dyspnea, 60% were not hypoxic.[413]

Studies evaluating oxygen compared with air for relief of dyspnea in hypoxemic and nonhypoxemic adults have shown no clear superiority of oxygen over air.[414-417] An explanation for the ability to compare flowing oxygen and air in relieving dyspnea is based on their capacity to stimulate mechanoreceptors in the trigeminal nerve. Receptors in the distribution of the trigeminal nerve appear to influence induced dyspnea in normal subjects.[418] In addition, administration of cold air appears to improve dyspnea in patients with chronic obstructive pulmonary disease (COPD).[419] Therefore, provision of flowing air or oxygen might reduce dyspnea through this mechanism. Trigeminal nerve stimulation may explain why being exposed to cool moving air provided by a fan or open window also seems to reduce dyspnea.

Anxiolytics

Although anxiety may worsen perceived dyspnea, and dyspnea may induce anxiety, evidence to date does not support the routine use of anxiolytics for dyspnea, particularly not as a first-line agent. Dyspnea is a common symptom in panic attacks or anxiety disorder. However, anxiety may contribute less to coexisting dyspnea than has been traditionally thought. Dudgeon and Lertzman's work[413] has revealed that in adults with advanced cancer, anxiety explains only 10% of the variance in dyspnea. Use of an anxiolytic to alleviate anxiety may be appropriate when anxious symptoms are particularly prominent and thought to influence a patient's interpretation of the sensation of dyspnea significantly. Anxiolytics may also be indicated for sedation to manage escalating dyspnea at the end of life (see Chapter 30).

Nonpharmacologic Interventions

To the extent that the cerebral cortex mediates the sensation of dyspnea, interventions that modify cognitive and emotional factors, such as breathing and relaxation training that influence the interpretation of dyspnea, may be helpful. In healthy adults undergoing induced dyspnea, the distraction of subjects did not change dyspnea severity ratings but decreased the perceived unpleasantness of the dyspnea.[420] Increased support, such as that provided in the nurse-run dyspnea clinic studied by Bredin[420a] and the one described by Booth and associates,[421] may reduce dyspnea by providing education, cognitive-behavioral training, and psychosocial support.

Escalating Dyspnea

The symptom of dyspnea may escalate at the end of life. Respiratory changes and the development of secretions are discussed in Chapter 30. Escalating dyspnea, such as that which may occur at the end of life, is an indication for consideration of palliative sedation (see Chapter 30).

Future Directions

Much remains to be learned regarding the physiology and mechanisms of dyspnea. Once these are better understood, targeted interventions to ameliorate this challenging symptom with relatively few treatment options may be developed. Within the pediatric realm, better understanding of how children sense and interpret this highly subjective symptom is needed. This in turn may enable the development of methods to measure and assess dyspnea, allowing for the care team to develop a better understanding of how it affects children and to evaluate dyspnea-directed interventions.

COUGH

Cough may be a distressing symptom and may lead to dyspnea, vomiting, sleep disruption, and chest or throat pain. Topical antitussives act on receptors in the respiratory tree to reduce cough. Nebulized lidocaine has been described for intractable cough at the end of life.[422] Symptomatic treatment for significant cough usually entails the administration of an opioid to suppress the cough reflex in the medulla. Dextromethorphan and codeine are most commonly used, although all opioids have antitussive activity.

FATIGUE

Cancer-related fatigue has been defined by the NCCN as a "distressing persistent, subjective sense of tiredness or exhaustion related to cancer or cancer treatment that is not proportional to recent activity and interferes with usual functioning."[423] Fatigue is a complex symptom that may have physical, cognitive, and emotional components. In addition, fatigue is subjective and highly individualized so that patients may experience and interpret fatigue differently. They may have varied descriptions of fatigue (Box 31-3). Adults with cancer-related fatigue almost universally report that it is unresponsive to rest and not proportional to activity, and pervades many areas of their lives. Clearly, this type of fatigue is not the fatigue of everyday life. Studies in adult cancer survivors have revealed that fatigue may be long-lived, lasting for months to years after cancer-directed treatment has been completed.[424,425] In pediatric cancer survivors, fatigue is the only factor associated with poor physical and psychosocial health-related quality of life.[426]

Impact

It is well established that fatigue is the most common symptom in patients with cancer.[427,428] One survey of published studies on cancer-related fatigue in adults has found that fatigue is present in 50% to 75% of patients at diagnosis, with the prevalence increasing to 80% to 96% in patients undergoing chemotherapy and to 60% to 93% in patients receiving radiotherapy.[429] In children, fatigue is less well studied but has been shown to be the most common symptom.[3] For example, Wolfe and coworkers have found that fatigue is the most common symptom in children with advanced cancer, with 96% of children expe-

| Box 31-3 | **Manifestations of Fatigue** |

PHYSICAL

Weakness
Physical tiring
Heaviness

COGNITIVE

Mental clouding
Poor concentration
Impaired memory

EMOTIONAL

Depression
Apathy
Irritability
Decreased motivation

ENERGY

Tiredness
Lethargy
Low energy
Decreased endurance

SLEEP

Insomnia
Hypersomnia
Somnolence
Nonrestorative sleep

From Ullrich C, Mayer O. Assessment and management of fatigue and dyspnea in pediatric palliative care. Pediatr Clin North Am. 2007;54:735-756.

riencing fatigue.[3] Collins and colleagues[1] have also found that in a cross-sectional study of children aged 10 to 18 years, with current or previous cancer, lack of energy is the most common symptom, affecting 49.7%.

According to adult patients with cancer, fatigue is the most distressing of all the symptoms that they experience, creating profound physical, psychological, and financial burdens that can impair quality of life and diminish hope.[430] It not only leads to a decrement in physical ability, but also to a sense of loss of control, loneliness, and isolation. In the Fatigue II study of 379 adults undergoing treatment for cancer, 60% ranked fatigue as the symptom most affecting their lives.[430] According to the parents in Wolfe and associates' study,[3] fatigue caused "a great deal" or "a lot" of suffering in 57% of children approaching the end of life. In another study, Jalmsell and coworkers[4] have reported that of 449 parents of children who had died from cancer, 86% reported that fatigue significantly affected their child's well-being. Adolescents with cancer also have reported that fatigue significantly affects their physical, social, and psychological well-being.[431]

In addition to causing suffering, concerns regarding fatigue as a side effect of disease-directed or symptom-directed treatment may limit therapy. Fatigue is documented to be the most common side effect of chemotherapy and radiotherapy in adults.[429,432] In adults, treatment-related fatigue can be severe enough to prevent maximal treatment and disease control[423,433]; however, in children, fatigue is rarely cited as a reason to reduce

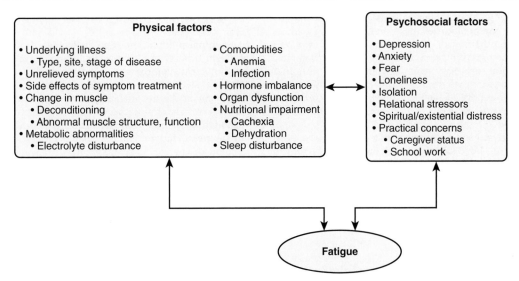

FIGURE 31-5. Conceptual model of fatigue.

therapy. In terms of symptom-related treatment, pain may be inadequately relieved when concerns regarding opioid-related fatigue or sedation inhibit optimal opioid administration.[434,435] When fatigue is not controlled, patients are forced to choose between adequate analgesia with somnolence and mental clouding, and less sedation at the price of increased pain.

Approach

Despite its prevalence and impact, fatigue frequently is not addressed by clinicians and patients. In a large multicenter study of 1,317 adults with cancer, 52% of those with fatigue reported it to their physician.[436] One significant barrier to addressing fatigue is the perception on the part of the care team that fatigue, although undesirable, does not adversely affect patients significantly. The Fatigue I study has found that although oncologists think that pain adversely affects their patients to a greater degree than fatigue (61% vs. 37%), cancer patients thought that fatigue adversely affects their daily lives more than pain (61% vs. 19%).[428] This may be caused in part by clinicians' personal understanding of daily fatigue, which leads them to believe that they understand the reality of cancer-related fatigue. Other barriers to addressing fatigue may include the following: (1) a belief that fatigue is normal or to be expected in a cancer patient; (2) paucity of descriptors available for patients to convey the various manifestations of fatigue adequately; (3) lack of familiarity on the part of the clinician with options to ameliorate fatigue; (4) disease-directed focus to the exclusion of attention to symptoms; and (5) system-related problems, such as time pressures or reimbursement difficulties.

Measurement and Assessment

The NCCN provides guidelines for fatigue management in adults and children that calls for screening for fatigue at every visit using a 1 to 10 scale.[423] Although use of such a scale has not been validated in children, numerical scales may generally be used reliably in children aged 7 years and older.

Once screening identifies fatigue, it should be further assessed, although there are no universally accepted means for assessing fatigue in adults and children. Several unidimensional and multidimensional scales for assessment in adults are available and two instruments are available for children. One, developed by Hockenberry-Eaton and colleagues,[437] is for children with cancer. Although it is part of a series of instruments that evaluate fatigue in pediatric oncology patients from the child's, parent's, and staff's perspective, it was derived from interviews with only 13 children and needs to be prospectively evaluated. The other instrument, the PedsQL Multidimensional Fatigue Scale, measures the child's and parent's perceptions of fatigue in pediatric patients. This instrument has been studied in healthy children and children with cancer.[438]

Even when a formal assessment instrument is not used to assess fatigue, clinicians should explore various possible manifestations of fatigue that may be identified by the child or adolescent and adult caregiver (see Box 31-3). Exacerbating and alleviating factors, pattern of fatigue, and degree to which the symptom is affecting the child's life can then be explored. In assessing fatigue, it may be helpful to bear in mind that children tend to conceptualize fatigue as a physical sensation, although adolescents alternate or merge the physical concept with mental tiredness.[439] Conversely, parents and staff conceptualize fatigue as a symptom that interferes with the child's ability to participate in various activities and may be manifested by physical, emotional, and mental changes. Investing the time to assess a report of fatigue fully may frequently yield important clues regarding the cause of the fatigue; this is valuable because there are few diagnostic tests available to determine the cause of fatigue.

Associated Factors

Fatigue may stem from concomitant interrelated causes including physical and psychological factors (Fig. 31-5). Studies aiming to uncover the cause of fatigue have been carried out only in adults and consist of retrospective and prospective analyses of factors associated with fatigue. There are no published studies evaluating objective factors associated with fatigue in children with cancer.

For simplicity, factors considered to be associated with fatigue may be categorized into physical and psychosocial factors, recognizing that many patients experience fatigue resulting from a combination of these. For example, in adults undergoing chemotherapy or radiotherapy, fatigue correlates with physical factors (symptom distress) and psychological factors (depression, anxiety, anger or confusion).[440] Another study of adult cancer patients has similarly determined that physical factors (severity of pain, dyspnea) and psychological symptoms (anxiety, depression) are associated with the experience of fatigue.[427]

In adults, certain sociodemographic factors are also associated with fatigue. For example, the demographic factors of being employed or living alone were significantly associated with the symptom of fatigue.[441] Although children are unlikely to experience fatigue related to these exact sociodemographic considerations, the stress induced by situational concerns can affect children and the fatigue that they experience.

Physical Factors

Physical factors contributing to fatigue include direct effects of the underlying disease and side effects of treatment of the underlying illness. Unrelieved symptoms are also likely to contribute to a patient's fatigue. In adults, overall symptom distress is associated with the report of fatigue.[442] Conversely, treatment for symptoms such as pain or dyspnea may also contribute to fatigue. Because various medications, including benzodiazepines, opioids, and antihistamines, may cause fatigue, thoroughly reviewing the patient's medications may reveal agents that can cause fatigue. Finally, various comorbidities, such as organ dysfunction (e.g., renal, hepatic, cardiac, pulmonary, endocrine), electrolyte imbalance, poor nutritional status, and infection may contribute to fatigue.

Anemia is a well-established cause of fatigue in various patient populations. In adults with cancer, it has been demonstrated to be associated with fatigue and impaired quality of life. In some adults with advanced cancer, anemia is not significantly related to fatigue.[443,444] Thus, anemia may not fully account for the fatigue experienced by some patients, suggesting that at least in some patients factors other than anemia are contributing to fatigue.

Like anemia, hypothyroidism is associated with fatigue in patients with and without cancer. Other endocrine abnormalities associated with the experience of fatigue include hypothalamus-pituitary axis alterations[445] and hypogonadism, which is also associated with negative mood and cachexia.[446-448]

Deconditioning from decreased activity may lead to fatigue, which in turn lessens activity and may further exacerbate fatigue. Various muscle abnormalities have been described in patients with cancer and may be associated with fatigue.[449] Finally, muscle wasting (cachexia) is associated with fatigue. This may be caused by the cytokines proposed to mediate cachexia such as tumor necrosis factor, which are also thought to contribute to the sensation of fatigue.[445]

Psychosocial Factors

Psychosocial factors such as depression and anxiety, existential or spiritual suffering, and stress from practical concerns may all be related to fatigue. When psychological factors such as fatigue and depression coexist, depressed mood may be a contributor or a consequence of fatigue. For example, fatigue, when characterized by withdrawal and decreased participation in activities in an adolescent, may be a manifestation of depression. On the other hand, the experience of fatigue may lead to isolation, decreased engagement in activities, and impaired quality of life, all of which may contribute to depression.

Sleep Impairment

Sleep impairment, manifested as decreased quantity or quality of sleep, has various causes, including unrelieved physical or psychological symptoms or environmental factors, such as distortion of sleep architecture by medications or sleep disruptions that occur in the hospital. Impaired sleep may in turn worsen physical or psychological distress experienced by patients. Although a decrement in the quantity or quality of sleep may contribute to fatigue, cancer-related fatigue may occur independent of changes in sleep.[450]

Interventions

An algorithm for approaching the symptom of fatigue is presented in Figure 31-6. Although fatigue is frequently multifactorial, targeting underlying factors suspected to contribute to fatigue can improve this symptom. Even when no particular contributing factor is identified, nonspecific interventions may ameliorate fatigue. For example, exercise and stimulants are effective interventions that reduce fatigue. Educating the patient and family about fatigue is important in helping them understand fatigue and its impact, as well as the available options for addressing it. Strategies to optimize function and facilitate adaptation to fatigue such as realistic goal setting, modifying activities, and conserving energy should also be reviewed.

Exercise

Curtailing activity is a natural reaction to fatigue, and oncologists report recommending activity in response to the complaint of fatigue.[428] Several randomized controlled trials in adults have demonstrated that exercise actually reduces fatigue, and in some cases also ameliorates psychological symptoms such as depression and anxiety. For example, a 6-week walking program for women undergoing radiotherapy for breast cancer improved fatigue as well as anxiety, depression, and sleep disturbance.[451] Finally, exercise can also provide physical benefits, including improved strength and function.

Psychosocial Interventions

Strategies to address psychological factors include pharmacologic and nonpharmacologic approaches. Psychological interventions such as psychotherapy and support group participation may reduce fatigue,[452] as can increased support from clinicians, such as intensive nursing support.[453] If depression or anxiety is suspected to contribute to fatigue, a trial of a pharmacologic agent such as an antidepressant or anxiolytic may be of benefit, recognizing that some drugs in each of these classes may exacerbate sedation and fatigue If other stressors are uncovered, such as spiritual suffering or concerns about practical matters, professionals such as a chaplain, resource specialist, or staff at school should be approached for assistance.

Sleep

If sleep disturbance is suspected, reducing factors that impair sleep and strategizing with patients to improve sleep hygiene are a necessary first step. If indicated by persistent or severe sleep impairment, pharmacologic interventions such as benzodiazepines, benzodiazepine receptor agonists, and antidepressant with sedating qualities (e.g., TCAs, trazodone, mirtazapine) may be tried. It is important to keep in mind, however, that benzodiazepines and antihistamines in particular may have paradoxical effects in children and that the benzodiazepine receptor agonists have not yet been well studied in young children.

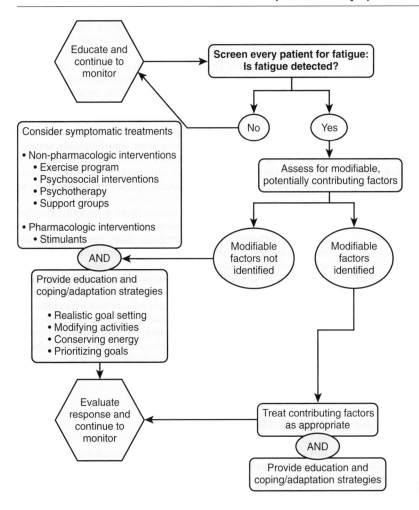

FIGURE 31-6. Algorithm for managing fatigue.

Pharmacologic Interventions

Correction of Anemia

Correcting anemia associated with cancer or chemotherapy with erythropoietin is a strategy often used in adult oncology. Some studies have supported this practice in adults, demonstrating that improving anemia may also improve fatigue and quality of life.[454] However, correction of anemia with erythropoietin has not been as widely pursued in pediatric oncology practice, in part because there is no evidence that treatment of anemia with erythropoietin improves quality of life. The one study published in children examining this question has failed to show that health-related quality of life improves with correction of anemia.[455] The authors provided several possible explanations for this finding, but the lack of association between correction of anemia and quality of life and fatigue suggests that focusing on anemia at the exclusion of other suspected causes of fatigue and decreased quality of life may lead to inadequate treatment of fatigue. If erythropoietin is used, concerns that it is associated with more rapid tumor progression, thrombosis, and increased mortality in adults[456-458] should be kept in mind. If anemia is suspected as a cause of fatigue, transfusion support is an alternative to erythropoietin therapy.

Stimulants

The stimulant with the best-established efficacy in ameliorating fatigue in adults is methylphenidate. This agent reduces fatigue in adults with cancer and HIV, regardless of the underlying cause.[459,460] In a study of adults with cancer-related fatigue, patients had significantly less fatigue after starting methylphenidate.[461] Methylphenidate is also advantageous in that it improves cognition and exerts direct analgesic and antidepressant actions.[459,461] One study has reported success in improving cognition in children who survived cancer.[462] A case series documenting successful treatment of opioid-related sedation in children with cancer with methylphenidate has been published,[463] but currently there are no published randomized controlled trials of its efficacy for fatigue in children with cancer.

Methylphenidate has a history of extensive use in children with attention-deficit/hyperactivity disorder (ADHD)[464] and has a well-established record in terms of being safe and well tolerated by children. The most prevalent side effect of methylphenidate is decreased appetite, which we approach by giving the first dose after breakfast. Despite concerns that methylphenidate should be used with caution in children at risk for seizure, open-label and controlled trials in adults and children with ADHD and epilepsy have not supported this (reviewed by Baptista-Neto and colleagues[465]). For example, a study in children with epilepsy has found no increase in seizure frequency and observed beneficial electroencephalographic changes with methylphenidate.[466] Modafinil may be considered as an alternative to methylphenidate, although there is significantly less pediatric experience with this agent. Modafinil has been used with success to treat adults with fatigue associated with multiple sclerosis or sedation caused by opioids,[467,468] but no studies

Options for medical interventions for depression include tricyclic antidepressants (TCAs), selective serotonin reuptake inhibitors (SSRIs), and newer selective serotonin-norepinephrine reuptake inhibitors. TCAs are rarely used for depression because of their anticholinergic side effects and the lack of efficacy data in children. SSRIs appear to be the most commonly prescribed class of antidepressants in pediatric oncology.[509,510]

No particular antidepressant has been demonstrated to be superior to another in the pediatric cancer population. Instead, the choice of antidepressant should be determined by the characteristics, including side effect profiles, of different agents. For example, mirtazapine may be an optimal agent for a child with anorexia or difficulty sleeping. Similarly, a tricyclic TCA may be the treatment of choice for a child with concomitant neuropathic pain. A modest increase in suicidal ideation has been noted in studies evaluating children treated with SSRIs compared with placebo.[511] The FDA now requires labeling of all antidepressants warning clinicians of such a risk.[512] Although the meaning of the increased risk is unclear, initiation of an antidepressant warrants discussion of the risks and benefits with families as well as close monitoring of children for worsening depression or signs of suicidality. Some medications such as tramadol, triptans, and linezolid interact with SSRIs, increasing the risk of serotonin syndrome. Children with depression not responding to these measures, and those with suicidal ideation or complex psychological symptoms, should be referred for formal psychiatric evaluation.

Evaluation of screening for depression, longitudinal studies of mood disorders and their predictors, and prospective evaluation of interventions for children with cancer and depressive symptoms are clearly needed to understand and ameliorate depression better in children with cancer.

Anxiety

Children with cancer may experience anxiety that is situation-dependent (e.g., related to treatment). Such anxiety may respond to anxiolytic medications administered prior to treatment as well as cognitive-behavioral interventions. Such nonpharmacologic interventions have been described in more detail earlier (see "Pain"). Other types of anxiety in children should be approached with an exploration of potentially contributing factors (e.g., stress related to family or school) and referral for increased psychosocial support. A child with anxiety meeting criteria for a psychiatric anxiety disorder (e.g., generalized anxiety disorder, panic disorder) or a child whose anxiety significantly impairs his or her function should be referred for psychiatric evaluation.

Delirium

Delirium is a state of disturbed consciousness or level of arousal characterized by an inability to focus or maintain or divert attention. It is of rapid onset and results in significant confusion for the patient. Delirious patients may have mumbling speech, perceptual disturbances with delusion or hallucinations, or alterations in their sleep-wake cycle. Patients may exhibit hyperalert-hyperactive delirium, with anxiety, agitation, or even aggression. Alternatively, patients may have hypoalert-hypoactive delirium, characterized by slowed reactions and difficulty focusing. Delirium is a disturbing symptom for patients and may be extremely distressing for caregivers.[513]

Delirium may be caused by metabolic disturbances (e.g., hypoglycemia, electrolyte abnormalities), medications, CNS pathology, liver or kidney dysfunction, infection, constipation, or urinary obstruction. The most common cause of delirium is drug effect. The most common offending medications are anticholinergics, corticosteroids, benzodiazepines, and opioids. Thus, delirium should never be treated with escalation of opioid therapy, unless uncontrolled pain is suspected to be the cause. Instead, the opioid dose should be decreased or converted to an alternative opioid. In addition, psychoactive medications such as benzodiazepines should be discontinued, if possible, and a neuroleptic such as haloperidol should be initiated. In fact, a randomized controlled trial of haloperidol versus chlorpromazine or lorazepam for adults with HIV and delirium was halted early because of adverse effects in the lorazepam arm. Haloperidol should be initiated by dose escalation similar to the process used for treating pain.

Atypical antipsychotic medications have also been used successfully in adults with delirium, although there are no trials comparing them with haloperidol.[514] For delirium with significant agitation, benzodiazepines may be considered, but they may cause paradoxical exacerbation of symptoms. Regardless of the pharmacologic agent used, concomitant nonpharmacologic interventions should always be used. Measures to reduce stimulation in the environment or to orient the patient, such as a familiar person remaining with the patient and frequent orientation to time and place, may be helpful.

REFERENCES

1. Collins JJ, Byrnes ME, Dunkel IJ, et al. The measurement of symptoms in children with cancer. J Pain Symptom Manage. 2000;19:363-377.
2. Collins JJ, Devine TD, Dick GS, et al. The measurement of symptoms in young children with cancer: the validation of the Memorial Symptom Assessment Scale in children aged 7-12. J Pain Symptom Manage. 2002;23:10-16.
3. Wolfe J, Grier HE, Klar N, et al. Symptoms and suffering at the end of life in children with cancer. N Engl J Med. 2000;342:326-333.
4. Jalmsell L, Kreicbergs U, Onelov E, et al. Symptoms affecting children with malignancies during the last month of life: a nationwide follow-up. Pediatrics. 2006;117:1314-1320.
5. Goldman A, Hewitt M, Collins GS, et al. Symptoms in children/young people with progressive malignant disease: United Kingdom Children's Cancer Study Group/Paediatric Oncology Nurses Forum survey. Pediatrics. 2006;117:e1179-e1186.
6. National Comprehensive Cancer Network Clinical Practice Guidelines in Oncology. Pediatric Cancer Pain, 2007. Available at http://www.nccn.org/professionals/physician_gls/PDF/pediatric_pain.pdf
7. NIH State-of-the-Science Statement on symptom management in cancer: pain, depression, and fatigue. NIH Consens State Sci Statements. 2002;19:1-29.
8. Merskey H. Pain terms. Pain. 1986;(Suppl 3):S215-S221.
9. van den Beuken-van Everdingen MH, de Rijke JM, Kessels AG, et al. Prevalence of pain in patients with cancer: a systematic review of the past 40 years. Ann Oncol. 2007;18:1437-1449.
10. Enskar K, Carlsson M, Golsater M, et al. Life situation and problems as reported by children with cancer and their parents. J Pediatr Oncol Nurs. 1997;14:18-26.
11. Anand KJ, Hickey PR. Pain and its effects in the human neonate and fetus. N Engl J Med. 1987;317:1321-1329.
12. Zernikow B, Meyerhoff U, Michel E, et al. Pain in pediatric oncology—children's and parents' perspectives. Eur J Pain. 2005;9:395-406.
13. Hewitt M, Goldman A, Collins GS, et al. Opioid use in palliative care of children and young people with cancer. J Pediatr. 2008;152:39-44.
14. Ljungman G, Gordh T, Sorensen S, Kreuger A. Pain variations during cancer treatment in children: a descriptive survey. Pediatr Hematol Oncol. 2000;17:211-221.

15. World Health Organization: Cancer Pain Relief and Palliative Care in Children. Geneva, World Health Organization, 1998.

16. Mense S. Nervous outflow from skeletal muscle following chemical noxious stimulation. J Physiol. 1977;267:75-88.

17. Scott D Jr. Aspirin: action on receptor in the tooth. Science. 1968;161:180-181.

18. Harris MB. Palliative care in children with cancer: which child and when? J Natl Cancer Inst Monogr. 2004:144-149.

19. Himelstein BP. Palliative care for infants, children, adolescents, and their families. J Palliat Med. 2006;9:163-181.

20. Franck LS, Greenberg CS, Stevens B. Pain assessment in infants and children. Pediatr Clin North Am. 2000;47:487-512.

21. Cheng SF, Foster RL, Hester NO. A review of factors predicting children's pain experiences. Issues Compr Pediatr Nurs. 2003; 26:203-216.

22. Weisman SJ, Bernstein B, Schechter NL. Consequences of inadequate analgesia during painful procedures in children. Arch Pediatr Adolesc Med. 1998;152:147-149.

23. Treadwell MJ, Franck LS, Vichinsky E. Using quality improvement strategies to enhance pediatric pain assessment. Int J Qual Health Care. 2002;14:39-47.

24. Bovier PA, Charvet A, Cleopas A, et al. Self-reported management of pain in hospitalized patients: link between process and outcome. Am J Med. 2004;117:569-574.

25. Beyer JE, McGrath PJ, Berde CB. Discordance between self-report and behavioral pain measures in children aged 3-7 years after surgery. J Pain Symptom Manage. 1990;5:350-356.

26. Chambers CT, Reid GJ, Craig KD, et al. Agreement between child and parent reports of pain. Clin J Pain. 1998;14:336-342.

27. Goodenough B, Addicoat L, Champion GD, et al. Pain in 4- to 6-year-old children receiving intramuscular injections: a comparison of the Faces Pain Scale with other self-report and behavioral measures. Clin J Pain. 1997;13:60-73.

28. Romsing J M-SJ, Hertel S, Rasmussen M. Postoperative pain in children: comparison between ratings of children and nurses. J Pain Symptom Manage. 1996;11:42-46.

29. Abu-Saad H. Assessing children's responses to pain. Pain. 1984; 19:163-171.

30. Hester NK. The preoperational child's reaction to immunization. Nurs Res. 1979;28:250-255.

31. Wong DL Baker CM. Pain in children: comparison of assessment scales. Pediatr Nurs. 1988;14:9-17.

32. Bieri D, Reeve RA, Champion GD, et al. The Faces Pain Scale for the self-assessment of the severity of pain experienced by children: development, initial validation, and preliminary investigation for ratio scale properties. Pain. 1990;41:139-150.

33. von Baeyer CL. Children's self-reports of pain intensity: scale selection, limitations and interpretation. Pain Res Manag. 2006; 11:157-162.

34. Grunau RV, Johnston CC, Craig KD. Neonatal facial and cry responses to invasive and noninvasive procedures. Pain. 1990;42: 295-305.

35. Stevens B, Johnston C, Petryshen P, Taddio A. Premature Infant Pain Profile: development and initial validation. Clin J Pain. 1996;12:13-22.

36. Hunt A, Mastroyannopoulou K, Goldman A, Seers K. Not knowing—the problem of pain in children with severe neurological impairment. Int J Nurs Stud. 2003;40:171-183.

37. Hunt A, Goldman A, Seers K, et al. Clinical validation of the paediatric pain profile. Dev Med Child Neurol. 2004;46:9-18.

38. Solodiuk J, Curley MA. Pain assessment in nonverbal children with severe cognitive impairments: the Individualized Numeric Rating Scale (INRS). J Pediatr Nurs. 2003;18:295-299.

39. Merkel SI, Voepel-Lewis T, Shayevitz JR, Malviya S. The FLACC: a behavioral scale for scoring postoperative pain in young children. Pediatr Nurs. 1997;23:293-297.

40. Voepel-Lewis T, Merkel S, Tait AR, et al. The reliability and validity of the Face, Legs, Activity, Cry, Consolability observa-

tional tool as a measure of pain in children with cognitive impairment. Anesth Analg. 2002;95:1224-1229.

41. Malviya S, Voepel-Lewis T, Tait AR, et al. Pain management in children with and without cognitive impairment following spine fusion surgery. Paediatr Anaesth. 2001;11:453-458.

42. Krebs EE, Carey TS, Weinberger M. Accuracy of the pain numeric rating scale as a screening test in primary care. J Gen Intern Med. 2007;22:1453-1458.

43. Jadad AR, Browman GP. The WHO analgesic ladder for cancer pain management. Stepping up the quality of its evaluation. JAMA. 1995;274:1870-1873.

44. Meuser T, Pietruck C, Radbruch L, et al. Symptoms during cancer pain treatment following WHO-guidelines: a longitudinal follow-up study of symptom prevalence, severity and etiology. Pain. 2001;93:247-257.

45. Zech DF, Grond S, Lynch J, et al. Validation of World Health Organization Guidelines for cancer pain relief: a 10-year prospective study. Pain. 1995;63:65-76.

46. Maltoni M, Scarpi E, Modonesi C, et al. A validation study of the WHO analgesic ladder: a two-step vs three-step strategy. Support Care Cancer. 2005;13:888-894.

47. Marinangeli F, Ciccozzi A, Leonardis M, et al. Use of strong opioids in advanced cancer pain: a randomized trial. J Pain Symptom Manage. 2004;27:409-416.

48. Stockler M, Vardy J, Pillai A, Warr D. Acetaminophen (paracetamol) improves pain and well-being in people with advanced cancer already receiving a strong opioid regimen: a randomized, double-blind, placebo-controlled cross-over trial. J Clin Oncol. 2004;22:3389-3394.

49. Axelsson B, Borup S. Is there an additive analgesic effect of paracetamol at step 3? A double-blind randomized controlled study. Palliat Med. 2003;17:724-725.

50. Vetter TR, Heiner EJ. Intravenous ketorolac as an adjuvant to pediatric patient-controlled analgesia with morphine. J Clin Anesth. 1994;6:110-113.

51. Eisenberg E, Berkey CS, Carr DB, et al. Efficacy and safety of nonsteroidal antiinflammatory drugs for cancer pain: a meta-analysis. J Clin Oncol. 1994;12:2756-2765.

52. Goldstein JL, Silverstein FE, Agrawal NM, et al. Reduced risk of upper gastrointestinal ulcer complications with celecoxib, a novel COX-2 inhibitor. Am J Gastroenterol. 2000;95:1681-1690.

53. Leese PT, Hubbard RC, Karim A, et al. Effects of celecoxib, a novel cyclooxygenase-2 inhibitor, on platelet function in healthy adults: a randomized, controlled trial. J Clin Pharmacol. 2000;40: 124-132.

54. Birmingham PK, Tobin MJ, Fisher DM, et al. Initial and subsequent dosing of rectal acetaminophen in children: a 24-hour pharmacokinetic study of new dose recommendations. Anesthesiology. 2001;94:385-389.

55. Anderson BJ, Holford NH, Woollard GA, et al. Perioperative pharmacodynamics of acetaminophen analgesia in children. Anesthesiology. 1999;90:411-421.

56. Collins JJ, Grier HE, Kinney HC, Berde CB. Control of severe pain in children with terminal malignancy. J Pediatr. 1995;126: 653-657.

57. Gupta K, Kshirsagar S, Chang L, et al. Morphine stimulates angiogenesis by activating proangiogenic and survival-promoting signaling and promotes breast tumor growth. Cancer Res. 2002; 62:4491-4498.

58. Singleton PA, Lingen MW, Fekete MJ, et al. Methylnaltrexone inhibits opiate and VEGF-induced angiogenesis: role of receptor transactivation. Microvasc Res. 2006;72:3-11.

59. Farooqui M, Li Y, Rogers T, et al. COX-2 inhibitor celecoxib prevents chronic morphine-induced promotion of angiogenesis, tumour growth, metastasis and mortality, without compromising analgesia. Br J Cancer. 2007;97:1523-1531.

60. Blanco JG, Harrison PL, Evans WE, Relling MV. Human cytochrome P450 maximal activities in pediatric versus adult liver. Drug Metab Dispos. 2000;28:379-382.

61. Tegeder I, Lotsch J, Geisslinger G. Pharmacokinetics of opioids in liver disease. Clin Pharmacokinet. 1999;37:17-40.

62. Williams DG, Patel A, Howard RF. Pharmacogenetics of codeine metabolism in an urban population of children and its implications for analgesic reliability. Br J Anaesth. 2002;89:839-845.

63. Clark E, Plint AC, Correll R, et al. A randomized, controlled trial of acetaminophen, ibuprofen, and codeine for acute pain relief in children with musculoskeletal trauma. Pediatrics. 2007;119:460-467.

64. St. Charles CS, Matt BH, Hamilton MM, Katz BP. A comparison of ibuprofen versus acetaminophen with codeine in the young tonsillectomy patient. Otolaryngol Head Neck Surg. 1997;117:76-82.

65. Kaiko RF, Foley KM, Grabinski PY, et al. Central nervous system excitatory effects of meperidine in cancer patients. Ann Neurol. 1983;13:180-185.

66. Vetter TR. Pediatric patient-controlled analgesia with morphine versus meperidine. J Pain Symptom Manage. 1992;7:204-208.

67. Warfield CA. Controlled-release morphine tablets in patients with chronic cancer pain: a narrative review of controlled clinical trials. Cancer. 1998;82:2299-2306.

68. Bartlett SE, Dodd PR, Smith MT. Pharmacology of morphine and morphine-3-glucuronide at opioid, excitatory amino acid, GABA and glycine binding sites. Pharmacol Toxicol. 1994;75:73-81.

69. Paul D, Standifer KM, Inturrisi CE, Pasternak GW. Pharmacological characterization of morphine-6 beta-glucuronide, a very potent morphine metabolite. J Pharmacol Exp Ther. 1989;251:477-483.

70. Hanks GW, Hoskin PJ, Aherne GW, et al. Explanation for potency of repeated oral doses of morphine? Lancet. 1987;2:723-725.

71. Reid CM, Martin RM, Sterne JA, et al. Oxycodone for cancer-related pain: meta-analysis of randomized controlled trials. Arch Intern Med. 2006;166:837-843.

72. Fahnenstich H, Steffan J, Kau N, Bartmann P. Fentanyl-induced chest wall rigidity and laryngospasm in preterm and term infants. Crit Care Med. 2000;28:836-839.

73. Flacke JW, Flacke WE, Bloor BC, et al. Histamine release by four narcotics: a double-blind study in humans. Anesth Analg. 1987;66:723-730.

74. Allan L, Hays H, Jensen NH, et al. Randomised crossover trial of transdermal fentanyl and sustained release oral morphine for treating chronic noncancer pain. BMJ. 2001;322:1154-1158.

75. van Seventer R, Smit JM, Schipper RM, et al. Comparison of TTS-fentanyl with sustained-release oral morphine in the treatment of patients not using opioids for mild-to-moderate pain. Curr Med Res Opin. 2003;19:457-469.

76. Finkel JC, Finley A, Greco C, et al. Transdermal fentanyl in the management of children with chronic severe pain: results from an international study. Cancer. 2005;104:2847-2857.

77. Solassol I, Caumette L, Bressolle F, et al. Inter- and intra-individual variability in transdermal fentanyl absorption in cancer pain patients. Oncol Rep. 2005;14:1029-1036.

78. Larsen RH, Nielsen F, Sorensen JA, Nielsen JB. Dermal penetration of fentanyl: inter- and intraindividual variations. Pharmacol Toxicol. 2003;93:244-248.

79. Koehntop DE, Rodman JH. Fentanyl pharmacokinetics in patients undergoing renal transplantation. Pharmacotherapy. 1997;17:746-752.

80. Ahmedzai S, Brooks D. Transdermal fentanyl versus sustained-release oral morphine in cancer pain: preference, efficacy, and quality of life. The TTS-Fentanyl Comparative Trial Group. J Pain Symptom Manage. 1997;13:254-261.

81. Donner B, Zenz M, Tryba M, Strumpf M. Direct conversion from oral morphine to transdermal fentanyl: a multicenter study in patients with cancer pain. Pain. 1996;64:527-534.

82. Payne R, Mathias SD, Pasta DJ, et al. Quality of life and cancer pain: satisfaction and side effects with transdermal fentanyl versus oral morphine. J Clin Oncol. 1998;16:1588-1593.

83. Schechter NL, Weisman SJ, Rosenblum M, et al. The use of oral transmucosal fentanyl citrate for painful procedures in children. Pediatrics. 1995;95:335-339.

84. Coluzzi PH, Schwartzberg L, Conroy JD, et al. Breakthrough cancer pain: a randomized trial comparing oral transmucosal fentanyl citrate (OTFC) and morphine sulfate immediate release (MSIR). Pain. 2001;91:123-130.

85. Christie JM, Simmonds M, Patt R, et al. Dose-titration, multicenter study of oral transmucosal fentanyl citrate for the treatment of breakthrough pain in cancer patients using transdermal fentanyl for persistent pain. J Clin Oncol. 1998;16:3238-3245.

86. Toombs JD, Kral LA. Methadone treatment for pain states. Am Fam Physician. 2005;71:1353-1358.

87. Inturrisi CE, Colburn WA, Kaiko RF, et al. Pharmacokinetics and pharmacodynamics of methadone in patients with chronic pain. Clin Pharmacol Ther. 1987;41:392-401.

88. Grochow L, Sheidler V, Grossman S, et al. Does intravenous methadone provide longer lasting analgesia than intravenous morphine? A randomized, double-blind study. Pain. 1989;38:151-157.

89. Ripamonti C, De Conno F, Groff L, et al. Equianalgesic dose/ratio between methadone and other opioid agonists in cancer pain: comparison of two clinical experiences. Ann Oncol. 1998;9:79-83.

90. Ripamonti C, Groff L, Brunelli C, et al. Switching from morphine to oral methadone in treating cancer pain: what is the equianalgesic dose ratio? J Clin Oncol. 1998;16:3216-3221.

91. Crettol S, Deglon JJ, Besson J, et al. ABCB1 and cytochrome P450 genotypes and phenotypes: influence on methadone plasma levels and response to treatment. Clin Pharmacol Ther. 2006;80:668-681.

92. Crettol S, Deglon JJ, Besson J, et al. Methadone enantiomer plasma levels, CYP2B6, CYP2C19, and CYP2C9 genotypes, and response to treatment. Clin Pharmacol Ther. 2005;78:593-604.

93. Maremmani I, Pacini M, Cesaroni C, et al. QTc interval prolongation in patients on long-term methadone maintenance therapy. Eur Addict Res. 2005;11:44-49.

94. Chugh SS, Socoteanu C, Reinier K, et al. A community-based evaluation of sudden death associated with therapeutic levels of methadone. Am J Med. 2008;121:66-71.

95. Package insert. Avinza (morphine sulfate) LP, February 2003. San Diego, Calif, Ligand Pharmaceuticals, 2003.

96. Amabile CM, Bowman BJ. Overview of oral modified-release opioid products for the management of chronic pain. Ann Pharmacother. 2006;40:1327-1335.

97. Wilkinson TJ, Robinson BA, Begg EJ, et al. Pharmacokinetics and efficacy of rectal versus oral sustained-release morphine in cancer patients. Cancer Chemother Pharmacol. 1992;31:251-254.

98. Beaver WT, Feise GA. A comparison of the analgesic effect of oxymorphone by rectal suppository and intramuscular injection in patients with postoperative pain. J Clin Pharmacol. 1977;17:276-291.

99. Bruera E, Fainsinger R, Moore M, et al. Local toxicity with subcutaneous methadone. Experience of two centers. Pain. 1991;45:141-143.

100. Pillitteri LC, Clark RE. Comparison of a patient-controlled analgesia system with continuous infusion for administration of diamorphine for mucositis. Bone Marrow Transplant. 1998;22:495-498.

101. Berde CB, Lehn BM, Yee JD, et al. Patient-controlled analgesia in children and adolescents: a randomized, prospective compari-

son with intramuscular administration of morphine for postoperative analgesia. J Pediatr. 1991;118:460-466.

102. Collins JJ, Geake J, Grier HE, et al. Patient-controlled analgesia for mucositis pain in children: a three-period crossover study comparing morphine and hydromorphone. J Pediatr. 1996;129: 722-728.

103. Dunbar PJ, Buckley P, Gavrin JR, et al. Use of patient-controlled analgesia for pain control for children receiving bone marrow transplant. J Pain Symptom Manage. 1995;10: 604-611.

104. Anghelescu DL, Burgoyne LL, Oakes LL, Wallace DA. The safety of patient-controlled analgesia by proxy in pediatric oncology patients. Anesth Analg. 2005;101:1623-1627.

105. Portenoy RK, Payne D, Jacobsen P. Breakthrough pain: characteristics and impact in patients with cancer pain. Pain. 1999;81: 129-134.

106. Friedrichsdorf SJ, Finney D, Bergin M, et al. Breakthrough pain in children with cancer. J Pain Symptom Manage. 2007;34: 209-216.

107. Fisher K, Stiles C, Hagen NA. Characterization of the early pharmacodynamic profile of oral methadone for cancer-related breakthrough pain: a pilot study. J Pain Symptom Manage. 2004;28:619-625.

108. Sabatowski R, Kasper SM, Radbruch L. Patient-controlled analgesia with intravenous L-methadone in a child with cancer pain refractory to high-dose morphine. J Pain Symptom Manage. 2002;23:3-5.

109. Drake R, Longworth J, Collins JJ. Opioid rotation in children with cancer. J Palliat Med. 2004;7:419-422.

110. Trujillo KA, Akil H. Inhibition of morphine tolerance and dependence by the NMDA receptor antagonist MK-801. Science. 1991;251:85-87.

111. Flogegard H, Ljungman G. Characteristics and adequacy of intravenous morphine infusions in children in a paediatric oncology setting. Med Pediatr Oncol. 2003;40:233-238.

112. Ross JR, Riley J, Taegetmeyer AB, et al. Genetic variation and response to morphine in cancer patients: catechol-O-methyltransferase and multidrug resistance-1 gene polymorphisms are associated with central side effects. Cancer. 2008; 112:1390-1403.

113. Gilron I, Bailey JM, Tu D, et al. Morphine, gabapentin, or their combination for neuropathic pain. N Engl J Med. 2005;352: 1324-1334.

114. Hemstapat K, Monteith GR, Smith D, Smith MT. Morphine-3-glucuronide's neuro-excitatory effects are mediated via indirect activation of N-methyl-D-aspartic acid receptors: mechanistic studies in embryonic cultured hippocampal neurones. Anesth Analg. 2003;97:494-505.

115. Walker SM, Cousins MJ. Reduction in hyperalgesia and intrathecal morphine requirements by low-dose ketamine infusion. J Pain Symptom Manage. 1997;14:129-133.

116. McQuay HJ, Moore RA. Using numerical results from systematic reviews in clinical practice. Ann Intern Med. 1997;126:712-720.

117. Lin C, Durieux ME. Ketamine and kids: an update. Paediatr Anaesth. 2005;15:91-97.

118. Smith TJ, Staats PS, Deer T, et al. Randomized clinical trial of an implantable drug delivery system compared with comprehensive medical management for refractory cancer pain: impact on pain, drug-related toxicity, and survival. J Clin Oncol. 2002; 20:4040-4049.

119. Clemente C. Anatomy. A Regional Atlas of the Human Body, 3rd ed. Baltimore, Urban & Schwarzenberg, 1987, Plate 564.

120. Jay SM, Elliott CH, Ozolins M, et al. Behavioral management of children's distress during painful medical procedures. Behav Res Ther. 1985;23:513-520.

121. Ellis JA, Spanos NP. Cognitive-behavioral interventions for children's distress during bone marrow aspirations and lumbar

punctures: a critical review. J Pain Symptom Manage. 1994;9: 96-108.

122. Jay S, Elliott CH, Fitzgibbons I, et al. A comparative study of cognitive behavior therapy versus general anesthesia for painful medical procedures in children. Pain. 1995;62:3-9.

123. Rusy LM, Weisman SJ. Complementary therapies for acute pediatric pain management. Pediatr Clin North Am. 2000;47: 589-599.

124. Liossi C, Hatira P. Clinical hypnosis versus cognitive behavioral training for pain management with pediatric cancer patients undergoing bone marrow aspirations. Int J Clin Exp Hypn. 1999;47:104-116.

125. Liu RW, Mehta P, Fortuna S, et al. A randomized prospective study of music therapy for reducing anxiety during cast room procedures. J Pediatr Orthop. 2007;27:831-833.

126. Sparber A, Bauer L, Curt G, et al. Use of complementary medicine by adult patients participating in cancer clinical trials. Oncol Nurs Forum. 2000;27:623-630.

127. Bardia A, Barton DL, Prokop LJ, et al. Efficacy of complementary and alternative medicine therapies in relieving cancer pain: a systematic review. J Clin Oncol. 2006;24:5457-5464.

128. Bruera E, Roca E, Cedaro L, et al. Action of oral methylprednisolone in terminal cancer patients: a prospective randomized double-blind study. Cancer Treat Rep. 1985;69:751-754.

129. Langer SW, Sehested M, Jensen PB. Treatment of anthracycline extravasation with dexrazoxane. Clin Cancer Res. 2000;6: 3680-3686.

130. Mouridsen HT, Langer SW, Buter J, et al. Treatment of anthracycline extravasation with Savene (dexrazoxane): results from two prospective clinical multicentre studies. Ann Oncol. 2007;18: 546-550.

131. Bomgaars L, Geyer JR, Franklin J, et al. Phase I trial of intrathecal liposomal cytarabine in children with neoplastic meningitis. J Clin Oncol. 2004;22:3916-3921.

132. Socie G, Selimi F, Sedel L, et al. Avascular necrosis of bone after allogeneic bone marrow transplantation: clinical findings, incidence and risk factors. Br J Haematol. 1994;86:624-628.

133. Wong R, Wiffen PJ. Bisphosphonates for the relief of pain secondary to bone metastases. Cochrane Database Syst Rev. 2002;2: CD002068.

134. Kubista E, Glaspy J, Holmes FA, et al. Bone pain associated with once-per-cycle pegfilgrastim is similar to daily filgrastim in patients with breast cancer. Clin Breast Cancer. 2003;3:391-398.

135. Gudi R, Krishnamurthy M, Pachter BR. Astemizole in the treatment of granulocyte colony-stimulating factor-induced bone pain. Ann Intern Med. 1995;123:236-237.

136. Shenep JL, Kalwinsky DK, Hutson PR, et al. Efficacy of oral sucralfate suspension in prevention and treatment of chemotherapy-induced mucositis. J Pediatr. 1988;113:758-763.

137. Cruz LB, Ribeiro AS, Rech A, et al. Influence of low-energy laser in the prevention of oral mucositis in children with cancer receiving chemotherapy. Pediatr Blood Cancer. 2007;48:435-440.

138. Gandemer V, Le Deley MC, Dollfus C, et al. Multicenter randomized trial of chewing gum for preventing oral mucositis in children receiving chemotherapy. J Pediatr Hematol Oncol. 2007;29:86-94.

139. Bensadoun RJ, Schubert MM, Lalla RV, Keefe D. Amifostine in the management of radiation-induced and chemo-induced mucositis. Support Care Cancer. 2006;14:566-572.

140. Spielberger R, Stiff P, Bensinger W, et al. Palifermin for oral mucositis after intensive therapy for hematologic cancers. N Engl J Med. 2004;351:2590-2598.

141. Peterson DE, Jones JB, Petit RG 2nd. Randomized, placebo-controlled trial of Saforis for prevention and treatment of oral mucositis in breast cancer patients receiving anthracycline-based chemotherapy. Cancer. 2007;109:322-331.

142. Nicholson AB. Methadone for cancer pain. Cochrane Database Syst Rev. 2007;4:CD003971.

143. Raskin P, Donofrio PD, Rosenthal NR, et al. Topiramate vs placebo in painful diabetic neuropathy: analgesic and metabolic effects. Neurology. 2004;63:865-873.

144. Lesser H, Sharma U, LaMoreaux L, Poole RM. Pregabalin relieves symptoms of painful diabetic neuropathy: a randomized controlled trial. Neurology. 2004;63:2104-2110.

145. Caraceni A, Zecca E, Bonezzi C, et al. Gabapentin for neuropathic cancer pain: a randomized controlled trial from the Gabapentin Cancer Pain Study Group. J Clin Oncol. 2004;22:2909-2917.

146. Vecht CJ, Haaxma-Reiche H, van Putten WL, et al. Initial bolus of conventional versus high-dose dexamethasone in metastatic spinal cord compression. Neurology. 1989;39:1255-1257.

147. Wilkins KL, McGrath PJ, Finley GA, Katz J. Phantom limb sensations and phantom limb pain in child and adolescent amputees. Pain. 1998;78:7-12.

148. Krane EJ, Heller LB. The prevalence of phantom sensation and pain in pediatric amputees. J Pain Symptom Manage. 1995;10:21-29.

149. Rusy LM, Troshynski TJ, Weisman SJ. Gabapentin in phantom limb pain management in children and young adults: report of seven cases. J Pain Symptom Manage. 2001;21:78-82.

150. Harden RN, Houle TT, Remble TA, et al. Topiramate for phantom limb pain: a time-series analysis. Pain Med. 2005;6:375-378.

151. Weiss T, Miltner WH, Adler T, et al. Decrease in phantom limb pain associated with prosthesis-induced increased use of an amputation stump in humans. Neurosci Lett. 1999;272:131-134.

152. Barker CC, Anderson RA, Sauve RS, Butzner JD. GI complications in pediatric patients post-BMT. Bone Marrow Transplant. 2005;36:51-58.

153. Akpek G, Chinratanalab W, Lee LA, et al. Gastrointestinal involvement in chronic graft-versus-host disease: a clinicopathologic study. Biol Blood Marrow Transplant. 2003;9:46-51.

154. Treister NS, Cook EF Jr, Antin J, et al. Clinical evaluation of oral chronic graft-versus-host disease. Biol Blood Marrow Transplant. 2008;14:110-115.

155. Treister NS, Woo SB, O'Holleran EW, et al. Oral chronic graft-versus-host disease in pediatric patients after hematopoietic stem cell transplantation. Biol Blood Marrow Transplant. 2005;11:721-731.

156. Stratton P, Turner ML, Childs R, et al. Vulvovaginal chronic graft-versus-host disease with allogeneic hematopoietic stem cell transplantation. Obstet Gynecol. 2007;110:1041-1049.

157. Spiryda LB, Laufer MR, Soiffer RJ, Antin JA. Graft-versus-host disease of the vulva and/or vagina: diagnosis and treatment. Biol Blood Marrow Transplant. 2003;9:760-765.

158. Greco C, Berde C. Pain management for the hospitalized pediatric patient. Pediatr Clin North Am. 2005;52:995-1027.

159. Greco C, Berde C. Pediatric acute pain management. In Ballantyne JC (ed). Bonica's Management of Pain, 4th ed. Philadelphia, Lippincott Williams & Wilkins, 2008.

160. Cravero JP, Blike GT. Review of pediatric sedation. Anesth Analg. 2004;99:1355-1364.

161. Cote CJ, Wilson S. Guidelines for monitoring and management of pediatric patients during and after sedation for diagnostic and therapeutic procedures: an update. Pediatrics. 2006;118:2587-2602.

162. Eriksen J, Sjogren P, Bruera E, et al. Critical issues on opioids in chronic noncancer pain: an epidemiological study. Pain. 2006;125:172-179.

163. Miaskowski C, Dodd M, West C, et al. Randomized clinical trial of the effectiveness of a self-care intervention to improve cancer pain management. J Clin Oncol. 2004;22:1713-1720.

164. Rubenstein EB, Slusher BS, Rojas C, Navari RM. New approaches to chemotherapy-induced nausea and vomiting: from neuropharmacology to clinical investigations. Cancer J. 2006;12:341-347.

165. Hornby PJ. Central neurocircuitry associated with emesis. Am J Med. 2001;111(Suppl 8A):106S-112S.

166. Hawthorn J, Ostler KJ, Andrews PL. The role of the abdominal visceral innervation and 5-hydroxytryptamine M-receptors in vomiting induced by the cytotoxic drugs cyclophosphamide and cis-platin in the ferret. Q J Exp Physiol. 1988;73:7-21.

167. Cubeddu LX. Mechanisms by which cancer chemotherapeutic drugs induce emesis. Semin Oncol. 1992;19(Suppl 15):2-13.

168. Hesketh PJ. Understanding the pathobiology of chemotherapy-induced nausea and vomiting. Providing a basis for therapeutic progress. Oncology (Williston Park). 2004;18(Suppl 6):9-14.

169. Grunberg SM, Hesketh PJ. Control of chemotherapy-induced emesis. N Engl J Med. 1993;329:1790-1796.

170. Dupuis LL, Nathan PC. Options for the prevention and management of acute chemotherapy-induced nausea and vomiting in children. Paediatr Drugs. 2003;5:597-613.

171. Bianchi C, Beani L, Crema C. Effects of metoclopramide on isolated guinea-pig colon. 2. Interference with ganglionic stimulant drugs. Eur J Pharmacol. 1970;12:332-341.

172. Fontaine J, Reuse JJ. Pharmacological analysis of the effects of metoclopramide on the guinea-pig ileum in vitro. Arch Int Pharmacodyn Ther. 1973;204:293-305.

173. Higgins GA, Kilpatrick GJ, Bunce KT, et al. 5-HT3 receptor antagonists injected into the area postrema inhibit cisplatin-induced emesis in the ferret. Br J Pharmacol. 1989;97:247-255.

174. Miner WD, Sanger GJ, Turner DH. Evidence that 5-hydroxytryptamine-3 receptors mediate cytotoxic drug and radiation-evoked emesis. Br J Cancer. 1987;56:159-162.

175. Costall B, Kelly ME, Naylor RJ, et al. 5-Hydroxytryptamine M-receptor antagonism in the hypothalamus facilitates gastric emptying in the guinea-pig. Neuropharmacology. 1986;25:1293-1296.

176. Costall B, Domeney AM, Naylor RJ, Tattersall FD. Emesis induced by cisplatin in the ferret as a model for the detection of anti-emetic drugs. Neuropharmacology. 1987;26:1321-1326.

177. Kamato T, Ito H, Nagakura Y, et al. Mechanisms of cisplatin- and *m*-chlorophenylbiguanide-induced emesis in ferrets. Eur J Pharmacol. 1993;238:369-376.

178. Fukui H, Yamamoto M, Sato S. Vagal afferent fibers and peripheral 5-HT3 receptors mediate cisplatin-induced emesis in dogs. Jpn J Pharmacol. 1992;59:221-226.

179. Preziosi P, D'Amato M, Del Carmine R, et al. The effects of 5-HT3 receptor antagonists on cisplatin-induced emesis in the pigeon. Eur J Pharmacol. 1992;221:343-350.

180. Barnes NM, Barry JM, Costa B, et al. Antagonism by parachlorophenylalanine of cisplatin-induced emesis. Br J Pharmacol. 1987;92:649P (abstract).

181. Cubeddu LX, Hoffmann IS, Fuenmayor NT, Malave JJ. Changes in serotonin metabolism in cancer patients: its relationship to nausea and vomiting induced by chemotherapeutic drugs. Br J Cancer. 1992;66:198-203.

182. Barnes JM, Barnes NM, Costall B, et al. Identification and distribution of 5-HT3 recognition sites within the human brainstem. Neurosci Lett. 1990;111:80-86.

183. Hesketh PJ, Van Belle S, Aapro M, et al. Differential involvement of neurotransmitters through the time course of cisplatin-induced emesis as revealed by therapy with specific receptor antagonists. Eur J Cancer. 2003;39:1074-1080.

184. Navari RM. Pathogenesis-based treatment of chemotherapy-induced nausea and vomiting—two new agents. J Support Oncol. 2003;1:89-103.

185. Diemunsch P, Grelot L. Potential of substance P antagonists as antiemetics. Drugs. 2000;60:533-546.

186. Bountra C, Bunce K, Dale T, et al. Anti-emetic profile of a nonpeptide neurokinin NK1 receptor antagonist, CP-99,994, in ferrets. Eur J Pharmacol. 1993;249:R3-R4.

187. Tattersall FD, Rycroft W, Hargreaves RJ, Hill RG. The tachykinin NK1 receptor antagonist CP-99,994 attenuates cisplatin

induced emesis in the ferret. Eur J Pharmacol. 1993;250:R5-R6.

188. Kris MG, Gralla RJ, Clark RA, et al. Incidence, course, and severity of delayed nausea and vomiting following the administration of high-dose cisplatin. J Clin Oncol. 1985;3:1379-1384.

189. Kris MG, Gralla RJ, Tyson LB, et al. Controlling delayed vomiting: double-blind, randomized trial comparing placebo, dexamethasone alone, and metoclopramide plus dexamethasone in patients receiving cisplatin. J Clin Oncol. 1989;7:108-114.

190. Hickok JT, Roscoe JA, Morrow GR, et al. Nausea and emesis remain significant problems of chemotherapy despite prophylaxis with 5-hydroxytryptamine-3 antiemetics: a University of Rochester James P. Wilmot Cancer Center Community Clinical Oncology Program Study of 360 cancer patients treated in the community. Cancer. 2003;97:2880-2886.

191. Goedhals L, Heron JF, Kleisbauer JP, et al. Control of delayed nausea and vomiting with granisetron plus dexamethasone or dexamethasone alone in patients receiving highly emetogenic chemotherapy: a double-blind, placebo-controlled, comparative study. Ann Oncol. 1998;9:661-666.

192. The Italian Group for Antiemetic Research. Dexamethasone alone or in combination with ondansetron for the prevention of delayed nausea and vomiting induced by chemotherapy. N Engl J Med. 2000;342:1554-1559.

193. Grunberg SM, Deuson RR, Mavros P, et al. Incidence of chemotherapy-induced nausea and emesis after modern antiemetics. Cancer. 2004;100:2261-2268.

194. Fabi A, Barduagni M, Lauro S, et al. Is delayed chemotherapy-induced emesis well managed in oncological clinical practice? An observational study. Support Care Cancer. 2003;11:156-161.

195. Bloechl-Daum B, Deuson RR, Mavros P, et al. Delayed nausea and vomiting continue to reduce patients' quality of life after highly and moderately emetogenic chemotherapy despite antiemetic treatment. J Clin Oncol. 2006;24:4472-4478.

196. Pinkerton CR, Williams D, Wootton C, et al. 5-HT3 antagonist ondansetron—an effective outpatient antiemetic in cancer treatment. Arch Dis Child. 1990;65:822-825.

197. Dupuis LL, Lau R, Greenberg ML. Delayed nausea and vomiting in children receiving antineoplastics. Med Pediatr Oncol. 2001;37:115-121.

198. Morrow GR. Clinical characteristics associated with the development of anticipatory nausea and vomiting in cancer patients undergoing chemotherapy treatment. J Clin Oncol. 1984;2:1170-1176.

199. Morrow GR. Prevalence and correlates of anticipatory nausea and vomiting in chemotherapy patients. J Natl Cancer Inst. 1982;68:585-588.

200. Morrow GR. Susceptibility to motion sickness and the development of anticipatory nausea and vomiting in cancer patients undergoing chemotherapy. Cancer Treat Rep. 1984;68:1177-1178.

201. Chin SB, Kucuk O, Peterson R, Ezdinli EZ. Variables contributing to anticipatory nausea and vomiting in cancer chemotherapy. Am J Clin Oncol. 1992;15:262-267.

202. Dolgin MJ, Katz ER, McGinty K, Siegel SE. Anticipatory nausea and vomiting in pediatric cancer patients. Pediatrics. 1985;75:547-552.

203. Stockhorst U, Spennes-Saleh S, Korholz D, et al. Anticipatory symptoms and anticipatory immune responses in pediatric cancer patients receiving chemotherapy: features of a classically conditioned response? Brain Behav Immun. 2000;14:198-218.

204. Tyc VL, Mulhern RK, Barclay DR, et al. Variables associated with anticipatory nausea and vomiting in pediatric cancer patients receiving ondansetron antiemetic therapy. J Pediatr Psychol. 1997;22:45-58.

205. Ihbe-Heffinger A, Ehlken B, Bernard R, et al. The impact of delayed chemotherapy-induced nausea and vomiting on patients, health resource utilization and costs in German cancer centers. Ann Oncol. 2004;5:526-536.

206. Osoba D, Zee B, Warr D, et al. Effect of postchemotherapy nausea and vomiting on health-related quality of life. The Quality of Life and Symptom Control Committees of the National Cancer Institute of Canada Clinical Trials Group. Support Care Cancer. 1997;5:307-313.

207. O'Brien BJ, Rusthoven J, Rocchi A, et al. Impact of chemotherapy-associated nausea and vomiting on patients' functional status and on costs: survey of five Canadian centres. CMAJ. 1993;149:296-302.

208. Rusthoven JJ, Osoba D, Butts CA, et al. The impact of postchemotherapy nausea and vomiting on quality of life after moderately emetogenic chemotherapy. Support Care Cancer. 1998;6:389-395.

209. Decker GM, DeMeyer ES, Kisko DL. Measuring the maintenance of daily life activities using the functional living index-emesis (FLIE) in patients receiving moderately emetogenic chemotherapy. J Support Oncol. 2006;4:35-41, 52.

210. Roscoe JA, Morrow GR, Hickok JT, Stern RM. Nausea and vomiting remain a significant clinical problem: trends over time in controlling chemotherapy-induced nausea and vomiting in 1413 patients treated in community clinical practices. J Pain Symptom Manage. 2000;20:113-121.

211. Morrow GR. A patient report measure for the quantification of chemotherapy-induced nausea and emesis: psychometric properties of the Morrow assessment of nausea and emesis (MANE). Br J Cancer Suppl. 1992;19:S72-S74.

212. Rhodes VA, Watson PM, Johnson MH. Development of reliable and valid measures of nausea and vomiting. Cancer Nurs. 1984;7:33-41.

213. Keller VE, Keck JF. An instrument for observational assessment of nausea in young children. Pediatr Nurs. 2006;32:420-426.

214. Dupuis LL, Taddio A, Kerr EN, et al. Development and validation of the pediatric nausea assessment tool for use in children receiving antineoplastic agents. Pharmacotherapy. 2006;26:1221-1231.

215. Zeltzer LK, LeBaron S, Richie DM, et al. Can children understand and use a rating scale to quantify somatic symptoms: assessment of nausea and vomiting as a model. J Consult Clin Psychol. 1988;56:567-572.

216. McGrath PA, Seifert CE, Speechley KN, et al. A new analogue scale for assessing children's pain: an initial validation study. Pain. 1996;64:435-443.

217. Hinds PS, Quargnenti AG, Wentz TJ. Measuring symptom distress in adolescents with cancer. J Pediatr Oncol Nurs. 1992;9:84-86.

218. Lo LH, Hayman LL. Parents associated with children in measuring acute and delayed nausea and vomiting. Nurs Health Sci. 1999;1:155-161.

219. Zeltzer L, LeBaron S, Zeltzer PM. The effectiveness of behavioral intervention for reduction of nausea and vomiting in children and adolescents receiving chemotherapy. J Clin Oncol. 1984;2:683-690.

220. Zeltzer LK, LeBaron S, Zeltzer PM. A prospective assessment of chemotherapy-related nausea and vomiting in children with cancer. Am J Pediatr Hematol Oncol. 1984;6:5-16.

221. Tyc VL, Mulhern RK, Fairclough D, et al. Chemotherapy-induced nausea and emesis in pediatric cancer patients: external validity of child and parent emesis ratings. J Dev Behav Pediatr. 1993;14:236-241.

222. Morrow GR. Methodology in behavioral and psychosocial cancer research. The assessment of nausea and vomiting. Past problems, current issues and suggestions for future research. Cancer. 1984;53(Suppl):2267-2280.

223. de Wit R, Schmitz PI, Verweij J, et al. Analysis of cumulative probabilities shows that the efficacy of 5HT3 antagonist prophylaxis is not maintained. J Clin Oncol. 1996;14:644-651.

224. Gralla RJ, Osoba D, Kris MG, et al. Recommendations for the use of antiemetics: evidence-based, clinical practice guidelines. American Society of Clinical Oncology. J Clin Oncol. 1999;17:2971-2994.

225. Pollera CF, Giannarelli D. Prognostic factors influencing cisplatin-induced emesis. Definition and validation of a predictive logistic model. Cancer. 1989;64:1117-1122.

226. ASHP Therapeutic Guidelines on the Pharmacologic Management of Nausea and Vomiting in Adult and Pediatric Patients Receiving Chemotherapy or Radiation Therapy or Undergoing Surgery. Am J Health Syst Pharm. 1999;56:729-764.

227. Roila F, Tonato M, Basurto C, et al. Protection from nausea and vomiting in cisplatin-treated patients: high-dose metoclopramide combined with methylprednisolone versus metoclopramide combined with dexamethasone and diphenhydramine: a study of the Italian Oncology Group for Clinical Research. J Clin Oncol. 1989;7:1693-1700.

227a. Nathan PC, Tomlinson G, Dupuis LL, et al. A pilot study of ondansetron plus metopimazine vs ondansetron monotherapy in children receiving highly emetogenic chemotherapy: a Bayesian randomized serial N-of-1 trials design. Support Care Cancer. 2006;14:268-276.

228. Burris H, Hesketh P, Cohn J, et al. Efficacy and safety of oral granisetron versus oral prochlorperazine in preventing nausea and emesis in patients receiving moderately emetogenic chemotherapy. Cancer J Sci Am. 1996;2:85-90.

229. Marty M, Pouillart P, Scholl S, et al. Comparison of the 5-hydroxytryptamine-3 (serotonin) antagonist ondansetron (GR 38032F) with high-dose metoclopramide in the control of cisplatin-induced emesis. N Engl J Med. 1990;322:816-821.

230. Heron JF, Goedhals L, Jordaan JP, et al. Oral granisetron alone and in combination with dexamethasone: a double-blind randomized comparison against high-dose metoclopramide plus dexamethasone in prevention of cisplatin-induced emesis. The Granisetron Study Group. Ann Oncol. 1994;5:579-584.

231. Bonneterre J, Chevallier B, Metz R, et al. A randomized double-blind comparison of ondansetron and metoclopramide in the prophylaxis of emesis induced by cyclophosphamide, fluorouracil, and doxorubicin or epirubicin chemotherapy. J Clin Oncol. 1990;8:1063-1069.

232. Hainsworth J, Harvey W, Pendergrass K, et al. A single-blind comparison of intravenous ondansetron, a selective serotonin antagonist, with intravenous metoclopramide in the prevention of nausea and vomiting associated with high-dose cisplatin chemotherapy. J Clin Oncol. 1991;9:721-728.

233. Jorgensen M, Victor MA. Antiemetic efficacy of ondansetron and metoclopramide, both combined with corticosteroid, in malignant lymphoma patients receiving noncisplatin chemotherapy. Acta Oncol. 1996;35:159-163.

234. Chevallier B, Cappelaere P, Splinter T, et al. A double-blind, multicentre comparison of intravenous dolasetron mesilate and metoclopramide in the prevention of nausea and vomiting in cancer patients receiving high-dose cisplatin chemotherapy. Support Care Cancer. 1997;5:22-30.

235. Koseoglu V, Kurekci AE, Sarici U, et al. Comparison of the efficacy and side-effects of ondansetron and metoclopramide-diphenhydramine administered to control nausea and vomiting in children treated with antineoplastic chemotherapy: a prospective randomized study. Eur J Pediatr. 1998;157:806-810.

236. Madej G, Krzakowski M, Pawinski A, et al. A report comparing the use of tropisetron (Navoban), a 5-HT3 antagonist, with a standard antiemetic regimen of dexamethasone and metoclopramide in cisplatin-treated patients under conditions of severe emesis. Semin Oncol. 1994;21(Suppl 9):3-6.

237. Mehta NH, Reed CM, Kuhlman C, et al. Controlling conditioning-related emesis in children undergoing bone marrow transplantation. Oncol Nurs Forum. 1997;24:1539-1544.

238. Dick GS, Meller ST, Pinkerton CR. Randomised comparison of ondansetron and metoclopramide plus dexamethasone for chemotherapy induced emesis. Arch Dis Child. 1995;73:243-245.

239. Luisi FA, Petrilli AS, Tanaka C, Caran EM. Contribution to the treatment of nausea and emesis induced by chemotherapy in children and adolescents with osteosarcoma. Sao Paulo Med J. 2006;124:61-65.

240. Hirota T, Honjo T, Kuroda R, et al. [Antiemetic efficacy of granisetron in pediatric cancer treatment—(2).Comparison of granisetron and granisetron plus methylprednisolone as antiemetic prophylaxis.] Gan To Kagaku Ryoho. 1993;20:2369-2373.

241. Alvarez O, Freeman A, Bedros A, et al. Randomized double-blind crossover ondansetron-dexamethasone versus ondansetron-placebo study for the treatment of chemotherapy-induced nausea and vomiting in pediatric patients with malignancies. J Pediatr Hematol Oncol. 1995;17:145-150.

242. Culy CR, Bhana N, Plosker GL. Ondansetron: a review of its use as an antiemetic in children. Paediatr Drugs. 2001;3:441-479.

243. Parker RI, Prakash D, Mahan RA, et al. Randomized, double-blind, crossover, placebo-controlled trial of intravenous ondansetron for the prevention of intrathecal chemotherapy-induced vomiting in children. J Pediatr Hematol Oncol. 2001;23:578-581.

244. Perez EA. Review of the preclinical pharmacology and comparative efficacy of 5-hydroxytryptamine-3 receptor antagonists for chemotherapy-induced emesis. J Clin Oncol. 1995;13:1036-1043.

245. Hesketh P, Navari R, Grote T, et al. Double-blind, randomized comparison of the antiemetic efficacy of intravenous dolasetron mesylate and intravenous ondansetron in the prevention of acute cisplatin-induced emesis in patients with cancer. Dolasetron Comparative Chemotherapy-induced Emesis Prevention Group. J Clin Oncol. 1996;14:2242-2249.

246. Gralla RJ, Navari RM, Hesketh PJ, et al. Single-dose oral granisetron has equivalent antiemetic efficacy to intravenous ondansetron for highly emetogenic cisplatin-based chemotherapy. J Clin Oncol. 1998;16:1568-1573.

247. Perez EA, Hesketh P, Sandbach J, et al. Comparison of single-dose oral granisetron versus intravenous ondansetron in the prevention of nausea and vomiting induced by moderately emetogenic chemotherapy: a multicenter, double-blind, randomized parallel study. J Clin Oncol. 1998;16:754-760.

248. Chua DT, Sham JS, Kwong DL, et al. Comparative efficacy of three 5-HT3 antagonists (granisetron, ondansetron, and tropisetron) plus dexamethasone for the prevention of cisplatin-induced acute emesis: a randomized crossover study. Am J Clin Oncol. 2000;23:185-191.

249. Audhuy B, Cappelaere P, Martin M, et al. A double-blind, randomised comparison of the anti-emetic efficacy of two intravenous doses of dolasetron mesilate and granisetron in patients receiving high dose cisplatin chemotherapy. Eur J Cancer. 1996;32A:807-813.

250. National Comprehensive Cancer Network Clincial Practice Guidelines in Oncology. Antiemesis, 2008. Available at http://www.nccn.org/professionals/physician_gls/PDF/antiemesis.pdf.

251. Roila F, Hesketh PJ, Herrstedt J. Prevention of chemotherapy- and radiotherapy-induced emesis: results of the 2004 Perugia International Antiemetic Consensus Conference. Ann Oncol. 2006;17:20-28.

252. Walsh T, Morris AK, Holle LM, et al. Granisetron vs ondansetron for prevention of nausea and vomiting in hematopoietic stem cell transplant patients: results of a prospective, double-blind, randomized trial. Bone Marrow Transplant. 2004;34:963-968.

253. Fox-Geiman MP, Fisher SG, Kiley K, et al. Double-blind comparative trial of oral ondansetron versus oral granisetron versus IV ondansetron in the prevention of nausea and vomiting associated with highly emetogenic preparative regimens prior to stem cell transplantation. Biol Blood Marrow Transplant. 2001;7:596-603.

254. Jaing TH, Tsay PK, Hung IJ, et al. Single-dose oral granisetron versus multidose intravenous ondansetron for moderately emetogenic cyclophosphamide-based chemotherapy in pediatric outpatients with acute lymphoblastic leukemia. Pediatr Hematol Oncol. 2004;21:227-235.

255. Roila F, Aapro M, Stewart A. Optimal selection of antiemetics in children receiving cancer chemotherapy. Support Care Cancer. 1998;6:215-220.

256. Hesketh PJ, Beck T, Uhlenhopp M, et al. Adjusting the dose of intravenous ondansetron plus dexamethasone to the emetogenic potential of the chemotherapy regimen. J Clin Oncol. 1995;13: 2117-2122.

257. Needles B, Miranda E, Garcia Rodriguez FM, et al. A multicenter, double-blind, randomized comparison of oral ondansetron 8 mg b.i.d., 24 mg q.d., and 32 mg q.d. in the prevention of nausea and vomiting associated with highly emetogenic chemotherapy. S3AA3012 Study Group. Support Care Cancer. 1999;7:347-353.

258. Hainsworth JD, Hesketh PJ. Single-dose ondansetron for the prevention of cisplatin-induced emesis: efficacy results. Semin Oncol. 1992;19(Suppl 15):14-19.

259. Beck TM, Hesketh PJ, Madajewicz S, et al. Stratified, randomized, double-blind comparison of intravenous ondansetron administered as a multiple-dose regimen versus two single-dose regimens in the prevention of cisplatin-induced nausea and vomiting. J Clin Oncol. 1992;10:1969-1975.

260. Khojasteh A, Sartiano G, Tapazoglou E, et al. Ondansetron for the prevention of emesis induced by high-dose cisplatin. A multicenter dose-response study. Cancer. 1990;66:1101-1105.

261. Tsavaris N, Kosmas CH, Vadiaka M, et al. Efficacy of ondansetron treatment for acute emesis with different dosing schedules 8 vs 32 mg. A randomized study. J Exp Clin Cancer Res. 2001; 20:29-34.

262. Tsavaris N, Kosmas C, Vadiaka M, et al. Ondansentron and dexamethasone treatment with different dosing schedules (24 versus 32 mg) in patients with nonsmall-cell lung cancer under cisplatin-based chemotherapy: a randomized study. Chemotherapy. 2000;46:364-370.

263. Walker PC, Biglin KE, Constance TD, et al. Promoting the use of oral ondansetron in children receiving cancer chemotherapy. Am J Health Syst Pharm. 2001;58:598-602.

264. Krzakowski M, Graham E, Goedhals L, et al. A multicenter, double-blind comparison of i.v. and oral administration of ondansetron plus dexamethasone for acute cisplatin-induced emesis. Ondansetron Acute Emesis Study Group. Anticancer Drugs. 1998;9:593-598.

265. White L, Daly SA, McKenna CJ, et al. A comparison of oral ondansetron syrup or intravenous ondansetron loading dose regimens given in combination with dexamethasone for the prevention of nausea and emesis in pediatric and adolescent patients receiving moderately/highly emetogenic chemotherapy. Pediatr Hematol Oncol. 2000;17:445-455.

266. Cohen IJ, Zehavi N, Buchwald I, et al. Oral ondansetron: an effective ambulatory complement to intravenous ondansetron in the control of chemotherapy-induced nausea and vomiting in children. Pediatr Hematol Oncol. 1995;12:67-72.

267. Davidson NG, Paska W, Van Belle S, et al. Ondansetron suppository: a randomised, double-blind, double-dummy, parallel-group comparison with oral ondansetron for the prevention of cyclophosphamide-induced emesis and nausea. The Ondansetron Suppository emesis study group. Oncology. 1997;54:380-386.

268. Eisenberg P, MacKintosh FR, Ritch P, et al. Efficacy, safety and pharmacokinetics of palonosetron in patients receiving highly emetogenic cisplatin-based chemotherapy: a dose-ranging clinical study. Ann Oncol. 2004;15:330-337.

269. Grunberg SM, Koeller JM. Palonosetron: a unique 5-HT3-receptor antagonist for the prevention of chemotherapy-induced emesis. Expert Opin Pharmacother. 2003;4:2297-2303.

270. Gralla R, Lichinitser M, Van Der Vegt S, et al. Palonosetron improves prevention of chemotherapy-induced nausea and vomiting following moderately emetogenic chemotherapy: results of a double-blind randomized phase III trial comparing single doses of palonosetron with ondansetron. Ann Oncol. 2003;14: 1570-1577.

271. Eisenberg P, Figueroa-Vadillo J, Zamora R, et al. Improved prevention of moderately emetogenic chemotherapy-induced nausea and vomiting with palonosetron, a pharmacologically novel 5-HT3 receptor antagonist: results of a phase III, single-dose trial versus dolasetron. Cancer. 2003;98:2473-2482.

272. Aapro MS, Grunberg SM, Manikhas GM, et al. A phase III, double-blind, randomized trial of palonosetron compared with ondansetron in preventing chemotherapy-induced nausea and vomiting following highly emetogenic chemotherapy. Ann Oncol. 2006;17:1441-1449.

273. D'Olimpio JT, Camacho F, Chandra P, et al. Antiemetic efficacy of high-dose dexamethasone versus placebo in patients receiving cisplatin-based chemotherapy: a randomized double-blind controlled clinical trial. J Clin Oncol. 1985;3:1133-1135.

274. Aapro MS, Alberts DS. High-dose dexamethasone for prevention of cisplatin-induced vomiting. Cancer Chemother Pharmacol. 1981;7:11-14.

275. Cassileth PA, Lusk EJ, Torri S, Gerson SL. Antiemetic efficacy of high-dose dexamethasone in induction therapy in acute nonlymphocytic leukemia. Ann Intern Med. 1984;100:701-702.

276. Markman M, Sheidler V, Ettinger DS, et al. Antiemetic efficacy of dexamethasone. Randomized, double-blind, crossover study with prochlorperazine in patients receiving cancer chemotherapy. N Engl J Med. 1984;311:549-552.

277. Aapro MS, Plezia PM, Alberts DS, et al. Double-blind crossover study of the antiemetic efficacy of high-dose dexamethasone versus high-dose metoclopramide. J Clin Oncol. 1984;2:466-471.

278. Roila F, Basurto C, Minotti V, et al. Methylprednisolone versus metoclopramide for prevention of nausea and vomiting in breast cancer patients treated with intravenous cyclophosphamide methotrexate 5-fluorouracil: a double-blind randomized study. Oncology. 1988;45:346-349.

279. Jones AL, Hill AS, Soukop M, et al. Comparison of dexamethasone and ondansetron in the prophylaxis of emesis induced by moderately emetogenic chemotherapy. Lancet. 1991;338:483-487.

280. Ahn MJ, Lee JS, Lee KH, et al. A randomized double-blind trial of ondansetron alone versus in combination with dexamethasone versus in combination with dexamethasone and lorazepam in the prevention of emesis due to cisplatin-based chemotherapy. Am J Clin Oncol. 1994;17:150-156.

281. Olver I, Paska W, Depierre A, et al. A multicentre, double-blind study comparing placebo, ondansetron and ondansetron plus dexamethasone for the control of cisplatin-induced delayed emesis. Ondansetron Delayed Emesis Study Group. Ann Oncol. 1996;7:945-952.

282. Koo WH, Ang PT. Role of maintenance oral dexamethasone in prophylaxis of delayed emesis caused by moderately emetogenic chemotherapy. Ann Oncol. 1996;7:71-74.

283. Kirchner V, Aapro M, Terrey JP, Alberto P. A double-blind crossover study comparing prophylactic intravenous granisetron alone or in combination with dexamethasone as antiemetic treatment in controlling nausea and vomiting associated with chemotherapy. Eur J Cancer. 1997;33:1605-1610.

284. The Italian Group for Antiemetic Research. Dexamethasone, granisetron, or both for the prevention of nausea and vomiting during chemotherapy for cancer. N Engl J Med. 1995;332: 1-5.

285. Joss RA, Bacchi M, Buser K, et al. Ondansetron plus dexamethasone is superior to ondansetron alone in the prevention of emesis in chemotherapy-naive and previously treated patients. Swiss

Group for Clinical Cancer Research (SAKK). Ann Oncol. 1994;5:253-258.

286. Sorbe BG. Tropisetron (Navoban) alone and in combination with dexamethasone in the prevention of chemotherapy-induced emesis: the Nordic experience. Semin Oncol. 1994;21(Suppl 9):20-26.

287. Stephens SH, Silvey VL, Wheeler RH. A randomized, double-blind comparison of the antiemetic effect of metoclopramide and lorazepam with or without dexamethasone in patients receiving high-dose cisplatin. Cancer. 1990;66:443-446.

288. Ozkan A, Yildiz I, Yuksel L, et al. Tropisetron (Navoban) in the control of nausea and vomiting induced by combined cancer chemotherapy in children. Jpn J Clin Oncol. 1999;29:92-95.

289. Carmichael J, Bessell EM, Harris AL, et al. Comparison of granisetron alone and granisetron plus dexamethasone in the prophylaxis of cytotoxic-induced emesis. Br J Cancer. 1994;70: 1161-1164.

290. Jochelson MS, Tarbell NJ, Weinstein HJ. Unusual thoracic radiographic findings in children treated for Hodgkin's disease. J Clin Oncol. 1986;4:874-882.

291. Pezner RD, Bertrand M, Cecchi GR, et al. Steroid-withdrawal radiation pneumonitis in cancer patients. Chest. 1984;85:816-817.

292. Wilkinson ID, Jellineck DA, Levy D, et al. Dexamethasone and enhancing solitary cerebral mass lesions: alterations in perfusion and blood-tumor barrier kinetics shown by magnetic resonance imaging. Neurosurgery. 2006;58:640-646.

293. Gralla RJ. Antiemetic treatment. Eur J Cancer Clin Oncol. 1985;21:155-157.

294. Strum SB, McDermed JE, Pileggi J, et al. Intravenous metoclopramide: prevention of chemotherapy-induced nausea and vomiting. A preliminary evaluation. Cancer. 1984;53:1432-1439.

295. Strum SB, McDermed JE, Streng BR, McDermott NM. Combination metoclopramide and dexamethasone: an effective antiemetic regimen in outpatients receiving noncisplatin chemotherapy. J Clin Oncol. 1984;2:1057-1063.

296. Bishop JF, Wolf M, Matthews JP, et al. Randomized, double-blind, cross-over study comparing prochlorperazine and lorazepam with high-dose metoclopramide and lorazepam for the control of emesis in patients receiving cytotoxic chemotherapy. Cancer Treat Rep. 1987;71:1007-1011.

297. O'Brien ME, Cullen MH, Woodroffe C, et al. The role of metoclopramide in acute and delayed chemotherapy induced emesis: a randomised double blind trial. Br J Cancer. 1989;60:759-763.

298. Allen JC, Gralla R, Reilly L, et al. Metoclopramide: dose-related toxicity and preliminary antiemetic studies in children receiving cancer chemotherapy. J Clin Oncol. 1985;3:1136-1141.

298a. Sallan SE, Cronin C, Zelen M, Zinberg NE. Antiemetics in patients receiving chemotherapy for cancer: a randomized comparison of delta-9-tetrahydrocannabinol and prochlorperazine. N Engl J Med. 1980;302:135–138.

299. Cichewicz DL. Synergistic interactions between cannabinoid and opioid analgesics. Life Sci. 2004;74:1317-1324.

300. Navari RM, Reinhardt RR, Gralla RJ, et al. Reduction of cisplatin-induced emesis by a selective neurokinin-1-receptor antagonist. L-754,030 Antiemetic Trials Group. N Engl J Med. 1999;340:190-195.

301. Campos D, Pereira JR, Reinhardt RR, et al. Prevention of cisplatin-induced emesis by the oral neurokinin-1 antagonist, MK-869, in combination with granisetron and dexamethasone or with dexamethasone alone. J Clin Oncol. 2001;19:1759-1767.

302. Van Belle S, Lichinitser MR, Navari RM, et al. Prevention of cisplatin-induced acute and delayed emesis by the selective neurokinin-1 antagonists, L-758,298 and MK-869. Cancer. 2002;94:3032-3041.

303. Oechsle K, Muller MR, Hartmann JT, et al. Aprepitant as salvage therapy in patients with chemotherapy-induced nausea and emesis refractory to prophylaxis with 5-HT(3) antagonists and dexamethasone. Onkologie. 2006;29:557-561.

304. de Wit R, Herrstedt J, Rapoport B, et al. Addition of the oral NK1 antagonist aprepitant to standard antiemetics provides protection against nausea and vomiting during multiple cycles of cisplatin-based chemotherapy. J Clin Oncol. 2003;21:4105-4111.

305. Smith AR, Repka TL, Weigel BJ. Aprepitant for the control of chemotherapy induced nausea and vomiting in adolescents. Pediatr Blood Cancer. 2005;45:857-860.

306. de Jonge ME, Huitema AD, Holtkamp MJ, et al. Aprepitant inhibits cyclophosphamide bioactivation and thiotepa metabolism. Cancer Chemother Pharmacol. 2005;56:370-378.

307. McCrea JB, Majumdar AK, Goldberg MR, et al. Effects of the neurokinin1 receptor antagonist aprepitant on the pharmacokinetics of dexamethasone and methylprednisolone. Clin Pharmacol Ther. 2003;74:17-24.

308. Massaro AM, Lenz KL. Aprepitant: a novel antiemetic for chemotherapy-induced nausea and vomiting. Ann Pharmacother. 2005;39:77-85.

309. Blum RA, Majumdar A, McCrea J, et al. Effects of aprepitant on the pharmacokinetics of ondansetron and granisetron in healthy subjects. Clin Ther. 2003;25:1407-1419.

310. Depre M, Van Hecken A, Oeyen M, et al. Effect of aprepitant on the pharmacokinetics and pharmacodynamics of warfarin. Eur J Clin Pharmacol. 2005;61:341-346.

311. Laszlo J, Clark RA, Hanson DC, et al. Lorazepam in cancer patients treated with cisplatin: a drug having antiemetic, amnesic, and anxiolytic effects. J Clin Oncol. 1985;3:864-869.

312. Kris MG, Gralla RJ, Clark RA, et al. Consecutive dose-finding trials adding lorazepam to the combination of metoclopramide plus dexamethasone: improved subjective effectiveness over the combination of diphenhydramine plus metoclopramide plus dexamethasone. Cancer Treat Rep. 1985;69:1257-1262.

313. Clerico M, Bertetto O, Morandini MP, et al. Antiemetic activity of oral lorazepam in addition to methylprednisolone and metoclopramide in the prophylactic treatment of vomiting induced by cisplatin. A double-blind, placebo-controlled study with crossover design. Tumori. 1993;79:119-122.

314. Malik IA, Khan WA, Qazilbash M, et al. Clinical efficacy of lorazepam in prophylaxis of anticipatory, acute, and delayed nausea and vomiting induced by high doses of cisplatin. A prospective randomized trial. Am J Clin Oncol. 1995;18:170-175.

315. Gordon CJ, Pazdur R, Ziccarelli A, et al. Metoclopramide versus metoclopramide and lorazepam. Superiority of combined therapy in the control of cisplatin-induced emesis. Cancer. 1989;63: 578-582.

316. Buzdar AU, Esparza L, Natale R, et al. Lorazepam-enhancement of the antiemetic efficacy of dexamethasone and promethazine. A placebo-controlled study. Am J Clin Oncol. 1994;17:417-421.

317. Longo DL, Wesley M, Howser D, et al. Results of a randomized double-blind crossover trial of scopolamine versus placebo administered by transdermal patch for the control of cisplatin-induced emesis. Cancer Treat Rep. 1982;66:1975-1976.

318. Meyer BR, O'Mara V, Reidenberg MM. A controlled clinical trial of the addition of transdermal scopolamine to a standard metoclopramide and dexamethasone antiemetic regimen. J Clin Oncol. 1987;5:1994-1997.

319. Thiele EA, Riviello JJ. Scopolamine patch-induced unilateral mydriasis. Pediatrics. 1995;96(Pt 1):525.

320. Tsavaris N, Zamanis N, Zinelis A, et al. Diphenhydramine for nausea and vomiting related to cancer chemotherapy with cisplatin. J Pain Symptom Manage. 1991;6:461-465.

321. Tsavaris NB. Diphenhydramine for nausea and vomiting related to cancer chemotherapy with cisplatin. J Pain Symptom Manage. 1992;7:440-442.

322. Navari RM, Einhorn LH, Loehrer PJ Sr, et al. A phase II trial of olanzapine, dexamethasone, and palonosetron for the prevention of chemotherapy-induced nausea and vomiting: a Hoosier oncology group study. Support Care Cancer. 2007;15:1285-1291.

323. Guttuso T Jr, Roscoe J, Griggs J. Effect of gabapentin on nausea induced by chemotherapy in patients with breast cancer. Lancet. 2003;361:1703-1705.

324. Navari RM, Madajewicz S, Anderson N, et al. Oral ondansetron for the control of cisplatin-induced delayed emesis: a large, multicenter, double-blind, randomized comparative trial of ondansetron versus placebo. J Clin Oncol. 1995;13:2408-2416.

325. Kaizer L, Warr D, Hoskins P, et al. Effect of schedule and maintenance on the antiemetic efficacy of ondansetron combined with dexamethasone in acute and delayed nausea and emesis in patients receiving moderately emetogenic chemotherapy: a phase III trial by the National Cancer Institute of Canada Clinical Trials Group. J Clin Oncol. 1994;12:1050-1057.

326. Friedman CJ, Burris HA 3rd, Yocom K, et al. Oral granisetron for the prevention of acute late onset nausea and vomiting in patients treated with moderately emetogenic chemotherapy. Oncologist. 2000;5:136-143.

327. Latreille J, Pater J, Johnston D, et al. Use of dexamethasone and granisetron in the control of delayed emesis for patients who receive highly emetogenic chemotherapy. National Cancer Institute of Canada Clinical Trials Group. J Clin Oncol. 1998;16:1174-1178.

328. Gandara DR, Harvey WH, Monaghan GG, et al. Delayed emesis following high-dose cisplatin: a double-blind randomised comparative trial of ondansetron (GR 38032F) versus placebo. Eur J Cancer. 1993;29A(Suppl 1):S35-S38.

329. Pater JL, Lofters WS, Zee B, et al. The role of the 5-HT3 antagonists ondansetron and dolasetron in the control of delayed onset nausea and vomiting in patients receiving moderately emetogenic chemotherapy. Ann Oncol. 1997;8:181-185.

330. Sorbe BG, Berglind AM, Andersson H, et al. A study evaluating the efficacy and tolerability of tropisetron in combination with dexamethasone in the prevention of delayed platinum-induced nausea and emesis. Cancer. 1998;83:1022-1032.

331. The Italian Group for Antiemetic Research. Ondansetron versus metoclopramide, both combined with dexamethasone, in the prevention of cisplatin-induced delayed emesis. J Clin Oncol. 1997;15:124-130.

332. Aapro MS, Thuerlimann B, Sessa C, et al. A randomized double-blind trial to compare the clinical efficacy of granisetron with metoclopramide, both combined with dexamethasone in the prophylaxis of chemotherapy-induced delayed emesis. Ann Oncol. 2003;14:291-297.

333. Kris MG, Tyson LB, Clark RA, Gralla RJ. Oral ondansetron for the control of delayed emesis after cisplatin. Report of a phase II study and a review of completed trials to manage delayed emesis. Cancer. 1992;70(Suppl):1012-1016.

334. Grote T, Hajdenberg J, Cartmell A, et al. Combination therapy for chemotherapy-induced nausea and vomiting in patients receiving moderately emetogenic chemotherapy: palonosetron, dexamethasone, and aprepitant. J Support Oncol. 2006;4:403-408.

335. Scarantino CW, Ornitz RD, Hoffman LG, Anderson RF Jr. Radiation-induced emesis: effects of ondansetron. Semin Oncol. 1992;19(Suppl 15):38-43.

336. The Italian Group for Antiemetic Research in Radiotherapy. Radiation-induced emesis: a prospective observational multicenter Italian trial. Int J Radiat Oncol Biol Phys. 1999;44:619-625.

337. Scarantino CW, Ornitz RD, Hoffman LG, Anderson RF Jr. On the mechanism of radiation-induced emesis: the role of serotonin. Int J Radiat Oncol Biol Phys. 1994;30:825-830.

338. Priestman TJ, Roberts JT, Lucraft H, et al. Results of a randomized, double-blind comparative study of ondansetron and metoclopramide in the prevention of nausea and vomiting following high-dose upper abdominal irradiation. Clin Oncol (R Coll Radiol). 1990;2:71-75.

339. Priestman TJ, Roberts JT, Upadhyaya BK. A prospective randomized double-blind trial comparing ondansetron versus prochlorperazine for the prevention of nausea and vomiting in patients undergoing fractionated radiotherapy. Clin Oncol (R Coll Radiol). 1993;5:358-363.

340. Lippens RJ, Broeders GC. Ondansetron in radiation therapy of brain tumor in children. Pediatr Hematol Oncol. 1996;13:247-252.

341. Bey P, Wilkinson PM, Resbeut M, et al. A double-blind, placebo-controlled trial of i.v. dolasetron mesilate in the prevention of radiotherapy-induced nausea and vomiting in cancer patients. Support Care Cancer. 1996;4:378-383.

342. Wong RK, Paul N, Ding K, et al. 5-hydroxytryptamine-3 receptor antagonist with or without short-course dexamethasone in the prophylaxis of radiation induced emesis: a placebo-controlled randomized trial of the National Cancer Institute of Canada Clinical Trials Group (SC19). J Clin Oncol. 2006;24:3458-3464.

343. Maranzano E, Feyer P, Molassiotis A, et al. Evidence-based recommendations for the use of antiemetics in radiotherapy. Radiother Oncol. 2005;76:227-233.

344. Aouad MT, Siddik SS, Rizk LB, et al. The effect of dexamethasone on postoperative vomiting after tonsillectomy. Anesth Analg. 2001;92:636-640.

345. Subramaniam B, Madan R, Sadhasivam S, et al. Dexamethasone is a cost-effective alternative to ondansetron in preventing PONV after paediatric strabismus repair. Br J Anaesth. 2001;86:84-89.

346. Henzi I, Walder B, Tramer MR. Dexamethasone for the prevention of postoperative nausea and vomiting: a quantitative systematic review. Anesth Analg. 2000;90:186-194.

347. Gan TJ, Meyer T, Apfel CC, et al. Consensus guidelines for managing postoperative nausea and vomiting. Anesth Analg. 2003;97:62-71.

348. Tramer MR, Reynolds DJ, Moore RA, McQuay HJ. Efficacy, dose-response, and safety of ondansetron in prevention of postoperative nausea and vomiting: a quantitative systematic review of randomized placebo-controlled trials. Anesthesiology. 1997;87:1277-1289.

349. White PF, Tang J, Song D, et al. Transdermal scopolamine: an alternative to ondansetron and droperidol for the prevention of postoperative and postdischarge emetic symptoms. Anesth Analg. 2007;104:92-96.

350. Diemunsch P, Gan TJ, Philip BK, et al. Single-dose aprepitant vs ondansetron for the prevention of postoperative nausea and vomiting: a randomized, double-blind phase III trial in patients undergoing open abdominal surgery. Br J Anaesth. 2007;99:202-211.

351. Gan TJ, Apfel CC, Kovac A, et al. A randomized, double-blind comparison of the NK1 antagonist, aprepitant, versus ondansetron for the prevention of postoperative nausea and vomiting. Anesth Analg. 2007;104:1082-1089.

352. Hardy J, Daly S, McQuade B, et al. A double-blind, randomised, parallel group, multinational, multicentre study comparing a single dose of ondansetron 24 mg p.o. with placebo and metoclopramide 10 mg t.d.s. p.o. in the treatment of opioid-induced nausea and emesis in cancer patients. Support Care Cancer. 2002;10:231-236.

353. Mercadante S, Sapio M, Serretta R. Ondansetron in nausea and vomiting induced by spinal morphine. J Pain Symptom Manage. 1998;16:259-262.

354. Cepeda MS, Alvarez H, Morales O, Carr DB. Addition of ultralow dose naloxone to postoperative morphine PCA: unchanged analgesia and opioid requirement but decreased incidence of opioid side effects. Pain. 2004;107:41-46.

355. Maxwell LG, Kaufmann SC, Bitzer S, et al. The effects of a small-dose naloxone infusion on opioid-induced side effects and analgesia in children and adolescents treated with intravenous patient-controlled analgesia: a double-blind, prospective, randomized, controlled study. Anesth Analg. 2005;100:953-958.

356. DiBaise JK, Lyden E, Tarantolo SR, et al. A prospective study of gastric emptying and its relationship to the development of nausea, vomiting, and anorexia after autologous stem cell transplantation. Am J Gastroenterol. 2005;100:1571-1577.

357. Eagle DA, Gian V, Lauwers GY, et al. Gastroparesis following bone marrow transplantation. Bone Marrow Transplant. 2001; 28:59-62.

358. Brand RE, DiBaise JK, Quigley EM, et al. Gastroparesis as a cause of nausea and vomiting after high-dose chemotherapy and haemopoietic stem-cell transplantation. Lancet. 1998;352:1985.

359. Kim SW, Shin IS, Kim JM, et al. Mirtazapine for severe gastroparesis unresponsive to conventional prokinetic treatment. Psychosomatics. 2006;47:440-442.

360. Pae C-U. Low-dose mirtazapine may be successful treatment option for severe nausea and vomiting. Prog Neuropsychopharmacol Biol Psychiatry. 2006;30:1143-1145.

361. Teixeira FV, Novaretti TM, Pilon B, et al. Mirtazapine (Remeron) as treatment for nonmechanical vomiting after gastric bypass. Obes Surg. 2005;15:707-709.

362. Guclu S, Gol M, Dogan E, Saygili U. Mirtazapine use in resistant hyperemesis gravidarum: report of three cases and review of the literature. Arch Gynecol Obstet. 2005;272:298-300.

363. Hallenbeck J. Fast Fact and Concepts 005: Causes of Nausea and Vomiting (V.O.M.I.T.). 2nd ed, August 2005. Treatment of Nausea and Vomiting. End-of-Life/Palliative Education Resource Center. Available at http://www.eperc.mcw.edu/fastFact/ff_005.htm.

364. Reeves JJ, Shannon MW, Fleisher GR. Ondansetron decreases vomiting associated with acute gastroenteritis: a randomized, controlled trial. Pediatrics. 2002;109:e62.

365. Shen J, Wenger N, Glaspy J, et al. Electroacupuncture for control of myeloablative chemotherapy-induced emesis: A randomized controlled trial. JAMA. 2000;284:2755-2761.

366. Wang XS, Giralt SA, Mendoza TR, et al. Clinical factors associated with cancer-related fatigue in patients being treated for leukemia and nonHodgkin's lymphoma. J Clin Oncol. 2002;20: 1319-1328.

367. Roscoe JA, Morrow GR, Hickok JT, et al. The efficacy of acupressure and acustimulation wrist bands for the relief of chemotherapy-induced nausea and vomiting. A University of Rochester Cancer Center Community Clinical Oncology Program multicenter study. J Pain Symptom Manage. 2003;26:731-742.

368. Ezzo J, Vickers A, Richardson MA, et al. Acupuncture-point stimulation for chemotherapy-induced nausea and vomiting. J Clin Oncol. 2005;23:7188-7198.

369. Jacknow DS, Tschann JM, Link MP, Boyce WT. Hypnosis in the prevention of chemotherapy-related nausea and vomiting in children: a prospective study. J Dev Behav Pediatr. 1994;15: 258-264.

370. Morrow GR, Morrell C. Behavioral treatment for the anticipatory nausea and vomiting induced by cancer chemotherapy. N Engl J Med. 1982;307:1476-1480.

371. Molassiotis A, Yung HP, Yam BM, et al. The effectiveness of progressive muscle relaxation training in managing chemotherapy-induced nausea and vomiting in Chinese breast cancer patients: a randomised controlled trial. Support Care Cancer. 2002;10: 237-246.

372. Edwards JN, Herman JA, Wallace BK, et al. Comparison of patient-controlled and nurse-controlled antiemetic therapy in patients receiving chemotherapy. Res Nurs Health. 1991;14: 249-257.

373. Dix S, Cord M, Howard S, et al. Safety and efficacy of a continuous infusion, patient-controlled anti-emetic pump to facilitate outpatient administration of high-dose chemotherapy. Bone Marrow Transplant. 1999;24:561-566.

374. Jones E, Koyama T, Ho RH, et al. Safety and efficacy of a continuous infusion, patient-controlled antiemetic pump for children

375. receiving emetogenic chemotherapy. Pediatr Blood Cancer. 2007;48:330-332.

375. Mancini I, Bruera E. Constipation in advanced cancer patients. Support Care Cancer. 1998;6:356-364.

376. Tuteja AK, Talley NJ, Joos SK, et al. Is constipation associated with decreased physical activity in normally active subjects? Am J Gastroenterol. 2005;100:124-129.

377. Radbruch L, Sabatowski R, Loick G, et al. Constipation and the use of laxatives: a comparison between transdermal fentanyl and oral morphine. Palliat Med. 2000;14:111-119.

378. Mancini IL, Hanson J, Neumann CM, Bruera ED. Opioid type and other clinical predictors of laxative dose in advanced cancer patients: a retrospective study. J Palliat Med. 2000;3:49-56.

379. Solomon R, Cherny NI. Constipation and diarrhea in patients with cancer. Cancer J. 2006;125:355-364.

380. Goodman M, Low J, Wilkinson S. Constipation management in palliative care: a survey of practices in the United kingdom. J Pain Symptom Manage. 2005;29:238-244.

381. Yuan CS, Foss JF. Oral methylnaltrexone for opioid-induced constipation. JAMA. 2000;284:1383-1384.

382. Yuan CS, Foss JF, O'Connor M, et al. Methylnaltrexone for reversal of constipation due to chronic methadone use: a randomized controlled trial. JAMA. 2000;283:367-372.

383. Mystakidou K, Tsilika E, Kalaidopoulou O, et al. Comparison of octreotide administration vs conservative treatment in the management of inoperable bowel obstruction in patients with far advanced cancer: a randomized, double-blind, controlled clinical trial. Anticancer Res. 2002;22:1187-1192.

384. Mercadante S, Ferrera P, Villari P, Marrazzo A. Aggressive pharmacological treatment for reversing malignant bowel obstruction. J Pain Symptom Manage. 2004;28:412-416.

385. Ripamonti C, Mercadante S, Groff L, et al. Role of octreotide, scopolamine butylbromide, and hydration in symptom control of patients with inoperable bowel obstruction and nasogastric tubes: a prospective randomized trial. J Pain Symptom Manage. 2000;19:23-34.

386. Benson AB 3rd, Ajani JA, Catalano RB, et al. Recommended guidelines for the treatment of cancer treatment-induced diarrhea. J Clin Oncol. 2004;22:2918-2926.

387. Sale GE, Shulman HM, McDonald GB, Thomas ED. Gastrointestinal graft-versus-host disease in man. A clinicopathologic study of the rectal biopsy. Am J Surg Pathol. 1979;3:291-299.

388. Alimonti A, Gelibter A, Pavese I, et al. New approaches to prevent intestinal toxicity of irinotecan-based regimens. Cancer Treat Rev. 2004;30:555-562.

389. Takasuna K, Hagiwara T, Hirohashi M, et al. Involvement of beta-glucuronidase in intestinal microflora in the intestinal toxicity of the antitumor camptothecin derivative irinotecan hydrochloride (CPT-11) in rats. Cancer Res. 1996;56:3752-3757.

390. Zidan J, Haim N, Beny A, et al. Octreotide in the treatment of severe chemotherapy-induced diarrhea. Ann Oncol. 2001;12: 227-229.

391. Ippoliti C, Champlin R, Bugazia N, et al. Use of octreotide in the symptomatic management of diarrhea induced by graft-versus-host disease in patients with hematologic malignancies. J Clin Oncol. 1997;15:3350-3354.

392. Sergio GC, Felix GM, Luis JV. Activated charcoal to prevent irinotecan-induced diarrhea in children. Pediatr Blood Cancer. 2008;51:49-52.

393. Gupta D, Lis C, Grutsch J. The relationship between dyspnea and patient satisfaction with quality of life in advanced cancer. Supportive Care Cancer. 2007;15:533-538.

394. Booth S, Silvester S, Todd C. Breathlessness in cancer and chronic obstructive pulmonary disease: using a qualitative approach to describe the experience of patients and carers. Palliat Support Care. 2003;1:337-344.

395. Reuben DB, Mor V. Dyspnea in terminally ill cancer patients. Chest. 1986;89:234-236.

396. Hardy JR, Turner R, Saunders M, A'Hern R. Prediction of survival in a hospital-based continuing care unit. Eur J Cancer. 1994;30A:284-288.

397. Thomas JR, von Gunten CF. Clinical management of dyspnoea. Lancet Oncol. 2002;3:223-228.

398. Schwartzstein RM, Manning HL, Weiss JW, Weinberger SE. Dyspnea: a sensory experience. Lung. 1990;168:185-199.

399. Adams L, Chronos N, Lane R, Guz A. The measurement of breathlessness induced in normal subjects: validity of two scaling techniques. Clin Sci (Lond). 1985;69:7-16.

400. Borg GA. Psychophysical bases of perceived exertion. Med Sci Sports Exerc. 1982;14:377-381.

401. Tanaka K, Akechi T, Okuyama T, et al. Prevalence and screening of dyspnea interfering with daily life activities in ambulatory patients with advanced lung cancer. J Pain Symptom Manage. 2002;23:484-489.

402. McGrath PJ, Pianosi PT, Unruh AM, Buckley CP. Dalhousie dyspnea scales: construct and content validity of pictorial scales for measuring dyspnea. BMC Pediatr. 2005;5:33.

403. Bruera E, MacEachern T, Ripamonti C, Hanson J. Subcutaneous morphine for dyspnea in cancer patients. Ann Intern Med. 1993;119:906-907.

404. Bruera E, Macmillan K, Pither J, MacDonald RN. Effects of morphine on the dyspnea of terminal cancer patients. J Pain Symptom Manage. 1990;5:341-344.

405. Mazzocato C, Buclin T, Rapin CH. The effects of morphine on dyspnea and ventilatory function in elderly patients with advanced cancer: A randomized double-blind controlled trial. Ann Oncol. 1999;10:1511-1514.

406. Allard P, Lamontagne C, Bernard P, Tremblay C. How effective are supplementary doses of opioids for dyspnea in terminally ill cancer patients? A randomized continuous sequential clinical trial. J Pain Symptom Manage. 1999;17:256-265.

407. Abernethy AP, Currow DC, Frith P, et al. Randomised, double blind, placebo-controlled crossover trial of sustained release morphine for the management of refractory dyspnoea. BMJ. 2003;327:523-528.

408. Graff GR, Stark JM, Grueber R. Nebulized fentanyl for palliation of dyspnea in a cystic fibrosis patient. Respiration. 2004;71:646-649.

409. Janahi IA, Maciejewski SR, Teran JM, Oermann CM. Inhaled morphine to relieve dyspnea in advanced cystic fibrosis lung disease. Pediatr Pulmonol. 2000;30:257-259.

410. Coyne PJ, Viswanathan R, Smith TJ. Nebulized fentanyl citrate improves patients' perception of breathing, respiratory rate, and oxygen saturation in dyspnea. J Pain Symptom Manage. 2002;23:157-160.

411. Bruera E, Sala R, Spruyt O, et al. Nebulized versus subcutaneous morphine for patients with cancer dyspnea: a preliminary study. J Pain Symptom Manage. 2005;29:613-618.

412. Jennings AL, Davies AN, Higgins JP, Broadley K. Opioids for the palliation of breathlessness in terminal illness. Cochrane Database Syst Rev. 2001;4:CD002066.

413. Dudgeon DJ, Lertzman M. Dyspnea in the advanced cancer patient. J Pain Symptom Manage. 1998;16:212-219.

414. Bruera E, de Stoutz N, Velasco-Leiva A, et al. Effects of oxygen on dyspnoea in hypoxaemic terminal-cancer patients. Lancet. 1993;342:13-14.

415. Bruera E, Sweeney C, Willey J, et al. A randomized controlled trial of supplemental oxygen versus air in cancer patients with dyspnea. Palliat Med. 2003;17:659-663.

416. Booth S, Kelly MJ, Cox NP, et al. Does oxygen help dyspnea in patients with cancer? Am J Respir Crit Care Med. 1996;153:1515-1518.

417. Philip J, Gold M, Milner A, et al. A randomized, double-blind, crossover trial of the effect of oxygen on dyspnea in patients with advanced cancer. J Pain Symptom Manage. 2006;32:541-550.

418. Schwartzstein RM, Lahive K, Pope A, et al. Cold facial stimulation reduces breathlessness induced in normal subjects. Am Rev Respir Dis. 1987;136:58-61.

419. Spence DP, Graham DR, Ahmed J, et al. Does cold air affect exercise capacity and dyspnea in stable chronic obstructive pulmonary disease? Chest. 1993;103:693-696.

420. von Leupoldt A, Seemann N, Gugleva T, Dahme B. Attentional distraction reduces the affective but not the sensory dimension of perceived dyspnea. Respir Med. 2007;101:839-844.

420a. Bredin M, Corner J, Krishnasamy M, et al. Multicentre randomised controlled trial of nursing intervention for breathlessness in patients with lung cancer. BMJ. 1999;318:901-904.

421. Booth S, Farquhar M, Gysels M, et al. The impact of a breathlessness intervention service (BIS) on the lives of patients with intractable dyspnea: a qualitative phase 1 study. Palliat Support Care. 2006;4:287-293.

422. Lingerfelt BM, Swainey CW, Smith TJ, Coyne PJ. Nebulized lidocaine for intractable cough near the end of life. J Support Oncol. 2007;5:301-302.

423. National Comprehensive Cancer Network Clincial Practice Guidelines in Oncology. Cancer-Related Fatigue, 2008. NCCN website. Available at http://www.nccn.org/professionals/physician_gls/PDF/fatigue.pdf.

424. Bower JE, Ganz PA, Desmond KA, et al. Fatigue in long-term breast carcinoma survivors: a longitudinal investigation. Cancer. 2006;106:751-758.

425. Loge JH, Abrahamsen AF, Ekeberg O, Kaasa S. Hodgkin's disease survivors more fatigued than the general population. J Clin Oncol. 1999;17:253-261.

426. Meeske KA, Patel SK, Palmer SN, et al. Factors associated with health-related quality of life in pediatric cancer survivors. Pediatr Blood Cancer. 2007;49:298-305.

427. Stone P, Hardy J, Broadley K, et al. Fatigue in advanced cancer: a prospective controlled cross-sectional study. Br J Cancer. 1999;79:1479-1486.

428. Vogelzang NJ, Breitbart W, Cella D, et al. Patient, caregiver, and oncologist perceptions of cancer-related fatigue: results of a tripart assessment survey. The Fatigue Coalition. Semin Hematol. 1997;34(Suppl 2):4-12.

429. Stasi R, Abriani L, Beccaglia P, et al. Cancer-related fatigue: evolving concepts in evaluation and treatment. Cancer. 2003;98:1786-1801.

430. Curt GA, Breitbart W, Cella D, et al. Impact of cancer-related fatigue on the lives of patients: new findings from the Fatigue Coalition. Oncologist. 2000;5:353-360.

431. Gibson F, Mulhall AB, Richardson A, et al. A phenomenologic study of fatigue in adolescents receiving treatment for cancer. Oncol Nurs Forum. 2005;32:651-660.

432. Iop A, Manfredi AM, Bonura S. Fatigue in cancer patients receiving chemotherapy: an analysis of published studies. Ann Oncol. 2004;15:712-720.

433. Malik UR, Makower DF, Wadler S. Interferon-mediated fatigue. Cancer. 2001;92(Suppl):1664-1668.

434. Shaiova L. The management of opioid-related sedation. Curr Pain Headache Rep. 2005;9(4):239-242.

435. Bourdeanu L, Loseth DB, Funk M. Management of opioid-induced sedation in patients with cancer. Clin J Oncol Nurs. 2005;9:705-711.

436. Stone P, Richardson A, Ream E, et al. Cancer-related fatigue: inevitable, unimportant and untreatable? Results of a multi-centre patient survey. Cancer Fatigue Forum. Ann Oncol. 2000;11:971-975.

437. Hockenberry MJ, Hinds PS, Barrera P, et al. Three instruments to assess fatigue in children with cancer: the child, parent and staff perspectives. J Pain Symptom Manage. 2003;25:319-328.

438. Varni JW, Burwinkle TM, Katz ER, et al. The PedsQL in pediatric cancer: reliability and validity of the Pediatric Quality of Life

Inventory Generic Core Scales, Multidimensional Fatigue Scale, and Cancer Module. Cancer. 2002;94:2090-2106.

439. Hinds PS, Hockenberry-Eaton M, Gilger E, et al. Comparing patient, parent, and staff descriptions of fatigue in pediatric oncology patients. Cancer Nurs. 1999;22:277-288.

440. Irvine D, Vincent L, Graydon JE, et al. The prevalence and correlates of fatigue in patients receiving treatment with chemotherapy and radiotherapy. A comparison with the fatigue experienced by healthy individuals. Cancer Nurs. 1994;17:367-378.

441. Akechi T, Kugaya A, Okamura H, et al. Fatigue and its associated factors in ambulatory cancer patients: a preliminary study. J Pain Symptom Manage. 1999;17:42-48.

442. Tranmer JE, Heyland D, Dudgeon D, et al. Measuring the symptom experience of seriously ill cancer and noncancer hospitalized patients near the end of life with the memorial symptom assessment scale. J Pain Symptom Manage. 2003;25:420-429.

443. Holzner B, Kemmler G, Greil R, et al. The impact of hemoglobin levels on fatigue and quality of life in cancer patients. Ann Oncol. 2002;13:965-973.

444. Munch TN, Zhang T, Willey J, et al. The association between anemia and fatigue in patients with advanced cancer receiving palliative care. J Palliat Med. 2005;8:1144-1149.

445. Gutstein HB. The biologic basis of fatigue. Cancer. 2001; 92(Suppl):1678-1683.

446. Shafqat A, Einhorn LH, Hanna N, et al. Screening studies for fatigue and laboratory correlates in cancer patients undergoing treatment. Ann Oncol. 2005;16:1545-1550.

447. Strasser F, Palmer JL, Schover LR, et al. The impact of hypogonadism and autonomic dysfunction on fatigue, emotional function, and sexual desire in male patients with advanced cancer: a pilot study. Cancer. 2006;107(12):2949-2957.

448. Stone P, Hardy J, Huddart R, et al. Fatigue in patients with prostate cancer receiving hormone therapy. Eur J Cancer. 2000; 36:1134-1141.

449. Bruera E, Brenneis C, Michaud M, et al. Muscle electrophysiology in patients with advanced breast cancer. J Natl Cancer Inst. 1988;80:282-285.

450. Fernandes R, Stone P, Andrews P, et al. Comparison between fatigue, sleep disturbance, and circadian rhythm in cancer inpatients and healthy volunteers: evaluation of diagnostic criteria for cancer-related fatigue. J Pain Symptom Manage. 2006;32: 245-254.

451. Mock V, Dow KH, Meares CJ, et al. Effects of exercise on fatigue, physical functioning, and emotional distress during radiation therapy for breast cancer. Oncol Nurs Forum. 1997; 24:991-1000.

452. Forester B, Kornfeld DS, Fleiss JL, Thompson S. Group psychotherapy during radiotherapy: effects on emotional and physical distress. Am J Psychiatry. 1993;150:1700-1706.

453. Given B, Given CW, McCorkle R, et al. Pain and fatigue management: results of a nursing randomized clinical trial. Oncol Nurs Forum. 2002;29:949-956.

454. Demetri GD, Kris M, Wade J, et al. Quality-of-life benefit in chemotherapy patients treated with epoetin alfa is independent of disease response or tumor type: results from a prospective community oncology study. Procrit Study Group. J Clin Oncol. 1998;16:3412-3425.

455. Razzouk BI, Hord JD, Hockenberry M, et al. Double-blind, placebo-controlled study of quality of life, hematologic end points, and safety of weekly epoetin alfa in children with cancer receiving myelosuppressive chemotherapy. J Clin Oncol. 2006;24: 3583-3589.

456. Leyland-Jones B, Semiglazov V, Pawlicki M, et al. Maintaining normal hemoglobin levels with epoetin alfa in mainly nonanemic patients with metastatic breast cancer receiving first-line chemotherapy: a survival study. J Clin Oncol. 2005;23:5960-5972.

457. Wright JR, Ung YC, Julian JA, et al. Randomized, double-blind, placebo-controlled trial of erythropoietin in nonsmall-cell lung cancer with disease-related anemia. J Clin Oncol. 2007;25: 1027-1032.

458. U.S. Food and Drug Administration. Information on Erythropoiesis-Stimulating Agents (ESA) (Marketed as Procrit, Epogen, and Aranesp), 2007. Available at http://www.fda.gov/cder/drug/infopage/RHE.

459. Bruera E, Miller MJ, Macmillan K, Kuehn N. Neuropsychological effects of methylphenidate in patients receiving a continuous infusion of narcotics for cancer pain. Pain. 1992;48:163-166.

460. Breitbart W, Rosenfeld B, Kaim M, Funesti-Esch J. A randomized, double-blind, placebo-controlled trial of psychostimulants for the treatment of fatigue in ambulatory patients with human immunodeficiency virus disease. Arch Intern Med. 2001;161: 411-420.

461. Bruera E, Driver L, Barnes EA, et al. Patient-controlled methylphenidate for the management of fatigue in patients with advanced cancer: a preliminary report. J Clin Oncol. 2003;21:4439-4443.

462. Thompson SJ, Leigh L, Christensen R, et al. Immediate neurocognitive effects of methylphenidate on learning-impaired survivors of childhood cancer. J Clin Oncol. 2001;19:1802-1808.

463. Yee JD, Berde CB. Dextroamphetamine or methylphenidate as adjuvants to opioid analgesia for adolescents with cancer. J Pain Symptom Manage. 1994;9:122-125.

464. Greenhill LL, Pliszka S, Dulcan MK, et al. Summary of the practice parameter for the use of stimulant medications in the treatment of children, adolescents, and adults. J Am Acad Child Adolesc Psychiatry. 2001;40:1352-1355.

465. Baptista-Neto L, Dodds A, Rao S, et al. An expert opinion on methylphenidate treatment for attention deficit hyperactivity disorder in pediatric patients with epilepsy. Expert Opin Investig Drugs. 2008;17:77-84.

466. Gucuyener K, Erdemoglu AK, Senol S, et al. Use of methylphenidate for attention-deficit hyperactivity disorder in patients with epilepsy or electroencephalographic abnormalities. J Child Neurol. 2003;18:109-112.

467. Rammohan KW, Rosenberg JH, Lynn DJ, et al. Efficacy and safety of modafinil (Provigil) for the treatment of fatigue in multiple sclerosis: a two-centre phase 2 study. J Neurol Neurosurg Psychiatry. 2002;72:179-183.

468. Webster L, Andrews M, Stoddard G. Modafinil treatment of opioid-induced sedation. Pain Med. 2003;4:135-140.

469. Bardia A, Greeno E, Bauer BA. Dietary supplement usage by patients with cancer undergoing chemotherapy: does prognosis or cancer symptoms predict usage? J Support Oncol. 2007;5: 195-198.

470. Cruciani RA, Dvorkin E, Homel P, et al. Safety, tolerability and symptom outcomes associated with L-carnitine supplementation in patients with cancer, fatigue, and carnitine deficiency: a phase I/II study. J Pain Symptom Manage. 2006;32:551-559.

471. Barton DL, Soori GS, Bauer B, et al. 2007 ASCO Annual Meeting Proceedings, Part I. J Clin Oncol. 2007;25:9001.

472. Krajnik M, Zylicz Z. Understanding pruritus in systemic disease. J Pain Symptom Manage. 2001;21:151-168.

473. Agero AL, Dusza SW, Benvenuto-Andrade C, et al. Dermatologic side effects associated with the epidermal growth factor receptor inhibitors. J Am Acad Dermatol. 2006;55:657-670.

474. Kranke P, Koetter K. Interventions for the treatment of opioid-induced pruritus (itching). Cochrane Database Syst Rev. 2004;2: CD004841.

475. Choi CJ, Nghiem P. Tacrolimus ointment in the treatment of chronic cutaneous graft-vs-host disease: a case series of 18 patients. Arch Dermatol. 2001;137:1202-1206.

476. Bergasa NV, Alling DW, Talbot TL, et al. Effects of naloxone infusions in patients with the pruritus of cholestasis: a double-blind, randomized, controlled trial. 1995;123:161-167.

477. Terg R, Coronel E, Sorda J, et al. Efficacy and safety of oral naltrexone treatment for pruritus of cholestasis, a crossover, double blind, placebo-controlled study. J Hepatol. 2002;37:717-722.

478. Wolfhagen FH, Sternieri E, Hop WC, et al. Oral naltrexone treatment for cholestatic pruritus: a double-blind, placebo-controlled study. Gastroenterology. 1997;113:1264-1269.

479. Raderer M, Muller C, Scheithauer W. Ondansetron for pruritus due to cholestasis. N Engl J Med. 1994;330:1540.

480. Schworer H, Hartmann H, Ramadori G. Relief of cholestatic pruritus by a novel class of drugs: 5-hydroxytryptamine type 3 (5-HT3) receptor antagonists: effectiveness of ondansetron. Pain. 1995;61:33-37.

481. Muller C, Pongratz S, Pidlich J, et al. Treatment of pruritus in chronic liver disease with the 5-hydroxytryptamine receptor type 3 antagonist ondansetron: a randomized, placebo-controlled, double-blind cross-over trial. Eur J Gastroenterol Hepatol. 1998; 10:865-870.

482. Prommer E. Re: Pruritus in patients with advanced cancer. J Pain Symptom Manage. 2005;30:201-202.

483. Ashmore SD, Jones CH, Newstead CG, et al. Ondansetron therapy for uremic pruritus in hemodialysis patients. Am J Kidney Dis. 2000;35:827-831.

484. Balaskas EV, Bamihas GI, Karamouzis M, et al. Histamine and serotonin in uremic pruritus: effect of ondansetron in CAPD-pruritic patients. Nephron. 1998;78:395-402.

485. Peer G, Kivity S, Agami O, et al. Randomised crossover trial of naltrexone in uraemic pruritus. Lancet. 1996;348:1552-1554.

486. Pauli-Magnus C, Mikus G, Alscher DM, et al. Naltrexone does not relieve uremic pruritus: results of a randomized, double-blind, placebo-controlled crossover study. J Am Soc Nephrol. 2000;11: 514-519.

487. Juneja MM, Ackerman WE 3rd, Bellinger K. Epidural morphine pruritus reduction with hydroxyzine in parturients. J Ky Med Assoc. 1991;89:319-321.

488. Gan TJ, Ginsberg B, Glass PS, et al. Opioid-sparing effects of a low-dose infusion of naloxone in patient-administered morphine sulfate. Anesthesiology. 1997;87:1075-1081.

489. Katcher J, Walsh D. Opioid-induced itching: morphine sulfate and hydromorphone hydrochloride. J Pain Symptom Manage. 1999;17:70-72.

490. Goodarzi M. Comparison of epidural morphine, hydromorphone and fentanyl for postoperative pain control in children undergoing orthopaedic surgery. Paediatr Anaesth. 1999;9:419-422.

491. Kyriakides K, Hussain SK, Hobbs GJ. Management of opioid-induced pruritus: a role for 5-HT3 antagonists? Br J Anaesth. Mar 1999;82:439-441.

492. Yeh HM, Chen LK, Lin CJ, et al. Prophylactic intravenous ondansetron reduces the incidence of intrathecal morphine-induced pruritus in patients undergoing cesarean delivery. Anesth Analg. 2000;91:172-175.

493. Borgeat A, Stirnemann HR. Ondansetron is effective to treat spinal or epidural morphine-induced pruritus. Anesthesiology. 1999;90(2):432-436.

494. Arai L, Stayer S, Schwartz R, Dorsey A. The use of ondansetron to treat pruritus associated with intrathecal morphine in two paediatric patients. Paediatr Anaesth. 1996;6:337-339.

495. Charuluxananan S, Kyokong O, Somboonviboon W, et al. Nalbuphine versus ondansetron for prevention of intrathecal morphine-induced pruritus after cesarean delivery. Anesth Analg. 2003;96:1789-1793.

496. Bigliardi PL, Stammer H, Jost G, et al. Treatment of pruritus with topically applied opiate receptor antagonist. J Am Acad Dermatol. 2007;56:979-988.

497. Hariharan B, Rajagopal MR. Re: Paroxetine in the treatment of severe nondermatological pruritus. J Pain Symptom Manage. 2005;29:115.

498. Michalowski M, Ketzer C, Daudt L, Rohde LA. Emotional and behavioral symptoms in children with acute leukemia. Haematologica. 2001;86:821-826.

499. Noll RB, Gartstein MA, Vannatta K, et al. Social, emotional, and behavioral functioning of children with cancer. Pediatrics. 1999;103:71-78.

500. Allen R, Newman SP, Souhami RL. Anxiety and depression in adolescent cancer: findings in patients and parents at the time of diagnosis. Eur J Cancer. 1997;33:1250-1255.

501. Frank NC, Blount RL, Brown RT. Attributions, coping, and adjustment in children with cancer. J Pediatr Psychol. 1997;22: 563-576.

502. Phipps S, Fairclough D, Mulhern RK. Avoidant coping in children with cancer. J Pediatr Psychol. 1995;20:217-232.

503. Wedding U, Koch A, Rohrig B, et al. Requestioning depression in patients with cancer: contribution of somatic and affective symptoms to Beck's Depression Inventory. Ann Oncol. 2007; 18:1875-1881.

504. Hedstrom M, Kreuger A, Ljungman G, et al. Accuracy of assessment of distress, anxiety, and depression by physicians and nurses in adolescents recently diagnosed with cancer. Pediatr Blood Cancer. 2006;46:773-779.

505. Varni JW, Katz E. Stress, social support and negative affectivity in children with newly diagnosed cancer: a prospective transactional analysis. Psychooncology. 1997;6:267-278.

506. Last BF, van Veldhuizen AM. Information about diagnosis and prognosis related to anxiety and depression in children with cancer aged 8-16 years. Eur J Cancer. 1996;32A:290-294.

507. Zebrack BJ, Zeltzer LK, Whitton J, et al. Psychological outcomes in long-term survivors of childhood leukemia, Hodgkin's disease, and non-Hodgkin's lymphoma: a report from the Childhood Cancer Survivor Study. Pediatrics. 2002;110(Pt 1):42-52.

508. Schultz KA, Ness KK, Whitton J, et al. Behavioral and social outcomes in adolescent survivors of childhood cancer: a report from the childhood cancer survivor study. J Clin Oncol. 2007; 25:3649-3656.

509. Pao M, Ballard ED, Rosenstein DL, et al. Psychotropic medication use in pediatric patients with cancer. Arch Pediatr Adolesc Med. 2006;160:818-822.

510. Kersun LS, Kazak AE. Prescribing practices of selective serotonin reuptake inhibitors (SSRIs) among pediatric oncologists: a single institution experience. Pediatr Blood Cancer. 2006;47:339-342.

511. Hammad TA, Laughren T, Racoosin J. Suicidality in pediatric patients treated with antidepressant drugs. Arch Gen Psychiatry. 2006;63:332-339.

512. U.S. Food and Drug Administration. Antidepressant Use in Children, Adolescents, and Adults, 2007. Available at http://www.fda. gov/cder/drug/antidepressants/default.htm.

513. Buss MK, Vanderwerker LC, Inouye SK, et al. Associations between caregiver-perceived delirium in patients with cancer and generalized anxiety in their caregivers. J Palliat Med. 2007;10: 1083-1092.

514. Ozbolt LB, Paniagua MA, Kaiser RM. Atypical antipsychotics for the treatment of delirious elders. J Am Med Dir Assoc. 2008;9:18-28.

Lisa B. Kenney and Lisa Diller

Advances in the treatment of childhood cancer have resulted in increasing numbers of children cured of this once universally fatal diagnosis. As a result, more children and young adults are childhood cancer survivors. Although children and adults who are long-term survivors are considered cured, it is widely recognized that the diagnosis and treatment of cancer during childhood and adolescence have lifelong implications for the survivor's health and well-being. The care of the child or adolescent diagnosed with cancer does not end with the completion of therapy, but rather continues on a trajectory into adulthood. Consequently, the clinical focus shifts from treatment of the primary cancer and screening for its recurrence to prevention and management of adverse consequences of prior therapy.

Cancer therapy administered to children and adolescents during critical periods of growth and development render childhood cancer survivors vulnerable to various physical and emotional disorders, often referred to as late effects. Some late effects can be diagnosed soon after completion of therapy and others may not manifest until decades later. The severity of late effects ranges from minor disabilities to life-threatening morbidities, including second cancers, cardiac disease, and pulmonary dysfunction. Severe late effects can reduce a survivor's life expectancy. Remarkable progress has been made in advancing our understanding of the adverse health outcomes associated with treatment for childhood cancer. Despite this, survivors continue to experience significant long-term morbidity related to late effects. Much remains to be learned about the early detection and management of the unintentional consequences of treatment. Ultimately, ongoing research may result in the reduction or even elimination of late effects and in improved quality of life for childhood cancer survivors.

HISTORY AND OVERVIEW

Prior to 1950, children and adolescents rarely survived a cancer diagnosis. The first generation of survivors primarily consisted of children with Hodgkin's lymphoma, sarcoma, and Wilms' tumor who were successfully treated with surgery and high-dose, large-field radiation therapy.[1-4] The widespread use of multiagent chemotherapy in the 1970s resulted in dramatic increases in survival for the most common childhood cancer, acute leukemia, and continued improvement in survival for other pediatric cancers as well.[5] By the mid-1970s, many forms of childhood cancer became treatable, and often curable. Continuing advances in treatment for childhood cancer, including dose and time intensification of chemotherapy regimens, the introduction of new chemotherapeutic agents, refinements in surgical techniques, and the use of alternative modes of delivering radiotherapy, have continued to improve survival. Children with cancer have also benefited from improvements in diagnostic testing, resulting in earlier and more precise diagnosis and more timely delivery of necessary treatment. Enhanced supportive care, including advances in intensive care, blood banking, and management of infectious disease, has also contributed to successful treatment. Currently, the overall 5-year survival for childhood cancer approaches 75%, and for some cancer diagnoses the 5-year survival is above 95% (Fig. 32-1A).[6] Based on these survival statistics, there are an estimated 250,000 young adult survivors of childhood cancer in the U.S. population, and this number continues to grow by approximately 10,000 survivors each year.[6]

Recognition of Late Effects

Along with these truly remarkable advances in survival, there was a growing recognition that treatment for childhood cancer is associated with long-term complications or late effects. Late effects can be defined as adverse health outcomes experienced by childhood cancer survivors associated with previous curative therapy that reduce survival or affect the quality of survival. Some late effects, such as second cancers and cardiac disease, are life-threatening and contribute to the increased mortality rates observed in adults who are long-term survivors of childhood cancer. Other late effects, such as neurocognitive impairment, physical deformity, and infertility, can limit survivors' social or economic opportunities and impair their overall quality of life. In contrast, some late effects may be positive effects, such as an increase in psychological resiliency, decrease in smoking rates, and decrease in other high-risk behaviors in survivors compared with control populations.[7,8]

Second cancers, cardiopulmonary disease, and infertility were among the first treatment-associated late effects observed in childhood cancer survivors. These first descriptions were based on clinical observations in small numbers of the earliest survivors of childhood cancer treated primarily with surgery and radiation in the 1960s.[9-11] These early clinical observations created awareness about late effects and identified the need for future research to define treatment-related health outcomes for growing numbers of survivors.

Early Mortality

Follow-up studies of the earliest cohorts led to the observation that childhood cancer survivors are at risk for early mortality. These studies have shown that late recurrence of the primary cancer and treatment-associated complications result in decreased long-term survival: 80% at 20 years after diagnosis compared with 97% expected survival in the age-matched general population.[12,13] Most premature deaths observed in survivors in these early studies were attributed to late relapse, whereas treatment-associated second cancers and major organ toxicity accounted for 30% of deaths.[12-15] It was also recognized that the risk of dying from a treatment-related cause increased with increasing intensity of therapy. Modern therapy has succeeded in reducing the overall risk for late mortality observed in survivors, mostly as a result of reduction in deaths caused by primary cancer recurrence (90% survival at 20 years; see Fig. 32-1B).[16,17] Although late recurrence accounts for most premature deaths observed in childhood cancer survivors, the risk of relapse diminishes over time, whereas the risk of therapy-related mortality persists beyond 25 years of follow-up.[17,18] It remains to be determined whether current treatment protocols that are specifically designed to reduce late effects will continue to improve very long-term survival by reducing the risk of therapy-related mortality.

Identifying Risk Factors for Late Effects

Following the early descriptive studies, registry-based investigations of larger groups of childhood cancer survivors were undertaken with the aim of identifying specific risk factors for late effects. These included the following: the National Cancer Institute's Five Center Study, a registry-based cohort that enrolled 2490 adult 5-year survivors younger than 20 years treated from 1945 to 1975 for cancer who were followed prospectively for reproductive outcomes, second cancers, and mor-

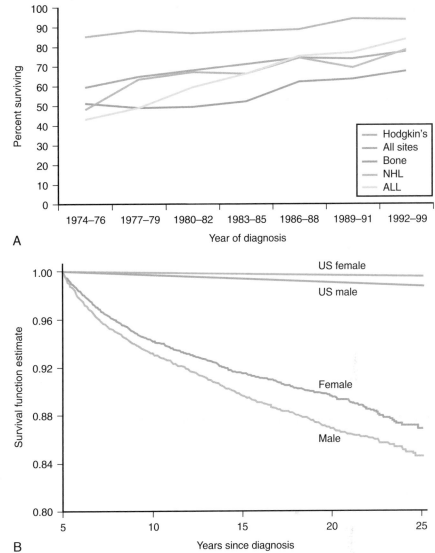

FIGURE 32-1. A, Trends in 5-year cancer survival by selected diagnosis, age younger than 20 years, 1974-1999. **B,** Gender-specific survival, all causes of mortality, 5-year survivors of childhood cancer diagnosed 1970-1986, age younger than 21 years. ALL, acute lymphoblastic leukemia; NHL, non-Hodgkin's lymphoma. *(A adapted from Ries LAG, Eisner MP, Kosary CL, et al. SEER Cancer Statistics, 1975-2000. Bethesda, Md, National Cancer Institute, 2000; **B** adapted from Mertens AC, Yasui Y, Liu Y, et al. Pulmonary complications in survivors of childhood and adolescent cancer: a report from the Childhood Cancer Survivor Study. Cancer. 2002;95:2431-2441.)*

tality[19]; the Late Effects Study Group, a multi-institution–based cohort, which analyzed the occurrence of second cancers in 9170 2-year survivors of childhood cancer diagnosed from 1936 to 1979[20]; and cancer registry–based studies in the United Kingdom,[21] and the Netherlands,[22] and Denmark, Finland, Iceland, Norway, and Sweden[23] from the same early treatment era and beyond. These epidemiologic studies analyzed the association between specific treatments and the adverse health outcomes of interest. Relative risks were calculated to compare rates of a particular outcome in cancer survivors with rates of the outcome in a control population. Collectively, these investigations made significant contributions to the understanding of late effects, but their limitations should be noted. First, the cohorts under investigation were often not large enough to address the relationship between details of treatment, such as range of doses, and rare outcomes of interest. Second, the late effects observed in these cohorts were usually associated with historical treatments that had already been replaced by modern modalities. Last, recruitment for these follow-up studies of late-occurring outcomes was often incomplete, resulting in a possible overrepresentation of childhood cancer survivors who were experiencing health conditions related to their prior therapy.

Despite these limitations, these studies were able to identify the relationships, now well accepted, between cancer therapy and early mortality, radiation therapy and secondary cancers, and alkylating agents and gonadal dysfunction.[15,19,24,25]

To address the limitations of prior studies, the development of survivor cohorts prospectively followed was undertaken by investigators in North America and Europe. In the United States, a multi-institutional follow-up study of a cohort of over 14,000 childhood cancer survivors, the Childhood Cancer Survivor Study (CCSS), was created to evaluate late effects in survivors treated with modern therapies (1970 to 1986).[26] The CCSS uses self-reported questionnaires to obtain health outcomes and analyzes the association between outcome and treatment variables documented in abstracted medical records. The primary end points investigated by the CCSS include second cancers, mortality, and heart disease. Large registry-based cohort studies of childhood cancer survivors treated in Britain, the Netherlands, and Denmark are ongoing and continue to contribute to our understanding of survivorship.[27,28] These cohorts have the advantage of national health care systems, in which medical records are centralized; diagnosis, treatment, and outcomes can be efficiently linked and self-reported outcomes validated. The high prevalence of chronic disease and the poor health status observed in survivors participating in these large cohorts have resulted in a change in thinking about childhood cancer as a curable disease to considering childhood cancer as a lifelong condition.

Interpreting Late Effects Research

Advances continue to be made in recognizing and categorizing late effects in childhood cancer survivors. However, the study of late effects in cancer survivors has inherent challenges that must be considered when interpreting research findings. First, there is no consensus on the definition of cancer survivor. The definition chosen by investigators determines eligibility for studies and influences how results can be interpreted and generalized to specific populations of survivors. The U.S. Office of Cancer Survivorship at the National Cancer Institute considers an individual a cancer survivor from the moment of cancer diagnosis through the remainder of his or her life, regardless of degree of cancer control.[29] Although this definition is meaningful from an advocacy perspective, it is not useful for the purposes of understanding late outcomes in a cured population. Survival 5 years beyond cancer diagnosis is the definition of cancer survivor that is most often, but not universally, used for the purpose of research on late effects.

Another consideration is how investigators measure the late effect of interest. Self-report is frequently used to measure outcomes in epidemiologic studies of late effects. Although cost-effective, self-report can lead to reporting bias that results in inaccurate measures of the incidence or severity of outcomes. Studies of smaller groups of survivors using direct observation to delineate outcomes help confirm self-reported outcomes, refine our understanding of these outcomes, and allow direct measurement of asymptomatic or early morbidity that is not evident by self-report. The disadvantages of this type of clinical studies are cost, complexity, and small sample size, which can limit the interpretation of results.

The timing of assessments can also influence the results and interpretation of late effects research. It is most efficient to recruit survivors for follow-up studies during or soon after treatment. However, late effects often are not observed until decades after initial therapy. Studies with inadequate periods of follow-up might yield results that underestimate or overestimate late effects. Retaining survivors in observational cohorts over long periods of follow-up is challenging and results are biased toward retention of patients experiencing the outcomes under investigation. Duration of follow-up is particularly important when applying results to populations of pediatric survivors, in whom late effects may emerge in the course of developmental change.

Another challenge when interpreting the results of late effects studies is that most results are reported as relative risks, the rate of an outcome observed in a cohort of survivors relative to the rate of the outcome observed in a control population. Elevated relative risks must be interpreted and communicated with caution, because even the smallest increase in an otherwise rare outcome results in a large relative risk; however, even a small or statistically insignificant increase in relative risk might have important clinical implications.

Finally, an inherent difficulty with studying late effects in survivors is that treatments for cancer continue to evolve, so the health outcomes of interest in follow-up studies are often reflective of historical or outdated treatments. Methodology does not exist to address this issue, so treatment period must be taken into consideration when interpreting the results of these investigations. Duration of follow-up, treatment era, cohort eligibility, and outcome measures are all aspects of study design that merit careful consideration when interpreting results of late effects research studies.

Box 32-1	**Risk Factors for Late Effects in Childhood Cancer Survivors**

TREATMENT FACTORS

Time since treatment
Modality, dose, and intensity of treatment
Concurrent treatments
Prior treatment toxicities

INDIVIDUAL FACTORS

Age
Developmental stage
Gender
Genetic predisposition
Health behaviors
Comorbidities

General Principles of Late Effects

Epidemiologic studies investigating the association between treatment and risk of adverse health outcomes have led to general principles that contribute to our thinking about an individual survivor's potential for developing late effects (Box 32-1). A childhood cancer survivor's risk for developing late effects depends on the nature of prior treatment and individual characteristics that can modify risk for treatment toxicity.

First, the dose and intensity of the treatment are directly correlated with the risk for late effects. In general, survivors exposed to larger doses of therapy have worse outcomes. For example, risk of male infertility after treatment with gonadotoxic chemotherapy is directly related to dose; males exposed to the highest cumulative doses have the greatest risk for future infertility.[30] In addition, a survivor's likelihood for late effects is increased if there is exposure from more than one modality with related toxicities. For example, survivors treated concurrently with mediastinal irradiation and cardiotoxic chemotherapy are at greater risk for cardiac late effects than those treated with either of those modalities alone.[31]

Organ toxicity associated with a single treatment exposure can manifest clinically as different late effects, depending on the timing of the clinical assessment. For example, consider a postmenarchal female adolescent treated with gonadotoxic chemotherapy. During treatment, she might experience acute reversible amenorrhea. Years later, after resolution of acute menorrhea, the woman might experience infertility secondary to premature menopause. Over time, the same woman might have osteoporosis as a secondary late effect of chronic estrogen deficiency. Neurocognitive impairment after central nervous system (CNS) therapy provides another example of how the timing of assessment influences detection of late effects. Children treated with CNS therapy might not manifest treatment-related neurocognitive deficits until they reach a time when schoolwork, employment responsibilities, or social interactions require more complex cognitive function. The clinical manifestations of a single toxic treatment exposure can change over time and are influenced by the physical, emotional, and social needs of the individual survivor.

Duration of follow-up also influences the potential for late effects. Some radiation-associated late effects, especially secondary malignancies, have long latency periods, with increases in cumulative incidence over time. In contrast, other treatment-related toxicities can be acute and resolve (bone marrow suppression), or occur late and be progressive (pulmonary fibrosis). The leukemogenic potentials of specific forms of chemotherapy appear to be associated with fairly discrete time frames after exposures; topoisomerase inhibitors are associated with the development of secondary leukemias within months of exposure and almost never beyond 5 years, whereas alkylating agents are associated with a later onset and a later but still predictable plateau in cumulative incidence at 10 years after exposure.[32] Acute chemotherapy organ toxicity can sometimes predict late toxicity. For example, chemotherapy-associated acute cardiomyopathy diagnosed during therapy can sometimes persist as a chronic condition or resolve and be diagnosed again decades after treatment. However, chemotherapy-associated late-onset cardiomyopathy can also be observed in the absence of acute toxicity.

Although treatment exposures are the largest determinants of future late effects, medical history, family history, and personal habits can modulate a survivor's risk. A survivor's age or developmental stage during cancer treatment, his or her gender, family history, health behaviors, and existing comorbidities can all contribute to the risk for late effects. In general, younger age at treatment is associated with a higher risk and/or greater severity of late effects. Children treated with cranial irradiation during the critical period of rapid brain development (younger than 2 years) are at greater risk for neurocognitive late effects than children treated when they are older.[33] In addition, female survivors are at greater risk than males for some late effects, including chemotherapy-associated cardiomyopathy, neurocognitive impairment, and second cancers, although the explanation for this gender difference is not clear.[34-37]

An underlying genetic predisposition for cancer, contributing as a causative factor in the primary cancer occurrence, will influence the risk of secondary cancers, as has been observed in hereditary retinoblastoma and nevoid basal cell carcinoma syndrome. In some patients, the only marker of this predisposition will be family history or the features of the primary tumor itself (e.g., young age at occurrence, occurrence in paired organs). Those survivors with a genetic predisposition to chronic medical conditions, such as heart disease, may be at greater risk for those treatment-associated chronic conditions, such as radiation-associated coronary artery disease.[38] Similarly, medical comorbidities such as hypertension or hypercholesterolemia may contribute to a survivor's risk for various medical late effects, including chronic renal disease, heart disease, and cerebral vascular disease. Modifiable health behaviors such as diet, exercise, smoking, and sun exposure may also modulate a survivor's risk for late effects.

SPECIFIC LATE EFFECTS

The following section provides an overview of the common late effects experienced by survivors of childhood cancer. The current understanding of pathophysiology, incidence, risk factors, evaluation, and management of late effects is presented. A summary of the risk estimates for selected treatment-associated late effects is presented in Table 32-1.

Second Cancers

Second cancers are the leading cause of treatment-related mortality in long-term survivors. In the CCSS cohort, second

cancers accounted for 13% of deaths overall and 60% of deaths defined as treatment-related.[16] Usually, a new cancer diagnosed in a survivor can be associated with a prior treatment exposure, such as radiation therapy or alkylating agent chemotherapy. Genetic cancer predisposition may also contribute to a survivor's risk for subsequent cancers. In addition, survivors are at risk for cancers unrelated to prior treatment or known genetic predisposition, and these cancers will become more prevalent as the childhood cancer survivor population ages. To date, there are no data that address the comparative morbidity and mortality from these adult-onset cancers and whether survivors will be compromised in their ability to receive or respond to known effective therapies.

Overall, the likelihood of a childhood cancer survivor being diagnosed with a second primary cancer is six times greater than the risk in the age-matched general population.[6,39-41] At 20 years after diagnosis, the cumulative incidence of second cancers in childhood cancer survivors is estimated at 3.2% to 4.2%. Treatment factors that increase the risk of second cancers include exposure to radiation and chemotherapy with alkylating agents or epipodophyllotoxins. Other cancer treatments that have been associated with an increased risk of secondary malignancy include anthracycline chemotherapy[42-44] and splenectomy.[45,46] As with many late effects, females and those diagnosed at the youngest age are at greatest risk for a second malignant neoplasm. Diagnoses that confer the greatest risk for subsequent cancers include Hodgkin's lymphoma (relative risk [RR] = 10), sarcomas (RR = 14), and retinoblastoma (RR = 15).[39,40]

A genetic predisposition for second cancers results from an inherited or spontaneous germline mutation in a known or presumed cancer susceptibility gene. Characteristic findings in family cancer predisposition syndromes are younger age at cancer diagnosis, cancer in two or more generations, two or more cancers in an individual, and rare forms of cancer in combination.[47,48] An example of a rare cancer predisposition syndrome associated with pediatric malignancies is Li-Fraumeni syndrome, which results from mutations in the tumor suppressor gene *TP53*. It is inherited as an autosomal dominant trait and has a high penetrance, with a cancer risk of 50% by age 40 years. The cancers most commonly observed in Li-Fraumeni syndrome are soft tissue sarcomas, breast cancer, leukemia, osteosarcoma, adrenocortical cancer, and brain tumors.

Survivors with an underlying genetic predisposition for cancer may be more susceptible to treatment-associated secondary malignancies. This is demonstrated in survivors of retinoblastoma who carry a mutation in the *RB1* gene. Those with hereditary retinoblastoma treated with radiation for their primary cancer have a cumulative risk of second cancers of 58% at 50 years, compared with 26% if not treated with radiation.[49] There are other rare genetic syndromes associated with an increased susceptibility to pediatric cancers and subsequent adult-onset cancers, including Cowden's syndrome, neurofibromatosis types 1 and 2, familial polyposis, ataxia telangiectasia, xeroderma pigmentosum, Beckwith-Wiedemann syndrome, Bloom syndrome, Fanconi's anemia, Bannayan-Riley-Ruvalcaba syndrome, Turcot syndrome, Carney complex, Gorlin's syndrome, and tuberous sclerosis.[50] Survivors with a history suggestive of an underlying cancer predisposition syndrome should be referred for genetic counseling and have ongoing surveillance for syndrome-associated cancers and treatment-related secondary cancers.

Secondary Solid Tumors

Cancer that develops in a prior radiation field is the most common type of second cancer observed in survivors.[39,40] Risk

TABLE 32-1	**Risk of Selected Late Effects by Treatment Exposure**		
Treatment	**Late Effect**	**Risk Estimates***	**Comments**
Alkylating agents (busulfan, carmustine, lomustine, mechlorethamine, procarbazine, cyclophosphamide, ifosfamide, dacarbazine, melphalan)	Secondary leukemia, myelodysplasia[20,21,24,40,108]	RR = 1.6-20; CI = 0.2%-2.9% at 15 yr	Melphalan and mechlorethamine more leukemogenic than cyclophosphamide; median latency 4-6 yr; dose-response relationship
	Premature menopause[255,256]	RR = 2.3-9.2; CI = 10%-15% by age 40	Risk factors: high cumulative total dose, concurrent pelvic radiation; myeloablative doses associated with ovarian failure
	Male infertility[19,30,260]	Prevalence, 20%-60%	Azoospermia detected at cumulative cyclophosphamide dose > 5 g/m^2; cyclophosphamide > 20 g/m^2 associated with diminished testosterone production
Anthracyclines (daunorubicin, doxorubicin, mitoxantrone, idarubicin)	Clinical heart failure[37,117-119]	RR = 4.5-12; CI = 4%-5% at 20 yr	Risk factors: female gender, age < 5 yr, cumulative equivalent dose > 300 mg/m^2, concurrent radiation
Bleomycin, BCNU, busulfan carmustine (pulmonary toxic chemotherapies)	Pulmonary fibrosis[160]	RR = 1.4-2.1; CI = 0.8% at 20 yr	Usually preceded by acute pneumonitis; no plateau in incidence observed
Platinum compounds (cisplatin, carboplatin)	High-frequency hearing loss[241,244,246]	Prevalence, 50%	Cumulative dose cisplatin > 450 mg/m^2; risk factors: dose, age < 5 yr; carboplatin ototoxic at myeloablative dose
	Speech frequency hearing loss[241,244,246]	Prevalence, 20%-25%	Cumulative dose cisplatin > 720 mg/m^2; rarely observed cumulative dose cisplatin < 360 mg/m^2; Risk factors: dose, age < 5 yr; carboplatin ototoxic at myeloablative dose
Topoisomerase II inhibitors (epipodophyllotoxins, anthracyclines)	Secondary leukemia[21,44,109,111,112,114]	RR = 3.4-40; CI = 4% at 6 yr	Median latency, 1-3 yr; frequent administration increases risk (weekly, twice weekly); dose-response relationship
Radiation (any type)	Secondary sarcoma[40,42,54,57,58,92-95]	RR = 9-40; CI = 1%-3% at 30 yr	Risk factors: high radiation dose (40-60 Gy), concurrent alkylating agent therapy, young age at diagnosis, primary diagnosis of sarcoma or retinoblastoma
	Nonmelanomatous skin cancer[106]	RR = 6.3	50% of survivors will have multiple lesions
	Melanoma[39,104]	SIR = 5-9	Risk factors: radiation dose > 15 Gy, prior history melanoma, retinoblastoma, familial melanoma
Cranial, head and neck radiation (including TBI)	Growth hormone deficiency[162,168,169]	Prevalence, 85%-100%	Median dose, 45-55 Gy; observed at 18-24 Gy, with lower prevalence and longer latency
	Obesity[206]	OR = 1.9-2.6	Risk factors: ≥20 Gy cranial radiation, female gender, age < 5 yr
	Hypothyroidism[77,162,168]	RR = 17 CI = 30-50% at 20 yrs	Direct neck radiation ≥ 10 Gy; central hypothyroidism, cranial dose > 35 Gy; dose-response relationship with no plateau in incidence observed after neck radiation
	Thyroid cancer[77-83]	SIR = 10-35 CI = 5% at 30 yr	Risk factors: radiation dose 20-30 Gy, young age at treatment, female gender
	Brain tumors[36,39,40,97-99]	SIR = 10-20 CI = 3% at 30 yr	Meningioma: median latency = 20 yr; glioma: median latency = 9 yr; risk factors: increasing radiation dose, age < 5 yr at treatment, CNS leukemia at diagnosis
	Head and neck carcinoma[40,60]	SIR = 13-27	Parotid gland carcinoma most common secondary head and neck carcinoma
	Stroke[154]	RR = 6.4-29	Mean cranial radiation dose ≥ 30 Gy—increased risk for both leukemia and brain tumor survivors; highest risk after cranial dose ≥ 50Gy
	Dental abnormalities[315-317]	Prevalence, 50%-94%	Risk factors: age at diagnosis < 5 yr, higher dose radiation
Chest radiation (chest, mantle, lung, mediastinal, TBI)	Coronary artery disease[28,31,137,138,140]	RR = 5-40; prevalence, 14%-20%	Risk factor: dose > 30 Gy
	Cardiac valve disease[38,145]	Prevalence, 16%-42%	Risk factor: dose > 40 Gy
	Breast cancer[24,55,65-72]	SIR = 15-30; CI = 12%-35% at 20 yr	Risk factor: radiation dose > 20 Gy; latency 10-15 yr Ovarian failure reduces risk
	Lung fibrosis[154,158,160]	RR = 4.3; CI = 3.5% at 20 yr	Risk factors: younger age at exposure, concurrent pulmonary toxic chemotherapy
	Lung cancer[40,59,60,78]	SIR = 4-27	Increased risk in smokers
	Thyroid cancer[77-83]	SIR = 10-35; CI = 5% at 30 yr	Risk factors: radiation dose 20-30 Gy, young age at treatment, female gender
	Hypothyroidism[77,162,168]	RR = 17; CI = 30%-50% at 20 yr	Dose-response relationship; no plateau in incidence observed

TABLE 32-1	Risk of Selected Late Effects by Treatment Exposure—cont'd		
Treatment	**Late Effect**	**Risk Estimates***	**Comments**
Abdominal radiation (abdominal, periaortic, flank)	Gastrointestinal cancer[40,60,61]	SIR = 2.5-15	Risk factor: dose > 30 Gy
Pelvic radiation (pelvic, inverted Y, TBI)	Genitourinary tract cancer[40,60]	SIR = 1.4-3.1	Not statistically significant increased risk
	Premature menopause[187,255,256]	RR = 3.7-5.7; CI = 30%-40% by age 40 yr	Risk factors: dose (1-20 Gy), concurrent alkylating agent chemotherapy; pelvic radiation > 20 Gy associated with ovarian failure

*Risk estimates presented in this table represent a summary of data available in the medical literature. Rate ratios (relative risk, odds ratio) are calculated by comparing incidence and prevalence of the late effect reported or observed in a survivor cohort to incidence and prevalence reported or observed in a control population (most often sibling or nonexposed survivors). Standardized incidence ratios are calculated by comparing frequency of late effect observed in survivor cohort to frequency expected in age-matched general population.

CI, cumulative incidence; CNS, central nervous system; OR, odds ratio; RR, relative risk; SIR, standardized incidence ratio; TBI, total-body irradiation.

estimates for second cancers have been reported from populations of survivors treated with radiation during historical treatment eras, when the modes of radiation therapy routinely used in clinical practice were different from those used at present. In current oncology practice, megavoltage radiation has replaced orthovoltage radiation, thus reducing radiation doses to nontumor tissues such as skin, bones, and soft tissue. Large-dose extended-field radiotherapy is increasingly being replaced by involved-field lower dose radiotherapy or conformal radiotherapy, often in combination with chemotherapy. It is assumed that this change in clinical practice aimed at reducing exposure to radiation will result in a lower incidence of radiogenic cancer. However, no safe dose of therapeutic radiation has been established and radiation-associated cancers have been observed at what would be considered the lowest treatment doses.[51,52] Encouraging data are available from a study that compared second cancer risk associated with typical therapy using a mantle field to current involved-field radiotherapy by using dosimetric risk modeling. This study predicted a 35% to 65% reduction in relative risk of secondary cancers in Hodgkin's disease survivors.[53] It is still uncertain whether these data derived from predictive models will accurately reflect what will be observed clinically in radiation treated survivors over time.

In general, risk factors for radiation-associated second cancers include treatment with radiation doses higher than 30 Gy, radiation therapy in combination with alkylating agent or anthracycline chemotherapy, young age at exposure, more than 10 years beyond treatment, and the presence of a cancer predisposition syndrome.[22,24,42,54] Of particular concern is the observation that the cumulative incidence of radiation-associated cancers does not plateau in groups of survivors followed for up to 50 years after treatment for childhood cancer.[24,55-58] Second cancer risk is modulated by lifestyle choices; for example, survivors who smoke after exposure to chest irradiation have a 20-fold greater risk of secondary lung cancer compared with survivors who are nonsmokers.[56,59] This finding supports the notion that accumulation of further DNA damage after initial radiation-induced insult contributes to the pathogenesis of secondary cancers in survivors. Survival after a diagnosis of secondary radiogenic cancer may be lower than that observed in population-based cancers because, biologically, these cancers may be more resistant to therapy, and organ toxicity from prior therapy may limit treatment options.

All tissues and organs are vulnerable to cancer induction after exposure to radiation. However, some tissues, such as thyroid and breast tissue, have greater sensitivity to radiation. Excluding low-grade nonmelanomatous skin cancer and (benign) meningiomas, the most frequently reported radiation-associated second cancers in 5-year survivors of childhood cancer followed in the CCSS are, in order: breast cancer, thyroid cancer, central nervous system cancers, soft tissue sarcomas, and bone sarcomas.[39] Additional radiation-associated second cancers reported in survivors include carcinomas of the head and neck (especially parotid gland), colon cancer, other gastrointestinal cancers, lung cancer, and carcinomas of the genitourinary tract.[60-64] The most common second cancers observed in childhood cancer survivors will be described below.

Breast Cancer

Breast cancer is one of the most frequently diagnosed radiation-associated second cancers in childhood cancer survivors. Women treated with mantle, mediastinal, chest, whole-lung, and total-body irradiation during childhood or adolescence are at risk for secondary breast cancer.[24,55,56,61,65-70a] Large cohort studies of childhood Hodgkin's lymphoma survivors have reported a 15- to 30-fold increased risk of radiation-associated secondary breast cancer compared with the age-matched general population. Risk estimates vary by characteristics of the cohort, including radiation dose, age at therapy, and duration of follow-up. The cumulative incidence of secondary breast cancer is estimated to be between 12% to 35% 20 years after therapy for Hodgkin's lymphoma, and the incidence does not plateau with longer duration of follow-up.

Female survivors at greatest risk for secondary breast cancer are those treated between the ages of 10 and 30 years with chest radiation doses greater than 20 Gy.[67,71] Studies have demonstrated a dose-response relationship between radiation dose and risk of secondary breast cancer; higher mediastinal doses are associated with a greater relative risk.[72] The typical latency of radiation-associated breast cancer is 10 to 15 years after therapy, but secondary breast cancer has been reported in women as young as 20 years of age and as soon as 6 years after therapy. Secondary breast cancer is most often associated with chest radiation for Hodgkin's lymphoma; however, it is important to recognize that women treated with chest irradiation for any childhood cancer diagnosis have an increased risk for subsequent breast cancer (Fig. 32-2).[55] Survivors of primary sarcomas not treated with chest radiation also have an increased risk of secondary breast cancer (RR = 7) (Fig. 32-2). Breast cancer in sarcoma survivors has a shorter latency period (5 to 9 years), suggesting an underlying genetic predisposition for breast cancer in these women. Interestingly, survivors with therapy-induced ovarian dysfunction have a relative decreased risk of radiation-associated breast cancers compared with survivors with normal ovarian function. Although very rare,

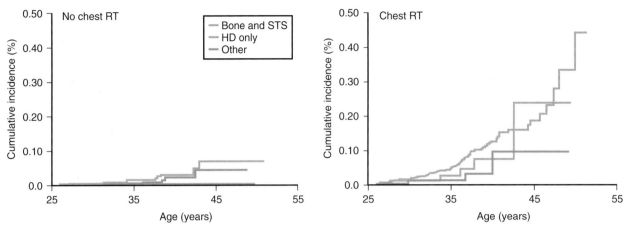

FIGURE 32-2. Cumulative incidence of breast cancer in survivors of Hodgkin's lymphoma, sarcomas, and other diagnoses exposed and not exposed to chest radiation therapy (RT), as a function of attained age. HD, Hodgkin's disease; STS, soft tissue sarcomas. *(Adapted from Kenney LB, Yasui Y, Inskip PD, et al. Breast cancer after childhood cancer: a report from the Childhood Cancer Survivor Study. Ann Intern Med. 2004;141: 590-597.)*

sporadic cases of male breast cancer have been reported in men treated with whole-lung radiation as children.[73]

The most common type of breast cancer diagnosed in survivors is invasive ductal carcinoma positive for estrogen receptors.[55,65,74] Similar to the general population, secondary breast cancer is detectable by radiographic imaging and has an excellent prognosis when treated in the earliest stages. Breast cancer treatment options for survivors can be limited by the therapy given for their childhood cancer. Specifically, prior anthracycline exposure and concern for potential cardiotoxicity may limit the use of adjuvant systemic chemotherapy with doxorubicin, and the concern for tissue necrosis with repeated exposure to chest irradiation limits the option of breast-conserving surgery for some women.

Current screening recommendations for childhood cancer survivors treated with chest radiation published by the Children's Oncology Group include monthly self-breast examination, annual clinical breast examination, and mammography starting 8 years after treatment or age 25, whichever comes last.[75] Guidelines published by the American Cancer Society advocate annual breast magnetic resonance imaging (MRI) in addition to these recommendations for all women at high risk for breast cancer, including those treated between ages 10 and 30 years with chest irradiation.[76] These recommendations reflect current expert consensus based on available knowledge and information, and have not been tested for efficacy in terms of reduction in secondary breast cancer mortality.

Thyroid Cancer

Radiation of the head, neck, and upper thorax places childhood cancer survivors at risk for subsequent thyroid cancers. Large cohort studies of childhood cancer survivors have estimated the relative risks of secondary thyroid cancer as between 10 and 35, with a cumulative incidence of 4.4% at 30 years reported in Hodgkin's disease survivors.[68,77-81] Well-differentiated papillary carcinoma is the most common pathology; however, follicular carcinomas have also been observed.[81,82] The minimum latency period for secondary thyroid carcinoma is 5 years, but the risk of thyroid carcinoma is increased beyond 20 years after irradiation for primary cancer; a plateau in incidence has not been observed beyond 40 years of follow-up.[78,83,84] The risk of thyroid cancer is related to radiation dose but, unlike most other radiation-induced second cancers, the risk of thyroid cancer is greatest at lower doses, 20 to 29 Gy; beyond

30 Gy there is a decline in risk.[80,81,85] This finding demonstrates that thyroid tissue has enhanced sensitivity to radiation toxicity and supports the cell kill hypothesis; this suggests that higher doses of radiation cause cell death, which reduces the initiation of carcinogenesis observed at lower doses. Chemotherapy does not appear to modify the risk of secondary thyroid cancer. Secondary thyroid cancer is more common in females, and young age at treatment is an independent risk factor.[78]

Radiation-induced thyroid cancer in young survivors has an excellent prognosis; therefore, many experts have recommended clinical screening. Appropriate screening schedules for secondary thyroid cancers and recommended modality for screening are controversial.[86-89] At a minimum, annual palpation of the thyroid for nodules by an experienced examiner is recommended.[75] Routine screening to detect subclinical thyroid nodules with high-resolution ultrasound has been recommended by some investigators, but remains controversial. Ultrasound screening has the benefit of detecting smaller nonpalpable nodules, but has the consequence of false-positive findings and potential for unnecessary biopsies. Thyroid nodules have ultrasound characteristics that are of concern for malignancy (e.g., hypoechogenicity, irregular margins, microcalcification); however, these findings are not diagnostic. Because ultrasound findings are not diagnostic, fine-needle aspiration (FNA) of nodules larger than 1.0 cm or with suspicious features is usually necessary to evaluate for malignancy. Serial ultrasound is then recommended to monitor thyroid nodules that are small or benign on biopsy.[90] Routine ultrasound screening of asymptomatic survivors remains controversial and should only be considered for high-risk irradiated patients after a discussion of the potential risks and benefits.

In general, radiation-associated thyroid cancer is treated the same as other thyroid cancers, with an excellent prognosis. Thyroid surgery is indicated for nodules that are enlarging, are of indeterminate pathology on FNA, or have FNA results positive for malignancy.[90] Total thyroidectomy is often recommended to survivors because radiation-associated thyroid cancers can be multicentric, and benign nodules can accompany clinically undetectable malignant lesions. Finally, there is indirect evidence to support the finding that exogenous thyroid hormone use reduces the risk of secondary thyroid cancer by suppressing thyroid-stimulating hormone (TSH)–induced proliferation of thyroid nodules. Although not proven to reduce the risk of thyroid cancer, the use of exogenous thyroid hormone to suppress thyroid proliferation is supported by studies that have shown a decrease in incidence of new thyroid nodules in patients treated with exogenous thyroid hormone after partial thyroidectomy (34% vs. 14%).[91]

Sarcomas

Survivors treated with radiation are at increased risk for secondary cancer of the bone and soft tissue in the radiation field. Although secondary sarcomas are most often associated with radiation, survivors of primary sarcoma and hereditary retinoblastoma not treated with prior radiation also have an increased risk, suggesting a genetic predisposition.[42,49,92] Risk estimates for secondary sarcoma vary by type of sarcoma and composition of the study cohort.[42,57,93-95] The CCSS cohort, which did not include survivors of retinoblastoma (RB), has reported an overall ninefold increased risk of secondary sarcomas, with a 30 year cumulative incidence of 1.03% for irradiated survivors. The Late Effects Study Group, which included survivors of retinoblastoma, reported an overall RR of 133 for secondary bone sarcomas, with a cumulative incidence of 2.8% at 20 years.[57] The British survivors cohort, which also included retinoblastoma survivors, reported a RR of 43 for secondary bone sarcomas, with a cumulative incidence of 0.9% at 20 years.[93] The median latency for secondary sarcomas is 11 years, with increased risk persisting beyond 20 years.[42,57] Risk factors for subsequent sarcomas include higher doses of radiation, primary diagnosis of sarcoma or retinoblastoma, younger age at diagnosis, concurrent alkylating agent exposure, family history of sarcoma, and possibly anthracycline exposure.[94-96] Gender does not appear to modify risk. In a study of bone sarcomas after childhood cancer from the LEFS, Tucker and colleagues[57] demonstrated a radiation dose-response gradient. In this study, no sarcomas were observed in survivors treated with less than 10 Gy and a significantly increased risk was noted for survivors who had a treatment dose higher than 40 Gy. This and other studies have also shown that alkylating agent exposure potentiated the risk of bone sarcomas, because the risk of bone sarcomas increases linearly with cumulative dose of alkylating agent.[57,93]

For survivors of hereditary retinoblastoma treated with radiation, the risk of subsequent bone sarcomas is as high as 400-fold, with a cumulative incidence at 20 years of 14.1%, and the relative risk for soft tissue sarcomas is 140, with a 50-year cumulative incidence of 13%.[57,92,93] As illustrated in Figure 32-3, which compares the cumulative incidence of secondary sarcomas in hereditary versus nonhereditary RB survivors and irradiated versus nonirradiated hereditary RB survivors, radiation exposure and underlying genetic predisposition both contribute to the risk of secondary sarcomas in retinoblastoma survivors.

Routine radiographic screening for secondary sarcomas is currently not recommended, although experimental protocols using positron emission tomography (PET) scanning or MRI imaging for survivors with hereditary retinoblastoma or Li-Fraumeni syndrome are under consideration (D. Malkin and L. Diller, personal communication, 2007). Survivors at risk for secondary sarcomas should be counseled to report new pain, lesions, or masses in the radiation field and should be promptly evaluated for any signs or symptoms suggestive of a secondary sarcoma. As survivors enter follow-up care, providers should consider obtaining baseline imaging of any previously irradiated site, so that these studies will be available for comparison if symptoms suggestive of a new malignancy develop.

Central Nervous System Tumors

Past exposure to cranial irradiation is associated with secondary CNS malignancies. The most common pathologies include meningiomas and gliomas but other pathologies, such as primitive neuroectodermal tumors and CNS lymphomas, have been reported.[36,97] The relative risk of secondary brain tumors in survivors treated with cranial radiation is between 10 and 20.[36,40,98] The median latency is shorter for secondary gliomas, 9 years, compared with 20 years for meningiomas. There is a well-established dose-response relationship between cranial radiation dose and incidence of secondary CNS tumors. In a St. Jude Children's Research Hospital cohort study of 1251 acute lymphoblastic leukemia (ALL) survivors treated with cranial irradiation,[97] the 20-year cumulative incidence of CNS tumors was 1.36% overall. Further analysis has shown a dose-response relationship, because the 20-year cumulative incidence of CNS tumors increased with radiation dose—1% at 10 to 21 Gy, 1.65% at more than 21 to 30 Gy, and 3.2% at more than 30 Gy. In a recent updated report on the same cohort,[99] the overall 30-year cumulative incidence of CNS malignancies after radiation was found to have reached 3.0%. In the CCSS cohort, Neglia and associates[36] have reported an excess relative risk of 1.06/Gy of cranial x-ray therapy for meningiomas and 0.3/Gy for gliomas. Additional risk factors for secondary CNS tumors are treatment in those younger than 5 years and CNS leukemia at diagnosis.[36,97] The contribution of chemotherapy to the risk of CNS malignancies is controversial. Laboratory investigations have suggested an association between radiation-induced brain tumors and thiopurine-based chemotherapy related to a deficiency in the enzyme thiopurine methyltransferase (TPMT).[100] In the CCSS cohort, after adjusting for radiation dose, chemotherapy did not alter survivors' brain tumor risk.[36]

Survivors of hereditary retinoblastoma are at risk for trilateral retinoblastoma, an intracranial neuroblastic tumor usually a pineal tumor, but also found in the suprasellar or parasellar region. This tumor does not appear to be treatment-associated; in contrast, a possible protective effect of systemic chemotherapy used to treat retinal tumors has been observed.[101] The prognosis of trilateral retinoblastoma is dependent on tumor size at diagnosis, so aggressive screening of survivors of hereditary retinoblastoma during the period of greatest risk is advised.[102] Based on data from a meta-analysis by Kivela,[102] MRI neuroimaging is recommended every 3 months for the first year after diagnosis of retinoblastoma and then twice a year for 3 years or until age 5 years, whichever comes first.

Routine surveillance for secondary CNS tumors with neuroimaging is currently not recommended.[75] However, in a prospective study of 76 survivors of acute lymphoblastic leukemia (ALL) treated with cranial radiation who were screened with MRI every 3 to 6 years for 20 years, Goshen and coworkers[103] have found 16 meningiomas (15 asymptomatic) and 1 glioma. Cumulative incidence in this screened population was 14.8% at 20 years. Surgical resection was recommended for 12 of the 16, with one surgical complication reported. The authors concluded that early detection of small meningiomas by routine MRI surveillance might reduce morbidity by facilitating surgical resection and minimizing neurologic complications for those whose tumors require surgical intervention. Survivors with a prior history of cranial radiation should be educated about this potential late-occurring complication and instructed to report new or persistent neurologic signs or symptoms.

Skin Cancer

Melanoma and nonmelanomatous skin cancers have been reported with increased incidence in survivors. The relative risk of melanoma is 5.0 to 9.0 in childhood cancer survivors, with a median latency of almost 15 to 18 years.[39,104] Survivors of

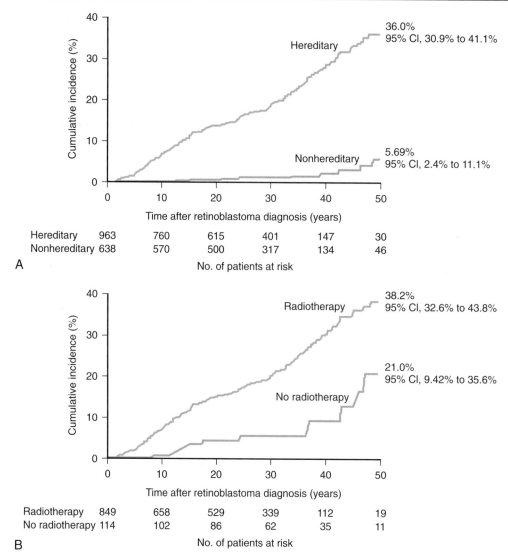

FIGURE 32-3. **A,** Cumulative incidence of new cancers in survivors of hereditary and nonhereditary retinoblastoma, by time since diagnosis. **B,** Cumulative incidence of new cancers in survivors of hereditary retinoblastoma exposed and not exposed to radiotherapy, by time since diagnosis. CI, confidence interval. *(Adapted from Kleinerman RA, Tucker MA, Tarone RE, et al. Risk of new cancers after radiotherapy in long-term survivors of retinoblastoma: an extended follow-up. J Clin Oncol. 2005;23:2272-2279.)*

hereditary retinoblastoma, familial melanoma syndromes, and those with a prior history of melanoma all have an increased risk of subsequent melanoma, independent of radiation.[6,40,50,92,105] Although the association between therapeutic radiation and melanoma is not firmly established, a case-control study of 16 survivors with secondary melanoma in a European cohort of 4000 childhood cancer survivors found an association between melanoma occurrence and exposure to more than 15 Gy radiation.[104] In contrast, basal cell carcinomas and squamous cell carcinomas are known to be more common in radiation-exposed survivors (RR = 6.3), with 90% of all nonmelanomatous skin cancers diagnosed in previously irradiated fields.[99,106] Also, these low-grade skin cancers can recur, and almost half of survivors diagnosed will have multiple lesions.[106] The prognosis for secondary skin cancers is excellent with early diagnosis; therefore, routine screening with skin examination is recommended.[107] Ultraviolet radiation from the sun is known to contribute to skin cancer risk; patients should be routinely educated about preventive strategies, such as aggressive sun exposure protection.

Hematologic Malignancies

Acute leukemias and myelodysplasia are associated with exposure to high cumulative doses of alkylating agents and with topoisomerase II inhibitors, including epipodophyllotoxins and anthracyclines. The alkylating agents presenting the greatest concern for secondary leukemias are melphalan and mechlorethamine, compared with cyclophosphamide and ifosfamide.[20,22,108] Secondary leukemias induced by exposure to high-dose alkylating agents can be preceded by myelodysplasia, have a median latency of 4 to 6 years, are more often diagnosed in older children, and are often associated with deletions of chromosomes 5 and 7.[32] Topoisomerase II–induced leukemias typically do not have an indolent course, have a relatively short latency (median, 1-3 years), are diagnosed in younger children, and are associated with balanced chromosomal translocation of 11q23 and, less frequently, 21q22.[21,32,109,110]

Secondary leukemias are usually resistant to therapy and in general have a poor prognosis.[32,109] The contributory role of therapeutic doses of radiation in the development of secondary leukemia is debated. Although some studies have found no association between leukemia and exposure to radiation therapy,[40,111,112] other studies have documented subsequent leukemia in survivors after exposure to radiation in the absence of chemotherapy.[21,32,111] Thus, therapeutic radiation is likely, in some part, to contribute to leukemogenesis in survivors.

Overall, the relative risk of secondary acute leukemia in childhood cancer survivors is between 7 to 20.[20,21,39,40,61,68,111,113] The reported cumulative incidence of secondary leukemia after solid tumors is 0.2% to 2.9% at 15 years[111] and as high as 3.8% at 6 years in ALL survivors treated with topoisomerase II inhibitors.[112] In contrast to radiation-associated malignancies, the latency period for leukemogenesis associated with chemotherapy is the first 10 years after treatment, with the greatest risk observed in the first 5 years off therapy. In a European study of 4202 3-year survivors of childhood solid tumors, the relative risk of leukemia was 20 at 3 to 5 years and then decreased to 2.2 by 10 years off therapy.[111] Of interest, in this same study, a second peak in incidence of secondary leukemia was after 20 years or more of follow-up, with a relative risk of 14.8. This finding has not been observed in studies with shorter follow-up periods.[21,39,56] A dose-response relationship has been demonstrated for both alkylating agent and topoisomerase II–associated leukemias.[22] In a case-control study of 61 cases of secondary leukemia in childhood survivors, Le Deley and colleagues have shown a more than 20-fold increased risk of leukemia after exposure to more than 6 g/m^2 of an epipodophyllotoxin and a sevenfold increased risk after exposure to 1.2 to 6 g/m^2 of an epipodophyllotoxin or more than 170 mg/m^2 of an anthracycline, compared with lower doses of these agents.[44] The schedule of administration of epipodophyllotoxins also appears to contribute to the risk of secondary leukemia, because prolonged infusions (twice weekly or weekly) were found to be an independent risk factor for leukemia.[112,114] Interestingly, more recent pediatric studies have not demonstrated an increased risk of leukemia after alkylating agent exposure,[44,111] which had been previously documented.[20,21] This finding most likely indicates that current patient populations are less likely to be treated with the most leukemogenic alkylating agents, including melphalan and mechlorethamine.

ORGAN SYSTEM LATE EFFECTS

Cardiovascular System

The leading cause of noncancer mortality observed in childhood cancer survivors is cardiac disease. Cardiac late effects account for 4.5% of the mortality observed in 5-year survivors of childhood cancer in the CCSS cohort, and 21% of the treatment-related mortality.[16] Cardiovascular toxicity has been observed after radiation to the thorax and after exposure to all anthracyclines, including doxorubicin, daunorubicin, idarubicin, and mitoxantrone. Anthracycline therapy is directly toxic to myocardial cells and results in cardiomyopathy and arrhythmias. Risk factors for late anthracycline cardiotoxicity (occurring 1 year beyond completion of therapy) include cumulative dose (more than 300 mg/m^2), history of acute cardiac toxicity, combination with other cardiotoxic therapy, female gender, young age at exposure (younger than 5 years), and duration of follow-up.[37,115-119] Irradiation of the heart as a consequence of radiation to the chest for treatment of childhood cancer can cause functional and anatomic cardiac disease. Mantle field, whole-lung field, left abdominal, spinal irradiation, and total body irradiation (TBI) all put a survivor at risk for cardiac late effects.[31,117,120-122] Radiation-associated cardiac late effects include constrictive pericarditis,[123] myocardial fibrosis,[124] cardiomyopathy, coronary artery disease, valvular abnormalities, conduction disturbances, and vascular disease.[31,38,117] Similar to other radiation-associated late effects, cardiac toxicity is observed more frequently in those survivors treated at the youngest age who received higher radiation dose volumes to the heart and were followed the longest.[31,120] Modern radiation techniques designed to reduce the dose to the heart will hopefully reduce survivors' future risk of cardiac effects, although longer follow-up is necessary for this to be confirmed.

The spectrum and nature of cardiac late effects experienced by childhood cancer survivors suggest a need for regular screening with one or more cardiac imaging modalities. Risk-based screening recommendations for childhood cancer survivors exposed to cardiotoxic therapies have been published by the Children's Oncology Group (COG) as part of the Long-Term Follow-Up Guidelines for Survivors of Childhood, Adolescent and Young Adult Cancers.[75] However, these guidelines have not been tested for efficacy in terms of reduction of cardiac mortality or morbidity. Management of cardiovascular disease in survivors is similar to management of cardiovascular disease in the general population; however, there are some therapeutic challenges unique to survivor populations (see below). Survivors exposed to cardiotoxic therapy should be informed about their risk for heart disease and should also be made aware of activities that present potential stressors to already impaired cardiac function, including isometric exercise (such as weight lifting), smoking, pregnancy, and anesthesia.[75]

Cardiomyopathy

Cardiomyopathies diagnosed in childhood cancer survivors after completion of therapy are associated with thoracic radiation and anthracycline chemotherapy. Survivors are at risk for both systolic and diastolic left ventricular dysfunction, which can lead to clinical heart failure.[125-127] Acute cardiotoxicity and late-onset cardiomyopathy are both associated with anthracycline therapy.[128] Anthracyclines are directly toxic to cardiac myocytes, resulting in reduced myocyte mass and impaired function of cardiac muscle. Subclinical anthracycline cardiotoxicity is measured as diminished left ventricular contractility and a thinning of the left ventricular wall. Thinning of the ventricular wall causes elevated wall stress, which increases afterload, and ultimately can progress to symptomatic left ventricular failure. In children, loss of cardiac myocytes at a young age can result in impaired cardiac growth and function relative to somatic growth, which contributes to the observed decrease in left ventricular systolic function.[37,129]

Anthracycline-associated late cardiac toxicity can manifest as asymptomatic cardiac dysfunction detected by echocardiography, or symptomatic dysfunction, which is associated with the classic signs of heart failure.[117,118] Longitudinal data have supported that cardiac abnormalities diagnosed in childhood cancer survivors treated with anthracyclines are persistent and progressive.[130] In a Dutch cohort of over 800 anthracycline-exposed childhood survivors, the cumulative incidence of anthracycline-induced clinical heart failure increased with the duration of follow-up—a cumulative incidence of 2.6% at 10 years and 5.5% at 20 years, with no evidence of plateau in incidence with longer duration of follow-up.[119] Of further concern, the incidence of asymptomatic left ventricular dysfunction detected by cardiac screening is reported to be as high as 50% to 60%.[115] Longitudinal data have confirmed that asymptomatic anthracycline-associated cardiac dysfunction is persistent and sometimes progressive, but the trajectory of progression of asymptomatic dysfunction to overt clinical heart failure has not been determined.[130]

TABLE 32-2 Calculation of Anthracycline (Doxorubicin) Dose Equivalents

Anthracycline	Conversion Factors
Doxorubicin	Total dose (mg/m²) × 1
Daunorubicin	Total dose (mg/m²) × 0.75
Mitoxantrone	Total dose (mg/m²) × 2.5
Idarubicin	Total dose (mg/m²) × 3

Estimation of cardiotoxic equivalents for commonly used anthracyclines, developed by P. Blanding, Pediatric Oncology, Dana-Farber Cancer Institute, Boston, Mass. Note: Estimates do not factor in clinical variations such as age at treatment, previous chest radiation, or use of cardioprotectants.

Many risk factors for anthracycline-associated cardiomyopathy have been identified, including cumulative dose, female gender, and age at exposure, which is related to length of subsequent survival and remaining somatic growth.[37,117,118] In addition, cardiotoxicity diagnosed during or within 1 year of completion of therapy is considered a risk factor for late cardiotoxicity. The major risk factor for anthracycline cardiomyopathy is cumulative dose (doxorubicin equivalent). Equivalent dose takes into consideration exposure to different anthracyclines and can be calculated using conversion factors (Table 32-2). Survivors exposed to cumulative doses of doxorubicin equivalents more than 300 mg/m² are at greatest risk for cardiomyopathy.[18,37,119,131] The dose-dependent relationship between anthracyclines and subsequent congestive heart failure (CHF) was demonstrated in the Dutch cohort, in which the greatest risk of CHF was at a dose more than 300 mg/m² (RR = 8), and no CHF was observed at doses lower than 150 mg/m².[119] Although exposure to more than 300 mg/m² is consistently associated with the greatest risk for cardiomyopathy, studies have shown that survivors treated with the lowest cumulative dose (45 mg/m²) also have asymptomatic cardiac abnormalities detectable by echocardiography, confirming that exposure to anthracycline at any dose poses a risk for late cardiotoxicity.[130] Furthermore, survivors exposed to anthracycline therapy and concurrent mediastinal radiation are considered to be at risk for cardiomyopathy at a lower total anthracycline dose, more than 200 mg/m².[120]

Interventions to prevent or reduce long-term anthracycline-associated cardiotoxicity in childhood cancer survivors have included limiting anthracycline doses in most therapeutic regimens to lower than 300 mg/m², adding cardioprotectants such as dexrazoxane to anthracycline-based regimens, and prescribing afterload-reducing agents to prevent progression of asymptomatic dysfunction to overt heart failure. Encouraging data from clinical trials in childhood ALL have shown that the addition of cardioprotectants does not adversely affect survival and reduces cardiac injury as measured by serum troponin T.[132,132a] However, early analysis of a Pediatric Oncology Group clinical trial of an anthracycline-containing regimen for Hodgkin's disease, which randomized the use of dexrazoxane as a cardioprotectant, has shown no change in cancer-free survival but a possible increase in second cancers when dexrazoxane was used in combination with etoposide.[133] Longer follow-up is necessary to determine the efficacy and safety of cardioprotectants in children. Childhood cancer survivors diagnosed with anthracycline-associated left ventricular (LV) dysfunction are often treated with angiotensin-converting enzyme (ACE) inhibitors with the aim of reducing afterload and preventing the progression of LV dysfunction to heart failure. In a longitudinal study of 18 survivors with LV dysfunction treated with enalapril, and followed for a median of 10 years, all initially showed improvement in LV function. The effects, however, were transient, lasting 6 to 10 years, and were followed by deterioration

of LV function over time.[134] Although medical management improved symptoms, it did not prevent progression. Future investigations should be directed at testing interventions to prevent cardiac injury during therapy and progression of asymptomatic left ventricular dysfunction to overt cardiac disease.

Radiation-associated cardiomyopathy is most often restrictive, with impaired diastolic function, although systolic dysfunction may also be observed.[123,124] Radiation is thought to induce injury to the myocardial microvasculature, which in turn causes myocardial ischemia and ultimately myocardial fibrosis, resulting in diastolic dysfunction. Although clinical heart failure is uncommon in survivors treated with radiation only, studies have demonstrated a significant incidence of diastolic dysfunction in asymptomatic patients treated with radiation therapy.[31,135,136] A small cohort of Hodgkin's disease survivors was treated with a median mediastinal dose of 35 Gy and evaluated at a mean of 9 years after therapy; 20% had evidence of diastolic dysfunction on cardiac imaging.[135] The extent to which these changes are progressive, and whether subclinical dysfunction will result in clinical heart failure over time is unknown. As noted, the exposure to both anthracyclines and radiation compounds the risk for cardiotoxicity.[31,137]

Screening for cardiomyopathy with serial echocardiography is recommended for survivors treated with anthracyclines and/or thoracic radiation therapy.[75] The frequency of echocardiographic screening depends on the individual survivor's risk of cardiomyopathy, as determined by the survivor's age at exposure, treatment dose, and concurrent exposure to thoracic radiation. Screening has been recommended for survivors exposed to cardiotoxic therapy because late-onset cardiomyopathy is relatively common, has defined risk factors, and subclinical changes in cardiac function are detectable before clinical heart failure. The extent to which screening will result in a reduction in cardiac morbidity and mortality in survivors remains unknown.

Coronary Artery Disease

Survivors treated with thoracic radiation are at increased risk of radiation-associated coronary artery disease (CAD), which is an established cause of early mortality.[91,138] Radiation injury to the coronary arteries is caused by endothelial damage and subsequent acceleration of atherosclerosis.[120] Radiation-associated coronary artery stenosis is most common in the proximal coronary arteries, which are not necessarily shielded during cardiac blocking.[139] A historical cohort of childhood Hodgkin's lymphoma survivors, treated with more than 40 Gy of mediastinal radiation, had a 40-fold excess risk of fatal myocardial infarction compared with the age-matched general population.[140] A Dutch cohort, which included 314 Hodgkin's lymphoma survivors treated when they were younger than 20 years, found a fivefold increased risk of myocardial infarction at a median of 19 years after treatment.[137] A British cohort, which included 2158 Hodgkin's lymphoma survivors treated when they were younger than 25 years, found a 19-fold increased risk of death from myocardial infarction.[28] Modern radiation techniques are likely to reduce radiation to the coronary arteries, although this is not certain. In addition, a recent pilot study has provided evidence that anthracyclines also damage vascular endothelium directly, and perhaps contribute to late CAD observed in survivors.[141]

The risk of asymptomatic CAD in survivors is described in many studies, but optimal screening and interventions to detect and treat radiation-associated cardiovascular disease have not been determined. Survivors at risk for radiation-associated CAD are advised to adopt preventive measures commonly used to reduce the risk of atherosclerotic CAD in the general population (e.g., aggressive treatment of hypertension, diabetes, obesity, dyslipidemias). Although efficacy of these measures has not been proven in this population, at least one cardiac risk factor was present in all survivors who developed CAD in a single-institution study of 400 Hodgkin's disease survivors. These data suggest that standard cardiovascular risk-reducing strategies might be beneficial to survivors.[38]

Stress echocardiograms can be used as a noninvasive method to detect asymptomatic ischemic heart disease by observing stress-induced wall motion abnormalities. Noninvasive nuclear scintigraphy has also been considered to screen survivors for asymptomatic CAD. A recent report of screening 294 asymptomatic Hodgkin's lymphoma survivors treated at a median age of 25 years with more than 35 Gy has found that 20% have electrocardiographic findings consistent with prior ischemia, and 14% have abnormal stress echocardiograms or stress-induced perfusion defects by nuclear scintigraphy.[142] The survivors with abnormal nuclear perfusion studies who went on to cardiac catheterization were diagnosed with radiation-induced microvascular damage in the myocardium not amenable to surgical intervention.[142] This study has shown that the increased sensitivity of adding perfusion scanning to stress echocardiography is at the expense of decreased specificity, with false-positive detection of small coronary artery disease not amenable to intervention. This calls into question the benefit of adding nuclear studies to routine screening of asymptomatic survivors for CAD.

Surgical treatment of CAD in survivors with prior radiation exposure can be complicated by mediastinal fibrosis, myocardial fibrosis, and the coexistence of other radiation-associated morbidities, including valvular disease, conduction abnormalities, and pulmonary dysfunction. Consideration should be given to repairing multiple radiation-associated cardiac morbidities simultaneously, even those not yet determined to be severe enough for surgical intervention, because repeated surgeries in chest-irradiated survivors may increase the risk of complications.[143]

Arrhythmias

A full spectrum of cardiac arrhythmias and conduction disturbances have been reported in childhood cancer survivors treated with both radiation and anthracyclines. These include atrioventricular nodal bradycardia, sick sinus syndrome, complete and incomplete heart block, prolonged QT interval, and serious ectopy (ventricular tachycardia).[144] In a series of 48 survivors of pediatric Hodgkin's disease treated with mediastinal radiation (median dose, 40 Gy), 75% were found to have conduction abnormalities.[145] The most frequent conduction disturbance was right anterior bundle branch block, the most anterior structure in the conduction system.[145] These arrhythmias are rarely symptomatic; however, the concern is that conduction abnormalities may be progressive. Because conduction abnormalities typically are asymptomatic, they usually are detected in association with other radiation-induced cardiac abnormalities.

Valvular Disease

The mitral, aortic, and tricuspid valves can all be affected by radiation-associated fibrous endocardial thickening. Valvular insufficiency is more common than valvular stenosis, but stenosis tends to be more severe, requiring intervention.[38,146,147] The frequency of left-sided valvular regurgitation is reported to be 16% to 24% in chest-irradiated survivors of Hodgkin's disease screened by echocardiography at a median of 10 years, and valvular dysfunction was not observed at a radiation dose less than 30 Gy.[147,148] A cohort of 48 survivors of pediatric Hodgkin's disease (median age, 16 years; median dose, 40 Gy), showed a slightly higher frequency of left-sided regurgitation,

36%, and valvular defects were detected in 42% of survivors screened.[145]

Although radiation-associated valvular defects are frequently observed in survivors, they are often clinically insignificant. Valvular defects can be progressive, which is of particular concern for young survivors.[146] In a single-institution series of 415 survivors of Hodgkin's lymphoma who received mediastinal irradiation, clinically significant valvular dysfunction developed in 6.2% at a median of 22 years.[38] In this cohort, aortic stenosis was the most common clinically significant valve lesion and compared with the age-matched general population, the relative risk of needing valve surgery was eightfold higher in survivors. The only treatment risk identified for significant valvular disease in this cohort was radiation technique that resulted in a higher total dose to the heart.[38]

Symptoms of valvular heart disease are the same in survivors as in the general population, and valve function can be monitored by routine echocardiographic screening.

Pericarditis

The incidence of late-occurring radiation-associated pericarditis has been significantly reduced by modern radiation techniques.[149,150] In historical cohorts of children treated with orthovoltage mediastinal radiation, 7% to 15% developed symptomatic constrictive pericarditis, compared with 0% to 2.5% of children treated with megavoltage therapy.[150-153] Although the incidence of pericarditis has been significantly reduced in recent cohorts, older childhood cancer survivors continue to be at risk for pericarditis. Presenting signs and symptoms include pleuritic chest pain, shortness of breath, a friction rub, and electrocardiographic changes. A survivor presenting with symptomatic pericarditis is at risk of progressing to cardiac tamponade.[145] Management includes pericardiocentesis and pericardiectomy, which are high-risk procedures in this patient population with known risks for other radiation-associated cardiac morbidities.

Vascular Disease

Clinically significant premature cerebrovascular disease and carotid artery disease occur in survivors treated with cranial, head and neck, and thoracic radiation.[154] A recent pilot study has shown that anthracyclines can also damage vascular endothelium and perhaps contribute to late vascular disease observed in survivors.[141] Data from the CCSS have shown an increased risk of stroke in survivors of brain tumors (RR = 29) and leukemia (RR = 6.4) when compared with sibling controls, and the risk of stroke was associated with a mean cranial radiation dose greater than or equal to 30 Gy.[154] The prevalence and risk factors for premature radiation-associated vascular disease in pediatric populations has not been determined. Based on current data, routine screening for carotid and cerebrovascular disease in asymptomatic survivors has not been recommended.[75]

Pulmonary System

Childhood cancer survivors have a ninefold increased risk of death from pulmonary complications.[16] The late effects of radiation therapy on the respiratory system include pulmonary fibrosis, often preceded by acute radiation pneumonitis, reduced lung volumes, and decreased chest wall growth. Risk factors for radiation-induced pulmonary late effects are younger age at exposure, concurrent pulmonary toxic chemotherapy, lung radiation dose higher than 15 Gy, spinal irradiation, and total body irradiation.[155-157] Treatment with chemotherapy, including bleomycin, mitomycin C, busulfan, and nitrosoureas, can also cause late pulmonary fibrosis that, like radiation-associated fibrosis, is often preceded by an acute-phase interstitial lung injury.[158,159]

Data from the CCSS study[160] have shown an increased risk of pulmonary fibrosis (RR = 4.3) and emphysema (RR = 2.0) in those exposed to chest irradiation, and increased risk of pulmonary fibrosis in those exposed to bleomycin (RR = 1.4), carmustine (BCNU; RR = 1.6), and busulfan (RR = 2.1). At 20 years, the cumulative incidence of pulmonary fibrosis is 3.5% after radiation and 0.75% after pulmonary toxic chemotherapy. A plateau in cumulative incidence of pulmonary fibrosis was not observed up to 15 years after diagnosis in survivors treated with chemotherapy alone or in combination with radiation.

Survivors with significant risk factors for late pulmonary toxicity should be monitored with periodic pulmonary function tests for symptoms or signs of progressive pulmonary dysfunction. Smoking is known to contribute to risk for pulmonary diseases in the general population and, although not documented, tobacco use likely increases the risk of lung disease in survivors treated with modalities causing pulmonary toxicity. Reports of worsening bleomycin-associated pulmonary fibrosis after exposure to 100% oxygen have suggested that survivors receive pulmonary evaluation prior to undergoing anesthesia and avoid situations with increased oxygen concentrations, such as scuba diving.[161]

Endocrine System

Hypothalamic-Pituitary Dysfunction

Hypothalamic pituitary dysfunction is a potential late effect in childhood cancer survivors treated with radiation for CNS malignancies or for orbital, facial, or nasopharyngeal cancers. Central nervous system tumors of the optic pathway, hypothalamus, or suprasellar region can also cause long-term hypothalamic-pituitary dysfunction as a result of hypothalamic injury from tumor growth or surgical resection. The incidence of pituitary hormone deficiencies after cranial radiation varies by radiation dose and other treatment factors such as age at therapy and duration of follow-up.[162] The range in prevalence of anterior pituitary deficiencies reported in the literature after a median dose of 45 to 55 Gy cranial radiation is as follows: growth hormone (GH) 85% to 100%; TSH, 3% to 60%; luteinizing hormone–follicle-stimulating hormone (LH-FSH); 5% to 40%; and adrenocorticotropic hormone (ACTH), 4% to 30%.[162] The GH pathway is the most sensitive to radiation and therefore GH deficiency is the most likely manifestation of hypothalamic hypopituitarism in survivors treated with cranial radiation. The pituitary-thyroid, gonadal, and adrenal axes are less sensitive to late-onset radiation toxicity. As such, centrally mediated deficiencies of these hormones are usually not observed in survivors treated with cranial radiation below the range of 35 to 50 Gy.[135,163-167]

Growth Hormone Deficiency

The severity and latency of growth hormone deficiency (GHD) diagnosed in survivors is related to cranial radiation dose. GHD can be observed after doses as low as 18 to 24 Gy, with late onset typically more than 10 years after therapy, whereas a cranial dose of more than 30 Gy can result in GHD within 5 years after treatment.[168] This suggests that after a dose threshold of 18 to 25 Gy, the incidence of GHD increases with increased duration of follow-up.[169,170] Clinical features of growth hormone deficiency (GHD) in survivors treated with cranial radiation can include poor growth, increased fat mass, reduc-

tion in lean body mass, decreased strength and exercise tolerance, adverse lipid profile, and decreased bone mineral density. All these can be improved by GH replacement[171]; however, the benefit of GH replacement in GH deficient survivors after they obtain final height is controversial.[169] A small randomized study of GH-deficient ALL survivors who stopped GH replacement therapy after attaining their final height has shown an increase in fat mass and decrease in lean body mass 1 year after stopping therapy; these findings were reversed in 19 survivors after resuming GH replacement.[172] It remains to be determined whether survivors need lifelong follow-up for GHD and if those receiving GH replacement should continue after final height attainment.

The safety of GH replacement in survivors is controversial, particularly with respect to disease recurrence and second neoplasms. In the CCSS cohort, there was no documented increased risk of disease recurrence in GH-treated survivors; however, the rate ratio of second cancers for GH-treated survivors was significantly higher, with a relative risk of 3.4.[173,174] In another study,[175] which compared recurrence rates in a cohort of 180 GH-treated brain tumor survivors with 891 brain tumor survivors not treated with GH, there was no increased risk of brain tumor recurrence over time. Based on available data, GH replacement therapy appears to be safe with respect to disease recurrence; however, it might increase the risk of new primary cancers. The frequency and duration of screening for GHD in childhood cancer survivors, the long-term effects and safety of GH replacement therapy, and the usefulness of replacement therapy beyond attainment of final height needs further investigation.

Bone Disorders

Loss of bone mineral density (BMD) is a common complication of treatment for childhood cancer that is probably underdiagnosed in survivors. Bone mass is dependent on peak bone density attained during puberty and young adulthood, as well as the rate of bone loss. Failure to achieve peak bone density puts survivors at risk for osteopenia (BMD higher than 1 and less than 2.5 SD below mean) and osteoporosis (BMD higher than 2.5 SD below mean). In the general population, osteoporosis is a major cause of fractures, resulting in significant morbidity and mortality. The long-term risk of osteoporosis-associated fractures has not been documented in survivors. Risk factors for reduced BMD in childhood cancer survivors include prior treatment with corticosteroids and methotrexate, direct skeletal radiation, cranial radiation, hormonal deficiencies, nutritional deficiencies during and after therapy, and prolonged immobilization or physical inactivity.[176-178] Female survivors with treatment-induced gonadal dysfunction during their teenage years and young adulthood are known to have an especially high risk for reduced BMD during adulthood.[168] Male survivors are also at risk for reduced BMD, especially those with treatment-associated hypogonadism because of the known correlation between serum testosterone and BMD.[179]

Bone density evaluation with dual-energy x-ray absorptiometry (DEXA) scan has been recommended for adult survivors of childhood cancer with a treatment risk for low BMD.[75] Measurement of bone mineral density in children who have not reached peak bone mass is not standardized and treatment for low BMD in children is not established. Nutritional evaluation and exercise are recommended for survivors with risk for low BMD, and calcium and vitamin D supplements are recommended for survivors diagnosed with osteopenia. Treatment of hypogonadism with hormone replacement therapy is also suggested to improve bone health. However, data are not available to guide the use of hormone replacement therapy in survivors, so even low-dose therapy must be weighed against risk in these patients.[180]

Osteonecrosis of the capital femoral epiphysis is a known late toxicity of treatment for childhood cancer, which can result in pain, loss of function, and joint collapse requiring surgical intervention.[181-183] Other lower extremity joints can also be affected by osteonecrosis (ON), including the knee and ankle. In a recent report on children treated with European protocols for ALL, the 5-year cumulative incidence of osteonecrosis was 1.8%.[182] A prospective study of osteonecrosis in a Nordic cohort of ALL survivors has identified MRI evidence of lower extremity ON in 24% of those studied; risk factors identified in this study were increased BMI, female gender, older age at diagnosis (older than 10 years) and higher cumulative dose of dexamethasone.[181] Molecular studies have shown an association between genetic variation in the *PAI-1* gene and risk for osteonecrosis in ALL survivors older than 10 years treated with dexamethasone.[183a] Management for osteonecrosis is primarily symptomatic; however, surgical intervention is sometimes necessary to improve pain or preserve or restore function.[183]

Bone and soft tissue in treatment fields are vulnerable to radiation-induced hypoplasia and fibrosis, resulting in reduced or uneven skeletal growth. Survivors treated with radiation that included the spine (more than 12 Gy) and long bones are at risk for scoliosis, shortened trunk height, and growth asymmetry.[184,185]

Thyroid Disorders

The thyroid gland is extremely sensitive to radiation toxicity; subsequently, thyroid abnormalities are among the most common radiation-induced morbidities after childhood cancer therapy. Childhood cancer survivors exposed to thyroid radiation as a consequence of direct neck radiation for Hodgkin's lymphoma, sarcomas, nasopharyngeal or oropharyngeal carcinomas, and other tumors are at risk for thyroid abnormalities, including hypothyroidism, hyperthyroidism, thyroid nodules, and cancer. Because even low doses and scatter radiation can damage thyroid tissue, survivors who received seemingly distant radiation such as whole-lung, craniospinal, and total-body irradiation for bone marrow transplantation are at risk for thyroid abnormalities.

Primary hypothyroidism (low thyroxine [T_4] level, with elevated TSH or compensated normal T_4 with elevated TSH) is the most common thyroid abnormality observed after thyroid radiation.[77] Survivors in the CCSS cohort had a 17-fold increased risk of hypothyroidism compared with siblings. The incidence of hypothyroidism increases with increasing radiation dose; at 20 years after treatment with 35 to 44.99 Gy, the cumulative incidence is 35%, and with 45 Gy or more, the cumulative incidence is 50%. Risk factors identified for hypothyroidism are larger dose of radiation, older age at diagnosis, and female gender. Although the greatest risk of hypothyroidism occurs the first 5 years after treatment, no plateau for thyroid disease has been observed and cumulative incidence continues to rise beyond 20 years of follow-up. Hyperthyroidism is a less common late effect and is usually only observed after doses of thyroid radiation more than 35 Gy. Radiation-induced thyroid nodules are commonly detected in survivors treated with head and neck radiation. One cohort study has shown that the median latency of nodules is 10 years (range, 1 to 25 years) after therapy, and only 10% detected by physical exam or screening ultrasound were malignant.[186]

Recommended screening for survivors at risk for radiation-associated thyroid disease include annual palpation of the thyroid by a skilled examiner and annual measurements of serum thyroid hormones beginning 1 year after completion of therapy.[75,77] Thyroid replacement therapy is successful in treat-ing radiation-associated hypothyroidism. Treatment with thyroxine to suppress elevated TSH has also been recommended to reduce the frequency of benign nodules.[187] Routine ultrasound screening of asymptomatic survivors is not generally advocated, because most thyroid nodules detected in survivors have an indolent course and only a small percentage are malignant.[186] Survivors with palpable thyroid nodules are recommended to have a high-resolution thyroid ultrasound with FNA of any large or suspicious nodules. Nodules with benign pathology can be followed by serial ultrasound and rebiopsied if there is an interval change; nodules that have indeterminate or malignant pathology are referred for thyroidectomy. Total thyroidectomy is often recommended to survivors because radiation-associated thyroid cancers can be multicentric, and benign nodules can accompany clinically undetectable malignant lesions.[90]

Parathyroid Disorders

Neck radiation is associated with an increased incidence of hyperparathyroidism. Studies of adults treated with head and neck radiation for nonmalignant conditions during childhood have shown a 2.5-fold increased risk of hyperparathyroidism, with a prolonged latency of 25 to 50 years.[162,188-190] The risk of hyperparathyroidism in survivors treated with radiation for malignant disease has not been reported. Because this is a potential late-occurring complication, survivors treated with neck radiation as children should have routine monitoring of their calcium as they approach older adulthood.

Growth Disturbances

Short Stature

Many factors can cause growth disturbances in childhood cancer survivors. Because the process of normal growth is complex, it is often challenging to isolate a specific cause for diminished height in an individual child. Final height in survivors can be directly affected by cancer therapy and indirectly affected by treatment-related hormonal deficiencies and poor nutrition. Studies have identified independent risk factors for diminished final height in childhood cancer survivors, including treatment with cranial radiation (related to growth hormone deficiency), and age at diagnosis younger than 13 years, with children younger than 4 years at greatest risk.[191-194]

Radiation-associated bone hypoplasia and fibrosis can directly impede skeletal growth, so that radiation fields that include the spine or lower extremities can result in diminished adult final height.[193,195,196] Radiation-associated spinal deformities (kyphosis or scoliosis) can also diminish survivors' final adult height.[184,185,195,196] Prolonged use of corticosteroids for antineoplastic therapy, immunosuppression, or symptom management can impair longitudinal growth and reduce final adult height. The mechanism of steroid-induced growth suppression includes suppression of pituitary growth hormone secretion, reduction of insulin-like growth factor I (IGF-I) production by the liver, and possibly impaired action of IGF-I on bone, all of which contribute to diminished growth.[177,195,197] Antimetabolite chemotherapy has also been associated with decreased bone growth and diminished final height in some clinical studies. This finding is supported by animal and in vitro models, which have demonstrated that antimetabolite chemotherapy damages growth plate chondrocytes and impairs growth.[198]

Loss of height velocity without subsequent catch-up growth during a prolonged course of treatment can also result in diminished final attained height. Interruption of growth during the active treatment period can be related to the malignant process itself, poor nutrition, or growth suppression by therapy.[192,199] In a single-institution study of final height in survivors of childhood ALL, decrease in height growth scores in children undergoing active treatment was noted as soon as 6 months after beginning therapy.[192] Thus, loss in height velocity during treatment, followed by inadequate catch-up growth, can result in diminished final height observed in survivors.

Treatment-induced deficiencies of growth hormone, thyroid hormone, testosterone, and estrogen can all contribute to reduced final height in survivors. The effect of hormone deficiencies on final height can be minimized by early recognition and use of hormone replacement therapy.[200,201] Precocious puberty, a late effect observed after cranial irradiation, can also indirectly result in diminished final height by decreased interval of prepubertal growth.[202] Cranial radiation for central nervous system leukemia prophylaxis (18 to 24 Gy) is associated with relatively early and precocious puberty in girls, and higher doses of cranial radiation often used to treat brain tumors can precipitate early puberty in both genders.[202]

All childhood cancer survivors should be monitored for appropriate growth during and after therapy because some causes of growth disturbances are treatable, and early intervention can positively influence final attained height.

Obesity

Obesity has been reported as a potential late complication in survivors of childhood cancer. Obesity is usually defined as body mass index (BMI) higher than 95th percentile for age, or higher than or equal to 30 after 21 years of age.[187] Children treated for ALL and CNS malignancies appear to be at greatest risk for this complication. Children are at risk for excessive weight gain at the end of therapy, during early follow-up, at the time of final height attainment, and possibly into their adult years.[77,203] Radiation-induced hypothalamic damage has been implicated in the pathogenesis of obesity in childhood cancer survivors, resulting in impaired growth, low metabolic rate, altered body composition, and dysregulation of eating behaviors.[191,204,205] A study of 1765 young adult ALL survivors enrolled in the CCSS identified female gender, younger age at diagnosis (younger than 4 years), and treatment with more than 20 Gy of cranial radiation as risk factors for obesity (RR: females, 2.6; males, 1.9).[206] Treatment with lower dose radiotherapy or chemotherapy only, representative of current ALL therapy, was not associated with an increased risk of obesity in this study. In contrast, a prospective study[207] measuring BMI of 422 children with ALL and non-Hodgkin's lymphoma (NHL) before, during, and after completion of therapy has found no difference in the rate of BMI increase between radiated and nonradiated children. It was concluded that high BMI at diagnosis is the best predictor of adult obesity in ALL and NHL survivors.

Metabolic syndrome, which includes obesity, insulin resistance, hyperglycemia, and dyslipidemia, has also been observed in young survivors.[208-210] Risk factors for metabolic syndrome are cranial radiation and prolonged steroid therapy. Case-control studies of small cohorts of young survivors have demonstrated that cranially irradiated survivors have significantly higher weight, body fat, fasting glucose and insulin levels, and significantly decreased high-density lipoprotein cholesterol (HDL-C). Metabolic syndrome is an established risk factor for adult diabetes and cardiovascular disease, which has concerning implications for survivors' future health.

Physical inactivity as a consequence of treatment-associated morbidities, including cardiopulmonary disease that limits exercise tolerance, neurocognitive disabilities that limit coordination and participation, chronic pain, genetic factors, and social factors all likely contribute to the obesity observed

in survivors. Survivors should be educated about the long-term health consequences of obesity and given support to reduce their modifiable risk factors for this late effect.

Central Nervous System

Therapy for childhood cancer can result in long-term adverse sequelae on CNS and sensory organ function. Surgery, radiation, and chemotherapy used to treat brain tumors and solid tumors in the head and neck region, and cranial radiation and chemotherapy used as CNS prophylaxis for leukemia and lymphoma, can all contribute to the neurologic, cognitive, and sensory deficits observed in survivors.

Neurocognitive Impairment

Neurocognitive impairment is most commonly observed in survivors treated with cranial irradiation. Methotrexate, administered intrathecally as CNS prophylaxis or at high doses systemically (single dose more than 1000 mg/m^2), is also associated with neurocognitive late effects.[211,212] Brain tumor survivors treated with surgery alone are at risk for neurocognitive impairment attributable to direct brain injury from tumor growth, surgical resection, hydrocephalus, and seizures.[213] There is a broad spectrum of neurocognitive impairments observed in childhood cancer survivors. These include deficits in executive functioning (planning and organization), sustained attention, memory (visual sequencing and temporal memory), processing speed, and visual-motor integration. As a result of these deficits, survivors experience learning difficulties in mathematics and reading comprehension, diminished intelligence, academic failure, and behavioral changes.[33,211,214-219]

Risk factors for neurocognitive impairment in childhood cancer survivors treated with radiation include higher dose, young age at exposure (younger than 3 years), female gender, and personal or family history of learning disabilities.[33,215-217,220,221] Additional risk factors include concurrent treatment with dexamethasone, TBI, methotrexate, and cytarabine.[215] Lower dose cranial radiation as CNS prophylaxis for leukemia or lymphoma (18 to 24 Gy) is more commonly associated with information processing or learning disabilities,[33] whereas higher dose cranial radiation necessary to treat brain tumors is more often associated with global cognitive impairments and diminished intelligence.[216] Neurocognitive deficits are persistent and new deficits may emerge over time, particularly during periods of increasing cognitive demands, which is of particular concern to the older survivor.[215]

Formal neurocognitive testing is used to diagnose impairments. A full battery of tests administered by specially trained psychologists is indicated to evaluate the full spectrum of potential deficits. Survivors diagnosed with neurocognitive impairments should be referred to specialized services at the treating center or in the community to facilitate access to educational, rehabilitation, social, and vocational resources. Cognitive remediation, educational interventions with individualized learning programs, and family support that addresses survivor-specific needs are all necessary for survivors to attain their full educational potential.[215,222]

Neurologic Disorders

Surgery for brain tumors and head and neck cancers can result in permanent neurologic deficits specific to the location of the primary cancer. For example, postoperative cerebellar mutism may persist years beyond the surgical resection of a posterior fossa tumor.[223] In addition, postoperative hydrocephalus, infections, and seizures can evolve into chronic neurologic conditions, resulting in neurologic deficits that can be stable or progressive over time.[35]

Leukoencephalopathy, presenting as spasticity, ataxia, dysarthria, dysphagia, hemiparesis, and seizures, is associated with cranial radiation more than 18 Gy and chemotherapy with methotrexate and dexamethasone. Signs and symptoms of leukoencephalopathy may present without imaging abnormalities (brain MRI, MR angiography, computed tomography [CT]); conversely, findings on neuroimaging (white matter changes, cerebral lacunae, atrophy, dystrophic calcifications, mineralizing microangiopathy) do not necessarily correlate with clinical severity.[224-226] Leukoencephalopathy has also been described as a late manifestation of childhood histiocytic syndromes, with no known treatment association.[227]

Peripheral sensory and motor neuropathy presenting as weakness, paresthesias, or pain, and episodic vasospasm of the digits (Raynaud's phenomenon) are potential late effects associated with vincristine and vinblastine therapy.[228-230] Treatment-induced neuropathy might restrict survivors from physical activity; however, impaired motor performance, measured in a cohort of 128 childhood cancer survivors, was not associated with cumulative vincristine dose[231] nor was prolonged vincristine exposure associated with physical inactivity observed in ALL survivors in the CCSS cohort.[232] Management of these late effects is primarily symptomatic, and a trial of agent used to treat neuropathic pain or prevent peripheral vascular spasm can be considered.[75,228]

Rare neurologic late effects of radiation therapy typically associated with higher doses of cranial radiation (more than 50 Gy) include focal brain necrosis, spinal cord myelitis, and cerebrovascular disease, including vasculitis, moyamoya, cavernomas, and large-vessel stroke.[233-235a] Late onset of seizures was reported in 6.5% of brain tumor survivors in the CCSS cohort and cortical radiation of more than 30 Gy was associated with a twofold risk of this complication.[35] These late-onset neurologic complications can present with various nonspecific neurologic symptoms, including headache, seizure, hemiparesis, and other focal findings. Neuroimaging is indicated for diagnostic assessment. Survivors with prior exposure to high-dose cranial radiation often receive periodic screening with MRI to monitor for these late effects; however, there are no data to support the concept that screening asymptomatic survivors reduces morbidity or mortality from neurologic complications.

Vision Impairment

Childhood cancer survivors' vision may be impaired by surgery, radiation, TBI, or chemotherapy with corticosteroids. Visual late effects are anatomic and functional, including cataracts, orbital hypoplasia, lacrimal gland atrophy, conjunctival corneal damage, retinopathy, glaucoma, and optic nerve damage.[35,236-238] Cataracts are a visual late effect frequently diagnosed in bone marrow transplant survivors and survivors treated with cranial radiation. Bone marrow transplantation–conditioning regimens that include TBI are associated with a significant risk for cataract development and can require surgical intervention.[239,240] Chemotherapy-based conditioning regimens are not as likely to induce cataracts, and those that develop are usually less severe and usually do not require intervention. Survivors with visual symptoms or a history of an ocular tumor, those who received TBI or treated with cranial, orbital, or ocular radiation are at highest risk for late-onset ocular complications and should receive ongoing follow-up by an ophthalmologist.[35,75,238,239]

Hearing Loss

Hearing loss is a late effect experienced by childhood cancer survivors exposed to head and neck radiation and platinum-based chemotherapy. Radiation fields that include the temporal bone and adjacent soft tissues can cause impaired auditory function.[35] Cranial irradiation alone is unlikely to cause hearing loss; however, sensorineural hearing loss can occur at cranial doses more than 50 Gy and at lower doses (40 to 50 Gy) when combined with ototoxic chemotherapy, especially when the treatment sequence is chemotherapy administered after radiation.[35,241,242] In a series of 157 children with brain tumors treated with radiation only (median dose, 54 Gy), the cumulative incidence of hearing loss in the speech frequency range was 27% at 5 years after therapy.[243] The cumulative incidence of hearing loss steadily increased over the 9-year follow-up period, and no plateau was observed.

The effect of cisplatin chemotherapy on ototoxicity is dose- and age-dependent. Children treated at a younger age (younger than 5 years) are more vulnerable to cisplatin ototoxicity at any dose level.[244,245] The incidence of high-frequency hearing loss (4000 to 8000 Hz) was found to be up to 50% in children treated with more than a 450 mg/m^2 cumulative dose of cisplatin.[244] Hearing loss in the speech range (500 to 3000 Hz) is rarely observed at cumulative cisplatin dosages less than 360 mg/m^2, and the incidence is as high as 22% to 25% at cumulative dosages more than 720 mg/m^2.[241,244] Cisplatin ototoxicity is typically bilateral and irreversible, and children with normal hearing at the completion of platinum therapy who have not received cranial radiation are unlikely to have subsequent loss of hearing. Survivors treated with carboplatin in nonmyeloablative doses do not appear to be at risk for hearing loss.[246,247]

During cancer therapy, survivors might also have had prolonged or periodic exposure to other ototoxins, including aminoglycoside antibiotics and furosemide. Prior and current exposure to all ototoxic agents should be considered in the assessment of auditory function. The contribution of environmental factors (e.g., use of headphones, occupational exposures) to hearing loss in the young survivor population has not been documented.[247] Survivors with treatment exposures that put them at risk for hearing loss or those with symptoms of hearing impairment should have serial auditory evaluations. Those diagnosed with hearing impairments should be prescribed hearing aids and provided with classroom or workplace accommodations, as indicated. Early intervention for auditory problems is particularly important in the survivor population because hearing loss has the potential to compound already existing social, developmental, and cognitive impairments.

Reproductive System

Male and female childhood cancer survivors' reproductive function can be impaired by radiation and chemotherapy. Survivors treated with gonadotoxic therapy are at risk for treatment-related infertility and diminished sex hormone production. Chemotherapy-induced gonadotoxicity is directly related to dose and specific agent. The alkylating agents cyclophosphamide and procarbazine pose a greater risk for gonadal dysfunction than cisplatin and dacarbazine.[30,248-250] In general, the ovary is less vulnerable to chemotherapy-induced damage than the testis. As with other late effects, radiation-associated toxicity to the ovaries and testes is dependent on dose and field of radiotherapy.

Females

Late ovarian dysfunction experienced by childhood cancer survivors can be a result of acute toxicity that persists or premature ovarian failure. Most prepubertal and adolescent girls receiving standard-dose chemotherapy will retain or recover ovarian function, and those receiving high-dose alkylating agents, conditioning for bone marrow transplantation, or exposed to pelvic radiation are at greatest risk for irreversible ovarian toxicity, which includes estrogen deficiency and infertility.[180,195,251,252] Radiation to the pelvis, abdomen, or spine may include the ovaries in the field. Doses greater than 20 Gy can result in complete ovarian failure, requiring hormone replacement therapy.[253] Survivors treated with both radiation and gonadotoxic chemotherapy have a worse prognosis for ovarian function.[254,255]

Survivors who retain or recover ovarian function after completing therapy are at risk for premature menopause, defined as cessation of menses prior to age 45 years. Risk factors for premature menopause include increasing age, older age at treatment, increasing radiation dose to the ovaries, and increasing cumulative dosage of alkylating agents.[254,255] The pathophysiology of therapy-induced premature menopause is reduction in the number of ovarian follicles, which explains the finding that prepubertal girls who have the greatest reserve of follicles are less vulnerable to premature ovarian failure than older survivors. In the historic five-center study, which included 1067 female survivors, the risk of reaching early menopause (age younger than 25 years) for those treated between the ages of 13 and 19 years was four times greater than sibling controls.[256] Increased risk of premature menopause was observed in survivors treated with radiation below the diaphragm (RR = 3.7), alkylating agents (RR = 9.2), or both (RR = 27). In this study, 42% of women treated with radiation below the diaphragm and alkylating agents had reached menopause by age 31 years.[256] The overall relative risk for premature menopause in survivors in the CCSS cohort was 13-fold higher than sibling controls, with a cumulative incidence (CI) of 8% by age 40.[255] In this study, the cumulative incidence of menopause for survivors exposed to alkylating agents only was 5% at age 35 years, which increased to 15% by age 40 years. Survivors exposed to radiation and alkylating agents had a cumulative incidence of menopause of 15% at age 30 years, which increased to 30% by age 40. A threshold dose of cumulative alkylating agent exposure for preserving ovarian function has not been determined, and even the lowest doses of pelvic radiation (1 to 99 cGy) are associated with increased risk of premature menopause.[255]

Although risk factors for premature menopause have been described in populations of survivors, an individual survivor's risk for premature or impending menopause cannot be measured clinically for the purpose of fertility counseling. A Danish sample of 21 survivors with regular menstrual cycles and FSH lower than 10 IU/L were shown to have a lower total number of follicles per ovary as measured by ultrasound compared with normal controls. Although not proven, this measure is possibly predictive of diminished ovarian reserve and shortened reproductive span.[257] Women at risk for premature menopause should be educated about their potentially reduced window of fertility and, if interested in having children, should be counseled against delaying childbearing. Cryopreservation of fertilized embryos during the period of ovarian function has been proposed as a means to preserve the option for future pregnancy.[258] No reliable measures to predict duration of fertility are currently available, nor are there interventions that could prolong ovarian function and delay the onset of menopause.

Males

Males treated with alkylating agent chemotherapy as children and adolescents are at risk for infertility secondary to impaired testicular germ cell function and low testosterone resulting from Leydig cell insufficiency. Alkylating agent gonadotoxicity is dose-dependent, and pubertal status or age at exposure is not protective.[30,164,259] A significant risk of azoospermia has been observed with a cumulative cyclophosphamide dosage greater than 5 to 7.5 g/m^2. Subclinical Leydig cell insufficiency (elevated serum LH, normal testosterone) or Leydig cell failure (elevated LH, low testosterone) is usually not detected at total cyclophosphamide dosages less than 20 g/m^2.[30,260,261] Most male survivors with alkylating agent–induced infertility will have normal testosterone production, with normal sexual function and secondary sexual characteristics. Male survivors with azoospermia diagnosed soon after completion of therapy have the potential to recover spermatogenesis many years later.[261,262] Thus, a sexually active survivor who is not contemplating paternity must be counseled about birth control, even if he has had an abnormal semen analysis in the past. Survivors treated with unilateral orchiectomy and not exposed to additional gonadotoxic therapy usually maintain adequate testicular function.[263,264] Although reduced testicular volume on physical examination and elevated serum gonadotropins (FSH) suggest infertility, the only definitive measures of a survivor's potential fertility is by semen analysis or paternity.

A survivor's risk for radiation-induced testicular function depends on radiation dose and age at exposure. Testicular germ cells are very sensitive to radiation damage. Changes in spermatogenesis can be observed after doses as low as 0.1 Gy and irreversible azoospermia usually occurs after doses more than 2 Gy.[251] In contrast, testicular testosterone production is usually preserved with doses up to 20 Gy. Irreversible damage to testicular germ cell and endocrine function usually occurs after exposure to more than 20 Gy of radiation, requiring androgen replacement therapy. However, survivors who are beyond puberty at the time of diagnosis can usually tolerate higher doses of radiation before loss of testicular endocrine function occurs.[265]

Pregnancy

Women treated with abdominal or pelvic radiation who can conceive children are at risk for treatment-associated complications of their pregnancy and delivery. Radiation-induced damage to uterine muscle and blood flow adversely affects survivors' prognosis for a healthy full-term pregnancy.[266] Pelvic radiation and abdominal fields that include the uterus are associated with pregnancy complications, including spontaneous abortions, preterm labor, low birth weight infants, and small for gestational age (SGA) infants.[267-270] A report of more than 4000 pregnancies in childhood cancer survivors has shown that the only risk factor for adverse pregnancy outcomes is pelvic radiation, which was associated with low birth weight infants (RR = 1.84). No other treatment factor was a risk for any adverse pregnancy outcome in this large cohort.[267,268] When the analysis was restricted to 2201 live-born children of 1264 survivors in the CCSS cohort, maternal uterine radiation (more than 5 Gy) was associated with prematurity (OR = 3.5), low birth weight (OR = 6.8), and SGA infants (OR = 4.0).[269] Estrogen therapy prescribed in attempts to restore uterine function after radiation injury increases uterine size and stimulates blood flow, but it has not been shown to improve uterine muscular function.[271]

Survivors with therapy-associated cardiac toxicity (subclinical or overt) are at risk for pregnancy-associated congestive heart failure and should be monitored prior to pregnancy, during pregnancy, and after delivery by obstetricians aware of potential complications.[119,272] Peripartum acute congestive heart failure (A-CHF) has been described in survivors treated with anthracyclines and chest radiation, but the incidence has not been determined.[119,272] One study of 37 anthracycline-exposed pregnant women has shown that prepregnancy LV dysfunction is a risk factor for A-CHF during pregnancy, supporting the need to monitor at-risk survivors closely.[272] Survivors with risks for other organ toxicities, such as endocrinopathies, pulmonary fibrosis, and renal insufficiency, should also be meticulously evaluated and monitored prior to pregnancy, during pregnancy, and after delivery.

Offspring

Many studies have investigated the possible association between exposure to cancer therapy during childhood and a mutagenic or teratogenic effect on future offspring. Fortunately, no study to date has found an increased risk of congenital anomalies or cancer in the offspring of adult survivors of nonhereditary childhood cancer treated prior to conception.[30,273-279] This is true for male and female survivors of childhood cancer and survivors treated with chemotherapy and radiation therapy. Survivors of childhood cancers associated with genetic syndromes and hereditary cancer predisposition (e.g., Cowden's syndrome, Li-Fraumeni syndrome, retinoblastoma) are at increased risk of their offspring being diagnosed with cancer. These survivors should be referred for genetic counseling and genetic testing, as desired and appropriate. Preimplantation genetic testing is available to survivors with known retinoblastoma or Li-Fraumeni–associated gene mutations who are contemplating pregnancy.[280,281]

Renal System

Chronic renal insufficiency is a late effect associated with radiation to the kidneys as part of abdominal field radiation or TBI, chemotherapy with ifosfamide and high-dose cisplatin, and nephrectomy, especially when in association with other nephrotoxic therapy. The pathophysiology of radiation injury to the kidney is progressive arteriolonephrosclerosis, resulting from radiation injury of the renal microvasculature, with subsequent secondary damage to the glomeruli and tubules. Radiation-associated renal injury is dose-related and the threshold dose is approximately 15 Gy. However, nephrectomy and exposure to other nephrotoxic agents lower that threshold.[282,283]

Chemotherapy with cisplatin at doses greater than 200 mg/m^2 can cause nephropathy secondary to glomerular or tubular injury. This injury is usually acute and reversible; however, it can be stable or progressive.[284] Carboplatin does not appear to be associated with long-term nephrotoxicity.[285] Ifosfamide nephrotoxicity is also a result of glomerular or tubular injury and presents most often as renal tubular acidosis.[286] The greatest risk for ifosfamide nephrotoxicity is at a total dose greater than 45 g/m^2 and age younger than 3 years.[286] Combination nephrotoxic chemotherapy, nephrectomy, and therapy with nephrotoxic antibiotics all contribute to survivors' risk for long-term renal damage.[287-290]

In a cohort of survivors of childhood Wilms' tumor, the cumulative incidence of renal failure at 15 years was 0.6% for patients with unilateral disease and 13% for patients with bilateral disease.[291,292] Survivors of Wilms' tumor with the highest cumulative incidence of chronic renal failure at 20 years are survivors with predisposition syndromes such as Denys-Drash (74%), WAGR (*W*ilms' tumor, *a*niridia, *g*enitourinary anomalies, and mental *r*etardation; 36%), genitourinary abnormalities (7%), and survivors with bilateral disease (12%). Survivors of Wilms' tumor with progressive tumor in the contralateral kidney or nephrogenic rests and survivors treated with radiation have also been identified as having an increased risk of renal dysfunction.[291,293,294] In a study of bone marrow transplantation survivors treated with fractionated TBI, 12 to 14 Gy over 3 to 4 days, late renal dysfunction was reported in 35% of ALL survivors and 71% of neuroblastoma survivors.[295] Modern conditioning regimens with altered fractionation should reduce the incidence of renal insufficiency in transplantation survivors.

The risk of chronic renal failure in survivors treated with unilateral nephrectomy alone appears to be minimal.[292] However, studies have suggested that patients treated with unilateral nephrectomy manifest subclinical evidence of early reversible renal injury detectable by elevated urine microalbumin.[296,297] A study linking Wilms' tumor survivors in the NWTSG to the U.S. End-Stage Renal Disease registry, followed for a median of 11 years, has shown a low risk of end-stage chronic renal failure in nonsyndromic Wilms' tumor survivors (cumulative incidence [CI] = 0.6% at 20 years). These data suggest that Wilms' tumor survivors with clinically detectable renal dysfunction will not routinely progress to end-stage renal disease.[292] This cohort has not reached an age when survivors might be at the greatest risk of chronic renal failure.

Survivors treated with potentially nephrotoxic therapy should be routinely monitored for early signs of renal dysfunction, including hypertension, proteinuria, and elevated serum creatinine. Survivors with the earliest signs of renal injury, microalbuminuria, might benefit from therapeutic interventions with ACE inhibitors to reverse or halt progression of renal injury. Survivors with a single kidney should be counseled to adopt health behaviors to maintain kidney health, including hydration, salt reduction, avoidance of prolonged use of nonsteroidal anti-inflammatory drugs (NSAIDs) and acetaminophen, prompt treatment for urinary tract infections, and meticulous control of coexisting diabetes and hypertension.[75]

Genitourinary System

In addition to the renal late effects discussed, survivors of childhood cancer are also at risk for toxicity to the genitourinary system from surgery, treatment with pelvic and whole-abdomen radiation, and alkylating agent chemotherapy. Genitourinary surgery can result in long-term functional impairments, including urinary incontinence, and sexual dysfunction. The primary late effects associated with radiation include fibrosis or hypoplasia of the anatomic components of the male and female genitourinary systems, including urinary bladder, ureter, urethra, prostate, vagina, and uterus, resulting in chronic pain or dysfunction. Survivors experiencing anatomic or functional genitourinary late effects, including sexual dysfunction, should be referred to a urologist or gynecologist, as indicated, for evaluation and management of their symptoms.

Chemotherapy with cyclophosphamide and ifosfamide has been associated with protracted hemorrhagic cystitis and bladder fibrosis, although this late effect has been reduced by concurrent therapy with mesna.[298,299] Hemorrhagic cystitis that develops beyond the time of therapy more often has a viral cause or is associated with chronic graft-versus-host disease (GVHD) in transplantation survivors.[300] There have been reports of bladder cancer after cyclophosphamide, and the risk appears to be dependent on dose and duration of therapy.[301-303] An adult series of over 6000 NHL survivors treated with cyclophosphamide has reported 31 cases of bladder cancer (RR = 4), and no significantly increased risk was observed at doses less than 20 g/m^2.[302] In another series of adults treated with prolonged cyclophosphamide for nonmalignant disease, 5% developed secondary bladder cancer at a median of 8.5 years; all diagnoses were preceded by symptoms of microscopic hematuria.[304] The risk of bladder cancer is probably lower in survivors treated as children, who in general receive lower does and shorter courses of cyclophosphamide. Nonetheless, routine monitoring by urinalysis of survivors exposed to cyclophosphamide is clinically indicated.[75]

Gastrointestinal System

Potential late effects of cancer therapy on the gastrointestinal system are late-onset surgical complications such as adhesions, small bowel obstruction, and fecal incontinence,[305] radiation-induced functional impairment such as chronic diarrhea, and secondary neoplasms of the gastrointestinal tract and liver.[60] Hepatic fibrosis is a rare late complication of anti-metabolite chemotherapy (methotrexate, mercaptopurine, thioguanine), and the fibrosis typically follows acute hepatic toxicity, such as veno-occlusive disease.[306,307] As with other organ systems, radiation can result in functional impairment and second cancers of the gastrointestinal organs consequently exposed to radiation as a result of location in a treatment field. The relative risk of radiation-associated colorectal cancer reported in the literature is between 3.6 to 13, and 7.0 for other gastrointestinal cancers.[40,60,61] These late effects are usually observed after higher doses of radiation therapy (more than 30 Gy). The clinical spectrum of radiation-induced gastrointestinal toxicity that has been reported includes salivary gland dysfunction, esophageal stricture, hepatitic fibrosis and cirrhosis, cholelithiasis, and chronic enterocolitis.

Common gastrointestinal symptoms reported by a childhood cancer survivor, such as abdominal pain and heartburn, should be evaluated in the context of his or her treatment history. A survivor's risk for serious gastrointestinal pathology should be considered when planning a diagnostic workup and therapy for common symptoms. Children requiring abdominal surgery as part of their cancer therapy are at risk for late-onset small bowel obstruction and should be educated about this late effect.[308] Because survivors exposed to abdominal radiation (more than 30 Gy) are considered to be at higher risk for colon cancer, they are advised to begin colon cancer screening earlier than what is recommended for the general population (10 years after completing radiation therapy or age 35 years, whichever comes last).[60,75]

OTHER LATE EFFECTS

Infections

Late-occurring infectious complications can result from surgery, transfusions, immunosuppression, and radiation therapy. Childhood cancer survivors who have had a surgical splenectomy as part of their staging for Hodgkin's lymphoma are at lifelong risk for potentially fatal bacterial sepsis with encapsulated organisms. Survivors who received more than 40 Gy of abdominal or left flank radiation are considered functionally asplenic and have a similar risk for sepsis.[309] These survivors must be continually reminded of their risk and educated to receive immediate medical evaluation and prophylactic antibiotic therapy for fever or other signs of sepsis. Immunizations

against *Streptococcus pneumoniae*, *Haemophilus influenzae*, and meningococcus are also recommended for this high-risk group (Table 32-3).[310] Bone marrow transplantation survivors receiving immunosuppression for chronic GVHD are also at risk for ongoing infectious complications and should be considered for prophylactic antibiotics.[311] Older survivors treated in the United States are at risk for transfusion-acquired chronic hepatitis B if they received blood products prior to 1972, hepatitis C if they received blood products prior to 1993, and HIV if they received blood products between 1977 and 1985.[312] Radiation to the sinuses for a primary sarcoma or CNS tumor at doses greater than 30 Gy is associated with chronic bacterial sinusitis that might require surgical intervention.[313] Survivors who underwent therapy associated with a risk for pulmonary disease, such as lung radiation or TBI, and those with cardiac disease should receive an annual influenza vaccination. Survivors with known radiation-associated valve disease should receive appropriate subacute bacterial endocarditis (SBE) antibiotic prophylaxis.[314] Survivors at risk for infectious complications should be educated about their risk and informed of the necessity for preventive strategies.

Dental Problems

Dental late effects are reported frequently in childhood cancer survivors. Survivors treated with head and neck radiation are at risk for root stunting, microdontia, hypodontia, and craniofacial abnormalities, resulting in severe cosmetic or functional impairment necessitating surgical or orthodontic intervention.[315-317] The risk for dental facial abnormalities is greatest in survivors treated at the youngest age and with higher doses of radiation. Survivors treated with chemotherapy prior to the complete eruption of their permanent teeth are at risk for tooth agenesis, root thinning or shortening, and enamel dysplasia.[317,318] Neuroblastoma survivors and leukemia survivors treated with cranial radiation or TBI have a particularly high incidence of dental abnormalities (71% and 94%, respectively), most likely associated with young age at treatment.[316,317] All childhood cancer survivors should be advised to have regular dental care, which includes cleaning, fluoride applications, and Panorex films to evaluate tooth development.[75]

Psychosocial Function

The experience of having childhood cancer and its associated treatment can have long-term effects on a survivor's emotional and social functioning. Common disorders of emotional function, such as depression, anxiety, and post-traumatic stress disorder, are reported more frequently in populations of childhood cancer survivors than in their siblings and the general population.[319,320] Serious emotional distress, such as suicidal symptoms, are also reported more commonly in survivors. In a cohort of 226 adult survivors of childhood cancer, 13% reported suicidality, and there were associations among suicidal symptoms and impaired physical functioning, pain, and self-perceived altered physical appearance.[321] Although this observed prevalence of suicidality is a finding of concern, the identification of risk factors presents an opportunity for intervention. There is no known increased incidence of psychiatric disorders such as schizophrenia or other psychoses in childhood cancer survivors, with the exception of survivors of brain tumors. A Dutch study of over 3700 childhood cancer survivors has found that brain tumor survivors have an excess risk for psychiatric hospitalizations for diagnoses that included psychoses of somatic and cerebral causes, psychiatric disorders in somatic disease, and schizophrenia.[322]

TABLE 32-3	Immunization Schedule for Asplenic Survivors[310]
Vaccine	**Frequency**
Pneumococcal	Every 5 yr
Haemophilus influenzae type B conjugate	Once after splenectomy
Meningococcal	Every 5 yr
Influenza	Yearly, seasonal

Challenges to normal social functioning such as educational remediation, employment discrimination, insurance discrimination, marital dissatisfaction, social isolation, and poor health-related quality of life have all been reported more frequently in survivors of childhood cancer.[323-332] Most childhood cancer survivors will not experience significant psychosocial dysfunction as a result of their cancer experience or cancer therapy; however, survivors of childhood CNS malignancies and those treated with cranial irradiation are more vulnerable to psychosocial morbidity. These survivors, in particular, should be routinely monitored for emotional distress and social disability.

FOLLOW-UP CARE OF CHILDHOOD CANCER SURVIVORS

Systems of Care

The need for specialized follow-up care for childhood cancer survivors is evident, given the numerous morbidities associated with childhood cancer treatment and the potential for survivors to develop complications decades after treatment. The prevalence of chronic health conditions observed in adult survivors of childhood cancer was 62% in the CCSS cohort and 58% in a single-institution cohort of survivors from the United Kingdom.[333,334] In the CCSS, almost a third of patients had a severe or life-threatening health condition and the cumulative incidence of a severe or disabling health condition approached 50% at 30 years after the diagnosis of childhood cancer.[333] Survivors' self-reported health status, including self-assessment of functional health, general health, mental health, and pain, has been described in several studies of young adult survivors of childhood cancer. Impaired health status has been reported in more than 75% of adult survivors surveyed in Canada, 58% of adult survivors in a British cohort, and 48% of adult survivors in the CCSS.[334-336] In these studies, survivors who reported impaired health status were more likely to have lower educational attainment, lower income, and a childhood diagnosis of brain tumor, bone tumor, or sarcoma. These findings demonstrate the high prevalence of morbidity in childhood cancer survivors overall and identify high-risk groups of survivors who might especially benefit from specialized survivor-oriented services and interventions.

Although childhood cancer survivors are at risk for various treatment-related health conditions as they age, they are not necessarily knowledgeable about the specifics of their cancer diagnosis and treatment, nor are they proactive about their future health. Of the young adult survivors surveyed in the CCSS cohort, only 72% could accurately report their diagnosis. Although most were knowledgeable about the general type of therapy they received (chemotherapy, surgery, radiation), only 70% of those receiving radiation could report the site.[337] An analysis of cancer screening practices of the young adults in the CCSS cohort has shown that compliance is not optimal and risk factors for poor compliance with screening recommendations are low level of educational attainment, lack of health insurance, lack of concern for future health, and young age.[338] These data suggest that young adult survivors are not necessarily knowledgeable about their cancer history and future health risks.

The high prevalence of chronic health conditions, poor health status, knowledge deficits, and suboptimal screening behaviors all support the need for comprehensive and specialized follow-up care of childhood cancer survivors, including provision of health care services and risk education. The optimal patterns and models of care for childhood cancer survivors have

not been well studied. Historically, childhood cancer survivors received follow-up care from a pediatric oncology provider. The frequency, quality, and duration of follow-up varied, and some centers "discharged" patients as they aged to primary care. More recently, designated long-term follow-up programs have been developed as models for delivery of comprehensive survivor care. In general, these comprehensive center-based programs have the advantage of providing multidisciplinary expertise and survivor education, and have facilities available for research in cancer survivorship. Despite these strengths, in a survey of 24 U.S. children's hospitals or cancer centers with comprehensive survivor programs, Aziz and colleagues[339,340] identified some common challenges faced by these designated programs in providing ideal care for all survivors. The specific challenges identified include the required commitment of significant financial and personnel resources, inadequate capacity to meet the needs of growing numbers of survivors, and limitation of access because of geography, insurance, or lack of awareness on the part of the primary care providers or the individual survivor. Consensus opinion has suggested that all survivors of childhood cancer receive regular follow-up care that includes surveillance for primary cancer recurrence, risk-based assessment for potential late effects, and counseling about future health risks and preventive measures.[341]

In 2003, the U.S. Institute of Medicine published a report[341] on childhood cancer survivorship that included recommendations to improve the care and quality of life for survivors. Included in the report was a description of the components of an ideal follow-up system and a challenge to define the minimal essential components of a follow-up system. A model endorsed by leaders of existing pediatric long-term follow-up clinics contains the following elements: clinic services under the direction of a pediatric oncologist with expertise in survivorship care; staffing by advanced degree nurses to provide and coordinate patient care; and access to social workers, psychologists, and a referral network of medical and surgical specialists with survivorship expertise. The spectrum of clinical services should include surveillance for primary cancer recurrence, late effects screening, and education for survivors. Clinical evaluations would occur annually or at an interval as determined by risk, and would be located in an academic center. Ongoing care would be provided in the community, with periodic center-based follow-up.[339] This model assumes frequent bidirectional communication among survivors, primary care providers, and oncologists, with clear delineation of responsibilities for ongoing care. These and other alternative models for extending and improving care delivered to childhood cancer survivors have been proposed but have not been formally evaluated in terms of feasibility and efficacy.

Finally, pediatric transition programs are an emerging trend in pediatric cancer care. These programs are designed to educate survivors who have recently completed therapy regarding treatment-related risks and to introduce issues related to survivorship early after cancer treatment. The goal of these programs is to bridge the period between active therapy and survivorship follow-up care, and subsequently reduce the knowledge deficit and loss to follow-up seen in prior cohorts of long-term survivors.[342]

Comprehensive Clinical Evaluation

Independent of the setting in which it occurs, the clinical evaluation of the childhood cancer survivor should include a comprehensive treatment summary, thorough physical examination, and diagnostic or screening tests, as indicated. The results of the evaluation should be summarized, documented, and communicated to the survivor and all health care providers participating in the survivor's care.

Treatment Summary

Information about prior diagnosis and treatment is necessary for a health care provider to begin a comprehensive childhood cancer survivor's evaluation. This critical information is likely contained in a pediatric oncology "treatment summary." Details about diagnosis that are necessary for the survivor follow-up evaluation include age at diagnosis, presenting symptoms, results of diagnostic and staging evaluation, and pathology. Specifics of radiation therapy (field and dose), chemotherapy (specific agents and cumulative doses), surgeries (splenectomy, organ resections, and biopsies), and blood transfusions are all important components of a survivor's treatment history that contribute to the assessment of future health risks. Information about any required modifications in treatment, major acute complications of therapy, and ongoing treatment-related issues, such as chronic GVHD, should be available at the time of evaluation. For a provider not familiar with a survivor's prior therapy, a treatment summary can usually be obtained from the treating institution. A sample treatment summary is provided in Figure 32-4. A summary of late effects associated with curative treatments for the most common childhood cancer diagnoses is presented in Table 32-4.

Medical History and Physical Examination

As with all medical assessments, obtaining and documenting a history of current and past medical problems is important to the childhood cancer survivor evaluation. Past medical history, including birth history, surgeries, and medical conditions that preceded the cancer diagnosis may be pertinent. For older survivors, menstrual history, reproductive history, and obstetric history all contribute important information to the follow-up

TREATMENT SUMMARY		
Current name: *Sarah Brown*	Medical record number: *075-623*	
Name at diagnosis: *same*	Date of birth: *5/12/84*	
Diagnosis: *ALL*	Site(s): *CNS negative*	
Presenting symptoms: *Fever, lymphadenopathy*		
Date of diagnosis: *7/9/88*	Protocol: *Standard risk - ALL*	
Date of recurrence:	Site(s):	
Relapse protocol:	Date of treatment completion: *9/90*	
Complications during treatment: *Fever/neutropenia*		
Chemotherapy		
Agent: *Doxorubicin*	Total dose: *360 mg/m2*	
Agent: *Vincristine*	Total dose:	
Agent: *Corticosteroids*	Total dose:	
Agent: *Mercaptopurine*	Total dose:	
Agent: *Methotrexate IM/IT*	Total dose:	
Radiotherapy		
Date *8/88*	Site: *Cranial*	Dose: *18 Gy*
Bone marrow transplant		
Date	Allo/auto	Allo donor/HLA matching
Chemotherapy conditioning (include doses)		
TBI/other radiotherapy	Site	Dose	Fractions
Acute GvHD (grade, site)	Chronic GvHD (grade, site)	Treatment
Surgery		
Site: *Central line placement*	Date: *7/88*	
Medical history		
Complications after treatment completion: *Learning disability*		
Familial history: *Depression/cardiovascular disease*		
Recent studies		
Test: *Echocardiogram*	Date *9/07*	Results: *Normal/EF-45%*

FIGURE 32-4. Example of childhood cancer survivor treatment summary. (*Adapted from Skinner R, Wallace WHB, Levitt GA [eds]. Therapy Based Long Term Follow-up Practice Statement. United Kingdom Children's Cancer Study Group, 2nd ed, 2005.*)

TABLE 32-4 Potential Late Effects Associated with Curative Therapies for Common Childhood Cancers

CATEGORIES OF TREATMENT-ASSOCIATED LATE EFFECTS BY PRIMARY CANCER

Primary Cancer	Secondary Malignancy	Cardiovascular and Pulmonary	Musculoskeletal	Neurologic and Developmental	Endocrine and Reproductive	Other
Leukemia	MDS, leukemia (alkylating agents, topoisomerase inhibitors) Skin cancer, meningiomas, CNS tumors (cranial radiation)	Cardiomyopathy, arrhythmias (anthracyclines)	Osteopenia, osteoporosis (corticosteroids, MTX) Osteonecrosis (corticosteroids) Short stature (corticosteroids, cranial radiation) Dental abnormalities (cranial radiation)	Learning disabilities (cranial radiation, intrathecal therapy) Vasculopathy (cranial radiation) Cataracts (corticosteroids, cranial radiation) Peripheral neuropathy, Raynaud's syndrome (vincristine)	GH deficiency, obesity (cranial radiation) Hypogonadism, azoospermia (testicular radiation) Infertility, hypogonadism (alkylating agents)	Alopecia (cranial radiation)
Brain tumor	CNS tumors, meningiomas, skin cancer (cranial, spinal radiation) MDS, leukemia (alkylating agents, topoisomerase inhibitors)	Cardiac dysfunction (spinal radiation)	Scoliosis, short stature (cranial, spinal radiation) Dental abnormalities (cranial radiation)	Learning disabilities (cranial radiation, neurosurgery) Cataracts, neurosensory deficits, vasculopathy (cranial radiation) Seizures, hydrocephalus (neurosurgery) Hearing loss (platin compounds, cranial radiation) Peripheral neuropathy, Raynaud's syndrome (vincristine)	Hypothalamic hypopituitarism, GH deficiency, obesity (cranial radiation) Infertility, hypogonadism (alkylating agents)	Renal insufficiency (platin compounds, ifosfamide) Alopecia (cranial radiation)
Hodgkin's lymphoma	Thyroid cancer, breast cancer, lung cancer, upper GI cancer, sarcomas, skin cancer (mantle radiation) Colon cancer, GU cancers, skin cancer (abdominal, pelvic radiation) MDS, leukemia (alkylating agents, topoisomerase inhibitors)	Carotid artery stenosis, coronary artery disease, valvular heart disease, cardiomyopathy, pericardial fibrosis, arrhythmias (mantle radiation) Cardiomyopathy, arrhythmias (anthracyclines)	Scoliosis, short stature (thoracic radiation) Osteopenia, osteoporosis (corticosteroids)		Thyroid disease (mantle radiation) Infertility, hypogonadism (pelvic radiation, alkylating agents)	High-risk pregnancy (radiation, anthracyclines) Life-threatening bacterial sepsis (splenectomy) GI strictures (mantle radiation) Pulmonary fibrosis (mantle radiation, bleomycin)

Continues

TABLE 32-4 Potential Late Effects Associated with Curative Therapies for Common Childhood Cancers—cont'd

Primary Cancer	CATEGORIES OF TREATMENT-ASSOCIATED LATE EFFECTS BY PRIMARY CANCER					
	Secondary Malignancy	Cardiovascular and Pulmonary	Musculoskeletal	Neurologic and Developmental	Endocrine and Reproductive	Other
Neuroblastoma	Skin cancer, sarcomas (any radiation) Breast cancer, thyroid cancer (thoracic radiation) MDS, leukemia (alkylating agents, topoisomerase inhibitors)	Cardiomyopathy, arrhythmias (anthracycline)	Scoliosis, short stature (thoracic radiation, TBI)	Hearing loss (platin compounds)	Thyroid disease (thoracic radiation) Infertility, hypogonadism (alkylating agents)	Renal insufficiency (platin compounds, ifosfamide, abdominal radiation) Pulmonary fibrosis (thoracic radiation) Small bowel obstruction (abdominal surgery) Horner's syndrome, scoliosis (thoracic surgery)
Wilms' tumor	Colon cancer, skin cancer, sarcoma (abdominal radiation) Skin cancer, breast cancer, thyroid cancer, lung cancer (lung radiation)	Cardiomyopathy, arrhythmias (anthracycline)	Scoliosis, short stature (abdominal radiation)	Peripheral neuropathy, Raynaud's syndrome (vincristine)	Infertility, hypogonadism (alkylating agents) Thyroid disease (lung radiation)	Small bowel obstruction (abdominal surgery) Renal insufficiency, nephrectomy (abdominal radiation) Pulmonary fibrosis (lung radiation) High-risk pregnancy (radiation, anthracyclines)
Sarcoma	MDS, leukemia (alkylating agents, topoisomerase inhibitors) Cancer of the skin, bone, soft tissue, organs in the treatment field (radiation)	Cardiomyopathy, arrhythmias (anthracycline)	Hypoplasia of the bone, soft tissue in radiation field (radiation) Deformity of bone, soft tissue (surgery) Dental abnormalities (radiation)	Hearing loss (platin compounds) Peripheral neuropathy, Raynaud's syndrome (vincristine)	Infertility, hypogonadism (alkylating agents)	Renal insufficiency (platin compounds, ifosfamide) High-risk pregnancy (radiation, anthracyclines) Dysfunction of organs in treatment field (radiation)

CNS, central nervous system; GH, growth hormone; GI, gastrointestinal; GU, genitourinary; MDS, myelodysplastic syndrome; MTX, methotrexate.

evaluation. Information about current medications and chronic medical conditions should also be obtained. Survivors should specifically be asked about any late effects diagnosed or treated to date, including subsequent cancers.

Family history of chronic diseases and family cancer history are also an important part of the comprehensive survivor evaluation. Cancer diagnosed in first-degree relatives (parents, offspring, siblings) in a pattern suggestive of a hereditary cancer predisposition syndrome should be noted and appropriate referrals to cancer geneticists considered. A family history that includes other children with cancer raises particular concerns about hereditary cancer syndromes, as does a family history of genetic syndromes associated with cancer predisposition, such as Fanconi's anemia, neurofibromatosis, and immunodeficiency syndromes. A survivor's family history of common chronic diseases should be noted, with special attention to conditions for which the survivor may have treatment-related risk factors, such as heart disease, osteoporosis, or depression. Family history should be updated and reassessed at each subsequent evaluation.

All survivors should be asked about educational attainment and special education services or needs. For older survivors, employment history and insurance status are also critical to determining health care needs. Health behaviors, including exercise, diet, sleep, tobacco use, alcohol use, and nonprescription drug use are also important aspects of the follow-up assessment. To evaluate a survivor's emotional and physical needs that are not addressed in a medical history, survivors should be asked about their relationships with family and peers, sexual activity, and current living arrangements.

A comprehensive childhood cancer survivor's evaluation also includes a review of current and recent symptoms. This review of symptoms should include special consideration of symptoms known to be associated with specific late effects. Symptoms should be evaluated in light of the increased prior probability of significant morbidity compared with patients of a similar age. For example, a complaint of chronic headaches or sinus problems in a patient with a history of head and neck radiation should be evaluated in light of the risk of radiogenic tumors, and a young patient with dyspnea or chest pain might undergo a cardiac evaluation with a lower threshold than a patient who was not exposed to cardiotoxic therapies as a child.

A thorough physical examination, including skin and neurologic examinations, is also part of a childhood cancer survivor's routine evaluation. Radiation fields in particular should be examined carefully for any skin changes, masses, or lesions. A careful thyroid examination is indicated, in particular for patients who have received radiation to the head, neck, chest, or upper spine. Head, trunk, and limbs should be examined for growth disturbances related to surgery or radiation, such as limb length discrepancies, spinal deformity, and facial bone deformity. Major organ toxicities associated with specific chemotherapy agents and radiation fields commonly used to treat pediatric cancers are shown in Figure 32-5. Transplantation survivors should be examined for signs of chronic GVHD.

Diagnostic and Screening Tests

The health care provider evaluating the childhood cancer survivor should arrange for diagnostic or screening tests and subspecialty consultations based on the survivor's treatment risks, symptoms, or other findings. The provider should recommend surveillance studies assessing primary disease recurrence, if indicated, studies to assess organ function in any organs potentially affected by cancer therapy, and specialist consultation to evaluate findings or potential health risks. Depending on expo-

sures, age, and gender, screening studies to assess for second cancers, such as mammography or colonoscopy, should be considered. Clinical guidelines developed by the Children's Oncology Group are available to help direct clinicians in the evaluation of survivors of childhood, adolescent, and young adult cancers (available at www.survivorshipguidelines.org).[75] These risk-based treatment-related guidelines are intended to provide screening recommendations for late effects commonly observed in survivors.

Assessment and Follow-up Plan

A childhood cancer survivor's risk for each late effect should be interpreted in light of his or her treatment history, past medical history, family history, symptoms, and physical examination. All findings and test results from the comprehensive survivor evaluation should be summarized, and recommendations and plans for follow-up documented and communicated to the patient and all providers involved in the patient's care. Acknowledging the complexity of the issues, the provider should prioritize the follow-up recommendations for the survivor and family, and emphasize that this advice is limited by our current knowledge of late effects and is based on future probabilities.

In summary, the successful follow-up care for the childhood cancer survivor depends on thorough evaluation, with attention to possible late effects and effective communication with patient, family, and other providers involved in ongoing care.

SPECIAL CONSIDERATIONS FOR THE HEMATOPOIETIC STEM CELL TRANSPLANT SURVIVOR

The comprehensive clinical evaluation of the hematopoietic stem cell transplant (HSCT) survivor requires that the clinician consider all aspects of the survivor's pretransplant history, transplant course, post-transplant immune function, and disease status. In assessing a survivor of HSCT, both the treatments associated with the condition that led to the transplant and the therapies associated with the transplant must be considered. The modality, dose, and intensity of the conditioning regimens for HSCT are major factors that determine survivors risk for late effects. Total body radiation used as conditioning for HSCT may contribute to the organ-specific toxicity of prior chemotherapy such as cardiotoxicity from anthracyclines,[137] ototoxicity from platinum agents,[242] and gonadotoxicity of alkylating agents.[254] The transplant history should be reviewed for complications that occurred during the course of transplant, such as acute pneumonitis or renal failure, which might add to the survivor's risk for late onset organ toxicity.[159,283] The source of the stem cells also is a factor in a HSCT survivor's risk for late effects. Survivors who received an allogeneic HSCT are at risk for chronic graft-versus-host disease (CGVHD) that can be associated with severe chronic illness. Long-term consequences of CGVHD can include joint contractures, polymyositis, vaginal stenosis, alopecia, vitiligo, scleroderma, lichenoid skin lesions, xerostomia, lichenoid or atrophic oral lesions, xerophthalmia, keratoconjunctivitis, esophageal strictures, malabsorption, cholestasis, bronchiolitis obliterans, and obstructive airway disease.[342a] Survivors with CGVHD and those on chronic immunosuppressive regimens have an increased risk of infection.[311] Comprehensive assessment of the HSCT must also include post-transplant immunization history to assure revaccination was accomplished at appropriate intervals after transplant.

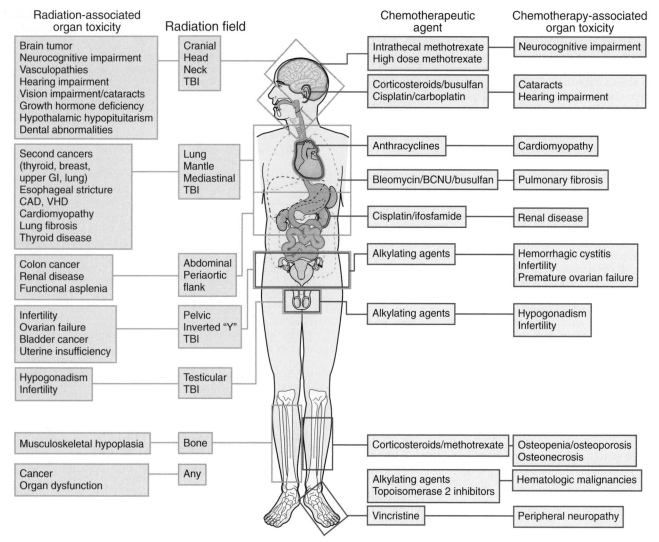

FIGURE 32-5. Late effects associated with common treatments for childhood cancer by organ system. GI, gastrointestinal; TBI, total-body irradiation; CAD, coronary artery disease; VHD, valvular heart disease.

FUTURE DIRECTIONS

Advances in the treatment of childhood cancer have resulted in growing numbers of survivors. Epidemiologic studies have shown that survivors of childhood cancer are likely to experience adverse health-related consequences of their treatment and the potential to develop late effects appears to be lifelong. Although remarkable progress has been made in describing the late effects experienced by childhood cancer survivors and their associated risk factors, future research is needed. This will help decrease incidence and morbidity and improve the quality of life for current and future survivors. In response, survivorship research is focused on three main areas: (1) changes in primary cancer therapy focused on decreasing the incidence of late toxicity; (2) improvements in care to decrease the incidence or severity of a particular late effect; and (3) changes in health care systems to ensure that all survivors have access to best practices to detect and manage late effects.

Current treatment protocols for childhood cancer are designed to minimize late effects without compromising survival. The strategies that have been investigated, or are under investigation, include eliminating or reducing exposure to

specific chemotherapies with known late toxicities, such as anthracyclines and alkylating agents, reducing radiation dose and field, and delaying radiation therapy for very young children.[343-349] Studies to quantify the efficacy of these strategies to obviate late effects while maintaining survival are forthcoming. Current strategies for primary treatment of standard-risk ALL, localized Hodgkin's lymphoma, Wilms' tumor, and neuroblastoma designed to reduce late effects have currently resulted in excellent outcomes, with a low incidence of recurrence and treatment-related late effects.[132,346,349,350]

Another strategy to reduce late morbidity in childhood cancer survivors is the identification of individuals with heightened susceptibility for specific treatment-associated late effects. One potential method of identification is genetic polymorphism testing, which identifies individuals with a genotype known to increase susceptibility to treatment-associated toxicity, such as second cancers, obesity, and cardiac disease.[100,351-354] Testing could be done prior to cancer treatment and the results used to modify treatment plans to account for an individual's genetic susceptibility to late effects. For example, lower dose radiation therapy might be indicated for an individual identified by genetic polymorphism testing as having a genotype associated with radiation-induced second cancers. Similarly, genetic polymorphism testing could be done decades after therapy to identify survivors at risk for late effects, which would inform screening recommendations and eligibility for preventive interventions.

Health services research focused on understanding cancer survivor care and studying improvements in care is ongoing. As the current population of childhood cancer survivors ages, health care delivery to this group will become more complex, and will include integration of treatment-related risks and adult-onset morbidity. Optimal and innovative methods of patient and health care provider education that achieve this integration will need to be elucidated and disseminated to ensure the best possible quality of life for survivors of childhood cancer.

SUMMARY

The care of the child diagnosed with cancer does not end with the completion of therapy. Consequently, pediatric oncology providers need to have a working knowledge of the potential late effects of curative therapy for childhood cancer, and are responsible for communicating information about late effects to survivors, their families, and other health care providers involved in the care of the childhood cancer survivor. Pediatric survivorship research has made significant contributions which advance our understanding of long-term treatment-associated morbidities, and current therapeutic protocols are designed with the intention of minimizing known late effects. However, despite progress, childhood cancer survivors remain vulnerable to many long-term treatment-related morbidities. Ongoing efforts in research and clinical care for childhood cancer survivors must be directed at improving and extending follow-up care, developing interventions for individuals identified as being at risk for specific late effects, and optimizing management of late effects, with the ultimate aim of improving quality of life for all current and future childhood cancer survivors.

REFERENCES

1. D'Angio GJ. Management of children with Wilms' tumor. Cancer. 1972;30:1528-1533.
2. Tan C, D'Angio GJ, Exelby PR, et al. The changing management of childhood Hodgkin's disease. Cancer. 1975;35:808-816.
3. Ghavimi F, Exelby PR, D'Angio GJ, et al. Multidisciplinary treatment of embryonal rhabdomyosarcoma in children. Cancer. 1975;35:677-686.
4. Hayles AL, Dahlin DC, Coventry MB. Osteogenic sarcoma in children. JAMA. 1960;174:1174-1177.
5. Nesbit ME, Krivit W, Robison L. A follow-up report on long-term survivors of childhood acute lymphoblastic or undifferentiated leukemia: a report for Children's Cancer Study Group. J Pediatr. 1979;95:727-730.
6. Ries LAG, Melbert D, Krapcho M, et al. SEER Cancer Statistics Review, 1975-2004 (based on November 2006 Surveillance Epidemiology and End Results (SEER) data submission) Available at http://seer.cancer.gov/csr/1975_2004.
7. Clarke SA, Eiser C. Health behaviours in childhood cancer survivors: a systematic review. Eur J Cancer. 2007;43:1373-1384.
8. Mulhern RK, Tyc VL, Phipps S, et al. Health-related behaviors of survivors of childhood cancer. Med Pediatr Oncol. 1995;25:159-165.
9. Li FP, Cassady R, Jaffe N. Risk of second tumors in survivors of childhood cancer. Cancer. 1975;35:1230-1235.
10. Meadows AT, D'Angio GJ, Evans AE, et al. Oncogenesis and other late effects of cancer treatment in children. Radiology. 1975;114:175-180.
11. D'Angio GJ. The late consequences of successful cancer treatment given children and adolescents. Radiology. 1975;114:145.
12. Li FP, Myers MH, Heise HW, Jaffee N. The course of five-year survivors of cancer in childhood. J Pediatr. 1978;93:185-187.
13. Hawkins MM, Kingston JE, Kinnier Wilson LM. Late deaths after treatment for childhood cancer. Arch Dis Child. 1990;65:1356-1363.
14. Nicholson HS, Fears TR, Byrne J. Death during adulthood in survivors of childhood and adolescent cancer. Cancer. 1994;73:3094-3102.
15. Robertson CM, Hawkins MM, Kingston JE. Late deaths and survival after childhood cancer: implications for cure. BMJ. 1994;309:162-166.
16. Mertens AC, Yasui Y, Neglia JP, et al. Late mortality experienced in five-year survivors of childhood and adolescent cancer: the Childhood Cancer Survivor Study. J Clin Oncol. 2001;19:3163-3172.
17. Moller TR, Garwicz S, Barlow L, et al. Decreasing late mortality among five-year survivors of cancer in childhood and adolescence: a population-based study in the Nordic countries. J Clin Oncol. 2001;19:3173-3181.
18. Cardous-Ubbink MC, Heinen RC, Langeveld NE, et al. Long-term cause-specific mortality among five-year survivors of childhood cancer. Pediatr Blood Cancer. 2004;42:563-573.
19. Byrne J, Mulvihill JJ, Myers MH, et al. Effects of treatment of fertility in long-term survivors of childhood or adolescent cancer. N Engl J Med. 1987;317:1315-1321.
20. Tucker MA, Meadows AT, Boice JD, et al. Leukemia after therapy with alkylating agents for childhood cancer. J Natl Cancer Inst. 1987;78:459-464.
21. Hawkins MM, Kinnier Wilson LM, Stovall MA, et al. Epipodophyllotoxins, alkylating agents, and radiation and risk of secondary leukemia after childhood cancer. BMJ. 1992;304:951-958.
22. van Leeuwen FE, Chorus AMJ, van den Belt-Dusebout AW, et al. Leukemia risk following Hodgkin's disease: relation to cumulative dose of alkylating agents, treatment with teniposide combinations, number of episodes of chemotherapy, and bone marrow damage. J Clin Oncol. 1994;12:1063-1073.
23. Olsen JH, Garwicz S, Hertz H, et al. Second malignant neoplasms after cancer in childhood or adolescence. Nordic Society of Pediatric Hematology and Oncology Association of the Nordic Cancer Registries. BMJ. 1993;307:1030-1036.
24. Bhatia S, Robison LL, Oberlin O, et al. Breast cancer and other second neoplasms after childhood Hodgkin's disease. N Engl J Med. 1996;334:745-751.
25. Green DM, Gingell RL, Pearce J, et al. The effect of mediastinal irradiation on cardiac function of patients treated during childhood and adolescence for Hodgkin's disease. J Clin Oncol. 1987;5:239-245.
26. Robison LL, Mertens AC, Boice JD, et al. Study design and cohort characteristics of the Childhood Cancer Survivors Study: a multi-institutional collaborative project. Med Pediatr Oncol. 2002;38:229-239.
27. van der Pal HJH, van Dalen EC, Kremer LCM, et al. Risk of morbidity and mortality from cardiovascular disease following radiotherapy for childhood cancer: a systematic review. Cancer Treat Rev. 2005;31:173-185.
28. Swerdlow AJ, Higgins CD, Smith P, et al. Myocardial infarction mortality risk after treatment for Hodgkin's disease: a collaborative British cohort study. J Natl Cancer Inst. 2007;99:206-214.
29. Hewitt M, Greenfield S, Stovall E (eds). From Cancer Patient to Cancer Survivor Lost in Translation. Washington, DC, National Academic Press, 2006.

30. Kenney LB, Laufer MR, Grant FD, et al. High risk of infertility and long-term gonadal damage in males treated with high-dose cyclophosphamide for sarcoma during childhood. Cancer. 2001; 91:613-621.

31. Adams MJ, Lipshultz SE, Schwartz C, et al. Radiation-associated cardiovascular disease: manifestations and management. Semin Radiat Oncol. 2003;13:346-356.

32. Smith SM, Le Beau MM, Huo D, et al. Clinical-cytogenetic associations in 306 patients with therapy-related myelodysplasia and myeloid leukemia: the University of Chicago series. Blood. 2003;102:43-52.

33. Butler RW, Copeland DR. Neuropsychological effects of central nervous system prophylactic treatment in childhood leukemia: methodological considerations. J Pediatr Psychol. 1993;18:319-338.

34. Pui CH, Cheng C, Leung W, et al. Extended follow-up of long-term survivors of childhood acute lymphoblastic leukemia. N Engl J Med. 2003;349:640-649.

35. Packer RJ, Gurney JG, Punyko JA, et al. Long-term neurologic and neurosensory sequelae in adult survivors of a childhood brain tumor: childhood Cancer Survivor study. J Clin Oncol. 2003;21:3255-3261.

36. Neglia JP, Robison LL, Stovall M, et al. New primary neoplasms of the central nervous system in survivors of childhood cancer: a report from the Childhood Cancer Survivor Study. J Natl Cancer Inst. 2006;98:1528-1537.

37. Lipshultz SE, Lipsitz SR, Mone SM, et al. Female sex and drug dose as risk factors for late cardiotoxic effects of doxorubicin therapy for childhood cancer. N Engl J Med. 1995;332:1738-1743.

38. Hull MC, Morris CG, Pepine CJ, Mendenhall NP. Valvular dysfunction and carotid, subclavian, and coronary artery disease in survivors of Hodgkin lymphoma treated with radiation therapy. JAMA. 2003;290:2831-2837.

39. Neglia JP, Friedman DL, Yasui Y, et al. Second malignant neoplasms in five-year survivors of childhood cancer: Childhood Cancer Survivor Study. J Natl Cancer Inst. 2001;93:618-629.

40. Inslap PD, Reis LAG, Cohen RJ, Curtis RE. New malignancies following childhood cancer. In Curtis RE, Freedman DM, Ron E (eds). New malignancies among cancer survivors: SEER Cancer Registries, 1973–2000. Bethesda, Md, National Cancer Institute, 2006, pp 465–482.

41. Jenkinson HC, Hawkins MM, Stiller CA, et al. Long-term population-based risk of second malignant neoplasms after childhood cancer in Britain. Br J Cancer. 2004;91:11905-11910.

42. Henderson TO, Whitton J, Stovall M, et al. Secondary sarcomas in childhood cancer survivors: a report from the Childhood Cancer Survivor study. J Natl Cancer Inst. 2007;99:300-308.

43. Breslow NE, Takashima JR, Whitton JA, et al. Second malignant neoplasms following treatment for Wilms' tumor: a report from the National Wilms' Tumor Study Group. J Clin Oncol. 1995;13:1851-1859.

44. Le Deley MC, Leblanc T, Shamsaldin A, et al. Risk of secondary leukemia after a solid tumor in childhood according to the dose of epipodophyllotoxins and anthracyclines: a case-control study by the French Society of Pediatric Oncology. J Clin Oncol. 2003;15:1074-1081.

45. Dietrich PY, Henry-Amar M, Cosset JM, et al. Second primary cancers in patients continuously disease-free from Hodgkin's disease: a protective role for the spleen? Blood. 1994;84:1209-1215.

46. Meadows AT, Obringer AC, Marrero O, et al. Second malignant neoplasms following childhood Hodgkin's disease: treatment and splenectomy as risk factors. Med Pediatr Oncol. 1989;17:477-484.

47. Hisada M, Garber J, Fung CY, et al. Multiple primary cancers in families with Li-Fraumeni syndrome. J Natl Cancer Inst. 1998;90:606-611.

48. Lustbader ED, Williams WR, Bondy ML, et al. Segregation analysis of cancer in families of childhood soft-tissue-sarcoma patients. Am J Hum Genet. 1992;51:344-356.

49. Wong FL, Boice JD Jr, Abramson DH, et al. Cancer incidence after retinoblastoma. Radiation dose and sarcoma risk. JAMA. 1997;278:1262-1267.

50. Garber JE, Offit K. Hereditary cancer predisposition syndromes. J Clin Oncol. 2005;23:276-292.

51. Modan B, Chetrit A, Alfandary E, Katz L. Increased risk of breast cancer after low-dose irradiation. Lancet. 1989;25:629-631.

52. Sadetzki S, Chetrit A, Freedman L, et al. Long-term follow-up for brain tumor development after childhood exposure to ionizing radiation for tinea capitis. Radiat Res. 2005;163:424-432.

53. Koh ES, Tran TH, Heydarian M, et al. A comparison of mantle versus involved-field radiotherapy for Hodgkin's lymphoma: reduction in normal tissue dose and second cancer risk. Radiat Oncol. 2007;2:13.

54. Hawkins MM, Wilson LM, Burton HS, et al. Radiotherapy, alkylating agents, and risk of bone cancer after childhood cancer. J Natl Cancer Inst. 1996;88:270-278.

55. Kenney LB, Yasui Y, Inskip PD, et al. Breast cancer after childhood cancer: a report from the Childhood Cancer Survivor Study. Ann Intern Med. 2004;141:590-597.

56. Ng AF, Bernardo MV, Weller E, et al. Second malignancy after Hodgkin disease treated with radiation therapy with or without chemotherapy: long-term risks and risk factors. Blood. 2002;100:1989-1996.

57. Tucker MA, D'Angio GJ, Boice JD Jr, et al. Bone sarcomas linked to radiotherapy and chemotherapy in children. N Engl J Med. 1987;317:588-593.

58. Kleinerman RA, Tucker MA, Tarone RE, et al. Risk of new cancers after radiotherapy in long-term survivors of retinoblastoma: an extended follow-up. J Clin Oncol. 2005;23:2272-2279.

59. Travis LB, Gospodarowicz M, Curtis RE, et al. Lung cancer following chemotherapy and radiotherapy for Hodgkin's disease. J Natl Cancer Inst. 2002;94:182-192.

60. Bassal M, Mertens AC, Taylor L, et al. Risk of selected subsequent carcinomas in survivors of childhood cancer: a report from the Childhood Cancer Survivor Study. J Clin Oncol. 2006;24:476-483.

61. Metayer C, Lynch CF, Clarke EA, et al. Second cancers among long-term survivors of Hodgkin's disease diagnosed in childhood and adolescence. J Clin Oncol. 2000;18:2435-2443.

62. Densmore TL, Langer JC, Molleston JP, et al. Colorectal adenocarcinoma as a second malignant neoplasm following Wilms' tumor and rhabdomyosarcoma. Med Pediatr Oncol. 1996;27:556-560.

63. Scaradavou A, Heller G, Sklar CA, et al. Second malignant neoplasms in long-term survivors of childhood rhabdomyosarcoma. Cancer. 1995;76:1860-1867.

64. Stites Whatley W, Thompson JW, Rao B. Salivary gland tumors in survivors of childhood cancer. Otolaryngol Head Neck Surg. 2006;134:385-388.

65. Yahalom J, Petrek JA, Biddinger PW, et al. Breast cancer in patients irradiated for Hodgkin's disease: a clinical and pathologic analysis of 45 events in 37 patients. J Clin Oncol. 1992;10:1674-1681.

66. Travis LB, Hill DA, Dores GM, et al. Breast cancer following radiotherapy and chemotherapy among young women with Hodgkin disease. JAMA. 2003;290:465-475.

67. van Leeuwen FE, Klokman WJ, Stovall M, et al. Roles of radiation dose, and hormonal factors in breast cancer following Hodgkin's disease. J Natl Cancer Inst. 2003;95:971-980.

68. Sankila R, Garwicz S, Olsen JH, et al. Risk of subsequent malignant neoplasms among 1,641 Hodgkin's disease patients diagnosed in childhood and adolescence: a population-based cohort

study in the five Nordic countries. J Clin Oncol. 1996;14: 1442-1446.

69. Swerdlow AJ, Barber JA, Hudson GV, et al. Risk of second malignancy after Hodgkin's disease in a collaborative British cohort: the relation of age to treatment. J Clin Oncol. 2000;18: 498-509.

70. Green DM, Hyland A, Barcos MP, et al. Second malignant neoplasms after treatment for Hodgkin's disease in childhood or adolescence. J Clin Oncol. 2000;18:1492-1499.

70a. Friedman DL, Rovo A, Leisenring W, et al. Increased risk of breast cancer among survivors of allogeneic hematopoietic cell transplantation: a report from the FHCRC and the EBMT—Late Effect Working Party. Blood. 2008;111:939–944.

71. Travis LB, Hill D, Dores GM, et al. Cumulative absolute breast cancer risk for young women treated for Hodgkin lymphoma. J Natl Cancer Inst. 2005;97:1428-1437.

72. Guibout C, Adjadj E, Rubino C, et al. Malignant breast tumors after radiotherapy for a first cancer during childhood. J Clin Oncol. 2005;23:197-204.

73. Li CI, Malone KE, Daling JR. Difference in breast cancer stage, treatment, and survival by race and ethnicity. Arch Intern Med. 2003;163:49-65.

74. Wolden SL, Hancock SL, Carlson RW, et al. Management of breast cancer after Hodgkin's disease. J Clin Oncol. 2000;18: 765-772.

75. Children's Oncology Group. Long-Term Guidelines for Survivors of Childhood, Adolescent, and Young Adult Cancers, and related Health Links. Available at www.survivorshipguidelines. org.

76. Saslow D, Boetes C, Burke W, et al. American Cancer Society guidelines for breast screening with MRI as an adjunct to mammography. CA Cancer J Clin. 2007;57:75-89.

77. Sklar C, Whitton J, Mertens A, et al. Abnormalities of the thyroid in survivors of Hodgkin's disease: data from the Childhood Cancer Survivor Study. J Clin Endocrinol Metab. 2000;85: 3227-3232.

78. Bhatia S, Yasui Y, Robison LL, et al. High risk of subsequent neoplasms continues with extended follow-up of childhood Hodgkin's disease: report from the Late Effects Study Group. J Clin Oncol. 2003;21:4386-4394.

79. van Leeuwen FE, Klokman WJ, van't Ver MB, et al. Long-term risk of second malignancy in survivors of Hodgkin's disease treated during adolescence or young adulthood. J Clin Oncol. 2000;18:487-497.

80. Sigurdson AJ, Ronckers CM, Mertens AC, et al. Primary thyroid cancer after a first tumor in childhood (the Childhood Cancer Survivor Study): a nested case-control study. Lancet. 2005;365: 2014-2023.

81. Acharya S, Sarafoglou K, LaQuaglia M, et al. Thyroid neoplasms after therapeutic radiation for malignancies during childhood or adolescence. Cancer. 2003;97:2397-2403.

82. Black P, Straaten A, Gutjahr P. Secondary thyroid carcinoma after treatment for childhood cancer. Med Pediatr Oncol. 1998; 31:91-95.

83. Tucker MA, Jones PH, Boice JD, et al. Therapeutic radiation at a young age is linked to secondary thyroid cancer. The Late Effects group. Cancer Res. 1991;51:2885-2888.

84. Schneider AB, Ron E, Lubin J, et al. Dose-response relationships for radiation-induced thyroid cancer and thyroid nodules: evidence for the prolonged effects of radiation on the thyroid. J Clin Endocrinol Metab. 1993;77:362-369.

85. Ronckers CM, Sigurdson AJ, Stovall M, et al. Thyroid cancer in childhood cancer survivors: a detailed evaluation of radiation dose response and its modifiers. Radiat Res. 2006;166:618-628.

86. Crom DB, Kaste SC, Tubergen DG, et al. Ultrasonagraphy for thyroid screening after head and neck irradiation in childhood cancer survivors. Med Pediatr Oncol. 1997;28:15-21.

87. Schneider AB, Bekerman C, Leland J, et al. Thyroid nodules in the follow-up of irradiated individuals: comparison of thyroid ultrasound with scanning and palpation. J Clin Endocrinol Metab. 1997;82:4020-4027.

88. Eden K, Mahon S, Helfand M. Screening high-risk populations for thyroid cancer. Med Pediatr Oncol. 2001;36:583-591.

89. Metzger ML, Howard SC, Hudson MM, et al. Natural history of thyroid nodules in the survivors of pediatric Hodgkin lymphoma. Pediatr Blood Cancer. 2006;46:314-319.

90. Schneider SB, Sarne DH. Long-term risks for thyroid cancer and other neoplasms after exposure to radiation. Nat Clin Pract Endocrinol Metab. 2005;1:82-91.

91. Subbiah S, Collins BJ, Schneider AB. Factors related to the recurrence of thyroid nodules after surgery for benign radiation-related nodules. Thyroid. 2007;17:41-47.

92. Kleinerman RA, Tucker MA, Abramson DH, et al. Risk of soft tissue sarcomas by individual subtype in survivors of hereditary retinoblastoma. J Natl Cancer Inst. 2007;99:24-31.

93. Hawkins MM, Kinnier Wilson L, Burton HS, et al. Bone cancer after childhood cancer. J Natl Cancer Inst. 1996;88:270-278.

94. Le Vu B, de Vathaire F, Shamsaldin A, et al. Radiation dose, chemotherapy and risk of osteosarcoma after solid tumors during childhood. Int J Cancer. 1998;77:370-377.

95. Kuttesch JF Jr, Wexler LH, Marcus RB, et al. Second malignancies after Ewing's sarcoma: radiation dose-dependency of secondary sarcomas. J Clin Oncol. 1996;14:2818-2825.

96. Newton WA Jr, Meadows AT, Shimada H, et al. Bone sarcomas as second malignant neoplasms following childhood cancer. Cancer. 1991;67:193-201.

97. Walter AW, Hancock ML, Pui CH, et al. Secondary brain tumors in children treated for acute lymphoblastic leukemia at St. Jude Children's Research Hospital. J Clin Oncol. 1998;16: 3761-3767.

98. Loning L, Zimmermann M, Reiter A, et al. Secondary neoplasms subsequent to Berlin-Frankfurt-Munster therapy of acute lymphoblastic leukemia in childhood: significantly lower risk without cranial radiotherapy. Blood. 2000;95:2770-2775.

99. Hijaya N, Hudson MM, Lensing S, et al. Cumulative incidence of secondary neoplasms as a first event after childhood acute lymphoblastic leukemia. JAMA. 2007;297:1207-1215.

100. Relling MV, Rubnitz JE, Rivera GK, et al. High incidence of secondary brain tumors after radiotherapy and antimetabolites. Lancet. 1999;354:34-39.

101. Shields CL, Meadows AT, Shields JA, et al. Chemoreduction for retinoblastoma may prevent intracranial neuroblastic malignancy (trilateral retinoblastoma). Arch Ophthalmol. 2001;119:1269-1272.

102. Kivela T. Trilateral retinoblastoma: a meta-analysis of hereditary retinoblastoma associated with primary ectopic intracranial retinoblastoma. J Clin Oncol. 1999;17:1829-1837.

103. Goshen Y, Stark B, Kornreich L, et al. High incidence of meningioma in cranial irradiated survivors of childhood acute lymphoblastic leukemia. Pediatr Blood Cancer. 2007;49:294-297.

104. Goshen Y, Stark B, Kornreich L, et al. Radiation dose as a risk factor for malignant melanoma following childhood cancer. Eur J Cancer. 2003;39:2379-2386.

105. Bishop JN, Harland M, Randerson-Moor J, Bishop DT. Management of familial melanoma. Lancet Oncol. 2007;8:46-54.

106. Perkins JL, Liu Y, Mitby PA, et al. Nonmelanoma skin cancer in survivors of childhood and adolescent cancer: a report from the Childhood Cancer Survivor study. J Clin Oncol. 2005;23:3733-3741.

107. Wolfe JT. The role of screening in the management of skin cancer. Curr Opin Oncol. 1999;11:123-128.

108. Schellong G, Riepenhausen M, Creutzig U, et al. Low risk of secondary leukemias after chemotherapy without mechlorethamine in childhood Hodgkin's disease. German-Austrian Pediatric

Hodgkin's Disease Group. J Clin Oncol. 1997;15(6):2247-2253.

109. Pui CH, Relling MV, Rivera GK, et al. Epipodophyllotoxin-related acute myeloid leukemia: a study of 35 cases. Leukemia. 1995;9:1990-1996.

110. Felix CA. Leukemias related to treatment with DNA topoisomerase II inhibitors. Med Pediatr Oncol. 2001;36:525-535.

111. Haddy N, Le Deley MC, Samand A, et al. Role of radiotherapy and chemotherapy in the risk of secondary leukemia after a solid tumor in childhood. Eur J Cancer. 2006;42:2757-2764.

112. Pui CH, Ribeiro RC, Hancock ML, et al. Acute myeloid leukemia in children treated with epipodophyllotoxins for acute lymphoblastic leukemia. N Engl J Med. 1991;325:1682-1687.

113. Neglia JP, Meadows AT, Robison LL, et al. Second neoplasms after acute lymphoblastic leukemia in childhood. N Engl J Med. 1991;325:1330-1336.

114. Le Deley MC, Vassal G, Taibi A, et al. High cumulative rate of secondary leukemia after continous etoposide treatment for solid tumors in children and young adults. Pediatr Blood Cancer. 2005;45:25-31.

115. Lipshultz SE, Colan SD, Gelber RD, et al. Late cardiac effects of doxorubicin therapy for acute lymphoblastic leukemia in childhood. N Engl J Med. 1991;324:808-815.

116. Grenier MA, Lipshultz SE. Epidemiology of anthracycline cardiotoxicity in children and adults. Semin Oncol. 1998;25:72-85.

117. Green DM, Grigoriev YA, Nan B, et al. Congestive heart failure after treatment for Wilms' tumor: a report from the National Wilms' Tumor Study group. J Clin Oncol. 2001;19:1926-1934.

118. Kremer LCM, van Dalen EC, Offinga M, et al. Anthracycline-induces clinical heart failure in a cohort of 607 children: long-term follow-up study. J Clin Oncol. 2001;19:191-196.

119. van Dalen EC, van der Pal HJH, Kok WEM, et al. Clinical heart failure in a cohort of children treated with anthracyclines: a long-term follow-up study. Eur J Cancer. 2006;42:3191-3198.

120. Adams MJ, Lipshultz SE. Pathophysiology of anthracycline- and radiation-associated cardiomyopathies: implications for screening and prevention. Pediatr Blood Cancer. 2005;44:600-606.

121. Jakacki RI, Goldwein JW, Larsen RL, et al. Cardiac dysfunction following spinal irradiation during childhood. J Clin Oncol. 1993;11:1033-1038.

122. Eames GM, Crosson J, Steinberger J, et al. Cardiovascular function in children following bone marrow transplant: a cross-sectional study. Bone Marrow Transplant. 1997;19:61-66.

123. Stewart JR, Fajardo LF, Gillette SM, Constine LS. Radiation injury to the heart. Int J Radiat Oncol Biol Phys. 1995;31:1205-1211.

124. Lipshultz SE, Sallan SE. Cardiovascular abnormalities in long-term survivors of childhood malignancy. J Clin Oncol. 1993;11:1199-1203.

125. Krischer JP, Epstein S, Cuthbertson DD, et al. Clinical cardiotoxicity following anthracycline treatment for childhood cancer: the Pediatric Oncology Group experience. J Clin Oncol. 1997;15:1544-1552.

126. Lipshultz SE. Heart failure in childhood cancer survivors. Nat Clin Pract Oncol. 2007;4:334-335.

127. Lipshultz SE. Exposure to anthracyclines during childhood causes cardiac injury. Semin Oncol. 2006;33:S8-S14.

128. Lipshultz SE, Vlach SA, Lipsitz SR, et al. Cardiac changes associated with growth hormone therapy among children treated with anthracyclines. Pediatrics. 2005;115:1613-1622.

129. Nysom K, Colan SD, Lipshultz SE, et al. Late cardiotoxicity following anthracycline therapy for childhood cancer. Prog Pediatr Cardiol. 1998;8:121-138.

130. Lipshultz SE, Lipsitz SR, Sallan SE, et al. Chronic progressive cardiac dysfunction years after doxorubicin therapy for childhood

131. Sorensen K, Levitt GA, Bull C, et al. Late anthracycline cardiotoxicity after childhood cancer: a prospective longitudinal study. Cancer. 2003;97:1991-1998.

132. Moghrabi A, Levy DE, Asselin B, et al. Results of the Dana-Farber Cancer Institute ALL Consortium Protocol 95-01 for children with acute lymphoblastic leukemia. Blood. 2007;109:896-904.

132a. Lipshultz SE, Rifai N, Dalton VM, et al. The effect of dexrazoxane on myocardial injury in doxorubicin-treated children with acute lymphoblastic leukemia. N Engl J Med. 2004;351:145-153.

133. Tebbi CK, London WB, Friedman D, et al. Dexrazoxane-associated risk for acute myeloid leukemia myelodysplastic syndrome and other secondary malignancies in pediatric Hodgkin's disease. J Clin Oncol. 2007;25:493-500.

134. Lipshultz SE, Lipsitz SR, Sallan SE, et al. Long-term enalapril therapy for left ventricular dysfunction in doxorubicin-treated survivors of childhood cancer. J Clin Oncol. 2002;20:4517-4522.

135. Constine LS, Schwartz RG, Savage D, et al. Cardiac function, perfusion, and morbidity in irradiated long-term survivors of Hodgkin's disease. Int J Radiat Oncol Biol Phys. 1997;39:897-906.

136. Guldner L, Haddy N, Pein F, et al. Radiation dose and long-term risk of cardiac pathology following radiotherapy and anthracycline for a childhood cancer. Radiother Oncol. 2006;81:47-56.

137. Aleman BMP, van den Belt-Dusebout AW, De Bruin ML, et al. Late cardiotoxicity after treatment for Hodgkin lymphoma. Blood. 2007;19:1878-1886.

138. Hancock SL, Donaldson SS, Hoppe RT. Cardiac disease following treatment of Hodgkin's disease in children and adolescents. J Clin Oncol. 1993;11:1208-1215.

139. Halprin EC. Pediatric Radiation Oncology. Philadelphia, Lippincott Williams & Wilkins, 2005.

140. Hancock SL, Tucker MA, Hoppe RT. Factors affecting late mortality from heart disease after treatment for Hodgkin's disease. JAMA. 1993;270:1949-1955.

141. Chow AY, Chin C, Dahl G, Rosenthal DN. Anthracyclines cause endothelial injury in pediatric cancer patients: a pilot study. J Clin Oncol. 2006;24:925-928.

142. Heidenreich PA, Schnittger I, Stauss HW, et al. Screening for coronary artery disease after mediastinal irradiation for Hodgkin's disease. J Clin Oncol. 2007;25:43-49.

143. Handa N, McGregor CG, Danielson GK, et al. Coronary artery bypass grafting in patients with previous mediastinal radiation therapy. J Thorac Cardiovasc Surg. 1999;117:1136-1142.

144. Orzan F, Brusca A, Gaita F, et al. Associated cardiac lesions in patients with radiation-induced complete heart block. Int J Cardiol. 1993;39:151-156.

145. Adams MJ, Lipsitz SR, Colan SD, et al. Cardiovascular status in long-term survivors of Hodgkin's disease treated with chest radiotherapy. J Clin Oncol. 2004;22:3139-3148.

146. Carlson RG, Mayfield WR, Normann S, Alexander JA. Radiation-associated valvular disease. Chest. 1991;99:538-545.

147. Lund MB, Ihlen H, Voss BM, et al. Increased risk of heart valve regurgitation after mediastinal radiation for Hodgkin's disease: an echocardiographic study. Heart. 1996;75:591-595.

148. Glanzmann C, Huguenin P, Lütolf UM, et al. Cardiac lesions after mediastinal irradiation for Hodgkin's disease. Radiother Oncol. 1994;30:43-45.

149. Stewart JR, Fajardo LF. Radiation-induced heart disease: an update. Prog Cardiovasc Dis. 1984;27:173-194.

150. Greenwood RD, Rosenthal A, Cassady R, et al. Constrictive pericarditis in childhood due to mediastinal irradiation. Circulation. 1974;50:1033-1039.

151. Applefeld MM, Slawson RG, Spicer KM, et al. Long-term cardiovascular evaluation of patients with Hodgkin's disease treated

by thoracic mantle radiation therapy. Cancer Treat Rep. 1982; 66:1003-1013.

152. Mauch PM, Weinstein H, Botnick L, et al. An evaluation of long-term survival and treatment complications in children with Hodgkin's disease. Cancer. 1983;51:925-932.

153. Donaldson SS, Kaplan HS. Complications of treatment of Hodgkin's disease in children. Cancer Treat Rep. 1982;66:977-989.

154. Bowers DC, Mulne AF, Reisch JS, et al. Nonperioperative strokes in children with central nervous system tumors. Cancer. 2002;94:1094-1101.

155. Griese M, Rampf U, Hofmann D, et al. Pulmonary complications after bone marrow transplantation in children: twenty-four years of experience in a single pediatric center. Pediatr Pulmonol. 2000;30:393-401.

156. Wohl ME, Griscom NT, Traggis DG, Jaffee N. Effects of therapeutic irradiation delivered in early childhood upon subsequent lung function. Pediatrics. 1975;55:507-516.

157. Jakacki RI, Schramm CM, Donahue BR, et al. Restrictive lung disease following treatment for malignant brain tumors: a potential late effect of craniospinal irradiation. J Clin Oncol. 1995;13: 1478-1485.

158. Kreisman H, Wolkove N. Pulmonary toxicity of antineoplastic therapy. Semin Oncol. 1992;19:508-520.

159. O'Driscoll BR, Hasleton PS, Taylor PM, et al. Active lung fibrosis up to 17 years after chemotherapy with carmustine (BCNU) in childhood. N Engl J Med. 1990;323:378-382.

160. Mertens AC, Yasui Y, Liu Y, et al. Pulmonary complications in survivors of childhood and adolescent cancer: a report from the Childhood Cancer Survivor Study. Cancer. 2002;95:2431-2441.

161. Goldiner PL, Carlon GC, Cvitkovic E, et al. Factors influencing postoperative morbidity and mortality in patients treated with bleomycin. BMJ. 1978;1:1664-1667.

162. Cohen LE. Endocrine late effects of cancer treatment. Endocrinol Metab Clin N Am. 2005;34:769-789.

163. Livesey EA, Hindmarsh PC, Brook CGD, et al. Endocrine disorders following treatment of childhood brain tumors. Br J Cancer. 1990;61:622-625.

164. Shalet SM, Hann IM, Lendon M, et al. Testicular function after combination chemotherapy in childhood for acute lymphoblastic leukemia. Arch Dis Child. 1981;56:275-278.

165. Lando A, Holm K, Nysom K, et al. Thyroid function in survivors of childhood acute lymphoblastic leukemia: the significance of prophylactic cranial radiation. Clin Endocrinol (Oxf). 2001;55: 21-25.

166. Rose SR, Danish RK, Kearney NS, et al. ACTH deficiency in childhood cancer survivors. Pediatr Blood Cancer. 2005;45: 808-813.

167. Littley MD, Shalet SM, Beardwell CG, et al. Radiation-induced hypopituitarism is dose-dependent. Clin Endocrinol (Oxf). 1989; 31:363-373.

168. Sklar CA. Endocrine complications of the successful treatment of neoplastic diseases in childhood. Growth Genet Horm. 2001; 17:37.

169. Brennan BM, Rahim A, Mackie EM, et al. Growth hormone status in adults treated for acute lymphoblastic leukemia in childhood. Clin Endocrinol (Oxf). 1998;48:777-783.

170. Merchant TE, Goloubeva O, Pritchard DL, et al. Radiation dose-volume effects on growth hormone secretion. Int J Radiat Oncol Biol Phys. 2002;52:1264-1270.

171. Ogilvy-Stuart AL, Shalet SM. Growth and puberty after growth hormone treatment after irradiation for brain tumors. Arch Dis Child. 1995;73:141-146.

172. Vahl N, Juul A, Jorgensen JO, et al. Continuation of growth hormone (GH) replacement in GH-deficient patients during transition from childhood to adulthood: a two-year placebo-controlled study. J Clin Endocrinol Metab. 2000;85:1874-1881.

173. Sklar CA, Mertens AC, Mitby P, et al. Risk of disease recurrence and second neoplasms in survivors of childhood cancer treated with growth hormone: a report from the Childhood Cancer Survivor study. J Clin Endocrinol Metab. 2002;87:3136-3141.

174. Ergun-Longmire B, Mertens AC, Mitby P, et al. Growth hormone treatment and risk of second neoplasms in the childhood cancer survivor. J Clin Endocrinol Metab. 2006;91:3494-3498.

175. Swerdlow AJ, Reddingius RE, Higgins CD, et al. Growth hormone treatment of children with brain tumors and risk of tumor recurrence. J Clin Endocrinol Metab. 2000;85:4444-4449.

176. Jarfelt M, Fors H, Lannering B, Bjarnason R. Bone mineral density and bone turnover in young adult survivors of childhood acute lymphoblastic leukemia. Eur J Endocrinol. 2006;154: 303-309.

177. van Leeuwen BL, Kamps WA, Jansen HW, Hoekstra HJ. The effect of chemotherapy on the growing skeleton. Cancer Treat Rev. 2000;26:363-376.

178. Kaste SC. Bone-mineral density deficits from childhood cancer and its therapy: a review of at-risk patient cohorts and available imaging methods. Pediatr Radiol. 2004;34:373-378.

179. Holmes SJ, Whitehouse RW, Clark ST, et al. Reduced bone mineral density in men following chemotherapy for Hodgkin's disease. Br J Cancer. 1994;70:371-375.

180. Mulder JE. Benefits and risks of hormone replacement therapy in young adult cancer survivors with gonadal failure. Med Pediatr Oncol. 1999;33:46-52.

181. Niinimaki RA, Harila-Saari AH, Jartti AE, et al. High body mass index increases the risk of osteonecrosis in children with acute lymphoblastic leukemia. J Clin Oncol. 2007;25:1498-1504.

182. Bürger B, Beier R, Zimmermann M, et al. Osteonecrosis: a treatment-related toxicity in childhood acute lymphoblastic leukemia (ALL)—experiences from trial ALL-BFM 95. Pediatr Blood Cancer. 2005;44:220-225.

183. Karimova EJ, Rai SN, Howard SC, et al. Femoral head osteonecrosis in pediatric and young adult patients with leukemia or lymphoma. J Clin Oncol. 2007;25:1525-1531.

183a. French D, Hamilton LH, Mattano LA Jr., et al. A PAI-1 (SERPINE1) polymorphism predicts osteonecrosis in children with acute lymphoblastic leukemia: a report from the Children's Oncology Group. Blood. 2008;111:4496–4498.

184. Paulino AC, Mayr NA, Simon HJ, Buatti JM. Locoregional control in infants with neuroblastoma: role of radiation therapy and late toxicity. Int J Radiat Oncol Biol Phys. 2002;52: 1025-1031.

185. Fletcher BD. Effects of pediatric cancer therapy on the musculoskeletal system. Pediatr Radiol. 1997;27:623-636.

186. Metzger ML, Howard SC, Hudson MM, et al. Natural history of thyroid nodules in survivors of pediatric Hodgkin lymphoma. Pediatr Blood Cancer. 2006;46:314-319.

187. Gleeson HK, Darzy K, Shalet SM. Late endocrine, metabolic and skeletal sequelae following treatment of childhood cancer. Best Pract Res Clin Endocrinol Metab. 2002;16:335-348.

188. Rao SD, Frame B, Miller MJ, et al. Hyperparathyroidism following head and neck irradiation. Arch Intern Med. 1980;140: 205-207.

189. Stephen AE, Chen KT, Milas M, Siperstein AE. The coming of age of radiation-induced hyperparathyroidism: evolving patterns of thyroid and parathyroid disease after head and neck irradiation. Surgery. 2004;136:1143-1153.

190. Cohen J, Gierlowski TC, Schneider AB. A prospective study of hyperparathyroidism in individuals exposed to radiation in childhood. JAMA. 1990;264:581-584.

191. Muller HL, Klinkhammer-Schalke M, Kuhl J. Final height and weight of long-term survivors of childhood malignancies. Exp Clin Endocrinol Diabetes. 1998;106:135-139.

192. Dalton VK, Rue M, Silverman LB, et al. Height and weight in children treated for acute lymphoblastic leukemia: relationship to CNS treatment. J Clin Oncol. 2003;21:2953-2960.

193. Gurney JB, Ness KK, Stovall M, et al. Final height and body mass index among adult survivors of childhood brain cancer:

Childhood Cancer Survivor study. J Clin Endocrinol Metab. 2003;88:4731-4739.

194. Sklar C, Mertens A, Walter A, et al. Final height after treatment for childhood acute lymphoblastic leukemia: comparison of no cranial irradiation with 1800 and 2400 centigrays of cranial radiation. J Pediatr. 1993;123:59-64.

195. Gleeson HK, Stoeter R, Ogilvy-Stuart AL, et al. Improvements in final height over 25 years in growth hormone (GH)—deficient childhood survivors of brain tumors receiving GH replacement. J Clin Endocrinol Metab. 2003;88:3682-3689.

196. Wallace WH, Shalet SM, Morris-Jones PH, et al. Effect of abdominal irradiation on growth in boys treated for a Wilms' tumor. Med Pediatr Oncol. 1990;18:441-446.

197. Nivot S, Benelli C, Clot JP, et al. Nonparallel changes in growth hormone (GH) and insulin-like growth factor-I, insulin-like growth factor binding protein-3, and GH-binding protein, after craniospinal irradiation and chemotherapy. J Clin Endocrinol Metab. 1994;78:597-601.

198. Robson H, Anderson D, Eden OB, et al. Chemotherapeutic agents used in the treatment of childhood malignancies have direct effects on growth plate chondrocyte proliferation. J Endocrinol. 1998;157:225-235.

199. Shalet SM, Gibson B, Swindell R, Pearson D. Effect of spinal irradiation on growth. Arch Dis Child. 1987;62:461-464.

200. Clarson CL, Del Maestro RF. Growth hormone after treatment of pediatric brain tumors. Pediatrics. 1999;103:E37.

201. Brownstein CM, Mertens AC, Mitby PA, et al. Factors that affect final height and change in height standard deviation scores in survivors of childhood cancer treated with growth hormone: a report from the Childhood Cancer Survivor Study. J Clin Endocrinol Metab. 2004;89:4422-4427.

202. Ogilvy-Stuart AL, Clayton PE, Shalet SM. Cranial irradiation and early puberty. J Clin Endocrinol Metab. 1994;78:1282-1286.

203. Craig F, Leiper AD, Stanhope R, et al. Sexually dimorphic and radiation dose dependent effect of cranial irradiation on body mass index. Arch Dis Child. 1999;81:500-504.

204. Brennan BM, Rahim A, Blum WF, et al. Hyperleptinaemia in young adults following cranial irradiation in childhood: growth hormone deficiency or leptin insensitivity. Clin Endocrinol (Oxf). 1999;50:163-169.

205. Lustig RH. Hypothalamic obesity: the sixth cranial endocrinopathy. Endocrinologist. 2002;12:210.

206. Oeffinger KC, Mertens AC, Sklar CA, et al. Obesity in adult survivors of childhood acute lymphoblastic leukemia: a report from the Childhood Cancer Survivor Study. J Clin Oncol. 2003;21:1359-1365.

207. Razzouk BI, Rose SR, Hongeng S, et al. Obesity in survivors of childhood acute lymphoblastic leukemia and lymphoma. J Clin Oncol. 2007;25:1183-1189.

208. Link K, Moell C, Garwicz S, et al. Growth hormone deficiency predicts cardiovascular risk in young adults treated for acute lymphoblastic leukemia in childhood. J Clin Endocrinol Metab. 2004;89:5003-5012.

209. Gurney JG, Ness KK, Sibley SD, et al. Metabolic syndrome and growth hormone deficiency in adult survivors of childhood acute lymphoblastic leukemia. Cancer. 2006;107:1303-1312.

210. Talvensaari K, Knip M. Childhood cancer and later development of the metabolic syndrome. Ann Med. 1997;29:353-355.

211. Spiegler BJ, Kennedy K, Maze R, et al. Comparison of long-term neurocognitive outcomes in young children with acute lymphoblastic leukemia treated with cranial radiation or high-dose or very high-dose intravenous methotrexate. J Clin Oncol. 2006;24:3858-3864.

212. Copeland DR, Moore BD, Francis DJ, et al. Neuropsychologic effects of chemotherapy with cancer: a longitudinal study. J Clin Oncol. 1996;14:2826-2835.

213. Glauser TA, Packer RJ. Cognitive deficits in long-term survivors of childhood brain tumors. Childs Nerv Syst. 1991;7:2-12.

214. Brouwers P, Riccardi R, Fedio P, Poplack DG. Long-term neuropsychologic sequelae of childhood leukemia: correlation with CT brain scan abnormalities. J Pediatr. 1985;106:723-728.

215. Butler RW, Mulhern RK. Neurocognitive interventions for children and adolescents surviving cancer. J Pediatr Psychol. 2005;30:65-78.

216. Ris MD, Noll RB. Long-term neurobehavioral outcome in pediatric brain-tumor patients: review and methodological critique. J Clin Exp Neuropsychol. 1994;16:21-42.

217. Palmer SL, Goloubeva O, Reddick WE, et al. Patterns of intellectual development among survivors of pediatric medulloblastoma: a longitudinal analysis. J Clin Oncol. 2001;19:2302-2308.

218. Langer T, Martus P, Ottensmeier H, et al. CNS late-effects after ALL therapy in childhood. Part III: neuropsychological performance in long-term survivors of childhood ALL: impairments of concentration, attention, and memory. Med Pediatr Oncol. 2002;38:320-328.

219. Rowland JH, Glidewell OJ, Sibley RF, et al. Effects of different forms of central nervous system prophylaxis on neuropsychologic function in childhood leukemia. J Clin Oncol. 1984;2:1327-1335.

220. Ris MD, Packer R, Goldwein J, et al. Intellectual outcome after reduced-dose radiation therapy plus adjuvant chemotherapy for medulloblastoma: a Children's Cancer Group study. J Clin Oncol. 2001;19:3470-3476.

221. Palmer SL, Gajjar A, Reddick WE, et al. Predicting intellectual outcome among children treated with 35-40 Gy craniospinal irradiation for medulloblastoma. Neuropsychology. 2003;17:548-555.

222. Spencer J. The role of cognitive remediation in childhood cancer survivors experiencing neurocognitive late effects. J Pediatr Oncol Nurs. 2006;23:321-325.

223. Robertson PL, Muraszko KM, Holmes EJ, et al. Incidence and severity of postoperative cerebellar mutism syndrome in children with medulloblastoma: a prospective study by the Children's Oncology Group. J Neurosurg. 2006;105:444-451.

224. Duffner PK. Long-term effects of radiation therapy on cognitive and endocrine function in children with leukemia and brain tumors. Neurologist. 2004;10:293-310.

225. Fouladi M, Chintagumpala M, Laningham FH, et al. White matter lesions detected by magnetic resonance imaging after radiotherapy and high-dose chemotherapy in children with medulloblastoma or primitive neuroectodermal tumor. J Clin Oncol. 2004;22:4551-4560.

226. Matsumoto K, Takahashi S, Sato A, et al. Leukoencephalophathy in childhood hematopoietic neoplasm caused by moderate-dose methotrexate and prophylactic cranial radiotherapy—an MR analysis. Int J Radiat Oncol Biol Phys. 1995;32:913-918.

227. Prayer D, Grois N, Prosch H, et al. MR imaging presentation of intracranial disease associated with Langerhans cell histiocytosis. Am J Neuroradiol. 2004;25:880-891.

228. Lehtinen SS, Huuskonen UE, Harila-Saari AH, et al. Motor nervous system impairment persists in long-term survivors of childhood acute lymphoblastic leukemia. Cancer. 2002;94:2466-2473.

229. Vogelzang NJ, Bosl GJ, Johnson K, Kennedy BJ. Raynaud's phenomenon: a common toxicity after combination chemotherapy for testicular cancer. Ann Intern Med. 1981;95:288-292.

230. McGuire WA, Passo MH, Weetman RH. Chemotherapy-associated Raynaud's phenomenon in a two-year-old girl. Med Pediatr Oncol. 1985;13:392-394.

231. Hartman A, van den Bos C, Stijnen T, Pieters R. Decrease in motor performance in children with cancer is independent of the cumulative dose of vincristine. Cancer. 2006;106:1395-1401.

232. Florin TA, Fryer GE, Myoshi T, et al. Physical inactivity in adult survivors of childhood acute lymphoblastic leukemia: a report

from the Childhood Cancer Survivor study. Cancer Epidemiol Biomarkers Prev. 2007;16:1356-1363.

233. Rottenberg DA, Chernik NL, Deck MD, et al. Cerebral necrosis following radiotherapy of extracranial neoplasms. Ann Neurol. 1977;1:339-357.

234. Marcus RB Jr, Million RR. The incidence of myelitis after irradiation of the cervical spinal cord. Int J Radiat Oncol Biol Phys. 1990;19:3-8.

235. Fung LW, Thompson D, Ganesan V. Revascularisation surgery for paediatric moyamoya: a review of the literature. Childs Nerv Syst. 2005;21:358-364.

235a. Lew SM, Morgan JN, Psaty E, et al. Cumulative incidence of radiation-induced cavernomas in long-term survivors of medulloblastoma. J Neurosurg. 2006;104:103–107.

236. Oberlin O, Rey A, Anderson J, et al. Treatment of orbital rhabdomyosarcoma: survival and late effects of treatment—results of an international workshop. J Clin Oncol. 2001;19:197-204.

237. Weaver RG Jr, Chauvenent AR, Smith TJ, Schwartz AC. Ophthalmic evaluation of long-term survivors of childhood acute lymphoblastic leukemia. Cancer. 1986;58:963-968.

238. Raney RB, Anderson JR, Kollath J, et al. Late effects of therapy in 94 patients with localized fhabdomyosarcoma of the orbit: Report from the Intergroup Rhabdomyosarcoma Study (IRS)-III, 1984-1991. Med Pediatr Oncol. 2000;34:413-420.

239. Holmström G, Borgström B, Calissendorff B. Cataract in children after bone marrow transplantation: relation to conditioning regimen. Acta Ophthalmol Scand. 2002;80:211-215.

240. Fahnehjelm KT, Törnquist AL, Olsson M, Winiarski J. Visual outcome and cataract development after allogeneic stem-cell transplantation in children. Acta Ophthalmol Scand. 2007;85(7):724-733.

241. Raney RB, Asmar L, Vassilopoulou-Sellin R, et al. Late complications of therapy in 213 children with localized, nonorbital soft tissue sarcoma of the head and neck: a descriptive report from the Intergroup Rhabdomyosarcoma Studies (IRS)-II and -III. IRS Group of the Children's Cancer Group and the Pediatric Oncology Group. Med Pediatr Oncol. 1999;33:362-371.

242. Kretschmar CS, Warren MP, Lavally BL, et al. Ototoxicity of preradiation cisplatin for children with central nervous system tumors. J Clin Oncol. 1990;87:1191-1198.

243. Williams GB, Kun LE, Thompson JW, et al. Hearing loss as a late complication of radiotherapy in children with brain tumors. Ann Otol Rhinol Laryngol. 2005;114:328-331.

244. Schell MJ, McHaney VA, Green AA, et al. Hearing loss in children and young adults receiving cisplatin with or without prior cranial irradiation. J Clin Oncol. 1989;7:754-760.

245. Li Y, Womer RB, Silber JH. Predicting cisplatin ototoxicity in children: the influence of age and the cumulative dose. Eur J Cancer. 2004;40:2445-2451.

246. Parsons SK, Neault MW, Lehmann LE, et al. Severe ototoxicity following carboplatin-containing conditioning regimen for autologous marrow transplantation for neuroblastoma. Bone Marrow Transplant. 1998;22:669-674.

247. Bertolini P, Lassalle M, Mercier G, et al. Platinum compound-related ototoxicity in children: long-term follow-up reveals continuous worsening of hearing loss. J Pediatr Hematol Oncol. 2004;26:649-655.

248. Whitehead E, Shalet SM, Jones PH, et al. Gonadal function after combination chemotherapy for Hodgkin's disease in childhood. Arch Dis Child. 1982;57:287-291.

249. Wallace WH, Shalet SM, Crown EC, et al. Gonadal dysfunction due to cisplatinum. Med Pediart Oncol. 1989;17:409-413.

250. Howell SJ, Shalet SM. Effect of cancer therapy on pituitary-testicular axis. Int J Androl. 2002;25:269-276.

251. Brennan BM, Shalet SM. Endocrine late effects after bone marrow transplant. Br J Haematol. 2002;118:58-66.

252. Mills JL, Fears TR, Robison LL, et al. Menarche in a cohort of 188 long-term survivors of acute lymphoblastic leukemia. J Pediatr. 1997;131:598-602.

253. Wallace WH, Shalet SM, Hendry JH, et al. Ovarian failure following abdominal irradiation in childhood: the radiosensitivity of the human oocyte. Br J Radiol. 1989;62:995-998.

254. Byrne J. Infertility and premature menopause in childhood cancer survivors. Med Pediatr Oncol. 1999;33:24-28.

255. Sklar CA, Mertens AC, Mitby P, et al. Premature menopause in survivors of childhood cancer: a report from the Childhood Cancer Survivor Study. J Natl Cancer Institute. 2006;98:890-896.

256. Byrne J, Fears TR, Gail MH, et al. Early menopause in long-term survivors of cancer during childhood and adolescence. Am J Obstet Gynecol. 1992;166:788-793.

257. Larsen EC, Muller J, Rechnitzer C, et al. Diminished ovarian reserve in female childhood cancer survivors with regular menstrual cycles and basal FSH < 10 IU/l. Hum Reprod. 2003;18:417-422.

258. Lee SJ, Schover LR, Partridge AH, et al. American Society of Clinical Oncology Recommendations on Fertility Preservation in Cancer Patients. J Clin Oncol. 2006;24:2917–2931.

259. Jaffe N, Sullivan MP, Ried H, et al. Male reproductive function in long term survivors of childhood cancer. Med Pediatr Oncol. 1988;16:241-247.

260. Bramswig H, Heimes U, Heiermann E, et al. The effects of different cumulative doses of chemotherapy on testicular function. Cancer. 1990;65:1298-1302.

261. Howell SJ, Radford JA, Ryder WDJ, Shalet SM. Testicular function after cytotoxic chemotherapy: evidence of Leydig cell insufficiency. J Clin Oncol. 1999;17:1493-1498.

262. Buchanan JD, Fairley KF, Barrie JU. Return of spermatogenesis after stopping cyclophosphamide therapy. Lancet. 1975;26:156-157.

263. Lin WW, Kim ED, Quesada ET, et al. Unilateral testicular injury from external trauma: evaluation of semen quality and endocrine parameters. J Urol. 1998;159:841-843.

264. Meistrich ML, Chawla SP, Da Cunha MF, et al. Recovery of sperm production after chemotherapy for osteosarcoma. Cancer. 1989;63:2115-2123.

265. Sklar C. Reproductive physiology and treatment-related loss of sex hormone and production. Med Pediatr Oncol. 1999;33:2-8.

266. Critchley HO, Bath LE, Wallace WH. Radiation damage to the uterus: review of the effects of treatment of childhood cancer. Hum Fertil. 2002;5:61-66.

267. Green DM, Peabody EM, Nan B, et al. Pregnancy outcome after treatment for Wilms' tumor: a report from the National Wilms' Tumor Study group. J Clin Oncol. 2002;20:2506-2513.

268. Green DM, Whitton JA, Stovall M, et al. Pregnancy outcome of female survivors of childhood cancer: a report from the Childhood Cancer Survivor study. Am J Obstet Gynecol. 2002;187:1070-1080.

269. Signorello LB, Cohen SS, Bosetti C, et al. Female survivors of childhood cancer: preterm birth and low birth weight among their children. J Natl Cancer Inst. 2006;98:1453-1461.

270. Blatt J. Pregnancy outcome in long-term survivors of childhood cancer. Med Pediatr Oncol. 1999;33:29-33.

271. Critchley HO, Wallace WH. Impact of cancer treatment on uterine function. J Natl Cancer Inst Monogr. 2005;34:64-68.

272. Bar J, Davidi O, Goshen Y, et al. Pregnancy outcome in women treated with doxorubicin for childhood cancer. Am J Obstet Gynecol. 2003;189:853-857.

273. Boice J Jr. Cancer following irradiation in childhood and adolescence. Med Pediatr Oncol. 1996;1:29-34.

274. Green DM, Fine WE, Li FP. Offspring of patients treated for unilateral Wilms' tumor in childhood. Cancer. 1982;49:2285-2288.

275. Green DM, Fiorello A, Zevon MA, et al. Birth defects and childhood cancer in offspring of survivors of childhood cancer. Arch Pediatr Adolesc Med. 1997;151:379-383.

276. Sankila R, Olsen JH, Anderson H, et al. Risk of cancer among offspring of childhood cancer survivors. N Engl J Med. 1998; 338:1339-1344.

277. Hawkins MM, Draper GJ, Winter DL. Cancer in the offspring of survivors of childhood leukemia and non-Hodgkin's lymphomas. Br J Cancer. 1995;71:1335-1339.

278. Byrne J, Rasmussen SA, Steinhorn SC, et al. Genetic disease in offspring of long-term survivors of childhood and adolescent cancer. Am J Hum Genet. 1998;62:45-52.

279. Li FP, Gimbrere K, Gelbar R, et al. Outcome of pregnancy in survivors of Wilms' tumor. JAMA. 1987;257:216-219.

280. Rechitsky S, Verlinsky O, Chistokhina A, et al. Preimplantation genetic diagnosis for cancer predisposition. Reprod Biomed Online. 2002;5:148-155.

281. Avigad S, Peleg D, Barel D, et al. Prenatal diagnosis in Li-Fraumeni syndrome. J Pediatr Hematol Oncol. 2004;26:541-545.

282. Cassidy JR. Clinical radiation nephropathy. Int J Radiat Oncol Biol Phys. 1995;31:1249-1256.

283. Tarbell NJ, Guinan EC, Niemeyer C, et al. Late onset of renal dysfunction in survivors of bone marrow transplantation. Int J Radiat Oncol Biol Phys. 1988;15:99-104.

284. Bianchetti MG, Kanaka C, Ridolfi-Lüthy A, et al. Persisting renotublar sequelae after cisplatin in children and adolescents. Am J Nephrol. 1991;11:127-130.

285. Stern JW, Bunin N. Prospective study of carboplatin-based chemotherapy for pediatric germ cell tumors. Med Pediatr Oncol. 2002;39:163-167.

286. Loebstein R, Atanackovic G, Bishai R, et al. Risk factors for long-term outcome of ifosfamide-induced nephroxicity in children. J Clin Pharmacol. 1999;39:454-461.

287. Arndt C, Morgenstern B, Hawkins D, et al. Renal function following combination chemotherapy with ifosfamide and cisplatin in patients with osteogenic sarcoma. Med Pediatr Oncol. 1999;32:93-96.

288. Loebstein R, Koren G. Ifosfamide-induced nephrotoxicity in children: critical review of predictive risk factors. Pediatrics. 1998;101:E8.

289. Skinner R. Chronic ifosfamide nephrotoxicity in children. Med Pediatr Oncol. 2003;41:190-197.

290. Marina NM, Poquette CA, Cain AM, et al. Comparative renal tubular toxicity of chemotherapy regimens including ifosfamide in patients with newly diagnosed sarcomas. J Pediatr Hematol Oncol. 2000;22:112-118.

291. Ritchey ML, Green DM, Thomas PR, et al. Renal failure in Wilms' tumor patients: a report from the National Wilms' Tumor Study Group. Med Pediatr Oncol. 1996;26:75-80.

292. Breslow NE, Collins AJ, Ritchey ML, et al. End-stage renal disease in patients with Wilms' tumor: results from the National Wilms' Tumor Study Group and the United States Renal Data System. J Urol. 2005;174:1972-1975.

293. Bailey S, Roberts A, Brock C, et al. Nephrotoxicity in survivors of Wilms' tumours in the North of England. Br J Cancer. 2002;87:1092-1098.

294. Breslow NE, Takashima JR, Ritchey ML, et al. Renal failure in the Denys-Drash and Wilms' tumor-aniridia syndromes. Cancer Res. 2000;60:430-4032.

295. Tarbell NJ, Guinan EC, Niemeyer C, et al. Late onset of renal dysfunction in survivors of bone marrow transplantation. Int J Radiat Oncol Biol Phys. 1988;15:99-104.

296. Chevallier C, Hadj-Aissa A, Brunat-Metigny M, et al. Renal function after nephrectomy for Wilms' tumor. Arch Pediatr. 1997;4:639-677.

297. Di Tullio MT, Casale F, Indolfi P, et al. Compensatory hypertrophy and progressive renal damage in children nephrectomized for Wilms' tumor. Med Pediatr Oncol. 1996;26:325-328.

298. Stillwell TJ, Benson RC Jr. Cyclophosphamide-induced hemorrhagic cystitis: a review of 100 patients. Cancer. 1988;61:451-457.

299. Hale GA, Rochester RJ, Heslop HE, et al. Hemorrhagic cystitis after allogeneic bone marrow transplantation in children: clinical characteristics and outcome. Biol Blood Marrow Transplant. 2003;9(11):698-705.

300. Kondo M, Kojima S, Kato K, Matsuyama T. Late-onset hemorrhagic systitis after hematopoietic stem cell transplantation in children. Bone Marrow Transplant. 1998;22:995-998.

301. Kersun LS, Wimmer RS, Hoot AC, Meadows AT. Secondary malignant neoplasms of the bladder after cyclophosphamide treatment for childhood acute lymphocytic leukemia. Pediatr Blood Cancer. 2004;42:289-291.

302. Travis LB, Curtis RE, Glimelius B, et al. Bladder and kidney cancer following cyclophosphamide therapy for non-Hodgkin's lymphoma. J Natl Cancer Inst. 1995;87:524-530.

303. Gossmann J. Cyclophosphamide-induced bladder cancer. Ann Intern Med. 1997;126:86.

304. Talar-Williams C, Hijazi YM, Walther MM, et al. Cyclophosphamide-induced cystitis and bladder cancer in patients with Wegener granulomatosis. Ann Intern Med. 1996;124:477-484.

305. Paulino AC, Wen BC, Brown CK, et al. Late effects in children treated with radiation therapy for Wilms' tumor. Int J Radiat Oncol Biol Phys. 2000;46:1239-1246.

306. Broxson EH, Dole M, Wong R, et al. Portal hypertension develops in a subset of childred with standard risk acute lymphoblastic leukemia treated with oral 6-thioguanine during maintenance therapy. Pediatr Blood Cancer. 2005;44:226-231.

307. McIntosh S, Davidson DL, O'Brien RT, Pearson HA. Methotrexate hepatotoxicity in children with leukemia. J Pediatr. 1997;90:1019-1021.

308. Ritchey ML, Kelalis PP, Etzioni R, et al. Small bowel obstruction nephrectomy for Wilms' tumor. A report of the National Wilms' Tumor Study-3. Ann Surg. 1993;218:654-659.

309. Colman CN, McDougall IR, Dailey MO, et al. Functional hyposplenia after splenic irradiation for Hodgkin's disease. Ann Intern Med. 1982;96:44-47.

310. Castagnola E, Fioredda F. Prevention of life-threatening infections due to encapsulated bacteria in children with hyposplenia or asplenia: a brief review of current recommendations for practical purposes. Eur J Haematol. 2003;71:319-326.

311. Maury S, Mary JY, Rabian C, et al. Prolonged immune deficiency following allogeneic stem cell transplantation: risk factors and complications in adult patients. Br J Haematol. 2001;115:630-641.

312. Dodd RY. The risk of transfusion-transmitted infection. N Engl J Med. 1992;327:419-421.

313. Ellingwood KE, Million RR. Cancer of the nasal cavity and ethmoid/sphenoid sinuses. Cancer. 1979;43:1517-1526.

314. Soxman JA. Subacute bacterial endocarditis: considerations for the pediatric patient. J Am Dent Assoc. 2000;131:668-669.

315. Kaste SC, Hopkins KP, Bowman LC. Dental abnormalities in long-term survivors of head and neck rhabdomyosarcoma. Med Pediatr Oncol. 1995;25:96-101.

316. Kaste SC, Hopkins KP, Bowman LC, Santana VM. Dental abnormalities in children treated for neuroblastoma. Med Pediar Oncol. 1998;30:22-27.

317. Sonis AL, Tarbell N, Valachovic RW, et al. Dentofacial development in long-term survivors of acute lymphoblastic leukemia: a comparison of three treatment modalities. Cancer. 1990;66:2645-2652.

318. Duggal MS, Curzon MEJ, Bailey CC, et al. Dental parameters in the long term survivors of childhood cancer compared with siblings. Oral Oncol. 1997;33:348-353.

319. Hobbie WL, Stuber M, Meeske K, et al. Symptoms of posttraumatic stress in young adult survivors of childhood cancer. J Clin Oncol. 2000;18:4060-4066.

320. Zeltzer LK, Chen E, Weiss R, et al. Comparison of psychologic outcome in adult survivors of childhood lymphoblastic leukemia versus sibling controls: a Cooperative Children's Cancer Group and National Institutes of Health Study. J Clin Oncol. 1997;15:547-556.

321. Recklitis CJ, Lockwood RA, Rothwell MA, Diller LR. Suicidal ideation and attempts in adult survivors of childhood cancer. J Clin Oncol. 2006;24:3852-3857.

322. Ross L, Johansen C, Oksbjerg S, et al. Psychiatric hospitalizations among survivors of cancer in childhood or adolescence. N Engl J Med. 2003;349:650-657.

323. Hays DM, Landsverk J, Sallan SE, et al. Educational, occupational, and insurance status of childhood cancer survivors in their fourth and fifth decades of life. J Clin Oncol. 1992;10:1397-1406.

324. Park ER, Li FP, Liu Y, et al. Health insurance coverage in survivors of childhood cancer: the Childhood Cancer Survivor Study. J Clin Oncol. 2005;23:9187-9197.

325. Byrne J, Fears TR, Steinhorn SC, et al. Marriage and divorce after childhood and adolescent cancer. JAMA. 1989;262:2693-2699.

326. Ness KK, Mertens AC, Hudson MM, et al. Limitations on physical performance and daily activities among long-term survivors of childhood cancer. Ann Intern Med. 2005;143:639-647.

327. Haupt R, Fears TR, Robison LL, et al. Educational attainment in long-term survivors of childhood acute lymphoblastic leukemia. JAMA. 1994;272:1427-1432.

328. Mitby PA, Robison LL, Whitton JA, et al. Utilization of special education services and educational attainment among long-term survivors of childhood cancer: a report from the Childhood Cancer Survivor Study. Cancer. 2003;97:1115-1126.

329. Nagarajan R, Neglia JP, Clohisy DR, et al. Education, employment, insurance, and marital status among 694 survivors of pediatric lower extremity bone tumors: a report from the Childhood Cancer Survivor Study. Cancer. 2003;97:2554-2564.

330. Hays DM. Adult survivors of childhood cancer. Employment and insurance issues in different age groups. Cancer. 1993;71(Suppl 10):3306-3309.

331. Speechley KN, Barrera M, Shaw AK, et al. Health-related quality of life among child and adolescent survivors of childhood cancer. J Clin Oncol. 2006;24:2536-2543.

332. Rauck AM, Green DM, Yasui Y, et al. Marriage in the survivors of childhood cancer: a preliminary description from the Childhood Cancer Survivor Study. Med Pediatr Oncol. 1999;33:60-63.

333. Oeffinger KC, Mertens AC, Sklar CA, et al. Chronic health conditions in adult survivors of childhood cancer. N Engl J Med. 2006;355:1572-1582.

334. Stevens MCG, Mahler H, Parkes S. The health status of adult survivors of cancer in childhood. Eur J Cancer. 1998;34:694-698.

335. Pogany L, Barr RD, Shaw A, et al. Health status in survivors of cancer in childhood and adolescence. Qual Life Res. 2006;15:143-157.

336. Hudson MM, Mertens AC, Yasui Y, et al. Health status of adult long-term survivors of childhood cancer: report from the Childhood Cancer Survivor Study. JAMA. 2003;24:1583-1592.

337. Kadan-Lottick NS, Robison LL, Gurney JG, et al. Childhood cancer survivors' knowledge about their past diagnosis and treatment: Childhood Cancer Survivor Study. JAMA. 2002;287:1832-1839.

338. Yeazel MW, Oeffinger KC, Gurney JG, et al. The cancer screening practices of adult survivors of childhood cancer: a report from the Childhood Cancer Survivor Study. Cancer. 2004;100:631-640.

339. Aziz NM, Oeffinger KC, Brooks S, Turoff AJ. Comprehensive long-term follow-up programs for pediatric cancer survivors. Cancer. 2006;107:841-848.

340. Oeffinger KC, Mertens AC, Hudson MM, et al. Health care of young adult survivors of childhood cancer: a report from the Childhood Cancer Survivor Study. Ann Fam Med. 2004;2:61-70.

341. Hewitt M, Weiner SL, Simone JV (ed). Childhood Cancer Survivorship: Improving Care and Quality of Life. Washington, DC, National Academic Press, 2003.

342. Duffey-Lind EC, O'Holleran E, Healey M, et al. Transitioning to survivorship: a pilot study. J Pediatr Oncol Nurs. 2006;23:335-343.

342a. Faraci M, Bèkassy AN, DeFazio V. Non-endocrine late complications in children after allogeneic haematopoietic SCT. Bone Marrow Transplant. 2008;41:S49–S51.

343. Warren KE, Packer RJ. Current approaches to CNS tumors in infants and very young children. Expert Rev Neurother. 2004;4:681-690.

344. Mulhern RK, Kepner Jl, Thomas PR, et al. Neuropsychologic functioning of survivors of childhood medulloblastoma randomized to receive conventional or reduced-dose craniospinal irradiation: a Pediatric Oncology Group study. J Clin Oncol. 1998;16:1723-1728.

345. Donaldson SS, Link MP, Weinstein HJ, et al. Final results of a prospective clinical trial with VAMP and low-dose involved-field radiation for children with low-risk Hodgkin's disease. J Clin Oncol. 2007;25:332-337.

346. Donaldson SS, Hudson MM, Lamborn KR, et al. VAMP and low-dose, involved-field radiation for children with adolescents with favorable, early-stage Hodgkin's disease: results of a prospective clinical trial. J Clin Oncol. 2002;20:3081-3087.

347. Schrappe M, Reiter A, Ludwig WD, et al. Improved outcome in childhood acute lymphoblastic leukemia despite reduced use of anthracyclines and cranial radiotherapy: results of trial ALL-BFM 90. German-Austrian-Swiss ALL-BFM Study Group. Blood. 2000;95:3310-3322.

348. Tebbi CK, Mendenhall N, London WB, et al. Treatment of stage I, IIA, IIIA1 pediatric Hodgkin disease with doxorubicin, bleomycin, vincristine and etoposide (DBVE) and radiation: a Pediatric Oncology Group (POG) study. Pediatr Blood Cancer. 2006;46:198-202.

349. Breslow NE, Beckwith JB, Haase GM, et al. Radiation therapy for favorable histology Wilms' tumor: prevention of flank recurrence did not improve survival on National Wilms' Tumor Studies 3 and 4. Int J Radiat Oncol Biol Phys. 2006;65:203-209.

350. Bagatell R, Rumcheva P, London WB, et al. Outcomes of children with intermediate-risk neuroblastoma after treatment stratified by MYCN status and tumor cell ploidy. J Clin Oncol. 2005;23:8819-8827.

351. Shah SH. Gene polymorphisms and susceptibility to coronary artery disease. Pediatr Blood Cancer. 2007;48:738-741.

352. Mertens AC, Mitby PA, Radloff G, et al. XRCC1 and glutathione-S-transferase gene polymorphisms and susceptibility to radiotherapy-related malignancies in survivors of Hodgkin disease. Cancer. 2004;101:1463-1472.

353. Ross JA, Oeffinger KC, Davies SM, et al. Genetic variation in the leptin receptor gene and obesity in survivors of childhood acute lymphoblastic leukemia: a report from the Childhood Cancer Survivor study. J Clin Oncol. 2004;22:3558-3562.

354. Blanco JG, Leisenring WM, Gonzalez-Covarrubias VM, et al. Genetic polymorphisms in the carbonyl reductase 3 gene CBR3 and the NAD(P)H: quinone oxidoreductase 1 gene NQO1 in patients who developed anthracycline-related congestive heart failure after childhood cancer. Cancer. 2008;112:2789–2795.

33

Psychosocial Care of Children and Families

Christopher J. Recklitis, Robert L. Casey, and Lonnie Zeltzer

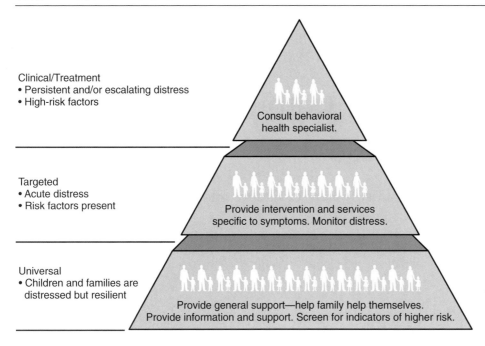

Clinical/Treatment
• Persistent and/or escalating distress
• High-risk factors

Consult behavioral health specialist.

Targeted
• Acute distress
• Risk factors present

Provide intervention and services specific to symptoms. Monitor distress.

Universal
• Children and families are distressed but resilient

Provide general support—help family help themselves. Provide information and support. Screen for indicators of higher risk.

FIGURE 33-1. Pediatric psychosocial preventive health model. *(Redrawn from Kazak AE, Pediatric psychosocial preventive health model (PPPHM): research, practice, and collaboration in pediatric family systems medicine. Fam Syst Health. 2006;24:381-395. Copyright © 2005 by the Center for Pediatric Traumatic Stress, Children's Hospital of Philadelphia.)*

INTRODUCTION

The diagnosis and treatment of cancer represents a major set of challenges to the family and the individual child. For most families, coping with a child's cancer will be the most stressful and difficult experience they will face. The majority make adequate adjustments,[1-4] but confronting the diagnosis and finding ways of coping with the many challenges of treatments is a difficult and demanding process.[5-9] In this chapter we address the emotional and psychosocial needs of children and their families as they go through cancer therapy, and we describe some of the resources and interventions that may be useful for them. The chapter is intended primarily for oncologists, nurse practitioners, and other medical professionals working to understand and attend to the psychosocial needs of children with cancer. In each section we highlight the issues facing children and their families and suggest supportive strategies. A description of the psychosocial clinician's role is included in certain sections so that oncology providers can better understand and collaborate with psychosocial clinicians, but readers looking for detailed descriptions of psychosocial assessment and treatment techniques will have to look beyond this chapter for more comprehensive discussions of the subject.[10,11] Given the great variability in oncology diagnoses and treatments, as well as individual differences among children and families, we focus on the issues that are most common in these populations. Beginning with the crisis of diagnosis and proceeding chronologically through the treatment period to the end of therapy, we address the expectable issues that arise for most families.

Conceptual Models Guiding the Psychosocial Care of Children and Families

In approaching the topic of psychosocial care for the child and family, we have adopted a conceptual model developed by Anne Kazak[12] that illustrates the various levels of need seen in the families of pediatric cancer patients (Fig. 33-1). In this model, adapted from the preventive mental health model,[12]

Kazak represents the distribution of families along the continuum of needs in the form of a pyramid, with least acute needs at the bottom and most acute needs at the top. The largest section of the pyramid at the bottom represents the majority of patients and families, who have expectable levels of distress but who generally have adequate resources and may benefit from information and psychosocial support. Moving up the pyramid, the second largest group of families represented has more significant needs, according to Kazak, because of existing risk factors or the presence of more acute distress. Finally, at the top of the pyramid is the smallest group of families; their level of distress is in the clinical range, and significant behavioral or psychiatric intervention is required. The focus of this chapter is on describing the needs of the largest group of families, those who have universal; or expectable, needs and on discussing the support strategies and interventions that can be helpful for them. In addition, we address some of the special issues that are likely to be seen in the targeted group of families, such as noncompliance or marital conflicts that are not typical but that the treatment team should be aware of and prepared to address. The less common situations in which patients or parents require significant mental health interventions require referrals to specialists, and these situations are discussed briefly at the end of this chapter.

Two other perspectives essential for understanding the experiences of children and families going through cancer therapy are the ecologic and developmental perspectives. Urie Bronfenbrenner (1917-2005) created the modern concept of the ecology of human development.[13] In his model, no single factor operates in isolation, and the biopsychosocial model is considered in a developmental context. There are genetic and environmental influences on children's emotions, cognition, and behaviors. Children's views of and reactions to the environment influence their emotions, thoughts, and behaviors and, in turn, their own characteristics influence their microenvironments.[14,15] For example, children who are fearful of new situations and transitions react to exposure to new medical experiences differently from children who are less fearful, and their behaviors influence the ways in which medical personnel react to them and treat them. This transactional model of child development and behavior must also be considered within the

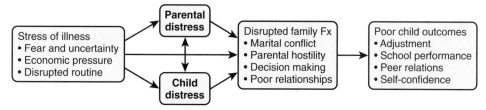

FIGURE 33-2. Family stress model. *(Adapted from Conger KJ, Rueter MA, Conger RD. The role of economic pressure in the lives of parents and their adolescents: the family stress model. In Crockett LJ, Silbereisen RJ [eds]. Negotiating Adolescence in Times of Social Change. Cambridge, England, Cambridge University Press, 2000, pp 201-233. Copyright © 2000 by Cambridge University Press.)*

larger context of the family. Factors such as family composition, parents' emotional states and the status of marital relationships, socioeconomic status, and other family stressors, including work and, for the child and siblings, school, also influence children's experiences of illness.[16-19] For example, maternal depression might reduce the extent of nurturing and support that mothers can provide for children with cancer. Marital conflicts create added stress, especially if each parent has a different coping style, a different way of interacting with the health care team, and a different approach to decision-making situations regarding children's care. Family-centered care has been proposed as the primary model of care for children in a health care setting, as noted in an extensive report by the American Academy of Pediatrics' Task Force on the Family.[18] The family stress model[20] suggests that stress in the family impacts children's stress levels and their behavior (Fig. 33-2).

Finally, racial, ethnic, community, and cultural factors impact the entire family-child system.[21] In this model (Fig. 33-3), clearly the families have to be a target of attention as much as the children. Within this perspective, Kazak[22] offers a systems and socioecologic model of understanding the needs of children and families. She and colleagues place this model in the unique framework of the traumatic stress that a diagnosis and treatment for cancer can create for both children and their families.[23,24] Good communication with the parents and children effect better care outcomes, as noted within the family systems model of care.[25] Such communication efficacy can not only impact parental decision making about treatment[26,27] but can also help the clinical team learn about other treatments such as complementary therapies that parents are including in their children's treatment armamentaria.[28]

Children go through stages of development, from newborn period to adulthood, that are typically divided into five periods: infant, toddler, preschool, school age, and adolescence. Different developmental tasks are associated with each and the needs for information, support, and care vary according to developmental stage. A review of communication methods to be used with sick children during various developmental stages is provided by Rushforth.[29] Pediatric providers are accustomed to tailoring their approaches to patients and families according to the children's developmental stages, and the care of oncology patients draws on these skills. For example, infants need significant parental soothing and physical contact as do toddlers, yet toddlers also need explanations and consistency in the environment. Preschool children can understand simple information that reduces fears of the unknown, whereas school age children need opportunities for peer interaction as well as clear communication. By adolescence, there is a need for the development of autonomy and for identity formation. The drive for independence, when little room for individual choice is perceived by the adolescent, can lead to maladaptive coping, such as nonadherence to medications or refusals to go to the clinic or to undergo medical procedures. Adolescents with cancer become by necessity more dependent upon their parents for

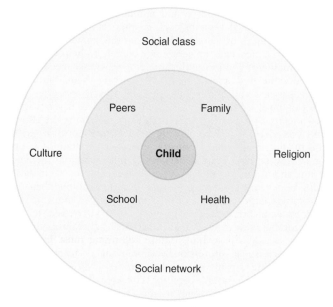

FIGURE 33-3. Child health from an ecological perspective. *(Adapted from Kazak AE. Pediatric psychosocial preventative health model (PPPHM): research, practice, and collaboration in pediatric family systems medicine. Fam Syst Health. 2006;24:381-395. Copyright © 2005 by the Center for Pediatric Traumatic Stress, Children's Hospital of Philadelphia.)*

physical and emotional needs and may have self-image issues related to weight loss or baldness because this is a developmental period during which peer acceptance is important and sexuality develops.[30,31] The specific needs of the adolescent patient are discussed later.

Professional Roles and a Team Approach to Psychosocial Care

No single individual is capable of fulfilling all the psychosocial needs of children and families going through cancer therapy. Many pediatric oncology settings use a team approach,[32-35] with the team comprising both medical and psychosocial providers. The medical team generally includes an attending oncologist, a surgeon, and a radiation oncologist (if these treatment modalities are indicated) as well as other oncology providers, such as an oncology fellow, a nurse practitioner or physician's assistant, and an oncology nurse. The psychosocial team may include a resource specialist, social worker, psychologist, child life specialist, or psychiatrist. Variation in the professions included in the psychosocial support team in a particular treatment setting generally has more to do with local culture and tradition than with the specific training or skills of a particular profession. Each psychosocial discipline has its particular focus or specialized skill set[36-43] (e.g., prescriptive authority, psychological testing) for working with pediatric oncology patients and families, but there is likely to be considerable overlap in their roles.

Psychosocial professionals have several important roles on the care team. The primary role may be as a consultant to other members of the team, including the patients and their families.[44-47] All team members interact and provide some level of information and support, so it is essential that they develop a consistent approach to supporting families.[48] As consultants, the psychosocial team members should conduct preliminary assessments of the children and families to understand their histories, preferred ways of coping, important supports, and potential sources of vulnerability. Using this knowledge of the families, psychosocial providers may be able to help the other team members understand families' individual needs and consider the best approaches to supporting them. Similarly, when patients and families have questions and concerns that are not resolved in the course of routine care, psychosocial providers may help them solve problems concerning the issues and consider ways of helping them raise their concerns with the medical team. The emphasis of these consultations is on improving communication between families and the medical teams and in most instances these consultations focus on clarifying issues and correcting misunderstandings rather than on resolving conflicts. In cases in which families are reluctant to address a concern to medical teams and when there is a significant conflict with medical teams, psychosocial team members may be asked to play more formal consulting roles. In these cases psychosocial professionals should make clear that the "client" in the consultation is the team as a whole, including the family, and should carefully consider the goal of the consultation. Often the goal is not to resolve an underlying disagreement between the family and medical staff but to repair the working relationship between the family and the medical staff and allow the treatment to move forward. The family and staff may agree to disagree about some significant issue, such as appropriate discipline or a recommendation for therapy or counseling, but may be able to work together in providing care to the child.

A second role that psychosocial team members fulfill is the provision of direct services to patients and the families. Typically this process begins with several preliminary meetings to conduct formal assessments and to offer guidance and support at the time of diagnosis. Depending on the setting and the needs of particular patients and families, psychosocial providers may set up individual or family meetings to offer support to the parents, patients, and families as well as to educate them and prepare them for surgery and other medical procedures. Support groups run by psychosocial or nursing staff in an inpatient or outpatient setting may be helpful in meeting families' educational and emotional needs.[49-52] If the medical team has questions or concerns about patients' or families' adjustment or emotional states, they may request that the psychosocial team conduct an assessment or provide a particular service, but in most cases the need for direct services is considered and ultimately determined by the patients and families.

Finally, psychosocial providers' roles often include consultation and liaison with outside agencies and community resources.[53-56] This function may include assisting families in accessing financial and insurance resources; contacting schools, tutors, and other childcare agencies; and helping to identify additional support services in the community, including referrals for psychotherapy when appropriate. In striving to fill these various roles, psychosocial providers need to work closely with families and other team members, remembering that their job is not to provide all the support directly but to maximize the potential for all interactions with the families to be as supportive as possible.

THE CRISIS OF CANCER DIAGNOSIS

Cancer diagnosis and the events leading up to it are typically frightening, complex, and unfamiliar.[7,8,57] The diagnosis period, which can be thought of as beginning when children first come to medical attention and lasting until clear diagnoses and treatment plans have been made, is primarily a period of uncertainty. At some point in this period, parents are told that diagnosis of cancer is possible or even likely, but it may be days or even longer until a definitive diagnosis is made. During this period children's symptoms may persist and usually, painful diagnostic tests and procedures must be faced.

Until their child has been diagnosed, most families have never thought about childhood cancer and don't know anyone who has had to face it. Although families facing common stressful life events can be guided by their prior experiences and the experiences of their friends and families, the cancer diagnosis pushes them beyond the realm of ordinary experience. It is not surprising that parents are typically overwhelmed emotionally as well as cognitively as they try to understand their child's illness. In addition, parents may describe feelings of unreality such as "this is not really real." Children's immediate reactions to illness depend largely on their age, their symptoms, and the medical procedures they have had to undergo. Except in cases of older adolescents, it is most commonly the parents who are most eager to learn the diagnosis, and they are the first ones to be informed of a diagnosis of cancer. In this section we consider parents' immediate reactions to such diagnoses and the supportive interventions that can be most helpful to them and to families as a whole.

Parents' Reactions to Children's Illness

Many factors can contribute to the overwhelming nature of cancer diagnoses. The word *cancer* continues to have a significant social stigma[58-63] as well as personal connotations. For many parents, personal experiences with cancer may be limited to relatives who were diagnosed later in life and may not have survived long after diagnosis. It can be helpful to learn about these personal associations with cancer, and it is important to correct parents' explicit or implicit assumptions as they apply to their child's illness. Families who have lost family members to cancer may need explicit explanations that the term *cancer* represents a group of related diseases and that parents' or grandparents' experiences with prostate or lung cancer may have little in common with children's diagnoses of cancer.

In the context of a new diagnosis, most parents experience many intense emotional reactions and may even report psychiatric symptoms of acute stress.[5,64] They are typically frightened and anxious about their child's prognosis and distraught about the thought of their child's physical suffering. If many days or weeks elapse between the child's initial symptoms and the diagnoses, parents may feel angry at medical providers whom they feel "missed the diagnosis" or did not listen to them or to their children. Parents' beliefs that there was a delay in diagnosis may also contribute to their feeling angry at themselves. Parents are ordinarily active agents in shaping every aspect of their children's care and well-being and may feel dismayed about how helpless they feel to protect their ill children. This sense of responsibility may lead many parents to feel responsible for their child's situation, perhaps blaming themselves for not bringing the child to medical attention earlier or for not understanding the significance of their child's initial symptoms.[2,7,8,65,66] In some cases this sense of responsibility and the need to understand the cause of the child's illness may make parents (or other family members) wonder if they themselves are responsible for the cancer. Examples of these thoughts, many of which are not entirely rational, might be parents' wondering whether allowing their children to use certain electrical devices or bringing some kind of contamination into the home from a work site may have contributed to the cancer.[2,7,8,66]

Listening to families in crisis and providing reassurance can be the most useful responses for all members of the care team. Normalizing parents' reactions by letting them know that parents almost universally feel overwhelmed and that intense emotional reactions are normal responses to their children's illnesses can help to reassure them they are not "going crazy" and that they won't be judged for their reactions by the care team.[2,3,7,49,67,68] One reason parents feel overwhelmed is their awareness that they are facing more complicated, frightening, and demanding challenges than they have ever faced before. It is helpful to acknowledge the feeling of facing this seemingly overwhelming challenge, but it is also useful to let parents know that families do cope well and, with some assistance and support, there is every reason to believe that their own families will cope successfully, even though that may be difficult to imagine at the beginning of treatment.[57,69-72]

During the crisis of diagnosis, many families benefit from concrete structuring by the care team. Parents often need to be encouraged to focus on their own self-care, including taking time to sleep and eat adequately, as well as taking brief breaks from the hospital and seeking their own emotional support. Along with encouraging these behaviors, it can be helpful to remind them that cancer therapy is often a challenge lasting weeks or months or years, and part of the challenge is finding ways to take care of themselves and maintain their strength for a prolonged period. In addition, they may need help mobilizing their social supports and other resources, such as arranging extended time away from work or asking friends and extended family to help with meals, childcare for well siblings, and other concrete tasks. This may be a challenge for some parents, especially those not used to asking for assistance from others. These parents in particular may benefit from some active problem solving,[57,67,73-75] with staff helping them to identify needs, generate possible solutions, and then select and implement potential solutions. Social workers and resource specialists on the care team may be helpful in identifying sources of practical support (e.g., transportation, meals, lodging), sorting through insurance issues, and helping to solve problems about meeting patients' and families' needs.

Other parents may have very strong needs to act and may make decisions that can be premature or even impulsive. For example, some parents have quit their jobs, mortgaged their homes, or changed their residences even before knowing the details of their children's treatments and before taking time to consider these major life decisions. Parents must decide for themselves how their families will adjust and cope with the demands of the children's illnesses and treatments, but it is appropriate for members of the care team to caution against impulsive decisions. Part of encouraging families to take long views of illnesses is helping them to avoid feeling they need to know every detail of the challenges that lie ahead but can cope successfully by focusing on the immediate challenges while anticipating the challenges that lie ahead. A metaphor attributed to E. L. Doctorow may be particularly useful for parents faced with long and complicated treatments for their children: "[it] is like driving a car at night. You can see only

as far as your headlights, but you can make the whole trip that way."[76]

During the crisis period parents can experience a wide range of intense emotional reactions. In most cases parents' reactions can be managed by education and support from the care team. Specialized services by a psychosocial provider, usually a psychologist or social worker, can be particularly useful in helping parents to identify and begin to cope with their emotional reactions.[67,77-79] Many of these reactions are of short duration because parents commonly report feeling less overwhelmed after they have heard a definitive diagnosis and can focus on the demands of definitive treatment plans. In rare cases parents may have emotional reactions that are more enduring or problematic,[2,80-82] and they may require more targeted intervention during the crisis period. Situations involving confusion about a child's diagnosis or requiring prolonged diagnostic evaluation periods are more stressful for parents and may be more likely to cause significant distress. Similarly, parents who are managing other significant stressors such as having a parent or other family member with medical needs and parents who have preexisting psychological problems are more likely to have symptoms that interfere with their abilities to function (Box 33-1).[2,80] Examples of these problematic

---

| Box 33-1 | **Factors Associated with Increased Psychosocial Distress** |

FAMILY FACTORS

Single parent
Preexisting chronic or mental health problems
Concurrent illness or injury (e.g., parent or sibling illness)
Marital problems (e.g., separation or divorce)
Family problems (e.g., emotional or learning difficulties)
Recent stressful life events (e.g., job or school problems, move or relocation)

DISEASE FACTORS

Unclear diagnoses
Poor prognoses
Prolonged or intense treatments (e.g., bone marrow transplant)
Disfiguring disease or treatments (e.g., amputation)
Disease status (e.g., relapse, recurrence)

ENVIRONMENT AND RESOURCE FACTORS

Financial problems (e.g., job loss, debts)
Isolation (e.g., lack of family and peer support)
Language differences (e.g., foreign national or immigrant)
Transportation (e.g., no car to get to the hospital)
Minimal or no health insurance

Adapted from Hersh SP, Wiener LS. Psychosocial support for the family of the child with cancer. In Pizzo PA, Poplack DG (eds). Principles and Practice of Pediatric Oncology. Philadelphia, JB Lippincott, 1989, pp 897-913; Kazak AE, Cant MC, Jensen MM, et al. Identifying psychosocial risk indicative of subsequent resource use in families of newly diagnosed pediatric oncology patients. J Clin Oncol. 2003;21:3220-3225; Lansky SB, List MA, Ritter-Sterr C. Psychiatric and psychological support of the child and adolescent with cancer. In Pizzo PA, Poplack DG (eds). Principles and Practice of Pediatric Oncology. Philadelphia, JB Lippincott, 1989, pp 885-896.

reactions include parents who manifest signs of clinical depression or anxiety, those who are not able to care for themselves adequately (i.e., not sleeping or eating), and those who are so frustrated and angry that they cannot consistently collaborate with medical providers. In these situations, in which parents' reactions will have negative impacts on the children and have the potential to interfere with treatment processes, it is important to address the parents' problems directly and make appropriate referrals for intervention.

Addressing these issues with parents can be a delicate matter, especially when parents are angry and agitated. One approach that may be helpful is to elicit feedback from parents, asking them how they think things are going, how they feel they and their children are doing, and how they feel the team is working with them. Many times, in the context of this discussion, parents will mention their own difficulties in working with the treatment team, thus providing an opportunity for the providers to discuss the issues. In the discussion it is helpful to remind parents that the well-being of patients and the families is the primary concern, and the team is invested in supporting that particular family through the crisis of a cancer diagnosis. If parents are not meeting the team's expectations in some ways, such as not being available for meetings or being disruptive in the medical setting, it is important to state this clearly and without reproach. The emphasis should be on informing parents about the team's expectations and finding ways to help the parents meet them. It is often useful to talk explicitly about working together with the parents and patients as part of the team and to reinforce the critical roles that parents will play.

Interventions for parents experiencing these problematic reactions may require more intensive services from some member of the care team, as well as consultation with and referral to other individuals. The underlying problems may be longstanding, but intervention during the crisis of diagnosis may focus appropriately on the alleviation of symptoms. Parents showing signs of severe distress should be evaluated by an appropriate psychosocial team member or referred to a mental health provider who can assess psychological status and make referrals for any urgent interventions they may need. Psychopharmacologic intervention may be particularly helpful for parents with severe anxiety or depressive reactions, those with severe sleep disturbance,[83,84] and those with preexisting psychopathology. Pastoral counseling may be useful for parents whose faith is an important source of support as well as for those experiencing a crisis of faith as they struggle to find meaning in their children's illnesses.[85-87] For families experiencing intense frustration and anger with the medical system or the care team in particular, it can be useful to engage a third party who is responsible for hearing such complaints, such as an ombudsman or patient-relations specialist.[88]

Giving parents an appropriate place to report problems with patient care may help them to feel that their concerns about these issues have been heard, to express their anger, and to leave them more able to engage with the care team subsequently. In the context of a medical crisis, some parents may be able to "agree to disagree" or at least to temporarily table issues of conflict between themselves and the care team. For these parents it can be useful for medical and psychosocial providers to acknowledge the conflict and its seriousness but suggest that for a discrete period of time, the team and the parents concentrate on working together to get through a particular phase of care (e.g., completing diagnostic workups or specific treatments) but plan to revisit the issue and evaluate it at a later time. There may be a tendency to withdraw from angry parents, and this reaction on the part of the care team should be guarded against; otherwise, already angry parents may legitimately add neglect to their list of complaints. Main-taining an open dialogue with parents and empathizing with their frustrations are more effective in helping families with their anger than is avoidance. If lapses occur in patient care or communication with families, appropriate apologies from the providers involved can be particularly relieving to parents.[89,90]

Children's Reactions to Illness

Children react to a diagnosis and initial treatments according to their developmental levels, their own individual temperaments and past experiences and, to a large degree, how their parents cope with the new diagnoses and treatment plans.[91,92] Typically, infants, toddlers, and especially preschoolers are more concerned about changes in routine and normal home environments, separation from family, especially the primary caregiver, and bodily intrusion through physical examinations and medical procedures for diagnostic or treatment purposes. Strange environments disrupt normal wake/sleep patterns, and sleep deprivation can reduce children's normal effectiveness in self-regulation. For example, infants who had been able to sleep through the night at home might have constant awakenings. Separation from primary caregivers then becomes an even larger issue if the parents are not present during the night or to help comfort children during episodes of bodily intrusion. Clearly, this need for the parents suggests that when possible, it is better for parents to create shifts so they can be with their children as much as possible, day and night. Such parental support also means that the issue of support for parents, both emotionally and in practical ways, must be addressed.[93] Stressed parents who cope poorly are not able to help their children soothe themselves.[13,94]

One issue that the medical team can address is the manner in which examinations and procedures are carried out. For example, Chen and colleagues[95,96] found that children had memories of stressful and painful procedures that impacted their experiences and behaviors during subsequent procedures. Asking parents to leave when a team of doctors and nurses in white coats enters children's rooms to carry out examinations is more likely to create uncooperative children who will become conditioned to be anxious around all those with white coats. Having one member of the team develop a relationship with the children, whether toddlers or adolescents, is helpful in establishing children's trust in the nonfamily team. In very young children, procedures that can be performed competently and quickly while distracters are present (e.g., soap bubbles, party blowers, cartoons, stories) can reduce fear of future procedures and help children develop a sense of control and cooperation (which helps procedures to be performed efficiently and effectively). After all procedures, some type of positive reinforcement is helpful, whether it is verbal praise or stickers or the choice of a surprise from a toy box (the toys can be small and inexpensive items). The goal is to pair scary, novel, and intrusive experiences with positive, pleasurable experiences. Novelty can create fear (e.g., a new treatment room) and also a focus of attention and curiosity (e.g., "I wonder what is in this special box?"). Providing parents with ways in which they can help support their children in these novel and intrusive situations can help the children develop a sense of security and mastery. In addition, it may be useful to encourage families to bring in transitional objects for their children. There might be favorite blankets or stuffed animals that provide comfort to their children at home and can provide a sense of familiarity in the hospital. Favorite stories told by the parents in the hospital or favorite CDs or other music and songs can also provide transitional objects for children, as can placing pictures of their families and pets in the room. In a study of memory revaluation in children with cancer undergoing lumbar punctures, Chen and colleagues[97] found that helping children to remember positive aspects of coping during previous procedures and providing children with brightly colored cards to take to the next procedure as reminders of the children's successful coping during the previous procedures helped to reduce subsequent distress.

School-age children often ask questions in concrete ways that require specific answers. For example, they ask why they are going to the hospital, what the reasons are for the examinations, and what the doctors are going to do. It is important to provide brief descriptions of the various procedures so that there are no surprises. If parents typically avoid direct responses to their children or avoid discussing uncomfortable subjects, their children learn to avoid asking the questions that are active in their minds. Their own mentally created "answers" are often far more frightening to them than the actual direct responses of their parents. Children need to know that they have serious illnesses, that the tests determine the best ways to treat their illnesses, and that there are treatments for their illnesses.[98] If they ask, "Am I going to die?" parents should answer that question in the right way, according to the children's diagnoses and medical conditions.[99] For example, at diagnoses and at the beginning of treatments, the response is that the doctors have a treatment for your illness to make you well and healthy again. If children are in relapse or have serious concomitant infections or treatment side effects, the responses should involve not yes or no answers but explorations into what they think and what their fears are about dying. Responses should also provide explanations that let the children understand that you will continue to be there and will not leave them.[100] This often becomes most difficult for adolescents who may want to know many more details than younger children who think more concretely. Children and adolescents often gain a sense of mastery from knowing the names of their conditions and treatments and other "medical lingo." In the following section, approaches to informing patients and families about cancer diagnoses and treatment plans are discussed.

School-age children need plans for re-entering school and social activities following diagnosis and initiation of treatment. Normalizing activities as much as is possible is helpful in re-creating a sense of normalcy for children following diagnosis and treatment initiation. Children and adolescents who have formed relationships with members of the treating team can ask questions of those team members that might seem difficult to ask parents.[101,102] Some adolescents feel a need to protect their parents from more stress by not acknowledging to their parents their own fears, anger, and worries. Team members can facilitate adolescent-parent communication so that it is as good as possible.

Finally, children of all ages often regress when they are scared, and parents need to know that changes in their children's behaviors are not unusual.[103] Parents may need help in learning how best to address the behaviors as well as how to handle their child's anxiety, anger, or withdrawal. Facilitating night-time sleep is essential when possible, whether at home or in the hospital.[104] Setting up a routine in the hospital as soon as possible helps; story times can be useful, and medication can be used if needed. Having social interactions during the days in the hospital can also facilitate coping, and this is why, among other reasons, child life programs and playrooms are so important.[105] The following are some guidelines related to children's reactions to diagnosis and treatment.[106]

- Many parents need help talking to their children, who are often scared and need explanation and education by parents.
- A variety of disciplines, such as child life, nursing, social work, and psychology, can all be helpful to parents, siblings,

and child patients. Child life specialists can help to normalize daily social, physical, and educational activities and can often provide psychological preparatory and interventional supports for medical procedures. Nurses are at the bedside and can develop more intimate relationships with parents and patients because of this ongoing contact. These relationships can be helpful in supporting both parents and patients. Social work can assess parental support and care-giving burdens and can assist with both. Finally, there are times when psychological intervention can be especially useful to help the subgroup of parents and patients who need added expertise to cope.
- Connections with other children and families are helpful.
- Getting through diagnostic procedures: the goal is good preparation and good pharmacologic and psychological management of pain and anxiety.

Presenting Diagnoses and Plans for Treatment: The Day One Talk

The diagnostic period comes to a close when the treatment team has made a clear diagnosis and communicates the diagnosis and the related treatment plans to the patient and the family. Often referred to as the "Day One Talk," this conversation with family members usually takes place in the form of a treatment conference between a family and several members of the care team, including physicians, nurses, and psychosocial providers. During the diagnostic period there typically would have been several prior conversations between the physicians and the family about the likelihood of cancer and the diagnostic tests being conducted, but the Day One Talk is a more comprehensive discussion and is usually the first to address the child's prognosis and specific treatment recommendations. For many families this meeting is a pivotal event in their lives, marking the real beginning of their child's cancer. Throughout the diagnostic phase most families maintain hope that their child does not in fact have cancer, so the Day One Talk is similar to other situations in which physicians must communicate bad news to families. The literature concerning communicating bad news about children's health[107-111] may be relevant, and recommendations from these noncancer settings may be instructive. Box 33-2 provides a summary of essential points to address when communicating diagnoses.

The medical details discussed vary with circumstances, but there are challenges in communicating diagnostic, prognostic, and treatment information that are consistent across families and can be considered and planned for.[112-115] Planning is essential for successful meetings with families, and although there may be pressure from family members or medical staff to have the conversation as soon as possible, a certain amount of scheduling and organization are required. A written protocol for communicating diagnoses has been recommended,[114] with the expectation that it will be tailored to meet the needs of the patients and family. A private space free of interruptions is important, as is scheduling the meeting so that the important members of the family and care teams can attend. In addition to the oncologists directly caring for the patients, this meeting should include nurses and psychosocial caregivers whenever possible.[116,117] The organization of, and the roles of, a medical center's staff are often confusing to families, and taking the time to introduce the various members of the team and describe their roles is essential. Both parents should attend, and they should be offered the opportunity to include other family members involved in the care of the child. Whether to include the child in all or part of this session or to arrange

STRUCTURE—ORGANIZATION

- Establish an initial plan for communication.
- Communicate in a private and comfortable space where interruptions are minimized.
- Communicate with the parents, children, and other family members, if desired. Nursing staff and psychosocial workers should also be included whenever possible.
- Hold separate sessions with children if they are not present during the initial communication.

CONTENT—INFORMATION TO DISCUSS

- Solicit questions from parents and children, especially regarding their understanding of the present illness.
- Share information about the diagnoses, treatments, and plans for cure or goals of treatment.
- Share information on lifestyle and psychosocial issues, particularly surrounding causation (e.g., the cancer is neither the children's nor the families' fault!).

PROCESS—COMMUNICATION

- Communicate immediately at diagnoses and follow up later.
- Communicate at a pace families can follow, allowing the children's or families' emotional reactions to guide the flow of the conversation.
- Communicate in ways that are sensitive to cultural differences (e.g., for families who are not native English speakers, arrangements should be made for an interpreter).
- Encourage the entire family to talk together.

Adapted from Krahn GL, Hallum A, Kime C. Are there good ways to give bad news? Pediatrics. 1993;91:578-582; Mack JW, Grier HE. The day one talk. J Clin Oncol. 2004;22: 563-566; Masera G, Chesler MA, Jankovic M, et al. SIOP Working Committee on psychosocial issues in pediatric oncology: guidelines for communication of the diagnosis. Med Pediatr Oncol. 1997;28:382-385.

for a separate session for the child depends largely on the ages of the child and on parental preference. A smaller meeting of parents and one or two medical professionals held subsequently may be more appropriate for younger children,[118-120] but including adolescents in the Day One Talk can help them to develop trust in the medical team and to invest in their own care.[113,121]

The principal goal of the meeting is to provide families with overviews of their child's diagnosis, the treatment recommendations, and the prognosis. It is important to elicit questions the patient and family may have and to provide sufficient time to discuss their concerns. Mack and Grier[113] emphasize the importance of the opportunity to address the families' questions about what may have caused the children's cancers and particularly to correct misconceptions that may lead to a sense of blame or responsibility for the cancer. Communicating prognostic information to families is critical because it is likely to

have an impact on their understanding of the treatment recommendations,[122,123] but delivering this information can be difficult, especially when the prognosis is guarded or poor. How much to rely on numeric presentations of this information is a question that arises in many cases, and there is some evidence that patients may misunderstand the information if it is not carefully explained.[124-126] Numeric information about risks such as 5-year survival rates should not be avoided altogether because many families want this information,[127] but care should be given to ensure that parents receive information in the ways they find most useful and that they understand the information given. Recommendations for treatment should be presented, beginning with a general overview of the modalities used and the timing and settings for treatments. The introduction of consent forms and discussion of known and likely side effects (short- and long-term) should follow, once families have understood the general outline of the treatments.

In separate sessions for children, the same general information about diagnosis, prognosis, and treatment plans should be covered. The information will have to be tailored to the developmental levels and the particular concerns of patients, such as the ability to return to home and school, to see friends, and to participate in sports and other activities.[121] Children should be told about specific expectable side effects such as hair loss, with an emphasis on concrete ways in which these effects may affect their appearance or activities. Older children and adolescents may be able to engage directly with the medical providers, but younger children may be more comfortable talking with their parents, who can elicit their questions and reinforce what medical providers have communicated directly.

Most professionals emphasize the importance of children's knowing the names of their disease and that they have cancer. Parents may initially shy away from this direct approach and from particular words like *cancer* and may need some preparation before talking with their children so they know the words to use. Understandably, many parents feel protective toward their children and may wish to avoid using the word *cancer* or *leukemia*. It is important to help parents understand that honesty, even about potentially frightening information, is containing and supportive for children in the long term because they can grow to trust that adults are not withholding information and that they need not fear unpleasant surprises. Similarly, it is important to explain that the word *cancer* is commonly used with pediatric patients and that it is important for children not to feel that any condition is so frightening that it can't be named or spoken about. It can be helpful to share with parents that the climate of open communication with children who are patients is based on lessons learned in past eras when communication was not open; it was found that the lack of frankness contributed to children's anxieties and fears about their disease. With this sort of preparation, most parents can begin to feel comfortable with open communication with their children. Parents from certain cultural backgrounds,[120,128,129] and those who are unused to open discussions of illness, may not easily accept this openness and naming of the disease, and it may take some careful negotiation and compromise to reach an agreement about which words to use and which topics to discuss with their children. Over time, families themselves may become more comfortable about being open with their children as they meet other families and children and see that they are comfortable with this kind of open discussion.

In our experience it is rare that, with some time and effort, families and treatment teams cannot agree on a mutually acceptable approach to talking with children. This may mean coming to some initial agreement about what will, and will not, be discussed with the children initially, and agreeing to revisit this issue over time. Parents who are reluctant to disclose diagnoses or prognoses to children are attempting to protect the children and act in their best interests, and it is important for providers to acknowledge this. Parents who feel their positions are respected may come to trust the treatment team and even accept some increased openness in discussion with their children. But in extreme cases, for example if parents were to refuse to let providers discuss even basic information with adolescent patients, or were to ask providers to communicate false information, teams may feel they are faced with an ethical dilemma,[121,130-133] and should seek consultation concerning the ethical and legal questions involved.[134]

Families typically find the Day One Talk overwhelming[113,135-137] and may not remember many of the details discussed. To help families manage this information overload, several steps can be taken. Some practitioners recommend providing a tape recording of the meeting for the parents to review subsequently,[136,138-140] and this has been shown to be effective in other oncology populations.[141] Reassuring families that they are not expected to remember all the details discussed can reduce their sense of information overload, as does making explicit the critical pieces of information they are being asked to focus on. Providing written material to be reviewed after the meeting, and emphasizing the availability of the team for future conversations about diagnoses and treatment plans, are also of value. Reminding families of the various roles of the providers on the care team at this point can also help families to feel comfortable addressing them with appropriate questions in the future.

In an elegant description of the Day One Talk in pediatric oncology, Mack and Grier highlight the importance of an alliance between the families and medical providers, and discuss the ways in which this alliance can affect adjustment to diagnoses. In particular, they emphasize the importance of listening closely, making emotional connections with the families, and acknowledging the overwhelming impact of such diagnoses on every aspect of the families' lives. The authors offer specific guidelines for discussing the necessary information but conclude that "... listening and the openness of silence may be more important than the words themselves."[113]

ADJUSTING TO TREATMENT

As children and families come to understand their treatment plans, their focus begins to shift from managing uncertainty to coping with the demands of treatment. Parents in particular will continue to worry about their children's prognoses for years to come, but the day-to-day demands of treatment combined with the other demands of work and family life become increasingly salient. Families often experience a sense of relief associated with the reduction in uncertainty, but they may also feel an increased burden. During the crises of new diagnosis, parents usually take time off from work and temporarily set aside many practical concerns. With the initiation of treatment, parents and children typically have to return to their regular roles and responsibilities while also taking on the new responsibilities associated with treatment. During this period of adjusting to treatment, families often benefit from continued psychosocial assessment, education, and support. In actual practice, encounters with patients and families blend these three objectives, especially at the initiation of treatment, but they are discussed separately here for clarity of presentation.

Psychosocial Assessment of Patients and Families

In many cases, a formal assessment of the patient and family may be deferred until a definitive diagnosis is made. Once a treatment plan has been developed, psychosocial assessment can focus more effectively on how the families will cope with the upcoming demands of treatments and can offer more targeted support. Regardless of when it is completed, a psychosocial assessment is critical for planning and organizing a family's care. The assessment is usually completed in one to three meetings during which psychosocial providers, typically social workers or psychologists, interview the patients and parents. The assessment should be summarized in a written report that is shared with the treatment teams and that describe the family's constellation and history and their particular strengths and vulnerabilities relevant to the child's illness and provide recommendations and plans to provide support or intervention for the family.

Depending on how involved the psychosocial providers have been previously, the assessment interviews may be the first opportunity for scheduled and extended conversations with the patient and parents. These conversations will form the basis of the assessment, although intake forms and rating scales may be used to collect preliminary information or to supplement the interviews. For example, rating scales[142,143] assessing children's behavior prior to cancer diagnoses can be useful in some cases, and Anne Kazak and her colleagues have developed a cancer-specific instrument that is a promising addition to the assessment of family resources.[144,145]

Experienced providers generally have ways of conducting assessments that are comfortable for them and generate the relevant information. For illustrative purposes, one approach to assessment interviews is discussed here, and additional suggestions are summarized in Box 33-3. The process of the interview should include time for the family members to speak about their concerns, but providers should actively direct the conversations to ensure that the necessary topics are covered. In an interview with both parents, if possible, providers may begin by asking about family constellation, the names and ages of family members living at home, and the involvement of extended family. Focusing on premorbid functioning, developmental histories of the patient and relevant history of any other children can then follow. Details of the patient's functioning at school, in relationships with peers and siblings should be asked about specifically. It is particularly useful to know how children have coped with previous challenges and frustrations and whether there have been any behavioral, developmental, or emotional concerns prior to the cancer diagnosis. To learn more about the parents, it is useful to know the basic outline of their families of origin, their education and present employment status, and their marital relationship. If parents are divorced or not married, understanding this history, as well as the practical and legal aspects of any custody arrangements, is critical. Understanding how families have coped with any previous illnesses or other major life events can be useful in anticipating how families may respond to current illness. It is important to know whether families are also facing any other significant stressors and whether there are any other significant medical or emotional problems in the family at present. Providers should ask about important traditions and values, especially religious and cultural traditions that may be involved in their coping with illness.

Understanding families' practical and social resources is also an important component of the assessment. A child's cancer often results in significant costs to families in terms of

---

| Box 33-3 | **Psychosocial Assessment Interview of Patients and Families** |

STRUCTURE OF INTERVIEW

- One to three intake meetings with patients and parents, conducted by a mental health professional
- Meetings held in a relaxed, nonthreatening setting
- Written summary of assessment to be shared with the treatment team

CONTENT OF ASSESSMENT

Context of Illness

- Initial presentation of the illness
- Diagnoses, prognoses, and anticipated treatments
- Previous children's and families' experiences with physical health problems and behavioral problems
- Families' coping abilities, especially cohesiveness, communication style, and ways of resolving conflicts

Patients

- History
  Developmental: milestones, temperament, delays
  Medical: previous diagnoses and responses to medical care
  Behavioral: energy levels, moods, sleeping and eating habits pre- and postillness
  School and social: relationships with parents, siblings, peers
  Education: history and functioning in school
- Response to diagnosis; coping style

Parents and Families

- Background and history
  Basic structure and involvement of extended family
  Sources of social support
  Relationships, sources of conflicts and cohesion
  Physical and mental health
  Sibling relationships
  Parent education and employment
  Religious beliefs and cultural traditions
  Parenting styles
- Initial responses to the diagnoses
  Knowledge and understanding of diagnoses
  Level of distress: emotional and physical symptoms
  Strength and vulnerabilities during the crisis
  Coping styles and experienced need for support
  Expectations and sources of stress and anxiety

RESOURCES

- Housing
- Names and ages of family members living at home (siblings, grandparents, etc.)
- Available support for work, neighborhood, and school
- Financial status
- Health insurance
- Involvement within the community and social supports
- Travel time and transportation to treatment center
- Resources available during children's ongoing medical treatments

Adapted from Hersh SP, Wiener LS, Figueroa V, Kunz JF. Psychiatric and psychosocial support for the child and family. In Pizzo PA, Poplack DG (eds). Principles and Practice of Pediatric Oncology, 3rd ed. Philadelphia, Lippincott-Raven, 1997, pp 1241-1266.

---

both lost income and unreimbursable expenses,[64] making it important to assess sources of financial support and health insurance as well as the adequacy of their housing and transportation. Social resources, including emotional and practical support available from family members and friends as well as community and work groups, should also be explored with parents. It may also be important to underscore the importance of parental self-care at this point and to encourage parents to think about the resources they have to meet the challenges of a child's ongoing medical treatment. As mentioned in the section on diagnosis, families may need help in mobilizing their social supports and asking for concrete help or emotional support. This is an area in which some anticipatory guidance about expectable challenges and possible solutions may be useful. Families who have significant financial difficulties or problems with other practical aspects of preparing for treatment (e.g., transportation, meals and lodging, insurance) may be referred to other providers such as resource specialists for additional help in identifying sources of practical support.

Assessments of children vary significantly with the children's ages and medical status. An infant or toddler will be seen along with the parents, and the goals may be to observe parent-child interaction, appreciate the child's temperament and reactions to the medical setting, and establish the psychosocial provider as a friendly and nonthreatening presence. With older children, the goals may include these as well as the goal of directly assessing the children's reactions to their illnesses as they are able to express them verbally or in play. Children have

typically met many health care providers in the hospital or clinic, so it is important for psychosocial providers to begin by introducing themselves and explaining the purposes of the meetings; reassuring the children that there will be no medical examinations or needles in this meeting can be essential. With most children, assessment is greatly facilitated by including action, such as unstructured play, a walk in the hospital, a craft, or a game. Even with older adolescents who may be able to express themselves verbally quite clearly, exchanges are often made easier by simultaneously engaging in some shared activity.

Preschool and even school-age children may be hesitant to be interviewed without the presence of parents, and parents may be reluctant to leave their children alone for the interview. This is not an essential point, but it can be helpful to interview children alone, and family members learning to separate from each other in medical settings can be a useful skill to develop. Being careful not to increase families' anxiety and distress, providers can often finesse this issue by showing children where their parents will be waiting nearby or by negotiating a short separation of a few minutes before the parents return to check in, and ask "permission" to remain or leave again. With preschool and school-aged children, familiar activities such as drawing or symbolic play with dolls or puppets can serve the dual purpose of engaging them and providing an expressive medium through which they can relate their concerns. For children who engage in this kind of play, much of the meeting may be used productively in this manner, with the provider observing or participating in the play and asking questions to gain insight into how the children are coping and what issues may be on their minds. It is also important to devote some part of the meeting to direct questions to the child about their illness, their medical care, and how they are coping. Asking explicitly about what have been the hardest or the easiest parts of being a patient can be important, as is brainstorming with patients about what might help them to cope with the challenges of their medical treatment. This discussion may bring to light questions and misunderstandings that can be corrected or identified so they can be addressed later. In ending sessions with children it is important for providers to restate their roles as people who help children and families cope with being sick and needing medical care, and to reaffirm that they themselves, or others, will be available to help the children and their families if questions or difficulties arise.

Older children and adolescents may have both greater ability and less inclination to engage in discussions of their illness and how they are coping. They may respond to the loss of control and autonomy that typically comes with the patient role by emotionally withdrawing or even refusing any meetings not required for their treatment. Except in extraordinary cases in which a question of serious psychological illness or safety has been raised, insisting on meeting with patients is ill advised. An approach that empathizes with patients and shows a willingness to acknowledge their rights and abilities to refuse will be more successful. One approach may be to respect their autonomy by rescheduling the meeting at a preferable time, or providers may successfully bargain with patients for access by requesting a small amount of time (e.g., 15 minutes) and agreeing to renegotiate for more time after that. Both parents and children should understand the limits of confidentiality of the information shared during children's assessments, and children should be encouraged as far as is reasonable to feel comfortable sharing personal information. It is important to help most older children understand how the assessment can be concretely useful to them by explaining that the assessment helps the care team get to know them better and learn the best ways of interacting with them, and means that each provider will not have to ask the same questions, thus sparing them from repeated inquiries from several people.

Once engaged in the assessment process, older children and adolescents will generally be forthcoming about the course of their illness and their care, especially if given the opportunity to vent their frustrations. Asking questions about older children's lives in general, including friends, hobbies, and school activities, can be a good starting place before asking about their illness and how they are coping with their medical care. It is important to ask older children what they are concerned about and how the adults involved in their care can best help and support them. Direct inquiry about their worries, anxieties, and any symptoms of depression or hopelessness should be included. Adolescents may have very personal concerns about how their illnesses will affect them, such as missing upcoming social events, that may not be immediately apparent to parents or medical teams. Asking explicitly about what adolescents anticipate will be difficult about their treatment plans is an important part of assessments, as is inquiring about the ways they think they will deal with the challenges of treatment. During their treatments, adolescents are typically more dependent on their parents and spend more time with them than they normally would. For that reason it can be helpful to inquire about their premorbid relationships with parents and other important adults in the family system, and about how they have been getting along with these adults since their diagnosis. Family systems often shift in response to children's illness and it can be important to understand the changes adolescents may have experienced and how those changes are affecting them.

When concluding the assessment meeting, older children should be asked about any concerns they have that have not been addressed and about any information about those concerns that the care team should be asked to keep in mind. Providers should restate their roles in the care team, explaining how they, or others, will be available to help the children if questions or difficulties arise and informing the patients about what information will be shared with their parents and the care team, including any additional recommendations that will be made for their care.

After concluding interviews with the patients, it is important to give feedback to the parents about what was discussed, what the children's main concerns are, and generally how the patients are coping with their illness and the demands of the treatment. If there are specific recommendations for further assessment or intervention, those recommendations should be explained to the parents and the patients. For illustrative purposes, this description has emphasized the information that should be gathered in an assessment, but the process of the interviews should accommodate both the goals of assessment and the goals of education and support. Ideally, providers should gain better understanding of the family and their history and also develop better relationships and rapport. As areas of concern arise in the interview, such as problems with financial resources or concerns about schoolwork, providers should attend to those concerns during the interviews or should inform the family members how those concerns will be attended to in the future. Questions about managing side effects may be directed to the medical or nursing staff (see later material). Social and emotional concerns, such as questions about patients' behavior, worries about siblings or questions about how to talk with friends and family about the illness, may be opportunities for psychosocial providers to listen empathically and offer some anticipatory guidance. Modeling ways of assessing and solving problems in the medical environment can create important roles for psychosocial providers and can help families to take on these functions themselves. Finally, letting patients and parents know that their concerns are common and offering suggestions for coping, including examples of how other families have successfully coped, should be incorporated into assessment processes whenever possible.

Education and Information About Treatment

Most treatment regimens put enormous information burdens on the families. Children are commonly treated by several modalities (surgery, radiation, chemotherapy) and may receive a large number of medications and undergo a variety of blood tests and other diagnostic procedures. Adolescents may be active in their own care to some extent, but parents are responsible for understanding and managing their children's treatments. This may be especially true during outpatient phases of treatment when parents will have to work with home care agencies, administer treatments themselves, and monitor their children's health. To meet these demands, parents require detailed information about their children's treatment regimens and the expectable reactions.[77,78,146,147] Most of this detailed information is provided by nursing and medical providers. Many centers give parents treatment notebooks that include information about the diagnoses and treatments, teaching sheets about interpreting blood counts and other diagnostic tests, and information about nutrition, caring for a central line, and managing children's behaviors. Parents and older children should be oriented to this information and be given opportunities to ask questions and talk about any concerns they have about their roles in the treatment processes. Patients and families are generally quite resilient and successfully accommodate even the most demanding treatment regimens, but initial apprehension about being able to understand and take on these demands is common. Staff may have to present information several times and reinforce verbal exchanges with written materials. While remaining optimistic and encouraging families to develop competence, it is also important for providers to recognize the complexity and the burden of the functions they are asking of families. Normalizing family concerns by making it clear that feeling anxious and overwhelmed are common first reactions may be helpful. Talking with other families who are undergoing similar treatments can be particularly helpful,[78,79,146,148,149] and many centers offer education and support groups for new patients and families. In addition, a wide variety of books useful to parents,[150-155] patients, and siblings[156-167] may be available from hospitals, as well as from libraries and booksellers.

Psychosocial providers can be of assistance by empathizing with parents' feelings of "information overload" and by problem solving with them about adapting family routines to meet the new demands of treatments. For some parents and older children it can be helpful to talk about their preferred styles of receiving information. Do they prefer detailed information about how the treatments work, or would they rather focus on the concrete aspects of what to do and when to do it? Do they appreciate being reminded of long-term treatment plans, or would focusing on the current phase of treatment be more helpful and reassuring? If families are encouraged to ask for the specific types of information they find helpful, that may guide their care teams in providing the most appropriate information and increase parents' experiences of self-efficacy and control.

Children have their own particular needs when adjusting to new routines and the demands of ongoing treatment. For many children, the start of cancer therapy, particularly if it requires an inpatient stay, signals that their involvement with the medical system will not be short-lived. They may feel their lack of control and autonomy more acutely and may become more upset, anxious, or oppositional. With the increase in anxiety and the decrease in opportunities for autonomy, young children often regress, displaying behaviors such as talking in baby talk or sucking their thumbs that they have not displayed for some time. For these young children opportunities to incorporate medical themes and materials into their play provide important ways for children to express themselves and receive new information about their own care.[168-170] In some settings child life specialists may be available to work with children individually or in groups to familiarize them with medical routines and procedures, and to help them develop new coping mechanisms, including relaxation and distraction. Young children tend to be more focused on the here-and-now and may benefit from having new routines explained to them as they arise, with less focus on planning for events far in the future. To the extent possible, children should be given age-appropriate opportunities for choice and autonomy and for participation in their own self-care, such as filling or pushing syringes, counting pills, or deciding the order in which to take medications.

Older children and adolescents can be highly variable in their interest in and openness to learning more about their illness and treatment. With more developed cognitive and language abilities, older children can ask more questions and understand more about their treatment and, like parents, they may receive educational information from nursing staff, as described earlier. To whatever extent they are able, adolescents should be encouraged to participate in their own treatment by learning about their medications and the schedules for taking them, by helping with simple self-care such as the routine care of central lines, and by learning the best ways of coping with side effects and medical procedures. In some cases, however, adolescents may not be interested in some of this information or may feel disinclined to take on even basic self-care responsibilities. Because older children and adolescents typically experience the greatest loss of autonomy while ill, they may feel angry and upset at being placed in the "sick role," but at the same time feel helpless to be actively involved in care, which is so often highly regimented. It can be helpful to empathize with adolescents' plight of feeling pushed around, while actively working with them to develop adaptive coping strategies that may make them feel less helpless. It is often important to point out that many aspects of the situation cannot be changed (i.e., you have cancer, you need treatment, the treatment will cause you to miss school), but that some can (i.e., you can try to keep up with friends by phone or Internet or visits; you can keep up with some school work; and you can plan some events such as parties to celebrate an upcoming treatment milestone). Many adolescents feel overwhelmed by information and by talk about their condition, particularly when they may be trying to maintain developing a sense of themselves separate from those of their parents and from their identity as a patient. It may be particularly important for psychosocial providers to help them to think about their own information preferences and to talk with their parents and care teams about them. For example, do they want to be reminded of upcoming appointments and procedures far in advance, or do they prefer to be reminded only a day or so in advance? Similarly, are they interested in hearing more about their conditions and treatments from providers and parents, or do they feel these conversations are intrusive and prefer to hear only the essential information, presented briefly? Parents and providers who wish to include adolescents in their own care may need encouragement to respect the adolescents' wishes and to understand that limiting the conversations and information shared with adolescents may be a way of supporting their choices and their autonomy.

Support for Parents and Families During Treatment

Families may require varying levels of psychosocial support during treatments, and even within a single family, needs vary over time. Ideally, psychosocial support can be offered to patients and families in flexible ways that can be tailored to their individual needs. This requires ongoing assessments of and communications with families about their coping skills and adjustments as well as the ability quickly to adjust the level of services offered to families. Typically, families require more intensive involvement by psychosocial providers during diagnostic periods and the beginning of treatment.[171,172] Some families may continue to have high levels of emotional distress or ongoing problems while adjusting to treatments (see Box 33-1), and they require continual, regular meetings with psychosocial providers, but many families do not. In families that are adjusting adequately to the routines of treatments, the need for psychosocial care often decreases. In these families, psychosocial providers may briefly check in with patients and parents in the context of regular medical care. These brief visits may be useful for assessing adjustment as well as for reinforcing previously offered suggestions and interventions. Psychosocial teams may also offer educational and support groups, which can be particularly helpful for parents adjusting to their children's treatments.

With any decrease in the intensity of direct psychosocial involvement, care should be taken to ensure that patients and families do not feel abandoned by psychosocial providers. In most clinical settings, the nurses and physicians treating patients actively monitor the children's and families' adjustment and consult with the psychosocial providers as needed. This team model should be reiterated to patients and families, and the ways in which psychosocial providers work closely with the medical providers and the families should be explained. Patients and families should be told what to expect in terms of the frequency and duration of contact with the psychosocial providers. Parents in particular should be informed of the expected challenges that may arise during the course of treatments (described in the next section) and should be encouraged to contact the psychosocial providers if they need assistance with these or other issues that arise. Over the course of treatment, if some adjustment problems arise, such as problems at school or difficulties with discipline, the psychosocial providers should offer symptom-focused intervention, such as educational support, behavioral intervention, or other counseling. Typically, these interventions involve a small number of sessions delivered as part of the patients' regular medical visits or as referrals for short-term therapy in the treating institution or in the community. As the presenting issue is resolved, children and families typically return to their previous levels of adjustment, and the interventions can be tapered off and discontinued.

Some families experience brief periods of intense emotional distress related to the stress of cancer treatments. They may occur when facing painful or unpleasant therapies or when treatment complications arise. For the majority of families, episodes of severe distress are naturally time-limited and respond to improving external circumstances as well as to psychosocial interventions provided in cancer treatment settings. Even moderate distress that is persistent or is not responsive to intervention may require more intensive interventions. It may involve an increase in the intensity of routine psychosocial support services and consultations with additional mental health providers to provide crisis intervention, psychiatric assessment, and psychopharmacology for patients or other family members. In outpatient settings, referral to outpatient providers in the community are also important. For example, it is not uncommon for parents to have trouble sleeping or to report symptoms of anxiety and depression that may benefit from referral to primary care physicians or psychiatrists for psychopharmacologic treatment, particularly if the symptoms last beyond the initial diagnostic period or interfere with the parents' functioning.

Some children and families require more intensive levels of psychosocial care consistently throughout treatment. In most cases, these are families with high emotional distress levels, multiple stressors, or limited resources, which can often be recognized during the psychosocial assessments (see previous section). For most of these children and families, regular, ongoing psychosocial services should be provided for much or all of the treatment period. In these cases psychosocial providers should consider several types of interventions. Care delivered as part of regular medical visits, whether brief visits in the treatment area or scheduled counseling sessions in providers' offices, has the advantage of capitalizing on patients' treatment schedules and may be particularly helpful in addressing behaviors directly related to compliance with medical care. Referral to other specialists, either within the treating medical center or in the community, is useful when specialized services are needed (e.g., psychopharmacology) and the children or families need more intensive treatment than can be accommodated within the oncology clinic. Referral to outside services, such as psychopharmacology and individual or family therapy, is particularly useful in cases

of preexisting mental illnesses, family conflicts, or multiple major stressors.

A few families present with psychological distress or behavioral problems that cannot be successfully managed by routine psychosocial care along with provisions for brief intensive interventions.[12] Often these are families that include an individual with a preexisting psychiatric disorder, such as major mental illness, developmental delay, substance abuse, or severe personality disorder. Preexisting psychiatric disorders should be evaluated as part of the psychosocial assessments. Vulnerable individuals at high risk for symptom worsening or relapse should be referred for mental health treatment or counseled about the need to access treatment quickly if symptoms recur. Communication between the psychosocial providers on the oncology team and outside mental health providers can be helpful for sharing a common understanding of the status of a child's cancer treatment and updates about the mental health status of the family member in treatment, but the communication must be made in limited ways that preserve privacy.

Families with consistently active psychosocial needs can present challenges for the care team because of the emotional distress and the demands they may make on staff time. By providing consultation to the nursing and oncology staffs, psychosocial providers can help treatment teams to formulate understanding of families' needs and coordinate appropriate and consistent responses.

EXPECTABLE CHALLENGES DURING TREATMENT

Psychosocial needs vary considerably among families, but certain challenges arise commonly as children go through cancer treatment. Some of these challenges are directly related to coping with the demands of treatment, whereas others have to do with managing the ongoing demands of work, school, and family life while also managing the added stressors of cancer and its treatment. Understanding these expectable challenges can help families to anticipate when and how they may need to mobilize their resources. As part of the assessment, psychosocial providers should try to help families anticipate the particular challenges they may face during the course of cancer therapy and should offer anticipatory guidance if appropriate. Doing so may help families cope successfully with the challenges and may also facilitate their accessing additional psychosocial support should they require it.

Coping with Treatment and Side Effects

About 25 years ago, adolescents with cancer reported that the treatments and their side effects were the worst things about having cancer.[173] The nausea and vomiting resulting from chemotherapy and the pain associated with procedures such as lumbar punctures and bone marrow aspirations were reported to be particularly distressing.[174-177] The treatment of these side effects has significantly improved since then. There are fairly effective antiemetics, and in most patients procedures are carried out under light or deep sedation or under general anesthesia. Despite these advances, children still find chemotherapy, radiation therapy, and various procedures to be very unpleasant and sources of significant apprehension and distress.[178-183] A variety of studies document the usefulness of hypnotherapy, memory evaluation, and other behavioral therapies in reducing side effects in this population.[96,184-191] Reducing procedure-related pain and anxiety and the nausea and vomiting associated with chemotherapy and radiation therapy is critically important to the reduction of risk factors for post-traumatic stress disorder, long-term pain, and psychological distress in survivors and because it is the right thing to do.[1,81,192-203] The topics of pain and symptom management are treated more extensively in Chapter 31.

Transitions and Changes in Care

As families transition from one phase of cancer care to the next, they may experience the change as a loss. In each phase of treatment, children and families adapt, even if unwittingly, to the difficult circumstances of treatment. When these circumstances change, they feel their new routines and habits have been disrupted. Parents may be particularly susceptible and often appreciate the irony of having spent days or weeks feeling "trapped" in the hospital, only to find themselves later terrified to leave it. Children may miss special care they received in certain settings, the reassurance and attention from nursing staff, the relationships with other children, and the relaxed expectations that may apply while they are undergoing intensive treatment. Many kinds of transitions in care can be challenging to families, but discharges from the hospital and the transition from active treatment to going off therapy may be among the most stressful.[204-208] During these transitions it is especially important for providers to be sensitive to the likelihood that families will feel anxious and unsure, even as the treatment is progressing. Providers may naturally tend to emphasize only the positive aspects of transitions, but this is likely to increase feelings of anxiety and isolation. Providers should normalize families' feelings by asking about uncertainty or ambivalence related to moving to a new phase of treatment and should reassure them that such reactions are common. Asking, "How does it feel now that you are going home?" is much more useful to families than a well-intentioned statement such as, "Oh, you must be so happy to be going home." Acknowledging that the transition may require patients and families to adapt to new routines and providers and to manage aspects of the medical care more independently is important, as is reassuring families that there will be continued support for them during the transition period.

For families beginning new phases of treatment, such as outpatient radiation or chemotherapy, tours of new treatment areas, introductions to new providers, and opportunities to meet other children and families can be very helpful. Child life specialists can be particularly useful in acclimating children to new treatment settings and modalities. Families transitioning from active therapy to off-treatment care can experience significant uncertainty and emotional distress, especially when treatment has lasted for a year or longer. Some families find the end of therapy a great relief, but many families are surprised to find themselves experiencing anxiety, uncertainty, and feelings of helplessness reminiscent of the feelings they had during the crisis period of diagnosis.[205] It is helpful to normalize these families' reactions by helping them to understand that during active therapy, their anxieties were kept at bay by the demands of treatment, the frequent contact with providers, and the rituals of medical care. As the demands of treatment decrease, they may find themselves looking back and reflecting on all they have been through since diagnosis. In addition, the cessation of treatment raises concerns about the possibility of relapse, and less frequent visits to the oncologist may make parents in particular worry about how their children's health is to be monitored. Because off-therapy transitions can be a time of increased stress and uncertainty for many families, it is helpful to anticipate their needs by offering additional psychosocial support, either in individual meetings with families or in support groups for parents. In addition to providing increased emotional support, effective reduction of parents' anxieties and uncertainties can be achieved by offering programs that provide medical information tailored to families ending treatment, such as summaries of children's treatments and their schedules for off-treatment and follow-up care.[205]

Home Care

Children's cancer treatments commonly require that some specialized care be provided in the home. Depending on the specifics of the treatments, such care may include giving oral medications or nutrition supplements, caring for a central venous line, and administering injections or intravenous medications. Care in the home is critical to allowing children and families to leave the medical setting and return to normal routines, but it also represents a significant new responsibility for parents and children.[209,210] Over time, providing care in the home can give both parents and patients ways of feeling active and competent in managing the care, but at least initially it can be a source of burden and anxiety. Parents may feel overwhelmed by the technical aspects of home care they must learn, such as flushing a central venous line or giving an injection, as well as by the sense of responsibility they have to monitor their children's health. Children can feel confused about why their homes are being "invaded" by the medical world they had hoped to leave behind in the hospital, and some resistance to treatment may emerge. Receiving care from parents rather than medical providers can be a relief for some children but may raise problems for others. Parents' discomfort and lack of familiarity with the techniques can be unsettling for children and seeing parents become medical providers can be an awkward change of roles in the family. Young children may have difficulty having parents shift from emotionally supportive roles to hands-on people providing their care and may become resistant to certain aspects of their care such as taking oral medications. Older children and adolescents may want to assert their independence and be directly involved in their care but may not be sure how to do so. They may also be ambivalent, sometimes striving for independence, other times feeling dependent and passive.

Practical education by nursing staff is vital for parents and children assuming responsibility for home care.[25,209] The availability of home care nurses to provide some of this care, monitoring, and education is also critical. Nursing and psychosocial professionals can also offer important emotional support by normalizing feelings of uncertainty and responsibility and by helping patients and families to develop a sense of competence. For children of every age it is useful for parents and providers to consider how the children can be involved in their own care in ways that will help them feel some mastery and sense of control. If problems with compliance are anticipated or develop once home, psychosocial providers should work with families to develop behavioral plans to address the problems. Supporting parents in their role, helping them to set clear and consistent expectations, implementing a reward system with tokens, and helping children to find ways of being appropriately active in their own care can all be useful interventions. For older children and adolescents a token reward system such as a sticker chart is less likely to be effective, and some negotiation of roles and responsibilities is likely to be more helpful. Family members may have to be encouraged to be more flexible and try involving different family members or using different schedules to manage the home care. In these cases psychosocial providers may want to involve other members of the treatment team, such as nurses, nutritionists, and pharmacists, in considering how the home care plan can be adapted to the needs of a particular family.

Peer support from other families and patients may also be helpful.

Maintaining Children's and Families' Routines

Basic Needs

In the aftermath of a pediatric cancer diagnosis, family members must find ways of attending to their own basic needs and responsibilities. Although this process can be difficult, family members must eventually shift their focus from the diagnosed child and the isolation of hospital rooms, to life outside of the hospital. For many, this process may include working to understand their insurance coverage and medical costs or negotiating with employers about the use of vacation days and sick leave to care for their children. Grocery shopping, cleaning the house, paying bills, and keeping up with the laundry are additional activities that make up a typical week for the average family, activities that were probably ignored or attended to by others during the early stages of diagnosis and treatment.

For some, the transition from managing a medical crisis to managing the more mundane tasks of everyday life can be challenging. For others, this transition may come as a welcome relief because the resumption of these activities can reintroduce a sense of normalcy. For most, it is a combination of the two. One factor that can necessitate this transition is the financial pressure that typically increases in the weeks and months following initial diagnosis. Even with excellent insurance coverage, the costs associated with treatment can be significant. These costs can feel especially overwhelming for parents and caregivers who have been away from work since the diagnosis and are now feeling internal or external pressure to return. Other costs, such as parking at the medical center and dining in the hospital cafeteria, can add to the financial burden.

After the initial phase of treatment, parents and caregivers typically attempt to piece together plans that allow families to function effectively and attend to basic needs. This plan takes into account children's medical appointments (both scheduled and unscheduled), children's school re-entry and ongoing attendance, parents' work responsibilities, attention to the academic and social needs of children and their siblings, and other family commitments and responsibilities. Families' abilities to develop and implement these plans successfully are dependent upon a number of factors, including characteristics of individual family members (e.g., coping styles, organizational skills, cognitive abilities); the functioning of the family as a whole (e.g., cohesion, adaptability, flexibility); and the responses of community members (e.g., supportive networks of friends, flexibility of employers, commitment of school personnel).

Attending to basic needs and securing resources is crucial to the successful treatment of children and the overall functioning of families. Thus, it is essential that whenever possible, members of the medical team support families in their efforts to meet basic needs. Such support might include the timely completion of medical forms that will facilitate the implementation of educational services, securing appropriate financial resources for eligible families, allowing for flexibility in the scheduling of appointments to accommodate a long commute to the clinic, or simply being willing to listen empathically when parents discuss the challenges they face.

Discipline

The diagnosis and treatment of pediatric cancer can disrupt every facet of family functioning, including expectations parents have about their children's behavior and their ability to set effective limits and exercise appropriate discipline. Understandably, many parents and caregivers are unable or unwilling to discipline their children, given the difficult medical circumstances in which the children find themselves. Children's behavioral outbursts, which may include hitting, kicking, and screaming, are seen as natural consequences of the very difficult and unnatural situations the children are in. Disruptions of daily routines, undergoing invasive medical procedures, experiencing medications' side effects, and just "feeling lousy," can provide more than sufficient rationale to let children's behavior remain unchecked. In addition, parents and caregivers may be wrestling with their own feelings of guilt, sadness, anxiety, and exhaustion, which can make it difficult to impose behavioral expectations, even for parents who had previously demonstrated consistent and appropriate behavior management techniques with their children.

For children whose parents or caretakers are unable to provide effective discipline during treatment, the short-term and long-term consequences can be disastrous. For example, children who do not experience appropriate limit setting may feel out of control and unsafe, which leads to further behavioral disruption. Outbursts and noncompliance can interfere with medical care and impact effective working relationships with staff. Inappropriate behavior can spread quickly to siblings, who learn through observation that parental authority has been eroded, increasing the overall chaos within a family system. By the time treatment ends months or years later, it can be extremely difficult, if not impossible, to reestablish expectations of appropriate behavior.

In order to avoid these short- and long-term consequences, parents and caregivers should provide clear and consistent expectations of children's behavior as soon as possible after diagnosis. It is essential to acknowledge to children that the pain and disruption associated with diagnosis and treatment often cause frustration, sadness, anger, and despair, and that they are to be expected. However, it is equally essential to convey to children that expressing emotions through appropriate means is imperative.

Members of medical teams should work with parents to re-establish appropriate discipline practices. During the initial phases of treatments, the team's assessment of the families should include questions about the parents' approach to discipline and strategies that are effective and ineffective in managing their child's behavior. Understanding parenting styles[211] and children's prior experiences with discipline can be extremely helpful in predicting possible reactions in both children and parents. For example, authoritative parents who use clear, firm limit setting coupled with appropriate encouragement of independence are likely to have children who are successful in negotiating the difficulties associated with diagnosis and treatment. Authoritarian parents who are punitive, restrictive, and demand compliance without giving their children a voice are likely to increase the anxiety and fear the children are already experiencing. And indulgent or permissive parents who fail to use appropriate behavioral controls foster noncompliance and increased disrespect of others, a combination that can greatly affect the management of children's illnesses.

A number of behavioral techniques can be used to increase children's compliance and to minimize disruptive behavior. First, taking parents aside, acknowledging the challenges of disciplining sick children, and offering suggestions is more effective than openly criticizing parents' poor behavior management in front of the children. When children's behavior interferes with medical care, staff should encourage and support authoritative parenting. This might include staff modeling of behavior management techniques, such as giving children clear instructions ("You have to sit on the table, and you can hold

Dad's hand"); praise ("I really appreciate how you answered my questions, you've done a great job"); and attention ("Because you were so cooperative and we finished your dressing change so quickly, I have a few minutes to look at your baseball cards, if you'd like to show them to me"). Praise and attention are examples of positive reinforcement, approaches that increase the likelihood that children will behave the same way in the future.

Behavior-controlling techniques such as using sticker charts can be implemented with the help of mental health practitioners or child life specialists. Developing sticker charts includes identifying behaviors the team wants children to perform (e.g., swallowing pills) and finding a reward that increases children's willingness to engage in the behaviors. Each time children behave appropriately, a sticker is applied to the chart and, after a specified number of stickers have been earned, a predetermined reward is given. Deciding on the reward is not always easy because it has to be significant enough to sustain children's behavior over time (e.g., 10 to 15 stickers may take several days to earn) but not so significant that its cost is prohibitive. The reward must be given frequently enough that the children experience the benefits of their efforts. When available, these techniques should be used in conjunction with psychosocial services provided by mental health practitioners familiar with the treatment of medically compromised children. Education and guidance for parents, as well as counseling or psychotherapy, can be helpful in supporting parents and caregivers in maintaining discipline while providing children with appropriate outlets for their feelings. Many parents benefit from referral to parenting support groups and to books that are guides to effective discipline.[212-214]

School

Shortly after diagnosis, questions arise regarding children's academic needs and how those needs will be met. Will the child be able to attend school or will tutors be provided until the child is able to return to the classroom? How are the treatment courses likely to interfere with children's abilities to succeed academically? Will the child meet the academic requirements necessary to be promoted the next grade or is it likely the child will have to repeat a grade? These are the types of questions that families, schools, and medical teams must address.

School is an important locus for children's cognitive, social, and emotional development, so maintaining ties or reconnecting with school should be a priority in planning children's treatment and care.[215,216] For children, resuming school responsibilities can feel overwhelming, given the demands of treatment. Nausea and fatigue may make it difficult to maintain consistent concentration and achieve academic progress. In addition, if children's days have been filled with video games and countless hours of television watching during the early stages of treatment, the transition back to school can be challenging. For this reason, it is recommended that school assignments resume as soon as possible, so as to minimize the disruption of academic progress and to maximize the children's ability to reengage in school-related tasks. Many children will be unable to attend school for at least some part of their treatment, so home- or hospital-based tutoring, along with structured schedules that provide children with the exact times and durations of school-related work, often promote compliance.

Parents and caregivers must commit themselves to providing the necessary structure and support to promote children's academic progress, even when juggling numerous other responsibilities. Reminding children when tutors will arrive and what will occur at that time can be helpful in transitioning children

to school-related tasks. For example, informing children that the television will be turned off and games will be put aside just prior to the arrival of the tutor may increase compliance and overall success. Assisting children in completing math problems or reading assignments is often best left to the tutors responsible for the children's learning, but parents and caregivers should encourage and praise children for successfully attending to academic work, just as they would normally. For children who have a particularly difficult time returning to school tasks, positive reinforcement techniques can be implemented with the help of tutors or psychosocial providers to increase compliance.

Medical teams are often called upon to provide schools with relevant information about children's abilities to attend to academic responsibilities and any vulnerabilities children may have as a result of treatment (e.g., risk for infection, susceptibility to illness, potential cognitive or physical deficits). School personnel may be especially anxious when children initially return to school, and may make multiple calls to treating physicians. Parents play critical roles in educating the school about children's situations and advocating for their needs. Parents may find schools are initially uncertain how best to accommodate their children, and some may even feel the schools are being unresponsive. In these cases parents may want to meet with several members of the school staff, including classroom teachers, school nurses, principals, and special education directors. Parents can find themselves frustrated with the amount of time and the number of meetings involved, and animosity toward the school can develop. Most parents find that persistence and tact, rather than direct confrontation, are the most beneficial approaches to take whenever possible. Many parents benefit from some consultation with psychosocial providers about how best to negotiate the return to school and often find written guides for parents[154,155] to be helpful. Input from medical teams is also essential, and this may involve a telephone call to the teachers or school nurses, written instructions for care at school, and the presence of a member of the treatment team at a school meeting. Some clinics have established school reentry programs in which staff members (e.g., from the child life, nursing, and mental health departments) visit schools to present information to teachers and classmates about children's diagnoses and treatments.[217-219] This proactive approach can be effective in providing medical information to school nurses and other staff, and can help to answer questions that teachers and classmates may have about returning children's conditions and needs. In most cases, these efforts result in plans for school reentry that is appropriate and comfortable for children.

For children who need specialized instruction because of their illnesses or the consequences of their treatments, individual education plans (IEPs) are required. Federal laws as well as the laws in several states require that children with disabilities be accommodated in their schools,[220-222] and parents who suspect that their children will need some accommodation should speak with schools' special education directors and refer to their states' departments of education Websites for information about the special education procedures in their locations. In most cases, parents begin the process by making written requests for evaluations. The evaluations are carried out by the schools, often with significant input from the medical and psychosocial providers involved in the children's cancer treatment. If the evaluation finds that children are eligible for special education services, IEPs are developed and implemented by the schools. If children do not qualify for specialized education services, they may still qualify for accommodations under the Federal Rehabilitation Act, often referred to as a 504 plan.[223] Such a plan ensures appropriate accommodation of problems with physical mobility, fatigue, attendance, and other needs of children that affect school performance but do not require specialized instruction. Parents should be encouraged to consider the advantages of these formal 504 plans over informal accommodation by schools because they often have the advantage of offering monitoring for compliance, and may offer additional protections for children's rights to accommodation in the classroom. The IEP process can be time-consuming and frustrating for parents who have already had to negotiate complex health and insurance systems for their children. In most cases persistence produces educational plans that are acceptable to all parties. When acceptable plans cannot be arranged with schools, parents may have to pursue formal appeal or grievance procedures against schools. Parents in this situation have to educate themselves about their states' education laws and the federal laws that govern accommodation of children with medical conditions and disabilities,[221,222,224] and may want to consider the services of educational advocates[225,226] to assist them in negotiating with their schools.

Siblings

The siblings of children diagnosed with cancer have difficult roads to travel from the moment a brother or sister is diagnosed with cancer. The road may start when the sibling arrives home from school to find a visibly distraught relative or neighbor who explains, "Your sister is sick. Your parents are at the hospital and will call later." Thus begins the long process of waiting for a parent to come home from the hospital, for the ill brother or sister to get well, for the attention and affection that had once been the norm, and for life to return to normal. Although parents may work diligently to attend to the needs of all of their children, they are often overwhelmed and overburdened, leaving the siblings of diagnosed children feeling ignored and excluded.[227] The types of challenges and how siblings respond are greatly dependent on developmental level. For example, preschoolers may experience significant anxiety related to prolonged separation from caregivers who remain at the hospital with patients, whereas adolescents may be more concerned about details of their sibling's treatments and prognoses.

Siblings of children with cancer have been the subjects of numerous studies designed to investigate adjustment and adaptation following the diagnosis of brothers or sisters.[228-232] Findings suggest that most siblings experience some level of stress associated with the treatment of ill children, especially during the first few months,[172,233] and that this stress may lead to deterioration in normal functioning. Siblings may demonstrate a range of externalizing and internalizing problems, including withdrawal from friends and activities, disturbances in eating and sleeping, temper tantrums, depressed mood, and anxiety.[230,231,234-238] A few studies have documented positive effects, particularly in older siblings who may exhibit high levels of empathy and maturity.[239-241]

Despite years of research highlighting the challenges encountered by siblings of children with cancer, there remain relatively few targeted interventions for this group. Ideally, interventions should address sibling adjustment throughout the treatment process rather than at specific phases (e.g., diagnosis, bone marrow transplantation).[242] General guidelines for improving sibling adjustment include involving siblings in developmentally appropriate discussions as early as possible, educating siblings about the illness and treatment course, encouraging siblings to visit the hospital, and providing opportunities for supportive interactions (e.g., sibling support groups, individual counseling, summer camp experiences).[227,243] Programs such as SuperSibs, a nonprofit organization for siblings of pediatric cancer patients,[244] provide opportunities for siblings to feel valued and heard through activities and services. Feelings of frustration, anger, jealousy, or guilt need to be acknowledged and normalized, and younger siblings may need to be reassured that the illnesses of their brothers or sisters are in no way attributable to anything they themselves may have said or done. Having siblings maintain normal routines by attending school or daycare, socializing with friends, and engaging in various extracurricular activities provides structure and a sense of normalcy during a very challenging time for families; doing so also increases opportunities for social support when parents and caregivers are busy attending to ill children. For siblings who demonstrate ongoing emotional distress or significant difficulties in returning to regular school, family, and social routines, consultation with psychosocial providers should be recommended. Depending on siblings' needs and the available resources, providers may be able to offer short-term supportive therapy or make referrals to community- or school-based resources.

Peer Relationships

At any developmental level, relationships with peers provide children and adolescents with crucial components of successful adaptation, including a sense of connection, friendship, and support. This is equally true for children diagnosed with cancer and for their healthy peers. Several research studies have focused on the role of peer relationships in the coping and adjustment of children and adolescents with cancer.[245-249] Although parents have been identified as the primary source of nurturance, support, and information for pediatric cancer patients,[247] research findings suggest that relationships with healthy peers, and with peers diagnosed with cancer, are also extremely important. For example, adolescents diagnosed with cancer who report close friendships have been noted to experience increased social support,[246,250] increased feelings of hope,[251] and greater ease in communicating about their cancer experiences.[247] Additional research suggests that adolescent cancer patients view peer relationships as being vital to the continued development of their independence and identity, areas that can easily be derailed by illness.[248,252]

Studies examining other aspects of peer interactions reveal somewhat mixed results. Some findings have suggested that both children and adolescents diagnosed with cancer have fewer friends than their peers,[247,253] and that this trend may continue after treatment has been completed.[254-255] Other findings have indicated that children diagnosed with cancer may be socially isolated and withdrawn,[256] despite the fact that their popularity and number of friendships is comparable to those of peers.[257] Whether these results reflect a change in the nature or quality of peer interactions because of illness-related factors (e.g., prolonged hospitalizations, significant school absences, inability to engage in recreational activities) is difficult to determine.

Given the importance of peer relationships in the course of normal development, and the potential for disruption of these relationships during diagnosis and treatment, members of medical teams must support connections with peers whenever possible.[258] Support may include encouraging parents to facilitate peer interactions at home and at the hospital, and to work with educators to establish opportunities for children to visit school for lunch, or to attend a single class, so that peer connections can continue even when children are not well enough to attend school regularly. When appropriate, medical staff can also support adolescent patients who may wish to share clinic experiences with friends by inviting them to attend an outpatient appointment. These opportunities, although often limited by the impact of treatment, help pediatric cancer patients and their peers maintain crucial relationships that will improve post-treatment adjustment.

SPECIAL ISSUES THAT MAY ARISE DURING TREATMENT

Marital Adjustment

A diagnosis of pediatric cancer has immediate and significant consequences for those connected to the ill child, most notably the parents. Although the level of care children require through the treatment process depends on several factors, including the severity of illness and the children's developmental levels, most children undergoing cancer treatment require significant support from at least one parent or caregiver. Many families find that managing children's hospitalizations, clinic visits, daily medications, side effects, and other illness-related factors to be a full-time job, often leaving the responsible adult feeling overwhelmed. With one parent dedicated to caring for the ill child, the other parent is often left to support the family financially, attend to the other children, and ensure that the household continues to function effectively. Not surprisingly, these circumstances can present significant challenges to all aspects of family functioning and can test marital relationships. Understanding how these circumstances affect children and their families is complex and necessitates the consideration of several factors, such as parental coping, family cohesion and organization, emotional expression, and marital satisfaction.[259]

Given the challenges that parents must face after a child has been diagnosed, one might predict that marital relationships would suffer as a result. Research has suggested that although parents of children with cancer were no more likely to divorce than other parents, and that marriages remain stable,[260-262] marital dissatisfaction and distress do increase.[263-265] Specifically, Hoekstra-Weebers and colleagues[263] noted that marital dissatisfaction was associated with higher levels of psychological distress 6 and 12 months after diagnosis but not at the time of diagnosis. Schuler and colleagues[264] found that parents, especially mothers, experienced distress around adjusting to new demands. Similarly, Dahlquist and colleagues[69,265] reported that marital distress was predicted by general emotional distress and a discrepancy between the couple's perceived anxiety levels. Although pediatric cancer may strain marital relationships and accentuate differences in parental coping styles, these results suggest that couples are committed to remaining in their marriages, perhaps to minimize any additional disruption to their families and to the diagnosed children. Given that marital distress appears to increase over the course of children's treatments and may not be evident at diagnosis when clinical assessments are initiated, it may be helpful for medical staff to monitor parental functioning over time and to seek consultation from mental health colleagues when marital tension is evident and could potentially impact the emotional adjustment of children and families.

Noncompliance by Patients

The ability of children and adolescents to comply with intensive cancer treatments is often in question.[266] In one study, at least some noncompliance with treatment was found in nearly 60% of adolescents, and in 33% of children younger than 13 years of age who required oral medications for their cancer treatments.[267] The higher rate of noncompliance in adolescents may result from adolescents' limited or developing sense of autonomy, as well as from miscommunication between parents and children about who is responsible for ensuring compliance with treatment.[266] Parents monitor medication intake for younger children, but adolescents often resent parental monitoring, adopting the stance that they can care for themselves. Parents must ensure successful treatment coupled with adolescents' needs to exert some level of independent functioning; the combination can increase conflict and noncompliance. The impact of this noncompliance can be significant and can include inaccurate conclusions regarding medication efficacy, skewed research findings for experimental protocols, and an even decreased chance for survival.

A number of individual, family, and treatment characteristics have been linked to noncompliance with treatment. To summarize, Die-Trill and Stuber[267] found that noncompliance was positively correlated with such children's characteristics as behavioral problems, poor self-image, poor insight regarding prognosis, and poor coping mechanisms. Family characteristics that predict noncompliance included increased parental depression and a large number of siblings. Treatment intensity and the number of medications needed for effective treatment also increase noncompliance. Die-Trill and Stuber identified additional factors that promote treatment adherence, including increased anxiety in female patients and increased obsessive-compulsive behaviors in parents of male patients. Manne, Bakeman, and Jacobsen[268] found that younger children evidenced greater difficulty complying with more invasive medical procedures (e.g., lumbar punctures), as did children from families from lower socioeconomic backgrounds. Supportive parenting styles that promoted the sense that the children were being heard and understood led to greater compliance.

Given that compliance is essential for the successful treatment of pediatric cancer, a number of behavioral interventions have been developed to increase children's abilities to comply with medication intake and invasive treatment procedures. Overall, positive reinforcement, response cost, and verbal reprimands have been found to be effective in promoting compliance.[269] Parents of children with cancer were less tolerant of punishment techniques such as time-outs than nurses or parents of medically well children. Parents of children with cancer appear to feel that their children are suffering enough and should not be subjected to further punishing experiences. These parents often struggle to set effective limits in order to avoid conflict with their children, even if the child's behavior is jeopardizing the overall prognosis. Additional interventions to increase compliance have focused on educating parents about the prescribed medical treatment and helping parents to develop supportive relationships with their children that will allow for the use of appropriate behavioral techniques. Prior to the implementation of any behavioral approach, assessment of the parents' willingness to accept and use the approach is essential. Approaches to helping parents provide discipline for their children during cancer therapy are described earlier.

Depression and Anxiety

Given the many challenges that children and adolescents face during the course of cancer treatments, many investigators have hypothesized that pediatric cancer patients are at risk for higher levels of depression and anxiety. Research findings to date are mixed, with some studies suggesting emotional and behavioral maladjustments that include depression and anxiety in pediatric cancer patients,[270-272] and others showing less behavior or emotional disruption in these children.[273,274]

Difficulties associated with accurately diagnosing depression and anxiety in children and adolescents, especially those with serious or chronic illnesses, have contributed to the variability in findings. Psychological assessment is further complicated by the need to determine whether the pediatric patients' physical symptoms are secondary to their cancers or whether they are evidence of psychological disturbance.[275-277] Hedstrom and colleagues[278] found that medical and nursing staff underestimated the level of depression and anxiety in adolescent oncology patients, calling into question how often depression and anxiety may go untreated.

Given the emotional distress associated with the diagnosis and treatment of pediatric cancer, some level of heightened anxiety and depression is to be expected, although these symptoms may not be of sufficient intensity to reach clinical significance, and the constellation of children's symptoms may not be consistent with psychiatric diagnoses. Nonetheless, it is essential for the medical team to monitor closely the psychological adjustment of children and to consider a broad range of behavioral symptoms that may indicate emotional difficulty. The inability to attend school, participate in extracurricular activities, and socialize with friends, coupled with invasive procedures, nausea, and hair loss, would leave even the most well-adjusted children and adolescents struggling to maintain appropriate functioning. Periodic sleep disturbances, anhedonia, irritability, and social isolation are not uncommon in children struggling with the realities associated with pediatric cancers. Given the likelihood that most patients experience at least some transient symptoms of anxiety and depression, the tasks of providers and parents are to identify symptoms that are so intense or enduring that they warrant further assessment by a mental health provider.

The identification of clinically significant levels of anxiety and depression commonly occurs when patients' compliance with medical care is compromised or children are unable to engage in essential activities such as attending school. For these children, formal psychological assessments are often sought and treatment is provided. However, in children who are compliant and whose symptoms are more subtle, the ability to diagnose depression and anxiety accurately is more difficult, but no less important. Medical teams, with the assistance of parents or caregivers, should consistently assess children's moods and behaviors for signs of emotional difficulties, comparing current functioning with functioning prior to diagnosis. Teams may find themselves asking why children are no longer playing their favorite video games, are being disrespectful to nursing staff, are refusing physical therapy, or are ignoring visitors. These types of symptoms may indicate more serious psychological problems that require assessment by a mental health professional and referral for intervention such as psychotherapy or medication if needed. The psychosocial assessments performed at the start of treatment (described earlier) should identify any prior symptoms of anxiety and depression, and provide baseline assessments of children's functioning against which later functioning can be compared to determine whether there have been significant deviations from children's baseline behaviors.

Although rates of diagnosable depression and anxiety may not be significantly elevated in pediatric cancer patients, many children do struggle with some symptoms of depression and anxiety, and it is the responsibility of the medical teams to assess accurately children's functioning to ensure that appropriate interventions are in place. The physical effects of treatment may mimic depression or anxiety (e.g., fatigue, pain, nausea) and hence interfere with accurate diagnosis. Social support and effective parenting throughout treatment appear to provide protection from the adversity encountered by children with cancer. Noll and colleagues[274] report that intensive support and positive social interactions with parents and medical staff are key to children's adjustment and conclude that children may be protected from the adverse effects of treatments when parents' functioning remains high and damage to the children's central nervous systems is low.

Adolescent Patients

Traditionally, adolescence is seen as a time of transition and growth in independence. The diagnosis of cancer during this developmental stage has the potential to disrupt normal functioning and limit the attainment of specific goals that move adolescents from childhood into adulthood. Research has considered several important areas related to the psychosocial adjustment of adolescent cancer patients, including family factors, psychological factors, and socialization factors.[31,203]

Mental health professionals have noted that children and adolescents commonly function as well or as poorly as their parents do during stressful life events. The psychological adjustment of adolescent cancer patients was noted to be better when maternal distress was low[279] and maternal adjustment was high.[280] In addition, adolescents benefited from the ability of family members to introduce a sense of normalcy and felt more supported during treatment when family members demonstrated flexibility.[250] Some adolescents noted that stressful family relationships impeded successful adjustment to illness.[281] These data taken together suggest that adolescents' families are crucial to adolescents' successful management of, and coping with illness. Medical teams should encourage open communication among family members that will promote positive interactions and allow for ongoing assessment of individual functioning. Psychosocial support should extend beyond adolescent patients to all family members to ensure the healthy functioning of the entire family system. When problems in adolescents' behavior or coping are identified, providers should be mindful that some family-focused assessments and interventions may be indicated.

Psychologically, adolescents typically possess cognitive abilities that allow for more sophisticated understanding of their illnesses and treatments than would be found in younger children. Adolescents often seek information[78,146] and feel empowered by their understanding, which may in turn facilitate their active participation in treatment decisions, thereby increasing their use of effective coping strategies and their overall sense of control.[30] However, the ability to understand illness-related information does not guarantee increased psychological adjustment. In fact, some adolescents may feel overwhelmed by extensive medical information and corresponding treatment decisions, which increases the levels of stress and potential psychological maladjustment. To ensure that adolescents are appropriately informed, careful assessments must be conducted to evaluate how information is processed and understood by the adolescents, and the amounts and types of information that will be most helpful. Adolescents may feel that opportunities to achieve increased independence (e.g., attaining a driver's license) are limited by their illnesses, so including them in discussions about treatments, facilitating effective coping strategies, and encouraging participation in decision-making processes may promote an increased sense of autonomy.

Adolescents' abilities to engage with peers, participate in extracurricular activities, or attend school while undergoing treatment are often very limited. Immediately after diagnosis, extensive support may be available to adolescents and their families. However, as treatments progress and the initial shock associated with diagnosis decreases, support by friends, teachers, and others in the community may be less consistent. Over time, friends may return their focus to school and other activities, leaving diagnosed adolescents feeling isolated and left out.[146,203,255,282] Evan and Zeltzer[30] suggest that developmental levels play significant roles in the type of support that adolescents both provide and seek. Research findings suggest that adolescent cancer patients seek social support from same-aged peers encountering similar developmental issues,[283] and from parents and other adults who have a wider range of life experiences that may be relevant to overcoming their illnesses.[282]

Studies have considered several factors related to the development of successful adolescent social relationships, including the importance of self-esteem and sexual identity.[31,284-289] For example, findings suggest that adolescents who are absent from school may begin to experience academic difficulties that negatively impact their self-confidence and self-esteem. This decrease in self-confidence and self-esteem undermines adolescents' attempts to form and sustain social relationships. Other findings highlight sexual identity and the significant role sexual identity plays in adolescent relationships and in developing self-esteem.[31] Adolescents diagnosed with cancer may have negative body images resulting from treatment-related side effects (e.g., hair loss, procedural and surgical scars, weight gain or loss),[290,291] and they have limited opportunities for both formal and informal sex education, impeding healthy sexual development and positive self-esteem.[292] Evan and colleagues[31] suggest assessing adolescents' cognitive, social, developmental, and family functioning to determine the most appropriate paths to sexual health and self-esteem and recommend creating opportunities to assume personal control and interact with other adolescents who may be encountering similar experiences.

Social support and social relationships are essential to successful adjustment during the treatment course and beyond. Although parents and other family members typically provide the primary day-to-day support needed by adolescent patients to complete treatment successfully, peer relationships are equally valuable because they allow adolescents to remain connected to other key aspects of their lives that exist outside of their treatments. Members of the medical staff can also provide important interpersonal connections that can greatly improve adolescents' social functioning. Medical teams should encourage peer interactions by supporting adolescents' return to school and participation in peer-related activities when feasible and by permitting adolescent patients to take a friend to an occasional clinic appointment when possible.

Relapse and Recurrence

Patients and families who experience relapse or recurrence of cancer can be expected to enter a second crisis period. As in the initial crisis of diagnosis, families experience cognitive and emotional overload, and are overwhelmed by fear and anxiety at the same time they are trying to understand the medical implications of the return of the cancer. Families typically feel shocked by news of relapse. For many families, faith in the medical care, trust in the world, and hope for future treatment are severely challenged.

The initial approach to this new crisis should draw on the same elements of psychosocial support described in the section about the crisis of diagnosis, including provision of psychosocial support and participation in a new treatment conference, or Day One Talk. In the context of relapse, emotional distress and disbelief are to be expected, and parents as well as older patients may be distraught. Presenting information about prognosis after relapse can be even more difficult because the prognoses are typically less favorable, and patients and families who may have previously been reassured may now have to be told that cure is less likely, or even that it is not to be expected. Accurate medical information must be presented to families in ways they can understand, but it is perhaps just as important that they feel that the physicians and other providers are committed to continuing to care for them. For some patients and families, recurrence may be experienced as personal failure, and the team should be careful to readdress this issue of blame and

causality in the context of relapse or recurrence. In cases in which new treatment plans mean transferring care to a new clinical service (e.g., in the case of a bone marrow transplant) or referral to a new care team or hospital, great care should be taken to ensure that patients and families do not feel abandoned.

The psychosocial challenges facing patients and families after relapse are determined to a large extent by the subsequent treatments that are planned and the extent to which cure remains the goal of treatment. When potentially curative treatments are planned, patients face the challenge of re-engaging with new and often more intensive therapy regimens. Patients and families already burdened by initial treatments may have more trouble adjusting to new demands along with increased anxiety and the psychological experience of starting over with new treatments. Psychosocial providers should be prepared to reassess patients and families in these new contexts and offer emotional support and crisis intervention. Psychosocial providers should also anticipate new issues that could emerge, such as financial stress, parents' depression, patients' behavioral problems, or emotional distress, and should be prepared to help families address them.

For some patients, the likelihood of cure after relapse or recurrence is remote. For these patients, treatment options may include palliative care or experimental therapies. Learning that cures are unlikely and that patients may be expected to die of their diseases is devastating for families. Parents and patients are likely to be terrified and overwhelmed, and care providers may feel unsure how to help these families. Communication between the physicians and other members of the team is especially important at this juncture,[127] and care should be taken to communicate directly with patients as well as parents, and to provide honest information in a sensitive manner. Psychosocial providers should participate in team meetings with the families, assess the needs of the patients, parents, and other family members, and offer crisis intervention and emotional support. They should anticipate that symptoms of depression, hopelessness, and anxiety may become significant in one or more family members, and should be prepared to offer clinical care and referrals to other specialists or community agencies. A more comprehensive discussion of care for dying children is included in Chapter 30.

REFERENCES

1. Kazak AE, Alderfer M, Rourke MT, et al. Posttraumatic stress disorder (PTSD) and posttraumatic stress symptoms (PTSS) in families of adolescent childhood cancer survivors. J Pediatr Psychol. 2004;29:211-219.
2. Kupst MJ, Natta MB, Richardson CC, et al. Family coping with pediatric leukemia: ten years after treatment. J Pediatr Psychol. 1995;20:601-617.
3. Fife B, Norton J, Groom G. The family's adaptation to childhood leukemia. Soc Sci Med. 1987;24:159-168.
4. Patenaude AF, Kupst MJ. Psychosocial functioning in pediatric cancer. J Pediatr Psychol. 2005;30:9-27.
5. Patiño-Fernández AM, Pai AL, Alderfer M, et al. Acute stress in parents of children newly diagnosed with cancer. Pediatr Blood Cancer. 2008;50:289-292.
6. Han HR. Korean mothers' psychosocial adjustment to their children's cancer. J Adv Nurs. 2003;44:499-506.
7. Hersh SP, Wiener LS. Psychosocial support for the family of the child with cancer. In Pizzo PA, Poplack DG (eds). Principles and Practice of Pediatric Oncology. Philadelphia, JB Lippincott, 1989, pp 897-913.
8. Hersh SP, Wiener LS, Figueroa V, Kunz JF. Psychiatric and psychosocial support for the child and family. In Pizzo PA,

Poplack DG (eds). Principles and Practice of Pediatric Oncology, 3rd ed. Philadelphia, Lippincott-Raven, 1997, pp 1241-1266.

9. Michael BE, Copeland DR. Psychosocial issues in childhood cancer: an ecological framework for research. Am J Pediatr Hematol Oncol. 1987;9:73-83.

10. Brown RT. Comprehensive Handbook of Childhood Cancer and Sickle Cell Disease: A Biopsychosocial Approach. New York, Oxford University Press, 2006.

11. Holland JC (ed). Psycho-Oncology. New York, Oxford University Press, 1998.

12. Kazak AE. Pediatric psychosocial preventative health model (PPPHM): research, practice, and collaboration in pediatric family systems medicine. Fam Syst Health. 2006;24:381-395.

13. Ceci SJ. Urie Bronfenbrenner (1917-2005). Am Psychol. 2006;61:173-174.

14. Bronfenbrenner U, Ceci SJ. Nature-nurture reconceptualized in developmental perspective: a bioecological model. Psychol Rev. 1994;101:568-586.

15. Grzywacz JG, Fuqua J. The social ecology of health: leverage points and linkages. Behav Med. 2000;26:101-115.

16. Rutter M, Dunn J, Plomin R, et al. Integrating nature and nurture: implications of person-environment correlations and interactions for developmental psychopathology. Dev Psychopathol. 1997;9:335-364.

17. Reiss D, Neiderhiser JM. The interplay of genetic influences and social processes in developmental theory: specific mechanisms are coming into view. Dev Psychopathol. 2000;12:357-374.

18. Schor EL. Family pediatrics: report of the task force on the family. Pediatrics. 2003;111:1541-1571.

19. Robinson KE, Gerhardt CA, Vannatta K, Noll RB. Parent and family factors associated with child adjustment to pediatric cancer. J Pediatr Psychol. 2007;32:400-410.

20. Conger KJ, Rueter MA, Conger RD. The role of economic pressure in the lives of parents and their adolescents: the family stress model. In Crockett LJ, Silbereisen RJ (eds). Negotiating Adolescence in Times of Social Change. Cambridge, England, Cambridge University Press, 2000, pp 201-233.

21. Atzaba-Poria N, Pike A, Deater-Deckard K. Do risk factors for problem behavior act in a cumulative manner? An examination of ethnic minority and majority children through an ecological perspective. J Child Psychol Psychiatry. 2004;45:707-718.

22. Kazak AE. Families of chronically ill children: a systems and social-ecological model of adaptation and challenge. Consult Clin Psychol. 1989;57:25-30.

23. Kazak AE, Kassam-Adams N, Schneider S, et al. An integrative model of pediatric medical traumatic stress. J Pediatr Psychol. 2006;31:343-355.

24. Pai AL, Kazak AE. Pediatric medical traumatic stress in pediatric oncology: family systems interventions. Curr Opin Pediatr. 2006;18:558-562.

25. Corlett J, Twycross A. Negotiation of parental roles within family-centered care: a review of research. J Clin Nurs. 2006;15:1308-1316.

26. Pyke-Grimm KA, Stewart JL, Kelly KP, Degner LF. Parents of children with cancer: factors influencing their treatment decision-making roles. J Pediatr Nurs. 2006;21:350-361.

27. Stewart JL, Pyke-Grimm KA, Kelly KP. Parental treatment decision-making in pediatric oncology. Semin Oncol Nurs. 2005;21:89-97.

28. Gagnon EM, Recklitis CJ. Parents' decision-making preferences in pediatric oncology: the relationship to health care involvement and complementary therapy use. Psychooncology. 2003;12:442-452.

29. Rushforth H. Practitioner review: communicating with hospitalized children: review and application of research pertaining to children's understanding of health and illness. J Child Psychol Psychiatry. 1999;40:683-691.

30. Evan EE, Zeltzer LK. Psychosocial dimensions of cancer in adolescents and young adults. Cancer. 2006;107:1663-1671.

31. Evan EE, Kaufman M, Cook AB, Zeltzer LK. Sexual health and self-esteem in adolescents and young adults with cancer. Cancer. 2006;107:1672-1679.

32. Earle CC. Failing to plan is planning to fail: improving the quality of care with survivorship care plans. J Clin Oncol. 2006;24:5112-5116.

33. Fleissig A, Jenkins V, Catt S, Fallowfield L. Multidisciplinary teams in cancer care: are they effective in the UK? Lancet Oncol. 2006;7:935-943.

34. Hicks MD, Lavender R. Psychosocial practice trends in pediatric oncology. J Pediatr Oncol Nurs. 2001;18:143-153.

35. Penson RT, Kyriakou H, Zuckerman D, et al. Teams: communication in multidisciplinary care. Oncologist. 2006;11:520-526.

36. Baillet F. The organization of psycho-oncology. Cancer Radiother. 2002;6:214-218.

37. Blackburn KM. Roles of advanced practice nurses in oncology. Oncology. 1998;12:591-598.

38. Christensen J, Akcasu N. The role of the pediatric nurse practitioner in the comprehensive management of pediatric oncology patients in the inpatient setting. J Pediatr Oncol Nurs. 1999;16:66-67.

39. Gwyther LP, Altilio T, Blacker S, et al. Social work competencies in palliative and end-of-life care. J Soc Work End Life Palliat Care. 2005;1:87-120.

40. Jones BL. Pediatric palliative and end-of-life care: the role of social work in pediatric oncology. J Soc Work End Life Palliat Care. 2005;1:35-61.

41. Maloney AM, Volpe J. The inpatient advanced practice nursing roles in Canadian pediatric oncology unit. J Pediatr Oncol Nurs. 2005;22:254-257.

42. Pao M, Ballard ED, Rosenstein DL, et al. Psychotropic medication use in pediatric patients with cancer. Arch Pediatr Adolesc Med. 2006;160:818-822.

43. Wittmeyer H, Clauss-Euler I, Dorr C, Kaufmann U. Psychosocial management in pediatric oncology: presentation of a cooperative team model. Psychother Psychosom Med Psychol. 1989;39:411-417.

44. Kissane DW, Smith GC. Consultation-liaison psychiatry in an Australian oncology unit. Aust N Z J Psychiatry. 1996;30:397-404.

45. Kusch M, Vetter C, Bode U. Inpatient psychological management in pediatric oncology: the concept of liaison management. Prax Kinderpsychol Kinderpsychiatr. 1993;42:316-326.

46. Pendlebury SC, Snars J. Role of a psychiatry liaison clinic in the management of breast cancer. Australas Radiol. 1996;40:283-286.

47. Weis J, Heckel U, Muthny F, et al. Experiences with psychosocial liaison service on oncologic units of an acute clinic. Psychother Psychosom Med Psychol. 1993;43:21-29.

48. Masera G, Spinetta JJ, Jankovic M, et al. Guidelines for a therapeutic alliance between families and staff: a report of SIOP Working Committee on psychosocial issues in pediatric oncology. Med Pediatr Oncol. 1998;30:183-186.

49. Amico J, Davidhizar R. Supporting families of critically ill children. J Clin Nurs. 1994;3:213-218.

50. Kazak AE. Evidence-based interventions for survivors of childhood cancer and their families. J Pediatr Psychol. 2005;30:29-39.

51. Kazak AE, Simms S, Alderfer MA, et al. Feasibility and preliminary outcomes from a pilot study of a brief psychological intervention for families of children newly diagnosed with cancer. J Pediatr Psychol. 2005;30:644-645.

52. Phillips M. Support groups for parents of chronically ill children. Pediatr Nurs. 1990;16:404-406.

53. Mitchell W, Clarke S, Sloper P. Care and support needs of children and young people with cancer and their parents. Psychooncology. 2006;15:805-816.

54. Kash KM, Mago R, Kunkel EJ. Psychosocial oncology: supportive care for the cancer patient. Semin Oncol. 2005;32:211-218.

55. Shelby RA, Taylor KL, Kerner JF, et al. The role of community-based and philanthropic organizations in meeting cancer patient and caregiver needs. CA Cancer J Clin. 2002;52:229-246.

56. Weis J. Support groups for cancer patients. Support Care Cancer. 2003;11:736-768.

57. Pollin I, Kanaan SB. Medical Crisis Counseling: Short-Term Therapy for Long-Term Illness. New York, WW Norton, 1995.

58. Bloom JR, Kessler L. Emotional support following cancer: a test of the stigma and social activity hypotheses. J Health Soc Behav. 1994;35:118-133.

59. Ehrmann-Feldmann D, Spitzer WO, Del Greco L, Desmeules L. Perceived discrimination against cured cancer patients in the work force. CMAJ. 1987;136:719-723.

60. MacDonald LD, Anderson HR. Stigma in patients with rectal cancer: a community study. J Epidemiol Community Health. 1984;38:284-290.

61. Muzzin LJ, Anderson NJ, Figueredo AT, Gudelisso SO. The experience of cancer. Soc Sci Med. 1994;38:1201-1208.

62. Peters-Golden H. Breast cancer: varied perceptions of social support in the illness experience. Soc Sci Med. 1982;16:483-491.

63. Rosman S. Cancer and stigma: experience of patients with chemotherapy-induced alopecia. Patient Educ Couns. 2004;52:333-339.

64. Sloper P. Needs and responses of parents following the diagnosis of childhood cancer. Child Care Health Dev. 1996;22:187-202.

65. Lansky SB, List MA, Ritter-Sterr C. Psychiatric and psychological support of the child and adolescent with cancer. In Pizzo PA, Poplack DG (eds). Principles and Practice of Pediatric Oncology. Philadelphia, JB Lippincott, 1989, pp 885-896.

66. Ruccione KS, Waskerwitz M, Buckley J, et al. What caused my child's cancer? Parents' responses to an epidemiology study of childhood cancer. J Pediatr Oncol Nurs. 1994;11:71-84.

67. Morrow GR, Hoagland AC, Morse IP. Sources of support perceived by parents of children with cancer: implications for counseling. Patient Couns Health Educ. 1982;4:36-40.

68. Ross JW. Social work intervention with families of children with cancer: the changing critical phases. Soc Work Health Care. 1978;3:257-272.

69. Dahlquist LM, Czyzewski DI, Jones CL. Parents of children with cancer: a longitudinal study of emotional distress, coping style, and marital adjustment two and twenty months after diagnosis. J Pediatr Psychol. 1996;21:541-554.

70. Grootenhuis MA, Last BF. Adjustment and coping by parents of children with cancer: a review of the literature. Support Care Cancer. 1997;5:466-484.

71. Taanila A, Jarvelin MR, Kokkonen J. Parental guidance and counseling by doctors and nursing staff: parents' views of initial information and advice for families with disabled children. J Clin Nurs. 1998;7:505-511.

72. Taanila A, Syrjala L, Kokkonen J, Jarvelin MR. Coping of parents with physically and/or intellectually disabled children. Child Care Health Dev. 2002;28:73-86.

73. Caine RM. Families in crisis: making the critical difference. Focus Crit Care. 1989;16:184-189.

74. Hendricks-Ferguson VL. Crisis intervention strategies when caring for families of children with cancer. J Pediatr Oncol Nurs. 2000;17:3-11.

75. Ross JW. Coping with childhood cancer: group intervention as an aid to parents in crisis. Soc Work Health Care. 1979;4:381-391.

76. Lamott A. Bird by Bird: Some Instructions on Writing and Life. New York, Anchor Books, 1995.

77. Kerr LM, Harrison MB, Medves J, Tranmer J. Supportive care needs of parents of children with cancer: transition from diagnosis to treatment. Oncol Nurs Forum. 2004;31:116-126.

78. Ljungman G, McGrath PJ, Cooper E, et al. Psychosocial needs of families with a child with cancer. J Pediatr Hematol Oncol. 2003;25:223-231.

79. McGrath P. Identifying support issues of parents of children with leukemia. Cancer Pract. 2001;9:198-205.

80. Kazak AE, Cant MC, Jensen MM, et al. Identifying psychosocial risk indicative of subsequent resource use in families of newly diagnosed pediatric oncology patients. J Clin Oncol. 2003;21:3220-3225.

81. Kazak AE, Boeving CA, Alderfer MA, et al. Posttraumatic stress symptoms during treatment in parents of children with cancer. J Clin Oncol. 2005;23:7405-7410.

82. Santacroce S. Uncertainty, anxiety, and symptoms of posttraumatic stress in parents of children recently diagnosed with cancer. J Pediatr Oncol Nurs. 2002;19:104-111.

83. Barrera M, D'Agostino NM, Gibson J, et al. Predictors and mediators of psychological adjustment in mothers of children newly diagnosed with cancer. Psychooncology. 2004;13:630-641.

84. Boman K, Lindahl A, Bjork O. Disease-related distress in parents of children with cancer at various stages after the time of diagnosis. Acta Oncol. 2003;42:137-146.

85. Feudtner C, Haney J, Dimmers MA. Spiritual care needs of hospitalized children and their families: a national survey of pastoral care providers' perceptions. Pediatrics. 2003;111:67-72.

86. Fina DK. The spiritual needs of pediatric patients and their families. AORN J. 1995;62:556-564.

87. Still JV. Spiritual care. How to assess spiritual needs of children and their families. J Christ Nurs. 1984;1:4-6.

88. Heller KS, Solomon MZ. Continuity of care and caring: what matters to parents of children with life-threatening conditions. J Pediatr Nurs. 2005;20:335-346.

89. Lazare A. Apology in medical practice: an emerging clinical skill. JAMA. 2006;296:1401-1404.

90. Leape LL. Full disclosure and apology: an idea whose time has come. Physician Exec. 2006;32:16-18.

91. Earle EA, Eiser C. Children's behavior following diagnosis of acute lymphoblastic leukemia: a qualitative longitudinal study. Clin Child Psychol Psychiatry. 2007;12:281-293.

92. Woodgate RL, Degner LF. "Nothing is carved in stone!": uncertainty in children with cancer and their families. Eur J Oncol Nurs. 2002;6:191-202.

93. Melnyk BM, Alpert-Gillis L, Feinstein NF, et al. Creating opportunities for parent empowerment: program effects on the mental health/coping outcomes of critically ill young children and their mothers. Pediatrics. 2004;113:597-607.

94. Liossi C, White P, Franck L, Hatira P. Parental pain expectancy as a mediator between child expected and experienced procedure-related pain intensity during painful medical procedures. Clin J Pain. 2007;23:392-399.

95. Chen E, Craske M, Katz ER, et al. Pain-sensitive temperament: does it predict procedural distress and response to psychological treatment among children with cancer? J Pediatr Psychol. 2000;25:269-278.

96. Chen E, Zeltzer LK, Craske MG, Katz ER. Alteration of memory in the reduction of children's distress during repeated aversive medical procedures. J Clin Consult Psychol. 1999;67:481-490.

97. Chen E, Zeltzer LK, Craske MG, Katz ER. Children's memories of painful cancer treatment procedures: implications for distress. Child Dev. 2000;71:933-947.

98. Crisp J, Ungerer JA, Goodnow JJ. The impact of experience on children's understanding of illness. J Pediatr Psychol. 1996;21:57-72.

99. Poltorak DY, Glazer JP. The development of children's understanding of death: cognitive and psychodynamic considerations. Child Adolesc Psychiatr Clin North Am. 2006;15:567-573.

100. Clunies-Ross C, Lansdown R. Concepts of death, illness and isolation found in children with leukemia. Child Care Health Dev. 1988;14:373-386.

101. Kreicbergs U, Valdimarsdottir U, Onelov E, et al. Talking about death with children who have severe malignant disease. N Engl J Med. 2004;351:1175-1186.

102. Stuber ML, Houskamp BM. Spirituality in children confronting death. Child Adolesc Psychiatr Clin North Am. 2004;13: 127-136.

103. Forinder U, Lof C, Winiarski J. Quality of life following allogeneic stem cell transplantation, comparing parents' and children's perspective. Pediatr Transplant. 2006;10:491-496.

104. Gedaly-Duff V, Lee KA, Nail L, et al. Pain, sleep disturbance, and fatigue in children with leukemia and their parents: a pilot study. Oncol Nurs Forum. 2006;333:641-646.

105. Eiser C, Eiser JR, Stride CB. Quality of life in children newly diagnosed with cancer and their mothers. Health Qual Life Outcomes. 2005;283:29.

106. Power N, Liossi C, Franck L. Helping parents to help their child with procedural and everyday pain: practical, evidence-based advice. J Spec Pediatr Nurs. 2007;12:203-209.

107. Bartolo PA. Communicating a diagnosis of developmental disability to parents: multiprofessional negotiation frameworks. Child Care Health Dev. 2002;28:65-71.

108. Jedlicka-Kohler I, Gotz M, Eichler I. Parents' recollection of the initial communication of the diagnosis of cystic fibrosis. Pediatrics. 1996;97:204-209.

109. Krahn GL, Hallum A, Kime C. Are there good ways to give bad news? Pediatrics. 1993;91:578-582.

110. Lucas PJ, Lucas AM. Down's syndrome: breaking the news to Irish parents. Ir Med J. 1980;73:248-252.

111. Sharp MC, Strauss RP, Lorch SC. Communicating medical bad news: parents' experiences and preferences. J Pediatr. 1992;121: 539-546.

112. Garwick AW, Patterson J, Bennett FC, Blum RW. Breaking the news. How families first learn about their child's chronic condition. Arch Pediatr Adolesc Med. 1995;149:991-997.

113. Mack JW, Grier HE. The day one talk. J Clin Oncol. 2004;22: 563-566.

114. Masera G, Chesler MA, Jankovic M, et al. SIOP Working Committee on psychosocial issues in pediatric oncology: guidelines for communication of the diagnosis. Med Pediatr Oncol. 1997;28:382-385.

115. Rahi JS, Manaras I, Tuomainen H, Hundt GL. Meeting the needs of parents around the time of diagnosis of disability among their children: evaluation of a novel program for information, support, and liaison by key workers. Pediatrics. 2004;114: 477-482.

116. Dunniece U, Slevin E. Nurses' experiences of being present with a patient receiving a diagnosis of cancer. J Adv Nurs. 2000;32: 611-618.

117. Seo M, Tamura K, Shijo H, et al. Telling the diagnosis to cancer patients in Japan: attitude and perception of patients, physicians and nurses. Palliat Med. 2000;14:105-110.

118. Levenson PM, Pfefferbaum BJ, Copeland DR, et al. Information preferences of cancer patients ages 11-20 years. J Adolesc Health Care. 1982;3:9-13.

119. Levenson PM, Pfefferbaum B, Silberberg Y, Copeland DR. Sources of information about cancer as perceived by adolescent patients, parents, and physicians. Patient Couns Health Educ. 1982;3:71-76.

120. Parsons SK, Saiki-Craighill S, Mayer DK, et al. Telling children and adolescents about their cancer diagnosis: cross-cultural comparisons between pediatric oncologists in the US and Japan. Psychooncology. 2007;16:60-68.

121. Spinetta JJ, Masera G, Jankovic M, et al. Valid informed consent and participative decision-making in children with cancer and their parents: a report of the SIOP Working Committee on psychosocial issues in pediatric oncology. Med Pediatr Oncol. 2003;40:244-246.

122. Weeks JC, Cook FF, O'Day SJ, et al. Relationship between cancer patients' predictions of prognosis and their treatment preferences. JAMA. 1998;279:1709-1714.

123. Wolfe J, Klar N, Grier HE, et al. Understanding of prognosis among parents of children who died of cancer: impact on treatment goals and integration of palliative care. JAMA. 2000;284: 2469-2475.

124. Lobb EA, Butow PN, Kenny DT, Tattersall MH. Communicating prognosis in early breast cancer: do women understand the language used? Med J Aust. 1999;20:290-294.

125. Mackillop WJ, Stewart WE, Ginsburg AD, Stewart SS. Cancer patients' perceptions of their disease and its treatment. Br J Cancer. 1988;58:355-358.

126. Quirt CF, Mackillop WJ, Ginsburg AD, et al. Do doctors know when their patents don't? A survey of doctor-patient communication in lung cancer. Lung Cancer. 1997;18:1-20.

127. Mack JW, Wolfe J, Grier HE, et al. Communication about prognosis between parents and physicians of children with cancer: parent preferences and the impact of prognostic information. J Clin Oncol. 2006;24:5265-5270.

128. De Trill M, Kovalcik R. The child with cancer: influence of culture on truth-telling and patient care. Ann N Y Acad Sci. 1997;20:197-210.

129. Surbone A. Cultural aspects of communication in cancer care. Recent Results Cancer Res. 2006;168:91-104.

130. Higgs R. Case conference: a father says, "Don't tell my son the truth." J Med Ethics. 1985;11:153-158.

131. Kunin H. Ethical issues in pediatric life-threatening illness: dilemmas of consent, assent, and communication. Ethics Behav. 1997;7:43-57.

132. Midwest Bioethics Center Task Force on Health Care Rights for Minors. Health care treatment decision-making guidelines for minors. Bioethics Forum. 1995;11:A1-A6.

133. Sigman GS, Kraut J, La Puma J. Disclosure of a diagnosis to children and adolescents when parents object: a clinical ethics analysis. AJDC. 1993;147:764-768.

134. van Straaten J. The minor's limited right to confidential health care and the inverse of confidentiality: a parent's decision not to disclose illness status to a minor child. Child Leg Rights J. 2000;20:46-54.

135. Clarke JN, Fletcher P. Communication issues faced by parents who have a child diagnosed with cancer. J Pediatr Oncol Nurs. 2003;20:175-191.

136. Eden OB, Black I, MacKinlay GA, Emery AE. Communication with parents and children with cancer. Palliat Med. 1994;8: 105-114.

137. Levi RB, Marsick R, Drotar D, Kodish ED. Diagnosis, disclosure, and informed consent: learning from parents of children with cancer. J Pediatr Hematol Oncol. 2000;23:3-12.

138. Eden OB, Black I, Emery AE. The use of taped parental interviews to improve communication with childhood cancer families. Pediatr Hematol Oncol. 1993;10:157-162.

139. Johnson IA, Adelstein DJ. The use of recorded interviews to enhance physician-patient communication. J Cancer Educ. 1991;6:99-102.

140. Masera G, Beltrame F, Corbatta A, et al. Audiotaping communication of the diagnosis of childhood leukemia: parents' evaluation. J Pediatr Hematol Oncol. 2003;25:368-371.

141. Ong LM, Visser MR, Lammes FM, et al. Effect of providing cancer patients with the audiotaped initial consultation on satisfaction, recall, and quality of life: a randomized, double-blind study. J Clin Oncol. 2000;18:3052-3060.

142. Achenbach TM, Rescorla LA. Manual for the ASEBA School-Age Forms and Profiles. Burlington, VT, University of Vermont, Research Center for Children, Youth, and Families, 2001.

143. Reynolds CR, Kemphaus RW. Behavior Assessment System for Children (BASC). Circle Pines, MN, American Guidance, 1992.

144. Kazak AE, Prusak A, McSherry M, et al. The Psychosocial Assessment Tool (PAT)©: pilot data on a brief screening instrument for identifying high-risk families in pediatric oncology. Fam Syst Health. 2001;19:303-317.

145. Pai AL, Drotar D, Zebracki K, et al. A meta-analysis of the effects of psychological interventions in pediatric oncology on outcomes of psychological distress and adjustment. J Pediatr Psychol. 2006;31:978-988.

146. Ishibashi A. The needs of children and adolescents with cancer from information and social support. Cancer Nurs. 2001;24: 61-67.

147. Nathanson MN, Monaco GP. Meeting the educational and psychosocial needs produced by a diagnosis of pediatric/adolescent cancer. Health Educ Q. 1984;10:67-75.

148. Neil-Urban S, Jones JB. Father-to-father support: fathers of children with cancer share their experience. J Pediatr Oncol Nurs. 2002;19:97-103.

149. Monaco GP. Parent self-help groups for the families of children with cancer. CA Cancer J Clin. 1988;38:169-175.

150. Hermann JF, Wojkowiak SL, Houts PS, Kahn SB. Helping People Cope: A Guide for Families Facing Cancer. Harrisburg, PA, Pennsylvania Department of Health, 1988.

151. Sourkes BM. Armfuls of Time: The Psychological Experience of the Child with a Life-Threatening Illness. Pittsburgh, PA, University of Pittsburgh Press, 1995.

152. Carroll WL, Reisman J. 100 Questions and Answers about Your Child's Cancer. Sudbury, MA, Jones and Bartlett, 2005.

153. Woznick LA, Goodheart CD. Living with Childhood Cancer: A Practical Guide to Help Families Cope. Washington, DC, American Psychological Association, 2002.

154. Fromer MJ. Surviving Childhood Cancer: A Guide for Families. Washington, DC, American Psychiatric Press, 1995.

155. Keene N. Educating the Child with Cancer: A Guide for Parents and Teachers. Kensington, MD, Candlelighters Childhood Cancer Foundation, 2003.

156. Carney KL. What is Cancer, Anyway? Explaining Cancer to Children of All Ages. Wethersfield, CT, Dragonfly, 2001.

157. Chamberlain S. My ABC Book of Cancer. San Francisco, Synergistic Press, 1990.

158. Duncan D, Ollikainen N. When Molly was in the Hospital: A Book for Brothers and Sisters of Hospitilized Children. Windsor, CA, Rayve Productions, 1994.

159. Gaes J. My Book for Kids with Cansur: A Child's Autobiography of Hope. Aberdeen, SD, Melius Publishing, 1987.

160. Peterkin AD, Middendorf F. What About Me? When Brothers and Sisters Get Sick. Washington, DC, American Psychological Association, 1992.

161. Richmond C. Chemo Girl: Saving the World One Treatment at a Time. Sudbury, MA, Jones and Bartlett, 1997.

162. Rogers F, Judkis J. Going to the Hospital. New York, Penguin Young Readers Group, 1988.

163. Schulz CM. Why, Charlie Brown, Why? New York, Topper Books, 1990.

164. de Garis B. The Adventures of Captain Chemo and Chemo Command. The Captain Chemo Website. www.royalmarsden. org/captchemo/. Accessed May 5, 2008.

165. Rogers F. Some Things Change and Some Things Stay the Same. Atlanta, GA, The American Cancer Society, 1989.

166. Gravelle K, John BA. Teenagers Face to Face with Cancer. New York, Simon & Schuster, 1986.

167. Gill KA. Teenage Cancer Journey. Pittsburgh, PA, Oncology Nursing Society; 1999.

168. Haiat H, Bar-Mor G, Shochat M. The world of the child: a world of play even in the hospital. J Pediatr Nurs. 2003;18:209-214.

169. D'Antonio IJ. Therapeutic use of play in hospitals. Nurs Clin North Am. 1984;19:351-359.

170. Kuntz N, Adams JA, Zahr L, et al. Therapeutic play and bone marrow transplantation. J Pediatr Nurs. 1996;11:359-367.

171. Dolgin MJ, Phipps S, Fairclough DL, et al. Trajectories of adjustment in mothers of children with newly diagnosed cancer: a natural history investigation. J Pediatr Psychol. 2007;32:771-782.

172. Houtzager B, Oort F, Hoekstra-Weebers J, et al. Coping and family functioning predict longitudinal psychological adaptation of siblings of childhood cancer patients. J Pediatr Psychol. 2004;29:591-605.

173. Zeltzer LK, LeBaron S. Hypnosis and nonhypnotic techniques for reduction of pain and anxiety during painful procedures in children and adolescents with cancer. J Pediatr. 1982;101: 1032-1035.

174. Dolgin MJ, Katz ER, Zeltzter LK, Landsverk J. Behavioral distress in pediatric cancer patients receiving chemotherapy. Pediatrics. 1989;84:103-110.

175. LeBaron S, Zeltzer LK, LeBaron C, et al. Chemotherapy side effects in pediatric oncology patients: drugs, age, and sex as risk factors. Med Pediatr Oncol. 1988;16:263-268.

176. Zeltzer LK, LeBaron S, Zeltzer PM. Paradoxical effects of prophylactic phenothiazine antiemetics in children receiving chemotherapy. J Clin Oncol. 1984;2:930-936.

177. Zeltzer LK, LeBaron S, Zeltzer PM. A prospective assessment of chemotherapy related nausea and vomiting in children with cancer. Am J Pediatr Hematol Oncol. 1984;6:5-16.

178. Docherty SL. Symptom experiences of children and adolescents with cancer. Annu Rev Nurs Res. 2003;21:123-149.

179. Collins JJ, Byrnes ME, Dunkel IJ, et al. The measurement of symptoms in children with cancer. J Pain Symptom Manage. 2000;19:363-377.

180. Hockenberry M, Hooke MC. Symptom clusters in children with cancer. Semin Oncol Nurs. 2007;23:152-157.

181. Walco GA, Conte PC, Labay LE, et al. Procedural distress in children with cancer: self-report, behavioral observations, and physiological parameters. Clin J Pain. 2005;6:484-490.

182. Williams PD, Schmideskamp J, Ridder EL, Williams AL. Symptom monitoring and dependent care during cancer treatment in children: pilot study. Cancer Nurs. 2006;29:188-197.

183. Woodgate RL, Degner LF. Expectations and beliefs about children's cancer symptoms: perspectives of children with cancer and their families. Oncol Nurs Forum. 2003;30:479-491.

184. Hockenberry M. Symptom management research in children with cancer. J Pediatr Psychol. 2004;21:188-197.

185. Ladas EJ, Post-White J, Hawks R, Taromina K. Evidence for symptom management in the child with cancer. J Pediatr Hematol Oncol. 2006;28:601-615.

186. Liossi C, Hatira P. Clinical hypnosis in the alleviation of procedure-related pain in pediatric oncology patients. Int J Clin Exp Hypn. 2003;51:4-28.

187. Liossi C, White P, Hatira P. Randomized clinical trial of local anesthetic versus a combination of local anesthetic with self-hypnosis in the management of pediatric procedure-related pain. Health Psychol. 2006;25:307-315.

188. Myers CD, Stuber ML, Bonamer-Rheingans JI, Zeltzer LK. Complementary therapies and childhood cancer. Cancer Control. 2005;12:172-180.

189. Rheingans JI. A systematic review of nonpharmacologic adjunctive therapies for symptom management in children with cancer. J Pediatr Oncol Nurs. 2007;24:81-94.

190. Zeltzer LK, LeBaron S, Zeltzer PM. The effectiveness of behavioral intervention for reducing nausea and vomiting in children

and adolescents receiving chemotherapy. J Clin Oncol. 1984;2: 683-690.

191. Zeltzer LK, Dolgin MJ, LeBaron S, LeBaron C. A randomized, controlled study of behavioral intervention for chemotherapy distress in children with cancer. Pediatrics. 1991;88:34-42.

192. Casillas JN, Zebrack BJ, Zeltzer LK. Health-related quality of life for Latino survivors of childhood cancer. J Psychosoc Oncol. 2006;24:125-145.

193. Glover DA, Stuber M, Poland RE. Allostatic load in women with and without PTSD symptoms. Psychiatry. 2006;69:191-203.

194. Nagarajan R, Clohisy DR, Neglia JP, et al. Function and quality of life of survivors of pelvic and lower extremity osteosarcoma and Ewing's sarcoma: the Childhood Cancer Survivor Study. Br J Cancer. 2004;91:1858-1865.

195. Nathan PC, Jovcevska V, Ness KK, et al. The prevalence of overweight and obesity in pediatric survivors of cancer. J Pediatr. 2006;149:518-525.

196. Nathan PC, Ness KK, Greenberg ML, et al. Health-related quality of life in adult survivors of childhood Wilms' tumor or neuroblastoma: a report from the Childhood Cancer Survivor Study. Pediatr Blood Cancer. 2007;49:704-715.

197. Phipps S, Long A, Hudson M, Rai SN. Symptoms of post-traumatic stress in children with cancer and their parents: effects of informant and time from diagnosis. Pediatr Blood Cancer. 2005;45:952-959.

198. Robison LL, Green DM, Hudson M, et al. Long-term outcomes of adult survivors of childhood cancer: results from the Childhood Cancer Survivor Study. Cancer. 2005;104:2557-2564.

199. Seitzman RL, Glover DA, Meadows AT, et al. Self-concept in adult survivors of childhood acute lymphoblastic leukemia: a cooperative Children's Cancer Group and National Institutes of Health study. Pediatr Blood Cancer. 2004;42:230-240.

200. Taieb O, Moro MR, Baubet T, et al. Posttraumatic stress symptoms after childhood cancer. Eur Child Adolesc Psychiatry. 2003;12:255-264.

201. Zebrack BJ, Zeltzer LK, Whitton J, et al. Psychological outcomes in long-term survivors of childhood leukemia, Hodgkin's disease, and non-Hodgkin's lymphoma: a report from the Childhood Cancer Survivor Study. Pediatrics. 2002;110:42-52.

202. Zebrack B, Gurney JG, Oeffinger K, et al. Psychological outcomes in long-term survivors of childhood brain cancer: a report from the Childhood Cancer Survivor Study. J Clin Onc. 2004;22:999-1006.

203. Zebrack BJ, Zevon MA, Turk N, et al. Psychological distress in long-term survivors of solid tumors diagnosed in childhood: a report from the Childhood Cancer Survivor Study. Pediatr Blood Cancer. 2006;49:47-51.

204. Labay LE, Mayans S, Harris MB. Integrating the child into home and community following the completion of cancer treatment. J Pediatr Oncol Nurs. 2004;21:165-169.

205. Keene N, Hobbie WL, Ruccione K. Childhood Cancer Survivors: A Practical Guide to Your Future. Cambridge, MA, O'Reilly Media, 2000.

206. Arnold EM. The cessation of cancer treatment as a crisis. Soc Work Health Care. 1999;29:21-38.

207. Haase JE, Rostad M. Experiences of completing cancer therapy: children's perspectives. Oncol Nurs Forum. 1994;21:1483-1492.

208. Duffey-Lind EC, O'Holleran E, Healey M, et al. Transitioning to survivorship: a pilot study. J Pediatr Oncol Nurs. 2006;23:335-343.

209. James K, Keegan-Wells D, Hinds PS, et al. The care of my child with cancer: parents' perceptions of caregiving demands. J Pediatr Oncol Nurs. 2002;19:218-228.

210. Kirk S. Negotiating lay and professional roles in the care of children with complex health care needs. J Adv Nurs. 2001;34:593-602.

211. Baumrind D. Current patterns of parental authority. Dev Psychol Monograph. 1971;4:1-103.

212. Phelan TW. 1-2-3 Magic: Effective Discipline for Children 2-12. Glen Ellyn, IL, Parentmagic, 2004.

213. Clarke L. SOS! Help For Parents: A Practical Guide for Handling Common Everyday Behavior Problems. Bowling Green, KY, Parents Press, 1985.

214. Crary E. Without Spanking or Spoiling. Seattle, WA, Parenting Press, 1993.

215. Armstrong FD, Briery BG. Childhood cancer and the school. In Brown RT (ed). Handbook of Pediatric Psychology in School Settings. Mahwah, NJ, Lawrence Erlbaum Associates, 2004, pp 263-281.

216. Katz ER, Madan-Swain A. Maximizing School, Academic, and Social Outcomes in Children and Adolescents with Cancer. In Brown RT (ed). Comprehensive Handbook of Childhood Cancer and Sickle Cell Disease: a Biopsychosocial Approach. New York, Oxford University Press 2006, pp 313-338.

217. Armstrong D, Gannon B. Returning to School after Treatment for Childhood Cancer. (Website): www.cancercare.org. Accessed September 27, 2007 (teleconference).

218. Leigh LD. School re-entry. In Keene N (ed). Educating the Child with Cancer: A Guide for Parents and Teachers. Kensington, MD, The Candlelighters Childhood Cancer Foundation, 2003:41-55.

219. Prevatt FF, Heffer RW, Lowe PA. A review of school reintegration programs for children with cancer. J Sch Psychol. 2000;38:447-467.

220. Monaco GP, Smith GP. Special education: the law. In Keene N (ed). Educating the Child with Cancer: A Guide for Parents and Teachers. Kensington, MD, The Candlelighters Childhood Cancer Foundation, 2003, pp 193-215.

221. Seigel L. The Complete IEP Guide: How to Advocate for Your Special Ed Child. Hartfield, VA, Harbor House Law Press, 2001.

222. Wright PW, Wright PD. Wrightslaw: Special Education Law, 2nd ed. Hartfield, VA, Harbor House Law Press, 2007.

223. Handmaker SD. Developing and implementing a 504 plan. In Betz CL, Nehring WM (eds). Promoting Health Care Transitions for Adolescents with Special Health Care Needs and Disabilities. Baltimore, MD, Paul H Brooks, 2007, pp 205-216.

224. Wright PD, Wright PW. Wrightslaw: The Special Education Survival Guide: From Emotions to Advocacy, 2nd ed. Hartfield, VA, Harbor House Law Press, 2006.

225. Council of Parent Attorneys and Advocates (COPAA). (Website): www.copaa.net/about/index.html. Accessed May 5, 2008

226. The Childhood Brain Tumor Services. The Childhood Brain Tumor Foundation. (Website): www.childhoodbraintumor.org/index.php/services.html. Accessed May 5, 2008.

227. Spinetta J, Momcilo J, Eden T, et al. Guidelines for assistance to siblings of children with cancer; report of the SIOP Working Committee on psychosocial issues in pediatric oncology. Med Pediatr Oncol. 1999;33:395-398.

228. Norbis M, Enskar K, Hellstrom AL. Experience of siblings of children treated for cancer. Eur J Oncol Nurs. 2007;11:106-112.

229. Massimo LM, Wiley TJ. Young siblings of children with cancer deserve care and a personalized approach. Pediatr Blood Cancer. 2008;50:708-710.

230. Murray JS. Siblings of children with cancer: a review of the literature. J Pediatr Oncol Nurs. 1999;16:25-35.

231. Ross-Alaolmolki K, Heinzer M, Howard R. Impact of childhood cancer on siblings and family: family strategies for primary health care. Holistic Nurs Pract. 1995;9:66-75.

232. Kinrade LC. Preventative group intervention with siblings of oncology patients. Child Health Care. 1985;14:110-113.

233. Houtzager BA, Grootenhuis MA, Hoekstra-Weebers J, Last BF. One month after diagnosis: quality of life, coping and previous

functioning in siblings of children with cancer. Child Care Health Dev. 2005;31:75-87.

234. Sahler OJ, Roghmann KJ, Carpenter PJ, et al. Sibling adaptation to childhood cancer collaborative study: prevalence of sibling distress and definition of adaptation levels. J Dev Behav Pediatr. 1994;15:353-366.

235. Tritt S, Esses L. Psychosocial adaptation of siblings of children with chronic mental illnesses. Am J Orthopsychiatry. 1988;58: 211-219.

236. Walker C. Stress and coping in siblings of childhood cancer. Nurs Res. 1988;37;208-212.

237. Cairns N, Clark G, Smith S, Lansky S. Adaptation of siblings to childhood malignancy. J Pediatr. 1979;95:484-487.

238. Zeltzer LK, Dolgin MJ, Sahler OJ, et al. Sibling adaptation to childhood cancer collaborative study: health outcomes of siblings of children with cancer. Med Pediatr Oncol. 1996;27: 98-107.

239. Barbarin O, Sahler O, Carpenter P. Sibling adaptations to childhood cancer collaborative study: parental views of pre- and post-diagnosis adjustment of siblings of children with cancer. J Psych Oncol. 1995;13:1-20.

240. Harverman T, Eiser C. Siblings of a child with cancer. Child Care Health Dev. 1994;20:309-322.

241. Lobato D, Faust D, Spirito A. Examining the effects of chronic disease and disability on children's sibling relationships. J Pediatr Psychol. 1988;13:389-407.

242. Sidhu R, Passmore A, Baker D. The effectiveness of a peer support camp for siblings of children with cancer. Pediatr Blood Cancer. 2006;47:580-588.

243. Ballard KL. Meeting the needs of siblings of children with cancer. Pediatr Nurs. 2004;30:394-401.

244. SuperSibs! (Website): www.supersibs.org/aboutUs.html. Accessed May 5, 2008.

245. Decker C. Social support and adolescent cancer survivors: a review of the literature. Psychooncology. 2007;16:1-11.

246. Richie M. Sources of emotional support for adolescents with cancer. J Pediatr Oncol Nurs. 2001;18:105-110.

247. Enskar K, Carlsson M, Golsater M, Hamrin E. Symptom distress and life situation in adolescents with cancer. Cancer Nurs. 1997;20:23-33.

248. Dunsmore J, Quine S. Information, support and decision-making needs and preferences of adolescents with cancer: implication for health professionals. J Psych Oncol. 1995;13:39-55.

249. Nichols M. Social support and coping in young adolescents with cancer. Pediatr Nurs. 1995;21:235-240.

250. Kyngas H, Mikkonen R, Nousiainen E, et al. Coping strategies and resources of young people with cancer. Eur J Cancer Care. 2001;10: 6-11.

251. Saba D. Fostering hope in adolescents with cancer: do friends make a difference? J Pediatr Oncol Nurs. 1991;8:85-86.

252. Zebrack B, Bleyer A, Albritton K, et al. Assessing the health care needs of adolescent and young adult cancer patients and survivors. Cancer. 2006;107:2915-2923.

253. Deasy-Spinetta P. School and the child with cancer. In Spinetta JJ, Deasy-Spinetta P (eds). Living with Childhood Cancer. St Louis, CV Mosby, 1981, pp 153-168.

254. Vannatta K, Gartstein M, Short A, Noll R. A controlled study of children surviving brain tumors: teacher, peer, and self ratings. J Pediatr Psychol. 1998;23:279-287.

255. Noll R, Bukowski W, Davies W, et al. Adjustment in the peer systems of adolescents with cancer. J Pediatr Psychol. 1993;18: 351-364.

256. Noll R, Bukowski W, Rogosch F, et al. Social interactions between children and their peers: teaching ratings. J Pediatr Psychol. 1990;15:43-56.

257. Noll R, LeRoy S, Bukowski W, et al. Peer relationships and adjustment in children with cancer. J Pediatr Psychol. 1991;1: 307-326.

258. Stam H, Hartman E, Deurloo J, et al. Young adult patients with a history of pediatric disease: impact on course of life and transition into adulthood. J Adolesc Health. 2006;39:1-2.

259. Brown R, Kaslow N, Hazzard A. Psychiatric and family functioning in children with leukemia and their parents. J Am Acad Child Adolesc Psychiatry. 1992;31:495-502.

260. Barbarin O, Hughes D, Chelser M. Stress, coping and marital functioning among parents of children with cancer. J Marriage Fam. 1985;47:473-480.

261. Lansky S, Cairns N, Hassanein R. Childhood cancer: parental discord and divorce. J Pediatr. 1978;62:184-188.

262. Stehbens A, Lascani A. Psychological follow-up of families with childhood leukemia. J Clin Psychol. 1974;30:394.

263. Hoekstra-Weebers J, Jaspers J, Kamps W, Klip E. Marital dissatisfaction psychological distress, and coping in parents of pediatric cancer patients. J Marriage Fam. 1998;60:1012-1021.

264. Schuler D, Bakos M, Zsambor C, et al. Psychosocial problems in families of children with cancer. Med Pediatr Oncol. 1985;13:173-179.

265. Dahlquist L, Czyzewski D, Copeland C, et al. Parents of children newly diagnosed with cancer: anxiety, coping, and marital distress. J Pediatr Psychol. 1993;18:365-376.

266. Tebbi C. Treatment compliance in childhood and adolescence. Cancer. 1993;71:3441-3449.

267. Die-Trill M, Stuber M. Psychological problems of curative cancer treatment. In Holland J (ed). Psycho-Oncology. New York, Oxford University Press, 1998, pp 897-906.

268. Manne SL, Bakeman R, Jacobsen PB, et al. Adult-child interaction during invasive medical procedures. Health Psychol. 1992;11:241-249.

269. Miller D, Mann S, Palevsky S. Brief report: acceptance of behavioral interventions for children with cancer: perceptions of parents, nurses and community controls. J Pediatr Psychol. 1998;23:267-271.

270. Kashani J, Hakami N. Depression in children and adolescents with malignancy. Can J Psychiatry. 1982;27:474-477.

271. van Dongen-Melman J, Sanders-Wondstra J. Psychological aspects of childhood cancer: a review of the literature. J Child Psychol Psychiatry. 1986;27:145-180.

272. Eiser C. Choices in measuring quality of life in children with cancer: a comment. Psychooncology. 1995;4:121-131.

273. Allen L, Zigler E. Psychological adjustment of seriously ill children. J Am Acad Child Psychiatry. 1986;25:708-712.

274. Noll R, Gartstein M, Vannatta K, et al. Social, emotional and behavioral functioning of children with cancer. Pediatrics. 1999;103:71-78.

275. Shemesh E, Bartell A, Newcorn J. Assessment and treatment of depression in medically ill children. Curr Psychiatry Rep. 2002;4:88-92.

276. Shemesh E, Annunziato R, Shneider B. Parents and clinicians underestimate distress and depression in children who had a transplant. Pediatr Transplant. 2005;9:673-679.

277. Reuter K, Harter M. The concepts of fatigue and depression in cancer. Eur J Cancer Care. 2004;13:127-134.

278. Hedstrom M, Krueger A, Ljungman G. Accuracy of assessment of distress, anxiety and depression by physicians and nurses in adolescents recently diagnosed with cancer. Pediatr Blood Cancer. 2006;46:773-779.

279. Manne S, Miller D. Social support, social conflict and adjustment among adolescents with cancer. J Pediatr Psychol. 1998;23: 121-130.

280. Barrera M, Wayland L, D'Agostino N, et al. Developmental differences in psychological adjustment of health-related quality of life in pediatric cancer patients. Child Health Care. 2003;32: 215-232.

281. Stern M, Norman S, Zevon M. Adolescents with cancer: self-image and perceived social support as indexes of adaptation. J Adolesc Res. 1993;8:124-142.

282. Palmer L, Erickson S, Shaffer T, et al. Themes arising in group therapy for adolescents with cancer and their parents. Int J Rehab Health. 2000;5:43-54.

283. Daum A, Collins C. Failure to master early developmental tasks as a predictor of adaptation to cancer in the young adults. Oncol Nurs Forum. 1992; 19:1513-1518.

284. Newby W, Brown R, Pawletco T, et al. Social skills and psychological adjustment of child and adolescent cancer survivors. Psychooncology. 2000;9:113-126.

285. Challinor J, Miaskowski C, Moore I, et al. Review of research studies that evaluated the impact of treatment for childhood cancers on neurocognition and behavioral and social competence: nursing implications. J Soc Pediatr Nurs. 2000;5:57-74.

286. Gavaghan M, Roach J. Identity development of adolescents with cancer. J Pediatr Psychol. 1987;12:203-213.

287. Eccles J, Midgley C, Wigfield C. Development during adolescent: the impact of stage-environment fit on young adolescents' experiences in schools and families. Am Psychol. 1993;48: 90-101.

288. Simmons R, Blythe D. Moving into Adolescence: The Impact of Pubertal Change and School Context. Hawthorne, NY, Aldine de Grutyer, 1987.

289. Derevensky J, Tsanos A, Handman M. Children with cancer: an examination of their coping and adaptive behavior. J Pediatr Psychol. 1998;16:37-61.

290. Pedley J, Dahlquist L, Dreyer Z. Body image and psychosocial adjustment in adolescent cancer survivors. J Pediatr Psychol. 1997;22:29-43.

291. Madan-Swain A, Brown R, Sexson S, et al. Adolescent cancer survivors: psychosocial and familial adaptation. Psychosomatics. 1994;35:453-459.

292. Felder-Puig R, Formann A, Mildner A. Quality of life and psychosocial adjustment of young patients after treatment of bone cancer. Cancer. 1998;83:69-75.

34

Ethical Considerations in Pediatric Oncology Clinical Trials

Raymond C. Barfield and Eric Kodish

Ethical decision making is a fundamental goal common to clinical medicine and clinical research trials of all types. Broad attempts have long been made to explicate the elements of ethical decision making common to both settings thoroughly. However, this goal has been pursued with increased vigor since the exposure of human moral abuses in the U.S. Public Health Service–sponsored Tuskegee Syphilis Study and by the Nuremberg trials and President Clinton's Advisory Committee on Human Radiation Experiments.[1] The practical yield has been the production of highly influential documents such as the Belmont Report, the Declaration of Helsinki and its several versions, Guidelines Produced for the International Arena by the Council for International Organizations of Medical Sciences (CIOMS) and, most recently, the adoption of the Universal Declaration of Bioethics and Human Rights by the United Nations Educational, Scientific and Cultural Organization in October 2005.[2] Common to these efforts are ethical principles such as respect for persons, beneficence, and justice. Table 34-1 lists selected guidelines for research ethics. But, how do general principles translate into practical action that is ethically sound for the practitioner faced with a particular clinical situation, for the clinical research physician considering whether to offer a phase I trial to a patient, and for the investigator whose nontherapeutic trials pose some risks?

The issues become considerably more complex when the patient or research participant is a child, and the decision maker is not the person facing the possibility of risk or benefit. This issue poses special challenges for pediatric clinical medicine and pediatric clinical research. The challenges are made more acute by the fact that they are dynamic, not static. The considerations change as a child grows in age and experience and as we move from standard of care therapy to clinical trials, which, as recently argued, involve the standard of care for future children. Furthermore, the issues do not remain static across all types of clinical trials.[3] A child enrolled in a phase III clinical trial for newly diagnosed, standard-risk leukemia faces a situation quite different from that of a child who has had multiple relapses of leukemia, and whose family must choose between a phase I trial and, for example, a Make A Wish trip to the Grand Canyon.

This chapter begins with a brief historical review of the unique issues in pediatric medicine and pediatric clinical trials. It then moves to issues of parental permission and assent issues that draw on, but are not fully informed by, the many studies of informed consent in adults. The differences in language and approach required as patients progress from phase III to phase I trials and palliative care are examined. We will consider more specific questions, such as those raised by autopsy, stem cell transplantation, advances in technology, conflict of interest, insurance, ethics consultation, and international bioethics.

HISTORICAL PERSPECTIVE

For hundreds of years, medical research has involved children as subjects.[4] Edward Jenner first used experimental smallpox vaccine on his own 1-year-old son at the end of the 18th century. At the end of the 19th century, a 9-year-old child was the first human recipient of Louis Pasteur's rabies vaccine.[5] It was not until the first half of the 20th century, however, that regulations governing such experimental therapy began to be established and the importance of consent and parental permission became more clear.

The informed consent of human research subjects was first officially advocated in the Nuremberg Code, a code of ethics that grew out of the trial of German physicians who conducted human experiments in Nazi concentration camps. However, because this important code emphasized the absolute require-

TABLE 34-1	Selected Guidelines on Ethics of Biomedical Research with Human Subjects	
Guideline	**Source**	**Year and Revisions**
Nuremberg Code	Fundamental; Nuremberg Military Tribunal decision in *United States v Brandt*	1947
Declaration of Helsinki	World Medical Association	1964, 1975, 1983, 1989, 1996
Belmont Report	National Commission for the Protection of Human Subjects of Biomedical and Behavioral Research	1979
International Ethical Guidelines for Biomedical Research Involving Human Subjects	Council for International Organizations of Medical Sciences in collaboration with World Health Organization	Proposed in 1982; revised, 1993
45 CFR 46, Common Rule	Other: U.S. Department of Health and Human Services (DHHS) and other federal agencies	DHHS guidelines in 1981; Common Rule, 1991
Guidelines for Good Clinical Practice Trials on Pharmaceutical Products	World Health Organization	1995
Good Clinical Practice: Consolidated Guidance	International Conference on Harmonisation of Technical Requirements for Registration of Pharmaceuticals for Human Use	1996
Convention of Human Rights and Biomedicine	Council of Europe	1997
Guidelines and Recommendations for European Ethics Committees	European Forum for Good Clinical Practice	1997
Medical Research Council Guidelines for Good Clinical Practice in Clinical Trials	Medical Research Council, United Kingdom	1998
Guidelines for the Conduct of Health Research Involving Human Subjects in Uganda	Uganda National Council for Science and Technology	1998
Ethical Conduct for Research Involving Humans	Tri-Council Working Group, Canada	1998
National Statement on Ethical Conduct in Research Involving Humans	National Health and Medical Research Council, Australia	1999

CFR, Code of Federal Regulations.
From Emanuel EJ, Wendler D, Grady C. What makes clinical research ethical? JAMA. 2000;283:2701-2711.

ment of informed consent, it implicitly excluded children—who cannot give informed consent—from participating in research on human subjects.[6]

The issue was more explicitly addressed in 1964, when the World Medical Association adopted a set of research ethics principles now known as the Declaration of Helsinki.[7,8] This set of principles established the priority of the human subjects' interests over those of science and society, and it sanctioned the participation of children in research if permission was given by the child's responsible guardian.

Interestingly, experiments were performed on children after the publication of the Nuremberg Code, which implicitly excluded children from research, and before the Declaration of Helsinki, which explicitly allowed such research under specific conditions. One of the most important of these was a series of radiation exposure experiments.[9,10] Among participating institutions was the Fernald School, in which children deemed mentally retarded were fed radioactive iron and calcium in their cereal. President Clinton's advisory committee on human radiation experiments revealed the inadequacy of parental permission in these experiments.

Another important set of experiments on children at that time occurred at the Willowbrook institution[10] and was designed to follow the natural history of hepatitis in children deemed mentally retarded. Children were infected with hepatitis virus. Participating children were kept in a special unit with better conditions and nutrition, and children whose parents agreed that they could participate were admitted more rapidly. The lead investigator required a thorough consent process that included a 2-week waiting period for full deliberation. Because Willowbrook was so crowded, however, critics subsequently argued that the expedited admission and special treatment amounted to coercion. These two cases underscored the need for ethical review and oversight of human subjects research involving children, even when parental permission is obtained.

Congress became increasingly concerned about research ethics during the early 1970s, in part because of the Tuskegee Syphilis Study involving poor black men. As a result, the National Commission for the Protection of Research Subjects of Biomedical and Behavioral Research was formed, and it published the Belmont Report in 1979.[11] This report embraced three principles that are now familiar and accepted as crucial for research involving human subjects: respect for persons, beneficence, and justice. The principle of beneficence acknowledges the Hippocratic maxim "do no harm" and extends it to include maximizing the possible benefits and minimizing the possible harms to research subjects; minimizing harms is often formulated separately as a fourth principle, nonmaleficence.[12] The principle of beneficence is operative in any discussion weighing the risks and benefits of human subjects research, especially when the subject is a minor. The principle of justice concerns the right and fair distribution of the benefits of research as well as the burdens, an issue that has particular urgency when clinical treatment and research are considered globally. The concept of respect for persons includes two principles, that individuals be treated as autonomous agents and that those with less autonomy are entitled to protection. The latter principle is especially relevant in pediatrics and is somewhat fluid in its definition because of the growing autonomy of pediatric patients as they approach adulthood.

Given past abuses of research subjects who were harmed in studies that they did not understand and for which they had not given meaningful permission, it is understandable that informed consent has become the dominant concept in any discussion about ethical research on human subjects. However, recent arguments have stated that informed consent is not always necessary for ethical clinical research, nor is it sufficient

to qualify research as ethical. Reviews of major codes and declarations relating to human subjects research have led to the proposal that there are six requirements for ethical clinical research[8,13-15]:

1. The research must lead to enhancement of health or knowledge.
2. It must be methodologically rigorous.
3. Selection of study sites and of individual subjects should be determined by scientific objectives and the potential for and distribution of risks and benefits.
4. Given standard clinical practice and the research protocol, risks should be minimized, the potential for benefits should be enhanced, and risks must be outweighed by potential benefits to individuals and knowledge for society.
5. Individuals should be informed about the research and provide voluntary consent.
6. Research subjects should have their privacy protected, have the opportunity to withdraw, and have their well-being monitored.

These requirements are thorough and persuasive, but still they must be adapted to the conditions under which the research is conducted. Factors of health, economy, culture, religion, and technology will affect how these requirements are translated into concrete ethical action. For this reason, living ethical deliberation and the specific context will always be important.

Ethical decision making in therapeutic and research efforts for children comprise all the considerations discussed, plus the profoundly salient fact that the recipient of the risk or benefit is not the person who makes the decisions. The minor may not be capable of assimilating sufficient information to meaningfully participate in an informed choice. One need not enter the arena of international bioethics to find challenges to the role of autonomy in ethical decision making: such challenges are the daily fare in pediatric medicine and research, because children's autonomy is an issue that changes from day to day.

CONSENT AND PARENTAL PERMISSION

What Is "Consent" in Pediatrics?

The Nuremberg Code provided a starting point for understanding the meaning and importance of informed consent. The statement in this code that "the voluntary consent of human subjects is absolutely essential" has been interpreted as legal capacity, a power of free choice based on knowledge and comprehension.[16] Consent, once seen as a single event, has come to be understood to be more of a process.[17] Not unsurprisingly, with the development of guidelines and goals for consent, the process has become more intentional and more highly scrutinized.

The dominant theoretical framework for morally valid informed consent requires that four criteria be met—disclosure, understanding, voluntariness, and competence.[12] Briefly, the core set of information that must be disclosed includes the following: (1) facts (e.g., risks, benefits and alternatives) that patients and providers believe are relevant to the decision; (2) the recommendation of the professional; and (3) the purpose, nature, and limitations of consent. Understanding goes beyond disclosure because, although the elements disclosed can be objectively stated, true understanding involves many variables and is more difficult to assess. Establishing and documenting understanding remains a great challenge, because information that has been disclosed but not understood contributes little to the ideal paradigm of informed consent. Voluntariness, another complex notion open to interpretation, means at least that a decision is made without constraints of coercion or manipulation. Finally, competence, which is conventionally understood as the ability to perform a task, has also become a complex concept whose definitions are derived from law, psychiatry, and philosophy. A person's competence to make a particular decision relates to the person's ability to understand and think logically about available choices and to use that understanding and logic to make a decision.

In the context of complex pediatric medical therapy and research, the process of consent is influenced by the fact that parents are making high-stakes decisions for their own child. The Children's Cancer Group (CCG) has conducted studies that show that a sense of pressure is perceived by parents when making the consent decision for intervention in the context of childhood cancer.[18] A more recent study, however, has indicated that despite significant dissatisfaction with the consent process among CCG clinician investigators, most parents are satisfied with it.[19] The same study indicated that the parents' satisfaction did not constitute adequate informed consent.

Even among clinicians, assessment of the process of informed consent varies. The experience of the clinician is relevant in this assessment. Simon and colleagues[20] have found that clinicians with 10 or fewer years of experience are more likely to say that the most important goal of informed consent is to explain the disease and treatment and more likely to suggest to parents that other children might benefit from the research. The same study found that in the end, when reports from clinicians and parents are compared, clinicians are dissatisfied with aspects of consent with which parents seem far more satisfied. For example, clinicians expressed concern about information overload and about the fact that the consent discussion often occurs while the parents are still in a state of shock about the diagnosis.

Further insights into this difference have been gained from a number of studies addressing the perspectives of parents of children with cancer. One such study used three focus groups of parents of children with cancer[21] to examine their perceptions of the informed consent process retrospectively. High levels of stress were consistently reported; these were attributed to efforts to cope with multiple demands, including assimilating their child's diagnosis, nurturing and supporting the child, understanding the information given to them about the diagnosis and treatment, getting to know an entirely new group of people involved in the child's care, and participating in the child's treatment. Another important point was that the parents did not consistently distinguish research from their child's medical treatment. This finding underscores the importance of clearly explaining that research is optional during the process of informing. If no distinction is made between research and treatment, one might question whether the goal of informing has been met. Physician investigators often experience tension between their role as the patient's physician and their role as a researcher offering an unproven alternative to standard therapy. The results of this study suggest that a professional other than the study investigator should conduct the consent process and that the nature of research and the difference between research and standard therapy may be difficult for parents to grasp.

These conclusions were supported by a second study, in which parents of children with newly diagnosed cancer were interviewed.[22] All the participants recalled the diagnosis and most (80%) recalled survival statistics. Only slightly more than 50%, however, knew that the treatment protocol involved research and understood the concept of randomization. This finding is striking when coupled with the fact that 75% of the parents thought that alternatives to enrollment in a randomized protocol had been insufficiently discussed. Because randomization is such an important tool for answering certain clinical questions, this finding suggests that greater emphasis be placed

on explaining unfamiliar concepts during the process of informing. Again, in this study, most participants were satisfied with the consent process.

A study by Kodish and associates[23] has confirmed the difficulty of effectively conveying the meaning of randomization during the consent process in pediatric leukemia trials. In this multisite study, informed consent conferences were observed and audiotaped and then compared with information acquired in interviews with parents shortly after the conference. The investigators found that although randomization was explained in 83% of cases, 50% of the parents did not understand it. Furthermore, parents who did not understand randomization were more likely to consent to the randomized study than those who did understand it, although this difference was not statistically significant ($P = .07$). These findings led to several recommendations for improving understanding, including a clear explanation of the differences between the randomized trial and off-study therapy, assessment of parental understanding of randomization, and further explanation when the idea was still not grasped.

Other efforts have been made to improve the process of informed consent in pediatrics, especially in the case of complex clinical trials. For example, a study by the Children's Cancer Group assessed the possibility of staged consent; investigators had the option of obtaining consent over a 28-day period using a staged approach.[24] This option allowed parents and patients more time to discuss and absorb facts about the disease, the purpose of the trial, the design of the study, and the potential risks. Several measures in this study suggested benefit from the staged approach. There was greater understanding of treatment choices and of the distinction between a randomized controlled trial and standard therapy with the staged approach (80% understanding) than in the other studies (62.5%; $P = .05$).

Contemporary medicine will require the introduction of new methods of informing patients and parents to meet the ethical imperative of informed consent in pediatric trials. Informed consent documents for cancer clinical trials are sometimes long and difficult to understand, with language that serves less to protect human subjects than to decrease institutional liability.[25] Therefore, some advances may take the form of technologic and educational methods to explain ever more complex medicine and research to people not formally trained in a medical discipline. One such example is a device known as the Informed Consent (IC) Team Link (Fig. 34-1). This device was designed to help families understand phase I trials, which present daunting challenges to fully informed consent. The design was based on information from focus groups of parents, physicians, nonphysician health care workers, and teenage patients. Among the elements considered important were (1) the need for a big picture overview that would create a context for details, (2) delivery of information in small chunks, (3) use of multiple modes of information delivery, and (4) prioritization of information. Such basic observations provided a basis for the design of a device that uses interactive technology, voice, animation, and health education principles to deliver information about phase I trials. Because of children's apparently natural affinity for interactive electronic devices, this approach may be helpful in addressing assent as well.

Concepts about the nature of consent in pediatrics are evolving with changes in contemporary medicine. For example, some have argued that informed consent may be too restrictive a concept and that valid consent should be substituted.[26] The three aspects of valid consent are personal competence (Does the patient have the capacity to make the decision?), procedural competence (Is the consent given correctly?), and material competence (Is the procedure consented to appropriate for valid consent?). The concept of valid consent has been explored in the pediatric context by the SIOP working committee on

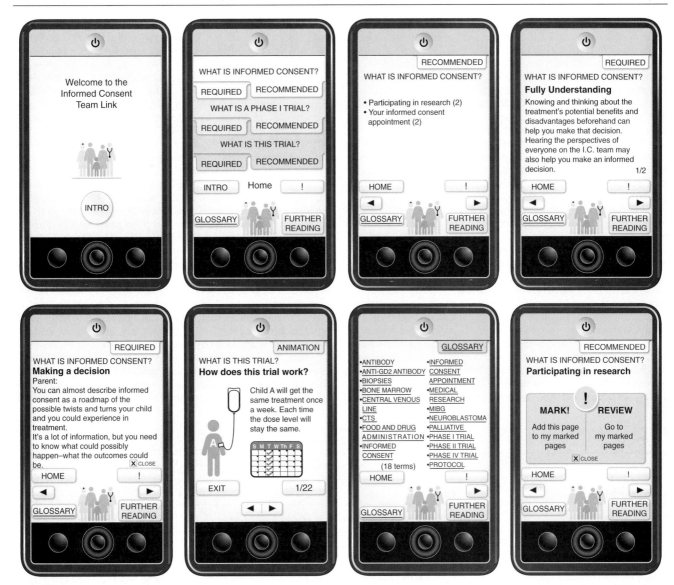

FIGURE 34-1. The Informed Consent Team Link, a prototype device to augment the process of informed consent in phase I trials. This device was developed through multidisciplinary user-centered research and design. The aim of such efforts is to use technologic and educational advances to address the widening gap between the average capacity to understand concepts and the advances in medical technology and research.

psychosocial issues in pediatric oncology.[27] The value of this notion, they have suggested, is that it emphasizes the patient's or parents' understanding of what is being consented to and recognizes that there are rational and nonrational aspects to the decision making process that must be understood. The underlying concern is that informed consent has come to mean legally signed documentation rather than real understanding, insofar as that is possible. Because parents come from different backgrounds and because children of different ages differ in their ability to grasp complex concepts, the level of understanding that is attainable may vary from situation to situation. The notion of valid consent acknowledges this and attempts to resist the idea that a signed document is equivalent to informed consent.

The four elements of informed consent mentioned—disclosure, understanding, voluntariness, and competence—are useful for informed consent in adults, but informed consent in pediatrics is complicated by the fact that three parties are involved (parent, child, and clinician investigator) and that the research subject is the child. In pediatrics, it is not autonomy

(the basis of the four components of consent) that takes precedence but rather the best interest of the child.[28] The best interests notion is clearer in a purely clinical setting than in a research setting, in which interventions are designed to contribute to general knowledge. Despite the difficulty of approximating truly informed consent in the setting of pediatrics, and especially pediatric research, the obligation to advance pediatric medicine lends urgency to continued efforts to offer the closest possible approximation to informed consent.

One important aspect of the difference between informed consent in adult and pediatric medicine and research is the fact that in pediatrics, informed consent is better thought of as a combination of parental permission and, as appropriate, the more complex concept of the assent of the child.

Assent in Childhood Cancer Trials

The ethics of assent is one of the most difficult issues faced in pediatric clinical trials. Many adolescents, and even some younger children, possess the elements of competence (setting aside for the moment the legal definitions, which hinge on age rather than capacity). This is especially true, perhaps, of those who are exposed to long-term clinical trials and to the environment of a children's hospital for long periods. Certainly, younger children are not developmentally capable of comprehending complex protocols, but they do have some level of understanding that increases with age and experience.[29] How should assent be understood and when should it be required?

Far less is known about assent than about consent. Much remains to be learned about the practices of institutional review boards (IRBs), the perceptions of parents, clinicians, and children about consent, and the methods that might be most effective in the process of assent. Several studies have looked into these issues and documented the need for further work. Two recent studies have found variability in IRB practices and the implementation of assent. One study has found that half of IRBs have a method that they require investigators to follow when determining which children are capable of assent, but half have no such method, and most IRBs rely on investigators' judgment.[30] IRBs need guidance on the implementation of requirements regarding assent. A second study has compared standards for assent as well as consent forms approved by 55 local IRBs reviewing three standardized, multicenter research protocols.[31] Standards varied widely; 35 had separate forms and simplified language for assent, and 31 specified lower age ranges for obtaining assent in three studies. For a hypertension study, the age at which assent was required ranged from 6 to 15 years, for a pain study, the age range was 6 to 12 years and, for a

respiratory failure study, the range was 7 to 12 years. It is not clear why some IRBs consider a child of 6 capable of assent whereas others do not require assent until a child is 15 years old.

Do the regulations help us understand assent? Most research on children is governed by subpart D of 45 Code of Federal Regulations (CFR) 46, which provides additional protections for children, as vulnerable subjects, beyond those specified in subpart A of 45 CFR 46. Subpart D, added in 1983, outlined three categories of research that a local IRB can approve: research not involving greater than minimal risk to participants (45 CFR 46.404), research involving greater than minimal risk but with the prospect of direct benefit to individual participants (45 CFR 46.405), and research involving no greater than a minor increase over minimal risk (with no prospect of direct benefit) but likely to provide generalizable knowledge of the subject's condition or disorder that is vital to understanding or ameliorating it (45 CFR 46.406; Table 34-2).[32] Local IRBs cannot approve research that does not fall into one of these categories, and performance of the research is possible only if two conditions are met: (1) the local IRB finds that the research provides a reasonable opportunity to further the understanding, prevention, or alleviation of a serious problem affecting the health and welfare of children; and (2) the protocol is approved by the Secretary of Health and Human Services, after soliciting the opinions of an expert panel and providing for a period of public comment (45 CFR 46.407). According to these regulations governing research on children, assent means "a child's voluntary affirmative agreement to

TABLE 34-2	Categories of Pediatric Research and Requirements for Institutional Review Boards (IRB) Approval	
	PROSPECT OF DIRECT BENEFIT	
Level of Risk	**No**	**Yes**
Minimal risk	Approval by IRB permitted (46.404), conditioned on: • Permission from one parent or guardian • Assent of child, unless waived on capacity grounds	
Greater than minimal risk	Approval by IRB permitted (46.406), conditioned on: • Minor increase over minimal risk • Research involves experiences commensurate with those inherent in children's actual or expected medical, dental, psychological, social or educational circumstances • Intervention or procedure is likely to yield generalizable knowledge about the subject's disorder or condition that is of vital importance for understanding or ameliorating that condition or disorder • Permission from both parents, if reasonably available • Assent of child, unless waived on capacity grounds	Approval by IRB permitted (46.405), conditioned on: • Risks are justified by anticipated benefit to subjects • Relation of anticipated benefit to risk is at least as favorable as that presented by available alternatives • Permission from one parent or guardian • Assent of child, unless waived on capacity grounds or grounds of prospect of direct benefit that "is available only in the context of the research"
Not otherwise approvable, but presents opportunity to understand, prevent, or alleviate a serious problem affecting the health or welfare of children	Approval requires U.S. Department of Health and Human Services approval after consultation with an expert panel and opportunity for public review and comments (46.407), conditioned on: • Research presents reasonable opportunity to further understanding, prevention, or alleviation of a serious problem affecting health or welfare of children • Permission from both parents, if reasonably available • Assent of child, unless waived on capacity grounds	

From Joffe S, Fernandez CV, Pentz RD, et al. Involving children with cancer in decision-making about research participation. J Pediatr. 2006;149:862-868.

participate in research" (45 CFR 46.402). If the IRB determines that the participants in certain categories of age and maturity are capable of providing assent, investigators must obtain it to proceed. When assent is required, a child's refusal is binding.

Can an IRB waive the requirement for assent? This can be done, but only in the following situations: (1) if the intervention or procedure offers the possibility of direct benefit that is important to the health or well-being of the child and this intervention or procedure is only available in the research context (45 CFR 46.408(a)); or (2) the IRB determines that children below a certain age in a certain situation or with a certain condition have such a limited capacity to participate in the decision that they cannot reasonably be consulted.[6]

The requirements are difficult to apply, especially in the context of clinical trials for childhood cancer. Most of the children are enrolled in research studies in which the therapy is prolonged and carried out in the context of profound physical, spiritual, and psychological stress. The Bioethics Committee of the Children's Oncology Group (COG) convened an international multidisciplinary task force to address assent in 2003. This group identified a number of problems with the regulatory framework.[33] In brief, the regulations do not take adequate account of the dynamic moral and cognitive development of children and therefore allow a child either to have no formal role in decision making or to have the power of veto. Also, the guidelines do not make clear what constitutes meaningful assent, and consequently leave IRBs and investigators uncertain about when they have or have not hit the mark, although other groups have provided guidance in this area.[34,35] The regulations do not take into account the fact that some clinical research is more complex than other research, and thus some may be more accessible to the understanding of children than others. The regulations state that permission from the guardians and assent from the child are distinct decisions, and they do not take into account the manner in which parents and children make decisions together. Finally, cultures in which autonomy is less emphasized are not accommodated by a regulation that potentially sets parental prerogatives against a child's veto power.[36]

Taking into account these factors, the COG task force offered three principles governing children's participation in research decisions (Box 34-1).[33] A number of specific recommendations followed from these principles. The task force acknowledged that in some settings, the principles offered will sometimes conflict. Therefore, the recommendations emphasize the importance of establishing procedures for the resolution of conflict rather than attempting to define universal rules. In that way, the absence of universal rules governing decisions in families with, perhaps, different cultural backgrounds and assumptions does not end conversation and negotiation. This approach is especially valuable in an increasingly pluralistic society and a global culture of information sharing. Much work remains to be done to understand the processes of communication and learning and the interactions that comprise the permission and assent process.

The flexibility of the approach using conflict resolution acknowledges that the obligation to obtain assent may change, depending on the time and situation, even for the same child. For example, assent considerations may differ between a 9-year-old child with standard-risk leukemia who may obtain considerable benefit from enrollment on a phase III leukemia trial and a 9-year-old child with leukemia who has relapsed multiple times and for whom a phase I trial is being considered. Similarly, a child at the beginning of a 2½-year course of therapy for leukemia will be different in age, maturity, vocabulary, experience, and capacity to understand by the end of that course of therapy (Fig. 34-2). Developmentally appropriate

| Box 34-1 | **Principles Governing Children's Participation in Research Decisions** |

1. Investigators should always respect children as persons. In particular, investigators together with parents should honor children's developing autonomy in decisions about research.
2. Investigators should respect parents' roles in guiding their children's moral development and assessing their best interests. For example, parents should have discretion to determine the degree to which children should be encouraged to participate in activities that benefit others.
3. Policies regarding assent, as well as IRBs' decisions with respect to particular protocols, should be sufficiently flexible to accommodate the wide range of medical, psychological, and contextual circumstances seen in pediatric oncology.

From Joffe S, Fernandez CV, Pentz RD, et al. Involving children with cancer in decision making about research participation. *J Pediatr.* 2006;149:862-868.

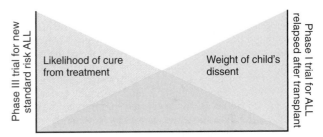

FIGURE 34-2. The weight of childhood dissent changes as the likelihood for direct benefit, in the form of cure or extension of life, diminishes. For example, this would apply to a patient who goes through a phase III trial for standard-risk leukemia, relapses, is transplanted in second remission, relapses, and goes on to consider phase I trials. ALL, acute lymphocytic leukemia.

approaches to help the child understand the experience do not have the restrictions and limitations that accompany the binding aspects of assent.

For older adolescents, assent should be approached in the same way as adult informed consent, even though parental consent is required.[37,38] Some adolescents may have the capacity for consent but may choose to have their parents make decisions about their participation in research.[39] Several studies have assessed assent in adolescents.[40,41] Our understanding of the differences between parents' and adolescents' perceptions of research is growing as we learn more about the assessment of risk (i.e., concern for physical safety) versus aversion (psychological discomfort).[42] More than 3000 adolescents in the United States alone die of chronic illness and cancer each year. In such situations, when adolescents meet the criteria for functional competence, the broad ethical consensus is that decisional authority should be granted to them, regardless of their legal decisional status.[43]

PEDIATRIC CLINICAL TRIALS

Most children with cancer are enrolled in clinical trials.[44] This systematic evaluation of interventions is largely responsible for the dramatic improvement in survival over the past 30 years. A number of important ethical concepts have influenced the design and execution of these trials. Consent and assent have been discussed earlier. Other important issues include the distinction between therapeutic and nontherapeutic research, the corollary concepts of minimal risk and clinical equipoise, and the considerations that set phase I and II trials apart from phase III trials.

As described above, and in Table 34-2, reports published by the National Commission for Subjects of Biomedical and Behavioral Research have formed the basis of current regulations governing research with human subjects, including children. One of the most important distinctions made was that between research that does and does not offer the prospect of direct benefit to the child. Some elements of a clinical trial may offer the prospect of direct benefit (e.g., chemotherapy for acute lymphoblastic leukemia) whereas other elements may not (e.g., biologic and pharmacokinetic studies designed to improve future trials). There are some general criteria that can be used to determine whether the latter types of research are permissible.

Minimal Risk

The central ethical concept that guides discussion of pediatric research that has no prospect of direct benefit is minimal risk. The Belmont Report has defined minimal risk as "the probability and magnitude of physical or psychological harm that is normally encountered in the daily lives, or in the routine medical or psychological examination, of healthy children." The question that immediately arises is which children's lives should be the basis for deciding what is normally encountered in daily life. These risks can vary widely, not only from country to country but within subgroups in a single country. Even if the notion of harms or discomforts that average, healthy, normal children may encounter, as clarified by the National Bioethics Advisory Commission, can be roughly agreed on as a standard, the question remains whether it is ever acceptable for a parent to give permission for any risk greater than minimal risk in the absence of direct benefit to the child.

Because of concern that the minimal risk standard would exclude some pediatric research that is important and appropriate, the National Commission has allowed parental discretion in giving permission for research that exposes children to a minor increase over minimal risk, given the fact that parents routinely permit their children to participate in activities, such as contact sports, that present more than a minimal risk, and given the potential benefits of such research to others. Therefore, a minor increase over minimal risk is permissible if the proposed research involves only procedures that such children might normally experience because of their medical condition, and if the proposed research has the potential to yield vitally important knowledge for understanding or ameliorating the child's particular condition. This position has been criticized, given that the children for whom acceptable risk is being redefined are already at higher risk because of their illness.[45]

The permissibility of a minor increase over minimal risk provides a conceptual way to avoid crippling important pediatric research. However, a difficult question remains: exactly what constitutes a minor increase? The term is used in the federal regulations, but is not defined. Wendler and Emanuel[46] have proposed five possible standards for defining minor increase consistently among IRBs: (1) a fixed percentage above daily risks; (2) the confidence intervals around the risks of daily life; (3) the risks an ill child might encounter in an examination; (4) the "scrupulous parent" standard, in which minor risks are sufficiently similar to the child's past experiences in daily life; and (5) the "socially acceptable" risk standard.

Wendler and Emanuel have argued that the fifth standard is the most reasonable one. The socially acceptable risk standard takes as its starting point the fact that some children encounter greater risks in daily life than others. The socially acceptable risk standard allows risks that are greater than those faced every day by healthy children, but it limits the risks to those that are socially acceptable. The socially acceptable risks that are greater than those experienced by the average healthy child may be more closely defined through research. In any case, this standard tethers the concept of minor increase over minimal risk to a standard that is nonarbitrary, that does not cripple important beneficial research, and that does not justify greater risks for ill children simply because their daily lives are filled with more risk.

Phase I and II Trials in Pediatric Oncology

Phase I studies have the unique primary objective of assessing the maximum tolerated dose (MTD) and estimating toxic effects in human subjects, in contrast to phase II and phase III studies, which explicitly assess the efficacy and relative safety of interventions. Phase I studies in children are important, because the pharmacokinetics and toxic effects of drugs differ between children and adults. Therefore, if drugs were used in the general pediatric population without phase I testing in children, any adverse effects would occur to a greater number of children. Additionally, some diseases are unique, or almost unique, to the pediatric population, including a number of pediatric cancers.[47] Prohibition of phase I studies in children would limit our ability to develop new drugs that target uniquely pediatric diseases.

Phase I studies are typically dose escalation trials in which some children receive a dose unlikely to be of any benefit whereas others receive a dose that is toxic. Therefore, phase I studies do not fit the category of minimal risk nor, many would argue, of a minor increase over minimal risk. Much of the controversy about phase I studies in children, therefore, centers on whether they offer sufficient direct benefit to justify the risks, both from a purely ethical point of view and from the regulatory point of view.

What is the likelihood of harms and benefits in phase I trials? A review of abstracts and reports of the results of phase I cancer trials submitted to the American Society of Clinical Oncology from 1991 to 2002 found that the death rate from toxicity was 0.54%, with an overall objective response rate of 3.8%, and that risks decreased over time.[48] A more recent National Cancer Institute (NCI)–sponsored study of adult phase I oncology trials between 1991 and 2002 found an overall response rate of 10.6%. The response rates in classic single-agent phase I trials were lower (4.4%), whereas those that included at least one U.S. Food and Drug Administration (FDA)–approved anticancer agent had a response rate of 17.8%.[49] The overall rate of death caused by toxicity was 0.49%. In pediatric oncology phase I trials, the overall objective response rate has been reported to be 7.9%. The overall rate among phase I trials differs among diseases: neuroblastoma, 17.7%; acute myelogenous leukemia, 11.6%; and osteosarcoma and rhabdomyosarcoma, less than 3%.[50] The overall death rate from drug toxicity was 0.7%. That said, in any single phase I trial centered around a single drug, there can be considerable variability in outcomes among the patients recruited. Can phase I trials be viewed as offering a prospect of direct benefit in the context of pediatric oncology? The pediatric medical and bioethics communities are divided on this question. Most people who enroll in phase I trials hope for personal benefit, although they know that the trial is designed to test toxicity.[51,52] There is concern that such a therapeutic misconception might encourage false hope for cure and lead parents to make decisions that do not take into account all the elements that make up the child's best interest.[53,54] Conversely, because only patients for whom known therapies have failed are usually eligible for phase I trials, these trials may be viewed as offering a relative prospect of direct benefit, although the chance of controlling the disease is small.[55] Such a view would bring phase I research under CFR 46.405 of the federal regulations, but it has been criticized because such a classification, in which risk is justified by potential benefit, fails to take into account the researcher's focus on safety rather than efficacy. From the latter point of view, phase I research would be approvable only under CFR 46.407, in which the research is reviewed and approved by a panel appointed by the Secretary of the Department of Health and Human Services, a time-consuming effort that requires national and local IRB review.

One critic of the direct benefit argument[56] has also questioned the approval of phase I trials under CFR 46.407, because the required review process delays providing benefit to children and adds little to the meaningful protection of children. It was suggested that a new category of research offering the potential for secondary direct benefit be added to the regulations. Such a category would require the following: (1) that the risks be justified by the likelihood that the research will yield generalizable knowledge; (2) that the research be commensurate with the lived experience of those with the disease or condition; (3) that the research offer a potential secondary benefit that is otherwise not available (a potential therapeutic benefit, even though the trial lacks therapeutic intent); and (4) that consent requirements be met. Work that addresses gaps in the understanding of phase I trials and the federal regulations governing them should take high priority in pediatric medical ethics research.

Phase II trials play an important role in all areas of cancer therapy; they provide the initial assessment of treatment efficacy and identify agents for further investigation in phase III studies.[57] Phase II studies are likely to increase in number as high-throughput screening of compounds identifies more candidate anticancer drugs. This will raise many important ethical questions in pediatric clinical trials, because phase II studies specifically evaluate drug efficacy before there is clear demonstration of benefit. Therefore, it is vital that families and patients be fully informed about alternatives.

Phase III Trials and Clinical Equipoise

If the concept of minimal risk demarcates the upper limit of nontherapeutic research, the notion of clinical equipoise is central, although not unproblematic, to ethical thought about randomization in clinical research. Clinical equipoise requires that if patients are to be randomly assigned to one of two interventions in a clinical trial, there must be real doubt—in the medical community as a whole, if not in the mind of the investigator—about which of the two interventions is superior. This requirement is said to provide one answer to the possible conflict of interest that clinical investigators can experience in the dual role of researcher and physician.[58] However, there is no complete agreement about whether the physician's therapeutic obligation requires the provision of the best possible care or simply of competent care.[59] Furthermore, the concept of clinical equipoise has been challenged from a number of perspectives. Some critics have argued that therapeutic medicine and

clinical research are distinct types of activity that require distinct ethical frameworks, and that the concept of clinical equipoise cannot provide a unifying ethical framework.[60,61] Clinical equipoise has also been criticized as being especially problematic in developing countries, in which the lack of resources may not support trials that test new treatments against established therapies or placebo. The requirement for clinical equipoise could make it difficult to justify the search for interventions that, although they provide significant benefit for less money, are known not to be the most effective interventions.[62,63]

Several other considerations are important in evaluating the concept of clinical equipoise. First, the conditions for establishing true equipoise are not objective, because they are based on unverified judgments that are open to bias.[64,65] Second, if clinical equipoise is not always a reliable foundation for randomized studies, how do we resolve the conflicts that could be posed by clinical investigators' dual roles? Finally, although adults may be able to negotiate the ambiguities of clinical equipoise in a clinical trial, children cannot. In view of the earlier discussion regarding the best interest of the child—or the attempt to avoid harm to the child—no phase III randomized pediatric trial should be conducted unless there is genuine doubt about which of two or more alternatives is better.

CANCER TRIALS USING ALLOGENEIC HEMATOPOIETIC STEM CELL TRANSPLANTATION

Many patients with high-risk cancers, especially leukemias, that are resistant to standard chemotherapy can be cured with hematopoietic stem cell transplantation (HSCT). As in other areas of pediatric oncology, most such patients are treated through research protocols or treatment plans recently derived from research protocols. Because of the continuing rapid changes in the field of HSCT, ethical considerations, such as the specifics of the risk-benefit analysis, are rapidly changing as well.

The issues that apply to pediatric oncology trials in general are also relevant to those that include HSCT. However, HSCT raises additional questions. Unlike most phase III trials, transplantation is usually a second medical procedure aimed at cure. Common indications for transplantation in patients with malignant disease include lack of response to conventional chemotherapy and a known high risk of relapse, despite conventional therapy. In both cases, patients have been treated prior to transplantation, and the education received in this experience will be relevant to the consent process (the same, of course, can be said for phase I trials). Patients' and parents' familiarity with the language of pediatric oncology makes the discussion about transplantation easier in some ways than the discussion about a phase III trial in the context of a newly diagnosed childhood malignancy. However, these considerations are primarily cognitive. There are other issues involved as well.

No studies have examined noncognitive considerations in consent for pediatric HSCT, but one study has addressed the relative value of receiving full information in decision making in adult patients.[66] The findings provide interesting information that might partly guide future assessments of the unique characteristics of consent and assent in pediatric HSCT. The study had an unusual hypothesis—in the context of a potentially lifesaving procedure, when there are no treatment alternatives that have a reasonable chance of cure, factors other than the effort to inform fully have the greatest influence on the patient's decision making process. The notion of voluntary action is complex in such cases, because the patients' life-threatening illness has forced them to consider HSCT as an option. Four factors were considered by patients, according to this study: (1) a full understanding of the treatment; (2) trust in the physician; (3) trust in the treatment team; and (4) the best chance for a good outcome. The most important factor was best chance for a good outcome and the least important factor was a full understanding of the treatment.

The above finding is relevant to any high-risk, complex intervention such as transplantation, in which the patient's life is at stake. The lack of alternative therapies that offer the real possibility of cure limits the voluntariness of the decision, and trust in the physician and health care team become more significant than understanding of the treatment. Given the vulnerability of these patients, this fact underscores the importance of careful attention to the therapeutic rationale of treatment, especially when the intervention has not been established as the standard of care.

Another significant difference between cancer chemotherapy trials and those using allogeneic HSCT is the fact that HSCT involves two patients, the recipient and the donor. Different issues arise, depending on whether the donor is a matched unrelated, matched related, or haploidentical donor. These differences are partly based on the fact that the matched unrelated donor is a stranger, the matched related donor is a brother or sister, and the haploidentical donor is usually a parent. The patient's course and outcome affect the donor in various ways, depending on the relationship of the donor to the patient, and this effect is relevant to the ethical issues involved in HSCT cancer clinical trials.

More than 7 million people are registered as potential bone marrow or peripheral blood stem cell (PBSC) donors[67] for the 70% of candidates for HSCT who do not have a matched sibling donor. The risks of bone marrow donation are small; life-threatening complications occur in approximately 0.1% of healthy donors.[68] Ninety-five percent of PBSC donors do well with only minor complaints.[69] In matched unrelated donor transplantation, one must consider the donor's rights as well as the patient's rights. These issues were outlined in a review by the WMDA (World Marrow Donor Association).[70] First, donor autonomy must always be honored. At a minimum, this means that the consequences of each act in the process, as they bear on both the donor and patient, must be explained to the donor. The informed consent process and document must stipulate the donor's right to withdraw at any time, even during the pretransplantation conditioning, and must state the possible consequences of withdrawal. The donor registry cannot pressure or coerce donors, although the center or registry has the right to exclude a donor.

No one is obligated to join a donor registry, but a donor who does join a registry with clear knowledge of the expectations voluntarily incurs some moral obligation. This obligation grows as the process continues: a donor at the point of donation for a patient who is being conditioned has a greater obligation than a person who is only at the stage of registering. Therefore, donor centers are obligated to communicate clearly with donors to avoid disrupting the recipient's treatment plan, if possible.

There are limits to a donor's obligation. Sometimes, the clinical situation is such that optimal care of a patient would require additional cell products from the donor, such as T cells or additional stem cells. The donor does not have an obligation to continue donating cells or bone marrow after the original donation.

Donor unavailability remains a problem that affects decision making because the therapy is dependent on such variables. When donor unavailability rates over 1 year were examined by the National Marrow Donor Program (NMDP), the worldwide registry of volunteer unrelated stem cell donors,

some interesting facts were discovered.[71] Initially, when a donor search is started there is a request for confirmatory typing. Over the course of the study (March 1, 1999 to February 29, 2000), 20% of all donors were permanently deferred at the time of confirmatory testing and another 12% were temporarily unavailable, because of such factors as pregnancy, high-risk exposure, job change, and location change. Donation centers differed considerably. The likelihood that the donor would be available when requested was affected by the self-identified racial or ethnic group of the donor. These findings suggest important areas in which practical improvement might be achieved: better medical screening, better collection of contact information, better education about the details of the commitment, and movement toward a pressure-free environment. Other important issues that affect ethical decision making, such as cultural sensitivity and route of contact, must be studied further. The overall goal is to structure the donor registry in such a way that donor availability is maximized through better recruitment, retention, and contact.

A second important source of hematopoietic stem cells in pediatric oncology transplantation trials is the sibling donor, many of whom are minors. Although there is minimal coercion of unrelated donors, sibling donors may experience various pressures. The ethical questions center on the coercion of an anxious child who is dependent on the parents who consent to the donation and the question of what, if anything, constitutes a benefit to the donor. The sibling donor can experience psychological, spiritual, and physical stress such as that experienced by the HSCT recipient. The pain and anxiety among adult sibling donors of bone marrow or PBSC has been described.[72-75] Furthermore, refusal to donate can be perceived as resulting in the loss of a sibling, even though the loss is actually caused by the underlying disease. Because the variable of developmental age is added in pediatrics, the issue is more complex. If the sibling dies, the complexity is compounded.[76] In many areas of family life, parents are allowed to give more weight to the interest of one child than to those of another or of the family in general. Therefore, some have advocated leaving the decision of whether a minor child should donate bone marrow to a sibling in the hands of the parents.[77] Regardless of how such issues are ultimately resolved, sibling donors clearly deserve all developmentally appropriate information at the beginning of the process and full psychological support throughout and after the procedure.

Sibling donor interviews provide helpful information. Irrespective of transplant outcome, pediatric sibling donors have reported a perception of having no choice about becoming a donor, whether the sense of constraint is derived from outside pressure (indicated by participants' use of the words guilt, propaganda, privileged, and conned) or from the donor's own beliefs.[78] Hesitancy arises not from a lack of concern for the patient's health, but rather from fear of the procedure and of pain. Donors whose recipient sibling died offered a unique perspective. Anger, guilt, and blame were common emotions expressed. These seemed to be most difficult in cases in which the death was directly related to graft failure or to graft-versus-host disease (GVHD). These issues have not been studied enough to draw substantial conclusions, but enough is known to raise questions about competence to consent, the weight accorded to a child's refusal to donate, the limits of the parents' decision making power, and the worrisome specter of what might constitute battery in the face of a child's refusal. One might override the refusal of a 5-year-old, but what about that of a 10-year-old, 13-year-old, or 17-year-old?

Another important issue in the case of sibling donors for pediatric HSCT is that siblings who are not chosen as donors are susceptible to ambivalent feelings of relief, disappointment, and guilt.[79] If siblings are involved in the screening process, issues of psychological well-being and respect for persons are complex. In one study that compared sibling donors with sibling nondonors, nondonors had more school problems than donors, and a third of siblings in both groups reported moderate to severe post-traumatic stress.[80-82] Medical encounters with a nondonor sibling may show suffering that would not have occurred apart from the process of being screened for stem cell donation. Caregivers owe this person as much respect as they owe any patient.

A third and increasingly prominent source of stem cells is cord blood. Initial concerns about early clamping of the umbilical cord to obtain the maximum number of cells have been allayed,[83] but other ethical questions remain. Should the cord blood be linked to the identity of the donor so that unsafe units can be identified if the donor is later disqualified (e.g., by genetic testing)? The controversy centers on concerns about loss of privacy for donors. Because the cord blood DNA holds genetic information (the social implications of which are not clear at present), the donor is potentially vulnerable to inappropriate disclosure.[84] A related issue concerns what the limits for cord blood testing ought to be and what should be done with the results. Clearly, some testing is needed to avoid unnecessary risk to the recipient. However, in 1994, the Institute of Medicine recommended that children should not be tested for abnormal genes unless the disease has an effective curative or preventive treatment that must be initiated early in life.[85] Thus, it may be that samples should be tested broadly to protect the recipient, but that the testing should be done in a blinded way to protect the donor. The details of this issue will require further consideration and debate as more is learned about the human genome and prediction of disease.

The fourth source of stem cells used in pediatric clinical oncology trials is the haploidentical donor, usually a parent. The advantage of this type of transplant is the ready availability of a partially matched donor. No research has been done on the impact of this type of transplant on parents and families, but it would not be surprising if the issues seen with sibling donation are compounded when the parent is the donor, including feelings of guilt when the child has severe GVHD or graft failure. Another important question is whether there is a limit to acceptable parental sacrifice and, if so, what it is. For example, one would not allow a parent to donate his or her heart, but intermediate scenarios include those in which a parent donates a portion of lung, kidney, or liver in the face of post-transplantation complications.

MODELS AND TOOLS FOR ETHICAL DECISION MAKING

The individual issues (e.g., consent, assent, clinical equipoise) are important, but they make the most sense in clinical and research settings when they are considered within a larger framework for ethical decision making. Such a framework takes into account fundamental principles, such as respect for persons, individual and cultural variation, the importance of full information, and the relevance of an individual's experience of illness to the concrete process of decision making.

The individualized care planning and coordination (ICPC) model for ethical decision making developed by Baker and coworkers[86] combines the various elements of decision making so that they are intentionally and systematically addressed (nothing is missed) and revisited using the care model (so that changes over time are acknowledged and addressed). The model begins by establishing a foundation based on the principles of competence, empathy, compassion, communication, and quality (Fig. 34-3). The aims of this model are to attend

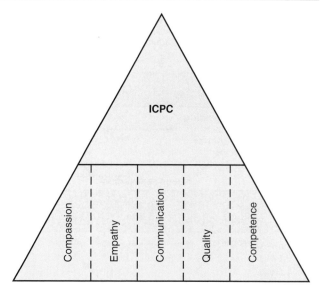

FIGURE 34-3. Foundation of the individualized care planning and coordination (ICPC) model. *(Adapted from Baker JN, Barfield RC, Hinds PS, Kane JR. A model to facilitate decision making in pediatric stem cell transplantation: the individualized care planning and coordination model. Biol Blood Marrow Transplant. 2007;13:245-254.)*

to quality of life, healing, and suffering from the beginning of a life-threatening illness. The ICPC model has three steps, each of which has three components (Fig. 34-4; Table 34-3).

The first step, relationship, is made up of three interrelated components—understanding the illness experience, sharing relevant information, and needs assessment. Without comprehending the illness experience of the child and the family, the clinician will be unable to proceed to seeking the best interest of the child and the decision making process. This may be especially true at the extreme of consideration of phase I clinical trials, toward the end of the child's life. Similarly, no decision can realistically address the best interest of the child unless all involved in the decision making process have the needed information. This issue can be difficult when the relevant information is bad news; several studies have shown that the bearer of bad news can elicit strong negative reactions from family members that in turn make the clinician reluctant to deliver bad news (known as the "MUM effect").[87-89] Communication of sufficient information for ethical decision making can also be truncated in approximately 10% of cases by lack of training and communication of the pediatric oncologist.[90] A comprehensive needs assessment, not just assessment of medical needs, is also vital to the process of ethical decision making in clinical medicine and clinical oncology trials (see Table 34-3). Such comprehensive assessments can inform the decision making processes by incorporating relevant changes in a patient's needs.

The second step in the ICPC model is negotiation, in which goals, prognoses, and treatment options are considered. Although the prognosis for cure can be dynamic because of advances in pediatric oncology clinical trials, this information is helpful to patients and families in decision making in all clinical trials, and perhaps especially in phase I and II trials, in which the response rate and progression-free survival are low.[91,92] Another relevant consideration is that there is more than one relevant prognosis—more, that is, than the prognosis for cure. There are, for example, the prognosis for life prolongation and the prognosis for relief of suffering. These two prognoses are relevant and relate intimately to the goals of care,

INDIVIDUALIZED CARE PLANNING

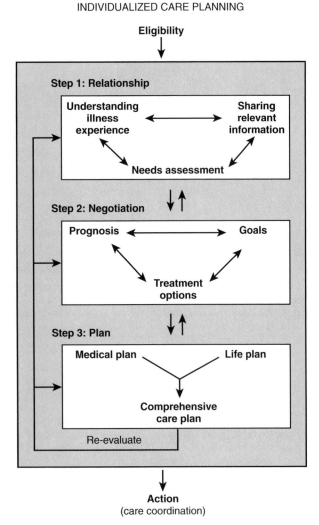

FIGURE 34-4. The three-step individualized care planning and coordination model. *(Adapted from Baker JN, Barfield RC, Hinds PS, Kane JR. A model to facilitate decision making in pediatric stem cell transplantation: the individualized care planning and coordination model. Biol Blood Marrow Transplant. 2007;13:245-254.)*

TABLE 34-3	Domains of Interdisciplinary Needs Assessment	
Assessment Domain	**Examples**
Structure and process of care	Specialty-level trained symptom management experts are available.
	The setting of care should meet the preferences, needs, and circumstances of the patient and family.
	The care plan is based on a comprehensive interdisciplinary assessment.
Physical aspects of care	Symptoms and side effects are assessed and managed in a timely, safe, and effective manner.
	Symptoms and side effects are assessed and managed in a manner that is patient and family-centered.
Psychological and psychiatric aspects of care	Psychological and psychiatric needs are assessed and managed in a timely, safe, and effective manner.
	Grief and bereavement program is available to assess and manage patient, family, and staff grief.
Social aspects of care	Comprehensive interdisciplinary assessment identifies the social needs of patients and families.
Spiritual, religious, and existential aspects of care	Spiritual and existential dimensions are assessed and responded to based on the best available evidence.
	Spiritual and existential dimensions are approached in a manner that is acceptable to the patient and family as they pertain to the patient's illness.
Cultural aspects of care	Needs are assessed in a culturally sensitive manner.
	Specific patient and family cultural needs are assessed.
Care of the imminently dying	During this stage of the illness trajectory, the comprehensive needs assessment continues.
	Signs and symptoms of impending death are assessed, recognized, communicated, and treated as needed.
Ethical and legal aspects of care	Health care professionals assess and attempt to incorporate the values, goals, and preferences of each patient and family.
	Need for ethics consultation should be assessed based on the comprehensive needs assessment and discordant steps in the process (i.e., cure as primary goal in end-stage cancer).
Informational aspects of care	Comprehensive interdisciplinary assessment identifies the informational and educational needs of patients and families.
	Specific patient and family information is provided in a timely manner.
Relational aspects of care	As a part of the generation of a life plan, the relational needs of the patient and family are assessed.
	Relationships are assessed and augmented throughout the illness trajectory

(From Baker JN, Barfield RC, Hinds PS, Kane JR. A model to facilitate decision making in pediatric stem cell transplantation: the individualized care planning and coordination model. Biol Blood Marrow Transplant. 2007;13: 245-254.)

which are profoundly important aspects of ethical decision making in pediatric clinical oncology trials.

After the range of prognostic elements has been considered, it is possible to move on to a discussion of what the goals are to be, goals that may change as the prognosis changes (Fig. 34-5).[93] In a phase III clinical trial, cure may be the dominant goal. For a child who has had multiple relapses and whose family is considering a phase I trial, however, ethical decision making will involve a reassessment of goals in view of the best interest of the child, including a reassessment of the child's expressed values. Assessment and prioritization of the values of the child, especially perhaps in the context of a low probability of cure, is an area in which much research remains to be done. Among novel projects being assessed is the use of interactive technologies (tapping into the video game culture) to augment the expressive ability of younger children (Fig. 34-6).

Each potential goal, with its associated prognosis, is related in turn to a treatment option aimed at achieving the goal as

GOALS OF CARE

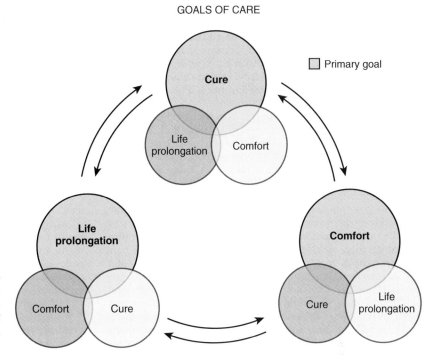

FIGURE 34-5. Goals of care. *(Adapted from Baker JN, Barfield RC, Hinds PS, Kane JR. A model to facilitate decision making in pediatric stem cell transplantation: the individualized care planning and coordination model. Biol Blood Marrow Transplant. 2007;13:245-254.)*

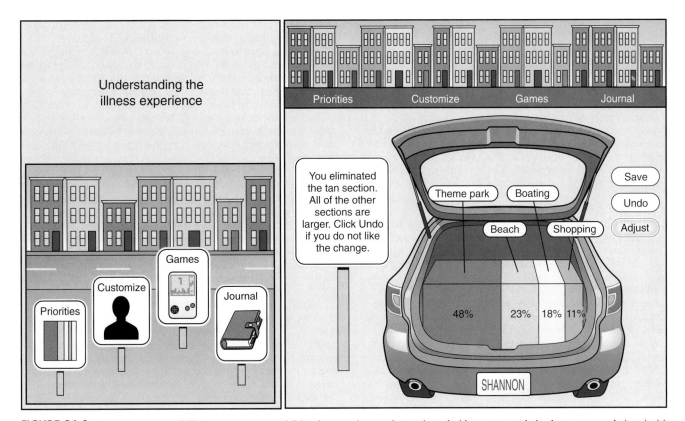

FIGURE 34-6. The "treasure box." This prototype uses children's attraction to electronic and video games to help them express their priorities and values in the context of ethical decision making regarding phase I trials.

efficaciously as possible (i.e., as limited by progress). If families see that supportive care is available to help them achieve their goals, they are less likely to feel abandoned and fear discontinuation of certain therapies.[94] Ethical decision making takes into account prognoses, goals, and treatment options and involves shared decision making by the family, patient, and clinicians. This process leads to the third step of the ICPC, the comprehensive care plan.

The ethical decision making process that yields a comprehensive plan takes into account consent, assent, full disclosure of information, and attention to the various ways that families and individuals prioritize values. The comprehensive care plan includes a medical plan (decisions about medical treatment and symptom management) and a life plan (addressing personal goals and family needs). The former might carry more weight when the goals emphasize cure, and the latter might carry more weight for a patient with incurable disease.[95]

The value of such an approach is that it can clarify complex ethical decision making in settings such as the intensive care unit (with the extraordinary advances in sustaining biologic life) and can clarify the goals of care. A useful tool that complements the ICPC is the four-box method developed by Jonsen and colleagues[96] that offers specific questions that can add content to the information categories relevant to comprehensive ethical decision making. This more detailed set of questions in the categories of medical information, family preferences, contextual details, and quality of life expands those put forward in 1983 by the President's Commission.[97] The five considerations offered for determining the best interest of the child in such situations are the amount of suffering and potential for relief, severity of dysfunction or potential for restoration of function, expected duration of life, potential for personal satisfaction and enjoyment of life, and potential to develop a capacity for self-determination.

CHALLENGES OF TECHNOLOGY, GLOBALIZATION, AND ECONOMIC DISPARITY

The past two decades have seen an unprecedented worldwide increase in the sharing of information and ideas. This has allowed more rapid dissemination of useful information and has increasingly uncovered disparities in access to technology, availability of resources, and ethical values. All of these have an effect on the ethics of pediatric clinical oncology trials when considered from a global perspective.

Technologic advances that are revolutionizing the diagnosis and treatment of childhood cancer and other childhood disorders bring with them new ethical issues.[98] These complex questions challenge us to develop a coherent approach that accommodates the diversity of political, religious, cultural, philosophical, and vocational backgrounds involved in the discussion.

Bioinformatics is one area showing rapid advances; it attempts large-scale organization of information, including genomic data, protein expression data, and molecular interactions.[99] Genomics is revolutionizing the diagnosis and treatment of cancer.[100] High-throughput microarrays can profile the expression patterns of tens of thousands of genes simultaneously.[101] This technology offers much promise, and also raises a number of important ethical questions. If a disease gene or disease susceptibility gene profile is discovered, should the subject be notified? Should the subject's family also be notified or is this a breach of confidentiality?[102]

The American Society of Clinical Oncology (ASCO) has recommended that genetic testing for cancer predisposition be offered when (1) the individual has a personal history, family history, or features suggestive of genetic cancer susceptibility, (2) the test can be adequately interpreted, and (3) the result will aid in diagnosis or in the medical or surgical management of a patient or family member who has a hereditary risk for cancer.[103] ASCO has also recommended that the regulatory oversight of laboratories providing such tests be strengthened and that federal laws be established to prohibit discrimination by health care providers, employers, and insurance agencies on the basis of such information. Although some maintain that genetic discrimination will not affect insurance coverage, several surveys have shown that the public fears this possibility.[104-106]

In pediatric oncology, the ethical issue is even more complex because decisions that may affect the research subjects' future employability, insurability, and privacy are made by surrogate decision makers. Furthermore, as technology grows more complex, the gap between technology and meaningful understanding on the part of the family and patient widens, a growing challenge to informed consent. Can the surrogate decision makers understand fully the implications of their decision? How much can be expected of a parent without special training?

Pharmacogenomics is the subcategory of genomics research that has perhaps the most immediate potential impact on pediatric clinical oncology trials. This area has enormous potential to benefit children but also creates the potential for social and economic discrimination, nationally and internationally, and abuse of information in genomic databases. Pharmacogenomics combines human genomics with pharmacogenetics to study the role of the individual's genetic makeup in his or her response to a drug.[107] The promise of this approach is that patients can receive individually tailored medical therapy and dosing. This technology advances the important concept of risk stratification, which has historically led to better protection of children with lower risk cancers from excess toxicity while ensuring that children with higher risk disease are not undertreated.

Pharmacogenomics raises several ethical questions. For example, there is an economic question. Might pharmacogenomic criteria eventually become regulatory requirements for the development and testing of medicines?[108] Because the pharmaceutical industry functions on a business model, it is unlikely to develop medicines that will benefit only a small, narrowly defined group of patients. This dilemma is familiar to investigators in pediatric oncology. Orphan drugs might therefore become more common. How should economic risk be weighed against the potential clinical benefit for a small group of patients? Second, if pharmacogenomics information suggests only that a child is more or less likely to benefit from a drug, what likelihood threshold would exclude the child from the use of a drug—10%, 30%? If a child is less likely to respond to a drug, is an insurance company obligated to pay for the drug?[109] If genetic variance peculiar to an ethnic group is found, what are the political, social, and economic implications? Might these be used to decide whether to develop certain medicines for certain populations?[110]

Such questions about the impact of technology present a contrast to the ethical issues involved in pediatric oncology trials in low-income countries.[111] The cure rates of many diseases in children differ substantially between high- and low-income countries.[112] The interventions that have the greatest impact in such countries are often not therapies per se but are rather aimed at reducing the substantial relapse rate caused by, for example, abandonment of treatment, the main cause of treatment failure in low-income countries. Remedial interventions can have significant impact.[113] St. Jude Children's Research Hospital has collaborated with a pediatric cancer center in Recife, Brazil, to reduce abandonment of therapy by

CHILDHOOD ALL SURVIVAL GAP

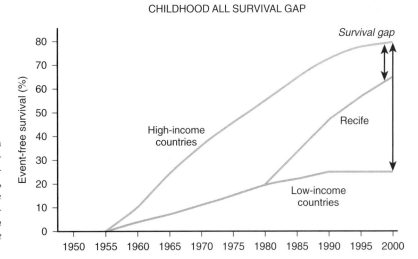

FIGURE 34-7. Event-free 5-year survival of children with acute lymphoblastic leukemia (ALL) in high-income countries versus low-income countries. Interventions to reduce loss of patients to follow-up (e.g., making work available near the hospital so that the parents could earn sufficient income to feed other children) increased survival in Recife, Brazil. *(Adapted from Howard SC. Delivering global oncology care. Available at www.cure4kids.org/public/873.)*

providing family support, such as housing, work, and food; the 5-year event-free survival rate of children with acute lymphoblastic leukemia rose from 32% in the 1980s to 63% in 2000 (Fig. 34-7).[114] Similarly, in El Salvador, the 4-year survival rate for children with acute lymphoblastic leukemia increased from 5% to 46% for high-risk cases and 69% for standard-risk cases.[115] Such success has underscored the promise of international collaborative clinical care and research for children with cancer, but there are many challenges remaining.

One important challenge is that of ethical oversight of international research in pediatric oncology. Researchers in low-income countries often have little or no access to a functional research ethics committee. However, institutions in high-income countries require, in part under the guidance of governmental regulations, that adequate ethical oversight be in place as a prerequisite for cooperative clinical research. Collaborative research that uses the strategy of twinning institutions in high-income countries with those in low-income countries can produce important advances, as described earlier, but the lack of ethical oversight can preclude these collaborations. Also, researchers cannot report such work in high-profile journals, because the International Committee of Medical Journal Editors requires that reports of research involving human subjects document established mechanisms of human subject protection.

The Council for International Organizations of Medical Sciences guidelines state that researchers and institutions in high-income countries sponsoring research in low-income countries have an ethical obligation to improve the capacity for human participant protection in these countries. However, in a survey of 203 clinical researchers in low-income countries, 44% have reported that their studies are not reviewed by the country's ministry or department of health and 25% have reported that their studies undergo no ethical review by a research ethics committee, IRB, or ministry or department of health.[116]

Federal regulations require that clinical trials conducted in low-income countries in collaboration with U.S. institutions must meet the ethical standards for trials based in the United States. However, within the framework of these ethical standards, the research procedures can be adapted to local needs, conditions, and culture.[117] Advancing the development of research ethics in developing countries will open future possibilities for international collaboration that can increase the

survival of children with cancer worldwide. Such trials do not necessarily require advanced technology to address the root causes of the disparate survival rates of children in low- versus high-income countries. Addressing this disparity is itself an ethical imperative.

CONCLUSION

Pediatric clinical trials present some of the most challenging ethical issues in modern medicine. Children are inherently vulnerable, yet they are in need of the best, most effective, and least toxic therapies; therefore, much is at stake in the field of childhood cancer. New therapies are developed through research, but in pediatric trials the person experiencing the risk is not the same person who is deciding whether the child participates. There are many questions that will require further thought, discussion and, for those questions amenable to such approaches, empirical research. Children do not have legal status as decision makers; those who care for children in pediatric clinical trials know how mature a child's perception can be, even a young child. What weight should be given to their opinions? From an international perspective, how should we respond to disparity of wealth in prioritizing pediatric research goals, even within the boundaries of a developed nation? How should we navigate cultural and political differences that influence the ethical considerations in international clinical trials?

Globally advancing the excellent care of children with catastrophic diseases such as cancer depends on clinical trials. Good clinical trials require ethical decision making at every level. There are two questions regarding advances in therapy for childhood cancer that must always be asked at the same time: "What can be done next?" and "What should be done next?" The means for answering the first question is scientific. The means for answering the second question is often more philosophical, drawing on many sources of wisdom and insight that are not intrinsically scientific in their approach. History has taught us that scientific advances without ethical considerations can become horrific. Similarly, wisdom without scientific advances cannot further the effort to cure sick children. Medical science committed to ethical research, however, offers the best possibility for continuing the advancement of cures for childhood cancer through well-designed clinical trials.

REFERENCES

1. Moreno JD. Undue Risk. Florence, Ky, Routledge, 2000.
2. Brody BA. Ethics of Biomedical Research: An International Perspective. New York, Oxford University Press, 1998.
3. Barfield RC, Church C. Informed consent in pediatric clinical trials. Curr Opin Pediatr. 2005;17:20-24.
4. Lederer SE. Children as guinea pigs: historical perspective. Account Res. 2003;10:1-16.
5. Fisher DJ. Resurgence of rabies. A historical perspective on rabies in children. Arch Pediatr Adolesc Med. 1995;149:306-312.
6. Diekema DS. Conducting ethical research in pediatrics: a brief historical overview and review of pediatric regulations. J Pediatr. 2006;149:S3-S11.
7. Levine RJ. International codes of research ethics: current controversies and the future. Indiana Law Rev. 2002;35:557-567.
8. Zion D, Gillam L, Loff B. The Declaration of Helsinki, CIOMS and the ethics of research on vulnerable populations. Nat Med. 2000;6:615-617.
9. Krugman S. The Willowbrook hepatitis studies revisited: ethical aspects. Rev Infect Dis. 1986;8:157-162.
10. Krugman S. Experiments at the Willowbrook State School. Lancet. 1971;1:966-967.
11. National Commission for the Protection of Human Subjects of Biomedical and Behavioral Research. The Belmont Report. Washington, DC, U.S. Government Printing Office, 1979.
12. Beauchamp TL, Childress JF. Principles of Biomedical Ethics, 5th ed. New York, Oxford University Press, 2001.
13. Emanuel EJ, Wendler D, Grady C. What makes clinical research ethical? JAMA. 2000;283:2701-2711.
14. Grodin MA, Annas GJ. Legacies of Nuremberg. Medical ethics and human rights. JAMA. 1996;276:1682-1683.
15. Katz J. The Nuremberg Code and the Nuremberg Trial. A reappraisal. JAMA. 1996;276:1662-1666.
16. Levine RJ. Ethics and Regulation for Clinical Research, 2nd ed. New Haven, Conn, Yale University Press, 1986, p 98.
17. Katz J. The Silent World of Doctor and Patient. New York, Free Press, 1984.
18. Ruccione K, Kramer RF, Moore IK, Perin G. Informed consent for treatment of childhood cancer: factors affecting parents' decision making. J Pediatr Oncol Nurs. 1991;8:112-121.
19. Kodish ED, Pentz RD, Noll RB, et al. Informed consent in the Childrens Cancer Group: results of preliminary research. Cancer. 1998;82:2467-2481.
20. Simon C, Eder M, Raiz P, et al. Informed consent for pediatric leukemia research: clinician perspectives. Cancer.2001;92:691-700.
21. Levi RB, Marsick R, Drotar D, Kodish ED. Diagnosis, disclosure, and informed consent: learning from parents of children with cancer. J Pediatr Hematol Oncol. 2000;22:3-12.
22. Kupst MJ, Patenaude AF, Walco GA, Sterling C. Clinical trials in pediatric cancer: parental perspectives on informed consent. J Pediatr Hematol Oncol. 2003;25:787-790.
23. Kodish E, Eder M, Noll RB. et al. Communication of randomization in childhood leukemia trials. JAMA. 2004;291:470-475.
24. Angiolillo AL, Simon C, Kodish E, et al. Staged informed consent for a randomized clinical trial in childhood leukemia: impact on the consent process. Pediatr Blood Cancer. 2004;42:433-437.
25. Grossman SA, Piantadosi S, Covahey C. Are informed consent forms that describe clinical oncology research protocols readable by most patients and their families? J Clin Oncol. 1994;12:2211-2215.
26. Syse A. Norway: valid (as opposed to informed) consent. Lancet. 2000;356:1347-1348.
27. Spinetta JJ, Masera G, Jankovic M, et al. Valid informed consent and participative decision making in children with cancer and their parents: a report of the SIOP Working Committee on psychosocial issues in pediatric oncology. Med Pediatr Oncol. 2003;40:244-246.
28. Kodish E. Informed consent for pediatric research: is it really possible? J Pediatr. 2003;142:89-90.
29. Nelson RM, Reynolds WW. We should reject passive resignation in favor of requiring the assent of younger children for participation in nonbeneficial research. Am J Bioeth. 2003;3:11-13.
30. Whittle A, Shah S, Wilfond B, et al. Institutional review board practices regarding assent in pediatric research. Pediatrics. 2004; 113:1747-1752.
31. Kimberly MB, Hoehn KS, Feudtner C, et al. Variation in standards of research compensation and child assent practices: a comparison of 69 institutional review board-approved informed permission and assent forms for three multicenter pediatric clinical trials. Pediatrics. 2006;117:1706-1711.
32. Department of Health and Human Services. Additional protections for children involved as subjects in research. Final rule. Fed Regist. 1983;48:9814-9820.
33. Joffe S, Fernandez CV, Pentz RD, et al. Involving children with cancer in decision making about research participation. J Pediatr. 2006;149:862-868.
34. Committee on Bioethics, American Academy of Pediatrics. Informed consent, parental permission, and assent in pediatric practice. Pediatrics. 1995;95:314-317.
35. National Commission for the Protection of Human Subjects of Biomedical and Behavioral Research. Report and Recommendations Research Involving Children (DHEW Publication No. [OS] 77-0004). Washington, DC, U.S. Department of Health, Education, and Welfare, 1977.
36. Blackhall LJ, Murphy ST, Frank G, et al. Ethnicity and attitudes toward patient autonomy. JAMA. 1995;274:820-825.
37. Rossi WC, Reynolds W, Nelson RM. Child assent and parental permission in pediatric research. Theor Med Bioeth. 2003;24:131-148.
38. Committee on Drugs, American Academy of Pediatrics. Guidelines for the ethical conduct of studies to evaluate drugs in pediatric populations. Pediatrics. 1995;95:286-294.
39. National Commission for the Protection of Human Subjects of Biomedical and Behavioral Research. Report and Recommendations: Research Involving Those Institutionalized as Mentally Infirm (DHEW Publication No. [OS] 78-0006). Washington, DC, U.S. Government Printing Office, 1978.
40. Olds RS. Informed-consent issues with adolescent health behavior research. Am J Health Behav. 2003;27 Suppl 3:S248-S263.
41. Lothen-Kline C, Howard DE, Hamburger EK, et al. Truth and consequences: ethics, confidentiality, and disclosure in adolescent longitudinal prevention research. J Adolesc Health. 2003;33:385-394.
42. Brody JL, Scherer DG, Annett RD, Pearson-Bish M. Voluntary assent in biomedical research with adolescents: a comparison of parent and adolescent views. Ethics Behav. 2003;13:79-95.
43. Freyer DR. Care of the dying adolescent: special considerations. Pediatrics. 2004;113:381-388.
44. Bleyer WA. The U.S. pediatric cancer clinical trials programmes: international implications and the way forward. Eur J Cancer. 1997;33:1439-1447.
45. Kopelman LM. When is risk minimal enough for children to be research subjects? In Kopelman LM, Moskop JC (eds). Children and Health Care: Moral and Social Issues. Boston, Kluwer Academic, 1989, pp 89-99.
46. Wendler D, Emanuel EJ. What is a "minor" increase over minimal risk? J Pediatr. 2005;147:575-578.
47. American Society of Clinical Oncology. Critical role of phase I clinical trials in cancer treatment. J Clin Oncol. 1997;15:853-859.
48. Roberts TG Jr, Goulart BH, Squitieri L, et al. Trends in the risks and benefits to patients with cancer participating in phase 1 clinical trials. JAMA. 2004;292:2130-2140.

49. Horstmann E, McCabe MS, Grochow L, et al. Risks and benefits of phase 1 oncology trials, 1991 through 2002. N Engl J Med. 2005;352:895-904.

50. Shah S, Weitman S, Langevin AM, et al. Phase I therapy trials in children with cancer. J Pediatr Hematol Oncol. 1998;20:431-438.

51. Agrawal M, Emanuel EJ. Ethics of phase 1 oncology studies: reexamining the arguments and data. JAMA. 2003;290:1075-1082.

52. Daugherty C, Ratain MJ, Grochowski E, et al. Perceptions of cancer patients and their physicians involved in phase I trials. J Clin Oncol. 1995;13:1062-1072.

53. Appelbaum PS, Roth LH, Lidz CW, et al. False hopes and best data: consent to research and the therapeutic misconception. Hastings Cent Rep. 1987;17:20-24.

54. Ulrich CM, Grady C, Wendler D. Palliative care: a supportive adjunct to pediatric phase I clinical trials for anticancer agents? Pediatrics. 2004;114:852-855.

55. Kodish E. Pediatric ethics and early-phase childhood cancer research: conflicted goals and the prospect of benefit. Account Res. 2003;10:17-25.

56. Ross L. Phase I research and the meaning of direct benefit. J Pediatr. 2006;149:S20-S24.

57. Mariani L, Marubini E. Content and quality of currently published phase II cancer trials. J Clin Oncol. 2000;18:429-436.

58. Freedman B. Equipoise and the ethics of clinical research. N Engl J Med. 1987;317:141-145.

59. Miller PB, Weijer C. Rehabilitating equipoise. Kennedy Inst Ethics J. 2003;13:93-118.

60. Miller FG, Brody H. The internal morality of medicine: an evolutionary perspective. J Med Philos. 2001;26:581-599.

61. Miller FG, Brody H. A critique of clinical equipoise. Therapeutic misconception in the ethics of clinical trials. Hastings Cent Rep. 2003;33:19-28.

62. London AJ. The moral foundations of equipoise and its role in international research. Am J Bioeth. 2006;6:48-51.

63. London AJ. Equipoise and international human-subjects research. Bioethics. 2001;15:312-332.

64. Veatch RM. Indifference of subjects: an alternative to equipoise in randomized clinical trials. Soc Philos Policy. 2002;19:295-323.

65. Veatch RM. Why researchers cannot establish equipoise. Am J Bioeth. 2006;6:55-57.

66. Jacoby LH, Maloy B, Cirenza E, et al. The basis of informed consent for BMT patients. Bone Marrow Transplant. 1999;23:711-717.

67. Gahrton G. Goals and activities of the WMDA. World Marrow Donor Association. Int J Hematol. 2002;76(Suppl 1):384-385.

68. Buckner CD, Peterson FB, Bolonesi BA. Bone marrow donors. In Forman SJ, Blume KG, Thomas ED (eds). Bone Marrow Transplantation. Boston, Blackwell Scientific, 1994, pp 259-269.

69. Egeland T, Lie J, Persson U, et al. Donor and liability insurance of donor registries, donor centers, and collection centers—recommendations. Bone Marrow Transplant. 2004;33:467-470.

70. Bakken R, van Walraven AM, Egeland T. Donor commitment and patient needs. Bone Marrow Transplant. 2004;33:225-230.

71. Confer DL. The National Marrow Donor Program. Meeting the needs of the medically underserved. Cancer. 2001;91:274-278.

72. Fortanier C, Kuentz M, Sutton L, et al. Healthy sibling donor anxiety and pain during bone marrow or peripheral blood stem cell harvesting for allogeneic transplantation: results of a randomised study. Bone Marrow Transplant. 2002;29:145-149.

73. Auquier P, Macquart-Moulin G, Moatti JP, et al. Comparison of anxiety, pain and discomfort in two procedures of hematopoietic stem cell collection: leukocytopheresis and bone marrow harvest. Bone Marrow Transplant. 1995;16:541-547.

74. Munzenberger N, Fortanier C, Macquart-Moulin G, et al. Psychosocial aspects of haematopoietic stem cell donation for allogeneic transplantation: how family donors cope with this experience. Psychooncology. 1999;8:55-63.

75. Switzer GE, Dew MA, Magistro CA, et al. The effects of bereavement on adult sibling bone marrow donors' psychological well-being and reactions to donation. Bone Marrow Transplant. 1998;21:181-188.

76. Weisz V, Robbennolt JK. Risks and benefits of pediatric bone marrow donation: a critical need for research. Behav Sci Law. 1996;14:375-391.

77. Mumford SE. Donation without consent? Legal developments in bone marrow transplantation. Br J Haematol. 1998;101:599-602.

78. MacLeod KD, Whitsett SF, Mash EJ, Pelletier W. Pediatric sibling donors of successful and unsuccessful hematopoietic stem cell transplants (HSCT): a qualitative study of their psychosocial experience. J Pediatr Psychol. 2003;28:223-230.

79. Packman W. Psychosocial impact of pediatric BMT on siblings. Bone Marrow Transplant. 1999;24:701-706.

80. Packman W, Greenhalgh J, Chesterman B, et al. Siblings of pediatric cancer patients: the quantitative and qualitative nature of quality of life. J Psychosoc Oncol. 2005;23:87-108.

81. Packman W, Gong K, Van Zutphen K, et al. Psychosocial adjustment of adolescent siblings of hematopoietic stem cell transplant patients. J Pediatr Oncol Nurs. 2004;21:233-248.

82. Packman WL, Crittenden MR, Schaeffer E, et al. Psychosocial consequences of bone marrow transplantation in donor and non-donor siblings. J Dev Behav Pediatr. 1997;18:244-253.

83. Bertolini F, Battaglia M, De IC, et al. Placental blood collection: effects on newborns. Blood. 1995;85:3361-3362.

84. Sugarman J, Kaalund V, Kodish E, et al. Ethical issues in umbilical cord blood banking. Working Group on Ethical Issues in Umbilical Cord Blood Banking. JAMA. 1997;278:938-943.

85. Marshall E. Clinical promise, ethical quandary. Science. 1996;271:586-588.

86. Baker JN, Barfield RC, Hinds PS, Kane JR. A model to facilitate decision making in pediatric stem cell transplantation: the individualized care planning and coordination model. Biol Blood Marrow Transplant. 2007;13:245-254.

87. Contro N, Larson J, Scofield S, et al. Family perspectives on the quality of pediatric palliative care. Arch Pediatr Adolesc Med. 2002;156:14-19.

88. Kim SS, Kaplowitz S, Johnston MV. The effects of physician empathy on patient satisfaction and compliance. Eval Health Prof. 2004;27:237-251.

89. Tesser A, Rosen S, Waranch E. Communicator mood and the reluctance to transmit undesirable messages (the Mum effect). J Commun. 1973;23:266-283.

90. Hilden JM, Emanuel EJ, Fairclough DL, et al. Attitudes and practices among pediatric oncologists regarding end-of-life care: results of the 1998 American Society of Clinical Oncology survey. J Clin Oncol. 2001;19:205-212.

91. Hinds PS, Kelly KP. Studying clinical decision making by patients, parents, and health care providers in pediatric oncology. J Pediatr Oncol Nurs. 1998;15:1-2.

92. Hinds PS, Oakes L, Furman W, et al. End-of-life decision making by adolescents, parents, and healthcare providers in pediatric oncology: research to evidence-based practice guidelines. Cancer Nurs. 2001;24:122-134.

93. Kane JR, Primomo M. Alleviating the suffering of seriously ill children. Am J Hosp Palliat Care. 2001;18:161-169.

94. Kane JR, Hellsten MB, Coldsmith A. Human suffering: the need for relationship-based research in pediatric end-of-life care. J Pediatr Oncol Nurs. 2004;21:180-185.

95. Whitney SN, Ethier AM, Fruge E, et al. Decision making in pediatric oncology: who should take the lead? The decisional priority in pediatric oncology model. J Clin Oncol. 2006;24:160-165.

96. Jonsen AR, Siegler M, Winslade WJ. Clinical Ethics: A Practical Approach to Ethical Decisions in Clinical Medicine, 6th ed. New York, McGraw-Hill, 2006.

97. President's Commission for the Study of Ethical Problems in Medicine and Biomedical and Behavioral Research. Deciding to Forgo Life-Sustaining Treatment: Ethical, Medical and Legal Issues in Treatment Decisions. Washington, DC, U.S. Government Printing Office, 1983.

98. Feigin RD. Prospects for the future of child health through research. JAMA. 2005;294:1373-1379.

99. Hocquette JF. Where are we in genomics? J Physiol Pharmacol. 2005;56(Suppl 3):37-70.

100. Segal E, Friedman N, Kaminski N, et al. From signatures to models: understanding cancer using microarrays. Nat Genet. 2005;37 Suppl:S38-S45.

101. Joos L, Eryuksel E, Brutsche MH. Functional genomics and gene microarrays—the use in research and clinical medicine. Swiss Med Wkly. 2003;133:31-38.

102. D'Ambrosio C, Gatta L, Bonini S. The future of microarray technology: networking the genome search. Allergy. 2005;60: 1219-1226.

103. American Society of Clinical Oncology. American Society of Clinical Oncology policy statement update: genetic testing for cancer susceptibility. J Clin Oncol. 2003;21:2397-2406.

104. Thomas SM. Society and ethics—the genetics of disease. Curr Opin Genet Dev. 2004;14:287-291.

105. Nowlan W. Human genetics. A rational view of insurance and genetic discrimination. Science. 2002;297:195-196.

106. Rothenberg KH, Terry SF. Human genetics. Before it's too late—addressing fear of genetic information. Science. 2002;297: 196-197.

107. Weinshilboum R, Wang L. Pharmacogenomics: bench to bedside. Nat Rev Drug Discov. 2004;3:739-748.

108. Breckenridge A, Lindpaintner K, Lipton P, et al. Pharmacogenetics: ethical problems and solutions. Nat Rev Genet. 2004;5: 676-680.

109. Service RF. Genetics and medicine. Recruiting genes, proteins for a revolution in diagnostics. Science. 2003;300:236-239.

110. Lipton P. Pharmacogenetics: the ethical issues. Pharmacogenomics J. 2003;3:14-16.

111. Caniza MA, Clara W, Maron G, et al. Establishment of ethical oversight of human research in El Salvador: lessons learned. Lancet Oncol. 2006;7:1027-1033.

112. Nandakumar A, Anantha N, Venugopal T, et al. Descriptive epidemiology of lymphoid and haemopoietic malignancies in Bangalore, India. Int J Cancer. 1995;63:37-42.

113. Metzger ML, Howard SC, Fu LC, et al. Outcome of childhood acute lymphoblastic leukaemia in resource-poor countries. Lancet. 2003;362:706-708.

114. Howard SC. Delivering global oncology care. Available at www. cure4kids.org/public/873.

115. Howard SC, Pedrosa M, Lins M, et al. Establishment of a pediatric oncology program and outcomes of childhood acute lymphoblastic leukemia in a resource-poor area. JAMA. 2004;291: 2471-2475.

116. Hyder AA, Wali SA, Khan AN, et al. Ethical review of health research: a perspective from developing country researchers. J Med Ethics. 2004;30:68-72.

117. Shapiro HT, Meslin EM. Ethical issues in the design and conduct of clinical trials in developing countries. N Engl J Med. 2001; 345:139-142.

Index

Note: Page numbers followed by f, t, or b denote figures, tables, or boxes, respectively.